LEWIS'S CHILD AND ADOLESCENT PSYCHIATRY

A Comprehensive Textbook

FIFTH EDITION

LEWIS'S CHILD AND ADOLESCENT PSYCHIATRY

A Comprehensive Textbook

FIFTH EDITION

Editors

Andrés Martin, MD, MPH
Riva Ariella Ritvo Professor
Child Study Center
Yale School of Medicine
New Haven, Connecticut

Michael H. Bloch, MD, MS
Associate Professor
Child Study Center
Yale School of Medicine
New Haven, Connecticut

Fred R. Volkmar, MD
Irving B. Harris Professor of Child Psychiatry, Pediatrics, and Psychology
Child Study Center
Yale School of Medicine
New Haven, Connecticut

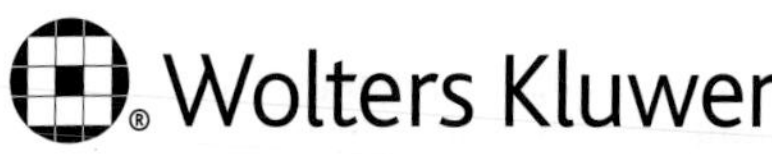

Philadelphia • Baltimore • New York • London
Buenos Aires • Hong Kong • Sydney • Tokyo

Acquisitions Editor: Chris Teja
Product Development Editor: Ashley Fischer
Editorial Coordinator: David Murphy
Editorial Assistant: Brian Convery
Marketing Manager: Rachel Mante Leung
Production Project Manager: David Saltzberg
Design Coordinator: Elaine Kasmer
Manufacturing Coordinator: Beth Welsh
Prepress Vendor: Aptara, Inc.

5th edition

9 8 7 6 5 4 3 2 1

Printed in China

Library of Congress Cataloging-in-Publication Data

Names: Martin, Andrés, editor. | Volkmar, Fred R., editor. | Bloch, Michael (Michael Howard), editor.
Title: Lewis's child and adolescent psychiatry : a comprehensive textbook / editors, Andrés Martin, Fred R. Volkmar, Michael Bloch.
Other titles: Child and adolescent psychiatry
Description: Fifth edition. | Philadelphia : Wolters Kluwer, [2018] | Includes bibliographical references.
Identifiers: LCCN 2017025399 | ISBN 9781496345493
Subjects: | MESH: Mental Disorders | Infant | Child | Adolescent
Classification: LCC RJ131 | NLM WS 350 | DDC 618.92/89–dc23
LC record available at https://lccn.loc.gov/2017025399

LWW.com

We dedicate this book

To our wives:
Rebecca, Angie, and Lisa;
To our children:
Max, Ariela, Gabriela, and Jacob Donald; Rachel, Sam, and Tom; and
Lucy and Emily;
To the teachers and mentors from whom we have received so much;
To the patients, families, students and colleagues
to whom we hope in some measure to have given back;
To all those dedicated to child and adolescent mental health,
working each day to make a difference.

As editors we are proud to donate our royalty proceeds,
in loving memory of our teacher and friend, the late Melvin Lewis,
to the Break the Cycle initiative of
the American Academy of Child and Adolescent Psychiatry.
The Academy continues to support efforts in education, training, and research
for the next generation of practitioners, a mission that was near and dear to Mel.
We ourselves have been the grateful recipients of such support,
and are honored to contribute so that others may benefit like we did.

CONTRIBUTING AUTHORS

Jean A. Adnopoz, MPH
Clinical Professor
Director In-Home Services
Child Study Center
Yale School of Medicine
New Haven, Connecticut

Robert R. Althoff, MD, PhD
Vermont Center for Children, Youth, and Families
University of Vermont College of Medicine/
Fletcher Allen Health Care
Burlington, Vermont

Thomas F. Anders, MD
Distinguished Professor Emeritus
UC Davis School of Medicine
Davis, California

George M. Anderson, PhD
Senior Research Scientist
Child Study Center and the Department of Laboratory Medicine
Yale School of Medicine
New Haven, Connecticut

Adrian Angold, MRCPsych
Professor Emeritus
Department of Psychiatry and Behavioral Sciences
Duke University Medical Center
Durham, North Carolina

Eugene L. Arnold, MD, MEd
Professor Emeritus
Department of Psychiatry and Behavioral Health
Ohio State University
Columbus, Ohio

Peter Ash, MD
Professor and Director
Psychiatry and Law Service
Department of Psychiatry and Behavioral Sciences
Emory University
Atlanta, Georgia

Andrea G. Asnes, MD, MSW
Associate Professor of Pediatrics
Yale School of Medicine
New Haven, Connecticut

David A. Axelson, MD
Professor
Department of Psychiatry and Behavioral Health
The Ohio State University College of Medicine
Chief of Psychiatry and Behavioral Health
Nationwide Children's Hospital
Columbus, Ohio

Kathleen M.B. Balestracci, PhD, MSW
Assistant Clinical Professor
Child Study Center
Yale School of Medicine
New Haven, Connecticut

Argelinda Baroni, MD
Assistant Professor
The Child Study Center at NYU Langone Medical Center
New York, New York

Steven J. Barreto, PhD
Clinical Associate Professor
Warren Alpert Medical School of Brown University
Department of Psychiatry and Behavioral Medicine
Bradley Hospital
East Providence, Rhode Island

Karen Bearss, PhD
Assistant Professor
Marcus Autism Center
Department of Pediatrics
Emory University
Atlanta, Georgia

Myron L. Belfer, MD, MPA
Professor of Psychiatry
Harvard Medical School
Senior Associate in Psychiatry
Boston Children's Hospital
Boston, Massachusetts

Eugene V. Beresin, MD, MA
Executive Director
The Clay Center for Young Healthy Minds
Senior Educator in Child and Adolescent Psychiatry
Massachusetts General Hospital
Professor of Psychiatry
Harvard Medical School
Boston, Massachusetts

Chad Beyer
Stellenbosch University Stellenbosch
South Africa

Boris Birmaher, MD
Professor of Psychiatry
Endowed Chair in Bipolar Disorder
University of Pittsburgh Medical Center
Western Psychiatric Institute and Clinic
Pittsburgh, Pennsylvania

Joseph C. Blader, PhD
Meadows Foundation and Semp Russ Professor of Child Psychiatry
Departments of Psychiatry and Pediatrics
University of Texas Health Science Center at San Antonio
San Antonio, Texas

Efrain Bleiberg, MD
Professor
Menninger Department of Psychiatry and Behavioral Sciences
Baylor College of Medicine
Houston, Texas

Michael H. Bloch, MD, MS
Associate Professor
Child Study Center
Yale School of Medicine
New Haven, Connecticut

John R. Boekamp, PhD
Department of Psychiatry and Human Behavior
Alpert Medical School of Brown University
Emma Pendleton Bradley Hospital
East Providence, Rhode Island

Jeff Q. Bostic, MD, EdD
Associate Clinical Professor
Department of Psychiatry
Harvard Medical School
Boston, Massachusetts

Eric N. Boyum, MD
Adjunct Clinical Assistant Professor
Child and Adolescent Psychiatry
University of Iowa Hospitals and Clinics
Iowa City, Iowa

David A. Brent, MD
Academic Chief
Child and Adolescent Psychiatry
Western Psychiatric Institute and Clinic
University of Pittsburgh Medical Center
Professor of Psychiatry, Epidemiology, Pediatrics, and Clinical Translational Science
Department of Psychiatry
University of Pittsburgh School of Medicine
Pittsburgh, Pennsylvania

Rachel Margaret Ann Brown, MBBS, MPhil
Professor of Clinical Psychiatry
Department of Psychiatry
University of Missouri School of Medicine
Columbia, Missouri

Catherine Brownstein, MPH, PhD
Division of Genetics and Genomics
Boston Children's Hospital
Instructor, Department of Pediatrics
Harvard Medical School
Scientific Director
Manton Center for Orphan Disease Research
Boston, Massachusetts

T. Lindsey Burrell, PhD
Assistant Professor
Marcus Autism Center
Department of Pediatrics
Children's Healthcare of Atlanta
Emory University
Atlanta, Georgia

John V. Campo, MD
Sinsabaugh Professor and Chair
Department of Psychiatry and Behavioral Health
The Ohio State University
Wexner Medical Center
Columbus, Ohio

Laurie Cardona, PsyD
Assistant Professor
Child Study Center
Yale School of Medicine
New Haven, Connecticut

Lee Combrinck-Graham, MD
Medical Director
LifeBridge Community Services
Bridgeport, Connecticut

Kathryn A. Coniglio, BA
Clinical Research Coordinator
Department of Psychiatry
Massachusetts General Hospital
Boston, Massachusetts

Daniel F. Connor, MD
Lockean Distinguished Professor of Psychiatry and Chief, Division of Child and Adolescent Psychiatry
University of Connecticut School of Medicine
Farmington, Connecticut

Kate L. Conover, BA
SDSU-UC San Diego Joint Doctoral Program in Clinical Psychology
San Diego, California

Elizabeth Jane Costello, PhD
Professor
Department of Psychiatry and Behavioral Sciences
Duke University School of Medicine
Durham, North Carolina

Peter T. Daniolos, MD
Clinical Professor and Training Director
Child and Adolescent Psychiatry
University of Iowa Hospitals and Clinics
Iowa City, Iowa

Mary Lynn Dell, MD, DMin
Professor of Clinical Psychiatry and Pediatrics
Nationwide Children's Hospital and the Ohio State University
Columbus, Ohio

Annelou L. C. de Vries, MD, PhD
Department of Child and Adolescent Psychiatry
Center for Expertise on Gender Dysphoria
VU University Medical Center
Amsterdam, The Netherlands

Deborah Blythe Doroshow, MD, PhD
Section of the History of Medicine
Yale School of Medicine
New Haven, Connecticut

Jana K. Dreyzehner, MD
Child Psychiatrist
Tennessee School for the Deaf
Knoxville, Tennessee

Elisabeth M. Dykens, PhD
Professor
Psychology and Human Development
Vanderbilt University
Nashville, Tennessee

Helen Egger, MD
Professor and Chair
Department of Child and Adolescent Psychiatry
The Child Study Center at NYU Langone Medical Center
New York, New York

Leon Eisenberg, MD[†]
Professor of Social Medicine and Psychiatry, Emeritus
Harvard Medical School
Boston, Massachusetts

[†]Deceased.

Maurice Eisenbruch, MD
Professor
Department of Psychiatry
Monash University
Melbourne, Victoria, Australia
Emeritus Professor
Royal Phnom Penh University
Phnom Penh, Cambodia

Thomas V. Fernandez, MD
Associate Professor
Child Study Center and Department of Psychiatry
Yale School of Medicine
New Haven, Connecticut

Matia Finn-Stevenson, PhD
Research Scientist
Edward Zigler Center in Child Development and Social Policy
Child Study Center
Yale School of Medicine
New Haven, Connecticut

Michael B. First, MD
Professor of Clinical Psychiatry
Division of Clinical Phenomenology
Columbia University/New York State Psychiatric Institute
New York, New York

Carmel A. Foley, MD
Associate Professor
Hofstra Northwell Medical School
Department of Psychiatry
Cohen Children's Medical Center of New York
New Hyde Park, New York

Eric Fombonne, MD
Professor
Department of Psychiatry
Director of Autism Research, Institute for Development and Disability
Oregon Health and Science University
Portland, Oregon

Emily A. Fox, BA
Clinical Research Associate
Seattle Children's Autism Center
Seattle, Washington

Geraldine S. Fox, MD, MHPE
Professor of Clinical Psychiatry
Assistant Dean of Graduate Medical Education
Director of Psychiatry Medical Student Education
Department of Psychiatry
University of Illinois at Chicago/Institute for Juvenile Research
Chicago, Illinois

Gregory K. Fritz, MD
Professor
Director of Child and Adolescent Psychiatry
Vice Chair
Department of Psychiatry and Human Behavior
Alpert School of Medicine at Brown University
Academic Director
Bradley Hospital
Providence, Rhode Island

Ruth S. Gerson, MD
Director
Children's Comprehensive Psychiatric Emergency Program at Bellevue Hospital
Clinical Assistant Professor
Department of Child and Adolescent Psychiatry
NYU School of Medicine
New York, New York

Walter S. Gilliam, PhD
Professor of Child Psychiatry and Psychology
Director
Edward Zigler Center in Child Development and Social Policy
Child Study Center
Yale School of Medicine
New Haven, Connecticut

John P. Glazer, MD
Pediatric Psychiatry Consultation Service
Boston Children's Hospital
Lecturer in Psychiatry
Harvard Medical School
Boston, Massachusetts

Mary Margaret Gleason, MD
Associate Professor
Department of Psychiatry and Behavioral Sciences
Tulane University School of Medicine
New Orleans, Louisiana

Jeffrey A. Gliner, PhD
Professor Emeritus of Occupational Therapy
Colorado State University
Fort Collins, Colorado

Pauline Goger, BA, MA
SDSU-UC San Diego Joint Doctoral Program in Clinical Psychology
San Diego State University
San Diego, California

Nitin Gogtay, MD
Director
Office of Clinical Research
National Institutes of Mental Health
Bethesda, Maryland

Karen A. Goldberg, MD, AACAP
Assistant Professor of Psychiatry
Director, Deaf Mental Health
Department of Psychiatry and Behavioral Neurosciences
University of South Florida
Tampa, Florida

Tina Goldstein, PhD
Associate Professor
Child Psychiatry
Western Psychiatric Institute and Clinic
Pittsburgh, Pennsylvania

Joseph Gonzalez-Heydrich, MD
Director, Developmental Neuropsychiatry Clinic
Boston Children's Hospital
Associate Professor of Psychiatry
Harvard Medical School
Boston, Massachusetts

Sandra Gossart-Walker, MSW
Assistant Clinical Professor
Child Study Center
Yale School of Medicine
New Haven, Connecticut

Elena L. Grigorenko, PhD
Hugh Roy and Lillie Cranz Cullen Distinguished Professor of Psychology
Developmental, Cognitive, Neuroscience, and Clinical Psychology
Director of Human Genetics Lab
University of Houston
Professor
Molecular Human Genetics and Pediatrics
Baylor College of Medicine
Houston, Texas

Abha R. Gupta, MD, PhD
Assistant Professor
Department of Pediatrics and Child Study Center
Yale School of Medicine
New Haven, Connecticut

Katherine A. Halmi, MD
Professor Emerita, Psychiatry
Weill Cornell Medical College
New York, New York

John Hamilton, MD, MSc
Teaching Associate in Psychiatry
Department of Psychiatry
Cambridge Health Alliance
Harvard Medical School
Cambridge, Massachusetts

Hesham M. Hamoda, MD, MPH
Staff Psychiatrist
Boston Children's Hospital
Assistant Professor
Harvard Medical School
Boston, Massachusetts

Robert J. Harmon, MD[†]
Department of Psychiatry
University of Colorado at Denver and Health Sciences Center
Denver, Colorado

Lesley Hart, PhD
Associate Research Scientist
Child Study Center
Yale School of Medicine
New Haven, Connecticut

Jennifer F. Havens, MD
Vice Chair for Public Psychiatry
Department of Child and Adolescent Psychiatry
NYU School of Medicine
Director and Chief of Service
Department of Child and Adolescent Psychiatry
Bellevue Hospital Center
New York, New York

Karen R. Hebert, PhD
Adjunct Professor
Department of Psychology
Columbia University
New York, New York

Schuyler W. Henderson, MD, MPH
Deputy Director
Child and Adolescent Psychiatry
Bellevue Hospital
New York, New York

Jesse D. Hinckley, MD, PhD
Department of Psychiatry
University of Colorado
Aurora, Colorado

Robert M. Hodapp, PhD
Professor
Director, Center for the Advancement of Children's Mental Health
Department of Special Education
Vanderbilt University
Nashville, Tennessee

Ellen J. Hoffman, MD, PhD
Assistant Professor
Child Study Center
Yale School of Medicine
New Haven, Connecticut

Daniel Hoover, PhD
Center for Child and Family Traumatic Stress
Kennedy Krieger Institute
Department of Psychiatry
Johns Hopkins School of Medicine
Baltimore, Maryland

Sharon A. Hoover, PhD
Associate Professor, Co-Director
Department of Child and Adolescent Psychiatry
National Center for School Mental Health
University of Maryland School of Medicine
Baltimore, Maryland

Christian Hopfer, MD
Professor
Department of Psychiatry
University of Colorado School of Medicine
Aurora, Colorado

James J. Hudziak, MD
Professor of Psychiatry, Medicine, Pediatrics and Communication Sciences & Disorders
Director of the Vermont Center for Children, Youth, and Families and the Division of Child Psychiatry
Thomas M. Achenbach Endowed Chair of Developmental Psychopathology
University of Vermont College of Medicine/ Fletcher Allen Health Care
Burlington, Vermont

Shashank V. Joshi, MD
Associate Professor of Psychiatry, Pediatrics, and Education
Faculty Research Fellow
Center for Comparative Studies in Race and Ethnicity (CCSRE)
Stanford University
Stanford, California

Joan Kaufman, PhD
Center for Child and Family Traumatic Stress
Kennedy Krieger Institute
Department of Psychiatry
Johns Hopkins School of Medicine
Baltimore, Maryland

Robert A. King, MD
Professor
Child Study Center
Yale School of Medicine
New Haven, Connecticut

Martin Knapp, PhD
Professor of Social Policy
Personal Social Services Research Unit
London School of Economics and Political Science
London, United Kingdom

Nathaniel Laor, MD, PhD
Director, Donald J. Cohen & Irving B. Harris Resilience Center
Professor, Departments of Psychiatry and Philosophy
Tel Aviv University
Tel Aviv, Israel

[†]Deceased.

Eli R. Lebowitz, PhD
Assistant Professor
Child Study Center
Yale School of Medicine
New Haven, Connecticut

James F. Leckman, MD
Neison Harris Professor of Child Psychiatry, Psychology and Pediatrics
Child Study Center
Yale School of Medicine
New Haven, Connecticut

Jessica B. Lennington, PhD
Child Study Center
Yale School of Medicine
New Haven, Connecticut

Robert J. Levine, MD
Professor of Medicine and Lecturer in Pharmacology
Co-Director, Interdisciplinary Center for Bioethics
Department of Internal Medicine
Yale School of Medicine
New Haven, CT

Paul J. Lombroso, MD
Elizabeth Mears and House Jameson Professor in the Child Study Center and Professor of Neuroscience and of Psychiatry
Director, Laboratory of Molecular Neurobiology
Yale School of Medicine
New Haven, Connecticut

Suniya S. Luthar, PhD
Foundation Professor of Psychology
Department of Psychology
Arizona State University
Tempe, Arizona

Megan C. Lyons, MS, CCC-SLP
Child Study Center
Yale School of Medicine
New Haven, Connecticut

Mollie Marr, BFA
Oregon Health and Science University
Portland, Oregon

Andrés Martin, MD, MPH
Riva Ariella Ritvo Professor
Child Study Center
Yale School of Medicine
New Haven, Connecticut

Linda C. Mayes, MD
Arnold Gesell Professor of Child Psychiatry, Pediatrics and Psychology
Director
Child Study Center
Yale School of Medicine
New Haven, Connecticut

David McDaid, MSc
Associate Professorial Research Fellow
Personal Social Services Research Unit
London School of Economics and Political Science
London, United Kingdom

Edwin J. Mikkelsen, MD
Associate Professor of Psychiatry
Harvard Medical School
Boston, Massachusetts

Mendy Boettcher Minjarez, PhD
Assistant Professor
Psychiatry and Behavioral Sciences
University of Washington School of Medicine
Seattle, Washington

Samantha J. Moffett, BA
Child Study Center
Yale School of Medicine
New Haven, Connecticut

Rachel A. Montague, PhD
Clinical Psychologist
Department of Psychiatry and Behavioral Medicine
Seattle Children's Hospital
Seattle, Washington

George A. Morgan, PhD
Professor Emeritus, Education and Human Development
Colorado State University
Fort Collins, Colorado

Nancy E. Moss, PhD
Clinical Assistant Professor
Child Study Center
Yale School of Medicine
New Haven, Connecticut

Corinne Moss-Racusin, PhD
Assistant Professor
Department of Psychology
Skidmore College
Saratoga Springs, New York

Megan M. Mroczkowski, MD
Program Medical Director
Pediatric Psychiatry Emergency Service
Department of Psychiatry
Columbia University Medical Center
New York, New York

Laura Mufson, PhD
Co-Director of Clinical Psychology
Department of Psychiatry
Columbia University Medical Center
Columbia University College of Physicians and Surgeons
New York, New York

Kaizad Munshi, MD, MPH
Department of Psychiatry Boston Children's Hospital
Instructor in Psychiatry
Harvard Medical School
Boston, Massachusetts

Robert A. Murphy, PhD
Associate Professor
Department of Psychiatry and Behavioral Sciences
Duke University School of Medicine
Durham, North Carolina

Kathleen Myers, MD, MPH, MS, DFAACAP
Professor
University of Washington
Director
Telemental Health
Department of Psychiatry and Behavioral Medicine
Seattle Children's Hospital
Seattle, Washington

Barry Nurcombe, MD
Professor Emeritus
Department of Child and Adolescent Psychiatry
The University of Queensland
Brisbane, Australia

Karen E. O'Donnell, PhD
Director of Prevention and Global Initiatives
Center for Child and Family Health
Durham, North Carolina

Jessica R. Oesterheld, MD
Lecturer
Department of Psychiatry
Tufts University School of Medicine
Boston, Massachusetts

Kerry O'Loughlin, PhD
Vermont Center for Children, Youth, and Families
University of Vermont College of Medicine/Fletcher Allen Health Care
Burlington, Vermont

Anna E. Ordóñez, MD, MAS
Deputy Director
Office of Clinical Research
National Institutes of Mental Health
Bethesda, Maryland

Margaret Paccione-Dyszlewski, PhD
Alpert Medical School of Brown University
Emma Pendleton Bradley Hospital
East Providence, Rhode Island

Maryland Pao, MD
Clinical Director and Deputy Scientific Director
NIMH National Institutes of Health
Bethesda, Maryland

Rhea Paul, PhD, CCC-SLP
Professor and Chair
Department of Speech-Language Pathology
Sacred Heart University
Fairfield, Connecticut

Mani Pavuluri, MD, PhD
Berger-Colbeth Chair in Child Psychiatry
Professor and Director
Pediatric Mood Disorders Clinic
Colbeth Child and Adolescent Psychiatry Clinic and Institute for Juvenile Research
Department of Psychiatry
University of Illinois at Chicago
Chicago, Illinois

Cynthia R. Pfeffer, MD
Professor of Psychiatry
Weill Cornell Medicine and New York Presbyterian Hospital
White Plains, New York

John Piacentini, PhD
Director of the Child OCD, Anxiety, and Tic Disorders Program
UCLA Semel Institute for Neuroscience and Human Behavior
Los Angeles, California

Yann B. Poncin, MD
Assistant Professor
Yale School of Medicine
New Haven, Connecticut

Valentina Postorino, PhD
Marcus Autism Center
Department of Pediatrics
Children's Healthcare of Atlanta
Emory University
Atlanta, Georgia

Mona P. Potter, MD
Instructor in Psychiatry
Department of Child and Adolescent Psychiatry
Harvard Medical School
McLean Hospital
Belmont, Massachusetts

Kelly K. Powell, PhD
Associate Research Scientist
Child Study Center
Yale School of Medicine
New Haven, Connecticut

Laura M. Prager, MD
Assistant Professor
Department of Psychiatry
Harvard Medical School
Boston, Massachusetts

Kyle D. Pruett, MD
Clinical Professor of Psychiatry and Nursing
Child Study Center
Yale School of Medicine
New Haven, Connecticut

Andres J. Pumariega, MD
Professor and Chair
Department of Psychiatry
Cooper Medical School of Rowan University and Cooper Health System
Camden, New Jersey

Gary R. Racusin, PhD
Assistant Clinical Professor
Child Study Center
Yale School of Medicine
New Haven, Connecticut

Gautami K. Rao, MD
North East Regional Epilepsy Group at Pascack Valley Hospital
Westwood, New Jersey

Elizabeth L. Reichert, PhD
Clinical Instructor
Division of Child and Adolescent Psychiatry
Department of Psychiatry and Behavioral Sciences
Stanford University School of Medicine
Stanford, California

Joseph M. Rey, MBBS, PhD
Honorary Professor of Psychiatry
University of Sydney
Adjunct Professor
Notre Dame University Medical School
Sydney, Australia

Mark A. Riddle, MD
Professor of Psychiatry and Pediatrics
Johns Hopkins University School of Medicine
Baltimore, Maryland

Paula Riggs, MD
Professor and Director
Division of Substance Dependence
Department of Psychiatry
University of Colorado School of Medicine
Aurora, Colorado

Rachel Z. Ritvo, MD
Assistant Clinical Professor of Psychiatry and Behavioral Sciences
George Washington School of Medicine and Health Sciences
Washington, DC

Alexander Rotenberg, MD, PhD
Director of the Neuromodulation Program
Boston Children's Hospital
Associate Professor of Neurology
Harvard Medical School
Boston, Massachusetts

David E. Roth, MD, FAAP, FAPA
President
Mind & Body Works, Inc.
Honolulu, Hawaii

Melisa D. Rowland, MD
Associate Professor
Department of Psychiatry and Behavioral Sciences
Medical University of South Carolina
Charleston, South Carolina

Helena J. V. Rutherford, PhD
Assistant Professor
Child Study Center
Yale School of Medicine
New Haven, Connecticut

Lawrence Scahill, MSN, PhD
Marcus Autism Center
Department of Pediatrics, Children's Healthcare of Atlanta
Emory University
Atlanta, Georgia

Steven C. Schlozman, MD
Assistant Professor
Department of Psychiatry
Harvard Medical School
Boston, Massachusetts

Elizabeth Schoen Simmons, MS, CCC-SLP
Speech-Language Pathologist
Child Study Center
Yale School of Medicine
New Haven, Connecticut

David J. Schonfeld, MD, FAAP
Director
National Center for School Crisis and Bereavement
Professor of the Practice in the School of Social Work at the University of Southern California
Department of Pediatrics
Children's Hospital Los Angeles
Los Angeles, California

Mary Schwab-Stone, MD
Professor Emerita,
Child Study Center
Yale School of Medicine
New Haven, Connecticut

Richard I. Shader, MD
Professor Emeritus
Department of Integrative Physiology and Pathobiology
Department of Psychiatry
Tufts University School of Medicine
Boston, Massachusetts

Michael Shapiro, MD
Assistant Professor
Department of Psychiatry
University of Florida
Gainesville, Florida

Carla Sharp, PhD
Professor and Director of Clinical Training
Department of Psychology
University of Houston
Houston, Texas

G. Pirooz Sholevar, MD
Clinical Professor, Child Psychiatry
Department of Psychiatry
Jefferson Medical College
Philadelphia, Pennsylvania

Wendy K. Silverman, PhD
Alfred A. Messer Professor of Child Psychiatry
Child Study Center
Yale School of Medicine
New Haven, Connecticut

Adrian Sondheimer, MD
Clinical Assistant Professor
Department of Psychiatry
SUNY at Buffalo School of Medicine
New York, New York

Laura Stout Sosinsky, PhD
Research and Evaluation Consultant
Chadds Ford, Pennsylvania

Cesar A. Soutullo, MD, PhD
Assistant Professor
Department of Psychiatry
University of Navarra College of Medicine
Pamplona, Spain

Lacramioara Spetie, MD
Assistant Professor
Nationwide Children's Hospital
The Ohio State University Behavioral Health Services
Westerville, Ohio

Hanna E. Stevens, MD, PhD
Assistant Professor
Department of Psychiatry
University of Iowa Carver College of Medicine
Iowa City, Iowa

Dorothy E. Stubbe, MD
Associate Professor and Training Director
Child Study Center
Yale School of Medicine
New Haven, Connecticut

Denis G. Sukhodolsky, PhD
Associate Professor
Child Study Center
Yale School of Medicine
New Haven, Connecticut

Jerome H. Taylor, MD
Child Study Center
Yale School of Medicine
New Haven, Connecticut

Laine Taylor, DO, MBA
Assistant Professor
Child Study Center
Yale School of Medicine
New Haven, Connecticut

Cynthia J. Telingator, MD
Assistant Professor
Department of Psychiatry
Harvard Medical School
Cambridge, Massachusetts

Christopher R. Thomas, MD
Robert L. Stubblefield Professor of Child Psychiatry
Department of Psychiatry and Behavioral Sciences
University of Texas Medical Branch
Galveston, Texas

Jennifer J. Thomas, PhD
Associate Professor of Psychology (Psychiatry)
Department of Psychiatry
Harvard Medical School
Boston, Massachusetts

Amalia Londono Tobon, MD
Child Study Center
Yale School of Medicine
New Haven, Connecticut

Simone Tomasi, MD, PhD
Associate Research Scientist
Child Study Center
Yale School of Medicine
New Haven, Connecticut

Kenneth E. Towbin, MD
Chief, Clinical Child and Adolescent Psychiatry
Emotion and Development Branch
National Institute of Mental Health, National Institutes of Health
US Department of Health and Human Services
Rockville, Maryland

Katherine D. Tsatsanis, PhD
Assistant Clinical Professor
Child Study Center
Yale School of Medicine
New Haven, Connecticut

Jack L. Turban III, BA
Child Study Center
Yale School of Medicine
New Haven, Connecticut

Flora M. Vaccarino, MD
Harris Professor
Child Study Center and Department of Neuroscience
Yale School of Medicine
New Haven, Connecticut

Gerrit I. van Schalkwyk, MB, ChB
Child Study Center
Yale School of Medicine
New Haven, Connecticut

Brent van der Wyk, PhD
Assistant Professor
Child Study Center
Yale School of Medicine
New Haven, Connecticut

Fred R. Volkmar, MD
Irving B. Harris Professor of Child Psychiatry, Pediatrics, and Psychology
Child Study Center
Yale School of Medicine
New Haven, Connecticut

Casey Walsh, MSW, LCSW
Doctoral Fellow
Institute for Collaborative Health Research and Practice
School of Social Work
University of Texas at Austin
Austin, Texas

Garry Walter, MBBS, PhD
Professor of Psychiatry
Sydney Medical School and Centre for Values, Ethics and the Law in Medicine (VELiM)
The University of Sydney
Sydney, Australia

V. Robin Weersing, PhD
SDSU-UC San Diego Joint Doctoral Program in Clinical Psychology
San Diego State University
San Diego, California

Daniel T. Williams, MD
Special Lecturer
Department of Psychiatry
Columbia College of Physicians and Surgeons
New York, New York

Emma Wilson, MSc
Learning Technology and Innovation
London School of Economics and Political Science
London, United Kingdom

Nancy C. Winters, MD
Associate Professor
Residency Training Director
Department of Psychiatry
Oregon Health and Science University
Portland, Oregon

Leo Wolmer, PhD
Director of Psychology Research
Donald J. Cohen & Irving B. Harris Resilience Center
Tel-Aviv, Israel
Baruch Ivcher School of Psychology
Herzlyia Inter-Disciplinary Center
Herzlyia, Israel

Joseph L. Woolston, MD
Albert J. Solnit Professor
Child Study Center
Yale School of Medicine
New Haven, Connecticut

Jami F. Young, PhD
Associate Professor of Clinical Psychology
Graduate School of Applied and Professional Psychology
Rutgers University
Piscataway, New Jersey

Charles H. Zeanah, MD
Professor
Psychiatry and Behavioral Sciences
Tulane University School of Medicine
New Orleans, Louisiana

Bradley J. Zebrack, PhD, MSW, MPH
Professor
School of Social Work
University of Michigan
Ann Arbor, Michigan

Edward F. Zigler, PhD
Professor Emeritus of Psychology
Director, Emeritus
Edward Zigler Center in Child Development and Social Policy
Child Study Center
Yale School of Medicine
New Haven, Connecticut

Kenneth J. Zucker, PhD
Professor
Department of Psychiatry
University of Toronto
Toronto, Ontario

■ FOREWORD TO THE FOURTH EDITION

A WORD is dead
When it is said,
Some say.
I say it just
Begins to live
That day.
— Emily Dickinson

The Belle of Amherst hit the nail on the head. Words are living things. And Emily Dickinson gave them meaning, with a new style, well ahead of its time. Words give meaning to our work, too. They form our knowledge base, which is itself a life in words that is always evolving. Yet basic developmental principles beneath that changing knowledge base offer continuity as well. Change mixed with continuity. That's what a textbook should offer.

The original *Child and Adolescent Psychiatry: A Comprehensive Textbook* was the first one published in our field since Leo Kanner's classic *Child Psychiatry* half a century before. Since then a number of other texts have been published, forming the excellent selection available today. But the latest edition of this volume continues to be the cornerstone of my library, and the first choice of many other child and adolescent psychiatrists. Its encyclopedic scope offers a broad reference that serves as a foundation for our field, as well as offering answers to the questions of everyday clinical practice and posing new ones that have yet to be answered.

A word about its development: Melvin Lewis, the pioneering editor of the first three editions of the *Textbook,* has given over responsibility for its fourth edition to the next generation—to a pair of valued colleagues with whom he has worked for years. The first, Andrés Martin, also follows in Lewis's footsteps as editor of the *Journal of the American Academy of Child and Adolescent Psychiatry,* a periodical that contains the cutting edge of research in our field. He is joined by coeditor Fred Volkmar, a distinguished scholar and world-renowned researcher in the area of autism. Together, they have assembled an impressive list of experts as contributors to this fourth edition.

A published book is a finished product, but it doesn't begin to live until its words are read and discussed, its inaccuracies debated and corrected, its truths corroborated and its hypotheses tested. *Lewis's Child and Adolescent Psychiatry: A Comprehensive Textbook, Fourth Edition* illustrates so well the changes in child and adolescent psychiatry, but it also insists upon the continuity of our field, teaching us how to listen to the young voices who are just setting on their course. Its words are alive; in them are both the continuity and the changes that are our field.

John F. McDermott, MD
Professor of Psychiatry Emeritus
University of Hawaii School of Medicine
Editor Emeritus
Journal of the American Academy of Child and Adolescent Psychiatry

PREFACE TO THE FIFTH EDITION

Lewis's Fifth

It has been exactly a decade since the publication of *Lewis's* last edition. We are delighted to present this latest iteration, its fifth. We have sought to maintain and expand in it the changes introduced in the previous edition, which represented a large departure from the three initial versions that Mel Lewis so diligently brought to life. Notwithstanding its changes, the current edition is true to Mel's original spirit and expands on the trajectory he began a quarter century ago, back in 1991. For the reader getting first acquainted with *Lewis's Textbook*, we have next included the preface to the fourth edition, in which we review the evolution of the imprint.

The changes in this edition are subtler than in the last. Most chapters have been updated and a select few have been left behind. Many have been entirely rewritten by new authors. The chapter on telepsychiatry introduces a topic that was in its infancy 10 years ago and has become all but standard today. The fifth edition of another book, the Diagnostic and Statistical Manual (DSM-5), also makes its first appearance in this edition, as does the Research Domain Criteria (RDoC) approach advanced by the National Institute of Mental Health over the past decade. A large and unwieldy chapter on psychopharmacology from the fourth edition has been carved out into five thematically linked, updated and more manageable component pieces. In a salute to our tradition and legacy, just as much to our field's vibrant practice and exciting future, we have left two meaningful components entirely unchanged: the foreword to the fourth edition, by the late Jack McDermott, and "Looking back, dreaming forward," the cautionary postscript by the late Leon Eisenberg.

One noteworthy change is the expansion of our original editorial duo. In this edition we have been joined by Michael H. Bloch—a younger colleague who did not have the privilege of getting to know and work with Mel Lewis like we did, and who is now enlisted, along both of us and so many of the authors herein, to carry on Mel's legacy into the future. The three of us wish to express our gratitude to the Wolters Kluwer team superbly orchestrated by Ashley Fischer, Rebecca Gaertner, and Chris Teja on the editorial side, and to Linda Francis and David Saltzberg on the production side. Finally, and as noted in the dedication page, we are proud as editors to direct our royalties to the American Academy of Child and Adolescent Psychiatry, an organization that Mel served so well and for so long. We hope this will not only honor his memory, but help in very tangible ways to further the overall goal of *Lewis's Textbook*: to train and inspire a new generation of clinicians whose life's work is easing the burden of mental illness and improving the lives of children and families everywhere.

Andrés Martin
Michael H. Bloch
Fred R. Volkmar
Child Study Center
Yale School of Medicine
New Haven, Connecticut

PREFACE TO THE FOURTH EDITION

Lewis's Fourth

> *[T]he mission . . . is not to pass on an unchanged truth through a succession of the learned but to host the endless labor, carried on from generation to generation, needed to come closer to the truth: the work of challenging the adequacy of what currently passes for the truth, attempting to seize it more fully, and making that understanding available to others so they can move beyond it to a yet fuller realization.*
>
> —Richard Broadhead: Free Speech and its Discontents (2004)

Readers acquainted with the three earlier editions of this volume are as likely to be reassured as they are to be disoriented on seeing this latest version. The reassurances will come from the textbook's signature heft and color, a similar breadth in scope and depth in coverage, and the welcome resurfacing of many familiar names within. The disorientation should be slight but significant, perhaps beginning with the very name of the book, subtly but most certainly different from its predecessors'. The landmark *Child and Adolescent Psychiatry: A Comprehensive Textbook* that first appeared in 1991 had reached second and third editions within just eleven years (in 1996 and 2002, respectively). Today, 16 years after it first appeared onstage to set a new standard in the field, its latest edition comes forth, under the slightly altered title of *Lewis's Child and Adolescent Psychiatry: A Comprehensive Textbook.* The one-word change is at once subtle and momentous.

In this fourth edition, Melvin Lewis, for whom this landmark text has been a labor of love, makes way for two of his colleagues and students (not to mention admirers and friends) to continue his editorial vision and commitment. The book's new title reflects more than a semantic detail: in a fundamental way, *Lewis* embodies Mel's legacy and the values he has held dear for decades. His has been a model of professional and scholarly comportment that the two of us emulate each day. We are grateful for the opportunity granted us, and aware of the responsibility implicit in the stewardship we have been entrusted. We have strived for a new edition that includes the best of our science; that translates and makes it accessible and applicable; that provides cohesion for a rapidly evolving discipline; that welcomes and guides the novice as much as reminds the veteran of the richness of our work. An edition, in brief, that by becoming a vehicle to improve the mental health of children and adolescents will make Melvin Lewis proud.

This fourth edition's title and cover art are the first and most apparent differences, but not the only ones. Indeed, it is in its substantially revised, updated and reorganized inner structures that the book is very much a new edition. The better testament to *Lewis's* ability to advance Mel's legacy may be in how different, rather than in how similar, it is from earlier versions. An evolving discipline is reflected in organically changing books that refuse to become definitive: Gauging from the changes to this tome from a mere five years ago, our field is a lively and thriving one.

An Approach to the Discipline, the first of seven sections, sets the tone for the volume as a whole. If there has been a guiding principle in assembling this textbook, it has been our effort to trace the links between multiple components of our field. We sought to identify continuities across the domains of clinical practice, research, training, and policy—a mutually enriching interplay at times more aspired to than real. We have opted for a reorganized structure in which aspects as varied as economics, diversity, or evidence-based practice are not treated as afterthoughts. To the contrary, we see such topics as a necessary foundation upon which to build. We have been deliberate in our choice of a first chapter that begins with the clinical care of a single child and ripples outward toward familial and societal dimensions: The care of children and families remains not only our foremost concern, but the place from where our major insights have almost invariably come.

The second section, *Scientific Foundations,* synthesizes three major domains of critical relevance to advance our knowledge base in childhood psychiatric disorders: epidemiology and prevention, genetics, and neuroscience. While this section could never be all-inclusive, it does aim to provide a basic level of scientific literacy required to be an informed consumer of the literature; one aware that today's arcane and seemingly esoteric finding may hold the key to tomorrow's breakthrough intervention. To provide a framework for understanding these or any other pertinent scientific approaches, the section includes an overarching chapter on research methodology and statistics.

We pause here to note with sadness the untimely passing of our colleague Robert Harmon during the making of this book. The very first chapter that we received came from Bob and his colleagues in Colorado. *Methodology and Statistics: A Relevant Primer and Overview* arrived with a characteristically encouraging and upbeat message from Bob. Of note, it appeared in our inboxes a full two days before the very first deadline, one so fashionably ignored by the other authors—ourselves included. We remember Bob with affection, and thank him not only for teaching and writing skills we all admire, but for punctuality that is an editor's dream.

The third section, *A Developmental Framework,* chronologically follows normal development from the prenatal period through late adolescence. While incorporating the more relevant theories of human development, its chapters have a stronger emphasis on clinical applicability than encyclopedic coverage of specific milestones or schools of thought. The section is very much in line with our experience of Mel's teaching and is capped with a review of developmental psychopathology, addressing the ways in which genetic endowment and environmental conditions can interact along the dimension of time to increase the likelihood of resilient or pathologic outcomes.

A fourth section on *Nosology, Classification, and Diagnostic Assessment* starts with an overview of the different ways in which child psychopathology has been historically classified. This chapter identifies differences across, and within, the major nosological schemes: the European ICD versus the American DSM, and the various iterations of the latter. Although this discussion will eventually be eclipsed by the arrival of the forthcoming DSM-5, the more relevant point to make here is that this volume is not beholden to any given system: we have not imposed editorial consistency at this level, realizing that such classification schemes are fluid and perfectible products. Thus, some chapters stay within well-demarcated diagnostic lines, others see the limitations in existing criteria, while yet others take whatever is useful from different classifications. The longer part of this section is dedicated to the diagnostic and clinical assessment process, and includes chapters that range from specific forms of assessment to the integration of the rich complexity inherent in child psychiatric practice.

Specific Disorders and Syndromes is the fifth and longest section. We should note here that for many conditions we have followed groupings that made good clinical sense to us, even if our organization scheme was not necessarily the most traditional. The same can be said of the part on treatment in the sixth section, where we created a *Continuum of Care and Location-Specific Interventions* category that, while wordily titled, brings together aspects that are often as poorly articulated in textbooks as they are out in the community.

The seventh and final section encompasses the very broadly ambassadorial *Interface Areas of Child and Adolescent Psychiatry*. Specifically, it includes our discipline's work on the borders—and often well within the territories—of pediatrics, schools, and the law.

Lewis comes up to 87 chapters, 155 contributing authors and over 1000 pages of text. What if anything can we make of these summary and impressive statistics? And what can we make of the fact that it has 46 *fewer* chapters and a significantly different line-up and content than its previous edition? More importantly, how does a discipline know that its knowledge base is moving in the right direction? When its truths become pickled into canonical and unchanging texts, or when they squirm out of our grasp and refuse to be fixed? When their tomes become thicker? When they become leaner? Perhaps it is when the tomes disappear altogether?

These questions are not rhetorical, nor are they simply meant to provoke. The fact is that books today are not what they used to be just a decade ago, and the place and function of the academic textbook needs to be reconsidered in light of today's hegemony of the internet as a source of living and constantly shifting knowledge. Knowledge that in turn brings up a whole new set of questions about the information available to clinicians, practitioners, and patients: What is the least disorienting and most reassuring source of information after all? Do not get us wrong: neither one of us is a pessimist. We are proud of this book and confident that it will teach and, we hope, inspire the readers it reaches, that it can provide a sense of overarching coherence one would be hard-pressed to find elsewhere. But we are realists and aware that some of the information contained in these pages will be out of date even before the book sees the light of day and that some more will gradually decay like so much radioactive material. The problem we now face is finding some sort of effective rapprochement between nimble cybernetics, with its propensity to conflate the constructive and responsible with the misleading and reckless through a simple mouse click, and the solid consensus of the textbook, where rigorous methodology and transparent use of science and sources also risk reifying what is incorrect as authoritative.

Lewis's previous edition was already available as an e-book that included hypertext links. This new edition follows suit with updated technology, and a shorter, pocket companion version with self-assessment questions is planned. In these ways, this traditional textbook will continue to advance into electronic territory. As we look at the first three editions sitting on our shelves, we think back to the shelf of Professor Victor McCusick, father of modern human genetics and editor of the classic *Mendelian Inheritance in Man* first published in 1966. During the years under his watch, genetic information exploded, such that his svelte single tome evolved into a massive three-volume 12th edition by 1998. Paper stock and wet forests shuddered at the thought of what the next edition might entail. As it turns out, it entailed very little, at least by ways of paper: By then the resource had all but ceased to be a book, having migrated almost entirely to the web as OMIM (http://www.ncbi.nlm.nih.gov/omim).

Even as this and other textbooks are likely to continue merging, blending, and otherwise becoming complementary with electronic resources, we do not hold our breath for a complete migration to the web. But even if there is one, we wager that there are abiding values and clinical wisdom in these pages that will continue to hold true and guide our practice for years to come. The very first and the very last contributions to this communal effort reassure us of as much: we are indebted to Jack McDermott for his foreword, to Leon Eisenberg for his postscript, and to both for standing as beacons who direct us toward values and principles worth holding dear.

We are grateful to the superb lineup of contributing authors for their engagement, responsiveness and excellent work. We thank our advisory board members for their input and sage advice at critical junctures en route to the palpable reality of this book. We express special thanks to a Lippincott Williams and Wilkins team superbly orchestrated by Charley Mitchell. And to end as we began, our gratitude and deep appreciation to Melvin Lewis, whose passion and vision were the original ingredients for this textbook's secret recipe. Grateful though we are, we humbly recognize that the success of this edition should be measured by how much it helps move our field toward the fuller realization of helping children and families everywhere.

Andrés Martin
Fred R. Volkmar
Child Study Center
Yale School of Medicine
New Haven, Connecticut

CONTENTS

SECTION IV: CLINICAL ASSESSMENT AND NOSOLOGY

SECTION V: SPECIFIC DISORDERS AND SYNDROMES

SECTION VII: INTERFACE AREAS OF CHILD AND ADOLESCENT PSYCHIATRY

SECTION I
AN APPROACH TO THE DISCIPLINE

CHAPTER 1.1 ■ THE ART OF A CHILD, FAMILY, AND SYSTEMS-CENTERED SCIENCE

KYLE D. PRUETT

> *I keep picturing all these little kids playing some game in this big field of rye... Thousands of little kids and nobody's around—nobody big, I mean—except me... What I have to do, I have to catch everybody if they start over the cliff.*
>
> —J.D. Salinger, *The Catcher in the Rye*

INVITATION TO THE PRACTICE OF CHILD AND ADOLESCENT PSYCHIATRY

Like many medical students before me, I had been moved and troubled by my first encounters with the mind-shattering onset of schizophrenia in adolescence: such pain and disorientation during such a promising era of life. There had to be better ways to understand and reduce the morbidity of such illnesses for these young people and their families, or at least to catch them before they edged Holden Caulfield's cliff.

Such thinking diverted me from pediatrics and adult psychiatry toward working with ever younger children, looking earlier and earlier for how to be of use. I eventually found myself standing by NICU bassinettes of poorly thriving infants with anyone I could corral to help me fathom how things could go so wrong, so soon, and too often with the very young. I found smart, humane mentors in child psychiatrists Al Solnit (Yale Child Study Center), pediatricians Sydney Gellis (Boston Floating Hospital) and Sally Provence (Yale Child Study Center); each one discouraging simplistic formulations and helping me embrace the complexity of early experience with all the rigor I could muster.

It struck me that child and adolescent psychiatry had it right. The earlier the better—for diagnosis, treatment, parent guidance, cost–benefit ratios, and whatever we could do to help families support, and grow with, their vulnerable and promising children. It also struck me as shortsighted to dissect the child out—even intellectually—from its family for diagnostic studies, economies of time, convenience of intervention, ease of insurance, billing or cost containment. Such a myopic approach was like a celestial navigator trying to identify a constellation by fixing a solitary star with his sextant; then as now, a guaranteed way to get good and lost.

So, how to stay on course in this odyssey to effective intervention and prevention? We now know, thanks to the advances in epigenetics, that we must consult both the gene map (nature) *and* family tree (nurture) and experiences that bridge them to stay on course. From the beginning of developmental mental health explorations in the 1920s and 30s, child psychiatry distrusted the facile nature versus nurture dichotomy offered up as dogma by so many behavioral scientists. Careful clinical investigations and longitudinal inquiry repeatedly fell short of affirming it as the best way to formulate helpful interventions.

Contemporary science has all but eliminated this distraction, helping us to conceptualize the dichotomy less as competition, and more as a transaction (1). It has proven more illuminating to investigate how we nurture nature than to officiate at the face-off between the two. Tienari et al. (2) highlight clearly the interaction between environment and genome as accounting for more of the variance in clinical outcomes of illness than either genetics or environment alone. The compelling early studies by Caspi et al. of G(ene) × E(xperience) (3), and Kaufman et al. (4), and more recently Yehuda et al. (5) and Meaney (6) of gene interactions and environmental modifiers of depression in children provide elegant empirical grounding to that effect. Taken together, their work addressing G × E interactions between severity of child abuse, 5HT transporter polymorphisms, and outcomes of depression and conduct disorder have profound implications for societal and mental health intervention.

The outcomes of well-designed longitudinal studies of young children and families at risk also encourage us to focus on this discourse between gene and environment to design more effective and relevant service, policy, and research agendas (7). Sroufe et al. (8) concluded from his classic *Minnesota Study of Risk and Adaptation from Birth to Adulthood* that "early history is not destiny, important as it is…[D]ata suggest a renewed focus on the lived experience of the child and [less] preoccupation with inherent biologic variations."

This perspective can save us from a too myopic focus on the behavior of the child as we struggle to understand ways to decrease the morbidity of psychopathology and increase resilient contexts which, in turn, lessen comorbidities. Hechtman's (9) discussion of research into long-term outcomes of childhood disorders encourages us to cast a broad net in our search for the salient factors affecting outcome which extend beyond behavior. She reminds us to look beyond age, gender, IQ, comorbid conditions, physical, and emotional health to include socioeconomic status, family function, and composition, and child rearing practices. Felitti and Robert's (10) work on the long-term negative health sequelae of adverse childhood experiences makes a most compelling case for this approach.

It is the ability to embrace this complexity—not avoid or oversimplify it—that defines child psychiatric clinical competence. Authors have tried to conceptualize this visually by drawing concentric circles outward from the child to include all the factors that shape development, per se; particularly when we adhere to classical definitions of development as the melding of genetic predisposition, or maturation, with experience. But such visuals typically fall short, because as Spitz (11) so efficiently summarized four decades ago, "Maturation is a useful concept, but in reality there is only development." Ultimately, it is the environment that processes any given child's genetic blueprint, through maturation, into lived experience.

The core purpose in diagnostic and intervention strategies is to encompass and embrace the complexity of the child's experience to understand and treat, while fully incorporating the hegemony of age (chronologic and developmental) and circumstance. This is precisely what obligates the researching and treating physician to employ the child-, family-, and systems-centered approach embraced throughout this textbook.

Families render humans human. Era-specific developmental forces within the family and the child jointly define the salient relationships and intimacies that draw the infant in one human transaction at a time. The family in all its permutations ultimately embraces that particular child's maturational promise and, through powerful reciprocal forces, converts tissue, synaptic connection, and instinct into human development. Although family processes seem linear (from birth and growth to decline and death, repeated ad libitum), family process itself seems more helical in form. Each generation must accommodate its own unique life cycle agenda. Consequently, it may be more helpful to visualize family processes as intertwined developmental courses, not unlike Watson, Crick, and Franklin's double helix. Winding side by side, the generations develop together, intimately connected with, but nevertheless distinct from, other generations in the family.

This helical image of family development consists of two distinct conceptual strands. One strand is the family's trail of generational myths, expectations, attributes, memories, and secrets—the family's "givens." This is the family's narrative about itself, eloquently described by Pincus and Dare (12) and Vangelisti (13). The narrative evolves much like folk songs in the oral tradition, passed on at home, as children are taught who and what their family has been, and is hoped or expected to be.

The other strand is the family's forward progression through time in the here and now. This encompasses the usual stresses and opportunities of the family's children's developmental requirements and the intrusion of "fateful events," both positive and negative. How the family copes with the course of development, accidents, and intrusions from outside and within is determined in part by whether these two strands intersect at strong or weak points. Real trouble seems most likely when a vulnerable stretch on the transgenerational strand intersects with an equally vulnerable stretch on the developmental strand.

For example, the Jones family narrative carries the myth/expectation that "Jones boys always marry wild women" at a time when, on the developmental strand, the Jones' first born son is starting his adolescence by easing up on his typical and historic academic discipline and atypically, for him, testing behavioral boundaries. He tells his parents progressively less about his life and whereabouts (appropriately), especially where girls are concerned and voilà—his and his family's fantasies about "wild women" fuse and sparks fly. Unless the clinician has some awareness of this fraught intersection of the Jones' family brand of developmental and transgenerational vulnerabilities, he or she may be too quick to assign an impulse or other behavior disorder label, which in turn, might lead to ineffective or inappropriate intervention.

Family development as a dynamic phenomenon is particularly hard to fathom because clinicians tend to encounter families at but one nodal point in time, denying them a critical longitudinal perspective. Classic and current research suggests strong links between early loss, trauma, and disturbance in the family and later interpersonal dysfunction (14–16). At any given time in our interaction with a family, we may be uncertain about which direction the causal links may be moving (such as whether a vulnerable child destabilizes the family, or vice versa) (17); most mental illnesses are not the result of a sole inborn factor, or some single extraneous perturbation, but rather the multiply determined end result of human development gone (momentarily, one hopes) awry.

THE EVOLVING FAMILY SYSTEM

Most sociologists opine that the range of family structure continues to evolve. Lower birth rates, substantial (though stabilizing) divorce rates, older age of first child births (26 in 2015 compared to 21 in 1970) increasing remarriage rates, accelerated same-sex marriage and step-family rates, and longer life expectancies have all reduced childbearing from being the major occupation of parents to what is now less than 50% of parents' lifelong commitment (18).

Typically, historians urge caution whenever referring to "unprecedented change." Demos (19), and Laslette and Wall (20), dispelled the myth of the ideal three-generational family holding sway in preindustrial family life, citing instead a social process over the past several hundred years, and in particular over the past few decades, that has effected major changes in family functioning. Hareven (21) summarizes "Through a process of differentiation, the family gradually surrendered functions previously concentrated within it to other social institutions. During the pre-industrial period, the family not only reared children, but also served as a workshop, a school, a church, and an asylum." The difficulties faced by contemporary families are rooted in this diminished capacity to adapt and cope (partly because of smaller size) and the further narrowing in the range of the family's socioeconomic functions and independence.

The declining maternal and child death rates of the 1950s, combined with a higher marriage rate and longer life span created a higher percentage of children growing up in stable, two-parent families than had ever occurred in America's history. Beginning with the 1960s, however, multiply determined trends began to reshape the ideal and real traditional nuclear family. The sexual revolution uncoupled the societal association of sexual and reproductive behavior, particularly for women. From 1971 to 2002, the percentage of unmarried American girls 15 to 19 years of age who engaged in sexual intercourse rose from 28% to 60%. Second, married women with children moved into the paid workforce: There was an increase from the 1960 level of 19% of married women with children younger than 6 years of age in the labor force to a real figure of 66% in 2001. Historian Robert Griswold (22) noted that these forces, combined with attitudinal changes toward co-parenting, have brought increasing numbers of fathers into the nurturing domain, whether or not they want to be there.

Fertility and fecundity also declined in the United States beginning in the 1960s. We are now at levels lower than those necessary for the replacement of the population, having moved from an average of 3.7 children per woman in 1960 to 1.83 (23). Increased child survival over the last century, combined with women having their first children later in their reproductive years, may also be contributing to families having fewer children.

The divorce rate in America, though currently stable at roughly 38%, brought us past a landmark in 1974, when for the first time in our history, more marriages concluded in divorce than in the death of a spouse (18). The percentages of unmarried couples, same-sex couples, serial and stepfamilies, and single-parent families (single by choice or not) have all increased, whereas nuclear unit percentages continue to decrease.

Finally, many clinicians and researchers share the opinion that the quality of life for children in the past 40 years has not improved at the same rate as it has for adults. Also, rates of distress seem to be on the rise. Achenbach and Howell (24) studied the changes over 13 years in the prevalence of children in the general population with behavioral/emotional problems. They found more untreated children who needed psychological intervention in the 1989 sample than in the 1976 sample. The 2014 Kids Count Report by the Annie E. Casey Foundation documented a continuing downturn in child well-being trends with increasing child poverty and obesity, infant low birth weight and mortality, and a teen death rate increase over the previous 5-year report. This suggests that the trend noted by Achenbach has yet to reverse itself (25).

Though family structure continues to evolve to include different constellations within and across generations, most children continue to long for meaningful relationships with both biologic parents in his or her life (26). The family structure that is most influential in the child's development, however, is the one perceived by the child as his or her family, not the one perceived by the Census Bureau or any given research protocol.

Many contemporary statistics illustrate an important, irreducible fact about ongoing change in the American family: Most moms work some or full time (71%, 2015). The 2003 U.S. Bureau of Labor Statistics report (27) documented that 16% of all married couple families have a wage-earning father and a stay-at-home mother; that number was 67% in 1940. Child rearing families also tend to receive more societal and economic support when both parents are committed to the job in all its complexity. Families have changed, particularly in expectations around co-parenting and paternal engagement, according to a recent *Zero to Three* Survey (28) yet the institutions the families rely on most heavily—schools, health care, and the workplace—have been slow to respond to these changes.

MOTHERHOOD AND FATHERHOOD

Each child who enters the family changes it permanently, rendering each child's perception of their family as unique in, and to, their own experience. Sameroff and Fiese have moved us away from the restrictions of the linear, interactional model of child development, and toward one that better encompasses the progressive, dynamic, reciprocal forces that have helped children change families and vice versa (1). Their "transactional model" emphasizes the need for incorporating social and economic as well as biologic forces, proposing instead a "continuum of caretaking causality," with increased emphasis on the qualitative aspects of the nurturing domain. It encourages clinicians and researchers to think anew about who in the family is doing what with the children, and not simply how long they are doing it.

The Berkeley Adult Attachment Interview (29) in its application to family development (30) is an example of our growing skills in assessing the mother's and father's separate states of mind (and not simply their behavior) with regard to attachment to their children, and vice versa. As such it exemplifies how we are returning to the exploration of the overriding significance of the quality, sensitivity, and intent of the nurturing interaction, and not merely the biologic predispositions of the interactors. Mothers, fathers, grandparents, aunts, uncles, and siblings—all form unique attachments that, in formative settings, are welcomed and easily integrated by the child into a mosaic of consistent, predictable, stabilizing internalizations of the nurturing experience. We are now aware that attachment behavior between mother and child is obvious within the first months of life and is centered on establishing a sense of comfort and security, especially when the child is stressed. Attachment behavior between fathers and children becomes defined later in development, when the child is more mobile and more likely to test the limits of safety through risk taking. Managing the excitement of novel exploration and remaining safe when doing so is more typical of paternal attachment behavior than of maternal attachment behavior (31,32). Internalization of the nurturing experience, be it positive or negative, is not merely the result of a single adult attachment, but rather of the mosaic of the infant's experience with meaningful relationships over time.

Optimal family development, as perceived by the child, begins with a secure individual relationship, which the infant typically makes with its primary caregiver, typically the mother. Fathers can also form such attachments, rearing their children without placing them at developmental risk (33–35). Radin and Harold-Goldsmith (36) and Pruett (35) cite the advantages to young children of paternal involvement, independent of the reasons for the father's presence (29). The other optimal phenomenon for promoting development in the family network consists of the capacity of mothers and fathers to form reciprocal, empathic, and unique relationships with the child, aided by a broad and complete range of affective expression. Both parents must be ready to accept developmental progression and change, because it comes rapidly, particularly in the first year, aided by appreciation for the child's idiosyncratic traits, temperament, skills, and vulnerabilities.

Much clinical literature, however, falls short in clarifying distinct maternal and paternal antecedents to psychological syndromes (37). When Bezirganian et al. (38) found that maternal overinvolvement, paired with maternal inappropriateness, combined to form pathogenic predispositions toward borderline personality disorder in children, paternal measures, which were included, were not commented on in their discussion. Despite the dramatic increase in the number of publications on fathering since the mid-1980s (39), fathers continue to be vastly underrepresented in the clinical and research literature, though fathers are now more engaged with their young children than in any era since the Industrial Revolution; the father's share of childcare more than doubled between 1965 and 1998 (40). A typical example of how this remains neglected in the literature: A major prospective, longitudinal study on parental psychopathology, and parenting styles as related to the risk of social phobia in children failed to include any data on fathers (41). Panter-Brick's (42) important global review of paternal engagement literature found that the vast majority of published literature in peer-reviewed journal rarely includes paternal measures or variables, much less correlative findings, even when "parents" is in the title of the paper.

Phares and Compas (43) reviewed research papers in the major journals dealing with clinical child development published from 1984 to 1991 and found that nearly half of all studies involved mothers only. Nearly one-fourth of the remaining studies did include father-related material, but did not differentiate its effects. The final one-fourth did measure father–child effects and found them consistently present. So, when researchers do bother to look for father effects, they typically find them. The authors suggested that the overreliance on mothers as research participants has fostered not only an incomplete data set with regard to child development, but also one that is heavily gender biased because "relations cannot be found among variables that are not investigated (43)."

EVALUATING THE FAMILY

As child psychiatrist works to understand the child's experience despite such lacunae in the literature, he or she is best served by viewing the family as a system, in which change in one segment of the family resonates throughout the system; promoting or discouraging development in other family members. Families must "raise the children" while socializing their young, balancing risk and protective factors (44), and simultaneously meeting the demands of rapidly evolving maturational forces in the child. It is crucial, then, to appropriately evaluate the family system's potential for preparing its children for adulthood.

Skinner et al. (45) created the classic Family Assessment Measure, consisting of a general and dyadic scale to distinguish reliably between normal and problem families. Mrazek et al. (46) developed the Parenting Risk Scale, which uses a semistructured interview to rate difficulties and concerns regarding parental commitment, knowledge base, control, psychiatric disturbance, and emotional availability. The McMaster Family Assessment Device is a questionnaire filled out by both parents to assess seven categories of family functioning (47). Fleck (48) described an efficient, five-factor method, based on a family interview, for assessing the family's capacity to support the development of its children across its life cycle, consisting of (a) leadership, (b) boundaries, (c) emotional climate, (d) communication, and (e) the establishment and accomplishment of goals and tasks throughout the life cycle.

Leadership is the decision making, facilitating source of power and discipline used by the parents to lead the family forward (or not). It is shaped by the presence or absence of mutual support and regard, and by the effectiveness of the communication between the leaders of the family unit. Leadership itself is complex, as seen in the work of Minuchin and Fishman (49), who have tracked its migration between family members and generations, depending on the particular mix of strengths, vulnerabilities, or developmental demands that are preoccupying the family at any given moment.

Family boundaries refer to boundaries (a) within the individual that define the self, (b) between generations, and (c) between the family and the community. It is important that these boundaries be semipermeable, permitting contact and discourse with others outside the family boundary. Self and generational boundaries tend to remain stable throughout the life cycle, whereas family/community boundaries must become increasingly permeable as children cross them with increasing frequency to participate in the community around them.

The emotional climate, or affectivity, of the family unit is the connective tissue that binds the family together as a functioning unit. It sustains—or erodes—the family's capacity to care for and support itself and one another, especially since the family has ceased to be such a self-contained economic unit. Chronic scapegoating of a family member, child abuse, interpersonal violence between parents, and neglect are classic signs of failure in the family's emotional climate.

Communication within families is obviously both verbal and nonverbal. Communicative language and its uses for deepening relationships are learnt best within the family, assuming a healthy emotional climate. Experiences and affect are shared through the medium of language verbal and nonverbal, whereas values and culture are differentiated and reinforced by the consistency, tone, and content of communication within the family.

Finally, the expectation that families will nurture and socialize their young so that they develop into contributing members of society is the moral obligation placed on these functions. The success or failure of this expectation is determined by the way the family achieves its goals for individual members and sets the members' tasks toward reaching those goals. Goals and tasks throughout the life cycle change and evolve in complex ways and, unlike communication or boundaries, seem not to diminish in significance over time.

Cultural influences powerfully shape the tasks of the family across the life span. As child-rearing domains become increasingly complex, it is essential that clinicians and researchers remain vigilant for the health-promoting cultural and functional forces that frame a particular family's expectations, resources, strengths, and vulnerabilities in their context (35,50,51). Values about dependability, family loyalty, intimacy, privacy, autonomy, and extended family access vary widely and normatively across the whole range of families created by adoption and assisted reproductive technologies (52,53).

Appreciating particular values in context is critical for the growing number of children raised in families shaped by multiple cultural influences. Social and cultural isolation of such children and their parents can frustrate the resilience and strength so common in the families that adopt cross-racially, or a multiply fostered child, making their task unnecessarily more complex. Same-sex parenting partners and their children can experience conflict in certain communities stemming from the failure to appreciate such a family's contextual needs and competencies (54), rendering the children at greater risk in certain developmental stages, especially the transition to adolescence (55).

THE ARTS OF CHILD PSYCHIATRY

Having defined the parameters of the task, we can look in greater detail at the skills on which child psychiatrists rely to help them accomplish their goals, and what, if anything, is contributed by an artful or humanistic approach to their work. Child psychiatry as a field has had a historical influence on the country's general attitudes toward the needs of its children that is out of proportion to its number of practitioners. Child psychiatrists figure so prominently in the creation of the fields of mental health consultation and crisis intervention that one may ask "Why them?" Why have they consistently held seminal leadership positions in public policy, from the landmark Joint Commission on the Mental Health of Children in 1965 right up to the Neurons to Neighborhoods Report of the National Institutes of Medicine in 2002? Why did the nation's media turn to them for consultation and guidance following the events of 9/11/01, the mass shootings in Newtown, CT, and more recent acts of terrorism, both local and global? Why this trusted provenance in the well-being of all children, and not simply the mentally ill, from this medical subspecialty at the local and national level?

Attempts at defining *art* are instructive in understanding this penchant for hard-headed soft-heartedness among child and adolescent psychiatrists. The OED's "skill in doing anything as a result of knowledge or practice" definition suggests that medical training in and of itself prepares and predisposes these practitioners and researchers to embrace interdisciplinary thinking automatically. Such thinking is essential to understanding child development, as one is constantly juggling competing theories to understand a particular child and family's vulnerability, be it behavioral, psychodynamic, cognitive, or all of the above. So, when it comes to working with a team on an inpatient unit, a military base or in school consultation, it is already second nature to welcome and be informed by other "systems" of understanding. It is likewise second nature to be thinking differentially about case-based diagnostic and symptomatic material the moment it is encountered.

A further OED definition of *art* reads, "human workmanship as opposed to natural [ability]." The ability to listen with nonjudgmental patience, discriminating care, and open mindedness to children's verbal *and* nonverbal communication is one of the hallmarks of this specialty's competence. So many of our young patients trust us because they feel heard by us. This skill at listening to behavior, symptoms, play, artwork, or rationalizations develops over time in the clinic, supervision, team meetings, emergency departments, the movie theater or the waiting room, and eventually starts to resemble a "knack." However, as a teacher and supervisor of hundreds of practitioners in this field for over three decades, I am more persuaded by the "work(wo)manship" argument for developing the "knack" than the "nature" one.

This particular skill or "intellectual instrument" undergirds the child psychiatrists' reputation for being among the best interviewers in medicine, whether the subject is child or adult. The daily experience with children and their families shapes one's judgment over time about what to ask and when, in investigating and fathoming the child's distress. The clinician knows that questions are never simply queries, but rather a medium for judgment, concern, comprehension, or indifference, depending on how and when they are asked, and how carefully they attend to the answers. It is in the art of the interview itself that the potentially caring/healing relationship is first introduced and subsequently shaped, and the empathic apprehension of the skilled listener/observer is established, whether with an individual child/infant, parent, couple, or entire family system.

Outside the interviewing domain, however, child psychiatrists also respect and embrace the complexity of the context in which the child of concern lives his or her daily life. It is this appreciation for contextual symptom expression that makes them so useful to the institutions that serve the needs of children in the community, and such effective advocates for policies that increase care and well-being of society's most vulnerable; hence, their pioneering role in establishing mental health consultation in community agencies and schools (56,57), and crisis intervention in the first place.

This predilection for contextual information also renders typical child psychiatrists slower than the average general practitioner to prescribe medications with the potential to change behavior, understanding as they do the power of context, positive and negative, to influence behavior (58). The longer amount of time with the child and family utilized by the child psychiatrist may predispose toward this difference, but it remains more a perceptual than a time management issue.

Another perceptual distinction that defines the child psychiatrist's unique approach to understanding and studying mental health and illness is the enduring respect for the power of development to predispose to health. Child psychiatrists, therefore, habitually embed their understanding of a particular child's clinical presentation into the proper era/context of child and family development.

Family development itself is somewhat arbitrarily divided into sequential stages for better understanding of the predictable developmental phenomena typical of a certain era. This approach risks oversimplifying the complexity of the relationship system which expands or contracts to support the entrance, development, and exit of family members emotionally, culturally, and historically. I review these stages with an eye to the contributions made by the nurturers and the "nurturants," examining the unique and differing roles of mothers and fathers as participants and facilitators of normal development across the life cycle.

THE DEVELOPMENTAL APPROACH

Coupling and Family Formation

Making a deliberate decision about family formation predisposes toward child and family well-being, just as an unconscious, nonconjoint decision predisposes to developmental risk. One of the stronger unconscious motivations toward coupling is the wish to acquire in one's mate a longed-for or unfinished aspect of oneself. This can strongly predispose toward stability in a marriage and may have an ameliorating effect on eventual family formation despite previous negative experiences, particularly on the part of the mother in her own childhood nurturing interactions. Eichberg has found in her research using the Adult Attachment Inventory that the father's role is positively ameliorative of a mother's negative experience with her own parents (59,60).

When the coupling results in a stable, long-term relationship or marriage, it is a joining of two complex historical, interpersonal, emotional, and economic systems. Couples are marrying later and postponing birthing their children: the average age of first marriage for women in 2004 was 23.1 and for men 24.9 years, and the birth of their first child came on average 1 year and 11 months later. In 2014 it was 26 for women and 27 for men. The rise in cohabitation rates, both planned and unplanned, however has kept first child age cohorts stable over the last 20 years (61). These numbers imply there is a relatively short time given to adjusting to this phase of life, and sociologists note that there is a relatively narrow window for the timing of this family preparation phase. Women are twice as likely to divorce if they marry before the age of 20 years as if they marry during their 20s. They are half again as likely to divorce if they marry after 30 years of age than if they marry during their 20s (62).

A variety of other factors also can contribute to difficulty at this life cycle transition: (a) the couple resides at either great distance or close proximity to either family of origin; (b) the couple meets or marries in close proximity to a significant loss; (c) the couple marries after knowing each other for fewer than 6 months or an engagement lasting over 3 years; (d) the wedding is performed without family or friends; and (e) the wife becomes pregnant before or within the first year of marriage (63,64). It does seem that the rise in women's socioeconomic and political status is correlated (though not necessarily causally) with some degree of marital destabilization and with the increasing, although not absolute, marital dissatisfaction of their husbands. We are clearly in a transition toward more egalitarian relationships, and the educational and occupational equity of the sexes can be a creative catalyst (65). In the recent revision of her classic sociology of marriage, Stephanie Coontz [2016] (66) summarizes, *"There is* ***not*** *growing estrangement or a widening gender gap in what women and men want from each other. Most men and women are moving in the same direction in terms of their values... Tensions between men and women today stem* *less from different aspirations than from the difficulties they face translating their **ideals** into practice."*

How people are choosing partners, and who they are choosing has also changed, most remarkably with the use of online relationship brokerage, as trends in miscegenation and same-sex partnerships show, which brings new challenges, opportunities, strengths and stressors to the new family.

First Conception, Birth, and Nurturance

This era begins with conception and ends at the end of the child's first year. There is much psychological work to be done by both parents in preparing for and dealing with conception. There also is enormous variability in the amount of conscious deliberation devoted to the decision to conceive a child. Once conception does take place, planned or unplanned, complex psychological responses follow in both wife and husband. The mother struggles with profound changes occurring in most of the organ and hormonal systems in her body during pregnancy and after delivery. Fathers also undergo physiologic (hormonal and body mass) changes during pregnancy and the perinatal periods, most notably in increased in oxytocin and estrogen secretion and decreased testosterone production (67).

Meanwhile, much of the psychological work is fueled by a conscious reassessment of the couple's own family experience. A new identity comes to fruition, that of being a parent, not just of having one (68). What makes this riveting is that both maternal and paternal identifications are deeply rooted in each parent. The mother prepares herself psychologically for the coming attachment to her infant by drawing her attention to her own inner experience and her growing fetus, as her preoccupation with the outside world decreases.

Fathers are involved in psychological work of a different sort, albeit active and equally important in terms of preparation. Food cravings, somatic preoccupations such as vague gastrointestinal disorders, and nutritional changes are widely reported. Concern about his adequacy as a provider and protector may erode an expectant father's self-esteem. Mood changes, frequently expected in mothers, also occur in fathers: "Even before the birth of his child, the father's life, his body, and his mind are busy making ready in ways of which he may only have a passing awareness (34)." Birth preparation and perinatal classes may be helpful and supportive to both mothers and fathers in promoting a sense of mutual commitment and in explaining the universal pleasures and fears during the pregnancy and birth phase. Both mothers and fathers have complex mental images of their children (often crystallized with the help of well pixilated ultrasound images) long before the child sees the light of day.

Few human experiences rival birth itself, with first contact feeling so powerful for both mothers and fathers. Attachment and bonding research has clearly articulated the importance of the parent–infant haptic involvement in the hours and days following birth. Fathers who are present at the birth are more verbal about their babies, more accurate in describing them, and are more intimately attached to them at follow-up (35).

The newborn's job is no less salient—though more complex neurobiologically—than that of the parents (69). The neonate must first stabilize and regulate themselves neurobiologically in order to perceive and respond to events in the external world by processing sensory, vestibular, and human interaction (70). Next, newborns must use their repertoire of skills and intrinsic reflexes to try to elicit sensitive nurturing experiences from the human world, which then facilitates their entering the dynamic, reciprocating intimacies of relating pleasurably to, and accurately with, their caregivers (71).

Finally, infants must communicate in a meaningful, intimate way so that they will be stimulated, fed, entertained, and cared for physically. Both mothers and fathers, whether or not they have had prior experience, learn by on-the-job training to read, as well as anticipate, their infant's signals. Empathic connections and the capacity to comfort, soothe, woo, distract, and entertain are tasks common to both sensitive mothering and fathering. Qualitative differences are present, however, in the idiosyncratic ways in which mothers and fathers respond (35). Mothers tend to respond to their babies on a more intimate scale, facilitating fine motor development and affective differentiation. Fathers tend to be more activating and gross-motor involved. Nevertheless, as shown by Parke, fathers are able to feed and comfort their babies as effectively and efficiently, although somewhat differently stylistically, as their partners (all couples in the study were married) (72).

Infants also appear interested in, and responsive to, the differences between paternal and maternal interactive styles (73). Yogman (74) noted that by the time infants were 8 weeks old, they were responding differentially to their fathers and mothers. At 8 weeks, infants hunched their shoulders and lifted their eyebrows when their fathers appeared in their visual field. The same infants, when they saw or heard their mother's approach, seemed to expect more routine functional handling, such as feeding or diapering and became settled with relaxed shoulders, lowered eyebrows, and more regular breathing rather than become animated.

The involvement in the first year of life of two caring and competent adults appears to have a positive effect on overall cognitive development. Pedersen et al. (75) found that the more actively involved a 6-month-old had been with his or her father, the higher the infant's scores on the Bailey test of mental and motor development. Parke (72), in examining children over the first 8 weeks of life, found that the more fathers were involved in everyday, repetitive aspects of care, such as bathing, feeding, dressing, and diapering, the more socially responsive the infants were.

It is in the mutual pleasures of this early experience that the adults, who have now moved up a generation and become caretakers to the younger generation, feel their own personal development frequently propelled forward to new levels of empathic—even altruistic—connections, not only with their children but also with other important objects in their lives.

Given these important health-promoting interactions in the first year of life, we are wise to take seriously the potential effects on the infant of time-sensitive adult vulnerabilities during this era, such as postpartum depression. The prevalence of maternal postpartum depression and its potentially negative effects, if untreated, on the infant is well-known. Recent research draws our attention to the unexpectedly high incidence of paternal postpartum depression in fathers, once researchers began to investigate it (76). Untreated, this can further complicate comorbidity in the mother and potentially further threaten the infant's well-being in the first year (77).

Toddlerhood and Individuation within the Family

The child's astounding increase in mental and physical resources propels him or her out of the less differentiated omnipotence of the first year of life into a much more social context, in which new skills permit more active participation and shaping of the need-satisfying environment. The development of language, increasing sophistication in cognitive structures, mastery over motility and sphincters, and the incorporation of gender awareness all prepare the child for the complex sequences of the vital separation–individuation process (78). Parents are alternately challenged through intense clinging and contentious interchange, giving this era *ambivalence* as its marquee. Aggression, caretaking, affection, anger, and sensuous intimacy are now part of the toddler's repertoire (49). This makes limit setting a vital companion to the toddler's adventurous experimentation with challenging, aggressive, and seductive behaviors. The parent is wise to be led by, rather than attempt to lead the toddler (79). Fathering styles are more differentiated from mothering styles of interaction, with fathers initiating more rough-and-tumble, unpredictable, physical, and stimulating forms of play. Biller and Meredith noted that mothers tended to engage in more conventional, toy-mediated play, picking up their children to engage in caretaking and nurturing activities more often than fathers (80).

The child's increased level of mastery over the internal environment leaves more energy available to explore the boundaries of the external environment, giving separation tasks more salience during this era. Adjustments to the toddler's new, if clumsy, drive for autonomy are necessary to avoid prolonging the child's functional dependency. Because separation from the mother sometimes is the fuel for the sleep disturbances that are common during the second year of life, the father can help decrease the virulence of nighttime disruption by being the one who soothes and settles the child. This spares the child from yet another separation from the mother, while also helping the child feel safe and secure.

Clearly, the child's unique temperament and style interact with parental values and experience with regard to personal autonomy, separateness from family of origin, and impulse and bodily control. The unique contributions of the father during these years have been increasingly recognized as important to the success of this developmental era (81), and need to become a more routine part of the health professionals approach to, and their systems and routines of care of, children from early on (82).

The Preschooler

The preschool child's appropriate use of personal pronouns, ability to say "no," and increasingly adaptive capacities all draw the family as a whole further into this new domain characterized by three-party, rather than two-party, relationships. Curiosity, assertiveness, and the capacity to begin to delay gratification help the child regulate and moderate intense instinctual impulses and affects. Cognitive growth, meanwhile, assists the child in learning and remembering what the important objects in his or her life will or will not tolerate. Appropriate, predictable limit setting, counting to 10, and humor play important roles in helping both the child and parent withstand the heavy weather of strong, rivalrous feelings. By now, parents are able to yield most control over bodily functions to the child, relinquishing him or her as a physical possession, and become more admiring and encouraging of his or her attributes as a separate, human being who is becoming aware of the benefits of the delay of gratification. During these preschool years, fathers interact with their children mainly through play, limit-setting, and productivity. Through role modeling, the father provides opportunities for children of both sexes to build increasingly positive self-esteem (83).

We are now aware that maternal and paternal styles of attachment behavior differ from one another; maternal attachment behavior is designed to provide comfort and security to the young during periods of stress and distress. Paternal attachment provides security during monitored controlled excitement through sensitive and challenging support *"when child's exploratory system is aroused"* (84). Such dynamic distinctions show the benefit of positive and consistent involvement of both parents in supporting the separation/individuation tasks faced by the child during this particular era.

The press of such developmental needs during this period, highlighted in research, shows us a critical relationship between marital satisfaction and parental involvement. Marital satisfaction can be at its lowest ebb during the childbearing years (85). Waldron and Routh (86) note that marital satisfaction follows a U-shaped graph, with higher levels of marital comfort before children are born and again after they leave home. Frequently, children place such significant demands on the couple that there is little energy left to fuel, let alone sustain, the marital relationship, though it is not suggested that children destroy marriages. Rapoport et al. (87) report that marriage often is experienced by fathers as better than by mothers during this nadir of marital satisfaction because it is mothers who usually have more negative experiences with their children, feel more isolated, and are more vulnerable to psychosomatic stress ailments, including fatigue. Although the discrepancies between maternal and paternal experience can be problematic, including occasional envy and jealousy on the part of the parent who is having the more difficult and challenging time with the preschool child, the long-term effects of having both parents involved intimately during this phase are strongly positive. Awareness of the positive effects of co-parenting on the parental relationship seems to be on the increase, as documented by current surveys of parental wishes and expectations (28).

One of the more dramatic findings in the father–infant care research is the relationship between early involvement and subsequent sexual abuse. If a man is involved in the physical care of his child before the age of 3 years, there is a dramatic drop in the probability that man will be involved later on in life with sexual abuse of his own or anyone else's children (88).

School Age and Family Unity

The timely differentiation of the child–parent relationship from interdependent dyad to more intergenerational autonomy allows the child to make powerful psychological investments in nonparental adults. An unexpected sequela of this change is the potential for the first disillusionment in one's parents. Just as the child's body is relinquished from parental control, so is the child's mind. The family now helps the child separate for most of his or her waking hours to attend school and confront social and cognitive challenges. Interest grows exponentially in relating to other children and adults, as well as for learning and problem-solving. The integration of family and tradition, as guided by societal mythology, serves as the hallmark of this period of development. It often becomes easier for a family to spend prolonged, uninterrupted segments of time with one another for community or neighborhood activities or projects, and simple travel or leisure activities. Girls may have only one or two friends they would call "best," whereas boys may name six or seven friends, who usually turn out to be somewhat more casual acquaintances with whom they "do things... hang out." The opportunity for shared activities and mastery experiences with adults of the same sex is extremely important in terms of the solidification of gender role behavior and gender identity itself. During the school-age period, a father may serve as a confidant, a pal, even a friend, or teacher (89). Father absence, however (90), leads teachers to rate both boys and girls as more aggressive relative to mother–father families. Especially poignant was the finding that the protective factors for mother–father families were less apparent among low-income families.

Adolescence and Generational Redefinition

Families of adolescents craft boundaries that are qualitatively different from families with younger children. These boundaries assist the children in managing their own impulses because parents no longer have the unquestioned authority they once enjoyed. The boundaries between the family and the outside world must become more permeable, hence the normal careening and ambivalence between independence and dependence. The adolescent's sense of self is beginning to be consolidated and shaped by the search for pleasure and purpose with goals and tasks that can stretch far into the future and at other times be more immediate and impulse-driven. They are intensely interested in and preoccupied by their constantly changing bodies and moods. Meanwhile, accepted family values such as "do unto others as you would have them do unto you" [beliefs more typical of middle childhood] are subjected to greater scrutiny.

Developmental stress does not necessarily doom the family to turmoil during this phase, but profound physical and psychological changes not seen since toddlerhood threaten the previous level of homeostasis. Adolescents notice weaknesses and vulnerabilities in their family, as well as in their own psychological functioning, but these may also be seen as possible points of departure for new adaptive functioning. Uncertainty about where strengths and weaknesses lie, and intergenerational disagreement about their relevance can lead to disputes. And adolescent observations are notoriously selective; bulimic teenagers and young adults rated their fathers as showing less affection and more control toward them than their nonbulimic siblings, suggesting that the paternal relationship may be a source of nonshared environmental experience associated with bulimia (91).

Adolescence can be a period of significant stress in the family because both the adolescents and their parents are often experiencing physiologic and mental changes simultaneously. Both generations may be scrutinizing their primary relationships anew and questioning their value and trustworthiness. Just as adolescents are beginning to make choices regarding values and life goals, their parents are often needing to accept that certain of their own cherished goals may never be achieved, becoming preoccupied with the limited time left in their lives.

As adolescents pull further away from the nurturing domain by taking a job or starting college, the parental response can be one of either pride in their child's capacity to cope with life's new challenges, or sadness over what appears to be their increasing absence from family life. An adolescent's need to extract his or her autonomy from the parental nurturing domain can be a strong challenge to a family's homeostatic balance.

THE LATTER STAGES

Young adulthood emancipation, the marriage of offspring (the "middle family"), and, finally, aging and senescence are the last three phases of family development. The kind of influence parents now have on their children is largely encompassed by their ability to provide resources, availability for discussion and advice and by bearing witness to their children's integrity, while being careful to support their own autonomy. Grandchildren may come next, providing an opportunity for rejuvenation of spirit and body (and hints of immortality). The potential relaxations of retirement, the consolidation of the family around a patriarch or matriarch, and finally, the privileges and honor of the emerita/emeritus define the tableau of the senior family era.

The developmental tasks faced by the child and the child's caregivers are the same whether the structure of the family is nuclear or not, same-sex or heterosexual. The energy and resources, both emotional and physical, to attend to those tasks are strongly influenced, however, by a particular family's resources, limits, and flexibility. Adoptive, single-parent, foster, and recombined family groupings are all subject to the same leadership, boundary, affectivity, communicative, and task and goal requirements. The issues of attachment, separation, emancipation, loss, and response to change are largely the same. Each exerts its own particular spin on normal development, but none is doomed to trouble by dint of family structure alone.

Adoptive families often do not have the same biologic preparation time, but given support, and some measure of good fortune, they usually follow a similar psychological preparation sequence. The separate biologic parents' narrative can be integrated into the family's mental history of itself over time, ensuring continuity to the child's narrative of how he or she became themselves. Single-parent families, whether male- or female-headed, face depletion and isolation early and often and work best when social and medical support systems are available early and are flexible enough to supplement parental and child needs.

Recombined and reconstituted families—when a divorced, widowed, or never-married single parent forms a new household with a new partner who may or may not be a parent—are also increasing. Depending on the mode of single parenthood (death, divorce, abandonment), the new parent may be seen as a threat, or solution, to intimacy between parent and child. Rivalry and jealousy frequently stimulate guilt and anxiety. Interestingly, Black and Pedro-Carroll (92) have shown that the effects of interparental conflict on the psychological well-being of children were mediated more by the overall quality of parent–child relationships than by inter-adult conflict itself. Stepparents frequently are in risk situations, being tested by their "new" children while feeling special loyalty to their "old" children, and simultaneously trying to grow and sustain a new spousal relationship. Time (measured in years), patience, and liberal, frequent communication (sometimes new to everyone as a process) plus permission to co-parent are all essential. Society's myths are of little help; *stepmother* in English conjures up Cinderella's stepmother, and stepfather in Spanish is *padrastro,* which also can mean hangnail. On a smaller scale, all families face similar issues because families are always reconstituting biologically and psychologically. Because of the relentless push of developmental and maturational forces in the individuals of our species, like the river, one can never step into one family in the same place twice.

IN SUMMARY

As we review these developmental trajectories for families, we note the parallel processes at work in the developmental trajectory of the career of the child psychiatrist. How is the art of the practice itself woven over time into the child psychiatrist's personal growth and development? Their own personal context shapes their practice, and their personal attitude toward it, in countless ways. For example, they do or do not become parents themselves, struggle with the same universal doubts, joys, slings, and arrows of either path. I have heard my students wish aloud that they could revise some old piece of advice given or judgment made through the lens of their own personal experience of parenting or not. On the other hand, those who do have children may at times carry the burden of self-doubt as a useless "expert" when they have no idea about how to help their own distressed offspring or despairing spouse manage some interpersonal or intrapsychic skirmish.

Child psychiatrists struggle with their own health issues, emotional and physical, suffer personal losses, and experience their own 15 minutes of fame, or not, all the while trying to listen with mustered patience, during times when they are feeling unheard themselves. This is one of the compelling reasons that vigilance, supervision, and collegial support throughout one's professional life should be the rule, not the exception.

Such vigilance is especially germane if the clinician holds to the standard, "treat others as you would have them treat you." Desirable as this standard may be, it occasions personal depletion at a rapid clip. A lifelong trajectory of repletion through reflective supervision, real continuing education [not simply CMEs], restorative play (mental and physical), and diversion will protect and preserve that "knack" for listening for meaning in what matters to our patients and their families.

Over time I have grown less judgmental, more patient, and I hope more reflective, effective, and efficient with age. I am freer with my doubts, humor, and compassion, and more grateful for what I have learned from my patients' shared experiences in our work together. I assume from the beginning that my patients—child and family—are doing the best they can, regardless of how troubled the results of those efforts to date may at first appear.

At the same time, I feel more demanding of myself and my patients, trusting our skills and creativities more than I did at the beginning of my career, when I thought life might somehow be more perfectible. Innovations seem to arise in more and more cases, partly as a function of the extraordinary pace of science's advance in our field. In fact, as I reflect on the beginning of my career, I wonder if we as a medical specialty got so good at asking questions because there were so few answers; this may be less the case today with the arrival of each new online journal. It is hard to imagine a medical specialty with a broader intellectual horizon than ours (a strong recruitment talking point whenever I get the chance).

That is precisely why I am simultaneously enthusiastic and concerned about our ongoing preoccupation with evidence-based medicine. On one hand, it can upgrade the quality of evidence that we use and generate, and upon which we rely to make diagnoses and develop treatment plans. On the other hand, "evidence" for its own sake or in isolation falls short of helping the clinician "do the right thing" because the patient's needs are embedded in the complex context of their culture-specific, value-laden, intergenerational "system" of beliefs and hopes [as are the clinicians!]. Few have said it better than Jeree Pawl (93):

> We learn over time that everything we think we know is a hypothesis; that we have ideas, but that we don't have truth. We learn that those [patients] with whom we work have all of the information we need, and that this is what we will work with. When we know this, our attitude conveys it; and the child and family sense themselves as sources, not objects. In this context, they become aware of a mutual effort; they do not feel weighed, measured, or judged. They feel listened to, seen and appreciated.

If the reader is interested in such support in a narrative form, I commend my mentor, Kenneth Robson's brief and wonderful book, «The Children's Hour; A life in child psychiatry (94)»

References

1. Sameroff A, Fiese B: Transactional Regulation: the developmental ecology of early intervention. In: Shonkoff J, Meisels S (eds): *Handbook of Early Childhood Intervention.* 2nd ed. New York, NY, Cambridge University Press, 135–159, 2000.
2. Tienari P, Wynne LC, Sorri A, et al.: Genotype-environment interaction in schizophrenia-spectrum disorder: long-term follow-up of Finnish adoptees. *Brit J Psychia* 184:216–222, 2004.
3. Caspi A, Sugden K, Moffitt TE, et al.: Influence of life stress on depression: moderation by a polymorphism in the 5_HTT gene. *Science* 301: 386–389, 2003.
4. Kaufman J, Yang BZ, Douglas-Palumberi H, et al.: Brain-derived neurotrophic factor-5-HTTLPR gene interaction and environmental modifiers of depression in children. *Biol Psychiatry* 59:958–965, 2006.
5. Yehuda R, Daskalakis NP, Lehrner A, et al.: "Influences of maternal and paternal PTSD on epigenetic regulation of the glucocorticoid receptor gene in Holocaust survivor offspring." *Am J Psychiatry* 171(8):872–880, 2014.
6. Meaney MJ: Epigenetics and the biological definition of gene x environment interactions. *Child Dev* 81(1):41–79, 2010.
7. Provencal N, Binder EB: The effects of early life stress on the epigenome: from the womb to adulthood and even before. *Exp Neurol* 268:10–20, 2015.
8. Sroufe LA, Egeland B, Carlson E, et al.: *The Development of the Person: Minnesota Study of Risk and Adaptation from Birth to Adulthood.* New York, Guilford Press, 2005.
9. Hechtman L (ed): *Do They Grow Out of It? Long-term Outcomes of Childhood Disorders.* Washington, DC, American Psychiatric Press, 1996.
10. Felitti VJ, Anda RF: The relationship of adverse childhood experiences to adult medical disease, psychiatric disorders and sexual behavior: Implications for healthcare. In: Lanius R, Vermetten E, Pain C (eds): *The Impact of Early Life Trauma on Health And Disease: The Hidden Epidemic.* Cambridge, UK, Cambridge University Press, 77–87, 2010.
11. Spitz RA: *The First Year of Life: A Psychoanalytic Study of Normal and Deviant Development of Object Relations.* New York, International Universities Press, 1965.
12. Pincus L, Dare C: *Secrets in the Family.* New York, Pantheon, 1978.
13. Vangelisti AL: Family secrets: forms, functions, and correlates. *J Social Pers Relationships* 11:113–135, 1994.
14. Ainsworth M, Eichberg C: Effects on infant-mother attachment of mother's unresolved loss of an attachment figure or other traumatic experience. In: Morris P, Parks C, Hinde R (eds): *Attachment Across the Life Cycle.* New York, Routledge Press, 160–186, 1991.
15. Borkowski J, Ramey S: *Parenting and the Child's World: Influences on Academic, Intellectual and Socioeconomic Development.* New York, Erlbaum Press, 2001.
16. Bowen M: *Family Therapy in Clinical Practice.* New York, Aronson, 1978.
17. Wamboldt MZ, Wamboldt FS: Role of the family in the onset and outcome of childhood disorders: selected research findings. *J Am Acad Child Adolesc Psychiatry* 39:1212–1219, 2000.
18. DiFonzo JH, Ruth CS: Breaking the mold and picking up the pieces: Rights of parenthood and parentage in nontraditional families. *Family Court Review* 51(1): 104–118, 2013.
19. Demos J: *A Little Commonwealth: Family Life in Plymouth Colony.* New York, Oxford University Press, 1970.
20. Laslette P, Wall R (eds): *Household and Family in Past Time.* Cambridge, Cambridge University Press, 1972.
21. Hareven T: American families in transition: historical perspectives on change. In: Walsh F (ed): *Normal Family Processes.* New York, Guilford, 446–466, 1982.
22. Griswold R: *Fatherhood in America: A History.* New York, Basic Books, 1993.
23. Achenbach T, Howell C: Are American children's problems getting worse? A 13-year comparison. *J Am Acad Child Adolesc Psychiatry* 32:1145–1154, 1993.
24. Center for Disease Control and prevention: *National Vital Statistics System—National Center of Health Statistics, Birth data.* 2014. Available at: https://www.cdc.gov/nchs/nvss/births.htm
25. Bilancia SD, Rescorla L: "Stability of behavioral and emotional problems over 6 years in children ages 4 to 5 or 6 to 7 at time 1." *J Emot Behav Disord* 18(3):149–161, 2010.
26. Galinsky E: Family life and corporate policies. In: Yogman M, Brazelton B (eds): *In Support of Families.* Cambridge, MA, Harvard University Press, 108–118, 1986.
27. U.S. Bureau of Labor Statistics report, National Survey of Parents as Wage-Earners, 2003. Available at: https://www.bls.gov/opub/ted/2017/employment-in-families-with-children-in-2016.htm
28. George C, Kaplan N, Main M: *The Berkeley Adult Attachment Interview.* Berkeley, CA, University of California, Department of Psychology, 1985.
29. Zero To Three: National Parent Survey, June 2016. Available at: www.zerotothree.org/resources
30. Main M, Kaplan N, Cassidy J: Security in infancy, childhood and adulthood: a move to the level of representation. *Monogr Soc Res Child Dev* 50:66–104, 1985.
31. Cowan P, Cowan C: Attachment theory; Seven unresolved issues and questions for future research. *Res Hum Dev* 4(3–4):181–201, 2007.
32. Bretherton I: Fathers in attachment theory and research: a review. *Early Child Dev Care* 180(1–2):9–23, 2010.
33. Pruett K: Infants of primary nurturing fathers. *Psychoanal Study Child* 40:257–277, 1983.
34. Pruett K: *The Nurturing Father.* New York, Warner, 1987.
35. Pruett K: *Fatherneed: Why Father Care Is as Essential as Mother Care for Your Child.* New York, Free Press, 2000.
36. Radin N, Harold-Goldsmith R: The involvement of selected unemployed and employed men with their children. *Child Dev* 60;454–459, 1989.
37. Raeburn P: *Do Fathers Matter? What Science Is Telling Us about the Parent We've Overlooked.* Strauss, Giroux, New York, Scientific American/Farra, 2014.
38. Bezirganian S, Cohen P, Brook J: The impact of mother-child interaction on the development of borderline personality disorder. *Am J Psychiatry* 150:1836–1842, 1993.
39. Lamb M: *The Role of the Father in Child Development.* 3rd ed. New York, John Wiley & Sons, 1997.

40. Yeung W, Sandberg J, Davis-Kean P, Hofferth S: Children's time with fathers in intact families. *J Marriage Fam* 63:136–154, 2000.
41. Lieb R, Wittchen H, Hofler M, et al.: Parental psychopathology, parenting styles, and the risk of social phobia in offspring. *Arch Gen Psychiatry* 57:859–865, 2000.
42. Panter-Brick C, Burgess A, Eggerman M, McAllister F, Pruett K, Leckman JF: "Practitioner review: engaging fathers—recommendations for a game change in parenting interventions based on a systematic review of the global evidence." *J Child Psychol Psychiatry* 55(11):1187–1212, 2014.
43. Phares V, Compas BE: The role of fathers in child and adolescent psychopathology: make room for daddy. *Psychol Bull* 111:387–412, 1992.
44. Werner E: Protective factors and individual resilience. In: Shonkoff J, Meisels S (eds): *Handbook of Early Childhood Intervention.* 2nd ed. New York, Cambridge University Press, 2000.
45. Skinner HA, Steinhauer PD, Santa-Barbara J: The Family Assessment Measure. *Can J Ment Health* 2:91–105, 1983.
46. Mrazek D, Mrazek P, Klinnert M: Clinical assessment of parenting. *J Am Acad Child Adolesc Psychiatry* 34:272–282, 1995.
47. Epstein NB, Baldwin LM, Bishop DS: The McMaster family assessment device. *J Marital Fam Ther* 9(2):171–180, 1983.
48. Fleck S (ed): *Psychiatric Prevention and the Family Life Cycle.* New York, Brunner/Mazel, 1989.
49. Minuchin S, Fishman H: *Family Therapy Techniques.* Cambridge, MA, Harvard University Press, 2009.
50. Johnson-Powell G, Yamamoto J (eds): *Transcultural Child Development.* New York, John Wiley & Sons, 1997.
51. Pruett K: *Me, Myself and I; How Children Build Their Sense of Self.* New York, Goddard, 1999.
52. Coll C, Magnuson K: Cultural differences as sources of developmental vulnerabilities and resources. In: Shonkoff J, Meisels J (eds): *Handbook of Early Childhood Intervention.* 2nd ed. New York, Cambridge, 2000.
53. Rey J, Peng R, Morales-Blanquez C, Widyawati I, Peralta V, Walter G: Rating the quality of family environment in different cultures. *J Am Acad Child Adolesc Psychiatry* 39:1168–1174, 2000.
54. D'Augelli A, Patterson C: *Lesbian, Gay, and Bisexual Identities over the Lifespan: Psychological Perspectives.* New York, Oxford University Press, 1995.
55. Lock J, Steiner H: Gay and lesbian, and bisexual youth risks for emotional, physical, and social problems: results from a community-based survey. *J Am Acad Child Adolesc Psychiatry* 38:297–304, 1999.
56. Pruett K, Cotton P: The affective experience of residency training in community psychiatry. *Am J Psychiatry* 132(3):57–63, 1975.
57. Pruett K: Home treatment of two infants who witnessed their mother's murder. *J Amer Acad Child Psychiatry* 18:647–658, 1979.
58. Pruett KD, Joshi SV, Martin A: Thinking about prescribing: the psychology of psychopharmacology. In: Martin A, Scahill L, Kratochvil C (eds): *Pediatric Psychopharmacology: Principles and Practice.* New York, Oxford University Press, 422–433, 2010.
59. Eichberg C: Quality of infant-parent attachment: related to mother's representation of her own relationship history. Presented at the meeting of the Society for Research in Child Development. Baltimore, MD, 19–22, April 1987.
60. Main M, Goldwyn R: Adult attachment classification system. In: Main M (ed): *A Typology of Human Attachment Organization: Assessed in Discourse, Drawings and Interviews.* New York, Cambridge University Press, 134–149, 1992.
61. Manning WD, Brown SL, Payne KK: "Two decades of stability and change in age at first union formation." *J Marriage Family* 76(2):247–260, 2014.
62. Glick P, Norton A: Marrying, divorcing, and living together in the US today. *Pop Bull* 38:3–38, 1978.
63. Bacon L: Early mother Oxytocinhood, accelerated role transition and social pathologies. *Soc Forces* 52:333–341, 1974.
64. Becker G: Economics of marital instability. *J Polit Econ* 85:1141–1187, 1987.
65. Burke R, Weir T: The relationships of wives' employment status to husband, wife and peer satisfaction. *J Marriage Fam* 2:279–287, 1976.
66. Coontz S: *Marriage: A History—How Love Conquered Marriage.* Penguin. 2nd Ed. New York, NY, Penguin Books, 2016.
67. Feldman R, Gordon I, Zagoory-Sharon O: Maternal and paternal plasma, salivary, and urinary oxytocin and parent-infant synchrony: considering stress and affiliation components of human bonding. *Dev Sci* 14(4):752–761, 2011.
68. Cowan C, Cowan P: *When Partners Become Parents.* Mahwah, NJ, Earlbaum Associates Publishers, 2000.
69. Shonkoff J: *Neurons to Neighborhoods.* Bethesda, MD, National Institutes of Medicine, 2002.
70. Ramey C, Ramey S: *Right from Birth.* New York, Goddard Press, 1999.
71. Leckman J, Mayes L: Primary parental preoccupation: circuits, genes, and the crucial role of the environment. *J Neural Trans* 111:753–771, 2004.
72. Parke RF: *Fathers.* Cambridge, MA, Harvard University Press, 1981.
73. Feldman R: Infant-mother and infant-father synchrony: the co-regulation of positive arousal. *Infant Mental Health J* 24:1–23, 2003.
74. Yogman M: Development of the father–infant relationship. In: Fitzgerald G, Lester F, Yogman M (eds): *Theory and Research in Behavioral Pediatrics.* Vol 1. New York, Plenum, 221–297, 1982.
75. Pedersen F, Rubinstein J, Yarrow L: Infant development in father-absent families. *J Genet Psychol* 135:51–61, 1979.
76. Ramchandani PG, Stein A, O'Connor TG, Heron JO, Murray L, Evans J: Depression in men in the postnatal period and later child psychopathology: a population cohort study. *J Am Acad Child Adolesc Psychiatry* 47(4):390–398, 2008.
77. Ramchandani P, Stein A, Evans J, O'Connor T: Paternal depression in the postnatal period and child development: a prospective longitudinal study. *Lancet* 365:2158–2159, 2005.
78. Zeanah C, Larrieu J, Heller S: Developmental assessment of infants and toddlers. In: Zeanah C (ed): *Handbook of Infant Mental Health.* 2nd ed. New York, Guilford Press, 222–235, 2000.
79. Lieberman A: *The Emotional Life of the Toddler.* New York, Free Press, 1993.
80. Biller H, Meredith D: *Father Power.* New York, David McKay, 1974.
81. Greenspan S: The second other: the role of the father in early personality formation. In: Cath S, Gurwitt A, Ross JM (eds): *Father and Child: Developmental and Clinical Perspectives.* Boston, MA, Little Brown, 123–138, 1982.
82. Yogman M, Garfield CF, Committee on Psychosocial Aspects of Child and Family Health: Fathers' roles in the care and development of their children: the role of pediatricians. *Pediatrics* 138(1):e20161128, 2016.
83. Sarnoff C: The father's role in latency. In: Cath S, Gurwitt A, Ross J (eds): *Father and Child: Developmental and Clinical Perspectives.* Boston, MA, Little Brown, 253–264, 1982.
84. Cowan PA, Cowan CP: Couple relationships: a missing link between adult attachment and children's outcomes. *Attach Hum Dev* 11(1):1–4, 2009.
85. Glenn G, McLanahan S: Children and marital happiness: a further specification of the relationship. *J Marriage Fam* 44:63–72, 1982.
86. Waldron H, Routh D: The effect of the first child on the marital relationship. *J Marriage Fam* 43:785–788, 1981.
87. Rapoport R, Rapoport R, Strelitz Z: *Fathers, Mothers and Society.* New York, Basic Books, 1977.
88. Parker H, Parker S: Cultural roles, rituals and behavior regulation. *Am Anthropol* 86:584–600, 1984.
89. Benson L: *Fatherhood: A Sociological Perspective.* New York, Random House, 1968.
90. Pearson JL, Ialongo NS, Hunter AG, et al.: Family structure and aggressive behavior in a population of urban elementary school children. *J Am Acad Child Adolesc Psychiatry* 33:540–548, 1994.
91. Wonderlich S, Ukestad L, Perzacki R: Perceptions of nonshared childhood environment in bulimia nervosa. *J Am Acad Child Adolesc Psychiatry* 33:140–141, 1994.
92. Black A, Pedro-Carroll J: Role of parent–child relationship in mediating the effects of marital disruption. *J Am Acad Child Adolesc Psychiatry* 32:1019–1027, 1993.
93. Pawl J: The interpersonal center of the work that we do. *Zero Three* 20(4):5–7, 2000.
94. Robson KS: *The Children's Hour; A Life in Child Psychiatry.* West Hartford, CT, Lyre Books, 2010.

CHAPTER 1.2 ■ ETHICS

ADRIAN SONDHEIMER

The assertion that Mel Brooks is arguably the finest, and paradoxically the longest-living (traversing numerous cultures and eras over many centuries) American Jewish philosopher of the second half of the 20th century (1), might be open to disagreement by some. It is offered as an opinion, quite possibly not universally shared. Further, Mr. Brooks' assertion that "it is good to be the king" (2), while often a truism due to its emphasis on noblesse oblige (though others might disagree, viz. Kings Charles I, Louis XVI, Conraden of Italy, who all literally lost their heads while in office), speaks to the benefits of privilege by virtue of position, the exact opposite of what other philosophers would generally agree to be universal values that apply to all human beings. Such musings, encompassing history, human behaviors, and senses of humility (and humor) or the lack of them, lead naturally to a discussion of ethics, a branch of moral philosophy the study of which also transcends millennia. Simply put, such study attempts to determine the rightness and wrongness of human behaviors. The Golden Rule and the Ten Commandments are commonly known efforts, in the near Eastern and Western worlds, to create such ethically universal rules, though they may often be limited by parochial concerns.

The English word *ethics* derives from the Greek *etikos,* commonly understood to refer to "character," as used in the judgment of an individual's honesty, virtue, trustworthiness, and personal conduct. Ethical thinking thus strives to define norms or standards of desirable human behaviors that would be applicable in all circumstances and are not, by contrast, situation dependent. These standards are pertinent independent of the professional discipline to which they might be applied, as in *medical* (as distinct from, e.g., legal, business or educational) *ethics*. In other words, universal ethical principles do not change because they are applied specifically to medical practice, while medicine as a discipline is required to work with these principles by applying them to its practice. Psychiatry is a branch of medicine, child and adolescent psychiatry (CAP) is a subspecialty of general psychiatry, and, it follows, to do good work, ethical thought must be applied to CAP practice.

CODES OF ETHICS

For millennia, societies have designated specified individuals within their communities as professional healers who might be known, for example, as shamans, witches, physicians, and/or doctors. The communities have always expected their healers to have mastery of the knowledge of their profession and to pursue, as their primary interest and obligation, the betterment of the welfare of the individuals seeking help from these professionals. Consequently, over all these years, societies have created numerous codes designed to guide proper practice by their healers. Executed by the healers themselves or in concert with other informed members, the codes have derived from the moral, philosophic, and religious ideas embedded in the community, and they served as the bases for standards of conduct the communities expected of their practitioners (3). Almost invariably, these medical codes touched upon several or more of the following topics: respect for human life; provision of benefit and avoidance of harm; the need for personal virtue; acknowledgement of duty to, and responsibility for, the patient; financial considerations; diagnostic methodologies; therapeutic choices; confidentiality of patient–physician communications; prohibition of sexual contact with patients; and, punishment or sanctions for poor technical performance.

ETHICAL PRINCIPLES

The knowledge and attitudes of these societies would undoubtedly change over time, leading to changes in what might be considered, at any particular point in time, right or wrong behaviors. However, certain principles evolved that were considered to be immutable. These have recurred as constants in emerging and evolving codes. Thus, ***beneficence***, within the medical context, refers to the obligation to contribute to the health and welfare of patients and to further their legitimate interests. Its converse, ***nonmaleficence***, cautions against the infliction of evil or harm. The cardinal medical maxim, *primum non nocere* (i.e., above all, do no harm), appears in the Hippocratic Oath, a commonly cited and utilized Western medical code established ca. 400 BC. This maxim is directly based on the underlying ethical principle of nonmaleficence. It should be noted, though, that at the time of its initial promulgation, a major intention, when considering this principle, was to warn against the performance of surgery by most current physicians. ***Autonomy*** refers to the notion that individuals are due, by inherent right, freedom of action and choice, provided that such choices do not infringe on the rights of others. Within the medical context autonomy implies the patient's right to make decisions for oneself, even in the face of opposition by others, for example, the physician. ***Justice*** implies fairness. This principle demands that all individuals are to be treated equally and fairly, unless the differences between them rationally justify differential treatment. Additional universal principles have been proposed. Thus, for example, ***fidelity***, which encompasses the obligation to be faithful and loyal to persons and their needs, and ***veracity***, emphasizing the obligation of truth-telling, inclusive of misleadings consequent to the omissions of facts. In any case, these principles stand as unique bases, covering proper practitioner conduct (4). They are considered universalizable, that is, applicable in all conceivable circumstances, and overriding, that is, taking precedence over personal and group values.

ETHICAL REASONING PROCESS

When faced with ethical dilemmas, whether in the clinical, educational, administrative, or research spheres, the fundamental ethical principles are employed in a reasoning process designed to enable practitioners to arrive at least damaging resolutions via an objective risk–benefit analysis. Described simply, the process involves the initial encounter with a problem, followed by the recognition of underlying ethical conflicts. The practitioners should rapidly identify their immediate affective responses and inclinations for action in order to then set them aside, allowing the practitioners instead time to reflect. Doing so provides the opportunity to obtain a sense of prevalent current practice concerning the matter and greater cognizance of one's own value systems and their derivations, to incorporate the views of others involved in the subject of concern and, finally, to employ the previously cited principles which, not infrequently, may conflict with each other. ***To illustrate:*** the Hippocratic Oath, emphasizing the avoidance of harm, meant, in its day, "do not do surgery." In that era's absence of both anesthesia and sterile technique surgery was commonly an exercise in maleficence, despite the physician's beneficent intentions. Thus, in the ethical reasoning process, one principle will predominate over another. However, with changes over time in medical knowledge and expertise in provision of care, reversals of these priorities can and should occur, and they have.

HISTORY AND CHILDREN

Societies' desires for healers go back millennia. While initial writings focused exclusively on somatic concerns, comments about mental disturbance first appeared in works by Hippocrates in Greece and, several centuries later, Galen in Rome. The etiologies underlying manifestations of mental disturbance and its proposed treatments were debated in those days and have been ever since. Of note, however, all of these writings, until relatively recently, centered exclusively on adults and their needs. Children, by contrast, were generally viewed in society as objects, owned by their parents. In exchange for housing and food, the children were expected to provide service upon achievement of physical capability. Notions of formal education of children did not emerge until the 17th century, and, at that time, their applications were limited to the privileged classes (5). Gradually changing impressions, and the development of new technologies, led to an increase in educational opportunities for wider groups of children and of perceptions of children as developing individuals with their own rights, rather than as "little adults." Consequent to these changing perspectives, pediatrics first emerged as a medical specialty in the last decades of the 19th century. During the following century, various agencies were created and legal precedents established, in both the USA and England, designed to aid and protect children, including, for example, the first juvenile courts, Federal Children's Bureau, U.S. Supreme Court decision In re: Gault, and Britain's Guardianship of Infants' Act.

These evolutionary societal changes were paralleled in medical and psychiatric practice. In the USA, 3 years prior to the establishment of the American Medical Association in 1847, 13 superintendents of American "insane asylums" banded together to form an organization that served as the foundation, eight decades later, for the formation of the American Psychiatric Association. That organization, in turn, created training standards for its trainees. Mirroring the public's newfound concerns for youngsters, a group of psychiatrists and other fellow professionals, with shared interests in children, created the American Academy of Child Psychiatry (AACP) in 1953. The AACP formulated training standards for child psychiatrists, and created its first Code of Ethics in 1980 (6). That code has since undergone several revisions to bring it in line with current knowledge and attitudes (7). Education in ethics is mandated by CAP training requirements as the specialty's residents are inevitably exposed to varieties of ethical dilemmas. These dilemmas serve to sensitize the trainees to conflicts they will undoubtedly face during the rest of their careers. The AACAP Code of Ethics thus serves as a valuable potential resource, in perpetuity, to CAPs that are destined, periodically, to encounter perplexing ethical problems. International codes, discussed later, hold the same importance.

CHILDREN, ETHICS AND LAW

Children are not little adults. They developmentally mature over time, in the physiological, cognitive, language and affective spheres, as well as in their social relationships with others. As a group, children are best not viewed as a single unit. Rather, they must be differentiated at distinct developmental stages, beginning with infancy and advancing through the preschool, school-age, adolescent, and transitional-age youth phases. Concomitantly, the application of ethical reasoning must attend to the individual child's developmental attainments within his or her specific phase. ***To illustrate***: A 2½- and a 17-year old may refuse a recommended and sensible medical intervention. As their cognitive capacities differ greatly from each other, given their ages, it is much more likely that the practitioner will respect the autonomy rights due the adolescent in contrast to those of the toddler. Similarly, the clinician is less likely to respect the autonomy of the 15-year old suicidal adolescent when compared to that of her relatively mentally healthy peer.

Of note, with the exception of the transitional-age youth, a child or adolescent commonly does not possess the legal right to refuse a medical intervention. Legal consent to proposed care resides with the youngster's adult guardian, most commonly a parent. The contrast of the law with ethical considerations is important, and the CAP should not confuse one with the other. To that end, ethical codes embody broad standards of preferred conduct. Ethical reasoning, employing fundamental principles, similarly serves as a guide to making moral choices. The law, by contrast, tends to be definitive, with little elasticity. CAP practitioners are ethically obligated to be aware of relevant laws, but the ethical choices that are made might, depending on the dilemma, conflict or agree with the law as written. For example, laws mandating distant biological relatives as the primary options to provide guardianship for neglected or abused children might conflict with the emotional needs of children who have experienced valued long-term "temporary" care with biologically unrelated foster parents.

ETHICAL REASONING AND CHILD-RELATED CONCERNS

Ethical considerations regarding children differ from those affecting adults in three major ways. As previously noted, children live in a state of developmental flux. With each child, the degree of developmental attainment must be determined, while acknowledging that the youngster has not matured to the level at which adult rights are accorded. Second, while children's opinions and desires deserve respect, it falls to adult guardians to make definitive choices about the youngsters' care, and not to the children themselves. Clearly, the child's and guardian's views may coincide or conflict. When the latter occurs, practitioners face dilemmas. A common question ensues—to whom does the practitioner owe fidelity? And third, the nature of child care often involves multiple parties. These may include guardians, parents, school systems, physicians, social agencies, courts, and other interested caregivers. Information about the child is often needed, requested, and exchanged. The nature and degree of those exchanges, as well as the navigation of permissions for the information transmission, commonly raise concerns about the information content, intents of the recipients, and the extent to which the child's privacy is maintained.

Context affects ethical reasoning as well. Well-endowed parents, communities, and countries are capable of providing more assets for their children than those with limitations on available resources. Thus, recommendations for special education, medications, or legal assistance might frequently be indicated, but their provision would be impossible in specific contexts. To ignore those realities but nevertheless make such recommendations in impoverished settings, thus heightening uncalled-for hopes, would ultimately negatively impact the intended recipients, producing maleficent impact. Relatedly, indicated resources allotted to one individual could render such supplies unavailable for another, equally needy, child. These considerations commonly raise the issue of balancing the needs of the individual with those of the larger society (8).

Cultural considerations may also affect ethical reasoning. One society might encourage and support children who challenge the status quo while another urges unquestioned obedience to elders. One culture might support unrestrained access to care while another defunds or stigmatizes it. While practitioners must always consider contextual and cultural factors in their deliberations, two criteria, as well as the four primary ethical principles, demand universal applicability in the ethical reasoning process, independent of culture and context. First is the assurance that children's safety must have priority over all other considerations. Second is the requirement that practitioners employ deep reflection and careful and rigorous thought when they attempt to resolve ethical problems.

ETHICAL CONCERNS ABOUT CHILDREN AND CARE

Children brought to psychiatric attention require thorough evaluations. When the evaluations are completed, recommendations are made and commonly implemented. Reports are written and documents are created, transmitted, and stored. Stored electronically, these documents have long lives. They have the potential to affect the child's care for years, and practitioners are ethically bound to use caution in their wording and dissemination. Thus, CAPs are ethically obliged to bear children's short- and long-term interests constantly in mind. If it is determined, in the course of an evaluation, that a child lacks competent adult supports, the CAP has the additional ethical responsibility to act as advocate on the child's behalf. *Advocacy* as an obligation differentiates CAPs from professionals who provide care to patients who have reached the age of majority and who, therefore, bear full adult responsibilities for themselves (9).

ADVOCACY

Work with children invariably involves the children's caretakers. Provision of *beneficence* for the child requires the CAP to be aware of the child and the pertinent guardians, and the importance of the latter to the former. However, when push comes to shove, the CAP must prioritize the needs of the child over familial, agency, or societal counterpressures. Notably, the CAP as forensic evaluator is sometimes cited as an exception to this general rule, as that professional role has the primary obligation of rendering sound scientific opinion to the entity requesting the information. Even in those situations, however, the CAP is mandated to actively consider the full range of needs of the child (ibid. 7 – Principle II). *Nonmaleficence* refers to the obvious expectation of CAPs that they will not engage in harmful or exploitative behaviors toward children under their care. A stipulated corollary is the expectation that the CAP will act to prevent harmful or exploitative acts, directed by others, at the child receiving professional attention. Insofar as the *justice* principle urges the CAP to continuously consider how care might be improved and how relevant injustices might be countered, these three principles (beneficence, nonmaleficence, and justice) combine to promote a major CAP responsibility, that of *advocacy* for the minor. Periodically, a child or children may lack adults who act in their best interests, be they guardians, social agencies, or legal representatives. It becomes the ethical responsibility of CAPs, at those times, to advocate for the minors' needs, as individuals and as a group, as the children themselves are deemed cognitively and politically incapable of competently defending their interests.

DOCTOR–PATIENT RELATIONSHIP; ASSENT AND CONSENT

Basic to physician–patient interactions is the existence of mutual *trust*. When working with children, the CAP–patient relationship is actually created between the CAP and two entities—the child and the guardians. Both of the latter have interests in the process, and it is with both entities that trust ideally is established. The relationship begins when the guardians, child, and physician first meet. While the physician–patient relationship is a legal one, and violation of that relationship could lead to legal sanctions against the professional, the primary basis for the relationship is the faith invested by the child in the physician. That patient has the complete right to expect that his or her best interests will always be the primary guide to recommended interventions and that the healer will avoid pursuing goals that primarily benefit the physician. ***To illustrate:*** "You told me that if I threaten to harm others or myself you'd tell my parents; all the other stuff is between you and me. Well, during the last few weeks I've done ecstasy twice. I don't want them to know—you going to tell them?" Response with a simple yes or no, accompanied by the CAP's justifications, quickly obscures the primary issue—can the adolescent trust the CAP to think through the matter carefully, with the patient and independently, and ultimately advise a course of action that does not undermine the faith and confidence of the patient in the physician? That element is the one most crucial to the outcome.

Except in cases of true emergencies, when safety of the child becomes the prime consideration, it falls to the adults to provide ***consent*** for the medical procedures which follow, be they the initiations of evaluations, research studies, or continuations of treatment. Children below age 18 cannot legally consent to these procedures though they may request, ***assent*** to, or ***dissent*** from, them (10). Minors, in general, are not considered legally endowed with *competence*, that is, the attribute ascribed to adults of the capacity to appreciate the contexts and effects of their behaviors. Legal exceptions for minors are made for emancipated adolescents and in some instances surrounding a minor's pregnancy.

Consent should always be informed, that is, all the parties, including the minor, need to know the nature of a diagnosed condition and the risks or benefits to be derived from accepting or forgoing treatment. Relatedly, coercion of the parties to comply with proposed care should generally be avoided. In the event of interparental dissent, as could occur with, for example, divorced parents, one must determine which parent(s) have legal medical decision-making rights concerning the child. In any case, independent of age, the children's desires or refusals are always to be acknowledged, and their assent should be obtained free from coercion. The degree to which the minor's wishes are seriously considered, however, will depend on the individual child's age and cognitive maturity as well as the clinical circumstances.

Assent is always preferred and desirable as the child is more likely to cooperate with proffered care; communication between all the pertinent parties is facilitated; mutual respect is better maintained; and the child experiences a greater sense of control of the process. On the other hand, on occasion treatment can, and sometimes must, be provided to children in the face of their dissent. Safety considerations should trump the wishes of suicidal youngsters who oppose hospitalization, as should mature adult cognitions prevail over the squalling tantruming of the preschooler who, for example, might dissent from entering a classroom. Thus, respect for autonomous dissent also requires sensible limits.

AGENCY

The CAP is commonly exposed to multiple stakeholders when dealing with problematic cases. While aware of the need to serve as the child's advocate other interested parties, including guardians, regulatory entities, social agencies, schools, faculty hierarchies, health insurance companies, and sponsors of research, may apply pressures, based on economic or other concerns, and demand the CAP's attention.

To illustrate: A second-year psychiatry resident, performing a 3-month CAP rotation, informs the faculty CAP supervisor that she intends to call the state's child protective services agency (CPS) to report abuse by the foster parent of a 10-year old girl in temporary care. The girl mentioned, in an outpatient treatment session, that the parent had hit her thrice on her legs with a broom handle as punishment for returning home half an hour late from school. This physical reprimand left faint bruise marks on her skin. The resident noted that the girl had previously resided, with rapid turnover, in three foster homes, had lived with the current guardian for the past 3/4 year, the guardian and the girl had developed a warm mutual relationship, and this temporary foster parent had recently spoken of her intention to seek permanent adoption of the girl.

For whom is the CAP supervisor an agent? Is the faculty CAP's major obligation to provide quality education for the resident? As safety is always the primary consideration, the CAP must consider whether the child is at risk for near- or longer-term harm. Would the child benefit from removal to another foster care placement or could the current situation be maintained, salvaged, and improved? Would it be possible to accomplish the latter if CPS were to be notified and subsequently intervened? Might such a move and intervention wreck the possibility of adoption, by the seemingly loving temporary foster parent, from going forward? Might contact with CPS prevent future abuses of the girl? And what of the statutory mandate to report abuse to the designated authorities? What might the impact be on a trainee who observes a faculty member following through on this reportage obligation, possibly followed by damage to, or the severance of, the girl's relationship with her foster parents? Or, to the contrary, of receiving advice from the attending, due to this concern, that they should abstain from reporting, thus encouraging a trainee's violation of the law? The CAP must consider all of these possibilities and the competing interests of these parties. Acceding to the demands or expectations of some will undoubtedly alienate others. But, after weighing these competing interests, the CAP must ultimately decide on an approach that will keep the child's best interests as paramount. Thus, despite feeling beholden as an agent with partial obligations to multiple entities, the fundamental choice must devolve to that of advocate for the most vulnerable entity, the child. In addition, in the course of intervention, the CAP ideally engenders discussion with, and possibly between, the involved parties. Acting thus as facilitator, the CAP propagates potentially greater "buy-in" and collaboration from all those affected by a case, even as their cultures and views may clash with each other. But, in the end, with or without discussion, the CAP's obligation remains to act as the child's agent.

CONFIDENTIALITY

Confidentiality of communications between patient and physician is a bedrock for the development of mutual trust between the two. The patient has the assurance that what has been revealed to the CAP remains between them, not to be divulged without the patient's permission, with an exception provided in the event the patient indicates imminent danger to self or others. Work with young children does not ordinarily pose a problem as they often expect, and are even desirous of, communication of their thoughts by the physician to their guardians. However, not infrequently, adolescents and transitional age youth will test, via provocative communications, the CAP's capacity to live silently with ambiguity and worry.

As a separate matter, interactions between the CAP and children's guardians are, not infrequently, complicating factors. A good relationship between the CAP and the guardians is commonly crucial to the continued treatment of the child. The guardians usually want, and are entitled, to know about matters relating to their child, and the CAP must provide them with pertinent information without violation of the patient's confidentiality concerns.

The phases of children's growth coincide with gradual development of prefrontal cortical neuronal architecture. Impulsive behaviors and inadequate self-control are associated consequences of immature brain development observed in youth (11). Thus, with regularity, CAPs are informed by their adolescent and younger transitional age youth patients of, for example, illicit drug ownership and use, sexual activity, cessation of prescribed medication use, intemperate physical and verbal outbursts, and contemplation of or engagement in behaviors that skirt or violate the law. If the CAP were to discuss these matters with the youngsters' guardians it is likely that, after an experience of initial upset, the adults would be appreciative and seek to remedy the situation. However, if the information were conveyed without prior notice to the youths, or without their assent, the patients would likely feel alienated and quite possibly terminate care.

Approaching cases with a family-centered approach, where possible, manages to contain many of the concerns around confidentiality (12). This method, described to the participants at the outset, reconciles the guardians' desires for information with the patient's need for confidentiality. The concept of confidentiality and its breadth and limits are briefly mentioned but, much more importantly, the desirability of cross-communication, transparency, and the utility of trust in the physician to keep the best interests of the child foremost, while including employment of judicious exchange of information among all parties, is emphasized.

Limits on confidentiality, in professional contexts other than the therapeutic setting, must be acknowledged. Forensic CAP examiners must inform the child under evaluation, and the child's guardians, that none of the material obtained during the course of the interviews has confidentiality protections, and that the obtained information will be shared with the requesting parties. On the other hand, all patient-related notes, in addition to those taken during forensic evaluations, should contain no extraneous data, and care must always be taken to ensure that exposure of the written material is limited to previously designated and approved pertinent recipients. Research subjects are entitled to anonymity, without identifiable attributes, while their data is grouped together with that of other subjects in a cohort. Not uncommonly, clinicians, CAP trainees, and faculty will orally present or publish material centering on patient cases. It is incumbent on these presenters and authors to disguise inconsequential descriptive attributes that could contribute to the identification of specific patients by others. In addition, it is preferable to obtain permission from a patient (or the guardian, in the instance of a minor) in order to publish material descriptive of a child when significant disguise would result in the distortion of important and germane data. This is all the more true for visual material, itself difficult to disguise, and therefore requiring assent from the minor and consent from the guardian.

ASSESSMENT, DIAGNOSIS, AND TREATMENT

Competent assessments should result in accurate diagnoses followed by, when indicated, appropriate treatments. To what extent, however, might psychiatrically evaluated children subsequently be stigmatized by their diagnosis? How verifiable are the proposed diagnoses, who is performing the diagnostic process, and with what degree of accuracy? Who has a stake, beyond the child him- or herself, in treatment interventions—that is, to what extent are pressures from family, schools, health insurance companies, and the pharmaceutical industry encouraging, recommending, or demanding specific kinds of interventions? Raising these questions in no way diminishes the value of the diagnostic process, which must underlie treatment interventions. Their answers, however, should indicate whether the sought-after benefit is primarily intended for the patient or, by contrast, for the other parties involved in the clinical picture. Should the latter's interests predominate, a different and new diagnostic process would be ethically required.

The practice of medicine developed over millennia. Progressively, clinical observation, coupled with the incorporation of historical data and later the results of laboratory tests, all of which would be passed through the sieve of comparisons to similar phenomenologic manifestations in other individuals, led to classifications of illness and the desirability of verifiable and reproducible treatment results. This systematic problem-solving approach became the medical model that provided the basis for illness identification and its treatment. This model, itself resting on the scientific method, was incorporated into psychiatry, with the advent of the DSM-III in 1980, in considerably more structured fashion. If, prior to that time, the diagnostic process was conceptualized primarily as established on etiologic theories, it now began to base itself on observed, consensually agreed-to data. This development was a boon to CAP in particular as a significant number of psychiatric disorders clearly present first in children, including those comprising intellectual disabilities and neurodevelopmental disorders. The latter include disturbances of communication, autism spectrum, attention deficit, learning, and motor disorders. Schizophrenia spectrum, bipolar, depression, anxiety, eating, elimination, sleep-wake, gender dysphoria, and conduct disorders usually manifest before the mid 20s and often much earlier. Accurate diagnosis allows for earlier interventions with appropriate specific treatments, preferably sooner rather than later, thus promoting earlier improvement in the child's condition rather than prolongation of the child's distress and suffering (13). Thus, correct diagnosis, followed by scientifically supported integrated medical interventions, ought ordinarily to be an ethically indicated, desirably beneficent, approach.

The treatment armamentarium of CAPs is limited to environmental manipulation, coordination of care, verbal therapies, pharmacologic interventions and, rarely, other somatic approaches. While the knowledge base underlying treatment provision improves and enlarges over time, the multifaceted problems with which children present commonly necessitate use of more than one of the above, if not the majority, of the cited modalities. Ethical treatment requires sound reasoning for the employment of any of the modalities and, foremost, avoidance of interventions that might prove harmful. Recommendations for inpatient versus outpatient care, residential placement, special versus mainstreamed education, and the choices of specific psychotherapeutic modalities and/or pharmacologic agents all carry potential risks and benefits for the child. These choices may raise questions about third-party influences on, and potential conflicts of interest for, the CAP. Does the CAP receive financial support from any relevant parties to the case, be they the guardians, health insurance providers, schools, or court systems? Are any of these entities suggesting their preferred courses of action to the CAP? Does the CAP, directly or at a distance, benefit from pharmaceutical company largesse? Does referral for psychotherapy to a nonmedical colleague or employee encourage return benefit to the CAP? To what extent, and with what degree of openness, does the CAP address these questions? To what extent does the CAP declare potential conflicts of interest to the patient and family? To what degree does the CAP employ evidence-based knowledge in making therapeutic choices and, when doing so, is informed assent and consent provided? Modes of psychotherapy and pharmaceutics are not inherently good or bad—they both have the potential to improve, maintain, damage, or have no effect on the child's condition. When the above questions are posed and answered honestly and transparently, and a risk/benefit analysis is supplied to the recipient concerning the proposed interventions, treatment can be instituted on a sound ethical basis (14).

For the CAP prescribing or directly providing treatment the ethical imperative is to be knowledgeable, in a comprehensive manner, concerning the range of available therapeutics. Thus, knowledge of medications implies learned awareness of a variety of chemical classes and entities, their indications, benefits, side effects, possible long-term impacts on developing brains and potentials for off-label uses, as well as the necessity to ascertain a patient's current use of "alternative" or "complementary" medicines. The same degree of knowledge holds true for the potential contributions of the psychotherapies. Thus, familiarity with the concepts and the application of psychodynamic, behavioral, familial, and cognitive-behavioral approaches should be expected of the practitioner, whether or not the CAP provides such care directly or refers patients to nonmedical providers for this care. Ineptitude in the provision of verbal therapies holds the potential to be as dangerous to the child as the prescription of inappropriate medication or child placement in an unsuitable facility. In other words, when it comes to providing treatment, the primary commandment is to "above all, do no harm."

RESEARCH

Investigations designed to elucidate disease mechanisms, improve current care, and develop new treatment interventions are imperatives for all medical specialties. Research is crucial for the development of the field of CAP. As the specialty's focus is on children, however, safety concerns accrue beyond those impacting adult populations and additional safeguards are required in the course of the research efforts in this field.

All research requires the balance of potential benefits versus the risks to the research subjects, and equal risk to benefit ratios are commonly applied to research studies with adults. In contrast to these ratios, United States federal guidelines for research with children require that the benefit to risk ratio be directly favorable to the child participants (15). In thorough and painstaking fashion, proposed research is divided into the categories of "minimal risk," "more than minimal risk, but with the prospect of direct benefit," "more than minimal risk, with no prospect of direct benefit, but likely to yield disorder-relevant knowledge," and "research not otherwise approvable" (16). As might be expected, these categories are often the subject of debates between researchers and oversight bodies, but their thrust is clear—to avoid harm befalling individual child subjects. Secondly, the potential risks and benefits of proposed research requires developmentally appropriate explanation to the child, out of respect to the child's autonomy and geared to the level of the child's cognitive maturation. In addition, both the parents and children must be alerted in advance to distinctions made between studies that offer definite versus possible exposure of the child to a therapeutic agent, for example, in placebo studies. Thus, honest and transparent descriptions of study protocols are required for truly informed assent and consent.

As children are legally minors and therefore unable to provide legal consent, it is required that they assent to their participation in research studies. Legal consent is required from the guardians for the child's participation but, even if that is supplied, a child's dissent is binding, and the child's subsequent nonparticipation in a study would therefore be assumed. A child might experience coercion, from guardians or researchers, to participate in research efforts. Assent provided under such circumstances would be considered obtained in violation of the child's autonomous rights and consequent to undue attempts at influence, and therefore be deemed unethically acquired and nonbinding.

Finally, strong confidentiality safeguards are required, regarding the information obtained from individual children in research studies, related to the filing and later dissemination of collected data. Furthermore, it is ethically required that the aggregated and anonymous data be made public, independent of the nature of the findings and the sources of the funding or other sponsorship of the research efforts, and that the authorial conclusions be accurately based on the study's data-driven results.

EMERGING LOCI OF CONCERN

While fundamental ethical principles remain immutable, they are applied to the analyses of dilemmas that arise in a constantly changing world. A variety of relatively recent scientific advances have brought both benefits and new conundrums. Four areas will each receive brief address—genomics, treatment of psychiatric prodromes, impacts of social media, and potentials for brain enhancement.

GENOMICS

The entire DNA sequence of a human being's chromosomes was first decoded 15 years ago. Prior to that time and since, numerous single gene anomalies were and have been correlated with specific disease expressions. More recently, however, multiple genetic risk factors have been associated with the emergence of psychiatric disorders which are in turn associated with, for example, alterations in calcium-channel signaling (17). These, in turn, might be related to the degree of production, release, and reception of neurotransmitters at specific brain sites. Unlike Huntington Disorder, an illness with psychiatric components whose expression is consequent to the presence of a single defective gene, the prevailing view of the psychiatric research community holds that psychiatric disease expression is likely polygenic in origin and vulnerability, and that the development of the disorders probably stems from a combination of environmental influences and underlying genomic structure. It appears that continued investigation is likely to result in progressively greater elucidation of genetic vulnerabilities to, and bases for, disease expression. Should this happen, as much psychiatric illness first emerges in child populations, targeted interventions, perhaps primarily pharmacologic, will hopefully prove to be useful to CAPs and their patients.

Conjectured screenings of children for genetically based disorders infer ethical risks, however. Medical records containing specific genetic data, both about the children and their parents, could precipitate stigma when the information is made available to health insurers or local communities. Approaches to assent and consent would likely require revision in light of this potential and, as well, in response to the possible development of entirely new treatment methods (18).

PSYCHIATRIC PRODROMES

Presaging the identification of specific genetic markers, the identification of subclinical aberrant behavioral or cognitive phenomena, often coupled with documentation of disturbed family genealogies, led to the suggestion of treatment for psychiatric prodromal symptomatology before its postulated full-blown expression in frank disorders. In other words, full disease expression might be headed off, thus sparing the child, and later the adult, the burden of chronic disease. Focusing largely on schizophrenia, research institutions have studied the effects of interventions, with neuroleptic medications and at times family interventions, on individuals exhibiting schizotypal symptoms with positive family histories for the disease. While the intentions are noble, that is, to spare children distress by providing pre-emptive treatment, thoughtful critiques have accompanied the efforts (19,20). Aside from obvious ethical concerns about the potentially debilitating effects associated with the introduction of neuroleptic medications, it is clear that determination of disease prevention is difficult to ascertain as in no way could one conclude which specific individual was in fact destined to develop severe illness. Thus, for example, the individual who has been so treated and does not develop psychosis years later may never have been destined to do so in the first place.

Despite such cautions, these preventive approaches continue in designated settings and may gain strength with advances in genetic understandings of psychiatric disease mechanisms. As many psychiatric disorders first emerge in childhood, proposals to treat any number of them pre-emptively are likely to be made. The ethical risk-benefit analysis called for at those times would need to be based on the nature of the then-current scientific knowledge base, potential benefits of new and positive interventions, and possible negative impacts. Given children's cognitive immaturities, CAPs would need to be very aware of the latent deleterious impacts on future brain and motor development, while desperate families might want to focus exclusively on the potential benefits.

SOCIAL MEDIA (BOUNDARIES AND PROFESSIONALISM)

For the older practitioner, social media is a novel technology to be mastered or approached gingerly. For the younger practitioner, and most definitely for the child through TAY population, social media have "always" been there and fluency with their use is a given. Vast majorities of populations worldwide are adept at communicating electronically via e-mail, Twitter, Instagram, Facebook, and the like. This widespread employment of digital communications requires CAPs' awareness of potential ethical pitfalls in their electronic dealings with patients and their families, and of ethical considerations as a component of practitioners' adherence to professional behavior.

Roberts and Dyer view professionalism as a concept expressed via ethical behavior and thought, that is, as applied ethics (21). Ideally, the physician's professional behavior encourages the patient's trust in the practitioner and solidification of the physician–patient relationship. Professionally set boundaries serve as an envelope that promotes and enforces pro-therapeutic behaviors; transgressions or frank violations of these boundaries pose the major threats to this supremely important relationship. These boundaries, some discussed earlier and all of which are subject to transgression, include patient's confidentiality rights, practitioner conflicts of interest and eschewing of transparency, child exploitation, provision of informed assent and respect for dissent, and inappropriate romantic or physical contact with the patient and the patient's relatives (22,23). The ethical considerations surrounding electronic communications and boundary violations, however, can seem new and become quite complicated, particularly for the unwary CAP (24).

It is crucial for CAPs to know that internet use has been adopted by huge numbers of people, their access to countless quanta of digital communications is easily achieved, and these communications, therefore, however they might be intended, are not private and are recorded in perpetuity. Further, CAPs' blog posts concerning patients may violate their legitimate expectations of confidentiality; practitioners' personal information is readily accessible to patients; information about patients and their families exists in the public domain, is open to exploration by the CAP, and might possibly be obtained without the patient's knowledge and consent; and electronic communications between CAPs and their patients or family members can easily become public, by unintended breach or error, and, dependent on the nature of their interpretation, could potentially lead to professional liability. Liability concerns could include errors committed by practitioners secondary to receipt or sending of inadequate evaluation information; patient responses based on recommendations received via electronic versus face-to-face meetings; practice of medicine across states while lacking proper medical licensure; and inadequate documentation of electronic communications in the medical record. The not unusual, delicate dance of ethically balancing a patient's privacy rights with those of the parent's right to know can become all the more complicated when both parties are permitted, encouraged, or expected to engage electronically, but separately, with the practitioner. Given all of these scenarios the CAP is strongly advised to be knowledgeable about electronic communications, use them judiciously but not as a substitute for face-to-face contact, and be aware of the need to maintain professional demeanor while simultaneously remaining alert to legal liability potentials.

NEUROETHICS

Research efforts have consistently indicated that central nervous system stimulant medications are the treatments of choice for children competently and accurately diagnosed with attention deficit hyperactivity disorder (ADHD). Appropriate use of the medications benefits these youngsters by increasing their abilities to attend and concentrate, and improving their time management and executive functioning. In this fashion deficited youngsters are enabled to compensate for their diagnosed impairments and can learn and participate with peers in more equal fashion. However, research efforts also indicate that not only youngsters with ADHD benefit from this medical intervention but that segments of nondisordered, or "healthy," individuals, respond similarly (25). Thus, "normal range" individuals who access such medications may have their skills "artificially" enhanced, possibly advantaging them over their peers who do not use, or have access to, these resources. The emerging field of neuroethics engages in considerations and analyses of these conundrums (26).

How might pharmacologic agents be used? Are they intended only for the disabled or also for healthy individuals, possibly to enhance not only cognitions but mood as well? Ordinarily, CAPs must be alert to the potential deleterious effects of pharmacologic interventions with their patients, both for the immediate-term, for example, overt negative side effects, and longer-term, for example, the yet-to-be-known impacts of chronically administered neuropharmacologic medications on developing brain. But the potential benefits of the administration of such medications for "normal range" children raise additional and different sets of issues.

From the *justice* perspective—would such medications be available to all, or not? Might such cognitive enhancers, by artificially facilitating achievement, negatively impact the expectation of sustained effort expenditure in the pursuit of goals, a positively valued personality trait commonly encouraged during character formation in childhood? In 2012, 13% of the U.S. adult population was prescribed antidepressant medication in order to improve mood (27). Might an eventual generalized introduction of mood enhancers produce a happier or better-functioning society, or simply a more compliant one (28)? How would one measure the quality of outcomes when comparing results between medication-enhanced and -naïve students or athletes? Some of these questions are commonly debated in the larger society, about which, respectively, CAPs must be aware and to which they belong. For the moment, perhaps society's predominantly negative response to athletic-ability enhancement, on the part of professional athletes, is the best indicator of popular sentiment regarding medication-induced mood and cognitive enhancement for the "well."

INTERNATIONAL ETHICS

The United States, wedged between two large oceans, has periodically functioned as a country reluctantly forced to engage with the larger world. In this era of rampant globalization, however, that stance often becomes untenable. As is true across a variety of global matters, an openness to worldwide ethical concerns is crucial to America. While the fundamental ethical principles, discussed earlier, are universally acknowledged, their applicability must take cognizance of culture, context, and locale. Thus, political, geographic, economic, and religious influences and mores must be strongly considered by those individuals who suggest approaches to the provision of mental health care for children (29,30).

International efforts to create ethical codes intended for physicians worldwide include the World Medical Association's (WMA) International Code of Medical Ethics, established in 1949 and subsequently revised, and the World Psychiatric Association's declarations, originally produced in 1996 and enhanced repeatedly since, that created ethical guidelines for psychiatric practice. In addition to ethical matters of expected address, such as concerns surrounding confidentiality, professional boundaries, and responsibilities to patients, the WMA's declarations specifically embrace prohibitions against participation in torture, enjoin discriminatory behaviors against ethnicities and cultures, endorse patients' rights to information about their diagnoses and the bases for prescribed treatments, and exhort avoidance of politically induced conflicts of interest. Specific child-centered concerns have similarly been addressed by international bodies. Thus, the United Nations Convention on the Rights of the Child (1989) delineated children's rights to survival, protection, and maturation, inclusive of the right to live with their families. The United Nations Convention on the Rights of Persons with Disabilities (2008) specifically includes children as it discusses those individuals afflicted by psychiatric disturbance.

The International Association for Child and Adolescent Psychiatry and Allied Professions (IACAPAP) created ethical guidelines in 2006 for practitioners worldwide that, in addition to setting out basic principles and expectations of proper patient care behaviors, highlighted concerns about potential child exploitation, sexual engagements, publication ethics, and multidisciplinary collaboration. IACAPAP's Declaration of Berlin (2004) focused, in part, on research approaches with children, declaring the priority of the individual child's welfare over other research goals, prohibition of involuntary child participation, and the imperative of proper assent and consent procedures.

Democratic forces, pitted in the past against totalitarian and authoritarian governments and responding to their cruel treatments of civilians, were pivotal in the creation of these documents. Medical support of, and collaboration with, the murderous Nazi machine of mid-twentieth century wartime Europe, and the creation of bogus diagnoses (e.g., the Soviet Union's use of "sluggish schizophrenia" to imprison political dissidents in psychiatric hospitals and mistreat them against their will), subsequently galvanized medical and psychiatric communities to create ethical standards in the effort to forestall similar future medical embarrassments. Current newspapers' front pages, replete with articles describing governmental-, tribal-, and religion-inspired chaos and mayhem that evinces no regard by its perpetrators for the rights of innocent civilians, as well as a democratic government's sponsorship, directly and indirectly, of state-supported torture (i.e., the United States and its international prisoners at Guantanamo [Cuba] prison as well as its secret international prisoner renderings to foreign governments), might seem to make a mockery of these noble declarations and documents. On the other hand, these documents continue to shine a positive light on medicine's and psychiatry's most honorable ethical aspirations, with the hope that they might prevail during or after the direst of circumstances.

Apart from political contexts, economic factors have played large roles in the creation of these documents. As global studies indicate that up to 20% of child populations suffer from mental health disturbance, it is noteworthy that, in many countries, these children are homeless, often refugees living with or without their families, orphans, and abuse victims (31). A majority of these children live in resource-poor countries. Recently, though, many more have inundated relatively resource-rich Europe, having arrived from the Middle East and Africa and achieved at least temporary residence. Their needs are great. The ethical imperatives to provide for those needs and to avoid harm, endorsed by these above documents, continue to operate, independent of locale.

In most countries, the ability to prescribe best interventions for the individual child patient, as well as for children viewed as a group, is limited by the available resources. Thus, in certain locales custodial institutions may be the only prescriptive possibility for an autistic child, versus possible accessibility, in well-endowed settings, of therapeutic schooling, school-based aides, occupational and other therapeutic guidance, and additional state-funded programs. Similarly, psychotropic medications of differing chemical classes might be missing entirely from formularies in resource-poor countries. Differing cultures also affect ethical choices. Thus, cultures that place greater emphasis on the value of societal maintenance in contrast to the needs of the individual will probably unconsciously influence the ethical reasoning processes of the conflicted child care practitioner. As well, the CAP working in settings with limited available resources is likely to focus on mental health applications that can be applied to groups, while focusing training in mental health care on nonmedical child care workers in order that they be enabled to provide care for individual children (32–34). Finally, it is of interest that while differences exist between countries with regard to resources, measurements of the incidence of psychiatric illness, and treatment approaches, by contrast it appears that the values ascribed to fundamental ethical principles are similarly shared and respected across disparate borders (35).

ETHICS, FORENSICS, AND THE LAW

Ethical thought is intended to help guide individuals' behaviors in directions that benefit fellow human beings and their societies while respecting each individual's autonomy. Ethical exhortations of clearly preferred behaviors are usually presented in flexible fashion that allows for differing choices in their implementation. By contrast, the law's intent is to codify these ethical goals within relatively firm and defined limits. To wit, Potter Stewart, a former associate justice of the U.S. Supreme Court, breezily distinguished between the two disciplines: "Ethics is knowing the difference between what you have a [legal] right to do and what is right to do."

Principle X (tenth), a recent addition to AACAP's Code of Ethics (7), deems it an ethical imperative, for the properly practicing CAP, to be fully cognizant of the laws governing medical and psychiatric practice of the jurisdictions in which the physician works. Thus, in addition to knowledge of generic legislations regarding medical responsibilities and negligence, documentations of care, and information release, CAPs are expected to be cognizant of the operative laws regarding custodial arrangements and responsibilities, child abuse and neglect, reportage requirements, responses to patients' expressions of harm directed against self or others, and assent and consent to medical care. While ethical inclinations and legal requirements often coincide, in some circumstances they may conflict. At those times, it is ethically incumbent on the CAP to recognize these conflicts and the various implications, for the patient and the physician, of the choices subsequently made by the psychiatrist.

In addition to responsibility for knowledge of relevant laws, the following comments address a smattering of other legal matters that may crop up in the course of CAP practice. Patients and their guardians must be alerted, by CAPs, to factors that distinguish between forensic and psychiatric evaluations (36). The former is intended to be impartial, objective, and not therapeutic. The evaluating CAP owes primary responsibility to the requesting party, commonly the juvenile justice or school systems, to render a sound medical opinion. That opinion may run counter to the child's preferences, though the evaluator is expected simultaneously to consider and acknowledge the child's needs. By contrast, a treating CAP has an ethical responsibility to make the needs of the child patient paramount. Furthermore, confidentiality rights do not apply in the forensic setting. The forensic evaluator must include all relevant data, inclusive of the patient's verbalizations, in the forensic report, and must utilize this data to substantiate the rendered opinions. By comparison, the treating psychiatrist is bound by the patient's confidentiality rights. A treating CAP, therefore, should avoid adopting a forensic role with the CAP's patient as combining the two roles potentially creates clear conflicts of interest, endangers the CAP's objectivity, diminishes the acceptability of the report, and could create havoc in the therapeutic relationship (37).

As a separate matter, when presenting release of information forms for guardian signature or responding to requests for information, CAPs have the ethical obligation to request or provide only that information necessary for the provision of care. Request or provision of more information than needed could be viewed as negligent practice. In related fashion, CAPs have ethical and professional responsibilities, to themselves and their patients, to be honest in their dealings, even in the face of health insurance companies whose primary motives appear to be solely financially driven. Therefore, CAPs must complete insurance forms, including diagnostic codes, honestly, even when doing so might negatively impact their patient's welfare.

Finally, complaints are periodically addressed to the AACAP's Ethics Committee concerning alleged violations of professional ethics by CAPs. To date, the committee has largely functioned in an educational role for the parent organization, though more recently it is seeking an advisory role as well. The committee has not, however, due to a paucity of resources, ever engaged in investigational or quasi-judicial activities. In the event of the receipt of nonanonymous allegations of ethical violations against members, complainants are referred by AACAP's ethics committee to the ethics committees of the American Psychiatric Association's district branches and to state medical licensing boards. Following their investigations, subsequent ethical and legal decisions range from "no findings" to such sanctions as the loss of medical licensure to practice, with intermediary penalties inclusive of formal reprimands and temporary license suspensions. The loss of medical licensure by a CAP under these circumstances automatically leads to loss of membership in the AACAP.

CONCLUSION

Ethical thought provides the bedrock for guidelines and standards created for the practice of medicine and the profession of CAP. Professional conduct requires adherence to these standards and encourages awareness of these matters in the course of daily practice. Commonly, practitioners are not consciously aware of ethical dilemmas until they find themselves experiencing sticky situations. Those are ideal times to consult the AACAP Code of Ethics, members of the AACAP Ethics Committee, and respected colleagues. Often, optimal ethical results follow from the physician's opting to view dilemmas from a patient's perspective and following that lead (38).

References

1. Reiner C, Brooks M: *The 2000 Year Old Man—The Complete History.* Shout! Factory 826663-11525-B1, 2009.
2. Brooks M: *History of the World—Part I.* Director: Mel Brooks. Distribution: 20th Century Fox, 1981.
3. Bloch S, Pargiter R: Codes of ethics. In: Bloch S, Green S (eds): *Psychiatric Ethics.* 4th ed. Oxford, Oxford University Press, 151–173, 2009.
4. Beauchamp T, Childress J: *Principles of Biomedical Ethics.* 7th ed. Oxford, Oxford University Press, 2012.
5. Aries P: *Centuries of Childhood.* New York, Random House, 1962.
6. Enzer N: Ethics in child psychiatry—an overview. In: Schetky D, Benedek E (eds): *Emerging Issues in Child Psychiatry and the Law.* New York, Brunner/Mazel, 3–21, 1985.
7. American Academy of Child and Adolescent Psychiatry: Code of Ethics. https://www.aacap.org/App_Themes/AACAP/docs/about_us/transparency_portal/aacap_code_ of_ethics_2012.pdf. Accessed January 18, 2016.
8. Sondheimer A: Ethics and international child and adolescent psychiatry. In: Rey J (ed): *IACAPAP e-Textbook of Child and Adolescent Mental Health.* Geneva, International Association for Child and Adolescent Psychiatry and Allied Professions, 1–26, 2012.
9. Rosenfeld A, Pilowsky D, Fine P, et al.: Foster care: an update. *J Am Acad Child Adol Psychiat* 36:448–457, 1997.
10. Leikin S: Minors' assent or dissent to medical treatment. *J Pediat* 102: 169–176, 1983.
11. Lenroot R, Giedd J: Brain development in children and adolescents: insights from anatomical magnetic resonance imaging. *Neurosci Biobehav Rev* 30:718–729, 2006.
12. Sondheimer A: Ethics and child and adolescent psychiatry: avoiding confidentiality conflicts. *Psychiat Times* 27:28,39, 2010.
13. Fritz G: Child and adolescent psychiatry in the era of health care reform. *J Am Acad Child Adol Psychiat* 56:3–6, 2016.
14. Klykylo W: General principles of psychopharmacotherapy with children and adolescents—ethical issues in child and adolescent psychopharmacology. In: Klykylo W, Bowers R, Weston C, Jackson J (eds): *Green's Child and Adolescent Psychopharmacology.* 5th ed. Philadelphia, PA, Lippincott Williams & Wilkins, 14–16, 2014.
15. Department of Health and Human Services: Protection of human subjects: research involving children. *Fed Regist* 48:9814–9820, 1983.
16. Department of Health and Human Services: OPRR Reports: protection of human subjects. *Fed Regist* 46:115–408, 1991.
17. Cross-Disorders Group of the Psychiatric Genomics Consortium: Identification of risk loci with shared effects on five major psychiatric disorders: a genome-wide analysis. *Lancet* 381:1371–1379, 2013.
18. Hinshaw S: The stigmatization of mental illness in children and parents: developmental issues, family concerns, and research needs. *J Child Psychol Psychiat* 46:714–734, 2005.
19. Cornblatt B, Lencz T, Kane J: Treatment of the schizophrenia prodrome: is it presently ethical? *Schizophr Res* 51:31–38, 2001.
20. Appelbaum P: Ethical challenges in the primary prevention of schizophrenia. *Schiz Bull* 41:773–775, 2015.
21. Roberts L, Dyer A: Ethics: Principles and Professionalism. In: Roberts L, Dyer A (eds): *Ethics in Mental Health Care.* Washington, DC, American Psychiatric Publishing, 1–17, 2004.
22. Gabbard G, Nadelson C: Professional boundaries in the physician-patient relationship. *JAMA* 273:1445–1449, 1995.
23. Schetky D: Boundaries in child and adolescent psychiatry. In: Schetky D (ed): *Child and Adolescent Psychiatric Clinics of North America.* Philadelphia, PA, Saunders, 4:769–778, 1995.
24. DeJong S: Professionalism and adolescent psychiatry in the digital age. *Adol Psychiat* 4:1–9, 2014.
25. Smith M, Farah M: Are prescription stimulants "smart pills"? The epidemiology and cognitive neuroscience of prescription stimulant use by normal healthy individuals. *Psychol Bull* 137:717–741, 2011.
26. Illes J (ed): *Neuroethics: Defining the Issues in Theory, Practice and Policy.* Oxford, Oxford University Press, 2006.
27. Kantor E, Rehm C, Haas J, Chan AT, Giovannucci EL: Trends in prescription drug use among adults in the United States from 1999–2012. *JAMA* 314:1818–1831, 2015.
28. Huxley A: *Brave New World.* London, Chatto & Windus, 1932.
29. Belfer M, Eisenbruch M: International child and adolescent mental health. In: Martin A, Volkmar F (eds): *Lewis's Child and Adolescent Psychiatry.* Philadelphia, PA, Wolters Kluwer, 87–101, 2007.
30. Leckman J, Leventhal B: A global perspective on child and adolescent mental health. *J Child Psychol Psychiat* 49:221–225, 2008.
31. Desjarlais R, Eisenberg L, Good B, Kleinman A: *World Mental Health: Problems and Priorities in Low-Income Countries.* Oxford, Oxford University Press, 1995.
32. Wolmer L, Laor N, Yazgan Y: School reactivation programs after disaster: could teachers serve as clinical mediators? In: Lewis M, Laor N, Wolmer L (eds): *Child and Adolescent Psychiatric Clinics of North America.* 12:363–381, 2003.
33. Omigbodun O: Developing child mental health services in resource-poor countries. *Int Rev Psychiat* 20:225–235, 2008.
34. Betancourt T: Attending to the mental health of war-affected children: the need for longitudinal and developmental research perspectives. *J Am Acad Child Adol Psychiat* 50:323–325, 2011.
35. Lindenthal J, Thomas C, Ghali A: A cross-cultural study of confidentiality. *Soc Psychiat Psychiat Epidem* 20:140–144, 1985.
36. Kraus L, Thomas C: Practice parameter for child and adolescent forensic evaluations. *J Am Acad Child Adol Psychiat* 50:1299–1312, 2011.
37. Strasburger L, Gutheil G, Brodsky A: On wearing two hats: role conflict in serving as both psychotherapist and expert witness. *Am J Psychiat* 154:448–456, 1997.
38. Brewin T: How much ethics is needed to make a good doctor? *Lancet* 341:161–163, 1993.

CHAPTER 1.3 ■ A HISTORY OF CHILD PSYCHIATRY

DEBORAH BLYTHE DOROSHOW

INTRODUCTION

Most discussions of the history of modern child psychiatry describe a haphazard process by which many different intellectual and therapeutic movements directed toward the mental health of children coexisted and ultimately coalesced. Leo Kanner (1), considered by many to be the father of child psychiatry, lamented in 1971 that "child psychiatry is the result of the convergence of a number of interests which for about half a century have existed alongside each other, with only sporadically and tenuously maintained areas of mutual contact." In one lecture, Kanner described the "parade of segments" as they passed by, from the care of intellectually disabled children to the creation of intelligence testing, the formation of the field of developmental psychology, the rise of psychoanalysis, the child guidance movement, and finally his own arrival among pediatricians at the Harriet Lane Home of the Johns Hopkins School of Medicine. Neither was this parade an organized one. As Kanner (2) later described, "Collections of different shapes and sizes of building stones, for a long time not even conceived as such, were piled up at some distance from each other, then brought haphazardly into casual relationship, and eventually carried together to become parts of an integral edifice."

TROUBLED CHILDREN IN THE NINETEENTH CENTURY

Professional discussion of mental illness in children during the nineteenth century was negligible, if only because it was generally believed (and famously stated by American psychiatrist Benjamin Rush) that children's minds were too unformed to absorb the permanent disfiguration required by insanity (3). Primarily, such children were discussed as case reports of extraordinary children with bizarre behavior. For example, British psychiatrist Alexander Walk (4) described one 4-year-old boy reported in 1846 to "[have] been refused an outing and on becoming excited over this was punished; he then went into paroxysms of terror, was violent, and finally passed into a state of stupor described as 'idiocy'." Although large numbers of mentally ill adults resided in public and private asylums by the mid-nineteenth century in both Europe and the United States, few children resided in these institutions (5).

Although the practical aspects of care of mentally ill children are unclear, many physicians were writing about the concept of what they then referred to as "insanity" in young people. For example, prominent British psychiatrist Henry Maudsley (6) devoted an entire chapter of his renowned 1867 textbook to the subject. Maudsley's work set a standard for such textbooks, in which childhood insanity would more frequently be considered separately from "feeblemindedness" and neurologic disorders like epilepsy. Still, childhood insanity was believed to be very rare. Maudsley (7) himself commented: "How unnatural! is an exclamation of pained surprise which some of the more striking instances of insanity in young children are apt to provoke…[but] Anomalies, when rightly studied, yield rare instruction."

INTELLECTUAL DISABILITY AND THE RISE OF INTELLIGENCE TESTING

Professional work on intellectually disabled children, described as "mentally defective," "feebleminded," or "idiots," was much more common, as well as more organized. In France, Jean-Étienne Esquirol and his colleague Edouard Seguin worked intensely with this population. By the late twentieth century, many such children were institutionalized in the United States (8,9). This population would become critical to the development of intelligence tests in the United States. French researcher Alfred Binet and his student Theodore Simon developed the first modern intelligence test in 1905 when Binet was commissioned by the French government to create a means of separating out intellectually disabled children for special schooling when compulsory public education became law. The test was unusual in that it attempted to quantify intelligence and was based on data from real children, representing a departure from strict theorizing. In 1916, Lewis Terman modified Binet's original intelligence test and introduced the Stanford-Binet revised edition for use in the United States (10).

American psychologist Henry Goddard appropriated and popularized this test in the United States. Previously, physicians had used a number of competing classification systems to identify intellectually disabled children, ranging from their degree of impairment to physical symptoms, the supposed etiology of impairment, or a child's ability to function socially. As the psychologist at the Training School for Feeble-Minded Girls and Boys in Vineland, NJ, Goddard demonstrated that Vineland students' scores on Binet's tests correlated well with teachers' assessments of their performance. In the process, he redefined "feeblemindedness" as a lack of intelligence, as opposed to a vague hereditary condition. In Philadelphia and Boston, psychologist Lightner Witmer and physician Walter Fernald conducted similar research on intellectually disabled children, focusing on how intelligence testing could be used to measure degrees of intellectual disability.

Intelligence testing in early twentieth-century America was an inherently eugenicist project. This was only natural for a project that intended to sort normal from abnormal; eugenics was at its heart an attempt to identify the best specimens of the human race and do away with the worst. For example, Henry Goddard and Lewis Terman were strong supporters of eugenics; Goddard even promoted the passage of eugenic sterilization laws in his home state of New Jersey. In his most famous case study, *The Kallikak Family*, Goddard did extensive pedigree work to argue that a girl at his training school whom he described as feebleminded had become such due to a long family history of intellectual disability, poverty, and crime. Thus, he argued, intellectual disability was fundamentally heritable (11).

CHILD STUDY AND THE DESCRIPTION OF NORMAL DEVELOPMENT

As researchers like Goddard focused on identifying abnormal children, other researchers directed their attention to understanding the processes of normal child development. As childhood began to be recognized as a special stage of life in the late nineteenth century, these researchers described the period as encompassing multiple stages of development through which all children had to pass sequentially. These efforts took place under the umbrella of the child study movement, which quickly grew to involve not only pediatricians and psychologists, but also mothers who were anxious to implement the latest scientific knowledge into their childrearing practices. The professional figurehead of the movement was Clark University psychologist G. Stanley Hall, who identified the period of adolescence as a transitional one between childhood and adulthood in his most famous work, the 1904 study *Adolescence*. In the same study, he famously argued that the stages of child development recapitulated human evolution (12).

Hall's graduate student Arnold Gesell took an even more granular approach to child development, describing a series of emotional and physical milestones by which every physician and parent could assess a child's progress. Gesell put his theoretical work into practice in 1911 when he founded the Yale Clinic of Child Development, which later became what is known today as the Yale Child Study Center. His work was especially novel in that he employed new technologies, namely one-way mirrors and films, to observe and record children's behavior. Mothers were active participants in the Child Study Movement as well. Through the Child Study Association of America, middle class women studied G. Stanley Hall's writings together and kept detailed records of their childrearing which they sought to understand using the latest psychological principles. In the 1920s and 1930s, so-called child study groups enabled mothers to share their experiences with one another using the psychological framework of child development. These groups provided a safe space for mothers to discuss their anxieties and uncertainties about childrearing. In the 1940s, efforts to educate women in normal childhood development expanded through local PTAs, home economics courses, and classes for expectant women (13).

Child researchers like Gesell not only sought to describe child development; they also became coveted sources of advice for new parents during the rise of what historian Rima Apple has called "scientific motherhood," or the idea that mothers were incapable of raising their children properly without consulting expert scientific advice on the matter. This concept dated to the late nineteenth century. In 1894, pediatrician Luther Emmett Holt advised a strict approach to childrearing in his *Care and Feeding of Children*, including early toilet training and strict discipline. Meanwhile, the United States Children's Bureau published regular pamphlets on infant care which stressed the importance of scheduling feedings, promoting a child's ability to self soothe, and addressing bad habits early. In the 1920s, the dominant figure in the child-advice field was behaviorist psychologist John Watson, who published a widely read book entitled *Psychological Care of Infant and Child* that encouraged parents to use conditioning to rid their children of bad habits, and warned mothers not to coddle their infants by kissing or hugging them excessively. In many ways, his work was a logical continuation of the advice given by Holt and later by the Children's Bureau. Watson's advice gained great popularity in the 1920s as a highly scientific, straightforward approach to child rearing. Discipline, Watson explained, should occur not by traditional means like spanking, but by reinforcing good behavior and ignoring or isolating a child in response to bad behavior.

By the 1930s and 1940s, childrearing advice had softened, using a more child-centered approach in which parents would encourage their child's natural development, taking cues from their children rather than imposing schedules and behaviors upon them. Pediatrician C. Anderson Aldrich and Mary Aldrich were some of the first to advocate so-called "permissive" child rearing in their 1938 *Babies are Human Beings*, followed by Yale professor Arnold Gesell and his colleague Frances Ilg in their popular 1943 work, *Infant and Child in the Culture of Today*. By the time psychoanalyst and pediatrician Benjamin Spock reassured parents that "you know more than you think you do" in the first edition of his 1946 bestseller *Common Sense Book of Baby and Child Care*, permissiveness was here to stay (14).

PEDIATRICS AND THE HEALTHY MIND

As the parental advice industry flourished, pediatrics was developing as a medical specialty focused not on a specific organ system but on an age group. Although physicians like Abraham Jacobi had focused their medical practices on children since the 1860s, pediatrics was first formalized when the American Medical Association inaugurated a Section on the Diseases of Children in 1880, acknowledging that children were fundamentally different, physically and emotionally, from adults. In 1930, the American Academy of Pediatrics was founded and by 1933 there existed a formal licensing board. In the realm of clinical practice, well baby clinics flourished after World War I, a natural outgrowth of milk stations which provided quality-controlled milk and health advice to mothers at the turn of the century. While child study experts were providing detailed charts describing normal childhood development in the 1920s and 1930s, their counterparts (and sometimes even those same experts, like Gesell) provided charts detailing normal heights and weights (15).

In the midst of this focus on normal children arrived Leo Kanner, a psychiatrist trained under the formidable Adolf Meyer at Johns Hopkins. In 1930, the White House had convened a special Conference on Child Health and Protection, for which a subcommittee was assigned to study "Psychology and Psychiatry in Pediatrics." The subcommittee concluded not that psychiatrists should see children, but that there was a great need for general doctors to understand the basics of psychiatry (16). That same year, Meyer dreamed up the idea of setting up a psychiatric consultation service at the Harriet Lane Home, the epicenter of pediatric activity at Johns Hopkins. His goal was to examine "the rank and file of patients in the pediatric clinics for the formulation of psychiatric problems"—essentially, to learn about the psychology of children not through examining selected mentally ill children, but by observing every child who walked in the door of the pediatrics department (17). It was through this unusual one-man project that Kanner observed and treated children, both normal and abnormal, gleaning the information with which he would write the first textbook of child psychiatry in 1935.

Although Kanner certainly considered himself the founder of the field, this is a shortsighted view. His work at the Harriet Lane Home was certainly an important moment of interaction between pediatrics and psychiatry, but it was a much longer tradition of child saving, juvenile justice, and child guidance that gave rise to the profession of child psychiatry we know today.

CHILD SAVING AND THE MENTAL HYGIENE MOVEMENT

Beginning in the mid-nineteenth century, an enthusiastic generation of reformers, many of them women, became concerned with ensuring the physical and emotional well-being of neglected or mistreated children. They founded organizations opposing the cruelty of children, built lodging houses for working boys and girls, and sent poor children to live with families in rural areas in the so-called "Orphan Train" movement (18). Until then, many unwanted or dependent children had lingered in houses of refuge, where they were often subject to abuse and horrid physical conditions. In the mid-nineteenth century, reformers constructed orphanages to provide a more kindly (yet still relatively custodial) place for children to stay (19). Even reformatories, custodial institutions introduced in the 1820s for "delinquent" children, were increasingly concerned with engendering proper moral values (20,21).

By the late nineteenth century, reform efforts swelled into a full-fledged "child saving" movement, which focused on improving the welfare of dependent and neglected children by ending child labor, promoting compulsory progressive education, providing school lunches, and creating a multitude of agencies designed to help dependent children (22). In 1912, the federal government announced its involvement in child saving with the creation of the United States Children's Bureau. The Bureau, administered by a group of highly educated, single women, quickly became an authoritative voice on child welfare. Among a wide range of activities, the Bureau's staff worked to end child labor, conducted studies on the social factors contributing to infant mortality, and advised new parents on prenatal and infant care (23). The work of the Children's Bureau culminated in the 1921 Sheppard-Towner Maternity and Infancy Act, which provided federally funded preventive health care to mothers and children for the first time.

Meanwhile, the mental hygiene movement was bringing psychiatry out of the asylum and into the larger community, shifting its attention from treatment to prevention. New leaders, like Johns Hopkins psychiatrist Adolf Meyer, suggested that mental illness might be influenced by both heredity and environment (24). If a person's early environment could be modified, perhaps mental illness might be prevented entirely. Because of its preventive focus, mental hygiene was especially directed toward children, who were deemed the most vulnerable and most promising sector of American society (25). Juvenile delinquency was first on the agenda. At the turn of the twentieth century, delinquency was still considered a fundamentally legal problem, often stemming from inherited degeneracy. Many children deemed delinquent or at risk for delinquency, continued to be sent to reformatories, which often remained prison-like even with the introduction of cottages and housemothers.

A new approach emerged in 1899 with the creation of the first juvenile court in Chicago. Juvenile courts, which emerged throughout the United States in the first two decades of the century, were not just courts for minors but rehabilitative agencies. Children, usually from the working class, were brought in for status offenses like truanting or running away from home, petty and serious crimes, and age-inappropriate behaviors like drinking or gambling. In the court, which had no jury or lawyers, the judge would offer individualized guidance, and a probation officer would serve as the child's mentor. Reality often proved sobering, as some juvenile courts became mere detention centers or distribution centers for unwanted children. Yet the juvenile justice system signified an important shift in the way delinquency was understood. No longer the straightforward act of breaking the law, delinquency was starting to become an expression of both psychological and socioeconomic stressors, a reconceptualization that would only continue over the next several decades. Chicago psychiatrist William Healy was also instrumental in changing this perception; in his 1915 book, *The Individual Delinquent,* Healy stressed the importance of understanding each individual child as a product of his or her environment and used psychological language to understand the motives of a "delinquent" child (26).

Mental health experts at the National Committee for Mental Hygiene (NCMH), which was the flagship organization of the mental hygiene movement, hoped to use their institutional clout to create programs that would not only treat, but also prevent delinquency. In 1922, NCMH director Thomas Salmon teamed up with the Commonwealth Fund, a philanthropic organization that was hoping to start a child welfare initiative, to find a Program for the Prevention of Delinquency. In an effort to approach juvenile delinquency from as many angles as possible, the program placed social workers in schools to identify children in need of help, created a Bureau of Children's Guidance in New York City to train psychiatric social workers, offered psychiatric consultation to juvenile courts, and used public outreach to raise awareness of the importance of good mental hygiene. As part of the program, the Fund and the NCMH set up demonstration clinics to treat delinquent children based on a new model that had emerged a decade earlier at William Healy's Chicago Juvenile Psychopathic Institute. When the Commonwealth Fund and NCMH began to set up similar clinics in seven new cities starting in 1922, only one other clinic, the Judge Baker in Boston, existed. By 1942, the Fund had helped set up 60 child guidance clinics across the country (27).

CHILD GUIDANCE AND RESIDENTIAL TREATMENT

Initially child guidance clinics were intended to treat delinquent, typically working class children, who were referred there from juvenile courts. Almost immediately, however, clinic professionals began to identify a new population of patients: "predelinquent" children. These typically middle class "troublesome" or "problem" children had minor emotional and behavioral problems ranging from enuresis to temper tantrums and truancy. Most importantly, they had a better prognosis than delinquent children, many of whom came from poverty and tended to be repeat offenders. In order to treat them, teams of psychiatrists, psychologists, and social workers worked with child and parents to understand the origin of the problematic emotions or behavior, often tracing it to the child's relationships with his parents, especially his mother. Often, a child's problems were gendered in tone—a teenage girl might be brought to a clinic because of her sexual activity, for example. At the clinic, each team member played a different role. The psychiatrist interviewed the child, while the psychologist conducted a battery of tests and the social worker spoke to the parent(s). These roles were rigid and by no means equal; the psychiatrist was typically male and led the team, while the social worker, usually a woman, played a subservient role. Despite their appeal to a middle-class population struggling with the birth of a new peer culture amongst children and adolescents, child guidance clinics had many limitations. Most significantly, children with serious or intractable conditions like epilepsy, intellectual disability, or schizophrenia were not welcome (28).

The efforts of mental hygiene experts, including child guidance professionals, to identify and treat a vast, previously unidentified population of "troublesome" children had many consequences, both expected and unexpected. With increased preventive work and efforts to identify and work with "problem children," experts identified a large number of children requiring help. One psychiatrist observed in 1935 that "With the excellent work accomplished by [child guidance], or rather in spite of it, there is a steadily increasing number of children under 15 years of age requiring ... treatment" (29). This phenomenon, he explained, might also be due to a gross increase in the number of children with problems. However, it seems likely that the active work of the NCMH and other mental hygiene organizations to promote mental health and identify at-risk children in schools contributed to the perception of this increase.

Throughout the 1930s, 1940s, and 1950s, mental health professionals struggled to find a place for children who did not fit the mold of any existing community resources. These children had been rejected by their families, their schools, and their communities for being unruly, unmanageable, and incomprehensible. Before the mid-twentieth century, many of them would have been sent to custodial institutions after failed attempts to help them at home, at school, and in the community. In their midst arose residential treatment centers (RTCs), a heterogeneous group of institutions often transformed from punitive training school, orphanages, and other custodial institutions to meet the need of a new population of seriously troubled children now defined as "emotionally disturbed." Some RTCs were affiliated with universities, some with private philanthropic institutions, and others with state mental health systems. Despite their differences, all RTCs shared the mission of caring for this population of deeply troubled, rejected children. They also shared a commitment to the concept of the therapeutic milieu, an idea first introduced in postwar England among troubled war veterans. Professionals who adopted the therapeutic milieu approach fundamentally believed that every aspect of a child's stay, from meals to games, bedtime routines, and interactions with staff members, had the potential to be therapeutic (30).

RTCs also generally shared a commitment to a psychodynamic, or modified psychoanalytic, context (31). Psychoanalysis, based in large part upon Freudian concepts, had become central to American psychiatry in the first two decades of the twentieth century (32,33). In the late 1920s, Anna Freud in Vienna and Melanie Klein in London, among others, had begun to write about and practice psychoanalysis on young children (34). During World War II in Britain, the evacuation of children to the countryside and the involvement of many mothers and fathers in military work meant that parents and children were often separated. This phenomenon provided fertile ground for psychoanalysts studying the effects of separation and war on anxiety, personality development, and behaviors like bedwetting and delinquency (35). In the United States, the application of psychoanalytic concepts to children would influence not only child guidance, but residential treatment as well. Whereas professionals in both arenas employed analysis as a means of understanding children, in many ways residential treatment embodied the practical application of psychoanalytic tools for daily interaction beyond the therapy hour.

INSTITUTIONALIZING A NEW PROFESSION

In the 1920s, psychiatrists who wanted to work with children could have participated in training programs associated with child guidance clinics, funded by the mental hygiene-oriented Commonwealth Fund and the Rockefeller Foundation. By 1940, the two organizations were funding training programs for 138 young psychiatrists. In addition to their work in child guidance clinics, many trainees also spent time training in pediatrics, neurology, and in psychoanalysis, which had become a standard part of any psychiatrist's training. Psychiatrists played an important role during World War II, helping to eliminate draftees whom they felt were "unfit" for service. As a result, the profession grew in size and prominence. After the war, the 1946 National Mental Health Act provided new federal training grants for psychiatrists, contributing to significant growth of the profession. Child psychiatrists were among those affected, and child guidance clinics continued to grow in number and size (36).

At the same time, child psychiatrists were building institutions to more formally organize their profession. This began in 1924 with the founding of the American Orthopsychiatric Association, an interdisciplinary group of child psychiatrists, psychologists, and social workers. During annual meetings of the group, clinic directors began to meet informally, gradually including more and more clinic staff. In 1945, this offshoot formally named itself the American Association of Psychiatric Clinics for Children and in 1947, established formal guidelines for child guidance clinics providing training in child psychiatry (37). In 1953, the American Academy of Child Psychiatry was founded, and in 1957 the American Board of Psychiatry and Neurology recognized child psychiatry as a subspecialty and established training standards for all new child psychiatrists (38). Although these events formally announced child psychiatry as its own subspecialty, in many ways they were merely capstones for a new style of practice that had been developing over the previous 30 years.

A MENTAL HEALTH "CRISIS"

Only 12 years after child psychiatry was recognized as a subspecialty, mental health policymakers announced that there was a crisis in child mental health. In the 1969 report of the Joint Commission on Mental Health of Children, *Crisis in Child Mental Health,* the authors estimated that there were 1.4 million American children in need of mental health care, more than two thirds of whom were not receiving any treatment (39). In part, the perception of a crisis was based on the discovery of the Warren Commission that Lee Harvey Oswald, President John F. Kennedy's assassin, had been an "emotionally disturbed" child who had failed to receive adequate treatment (40). How many other Oswalds might exist among America's children, who might pose harm to themselves or others if they did not receive the treatment they desperately needed? The "crisis" in child mental health, experts believed, was primarily due to a large number of troubled children who were racial minorities from socioeconomically disadvantaged backgrounds. In part, this concept—and the sudden recognition that there were now millions of untreated mentally ill children in the United States—was driven by the theory that these children were raised in a "culture of poverty" characterized by pathologic families who deprived their children of the sensory and cultural stimuli required for normal development (41). It was no wonder, culture of poverty proponents argued, that these children became mentally ill.

Crisis or not, the identification of a large population of troubled children was problematic for a system largely unequipped to handle them. RTCs, child guidance centers, and child psychiatry units in hospitals were simply too few and too small to treat thousands of primarily poor, minority children. Furthermore, funding for existing infrastructure was declining rapidly as psychiatric institutions fell out of favor. One tragic result was the ascendance of the juvenile justice system as the primary caretaker for many mentally ill children, especially those from minority or low income backgrounds (42). Another was a greater reliance on shorter hospital stays and on using medications to treat childhood mental illness.

A BIOLOGIC APPROACH

Psychopharmaceuticals were latecomers to child psychiatry. The first modern psychopharmaceuticals were introduced into adult psychiatry in the 1950s. Yet few psychiatrists were employing medications for children until the 1980s, perhaps because treatment models remained focused on family dynamics and in many cases, retained an analytic grounding. By the 1990s, medications had become a routine part of child psychiatric practice (43). It was during this same time that both adult and child psychiatrists devoted new efforts to understanding the biologic basis of mental illness, looking for its basis in genetic inheritance and documenting its fundamental alteration of neurologic function (44). Starting in the 1980s, efforts to trace the heritability of childhood mental illness were particularly prominent in the field of autism research (45). In the 1990s, efforts to use advanced brain imaging to better understand psychiatric disorders in adults became a topic of interest in child psychiatry as researchers looked to imaging as one tool that might help them better understand both normal and abnormal development. These efforts, although novel, did not preclude study of the multiple, interrelated etiologies of childhood mental illness. In fact, the biopsychosocial model, introduced in the 1950s to emphasize the biologic aspect of mental illness and reintroduced in the 1970s to emphasize the psychosocial aspect of medical illness, remains a dominant concept in child psychiatry (46).

Modern child psychiatry is a flourishing subspecialty comprised of physicians who work in interdisciplinary teams to serve children with complex psychosocial needs. Yet its biggest challenge remains providing necessary care to all the children who need it. As a June 2003 policy statement by the American Academy of Child and Adolescent Psychiatry (47) explained, "Despite the dramatic advances in scientific knowledge regarding childhood mental illnesses and their treatment over the past 20 years, only a small fraction of children suffering from mental illnesses receive treatment." The inability to provide mental health services to children who need them most is a function of multiple factors, including a shortage of child psychiatrists, lack of insurance parity, and reduced public funds available to children without the means to otherwise obtain treatment. Despite these challenges, promising changes like mental health parity provisions in the Affordable Care Act and programs which encourage medical students to consider careers in child psychiatry, as well as novel therapies for childhood mental illness, ensure that the history of child psychiatry will continue to be a rich one characterized by service to some of society's most vulnerable citizens.

References

1. Kanner L: Introduction: Trends in child psychiatry. In: Howells JG (ed): *Modern Perspectives in International Child Psychiatry.* New York, Brunner/Mazel Publishers, 1971.
2. Kanner L: Child psychiatry: retrospect and prospect. *Am J Psychiatry* 117:15–22, 1960.
3. Brandon S: The early history of psychiatric care of children. In: Cule J, Turner T (eds): *Child Care Through the Centuries.* Cardiff, STS Publishing, 1986.
4. Walk A: The pre-history of child psychiatry. *Br J Psychiatry* 110:756, 1964.
5. Parry-Jones WL: Annotation: the history of child and adolescent psychiatry: its present day relevance. *J Child Psychol Psychiatry* 30(1):3–11, 1989.
6. Maudsley H: *The Pathology of Mind: A Study of its Distempers, Deformities and Disorder.* London, Macmillan, 1867.
7. Maudsley H, quoted in Kanner: Introduction: Trends in child psychiatry. 2–3.
8. Tyor PL, Bell LV: *Caring for the Retarded in America: A History.* Westport, Conn., Greenwood Press, 1984.
9. Trent JW: *Inventing the Feeble Mind: A History of Mental Retardation in the United States.* Berkeley, University of California Press, 1994.
10. Sokal MM: *Psychological Testing and American Society, 1890–1930.* New Brunswick, Rutgers University Press, 1990.
11. Zenderland L: *Measuring Minds: Henry Herbert Goddard and the Origins of American Intelligence Testing.* New York, Cambridge University Press, 3, 1997.
12. Kett JF: *Rites of Passage: Adolescence in America, 1790 to the Present.* New York, Basic Books, 1977.
13. Grant J: *Raising Baby by the Book: The Education of American Mothers.* New Haven, CT, Yale University Press, 1998.
14. Apple RD: *Perfect Motherhood: Science and Childrearing in America.* New Brunswick, NJ, Rutgers University Press, 2006.
15. Halpern SA: *American Pediatrics: The Social Dynamics of Professionalism, 1880–1980.* Berkeley, University of California Press, 1988.
16. White House Conference on Child Health and Protection Committee on Medical Care for Children: *Psychology and Psychiatry in Pediatrics: the Problem; Report of the Subcommittee on Psychology and Psychiatry.* New York, The Century Co., 1932.
17. Kanner L: Child psychiatry: Retrospect and prospect. *Am J Psychiatry.* 117:20, 1960.
18. O'Connor S: *Orphan Trains: The Story of Charles Loring Brace and the Children He Saved and Failed.* Boston, MA, Houghton Mifflin Company, 2001.
19. Hacsi TA: *Second Home: Orphan Asylums and Poor Families in America.* Cambridge, Mass, Harvard University Press, 1997.
20. Schneider EC: *In the Web of Class: Delinquents and Reformers in Boston, 1810s-1930s.* New York, New York University Press, 1992.
21. Mennel RM: *Thorns & Thistles; Juvenile Delinquents in the United States, 1825–1940.* Hanover, University Press of New England, 1973.
22. Ashby L: *Saving the Waifs: Reformers and Dependent Children, 1890–1917.* Philadelphia, PA, Temple University Press, 1984.
23. Lindenmeyer K: *A Right to Childhood: The U.S. Children's Bureau and Child Welfare, 1912–46.* Urbana, University of Illinois Press, 1997.
24. Lamb SD: *Pathologist of the Mind: Adolf Meyer and the Origins of American Psychiatry.* Baltimore, MD, Johns Hopkins University Press, 2014.
25. Richardson TR: *The Century of the Child: The Mental Hygiene Movement and Social Policy in the United States and Canada.* State University of New York Press, 1989.
26. Schlossman SL: *Love and the American Delinquent: The Theory and Practice of "Progressive" Juvenile Justice, 1825–1920.* Chicago, University of Chicago Press, 1977.
27. Horn M: *Before It's Too Late: The Child Guidance Movement in the United States, 1922–1945.* Philadelphia, PA, Temple University Press, 1989.
28. Jones KW. *Taming the Troublesome Child: American Families, Child Guidance, and the Limits of Psychiatric Authority.* Cambridge, Mass, Harvard University Press, 1999.
29. O'Donnell LP: Prevision of the development of the new children's unit of Rockland State Hospital. *Psychiatric Quarterly* 9(3):426–435, 1935.
30. Doroshow DB: Residential Treatment and the Invention of the Emotionally Disturbed Child in Twentieth-Century America. *Bull Hist Med* 90(1):92–123, Spring 2016.
31. Horn M: *Before It's Too Late: The Child Guidance Movement in the United States, 1922–1945.* Philadelphia, PA, Temple University Press, 1989.
32. Hale NG: *Freud and the Americans: The Beginnings of Psychoanalysis in the United States, 1876–1917.* New York, Oxford University Press, 1971.
33. Hale NG: *The Rise and Crisis of Psychoanalysis in the United States: Freud and the Americans, 1917–1985.* New York, Oxford University Press, 1995.
34. Makari G: Chapter 11. Freud took a more empirical approach, emphasizing winning the child's trust and focusing on traumatic events in the child's life, whereas Klein argued that even the very young child had unconscious impulses that might be uncovered through play therapy and transference. *Revolution in Mind: The Creation of Psychoanalysis.* New York, HarperCollins, 2008.
35. Shapira M: *The War Inside: Psychoanalysis, Total War, and the Making of the Democratic Self in Postwar Britain.* New York, Cambridge University Press, 2013, Chapter 2.
36. Kirkpatrick ME: Fellowship training in orthopsychiatry. In: Lowrey LG, Sloane V (eds): *Orthopsychiatry, 1923–1948, Retrospect and Prospect.* New York, American Orthopsychiatric Association, 83–99, 1948.
37. American Association of Psychiatric Clinics for Children: *History, Purposes, and Organization of The American Association of Psychiatric Clinics for Children.* New York, American Association of Psychiatric Clinics for Children, 1957.
38. The history of the American academy of child psychiatry. *J Am Acad Child Psychiatry* 1(1):196–202, 1962.
39. Joint Commission on Mental Health of Children: *Crisis in Child Mental Health: Challenge for the 1970's.* Washington, DC, Joint Commission on Mental Health of Children, 1969.
40. United States, *Report of the President's Commission on the Assassination of President John F. Kennedy.* Washington, United States Government Printing Office, 1964.
41. Mical Raz: *What's Wrong with the Poor? Psychiatry, Race, and the War on Poverty.* Chapel Hill, University of North Carolina Press, 2013.
42. See Chapter 7, Doroshow D: *Emotionally Disturbed: Residential Treatment, Child Psychiatry, and the Creation of Normal Children in Mid-Twentieth Century America.* Ph.D. Diss., Yale University, 2012.
43. Bolman WM: Pharmacologic advances in residential treatment. *Resid Treat Child Youth* 13(2): 279–283, 1995.
44. Andreasen NC: *The Broken Brain: The Biological Revolution in Psychiatry.* New York, Harper & Row, 1984.
45. Smalley SL, Asarnow RF, Spence MA: Autism and genetics. A decade of research. *Arch Gen Psychiatry* 45(10):953–961, 1988.
46. Ghaemi SN: The rise and fall of the biopsychosocial model. *Br J Psychiatry* 195(1):3–4, 2009.
47. American Academy of Child and Adolescent Psychiatry: *Parity and Access for Child and Adolescent Mental Health Care.* 2003, available at http://www.aacap.org/aacap/policy_statements/2003/Parity_and_Access_for_Child_and_Adolescent_Mental_Health_Care.aspx.

CHAPTER 1.4 ■ EDUCATION AND TRAINING

DOROTHY E. STUBBE AND EUGENE V. BERESIN

Education is the most powerful weapon that you can use to change the world.

—Nelson Mandela

BACKGROUND AND CONTEXT

There is a national shortage of child and adolescent psychiatrists to care for the nation's youth with serious mental health needs and their families (1–5). Epidemiologic studies suggest that up to 9% to 13% of U.S. children and adolescents, ages 9 to 17, meet the definition of "serious emotional disturbance," with 5% to 9% suffering from "extreme functional impairment" (6–8). For adolescents, the estimates are even higher. The National Comorbidity Study of Adolescents reported 22% of adolescents aged 13 to 18 experienced severe impairments from emotional disorders (9). The approximately 8,500 practicing child and adolescent psychiatrists in the United States are considerably fewer than the estimated 20,000 needed to provide the psychiatric care of seriously psychiatrically ill children and youth within a multidisciplinary system of care (5). Child and adolescent psychiatry researchers are similarly insufficient to meet the need to advance our understanding of the etiology and treatment of these disorders (10–12).

Recruiting, training, and mentoring the next generation of child and adolescent psychiatrists is one of the major challenges, as well as one of the prime opportunities, of the field. Graduates face a plethora of career opportunities in clinical practice, academics, and research. Lifestyle and improving remuneration also draw medical graduates to the field (13). Yet there are many challenges facing training programs and obstacles to recruitment. Enhanced training requirements, a paucity of funding for graduate medical education (GME) of subspecialties, and depleted faculty time to provide the required mentorship and teaching are ongoing challenges. The vigor, rejuvenation, and satisfaction of training the next generation of superior physician clinicians and scientists are the enduring rewards (14).

CHILD AND ADOLESCENT PSYCHIATRY RESIDENCY TRAINING IN THE UNITED STATES

Historical Note

Child psychiatry in the United States began with the establishment of the child guidance clinics, the first of which was the Juvenile Psychopathic Institute in Chicago, established by Dr. William Healy in 1909. As child guidance clinics grew in number and in size, it became clear that psychiatrists who worked with children required training that was more extensive and specific than that obtained in their general psychiatry residency. The Commonwealth Fund sponsored a major conference in 1944 which resulted in a standard set of skill areas that should be mastered by psychiatrists who treat children and their families. These skill areas included growth and development, psychodynamics, working with parents, administration, and community organizations (15).

In 1946, World War II was over and there was a renewed vigor to provide for the children of the new baby boom. The Mental Health Act of 1946 provided funding for the training of child psychiatrists. Additionally, the American Association of Psychiatric Clinics for Children (AAPCC) was formed. The AAPCC training committee provided an approval process for potential training sites, including an application and survey. About half of the child guidance clinics were approved as training sites in this manner.

The American Academy of Child Psychiatry (AACP), founded in 1953, was initially a by-invitation-only organization. The AACP was committed to ensuring training accreditation within the medical specialty, not only through child guidance clinics. After a debate of whether child psychiatry was more appropriately a pediatric or psychiatric subspecialty, the choice was made for psychiatry. The American Board of Medical Specialties (ABMS) approved the subspecialty in 1959 (16), and a total of 11 child psychiatry fellowship programs were accredited. The field has grown. As of 2016, there were 126 accredited child and adolescent psychiatry fellowship programs in the United States, and 827 filled fellowship positions in child and adolescent psychiatry (17).

Inextricably linked to subspecialty certification are standardized training criteria formulated through the Accreditation Council for Graduate Medical Education (ACGME). The ACGME Residency Review Committee (RRC) in Psychiatry oversees periodic surveys and determines the accreditation status of each training program. This approach was much more medically oriented than the earlier AAPCC reviews. The ACGME demanded that child psychiatry training programs be linked to accredited general psychiatry residency programs and to medical centers approved by the Joint Commission on the Accreditation of Hospitals. These requirements forced the child guidance clinics interested in training to abscond from their exclusive community roots and to become attached to medical schools. It also stimulated the development of new child psychiatry training programs that were situated in medical centers, rather than freestanding in the community.

In 1969, AACP opened its doors to all child psychiatrists who graduated from, or who were in training in, ACGME-approved programs. With the expansion of the specialty to capture the treatment of adolescents into its purview in 1989, AACP changed its name to the American Academy of Child and Adolescent Psychiatry (AACAP). The American Association of Directors of Psychiatric Residency Training (AADPRT) and the Association for Academic Psychiatry (AAP) are more recently formed organizations specifically devoted to education and training (15).

As with all of medicine, training and education is both an art and a science. A good program director (PD) serves as the conductor for the symphony—transmitting a serious and passionate commitment to the highest standards of comprehensive care for children, adolescents, and families; a dedication to residents and their personal and professional growth and excellence as physicians; and a vision of the field—where it is now and where it needs to go. In each institution, the instrumentation and symphonic music will vary, but the basic principles apply. Excellence in training requires coordinated and well-constructed training experiences that adhere to all training requirements, within multiple systems (medical school, hospital, clinics), synchronized with the goals and structure of the broader administration (Dean, hospital administration, Chair of Department of Psychiatry, Child and Adolescent Psychiatry Division Head or Chair, Program Directors of Residency Training, and Designated Institutional Official) and harmonized with the resources and needs of the Division and Department.

Recruitment, Portals of Entry, and Training Program Types (Traditional and Novel)

Recruitment and Workforce Issues

A survey by Beresin and Borus of accredited child and adolescent psychiatry fellowships identified a shortage of recruits for residency and faculty positions in child and adolescent psychiatry in the late 1980s (18). This shortage has continued (5). Lack of exposure to child and adolescent psychiatry during medical school education, increasing levels of educational debt burden, long years of residency training, and relatively smaller income potential in the field of psychiatry, as well as in child and adolescent psychiatry, are factors that may influence a medical student's career decision (19,20). Other obstacles to recruitment include inadequate support in academic institutions, decreasing GME funding, and decreasing clinical revenues in the managed care environment (21).

In spite of the shortages, child and adolescent psychiatry has made impressive progress in its scientific knowledge base through research, especially in neuroscience, developmental science, and genetics (22). Additionally, there is a growing recognition of the need for child and adolescent psychiatry by policymakers and the public at large. The Surgeon General's Conference on Children's Mental Health in 2000 (3), and the President's New Freedom Commission on Mental Health in 2003 (4), have both acknowledged the shortage as a national crisis. There is increasing media coverage on mental health problems of children and adolescents, as the public becomes more aware and concerned about these vital issues facing our youth. The public has become increasingly interested in issues of mental health and effective interventions, as the aftermaths of such disasters as Hurricane Katrina in the Gulf Coast in August 2005 and the shootings at the Sandy Hook Elementary School in December of 2012 have left not only physical, but also mental health scars on the population.

Recruitment efforts in child and adolescent psychiatry focus on three salient areas: (1) ensuring that talented, interested physicians have positive exposure and engagement early in medical training to the field of child and adolescent psychiatry; (2) providing training opportunities that are appealing and ensure ongoing engagement of the psychiatry resident and child and adolescent psychiatry fellow in work with children and families; and (3) the positive aspects of lifestyle, remuneration, and the plethora of job opportunities for individuals seeking a career in the field.

Traditional and Innovative Child and Adolescent Psychiatry Training Models

There has been an ongoing debate about the most effective, efficient, and appealing methods to train competent child and adolescent psychiatrists. There were early proposals that child and adolescent psychiatry should split from general psychiatry, as did pediatrics from internal medicine. There have been numerous other proposals, as well. The primary impetus for new and more innovative training portals are twofold: (1) a philosophy of training that endorses innovative training tracks to more fully ensure quality education of competent graduates by optimizing training methods; and (2) enhancing recruitment into the field by providing a variety of attractive and novel training portals. Figure 1.4.1 summarizes the current training pathways for child and adolescent psychiatry training.

Existing Portals

Traditional Child and Adolescent Psychiatry Training. Training in child and adolescent psychiatry generally occurs after medical school; after a first post graduate (PG-1) year that includes at least 4 months of general medicine or pediatrics and 2 months of neurology; and following the completion of at least 2 years of general psychiatry training. However, child and adolescent psychiatry training may commence any time after the PG-1 year. Training in child and adolescent psychiatry is for 2 years, and the first year of training may count for the last (PG-4) year of general psychiatry training. Thus, traditional training in child and adolescent psychiatry may be completed in either 5 years (referred to as "fast-tracking" when CAP

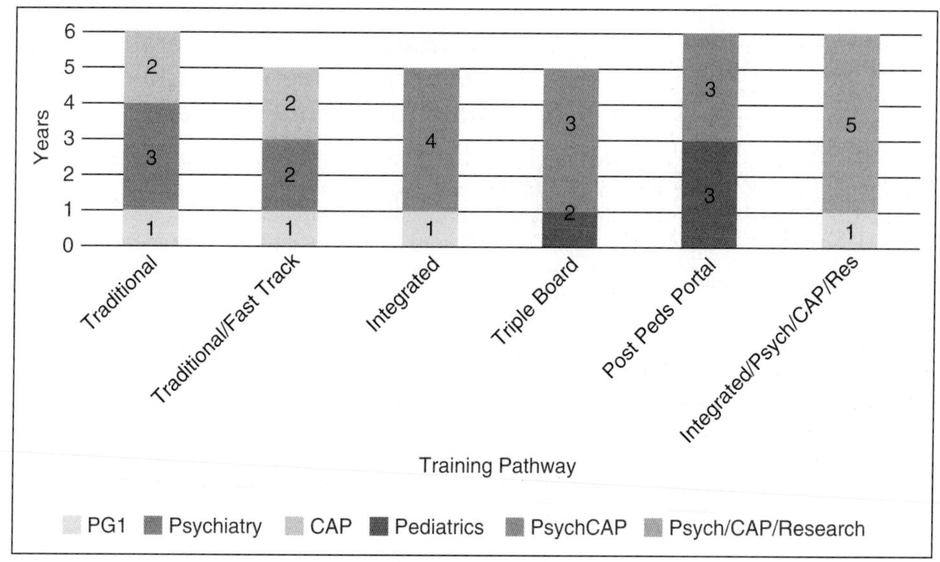

FIGURE 1.4.1. Training pathways in child and adolescent psychiatry.

training begins in the PG-4 year) or 6 years (when CAP training begins in the PG-5 year following completion of the full 4 years of psychiatry residency). A majority of residents enter in the PG-4 year. These residents are eager to work with children and families more intensively, and they may experience pressures to finish training: to address family, finances, and career development issues, and for some, to plan ahead toward further training, such as forensics, addictions, or research fellowships. Other residents prefer to complete the full 4 years of general psychiatry training prior to starting child and adolescent psychiatry residency to take advantage of the opportunity for elective experiences, chief residency, and/or to consolidate skills in their work with adults (14).

Integrated Training

Triple Board. An innovative 5-year training sequence in pediatrics, general psychiatry, and child and adolescent psychiatry, better known as the "Triple Board," began as a pilot training experiment in 1985 and was approved nationwide as a combined residency in 1992 (23). The "Triple Board" concept was to create an alternative pathway of training to become a child and adolescent psychiatrist that would combine pediatric, general psychiatry, and child and adolescent psychiatry training and would allow a path shorter than would be required in the conventional (additive) training sequence of 7 or 8 years. One of the goals of the combined training program was to create a nucleus of academically based child and adolescent psychiatrists who were trained and socialized as pediatricians, thus serving to bridge a gap between the pediatric and the child and adolescent psychiatry communities. Additionally, it was hoped that this core of "Triple Boarders" could serve as a magnet in the academic environment to attract medical students to the specialty field of child and adolescent psychiatry. This track is sponsored by the American Board of Psychiatry and Neurology (ABPN), the ABPN Committee on Certification in Child and Adolescent Psychiatry, and the American Board of Pediatrics (16). Follow-up suggests that this training track has trained competent and successful clinicians and scientists, most of whom practice predominantly child and adolescent psychiatry, although often in a setting with medically compromised children (24). The rotations and integration of the three specialties varies from program to program, but all programs provide 24 months of pediatrics and 18 months each of general and child and adolescent psychiatry. Upon completion of training, residents may sit for Board examinations in all three disciplines. There are presently 10 approved Triple Board training programs.

Post Pediatric Portal Program. A newly initiated training model utilizes the Triple Board model for training physicians who have completed a core 3-year ACGME-accredited pediatric residency. The Post Pediatric Portal Program (PPPP) is a 3-year combined training program in general psychiatry and child and adolescent psychiatry which is formally approved and overseen by the ABPN. Graduates are Board eligible in both general and child and adolescent psychiatry. The PPPP allows newly graduated pediatricians or pediatricians who have been in practice for a number of years and wish to retool in child and adolescent psychiatry to do so in 3 years, rather than the usual 4. Currently, there are four PPPP training programs (25).

Other Integrated Training Tracks. Integrated training specifies a residency that combines training in two or more disciplines in a contiguous, rather than consecutive, training model. This approach, initially developed and implemented in the 1970s at the University of Pittsburgh by Peter Henderson, M.D., combined child and general psychiatry training from the onset of training. Since that time, a few more institutions have adopted similar models of integrated training. Other programs have the flexibility to initiate a variety of child and adolescent psychiatry clinical experiences within the general psychiatry residency for individuals with a declared interest. Although programs vary in the specific manner in which they configure training requirements, all share in common the principle of exposing residents early and continuously to children and childhood pathology (15).

Training programs with an integrated track meet all existing program requirements for residency education in both general psychiatry and child and adolescent psychiatry. Programs with integration seek to allow knowledge, skills, and attitude building in a developmental context of patient care, and to solidify the trainee's identity as a child psychiatrist early on. Most integrated training occurs within the context of a 5-year clinical training program.

Academic Integrated Training Tracks. In the United States, there is a dearth of academic child and adolescent psychiatrists to propagate the research base on the etiologies and effective treatments of childhood psychiatric disorders (3,10). Integrated training in general psychiatry, child and adolescent psychiatry, and research allows medical students to move directly into an integrated child–adult psychiatric residency and research training program that is constructed to do justice to the basic developmental sciences and efficacious interventions while not neglecting the fundamentals of psychiatry. The major goal of this alternative training route is to provide a national model to increase the number and quality of child and adolescent psychiatrists in research careers.

In response to the Institute of Medicine's report on the shortage of psychiatrist researchers, the National Institute of Mental Health established the National Psychiatry Training Council (NPTC) (26). With the support of the NPTC, of which he was co-chair, Dr. James Leckman and others proposed 6-year integrated child and adolescent psychiatry academic track (10) that has become a reality at the Yale Child Study Center, the University of Colorado, and the University of Vermont and is being considered in other institutions. This program highlights three basic principles: (1) early identity formation as a child and adolescent psychiatric researcher; (2) the developmental continuity of training; and (3) individualization of training and "tooling" opportunities to prepare the trainee for a research career. The program has an internship year that includes pediatric medicine, followed by a cohesive curriculum that includes identification of a research team and mentor(s), and integration of full general psychiatry and child and adolescent psychiatry clinical training with research training over the subsequent 5 years (27).

The Transition from General Psychiatry Residency to Child and Adolescent Psychiatry

By the time a resident enters child and adolescent fellowship training he/she has had at least three initiations into new territory: medical school, internship, and general psychiatry residency. The entry into child and adolescent residency training is yet another "beginning," with the attendant narcissistic challenge of starting over and having to master new skills, having just achieved competence and confidence with adults. The loss of working with adults threatens losing skills acquired over 3 to 4 years.

Child and adolescent fellows working clinically with children use nonverbal skills, deal with primitive defenses, and manage behavior in individuals who are far less able to use advanced cognitive skills and concepts than the adults with whom they previously were quite comfortable. They also have to manage new and complex countertransference problems, such as the wish to "adopt" their patients, undo the actions of "incompetent" parents, and the susceptibility to overidentify with their child patients. They are mandated reporters, and must "turn in" parents to authorities. And they now must serve as authorities for schools, courts, and social service agencies in making decisions that have a profound effect on the child and family, including decisions about custody, placement, and incarceration—all at a time when they have relatively limited knowledge and skill in the field. They must shoulder the responsibility of working with dying children and grieving parents. At a less intense level, they have to answer complex developmental and behavioral questions from parents, pediatricians, and allied professionals when they are themselves novices. The new fellows have to face all this in the context of increased time demands for calls, emails, documentation, and meetings. They need to help deeply troubled children and families at a time when there are limited resources for outpatient and inpatient care, and far too few clinicians in all child-related healthcare disciplines to take on referrals for the comprehensive care of the children and families they serve. Child and adolescent psychiatry is more demanding than general psychiatry, in that fellows need to embrace a developmental model that requires greater integration of the many factors that impact child development, such as genetics, family, culture, educational systems, and social forces. Additionally, child psychiatry training occurs at a time when many fellows are attempting to, or have established, new love relationships and families, and struggle to find precious time to spend with them.

Training programs need to appreciate the difficulty of the transition, and promote means for fellows to cope with these stresses. The effective collaboration between the fellowship program coordinator and the PD is crucial to this task. At the admissions level, screening for the most mature, adaptive, and resilient candidates is helpful. Trying to assemble a fellowship class that is cohesive and supportive is also useful. The program should provide time for residents to meet with faculty and discuss the issues and problems involved in the transition. Alerting the faculty to these transition issues is vital, so they may be addressed in individual supervision. Finding many opportunities to have fellows observe faculty treating children and families and serving as consultants provides the means for them to learn skills and have working role models for identification. It may be valuable for some fellows to continue treating adult patients, either in the program or through moonlighting, to help preserve previously acquired skills.

Milestones: Competency-Based Assessment in Child and Adolescent Psychiatry Training

The Core Competencies

The training of competent physicians is the goal of all residency training. In 1999, the ACGME (27) identified six core domains in which each resident is required to obtain competence (Patient Care; Medical Knowledge; Systems-Based Practice; Practice-Based Learning and Improvement; Professionalism; and Interpersonal and Communication Skills). Training programs must define the specific knowledge, skills, and attitudes required for competence in each of the six Core Competencies, and provide educational experiences as needed in order for residents to demonstrate competence (28–30).

The Next Accreditation System: Milestones

The Next Accreditation System (NAS) is a process initiated in 2009 by which the ACGME restructured its accreditation system to be based on educational outcomes (Milestones) of the six Core Competencies for all medical specialties. "The aims of the NAS are threefold: to enhance the ability of the peer-review system to prepare physicians for practice in the 21st century, to accelerate the ACGME's movement toward accreditation on the basis of educational outcomes, and to reduce the burden associated with the current structure and process-based approach" (31) (p. 1051). A key element of the NAS is the measurement and reporting of outcomes through the educational milestones: developmentally based, specialty-specific achievements that residents are expected to demonstrate at established intervals as they progress through training. In each specialty, the Milestones for each of the Core Competencies have been formulated through a collaboration of the ABMS certifying boards (the ABPN for psychiatry and its subspecialties), the RRC, medical specialty organizations, PD associations (for psychiatry, the American Association of Directors of Psychiatry Residency Training [AADPRT]), and trainees.

The NAS initiated a progressive rollout of Milestones and NAS indicators of program quality to GME programs in 2013. In July of 2014, general psychiatry programs began to implement psychiatry-specific Milestone monitoring, and in July of 2015, child and adolescent psychiatry training programs began to implement the Milestone performance data for each program's fellows to determine whether fellows overall are progressing. The ACGME Milestones provide five levels of competence, with specific behavioral skill anchors tied to each level. Tracking from level 1 to level 5 is synonymous with moving from novice to expert in the specialty. Level 4 is designed as the graduation target, although graduation has not been specifically linked to Milestone metrics. Level 5 serves as an "aspirational" goal for which it is expected that only a few exceptional fellows will reach prior to graduation (32,33). Upon completion of fellowship training, the PD must verify that the fellow has demonstrated sufficient competence to enter practice without direct supervision (34). Milestone metrics for each trainee are assessed by the program's Clinical Competency Committee (CCC) and entered semi-annually into the ACGME Accreditation Data System (ADS)—they are not currently being utilized for program accreditation purposes. Table 1.4.1 summarizes Competencies and associated Milestones.

The Next Accreditation System: Clinical Learning Environment Review

Another component of NAS is the Clinical Learning Environment Review (CLER). This is a periodic site visit of ACGME-accredited institutions by national field representatives. The CLER review provides feedback to the core training institution on the residency learning environment that addresses the following 6 areas: patient safety, healthcare quality, care transitions, supervision, duty hours and fatigue management and mitigation, and professionalism (35). The feedback provided by the CLER program is designed to encourage clinical sites to improve engagement of resident and fellow physicians in learning to provide safe, high-quality patient care. The CLER program is separate from the accreditation process.

The Next Accreditation System: Program and Institutional Accreditation

Training in all of the medical specialties is well regulated for quality, to ensure that the training program is providing the full scope of experiences, didactics, and supervision in a suitable environment. The ACGME is responsible for setting training requirements for all specialties and subspecialties approved by the ABMS.

The General or Institutional Requirements are the same regardless of the specialty being reviewed. They are concerned less with the particular training area than with the

TABLE 1.4.1

CORE COMPETENCIES AND MILESTONES IN CHILD AND ADOLESCENT PSYCHIATRY (CAP) FELLOWSHIP TRAINING

Competency	Definition	CAP Milestones
Patient Care	Compassionate, appropriate, and effective treatment of patients, which serves to promote health and recovery	PC1: Psychiatric Evaluation PC2: Formulation and Differential Diagnosis PC3: Treatment Planning and Management PC4: Psychotherapy PC5: Somatic Therapies
Medical Knowledge	Established and evolving biomedical, clinical, and cognate sciences, as well as the application of this knowledge to patient care	MK1: Development MK2: Psychopathology and Wellness MK3: Clinical Neuroscience and Genetics MK4: Psychotherapy MK5: Somatic Therapies MK6: Practice of Psychiatry
Systems-Based Practice	Actions that demonstrate an awareness of and responsiveness to the larger context and system of health care, as well as the ability to call effectively on other resources in the system to provide optimal health care for patients	SBP1: Patient Safety and the Health Care Team SBP2: Resource Management SBP3: Community-based Care SBP4: Consultation to and Integration with Nonpsychiatric Providers
Practice-Based Learning and Improvement	Investigation and evaluation of care for patients, the appraisal and assimilation of scientific evidence, and accessing of the evidence base for treatments to improve patient care	PBLI1: Development and Execution of Lifelong Learning PBLI2: Teaching
Professionalism	Commitment to carrying out professional responsibilities, adherence to ethical principles, and sensitivity to patients of diverse backgrounds	PROF1: Compassion, Respect, Adherence to Ethical Principles PROF2: Accountability to Self, Patients, Colleagues, Profession
Interpersonal and Communication Skills	Effective exchange of information and collaboration with patients, their families, and other allied health professionals	ICS1: Relationship Development and Conflict Management ICS2: Information Sharing and Record Keeping

overall support and surveillance provided by the medical center in which the training program is embedded. These issues include requirements for the selection of trainees and assurance that there are procedures for evaluation, feedback, grievance reporting, duty hours, and due process. There also must be adequate compensation, an emphasis on education rather than on service, and acculturation help for those trainees who need it (34).

The Special Requirements are the essential training components that are specific to a particular specialty or subspecialty. They are revised every 5 to 10 years, although discrete changes or "minor revisions" may be made between revisions. The revisions of the Special Requirements and the evaluation of the ACGME surveys are the responsibility of the RRC for each specialty. RRC members for psychiatry are nominated by three organizations: the American Medical Association (AMA), the ABPN, and the American Psychiatric Association (APA).

In the NAS, program accreditation has changed from "an episodic 'biopsy' model" (in which compliance is assessed every 5 years for programs in good standing) to annual data collection (31). The Psychiatry RRC performs an annual evaluation of trends in key performance measurements for each accredited training program. In addition to the Milestones, other data elements for annual surveillance include the ACGME resident and faculty surveys and annual program information that is entered by the PD into the ACGME ADS. Programs conduct a self-study before the accreditation site visit, which is scheduled for every 10 years unless the annual metrics suggest concerns that require assessment by a more immediate on-site review. Programs are informed annually about accreditation status, any citations or areas for improvement (AFI) for noncompliance with training requirements. Accreditation with warning or probationary status may be conferred to programs with serious lapses in the required training components, or accreditation may be withdrawn for egregious violations.

Evaluation: Formative and Summative Assessments

Professional competence includes multiple skill dimensions that must be integrated in the care of patients. Epstein and Hundert (36) have defined this as "the habitual and judicious use of communication, knowledge, technical skills, clinical reasoning, emotions, values, and reflection in daily practice for the benefit of the individual and the community being served" (p. 226). They conceptualize competence as more than simply a demonstration of specific knowledge, skills and attitudes, but rather as the integration of ways of thinking, feeling and behaving that are synthetic, ongoing, context dependent, mindful, and in continuous development.

It is useful to conceptualize competency evaluation as formative or summative. Formative assessment, performed as a trainee learning tool, is optimally done early and often so that areas of strength or deficiency may be identified. This allows an ongoing means for constructive change, and serves as a tool to evaluate effectiveness of targeted learning interventions. Summative assessment evaluates the attainment of skills, usually at the completion of an educational experience such as a rotation, didactic seminar, or at the end of a training year. Summative assessments include annual examinations, such as the Child Psychiatric In-Training Examination (Child PRITE), a multiple-choice exam modeled after the ABPN Board Examination and with nationally normed scores. Another example of a summative examination is the annual clinical skills assessment, typically an assessed oral examination of competence of each trainee in diagnostic interviewing, formulation, and treatment planning. The specialty-specific Milestones are used as one of the tools to ensure fellows are able to practice core professional activities without supervision upon completion of the program (34).

The cornerstone of formative assessment is feedback. Feedback is defined as an information exchange between trainee and faculty describing performance in a particular activity. It is intended to assist in the acquisition of knowledge, skills, and attitudes. If executed properly, feedback should be done once specific goals and objective have been defined. It should be timely, ongoing, face-to-face, based on first-hand data, objective, nonjudgmental, and allow a discussion of the process (37). Far too often in our medical schools and residency training programs, feedback is neglected, and residents receive either subjective superlative reviews (e.g., "great job!") or hear about their daily performance only if something goes wrong.

Clinical Skills Verification (CSV) assessments may be conceptualized as both formative and summative. These exams are patient interviews that assess a fellow's competence on the following skills: (1) physician–patient relationship; (2) conduct of the psychiatric interview; and (3) case presentation. Fellows must pass three CSVs at the competence level of a practicing physician with patients of age least two different age groups (preschool, school-age, or adolescent), and with at least two different Board Certified child and adolescent psychiatrist examiners as one component of eligibility to sit for the child and adolescent psychiatry Board Certifying Examination. Because these interviews may be embedded in the course of normal clinical care activities, may be completed multiple times, and have nationally approved rating forms with skill anchors, they may serve as an excellent method of providing feedback on important clinical interviewing skills, as well as being used as a summative assessment of eligibility to sit for the ABPN certifying exam.

One of the important consequences of a highly successful evaluation methodology is that it may provide an alternative model to the one used currently in residency training (38). Many of the ACGME requirements for residency training are timed: They require a certain period of time on a service or rotation for successful completion. This allows for a relatively stable and predictable process for training programs, but decreases flexibility for an individual resident. In a purely milestone competency-based training model, if a resident can demonstrate competency at a relatively early stage of training in a given area, more time could be devoted to other, more advanced or elective experiences. This could open up the training process to facilitate specialty training in a wide range of clinical, academic, or research endeavors.

Remediation

The enormous personal investment, as well as institutional and national investment in each physician, provides a crucial impetus to ensure that each resident competently complete training and enters the workforce to care for the large number of underserved children and families in need.

A failure to meet the core competency criteria in knowledge or skills in any of the six competencies can be described as a "deficiency" that must be made up, for example, through access to a missed learning opportunity or repetition of previously offered material (39,40). In contrast, the "remediation" of attitudes is a more difficult definition, which suggests that a change is required in a resident's outlook (41). Health impairments, due to physical, psychiatric, or substance abuse problems, are special challenges to remediation, and have federal and state guidelines that must be followed regarding the impaired physician and the safety of the public.

Remediation of competence is embedded within the overall philosophy of lifelong learning and improvement. At the start of any educational or training endeavor, the novice does not yet possess the knowledge, skills, and attitudes required for competence. Remediation is the act of identifying areas that are not yet performed competently and addressing them. Learners who are not making the progress expected of a resident at their level of training require remediation to ensure that the skill level is consistent with the expertise needed to perform the tasks with competence.

Competency-based training, assessment, and remediation utilize a skills-attainment model rather than an apprentice model of training. Except for the very rare circumstance in which a trainee has such an egregious violation of ethics and practice that termination is required, fellows should receive constructive feedback on strengths and relative weaknesses in their skill set, and be engaged and motivated for self-improvement on an ongoing basis. From this theoretical stance, training and supervision may be conceptualized as ongoing remediation—or remediation may be conceptualized as ongoing improvement of medical practice. Remediation is not discipline. It is only when a resident does not meet required expectations for improvement of practice that the process may move forward into a more disciplinary procedure.

If a trainee displays deficiencies in competence that are severe, pose a danger to the public, or have not been modified by a concerted and comprehensive remediation plan, the mediation process may need to enter into a disciplinary phase. Each institution has a Due Process procedure in place for trainees, and the PD should be familiar with the process and ensure that all fellows are informed of them, as well.

PDs of residency training are charged with the task of ensuring competent graduating physicians. The courts have strongly supported the academic judgment of professional faculty unless evidence of discrimination or other wrongdoing by the faculty exists. The courts view residents as clinician/faculty rather than students as far as disciplinary actions are concerned. As a matter of public policy, the courts support disciplinary actions, including dismissal of a resident physician, in the interest of public safety in the course of patient care (36). Component of competency-based assessment and remediation are shown in Table 1.4.2.

Faculty Development in the Age of Competencies

The incorporation of a competency-based curriculum in medical education requires new challenges to the faculty. First, they need to understand the conceptual basis for looking at outcomes in the educational process, assimilate the new language of the competency. Milestones into their lexicon, and embrace the process as not simply additional bureaucratic burdens, but rather a more effective approach to the educational mission. There is no doubt that building ongoing assessment into the daily process of working with trainees will be more time-consuming.

The faculty needs to learn how to provide ongoing objective feedback and begin doing so. This will involve increased direct observation of trainee–patient interactions, as well

TABLE 1.4.2

COMPETENCY-BASED ASSESSMENT AND REMEDIATION: STEPS AND EXAMPLE

1. Clarify educational goals and instructional learning objectives for each rotation
2. Ensure educational outcomes are related to identified objectives that are observable and measurable
3. Identify trainee strengths and areas for improvement in the relevant Core Competencies (examples provided, but the table should be specific to the trainee)
4. Choose the Competency(ies) that requires remediation
5. Formulate a remediation plan that is specific and measurable, with a timeline
6. Consider assigning a Program Mentor that is not a direct supervisor/evaluator, to assist with remediation implementation
7. Agree upon the plan via joint signatures

Trainee: Dr. Smith	**Date: November 15**
Areas of Strength	**Areas for Improvement**
Interpersonal and Communication Skills	
Has demonstrated superior ability to communicate with patients around diagnosis, medication risks, and benefits	Has not demonstrated adequate problem-solving or effective communication in situations in which there are questions about coverage, vacations, or call
Is prepared and actively participates in Inpatient Rounds	Has avoided communicating with colleagues when there are areas of conflict
Calls outpatient treaters and communicates with referral sources	Has utilized ineffective or inappropriate means of communication—e.g., using e-mails and texts to publicly air grievances about a colleague or the program
Patient Care	
Clear commitment to patients and excellent care	Intermittent incomplete sign-outs to colleagues may adversely impact patient care
Professionalism	
High ethical principles for patient care	At times, avoidance of speaking directly with colleagues has negatively impacted professionalism
Patient care comes before self-interest	Has spoken negatively about colleagues in a public venue
Medical Knowledge	
Excellent knowledge base	
Usually very engaged in didactics	Inconsistent participation in didactics
Systems-Based Practice	
Generally collaborates well	Interpersonal conflicts have hindered team collaboration at times
Practice-Based Learning and Improvement	
Keeps up with the literature	Has avoided receiving feedback to improve performance

REMEDIATION PLAN: Competency–Interpersonal and Communication Skills

Dr. Smith (trainee) will collaborate with Program Mentor, Dr. Jones, on the following objectives to meet basic competency criteria prior to March 31. A reevaluation of competence will occur on or before March 31 to review progress and make a plan regarding promotion to second year.

1. **Dr. Smith will demonstrate consistent effective communication with colleagues, faculty, and collaborators around all aspects of residency duties.**
   a. Methods: Dr. Smith will
      i. discuss changes in schedules with appropriate colleagues, chief residents, and faculty, to ensure appropriate coverage;
      ii. ensure that all pertinent staff and colleagues are included in communication links;
      iii. talk to all collaborators;
      iv. meet for supervision and group meetings, as scheduled;
      v. problem-solve issues with other fellows, etc., utilizing meeting resources/supports provided;
      vi. communicate regarding needs and requests at the time that decisions are being made;
      vii. communication ideas and suggestions for positive change, and refrain from negative communication that may interfere with the educational experience of others.
2. **Dr. Smith will demonstrate an attitude of interest in feedback and self-improvement**
   a. **Methods: Dr. Smith will**
      i. meet twice monthly with Program Mentor, who will assist with skill acquisition via discussion, readings, feedback—with reporting back to Clinical Competence Committee on participation;
      ii. utilize direct feedback from Program Mentor and supervisors on communication effectiveness for gaining positive communication/interpersonal skills;
      iii. complete two Clinical Skills Exams with different attendings, and utilize feedback provided;
      iv. optional, but recommended—consultation with a therapist, psychiatrist in the community, or hospital Employee Assistance Program for support.

Program Director Fellow

as codifying ways of observing them. Training to improve interrater reliability among faculty members may improve consistency of assessments. Other standardized techniques, such as chart reviews and checklists for resident presentations, are needed. The faculty will increasingly be involved in multirater evaluations (formerly called 360-degree evaluations), and help implement these by engaging staff from other disciplines, and inviting patients and families to contribute. The faculty and residents will need to be more comfortable and familiar with the use of videotaped sessions, an excellent means of observing their interactions with patients. In-service programs are needed to help faculty learn new ways of teaching the core competencies. Examples include innovative collaborative rounds with pediatricians and schools in the care of patients with complex disorders as an effective method to teach systems-based practice. The Kalamazoo Consensus Statement on Communication Skills may be an effective means of learning to teach and assess Interpersonal and Communication Skills (42). Engaging faculty and residents in the creative endeavor of training keeps faculty up to date and fresh, as well as provides an optimal training environment for residents.

The competency movement and need for increased faculty training and participation comes at a time when the faculty is stretched more than ever—and at risk of providing suboptimal teaching. Lieff (43) has described a faculty development philosophy of "meaningful and aligned work." This conceptualization encourages faculty to reflect upon the aspects of their work that are most meaningful and align their career trajectories accordingly. Despite the multiple productivity demands, faculty that practice this career reflection, and model it for trainees, tend to be the most effective academic mentors, teachers, and clinicians.

Board Certification in Child and Adolescent Psychiatry

Original Certification

It is the RRC's responsibility to accredit training programs, but it is the ABPN that certifies individuals as competent to practice as specialists. The ABPN determines the accuracy of the applicant's credentials in regard to schooling and residency. To be a candidate for certification in child and adolescent psychiatry, one must have competently completed at least 3 postgraduate years of ACGME-approved residency in general psychiatry, including three clinical skills examinations on clinical interviewing skills; completed 2-year approved fellowship in child and adolescent psychiatry, including three clinical skills examinations with children and adolescents of at least two age groups, and one must have passed the ABPN examination in general psychiatry (16).

Maintenance of Certification

In 1995, the ABPN moved from an unlimited certification to a time-limited certification that requires recertification every 10 years. As posited by the ABMS, of which the ABPN is a member, each physician must engage in the process of maintenance of certification (MOC) that includes strategies that ensure a continuum of learning, self-assessment, professionalism, and cognitive growth through the MOC program. The ultimate goal is to assure the public of continued physician competence.

For child and adolescent psychiatry, MOC has four components: (1) professional standing, including holding an unrestricted medical license; (2) self-assessment and CME to enhance life-long learning; (3) cognitive performance, which includes passing a multiple-choice exam every 10 years; and (4) performance in practice (PIP)—one PIP unit per 3-year stage, which includes a chart-reviewed assessment of practice patterns. Beginning in 2016, a Patient Safety course is also required (16).

CHILD AND ADOLESCENT PSYCHIATRY TRAINING WITHIN BROADER MEDICAL EDUCATION

Medical Student Education in Child Psychiatry and Human Development

Lack of exposure to child and adolescent psychiatry has been identified as one of the major obstacles to recruitment into the field (1,19). Medical schools vary considerably in their curricula and in the utilization of their child and adolescent psychiatry faculty. Some schools have faculty contributing to required courses in human development, but child psychiatry didactics are rare throughout medical school curricula. Most clerkships are heavily geared to teaching psychiatry in adult settings and medical students may receive few opportunities to see children and families—certainly not enough exposure in most schools to stimulate interest in the field (44). The Association of Directors of Medical Student Education in Psychiatry (ADMSEP) has developed a core group of child and adolescent psychiatry educators who are attempting to change this pattern, with recommendations and models of increasing medical student exposure to child psychiatry (45). Medical students who have an interest in development and in the psychosocial issues of children and families may choose elective opportunities in community settings, schools, child and adolescent inpatient or residential programs, or in clinical settings around the United States and abroad. There are many opportunities, but much has been relegated to the creativity of students and their mentors.

One important and innovative program is the Klingenstein Third Generation Foundation Fellowship (KTGF) in Child and Adolescent Psychiatry. Begun at Yale School of Medicine, the Klingenstein Fellowship serves to mentor interested medical students in child and adolescent psychiatry from their first year through graduation. The program has been replicated to currently include 14 programs nationally. Students accepted into the program are assigned a child and adolescent psychiatrist mentor based on their particular interests in the field. Students generally "shadow" faculty members in their work in a variety of clinical service areas. On a monthly basis, the students at each medical school spend an evening with faculty that may involve clinical discussions, movies, or didactic presentations. Additional opportunities for mentoring, observing clinical work, or doing elective academic projects, including engaging in research are encouraged (27). Annually, the programs meet to share experiences and collaborate in active learning and leisure activities.

The Continuum from Medical School through Residency Training

For residents who choose a traditional portal of entry into child and adolescent psychiatry and who did not have the good fortune of a KTGF or comparable fellowship experience, there is limited continuity in education and training from medical school through general psychiatry residency into child and adolescent psychiatry training. Most medical students interested in child and adolescent psychiatry have an interest in pediatrics. In fact, many struggle with the career decision between child psychiatry and pediatrics. Such students take many pediatric electives, though there may be few training opportunities in child psychiatry or the psychosocial aspects of pediatrics (44).

The general psychiatry residency requirement for child and adolescent psychiatry is for 2 months of clinical work with children and families. This may be done in inpatient, partial hospital, or outpatient settings. General psychiatry residents may also take one of their two months of consultation psychiatry in child psychiatry and may take one of their two required months of neurology in pediatric neurology. In addition, the requirements for forensic and addictions may be completed with child and adolescent patients and 20% of outpatients may be youth. For residents interested in child and adolescent psychiatry early on, if their program offers the opportunity, they may be able to have considerable child psychiatry training before their child and adolescent psychiatry fellowship. For others, particularly the ones who discover child and adolescent psychiatry later in their generally psychiatry residency, there may be limited continuity between child and adolescent and general psychiatric residency training.

The Relationship between Child and Adolescent Psychiatry and Pediatrics

Collaborative Care Models

Pediatric residencies are required to teach 2 months of Developmental Behavioral Pediatrics within their 3 years of training. This is taught largely within pediatric programs themselves, although some may use affiliated child and adolescent psychiatry faculty to train their residents. All child and adolescent psychiatry programs have a formal rotation in consultation-liaison to pediatrics (34).

It is crucial for child and adolescent psychiatry and pediatric programs to develop and foster a close collaborative relationship. The Patient-Centered Medical Home, in which the primary care provider is the hub, and specialists, including child and adolescent psychiatrists, provide consultative services, is expected to proliferate under the Patient Protection and Affordable Care Act (46). This model of care is designed to improve access to care and integrate the full spectrum of health and mental health services to improve patient health outcomes. Additionally, the passage of the Mental Health Parity and Addiction Equity Act of 2008 (47), reflects the growing recognition of the legitimacy of mental illness as a health issue and societal acceptance of a principle of nondiscrimination in regard to the financing and provision of mental health services. The policy changes resulting from these statutes have set in motion a process of change in the healthcare system with significant implications for the professional role of child and adolescent psychiatrists—conferring a much more active role in the collaborative care environment (48,49). Child and adolescent psychiatry fellowship programs must anticipate these changes and begin to train the next generation of child and adolescent psychiatrists in the competencies required for optimal collaboration, consultation, and system-based practice within the patient-centered medical home setting (50,51). However, we must be sure not to "throw out the baby with the bath water." As a relationship-based specialty, child and adolescent psychiatry training programs must maintain an emphasis on therapeutic engagement and the healing attributes of the doctor–patient relationship.

SPECIAL ISSUES IN EDUCATION AND TRAINING: MENTORSHIP, MORALE, LEADERSHIP, LIFESTYLE, AND COMMUNITY

Professional Identity Formation: The Role of Mentors

Mentoring is frequently cited by trainees and early career psychiatrists as one of the most powerful influences in career development. Williams et al. (52), in a focus group study of mentor–mentee relationships, identified qualities that mentors and mentees should possess that facilitate good mentoring relationships. "Specifically, mentors must be compatible on a personal level, active listeners, able to identify potential strengths in their mentees, and able to assist mentees in defining and reaching goals. Mentees must be proactive, willing to learn, and be selective in accepting advice from their mentors." (p. 113)

Mentorship is an active process, which, when the key elements are present, may be a life-changing experience for both the mentor and the mentee. It is the power of the relationship that promotes development—the mentor's ability to envision in the mentee strengths, weaknesses, and growth potential—not just what he/she is at the time, but what he/she has the potential to become (53). Idealization of the mentee by the mentor and vice versa makes for a powerful bond. However, there is much more than idealization. Realistic appraisal, insight, motivation, and career expertise are other qualities of mentorship that are required to effectively assist the mentee in genuine growth.

Mentorship has been acknowledged as a crucial element of research careers, as demonstrated by the National Institutes of Health (NIH) Mentored Career Development Awards. However, mentorship may help launch clinical, administrative, teaching, and other career paths as well. Mentors may be assigned or developed on the basis of mutual identification in a less formal process. A study by Ragins and Cotton (54) suggests that informal mentored relationships, developed on the basis of mutual identification, led to greater benefits for protégés than formal arrangements. Formally arranged mentorship arrangements typically last between 6 months and 1 year (55); informal ones between 3 and 6 years (56). Martin (53) has noted that "it is less physical proximity than meaningful intellectual, personal, and emotional connections that count most" (p. 1226) in the mentor–mentee relationship. "More than duration, internalization can be seen as providing a useful metric for the success of the experience. Those individuals capable of invoking and making use of the other (whether spontaneously or through active effort) have been effectively mentored." (p. 1228)

The risks inherent in the mentorship relationship are those that come with a power differential in a personal and intimate relationship. To be optimally successful, early and clear articulation of expectations of the work together in the mentorship relationship may provide the template and the scaffolding to build a relationship that launches a successful career. Frequent reassessment of the working relationship to ensure alignment of goals and expectations reinvigorates the work, and ensures the optimal effectiveness of the mentor–protégé bond. It is the sign of a successful mentorship relationship when the protégé becomes a mentor to others, thus rejuvenating and promulgating the transmission of values from generation to generation (53,55).

Physician Well-being: Promoting Resilience and Values in Our Students, Residents, and Faculty

While training departments may differ in their healthcare delivery system, the size and nature of the faculty, and in the population served, the core values and philosophy of child and adolescent psychiatry fellowship programs remain the same: We share a profound and passionate commitment to providing the highest standard of care for the children, adolescents, and families we serve. To optimally achieve this, departments must provide a culture in which students, residents, and faculty are treasured, where teaching is cherished, where deficiencies in individuals and in the program are sensitively remediated, and where deep trust and honest, open communication are shared and encouraged between all members of the community (57).

However, physician well-being and prevention of "burnout" is a very real concern. Physicians demonstrate higher rates of anxiety, depression, suicide, divorce, stress, and emotional exhaustion than other segments of the population (58). Burnout (emotional exhaustion, depersonalization, and feelings of worthlessness) results in poor patient care, poor self-care and physical health, diminished empathy, and medical errors (59). Morale may be diminished by many of the stresses facing modern healthcare systems: regulatory and managed care pressures; increasing faculty and fellow demands to provide clinical care and productivity demands; financial pressures and educational debt; and documentation requirements that may decrease time available to spend with children, families, and collaborators. All of these forces can breed demoralization among faculty and disappointment among the trainees, who in many institutions have had to shoulder increased caseloads and less direct supervision and mentoring. "These challenges are compounded by our profession's hidden curriculum—the reluctance to admit weakness, expose our shame of suffering from the stigma of a psychiatric disorder, or even discuss the pressures we share." (58) (p. 9)

How then can well-being, morale, and maintenance of the esteemed values of residency training and education be fostered? First and foremost, the PD must be fully aware of the service needs, administrative structures, and emotional climate within the institution and training sites. The PD needs to have a close working relationship with the director of GME, chair of the department, and division chief of child and adolescent psychiatry in order to make problems in the residency known and viewed as a priority. The ACGME has strengthened its mandates on the institution to provide support for the residency training mission, with monitoring via regular CLER. For serious issues related to the training program's learning environment, the medical school and/or hospital may be a source of needed resources. While the PD has no hiring or firing power over the faculty, he/she has significant authority, especially if his/her word is viewed by all as one with that of the Chair.

Beresin et al. (58) contend that, "State-of-the-art and well-evidenced education will impart not only medical knowledge but also a tool-box of coping skills.... The evidence needs to be marshaled to shift the hidden curriculum so that caring for oneself, maintaining cognitive and emotional acuity, and seeking fulfillment are considered professional obligations and preconditions for optimal patient outcomes" (p. 10). Improving physician well-being and satisfaction has been found to improve patients' satisfaction with the care they receive (57,60). Table 1.4.3 provides suggestions to promote physician well-being.

TABLE 1.4.3

ACTIVITIES TO PROMOTE PHYSICIAN RESILIENCE AND WELL-BEING

1. Engagement activities to facilitate group cohesion:
   - Social or topic-related opportunities for relationship building
   - Retreats, meetings, conferences, with active listening and mutual feedback
   - Participation in small, process-oriented, longitudinal reflective seminars that discuss the emotional, physical, and social impacts of the practice of medicine
2. Ensure time in curriculum to discuss residency topics related to becoming an independently functioning physician:
   - Managing uncertainty and ambiguity
   - Caring for the difficult or hateful patient
   - Optimizing team functioning
   - Understanding medical errors and importance of apology
   - Discovering personal sources of renewal
   - Finding meaning in work
   - Fighting "burnout"
3. Skill building to become a reflective practitioner:
   - Practice writing and sharing reflective essays
   - Healthcare humanities book-clubs and readings
   - Mindfulness training
   - Participation in reflective seminars that discuss the emotional, physical, and social impacts of the practice of medicine
4. Curricular modules on Wellness:
   - Self-care, mindful meditation, and healthy lifestyle
   - Education about signs and symptoms of burnout and resources for professional help
5. Actively promote career and life goal setting:
   - Self-reflective activities and discussions to assist with defining career-life priorities
   - Facilitate specific opportunities—personal introductions to others in the field, nominating for committees, awards and fellowships, etc.
   - Regularly acknowledge accomplishments, joys, sorrows, and personal value of each trainee

Faculty morale and well-being optimizes the learning environment for the fellows. Faculty that feel respected, valued, and connected to the mission of the department and the training program will improve the morale of the trainees and the institution. Frequent group and individual meetings of the PD with the teaching faculty are essential, as is being a direct conduit to the chief and chair. The PD may not be able to increase reimbursement for services or salaries, but can help the faculty in being recognized as key members of the academic program through providing and acknowledging educational contributions (e.g., teaching awards, notices of local and national presentations, and publications), and support of promotions. Regular faculty development workshops, retreats, and social gatherings are valuable ways to help foster a sense of group cohesion, even in times of increasing fragmentation. Most programs now have software for a common portal that allows for schedules, evaluations, and posting articles. These sites may serve a function of faculty engagement, in addition to information sharing.

Morale in a fellowship class is critical for the functioning of a training program. A class that is tight, supportive, smooth functioning, and just plain fun is instrumental to the personal and professional development of the residents. Fellows need the proper balance of supervision, mentoring, guidance, autonomy, time with each other, and time with friends and family. Morale is high when residents and faculty can truly say that they work hard, and play hard, and that they feel like family—and as in most families, there will be struggles and differences, but above all, unconditional love and support (58).

Teaching How to Teach: Leadership Development, Professional, and Public Education

The goal of child and adolescent psychiatry residency training is to train competent physicians and the next generation of leaders in the field. Integration of components of leadership training into the curriculum enhances this mission.

Graduates have identified lack of training in administrative, supervisory, and financial/managed care issues to be the areas of most deficiency in their training (61). Many child and adolescent psychiatrists are hired as team leaders and medical directors upon graduation. Thus, development of a high skill level in leadership, management, and teaching is needed in training.

Leaders may be defined as individuals who inspire others to go beyond what they think they are capable of doing, making it possible for a group to attain a goal that was previously thought unattainable by (1) inspiring trust, (2) acting consistently, and (3) motivating with words and deeds.

Components of training in leadership skills and enhancing leadership potential may be categorized into six primary arenas: (1) value transmission and formation of an identity as a leader; (2) competency in core knowledge and skills; (3) effective listening, learning, and integrating skills; (4) promoting creativity; (5) effective communication and collaboration skills; and (6) promoting by words and actions sacrifice for the greater goal (62,63).

Programs have embedded components of leadership and management training to varying degrees. However, a more focused curriculum in leadership is needed. Teaching (public speaking skills, how to put together a presentation, making presentations more interactive, mentored teaching experiences), a high level of collaborative skills, team building, and a deep and abiding vision are required for truly effective leadership. Providing team leadership experiences, seminars on teaching, effective supervision and mentorship—all of these are curricular aspects of promoting leadership skills in trainees. Other components of a training curriculum to promote leadership development include interactive and experiential seminars on effective listening, learning and integrating, with constructive feedback on these skills by supervisors and others. A professional development seminar, working in and learning about systems, meeting creative leaders in the field to learn about their lives, career trajectories, motivations and advice, and ample elective time to explore areas of interest and promote creative projects are other options for promoting leadership within the residency training program. The options are numerous, and call on the creativity and resources of each program to individualize the professional development curriculum to the training mission of the institution.

Public education is a core professional responsibility of all physicians. Education begins in the office and hospital units with our patients, parents, and families. A parent and child need to understand principles of normal development and psychopathology and its treatment for a sound therapeutic alliance and effective collaboration with the physician. Child and adolescent psychiatrists are also frequently asked to speak at schools, religious organizations, and other community groups. Many of these talks help educate the public about normal development and its variations, as well as psychiatric problems and their treatment. Residencies are required to instruct residents in these patient-care–centered and public educational venues (34).

Research shows that Americans get much, if not most, of their mental health information from media news, including the Internet, and from public entertainment. Some programs perpetuate myths and misinformation. Others present controversial information that scares parents away from certain treatments. For example, the Federal Drug Administration's black box warnings on certain antidepressants and stimulants frighten parents, are often misrepresented by certain groups in the media, and cast doubt on some treatments frequently used by child and adolescent psychiatrists. Our residents and future practitioners need to be prepared to discuss these issues with patients and with the media. When used well, the many forms of mass and targeted media—including newspapers, radio, television, and the Internet—can counter inaccurate reports and destructive stereotypes. They can also provide information, reassurance, and perspective that can transform the lives of our patients and their families (64).

The expansion of mass media offers child and adolescent psychiatrists a new opportunity to influence public opinion and policy, and educate parents, teachers, and allied professionals who work with children and families. However, few residency programs prepare residents on how to interact with media. Residents benefit from seminars that help them appreciate the complex interests and motivations of journalists and how different forms of the mass media operate; learn ways of ordering priorities for public presentations as opposed to professional lectures and seminars; acquire specific skills needed for managing different forms of media and using mass media as an extension of their clinical practice; and have ample opportunity to practice these skills with teachers who have experience in interactions with the media (64,65).

Community in Education: The Role of Local, Regional, and National Organizations

Parker J. Palmer noted that "To teach is to create a space in which the community of truth is practiced" (66). Our community of truth is established by the close ties child and adolescent psychiatrists, pediatricians, and allied health professionals develop. Teaching requires a personal, inner commitment and devotion to our students, but cannot be separated from our community of practicing clinicians, researchers, educators, and administrators. How we establish "truth" is complex and communal. How we transmit, assess, and regulate the material of our field requires community. Sharing our research, empirical findings, clinical perspectives, standards of care, or educational models requires a community of professionals who are in continual dialogue. In this way, we advance child and adolescent psychiatry.

As our field moves more toward outcomes-based curricula, predicated on the acquisition of competencies, and as the attainment of knowledge, skills, and attitudes are viewed and assessed in a developmental context, we need ongoing collaboration between the national organizations that oversee educational programs. The Liaison Committee on Medical Education (LCME) and the Association of American Medical Colleges (AAMC), which oversee medical school education; the Accreditation Council for Continuing Medical Education (ACGME) and the ABMS, which oversee GME and certification; and the ABMS and the ACCME, which oversee continuing education and recertification, should actively work together to ensure that there is a real continuum between all levels of medical education.

At local and regional levels, medical schools and residencies should share precious educational resources. Beyond exchanging teachers, examinations such as the "Mock Board" annual clinical exam could be shared between programs. Regional associations of our national organizations often have special events for medical students, residents, and faculty, and these enterprises should continue. It is not hard to offer mentors in a region for an interested medical student or resident. There are endless possibilities for developing and nurturing our educational community in child and adolescent psychiatry—for students, residents, faculty, and practicing clinicians. We must also not forget that our community has largely been confined to our medical schools and residencies. However, there are many allied professional schools, such as nursing, dental, public health, education, business, and law among others, that can prove invaluable by our facilitating cross-fertilization of students and faculty. Beyond this, an untapped resource in our local community is the university, with its undergraduate college and graduate schools of arts and sciences. Medicine has remained rather distant from these campuses. However, our faculty could provide excellent teaching for undergraduates, as is occurring in many colleges—including a minor in child and adolescent mental health studies (67). Further we are greatly underutilizing the many excellent faculty in the humanities, neuroscience, and social sciences that may make a new and important contribution to the training and education of our students and residents, while expanding and enriching our community of scholars.

Lifestyle Issues

Child and adolescent psychiatry, as one of the most underserved medical specialties, provides for a plethora of job opportunities for graduates. Child and adolescent psychiatry also fared extremely well in graduates' ratings of diversity of practice options, work–life balance, and flexibility (68).

Child and adolescent psychiatrists have widely diverse and varied practice options, including academics, research, clinical practice in a variety of settings (private practice, group practice, clinics, and within a continuum of care from outpatient, day treatment programs, residential treatment programs, and inpatient hospitalization). Consultations to schools, courts, hospitals, pediatric settings, and other agencies are common. Additionally, advocacy and public policy initiatives may be a formal or informal aspect of many child and adolescent psychiatry careers.

Child and adolescent psychiatry offers a unique opportunity to spend time with your patients and to watch them grow and develop over time and to their best potential. In a survey of early career child and adolescent psychiatrists, job satisfaction was rated very high overall—with a median overall career satisfaction rating of 5 on a 6-point Likert scale (13).

Lifestyle issues are being considered seriously by medical graduates when choosing a specialty. A carefully crafted career in child and adolescent psychiatry provides flexibility in work hours to allow a balance between career and family or other interests. Salaries are highly competitive. There are jobs in all parts of the country, allowing for geographic flexibility. Most institutions and agencies pay a higher salary to psychiatrists who have completed child and adolescent psychiatry training. According to 2016 survey data, the median income for child and adolescent psychiatrists was almost $200,000 (68,69).

Child and adolescent psychiatry remains a medical specialty with a serious shortage of physicians. However, the training and mentorship enterprise is thriving, with recruitment efforts starting from early in training. The superior training of the next generation of effective leaders in the field is the mission of PDs in child and adolescent psychiatry training programs. However, it "takes a village" to train a superior child and adolescent psychiatrist. Physicians, allied professionals, residency training coordinators, and patients and their families are all part of that village.

References

1. Kim WJ: Child and adolescent psychiatry workforce: a critical shortage and national challenge. *Acad Psychiatry* 27:277–282, 2003.
2. Sierles FS, Yager J, Weissman SH: Recruitment of U.S. medical graduates into psychiatry: reasons for optimism, sources of concern. *Acad Psychiatry* 27:252–259, 2003.
3. U.S. Public Health Service: *Report of the Surgeon General's Conference on Children's Mental Health: A National Action Agenda*. Washington, DC, Department of Health and Human Services, 2000.
4. New Freedom Commission on Mental Health: *Achieving the Promise: Transforming Mental Health Care in America. Final Report*. Rockville, MD, Department of Health and Human Services, 2003.
5. Brown L, Zhang S, Schuppe J: Decades into crisis, kids still suffer from shortage of psychiatrists. NBC News 6/18/2016. Available at: http://www.nbcnews.com/news/us-news/decades-crisis-kids-still-suffer-shortage-psychiatrists-n581276. Accessed June 19, 2016.
6. U.S. Department of Health and Human Services: *Mental Health: A Report of the Surgeon General*. Rockville, MD, U.S. Department of Health and Human Services, 1999.
7. Costello EJ, Egger H, Angold A: 10-year research update review: the epidemiology of child and adolescent psychiatric disorders: I. Methods and public health burden. *J Am Acad Child Adolesc Psychiatry* 44:972–986, 2005.
8. Merikangas KR, He JP, Brody D, Fisher PW, Bourdon K, Koretz DS: Prevalence and treatment of mental disorders among US children in the 2001-2004 NHANES. *Pediatrics* 125:75–81, 2010.
9. Merikangas KR, He JP, Burstein M, et al.: Lifetime prevalence of mental disorders in U.S. adolescents: results from the National Comorbidity Survey Replication–Adolescent Supplement (NCS-A). *J Am Acad Child Adolesc Psychiatry* 49(10):980–989, 2010.
10. Institute of Medicine: *Research in Training in Psychiatry Residency: Strategies for Reform*. Washington, DC, The National Academies Press, 2003.
11. Fenton W, James R, Insel T: Psychiatry residency training, the physician scientist, and the future of psychiatry. *Acad Psychiatry* 28:263–266, 2004.
12. Kupfer DJ, Hyman SE, Schatzberg AF, Pincus HA, Reynolds CF: Recruiting and retaining future generations of physician scientists in mental health. *Arch Gen Psychiatry* 59:657–660, 2002.
13. Stubbe DE, Thomas WJ: A survey of early-career child and adolescent psychiatrists: professional activities and perceptions. *J Am Acad Child Adolesc Psychiatry* 41(2):123–130, 2002.
14. Beresin EV: The administration of residency training programs. *Child Adolesc Psychiatric Clin N Am* 11:67–89, 2002.
15. Schowalter JE: Child and adolescent psychiatry comes of age. In: Menninger R, Nemiah J (eds): *American Psychiatry After World War II (1944–1994)*. Washington, DC, American Psychiatric Press, 461–480, 2000.
16. Brooks BA, Mrazek DA: Child and adolescent psychiatry. In: Amineff JJ, Faulkner LR (eds): *The American Board of Psychiatry and Neurology: Looking Back and Moving Ahead*. Washington, DC, American Psychiatric Publishing, 129–134, 2005.
17. Accreditation Council for Graduate Medical Education: *ACGME Annual Survey*. Chicago, IL, ACGME, 2016.
18. Beresin EV, Borus JF: Child psychiatry fellowship training: a crisis in recruitment and manpower. *Am J Psychiatry* 146:759–763, 1989.
19. Martin VL, Bennet DS, Pitale M: Medical students' perceptions of child psychiatry: pre- and post-psychiatry clerkship. *Acad Psychiatry* 29:362–367, 2005.
20. Szajnberg NM, Beck A: Medical student attitudes toward child psychiatry. *J Am Acad Child Adolesc Psychiatry* 33(1):145, 1994.
21. Beresin EV: Child and adolescent psychiatry residency training: current issues and controversies. *J Am Acad Child Adolesc Psychiatry* 36:1339–1348, 1997.
22. Eisenberg L: The past 50 years of child and adolescent psychiatry: a personal memoir. *J Am Acad Child Adolesc Psychiatry* 40:743–748, 2001.
23. Schowalter JE: Tinker to evers to chance: triple board update. *J Am Acad Child Adolesc Psychiatry* 32:243, 1993.
24. Schowalter JE, Friedman CP, Scheiber SC, Juul D: An experiment in graduate medical education: combined residency training in pediatrics, psychiatry, and child and adolescent psychiatry. *Acad Psychiatry* 26:237–244, 2002.
25. Stetka B, Findling RL, Thomas TC: Child psychiatrists needed! Are pediatricians the answer? *Medscape Psychiatry* 2011.
26. Yager J, Greden J, Abrams M, Riba M: The Institute of Medicine's report on research training in psychiatry residency: strategies for reform—background, results and follow up. *Acad Psychiatry* 28:267–274, 2004.
27. Martin A, Bloch M, Stubbe D, et al.: From too little too late to early and often: child psychiatry education in medical school (and before and after). *Child Adolesc Psychiatric Clin N Am* 16(1):17–43, 2007.
28. Accreditation Council for Graduate Medical Education (ACGME) Outcome Project: *ACGME General Competencies Version 1.3*. Chicago, IL, ACGME, 2000.
29. Sargent J, Sexson S, Cuffe S, et al.: Assessment of competency in child and adolescent psychiatry training. *Acad Psychiatry* 28:18–26, 2004.
30. Sexson S, Sargent J, Zima B, et al.: Sample core competencies in child and adolescent psychiatry training: a starting point. *Acad Psychiatry* 25:201–213, 2001.

31. Nasca TJ, Philibert I, Brigham T, Flynn TC: The next GME accreditation system—rationale and benefits. *New Engl J Med* 366(11):1051–1056, 2012.
32. The psychiatry milestone project. *J Grad Med Educ* 6(1 Suppl 1):284–304, 2014.
33. ACGME, ABPN: The child and adolescent psychiatry milestone project. 2015. Available at: www.acgme.org/portals/0/pdfs/milestones/childand adolescentpsychiatrymilestones.pdf. Accessed August 13, 2016.
34. ACGME: Program requirements for graduate medical education in child and adolescent psychiatry. ACGME-approved: February 9, 2015; effective: July 1, 2015 Revised Common Program Requirements effective. 2016. Available at: https://www.acgme.org/Portals/0/PFAssets/Program-Requirements/405_child_and_adolescent_psych_2016.pdf. Accessed June 10, 2016.
35. Weiss KB, Bagian JP, Nasca TJ: The clinical learning environment: the foundation of Graduate Medical Education. *JAMA* 309:1687–1688, 2013.
36. Epstein R, Hundert EM: Defining and assessing professional competence. *JAMA* 287:226–235, 2002.
37. Ende J: Feedback in clinical medical education. *JAMA* 250:777–781, 1983.
38. Swing SR, Cowley DS, Bentman A: Assessing resident performance on the psychiatry milestones. *Acad Psychiatry* 38:294–302, 2004.
39. Boiselle PM: A remedy for resident evaluation and remediation. *Acad Radiol* 12:894–900, 2005.
40. Schwind CJ, Williams RG, Boehler ML, Dunnington GL: Do individual attendings' post-rotation performance ratings detect residents' clinical performance deficiencies? *Acad Med* 79:453–457, 2004.
41. Hays RB, Jolly BC, Caldon LJ, et al.: Is insight important? Measuring capacity to change performance. *Med Educ* 36:965–971, 2002.
42. Bayer-Fetzer Conference on Physician-Patient Communication in Medical Education: Essential elements of communication in medical encounters: the Kalamazoo Consensus Statement. *Acad Med* 76:390–393, 2001.
43. Lieff SJ: The missing link in academic career planning and development: pursuit of meaningful and aligned work. *Acad Med* 84:1383–1388, 2009.
44. Schlozman SC, Beresin EV: Frustration and opportunity: teaching child and adolescent psychiatry throughout medical education. *Acad Psychiatry* 34:172–174, 2010.
45. Fox GS, Stock S, Briscoe GW, et al.: Improving child and adolescent psychiatry education for medical students: an inter-organizational collaborative action plan. *Acad Psychiatry* 36(6):461–464, 2012.
46. United States Department of Health and Human Services. *The Affordable Care Act.* 2010. Available at: http://www.hhs.gov/healthcare/rights/law/index.html. Accessed May 3, 2016.
47. United States Department of Labor: *Mental Health Parity and Addiction Equity Act of 2008.* Available at: http://www.dol.gov/ebsa/mentalhealthparity/. Accessed May 1, 2016.
48. Gabel S: The integration of mental health into pediatric practice: pediatricians and child and adolescent psychiatrists working together in new models of care. *Pediatrics* 157(5):848–851, 2010.
49. Sarvet BD, Wegner L: Developing effective child psychiatry collaboration with primary care: leadership and management strategies. *Child Adolesc Psychiatric Clin N Am* 19:139–148, 2010.
50. Rickerby ML, Roesler TA: Training child psychiatrists in family-based integrated care. *Child Adolesc Psychiatric Clin N Am* 24:501–515, 2015.
51. McGinty KL, Larson JJ, Hodas G, Musick D, Metz P: Teaching patient-centered care and systems-based practice in child and adolescent psychiatry. *Acad Psychiatry* 36(6):468–472, 2012.
52. Williams LL, Levine JB, Malhotra S, Holtzheimer P: The good-enough mentoring relationship. *Acad Psychiatry* 28:111–115, 2004.
53. Martin A: Ignition sequence: on mentorship. *J Am Acad Child Adolesc Psychiatry* 44:1225–1229, 2005.
54. Ragins BR, Cotton JL: Mentor functions and outcomes: a comparison of men and women in formal and informal mentoring relationships. *J Appl Psychol* 84:529–550, 1999.
55. Kram KE: *Mentoring At Work: Developmental Relationships in Organizational Life.* Glenview, IL, Scott Foresman, 1985.
56. Murray M: *Beyond the Myths and Magic of Mentoring: How to Facilitate an Effective Mentoring Program.* San Francisco, CA, Jossey-Bass, 1991.
57. Goitein L: Physician well-being: addressing downstream effects, but looking upstream. *JAMA Int Med* 174:533–534, 2014.
58. Beresin EV, Milligan TA, Balon R, Coverdale JH, Louie AK, Roberts LW: Physician wellbeing: a critical deficiency in resilience education and training. *Acad Psychiatry* 40:9–12, 2016.
59. Krasner MS, Epstein RM, Beckman H, et al.: Association of an educational program in mindful communication with burnout, empathy, and attitudes among primary care physicians. *JAMA* 302:1284–1293, 2009.
60. DeVoe J, Fryer GE, Straub A, McCann J, Fairbrother G: Congruent satisfaction: is there geographic correlation between patient and physician satisfaction? *Med Care* 45:88–94, 2007.
61. Stubbe DE: Preparation for practice: child and adolescent psychiatry graduates' assessment of training experiences. *J Am Acad Child Adolesc Psychiatry* 41(2):131–139, 2002.
62. Goleman D: Leadership that gets results. *Harvard Business Rev* 78:78–90, 2000.
63. Heifetz R: *Leadership Without Easy Answers.* Cambridge, MA, Harvard University Press, 1994.
64. Kutner L, Beresin EV: Reaching out: mass media techniques for child and adolescent psychiatrists. *J Am Acad Child Adolesc Psychiatry* 39:1452–1454, 2000.
65. Olson CK, Kutner LA: Media outreach for child psychiatrists. *Child Adolesc Psychiatric Clin N Am* 14:613–623, 2005.
66. Palmer PJ: *The Courage to Teach: Exploring the Inner Landscape of a Teacher's Life.* San Francisco, CA, Jossey-Bass, 90, 1998.
67. Shatkin JP, Koplewicz HS: The child and adolescent mental health studies (CAMS) minor at New York University. *Acad Psychiatry* 32(5):438–445, 2008.
68. Nolan JA, Forte GJ, Salsberg ES: *Physician Supply and Demand Indicators in New York and California: A Summary of Trends in Starting Income, Relative Demand, and GME Graduates in 35 Medical Specialties.* Albany, NY, SUNY School of Public Health, 2003.
69. Fox G: Choosing child and adolescent psychiatry as a career: the top ten questions. Available at: http://www.aacap.org/training/DevelopMentor/Content/2005Fall/f2005_a2.cfmhttp://www.aacap.org/training/DevelopMentor/Content/2005Fall/f2005_a2.cfm. Accessed August 31, 2016.

CHAPTER 1.5 ■ GLOBAL CHILD AND ADOLESCENT MENTAL HEALTH

MYRON L. BELFER, HESHAM M. HAMODA, AND MAURICE EISENBRUCH

GOAL

This chapter delineates areas of concern in global child and adolescent mental health and focuses on issues of particular clinical import to child and adolescent psychiatrists and other child mental health clinicians. Many of the topics that are addressed are now relevant to domestic practice given widespread global immigration patterns.

OVERVIEW

The concept of Global Mental Health is relatively recent embracing concerns for accessing evidence-based care, utilizing nonprofessional providers and engaging consumers. It should be noted that the concern for an international understanding of psychopathology in children goes back to the 1970s with seminal articles on child psychiatry in developing countries (1–3). As stated by Whitley (4) the origin can be traced back to 2007 when a series of articles in the *Lancet* discussed in detail the impact of mental health on health and well-being. The original articles did not address child and adolescent mental health concerns in a meaningful manner and it was not until 2011 that the *Lancet* published a comprehensive paper on global child and adolescent mental health (5). The various parties invested in global mental health established a Movement for Global Mental Health. The Movement and its associated initiatives have not been without some controversy. However, the goal to improve services for people living with mental health problems and psychosocial disabilities, particularly in low and middle income countries (LAMI) has brought about a global dialogue that has been beneficial in a number of ways. While the emphasis on global mental health has highlighted problems in access to care, diagnosis, and treatment more broadly it has been an ongoing challenge to have child mental health seen as a priority despite the overwhelming evidence of the early roots of mental illness and the impact of mental ill health on a host of social issues.

Global child and adolescent mental health embraces the world view on the place of children in society, the appreciation of diverse behavioral styles, the identification of psychopathology, and the setting of priorities for the use of scarce resources. Child and adolescent mental health is influenced by the economics of countries and societies within countries, by the internal and external displacement of children and adolescents through war and natural disasters, by the role of the child in the family, and by the place of women in society. New knowledge and greater recognition of the impact on children of exposure to trauma, sexual and physical abuse, inhumane living and working situations, inadequate health care, and drug abuse have heightened interest in approaches to ameliorating the impact on child and adolescent health and mental health of these potentially pathogenic influences. It is a challenge to child and adolescent psychiatrists and allied professionals to be active participants in understanding the nature of the problems faced and in being a part of the solution (6).

The overall health and well-being of children are global concerns. All countries with the exception of the United States of America have ratified the 1989 United Nations Convention on the Rights of the Child (7,8). It commits countries to "ensure that all children have the right to develop physically and mentally to their full potential, to express their opinions freely, and to be protected against all forms of abuse and exploitation." The concern among some countries was the perception that ratification of the treaty would intrude on sovereign rights and/or traditional views of the child in a dependent position in society. In the end these concerns did not impede ratification but do impact implementation. In some countries that are party to the treaty, the affirmation of the rights of children has not resulted in benign policies toward the protection of children from harm or the fostering of positive development.

In the global arena, and increasingly in multicultural societies, child mental health and child psychopathology cannot be gauged solely from a Western perspective. It is simplistic to state, but meaningful to understand, that what may appear pathologic in one country or society, or to one cultural or subcultural group within a country, may be deemed normative or adaptive in another. This does not imply that it may not be helpful to have a consensus about a frame of reference regarding psychopathologic conditions, but the interested party must keep an open mind in attributing cause to behaviors, interpreting responses to events, or judging parental or familial interactions with children. The complexity of understanding children and adolescents embraces anthropologic, social, psychological, political, and rights dimensions. For the domestic practitioner, understanding the cultural context of the individual and family is important. For example, Murthy (9) reports that studies have found that suicide rates among immigrants are more closely aligned to the rates in the country of origin than to the rates in the country of adoption. Generally, suicide rates of immigrant populations are higher than in the country of origin. The methods of suicide are those used traditionally in the culture of origin. Canino et al. (10) also documented the persistence of the importance of culture-bound syndromes.

In many resource-poor countries, educational institutions represent the most coherent system for providing services to children and adolescents. As never before, the value placed on education in societies is being emphasized as agrarian pursuits have diminished in favor or more lucrative employment in other sectors or due to restrictive land policies. In resource-poor countries, the impact of technology is offering new opportunities but at the same time widening the gulf between rich and poor, educated and uneducated. Urbanization combines with the technology revolution further to challenge accustomed ways that may stress individuals and families including the erosion of the extended family for support (11). Children and adolescents, as students or as part of a family, experience new stresses that convey either advantage or disadvantage, depending on access, intelligence, and resources. In response to these changes in society, resilience-building programs in schools, along with primary care health programs in communities, have evolved. While the emphasis on education may be profound in urban settings in resource-poor countries, the role of traditional healing for child mental health disorders, especially in rural settings, remains powerful (12–17). For instance, in Cambodia, the taxonomies and explanatory models of childhood illnesses are embedded in powerful beliefs about the role of ancestral spirits and the child's previous incarnation (18,19).

The role and responsibilities of child and adolescent psychiatrists and other child mental health professionals vary in resource-poor countries. The competencies of the child and adolescent psychiatrist must fit the needs of the society in which they exist (20,21). For example, epilepsy and intellectual disability clearly fall within the expected clinical competencies of child and adolescent psychiatrists in resource-poor countries but not in resource-rich countries. The infrastructure in some countries post conflict may have decimated the child mental health workforce. In Cambodia, for example, where the country's entire infrastructure, including the health system, was destroyed during the Khmer Rouge regime none of 43 surviving medical doctors in Cambodia were psychiatrists (22). When child psychiatry is a very scarce resource, there may be the opportunity for only a consultative role, limited diagnostics, and an inability to be part of or to stimulate discussion of national policy. Child and adolescent psychiatrists coming to resource-poor countries may play a vital role in educating others but must be willing to increase their cultural competence, self-reflection and in this way to increase their mindfulness of the local cultural context, inherent capacity of the existing systems, and ways to ensure the provision of appropriate education. "Dropping in" to provide Western-oriented psychiatric education or consultation may do more harm than good.

In understanding the impact of child and adolescent psychiatric disorders, it is not sufficient to understand diagnosis alone. Significant gains have been made in raising the consciousness about the mental health of children and adolescents, as well as adults, by bringing attention to the "burden" of mental illness (23). The global burden of disease is now most often measured in disability-adjusted life-years (DALYs). This approach makes possible a more standardized assessment of the burden of disease as measured by lost opportunity, diminished function, and the cost of treatment and rehabilitation, and it has gained a supportive response from policymakers. From the child mental health perspective, DALYs have limitations in that they do not quantify negative or positive effects of behaviors but only address outcomes. As a result, the importance of behaviors that start during childhood and adolescence but result in disease and death only later in life may be underestimated by this approach.

While global partnerships and international collaboration is essential in advancing child mental health, efforts in this regard are still in their infancy. Hamoda and Belfer (24) note that the global health scene, including that of global child mental health is characterized by fragmentation, lack of coordination, and even confusion. Many global health initiatives have been criticized as being narrowly focused on specific diseases rather than systems-wide strengthening, tend to be "top-down" in nature and are largely driven by donor agendas rather than the country's own needs and priorities (25). Many of the initiatives also lack mechanisms of accountability, transparency, and evaluation (26).

CONTEXTUAL CONCERNS ASSOCIATED WITH MENTAL DYSFUNCTION

Displacement

The global problem of displacement from family, home, community, and country are of enormous importance to the mental health of populations. Displacement by war resulted in approximately 60 million refugees, and displaced people in 2015 many of whom are children and women (27). Fullilove (28) emphasizes the importance of "place" in the healthy development of individuals and clearly the displacement resulting from war, ethnic conflict, and famine undermine the ability to establish "place." Sampson et al. (29) specifically address the importance of the community as a mitigating influence on violence impacting children and adolescents. "Collective efficacy" and individual "agency" in communities are important concepts when one considers the impact of imposed poverty, housing disruption, and displacement in ethnic conflicts affecting previously closely aligned groups. In resource-poor countries, the notion of "place" and community are of equal or greater importance. Forced emigration and the loss of parents and relatives in war often mean abandonment or orphaning of children and adolescents. Although these stressors may serve to demonstrate the enormous resiliency of youth it must be recognized that there are significant psychological consequences that can lead to depression, suicide, and a range of stress responses that require informed intervention.

The problems of displacement from homes, families, communities, and countries affect children in a host of ways. Zivcić (30), in a study of Croatian children during war, found significantly higher depressive and phobic symptoms in displaced refugee children than in local children in stable social conditions. Laor et al. (31), in a developmental study of Israeli children exposed to Scud missile attacks, found higher externalizing and stress symptoms in displaced children as opposed to those able to maintain family and community connections. Children in these circumstances may find themselves without the protection and support of parents at critical junctures in their lives. Children are forced to act in more mature ways far earlier than normal development would dictate or allow. Displaced children are faced with exposure to war and violence that may have included seeing family members murdered. Less often, but even more horrific, some children have been forced into being the murderers of their family or conscripted to serve as child soldiers. Displaced children who need to survive on urban streets engage in survival tactics that include criminal activity and prostitution. In an effort to find a context for survival, the formation of youth gangs is increasingly evident, especially in societies where there is a lapse in government organization and control. More often than not, the children are the victims rather than the perpetrators.

Many refugees live in camps that have become "total institutions" with the attendant "process of mortification" (32). Dependency is a feature in many camps and especially in those that reproduce the authoritarian regimes from which the refugees escaped (33). Others are suffering from the multiple traumatic effects of torture. An outbreak of peace may mean fewer violent deaths, but entering the repatriation and resettlement phase of the cycle is yet another challenge for the disempowered (34,35).

Children Exposed to Conflict

The priority concern of global child and adolescent mental health is often the acute and continuing tragedies that involve youth in armed conflict or its aftermath. Eighty percent of the victims of war are reported to be children and women (36). The result of armed conflict is often displacement externally as refugees or asylum seekers or internally within settings of civil war. Thabet and Vostanis (37) investigated anxiety symptoms and disorders in children living in the Gaza strip and their relation to social adversities. Children reported high rates of significant anxiety problems and teachers reported high rates of mental health problems that would justify clinical assessment. Anxiety problems, particularly negative cognitions, increased with age and were significantly higher among girls. Low socioeconomic status (father unemployed or unskilled worker) was the strongest predictor of general mental health problems. Living in inner city areas or camps, both common among refugees, was strongly associated with anxiety problems. Among Syrian refugees displaced internally or as refugees more than half are children, and of these, nearly 75% are less than 12 years old (38).

Thabet et al. (39) examined the mental health profile among 322 Arab children living in the Gaza strip. Western categories of mental health problems did not clearly emerge from the factor analysis, the main difference appearing to operate in parents' perceptions of emotional problems in preschool children. The authors warn of the need to establish indigenously meaningful constructs within this population and culture, and subsequently revise measures of child mental health problems.

More attention is needed to culturally appropriate trauma therapy for children. Culture mediates the possible range of child responses (40). In older studies more than half of children exposed to war meet the criteria of posttraumatic stress disorder (PTSD) (41). With more experience the need to be cautious about the diagnosis of PTSD in children has emerged. Anxiety and depression are the disorders of primary concern. Symptoms should not be mistaken for disorders. Panter-Brick et al. (42) showed in her study of children exposed to war and violence in Afghanistan that the overwhelming concern of children even when witnessing death was the day-to-day anxieties associated with family issues, school, and peers. Cartwright et al. (43) found that among a sample of Syrian refugee children in Turkey nearly half had clinically significant levels of anxiety or withdrawal, and almost two thirds were fearful. Several reports (44–47) have shown a variety of psychosocial difficulties among Syrian refugee children including insomnia, sadness, grieving and depression, aggression and behavioral problems, nervousness, regression, hyperactivity, speech problems, and somatic symptoms.

"Child Soldiers" and Exploitation of Children

In the turmoil of some resource-poor countries, children are now being forced to become child soldiers, and others are drawn into the conflict as sexual slaves. Child soldiers reportedly suffer PTSD (48–53). Somasundaram states that to prevent children becoming soldiers we need first to understand why children choose to fight due to push factors (traumatization, brutalization, deprivation, institutionalized violence, and sociocultural factors) and pull factors (military drill from early childhood), as well as society's complicity (54).

These horrific experiences place an as yet undefined burden on the psychological development of the victim. Understanding these experiences may shed additional light on the extremes to which resiliency may allow future healthy development, but perhaps more likely it will demonstrate the more permanent scarring evidenced in disturbed interpersonal relationships, distorted defenses, heightened aggression, reduced empathy, and self-destructive behavior. The data are not yet available to ascertain whether these young people evidence PTSD in the classic sense or whether, because of the early age of induction into the culture of war, they develop in a different way as a survival response. Huge challenges face child mental health clinicians in helping to reclaim the lives of former child soldiers (55,56).

As for trafficking in children, worldwide, in 2015 an estimated 1.2 million children are forced into prostitution or trafficked every year and the total number of prostituted children could be as high as 10 million (57). Children are trafficked worldwide (58–66). The most urgent attention is paid to combating the trafficking (67), but the management of the psychological sequelae for the children will need to be given further attention. Nongovernmental organizations have been taking a lead in developing programs for children and adolescents freed from trafficking. Another issue of concern is the trafficking of children for child labor and other forms of exploitation. The International Labor Organization has taken this up as a major concern (68). The psychological consequences of child labor are complex, involving distorted relationships of children to their families and the assumption of adult roles prematurely.

HIV/AIDS

In sub-Saharan Africa, Russia, and parts of Asia, acquired immunodeficiency syndrome (AIDS) continues to be a major health concern (69). As documented by Carlson and Earls (70), whether through social policy as evidenced in the Leagane children of Romania, or as the consequence of the pandemic of AIDS, the rearing of children in orphanages or in other situations that deprive children of appropriate stimulation and nurturance has potentially long-lasting consequences for societies. Those infected but struggling with the illness face the prospect of having to adjust to declining physical and mental functioning and often living isolated lives. Thus, the mental health consequences of AIDS as a chronic and pervasive illness must be considered. There is the obvious concern with the direct effect of AIDS on the youth with manifestations of neuropsychological dysfunction including dementia, depression, and other disorders, which go largely untreated. Access to antiretroviral drugs is often denied or difficult to access due to economic or discriminatory policies. Special attention needs to be given to the consequences of AIDS on children and youth. The direct impact on children and adolescents is evident in India, other parts of Asia, and Africa, where sexual exploitation has led to a high incidence of youth infected. With wider use of antiretroviral medications the challenge has shifted to provide for a healthy living environment for those who are often discriminated against.

Substance Abuse

Substance abuse in children and adolescents is a worldwide problem (71). In resource-poor countries, the problem is of no less importance than in Western countries and exacts a tremendous toll in terms of morbidity and mortality. Illicit drugs and psychoactive substances not defined as drugs of abuse (such as khat, inhalants, and alcohol) are used by youth regardless of economic circumstance or religious prohibition. Risk factors, while sharing features in common, vary by cultural context, for example in Turkey (72) or Lebanon (73). Due to prohibition in some Muslim countries official data on alcohol use and abuse is very limited. Remarkably in some Muslim countries, alcohol use and abuse are significant contributors to psychological morbidity (74). Khat or miraa (Catha edulis) is used extensively in East Africa and the Middle East. In Somalia, Ethiopia, and Kenya, the leaves of khat are chewed at all levels of society from about the age of 10 (75). Khat may induce a mild euphoria and excitement that can progress to hypomania. In youth, khat use, especially if it is combined with the use of other psychoactive substances, may lead to psychosis.

Homeless street children are now found worldwide and appear particularly vulnerable to substance abuse and other high-risk behavior (76). Senanayake et al. (77) studied the background, life styles, health, and prevalence of abuse of street children in Colombo. Family disintegration was mentioned as the cause for life on the streets by 36%; child labor was reported in 38%; 16% admitted to being sexually abused; 20% were tobacco smokers. Homeless children also are prominent among those groups using inhalants and who are caught in cycles of physical and sexual abuse, often under the influence of drugs. Road accidents among those using drugs are also high.

Solvent and inhalant use is associated with poor economies. In South America, inhalant use is a dominant factor in the presentation of youth affected by psychoactive substances. In São Paolo, Brazil it is reported that up to 25% of children age 9 to 18 years abuse solvents (78). In the Sudan, gasoline is the inhalant of choice, whereas in Mexico, Brazil, and elsewhere in Latin America, paint thinner, plastic cement, shoe dye, and industrial glue are often used. Solvent use is also found among the aboriginal groups in Australia and on Native Canadian reservations (79). In Mexico, 3 of every 1,000 people between the ages of 14 and 24 years use inhalants on a regular basis (80). These figures do not include two high-risk groups, the homeless population and those less than 14 years old, whose rates of inhalant abuse are much greater. Several community studies carried out in different parts of Mexico show that starting ages are as young as 5 or 6 years (80). Data suggest that the percentage of young people using inhalants decreases with age, as other substances such as alcohol and marijuana are substituted. Inhalant use decreases as educational level increases (81).

Wittig et al. (82) examine the hypothesis that drug use among Honduran street children is a function of developmental social isolation from cultural and structural influences. Data from 1,244 children working and/or living on the streets of Tegucigalpa are described, separating "market" from "street" children. The latter group is then divided into those who sniff glue and those who do not to identify salient distinguishing factors. Family relations, length of time on the street, and delinquency are the most important factors.

Forster et al. (83) studied the self-reported activities engaged in by children found wandering on the streets of Porto Alegre, Brazil, aiming to describe their drug abuse habits and practice of thefts or mendicancy. Regular abuse of inhalants was reported much more frequently by the street subgroup of children, reaching a prevalence of 40%. The practice of theft was self-reported mainly by the children from the street group and only by the ones who used illicit drugs. These results show that very poor children might spend many hours of the day by themselves in the streets of a big city accompanied by children who are never under adult supervision. In spite of being alone for some hours a day and making friends with others who might use drugs, having a family and regularly attending school decreases the risk of delinquent acts and drug use.

Violence and Abuse

Violence to and by children and adolescents now appears to be all too prevalent worldwide (84). Bullying, corporal punishment, victimization of parents by children and adolescents has now been reported worldwide. It is beyond the scope of this chapter to address all forms of violence; it will focus on specifics related to child abuse. Understanding child abuse requires understanding the vast cultural diversity in which children and adolescents live, and there is a need for greater attention to be given to possible country-specific interventions (85). What is termed abuse varies between cultures.

There are differences in cross-cultural definitions, incidence in developed and developing countries across continents, and measures that have been instituted to prevent and manage child maltreatment (86). The literature suggests that child maltreatment is less likely in countries in which children are highly valued for their economic utility, for perpetuating family lines, and as sources of emotional pleasure and satisfaction. However, even in societies that value children, some children are valued more than others (87). Ethnicity has been found to play a role in the epidemiology of pediatric injury (88). There is a diverse culture-specific literature on abuse (89–91).

There are reports of structural models of the determinants of harsh parenting, for example, among Mexican mothers, where cultural beliefs play a major role in parenting within the framework of Mexican family relations (92). Changing cultural norms and attitudes in a given setting (e.g., Korea) can lead to children being at risk of abuse in the name of discipline or other seemingly appropriate parental or authority responses (93–95). Child abuse might increase in certain cultural groups as a result of cultural change rather than emerging from their traditions (96). Child psychiatrists with insufficient awareness about normative practices by parents, for example, dermabrasion or cao gao in Vietnam (97), may jump to the conclusion that hematomas around the child's head, neck, or chest signal that the parents may have been wrongdoers who abused their child. A culturally competent child psychiatrist, while not dismissing abuse out of hand, would also evaluate the alternative possibility, that the parents, with the best interests of the child in mind, submitted him/her to ritual treatment, for which the bruising acts as a public signal to the community that the child has been unwell.

Shalhoub-Kevorkian (98) reported a survey of victims of sexual abuse among Palestinian Israeli girls aged 14 to 16 years. Data revealed that the girls' attitudes not only conformed to general findings on disclosure of sexual abuse but also reflected sociopolitical fears and stressors. Helpers struggled between their beliefs that they should abide by the state's formal legal policies and their consideration of the victim's context. The study reveals how decontextualizing child protection laws and policies can keep sexually abused girls from seeking help.

The legal implications of child abuse are affected by practices which may be normative in certain cultural settings, for example, female genital mutilation (99). Some ethnic groups may carry out procedures on their children as a sign of caring rather than as a punitive measure. For instance in Cambodian and Vietnam there are cases with facial burns associated with what was termed "innocent cultural belief" (100). Thus, factors that lead to underreporting by physicians have included ethnic and cultural issues (101). Ethnographic data point to the importance of the social fabric in accounting for differences in child maltreatment report rates by predominant neighborhood ethnicity (102). There can be mismatches between the definition of child abuse between the culture of the professional and the culture of the families (103). There is much to be learned about the use of cultural evidence in child maltreatment law (104).

Case Illustration

Child abuse is subject to the definitions of various audiences rather than being intrinsic to the act. There are a few studies concerning the effect of culture and context of the professionals (as opposed to the families)—as in a study of Palestinian health/social workers where people agreed on what was child abuse but disagreed on when it should be reported. The results indicated a high level of agreement among students in viewing situations of abuse as well as neglect as maltreatment. Differences were found in their willingness to report situations of maltreatment. An inclination was found among students to minimize social and cultural factors as risk factors and to disregard signs that did not contain explicit signals of danger as characteristics of maltreated children (105). Baker and Dwairy (106) examined intervention in sexual abuse cases among the Palestinian community in Israel. They suggest that in many collective societies people live in interdependence with their families. Enforcing the laws against sexual perpetrators typically threatens the unity and reputation of the family, and therefore this option is rejected and the family turns against the victim. Instead of punishing the perpetrator, families often protect him and blame the victim. The punishment of the abuser results in the re-victimization of the abused since the family possesses authority. Baker and Dwairy (106) suggest a culturally sensitive model of intervention that includes a condemning, apologizing, and punishing ceremony. In this way, exploiting the power of the family for the benefit of the victim of abuse before enforcing the law may achieve the same legal objectives as state intervention, without threatening the reputation and the unity of the family, and therefore save the victim from harm.

TAXONOMY AND CLASSIFICATION

Munir and Beardslee (107) are critical of DSM approaches and propose a developmental and psychobiologic framework for understanding the role of culture in child and adolescent psychiatry. Kriegler (108), taking a social constructivist perspective on the potential relevance of DSM-5 disorders for South African children and youth, regarding PTSD and attention deficit hyperactivity disorder (ADHD), demonstrates that these psychiatric labels are impracticable and irrelevant in a postcolonial developing country, where mental health care is delivered in the context of scarce services and unequal access. Beauchaine (109) notes that developmental psychopathologists have criticized categorical classification systems for their inability to account for within-generation heterogeneity in cultural influences on behavior. Novins et al. (110) attempted cultural case formulations for four American Indian children and identified several gaps concerning cultural identity and cultural elements of the therapeutic relationship.

Culture and Assessment

There has been a growing recognition in child psychiatry in Western settings to consider cultural context in the assessment of psychopathology (10). A culturally competent framework for assessment in resource-poor countries, while sorely needed, has not been developed. A simplistic attribution to culture of seemingly bizarre symptoms that in fact represent treatable mental illness would deflect energy from the development of effective treatment and prevention efforts. At the same time, an understanding of the cultural construction of major psychiatric disorders (including culture-bound disorders affecting young people) would minimize inaccurate diagnoses. This view has to be balanced with the understanding of less severe psychopathology, in which the observation of Neki (111) holds true, that ethnodynamics determine psychodynamics. In India, where the cultural ideal of an independent adult is not an autonomous adult, dependency is inculcated from childhood through a prolonged dependency relationship between mother and child. Dependency has a negative, pejorative connotation in Western thought, which is not so in the Indian context. The fostering of dependency is coupled with a high degree of control, low autonomy, and strict discipline, enforced within the broad framework of the family system. When this is identified by clinicians as representing a degree of pathology, decreased emphasis on the expression of thoughts and emotions in children could explain the greater preponderance of neurotic, psychosomatic, and somatization disorders (112). Thus, cultural context influences the definition of normalcy or disorder. It proscribes the values and ideals for the behavior of individuals, it determines the threshold of acceptance of pathology, and it provides guidelines for the handling of pathology and its correction (113).

Cultural issues also affect assessment because of problems with cultural validation of instruments. A German study showed problems in applying the United States factor structure of the Conners Parent Rating Scale (CPRS), with lack of correspondence of the impulsiveness/hyperactivity scale (114). The factor structure of scores of the CPRS has been examined among Nepali children (115). A Greek study of the Conners-28 teacher questionnaire in a Greek community sample of primary schoolchildren found that the factor structure was similar to that originally reported by the United States, with a high level of discrimination between the referred and nonreferred sample, especially for the inattentive-passive scale (116).

Rey et al. (117) noted the lack of simple, reliable measures of the quality of the environment in which a child was reared which could be used in clinical research and practice. They developed a global scale to appraise retrospectively the quality of that environment and found good interrater reliability with clinicians from Australia, Hong Kong, and the People's Republic of China. Goodman et al. (118) developed a computerized algorithm to predict child psychiatric diagnoses on the basis of the symptom and impact scores derived from Strengths and Difficulties Questionnaire (SDQ) completed by parents, teachers, and young people. The predictive algorithm generates ratings for conduct disorders, emotional disorders, hyperactivity disorders, and any psychiatric disorder. The algorithm was applied to patients attending child mental health clinics in Britain and Bangladesh. SDQ prediction for any given disorder correctly identified 81% to 91% of the children who had that diagnosis.

Epidemiology

Determining the epidemiology of childhood mental disorders in Western society is a challenge. On the international scene, the ability to determine the precise magnitude of mental disorders is even more complex. Reporting systems are inadequate, the definition or recognition of disorders varies or has variable interpretations, and the cultural component of what constitutes a disorder is only now being more fully appreciated by epidemiologists and researchers. Of significance in resource-poor countries is that any measure of mental disorder takes place against a background of child and adolescent mortality and morbidity that makes the epidemiology of psychiatric disorder is not only inaccurate, but often of a lower priority. Thus, in studying the epidemiology of psychiatric disorder in children and adolescents in resource-poor countries, it is important to define not only the prevalence and incidence of the disorders, but also the degree of impairment and burden of disease. No single study or consistent set of independent studies on the epidemiology of child and adolescent disorders since 1980 can be identified as definitive or relevant across societies. Those studies carried out in the 1980s reflect the deficiencies noted earlier and certainly do not reflect the current realities of the countries from which the data were reported (119,120). Weiss has defined a new epidemiological approach combining qualitative study with classic epidemiologic methods (121–123). This new "cultural epidemiologic" approach has not yet been applied to child and adolescent mental disorders but holds the promise of gaining a more satisfactory understanding of the nature and extent of child and adolescent mental disorders worldwide.

Until now, when one has been faced with the realities of resource-poor countries, as noted, there is the danger of becoming a diagnostic nihilist in attempting to understand mental disorders in youth. However, for example, responsible investigators in Western Ethiopia clearly identified disordered mental functioning that meets a set of defined criteria (124). There is clear evidence that depression, psychosis, and mania can be defined and treated. The problem arises when one considers the context for the presentation of child and adolescent mental disorders. Is a hallucination during a ritual a disturbance in need of treatment? If the hallucination persists, should it be treated? What diagnostic label is appropriate? Giel and Van Luijk (125) found, in the pre-HIV/AIDS era, and counter to prevailing belief, that mental disorders were diagnosed more frequently than infectious diseases in the health centers in Africa that they studied. Until reporting is adequate and accurate, it cannot be assumed that the current state of mental health in the developing world actually supports the too prevalent minimalist and optimistic view. This sense is supported by the finding from WHO studies of primary care clinicians that showed that many patients seeking care had mental disorders, and their communities were aware of the problem (126). In the current era, Omigbodun (127) documented the psychosocial problems in a child and adolescent psychiatric clinic population in Nigeria: 62.2% of new referrals to the clinic had significant psychosocial stressors in the year preceding presentation. Problems with primary support, such as separation from parents to live with relatives, disruption of the family, abandonment by the mother, psychiatric illness in a parent, and sexual/physical abuse occurred in 39.4%. Significantly more children and adolescents with disruptive behavior disorders and disorders like enuresis, separation anxiety, and suicidal behavior had psychosocial stressors when compared to children with psychotic conditions, autistic disorder, and epilepsy.

Prevalence

Although it is interesting to consider epidemiological reports of more esoteric disorders, these are a distraction from the significant burden of disease that needs to be addressed in the mainstream of care. In most studies, the methodological inadequacies and other constraints do not permit these studies to be of use for program planning nor needs assessment. However, most countries today have access to appropriate epidemiologic study guidelines, and it is a matter of setting a national priority and allocating resources to ascertain the data.

What of the disorders that now occupy considerable attention in developed countries such as ADHD, autism, and anorexia nervosa? The diagnosis and treatment of these disorders highlight both weakness and strength of having an international perspective. The recognition and labeling of disorders come as a result of improved international communication. However, the process of assessment must take into account a host of cultural as well as formal diagnostic criteria, and this is too often ignored. Cultural concepts of what is normal or abnormal and how parents perceive the presence or absence of a diagnosable disorder are essential to consider (128). In the case of eating disorders, there is clear evidence that the incidence may be affected by Western influences (129). In the diagnosis of ADHD pharmaceutical companies are now a primary source of both public and professional education and they often focus on the use of the diagnosis for the purpose of implementing a pharmacological intervention. This trend may provide an indirect incentive for the overdiagnosis of disorders such as ADHD and bipolar disorder. The understanding of the influence of increased public education on diagnosis requires further study (130).

Fayyad et al. (131), discussing the development of systems of care in resource-poor countries, focuses on ADHD and the development of a comprehensive system of care around it in Lebanon. In a study of adolescents in Bahrain diagnosed with adjustment disorder, al-Ansari and Matar (132) examined the type of life stressors that initiated their referrals to a child psychiatry unit. Disappointment in relationships with a family member or with a friend of the opposite sex was found to be the main stressor. Eating disorders classically are rare in resource-poor countries such as India (133), but anecdotal evidence suggests that with globalization and migration the rates are increasing (134–137). Autism is reported around the world, including in resource-poor countries (138–140), and with a cross-national consistency (141,142).

Specific Mental Disorders

In an earlier version of this chapter considerable attention was devoted to individual mental disorders as seen in countries around the world. It is now evident that with comparable methodologies there is little variation between countries in terms of formal diagnoses. Giel et al. (128) demonstrated in four countries (Sudan, Philippines, Colombia, and India) that between 12% and 29% of children aged 5 to 15 years showed mental health problems. The types of disorder identified in these resource-poor countries were reported as being no different from those encountered in industrialized countries. Thabet and Vostanis (37) state that their findings do not support the commonly held belief that in non-Western societies anxiety and other mental health symptoms are predominantly expressed through somatizing symptoms. Citing Nikapota, Thabet and Vostanis (37) state that child mental health symptoms do not differ significantly across cultures and culture-specific mental health disorders are rare. A cross-cultural evaluation of depression in children in Egypt, Kuwait, and the United States showed similar clinical patterns (143).

More important is an understanding that the current diagnostic nomenclatures are limited in given full expression to the nature of distress and the degree of impairment experienced. Furthermore, considerable attention needs to be paid to specific cultural overlays on the disorders seen. Developing countries give added insight to understanding the importance of considering dimensional as opposed to categorical diagnoses.

The impact of "big pharma" in developing countries—which has been called "Bad Pharma, Bad Karma" (144) has often skewed the assessment of the true prevalence of disorders and influenced the diagnoses of disorders. There needs to be a balance between an understanding of the beneficial effects of medication and the need to provide "rational" care, that is, the use of psychosocial treatments as a first line of care.

Of concern is the implementation of clinical interventions that may inadvertently lead to an exacerbation or prolongation of symptoms: For example, the use of "ventilation" and retelling of the trauma through various means has been shown to have negative effects (145), whereas reestablishing families and returning to normal routines, including school attendance, has a salutary impact.

Suicide

Suicide in youth is a pervasive world mental health problem. In Western cultures, suicide is overwhelmingly associated with defined mental illness. Suicide is the second leading cause of death for American Indian and Alaska Native youth (146). Elsewhere in the world, it may be very difficult to identify the mental illness associated with the suicidal act—and in the face of overwhelming helplessness; suicide may appear from the perspective of the protagonists as the only way out, with no clearly labeled mental illness. Doing qualitative research on suicide in a developing country poses special challenges (147). Studies of suicide in the West have focused on risk factors associated with cognitive distortions, substance use, and familial factors (148). In trying to assess the high rates of suicide in some resource-poor countries, it appears that the balance in determining suicidal risk may rest with environmental stressors and the perception of no way out. Expectations may often be more determinant of suicidal angst than reality (149). According to one view expressed by Murthy (150), the traditional protective effect of religion in certain cultures seems not to operate among the younger generation.

Chan et al. (151) consider suicide in China as a response to change due to globalization, in which Chinese values are more closely identified with the global culture. The high suicide rate is thus not seen as a reflection of psychiatric disorder but of sociocultural factors. It seems more apparent that suicide is viewed by those without demonstrable mental illness as a solution to social and personal dilemmas that bring with them thwarted expectations for a happy or successful life. For example, from this perspective, in India and in other resource-poor countries, the focus of the suicidal individual is not on achieving some exalted goal, but on being able to have enough of a dowry to be married, to not be isolated because of rape, or to be successful in passing a school advancement examination. This relative alteration in emphasis is important in the consideration of intervention strategies and in the training of workers to perform triage and to treat suicidal children and adolescents. A survey of adolescent health in nine Caribbean countries identified risk and protective factors predisposing to suicide attempts (152). In Hong Kong, amid the impressive high-rise buildings and fancy stores, reside families barely able to subsist. In this context of economic hardship, the result in part of massive economic adjustment in the Far East, the phenomenon of family suicide exists. Chan reports that families come together and, in a well-planned manner, seal themselves in their small apartments and light a charcoal heater (153). In a relatively brief time, the members of the family are asphyxiated. This has become an acceptable form of suicide in that the bodies remain intact and have an attractive appearance because of the monoxide poisoning. To the extent that it has been possible to determine the psychological state of the family before the suicides, major psychiatric disturbance has not been reported.

In a review Lester (154) notes that suicide rates have been reported to be lower in Muslims than in those of other religions even in countries that have populations belonging to several religious groups. However, rates of attempted suicide, on the other hand, do not appear to be lower in Muslims as compared to non-Muslims. The reports of suicide being lower in Muslim countries has been challenged though by the notion that suicide has been poorly studied in these countries and that some Muslim countries do not collect such data and/or do not report them to the WHO (155). Similar questions have also been raised about lower suicide rates in Catholic countries. Kelleher et al. (156) note that the average reported rates of suicide for countries with religious sanctions are lower than those for countries without religious sanctions. However, recording and reporting for those countries may be affected by the existence of sanctions, thus diminishing the reliability of reported rates.

Case Illustration

In India, four sisters aged 16 to 24 years committed suicide by hanging after an evening during which they bought sweet cakes and samosas and played word games. The context was that they were part of a once prosperous family in which the father died of tuberculosis for lack of medical treatment. Now they were periodically without sufficient food, but with a mother too proud to ask for help. This family was socially isolated because of parental marriage across religious lines, and they had suffered an unexpected financial downturn as a result of a road-widening project that took their once-fertile land. Suicide rates in India, although lower than the international average of 16 per 100,000, have been steadily rising. Psychiatrists believe this is in part a result of the accelerating pace of social and economic change. Whereas the biggest risk factor in the West is mental illness, studies in India have consistently found that the dominant risk factor is a combination of social and economic strain. Farmers in debt may take pesticide, and ostracized women who are victims of the dowry system in economically stretched circumstances might immolate themselves (157).

Disabilities, Intellectual Disability, and Epilepsy

Disability—whether physical or mental—is all too common in resource-poor countries, especially those post conflict. In Cambodia, for example, between 2% and 3% of the population, or about 1 out of every 40 Cambodians, have physical disabilities (including 50,000 landmine survivors, many of them young people; 60,000 with paralysis from polio; 100,000 who are blind; 120,000 who are deaf; 102,000 to 178,500 with intellectual disability; 20,400 to 40,800 people with severe mental disorders; and 154,000 to 408,000 people with epilepsy) (158,159).

Intellectual disability and epilepsy are major disorders that often dominate the services of child mental health and pediatric professionals in resource-poor countries. Intellectual disability and epilepsy are the most common mental disorders in India (160). The rate of serious intellectual disability in some resource-poor countries ranges from 5 to 16.2 per 1,000 population (161,162), significantly higher than the rate in the West. Cerebral palsy and postnatal causes of intellectual disability are much more common in transitional societies than in developed countries. Untreated epilepsy limits a person's potential to participate in society. Unfortunately, although the cost of medication is relatively low, access to care is often limited. The care of the intellectually disabled varies widely in resource-poor countries. In some countries, special effort is made to provide for productive lives with meaningful vocational education, especially in agrarian economies. All too often, the moderately and severely retarded are housed in minimal care institutions where premature death and illness are common.

Kim and Kumar (163) describe Dohsa-hou as a Japanese psychological rehabilitation method widely used in Japan for children with intellectual disability, cerebral palsy, and autism. The focus is to improve bodily movements and posture as well as to introduce social support to patients and their first-degree relatives. Analysis showed mothers got more social support interacting with their child's trainer and supervisor during Dohsa-hou. Trainers were more interactive than mothers in the Indian group, followed by the Japanese and Korean cultural groups.

Children with disability such as epilepsy are among the most marginalized in many resource-poor countries. In Cambodia, for example, they have limited access to education, vocational training, employment, and income-generating opportunities and other services. Childhood epilepsy is viewed traditionally as caused by the attack of the preceding mother from the previous incarnation of the infant, and treatment may be sought by parents from kruu, or traditional healers, to ward off her attacks. The children may be cared for in the Buddhist temple, or kept indoors out of the sight of neighbors.

SERVICES

The World Health Organization (WHO), through the Atlas project, has developed the first objective profile of resources for services related to child and adolescent mental health (164). The findings confirm the worldwide gap in services to address child and adolescent mental health (165); the gaps exist in both resource-poor and resource-rich countries. The lack of services is tied to insufficient and unstable financing, lack of trained professionals, and lack of policy to support the development of child and adolescent mental health services.

Resource-poor countries lack the child mental health personnel to mount large-scale programs of treatment with fully trained staff members. The prospect of training large numbers of child mental health workers remains a continuing goal, whereas the training of child and adolescent psychiatrists to meet the potential need is beyond the realm of possibility. In the interim, what can be done to provide a way to intervene for the promotion of child mental health? Obviously, one focus is on developing prevention programs in general health and education systems. Second, training primary care practitioners from numerous disciplines is needed to provide basic child mental health services. Basic assessment and treatment are possible, with triage of the most severely disturbed. In a WHO Atlas project focusing on the Eastern Mediterranean Region (166) it was noted that only 67% of countries surveyed had a system for providing inpatient mental health care for children and adolescents, only 53% of the reporting countries include information about child and adolescent mental health in their annual health reports and the majority of countries in the region lack national standards of car for child and adolescent mental health.

McKelvey et al. (167) illustrate the differing priorities for child psychiatric services in Vietnam, where there is a focus on infectious diseases and malnutrition. Treatment is reserved for the most severely afflicted, especially patients with epilepsy and intellectual disability. Specialized care is available in only a few urban centers. In rural areas treatment is provided by allied health personnel, paraprofessionals, and community organizations.

In some countries, the lack of child mental health personnel has stimulated some remarkable efforts to train persons from diverse backgrounds to be effective in identifying and intervening to ameliorate child mental health problems. In Alexandria, Egypt, child counselors have been trained to develop sophisticated interventions in schools (168).

Program Illustration

In Alexandria, the Department of Community Medicine has supported the development of a cadre of school counselors.

These counselors come from the ranks of volunteers, social workers, and psychologists. Without prior child mental health training, the workers are provided with coursework on common child mental health problems and then are supervised in field placements. The counselors work with parents around children identified by both the school and parents as having some type of behavioral problem. They also serve as contact points for the school, parents, or pediatricians to bring children with more severe behavioral disturbance to the attention of the few fully trained mental health professionals.

Leaders in child mental health programming in resource-poor countries are emphatic when faced with the reality of program implementation that Western models of care by specialists are neither feasible nor desirable. Indigenous methods and models of care need to be developed that are not dependent on specialists. Conversely, the development of these models that use parents, teachers, pediatricians, and others can be informed by the best thinking of child psychiatrists and other specialists. This has led to an emphasis on the training of primary care practitioners. Furthermore, short-term, focused training in specific areas related to diagnosis or intervention can be provided by specialists or through specialized child psychiatric centers that have a broad regional or national area of responsibility.

The development of child mental health training for primary care practitioners is well established in many sites, but the WHO Atlas documents and other studies document that the utilization of primary care providers falls far short of the goal in both developing and developed countries (164,169). Murthy (9) describes the use of primary health care providers in resource-poor countries. In India, with 1.5 billion people, there are only 5,000 mental health providers—of whom only a fraction are psychiatrists—35,000 psychiatric beds, and a dearth of emergency services. The primary care provider, when adequately trained, is a valuable and essential point of contact and treatment for the mentally ill. In India, it has been demonstrated that primary care providers can provide a level of professional care that reduces morbidity and mortality. However, without appropriate training, primary practitioners have been shown to have a poor record of recognizing mental disorders. Giel et al. (169) report in their study in resource-poor countries that primary care practitioners identified only 10% to 20% of the disorders that the researchers were able to diagnose. WHO has devoted considerable efforts to the development and distribution of training manuals to aid primary care practitioners in the recognition of child mental disorders (170,171).

Moreover, India has developed the anganwadi system to provide basic nutrition and educational support in villages. This is both an appropriate preventive intervention and a way to assess youngsters presenting with disorders (172). The anganwadi system focuses on providing essential services to very young children. Like Head Start, the program provides nutrition, basic education, socialization, and a venue for more specialized intervention for children perceived to be at risk or in need of additional services (172). There must be a concern in the development of these indigenous systems of care that not too much dependence be placed on family structure and support at a time when urbanization and industrialization are eroding the traditional family structure. With the absence of security, and often living at a subsistence level, the new nuclear family faces previously unknown challenges and may be particularly vulnerable over this and the next generation.

Some programs are international in scope. For instance, WHO, as part of its Program on Mental Health, fostered the use of life skills education (173). The goal of the Life Skills Program is to foster psychosocial competence. For children and adolescents, the Life Skills Program is taught in schools. The program itself as promulgated by WHO is based on the social learning theory of Bandura (174). Many similar models are operative throughout the world. A "training the trainer" component affects the overall resource of a community to provide for the mental health needs of some children and adolescents who are at risk. The "training the trainer" model has now been critiqued in an effort to improve outcomes from such programs (175). Among the obvious limitations in the developing world are the absence of universal education and the capacities of the teachers to go beyond essential educational tasks. Kapur et al. (176) demonstrate that the training of teachers as counselors was effective in India.

The prospect for the future of child mental health practice in resource-poor countries is tied to economic growth, health literacy, and reduction of stigma. The creative efforts to develop programs to reach children and adolescents in resource-poor countries need to be supported. Child and adolescent psychiatry will remain a scarce resource to be used in ways that will have a duplicative impact. This means that the training of volunteers, the training of peers, the support of family intervention programming, and the use of community-based early intervention need to be the focus of attention. Kim (177) proposed a curriculum guideline of cultural competence for child and adolescent psychiatric residencies. These guidelines stress ethnogeneric and developmental perspectives, which can be expanded further to include ethnospecific issues depending on the needs of each training program.

The notion of a continuum of care as advocated as a goal in developed countries is but a fantasy in the developing world, where there remains a reliance on inpatient care for the most seriously disturbed, and where outpatient care is often sparse. In some developing countries the Western model of managed care and the institution of various insurance schemes are underway. Unfortunately, the negative consequences of these aspects of care systems are too often unrecognized. In some countries the introduction of insurance has had the unintended consequence of reducing access for uncovered populations and has led to flight of health professionals into the private sector.

RESEARCH

Ordóñez and Collins (178) call for advancing research to action in global child mental health. They point out that although 90% of the world's children live in developing countries, only 10% of randomized control trials testing mental health interventions for children. The grand challenges included the development of locally appropriate strategies to eliminate childhood abuse and enhance protection and to reduce the duration of illness by developing culturally sensitive interventions across settings. Cullins and Mian (179) adduce evidence for the integration of culture into meeting the global challenges in child and adolescent mental health. Techniques include task shifting and the incorporation of culture into evidence-based research and into its implementation.

Patel and Kim (180) reviewed original research contributions from LAMI countries published over a 3-year period in the six highest-impact general psychiatry journals and found that only 3.7% of published research comes from LAMI countries, which account for over 80% of the global population. The authors proposed several explanations for their findings including the low proportion of submissions from LAMI countries, the possibility that authors might be choosing local journals for their research, and the low research output and research capacity in these countries. In addition the authors suggested other potential explanations on why articles from LAMI countries are more likely to be rejected including the quality of the research and editorial and reviewers attitudes toward articles from these countries, a view shared by others (181).

Earls and Eisenberg (182) highlight three areas for enhanced research activity in relation to child and adolescent mental health. First is research to understand how the changes in contemporary society are reflected in the prevalence and incidence of mental disorders. Second is research to enhance the understanding of how different childrearing methods affect normal and deviant behavioral and emotional development. Third involves research on the design and delivery of mental health services. Mohler (183) describes and discusses the major challenges in cross-cultural research on child mental health. Nelson and Quintana (184) present strategies for designing and conducting qualitative investigations, and address ethical issues involved in conducting qualitative research with minors. International child development and mental health studies often call for a mixed-methods approach (185).

Hamoda and Belfer (24) note that while the obstacles to collaboration internationally are understandable they can be overcome with careful planning, development of trusting relationships, and attention to seemingly mundane impediments, such as, language, financial transactions, International Review Board approvals, among others. Eisenbruch (186) has defined a template for the steps needed to ensure cultural competence in research, namely cultural competence in community engagement, communicating with research subjects, design, cross-cultural validation of research instruments, sampling, calibrating diversity variables, demographic variables measured in datasets, research ethics, data collection techniques, data processing and analysis, and dissemination and action. Culturally competent community engagement by the researcher, for example, depends on (a) building community partnerships; (b) developing interventions that are acceptable and relevant; (c) promoting successful recruitment, participation, and retention of participants; and (d) developing a diverse, cohesive, and committed research team and effective managerial information support systems. International child psychiatry research program should pay attention to participation from the perspective of community members (187). International child psychiatric research should avoid sampling barriers among culturally diverse communities to do, for example, with lack of tolerance of diverse groups, social stigma, concern for issues of confidentiality, and fear of exposure because of possible threats to security (188,189). The research should avoid the use of instruments developed in one culture transferred to another given the cultural differences in the interpretation of certain items. The research should avoid definition of diversity with only a single variable. Cultural, racial, religious, and immigrant groups are not homogeneous (190). For example, any one population includes native-born, migrant, and immigrant peoples with distinctive national origins and regional settlement patterns, and varied and complex demographic structures. Data collection should be clear about descriptions of ethnic or racial measurement and reasons for including or excluding clearly defined populations. The research should be open to innovative recipes for data collection, for example, as proposed by Roszak (191) with clarity about (1) who provides information; (2) when data are collected; (3) which racial and ethnic categories are used—all hospitals should use standard racial and ethnic categories; (4) how data are stored; and (5) responses to patients' concerns. Nikapota (1) underscores the importance of determining "culture-appropriate" criteria to permit consistency in diagnosis. In doing research, it is important to consider the characteristics of the interviewer as well as the informant.

Fontes (192), drawing on his experiences conducting research on sexual abuse in a shantytown in Chile and with Puerto Ricans, examined ethical issues in cross-cultural research on family violence. It was emphasized that special attention needs to be given to informed consent, definition of the sample, composition of the research team, research methods, and potential harm and benefit. Munir and Earls (193) articulate a set of ethical parameters for research that must be considered in doing research among children and adolescents of resource-poor countries. To apply a different standard justified by the difficulty of implementing protocols would violate the very support of a rights framework so essential for progress to be made on behalf of children in resource-poor countries.

An area of great interest is the development of assessment tools that incorporate the diversity of cultural parameters. Increasing numbers of instruments have been translated and back-translated for use in cross-cultural studies. Instruments exist for the assessment of depression, anxiety, PTSD, quality of life, and other conditions. It remains for there to be a sufficient body of cross-cultural research with modern standards for the conduct of the research that yields information on the reliability and validity of the instruments in their revised versions. Few instruments meet an agreed standard for use across all cultures in their current form.

As described by Earls (194) compulsory schooling leads to the need to understand the impact of learning disorders better. The appropriate diagnosis and remediation of these disorders are first-order priorities in countries where technologic advance places a premium on knowledge acquisition and use. As yet, research in this area has not been implemented in resource-poor countries, but the pressure to implement such studies is mounting.

Research into the understanding of the differential impact of childrearing methods should be an area of collaborative inquiry between those interested in mental health and those concerned with the role of women and the family in evolving societies. It is not evident that any one method of childrearing is superior to another. Perhaps developing and developed societies can learn from one another about the optimal methods for childrearing in the presence of the evolution of individual societies. The experience with the effects of urbanization, industrialization, changing roles of women, and increased survivorship of children in developed countries may form the basis for translation into the programs for resource-poor countries. Conversely, the healthy development of youngsters growing up in adversity in resource-poor countries may provide information on how to enhance understanding and to develop new interventions for children at risk in developed countries.

Attention needs to be focused on the important developments in global and international child mental health that are published in peer reviewed journals in languages other than English. A mechanism is needed to ensure that these key findings are not lost to the English-speaking world (195).

PREVENTION

It appears that prevention of mental disorders is the way to approach the problem of reducing the toll of mental illness in resource-poor countries. Many of the mental health issues that need to be addressed are inextricably related to contextual issues, as noted earlier. One area too often overlooked in considering a way in which mental health problems can be prevented is through the overall reduction in malnutrition. The effect of malnutrition in societies impacts both the child directly and the parent who cares for the child. Both lead to significant mental health consequences that are preventable. The consequences from malnutrition can be delayed cognitive development, but also more subtle behavioral manifestations with attentional problems and learning disabilities (196,197). Some studies suggest that the behavior disorders associated with malnutrition are secondary to impaired maternal capacities and not to the malnutrition itself, because malnutrition does not appear to contribute to behavioral disturbance later in life although this remains an open question due to lack of a sufficient number of longitudinal studies (198,199). Thus, mental health professionals working in the international arena must be mindful of this issue and consider it in their assessment of mental functioning, as well as advocating for proper nutrition as a preventive measure (200). There is an opportunity to reduce some behavioral and cognitive problems through a reduction in malnutrition.

Maternal depression associated with malnutrition, poor health, social deprivation, abuse, or other stressors affects the child and adolescent as well as the mother. This too is a preventable cause of childhood mental disorder, as demonstrated by Beardslee et al. (201). Using a family-based approach, Beardslee and colleagues sought to reduce risk factors and enhance protective factors for early adolescents. They demonstrated that providing parents with information about their affective state, equipping them with enhanced communication skills, and fostering parent–child dialogue led to an improvement in children's self-understanding and children's depressive symptomatology. This program is now being replicated in Finland, Costa Rica, and elsewhere (202).

Life skills education promoted by the WHO is the backbone of prevention programming in many resource-poor countries (203). Life skills training is provided in the context of the school curriculum as a program to enhance psychosocial competencies. The training focuses on basic, generic skills such as decision-making and problem-solving, creative and critical thinking, communication and other interpersonal skills, self-awareness and empathic skills, and coping with stress and with emotions. The aims are to promote mental well-being and to enable children to take more responsibility for their lives and feel more effective (205).

The World Psychiatric Association Presidential Global Program for Child Mental Health identified school dropout as a major issue in both developing and developed countries. Intervention to prevent dropout was considered to be an important preventive strategy related to child mental health. The program conducted research on school dropout and prepared materials for use by clinicians and educators (206). The Global Program has produced other materials to support preventive intervention in resource poor countries (206).

Schools have an important role to play in mental health promotion, prevention, and early identification of children in need of services. Programs that focus on social, emotional and academic learning from kindergarten through high school have been found to improve school attitudes, behavior, and academic performance (207). Social development, including meaningful peer relationships, can improve academic achievement and motivation, while negative peer pressure or social disapproval toward school work might lead some students to drop out (208). Not only is effective social and affective education of direct benefit to academic attainment, it also improves teacher effectiveness and satisfaction (209). These findings from a host of educational initiatives have been difficult to adopt in countries where the metric for success is often dependent on rote learning and performance on examinations.

SYSTEMIC ISSUES

Throughout the world, it is rare to see child mental health being incorporated into national health policy (210). This lack of policy was documented in 2005 (164) and in the ensuring decade relatively little progress has been made despite the recognition of the importance of policy for good governance and program development. In many countries, developed or developing, no coherent health policy exists that would provide a framework for program development. In countries with a health policy, child mental health rarely rises to a prominent position. Until child mental health becomes integrated into health policy, stable budgetary support for child and adolescent mental health programs will not be realized.

Advocacy for child and adolescent mental health is evident throughout the world, but competition with other interests often forces the issue off the policy agenda. Intersectoral competition and lack of collaboration is too often the limiting factor in developing the type of collaborative programming needed for children and adolescents with mental health problems. When crises involve children, such as child soldiers in the Sudan or female genital mutilation, the issue of child mental health, for a time, gains the spotlight. Unfortunately, the advocacy and concern diminish with time and rarely find a sustaining constituency.

Nongovernmental organizations play an important role in promoting child mental health, in disseminating information, in providing a forum for professional exchange, and in advocating for specific causes. The constituent base of these organizations differs, but they generally have broad representation and provide an opportunity for interested persons to learn more about specific topics or develop ideas in a context of knowledgeable individuals. Many of the nongovernmental organizations have affiliated regional organizations that permit ongoing local involvement. However, from a policy perspective NGOs may allow governments to avoid their responsibility to support capacity building or to allow special interests or disorder specific initiatives to skew the development of rational care programs. National organizations have often taken leadership roles in advocacy efforts and crisis response. The following are some of the more established international nongovernmental organizations focused on child and adolescent mental health: the International Association for Child and Adolescent Psychiatry and Allied Professions, the World Association for Infant Mental Health, the International Association for Adolescent Psychiatry and Psychology, and the World Federation for Mental Health.

It is important for child mental health to be recognized in the various global initiatives seeking to reduce mortality, foster mother and child development, and otherwise to aid human development. The Millennium Development Goals promulgated by the United Nations highlighted important goals for reducing maternal mortality, and a host of other conditions. The framework provided a benchmark for countries. Mental health was not identified in these development goals, but improving mental health was important to reaching the goals in many areas. Recently the UN Sustainable Development Goals have been promulgated for the next decade (211). The Sustainable Development Goals for the first time identify mental health–related goals; however, again child mental health is not identified as a standalone area.

The lack of trained individuals in resource-poor countries and the maldistribution of professionals in developed countries is a significant impediment to the development of child and adolescent mental health services. The WHO mhGAP (212) program has for almost a decade provided a comprehensive set of guidelines for the closing the treatment gap, particularly in LAMI. mhGAP has emphasized the need for developing primary care provider competencies and for the implementation of task shifting. The guidance and associated training is now widely available. Child mental health is recognized in mhGAP but not as a primary focus.

The limitation for program implementation is the availability of trained persons as recognized in mhGAP for leadership and "training of the trainer." However, it is increasingly recognized that the training must be more sophisticated in its implementation and more sustained that was initially thought. Bolton et al. identified the "apprenticeship model" for training and most recently suggested a "common elements treatment approach" (213). Both seek to ensure quality training that will be sustained. This can counter the too-facile adoption of interventions and strategies that do not fully appreciate local culture and the appropriate utilization of available resources. Further, there is the need for these programs to be able to access tertiary diagnostic and treatment services for those with manifest psychiatric disorder and in this regard new efforts at telepsychiatry and the use of mobile diagnostic devices hold promise. Efforts to support training are now ongoing through many nongovernmental and governmental efforts. The training of a sufficient number of individuals to implement appropriate, accessible care will be an ongoing challenge.

LESSONS TO BE LEARNED

It would be wrong to focus only on the areas where it appears that more could be done to enhance child and adolescent mental health services. Western mental health professionals and program developers can learn from the programmatic necessities and innate capacities of individuals and families in resource-poor countries.

Family participation in the care of the mentally ill or retarded children in resource-poor countries is impressive by any standard. The acceptance by communities of the special needs of affected families is often dramatic. Likewise, the willingness and ability of families to care for children, including the appropriate use of medication, for children with epilepsy and other disorders challenge Western concepts of continuity of care and the role of providers.

While the West has flirted with the enhanced use of primary care providers in the delivery of mental health services, but in resource-poor countries, necessity has led to impressive models for the training of primary care practitioners, as noted earlier. Primary care training for specific mental health interventions is also part of a WHO mhGAP strategy (214).

Conversely, there is a global trend toward the imposition of managed care on mental health services. This is occurring in countries, such as China and Eastern Europe, which have hardly met their child and adolescent mental health needs. The need is felt to control the cost of mental health services. Perhaps uncritically, economies throughout the world are adopting managed mental health care. From a Western perspective, it is obvious that although all mental health services suffer in a managed-care environment, child and adolescent mental health services are often most vulnerable to reductions and the use of the lowest common denominator service. Research into managed care and health services has not had the beneficial impact of stimulating the development of innovative systems of care. Unfortunately the investment needed to foster these systems of care and the social network needed to provide "wraparound" services do not exist in resource-poor countries. It remains to be seen whether traditional systems of care can be integrated into a meaningful continuum.

EMERGING ISSUES

The impact of globalization and political change underpins much of this chapter. Globalization and modernization bring new challenges to the attention of child and adolescent mental health professionals. On the positive side for child mental health is growing support for a democratic process within the family, the public awareness that children have a mental life and that they can suffer from depression and other disorders, a reduction in the stigma associated with seeking professional help, the passage of laws assuring basic children's rights, the many initiatives for capacity building in developing countries, reforms in education, and the enhanced training of mental health professionals in many countries. International adoption, the use of telepsychiatry in the developing and developed world, the role of industry and the for-profit sector in program development and education, and the increased recognition of the need to address the mental health consequences of conflict and natural disaster will be an ongoing challenge to professionals and those impacted by mental illness.

CONCLUSION

Global child and adolescent mental health is no longer an exotic topic for theoretical discussion. With our global village, knowledge of child and adolescent mental health problems throughout the world is an important part of the education of all child and adolescent psychiatrists and allied professionals. The perspective gained from appreciating the stressors of children and adolescents in parts of the world embroiled in conflict and the nature of the responses offers the opportunity to learn more about the resilience of children and adolescents and about what we must do to develop more effective intervention programs.

The dearth of trained child and adolescent psychiatrists and allied professionals in developing countries challenges us to find the most effective means for inculcating knowledge and providing meaningful services. It is unrealistic to assume that any effort will meet the needs of child and adolescent psychiatry as determined by conventional planning assumptions. As services evolve in developed countries, there is probably much that can be learned from the way in which less developed countries have found the means to support families and individual persons to be relatively self-sufficient even when they are affected by mental disorders.

Given the enormity of the challenge to extend child mental health in a meaningful manner globally there will be a need to adopt a more public health approach to addressing the mental health needs of children and adolescents (215). Likely, there will never be enough fully trained child and adolescent psychiatrists globally so finding the way to provide quality care through effective training will be a challenge. Recent movements toward task shifting and task sharing will need to be studied and the way in which more highly trained individuals can impact this trend will need to be monitored.

References

1. Nikapota AD: Child psychiatry in developing countries. [Review] [70 refs]. *Brit J Psychiatr* 158:743–751, 1991.
2. Velasco D: [Child psychiatry in developing countries] [French]. *Ann Med Psychol (Paris)* 139(6):626–628, 1981.
3. Minde K: Child psychiatry in developing countries. *J Child Psychol Psychiatr* 17(1):79–83, 1976.
4. Whitley R: Global Mental Health: concepts, conflicts and controversies. *Epidmiol Psychiatr Sci* 24(4):285–291, 2015.
5. Kieling C, Baker-Henningham H, Belfer M, et al.: Child and adolescent mental health worldwide: evidence for action. *Lancet* 378:1515–1525, 2011.
6. Sugar JA, Kleinman A, Eisenberg L: Psychiatric morbidity in developing countries and American psychiatry's role in international health. *Hosp Community Psychiatry* 43(4):355–360, 1992.
7. United Nations, Centre for Human Rights, UNICEF: *The Convention on the Rights of the Child, adopted by the General Assembly of the United Nations 20 November 1989.* London, UNICEF, 1990.
8. United States, Congress, Senate, Committee on Foreign Relations: *The Optional Protocol to the Convention on the Rights of the Child on the Sale of Children, Child Prostitution and Child Pornography and the Optional Protocol to the Convention on the Rights of the Child on the Involvement of Children in Armed Conflict—Report (to accompany Treaty doc. 106-37).* Washington, DC, U.S. GPO, 2002.
9. Murthy RS: Rural psychiatry in developing countries. *Psychiatr Serv* 49(7):967–969, 1998.
10. Canino I, Chou JC, Christmas JJ, et al.: Cross-cultural issues and treatments of psychiatric disorders. *Am J Psychiatr* 148(4):543–544, 1991.

11. Rahim SI, Cederblad M: Effects of rapid urbanization on child behaviour and health in a part of Khartoum, Sudan: II. Psycho-social influences on behaviour. *Soc Sci Med* 22(7):723–730, 1986.
12. Adelekan ML, Makanjuola AB, Ndom RJ: Traditional mental health practitioners in Kwara State, Nigeria. *East African Med J* 78(4):190–196, 2001.
13. Reynolds P: *Traditional healers and childhood in Zimbabwe*. Athens, Ohio, University Press, 1996.
14. Manci M: Clinical experience of treating STD's with traditional medicines, leading to treatment and prevention of HIV/AIDS. *Int Conf AIDS* 10:215, 1994.
15. Robertson BA, Kottler A: Cultural issues in the psychiatric assessment of Xhosa children and adolescents. *S Afr Med J* 83(3):207–208, 1993.
16. Somasundaram DJ, van de Put WA, Eisenbruch M, et al.: Starting mental health services in Cambodia. *Soc Sci Med* 48(8):1029–1046, 1999.
17. Suryani LK, Jensen GD: Psychiatrist, traditional healer and culture integrated in clinical practice in Bali. *Med Anthropol* 13(4):301–314, 1992.
18. Eisenbruch M: The ritual space of patients and traditional healers in Cambodia. *Bull de l'École Française d'Extrême-Orient* 79[2]:283–316, 1992.
19. Eisenbruch M: Children with failure to thrive, epilepsy and STI/AIDS: Indigenoustaxonomies, attributions and ritual treatments. *Clin Child Psychol Psychiatr* 3:505–518, 1998.
20. Ahmed HU, Alam MT, Hossain T, et al.: Child psychiatry services in Bangladesh: issues and concerns. *Euro Psychiatr* 309(Suppl 1):696.
21. Lim CG, Vitiello B: Child psychiatry services in Asia: evolving state of affairs? *Child Adolesc Psychiatry Ment Health* 9:12, 2015.
22. Savin D: Developing psychiatric training and services in Cambodia: psychiatric services. *J Am Psychiatr* 51(7):935, 2000.
23. Desjarlais R, Eisenberg L, Good B, et al.: *World mental health: Problems and priorities in low-income countries*. 10th ed. New York, Oxford University Press, 1995.
24. Hamoda HM, Belfer ML: Challenges in international collaboration in child and adolescent psychiatry. *J Child Adolesc Ment Health* 22(2): 83–89, 2010.
25. Sridhar D, Khagram S, Pang T: Are existing governance structures equipped to deal with today's global health challenges towards systematic coherence in scaling up? *Glob Health Gov* 2:1–25, 2009.
26. Shridhar D, Batniji R. Misfinancing global health: A case for transparency in disbursements and decision making. *Lancet* 372:1185–1191, 2008.
27. UNHCR: Global Peace Index 2015.
28. Fullilove MT: Psychiatric implications of displacement: Contributions from the psychology of place. *Am J Psychiatr* 153:1516–1523, 1996.
29. Sampson RJ, Raudenbush SW, Earls F: Neighborhoods and violent crime: A multilevel study of collective efficacy. *Science* 277(5328):918–924, 1997.
30. Zivcić I. Emotional reactions of children to war stress in Croatia. *J Am Acad Child Adolesc Psychiatr* 32(4):709–713, 1993.
31. Laor N, Wolmer L, Mayes LC, et al.: Israeli preschoolers under SCUD missile attacks. A developmental perspective on risk-modifying factors. *Arch Gen Psychiatr* 53(5):416–423, 1996.
32. Goffman I: Asylums. Garden City, Anchor of Doubleday, 1961.
33. Marsella AJE, Bornemann TE, Ekblad SE, et al.: *Amidst peril and pain: The mental health and well-being of the world's refugees*. 20th ed. Washington, DC, American Psychological Association, 1994.
34. Eisenbruch M: The cry for the lost placenta: cultural bereavement and cultural survival among Cambodians who resettled, were repatriated, or who stayed at home. In: van Tilburg M, Vingerhoets A (eds): *Home is where the heart is: The psychological aspects of permanent and temporary geographical moves*. Tilburg, Tilburg University Press, 1997:119–142.
35. Tseng WS, Cheng TA, Chen YS, et al.: Psychiatric complications of family reunion after four decades of separation. *Am J Psychiatr* 150(4):614–619, 1993.
36. Lee I: Second International Conference on Wartime Medical Services. *Med War* 7(2):120–128, 1991.
37. Thabet AA, Vostanis P: Social adversities and anxiety disorders in the Gaza Strip. *Arch Dis Child* 78(5):439–442, 1998.
38. United Nations High Commissioner for Refugees: *The future of Syria: Refugee Children in Crisis*. Geneva, UNHCR, 2014.
39. Thabet AA, Stretch D, Vostanis P: Child mental health problems in Arab children: application of the strengths and difficulties questionnaire. *Int J Soc Psychiatr* 46(4):266–280, 2000.
40. Aptekar L, Stocklin D: Children in particularly difficult circumstances. In: Berry JW, Saraswathi TS, Dasen PR (eds): *Handbook of cross-cultural psychology*, Vol. 1. Boston, MA, Allyn & Bacon, 377–412, 1997.
41. Allwood MA, Bell-Dolan D, Husain SA: Children's trauma and adjustment reactions to violent and nonviolent war experiences. *J Am Acad ChildAdolesc Psychiatr* 41(4):450–457, 2002.
42. Panter-Brick C, Eggerman M, Gonzalez V, et al.: Violence, suffering, and mental health in Afghanistan: a school-based survey. *Lancet* 374:807–816, 2009.
43. Cartwright K, El-Khani A, Subyan A, et al.: Establishing the feasibility of assessing the mental health of children displaced by the Syrian conflict. *Glob Ment Health* 2:28, 2015.
44. Hassan G, Kirmayer LJ, Mekki-Berrada A, et al.: *Culture, Context and the Mental Health and Psychosocial Wellbing of Syrians: A review for Mental Health and Psychosocial Staff Working with Syrians Affected by Armed Conflict*. Geneva, UNHCR, 2015.
45. International Medical Corps, UNICEF: *Mental health, psychosocial and child protection for Syrian adolescent refugees in Jordan*. Amman, Jordan, IMC and UNICEF, 2014.
46. International Medical Corps: *Rapid gender and protection assessment report*. Turkey, Kobane Refugee Population, Suruc, 2014. https//data.unhcr.org/Syrian refugees/download.php?id=7318.
47. James L, Sovcik A, Garoff F, et al.: The mental health of Syrian refugee children and adolescents. *Forced Migration Rev* 47:42–44, 2014.
48. Singh S: Post-traumatic stress in former Ugandan child soldiers [comment]. *Lancet* 363(9421):1648, 2004.
49. Kuruppuarachchi K, Wijeratne LT: Post-traumatic stress in former Ugandan child soldiers.[comment]. *Lancet* 363(9421):1648, 2004.
50. Magambo C, Lett R: Post-traumatic stress in former Ugandan child soldiers. [comment]. *Lancet* 363(9421):1647–1648, 2004.
51. McKay S, Wessells MG: Post-traumatic stress in former Ugandan child soldiers.[comment]. *Lancet* 363(9421):1646–1647, 2004.
52. Derluyn I, Broekaert E, Schuyten G, et al.: Post-traumatic stress in former Ugandan child soldiers.[see comment]. *Lancet* 363(9412):861–863, 2004.
53. Moszynski P: Child soldiers forgotten in Angola. *BMJ* 326(7397):1003, 2003.
54. Somasundaram D: Child soldiers: understanding the context. [Review] [11 refs]. *BMJ* 324(7348):1268–1271, 2002.
55. Lamberg L: Reclaiming child soldiers' lost lives. *JAMA* 292(5):553–554, 2004.
56. Bracken PJ, Giller JE, Ssekiwanuka JK: The rehabilitation of child soldiers: defining needs and appropriate responses. *Med, Conflict Survival* 12(2):114–25, 1996.
57. Willis BM, Levy BS: Child prostitution: global health burden, research needs, and interventions. *Lan Lancet* 359(9315):1417–1422, 2002.
58. UNICEF, Innocenti Research Centre: *Trafficking in human beings, especially women and children, in Africa*. Florence, Italy, UNICEF Innocenti Research Center, 2003.
59. International Organization for Migration: *Trafficking in women and children from the Republic of Armenia: A study*. Yerevan, International Organization for Migration, 2001.
60. Jalalza'i MK: *Children trafficking in Pakistan*. Karachi, Royal Book Co, 2003.
61. Subedi G, Trafficking iC, International Labour Org: *Trafficking and Sexual Abuse among Street Children in Kathmandu*. 1st ed. Kathmandu International Labour Organization, 2002.
62. Sorajjakool S: *Child Prostitution in Thailand: Listening to Rahab*. New York, Haworth Press, 2003.
63. Rozario MR, Kesari P, Rasool J: *Trafficking in Women and Children in India: Sexual Exploitation and Sale*. New Delhi, Uppal Public House, 1988.
64. International Office for Migration: *Victims Trafficking in the Balkans: A study of Trafficking in Women and Children for Sexual Exploitation to, through, and from the Balkan Region*. Vienna, Geneva, IOM International Organization for Migration, 2001.
65. Commission of the European Communities: *Combating Trafficking in Human Beings and Combating the Sexual Exploitation of Children and Child Pornography*. Brussels, Commission of the European Communities, 2001.
66. Inter-American Commission of Women: Trafficking of women and children for sexual exploitation in the Americas—An introduction to trafficking in the Americas, 2001.
67. Asian DB: *Combating Trafficking of Women and Children in South Asia—Regional Synthesis Paper for Bangladesh, India, and Nepal*. Manila, Asian Development Bank, 2003.
68. International Labour Organisation, International Programme on the Elimination of Child Labour. Combating trafficking in children for labour exploitation in the Mekong sub-region: A proposed framework for ILO-IPEC action and proceedings of a Mekong sub-regional consultation. ILO/IPEC, 1998.
69. Munir K, Belfer ML: HIV and AIDS: global and United States perspectives. In: Wiener JM, Dulcan MK (eds): *Textbook of child and adolescent psychiatry*. 3rd ed. Washington, DC, American Psychiatric Publishing, Inc, 869–889, 2004.
70. Carlson M, Earls F: Psychological and neuroendocrinological sequelae of early social deprivation in institutionalized children in Romania. In: Carter CS, Lederhendler II, Kirkpatrick B (eds): *The integrative neurobiology of affiliation*. New York, AcadSci, 1997:419–28.
71. Belfer M, Heggenhougen K: Substance abuse. In: Desjarlais R, Eisenberg L, Good B, et al., (eds): *World Mental Health: Problems and Priorities in Low-income Countries*. New York, Oxford University Press, 87–115, 1995.
72. Pumariega AJ, Burakgazi H, Unlu A, et al.: Substance abuse: risk factors for Turkish youth. *Bull Clin Pharmacol* 24:5–14, 2014.
73. Badr L, Taha A, Dee V: Substance Abuse in middle eastern adolescents living in two different countries: spiritual, cultural, family and personal factors. *J Religion Health* 53:1060–1074, 2014.

74. AlMarri TS: Oei TP Alcohol and substance use in the Arabian Gulf region: a review. *Int J Psychol* 44(3):222–233, 2009.
75. Alem A, Kebede D, Kullgren G: The prevalence and socio-demographic correlates of khat chewing in Butajira, Ethiopia. *Acta Psychiatr Scand Supp* 397:84–91, 1999.
76. Raffaelli M, Larson RW: *Homeless and Working Youth Around the World—Exploring Developmental Issues*. San Francisco, CA, Jossey-Bass, 95, 1999.
77. Senanayake MP, Ranasinghe A, Balasuriya C: Street children—A preliminary study. *Ceylon Med J* 43(4):191–193, 1998.
78. Carlini-Cotrim B, Carlini EA: The use of solvents and other drugs among children and adolescents from a low socioeconomic background: a study in São Paulo, Brazil. *Int J Addict* 23(11):1145–1156, 1988.
79. Cameron FJ, Debelle GD: No more Pacific island paradises. *Lancet* 1(8388):1238, 1984.
80. Belasso G: The international challenge of drug abuse: the Mexican experience. In: Petersen RC, National Institute on Drug Abuse (eds): *The International Challenge of Drug Abuse*. 19th ed. Rockville, MD, Dept. of Health, Education, and Welfare, Public Health Service, Alcohol, Drug Abuse, and Mental Health Administration, National Institute on Drug Abuse, Division of Research, 1978.
81. Cravioto P, Anchondo R-L, de la Rosa B: Risk factors associated with inhalant use among Mexican juvenile delinquents. In: National Institute on Drug Abuse, Community Epidemiology Work Group, Johnson B&S (eds): *Epidemiologic Trends in Drug Abuse*. Rockville, MD, U.S. Dept. of Health and Human Services, Public Health Service, Alcohol, Drug Abuse, and Mental Health Administration, Division of Epidemiology and Prevention Research, National Institute on Drug Abuse, 472–477, 1992.
82. Wittig MC, Wright JD, Kaminsky DC: Substance use among street children in Honduras. *Subst Use Misuse* 32(7–8):805–827, 1997.
83. Forster LM, Tannhauser M, Barros HM: Drug use among street children in southern Brazil. *Drug Alcohol Depend* 43(1–2):57–62, 1996.
84. World Health Organization: *World Report on Violence and Health*. Geneva, Switzerland, 2002.
85. Djeddah C, Facchin P, Ranzato C, Romer C: Child abuse: Current problems and key public health challenges. *Soc Sci Med* 51(6):905–915, 2000.
86. Ohtsuji M, Ohshima T, Kondo T, et al.: [Fatal child abuse in Japan and Germany. Comparative retrospective study] [German]. *Archiv für Kriminologie* 202(1–2):8–16, 1998.
87. D'Antonio IJ, Darwish AM, McLean M: Child maltreatment: International perspectives. *Maternal Child Nurs J* 21(2):39–52, 1993.
88. Mazurek AJ: Epidemiology of paediatric injury. *J Accid Emerg Med* 11(1):9–16, 1994.
89. Marzouki M, Hadh Fredj A, Chelli M: Child abuse and cultural attitudes: The example of Tunisia. *Child Abuse Negl* 11(1):137–141, 1987.
90. Agathonos H, Stathacopoulou N, Adam H, et al.: Child abuse and neglect in Greece: Sociomedical aspects. *Child Abuse Negl* 6(3):307–311, 1982.
91. Santana-Tavira R, Sanchez-Ahedo R, Herrera-Basto E: [Child abuse: a world problem]. *Salud Publica Mex* 40(1):58–65, 1998.
92. Frias-Armenta M, McCloskey LA: Determinants of harsh parenting in Mexico. *J Abnormal Child Psychol* 26(2):129–139, 1998.
93. Doe SS: Cultural Factors in Child Maltreatment and Domestic Violence in Korea. *Child Youth Serv Rev* 22(3–4):231–236, 2000.
94. Qureshi B: Cultural aspects of child abuse in Britain. *Midwife, Health Visit Community Nurse* 24(10):412–413, 1988.
95. Reid S: Cultural difference and child abuse intervention with undocumented Spanish-speaking families in Los Angeles. *Child Abuse Negl* 8(1):109–112, 1984.
96. Loening W-EK: Child abuse among the Zulus: a people in cultural transition. *Child Abuse Negl* 5(1):3–7, 1981.
97. Davis RE: Cultural health care or child abuse? The Southeast Asian practice of cao gio. *J Am Acad Nurse Practition* 12(3):89–95, 2000.
98. Shalhoub-Kevorkian N: Disclosure of child abuse in conflict areas. *Violence Against Women* 11(10):1263–1291, 2005.
99. Hopkins S: A discussion of the legal aspects of female genital mutilation. *J Adv Nurs* 30(4):926–933, 1999.
100. Ho WS, Ying SY, Wong TW: Bizarre paediatric facial burns. *Burns* 26(5):504–506, 2000.
101. Warner JE, Hansen DJ: The identification and reporting of physical abuse by physicians: a review and implications for research. *Child Abuse Negl* 18(1):11–25, 1994.
102. Korbin JE, Coulton CJ, Chard S, et al.: Impoverishment and child maltreatment in African American and European American neighborhoods. *Dev Psychopathol* 10(2):215–233, 1998.
103. Maitra B: Child abuse: a universal "diagnostic" category? The implication of culture in definition and assessment. *Int J Soc Psychiatr* 42(4):287–304, 1996.
104. Levesque RJ: Cultural evidence, child maltreatment, and the law. *Child Maltreat* 5(2):146–160, 2000.
105. Haj YM, Shor R: Child maltreatment as perceived by Arab students of social science in the West Bank. *Child Abuse Negl* 19(10):1209–1219, 1995.
106. Baker KA, Dwairy M: Cultural norms versus state law in treating incest: a suggested model for Arab families.[see comment]. *Child Abuse Negl* 27(1):109–123, 2003.
107. Munir KM, Beardslee WR: A developmental and psychobiologic framework for understanding the role of culture in child and adolescent psychiatry. *Child Adolesc Psychiatr Clinics North Am* 10(4):667–677, 2001.
108. Kriegler SA: Social constructivist perspective on the potential relevance of selected DSM-5 disorders for South African children and youth. *Child Soc* 29:604-614, 2015.
109. Beauchaine TP: Taxometrics and developmental psychopathology. [Review] [198 refs]. *Dev Psychopathol* 15(3):501–527, 2003.
110. Novins DK, Bechtold DW, Sack WH, et al.: The DSM-IV outline for cultural formulation: a critical demonstration with American Indian children. *J Am Acad Child Adolesc Psychiatr* 36(9):1244–1251, 1997.
111. Neki JS: An examination of the cultural relativism of dependence as a dynamic of social and therapeutic relationships. I. Socio-developmental. *Brit J Med Psychol* 49(1):1–10, 1976.
112. Malhotra S, Malhotra A, Varma VK: *Child mental Health in India*. Delhi, Macmillan India Limited, 1992.
113. Malhotra S: Challenges in providing mental health services for children and adolescents in India. In: Young JG, Ferrari (eds): *Designing Mental Health Services for Children and Adolescents—A Shrewd Investment*. Philadelphia, PA, Brunner/Mazel, 1988:321–334.
114. Huss M, Iseler A, Lehmkuhl U: [Cross-cultural comparison of Conners Scales: Can the US-American factorial structure be replicated on German clinical sample?] [German]. *Zeitschrift fur Kinder-und Jugendpsychiatrie und Psychotherapie* 29(1):16–24, 2001.
115. Pendergast LL, Vandiver BJ, Schaefer BA, et al.: Factor structure of scores from the Conners' Rating Scales—revised among Nepali children. *Int J School Educ Psychol* 2:261–270, 2014.
116. Roussos A, Richardson C, Politikou K, et al.: The Conners-28 teacher questionnaire in clinical and nonclinical samples of Greek children 6–12 years old. *Euro Child Adolesc Psychiatr* 8(4):260–267, 1999.
117. Rey JM, Singh M, Hung SF, et al.: A global scale to measure the quality of the family environment. [see comment]. *Arch Gen Psychiatr* 54(9):817–822, 1997.
118. Goodman R, Renfrew D, Mullick M: Predicting type of psychiatric disorder from Strengths and Difficulties Questionnaire (SDQ) scores in child mental health clinics in London and Dhaka. *Eur Child Adolesc Psychiatr* 9(2):129–134, 2000.
119. Odejide AO, Oyewunmi LK, Ohaeri JU: Psychiatry in Africa: an overview. *Am J Psychiatr* 146(6):708–716, 1989.
120. Hackett R, Hackett L: Child psychiatry across cultures. *Int Rev Psychiatr* 11(2):225–235, 1999.
121. Taeb O, Heidenreich F, Baubet T, et al.: [Finding a meaning for illness: from medical anthropology to cultural epidemiology]. *Med et maladies Infect* 35(4):173–185, 2005.
122. Raguram R, Raghu TM, Vounatsou P, et al.: Schizophrenia and the cultural epidemiology of stigma in Bangalore, India. *J Nerv Mental Dis* 192(11):734–734, 2004.
123. DiGiacomo SM: Can there be a "cultural epidemiology"? *Med Anthropol Q* 13(4):436–457, 1999.
124. Tadesse B, Kebede D, Tegegne T, et al.: Childhood behavioural disorders in Ambo district, western Ethiopia. I. Prevalence estimates. *Acta Psychiatrica Scandinavica Suppl* 397:92–97, 1999.
125. Giel R, Van Luijk JN: Psychiatric morbidity in a small Ethiopian town. *RevMed Psychosom Psychol Med* 11(4):435–456, 1969.
126. Harding TW, De Arango MV, Baltazar J, et al.: Mental disorders in primary health care: A study of their frequency and diagnosis in four developing countries. *Psychol Med* 10(2):231–241, 1980.
127. Omigbodun OO: Psychosocial issues in a child and adolescent psychiatric clinic population in Nigeria. *Soc Psychiatr Epi* 39(8):667–672, 2004.
128. Giel R, de Arango MV, Clement CE, et al.: Childhood mental disorders in primary health care: results of observations in four developing countries. *Pediatrics* 68:677–683, 1981.
129. Becker AE: *Body, Self and Society—The View from Fiji*. Philadelphia, PA, University of Pennsylvania Press, 1995.
130. Eisenberg L, Belfer M: Prerequisites for child and adolescent mental health. *J Child Psychol Psychiatr* 50(1–2):26–35, 2009.
131. Fayyad JA, Jahshan CS, Karam EG: Systems development of child mental health services in developing countries. *Child Adolesc Psychiatric Clin North Am* 10(4):745–762, 2001.
132. al-Ansari A, Matar AM: Recent stressful life events among Bahraini adolescents with adjustment disorder. *Adolescence* 28(110):339–346, 1993.
133. Khandelwal SK, Sharan P, Saxena S: Eating disorders: an Indian perspective. *Int J Soc Psychiatr* 41(2):132–146, 1995.
134. Littlewood R: Psychopathology and personal agency: modernity, culture change and eating disorders in South Asian societies. *Brit J Med Psychol* 68(1):45–63, 1995.
135. Hill AJ, Bhatti R: Body shape perception and dieting in preadolescent British Asian girls: links with eating disorders. *Int J Eat Disord* 17(2):175–183, 1995.
136. Bryant WR, Lask B: Anorexia nervosa in a group of Asian children living in Britain [see comments]. *Brit J Psychiatr* 158:229–233, 1991.
137. le Grange D, Telch CF, Tibbs J: Eating attitudes and behaviors in 1,435 South African Caucasian and non-Caucasian college students. [see comment]. *Am J Psychiatr* 155(2):250–254, 1998.
138. Gupta N: Autism: some conceptual issues.[comment]. *Indian Ped* 38(9):1065–1067, 2001.

139. Yeargin-Allsopp M, Boyle C: Overview. The epidemiology of neurodevelopmental disorders. *Ment Retard Dev Disabilities Res Rev* 8(3):113–116, 2002.
140. Lotter V: Childhood autism in Africa. *J Child Psychol Psychiatr* 19(3):231–244, 1978.
141. Chung SY, Luk SL, Lee PW: A follow-up study of infantile autism in Hong Kong. *J Autism Dev Disord* 20(2):221–232, 1990.
142. Takei N: Childhood autism in Japan.[comment]. *Brit J Psychiatr* 169(5):671–672, 1996.
143. Abdel-Khalek AM, Soliman HH: A cross-cultural evaluation of depression in children in Egypt, Kuwait, and the United States. *Psychol Rep* 85(3 Pt. 1): 973–980, 1999.
144. Boer MD, Morgan R. Bad Pharma, Bad Karma; The Pharmaceutical Industry in Developing Countries. 2014
145. Responding to Emergency Situations, Geneva, World Health Organization, Department of Mental Health and Substance Abuse. 2005.
146. Borowsky IW, Resnick MD, Ireland M, et al.: Suicide attempts among American Indian and Alaska Native youth: risk and protective factors. *Arch Ped Adolesc Med* 153(6):573–580, 1999.
147. Mugisha J, Knizek BL, Birthe L, et al.: Doing qualitative research on suicide in a developing country: practical and ethical challenges. *Crisis: J of Crisis Intervention and Suicide Prev* 32(1):15–23, 2011.
148. Shaffer D: The epidemiology of teen suicide: an examination of risk factors. *J Clin Psychiatr* 49:36–41, 1988.
149. Bertolote J: *Department of Mental Health and Substance Abuse, World Health Organization.* Geneva, Switzerland, Personal communication, 2003.
150. Murthy RS: Approaches to suicide prevention in Asia and the Far East. In: Hawton K, Van Heeringen K (eds): *International Handbook of Suicide and Attempted Suicide.* London, Wiley, 2000:625–637.
151. Chan KP, Hung SF, Yip PS: Suicide in response to changing societies. *Child Adolesc Psychiatr Clin North Am* 10(4):777–795, 2001.
152. Blum RW, Halcon L, Beuhring T, et al.: Adolescent health in the Caribbean: Risk and protective factors. *Am J Pub Health* 93(3):456–460, 2003.
153. Chan K: *Hong Kong, China. Personal communication.* 2003.
154. Lester D: Suicide and islam. *Arch Suicide Res* 10(1):77–97, 2006.
155. Shah A, Chandia M: The relationship between suicide and Islam: a cross-national study. *J Inj Violence Res* 2(2):93–97, 2010.
156. Kelleher MJ, Chambers D, Corcoran P, et al.: Religious sanctions and rates of suicide worldwide. *Crisis* 19(2):78–96, 1998.
157. Dugge C: A mirror for India: Suicide of 4 sisters. *Int Herald Tribune* 2000.
158. United Nations, Economic and Social Commission for Asia and the Pacific: *Focus on ability, celebrate diversity—Highlights of the Asian and Pacific decade of disabled persons, 1993-2003.* New York, United Nations, 2003.
159. Belmont L: *The international pilot study of severe childhood disability—Final report—Screening for Severe Mental Retardation in Developing Countries.* Utrecht, Bishop Bekkers Institute, 1984.
160. Narayanan H: A study of the prevalence of mental retardation in Southern India. *Int JMental Health* 10:128–136, 1981.
161. Tao K: Mentally retarded persons in the People's Republic of China: A review of epidemiological studies and services. *Am J Mental Retardation* 93:193–199, 1988.
162. Stein Z, Durkin M, Belmont L: "Serious" mental retardation in developing countries: An epidemiologic approach. *Annal New York Acad Sci* 477:8–21, 1986.
163. Kim YS, Kumar S: Cross-cultural examination of social interactions during a one-week dousa-hou (Japanese psychorehabilitation) camp. *Psychol Rep* 95(3 Pt. 1):1050–1054, 2004.
164. *Atlas on child and adolescent mental health resources—Global concerns: Implications for the future.* Geneva, Switzerland, World Health Organization; 2005.
165. Belfer ML, Saxena S: WHO Child Atlas Project. *Lancet* 367:551–552, 2006.
166. Atlas: Child, Adolescent and Maternal Mental Health in the Eastern Mediterranean Region. Eastern Mediterranean Regional Office, World Health Organization, Technical Publications Series. 39:1–48, 2013.
167. McKelvey RS, Sang DL, Tu HC: Is there a role for child psychiatry in Vietnam? *AustNew Zealand J Psychiatr* 31(1):114–119, 1997.
168. El-Din A, Moustafa A, Mohit A: A multi-sectoral approach to school mental health, Alexandria, Egypt. II. *Health Serv J East Medit Reg* 7(34):40, 1993.
169. Giel R, De Arango MV, Climent CE, et al.: Childhood mental disorders in primary health care: results of observations in four developing countries. A report from the WHO Collaborative Study on Strategies for Extending Mental Health Care. *Pediatrics* 68(5):677–683, 1981.
170. Graham P, Orley J: WHO and the mental health of children. *World Health Forum* 19(3):268–272, 1998.
171. Nikapota AD: *Recognition and Management of Children with Functional Complaints—A Training Package for the Primary Care Physician.* New Delhi, WHO Regional Office for South-East Asia, 1993.
172. Mathur G, Mathur S, Singh Y: Detection and prevention of childhood disability with the help of anganwadi workers. *Indian Ped J* 32:773–777, 1995.
173. World Health Organization Division of Mental Health: *Life skills education in schools.* Geneva, World Health Organization, 1994.
174. Bandura A: *Social Learning Theory.* Englewood Cliffs, NJ, Prentice Hall, 1977.
175. Murray LK, Dorsey S, Bolton P, et al.: Building capacity in mental health interventions in low resource countries: an apprenticeship model for training local providers. *Int J Ment Health Syst* 5(1):30, 2011
176. Kapur M, Cariapa I, Parthasarathy R: Evaluation of an orientation course for teachers on emotional problems amongst school children. *Indian J Clin Psychol* 7(2):103–107, 1980.
177. Kim WJ: A training guideline of cultural competence for child and adolescent psychiatric residencies. *Child Psychiatr Human Dev* 6(2): 125–136, 1995.
178. Ordóñez AE, Collins PY: Advancing research to action in global child mental health. *Child Adolesc Psychiatr Clin N Am* 24:679–697, 2015.
179. Cullins LM, Mian AI: Global child and adolescent mental health: a culturally informed focus. *Child Adolesc Psychiatr Clin N Am* 24:823-830, 2015.
180. Patel V, Kim Y: Contribution of low and middle income countries to research published in leading general psychiatry journals, 2002-2004. *Brit J Psychiatr.* 190:77–78, 2007.
181. Tyrer P: Combating editorial racism in psychiatric publications. *Brit J Psychiatr* 186:1–3, 2005.
182. Earls F, Eisenberg L: International perspective in child psychiatry. In: Lewis M (eds): *Child and Adolescent Psychiatry—A Comprehensive Textbook.* Baltimore, MD, Williams & Wilkins, 1991:1189–1196.
183. Mohler B: Cross-cultural issues in research on child mental health. *Child Adolesc Psychiatr Clin N Am* 10(4):763–776, 2001.
184. Nelson ML, Quintana SM: Qualitative clinical research with children and adolescents. [Review] [60 refs]. *J Clin Child Adoles Psychol* 34(2):344–356, 2005.
185. Weisner TS: *Discovering Successful Pathways in Children's Development—Mixed Methods in the Study of Childhood and Family Life.* Chicago, University of Chicago Press, 2005.
186. Eisenbruch M: *The lens of culture, the lens of health: Toward a framework and toolkit for cultural competence. Resource document, for UNESCO Asia-Pacific Regional Training Workshop on Cultural Mapping and Cultural Diversity Programming Lens to Safeguard Tangible and Intangible Cultural Expressions and Protect Cultural Diversity, Bangkok, 15–19 December 2004; pp. 1–248.*
187. Lindenberg CS, Solorzano RM, Vilaro FM, et al.: Challenges and strategies for conducting intervention research with culturally diverse populations. [Review] [30 refs]. *J Transcult Nurs* 12(2):132–139, 2001.
188. Lindgren T, Lipson JG: Finding a way: Afghan women's experience in community participation. *J Transcult Nurs* 15(2):122–130, 2004.
189. Penrod J, Preston DB, Cain RE, et al.: A discussion of chain referral as a method of sampling hard-to-reach populations. *J Transcult Nurs* 14(2):100–107, 2003.
190. Portillo CJ, Villarruel A, de Leon Siantz ML, et al.: Research agenda for Hispanics in the United States: a nursing perspective. [Review] [70 refs]. *Nurs Outlook* 49(6):263–269, 2001.
191. Roszak DJ: To eliminate racial/ethnic disparities, hospitals must standardize data collection. *Hosp Health Netw* 78(6):78, 2004.
192. Fontes LA: Ethics in family violence research: cross-cultural issues: family relations. *J Applied Family Child Studies* 47(1):53–61, 1998.
193. Munir K, Earls F: Ethical principles governing research in child and adolescent psychiatry. *J Am Acad Child Adolesc Psychiatry* 31(3):408–414, 1992.
194. Earls F: Child psychiatry in an international context: with remarks on the current status of child psychiatry in China. In: Super CM (ed): *The Role of Culture in Developmental Disorder.* San Diego, Academic Press; 1987:235–248.
195. Patel V, Sumathipala A: International representation in psychiatric literature: Survey of six leading journals. *Brit J Psychiatr* 178:406–409, 2001.
196. Galler JR, Ramsey F, Solimano G, et al.: The influence of early malnutrition on subsequent behavioral development. I. Degree of impairment in intellectual performance. *J Am Acad Child Psychiatry* 22(1):8–15, 1983.
197. Agarwal DK, Upadhyay SK, Agarwal KN, et al.: Anaemia and mental functions in rural primary school children. *Ann Trop Paediatr* 9(4):194–198, 1989.
198. Galler JR, Ramsey F: A follow-up study of the influence of early malnutrition on development: Behavior at home and at school. *J Am Acad Child Adolesc Psychiatr* 28(2):254–261, 1989.
199. Miranda CT, Paula CS, Santos L, et al.: Association between mother–child interaction and mental health among mothers of malnourished children. *J Trop Ped* 46(5):314, 2000.
200. Gillespie S, McLachlan M, Shrimpton R, et al.: *Combating Malnutrition—Time to Act.* Washington, DC, World Bank, 2003.
201. Beardslee WR, Gladstone TR, Wright EJ, et al.: A family-based approach to the prevention of depressive symptoms in children at risk: evidence of parental and child change. *Pediatrics* 112(2):119–313, 2003.
202. Beardslee: *Personal communication,* 2005.
203. Graham P, Orley J: WHO's activities related to psychosocial aspects of health (including child and adolescent health and development). In: de Girolamo G, Sartorius N (eds): *Promoting Mental Health Internationally.* London, Gaskell, 1999:117–131.

204. Focusing Resources on Effective School Health: A FRESH Start to Enhancing the Quality and Equity of Education. <www.unesco.org/education?index.shtml>; <www.unicef.org/programme/lifeskills/mainmenu.html>; <www.who.int/hpr.fshi/index.htm>; <www.schoolsandhealth.org>.
205. Remschmidt H, Belfer ML: Mental health care for children and adolescents worldwide: a review. *World Psychiatry* 4(3):147–153, 2005.
206. International Association for Child and Adolescent Psychiatry and Allied Professions Webpage <www.iacapap.org>.
207. Zins JE, Weissberg RP, Wang MC, et al.: *Building academic success on social and emotional learning: What does the research say?* New York, Teachers College Press, 2004.
208. Stewart EB: School structural characteristics, student effort, peer associations, and parental involvement: The influence of school- and individual-level factors on academic achievement. *Edu Urban Soc* 40(2):179–204, 2008.
209. Weare K: *Promoting Mental, Emotional and Social Health*. London, Routledge, 2000.
210. Shatkin JP, Belfer, ML: The global absence of child and adolescent mental health policy. *Child Adolesc Mental Health* 9:104–108, 2004.
211. Maurice J: UN set to change the world with new development goals. *Lancet* 386:1121–1124, 2015.
212. mhGAP: Mental Health Gap Action Programme: *Scaling Up Care for Mental, Neurological and Substance Abuse Disorders*. Geneva, World Health Organization, 2008.
213. Murray LK, Dorsey S, Haroz E, et al.: A common elements treatment approach for adult mental problems in low- and middle-income countries. *Cogn Behav Pract* 21(2):111–123, 2014.
214. Gureje O, Abdulmalik J, Kola L, et al.: Integrating mental health inot primary care in Nigeria: report of a demonstration project using the mental health gap action programme intervention guide. *BMC Health Serv Res* 15:242, 2015.
215. Belfer ML: Child Mental Health in the 21st Century: Universal Challenges. In: Sorel E (ed): *21st Century Global Mental Health*. Burlington, MA, Jones and Bartlett, 153–170.

CHAPTER 1.6 ■ CHILD AND FAMILY POLICY: A ROLE FOR CHILD PSYCHIATRY AND ALLIED DISCIPLINES

WALTER S. GILLIAM, MATIA FINN-STEVENSON, LAINE TAYLOR, AND EDWARD F. ZIGLER

Child and adolescent psychiatrists and their allied discipline colleagues have long understood many of the family and societal factors that impact children's development and functioning (e.g., poverty, community violence, substance abuse, substandard education, family discord). Many of these contributors to psychiatric impairment have been the focus of public concern, debate, and often policy development. Although child and adolescent psychiatrists and other mental health professionals have much to contribute to thinking about population-wide efforts to address these problems, few receive any training on how to understand effective policy development or their role in it.

In this chapter, we discuss some of the social changes we experience in our society, their impact on children and families, and policy responses to address these. We also discuss the role of mental health professionals in the policy arena. As will become apparent in the course of this chapter, there are benefits as well as challenges inherent in the utilization of mental health research in policy settings. A number of opportunities exist for mental health professionals to contribute to the development of policies for children and families. However, their effectiveness is dependent not only on their scientific and clinical knowledge but also on their familiarity with the social policy process and their ability to work with policymakers.

WHAT IS POLICY?

Policy is any agreed-upon set of principles used to guide decisions or procedures. Policies often are codified in written forms, such as laws, governmental regulations, or organizational procedures. In many cases, however, policies are not explicated formally and exist simply as implicit assumptions about "the way things are done." In democratic societies, the most formal type of policy is legislation—the laws enacted by state and federal governments that create and fund service programs (e.g., health care, public-funded prevention services, entitlement services for persons with disabilities), establish or alter rules for government services (e.g., procedures for arbitrating disputes regarding special education), and regulate the way individuals and private businesses may interact (e.g., mental health parity laws regarding insurance providers, laws regarding domestic violence and protection). Regulations, as opposed to legislation, are governmental procedures and definitions that are developed by executive branch staff to guide the provision of their services, but do not rise to the formalized level of legislation. What differentiates policies is the degree to which they have been formalized, who they regulate, the consequences that can be imposed for breaking them, and how difficult it is to change them. What all policies have in common is that in all cases someone first envisioned the need for a policy, someone decided what the policy should be, and some individuals actively or implicitly agreed to it. In many cases the persons writing and deciding policies understand the policy process very well, but may have little or no knowledge of the systems they are regulating or the implications of their policies.

Over recent decades, researchers and clinicians in psychiatry, developmental psychology, and other disciplines related to mental health, as well as professional organizations representing these professionals, have become increasingly involved in the shaping of policies and legislation designed to address the mental health challenges of children and youth. While the focus of legislative action on behalf of children is not new, the presence of researchers and clinicians in the debate has added a different dimension, offering new opportunities for interaction between research and policy.

The interest in social policy among mental health professionals was precipitated by a number of developments. One of these was the recognition that children develop within the social context; they are influenced by various aspects of their immediate environment as well as by the more remote social institutions such as the school, the workplace, government, and media (1). This led to policy responses and the development of programs to address the health and mental health needs of children. An example is the implementation during the 1960s and 1970s of federally sponsored social programs such as Project Head Start (2). The proliferation of such programs, and the funds made available for them, enabled researchers and clinicians to apply their knowledge and training to such areas as program development as well as become involved in and refine the understanding of policy and program evaluation (3). The integration of child development research and social policy has become so entwined in both the research and policy arenas that in order to secure funding for research, it has become necessary to demonstrate the practical application of findings and their potential to address unmet needs (4).

The problem of unmet psychiatric needs in children has been acknowledged for decades, as well as the contributory societal forces needed for proactive policy remedies (5). Between 10% and 20% of US children experience some form of diagnosable mental illness, and the aggregate cost of mental illness in terms of both direct and indirect costs to US taxpayers continues to climb (6). However, only a small proportion of the overall health budget is directed to children (7). Also, the recent health care reforms that have replaced fee-for-service care with managed care have had both a positive and negative impact on mental health care for children and adolescents. Although access to health services in general has increased for young people (8), with the emphasis on brief, problem-oriented approaches, it has become more difficult for children with serious emotional disorders to obtain the level of needed care. Additionally, 90% of health care expenditures for children are consumed by the 15% of children who have chronic illness and disability, leaving little for mental health care for the vast majority of children who need it.

WHO SHAPES POLICY?

Within the world of health care, there are several types of individuals whose work are critical in shaping policy and helping to move proposed bills into law. There are even more individuals involved in assuring that those policies that require funding receive appropriations. Researchers and clinicians have an opportunity to inform the policy process through various activities, such as conducting policy-relevant research, providing expert testimony, and informing policymakers of social and economic trends that may contribute to child and adolescent health problems and require a policy response.

Policy Analysts

These are individuals who most commonly hold a masters degree, juris doctorate, or PhD and work for government or policy think tanks. A think tank is an organization who is endowed or funded to work on specific issues (i.e., health care, housing, and defense). Think tanks employ policy analysts to do research on these topics that are later used to inform policy (9). An example of a think tank that focuses much of its research on health care policy is the RAND Corporation. This corporation is primarily federally funded. The U.S. Department of Defense, branches of the U.S. military and the Department of Health and Human Services contribute the largest percentages of the organization's funding. RAND develops research to evaluate existing policies and identify policy gaps. Within organizations such as RAND, policy analysts are employed to review extant research and complete studies with the aim of scientifically informing policy (for our purposes, health policy specifically) that often directly impact policy language and funding of legislation (10). These individuals spend their days researching topics in health care, collecting and analyzing data, and publishing papers that help translate scientific results into policy language.

Lobbyists

A lobbyist is a person who works for an organization either for pay or pro bono to influence legislation directly. Lobbyists may work directly with legislators to influence language and initiation of bills or they may work to have constituents contact legislators on specific raised bills. In addition to meeting with legislators, they also analyze, research, and educate others about issues pertinent to the raised legislation. Lobbyists have no specific educational requirements, but most have at least a bachelor's degree and have completed internships with lobbying groups or in government (11). While there are no educational requirements, there are laws that regulate the activities of lobbyists, amount of time an organization can lobby, and the amount of money that can be spent on lobbying activities. Lobbyists must be registered with state and federal governments. This registration monitors the activities of the lobbyist and for whom they work. California requires lobbyists to participate in an ethics course.

Advocates

The terms *advocate* and *lobbyist* are often used interchangeably. However, there is a distinction between the two. As we have covered, lobbyists work to directly influence specific legislation. An advocate is an individual who supports or promotes dissemination of information on a particular topic or issue. Advocates work to promote awareness about issues through direct discussion with law makers, supporting activities, educating the public, and creating networks of influence. Both advocates and lobbyists have relationships with legislators and influence policy, but advocates often focus on an issue, while lobbyists often focuses mostly on a specific piece of legislation. There is no specific education or registration for policy advocates (11).

Policy Consultants

A public policy consultant serves to inform the public and the organization on a particular issue. They may inform a community on issues of child mental health through partnerships with community organizations, developing outreach programs, or working with various media outlets. They inform the organization about policy relevant to the organization and research the impact that the organization has on their community. A policy consultant usually has a master's degree in a policy-related field. The consultant influences policy through the organization's influence in their community and through relationships with policy makers (11).

CONTRIBUTORY FACTORS AMENABLE TO POLICY IMPACT

Many social and environmental risk factors are implicated in the onset of mental dysfunction. Included among these risk factors are prolonged separations between the parent and child, physical or sexual abuse, poverty, marital discord, parental psychopathology, instability in the family environment, and a variety of other stressors related to family life. Children who experience one of these risk factors may not be any more likely to suffer serious consequences than children with no risk factors (12). However, the more risks or stressors that are present in children's lives, the greater the probability of damaging outcomes. Also, some risk factors compound other problems. For example, low birth weight and central nervous system difficulties in isolation often may have no discernable negative effects, but may be exacerbated if the child is raised in an unstable, low-income, or stressful or unresponsive family environment (13).

Access to Health Care

The Affordable Care Act (ACA) was comprehensive health care legislation passed in 2010 that aimed to increase access and affordability of health care for all US citizens. Its comprehensive nature precludes many from understanding how it pertains to them as an individual health care consumer or practitioner. Therefore, we will cover aspects of the ACA that are particularly pertinent to the practicing child and adolescent psychiatrist.

The first area to discuss is the expansion of coverage. This is important for child and adolescent psychiatrists as many more children seeking mental health care will have private insurance. The number of individuals with insurance overall has increased and the reinforcing mental health parity act means that more children will also have mental health coverage (14). Prior to this law, many children were not covered by any insurance (including Medicaid) leaving the costs of treatment in the hands of parents or hospitals in the form of indigent care provisions.

In order to enforce this coverage expansion, the federal government established incentives and penalties. One incentive for states is that they will get federal support for Medicaid programs to start mandatory health care exchanges. An exchange is an online health insurance marketplace where consumers can compare various policies and be informed about their individual incentive-tax credits. The government provides for graduated tax credits for individual incomes at 100% to 400% of the federal poverty level (15). The programs receiving federal support include Medicaid and the Children's Health Insurance Program (CHIP). Medicaid coverage was expanded to individuals at or below 133% of the federal poverty level (this was $24,300 for a family of four in 2016). CHIP is a program created by the balanced budget act of 1997. CHIP expands health coverage for children through a federal fund match for state Medicaid and increases the wage limit for children to access Medicaid insurance (16). If individuals and families are not insured through their employer or the exchanges, with some exceptions, then there is a tax penalty ranging from $695 to $2,085 and based on household income.

In addition to an increase in the numbers of individuals with increased access to health insurance, individuals saw differences in the ways that they were able to use their insurance and what their insurance covered. Firstly, insurance companies now have to report the percentage of collected premiums used on clinical services. If this is under 85%, then the insurance company is required to provide a rebate to their customers. Second, there may no longer be lifetime or annual limits on insurance use and an individual may not be excluded from being insured based on a pre-existing condition (17). The importance of this is that those with mental health disorders were hit hardest by these limits. For example, some insurance companies may stipulate only 30 days of inpatient psychiatric treatment per year. This would not impact some, but those with chronic and treatment resistant illness would reach a period in which their insurance would not pay, regardless of need. Thirdly, there are limits on the deductible that may be charged by the insurance company. This is $2,000 for an individual and $4,000 for a family. Also, insurance companies now must cover certain preventative health interventions. Finally, the Centers for Medicaid and Medicare Services may receive a 17.1% reduction in costs from pharmaceutical companies for medications exclusively developed for pediatric populations (17).

There were three important provisions of the ACA impacting children and pediatric providers that are not insurance related. One is that it reinforced the Mental Health Parity Addiction Equity Act of 2008. This law stated that mental health and addiction services must have equal coverage and reimbursement to medical services of a similar level. This landmark legislation is not yet fully enacted in many states as it is the responsibility of the state to ensure that this is occurring (18). The second provision is for an increase in funding to community- and school-based health centers. Finally, there was an expansion of funding for the National Health Service Corps (NHSC) to increase the recruitment of primary care practitioners (17). House bill 2646 seeks to have child psychiatrists included amongst the NHSC practitioners, and this bill currently is making its way through the legislation process at the time that this chapter was written.

Poverty

Numerous programs designed to mitigate the negative outcomes associated with poverty have been implemented over the years. Nevertheless, poverty's impact on children remains a grave concern. One in five children ages 18 and under live in poverty (19). Several contributing factors, such as single-parent families are noted. Other historically contributing factors are related to ebbs and flows in the economy, leading to cuts in public assistance and the decline in the real value of family income (20). The ramifications of living in poverty are numerous and include assaults on children's physical and mental health (21), brought on by unsteady access to health care, a lack of money to spend on health-promoting activities, poor nutrition, lack of transportation, and inadequate housing (22). As a result, children in poverty have a higher mortality rate and experience greater health and mental health challenges (23), with the major pathways occurring indirectly through environmental stresses and feelings of powerlessness and frustration that often accompany poverty (24). The economy's impact on all families, not only those in poverty, can be significant. For example, the Great Recession of 2008 left many without jobs, and while its repercussions on individuals and families are still unfolding (25), impacts have contributed to an increase in child maltreatment cases (26).

The United States provides far less public income assistance to poor and single-parent families than many other industrialized nations. Instead, welfare reform initiatives, particularly those of the late 1990s, emphasize labor force participation as the route out of poverty. More recently, increases in the minimum wage have occurred, but wage rates remain low, particularly for less-skilled workers, and contribute to poverty. For two-parent families, low wages have been partly offset by the entry of increasing numbers of women into the labor force, but for single-parent families the escape from poverty is more difficult. The decline in real income affects adults and children. However, for children the consequences are particularly serious because a significant percentage of families in poverty are those with young children.

Sometimes new policies and legislation create new challenges. The most dramatic piece of US legislation for low-income children and families during the past 40 years was the Personal Responsibility and Work Opportunity Reconciliation Act of 1996, which included provisions for job training. This resulted in a 40% of reduction in the numbers of dependent families, along with a substantial increase in labor force participation by mothers (17). However, a primary implication of increased employment, particularly for mothers, was the need for child care. Many parents lack access to high-quality care for their children, either through availability or cost. A second implication of the welfare reform emphasis on employment was that some parents who have difficulty maintaining employment, often those with mental illness or substance abuse problems, were rendered ineligible for financial assistance, thus increasing the poverty of their family. Thirdly, welfare and immigration legislation has reduced access to noncash services such as Medicaid and food-assistance programs, affecting 20% of US children, increasing the effective child poverty rate (27).

Community and Domestic Violence

Although exact numbers are hard to quantify, there is little doubt that a large number of children are exposed to violence in their homes, schools, and communities as victims, observers, or perpetrators. Violence in schools received much media attention during the past decade, but despite several tragic incidents, has actually been declining (28), due in part to the provision of federal and state funding for after-school programs which provide supervised recreational and educational activities for children and youth during times when school is out (29).

However, increasing numbers of children and youth are exposed to violence in other settings. In 2014, more than two thirds of children ages 17 and younger were exposed to violence within the past year, or at some time during their lives, either as victims or witnesses and were more likely than adults to be exposed to violence and crime (30). Such findings are troubling not only because of the threat to children's safety, but because of the short- and long-term impact on their healthy development (31). A key protective factor is a relationship with a caring, responsible adult, usually a parent (32). However, in some instances, parents may be emotionally or practically unavailable to their children, because they themselves may be the victims or perpetrators of violence. Therefore, the resources of other adults in the community need to be tapped, creating a great potential for community partnerships and school-based programs to lead the way in reducing violence among young people and to promote resilience.

Unfortunately, many children also experience violence in their own homes. While the issue of domestic violence has been on the policy and research agenda for several decades, the impact on children has received less attention. Such violence cuts across social strata, but is more prevalent among families living in poverty and is associated with multiple stressors, including substance abuse; in 30% to 60% of families experiencing domestic violence, child maltreatment is also present (33). Possible consequences for these children include behavioral and academic problems and depression, and in adulthood they may develop low self-esteem, and resort to violence and criminal behavior (34). Innovative approaches to address the needs of children involved in violence have been developed. One example of these is a collaboration among police departments and mental health professionals to identify children experiencing violence as well as provide needed clinical services and follow-up home visits (35). Another example is the use of canine-assisted therapy in schools to help calm the children and enhance their self-esteem and ability to cope (36).

Divorce

Divorce has become the norm for the majority of families. Although the divorce rate has peaked, most US children experience the remarriage of one or both of their parents or live in reconstituted families (37). While divorce is not necessarily insurmountable for children, stresses arising from the disruption and subsequent remarriage of parents can lead to psychological difficulties among children (38). The long-term effects of divorce and remarriage are related to a number of factors, including the child's developmental status, gender, and temperament; the quality of the home environment; mental health status of the parents; and availability of support systems both to the parents and the child (39). Particular concern is noted for children whose custodial parent experiences extreme economic difficulties for an extended period of time and/or whose noncustodial parent fails to pay for child support (40). At substantial risk are children who are involved in prolonged custody fights. Many judges and lawyers are ill-prepared for the arduous task of determining the best interests of the child, not trained to consider children's needs and concerns or weigh the urgency of their condition and circumstances (41). Today, all states have statutes requiring that in all child custody cases, as well as in proceedings for termination of parental rights, decisions be made on the basis of the best interests of the child (42). Since such determination is often difficult to make, the courts often seek guidance from mental health professions (43).

Knowledge about how divorce affects children and parents should be disseminated not only among policymakers and those in the legal profession but also among other professionals who work with children, such as teachers. One important policy development has been the use of mediation services in divorce cases. These services are staffed by mental health professionals who have access to legal advice. Although initially begun as a way to curtail the high costs of divorce, families who have used mediation services note that one of the major benefits of the services is the availability of psychological support (44). Several successful support programs for children of divorce have been developed in schools across the United States (45). However, they are few in number and meet the needs of only a small percentage of the children who stand to benefit from such programs (46). Given the number of children who need such support, these programs should be made available in all schools, or at least in some schools in every community. The federal government can take a leadership role by making available funds that would finance the development of such programs.

Child Care, Work-Life Balance, and Family Leave Policy

Although numerous societal changes and potential problems are associated with women's participation in the labor force, none are as significant as the unprecedented demand for child care services. Today, the need for high quality, affordable child care is one of the most widely recognized social issue and has been a major problem for several decades. At the 1970 White House Conference on Children, the need for child care services was noted as the number one priority for the nation to address. However, two obstacles—ideological arguments against the use of child care, as well as the lack of public awareness of the need for child care services—stood in the way of policy action on the issue (47). As a result, the problem worsened, reaching crisis proportions as more mothers, especially those with infants and young children, joined the labor force.

There are numerous facets to the child care problem, one of these being the high cost of services. From a policy perspective, the high cost of care is significant for at least two other reasons. First, child care costs are a major expenditure for families, and the amount of money families spend on child care is directly related to their income (48). Low-income families spend less on child care in absolute terms than do higher income families, but the proportion of the family budget that is taken up by child care costs is greater among low-income families, who have to allocate as much as 27% of their earnings to child care (49). Even for middle-income families, the burden of child care costs is great, as they do not qualify for state subsidies and pay higher taxes on their earnings (50). Second, there is a relationship between the cost and quality of care, with good-quality care costing substantially more than poor quality, custodial care. This being the case, there are inequalities in the quality of child care children experience depending on their family's income. The fact that good-quality care is a privilege that only some children are enjoying is of concern, because child care is an environment where children spend a large portion of every day and has significant effects on children's development and well-being (51).

The high cost of child care and lack of good quality care is an issue not only due to the possible harm to children, but also because it is a source of stress for parents. This has prompted discussions of the need to make changes in the workplace to create conditions that are supportive of family life, such as corporate support of child care services. Also, some corporations implement flexible schedules to allow employees time for child-rearing responsibilities (52).

Related to flexible work schedules is the need for family leave policies that would enable parents to spend time with their infants during the first several months after birth. The first few months of life represent a critical period for the development of attachment between parents and the infant, and within the context of a secure parent–infant relationship babies thrive and become increasingly autonomous (53). The first few months of life also represent a very stressful period that necessitate the adjustment of all family members to the newborn (54). Although the importance of such leave has been noted on the basis of medical and social science research for over three decades (55), adequate parental leave is still not available to most US parents. The Family and Medical Leave Act (FMLA) was enacted in 1993, granting 12 weeks of unpaid leave in any 12-month period to employees in companies of 50 or more workers. Its impact was limited by prior state legislation and exemptions for many employers (56,57). Furthermore, the leave was unpaid, and research shows that many have been discouraged from taking leave for financial reasons (58).

EFFECTING POLICY CHANGE

In order to effect positive policy change on behalf of children and families, it is important to note both the promise and problems inherent in research-informed policy decisions, as well as the need for a cadre of professionals well trained to work at the intersect of clinical knowledge, research, and policy development.

Promise and Problems in Research-Informed Policy Decisions

There are numerous contributions that mental health professionals have made. For example, school-based programs have been developed by psychiatrists such as James Comer in an effort to prevent affective disorders in children and ensure responsivity to children's mental health needs. The authors of this chapter have also developed a school-based early care and family support program, known as the School of the 21st Century (21C). The program has been implemented in over 1,300 schools across the country (59) and has paved the way for a range of other programs that utilize the school building to provide academic as well as nonacademic support services for both children and families. 21C also inspired a renewed focus on the community school and the importance of addressing the needs of the whole child—focusing on all developmental pathways, including cognitive, social, emotional, and physical development. This point was noted by the National Institute of Health and is reflected in the 2015 Reauthorization of the Elementary and Secondary Education Act. This legislation, recently reauthorized as the Every Child Succeeds Act (ESSA), opens the door to assessing the school's climate and providing mental health and other support services.

Indeed, as a result of their involvement in program development and evaluation, mental health researchers have accumulated a vast amount of knowledge that "totally transforms the nation's capacity to improve outcomes for vulnerable children" (60). This knowledge, derived from over three decades of program development and evaluation, includes evidence of the effectiveness of a number of programs that reduce the burdens of risk factors in childhood, thereby reducing the probability of later damage (61). Fortunately, it is not necessary to change everything—the structure of opportunity, the neighborhood environment, and other aspects of the child's life—in order to make a crucial difference for children at risk.

The failure to utilize research to impact policy stems from several problems. One such problem is that the information on effective programs is generally not shared with the public or with policymakers (62). Even in cases where programs' potential benefits are known, there is skepticism that such programs, once they are replicated, will continue to be effective. Although this is a valid concern, successful programs can be built upon if we can attract and train enough skilled and motivated individuals, if we devise a variety of replication strategies, and if we resist the lure of replication through dilution. In efforts to serve as many children as possible or due to lack of sufficient funds, programs often are diluted, thus diminishing their quality and potential benefits (63).

Although an increasing number of mental health researchers are working in the policy arena, there is still a rather uneasy relationship between them and policymakers. Policymakers often regard researchers as impractical (64). From their perspective, they may be skeptical of policy recommendations coming from researchers who do not seem to understand the complexities of achieving a consensus among rival constituencies. Researchers, on the other hand, seem to regard policymakers as disingenuous and too willing to compromise even when the research evidence does not justify such action. Part of the tension and mistrust between policymakers and mental health researchers emanates from the assumption that knowledge from research is value free, whereas policies are made in a complex value-laden context (65). However, this characterization of research and policy is misleading. Often, scientific research takes on the values of the investigators, as is evident in the questions asked, methodologies employed, and the interpretation and presentation of the findings.

Problems such as these impede the utilization of research in policy settings. The problems are further exacerbated by the fact that researchers are often perceived as unable to provide clear answers to policy questions, or, looked at from another perspective, that policymakers are unable to ask questions in a way that would lead to valid and reliable research. In part, this problem stems from the unrealistic expectations among policymakers and the inability of many of them to appreciate that single studies cannot, in and of themselves, provide definitive answers to questions. But researchers also contribute to the problem. Often researchers are unfamiliar with the policy process or are unable to "read" political issues. They hold to long, slow standards of proof and refutation that are, in the policy arena, "obstructive and nihilistic" (66). Although it is imperative that researchers uphold their professional standards and credibility as scientists (67), there are times when findings from the research, even if they are not entirely conclusive, can nonetheless provide a direction for policy. For example, the research on the effects of child care on children's development was controversial, yielding conflicting findings that served to confuse the public and policymakers (68). Although research on the topic continues, researchers were able to convene and come to a consensus that indicated that as long as young children are in a good-quality child care settings, they will not be adversely affected by their experiences in child care. This led to a policy recommendation for efforts to monitor the quality of care children receive and ensure that all children receive care that is conducive to optimal development (69). It is apparent that there are circumstances, such as the increasing number of children in child care, when awaiting definitive conclusions from the research is counterproductive, especially when action can be taken at the same time that research on a particular issue is continuing.

A different problem occurs when research findings are misused by academics or the media to support a vested policy interest. An example is the controversial issue of the importance of the early years in child development. The findings on brain research have been illuminating, although in many cases preliminary, and have shown the developmental importance of the first three years of life. Such studies have captured media and policy attention. Some researchers, excited by the window of opportunity for action on behalf of children, made exaggerated and distorted claims not substantiated by the research (70). The debate has been taken up by the national media, with viewpoints expressed through sound bites, undermining the complex scientific findings of decades of research (71).

Training the Next Generation of Policy Shapers

Understanding what impedes the use of research in policy is important if mental health researchers are to have an impact in the policy arena. To encourage the use of research in carving out policy directions, researchers should (a) be concerned in a nonpartisan way with the values and interests of society in general and children in particular, (b) take a practical approach and suggest policies that are feasible and have a chance of attracting widespread political and public support, (c) respond to the needs of policymakers and provide them with recommendations for action on the basis of research findings, and (d) become cognizant of and responsive to the policy process (72). Researchers also should make serious attempts to disseminate their findings to the greater world outside of academia, not only to policymakers but also to the general public. No society acts until it has a sense of the immediacy of the problem (73). Unfortunately, many professionals who understand the needs of children and families best have little or no training or experience in the media and policy arenas.

Fortunately, child and adolescent psychiatrists, developmental psychologists, and other mental health professionals are becoming aware of the need for public education on the needs of children (74). And, in a departure from their past practices, many mental health professionals are no longer satisfied with simply sharing information with one another. Rather, they disseminate their knowledge not only by presenting their findings directly to policymakers but also by taking steps to ensure that the information is covered in the popular media. Indeed, the dissemination of research in the context of the popular media has come to be accepted as an important aspect of the training received by some, yet still far too few, professionals in the field of mental health.

Some mental health professionals are also receiving training in the integration of child development research and social policy, learning not only about the policy process but also about some of the ways to merge their knowledge with that of policymakers in the formation of programs and policies for children. For example, in 1978 with support from the Bush Foundation in Minnesota, four university-based child development and social policy training centers were established, one of which is the Edward Zigler Center in Child Development and Social Policy at Yale University. The Zigler Center has prepared doctoral students and postdoctoral fellows in a variety of disciplines related to mental health to apply their knowledge in the policy arena. Many graduates of the Zigler Center have gone on to work in the policy arena or in other universities where they have established courses and programs on the integration of child development research and social policy. The success of the training centers is evident not only in the increased number of researchers who apply their work to the policy arena, but also in the numerous issues, such as child care, parental leave, and the need for family support services, that only a few years ago were not discussed but that now command national attention. The success of these efforts is further evident in that an increasing number of policymakers are now acknowledging the importance of research in the formulation of policies and are actively seeking the collaboration of professionals in the field of mental health. If mental health professionals and policymakers continue to work together in this spirit of collaboration, we will be able to bring about much-needed changes that will assist family life.

References

1. Bronfenbrenner U: *The Ecology of Human Development*. Cambridge, MA, Harvard University Press, 1979.
2. Zigler E, Styfco S: *Head Start and Beyond: A National Plan for Extended Childhood Intervention*. New Haven, CT, Yale University Press, 1993.
3. Phillips D: *Quality Child Care: What Does the Research Tell Us?* Washington, DC, National Association for the Education of Young Children, 1987.
4. Zigler E: A place of value for applied and policy studies. *Child Dev* 69: 532–542, 1998.
5. *Institute of Medicine Research on Children and Adolescents with Mental, Behavioral and Developmental Disorders*. Washington, DC, National Academy Press, 1989.
6. Insel TR: Editorial: assessing the economic costs of serious mental illness. *Am J Psychiatry* 165:663–665, 2008.
7. Deal LW, Shiono PH, Behrman RE: Children and managed healthcare: analysis and recommendations. *Future Child* 8(2):4–24, 1998.
8. Stroul BA, Pires SA, Armstrong MI, et al.: The impact of managed care on mental health services for children and their families. *Future Child* 8(2):119–133, 1998.
9. Blanchard S: Policy analysts: shaping society through research. *Occup Outlook Q* 20–25, 2007.
10. RAND Corporation: Access June 2016, http://www.rand.org/about.html
11. Brown L: *Life after Law: Finding Work You Love with the J. D. You Have*. Brookline, MA, Bibiliomotion, 2013.
12. Rutter M: *Changing Youth in a Changing Society*. Cambridge, MA, Harvard University Press, 1980.
13. Hughes D, Simpson L: The role of social change in preventing low birthweight. *Future Child* 5(1):87–102, 1995.
14. *Mental Health Parity and Addiction Equity Act*. Washington, DC, U.S. Department of Health and Human Services. Accessed June 2016, https:// www.cms.gov/CCIIO/Programs-and-Initiatives/Other-Insurance-Protections/mhpaea_factsheet.html
15. *Children's Health Insurance Program*. Washington, DC, National Conference of State Legislators. Accessed June 2016, http://www.ncsl.org/research/health/childrens-health-insurance-program-overview.aspx
16. *Summary of the Affordable Care Act*. Menlo Park, CS, Henry J. Kaiser Family Foundation. Accessed June 2016, http://kff.org/health-reform/fact-sheet/summary-of-the-affordable-care-act/
17. Blum BB, Berrey EC: *Welfare Research Perspectives: Past, Present and Future*. New York, National Center for Children in Poverty, 1999.
18. Barry C, Huskamp H, Goldman H: A political history of federal mental health and addiction insurance parity. *Milbank Q* 88:404–433, 2010.
19. U.S. Bureau of the Census: *Income and Poverty in US 2014 Report*. Report # P60-252. Washington, DC, U.S. Bureau of the Census, 2015.
20. Blank RM: *It Takes a Nation: A New Agenda for Fighting Poverty*. New York, RussellSage, 1997.
21. Wolfe B: Economic issues of healthcare. In: Chase-Lansdale PL, Brooks-Gunn J (eds): *Escape from Poverty: What Makes a Difference to Children?* New York, Cambridge, 1995:170–188.
22. Klerman L: *Alive and Well? Health Care for Children in America*. New York, National Center for Children in Poverty, 1991.
23. Webster-Stratton C: Preventing conduct problems in Head Start children: Strengthening parenting competencies. *J Consult Clin Psychol* 66:715–730, 1998.
24. Albee GW, Gullotta TP: *Primary Prevention Works*. Thousand Oaks, CA, Russell Sage, 1997.
25. Grusky DM, Western B, Wimer C (eds): *The Great Recession*. New York, Russell Sage, 2011.

26. Brooks-Gunn J, Schneider W, Waldfogel J: The Great Recession and the risk for child maltreatment. *Child Abuse Negl* 37:721–729, 2013.
27. Aber L, Brooks-Gunn J, Maynard R: The effects of welfare reform on teenage parents and their children. *Future Child* 5(2):53–71, 1995.
28. U.S. Department of Education, National Center for Education Statistics: *Indicators of School Crime and Safety: 2014 (NCES 2015-072).* Washington, DC, U.S. Department of Education, 2015.
29. Sandoval J, Brock S, Knifton K: Acts of violence. In: Sandoval J (ed): *Handbook of Crisis Counseling, Intervention and Prevention in Schools.* 3rd ed. New York, Routledge, 212–228, 2013.
30. Finkelhor D, Turner H, Shattcuk A, et al.: Prevalence of childhood exposure to violence, crime, and abuse: results from the national survey of children's exposure to violence. *Pediatrics* 169:756–754, 2015.
31. Marans S, Schaefer MC: Community policing, schools and mental health: the challenge of collaboration. In: Elliott DE, Hamburg BA, Williams KR (eds): *Violence in American Schools: A New Perspective.* New York, Cambridge University Press, 1998.
32. Gunnar M: *Quality Care and the Buffering of Stress Physiology: Its Potential in Protecting the Developing Human Brain.* Minneapolis, University of Minnesota, Institute of Child Development, 1996.
33. Edelson JL: The overlap between child maltreatment and woman battering. *Violence Against Women* 5:134–154, 1999.
34. *Future Child: Domestic Violence and Children* 9(3), 1999 [entire issue].
35. Marans S, Beckman M: Police-mental health collaboration on behalf of children exposed to violence. In: Lightburn A, Sessions P (eds): *Handbook of Community-Based Clinical Practice.* New York, Oxford, 2015.
36. Finn-Stevenson M: The transformative power of the dog: the growing use of canine-assistants in therapeutic interventions and school settings. *J Am Acad Child Adolesc Psychiatry* 55:437–438, 2016.
37. Emery RE: *Marriage, Divorce, and Children's Adjustment.* 2nd ed. Thousand Oaks, CA, Sage, 1999.
38. Twaite JA, Silitsky D, Luchow AK: *Children of Divorce: Adjustment, Parental Conflict, Custody, Remarriage, and Recommendations for Clinician.* Lanham, MD, Jason Aronson, 1998.
39. Hetherington EM, Hagan MS, Anderson ER: Marital transition: a child's perspective. *Am Psychol* 44:303–312, 1989.
40. Haskins R, Schwartz JB, Akin JS, et al.: How much support can absent fathers pay? *Policy Studies* 14:201, 1985.
41. Wallerstein J: Child of divorce: an overview. *Behav Sci Law* 4:105–118, 1986.
42. U.S. Administration for Children, Youth and Families, Children's Bureau: *Determining the Best Interests of the Child.* Washington, DC, Author, 2012.
43. Hetherington EM, Camara KA: Families in transition: the process of dissolution and reconstitution. In: Parke RD (ed): *Review of Child Development Research.* Vol 7: The Family. Chicago, University of Chicago Press, 1984.
44. Bahr SJ: An evaluation of court mediation: a comparison in divorce cases with children. *J Fam Issues* 2:39–60, 1981.
45. Weiss HB: *State Leadership in Family Support Programs.* Cambridge, MA, Harvard Family Research Project, Harvard University, 1989.
46. Emory R: *Renegotiating Family relationships: Divorce, Child Custody and Mediation.* New York, Guildford, 2012.
47. Nelson JR: The politics of federal day care regulation. In: Zigler E, Gordon E (eds): *Day Care: Scientific and Social Policy Issues.* Boston, MA, Auburn House, 1982.
48. *Future Child: Financing Child Care* 6(2), 1996 [entire issue].
49. Kagan SL, Cohen N: *Funding and Financing Early Care and Education.* New Haven, CT, Bush Center on Child Development and Social Policy, Yale University, 1997.
50. Betson DM, Michael RT: Why so many children are poor. *Future Child* 7(2): 25–39, 1997.
51. Newman S, Brazelton TB, Zigler E, et al.: *America's Child Care Crisis: A Crime Prevention Tragedy.* Washington, DC, Fight Crime: Invest in Kids, 2000.
52. U.S. Bureau of National Affairs: *Special Report. Work and Family: A Changing Dynamic.* Rockville, MD, Author, 1986.
53. Cicchetti D, Cummings M, Greenberg M, et al.: An organizational perspective on attachment beyond infancy: implications for theory, measurement, and research. In: Greenberg M, Cicchetti D, Cummings M (eds): *Attachment in the Preschool Years: Theory, Research, and Intervention.* Chicago, University of Chicago Press, 1990.
54. Brazelton TB: Issues for working parents. *Am J Orthopsychiatry* 56: 14–25, 1985.
55. Hopper P, Zigler E: The medical and social science basis for a national infant care leave policy. *Am J Orthopsychiatry* 58:324–338, 1988.
56. Finn-Stevenson M, Trzcinski E: Mandated leave: an analysis of federal and state legislation. *Am J Orthopsychiatry* 61:567–575, 1991.
57. U.S. Department of Labor, Commission on Family and Medical Leave: *A Workable Balance: Report to the Congress on Family and Medical Leave Policies.* Washington, DC, U.S. Department of Labor, Women's Bureau, 1996.
58. Waldfogel J: The impact of the family and medical leave act. *J Pol Anal Manag* 18:281–302, 1999.
59. Finn-Stevenson M, Zigler E: *Schools of the 21st Century: Linking Child Care and Education.* Boulder, CO, Westview Press, 1999.
60. Schorr LB, Schorr D: *Within Our Reach: Breaking the Cycle of Disadvantage.* New York, Doubleday, 1988.
61. Price RH, Cowen EL, Lorion RP, et al., (eds): *Fourteen Ounces of Prevention: A Casebook for Practitioners.* Washington, DC, American Psychological Association Press, 1988.
62. Zervigon-Hakes A: Culture clash: translating research findings into public policy. In: Barnett WS, Boocock SS (eds): *Early Care and Education for Children in Poverty: Promises, Programs, and Long-Term Results.* New York, State University of New York Press, 1998.
63. Zigler E, Berman W: Discerning the future of early childhood intervention. *Am Psychologist* 38:894–906, 1983.
64. Maccoby EE, Kahn A, Everett BA: The role of psychology research in the formation of policies affecting children. *Am Psychologist* 38:80–84, 1983.
65. Meltsner AI: The seven deadly sins of policy analysis. *Knowledge: Creation, Diffusion, Utilization* 7:367–382, 1986.
66. Thompson R: Developmental research and legal policy: toward a two-way street. In: Cicchetti D, Toth S (eds): *Child Abuse, Child Development and Social Policy.* Norwood, NJ, Ablex, 1993.
67. Zigler E, Finn-Stevenson M: Applied developmental psychology. In: Lamb M, Bornstein M (eds): *Developmental Psychology: An Advanced Textbook.* Hillsdale, NJ, Erlbaum, 1987.
68. Clarke-Stewart KA: Infant day care: maligned or malignant? *Am Psychologist* 44:266–273, 1989.
69. National Center for Clinical Infant Programs: *Who Will Mind the Babies?* Washington, DC, National Center for Clinical Infant Programs, 1988.
70. Bruer JT: *Myth of the First Three Years: A New Understanding of Early Brain Development and Lifelong Learning.* New York, Free Press, 1999.
71. Zigler E, Finn-Stevenson M, Hall N: *The First Three Years and Beyond: Brain Development and Social Policy.* New Haven, CT, Yale University Press, 2004.
72. Lindblom CE: Who needs what social research for policy making? *Knowledge: Creation, Diffusion, Utilization* 7:345–366, 1986.
73. Zigler E, Finn M: From problem to solution: changing public policy as it affects children and families. *Young Child* 36:31–59, 1981.
74. McCall RB, Gregory TG, Murray JP: Community developmental research results to the general public through television. *Dev Psychol* 20:45–54, 1984.

CHAPTER 1.7 ■ MONEY MATTERS: FUNDING CARE

MARTIN KNAPP, DAVID MCDAID, AND EMMA WILSON

INTRODUCTION

The primary concerns of anyone working with children and adolescents with mental health issues are alleviation of symptoms, promotion of quality of life, support for families, and improvement of broad life chances. These should also be the primary concerns of anyone with responsibility for resource allocation, whether it is deciding how much funding can be made available, how it is shared between competing uses, or how to improve efficiency in its use. These latter concerns can be seen as economic questions, but they cannot be answered without a clear understanding of child and family needs and preferences, and the expected outcomes of interventions.

Interventions for children and adolescents include primary prevention of behavioral and emotional problems, services that respond to the emergence of such problems, treatments that directly address symptoms and their immediate consequences, and actions targeted on longer-term, broader implications for individuals and communities. For almost any such intervention to be successful—indeed, for it to be initiated—skilled staff are needed, supported by appropriate capital and other resources. Underpinning this process should be meaningful input from children and adolescents during the design, development, delivery, and evaluation of any intervention. In turn, because little in life is free, this requires commitment of the necessary finances.

The purpose of this chapter is to explore the links just outlined between finances, resources, and achievements. We first introduce a conceptual framework that summarizes the main connections linking resources to outcomes. One source of complexity that runs throughout the arguments in this chapter is that many children and adolescents have multiple needs, often prompting multiple responses—from health care, education, social work, criminal justice, and other services. Each service sector has its own funding streams and associated arrangements for allocating resources; we consider this mixed economy in the third section and the importance of integrated services, including both mental and physical. We then turn to a discussion of financing arrangements: How are child and adolescent mental health services funded? In judging whether financing arrangements are delivering the services and outcomes needed and wanted, we refer to two widely discussed performance criteria: efficiency (the balance between outcomes and what it costs to achieve them) and equity (whether outcomes, access, and burdens are fairly distributed). Achieving better performance by those criteria is often hampered. We therefore next discuss the resource barriers in the way of progress and the opportunities moving forward. The concluding section summarizes the key messages.

THE PRODUCTION OF WELFARE

As a starting point, it is helpful to explicate the links between budgets, staff, and other resources hired or purchased, treatments and other services thereby delivered, and health and quality of life improvements hopefully experienced by children, families, and communities. A simple representation of a treatment and care system helps to identify the probable connections between key entities (Figure 1.7.1):

- *Revenue collection* is the process by which health, education, social care, and other systems receive money from individuals, households, employers, and other organizations. The funds thereby available to those systems are the *purchasing budgets,* to be allocated between competing needs and demands.
- *Commissioning* is the process by which purchasers (e.g., insurance funds and government departments) transfer funds to service providers in return for (usually) contractually agreed services.
- *Provider budgets* are the funds available to the bodies that actually deliver services, such as the operating budget of a hospital or citywide community program.
- For those services to be delivered (whether administering referrals, assessment, treatment, or supervision), *resource inputs* are employed: staff, buildings, equipment, medications, and other consumables.
- Some resources are not bought and sold in markets, such as family care, volunteer inputs (such as befriending or peer-mentoring), and support from faith and community groups. But these inputs are not really "free": using them in one activity (in supporting children with behavioral problems, say) means they are unavailable for other uses (such as a volunteer or parent getting a paid job). In other words, there are *opportunity costs.*
- Services produced from combinations of the resource inputs can be labeled *intermediate outputs.* They indicate success: deploying funds to hire staff to deliver services is an achievement in its own right. But they are not the ultimate goals of mental health systems (which are usually expressed in terms of health and quality of life improvement). Relevant questions about these intermediate outputs concern volume (How many patients attend their appointments? How many therapy sessions are delivered? How many children are supported in a

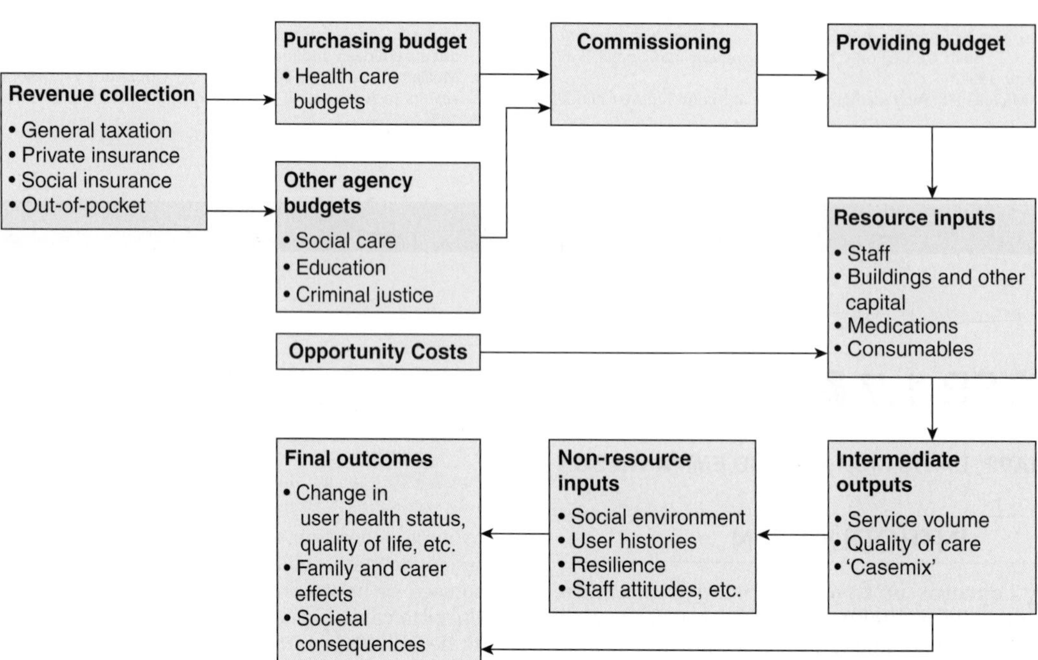

FIGURE 1.7.1. The production of welfare framework, revenue collection, and commissioning.

school-based program?), quality of care, and the characteristics of service users ("case-mix" in health care parlance).

- *Final outcomes* are the focal point of the whole system: symptom alleviation, fewer behavioral problems, improved functioning, educational attainment, and quality of life enhancement. Potentially, there are also outcomes for communities. Some final outcomes take years to reveal themselves fully. Few can be assessed adequately without asking the individuals themselves about their experiences.
- In between services (intermediate outputs) and outcomes are a number of mediating factors, such as the care-setting social milieu, young people's care histories, individual and family resilience, and staff attitudes. Although potentially very influential in determining the success of an intervention, they do not have a readily identified cost (since they are not usually marketed) and so they might get overlooked when attention focuses on how services are financed and what they achieve. These can be called *nonresource inputs.*

This representation was originally called the production of welfare framework (1) and developed to underpin discussion of the economics of care systems because (loose) analogies could be drawn between production processes as studied in mainstream economics and treatment and support approaches found in health, social care, and education to improve individual and family well-being. The stylized framework in Figure 1.7.1 has the signal virtues of highlighting the core connections between what goes into this system (finances, resource inputs thereby purchased, and unfunded contributions of family members and volunteers) and what comes out (services delivered, and improved outcomes for children, adolescents, and families). Although it looks highly simplified to anyone familiar with psychiatric, education, social care, or justice systems, in fact this representation is more complicated than often assumed by strategic decision makers looking for "quick fixes." Pumping more money into a system will only generate better outcomes for children, adolescents, and families if all the necessary links are in place and are functioning properly. Thus, revenue generation or collection needs to be planned carefully to avoid creating perverse incentives (see below), and skilled staff need support from other resources if they are to deliver quality services. Equally, organization of those services and the therapeutic approaches they employ should be chosen carefully to maximize the chances of successful resolution. This means looking not only at whether there is evidence of therapeutic effectiveness but also at cost-effectiveness.

Succinctly expressed, the success of a child and adolescent mental health system in improving health and quality of life will depend on the mix, volume, and deployment of resource inputs and the services they deliver, which in turn are dependent on available finances.

A MIXED ECONOMY

Child and adolescent mental health services as narrowly defined and conventionally viewed sit in a complex, multiservice, multibudget world. This is because children and adolescents with behavioral or emotional problems and their families often have multiple needs. In well-developed, well-resourced systems, these needs could be identified, assessed, and addressed by a number of different agencies (including pediatrics, child psychiatry, education, social work, and youth justice), and could have wide-ranging impacts.

For example, in the United States Costello et al., using survey data, documented if and what type of services were used by adolescents diagnosed with psychiatric disorders in a 1-year period. Of the 45% of adolescents who received any treatment, most were likely to receive care in an educational setting (23.6%) or specialty mental health services (22.8%), with just 10.1% supported by primary care services (2). Glied and Evans Cuellar (3) describe how 92% of children with serious emotional disturbances in another US study received services from more than two systems, and 19% from more than four. In England, around 50% of looked-after children (i.e., formally in the social care system managed by municipalities) were reported having emotional and mental health problems that would likely require inputs from the health care sector (4). Snell et al. (5) found that the education system bears by far the largest share (89%) of the costs of services used by children aged 5 to 15 with psychiatric disorders in Britain (compared to 7% for the health system, and 4% for social care). In contrast, in France inpatient and outpatient hospital services remain the mainstay of child and adolescent mental health services (6). Survey data in Australia indicated that 49% of adolescents with mental disorders made use of school-based services in the previous 12 months; 42% and 21% had visited a primary care doctor or psychiatrist at least once, but only 6% had made use of hospital and specialist mental health services (7). A study of the impact of youth mental illness on the United States economy showed how a range of services contributed substantially to the $247 billion estimate, alongside costs associated with lost productivity in employment and crime (8).

Multiple Provider Sectors

The resources described in Figure 1.7.1 might therefore come from any number of different systems. These services could be delivered by government (public sector), for-profit, or nonprofit organizations. Indeed, most countries have a thriving mixed economy of provision. There are additionally the multifarious contributions of parents, other family caregivers, and volunteers. Even health promotion strategies, which tend to be coordinated by public bodies, still need inputs from others, such as local communities (linked to the social capital effect).

Do these provider distinctions matter? Entities with different legal forms often behave differently in response to different incentives, and might be motivated by different goals. For instance, a government hospital may have different objectives and constraints from a for-profit hospital or a charitable hospital linked to a faith community. A school that provides emotional and behavioral health services may be focused primarily on pedagogical issues such as educational attachment or risk of classroom disruption by children with mental health difficulties. This may affect their modus operandi, patterns of resource dependency, and styles of governance. Distinctive motivations could influence how they respond to changes in funding levels and routes, market prices for staff or medications, competition or curriculum/time pressures on school teaching staff, with implications for costs, case-mix, quality of care, and outcomes (9).

Multiple Funding Sources

Another reason for distinguishing between provider types and the sectors in which they are located is because they are likely to have different funding bases. A treatment facility in the public sector—where most are located in the United Kingdom, for example—is likely to be heavily reliant on tax revenues or mandatory heavily regulated health insurance premiums, whereas a for-profit provider will probably receive more of its funding from private insurance plans or user fees. School-based behavioral health and social work services in some countries may be funded through the general education budget, which itself is usually funded through some form of taxation and whose use may even be at the discretion of the school principal. Services run by nonprofit and faith organizations might be funded under contract from government and by insurance payments, but could also receive charitable donations. Family caregivers, although ostensibly unpaid, might actually receive social security support or disability allowances tied to children's needs. Matching the diversity in provision, therefore, is a mixed economy of funding.

Interconnections: Transaction Types

Cross-classifying the main funding and provider types generates a large number of possible interconnections (Figure 1.7.2). This matrix describes just the broadest categorization of provider sectors and funding sources, but immediately demonstrates that the mixed economy of child mental health care is a highly pluralist system. Moreover, each combination of funding arrangement and provider sector could apply to the health, education, social care, criminal justice, and other systems.

There are many transaction types reflected in the links captured by this matrix. For example, tax revenues that support for-profit providers could be linked through performance-related contracts, tax breaks, or lump-sum cash subsidies. Payments from insurance companies to providers could be made through fee-for-service (FFS), capitation, or other mechanisms. Each transaction type will therefore have accompanying needs for regulatory frameworks for quality, probity, and perhaps efficiency in resource use.

Charting the broad contours of the mixed economy in this way helps identify the range and volume of services potentially available to children, adolescents, and families, and the means by which they are funded. It also emphasizes the inherent financial interdependence of different services and agencies. When the "expanded school mental health framework" initiated by the US government in the early 2000s encouraged education services to liaise with community mental health centers, health departments, hospitals, and others to broaden mental health promotion and intervention, implementation was hampered by "patchy and tenuous" (10) funding. In England, a taskforce set up to look at how to protect and promote child mental health put an emphasis on collaboration and joint working between health service commissioners, local government, children and young people, their families and schools (11), including training programs to support lead contacts in schools. It is up to schools to decide on the extent to which they will fund and provide most school-based mental health services, including counselling (12).

Coordination

Good interagency coordination increases the likelihood that individual and family needs will be met, which in turn might require collaborative approaches to financing to avoid yawning gaps in the spectrum of support. Even in well-resourced care systems there are large numbers of young people whose needs go unrecognized or undertreated, as we have already noted. This has also been highlighted by an independent Mental Health Taskforce in England, which recommended to NHS England that 70,000 more children and young people have access to high-quality support by 2020/21 by placing greater emphasis on prevention and early identification (13). Wasteful duplication of effort is another possibility. National/federal, regional, and local levels of administration differ in their service and agency definitions, responsibilities and arrangements,

Revenue collection (funding)	Mode or sector of provision			
	Public/government sector	Non-profit/NGO sector	For-profit sector	Informal sector
Tax-based				
Mandatory health insurance				
Voluntary health insurance				
Charitable donations				
Foreign aid				
Out-of-pocket payments				
No monetary exchange				

FIGURE 1.7.2. The mixed economy. (Adapted from Knapp M: *The Economics of Social Care*. London, Macmillan, 1984.)

and therefore in their interagency boundaries and the potential connected action that could span them. A major organizational resource challenge is to coordinate service funding in ways that are effective, cost-effective, and fair. Cost-shifting and problem-dumping between agencies will not help children and families. Recognition of economic symbiosis has helped decision makers in some contexts, most notably in the Nordic countries, respond better to needs through intersectoral partnership arrangements, including jointly commissioned programs between the health and education sectors, pooled budgets, and other system-wide initiatives (3,14,15).

FINANCING ARRANGEMENTS

Accessing health care services is not like buying groceries, which is why most high- and middle-income countries rely on prepayment systems of revenue collection. Prepayment is organized through some combination of tax, mandatory and/or voluntary insurance contributions. Prepayment is preferable to out-of-pocket payments. An individual's risk of needing health care is very uncertain, but when the need arises, the attendant costs (of treatment) and losses (of earnings) could be catastrophic. Prepayment contributions pool risks, and have the potential to redistribute benefits toward people with greater health needs. They can also be made progressive, so that poorer individuals pay less for equivalent health care than wealthier people. Out-of-pocket-payment systems cannot achieve such targeting unless accompanied by well-informed systems of payment exemptions that are closely monitored to ensure implementation and prevent abuse.

Prepayment systems have their problems. If there is no charge at the point at which a service is used there may be excessive utilization; this "moral hazard" problem might be addressed by introducing copayments at point of use. Another potential difficulty is adverse selection: In countries relying on voluntary insurance high-risk individuals may be at risk of being denied coverage or face unaffordable premiums. In attempts to cap expenditures, some insurance or managed care arrangements could exclude mental health coverage, with predictable consequences for access, knock-on costs, societal inefficiencies, and inequity. Legal and regulatory measures, including guaranteed enrollment, controls on premium levels, and risk-equalization between insurers, may be needed as countermeasures, as well as safety-net universal coverage guaranteed by public financing.

Whatever the merits of prepayment systems, there are obstacles to their wider use in low-income countries, including the state of the economy, unstable governance structures, and the informality of much employment, making revenue collection impractical. Consequently, out-of-pocket payments dominate in many low-income countries (16), where there may also be some reliance on foreign donors for additional but very limited resources (17).

Financing can be public or private. There are many different financing models, but public systems will normally rely on some combination of tax and mandatory insurance contributions, while private systems will rely more on voluntary health insurance (VHI) contributions. Voluntary insurance packages may also provide additional coverage for services not included in the basic package of services provided by the public health system. Both systems will make use to differing extent of out-of-pocket payments. Mandatory health insurance systems (often known as social health insurance systems because of guaranteed enrolment and without risk-rated premiums), which are common in parts of continental Europe, are often quasi-public, as funding is often collected and managed by insurance agencies established by government. The picture is however complex; governments have relied on private insurers to offer mandatory insurance packages in some countries for many years, (one example is Germany) while recent reforms in countries such as the Netherlands mean that citizens must now enroll with a private insurer; but the government continues to ensure that all insurers cover the same standard package of care and charge the same premium regardless of individual risk.

Globally, and looking at health systems as a whole, the most common method of financing in OECD countries is tax-based (37%), followed by mandatory insurance (36%), out-of-pocket payments (19%), and voluntary insurance (6%) (18). As far as mental health systems are concerned, almost every country has a mix of public and private funding.

Tax-Based Financing

Many health, education, and other systems are funded from national, regional, or local taxes. Income tax is usually described as progressive because it can be structured to capture progressively larger income shares from wealthier individuals. Indirect taxes such as sales tax tend to be regressive, because poorer individuals generally contribute larger proportions of their incomes. Tax-based systems of health financing are seen as the most progressive and equitable (19). Payments are mandatory, and scale economies can be achieved in administration, risk management and purchasing power (20). For those who advocate health as a right, taxation-based health systems fit the bill, while those with conservative leanings might view such arrangements as an erosion of personal responsibilities and freedom.

Tax-based systems have limitations. Health care funding levels may fluctuate with the state of the national economy, so that when an economy is not doing well, there may be cutbacks to public programs (21,22). Competing political and economic objectives also make a tax-based system less transparent, and bureaucracy can cause inefficiency, reflected perhaps in long waiting lists (although these are also symptomatic of underfunding). Patients tend to view tax-based systems as offering them less choice, but uninsured individuals in other financing systems might argue that they face no choice whatsoever.

With an annual budget of $59 billion the largest publicly-funded health care system in the United States is run by the Veterans Administration (VA), but its focus is on more than nine million enrolled military veterans, and to a lesser extent their families. Most other publicly funded mental health care in the United States that would be relevant to children is delivered through privately owned/managed health maintenance organizations (HMOs), preferred provider organizations (PPOs), or physicians in private practice. In contrast, the tax-funded Swedish health system channels its mental health expenditure through individual counties, ensuring considerable decentralization (18). Child and adolescent mental health systems in countries such as the United Kingdom, Canada, Italy, and Hong Kong are also mainly delivered through public institutions (23).

The tax-based part of the US health system is organized at state level but delivered primarily through nongovernment providers. Medicaid is one such approach, supporting low-income individuals, financed jointly by the federal government and the states, and covering a substantial proportion of all child and adolescent mental health expenditure across the country (3). There have been significant developments in recent years: The Mental Health Parity and Addiction Equity Act 2008 (MHPAEA), expansion of the State Children's Health Insurance Program and the Affordable Care Act (ACA) have made large strides in expanding health insurance, including mental health coverage, to more children from low-income families across the United States. ACA mandates that Medicaid benchmark plans and state-based insurance exchanges cover behavioral health services as part of an essential benefits package (24); Early and Periodic Screening, Diagnosis, and Treatment (EPSDT) services have been extended to all young people covered by Medicaid; and Medicaid covers all children and adolescents under 18 with incomes up to 133% of the Federal Poverty Level (FPL) (25). Furthermore, children in families between 100% and 400% of the FPL qualify for subsidies in the health insurance marketplace. Nonetheless, it remains to be seen whether ACA will provide greater protection for those experiencing mental health issues. The provisions concerning Medicaid are voluntary for state implementation; as of December 2015, there was uptake by 31 states (26). Research also suggests the expansion of Medicaid has not greatly increased utilization rates for people with mental health issues, highlighting the importance of tracking the barriers to mental health care (27).

Mandatory Health Insurance

Health and other systems based on mandatory health insurance generate their revenues from salary-based contributions, either administered and managed by quasi-public bodies (sometimes called sickness funds) or alternatively by private health insurance providers. Employers also make contributions, and transfers are made from general taxation to insurance funds to provide cover for unemployed, retired, and other disadvantaged or vulnerable people, which is clearly pertinent for families where there is someone with mental health issues. In nearly all countries in Europe that have mandatory health insurance tax revenues are used to cover shortfalls in funding or cover the costs of long-term hospitalization.

Enrollment is usually mandatory, although in some systems, for example, Germany, some citizens can opt out and obtain separate insurance, while in the Netherlands individuals can register as conscientious objectors to mandatory insurance and avoid enrollment. Although premiums are not risk-adjusted, they tend to be linked to income so that pooling allows for redistribution according to need and income.

Entitlement to health care services through taxation or social insurance is commonplace in European countries, and in fact accounts for over 70% of total health spending in most western European states. In some low- and middle-income countries, where tax compliance and collection are difficult, mandatory insurance has been seen as a viable alternative for health care funding (28). However, the link between health financing and employment constrains job mobility and hence economic competitiveness. Both tax-based and mandatory insurance-dominated systems take account of ability to pay and cover vulnerable and low-income groups (19).

Even where universal entitlement under tax or insurance predominates, entitlement to mental health services may be limited, and arguably inequitable. Until 2011 in Austria, mandatory health insurance excluded most mental disorders on the grounds that they were chronic rather than curable. Diagnosis and treatment, including psychotherapy are now covered, but much long-term care including rehabilitation is funded separately through pension fund contributions (29) and private out-of-pocket payments (30). Where services have been shifted out of the health sector, for instance to the social welfare sector, there are greater possibilities for copayments that could inhibit access (31). By contrast, the Netherlands now has expanded coverage for primary and secondary mental health care services within the standard (and compulsory) health insurance package that private insurers must offer. Since 2015 long-term mental health care is now only covered by a separate mandatory long-term care insurance after 3 years rather than 1 year. However, 2015 also saw the transfer of responsibility of mental health services for children to the municipalities; these are no longer funded or covered by the basic insurance package.

Voluntary Health Insurance

VHI can be taken up and paid for at the discretion of individuals (or employers on behalf of individuals) and offered by public, quasi-public, for-profit, or nonprofit organizations. Generally speaking, VHI plays only a marginal role in Europe. We have already noted that in Germany some individuals traditionally could opt out of mandatory insurance and use private VHI schemes instead. Elsewhere it is used as a complement to tax or mandatory health insurance funding. In France it is predominantly used to cover the costs of co-payments, while in Ireland VHI insurance can provide additional "hotel" services, allow for more rapid care and limit some co-payments for services provided by the public sector health care system. In the Netherlands VHI provides coverage for services not covered by the basic insurance package.

In contrast, VHI accounts for two-thirds of health care expenditure in the United States (32), and 60% of children aged under 18 access health care through private (employer-sponsored) insurance (33). As mentioned above, the ACA updated the MHPAEA 2008, so that group health plans and insurance companies cannot impose treatment limitations and financial requirements (including co-payments and deductibles) for "behavioral health" which are more restrictive than all other medical/surgical benefits (34). There are several other positive changes for young people: Children cannot be excluded from coverage due to a mental health diagnosis; young people can remain on their parents' insurance policy until age 26; there are no annual limits on the amount insurance providers can pay for basic health care; and lower deductibles (25).

Despite these changes, obstacles still remain. Some groups will not benefit from ACA, including those in employer-sponsored plans that do not offer behavioral health benefits, as well as undocumented immigrants (33). It is also essential that delivery systems such as Accountable Care Organizations take into account the behavioral health perspective when facilitating integration within the private insurance system (24). As far as children's mental health services are concerned, because they have been underdeveloped and poorly coordinated in some states for many years, the effect of ACA has been modest in some localities, although there appears now to be greater recognition of the consequences of inadequate service systems and the need to take action (35).

People individually purchasing insurance have lower bargaining power, which affects the premium paid and/or the benefits covered. Inherent also in this financing system are disadvantages like adverse selection and cream skimming: Higher-risk groups (such as those with mental health issues) may find insurance unaffordable, especially as mental illness is more prevalent among lower income groups, and lower-risk groups may feel that their own premiums are too high. Most insurance plans also exempt existing conditions from the benefit packages.

Out-of-Pocket Payments

In prepayment systems, out-of-pocket payments may be co-payments (specific amount to be paid), coinsurance (agreed percentage of expenses) or deductibles (agreed amount to be paid before insurance kicks in). Though the objectives for introducing out-of-pocket payments differ, the impact remains common everywhere in adversely affecting access and equity. An argument for out-of-pocket payments is that they discourage unnecessary service use (moral hazard) and create price sensitivity that might help direct patients to more cost-effective and appropriate treatments. On the other hand, out-of-pocket payments might defeat the very purpose of cost efficiency, as delayed treatments might substantially increase longer-term costs. Given the stigma associated with mental health issues, their chronicity, and the damage they can cause, heavy reliance on out-of-pocket funds is surely inadvisable.

A 2011 study of six western European countries found 41% of citizens paying some out-of-pocket charges for specialist mental health services, rising to 87.9% in Belgium and 61.7% in Italy (36), although some will get reimbursed under current insurance schemes. They are even more prevalent in parts of central and eastern Europe (37,38), and are often the only means of health finance in low-income countries (39). In the United States, Medicaid expansions between 1998 and 2011 significantly lowered out-of-pocket spending for mental health amongst adults (27).

Commissioning

In order to move revenues collected from taxes or insurance premiums to service providers, a variety of commissioning or purchasing mechanisms can be used. Provider reimbursements can be retrospective (such as FFS) or prospective (capitation and/or fixed budgets). Historically, FFS arrangements dominated health care commissioning, and although they encourage productivity, they also perversely encourage resource consumption through unnecessary visits, diagnostic investigations, and hospitalizations, and so push up overall costs. Consequently, prospective payments have increasingly been substituted, particularly as part of managed care developments, to encourage cost consciousness among providers. Capitation is one such method: A fixed payment is made for a defined set of benefits (in input and/or outcome terms). It encourages efficiency, but risks adverse selection and cream-skimming. Providers might narrow their practice and undermine the objectives of managed care to provide primary and preventive interventions (40). Such behavior shifts costs onto other providers. Some prospective payment methods use diagnosis-related groups (DRGs), a case-mix classification system that groups patients with a similar clinical diagnosis and treatment process to calculate the funds to be allocated. DRG-based pricing can help save costs but to get around this providers might resort to up-coding or "DRG creep," which is the practice of billing using a DRG code that provides a higher payment rate than the DRG code that accurately reflects the service furnished to or needed by the patient.

Some public financing systems adopted commissioning methods from the private insurance market, with emphasis on managed plans. In the United States earlier experience with Medicaid, for example, showed that enrollment in some form of managed care shifted the balance of treatment away from inpatient treatment (41), but perhaps increased the risk that seriously ill children would be undertreated (3). A study comparing three different arrangements (FFS, HMO, and carved-out managed care plans) found no significant differences in access rates, but the FFS plan was favorable for children with an increased risk profile (42). Another study found that satisfaction ratings were much higher in Medicaid for FFS than for managed plans (43).

TARGETING, EFFICIENCY, AND EQUITY

There are never likely to be enough resources to meet all mental health needs. Choices must be made. For example, to what extent should child psychiatric services be delivered from a hospital base or from a community clinic? If there are more children and adolescents needing to see specialist staff than there are treatment sessions available, who should get priority? What proportion of a mental budget should be diverted away from treating identified needs in order instead to uncover previously unrecognized needs? What investment should be made to support a broader health promotion strategy? When does it make sense to stop treating or supporting one particular child or family and to use the time to initiate a treatment program for a newly referred child?

Decision makers—from those who control the budgets to those who actually deliver the services—need to be clear about the basis upon which they choose one option over another. In a world that is increasingly seeking evidence-based approaches to policy and practice while recognizing resource scarcity, a number of resource-related criteria are likely to be invoked to guide such decisions, maximizing therapeutic impact from available resources, integrating more children with behavioral problems into mainstream education, broadening access to effective therapies, improving fairness in what families have to pay for treatment, and improving targeting of services on needs. Many of these resource-related criteria fall into two groups: efficiency and equity.

Efficiency

Efficiency means achieving the maximum effects in terms of services delivered or outcomes achieved (such as needs met, wants satisfied, or quality of life improved) from a specified volume of resources (such as an annual budget).

Many factors might prevent a mental health system from being fully efficient. Perhaps too many resources are tied up in the administration of the system itself: Are there, for example, too many managers supervising the people who actually deliver treatment? Another source of inefficiency could be that resources are used in inappropriate combinations: A child psychiatrist is likely to be more effective, for example, if they can access a range of therapies supported by a multidisciplinary team. Or there may be poor target efficiency in that available services are not provided to the people with greatest needs, because insufficient efforts are made to identify and prioritize needs or to encourage families to seek treatment. Another reason for inefficiency could simply be that little is known about the relationship between resources, services, and outcomes.

Cost-Effectiveness Evidence

When considering whether to use or recommend a particular treatment for a specified problem, decision makers must first get an answer to the central clinical question: Is the treatment effective in improving health and quality of life? They will then usually want an answer to the second question: Does the treatment achieve the outcomes at a cost that is worth paying? Not surprisingly, the second question—the economic question—can generate howls of concern that it encourages rationing or in some way denies people access to services or better quality of life.

Cost-effectiveness analysis compares the two parts of the chain in Figure 1.7.1 that link what gets spent (resources and costs) to what is achieved (outcomes). While it is always likely to be necessary to reformulate the clinical and economic questions in ways that make them answerable with empirical research, we should not forget their inherently straightforward intent.

Given what we have already discussed in relation to the broad mixed economy of provision and financing, it is obvious that we will generally need to view both costs and outcomes in quite broad terms:

- There are many inputs to a child and adolescent mental health system—health, social services, education, criminal justice, and so on—plus economic impacts in terms of lost productivity, premature mortality, and family burden. Each of these has associated costs (5,8).

- Good mental health care is not just about tackling clinical symptoms, but about improving someone's ability to function in ways that are valued by them and about promoting quality of life. There are also likely to be impacts on parents, siblings, classmates, and communities.

There have been relatively few studies of cost-effectiveness of interventions for children and adolescents with mental health problems. Most have been undertaken in North America, Western Europe, or Australia. This geographical unevenness needs emphasis because the results of economic evaluations may not transfer readily from one country to another: Differences in health systems, financing arrangements, incentive structures, and relative prices hamper generalization.

A recent review of the international literature found 67 studies reporting costs or cost-effectiveness analyses, with half coming from the United States (44). The most commonly studied areas were autism spectrum disorder (23 papers), attention deficit hyperactivity disorder (15 papers), conduct disorder (7 papers), and anxiety or depression (8 papers). The great majority were narrowly focused on health care costs (which is a major limitation, given the important service contributions from the education and social care sectors, the impacts often on criminal justice, and the unpaid contributions from families). Full cost-effectiveness analyses remain relatively rare, however.

Equity

Equity relates to the distribution of outcomes, access, and payment. One very relevant equity question is whether individual financial contributions are linked to ability to pay, indeed whether there needs to be a redistributive effort so that families with lower incomes contribute proportionately lower amounts. We touched on this question in discussing financing, and arrangements can be made to improve distribution. Equity in relation to outcomes is another matter. Certainly, equity in final outcomes is a laudable but ambitious goal, primarily because those outcomes are influenced by so many factors over and above the resources devoted to mental health care, including socioeconomic position, family resources and dynamics, housing and community environments, and individual lifestyle and personality. Consequently, equity in access—perhaps expressed as equal access to treatment for equal need—is more frequently discussed as a policy criterion, yet is still of course very hard to achieve.

It is clear that rates of service utilization by children and adolescents with mental health problems remain low across many countries, and that patterns of access are unevenly distributed (45,46). From an egalitarian standpoint it could be argued that utilization should not be influenced by "extraneous" factors such as ability to pay or geographical location.

Why do children, adolescents, and families not use services? One enduring reason is the stigma widely associated with mental illness. Another is the low rate of identification of needs. A third, obviously, is inability to pay for treatments. Many factors therefore contribute to inequality and numerous solutions have been propounded, including actions to improve public awareness and reduce discrimination, and redistributive financing arrangements that are less disadvantageous to poor families.

BARRIERS AND OPPORTUNITIES

Even when there is an evidence base—that is, even when there is a good appreciation of how to enhance child and family health and quality of life, or improve system efficiency, or improve the distribution of payments or access—there could be resource barriers in the way (47). These barriers challenge child and adolescent mental health systems across the world.

Resources

One of the most insidious and seemingly insurmountable barriers is resource insufficiency. This is clearly a major issue for countries where the proportion of national income devoted to health care is low, as in most low-income countries, or where the proportion of the health budget allocated to child and adolescent mental health is minimal. Without funds, it is difficult to build any kind of service system. Resource insufficiency leads inevitably to shortages of skilled staff (3,45) and difficulties in recruiting and training appropriate personnel. Such shortages might energize the search for treatment modalities that make more cost-effective use of what is actually available, but there are limits to what can be achieved.

Increasing the resources available for child and adolescent mental health care would help overcome these challenges. But even when resources are committed, available services might be poorly distributed, available at the wrong place or time relative to the distribution of needs. They may be available only if delivered by specialist clinics or particular schools, or concentrated in major cities, or available only to certain population groups (usually those with higher incomes). This resource distribution barrier is often related to the fundamental way in which a health or education system is financed or structured. In centrally coordinated systems, resources could perhaps be allocated according to need, but systems built on private insurance and out-of-pocket financing have few such opportunities.

Inappropriate Use of Services and Personalized Care

A more general difficulty is resource inappropriateness: Available services do not match what is needed or preferred. Treatment arrangements may be too rigidly organized, leaving service systems unable to respond to differences in individual needs or preferences, or to community circumstances. Such inflexibility is common when there is scant information on population or individual needs, or when families have few opportunities to participate in treatment decisions. There may also be a deep-rooted reluctance to move away from hospital-based services.

More research is needed on less conventional evidence-based therapy such as mHealth (online therapy), mindfulness, and various community-based interventions. For example, a recent study of a parenting intervention for reducing anxiety in children has shown encouraging cost-effectiveness results (48). Personalization of treatment might include using personal budgets, giving young people and their families more control over how their health and other needs are met. This has been trialled in the United Kingdom, for example (49). Ultimately, better quality services and improved outcomes will require input from mental health service users and carers—and a framework to support such engagement (50).

Co-ordination

A linked challenge is resource dislocation. Services may potentially be available to meet individual and family needs, but they are poorly coordinated (13). Such a situation can be compounded by professional rivalry, performance assessment regimes, stultifying bureaucracy or "silo budgeting" (resources held in one agency's "silo" cannot be allocated to other uses), and some forms of managed care. Improved coordination might be achieved by reducing budgetary conflicts between agencies, rewarding efficiency and equity improvements, and encouraging individual and family participation in decision making. These arrangements have their own (transaction) costs, of course, and a careful spending balance must be struck between using resources to deliver services and using them simply to coordinate. In England, it is hoped that Local Transformation Plans, which encourage joined up working between national government and local agencies, will promote greater integration of children's services—thus providing a more responsive and efficient system for supporting children's mental health (51).

Short-Term vs. Long-Term Effects

The timing problem can be quite insidious. For a start, most intended improvements to practice take a long time to work their way through to improved health outcomes, cost-effectiveness gains, or fairer access. Moreover, evidence for improved practice may have been gathered under experimental circumstances and the advantages suggested by research may not actually get realized in real-world settings. There could be transitional or longer-term difficulties recruiting suitable professionals, or opening new facilities. Decision makers must also be encouraged to think long, for the immediate consequences of many interventions could be modest, but the long-term benefits immense (52–54).

Stigma and Attitudes

Negative and stigmatizing attitudes towards mental illness can put up other barriers, leading to disadvantages in relationships, education, and work (55). Such attitudes may also contribute toward premature mortality for individuals with comorbid mental and physical health problems (56). There have been attempts to alleviate experienced discrimination such as through social contact (57), and through anti-stigma campaigns such as Bring Change 2 Mind or Time to Change in the United Kingdom, but greater research is needed for determining the best intervention for reducing stigma in young people (58).

New Technologies

Attention must briefly be given to the barriers and opportunities linked with social media, the internet and mobile/cell phone technology. Whilst the online world has its dangers (unmonitored online forums, cyberbullying, unwanted sexual messaging, psychosocial risk factors (59)), there are also opportunities: individual choice (of support), mobile phone apps for symptom monitoring (60), information on mental health conditions, and complementary interventions to cognitive behavior therapy (61). Workforce shortages, geographical barriers to service provision, and the difficulties of engaging with certain minority groups could see e-health innovations providing cost-effective benefits, although problems of equity may arise if the already disadvantaged poorer population cannot reap the benefits of high-tech interventions (62).

CONCLUSION

Child and adolescent mental health systems—interpreting this term broadly to include health, education, social work, and criminal justice components—are often in a state of flux. It may be a shift of emphasis from inpatient to community-based services, or the broadening of treatment eligibility criteria, or the expansion of insurance coverage. It could be the reconfiguration of multiprofessional staff teams, or new school-based proposals for identifying need. Changes of this kind usually raise economic questions. How are these initiatives to be financed? What cost implications will they have? Are they affordable? Will they prove cost-effective? What will they imply for the distribution of payment, access, and outcome?

There are many ways to raise and distribute funds for child and adolescent mental health services, but there is no agreement on the best form of prepayment system, and the balance between tax and different models of insurance based funding. It is also important to consider whether out-of-pocket payments create appropriate incentives, or whether fee-for-service, capitation, or some other mechanism is the best way to pay service providers. There is growing experience of using these approaches, and growing evidence about what they might imply in particular for children and families affected by emotional or behavioral problems.

Given the comparatively high prevalence of these problems among poorer groups in the population and the often high costs of accessing effective treatments, governments need to make commitments to redistributive policies. They need to set in place the structures that encourage efficient and equitable links between the fundamental aims of improving the lives of children, adolescents, and families; the services and interventions that can deliver those improvements; and the financing mechanisms and purchasing systems that get the funds to providers. And they need to do so across many service sectors—certainly looking at specialist mental health, general medical care, education, social work, supported housing, social security, and criminal justice.

References

1. Knapp M: *The Economics of Social Care.* London, Macmillan, 1984.
2. Costello EJ, He JP, Sampson NA, Kessler RC, Merikangas KR: Services for adolescents with psychiatric disorders: 12-month data from the National Comorbidity Adolescent. *Psychiatr Serv* 65(3):359–366, 2014.
3. Glied S, Evans Cuellar A: Trends and issues in child and adolescent mental health. *Health Aff* 22:39–50, 2003.
4. Department of Education: *Statistical First Release, SFR 49/2014: Outcomes for children looked after by local authorities in England as at 31 March 2014.* London, Department of Education, 2014. Available at https://www.gov.uk/government/uploads/system/uploads/attachment_data/file/384781/Outcomes_SFR49_2014_Text.pdf. [accessed 23.02.2016]
5. Snell T, Knapp M, Healey A, et al.: Economic impact of childhood psychiatric disorder on public sector services in Britain: estimates from national survey data. *J Child Psychol Psychiatry* 55(6):714–732, 2013.
6. Delamare C, Ibeziako P: A comparison of child mental health systems in France and the United States. *Adolesc Psychiatry* 3:5–9, 2013.
7. Lawrence D, Johnson S, Hafekost J, et al.: The Mental Health of Children and Adolescents. Report on the second Australian Child and Adolescent Survey of Mental Health and Wellbeing. Canberra, Department of Health, 2015.
8. National Research Council and Institute of Medicine: Preventing mental, emotional, and behavioral disorders among young people: progress and possibilities. In: O'Connell M, Boat T, Warner K (eds): *Board on Children, Youth, and Families, Division of Behavioral and Social Sciences and Education.* Washington, DC, National Academies Press, 2009.
9. Frank RG, McGuire T: Economics and mental health. In: Culyer AJ, Newhouse JP (eds): *Handbook of Health Economics.* Amsterdam, Elsevier, 2000.
10. Weist MD, Goldstein J, Evans SW, et al.: Funding a full continuum of mental health promotion and intervention programs in the schools. *J Adolesc Health* 32:S70–S78, 2003.
11. Department of Health: *Future in Mind. Promoting, Protecting and Improving Our Children and Young People's Mental Health and Wellbeing.* London, Department of Health, 2015.
12. Department of Education: *Counselling in Schools: A Blueprint for the Future.* London, Department of Education, 2016. Available at: https://www.gov.uk/government/publications/counselling-in-schools. [accessed: 28.03.16]

13. Mental Health Taskforce: *The Five Year Forward View for Mental Health: A Report From the Independent Mental Health Taskforce to the NHS in England.* London, 2016. Available at: https://www.england.nhs.uk/wp-content/uploads/2016/02/Mental-Health-Taskforce-FYFV-final.pdf. [accessed: 28.03.2016]
14. Rampazzo L, Mirandola M, Davis R, et al.: *Joint Action on Mental Health and Wellbeing. Mental Health and Schools.* Brussels, Joint Action on Mental Health and Wellbeing, 2015.
15. McDaid D: Joint budgeting: can it facilitate intersectoral action? In: McQueen D, Wismar M, Lin V, Jones C, Davies M (eds): *Intersectoral governance for health in all policies. Structure, actions and experiences.* Copenhagen, World Health Organization, 111–128, 2012.
16. De Menil V, Ndetei D, Waruguru M, Knapp M, McDaid D: A hidden face of community mental healthcare in Kenya: specialist care from private providers. *World Psychiatry* 13(1):100, 2014.
17. Gilbert BJ, Patel V, Farmer P, Lu C: Assessing development assistance for mental health in developing countries: 2007–2013. *PLoS One* 12(6):e1001834, 2015.
18. OECD. Financing of health care: In: *Health at a Glance 2015: OECD Indicators.* Paris, OECD Publishing, 2015. Available at: http://www.oecd.org/health/health-systems/health-at-a-glance-19991312.htm. [accessed 23.02.2016]
19. Mossialos E, Dixon A, Figueras J, Kutzin J (eds): *Funding Health Care: Options for Europe.* Buckingham, Open University Press, 2002.
20. Savedoff W: *Tax Based Financing for Health Systems: Options and Experiences.* Geneva, World Health Organization, 2004.
21. Stuckler D, Basu S, Suhrcke M, Coutts A, McKee M: Effects of the 2008 recession on health: a first look at European data. *Lancet* 378:124–125, 2011.
22. Wahlbeck K, McDaid D: Actions to alleviate the mental health impact of the economic crisis. *World Psychiatry* 11:139–145, 2012.
23. Ghodse H (ed): *International Perspectives on Mental Health.* London, RCPsych Publications, 2011.
24. Barry C, Huskamp A: Moving beyond parity—mental health and addiction care under the ACA. *N Engl J Med* 365:973–975, 2011.
25. *Compilation of Patient Protection and Affordable Care Act, as amended through May 1, 2010. Public Law 111–148.*
26. Henry J: *Kaiser Family Foundation: Status of State Action on the Medicaid Expansion Decision.* Available at: http://kff.org/health-reform/state-indicator/state-activity-around-expanding-medicaid-under-the-affordable-care-act/. Accessed February 23, 2016.
27. Golberstein E, Gonzales G: The effects of Medicaid eligibility on mental health services and out-of-pocket spending for mental health services. *Health Serv Res* 50(6):1734–1750, 2015.
28. Carrin G: Social health insurance in developing countries: a continuing challenge. *Int Soc Sec Rev* 55:57–69, 2002.
29. Hofmarcher M: Austria. Health systems review. *Health Syst Transit* 15(7):1–331, 2013.
30. Zechmeister I, Osterle A: Distributional impacts of mental health care financing arrangements: a comparison of the UK, Germany and Austria. *J Ment Health Policy Econ* 9(1):35–44, 2006.
31. Knapp M, McDaid D: Economic realities: financing, resourcing, challenging, resolving. In: Knapp M, McDaid D, Mossialos E, Thornicroft G (eds): *Mental Health Policy and Practice Across Europe.* Buckingham, Open University Press, 2007.
32. DeNavas-Walt C, Proctor BD, Smith JC: *U.S. Census Bureau, Current Population Reports, P60-235.Income, Poverty, and Health Insurance Coverage in the United States: 2007.* Washington, DC, U.S. Government Printing Office, 2008.
33. U.S. Census Bureau: *Current Population Survey, 2010 Annual Social and Economic Supplement.* Available at: http://www.census.gov/hhes/www/cpstables/032010/health/h08_000.htm. [accessed 23.02.2016]
34. U.S. Department of Labor, Employee Benefits Security Administration: *The Mental Health Parity and Addiction Equity Act 2010 Fact Sheet.* Available at: http://www.dol.gov/ebsa/newsroom/fsmhpaea.html. [accessed 23.02.2016]
35. Behrens D, Graham Lear J, Acosta Price O: *Improving Access to Children's Mental Health Care: Lessons from a Study of Eleven States.* Washington, DC, George Washington University, 2013.
36. Sevilla-Dedieu C, Kovess-Masfety V, Gilbert F, et al.: Mental health care and out-of-pocket expenditures in Europe: results from the ESEMeD project. *J Ment Health Policy Econ* 14(2):95–105, 2011.
37. Balabanova D, Roberts B, Richardson E, Haerpfer C, McKee M: Health care reform in the former Soviet Union: beyond the transition. *Health Serv Res* 47(2):840–864, 2012.
38. Zaluska M, Suchecka D, Traczewska J, Paszko J: Implementation of social services for the chronically mentally ill in a Polish health district: consequences for service use and costs. *J Ment Health Policy Econ* 8:37–44, 2005.
39. Dixon A, McDaid D, Knapp M, Curran C: Financing mental health: equity and efficiency concerns for low and middle income countries. *Health Policy Plan* 21:171–182, 2006.
40. Robinson CJ: Theory and practice in the design of physician payment incentives. *Milbank Q* 79:2, 2001.
41. Simpson L, Zodet MW, Chevarley FM, Owens PL, Dougherty D, McCormick M: Health care for children and youth in the United States: 2002 report on trends in access, utilization, quality and expenditures. *Ambul Pediatr* 4:131–53, 2004.
42. Mandell DS, Boothroyd RA, Stiles PG: Children's use of mental health services in different Medicaid insurance plans. *J Behav Health Serv Res* 30:230–240, 2003.
43. Heflinger CA, Simpkins CG, Scholle SH, Kelleher KJ: Parent/caregiver satisfaction with their child's Medicaid plan and behavioral health providers. *Ment Health Serv Res* 6:23–32, 2004.
44. Beecham J: Child and adolescent mental health interventions: a review of progress in economic studies across different disorders. *J Child Psychol Psychiatry* 55(6):714–732, 2014.
45. Levav I, Jacobsson L, Tsiantis J, Kolaitis G, Ponizovsky A: Psychiatric services and training for children and adolescents in Europe: results from a country survey. *Eur Child Adolesc Psychiatry* 13:395–401, 2004.
46. Knapp M, Snell T, Healey A, et al.: How do child and adolescent mental health problems influence public sector costs? Interindividual variations in a nationally representative British sample. *J Child Psychol Psychiatry* 56(6):667–676, 2015.
47. Knapp M, Funk M, Curran C, Prince M, Gibbs M, McDaid D: Mental health in low- and middle-income countries: economic barriers to better practice and policy. *Health Policy Plan* 21:157–170, 2006.
48. Mihalopoulos C, Vos T, Rapee RM, et al.: The population cost-effectiveness of a parenting intervention designed to prevent anxiety disorders in children. *J Child Psychol Psychiatry* 56(9):1026–1033, 2015.
49. Forder J, Jones K, Glendinning C, et al.: Evaluation of the personal health budget pilot programme. *PSSRU Discussion Paper, vol. 2840_2. Canterbury: PSSRU University of Kent,* 2012.
50. Carman K, Dardess P, Maurer M, Sofaer S, Adams K, Bechtel C: Patient and family engagement: a framework for understanding the elements and developing interventions and policies. *Health Aff* 32(2):223–231, 2013.
51. Mental Health Taskforce: *The Five Year Forward View for Mental Health: A report from the independent Mental Health Taskforce to the NHS in England.* London, 2014. Available at: https://www.england.nhs.uk/wp-content/uploads/2016/02/Mental-Health-Taskforce-FYFV-final.pdf. [accessed: 23.02.2016]
52. Fergusson DM, Horwood LJ, Ridder EM: Show me the child at seven: the consequences of conduct problems in childhood for psychosocial functioning in adulthood. *J Child Psychol Psychiatry* 46:837–849, 2005.
53. Goodman A, Joyce R, Smith JP: The long shadow cast by childhood physical and mental problems on adult life. *Proc Natl Acad Sci U S A* 108(15):6032–6037, 2013.
54. Knapp M, King D, Healey A, Thomas C: Economic outcomes in adulthood and their associations with antisocial conduct, attention deficit and anxiety problems in childhood. *J Ment Health Policy Econ* 14:122–132, 2011.
55. Thornicroft G: *Shunned: Discrimination Against People with Mental Illness.* Oxford, Oxford University Press, 2006.
56. Thornicroft G: Premature death among people with mental illness. *Br Med J* 346:f2969, 2013.
57. Corker E, Hamilton S, Henderson C, et al.: Experiences of discrimination among people using mental health services in England 2008–2011. *Br J Psychiatry* 202(55):58–63, 2013.
58. Evans-Lacko S, Courtin E, Fiorillo A, et al.: The state of the art in European research on reducing social exclusion and stigma related to mental health: a systematic mapping of the literature. *Eur Psychiatry* 29(6):381–389, 2014.
59. Livingstone S, Smith PK: Annual research review: Harms experienced by child users of online and mobile technologies: the nature, prevalence and management of sexual and aggressive risks in the digital age. *J Child Psychol Psychiatry* 55(6):635–654, 2014.
60. Majeed-Ariss R, Baildam E, Campbell M, et al.: Apps and adolescents: a systematic review of adolescents' use of mobile phone and tablet apps that support personal management of their chronic or long-term physical conditions. *J Med Internet Res* 17(12):e287, 2015.
61. Kobak K, Mundt J, Kennard B: Integrating technology into cognitive behaviour therapy for adolescent depression: a pilot study. *Ann Gen Psychiatry* 14:37, 2015.
62. Blanchard M, Hosie A, Burns J: Embracing technologies to improve wellbeing for young people: an Australian view of evidence and policy implications in commonwealth health partnerships 2013. Available at: https://www.youngandwellcrc.org.au/knowledge-hub/publications/embracing-technologies-improve-wellbeing-young-people/ [accessed 24.02.2016]

SECTION II
A DEVELOPMENTAL FRAMEWORK

2.1 ■ NORMAL DEVELOPMENT

CHAPTER 2.1.1 ■ THE INFANT AND TODDLER

LINDA C. MAYES, WALTER S. GILLIAM, AND LAURA STOUT SOSINSKY

The role of child psychiatry in care of infants and toddlers is expanding especially as the diagnostic nosology for serious early development disorders such as autism or attachment disorders becomes increasingly refined. Further, as child psychiatrists collaborate actively with pediatricians (1), they often are called upon to assess infants and toddlers for apparent developmental delays, behavioral difficulties, or parent–child problems. The interface between child psychiatry and pediatrics also means child psychiatrists may consult with parents during their pregnancy or as they anticipate their older child's response to the birth of a new sibling. As child psychiatrists also provide consultation to a range of child care and early education settings, they are more often consulting with parents about child care decisions and settings. Each of these consultative settings requires that child psychiatrists have a solid understanding of normative early development. In this chapter, we provide guidelines for thinking about normal early development and the basic phases of infant and toddler development especially as these are relevant to the clinical practice of child psychiatry. We also provide an overview of salient issues regarding the environments of infants and toddlers again as these are relevant to clinically salient issues in the development of young children.

Most scientists and clinicians define the periods of infancy and toddlerhood as being the first 3 years of postpartum life. More specifically, infancy refers to the time before the beginning of expressive verbal communication that occurs at about 18 months. The developmental shift that occurs at this time has a dramatic transformational impact on the child's ability to reason cognitively, deepen elaborate social relationships, and mediate emotional experiences linguistically. Toddlerhood is a period of increasing autonomy in which the child uses his or her new skills to explore their world, physically, cognitively, and socially. Regardless of the exact chronological time frame, infancy and toddlerhood encompass the most rapid and contextually transactional period of neurodevelopmental change throughout the postpartum life span. Therefore, all clinical work in child psychiatry with infants and toddlers is framed by the context of rapidly changing, growing systems that may be in or out of synchrony with one another.

NORMATIVE DEVELOPMENTAL FORCES

Development is characterized by processes by which each individual uniquely adapts and integrates his or her own nature with the opportunities and limitations of his or her experience across time. The developmental transactional ecological framework posits a child's behavior at any point in time as a product of reciprocal transactions among the child's characteristics (genetic/biological/physical, cognitive/linguistic, and social/emotional competencies) and the caregiving environment (dynamic interrelationships among child behavior, caregiver responses to such behavior, and the dyadic relationship) and the broader ecological context (multiple levels of social organization, including family, neighborhood, and child care) (2–7).

Developmental psychopathology is similarly characterized by patterns of behavioral adaptation over time and in context, rather than by static, isolated, or domain-specific problems (7–9). The average environment often can sufficiently compensate for problems when they occur. But when a child's unique needs or difficulties are present in an environment lacking adequate nurturance and support, they combine to produce "initial patterns of maladjustment which then spin their way into diagnosable pathology" (7).

Interacting Factors in Development

There are several interacting factors that drive or moderate developmental processes. Indeed, clinical assessment of infants and their families represents a process of gaining a better understanding of these interacting forces. Five specific areas are discussed: (a) the interaction of innate and experiential factors, (b) maturational processes, (c) the essential role of relationships with others for healthy development; (d) the broader context of relationships and the environment; and (e) developmental stages and critical or sensitive periods. While each of these areas is interrelated, there are points that are unique to each.

The Interaction of Innate and Experiential Factors

The interactive balance between innate and experiential factors is a well-worn controversy in developmental science, and even now it is possible to find proponents emphasizing the singular importance of one over the other. Rarely are these issues clearly distinguishable in a clinical evaluation. At the least, infants bring a set of innate capacities that influence how they respond to the environment and how it responds to them. The clinician is always faced with considering how intrinsic and extrinsic factors have interacted to contribute to an infant's developmental difficulties or strengths. Infants are more vulnerable to developmental dysfunction, even with a supportive environment, if there is biological dysfunction, as in genetic disorders or severe prematurity. Conversely, even "well endowed" infants are at risk for developmental dysfunction if their environment provides inadequate or inconsistent nurturing. A combination of an impoverished or dangerous environment combined with biological or genetic risks is a significant predictor of developmental dysfunction, and as the number of risk factors increase so increases the likelihood for poor outcomes (10,11). Indeed, genes, the environment, and the interaction of these two forces each play a large role in cognitive development (12). This transactional model of child development, which stresses the dynamic interplay between individual- (genes, experience) and contextual-level (aspects of environment, culture) factors, is the prevailing paradigm (13) and there are now several compelling examples of apparent gene–environment interaction including, for example, in utero effects of stress on later cognitive development (14).

Maturational Processes

Depending on the clinician's frame of mind, maturation, or the progressive unfolding and differentiation of intrinsic capacities, presents either a complication or a challenge in the process of developmental assessment. Infants change rapidly, and the appearance of behaviors and responses can be highly variable despite certain expected sequences. Also, although very young infants begin life in a relatively undifferentiated state, within the first months, perceptual and motor systems differentiate rapidly. Implicitly, a stage-based model of infant development guides much of clinical perspectives by acknowledging that sequences of development *generally* are based upon orderly maturational steps that have been well described and defined. This sequence and the knowledge of when children typically achieve certain skills can be used to establish norms, against which an individual infant's developmental skills can be contrasted. As Provence (15) has stated, "Maturation…is a necessary construct, an invisible process represented by observable behaviors."

As described above, environment, genetic predisposition, and the interaction of both can alter maturational forces significantly. For example, we expect grasping patterns to follow an expectable, regular sequence of neurologic maturation but know that the timetable for infants' use of a particular grasp to hold a toy or explore a box is individually variable and can be highly related to the infant's exposure. Or, although the infant may have the neurological capacity for a responsive smile and the perceptual–motor integration to extend his or her arms toward an adult, experience in interaction with the environment is a necessary factor for such observable behaviors to emerge. Also, it is true that variants of typical maturational processes exist that are not necessarily associated with later problems. For example, it is typical for infants to learn to crawl on hands and knees at 8 to 9 months old and then walk at 12 months. However, various alternative pathways of infant locomotion are fairly common and are not necessarily related to underlying problems, and researchers have long known that age of walking alone is not a good predictor of developmental outcomes (16).

It is important to draw a distinction between developmental processes that are primarily delayed versus those that represent a qualitative deviation from the typical progression of skills. For example, some infants and young children present a pattern of development that approximates the typical orderly progression of developmental skills, but are nonetheless developing along that track at a pace significantly behind their same-age peers. Others, however, may evidence patterns of development that are substantially different from the normal progression or show signs of qualitative differences in neuromuscular development (localized or diffuse hypotonia, abnormal reflex patterns). Significantly deviant patterns of development appear to be more common in children whose overall development is very delayed relative to chronological age expectations.

Relationships

It is impossible to overstate the role of human relationships in development. The essential role of stable and nurturing human relationships is well established and universally acknowledged among researchers (17). However, most formal infant assessment techniques were developed to focus exclusively on the measurement of maturational forces, as if assuming that development proceeds relatively independent of environmental input. Thus, it is important to emphasize *that every infant assessment* must consider the other individuals in that infant's life. Understanding normal, delayed, or deviant development requires some understanding of the infant's experiences with adults. The younger the child, the more central are such individuals to the child's safety and total well-being. Such serious events as traumatic separation, physical abuse, witnessing violence, deprivation, loss, and neglect often have devastating effects on a child's development (18). Moreover, less extreme variations in children's environments have profound effects on every aspect of early development, with relationships and interactions with primary caregivers being of acute importance in the very early years.

Understanding the early environment in which infants and toddlers develop is a vast topic that encompasses individual differences in parenting style, the impact of parental psychopathology such as depression, family disruption such as divorce, and how parents adapt their behaviors to the emerging developmental skills of the infant, each area of extensive clinical scholarship and research. In this section are highlighted the areas most relevant for child psychiatrists beginning to evaluate a young child or work with the parents of an infant or toddler.

Relationships and interactions with primary caregivers, most often the mother and/or father, directly affect and dynamically interact with multiple domains of child development. These domains include attachment and social-emotional development; behavior, cooperation, and development of morality; early learning, exploration, and cognitive and language development; and health and physical development. Parents also indirectly transmit to their children, through their impact on caregiving behaviors, the effects of more distal environmental factors such as poverty (19–21), parental life circumstances (21,22), and parental beliefs and attitudes (23). Parents can also shape their child's environment indirectly through provision of stimulating and supportive social and material resources in the home environment, through choice of neighborhood, and, most crucially in early childhood, through their decisions regarding nonparental child care (21,24–26). Furthermore, the same distal environmental factors, like poverty, that affect parenting also limit parents' ability to choose and shape their child's home, neighborhood, and childcare environments (17,20,21,25,26).

Infants are strongly motivated and primed to develop attachments with adult caregivers to ensure close, protective, and nurturing contact. When parenting (or primary caregiving) is reliably sensitive and contingently responsive to a child's cues and needs, the child is more likely to develop a secure attachment. Secure attachment behaviors include using the parent as a secure base from which to comfortably explore, monitoring and seeking proximity with the parent, seeking contact eagerly after separation or if frightened, and evidence of trust and delight in the parent. When parenting is detached, intrusive, erratic, inconsistent, or rejecting, children are more likely to develop an insecure attachment, characterized by disrupted play, preoccupation with the parent's presence, avoidance or resistance to contact and distress or anger at reunion after separation, or difficulty being comforted. Secure attachment has been associated longitudinally with development of social and emotional competence, a child's confidence and sense of efficacy in novel or challenging situations and ability to manage stress, and greater self-efficacy, and is shown to set the stage for future positive relationships with others (16,27,28).

Adequate care and nurturing for an infant involves a balance among gratification, comfort, and support and the frustration inevitable in all developmental phases. Adequacy in caregiving, difficult as it is to define, generally includes attempts to mediate painful, tension-producing situations and to adjust the balance between comfort and frustration. The appropriate balance varies depending on the child's age. For example, the infant's frustration at not being fed immediately is different from the toddler's frustration at being unable to reach a favorite toy, and each requires a different response from the parents. In one instance, frustration may produce a painful, tense state; in another, it may lead to an adaptive solution that enhances further learning and appropriate individuation and independence.

Parenting is associated powerfully with other domains of child development beyond attachment, although the lines between various parenting behaviors and areas of child development are blurred by dynamic transactions and integration over time. Sensitivity, contingent, appropriate responsiveness, and consistency are associated with all areas of social-emotional development (including competencies such as sustained attention, compliance, empathy, prosocial peer interactions, and emotion regulation) and also support children's early learning. Parents promote their child's language and cognitive abilities when they understand their child's current abilities and structure learning opportunities accordingly, provide a rich verbal environment, and adjust their support and stimulation as the child's capacities emerge (16,29).

Furthermore, while encouragement rather than restriction of exploration is helpful, limit setting and consistent and firm standards are also important especially for a toddler's development of cooperation, behavioral control, and sense of conscience. Authoritative (rather than harsh or permissive) setting and enforcement of limits, incentives, and punishments, modeling of desired behaviors, and consistent routines all positively affect child's behavioral development. Rather than a static "parenting style," these behaviors are dynamic, adjust for changing child characteristics, and involve give and take. Toddlers' developing cognitive capacities integrate parental expectations and standards, in turn affecting development of self-regulation, conflict management, empathy, cooperation, and awareness of the feelings and perspectives of others (16,29).

Often clinicians are not always dealing with gross parenting deficits or failures, such as in serious abuse and neglect (30). For many infants and young children, there are crucial experiences that may have adverse effects that are much harder to identify. For example, we are only beginning to understand the critical effect of maternal depression in the first month to 1 year, when the mother is psychologically and sometimes physically unavailable to her infant (22,31,32). A growing body of research on the issue of caregiver mental illness, however, suggests that serious psychopathology in caregivers can significantly alter dyadic and familial interaction patterns, which in turn lead to altered developmental courses for infants. Caregiver psychopathology is a forceful example of how parental life circumstances might alter parenting and, thereby, infant and toddler development. Other factors internal to the parent—such as parenting stress (negative perceptions of child behavior, the parent–child relationship, and the self as parent) and child-rearing beliefs (nonauthoritarian or progressive child-centered child-rearing beliefs, such as belief that children learn actively vs. traditional or adult-centered child-rearing beliefs, such as approval of uniform treatment and encouragement of obedience to authority)—also shape parenting behaviors. Life circumstances, such as single parenthood, low parental education, substance abuse, and, most pervasively, poverty, can strain the parent's ability to respond sensitively and contingently to their infant's cues and needs (17,20,21). Caregivers, however articulate and enlightened, may be unaware of their own difficulties in responding to their infants, or of how their mood states, worries, and frustrations affect their parental responsiveness. It is at this level that the importance of establishing a working relationship between parents and evaluator is clearest.

Broader Context and Environment

The early environment in which infants and toddlers develop is influenced by the broader ecological context. The broader ecological context includes the home environment, other caregiving environments such as nonparental child care, broader family circumstances and risks, and the neighborhood. These contextual influences on child development may be direct, as in the case of a nonparental caregiver's interactions with the child, indirect, as in the effect of poverty on parenting behaviors and available resources, or both direct and indirect, as when poverty limits a parent's child care choices, thus exposing the child to poorer quality child care.

The Home Environment. Within the family setting, the materials, activities, and transactions that are supportive of early learning have been shown to be associated with children's IQ, cognitive and language development, and later school performance (24). The supportiveness and stimulation of home environments vary greatly by family socioeconomic and ethnic status, and such variations, even in the very early years, demonstrate differential effects on child outcomes. Parents' provision of social resources, such as opportunities to interact with peers, also influence child development (17,20,21).

Understanding a young child's typical "environment" is a crucial part of any thorough child psychiatric assessment. Who cares for the infant during the day? Is there a live-in nanny or do the parents take their baby to grandparents, older aunt or uncle, or a family childcare program neighbor? Often these individuals may actually spend more direct care time with a young infant than parents themselves and in addition to being able to provide extensive history about the infant's daily routines and emerging skills, are also important attachment figures for the infant. Furthermore, infants and toddlers adapt differently to different caregivers and not uncommonly, may behave differently with different adults or show fewer or more symptoms depending on the adult caring for them at the time. Hence, it is very important to have multiple informants regarding an infant or young child's development and behavior when she or he is being evaluated.

Nonparental Child Care. A very young child's relationship and interactions with his or her parent (or primary caregiver) may be most salient and central to early development, but other caregiving experiences also impact child well-being. For the vast majority of young children today in the United States, nonparental child care is "second only to the immediate family" as a developmental context (17). The impact of relationships and interactions with nonparental childcare providers on child development is similar in many ways to the influence of parental relationships. Children can form attachment bonds with nonparental caregivers and receive supports for early learning and language development. In addition, in many settings, young children experience peer interactions and a school-like environment.

To put the scope of child care environments in context, about 20.4 million young children are regularly in care by someone other than their parents, largely due to the vast increase in employment of mothers of young children in recent decades. The largest increase in the last decade and a half has been in child care use by infants and toddlers, with nearly half of all children under the age of 3 in the United States spending some time in child care (17). Child care settings, which vary widely, fall into four broad categories, listed from the least to the most formal: relative care, in-home nonrelative care (nannies, au pairs), family day care, and center-based care. Parents more often utilize home-based care for infants and toddlers, in part due to greater preference, flexibility, and availability, and sometimes to lower cost. Almost one-third of infants and toddlers in care are in family day care homes.

The quality, as well as the quantity and type, of child care experienced by young children contributes to child development. High quality child care is characterized by warm, responsive, and stimulating interactions between children and caregivers. For example, high-quality interactions are characterized by caregivers who express positive feelings in interactions with children, are emotionally involved, engaged, and aware of the child's needs and sensitive and responsive to their initiations, speak directly with children in a manner that is elaborative and stimulating while being age-appropriate, and ask questions and encourage children's ideas and verbalizations. Structural and regulatable quality features of the setting, including ratio of children to adults, group size, and caregiver education and training, act indirectly on child outcomes by facilitating high-quality child–caregiver interactions. To illustrate, it would be difficult for even the most sensitive and stimulating provider to provide high-quality interactions with each child if she was the sole caregiver of 10 toddlers (33). Furthermore, given the unique developmental characteristics of infants and toddlers, a specific focus on developing and supporting relationships between young children and their caregivers can give babies opportunities and time to establish strong relationships with their child care teachers (34–36).

Disentangling the effects of nonparental caregiving on child development is complex, as the type, quantity, and quality of child care to which children are exposed is not random but selected by parents. Recent research, especially the NICHD Study of Early Child Care and Youth Development, have made strides in this direction (33). Furthermore, as parents choose child care, it can be considered indirect parenting (even by many parents) (37), and is another important avenue by which parents impact their young children's early development. The magnitude of the effects of parenting and family factors on child development is about twice that of child care factors (38). However, after adjusting for family characteristics, child care retains unique influence on child development, with one study finding child care's influence up to about half the magnitude of the effect of parenting. The greater strength of effect of parenting is to be expected, as biologic parents share genetic characteristics with their children, which most nonparental child caregivers do not (or share less genetic similarity, in the case of grandparents or other relatives). Plus, parents (whether biologic parents or not) are typically stable, consistent, central presences in their children's early years, whereas most nonparental caregivers come in and out of the children's lives, and many times children have multiple caregivers (and even multiple arrangements) simultaneously. The effects of child care characteristics on child development are highlighted next.

A child's experience of child care per se is not related to better or worse outcomes for children compared to child's experience of exclusive maternal care (39). Earlier research suggested that child care exposure in the first year of life may interfere with the mother–child attachment bond (40). However, one subsequent study demonstrated that only when combined with low maternal sensitivity and responsiveness did poor-quality child care, larger quantities of child care, or multiple child care arrangements predict greater likelihood of insecure attachment (41). Beyond the question of attachment, the longitudinal effects of child care quality, quantity, and type on child outcomes have been examined extensively, demonstrating that child care quality is a consistent and modest predictor of child outcomes across most domains of development, child care quantity is a consistent, modest predictor of social behavior, and child care type is an inconsistent, modest predictor of cognitive and social outcomes, adjusting for family factors (parental income, education, and race/ethnicity, family structure, parental sensitivity; 42,43). In general, children who experienced higher quality child care performed better than other children on cognitive, language, and academic skill tests and, at some points in early childhood, were rated as showing more prosocial skills and fewer behavior problems and negative peer interactions.

The disturbing fact is that, despite the importance of high-quality child care for child development, several large studies have found that most child care is of "poor to mediocre" quality (33,41,42). Observed quality in infant and toddler settings is low in general and often lower than in preschool settings (44,45). In one study, only 14% of centers (8% of center-based infant care) were found to provide developmentally appropriate care, while 12% scored at minimal levels that compromised health and safety (40% for infant care) (41). Similarly, in another study, 58% of family day care homes provided adequate or custodial care, and only 8% provided good care (42). Unfortunately, children with the greatest amount of family risk may be the most likely to receive child care that is substandard in quality. However, many children from lower risk families also receive lower quality care, and despite their advantages at home, these children may not be protected from the negative effects of poor-quality care (46).

In addition, changes in nonparental care can be disruptive for young children, and are important factors for clinicians to consider in assessment and treatment. In one early study, children who changed caregivers before 2 years of age were less securely attached to their caregivers and were more aggressive compared to children who remained with their caregivers (46). Toddlers 18 to 30 months of age who experience multiple caregivers or multiple child care arrangements over the course of a day are more likely to have more behavioral problems (47,48).

For most parents, finding child care that they can afford, access, manage, and accept as a good environment for their child is a very difficult process, and one many parents find distressing (25,49). Not only is affordable and accessible child care hard to find, many parents are worried about how their child will fare in child care. Many parents worry that their child will feel distressed by group settings, will suffer from separation from the parents, or will even be subjected to neglect or abuse. This worry is especially likely among low-income parents with fewer family and community resources to draw upon (50). A smaller proportion of parents may think of child care only as babysitting, and may not consider consequences for their child's development so long as the child is safe and warm. These parents may be less likely to select a high-quality child care arrangement, which is especially problematic, if the family is facing socioeconomic challenges that already place them at risk of receiving lower quality care for their children (51). Complicating the problem, many parents feel that little organized, helpful professional guidance in choosing child care is available (25). Furthermore, parents are the purchasers but not the recipients of care, and are not in the best position to judge its quality. In addition, many parents are first-time consumers of child care with little experience and very immediate needs, selecting care in a market that does little to provide them with useful information about child care arrangements (50).

Importantly, children may be in the same child care setting, but they may have very different experiences depending on their individual characteristics, dispositions, and even physiological responses to the environment (52). Parents and child mental health practitioners need to know more about the individual child's own environment and how the child acts and interacts in that environment, and must do so in micro-contexts throughout the day (i.e., morning and afternoon, during transitions, during group time and individual time, with each caregiver if more than one, etc.; 53).

Child professionals may be many parents' only source of professional consultation regarding their child. Child psychiatrists can emphasize the importance of high quality care for an infant's or toddler's development, describe how it looks and provide referrals and information on how to find and select high-quality child care. Furthermore, child psychiatrists can help parents determine how to adjust child care arrangements to best meet their child's specific needs (eating and sleeping habits, enhanced language classrooms). Parents may also request a child psychiatrist's assistance in evaluating a program for their child. Child psychiatrists may find it important to see an infant or toddler in their child care setting and to meet the teachers and staff. Increasingly child psychiatrists are called upon to serve as consultants to such settings, both to evaluate individual children and also to consult to the teachers and staff about program development and continued staff education.

Developmental Stages and Critical Periods

Historically, theories of development have conceptualized the phenomena as primarily either quantitative or qualitative. A quantitative conceptualization portrays development primarily as a continuous orderly accumulation of skills, dependent on the mastering of prerequisite skills. Qualitative conceptualizations, in contrast, stress the importance of various developmental stages that are each qualitatively different and represent a marked shift in the manner in which the person perceives, understands, and interacts with the environment. In short, the quantitative conceptions represent development as a continuous process, whereas qualitative theories propose that development is a process marked by periodic discontinuities or reorganizations. The concept of developmental stages involves such theories as Freud theory of psychosexual stages, Erikson theory of psychosocial stages, and Piaget's theories of cognitive stages. Clinically, the concept is a valuable one in that it provides schemata for understanding development. Extant research provides some support for both conceptualizations, and the developmental continuity versus discontinuity debate continues.

Research suggesting the existence of certain *critical periods* in human development has provided some support for conceptualizing development as occurring in qualitative different stages. The concept of critical periods for the optimal development of different functions suggests that certain capabilities are optimally mastered at certain times, and difficulties arise when this optimal period is disrupted. Although the concept of critical periods was first clearly established in animal models, it has been demonstrated in humans, especially in the areas of social competence and language acquisition. Indeed, it appears clinically true that when the critical period passes without optimal organization of a given function, mastery is fully achieved with far more difficulty, if ever. It is also a clinical truism that when a function is newly emerging, it is most vulnerable to environmental stresses. This statement is supported by the common observation that an infant may stop talking if hospitalized just as the first words appear. Similarly, for an infant, chronic environmental stressors may result in a delay of appearance of age-appropriate skills. For example, a parent's anxiety over a toddler's growing motoric independence may slow the development of motor skills and the elaboration of exploration. An infant's particular stage of development may influence which issues are most salient and most vulnerable to stress. During an *evaluation* session, stage-specific developmental characteristics also may influence not only the child's ability to demonstrate mastery of certain developmental skills, but also how the infant approaches challenges, including challenges elicited during a developmental assessment. For example, toddlers struggling with emerging independence may react differently to an evaluator's *assessment* tasks than would the younger infant who is focused more establishing social reciprocity and engaging his or her surrounding environment.

Reviewing research over the past decade, Zeanah et al. (54) concluded that there exist four distinct stages of qualitative reorganization during the first 3 years of life. [See also Greenspan (55).] Although their perspective is primarily focused on social-emotional aspects of development and draws from recent research and theory, the stages correspond rather closely to those of earlier developmentalists, especially Piaget and Inhelder (56). Indeed, many of the qualitative changes in cognitive development first proposed by Piaget seem to provide the prerequisites for qualitative changes in social and emotional functioning now being proposed. The following description of different stages during infancy and toddlerhood illustrate these qualitative changes, as well as the dynamic interaction between maturational processes and social relationships and the interactive nature of development across cognitive, sensorial, social, linguistic, and motoric domains.

Five Qualitative Stages of Infancy and Toddlerhood

The Stage 1 Prenatal Development

Although infants with birth defects or malformations are not routinely brought to child psychiatry as the first referral, child psychiatrists working with young children and their families necessarily consider the child's pregnancy. In instances of developmental delays, careful histories regarding exposures to illness or toxins during pregnancy, rate of maternal weight gain, ease or difficulty of delivery, or immediate postnatal complications are important landmarks for charting the health of the pregnancy. Additionally, and especially relevant to child psychiatry, are parental expectations and wishes for the unborn infant. Does the pregnancy come at an optimal or a stressful time for the parent or parents? Have there been major life events during the pregnancy that the parents now associate with their child's development such as the illness of an elderly parent, a job loss, a sudden move? How do the parents imagine their infant to be (a process sometimes referred to as developing a mental portrait of the baby)? This may include imagined personality or physical characteristics, attributions to the fetal patterns of movement during the day (This is going to be a very active baby—kicks all the time), or perceptions of how the fetus is apparently responding to the parents' likes and dislikes such as to favorite foods or music. Does the parent perceive the pregnancy as a burden and the fetus as complicating unnecessarily the parent's life, or is the pregnancy viewed as a positively life-changing event, transforming the parent's views of self and of life in general? The "psychological background" of a pregnancy is critical information for understanding how that infant fits into the family and the parents' perceptions and expectations for that child, especially when young children are referred for behavioral or early regulatory difficulties. These mental portraits are equally important information in instances when infants are severely compromised medically (57).

The Stage 2 Infant (0 to 2 Months)

During the first couple of months postpartum, infants work primarily toward achieving homeostasis, or the capacity for maintaining physiological equilibrium, in the face of internal and external stimulation. However, they are also surprisingly active and sophisticated learners, capable of cross-modally exploring and perceiving his or her environment, visually tracking objects as they move through space, habituating to invariant stimuli, discriminating novelty, and even anticipating caregiver actions (58).

The Stage 3 Infant (2 to 7 Months)

The second stage (2 to 7 months) is marked primarily by increased social reciprocity between the infant and caregiver(s). This qualitative change follows increased awareness of the external world (made possibly by greatly enhanced visual abilities) and improved coordination of sensory input and nonreflexive (voluntary) motor output occurring at about 1 month of age. During the second stage, the infant's responsive cooing, repertoire of increasingly differentiated emotional responses, and a proclivity toward direct imitation of others' behaviors starting at about 4 months serve to facilitate reciprocal or contingent social interactions. During the latter half of the second stage (beginning as early as about 4½ months), infants start to show an understanding of *object permanence* (the understanding that objects and people continue to exist even when they are no longer within sight or sound) and a rudimentary understanding of the principles of *cause and effect.* These two epiphanies transform the infant's perception of the world and provide the requisite abilities for all future social-cognitive development. The concept of object permanence allows the infant to create mental representations of objects and others. It is therefore a prerequisite skill for imagining and for visual differentiation between caregivers and strangers. Cause-and-effect reasoning leads to increased intentionality of actions. Both of these newfound cognitive abilities make possible simple interactive games between infants and caregivers, such as peek-a-boo.

The Stage 4 Infant (7 to 18 Months)

At about 7 to 9 months another qualitative shift occurs with profound impacts on reciprocal communication and social preference or familial belonging. At this time infants develop a sense of *intersubjectivity,* the understanding that their thought, feelings, gestures, and sounds can be understood by others. Also, at about this age, most infants begin to demonstrate means–end reasoning leading to goal-directed behavior. They can string together several behaviors (more than one) in order to achieve a final outcome, often the attainment of some desired object. Through intersubjectivity and means–ends reasoning, the infant is able to consider caregivers as objects that can be used to get their needs and wants met. (And the stage 3 infant's now solid grasp of object permanence gives him or her a large inventory of these wants and needs.) Together, intersubjectivity and means–end reasoning lead to the beginning of *communicative gesturing* (e.g., the moment when stretching for an object just out of reach becomes pointing to that object while looking at the caregiver in order to request assistance). In the context of all of these qualitative changes in the way in which the infant interacts with others, social preferences are established and become increasingly salient. At about 6 to 8 months of age, *separation anxiety* is first observable with most infants, peaking at about 14 to 18 months and declining thereafter (59). Relatedly, *stranger anxiety* appears to begin at about 8 months, peaks at about 24 months, and steadily declines thereafter.

By the second half of stage 3 (starting at about 12 months), several new skills in the cognitive, language and motor domains create profound changes. At about 12 months, infants typically first learn to walk, and this new form of independent locomotion, more so than crawling, heralds increased independence and a broadening world. Cognitively, the infant's reasoning becomes strikingly less rigid and more open to alternative solutions. For example, prior to about 12 months, infants who learn that an object is hidden in a particular place will persist in looking for that object at that same location even after watching someone relocate that object to a different location. This is commonly referred to as the AB error. However, after about 12 months the infant's ability to hold increasingly larger amounts of information and to discard outdated information allows for a fluidity of reasoning such that the AB error diminishes or disappears. Given this increased cognitive capacity and fluidity of reasoning, *trial-and-error problem solving* begins to replace conditioned response learning. Also, from about 12 to 18 months, infants develop rudimentary communicative speech. By 12 months most infants understand the meaning of several words and may have an expressive vocabulary of about five or six words. By the time they reach 18 months of age, infants typically understand the meaning of an amazing number of words, can communicate in one-word sentences, and have doubled their expressive vocabulary to about 10 words. Their melodic, jargoned speech patterns now closely resemble the inflections and turn-taking pauses observed in conversation.

The Stage 5 Infant (18 to 36 Months)

At about 18 months an increased ability to use *symbolic representation* transforms the infant's cognitive and social world. About 12 months earlier, object permanence marked the beginning of the infant's ability to hold in the mind mental representations of objects. The stage 4 infant is now well able to allow symbols to stand for objects, heralding greatly increased language proficiency. The use of words marks a qualitative change in the way infants think about the world and interact with others, and, likely, the reverse is true as well (60). The beginning of this transformation appears to be marked by a move from direct imitation of others to *deferred imitation,* where the behaviors of others are remembered and then practiced later. *Symbolic play* appears as the infant uses a doll to symbolize a baby, and the infant begins to combine words and gestures in order to label objects in his or her world or make needs and wants known to caregivers. By 18 months these skills are becoming solidified, and the infant's interactions with others change dramatically. Additionally, at about 18 to 24 months, *internal problem solving* begins to replace trial-and-error problem solving, as the infant's ability to mentally hold and manipulate internal representations increases. From 18 to 24 months, toddlers' expressive vocabularies typically increase from about

10 words to about 50 to 75 words. By 30 months, the toddler's expressive vocabulary has increased to nearly 300 words, and by 36 months many toddlers have an expressive vocabulary of 500 to 1,000 words and typically speak in three- to four-word sentences (61).

FORCES THAT MAY COMPROMISE NORMATIVE DEVELOPMENT

A variety of both endogenous and exogenous forces may compromise normal infant and toddler development. These are described briefly below and listed in Table 2.1.1.1.

Regulatory Disturbances

These include disturbances in self-regulatory capacities, such as sleep or eating disturbances, including food refusal, night terrors, repeated waking, or problems in impulse control such as excessively aggressive behavior. Low frustration tolerance is another mark of regulatory difficulties. Self-stimulatory behaviors, such as rocking or head banging, may indicate a variety of social or regulatory difficulties, may be a manifestation of environmental stress, or may signify more profound difficulties in relatedness, as in pervasive developmental disorder.

TABLE 2.1.1.1

FORCES THAT MAY COMPROMISE NORMATIVE DEVELOPMENTAL PROCESSES

1. **Regulatory Disturbances**
   A. Sleep disturbances (frequent waking)
   B. Excessive crying or irritability
   C. Eating difficulties (finicky eating or food refusal)
   D. Low frustration tolerance
   E. Self-stimulatory/unusual movements (rocking, head banging, excessive finger sucking)
2. **Social/environmental Disturbances**
   A. Failure to discriminate caregiver
   B. Apathetic, withdrawn, no expression of affect or interest in social interaction
   C. Excessive negativism
   D. No interest in objects or play
   E. Abuse, neglect, or multiple placements or caregivers
   F. Repeated or prolonged separations from caregivers
3. **Psychophysiological Disturbances**
   A. Nonorganic failure to thrive
   B. Recurrent vomiting or chronic diarrhea
   C. Recurrent dermatitis
   D. Recurrent wheezing
4. **Developmental Delays**
   A. Specific delays (gross motor, language)
   B. General delays or arrested development
5. **Genetic and Metabolic Disorders with Known Neurodevelopmental Sequelae**
   A. Down syndrome
   B. Fragile X syndrome
   C. Inborn errors of metabolism
6. **Exposure to Toxins**
   A. Fetal alcohol syndrome
   B. Lead poisoning
7. **Central Nervous System Damage**
   A. Traumatic brain injuries
   B. Intraventricular hemorrhages
8. **Prematurity and Serious Illnesses Early in Life**

Social/Environmental Disturbances

Disturbances in social development and/or the caregiving environment, including serious and profound problems in differentiating mother or caregiver, such as might be seen in pervasive developmental disorder or infantile autism, and disturbances in predominant mood. Infants who are predominantly withdrawn and apathetic are at great risk for developmental difficulties. In this category are also included environmental conditions such as repeated or prolonged separations or neglect, abuse, and exposure to violence, all of which place infants at risk for social and affective disturbances (30).

Psychophysiological Disturbances

These include, among others, failure to thrive, recurrent vomiting, wheezing, or chronic skin rashes. The younger the child, the more likely the response to an environmental stress will be a global one involving several organ systems (e.g., failure to thrive). Clearly, any one of these problems may have physical causes, but clinicians should be alert to the close connection between physiological and psychological adjustment in young children.

Developmental Delays

Delays in specific areas of development, including motor development and activity, language and communication, awareness of others and degree of relatedness to others (seen often together with language delay), or delays in more than one of these areas. Such delays may be more common among infants with complicated perinatal courses such as those born severely premature or following parental substance abuse and prenatal exposure to alcohol, cocaine, or other drugs. Thus, infants with such histories will more often be referred for assessments early in order to plan for appropriate interventions.

Genetic and Metabolic Disorders with Known Neurodevelopmental Sequelae

Various genetic and metabolic disorders have known neurodevelopmental sequelae. These include, but are not limited to, Down syndrome, fragile X, Prader–Willi, certain sex chromosome anomalies (e.g., Klinefelter syndrome), and poorly managed phenylketonuria (PKU) (62). Although certain developmental and behavioral sequelae are associated with these conditions, the extent can often vary considerably, and developmental assessment can be useful to document its course and better target psychosocial interventions.

Exposure to Toxins

Exposure to environmental toxins, such as the case with fetal alcohol syndrome and lead poisoning, has been associated with both developmental delays and behavioral dysregulation. Though useful in treatment planning, assessments are not able to determine the proportion of the developmental presentation attributable to these potential causal factors.

Central Nervous System Damage

Central nervous system damage (e.g., traumatic brain injuries and intraventricular hemorrhages) can, of course, lead to developmental sequelae, and follow-up with a developmentalist can be invaluable in understanding the level of functional impairment and tracking recovery.

Prematurity and Early Illnesses

Prematurity and other serious medical conditions that may result in hospitalization or other restriction of appropriate stimulation early in a child's life, may lead to altered parent–child interaction and adversely affect development (63).

Extant research suggests that the specific disturbances and conditions listed above are highly interrelated and mediated by the social context of the child (64). For example, failure to thrive may also indicate social (the family and caregiver–child dyadic relationships) and/or environmental disturbances, or general developmental delay may occur with repeated separations or in a withdrawn, apathetic child. A particular developmental profile, such as delayed language skills but age-appropriate motor and problem-solving skills, may occur with different presenting difficulties, and thus it is not possible to specify a characteristic diagnostic developmental pattern for failure to thrive, sleep disturbances, or the other problems listed in the table.

In addition to the above caveats, three general points are important to remember. First, language and communication skills are particularly vulnerable to biological and environmental stresses. Moreover, problems in communication also affect personal-social development. For most of the problems listed under social/environmental disturbances, the infant will likely show minimally delayed language and personal-social development. Also, any adaptive or motor items that require interaction with the examiner will be affected by disturbances in relatedness, and the child's skills in these areas will appear scattered not necessarily because of motor impairment but because of the necessity for social interaction for administering the item. Second, it is possible for an infant presenting with some of the difficulties outlined in the table to have an age-appropriate developmental profile in terms of what things the child can and cannot do. In this case, the qualitative observations of how the infant approaches the setting are crucial. The qualitative aspects of the child's interactions with the caregiver and the evaluator, motivations, problem-solving processes, and mood state are infinitely more important than a simple inventory of the infant's skills. Third, an infant's or toddler's level of developmental functioning may vary considerably between domains. Infants with psychophysiological disturbances often show such a "scattered" developmental profile. Qualitative observations are again important with this kind of profile, as well as repeated assessments over time in order to gain a better sense of the child's developmental trajectory.

Generally, a comprehensive assessment of a young child provides a description of the child's functional capacities, the relationships among the various domains such as language and socialization, the child's ability to adapt, and the range of coping strategies. For the very young infant, developmental assessments describe neurodevelopmental functioning and individual regulatory capacities. For caregivers, the evaluation provides information about both their child and the potential therapeutic value of the alliance established with the clinician. For the referring clinician, the assessment may provide a more integrated view of the infant's psychological as well as physical status. Finally, infant assessments often serve the purpose of facilitating referrals to appropriate educational or rehabilitative services. In such cases, the useful question is not whether or not the infant is delayed or has problems, but what are the most appropriate services to ameliorate these problems or to compensate for these conditions. In cases such as these, the evaluating clinicians will need to be collaborators themselves with individuals directing intervention and educational services for infants. [Several excellent reviews of the effectiveness of early intervention services for infants are available (64–66).]

SUMMARY

Infant psychiatry is a developing field that brings child psychiatrists into closer work with very young children and their parents. Disorders such as autism have long been recognized as specific developmental disorders requiring intensive child psychiatric care but more recently, early regulatory disturbances, disruptions in attachments, prematurity, and other biologic disruptions have come into the purview of child psychiatrists. Working with infants and toddlers brings child psychiatrists into close contact with rapidly developing systems and infant psychiatry requires a detailed appreciation of the range of normative as well as abnormal development and an understanding of how different caregiving environments may dramatically alter developmental trajectories, especially in the first years of life. The child psychiatrist with a special interest in infancy and early childhood by virtue of his or her medical training has a special appreciation of the biological aspects of early development. The contemporary infant psychiatrist has available the wealth of data from many infant observational studies, from genetic and neurobiologic perspectives, and from a rich multidisciplinary environment of professionals working with infants, toddlers, and their families that includes developmental psychologists, social workers, pediatricians, geneticists, and developmental neurobiologists. Further, the infant psychiatrist is constantly integrating biology with an understanding of the infant's adult caring environment and assessing the relationship between infant and family as much as the developmental integrity of the infant.

References

1. Mayes LC: Collaboration between child psychiatrists and pediatricians. In: Cavenar JO (ed): *Psychiatry (Revised Edition).* Ch. 73. Philadelphia, PA, J.B. Lippincott, 1992.
2. Bronfenbrenner U: Contexts of child rearing: problems and prospects. *Am Psychol* 34(10):844–850, 1979.
3. Bronfenbrenner U: Ecology of the family as a context for human development: research perspectives. *Dev Psychol* 22(6):723–742, 1986.
4. Bronfenbrenner U: Environments in developmental perspective: theoretical and operational models. In: Friedman SL, Wachs TD (eds): *Measuring Environment Across the Life Span: Emerging Methods and Concepts.* Washington, DC, American Psychological Association, 3–28, 1999.
5. Sameroff AJ: Transactional models in early social relations. *Human Dev* 18(1–2):65–79, 1975.
6. Sameroff AJ: The social context of development. In: Eisenberg N (ed): *Contemporary Topics in Development.* New York, Wiley, 1987.
7. Sameroff AJ: Developmental systems and psychopathology. *Dev Psychopathol* 12(3):297–312, 2000.
8. Sroufe LA, Rutter M: The domain of developmental psychopathology. *Child Dev* 55(1):17–29, 1984.
9. Cicchetti D: Developmental psychopathology: reactions, reflections, projections. *Dev Rev* 13(4):471–502, 1993.
10. Sameroff AJ, Chandler MJ: Reproductive risk and the continuum of caretaking causality. In: Horowitz FD, Hetherington M, Scarr-Salapatek S, et al., (eds): *Review of Child Development Research.* Vol. 4. Chicago, IL, University of Chicago Press, 187–244, 1975.
11. Peck S, Sameroff A, Ramey S, Ramey C: Transition into school: ecological risks for adaptation and achievement in a national sample. In: *Paper presented at: Biennial Meeting of the Society for Research in Child Development; April, 1999;* Albuquerque, NM.
12. Keating DP: Transformative role of epigenetics in child development research: commentary on the special section. *Child Dev* 87:135–142, 2016.
13. Bock J, Wainstock T, Braun K, Segal M: Stress in utero: prenatal programming of brain plasticity and cognition. *Biol Psychiatry* 78:315–326, 2015.
14. Kaufman J, Yang BZ, Douglas-Palumberi H, et al.: Brain-derived neurotrophic factor-5-HHTLPR gene interactions and environmental modifiers of depression in children. *Biol Psychiatry* 59(8):673–680, 2006.
15. Provence S: Developmental assessment: principles and process. In: Brennemann (ed): *Practice of Pediatrics.* Vol. 1. Hagerstown, MD, Harper & Row, 1972.

16. McGraw MB: From reflex to muscular control in the assumption of an erect posture and ambulation of the human foot. *Child Dev* 3:291–297, 1932.
17. Mulligan GM, Brimhall D, West J: *Child care and early education arrangements of infants, toddlers, and preschoolers: 2001 (NCES 2006–039).* Washington, DC, U.S. Government Printing Office, 2005.
18. Rogeness GA, Amrung SA, Macedo CA, Harris WR, Fisher C: Psychopathology in abused children. *J Am Acad Child Adolesc Psychiatry* 25:659–665, 1986.
19. Brooks-Gunn J, Duncan GJ: The effects of poverty on children. *Future Child* 7(2):55–71, 1997 Summer-Fall.
20. Bornstein MH, Bradley RH. *Socioeconomic Status, Parenting, and Child Development.* Mahwah, NJ, Lawrence Erlbaum Associates, 2003.
21. Aber JL, Jones SM, Cohen J. The impact of poverty on the mental health and development of very young children. In: Zeanah CH (ed): *Handbook of Infant Mental Health.* New York, Guilford Press, 2000.
22. Cicchetti D, Rogosch FA, Toth SL: Maternal depressive disorder and contextual risk: Contributions to the development of attachment insecurity and behavior problems in toddlerhood. *Dev Psychopathol* 10(2):283–300, 1998.
23. Kochanska G: Maternal beliefs as long-term predictors of mother–child interaction and report. *Child Dev* 61(6):1934–1943, 1990.
24. Bradley RH, Caldwell BM: Home observation for measurement of the environment: a revision of the preschool scale. *Am J Ment Defic* 84(3): 235–244, 1979.
25. Pungello EP, Kurtz-Costes B: Why and how working women choose child care: a review with a focus on infancy. *Dev Rev* 19(1):31–96, 1999.
26. Gable S, Cole K: Parents' child care arrangements and their ecological correlates. *Early Educ Dev* 11(5):549–572, 2000.
27. Oates J, Lewis C, Lamb ME: Parenting and attachment. In: Ding S, Littleton K (eds): *Children's Personal and Social Development.* Wiley-Blackwell, 12–51, 2005.
28. Baumwell L, Tamis-LeMonda CS, Bornstein MH: Maternal verbal sensitivity and child language comprehension. *Infant Behav Dev* 20(2):247–258, 1997.
29. Kochanska G, Thompson RA: The emergence and development of conscience in toddlerhood and early childhood. In: Grusec JE, Kuczynski L (eds): *Parenting and Children's Internalization of Values: A Handbook of Contemporary Theory.* New York, John Wiley & Sons, Inc, 53–77, 1997.
30. Kaufman J, Henrich C: Exposure to violence and early childhood trauma. *Handbook of infant mental health* 2:195–207, 2000.
31. Garrison WT, Earls FT: Epidemiology and perspectives on maternal depression and the young child. In: Tronick E, Field T (eds): *Maternal Depression and Infant Disturbance.* San Francisco, CA, Jossey-Bass New Divisions for Child Development, 13–30, 1986.
32. Murray L, Cooper PJ: *Postpartum Depression and Child Development.* New York, Guilford Press, 1997.
33. NICHD Early Child Care Research Network. *Child Care and Child Development: Results From the NICHD Study of Early Child Care and Youth Development.* New York, Guilford Press, 2005.
34. Sosinsky LS, Ruprecht K, Kriener-Althen K, Vogel C, Halle T: *Including relationship-based care practices in infant-toddler care: Implications for practice and policy.* (manuscript under review).
35. Dombro AL, Lerner C: Sharing the care of infants and toddlers. *Young Child* 61:29–33, 2006.
36. McMullen MB, Dixon S: In support of a relationship-based approach to practice with infants and toddlers in the United States. In: Brownlee J (ed): *Participatory Learning and the Early Years.* London: Routledge, 109–128, 2009.
37. Uttal L: Custodial care, surrogate care, and coordinated care: employed mothers and the meaning of child care. *Gen Soc* 10(3):291–311, 1996.
38. NICHD Early Child Care Research Network: Child-care effect sizes for the NICHD study of early child care and youth development. *Am Psychol* 61(2):99–116, 2006.
39. Belsky J, Rovine MJ: Nonmaternal care in the first year of life and the security of infant–parent attachment. *Child Dev* 59(1):157–167, 1988.
40. Ahnert L, Pinquart M, Lamb ME: Security of children's relationships with nonparental care providers: a meta-analysis. *Child Dev* 77:664–679, 2006.
41. Helburn SW (ed): *Cost, Quality, and Child Outcomes in Child Care Centers: Public Report.* 2nd ed. Denver, CO, Department of Economics, Center for Research in Economic and Social Policy, University of Colorado, 1995.
42. Kontos S, Howes C, Shinn M, Galinsky E: *Quality in Family Child Care and Relative Care.* New York, Teachers College Press, 1995.
43. Peisner-Feinberg ES, Burchinal MR: Relations between preschool children's child-care experiences and concurrent development: The cost, quality, and outcomes study. *Merrill Palmer Q* 43(3):451–477, 1997.
44. Phillips D A, Lowenstein AE: Early care, education, and child development. *Annu Rev Psychol* 62:483–500, 2011.
45. Vogel CA, Boller K, Xue Y, et al.: *Learning as we go: A first snapshot of early Head Start programs, staff, families, and children.* OPRE Report #2011–7. Washington, DC, Office of Planning, Research, and Evaluation, Administration for Children and Families, U.S. Department of Health and Human Services, 2011.
46. Howes C, Hamilton C: The changing experience of child care: changes in teachers and in teacher-child relationships and children's social competence with peers. *Early Child Res Q* 8:15–32, 1993.
47. deSchipper J, van Izendoorn M, Tavecchio L: Stability in center day care: relations with children's well-being and problem behavior in day care. *Soc Dev* 13:531–550, 2004.
48. Morrissey T: Multiple child care arrangements and young children's behavioral outcomes. *Child Dev* 80:59–76, 2009.
49. Farkas S, Duffet A, Johnson J: *Necessary Compromises: How Parents, Employers, and Children's Advocates View Child Care Today.* Washington, DC, Public Agenda, 2000.
50. Sosinsky LS: *Parental Selection of Child Care Quality: Income, Demographic Risk, and Beliefs About Harm of Maternal Employment to Children* [Dissertation]. New Haven, CT, Department of Psychology, Yale University, 2005.
51. Helburn SW: Preface. *Ann Am Acad PolSoc Sci* 563(1):8–19, 1999.
52. Curby TW, Stuhlman M, Grimm K, et al.: Within-day variability in the quality of classroom interactions during third and fifth grade. *Elem Sch J* 112:16–37, 2011.
53. Phillips DA, Fox NA, Gunnar MR: Same place, different experiences: Bringing individual differences to research in child care. *Child Dev Perspect* 5:44–49, 2011.
54. Zeanah CH, Boris NW, Larrieu JA: Infant development and developmental risk: a review of the past 10 years. *J Am Acad Child Adolesc Psychiatry* 36:165–178, 1997.
55. Greenspan S: *Psychopathology and Adaptation in Infancy and Early Childhood.* New York, International Universities Press, 1981.
56. Piaget J, Inhelder B: *La Psychologie De L'enfant [The Psychology of the Child].* Paris, Presses Universitaires de France, 1966.
57. Mayes LC: The assessment and treatment of the psychiatric needs of medically compromised infants: consultation with preterm infants and their families. *Child Adoles Psychiatric Clin N Am* 4(3):555–569, 1995.
58. Bremner G, Fogel A: *The Blackwell Handbook of Infant Development.* Oxford, Blackwell Publishing, 2004.
59. Kagan J. Emergent themes in human development. *Am Sci* 64:190, 1976.
60. Hollich GJ, Hirsh-Pasek K, Golinkoff RM: Breaking the language barrier: An emergentist coalition model for the origins of word learning. *Monogr Soc Res Child Dev* 65(3), 2000.
61. Ulrey G: Assessment considerations with language impaired children. In: Ulrey G, Rogers SJ (eds): *Psychological Assessment of Handicapped Infants and Young Children.* New York, Thieme-Stratton, 1982.
62. Madrid A, Marachi JP: Medical assessment: its role in comprehensive psychiatric evaluation. *Child Adoles Psychiatric Clin N Am* 8:257–270, 1999.
63. Minde K: Prematurity and serious medical conditions in infancy: implications for development, behavior, and intervention. In: Zeanah J (ed): *Handbook of Infant Mental Health.* 2nd ed. New York, Guilford Press, 176–194, 2000.
64. Clarke-Stewart K, Fein GG: Early childhood programs. In: Haith MM, Campos JJ (eds): *Handbook of Child Psychology.* Vol 2. New York, Wiley, 917–999, 1983.
65. Guralnick MJ (ed): *The Effectiveness of Early Intervention.* Baltimore, MD, Brookes, 1997.
66. Shonkoff JP, Meisels SJ: Early childhood intervention: the evolution of a concept. In: Meisels SJ, Shonkoff J (eds): *Handbook of Early Childhood Intervention.* New York, Cambridge University Press, 3–31, 1990.

CHAPTER 2.1.2 ■ THE PRESCHOOL CHILD

LAURA STOUT SOSINSKY, WALTER S. GILLIAM, AND LINDA C. MAYES

Between the ages of 2 and 5 years and under average conditions, children's cognitive, social, and emotional worlds are rapidly expanding and changing (1). Their language abilities expand their capacity for imagination and symbolic thinking and for enlarging social relationships. Their changing cognitive capacities expand their ability for problem-solving and learning about the world. They develop the ability to name their own and others' feelings and to relate behavior to emotional states and expressions. During the preschool period of development, children are even more commonly in broader social worlds, such as child care and early childhood education programs, and may also experience the birth of a new sibling. While pediatricians remain the most likely professional to be consulted by parents when they are concerned about their 2- to 5-year-old child's health and development (throughout this chapter, the use of the word "parent" is inclusive of all adults that assume an important and regular role in providing care to the child), a number of other professionals are very likely to be involved in a preschooler's life, including child care and educational professionals. Also, this developmental period marks the beginning of more common referrals to child psychiatrists. These referrals come from teachers, parents, and pediatricians most commonly for behavioral problems, especially excessive aggression with peers or other adults, separation difficulties when faced with school and child care programs, developmental delays, especially of speech and language, and concerns about social delays, especially as these relate to social disabilities such as autism.

Development of behavior and competencies is a process of change over time as a child's characteristics reciprocally transact with the immediate caregiving environment and the broader ecological context, as discussed in the previous chapter on infant and toddler development (2–6; see Chapter 2.1.1). In the preschool years, specific features of these elements that differ from the earlier infancy and toddlerhood period include, for most preschoolers, increasing sophistication and capacity of cognitive, communicative, and social-emotional skills, a longer history of more varied experiences with parents and primary caregivers, and the high likelihood of exposure, often extensive, to nonparental early care and education contexts, perhaps for the first time.

As with infancy and toddlerhood, the diagnostic nosology for specific disorders among preschool children is only beginning to emerge and only a few diagnostic labels, such as autism and the related social disabilities, are commonly used. Furthermore, social-emotional well-being has received lesser emphasis relative to the impact of cognitive and linguistic competencies on later child outcomes. In addition, developmental change in early childhood is rapid, and assessment of normal and problematic behaviors can be challenging. However, there is a growing body of research evidence that social-emotional and behavioral problems in early childhood are real, not transient, and that occurrence and persistence are associated both with co-occurrence of other problems and with family and parenting difficulties (7). From this and other work, there is general consensus that the understanding of a child's development requires an appreciation of the caregiving contexts which support, protect, and nurture the child during this period of dependence on adults (8).

In this chapter, we review several areas relevant to preschool children's development and those issues about which child psychiatrists may be most often called upon to consult with families and teachers. The basic developmental areas of normative preschool development include (a) robust language learning, including the word-learning explosion and use of language to express emotions and convey more complex or hypothetical information; (b) emerging thinking and learning capacities, including executive functioning skills as well as the young child's emerging ability to reflect on his own and others' mental activities—feelings, dreams, beliefs, and thoughts; (c) emerging peer relationships and the capacity for imaginary play (and imaginary friends); and (d) normative issues regarding separation and individuation. Consideration is given to each of these areas' transactions over time with each other, with caregiving, and with the broader environmental context. Understanding these basic developmental areas is key to a child psychiatrist's ability to consult effectively when parents and teachers bring developmental concerns about a young child.

In terms of specific consultative questions, we cover three areas in brief—fears and apparent anxiety, aggressive behavior, and child psychiatric consultation to preschool settings as examples of the more common reasons for child psychiatric involvement with preschool children. Specific diagnoses including autism, conduct or oppositional difficulties, attentional problems, and assessment for developmental delay are covered elsewhere in this volume.

LANGUAGE

A word-learning language explosion begins at about 18 months and continues through the preschool years, during which children learn on average about nine words per day. Language acquisition is robust, with children learning vocabulary and the fundamentals of linguistic semantics by age 4 or 5, even with very little environmental support (as exemplified by deaf children's early communication even without language input). However, there appears to be a sensitive period for language proficiency. The specific language a child learns and linguistic qualities such as morphology, grammar, phonology, verbal expression of emotions, and conveyance of information about past, present, or hypothetical events are best learned by the preschool period. The difference among children of differing language proficiency levels on these linguistic qualities is not as much whether or not they can use these linguistic skills, but in the frequency and effectiveness with which they use them in their daily lives. The ease at which these skills can be learned begins to decline at about 6 or 7 years of age (9).

As language proficiency is pivotal for subsequent cognitive and social development, especially school readiness and success, the contributors to development of language proficiency are of great interest. There is evidence that the amount of talk caregivers (usually mothers) direct toward their young children is associated with vocabulary growth and preliteracy skills. The amount and richness of the vocabulary children are exposed to, both child- and other-directed, is also related to language development (10). The genetic contribution of parents is of course important, but so is the family's socioeconomic status, with children of lower income, less-educated parents receiving less quantity and quality of linguistic exposure and demonstrating lower levels of language proficiency (9). Indeed, recent research finds that, by 2 years of age, the disparities between children from higher- and lower-SES families are equivalent to a 6-month gap in both language processing skills and vocabulary knowledge (11).

EMERGING MINDS

Beginning around 2 years of age, young children start to form more stable concepts of the world around them. They begin to think symbolically—to use one object to stand for others. For example, young children use scribbled drawings to represent houses, people, animals—and to tell stories using these scribbled bits.

Moreover, in the preschool period, there begin to be vast individual differences in children's executive functioning—a child's capabilities to self-regulate, sequence, plan, and organize. The development of these executive controls has a global and lasting effect on later competencies, and problems in executive functioning can lead to later school problems. In contrast, there is little individual variation in normally developing preschoolers' disposition toward a positive motivation. Young children are intrinsically motivated to explore, try, and learn. In the preschool period, this intrinsic motivation is related to self-attributions about their abilities that are indiscriminately positive. Typically developing preschoolers often perceive themselves as being the best at everything, and to be getting better and better everyday. This disposition often declines on school entry, which may be related to improved cognitive abilities of self-appraisal and social comparison, but is also likely associated with a greater exposure to peers and the increased judgment and potential for criticism in formal school environments. Early education, whether formal or informal by parents and caregivers, should have as a goal encouragement of a child's natural inclination to explore and learn, not only to foster cognitive skills but also a positive motivation toward learning (9).

The preschool period is also marked by the beginnings of concerted attention to a child's skills and abilities considered basic to school readiness, as well as basic self-care skills. Children acquire skills best when caregivers present them with tasks that are just a bit too difficult to accomplish independently, but are possible with appropriate assistance, or "scaffolding." This highly effective approach to teaching young children requires a certain degree of sensitivity to the child's developmental level, often referred to as the child's "zone of proximal development" (12). In addition to this type of parent–child interaction, parents encourage their child's preliteracy and premath skills with activities such as reading (13), quantitative games, and provision of opportunities such as trips to the library. These activities are most influential when undertaken in warm and nurturing routines. Being read to has the most impact when the child is comfortably and regularly cuddled in a parent's lap for a bedtime story (9).

By the time children are 4 to 5 years old, they have acquired the ability to understand that their thoughts, beliefs, and feelings are their own and that others may feel differently, even believe differently from them. Interpreting the behaviors and words of others as being a part of their feelings and thoughts is a major part of being human and getting along in a social world. This capacity is a remarkable developmental achievement covered broadly under the term *developing theory of mind*—the notion that a part of social development is seeing the world in both physical and nonphysical terms, with the latter being invisible or imagined states of thoughts, feelings, and beliefs. There is a large literature on the emerging theory of mind in young children, especially as a capacity that does not develop fully in autistic children, and several have proposed distinct stages in this developmental progression—from a physical stance (the world is as we see it, and we predict the world based on the laws of nature) to an intentional stance in which we understand and predict the world at the level of mental states—beliefs, feelings, fears, worries. The boy is crying because he misses his grandmother, or the girl is happy because she got the present she was hoping to receive.

Once children begin to see the world through the lens of mental states, their understanding of their own self and others greatly expands. They are capable then, for example, of playful deceit—hiding something in a way that sends another person down the wrong path because they understand that by providing deceptive clues, the other person develops a false belief as to the whereabouts of an object. They become capable of subtle sarcasm, understanding that just by a change in a tone of voice, someone else reads their intent and not just the meaning of their words. However, during the preschool years, these capacities are just emerging and tend to disappear at moments of fatigue or stress. Thus, a clinician working with a 4-year-old who has been remarkably clear about his feelings and the feelings of others may be very surprised when a usually competent boy melts in disappointment or anger because he was sure his mother knew exactly what he was thinking about for his birthday. Further, under stress or unusually severe trauma and neglect, it is very difficult for children to fully develop or allow themselves to imagine the intentions of others who may have been hurtful or neglectful and thus, clinicians working with severely disadvantaged populations may see a delay in the appearance of these very important social perspective-taking capacities. Thus, in addition to understanding where their patients are in basic developmental domains such as cognition, language, fine and gross motor, child psychiatrists working with young children need also to evaluate where their preschool patient is in his/her capacity to think about his own feelings and beliefs as well as those of others. This is most evident in their play (see next section) and less often through direct questions of "How do you feel?" or "What do you think?" though they may answer such questions indirectly about characters in a story or in a play sequence of their own.

PLAY

Play, broadly defined, covers many activities. One is the rough and tumble play of children running, jumping, chasing, and wrestling with one another. This form is universal across most cultures, and even across different species. Play also includes verbal forms that are uniquely human, in which children play with sounds and words, even inventing their own language and rhymes—and it is this capacity that is most central to a child psychiatrist's ability to communicate with younger children through the special language of play. Manipulating and exploring toys and other objects is a form of play that gives young children a chance to learn by looking, feeling, tasting, listening—a form of trial and error, hands-on learning.

Pretend Play

Children's pretend play varies remarkably in quality, content, intensity, and engagement with other children and adults.

In part, their developmental maturity defines the type of play they are capable of creating. Pretend play begins around age 2, or just before children are able to let a real object stand for another or for something imaginary. When a toddler begins to brush a doll's hair, this is the very beginning of her ability to pretend. She is using a toy (a doll) with a real object (a brush) to represent a real action. When she starts to feed the doll with a spoon, making lip-smacking noises and blowing on the spoon to cool the soup, she has gone one step further. She is "representing" imaginary food. And when she offers that food to another doll or an adult, the full ability to pretend—to represent her mental world through play—is in evidence.

The ability to pretend requires the ability to symbolize—to let one thing stand for another, just as a picture of a car stands for a real car. The ability to create symbols or representations is part of entering a more complex and layered world of social communication. There are several different levels or stages in learning to use symbols. In the earliest, a baby picks up a spoon and touches it to the edge of a bowl. She thus shows she understands this object's use—what actions a spoon is associated with, even when she is not using it for that action. A variant on this later stage is when a child "eats" from an empty spoon and looks with a smile to her father as she nibbles. Similarly, a toddler can act out sleep, closing his eyes for a few seconds before looking to see if a parent is watching. When a preschooler pretends to feed a doll and read it a story, he shows he is capable of a more complicated level of pretense. And when children begin turning one representation into another, such as having a cup be a hat, their pretend abilities are at an even more sophisticated level. That opens up more avenues for expression.

Peer Play

Play with peers and establishing relationships with other children is "one of the major developmental tasks of early childhood" (9). Both the type and the complexity of play have been studied, specifically in regard to prosocial play, engaged behavior, and emotional expression during play. A child's acceptance among peers also begins to vary in the preschool years, although peer like- or dislike-nominations are very unstable at this time. A striking increase in social skills occurs in the preschool years, and peer play increasingly involves pretense (described further below) and expanded numbers of children.

Very young children under 3 years of age often play alone with a toy or other object. They may roll a truck around and make authentic truck sounds. But they make no special effort to invite others to join their play. In "parallel play," which is also characteristic of children 3 years of age and younger, two or more children play by themselves but close to each other. They may even use similar toys, such as a bucket and sand, but they are not playing with one another. They are simply in close proximity.

Children 3 to 4 years old begin to engage one another. They share toys, pass them back and forth, even talk about the same activity and follow one another. Their play is still not completely cooperative, however. If preschoolers have no real companion nearby, they may engage an imaginary friend as a playmate. When children are around 4 years and older, they begin to engage one another in games in which they must share a goal and a story. They assign roles, direct action, even carry stories and games from day to day.

Peer play is influenced by caregivers. Secure attachment relationships have been associated with higher levels of social competence, greater preschool popularity, and more positive friendships (14,15). In addition, parents' role in helping children play well with others and provision of peer play opportunities, monitoring of peer interactions, modeling and coaching acceptable behaviors, and discouraging unacceptable behaviors are all associated with more positive peer relationships (9).

A child's temperament is also related to his or her peer interactions. Inhibition hinders children's peer interactions, although excessive exuberance can also cause difficulties. More importantly, the child's ability to regulate his or her individual temperament is associated with peer-interaction skills. A child's competencies at sustained attention, controlled expression of negative emotion, and ability to inhibit certain actions are more related to positive peer interactions and relationships than is underlying temperament as such (9).

Clinical Use of Play

One of the important skills for a child psychiatrist working with younger children is learning how to use play therapeutically and as a means of communicating with young children about what is uppermost in their minds. Often children who have been neglected or otherwise stressed and traumatized are unable to use play adaptively and unable to engage in imaginative fantasy play. If we consider play as a special language for communication with younger children, it is appropriate to work with a young child to enhance their ability to play as a means of expression of anxieties and worries (though play should never be taken as a veridical account of children's past experiences). To use play therapeutically requires different techniques from simply joining in with children's play. For one, the child psychiatrist is always trying to understand what a child may be conveying through his or her play—why this burst of anger in the animals surrounding the house? why the lonely child whose cries are never heard? At the same time, direct interpretation of play, that is, taking the imaginary action and translating it into questions about the child's own experiences, is not always effective inasmuch as young children are not always able or aware of using play characters and themes to tell stories directly reflective of their own experiences. Their play may reflect what is concerning to them—how to handle being angry or feeling lonely—but this is not the same as interpreting, for example, the lonely crying child in the play as being a direct statement of an experience the patient must have had. Thus, while there is a considerable literature on this issue, child psychiatrists using play as a therapeutic technique may be more effective by staying "within the play" and, for example, introducing another character who also feels very lonely and lost and does not know what to do or a character who comes along to help. Either way, the therapist is working within the child's story to try to help the child expand his expression of his feelings and his beliefs in a way that helps the therapist better understand the patient.

Many preschool children—up to half, according to some surveys—create imaginary companions and insist on their reality. For children under 5, the boundary between fact and fantasy is often more fluid. But if pressed, most preschoolers will agree that their friends are not really visible, not really hungry, not really sleeping beside them. Imaginary friends seem to serve a number of normative purposes including companionship. Indeed, the forms that imaginary friends take often reflect children's concerns and anxieties, just as their games do. An imaginary friend can offer a child psychological protection from her worries by taking on magical powers, or even by succumbing to dangers in the child's place. Child psychiatrists are often faced with distinguishing between the normative use of an imaginary friend and a young child's more than expected difficulty in distinguishing real from pretend. With younger children, this distinction may be especially difficult and requires seeing the child in more than one setting and over time.

SEPARATION

Typically developing preschool-aged children are struggling between independence and dependence, to be both "grown up" and at the same time able to turn to their parents. Especially around separations and transitions, preschoolers are often unpredictable and emotionally labile. They can effortlessly separate for child care one day and the next tearfully cling to their parents. An outside stress, such as the birth of a new baby, may make separation more difficult. Many preschoolers have had some successful experiences with separations, such as going to child care or staying at home with a babysitter. Each separation successfully weathered enhances the preschooler's ability to withstand the next.

Preschoolers often struggle to deal with separations because their repertoire of coping abilities is still developing. Older children can call on their increased cognitive abilities and a repertoire of past experiences, but preschool children do not always have the cognitive abilities to reassure themselves that each separation will work out. This is why it is very common for a preschool child to question her parents repeatedly, even about daily experiences like child care, and ask to be reassured about when parents will return, where they will be during the day, and who will pick them up. Parents often feel confused, frustrated, and guilty hearing these questions repeated, but preschool children ask because they are using their newfound language skills to deal with uncertainty.

Preschool children's emerging symbolic capacities also help them cope with separations—a stuffed animal or other favorite toy, a picture, or even something belonging to their parent can stand for a person they miss. Preschoolers' use of symbolic possessions also shows their newfound capacity for "object constancy," the knowledge that something can be out of sight but nonetheless continue to exist. Preschool children are just beginning to grasp this idea as it pertains to people. They are starting to create mental images of their absent parents and to wonder what people are doing when they are not with them. Nearly every young child worries about being left alone or separated from his parents. This is true no matter how thoughtful or careful parents have been or even if they have not been separated from their preschoolers. Children especially need their parents close when they are afraid, feeling sick, or going through important changes, such as moving or starting a new school.

Parents are often surprised at how hard it is for a preschooler to say goodbye to a favorite teacher at the end of the year, or accept a new teacher the following year. Children this age also mourn the loss of a regular babysitter or nanny, and do not easily replace that person with someone new. Preschoolers need help in mastering the experience of parting with people outside the family. They need to be reassured that their caregiver did not leave because of them. Visits with an old nanny or teacher after the farewell are helpful, as are pictures, letters, and phone calls. Sometimes parents think continued contact will make it harder for their children to get used to a new teacher or nanny, and feel that it is best for the child to experience a "clean break" with their previous teacher or nanny. This approach, however, rarely helps preschoolers. Even years later, children may mention an early teacher or babysitter parents had long forgotten. They return time and time again to rework the separation and think about what that person meant in their lives.

An especially difficult separation for young children may be during parental separation and divorce (16). How does the nearly inevitable conflict between parents that accompanies divorce affect a young child still concerned about consistency and object constancy? What is the impact of parental loss versus shared custody? Goldstein et al. (17) emphasized the critical roles of clinical expertise and opinion in serving the best interests of young children in custody disputes, and it is an increasingly common consultation for child psychiatrists to be asked either by a court or by parents to consult about how best to help a young child in the instance of parental conflict and divorce.

The principle of continuity of care, so often stressed for young children as essential for their ability to deal with separation, comes into practical application in two major decisions during divorce—custody and visitation. By and large, for preschool children, single-parent—rather than two-parent—custody remains the most common decision of courts but joint custody is increasing as fathers want to be more involved in their children's lives and more mothers face the difficulties of working full time and raising a family. While there is no firm empirical evidence to support either alternative, experiential case reports do suggest that younger children do better when parents are able to minimize the degree of discord and conflict and/or avoid catching the child in the middle of their disputes. Similarly, there are few to no systematic data about appropriate visitation models but it is clear that consistency, structure, and predictability are keys, especially as preschoolers are highly dependent on routines and dependable structure. Child psychiatrists specializing in work with younger children may be involved not only in consultation to the court but also in ongoing consultation to one or both parents for how best to care for their child and how both parents, if they so desire or if appropriate, may have a role in their child's life.

FEARS AND ANXIETY

Fears, worries, and anxiety are often more evident in children's second and third years, even as separation and stranger anxiety wane. This fearfulness and caution is normative. It keeps a very young, very small child from straying too far. While it may sound paradoxical, children who are well cared for are more able to experience normal fear and worry and thus to run back to their parents for comfort and reassurance. Children who have been neglected and abused are more often heedless of danger. They cannot easily recognize normal feelings of fear and worry as protective signals (18).

Despite their energy and enormous interest in the world, 2- and 3-year-old children are still quite dependent on adults and are still often preoccupied, even in the most optimal of situations, with the constancy of the important people in their lives. They feel apprehensive not just about new things they encounter but also about what appears in their thoughts and fantasies. They may feel particularly uneasy at bedtime when they are about to be left alone. Preschool children soothe their worries through constancy and routines. Indeed, such rituals are the essence of this age. If a child can keep things around her unchanging and predictable, the world seems a little less uncertain and daunting. For the child psychiatrist asked to evaluate a young child who becomes inconsolable with the slightest change in routine, the question is how normative versus how rigid such routines are, what purpose they serve, and how they fit in the child's daily routine.

Fears and worries also become more evident in the preschool years because, as discussed earlier, this is when the capacities for imagination greatly expand—and usually what young children imagine is far more frightening than their actual experiences. Their bad dreams seem real, and for them there is only a thin line between scary thoughts and actual events. Playing about monsters, they may suddenly become quite scared when they hear a door open elsewhere in the house. Two- and three-year-olds are certain that just by thinking about scary things, they can sometimes make them happen. They are sure that everyone knows about their occasionally angry thoughts, and that such anger can actually harm others. Young children thus feel simultaneously powerful and helpless, at the center of their world and insignificant. They have the power to make things happen and, at the same time, are so small in the face of the bad things they can imagine in the world. All this is cause for normal anxieties but once again, often poses a diagnostic challenge for a child psychiatrist who must distinguish between what is usual for age and what has gone beyond the bounds of normative to be constrictive and maladaptive.

Unlike older children and adults, preschoolers cannot always talk explicitly about their worries or try to avoid the thoughts or situations that frighten them. Often, therefore, they show their fears in paradoxical ways. Afraid of the vacuum cleaner, they may actively avoid it, or they may constantly try to explore and master it. Fearing the dark, they may play with turning the lights on and off or be frantic whenever they are left alone in their beds at night. They may become ever more insistent on certain rituals. Some preschoolers meet any change in their routine with irritability. Young children going through a particularly worrisome time may have routines about food, clothing, bathing, and going to school. These routines are soothingly predictable whenever the child feels uncertain and confused. At the same time, insistence on sameness is a characteristic of a number of early developmental disorders and the consulting child psychiatrist faces, as with other issues raised in this chapter, the dilemma of sorting normative from maladaptive.

Often young children show their worry and fear in ways that seem unexpected, such that the more anxious they are, the more active and uncontrollable they become. Often they are so excited that they cannot heed their parents' or teachers' efforts to help them. Some adults might interpret this behavior as willful or oppositional, but it often reflects a state of such internal overstimulation and anxiety that the child simply cannot control himself. For some children, worries and fears are not simply responses to developmental pressures or the stresses of ordinary living. Rather, their strong, often overwhelming feelings grow out of proportion to their experiences. Anxieties interfere with their lives at school and home, with their friendships, and with their pleasure in play. This increase in worry can be a part of a stressful life event, such as the birth of a new sibling, an illness, or a death in the family.

AGGRESSION

Aggression is a complex set of behaviors, especially in preschool children that reflects a balance between response to frustration versus assertiveness and individuation. Aggressive behavior is one of the more common reasons for child psychiatry consultation, especially in the context of a young child's placement in a child care or educational setting. Furthermore, out of control, aggressive behavior may be one of the most common difficulties between young children and their parents that prompt families to seek mental health consultation. Thus, understanding aggression as both a normative developmental requirement and a possible symptom is the key to effective child psychiatric consultation.

Aggressive behavior in young children has many roots and serves some important social roles. Furthermore, adults have considerable influence over how children view and express their aggressive thoughts. While some variables in a child's aggression, such as her basic tolerance for frustration, may depend in part on genetic endowment and/or early experience, many others are shaped by what he or she learns from her experiences with parents and teachers.

At the very least, aggressive behaviors always express some needs and feelings of the child. Also, children who enter their second year of life with few words sometimes may exhibit greater levels of physical aggression than their more verbose peers because they have no other means to express their needs and frustrations. Some children rarely, if ever, express themselves through aggressive behaviors, while others find aggressive behaviors a ready and comfortable way of communicating. Reliance on aggressive behaviors to meet needs can be modeled by parents, other adults, peers, and siblings, and screen media (television, videos, movies, computer games).

For very young children, aggressive behavior is also a way of expressing independence, as in "Mine!" "Me do!" and "Go away!" These firm statements may be unpleasant, even hurtful, to another person or anger an adult. Toddlers' temper tantrums, while surely tempestuous and irritating for parents, are statements of frustration. These young children often feel small, dependent, and powerless, but as they grow, their need for independence grows too. Thus, developmentally, temper tantrums begin as children start to experiment with separation from their parents. The more they move away from the emotionally secure base of the parent, the more dependent and little they may feel, and the more vulnerable to frustration and tantrums they may become.

Aggressive feelings and thoughts, not necessarily expressed in behavior, are also a central part of young children's fantasy lives. They are small and dependent upon a much larger, stronger adult world. They struggle for independence—to be "grown up." Pretending to be very powerful, even scary and aggressive, is one way to play with getting bigger. In preschool children, aggressive behaviors have different intents, causes, and outcomes.

In trying to figure out why a child is biting or hitting, it is important for the child psychiatrist to ask where she directs her violence: toward other people or only toward inanimate objects? In other words, does she kick and break toys or kick and hurt her classmates, siblings, and parents? What typically starts the aggressive behavior? Is she frustrated by wanting a toy she cannot have, or by wishing to be hugged by a very busy parent or teacher? Is she very tired or very excited—at the end of the day or just after a puppeteer has visited the child care center? Is she reacting to another child's teasing about her hair, how she fell on the playground, or how she cried when her father left? Did another child hit or push her? It is also wise to consider the apparent intent of a child's aggressive behavior. Is it a means to an end—to get the desired toy or make a place on the teacher's lap? Is it to create a personal space—a kind of "don't tread on me" signal? Does the goal seem to injure or destroy, or is it really to gain another's attention, to win in a game, or get the best seat in circle time? No child acts aggressively in the same way for the same reasons in every situation. By identifying what a child really wants, her caregivers can tell her not to push or hit while also showing her a better way to achieve her aim, thus reducing her frustration and need to act out.

When evaluating a child's aggression, it is also important to consider how it might be linked to his fears and worries. Such behavior may be a way for him to express how he is really worried deep down without acting fearful. Not all aggressive feelings in children reflect deeper fears and anxiety, but when they do, it is very important for parents and teachers to be made aware of these fears and worries. For most young children, physically aggressive behavior—hitting, biting, pushing, kicking—begins to subside by their third, or at the latest their fourth, birthdays. On the other hand, verbal aggression—shouting, yelling, name-calling—increases between the ages of 2 and 4 years as children gain more language skills. Most often, all kinds of hostile behaviors, verbal and physical, diminish in frequency by 5 or 6 years of age when children enter first and second grade. Younger children are most aggressive around asserting their physical needs and wants. Older children, in contrast, focus their aggression on social situations and needs. Indeed, as children get older, their aggression is more often related to a perceived hurt or slight; they want to pay back an insult to their self-esteem which they perceive from a particular person. Thus, paradoxically, as children get older, they are far less aggressive, but when they are, their actions may be more often intended to harm another person.

Although significant behavior problems during the early years are often stable and predictive of later behavioral difficulties (7), it is not guaranteed that an aggressive preschooler will grow into an aggressive school-age child. Despite parents' and teachers' concerns, the hitting, kicking, biting 3-year old is not guaranteed to become an aggressive school-age child. What matters most is how adults understand and meet aggressive behavior in younger children. By finding methods for young children to strive for mastery, self-assertion, and self-protection, adults support these important developmental tasks without encouraging hostile or violent behavior. Aggression met with aggression is far more likely to convey the message that people can express frustration and anger only through shouting, name-calling, or physical action. Aggression met with an effort to understand what a young child is trying to communicate shows that when people feel frustrated and angry, they can think about how to express those feelings in ways other people understand.

CHILD PSYCHIATRIC CONSULTATION IN PRESCHOOL SETTINGS

There are more preschoolers enrolled in early education and child care programs than ever before (19,20). The recent increase in the number of preschoolers enrolled in formal care outside means that a greater number of young children are coming into contact with potential referral agents (preschool teachers, child care providers), which translates into more psychiatric referrals at lower ages than ever. Rather than simply waiting for these young children and their families to present at the child psychiatrist's office, many child psychiatrists and clinicians of other disciplines have sought to address the referral issues in the child care or preschool setting (21,22).

There are many advantages to providing child psychiatric services as part of a consultative service to early care and education programs (23). Consultative delivery models afford the clinician an opportunity to observe the patient in a natural setting (e.g., the child care program), observe interactions with often several peers, obtain information about the child's functioning from other adults in addition to the parents, and enlist the assistance of many adults in supporting treatment recommendations. Additionally, children often behave very differently at home versus in their child care programs, where the degree of structure and behavioral expectations may vary considerably. The opportunity to observe the child across these different settings is often invaluable as a way of better understanding potential environmental triggers for the behavioral concerns and understanding the child's capacity to modulate her behavior to match different environmental contexts.

Mental health consultation in early education programs can take many forms. Consultation can be focused solely on classroom-specific reduction of particular behaviors that the teacher finds difficult to manage (peer aggression, tantruming, running out of the classroom), or it can be more global in focus, such as using the classroom experiences to create opportunities for the child to develop competencies that can lead to increased self-efficacy. Sometimes the consultation is focused specifically on the child, but often the consultation may include systemic assistance to the teaching staff regarding how to improve the overall mental health climate in the classroom, facilitating teachers' understanding of children's behaviors and teacher behavior management skills, creating a more efficient and effective system of screening and identifying children in need of assistance, and sometimes even addressing mental health needs in the teaching staff.

Attention paid to the overall functioning of preschool and child care classroom (from the physical setting to interactions between teachers and children) can provide clues to understanding the child's behavior and how best to intervene. When a child and family presents in a psychiatric office, it is essential to understand the effect of familial psychopathology on the young child (24). Similarly, the mental health of preschool teachers, who sometimes spend as many or more waking hours with a preschooler than do his parents, can impact child–adult interactions and contribute to emotional and behavioral difficulties. For example, child care provider depression has been associated with child care that is less sensitive, more detached from the children, and (when not detached) more intrusive or negative (25). Also, child care teachers who report elevated levels of depression or job stress, or depressed levels of job satisfaction, are more likely to report having expelled a preschooler from their classroom in the past year (26). Of course, low wages and relatively high levels of job turnover in the child care workforce (27) may contribute significantly to teacher burnout. Unfortunately, mental health consultation in child care settings may often ignore adult functioning.

SUMMARY

Between 2 and 5 years of age is a time of very rapid development, especially in social and cognitive skills that expand the world for preschool children. They gradually acquire the ability to think in terms of mental states such as feelings and beliefs, to understand others' intentionality, and to play symbolically and imaginatively. Increasingly, they are venturing further from the home, forming relationships with peers and nonfamilial adults in child care and early education settings. Child psychiatrists working with children of this age are often faced with distinguishing normative heightened anxiety, preference for routines, and aggression from presentations in which these same characteristics are maladaptive and in need of intervention. Hence, this developmental period especially calls for a thorough understanding of normal as well as abnormal development. Further, as with infancy, this period of development also brings child psychiatrists in close collaboration and consultation with pediatricians and early childhood education settings.

References

1. Goswami U: *Blackwell Handbook of Childhood Cognitive Development*. Oxford, Blackwell Publishing, 2004.
2. Bronfenbrenner U: Contexts of child rearing: Problems and prospects. *Am Psychol* 34:844–850, 1979.
3. Bronfenbrenner U: Ecology of the family as a context for human development: research perspectives. *Dev Psychol* 22:723–742, 1986.
4. Bronfenbrenner U: Environments in developmental perspective: theoretical and operational models. In: Friedman SL, Wachs TD (eds): *Measuring Environment across the Life Span: Emerging Methods and Concepts*. Washington, DC, *American Psychological Association*, 1999, 3–28.
5. Sameroff AJ: Transactional models in early social relations. *Hum Dev* 18:65–79, 1975.
6. Sameroff AJ: The social context of development. In: Eisenberg N (ed): *Contemporary Topics in Development*. New York, Wiley, 1987.
7. Briggs-Gowan MJ, Carter AS, Bosson-Heenan J, Guyer AE, Horwitz SM: Are infant-toddler social-emotional and behavioral problems transient? *J Am Acad Child Adolesc Psychiatr* 45:849–858, 2006.
8. Carter AS, Briggs-Gowan MJ, Davis NO: Assessment of young children's social-emotional development and psychopathology: recent advances and recommendations for practice. *J Child Psychol Psychiatry* 45:109–134, 2004.
9. Shonkoff JP, Phillips DA: *From Neurons to Neighborhoods: The Science of Early Childhood Development*. Washington, DC, National Academy Press, 2000.

10. Hart B, Risley TR: *Meaningful Differences in the Everyday Experience of Young American Children*. Baltimore, MD, Paul H Brookes Publishing, 1995.
11. Fernald A, Marchman VA, Weisleder A: SES differences in language processing skill and vocabulary are evident at 18 months. *Dev Sci* 16:234–248, 2013.
12. Vygotsky L: Tool and symbol in child development and internalization of higher psychological functions. In: Cole M, John-Steiner V, Scribner S, Souberman E (eds): *L. Vygotsky, Mind in Society*. Cambridge, MA, Harvard University Press, 1978.
13. Dickinson DK, Griffith JA, Golinkoff RM, Hirsh-Pasek K: How reading books fosters language development around the world. *Child Dev Res* 2012:602807, 2012.
14. Howes C: The earliest friendships. In: Bukowski WM, Newcomb AF, Hartup WW (eds): *The Company They Keep: Friendship in Childhood and Adolescence*. New York, Cambridge University Press, 1996, 66–86.
15. Park KA, Waters E: Security of attachment and preschool friendships. *Child Dev* 60:1076–1081, 1989.
16. Mayes LC, Siegl AM: In: Galatzer-Levy R, Kraus L (eds): *The Scientific Basis of Child Custody Decisions*. New York, John Wiley and Sons, 188–204, 1999.
17. Goldstein J, Freud A, Solnit AJ: *Beyond the Best Interest of the Child*. New York, Free Press, 1973.
18. Crittenden PM, Ainsworth MDS: Child maltreatment and attachment theory. In: Cicchetti D, Carlson V (eds): *Child Maltreatment: Theory and Research on the Causes and Consequences of Child Abuse and Neglect*. New York, Cambridge University Press, 432–463, 1989.
19. Barnett WS, Carolan ME, Squires JH, Brown KC, Horowitz M: *The State of Preschool: 2014 State Preschool Yearbook*. New Brunswick, NJ, Rutgers University, National Institute for Early Education Research, 2015.
20. Gilliam WS, Zigler EF: A critical meta-analysis of all evaluations of state-funded preschool from 1977 to 1998: implications for policy, service delivery and program evaluation. *Early Child Res Q* 15:441–473, 2000.
21. Kaplan M: In: Mayes LC, Gilliam W (eds): *Child and Adolescent Psychiatric Clinics: Comprehensive Psychiatric Assessment of Young Children*. Philadelphia, PA, Saunders, 379–394, 1999.
22. Sosinsky LS, Gilliam WS: Child care: how pediatricians can support children and families. In: Kliegman RM, Stanton BF, St Geme JW, Schor NF, Behrman RE (eds): *Nelson Textbook of Pediatrics*. 19th ed. Philadelphia, PA, Elsevier, 45, 2011.
23. Donohue PJ, Falk B, Provet AG: *Mental Health Consultation in Early Childhood*. Baltimore, MD, Paul H. Brookes, 2000.
24. Cicchetti D, Rogosch FA, Toth SL: Maternal depressive disorder and contextual risk: contributions to the development of attachment insecurity and behavior problems in toddlerhood. *Dev Psychopathol* 10:283–300, 1998.
25. Hamre BK, Pianta RC: Self-reported depression in nonfamilial caregivers: prevalence and associations with caregiver behavior in child-care settings. *Early Child Res Q* 19:297–318, 2004.
26. Gilliam WS, Shahar G: Preschool and child care expulsion and suspension: Rates and predictors in one state. *Infant Young Child* 19:228–245, 2006.
27. Whitebook M, Sakai L: Turnover begets turnover: an examination of job and occupational instability among child care center staff. *Early Child Res Q* 18:273–293, 2003.

CHAPTER 2.1.3 ■ DEVELOPMENT OF SCHOOL-AGE CHILDREN

LEE COMBRINCK-GRAHAM AND GERALDINE S. FOX

FOREWORD TO THE FIFTH EDITION

In the 25 years since this chapter was originally drafted, there have been many changes that affect the way we view children, their development, and their health and mental health. This chapter in its current version still follows the lines of development outlined by our venerable ancestors, most significantly Erik Erikson and Jean Piaget. Erikson's eight stages of man, elaborated in Childhood and Society, not only offered a developmental template, but also located an individual child's development squarely in the social context in which the child was developing. Jean Piaget studied the evolution of thinking, and offered the sequence that seems to be a foundation for cognitive development. Other important contributions to our understanding of development either elaborate these two compatible lines or have since proven to be less helpful in understanding the process. However, there have been some significant shifts in viewpoint that may have affected children's progress through this period.

The recent developments we observe that have a profound effect on how children grow, learn, and develop means and strategies for advancing and solving intellectual, social, and emotional problems include the following: (1) An increased focus on psychopathology or learning differences that are seen as "disabilities," and (2) A focus, in school, on achievement measured by standardized tests.

Briefly, how do these changes in focus and understanding affect our view of school-aged children's development, or, indeed, their development itself? (1) Focus on "disability" distracts from looking at how children learn, cope, and problem-solve, and most importantly distracts from the fundamental drive for learning, curiosity. (2) Measuring achievement of children as representing the success of their teachers, schools, and school systems focuses their learning on taking tests and what is needed to pass a test. What is lost in this process for many children is the excitement of discovery. Further, it seems likely that the greater incidence of or recognition of "bullying" is associated with how kids perform in the eyes of other kids, how those who don't perform well may try to compensate by being bullies, and how those who focus on performing well may somehow be socially marginalized. Furthermore, this focus on individuals passing tests makes it difficult to have the kind of learning community that we describe as an essential part of the school-aged child's social and intellectual learning experience. More and more we see schools focusing on individual children and less on holding the peer group accountable for each child's participation and learning.

Considering the effects of the changes in these two areas offers reminders of the importance of social context to development in a way that we cannot ignore. It is not feasible to look at individual children behaving, learning, feeling, and thinking without also examining the contexts in which they do that. We said so in the original chapter, and as we look at the changes summarized above, we are even more struck by this fact.

Research is ongoing regarding the effects of these developments. We write about them to encourage the readers of this chapter to take what is presented as a basic direction of development and the essential accomplishments of development in this period, but to constantly question how our child patients are affected by current trends in the way children are viewed and treated. And how are we professionals affected by these changes as we identify strengths and liabilities in our work toward strengthening the children we see?

INTRODUCTION

The middle years of childhood, spanning the age from when a child enters primary school through the onset of adolescence (ages approximately 5 to 12 in Western cultures), are also referred to as "the school-age period" because of the critical importance of school in development in our society. Many classical theorists have classified this time as the period when a child enters society and begins to establish the basis for becoming a contributing member of his/her community.

Historically, Sigmund Freud, and other drive theorists, described middle childhood as a sexually dormant interlude between the mastery of Oedipal strivings with establishment of the superego, and the pubertal reawakening of sexual desire in a true genital phase. It has since been established that latency is a myth. Erik Erikson provided a more enduring characterization of this period when he described the critical psychological issue: "Industry versus Inferiority" (1). In formal schooling a child is attempting to master the basics of the industry of our society, to build on academic abilities. Failure to progress in school and in the peer context can establish a sense of inferiority, rather than support the momentum of a drive for competence. Neo-Freudians (Sullivan, Horney, Thompson) added an emphasis on social context as the critical shaping force on how this developmental period is negotiated. Harry Stack Sullivan, for example, observed that this "juvenile era" provides the first opportunity for society to "correct" the influence of the family.

Freud, Erikson, and Sullivan defined the important work of this period. Research into the details of cognitive, emotional, and social development confirm that civilization and being-in-society are the essentials of development in the school-age period. Thus, thinking about the child's psychological well-being must extend beyond the child to include not only the family but also the social, economic, and political contexts that define its functioning. Vygotsky's concept of "mind in society" and Bateson's "ecology of mind" point to the dynamic exchange of experience, accomplishment, and social response and effectiveness. In addition, ecologic theories such as Bronfenbrenner's (2) place development within a range of nested contexts: family as primary, school-as-work as connected and central, as well as larger cultural and societal contexts. Newer work has focused on the interplay basic developmental and contextual processes and links to policy and advocacy for children and teenagers (3).

The best way to emphasize the remarkable growth that occurs during middle childhood is to contrast the skills of children when they enter and exit grade school (Table 2.1.3.1).

Table 2.1.3.1 describes what can be seen in normal average children in the United States, whether they come from poor, inner city neighborhoods, rural settings, or more privileged and educated family backgrounds. Children may be more advanced if they have been provided with educationally stimulating experiences. Children who do not perform at the levels indicated in the table require closer examination to determine whether "delays" are due to disabilities, emotional factors, or contextual factors.

Abundant information supports a rich understanding of how the innate physical, cognitive, psychosexual, and moral maturation of children between the ages of 5 and 12 is meshed with the children's increasing presence in societies outside of the family: the school, the neighborhood, and the extended "family" of the family's community. Without the interaction of child in these societies in such a way that the child's presence and role is identified, confirmed, and appreciated, it is likely that the child will experience what Erikson saw as a developmental failure of this period, inferiority, and all of its consequences.

In this chapter, we will review current information about how children advance from preschool to preadolescence, examining the areas of central nervous system maturation, emotion, gender differences, moral development, social development, and cognition. These areas must be understood in the contexts of the child's internal life, and in relation to family, peers, and school. We will focus greater attention on issues of schooling because, since school-aged children spend most of their waking lives in school, the school environment is vital to every aspect of the child's development, including how the child views the family, how the family views itself in relation to the child, and ultimately how the child views himself.

MATURATION OF THE CENTRAL NERVOUS SYSTEM

The brain undergoes a period of rapid growth through age 2, then develops at a much slower rate until puberty. At birth the brain is estimated to be about 10% of adult volume. It grows to 90% of adult volume by age 5 and completes its growth slowly over the next 9 years. What is more significant than actual volume, however, is the modification of anatomical structures and myelinization, which is almost completed around the age of 7 (4). Synaptic pruning in the prefrontal cortex (the area affecting social judgment) continues as an ongoing process through adolescence (A).

MRI studies of school-aged children's brains have confirmed these observations. By the age of 7 the child's brain is about the size of the adult brain. Boys' brains are about 10% larger than girls' and this total volume difference persists into adulthood (5,6). Differences, too, are found in the basal ganglia, where the globus pallidus is larger in boys, while the caudate is larger in girls. Boys show a relatively greater increase in size of the amygdala, while girls have more growth of the hippocampus. These relative differences are consistent with findings of androgen receptors in the amygdala and of estrogen receptors in the hippocampus. There are also findings of greater lateral ventricular expansion in boys (4). Caveness et al. (7) found that subcortical gray structures are at adult volume in girls and are greater than their adult volumes in males, while the volume of central white matter is smaller in the female brain. As the frontal lobes develop, children become increasingly able to cognitively inhibit—that is, to focus their attention and refrain from being distracted by irrelevant stimuli (8) (B).

Some data on neurotransmitter development may further sharpen our view of the intrinsic maturational schedule of the child and elucidate the emergence of the abilities of school-age children. Noradrenergic systems develop early and exert early influence on the formation of the cortex. In contrast, dopaminergic systems (associated with attention regulation) and serotoninergic systems (associated with mood and aggression) have a more gradual effect on crucial connections between brainstem nuclei and cortical structures. Cholinergic systems, associated with memory and higher cortical functions, develop relatively late (9).

These refinements in brain structure and function result in the maturation of higher cortical functions, correlating with improved abilities in motor coordination, increased attention and focus, increased self-regulation, and expanded consideration for others (C). The speed of information processing increases significantly between 6 and 12 years of age, which parallels synaptic pruning and myelination (10). For example, tasks of writing, organizing work on a page, coordinating

TABLE 2.1.3.1

CHARACTERISTICS OF THE SCHOOL-AGED CHILD

Motor	Child entering first grade (5–6 years old) Hop, skip, jump, throw, catch, kick a ball Reasonable balance, able to stand still and hold arms steady; stands on one foot, left and right General sense of left and right, not always consistent Able to do rapid alternating movements Mild synkinesis on fine finger movements	Completing fifth grade (10–11 years old) Hop, skip, jump, throw, catch, and kick a ball with ease. Elaborates: e.g., dance steps; throw behind back or trick the receiver. Balance is good; tandem walking with ease. Accurate distinction of left and right. No synkinesis
Writing and drawing	Able to name and copy circle, square, triangle, and cross easily. Some copy diamond and asterisk. Five-pointed star is possible, if child has been exposed to this in kindergarten Draws person with body, arms, and legs. Can put detailed features, but often leaves them out. Can draw house and tree, as well.	Circle, square, triangle, diamond, asterisk, five-pointed star. Cube can be accomplished, but often only after shown how to draw it. Draws more detailed person with hands, feet, action figures. Girls with more decorative detail. Boys with more action detail.
Stories	About drawings, persons are largely self-referential. Even if a figure has a different name, the life circumstances are usually identical to the child's.	May draw someone who is not self and can have a story about another, even made-up family. Creates complex plots, using well-developed descriptive language.
Fund of knowledge (depends on exposure)	Recites alphabet; counts beyond 20, writes name, first and last. Recognizes printed letters and numbers (not cursive). Writes most letters and numbers. May have some reversals.	Reads aloud and to self with comprehension; performs double-digit addition and subtraction in head; multiplies, divides, and does fractions on paper; knows details about historical figures, geography, natural phenomena, body systems.
Cognitive	Egocentric; idiosyncratic definitions of "scientific" observations. centration, defining by only one dimension; beginning concrete operations: conservation and classification	Conservation of number, weight and volume; flexibility of operational skills, including reversibility
Moral	Defines right and wrong in terms of punishment and pain, or other personal and idiosyncratic rationales. Interested in how the world works, including life and death, religion; uses magical thinking.	Defines right and wrong through internal principles Has empathy and can weigh issues from another's position.
Social	Enjoys the company of other children. Names several friends. Interactional play with rules, often externally determined. Creative play is imitative. Peers judged by whether they are nice to child. Games of individual prowess. May play on team, but cooperates based on rules rather than complex strategizing.	Likely to have a best friend and a close circle of friends. Activities with peers are increasingly independent of parental supervision Able to create games and make up rules; consideration for others, particularly with girls. Increasing self-reliance and responsibility Peers judged by their qualities. Teamwork
Self-view	Dependent on others' descriptions	Dependent on view of success, competence, and evaluation by internal standards, as well as comparison with peers and social pressures. Selects from multiple available models to define standard for "cool" for self and select friends
Sex	Interested in sexual differences; pleasure from touching oneself; generally, play with same-sex friends but comfortable with organized co-ed activities	Secondary sexual changes from Tanner stages II–V, girls usually 2 years ahead of boys. Prefers same sex friends. Some awkwardness about growth (slouching, embarrassment about breast development and foot size). Wide range of pubertal onset in peer group may create challenges to individual self-esteem. Some admiration of individual members of the opposite sex versus thinking others are "yucky." Interest expressed through teasing, messages sent through others.
Family	Identification with parents or siblings, primarily same-sex Participates in family rituals and routines around meals and bedtimes	Compare parents with other adults, including teachers and other children's parents. More independent of family rituals and routines More responsibility for household tasks, own self-care, and homework

sounds with visual cues (e.g., deciphering words and spelling phonetically) require control in ear and eye–hand coordination. First graders who write letters or words backward, or who write their names with the correct letters but in a different order, are not necessarily showing signs of learning disability. Rather, they have not yet developed mastery of the conventions involving direction and order that are necessary to read and write and perform arithmetic functions. It is normal and expectable to not fully master these conventions until second grade.

MAJOR LINES OF DEVELOPMENT

Psychosexual Development

According to psychoanalytic theory, sexual development is biphasic, with a "latent" period during the school-age years. Freud believed that latency was a distinguishing feature of humans over animals, and hoped to discover anatomical evidence of this through then-promising studies of changes in the interstitial portions of the "sex glands" (11). However, contemporary studies of sex hormones do not support the biphasic theory. Infants have relatively high but varying proportions of sex hormones in cord blood. The levels of sex hormones fall after birth and begin to rise, due to endogenous production, during the school-age period (ages 7 to 8 in girls, and about 2 years later in boys). Sex hormones begin a gradual upsurge around age 8, continuing through the pubertal peak. Children engage in some sexual play with self and others. Some have postulated that school-age children's greater sexual awareness may be reflected in their expressed feelings of disgust and shame and the strong sense of modesty that develops during the school years. Others have reported that sex play among school children is a natural extension of that of preschoolers (12). Infants and toddlers masturbate; preschoolers also engage in mutual exploration.

Children often enter middle childhood with a few good friends of the opposite sex. Around age 8, however, the same-sex groupings become polarized, with the opposite sex having developing "cooties" and being generally avoided or teased (D). Moving toward preadolescence, however, the "yuckiness" of the opposite sex gradually gives way to admiring certain individuals from a distance (E). Older school-age girls' attraction to movie stars and rock idols serves a group interactional function, as well as helping to define identity. It is noteworthy that these developing interests and crushes are not sexually mature in nature. One must be alert to the fact that, as with preschoolers, if school-age children are preoccupied with sexual themes, it is wise to look for the possibility of sexually stimulating experiences, such as sexual abuse or witnessing of sex acts.

In middle childhood, socialization into gender role involves peer pressure and conforming to expectations, or else risking mockery. The individual also feels internal pressure to conform (13) (F).

There is a wide range of both timing and tempo of pubertal onset, and it begins for many girls near the end of what is traditionally termed middle childhood (G). Indeed, brain-related processes of puberty (including nighttime hormonal spiking and pituitary-hypothalamus feedback loop) starts for most young people during the ages of approximately 8 and 14. The visible onset of puberty from age 9 to 11, as measured through breast growth for girls, correlates with girls' positive body image, positive peer relationships, and superior adjustment (14). Conversely, a slower maturational pace may wreak havoc with social relationships, as peers re-align themselves with children who are perceived to possess more attractive or desirable traits.

It is well established that children adopt a firm gender identity by age 3 (15). This expression of their maleness or femaleness is manifested early by choices of role models and friends. With gender differences, as with so many of the other issues discussed in this chapter, the question of what is innate and what is the outcome of socialization remains intriguing.

A number of characteristics are associated with being male or female in the school-age period. Gilligan (16) (p. 9) cites Janet Lever's studies of 181 fifth-grade children at play. She observed that boys play outdoors in large and heterogeneous groups, and they play competitive games that last longer than those of girls (H). The games played by boys are full of disputes that seem to add interest to the interaction and do not derail the game. Similar observations of children playing led Jean Piaget to conclude that boys were more advanced in moral development because of their fascination with legal procedures and experience at generating fair arbitration of disputes. Many others concluded similarly that in the area of moral development and the development of the capacity to exert effective leadership in complex groups, boys preceded girls; few girls ever caught up.

In proposing that women listen to the demands of socialization and morality "in a different voice," Gilligan added new value to this "instrumental versus expressive" gender dichotomy. Gilligan's descriptions of different lines of moral development for boys and girls will be discussed later in the review of moral development during school age.

Recognizing that boys generally develop instrumental functions and girls expressive ones, has provided explanations for other observed differences between boys and girls. In academic achievement, for example, girls traditionally tend to do better in verbal areas, while boys have done better in math and science. Even as the causes of these differences are being explored, they are also being denied and re-characterized. Feminism apparently has had its effects on gender identity and gender role behaviors in both girls and their mothers. For example, the widely held view that boys are more mathematically capable than girls has been demonstrated to be more an effect of socialization than innate capability (I). Math anxiety was related to gender-stereotyped beliefs of parents, the mothers being most influential (17). Furthermore, gender differences in academic skills that had been previously noted are now not found on many tests of academic competence (18). It is likely that other so-called innate gender differences will be similarly reevaluated in the future. Still, Gilligan et al. (19) in a Harvard research study, describe "hitting the cultural wall," when preadolescent girls realize that society values appearances more than accomplishment, they become more self critical and worry about their weight. A negative body image was found to be associated with high IQ. In the American Association of University Women's "Shortchanging Girls, Shortchanging America," a study of 3,000 girls and boys in 4th through 10th grade concluded that girls lose their positive self esteem and switch to appearance as the primary way to measure themselves (20). Other studies (21,22) support that preadolescent girls are more likely to get depressed, have their IQ scores drop, and decline in math and science.

Cognitive Development

The standard by which school-age children's cognitive competence has been evaluated is the achievement of what Jean Piaget termed "concrete operations." The preschooler's pre-operational thought is a creative effort to grasp causality and make meaning of experience using idiosyncratic and egocentric logic. In contrast, school-age children master important operations that increase their objectivity and their ability to be conventional. Though we celebrate originality and creativity in our society, it can be argued that being able to be conventional enables children to participate effectively in their "society" whether it be peer group or the school at large. For example, many children who are referred to as "on the autistic spectrum," may be academically capable, even brilliant, but often may except themselves from listening to their classmates, doing their homework, or participating in classroom discussions. These exceptions may lead to increasing marginalization and eccentricity, and it appears that this is a highly sensitive time when such children recognize that they are different, may not have friends, as they would like, and become quite sad and depressed.

Classification and conservation are the two crucial achievements of concrete operational thinking (J). Classification is the ability to group objects or concepts; conservation is the ability to recognize constant qualities/quantities of material even when the material undergoes changes in morphology. The concrete logical operations enable the child to deal systematically with hierarchies and categories, series and sequences, alternative and equivalent ways of getting to the same place, and reciprocal relationships. They include:

1. Composition—combining elements leads to another class (e.g., red and blue leads to purple)
2. Associativity—combinations may be made in different orders with the same result;
3. Reversibility—being able to return mentally to an earlier point in the process;
4. Seriation—the ability to create an orderly sequence along a quantitative dimension such as height; and
5. Decentration—simultaneously relating several aspects of a problem. This includes the ability to mentally picture another's frame of reference, which affects not only spatial reasoning, but also the potential for increasingly empathic understanding of another's point of view (K) (23).

Logical operations are crucial to mastering basic reading and mathematics skills, and they are also necessary for conducting social interaction, with its increasing complexity of groups, games, and rules. Acquisition of the ability to do conventional and objective mental operations is associated with an interest in the scientific workings of the birth process, and a grasp of the finality, universality, and inevitability of death.

Successful school-age children have not just the ability to perform the specific concrete operations themselves but also the ability to communicate about them in conventional ways. They understand that there are conventions of conversation, response to questions on tests, and social comportment. With cognition, as with almost every other aspect of the school-age youngster's development, joining society and sharing conventions are the keys to success. This interest in conventions and rules is frequently accompanied by a fascination with ordering and ritual. For example, school-age children often develop favorite numbers, magical rituals (Step on a crack, break your grandmother's back), or the need to do things in even pairs (L). They may also become collectors of coins, stamps, insects, baseball cards, comic books, etc. and may spend a great deal of time reviewing and ordering their collections.

During middle childhood, attention becomes increasingly selective. The ability to plan before taking action also develops (24). The school-age child's theory of mind (metacognition) is increasingly sophisticated, viewing the mind as an active and reflective information processor (25). Children become aware of their own mental processes, private speech, and choice of memory strategies. However, school-age children are just beginning to develop cognitive self-regulation. One predictor of academic success is the ability to effectively self-regulate (M) (26).

Social Cognition and Morality

Along with the development of concrete operations during the middle childhood period of development comes the child's increasing ability to use these cognitive developmental changes to reflect on the self and on the social environment (27) (N). At approximately 7 or 8 years of age, social comparison becomes an important component of self and social cognition. Children's understanding of both social comparison and social relationships increases during this age period (27). A child's view of the self as comparable to or even ahead of peers on important dimensions will highlight belief in the self's agency and ability to be confidently "industrious," while a view of the self as lacking relative to the others can lead to feelings of inferiority (O).

Understanding of social relationships as described above leads to improvements in thinking about the complexity of social contracts, as well as moral and ethical obligations of the child and social group. A child's sense of morality, that is, the appreciation of consequences and justice, evolves from an egocentric idiosyncratic, and often harsh system of evaluations of behavior by punishment, to adopting internalized rules for evaluating behavior.

Piaget (28) posited that school-age children's morality is in the "interpretation of rules" stage. This accomplishment permits the child to understand the spirit of a rule and to make subjective moral judgments.

Kohlberg (29) described the moral development that most school-age children reach as the level of "conventional morality." Conventional morality contains two stages: "interpersonal concordance" and "orientation toward authority." In the stage of "interpersonal concordance" a child measures behavior and judges it on the basis of whether it pleases those he looks up to. These mutual interpersonal expectations are those of a "good girl" or "good boy," who wants to please her or his parents and teachers, and obeys the Golden Rule (Do unto others as you would have them do unto you) (P). The next stage in conventional morality, "orientation toward authority," reflects the societal values of duty, respect, and law and order. This differs from the stage of interpersonal concordance in that the child's moral compass is now set by the social system instead of the immediate social context of family, school, or neighborhood. The child supports the rules of society, believes that it is essential not to break these rules in order for society to function, and makes moral judgments based on how well an individual situation conforms to the rules of the social system (Q).

Gilligan's (19) studies of girls' and women's moral development led her to emphasize the importance of relationships. In contrast to the traditionally masculine, seemingly quasimathematical system for evaluating moral choices, Gilligan finds that girls use a form of narrative that evolves solutions within conversations and interpersonal action. Thus, Gilligan interprets the fifth-grade girls' play observed by Lever (described earlier) not as poorly developed or socially immature but as valuing different aspects of the social experience. Gilligan describes the different responses of an 11-year-old boy and an 11-year-old girl, both of whom were at the top of their sixth grade class in a private elementary school in an academic community. The moral test question was that of the man whose wife is gravely ill and whose survival depends on receiving a specific medicine. The medicine is too expensive and the pharmacist will not reduce the price. The man breaks into the pharmacy and steals the medicine for his wife. In responding to the question of what should happen to the man, the boy thoughtfully weighed the problem of laws against stealing and a higher law valuing life. The girl, on the other hand, felt that the various parties needed talk to each other, and could not render an opinion about what should happen to him. She was aware of the rules, but felt that the conflict was such that mediation was needed to reach a resolution.

There has been significant critical reanalysis of Gilligan's data and conceptualization of the gender differences in moral reasoning. For both girls and boys, the development of morality reflects conventional thinking and measuring their evaluations with the rules of their society, as they understand them. Although moral reasoning continues to evolve through and beyond adolescence, many of the standards that are developed for our own behavior during middle childhood are likely to remain internalized and used as self-evaluation measures into adulthood.

Stilwell et al., in a study of 132 students aged 5 to 17 years, describe moral development as a natural outgrowth of attachment, evolving through five stages (30). First, the child's sense of security and experience of empathic responsiveness become paired with a sense of moral obligation. Next, the caretaker's rules are incorporated. Then, an understanding develops of how empathy can modify strict rule following. Next, ideals and role models are selected that reflect earlier learning in attachment relationships. Finally, the self is visualized as a keeper of moral standards. These stages roughly correlate with Kohlberg's stages of morality, but emphasize the grounding of morality and conscience in the early and fundamental experience of attachment and secure base, out of which empathy develops.

EMOTIONAL DEVELOPMENT

The most significant emotional issues in the lives of school-aged children concern personal worth that is determined by a sense of competence and place (in family, peer group, and communities). Competence is reflected in all of the places a child may live, at home by accomplishing tasks of caring for self (completing dressing, including tying shoes) and at school by accomplishing the academic material presented (R). White (31,32) postulated a "drive" to competence that he felt to be as important as libidinal drives. In the school-age period, competence is not just experienced by the child succeeding at a task, but by others' evaluation of his or her performance. Self-concept is derived from the self-knowledge and social comparison developments discussed earlier; self-esteem is related to the *meaning* ascribed to one's competences and abilities (27) (S).

As Erikson warned, the emotional risk for the school-aged child is the possibility of feeling inferior if the child evaluates him or herself as not being able to accomplish tasks. This evaluation comes first from outside, from a teacher expressing disappointment or frustration, from other children laughing, from parents' disappointment with grades or a teacher's report. Increasingly through the school-aged period, children can evaluate their own performance and measure it against that of others. Failures in one area may be compensated by accomplishments in another, eventually, but the early school-aged child who has not yet learned about compensation, may just feel dejected. By the end of middle childhood, each child has constructed a composite evaluation of his or her own relative areas of competence and weakness, and has come up with his own answer to the questions, "What am I good at? Can I get the job done?" (T) It appears that emphasis on performance and assessment of one's self in comparison to others can lead to a sense of inferiority and to more divisive interactions between children as they jockey for recognition and "power," which is probably the source of bullying. How children negotiate these distracting competitive experiences lead to questions and feelings about themselves that tend to persist into adulthood.

The fears of a school-aged child are quite different from those of a preschooler. Because school-aged children are out and about in society, they are much more likely to witness or hear about catastrophic events that could happen to them (U). Their vulnerability to catastrophic fears is increased by the development, during the school-aged period, of understanding of the irreversibility and inevitability of death. Many school-aged children's dreams reflect efforts to master these fears by setting themselves up as heroes who save whole families or communities from robbers, murderers, fires, storms, or other disasters. Children who don't feel competent may be overwhelmed by these fears and have repeated dreams in which they are attacked and victimized and helpless.

Sullivan (33) was one of the first to emphasize the social influence on development. He described a series of internal processes by which the child gradually substitutes his or her own standards of evaluation for those of family members. Stimulated by models outside the family, these processes unfold throughout the early school period.

- *Social subordination* reflects a change in the child's acceptance of authority from the specifics of personal caretakers to general categories such as the principal, police, crossing guards, and teachers. The child first evaluates peers in terms of how they are regarded by these authority figures.
- *Social accommodation* is a process of acknowledging that there are differences between people. Early school-age children are intolerant of differences and can be cruel, but (with socialization and education) gradually differences may come to be respected.
- *Differentiation of authority figures* refers to the child's emerging ability to compare adults comparing parents to school-based authorities.
- *Control of focal awareness* refers to the child's response to social pressure to abandon some of his or her egocentric ideas and adopt a more conventional stance.
- *Sublimatory reformation* refers to the reorientation of focal awareness to the group-approved satisfactory behavior.
- *Supervisory patterns* reflect an awareness of one's behavior in groups. The supervisory patterns are almost like imaginary characters that develop in order to monitor oneself and eventually become internalized.

SELF IN SOCIETY

By the time they enter the school-age period, children have developed four basic areas of self-esteem: academic competence, social competence, physical/athletic competence, and physical appearance (34). As they progress through middle childhood, children continue to develop and refine their self-concept and sense of self-esteem, measuring and rating themselves within the context of their families, peers, and culture. The most salient achievement of the school-age period is a sense of oneself as a member of society. To accomplish this, maturation is required, as has been described. But the most significant arenas for advancing and refining the sense of self both in the present and in anticipating the future are the interpersonal arenas of family, peers, and school.

Home and Family

According to Heinz Kohut, the development of self occurs through a process of mirroring and idealization. In order to develop healthy narcissism, the child needs grown-ups to admire him and demonstrate attunement to his feelings (mirroring). The child also needs to be able to look up to his parents and other role models, and aspire to be like them without being unduly distracted by their faults and shortcomings (idealization).

Clearly, parents and teachers and other influential adults have important roles to play in how children view themselves. Baumrind (35) classified parenting styles according to "responsivity" (accurately assessing and responding to children's needs) and "demandingness" (setting high expectations) (V). Parents with high responsivity and high demandingness ("authoritative" style) tend to have the best outcome, with children who do well academically and socially. Low responsivity/low demandingness describes the neglectful or uninvolved parent; and high responsivity/low demandingness describes the permissive parent. Low responsivity/high demandingness is characteristic of an authoritarian style, which may be predictive of a positive outcome in some minority families. Inadequate parental monitoring correlates strongly with a risk of delinquent behaviors, while parental involvement positively contributes to the child's cognitive and social competence (36).

The parent's optimal role in middle childhood may be that of a consultant or facilitator, coaching the child's development of his or her own skills and opinions, assisting as needed when help is requested, but allowing mistakes to be made and independent striving to occur in a supportive environment whenever feasible. This approach is congruent with an authoritative style, in that high responsivity and high expectations can coexist with allowing self-exploration on the part of the child (W) (37).

The "goodness of fit" (38) between parenting style and child temperament is constantly in flux. As the child encounters new challenges and develops new competencies, the parallel parental challenge is to be sensitive to the child's ever-changing needs, providing progressive responsibility and supervised autonomy as appropriate (X) (39). Recent research on genotypes and family relationships suggests that parent–child interactions are genetically influenced. Children's genotypes evoke specific parental responses; similarly, parental response patterns evoked by their children's particular behaviors show evidence of heritability (40). Targeted interventions can favorably alter these parental responses to difficult behaviors (41) hopefully changing their expression. The familiar social context of the family and neighborhood (that also includes extended family and religious communities with which the family may be involved) are altered in the school-aged period through several processes. The first is a practical one: when children spend more time in school, parents may spend more time doing things other than caring for their children. For parents who were already working, or who remain at home caring for younger children, or who choose to home-school their children, this may not be a significant change. In general, however, this creates a significant shift from the family organized for care of itself and its young children, drawn inward by primarily centripetal forces, to the more outwardly oriented family of adolescent children, where forces seem to be centrifugal, drawing family members out into interactions with the society at large (Y). Combrinck-Graham (42) described the decreasing centripetal forces of the school-aged child's family as "a house in the summertime; it is sturdy but has doors and windows open for circulation. Everyone comes in to share the family meal, to take shelter from the rain, and to sleep" (p. 147) (Z).

A second process that changes the family environment is the evaluation that comes about from children bringing home their experiences with other children, other children's parents, and other adults whom they meet independently of their own families. Children make statements: John's mother lets him do this; Martha's mother doesn't do that; Sandy's father doesn't live with them (AA). Or they ask questions: Why doesn't Daddy stay home with us the way George's father does? How come you don't pick me up at school, Randy's mother does. Are we rich or poor? Are we Republican or Democrat? Why don't we celebrate Christmas? And so on. Or children reflect frank criticism: You don't know as much as my teacher. Smoking is bad for you; you shouldn't smoke.

A third process of family change is through children's relatively greater involvement in activities outside the home. Visits to friends, after-school activities, membership in clubs or participation on teams takes time out from family routines after school and on weekends. Adolescents are far more involved in activities outside the home, but most school-aged children's families have the opportunity to assemble for dinner and an evening routine that allows for completing homework and some form of age-appropriate bedtime routine (BB). Exceptions are largely due to complicated work schedules of caregivers who may work second shift or overtime. And in these situations, things go better if there is a reliable schedule, a supervising older person, and the opportunity to touch base during the evening.

A fourth process of family change is the possible social enrichment of all family life through involvement with the school as a community. This can be through socializing with families of other children, involvement in school and after-school activities, and through advocacy about school issues (e.g., PTA or participation on the school board). All family members, not just the children, usually become more involved in social experiences outside the family during the school-aged period.

Family/community relationships that have been stable prior to the school-aged period are subject to change in similar ways. In the early school-aged period children are developing skills that facilitate interaction with peers in the neighborhood (mastering a two-wheel bike; accomplishments in the pick-up sport of the neighborhood, such as soccer or basketball) (CC). Children may have different experiences with other children in the home area and in school. At home, in the neighborhood, a child may be included in a group of different-aged children and accepted because of familiarity or the relationships between the families. For example, children may be a part of a Sunday school group that is also part of the social context of the congregation. This peer group reflects the child's place in a family's place in a community. As the child grows older through school age in such a community, the child becomes more identified by distinct contributions to the community (such as participating in the music program, mastery of religious lessons, contributions to recreational activities) rather than just by membership in a family (DD).

Children may assume more distinct roles in their neighborhood society or Sunday school group as they develop in school, or they may be less involved, as they become more interested in other things. Hobbies and collections are characteristic passions of school-aged children and often become the basis for formation of new social groupings. Social contacts may be conducted online as children come together around a particular interest.

The roles of television, video games, and cell phones, access to the Internet, and texting are beginning to be evaluated (EE) (43). While these forms of occupation, entertainment, and communication now have an established place in the lives of American school children and their families, such activities tend to isolate children from the daily commerce with their families and peers, and may stimulate an increasingly unrealistic view of life, one's role in it, and one's abilities. These activities may be comforting to children who are otherwise struggling either with learning, attention, or socialization, though this comfort may further cut them off from activities that involve them in their society. Kramer (44) explored some concerns about the role of TV watching in interfering with the "function of brains... to interact with each other to form families and societies," when he wrote about the biology of family culture. Finally, such activities are sedentary and often accompanied by eating, and there is increasing concern about obesity, diabetes, and other health problems associated with this lifestyle. The family dinner where everyone participates in conversation, everyone expresses interest in what others are thinking or doing is a model for participating in a community and being a valued participant. Face-to-face conversations have a different and important function than side-by-side texting communications. And, as noted above, the permission to "participate" outside of interaction may be comforting to the child who is socially awkward, but does not add to that person's becoming more comfortably "conventional," and more able to contribute to his/her community.

Peers

The peer group can be one of the most facilitating influences in school-aged children's development, or it can be disastrously inhibiting. As with other developmental tasks, each child brings a particular pattern of prior experience to the task of developing a social self. There is considerable evidence that peers themselves have their own attractions and that a substantial if not primary influence over a child's social self-development comes from the outside, predominantly through peer culture and its particular draw on the child's drives for mastery and competence. Robert White's (31,32) description of the growth of competence drives in the school-age period includes how to get along with others in the sense of competing, compromising, learning the rules of the game, and protecting oneself from injury. Sullivan (33) points out that other children afford an opportunity to do something interesting with the environment and that gradually the world of contemporaries competes with the family circle. Bemporad (45) describes the juvenile era as a period between separation and procreation in which peers are the intermediaries. Erikson's focus on how children master industry overemphasizes individual achievement at the expense of cooperation. In a cross-cultural comparison, Kagan and Klein (46) credits the society of peers for advancing the development of children in San Marcos. He describes rural Guatemalan Indian infants and preschoolers who by all culturally relevant measures are "retarded" but who at 11 perform at the same level as American children in tests of cognitive functioning. The Guatemalan infant is unstimulated and left alone; only basic physical needs are attended to. Thus, Guatemalan infants do not have the assertive interaction with environment that is so prized in American infants and preschoolers. Kagan suggests that in the school-age period, where the relative neglect of these children by adults leaves them to form their own social groupings, Guatemalan youngsters begin to practice and learn assertiveness through jockeying for social position (FF). Grunebaum and Solomon (47) refer to Harry Harlow's studies, concluding that young rhesus monkeys leave their mothers because peer relationships are interesting, not because their mothers reject them. There has been debate about the relative influence of peer group versus parents on development, with some taking the view that the peer effect is significant while the parent effect is negligible (48).

Regardless of the relative weight placed on each of these factors, it seems that the drive for inclusion and acceptance, and the judgments of the other children that the child selects as his peer group, impact heavily on the school-age child's development of his own self-image and values. At the same time, the child's ongoing internal self-definition in turn influences his selection of peers to identify with and measure himself against. By around age 8, there has been a significant shift in a child's ability to assess his own skills in comparison to others, combined with feedback from parents, teachers, and peers. He begins to rank himself in various arenas, and combine these multiple assessments into his own ongoing "report card." This constant evaluation of self in social context becomes internalized into his own kinetic sense of identity. For better or worse, the opinions and descriptions we form of ourselves in middle childhood tend to continue throughout life. Personal "style," preferences, values, and self-assessment in comparison with others all have their foundation during the school-age period. How do children's attributions (explanations for why we act as we do) affect their self-esteem? Was their performance due to luck, ability, or effort? Children who make "mastery-oriented attributions" (49) give credit to their ability when they succeed (I'm great at math), and attribute failure to factors that are controllable (I need to study harder) or not fundamental (this was an especially tough exam). By contrast, children who attribute their failure to an innate lack of ability (learned helplessness) may develop a downward spiral in which they stop trying to succeed (50). Attribution retraining and help with self-regulation can be helpful, especially when started early (51).

Stages of peer development have been identified and described by Grunebaum and Solomon (52):

- Unilateral partners and one-way assistance—the preschool child,
- Bilateral partners and fair-weather cooperation—middle childhood, and
- Chumship and consensual exchange—preadolescence (pp. 288–291).

The first school-age phase is characterized by membership in peer groups and is based on playmates' willingness and ability to play the way the child wishes. The second school-age stage (from about age 9) advances friendship to a closeness that Sullivan referred to as "chumship" with a peer of the same sex with whom an intimacy is formed, which paves the way for heterosexual intimacy and caring beginning in adolescence (GG). A study that examined second, fifth, and eighth graders' attitudes and choices for companionship and intimacy found that family members were the most important sources for companionship for both second and fifth graders. Same-sex peers were important throughout school age, but were increasingly important as the subjects grew older. Girls tended to report intimate disclosure to peers earlier than boys, and possibly reflecting that girls may value intimacy more than boys (HH) (53).

As peer interaction and the view of self in relation to others are vital to cognitive and intellectual development, so cognitive operations are vital to a child's emerging social self in the school-age period. Minuchin (54) points out that children move from games such as "Simon Says," "Mother May I," and "Follow the Leader," in which the children in groups follow the directions of a leader, to games in which the rules are set and governed by the players themselves, to games that involve contributions to the efforts of a team. This evolution involves shifts in the ways in which others are evaluated. Children begin the period by deeming others good if they give them things and bad if they take things away, and move to recognizing skills and personal attributes, to finally acknowledging and valuing social attributes, such as fairness (II). This shift, in turn, requires the expansion of perspective, which permits a child to see a situation from another's point of view. This decentering may be seen as a cognitive component to empathy and the development of more sophisticated morality.

With social development, as with intellectual development, preparation and prior experience are substantial influences. Patterns of behavior involving aggression are established early, and generalized aggressive disposition and the tendency to exhibit aggression in the context of specific relationships are quite stable (55). Aggressiveness is also associated with social rejection in the school-age period (JJ) (56,57). One view of the stability of aggression is that it is constitutionally determined. Another view is that aggression develops and is maintained in interpersonal sequences. For example, one researcher reported that "early-timing" mothers, those whose first children are born when they are in their 20s, have more difficulty setting limits on their children than "late-timing" mothers do (58).

Children of early-timing mothers are more likely to be aggressive, and in the absence of good limit setting within the family, the aggression becomes less amenable to social intervention. It is most likely that aggression levels are determined by an ongoing interaction of biologic tendency with psychosocial context.

Sociometric studies of school-age children yield up to five groups: popular, average, rejected, neglected, and controversial (59). There are two subgroups of rejected children, those who undervalue themselves and have low self-esteem, even in comparison to their teachers' evaluations of them; and those who have a positive view of themselves but are seen as defensive and aggressive (56). When children in different sociometric groups were asked to evaluate themselves and one another, it was expected that aggressive children would show attributional biases not shown by nonaggressive children. But, in fact these children's evaluations of others were not out of line, even though other children clearly identified the reputation of rejected children. Additionally, negative reputation increasingly separates the rejected group at older ages (57). Aggression and consequent rejection and social isolation during middle childhood is a primary predictor of maladjustment in later years. Rejected children often form social groups with other unpopular peers, which unfortunately may compound the problem by reinforcing poor social skills (60).

Contemporary reviews of peer relationships in the middle years point to the difficulties in researching this ever-changing set of connections. For example, peer relationships occur in a context. The grouping of children in a classroom may not be the same as how these children seek each other's company and friendship out of school. Furthermore, how children relate to one another in the classroom is very much affected by whether the educational style facilitates interaction between the students or not.

How children group, how large is their network, how popularity is related to friendship, all of these conditions of peer relationships seem to evolve through the school-age period, but researchers are still not clear about what are the best tools for assessing and therefore understanding the processes of peer interaction (61–63).

SCHOOLING

Schooling refers to the ecologic setting in which children learn. It refers to the environment, the size, the philosophy, the characteristic transactions between teachers and students, and the culture of the school. How the child *can* function, what he or she can do, how the child perceives him or herself, especially in terms of competence and the accompanying confidence to be able to accomplish, and finally, how the child is a part of communities/societies, all of these are substantially forged and reshaped in the school environment.

We will discuss four aspects of schooling:

1. Preparation: the effects of prior experience;
2. Attunement to children's learning styles and needs;
3. Concordance or discordance with the patient's family/community ethos;
4. How the school serves as a model for a community in which a child finds a role?

The Effect of Experience and Preparation on Children's School Functioning

Children arrive at school with diverse experiences. Most dramatically different are the experiences of children from middle-class, educated families and those from poor, minority, inner-city families. The former are more likely to have attended educationally oriented preschools, have traveled at least in their own communities, have visited libraries and museums, and have been read to by their parents and teachers (KK), while the latter have more likely been involved with complex family and "adoptive" family relationships ("play" mamas and many "aunts" and "uncles"), have experienced comings and goings of people in their daily worlds, and have been exposed to situations of danger and hardship with little sense of control over these situations. Children from immigrant families may not speak English, or, alternatively, may be the only members of their family who do speak English. Some minority youngsters may never have seen a book or a piece of paper or a crayon by the time they enter school. But many of them may have been assuming responsibilities in the household, such as caring for younger children, getting meals, caring for themselves while adults are away, and translating for their parents. The former group has been prepared to enter school since toddlerhood, while the latter group is prepared to manage an entirely different set of experiences, which may not be compatible with what is expected in school (64–66).

There is abundant evidence that the parents' education is related to children's achievement. Davis-Kean (67) researched this premise and found that this relationship is true of both White and African-American families. For both races, there is the indirect relationship through reading and providing a warm and supportive environment. White families also added a measure of expectation that was an additional incentive for their children's achievement.

There has been considerable exploration of the relationship between attachment style and adjustment to school (68) Granot and Mayseless (69) examined the relationship between attachment styles and adjustment in school, as measured by teacher ratings and student sociograms. Their sample of nineteen 10 to 12 year olds in Israel found that 66% were secure, 15% avoidant, 6% ambivalent, and 13% disorganized. As expected, the secure children had the highest adjustment scores and the fewest negative nominations on the sociogram. The ambivalently attached children were intermediate in scholastic and emotional adjustment and had the highest number of negative nominations in the sociogram, corresponding with significantly lower levels of social adjustment than the secure children. Importantly, there was no relationship between attachment style and cognitive achievements.

Studies of the effects of model preschool programs and general application of Head Start programs for poor and minority children demonstrate that there is some advantage to having had a preschool experience, and this advantage is more dramatic and more lasting if the experience was in a model preschool program (70). In follow-up throughout the remainder of their school lives, children from model preschools were significantly less likely to be placed in special education programs than controls, but most often effects disappeared in 3 to 6 years, after the children entered formal public school (71). This suggests that preparation, alone, does not suffice to ensure a positive school experience. It is important to note that the most effective early education programs involved the parents in the school effort, so that the fit between home culture and school culture was enhanced.

Reading comprehension is largely thought to be text-based (i.e., content oriented) and interactional (i.e., develops within a relationship) (LL). It is increasingly evident that reading success is heavily influenced by the preparation of the reader, who brings to the task his or her expectations, prior knowledge of the content and structure of the material, and cultural background (72). Studies support this observation. One study reported that a group of 4 year olds given simple instructions in segmenting and blending words of two and three syllables 10 minutes a day for 13 weeks resulted in dramatically higher reading scores than those of children involved in nonspecific reading-related activities (73). Coles reported a study of the families of children with reading disabilities found that there is a significant lack of preparation of these children for reading. Other studies found that in some families, messages about expectations of failure were transmitted, while in others there were failures to provide exposure to preparatory material; in still others there was obvious evidence of "communication deviance" whereby the explanatory frameworks of language were so odd or idiosyncratic to the family that the child had unusual difficulty mastering conventional rules needed to learn to read (74). In addition to insufficient preparation, other etiologies of reading difficulty must be considered. These include learning disability (due to underlying processing deficits, auditory discrimination problems, decoding difficulties, etc.), intellectual disabilities, and knowledge deficits in oral language or vocabulary. Basic pre-reading skills include the ability to bring background knowledge to bear on a new situation, self-questioning behavior, and predictive skills.

Attunement to Children's Learning Styles and Needs

The second aspect of schooling involves the interaction around learning. Many use Vygotsky's ideas about the evolving mind in society to better understand how children learn successfully. In this framework, learning represents the transfer of responsibility for reaching a particular goal (75). This transfer takes place in the "zone of proximal development (ZPD)," which is defined as "the distance between the actual developmental level as determined by independent problem solving and the level of potential development as determined through problem solving under adult guidance or in collaboration with more capable peers" (Vygotsky, cited in Slavin (76) p. 1162). The ZPD is a useful measure of learning potential because it includes the instructional context (or, in the case of psychometrics, the relationship between child and examiner) as indispensable to the measured achievement. When children are presented with strategies, "strategy instruction" (whether children can adopt a strategy and apply it to other, similar situations without further instruction), those presented in the lower area of the ZPD are readily generalized, those in the midrange are adopted and gradually generalized, and those toward the higher end of the zone may not be adopted at all (MM) (70). The child's readiness, and the instructor's attunement to presenting material at a level that stretches already established abilities but is not so novel as to be overwhelming, are crucial to the "transfer of responsibility" that defines successful learning (NN).

Fellow students as well as teachers provide assistance with developing more sophisticated problem solving, as is stated in Vygotsky's definition of the ZPD. There are specific methods of peer involvement in learning that have come to be known as "cooperative learning." Cooperative learning refers to any number of types of student groupings for learning but differs from peer tutoring in that the material is presented by the teacher rather than by the peers. Students are given problems to solve or projects to complete, and the incentive to work together is encouraged by either rewarding the group's efforts, rewarding each individual child on the basis of the group's efforts, or rewarding the group on the basis of each child's achievement. Children can and will positively influence one another's progress. This is particularly true when some children in the group are more advanced than others, but it is also true when all children are struggling to master a new challenge. For example, using the Piagetian description of accomplishment of conservation, nonconserving children learn from peers who have mastered conservation, but they also progress in conservation skills when struggling with conservation problems with other nonconserving children (76). The process of working together must be specifically supervised and rewarded, because otherwise the more competent children take most of the responsibility for accomplishing the objectives or completing the project, while the less competent children do not contribute. But properly conceived, the value of cooperative teaching extends beyond the opportunities it creates for learning. It also provides a framework for learning about others, valuing differences, observing and utilizing the strengths of others, helping one another, and making a contribution to a community goal.

Regardless of the rate children learn and the specific strengths and weaknesses they may have in mastering certain materials, attunement to each child's ZPD and pitching the new material to the appropriate level will inevitably enhance not only the child's success but also enthusiasm for learning.

Gardner's (77) theory of multiple intelligences suggests eight areas of aptitude with different processing operations and skill sets. These areas include linguistic, logical-mathematical, musical, spatial, bodily-kinesthetic, naturalist, interpersonal, and intrapersonal (OO). By expanding the traditional narrow definition of intelligence, this view challenges families and schools to help realize each child's unique potential.

Gardner's theory of multiple intelligences is echoed in Mel Levine's neurodevelopmental profiling (78). In these and other approaches being utilized in innovative educational strategies, the principle is that different children have specific learning styles. According to these theories, it is incumbent upon the teacher to ask, "How does this particular child learn best?" and to design an educational strategy that utilizes the appropriate mode.

Concordance or Discordance with the Patient's Family/Community Ethos

Two facets of congruence between the style of school and family as interfacing systems have been studied. The first involves expectations in the areas of educational goals, what is expected of the child, rules, and areas of permissiveness. Since the education system has been established by the majority culture, generally goals are congruent between school and majority families. Parents expect their children to attend school regularly, to be respectful, to be motivated, and to achieve. Problems come up when children can't or don't fulfill these expectations, which are ordinarily shared by family and school systems. They also come up, however, when these expectations are not shared by family and school systems. Then the all-too-common complaint that the child misbehaves at school but is fine at home, or, less commonly, the reverse, is brought to the attention of a counselor or mental health professional. This type of problem is most likely to be found in children from ethnic and cultural minority families and can be ameliorated when parents are intimately involved in school life (79). The second facet concerns the congruence of the way school and family systems are organized. In general systems terms, interpersonal systems can be open and relatively closed, referring to characteristics of freedom of exchange with other systems, definition of system boundaries, and amount of variety that is encouraged or tolerated within the system. Some schools that have been founded around specific religions are examples of closed systems, and these often serve a specific population with shared rules and values, constituting a good fit (PP). Rules about conduct, limits, and privacy are consistent across school and family and may differentiate each from the rest of society. Some schools have a more closed system than many of the families of children attending. That is, the schools have clear rules and expectations about everything from dress to punctuality, while the families' own are more loosely organized. The school personnel tend to see these families as irresponsible and incompetent, and themselves as more capable caretakers. Open families sending their children to closed schools feel criticized and defensive, and a child is caught between the two systems, as he may want to conform to the school's expectations but depends upon the family to provide appropriate support. Open school systems allow for variability and have the potential of being flexible. But in many instances, open school systems interfacing with open family systems may have such a lack of definition that the children have no clear framework within which to define themselves. This kind of "congruence" between open family and open school systems often results in the involvement of the child with more systems, such as welfare, juvenile justice, or mental health (80).

Other aspects of the child and family's community relationships also support commitment to and investment in schooling. One study examining African-American students in different socioeconomic circumstances found that more important than poverty or prevalence of crime in a neighborhood was the effect of "collective socialization" (81). Collective socialization occurs in a community where adults recognize the children, speak to them, comment on their behavior, and will report to their parents or other authorities, if indicated (QQ). The study was primarily exploring the effect of collective socialization on conduct problems, and did note that in communities with collective socialization, there was a reduced risk for conduct problems. Schooling was a much more successful and valued part of the children's lives in these communities, as well.

How the School Serves as a Model for a Community in Which a Child Finds a Role?

A list of characteristics of effective schools includes strong leadership, an atmosphere that is orderly and not oppressive, teachers who participate in decision-making, school staff that has high expectations of students, and frequent monitoring of student progress (82). A specific aspect of school environment that has been studied is school size. It has been shown that large schools are often "overmanned," meaning that there are more students than role opportunities. This means that there are not enough opportunities in student government, arts, sports programs, or for individual distinction to recognize more than a very few children. In "undermanned" schools there are opportunities for students to be involved in activities and to take more initiative. The environmental role demands on the students in undermanned schools increase the levels of student participation so that they can contribute to the school community, develop identified roles in this community, and become known to themselves and each other as distinctive individuals. In large schools, there is the danger of anonymity and ultimately a high rate of dropping out and involvement in antisocial behavior and substance abuse. The movement to consolidate schools thus increases the chances that students will not have a positive experience in school, unless the student population is broken down into smaller units within which students experience a manageable-size community (82).

Summary of Salient Features of Schooling

For school to be most effective at supporting the crucial development in school-age children, there has to be attention to the preparation children have had prior to entering school, and assistance to those whose experience has not primed them to take advantage of the school experience. Second, each child's learning style and readiness need to be understood sufficiently that educational material is presented that stimulates a child's drive to competence, without being so overwhelming that the child gives up. Most curricula are established to meet the levels of most children in the grade. But there are always children who are either more advanced or slower to whom learning tasks need to be thoughtfully and individually offered (RR). Thirdly, attention needs to be placed on the congruence between expectations of school personnel and that of parents. Involving parents in school activities is the most effective way to collaborate and close any gaps that could cause confusion and loyalty conflicts for the children. Finally, schools need to form manageable sized communities in which children can distinguish themselves. Even if the total school size is very large, there are ways to subdivide into smaller communities.

We have increasingly come to think of the school as a Learning Community in which the students' membership and identity must be nurtured and respected. The desired emphasis on students learning together in optimally sized schools and classrooms that allow for the recognition of each student's unique place and contributions to the Learning Community, as described above, is unfortunately not a conscious part of many children's educational experience. Particularly with the No Child Left Behind legislation (83) school curriculum and teachers' concentration have been focused on individual children's performance, because both the schools' and teachers' evaluations and federal funding are based on this. This refocus puts this very important community function of schooling at great risk, in our view (84).

There are cultures where children learn the "industry" of their society other than in school, primarily through various forms of apprenticeship (SS). Schools in our society offer both the opportunity for learning the "industry" and for learning one's place in society. We would be remiss if we did not point out that children in our Western society are privileged to have time set aside in their development for schooling. Although child labor is almost nonexistent in the United States and Europe, there are currently 250 million child laborers in the world between the ages of 5 and 14 (90% in Asia and Africa), living in extreme poverty, engaged in repetitive and physically demanding tasks, who do not have the opportunity to go to school at all, and have limited opportunity to play and learn (85). One could argue that these children are also accomplishing the developmental task of learning the industry of their society.

FAILURES OF DEVELOPMENT IN THE SCHOOL-AGE PERIOD

From this discussion of normal developmental processes and influences on developmental outcome, understanding many failures of development is straightforward. Though maturational deviations or delays (such as developmental disabilities, or pervasive developmental disorders) may limit a child's developmental progress in all the spheres we have discussed, children with disabilities do and should achieve mastery of industry and the ability to participate in a community of school, peers, and subsequently adults at a level commensurate with their abilities (86). Though a family of children with disabilities may also develop differently, because of being more involved with their children and less open to the ebb and flow of peers and activities outside of the family, their children's school-age period does involve teachers, other educational professionals, and the families of other students, thus stretching the family very much as families are stretched for mainstream children. The challenge for mental health professionals who use a developmental approach in their work is to find arenas where handicapped children can be competent and interact socially. Lowering expectations of performance, providing ability-appropriate responsibilities for children to meet, and encouraging reciprocal social interaction are interventions that can maximize developmental accomplishments of these special youngsters.

Interference with learning may be on the basis of immaturity, or, as is more commonly diagnosed, due to disorders of focus, attention, impulse management, or specific learning dysfunction. Understanding the crucial developmental issues of establishing a view of oneself as a functioning person in a community can focus mental health consultant's attention on helping child, family, and teachers find strategies for managing areas of difficulty. Medication is often used to support such efforts, but is most effective when the child and the people closest to him or her are concentrating on competence and strategies for becoming competent.

Inferiority and defeat are the principal emotional pitfalls of school-aged children, because of the importance of mastery and recognition within the communities in which children participate. Depression is both a cause and an outcome of failure to progress in the manner that the child believes others expect. Assessment and treatment of depression in school-aged children must always include assessment of the developmental issues of competence and how a child is viewed by his or her peers so that in addition to psychotherapy and medication, assistance with social functioning and academic mastery will be included. Disabling anxiety may occur as a result of either separation fears or performance worries. Both of these scenarios require that the school-aged child learn how to reassure himself (TT). The developmental challenge is to find a secure sense of self, moving comfortably between his nuclear family and his peer group, and setting reasonable internal standards for success in the face of external expectations. Externalizing behavior disorders drastically interfere with children's developmental progress in this era by disrupting learning and social accomplishment. Many such behaviors may be viewed as a defense against a sense of failure and inferiority (better to be seen as bad than dumb). Developmental approaches to treatment must include attention to academic progress along with several approaches to helping such children be accountable for their behavior. Behavioral management may be helpful (UU), but will be more so in this age-group if there are exercises in putting oneself in others' places and developing empathy, so that these children can function in society (Table 2.1.3.2).

TABLE 2.1.3.2

VIDEO CLIPS CORRELATED WITH CHAPTER TOPICS, TO ILLUSTRATE TEACHING POINTS

The video clips cross-referenced below are part of Dr. Fox's Normal Development Video Series, a DVD curriculum resource that follows the development of her two children in the context of their family and community over 20 years. Clips referenced throughout the chapter are either from *Normal Development in the First Ten Years of Life—Complete Version (FTY), or Normal Development in Middle Childhood and Adolescence* (MCA). Further information and sample video clips may be viewed at Dr. Fox's faculty website: http://www.psych.uic.edu/ijr/gfox.

Chapter Reference	FTY	MCA	Clip #	Age	Clip Title
A		x	67	14½	Info needed before a date
B		x	34	12½	Helping 8 y/o brother with homework
C	x		166	8	Sarah reads her "All About Me" assignment to her second-grade class, and tests their recall
D	x		165	7¾	Sarah and girlfriend discuss how boys have cooties
E		x	5	11	Fifth-grade matchmaking and gossip
F		x	122	7½	Brian is teased for riding his sister's hand-me-down pink bike
G		x	28	12½	"Five guys are fighting over me"
H		x	130	8½	Driveway basketball game
I	x		168	8¼	Sarah demonstrates math regrouping in subtraction, cursive, spelling
J	x	x	201	7¼	David demonstrates conservation of liquid with Dr. Combrinck-Graham (compare with no.200 at age 5, preoperational).
	x	x			
	x				
			147	6¼	Coins versus money; conservation of length with pencils.
			168	8¼	Sarah demonstrates math regrouping in subtraction (using conservation)
			120	7½	Conservation of mass
			121	7½	Conservation of volume
K	x		196	5	Brian decides to let his pet "Tickles the Caterpillar" go
	x		173	9¼	Sarah writes and illustrates a story, "Sad Peggy," as a way to deal with losing her babysitter
L		x	128	8½	Lucky dice and home runs
		x	137	9½	Crime, restitution, conscience, and karma
M		x	20	12	Science homework rap
		x	25	12	Doesn't want to be viewed as "typical"
		x	46	13½	Positive self-talk to reassure and succeed
		x	142	11	Brian makes time smaller
N		x	37	13	How do other kids react to Sarah's awards?
O		x	153	12½	Brian reflects on his character traits and career goals
P	x		159	6¾	Sarah and two friends discuss moral dilemma (breaking plates)

TABLE 2.1.3.2

(CONTINUED)

Chapter Reference	FTY	MCA	Clip #	Age	Clip Title
Q	x		186	10½	Moral dilemma: should the church punish a reverend who conducted a gay marriage ceremony?
R	x	x	110	5	Brian learns to tie shoes
		x	112	5½	Brian reading aloud to self
			184	10½	Sarah shows her painting, discusses the process of making it
S	x		178	10	Doing homework with TV on, describes homework, test results, goals, creative writing.
	x		180	10	Discusses report card, focuses on the one grade that wasn't an "A"
T		x	71	15	Rewards for good grades—internal and external motivation
U	x	x	158	6½	Describes posttraumatic fears after home was burglarized
		x	17	11½	Mom soothing fears about going to sleep-away camp
			59	14	"If you had one week to live…"
V		x	22	12	Is Mom too lenient?
			129	8½	Brian gets allowance after cleaning his room
W		x	142	11	Brian makes time smaller (learning to manage his time on the weekend)
X		x	13	11½	Girls roam in packs, chase boys
		x	60	14	Is Sarah almost independent?
Y		x	62	14	Sarah never home, misses dinner
Z		x	87	16½	Studying together on porch during rainstorm
AA		x	15	11½	Girls plan outing, compare moms' rules
BB		x	123	8	Hates homework, loves Hedgie
CC		x	161	14	Makes high school soccer team, quits, rejoins
DD		x	23	12	Creates tap dance for school talent show
EE		x	118	7½	Turning off electronic games
		x	159	13½	Friends play Monster Hunter Freedom video game
		x	163	14½	Talk face-to-face or on Facebook?
FF	x		174	9½	Girls work out a group research project assignment
	x		177	10	Girls reading a play aloud, negotiating roles
GG	x	x	164	7½	Clapping game in pool with girlfriend and little brother
	x		181	10	Beth and Sarah sing "Stuff"—a song they made up
			21	12	Sarah and friend build hideout; Brian feels left out
HH		x	24	12	Does Sarah tell Mom everything?
II	x		167	8	Sarah receives $5 for a small box of candy, then refunds $4 because it was "too much"
JJ		x	16	11½	Why one girl is excluded
KK	x		76	1½	Reading Corduroy book with mom
	x		117	3	"Put-away time" at preschool
	x		137	4½	Sarah pretending to read to her new baby brother
LL	x		150	6½	Sarah reads Now I Am Six to mom
MM		x	127	8½	Brian divides by multiplying
NN	x		136	4½	Figuring out how to get hula hoop out of a tree
OO	x	x	155	6¾	Choreographs a dance on paper
	x	x	187	10½	Discusses art and tap interests, wants to be a teacher
			9	11	Tap class
			148	11½	Speed-stacking cups
PP	x		119	3	Teaching about charity at preschool—"Tzedakah" is the Hebrew word being defined
QQ		x	113	6	Skips Spanish class, gets caught in a lie
RR		x	37	13	How do other kids react to Sarah's awards?
SS		x	149	11½	First summer job at farmer's market
		x	150	12	Achieves lifetime goal as a kid
TT	x		157	6½	Sarah taught her beanie baby not to be afraid of heights, describes how she got over her own fear
UU		x	119	7½	Resists clean up after play date
		x	139	10	Kids describe their classroom behavioral management system

ACKNOWLEDGMENTS

The assistance of Margo McClelland and Roberta Paikoff Holzmueller, PhD in the preparation of this chapter is gratefully acknowledged.

References

1. Erikson E: *Childhood in Society.* New York, Norton, 1950.
2. Bronfenbrenner U: *The Ecology of Human Development.* Cambridge, MA, Harvard University Press, 1979.
3. Lerner RM, Steinberg L: The scientific study of adolescent development: Historical and contemporary perspectives. In: Lerner RM, Steinberg L, (eds): *Handbook of Adolescent Psychology Vol 1: Individual Bases of Adolescent Development.* 3rd ed. New York: Wiley, 3–14, 2009.
4. Shapiro T, Perry R: Latency revisited: the age of 7 plus or minus 1. *Psychoanal Study Child* 31:79–105, 1976.
5. Giedd JN, Castellanos FX, Jagath CR, et al.: Sexual dimorphism of the developing human brain. *Prog Neuropsychopharmacol Biol* 21:1185–1201, 1997.
6. Reiss AL, Abrams MT, Singer HS, et al.: Brain development, gender and IQ in children: a volumetric imaging study. *Brain* 119:1763–1774, 1996.
7. Caveness VS Jr, Kennedy DN, Richelme C, et al.: The human brain age 7–11 years: a volumetric analysis based on magnetic resonance images. *Cereb Cortex* 6:726–736, 1996.
8. Gogtay N, Giedd JN, Lusk L, et al.: Dynamic mapping of human cortical development during childhood through early adulthood. *Proc Nat Acad Sci* 101:8174–8179, 2004.
9. Coyle JT, Harris JC: The development of neurotransmitters and neuropeptides. In: Noshpitz J (ed): *Textbook of Child Psychiatry.* Vol 7. New York, Basic Books, 14–25, 1987.
10. Kail R: Speed of information processing: developmental change and links to intelligence. *J School Psychol* 38:51–61, 2000.
11. Buxbaum E: Between the Oedipus complex and adolescence: the "quiet" time. In: Greenspan SI, Pollock GH (eds): *Psychoanalytic Contributions Toward Understanding Personality Development.* Vol 2. Latency, Adolescence, and Youth. Rockville, MD, National Institute of Mental Health, 121–136, 1980.
12. Rutter M: Normal psychosexual development. *J Child Psychol Psychiatry* 11:259–283, 1971.
13. Ruble DN, Martin CL, Berenbaum S: Gender development. In: Kuhn D, Siegler R (eds): *Handbook of Child Sex Roles Psychology: Cognition, Perception and Language.* 6th ed. New York: Wiley, 2006.
14. Brooks-Gunn J: Antecedents and consequences of variation in girls' maturational timing. *J of Adol Health Care* 9:365–373, 1988.
15. Brill S, Rachel P: *The Transgender Child: A Handbook for Families and Professionals.* San Francisco, CA, Cleiss Press, 2008.
16. Gilligan C: *In a Different Voice: Psychological Theory and Women Development.* Cambridge, MA, Harvard University Press, 1982.
17. Eccles JS, Jacobs JE: Social forces shape math attitudes and performance. *Signs* 11:367–389, 1986.
18. Jacklin CN: Female and male: issues of gender. *Am Psychol* 44:127–133, 1989.
19. Gilligan C, Lyons N, Hanmer T (eds): *Making Connections: The Relational Worlds of Adolescent Girls at Emma Willard School.* Cambridge, MA, Harvard University Press, 1990.
20. Greenberg-Lake Analysis Group: *Shortchanging Girls, Shortchanging America: A Nationwide Poll of Students Ages 9–15. Research commissioned by American Association of University Women.* Washington, DC, American Association of University Women, 1991.
21. Debold E, Wilson M, Malave I: *Mother-Daughter Revolution: From Betrayal to Power.* New York, Addison-Wesley, 1993.
22. Sadker D: *Failing at Fairness: How Our Schools Cheat Girls.* New York, Simon & Schuster, 1995.
23. Piaget J, Inhelder B: *The psychology of the child.* New York, Basic Books, 1969.
24. Scholnick EK: *Knowing and Constructing Plans.* SRCD Newsletter, Fall issue, 17:1–2, 1995.
25. Kuhn D: Metacognitive development. *Curr Direct Psychol Sci* 9(5):178–181, 2000.
26. Joyner MH, Kurtz-Costes B: Metamemory development. In: Schneider W, Weinert FE (eds): *Memory Performance and Competencies: Issues in Growth and Development.* Hillsdale, NJ, Erlbaum, 275–300, 1997.
27. Harter S: The self. In: Damon W, Lerner RM (Series eds): *Handbook of Child Psychology,* 6th ed. Eisenberg N (Volume ed.) *Social, Emotional, and Personality Development.* New York: Wiley, 2006.
28. Piaget J: *The Moral Judgement of the Child.* New York, Free Press, 1948.
29. Kohlberg L: Stage and sequence: the cognitive-development approach to socialization. In: Goslin DA (ed): *Handbook of Socialization Theory and Research.* Chicago, Rand-McNally, 1969.
30. Stilwell B, Galvin M, Kopta SM, et al.: Moralization of attachment: a fourth domain of conscience functioning. *J Am Acad Child Adolesc Psychiatry* 36:1140–1147, 1997.
31. White RW: Motivation reconsidered: the concept of competence. *Psychol Rev* 66:297–333, 1959.
32. White RW: *Competence and the psychosexual stages of development.* In: *Nebraska Symposium on Motivation.* 1960:97–141.
33. Sullivan HS: *The Interpersonal Theory of Psychiatry.* New York, Norton, 1953.
34. Marsh HW: The structure of academic self-concept: the Marsh/Shavelson mode. *J Edu Psychol* 82:623–636, 1990.
35. Baumrind D: The discipline controversy revisited. *Fam Relat* 45:405–414, 1996.
36. Andrews DW, Dishion TJ: The microsocial structure underpinnings of adolescent problem behavior. In: Ketterlinus RD, Lamb ME (eds): *Theories of theories of mind.* Cambridge, England, Cambridge University, pp 184–199, 1994.
37. Parke RD, Buriel R: Socialization in the family: ethnic and ecological perspectives. In Damon W, Lerner RM (Series ed): *Handbook of Child Psychology.* 6th ed. Eisenberg N (Vol. ed.). *Social, Emotional, and Personality Development.* New York, Wiley, 2006.
38. Thomas A, Chess S: Genesis and evolution of behavioral disorders: from infancy to early adult life. *Am J Psychiatry* 141:1–9, 1984.
39. Goodnow JJ: From household practices to parents' ideas about work and interpersonal relationships. In: Harkness S, Super C (eds): *Parents' Cultural Belief Systems.* New York, Guilford, 313–344, 1996.
40. Reiss D: The interplay between genotypes and family relationships. *Curr Direct Psychol Sci* 14(3):139–143, 2005.
41. Bakermans-Kranenburg MJ, van Ijzendoorn MH, Juffer F: Less Is more: meta-analyses of sensitivity and attachment interventions in early childhood. *Psychol Bull* 129:195–215, 2003.
42. Combrinck-Graham L: A developmental model for family systems. *Fam Proc* 24:139–150, 1985.
43. Villani VS, Olson CK, Jellinek MS: Media literacy for clinicians and parents. *Child Adol Psychiat Clin N Am* 14(3):523–53, 2005.
44. Kramer DA: The biology of family culture. In: Combrinck-Graham L (ed): *Children in Family Contexts.* 2nd ed. New York, Guilford, 2006.
45. Bemporad JR: From attachment to affiliation. *Am J Psychoanal* 44:792–799, 1984.
46. Kagan J, Klein RE: Cross-cultural perspectives on early development. *Am Psychol* 28:947–961, 1973.
47. Grunebaum H, Solomon L: Toward a peer theory of group psychotherapy: I. On the developmental significance of peers and play. *Int J Group Psychother* 30:23–49, 1980.
48. Harris JR: *The Nurture Assumption: Why Children Turn Out the Way They Do.* New York, The Free Press, 1998.
49. Heyman GD, Dweck CS: Children's thinking about traits: Implications for judgments of the self and others. *Child Dev* 69:391–403, 1998.
50. Pomerantz EM, Saxon JL: Conceptions of ability as stable and self-evaluative processes: a longitudinal examination. *Child Dev* 72:152–173, 2001.
51. Eccles JS, Wigfield A, Schiefele U: Motivation to succeed. In: Eisenberg N (ed): *Handbook of Child Psychology.* Vol. 3. Social, emotional, and personality development. 5th ed. New York, Wiley, 1998, 1017–1095.
52. Grunebaum H, Solomon L: Toward a theory of peer relationships: II. On the stages of social development and their relationship to group psychotherapy. *Int J Group Psychother* 32:283–307, 1982.
53. Buhrmester D, Furman W: The development of companionship and intimacy. *Child Dev* 58:1101–1113, 1987.
54. Minuchin P: *The Middle Years of Childhood.* Belmont, CA, Brooks-Cole, 1977.
55. Cummings EM, Iannotti RJ, Zahn-Waxler C: Aggression between peers in early childhood: individual continuity and developmental change. *Child Dev* 60:887–895, 1989.
56. Boivin M, Begin G: Peer status and self-perception among early elementary school children: the case of the rejected children. *Child Dev* 60:591–596,1989.
57. Rogosch,FA, Newcomb AF: Children's perceptions of peer reputations and their social reputations among peers. *Child Dev* 60:597–610, 1989.
58. Hartup WW: Social relationships and their developmental significance. *Am Psychol* 44:120–126,1989.
59. Coie JD, Dodge KA, Coppotelli H: Dimensions and types of social status: a cross-age perspective. *Dev Psychol* 18:557–570, 1982.
60. Bagwell CL, Schmidt ME, Newcomb AF, Bukowski WM: Friendship and peer rejection as predictors of adult adjustment. In: Nangle DW, Erdley CA (eds): *The Role of Friendship in Psychological Adjustment.* San Francisco, Jossey-Bass, 25–49, 2001.
61. Gifford-Smith MD, Brownell CA: Childhood peer relationships: social acceptance, friendships, and peer networks. *J School Psychol* 41:235–284, 2003.
62. Sheridan SM, Buhs ES, Warnes ED: Childhood peer relationships in context. *J School Psychol* 41:285–292, 2003.
63. Brownell CA, Gifford-Smith ME: Context and development in children's school-based peer relations: Implications for research and practice. *J School Psychol* 41:305–310, 2003.
64. Heath SB: Oral and literate traditions among black Americans living in poverty. *Am Psychol* 44:367–373, 1989.
65. Miller-Jones D: Culture and testing. *Am Psychol* 44:360–366, 1989.
66. Wilson MN: Child development in the context of the black extended family. *Am Psychol* 44:380–385, 1989.
67. Davis-Kean PE: The influence of parent education and family income on child achievement: the indirect role of parental expectations and the home environment. *J Family Psychol* 19(2):294–304, 2005.

68. Humber N, Moss E: The relationship of preschool and early school age attachment to mother-child interaction. *Am J Orthopsychiatry* 75(1): 128–141, 2005.
69. Granot D, Mayseless O: Attachment security and adjustment to school in middle childhood. *Int J Behav Dev* 25(6), 530–541, 2001.
70. Haskins R: Beyond metaphor: the efficacy of early childhood education. *Am Psychol* 44:274–282, 1989.
71. Bradley RH, Caldwell BM, Rock SL: Home environment and school performance: a ten-year follow-up and examination of three models of environmental action. *Child Dev* 69:852–867, 1988.
72. Hall WS. Reading comprehension. *Am Psychol* 44:157–161, 1989.
73. Coles G: *The Learning Mystique.* New York, Pantheon, 1987.
74. Ditton P, Green RJ, Singer MT: Communication deviances: a comparison between parents of learning-disabled and normally achieving students. *Fam Process* 26:75–87, 1987.
75. Belmont JM: Cognitive strategies and strategic learning: the socio-instructional approach. *Am Psychol* 44:142–148, 1989.
76. Slavin R: Developmental and motivational perspectives on cooperative learnings: a reconciliation. *Child Dev* 58:1161–1167, 1987.
77. Gardner H: *Intelligence Reframed: Multiple Intelligences for the 21st Century.* New York, Basic Books, 1999.
78. Levine M, Hooper SR, Montgomery JW, et al.: Learning disabilities: an interactive developmental paradigm. In: Lyon GR, Gray DB (eds): *Better Understanding Learning Disabilities: New Voices from Research and Their Implications for Education and Public Policies.* Baltimore, Paul H. Brookes, 229–250, 1993.
79. Phinney J, Rotheram MJ: *Children's Ethnic Socialization: Pluralism and Development.* New York, Sage, 1986.
80. Rotheram MJ: The family and the school. In: Combrinck-Graham L (ed): *Children in Family Contexts.* New York, Guilford, 347–368, 1989.
81. Simons LG, Simons RL, Conger RD, Brody GH: Collective socialization and child conduct problems: a multilevel analysis with an African American sample. *Youth Soc* 35(3):267–292, 2004.
82. Linney JA, Siedman E: The future of schooling. *Am Psychol* 44:336–340, 1989.
83. Act, No Child Left Behind. PL 107–110. Washington, DC, US Department of Education, 2001.
84. Berliner D: Rational responses to high stakes testing: the case of curriculum narrowing and the harm that follows. *Cam J Educ* 41(3):287–302, 2011.
85. Jones PM: "From Childhood, A Life of Hard Labor" [Statistical sources: U.S. Department of Labor, International Labor Organization]. Chicago Tribune, p. 1, June 25, 2000.
86. Combrinck-Graham L: A life cycle approach to developmental disabilities. In: Dryden-Edwards RC, Combrinck-Graham L (eds): *Developmental Disabilities from Childhood to Adulthood.* Baltimore, MD, Johns Hopkins, 2010.

CHAPTER 2.1.4 ■ ADOLESCENCE

ROBERT A. KING AND HELENA J. V. RUTHERFORD

We are born, so to speak, twice over. Born in existence and born into life; born a human being and born a man.

—Rousseau, Emile

Adolescence in contemporary Western industrial society is shaped and defined by the interplay of complex biologic, cultural, economic, and historical forces. This lengthy transitional state, which may last a decade or more, is a distinctive period in which a youngster is no longer a child nor yet fully adult, but partakes of some of the challenges, privileges, and expectations of both epochs.

Adolescence is a period of paradoxes, as youngsters reach physical and sexual maturity well before they are fully cognitively and emotionally mature. On the one hand, a secular trend toward earlier puberty over the past century and a half means that defining maturational changes often begin by age 9 to 12, and that by 13 years of age, many youngsters are potentially fertile and sexually attuned, if not yet fully active. On the other hand, the educational demands of a complex modern economy have prolonged formal education and raised the age of mandatory school attendance to approximately 16 years, whereas social welfare concerns have abolished child labor and legally restricted adolescent employment, thus postponing entry into the world of work (1).

As a result, full economic emancipation usually is not possible until the later teens, at the earliest, and in the case of young people pursuing college or postgraduate education, often not until the middle to late twenties.

In the United States, the legal status of adolescents is a confusing mixture of privileges and strictures that attempts to balance the need for control and protection with the incremental granting of autonomy (2). For example, a 14 year old may fly a plane, but not legally drive a car, whereas a 17 year old may serve in the army, but not vote until 18 years of age, when he or she still is not legally allowed to drink. In many jurisdictions, a 14 year old may legally obtain an abortion without her parents' knowledge or consent but needs her parents' permission to be absent from school to do so.

Despite the restrictions on their full-time employment, young adolescent consumers are a potent economic force, controlling billions of dollars in disposable income annually. Teenagers, hence, comprise an eagerly sought-after demographic target for marketers, advertisers, and the broadcast, print, and electronic media. In turn, to attract and hold these young viewers and readers, media programming directed to them increasingly emphasizes sex and violence as prominent themes; sexual themes are estimated to make up approximately two-thirds of the content of prime time shows popular with teens (3).

Winnicott once remarked aphoristically: "There is no such thing as a baby," meaning that the baby could not be considered apart from its relationship with its mother (4). Although adolescence is the epoch *par excellence* of individuation and autonomy striving, it is similarly impossible to have a full understanding of adolescent development apart from its specific biologic, family, community, cultural, and historical contexts (5). Thus, while recent theoretical perspectives on adolescence acknowledge the development of *independence* and autonomy from parents, there is now an increased awareness of the complementary dynamic of the adolescent's developing capacity for *interdependence* and the ability to form and sustain mutually supportive relationships outside the family. Paralleling this relational perspective is an increased emphasis on the *ecologic* perspective, which sees individual adolescents and their relationships as embedded in the interconnected contexts of family, school, neighborhood, and culture (6).

The interactions among these factors are complex and multidirectional. Not only are adolescents influenced by their families, but they reshape their families' dynamics as they grow.

Although important aspects of adolescents' development are genetically and biologically determined, the effects of these determinants may be mediated or influenced by psychosocial factors. For example, family factors influence not only the impact of the timing of puberty but may actually affect the timing of puberty itself, with earlier and more rapid maturation in adolescents raised in more stressful, less supportive homes (7,8). Behavioral genetics studies that have revealed the importance of nonshared environmental factors suggest that adolescent siblings evoke different interactional and social environments even within the same family (9).

It is important to bear in mind the great diversity of social and family contexts in which today's adolescents grow up (10,11). In the United States, despite some commonalities, the experiences of adolescents who are immigrants; gay, lesbian, or gender-dysphoric; or growing up in poverty, foster care, single-parent, or other nontraditional family structures differ in important ways from the general patterns presented later in this chapter. Even greater differences exist between the majority culture of the West and more traditional societies, with less emphasis on individual autonomy and fewer expectations that adolescence should be a period of vocational choice or attaining full independence from families (12). Some anthropologic studies have concluded that in such preindustrial societies, there may be less adolescent turmoil and conflict with parents (13).

One important research question concerns the impact on adolescence as the processes of modernization (demographic shift to longer life span, smaller families, urbanization, shift from agrarian to manufacturing and service economies, etc.) and globalization (with development of the Internet and an "information society") expose more and more teenagers in such societies to the same media and cultural influences as in the West (11–13).

One facet of globalization transforming important aspects of adolescence is the near-ubiquitous availability, at least in the industrialized world, of various electronic media, such as TV, video games, cell phones, and the Internet (including texting, e-mail, streaming music and videos, and social networking sites, such as Facebook, Instagram, and Twitter) (3). The Youth Risk Behavior Survey (14) found that 42% of high school students reported three or more hours a day spent on an average school day playing video or computer games or using a computer for something other than school work. A recent Kaiser Family Foundation Study (15) documented the relative amounts of time youngsters, age 8 to 18 years old, spent daily on these activities: 7.5 hours using entertainment media (consuming 10.75 hours of content because of multitasking). In addition to this media use, the respondents reported 1.3 hours texting daily. Only about one-third reported that their parents set rules about time spent on TV, videogames, or the computer. Over and above the sheer number of hours spent on these various media and their impact on youngsters' attention and cognitive style, youngsters are now exposed, for good or ill, and often without much adult supervision, to a plethora of global influences and virtual subcommunities, ranging from pornography to fellow aficionados of various videogames, cultural, athletic, or intellectual interests. Many adolescents now live much of their lives in an "online social context" and how this will influence their emotional and social development remains a vast experiment in progress (3,16,17).

PHYSICAL CHANGES AT ADOLESCENCE

The term *puberty* (from the Latin *pubertas,* meaning "age of manhood") is used to refer to the physiologic and morphologic changes that mark the transition from childhood to adulthood.

Hormonally Mediated Changes

The most visibly dramatic aspects of adolescence relate to the hormonally mediated changes of puberty: the development of primary and secondary sexual characteristics; marked growth in stature, muscle mass, and strength; and increased sebaceous gland activity. These changes are the result of three different sets of hormonal changes: (1) adrenarche, (2) gonadarche, and (3) increased growth hormone secretion.

Adrenarche, the steady increase in adrenally produced androgens, begins as early as 6 to 8 years of age, leading to increased skeletal growth and the beginning appearance of body hair even before the surge of gonadal hormones associated with puberty proper.

Puberty proper is marked by *gonadarche,* in which the pulsatile release of gonadotropin-releasing hormone produces increased pituitary release of follicle-stimulating hormone and luteinizing hormone that in turn drive the production of gonadal hormones (primarily testosterone in boys, estrogen in girls) (7). Together with these gonadal hormones, increased release of growth hormone stimulates the pubertal growth spurt.

The triggers for this activation of the pituitary–gonadal axis are unclear, but have been speculated to include a variety of permissive signals, such as leptin or other metabolic indicators of adequate body weight/fat composition, interacting with a variety of genes and neural inputs (6,7,18).

The process of puberty takes approximately 4 to 5 years from start to finish, with girls (in the industrialized world) beginning the process on average at 9 to 11 years of age, approximately 2 years earlier than the average onset for boys. The various stages of this process, as indicated by pubic hair, breast development, height spurt, and menarche in girls, and pubic hair, penile and testicular growth, and height spurt in boys, have been classified by Tanner (19) into stages I through V.

The first harbinger of impending puberty usually is acceleration in linear growth, as much as 10 cm per year, which usually precedes increases in muscle mass and strength, thereby producing the gangling appearance of many early adolescents.

For girls, the initial stages of puberty are the beginnings of breast development (mean age 8.9 years [standard deviation (SD), 1.9] for African-American girls and 10.0 years [SD, 1.8] for white girls) and the appearance of pubic hair (mean age 8.8 years [SD, 2.0] and 10.5 years [SD 1.7], respectively) (20).

The clearest marker of puberty in girls is the onset of menses, or *menarche.* Girls' periods initially remain irregular for some time, and despite the high rates of early teen pregnancy, ovulation and full fertility may require 2 years to develop. Most modern girls have been well prepared for menarche by health classes, peers, and mothers, and news of who has (or has not) yet begun her periods is the topic of excited exchanges of confidences among middle school girls.

A critical body weight and fat/muscle ratio appears to be a necessary condition for menarche; hence, girls who train intensively for athletics or dance or who are anorectic may have delayed menarche. Probably related to the permissive role of adequate nutrition and body weight, there has been a steady secular decrease in the age of menarche since the Industrial Revolution, at the rate of approximately 2.3 months per decade (7,8). Currently, the average age of menarche is 12.9 years (SD, 1.2) in white girls and 12.2 years (SD, 1.2) in African-American girls (20). In recent years, there has been controversy about the appropriate norms for deciding at what age female pubertal development should be considered premature, since by age 7 to 8, a significant number of girls are already showing Tanner II breast or pubic hair development. Further study is needed as to whether this represents an increased prevalence of very early puberty in girls, and if so, what its causes and potential clinical implications are (7).

In boys, growth of the penis and testes and beginning spermatogenesis occur in early and middle adolescence. In contrast to menarche, however, "semenarche" or the beginning of ejaculation, whether by masturbation or spontaneous nocturnal emissions, usually remains a very private matter among Western boys (21).

Detailed longitudinal studies reveal considerable variation in the onset and progress of the various stages of puberty, both within and between genders. Thus, peak growth velocity in girls occurs approximately 2 years earlier than in boys, whereas pubic hair appearance often is only approximately 9 months earlier.

Much research has examined the question of the developmental impact on adjustment of early versus late maturation in boys and girls (8,22). In general, these studies show that, for boys, although earlier maturation has some advantages in terms of popularity, self-esteem, and intellectual abilities, it also confers mild-to-moderate increased risk for internalizing symptoms and externalizing problem behaviors in adolescence but less risk for conduct or substance abuse disorders than their later maturing peers. For girls, the picture is more complex, with early-maturing girls tending to have more adjustment difficulties (including lower self-image and greater vulnerability to depression, anxiety, and eating disorders) and greater likelihood of engaging in risky behaviors and experiencing early sexual intercourse. The impact of early versus late maturation in girls, however, also depends on social context variables such as social class, pubertal status of peers, cultural norms, and timing of concomitant changes (e.g., school transition), as well as prepubertal adjustment (8,23). These studies are complicated by the fact that family disruption or stress is also associated with earlier onset of puberty in girls (7,8).

Neurobiologic Changes in Adolescence

Greater availability of neuroimaging tools has provided the opportunity of a window into the dramatic changes in brain morphology and functioning during adolescence.

One of the most dramatic changes in adolescent brain reorganization is a massive elimination or "pruning" of cortical synapses, with an estimated loss of up to 30,000 synapses per second during adolescence (24,25).

Synaptic pruning occurs throughout the brain, with significant regional variation in the volume and time course of pruning (26,27). This extreme pruning is thought to be adaptive, ensuring optimal connectivity between different areas of the developing brain (28). Increasing connectivity has also been observed in the adolescent brain through linear increases in myelin—the substance that insulates axons and facilitates the transmission of electrical impulses through the neuron (27). This growth in myelination is thought to improve the efficiency of neural communication throughout the brain, with increasing white matter being associated with improvements in cognitive performance across development (29,30).

In addition to these structural brain changes observed during adolescence, neuroimaging techniques have evidenced important changes in brain activity during this developmental period. Several theoretical frameworks exist that bridge these functional brain changes to adolescent behavior (31–35), with all approaches evidencing agreement in the differential engagement of cortical and subcortical systems being central to adolescent behavior. In particular, these approaches posit that adolescence is a period characterized by delayed maturation of prefrontal and frontal cortices, neurobiologic regions that have been implicated in multiple cognitive control functions. Critically, concurrent to protracted frontal cortical development, increased activation in brain regions responsible for the processing of positive rewards have also been reported. One study found that adolescents, relative to children and adults, evidenced greater activation of the subcortical reward-processing structure, the nucleus accumbens (NAcc), in response to the receipt of large rewards (36). Reward-related activity in the NAcc has also been linked to an increased likelihood of engaging in risk-taking behavior across development (37). A recent longitudinal study also evidenced a peak in NAcc activity to reward during adolescence, with NAcc activity also being associated with risk-taking behavior as well as pubertal development and reward sensitivity (38). Consequently, this heightened responsivity to reward, coupled with decreased cognitive control, may represent underlying neurobiologic mechanisms subserving impulsivity, novelty-, and sensation-seeking behaviors typical of adolescence.

Neuroimaging studies have also evidenced increased reactivity of the subcortical emotion-processing region, the amygdala, to sources of negative emotions in adolescents. For instance, when viewing fearful as compared to neutral faces, amygdala activity was greater in adolescents as compared to adults and children (39,40). Furthermore, during an emotion regulation task, adolescents as compared to adults were less able to decrease amygdala reactivity to aversive stimuli through their employment of reappraisal strategies—with connectivity between the amygdala and prefrontal cortical regions during emotion regulation being associated with age (41). Therefore, delayed prefrontal cortical maturation may influence the capacity to downregulate emotional reactivity during adolescence. Critically, if these cortical regulatory functions are not fully developed, adolescents may be more susceptible to potential detrimental effects when experiencing negative emotions, including stress, which may be associated with the increased rates of psychopathology that have been observed during this developmental period. We will return to this potential source of adolescent vulnerability in the section on psychopathology.

Other Biologic Changes

Along with puberty come changes in appetite and sleep patterns.

Across species, the adolescence-associated growth spurt results in more time spent feeding and foraging for food. Most families with teenagers can attest to their youngsters' elevated metabolic rate and what has been termed *developmental hyperphagia* (18).

Adolescence also sees a shift in sleep patterns, with a sleep phase delay or tendency to fall asleep later and wake up later (42). On average, 10- to 12-year-old children sleep approximately 9.3 hours a night and awaken spontaneously. In contrast, the mean length of sleep for high school students is 7.5 hours per night, with one-fourth of students sleeping 6.5 hours or less per night. Laboratory studies, however, suggest that the actual average sleep need for high school students is closer to 10 hours per night (43).

Part of this phase shift appears to be biologic; later night-onset and later morning-termination of melatonin secretion make it difficult for the adolescent to go to sleep earlier or to wake up alert in time for school, which, deleteriously for many teenagers, may begin as early as 7:20 AM. This shift in sleep patterns also has a psychosocial component. Adolescents are given greater autonomy by their parents in controlling their own bedtimes, while the expansion of social contacts outside the home and increased social stimulation (in the form of cell phone and social media) keep the teenager up later.

As a result of both these environmental and neurobiologic factors, many adolescents suffer from "too little sleep at the wrong circadian phase," especially on school days, with consequent difficulty getting up, frequent daytime drowsiness, and impaired alertness and cognitive functioning (43). Such adolescents are also at increased risk of learning difficulties, impaired academic performance, depressed mood, and accident proneness (44). In recent years, there has been a strong movement advocating for later school start times for high school and middle school students (45).

COGNITIVE CHANGES IN ADOLESCENCE

Adolescence is marked by dramatic quantitative and qualitative growth in cognitive abilities (46) with increased hypothetico-deductive problem-solving abilities and a greater capacity for abstraction. Adolescents' cognitive abilities are characterized by growing complexity, the ability to think about possibilities, and increased speed and efficiency of information processing. As a result, adolescence often sees the flowering of passionate intellectual and aesthetic interests, with impressive achievements in areas such as music, mathematics, computer science, or physics. Interestingly, adolescent works of genius are more commonly in these abstract areas than in those involving the empirical sciences or the humanities.

These cognitive changes also have their counterpart in the adolescent's social cognition and moral development (47,48). The development of formal operational thinking permits a growth in social perspective-taking and a decline in childhood egocentrism; it enables the adolescent to contemplate better what a social situation might look like from another person's point of view. Moral reasoning becomes more complex and expands to include orientation to interpersonal relationships, maintenance of social order, notions of social contract and general rights, and, finally, reference to universal ethical principles.

Despite greater cognitive abilities, however, adolescents do not always use these capacities for sound decision-making, in part, perhaps, because their cognitive performance in real-life situations (as opposed to optimal test conditions) is more vulnerable to disruption by strong affects, everyday stresses, and peer influences (47,49–51).

On a practical level, the adolescent develops a more mature time sense, a greater awareness of the finality of death, and, along with wider knowledge of the outside world, a keener sense of the diversity and relativity of moral codes. This moral awakening may be accompanied by an intensified interest in and sophistication about politics, ideology, or religion. This wider vision, as most eloquently described in the work of Erik Erikson (52,53), provides both opportunities and hazards. Along with a penchant for philosophical musings, the adolescent may experience a sense of moral confusion and at least transient feelings of anomie. The anxieties of what Seltzer (54) has termed *frameworklessness* may lead some adolescents to a fanatical embrace of some ideology or religion on the one hand or a posture of nihilism on the other.

PSYCHOLOGICAL TASKS OF ADOLESCENCE

The physical, neurobiologic, and cognitive changes described previously herald dramatic shifts in the adolescent's relationship to his or her own body, appetites, parents, peers, and self-image. In this next section, we turn to the psychological tasks of adaptation these shifts impose on the developing teenager. Felice (55) has summarized these as:

- developing a satisfactory and realistic body image;
- developing increased independence from parents and adequate capacities for self-care and regulation;
- developing satisfying relationships outside the family;
- developing appropriate control and expression of increased sexual drives;
- identity consolidation, including a personal moral code and provisional plans for a vocation and economic self-sufficiency.

Coping with a Changing Body Image

Save for pregnancy or devastating illness, no other epoch sees such dramatic changes in the body and its self-representation as does adolescence. Although often welcome, these changes are also unsettling. Body and facial hair begins to grow. Menstrual discharges, erections, or ejaculation can occur at unexpected and embarrassing times. Acne and body odors make their appearance and are a source of anxiety. Boys' voices may break unexpectedly as they deepen. Changes in the distribution of fat and muscle alter body outlines. Not only must girls deal with breast development, but, to their embarrassment, many boys develop gynecomastia.

Adolescents compare their development carefully with that of their peers and are acutely aware of their self-perceived imperfections. Much time is spent brooding in front of the mirror, examining every potential blemish and trying to catch a glimpse of the self. A single pimple may seem to loom as large as the Matterhorn, its stigma increased by the sense that it is as glaringly obvious to everyone else as it is to the adolescent.

Boys and girls differ in the extent and ways in which social factors influence their body image and notions of body ideal. In Western society, girls in particular are very preoccupied with the body image ideal of thinness held up to them by the media (3,56). Girls' levels of satisfaction with their bodies and physical appearance decline as they pass through adolescence; this is especially problematic for girls who are earlier maturing. While girls generally regard thinness as a goal to be pursued regardless of their actual weight, boys usually regard muscularity as the ideal at which to aim.

The Youth Risk Behavior Survey (14) found that although 32% of high school boys and 27% of girls were overweight or at risk of being overweight (defined as having a body mass index equal to or greater than the 85th percentile for age and sex), only 25% of boys thought they were overweight, compared with 38% of girls; furthermore, only 31% of boys were trying to lose weight during the preceding 30 days, compared with 61% of girls. In addition to media representations, ethnicity, social class, and perceptions of schoolmates' weight and habitus are also important determinants of both boys' and girls' body self-perceptions (56).

Pathologic eating behaviors are common in adolescents, especially girls. For example, a survey of two private girls' secondary schools found that 18% of the girls reported at least one major symptom of an eating disorder: 8% to 15% thought about food all the time, 6% to 12% induced vomiting to control their weight, over 2% used laxatives for weight control, and 7% often fasted or starved to lose weight (57). The national Youth Risk Behavior Survey (58) found that within the past month, 4.5% of high school students (6.2% of girls and 2.9% of boys) reported vomiting or taking laxatives and 12.3% (16.5% of girls and 8.1% of boys) had fasted for at least 24 hours to lose or control weight. These endemically high levels of body dissatisfaction and pathologic eating attitudes and behaviors provide a large reservoir of vulnerable adolescents from whose ranks those with frank bulimia and anorexia are recruited.

More research is needed, however, to understand better the cultural factors that influence the wide variations in the prevalence of disordered eating attitudes and behaviors across different communities and ethnic groups and over time.

The adolescent's body is also a representation of the adolescent's self. Hence, not surprisingly, teenagers spend great amounts of time, energy, and money trying to make their appearance conform to some perceived ideal. Boys in middle adolescence may try to bulk up their gangling habitus or firm up a pudgy physique by weight lifting, bodybuilding, nutritional supplements, and even anabolic steroids in an effort to transform their self-image from weak, dependent, or vulnerable to that of a "hard body"—tough, masculine, and strong. Girls endlessly experiment with makeup and consult friends and websites regarding "makeovers." Both sexes may go through a dizzying panoply of clothing and hairstyles, trying on in rapid succession a kaleidoscope of fashions and styles that also represent possible social selves: punk, home-boy, preppie, slut, grunge, jock, goth, and so forth. Multiple body piercings and tattoos convey more permanent, but potentially disfiguring personal statements. (By tattooing on a lover's name, the bearer seeks self-reassuringly to reinforce the permanence of a relationship [49].)

Beyond its role as a source of anxiety or pleasure, the body also may be the vehicle for painful or self-destructive means of reducing psychic tension (e.g., through delicate cutting) or dealing with conflicts over dependency or instinctual longings (e.g., bulimia, anorexia nervosa) (60).

Changing Relations with Parents

Surveys such as those of Offer and Schonert-Reichl (61) have emphasized that most adolescents regard their relations with their parents as stable, trusting, and sustaining and continue to turn toward parents as important, primary sources of advice, comfort, and assistance. Although this appears to be objectively true for most adolescents, on a subjective level, there are important shifts in the emotional terms of the relationship for both the parents and youngster (23,62).

LOOSENING TIES TO PARENTS

Time spent with family decreases during adolescence, from 25% of waking hours for high school freshmen to only 15% for seniors (63). Furthermore, there is a shift in the affective tone of time spent with parents and in the adolescent's view of the parents.

The teenager's own parents often are de-idealized. This is a painful process for parents as their previously admiring child develops a keen (sometimes distorted, sometimes all-too-accurate) sense of their shortcomings. Even those many teens who retain warm and supportive relations with their parents experience an increased sense of loneliness because the youngster feels no longer able or willing to share many intimate concerns or longings as of old. The adolescent may alternate between wishes for autonomy and wishes to be taken care of. Feelings of dependency may have to be warded off with disparagement, indifference, or oppositionality (64). As a result, well-meaning parents often are bewildered as to which side of their child's ambivalence they are dealing with at any given moment (hence the titles to various guides for the parents of teens, such as *Get Out of My Life, but First Could You Drive Me and Cheryl to the Mall?* [65]).

CONFLICT WITH PARENTS

Csikszentmihalyi and Larson (63) remark that "friction appears to be an endemic feature of family life" in families with adolescents (p. 138), noting that "adults and adolescents live in separate, if overlapping, realities" (p. 140), often viewing the same events quite differently. This is true not only of specific events, but of family life in general, with adolescents tending to underestimate parental influence on them, and parents tending to overestimate their influence. Similarly, parents usually perceive the family's cohesion and adaptability as more satisfactory than do their teenagers who, in turn, report more conflicts with their parents than do the parents themselves (62,66).

Conflicts between parents and children increase with the beginning of adolescence. In early adolescence, these clashes concern household rules, chores, room cleaning, bedtime, diet, friends, dress, and hygiene; later in adolescence, issues such as dating and curfews become more prominent. Montemayor and Hanson's (67) naturalistic study of early adolescents found that conflicts with parents and siblings occurred at the rate of approximately 20 per month, or 1 every 3 days. Meta-analytic studies find that although the frequency of parent–child conflicts declines from early adolescence through late adolescence, the negative affective intensity of conflicts peaks in mid-adolescence (66).

Mothers appear to bear the brunt of most of these clashes, especially with early adolescent daughters (62,68); father–son clashes in particular take on greater affective intensity in mid-adolescence (66). Early maturation in girls and problems such as adolescent depression or substance abuse increase the likelihood of conflict (12).

This squabbling and bickering take a toll on the psychological well-being of the parents, as well as the adolescent, with many parents reporting difficulty adjusting to their teenager's strivings for autonomy (23).

The quality of daily family life thus becomes more turbulent in families with adolescents, with minor, but frequent "daily hassles"; for example, as boys approach puberty, there is a deterioration in family communication as both parents and child interrupt each other more frequently and explain themselves less (Steinberg, 1981, cited in 63). Time-sampling studies find that when with their families, adolescents' negative thoughts outnumber positive ones by 10 to 1 (63).

The apparent decrease in parent–child conflict in middle adolescence coincides with decreased time spent with parents and a turn toward greater involvement and reliance on peers, leading Laursen et al. (66) to speculate that "it is likely that parents and children disagree less simply because they are together less. Increases in conflict affective intensity coincide with increases in autonomy and emotional dysphoria that occur as adolescents spend more time alone and with peers" (p. 828).

Despite the mutual stresses of increased conflict, most parent–child relationships remain solid. As Arnett (11) notes, "Even amidst relatively high conflict, parents and adolescents tend to report that overall their relationships are good, that they share a wide range of core values, and that they retain a considerable amount of mutual affection and attachment" (p. 320).

Seen from one perspective, the immediate *causa belli* of many typical parent–adolescent clashes appear seemingly trivial (what John Hill [quoted in 62] labeled "garbage and galoshes" disputes): hairstyle, clothes, chores, curfew, or time spent on social media or videogames. The intensity of conflict, however, usually reflects the parents' or child's perception (accurate or not) that vital issues are at stake: for the parents, issues of loyalty, respect, responsibility, and the dangers of sex, substance abuse, or other risky behavior; for the adolescents, issues of autonomy, control of their own body, and connections to friends.

Adolescents whose parents are able to hold firm and maintain balance in the face of these upheavals, without being overly permissive, harshly authoritarian, or indifferent, appear to do best. Numerous studies conclude that what has been termed *authoritative parenting*—combining warmth and responsiveness on one hand with firmness and demandingness—is associated with a wide range of adolescent competencies, academic achievement, and positive outcomes (62).

By later adolescence, in most cases, volatility and strife decrease and some degree of equilibrium is restored to the parent–adolescent relationship, albeit on a newer and more egalitarian basis, with the youngster having more autonomy and involvement in family decision-making.

TRANSITION TO SELF-CARE

As adolescence progresses, youngsters gradually claim or are ceded greater control over their diet, hygiene, sleep schedule, and dress, as well as responsibility for their school work. Nonetheless, these remain topics of frequent minor skirmishes, at least in early adolescence, with much parental nagging about junk food, skipped meals, slovenly or inappropriate dress, time spent online or on social media, and the like.

Although adolescence is a time of general good physical health, it also is the period during which many attitudes and habits are established with respect to diet, exercise, substance use, smoking, driving, and sexual behaviors that will constitute long-term risk (or protective) factors for health in later life (69,70).

Ironically, for many youngsters with serious chronic illnesses, such as type 1 diabetes mellitus or cystic fibrosis, despite their greater cognitive understanding of the exigencies of their condition, the quality of their care frequently deteriorates as they take over the responsibility for adherence to their treatment regimen (71,72). Thus, many adolescent diabetic patients fail to adhere to their diet, blood glucose testing, and insulin regimen. Some chronically ill youngsters may stop their medication, including chemotherapy or immunosuppressant therapy, with potentially fatal consequences.

Unlike health-conscious adults, many adolescents perceive the need to pay extra attention to their physical condition as anxiety provoking, stigmatizing, or frighteningly threatening to their wish for autonomy and invulnerability; hence, rather than responding to their medical condition with heightened attentiveness, they may try to avoid thinking about or dealing with their illness altogether.

Developing Satisfying Relationships Outside the Family

As dependence on parents becomes less acceptable to adolescents, they turn increasingly to peers for companionship, advice, support, and intimacy (73). Csikszentmihalyi et al. (74) found that during the school year, adolescents spend one-third of their waking time talking with peers, but less than 8% of waking time talking with adults. Talking with friends was the activity that teens reported made them the happiest.

Parents may be bemused or annoyed by their adolescent's intense need to hang out with and be with peers, regardless of any family plans. This is not merely for the immediate pleasures of the event. Rather, the need for continuing access to peers is driven by an intense need to relate, to compare, and to try out aspects of the developing self. As Seltzer (54) points out, it is this developmental need that explains "why adolescents never seem to tire of being with one another.... [I]t is not the overt social activity or the content of the event (e.g., a rock concert, a football game, a dance) that feeds the drive. It is *being with one another*—looking, listening, and resultant comparing. Adolescents report details of who was there, what they did or said, and what they wore in far greater detail than they describe the content of the event" (p. 41).

With adolescence, the communicative, supportive, and intimate aspects of friendship take on increased importance. Although nonromantic opposite-sex friendships occur in later adolescence, close friendships in early adolescence tend to be with the same sex. Among girls, intimate conversations are most often the cement of friendships, whereas for boys, it tends to be shared activities. With age, the need for control and conformity decreases, and there is greater tolerance for differences between friends (23).

The choice of friends is a complex matter (73). Although the range of possibilities is defined by the given community and school population, the adolescent's specific choices of friends reflect an important and often fateful aspect of self-definition. Adolescents most often choose friends who share their behaviors, attitudes, interests, and identities (23,73). Friends, however, also may be chosen on many other grounds, including perceived virtues or aspects of the self that the adolescent consciously repudiates or feels he or she lacks. Friends may serve as sources of support or admiration, as collusive companions for regression or delinquency, objects of sexual or aggressive exploitation, targets for projection—the list is endless. The choice of friend may be used to try on or borrow self-attributes; for example, a girl who perceives herself as unattractive or unpopular may hang out with a girl whom she sees as beautiful or popular. A boy who feels himself to be overly compliant, timid, or passive may choose to hang out for a while with a more venturesome or delinquent peer. Friendships pursued out of such interests may be transient or unstable as the youngster comes to feel in greater possession of the desired attribute himself or herself, or repudiates the wish for it.

Empirical studies have examined what personal attributes of peers are most salient to adolescents. For example, Midwestern high school students were asked to rate a list of attributes as to the frequency with which they were noticed in age mates. The top 10 attributes most frequently rated as "always of interest" were (in decreasing order): cleanliness, loyalty to friends, clothes, dependability, trustworthiness, general physical appearance, maturity, popularity with opposite sex, figure/build/physique, and honesty. Despite some gender and age differences, appearance and dependability were widely viewed as very important, whereas specific skills and abilities were of little interest (54).

Over the course of high school, adolescents shift in the gender and group size with whom they associate (73). Thus, freshmen hang out predominantly in same-sex groups, sophomores in same-sex dyads, juniors in mixed-sex groups, and seniors predominantly in small groups of heterosexual couples (63). In early adolescence, the adolescent's crowd consists of a large group of peers with similar reputations and role stereotypes (e.g., preppies, goths, brains, jocks, nerds). Younger adolescents value crowd affiliation as fostering friendships, providing support, facilitating interactions, and providing a source of identity and status (according to where the adolescent's particular crowd fits in the school or community hierarchy). Attitudes toward being "part of a crowd" do, however, change over the course of adolescence (73). Older adolescents are more likely to be dissatisfied with the perceived conformity demands of crowds and prefer smaller, more intimate groups. By the later high school years, the salient peer group may be the clique, a smaller group of peers similar in terms of activities, attitudes, status, age, and race.

Ironically, many adolescents, while resisting parental advice in the name of autonomy, are slavishly compliant with the perceived tastes and values of peers, especially regarding fashions and preferences in dress, slang, music, television, and movies.

Peers, however, influence each other in positive ways, including prosocial behaviors and academic achievement, as well as in negative ways, such as delinquency or substance use (23). These influences are not necessarily coercive or conformist, but also stem from emulatory admiration and a community of attitudes and interests that form the basis for the friendship in the first place (73).

Adolescents' relationships with their parents are an important influence on peer relationships (62). Authoritative parenting styles appear to lessen the negative effects of peer influences;

conversely, teenagers from less cohesive families are more likely to be influenced by peers than by parents (23). A tendency to look to peers rather than to parents for guidance and values, especially when combined with a choice of peers with delinquent behavior, low academic aspirations, or with values markedly divergent from the adolescent's parents, is an important risk factor for a wide range of problem behaviors (75).

Sexual and Aggressive Drives

Adolescence sees the epochal development of experiencing sexual attraction toward others and perceiving oneself as the object of others' sexual desire. How these subjectivities unfold and are given individual and social meanings is a complex process with physiologic, cultural, and individual dimensions (76). The interplay of these factors has been the focus of much anthropologic, psychoanalytic, and developmental study (72,77,78).

After a period of fairly open genital interests and play during the preschool years, overt sexual behavior and interests diminish markedly during the school years (79). Although even in these years before adolescence, sexual interests are never completely latent, masturbation, if it continues, is more furtive, and the child becomes more modest and inhibited about discussing sexual and romantic matters.

Beginning at approximately 10 years of age, feelings of sexual awareness and attraction make their conscious appearance (76). This development, which appears to be linked to rising adrenal androgens, occurs even before the onset of gonadal puberty proper. The reticence of children at this age makes the phenomena difficult to study in Western culture, but in many preliterate cultures, sexual rites of passage, at least for boys, occur as early as 10 years of age (78). It is also around the age of 10 to 11 years that some children become aware of same-sex attractions and homoerotic fantasy; feelings of gender-dysphoria, which may have been present from a much earlier age, become more distressing (80).

In early adolescence, genital excitement and sexual interests often occur independently of liking, intimacy, or wish for emotional closeness. For young adolescent boys, the objects of sexual fantasy and masturbatory excitement frequently are media figures or Internet pornography, rather than actual acquaintances. In keeping with their burgeoning attunement to social relationships, early adolescent girls are usually intensely interested in the romantic relationships, real and fantasied, of their peers, with endless discussions of who is "going out" or has broken up with whom. However, the early teen boys who are their age-peers often are unpromising candidates as romantic partners, hence many girls' crushes and eroticized longings focus on media figures, such as the various "boy bands" marketed to this audience. Although movies and television have long provided the raw materials for adolescent sexual fantasy, it is not yet clear what the recent increases in the ubiquity, sexual explicitness, and violence of mass media (including now the Internet) will be on the sexual socialization of teens (76).

With adolescence, there also is a resurgence of overt sexual activity (76,79). The rate of explicit masturbation increases from approximately 10% at age 7 to approximately 80% at age 13 years, whereas that of heterosexual play rises to approximately 65% at age 13 years; homosexual play also is not uncommon in early adolescence, with 25% to 30% of 13-year-old boys reporting at least one episode of same-sex play.

The transition from childhood masturbation to that of adolescence involves more than an increased physiologic capacity for arousal and orgasm. Most teens report consciously fantasizing when masturbating to orgasm, and even those who do not seem aware of some sort of sexual imagery (77). Sexual fantasies (which also occur without overt masturbation) become an intense and important part of the adolescent's psychological inner life. Beyond serving as a source of pleasure and compensatory wish fulfillment in lieu of other sexual outlets, these fantasies provide the occasion for the adolescent to elaborate or explicate his or her idiosyncratic and personal erotic scripts: who, doing what, with whom, with what body parts, with what implicit and explicit emotional tone and interpersonal interactions, and with what admixture of dominance or submission, control or abandonment, sadism or masochism, and admiration or degradation. (Laufer [81] has coined the term *central masturbatory fantasy* to describe the organizing aspects of these not always fully conscious fantasies in relationship to arousal and orgasm.) These fantasies are more than just a form of rehearsal or anticipatory coping; they help the adolescent explore and become aware of what is pleasurable, anxiety provoking, transgressive, or deeply compelling in his or her longings and to become familiar with his or her own individual preconditions for erotic excitement and fulfillment.

A key task of adolescence is to bring these erotic longings adaptively into the interpersonal arena as a vehicle for intimacy, emotional closeness, and ultimately the formation of a stable partnership for the conception and rearing of the next generation.

Although early adolescence sees the transition from largely autoerotic sexual activity to sexual interactions with peers, this takes place at different rates in different social and ethnic groups and with different interpersonal meanings (72,76,77,82). The prevalence of ever having had sexual intercourse is about 24.1% in 9th grade and 58.1% by 12th grade, with higher rates among males (43.2%) than females (39.2%); the respective rates among black high school students are 48.5%, Hispanic students 42.5%, and white students 39.9% (14).

For girls, the relational aspect of sexual involvement usually is paramount, and girls may engage in petting, oral sex, or intercourse as an attempted means of winning or retaining a boy's perceived interest, affection, or commitment. For young adolescent boys, sexual activity often has a more exploitative nature, with less interest in the relational aspect of the activity. However, these gender distinctions are not universal (76).

Falling in love is an important part of adolescence, even when not accompanied by sexual intimacy (6,76,82). Adolescence's most intense longings, keenest pleasures, painful frustrations, and bitterest disappointments center on the quest for a reciprocated love that helps to define the still inchoate self and assuage the loneliness of individuation.

Adolescent sexuality stirs in adults a variable reactive mixture of envy, apprehension, or repressiveness. Parents who may be facing their own midlife crises must contend with their sons' or daughters' burgeoning sexuality. Many of the parent–child conflicts in mid-adolescence, such as those around clothes, friends, dating, curfews, social media, and driving, although seemingly trivial, have the subtext of the parents' attempts to control the pace, scope, and direction of their adolescent's sexual activity. (A few parents who are overidentified with their adolescent's sexuality or take too much vicarious excitement in it collusively encourage their teen's transition to sexual activity.)

Despite much forgetfulness about the travails of their adolescence, most adults retain evocative, bittersweet memories of their own adolescent romantic longings. It is not surprising then, that from *Romeo and Juliet* on, the pangs and passions of adolescent love, whether thwarted or fulfilled, have remained an enduring theme of plays, novels, poetry, movies, and songs.

Identity

In his seminal work *Childhood and Society,* Erik Erikson (52) describes the challenge of identity formation as follows:

> [I]n puberty and adolescence all samenesses and continuities relied on earlier are more or less questioned again.... The growing and developing youths, faced with [the] physiological revolution within them, and with tangible adult tasks ahead of them are now primarily concerned with what they appear to be in the eyes of others as compared with what they feel they are, and with the question of how to connect the roles and skills cultivated earlier with the occupational prototypes of the day.... [It is the ability] to integrate all identifications with the vicissitudes of the libido, with the aptitudes developed out of endowment, and with the opportunities offered in social roles. [The desired outcome] is the accrued confidence that the inner sameness and continuity prepared in the past are matched by the sameness and continuity of one's meaning for others (p. 261).

One of the most influential empirical extensions of Erikson's work was Marcia's taxonomy for classifying adolescents into four identity statuses: the *identity-diffused* subject who has not yet experienced an identity crisis or made a role commitment; the *identity-foreclosed* subject, who has made unexamined commitments, usually as received from parents and others; the *identity-moratorium* subject, who is actively struggling to define values and commitments; and the *identity-achieved* subject, who has resolved these crises (53,83). In contemporary Western middle-class society, many of these identity issues are not fully engaged until the college years or beyond (1).

Empirical research has shifted away from global notions of identity to focus more on the development of specific self-concepts (23,53,84). With their growing cognitive sophistication, adolescents' views of themselves become more differentiated and better organized. Harter (85) and others have examined the distinct dimensions of adolescents' self-concept across several realms, such as social relations, appearance, academics, athletics, and morality, and their relationship to global self-worth. Adolescents weigh these dimensions differently depending on whether they are interacting with peers, parents, or teachers, and it is only over time that that these discrepancies decline to produce a more consonant, better-integrated self-image. (Behavioral genetic studies of siblings suggest that heritable factors may exert more of an influence than do shared environmental factors on self-perceived scholastic and athletic competence, physical appearance, and general self-worth; self-perceived social competence appears to be primarily determined by nonshared environmental factors reflecting each sibling's unique family and social experiences [9,86].)

In addition to the generic categories of adolescent self-concept described by Harter, ethnic and sexual minority adolescents also must consolidate a sense of identity vis-á-vis both their minority group and the mainstream culture (23,53).

CLINICAL ASPECTS OF ADOLESCENCE

On the basis of many epidemiologic studies, it now appears that only approximately 20% of adolescents have diagnosable clinical disorders. However, it is equally clear that during adolescence, a substantial proportion of youngsters experience increased conflicts with parents and mood difficulties and engage in risk behaviors.

The Storm and Stress Debate Revisited

Historically, there has been a debate over the frequency and severity with which adolescent turmoil occurs and the extent to which it should be considered normative in American culture or universal across epochs and cultures (for a review of this issue, see Muus [83] and Arnett [12]).

Although, over the centuries, adolescents have at times been idealized for their beauty and grace or as bearing the hope of the future, they also have been regarded by their elders with deep misgivings and dismay as potentially disruptive and subversive, not only difficult to handle, but threatening to undermine society's strictures regarding sex, aggression, and respect for elders.

The term *adolescence* was coined as recently as 1904 by G. Stanley Hall (87), who saw adolescence as intrinsically a time of "storm and stress," with "a period of semicriminality [being] normal for all healthy [adolescent] boys" (vol. 1, p. 404, quoted in 11). Speaking of the internal emotional upheavals of adolescence, rather than overt deviant behavior, Anna Freud (64) noted, "the upholding of a steady equilibrium during the adolescent process is in itself abnormal" (p. 164). She observed that:

> it is normal for an adolescent to behave for a considerable length of time in an inconsistent and unpredictable manner; to fight his impulses and to accept them; to ward them off successfully and to be overrun by them; to love his parents and to hate them; to revolt against them and to be dependent on them...to thrive on imitation of and identification with others while searching unceasingly for his own identity; to be more idealistic, artistic, generous and unselfish than he will ever be again, but also the opposite—self-centered, egoistic, and calculating (pp. 164–165).

In more recent years, the view of adolescence as inherently tumultuous has come under attack as an inaccurate overgeneralization from mental health professionals' clinical samples, from a romantic notion of youthful struggle (88), or from popular authors' vivid portrayals of their own idiosyncratic adolescent experiences. In contrast, seminal surveys of nonclinical adolescent populations by Offer and colleagues (61,84) have led to the conclusion that "adolescence is not a time of severe disturbance for all adolescents. Moreover, ... a significant percentage of adolescents (80%) do not experience adolescent turmoil, relate well to their families and peers, and are comfortable with their social and cultural values.... [T]eenagers who exhibit little disequilibrium are normal... [and]... adolescence is a period of development that can be traversed without turmoil and that the transition to adulthood is accomplished gradually and without undue upheaval" (61, p. 1004).

This debate may turn on matters of degree (e.g., what type and severity of turmoil). In a review of the topic, Arnett (12, p. 324) concluded:

> [T]here is support for Hall's (1904) view that a tendency toward some aspects of storm and stress exists in adolescence. In their conflicts with parents, in their mood disruptions, and in their heightened rates of a variety of types of risk behavior, many adolescents exhibit a heightened degree of storm and stress compared with other periods of life. Their parents, too, often experience difficulty—from increased conflict when their children are in early adolescence, from mood disruptions during mid-adolescence, and from anxiety over the increased possibilities of risk behavior when children are in late adolescence. However...there are cultural differences in storm and stress, and within cultures there are individual differences in the extent to which adolescents exhibit the different aspects of it.
>
> [However], [e]ven amidst the storm and stress of adolescence, most adolescents take pleasure in many aspects of their lives, are satisfied with most of their relationships most of the time, and are hopeful about the future.

Having examined conflicts with parents, we turn to a more detailed consideration of mood problems and risk behaviors.

Mood Difficulties and Perceived Stress

Adolescence is a time of rising incidence for major depression, with the risk of depression and the preponderance of affected girls versus boys increasing not only with age, but more specifically with advancing pubertal status.

Only a minority of adolescents develop a full-blown affective disorder. Nonetheless, adolescence sees a marked increase in emotional lability, depressed mood, and negative emotions (e.g., anxiety and self-consciousness), with over one-third of adolescents in nonclinical samples reporting high levels of depressed mood (12,89–91). For example, the national Youth Risk Behavior Survey (14) of high school students found that, during the preceding year, 40% of girls and 20% of boys felt sad or hopeless almost every day for at least 2 weeks in a row that they stopped doing some usual activities and 23% and 12%, respectively, had seriously considered attempting suicide. Mood disruptions are associated with higher levels of negative life events (91,92). Comparing fifth graders and ninth graders, Larson and Richards (90) describe the dramatic decline in the proportion of time youngsters feel "very happy," "proud," or "in control" as an emotional fall from grace.

Girls appear especially prone to negative moods (91). For example, Offer and colleagues (84) found marked gender differences in emotional vulnerability across adolescence. Compared with boys, girls described themselves as moodier, sadder, lonelier, more prone to uncontrollable crying, more easily hurt, less autonomous and more other-directed, and more ashamed of their bodies.

Adolescents also report a substantial increase in the number of negative life events. It is difficult to determine to what extent this reflects a more stressful environment, greater sensitivity to events, or shifts in the types of situations that precipitate negative emotions (91,93,94). The nature and sources of perceived stress change over the course of adolescence, with early adolescents experiencing stress in relationship to peers and older adolescents with respect to academic issues. Especially in early adolescence, girls appear to experience more stress than at other ages and to perceive more stressful events than do boys (93,95,96).

Although significant life events, such as parental separations or unemployment, moves, or deaths, have a serious impact on adolescents, many of the fluctuations in adolescent mood reflect the less dramatic daily hassles—homework, tests, disagreements with friends—the minor disappointments, stresses, and embarrassments that form the fabric of adolescent life. It may be deceptive, however, to try to conceptualize and quantify these hassles as completely independent external variables because unlike many major life events, the intensity, valence, and even the occurrence of such episodes often lie largely in the eye of the adolescent beholder (63).

Time-sampling studies of adolescent mood in community samples find that, compared with adults, adolescents have greater mood variability as measured by both the width of their mood swings (between extreme highs and lows) and the evanescence of these extremes (63). In the nonclinical high school population studied, greater subjectively experienced mood lability was not associated with poorer adjustment or other pathologic processes.

As noted earlier, developmental neurobiologic factors (including hormonal ones [91]) also may influence the impaired mood regulation and increased stress reactivity observed in adolescence (41,50).

A longitudinal study by Angold and colleagues (97) found that reaching Tanner stage III was associated with increased levels of depression in girls; however, hormonal levels of testosterone and estradiol were more closely associated with levels of depression than age or Tanner stage per se. Although this suggests that it is not morphologic body changes themselves that render pubertal girls more prone to depression, it is unclear whether these findings reflect direct depressogenic endocrine influences on the central nervous system or hormonally mediated changes in responsivity to life events and stress.

Spear (18,28) proposed that age-related changes in the balance of dopamine regulation in the prefrontal cortex relative to mesolimbic brain regions lead to shifts in the incentive value and motivational power of different reinforcers. Drawing on both human and animal data, Spear proposes a transient relative "reward deficiency syndrome" or "adolescent anhedonia" that results in previously pleasurable activities being experienced as less rewarding and leads to a compensatory search for new and more intense forms of stimulation (e.g., greater novelty seeking, risk taking, and increases in consummatory behaviors, such as food and drugs). Adolescents' decision-making about risks may be as good as adults under affectively neutral conditions (so-called "cold" cognition); however adolescent's prefrontal cognitive functioning and inhibition is impaired under conditions of even mild stress or emotional arousal (so-called "hot" cognition) leading to difficulty suppressing responses to appetive social cues; other aspects of adolescent brain development may further amplify these stress-induced deficits (35,50,98).

Risk-Taking Behaviors

Adolescent risk-taking behavior is a significant source of morbidity and mortality in this otherwise healthy age group. In contrast to persons 25 years of age or older, for whom two-thirds of all deaths are due to cardiovascular disease and cancer, three-fourths of all deaths for youths 10 to 24 years of age are due to motor vehicle crashes, other unintentional injuries, homicide, and suicide. Behaviors that increase the risk of these adverse outcomes are common among teenagers. The national Youth Risk Behavior Survey (14) found that for the 30 days preceding the survey, 6% of high school students reported rarely or never wearing a seat belt, 18% had ridden with a driver who had been drinking and, among the 61% of adolescents who drove, 41% had texted or emailed while driving and 7.8% of adolescent drivers had driven a vehicle when they had been drinking and 22% had driven having used marijuana. Over all, in the preceding month, 16.2% of high school students had carried a weapon, 32.8% had drunk alcohol, 18.5% had smoked tobacco, 21.7% had used marijuana, and 8.6% had attempted suicide in the prior 12 months. Other health-impairing behaviors also were common. About 41% of the students had had sexual intercourse; of these, 43% had not used a condom at the last intercourse.

These risk behaviors are not uniformly distributed across the adolescent population. For example, among ninth graders, 22% are estimated to be at low risk, with no involvement with any risk behaviors such as substance use, sex, depression/suicide, antisocial behavior, school problems, unsafe vehicle use, or bulimia (99). Another 29% report only one such risk indicator, 18% report two, and 31% report three or more. High-risk youth (those reporting multiple risk behaviors) are characterized by early onset of high-risk behaviors, absence of nurturing parenting, child abuse, lack of involvement with school, susceptibility to peer influence, depression, disadvantaged neighborhoods, and lack of gainfully employed role models.

Certain patterns of autonomic reactivity may also predispose to increased risk taking under certain circumstances (100), and data from nonhuman primates suggest important interactions between genetically determined variations in neurotransmitter regulation and early rearing environment (see below).

It is important to distinguish between occasional experimentation and persistent patterns of dangerous behavior (23). Although most adolescents will experiment with alcohol or minor delinquent behaviors, in most cases these behaviors do not persist into adulthood. Studies in both human and nonhuman adolescents suggest that certain aspects of the neurobiology of the adolescent brain may make adolescents more vulnerable to substance abuse (101,102). (In turn, chronic alcohol, marijuana, or nicotine use during adolescence may have long-lasting deleterious effects on cognitive functioning). Human and animal research also suggests that certain personality and temperamental traits and genotypes may predispose adolescents to alcohol or nicotine abuse (102,103).

The prevalence of problem behaviors does increase in adolescence and early adulthood, but persistence in problem behaviors, such as substance use or antisocial behavior, usually is associated with difficulties in earlier childhood (104). The work of Jessor (75) and others (105) suggests that risk-taking behaviors such as sexual activity, substance use, reckless driving, and delinquency not only increase over adolescence but frequently are associated with each other and share common psychosocial antecedents. These behaviors are not simply arbitrary, perverse, or motivated only by sensation-seeking or exploratory motives, but are in part purposeful, meaningful, goal-oriented, and functional (106). For example, Jessor (75) observes that such behaviors also can serve the instrumental ends of gaining peer acceptance, establishing autonomy from parents, defying conventional authority, relieving anxiety or frustration, or affirming the transition to a more adult status.

Although the propensity to impulsivity, risk taking, and sensation seeking has important family and social determinants, it also appears to reflect the developmental immaturities in the neural mechanisms underlying inhibitory control, emotional processing, and executive functioning discussed earlier. Shifts in reward sensitivity occur early in adolescence and lead adolescents to seek higher levels of novelty and stimulation, while the more slow-maturing regulatory competencies that might check this novelty and stimulation seeking do not come online until later in adolescence (32,35,107).

ETHOLOGIC PERSPECTIVES

Examination of the transition from youth to adulthood in other mammalian (especially nonhuman primate) species suggests animal models for the counterpart of human adolescence. Like human adolescents, the young of other species exhibit increases in peer-directed social interactions and greater novelty-seeking and risk-taking behaviors (108). Spear (18,109) has suggested that these shared behavioral features represent ontogenetic adaptations that help individuals in this transitional period in "acquiring the necessary skills to permit survival away from parental caretakers. Increased affiliation with peers and the taking of risks via exploring novel areas, behaviors, and reenforcers may also help facilitate the dispersal of adolescents away from the natal family unit" (18, p. 418), with the adaptive goal of avoiding inbreeding. Similarly, human adolescents and many pubertal nonhuman primates spend increased time in social interactions with peers, including aggressive fighting, but also in reconciliatory and affiliative behaviors; paralleling this shift in social orientation from adults to peers is an increase in conflicts between the adolescent and parents, which also may help to encourage separation from the natal family unit (110,111). Increased risk taking also is seen across species, with increased exploratory behavior and novelty seeking, but also increased mortality. From an evolutionary perspective, such risk taking "may be—or at least once were—means of securing physical resources, attracting mates, and denying mating opportunities to competitors" (111, p. 117).

Research on nonhuman primates also provides clues about the complex interplay of heritable and environmental factors that shape risky behaviors during adolescence. Juvenile rhesus males with low CSF 5-HIAA are at increased risk to be expelled early from their natal troop and have very high mortality rates (46%) over a 4-year period compared to their peers with higher 5-CSF HIAA (0%) (112). Their high mortality rates (and unpopularity) reflect their excessively aggressive and impulsive behaviors, including inappropriate attacks on peers and higher-ranking adults and other risky behaviors, such as excessively dangerous leaps from tree to tree. Although 5-HIAA is a highly heritable trait in rhesus monkeys, it is also strongly influenced by early social experiences, especially attachment relationships, with peer-reared monkeys exhibiting lower CSF 5-HIAA levels throughout their life span than mother-reared counterparts. Gene x environment interactions are also apparent in the influence of early rearing conditions on the impact of other genotypes in adolescent nonhuman primates (103,113).

THE CLOSE OF ADOLESCENCE

The pubertal changes that are the hallmark of adolescence provide a relatively clear marker for the beginning of adolescence. In contrast, the close of adolescence in contemporary society is less clearly defined. At one time in the United States and even today in traditional societies, the end of adolescence and assumption of adult status was usually marked by a discrete event, such as marriage, beginning of full-time employment, or military service. Currently, however, the same forces that have helped to create adolescence as a distinctive period of life in industrial and postindustrial society also have blurred the end of adolescence (1,114). College and postgraduate education has become increasingly important, and the proportion of youth pursuing post–high school education has risen from 14% in 1940 to over 65% in 2014. Correspondingly, the median age of marriage in the United States rose from 21 years for women and 23 years for men in 1970 to 27 years for women and 29 years for men in 2010. Thus, for many young people, entry into adult roles regarding work, marriage, and parenthood is delayed until the late twenties or even early thirties.

Arnett (1,114) has proposed that the period from the late teens through the twenties be considered a distinctive period he terms *emerging adulthood*. In contrast to adolescents, 95% of whom live in a parental home, most young people age 18 years or older in the United States leave home, approximately one-third to live in a college setting and approximately 40% to live independently and work full time. Approximately two-thirds cohabit for a time with a romantic partner. However, despite high rates of residential mobility in the twenties, many young people retain some degree of dependence on their parents.

Hence, adolescence gives way to a prolonged period of quasi-autonomy and continued identity and vocational exploration that only gradually draws to a close in the third decade of life with the consolidation of an adult work identity, the capacity for adult friendships and a lasting intimate relationship, the emergence of a more mutual and equal relationship with parents, the integration of new attitudes toward time, and the beginning contemplation of parenthood (115).

References

1. Arnett JJ: Emerging adulthood: a theory of development from the late teens through the twenties. *Am Psychol* 55:469–480, 2000.
2. Woolard JL, Scott E: The legal regulation of adolescence. In: Lerner R, Steinberg L (eds): *Handbook of Adolescent Psychology*. Vol. 2. Hoboken, NJ, John Wiley & Sons, 345–371, 2009.

3. Roberts DF, Henriksen L, Foehr UG: Adolescence, adolescents, and media. In: Lerner R, Steinberg L (eds): *Handbook of Adolescent Psychology*. Vol. 2. Hoboken, NJ, John Wiley & Sons, 314–344, 2009.
4. Winnicott DW: Further thoughts on babies as persons. In: Hardenberg J (ed): *The Child and the Outside World: Studies in Developing Relationships*. London, England, Tavistock Publications Ltd, 134–140, 1957. (Original work published 1947).
5. Burton LM, Garrett-Peters R, Eaton SC: More than good quotations. How ethnography informs knowledge on adolescent development and context. In: Lerner R, Steinberg L (eds): *Handbook of Adolescent Psychology*. Vol. 1. Hoboken, NJ, John Wiley & Sons, 55–91, 2009.
6. Collins WA, Steinberg L: Adolescent development in interpersonal context. In: Damon W, Lerner RM (eds): *Handbook of Child Psychology*. Vol. 3. Hoboken, NJ, John Wiley & Sons, 1003–1067, 2006.
7. Lee Y, Stryve D: Influences on the onset and tempo of puberty in human beings and implications for adolescent psychological development. *Hormon Behav* 64:250–261, 2014.
8. Susman EJ, Dorn L: Puberty: its role in development. In: Lerner R, Steinberg L (eds): *Handbook of Adolescent Psychology*. Vol. 1. Hoboken, NJ, John Wiley & Sons, 116–151, 2009.
9. Reiss D: *The Relationship Code: Deciphering Genetic and Social Influences on Adolescent Development*. Cambridge, MA, Harvard University Press, 2000.
10. Larson R, Wilson S, Rickman A: Globalization, societal change, and adolescence across the world. In: Lerner R, Steinberg L (eds): *Handbook of Adolescent Psychology*. Vol. 2. Hoboken, NJ, John Wiley & Sons, 590–622, 2009.
11. Way N, Chu JY (eds): *Adolescent Boys: Exploring Diverse Cultures of Boyhood*. New York, University Press, 2004.
12. Arnett J: Adolescent storm and stress, reconsidered. *Am Psychol* 54: 317–326, 1999.
13. Schlegel A: Cross-cultural issues in the study of adolescent development. In: Lerner R, Steinberg L (eds): *Handbook of Adolescent Psychology*. Vol. 2. Hoboken, NJ, John Wiley & Sons, 570–589, 2009.
14. Centers for Disease Control and Prevention: Youth risk behavior surveillance—United States, 2015. *Morb Mortal Wkly Rep* 65(6):1–174, 2016.
15. Rideout VJ, Foehr UG, Roberts DF: Generation M^2: Media in the lives of 8–18 year-olds. A Kaiser Family Foundation Study. January, 2010. Available at: http://kff.org/other/report/generation-m2-media-in-the-lives-of-8-to-18-year-olds/. Accessed September 1, 2016.
16. Turkle S: *Alone Together: Why We Expect More from Technology and Less from Each Other*. New York, Basic Books, 2012.
17. Weisberg J: We are hopelessly hooked. *N Y Rev Books* 63(3), 2016.
18. Spear LP: The adolescent brain and age-related behavioral manifestations. *Neurosci Biobehav Rev* 24:417–463, 2000.
19. Tanner JM: Sequence and tempo in the somatic changes in puberty. In: Grumbach GG, Mayer FE (eds): *Control of the Onset of Puberty* New York, John Wiley & Sons, 448–470, 1974.
20. Herman-Giddens ME, Slora EJ, Wasserman RC, et al.: Secondary sexual characteristics and menses in young girls seen in office practice: a study from the Pediatric Research in Office Settings network. *Pediatrics* 99:505–512, 1997.
21. Stein JH, Reiser LW: A study of white middle-class adolescent boys' responses to "semenarche" (the first ejaculation). *J Youth Adolesc* 23:373–384, 1994.
22. Graber JA: Pubertal timing and the development of psychopathology in adolescence and beyond. *Hormon Behav* 64:262–269, 2013.
23. Steinberg L, Morris AS: Adolescent development. *Annu Rev Psychol* 52(1):83–110, 2001.
24. Bourgeois JP, Rakic P: Changes of synaptic density in the primary visual cortex of the macaque monkey from fetal to adult stage. *J Neurosci* 13:2801–2820, 1993.
25. Rakic P, Bourgeois JP, Goldman-Rakic PS: Synaptic development of the cerebral cortex: implications for learning, memory, and mental illness. *Prog Brain Res* 102:227–243, 1994.
26. Sowell E, Thompson PM, Holmes CJ, Jernigan TL, Toga AW: In vivo evidence for post-adolescent brain maturation in frontal and striatal regions. *Nat Neurosci* 2(10):859–861, 1999.
27. Lenroot RK, Giedd JN: Brain development in children and adolescents: insights from anatomical magnetic resonance imaging. *Neurosci Biobehav Rev* 30(6):718–729, 2006.
28. Spear LP: Adolescent neurodevelopment. *J Adolesc Health* 52(2): S7–S13, 2013.
29. Nagy Z, Westerberg H, Klingberg T: Maturation of white matter is associated with the development of cognitive functions during childhood. *J Cognit Neurosci* 16(7):1227–1233, 2004.
30. Mabbott DJ, Noseworthy M, Bouffet E, Laughlin S, Rockel C: White matter growth as a mechanism of cognitive development in children. *Neuroimage* 33(3):936–946, 2006.
31. Steinberg L, Albert D, Cauffman E, Banich M, Graham S, Woolard J: Age differences in sensation seeking and impulsivity as indexed by behavior and self-report: evidence for a dual systems model. *Dev Psychol* 44(6):1764, 2008.
32. Shulman E, Smith AR, Silva K, et al.: The dual systems model: review, reappraisal, and reaffirmation. *Dev Cogn Neurosci* 17:103–117, 2016.
33. Casey BJ, Getz S, Galvan A: The adolescent brain. *Dev Rev* 28(1):62–77, 2008.
34. Ernst M, Pine DS, Hardin M: Triadic model of the neurobiology of motivated behavior in adolescence. *Psychol Med* 36(3):299–312, 2006.
35. Casey BJ, Galván A, Somerville LH: Beyond simple models of adolescence to an integrated circuit-based account: a commentary. *Dev Cognit Neurosci* 17:128–130, 2016.
36. Galvan A, Hare TA, Parra CE, et al.: Earlier development of the accumbens relative to orbitofrontal cortex might underlie risk-taking behavior in adolescents. *J Neurosci* 26(25):6885–6892, 2006.
37. Galvan A, Hare T, Voss H, Glover G, Casey BJ: Risk-taking and the adolescent brain: who is at risk? *Dev Sci* 10(2):F8–F14, 2007.
38. Braams B, van Duijvenvoorde AC, Peper JS, Crone EA: Longitudinal changes in adolescent risk-taking: a comprehensive study of neural responses to rewards, pubertal development, and risk-taking behavior. *J Neurosci* 35(18):7226–7238, 2015.
39. Monk CS, McClure EB, Nelson EE, et al.: Adolescent immaturity in attention-related brain engagement to emotional facial expressions. *Neuroimage* 20(1):420–428, 2003.
40. Hare TA, Tottenham N, Galvan A, Voss HU, Glover GH, Casey BJ: Biological substrates of emotional reactivity and regulation in adolescence during an emotional go–no go task. *Biol Psychiatry* 63(10):927–934, 2008.
41. Silvers JA, Shu J, Hubbard AD, Weber J, Ochsner KN: Concurrent and lasting effects of emotion regulation on amygdala response in adolescence and young adulthood. *Dev Sci* 18(5):771–784, 2014.
42. Hagenauer MH, Lee TM: Adolescent sleep patterns in humans and laboratory animals. *Hormon Behav* 64(2):270–279, 2014.
43. Carskadon MA, Acebo C, Jenni OG: Regulation of adolescent sleep: implications for behavior. *Ann N Y Acad Sci* 1021:276–291, 2004.
44. Tarokh L, Saletin JM, Carskadon MA: Sleep in adolescence: physiology, cognition and mental health. *Neurosci Biobehav Rev* 70:182–188, 2016.
45. Adolescent Sleep Working Group; Committee on Adolescence; Council on School Health: Policy statement: school start times for adolescence. *Pediatrics* 134(3):642–649, 2014.
46. Kuhn D: Adolescent thinking. In: Lerner R, Steinberg L (eds): *Handbook of Adolescent Psychology*. Vol. 1. Hoboken, NJ, John Wilen & Sons, 152–186, 2009.
47. Eisenberg N, Morris AS, McDaniels B, Spinrad TL: Moral cognitions and prosocial responding in adolescence. In: Lerner R, Steinberg L (eds): *Handbook of Adolescent Psychology*. Hoboken, NJ, Wiley, 229–265, 2009.
48. Smetna JG, Villalobos M: Social cognitive development in adolescence. In: Lerner R, Steinberg L (eds): *Handbook of Adolescent Psychology*. Vol. 1. Hoboken, NJ, John Wiley & Sons, 187–228, 2009.
49. Dahl RE: The development of affect regulation: bringing together basic and clinical perspectives. *Ann N Y Acad Sci* 1008:183–188, 2003.
50. Arnsten AF, Shansky RM: Adolescence: vulnerable period for stress-induced prefrontal cortical function? *Ann N Y Acad Sci* 1021: 143–147, 2004.
51. Smith AR, Chein J, Steinberg L: Impact of socio-emotional context, brain development, and pubertal maturation on adolescent risk-taking. *Hormon Behav* 64(2):323–332, 2013.
52. Erikson EH: *Childhood and Society*. New York, Norton, 1963.
53. Cote JE: Identity formation and self-development in adolescence. In: Lerner R, Steinberg L (eds): *Handbook of Adolescent Psychology*. Vol. 1. Hoboken, NJ, John Wiley & Sons, 266–304, 2009.
54. Seltzer VC: *Psychosocial Worlds of the Adolescent: Public and Private*. New York, John Wiley & Sons, 1989.
55. Felice ME: Adolescence. In: Levine MD, Carey WB, Crocker AC (eds): *Developmental-Behavioral Pediatrics*. Philadelphia, PA, WB Saunders, 66, 1992.
56. Mueller AS: The role of school contexts in adolescents' weight-loss behaviors and self-perceptions of overweight. *Sociol Inquiry* 85(4): 532–555, 2015.
57. Hendren RL, Barber JK, Sigafoos A: Eating-disordered symptoms in a non-clinical population: a study of female adolescents in two private schools. *J Am Acad Child Psychiatry* 25:836–840, 1986.
58. Pisetsky EM, Chao YM, Dierker LC, May AM, Striegel-Moore RH: Disordered eating and substance use in high-school students: results from the Youth Risk Behaviour Surveillance System. *Int J Eat Disorder* 41:464–470, 2008.
59. Martin A: On teenagers and tattoos. *J Am Acad Child Adolesc Psychiatry* 36(6):860–861, 1997.
60. Ritvo S: The image and uses of the body in psychic conflict: with special reference to eating disorders in adolescence. *Psychoanal Study Child* 39:449–469, 1992.
61. Offer D, Schonert-Reichl KA: Debunking the myths of adolescence: findings from recent research. *J Am Acad Child Adolesc Psychiatry* 31:1003–1014, 1992.
62. Laursen B, Collins WA: Parent-child relationships during adolescence. In: Lerner R, Steinberg L (eds): *Handbook of Adolescent Psychology*. Vol. 2. Hoboken, NJ, John Wiley & Sons, 3–42, 2009.
63. Csikszentmihalyi M, Larson R: *Being Adolescent: Conflict and Growth in the Teenage Years*. New York, Basic Books, 1984.

64. Freud A: Adolescence. In: *The Writings of Anna Freud*. New York, International Universities Press, 136–166, 1958/1969 (1956–1965).
65. Wolf AE: *Get Out of My Life, but First Could You Drive Me and Cheryl to the Mall? A Parent's Guide to the New Teenager.* New York, Noonday Press, 1991.
66. Laursen B, Coy KC, Collins WA: Reconsidering changes in parent-child conflict across adolescence: a meta-analysis. *Child Dev* 69:817–832, 1998.
67. Montemayor R, Hanson E: A naturalistic view of conflict between adolescents and their parents and siblings. *J Early Adolesc* 5:23–30, 1985.
68. Graber JA, Brooks-Gunn J: Sometimes I think that you don't like me: how mothers and daughters negotiate the transition into adolescence. In: Cox MJ, Brooks-Gunn J (eds): *Conflict and Cohesion in Families: Causes and Consequences.* Mahwah, NJ, Lawrence Erlbaum, 207–242, 1999.
69. DiClemente RJ, Hansen W, Ponton LE (eds): *Handbook of Adolescent Health Risk Behavior.* New York, Plenum, 1996.
70. Ozer EM, Irwin CE Jr: Adolescent and young adult health: from basic health status to clinical interventions. In: Lerner R, Steinberg L (eds): *Handbook of Adolescent Psychology*. Vol. 1. Hoboken, NJ, John Wiley & Sons, 618–641, 2009.
71. King RA, Lewis M: The difficult child. *Child Adolesc Psychiatr Clin North Am* 3:531–541, 1994.
72. Brooks-Gunn J, Paikoff R: Sexuality and developmental transitions during adolescence. In: Schulenberg J, Maggs J, Hurrelmann K (eds): *Health Risks and Developmental Transitions During Adolescence.* Cambridge, Cambridge University Press, 190–219, 1997.
73. Brown BB, Larson J: Peer relationships in adolescence. In: Lerner R, Steinberg L (eds): *Handbook of Adolescent Psychology*. Vol. 2. Hoboken, NJ, John Wiley & Sons, 74–103, 2009.
74. Csikszentmihalyi M, Larson R, Prescott S: The ecology of adolescent activity and experience. *J Youth Adolesc* 6:281–294, 1977.
75. Jessor R: Risk behavior in adolescence: a psychosocial framework for understanding and action. *J Adolesc Health Care* 12:597–605, 1991.
76. Diamond LM, Savin-Williams RC: Adolescent sexuality. In: Lerner R, Steinberg L (eds): *Handbook of Adolescent Psychology*. Vol. 1. Hoboken, NJ, John Wiley & Sons, 479–523, 2009.
77. Katchadourian H: *Sexuality at the Threshold: The Developing Adolescent.* Cambridge, MA, Harvard University Press, 330–351, 1990.
78. Herdt G, McClintock M: The magical age of 10. *Arch Sex Behav* 29: 587–606, 2000.
79. Friedrich WN, Grambsch P, Broughton D, Kuiper J, Beilke RL: Normative sexual behavior in children. *Pediatrics* 88:456–464, 1991.
80. Steensma TD, Kreukels BP, de Vries AL, Cohen-Kettenis PT: Gender identity development in adolescence. *Hormon Behav* 64(2):288–297, 2013.
81. Laufer M: The central masturbation fantasy, the final sexual organization, and adolescence. *Psychoanal Study Child* 31:297–316, 1976.
82. Furman W, Brown B, Feiring C: *The Development of Romantic Relationships in Adolescence.* New York, Cambridge University Press, 1999.
83. Muus RE: *Theories of Adolescence.* New York, Random House, 1988.
84. Offer D, Ostrov E, Howard KI: *The Teenage World: Adolescents' Self-image in Ten Countries.* New York, Plenum Medical, 1988.
85. Harter S: *The Construction of the Self: A Developmental Perspective.* New York, Guilford Press, 1999.
86. McGuire S, Manke B, Saudino KJ, Reiss D, Hetherington EM, Plomin R: Perceived competence and self-worth during adolescence: a longitudinal behavioral genetic study. *Child Dev* 70:1283–1296, 1999.
87. Hall GS: *Adolescence: Its Psychology and Its Relation to Physiology, Anthropology, Sociology, Sex, Crime, Religion and Education.* Englewood Cliffs, NJ, Prentice Hall, 1904.
88. Rakoff VM: Nietzsche and the romantic construction of adolescence. *Adolesc Psychiatry Dev Clin Studies* 22:39–56, 1998.
89. Petersen AC, Compas BE, Brooks-Gunn J, Stemmler M, Ey S, Grant KE: Depression in adolescence. *Am Psychol* 48:155–168, 1993.
90. Larson R, Richards MH: *Divergent Realities: The Emotional Lives of Mothers, Fathers, and Adolescents.* New York, Basic Books, 1994.
91. Graber JA, Sontag LM: Internalizing problems during adolescence. In: Lerner R, Steinberg L (eds): *Handbook of Adolescent Psychology.* Vol. 1. Hoboken, NJ, John Wiley & Sons, 642–682, 2009.
92. Brooks-Gunn J: *How Stressful Is the Transition to Adolescence in Girls? Adolescent Stress: Causes and Consequences.* In: Coltern MD, Gore S (eds): Hawthorne, NY, Aldine de Gruyter, 131–149, 1991.
93. Wagner BM, Compas BE: Gender, instrumentality, and expressivity: moderators of the relation between stress and psychological symptoms during adolescence. *Am J Commun Psychol* 18:383–406, 1990.
94. Larson R, Asmussen L: Anger, worry, and hurt in early adolescence: an enlarging world of negative emotions. In: Colten ME, Gore S (eds): *Adolescent Stress: Causes and Consequences.* New York, Aldine de Gruyter, 21–41, 1991.
95. Vik P, Brown SA: Life events and substance abuse during adolescence. *Children of Trauma: Stressful Life Events and Their Effect on Adolescents,* 179–205, 1998.
96. Ge X, Lorenz FO, Conger RD, Elder GH, Simons RL: Trajectories of stressful life events and depressive symptoms during adolescence. *Developmental psychology* 30(4):467, 1994.
97. Angold A, Costello EJ, Erkanli A, Worthman CM: Pubertal changes in hormone levels and depression in girls. *Psychol Med* 29:1043–1053, 1999.
98. Casey BJ, Caudle K: The teenage brain: self control. *Curr Direct Psychol Sci* 22(2):82–87, 2013.
99. Dryfoos JG: *Safe Passage: Making it Through Adolescence in a Risky Society.* Oxford, Oxford University Press, 1998.
100. Liang SW, Jemerin JM, Tschann JM, Irwin CE Jr, Wara DW, Boyce WT: Life events, cardiovascular reactivity, and risk behavior in adolescent boys. *Pediatrics* 96:1101–1105, 1995.
101. Spear LP, Varlinskaya EI: Adolescence. Alcohol sensitivity, tolerance, and intake. *Recent Dev Alcohol* 17:143–159, 2005.
102. Chassin L, Hussong A, Beltran I: Adolescent substance use. In: Lerner RM, Steinberg L (eds): *Handbook of Adolescent Psychology*. Vol. 1. Hoboken, NJ, John Wiley & Sons, 723–763, 2009.
103. Suomi SJ: Gene-environment interactions and the neurobiology of social conflict. *Ann N Y Acad Sci* 1008:132–139, 2003.
104. Arnett J: Reckless behavior in adolescence: a developmental perspective. *Dev Rev* 12:339–373, 1992.
105. Igra V, Irwin CE Jr: Theories of adolescent risk-taking behavior. In: DiClemente HW, Ponton LE (eds): *Handbook of Adolescent Health Risk Behavior.* New York, Plenum, 1996:35–51.
106. Willoughby T, Good M, Adachi PJ, Hamza C, Tavernier R: Examining the link between adolescent brain development and risk taking from a social–developmental perspective. *Brain Cogn* 83(3):315–323, 2013.
107. Steinberg L: Risk taking in adolescence: what changes, and why? *Ann N Y Acad Sci* 1021:51–58, 2004.
108. Kelley AE, Schochet T, Landry CF: Risk taking and novelty seeking in adolescence. *Ann N Y Acad Sci* 1021:27–32, 2004.
109. Spear LP: Adolescent brain development and animal models. *Ann N Y Acad Sci* 1021:23–26, 2004.
110. Steinberg L: Pubertal maturation and parent-adolescent distance: an evolutionary perspective. In: Adams GR, Montemayor R, Gullotta TP (eds): *Advances in Adolescent Behavior and Development.* Newbury Park, CA, Sage Publications, 71–97, 1989.
111. Steinberg L, Belsky J: An evolutionary perspective on psychopathology in adolescence. In: *Rochester Symposium on Developmental Psychopathology. Adolescence: Opportunities and Challenges.* Vol. 7. Rochester, NY, University of Rochester Press, 93–124, 1996.
112. Higley JD, Mehlman PT, Higley SB, et al.: Excessive mortality in young free-ranging male nonhuman primates with low cerebrospinal fluid 5-hydroxyindoleacetic acid concentrations. *Arch Gen Psychiatry* 53:537–543, 1996.
113. Barr CS, Newman TK, Becker ML, et al.: The utility of the non-human primate model for studying gene by environment interactions in behavioral research. *Genes Brain Behav* 2(6):336–340, 2003.
114. Arnett JJ, Tanner JL (eds): *Emerging Adults in America: Coming of Age in the 21st century.* Washington, DC, American Psychological Association, 2006.
115. Colarusso CA: Adulthood. In: Sadock BJ, Sadock VA, Ruiz P (eds): *Kaplan and Sadock's Comprehensive Textbook of Psychiatry.* Vol. 2. Philadelphia, PA, Lippincott Williams & Wilkins, 3909–3931, 2009.

2.2 ■ DIVERSE POPULATIONS

CHAPTER 2.2.1 ■ CULTURAL CHILD AND ADOLESCENT PSYCHIATRY

G. PIROOZ SHOLEVAR AND SHASHANK V. JOSHI

INTRODUCTION

Cultural child and adolescent psychiatry consists of a body of theoretical and technical knowledge that informs high-quality psychiatric evaluation, treatment, and assessment of developmental process across cultural and language barriers to children, adolescents, and families. Clinicians are increasingly called upon to evaluate or treat patients from multiple cultural and linguistic groups. In our multicultural American society, treating a patient who speaks a different language or holds beliefs at variance with the majority culture requires the knowledge and skills that constitute cultural psychiatry (1). Cultural psychiatry defines the impact of culture on psychiatric evaluation and diagnosis, and provides guidelines for culturally competent and sensitive psychiatric treatment and systems of care (1–3). It is characterized by introducing the diversity of human experience into an understanding of the complexities of mental health and illness.

Cultural psychiatry has evolved consistently throughout the past century. Initially and at the beginning of the 20th century, it was primarily concerned with comparison of manifestations of mental disorders in different cultures and countries. It described the exotic and special features of different syndromes and disorders discovered in Africa, the Far East, and other non-Western countries. The descriptions were based on a universalist (and Western) viewpoint of psychiatry and mental disorders. In the mid-20th century, prominent anthropologists such as Ruth Benedict, Margaret Mead, and Bronislaw Malinowski incorporated psychoanalytic constructs into their cultural investigations of the impact of culture on personality development and disorders (4). This highly productive collaboration between psychiatry and anthropology also included Emile Durkhiem's landmark study on suicide and George Herbert Mead's Symbolic Interactionalist Theory.

The interest in sound methodologic measures in the mid-20th century resulted in the construction of a number of cross-culturally validated epidemiologic and diagnostic instruments. Recent findings based partially on such methodology have resulted in a gradual shift from a universalist viewpoint to a more culturally specific perspective (1,2,5).

The value orientation theory was originally proposed by Kluckhohn (6). It is based on variations in generalized cultural values. According to Kluckhohn, there are three possible variations in solution to the problems of time (past, present, future); activity (doing, being, being-in-becoming); relationship in groups (individual, collateral, linear); man–nature relationship (harmony-with-nature, mastery-over-nature, subjugated-to-nature); and basic nature of man (neutral/mixed, good, evil).

Cultures vary widely in these dimensions. For example, American culture emphasizes a future time orientation, a "doing" mode of activity, an "individualistic" relational orientation focusing on autonomy; mastery over nature; and the nature of man as neutral or mixed. Using this now-dated typology, Spiegel (7) pointed how Southern Italians in contrast are oriented toward present, being, collateral relational view, subjugation by nature, and a mixed view of human nature, while Southern Irish are oriented toward present, being, lineal relationships, subjugation by nature, and the evil nature of man. In their views, the contrast between variable value orientations can create interpersonal tension and conflicts, such as in a cross-cultural marriage.

The *cultural relativist* perspective of current cultural psychiatry is in contrast to the *universalist* one, and asserts that cultural values and meanings are relative to and embedded in their cultural context, and cannot be measured against a universal system. It uses locally meaningful categories to describe indigenous syndromes, their phenomenology, and native explanatory models based on an ethnographic perspective (8). They make strong attempts to avoid the categorical fallacy.

Category fallacy refers to the application of a category that is valid within one cultural context to a culture where the category has no diagnostic validity or relevance. It stems from a universalist approach to assigning meaning to behaviors transculturally. In contrast, cultural relativists propose that cultural meanings and values are relative and fundamentally embedded in their cultural context. The latter perspective is referred to as *emic,* in contrast to the former approach, known as *ethic,* which applies Western diagnostic categories to another cultural context (8).

Definitions

Culture consists of those patterns of behavior, acquired and transferred over time, which prescribe the norms, customs, roles, and values inherent in political, economic, religious, and social aspects of family life. Culture provides the set of rules and standards that guide people's actions, makes their behavior understandable to one another, and helps to explain individuals' relationships to their sociobiological context.

Ethnicity refers to the sense of belonging and having a rootedness in history that reaches beyond religion, race, or national or geographic origin. Ethnicity is our basic identity—who we are in relation to other human groups. It frames our manner of dress, style, and communication through language and rituals, as well as how we feel about life, death, and illness (9,10). The concept is derived from the Greek work *ethnos,* or people of a nation. We are born with an ethnic identity. Throughout life we experience and adopt different cultures, thereby living with expectations and values from both a majority culture (i.e., the American culture) and minority culture—our culture of origin. We carry with us both the values, assumptions, traditions, and worldviews transmitted over generations within our ethnic group and the concurrent—sometimes competing—view of the cultural context in which we live. As noted by McGoldrick et al. (10) and Herr (11), ethnic traditions still affect third and fourth generations in subtle ways and are often experienced as cultural conflicts between members of the younger generation.

Cultural context refers to the sociocultural environment in which people live and interact. The combination of ethnic origin and cultural context, together with the pressures imposed by cultural transitions and/or migration, inevitably creates difficulties that family groups must resolve. Landau (12) discusses the challenge minorities face in balancing the demands of living within two cultures—the culture of origin and the majority culture. She notes that if the stresses and differences are too great, the family network is too remote or too weak to help, the family must either adapt to the culture or turn inward on itself, becoming isolated and enmeshed as a family group. As a consequence of the ethnocentric defense, very often the family resists accepting help from outsiders unless their problems become too great to handle alone.

Cultural identity refers to the patient's cultural or ethnic reference group and the degree of involvement with both host culture and culture of origin. This internalized self-definition selectively incorporates values, beliefs, and historical elements from those available in the person's environmental values and contains self-experiences related to ethnicity, gender, values, and a wide range of beliefs.

Ethnic identity describes a sense of commonality transmitted over generations by the family and reinforced by the surrounding community (10). An ethnic group is defined as "those who conceive themselves as alike by virtue of their common ancestry, real or fictitious, and who are so regarded by others" (13). It is perceived as "we" in contrast to "they." Ethnic identity develops as the product of ethnic socialization by children acquiring the values, attitudes, behaviors, and perceptions of an ethnic group, and perception of themselves and others as members of the group (14).

Cultural mask, as described by Montalvo and Gutierrez (15), refers to the family's use of real elements in their culture to conceal their problematic behavior and interactions. For example, the family can use the rationale: "We are Latin, we are expected to have hot tempers." The family thus uses culturally sanctioned behavior in a defensive fashion in order to protect crucial underlying issues. The family presents to the therapist a view of who they are based on what they think is expected of them, instead of showing how they actually behave when trying to resolve problems or even interact with one another. Montalvo and Gutierrez caution the therapist to search for the problem-solving approach of the family and not get caught up in exotic or unusual behavior patterns unique to the family's culture.

Culture-Bound Syndromes

Culture-bound syndromes consist of disturbances in mood, behavior, or belief systems that appear restricted to a particular cultural context. They are frequently viewed as exotic or covert illness phenomena occurring in the context of a local culture. Many culture-bound syndromes have been described worldwide. For example, some syndromes can exhibit acute episodes of anxiety, such as *ataques de nervios* in Latin America or Koro in Malaysia. The former syndrome manifests by trembling, shouting, crying, fainting, seizure-like activity or suicidal gestures. The person may return to normal functioning rapidly. As with many similar syndromes, it is a pattern of behavior that is understood locally as a meaningful manifestation of distress, acceptable within the cultural context. Such symptoms signal distress and activate a culturally specific response to the situation. The symptoms are recognized and interpreted through the appropriate attribution, which is part of the common socialization process for the cultural subgroup (8).

Acculturation

Acculturation refers to the process of behavioral and attitudinal changes in a cultural subgroup as a result of exposure to the practices of a different dominant group (16). Initially, it was hypothesized that a high level of acculturation decreases stress and the risk of psychological disorder in members of cultural subgroups. Subsequent studies have further recognized the complexity of the process; the concurrent relationship between a high level of acculturation and increased psychological distress is likely due to social role conflicts and the partial loss of traditional support received from the original culture (1,17,18).

The culturally sensitive clinician can be well-served by paying close attention to the unique experiences of each individual in the acculturation process as it is manifested by intense rejection or blind acceptance of cultural elements of the host or original cultures, or a resistance to assimilation into the broader culture. The complexity of the acculturation process in child/adolescent and family psychiatry can be significant because of different levels of acculturation achieved by children and their parents. Children born in the host country can achieve a very high level of acculturation, while parents may adhere strongly to the practices of their original culture and reject the values of the host culture. Fathers may develop a much higher level of linguistic and cultural competence due to their workplace experiences in contrast to some mothers, who may not learn the new language and cultural practices if primarily functioning in the household. The level of acculturation of younger children may also differ significantly from that of older children, particularly if born and initially raised in the previous culture and exhibiting sharp differences from their younger and Americanized siblings. The degree and nature of the acculturation process can be determined by inquiry into age at immigration, number of years in the United States, language proficiency, and participation in the host culture's social activities and social networks (1,16). The term *enculturation* is also sometimes used to refer to this process in which children and teens learn about, and often incorporate, the societal norms in their cultural environment. This process may be influenced by peers, parents, and other adults. If the enculturation process is successful, the language, values, and rituals of that culture will be incorporated into the individual's worldview (72). Ideally, an optimal degree of biculturality will be achieved, whereby the young person incorporates the best of their parents' (or their own) culture of origin with those of the present (host) culture. Multiracial adolescents may face a more difficult challenge than their monoracial peers in that they must develop this new identity and decide how, or even if, they can reflect positive aspects of all heritages while also rejecting certain societal expectations and stereotypes (74–76). Often by adolescence, multiracial children have been made aware of any racial/ethnic differences between classmates and themselves. They may be reminded of these differences as they attend school and are asked questions such as "What are you?" from classmates puzzled or threatened by their racially or ethnically mixed appearance. These alienating questions often contribute to the feeling that no one understands them, not even their monoracial parents, as they may feel "stuck" between cultures (74,77). Concerns about not "fitting in" are magnified if multiracial adolescents find that they are no longer welcome in certain peer groups because of racial issues (e.g., family objections to interracial romantic relationships; 77,78). Additionally, some peers, and even their own parents, may pressure the adolescent to identify with only one ethnic background, prompting feelings of guilt or disloyalty (74,76,82).

Incongruent cultural values and language skills among immigrant parents and their acculturating offspring can lead to an acculturation "gap." This gap between parent and child has been termed acculturative family distancing, or AFD (83). AFD is defined as the distancing that occurs between parents and youth as a result of communication difficulties and cultural value incongruence, and has been studied extensively in Asian and Latino immigrant families, though it may have broad applicability to other cultural groups (83,84). AFD is intensified by parent–child acculturation differences. Specifically, parents and children may give up their heritage culture at different speeds and acquire the characteristics of the host culture at different rates. High AFD (i.e., a large acculturation gap) has been associated with increased intergenerational family conflict and decreased family cohesion in Asian American and Latino adolescents (85–87). AFD and its core domains (communication difficulties and cultural value incongruence) are hypothesized to increase over time and lead to distancing between parents and youth, thereby increasing risk for family conflict, which, in turn, increases risk for depression and other psychological problems (84–85). On the other hand, a sense of an integrated, bicultural self-concept may allow enculturated youth to persist through periods when they may experience rejection from one or both cultures (81,87). Several authors have highlighted important psychological features of healthy biculturalism (73,74,79,80) because it creates a sense of cultural self-efficacy within the institutional structure of society, along with a sense of pride and identification with one's ethnic roots. LaFromboise (79) proposes that it may also have much to do with parental modeling of this construct, and can be directly related to how well the parent has either *accommodated* the new culture (adopted certain aspects of the new culture, while still retaining important features of the root culture, or culture of origin) or *assimilated* the new culture (adopted most or all of the new culture, while having cast off the previous cultural values and belief system).

Effect of Culture and Ethnicity on Child Development

Recent trends have brought the cultural context of child and personality development into bold view. Among these are the global demographic trend toward cultural heterogeneity, and contributions from cross-cultural psychiatry and psychology. It is generally established now that culture influences the development of children and shapes personality from infancy through adulthood. The child-rearing practices of parents and family provide the infant with the basic nurturance needed for development. Equally important is the role of parents and family in transmitting cultural rules, standards, and values to the child through the process of socialization. Cultures vary widely and differ from each other in the way the tasks of socialization are carried out, the specific rules and values transmitted, and the behavioral and conceptual outcome of socialization process with regard to beliefs and worldviews adopted by the children (19,20,21,74).

It is also firmly established that much of our information on child and adolescent development is based on norms that are almost exclusively Western, middle-class, and male oriented. Most of the observations and studies have been conducted in Western settings and are nonrepresentative of the world's population. These studies perpetuate a given view of the universe and tell us little about how youth develop in so-called "minority cultures" in Western societies (22,23). Child-rearing practices vary widely in different cultural domains. In many cultures, particularly Western ones, the main parenting person is the mother, with the father assuming an important but secondary parental role. In African societies, older siblings assume a significant role in raising infants and young children. Other family members and grandparents assume important child-rearing roles in Asian and other cultures. Other caretakers offer the children a different or expanded view of the world (24,25). Socialization occurs not only through explicit teaching but also through day-to-day experience of childhood and through the structure of the settings where the children live and play.

Cultural Impact on Developmental Stages

Examinations of the influence of culture on differing developmental stages is gaining interest among investigators. We briefly review the investigations of several developmental stages.

Cross-Cultural Research on Infancy

A strong theme in literature is the "precocity" of babies from traditional, nonindustrialized societies. They may stand or sit 2 to 4 or more weeks earlier than American and European norms. At times, the precocity in Africa has been linked with reports of precocity at birth. The clusters of advanced behaviors are to a large degree correlated with environmental factors (26,27).

Putting aside the multiple and complex methodologic issues in many studies, it is generally established that African babies reared in relatively traditional ways achieve many motor functions, particularly in the first year of life, before their European and American counterparts. The findings from studies in Uganda have been subsequently supported by multiple studies in other African countries (26,27). The advanced skills frequently coincide with deliberate teachings of the infants by the mothers and other caretakers of how to walk, sit, and help the babies practice those skills. They may use props to facilitate those tasks. The encouragement of sitting and carrying the baby on the caretaker's back is more helpful in the development of trunk, buttocks, and thigh muscles in comparison to having the child sit on an infant seat (26,27,29). Similar findings have been reported in Asian countries, including India (28).

Lester and Brazelton (30) propose that African child-rearing practices are built on the infant's responsiveness to being handled in the neonatal period and facilitate motor precocity. Motor excitement of infants may elicit engagement and interpersonal handling from the caregiver, thus enhancing developmental progression. Normal infants in different traditional cultures appear to exhibit critical cognitive developmental levels at about the same time throughout the world (26,30).

Temperament

In studying temperament, cultural affiliation is a strong predictor of infant temperament in the first year of life and is exquisitely sensitive to environmental influences. McDermott (25) has proposed that temperament should be viewed as a constellation of traits with a threshold of expression that varies from culture to culture. Considering two broad clusters of temperament, namely rhythmicity and activity, significant cultural variations are evident. Chinese American, Japanese American, and Navajo Indians are temperamentally less excitable than other groups who exhibit lower levels of arousal and are easily consoled. Mexican Indians and Kenyan infants have smoother transitions from one state to another and maintain quiet, alert states for longer periods and are higher on motor maturity (25,31,32).

Examining the investigations of Jerome Kagan (33,34) on shyness and social/behavioral inhibition, McDermott (25) proposed that cultures impart meanings to the behavior but also determine how others perceive and react to the behavior. Inhibited and shy children are more readily accepted by mothers in the Chinese culture, in contrast to their North American counterparts. Shy–anxious children in China are valued and accepted by society and peers, and adjust well to their social environment (33–35). In the West, shyness and social withdrawal are associated with peer rejection and isolation, reflecting a stronger emphasis in the West on the need for self-expression and self-confidence (33–35). In contrast, the ready acceptance of these biologically determined traits and behaviors by parents, teachers, and peers in Asian culture reflects a low level of apprehension about these traits. McDermott proposes that Chess and Thomas's model of goodness-of-fit be applied at the cultural as well as the individual level.

The first large-scale investigation of children living in multiple cultures was undertaken by the anthropologic team of Beatrice and John Whiting (36,37). They compared the behavior of children and the adults' expectation of them in six different cultures: India, Kenya, Mexico, Okinawa, Philippines, and the United States. Children in nonindustrialized cultures were given tasks important to the well-being of the families, such as caring for younger siblings and tending to a goat so the family did not go without milk. Children showed nurturing and responsible behavior. Children in industrialized cultures were not expected to contribute to their family's survival, were more self-centered and dependent, and their self-centered orientation was tolerated by their families. The self-centeredness may be actually an asset in Western cultures and enhance the desire for personal profit (19). Whiting and Whiting found the influence of peers on young children to be very powerful and occur early. Additionally, parental efforts to control and redirect the aggression of their children emerged more strongly than their nurturance in all of the above cultures (25,36,37).

Attachment

Previous work in cross-cultural development and attachment has proposed that aspects of this construct may be very culturally dependent (74,107–109). For example, the degree of emotional intensity and its projection to a single primary parent, considered an underpinning of object relations theory, may be more typical of Western culture (versus multiple caretakers in many non-Western cultures) (107). Other outgrowths of Western concepts of attachment include the development of transitional objects (108) and the process of psychological hatching, or separation–individuation, as critical to psychological health (109). Evidence shows that all of these concepts in psychological development are variable across cultures, and in some cases even culture-bound. For example, Bornstein and colleagues (110) examined and compared characteristics of maternal responsiveness to infant activity during home-based naturalistic observations of mother–infant dyads in New York City, Paris, and Tokyo. They found that differences in maternal responsiveness across these cultures occurred in response to infant looking (at the mother) rather than infant vocalization, and in mothers emphasizing interactions within the mother–infant dyad, instead of outside or beyond the dyad (74,110).

Being part of a group, rather than individual assertiveness, is highly valued in many cultures. Being agreeable, respectful, emotionally mature, courteous, and self-controlled are considered major assets as they promote interdependence. Traditional Japanese culture, for example, views newborns as independent and making them dependent, bound to and part of the group, is considered a fundamental task of the family. The Japanese traditional practice of keeping young children close to the mother, including the practice of co-sleeping well into childhood, fosters a high level of social and personal closeness, interdependence, and other characteristics that are very different from American culture (19,38,111,112).

Preschoolers

Preschool Chinese children are expected to pay close attention during lessons, unlike American preschoolers. Chinese nursery school teachers initiate and organize most of the daily activities, while the children listen, follow directions, take turns, and share. The activity structure teaches the children the value of self-control, obedience, and cooperation with other children. In contrast, the American nursery school provides a wide range of toys that can be used by children in their own way in free play, transmitting the importance of self-expression and individuality in the American culture (19,38).

Children's inclination to compete or cooperate emerges as a signification differential point among Anglo-American and many non-Western or nonindustrialized cultures. Madsen used a cooperation game for two players, where only one child could partially win if s/he cooperated with the other person but both children lost if they competed. Madsen (34,40) found dramatic behavioral differences between urban Anglo-American and rural Mexican children. The Anglo-American children, particularly the older ones, were far more competitive even when it did not benefit them. The rural Mexican children were far more cooperative, even when they did not directly benefit. The strategies of both groups of children were adaptive within their culture (19).

Culture and School Achievement

Daily experiences of Japanese and many Asian children convey the high level of cultural value placed on formal education, which explains the much higher score of Japanese students on math and science in comparison to American students. Starting in elementary school, Japanese students spend many more hours in the classroom and doing homework than American students. They also receive extensive tutoring after hours for exams, and enrichment courses (19,38,40). The emphasis of Japanese parents on education reflects their cultural belief that achievement depends on effort; parents are rarely satisfied with their children's academic achievement and urge them to work harder. Until recently, many American parents have believed that academic success depends primarily on innate ability and assumed their children are doing their best (19). Recent research by Carol Dweck, Angela Duckworth, and others has highlighted the importance for teachers and parents to praise both effort and results of their students and children, and to cultivate a perseverance toward long-term goals. A *growth mindset* comes from the belief that one's basic qualities are things that can be cultivated through effort. And, although aptitude, talents, interests, or temperaments may differ, change and growth are possible through application, experience, and *grit* (113,114).

Transition to school is frequently difficult for children from a cultural subgroup attending a school representing the radically different social interactional pattern of the majority culture. Middle-class American children enter school already feeling very familiar and at ease with being asked many questions, particularly *test-type questions* with the answers already known by the adults. African-American children from a lower socioeconomic class were usually unfamiliar with this type of questions and more accustomed to *story-starter* or *accusation* or *analogy type questions* and acted unresponsively to the test-type questions (19,42). The same cultural mismatch between children's usual style of interacting with adults and the expected social style in school has been described with other minority groups, including Native American children and East Indian children in England. This cultural mismatch makes the transition to school more difficult for children from cultural subgroups. It interferes with the shift to decontextualized thought, learning to solve problems that are abstract, and removed from the immediate context by applying their informal problem-solving skills learned at home in everyday life (19,42). It can affect how much children can learn from their school experience and may help to explain the lower average achievement test scores for African-American and Latino children and their higher rate of school dropout and school failure in comparison to Anglo-Americans (43).

Cultural Bias in Testing Intelligence

Any test to measure intelligence (IQ test) is a product of a certain culture, and the level of knowledge of that culture affects how well one performs on that test. There are subtle ways in which cultural background can influence test scores. Cultures vary in their definition of intelligence and the preferred way of performing a cognitive task (44). The interpersonal setting and the racial or ethnic identity of the tester can reduce the accuracy of test results; children feel more comfortable being tested by members of their own ethnic group. Some children from cultural subgroups feel confused by an adult asking a series of questions when he already knows the answers to them.

To reduce the problem of cultural bias, *culture-free tests* (no culture-based content) and *culture-fair tests* have been developed. In one such test, the problems are presented visually to eliminate the use of language. However, the difference in performance scores on these tests for some cultural groups were unreliably high (44,45). Culture-fair IQ tests uses items that are appropriate to all cultures, but the problem of accurate assessment has remained unsolved. Therefore, intelligence tests remain an effective tool for comparison of intellectual ability within the same culture, but not for comparison across cultures (19).

Cross-Cultural Studies of Adolescence

Adolescence marks the transition from childhood to adult roles in different cultures and has been studied by multiple investigators since the initial observations of Margaret Mead in Samoa in the 1920s. The complexities of adult roles in Western industrialized societies require a very protracted period of learning to acquire the social and technical skills necessary to assume adult roles and gain privileges such as driving (in most states at age 16), voting (18), and drinking (21). Adolescents have to be dependent on their parents financially for a protracted period of time and feel as "marginal" people in a no-man's-land (46), denied full adult social and sexual roles (19). The inner feeling of frustration can lead to a period of conflictual relationship with parents.

In contrast to the experience of adolescents in industrialized societies, anthropologist Margaret Mead found the adolescent transition to adult roles in Samoan culture to be nonstressful and gradual; the adolescent's interests and activities matured progressively and without significant stress or conflicts (4). Her basic conclusions in this area have been supported by subsequent investigations (19).

In some cultures, such as certain tribes in Kenya, transition to adulthood is somewhat abrupt as the growing children's duties expand over a short period of time (19,35,46). Such societies have special ceremonies called "rites of passage" to mark entry into adult roles, which are anticipated by the children for years in advance (19).

The universally accepted dual developmental tasks of adolescence, namely preparation for adulthood and identity formation, follows differential patterns in different cultures. Western cultures tend to encourage achievement through academic endeavors and physical sports. In Confucian-influenced Asian cultures, emphasis is on self-discipline, subjugation of desires and self-refinement as the preferred methods of accomplishment of inner peace (46). Canino and Canino (47) point out that assertiveness, competitiveness, and independence, which are highly valued in Western culture, can be contradictory, for example, to core Puerto Rican values and may create conflict in Puerto Rican families who live in the mainland United States.

Puberty has been studied extensively cross-culturally. The major noticeable changes of puberty occur over a time span of 4 years and in girls between the ages 9 to 16. Girls in industrialized countries tend to reach menarche earlier than girls in nonindustrialized and developing countries because malnutrition and chronic illnesses are more common. The median age for menarche in North America, Japan, and Western Europe is 12.5 to 13.5, in contrast to Africa, where it is 14 to 17 years. Across a wide range of cultures and countries, girls from higher-income families with adequate nutrition reach menarche sooner than girls from lower-income families. There is no cross-cultural difference in the age of onset of menarche between girls in groups from comparable income families (19,48).

Multiculturalism in Clinical Care

Multiculturalism is based on the assumption that no single way exists to conceptualize human behavior or explain the realities and experiences of diverse cultural groups (89,92,115). In this framework, clinicians are asked to reflect on the observation that each individual has a unique story and that cultural meaning is woven into that story, and into each person, like a tapestry (88,93). Indeed, in every encounter with a patient, there are at least three separate cultures present and interacting: that of the patient and family, that of the provider, and that of the medical or institutional culture where the clinical work is occurring. In this tripartite model, proposed by Tseng and Streltzer (92), it becomes clear that every patient encounter involves mediating effectively ("cultural effectiveness") in relation to each cultural contribution that shapes the interaction (115).

One culture participating in the interaction is that of the patient. Patients come to the encounter with culturally shaped biases, assumptions, and beliefs that are not always known to the provider, but can influence the expectations and desired outcomes. The ethical principle of *Respect for Persons* is fulfilled when providers can effectively work with patients and families with cultural backgrounds different from the provider's (93). The patient's expectations of the psychiatrist, motivation for treatment, explanation for the emergence of symptoms, and adherence with treatment recommendations can all be influenced by the patient's cultural background (115).

The second culture to consider in this exchange is the culture of the health care provider. The social and demographic background, life experience, personal beliefs, and professional training of the provider will shape the interaction and communication with patients. Even when many aspects of the cultural background of the patient and family are similar to those of the clinician, differences are inevitable—and should be welcomed (115).

The culture of American medicine, and its expression in the clinical care institution, is the third factor in each doctor–patient interaction. Most physicians and other providers within an institution may become accustomed to both visible and invisible elements of the cultural environment of their workplace, and may be unaware of its collective influence on their practice (94). Child and adolescent psychiatry, furthermore, has its own subcultures that include traditions, regulations, and attitudes, not necessitated by specific psychiatric knowledge. For example, whether psychiatrist, nurse, and care manager work together as equal team members or in more hierarchical fashion depends on the past professional and training experiences of each member, as well as the cultural milieu and other influences in the clinical and societal setting. How patients and allied health personnel regard psychiatrists may vary by the dominant culture in that environment (115).

Given that many thousands of health care interactions occur each day and that each is affected by the culture of the patient, the psychiatrist, and the immediate context, the effectiveness of clinical care—as well as the ethics of clinical care—will be influenced by attentiveness to multiculturalism. Stated more negatively, failure to appreciate the impact of culture may render useless or inaccessible what would otherwise be excellent care resources. For instance, persons from other backgrounds may approach the American health care system differently than do persons who are well aligned with Western culture and may encounter significant barriers to care. Language differences serve as one example, but other less obvious barriers also exist related to lack of transportation, limited resources, inability to access and navigate health systems, and limited feelings of trust in health care institutions in the United States, based on prior life experiences (115).

Cross-cultural psychiatric evaluation and treatment describe the skills required to provide care across cultural and linguistic barriers when a clinician consults with a patient from a different cultural/ethnic group who holds a different system of belief values and may speak a different language. In addition to the goal of conducting a comprehensive clinical evaluation, the clinician should assess the contributions of culturally derived forces and stressors to the patient's symptomatology and the adequacy of protective factors in the patient's social environment to mediate stress and promote healthy adjustment. Training programs in child and adolescent psychiatry now have multiple resources, including model curricula and practice parameters which they can draw from when trying to incorporate organized didactic and scholarly experiences in cultural psychiatry (105,106).

Religion, faith, and healing are often so intertwined that in certain cultures, when a psychiatric condition occurs, diagnosis and remedy may be more influenced by spiritual rather than medical interpretation. For example, in Hispanic cultures there is a condition called *susto,* which describes a type of terror or fright that occurs consequent to some trauma. The victim of *susto* or trauma suffers a "soul loss" through fright. As in posttraumatic stress disorder (PTSD), the trauma can manifest clinically as anxiety, panic, fear, or depression. The cure consists of the intervention of a person skilled in healing—a *curandero,* or healer, who allows the patient to release fears and hostilities (17,49). Treatment consists of medicine, some ritual or ceremony with friends and relatives, and the support of a network of friends. Ultimately, the person is "reassured" through a type of transferential cure—a combined systemic approach that includes a spiritual orientation, the support of friends and family, and faith in the healer.

The evaluator should have an adequate understanding of the patient's culture of origin and the impact of the cultural—or immigration—issues on the child's developmental process. He should inquire about the expectations of parents from the psychiatric treatment, based on their culture of origin. Many immigrant patients may have initially tried folk healers, exorcists, and herbal medicine, prior to evaluation. Such efforts should be explored respectfully and with an accepting attitude. Many families only come for psychiatric evaluation under pressure from school, social agencies, or family court, and their ambivalence about treatment should also be respected (17,46,47). Frequently, there is a profound feeling of failure and alienation in the family because they have attempted unsuccessfully to solve the problem on their own for a prolonged period of time. The pain of the family should be acknowledged empathically, while countering their feelings of being a failure as a family; one should also disavow the family's view of themselves as a "mental illness family" rather than a family with a problem who are actively attempting to find a solution (46,47). The impact of the child's emotional disorder on the internal family environment, interpersonal dynamics, and weakening of the parental authority should be explored. The initial evaluative session serves the multiple tasks of forging a relationship with all family members, collecting data, and enlisting their active partnership in the treatment process. It requires continuous respect and empathy, particularly around inquiries into the parents' explanation for the child's behavior, and addressing their questions and fears. Clinicians can often perform these tasks more comfortably in separate sessions with parents and children. However, clinicians who are proficient in family and individual therapy can effectively accomplish these goals in child-centered conjoint family sessions.

Contrary to the initial view of many clinicians, the contemporary field of cultural psychiatry considers that comprehensive and meaningful evaluations across cultural boundaries can be performed by clinicians who are from a background radically different from a patient's culture as long as the principles and guideline outlined in this chapter are applied.

Clinical Interview

Interviews across the cultural barrier require a high level of attention and sensitivity to the establishment of rapport and empathy with the patient and the family. Respect and deference to elders and head of households can facilitate acceptance by patients and families. Comments on positive assets of family members, such as children's good manners, can enhance the sense of pride in all family members. The clinician should adopt the preferred communication style of the family; the patient may feel more comfortable with a formal conversational method of inquiry rather than an informal one, or with asking rapid-fire questions from a checklist. Some patients, particularly from more impacted families, should be allowed extra time initially to describe the symptoms in great detail; every daily call from the school about the child's disruptiveness; the child's poor eating habits; irregular sleeping routine; disrespect for the parents. This communication style should only be redirected in a way that avoids alienating the person. Certain content may carry stigma, such as discussion of overt aggression, suicidality, or sexuality with certain cultural groups. The patient's preference should be respected and handled with special tact, as if one were conducting a complex defense/resistance analysis.

Language proficiency as a barrier to health care is a formidable obstacle to the care of several cultural groups, particularly with the increasing number of immigrants in the United States. It is estimated that up to 50% of some cultural groups are monolingual and the level of language proficiency and language independence of many patients in the remaining half may fall short of what is needed for an accurate and comprehensive psychiatric assessment. Therefore, a variety of interpreters, specially trained translators, and cultural/linguistic consultants are engaged to facilitate the communication process between the clinician and the patient. The highest level of assistance can be rendered by cultural/linguistic consultants, who work closely with members of the clinical team, and are especially trained and sensitized to recognize rich affective and cognitive context accompanying the patient's verbal communication in order to arrive at the *connotative meaning* of their expressions, rather than just the literal ones. There are guidelines for the use of interpreters, using the necessary translation time to make additional observations about the patient's behavior, and also to recognize errors in translation based on a patient's response. Frequently, patients can recognize intuitively the translation errors of the interpreter and they should be empowered to point them out. The evaluator should have the necessary skills to recognize the patient/translator "transference," translator-patient "countertransference," and ways of avoiding splitting the authority (transference) between the translator and the clinician. Many fully bilingual patients—particularly Latinos—may choose to use an interpreter in the sessions in order to focus their efforts on describing their situation. They frequently correct the interpreter during translation errors. This phenomenon should not be misunderstood as a power-struggle maneuver, but as a preferred communication style. Furthermore, the language proficiency of a fully bilingual person can fall short during the description of traumatic events from the past that are laden with intense affect (50–53).

Cultural Formulation

Cultural formulation is a key concept in the biopsychosocial assessment and diagnosis of mental disorders, similar to psychodynamic or biologic formulations. The DSM-5 recommends inclusion of a number of components into such a formulation to make it serve as a sensitive instrument to address the requirements of a comprehensive assessment in culturally diverse or multicultural groups (1,53). The formulation should include (a) the cultural identity of the patient; (b) cultural explanations of the patient's illness; (c) cultural factors related to the psychosocial environment; (d) cultural elements of the physician–patient relationship; and (e) overall cultural assessment for diagnosis and treatment. Specific adaptations in the cultural formulation relevant to child and adolescent psychiatry are presented in a useful review by Aggarwal (95).

For immigrants, cultural formulations should include pre-immigration history, including educational or employment opportunities, as well as major conflicts, losses, or traumas that may have contributed to the immigration. For example, a 13-year-old girl who lived with her grandmother in Puerto Rico for most of her life was sent to the United States abruptly after she was severely abused by a relative. The trauma of the abuse, the abrupt loss of the relationship with her primary psychological caregiver, and the unpreparedness of the mother to care for the daughter after many years of separation were not included in the formulation. The American Psychiatric Association has now published highly practical guidelines for conducting interviews with diverse groups of patients and families. The Cultural Formulation Interview, CFI, is adapted for children, immigrants, the elderly, and other specific populations (96).

Mental Health and Psychiatric Care: Effect of Culture in Help-Seeking

Needs assessment surveys of the general population have consistently shown that most people with serious emotional problems do not seek professional help, particularly from mental health professionals. With a culturally diverse population, unique and powerful barriers are operative, which may explain the low level of utilization of mental health services by minorities and culturally diverse groups, as emphasized in the 2000 Surgeon General's report (54). Chief among them is fear of stigmatization and discrimination, which combines with attitudinal, demographic, and system-dependent factors.

The fear of discrimination, particularly due to linguistic barriers, is a formidable deterrent for many members of certain cultural groups. Equally significant is the fear of disregard, disrespect, or misunderstanding the patient's culture and customs. Fear of disregard for the status of parents and elders, and the importance of the children's respect for parents, parental values, and loyalty to the family keep many families from seeking help. Essential clinician variables are empathy, skillful perceptiveness, effective communication, straightforwardness, honesty, flexibility, intellectual curiosity, open mindedness, and tolerance for psychological challenges of adolescents and children (55,56). Adequate inquiry into parental views of the problems, their explanation for the behavior, their expectations of treatment outcome, keeping them informed of the treatment progress, and addressing crisis situations by involving the family can help forge a strong therapeutic alliance with the family. Rogler and colleagues (16) recommend the following requirements for providing mental health services to culturally diverse populations: (1) locating mental health services in minority neighborhoods and close to public transportation, as minority groups tend to congregate closely to each other; (2) employing mental health workers and clinicians who share the linguistic and cultural backgrounds of the patients; and (3) creating an ambiance that reflects the cultural heritage of the patient population in outpatient and hospital settings.

Culturally specific therapies are increasingly emerging in the clinical research literature and incorporate specific elements from the patient's native culture into therapeutic interventions (1). Such approaches modify conventional psychiatric treatments by incorporating folk rituals, herbs, and the patient's own cultural conception of the illness into therapeutic interventions.

A large number of patients in the majority culture tend to seek treatment for their emotional disorders from a primary care physician. In a seemingly parallel phenomenon, many members of minority groups tend to seek treatment relief and support from outside the mental health system from people such as a *curandero* and folk healers in Latino cultures. Mental health programs can penetrate the lay referral structure by assembling some credible members of the ethnic network into their professional structure (46,47). Informal and immediate registration of the patient for the initial contact with treatment can reduce the barrier to care (46,47,57).

The Social and Cultural Context of Psychopharmacology

As Lin and colleagues (97) have described, "pharmacotherapy is fundamentally a process of social transaction, and its outcome is determined by contextual factors impinging on the patient, [family], and the clinician by forces that powerfully shape their interactions." Furthermore, these investigators highlight the need for clinicians to acknowledge "that [they] are just as malleable, consciously and unconsciously, by their sociocultural environment and prevailing ideologies." They invite us to struggle against certain prevailing notions of modern pharmacotherapy, which can undermine effectiveness. These notions include that (1) the therapeutic effects of medications are determined exclusively by their biologic properties (2); the patient is a passive recipient of the prescription, and will be fully adherent with instructions; and (3) psychiatric and medical treatment represents (or is supposed to be) the only source of care available and used by the patient (97). Culture influences the same areas that are central to mental health, such as behavioral expectations and tolerance, language, emotion, attention, attachment, traumatic experiences, conduct, personality, motivation, limit setting, and other aspects of parenting in general. Cultural context plays an important role not only in structuring the environment in which children with emotional and behavioral disorders function, but also in the way such children are understood and treated (104).

Shame can be another cultural paradigm that enters the clinical setting (104). For both parent and (especially teenaged) patient, the stigma of mental illness may be further fed by being referred to the psychiatrist by the primary care provider (PCP). From the family/patient perspective, the implication is that the problems are so serious, too threatening, or so time consuming as to require a specialist, beyond what the PCP (who is often a trusted adult in the teen/child's life) can handle. Metzl (98) has described how clinicians should strive to promote an "open and honest exchange of affect," especially because patients and families are often "sent" to our offices "to relate deep and highly personal aspects of their lives to a total stranger" (p. 39). Broucek and Ricci (99) encourage us to "reduce the patient [and family's] shame and anxiety to levels more conducive to self-revelation. Intense shame [particularly among parents of some cultures] can be so aversive, noxious, and self-fragmenting that the [pharmacotherapist] may have to assist [them] in modulating it" (104, p. 435).

Another influential piece of writing comes from Havens (100,101), who describes the use of "psychological analgesics," which can be prescribed in much the same way as our medical predecessors may have told the patient to "take 2 aspirin and call me in the morning":

1. Protect self-esteem: the patient has been potentially affected by having to come to a psychiatrist, and the parent may feel guilty for having caused the illness through bad parenting, poor gene contribution, or both.
2. Emote a measure of understanding and acceptance: when this technique is successful, the patient's problem is grasped intellectually, and the patient's and family's predicament is understood from *their* point of view.
3. Provide a sense of future: many families have experienced frustration and failure in attempting to find solutions and may have lost hope. Discussion about and expectations for treatment that still acknowledges fears or even hopelessness may still preserve opportunities for change: "It may seem hopeless to you *for now*."

Sabo and Rand (102) emphasize the importance of spending adequate time with the patient (and family) in the initial evaluation. Patients too often feel as though they are merely "the next appointment" unless the doctor listens to the personal and unique elements of their story. Interpreters in the initial appointment can be crucial at this stage in the treatment relationship. Active empathic listening is necessary to create a special, common language between the patient and therapist. If a full workup cannot be completed in the first appointment, follow-up sessions (preferably within 1 to 2 weeks) may be necessary to sustain the developing alliance. This situation becomes especially true with those families sufficiently unfamiliar with mental health disorders and their treatment that they may be unsure of what to expect in terms of treatment planning and treatment response. In families from cultures in which somatization is a frequent way to present mental health symptoms, the attuned pharmacotherapist finds ways to selectively use the medical model or chemical imbalance explanation to gain buy-in, but may also use the opportunity to help families conceptualize how mental health problems can greatly impair daily function (e.g., school performance, peer and family relationships, self-worth). Choi (103) writes how "becoming familiar with the language for emotional distress and understanding cultural beliefs embedded in [certain cultural or culture-bound] expressions are critical steps for culturally competent communication between [clinicians] and adolescents" (104, p. 79).

Some cultural groups may hold a culturally shared belief that emotional disorders are somatically based and best treated with medication; they expect a rapid rate of recovery from target symptoms and are alarmed by side effects that they relate to "toxicity." Specific Asian groups, such as those of Chinese, Korean, and Japanese heritage, may require much lower medication doses, at times one-half or one-third of the conventional doses, to achieve therapeutic response (1,46). Therefore, cross-ethnic variations in drug responses ought to be a clinical focus.

Cytochrome P450 isoenzymes are key in the metabolism of psychotropic and nonpsychotropic drugs. The genetic anomalies in "poor metabolizers" are unequally distributed among ethnic populations. The percentage of CYP2D6 poor metabolizers is lower in Asians and higher in Caucasians. Similar interethnic variance exists in frequency of poor metabolizers of CYP2Cmp; low among whites (3%), intermediate for African Americans (18%), and higher in Asians (up to 20%). Immigrants and members of many subcultural groups commonly use herbal medicines. Inquiry into the use of the traditional herbal medicines of Asians, Latinos, and other immigrants to the United States is essential because many of these herbs possess psychoactive activities. Others such as ginseng may stimulate or inhibit cytochrome P450 enzymes (1,46).

The American Multicultural Society

At the start of the 21st century, American society and the global community have become increasingly heterogeneous with respect to racial, ethnic, and cultural composition. Global demographic trends reveal a world in which the majority is characterized by cultural heterogeneity rather than "ethnic purity." For the first time, the majority of the parents in the United States are raising their children in cultural settings other than those where they themselves were raised (57). The diverse profile of American and global families has given rise to the theoretical orientation of multiculturalism. Multiculturalism is based on the assumption that there is not a single way to conceptualize human behavior and to explain the realities and experiences of diverse cultural groups, and that no particular set of competencies have proven effective with every form of diversity (57,58,61).

Models of Culturally Informed Care

Multiple models have been proposed to guide clinicians in their professional roles. Here we adapt previously published work (115) and briefly discuss four models: the Cultural Competence Model (116), the Explanatory Models Approach (117), the LEARN Model (118), and the Culturally Competent Communications Model (119). All of these models highlight the role of culture in communication with patients and families, and focus on the development of treatment approaches that are respectful, helpful, and which avoid harm.

The Cultural Competence Model

Terry Cross and his colleagues introduced the term "Cultural Competence" in the 1980s to address the cultural needs of a growing population of diverse children and youth with serious emotional problems (116). They defined cultural competence as the state of being capable to serve people from diverse cultural and socioeconomic backgrounds. They outlined components of the knowledge, skill, attitudes, and values that both clinicians and their health care organizations should incorporate in order to operate effectively in a context of cultural difference.

While acknowledging that the concept of "cultural competence" may appeal to educators, some scholars point out that this term denotes a sort of end point, and that this "mastery of a body of knowledge and skills may insidiously lead us down the wrong path when applied to cross-cultural interactions. Culture is not a finite data set to be mastered, but instead a concept that is complex, dynamic and individual" (120).

Although our shared medical culture is based largely on achieving competence, we should take care when applying this term broadly to *mastering* other cultures (emphasis added). We may find that competency-based education can be applied more easily to the domains of knowledge and skills than to attitudes. Communication skills built upon the attitudes of openness, flexibility, self-reflection, and, yes, *humility* are ultimately what will make individuals responsive and sensitive to the delivery of care to diverse populations. This is the framework medical educators should be striving to introduce, model reinforce, and evaluate. This is the path of lifelong learning about oneself in relation to others that is most fruitful (120).

The term "cultural humility" (121,122) is consistent with the concepts of self-reflection and self-critique, instead of mastery of sets of information. The physician who can be responsive and attuned to cultural nuances and differences is most likely to incorporate information provided by patients and families, and is less likely to leave sociocultural misunderstandings unaddressed. In this way, the physician can emote an understanding of the patient's/family's situation from *their* point of view. Other authors caution against defining "culture" too narrowly (123).

The somewhat abstract nature of the term *culture* often results in a workplace definition of culture that is narrow and concrete, and may reduce culture to ethnic minorities (only). This type of thinking often leads to exempting providers from ethnic minority backgrounds from the responsibility of providing culturally competent care. It further leads to ignoring the need to provide culturally competent care to all groups, such as White men. Such a restricted notion of culture also fails to address the complexities in the relationships between an individual, his or her culture, and the culture of biomedicine, which is alien to most patients (p. 174).

The above models highlight that culturally informed approaches to medical care feature basic patient/provider communication skills that focus on a patient- and family-centered approach, openness to the experience of the other, flexibility, and self-reflection on the part of the provider.

The Explanatory Models Approach

In the field of anthropology, culture is seen as neither homogenous nor static (121,123). Culture is made up of multiple variables, affecting all aspects of experience. Medical anthropologist, Arthur Kleinman (117), states that culture "is inseparable from economic, political, religious, psychological and biological conditions. Culture is a process through which ordinary activities and conditions take on an emotional tone and a moral meaning for participants... Cultural processes frequently differ within the same ethnic or social group because of differences in age cohort, gender, political association, class, religion, ethnicity, and even personality." The shortcoming is that the medical field often falls into a categorical trap, and may *equate* culture with ethnicity, nationality and/or language. An example would be to assume that patients of a certain ethnicity are assumed to have a core set of beliefs about illness owing to ethnic traits.

Cultural "competency" (then) becomes a series of "do's and don't's" that define how to treat a patient of a given ethnic background. The idea of isolated societies with shared cultural meanings would be rejected by anthropologists today, since it leads to dangerous stereotyping—such as, "Chinese believe this, "Japanese believe that," and so on—as if entire societies or ethnic groups could be described by these simple slogans (p. 1673).

Kleinman introduced the Explanatory Models Approach as an interview technique that seeks to clarify how the social world affects and is affected by illness within the context of an individual's life. The aim of this approach is to more fully open clinicians to human communication and set their expert knowledge *alongside* the patient's own explanation and viewpoint.

The explanatory models approach does not ask, for example, "What do Mexicans call this problem?" It asks, "What do you call this problem?" and thus a direct and immediate appeal is made to the patient as an individual, not as a representative of a group... The one activity that even the busiest clinician should be able to find time to do is to routinely ask patients (and where appropriate, family members) what matters most to them in the experience of illness and treatment. The clinicians can then use that crucial information in thinking through treatment decisions and negotiating with patients (p. 1673).

This approach expands upon the DSM Cultural Formulation and allows clinicians to create a short ethnography-like formulation. "Ethnography" is a term from the field of anthropology that refers to the description of what life is like in the "local world" of the person (patient)—usually one different from the anthropologist's (physician's). It facilitates empathy with the patient/family's lived experience of the illness, and can lead to a narrative that ideally *conveys the clinical story* from the patient/family's worldview. The six steps in this ethnographic approach include (1): Asking about ethnic identity and whether it matters for the patient—e.g., whether it is an important part of the patient's sense of self (2); evaluating what is at stake for the patient/family and their loved ones. This can include inquiring about close relationships, financial/material resources, and religious/spiritual beliefs. It can shed light on the moral lives of patients/families (3); constructing the "illness narrative," based on a series of questions (Box 2.2.1.1) to understand the meaning of illness. Explanatory models can be used to open up a conversation on cultural meanings that have clinical relevance (4); considering the current stressors and social supports in patients/ families' lives (5); examining the influence of culture on the clinical relationship. An important ethnographic tool is self-reflection regarding the intersection of the world of the physician and the world of the patient. Kleinman reminds us that "teaching practitioners to consider the effects of the culture of biomedicine is contrary to the view of the expert as authority and to the media's view that technical expertise is always the best answer" (117), and (6) considering how relevant cultural issues are to a particular clinical situation. This important sixth step asks whether too much attention to potential cultural differences with the provider could be experienced by the patients and families as intrusive, and could even lead to a sense of being singled out and stigmatized, or lead to a misdiagnosis (124–126).

Another often-used model comes from the Family Practice literature, using the acronym *LEARN* (118). The authors created a process-oriented model by which cultural, social, and personal information relevant to a given illness episode could be elicited, discussed, and negotiated or incorporated (Box 2.2.1.2).

Teal and Street (119) have proposed that applying the cultural competency model to the medical encounter requires attention to the specific characteristics and circumstances of the individual patient and family (Fig. 2.2.1.1). The approach includes key communication skills such as the incorporation of cultural knowledge, recognition of potential differences,

BOX 2.2.1.1

THE EXPLANATORY MODELS APPROACH

What do you call this problem?
What do you believe is the cause of this problem?
What course do you expect it to take? How serious is it?
What do you think this problem does inside your body? How does it affect your body and your mind?
What do you most fear about this condition?
What do you most fear about the treatment?

(Kleinman A: *Rethinking Psychiatry: From Cultural Category to Personal Experience*. New York, The Free Press, 1988.)

BOX 2.2.1.2

THE LEARN MODEL OF CROSS-CULTURAL COMMUNICATION

***L**isten* with empathy to the patient's perception of the problem
***E**xplain* your perception of the problem
***A**cknowledge* and discuss both differences and similarities
Recommend treatment
Negotiate agreement

(Adapted from Berlin EA, Fowkes WC: A teaching framework for cross-cultural health care: application in family practice. *West J Med* 139:934–938, 1983.)

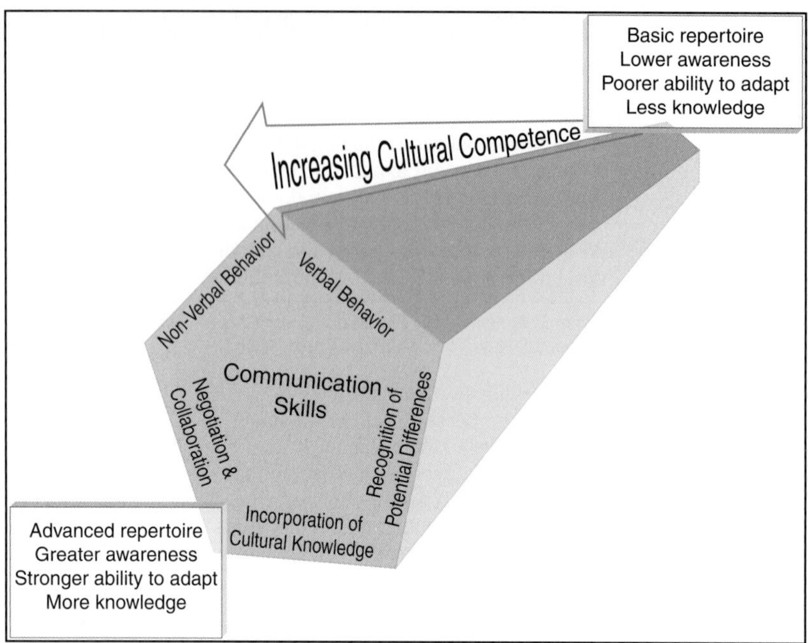

FIGURE 2.2.1.1. The Culturally Competent Communication Model. Reprinted, with permission, from Teal and Street (2009).

verbal and nonverbal behaviors, and negotiation and collaboration. These elements are seen as fundamental to acquisition of more skills and corresponds to increasing complexity and culturally competent communication.

The culturally competent communication model integrates existing frameworks for cultural competence and explanatory models including culture in patient care, with models of effective patient-centered communication. In this model, there are four critical elements of culturally competent communication in the medical encounter: communication repertoire, situational awareness, adaptability, and acknowledging core cultural issues.

In clinical situations where cultural elements present themselves as important elements of clinical care, it may be useful to consider obtaining a cultural consultation, where important insight and understanding may be gained by learning about the culture and history of a specific group. Discussion with a cultural broker to gain insight into a case where a cultural issue has the practitioner frustrated is very appropriate, and possibly essential. Furthermore, insights into that culture's model for disease and their perception of effective treatment may help clinicians to be more effective in understanding the perspective of their patients and families, and discussing treatment plans. Consultation on cultural issues may be considered similar to consulting with a health care colleague with a different specialty. Similarly, if a health care provider is working with many patients with a common experience, the provider can improve effectiveness by learning more about the realities and/or risks associated with that particular issue. For example, providers working with refugee patients would benefit greatly by learning about the experience of refugees, the common psychosocial circumstances refugees face, and the increased risks for adverse experiences and illness they have because of their experience (115).

CONCLUSIONS

Cultural child and adolescent psychiatry describes the body of theoretical and technical knowledge necessary for clinicians to provide competent psychiatric care across cultural and language barriers to children, adolescents, and families. It is based on the theoretical orientation of multiculturalism, which assumes that there are multiple ways to conceptualize human behavior and explain the realities and experience of various forms of cultural diversity, and that no particular set of competencies have proven effective in all cultural settings. The cultural relativist perspective asserts that cultural values and meanings are relative to and embedded in their cultural context, and cannot be measured against a universal system. It uses locally meaningful observations to examine the impact of cultural context on the developmental processes in children and their ultimate personality characteristics.

The increasingly multicultural American and global communities have acted as a compelling force for the growth of the field of cultural psychiatry and psychology. The incorporation of a vast body of cultural knowledge into descriptions of developmental processes, psychiatric diagnosis, clinical formulation, and culturally sensitive treatments have necessitated the expansion of our fundamental biopsychosocial model as described by George Engel 50 years ago. That model can be expanded into a *biopsychosociocultural model* to address the complexities of the clinical and developmental processes in a heterogeneous group with respect to their racial, ethnic, and cultural composition. It allows evaluation and description of the experience of individuals from one cultural group with another dominant culture, their acculturation process and tensions, and the opportunities created by their unique differences.

In this chapter, we have avoided organizing the sections into culturally specific categories, as online resources for culture-specific clinical strategies are easily accessible (127–129). Furthermore, while the practice of highlighting specific issues unique to ethnic, linguistic, and racial populations has its place in the medical literature, we agree with previous writers (115,117) that there is greater value in emphasizing more generalizable principles, knowledge, and skills for cultural effectiveness in clinical practice. Although some cultural groups have been highlighted more than others, these are meant to serve as examples of how to conduct culturally sensible practice, rather than to be focused on as broad assumptions about specific patients of a cultural group. We and others (103,105,130) are striving to change the "misguided perspective that the close relationship between culture and illness occurs strictly in the lives of ethnocultural minorities (only)." Rather, we believe this relationship and these connections are human ones, and occur in persons of all races, ethnicities, and backgrounds.

References

1. Trujillo M: Cultural psychiatry. In: Saddock B, Sadock V (eds): *Comprehensive Textbook of Psychiatry.* 7th ed. Baltimore, MD, Williams & Wilkins, ch. 44, 492–499, 2000.
2. Kleinman A: *Rethinking Psychiatry: From Cultural Category to Personal Experience.* New York, The Free Press, 1988.
3. Mezzich JE, Kleinman A, Fabrega H, Parron DL (eds.): *Culture and Psychiatric Diagnosis: A DSM-IV Perspective.* Washington, DC, American Psychiatric Press, 1996.
4. Mead M: *Coming of Age in Samoa.* New York: William Morrow, 1925/1939.
5. Alarcon R (ed.): Cultural psychiatry. *Psychiatry Clin North Am* 18:3, 1995.
6. Kluckhohn FR, Strodtbeck FL: *Variations in Value Orientations.* New York, Harper & Row, 1961.
7. Spiegel J: Ethnicity and family therapy: an overview. In: McGoldrick M, Pearce J, Giordano J (eds): *Ethnicity and Family Therapy.* 2nd ed. New York, Guilford Press, ch 1, 3–30, 1996.
8. Becker A, Kleinman A: Anthropology and psychiatry. In: Saddock B, Saddock V, (eds): *Comprehensive Textbook of Psychiatry,* 7th ed. Philadelphia, PA, Lippincott Williams & Wilkins, ch. 4.1, 463–475, 2000.
9. Giordano J, Giordano GP: *The Ethno-cultural Factor in Mental Health: A Literature Review and Bibliography.* New York, Institute on Pluralism and Group Identity, 1977.
10. McGoldrick M, Giordano J, Pearce JK (eds): *Ethnicity and Family Therapy.* 2nd ed. New York, Guilford Press, 1996.
11. Herr DM: Intermarriage. In: Thernstrom S, Orlov A, Handlin O (eds.): *Harvard Encyclopedia of American Ethnic Groups.* Cambridge, Harvard University Press, 1980.
12. Landau J: Therapy with families in cultural transition. In: McGoldrick M, Pearce JK, Giordano J (eds.): *Ethnicity and Family Therapy.* New York, Grune & Stratton, 1982:552–571.
13. Shibutani T, Kwan, KM: *Ethnic Stratification.* New York, Macmillan, 1965.
14. Rothernram MJ, Phinney JS: Introduction: definitions and perspectives in the study of children's ethnic socialization. In: Phinney JS, Rotheram MJ (eds.): *Children's Ethnic Socialization: Pluralism and Development.* Newbury Park, CA, Sage, 1986:10–28.
15. Montalvo B, Gutierrez M: A perspective for the use of the cultural dimension in family therapy. In: Hansen IJ, Falicov CJ (ed.): *Cultural Perspectives in Family Therapy.* Rockville, MD, Aspen Systems, 15–31, 1983.
16. Rogler LH, Gurak DT, Cooney RS: The migration experience and mental health: Formulation relevant to Hispanics and other immigrants. In: Gaviria M, Arana JD (eds.): *Health and Behavior: Research Agenda for Hispanics.* Chicago, Simon Bolivar Research Agenda for Hispanics I, University of Illinois, 1987.
17. Schwoeri L, Sholevar P, Combs, M: Impact of culture and ethnicity on family interventions. In: Sholevar GP, Schwoeri LA (eds.): *Textbook of Family & Couples Therapy: Clinical Applications.* Washington, DC, Amer Psychiatric Press, Inc., 725–745, 2003.
18. Escobar JI: Immigration and mental health: Why are immigrants better off. *Arch Gen Psychiatry* 55:781, 1998.
19. De Hart GB, Sroufe LA, Cooper RG: *Child Development: Its Nature and Course.* 4th ed. Boston, MA, McGraw Hill Co., 2000.
20. Bronfenbrenner U: *The Ecology of Human Development.* Cambridge, MA, Harvard University Press, 1979.
21. Bronfenbrenner U: Ecological systems theory. *Ann Child Dev* 6:187–249, 1989.
22. Nugent JK, Greene S, Wieczoreck-Deering D, Mazor K, Hendler J, Bombardier C: The cultural context of mother–infant play in the newborn period. In: Macdonald K (ed.): *Parent–Child Play.* Albany, NY, State University of New York Press, 367–389, 1993.
23. Nugent JJ, Lester BM, Brazelton TB: *The Cultural Context of Infancy.* Vol. 3. Norwood, NJ, Ablex, 1995.
24. Earls F: Cultural and national differences in the epidemiology of behavior problems of preschool children. *Cult Med Psychiatry* 6:45–56, 1982.
25. McDermott J: Effects of culture and ethnicity on child and adolescent development. In: Melvin L (ed.): *Child and Adolescent Psychiatry: A Comprehensive Textbook.* 3rd ed. Philadelphia, PA, Lippincott Williams & Wilkins, ch. 38, 494–498, 2002.
26. Super CM: Environmental effects on motor development: the case of African infant precocity. *Dev Med Child Neurol* 18:561–567, 1976.
27. Super CM: Behavioral development in infancy. In: Munroe RL, Munroe RH, Whiting BB (eds.): *Handbook of Cross-cultural Human Development.* New York, Garland Press, 1980.
28. Das VK, Sharma NL: Developmental milestones in a selective sample of Lucknow children: a longitudinal study. *Indian J Pediatr* 40:1–7, 1973.
29. Gerber M, Dean RF: The state of development of newborn African children. *Lancet* 272(1):1216–1219, 1957.
30. Lester BM, Brazelton TB: Cross-cultural assessment of neonatal behavior. In: Stevenson HW, Wagner DA (eds.): *Cultural perspectives on child development.* San Francisco, CA, Freeman, 1981.
31. Scarr-Salapatck S: An evolutionary perspective on infant intelligence: species patterns and individual variations. In: Lewis M (ed.): *Origins of Intelligence.* New York, Plenum, 1976.
32. De Vries M, Samaroff A. Culture and temperament: influences of infant temperament in three East African societies. *Am J Orthopsychiatry* 54:83–96, 1984.
33. LeVine RA: Human parental care: universal goals, cultural strategies, individual behavior. In LeVine RA, Miller PM, West MM (eds): *New Directions for Child Development: No. 40. Parental Behavior in Diverse Societies.* San Francisco, CA, Jossey-Bass, 1998.
34. Kagan S, Madsen M: Experimental analyses of cooperation and competition of Anglo-American and Mexican Children. *Dev Psychol* 6:49–59, 1972.
35. Chen X, Rubin K, Cen G, et al.: Child rearing attitudes and behavioral inhibition in Chinese and Canadian toddler: a cross cultural study. *Dev Psychol* 34:677–686, 1998.
36. Whiting BB, Edwards CP: *Children of Different Worlds.* Cambridge, MA, Harvard University Press, 1988.
37. Whiting B, Whiting J: *Children of Six Cultures: A Psycho-cultural Analysis.* Cambridge, MA, Harvard University Press, 1975.
38. Stevenson HW, Azuma H, Hakuta K: *Child Development and Education in Japan.* New York, Freeman, 1986.
39. LeVine RA: Parental goals: a cross-cultural view. *Teach Coll Rec* 76:226–239, 1974.
40. Madsen M: Development and cross-cultural differences in cooperative and competitive behavior of young children. *J Cross Cult Psychol* 2:365–371, 1971.
41. Stevenson HC: Missed, dissed, and pissed: Making meaning of neighborhood risk, fear and anger management in urban Black youth. *Cult Divers Mental Health* 3:37–52, 1997.
42. Tharp R: Psychocultural variables and constants: effects on teaching and learning. *Am Psychol* 44:349–359, 1989.
43. Goodnow JJ: The nature of intelligent behavior: questions raised by cross-culture studies. In: Resnick L (ed): *The Nature of Intelligence.* Hillsdale, NJ, Erlbaum, 169–1880, 1976.
44. Sternberg RJ: *Beyond IQ: A Triarchic Theory of Human Intelligence.* New York, Cambridge University Press, 1985.
45. Levine ES Padilla AM: *Crossing Cultures in Therapy: Pluralistic Counseling for the Hispanic.* Monterey, CA, Brooks/Cole, 1980.
46. Kim P: Culture and child and adolescent psychiatry. In: Tseng W, Streltzer J (eds): *Cultural Competence in Clinical Psychiatry.* Washington, DC, American Psychiatric Publishing, Inc., 125–145, 2004.
47. Canino IA, Canino G: Impact of stress on the Puerto Rican family: treatment considerations. *Am J Orthopsychiatry* 50:535–541, 1980.
48. Tseng W-S, McDermott J: *Culture, Mind and Therapy: An Introduction to Cultural Psychiatry.* New York, Brunner/Mazel, 1981.
49. Sholevar P: My child does not respect me. Presented at the Annual meeting of the American Academy of Child/Adolescent Psychiatry, Honolulu, HI, 2000.
50. Sholevar P: Mental health treatment of Latino patients. Annual Scientific meeting, Philadelphia Psychiatric Society, October 2005.
51. Marcos LR, Trujillo M: Culture, language and communicative behavior: the psychiatric examination of Spanish-Americans. In: Duran RP (ed.): *Latino Language and Communicative Behavior.* Norwood, NJ, Ablex Publishing, 1981.
52. Marcos LR: Linguistic dimensions in the bilingual patient. *AM J Psychoanal* 36:347, 1976.
53. Lu R, Mezzich, JE: Issues in the assessment and diagnosis of culturally diverse individuals. In: Oldham J, Riba M (ed.) *Annual Review of Psychiatry,* Vol. 14, Washington, DC, American Psychiatric Press, 1995.
54. U.S. Public Health Service: *Report of the Surgeon General's Conference on Children's Mental Health: A National Action Agenda.* Washington, DC, Department of Health and Human Services, 2000.
55. Canino IA, Spurlock J: *Culturally Diverse Children and Adolescents: Assessment, Diagnosis and Treatment.* New York, Guilford, 1994.
56. Flores JL: The utilization of a community mental health service by Mexican Americans. *Int. J Soc. Psychiatry* 24:271–275, 1978.
57. McLoyd VC: Changing demographics in the American population: Implications for research on minority children and adolescents. In: McLoyd VC, Steinberg L (eds.): *Studying minority adolescents: Conceptual, methodological, and theoretical issues.* Mahwah, NJ, Lawrence Erlbaum Associates, 3–28, 1998.
58. Day, JC: *Population Projections of the United States by Age, Sex, Race, and Hispanic Origin: 1995 to 2050, U.S. Bureau of the Census, Current Population Reports, P25–1130.* Washington, DC, U.S. Government Printing Office, 1996.
59. Nugent JK, Lester BM, Brazelton TB: *The Cultural Context of Infancy.* Vol. 3. Norwood, NJ, Ablex, 1995.
60. Bingham R, Porche-Burke L, James S, Sue D, Vazquez M: Report on the National Multicultural Conference and Summit II, in *Cult Divers Ethnic Minor Psychol* 8(2):75–87, 2002.
61. O'Hare W, Pollard K, Mann T, et al.: African Americans in the 1990s. *Popul Bull* 46:8–10, 1991.
62. Boyd-Franklin N: *Black Families in Therapy: A Multisystems Approach.* New York, Guilford, 1989.
63. Pinderhughes E: Afro-American families and the victim system. In: McGoldrick M, Pearce J (eds.): *Ethnicity and Family Therapy.* New York, Guilford, 108–122, 1982.
64. Billingsley A: *Black Families in White America.* Englewood Cliffs, NJ, Prentice-Hall, 1968.

65. Knox D: Spirituality: a tool in the assessment and treatment of black alcoholics and their families. *Alcohol Treat Q* 2(3/4):31–44, 1985.
66. Gonzalez D: *What Is the Problem with Hispanic? Just Ask a Latino.* New York Times, 1992.
67. Garcia-Preto N: Latino families: an overview. In *Ethnicity and Family Therapy.* 2nd ed. McGoldrick M, Giordano J, Pearce JK (eds.): New York, Guilford, 141–154, 846, 1996.
68. Comas-Diaz L: Lati Negra. *J Femin Family Ther* 5(3/4):35–74, 1994.
69. Lee E: A social system approach to assessment and treatment for Chinese-American families. In: McGoldrick M, Pearce JK, Giordano J (eds.): *Ethnicity and Family Therapy.* New York, Grune & Stratton, 552–571, 1982.
70. Shon SP, Ja DY: Asian families. In: McGoldrick M, Pearce JK, Giordano J (eds.): *Ethnicity and Family Therapy.* New York, Guilford, 208–228, 1982.
71. Uzee E: *Videotaped discussion of working with Asian-American families [Working With Minority Families].* Symposium conducted at the 142nd Annual Meeting of the American Psychiatric Association, San Francisco, CA, May 6–11, 1989.
72. Grusec, JE, Hastings PD: *Handbook of Socialization.* New York, NY, Guilford Press, 2007:547.
73. Northrup JC, Bean RA: Culturally competent family therapy with Latino Anglo-American adolescents: facilitating identity formation. *Am J Fam Ther* 35: 251–263, 2007.
74. Pumariega A, Joshi SV: Culture and development in children and youth. *Child Adolesc Psychiatric Clin N Am* 19:661–680, 2010.
75. Kerwin C, Ponterotto JG: Biracial identity development: theory and research. In: Ponterotto JP, Casas JM, Suzuki LA, et al., (eds): *Handbook of multicultural counseling.* Thousand Oaks, CA: Sage, 199–217, 1995.
76. Wehrly B, Kenney KR, Kenney ME: *Counseling Multiracial Families.* Thousand Oaks, CA, Sage Publications, 1999.
77. Root MP: Resolving "other" status: identity development of biracial individuals. In: Brown LS, Root MP (eds): *Diversity and Complexity in Feminist Therapy.* New York, Haworth, 185–205, 1990.
78. Diller JV: *Cultural Diversity: A Primer for the Human Services.* Toronto, Wadsworth Publishing Company, 1999.
79. LaFromboise T, Coleman HL, Gerton J: Psychological impact of biculturalism: evidence and theory. *Psychol Bull* 1993;114:395–412.
80. Rashid HM: Promoting biculturalism in young African-American children. *Young Child* 39:13–23, 1984
81. Rozek F: The role of internal conflict in the successful acculturation of Russian Jewish immigrants. *Dissert Abstracts Int* 41:2778, 1980. B. University Microfilms No. 8028799.
82. Cauce AM, Hiraga Y, Mason C, et al.: Between a rock and a hard place: social adjustment of biracial youth. In: Root MP (ed): *Racially mixed people in America.* Newbury Park, CA: Sage, 207–222, 1992.
83. Hwang WC: Acculturative family distancing: theory, research, and clinical practice. *Psychotherapy (Chic)* 43(4):397–409, 2006.
84. Hwang WC, Wood JJ: Acculturative family distancing: links with self-reported symptomatology among Asian Americans and Latinos. *Child Psychiatry Hum Dev* 40(1):123–138, 2009.
85. Hwang WC, Wood JJ, Fujimoto K: Acculturative family distancing (AFD) and depression in Chinese American families. *J Consult Clin Psychol* 78(5):655–667, 2010.
86. Farver JA, Narang SK, Bhadha BR: East meets West: Ethnic identity, acculturation, and conflict in Asian Indian families. *J Fam Psychol* 16(3):338, 2002.
87. Wang-Kraus SD, Loftus PD, Chu IM, Martin A, Hwang W-C, Joshi SV: *Acculturative Family Distancing (AFD) in Secondary School Students: An Examination of Family Cohesion, Ruminations, and Help-Seeking Behaviors in Relation to Depression; Presented at the American Academy of Child & Adolescent Psychiatry (AACAP) Annual Meeting,* 2014.
88. Sholevar GP: Cultural child and adolescent psychiatry. In: Martin A, Volkmar F (eds). *Lewis's child and adolescent psychiatry: a comprehensive textbook.* Philadelphia, PA: Lippincott Williams & Wilkins; 57–65, 2007.
89. McLoyd VC: Socioeconomic disadvantage and child development. *Am Psychol* 53(2):185–204, 1998.
90. McDermott JF: Effects of culture and ethnicity on child & adolescent development. In: Lewis M (ed): *Child and Adolescent Psychiatry—A Comprehensive Textbook.* 3rd ed. Philadelphia, PA: Lippincott, 494–498, 2002.
91. https://www.census.gov/newsroom/press-releases/2015/cb15-tps16.html; accessed 9–7–16.
92. Tseng WS, Streltzer J (eds): *Cultural Competence in Clinical Psychiatry,* Washington, DC, American Psychiatric Publishing, 2–6, 2004.
93. Comas-Diaz L: Cross-cultural mental health treatment. In Comas-Diaz L, Griffith E (eds.): *Clinical Guidelines in Cross-cultural Mental Health.* New York, Wiley, 335–361, 1988.
94. Betancourt J, Cervantes M: Cross-cultural Med Ed in the US: key principles and experiences. *Kaohsiung J Med Sci* 25(9), 471–478, 2009.
95. Aggarwal NK. Cultural formulations in child and adolescent psychiatry. *J Am Acad Child Adolesc Psychiatry* 49(4):306–309, 2010.
96. Lewis-Fernández R, Aggarwal NK, Hinton L, Hinton DE, Kirmayer LJ: *DSM-5® Handbook on the Cultural Formulation Interview* Washington, DC, American Psychiatric Press Inc, 2016.
97. Lin K-M, Smith MW, Ortiz V. Culture and psychopharmacology. *Psychiatr Clin N Am* 2001;24(3):523–538.
98. Metzl JA. Forming an effective therapeutic alliance. In: Tasman A, Riba MB, Silk KR (eds): *The Doctor-Patient Relationship In Pharmacotherapy: Improving Treatment Effectiveness.* New York, Guilford Press, 25–47, 2000.
99. Broucek F, Ricci W: Self-disclosure of self-presence? *Bull Menninger Clin* 26(4):427–438, 1998.
100. Havens L: Forming effective relationships. In: Havens L, Sabo A (eds): *The Real World Guide to Psychotherapy Practice.* Cambridge, MA: Harvard University Press, 17–33, 2000.
101. Joshi SV: Teamwork: the therapeutic alliance in pediatric pharmacotherapy. *Child Adolesc Psychiatr Clin N Am* 15:239–262, 2006.
102. Sabo A, Rand B: The relational aspects of psychopharmacology. In: Sabo A, Havens L (eds): *The Real World Guide to Psychotherapy Practice.* Cambridge, MA, Harvard University Press, 34–59, 2000.
103. Choi H: Understanding adolescent depression in ethnocultural context. *ANS Adv Nurs Sci* 25(2):71–85, 2002.
104. Malik M, Lawson WB, Lake J, Joshi SV: Culturally adapted pharmacotherapy and the integrative formulation. *Child Adolesc Psychiatric Clin N Am* 19:791–814, 2010.
105. Al-Mateen C, Mian A, Pumariega AJ, Cerda G, Carter D, members of the AACAP: *Diversity and Culture Committee: Diversity and Cultural Competency Curriculum for Child and Adolescent Psychiatry Training,* June 2011. Available at: https://www.aacap.org/AACAP/Resources_for_Primary_Care/Diversity_and_Cultural_Competency_Curriculum/Home.aspx, accessed on 9/7/2016.
106. Pumariega AJ, Rothe E, the AACAP Diversity and Culture Committee: *Practice Parameter for Culturally Competent Child & Adolescent Psychiatric Practice,* April 2013. Available at: http://www.aacap.org/App_Themes/AACAP/docs/practice_parameters/Cultural_Competence_Web.pdf; accessed 9/7/2016.
107. Klein M. *Love, Guilt, and Reparation & Other Works, 1921–1945.* New York, Free Press, 2002.
108. Winnicott D: Transitional objects and transitional phenomena—a study of the first not-me possession. *Int J Psycho-Anal* 34:89–97, 1953.
109. Mahler M: On the first three subphases of the separation–individuation process. *Psychoanal Contemp Sci* 3:295–306, 1974.
110. Bornstein M, Tamis-LeMonda C, Tal J, et al.: Maternal responsiveness to infants in three societies: the United States, France, and Japan. *Child Dev* 63:808–821, 1992.
111. Latz S, Wolf AW, Lozoff B: Cosleeping in Context: Sleep Practices and Problems in Young Children in Japan and the United States. *Arch Pediatric Adolesc Med* 153(4):339–346, 1999.
112. Shimizu M, Park H, Greenfield PM: Infant sleeping arrangements and cultural values among contemporary Japanese mothers. *Front Psychol* 5:718, 2014.
113. Dweck C: *Mindset: The New Psychology of Success.* New York, Ballantine, 2007.
114. Duckworth A: *Grit: The Power of Passion and Perseverence.* New York, Scribner, 2016.
115. Joshi SV, Pumariega A, Reicherter D, Roberts LW: Cultural issues in ethics and professionalism. In: Roberts L, Reicherter D (eds.): *Professionalism and Ethics: A Q & A Study Guide for Mental Health Professionals.* Washington, DC, American Psychiatric Press, Inc., 39–56, 2014.
116. Cross T, Bazron B, Dennis K, Isaacs M: *Towards a culturally competent system of care.* Vol. 1. Washington, DC: Child & Adolescent Service System Program, Tech Assistance Center; Georgetown University Child Development Center, 1989.
117. Kleinman A, Benson P: Anthropology in the clinic: the problem of cultural competency and how to fix it. *PLoS Med* 3(10):1673–1676, 2006.
118. Berlin EA, Fowkes WC: A teaching framework for cross-cultural health care: application in family practice. *West J Med* 139:934–938, 1983.
119. Teal CR, Street RL: Critical elements of culturally competent communication in the medical encounter: a review and model. *Soc Sci Med* 68(3):533–543, 2009.
120. Betancourt JR: Cultural competence—marginal or mainstream movement? *N Eng J Med* 351:953–954, 2004.
121. Dogra N, Karnik N: The Cultural Sensibility Model: a process-oriented approach for children and adolescents. *Child Adolesc Psychiatric Clin N Am* 19:719–737, 2010.
122. Hixon A: Beyond cultural competence. *Acad Med* 78(6):634, 2003.
123. Engebretson J, Mahoney J, Carlson ED: Cultural competence in the era of evidence-based practice. *J Prof Nurs* 24:172–178, 2008.
124. Lee SA, Farrell M: Is cultural competency a backdoor to racism? *Anthropol News* 47(3):9–10, 2006. Available at: http://raceproject.aaanet.org/pdf/rethinking/ lee_farrell.pdf; accessed 8 Feb 2014.
125. Green JW: On cultural competence. *Anthropol News* 47(5):3, 2006.
126. Lensing LA: Franz would be with us here. *Times Liter Suppl*:13–15, 2003.
127. American Psychiatric Association: Best practice highlights for treating diverse patient populations. Available at: https://www.psychiatry.org/psychiatrists/cultural-competency/treating-diverse-patient-populations; accessed 10–28–16.
128. American Psychological Association: Guidelines for providers of psychological services to ethnic, linguistic, and culturally diverse populations. Available at: http://www.apa.org/pi/oema/resources/policy/provider-guidelines.aspx; accessed 10–28–16.
129. DiversityRx: Cultural Competence 101. http://www.diversityrx.org/topic-areas/cultural-competence-101; accessed 10–28–16.
130. Joshi SV, Pumariega AJ: Preface: America's new kids. *Child Adolesc Psychiatric Clin N Am* 19(4):xv–xvii, 2010.

CHAPTER 2.2.2 ■ PSYCHIATRIC CARE OF THE DEAF, BLIND, OR DEAF-BLIND CHILD

KAREN A. GOLDBERG AND JANA K. DREYZEHNER

GENERAL CONSIDERATIONS

This chapter provides an overview of deafness and visual impairment conditions, which alone or in combination with other medical challenges, can have a significant impact on a child's development and mental well-being. Sensory-related loss does not cause psychiatric illness per se but may affect symptom presentation. Misdiagnosis of psychiatric disorders may occur if the diagnostician is unaware of the adaptive differences and, hence, the variability in timing and acquisition of developmental milestones. Misdiagnosis may also occur if the practitioner does not appreciate the impacts of communication challenges the deaf or blind child has with primary caregivers. The child's environment can shape the sequential acquisition of skills and the developmental process. Troubled behavior may represent independent psychiatric conditions or consist of acquired maladaptive compensatory behaviors. The influence of deafness or blindness on the developmental process as well as the presentation of psychiatric signs and symptoms and the context in which the child functions are pivotal to the psychiatric evaluation of the child with hearing loss or blindness.

The objectives of a psychiatric evaluation are accurate diagnosis and development of an appropriate treatment plan that addresses the multiple and complex problems identified (1). The nature and extent of impairments differ with etiology, age of onset, and other complicating factors. Fundamental considerations for evaluation of a deaf and/or blind child include:

a. The tremendous range and heterogeneity of the sensory loss;
b. Occurrence of multiple sensory losses (e.g., Deaf-blind conditions);
c. Co-occurring challenges (autism, intellectual disability);
d. Complex interdependence of the sensory-related issue with environment;
e. Caregiver response to having a deaf or blind child;
f. Differing potentials among children with similar sensory loss.

Comorbidities may occur from autism spectrum disorders, attention deficit hyperactivity disorder (ADHD), intellectual disabilities, neuropsychological disorders of learning, central nervous system syndromes, and traumatic brain injuries. Many children and adolescents who have comorbidities often do not fit neatly into a simple DSM-5 diagnosis, and should be categorized through a comprehensive biopsychosocial-developmental evaluation and presented in context of comorbid diagnoses. In addition, those who evaluate and work with youngsters who have degrees of deafness and blindness may lack awareness and understanding that many individuals with sensory-related losses with or without comorbidities lead successful and constructive lives. This point is important because professional attitudes and expectations can dramatically shape the evaluation and treatment outcomes.

Being a deaf, blind, or deaf-blind individual does not necessarily increase the risk of developing mental health problems. However, associated factors and presence of additional medical problems may increase the likelihood of mental health issues. Consequences of being deaf or visually impaired in a world that is oriented to the needs of hearing and sighted people may add to the burden of these individuals. The vast majority of deaf and visually impaired children are born into hearing and sighted families, and as such, it is important to consider the goodness of fit in meeting the needs of the child. Brain insults and other physical illnesses linked to the cause of deafness or blindness may confer additional neuropsychological vulnerabilities. Finally, children with deafness and visual sensory impairments are more vulnerable to all forms of abuse and neglect (2).

MODELS OF DEAFNESS, VISUAL IMPAIRMENT, AND DEAF-BLINDNESS: CULTURE AND DISABILITY

It is important that clinicians understand that there are two key models used in conceptualizing deafness and blindness: the medical model and the cultural model. These models are not necessarily in contrast with one another but may help clinicians in understanding the differing perspectives. Deafness and/or blindness not only affects how the child perceives the world, but how the world perceives the child and most importantly, how the child perceives him/herself.

Medical definitions of deafness and blindness focus on the sensory impairment including the etiology, severity, age of onset, and the presence or absence of additional disabilities. It also focuses on possible medical interventions to aid or correct the defect. The medical model provides a language for practitioners to communicate regarding the actual audiologic/ocular conditions but leaves out consideration of the context and cultural identity of the individual with the hearing or visual impairment. Medically accepted terms include sensory impairment, hearing impairment, hearing loss, and deafness as well as visual impairment, vision loss, and blindness.

Cultural models focus more on the richness and uniqueness of the social experience, as well as the connectedness among members sharing the sensory-related issue and their combined sense of purpose and group identity. The cultural model challenges the notion that deafness or blindness represents solely a sensory-related loss and rejects the notion that the person is disabled, impaired, or needs to be fixed. Deaf culture consists of a set of beliefs, unique language, and proud history shared by deaf individuals. Deaf with a capital D is used to connote this sense of cultural identity while the smaller case d, deaf, is used to connote the actual audiologic condition. Deaf cultural perspective rejects medical terminology that indicates impairment. Preferred terminology for the hearing loss is deaf, deafness or hard of hearing. Blind individuals and those with visual impairment share unique experiences with one another, but a specific blind culture does

TABLE 2.2.2.1

DEFINITIONS OF DEAFNESS AND BLINDNESS

Deafness	Blindness	Deaf-Blind
SEVERITY: Mild 21–40 dB Moderate 41–70 dB Severe 71–90 dB Profound 91+ dB	SEVERITY: Mild 20/70 or better Moderate 20/70–20/200 Severe 20/200–20/400 Blindness 20/400 or worse Legal blindness: Worse than 20/200	SEVERITY: Deafness + any degree blindness Legally blind + any degree deafness
AGE OF ONSET: Congenital Early onset Acquired/Late deafened Progressive	AGE OF ONSET: Congenital Early onset Acquired	AGE OF ONSET: Congenital Early onset Acquired
SITE: Conductive Sensorineural	SITE: Peripheral Central	SITE: Conductive or sensorineural deafness Peripheral or central blindness
DESCRIPTOR: Deaf: Profound deafness Hard of hearing: Moderate to severe deafness	DESCRIPTOR: Characterized by severity on the Snellen visual acuity test	DESCRIPTOR: Any combination of deafness combined with any degree of visual impairment
CULTURAL: Communication with common language (American Sign Language) Identification and unity with other deaf individuals Common experience of being minority community and history of oppression	CULTURAL: No distinct language apart from majority community Braille is translated majority language (not separate language) Shared experience of experiencing world with visual impairment	CULTURAL: Identify more with Deaf culture Common experience of communication with hand over hand signing or hands on finger spelling. Identification with other deaf-blind people and experience of oppression

not exist per se (3). Individuals who are both deaf and blind often align with Deaf culture and refer to themselves as Deaf-Blind persons. This chapter will attempt to present the material in a manner that is both culturally and linguistically affirmative, and as such, will utilize as much culturally preferred terminology as possible. Table 2.2.2.1 provides useful definitions.

The National Standards for Culturally and Linguistically Appropriate Services (National CLAS Standards) in Health and Healthcare were first developed by the Health and Human Services Office of Minority Health in 2000 with the aim of advancing health equity, improving quality, and helping eliminate health care disparities. It was designed as a blueprint for individuals and health care organizations to implement CLAS. The Enhanced Standards (2013) are a comprehensive series of guidelines that inform, guide, and facilitate practices related to culturally and linguistically appropriate health services (4).

There are several resources that would be useful for practitioners in working with deaf and blind children. The National Association of the Deaf (NAD) is the nation's premier civil rights organization of, by, and for deaf and hard of hearing individuals in the United States of America (www.NAD.org). Alexander Graham Bell Association is another resource for hearing loss with more focus on listening and spoken language (www.AGBELL.org). The American Foundation for the Blind (www.AFB.org) and the National Federation of the Blind (www.NFB.org) are two excellent resources for information regarding vision loss. The Helen Keller National Center for Deaf-Blind Youth and Adults (www.HKNC.org) is an excellent resource as well for the combined conditions.

THE ROLE OF THE CHILD AND ADOLESCENT PSYCHIATRIST

The role of the psychiatrist is unique as liaison to interface and interact with a multidisciplinary medical or rehabilitation team and the family, school, and community. The training of a child and adolescent psychiatrist permits the comprehensive integration of biologic, developmental, family/environmental, learning/educational, and psychodynamic/psychiatric issues in order to develop a diagnostic formulation. In both evaluation and treatment, the consulting psychiatrist needs to establish a collegial relationship with the parents and school staff. Frequently, the school or rehabilitation service requests a consultation in order to assess risk of suicide, psychopharmacologic management, or change in level of care or educational program. Current educational trends for sensory-related issues include early intervention assessments and therapeutic programs for infants and toddlers exhibiting developmental delays and integration of deaf and blind children into regular schools. These trends increase the probability that child psychiatrists lacking specialized experience may be asked to evaluate these youngsters. Referrals may come directly from schools where children are mainstreamed or from specialized schools (schools specific for deaf and/or blind students). In specialized schools, there is a need for initial triage, assessment of complex biopsychosocial issues, and managing the psychiatric care. Most cases of deafness or blindness are lifelong; hence, the initial involvement of the child psychiatrist often evolves into a long-term connection. Child and adolescent psychiatrists must accommodate comfortably to specialized settings and adapt innovative interviewing techniques in both assessment and treatment.

Learning manual sign language is very helpful in working with deaf and hard of hearing children, but difficult to master. A certified interpreter for deaf children and utilization of play with a blind child are feasible alternatives. Familiarity with the use and purpose of various assistive devices can facilitate rapport with the child and family. The child psychiatrist who is best able to approach the evaluation is knowledgeable in child development; looks for adaptational, problem-solving, and functional strengths; is aware that a sensory loss does not routinely result in psychological impairment; and seeks to identify the strengths and weaknesses within the child and his/her family. The questions, "How does the deafness or blindness interface with the developmental process and/or the environment and what have been the adaptive responses?" are very helpful. The goals of the examination should include looking for the child's level of independence, cognitive abilities, functional abilities, communication abilities, social adjustments, and psychological adaptations. Further, the examiner would want to consider why this case has been referred at this time; who made the referral; what is happening in the home, family, or school; for example, does the child need a new school or is the child aging out of the current school; has the child grown and developed to the point where previous management techniques are no longer possible and medications are being requested; and is there an underlying purpose for the referral, such as expediting removal of the child from the home, school, or changing the level of care? Assessment of the various domains of development is indicated in infants and toddlers. Further, the examiner would want to assess the child's ability to understand cause and effect relationships to modify his or her behavior. Reviewing various records and looking for the longitudinal patterns in addition to associated impairments answers some of these questions.

The psychiatrist who is educated about the medical and cultural aspects of the sensory-related condition would be in an ideal position to offer optimal service. The evaluating psychiatrist needs to ascertain the parents' expectations and from what sources they have received advice. The parent may have the view of the deaf or blind child as permanently damaged and this may be a contributor to the psychological distress that the child experiences. Alternatively, the parent may minimize or deny the reality of their child's circumstances, pursuing unrealistic treatments and goals. The level of the parental involvement and advocacy for their child are important predictors of the child's success. In many cases, the "validity" of the parental expectations can be determined only after the fact, retrospectively once the child has grown. Assessment of the environment and family of the deaf or blind child must be an integral component to the comprehensive psychiatric evaluation. The parents or primary caregivers may experience extreme demands on their time and energy in caring for the child, may experience pressure from family or community members on how best to deal with the situation, and may experience periods of emotional distress themselves. These strains could lead to deleterious interactions with the deaf or blind child and may negatively impact the bonding between child and parent. Family structure and alliances can become skewed, and the full dimensions of family life may be curtailed. Financial costs can further tax family resources. A gulf can grow between parents as polarized reactions occur. Siblings may feel excluded, jealous, or cheated while conflicted with the relief that they themselves are not dealing directly with the sensory-related issue. Many families are able to form healthy and constructive responses. The task of communicating one's findings and engaging the family and school toward recommended treatment and intervention is made more difficult if they have contributed to maladaptive behaviors and stunted development. Clinical sensitivity and expertise is required to help parents and other caregivers including school personnel recognize both their positive and negative influence on the process and outcome of treatment.

DEAF, HARD OF HEARING, AND HEARING LOSS

Definition

Hearing loss in children is divided into hard of hearing and profoundly deaf groups. Historically, the distinction was based on those youngsters who could utilize their diminished auditory perceptions for communication and those who could not. There was early pressure to mold these youngsters into the oral hearing world as much as possible. This drove the development and refinement of hearing-assistive devices such as cochlear implants, digital hearing aids, auditory loops, FM systems, and infrared systems. Early identification and expanded rehabilitation services has permitted an increasing number of children with significant hearing loss to effectively use their residual hearing. Hearing loss in children is also classified by the age of onset. "Prelingual" refers to onset of hearing loss before the use of spoken language, and "postlingual" to hearing loss occurring after spoken language has been acquired. Generally, a loss of hearing before 2 years of age is considered prelingual. The age of onset of hearing loss can have a significant impact on oral language acquisition.

Hearing deprivation has existed throughout history. Educators and religious figures who have taken on the task of instruction of deaf pupils have influenced Western European attitudes and practices. The controversy among proponents of manual, oral, and total communication (combination of both manual and oral language) has waxed and waned over time and are detailed in the *Oxford Handbook of Deaf Studies, Language, and Education*, Volume 2 by Marschark and Spencer (5). The Deaf culture movement has challenged the rights of parents, medical professionals, and educational systems to remove a child from the culture by assistive hearing devices such as cochlear implantation (which is often done by the age of 2 years old). Further, it has questioned the obligation of larger systems and even society's role in pressuring parents, particularly hearing parents, to pursue a means to "cure" deafness rather than present alternative perspectives in managing deafness (American Sign Language [ASL] and inclusion in Deaf culture). Deaf culture and the promotion of ASL have influenced implementation of the Individuals with Disabilities Education Act (IDEA). With the introduction of Public Law 94-142 in 1975, deaf and hard-of-hearing students have increasingly been taught and educated in regular schools largely populated by hearing children, although the extent of academic integration varies. The IDEA revision of 2004 further supported the movement of deaf and hard-of-hearing students into mainstream education where opportunities for bilingual (sign and oral language) education and an accommodation for various communication devices (language boards, computers, etc.) is an expectation. Public Law 99-457, which established early intervention programs, has done the same for children ages 0 to 3. The recommendations of the Commission on the Education of the Deaf also represent significant steps on behalf of the deaf to incorporate bilingual–bicultural (Bi-Bi) language approach.

Prevalence and Epidemiology

According to the Centers for Disease Control Early Hearing Detection and Intervention (EHDI) Program in 2013, the prevalence of hearing loss in all screened infants was 1.5 per 1,000 (6). Newborn hearing screening is conducted via otoacoustic emissions (OAEs) and Auditory Brainstem Response Test (ABR). The OAE Test operates as an objective measure of hearing by sending sound vibrations through the patient's ear canal and middle ear to the outer hair cells of the cochlea. If the middle ear is clear of fluid and infection and the cochlea working properly, then the outer hair cells will echo the sound back. The ABR is also an objective test that assesses the organs of hearing, auditory nerve, and auditory pathways to the level of the brainstem (7). Some infants who pass newborn hearing screening will later demonstrate permanent hearing loss (8). Although this loss may reflect delayed-onset hearing loss, both

ABR and OAE screening technologies will miss some hearing loss (e.g., mild or isolated frequency region losses).

By school age, approximately 6 to 7 per 1,000 can be expected to have a permanent hearing loss (9). Mehra et al. conducted a review of studies looking at prevalence of hearing loss in children and adolescents between 1958 and 1995 and found that the average prevalence of hearing impairment is 3.1% (10). According to the Annual Disability Statistics Compendium, the number of children with disabilities, ages 6 to 21, served in the public schools under the IDEA Part B in Fall 2013 was 5,693,441 (in the 50 states and DC) which reflected 8.4% of the resident population ages 6 to 21. Of these children, 65,502 (1.2%) received services for hearing impairment (11).

Morzaria et al. conducted a systematic review of etiology of bilateral sensorineural hearing loss in children in 2004 by reviewing 780 articles between 1966 and 2002 (12). They found that the most common etiology of bilateral sensorineural hearing loss is unknown, likely multifactorial. Of the known etiologies, nearly 30% were noted to be due to genetic etiologies including syndromic conditions such as Waardenburg syndrome, Velocardiofacial syndrome, Down syndrome, Goldenhar syndrome, Branchio-Oto-Renal syndrome and the remainder due to nonsyndromic genetic causes. There are many distinct genetic forms of hearing loss interfering with normal conversation. Mutations in the GJB2 gene are the most common cause of inherited congenital deafness (13). Of the prenatal etiologies, it was noted that the majority were due to infectious etiologies such as Rubella, CMV, and measles. Prematurity, kernicterus, and asphyxia accounted for the majority of perinatal etiologies. In childhood, recurrent otitis media with effusion accounts for the bulk of hearing loss which, if caught early and treated with myringotomy tubes, permanent damage can be minimized.

Developmental Considerations

Historically, the concern with hearing loss has been the deprivation of language, owing predominantly to the inability to acquire oral spoken language (14), particularly since more than 90% of deaf children are born to hearing parents (15). Deafness and its consequences on developing oral language can have a profound effect on other domains of development given its influence on cognition and social behaviors. During the developing preschool years, when hearing children gain sufficient mastery of spoken language to express needs, desires, and emotions, the deaf children of hearing families are confronted with tremendous obstacles.

This concern about oral language acquisition has been one of the reasons that roughly 40% of children who are born profoundly deaf receive a cochlear implant per the U.S. Food and Drug Administration. According to the Agency's analysis, as of December 2012, in the United States, approximately 96,000 cochlear implants were implanted in patients. This number constituted approximately 30% of all devices implanted in patients around the world. Also, in the United States, approximately 60% of the cochlear implants (N = 58,000) were implanted in patients who are 18 years of age and older, while the remaining 40% of the cochlear implants (N = 38,000) were implanted in pediatric patients who are 17 years of age and younger. Furthermore, approximately 26% of the cochlear implants (N = 25,000) were implanted in children aged 5 and younger (16).

Language Development

Language is the tool for formulating thoughts and is differentiated from speech (articulation) or communication (which is an interactive and reciprocal exchange). A deaf baby babbles at the same age as a hearing baby. The deaf baby ceases to babble when babbling becomes social and infants begin to model the sounds they produce on the sounds they hear. There are wide variations in the milestones of the onset of speech in hearing children. The deaf child's lack of response to sounds might be rationalized away. For the hearing parents, the delayed and startling diagnosis of deafness requires a dramatic reorientation of their conceptualization of their child. The parents are faced simultaneously with a major decision as to the type of language acquisition training including manual or sign language, oral language, or total communication which encompasses both, often in the face of conflicting professional opinions. The campaign against the use of manual language was based largely on the misconceptions that oral language is necessary for abstract thought and interacting with the hearing world, and that sign language is not a true language. Noam Chomsky's suggestion of an innate preprogramming for the process of language has been widely supported (17). Spontaneous sign systems observed in children of different cultures contribute to the understanding of the innateness of language in human infants (18). Observations that the syntactic structures and processes of language development of deaf and hearing children are similar lend support to the expanding use of sign. Stokoe et al. demonstrated sign language to be a true language through linguistic analysis of ASL and publication of the first dictionary of ASL that was based on linguistic principles in 1965 (19).

The hearing child with hearing parents learns spoken language through environmental interaction. The deaf child learns communicative language by visual means. The position of oral language proponents is that the deaf child will be unable to interact with the dominant hearing population without some spoken communication. Support for early auditory amplification and training is encouraged, so that the process of vocalization and babbling can be preserved and the concept of sound for communication and shaping of the vocalizations can be facilitated. The manual argument asserts that the vast majority of deaf people ultimately enter deaf culture for social and personal needs; therefore, they should feel comfortable with and accomplished in the language of their culture. The potential psychological conflicts in this dichotomy, which confront the consulting psychiatrist, are highly emotionally charged. This controversy is not dissimilar to the debates on bilingual education and accommodations to diversity and multiculturalism. Oral training is demanding; its proponents state that signing hinders its successful mastery. There remains great heterogeneity of achievement within both the oral and total communication groups and varying degrees of success in formal language acquisition. The tragedy of this politically charged controversy is that parents are required to make a lifelong decision for their child while facing emotional upheaval. Child psychiatrists' greatest value during the child's crucial cognitive and social development period may be to help parents teach acceptable behavior, including rules, compromise, and delayed gratification. This may be particularly difficult when the parent is dependent on only a "yes" or "no" response in exclusive oral communication.

The eventual language preference among deaf young adults balances the nature of the residual hearing, quality of early training, usefulness of communication, and cultural orientation of the individual toward the hearing world or deaf culture social groups. Many adults develop bilingualism in varying degrees but the issue of language and social isolation persists with varying psychological consequences. The deaf child in a hearing family tends to be isolated irrespective of communication. Deaf adolescents trying to function within the hearing environment particularly complain about their difficulty at parties and dances, where lowering of lights and background dance music makes communication and flirting almost impossible. To conceptualize such difficulties, consider the child who encounters any number of situations where vision and hearing are used and coordinated simultaneously, such as class note taking, talking at the dinner table, or honking cars warning of danger. Many children who later prefer to use sign but whose parents do not, often view the parents' lack of communication skills as evidence that they do not accept them. Sibling interactions with the deaf child also affect self-perceptions and social skills. Adolescents often try to fake hearing and discard aids with frequent negative consequence in self-concept.

Cognitive Processes and Theories

Cognition is linked to language acquisition. Areas of exploration, including memory, visual-motor and perceptual-motor functions and problem-solving strategies are being pursued with advanced technologies, an increased knowledge in the basic neuroscience, neuropsychology, and rehabilitation therapies. Reported intelligence quotient (IQ) scores and academic achievement are concerns for the child psychiatrist but scores can be misleading. The most commonly used tests among deaf children are the performance subscale of the Wechsler Intelligence Scale for Children, 4th edition (WISC-IV) and more recently the Wechsler Intelligence Scale for Children, 5th ed (WISC-V, 2014). The Leiter International Performance Scale, Wechsler Preschool and Primary Scale of Intelligence, 4th ed (WPPSI-IV, 2012), Goodenough Draw-a-Person Test, Kaufman Test of Educational Assessment, 2nd ed (KTEA-II), the nonverbal section of the Kaufman Assessment Battery for Children (K-ABC), Test of Nonverbal Intelligence (TONI) and Test of Early Reading Ability-Deaf or Hard of Hearing (TERA-D/HH) are also used for cognitive assessments in Deaf/Hard of Hearing children. The Wechsler scales were not designed for hearing, visual, or motor impairments. As stated in the WISC Manual, although one may prefer to place greater weight on the performance subtests to estimate the cognitive ability of a child with hearing loss, the WISC was not standardized with modifications. If sign language and other visual aids are necessary to give instructions to a deaf child, the evaluator and presumably the clinicians who are likely to use the tests scores should recall such alterations to have an impact on scores. For infants and preschoolers, developmental measures such as the Bayley Scales of Infant Development, 3rd Ed (BSID-III), Gesell Developmental Schedules, or Cattell Infant Intelligence Scales are used.

The following are considerations in the psychometric testing of deaf and hard of hearing children: The instrument should be nonverbal, because a verbal instrument can reflect language rather than cognition; there is greater likelihood that the instrument will report a falsely low score than a falsely elevated score; there is increased potential error when the test is administered by an examiner not familiar with hearing loss, unable to communicate instructions in the child's preferred mode; personality tests are difficult to interpret because subtlety of instructions might not have been communicated and responses may be limited or unintelligible; and testing of preschool children at whose age communication skills are only beginning to develop is vulnerable to error and underestimation of potential. Krouse and Braden investigated the validity of the WISC-IV and found that the scores are at least reliable in terms of internal consistency for deaf/hard of hearing students as they are for normal hearing students (20). Verbal tests of intelligence are not recommended for the cognitive assessment of deaf and hard of hearing individuals (21). Braden found little correlation of the nonverbal, WISC-R Performance Scale k(PS) IQ to academic achievement using the Stanford Achievement Test-Hearing Impaired Edition (22). This suggests that the criterion of academic achievement fails to be an accurate reflection of the deaf child's innate cognitive abilities. Currently, many schools for the deaf use total communication where the teacher articulates and uses sign. The educational outcome of impaired children who have been mainstreamed is still uncertain, as is the long-range achievement results for deaf children taught by total communication. However, it is most likely that the psychiatrist will evaluate a child with academic delays or unevenness in achievement.

Social Development

Language status influences social development and subsequent behavioral difficulties. The impact of deafness on child development can be readily observed in infants' orienting behaviors. Hearing children can hear their mother coo to them and orient toward their direction. They learn that crying attracts their mother's attention even out of sight. This experience is not available to the deaf child. Teaching social rules and concepts or right and wrong cannot be done easily by explanations, and the child often perceives limit setting as capricious. The child's developing theory of mind, as an interconnected network of beliefs, desires, and feelings influencing behavior, can be helpful in understanding social, emotional and cognitive development. Peterson and Siegal have developed a theory of mind from studies of prelingual signing deaf children (23). The influence of deafness on development can be understood in light of various theories of development, for example, Eriksonian developmental stages, Bowlby's attachment theories, and so on. Vaccari and Marschark have explored the role of effective parent–child communication in the social and emotional development of deaf children (24).

The prevalence of reported emotional and behavioral problems among deaf children is three times that of the general pediatric population. In summarizing various reports, Meadow and Trybus find deaf children to be described as hyperactive, immature, and impulsive (25). There is a general impression that a typical "deaf personality" exists. Personality features usually included are characteristics such as impulsivity, hyperactivity, rigidity, suspiciousness, and immaturity. Following other investigators who have challenged these suppositions, Chess et al. used a sample of 248 children with congenital rubella followed longitudinally from age 2.5 to 14 years. They concluded that deafness does not confer a "typical personality"; it is the behavioral symptomatology of those with neurologic damage that is largely responsible for such a stereotype in the rubella-deaf (26). Application of stress and coping models in studying adjustment indicate that social support is predictive of maternal adjustment and that maternal problem-solving skills are significant predictors of child adjustment (27).

Adolescent development poses different difficulties because information comes primarily from peers and the environment outside of the home, at the mall, pizza parlor, or street. By this age, deaf teens who are ASL users have a social network within the deaf community, obtaining information not accessed from hearing parents or other adults. Landsberger et al. conducted a study to look at psychiatric diagnoses and psychosocial needs of outpatient deaf children and adolescents compared to hearing counterparts. Over one-third of deaf youth had impaired family relationships, living situation, communication, judgment, and physical health (28). Charlson et al. have reported as an in-depth evaluation of successful deaf teenagers (29). All of their subjects reported some degree of isolation from hearing peers or family that was associated with communication difficulties. Their sample included deaf teenagers with deaf and hearing parents, and residential schools. Most of the students had developed a strategy for coping with the isolation, further raising the impact of parent's signing skill on adolescent social development, highlighting deafness as a significant variable in the task of developing sense of autonomy and competence.

Psychiatric Evaluation of a Deaf or Hard of Hearing Child or Adolescent

The evaluation, treatment, and management of deaf children with psychiatric disorder is intimately related to the child's communication (30). Beyond the general techniques of child psychiatry interviewing, the examiner should focus on the preferred mode of communication for the child and be prepared to function within that modality. Assessments should include the parent's ability to communicate in the child's preferred mode, the impact of the parent–child communication and alternative, nonverbal interactive strategies of parents and their deaf children (31). For preverbal and nonverbal children, a behavioral analysis with detailed information from long-term caregivers helps to interpret the child's behavior. The oral child relies on lip-reading cues; hence, the examiner should provide a continuous unobstructed view. To communicate with a deaf child, a gentle touch or waving the hand in the child's visual field is acceptable. The examiner should not sit with the sun or a bright light behind the back, creating shadows and eyestrain. If the child's preferred mode of communication is sign, a certified sign interpreter is required for an examiner with sign skills adaptable to the level of the child or adolescent. A family member is unacceptable, because the child is not free to communicate confidentially. The interpreter is best situated next to the examiner, allowing the child an unobstructed view of both examiner and interpreter.

The syntax and grammar of ASL, as with other languages, are completely different from those of English. ASL is a distinct language, not a codified form of English. When ASL is translated word for word, the language form appears fragmented and disorganized, and has been confused with psychotic processes (32). Formal language defects are often similar in sign language to those found among hearing populations, with changes in rate of production, echolalia, perseveration, and neologisms. The assessment of language and communication is fundamental to any psychiatric evaluation and particularly vulnerable to errors in assessing a child with hearing loss. Even good speech readers understand a limited percentage of the mouth and lip formations without cues. Effective communication requires constant concentration, guesses, adequate vocabulary level, quality training, and experience. The common use of idioms and slang in verbal conversations can present problems when working with oral (speech–reading dependent) youngsters. For example, an oral deaf adolescent boy considered to have excellent speech–reading skills responded with an inappropriate response to the quotation, "when push comes to shove." After a prolonged effort to understand and explore the bizarre response, it appeared that the youngster had speech read, "put it on the shelf" and that his response was congruent to that reading.

Proverbs that are used in psychiatric examination for the hearing are misleading. Many proverbs have no meaning to the deaf, such as, "The squeaky wheel gets all the grease." Many words and phrases routinely used in mental health settings adapted from physical medicine assume a mental health, context-dependent meaning. For example, "How are you feeling?" has elicited the response, "Nothing" from a crying deaf adolescent because she had no physical pain. A common vocabulary is important with children and adolescents; and a determination whether they know the sign "emotion" and its connotations is critical. The examiner might list for the child the signs of happy, sad, and the like, interspersed with some simple nouns to find if the patient can distinguish which are emotions. Deaf individuals have hallucinations, look into space, and even sign into space toward the source, but it is not helpful to pursue the question, "Are you hearing voices?" Some may report that people or sources such as loudspeakers are talking about them or commenting specifically to or about them. This must be distinguished from prevalent beliefs often true within deaf culture that hearing people talk about them behind their backs. Schneiderian first-rank symptoms can be elicited, but ideas of reference must be teased away from cultural belief systems and experience. The psychopathology of paranoia poses similar problems. Drawings can be helpful in finding psychodynamic material. The Goodenough Draw-a-Person Test can provide an estimated intelligence level. House-Tree-Person Test and Family Kinetic Drawings are helpful in gathering projective material and exploring relationships. It is best to interpret the drawings based on a story obtained about the drawing. Questions about what is happening, what the subject of the drawing is thinking, feeling, and hopes for the future prove richer than the usual theoretical interpretive formulations of symbolic meanings. Psychometrically sound functional scales specific to this population may further clarify symptoms and adaptive functioning.

Differential Diagnosis

Intellectual disabilities need to be ruled out in a deaf child or an adolescent with problem behavior. Autism spectrum disorders, childhood schizophrenia, ADHD, depression, conduct disorder, and parent–child conflict need careful consideration. ADHD occurs in 3% to 5% of the general childhood population and in 6.6% of children with hearing loss (33,34). Delays in academics or simple knowledge about the world may present as immaturity, dependency, or educational delay. Deaf children are accustomed to routine sequences of actions because their parents and mentors find it difficult to explain changes. They themselves may later insist on sameness, leading to a misdiagnosis of childhood schizophrenia, autism, or obsessive-compulsive personality disorder. In a deaf child, alternative causes must be considered for all these diagnoses.

Differential diagnosis of behavioral disturbances among deaf children requires the clinician to consider unusual presentations of conditions that exist in hearing children. Tinnitus that occurs among deaf children may be mistakenly diagnosed as hallucinations. The assessment of multiply disabled deaf children requires a large team of highly specialized evaluators including audiologists, speech–language pathologists, teachers of deaf/hard of hearing and certified sign language interpreters (certified ASL interpreter and certified deaf interpreter [CDI]). The position paper on recommended assessment procedures for these youngsters adopted by the Conference of Educational Administrators Serving the Deaf provides a useful and comprehensive listing of all the areas that need to be considered (35). IDEA and PL99-457 that establishes early intervention strategies for children 0 to 3 with developmental delays and handicapping conditions identify areas that need consideration. In evaluating a deaf child with comorbid diagnoses, the psychiatrist is cautioned from automatically placing the sensory-related issue as the primary issue. This could inadvertently underestimate other impairing conditions such as intellectual disability, ADHD, psychosis, central nervous system syndromes, and so on, which might more accurately dictate functional capacity, treatment, and prognosis.

Treatment and Management

Deaf and hard of hearing professionals have a vital role in providing mental health services to deaf children and adolescents. Intervention strategies utilizing evidenced-based approaches always should be considered. Offering services to support parents, enhance their coping skills, and develop their own support system is an integral part of providing services to this population. A developmental approach in providing services requires recognizing the parents' and children's varying needs at different ages and family stages. Management of the different developmental trajectories and unevenness in various developmental domains needs a wider array of viable modalities of communication, such as sign, play, art, movement, and so on. Prioritizing treatment and subsequent management is like that for other children presenting with psychiatric disorders.

Effective communication is a high priority for primary prevention and treatment of emotional–behavioral disorders in deaf and hard of hearing children. Child and adolescent psychiatrists who work in the field of deafness place a high priority on social/emotional development, psychosocial group identification and support, and a sense of self-identity, which is the core of deaf culture based on sign language. The well-versed practitioner is one who is able to help the family and patient weigh the benefits versus risks of which communication option to pursue, be it sign language or oral language or total communication. The selection of total communication or oral training depends on a number of factors, but it is best addressed by helping parents weigh the pros and cons of each. Parents are often not fully aware of the options as they are interfacing with the medical community and may have limited access or awareness of the Deaf community. To lead parents one way or the other may not ultimately be in the best interest of the child or the family (36).

Treatment focuses on the acquisition of acceptable behaviors for the developmental period, if the behavior problem is not owing to independent psychiatric conditions. Behavior modification has been successful with deaf children, as group psychotherapy has been with deaf adolescents. Group psychotherapy provides an avenue to share feelings and behavioral strategies, particularly around maturational and adjustment issues. Studies proving efficacy of individual psychotherapy in the language used by the child are limited only by the availability of therapists. Clinical reports on the value of psychotherapy tend to be single-case studies or highly selected samples. Hearing therapists are most successful if they use a transcultural model and acquaint themselves with the cultural beliefs of their clients. As in psychotherapy of the hearing patients, the therapist is advised to convey, "Teach me what your experience is like" rather than, "I know how you feel."

Evaluating psychopharmacologic agents and monitoring their desired and adverse effects is similar to hearing children with the same symptomatology or disorder, but with a warning. Psychoactive medications, especially neuroleptics, can be used successfully with deaf children for management, but the common anticholinergic side effects of psychoactive medications must be made clear, although they are difficult to communicate in sign language. The blurry vision often experienced with these drugs is intolerable for an individual dependent on vision and limits the usefulness of such medications.

Stimulant medications can be used effectively for ADHD in carefully diagnosed cases. Hyperactivity in hearing-impaired children may be confused with a reaction to poor communication or learning social cues and appropriately responding to them. The determination is complicated by reported impulsivity among deaf children. Cases referred for stimulant medications have identified overwhelmed parents lacking communication skills, having trouble setting limits, and overusing physical punishment to establish their authority. Kelly et al. evaluated a state residential school for the deaf and obtained ratings on 238 students using the Conners Parent Rating Scale and the Attention Deficit Disorder with Hyperactivity (ADD-H) Comprehensive Teacher Rating Scale (37). They found that the Conners ratings statistically differed from normative numbers for hearing children. Among those youngsters who were considered positive for ADD-H, hearing loss tended to be acquired (e.g., bacterial meningitis or congenital rubella). A wide range of management interventions, including stimulant medications, also was reported (38). The decision to use stimulant medication should consider that the chronic nature of the deafness often results in lifetime use of medications to maintain the child in the least restrictive environment. This dilemma can be addressed only on a cautious, case-by-case basis with careful monitoring and periodic assessments. Repeated failures at nonpsychopharmacologic intervention warrant a trial of medication including treatment goals and a time frame for the medication trial as well as a periodic review of the medications with a risk benefit analysis of optimum medication dosages.

Treatment and management includes counseling and supportive measures for the family. Emotional reactions of parents to a deaf child can interfere and/or limit their capacity to respond to their child's needs. A deaf child's temperament and the concept of goodness of fit should be considered (39). Siblings are a sadly neglected group requiring intervention and education. Family therapy with a hearing family and deaf child should use interpreters, even if the therapist can sign (40,41). Counseling for both the parents and siblings include teaching technical information in terms that can be understood clearly.

The first experimental cochlear implants on adults were performed in the early 1960s and clinical trials began in 1973. In 1984, the Food and Drug Administration (FDA) approved the devices in adults. The first implant trial on children was initiated in 1980 at the House Ear Institute in Los Angeles, California (42). By 1990, over 500 children, ranging in age from 2 to 17 years, had received the device when the FDA gave approval for implantation in children. Initially, the Subcommittee on Cochlear Implants of the American Academy of Otolaryngology stated that pediatric candidate selection required failure of benefit from appropriately fitted hearing aids and other devices, the absence of severe organic brain damage, psychosis, severe intellectual disability, personality traits that may interfere with training, and/or unrealistic expectations (43). Criteria and indication for cochlear implantation have changed over the years. For the most optimal benefit for oral language, there is still the recommendation for early implantation in prelingually deaf children and even additional disabilities are no longer considered contraindications (44). Cochlear implantation requires active long-term participation for parents and children. The decision to use this prosthesis is neither easy nor obvious (45). The concept that deafness is not a disability requiring intervention is a position held in deaf culture (46). Fink et al. developed the first longitudinal multicenter, national cohort study to evaluate systematically early cochlear implant (CI) outcomes in children called The Childhood Development after Cochlear Implantation (CDaCI) study. One of the key objectives of the CDaCI study was to better understand cognitive, social and emotional development as it relates to language acquisition. It was noted in the study that early cochlear implantation increased oral language communication skills and improved overall parent-child interactions. With improved oral communication skills, there is implications for overall positive outcome in social/emotional functioning (47).

BLINDNESS AND VISUAL IMPAIRMENT

Definition and Historical Note

Blindness was legally defined by the American Medical Association in 1934 as "central vision of 20/200 or less in the better eye with corrective glasses, and a visual field subtending an angular field of no greater than 20 degrees in the better eye." This definition, originally for the purpose of determining eligibility for federal insurance programs, has endured and is used in Public Law 94-142, 1975. "Legal blindness" remains a definition used by the US government to determine eligibility for vocational training, rehabilitation, schooling, disability benefits, low vision devices, and tax exemption programs. It is not a functional definition. A child who is legally blind may have residual useable vision, able to read large-type materials and learn through limited visual input (48). There are alternative definitions of blindness, low vision, and visual impairment that focus on functional capacities, rehabilitative potential, and the nature and quality of the residual vision on educational perspectives; however, there is no consensus about which criteria or classification system to use. Both the National Federation of the Blind and the American Foundation for the Blind indicate there is no generally accepted definition for "visual impairment" as it is a general term describing a wide range of visual function with many different definitions (48,49).

The child and adolescent psychiatrist in practice will likely encounter the World Health Organization's classification system in the International Classification of Diseases, 10th Revision, Clinical Modification (ICD-10-CM) for medical coding and reporting in the United States. The ICD-10-CM defines four levels of visual function: (1) Mild or no visual impairment (2) Moderate visual impairment (3) Severe visual impairment (4) Blindness. These levels are based on presenting distance visual acuity (in feet) and are further refined into nine categories by designation of monocular/binocular, no light perception, and unspecified. The levels of "severe visual impairment" (visual acuity worse than 20/200 but better than 20/400) and "blindness" (visual acuity worse than 20/400) meet the definition of "legal blindness" (50).

Prevalence and Epidemiology

The collection of statistics on prevalence and etiology of visual impairments is challenging due to inconsistent measuring criteria and the varying definitions of vision loss which include blindness, total blindness, legal blindness, visual impairment, low vision, functional limitation in seeing, and severe limitation in seeing (51). The United States does not keep a national register of blind or visually impaired people. Almost all statistics on blindness are estimated, meaning numbers found in a sample are extrapolated to the entire population. However, each year, the American Printing House for the Blind polls each state for the exact number of legally blind children through age 21 enrolled in elementary and high school to determine eligibility to receive free reading matter in Braille, large print, or audio format. The 2014 survey of the American Printing House for the Blind reported 60,393 students who were registered as legally blind. Of that group, 29.2% were classified as visual readers, 8.5% as Braille readers, 8.5% were in residential schools, and 2.3% were in programs for multi-handicapped individuals (52).

The WHO in 2006 has listed childhood blindness as the cause of 3.9% of blindness and visual impairment worldwide with cataract (47.9%) and glaucoma (12.3%) topping the list. "Vision 2020: The Right to Sight" is a global initiative with the mission to eliminate the main causes of all preventable and treatable blindness by the year 2020. Since its launch in 1999, a high priority has been eliminating the 45% of children with visual impairments and blindness from the avoidable or treatable causes of corneal scarring (mainly from Vitamin A deficiency and measles), cataract, retinopathy of prematurity, refractive error, and low vision (53,54). Two of the historically common causes of early vision impairment and blindness have decreased over time owing to medical advances: ophthalmia-neonatorum with the routine placement of silver nitrate solution drops in newborns eyes, and retinopathy of prematurity with careful use of oxygen in management of prematurity and earlier detection and intervention (53,55).

Vision loss in childhood caused by congenital, genetic, or prenatal congenital conditions represents approximately 50% of cases. Lymphocytic choriomeningitis causing chorioretinitis in utero is believed to be responsible for some (56). Other causes include optic atrophy, retinitis pigmentosa, optic nerve hypoplasia, cataracts, foveal hypoplasia, persistent hypoplastic vitreous, and microphthalmos. Uveitis potentially leading to blindness can develop in children with juvenile rheumatoid arthritis (57). Cortical visual impairment caused by a disturbance of the posterior visual pathways in the occipital lobe is most commonly caused by perinatal hypoxia, cerebral vascular accident, meningitis, and acquired hypoxia. Most children with cortical visual impairment have other associated neurologic abnormalities (58).

Developmental Considerations

Visual impairment has a significant and far reaching effect on all areas of development. Delay in all milestones is most evident in the preschool period, although obvious challenges remain in making progress at school. These delays are inevitable when consideration is given to the increased cognitive demand of tasks achieved without the benefit of the information provided by vision (e.g., the concept of object permanence and joint attention) (59). Children with vision limited to only awareness of light or light-reflecting objects show the greatest delay (60), between 1 and 2 years' delay compared to sighted peers.

Visually impaired children suffer the full range of clinical psychiatric syndromes. However, commonly observed behaviors in blind children, such as stereotypic rocking, passivity, and immobility, do not signify psychiatric illness, nor is late achievement of motor milestones reflective of cognitive problems. Such behaviors may be due to the visually impaired child's reliance on caregivers for environmental stimuli as well as insufficient environmental response. Developmental delays and maladaptive behavior among visually impaired children result from failure to learn adaptive skills or to correct maladaptive behaviors stemming from gaps in the teaching of social norms and behaviors given the paucity of incidental learning.

An additional consideration is the effect of the diagnosis of the child's visual impairment on the sighted parents who often react initially with shock and disbelief (61,62). Some parents experience considerable distress. It has been observed that parental depression and insufficient understanding of their baby's apparent lack of response can lead to decreased interaction between child and parent at a time when the infant is dependent on the parent for increased input and responsiveness from the environment to offset the lack of visual stimulation and feedback (63–65). Eventual positive parental adaptation to these reactions is usual, but may need appropriate support (66).

The quality of language used by parents is also affected by the presence of visual impairment. Parents have been found to be more directive and less contingent on their children's communicative cues (64) further decreasing the perception of control in the environment on the part of infant. Lowenfeld has observed the subtle but profound influence on the child's development that perception of control of their environment, and self in relation to it, can have (67). In the sighted child, seeing overcomes distances and provides a quick way to evaluate new or changing situations or emergencies. Vision provides the means for observing the behavior of others, especially parents or peers, and learning by imitation while obtaining immediate feedback through observing facial expressions or other nonverbal cues. Early face recognition and social smile by the infant along with eye-to-eye contact are important both to the infant and caretakers in establishing and developing affective bonds. Longitudinal studies of early development in children with visual impairment suggest that attachment formation may be significantly affected (64).

Moore and McConachie (68) found that mothers of blind children, when playing with their child, talked less about objects that their child was actually attending to at the time. The findings suggested that it is very difficult for parents to "think themselves into" what their child finds salient (69) and to ascertain what a blind child is actually focusing attention on and hence what to talk about. Blind parents of blind babies appear to have fewer obstacles to natural effective communication and have greater reliance on close proximity and touch (70). Given the child's dependence on gaining information through language, maintaining a "stream" of language (71), which is responsive to the child's activities and interests (72,73), appears important.

Vision provides the infant and young child with stimulation and observation to permit imitation and modeling, and to encourage and motivate exploration necessary for further development. This includes all domains of motor, language, cognitive, and social skills (74). The blind child is at a particular disadvantage with imitative learning. The constraints of lack of vision on learning are complex and the impact of delay in one area of development is likely to have secondary effects on other areas of development, so that the effects are cumulative (75).

Language Development

Language development for the blind and the sighted infant are essentially equivalent through the babbling stages but can be stunted without visual stimuli (76,77). Language development relies on an understanding of joint reference and developing the concept of symbolic understanding. The early opportunities that sighted children have to see objects and to establish joint reference to objects named by parents repeatedly in the first year of life before language develops is lost to the blind infant. Limited experience in general, and not only visual, may play a role in delaying language acquisition, as may parenting style including being more directive and less contingent on the child's communicative cues or withdrawing and having less interaction.

The visually impaired child must rely on verbal descriptions provided by the sighted to describe words that have a visual meaning. A blind hearing child can locate a bird by its sound but not describe its shape, size, or flight. Although the tactile sense can describe concrete objects that can be held in the hand, it does not help to describe clouds, stars, or colors, nor can the child experience a very large or small object. Without the experience of knowing through sight, verbalized descriptions repeated by the blind child can seem shallow or meaningless and are referred to as "verbalisms," the use of words whose concrete referent is unknown to the speaker. Rosel et al. have shown that all children regardless of their visual status, tend to use verbalisms in much the same way with frequency of use increasing with age but not affected by degree of sight or gender. This is interpreted as pointing to the positive capacity of children who are blind to adapt to the general linguistic behavior of the community in which they live. It also points to accepting that verbalisms in the language of children with visual impairments are normal rather than representing a cognitive or personality flaw or being a psychopathologic indicator as historically postulated by Cutsforth in 1951 (78,79).

Differences in the style of language development have also been described, for example, the use of multiword phrases, linked to familiar social routines, before the use of noun labels. This has been referred to as a more expressive rather than referential style of language use (80). Children with visual impairment also have a tendency to continue with immediate echolalia longer than sighted peers (81). Delays are also seen in the appropriate use of personal and other pronouns and the use of spatial–relational words (e.g., here-there) (82).

Motor and Perceptual Development

The early motor developmental milestones of the blind infant are similar to those of the sighted child until the age of 4 months (83). After this period, the lack of visual stimulation as motivator for the child to explore and interact with the environment can lead to delays in crawling, walking, reaching, grasping, and bilateral hand coordination. The blind child tends to lag behind the sighted in motor tasks where visual stimulation is a motivator, whereas there is little difference when the task is purely neuromuscular (e.g., sitting or standing alone) (84).

The environment may interact in limiting acquisition of skills when parents are more protective and cautious about giving their blind child the opportunities to explore. Temperamental factors in young children will also play a role; for example, a timid child, having learned to walk, may be more reluctant to "launch" herself into the world than a more adventurous one.

Developing reach and interest in play depend on developing concepts of sound localization and object permanence. Babies without vision require the support of their parents and caregivers to learn these concepts (85,86). Prolonged period of immobility and limited environmental stimulation for the blind infant can result in poor development, especially in the areas of initiative and self-confidence.

Cognitive Development

Cognitive development has been shown to be influenced by many variables including the severity of visual deficit, residual vision, timing of onset (congenital, early or late), personal experience, "innate IQ" and other factors such as motivation that are difficult to define and measure (64,87).

Cattaneo and Vecchi (87) review the neuroscience evidence that mental images or mental representations are important in the development of memory, reasoning, and creative problem solving, and that vision is not necessary for the development of this mental imagery so important in learning, navigation, and many other aspects of daily life. Evidence points to persons born without vision generating mental images similar to those of persons with sight, containing both accurate spatial relations and nonvisual sensory details (87). Cattaneo and Vecchi theorize that vision is not necessary for imagery formation as imagery is primarily spatial rather than visual. Multiple senses or modalities contribute to the generation of mental images. In sighted persons, vision is generally the dominant perceptual experience and is important in the development of multisensory integration or the interaction between the senses (87,88). In individuals without significant input from vision, the other senses play a greater role in perceptual input for mental images, but the multisensory integration is affected given the more sequential nature of the nonvisual sensory inputs (e.g., tactually examining a large object requires doing so one section at a time). Vision allows for easier simultaneous processing of sensory inputs (87,88).

Simultaneous rather than sequential cognitive processes may be a factor in modulating cognitive development. Cattaneo and Vecchi describe the case for sensory compensation or enhanced sensory acuity in the functioning senses through brain plasticity, which allows the functioning senses to recruit the portions of the visual cortex not receiving visual input (87). Occipital activation in blind subjects during Braille reading potentially reflects both sensory and higher-order (language-related) cognitive factors as some studies have suggested that early visual cortex recruitment during Braille reading tasks might actually reflect linguistic processing (87,89,90).

Learning to read through the use of Braille is potentially a more complex process than learning to read using vision, because it entails linguistic, motor, and spatial skills (64,91). Children with visual impairment may therefore make slower progress in the early stages of acquiring literacy, and this may also delay the recognition of other specific learning difficulties. The long-term follow-up study of children with visual impairment by Freeman et al. (92) found better than expected academic outcomes, with 76% having completed secondary education and 19% having attended or attending university.

Social and Emotional Development

Children with visual impairment face considerable challenges in social and emotional development (63,93,94). Attainment of social skills, such as learning to read nonverbal communication cues, initiating and maintaining interactions, and using eye gaze to regulate interactions (95) are highly visually dependent. Nonverbal social cues and body language are not available to the visually impaired child, complicating the development of peer and social relationships, as they are not able to see and learn the skills through observation (96,97). Despite this limited feedback from their environment, Mulford (98) found that most blind children (aged 5 to 6 years) had established a range of verbal and nonverbal communication strategies for establishing referential communication. However, Preisler (99) found that blind children rarely initiated and had difficulty maintaining social interactions and related much more to adults. Interactions with peers were more extended in structured play but they had more difficulty in free play settings. Children with visual impairment do not display a full range of play behaviors and demonstrate compromised social interactions, engaging more in solitary nonsocial play (96). The child's inability to imitate may inspire reluctance on the part of caretakers to introduce a wide variety of toys to the child, hence, social skills are hampered owing to the visually impaired child's paucity of interactive play experience. Adults' interventions to promote social contacts may focus the child's attention toward the adult and not the playmate.

The socially isolated child who is only around adults has no way to learn age-appropriate social behaviors. Despite this, many visually impaired children and adolescents are skillful at interpersonal manipulation. A long-term follow-up of children with visual impairment into adult life (92) found that half had a romantic relationship and 20% were in partnerships, all with sighted people.

Lowenfeld (67) describes four major concerns that present difficulty to the visually impaired adolescent: sexual curiosity, dating, mobility, and concern for the future. The inability to gather sexual information from observation or magazines might compel the sexually curious adolescent to behave in a manner that would violate cultural and social taboos. Dating is an important arena in which one develops self-confidence and asserts a gender role, but ability to date is dependent on meeting another person and engaging in rituals of flirtation and personal appearance. The visually impaired must rely on introductions and arrangements that diminish flexibility and self-confidence while invading privacy. Limited mobility reduces opportunities for the separation and individuation process to occur, which further limits autonomy. Concerns for the future that involve leaving a protective family or school setting, accepting vocational challenges, ensuring economic stability, worrying about marriage, and the genetic transmission of the visual impairments pose significant hurdles.

Psychiatric Evaluation of the Blind or Visually Impaired Child or Adolescent

As a general principal, the child and adolescent psychiatrist is cautioned against using a "deficit model," assuming that damage is inevitable with a perceptual impairment, or at best only partially compensated, and always results in personality and/or psychiatric disorder. The examiner should be aware of myths about the blind such as innate helplessness and total dependence, blindness as a punishment for sins, etiologic association with venereal disease, and belief of hyper acuity of other senses. Prior to the interview, the examiner should have knowledge of the child's medical history, degree of independence and cognitive level, events in the home, school adjustment, purpose of the referral, and the child's ability to modify behavior. The age of onset of blindness and presence of residual vision are major considerations.

The child psychiatrist evaluating a visually impaired child must be prepared to touch the child more than he or she would touch sighted children, asking for the child's permission when appropriate. Talking softly to orient the child toward the examiner before even touching or approaching the child helps sets the tone for the evaluation. The child should be led to the examining room, and the examiner may initially remain in continuous physical contact by holding his or her hand or touching the shoulder. The interview space, its layout—including where the child sits and all of the toys available to the child—should be described, so that valid conclusions can be drawn about activity selection. The child will often ask seemingly impertinent personal questions of the examiner, including appearance and marital status, some of which a sighted child or adolescent determines by observation. Whether answered or not, a friendly tone is essential. It is important to note that with sensory impaired children, and more so with the blind and multiply handicapped, any interaction presents an opportunity to teach and engage the child.

The vast majority of legally blind children are better described as low vision, thus lighting in the examining room is important. There are no fixed rules, but the examiner must be alert to the unique nature of the child's vision and maximize the residual capacities. Glare, background light and shadows, along with placement of objects in the visual field are considerations. A gooseneck lamp on the table enables the child to maximize vision while playing or drawing. Creating nonglare contrast can be helpful to increase visual perceptions. If drawing tasks are to be part of the evaluation, then the table surface should be free of glare. A dull light blue–gray table surface works well, contrasting both white and dark drawing paper or covering a white table with brown wrapping paper is a satisfactory solution. If white paper is used for drawings, then the standard pencil often does not provide sufficient contrast and a black felt-tipped pen or marker would provide better contrast. Some children prefer and respond better to dark drawing paper and a light-colored or white marker.

Play therapy can be used in the evaluation of blind children, but often the child must be taught how to play. The process of learning play through imitation often is not available to the blind child. The clinician can make some valuable observations about the child in the process of teaching a particular type of play. Blind children respond best to very realistic objects or toys. Play is better with utensils that the child routinely uses, such as real fork and spoons, rather than small toys, which have no meaning to the child. Similarly, dolls close to life size with molded realistic facial features and hair elicit more meaningful response as the child fingers the face than would the soft, more stylized, cloth dolls. Dollhouses with realistic figures of people and furniture can elicit helpful information about the home life of the child. The clinician might first have to teach the child how these small objects symbolize real people or furniture. In general, the child plays with toys that are for a younger age group. It is best to start with real props to develop "pretend" imaginative play as part of therapy. The children pretend play verbally by telling stories as opposed to acting out behaviors. The clinician can elicit psychodynamic material and dreams in a verbal form, but the content may seem to be lacking in affect. This lack of apparent substance or affective content or "verbalism" seems more related to the language acquisition process than to the potential for affective content and the alert clinician can piece together the affective web that binds the meaning for the child. The child's total body and other nonverbal responses including gestures as a communicative device need to be considered with the caveat that the child's facial expression may reveal less than he or she understands.

The visually impaired child may be slower to warm up than a typical sighted child. Long silences should be avoided and the child should be notified of the examiner's movements. Anticipated shifts of topic in the course of the evaluation should be announced so as not to confuse or contribute to disorientation. Echolalic language is relatively common and rarely pathologic. Self-stimulating behavior and stereotypic movements are frequently seen and not diagnostic of specific psychiatric conditions. The examiner should speak directly to the child and accept as an indication of relatedness that the child faces him or her with the ear and not the eyes. In an interesting protocol, Raver-Lampman (100) asked 50 subjects who were informed about blindness and in contact with the blind, to evaluate videotapes of two children without gaze direction and two with gaze direction as they answered questions from examiners sitting on either side of them. The tapes were presented in a random order and opposite recording positions. The results revealed that, when a visually impaired child used gaze direction toward the questioner, the responding subjects rated the child as being more intelligent and socially competent than when the child did not use gaze direction. This serves as a caution to the examiner to be alert to his or her personal bias and unconscious judgments, especially involving the child's body posture and direction of gaze during the evaluation.

It is helpful to indicate that several meetings with the child are normally required when accepting the referral. The clinician should initially be ready to teach the child tools necessary for a psychodynamic evaluation; for example, pretend play and drawing tasks. In effect, the assessment is a functional protocol looking at the child's strengths, learning, and problem-solving styles, and what if any, interfering psychiatric processes are present.

Differential Diagnosis

Differential diagnoses include intellectual disability; autistic spectrum disorder; ADHD; childhood schizophrenia; and conduct and personality disorders, including immaturity, over dependency, and obsessiveness. Repetitive rocking, swaying, or eyeball pressing and other "blindisms" are also seen in other child psychiatric entities, especially mental retardation and autism. When these behaviors are found among blind children, they should be differentiated from a symptom of other conditions.

Blind youngsters may not acquire factual information or develop learning skills without educational opportunities. Early social interaction may have been muted for blind youngsters, and care should be taken in assessing diminished interpersonal affective responses as indicating clinical psychiatric conditions. Superficial symptoms suggesting autism in a blind child often abate when meaningful personal interaction is offered. For reasons of convenience and safety, many parents and caretakers tend to provide unchanging sequences of activity to their children. An insistence on sameness or a severe negative reaction to a change in patterns and activities may be a nonpathologic adaptation to visual impairment and past learning.

Treatment

Early intervention programs with blind infants and preschoolers teach social skills and promote attainment of developmental milestones while supporting the family structure, thereby preventing psychiatric or behavioral problems. Providing a means of communication and socialization is the first consideration for preventing most conflicts. The blind child learns to speak in the usual manner, but the meaning of words that the youngster cannot experience (verbalisms) is difficult to convey and may cause frustration. Color and the contours of very large objects or very small ones are most difficult to describe. Checking self-appearance for neatness and simple rules of social behavior, such as chewing with lips closed, cannot be learned by imitation and must be demonstrated. Alternate strategies of adaptation to an invisible, barely discernible or at best blurred world must be taught so as to avoid confrontation, tantrums, and shame. A psychiatrist treating a blind child or adolescent may be involved in consultation and serve as a liaison to provide advice on management to parents, family, and the school.

The examiner's familiarity with specific technologies to help the visually impaired may be useful in guiding the family and school to meet the child or adolescent's developmental needs. Computerized magnification, Braille computer, and other literacy devices have been increasingly available to school-age children. Current advances in Global Positioning System via satellites and its application to cane technology have helped increase safe mobility, autonomy, and self-esteem. These new technologies have alleviated concerns and reassured parents and facilitated skill development. Behavior modification has been useful for both deaf and blind children. Changing specific behavior in order to gain acceptance is successful for motivated children. Sharing experiences, feelings, and problems in group therapy and counseling can be very helpful. Erin et al. (101) have provided a helpful review of literature regarding teaching social skills to the blind and visually impaired. They emphasize the value of social skills for a visually impaired child to be successful in mainstream programs. Studies strongly support success in teaching social skills using different approaches. There is the interesting question of whether the goal of social skills training should be to teach the blind behaviors of the sighted rather than other skills more appropriate to the blind. Individual psychotherapy can be invaluable for a visually impaired child or adolescent. The therapist must constantly be alert to the possibility of confusion in the use of language. Although blind individuals cannot follow a description of color, they do use many vision-related idioms, such as "I see" for "I understand." Transition-age youths with visual impairments experience barriers to a successful transition from secondary school environments to work. Interventions that were found to enhance employability skills and self-constructs were also identified in research as predictors of the successful employment of blind youth (102).

Medications can be employed with the same criteria as for nonhandicapped children and adolescents. Medications with the potential of interfering with residual vision should be avoided especially when some vision remains. Melatonin is helpful with treating circadian sleep–wake–rhythm disorders in children with vision impairment and has been shown to be safe and effective in long-term use (103,104). Stimulant medications can be used for ADHD, giving both child and caregiver an opportunity for better communication, education, and other interactions. Careful monitoring is necessary for adverse effects of increasing agitation or flattening of mood further decreasing the child's motivation for social interaction. Even more than in the nonperceptually impaired, psychopharmacologic intervention should be used judiciously as an adjunct in addition to other psychosocial interventions.

DEAF-BLINDNESS

All that has been said in the introductory sections under the heading of general considerations and role of the child and adolescent psychiatrist is even more pertinent in the case of deaf-blindness. In addition, attention should be given to the sections earlier in the chapter on children and adolescents with either one or the sensory-related loss. Having said that, it should be noted that the effects of a child with multiple sensory-related losses can have even more of an impact on the individual's development and communication abilities as well as the family dynamics than would be seen with a single condition.

Definition

The IDEA (2004) defines deaf-blindness as a condition with "concomitant hearing and visual impairments, the combination of which causes such severe communication and other developmental and educational needs that they cannot be accommodated in special education programs solely for children with deafness or children with blindness" (105). The definition is educational and does not focus on specific clinical presentations, however it does signify that the dual concomitant sensory impairments warrant additional specialized educational intervention above and beyond each condition alone.

Deaf-blindness does not refer to a total inability to see or hear. In reality, deaf-blindness is a condition in which there are varying degrees of vision loss in combination with hearing loss. The range included in the terminology of "deaf-blindness" is great. Barbara Miles, Ed.D, outlined the definition of deaf-blindness in her paper "Overview on Deaf-Blindness" (106). She notes that the deaf-blind child experiences the world in a much narrower perspective compared to individuals who can hear and see. With a child who is both totally blind and profoundly deaf, as was the case of Helen Keller, the "world extends only as far as the fingertips can reach" (106). These children are essentially alone when there is no physical contact with anyone or anything. Children with some residual hearing or usable vision would likely have an enlarged, yet still overall limited, view of their world.

The term "deaf-blind," although professionally widely used, might not accurately convey the individual client's circumstances. The imprecision in definition highlights the very nature of the clinical work, when the clinician's cumulative experience and knowledge is called to bear on a unique child or adolescent and his or her specific circumstances and needs. As indicated earlier in the chapter, the words "deaf" and "blind" have strong connotations and the combination can be overwhelming. Familiarity with resources and supports for sensory impaired children and their families is essential.

Prevalence and Epidemiology

The data from the National Child Count of Children and Youth who are Deaf-Blind is the first and longest running registry and knowledge base of children who are deaf-blind in the United States (107). Across the United States for the 2013 national count, there were 552 infants (birth to 2 years old old) and 8,847 children through young adulthood (3 years old to 21 years old) reported as deaf-blind. As such, there was a total of 9,454 infants, children and young adults who were identified as deaf-blind (107). The opportunity for early identification, intervention and the provision of instructional services aimed at the unique needs of young children and students who are deaf-blind is a critical component that cannot be lost.

There are many causes for deaf-blindness. There are genetic syndromes such as Usher syndrome, CHARGE Syndrome, Down Syndrome/Trisomy 21 and Trisomy 13 which have high correlations of deafness and blindness. Usher syndrome is an autosomal recessive disorder characterized by congenital deafness and retinitis pigmentosa (with progressive vision loss). It is the most frequent cause of deaf-blindness in adults and accounts for 3% to 6% of deaf children (108). CHARGE Syndrome is a rare genetic syndrome and is an acronym for a constellation of clinical features: coloboma, heart defects, choanal atresia, retardation (of growth and/or development), genitourinary malformation and ear abnormalities. It is associated with a mutation of the CHD7 gene (109). There are also other congenital anomalies associated with deaf-blindness including fetal alcohol syndrome, microcephaly, hydrocephaly and maternal drug use. Prenatal infectious exposure has been linked to deaf-blindness. Congenital rubella syndrome was the most common cause of congenital deaf-blindness but now is greatly reduced due to the use of immunization programs in past 20 years (110). The major causes of deaf-blindness are noted in Table 2.2.2.2 below (106,111).

Some trends were noted on the 2013 National Child Count of Children and Youth who are Deaf-Blind. The distribution of children/youth across age groups has remained relatively stable over the past 5 years, with a slight shift toward a younger overall population. There has been a slight overall decrease in the percentage of the total Deaf-Blind Child Count represented by infants, birth—2 years of age (6.2% to 5.9%). Early identification and referral to the deaf-blind programs continues to be an issue with less than 100 infants, birth to 1 year of age being included on the Deaf-Blind Child Count (107).

TABLE 2.2.2.2

MAJOR CAUSES OF DEAF-BLINDNESS

GENETIC SYNDROMES:
- Down Syndrome
- Usher Syndrome
- Trisomy 13
- CHARGE Syndrome

MULTIPLE CONGENITAL ANOMALIES:
- Fetal Alcohol Syndrome
- Hydrocephalus
- Microcephaly
- In Utero Substance Exposure
- Prematurity

CONGENITAL PRENATAL DYSFUNCTION:
- AIDS
- Rubella
- Toxoplasmosis
- Herpes
- Syphilis

POST-NATAL CAUSES:
- Asphyxia
- Traumatic Brain Injury
- Stroke
- Encephalitis
- Meningitis

Adapted from Etiologies and Characteristics of Deaf-Blindness, Heller and Kennedy (1994) and Overview on Deaf-Blindness: DB-LINK Fact Sheet, Miles (2008).

The number of children identified as having received cochlear implants has increased from 167 in 2005 to 914 in 2013, more than a fivefold increase during this time period. This increase spans the age ranges, from infants to young adults. Overall, the number of children/youth with additional disabilities has increased. In 2005, over 20% of the children/youth on the Deaf-Blind Child Count had no additional disabilities. In 2013, just over 10% had no additional disabilities. In 2005, just 13.1% of the children/youth on the count had four or more additional disabilities. In 2013, 43% of the children had four or more additional disabilities (107).

The prevalence of CHARGE syndrome continues to increase significantly. In 2013 there were 864 children and youth identified as having CHARGE Syndrome. The identified prevalence of Usher syndrome reached a peak in 2007 and has decreased over the past 3 years (107). As noted above, the rates of congenital rubella syndrome have been on the decline as rates of maternal infection have decreased due to effective immunization.

Developmental Considerations

Much of what has been addressed in prior sections regarding developmental challenges pertain to children with deaf-blindness, with the understanding that the child with multiple sensory-related issues faces challenges above and beyond having one impairment alone. This is why the emphasis is on early detection and involvement in early intervention programs. As such, the National Center on Deaf-Blindness has been committed to this initiative with the Early identification of infants who are Deaf-Blind for the past 10 years (112). With early identification of children in need, there is ability to intervene in a manner to reduce morbidity. Early identification can allow families and intervention specialists to develop appropriate team support for needs and access therapeutic specialists to address both developmental and educational needs (113). In addition, reporting children who are deaf-blind to the State Deafblind Centers for Education census (National Center on Deaf Blindness, 2014) allows continued national and state support and assistance for children with this low incidence condition as well as provides a mechanism to initiate technical assistance and supports for the families and Early Intervention providers (114). In 1966, Jan van Dijk developed child guided interaction strategies to engage, assess and teach deaf-blind children. The movement based approach was known as Coactive Movement and helped to develop language and acquire concepts for successful interaction with their world (115).

Psychiatric Evaluation of the Deaf-Blind Child or Adolescent

The diagnostic process is a collaborative team effort with psychologists, educators, and habilitation and rehabilitation specialists. Techniques for eliciting information, especially physical contact, lighting, and realistic props for toys, are similar to those described for blind children. Evaluation requires time, patience, and the use of an interpreter who is familiar with and to the child if a system of manual sign language has been developed. Meaningful evaluation requires gaining an understanding about the child's perceptions of the world. A child who is deaf-blind, has not had access to the experiences of the world, and therefore the natural incidental learning, that comes readily to the typical child.

Few centers are equipped to provide the comprehensive assessment that a deaf-blind child requires. The psychiatric evaluation has three potential pitfalls:

1. Failure to recognize visual or auditory loss when evaluating a child who is known to be either deaf or blind, but ascribing the behavioral difficulties to a clinical psychiatric illness, most commonly developmental delays, autism spectrum or intellectual disabilities;
2. Diagnosing a child as deaf-blind when only one sensory loss exists concurrently with a major clinical psychiatric syndrome;
3. Diagnosing cognitive disability, schizophrenia, autism, or organic brain syndrome in a deaf-blind child, based on an unusual presentation, without being fully aware of the child's potential strengths or problem-solving and adaptive abilities.

Miles and McLetchie (116) point to the importance of each experience in developing "concepts" or ideas that give meaning to our world, and caution evaluators not to assume that a child who is deaf and blind has understanding of even the most foundational concepts. Rather each experience within an evaluation can be viewed not only as eliciting information, but also as an opportunity to provide access to the world and contribute to concept development. Establishing mutual attention that is usually accomplished with pointing, often first needs to be through touch with children who are deaf-blind. Miles describes the technique of putting the examiner's hand alongside and gently under the last two fingers of the child's hand allowing for exploring through touch together without the examiner's hand on top forcing or directing movements (116).

Differential Diagnosis

The common differential psychiatric diagnoses in deaf-blind individuals include intellectual disability, autism spectrum disorder and other neurodevelopmental disorders, childhood schizophrenia, and reactive attachment disorder. One of the sensory impairments may be missed when a diagnosis of schizophrenia or autism already has been made. The converse might also occur if the clinician attributes behavior to the sensory impairments such as in a child diagnosed as deaf-blind who might be deaf-autistic, blind autistic, or sensory impaired with intellectual disability. Ritualistic acts are common in severe or profound mental retardation as well as in childhood autism, and both rigidity of behavior and perseveration may characterize deafness or blindness, as well as mental retardation or autism. Typical deaf-blind individuals easily stop the rituals if offered human contact or interaction.

Treatment

Data on treatment of deaf-blind individuals with reactive or more serious psychopathology are woefully lacking. Behavior therapy, psychotherapy, and counseling may each be useful but are dependent on meaningful communication and development of a therapeutic relationship. The use of medication that could affect residual hearing or diminish visual perception should be avoided, but can be useful for symptomatic treatment to assist in daily living. The remarkable achievement of Helen Keller is instructive and inspiring, but is not a good model because she acquired a language foundation of both sight and sound prior to the onset of her impairments. Some individuals who are deaf and blind fulfill their potential and lead competent lives. Deaf-blind youngsters who are aging out of the educational system often lack appropriate supportive services, including housing. There has been a shift in focus for adolescents to establish greater independence in the community rather than an abrupt transfer to adult rehabilitation facilities when they reach age 21.

Conclusion

Pivotal to the psychiatric evaluation and treatment of the child with hearing loss and/or blindness is understanding the influence and impact of the sensory loss(es) on both the developmental process and the presentation of psychiatric signs and symptoms. The deaf, blind, or deaf-blind child faces challenges learning about the physical and social world and him/herself in relation to others without the sensory information input readily available to typical peers, and in a world that is oriented to the needs of hearing and sighted people. The reality that many individuals with sensory-related losses lead successful and constructive lives is cause for optimism on the part of professionals and families that their efforts at enhancing the child's access to and interaction with their world can make a positive impact.

ACKNOWLEDGMENTS

The authors of this chapter wish to acknowledge Peter Hindley (4th Ed), Alison Salt (4th Ed), Stella Chess (3rd Ed) and Mayu PB Gonzalez (3rd Ed) who provided authorship to prior editions. Their contributions to the field of psychiatric care of deaf, blind and deaf-blind youth have been invaluable in advancing the evidence-based care to underserved communities.

References

1. American Academy of Child and Adolescent Psychiatry: Practice parameters for the psychiatric assessment of children and adolescents. *J Am Acad Child Adol Psychiatry* (Suppl36):10, 1997.
2. Jones L, Bellis MA, Wood S, et al.: Prevalence and risk of violence against children with disabilities: a systematic review and meta-analysis of observational studies. *Lancet* 380:899–907, 2012.
3. Weisleder P: No such thing as a "blind culture". *J Child Neurol* 27(6): 819–820, 2012.
4. National Standards for Culturally and Linguistically Appropriate Services in Health and Health Care Fact Sheet. Available at: www.ThinkCulturalHealth.hhs.gov. Accessed July 6, 2016.
5. Moores DF: The History of Language and Communication Issues in Deaf Education. In Marschark M, Spencer P (eds): *The Oxford Handbook of Deaf Studies, Language and Education*. Vol 2. New York, Oxford University Press, pp. 17–30, 2010.
6. Centers for Disease Control and Prevention: 2013 Annual Data Early Hearing Detection and Intervention (EHDI) Program. Available at: http://www.cdc.gov/ncbddd/hearingloss/ehdi-data2013.html. Accessed 7 July 2016.
7. Weill Cornell Medical College Department of Otolaryngology. Available at: http://cornellent.org/healthcare_services/hearing/oae.html. Accessed 7 July 2016.
8. Johnson JL, White KR, Widen JE, et al.: A multicenter evaluation of how many infants with permanent hearing loss pass a two-stage otoacoustic emissions/automated auditory brainstem response newborn hearing screening protocol. *Pediatrics* 116(3):663–672, 2005.
9. Bamford J, Fortnum H, Bristow K, et al.: Current practice, accuracy, effectiveness, and cost-effectiveness of the school-entry hearing screen. *Health Technol Assess* 11(32):1–168, 2007.
10. Mehra S, Eavey RD, Keamy DG Jr.: The epidemiology of hearing impairment in the United States: newborns, children, and adolescents. *Otolaryngol Head Neck Surg* 140(4):461–472, 2009.
11. Annual Disability Statistics Compendium. Special Education-Students Ages 6 to 21 Served under Individuals with Disabilities Education Act, Part B, as a Percentage of Population. Fall 2013. Available at: http://disabilitycompendium.org/statistics/special-education. Accessed 7 July 2016.
12. Morzaria S, Westerberg BD, Kozak FK: Systematic review of the etiology of bilateral sensorineural hearing loss in children. *Int J Pediatr Otorhinolaryngol* 68(9):1193–1198, 2004.
13. Green GE, Scott DA, McDonald JM, et al.: Carrier rates in midwestern US for GJB2 mutations causing inherited deafness. *JAMA* 28:2211–2216, 1999.
14. Meadow-Orlans K: An analysis of the effectiveness of early intervention programs for hearing-impaired children. In: Guralvick M, Bennett F (eds): *The Effectiveness of Early Intervention for At-Risk and Handicapped Children*. New York, Academic Press, 1987.
15. Mitchell RE, Karchmer MA: Chasing the mythical ten percent: parental hearing status of deaf and hard of hearing students in the United States. *Sign Language Studies* 4(2):138–163, 2004.
16. FDA Executive Summary: Prepared for the May 1, 2015 Meeting of the Ear, Nose, and Throat Devices Panel of the Medical Devices Advisory Committee.
17. Chomsky N: *Language and Mind*, 3rd Ed. New York, Cambridge University Press, 2006.
18. Goldin-Meadow S, Mylander C: Spontaneous sign systems created by deaf children in two cultures. *Nature* 391:279–281, 1998.
19. Stokoe WC, Casterline DC, Croneberg CG: *A Dictionary of American Sign languages on linguistic principles*. Washington, DC, Gallaudet College Press, 1965.
20. Krouse H, Braden J: The reliability and validity of the WISC-IV scores with deaf and hard of hearing children. *J Psychoeducat Assess* 29(3):238–248, 2010.
21. Braden JP, Kostrubala CE, Reed J: Why do deaf children score differently on performance vs. motor-reduced nonverbal intelligence tests? *J Psychoeducat Assess* 12, 357–363, 1994.
22. Braden J: The criterion-related validity of the WISC-R Performance Scale and other nonverbal IQ tests for deaf children. *Am Ann Deaf* 134:329–332, 1989.
23. Peterson CC, Siegal M: Deafness, conversation and theory of mind. *J Child Psychol Psychiatry* 36:459–474, 1995.
24. Vaccari C, Marschark M: Communication between parents and deaf children: implications for social-emotional development. *J Child Psychol Psychiatry* 38(7):793–801, 1997.
25. Meadow K, Trybus R: Behavior and emotional problems of deaf children: an overview. In: Bradford L, Hardy W (eds): *Hearing and Hearing Impairment*. New York, Grune & Stratton, 1979.
26. Chess S, Fernandez P, Korn S: The handicapped child and his family: Consonance and dissonance. *J Am Acad Child Psychiatry* 19:56–67, 1980.
27. Calderon R, Greenbert MT: Stress and coping in hearing mothers of children with hearing loss: factors affecting mother and child adjustment. *Am Ann Deaf* 144:7–16, 1999.
28. Landsberger S, Diaz DR, Spring NZ, et al.: Psychiatric diagnoses and psychosocial needs of outpatient deaf children and adolescents. *Child Psychiatry Hum Dev* 45(1):42–51, 2013.
29. Charlson E, Strong M, Gold R: How successful deaf teenagers experience and cope with isolation. *Am Ann Deaf* 137:261–270, 1992.
30. Roberts C, Hindley P: The assessment and treatment of deaf children with psychiatric disorders. *J Child Psychol Psychiatry* 40:151–167, 1999.
31. Vernon M, Alles B: Psychoeducational assessment of deaf and hard of hearing children and adolescents. In: Lazarus P, Strichart S (eds): *Psychoeducational Evaluation of Children and Adolescents with Low-Incidence Handicaps*. Orlando, FL, Grune & Stratton, 1986.
32. Evans J, Elliott H: The Mental Status Examination. In: Elliott H, Glass L, Evans J (eds): *Mental Health Assessment of Deaf Clients: A Practical Manual*. Boston, MA, Little Brown, 1987.
33. Barkley R: *Attention-deficit hyperactivity disorder: a handbook for diagnosis and treatment*. 2nd ed. New York, Guilford, 1998.
34. Schum R: Psychological assessment of children with multiple handicaps who have hearing loss. *The Volta Review* 104(4):237–255, 2004.
35. Conference of Educational Administrators of Schools and Programs for the Deaf (CEASD): Position paper on the full continuum of educational placements for all students who are deaf or hard of hearing. 2007.
36. Humphries T, Kushalnagar P, Mathur G, et al.: Language acquisition for deaf children: reducing the harms of zero tolerance to the use of alternative approaches. *Harm Reduct J* 9(16):1–9, 2012.
37. Kelly D, Forney J, Parker-Fisher S, et al.: The challenge of attention deficit disorder in children who are deaf or hard of hearing. *Am Ann Deaf* 138:343–348, 1993.
38. Kelly D, Forney J, Parker-Fisher S, et al.: Evaluating and managing attention deficit disorder in children who are deaf or hard of hearing. *Am Ann Deaf* 138:349–357, 1993.
39. Chess S, Fernandez P, Korn S: The handicapped child and his family: Consonance and dissonance. *J Am Acad Child Psychiatry* 19:56–67, 1980.
40. Harvey M: The influence and utilization of an interpreter for deaf persons in family therapy. *Am Ann Deaf* 127:821–827, 1982.
41. Culross RR: The use of interpreters in family therapy with deaf persons. *Contemporary Family Therapy* 18(4):507–512, 1996.
42. Eisenberg L, House W: Initial experience with the cochlear implant in children. *Ann Otol Rhinol Laryngol Suppl* 91(2):67–73, 1982.
43. Kveton J, Balkany T: Status of cochlear implantation in children. *J Pediatr* 118:1–7, 1991.
44. Sampaio A, Araujo M, Oliveria C: New criteria of indication and selection of patients to cochlear implant. *Int J Otolaryngol* 2011:573968, 2011.
45. Crouch RA: Letting the deaf be deaf: reconsidering the use of cochlear implants in prelingually deaf children. *Hastings Ctr Rep* 27:14–27, 1997.
46. Tucker BP: Deaf culture, cochlear implants and elective disability. *Hastings Ctr Rep* 28:6–14, 1998.
47. Fink NE, Wang N-Y, Visaya J, et al.: CDACI Investigative Team: childhood development after cochlear implantation (CDaCI) study: design and baseline characteristics. *Cochlear Implants Int* 8(2):92–116, 2007.
48. Low Vision and Legal Blindness Terms and Descriptions edited by Maureen A Duffy MS, CVRT. Available at: http://www.visionaware.org/info/your-eye-condition/eye-health/low-vision/low-vision-terms-and-descriptions/1235. Accessed 15 July 2016.
49. National Federation of the Blind. Available at: www.nfb.org/blindness-statistics. Accessed 15 July 2016.
50. ICD-10-CM – International Classification of Diseases, Tenth Revision, Clinical Modification. Available at: www.cdc.gov. Accessed 15 July 2016.

51. Kelly SM: Demographics of vision loss in the United States: dealing with definitions. *J Vis Impairment Blindness* 103(3):185–186, 2009.
52. American Printing House for the Blind, "Annual Report 2014: Distribution of Eligible Students Based on the Federal Quota Census of January 7, 2013 (Fiscal Year 2014)." Available at: http://www.aph.org. Accessed 17 July 2016.
53. Vision 2020: The Right to Sight GLOBAL INITIATIVE FOR THE ELIMINATION OF AVOIDABLE BLINDNESS ACTION PLAN 2006–2011.
54. Parikshit G, Clare G: Blindness in children: a worldwide perspective. *Comm Eye Health J* 20(62):32–33, 2007.
55. BlindBabies.org fact sheets. Available at: http://www.vabvi.org/five-leading-causes-of-visual-impairments-in-children-in-the-usa/. Accessed 15 July 2016.
56. Mets MB: Childhood blindness and visual loss: an assessment at two institutions including a "new cause." *Trans Am Ophtalmol Soc* 97:653–696, 1999.
57. Foster SC, Nguyen QD: Saving the vision of children with juvenile rheumatoid arthritis-associated uveitis. *JAMA* 280:113, 1998.
58. Lueck A: Cortical or cerebral visual impairment in children: a brief overview. *J Vis Impair Blindn* 104(10):585–592, 2010.
59. Bigelow AE: The development of joint attention in blind infants. *Dev Psychopathol* 15:259–275, 2003.
60. Sonksen PM, Dale N: Visual impairment in infancy: impact on neurodevelopmental and neurobiological processes. *Dev Med Child Neurol* 44:782–791, 2002.
61. Sonksen PM: Constraints on parenting: experience of a paediatrician. *Child: Care, Health Dev* 15:29–36, 1989.
62. Jan JE, Freeman RD, Scott EP: *Visual Impairment in Children and Adolescents*. New York, Grune & Stratton, 1977.
63. Fraiberg S: *Insights from the Blind: Comparative Studies of Blind and-Sighted Children*. New York, Basic Books, 1977.
64. Warren DH: *Blindness and Children: An Individual Differences Approach*. Cambridge, Cambridge University Press, 1994.
65. Sandler AM, Hobson RP: On engaging with people in early childhood: the case of congenital blindness. *Clin Child Psychol Psychiatry* 6:205–222, 2001.
66. Als H, Troninck E, Brazelton TB: Affective reciprocity and the development of autonomy: the study of a blind infant. *J Am Acad Child Psychiatry* 19:22–40, 1980.
67. Lowenfeld B: *Berthold Lowenfeld on Blindness and Blind People, Selected Papers*. New York, American Foundation for the Blind, 1981:39–67.
68. Moore V, McConachie H: Communication between blind and severely visually impaired children and their parents. *Br J Dev Psychol* 12: 491–502, 1994.
69. Preisler G: Early patterns of interaction between blind parents and their sighted infants. *Child Care, Health Dev* 17:65–90, 1991.
70. Rowbury C: *Referential communication between a blind mother and a blind child*. Cambridge, Paper presented at Developmental Section Conference, British Psychological Society, September, 1991.
71. Recchia SL: Play and concept development in infants and young children with severe visual impairments: a constructivist's view. *J Vis Impair Blindn* 91:401–406, 1997.
72. Rowland C: Patterns of interaction between three blind infants and their mothers. In: Mills AE (ed): *Language Acquisition in the Blind Child*. Beckenham, Croom Helm, pp. 114–132, 1983.
73. Peters AM: The interdependence of social, cognitive and linguistic development: evidence from a visually impaired child. In: Tager-Flusberg H (ed): *Constraints on Language Acquisition: Studies of Atypical Children*. Hillsdale, NJ, Lawrence Erlbaum, pp. 195–219, 1994.
74. O'Donnell LM, Livingston RL: Active exploration of the environment by young children with low vision: a review of the literature. *J Vis Impair Blindn* 85:287–291, 1991.
75. Sonksen PM: Vision and early development. In: Wybar R, Taylor D (eds): *Paediatric Ophthalmology: Current Aspects*. New York, Marcel Dekker; pp. 85–95, 1983.
76. Andersen ES, Dunlea A, Kekelis LS: Blind children's language: resolving some differences. *J Child Lang* 11:645–664, 1984.
77. Bigelow AE: Early words of blind children. *J Child Lang* 14:47–56, 1987.
78. Rosel J, Caballer A, Jara P, et al.: Verbalism in the narrative language of children who are blind and sighted. *J Vis Impair Blindn* 99(7):413, 2005.
79. Cutsforth TD: *The blind in school and society*. New York, American Foundation for the Blind, 1950.
80. Nelson K: Individual differences in language development: implications for development and language. *Dev Psychol* 17:170–187, 1981.
81. Prizant BM: Toward an understanding of language symptomatology of visually impaired children. In: Sykanda AM, Buchanan BK, Jan JE, Groenveld M, Blockberger SJ (eds): *Insight in sight: Proceedings of the fifth Canadian interdisciplinary conference on the visually impaired child*. Vancouver, CNIB, pp. 70–87, 1984.
82. Fraiberg S, Andelson E: Self representation in young blind children. In: Jastrzembska JS (ed): *The effects of blindness and other impairments on early development*. New York, American Foundation for the Blind, pp. 136–159, 1976.
83. Warren D: *Blindness and Early Childhood Development*. 2nd ed. New York, American Foundation for the Blind, 1984.
84. Sonksen PM, Levitt SL, Kitzinger M: Identification of constraints acting on motor development in young visually disabled children and principles of remediation. *Child Care Health Dev* 10:273–286, 1984.
85. Sonksen PM: The assessment of "vision for development" in severely visually handicapped babies. *Acta Ophthalmol Suppl* 157:82–90, 1983.
86. Bigelow AE: Locomotion and search behavior in blind infants. *Infant Behav Dev* 15:179–189, 1992.
87. Cattaneo Z, Vecchi T: *Blind vision: The neuroscience of visual impairment*. Cambridge, Mass, MIT Press, 2011.
88. Putzar LI, Goerendt K, Lange F, et al.: Early visual deprivation impairs multisensory interactions in humans. *Nature Neurosci* 10 (10):1243–1245, 2007.
89. Stilla R, Hanna R, Hu X, et al.: Neural processing underlying tactile microspatial discrimination in the blind: a functional magnetic resonance imaging study. *J Vision* 8(10):1–19, 2008.
90. Burton H, McLaren DG, Sinclair RJ: Reading embossed capital letters: an fMRI study in blind and sighted individuals. *Hum Brain Mapp* 27(4): 325–339, 2006.
91. Millar S: Reading without vision. In: Lewis V, Collis GM (eds): *Blindness and Psychological Development*. Leicester, BPS Books, pp. 86–98, 1997.
92. Freeman RD, Goetz E, Richards DP, et al.: Defiers of negative prediction: a 14-year follow-up study of legally blind children. *J Vis Impair Blindn* 85:365–370, 1991.
93. McGurk H: Affective motivation and development of communication competence in blind and sighted children. In: Mills AE (ed): *Language Acquisition in the Blind Child: Normal and Deficient*. London, Croom Helm, pp. 108–113, 1983.
94. Hobson R, Brown R, Minter EM, et al.: Autism "revisited": the case of congenital blindness. In: Lewis V, Collis GM (eds): *Blindness and Psychological Development*. Leicester, BPS Books, pp. 99–115, 1997.
95. Kekelis LS: Peer interactions in childhood: the impact of visual impairment. In: Sacks SZ, Kekelis LS, Gaylord-Ross RJ (eds): *The Development of Social Skills by Blind and Visually Impaired Students*. New York, American Foundation for the Blind, pp. 13–35, 1992.
96. Celeste M: Play behaviors and social interactions of a child who is blind: In theory and practice. *J Vis Impair Blindn* 100(2):75–90, 2006.
97. Salleh Norshidah Mohamad, Khalim Zainal: How and why the visually impaired students socially behave the way they do. *Procedia Soc Behav Sci* 9:859–863, 2010.
98. Mulford RC: Referential development in blind children. In: Mills AE (ed): *Language Acquisition in the Blind Child*. Beckenham, Croom Helm, pp. 89–107, 1983.
99. Preisler G: Social and emotional development of blind children: a longitudinal study. In: Lewis V, Collis GM (eds): *Blindness and Psychological Development*. Leicester, BPS Books, pp. 69–85, 1997.
100. Raver-Lampman SA: Effect of gaze direction on evaluation of visually impaired children by informed respondents. *J Vis Impair Blindn* 84: 67–70, 1990.
101. Erin JN, Dignan K, Brown PA: Are social skills teachable? A review of the literature. *J Vis Impair Blindn* 85:58–61, 1991.
102. Cavenaugh B, Giesen JM: A systematic review of transition interventions affecting the employability of youths with visual impairments. *J Vis Impair Blindn* 106:400–413, 2012.
103. Espezel H, Jan JE, O'Donnell ME, et al.: The use of melatonin to treat sleep-wake-rhythm disorders in children who are visually impaired. *J Vis Impair Blindn* 90:43–50, 1996.
104. Palm L: Long-term melatonin treatment in blind children and young adults with circadian sleep-wake disturbances. *Dev Med Child Neurol* 39:319–325, 1997.
105. U.S. Department of Education; Individuals with Disabilities Education Act; 34 CFR Section 300.8(c)(2); 2004. Available at: http://idea.ed.gov; accessed July 15, 2016.
106. Miles B: Overview on deaf-blindness. *DB-LINK*. Monmouth, OR, The National Clearinghouse on Children who are Deaf-Blind, 2008.
107. The 2013 National Child Count of Children and Youth who are Deaf-Blind; the National Center on Deaf-Blindness. September 2014.
108. Kaplan J, Gerber S, Bonneau D, et al.: A gene for usher syndrome type I (USH1A) maps to chromosome 14q. *Genomics* 4(14):979–987, 1992.
109. Hsu P, Ma A, Wilson M, et al.: CHARGE syndrome: a review. *J Paediatr Child Health* 7(50):504–511, 2014.
110. Abou-Elhamd K, ElToukhy HM, Al-Wadaani FA: Syndromes of hearing loss associated with visual loss. *Eur Arch Oto-Rhino-Laryngol* 4(271): 635–646, 2014.
111. Wolff Heller K, Kennedy C: *Etiologies and characteristics of deaf-blindness*. Monmouth, Teaching Research Publications, Western Oregon State College, 1994.
112. Malloy, P, Thomas, KS, Schalock, M, et al.: Early Identification of infants who are deaf-blind. National Consortium on Deaf-Blindness, 2009.
113. Wiley S, Parnell S, Belhorn T: Promoting early identification and intervention for children who are deaf or hard of hearing, children with vision impairment and children with deafblind conditions. *J Early Hear Detect Intervent* 1(1):26–33, 2016.
114. Wheeler L, Griffin H: A movement-based approach to language development in children who are deaf-blind. *Am Ann Deaf* 142(5):387–390, 1997.
115. VanDijk J: The first steps of the deaf-blind child towards language. *Int J Educ Blind* 15(4):112–114, 1966.
116. Miles B, McLetchie B: The National Information Clearinghouse on Children who are deaf-blind; Developing Concepts with Children Who Are Deaf-Blind, 2008. Available at: http://nationaldb.org. Accessed 20 July 2016.

CHAPTER 2.2.3 ■ SEXUAL MINORITY YOUTH: IDENTITY, ROLE, AND ORIENTATION

CYNTHIA J. TELINGATOR, ERIC N. BOYUM, AND PETER T. DANIOLOS

INTRODUCTION

The term sexual minority youth encompasses adolescents who are not exclusively heterosexual. It is challenging to write a chapter on sexual minority youth and avoid the trap of further entrenching a dichotomous discussion about sexuality, rather than advancing a discussion about the multidimensionality of an individual. Sexuality and gender are each complex entities which should be understood as being multidimensional, as well as individually experienced and expressed. Clinicians need to ask their patients about their experience in a developmentally sensitive manner in order to understand the meaning of these aspects of one's identity, and to help them to integrate their sexuality and gender with all the other aspects of their identity.

Sexual minority youth have joined with others who identify with a common label, such as "gay," "lesbian," "bisexual" to find acceptance and solidarity. Sexual minority youth across the country have lessened their isolation by finding community through the Internet and social media. These developments and other cultural influences have impacted young people who are increasingly resisting categorization. Creative and less rigid identity constructs have led to the development of new identities such as pansexual, polyamorous, and heteroflexible, to describe what has likely always been a more dynamic continuum of sexual experience and expression for individuals. In this chapter, we will use the term sexual minority to refer to youth with same sex attractions, relationships, or behaviors, regardless of their self-identification (1).

Although the categorization of gay, lesbian, and bisexual has been helpful in the past to find community, in many parts of the world it no longer is necessary to segregate oneself with others who label themselves in a similar way in order to find acceptance. Social change and the media have played an important role in redefining community for youth who are sexual minorities. Grassroots communities and school organizations such as Parents, Families, Friends, and Allies United with LGBTQ People (PFLAG), Gay, Lesbian, and Straight Education Network (GLSEN), and school-based Gay-Straight Alliances (GSA) have provided support to sexual minority youth, their families, friends and allies, irrespective of a youth's sexual identity. A decade ago, a *Washington Post*/Henry J. Kaiser Family Foundation/Harvard University sponsored survey noted that 57% of Washington, DC–area teens had a friend who is gay or lesbian (2). PFLAG now estimates that the rate is around 8 in 10 (3). The extensive media coverage, including social media, of recent legal and sociocultural advances supporting gay, lesbian, bisexual individuals, youth, and families provides an affirming backdrop in which sexual minority youth and all youth can explore their identities. A good example of the power of social media is the "It Gets Better Project," which features gay and straight individuals, some of whom are celebrities and political leaders, sharing hope-filled messages for youth struggling with their sexuality. Whether through journalism, popular television, music, or films, there has been a growing visibility of sexual minority youth and adults who partner, have children, and create a home and a life outside of a heterosexual construct.

The variation in adolescent sexual identity development is as complicated as any aspect of identity development; social and cultural factors are clearly not the only determinants of sexual identity. The biologic, environmental, psychological, and sociocultural influences leading to divergent pathways of psychosexual development have not been fully worked out.

Stressors adolescents may experience might lead an adolescent and/or a family to seek psychiatric consultation. While the problems these adolescents face require the full empathy and support of a trained professional, it is important to acknowledge that not all sexual minority adolescents face these challenges with the same degree of severity. There are many recognized cases of individuals whom, for whatever reason, whether it is a solid support system, a loving environment, or their own abilities to maneuver the many complex challenges most adolescents in these stages of development face, are able to enter adulthood fully self-accepting and secure in their feelings regarding their sexual identity. Sexual minority youth, like their heterosexual peers, have strengths and vulnerabilities that may contribute to the development of various physical or mental health conditions. Most sexual minority youth will never come to the attention of a mental health clinician.

As child and adolescent clinicians, we often see the most vulnerable youth, whose circumstances overwhelm—but do not eliminate—their capacity for resilience. This vulnerability occurs secondary to complex interactions of the child within a family, culture, and society. Although research findings often find higher rates of mental health risk in adolescent sexual minority populations, it is difficult to isolate what is due to internalized homophobia and external stressors that sexual minority youth experience, versus other biologic and psychosocial factors. The defenses used to cope with both internal and external stressors can lead to compartmentalization to protect this aspect of one's identity from being known. Youth may consciously and unconsciously do this as a shelter from stigma and shame, from rejection by family or friends, or from emotional and physical harm by family members, peers and/or communities.

THEORETICAL CONCEPTUALIZATIONS

Although in the literature and in clinical discussion definitions may vary, some core concepts are defined here and used within the chapter.

While extensive discussion of gender is beyond the scope of this chapter and will be presented elsewhere in this textbook, gender and sexuality as aspects of identity coexist and therefore gender definitions will be briefly reviewed. *Gender role or expression* refers to culturally underwritten masculine and feminine behaviors, attitudes, and personality traits, partly biologically driven, and partly shaped by environment. "Aspects of sex-typed behavior in childhood and adulthood are affected by hormones that were present very early in development, confirming findings in other mammalian species" (p. 839) (4). This is often noticeable as early as age 2 or 3, although it can be flexible throughout the life cycle.

Gender identity refers to the youngster's internally perceived gender, regardless of chromosomal constitution, gonadal/hormonal secretions, or genitalia. Most children develop a stable gender identity that is concordant with their natal or assigned sex by around the age of 3. For some, gender-variant roles/expression in childhood may coincide with a later homosexual identity. Adult homosexual men recall gender nonconformity in early childhood more commonly than adult homosexual women, while the rate of recalled gender nonconformity in early childhood is very low among heterosexual adults (5). Similar results were found when comparing gender expression in home videos of children who identified as homosexual adults to those who identified as heterosexual adults, although the difference between men and women was not observed (6).

Distinct from gender role or identity, *sexual orientation* is the predominance of erotic feelings, thoughts, and fantasies one has for members of one, both, or neither sex. *Sexual identity* is one's personal identity as a sexual being, a label used by youth in regard to themselves, for example "gay," "lesbian," "queer," "pansexual," or "asexual." As Thompson and Morgan point out, "although we would typically expect (sexual orientation and sexual identity) to generally inform one another, this is not always the case" (p. 16) (7).

Some theorists have considered sexual orientation to be biologically driven, immutable, and stable categorical entities, resistant to conscious control (8–10). Contemporary theorists, such as Lisa Diamond, have considered a more multidimensional model of sexual development. Diamond and Savin-Williams demonstrated, for example, how older models derived primarily from gay male populations did not readily apply to female sexual minority youth. They found that the context for sexual identity development was more likely to be emotionally oriented for female adolescents and sexually oriented for male adolescents. Their findings challenged the generalization at the time that homosexual attractions and self-identification were developed primarily around sexual contact–finding it held true less often for female youth (11). This upheld what has become a leading theory that "[i]n contrast to (the paradigm developed for homosexual males), female same-sex orientations often exhibit late and abrupt development, and inconsistencies among women's prior and current behavior, ideation and attractions have been extensively documented" (p. 1085) (12). Newer studies are beginning to include nonbinary descriptions of sexual orientation. For example, one study identified a group of predominantly women who identify as mostly heterosexual with some sexual minority aspects to their identities (13) and another identified a minority of individuals who display limited romantic feelings, attractions, or sexual behaviors toward either sex (14).

The idea of fluidity of sexual orientation is not limited to recent theorists. Sigmund Freud stated in *Analysis Terminable and Interminable* "We have come to learn, however, that every human being is bisexual in this sense and that his libido is distributed, either in a manifest or a latent fashion, over objects of both sexes" (pp. 211–253) (15). Kinsey first described a nonbinary understanding of sexual orientation as a spectrum with exclusive homosexuality on one end of a continuum and exclusive heterosexuality on the other. He found that for both men and women sexual behavior could be very fluid over time (16,17). Sexual orientation may not be within conscious control but may shift along a bisexual continuum for some, and for others remain in a fixed position.

In addition to sexual orientation, one's identity as a sexual minority can be malleable over time. Savin-Williams writes that sexual identity is most subject to conscious choice and thus fluid over time (8). Savin-Williams and Diamond posit that both sexual orientation and sexual identity exist along a continuum, with the possibility of a multitude of expressions over the lifespan of an individual. More recent research has identified some youth, particularly females, self-labeling as "mostly straight," adding to the diverse spectrum of sexual identity (7). Asexuality has become increasingly understood as a sexual orientation and identity. Although the meaning of this label can vary between individuals, most use it to denote an identity as someone who does not experience sexual attraction or desire, the need to engage in sexual behaviors, or the desire for romantic relationships with members of any sex (18).

Variability in the meaning of sexual orientation and identity can be related to a number of factors. Developmental stage is an important consideration. "The fluidity of sexual desire, behavior, and identity may be a fundamental characteristic of sexuality during the teenage years" (p. 323) (19). Shame and stigma, within cultural and social contexts, also play an important role with respect to both sexual orientation and sexual identity. For example, some African-American males take on a sexual identity known as "the Down Low," in which members typically self-identify as "straight" in daily life but may identify as "on the DL" with potential same-sex partners. Such males are often not in denial about bisexuality; rather, they face shame and stigma within the sexual minority community based upon their race, and within the African-American community based upon their sexual orientation (20,21). Joseph Carrier wrote about the youth in Guadalajara, Mexico, where sexual orientation is defined differently, both by gender behavior and sexual practices. "Feminine males are especially denigrated because it is unthinkable that a masculine male could be a 'real homosexual.' Generally speaking, only male receivers in homosexual intercourse are considered 'homosexual.'" He also notes that "all people exhibiting traits of the opposite sex are considered to be homosexual" (p. 290) (22).

HISTORICAL OVERVIEW AND EPIDEMIOLOGY

Although the existence of divergent attractions and sexual behaviors is not a new phenomenon, public and professional discourse have changed over time. It was only in 1973 that homosexuality was deleted from the *Diagnostic and Statistical Manual* (from DSM II to DSM III) of the American Psychiatric Association, following the work of Evelyn Hooker that did not find increased rates of psychopathology among homosexuals (23). The Stonewall Rebellion in 1969, when the visibility of the gay, lesbian, bisexual, and transgendered community was increased in the media, had an influence as well. The social movement that began at that time has accelerated with the help of popular culture in the United States in recent years. Youth today are rejecting the labels that have served to help identify community in the past, and those who need or want to affix a label to themselves are sometimes choosing broader categories as mentioned earlier.

In 1992, Gary Remafedi et al. conducted a survey of Minnesota junior and senior high school students. Of the 36,706 students, 52% reported having some heterosexual experience and 1% as having had a homosexual experience. In this early study Remafedi found that 1.6% of males and 0.9% of females identified themselves as either bisexual or predominantly homosexual, and more than 10% were "not sure." Interestingly only 27.1% of the students with homosexual experience self-identified as homosexual or bisexual. He also found that even though a larger number of adolescent boys reported a homosexual identification, more adolescent girls reported same-sex attractions and fantasies (24). This does not necessarily correlate with assuming a gay, lesbian, or bisexual identity. In a 1998 study sample of Massachusetts students, when asked about same-sex experiences rather than self-labels, 6.4% of sexually experienced students reported same-sex sexual contact. In addition, they found that an equal number of male and female adolescents had same-sex experiences (25).

Some ongoing large national surveys, such as the National Health and Nutrition Examination Surveys (NHANES), National Survey on Family Growth (NSFG), and the Youth Risk Behavior Survey (YRBS) have included questions aiming to estimate the prevalence of aspects of sexual orientation and/or identity within the general population. In the 20 years since Remafedi's early study, the number of youth reporting same-sex sexual encounters has increased dramatically. Using NHANES data, Liu et al. (26) found that 10.1% of females and 3.5% of males ages 14 to 19 reported at least one lifetime same-sex sexual partner. When adult respondents to the 1999 to 2012 NHANES surveys were categorized by 10-year birth cohorts, the rate of reporting a lifetime same-sex partner had doubled from the 1940 to 1949 cohort to the 1970 to 1979 cohort. Analysis of the NSFG data from 2002 to 2008 by Chandra et al. (27) yielded similar rates of same-sex experience as the NHANES data, around 11% for females and 2.5% for males age 15 to 19. Despite the increased reporting of same-sex sexual behavior over the past 20 years, the rates of adolescents reporting sexual minority identities in the 2005 to 2007 YRBS had increased only slightly from those observed by Remafedi in 1992, with 1.2% claiming a homosexual (gay or lesbian) identity, and 3.4% a bisexual identity (28). Similar to Remafedi's initial work, there was a low concordance between reported sexual identity and history of sexual behavior; only 21.4% of youth engaging exclusively with same-sex partners identified as a sexual minority, instead choosing to self-identify as heterosexual.

Data regarding traditional milestones in sexual orientation development were primarily developed through surveys of sexual minority youth involved in community programs. D'Augelli collected data in the late 1980s and again in the late 1990s in social and recreational programs for gay, lesbian, and bisexual youth in America and Canada. His final sample included 542 youths, 62% male, and 38% female. He found that 74% identified as gay or lesbian, and 20% reported being bisexual, but mostly gay or lesbian; and 6% said they were bisexual, but equally gay or lesbian and heterosexual. The bisexual group was significantly more represented by females. Notably, youth who identified as "bisexual but predominantly heterosexual" or "uncertain" were excluded from the sample. The sampled youth reported being aware of same-sex feelings around age 10 for males and age 11 for females. Self-labeling occurred on average 5 years after initial awareness. This is a significant decrease in the age that sexual minority youth are self-identifying from the literature of only a decade ago. More sexual minority youth are self-identifying while they are still of high school age and living at home even if they are not sexually active (19). D'Augelli found that even though society has become more accepting, "youths spent one-third of their lives aware of same-sex feelings but not revealing this to others" (19).

Floyd and Bakeman gathered data on a sample of 767 adult attendees of an LGBT festival in 2001, asking them to recall the age of certain milestones with respect to sexual orientation and identity development. They were able to compare milestone achievement between those who self-identified as a sexual minority before 1988, and after 1988. There was a change in both the age of disclosure of sexual orientation, which decreased over time from 20.7 to 17.9 years, and the period between self-identification and disclosure decreased from 6.1 years to 2 years (29).

Recent studies have shown that same-sex contact occurs a year or two prior to a boy's gay identification, while a girl is more likely to have her first same-sex contact after identifying as lesbian. The context for first same-sex sexual contact and self-labeling was found to be more emotionally or relationship oriented for young women and sexually oriented for young men (11). Although the data on this has varied, it probably represents diverse trajectories that sexual minority youth take in their development (22,30,31). Many adolescents begin to explore their sexuality during this developmental period. While this is normative for heterosexual youth, sexual minority youth may not have this experience, due to stigma and internalized homophobia, which may delay the exploration of their sexuality (1).

Sexual minority youth face similar and different developmental tasks than their heterosexual peers as they try to assimilate this aspect of their identity into their lives and their social and emotional relationships. Adolescents who are raised in families and communities where heterosexuality is considered normative often hide or deny their same-sex feelings and interests. The implications of this for identity development are unknown. Since many of these teens are being raised in families where the parents have a different sexual orientation, it is difficult to make use of parental identifications or count on parental support to help with the process of self-exploration (32). Most minorities can at least look to parents who have experienced similar stigmatization due to shared group membership, with exceptions including deaf and hard of hearing youth who have hearing parents, or minority youth adopted by majority parents.

A study of youth ages 14 to 21 involved in sexual minority programming in Utah, of whom 48% indicated a Mormon/LDS religious affiliation, noted that over 10% of youth identifying as gay or lesbian had steadily dated someone of the opposite sex in the past year, and that 14.6% had had sexual intercourse with someone of the opposite sex in the past year. The rates of self-identified straight individuals engaging in same-sex dating was much lower. However, the data also suggested that the range of romantic and sexual expressions amongst gay–lesbian youth with their same-sex partners and straight youth with their opposite-sex partners were essentially no different. These data suggest that even within a generally nonaccepting sociocultural context, sexual minority youth might be pressured to try to "pass" by engaging in heterosexual relationships, but also build and explore same-sex relationships in the same way that heterosexual youth build and explore opposite-sex relationships (33). The degree to which involvement in accepting community programming, or having accepting family experiences, mitigated the nonaccepting sociocultural context was not examined in this study.

In his study, D'Augelli found that half of the sexual minority adolescent males and three-quarters of the adolescent females had had heterosexual experiences, with more females having had heterosexual sex prior to having a same-sex experience. More males (84%) than females (60%) in this study were aware of their same-sex feelings prior to engaging in heterosexual sex (19). Sexual identity, sexual behavior, and sexual orientation are not stable or necessarily congruent for many adolescents during this period of development. This is particularly relevant for the mental health clinician who relies on the description of sexual behavior to define a patient's sexual orientation or sexual identity.

ADOLESCENT SEXUAL DEVELOPMENT

The development of sexual attractions, desires, behaviors, and self-identification is common among adolescents; yet, for both heterosexual and nonheterosexual youth these features of adolescent sexual development often are not stable and do not predict attractions, behaviors, or identities in adulthood (34).

TABLE 2.2.3.1

TROIDEN'S STAGES OF HOMOSEXUAL DEVELOPMENT

1. Sensitization	A sense of feeling different from childhood peers, typically only reaching awareness in retrospect. Children feel inadequate in their natal gender roles, including not sharing interests with peers of the same gender and boys experiencing warmth in relation to other males that is recalled as atypical.	Childhood
2. Identity Confusion	The suspicion one might be homosexual begins to arise, based on same-sex attractions and behaviors. Culturally assumed and mandated heterosexual identity is threatened. Youngsters may cope by trying to pass as heterosexual and may engage in heterosexual sex to prove to themselves and others that they are heterosexual.	Early Adolescence
3. Identity Assumption	Gradually, one begins to self-identify as homosexual and identify oneself as homosexual to others, usually in the context of social contact with other homosexuals. Youth in this stage are particularly vulnerable to stigmatization. Rural and minority youth may have a much harder time due to lack of role models and double discrimination for the latter.	Variable, but typically late adolescence
4. Commitment	Finding harmony between emotional, romantic, and sexual aspects of one's homosexual identity. Past ambivalence gives way to belief of one's identity as "natural" and "normal." People in this stage no longer try to "pass" as heterosexual, though may continue to "cover their homosexuality from looming too large." There is increasing disclosure to peers and to family. Management of stigma shifts from the personal to political and educational efforts in the broader community.	Early Adulthood

Currently, various models attempt to elucidate adolescent developmental pathways leading to sexual minority identities.

Early models used a linear stage theory perspective to describe "milestones" that sexual minority youth reached in sequential order on their way to becoming self-accepting sexual minorities in adulthood. Using data from primarily adult self-identified gay males, Troiden, Cass, and others helped to begin a dialogue in the field about "normal" development for sexual minorities, describing a linear stage model of sexual identity development that depicts a pathway to complete integration of one's sexual identity (Table 2.2.3.1) (10,35).

Contemporary theorists including Diamond, Garnets, Savin-Williams, Klein, and others have challenged these models of linear progression, and have introduced a multidimensional approach to sexual identity development (11,36,37). They critiqued earlier linear models for using male retrospective experiences as the norm, and not taking cultural factors into account (36,38). Diamond, for example, has argued that viewing sexual identity development in women as an evolving process may be more helpful in understanding their development with regard to both emotional and sexual attractions. In support of this, she showed that up to three quarters of self-identified sexual minority women had failed to progress linearly through Troiden's developmental stages, had experienced comparatively late and abrupt onset of development of same-sex attractions and had more often exhibited plasticity with respect attractions, behaviors, and self-identification (12,39). As Galatzer-Levy writes, "[i]n non-linear systems models, unlike epigenetic models, the fact that processes share initial and end points does not indicate that the paths joining these points are the same. Instead it leaves us free, in each case, to explore the path taken by the individual and suggests that there will often be multiple paths between various developmental points" (p. 432) (40). Fritz Klein developed the first alternative multidimensional model of sexual orientation, which includes a grid of seven variables: sexual attraction, sexual behavior, sexual fantasies, emotional preference, social preference, self-identification, and hetero/homosexual lifestyle, all plotted along a time course (11,16,17,41,42). Thus, these earlier linear models have given way to newer dimensional models of measuring how young people see themselves as sexual beings, regardless of sexual orientation (43).

Stigma and shame can deeply impact all aspects of human development, including that of sexual orientation and identity. Gay and lesbian youth who are consolidating their identities tend to use "impression management" skills, as described in the work of Goffman. His work has been expanded to help understand the experience of members of other stigmatized groups who use "covering" defenses to minimize the impact of stigma and the risk of rejection. Sexual minority youth do this by selectively disclosing to those most likely to be accepting, while minimizing disclosing to others aspects of their identity that they fear might lead to rejection. Goffman also described the process of "spoiled identities," as identity becomes reduced to the stigmatized aspects, denying membership in other aspects of the self, such as ethnicity and religious affiliation. This concept has been extended to sexual minority youth by authors such as Martin in his article *Learning to Hide: The Socialization of the Gay Adolescent*, and has been revisited by many others, including Yoshino's book on "covering" (44–46).

Some populations of sexual minorities have had significant struggles with respect to stigmatization. Rosario et al. looked at ethnic and racial differences in the coming-out process. They looked at a sample of Black, Latino, and white youths and found that there were no significant differences in the achievement of sexual developmental milestones, sexual orientation, sexual behavior, or sexual identity between groups. They found that cultural factors did not impede the formation of identity but instead impacted identity integration. Cultural factors (which include religious beliefs) may delay integration of a gay identity, as manifested by limiting involvement in gay-related social activities, increasing discomfort related to self-disclosure, and increasing negative attitudes toward homosexuality (internalized homophobia) due to the impact being affiliated with a stigmatized group. They reported that Black sexual minority youth were involved in fewer gay-related social activities, reported less comfort with others knowing about their sexual orientation, disclosed their sexual orientation less frequently to others and had fewer positive attitudes toward homosexuality at baseline than did white youth. Despite being similar to white youth in other measures, Latino youths disclosed to fewer people than white youth. The investigators found that despite having fewer positive attitudes than their white counterparts at the outset of the study, Black youth reported greater increases in positive attitudes regarding their sexual identity than did white youths over time, and by the end of the study there was no difference between the groups (47). Other studies have similarly demonstrated that negotiating multiple identities impacts sexual minority identity formation in males and females of varied ethnic backgrounds (48–50). Subsequent research by Jamil et al. indicated that the development of racial and sexual identity occurred concomitantly in so-called "double minority" youth, referencing Black or Latino sexual minority adolescents that he studied. It was not uncommon that these youths experienced maltreatment related to both their emerging racial and sexual identities; "[p]articipants who experienced oppression in the home reported experiencing particularly high levels of distress" (p. 11) (51). They found that such youth utilized community-based sexual minority organizations and peers for support in the process of self-identification, while learning to "...successfully navigate gay, White, and ethnic communities as a (sexual minority) person of color" (pp. 11–12) (51). For some racial and ethnic groups, cultural prohibitions present barriers to the expression of one's sexual identity, while others permit it within a defined construct.

Although context has been studied to some extent with respect to stigma, some recent literature has looked more closely at the immediate (e.g., familial) and larger (e.g., cultural, historical) contexts in which young people are exploring their sexuality. Phillip Hammack has proposed a life course theory of sexual identity formation, taking stock of biological, social, cultural, and historical contexts of the coming-out process and how "...individuals construct their own life course through the choices and actions they take within the opportunities and constraints of history and social circumstances" (p. 269) (52,53). Emphasis is on the cultural, social, and historical context in which the young person is experiencing partly biologically based sexual attractions, romantic feelings, and desires. In this model, individuals with same-sex attractions internalize social attitudes and identity labels, and make decisions about subsequent behavior based upon cultural possibilities and constraints. One ultimate goal of this line of research is to produce longitudinal narrative assessments of individuals to understand decision-making regarding sexual orientation and identity.

DEVELOPMENTAL CHALLENGES AND RESILIENCY

All adolescents face unique developmental challenges, heterosexual youth included, during this period of "storm and stress" (54). There has been debate in the literature about whether sexual minority youth are even more at risk. A growing number of studies has suggested this might be so for health risks (55), mental health symptoms (55–60), acting out (61), substance abuse (56,61), and suicidal thoughts and behaviors (56,57,59). Other investigators, however, have found similar rates of homosexuality in suicide victims to that of the general population (62), although some argue that difficulties in sampling and definitions of both suicidal events and sexual minority youth obscure these results (63).

Because of the evidence of a growing number of health disparities among sexual minorities, the Institute of Medicine (IOM) convened a panel to evaluate what is known about health status of sexual minorities, including sexual minority youth. The 2011 IOM report concluded that sexual minority youth indeed do face certain health disparities. Mental health and substance use disparities included increased rates of depression, suicidal behavior, and substance abuse. Suicidal behavior amongst sexual minority youth has been a concern for decades, though some have argued the risk has been overestimated. In 1989, the US government's report of the Secretary's Task Force on Youth Suicide showed that suicide was the leading cause of death among sexual minority youth. This report estimated that "up to" 30% of youth who committed suicide annually were sexual minorities. The author of this report went on to say that "...gay youth are 2 to 3 times more likely to attempt suicide than other young people" (64). Several private organizations convened an expert panel in 2007 to address the need for better understanding of suicide risk in sexual minorities, including sexual minority youth. They noted that sexual minority identification was more strongly predictive of suicide attempts in young males than in females, with the overall risk being 12% to 19% for males and less for females (65). After the IOM reviewed all available interim school-based, state-based, and national studies, the panel concluded that "...LGB youth and youth who report same-sex romantic attraction are at increased risk for suicidal ideation attempts, as well as depressive symptoms, in comparison with their heterosexual counterparts" (p. 147) (66). In addition to suicide, disproportionately high numbers of sexual minority youth have been found to use substances including tobacco, alcohol, and illicit drugs, with a younger age of first use compared to heterosexual youth. For unclear reasons, bisexual female youth are at the highest risk of illicit drug use. Methamphetamine use among gay male youth is a concern, especially when combined with other risk behaviors in social contexts such as Internet-related sexual contacts or bathhouses (66). Because adolescents who self-identify as a sexual minority still at times engage with opposite sex partners, they are at the same or increased risk of teen pregnancy (66). New cases of human immunodeficiency virus (HIV) infection are disproportionately high for among males under 25 who have sex with other males—regardless of self-identification; in fact, sexual minority youth comprise 60% of new diagnoses of HIV infections for those under age 25 (66). Between 14% and 15% of young urban men ages 18 to 22 who have sex with men reported being HIV positive in a recent survey (67). Additionally, the IOM notes that young men who have sex with men are the only demographic group with an increasing incidence of HIV/AIDS diagnoses, particularly high among young African-American gay men (66,68). Female sexual minority youth are not immune to the increased risk of HIV infection; adolescent girls reporting sexual minority identity frequently have had sexual contact with an opposite-sex partner at some point and often engage in higher risk sexual contact (66).

Some sexual minority youth face external stressors and distress related to their sexual minority status that may lead them to face increased health risk factors, both physical and emotional, as well as increased health risk behaviors (69). Increased risk is related to both external and internal stressors. External stress has been defined in the literature as experiences of violence, verbal abuse, rejection, and other acts that are perpetrated against sexual minority youth or those who are assumed to be sexual minority youth (70,71). Although the causal link between external stressors, risk behaviors, and poor outcomes is not fully established, ongoing research suggests that much of the excess risk of depression and suicidal behavior, substance abuse, and sex risk behaviors in adolescence and young adulthood is attributable to rejection, bullying, and other forms of victimization (72–75). Adolescents who disclose a sexual minority identity to their parents may experience increased family conflict, as well as family rejection, particularly sexual minority males (76). Sexual minority youth are heavily overrepresented among homeless youth in the United States, with 22% to 35% of some samples of homeless youth being sexual minorities, with self-identified gay male youth being at highest risk (66,77). In one study of sexual minority youth, Margaret Rosario found that 48% reported being homeless at least once, a full half of those having been evicted from their home by a parent, at a mean age of 14 (78). Once homeless, sexual minority youth are much more likely to engage in a number of health risk behaviors and develop mental health problems (66). Physical and verbal harassment and victimization, unfortunately, are commonly faced by sexual minority youth in the community, at school, and at times in the home. A study done by D'Augelli looked at gay, lesbian, and bisexual self-identified youth at community centers during two periods: 1987 to 1989 and 1995 to 1997. There was some geographic as well as cultural diversity in the sampling. He found that 81% of the 542 youths sampled reported verbal abuse related to being a sexual minority, 38% had been threatened with physical attacks, 22% had objects thrown at them, 15% had been physically assaulted, 6% had been assaulted with a weapon, and 16% had been sexually assaulted (19). All of these incidents were reported by the youth as being related to their sexual minority status. Some of this abuse occurred at school, some at home, and some in the community. Fear of being victimized was prevalent. Youth who were aware of their minority sexual orientation at earlier ages, self-identified earlier and self-disclosed earlier, reported more lifetime victimization. Some have reported that highly effeminate boys are targeted more than others as many have had atypical gender roles since childhood and have experienced social ostracism since an early age (79).

More recent retrospective data have been gathered on Adverse Childhood Events (ACEs) faced as youth by adult sexual minorities in comparison to their heterosexual peers, finding increased rates of verbal or physical abuse, physical or emotional neglect, household dysfunction, and school bullying (80). Both heterosexual and sexual minority men and women with gender nonconforming behaviors in childhood seem to be at increased risk of abuse, physical victimization, and emotional bullying, and later depression or PTSD symptoms (81,82).

Internal stress, plays a role in the excess risk of negative health outcomes for sexual minority youth, but the effect is less amenable to measurement and study. The internal stresses that sexual minority youth often face may shift, reflecting developmental factors at different life stages as well as different stages of the coming-out process, and tend to represent the internalization of society's negative attitudes toward homosexuality, termed *internalized homophobia* (83). In a case series of interviews retrospectively examining emotional angst faced in adolescence, Flowers and Buston describe a subject's account of distress through the coming-out process: "I remember going home at night and crying myself to sleep because I knew that I was different, and I was terrified of being different" (p. 54) (84). Another subject shared his experience of internalized homophobia: I felt different and yeah I suppose I knew I were gay, but I fought it, I really did fight it. Cos me mother is very very anti gay and me father is as well. I hated it. "I did not want to be gay, I did not want to be gay at all, ever. Because I, er, it made me an outcast. Everywhere I had to be constantly careful about what I did and I couldn't cope with it at all. I just didn't know about what to do or anything" (p. 55) (84). As Erik Erikson stated, "[t]he sad truth is that in any system based on suppression, exclusion, and exploitation, the suppressed, excluded, and exploited unconsciously accept the evil image they are made to represent by those who are dominant" (p. 445) (85). Newcomb and Mustanski completed a meta-analysis of over 5,800 adolescent and adult sexual minority subjects and found a small to moderate effect of internalized homophobia on depression and anxiety symptoms (86). As is the case for many minority populations, stigma and shame play powerful roles in the lives and mental well-being of lesbian, gay, bisexual, and questioning youth. Gay youth often learn to hide their homosexual orientation by attempting to present themselves as heterosexual. This facade can become a process of deception at all levels, living a lie in order to obtain acceptance in their larger peer group, and keeping a protective distance from peers and parents from whom they hide their homosexuality (44). As might be expected, lower rates of self-disclosure are correlated with increased distress among sexual minorities (87). As put by a subject in the Flowers and Buston series: "I mean you can...pretend to be heterosexual as much as you like, but, when push comes to shove,...(it is difficult) to like create this big lie all the time, you know, live this lie, you lose it every so often" (p. 57) (84).

In 1994, prior to many of the more recent societal changes taking place that have supported a sexual minority identity, Savin-Williams wrote: "In actuality, the vast majority of gay male, bisexual, and lesbian youths cope with their daily, chronic stressors to become healthy individuals who make significant contributions to their culture" (p. 262) (88). Andrew Anderson studied 77 gay male youth in cross section, finding that at the time of the study over 80% were A and B students, most had high self-esteem, a good sense of social support, and a high sense of competency (89). A recent prospective study of the psychological adjustment of sexual minority youth into young adulthood found that psychological distress decreases significantly through adolescence, with the trend continuing into adulthood (73). Although the strength and resilience required to negotiate adolescence and reach self-acceptance of a sexual minority identity is important and complex, relatively little research has been done in this area. Protective factors—which include self-acceptance and acceptance by families, peers, and communities—were commonly noted in early literature on vulnerabilities faced by sexual minority youth, yet the importance of these protective factors has not fully been explored (90). Although much historical research focused on negative interactions between families and sexual minority youth, newer research is more optimistic about the innate capacity of a family to accept their sexual minority loved one, as well as adapt over time to become more accepting (91).

The focus of several investigations has been on how personal psychological factors of sexual minority youth impact their well-being and risk. A study by Lewis et al. found that lesbian adults who had lower levels of "stigma consciousness" had fewer negative psychological and physical outcomes (92). Lasser and Tharinger, extending the work of Bandura on social learning theory, noted that gay, lesbian, and bisexual youth utilized a strategy termed "visibility management" to negotiate their environment (93). This refers to how these youths make decisions about to whom to disclose what, and how to go about disclosing their sexual orientation. This is similar to the work of Goffman regarding "impression management" skills often found among stigmatized groups where individuals might attempt to tone down traits or personal features which lead to discrimination (94). Assessments of risk and protection related to coping styles have consisted of cross-sectional studies to date, making the results hard to interpret since coping patterns in teenagers can change over time, sometimes in the face of stressors that sexual minorities often face (55,73,95).

Caitlin Ryan and her colleagues in the Family Acceptance Project have been working to understand the protection from risk afforded youth of generally accepting families (96). Sexual minority youth face a continuum of experiences including accepting, rejecting, or mixed behaviors and attitudes within a family, and the responses from parents and siblings may differ within each family.

Overall, the majority of sexual minority youth are well adjusted and not prone to health risk behaviors, mental health problems, suicide, or substance abuse and enter early adulthood as generally well-adjusted people. For some, "(the) experience of becoming gay (is) a difficult and painful journey of self-discovery and realization" (p. 60) (84). Scholar and psychoanalyst Galatzer-Levy, emphasizing that the vast majority of sexual minority youth emerge as healthy young adults, similar to their heterosexual peers, writes: "It is important that society as a whole come to terms with this new generation of well-adjusted, competent young men and women, who differ from their peers in terms of sexual orientation but little else" (p. 537) (97).

PSYCHOBIOLOGICAL THEORIES

Charlotte Patterson writes: "Is sexual orientation best thought of as an inborn characteristic determined by genetic factors? Or should it be regarded as socially constructed and malleable across the lifespan?" (p. 7) (98). The answer to this question is unknown. The development of a homosexual identity may be a complex and nonuniform interplay among genetics, in utero exposure to hormones, and neurodevelopmental, dynamic, and experiential factors. Given the breadth and fluidity of sexuality, one can theorize that there will never be a simple explanation for the development of sexual orientation (9,99–101).

Elevated concordance of homosexuality has been identified in several studies of identical male twins separated early in life and raised apart. Further, multiple twin studies have demonstrated that sexual orientation is highly heritable. Dean Hamer identified a sequence of markers at the tip of the X chromosome (Xq28) in 33 of 40 pairs of homosexual brothers; subsequent studies replicated this result, and also replicated that this finding is not present in lesbian twins (102). Recent attention has been paid to the genetics of female sexual orientation, gender nonconformity, and number of sexual partners, and found a heritable phenotype for homosexuality in women that provides evolutionary benefit, though no specific genetic locus was identified (101). While genes contributing to sexual orientation have not yet been discovered in humans, researchers are advancing further in determining genetic underpinnings of correlates in the fruit fly, *Drosophila melanogaster*. Early in genetic research of the fruit fly, researchers identified a gene they named *fru* in males with variant alleles of this locus who chose not to mate with females, courted both males and females, elicited courtship from other males, and attempted to copulate with wild-type males. Over the ensuing 50 years, researchers have been further elucidating the ways in which alternative splicing of the mRNA produced by this gene leads to male-specific and female-specific versions of the protein (103). A breakthrough came in 2005 when investigators showed that by altering *fru* and a related gene *tra* they were able to affect sexual orientation, behaviors, and sex roles (104). The degree to which there is a genetic "master switch" for homosexual behavior in humans remains unclear, though heritability in twin studies and the early onset of behavioral differences in young children who grow up to be sexual minorities suggests a genetic framework for sexual orientation exists.

It has long been hypothesized that differences in hormone exposure play a role in the development of homosexuality in humans. While in adulthood there is no consistent difference in masculine or feminine sex hormones between exclusively heterosexual and nonheterosexual males and females, investigators are exploring the role of prenatal sex hormones in the development of structural differences in the brain and sex-linked behaviors in humans. Exposure of the fetus to testosterone at six to 12 weeks' gestation alters the neuronal migration in the hypothalamus, preoptic area, corpus callosum, planum temporale, cerebellum, and amygdala. Gorski described an area in the hypothalamus of rats, which he labeled the "sexually dimorphic nucleus," that is eight times larger in males than in females. This has led to studies on the hypothalamic nuclei of humans with respect to differences in these areas not only between males and females, but also between people of the same sex assigned at birth with different sexual or gender identities. While a Dutch group conclusively showed that sex difference in the human hypothalamic uncinate nucleus was related to gender identity rather than sex assigned at birth (105), the results for humans with different sexual orientations has been less consistent. In 1991, LeVay found that the hypothalamic nucleus (INAH-3) was two to three times larger in heterosexual men than in women and homosexual men, who had similarly sized nuclei, and postulated that this was linked to prenatal testosterone levels. Byne et al. also showed a consistent trend toward more female-typical INAH-3 volume in homosexual men (106). No study has conclusively linked prenatal hormone exposure to the variation in this brain region (100). Some additional differences in brain structures–the origins of which are unclear–have been found to exist between heterosexual and homosexual men. Such differences include corpus callosum anatomy, patterns of cerebral asymmetry, and connectivity between brain regions (100).

In summary, biologic theories of the development of sexual orientation—including genetic, prenatal hormonal, and neurodevelopmental theories—remain in the preliminary stages. The interplay between biologic framework and life experience of sexual minority individuals has not yet been investigated. As Hines points out in her recent review on the role of hormones and sexual differentiation on gender and sexual orientation, "... social and cognitive developmental influences on children's activities could engage the same neural circuitry as underlies the effects of the early hormone environment," thus either synergizing with or reducing innate biologic influences on gender and sexual development (p. 81) (100).

EVALUATION AND INTERVENTION

There is no published or uniformly recommended evidence-based treatment strategy to assist youth with negotiating adolescence as a sexual minority youth (107). There is however a wealth of case based approaches, including family, psychodynamic, and cognitive-behavioral psychotherapeutic approaches, which have resulted in positive outcomes. This final section will review a range of recommendations for therapeutic approaches to sexual minority youth, their families, and—perhaps—their wider community. It is recommended that the reader also reference the current American Academy of Child and Adolescent Psychiatry's practice parameter on sexual minority youth.

The clinician should be aware of both the internal and external negotiations and compromises (reviewed in earlier sections of this chapter) that sexual minority youth need to face, and explore the adolescents' identity across the dimensions of emotional and physical attractions, intimate relationships, and behavior. The initial responsiveness and openness of the clinician will set the tone for the therapeutic encounter. Closed-ended questions will often foreclose on the possibility of developing trust and openness on the part of the sexual minority youth, as will a premature resolution of sexual identity. The patient is less likely to speak about same-sex attractions if the clinician assumes heterosexuality. Alternatively, identifying an adolescent with same-sex desires as gay or lesbian, without the adolescent labeling themselves as such, may prohibit exploration of other sexual orientations, identities, attractions or behaviors. The therapist can explore feelings that the adolescent is dealing with by creating a safe and nonjudgmental space. The adolescent is vulnerable to the internalization of the stigma associated with being a sexual minority youth, as detailed in earlier parts of the chapter. The therapist is similarly vulnerable both to impute stigma to the adolescent, and to feel stigmatized through the transference/countertransference interaction with the adolescent, possibly facilitated by projective identification. If he or she is unaware of this, it may impede both exploration and assimilation of this aspect of the patient's identity. Adolescents may not have conscious access to aspects of their sexual identity that are causing stress and emotional pain, but awareness may emerge through the creation of a safe therapeutic space. Dr. Hanley-Hackenbruck stated in her paper on *Coming Out and Psychotherapy* how "(g)iven that doctor and patient have society's attitudes in common, homophobia will be both a transference and counter transference issue" (108). Unfortunately, this initial step of gaining therapeutic rapport can be difficult, with client, therapist, and contextual factors all contributing to whether adolescents will later find that the therapy experience was helpful (109).

As with any patient, the therapist should assess the adolescent's safety, with an awareness of the risk factors involved. This should include a mental status exam and substance use history. The clinician needs to assess the use of Internet pornography and sexually focused chat rooms, offering discussion and education about Internet predators. The clinician should review the potential for violence directed toward the patient. The clinician should also address the possibility of self-harm, including cutting, eating disorders, substance abuse, suicidal ideation, and risk. Assessment of unsafe sexual practices, known or suspected pregnancy and history of STI testing including HIV testing is recommended, with education and referral for additional evaluation if concerns arise. It is important to assess victimization in the home, school, and community. It is also valuable to explore the youth's perception of support from friends, parents, school and/or community-based organizations or online websites. Sexual minority youth may be aware of supportive resources, so open-ended questions are helpful in allowing youth to take the lead in navigating affirming programs, with further clinician supported investigation of local organizations such as GSA, GLSEN, Parents, Families, Friends, and Allies United with LGBTQ People.

In some cases, the psychiatrist may be asked by the patient, family, or both to consult with the youth's school. While maintaining confidentiality around the patient's and family's struggles, it is important in this situation to educate relevant school personnel regarding the risks of victimization and the important protective effect of support from teachers and staff at school.

Sexual minority youth are emotionally vulnerable due to questions and concerns about disclosing their sexual minority status and the possible consequences on their lives from family, peers, and/or institutions (87). Because of their fear of rejection, discrimination, and violence, they often hide this aspect of their identity from their parents, teachers, and other important adults. Sexual minority youth might disclose their sexual identity to a therapist, without the youth's family, friends, school, religious organization, or larger community being aware of it. The therapist is faced with tolerating anxiety about knowing a core part of their patient's identity, which may still be a secret from the parents. Many gay youths are conflicted as they discover that their sexual orientation does not coincide with their own dreams, or their families' hopes and dreams for their future, which are typically socially constructed with respect to a heterosexual paradigm. In their case series on young gay men's angst during the coming-out process, Flowers and Buston write of one young man's account: "...I used to have this idea...(that) by the time I was 23, I would be married with so many kids...but then I was still fancying lads" (pp. 55–56) (84). The fear of needing to give up the fantasized future, causing psychic pain to themselves, as well as their parents, often contributes to the adolescent's decision to maintain this core aspect of their identity as a secret.

Internalized homophobia presents a significant challenge to the adolescent's psychological well-being, as referenced earlier in this chapter. Margolies, Becker, and Jackson-Brewer state in their paper *Internalized Homophobia: Identifying and Treating the Oppressor Within* that "[i]nternalized homophobia functions as a defense mechanism resulting from the ego's struggle between rules and desires. Rather than a single entity, internalized homophobia is comprised of a constellation of defense methods. Allowing for individual variations, the cluster usually includes rationalization, denial, projection, and identification with the aggressor" (pp. 229–242) (110). The form, intensity, and content of internalized homophobia will vary from adolescent to adolescent, and should be explored, in nonjudgmental terms, from genuine curiosity about the youth's experience (108). If the sexual minority identity of the patient is secret from the family, this binds the therapist and the patient together, but complicates work with the family. Bok speaks to the experience of secrets in psychotherapy (111), in which the therapist must remain mindful of both the protective and harmful aspects of secrets in a family. The therapist must respect the boundaries of confidentiality with the patient. When the adolescent wants to disclose his or her sexual identity to peers, siblings, and parents, the therapist may have a role in helping prepare their patient for the multitude of reactions he or she may face.

For some parents, their child's homosexual identity is experienced as a fundamental betrayal. Although still minimally represented in the literature, family accounts of their adolescent's coming-out process give valuable insight into parents' own beliefs, struggles, and capacity for acceptance. Parents' values are often part of the teenagers internalized value system, and both frequently derive from the larger sociocultural context in which the family lives. Not uncommonly, these values do not prepare a family to address such a revelation from their child in a healthy, accepting way. From her work with a community support group for parents of LGBT youth, Jessica Fields conducted in-depth parent interviews regarding their responses to their adolescents' disclosures about their sexual identities. Families commonly found that they did not have any "script" for handling the revelation and subsequent discussions about their child's sexual identity. "If people have been in a car accident we ask if they were hurt, how much damage there was to the car, whether or not it will be covered by insurance, [et cetera]. We had no script for this experience..." (p. 170) (112). Also, the parental fantasy about their adolescent's sexuality and sexual orientation is often infused with fantasies about their child's future relationships and creation of a family (113). This fantasy usually assumes heterosexuality, as "[s]exual orientation for gay men and lesbians is not recognized or acknowledged from birth, but is an achieved status rather than an ascribed status" (p. 437) (114). Recalling that some parents experienced the loss as similar to the death of a child, Fields quotes one mother as having said: "(I am) grieving here. I feel as if I lost my son. I wanted him to get married, have children—I want grandchildren—a house. But now [that is] not going to happen. I have lost all of those dreams I had for my son, because (they are) not going to come true. (He is) never going to have a wife and kids and a house like I wanted him to" (112). Parents also worried that they genuinely had, or would be judged as having had, done something to affect their children's sexual development. One mother wondered whether aspects of her own marriage caused her daughter's development of a lesbian identity. A father worried if a lack of gender-typical play contributed to his son's sexual minority identity: "I was never good at sports, for one thing. I (did not) play much with him—play ball or anything like that. And (then) he was never too good at sports" (p. 172) (112). Another narrative study of parents by Erika Grafsky noted that families typically saw themselves as functional and healthy at the time of disclosure (115). Most commonly, the parents she interviewed indicated a high degree of stress or emotionality at the time of the disclosure, even including anticipatory anxiety by both adolescent and parent leading up to the disclosure. When describing her son asking her to pull the car over because he needed to tell her something, one mother said: "At this point, (I am) getting a little nervous...his eyes start to get misty and (I am) like, Oh God, (he has) got a girl pregnant...[a]nd then he just looks at me and out of his mouth comes, (I am) gay. When I get taken by surprise I start to turn red from my chest up and I could feel heat and redness just rising; (I cannot) tell if (he is) joking, (I cannot) tell if [he is] serious. And I look at him and then I see the tears in his eyes. He starts crying and I start crying and (I am) just like, '(that is) all you had to tell me?'" (p. 8) (115). Even after disclosure, most parents in this study experienced a significant amount of anxiety: "I was petrified. I thought somebody would hurt him, I mean, all the horrors of...people not accepting him. Is life [going to] be hard? Afraid of him being harassed at school. How do I tell people? How are people going to treat him?" (p. 9) (115). These narratives from families give the therapist important insights, but limitations include that both studies were primarily or exclusively of Caucasian families in the United States, giving limited insight to the experience of racial and cultural minorities, or patients from or in other countries. Additionally, these studies recruited primarily parents of young gay men, although attempts were made to recruit parents of all sexual minorities.

Family acceptance is vital not only to the youth's self-esteem but also to the youth's psychological well-being in the short and long term (96). Caitlin Ryan's Family Acceptance Project has been developed to educate and encourage families to engage in highly accepting behaviors toward their sexual minority sons and daughters, both at the time of and following disclosure. Through this work, it became apparent that even the majority of parents who are perceived as rejecting, or engage in rejecting behaviors, want to help their child and maintain family stability and are motivated by genuine care and concern for their child (91). The interventions include a process of "meeting families where they are," similar to joining processes in other family therapy frameworks. This approach includes discussion of the overarching societal and cultural context in which the family lives, educating parents about the risks of family rejection, addressing common parent experiences of loss and shame, and addressing ongoing ambivalence and co-occurrence of accepting and rejecting behaviors by families (76,91,96). While the Family Acceptance Project does not yet have outcomes data as a health disparity intervention for sexual minority youth, the groundwork is promising.

For some families, the discovery of the adolescent's non-heterosexual orientation can lead them to want to change the young person's developmental trajectory, hoping that he or she might later assume a heterosexual identity, out of fear or misinformation that homosexuality is a mental disorder, or that the emergence of same-gender sexual desires among adolescents is abnormal or mentally unhealthy. While some programs propose to offer "conversion or reparative therapy" for sexual minority youth with this goal in mind, a recent report by the American Psychological Association reiterated previous denunciations of such sexual orientation change efforts. This report was supported by the American Academy of Pediatrics, American Psychiatric Association, the American Psychological Association, American Counseling Association, and the National Association of Social Workers (116). The United States Substance Abuse and Mental Health Services Administration (SAMHSA) released a report in October 2015 entitled "Ending Conversion Therapy: Supporting and Affirming LGBTQ Youth" (117). In this report, SAMHSA concludes that due to the significant risk of immediate and lasting harm to the young person, such sexual orientation change efforts are "inappropriate" (p. 26) (117). The most recent American Academy of Child and Adolescent Psychiatry practice parameter for working with sexual minority youth also states that "(c)linicians should be aware that there is no evidence that sexual orientation can be altered through therapy, and that attempts to do so may be harmful" (p. 967) (107). Thus, the consensus of the major mental health-related professional associations is that sexual orientation change efforts are strongly discouraged.

CONCLUSION

Due to massive and ongoing sociocultural shifts in many parts of the world, sexual minority youth increasingly have the opportunity to make life choices regardless of the gender of their partner(s), including marriage and having children. Here in the United States, the 2015 *Obergefell v. Hodges* Supreme Court decision affirming marriage as a right for all US citizens, not just heterosexual ones, has had a seismic impact (118). However, their path is complicated by the powerful forces of stigma, which can deeply impact their mental health, their core identity, and their sense of being a competent, "normal" sexual being, able to connect with others on an intimate level. Mental health professionals can offer a safe space in which such youth can find acknowledgment, support, and fortification, allowing them to continue navigating their life-course. Self-acceptance and family support play important roles in the psychological well-being of these adolescents (59,96).

Sexuality is a core aspect of identity. Sexual identity emerges over time, impacted by biologic, familial, cultural, and environmental forces. For those whose identity outcome is not acceptable in their communities and families, development can be strained. In addition, with adverse circumstances, the overwhelming psychic burden may contribute to the development of symptoms of emotional illness and at times serious psychopathology. For some, resilience and other factors may minimize the emotional challenges sexual minority youth face with regards to their sexual orientation, and/or sexual identity. For others, the impact of stigma leads to even greater resilience and capacity. As culture shifts and transforms, formerly ostracized minorities are increasingly finding themselves to be accepted members of society. This has allowed more sexual minority youth to exist without the same pressures to develop "covering" defenses, or to "pass" as heterosexual, thus spared the negative psychological impact of turning to such dysfunctional strategies. However, many others do not have this freedom due to cultural, regional, ethnic, familial, religious and/or intrapsychic factors.

The role of the child and adolescent psychiatrist is to understand the child regardless of what self-labels are used and to assist the family with accepting their child's developmental trajectory. The clinician is in a unique position to facilitate the integration of a youth's sexuality with other aspects of their identity. The hoped-for outcome is the emergence of a child less "spoiled" by stigma, and less "reduced" to any one aspect of their identity, a person well equipped for the emotional growth needed to emerge as a complex and multidimensional individual.

References

1. Russell ST, Consolacion TB: Adolescent romance and emotional health in the United States: beyond binaries. *J Clin Child Adolesc Psychol* 32(4):499–508, 2003.
2. Morin R: *What Teens Really Think, in Washington Post*. Washington, DC, pp. 14–19, 2005.
3. *About Straight for Equality*. 2015 [cited 2015 22 November]; Available at: http://www.straightforequality.org/About.
4. Pescovitz OH, Eugster EA (eds): *Pediatric Endocrinology: Mechanisms, Manifestations, and Management*. Lippincott Williams & Wilkins, 2004.
5. Bailey JM, Zucker KJ: Childhood sex-typed behavior and sexual orientation: a conceptual analysis and quantitative review. *Dev Psychol* 31(1):43–55, 1995.
6. Rieger G, Linsenmeier JA, Gygax L, Bailey JM: Sexual orientation and childhood gender nonconformity: evidence from home videos. *Dev Psychol* 44(1):46–58, 2008.
7. Thompson EM, Morgan EM: "Mostly straight" young women: variations in sexual behavior and identity development. *Dev Psychol* 44(1): 15–21, 2008.
8. Savin-Williams RC: *Adolescent Lives*. p. 272, 2005.

9. Savic I, Garcia-Falgueras A, Swaab DF: In: Savic I (ed): *Chapter 4—Sexual Differentiation of the Human Brain in Relation to Gender Identity and Sexual Orientation, in Progress in Brain Research*. Elsevier, p. 41–62, 2010.
10. Troiden RR: The formation of homosexual identities. *J Homosex* 17(1–2): 43–73, 1989.
11. Savin-Williams RC, Diamond LM: Sexual identity trajectories among sexual-minority youths: gender comparisons. *Arch Sex Behav* 29(6): 607–627, 2000.
12. Diamond LM: Development of sexual orientation among adolescent and young adult women. *Dev Psychol* 34(5):1085–1095, 1998.
13. Udry JR, Chantala K: Masculinity-femininity predicts sexual orientation in men but not in women. *J Biosoc Sci* 38(6):797–809, 2006.
14. Bogaert AF: Asexuality: prevalence and associated factors in a national probability sample. *J Sex Res* 41(3):279–287, 2004.
15. Freud S: *The Complete Psychological Works of Sigmond Freud*. 211–253, 1937.
16. Kinsey AC, Pomeroy WB, Martin CE: *Sexual Behavior in the Human Male*. p. 804, 1948.
17. Kinsey AC, I.f.S. Research: *Sexual Behavior in the Human Female*. p. 842, 1953.
18. Scherrer KS: Coming to an asexual identity: negotiating identity, negotiating desire. *Sexualities* 11(5):621–641, 2008.
19. Omoto AM, Kurtzman HS: *Contemporary Perspectives on Lesbian, Gay, and Bisexual Psychology*. p. 323, 2006.
20. Denizet-Lewis B: *Double Lives on the Down Low*. New York, New York Times, 28–33, 2003.
21. Sandfort TG, Dodge B: "And then there was the Down Low": introduction to Black and Latino male bisexualities. *Arch Sex Behav* 37(5):675–682, 2008.
22. Herdt GH, Boxer A: *Children of Horizons: How Gay and Lesbian Teens are Leading a New Way Out of the Closet*. p. 290, 1993.
23. Hooker E: The adjustment of the male overt homosexual. *J Proj Tech* 21(1):18–31, 1957.
24. Remafedi G, Resnick M, Blum R, Harris L: Demography of sexual orientation in adolescents. *Pediatrics* 89(4 Pt 2):714–721, 1992.
25. Faulkner AH, Cranston K: Correlates of same-sex sexual behavior in a random sample of Massachusetts high school students. *Am J Public Health* 88(2):262–266, 1998.
26. Liu G, Hariri S, Bradley H, Gottlieb SL, Leichliter JS, Markowitz LE: Trends and patterns of sexual behaviors among adolescents and adults aged 14 to 59 years, United States. *Sex Transm Dis* 42(1):20–26, 2015.
27. Chandra A, Mosher WD, Copen C, Sionean C: Sexual behavior, sexual attraction, and sexual identity in the United States: data from the 2006-2008 National Survey of Family Growth. *Natl Health Stat Report* (36):1–36, 2011.
28. Mustanski B, Birkett M, Greene GJ, Rosario M, Bostwick W, Everett BG. The association between sexual orientation identity and behavior across race/ethnicity, sex, and age in a probability sample of high school students. *Am J Public Health* 104(2):237–244, 2014.
29. Floyd FJ, Bakeman R: Coming-out across the life course: implications of age and historical context. *Arch Sex Behav* 35(3):287–296, 2006.
30. D'Augelli AR, Hershberger SL: Lesbian, gay, and bisexual youth in community settings: personal challenges and mental health problems. *Am J Community Psychol* 21(4):421–448, 1993.
31. Rosario M, Rotheram-Borus MJ, Reid H: Gay-related stress and its correlates among gay and bisexual male adolescents of predominantly Black and Hispanic background. *J Commun Psychol* 24(2):136–159, 1996.
32. Rotheram-Borus MJ, Fernandez MI: Sexual orientation and developmental challenges experienced by gay and lesbian youths. *Suicide Life Threat Behav* 25(Suppl):26–34, 1995; discussion 35–39.
33. Glover JA, Galliher RV, Lamere TG: Identity development and exploration among sexual minority adolescents: examination of a multidimensional model. *J Homosex* 56(1):77–101, 2009.
34. Savin-Williams RC, Ream GL: Prevalence and stability of sexual orientation components during adolescence and young adulthood. *Arch Sex Behav* 36(3):385–394, 2007.
35. Troiden RR: Becoming homosexual: a model of gay identity acquisition. *Psychiatry* 42(4):362–373, 1979.
36. Peplau LA, Spalding LR, Conley TD, Veniegas RC: The development of sexual orientation in women. *Annu Rev Sex Res* 10:70–99, 1999.
37. Garnets LD: Sexual orientations in perspective. *Cultur Divers Ethnic Minor Psychol* 8(2):115–129, 2002.
38. Chung YB, Katayama M: Assessment of sexual orientation in lesbian/gay/bisexual studies. *J Homosex* 30(4):49–62, 1996.
39. Diamond LM: A new view of lesbian subtypes: stable versus fluid identity trajectories over an 8-year period. *Psychol Women Quart* 29(2): 119–128, 2005.
40. Galatzer-Levy RM: Chaotic possibilities: toward a new model of development. *Int J Psychoanal* 85(Pt 2):419–441, 2004.
41. Fausto-Sterling A: *Sexing the Body: Gender Politics and the Construction of Sexuality*. p. 473, 2000.
42. Klein F: *Homosexuality/Heterosexuality: Concepts of Sexual Orientation*. p. 277–282, 1990.
43. O'Sullivan LF, Meyer-Bahlburg HFL, McKeague IW: The development of the sexual self-concept inventory for early adolescent girls. *Psychol Women Q* 30(2):139–149, 2006.
44. Martin AD: Learning to hide: the socialization of the gay adolescent. *Adolesc Psychiatry* 10:52–65, 1982.
45. Yoshino K: *Covering: The Hidden Assault on our Civil Rights*. p. 282, 2006.
46. Eliason MJ: Identity formation for lesbian, bisexual, and gay persons: beyond a "minoritizing" view. *J Homosex* 30(3):31–58, 1996.
47. Rosario M, Schrimshaw EW, Hunter J: Ethnic/racial differences in the coming-out process of lesbian, gay, and bisexual youths: a comparison of sexual identity development over time. *Cultur Divers Ethnic Minor Psychol* 10(3):215–228, 2004.
48. Dube EM, Savin-Williams RC: Sexual identity development among ethnic sexual-minority male youths. *Dev Psychol* 35(6):1389–1398, 1999.
49. Parks CA, Hughes TL, Matthews AK: Race/ethnicity and sexual orientation: Intersecting identities. *Cultur Divers Ethnic Minor Psychol* 10(3):241–254, 2004.
50. Consolacion TB, Russell ST, Sue S: Sex, race/ethnicity, and romantic attractions: multiple minority status adolescents and mental health. *Cultur Divers Ethnic Minor Psychol* 10(3):200–214, 2004.
51. Jamil OB, Harper GW, Fernandez MI; Adolescent Trials Network for HIV/AIDS Interventions: Sexual and ethnic identity development among gay-bisexual-questioning (GBQ) male ethnic minority adolescents. *Cultur Divers Ethnic Minor Psychol* 15(3):203–214, 2009.
52. Hammack PL: The life course development of human sexual orientation: an integrative paradigm. *Hum Dev* 48:267–290, 2005.
53. Hammack PL, Thompson EM, Pilecki A: Configurations of identity among sexual minority youth: context, desire, and narrative. *J Youth Adolesc* 38(7): 867–883, 2009.
54. Arnett JJ: Adolescent storm and stress, reconsidered. *Am Psychol* 54(5):317–326, 1999.
55. Lock J, Steiner H: Gay, lesbian, and bisexual youth risks for emotional, physical, and social problems: results from a community-based survey. *J Am Acad Child Adolesc Psychiatry* 38(3):297–304, 1999.
56. Fergusson DM, Horwood LJ, Beautrais AL: Is sexual orientation related to mental health problems and suicidality in young people? *Arch Gen Psychiatry* 56(10):876–880, 1999.
57. Russell ST, Joyner K: Adolescent sexual orientation and suicide risk: evidence from a national study. *Am J Public Health* 91(8):1276–1281, 2001.
58. Rosario M, Schrimshaw EW, Hunter J, Gwadz M: Gay-related stress and emotional distress among gay, lesbian, and bisexual youths: a longitudinal examination. *J Consult Clin Psychol* 70(4):967–975, 2002.
59. Hershberger SL, D'Augelli AR: The impact of victimization on the mental health and suicidality of lesbian, gay, and bisexual youths. *Dev Psychol* 31(1):65–74, 1995.
60. Hatzenbuehler ML, McLaughlin KA, Nolen-Hoeksema S: Emotion regulation and internalizing symptoms in a longitudinal study of sexual minority and heterosexual adolescents. *J Child Psychol Psychiatry* 49(12):1270–1278, 2008.
61. DuRant RH, Krowchuk DP, Sinal SH: Victimization, use of violence, and drug use at school among male adolescents who engage in same-sex sexual behavior. *J Pediatr* 133(1):113–118, 1998.
62. Shaffer D, Fisher P, Hicks RH, Parides M, Gould M: Sexual orientation in adolescents who commit suicide. *Suicide Life Threat Behav* 25 Suppl: 64–71, 1995.
63. Savin-Williams RC: Suicide attempts among sexual-minority youths: population and measurement issues. *J Consult Clin Psychol* 69(6):983–991, 2001.
64. Gibson P: *Report of the Secretary's Task Force on Youth Suicide: Prevention and Intervention in Youth Suicide*. U.S. Department of Health and Human Services, Editor. 1989.
65. Haas AP, Eliason M, Mays VM, et al.: Suicide and suicide risk in lesbian, gay, bisexual, and transgender populations: review and recommendations. *J Homosex* 58(1):10–51, 2011.
66. Institute of Medicine Committee on Lesbian, Gay, Bisexual and transgender: *The National Academies Collection: Reports funded by National Institutes of Health, in The Health of Lesbian, Gay, Bisexual, and Transgender People: Building a Foundation for Better Understanding*. Washington, DC, National Academies Press (US), National Academy of Sciences, 2011.
67. Oster AM, Johnson CH, Le BC, et al.: Trends in HIV prevalence and HIV testing among young MSM: five United States cities, 1994–2011. *AIDS Behav* 18(Suppl 3):S237–S247, 2014.
68. Centers for Disease Control and Prevention (CDC): Trends in HIV/AIDS diagnoses among men who have sex with men—33 states, 2001–2006. *MMWR Morb Mortal Wkly Rep* 57(25):681–686, 2008.
69. Bontempo DE, D'Augelli AR: Effects of at-school victimization and sexual orientation on lesbian, gay, or bisexual youths' health risk behavior. *J Adolesc Health* 30(5):364–374, 2002.
70. Garofalo R, Wolf RC, Kessel S, Palfrey SJ, DuRant RH: The association between health risk behaviors and sexual orientation among a school-based sample of adolescents. *Pediatrics* 101(5):895–902, 1998.
71. Bailey JM, Pillard RC, Dawood K, et al.: A family history study of male sexual orientation using three independent samples. *Behav Genet* 29(2):79–86, 1999.
72. Birkett M, Espelage DL, Koenig B: LGB and questioning students in schools: the moderating effects of homophobic bullying and school climate on negative outcomes. *J Youth Adolesc* 38(7):989–1000, 2009.

73. Birkett M, Newcomb ME, Mustanski B: Does it get better? A longitudinal analysis of psychological distress and victimization in lesbian, gay, bisexual, transgender, and questioning youth. *J Adolesc Health* 56(3):280–285, 2015.
74. Rosario M, Corliss HL, Everett BG, Russell ST, Buchting FO, Birkett MA: Mediation by peer violence victimization of sexual orientation disparities in cancer-related tobacco, alcohol, and sexual risk behaviors: pooled youth risk behavior surveys. *Am J Public Health* 104(6):1113–1123, 2014.
75. Russell ST, Ryan C, Toomey RB, Diaz RM, Sanchez J: Lesbian, gay, bisexual, and transgender adolescent school victimization: implications for young adult health and adjustment. *J Sch Health* 81(5):223–230, 2011.
76. Ryan C, Huebner D, Diaz RM, Sanchez J: Family rejection as a predictor of negative health outcomes in white and Latino lesbian, gay, and bisexual young adults. *Pediatrics* 123(1):346–352, 2009.
77. Kruks G: Gay and lesbian homeless/street youth: special issues and concerns. *J Adolesc Health* 12(7):515–518, 1991.
78. Rosario M, Schrimshaw EW, Hunter J: Risk factors for homelessness among lesbian, gay, and bisexual youths: a developmental milestone approach. *Child Youth Serv Rev* 34(1):186–193, 2012.
79. Remafedi G: *Death by Denial: Studies of Suicide in Gay and Lesbian Teenagers*. 1st ed. Boston, MA, Alyson Publications, 1994.
80. Zou C, Andersen JP: Comparing the rates of early childhood victimization across sexual orientations: heterosexual, lesbian, gay, bisexual, and mostly heterosexual. *PLoS One* 10(10):e0139198, 2015.
81. Roberts AL, Rosario M, Corliss HL, Koenen KC, Austin SB: Childhood gender nonconformity: a risk indicator for childhood abuse and posttraumatic stress in youth. *Pediatrics* 129(3):410–417, 2012.
82. Roberts AL, Rosario M, Slopen N, Calzo JP, Austin SB: Childhood gender nonconformity, bullying victimization, and depressive symptoms across adolescence and early adulthood: an 11-year longitudinal study. *J Am Acad Child Adolesc Psychiatry* 52(2):143–152, 2013.
83. Friedman RC, Downey JI: Homosexuality. *N Engl J Med* 331(14):923–930, 1994.
84. Flowers P, Buston K: "I was terrified of being different": exploring gay men's accounts of growing-up in a heterosexist society. *J Adolesc* 24(1):51–65, 2001.
85. Erikson EH: *Childhood and Society*. New York, Norton, 1993.
86. Newcomb ME, Mustanski B: Internalized homophobia and internalizing mental health problems: a meta-analytic review. *Clin Psychol Rev* 30(8):1019–1029, 2010.
87. Meyer IH: Prejudice, social stress, and mental health in lesbian, gay, and bisexual populations: conceptual issues and research evidence. *Psychol Bull* 129(5):674–697, 2003.
88. Savin-Williams RC: Verbal and physical abuse as stressors in the lives of lesbian, gay male, and bisexual youths: associations with school problems, running away, substance abuse, prostitution, and suicide. *J Consult Clin Psychol* 62(2):261–269, 1994.
89. Anderson A: Strengths of gay male youth: an untold story. *Child Adolesc Soc Work J* 15(1):55–71, 1998.
90. Remafedi G, Farrow JA, Deisher RW: Risk factors for attempted suicide in gay and bisexual youth. *Pediatrics* 87(6):869–875, 1991.
91. Substance Abuse and Mental Health Services Administration: *A Practitioner's Resource Guide: Helping Families to Support Their LGBT Children*. Rockville, MD, Substance Abuse and Mental Health Services Administration, 2014.
92. Lewis RJ, Derlega VJ, Clarke EG, Kuang JC: Stigma consciousness, social constraints, and lesbian well-being. *J Counsel Psychol* 53(1): 48–56, 2006.
93. Lasser J, Tharinger D: Visibility management in school and beyond: a qualitative study of gay, lesbian, bisexual youth. *J Adolesc* 26(2):233–244, 2003.
94. Goffman E: *Stigma; Notes on the Management of Spoiled Identity*. p. 147, 1963.
95. Bos H, van Beusekom G, Sandfort T: Sexual attraction and psychological adjustment in Dutch adolescents: coping style as a mediator. *Arch Sex Behav* 43(8):1579–1588, 2014.
96. Ryan C, Russell ST, Huebner D, Diaz R, Sanchez J: Family acceptance in adolescence and the health of LGBT young adults. *J Child Adolesc Psychiatr Nurs* 23(4): 205–213, 2010.
97. Cohler BJ, Galatzer-Levy RM: *The Course of Gay and Lesbian Lives: Social and Psychoanalytic Perspectives. 1st ed. Worlds of Desire: The Chicago Series on Sexuality, Gender, and Culture*. Chicago, IL, University of Chicago Press, 2000.
98. Patterson CJ: Sexual orientation and human development: an overview. *Dev Psychol* 31(1):3–11, 1995.
99. Hines M: Prenatal endocrine influences on sexual orientation and on sexually differentiated childhood behavior. *Front Neuroendocrinol* 32(2):170–182, 2011.
100. Hines M: Gender development and the human brain. *Ann Rev Neurosci* 34(1):69–88, 2011.
101. Burri A, Spector T, Rahman Q: Common genetic factors among sexual orientation, gender nonconformity, and number of sex partners in female twins: implications for the evolution of homosexuality. *J Sex Med* 12(4):1004–1111, 2015.
102. Ngun TC, Vilain E: The biological basis of human sexual orientation: is there a role for epigenetics? In Daisuke Y (ed): *Advances in Genetics*. Academic Press, pp. 167–184, 2014.
103. Yamamoto D: The neural and genetic substrates of sexual behavior in Drosophila. *Adv Genet* 59: 39–66, 2007.
104. Demir E, Dickson BJ: Fruitless splicing specifies male courtship behavior in Drosophila. *Cell* 121(5):785–794, 2005.
105. Garcia-Falgueras A, Swaab DF: A sex difference in the hypothalamic uncinate nucleus: relationship to gender identity. *Brain* 131(Pt 12):3132–3146, 2008.
106. Byne W, Tobet S, Mattiace LA, et al.: The interstitial nuclei of the human anterior hypothalamus: an investigation of variation with sex, sexual orientation, and HIV status. *Horm Behav* 40(2):86–92, 2001.
107. Adelson SL: Practice parameter on gay, lesbian, or bisexual sexual orientation, gender nonconformity, and gender discordance in children and adolescents. *J Am Acad Child Adolesc Psychiatry* 51(9):957–974, 2012.
108. Hanley-Hackenbruck P: 'Coming out' and psychotherapy. *Psychiatric Ann* 18(1):29–32, 1988.
109. Israel T, Gorcheva R, Burnes TR, Walther WA: Helpful and unhelpful therapy experiences of LGBT clients. *Psychother Res* 18(3):294–305, 2008.
110. Margolies L, Becker M, Jackson-Brewer K: In: Collectives (ed): *Internalized homophobia: identifying and treating the oppressor within., in Lesbian Psychologies: explorations and challenges*. Chicago, IL, University of Illinois Press, pp. 229–242, 1987.
111. Bok S: *Secrets: on the Ethics of Secrets and Revelation*. New York, Vintage, 1983.
112. Fields J: Normal queers: straight parents respond to their children's "coming out". *Symb Interact* 24(2):165–187.
113. Savin-Williams RC, Ream GL: Sex variations in the disclosure to parents of same-sex attractions. *J Fam Psychol* 17(3):429–438, 2003.
114. Weinberg MS, Williams CJ, Pryor DW: *Dual Attraction: Understanding Bisexuality*. New York, Oxford University Press, 1994.
115. Grafsky EL: Becoming the Parent of a GLB Son or Daughter. *J GLBT Fam Stud* 10(1–2):36–57, 2014.
116. APA: *Report of the Task Force on Appropriate Therapeutic Respones to Sexual Orientation*. Washington, DC, 2009.
117. Substance Abuse and Mental Health Services Administration: *Ending Conversion Therapy: Supporting and Affirming LGBTQ Youth.*, HHS, Editor. Rockville, MD, Substance Abuse and Mental Health Services Administration, 2015.
118. Obergefell v. Hodges. Oyez 2015 [cited 2015 22 December]. Available at: https://www.oyez.org/cases/2014/14-556.

CHAPTER 2.3 ■ DEVELOPMENTAL PSYCHOPATHOLOGY

SUNIYA S. LUTHAR

DEVELOPMENTAL PSYCHOPATHOLOGY DEFINED: MAJOR FEATURES

Developmental psychopathology is an integrative discipline, wherein principles from classical developmental theory are applied to investigate clinical and psychiatric phenomena (1–4). This integration of perspectives is invaluable because it promotes our understanding of atypical development and also illuminates understanding of normative developmental processes. To illustrate, applications of developmental theories such as those of Werner, Piaget, and Erikson provide critical insights into the organization and causes of different forms of maladjustment. Conversely, studies of pathology enhance our knowledge of normal development, particularly in terms of individual differences in development as well as risk and protective processes associated with different types of outcomes.

Whereas developmental and clinical psychology are integral elements in the field of developmental psychopathology, the scope of this integrative discipline extends beyond these areas. Theory and methods from these domains are integrated with those from various others, including epidemiology, biology, neuroscience, sociology, and anthropology. Such multidomain, multicontextual approaches to inquiry are essential in moving toward the long-term goal of a more comprehensive understanding of the development of psychopathology.

A final feature of developmental psychopathology is that it bridges the often wide span between empirical research and the application of knowledge, to benefit at-risk populations. Investigators in this tradition design and implement interventions that are based on developmental theory and research on risk and protective processes, such that they inform both preventive interventions and social policy.

To summarize, the four central characteristics that define the field of developmental psychopathology are (1) the use of classical developmental theory and research to inform issues of psychopathology, (2) the use of insights from at-risk or atypical populations to increase our understanding of normal developmental processes, (3) integration of developmental and clinical perspectives with those from other disciplines, and (4) the derivation of implications for preventive and therapeutic interventions, and for social policy.

RISK

In developmental psychopathology research, risk is defined in terms of statistical probabilities: A high-risk condition is one that carries high odds for measured maladjustment in critical domains (5). Exposure to community violence, for example, constitutes high risk given that children experiencing it reflect significantly greater maladjustment than those who do not (6). Similarly, maternal depression is a risk factor in that children of mothers with depressive diagnoses can be as much as eight times as likely as others to develop depressive disorders themselves by the adolescent years (7).

In addition to establishing discrete risk dimensions such as community violence, poverty, or parent mental illness, researchers have also examined composites of multiple risk indices such as parents' low income and education, their histories of mental illness, and disorganization in their neighborhoods. Seminal research by Rutter (8) demonstrated that when risks such as these coexist (as they often do, in the real world), effects tend to be synergistic, with children's outcomes being far poorer than when any of these risks existed in isolation. Use of this cumulative risk approach is well exemplified in work by Sameroff et al. (9,10). These authors computed a total risk score across 10 different dimensions, assigning for each one, a score of 1 (versus 0) if the child fell in the highest quartile of continuous risk dimensions, and for dichotomous dimensions such as single parent family status, if they were present in that child's life. An alternative approach, exemplified in work by Masten et al. (11), involves standardizing values on different risk scales and adding them to obtain a composite.

Decisions regarding the use of single- or multiple-risk indices in resilience research depend on the substantive research questions. The former is used, obviously, when applied researchers seek to identify factors that might modify the effects of particular environmental risks known to have strong adverse effects, so as to eventually derive specific directions for interventions. Examples are parental divorce or bereavement; knowledge of what ameliorates the ill effects of these particular adversities has been valuable in designing appropriate interventions (12,13). Additive approaches are more constrained in this respect, precluding identification, for example, of which of the indices subsumed in the composite are more influential than others. On the other hand, composite risk indices generally explain more variance in adjustment than do any of them considered alone, and as noted earlier, they may be more realistic in that many of these risks do co-occur in actuality (5,14).

Risk is rarely absolute; the potential for deleterious outcomes varies according to age as well as other child characteristics. Prolonged separation from the primary caregiver, for example, is more harmful for infants and toddlers than for older children, whereas community violence is less likely to affect preschoolers than older youth who are more able to move about the neighborhood independently. By the same token, there are some risks relatively unique to particular groups. An example is racial discrimination, which affects ethnic minority groups but not children of Caucasian heritage.

The same construct can connote risk in one setting but be relatively benign or even beneficial in others. An example is stringency of parent discipline. Whereas high levels of control and strictness are often seen as deleterious for children, a series of studies have shown that they are actually beneficial for youngsters living in dangerous inner-city neighborhoods (15–18).

DISORDER

In developmental psychopathology as in child psychiatry, the notion of disorder often represents psychiatric diagnoses. Researchers typically assess diagnoses via structured interviews such as the Schedule for Affective Disorders and Schizophrenia for School-Aged Children (K-SADS-PL) (19) or the Diagnostic Interview Schedule for Children (NIMH DISC-IV) (20), which are usually administered to the child aged 5 and older as well as the primary caregiver. For each diagnostic category, these interviews have a series of initial probes to determine the existence of a disorder, and if responses are in the affirmative, then additional probes are asked to determine if diagnostic criteria are met.

The other approach, also commonly used, is to assess overall children's symptom levels on different maladjustment domains, via instruments such as the Behavior Assessment System for Children (BASC), (21) or the Child Behavior Checklist (CBCL) (22) (and its variants, the Teacher Rating Form [TRF] and the Youth Self Report [YSR] (23)). These measures include a list of symptoms from diverse maladjustment domains which collectively yield scores on discrete subscales (such as attention, conduct, or depressive problems); in turn, composite scores across related subscales indicate overall maladjustment, such as internalizing and externalizing symptoms (CBCL), or overall dimensions of behavior and personality (BASC).

Such dimensional measures have two major advantages; they capture a wide range of functioning and are very well normed. With regard to the first of these features, symptom scales such as the CBCL and BASC characterize children in terms of varying severity of dysfunction as opposed to simply the presence or absence of diagnoses. From a research standpoint, this is a major advantage because the greater the variance on a particular dimension, the more likely it is that it will show statistical links with other constructs (such as potential causes or ramifications of the symptoms). The issue of norms, similarly, is critical in gauging children's adjustment levels relative to those of the average child of the same age. Instruments such as the CBCL have been administered to thousands of children from all over the country (and world) and as a result, we know the average symptom levels on these. Typically, average levels of problems correspond to a T score of 50 with a standard deviation of 10. Thus, if a child were to obtain a score of over 65 on the YSR, this would represent "much above average" dysfunction and a T score of 70 or more would indicate problems "very much above average."

Making such judgments about functioning vis-à-vis the average child is much more complicated with psychiatric disorders. There have been several large-scale epidemiologic studies on children's diagnoses, but there is some disagreement on rates of different disorders, with variations, for example, with the particular structured interview used. To illustrate, an NIMH study using the DISC reported that about 6% of adolescents suffer from depression (24), whereas a study using the K-SADS found the point prevalence to be 2.9% (25). At the same time, structured interviews remain the method of choice when the goal is specifically to assess the incidence of actual psychiatric diagnoses, rather than severity of symptoms.

A thorny problem in assessing childhood disorders—regardless of whether the approach involves diagnoses or symptom levels—is that there is considerable disagreement among respondents. The kappa statistic is commonly used to assess agreement across raters, with values above 0.75 representing high levels of agreement, values in the range from 0.40 to 0.75 representing moderate levels of agreement, and values below 0.40 representing low levels of agreement (26). In studies involving psychiatric diagnoses, agreement rates between parents and children have ranged from $k = 0.32$ for diagnoses of separation anxiety to $k = 0.22$ on diagnoses of general anxiety disorder to as low as $k = 0.17$ on ADHD (27, 28). Further demonstrating the disconnect between the child's and parents' understanding of the child's functioning, Roberts et al. (29) found that in measuring overall mental health, life satisfaction, happiness, and role strain, parent–child agreement was never above 0.20. On dimensional measures, similarly, the correlation between parents' reports and children's reports has ranged from $k = 0.02$ for anxious/depressed symptoms to $k = 0.14$ for delinquent behavior (30); there is generally more agreement among mother and father, but again, low consensus between parents and teachers (31).

Researchers have dealt with this disagreement in various ways. In the case of psychiatric diagnoses, a common approach is to use the "either/or" rule, assuming the child does in fact have a diagnosis if either the parent or the child indicates this is the case (32). An alternative strategy is by prioritizing adults' reports for some domains (conduct problems) and children's reports for others (depression), with the rationale that children are likely to underreport their own oppositional behavior, for example, or that parents are likely to know less about their child's inner life (33,34). Still others have separately considered parents' and children's reports, with the rationale that each reveals information not captured by the other (35–37).

A final comment about measurement of disorder: What is considered abnormal in one setting may be normative or even adaptive in another. This point is well illustrated in a paper by Richters and Cicchetti (38) entitled "Mark Twain meets DSM-III-R: Conduct disorder, development, and the concept of harmful dysfunction, with regard to definitions of conduct disorders." The authors argue that many inner-city youth might meet DSM criteria for conduct disorders but in their own subculture, being able to defend themselves physically can be quite adaptive. Accordingly, they exhort additional consideration of the notion of "harmful dysfunction," put forth by Wakefield (39–41). Wakefield argued that the DSM definition of mental disorders fails to distinguish adequately an individual's negative reactions to his problematic environment from a "true" mental disorder, and that a mental disorder is best conceptualized as a harmful dysfunction, where harm is a value judgment regarding the undesirability of a condition, and dysfunction is the failure of a system to function as designed by natural selection. Anchored in notions of evolutionary design, Wakefield specifically defines a harmful dysfunction as the "harmful failure of an internal mechanism to perform a natural function for which it was biologically designed" (42).[1]

RESILIENCE

A salient construct in developmental psychopathology is resilience: a phenomenon or process reflecting relatively positive adaptation despite experiences of significant adversity or trauma. Inherent in this definition lie two fundamental conditions: significant risk (or adversity) and positive adaptation. Thus, resilience is never directly measured, but is

[1]Subsequently, this notion has been criticized by some others. Lilienfield and Marino (1995), for example, argue that many mental disorders are not, as Wakefield claims, evolutionary adaptations but rather neutral byproducts of adaptation; they believe that Wakefield's sociobiological definition of disorder is too narrow in its conceptualization. Murphy and Woolfolk (2000) critique Wakefield's view from a different angle, arguing that it fails to account for those disorders that are not a result of malfunction and those disorders whose causes have no adaptive function.

indirectly inferred based on the evidence of the two subsumed constructs.

The notion of risk has already been discussed; positive adaptation, the second element in the construct of resilience, is defined as an outcome that is substantially better than what would be expected with respect to the risk circumstance being studied. In past studies of resilience across diverse risk circumstances, positive adaptation has been defined in terms of behaviorally manifested social competence, or success at meeting stage-salient developmental tasks (5,14,43). Among young children, for example, competence was operationally defined in terms of the development of a secure attachment with primary caregivers (44), and among older children, in terms of aspects of school-based functioning such as good academic performance and positive relationships with classmates and teachers (43,45).

In addition to being developmentally appropriate, indicators used to define positive adaptation must also be conceptually of high relevance to the risk examined in terms of both domains assessed and stringency of criteria used (46). When communities carry many risks for antisocial problems, for example, the degree to which children are able to maintain socially conforming behaviors is an appropriate indicator of success (47), whereas among children of depressed parents, the absence of depressive diagnoses would be of special significance (48,49). With regard to stringency of criteria, similarly, decisions must depend on the seriousness of the risks under consideration. In studying children facing major traumas, it is entirely appropriate to define risk-evasion simply in terms of the absence of serious psychopathology (psychiatric diagnoses) rather than superiority or excellence in everyday adaptation (50).

Regardless of whether competence is described as risk evasion or positive adaptation, competence must be defined across multiple spheres. The multilevel measurement of competence, therefore, differs from the measurement of risk, which may legitimately involve one or multiple negative circumstances. Doing well in only one domain cannot be conceptualized as connoting resilience, as overly narrow definitions can fallaciously convey a picture of "success in the face of adversity." Adolescents, for example, might be viewed very positively by their peers but at the same time, perform poorly academically, or even demonstrate conduct disturbances (51,52), such that peer popularity by itself cannot be seen as an indicator of overall risk evasion.

The major focus of resilience researchers is to identify vulnerability and protective factors that might modify the negative effects of adverse life circumstances, and having accomplished this, to identify mechanisms or processes that might underlie associations found (5,53–55). While researchers have debated how to delineate such factors statistically (14,56), the conceptual definitions are fairly straightforward. Vulnerability factors or markers encompass those indices that exacerbate the negative effects of the risk condition while protective factors modify the effects of risk in a positive direction.

In some instances, it is more appropriate to define positive adaptation in terms of the family or community rather than necessarily of the child him or herself. As Seifer (57) has argued, because infants' and toddlers' functioning is often regulated by their caregivers, it can be more logical to operationalize positive adjustment in terms of the mother–child dyad or family unit rather than in terms of the young child's behavior. Similarly, there are times when the label resilience is most appropriate for communities of well-functioning at-risk youth. Research on neighborhoods, for example, has demonstrated that some low-income urban neighborhoods reflect far higher levels of cohesiveness, organization, and social efficacy than others (58,59), with the potential, therefore, to serve as important buffers against negative socializing influences.

FACTORS AFFECTING RESILIENCE AND VULNERABILITY

In discussions that follow, we overview major factors that contribute to relatively positive or negative outcomes among at-risk children. These factors fall into three broad categories: aspects of families, features of communities, and attributes of the children themselves.

Familial Factors in Resilience and Vulnerability

The critical importance of strong family relationships has been emphasized in various studies of resilience; a plethora of studies identify supportive and responsive parenting as being among the most robust predictors of resilient adaptation (5,8,54,56,60–64). In particular, early family relationships are extremely important in shaping long-term resilient trajectories. In their comprehensive review of the early childhood literature, Shonkoff and Phillips (65) emphasized that "[relationships] that are created in the earliest years...constitute a basic structure within which all meaningful development unfolds." Early experience places people on probabilistic trajectories of relatively good or poor adaptation, shaping the lens through which subsequent relationships are viewed and the capacity to utilize support resources in the environment. Thus, if early attachments are insecure in nature, at-risk children tend to anticipate negative reactions from others and can eventually come to elicit these; these experiences of rejection further increase feelings of insecurity (66–68). Conversely, at-risk children with at least one good relationship are able to take more from nurturing others subsequently encountered in development (44,65,67,69). The protective potential of strong family relationship has been demonstrated for mothers, fathers, and siblings (70,71).

Whereas early relationships are fundamental in shaping the lens through which people view their subsequent interactions, a "faulty lens" can be corrected to some degree. In general, developmental psychopathologists maintain that there is continuity and coherence in development so that positive adaptation in early years determines, in a probabilistic rather than determinative fashion, the likely success at later stages (44,72,73). At the same time, scholars recognize that lawful discontinuities often do occur, and in the context of attachment status, such changes frequently derive from modifications in the caregiving environment (73–76). Intervention studies provide consistent evidence with regard to the possibility of shifting attachment status, as seen in work by Heinicke and Dozier. In both sets of studies, children's insecure early attachments were remediated to some degree by intervention services that fostered caregivers' positive qualities including nurturance, responsiveness, and their own attachment states of mind (77–79).

In terms of what defines "good parenting," warmth and appropriate control are the two core constructs that are most important in children's relationships with their primary caregivers. Each factor has protective functions and the benefits of each depend to some degree on levels of the other: Both high warmth with lax discipline and strict discipline without affection can be linked with poor adjustment. The authoritative parenting style, characterized by the appropriate balance of parental warmth and control (80), is generally optimal; authoritative parents are defined as those who "...are warm, supportive, communicative, and responsive to their children's needs, and who exert firm, consistent, and reasonable control and close supervision" (81).

In addition to warmth and control, limit-setting and monitoring are critical for resilient adaptation. Limit-setting refers to the use of appropriate rules and expectations in shaping socially desirable behavior in the child; the degree to which parents clearly define limits and consistently enforce rules is crucial in shaping the child's future compliance (82,83). Related to limit-setting and also important for resilient adaptation is the construct of parental monitoring, which is defined as a "set of correlated parenting behaviors involving attention to and tracking of the child's whereabouts, activities, and adaptations" (84). The salutary effects of consistent parental monitoring across various high-risk circumstances have been demonstrated from the elementary school years onward (85). The benefits of consistent parental monitoring are particularly pronounced among preadolescents and adolescents, who have increasing independence from parents and thus growing exposure to a host of risks in the peer and community environments. For example, a study of sixth graders with deviant peers showed that firm parental control inhibited the development of externalizing problems in later years (86–88).

Links between parent monitoring and adolescent adjustment are not always simple linear ones, but can depend on coexisting risks in the environment. To illustrate, Mason et al. (89) showed that in terms of ramifications for children's problem behaviors, optimal levels of control exerted by African-American parents varied according to negative influences in the community. When adolescents reported relatively high problem behaviors in their peer groups, for example, optimal levels of parental control tended to be higher than when children's peer problem behaviors were low. Regardless of circumstance, however, parental monitoring has emerged as a powerful construct in resilience research; in fact, among low-income 8 to 17 year olds, Buckner et al. (85) found that of several variables external to the child, only parental monitoring significantly differentiated resilient from nonresilient youths.

A relatively new construct related to limit-setting is parental "containment." Cavell (82) has emphasized the importance of an appropriate balance of warmth and discipline within the notion of parental containment, which is "any behavior that fosters in children a sense of restraint while not threatening their relationship security" (82). Recent studies have pointed to the protective potential of this construct. Building upon Cavell's (82) arguments on the significance of children's beliefs about the likelihood of being disciplined, Schneider et al. (83) defined perceived containment as the child's beliefs concerning the parent's capacity to enforce firm limits, and the likelihood that the parent will prevail in conflict. They found that children with a particularly strong sense of containment had mothers who applied effective discipline within the context of an emotionally positive relationship. Furthermore, high perceived containment was protective against externalizing behaviors as rated by parents and teachers (83).

The Importance of Genetic Factors

An interesting set of developments in the field of resilience is inquiry into the role of genetic contributions to vulnerability and protective mechanisms in the family, as is seen in research by Caspi et al. Two studies by this group identified specific genes implicated in protecting some maltreated children from developing psychopathology in adulthood. The first of these showed reduced likelihood of antisocial behavior in the presence of a genotype that confers high levels of the monoamine oxidase A enzyme (90), while the second study demonstrated that the likelihood of developing depression was lower in the presence of a genotype conferring the efficient transport of serotonin (91). Although the specific processes underlying the protective effects of such genetic factors are unknown, it is possible that they operate by shaping aspects of children's social–cognitive reactions to life stressors, as in their propensity to attributional biases, for example, or capacities for emotion recognition (92).

Further explicating the relationship between genetic factors and positive adaptation, a study by Kim-Cohen et al. (92) examined both genetic and environmental processes specifically within the resilience framework. The study involved an epidemiologic cohort of 1,116 twin pairs from low SES families. Two aspects of resilience were examined—behavioral and cognitive—and results of quantitative genetic models showed that additive genetic effects accounted for approximately 70% of the variation in children's behavioral resilience and 40% of the variation in cognitive resilience. Further analyses established protective effects of both maternal warmth and child's outgoing temperament, with each factor operating through both genetically and environmentally mediated effects.

A particularly critical conclusion drawn by these researchers, however, surrounds the implications for interventions: Heritability does not imply untreatability (93,94). As Kim-Cohen et al. (92) note, their study entailed "a genetically sensitive design (which demonstrated) that environmental effects can make a positive difference in the lives of poor children...Even child temperament promoted resilience through environmental processes." Of vital importance is their conclusion that if families confronting the myriad stresses of poverty are helped to move toward bestowing warm, supportive parenting, and providing stimulating learning materials, children can be helped to achieve greater behavioral and cognitive resilience.

Rutter (54,55) has outlined several important directions for future work involving gene–environment influences in resilience. Twin and adoptee studies of at-risk children can be used to (1) examine the relative contributions of genetic versus environmental influences in the ways that different protective and vulnerability factors operate; (2) uncover the mechanisms entailed in each of these (passive or active G–E mechanisms and critical influences underlying the environmental component); and (3) identify genetic markers that confer protection or vulnerability and better understand processes underlying their effects. Also needed are sibling studies illuminating the relative contributions of shared versus nonshared, extrafamilial environments on different outcomes. Finally, genetics research can also contribute to new developments in the study of resilience through precise quantification of risk. As noted in the first section of this chapter, risk is generally inferred based on statistical links between aspects of the environment (maltreatment or poverty) and children's maladjustment, but this "measure" of risk is imprecise at best. With knowledge that some children have genes conferring liability to particular disorders, examining factors in the lives of those who do not succumb could contribute vastly to our understanding of processes in resilience.

Community Factors in Resilience and Vulnerability

In the community domain, a primary conclusion from extant resilience research is that ongoing exposure to community violence is highly inimical not only for children but also their parents and other adults (56). Among those who fear for their very lives, it is unrealistic to expect psychological robustness: When physical survival is threatened, all developmental tasks and processes are jeopardized. In the case of such risks, therefore, there must be priority on eradicating these experiences in whatever ways possible.

In addition to family-level protective markers, community-level factors can mitigate the effects that risks have on a child's development. Mentors and informal support networks can serve critical protective functions. Evidence in this regard is seen in the Big Brothers Big Sisters of America (BBBSA) movement, where volunteers interact regularly one on one with youth from single-parent homes, and supervision is provided on a monthly basis for the first year, then subsequently on a quarterly basis. Compared to their nonparticipating peers, BBBSA youth reported more positive academic behaviors, had better relationships with their parents and peers, and were 46% less likely to initiate illegal drug use, 27% less likely to initiate alcohol use, and 52% less likely to skip school (95). Other studies have demonstrated that salutatory experiences can derive from religious affiliations (96–98) and other forms of social support (99,100), demonstrating the powerful potential that community-level factors can have in promoting resilience in adolescents.

Additionally, there are several studies corroborating the protective functions of supportive relationships with teachers (101–103). Assessing more than 3,000 teacher–child relationships, Howes and Ritchie (104) found that in a sample of toddlers and preschoolers with difficult life circumstances, the quality of attachment with teachers was significantly related to measures of behavior problems as well as social competence with peers. Among a group of aggressive second and third graders, African-American and Hispanic students benefited more than did Caucasian students from supportive relationship with their teachers (105). Noting that minority group students typically have lower access to positive relationships with school teachers, the authors suggested that they could be more responsive than Caucasians to supportive teachers when they are encountered (106). Finally, there are substantial benefits when classrooms reflect organized, predictable environments in which students participate in procedures governing their behaviors. Among African-American 7 to 15 year olds from low-income, mother-headed households, Brody et al. (87) demonstrated protective-stabilizing effects among children in such classrooms. Furthermore, positive classrooms were beneficial even when parent–child relationships were compromised as well as vice versa, indicating unique, significant contributions from both contexts in which children and adolescents spend appreciable amounts of time (87,107).

Individual Factors in Resilience and Vulnerability

Salient protective and vulnerability processes affecting at-risk children can occur not only at the familial and community level, but at the child level. For example, male gender can be a vulnerability marker among youth living in the ecology of urban poverty, as boys are typically more reactive than girls to negative community influences (108,109). In addition, lower levels of intelligence can act as a vulnerability factor in that among children experiencing severe and chronic life adversities, those with low intelligence are more vulnerable to adjustment difficulties over time than are others (5). Similarly, some personal attributes are linked with relatively positive outcomes among children facing adversities, such as internal locus of control (beliefs that events in one's life are largely determined by one's own efforts rather than by luck or chance) or feelings of self-efficacy (5,110–112). Studies have also suggested the protective potential of emotional intelligence, the ability to perceive and express emotions, to understand and use them, and to manage them to foster personal growth (113,114). Among adolescents, emotional intelligence is linked with relatively low likelihood of smoking cigarettes and drinking alcohol (115) and following the major life transition to beginning college, with greater likelihood of attaining high academic grades (116).

A critical caveat regarding "protective individual attributes" such as internal locus of control or intelligence is that they themselves are not fixed or immutable, but are highly influenced by the external environment. To consider intelligence as an example, Koenen et al. (117) have shown that even after controlling for genetic factors and externalizing and internalizing problems, exposure to domestic violence accounted for significant variation in children's IQs. Therefore, individual factors in resilience and vulnerability must be considered in relation to the environments in which they originate and operate.

Acknowledging the continued malleability of individual traits (especially among younger children), Luthar and Zelazo (56) argued that in considering the triad of protective and vulnerability factors in resilience, children's own attributes should be considered after aspects of their families and communities for three major reasons. From a basic research perspective, numerous studies have shown that many positive child attributes are themselves often dependent on processes in the proximal and distal environments. From an applied perspective, it is logical that interventions to foster resilience should focus less on what young children are able to do for themselves, and more on what adults must do to bolster the children's own efforts. From a policy perspective, finally, to place primary emphasis on child attributes could carry the risk that public debate will shift away from the major environmental risks that affect children, leading to decreased allocation of resources to ameliorate these risks (14,56).

Biologic Factors

The previous examples—like most of resilience research thus far—generally encompass psychological variables; also useful in scientific studies has been consideration of biologic indices, again, both as mediators of risk itself and as processes underlying vulnerability and protective factors (118,119). In terms of protective processes, the capacity to regulate or modulate negative emotions in the face of threats is of obvious importance for managing well in inauspicious situations (85,120,121) and here again, biologic processes can be salient. First, the capacity to recover relatively quickly from negative events experienced may be gauged by studying the startle reflex, which is a biologic and involuntary response (a fast twitch of facial and body muscles) to a sudden and intense visual, tactile, or acoustic stimulus (122). Studies have shown that adverse environmental influences not only affect the startle reflex, but the neural network that underlies this response (123). A second biologic mechanism that might be implicated is neuroendocrine in nature. Chronic exposure to stressful experiences tends to lead to excessive activation of the hypothalamic–pituitary–adrenal (HPA) axis, causing hypercortisolism, or elevations in the stress hormone cortisol. Hypercortisolism can result in pathogenic effects on neurons (124,125) and changes in the synthesis and reuptake of neurotransmitters and density of sensitivity of receptors (126,127). These findings point to the possibility that resilient individuals can be described in a neuroendocrine manner as those who, in the face of various stressors, tend to return relatively quickly to baseline levels of neuroendocrine functioning, and thus avoid the damage conferred by hypercortisolism.

SUMMARY OF EVIDENCE AND IMPLICATIONS FOR THE FUTURE

In concluding a review of almost half a century of work on resilience, Luthar summarized the major take-home message thus: "Resilience rests, fundamentally, on relationships. The desire to belong is a basic human need and positive connections with others lie at the very core of psychological development; strong, supportive relationships are critical for achieving and sustaining resilient adaptation" (128). The childhood years have emerged as especially significant, as a child's relationship with his or her primary caregiver forms a lens through which future interactions are interpreted. As a result, early attachments influence numerous nascent psychological attributes and the negotiation and resolution of major developmental tasks, and in turn, the likelihood of success at future tasks. Thus, serious disruptions in the early relationships with caregivers, whether in the form of physical, sexual, or emotional abuse, severely impair the chances of resilient adaptation later in life. On a more positive note, secure and healthy relationships with those in one's proximal circle act as invaluable protective processes, for children as well as adults (129). Over the years, "good relationships" have been conceptualized in terms of two broad components—warmth and support on the one hand, and appropriate control or discipline on the other. A central direction for interventions, therefore, is to foster the development and sustenance of positive parenting patterns among parents in high-risk circumstances. Additionally, there must be attention to the specific relationship ingredients that are particularly influential or important within the context of particular types of risk; in neighborhoods rife with community violence, for instance, strategies to ensure physical safety are clearly of unique importance.

While resilience research has labeled various community-level risk factors, the community can also be an important source of support when the child's own parents are constrained in this regard. High-quality child care is particularly valuable for children in the most at-risk families, as strong, supportive relationships with teachers can be highly beneficial for school-age children and adolescents. There is great potential to use K–12 schools as venues to foster resilient adaptation. Thus far, several school-based interventions based on social control and social learning theories—involving teachers as well as parents—have shown some success in randomized trials. Attachment-based interventions, where the emphasis is on developing close, supportive bonds with the teacher, have been insufficiently examined in school settings, though the positive effects of such programs are potentially far reaching. In addition to school-based initiatives, support provided by informal mentors (as in Big Brothers, Big Sisters) can serve important protective functions, especially when the relationships are of relatively long duration. Involvement in religion, similarly, can confer benefits via the availability of a stable support network and the promotion of relatively positive coping strategies. At the neighborhood level, cohesion and shared supervision of children are important positive influences, as is high participation in local and voluntary organization. Children benefit from participation in structured extracurricular activities, but unstructured settings (as in youth recreation centers) can exacerbate risks.

In terms of children's personal attributes, research on biological processes that confer significant vulnerability can be very useful for psychopharmacological interventions. Just as the environment sets confidence limits within which biology determines functioning, biology sets limits within which the environment determines adaptation levels. If a chemical imbalance in the brain predisposes a child or adolescent to depression, the threshold of tolerance to environmental stressors becomes considerably lower so that even stressors of moderate severity could precipitate a debilitating depression; awareness of such biologic vulnerabilities, therefore, is important for gaining complete understandings of risk exposure and positive adaptation. Even as we strive to promote the quality of children's family and community environments, careful pharmacologic interventions targeting the biology involved in psychiatric disorders—particularly among youth at high genetic risk by virtue of parent mental illness—will be critical in maximizing resilient adaptation among children and adolescents at high risk.

ACKNOWLEDGMENT

Thanks to Rebecca P. Prince for her contributions to an earlier version of this chapter.

References

1. Cicchetti D: Fractures in the crystal: developmental psychopathology and the emergence of the self. *Dev Rev* 11:271–287, 1993.
2. Luthar SS, Burack JA, Cicchetti D, Weisz JR (eds): *Developmental psychopathology: Perspectives on Adjustment, Risk and Disorder.* Cambridge, Cambridge University Press, 1997.
3. Rutter M: The developmental psychopathology of depression: Issues and perspectives. In: Rutter M, Tizard C, Read P (eds): *Depression in young people: Developmental and Clinical Perspectives.* New York, Guilford, 3–30, 1986.
4. Sroufe LA, Rutter M: The domain of developmental psychopathology. *Child Dev* 55:1184–1199, 1984.
5. Masten A: *Ordinary Magic: Resilience Processes in Development.* New York, Guilford, 2014.
6. Margolin G, Gordis EB: The effects of family and community violence on children. *Ann Rev Psychol* 51:445–479, 2000.
7. Wickramaratne PJ, Weissman MM: Onset of psychopathology in offspring by developmental phase and parental depression. *J Am Acad Child Adolesc Psychiatry* 37:933–942, 1998.
8. Rutter M: Protective factors in children's responses to stress and disadvantage. In: Kent MW, Rolf JE (eds): *Primary Prevention in Psychopathology: Social Competence in Children.* Vol. 8. Hanover, NH, University Press of New England, 49–74, 1979.
9. Gutman LM, Sameroff AJ, Cole R: Academic growth curve trajectories from 1st grade to 12th grade: effects of multiple social risk factors and preschool child factors. *Dev Psychol* 39:777–790, 2003.
10. Sameroff AJ, Gutman L, Peck SC: Adaptation among youth facing multiple risks: prospective research findings. In: Luthar SS (ed): *Resilience and Vulnerability: Adaptation in the Context of Childhood Adversities.* New York, Cambridge, 364–391, 2003.
11. Masten AS, Morison P, Pellegrini D, et al.: Competence under stress: risk and protective factors. In: Rolf J, Masten A, Cicchetti D, Neuchterlein K, Weintraub S (eds): *Risk and Protective Factors in Development of Psychopathology.* New York, Cambridge, 236–256, 1990.
12. Martinez CR Jr, Forgatch MS: Preventing problems with boys' noncompliance: effects of a parent training intervention for divorcing mothers. *J Consult Clin Psychol* 69:416–428, 2001.
13. Sandler I, Wolchik S, Davis C, et al.: Correlational and experimental study of resilience for children of divorce and parentally bereaved children. In: Luthar SS (ed): *Resilience and Vulnerability: Adaptation in the Context of Childhood Adversities.* New York, Cambridge, 213–240, 2003.
14. Luthar SS, Cicchetti D, Becker B: The construct of resilience: a critical evaluation and guidelines for future work. *Child Dev* 71:543–562, 2000.
15. Ceballo R, McLoyd VC: Social support and parenting in poor, dangerous neighborhoods. *Child Dev* 73:1310–1321, 2002.
16. Dearing E: The developmental implications of restrictive and supportive parenting across neighborhoods and ethnicities: exceptions are the rule. *J Appl Dev Psychol* 25:555–575, 2004.
17. Gonzales NA, Cauce AM, Friedman RJ, et al.: Family, peer, and neighborhood influences on academic achievement among African American adolescents: one year prospective effects. *Am J Commun Psychol* 24:365–388, 1996.
18. Lansford JE, Deater-Deckard K, Dodge KA, et al.: Ethnic differences in the link between physical discipline and later adolescent externalizing behaviors. *J Child Psychol Psychiatry* 45:801–812, 2004.
19. Kaufman J, Birmaher B, Brent D, et al.: Schedule for affective disorders and schizophrenia for school-age children—present and lifetime version (K-SADS-PL): initial reliability and validity. *J Am Acad Child Adolesc Psychiatry* 36:980–988, 1997.
20. Shaffer D, Fisher PS, Lucas CP, et al.: NIMH Diagnostic Interview Schedule for Children Version IV (NIMH DISC-IV): Description, differences from previous versions, and reliability of some common diagnoses. *J Am Acad Child Adolesc Psychiatry* 39:28–38, 2000.
21. Reynolds CR, Kamphaus RW: *Behavior Assessment System for Children.* Circle Pines, American Guidance Services, 1992.
22. Achenbach TM: *Manual for the Child Behavior Checklist/4–18 and 1991 Profile.* Burlington, University of Vermont Department of Psychiatry, 1991.
23. Achenbach TM, Rescorla LA: *Manual for the ASEBA School-Age Forms & Profiles.* Burlington, VT, University of Vermont, Research Center for Children, Youth, & Families, 2001.
24. Shaffer D, Fisher P, Dulkan MK, et al.: The NIMH Diagnostic Interview Schedule for Children version 2.3 (DISC-2.3): Description, acceptability, prevalence rates and performance in the MECA study. *J Am Acad Child Adolesc Psychiatry* 35:865–877, 1996.

25. Lewinsohn PM, Hops H, Roberts RE, et al.: Adolescent psychopathology: I. prevalence and incidence of depression and other DSM-III-R disorders in high school students. *J Abnormal Psychol* 102:133–144, 1993.
26. Fleiss JL: *Statistical Methods for Rates and Proportions*, New York, John Wiley & Sons, 1981.
27. Grills AE, Ollendick TH: Multiple informant agreement and the anxiety disorders interview schedule for parents and children. *J Acad Child Adolesc Psychiatry* 42:30–40, 2003.
28. Williams RJ, McDermitt DR, Bertrand LD: Parental awareness of adolescent substance use. *Addict Behav* 28:803–809, 2003.
29. Roberts RE, Alegria M, Roberts CR, et al.: Concordance of reports of mental health functioning by adolescents and their caregivers: a comparison of European, African and Latino Americans. *J Nerv Ment Dis* 193:528–534, 2005.
30. Yeh M, Weisz JR: Why are we here at the clinic? Parent–child (dis)agreement on referral problems at outpatient treatment entry. *J Consult Clin Psychol* 69:1018–1025, 2001.
31. Grietens H, Van Assche V, Prinzie P, et al.: A comparison of mothers', fathers' and teachers' reports on problem behavior in 5-to-6-year-old children. *J Psychopathol Behav Assess* 26:137–146, 2004.
32. Angold A, Costello EJ: The Child and Adolescent Psychiatric Assessment (CAPA). *J Am Acad Child Adolesc Psychiatry* 39:39–48, 2000.
33. Loeber R, Green SM, Lahey BB: Mental health professionals' perception of the utility of children, mothers, and teachers as informants on childhood psychopathology. *J Clin Child Psychol* 19:136–143, 1990.
34. Loeber R, Green SM, Lahey BB, et al.: Differences and similarities between children, mothers, and teachers as informants on disruptive child behavior. *J Abnorm Child Psychol* 19:75–95, 1991.
35. Achenbach TM, McConaughy SH, Howell CT: Child/adolescent behavioral and emotional problems: implications of cross-informant correlations for situational specificity. *Psychol Bull* 101:213–232, 1987.
36. Grills AE, Ollendick TH: Issues in parent–child agreement: the case of structured diagnostic interviews. *Clin Child Fam Psychol Rev* 5:57–83, 2002.
37. Hawley KM, Weisz JR: Child, parent, and therapist (dis)agreement on target problems in outpatient therapy: the therapist's dilemma and its implications. *J Consult Clin Psychol* 71:62–70, 2003.
38. Richters JE, Cicchetti D: Mark Twain meets DSM-III-R: conduct disorders, development, and the concept of harmful dysfunction. *Dev Psychopathol* 5:5–29, 1993.
39. Wakefield JC: The concept of mental disorder: on the boundary between biological facts and social values. *Am Psychol* 47:373–388, 1992.
40. Wakefield JC: Disorder as harmful dysfunction: a conceptual critique of DSM-III-R's definition of mental disorder. *Psychol Rev* 99:232–247, 1992.
41. Wakefield JC: Limits of operationalization: a critique of Spitzer and Endicott's (1978) proposed operational criteria for mental disorder. *J Abnorm Psychol* 102:160–172, 1993.
42. Wakefield JC, Horwitz AV, Schmitz M: Social disadvantage is not mental disorder: response to Campbell-Sills and Stein. *Canadian J Psychiatry* 50:324–326, 2005.
43. Masten A, Coatsworth JD: The development of competence in favorable and unfavorable environments: lessons from research on successful children. *Am Psychol* 53:185–204, 1998.
44. Yates TM, Egeland B, Sroufe LA: Rethinking resilience: a developmental process perspective. In: Luthar SS (ed): *Resilience and Vulnerability: Adaptation in the Context of Childhood Adversities*. New York, Cambridge, 243–266, 2003.
45. Wyman PA, Cowen EL, Work WC, et al.: Caregiving and developmental factors differentiating young at-risk urban children showing resilient versus stress-affected outcomes: a replication and extension. *Child Dev* 70:645–659, 1999.
46. Luthar SS: Annotation: methodological and conceptual issues in the study of resilience. *J Child Psychol Psychiatry* 34:441–453, 1993.
47. Seidman E, Pedersen S: Holistic, contextual perspectives on risk, protection, and competence among low-income urban adolescents. In: Luthar SS (ed): *Resilience and Vulnerability: Adaptation in the Context of Childhood Adversities*. New York, Cambridge, 318–342, 2003.
48. Beardslee WR: *Out of the Darkened Room: When a Parent is Depressed—Protecting the Children and Strengthening the Family*. New York, Little, Brown and Company, 2002.
49. Hammen C: Risk and protective factors for children of depressed parents. In: Luthar SS (ed): *Resilience and Vulnerability: Adaptation in the Context of Childhood Adversities*. New York, Cambridge, 50–75, 2003.
50. Masten AS, Powell JL: A resilience framework for research, policy, and practice: contributions from project competence. In: Luthar SS (ed): *Resilience and Vulnerability: Adaptation in the Context of Childhood Adversities*. New York, Cambridge, 1–25, 2003.
51. Luthar SS, Burack JA: Adolescent wellness: in the eye of the beholder? In: Cicchetti D, Rappaport J, Sandler I, Weissberg R (eds): *The Promotion of Wellness in Children and Adolescents*. Washington, DC, Child Welfare League of America, 29–57, 2002.
52. O'Donnell DA, Schwab-Stone ME, Muyeed AZ: Multidimensional resilience in urban children exposed to community violence. *Child Dev* 73:1265–1282, 2003.
53. Luthar SS, Cicchetti D: The construct of resilience: implications for interventions and social policies. *Dev Psychopathol* 12:857–885, 2000.
54. Rutter M: Resilience reconsidered: Conceptual considerations, empirical findings, and policy implications. In: Shonkoff JP, Meisels SJ (eds): *Handbook of Early Childhood Intervention*. 2nd ed. New York, Cambridge, 651–682, 2000.
55. Rutter M: Genetic influences on risk and protection: implications for understanding resilience. In: Luthar SS (ed): *Resilience and Vulnerability: Adaptation in the Context of Childhood Adversities*. New York, Cambridge, 489–509, 2003.
56. Luthar SS, Zelazo LB: Research on resilience: an integrative review. In: Luthar SS (ed): *Resilience and Vulnerability: Adaptation in the Context of Childhood Adversities*. New York, Cambridge, 510–549, 2003.
57. Seifer S: Young children with mentally ill parents: resilient developmental systems. In: Luthar SS (ed): *Resilience and Vulnerability: Adaptation in the Context of Childhood Adversities*. New York, Cambridge, 29–49, 2003.
58. Leventhal T, Brooks-Gunn J: The neighborhoods they live in: the effects of neighborhood residence on child and adolescent outcomes. *Psychol Bull* 126:309–337, 2000.
59. Sampson RJ, Raudenbush SW, Earls F: Neighborhoods and violent crime: a multilevel study of collective efficacy. *Science* 277:918–924, 1997.
60. Anthony EJ, Koupernik C (eds): *The Child in his Family: Children at Psychiatric Risk—III*. New York, Wiley, 3–10, 1997.
61. Garmezy N: The study of competence in children at risk for severe psychopathology. In: Anthony EJ, Koupernik C (eds): *The child in his Family: Children at Psychiatric Risk—III*. New York, Wiley, 547, 1974.
62. Murphy LB, Moriarty A: *Vulnerability, Coping, and Growth: From Infancy to Adolescence*. New Haven, Yale University Press, 1976.
63. Werner EE: Protective factors and individual resilience. In: Meisells R, Shonkoff J (eds): *Handbook of Early Intervention*. Cambridge, Cambridge, 115–132, 2000.
64. Werner EE, Smith R: *Kauai's Children Come of Age*. Honolulu, University of Hawaii Press, 1977.
65. Shonkoff JP, Phillips DA (eds): *From Neurons to Neighborhoods: The Science of Early Childhood Development*. Washington, DC, National Academy Press, 2000.
66. Allen JP, Hauser ST, Borman-Spurrell E: Attachment theory as a framework for understanding sequelae of severe adolescent psychopathology: an 11-year follow-up study. *J Consult Clin Psychol* 64:254–263, 1996.
67. Sroufe LA: From infant attachment to promotion of adolescent autonomy: prospective, longitudinal data on the role of parents in development. In: Borkowski JG, Ramey SL (eds): *Parenting and the Child's World: Influences on Academic, Intellectual, and Social-Emotional Development—Monographs in Parenting*. Mahwah, Lawrence Erlbaum, 187–202, 2002.
68. Weinfield NS, Sroufe LA, Egeland B: Attachment from infancy to early adulthood in a high-risk sample: continuity, discontinuity, and their correlates. *Child Dev* 71:695–702, 2000.
69. Conger RD, Cui M, Bryant M, et al.: Competence in early adult romantic relationships: a developmental perspective on family influences. *J Pers Soc Psychol* 79:224–237, 2000.
70. Black MM, Dubowitz H, Starr RH Jr: African American fathers in low income, urban families: Development, behavior, and home environment of their three-year-old children. *Child Dev* 70:967–978, 1999.
71. Brody GH: Siblings' direct and indirect contributions to child development. *Curr Dir Psychol Sci* 13:124–126, 2004.
72. Carlson EA, Sroufe LA, Egeland B: The construction of experience: A longitudinal study of representation and behavior. *Child Dev* 75:66–83, 2004.
73. Sroufe LA, Carlson EA, Levy AK, et al.: Implications of attachment theory for developmental psychopathology. *Dev Psychopathol* 11:1–13, 1999.
74. Egeland B, Sroufe LA: Attachment and early maltreatment. *Child Dev* 52:44–52, 1981.
75. Thompson RA: The legacy of early attachments. *Child Dev* 71:145–152, 2000.
76. Waters E, Weinfield NS, Hamilton CE: The stability of attachment security from infancy to adolescence and early adulthood: general discussion. *Child Dev* 71:703–706, 2000.
77. Dozier M, Albus K, Fisher P, et al.: Interventions for foster parents: Implications for developmental theory. *Dev Psychopathol* 14:843–860, 2002.
78. Dozier M, Stovall KC, Albus KE, et al.: Attachment for infants in foster care: the role of caregiver state of mind. *Child Dev* 72:1467–1477, 2001.
79. Heinicke CM, Rineman NR, Ponce VA, et al.: Relation-based intervention with at-risk mothers: outcome in the second year of life. *Infant Ment Health J* 22:431–462, 2001.
80. Baumrind D: Rearing competent children. In: Danon W (ed): *Child Development Today and Tomorrow*. San Francisco, Jossey-Bass, 349–378, 1989.
81. Hetherington EM, Elmore AM: Risk and resilience in children coping with their parents' divorce and remarriage. In: Luthar SS (ed): *Resilience*

and Vulnerability: Adaptation in the Context of Childhood Adversities. New York, Cambridge, 182–212, 2003.
82. Cavell TA: *Working with Parents of Aggressive Children: A Practitioner's Guide*. Washington, DC, American Psychological Association, 27–47, 2000.
83. Schneider WJ, Cavell TA, Hughes JN: A sense of containment: potential moderator of the relation between parenting practices and children's externalizing behaviors. *Dev Psychopatho* 15:95–117, 2003.
84. Dishion TJ, McMahon RJ: Parental monitoring and the prevention of child and adolescent problem behavior: a conceptual and empirical formulation. *Clin Child Fam Psychol Rev* 1:61–75, 1998.
85. Buckner JC, Mezzacappa E, Beardslee WR: Characteristics of resilient youths living in poverty: the role of self-regulatory processes. *Dev Psychopathol* 15:139–162, 2003.
86. Galambos NL, Barker ET, Almeida DM: Parents do matter: trajectories of change in externalizing and internalizing problems in early adolescence. *Child Dev* 74:578–594, 2003.
87. Brody GH, Murry VM, Kim S, et al.: Longitudinal pathways to competence and psychological adjustment among African American children living in rural single-parent households. *Child Dev* 73:1505–1516, 2002.
88. Lloyd JJ, Anthony JC: Hanging out with the wrong crowd: how much difference can parents make in an urban environment? *J Urban Health* 80:383–390, 2003.
89. Mason CA, Cauce AM, Gonzales N, et al.: Neither too sweet nor too sour: problem peers, maternal control, and problem behavior in African American adolescents. *Child Dev* 67:2115–2130, 1996.
90. Caspi A, McClay J, Moffitt TE, et al.: Role of genotype in the cycle of violence in maltreated children. *Science* 297:851–854, 2002.
91. Caspi A, Sugden K, Moffitt TE, et al.: Influence of life stress on depression: moderation by a polymorphism in the 5-HTT gene. *Science* 301:386–389, 2003.
92. Kim-Cohen J, Moffitt TE, Caspi A, et al.: Genetic and environmental processes in young children's resilience and vulnerability to socioeconomic deprivation. *Child Dev* 75:651–668, 2004.
93. Plomin R, Rutter M: Child development, molecular genetics, and what to do with genes once they are found. *Child Dev* 69:1223–1242, 1998.
94. Rutter M: Nature, nurture, and development: from evangelism through science toward policy and practice. *Child Dev* 73:1–21, 2002.
95. Tierney JP, Grossman JB, Resch NL: *Making a difference: An Impact Study of Big Brothers Big Sisters*. Philadelphia, PA, Public/Private Ventures, 1995.
96. Elder GH, Conger RD: *Children of the Land: Adversity and Success in Rural America*. Chicago, University of Chicago Press, 2000.
97. Miller L, Gur M: Religiosity, depression and physical maturation in adolescent girls. *J Am Acad Child Adolesc Psychiatry* 41:206–214, 2002.
98. Pearce MJ, Jones SM, Schwab-Stone ME, et al.: The protective effects of religiousness and parent involvement on the development of conduct problems among youth exposed to violence. *Child Dev* 74:1682–1696, 2003.
99. Burchinal MR, Follmer A, Bryant DM: The relations of maternal social support and family structure with maternal responsiveness and child outcomes among African-American families. *Dev Psychol* 32:1073–1083, 1996.
100. McLoyd VC, Jayaratne TE, Ceballo R, et al.: Unemployment and work interruption among African-American single mothers: effects on parenting and adolescent socioemotional functioning. *Child Dev* 65:562–589, 1994.
101. Hamre BK, Pianta RC: Early teacher–child relationships and the trajectory of children's school outcomes through eighth grade. *Child Dev* 72:625–638, 2001.
102. NICHD Early Child Care Research Network: Social functioning in the first grade: associations with earlier home and child care predictors and with current classroom experiences. *Child Dev* 74:1639–1662, 2003.
103. Reddy R, Rhodes JE, Mulhall P: The influence of teacher support on student adjustment in the middle school years: a latent growth curve study. *Dev Psychopathol* 15:119–138, 2003.
104. Howes C, Ritchie S: Attachment organizations in children with difficult life circumstances. *Dev Psychopathol* 11:251–268, 1999.
105. Meehan BT, Hughes JN, Cavell TA: Teacher–student relationships as compensatory resources for aggressive children. *Child Dev* 74:1145–1157, 2003.
106. Hughes JN, Cavell TA, Jackson T: Influence of the teacher–student relationship on childhood conduct problems: a prospective study. *J Clin Child Psychol* 28:173–184, 1999.
107. Way N, Robinson MG: A longitudinal study of the effects of family, friends, and school experiences on the psychological adjustment of ethnic minority, low-SES adolescents. *J Adolesc Res* 18:324–346, 2003.
108. Luthar SS: *Poverty and Children's Adjustment*. Thousand Oaks, Sage, 1999.
109. Spencer MB: Social and cultural influences on school adjustment: the application of an identity-focused cultural ecological perspective. *Edu Psychol* 34:43–57, 1999.
110. Luthar SS, Zigler E: Vulnerability and competence: a review of research on resilience in childhood. *Am J Orthopsychiatry* 61:6–22, 1999.
111. Rutter ML: Psychosocial adversity and child psychopathology. *Br J Psychiatry* 74:480–49, 1999.
112. Werner EE, Smith RS: *Overcoming the Odds: High Risk Children from Birth to Adulthood*. Ithaca, Cornell University Press, 1992.
113. Mayer JD, Salovey P, Caruso DR, et al.: Measuring emotional intelligence with the MSCEIT V2.0. *Emotion* 3:97–105, 2003.
114. Salovey P, Mayer JD, Caruso D, et al.: Measuring emotional intelligence as a set of abilities with the Mayer-Salovey-Caruso Emotional Intelligence Test. In: Lopez SJ, Snyder CR (eds): *Positive Psychological Assessment: A Handbook of Models and Measures*. Washington, DC, American Psychological Association, 251–265, 2003.
115. Trinidad DR, Johnson CA: The association between emotional intelligence and early adolescent tobacco and alcohol use. *Pers Individ Diff* 32:95–105, 2002.
116. Parker JDA, Summerfeldt LJ, Hogan MJ, et al.: Emotional intelligence and academic success: examining the transition from high school to university. *Pers Individ Diff* 36:163–172, 2004.
117. Koenen KC, Moffitt TE, Caspi A, et al.: Domestic violence is associated with environmental suppression of IQ in young children. *Dev Psychopathol* 15:297–311, 2003.
118. Cicchetti D: Experiments of nature: contributions to developmental theory. *Dev Psychopathol* 15:833–835, 2003.
119. Rutter M: The interplay of nature, nurture, and developmental influences: the challenge ahead for mental health. *Arch Gen Psychiatry* 59:996–1000, 2002.
120. Aspinwall LG, Taylor SE: A stitch in time: Self-regulation and proactive coping. *Psychol Bull* 121:417–436, 1997.
121. Eisenberg N, Champion C, Ma Y: Emotion-related regulation: an emerging construct. *Merrill-Palmer Quarterly* 50:236–259, 2004.
122. Davidson RJ: Affective style, psychopathology, and resilience: brain mechanisms and plasticity. *Am Psychol* 55:1196–1214, 2000.
123. Curtis WJ, Cicchetti D: Moving research on resilience into the 21st century: theoretical and methodological considerations in examining the biological contributors to resilience. *Dev Psychopathol* 15:773–810, 2003.
124. McEwen BS, Sapolsky RM: Stress and cognitive function. *Curr Opin Neurobiol* 5:205–216, 1995.
125. Sapolsky RM: Glucocorticoids and hippocampal atrophy in neuropsychiatric disorders. *Arch Gen Psychiatry* 57:925–935, 2000.
126. McEwen BS: Steroid hormone actions on the brain: when is the genome involved? *Hormon Behav* 28:396–405, 1994.
127. Watson C, Gametchu B: Membrane-initiated steroid actions and the proteins that mediate them. *Proc Soc Exper Biol Med* 220:9–19, 1999.
128. Luthar SS: Resilience in development: A synthesis of research across five decades. In: D. Cicchetti D, Cohen DJ (eds): *Developmental Psychopathology: Risk, Disorder, and Adaptation* (2nd ed). New York, Wiley, 739–795, 2006.
129. Luthar SS, Crossman EJ, Small PJ: Resilience and adversity. In: Lerner RM, Lamb ME (eds): *Handbook of Child Psychology and Developmental Science* (7th ed, Vol. III). New York, Wiley, 247–286, 2015.

SECTION III
SCIENTIFIC FOUNDATIONS

3.1 ■ RESEARCH METHODOLOGY

CHAPTER 3.1.1 ■ UNDERSTANDING RESEARCH METHODS AND STATISTICS: A PRIMER FOR CLINICIANS

GEORGE A. MORGAN, JEFFREY A. GLINER, AND ROBERT J. HARMON

INTRODUCTION

Purposes of Research

Research has two general purposes: (a) increasing knowledge within the discipline and (b) increasing your knowledge as a professional consumer of research in order to understand and evaluate research developments within your discipline. For many clinicians, the ability to understand research in one's discipline may be even more important than making research contributions. Dissemination of research occurs through an exceptionally large number of professional journals, workshops, and continuing education courses, as well as popular literature. Today's professional cannot simply rely on the statements in newspapers or of a workshop instructor to determine clinical practice. Even journal articles need to be scrutinized for weak designs, inappropriate data analyses, or incorrect interpretation of these analyses. Clinicians must have the research and reasoning skills to be able to make sound decisions. This chapter is intended to help clinicians be critical readers of the research literature.

Research Dimensions and Dichotomies

Self-Report Versus Researcher Observation

In some studies the participants self-report to the researcher about their attitudes, intentions, or behavior. In other studies the researcher directly observes and records the behavior of the participant. Sometimes instruments such as heart rate monitors are used by researchers to "observe" the participants' physiologic functioning. Self-reports may be influenced by biases such as the halo effect, or participants may have forgotten or not thought about the topic. Many researchers prefer observed behavioral data. However, sensitive, well-trained interviewers may be able to alleviate some of the biases inherent in self-reports.

Quantitative Versus Qualitative Research

We believe that this topic is more appropriately thought of as two related dimensions. The first dimension deals with philosophical or paradigm differences between the quantitative (positivist) approach and the qualitative (constructivist) approach to research (1). The second dimension, which is often what people mean when referring to this dichotomy, deals with the type of data, data collection, and data analysis. We think that, in distinguishing between qualitative and quantitative research, the first dimension is the most important.

Positivist Versus Constructivist Paradigms. Although there is disagreement about the appropriateness of these labels, they help us separate the philosophical or paradigm distinction from the data collection and analysis issues. A study could be theoretically positivistic, but the data could be subjective or qualitative. In fact, this combination is quite common. However, qualitative data, methods, and analyses often go with the constructivist paradigm, and quantitative data, methods, and analyses are usually used with the positivist paradigm. This chapter is within the framework of the positivist paradigm, but the constructivist paradigm provides us with useful reminders that human participants are complex and different from other animals and inanimate objects.

Quantitative Versus Qualitative Data, Data Collection, and Analysis. Quantitative data are said to be "objective," which indicates that the behaviors are easily and reliably classified or quantified by the researcher. Qualitative data are more difficult to describe. They are said to be "subjective," which indicates that they are hard to classify or score. Some examples are perceptions of pain and attitudes toward therapy. Qualitative/constructivist researchers usually gather these data from interviews, observations, or documents. Quantitative/positivist researchers also gather these types of data but usually translate such perceptions and attitudes into numbers. Qualitative researchers, on the other hand, usually do not try to quantify such perceptions; instead, they categorize them and look for themes.

Data analysis for quantitative researchers usually involves well-defined statistical methods, often providing a test of the null hypothesis. Qualitative researchers are more interested in examining their data for similarities or themes which might occur among all of the participants on a particular topic.

VARIABLES AND THEIR MEASUREMENT

Research Problems and Variables

Research Problems

The research process begins with a problem. A research problem is an interrogative sentence about the relationship between two or more variables. Prior to the problem statement, the scientist usually perceives an obstacle to understanding.

Variables

A variable must be able to vary or have different values. For example, gender is a variable because it has two values, female or male. Age is a variable that has a large number of potential values. Type of treatment/intervention is a variable if there is more than one treatment or a treatment and a control group. However, if one studies only girls or only 12-month-old infants, gender and age are not variables; they are constants. Thus, we define a *variable* as a characteristic of the participants or situation that has different values *in this study*.

Operational Definitions of Variables

An operational definition describes or defines a variable in terms of the operations used to produce it or techniques used to measure it. Demographic variables like age or ethnic group are usually measured by checking official records or simply by asking the participant to choose the appropriate category from among those listed. Treatments are described in some detail. Likewise, abstract concepts like mastery motivation need to be defined operationally by spelling out how they were measured.

Independent Variables

We do not restrict the term *independent variable* to interventions or treatments. We define an independent variable broadly to include any predictors, antecedents, or *presumed* causes or influences under investigation in the study.

Active Independent Variables. An active independent variable such as an intervention or treatment is *given* to a group of participants (experimental) but not to another (control group), within a specified period of time *during* the study. Thus, a pretest and posttest should be possible, even if not actually used.

Attribute Independent Variables. A variable that could not be manipulated is called an *attribute independent variable* because it is an attribute of the person (e.g., gender, age, and ethnic group) or the person's usual environment (e.g., abuse). For ethical and practical reasons, many aspects of the environment cannot be manipulated or given and are thus attribute variables. This distinction between active and attribute independent variables is important for determining what can be said about cause and effect. Research where an apparent intervention is studied after the fact is sometimes called *ex post facto*. We consider the independent variables in such studies to be attributes, and they do not justify cause and effect conclusions.

Dependent Variables

The dependent variable is the outcome or criterion. It is assumed to measure or assess the effect of the independent variable. Dependent variables are scores from a test, ratings on questionnaires, or readings from instruments (electrical diagram). It is common for a study to have several dependent variables (performance and satisfaction).

Extraneous Variables

These are variables that are not of interest in a particular study but could influence the dependent variable and need to be controlled. Environmental factors, other attributes of the participants, and characteristics of the investigator are possible extraneous variables.

Levels of a Variable

The word *level* is commonly used to describe the values of an independent variable. This does not necessarily imply that the values are ordered. If an investigator was interested in comparing two different treatments and a no-treatment control group, the study has one independent variable, treatment type, with three levels, the two treatment conditions and the control condition.

We have tried to be consistent and clear about the terms we use; unfortunately, there is not one agreed-upon term for many research and statistical concepts. At the end of most sections, we have included a table, similar to Table 3.1.1.1, that lists a number of key terms used in this chapter alongside other terms for essentially the same concept used by some other researchers. In addition to these tables of different terms for the same concept, we have appended a list of partially similar terms or phrases (such as independent variable vs. independent samples) which do not have the same meaning and should be differentiated.

Measurement and Descriptive Statistics

Measurement

Measurement is introduced when variables are translated into labels (categories) or numbers. For statistical purposes, we and many statisticians (2) do not find the traditional scales of measurement (nominal, ordinal, interval, or ratio) useful. We prefer the following: (a) *dichotomous* (a variable having only two values or levels), (b) *nominal* (a categorical variable

TABLE 3.1.1.1

SIMILAR RELATED TERMS ABOUT VARIABLES

- Active independent variable ≈ manipulated variable ≈ intervention ≈ treatment
- Attribute independent variable ≈ measured variable ≈ individual difference variable
- Dependent variable (DV) ≈ outcome ≈ criterion
- Independent variable (IV) ≈ antecedent ≈ predictor ≈ presumed cause ≈ factor
- Levels (of a variable) ≈ categories ≈ values ≈ groups ≈ samples

Note: The term we use most often is listed on the left. Similar terms (indicated by ≈) used by other researchers and/or us are listed to the right.

with three or more values that are not ordered), (c) *ordinal* (a variable with three or more values that are ordered, but not normally distributed), and (d) *normally distributed* (an ordered variable with a distribution that is approximately normal [bell-shaped] in the population sampled). This measurement classification is similar to one proposed by Helena Chmura Kraemer (personal communication, March 16, 1999).

Descriptive Statistics and Plots

Researchers use descriptive statistics to summarize the data from their samples in terms of frequency, central tendency, and variability. Inferential statistics, on the other hand, are used to make inferences from the sample to the population.

Central Tendency. The three main measures of the center of a distribution are mean, median, and mode (the most frequent score). The *mean* or arithmetic average takes into account all of the available information in computing the central tendency of a frequency distribution; thus, it is the statistic of choice if the data are normally distributed. The *median* or middle score is the appropriate measure of central tendency for ordinal level data.

Variability. Measures of variability tell us about the spread of the scores. If all of the scores in a distribution are the same, there is no variability. If they are all different and widely spaced apart, the variability is high. The *standard deviation* is the most common measure of variability, but it is appropriate only when one has normally distributed data. For nominal/categorical data, the measure of spread is the number of possible response categories.

Normal Curve

The normal curve is important because many of the variables that we examine in research are distributed in the form of the normal curve. Examples of variables that in the population fit a normal curve are height, weight, IQ, and many personality measures. For each of these examples, most participants would fall toward the middle of the curve, with fewer people at each extreme.

As shown in Figure 3.1.1.1, if a variable is normally distributed, about 68% of the participants lie within one standard deviation from either side of the mean, and 95% are within two standard deviations from the mean. For example, assume that 100 is the average IQ and the standard deviation is 15. The probability that a person will have an IQ between 85 and 115 is 0.68. Furthermore, only 5% (0.05) would be expected to have an IQ less than 70 or more than 130. It is important to be able to conceptualize area under the normal curve in the form of probabilities because statistical convention sets acceptable probability levels for rejecting the null hypothesis at 0.05 or 0.01.

Conclusions about Measurement and the Use of Statistics

Table 3.1.1.2 summarizes information about the appropriate use of various kinds of plots and descriptive statistics, given nominal, dichotomous, ordinal, or normal data. Statistics based on means and standard deviation are valid for normally distributed (normal) data. Typically, these data are used in the most powerful statistical tests, for example, analysis of variance, these statistical tests are called parametric statistics. However, if the data are ordered but grossly nonnormal (ordinal), means and standard deviations may not give meaningful answers. Then the median and a nonparametric test based on rank order would be preferred. Nonparametric tests have less power than parametric tests (they are less able to reject the null hypothesis when it should be rejected), but the sacrifice in power for nonparametric tests based on ranks usually is relatively minor. If the data are nominal (unordered), one would have to use the mode or frequency counts. In this case, there would be a major sacrifice in power. It would be misleading to use tests that assume the dependent variable is ordinal or normally distributed when the dependent variable is, in fact, nominal/not ordered. Table 3.1.1.3 provides examples of potentially confusing, essentially equivalent terms about measurement and descriptive statistics.

Measurement Reliability

Measurement reliability and measurement validity are two parts of overall research validity, the quality of the whole study. Reliability refers to consistency of scores on a particular instrument. It is incorrect to state that a test is reliable because reliability takes into account the sample that took the test. For example, there may be strong evidence for reliability for adults, but scores of depressed adolescents on this test may be highly inconsistent. When researchers use tests or other instruments to measure outcomes, they need to make sure that the tests provide consistent data. If the outcome measure is not reliable, then one cannot accurately assess the results.

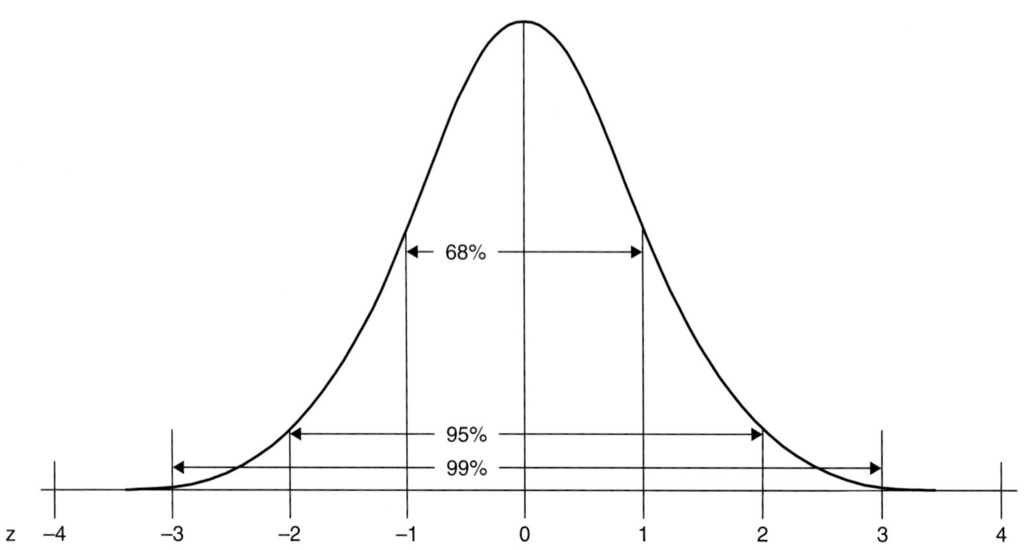

FIGURE 3.1.1.1. Frequency distribution and areas under the normal and standardized curve.

TABLE 3.1.1.2

SELECTION OF APPROPRIATE DESCRIPTIVE STATISTICS AND PLOTS

	Nominal	Dichotomous	Ordinal	Normal
Graphic Depiction (Plot)				
Frequency Distribution	Yes[a]	Yes	Yes	OK[b]
Bar chart	Yes	Yes	Yes	OK
Histogram	No[c]	No	OK	Yes
Frequency polygon	No	No	OK	Yes
Box and whiskers plot	No	No	Yes	Yes
Central Tendency				
Mean	No	OK	Of ranks, OK	Yes
Median	No	OK = mode	Yes	OK
Mode	Yes	Yes	OK	OK
Variability				
Range	No	Always 1	Yes	Yes
Standard deviation	No	No	Of ranks, OK	Yes
Interquartile range	No	No	OK	OK
How many categories	Yes	Always 2	OK	Not if truly continuous
Shape				
Skewness	No	No	Yes	Yes

[a]*Yes* means a good choice with this level of measurement.
[b]OK means OK to use, but not the best choice at this level of measurement.
[c]No means not appropriate at this level of measurement.

Conceptually, reliability is consistency. When evaluating instruments it is important to be able to express reliability numerically. The correlation coefficient, often used to evaluate reliability, is usually expressed as the letter *r*, which indicates the strength of a relationship. The values of *r* range between –1 and +1. A value of 0 indicates no relationship between two variables or scores, whereas values close to –1 or +1 indicate very strong relationships between two variables. A strong positive relationship indicates that people who score high on one test also score high on a second test. To say that a measurement is reliable, one would expect a coefficient between +0.7 and +1.0. Others have suggested even stricter criteria. For example, reliability coefficients of 0.8 are acceptable for research, but 0.9 is necessary for measures that will be used to make clinical decisions about individuals. However, it is common to see published journal articles in which one or a few reliability coefficients are below 0.7, usually 0.6 or greater. Although correlations of –0.7 to –1.0 indicate a strong (negative) correlation, they are totally unacceptable as evidence for reliability.

There are four different types of evidence for reliability, such as test–retest reliability, that are listed in Table 3.1.1.4, along with synonyms that you may see in the literature. In addition, there are many different methods to compute these different types of reliability. See Morgan, Gliner, and Harmon (3) for specifics about these approaches to assessing reliability.

TABLE 3.1.1.3

SIMILAR TERMS ABOUT MEASUREMENT

- Categorical variable ≈ usually nominal, but variables may have discrete ordered *categories*
- Dichotomous ≈ binary ≈ dummy variable ≈ nominal with two categories
- Interval scale ≈ numeric ≈ continuous variable ≈ quantitative ≈ scale data
- Mean ≈ average ≈ arithmetic average
- Median ≈ midpoint
- Normal ≈ (approximately) normally distributed variable ≈ interval and ratio data ≈ quantitative ≈ continuous
- Nominal scale ≈ unordered categorical variable ≈ qualitative ≈ discrete
- Ordered variable ≈ ordinal or interval scale
- Ordinal scale ≈ unequal interval scale ≈ discrete ordered categorical variable
- Range ≈ spread

Note: The term we use most often is listed on the left. Similar terms (indicated by ≈) used by other researchers and/or us are listed to the right.

Measurement Validity

Validity is concerned with establishing evidence for the use of a particular measure or instrument in a particular setting with a particular population for a specific purpose. Here we will

TABLE 3.1.1.4

SIMILAR TERMS ABOUT MEASUREMENT RELIABILITY

- Alternate forms reliability ≈ equivalent forms ≈ parallel forms ≈ coefficient of equivalence
- Internal consistency reliability ≈ interitem reliability ≈ Cronbach's alpha
- Interrater reliability ≈ interobserver reliability
- Measurement reliability ≈ reliability ≈ test, instrument, or score reliability
- Test–retest reliability ≈ coefficient of stability

Note: The term we use most often is listed on the left. Similar terms (indicated by ≈) used by other researchers and/or us are listed to the right.

TABLE 3.1.1.5

EVIDENCE FOR MEASUREMENT VALIDITY

Type of Evidence	Support for Validity Depends on
Evidence based on content—all aspects of the construct are represented in appropriate proportions	Good agreement by experts about the content and that it represents the concept to be assessed
Evidence based on response processes—participants' responses match the intended construct	Evidence that participants and raters are not influenced by irrelevant factors like social desirability
Evidence based on internal structure—relationships among items on the test consistent with the conceptual framework	Meaningful factor structure consistent with the conceptual organization of the construct(s)
Evidence based on relations to other variables	
Criterion-concurrent—test and criterion are measured at the same time	The effect size of the relationship[a]
Criterion-predictive—test predicts some criterion in the future	The effect size of the relationship[a]
Convergent—based on theory, variables predicted to be related are related	The effect size of the relationship[a]
Discriminant—variables predicted not to be related are not related	The effect size of the relationship[a,b]
Validity generalization—results using the measure generalize to other settings	Supportive meta-analytic studies
Evidence based on consequences—conducting the test produces benefits for the participants	Evidence that positive consequences outweigh unexpected negative ones in terms of the outcomes of therapy, job placement, etc.

[a]The strength or level of support for validity (weak, medium, strong) could be based on Cohen's (5) effect size guidelines, with the qualifications noted in the text.
[b]Depending on the data, the appropriate strength of association statistic will vary.

discuss what we call measurement validity; others might use terms such as *test validity, score validity,* or just *validity*. We use the *modifier measurement* to distinguish it from internal, external, and overall research validity and to point out that it is the measures or scores that provide evidence for validity. It is inappropriate to say that a test is "valid" or "invalid." Note also that an instrument may produce consistent data (provide evidence for reliability), but the data may not be a valid index of the intended construct.

In research articles, there is usually more evidence for the reliability of the instrument than for the validity of the instrument because evidence for validity is more difficult to obtain. To establish validity, one ideally needs a "gold standard" or "criterion" related to the particular purpose of the measure. To obtain such a criterion is often not an easy matter, so other types of evidence to support the validity of a measure are necessary.

Currently, the Standards (4) categorize evidence into five *types* that support the validity of a test or measure: (a) content, (b) response processes, (c) internal structure, (d) relations to other variables, and (e) the consequences of testing (4). Note that the five types of evidence are *not* separate types of validity and that any one type of evidence is insufficient. Validation should integrate all the pertinent evidence from as many of the five types of evidence as possible. Preferably validation should include some evidence in addition to content evidence, which is probably the most common and easiest to obtain. Table 3.1.1.5 expands the description of the five types of validity evidence and what information would be used to support each type of evidence.

Many researchers still classify evidence for validity into three types: content, criterion-related, and construct. Table 3.1.1.5 shows that the two types of criterion validity (concurrent and predictive) are now under evidence based on relations. Construct validity included convergent, discriminant, and factorial evidence; the latter is under evidence based on internal structure.

Evaluation of evidence for validity is often based on correlations with other variables, but there are no well-established guidelines. Our suggestion is to use Cohen's (5) guidelines for interpreting effect sizes, which are measures of the strength of a relationship. We describe several measures of effect size and how to interpret them. Cohen suggested that generally, in the applied behavioral sciences, a correlation of $r = 0.5$ could be considered a large effect, and in this context we would consider $r = 0.5$ or greater to be strong support for measurement validity. In general, an acceptable level of support would be provided by $r \geq 0.3$, and some weak support might result from $r \geq 0.1$, assuming that such an r was statistically significant. However, for concurrent, criterion evidence, if the criterion and test being validated are two similar measures of the same concept (e.g., IQ), the correlation would be expected to be very high, perhaps 0.8 or 0.9. On the other hand, for convergent evidence, the measures should not be that highly correlated because they should be measures of different concepts. If the measures were very highly related, one might ask whether they were instead really measuring the same concept.

The strength of the evidence for the measurement of validity is extremely important for research in applied settings because without measures that have strong evidence for validity the results of the study can be misleading. Validation is an ongoing, never fully achieved, process based on integration of all the evidence from as many sources as possible.

RESEARCH APPROACHES, QUESTIONS, AND DESIGNS

Quantitative Research Approaches

Our conceptual framework includes five quantitative research approaches (randomized experimental, quasiexperimental, comparative, associational, and descriptive). This framework is helpful because it provides appropriate guidance about inferring cause and effect.

Figure 3.1.1.2 indicates that the general purpose of four of the five approaches is to explore relationships between or among variables. This is consistent with the notion that all common parametric statistics are relational, and it is consistent with the typical phrasing of research questions and hypotheses as investigating the relationship between two or more variables. Figure 3.1.1.2 also indicates the specific

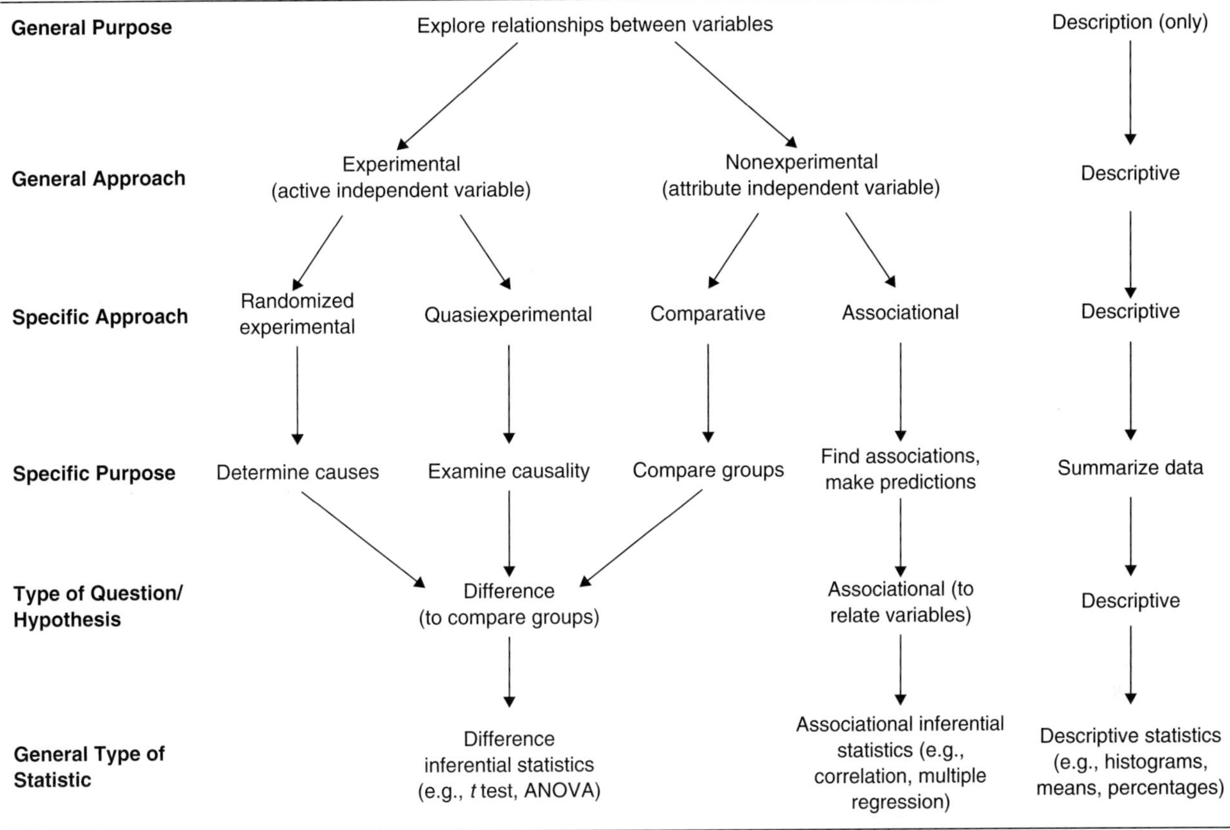

FIGURE 3.1.1.2. Schematic diagram showing how the general type of statistic and hypothesis or question used in a study corresponds to the purposes and the approach.

purpose, type of research question, and general type of statistic used in each of the five approaches.

Research Approaches with an Active Independent Variable

Randomized Experimental Research Approach. This approach provides the best evidence about cause and effect. For a research approach to be called randomized experimental, two criteria must be met. First, the independent variable must be active (be a variable that is *given* to the participant, such as a treatment). Second, the researcher must randomly assign participants to groups or conditions prior to the intervention; this is what differentiates experiments from quasiexperiments. More discussion of specific quasiexperimental and randomized designs is provided below.

Quasiexperimental Research Approach. Researchers do not agree on the definition of a quasiexperiment. Our definition is that there must be an active/manipulated independent variable, but the participants are not randomly assigned to the groups. In much applied research participants are already in groups such as clinics, and it is not possible to change those assignments and divide the participants randomly into experimental and control groups.

Nonexperimental Research Approaches

These approaches have attributed independent variables and are often called *observational studies* in the medical literature. We divide these nonexperimental approaches into comparative and associational. The distinctions between them are shown in Figure 3.1.1.2.

Comparative Research Approach. Like randomized experiments and quasiexperiments, the comparative approach, which is sometimes called *causal-comparative,* or *ex post facto,* usually has a few levels (typically two to four) or categories for the independent variable and makes comparisons between groups.

Associational Research Approach. This approach is similar to the comparative approach in that the independent variable is an attribute. In this approach, the independent variable is often continuous or has a number of ordered categories, usually five or more. We prefer to label this approach *associational* rather *correlational,* as used by some researchers, because the approach is more than, and should not be confused with, a specific statistic, the correlation coefficient.

Descriptive Research Approach

The term *descriptive research* refers to questions and studies that use only descriptive statistics, such as averages, percentages, histograms, and frequency distributions, which are not tested for statistical significance. This approach is different from the other four in that only one variable is considered at a time so that no comparisons or associations are determined. Although most research studies include some descriptive questions (at least to describe the sample), very few stop there; it is hard to find a purely descriptive study.

The approaches are based on the type of independent variable and research questions, so the whole study can and often does have more than one approach. For example, it is common for *survey research* to include both comparative and associational as well as descriptive research questions and therefore use all three approaches.

Research Questions and Hypotheses

Three Types of Basic Hypotheses or Research Questions

A *hypothesis* is a predictive statement about the relationship between two or more variables. Research questions are similar to hypotheses, but they are in question format. *Research questions* can be divided into three types: *difference questions, associational questions,* and *descriptive questions* (see Figure 3.1.1.2 again).

For difference questions, one compares groups or levels derived from the independent variable in terms of their scores on the dependent variable. This type of question typically is used with the randomized experimental, quasiexperimental, and comparative approaches. For an associational question, one associates or relates the independent and dependent variables. What we call descriptive questions are not answered with inferential statistics; they merely describe or summarize data.

As implied by Figure 3.1.1.2, it is appropriate to phrase any difference or associational research question as simply a *relationship* between the independent variable(s) and the dependent variable. However, we think that phrasing the research questions/hypotheses as a difference between groups or as a relationship between variables helps match the question to the appropriate statistical analysis. Table 3.1.1.6 shows the terms other researchers sometimes use that correspond to those for our research approaches and questions.

EXPERIMENTAL DESIGNS

We describe here specific designs for both quasiexperiments and randomized experiments. This should help the reader visualize the independent variables, levels of these variables, and whether the participants are assessed on the dependent variable more than once.

Quasiexperimental Designs

The randomized experimental and quasiexperimental approaches have an active independent variable, which has two or more values, called levels. The dependent variable is the outcome measure or criterion of the study.

In both randomized and quasiexperimental approaches, the active independent variable has at least one level that is some type of intervention given to participants in the experimental group during the study. Usually there is also a comparison or control group, which is the other level of the independent variable. There can be more than two levels or groups (e.g., two or more different interventions plus one or more comparison groups).

The key difference between quasiexperiments and randomized experiments is whether the participants are assigned randomly to the groups or levels of the independent variable. In quasiexperiments random assignment of the participants is not done; thus, the groups are always considered to be nonequivalent, and there are alternative interpretations of the results that make definitive conclusions about cause and effect difficult. For example, if some children diagnosed with attention-deficit/hyperactivity disorder were treated with stimulants and others were not, later differences between the groups could be due to many factors. Families who volunteer (or agree) to have their children medicated may be different, in important ways, from those who do not. Or perhaps the more disruptive children were given stimulants. Thus, later problem behaviors (or positive outcomes) could be due to initial differences between the groups rather than the stimulant.

Poor Quasiexperimental Designs

Results from these designs (sometimes called *pre-experimental*) are hard to interpret and should not be used. These designs lack a comparison (control) group, a pretest, or both.

Better Quasiexperimental Designs

Pretest–Posttest Nonequivalent Groups Design. As with all quasiexperiments, there is no random assignment of the participants to the groups in this design. First, measurements (O_1) are taken on the groups prior to an intervention. Then one group (E) receives a new treatment (X), which the other (comparison) group (C) does not receive (NX); often the comparison group receives the usual or traditional treatment. At the end of the intervention period, both groups are measured again (O_2) to determine whether there are differences between the two groups. The design is considered to be nonequivalent because the participants are not randomly assigned (NR) to one or the other group. Even if the two groups have the same mean score on the pretest, there may be characteristics that have not been measured that may interact with the treatment to cause differences between the two groups that are not due strictly to the intervention. The following diagram illustrates the procedures for the pretest–posttest nonequivalent groups design:

NR	E	O_1	X	O_2
NR	C	O_1	NX	O_2

Table 3.1.1.7 summarizes two issues that determine the strength (from weak to strong) of quasiexperimental designs. These designs vary, as shown, on whether the *treatments* are randomly assigned to the intact groups, such as clinics, and on the likelihood that the groups are similar in terms of attributes or characteristics of the participants. In none of the quasiexperimental designs are the *individual participants* randomly assigned to the groups, so the groups are always considered nonequivalent, but the participant characteristics may be similar if there was no bias in how the participants were assigned (got into) the groups.

Time-Series Designs. Time-series designs are different from the more traditional designs discussed above because they have multiple measurement (time) periods rather than just the pre- and postperiods. These designs often are referred to as *interrupted* time series because the treatment interrupts the baseline from posttreatment measures. The two most common types are single-group time-series designs and multiple-group time-series designs (6). Within each type, the treatment can be temporary or continuous. The logic behind any time-series design

TABLE 3.1.1.6

SIMILAR TERMS ABOUT RESEARCH APPROACHES AND QUESTIONS

- Associational approach ≈ correlational ≈ survey ≈ descriptive
- Associational questions ≈ correlational questions
- Comparative approach ≈ causal-comparative ≈ ex post facto
- Descriptive approach ≈ exploratory research
- Difference questions ≈ group comparisons
- Nonexperimental research (comparative, associational, and descriptive approaches) ≈ some writers call all three descriptive ≈ observational research

Note: The term we use most often is listed on the left. Similar terms (indicated by ≈) used by other researchers and/or us are listed to the right.

TABLE 3.1.1.7

ISSUES THAT DETERMINE THE STRENGTH OF QUASIEXPERIMENTAL DESIGNS

Strength of Design	Random Assignment of Treatments to Intact Groups	Participant Characteristics Likely to Be Similar
Poor (or pre)	No	No, because no comparison group or no pretest
Weak	No	Not likely, because participants decide which group to join (self-assign to groups)
Moderate	No	Maybe, because participants did not self-assign to groups and no known assignment bias
Strong	Yes	Maybe, because participants did not self-assign to groups and no known assignment bias

involves convincing others that a baseline (several pretests) is stable prior to an intervention so that one can conclude that the change in the dependent variable is due to the intervention and not due to other environmental events or maturation. It is common in time-series designs to have multiple measures before and after the intervention, but there must be multiple (at least three) pretests to establish a baseline. One of the hallmarks of time-series designs is the visual display of the data, which are often quite convincing. However, these visual displays also can be misleading due to the lack of independence of the data points, and therefore always must be statistically analyzed.

Randomized Experimental Designs

In randomized designs the participants are randomly assigned to the experimental and control groups. Random assignment of participants to groups should eliminate bias on all characteristics before the independent variable is introduced. This elimination of bias is one necessary condition for the results to provide convincing evidence that the independent variable caused differences between the groups on the dependent variable. For cause to be demonstrated, other biases in environmental and experience variables occurring during the study also must be eliminated.

Three types of randomized experimental designs are discussed. For each we describe and diagram the design and present some of the advantages and disadvantages. The diagrams and discussion are limited to two groups, but more than two groups may be used with any of these designs. The experimental group receives the intervention, and the "control" group(s) receives the standard (traditional) treatment, a placebo, and/or another (comparison) treatment. For ethical reasons, it is unusual and not desirable for the control group to receive no treatment at all, but it is difficult to decide which type of control group is appropriate. Here we call all such treatment options the *control group*.

Posttest-Only Control Group Design

The posttest-only control group design can be shown as follows:

R	E:	X	O
R	C:	NX	O

The sequential operations of the design are to randomly (R) assign participants to either an experimental (E) or control (C) group. Then the experimental group receives the intended intervention (X) and the control group does not receive it (NX). At the end of the intervention period, both groups are measured (O), using some form of instrumentation related to the study (dependent variable).

The key point for the posttest-only control group design is the random assignment of participants to groups. If participants are assigned randomly to one or the other group, the two groups should not be biased on *any* variable prior to the intervention. Therefore, if there are differences on the dependent measure following the intervention, it can be assumed that the differences are due to the intervention and not due to differences in participant characteristics.

Pretest–Posttest Control Group Design

The pretest–posttest control group design can be shown as follows:

R	E:	O_1	X	O_2
R	C:	O_1	NX	O_2

Reasons for using this design compared with the posttest-only control group design are to check for equivalence of groups before the intervention and to describe the population from which both groups are drawn. Another advantage of this design is that posttest scores could be adjusted statistically through analysis of covariance based on pretest score differences between the treatment and control groups. On the other hand, a problem could be created if a pretest is used. The pretest could bias the participants as to what to expect in the study, and practice on the pretest could influence the posttest (there could be carryover effects). Also, if the dependent variable is invasive (spinal tap), one would not want to use it as a pretest. Random assignment does mean that the groups will not differ substantially on the average, but this assurance is adequate only if the sample is large. In small-sample clinical research, it is not uncommon to find some large differences in important characteristics even when the participants were randomly assigned to groups.

Within-Subjects Randomized Experimental (or Crossover) Design

In the simplest case, this design has two levels and can be shown as follows:

		Condition 1	Test	Condition 2	Test
R	Order 1	X	O_1	NX	O_2
R	Order 2	NX	O_1	X	O_2

The participants are randomly assigned to order 1, which receives the experimental condition first and then the control condition, or to order 2, which receives the control condition and then the experimental. This type of design is frequently used in studies in which participants are asked to evaluate diets, exercise, and similar events assumed, from previous research, not to have carryover effects. The strength of this design is that participants act as their own control, which reduces error variance. This design can have problems if there are carryover effects from the experimental condition. Furthermore, one must be extremely cautious with this design when comparing a new treatment with a traditional treatment.

The problem, often referred to as *asymmetrical transfer effects,* occurs when the impact of one order (perhaps the traditional treatment before the new treatment) is greater than the impact of the other order (new treatment before the traditional treatment).

Many variants of the above quasiexperimental and experimental designs are discussed in Shadish, Cook, and Campbell (7).

GENERAL DESIGN CLASSIFICATIONS

General design classifications are important for determining appropriate statistical methods to be used in data analysis. Within the randomized experimental, quasiexperimental, and comparative approaches, all designs must fit into one of three categories or labels (between, within, or mixed). These design classifications do not apply to the associational or descriptive approaches.

Between-Groups Designs

Between-groups designs are defined as designs in which each participant in the research study is in one and only one condition or group. For example, in a study investigating the effects of medication on the number of symptoms in hyperactive children, there might be two groups (or conditions or levels) of the independent variable: the current medication and a new medication. In a between-groups design, each participant receives only one of the two conditions or levels: either the current medication or the new one.

Within-Subjects or Repeated-Measures Designs

Within-subjects designs, the second type of general design classification, are conceptually the opposite of between-groups designs. In these designs, each participant in the research receives or experiences all of the conditions or levels of the independent variable. If we use the hyperactive children example just given, there still would be two conditions or levels to the independent variable. In a within-subjects design, each participant would be given first one medication, then the second medication and would be measured for the number of symptoms on both conditions. Because each participant is assessed more than once (for each condition), these designs are also referred to as repeated-measures designs.

Within-subjects designs have appeal due to the reduction in participants needed and to reduction in error variance because each participant is in his or her own control. However, often these designs are less appropriate than between-groups designs because of the possibility of *carryover effects.* If the purpose of the study is to investigate conditions that may result in a long-term or permanent change, such as learning, it is not possible for a participant to be in one condition and then "unlearn" that condition to be in the same previous state to start the next condition. Within-subjects designs may be appropriate if the effects of order of presentation are negligible, as when participants are asked to evaluate several topics or when a medication effect would not be long lasting.

Matching is a second situation where a design is judged to be within subjects. When pairs of subjects in a comparison group and an experimental group are matched on key characteristics, the design is treated statistically as within subjects.

TABLE 3.1.1.8

SIMILAR TERMS ABOUT RESEARCH DESIGNS

- Between groups ≈ independent samples
- Comparison group ≈ control group ≈ placebo group
- Factorial design ≈ two or more independent variables ≈ complex design
- Poor quasiexperimental designs ≈ pre-experiments
- Random assignment to groups ≈ randomized design
- Randomized experiment ≈ true experiment ≈ randomized clinical trial ≈ randomized control trials ≈ RCT
- Single factor design ≈ one independent variable ≈ basic design
- Within subjects ≈ repeated measures ≈ related samples ≈ paired samples ≈ matched groups ≈ correlated samples ≈ within groups ≈ dependent samples

Note: The term we use most often is listed on the left. Similar terms (indicated by ≈) used by other researchers and/or us are listed to the right.

Mixed Designs

A mixed design has at least one between-groups independent variable and at least one within-subjects independent variable; thus there are a minimum of two independent variables. A between-groups independent variable is any independent variable that sets up between-groups conditions. A within-subjects independent variable is any independent variable that sets up within-subjects conditions.

Change Over Time (or Trials) as an Independent Variable

In within-subjects designs, there can be a third type (neither active nor attribute) of independent variable, called change over time or trials. This third type of independent variable is extremely important in randomized experimental and quasiexperimental designs because pretest and posttest are two levels of this type of independent variable. Longitudinal studies, in which the same participants are assessed at several time periods or ages, are another important case in which change over time is the independent variable.

Table 3.1.1.8 provides examples of terms for research designs sometimes used by other researchers that have meanings similar to ours.

DIMENSIONS OF RESEARCH VALIDITY

Research validity refers to the merit of the design of a whole study, as distinguished from validity of the measurement of a variable. Based on the work of Cook and Campbell (6), we (3) divide research validity into four key components:

1. *Measurement reliability and statistics.* We discussed the reliability above and will discuss the appropriate use and interpretation of statistics below.
2. *Internal validity* to be discussed below.
3. *Overall measurement validity of the constructs* which was discussed briefly above.
4. *External validity* which is how well the results of the study generalize to other populations, settings, treatments, and measures.

The next section describes briefly the issue of cause and effect, which is key to understanding internal validity.

Inferring Cause

A major goal of scientific research is to be able to identify a causal relationship between variables. Researchers note that even if they cannot identify all the causes or the most important causal factor of an outcome, they can identify a variable as one (or a partial) cause, under certain circumstances. Three criteria that must occur to infer a causal relationship: (a) the independent variable must precede in time the dependent variable; (b) there must be a relationship between the independent variable and the dependent variable (in the behavioral sciences this is usually determined statistically); and (c) there must be no plausible third (extraneous) variable that also could account for a relationship between the independent and dependent variables.

Four of the five specific research approaches (except the descriptive) attempt to satisfy the three prerequisites. All four can, but do not always, meet the first two criteria, the independent variable preceding the dependent variable and establishing a relationship between variables. The randomized experimental and, to a much lesser extent, the quasiexperimental approaches can be successful in meeting the third condition, elimination of extraneous variables. The comparative and associational approaches are not well suited to establishing causes, but things can be done to control for some extraneous variables. Although the comparative and associational approaches are limited in what can be said about causation, they can lead to strong conclusions about the differences between groups and about associations between variables, respectively. For example, strong associations (correlations) between variables can generate equations where knowing a score on one variable allows one to predict, with some degree of accuracy, the score on the other variable (linear regression). The descriptive approach, as we define it, does not attempt to identify causal relationships or, in fact, any relationships. It focuses on describing variables.

Internal Validity

Cook and Campbell (6) defined internal validity as "the approximate validity with which we can infer that a relationship is causal." Internal validity depends on the strength or soundness of the design and influences whether one can conclude that the independent variable or intervention caused the dependent variable to change. Although internal validity is often discussed only with respect to randomized and quasiexperiments, we believe the concept also applies to research with attribute independent variables (and nonexperimental studies).

We group the Shadish et al. (7) threats to internal validity into two main types: *equivalence of the intervention and control groups on participant characteristics prior to and during the intervention* and *control of extraneous experiences and environmental variables.*

Equivalence of Groups on Participant Characteristics

In research that compares differences among groups, a key question is whether the *groups* that are compared are *equivalent in all* respects prior to the introduction of the independent variable or variables. Using the randomized experimental approach, equivalence is approximately achieved through random assignment of participants to groups, especially if the sample size in each group is large. Random assignment of participants to the groups, which is characteristic of randomized experiments but not quasiexperiments, is the best way to ensure equivalent, or at least unbiased, groups. However, in quasiexperimental, comparative, or associational research, random assignment of participants to groups has not been or cannot be done.

TABLE 3.1.1.9

THREATS TO INTERNAL VALIDITY

Shadish, Cook, and Campbell (7)	Morgan, Gliner, and Harmon (3)
	Equivalence of Groups
Regression	Use of extreme groups
Attrition/mortality	Participant dropouts/attrition during the study
Selection	Bias in assignment to groups
	Control of Extraneous Variables
Maturation	Changes due to time or growth/development
History	Extraneous events
Testing	Repeated testing, carryover effects
Instrumentation	Measurement inconsistency
Additive and interactive threats	Combinations of two or more threats
Ambiguous temporal precedence	Did the independent variable occur before the dependent variable?

Control of Extraneous Experiences and Environment Variables

We have grouped several other "threats" to internal validity under a category that deals with the effects of extraneous (variables other than the independent variables) experiences or environmental conditions during the study. Thus, we have called this internal validity dimension *control of extraneous experiences and environment variables.* Many of these threats occur because participants gain information about the purpose of the study while the study is taking place. An important aspect of this dimension has to do with whether extraneous variables or events *affect one group more* than the other. For example, if participants learn that they are in a control group, they may give up or not try as hard, exaggerating differences between the intervention and control groups; or the opposite may occur and those in the control group overcompensate, eliminating differences between the two groups.

Control of extraneous experiences and the environment depends on the specific study, but it is generally better for randomized experiments and for studies done in controlled environments such as laboratories.

Threats to Internal Validity

Table 3.1.1.9 provides a current list of threats to interval validity as described by Shadish et al. (7). Some of the names for the various threats are confusing, but the concepts are important. We have added a column for our suggested names.

Sampling and Population External Validity

Sampling is the process of selecting part of a population of potential participants with the intent of generalizing from the smaller group, called the *sample,* to the *population.* If we are to make valid inferences about the population, we must select the sample so that it is *representative* of the population. With a few notable exceptions, modern survey techniques have proven to be quite accurate in selecting representative samples and making inferences about the population.

Steps in Selecting a Sample and Generalizing Results

There are many ways to select a sample from a population. The goal is to have an *actual sample* in which each participant

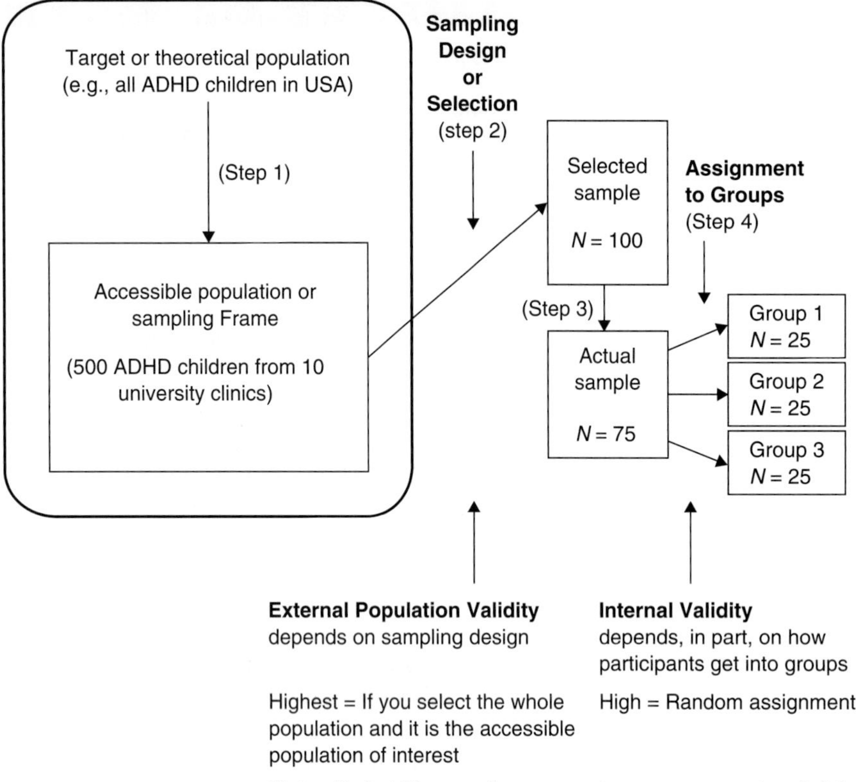

External Population Validity depends on sampling design	**Internal Validity** depends, in part, on how participants get into groups
Highest = If you select the whole population and it is the accessible population of interest	High = Random assignment
High = Probability sampling, e.g., simple random	Lower = groups already intact or groups based on attributes
Lower = Nonprobability sampling, e.g., convenience	Lowest = Self-selection based on knowledge of the treatment

FIGURE 3.1.1.3. Schematic diagram of the sampling process and the distinction between random sampling and random assignment.

represents a known fraction of the *theoretical* or *target population* so that characteristics of the population can be recreated from the sample. Obtaining a *representative sample* is not easy because things can go wrong at three stages of the research process. Figure 3.1.1.3 shows the key sampling concepts and the three steps (shown with arrows).

Types of Sampling

There are two major types of sampling designs that are used in obtaining the selected sample: probability (often considered unbiased sampling) and nonprobability (often considered biased sampling).

Probability Sampling. In probability sampling, every participant has a known, nonzero chance of being selected. The participants or elements of the population are usually people, but could be groups, animals, or events. With probability samples, researchers are able to make an estimate of the extent to which results based on the sample are likely to differ from what would have been found by studying the entire population. There are several types of probability sampling. The most basic is the *simple random sample,* which occurs when all participants have an equal and independent chance of being included in the sample. This technique can be implemented using a random number table to select participants from a list, the sampling frame, of the accessible population.

If some important characteristics of the accessible population such as gender or race are known ahead of time, one can reduce the sampling variation and increase the likelihood that the sample will be representative of the population by using *stratified random sampling.*

Nonprobability Sampling. These samples are ones in which the probability of being selected is unknown. Time and cost constraints lead many researchers to use nonprobability samples. The most common type of nonprobability sample is called a *convenience sample.* A sample is considered a convenience sample if the researcher selected either the accessible population or some participants from the accessible population based on convenience. An extended discussion of the types of sampling and the advantages and disadvantages of each can be found in Fowler (8).

How Many Participants?

The question, "How many participants are needed for this study?" is asked often. One part of the answer depends on whom you ask and their discipline (9). The size of the sample should be large enough so one does not fail to detect important findings, but a large sample will not necessarily help one distinguish the merely statistically significant from societally important findings. *Statistical power analysis* can help one compute the sample size needed to find a statistically significant result given certain assumptions (5).

Sampling and the Internal and External Validity of a Study

We have discussed the internal and external validity of a study and noted that external validity is influenced by the

TABLE 3.1.1.10

SIMILAR TERMS ABOUT SAMPLING

- Accessible population ≈ sampling frame
- Actual sample ≈ sample ≈ final sample
- Convenience sampling ≈ nonprobability sampling ≈ biased sampling
- Random selection ≈ random sampling ≈ probability sampling
- Response rate ≈ return rate ≈ percentage of selected sample participating
- Selected sample ≈ participants sampled
- Theoretical population ≈ target population ≈ population of interest

Note: The term we use most often is listed on the left. Similar terms (indicated by ≈) used by other researchers and/or us are listed to the right.

representativeness of the sample. Figure 3.1.1.3 also shows how the two uses of the word *random* have quite different meanings and different effects on internal and external validity. A probability sampling method such as *random selection* (Step 2) of who is asked to participate in the study is important for high external validity. On the other hand, *random assignment* or placement into groups of persons who agree to participate (Step 4), is important for high internal validity.

Table 3.1.1.10 provides alternate terms used by researchers for various aspects of the sampling process.

INFERENTIAL STATISTICS AND THEIR INTERPRETATION

Introduction to Inferential Statistics and Hypothesis Testing

There are two general approaches to performing quantitative research (10). One, the hypothesis testing approach, often referred to as null hypothesis significance testing (NHST), is the more traditional approach, and focuses on the outcomes of single studies. A second, more recent approach, referred to as the evidence based approach, focuses on conducting multiple studies and the reliability of a research finding. The two approaches are not independent of each other, and often NHST is included in the second approach but not always.

When performing research, rarely are we able to work with an entire population of individuals. Instead, we usually conduct the study on a sample of individuals from a population. It is hoped that if the sample is representative we can infer that the results from our sample apply to the population of interest. Inferential statistics involve making inferences from sample statistics, such as the sample mean and the sample standard deviation, to population parameters such as the population mean and the population standard deviation.

The Hypothesis Testing Approach

The goal of null hypothesis significance testing (NHST) is to reject the null hypothesis in favor of an alternative hypothesis. The *null hypothesis* states that the mean of the population of those who receive the intervention is equal to the mean of the population of those who do not. In other words, the intervention is not successful. An alternative hypothesis (our hypothesis of interest) states that the mean of the population of those who receive the intervention will be greater than the mean of the population of those who do not. If the null hypothesis is false, or rejected, the intervention is considered to be successful. Note that the null hypothesis was stated as a "no difference" null hypothesis, that is, that there is no difference between the population means of the treatment and control groups. However, especially in practical applications, the null hypothesis could be stated, but is not often, as some specific functionally important difference between the means of the two populations. In that case, to reject the null hypothesis, the treatment group would have to exceed the control group by an amount necessary to make a *functional* difference. This is referred to as a *nonnil null hypothesis.*

The hypothesis testing process can be summarized as a series of steps that the researcher takes to conduct the study. From the accessible population, a sample is selected. Participants in this sample are then assigned, randomly under the best circumstances, to one of two groups, an intervention group and a comparison group. (More than two groups could be used, such as two treatment groups and a comparison group.) Next, the participants in the intervention group undergo the new treatment and the participants in the comparison group receive the standard or traditional treatment. At the end of the treatment period, both groups are measured on the dependent variable and a comparison is made, usually between the means of the two groups.

How much of a difference between the two means is needed before one can conclude that there is a statistically significant difference? Inferential statistics provide an outcome (a statistic) that helps make the decision about how much of a difference is needed. However, even after performing inferential statistics, one is still making a decision with some degree of uncertainty.

An outcome that is highly unlikely (i.e., one that results in a low probability value) if the null hypothesis were true leads one to reject the null hypothesis. Most researchers set this probability value (alpha) as five times in 100, or 0.05. An outcome that is more likely (>0.05) will result in a failure to reject the null hypothesis.

Type I and Type II Errors

Although inferential statistics help one make a decision (e.g., reject or not reject the null hypothesis), there is still a possibility that the decision made may be incorrect because the decision is based on the *probability* of a given outcome. Figure 3.1.1.4 shows that four outcomes are possible; two of the outcomes are correct decisions and two are errors. The correct outcomes are (a) to not reject the null hypothesis when it is true (there is, in fact, no difference) and (b) to reject the null hypothesis when it is false (a correct decision that there is a difference). The error of commission is (c) to reject the null hypothesis when, in fact, it is true—type I error (saying that there is a difference when there really was no difference). The error of omission is (d) to not reject the null hypothesis when it is false—type II error (saying that there was no difference when there really was a difference).

Statistical Power

Statistical power is the probability of a correct decision to *reject the null hypothesis when it is false.* Conventionally, the desired statistical power of a study is 0.80. Because statistical power is inversely related to a type II error, that error would be 0.20 if power is 0.80.

Although there are numerous methods to increase statistical power, the most common is to increase the size of the sample. In order to determine how many participants to include in a study, one must know the significance level (usually established at 0.05), type of hypothesis (directional or

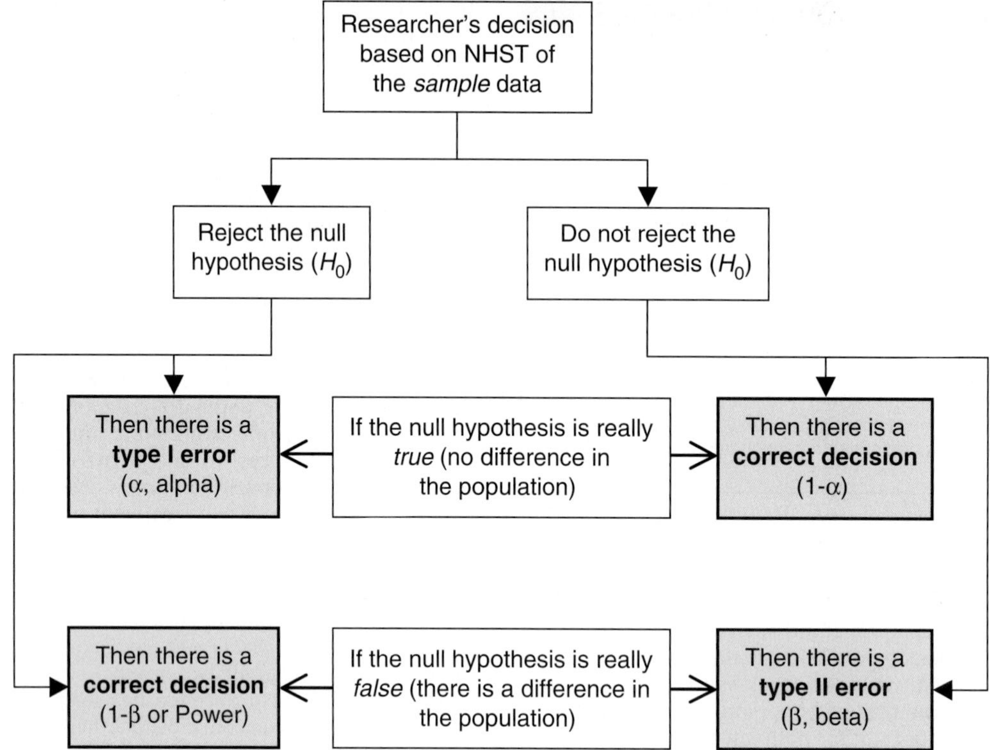

FIGURE 3.1.1.4. Flow chart showing the four possible outcomes (two correct and two errors, type I and type II) that could result from a decision to reject or not reject a null hypothesis.

nondirectional), desired power (0.8 if possible), and an estimate of the effect size (the strength of the relationship between the independent variable and the dependent variable, often stated in standard deviation units). Effect size information comes from a review of the literature on the topic. Most current research syntheses contain a meta-analysis that results in an effect size estimate.

Once the information (significance level, type of hypothesis, amount of power, and effect size) has been obtained, a power table or computer program can be used to determine the needed number of participants. Although increasing the number of participants in a study is a good way to increase statistical power, often this option is not possible. In program evaluation, frequently the number of participants is fixed, often below that desired for adequate power. There are other methods to increase power, such as using homogeneous groups, making sure the measure has strong evidence for reliability, and sometimes choosing a within-subjects design to reduce variability. Lipsey (11) and Cohen (5) provided valuable information on this topic.

More Points about Hypothesis Testing

Three more points about inferential statistics and hypothesis testing need to be considered. First, when the null hypothesis is not rejected, it is never actually accepted. There could be many reasons why the study did not result in a rejection of the null hypothesis. Perhaps another more powerful or better designed study might result in a rejection of the null hypothesis.

Second, testing the null hypothesis is a key part of all types of inferential statistical procedures used with all of our research approaches except the descriptive approach.

Last, in order to provide a fair test of the null hypothesis, there must be adequate statistical power. A power analysis should be planned prior to the study.

Practical Significance Versus Statistical Significance

A common misinterpretation is to assume that statistically significant results are practically or clinically important, but statistical significance is not the same as practical significance or importance. With large samples, statistical significance can be obtained even when the differences or associations are very small/weak. Thus, in addition to statistical significance, it is important to examine confidence intervals and/or the effect size.

An Evidence-Based Approach to Quantitative Research

While there have been numerous criticisms of NHST (10), perhaps the most important is the limited focus on a single study and its dichotomous outcome of whether the result was statistically significant or not. Furthermore, when we dichotomize statistical significance, we become removed from the actual data of our study. Underlying the evidence-based approach is the knowledge that a single study is not sufficient to use as evidence to substantiate a hypothesis or theory. The evidence-based approach relies less on statistical significance and more on confidence intervals and effect sizes.

Confidence Intervals

Confidence intervals (CI) use the same information that is needed to perform NHST. In the above section on NHST, we gave an example of comparing an intervention group who received therapy with a group that did not receive therapy. We stated that the mean of the population of those who receive the intervention will be greater than the mean of the population of those who do not receive the intervention. Using NHST, our outcome is expressed as a difference between sample means, and a statement of significance at a preset alpha level. With confidence intervals, our outcome is expressed as an interval around the sample mean with a lower and upper boundary and a level of confidence (usually 95%). Confidence intervals give an estimate of an interval that includes the actual population mean (or in many cases, an estimate of the difference between the intervention and control means). Unfortunately, the confidence interval derived from a single study does not necessarily include the population mean. Typically speaking, if 95% confidence intervals were developed on 100 studies, using the same sample size, independent and dependent variables, the confidence intervals in 95 of the studies would include the population mean and five would not. That is why confidence intervals are become more important for *multiple studies*.

If one increases the CI from 95% to 99%, and confidence that the true population mean (or difference between means) is in the interval also increases. However, other things being equal, the range (breadth) of the confidence interval also increases.

Effect Size

While confidence intervals always should be reported, they also have limitations. One of the problems is that the dependent variable from study to study must be the same to compare the different intervals. Unfortunately, exact replications of previous work are relatively rare because they are not rewarded by academic institutions. Therefore, replications of previous work are likely to involve some alteration of the independent variable, the dependent variable, or both. To solve this problem, researchers have added a second strategy to the evidence-based approach: effect size. As will be pointed out later in this chapter, numerous studies can be synthesized using effect sizes to provide an overall estimate of the effect on the independent variable (intervention) on the dependent variable (outcome).

A statistically significant outcome does not give information about the strength or size of the outcome or the effect. Effect size is the strength of the relationship between the independent variable and the dependent variable and/or the magnitude of the difference between levels of the independent variable with respect to the dependent variable. Statisticians have proposed effect size measures that fall mainly into three types or families: the *r* family, the *d* family, and measures of risk potency. We discuss these effect sizes and clinical significance in more detail below.

Steps in Interpreting Inferential Statistics

To fully interpret the results of an inferential statistic, the author should consider four issues.

First, decide whether to reject the null hypothesis, as discussed earlier.

Second, the direction of the effect should be stated. Difference inferential statistics compare groups, so which group performed better should be noted. For associational inferential statistics (e.g., correlation), the sign is very important, so whether the association or relationship is positive or negative should be clear.

Third, the effect size should be included in the description of the results or, at the least, the information to compute it should be presented. The interpretation of the effect size is subjective.

Fourth, the researcher or the consumer of the research (clinician and patient/client) should make a judgment about whether the result has practical or clinical significance or importance. To do so the effect size, the costs of implementing change, and the probability and severity of any side effects or unintended consequences need to be taken into account.

Examples of the Use and Interpretation of Statistics

In Figure 3.1.1.2 we divided research questions into difference questions and associational questions. *Difference questions* compare groups and utilize the statistics, which we call *difference inferential statistics* (e.g., *t* test and analysis of variance). *Associational questions* examine the association or relationship between two or more variables. They utilize *associational inferential statistics* (correlation and regression). Figure 3.1.1.5 is a decision tree that shows how researchers might make a decision about what type of inferential statistic to use. A clinician/reader might work backward from a reported statistic to understand a rationale for the choice of a statistic.

The following examples are from articles published in the *Journal of the American Academy of Child and Adolescent Psychiatry*. Readers can find the original study in the reference list or they can see an expanded version of our description of the study and how the cited statistic was interpreted in Morgan et al. (3).

Basic (Two Variable) Difference Questions and Statistics. For the *independent samples t test* and *one-way ANOVA*, the article we selected was by Herpertz et al. (12), who compared three groups of boys on psychophysiological and other measures (e.g., IQ). They had three levels of the independent variable, (ADHD, ADHD + CD, and a comparison group without ADHD), a between- or independent-groups design (unrelated children in each group), and a normally distributed dependent variable (IQ), so an appropriate statistic was one-way ANOVA to compare the three levels or groups. A nonparametric statistic could have been used to compare the three groups of boys if the ANOVA assumptions had been markedly violated. If Herpertz et al. had just compared two of the groups (e.g., ADHD and ADHD + CD) they could have used an independent samples *t* test.

To illustrate the *paired samples t test* and *repeated-measures ANOVA*, we chose an article by Compton et al. (13), who assessed the benefits of sertraline in adolescents with social anxiety disorder in an open 8-week trial. They applied the paired *t* test to assess whether there was a change from the baseline to the end of the trial on the behavior avoidance test. They used repeated-measures ANOVA to determine whether there was clinical improvement at 2, 4, 6, and 8 weeks compared to the baseline. These statistics were used because there was one group of adolescents assessed repeatedly (within-subjects design).

Basic (Two Variable) Associational Questions and Statistics. Dierker et al. (14) chose *Pearson correlations* to study the association or relationship between depression (CES-D scale) and anxiety (RCMAS). Note that both variables had many levels ranging from low to high, and these variables were at least approximately normally distributed.

A study by Wolfe et al. (15) was selected to illustrate the applicability of *chi-square*. They examined the relationship between family intactness (yes or no) and maltreatment classification (maltreated in the past or not). Note that both variables were dichotomous and produce a 2 × 2 contingency table. We will discuss risk potency effect size measures such as odds ratio (OR) and risk ratio (RR), which are commonly used to help researchers and clinicians interpret data from 2 × 2 tables.

Complex (Three or more Variable) Questions and Statistics. When there are three or more variables, we call the statistics complex rather than multivariate, because there is not unanimity about the definition of multivariate, and several such complex statistics (factorial ANOVA) are not usually classified as multivariate. It is possible to break down a complex research

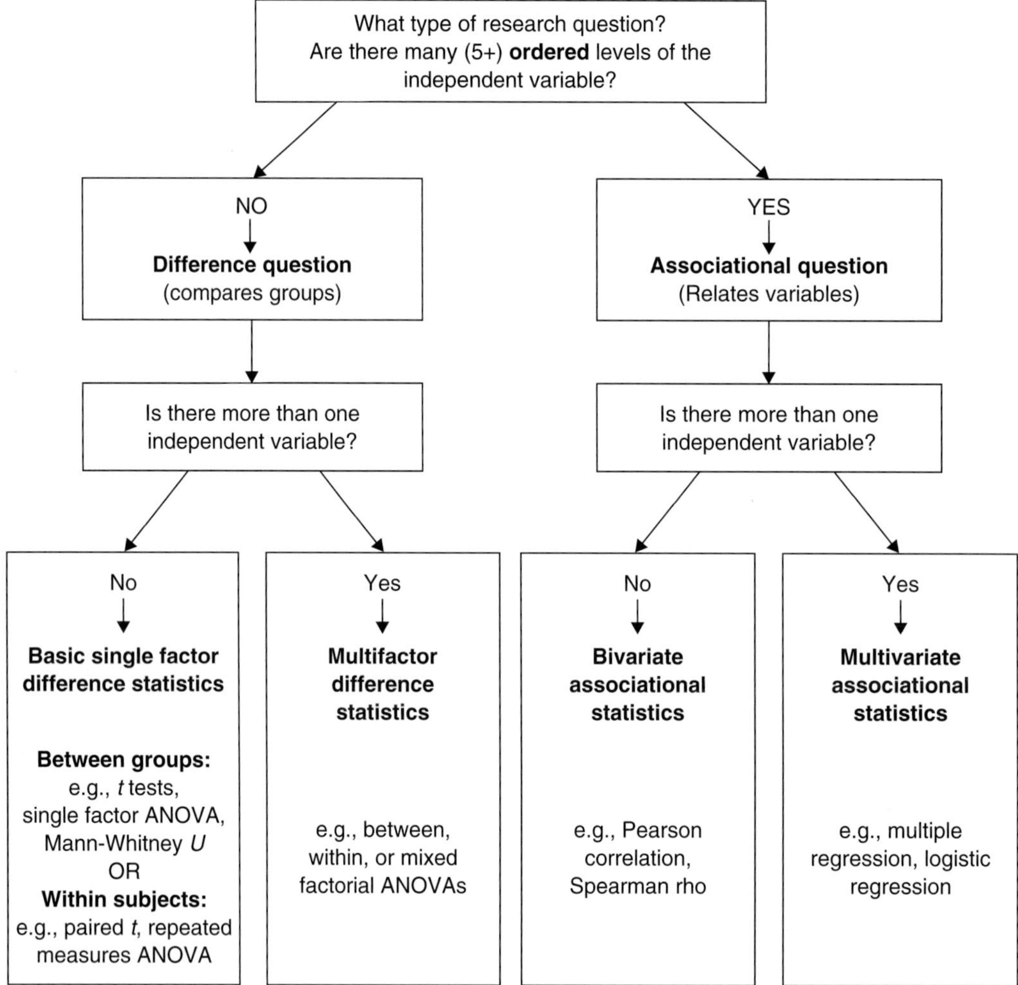

FIGURE 3.1.1.5. A decision tree for the selection of an appropriate inferential statistic.

problem or question into a series of basic (bivariate) questions and analyses as above. However, there are advantages to combining several bivariate questions into one complex analysis: Additional information is provided and a more accurate overall picture is obtained.

Conners et al. (16) selected *factorial ANOVA* to study the effects of four types of treatment and six treatment sites (a 4 × 6 factorial design) on a composite change or improvement scores in children with ADHD. Note that there are two between-groups independent variables (treatment type and site) and one dependent variable (improvement in ADHD symptoms).

Multiple regression was chosen by Logan and King (17) to study the extent of parents' ability to identify signs of depression in their adolescents (the dependent variable). They examined whether a combination of several independent variables would predict the degree to which parents could identify depression. Some of those independent variables were continuous and some were dichotomous.

Mick et al. (18) selected *logistic regression* to study whether children who had been diagnosed with ADHD or not (the dependent variable) seemed to be influenced by prenatal exposure to smoking, alcohol, and/or drug use. These and several of the "control" independent variables were dichotomous (parent smoked or did not smoke).

When there is a design similar to that appropriate for a *t* test or ANOVA but there are *two or more* normally distributed dependent variables that are moderately interrelated, it is desirable to consider treating the variables simultaneously with a *multivariate analysis of variance* (MANOVA). Marmorstein and Iacono (19) chose MANOVA to study differences between depression (yes or no) and conduct disorder (yes or no) on a linear combination of several dependent variables (grade point average, number of school suspensions, number of substance abuse symptoms) considered together.

The General Linear Model

Exploring the *relationship between variables can be addressed in two ways* as shown in Figure 3.1.1.6. Researchers choose to use either difference or associational statistics, but statisticians point out that the distinction between difference and associational statistics is artificial, as both serve the purpose of exploring and describing relationships (top box) and both are subsumed by the *general linear model* (middle box); that is, all common parametric statistics are relational. Thus, all of the methods used to analyze one continuous dependent variable and one or more independent variables, either continuous or categorical, are mathematically equivalent.

The bottom part of Figure 3.1.1.6 indicates that a *t* test or one-way ANOVA with a nominal or dichotomous independent variable is analogous to eta, which is a correlation coefficient for a nominal independent variable and a continuous dependent variable. Likewise, a one-way ANOVA with a continuous independent variable is analogous to bivariate

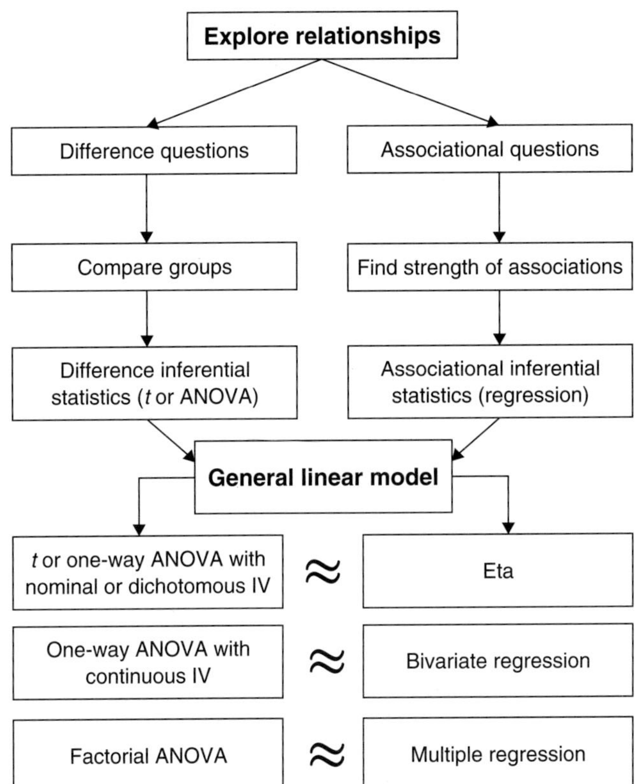

FIGURE 3.1.1.6. Schematic diagram showing how the general linear model is related to the purposes for and types of inferential statistics.

regression. Thus, if there is a continuous, normally distributed dependent/outcome variable and there are five or more levels of a normally distributed independent variable, it would be appropriate to analyze it with either regression or a one-way ANOVA. Finally, as shown in the lowest boxes in Figure 3.1.1.6, factorial ANOVA and multiple regression are analogous mathematically.

Although our distinction between difference and associational parametric statistics is a simplification, we think it is useful educationally. Table 3.1.1.11 provides a list of sometimes confusing statistical terms and alternative names for them. The appendix provides a list of some research terms which are partially similar (or overlapping), but need to be distinguished.

TABLE 3.1.1.11

SIMILAR TERMS ABOUT STATISTICS

- Alternative hypothesis ≈ research hypothesis ≈ H_1
- ANOVA ≈ *F* ≈ analysis of variance ≈ overall or omnibus *F*
- Associate variables ≈ relate ≈ predict → correlation or regression
- AUC ≈ probability of a superior (better) outcome
- Basic inferential statistics ≈ univariate statistics (one IV and one DV) ≈ also called bivariate statistics
- Compare groups ≈ test differences → *t* or ANOVA
- Complex inferential statistics ≈ multifactor statistics (more than one IV) ≈ multivariate statistics (usually more than one DV)
- Data mining ≈ fishing ≈ snooping ≈ multiple significance tests (without clear hypotheses)
- Multiple regression ≈ multiple linear regression
- Null hypothesis ≈ Ho
- Post hoc test ≈ follow-up tests ≈ multiple comparisons
- Repeated-measures ANOVA ≈ within-subject ANOVA
- Risk difference ≈ absolute risk reduction
- Significance level ≈ alpha level ≈ α
- Significance test ≈ null hypothesis significance test ≈ NHST
- Single-factor ANOVA ≈ one-way ANOVA

Note: The term we use most often is listed on the left. Similar terms (indicated by ≈) used by other researchers and/or us are listed to the right, and → means "leads to."

SUMMARIZING STATISTICAL OUTCOMES

Meta-analysis: Formulation and Interpretation

Meta-analysis is a research synthesis of a set of studies that uses a quantitative measure, effect size, to indicate the strength of relationship between the treatment or other independent variable and the dependent variables. Not all research syntheses are meta-analyses. Often, the purpose of a research synthesis is to provide a description of a subject area, illustrating the studies that have been undertaken. In other cases, the studies are too varied in nature to provide a meaningful effect size index. The focus of this section, however, is on research syntheses that result in a meta-analysis. (For a more detailed discussion see Lipsey and Wilson [20].)

One advantage of performing a meta-analysis includes the computation of a summary statistic for a large number of studies. This summary statistic provides an overall estimate of the strength of relationship between independent and dependent variables. A second advantage of meta-analysis is that it provides evidence of the reliability of a research finding. Researchers have more confidence in the findings of multiple studies than in the results of a single study. A third advantage is that it takes into account studies that failed to find statistical significance and may not have been published, perhaps because of a lack of statistical power (reduced sample size). A fourth advantage of meta-analysis is increased external validity. Many studies, strong in internal validity (design characteristics), do not use a representative sample of subjects. This limits the generalization of results. However, including many studies increases the variation of the sample and strengthens external validity.

Although there are many advantages to meta-analysis, there also has been considerable criticism. The most frequent criticism of meta-analysis is that it may combine "apples and oranges." Synthesizing studies that might differ on both independent and dependent variables brings into question the usefulness of the end product. Furthermore, many studies have similar independent and dependent variables, but differ in the strength of design. Should these studies be combined? Another criticism concerns small sample size. Introducing a large proportion of studies with inadequate statistical power into a meta-analysis could introduce bias into the overall effect size. Last, even though the statistics used in meta-analysis are quite sophisticated, the end product will never be better than the individual studies that make up the meta-analysis.

Criteria for Review

Although much of the focus of meta-analysis is on statistical procedures, perhaps the most important part of a meta-analysis is the planning of inclusion and exclusion criteria for selecting a study into the meta-analysis. These inclusion and exclusion criteria are often related to internal validity and external validity. Most researchers feel that meta-analyses composed of randomized control trials (RCTs) represent the gold standard for clinical research.

Statistical Computations for Individual Studies

Type of Effect Size. There are numerous types of effect size indices. Briefly, the *d* effect size indicates the strength of a relationship between an independent and dependent variable in standard deviation units. The most common effect size indices used in meta-analyses are *d*, *r*, and OR, although RR and number needed to treat (NNT) also have been used.

Number of Effect Sizes. Each study in the meta-analysis should yield at least one effect size. It is not uncommon, however, to observe studies that compare a treatment group with a control group on many measures. An effect size could be computed for each measure of the study. However, when studies have more than one measure, the measures are usually related or correlated. Thus, computing more than one effect size yields redundant information and gives too much weight to that particular study. Therefore, the researcher should select one representative measure from the study or use a statistical method to determine a representative measure.

Weights. For the most part, each study included in the meta-analysis is based on a different sample size. Studies with larger sample sizes are likely to be better estimates than studies with small sample sizes. Therefore, in order to take sample size into consideration when the effect sizes are averaged, a weight is computed for each effect size. Effect sizes also can be weighted by other important indices, such as quality of the study.

Computation of Combined Effect Size for Studies and Related Statistics

When all studies that meet the criteria for inclusion in the meta-analysis have been coded and effect size data entered, a *combined effect size* can be computed. Frequently there is an effect size computed for each construct. In addition to a mean effect size index computed for each construct, a confidence interval, usually 95%, also is obtained. Analyses also are performed to test for statistical significance, computing a *z* statistic, and to test for homogeneity, computing a *Q* statistic. If *Q* is statistically significant, the null hypothesis of homogeneity is rejected and the researcher assumes a heterogeneous distribution.

The most common follow-up procedure when a test for homogeneity of effect size distribution is statistically significant is to attempt to identify the variability that is contributing to the heterogeneity. Most often, the researcher has in mind, prior to the meta-analysis, certain hypotheses about which variables might contribute to variability in the mean effect size. These variables (such as strength of research design, sample subgroups, gender) are usually referred to as *moderator* variables.

Moderator variables are variables that interact with the independent variable to *cause* the change in the dependent variable. For example, gender might be a moderator variable that interacts with treatment such that there is only a success in women and not men. Moderator variables are often confused with *mediator* variables. Mediator variables are intervening variables between the independent and dependent variables that help explain the change in the dependent variable. For example, a meta-analysis might find class size (independent variable) is inversely related to student achievement (dependent variable). The mediator variable might be teacher attention, which intervenes between the independent and dependent variables.

Meta-analysis is a valuable tool for both the researcher and the clinician. Summarizing the results of many studies as an effect size index provides important strength of relationship information. Caution always should be used concerning the types of studies that went into the meta-analysis; especially, one should be aware of design issues.

Effect Sizes and Clinical Significance

Behavioral scientists are interested in answering three basic questions when examining the relationships between variables (21). First, should an observed result be attributed to chance or is it real (statistical significance)? Second, if the result is real, how large is it (effect size)? Third, is the result large enough to be meaningful and useful (clinical or practical significance)? In this chapter, we treat clinical significance as equivalent to practical significance.

Clinical Significance

The clinical significance of a treatment is based on external standards provided by clinicians, patients, and/or researchers. Judgments by the researcher and the consumers (clinicians and patients) regarding clinical significance should consider factors such as clinical benefit, cost, and side effects. Although there is no formal statistical test of clinical significance, we suggest using an effect size measure to assist in interpreting clinical significance. Each of these measures, however, has limitations that require the clinician to be cautious about interpretation.

Effect Size Measures

Statisticians have proposed many effect size measures. They fall mainly into three types or families: the *r* family, the *d* family, and measures of risk potency.

The *r* Family. One method of expressing effect sizes is in terms of strength of association, with statistics such as the Pearson product moment correlation coefficient, *r*, used when both the independent and the dependent measures are normally distributed. Such effect sizes vary between −1.0 and +1.0, with 0 representing no effect. This family of effect sizes also includes associational statistics such as the Spearman or Kendall rank correlation coefficients, and the multiple correlation coefficient (R).

The *d* Family. These effect sizes are used when the independent variable is binary (dichotomous) and the dependent variable is normally distributed. The *d* family effect sizes use different formulas, but they all express the mean difference in standard deviation units. Effect sizes for *d* range from minus to plus infinity, with zero indicating no effect; however, it is unusual to find *d* values in the applied behavioral sciences much greater than 1.

Measures of Risk Potency. These effect sizes are used when both the independent and the dependent variable are binary. There are many such effect sizes, but in this section we discuss five common ones: OR, RR, relative risk reduction (RRR), risk difference (RD), and NNT. ORs and RRs vary from 0 to infinity, with 1 indicating no effect. RRR and RD range from −1 to 1, with zero indicating no effect. NNT ranges from 1 to plus infinity, with very *large values* indicating no treatment effect.

AUC or Probability of a Superior Outcome. Finally we discuss an index that can be used when the independent variable is binary, but the dependent variable can be either binary or ordered. AUC stands for *area under the curve* but could be called the probability of a superior (better) outcome of one treatment over another. AUC integrates many of the other effect size indices and is directly related to clinical significance. Kraemer et al. (22) and Grissom and Kim (23) provide more information on this relatively new effect size.

Unfortunately, there is little agreement about which effect size to use for each situation. The most commonly discussed effect size in the behavioral sciences, especially for experiments, is *d*, but the correlation coefficient, *r*, and other measures of the strength of association are common in survey research. In medical journals, an OR is most common.

In the remainder of this section, we discuss the use and interpretation of each of the above measures and discuss the advantages and disadvantages of each as indicators of clinical significance. In this discussion, we focus on positive association only—that is, effect sizes ranging from the value that indicates no effect to the value indicating maximal effect.

Interpreting *d* and *r* Effect Sizes

Table 3.1.1.12 provides general guidelines for interpreting the size of the effect for five measures discussed in this section. Cohen (5) provided research examples of what he labeled small, medium, and large effects suggested by *d* and *r* values. Most researchers would not consider a correlation (*r*) of 0.5 to be very strong because only 25% of the variance in the dependent variable is predicted. However, Cohen argued that when the two variables measure different constructs, an *r* of 0.3 is typical and 0.5 is about as large as correlations are found in applied behavioral sciences. When, as in test–retest reliability measures, the two variables measure the same construct, typical correlations are much higher, for example, 0.7 or more.

Cohen (5) also pointed out that effects with a *d* of 0.8 are "grossly perceptible and therefore large differences...." Cohen's medium size effect is "visible to the naked eye. That is, in the course of normal experiences, one would become aware of an average difference." Kazdin and Bass (24), based on a review of psychotherapy research, found that *d* was approximately 0.8 when comparing a new active treatment against an inactive (treatment withheld) placebo. Comparing a new effective treatment with a usual or comparison treatment would produce a *d* of about 0.5.

The *d* and *r* guidelines in Table 3.1.1.12 are based on the effect sizes commonly found in studies in the applied behavioral sciences. They do not have absolute meaning; Cohen's "large," "medium," and "small" were meant to be relative to typical findings in behavioral research in general. For that reason, we suggest using "larger than typical" instead of "large," "typical" instead of "medium," and "smaller than typical" instead of "small." However, as suggested by the Kazdin and Bass (24) results, it is advisable to examine the research literature to see if there is information about typical effect sizes for those variables, in that context. The standards expressed in Table 3.1.1.12 then would need to be adjusted accordingly.

There are disadvantages of the *d* and *r* effect sizes as measures of clinical significance. First, they are relatively abstract, and consequently may not be meaningful to patients and clinicians, or even to researchers. They were not originally intended to be indices of clinical significance and are not readily interpretable in terms of how much *individuals* are affected by treatment.

Interpreting Measures of Risk Potency

Clinicians must make categorical decisions about whether or not to use a treatment (medication, therapy, hospitalization), and the outcomes also are often binary. For example, a child is classified as having ADHD or not, or being at risk for some negative outcome or not. In comparing two treatments, a positive outcome might indicate that the patient is sufficiently improved (or not) to meet the criteria for a clinically significant change. These binary decisions and outcomes provide data in a 2 × 2 contingency table. In some cases, a 2 × 2 table results when initially continuous outcome data are dichotomized (when responses on an ordered outcome measure in a clinical trial are reclassified as "success" and "failure"). Such dichotomization not only results in a loss of information, but, dichotomizing can result in inconsistent and arbitrary effect size indices due to different choices of the cut point or threshold for failure.

Odds Ratio. OR is the most commonly reported of these measures. However, a major limitation of the OR as an effect size index is that the magnitude of the OR may approach infinity if the outcome is rare or very common, even when the association is near random or no effect. The magnitude of the OR varies strongly with the choice of cut point.

Risk Ratio. Again, the choice of cut point and which RR (failure or success) is chosen change the magnitude of the RR, making it hard to interpret. Because the RR may approach infinity when the risk in the denominator approaches zero, there can be no agreed-on standards for assessing the magnitude or clinical significance of RR.

TABLE 3.1.1.12

INTERPRETATION OF THE STRENGTH (EFFECT SIZE) OF A POSITIVE RELATIONSHIP

General Interpretation of the Strength of a Relationship	The *d* Family: *d*	The *r* Family *r*	2 × 2 Associations *AUC*	*RD*	NNT
Much larger than typical	≥1.00	≥.70	≥76%	≥52%	≤1.9
Large or larger than typical	0.80	0.50	71%	43%	2.3
Medium or typical	0.50	0.30	64%	28%	3.6
Small or smaller than typical	0.20	0.10	56%	11%	8.9

Note: We interpret the numbers in this table as a range of values. For example, *d* greater than 0.90 (or less than –0.90) would be described as much "larger than typical," in the applied behavioral sciences, *d* between say 0.70 and 0.90 would be called "larger than typical," and *d* between say 0.60 and 0.70 would be "typical to larger than typical." We interpret the other columns similarly. AUC, Area under the curve, or probability of a superior outcome; RD, Risk difference; NNT, Number needed to treat.

Relative Risk Reduction. RRR can vary between 0 and 1.0. Because the "failure" RRR may be very small when the "success" RRR is large, RRR is difficult to interpret in terms of clinical significance, and there are no agreed-upon standards for judging its magnitude.

Risk Difference. RD, also called absolute risk reduction (ARR), can vary from 0% to 100%. When the RD is near zero, it indicates near random association. If the success or failure rates are extreme, the RD is likely to be near 0%. It is troublesome in terms of interpreting clinical significance that the RD is often very near zero when the OR and one of the RRs are very large.

Number Needed to Treat. NNT is a relatively new measure that has been recommended for improving the reporting of effect sizes, but it has not yet been widely used. NNT is the number of patients who must be treated to generate one more success or one less failure than would have resulted had all persons been given the comparison treatment. Mathematically, NNT is the reciprocal of the RD. A result of 1.0 means the treatment is perfect, that every treatment subject succeeds and every comparison subject fails. An NNT greater than 1.0 means that the treatment is less than ideally effective, and the larger the NNT, the relatively less effective the treatment.

AUC or the Probability of a Superior/Better Outcome. This relatively new effect size might substitute for either *d* family measures or measures of risk potency. It represents the probability that a randomly selected participant in the treatment group has a better result than a randomly selected one in the comparison group. As shown in Table 3.1.1.12, one can define guidelines for interpreting AUC that correspond to those for *d*. For example, a medium or typical effect size of $d = 0.5$ corresponds to AUC = 64%. Thus, when comparing a treatment subject against a comparison subject, 64% of the time the treatment subject would have a better response.

AUC is of special interest because it can be computed based on clinical judgments alone. One could randomly select pairs of subjects, one of each pair in the treatment and one in the comparison group, and submit their clinical records to experts with group membership masked. The experts would then be asked which of the two had a better outcome. The proportion of the pairs for which the experts said that the treatment group subject was better off is an estimate of AUC.

Conclusion

Nuovo et al. (25) pointed out that the Consolidated Standards on Reporting Trials (CONSORT) recommends reporting the NNT or the RD. However, often RD can seem unimpressively small, and NNT may seem very large, suggesting very little effect of treatment. In many such cases with small RD or large NNT, one of the RRs and one of the RRR measures and, most of all, the OR can give an inflated impression of the size of the effect, thus exaggerating apparent clinical significance. For this reason, our preferred effect size for understanding clinical significance would tend to be AUC (the probability of a superior outcome), but remember that *d*, NNT, and RD are all mathematically equivalent and can be converted to AUC.

We have provided some general guidelines for interpreting measures of clinical significance. It is not possible, however, to provide any fixed standards that a clinician could use to conclude that an effect size was clinically significant. It makes a difference whether the treatment is for a deadly disease or for the common cold, and whether the treatment is risky and costly or safe and free. The context in which an effect size is used matters in interpreting the size of the effect; the effect size only facilitates consideration of clinical significance.

EVALUATING THE DESIGN AND METHODS OF A RESEARCH STUDY

This concluding section provides an overview of the evaluation of *research validity,* the validity of the design and methods of a study as a whole.

Research Validity Versus Measurement Reliability and Measurement Validity

It is important to distinguish between evidence for the merit or worth of the whole study (*research validity*) as opposed to evidence in support of the quality of a specific instrument or test used in a study (*measurement validity*). Figure 3.1.1.7 shows that measurement reliability and validity (the upper two boxes) are different from, but related to, research reliability and validity (lower boxes), and the figure shows how all four fit into an overall conception of reliability and validity. The horizontal arrow indicates that measurement reliability is a necessary prerequisite for measurement validity (a measure cannot provide evidence for validity if it is not consistent/reliable). The vertical arrow indicates that the validity of a whole study depends to some extent on the reliability and validity of the specific measures or instruments used in the study.

Rating Scales to Evaluate Research Validity

A good study should have moderate to high internal *and* external validity. However, it is hard, in any given study, to achieve this goal. Using our research validity framework, a reader would evaluate a study from low to high on each of the four scales or dimensions shown in Figures 3.1.1.8 and 3.1.1.9. In Morgan et al. (3), we provide a comprehensive framework for evaluating the research validity of an article, including four additional rating scales.

Internal Validity

The top part of Figure 3.1.1.8 indicates the key features we use to rate the dimension of *equivalence of the groups on participant characteristics.* The bottom of Figure 3.1.1.8 shows the five issues that we use to rate the *control of experiences and the environment during the study,* that is, contamination.

External Validity

External validity broadly defined asks about generalizability to other populations, settings, treatment variables, and measurement variables. If a study is not rated high on external validity, the author should at least be cautious about generalizing the findings. We use the three issues in the top of Figure 3.1.1.9 to evaluate *population external validity* and the five issues listed in the bottom part of Figure 3.1.1.9 to evaluate *ecologic external validity,* whether the setting, testers, procedures, and timing of the study are natural and, thus, whether the result of the specific study can be generalized.

ACKNOWLEDGMENTS

This chapter draws heavily on our textbooks, *Understanding and Evaluating Research in Applied and Clinical Settings* (3)

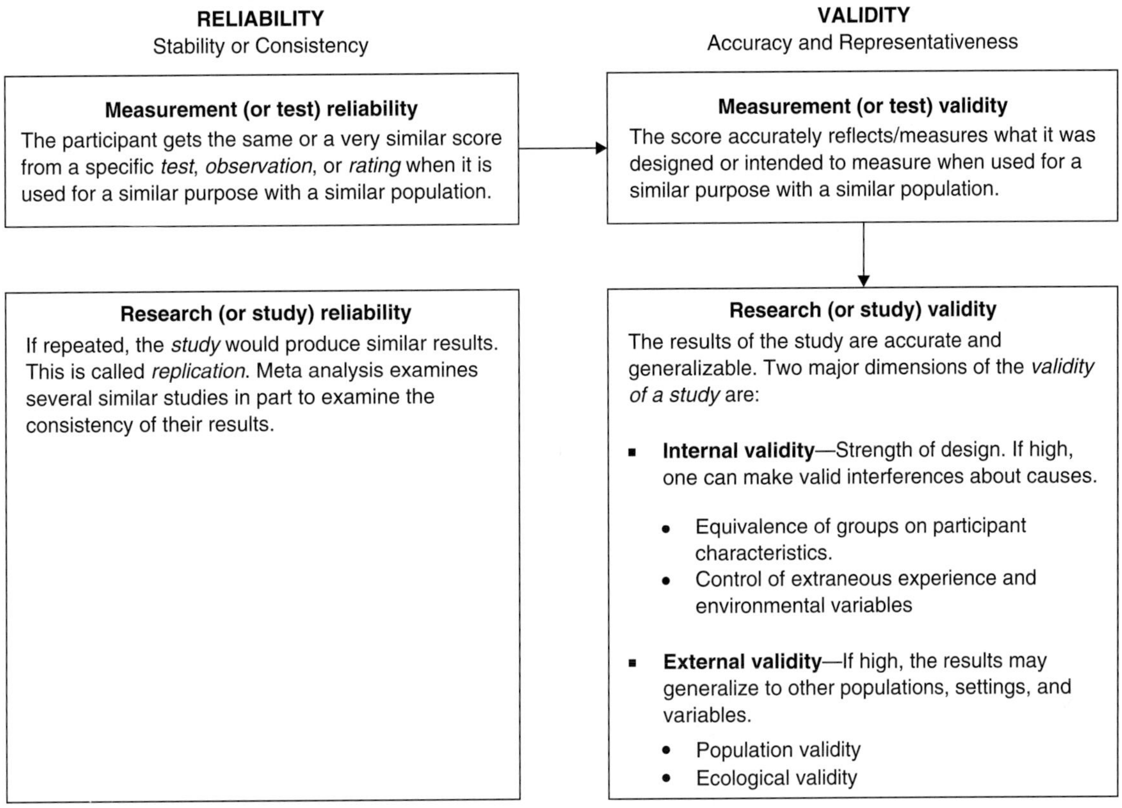

RELIABILITY
Stability or Consistency
VALIDITY
Accuracy and Representativeness
Measurement (or test) reliability
The participant gets the same or a very similar score from a specific test, observation, or rating when it is used for a similar purpose with a similar population.
Measurement (or test) validity
The score accurately reflects/measures what it was designed or intended to measure when used for a similar purpose with a similar population.
Research (or study) reliability
If repeated, the study would produce similar results. This is called replication. Meta analysis examines several similar studies in part to examine the consistency of their results.
Research (or study) validity
The results of the study are accurate and generalizable. Two major dimensions of the validity of a study are:
Internal validity—Strength of design. If high, one can make valid interferences about causes.
Equivalence of groups on participant characteristics.
Control of extraneous experience and environmental variables
External validity—If high, the results may generalize to other populations, settings, and variables.
Population validity
Ecological validity

FIGURE 3.1.1.7. Relationships and differences between measurement reliability and validity and research reliability and validity.

INTERNAL VALIDITY
Equivalence of Groups on Participant Characteristics
Based rating on:
a) Were the participants randomly assigned to the groups?
b) If not, were there adequate attempts to make groups similar (e.g., ANCOVA) or check similarity on a pretest?
c) If no randomization, were there adequate attempts to make groups similar or check similarity on other key variables?
d) Was retention during the study high and similar across groups?
LOW
MEDIUM
HIGH
Groups very different, marked differential attrition
Some attempts to equate groups or groups found to be similar
Random assignment to groups and low attrition
Control of Experiences and Environment Variables (Contamination)
Based rating on:
a) Was the study conducted in a controlled environment (e.g., a lab)?
b) Were extraneous variables that could affect one group more than the others controlled? Did the groups have the same type of environment?
c) Was there a no treatment group (placebo) or usual treatment group?
d) Were extraneous variables that could affect all groups and obscure the true effect controlled?
e) Were attempts to reduce other extraneous influences adequate?
LOW
MEDIUM
HIGH
Extraneous variables not controlled, no comparison group (field setting)
Attempts to control experiences and environment
All extraneous variables controlled, eliminated or balanced (controlled lab)

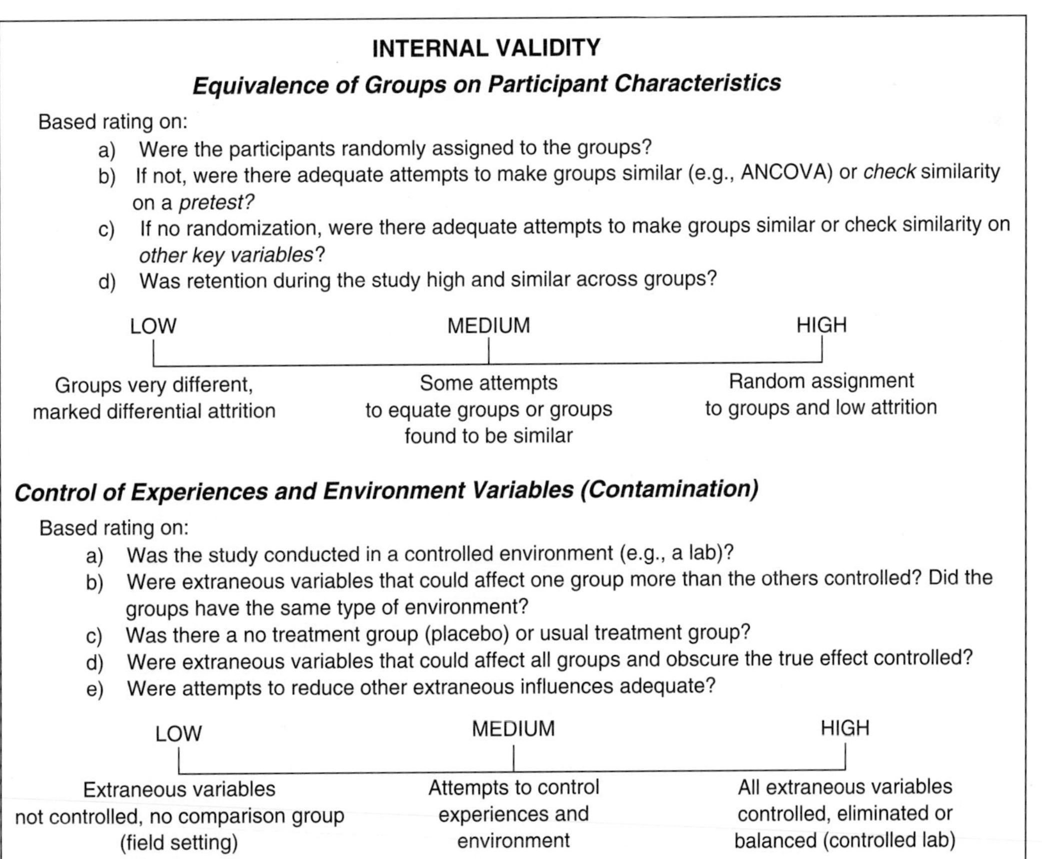

FIGURE 3.1.1.8. Rating scales to evaluate the internal validity of the findings of a study.

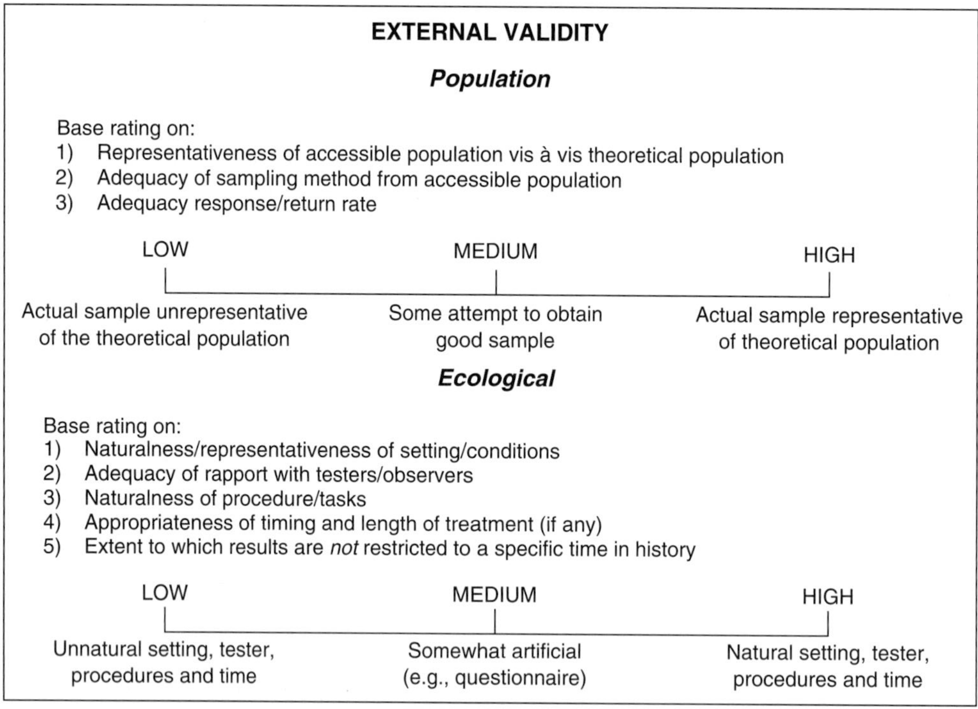

FIGURE 3.1.1.9. Rating scales to evaluate the external validity of the findings of a study.

and our current text Research Methods in Applied Settings (10). We appreciate permission to reprint or adapt from those books all the tables and figures used in this chapter.

Earlier versions of the tables, figures, and text were published as a series of articles, "Clinicians' Guide to Research Methods and Statistics," published between 1999 and 2003 in the *Journal of the American Academy of Child and Adolescent Psychiatry* (JAACAP) by Lippincott Williams & Wilkins. We especially appreciate the critiques and statistical advice on the JAACAP series from Helena Chmura Kraemer, professor of biostatistics at the Stanford University Medical School.

We also acknowledge the advice and encouragement of Andrés Martin, and we thank the Developmental Psychobiology Research Group (DPRG), Department of Psychiatry, University of Colorado School of Medicine, for support over many years. Dr. Harmon's unexpected death was a loss to us personally, and to the profession of child and adolescent psychiatry. We could not have completed the chapter without the word processing skills of Alana Stewart and Jessica Gerton.

APPENDIX: PARTIALLY SIMILAR TERMS FOR DIFFERENT CONCEPTS[1]

- Cronbach's *alpha* ≠ *alpha* (significance) level
- *Dependent* variable ≠ *dependent* samples design or statistic
- *Discriminant* analysis ≠ *discriminant* evidence for measurement validity
- *Factor* (i.e., independent variable) ≠ *factor* analysis
- Factorial *design* ≠ *factorial* evidence for measurement validity
- *Independent* variable ≠ *independent* samples
- *Levels* (of a variable) ≠ *level* of measurement
- *Odds* ratio ≠ *odds*
- *Outcome* (dependent) variable ≠ *outcome* (results) of the study
- Research *question* ≠ questionnaire *question* or item
- *Random* assignment of participants to groups ≠ *random* assignment of treatments to groups
- *Random* assignment (of participants to groups) ≠ *random* selection (or sampling of participants to be included in the study) ≠ random order
- Odds *ratio* ≠ risk *ratio*
- *Related* samples design ≠ variables that are *related*
- Random *samples* ≠ paired/related *samples* ≠ independent *samples*
- Measurement *scale* ≠ a rating *scale* ≠ summated/composite *scale*
- *Theoretical* research ≠ *theoretical* population
- Measurement *validity* ≠ research *validity*

[1]Italicized terms are listed alphabetically; ≠ means "not equal to."

References

1. Patton MQ: *Qualitative Research and Evaluation Methods.* 3rd ed. Thousand Oaks, Sage, 2002.
2. Velleman PF, Wilkinson L: Nominal, ordinal, interval, and ratio typologies are misleading. *Am Statistician* 47:65–72, 1993.
3. Morgan GA, Gliner JA, Harmon RJ: *Understanding and Evaluating Research in Applied and Clinical Settings.* Mahwah, Lawrence Erlbaum Associates, 2006.
4. American Educational Research Association; American Psychological Association; National Council on Measurement in Education: *Standards for Educational and Psychological Testing.* Washington, DC, American Educational Research Association, 1999.
5. Cohen J: *Statistical Power Analysis for the Behavioral Sciences.* 2nd ed. Hillsdale, Lawrence Erlbaum Associates, 1988.
6. Cook TD, Campbell DT: *Quasi-experimentation: Design and Analysis Issues for Field Settings.* Boston, MA, Houghton Mifflin, 1979.
7. Shadish WR, Cook TD, Campbell DT: *Experimental and Quasiexperimental Designs for Generalized Casual Influence.* Boston, MA, Houghton Mifflin, 2002.
8. Fowler FJ Jr: *Survey Research Methods.* 5th ed. Thousand Oaks, Sage, 2014.
9. Kraemer HC, Thiemann S: *How Many Subjects? Statistical Power Analysis in Research.* Newbury Park, Sage, 1987.
10. Gliner JA, Morgan GA, Leech NJ: *Research Methods in Applied Settings: An Integrated Approach to Design and Analysis.* New York, Routledge, 2017.

11. Lipsey MW: *Design Sensitivity: Statistical Power for Experimental Research*. Newbury Park, Sage, 1990.
12. Herpertz SC, Wenning B, Mueller B, et al.: Psychophysiological responses in ADHD boys with and without conduct disorder: implications for adult antisocial behavior. *J Am Acad Child Adolesc Psychiatry* 40:1222–1230, 2001.
13. Compton SN, Grant PJ, Chrisman AK, et al.: Sertraline in children and adolescents with social anxiety disorder: an open trial. *J Am Acad Child Adolesc Psychiatry* 40:564–571, 2001.
14. Dierker LC, Albano AM, Clarke GN, et al.: Screening for anxiety and depression in early adolescence. *J Am Acad Child Adolesc Psychiatry* 40:929–936, 2001.
15. Wolfe DA, Scott K, Wekerle C, et al.: Child maltreatment: risk of adjustment problems and dating violence in adolescence. *J Am Acad Child Adolesc Psychiatry* 40:282–289, 2001.
16. Conners CK, Epstein JN, March JS, et al.: Multimodal treatment of ADHD in the MTA: an alternative outcome analysis. *J Am Acad Child Adolesc Psychiatry* 40:159–167, 2001.
17. Logan DE, King CA: Parental identification of depression and mental health service use among depressed adolescents. *J Am Acad Child Adolesc Psychiatry* 41:296–304, 2002.
18. Mick E, Biederman J, Faraone SV, et al.: Case-control study of attention-deficit hyperactivity disorder and maternal smoking, alcohol use, and drug use during pregnancy. *J Am Acad Child Adolesc Psychiatry* 41:378–385, 2002.
19. Marmorstein NR, Iacono WG: Major depression and conduct disorder in a twin sample: gender, functioning, and risk for future psychopathology. *J Am Acad Child Adolesc Psychiatry* 42:225–233, 2003.
20. Lipsey MW, Wilson DB: *Practical Meta-analysis*. Thousand Oaks, Sage, 2000.
21. Kirk RE: Promoting good statistical practices: some suggestions. *Educ Psychol Meas* 61:213–218, 2001.
22. Kraemer HC, Morgan GA, Leech NL, et al.: Measures of clinical significance. *J Am Acad Child Adolesc Psychiatry* 42:1524–1529, 2003.
23. Grissom RJ, Kim JJ: *Effect Sizes for Research: Univariate and Multivariate Applications*. 2nd ed. New York, Routledge, 2011.
24. Kazdin AE, Bass D: Power to detect differences between alternative treatments in comparative psychotherapy outcome research. *J Consult Clin Psychol* 57:138–147, 1989.
25. Nuovo J, Melnikov J, Chang D: Reporting number needed to treat and risk difference in randomized controlled trials. *JAMA* 287:2813–2814, 2002.

CHAPTER 3.1.2 ■ EVIDENCE-BASED PRACTICE AS A CONCEPTUAL FRAMEWORK

JOHN HAMILTON

INTRODUCTION

Child and adolescent psychiatry is a unique discipline, often practiced within the context of a multiprofessional organization. Hence, this chapter begins with how various professional groups use the phrase "evidence based." It then proceeds to show how evidence-based processes achieve results significantly different than usual practice. It continues with common objections to EBP, with a rebuttal for each. The second part of this chapter presents selected elements of EBP within the context of pediatric mental health: tips on searching the most relevant databases, diagnostic approaches consistent with EBP, choosing a treatment, developing local data, and ideas about developing evidence-based systems. The definition of evidence-based practice used here is *feasible efforts to align clinical practice with valid, reliable, and relevant empirical results regards assessment and treatment in youth with the goal of reducing symptoms and improving functional outcomes—promptly, for extended periods, inexpensively and with few errors or adverse events using processes chosen by the youth and his or her parents or guardian.* This definition is idealistic—hence the adjective *feasible*—but it is useful in outlining the multiple and sometimes conflicting goals of EBP.

THREE STREAMS, ONE RIVER

Varied authors and groups have used "evidence-based" (EB) as a modifying phrase. Evidence-based practice, or EBP (1,2), is the term used here, but there is also evidence-based medicine, or EBM (3), evidence-based services, or EBSs (4), and evidence-based treatments, or EBTs (5). The phrase "empirically supported treatments," or ESTs, is often used interchangeably with EBT (6). To oversimplify, there are three groups. The first group, using the term EBM, is often associated with medication issues and child psychiatrists. The second group, using the term EBT, is associated with psychologists, psychosocial treatments, and the American Psychological Association (APA). The third group, EBS, is associated with systems striving to better use empirical results to improve outcomes. In this chapter, when we refer to EBP, we are including all three groups. These three groups share a common interest in making use of empirical data, both "local" data regards our own patients as well as data from published studies. Combining the work of all three groups produces a powerful flood of ideas.

There is considerable overlap between EBM, EBT, and EBS, but each retains its distinct flavor. EBM authors often focus on changing individual practitioner behavior. For example, EBM tries to interest practitioners in researching "answerable questions" regarding individual patients. Often examples used involve medications. Many well-known EBM leaders like David Sackett are epidemiologists or internists. On the other hand, EBT authors tend to focus more on studying specific manualized psychosocial treatments. EBT authors are often university-affiliated psychologists who study the effectiveness of a psychosocial intervention for a specific disorder, or who distill core elements of effective treatments from multiple studies into modules which can be employed flexibly with a multidisorder focus (7). They also study how a psychosocial intervention "travels" when it is "exported" to sites other than where it was developed. Finally, evidence-based services (EBSs) is a term used by clinicians in delivery systems trying to improve outcomes by better use of empirical evidence (8). In EBS a consensus-building group of providers, administrators, and consumers agrees on a menu of effective interventions including both EBTs and medications. These three empirical approaches are summarized in Table 3.1.2.1. The term evidence-based practices, or EBPs, used here is an umbrella term for processes based on all three groups while valuing patient preference and clinical expertise as well. EBP

TABLE 3.1.2.1

EVIDENCE-BASED MEDICINE (EBM), EMPIRICALLY SUPPORTED TREATMENTS (ESTs), AND EVIDENCE-BASED SYSTEMS (EBS)

	EBM	EST[a]	EBS
Origins	Many ideas developed at McMaster University in Ontario, Canada	American Psychological Association Task Force 12	State of Hawaii Child and Adolescent Mental Health Division (CAMHD)
Central Ideas	PICO (Population/Intervention/ Control or Comparison/Outcome) based on epidemiologic thinking is core idea; "Bringing the literature to the bedside"	Focus on efficacy and effectiveness of well-defined psychosocial interventions; laboratory–clinic gap a major hurdle	Feasible but proven treatments; extensive use of locally generated data; systemwide consensus on effective interventions
Frequent Members	University-based physicians	University-based psychologists	Large systems wanting improved results

[a]Also called Evidence-Based Treatments.

welcomes the use of clinical expertise, for example, in formulating the context of symptoms (9). And, while including both medication and psychosocial interventions, EBP is neutral in choosing between them, an advantage on a multidisciplinary team.

Significant boundaries between child psychology and child psychiatry have shaped these three streams of empiricism. Child psychologists and child psychiatrists typically belong to different professional organizations, attend different conventions, publish in different journals, and occupy different niches in clinical organizations such as state clinics or hospitals. These different worlds naturally evolve different ways of thinking, sometimes referred to as cognitive boundaries (10). In fact, the prevailing paradigm in each discipline may be so different that each discipline has distinct cognitive assumptions and may advance different claims to knowledge. At their worst, boundaries can be sufficiently extreme that there is no common ground for productive dialogue (11).

EBP is a helpful antidote to the tendency of practitioners to identify with a particular discipline or treatment. For example, a practitioner may think of himself as primarily a psychopharmacologist, or as a family therapist, a play therapist, a behavior therapist, or as an expert in delivering a specific manualized therapy. EBP as conceived here, on the other hand, is not attached to a specific treatment modality or profession. Instead, EBP chooses those feasible treatments proven in the most valid studies to deliver the most rapid, complete, and long-lasting improvement in functioning and symptoms with the least harm. A commitment to EBP therefore significantly changes the identity of practitioners: A commitment to finding and using both published and "local" evidence becomes a central value.

In a multidisciplinary team, the processes of making a diagnosis, choosing a treatment, and assessing its results are all significantly different in a team committed to EBP than in a team proceeding "as usual." Table 3.1.2.2 lists a chain of clinical processes fundamental to EBP, and highlights differences between the EBP approach and usual practice in defining the clinical population, in choosing an intervention, and in evaluating its effects relative to a comparison or control group. This order is the familiar PICO format derived from epidemiology: Population, Intervention (or Exposure), Control (or Comparison), and Outcome. Of course, a solo practitioner can also use many of these processes. For example, both the well-known PubMed site as well as the Internet site for the Journal of the American Academy of Child and Adolescent Psychiatry offer extensive resources for searching answerable questions. A major issue for practitioners, however, is how to offer ESTs that often require extensive training. To be competent to deliver Parent management training (PMT) for Oppositional Defiant Disorder, for example (12), or Cognitive Behavioral Treatment or Interpersonal Therapy for depression (13) requires training. Yet a practitioner may choose to obtain training in those ESTs which will be most useful in the practice she has developed. Informal subspecialization among community therapists is also an option.

WHY BOTHER? COMMON OBJECTIONS TO EBP, WITH REBUTTALS

Objections to EBP are inevitable. Here are some common ones; each is followed by a rebuttal.

There is not much evidence in child psychiatry anyway.

A variant of this complaint is *There aren't RCTs for everything.* Although this is certainly true, it is also true that there are a lot more now than when this objection was most popular. A wave of RCTs in the past decade means often there is a relevant RCT. Table 3.1.2.3 shows the increase in the number of RCTs in youth with ADHD or an anxiety disorder or depression or psychosis, searched as MeSH terms, published in PubMed (14). The growth in systematic reviews and meta-analyses has been similar. In addition, the EBP practitioner is committed to the judicious use of the most valid and relevant evidence available, not just RCTs, using a hierarchy of evidence to minimize bias, and RCTs are high up in that hierarchy. But if only case reports exist, then the EBP approach is to use them as evidence.

How closely are therapeutic relationship variables and outcomes associated in youth psychotherapy? Studies of the relationship between treatment outcomes and therapeutic alliance show a significant yet modest effect. A meta-analysis of individual psychotherapy with youth shows a weighted mean correlation of 0.22 ($k = 16$, $n = 1{,}306$, $p < 0.001$) between alliance and outcome (CI = +/–0.06) (15). Moreover, it is the changes in TA that robustly predict reduction in youth symptoms rather than initial alliance (16). And in community-based child therapy, a strong therapeutic relationship supported continuing to attend sessions (17). In addition, the parent–therapist alliance was associated with reductions in internalizing psychopathology, while a close child–therapist alliance assessed during treatment was associated with a reduction in anxiety symptoms (18,19).

In summary, the therapeutic alliance matters in promoting attendance, in dealing with externalizing, and internalizing disorders, as well as in community-based child therapy, and change in the therapeutic alliance robustly predicts symptom reduction. The therapist is an artist, and psychotherapy is a subjective human encounter with a unique youth that can never be captured in an RCT.

At least some therapists object to EBP because it examines outcomes for groups of youths and in the process loses the unique aspects of each individual youth. According to this

TABLE 3.1.2.2

FUNCTIONS AND PROCESSES: TREATMENT AS USUAL VERSUS EBP

Function or Process	Treatment as Usual	Team Committed to EBP
Defining characteristics of clinical population at intake	Highly variable, narrative intake note DSM-IV as guide	Functioning and psychopathology measured with defined instruments while clinical interview establishes alliance and context of symptoms
Defining primary outcome variable(s)	Usually not done	Preference for choosing primary outcome variable(s) at time of evaluation (or assessment)
Choosing an intervention	Chosen on basis of familiarity, ease of use, often clinician specific	Pyramid of evidence has central role, evidence updated regularly
Evaluating local effect of interventions proven elsewhere	Often ignored	Always an issue, addressed via collecting local data
Collecting and making use of composite local diagnostic and outcome data	Rarely done	Always done, including benchmarking results to compare with natural history and published outcomes
Use of outcome data to inform provider, consumer, and administrator	Case outcome often not tracked with reliable measure; minimal aggregate outcome data	Provider, administration, consumer all interested in outcome data, individual and aggregate
Teaching staff EBP	Minimally structured case conferences or traditional supervision	Staff learns EBP in programwide projects and has access to EBP instruction Culture welcomes fidelity monitoring and feedback from data
Linking providers to the literature	Conferences and reading	Conferences and reading; high-speed Internet connections to most useful databases; answerable questions searched often
Overall team culture	Multiple general practices; each clinician on her own	Clinicians specialize often; empirical results direct teamwide consensus

argument, EBP conclusions based on groups of youth fail to respond to each youth's uniqueness since no two youth share exactly the same genetic makeup, cultural heritage, social circumstances, developmental history, and family background. Yet it is a caricature of EBP interventions that they are applied indiscriminately without any interest in the individual. Consider an EBP psychosocial intervention as having a hard core but a soft exterior (20): Whereas the outside can be modified and individualized to make it easy to swallow, the hard inner core contains the essential components which create change.

In addition, newer generations of ESTs are sensitive to the criticism that a manualized treatment needs to be individualized as well as lively and engaging. Consider a recent study of collaborative problem solving in moody children with ODD (21). The design of this study allows for therapists providing the intervention to determine session content on the basis of their assessment of the clinical needs of the child and family. Other authors have also called for blending creativity and flexibility into a manualized treatment to allow individual variation within a defined intervention (22).

TABLE 3.1.2.3

INCREASING RCT EVIDENCE IN CHILD PSYCHIATRY, 1992–2015: PUBMED RCTs FOR ADHD, ANXIETY OR DEPRESSIVE DISORDER, OR PSYCHOSIS

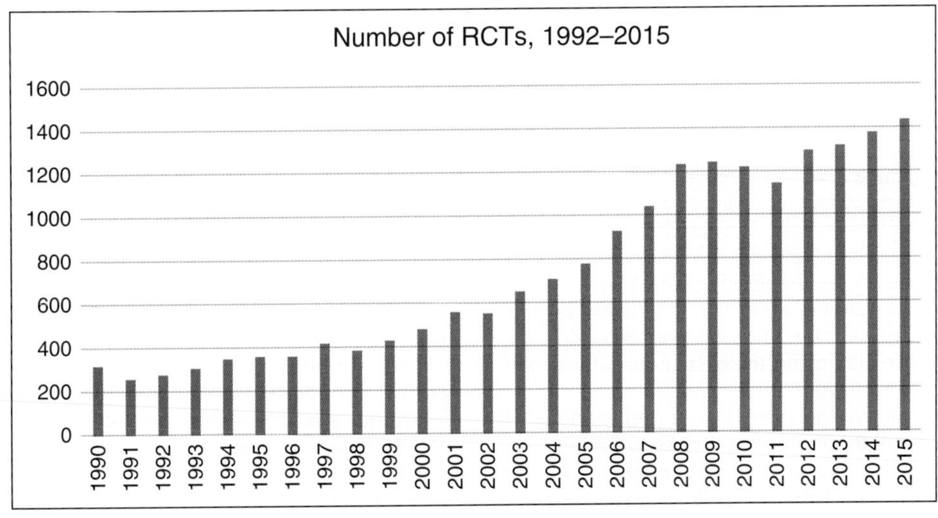

Finally, the first paradigm of the therapist as artist, working with the unique patient to create a unique solution, and the second paradigm of the therapist as adherent to the results of the best science, may be growing toward each other in recent years. For example, some recent EBM articles have softened their position toward the value of experience and clinical judgment (23), while the APA has hardened its position about the importance of randomized trials (24). And efforts to develop strategies based on individualizing treatments supported by research, called personalized interventions, blur usual distinctions (25). Both perspectives can be valued by a practitioner sensitive to multiple inputs: patient preference, his own experience, the nuances of each child, and the most valid available evidence.

THE CASE FOR EBP

Community care of clinically referred youth too often shows unimpressive results.

Two studies have shown that, in real-world practice settings, it is difficult for child mental health interventions to show an effect compared to a control group (26,27). In the first, a randomized study by Bickman et al. (26), one arm of the study received an increase in resources. Interviews were conducted for 2 years following collection of baseline data. Results in measures of symptoms and functioning showed that, while the arm with a considerable increase in resources did have improved access to care and in fact actually received more care, these access differences did not translate into improved clinical outcomes. In addition, children who did not receive any services improved at the same rate as treated children. This sobering conclusion is supported by Weisz and Jensen's review of the effectiveness of both medication and psychosocial intervention in the context of the real world of caring for clinically referred youth. The authors note that evidence, where available, on the effectiveness of such treatment is minimal when compared to the large body of evidence on efficacy. It seems reasonable to conclude that such null results suggest the need for change.

The evidence-based system in Hawaii's clinics appears to have improved outcome results.

In contrast to the sobering conclusions of these null results, committed efforts to build an evidence-based system of care in Hawaii's Child and Adolescent Mental Health Division (CAMHD) appear to have improved outcomes. This story begins in 1994 when federal courts charged the state with establishing a system of care to provide effective mental health and special education services for children and youth as required by federal law (8). The initial system responses to the court's decree included planning efforts and increases in service capacity, allowing more youth to access a wider variety of services, as well as increased quality monitoring and more interagency coordination. The statewide quality monitoring included basic quantitative feedback; this feedback demonstrated more youth being served by more services at a higher cost. Since stakeholders wanted assurances of efficiency, the focus turned to asking whether the increase in resources had led to improved symptomatic and functional outcomes with empirical results as the arbiter. In addition, CAMHD's leaders wanted the system to develop in a way that frontline decisions about patient care were based on the best available evidence. They focused, therefore, on linking the best and most relevant evidence to clinical decisions (8).

To accomplish this linking, the Hawaii Department of Health organized a task force on empirical services in October, 1999 (6); the only requirement for membership was, and remains today, regular attendance and willingness to read and review studies. Its membership has included clinicians from several disciplines, university faculty, parents, administrators, and CAMHD employees. This task force is charged with conducting ongoing multidisciplinary evaluation of psychosocial interventions for common disorders using methodology developed in the Clinical Division of the APA. Additional topics can be reviewed as well, such as the efficacy of seclusion procedures. Each search uses a structured methodology; results are evaluated with a five-level system ranking the efficacy and effectiveness of each intervention. (Effectiveness is based on the performance of the intervention under naturalistic, or real-world, conditions.) The task force begins with a literature-based approach but its diverse constituency tempers the results to fit local conditions.

The result of the task force's work has been a "menu" of recommended treatments distributed to clinicians on a single sheet of blue paper, creating the nickname "blue menu," summarizing recommended psychosocial treatments. It is also posted on the Internet. A one-page review of the task force's conclusions regarding psychotropic medications' efficacy and effectiveness for the children of Hawaii is also distributed and posted on the Internet. Both are updated biennially.

CAMHD also tracks its own results at case, clinic, and system levels wide as well with the Child and Adolescent Functional Assessment Scale, or CAFAS (28), the Child Behavior Check List, Teacher Report Form, and Youth Self-Report (29). Following individual cases allows clinical staff to identify whether or not a youth is improving. Documented ongoing progress leads to the recommendation of continuing the present treatment. If a youth is not improving, the clinicians can reexamine whether there is a problem in treatment selection; if so, a more favorable intervention is sought (8).

Quarterly outcomes based on parent, teacher, and clinician reports for Hawaiian youths treated improved significantly during the years 2001 through 2004, years when the system was actively moving toward EBP (30). The slope of mean improvement in functioning as rated by the CAFAS showed a 146% increase; the slope of mean improvement in CBCL showed a 271% increase, and the TRF a 50% increase over the course of the 3-year period (30). The proportion of youth showing a pattern of improvement during the service episode based on CBCL data rose from 54.7% to 68.2%, based on TRF data from 50.7% to 58.6%, and based on the CAFAS from 66.5% to 69.0%.

These results are consistent with the hypothesis that implementing EBSs significantly impacts both functional outcome and symptomatic outcome. Furthermore, the results are large and clinically significant. Whether the changes in functioning improvement and symptom reduction stabilize here or continue to improve requires continued study. Although this study did not control for such potentially confounding variables as diagnostic mix, gender, or ethnicity impacting the results, it nevertheless shows consistent and large results across three separate informant groups—parent, teacher, and clinician.

Rather than using manualized psychotherapies to integrate the evidence into practice, use "modules" of effective psychotherapy—central elements of multiple randomized trials distilled into a core practice, such as "exposure" or "relaxation training" or "psychoeducation."

In a randomized trial comparing usual care and an approach using modules—central elements of multiple randomized trials, distilled into modules—the modular approach significantly outperformed usual care as well as standard evidence-based treatments based on manuals proven in RCTs (7). A limitation to generalizability of the study's results to many clinics is the minimal use of combined psychotherapy and pharmacotherapy.

If EBP seems, therefore, well worth the effort, let's turn now to its core ideas.

CENTRAL CONCEPTS IN EBP

Number needed to treat, number needed to harm

The number needed to treat, or NNT, for any given intervention in a defined population, is the number of patients we need to treat with the intervention in order to prevent one additional bad outcome (31). This is calculated as follows:

NNT = 1/(Proportion of subjects in control group with bad outcome minus proportion of subjects in intervention group with bad outcome)

The denominator in the NNT equation is called the absolute risk reduction (ARR). Hence, a brief version of the formula is:

$$NNT = 1/ARR$$

As an example of NNTs, consider the Treatment for Adolescents with Depression Study (TADS). The "bad outcome" chosen was a failure to score either much improved or very much improved when assessed by an independent rater using the Clinical Global Impression (CGI) scale. Using this definition of bad outcome, 39.4% of subjects in the fluoxetine cell had a bad outcome versus 65.2% of subjects in the placebo cell. Thus:

$$NNT = 1(0.652 - 0.394) = 1/0.258 = 3.87$$

Therefore the NNT reported for fluoxetine alone was 4, with 95% CI 3 to 8 when response is defined as a CGI score of much improved or very much improved at the end of treatment. The calculated NNT for combined treatment with CBT and fluoxetine using the identical definition of response was 3, with 95% CI 2 to 4 (32). The value of adding CBT to fluoxetine is evident not only in the improved NNT but also in the much narrower confidence intervals. Table 3.1.2.4 calculates NNTs in child and adolescent psychiatry for a variety of other disorders as well. Note that, in general, these NNTs hold up well in comparison with many standard interventions in medicine: Sackett et al. (31) note that the NNT for preventing diabetic neuropathy with 6.5 years of intensive insulin treatment is 15, and that the risk of preventing a death over 5 weeks using streptokinase infusion in patients with acute myocardial infarction is 19. The NNTs in this table are a reflection of the progress made in recent decades in child and adolescent psychiatry.

TABLE 3.1.2.4

ABSOLUTE RISK REDUCTION (ARR) AND NUMBER NEEDED TO TREAT (NNT)[a] FOR SELECTED COMMON DISORDERS IN CHILD AND ADOLESCENT PSYCHIATRY

Disorder/Population	Intervention	Metric	Respond (%) Treatment	Respond (%) Control	ARR	NNT ≤
ADHD (MTA) (33)	Medication Behavioral R_x Both Community	SNAPIV[PT] <1.0[b]	56 34 68	25	31 9 43	3 11 2–3
MDD/Age 12–17 Outpatient TADS Team (32)	Fluoxetine CBT Fluox + CBT Placebo	CGI[c]	60.6 43.2 71.0	 34.8	25.8 8.4 36.2	4 12 3
MDD (34)	CBT Supportive Rx	BDI <9[d] 3 wks in a row	64.7	39.4	25.3	4
POTS (35)	CBT alone Sertraline alone CBT + sertraline Placebo	CY-BOCS <10	21.4 9.3 21.5 1.4 21.6 3.6	 3.6	17.8 5.7 17.9 7.8 17.10 0	3 6 2
ODD, Conduct Disorder (36)	PMT alone PSST alone Combined	CBCL Total Behavior Problems ≤90	38.9 33.3 64.0	Assume 0.0[e]	38.9 33.0 64.0	3 3 2
Mania (37)	Divalproex + quetiapine Divalproex + placebo	YMRS	87	53	34	3
Recurrent MDD (38)	Fluoxetine Placebo	Relapse over 32 wks	CDRS-R >40 + 2 wks doing poorly[f]	34 60	16	7

ADHD, attention deficit hyperactivity disorder; BPR, brief psychiatric rating—children; CBT, cognitive behavioral therapy; CD, conduct disorder; CDRS-R, children's depression rating scale—revised; CY-BOCS, children's Yale-Brown obsessive-compulsive scale; MDD, major depressive disorder; MTA, multimodal treatment of ADHD; ODD, oppositional defiant disorder; PMT, parent management training; POTS, Pediatric Obsessive-Compulsive Disorder Treatment Study; PSST, problem solving skills training; TADS, Treatment of Adolescent Depression Study; YMRS, Young Mania Rating Scale.
[a]How the NNT is calculated varies from study to study, and this needs to be considered when understanding what NNT means for that study (see below).
[b]SNAP-IV, Swanson, Nolan, Pelham, Version IV, parent and teacher rating scale, mean of parent and teacher score.
[c]CGI-Clinical Global Impression score, evaluator-rated, improved or very much improved.
[d]Control received nondirective supportive therapy.
[e]No control used; since the natural history of conduct disorder is that symptoms tend to persist over time, the assumption of no change in symptoms was assumed as the best estimate for a control (39).
[f]Or physician rater's impression of relapse.

By convention, NNT is always a whole number, rounded off to an integer. Note that NNT is impacted by several factors in addition to the effect of the intervention itself. First, how recovery is defined affects NNT; choosing a cutoff that makes it "easy" to achieve recovery produces a lower NNT. Second, how many in the control group spontaneously recover affects NNT; the more spontaneous recoveries in the control group, the more difficult it is to achieve a low NNT. Third, when the data are "sliced" to compare the intervention and comparison group may affect the NNT; time periods when the control and intervention groups diverge the most, such as longer follow-up times, produce lower NNTs. Ideally, NNTs are presented with 95% confidence intervals.

Note that classically, the NNT is calculated relative to a placebo group. However, some studies are purposefully designed without a placebo group for ethical or other reasons. Studies in Table 3.1.2.4 without a placebo arm are the MTA study, the Brent 1997 study, and the Kazdin 1992 study. Consider, for example, the MTA study, and the calculated NNT of 3 in the medication arm. This means it would be necessary to treat about 3 children with the carefully crafted medication management strategy in order to get 1 to reach the defined threshold for improvement who would not have reached that threshold if he had been treated in the community treatment arm. These studies, therefore, set an upper bound on the true NNT: the NNT relative to a true placebo, the formal definition of NNT. Therefore this column is indicated NNT ≤. The only exception to the upper bound rule is the study of PMT and PSST where no change is assumed as a control in the calculation, based on the natural history of the disorder.

The number needed to harm (NNH) is a useful measure of the frequency of undesired consequences from a treatment, and is calculated the same as the NNT, but based on the proportion of patients with the undesired consequence in the intervention group compared to the comparison group. For example, in the TADS study, 3.7% of the fluoxetine alone group had either an elevated mood, mania, or hypomania during the study, versus 1.78% of the placebo group (32). To put this number in context, however, it is important to note that adolescents with known bipolar disorder were excluded, and so were adolescents hospitalized for dangerousness to self or others within 3 months of consent or were deemed "high risk" for suicide. (The NNH regards a mood "switch" for fluoxetine in this sample is therefore 53.) In the same study, the adverse events of irritable or depressed mood including a worsening of depression or irritability or hypersensitivity or anger occurred in 4.6% of the fluoxetine group and 9% of the placebo group, generating an NNH of 22. One or more adverse events occurred in 18.3% of youth in the fluoxetine arm and 8.0% in the placebo group, for an NNH of 10 for at least one adverse event.

Both NNT and NNH are ideally stated with 95% confidence intervals. In practice, few parents wish to hear technical discussions of sample size and confidence intervals. Nevertheless, the issue of confidence intervals can be included with verbal statements like "this has been studied so well we are quite certain about this" if the confidence intervals are narrow. Alternatively, for large confidence intervals, the clinician may state something like "the studies so far have not been definitive, so there's a big range of possible answers once this gets studied in more detail."

Hierarchies of Evidence

If potential "evidence" in EBP is defined as "any empirical observation about the apparent relation between events," (40) then it is useful to have a system for rating such empirical observations about the relation between events, with the least biased studies at the top. In EBP, this is done by creating a vertical hierarchy: Each step of the hierarchy represents a certain level of bias within the research design. With each step downward on the hierarchy, more bias is introduced.

TABLE 3.1.2.5

A HIERARCHY OF STRENGTH OF EVIDENCE FOR TREATMENT DECISIONS

N of 1 randomized controlled trials
Systematic reviews of randomized trials
Single randomized trial
Systematic review of observational studies addressing patient-important outcomes
Single observational study addressing patient-important outcomes
Physiologic studies
Unsystematic clinical observations

(From Guyatt G, et al.: Introduction: the philosophy of evidence-based medicine. In: Guyatt G, Rennie D (eds): *Users' Guides to the Medical Literature: A Manual for Evidence-Based Clinical Practice*. Chicago, IL. AMA Press, 3–12, 2002, with permission.)

The hierarchy of evidence from EBM in Table 3.1.2.5 shows the weight given randomized controlled trials and the even higher weight given systematic reviews of such trials. The N of 1 randomized controlled trial is at the very top position, but it is useful only for certain kinds of interventions, such as a stimulant medication dose which can be randomized to "on" or "off" in the same patient during subsequent time periods. For stimulant dose trials, N of 1 trial data are very good evidence indeed, since they come directly from the patient of interest and concern the treatments under consideration. Unfortunately, however, most other treatments cannot be so easily studied in an N of 1 trial.

Guyatt's "classical EBM" hierarchy of evidence is only a beginning, however, in choosing a treatment. The APA's clinical division (Division 12) has established a hierarchy of evidence for rating psychosocial treatments with several levels. "Well established" requires two independent randomized trials with active controls. "Probably efficacious" requires 1 randomized trial with an active control or two trials with wait-list controls (6). Yet many questions remain in either of these approaches to creating a hierarchy. Even if a treatment is proven to have efficacy in two independent research studies, for example, the question of its effectiveness in a real-world setting remains.

Furthermore, treatment decisions depend not only on the strength of the methods used to establish efficacy or effectiveness, but also on a weighing of benefits against the risks and costs of treatment (41). Table 3.1.2.6 shows an approach to creating a hierarchy of recommendations about treatments based on combining the methodologic strength of the supporting evidence and the clarity of the balance between risk and benefit for that treatment. At the top of this hierarchy are treatments with excellent evidence for efficacy and/or effectiveness as well as clearly defined benefits outweighing clearly defined risks and costs. The number summarizes the clarity of the risk/benefit balance and the letter summarizes the likelihood that the supporting evidence is free from bias (or methodologic strength).

SEARCHING THE LITERATURE

General Tips on Searching

The most relevant databases for clinicians are Medline, PsycINFO, the Cochrane Library's Central Register of Controlled Trials (CENTRAL), the JAACAP website, and Google Scholar.

TABLE 3.1.2.6

GRADING TREATMENTS BASED ON RISK/BENEFIT CLARITY AND STRENGTH OF EVIDENCE

Grade	Clarity of Risks + Costs Versus Benefits	Strength of Evidence
1A	Clear	Multiple RCTs with no important flaws
1B	Clear	One or more RCTs with significant flaws and/or inconsistent results
1C+	Clear	No RCTs for this population, but RCT results can be extrapolated to the present patient *or* overwhelming evidence from observational studies Birth
1C	Clear	Observational studies
2A	Unclear	RCTs without significant limitations
2B	Unclear	RCTs with methodologic flaws and/or inconsistent results
2C	Unclear	Observational studies

Adapted from Guyatt et al. (41).

A clinician familiar with these four databases and how they work is able to quickly answer many useful questions. Table 3.1.2.7 demonstrates results from searching three of these sites for answers to varied answerable questions. Results are shown as the number of retrieved publications, or "hits." The first search in the table arose treating a 14-year-old boy with Tourette syndrome and ADHD. He was taking desipramine (DMI) after stimulants had greatly worsened his tics and atomoxetine had made him nauseous. When he started DMI his grades improved markedly, and he reported being able to focus. Four years later, he was continuing to do well, but his physician wondered whether there was new information regarding desipramine and sudden death in youth. He quickly found an article raising further concerns (42) and spoke with the family about retrying atomoxetine. The second search regards information on PMT began because a multidisciplinary team was looking for an EST to use with oppositional and defiant youth. The quotation marks around the phrase "parent management training" (PMT) greatly improve the specificity of the search, reducing hits from 299 to only 10 highly relevant ones. The quotation marks specify that these three words must be found as a phrase, rather than appearing individually throughout the title or abstract. The clinician in this case quickly found support for learning it (43).

Several Tips About Using These Four Databases are Helpful in Searching

1. *For efficiency, consider starting with searches yielding information high in the pyramid of evidence using the "Clinical Queries" feature of PubMed at https://www.ncbi.nlm.nih.gov/pubmed/clinical.* This feature allows you to access the most valid evidence quickly if your question is primarily about the efficacy of a therapy (44). Using the filters for a narrow, specific search is a good starting point in evaluating a therapy since the site will now retrieve only RCTs. If the result is negative, then move on to the "sensitive" search filter that will include

TABLE 3.1.2.7

"HITS" (RETRIEVED REFERENCES) IN SELECTED DATABASES ACCESSED VIA OVID[a]

Database	Search Terms	Limits	Hits	Comments
PubMed	Desipramine *and* death Desipramine *and* "Death, sudden" Parent Management Training "Parent Management Training"	Age 0 to 18 Last 5 yrs Age 0 to 18 No time limits Age 0 to 18 Last 5 yrs None	4 15 299 20	PubMed is a good place to begin for search terms like desipramine or atomoxetine, that is, for information regarding medications.
Clinical Queries at PubMed ("therapy" box)	"Parent Management Training"	Specific search Sensitive search	4 8	Clinical Queries' specific searches retrieve only randomized trials.
Cochrane Library's CCRCT via Ovid	Parent management training "Parent management training"	None None	7 7	The Cochrane Library databases are more difficult to use than these other Websites; they lack the "limits" options, for example, of other sites
PsycINFO (1985–2004 via Ovid)	"Parent management training"	None	79	PsycINFO is a good place to begin for search terms like "bullying" or "stepfamily problems."
	"Parent management training"	None	79	
Evidence-Based Mental Health Online	Desipramine Desipramine *and* death "Parent management training" "Parent management training"	None	16 1 9 2 2	Many references to child/adolescent literature. Requires subscription to search beyond first 150 words of article.

[a]Ovid accessed at www.ovid.com via The Permanente Medical Group portal, September 9, 2005 (except desipramine search done February 6, 2006).

nonrandomized studies as well; your search is moving down the pyramid of evidence. On the other hand, if time is not an issue, consider starting with a sensitive search and being as inclusive (sensitive) as possible; only later narrow the search by becoming increasingly narrow (specific).

2. *Consider with starting with low-bias, preappraised evidence form systematic reviews and meta-analyses.* A review qualifies as systematic if it explicitly states its inclusion and exclusion criteria, uses a comprehensive and transparent search strategy as well as explicit rules to summarize the data (45).

   Searching the PubMed Clinical Queries site, for example, with the terms "self-harm (children OR adolescents)" and the "Broad" filter retrieves 305 clinical studies, while the "Narrow" filter reduces that to 75 hits, a more manageable number to "hand search," the term used to briefly examine each abstract and assess its relevance and validity (46).
3. *Be familiar with Medical Subject Headings (MeSH) and how to "explode" or restrict MeSH subheadings, as well as how to use search tools such as Boolean operators and "wildcards."* Asking the search to explode a MeSH term means the program will now look for all subheadings of that MeSH term in addition to the term itself. At times this is useful; at other times, it is more useful to search only one or more specific subheadings of a MeSH term.

   Become familiar with how to use the MeSH "tree" of terms and subheadings, and note that PsycINFO does not use MeSH, but uses its own thesaurus. Become familiar as well with Boolean operators like "and," "or," and "not," which can quickly either expand or limit a search. Wildcards are useful in allowing searching with multiple terms in a single search. "Adolesc*" in Medline will retrieve, for example, articles on adolescence, adolescents, and adolescent. All databases have a tutorial function that explains its wildcards and its thesaurus; these are database specific.
4. *Understand the strengths and weaknesses of each database related to the journals it does and does not contain.* PubMed retrieves many references for medications but omits many significant journals in psychology. PsycINFO includes an extensive array of psychology journal articles of variable quality; this database has its own thesaurus of index terms as well. The JAACAP Website offers AACAP members full text access to articles published since 1995, but only from a single, albeit highly relevant, journal. The Cochrane Library's Central Register of Controlled Trials is helpful as a complete source for RCT data; its Systematic Reviews library rarely has completed reviews in child psychiatry. Table 3.1.2.7 summarizes characteristics of these databases.
5. *Understand which databases are available and whether each produces an abstract alone or a full text article.* Both Medline via Entrez PubMed at the National Center for Biotechnology Information (NCBI) and the Website of the Journal of the American Academy of Child and Adolescent Psychiatry are available to most child psychiatrists. The former is in the public domain and generates abstracts, while the latter is included in membership in the American Academy of Child and Adolescent Psychiatry. Three other databases often available via an institutional affiliation are the Cochrane Library's Central Register of Controlled Trials (CENTRAL), its database of Systematic Reviews, and the database PsycINFO from the APA. Most clinical "answerable questions" can be usefully searched using a combination of JAACAP, PubMed, CENTRAL, and PsycINFO. But in most organizational affiliations with Ovid, only some journals will supply full text access to the retrieved articles and abstracts. Hence, an advantage in searching the JAACAP site first is its access to full text articles; this avoids the frustration of finding excellent sources but being unable to obtain a full text copy immediately.
6. *Use branching out from a good specific reference whenever possible.* Look in the bibliography and expand from there. Look for other articles by the same author or by authors cited in the bibliography. Also note the MeSH subject term for a reference you find very helpful and use it for a MeSH search. This approach often quickly creates an expanding web of relevant references. One of the best examples of the "one good reference leads to another" strategy is Greenhalgh's review article on disseminating an innovation (20). Note also that databases like PubMed offer searching of "Relevant Articles" as a link.
7. *Search a single aspect of a multi-item search at a time, then combine sets of references using Boolean operators.* For example, in searching Medline for outbreaks of suicide attempts in adolescents, search the MeSH term for suicide attempts separately initially. Search the MeSH term for outbreaks separately as well. Only then combine the sets of references using the Boolean operator "and" to find references in both sets. Finally, add limits such as age, year of publication, language of publication, and publication type serially one at a time. The advantage of this approach is transparency. How many hits were achieved at each stage and the effect of combining sets, as well as the effect of each limit, is clear. This transparency is useful because, if necessary, you can immediately revise your search based on the results. Dropping references should also be done using a transparent methodology. Justifying each step of winnowing is worthwhile, since each such narrowing step means lost information. "Hand searching" simply means scanning the abstracts or even whole articles and deciding their relevance and quality for the purpose at hand. Hand searching is the final step after winnowing through limits.
8. *Know what to do when the search retrieves far too many references to examine.* In Medline, consider using the subheadings under MeSH terms to refine the search. For example, adding "Major" (abbreviated [MAJR]) after the term restricts the search to only those articles where the subject is a major topic heading in that journal article. Similarly, subheadings to MeSH terms like "prevention and control" or "statistics" can be helpful in limiting large searches if those are areas of primary concern. Using the "Limits" feature in databases also narrows the number of references. Common limits are either specifying a specific publication type, such as only meta-analyses or only RCTs, or only a specific age group such as adolescents, or only the most recent references from perhaps the last 5 or 10 years. Suppose, for example, a reader is interested in doing a comprehensive search on psychodynamic psychotherapy in children. He might start by searching the term "Psychotherapy [MeSH]" which uses the MeSH category psychotherapy, generating over 97,000 references. Limiting to age 6 to 12 reduces the number to about 14,000. Searching Medline with the term "psychodynamic" as a keyword and the limit of age 6 to 12 generates a more manageable 257. Combining these two sets generates a manageable list of 116 references to sort through. This list is a good start.

Tips on PubMed

To use PubMed well, it pays to understand MeSH terms, the National Library of Medicine's controlled vocabulary for medical subject headings. MeSH index words provide a consistent way to retrieve information even though articles may use varied terminology for the same concept. In other words, the MeSH term is the "official" term used by the database to organize all references relevant to a single subject that may be referred to using multiple words. Using MeSH terms in a search ensures that all references relevant to that subject are included. Furthermore, MeSH terms are organized as nested sets, becoming more and more specific; each term higher in the tree contains all the terms below it. Medline allows the searcher to visualize these nested sets of terms and choose the most specific term he can find for the subject of interest. This allows only highly specific articles to be retrieved. MeSH searches also allow the searcher to specify whether he wants articles retrieved if the MeSH term is found anywhere in the article, or whether he wants articles retrieved only if the MeSH term is a major heading in the article.

A therapist interested in alternatives to Dialectical Behavior Therapy (DBT), for example, searched "parasuicidal"—meaning frequent cutting or comparable low lethality self-harm attempts—in the MeSH tree of index terms. MeSH recognizes the term parasuicide, and suggests the term "Self-Injurious Behavior." This official MeSH term is defined as "behavior in which persons hurt or harm themselves without the motive of suicide or of sexual deviation" (47). The MeSH tree then looks like this:

- Self-Injurious Behavior (SIB)
  - Self-Mutilation
  - Suicide
    - Suicide, Assisted
    - Suicide, Attempted

The therapist might want to search "self-injurious behavior" as a MeSH term (simply put [MeSH] after the term). The therapist might choose not to explode the term (meaning the search also would include all four items nested underneath Self-Injurious Behavior) if the goal is to find alternatives to DBT. The unexploded term will be more specific because it will find articles based on the above definition of SIB only and not include the lower terms. The search Psychotherapy [MeSH] AND "Self-Injurious Behavior [MeSH:NoExp]" limited to the age group of adolescence generates 75 references which can be used as a base to answer the therapist's question. By contrast, a less specific search that allows the search to explode the SIB term and include subheadings retrieves over 792 references—far too many to hand search. In summary, exploding a MeSH term—meaning that all the MeSH terms underneath this item will also be searched—is only desirable if all the subheadings are of potential interest.

Tips on PsycINFO

PsycINFO is a database that includes nearly 2,000 journals as well as some books, book chapters, and dissertations. Operated by the APA, it is especially strong in searching questions related to psychosocial interventions.

A search generates abstracts and not full text articles. PsycINFO uses a thesaurus of index terms, providing a controlled vocabulary to structure the subject matter (20). The thesaurus includes more psychological terms than MeSH. "Pretend play," "Bullying," and "Parental involvement," for example, are legitimate thesaurus terms in PsycINFO. Yet in MeSH, "Bullying" has no suggested search strategy, and "Pretend play" in the MeSH tree returns "Play therapy" and "Play and playthings," a subset of Recreation. The PsycINFO thesaurus is available online.

However, not all searches do best with a thesaurus term. For example, searching the term "parent management training" in Ovid's PsycINFO thesaurus shows Parent Training as an index term which includes PMT. But because this index term also includes many forms of parent training, it retrieves 2,756 hits. A more successful strategy for a clinician seeking information about Patterson's well-known Parent Management Training is the keyword search for the phrase in quotes, "parent management training" (see Table 3.1.2.7). Options regards "limits" are also different than those in PubMed. PsycINFO, rather than offering a premade filter to choose only randomized trials, offers the filter "clinical trial" instead.

The searcher can search by index terms from the thesaurus or by keyword. PsycINFO also lists classification codes—large categories with an accompanying number such as "cognitive therapy" (3311) or "group and family therapy" (3313).

Searching by keywords is uncontrolled in that any search term can be tried. PsycINFO then searches for those words in the title or abstract. When building combined searches using more than one combination of keywords, classifications, or index terms, build the search one step at a time to maximize transparency of the process. For example, typing in "psychodynamic child psychotherapy" into the thesaurus, the index term is "child psychotherapy." The term itself generates 3,433 hits. Searching this index term exploded generates 4,732 hits. "Psychodynamic" searched in the Thesaurus returns "psychodynamics" as a thesaurus index term. Exploded, this term generates 8,049 hits.

Now combining this set with the results from exploding "child psychotherapy" with the Boolean "AND" creates a manageable set of 41 references. Another approach is to search "psychodynamic$" with "$" being a wildcard—it can represent any letter or combination of letters—and combine it with the results of exploding the index term "child psychotherapy": The result is 205 references.

Tips on Google Scholar

Google Scholar is a formidable search engine with the familiar Google logo and format. In 2012, it was estimated to have over 160,000,000 references in it. With its hip, colorful logo and familiar format, easy availability, and simple search box it is understandably popular. It is free, fast, and has an "Advanced" search box allowing for search by author, title, or date. Yet, while relatively stark and colorless, PubMed and PsycINFO have major advantages over Google Scholar in seeking low bias and complete results efficiently. First, PubMed and PsycINFO both have filters which function to narrow the search drastically based on the quality of the evidence using well-defined subject labels—MeSH in PubMed and Thesaurus in PsycINFO—in addition to well-defined classification systems for publication types, such as meta-analysis, review, or RCT. Therefore, it is possible to efficiently winnow results to a manageable number based on both publication type and subject label. No such classification has been done in Google Scholar, often resulting in an unwieldy set of references that is difficult to winnow toward the most valid results. And whereas PubMed and PsycINFO are transparent about their contents, Google Scholar is not. It is reassuring to know the boundaries and content of the ocean in which fishing is conducted. And whereas PubMed Clinical Queries filters retrieve a select group of studies chosen for low-bias design, Google Scholar, with its large size and no classification systems, can easily retrieve an unwieldy set of references that is difficult to winnow. Furthermore, since published meta-analyses typically retrieve their data from PubMed, CENTRAL, and PsycINFO and other bibliographic, defined sites, clinicians using these sites also align their own knowledge management procedures with those of definitive published knowledge.

The Cochrane Library

The Cochrane Central Register of Controlled Trials (CCRCT) is an efficient way to begin a search for those with access, because CCRCT strives to be complete, with over 350,000 registered controlled trials; importantly, it includes only controlled trials. Its advantage over a search for RCTs using the Clinical Queries PubMed site is that CCRCT attempts a search for any randomized trial published anywhere in the world (not just RCTs published in a journal indexed by PubMed). A parent seeking help regarding the usefulness of the Feingold diet could find a quick answer in CCRCT. A quick look for Feingold diet at the PubMed Clinical Query site, set for narrow searches, works equally well, and quickly reveals the same negative 1981 trial found in CCRCT. Moreover, the search options at the Clinical Queries PubMed site are easier to use, including the capacity to limit articles retrieved to only adolescents, for example. For this reason the Clinical Queries site may be more relevant for most clinicians unless no trials have been reported, in which case checking CCRCT may be worthwhile.

Historical Perspective: Archie Cochrane and the Virtual Library Named after Him

In 1972, the British epidemiologist Archie Cochrane wrote an influential book, Effectiveness and Efficiency: Random Reflections on Health Services, in which he pointed out that resources for health care would always be limited. Therefore, he concluded, using evidence from randomized controlled trials is critical, because the information they provide is more reliable than other sources of evidence. In 1979, he continued to advocate for the usefulness not only of RCTs, but also for efforts to summarize such trials in one place. "It is surely a great criticism of our profession," he wrote, "that we have not organized a critical summary, by specialty or subspecialty, adapted periodically, of all relevant randomized controlled trials." His remarks and influence were such that an international collaboration, the Oxford Database of Perinatal Trials (ODPT), developed around his way of thinking. The systematic review of randomized trials resulting from this collaboration became a centerpiece of what came to be called "the Cochrane approach": the structured method of presenting overview data summarizing multiple trials. This approach became a hallmark of the Cochrane Database of Systematic Reviews (CDSR), an online "library" that began in the 1980s with the ODPT. The Cochrane Collaboration was subsequently founded in 1993, 5 years after his death.

The symbol for the Cochrane Collaboration is two Cs facing each other and containing a closed circle with a central vertical line. The vertical line represents the null result, that is, an odds ratio of 1.0. Each horizontal line represents the results of a single randomized controlled trial. The length of the line represents the 95% confidence intervals for the primary outcome variable studied in that trial; the shorter the line, the more certain the results. Some horizontal lines cross the central vertical line, meaning that the null hypothesis was not refuted within 95% confidence intervals. The horizontal lines that do not cross the central vertical line represent a study inconsistent with the null hypothesis as regards the primary outcome variable at the 95% confidence level. This makes it easy to scan the figure visually to see which studies reached significance and which did not. Furthermore, at the bottom there is a small diamond just to the left of the central vertical line. The diamond summarizes the pooled effect estimate from summing over the results of all the trials within the circle.

The specific horizontal lines and diamond used in the Cochrane Collaboration logo (Figure 3.1.2.1) represent a meta-analysis of randomized trials as regards administering a short, inexpensive course of a corticosteroid to women about to give birth prematurely. The first of these RCTs was reported in 1972. The logo summarizes the evidence that would have been revealed had the available RCTs been reviewed systematically in about 1982; the position of the diamond demonstrates that corticosteroids reduce the risk of babies dying from the complications of immaturity. In fact, more modern estimates are that this treatment reduces the odds of premature infants dying from the complications of immaturity by 30% to 50% (48). But because no systematic review of these trials had been published until 1989, this evidence was not widely disseminated and many premature babies presumably died unnecessarily. Hence, the logo is a rather grim reminder of the high stakes in performing systematic, timely reviews of relevant randomized controlled trials.

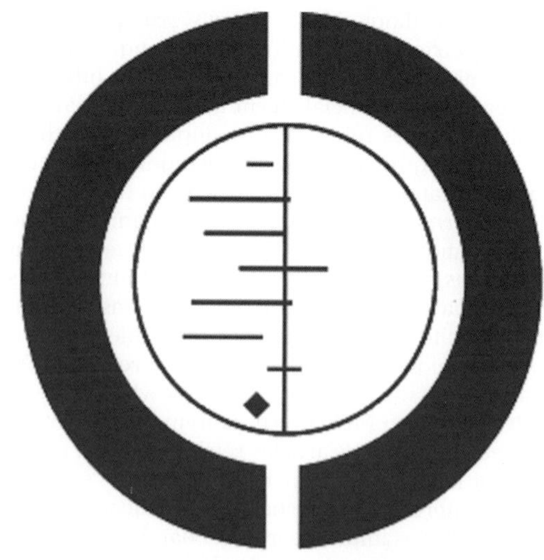

FIGURE 3.1.2.1. The Cochrane Collaboration logo. (Used with permission, courtesy of the Cochrane Colloquium.)

Abstracts of Cochrane systemic reviews are available for no charge (see Table 3.1.2.8) but access to the full text of the review usually occurs through affiliation with an institution that subscribes. The systematic reviews are updated regularly as more information becomes available, and in response to comments. The methodology is transparent. The "Library" exists only virtually in cyberspace. This system allows updates to include more recent studies and any criticism and comments (49). Comparisons with reviews in traditional journals have given the edge to the Cochrane Library versions (50). Cochrane systematic reviews are exclusively electronic and frequent review and openness to comments have been designed to take advantage of the electronic form (49).

The Cochrane Library thus developed a way of summarizing healthcare information that was systematic, completely electronic, up to date, open to criticism, and clearly distinguishing between trials based on their quality. The "system" used does not vary from review to review. Therefore once the consumer becomes accustomed to the format, he can quickly understand the results of any systematic review. Furthermore, the results are transparent, since each study's individual results are also summarized, as is the methodology. Finally, since the entire library is electronic, updating by teams working around the globe becomes feasible in a regular way through sharing the work in cyberspace. The Cochrane library has thus raised the bar for how medical knowledge is organized and disseminated, and been closely associated with the development of EBM.

TABLE 3.1.2.8

USEFUL DATABASES: URLs AND AVAILABILITY

Site/URL	Sources/Abstracts (A) Full Text (FT)	Classification System Used	Strengths	Weaknesses
PubMed http://www.ncbi.nlm.nih.gov/entrez/query.fcgi	Extensive medical journal base A, Some FT	MeSH terms	MeSH allows specific searching	DSM disorders not always MESH terms
PubMed Clinical Queries http://www.ncbi.nlm. nih.gov/entrez/query/static/clinical.shtml	Same as PubMed	Same	Filters allow either searching for RCTs only or more sensitive search	Systematic review less well defined than in CDSR
MeSH Database http://www.ncbi.nlm.nih.gov/entrez/query.fcgi?db=mesh	MeSH "tree" of terms	Branching "tree" of terms	Allows searching with controlled vocabulary	Excludes many less medical terms (e.g., bullying)
PsycINFO, PsycARTICLES http://www.psycinfo.com/psycarticles/	Extensive psychology journal base A, Fee-based FT	Index terms Classification Keywords	Allows very specific searching (e.g., bullying)	No RCT filter Variable quality "Publication type" filter not crisp
CRCT http://www.cochranelibrary.com/cochrane-database-of-systematic-reviews/	All RCTs No A or FT unless UK, Australia	Keyword	Immediate discovery of RCTs on subject; uniform data presentation	Mostly via institutions in United States No charge in UK, Australia, Latin America
CDSR http://www.cochranelibrary.com/about/central-landing-page.html	Only if SR completed A but no FT	Keyword	Uniform data presentation Updated	Limited regarding child psychiatry
JAACAP www.jaacap.com	JAACAP to 1995 A. FT also if AACAP member	Keyword	Full text option Highly specific Included in AACAP membership	Limited to one journal No filters
EBMH Online http://ebmh.bmjjournals.com/	EB Mental Health. First 150 words available; FT requires subscription	Keyword	Preappraised evidence only	Requires subscription for full access; mixed with adult literature

For answerable questions in child psychiatry, the CCRCT is often useful as a good place to start searching an answerable question. Paradoxically, the Cochrane Library of Systematic Reviews is often not useful to child psychiatrists, because a systematic review has most often not been done on the child psychiatric topic of interest. Searching for reviews on ADHD, for example, retrieves 13 reviews but none specifically devoted to ADHD. Searching for reviews on major depression in adolescents is similarly unfruitful. By contrast, searching the Clinical Query site of NCBI in the Find Systematic Reviews box retrieves 229 references with many devoted exclusively to ADHD and many highly relevant to a practitioner (see Table 3.1.2.8). Nevertheless, the Cochrane Library's emphasis on the importance to practitioners of systematic reviews, published in cyberspace and updated frequently, remains at the heart of EBM.

DIAGNOSTIC PATHS CONSISTENT WITH EBP PRINCIPLES

EBP differs significantly from conventional clinical practice in how it approaches differential diagnosis. Whereas clinicians often use an unstructured interview and their familiarity with the categories of DSM-IV TM, EBP encourages feasible routes to more definitive diagnoses compatible with research studies for that disorder. In other words, EBP supports the importance of test/retest and interrater reliability and the multiple forms of validity (51) in the diagnostic process, while also recognizing the process must be feasible. An EBP approach to diagnosis is not new at all; it is merely trying to make feasible the more rigorous diagnostic approaches used in research for some time. In this way EBP is a useful bridge between the culture of research and the culture of clinical care, striving to help clinicians find rigorous yet practical diagnostic methods. EBP also encourages a thorough yet feasible search in symptom domains other than the presenting problem, since comorbid disorders are common and easily missed (52). Let's begin with how EBM approaches arriving at a clear conclusion in the domain of a primary diagnostic concern and return to the issue of assessing comorbid disorders.

In diagnostic work, the EBM practitioner should try to create a link between his patient's disorders and the research base on effective treatments. It is important, therefore, that the diagnostic procedures are not idiosyncratic to that practitioner or clinic. The diagnostic system used must also generate data capable of becoming useful information when compiled. The EBS youth mental health clinics in Hawaii, for example, establish an initial baseline of functioning using the CAFAS (28). When the CAFAS is repeated 3 months later, its mean and median slope are useful measures of changes in functioning in the population served by these clinics (8).

The clinician may at times elect to use a component of a research-level instrument, especially in the domain of primary concern. For example, the K-SADS-P/L modules for selected diagnoses such as MDD, bipolar, bulimia nervosa, alcohol abuse, and multiple other disorders can be given as "standalone" modules within the context of a clinical interview as a compromise. Of course administration of the complete K-SADS provides a more thorough evaluation. This semistructured approach with clear anchor points to determine the presence or absence of symptoms is markedly less ambiguous than simply working from an open copy of DSM-IV. Furthermore, K-SADS modules are available free on the Internet (53). Another feasible research-level instrument is the computerized

Diagnostic Interview Schedule for Children (DISC), which can be administered only for the domain of interest or in multiple domains in a wide search for psychopathology (54).

Another approach is to use an instrument which has been studied as a proxy for a research-level instrument, and been shown to be a feasible substitute. For example, in pediatric bipolar disorder (PBD), the parent version of the Young Mania Rating Scale (P-YMRS) has been studied as a proxy for a semistructured interview (55). Higher scores on the P-YMRS predict increasing likelihood of PBD on semistructured interviews. In order to use these likelihood ratios, it is necessary to estimate the base rate of BPD among patients presenting to the clinic (56). Such a base rate can either be estimated using published data or from local data generated at the clinic itself. The latter process is recommended only if the diagnostic process used locally has been adequate. Using data from the literature to calculate a base rate for common disorders like ADHD, MDD, bipolar disorder, and substance abuse disorders has advantages: the sample sizes are larger, and use peer-reviewed data typically generated with well-defined diagnostic processes.

Bayes' theorem can be used to combine the information from an estimated base rate, family history, and parent-completed instrument assessing bipolar symptoms. Consider the example of a 9-year-old patient with episodes of extreme aggression, problems concentrating, and high levels of motor activity (56). To begin, the base rate for bipolar disorder in children entering community mental health center clinics is roughly 6%; this figure, therefore, becomes the initial estimated probability of bipolar disorder. Since this boy had a biologic father with bipolar I and a meta-analysis showed that children with a biologic parent with bipolar disorder are five times as likely to have a bipolar diagnosis themselves, Bayes' theorem allows the clinician to combine these two independent sources of information as follows (57):

Initial estimate of odds of bipolar disorder = Odds of having bipolar disorder in clinic × likelihood ratio from family history

Note that Bayes' theorem uses the odds, rather than the probability, of the boy having bipolar disorder. The information given as regards a base rate of 6% is actually a probability, which would need to be converted to odds for use in Bayes' theorem. A nomogram uses probabilities and avoids the clumsiness of converting probabilities to odds for use in Bayes' theorem and then back again to probability, the more familiar concept (see Figure 3.1.2.2). The nomogram shows that this boy's probability rises to 24% from 6% on the basis of his positive family history.

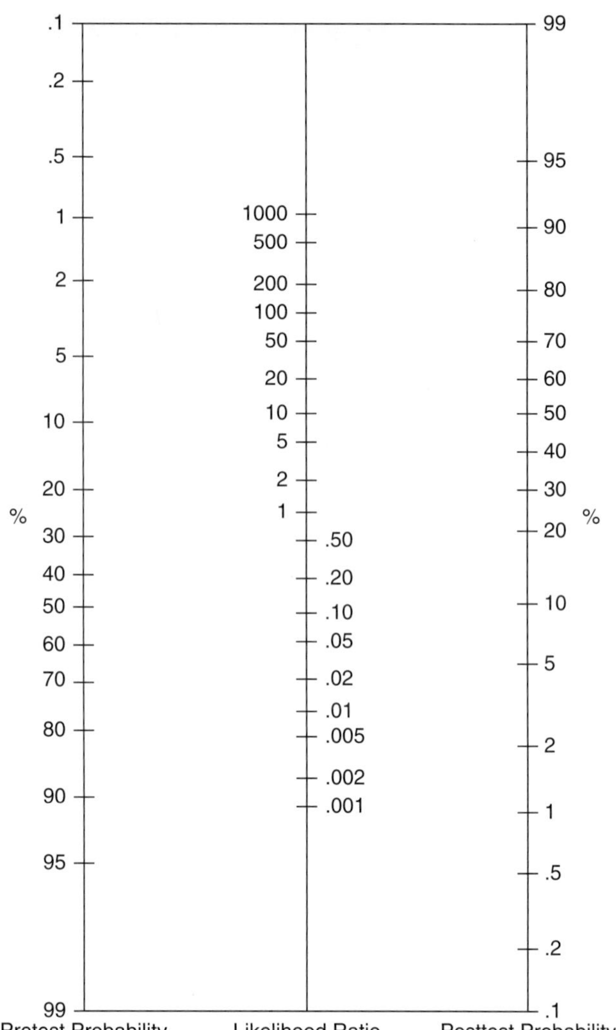

FIGURE 3.1.2.2. Nomogram for combining probability and likelihood ratio. (From Youngstrom EA, Youngstrom JK: Evidence-based assessment of pediatric bipolar disorder, Part II: incorporating information from behavior checklists. *J Am Acad Child Adolesc Psychiatry* 44:823–828, 2005, with permission.)

Bayes' theorem allows the clinician to further refine the probability of this boy's meeting diagnostic criteria for bipolar disorder by using his mother's reports of his symptoms as reported on the externalizing score on the Child Behavior Check List. This process is especially helpful in ruling out bipolar disorder, that is, showing that the probability of the boy meeting criteria for bipolar disorder is sufficiently low that no further testing is required. On the other hand, a high externalizing score on the CBCL should trigger use of a specific parent report regarding bipolar symptoms, such as the Parent Young Mania Rating Scale (P-YMRS). In such a case, continue to use Bayes' theorem with the boy in the example (58):

Refined odds of bipolar disorder = (Odds for probability of 24) × (likelihood ratio from that patient's score on P-YMRS)

Again, using a nomogram that translates probability into odds and back again to probability after the calculation makes things easier. With a likelihood ratio of 6 from his P-YMRS score, this boy's probability of having bipolar disorder jumps to 68.

This is not a diagnosis, but it is an easily arrived at probability which should trigger a full-scale evaluation for bipolar disorder (see Youngstrom's discussion [59]). This methodology can be used to estimate the probability for other disorders such as ADHD as well (56).

In addition to feasible but empirically supported approaches to a primary diagnosis, data support using a broad assessment of psychopathology and functioning. There are many possible instruments. Achenbach's multiple-informant System of Empirically Based Assessment (ASEBA) is one feasible approach, as is a computerized structured interview such as the parent and child versions of the DISC (54). Broad-based structured systems like ASEBA and the DISC are more likely to note comorbid anxiety disorders, substance abuse disorders, and the presence of multiple disorders than an unstructured clinical interview (59).

In comparing DISC diagnoses to diagnoses generated by clinicians in unstructured interviews, for example, agreement was higher for externalizing than for internalizing disorders, and clinicians were more likely than the DISC to assign a single diagnosis and less likely to assign no diagnosis. Systems like the ASEBA and DISC avoid the heuristic biases present in an unstructured diagnostic interview and their results are useful in building a local database. Such systems allow the interviewer more time and energy to pursue individual aspects

TABLE 3.1.2.9

FEASIBLE EVERYDAY INSTRUMENTS

Tracks or Aids Dx	Instrument	Reference	Informant
ADHD	SWAN	(61)	Teacher or Parent
Anxiety disorders	SCARED	(62)	Parent
Depressive disorders	Center for Epidemiologic Studies—Depression CES-D	(63)	Youth
Depressive disorders	Johns Hopkins Depression Scale	(64)	Parent
Functioning	Columbia Impairment Scale (CIS)	(65)	Parent or youth
Multiple categorical diagnoses	Diagnostic Interview Schedule for Children (DISC)	(54)	Parent or youth
Multiple scales of psychopathology	Achenbach System of Empirically Based Assessment (ASEBA)	(31)	Parent (CBCL) Youth (YSR) Teacher (TRF)
Pediatric bipolar disorders	Young Mania Rating Scale—Parent (YMRS-P)	(66)	Parent
Acute stress and posttraumatic symptoms	Child Stress Disorders Checklist	(67)[a]	Parent

[a]Actual instrument in Article Plus feature on JAACAP Website.

of that child's psychosocial functioning and the context of his symptoms—favorite Internet sites and bands, friendships with peers, relationships with parents and teachers, idealized heroes and heroines, and cell phone ring tone (60). In other words, broad-based, structured assessments can complement a clinical interview. The goal is to provide both a technically sound measure of psychopathology and function as well as a youth-friendly, youth-relevant experience.

In summary, there is no single diagnostic process consistent with EBP; there are many. The goals include a complete, wide-ranging assessment of functioning, impairment, and psychopathology that is unlikely to miss disorders with significant morbidity. The approach also ideally uses feasible methods to provide a solid empirical link to major studies in the field, as well as a baseline for tracking outcome and generating local data. Sound yet practical diagnostic and/or tracking tools useful in everyday practice are noted in Table 3.1.2.9; each is either in the public domain or reasonably priced.

ENACTING EVIDENCE-INFORMED CARE IN CLINICAL ORGANIZATIONS

The task of moving an organization from its current practices toward functioning with processes more consistent with EBP has been called implementation. But projects designed to do this have taken much longer than originally intended (11), creating an implementation gap. More recently, some have suggested the term enactment of evidence-informed health care as a replacement for the term implementation (11). The term enactment comes from enactment theory, which focuses on subjective issues in how organizations function rather than on formal organizational charts. A clinical team is, therefore, enacted by individuals based on their own social perceptions of a negotiated order based on repeated interpersonal processes (68).

Leading a multiprofessional organization toward EBP is complex, with many disputes about the meaning of the change. Furthermore, the available evidence in favor of any particular innovation is often ambiguous; it is inevitably open to at least some interpretation and will be contested. Varied professional groups each have their own way of thinking about what constitutes evidence and its meaning, leading inevitably to competing claims on the truth. Each professional group has its own paradigms and cognitive assumptions, leading to each advancing different claims to knowledge (69). As a result, it is often difficult to find common ground for productive dialogue. Instead, each discipline proceeds almost on its own path, resulting in a complex situation which actually allows the end-user clinician increased choice among the competing claims (11). In addition, managerial control over elite professional groups is limited, since autonomy over working practices is a core value for elite professionals (11).

Creating change in a multiprofessional healthcare organization is complex for several other reasons as well. First, the context of change efforts to enact EBP varies enormously from one organization to another, and varies over time even within the same organization (70). What external pressure is there on the organization to survive in a competitive market? How do union-management issues and interprofessional "turf" issues shape the organization? How does its history shape its culture? This series of questions is only a start. In other words, no context is discrete; complex connections and interactions are the rule. Assessing outcome is also complex. Basic issues as when change is assessed and what is measured can change results markedly. Also, large healthcare organizations respond not only to multiple professional groups inside the organization, but to accrediting bodies and government agencies outside its boundaries. Consider, for example, the complexity of disputes about the safety and benefits of selective serotonin reuptake inhibitors in depressed youth. Government agencies, the press, national professional organizations, and research evidence were all involved.

Tips on Enacting Evidence-Informed Health Care in Organizations

A review of six studies designed to implement EBP for varied medical conditions came to several conclusions. First, implementing change is facilitated by open access to membership in key groups that filter the literature and create guidelines and educational initiatives (8,71). In Hawaii's successful efforts to develop an EBS for youth mental health, groups of clinicians, administrators, and community members involved in the project had open membership; anyone willing to do the reading and attend regularly was allowed to join (4). Second, the hierarchical structure of the local team or hospital staff influences adoption of EBP; a more "flat" hierarchy offers less resistance to adoption. In a vertical hierarchy, junior staff members defer to more senior members regardless of the evidence, slowing adoption of EBP. Third, networks of social/professional relationships, rather than individuals, are central in whatever actions result from implementation efforts. Individuals live within and are a part of these networks.

From these studies, several useful guidelines appear for those interested in implementing EBP within the context of their own organization:

1. *An evidence-based perspective becomes reality only when it is enacted in local clinical settings by frontline clinicians.* Adopting a formal policy of committing to EBPs is insufficient by itself to create enactment by frontline clinical groups over which senior management has limited control (11).
2. *Think of context not as a stage for the action of change, but rather as an active element in the change process.* A shift toward EBP—like other organizational change processes—is highly context dependent (11), where context is defined as multidimensional, multifaceted configurations of forces, often developing historically as negotiated interpersonal patterns. Because these forces interact in complex ways, unexpected outcomes from a planned change are common (10). Individuals are influenced by the context of a network of social relationships beyond their immediate circle. Hence no context is discrete or separate.
3. *Key leaders are able to influence innovation toward EBP.* Although it is clear that the process is often complex, a senior, powerful, and skillful leader can stimulate innovation (10).
4. *Take into account the distinctive nature of the multiprofessional organization.* Boundaries—educational, cognitive, and social—between different professional groups inhibit the spread of EB ideas. Child psychiatrists may read only child psychiatry journals and not child psychology journals and vice versa, or attend only their own professional organizational meetings and vice versa. Knowledge can be powerful and threaten specific interest groups, which are then motivated to reject it (10).
5. *Use the extensive literature on "exporting" psychosocial interventions from development sites to practice sites and distilling components of effective treatments.* How to train practitioners to use manualized therapies developed at other sites is a topic that has been widely discussed elsewhere (71,72). Another approach is to use a process of distilling the common elements in evidence-based interventions and then match these with profiles of target symptoms from individual clients (73). This latter approach is novel and has great potential.
6. *Use multiple means to motivate practitioners to adopt EB processes.* A project to disseminate synthesized evidence to pediatric clinicians concluded that multiple routes of evidence are necessary to convince practitioners to apply evidence in daily patient care (74). An organization is more able to tip toward applying evidence to direct patient care when the organization recognizes a local problem in how it uses research results, and differentiates among classes of evidence. Data showing results from the state of Hawaii's efforts to implement EBP makes a compelling case for the value research can add to practice; it also illustrates how Hawaii's clinicians differentiate among classes of evidence (30). Established means of influencing practitioners' behaviors, such as "best practice" groups, are also useful means to convey EBP ideas (74). Building on such natural social groups is more likely to result in behavioral change in practitioners than efforts to impose major changes in a top-down approach (68).
7. *Because context is complex and multiple routes are necessary to persuade practitioners to change, enacting evidence-based approaches in child mental health needs to be uniquely tailored for each organization and each desired change.* Summaries of how organizations change to include new practitioner behavior more grounded in evidence suggest multiple processes or activities are necessary to create change (20,75). In brief, activities known to promote change successfully include skill-based training, evaluation of therapist fidelity and of programs, practice-based coaching, a facilitative administration, a well-defined implementation team, a high level of facilitator involvement, clarity in defining the core components being implemented, hiring practices, and organizational readiness. The latter is defined by a clear need for change, funding, the confidence of the implementation team, and the involvement of stakeholders (20).

Enacting Evidence-Informed Health Care: An Outpatient Team, an Individual Practitioner

Despite the conclusions that certain drivers of change within healthcare organizations are effective, there is no single way to implement EBP because context is all-important. For example, an opinion leader physician at an outpatient child psychiatry team chose to initiate and support context-sensitive efforts to improve the functioning and quality of life in a larger proportion of the youth served, to make these improvements more substantial, and to make them occur more quickly. Aware that organizational change processes like a shift to EBP are highly context dependent, she first made an effort to understand the team's context (76). One key aspect, she realized, was the multidisciplinary nature of the team—psychologists, physicians, and social workers. Such diverse professional groups do not share a universal, communal, and disinterested approach to knowledge; rather, each discipline displays distinct cognitive assumptions, often with clear boundaries around the discipline's knowledge, making knowledge often difficult to transfer from one discipline to another (77). Not only may the paradigms for generating knowledge in each profession be different, they may be so different that they lack common ground for productive dialogue. Each professional group may therefore produce bodies of knowledge that are not seen as authoritative within other groups (11).

She solved this by creating a work group open to anyone on the team willing to attend meetings and do the work required to complete the project. The group's first task would be to create a plan for how the team would approach youth with anxiety disorders. She led the group toward reviewing the work of the principal leaders in this field but also reviewing all published RCTs studying youth with panic disorder, generalized anxiety disorder, social anxiety disorder, separation anxiety disorder, or a phobia. Using the PubMed Clinical Queries site and limiting the search to recent publications focused on children or adolescents, she found a workable number of references for each disorder, and the group began its work. The work group's goal was to put together a short list of those core components appearing frequently in the most effective treatments. The group then chose those core components that both appeared frequently in effective treatments and were also feasible to use in the context of their setting, characterized by high volume and limited therapist availability. The work group stayed in touch via email and at team meetings with those staff members not participating in the literature review and feasibility discussions. The core components chosen as feasible within that context and supported by more than 1 RCT were exposure, relaxation training, cognitive restructuring, and fluoxetine. The approach she used—distillation of the literature into core components, and subsequently matching those components to a specific client in treatment—was well accepted by therapists. It helped that the process used was inclusive, open, and transparent; it may also have helped that the process respected therapists' autonomy and expertise in matching components and specific patients (73). The work group is currently developing ways to monitor fidelity to these core components.

Just as in organizations, there is no single path to implementing EBP among practitioners. Studies have shown that EBP is best learned in small group teaching experiences. Yet some practitioners may be able to improve their practice simply by being inquisitive, searching for evidence regards the answerable question as originally developed by EBM teachers (3). Resolving to improve his method of tracking response to treatment, for example, one practitioner began tracking symptoms in adolescents with anxiety disorders using an available instrument he uncovered through a Medline search (78). Similarly, he found that tracking responses of attention deficit/hyperactivity youth to stimulant treatment was inexpensive and feasible using an available brief report instrument (61) similar to the instrument used in the MTA study (79). This allowed him to build an alliance with parents by discussing likely outcomes. Parents appreciated the more thoughtful follow-up and their appreciation reinforced his change in behavior.

Solo practitioners can also benefit from joining the organization that uses their combined results to answer research questions, the Child and Adolescent Psychiatry Trials Network (79), allowing them to participate in research studies and inevitably piquing curiosity. In general, changing even an individual's practice begins with an action—a commitment to do something differently, be it a diagnostic process, a treatment decision, or choosing a follow-up methodology. Published summaries of EBP processes in child and adolescent psychiatry may be useful in reflecting on a starting point that is a good fit for a specific practitioner (80).

Errors, Child Psychiatry, and EBP

Error can be defined as "the failure of a planned action to be completed as intended or the use of a wrong plan to achieve an aim" (81). Like other physicians, child psychiatrists undoubtedly make errors. Yet in 2017 the search term "pediatrics" in PubMed and "medical errors" retrieves nearly 400 publications in the last 10 years whereas substituting the term "child psychiatry" for "pediatrics," only 7. Child psychiatrists may be less concerned than pediatricians about medical errors because our procedures do not include surgery, ICU care, chemotherapy, and similar invasive procedures, but also because our most frequent errors go unnoticed.

Developing a culture that is both rigorous *and* kind *and* searches for its own errors while focusing on systemic processes needing improvement is an important task in building and maintaining child mental health systems (82). EBP can help because it offers a metric for the effect of an error, the quality-adjusted life year. The QALY includes both any change in survival time for the patient as well as any change in the patient's quality of life and the duration of that change (83).

Errors of omission are undoubtedly common: An adolescent who has PTSD resulting from having been physically abused who receives only supportive treatment, or an oppositional child with ADHD who is treated with play therapy alone or treating an adolescent suffering from anorexia with supportive psychotherapy when more specific and proven treatments are available (84,85). Perhaps the most frequent error of omission is delay in treatment due to access problems or waiting lists. Delay increases the odds of diminished quality life years compared to anticipated outcomes from treatment.

In addition to making errors of omission, child psychiatrists can, of course, also make errors directly causing harm. Diagnostic errors during assessment can result in a drop in outcome results (86). Polypharmacy treatment with two or more antipsychotics may proceed with limited evidence of safety and efficacy (87), and excessive hospitalization in some states in the past have damaged youth with unnecessary stigma (88). With many possibilities both for errors of omission and errors in assessment and treatment, it makes sense for child mental health systems to build error detection into the core of their organizations. Vigorous error-detection systems can make a difference, such as a second opinion regards medications for outliers, fidelity monitoring, supervision, training, and specific technologies to support interventions (88,89).

CONCLUSION

Contemporary child psychiatry requires a practice model realistic enough to recognize the vast array of contexts in which evaluations and treatments are delivered, yet rigorous enough to insist that each youth receive the most proven diagnostic process and treatment feasible in that setting. Clearly this is vastly different from each clinicians relying on personal preference—it is more time consuming and more difficult than practice as usual. Results from the Hawaii group suggest it can make a substantial change in the bottom line of youth outcome, however, making the effort well worthwhile.

References

1. Guyatt GH, Rennie D (eds.): *Users' Guides to the Medical Literature*. Chicago, IL, AMA Press, 706, 2002.
2. Burns B, Hoagwood KE: Preface. *Child Adolesc Psychiatric Clin N Am* 13:717–728, 2005.
3. March JS, Chrisman A, Breland-Noble A, et al.: Using and teaching evidence-based medicine: The Duke University child and adolescent psychiatry model. *Child Adolesc Psychiatric Clin N Am* 14:273–296, 2005.
4. Chorpita BF, Yim LM, Donkervoet JC, et al.: Toward large-scale implementation of empirically supported treatments for children: a review and observations by the Hawaii empirical basis to services task force. *Clin Psychol Sci Pract* 9(2):166–190, 2002.
5. Kazdin A: Evidence-based treatments: challenges and priorities for practice and research. *Child Adolesc Psychiatric Clin N Am* 13(4):923–940, 2005.
6. Chorpita BF: *The Frontier of Evidence-Based Practice, in Evidence-Based Psychotherapies for Children and Adolescents, A.* In: Kazdin, Weisz J (eds). New York, Guilford Press, 42–59, 2003.
7. Weisz JR, Chorpita BF, Palinkas LA, et al.: Testing standarad and modular designs for psychotherapy treating depression, anxiety, and conduct problems in youth: A randomized effectiveness trial. *Arch Gen Psychiatry* 69(3):274–282, 2012.
8. Daleiden EL, Chorpita BF: From data to wisdom: quality improvement strategies supporting large-scale implementation of evidence-based services. *Child & Adoles Psychiatric Clin N Am* 14(2):329–350, 2005.
9. Jellinek M, McDermott J: Formulation: putting the diagnosis into a therapeutic context and treatment plan. *J Am Acad Child Adolesc Psychiatry* 43(7):913–916, 2004.
10. Ferlie E: Conclusion: From evidence to actionable knowledge? In: Dopson S, Fitzgerald L (eds): *Knowledge to Action? Evidence-Based Health Care in Context*. Oxford, Oxford University Press, 182–197, 2005.
11. Ferlie E, Dopson S: Studying complex organizations in health care. In: Dopson S, Fitzgerald L (eds): *Knowledge to Action? Evidence-Based Health Care in Context*. Oxford, Oxford University Press, 8–26, 2005.
12. Kazdin AE: *Parent Management Training Treatment for Oppositional, Aggressive, and Antisocial Behavior in Children and Adolescents*. Oxford, Oxford University Press, 2005.
13. Mufson L, Dorta KP, Olfson M, Weissman MM, Hoagwood K: *Interpersonal Psychotherapy for Depressed Adolescents*. 2nd ed. New York, Guilford, 2004.
14. PubMed accessed at Countway Library, B. 2017 [cited 2017 Feb 5]; MeSH terms (Meta-analysis OR Systematic review) AND (ADHD OR Anxiety Disorder OR Major Depression OR Psychosis)].
15. Shirk, SR, Karver MS, Borwn R: The alliance in child and adolescent psychotherapy. *Psychotherapy* 48(1):17-24, 2011.
16. Bickman L, de Andrade AR, Athay MM, Chen JI, et al.: The relationship between change in therapeutic alliance ratings and improvement in youth symptom severity: Whose ratings matter the most? *Adm Policy Ment Health* 39(1):78–89, 2012.

17. Garcia JA, Weisz JR: When youth mental health care stops: therapeutic relationship problems and other reasons for ending youth out-patient treatment. *J Consult Clin Psychol* 70(2):439–443, 2002.
18. Hawley K, Weisz J: Youth versus parent working alliance in usual clinical care: distinctive association with retention, satisfaction, and treatment out-come. *J Clin Child Adolesc Psychol* 34(1):117–128, 2005.
19. McLeod BD, Weisz JR: The therapy process observational coding system–alliance scale: measure characteristics and prediction of outcome in usual clinical practice. *J Consul Clin Psychol* 73(2):323–333, 2005.
20. Greenhalgh T, et al.: How to Spread Good Ideas: A systematic review of the literature on diffusion, dissemination and sustainability of innovations in health service delivery and organization, 2004. Available at: http://www.nets.nihr.ac.uk/data/assets/pdf_file/0017/64340/FR-08-1201-038.pdf. Accessed Jan 1, 2017.
21. Greene RW, Ablon JS, Goring JC, et al.: Effectiveness of collaborative problem solving in affectively dysregulated children with oppositional-defiant disorder: Initial findings. *J Consult Clin Psychol* 72(6):1157–1164, 2004.
22. Kendall PC, Chu B, Gifford A, Hayes C, Nauta, M: Breathing life into a manual: flexibility and creativity with manual-based treatments. *Cognit Behav Pract* 5:177–198, 1998.
23. Haynes RB, Devereaux PJ, Guyatt GH: Clinical expertise in the era of evidence-based medicine and patient choice. *ACP J Club* 136:A11–A14, 2002.
24. Levant RF: *Evidence-Based Practice in Psychology.* American Psychological Association, 2005. Available at: https://www.apa.org/practice/resources/evidence/evidence-based-report.pdf. Accessed Jan 19 2017.
25. Ng, MY, Weisz JR: Annual research review: Building a science of personalized intervention for youth mental health. *J Child Psychology and Psychiatry* 57(3):216–226, 2015.
26. Bickman L, Noser K, Summerfelt W: Long-term effects of a system of care on children and adolescents. *J Behav Health Services Res* 26(2):185–202, 1999.
27. Weisz JR, Jensen PS: Efficacy and effectiveness of child and adolescent psychotherapy and pharmacotherapy. *Ment Health Serv Res* 1:125–157, 1999.
28. Hodges K: *Child and Adolescent Functional Assessment Scale (CAFAS).* Ann Arbor, Michigan, Functional Assessment Systems, 1998.
29. Achenbach TM, McConaughy SH: *Empirically-Based Assessment of Child and Adolescent Psychopathology: Practical Applications.* Thousands Oaks, CA, Sage Publications, 1997.
30. Daleiden EL: *Child Status Measurement: System Performance Improvements.* During Fiscal Years 2002–2004. State of Hawaii Department of Health, Child and Adolescent Mental Health Division, 2004.
31. Sackett D, Richardson WS, Rosenberg W, Haynes RB: *Evidence-Based Medicine: How to Practice and Teach EBM.* London, Churchill Livingstone, 261, 2000.
32. March J, Silva S, Petrycki S, et al: Fluoxetine, cognitive-behavioral therapy, and their combination for adolescents with depression: treatment for adolescents with depression study. *JAMA* 292(7):807–820, 2004.
33. Swanson J, Kraemer HC, Hinshaw SP, et al.: Clinical relevance of the primary findings of the MTA: success rates based on severity of ADHD and ODD symptoms at the end of treatment. *J Am Acad Child Adolsec Psychiatry* 40(2):168–179, 2001.
34. Brent DA, Holder D, Kolko D, et al.: A clinical psychotherapy trial for adolescent depression comparing cognitive, family, and supportive therapy. *Arch Gen Psychiatry* 54(9):877–885, 1997.
35. POTS Team: Cognitive-behavior therapy, sertraline, and their combination for children and adolescents with obsessive-compulsive disorder: the pediatric OCD treatment study (POTS) randomized controlled trial. *JAMA* 292(16):1969–1976, 2004.
36. Kazdin A, Siegel T, Bass D: Cognitive problem-solving skills training and parent management training in the treatment of antisocial behavior in children. *J Consult Clinc Psychol* 60:733–747, 1992.
37. Delbello M, Schwiers ML, Rosenberg HL, Strakowski SM: A double-blind, randomized, placebo-controlled study of quetiapine as adjunctive treatment for adolescent mania. *J Am Acad Child Adolesc Psychiatry* 41(10):1216–1223, 2002.
38. Emslie GJ, Heiligenstein JH, Hoog SL, et al.: Fluoxetine treatment for prevention of relapse of depression in children and adolescents: a double-blind, placebo controlled study. *J Am Acad Child Adolesc Psychiatry* 43(11):1397–1405, 2004.
39. Robins L, Rutter M (eds): *Straight and Devious Pathways from Childhood to Adulthood.* London, Oxford University Press, 1990.
40. Guyatt G, Drummond R: Introduction: the philosophy of evidence-based medicine. In: Guyatt G, Rennie D (eds): *Users' Guides to the Medical Literature: A Manual for Evidence-Based Clinical Practice.* Chicago, IL. AMA Press, 3–12, 2002.
41. Guyatt G, Drummond R: Moving from evidence to action: grading recommendations—a qualitative approach. In: Guyatt G, Rennie D (eds): *Users' Guides to the Medical Literature: A Manual for Evidence-Based Clinical Practice.* Chicago, IL, AMA Press, 567–658, 2002.
42. Amitai Y, Frischer H: Excess fatality from desipramine in children and adolescents. *J Am Acad Child Adolesc Psychiatry* 45(1):54–60, 2006.
43. Mabe P, Turner M, Josephson A: Parent management training. *Child Adolesc Psychiatr Clin N Am* 10(3):451–464, 2001.
44. Medicine NLo, NCBI PubMed Clinical Queries. 2005. Available at: https://www.nlm.nih.gov/bsd/disted/pubmedtutorial/020_570.html. Accessed Jan 21, 2017.
45. Guyatt GH, Rennie D, Meade MO, Cook DJ, eds.: Moving from evidence to action. *Users' Guide to the Medical Literature: A Manual for Evidence-Based Clinical Practice,* Chicago, IL, 175–199, 2002.
46. Faraone S, Biederman J, Roe C: Comparative efficacy of Adderall and methylphenidate in attention-deficit/hyperactivity disorder: A meta-analysis. *J Clin Psychopharmacol* 6(2):43, 2002.
47. Medicine NLo, MeSH. 2005. NIH, Self-Injurious Behavior. Available at: https://meshb.nlm.nih.gov/#/record/ui?ui=D016728. Accessed Jan 21, 2017.
48. Cochrane Collaboration. Antenatal steroids for accelerating fetal lung maturation for women at risk of preterm birth. 1993. Available at: http://onlinelibrary.wiley.com/doi/10.1002/14651858.CD004454.pub2/abstract. Accessed Jan 21, 2017.
49. Starr M, Chalmers I. The evolution of the Cochrane Library, 1988-2003. Update Software: Oxford (www.update-software.com/history/clibhist.htm). Accessed October 6, 2004.
50. Jadad A, Cook DJ, Jones A, et al.: Methodology and reports of systematic reviews and meta-analyses: a comparison of Cochrane reviews with articles published in paper-based journals. *JAMA* 280:278–280, 1998.
51. Streiner DL, Norman GR: *Health Measurement Scales: A Practical Guide to Their Development and Use.* 2nd ed. Oxford, Oxford University Press, 231, 1995.
52. Doss AJ: Evidence-based diagnosis: Incorporating diagnostic instruments into clinical practice. *J Am Acad Child Adolesc Psychiatry* 44:947–952, 2005.
53. Kaufman J, Birmaher B, Brent D, et al.: *Kiddie-Sads-Present and Lifetime Version (K-SADS-PL).* Department of Psychiatry, University of Pittsburgh School of Medicine, 1997. Available at: http://www.psychiatry.pitt.edu/node/8233. Accessed Jan 22, 2017.
54. Shaffer D, Fisher P, Lucas CP, Dulcan MK, Schwab-Stone ME: NIMH diagnostic interview schedule for children version IV (NIMH DISC-IV): Description, differences from previous versions, and reliability of some common diagnoses. *J Am Acad Child Adolesc Psychiatry* 39(1):28–38, 2000.
55. Youngstrom E, Findling RL, Calabrese JR, et al.: Comparing the diagnostic accuracy of six potential screening instruments for bipolar disorder in youths aged 5 to 17 years. *J Am Acad Child Adolesc Psychiatry* 43:847–858, 2004.
56. Youngstrom EA, Duax J: Evidence-based assessment of pediatric bipolar disorder, Part I: Base rate and family history. *J Am Acad Child Adolesc Psychiatry* 44(7):712–717, 2005.
57. Friedland DJ (ed.): *Evidence-Based Medicine: A Framework for Clinical Practice.* Stamford, CT, Appleton & Lange, 263, 1998.
58. Youngstrom EA, Youngstrom JK: Evidence-based assessment of pediatric bipolar disorder, Part II: incorporating information from behavior checklists. *J Am Acad Child Adolesc Psychiatry* 44(8):823–828, 2005.
59. Jensen AL, Weisz JR: Assessing match and mismatch between practitioner generated and standardized interview-generated diagnoses for clinic referred children and adolescents. *J Consult Clinc Psychol* 70(1):158–168, 2002.
60. Rosenblum DS, Daniolos P, Kass N, Martin A: Adolescents and popular culture: a psychodynamic overview. In: Solnit AJ, et al. (eds): *Psychoanalytic Study of the Child.* New Haven, CT, Yale University Press, 1999, 319–338.
61. Swanson J, Schuck S, Porter M, et al. Categorical and Dimensional Definitions and Evaluations of Symptoms of ADHD: History of the SNAP and the SWAN Rating Scales. *Int J Educ Psychol Assess* 10(1):51–70,2012..
62. Birmaher B, Brent DA, Chiappetta L, Bridge J, Monga S, Baugher M: Psychometric properties of the screen for child anxiety related emotional disorders (SCARED): a replication study. *J Am Acad Child Adolesc Psychiatry* 38(10):1230–1236, 1999.
63. Radloff L: A CES-D Scale: A self-report depression scale for research in the general population. *Appl Psychol Meas* 1:385–401, 1977.
64. Joshi PT, Capozzoli JA, Coyle JT: The Johns Hopkins Depression Scale: Normative data and validation in child psychiatry patients. *J Am Acad Child Adolesc Psychiatry* 29(2):283–288, 1990.
65. Bird HR, Shaffer D, Fisher P, et al.: The Columbia Impairment Scale (CIS): Pilot findings on a measure of global impairment for children and adolescents. *Int J Methods Psych Res* 3:167–176, 1993.
66. Gracious BL, Youngstrom EA, Findling RL, Calabrese JR: Discriminative validity of a parent version of the young mania rating scale. *J Am Acad Child Adolesc Psychiatry* 41(11):1350–1359, 2002.
67. Saxe G, Chawla N, Stoddard F, et al: Child stress disorders checklist: a measure of ASD and PTSD in children. *J Am Acad Child Adolesc Psychiatry* 42(8):972–978, 2003.
68. Weick KE: *Making Sense of the Organization.* Malden, MA: Blackwell, 2001.
69. Burrell G, Morgan G: *Sociological Paradigms and Organizational Analysis.* London, Heinemann Educational Books, 1979.
70. Dopson S, Fitzgerald L: *The Active Role of Context, in Knowledge to Action? Evidence-Based Health Care in Context.* Fitzgerald L (ed): Oxford. Oxford University Press, 79–103, 2004.
71. Hoagwood KE: Making the translation from research to its application. *Clin Psychol Sci Pract* 9(2):210–213, 2002.

72. Schoenwald SK, Hoagwood K: Effectiveness, transportability, and dissemination of interventions: What matters when? *Psychiatr Serv* 52(9): 1190–1197, 2001.
73. Chorpita BF, Daleiden EL, Weisz JR: Identifying and selecting the common elements of evidence based interventions: a distillation and marching model. *Ment Health Serv Res* 7(1):5–20, 2005.
74. Lomas J: Retailing research: increasing the role of evidence in clinical services for childbirth. *Milbank Q* 71(3):439–475, 1993.
75. Fixsen DL, Naoom SF, Blase KA, Friedman RM, et al: *Implementation Research: A Synthesis of the Literature.* University of South Florida, Louis de la Parte Florida Mental Health Institute, The National Implementation Research Network (FMHI Publication #231), 2005.
76. Dopson S, Fitzgerald L: The active role of context. In: Dopson S, Fitzgerald L, (eds): *Knowledge to Action? Evidence-Based Health Care in Context.* Oxford, Oxford University Press: 79–103, 2005.
77. Fitzgerald L, Dopson S: Professional boundaries and the diffusion of innovation. In: Dopson S, Fitzgerald L, (eds): *Knowledge to Action? Evidence-Based Health Care in Context.* Oxford, Oxford University Press, 104–131, 2005.
78. Birmaher B, Khetarpal S, Brent D, et al.: The screen for child anxiety related emotional disorders (SCARED): scale construction and psychometric characteristics. *J Am Acad Child Adolesc Psychiatry* 36(4):545–553, 1997.
79. Group TMC: A 14-month randomized clinical trial of treatment strategies for attention-deficit/hyperactivity disorder. *Arch Gen Psychiatry* 56:1073–1086, 1999.
80. Hamilton J: Evidence-based practice for outpatient clinical teams. *J Am Acad Child Adolesc Psychiatry* 45(3):364–370, 2006.
81. Committee on Quality of Health Care in America, I.o.M. To Err Is Human: Building a Safer Health System. 2017 [cited 2017 Feb 3]; Available from: http://www.nap.edu/catalog/9728.html
82. Hamilton J, Daleiden E, Dopson S: Implementing evidence-based practices for youth in an HMO: The roles of external ratings and market share. *Adm Policy Ment Health* 38:203–210, 2011.
83. NCBI. Quality-Adjusted Life Years. 2017 [cited 2017 Feb 3]; Available from: https://www.ncbi.nlm.nih.gov/mesh/?term=quality+adjusted+life+year
84. Cohen J, Bukstein O, Walter H, et al.: Practive parameter for the assessment and treatment of children and adolescents with posttraumatic stress disorder. *J Am Acad Child Adolesc Psychiatry* 49(4):414–430, 2010.
85. Lock J, La Via MC; American Academy of Child and Adolescent Psychiatry (AACAP) Committee on Quality Issues (CQI): Practice parameter for the assessment and treatment of children and adolescents with eating disorders. *J Am Acad Child Adolesc Psychiatry* 54(5):412–425, 2015.
86. Jensen-Doss A, Weisz JR: Diagnostic agreement predicts treatment process and outcomes in youth mental health clinics. *J Consult Clin Psychol* 76(5):711–722, 2008.
87. Fontanella CA, Warner LA, Phillips GS, Bridge JA, Campo JV, et al., Trends in psychotropic polypharmacy among youths enrolled in Ohio Medicaid, 2002–2008. *J Am Acad Child Adolesc Psychiatry* 65(11):1132–1140, 2014.
88. Mohr WK: Experiences of patients hospitalized during the Texas mental health scandal. *Perspect Psychiatr Care* 34(4):5–17, 1998.
89. Novins DK, Green AE, Legha RK, Aarons GA: Dissemination and implementation of evidence-based practices for child and adolescent mental health: A systematic review. *J Am Acad Child Adolesc Psychiatry* 52(10):1009–1025, 2013.

CHAPTER 3.1.3 ■ RESPECT FOR CHILDREN AS RESEARCH SUBJECTS

ROBERT J. LEVINE

"So act as to treat humanity, whether in thine own person or in that of any other, in every case as an end withal, never as a means only." The German philosopher Immanuel Kant, writing late in the eighteenth century, provided this formal statement of the ethical principle of respect for persons. Persons are to be regarded as ultimate values in and of themselves; they are not to be used merely as means to another's goals.

Those who conduct research involving human subjects first define their goals and then identify persons whom they use as means to accomplish these goals. This is not unethical. What is proscribed is the use of persons merely as means—"as means only." To avoid this, researchers are required both ethically and legally to secure the approval of persons to be used as research subjects through a process called informed consent. If this approval entails acceptance of the researcher's goals, then the subject is not used merely as a means. Rather, the subject freely chooses to embrace the goals as his or her own and thus remains an end.

This chapter is concerned with informed consent and other issues related to the principle of respect for persons (e.g., privacy and confidentiality) as they relate to the involvement as research subjects of adolescents and children of various ages.

ETHICAL PRINCIPLES

The basic ethical principles identified by the National Commission for the Protection of Human Subjects of Biomedical and Behavioral Research (1) as those that should underlie the conduct of research involving human subjects are "respect for persons," "beneficence," and "justice." These principles were endorsed subsequently by the President's Commission for the Study of Ethical Problems in Medicine and Biomedical and Behavioral Research (2) as "basic values" for medical practice as well as for biomedical and behavioral research, calling them by somewhat different names: "respect," "well-being," and "equity." According to these authoritative commissions, research involving human subjects should be conducted in accord with norms or rules designed to uphold and embody these basic principles or values. These rules are assembled in federal regulations for the "protection of human research subjects"; most relevant to the present concerns are those of the Department of Health and Human Services (Code of Federal Regulations, Title 45, Part 46; hereafter abbreviated as 45 CFR 46)[1] and the Food and Drug Administration (FDA) (Code of Federal Regulations, Title 21, Parts 50 and 56; hereafter abbreviated as 21 CFR 50 and 21 CFR 56).

[1]SubPart A of 45 CFR 46, the basic DHHS regulations for the protection of human subjects are customarily referred to as the Common Rule because, with minor variations, they have been endorsed and adopted by almost all of the federal departments that conduct or support research involving human subjects. The other parts of the regulations providing special protections for fetuses and pregnant women (SubPart B), prisoners (SubPart C), and children (SubPart D) have not been adopted as part of the Common Rule. To avoid confusion in this chapter all DHHS regulations are referred to as 45 CFR 46. At the time of this writing, the DHHS Secretary's Advisory Committee on Human Research Protections is reviewing SubPart D with the aim of clarifying their definitions and the concepts. Their website is revised from time to time to show the current state of their deliberations (www.hhs.gov/ohrp/sachrp/index.html).

In this chapter there are frequent references to federal regulations. This is not intended to suggest that all ethical considerations are reflected adequately in the law. Rather, the regulations in this field generally represent a broad social consensus about what ought and ought not to be done. Even for research not covered by the regulations, they have come to be regarded as establishing a community standard, departures from which require justification (3). The regulations include both substantive and procedural rules (norms). A substantive rule specifies behaviors that are required (or forbidden) because they are morally right (or wrong). Some procedural rules specify procedures that should be performed to determine the most appropriate behavior when the behavior has not been specified by a substantive rule. Other procedural rules are designed either to assist in the adherence to the requirements of a substantive rule or to provide documentary evidence that research has been conducted in accord with the relevant substantive rules (3).

AN ILLUSTRATION

The principle of respect for persons requires that human persons must be treated as autonomous agents. The substantive norm that requires informed consent is a specification of one way in which this principle is to be made operational in the conduct of research involving human subjects. The procedural norm that requires review and approval by an institutional review board affords a method for determining what specific bits of information must be divulged to prospective subjects in a particular research protocol. Another procedural norm that requires the signing of a consent form provides documentary evidence that the behavior required by the substantive norm has been accomplished. The form itself assists the investigator's efforts to comply with the substantive rule.

> ***According to the National Commission:***
> Respect for persons incorporates at least two basic ethical convictions: First, that individuals should be treated as autonomous agents, and second, that persons with diminished autonomy and thus in need of protection are entitled to such protections. An autonomous person is . . . an individual capable of deliberation about personal goals and of acting under the direction of such deliberation (1).

To show respect for autonomous persons requires that we leave them alone, even to the point of allowing them to choose activities that might be harmful (e.g., hang gliding), unless they agree or consent that we may do otherwise. We are not to touch them or encroach on their private spaces unless such touching or encroachment is in accord with their wishes. Our actions should be designed to affirm their authority and enhance their capacity to be self-determining; we are not to obstruct their actions unless they are clearly detrimental to others. We show disrespect for autonomous persons when we either repudiate their considered judgments or deny them the freedom to act on those judgments in the absence of compelling reasons to do so.

Clearly, not every human being is capable of self-determination. The capacity for self-determination matures during a person's life; some lose this capacity partially or completely, owing to illness or mental disability or in situations that severely restrict liberty, such as prisons. Respect for the immature or incapacitated may require one to offer protection to them as they mature or while they are incapacitated.

Because the central focus of this chapter is on respect for persons, it is necessary to emphasize that the other two principles are of equal importance in the sense that they have equal moral force. Research involving human subjects can be considered ethically justified if, and only if, it is adequately responsive to each of the three basic ethical principles (3). As we shall see, considerations of justice and beneficence place constraints on, for example, whom we can ask to serve as research subjects and how much risk we may ask them to accept in the interests of research.

INFORMED CONSENT

Principle I of the Nuremberg Code (4) provides the definition of consent from which definitions supplied in all subsequent codes and regulations are derived:

> The *voluntary* consent of the human subject is absolutely essential.
>
> This means that the person involved should have *legal capacity* to give consent; should be so situated as to be able to exercise *free power of choice*, without the intervention of any element of force, fraud, deceit, duress, over-reaching or other ulterior form of constraint or coercion; and should have sufficient *knowledge* and *comprehension* of the elements of the subject matter involved as to enable him to make an understanding and enlightened decision [emphasis added].

Thus, consent is recognized as valid if it has each of these four essential attributes: It must be competent (legally), voluntary, informed, and comprehending (or understanding).

It is through informed consent that the investigator and subject enter into a relationship, defining mutual expectations and their limits. This relationship differs from ordinary commercial transactions in which each party is responsible for informing himself or herself of the terms and implications of any of their agreements. Professionals who intervene in the lives of others are held to higher standards. They are obligated to inform the layperson of the consequences of their mutual agreements.

It is worth noticing that the Nuremberg Code defines and requires "voluntary consent." Since 1957 this term has been replaced by "informed consent," a term that reflects an idealized vision of the person as a rational, self-determining agent (5).

Federal regulations identify "elements" of information that must be transmitted during the negotiations for informed consent (45 CFR 46.116a); these are:

1. A statement that the study involves research, an explanation of the purposes of the research, and the expected duration of the subject's participation, a description of the procedures to be followed, and identification of any procedures that are experimental
2. A description of any reasonably foreseeable risks or discomforts to the subject
3. A description of any benefits to the subject or others that may reasonably be expected from the research
4. A disclosure of appropriate alternative procedures or courses of treatment, if any, which might be advantageous to the subject
5. A statement describing the extent, if any, to which confidentiality of records identifying the subject will be maintained
6. For research involving more than minimal risk, an explanation as to whether any compensation and an explanation as to whether any medical treatments are available if injury occurs and, if so, what they may consist of or where further information may be obtained
7. An explanation of whom to contact for answers to pertinent questions about the research and research subjects' rights, and whom to contact in the event of a research-related injury to the subject
8. A statement that participation is voluntary, refusal to participate will involve no penalty or loss of benefits to

which the subject is otherwise entitled, and the subject may discontinue participation at any time without penalty or loss of benefits to which the subject is otherwise entitled

In addition, according to the regulations, the following elements must be provided "when appropriate" (45 CFR 46.116b):

1. A statement that the particular treatment or procedure may involve risks to the subject (or to the embryo or fetus, if the subject is or may become pregnant) that are currently unforeseeable
2. Anticipated circumstances under which the subject's participation may be terminated by the investigator without regard to the subject's consent
3. Any additional costs to the subject that may result from participation in research
4. The consequences of a subject's decision to withdraw from the research and procedures for orderly termination of participation by the subject
5. A statement that significant new findings developed during the course of the research that may relate to the subject's willingness to continue participation will be provided to the subject
6. The approximate number of subjects involved in the study

The regulations define only minimum standards for informed consent. In most cases it seems appropriate to supplement these basic requirements with additional elements of information (3). For example, prospective subjects should be told why they have been selected as invitees to participate in the research; ordinarily, this consists of a statement of the major inclusion and exclusion criteria for the protocol. In addition to the statement of "additional costs to the subject" required by the regulations, there should also be accurate statements of any cash payments or other economic advantages associated with participation in the research as a subject.

How does one determine whether any particular fact (e.g., any particular risk of injury) must be disclosed? The legal criterion for disclosure in the context of medical practice is "material risk," that is, any fact that is material to the patient's decision must be disclosed (3,6). The determination of which risks are material in that they must be disclosed may be accomplished according to three different standards or tests (3,7). Until recently, the prevailing standard was that of the "reasonable physician"; the determination of whether any particular risk or other fact should be disclosed was made on the basis of whether it was customary to do so in the community of practicing physicians.

The standard that is now applied most commonly is the "reasonable person" or "prudent patient" test. In the case of *Canterbury* v. *Spence* (8), the court held that the disclosure required was determined by the patient's right of self-decision, a right that can be effectively exercised only if the patient possesses enough information to enable an intelligent choice. A risk is thus material when a reasonable person, in what the physician knows or should know to be the patient's position, would be likely to attach significance to the risks or cluster of risks in deciding whether or not to forego the proposed therapy.

Some courts have adopted the rule that a risk is material if the particular patient making the choice or decision considers it material. Of the three standards, this rule, which some call the idiosyncratic person standard, is most responsive to the requirements of the ethical principle of respect for persons. It is, however, a highly impractical standard.

In the author's view, the reasonable person standard should determine the minimum amount of information that should be imparted by the researcher to each and every prospective subject. Then, in the course of the consent discussions, the researcher should attempt to learn from each prospective subject what more he or she would like to know.

Federal regulations permit "a consent procedure which does not include, or which alters, some or all of the elements of informed consent" or, in some cases, waiver of the entire requirement for informed consent, if:

> [a] The research involves no more than minimal risk to the subjects, [b] The waiver or alteration will not adversely affect the rights and welfare of the subjects, [c] The research could not practicably be carried out without the waiver or alteration, and [d] Whenever appropriate, the subjects will be provided with additional pertinent information after participation (45 CFR 46.116d).

Implicit in these conditions—particularly the second condition—is recognition of the standard of materiality. One may not withhold any material information without adversely affecting the rights of subjects. Waivers and alterations are commonly used in research involving medical records, "leftover" specimens of tissues and body fluids from which personal identifying information has been removed, survey research, and so on. It is more problematic when researchers propose to alter information for purposes of deceiving prospective research subjects (3).

The Department of Health and Human Services (DHHS) makes it clear that, "Nothing in these regulations is intended to limit the authority of a physician to provide emergency medical care, to the extent the physician is permitted to do so under applicable federal, state, or local law" (45 CFR 46.116f). Implicit in this rule is a recognition of two exceptions to the legal requirement for informed consent: the emergency exception and therapeutic privilege.[2]

The FDA permits waiver of the consent requirement for the use of investigational new drugs (or other regulated test articles) in the treatment of individuals in "life-threatening situations" in which "informed consent cannot be obtained...because of an inability to communicate with, or obtain legally effective consent from, the subject" (21 CFR 50.23). There is also a provision in FDA regulations for an exception from informed consent requirements for emergency research; this exception is designed for research activities in which most or all of the prospective subject population will be unable to consent and it will not be feasible (usually owing to lack of time) to get consent from a legally authorized representative (21 CFR 50.24).[3]

CONSENT FORMS

Thus far we have been considering informed consent, a process designed to show respect for subjects, fostering their interests by empowering them to pursue and protect their own interests. The consent form, by contrast, is an instrument designed to protect the interests of researchers and their institutions by defending them against civil or criminal liability. I believe that one of the reasons there has been so little successful litigation against investigators, as compared with practicing physicians, is the very formal and thorough documentation of informed consent on consent forms. Consent forms may be detrimental to the subject's interests not only in adversarial proceedings; signed consent forms in institutional records may lead to violations of privacy and confidentiality (3).

---

[2]For an authoritative commentary on these two exceptions, see Appendix 1 of the President's Commission's Report, Making Health Care Decisions (2). For a more concise discussion see Levine (3).

[3]There are further conditions specified by FDA in its regulations. For further discussion of 21 CFR 50.23, see Levine (3). For 21 CFR 50.24 see Brody (9).

DHHS regulations require:

> A written consent document that embodies the elements of informed consent.... This form may be read to the subject or the subject's legally authorized representative, but, in any event, the investigator shall give either the subject or the representative adequate opportunity to read it before it is signed (45 CFR 46.117).[4]

Although the primary purpose of the consent form is to protect the interests of researchers and their institutions, it is forbidden by federal regulations to:

> include any exculpatory language through which the subject or the representative is made to waive or appear to waive any of the subject's legal rights, or releases or appears to release the investigator, the sponsor, the institution or its agents from liability for negligence.[5]

DHHS requires that "[a] copy shall be given to the person signing the form" (45 CFR 46.117). The primary purpose of the form notwithstanding, it can and should be designed to be helpful to the subjects. Having a copy of the form will afford them an opportunity to continue to get more information as additional questions occur to them. It can also serve as a reminder of the plans they must follow in order to accomplish the purposes of research, of the symptoms they should watch for to protect their own safety, of the perils of omitting doses of drugs, and so on. It can serve as a guide to conversations they might choose to have with family, friends, personal doctors, and other trusted advisors about whether they should consent; in some cases such conversations should be recommended during the consent negotiations. In the use of these forms, however, the researcher should heed the words of the President's Commission (10): "Ethically valid consent is a process of shared decision-making based upon mutual respect and participation, not a ritual to be equated with reciting the contents of a form that details the risks of particular treatments."

No consent form can be designed so as to anticipate all of any particular prospective subject's wishes to be informed. The consent form is most effective when it is viewed by the researcher as a guide to the negotiations with the prospective subject. The consent form should contain at least the minimum amount of information and advice that should be presented during the negotiations. If any substantive new understandings are developed in the process of negotiations that have any bearing on the prospective subject's willingness to participate, these should be added to the consent form signed by that individual.

DHHS regulations (45 CFR 46.117) permit waiver of the requirement for documentation of informed consent if:

1. The only record linking the subject and the research would be the consent document and the principal risk would be potential harm resulting from a breach of confidentiality.
2. The research presents no more than minimal risk of harm to subjects and involves no procedures for which written consent is normally required outside of the research context.

In some cases in which the regulations permit waiver of the requirements for documentation, it may be advisable to provide subjects with information sheets. These documents provide a written account of all information that could serve subjects' interests in ways suggested earlier. They differ from consent forms primarily in that they are not signed by subjects and retained by researchers. Thus, they afford limited protection to the researcher and the institution.

JUSTIFICATION OF RESEARCH INVOLVING CHILDREN

Children, as a class of persons, lack the legal capacity to consent. Moreover, many of them, particularly the younger ones, are not only incapable of sufficient comprehension to meet the Nuremberg Code's standard but are also not "so situated as to be able to exercise free power of choice." It is necessary to rely on other devices to show respect for children because they cannot consent. Two of these devices are permission and assent.

Permission of one or both parents or of the legal guardian is closely related to what was formerly called proxy consent. With few exceptions, federal regulators regard permission as a necessary condition for authorizing the involvement of a child as a research subject; for children who cannot assent, it is usually a sufficient condition as well. The transactions involved in negotiating a valid permission are in all respects identical to those of informed consent.

Assent by the child should be as close an approximation of consent as the child's capabilities permit.

Before proceeding with our discussion of permission and assent, it is necessary to return to a consideration of the basic ethical principles.

Respect for persons requires that we treat individuals as autonomous agents only to the extent that they are autonomous. As noted earlier, "[p]ersons with diminished autonomy and thus in need of protection are entitled to such protections (1)." In response to this ethical conviction, there is established in federal regulations a standard called "minimal risk," which "means that the probability and magnitude of harm or discomfort anticipated in the research are not greater in and of themselves than those ordinarily encountered in daily life or during the performance of routine physical or psychological examinations or tests" (45 CFR 46).[6] Minimal risk serves as a threshold standard in that plans to involve children in research that presents more than minimal risk require special justification and procedural protections.

But many therapeutic procedures present far more than minimal risk, and it is not customary to obstruct children's access to them by calling for special procedural protections. The regulations make it clear that the minimal risk standard is applicable only to procedures that do not "hold out the prospect of direct benefit for the individual subjects" (45 CFR 46.405). Therapeutic procedures, by contrast, are to be authorized and justified precisely as they are in the practice of medicine. That is to say, the risk of any procedure is justified in terms of the benefit expected for the individual child-subject who will bear that risk. Also, as in medical practice, the relationship of anticipated benefit to the risk presented by the procedure must be at least as advantageous to the subject as that presented by any available alternative, unless, of course, the subject (or his or her parents) has considered and refused to accept a superior alternative. These rules are responsive to the ethical principle of beneficence, which as articulated by the National Commission (1) is expressed in the form of two general rules: "(1) Do no harm; and (2) maximize possible benefits and minimize possible harms."

Justice, as envisioned by the National Commission, requires a fair sharing of the burdens and benefits of society (1,3). In

---

[4]The Department of Health and Human Services regulations also permit use of a "short" form. Use of this form of documentation seems even more complicated and cumbersome than use of the standard consent form. Moreover, its use requires a witness to the consent discussion (3).

[5]Such language is also forbidden in the consent discussion (CFR 46.116).

[6]The term *minimal risk* presents many problems. As it is defined, it may be interpreted in several different ways. For a discussion of its deficiencies, see Levine (3) and Kopelman (11). For an excellent discussion relating the concept of risk to the child's level of development, see Thompson (41).

the distribution of these burdens and benefits, special consideration is to be given to those who are vulnerable or disadvantaged. Children are considered vulnerable and are to be protected from exploitation because they lack the capacity to consent. They are not to be involved in research that is irrelevant to the class of person of which they are representative. When appropriate, research should be done first on adults and then on older children before involving younger children and infants (3).

In summary, children and their parents are not completely free to do their own thing. There are constraints grounded in ethical considerations and enforced by regulations regarding whom researchers may invite to serve as subjects and how much risk they may be asked to assume for research purposes. With these constraints in mind, we now turn to further consideration of assent and permission.

ASSENT

Respect for children does not require that we leave them alone even to the point of allowing them to choose dangerous activities unless they agree that we may do otherwise. Young children have no such liberty rights. What they have instead is a right to custody (12). We show respect for them by fostering their well-being, protecting them from harm, and guiding them to become "the right kind of people."

As we have already noticed, federal regulations reflect the obligation to protect children from harm and to secure their well-being. Let us now consider the obligation to guide their moral and social development—an obligation not recognized explicitly in the regulations.

In the 1970s there was a spirited debate over the legitimacy of using persons who are incapable of consent ("unconsenting subjects") as research subjects. Paul Ramsey (13) argued that it is always morally wrong. Richard McCormick (14), arguing the opposing viewpoint, pointed out that members of a moral community have certain obligations. One of these is to contribute to the general welfare when to do so requires little or no sacrifice. In the case of children, one may presume that they would consent if they could; he calls this a "correctly construed consent." In his view, when supplemented with parental permission, correctly construed consent authorized the use of children as subjects in research that fulfilled an important social need and involved "no discernible risk."

At this point, Terrence Ackerman (15) entered the debate, arguing that we tend to fool ourselves with procedures designed to show respect for the child's very limited autonomy. He claims that the child tends to follow "the course of action that is recommended overtly or covertly by the adults who are responsible for the child's well-being." He further contends that, in general, this is as it ought to be. "Once we recognize our duty to guide the child and his inclination to be guided the task becomes that of guiding him in ways which will involve his well-being and contribute to his becoming the right kind of person."

Willard Gaylin (16) tells the story of a man who acted in accord with Ackerman's position. After directing his 10-year-old son to cooperate with a venipuncture for research purposes, he explained that his direction arose from his perceived moral obligation to teach his child that there are certain things one does to serve the interests of others even if it does cause a bit of pain:

> This is my child. I was less concerned with the research involved than with the kind of boy I was raising. I'll be damned if I was going to allow my child, because of some idiotic concept of children's rights, to assume that he was entitled to be a selfish, narcissistic little bastard.

Parenthetically, while it is appropriate to guide and persuade a 10-year-old boy to submit to a venipuncture for research purposes, it is not ethically defensible to command him to do so against his will; it is also contrary to the requirements of federal regulations. Guiding children to become the "right kind of persons" entails teaching them about and encouraging them to embrace the sense of obligation to the moral community discussed before. It further entails showing respect for their maturing capacities for self-determination; one hopes the child will learn to choose to do unto others as the child would wish them to do unto her or him.

At what age does a child become capable of assent? Federal regulations specify no age, leaving it to the discretion of the Institutional Review Board (IRB), taking into account not only the age but also the maturity and psychological state of the children involved.

As the assent regulation is written, it seems to reflect a presumption that the capability to assent is an all-or-none phenomenon; the child is either capable or incapable of assent. This presumption is incorrect (17,18) and, the author believes, unintended by the regulation writers. In the author's view the regulations are intended to be interpreted to permit a determination that prospective child-subjects may be capable of understanding some but not all of the elements of informed consent. Thus, for example, it may be appropriate to provide some children with "a description of any reasonably foreseeable risks or discomforts," without providing "an explanation as to whether any compensation [is] available if injury occurs."

It is possible to make some general comments on the capabilities to assent of children having normal cognitive development in various age groups. According to Lois Weithorn (17), who relates her empirical findings to Piaget's concepts of cognitive development:

> ...in general, developmental research suggests that most school-aged children are capable of meaningful assent for participation in most types of research studies. This means that the children probably are capable of comprehending the nature of the proposed procedures, the general purpose of the research, and of expressing a preference regarding participation. Research suggests that normal children ages 6 and older are quite capable of thoughtful and reasoned consideration of the types of information that investigators may provide.

Typically, at about age 11, children's cognitive development enters the "stage of formal operations," during which they become increasingly sophisticated in their capacities to reason about "possibility" and other abstract concepts. From ages 7 to 11, in the "stage of concrete operations," the child is more or less limited to thinking about matters that are not too far removed from concrete reality. Thus, there are those who argue that the "age of assent" should be around 6 or 7, and others who say it should be around 11 or 12.[7]

Weithorn (17) continues:

> Early empirical findings also suggest that, although they may not be legally authorized to provide independent consent for treatment or research in most jurisdictions, normal adolescents age 14 and older may be as capable as adults of making competent decisions about such participation, according to the more stringent legal standards of competency.

[7]According to the National Commission (19), a child with normal cognitive development becomes capable of meaningful assent at about the age of 7 years, although some may be younger and some older. The Department of Health and Human Services (DHHS) did not accept this recommendation. Rather, at the time the proposed regulations were published, DHHS solicited public comment on which of three options it should adopt for nontherapeutic procedures: either age 7, age 12, or leaving the age to the discretion of the IRB. The final regulations reflect the third of these options.

The authority of mature and emancipated minors to consent is discussed subsequently in this chapter.

PERMISSION

Parental permission is envisioned by the National Commission as a reflection of the collective judgment of the family that an infant or child may participate in research (3,19). In most cases the permission of one parent is sufficient; one may assume that he or she will represent the family's wishes satisfactorily.

When more than minimal risk is presented by a nontherapeutic procedure, the permission of both parents is required unless one is "deceased, unknown, incompetent, or not reasonably available, or when only one person has legal responsibility for the care or custody of the child" (45 CFR 46.408).

There are three additional criteria for justification of nontherapeutic procedures that present more than minimal risk (45 CFR 46.406): First, the degree of risk is limited to "a minor increase over minimal risk." Second, the procedure or intervention must be "likely to yield generalizable knowledge which is of vital importance for the understanding or amelioration of the subject's disorder or condition."[8] Third, the procedure or intervention must present "experiences to subjects that are reasonably commensurate with those inherent in their actual or expected medical, dental, psychological, social, or educational situations." This means that the procedures must be ones that they or others with the specific disorder or condition under study will ordinarily experience by virtue of their having or being treated for that disorder or condition. Thus, it might be appropriate to invite a child with leukemia who has had several bone marrow examinations to consider having another one for research purposes.

The requirement of commensurability reflects the National Commission's judgment that children who have had a procedure performed on them might be more capable than are those who are not so experienced of basing their assent on some familiarity with the procedure and its attendant discomforts; thus their decision to participate will be more knowledgeable.

Even though the parent gives permission, the child's refusal to assent to nontherapeutic interventions should be respected. Those who are incapable of assent may have some capacity to make their wishes known. The term *deliberate objection* is used to recognize that some children who are incapable of meaningful assent are able to communicate their disapproval or refusal of a proposed procedure. A 4 year old may protest, "No, I don't want to be stuck with a needle." However, an infant who might in certain circumstances cry or withdraw in response to almost any stimulus is not regarded as capable of deliberate objection. A child's deliberate objection usually should be regarded as a veto to his or her involvement in research (3,19).

In the case of therapeutic interventions or procedures, the situation is much different. Federal regulations state simply, the assent of children is not a necessary condition (45 CFR 46.408). Parents have both the right and responsibility to override the objection of school-age children to necessary therapy. With regard to teenagers, decisions regarding authorization of investigational therapies are about as complicated as they are in the practice of medicine. The law recognizes the authority of emancipated and some mature minors to consent to or refuse standard or accepted therapy; these rules are not recognized explicitly in federal regulations regarding investigational therapies.

In the practical world of decision making about who can authorize a therapeutic procedure, whether it is investigational or accepted, it rarely suffices to point to the law and thereby identify the person who has the legal right to make the decision. Many factors must be taken into account in reaching judgments about the capability of various persons to participate in and, in the event of irreconcilable disputes, prevail in such choices. In general, these judgments become more complicated as the child gets older or the stakes get higher (16,20).

IRBs have the authority to waive the requirement for permission when "it is not a reasonable requirement... provided an appropriate mechanism for protecting the children is substituted" (45 CFR 46.408). The regulations suggest as an example of research in which a requirement for parental permission might not be reasonable is that on "neglected or abused children." The National Commission (19) specified several other examples:

> Research designed to identify factors related to the incidence or treatment of certain conditions in adolescents for which, in certain jurisdictions, they may legally receive treatment without parental consent; research in which the subjects are "mature minors" and the procedures involved entail essentially no more than minimal risk that such individuals might reasonably assume on their own; research designed to meet the needs of children designated by their parents as "in need of supervision," and research involving children whose parents are legally or functionally incompetent.

THE NATIONAL COMMISSION (19) FURTHER ELABORATES:

> There is no single mechanism that can be substituted for parental permission in every instance. In some cases the consent of mature minors should be sufficient. In other cases court approval may be required. The mechanism involved will vary with the research and the age, status and condition of the prospective subject....
>
> Assent of... mature minors should be considered sufficient with respect to research about conditions for which they have the legal authority to consent on their own to treatment. An appropriate mechanism for protecting such subjects might be to require that a clinic nurse or physician, unrelated to the research, explain the nature and the purpose of the research... emphasizing that participation is unrelated to provision of care. Another alternative might be to appoint a social worker, pediatric nurse, or physician to act as surrogate parent when the research is designed, for example, to study neglected or battered children. Such surrogate parents would be expected to participate not only in the process of soliciting the children's cooperation but also in the conduct of the research, in order to provide reassurance for the subject and to intervene or support their desires to withdraw if participation becomes too stressful.

The recommendations of the National Commission reflected their assumption that the "normal" family is one in which the members stand in a loving relationship to one another and that the parents in such a family will strive to protect the interests and welfare of their children. This point notwithstanding, they were aware of the fact that there are exceptions. In obvious cases (e.g., neglected or abused children) they recommended that the IRB should have the authority to waive the requirement for parental permission. In the less obvious cases, of which there may be many, decisions as to whether the parents are

[8]What constitutes "minor increase" and "vital importance" is not defined in the regulations. Responsibility for deciding such matters in relation to particular research proposals is assigned to the IRB. If the IRB cannot decide or if it does decide that the degree of risk is more than a minor increase over minimal risk, it must refer the judgment to the Secretary of The Department of Health and Human Services (3).

loyal to their children and welfare require sophisticated professional judgment. The National Commission wisely refrained from recommending that IRBs engage in micromanagement of such cases. Implicitly, the responsibility for such judgments is assigned to the investigator. The National Commission provided a margin of safety by recommending special substantive and procedural protections in cases in which more than minimal risk is presented by interventions that do not hold out the prospect of direct benefit for the individual child-subject.

In recent years there has been increasing interest in giving mature minors independent authority to authorize their own participation in certain types of research without requiring permission of their parents or guardians. To some extent this interest reflects a general trend in public policy toward facilitating inclusion as research subjects members of groups who were previously excluded (21). This interest also represents a pragmatic response to problems presented by the AIDS pandemic; specifically, many, and perhaps most, adolescents will not enroll as research subjects if this necessarily entails allowing their parents or guardians to learn or even suspect certain details of their sexual or drug-taking experience (22).

Most of the current federal regulations for the protection of human subjects reflect the attitude that prevailed in the 1960s and 1970s when they were written, that investigational drugs and participation in research were dangerous and researchers were likely to exploit subjects. Since the mid-1980s, primarily as a consequence of the efforts of AIDS activists, this vision has been largely replaced by one that research participation and access to investigational drugs are both more beneficial than burdensome. As a result of this shift in perception, public policies that were designed to protect persons from harm and exploitation, particularly those persons who are considered vulnerable by reason of limitation in their capacity to give informed consent, are being reinterpreted or rewritten to assure the same classes of persons equitable access to the benefits of investigational drugs as well as to the benefits of participation in research (21).

It has long been known that restrictive policies on involvement of children in research have resulted in a class injustice. Children as a class have been deprived of the benefits of the new knowledge that could result from carrying out research involving children as subjects. This deprivation is exemplified by the fact that approximately 80% of the drugs approved by the FDA for commercial distribution are not labeled for use in children, usually because sufficient studies have not been conducted in children (23,24). In recent years agencies of the federal government have begun to respond to this class injustice. The National Institutes of Health now require that applications for grants or contracts to conduct research involving human subjects must include plans to enroll children unless the applicant can justify their exclusion (25). Similarly, the FDA requires inclusion of children in research done to support an application for a marketing permit unless the sponsor can justify their exclusion (26,27).

At the time of this writing, federal policies have not been revised to permit involvement of mature minors as research subjects on their own authority except as discussed earlier in this chapter. However, it seems reasonable to predict that in the near future there could be such changes in the relevant policies or their interpretation. Santelli et al. (28) and Levine (29) have published examples of specific proposals. Inclusion of children who are wards (e.g., of the state) in research in which more than minimal risk is presented by nontherapeutic interventions requires special procedural protections that are beyond the scope of this discussion (45 CFR 46.409) (3). Many states and cities have regulations designed to protect the interests of foster children.

Concern has been expressed recently that such regulations often create formidable bureaucratic barriers to involving such children in randomized clinical trials or gaining them access to investigational drugs. For two reasons this presents a special problem to children with AIDS: (a) A large percentage of such children are foster children; and (b) many apparently effective therapies for AIDS and its complications are investigational drugs (30).

DOCUMENTATION

The regulatory requirement for documentation of permission is exactly the same as it is for informed consent. In circumstances in which there is no requirement for permission because the minor is authorized to assent for himself or herself the same requirements for documentation obtain. Apart from this, when children are asked to sign forms, as they often and quite properly are, the principal purpose, in the author's view, is to enhance their sense of participation in the process.

PRIVACY AND CONFIDENTIALITY

Privacy is "the freedom of the individual to pick and choose for himself the time and circumstances under which, and most importantly, the extent to which, his attitudes, beliefs, behavior, and opinions are to be shared with or withheld from others" (31). Because this is the definition used in this chapter, some matters considered by the law to fall under the rubric of privacy are excluded (the right to abortion and contraception). In general, in clinical research, intrusions into individuals' privacy are permitted only with their informed consent. There is no invasion when an informed person allows a researcher into his or her private space.

Confidentiality is a term that is all too often used interchangeably with *privacy*. Confidentiality refers to a mode of management of private information; if a subject shares private information with (confides in) a researcher, the researcher is expected to refrain from sharing this information with others without either the subject's authorization or some other justification.

The ethical grounding for the requirement to respect the privacy of persons may be found in the principle of respect for persons. The ethical justification for confidentiality, according to Sissela Bok (32), is grounded in four premises, three of which support confidentiality in general; the fourth supports professional confidentiality in particular.

First and foremost, we must respect the individual's autonomy regarding personal information. To the extent they wish, and to the extent they are capable of doing so, they are entitled to have secrets. This facilitates their ability to live according to their own life plans.

Closely related is the second premise, which recognizes the legitimacy not only of having personal secrets but also of sharing them with whomever one chooses. This premise, which embodies an obligation to show respect for relationships among human beings and respect for intimacy, is exemplified by the marital privilege upheld in American law, according to which one spouse cannot be forced to testify against the other.

The third premise draws on the general requirement to keep promises. A pledge of confidentiality creates an obligation beyond the respect owing to persons and existing relationships. Once we are bound by a promise, we may no longer be fully impartial in our dealings with the promise.

These three premises, taken together, provide strong prima facie reasons to support confidentiality. That is to say, they are binding on those who have accepted information in confidence unless there are sufficiently powerful reasons to do otherwise—as, for example, when maintaining confidentiality would cause serious harm to innocent third parties.

Bok's fourth premise adds strength to the pledge of silence given by professionals. The professional's duty to maintain confidentiality goes beyond ordinary loyalty, "because of its utility to persons and to society...Individuals benefit from such confidentiality because it allows them to seek help they might otherwise fear to ask for" from doctors or others who can provide it.

Investigators, of course, are not necessarily professionals to whom individuals turn for professional help. Thus, only part of the fourth premise applies to investigators, the part that grounds the justification and requirement for confidentiality in its social utility. If researchers violated the confidence of their subjects, subjects would refuse to cooperate with them. This, in turn, would make it difficult, if not impossible, for researchers to contribute to the development of generalizable knowledge.

Over the millennia, the professions have viewed the obligation to maintain confidentiality as very important. The Hippocratic Oath requires, "What I may see or hear in the course of the treatment or even outside the treatment in regard to the life of men, which on no account one must spread abroad, I will keep to myself holding such things shameful to be spoken about."

Thomas Percival's *Code of Medical Ethics* (33), on which was based the first code of ethics of the American Medical Association, incorporated the following exhortation: "Patients should be interrogated concerning their complaints in a tone of voice which cannot be overheard."

In all states, the law not only recognizes the obligation of physicians and many other professionals to maintain confidentiality, it requires it. In many states, there are statutes granting testimonial privilege to information secured by physicians from patients in the course of medical practice (34). Testimonial privilege means that physicians cannot be compelled to disclose such information even under subpoena. Although the United States Supreme Court refused to extend the constitutional protections of privacy to physician–patient communications, the *Federal Rules of Evidence,* promulgated by the Judicial Conference, defer to state law on physician–patient privilege (34).

Most state laws on physician–patient privilege contain various exceptions, including mandatory reporting of information regarding battered and abused children, various communicable diseases, gunshot wounds, and certain proceedings concerned with health issues, including workers' compensation and insurance claims (34).

In 1974, in the case of *Tarasoff* v. *Board of Regents,* the supreme court of California ruled that a psychiatrist has a duty to protect the intended victim of a patient's threat of violence, if it is likely that such a threat would be carried out (35); this often but not always entails a duty to warn the intended victim. Subsequently, this duty has been recognized in many other states. The same principle is often invoked in debates over whether state laws should be changed to either permit or require doctors to warn sexual partners of persons infected with the HIV virus if they are unwilling to do so themselves (36).

It must be recognized that the right to confidentiality or privilege belongs to the patient. The patient may authorize sharing of private information for whatever purposes he or she chooses. In civil or criminal litigation where the patient makes the information in his or her medical record material to the support of his or her position, as so often happens in child custody cases or malpractice litigation, the court usually requires that the contents of the record be disclosed (35).

CONFIDENTIALITY IN RESEARCH

Most direct social injuries to research subjects result from breaches of confidentiality. An investigator may identify a subject as a drug or alcohol abuser, as a participant in various deviant sexual practices, as having any of a variety of diseases that may be deemed unacceptable by his or her family or social or political group, as having a higher or lower income than acquaintances might have predicted, as a felon, and so on. If certain individuals know such information, it might cost the subject his or her reputation, job, social standing, credit, or citizenship.

In recognition of these threats of social injury, federal regulations require the IRB to determine that "Where appropriate, there are adequate provisions to protect the privacy of subjects and to maintain the confidentiality of data" (45 CFR 46.111a).

How does one determine that provisions to maintain confidentiality are "adequate"? The first step is to become aware of the variety of factors that may pose threats to confidentiality in the research context. The second is to become aware of the various devices that are available to secure the confidentiality of research data.

The National Commission (37) offered some suggestions for safeguards of confidentiality: Depending on the degree of sensitivity of the data, appropriate methods may include coding or removal of individual identifiers as soon as possible, limitation of access to data, or the use of locked file cabinets. Researchers occasionally collect data that, if disclosed, would put subjects in legal jeopardy. Because research records are subject to subpoena, the National Commission suggests that when the identity of subjects who have committed crimes is to be recorded, the study should be conducted under assurances of confidentiality that are available from DHHS as well as the Department of Justice. For detailed information on these assurances of confidentiality, which provide immunity from subpoena, see (38).

CONSENT

As mentioned in the preceding, informed consent regulations require "a statement describing the extent, if any, to which confidentiality of records identifying the subject will be maintained." Statements about confidentiality of research records should not promise more than the researchers can guarantee. For most studies in which the private information to be collected is not especially sensitive, it suffices to state that the researchers intend to maintain confidentiality, that they will take precautions against violations, and that all reports of the research will be in the form of aggregated data and devoid of identifiers. When dealing with more sensitive information, it may be useful to specify some of the precautions; for example, videotapes will be destroyed within 60 days or, if the subject so requests, earlier; data will be kept in locked files; individuals will be identified by a code and only a small number of researchers will have access to the key that links code numbers to identifiers.

Plans to incorporate data in the subject's medical record should be made explicit. In general, when these data are relevant to patient management, they should be incorporated unless the subject objects. Incorporation of the results of nonvalidated diagnostic tests may lead to false diagnostic inferences, with adverse consequences to the patient's medical care or insurability. Most people do not understand the full implications of signing forms that release their medical records to insurance companies (39).

It is essential to disclose all serious threats of confidentiality breaches that can be anticipated. One such disclosure was used in a study of devices designed to encourage young children who are thought to have been abused sexually to speak freely of their experiences. A portion of the permission form for the normal control subjects reads as follows (3):

> Because this study is not intended to be related to either diagnosis or therapy for you or your child, you are entitled to decide whether the information obtained during this study should be entered into the medical record. If, however, during your child's interview, his or her behavior raises a concern of sexual abuse, a clinical evaluation of your child will be performed.... If after that evaluation the suspicion of sexual abuse persists, the case will be reported as mandated by law.

FDA regulations require (21 CFR 50.25a) "a statement describing the extent, if any, to which confidentiality of records identifying the subject will be maintained and notes the possibility that the [FDA] may inspect the records."

As noted earlier, federal regulations permit waiver of the informed consent requirement under certain conditions. These conditions are usually but not invariably met in studies of medical records (given adequate safeguards of confidentiality) or of "leftover" specimens obtained at autopsy, surgery, or collection for diagnostic purposes of body fluids such as blood or urine. In general, use of tissues or fluids without consent is justified if two conditions are satisfied (3): (a) No more tissue or fluid is removed than the amount needed to accomplish the medically indicated purpose of removal; and (b) the specimens are obtained by the researcher under conditions of anonymity (the diagnostic laboratory removes all personal identifiers before giving the specimens to the researcher).[9]

The practices just described are invasions of privacy. In such cases, patients are said to have a right of notice, that is, a right to be notified that such practices occur in the institution. These notices, which partially mitigate the invasion, are commonly printed in patient information brochures and on permission forms for surgery or autopsy. Although they are designed to afford patients opportunities to object, objections are rare. For examples of such notices, see Levine (3).

In some cases, with suitable justification, even the right of notice may be waived. Examples of such activities include collections of cord blood from neonates under conditions of anonymity in a nationwide study to determine the prevalence of HIV antibodies (3); monitoring for compliance in some randomized clinical trials (3); and covert observation or recording of public behavior (3). Further discussion of these activities and their justification is beyond the scope of this chapter. It must be noted that covert observation is a mild form of deception. In some cases even stronger forms of deception may be justified (3,40).

Researchers commonly use medical or laboratory records to identify patients who might be suitable subjects for their studies. Having identified them, they then contact them by telephone or mail with invitations to participate in research. Those who are contacted usually do not recall having read notices describing such activities in hospital brochures. Some will wonder why a stranger who knows his or her diagnosis is calling. Careful plans must be made to avoid offending patients in such activities (3).

CHILDREN AND PRIVACY

The concerns of young children about privacy are different from those of older children and adolescents (41). Young children first develop territorial privacy ("This is my room") and possessional privacy ("This is my tricycle") and only later begin to develop informational privacy (concerns about others' knowledge of one's activities, associations, and interests). Thus young children may not know that what they say to others may be detrimental to the privacy interests of their families.

DHHS regulations are responsive to this concern. There are several classes of research that are generally considered so free of complicated ethical problems that they are exempted from coverage by the regulations (45 CFR 46.101b). Two of these exemptions do not apply to research involving children: (a) research involving survey or interview procedures; and (b) research involving observation of public behavior in which the researcher is a participant. These activities are not exempt in cases in which they "could reasonably place the subject at risk of criminal or civil liability or be damaging to the subject's financial standing or employability."

Researchers often must secure the approval of various custodians of children to involve them in research. Such custodians may be teachers, daycare workers, camp counselors, and the like. At times it is important to withhold or disguise some of the purposes of the research in order to protect the family's privacy or to avoid prejudicial treatment of children. For example, one would generally avoid telling teachers that the children are selected because they are offspring of parents with emotional disturbances.

As mentioned, informed consent requires "an explanation of the purpose of research." Does this mean that parents must always receive a full disclosure of purposes? Suppose the purpose is—as it was in one study—to determine whether little boys with XYY chromosome patterns are more likely than those with XY patterns to develop violent behavior. Disclosure of such a purpose could become a self-fulfilling prophecy. For further discussion of withholding the purpose of research and its justification, see Levine (3).

As mentioned earlier, the requirement for parental permission may be waived in "research designed to identify factors related to the incidence or treatment of certain conditions in adolescents for which... they may legally receive treatment without parental consent." In general, the types of activities contemplated by this rule are treatment of sexually transmitted diseases, provision of contraceptive advice, and other matters that teenagers consider highly sensitive. We recognize the teenager's right to privacy, but how far should we go to protect it? Some of the factors that require consideration are illustrated in the following exchange.

Herceg-Baron (42) published a case study in which she detailed some of the special problems involved in research in the field of family planning involving minors as subjects. Many adolescents wish to seek advice about such matters as contraception without the awareness of such others as their parents. She details her institution's policy for protecting the minors' confidentiality. For instance, with regard to follow-up, investigators are required to offer various options, for example, telephone calls during certain hours when the minor knows she will be at home alone; contacts through school personnel such as nurses, teachers, or counselors; contacts by mail containing no agency letterhead or other identifying information; or leaving messages with friends.

In commenting on this case study, Carol Levine (43) raises several concerns. First, she suggests that many adolescents are ambivalent about clandestine sex and would, with some encouragement, welcome open discussion with their parents. The great concern with privacy seems to undermine the possibility for what could be valuable communication within the family. Levine is further concerned about the fact that the institution not only approves deception, but also it collaborates with the adolescent in deceiving her parents. This, she argues, sets a very poor example for the adolescent.

This brings us back to a point discussed in the preceding. Parents are not the only adults having responsibility

[9]In some cases it may be impossible to remove identifiers, as when the patient's physician is also the researcher. In such cases the requirement for consent may be waived if the research will not yield any information having diagnostic significance. For further discussion of this point, see Levine (3).

for guiding the child to become the "right kind of person." Professionals must be aware of the fact that children see them as models of proper behavior. Consciously or otherwise, they provide examples that children will emulate. Accordingly, they should be especially careful not to suggest by example that promises (e.g., of confidentiality), truthfulness, and other ethical matters discussed in this chapter are to be taken lightly. In short, they should help children understand the importance of showing respect for persons.

ACKNOWLEDGMENTS

This work was funded in part by grant 1 P30 MH 62294 01A1 from the National Institute of Mental Health and a grant from the Patrick and Catherine Weldon Donaghue Medical Research Foundation.

Portions of this chapter are excerpted or adapted from Levine RJ: *Ethics and Regulation of Clinical Research.* 2nd ed. New Haven, CT, Yale University Press, 1988.

References

1. National Commission for the Protection of Human Subjects of Biomedical and Behavioral Research: *The Belmont Report: Ethical Principles and Guidelines for the Protection of Human Subjects of Research.* (DHEW publication no. [OS] 78–0012). Washington, DC, U.S. Department of Health, Education, and Welfare, 1978.
2. President's Commission for the Study of Ethical Problems in Medicine and Biomedical and Behavioral Research. *Summing Up.* (stock no. 040–000–00475–1). Washington, DC, U.S. Government Printing Office, 1983.
3. Levine RJ: *Ethics and Regulation of Clinical Research.* 2nd ed. New Haven, Yale University Press, 1988.
4. *Nuremberg Code (in) Trials of War Criminals before the Nuremberg Military Tribunals*: Control Council Law no. 10 (vol. 2). Washington, DC, U.S. Government Printing Office, 181–182, 1949.
5. Katz J: *The Silent World of Doctor and Patient.* New York, Free Press, 1984.
6. Holder AR: *Medical Malpractice Law.* 2nd ed. New York, Wiley, 1978.
7. Curran WJ: Ethical issues in short term and long term psychiatric research. In: Ayd FJ (ed): *Medical, Moral, and Legal Issues in Mental Health Care.* Baltimore, MD, Williams & Wilkins, 1974.
8. *Canterbury* v. *Spence,* 464 F 2d 72, CA DC, 1972.
9. Brody B: Human subjects research, law, FDA rules. In: Murray TH, Mehlman MJ (eds): *Encyclopedia of Ethical, Legal and Policy Issues in Biotechnology.* New York, Wiley Interscience, 675–683, 2000.
10. President's Commission for the Study of Ethical Problems in Medicine and Biomedical and Behavioral Research: *Making Health Care Decisions: The Ethical and Legal Implications of Informed Consent in the Patient–Practitioner Relationship.* (stock no. 040–000–00459–9). Washington, DC, U.S. Government Printing Office, 1982.
11. Kopelman L: Children as research subjects: a dilemma. *J Med Philosophy Millennium Iss* 25(6):745–764, 2000.
12. Freedman B: A moral theory of informed consent. *Hastings Ctr Rep* 5(4):32–39, 1975.
13. Ramsey P: The enforcement of morals: nontherapeutic research on children. *Hastings Ctr Rep* 6(4):21–30, 1976.
14. McCormick RA: Proxy consent in the experimentation situation. *Perspect Biol Med* 18(2):2–20, 1974.
15. Ackerman TF: Fooling ourselves with child autonomy and assent in nontherapeutic clinical research. *Clin Res* 27:345–348, 1979.
16. Gaylin W: Competence: no longer all or none. In: Gaylin W, Macklin R (eds): *Who Speaks for the Child?* New York, Plenum, 27–54, 1982.
17. Weithorn LA: Children's capacities to decide about participation in research. *IRB: Rev Hum Subjects Res* 5(2):1–5, 1983.
18. Weithorn LA: Involving children in decisions involving their own welfare. In: Melton GB, Koocher GP, Saks MI (eds): *Children's Competence to Consent.* New York, Plenum, 235–260, 1983.
19. National Commission for the Protection of Human Subjects of Biomedical and Behavioral Research: *Research Involving Children: Report and Recommendations.* Washington, DC, U.S. Department of Health, Education, and Welfare. (DHEW publication no. [OS] 77–0004), 1977.
20. Thomasma DC, Mauer AM: Ethical complications of clinical therapeutic research on children. *Soc Sci Med* 16:913–919, 1982.
21. Levine RJ: The impact of HIV infection on society's perception of clinical trials. *Kennedy Inst Ethics J* 4:93–98, 1994.
22. Rogers AS, D'Angelo L, Futterman D: Guidelines for adolescent participation in research: current realities and possible resolutions. *IRB: Rev Hum Subjects Res* 16(4):1–6, 1994.
23. Guidelines for the ethical conduct of studies to evaluate drugs in pediatric populations. Committee on Drugs, American Academy of Pediatrics. *Pediatrics* 95:286–294, 1995.
24. Groopman J: The pediatric gap. Why have most medications never been properly tested on kids? *New Yorker* 32–37, 2005, (January 10).
25. National Institutes of Health: NIH policy and guidelines on the inclusion of children as participants in research involving human subjects. Available at: http://grants.nih.govgrantsguidenotice-filesnot 98–024.html, March 6, 1998.
26. Public Law 105–115: *Food and Drug Administration Modernization Act of 1997. Subtitle B. Section 111. Pediatric Studies of Drugs.*
27. Center for Drug Evaluation and Research: Frequently asked questions on pediatric exclusivity (505A), the pediatric "rule," and their interaction. Available at: http://www.fda.govcderpediatricfaqs.htm. Accessed May 24, 2017.
28. Santelli JS, Rogers AS, Rosenfeld WD, et al.: Guidelines for adolescent health research: a position paper of the Society for Adolescent Medicine. *Journal of Adolescent Health* 33:396–409, 2003.
29. Levine RJ: Adolescents as research subjects without permission of their parents or guardians: ethical considerations. *J Adolesc Health* 17:287–297, 1995.
30. *Secretary's Work Group on Pediatric HIV Infection and Disease: Final Report (NIH Publication no. 89–3063).* Washington, DC, Department of Health and Human Services, 1988.
31. Kelman HC: Privacy and research with human beings. *J Soc Issues* 33:169–195, 1977.
32. Bok S: *Secrets: On the Ethics of Concealment and Revelation.* New York, Pantheon, 1982.
33. Percival T: *Medical Ethics.* London, Russell, 1803. Reprint edited by Leake CD. Baltimore, MD, Williams & Wilkins, 1927.
34. Brennan TA: Research records. Litigation and confidentiality: the case of research on toxic substances. *IRB: Rev Hum Subjects Res* 5(5):6–9, 1983.
35. Holder AR: *Legal Issues in Pediatrics and Adolescent Medicine,* 2nd ed. New Haven, CT, Yale University Press, 1985.
36. Gostin LD: Public health strategies for confronting AIDS: legislative and regulatory policy in the United States. *JAMA* 261:1621–1630, 1989.
37. *National Commission for the Protection of Human Subjects of Biomedical and Behavioral Research: Institutional Review Boards: Report and Recommendations* (DHEW publication no; [OS] 78–0010). Washington, DC, U.S. Department of Health, Education, and Welfare, 1978.
38. Office for Human Research Protections (OHRP): *Guidance on Certificates of Confidentiality.* Available at: http://www.hhs.gov/ohrp/humansubjects/guidance/certconf.htm. February 25, 2003.
39. Siegler M: Confidentiality in medicine—a decrepit concept. *N Engl J Med* 307:1518–1521, 1982.
40. American Psychological Association: *Ethical Principles of Psychologists and Code of Conduct 2002.* Available at: http://www.apa.org/ethics/. Accessed May 24, 2017.
41. Thompson RA: Behavioral research involving children: a developmental perspective on research risk. *IRB: Rev Hum Subjects Res* 12(2):1–6, 1990.
42. Herceg-Baron R: Parental consent and family planning research involving minors. *IRB: Rev Hum Subjects Res* 3(9):5–8, 1981.
43. Levine C: Commentary: Teenagers, research and family involvement. *IRB: Rev Hum Subjects Res* 3(9):8, 1981.

3.2 ■ EPIDEMIOLOGY

CHAPTER 3.2.1 ■ EPIDEMIOLOGY

ERIC FOMBONNE

This chapter introduces the reader to basic concepts and terminology used in epidemiologic research. In the first part, we illustrate how epidemiologists measure disease occurrence, design studies, and select samples to identify risk factors, and evaluate data to establish the causal nature of statistical relationships. In the second part, some achievements of 40 years of epidemiologic research in child psychiatry are reviewed briefly. We first review issues specific to psychiatric epidemiology as they apply to the definition and assessment of child psychopathology in relation to the differentiation between normal and abnormal development, the use of dimensional or categorical approaches to case definition, the need to use impairment measures and to combine data from multiple informants, the need to take into account high rates of comorbidity between disorders, and the implications of pervasiveness or situational specificity of behaviors in estimating rates and risk associations for psychiatric disorders. Basic principles of measurement (reliability and validity) are defined as well as techniques used to screen and evaluate the performance of instruments. We then summarize findings on global psychiatric morbidity in children and adolescents as estimated from recent major population surveys and discuss issues relevant to special groups or new methodologies.

GENERAL EPIDEMIOLOGY

Definition and Historical Background

Epidemiology is the study of the distribution of diseases in human populations and of the factors that influence that distribution. The focus of epidemiology is to study patterns of disease occurrence in order to identify factors that are causally associated with the *onset* of disease in some individuals. Epidemiology relies essentially on *observational* (nonexperimental) methods. *Descriptive* epidemiology is mostly concerned with estimating rates of the disease for public health, or for administrative or monitoring purposes. *Analytical* or causative epidemiology concentrates on the identification of causes of disease occurrence in humans. *Clinical* epidemiology encompasses activities that use epidemiologic methods to study other aspects of a disease, such as its natural history, factors that facilitate offset or persistence of the disorder, or relapse or other outcomes (i.e., mortality). One part of clinical epidemiology employs *experimental* methods (randomized clinical trials), where investigators can manipulate (through randomization) variables (treatments to which patients will be exposed) in designs that facilitate the derivation of causal inferences. Other types of epidemiology (genetic, occupational, psychiatric, etc.) are defined both by the substantive area of research and by appropriate modifications of epidemiologic techniques and tools, although epidemiologic concepts and theories remain essentially the same across domains of application. The rest of the chapter is concerned with observational studies.

Epidemiology started in the nineteenth century with studies of infectious diseases, such as with the discovery of the infectious nature and mode of transmission of cholera in a London epidemic. In psychiatry, early efforts at the turn of the twentieth century helped to uncover the carential nature of the pellagra encephalopathy; or ecologic studies of suicide led to hypotheses linking suicide rates and social change. After World War II, major epidemiologic studies contributed to the understanding of the risk for cardiovascular disease or demonstrated the causal association between smoking and lung cancer. Explaining this relatively recent development, epidemiologic studies require the collection of large amount of data that may be difficult and costly to acquire. In the last 30 years, epidemiology has developed as an independent discipline, with its own set of concepts and approaches. Medical and biologic knowledge and statistical techniques are used by epidemiologists but epidemiology goes much beyond the statistical analysis of medical data.

Measures of Disease Occurrence

Several measures of disease occurrence are used by epidemiologists. We define here the three most commonly used: incidence rate, cumulative incidence or incidence proportion, and prevalence.

Incidence Rate and Cumulative Incidence

To calculate incidence, individuals initially free of the disease must be observed over a period of time. The example in Figure 3.2.1.1 illustrate new onsets of disease (or death, or relapse, or any other health event) among six individuals observed during a period of 10 units of time (i.e., months or years). Some individuals (subject 1) are observed for the whole observation period, whereas others (individuals 4 to 6) have reduced observation times as they join or leave the sample during the observation period. Three disease onsets (individuals 2, 3, and 5) are observed; for these individuals, the period of observation ceases when the event has occurred, as subsequently they are

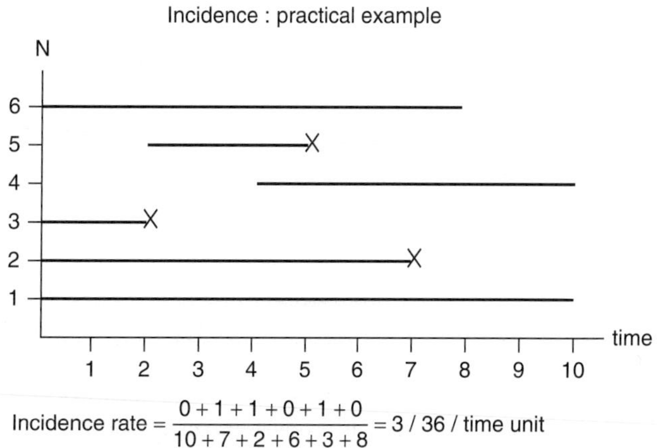

$$\text{Incidence rate} = \frac{0+1+1+0+1+0}{10+7+2+6+3+8} = 3\,/\,36\,/\,\text{time unit}$$

FIGURE 3.2.1.1. Calculating incidence.

no longer at risk of developing the disease and the observation time following the event becomes uninformative. The length of the line for each individual in Figure 3.2.1.1 represents the *person-time* experience of this individual and its own contribution to the denominator of the incidence rate. Only events occurring in individuals who are contributing to the person-time denominator are counted.

The incidence rate (IR) is calculated as follows:

$$IR = \frac{\text{N of new onsets of disease}}{\text{Sum of observation time across individuals}}$$

In the Figure 3.2.1.1 example, the incidence is IR = 3/36 = 0.083 time units^{-1}. IR can vary from 0 to infinite. It has the inverse of time as a unit (i.e., 0.083 per year) which, under some circumstances, can be interpreted as an average waiting time before disease onset. With a fixed number of events, the incidence increases if the person-time denominator decreases, as when the onset of new cases of disease occurs more rapidly, reflecting a faster penetration of the disease in the population. Calculation of incidence rates are more complex in real circumstances, depending on particular assumptions that hold true for the observed population (open [in steady state] or closed population, migration in or out, consideration of competing risks). Common examples of incidence rates are mortality rates, which have an easy intuitive meaning. For example, a young male suicide rate of 20/100,000/year or 0.0002/year means that, if one were to follow up 100,000 young males for a duration of 1 year each, 20 suicidal events would have been occurring during that observation period. However, the same incidence rate could be obtained with four suicidal deaths observed in following 2,000 subjects over a 10-year period. The numerical value of an incidence rate can therefore have different meanings depending on the study methodology.

Because incidence rates are not always that easy to interpret, epidemiologists use other measures of disease occurrence such as cumulative incidence (or incidence proportion). This measure is generally used for a closed population observed over a fixed period of time, all subjects being free of the disease at the beginning of the observation period. For example, if 9 of 100 siblings of autistic probands develop autism from birth (the beginning of the observation period) to age 3, the cumulative incidence of autism in this high-risk sample would be reported as 0.09 or 9% *over the first 3 years* of life. Unlike incidence rate, this figure is a proportion, dimensionless, and varying from 0 to 1. To be interpreted correctly, this cumulative incidence *must* be reported in conjunction to the length of the observation period, as the cumulative incidence will vary as a function of the follow-up time. In the previous example, if the sample is followed further from age 3 to 5, another six cases might be newly diagnosed with autism, leading to a cumulative incidence of 0.15 *over 5 years* of observation. The intuitive interpretation of cumulative incidence is that it represents the average risk of developing the disease in the population under study (i.e., the summation of individual risks across individuals from the study population). One variant of incidence proportion is survival proportion, which is the complement of incidence proportion (survival vs. death, no recurrence vs. recurrence) and is often used in clinical epidemiologic studies.

Prevalence

Prevalence focuses on disease *status* of individuals within a population rather than on the pattern of *onset* of new cases in that population. Prevalence is not a dynamic measure and, contrary to incidence rate or proportion, no passage of time is required for its calculation. Prevalence is calculated as the proportion of individuals in a population who, at a given point in time, have the disease. Prevalence (P) is a proportion[1] that is dimensionless and varies from 0 to 1. It is calculated as:

$$P = \frac{\text{N of subjects with the disease}}{\text{Population/sample size}}$$

Prevalence incorporates in its numerator recent and past onsets of the disease, and therefore the duration of the disease will influence the prevalence. If the disease is rapidly lethal or if it can be cured rapidly, the number of diseased individuals at any time point will drop and so will the prevalence. Thus, a prevalence rate reflects not only the incidence of the disease but factors that are associated with other aspects of the disease process (availability of treatments, natural history, lethality, etc.). The relationship of prevalence to incidence can be estimated, under some circumstances, as:

$$\frac{Nc}{N - Nc} \approx P \approx I \times D$$

where D is the average duration of the disease, I the incidence, Nc the number of cases in the population, N the population size, and P the prevalence proportion. If the prevalence is small enough (i.e., <0.10), the formula simplifies to: $P = I \times D$. As I and D have respectively time^{-1} and time as units, P is dimensionless; it is a proportion that varies from 0 to 1. Prevalence rates can be useful as descriptors of the morbidity due to specific causes. They are useful for planning health and educational services. In some circumstances, they may also help generate hypotheses about causal factors associated with disease onset.

In psychiatry, prevalence rates are often referred to specific time periods. For example, a subject who has experienced a major depressive episode during the last 12 months but has now remitted might still contribute to the numerator of a prevalence rate if prevalence in that study is defined as 12-month *period prevalence*. In this example, any individual who met criteria for depression at any time point during the 12 months preceding the survey date would be defined as a case that would contribute to the prevalence pool (the numerator). The most commonly used period prevalence rates are 3-, 6-, and 12-month prevalence rates. Prevalence rates for longer periods of time can be useful to capture events that are either rare or episodic. Because the onset of symptoms of psychiatric disorder is often difficult to determine, psychiatric epidemiologists have often used the concept of *lifetime* prevalence. Thus, any individual who would have experienced a major depressive episode at any point during his lifespan would be counted at the numerator of a lifetime prevalence rate estimate, irrespective of his current disease status, of the age of first onset, and of the total number of depressive episodes experienced by this individual over his lifespan.

Study Designs

The goal of epidemiologic studies is to examine whether or not particular variables are associated with a variation in disease occurrence. These variables are commonly referred to as exposures, as in the example of prenatal exposure to alcohol increasing the risk of neurodevelopmental and behavioral abnormalities in children. Exposures can be susceptibility genes, prenatal or later life exposure to biologic factors, a positive family history, psychosocial stressors, cognitive style or capacity, specific life events, and so on. When exposure to a variable of interest is associated with a demonstrated variation

[1]Technically, prevalence is a true proportion and not a rate (that implies different units of measurement for the numerator and denominator) although it is commonly referred to as a "rate," as we do later in the text.

A. Cohort study: design

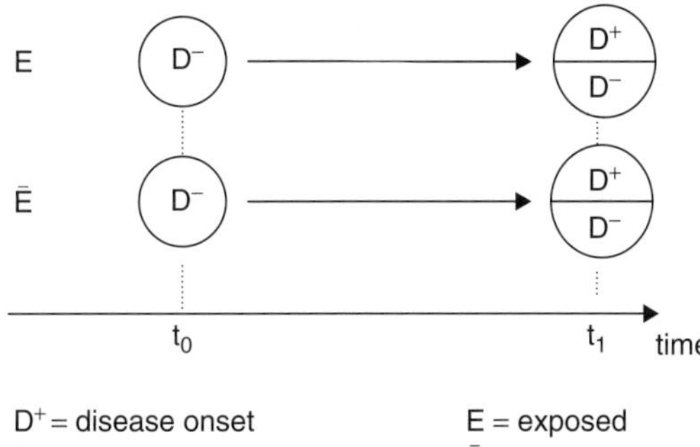

D^+ = disease onset
D^- = no disease onset
E = exposed
Ē = unexposed

B. Presentation of data

	Exposed	Unexposed
Events	a	b
Person – years denominator	N_e	$N_{\bar{e}}$

a/N_e = incidence among exposed subjects
$b/N_{\bar{e}}$ = incidence among unexposed subjects
IRR = incidence rate ratio $= \dfrac{a/N_e}{b/N_{\bar{e}}}$

FIGURE 3.2.1.2. Design (**A**) and presentation of data (**B**) in cohort studies.

in the risk of the disorder, this variable is referred to as a risk factor for that disorder. A risk factor is statistically associated with the disorder, but this relationship may or not be causal. The design and analysis of epidemiologic studies aims at identifying risk factors and at evaluating the causal nature of their association with the disorder of interest.

Cohort Study

In cohort (or incidence) studies, the starting point consists of selecting two cohorts of subjects initially all free of the disease (Figure 3.2.1.2A). One cohort has experienced the exposure (exposed cohort) whereas the other (reference) cohort has not experienced it (unexposed cohort). Then, the person-time experience is measured in each cohort and the incidence of the disease can be estimated in each. The incidence in the exposed and unexposed cohorts is then compared by calculating an *incidence rate ratio* (Figure 3.2.1.2B) that is not different from 1 if there is no association between the exposure and the incidence. Conversely, if the exposure is associated with an increased risk of the disease, the IRR will be higher than 1. When the measure of disease occurrence available is the cumulative incidence, the relative effect of exposure on the disease is estimated by the *risk ratio,* obtained by dividing the cumulative incidence in the exposed cohort by that from the unexposed cohort.

Cohorts are defined by the exposure status of their members. Sometimes, one single cohort will be available, but measurement of the exposure for each subject will allow the construction of two or several cohorts according to exposure levels (unexposed vs. exposed; or nil, medium, or high exposure). Cohort studies are difficult and costly to perform as they involve sometimes long periods of observation and therefore attrition can occur. One advantage of cohort studies is that several outcomes can be studied in relation to the initial exposure. Cohort studies are impractical if the disease incidence is low (rare disease), as the sample size required would be prohibitive. In some but not all studies, the investigator would be present at t_0 and wait for the cohort to mature (t_1) and live through the period at risk of developing the disease (*prospective cohort study*). In other studies (*retrospective cohort study*), the cohort study can be designed historically from data already collected. An example of this is the study showing a twofold increase in the risk of adult schizophrenia among subjects exposed to prenatal nutritional deficiency during the Dutch hunger winter in 1944–1945 (1), a finding recently replicated for the Chinese famine in 1959–1961 (2). Thus, the temporal position of the investigator regarding the data collection in a cohort study varies from study to study and is not what defines a cohort design. Knowledge of the biologic mechanisms that might underlie an association and of the disease model under investigation is critical in designing cohort studies. Some exposures might have a long induction period (e.g., parental loss in childhood in relation to adult female risk of depression), which must inform the precise delineation of the observational period and the data collection process.

Case–Control Study

In a case–control study, two groups are selected according to their present health status (with or without the disease of interest) and contrasted with respect to their past experiences of exposure to potential risk experiences (Figure 3.2.1.3A). Case ascertainment must be as complete as possible in order to represent the full spectrum of the disease and to avoid selection biases, particularly when case sampling is not independent of the exposure. Cases can be selected from the general population, but complete ascertainment may be difficult under these circumstances (i.e., identifying all cases of illness through hospitals, private clinics, and practices). Alternatively, cases may be selected in a cohort where more complete ascertainment can be achieved. Control selection is one of the most difficult design challenges in case–control studies. It is useful to conceptualize that controls should be selected from the same source population from which cases arose; in addition, selection of controls should remain strictly

A. Case–control study: design

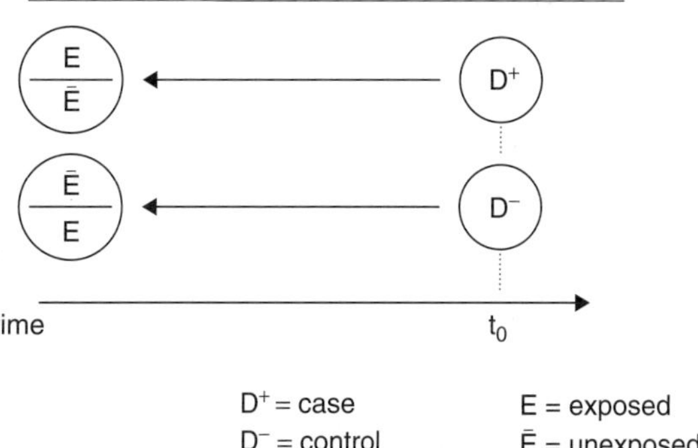

D^+ = case
D^- = control
E = exposed
Ē = unexposed

B. Case–control study: presentation of data

	Exposed	Unexposed
Cases	a	b
Controls	c	d

$$\text{OR} = \text{Odds–ratio} = \frac{a/b}{c/d} = \frac{a/c}{b/d} = \frac{a \times d}{b \times c}$$

FIGURE 3.2.1.3. Design (**A**) and presentation of data (**B**) in case–control studies.

independent from knowledge of their exposure status or level. Controls should therefore represent adequately the distribution of the exposure in the source population from which cases originated. Only when this is achieved can the case–control analysis evaluate if the exposure experience differs meaningfully between the cases and the controls. An implication for this conceptualization is that it is usually wrong to select controls among healthy volunteers who are likely to underrepresent the frequency of exposure (supernormal controls or healthy worker effect in occupational studies) in the source population and bias upward the estimates of association. Approaches to the selection of controls that rely on friends, neighborhood, or classroom controls are appealing due to their convenience but may also pose threats to the validity. Numerous examples of such problems are found in the psychiatric or psychological literature, when patient data are compared to healthy volunteer data (i.e., referred depressed adolescents compared to high school students) or other convenient series of controls (classmates, friends, etc.) leading to spurious "positive" findings (3).

To address the difficulty of control selection, two or more control groups may be selected that differ for their selection procedure and thus for the possible sampling biases that they each introduce. While intellectually appealing, this approach may be practically very labor intensive. Furthermore, there is no guarantee of the absence of bias when similar estimates are obtained when comparing the case series to each control group; conversely, if diverging estimates are obtained with each control group, the investigator is left with the difficult (and often impossible) task of determining where from and in which group the source of bias operates.

Exposure data are often (but not necessarily) collected retrospectively, making case-control the study vulnerable to measurement biases due to differential recall (or recall bias) or missing data. For example, when interviewed and compared to nondepressed controls, currently depressed individuals might overreport past negative life experiences simply because their threshold for remembering and evaluating as negative particular events might be affected by their current mood state.

Incidence rates are not available in a case–control study; estimates of the association between the candidate risk factor and the disease are calculated by comparing the odds of exposure among the cases and the controls (Figure 3.2.1.3B). One sometimes calculates the case/control ratio among exposed (a/c) and unexposed subjects (b/d), which leads mathematically to the same computation of the odds ratio. This calculation also illustrates how case–control studies converge toward cohort studies when controls provide an adequate representation of the exposure distribution in the source population (i.e., when c and d converge toward N_e and $N_{\bar{e}}$ (see Figures 3.2.1.2B and 3.2.1.3B)). The resulting odds ratio (OR) is an estimate of the incidence rate ratio obtained in cohort studies. Case–control studies can be performed more rapidly and are efficient. They are particularly indicated for rare diseases. Case–control studies also allow for the evaluation of several exposures in relation to a given disease.

Cross-Sectional Study

Cross-sectional studies are studies of large and representative samples of populations at a given point in time. Usually, disease status and exposure status are measured at the same time, and these data can then be used to calculate prevalence rates and prevalence rate ratios. Prevalence rates can be informative for planning and services purposes. Prevalence rates can also be compared in various subgroups of the population (males vs. females, high or low SES, rural vs. urban, etc.) in order to identify characteristics or risk factors associated with disease status. Limitations of cross-sectional studies are that duration of the disease and other factors (earlier diagnosis, efficacious treatments, etc.) unrelated to disease onset influence the size of the prevalence pool (see section on 'Prevalence').

Ecologic Study

In ecologic (or aggregate) studies, the unit of observation is the group rather than the individual. The level of analysis could be classrooms, schools, neighborhoods, municipalities, states, or countries. If both exposure and health outcome data are available at that level of analysis, their relationships can then be examined. For example, county suicide rates could be positively correlated with county unemployment rates, suggesting that unemployment leads to suicide. However, the joint distribution of exposure and disease is generally not known at the individual level, and it is possible that those individuals who commit suicide are not those who are unemployed (e.g., suicide might be occurring among young people, whereas unemployment would affect those over age 50). This interpretation problem has been identified as the *ecologic fallacy* or ecologic bias. In these studies, information about confounding factors (age, in the previous example) is usually very limited; in addition, the temporal sequence between disease events and exposure (that must precede the health outcome) can be difficult to determine. Ecologic studies have the advantage of being simple and cheap to perform considering the wide availability of vital statistics and sociodemographic indicators in many countries. Time trend analyses and cross-national comparisons are also forms of ecologic studies that may yield useful information not readily available otherwise. Ecologic analyses can also be informative in circumstances where levels of individual exposure lack variability (i.e., all individuals in a population are unexposed or all are exposed). For example, studies examining risk of autism in relation to exposure to vaccination might be uninformative if every child in the study population has been vaccinated. Comparing rates of autism in areas or time periods that *differ* for their rates of vaccine uptake (an ecologic comparison) might be the most informative approach. For example, rates of pervasive developmental disorders (PDDs) increased in Quebec from 1987 to 1998 but, as levels of exposure to thimerosal through vaccines varied from medium to high and then nil during the same period, investigators used this natural experiment to show that trends in PDD rates were unrelated to exposure to varying thimerosal levels (4). In some investigations, ecologic effects are also the focus of interest even when individual-level data are available. For example, one might want to examine the respective contribution to the individual risk of engaging in antisocial behavior from both child and familial characteristics (individual level) and of community characteristics (group level). Multilevel analyses of that kind have often been conducted in the social sciences.

Other Designs

Other study designs or mixed designs can be used in epidemiology. For example, a case–control study can be *nested* in a cohort study, which provides opportunities to ascertain a representative sample of cases and of controls and to rely on prospective (less biased) measurements of risk factors. In that instance, the case–control study would be referred to as a *prospective* case–control study owing to the fact that the measurement of risk factors *precedes* that of the onset of disease. Other study designs are discussed extensively elsewhere (5).

Issues of Sampling and Data Analysis

Sampling

In large population-based cross-sectional surveys that have been typical of psychiatric epidemiology in the last 40 years, sampling techniques vary from simple random sampling (SRS) to more complex stratified or cluster sampling strategies that aim to increase the precision of estimates, while optimizing survey resources and reducing costs. A typical example of a complex survey design would be a survey where two strata defined by the type of classrooms (special education vs. mainstream) are selected and children from special education classrooms are sampled with a higher sampling fraction than their counterparts. In addition, if all the subjects within each classroom are selected, the natural occurrence of these clusters must be taken into account, as observations are no longer independent (the same would apply to household surveys). For example, the same teachers would be providing data on several children who also happen to share common experiences that may be determinants of behavioral disorders (teaching quality, physical characteristics of the classroom).

In selecting children for inclusion in the study sample, it is crucial to note the probability of each child being selected, so that subsequently these probabilities can be used to weight back the observations (usually with weights that are the inverse of the sampling fraction) for extrapolation to the target population. This allows oversampling of some subgroups without distortion of the final estimates, provided that proper weights are devised and applied. Taking into account the clusters and strata used initially as sampling frames is also required in order to derive unbiased variance estimators. The analysis of two-phase or more complex survey designs is discussed further by Dunn et al. (6).

Registers or Population-Based Electronic Databases

Registers are data collection systems maintained by administrative or public health authorities over time to monitor health indicators. Several psychiatric case registers exist that have been used in epidemiologic investigations. When well maintained, they can provide an easy way to access potential participants and an efficient sampling source, from which various case–control or cohort studies can be derived in no time. Thus, national health and psychiatric registers available in Denmark or the General Practitioner Database in the United Kingdom have been invaluable tools for epidemiologists to allow them to test rapidly emerging hypotheses, such as on the risk of autism in relation to exposure to measles–mumps–rubella (MMR) vaccine, or to the thimerosal content of children's immunizations. Different research designs were used from those sources, and including cohort (7,8), case–control (9) or ecologic (10) studies, all of which failed to detect any association.

Sample Size and Precision

In each study, the goal is to estimate rates or measures of association with as much precision as possible. Precision is decreased by various sources of random error, including imperfect measurements of exposure or disease status (see below), or sampling errors. In order to limit the loss of precision due to sampling error, increasing the sample size is a common technique that involves detailed calculations at the designing stage of the study that consider cost of sampling, sample availability, and preliminary estimation (based on past studies or conceptual considerations) of the likely range of values for the rate differences or risk ratios to be estimated. A tradeoff between gaining more precision by increasing sample size and the expanding costs of the study is often a consideration. In some case–control studies, the study efficiency can be tremendously improved by selecting several controls for each case. This would apply to circumstances where the number of available cases is limited, more statistical power is required, and controls are ubiquitous and cheap to obtain. Matching up to four or five controls to each case would maximize the power of the study. Beyond that number, the gains of matching extra controls become rapidly smaller and not worth pursuing.

Missing Data

Methods for dealing with missing data are crucial and have been addressed more efficiently in recent surveys. Participation rates in child psychiatry surveys have generally been high, often well over 80%. Bias in the estimates of prevalence and risk associations might result, nevertheless, if those who do not participate have higher rates of disorders, more severe disorders, or disorders arising through different mechanisms. Empirical findings indicate that nonrespondents often differ systematically from respondents. For example, in a survey of school-age children, behavioral disturbances reported by teachers were 60% higher among nonparticipants than participants, but survey weights could be used to correct for this bias in the final prevalence estimation (11). Similarly, attrition bias in longitudinal studies may attenuate predictions regarding the persistence of disorders over time (12).

Missing data can also occur at the item level, with respondents omitting items on a checklist or failing to answer all questions in an interview. This may jeopardize data collection (if incomplete screens are deemed ineligible for further interview) or analysis (if incomplete interviews are not dealt with separately). Sophisticated statistical and imputation techniques are available to take account of missing data, different according to the reasons that they are missing (13,14).

Statistical Testing

Point estimates of disease occurrence (incidence, prevalence) and of measures of association (relative risks, such as rate, risk, and odds ratios) derive from the particular samples studied by investigators. The values obtained in one study are meant to be robust and unbiased estimators of the true population value, also called population parameters. In any one study, there is imprecision attached to each point estimate and epidemiologists communicate findings with 95% confidence intervals calculated around point estimates. For example, the odds ratio in a case control study could be expressed as: OR = 2.2 (95% confidence interval: 1.5–3.4). A 95% confidence interval can be construed around all measures of disease occurrence and of association reviewed earlier. Confidence intervals provide a range of values that are consistent with the true population parameter under the present study circumstances. For measures of association, a relative risk of 1 is the expected value under the null hypothesis of no association between the exposure and the disease. If a 95% confidence interval around a point estimate for the relative risk includes 1, the null hypothesis is not rejected. If 1 is not included in the 95% confidence interval (as in the above example), the null hypothesis is rejected at the 0.05 significance level. Too much emphasis is sometimes placed on statistical testing. Statistical testing is necessary in circumstances where decisions must be made (treat this patient or not). In most studies, epidemiologists are interested in evaluating causal relationships, and a probabilistic rather than a black and white (significant or not) approach to this problem is warranted. Suffice it to remember that a very small effect (OR = 1.2; 95% CI: 1.05–1.45) of unlikely biologic or clinical relevance could reach statistical significance only because the study has huge statistical power due to a very large sample size. Conversely, a larger, but statistically not significant, effect (OR = 2.9; 95% CI: 0.9–5.4) could point toward true associations of moderate magnitude. In those circumstances, epidemiologists who pursue causality will pay more attention to the strength of the association (the point estimate) and its interpretability in the larger context of the study design and findings. Causality assessment is better viewed as an ongoing, continuous, interpretative process that might be jeopardized with premature decision making rules embodied by classical statistical significance testing.

Bias and Confounding

Whereas sample size can influence the precision of a study, sample selection can limit the validity of the estimates obtained by introducing systematic (as opposed to random) error in the rate or risk ratio estimates. Various other sources of bias are well recognized in epidemiology, which are also briefly described here.

Selection Bias. Selection bias occurs when subjects who participate in the study differ systematically from the population that they represent for characteristics associated to the disease or exposure under study. Several examples have been discussed above. One other example of selection bias is selective attrition when, in a cohort study, subjects who are lost to follow-up differ from the cohort subjects with respect to the incidence of the disease. Migration in or out of a population or differential mortality are similarly potential sources of bias. When selection biases of that kind are suspected, it is critical for investigators to use baseline data to empirically test whether or not subjects lost to follow-up are systematically different from those who are not. Selection biases are a particular concern in case–control studies, especially with respect to the selection of controls.

Information Bias and Misclassification. A valid measure of the association between the exposure and the disease depends on the accuracy of measurement of both variables. Due to measurement error, a diseased subject could be classified as control, or an unexposed subject as exposed. Measurement errors on dichotomous classifications of exposure and disease status are described with concepts of sensitivity and specificity (see below). Classification errors are referred to as *misclassification* and a more general discussion of measurement principles and errors as it applies particularly to psychiatric research is provided below.

In an epidemiologic study where the goal is to estimate an association without bias, a critical feature of misclassification is whether or not it occurs independently of other variables. *Differential misclassification* occurs when the measurement error affects cases or controls, or exposed versus unexposed subjects, with different patterns. A typical example of differential misclassification is recall bias. For example, in a case–control study of a severe birth neurodevelopmental abnormality of unknown origin at the time, mothers of cases reported significantly more psychosocial stressors during pregnancy (financial difficulties, marital difficulties) than mothers of controls (15). This suggested that psychosocial stress could be a cause of the negative birth outcome. It turned out that the abnormality was Down syndrome, the chromosomal etiology of which was only discovered in the months that followed. The only explanation for the spurious association between Down syndrome and psychosocial stressors during pregnancy in Stott's study lies in the differential reporting by mothers of cases (in search of a cause for their child's anomaly) of their past psychosocial experiences. It is important to consider that measurement error itself is not the problem if it affects subjects across groups equally. The bias arises from the fact that cases and controls do not report their exposure experience in a comparable fashion. Recall bias is a well-recognized problem of retrospective case–control studies that can be addressed and prevented. For example, obtaining evidence from other sources of information, preferably collected before the onset of the disease (past medical or educational records), or through informants who are blind to the case status of study subjects, would limit the possibility of differential misclassification. Differential misclassification can inflate measures of association as in the previous example, or it may also attenuate them.

Nondifferential misclassification occurs when classification errors on exposure or on disease occur independently of each other. This type of misclassification almost always attenuates measures of association and biases the study results toward the null hypothesis of no association between the exposure and the disease. For example, in a case–control study free of measurement error of 200 depressed adolescents compared to 200 nondepressed controls, the presence of two or more negative life events (LE+) compared to one or less events (LE–) in the 12 months preceding the onset of depression is a risk factor for adolescent depression, with the ratio of exposure (LE+/LE–) being 80/120 in the cases and 40/160 in the controls, which translates into an odds ratio of 2.7 (see Figure 3.2.1.3B). If one assumes now that life events are measured with an imperfect questionnaire method that misclassifies 20% of subjects truly LE+ as LE– and 20% of subjects truly LE– as LE+, and that this occurs equally among cases and controls (the misclassification is nondifferential, as it is independent of disease status), the ratio of exposure (LE+/LE–) is now 88/112 in the cases and 64/136 in the controls, which translates into an odds ratio of 1.7. In this example, the odds ratio is biased toward the null value of no association due to an unwelcome mixture of exposed and unexposed subjects in both cases and controls that blurs the true contrast of exposure distribution that exists between cases and controls in the absence of measurement error. Similar biases would occur if nondifferential misclassification were applied to disease status. In general, therefore, nondifferential errors must be discussed in relation to negative studies or studies with associations of small magnitude. Differences in the error rate of measurement across studies may explain inconsistent or discrepant findings. In psychiatry, reliance on questionnaires and interviews, on lifetime measures of risk or disease experience, and on broad diagnostic groupings, are potential sources of considerable misclassification.

Confounding. Confounding factors are variables that may be responsible for a distortion of the relationship between the exposure and the disease. As such, confounding factors might over- or underestimate an association, and sometimes may even change the direction of the association. Confounding variables operate in all study designs, including in experiments. However, methods exist in experimental research (e.g., randomization) to limit the distorting effects of confounding factors. In nonexperimental designs, the control of confounding factors may be more difficult to achieve. To be a confounding factor, a variable must be shown (or known) to be associated with both the exposure and the disease independently. Furthermore, a confounding factor cannot merely be an intermediate variable in the causal chain linking exposure to disease. In a study where smoking during pregnancy is associated with later behavioral problems in the child, maternal antisocial behavior is a likely confounding factor. Maternal antisocial behavior is associated to smoking during pregnancy, and quite separately, it is associated with increased risk of child behavioral problems independently of its association to maternal prenatal smoking. Thus, the association between prenatal maternal smoking and later child behavioral problems could be entirely accounted by the confounding effects of maternal antisocial behavior. In other words, the co-occurrence of smoking and behavioral problems could be artefactual and entirely driven by their background association to maternal antisocial behavior.

Confounding factors must therefore be dealt with both at the planning and analysis stages of a study. When designing a study, it is important to include in the data collection careful and valid measurements of potential confounders. Confounders can be identified a priori by investigators based on past studies or on theoretical and biologic knowledge about the disease and risk mechanisms under scrutiny. Another strategy is to restrict the study to particular subgroups using exclusion criteria. For example, gender would be recognized as a potential confounding factor in a study examining the relationship between plasma levels of sex hormones and adolescent depressive symptomatology, since gender is associated with sex hormone levels and with the risk of depression. Restricting the study to females only is an effective solution but it has the disadvantage to limit the degree to which the findings can be generalized (nothing can be said about males). Another approach used by epidemiologists consists in stratifying the data at the analysis stage to obtain unconfounded stratum-specific estimates of the association that can be subsequently pooled together. Other techniques rely on statistical modeling, and techniques such as multiple logistic regression are often used to adjust the measures of association and remove the effects of confounders on the estimates. Detection, measurement, and adjustment on confounding factors is an important task of investigators that is never ending. Thus, it always remains possible in every study that an observed association is explained by residual confounding effects or by unobserved and unmeasured confounding variables. Thus, replication of associations across studies is important to offer additional evidence for the validity of an association.

Causality Assessment

Risk Association and Causality Assessment. Measures of association in epidemiologic studies (risk and odds ratios) are tested for statistical significance. When the risk or odds ratio departs sufficiently away from the value 1 that is expected under the null hypothesis, the null hypothesis of no association between the exposure and the disease under study can then be rejected. Two important features of this conclusion are to be noted. First, a significant association between exposure and disease reflects a statistical association between two variables. Demonstrating that this association is also causal is the ultimate goal of the epidemiologist, but requires several other types of evidence than a "statistically significant" result. Second, like statistical tests, the conclusion of epidemiologic studies is asymmetrical. When the study fails to detect an association (the null hypothesis is not rejected), it cannot be regarded as proof that no association exists in the nature. Rather, the lack of association could reflect poor research design, sampling bias, or nondifferential misclassification. Conversely, when a significant association is reported, epidemiologists reject the null hypothesis of no association but causality cannot generally be definitely inferred from that conclusion.

Hill's Criteria. Stronger evidence for a causal association can nevertheless be evaluated using different sets of criteria. Hill (16) laid out nine criteria that he proposed as guides for evaluating the causal nature of an association. There are: (1) strength of the association, where higher odds or risk ratios are more likely to indicate a causal relationship; (2) consistency, where an association is replicated in different samples studied with different methods; (3) specificity, where causality is more likely if the association between the exposure is confined to that disease, as opposed to leading to multiple, unrelated, negative outcomes; (4) dose–response, where the risk of the disease increases with increasing levels of exposure; (5) temporality, where the exposure must precede the onset of disease in order to be causal; (6) plausibility, whereby the association could be referred to a biologically plausible mechanism; (7) coherence, where the causal nature of the association must be consistent with other aspects of the biologic knowledge available about the disease; (8) experimental evidence, where the association is supported by the results of experimental manipulations of the exposure (in laboratory or human experiments, or field studies); and (9) analogy, when comparable associations can be identified in other domains of inquiry. Perhaps with the exception of the criterion of temporality, none of Hill's criteria is sufficient or necessary to establish causality. Thus, they should not be used as a mechanical checklist to "add" to the causal evidence, but simply as a set of arguments that may (or not) guide the interpretation of a given result.

Replication. An important argumentation for evaluating causality lies in the replication of findings across studies, preferably performed by different investigators, in different populations, and with different instrumentation. If findings converge (either for or against association) in studies that are otherwise likely to differ drastically in their potential sources of bias and imprecision, then the confidence in the interpretation increases substantially (although there remains no definite proof). For example, the recent hypothesis linking autism to exposure to the measles component of the MMR vaccine given to children in their second year of life was extensively tested by different epidemiologic approaches that included cohort (7), case–control (9,17), and ecologic (4) designs that failed to reject the null hypothesis of no association. The consistent failure across studies to find a positive association should be taken as stronger evidence of the lack of association than that deriving from each study taken in isolation. Conversely, consistent positive associations between an exposure and a disease across studies strengthen the argument for causality. Meta-analysis is a technique that provides a quantitative route toward evaluating jointly the evidence arising from separate studies.

Public Health Relevance of Epidemiology

Epidemiology is the fundamental discipline of public health insofar as both the research methodology and the substantive findings of epidemiologic studies are necessary to inform public health activities. Surveillance by public health agencies such as the Centers for Disease Control (CDC) is critical to the monitoring of the health of a population and for identifying variations in time and place in rates of disorders. Surveillance systems are also critical to respond to the emergence of new diseases (as in the AIDS example) or to changes in the incidence or prevalence of known illnesses or disorders (as suggested recently for autism). Vital statistics, including morbidity and mortality reports, have been traditional ways to monitor population health. They are often supplemented by specific and repeated surveys of disorders or events of importance for public health. Public health agencies also have the task to implement and evaluate universal or targeted preventive programs. Evaluation of models of service delivery, factors influencing access to health care, and more generally health services research, are public health activities that require the knowledge bases and contribution of epidemiologic methods and studies.

Examples of the contribution of child psychiatric epidemiologic studies to public health and surveillance programs are found easily. Several surveillance systems are in place in the United States to capture trends in child psychiatric disorders or problem behaviors. For example, as part of the Monitoring the Future Study, annual surveys of large samples of high school students have been conducted since the 1970s to monitor rates of marijuana and other drug use. From the early 1990s onward, the CDC Youth Risk Behavior Surveillance System (YRBSS) have performed national, state, and local school-based surveys conducted by education and health agencies to monitor several categories of health-risk behaviors, including unintentional injuries and violence, tobacco, alcohol and other drug use, risky sexual behaviors, and suicidal behaviors. These surveys have been instrumental in showing that annual rates of suicide attempts are around 8%, affecting a substantial minority of teenagers. Monitoring time trends in the incidence of disorders has also been possible with epidemiologic studies that relied on registers to identify cases over several decades. Thus, the Mayo Clinic register in Rochester, MN, has allowed investigators to detect changes in the incidence of disorders such as anorexia nervosa (18) or autism (19). Recently, the CDC has started a surveillance program of autism and related disorders in response to worldwide concerns about a possible increase in the incidence of autism spectrum disorders.

CHILD PSYCHIATRY EPIDEMIOLOGY

Brief History and Landmark Studies

Child psychiatric epidemiology started in the mid-'60s with the British Isle of Wight surveys (20,21). Prior to this landmark study, there had been few investigations of rates of behavioral problems in general population samples of children. One such survey emphasized the high prevalence of fears and worries and the discrepancies in rates of problems according to the informant (22). Most knowledge at the time relied on observations drawn from clinical case series. Behaviors were interpreted and theoretical inferences were made without having a proper calibration system of those behaviors that discriminated best between children seen in clinics and nonreferred children. Epidemiology, with its focus on general population samples and on comparisons between individuals with or without disorders, provided an obvious tool for the empirical investigation of child psychopathology.

The Isle of Wight surveys had key design characteristics that provided a model for surveys in the years after (23). A two-phase design was used with a systematic questionnaire screening of a large sample, followed by indepth assessments administered only to a subsample selected according to their positive and negative results at screening. Multiple informants were used at both phases, involving parents, teachers, and children. The value of asking direct questions to children was established and interviews subsequently replaced the old indirect techniques (projective tests and free play) as investigation tools. Questionnaires and diagnostic interviews of known reliability and validity were employed for the first time to gather data. *Caseness* was defined according to both a recognizable behavioral pattern *and* evidence of impairment in the child's functioning. The surveys also adopted longitudinal approaches to measure prospectively risk factors and chart the natural history of disorders, and to evaluate which behavioral outcomes were related to neurologic and educational risk factors (21). These methodologic advances have been developed further in surveys conducted since. Two-phase designs are cost-effective ways to conduct cross-sectional surveys of large population-based samples and they have been employed in numerous child psychiatry epidemiologic investigations (Table 3.2.1.1). However, the value of longitudinal studies has been increasingly recognized by developmental psychopathologists and, wherever feasible, cohort or longitudinal approaches are preferred to study causal mechanisms underlying the onset, persistence, and desistance of and from psychiatric disorders.

Measurement in Psychiatry

The planning of epidemiologic studies requires precise methods to ascertain "cases" of the disorder under study (40). A definition of "caseness" must be adopted at the outset. Its nature should be shaped by the goals of the survey. A survey of autism to identify representative cases for inclusion in genetic studies will require detailed phenotypic assessments, precise diagnostic subtyping, and exclusion of autistic syndromes associated with known medical disorders. If, on the other hand, the goal of the autism survey is to generate estimates of special educational needs for service planning, then a less restrictive and broader approach to caseness may be more suitable. Following the adoption of the most appropriate concept of the disorder, decisions must be made about the choice of various assessment procedures and instruments to evaluate caseness in study participants.

Definitions of Caseness

All epidemiologic surveys have shown the high frequency of individual emotional or behavioral difficulties (20,41). However, whereas some have a strong association with psychiatric disorder, others do not. Thus, in the Isle of Wight survey, thumb-sucking, nail-biting, and bilious attacks all had very weak associations with psychiatric disorder (20). Similarly, item scores for *Asthma* and *Allergy* have been removed from the computation of the total score of the Child Behavior Checklist after consistent evidence that these were not associated with psychiatric referral. By contrast, the symptom of *Depressed mood* has been shown to account for much of the variance in comparisons of matched samples of nonreferred and referred children (41,42).

However, continuities and discontinuities between individual symptoms and disorder may involve crucial transitions. Thus, depressed mood is experienced by about a third of adolescents in the general population (43) but the rate of depressive disorder is only about 5%. Similarly, some half of female adolescents diet, but anorexia nervosa occurs in less than 1% (44). The situation with substance use and abuse and with disruptive behavior is directly comparable. Many problem behaviors have a continuous distribution in the population and quantitative, rather than qualitative, deviance often defines psychopathology.

Dimensions and Categories

Because of this, most epidemiologic studies use a mixture of dimensional and categorical approaches. The former are needed both to assess symptom severity and to allow the adoption of different cutoffs for different purposes. The latter is required for clinical decision making with respect to individual diagnosis and service planning. The issues are not specific to psychopathology; rather, they apply throughout most of medicine (as exemplified by asthma, hypertension, diabetes—all of which have dimensional parallels). Sometimes it is assumed that dimensional measures are synonymous with questionnaires and categorical ones with interview assessments, but that is not so. All standardized interviews provide for various forms of quantification of severity or numbers of symptoms. Conversely, most questionnaires provide the means for deriving categories from dimensional scores with appropriate cutoff points.

Careful consideration of instruments characteristics is critical in planning an epidemiologic study (Table 3.2.1.2).

Obviously, that choice should be driven by the main purposes of the study. Questionnaires have all the advantages of economy and simplicity and may be the first preference if the goal involves only group differences and trends. They will almost always be used in the first screening phase of multistage studies. On the other hand, they are less suitable for individual diagnosis or for the assessment of uncommon disorders involving qualitative departures from normality. Standardized interviews have the opposite set of strengths and weaknesses. The chief decision issue with interviews is whether to use an investigator-based (semistructured) interview that obtains descriptions of behavior that are rated using a standardized research-driven concept or a respondent-based (structured) interview that obtains yes/no answers to carefully structured questions. Each has its own merits and researchers will need to consider carefully which is most likely to meet the needs for

TABLE 3.2.1.1

PREVALENCE FINDINGS FROM RECENT EPIDEMIOLOGIC SURVEYS

						Prevalence		
Authors/year	**Site**	**Age**	**N**	**Instruments/Diagnosis**	**Period**	**Any Emotional Disorder**	**Any Behavioral Disorder**	**Any Disorder**
Anderson et al., 1987 (24)	Dunedin, New Zealand	11	925	DISC-C/DSM-III	1 yr	7.3	11.6	17.6
Offord et al., 1987 (25)	Ontario, Canada	4–16	2,679	Structured interview/ DSM-III like	6 mo	—	—	18.1
Bird et al., 1988 (26)	Puerto Rico	4–16	777	DISC/DSM-III	6 mo	—	—	17.9
Esser et al., 1990 (27)	Mannheim, Germany	8	1,444	Clinical interview/ICD-9	6 mo	6	6	16.2
Morita et al., 1990 (28)	Gunma prefecture, Japan	12–15	1,999	Isle of Wight interview/ ICD-9	3 mo	—	—	15.0
Jeffers and Fitzgerald, 1991 (29)	Dublin, Ireland	9–12	2,029	Isle of Wight interview/ ICD-9	3 mo	—	—	25.4
Fergusson et al., 1993 (30)	Christchurch, New Zealand	15	986	DISC/DSM-III-R	—	—	—	22.1[C] 13.0[P]
Lewinsohn et al., 1993 (31)	Oregon, USA	16–18	1,710	K-SADS/DSM-III-R	Current	—	1.8	9.6
Fombonne, 1994 (11)	Chartres, France	6–11	2,441	ICD-9/Isle of Wight module	3 mo	5.9[P]	6.5[P]	12.4[P]
Costello et al., 1996 (32)	Great Smoky Mountains, North Carolina, USA	9, 11, 13	4,500	CAPA/DSM-III-R	3 mo	6.8	6.6	20.3
Verhulst et al., 1997 (33)	Nationwide, Netherlands	13–18	780	DISC C & P/DSM-III-R	6 mo	—	7.9[C or P] 0.9[C & P]	35.5[C or P] 4.0[C & P]
Simonoff et al., 1997 (34)	Virginia, USA	8–16	2,762	CAPA/DSM-III-R	3 mo	8.9	7.1	14.2
Steinhausen et al., 1998 (35)	Zurich, Switzerland	7–16	1,964	DISC-P/DSM-III-R	6 mo	—	6.5	22.5
Breton et al., 1999 (36)	Quebec, Canada	6–14	2,400	Dominic-DISC2/ DSM-III-R	6 mo	—	—	19.9[P] 15.8[C]
Ford et al., 2003 (37)	Nationwide, England and Wales	5–15	10,438	DAWBA/ICD-10	3 mo	4.3 0.9[a] 3.8[b]	5.9	9.5
Costello et al., 2003 (38)	Great Smoky Mountains, North Carolina, USA	9–16	6,674	CAPA, DSM-IV	3 mo	6.8[c,C or P]	7.0[C or P]	13.3[C or P]
Canino et al., 2004 (39)	Puerto Rico	4–17	1,897	DISC-IV/DSM-IV	12 mo	3.4[b,C or P] 6.6.9[c,C or P]	11.1[C or P]	16.4[C or P]

C, based on child as informant; P, based on parent as informant.
[a]Any depressive disorder;
[b]Any anxiety disorder.
[c]Any serious emotional disturbance.

the particular investigation to be undertaken. A further decision is needed on whether to choose a broad-based measure designed to tap all the common varieties of psychopathology or rather to use one or more focused instruments. The former will meet most needs but are less suitable for uncommon or unusual disorders such as autism, schizophrenia, or Tourette syndrome. Whatever the particular choice of instrument, investigators will usually need to test their chosen set of measures and data collection procedures in pilot studies of adequately sized samples to determine the procedural feasibility and its acceptability by respondents. Pilot studies should be analyzed carefully using quantitative methods whenever possible.

Situation Specificity, Multiple Informants

From the Isle of Wight studies onward, it has been evident that the agreement on childhood psychopathology between different informants is typically low, and is only moderate at best. Thus, in an epidemiologic survey of 6 to 11 year olds, only a quarter of children scoring above the cutoff on at least one screening measure were scoring above threshold on both parent *and* teacher questionnaires (45). In a meta-analysis of 119 studies, Achenbach et al. (46) found that the agreement was best (circa .60) when the pairs of informants had similar roles in relation to the child (such as with mother–father or

TABLE 3.2.1.2

CRITERIA FOR SELECTING AN INSTRUMENT

	Interview	Questionnaire
Purpose	Screening/Diagnosis	Screening/Assessment
Main use	Epidemiologic/clinical	Epidemiologic/clinical
Reliability	Test—retest Interrater	Test—retest Split-half, internal consistency
Validity	Content, discriminant, concurrent, predictive Cross-cultural	Content, discriminant, concurrent, predictive Factorial/construct validity Cross-cultural
Coverage/content	Diagnostic categories Number of disorders	Psychopathologic constructs Number of items
Method	Face-to-face interview	Self-report (usually) or other informant (parent, teacher, clinician)
Response format	Yes/No (highly structured) All informants' descriptions (semistructured)	Interval Likert scaling Visual analogue
Completion time	Long (hours)	Brief (minutes)
Informant	Subject Parent Other	Subject (over 10 yrs) Parent, teacher Clinician, interviewer, other
Time frame	Current (last 3 or 6 mo) Last year Lifetime	Current, last week Last 3 to 12 mo
Age assessed	Depends on informant and content	Depends on informant and content
Training	Required clinical for semistructured, basic for highly structured Availability of training packages Availability of manual	None (self-administered) or minimal (interviewer-assisted) Literacy requirement Availability of manual
Version	Paper & pencil Computer assisted Computer administered	Paper & pencil Computer administered
Data entry	Laborious (unless computerized)	Easy (optical forms)
Scoring	Diagnostic algorithms	Norms, centiles, cutoffs
Costs	High	Low
Repeat assessments	Modularity of the interview Scale scores available	Easy, demonstrated sensitivity to change
Extra features:		
other domains	That is, personal and family details, impairment, burden, etc.	That is, personal and family details, scholastic achievement, etc.
suitability for longitudinal studies	Adult diagnostic interviews	Parallel adult forms
observational assessments	Companion observational schedule	Parallel observational scale
cultural context	Availability in other languages Validity in different populations	Availability in other languages Validity in different populations

teacher–teacher), whereas the mean correlation fell to the .20s for other pair types (such as parent–child or parent–teacher).

There are many possible reasons for this low agreement between informants. These include random error in measurement; different perceptions of behavior according to the perspective of the observer; different frames of reference and variations in the child's behavior according to both setting and interpersonal features. The relative importance of these different possibilities is not known. However, it is clear that multiple informants are essential for any adequate epidemiologic study. That is partly because each informant contributes uniquely to the measurement of psychopathology (as well as contributing to shared variance); because when studying the correlates of disorder it is necessary to go across informants (or use composite ratings) in order to avoid halo effect artifacts; and because of the importance of differentiating between situation-specific and pervasive disorders.

That leaves open the crucially important (but largely unresolved) question of how to combine the data from different informants and from different settings. Although there is some evidence that different informants have different strengths, only rarely will it be desirable to adopt a hierarchical approach in which the report of one informant is automatically given precedence over those of others. Nevertheless, child self-reports are particularly important for the assessment of mood and other emotional disturbances. Conversely, they are of very limited use for the assessment of hyperactivity. Similarly, teachers are generally better at the assessment of disruptive behavior than they are of depressed mood. As the findings from Verhulst et al. (33) show dramatically (see Table 3.2.1.1), prevalence estimates are often hugely affected by how multiple ratings are dealt with.

Clinical interviewers usually use their "best" judgment in order to weigh the symptoms endorsed by each informant, resolving discrepancies by personal rules derived from a combination of experience and theoretical predictions. That is likely to result in different clinicians combining data in different ways. Another approach is trying to seek to resolve discrepancies between informants through a conjoint interview involving different informants (such as parent and child). This might be helpful in eliminating some errors due to miscomprehension and in "reconciling" the informants (47); however, the method is far from free of problems, most especially in giving rise to delicate situations that threaten to breach confidentiality. Nevertheless, this judgment method is recommended for some diagnostic interviews, such as the K-SADS (48), in order to allow the generation of a single unique score for each symptom rating. A third commonly used approach uses computer generation of diagnoses based on predefined algorithms. The method has the advantage of accuracy and speed. The algorithms must, however, deal with differences in reporting by informants according to specified rules. Usually, a symptom is counted as positive when it is reported by at least one informant—the so-called "or" rule (49). This technique typically leads to high numbers of generated diagnoses "comorbidity."

For dimensional assessments, Achenbach (50) has revised the data collected through his set of questionnaires in order to solve this cross-informant problem. Based on systematic analyses of the CBCL, the TRF, and the YSR, he identified common syndromes on each of these questionnaires, and core syndromes that appeared consistent across sex and age subgroups. Then, a set of cross-informant core syndromes that spanned at least two instruments was selected. These were subsequently scaled with the relevant normative samples. This approach does not resolve the problem of how to combine data from discrepant informants, but it helps in increasing the interpretability of a profile of scores for a given child (51,52). More sophisticated statistical techniques are available to researchers to deal with the measurement problems associated with multiple data sources and discrepancies between informants (see below), or are being developed (53).

Reliability and Validity Principles

At the core of medicine, and of any scientific inquiry, is the activity of measurement. Measurement theory (Figure 3.2.1.4) is concerned with defining and strengthening the relationships linking empirical or observable indicators (I1, I2, etc.) to the unobserved or latent constructs (V1, V2, etc.), that they intend to measure. In psychopathology, many constructs cannot be easily observed (such as self-esteem, personality traits, feelings of guilt, etc.). To address this gap, interviews, questionnaires or tests have been developed and evidence exists that their empirical results (whether those are signs, symptoms, algorithm or test scores) can be confidently related to the unobserved constructs of interest. Far from being a question restricted to research, the same requirements apply to everyday clinical practice. Clinical judgment is just one tool available to measure patient status, and as such, its measuring properties should be scrutinized and demonstrated. Thus, the choice is not between measuring or not (or between research and clinical practice), but rather between measuring with known and replicable procedures or with unspecified and imprecise approaches.

Two major properties, validity and reliability, are key features of assessment procedures (clinical or research instruments, but also the simple clinical judgment) for which Figure 3.2.1.4 provides a convenient representation. Data collected as part of clinical or research assessments can be seen as empirical indicators of the underlying (unobserved) constructs of interest.

Reliability is the tendency of measures to yield consistent results over repeated trials. Reliability concerns the replicability of measures and the extent to which each measurement is affected by random error. Reliability can therefore be examined

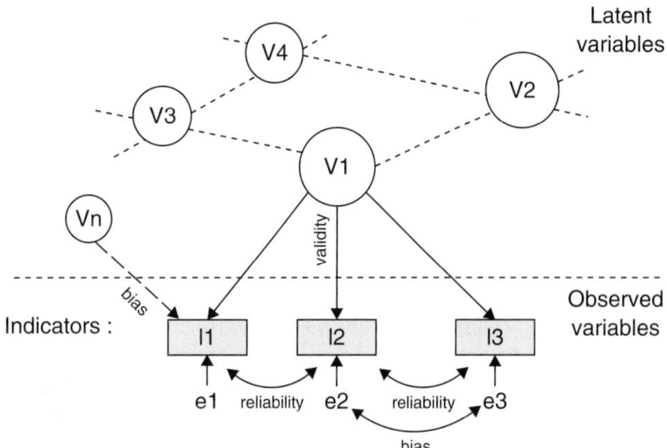

FIGURE 3.2.1.4. Measurement model.

empirically (see bottom level on Figure 3.2.1.4). Typical procedures to estimate reliability are the test–retest paradigm, interrater agreement, and techniques based on correlations between subsets of instruments (split-half reliability), or among items composing a questionnaire (internal consistency). The reliability of the measurement is assessed within each procedure by specific statistics such as the kappa coefficient for categorical measurements (54), the intraclass correlation coefficient for quantitative scores (55), and other statistics (e.g., Cronbach's (56) alpha coefficient). Reliability is a necessary condition, but not a sufficient one, for validity. If empirical indicators are unduly contaminated by random error (so that measurements cannot be replicated), then the question of their relationship to the constructs (the validity question) that they are purported to tap cannot even be assessed meaningfully. On the other hand, high replicability does not necessarily mean good validity.

Validity concerns the crucially important relationship between the empirical observables and the postulated latent construct (a diagnosis, a psychological concept, etc.) as represented by the connections between the bottom and top levels on Figure 3.2.1.4. Several types of validity have been described. *Content* validity is concerned with the extent to which an instrument is representative of the universe of empirical indicators that are related to the concept measured. It is usually assessed by reliance on experts or on agreement with established instruments tapping the same concept. *Criterion-related* validity is the most empirical form of validity. It allows an index or score to be compared to an independent external criterion thought to assess the same concept. This can be either *concurrent* (high stress predicts cortisol levels) or *predictive* (IQ predicts later academic achievement). *Construct* validity is the most elusive and theoretical type of validity. Basically, it concerns the extent to which individual items or measures intercorrelate or group together to produce derived higher order constructs. Factor analysis has often been used for this purpose in the field of psychopathology. Thus, numerous factor analyses of questionnaires have consistently identified separate dimensions (or constructs) of psychopathology (such as attention problems, conduct symptoms, or emotional disturbances). These tend to map onto a broad bipartite division into internalizing/emotional problems and externalizing/disruptive behaviors (57,58). Consistency of these factor analyses results has been taken as evidence of the construct validity of these psychopathology dimensions.

Diagnostic Reliability and Validity

In psychiatry, multiple efforts have been made to evaluate and improve the properties of psychiatric diagnosis. Since the first collaborative efforts sponsored by the World Health Organization to improve diagnosis in psychiatry, reliability studies have been undertaken to examine interrater agreement and to improve the definition, and thereby the diagnostic reproducibility, of disorders (59). In the late 1970s, with the development of research diagnostic criteria (60) and of standardized diagnostic interviews, emphasis was placed on the development of operational diagnostic criteria. This was embodied in the DSM-III (61) and its successors, and in the clinical and research versions of ICD-10 (62,63). Studies of the reliability of child psychiatric diagnoses have been conducted with various schemes and instruments, giving rise to broadly similar overall conclusions (59).

Diagnostic reliability involves three rather different potential sources of error or variability: *information* variation (how data are collected); *interpretation* variance (how data are weighted and put together); and *criterion* variance (how algorithms are used to produce diagnoses). The first may be examined through test–retest studies to examine the extent to which the same answers are obtained on two consecutive occasions. On the whole, the findings have been of moderate to good reliability that is higher for symptom dimensions than for categorical diagnoses (64). This is affected, however, by the tendency for informants to report less psychopathology on the second occasion (64,65). This is more pronounced with highly structured interviews but can be reduced somewhat by attention to both details of wording of questions and interview organization (66).

Interpretation variance can be assessed by determining the extent to which two informants agree (see above), or two investigators concur in their ratings of behavioral descriptions (67,68), or two different diagnostic instruments provide the same answer. Typically this form of variance is greater—particularly across informant and across instruments. *Criterion* variance needs to be evaluated by comparing different ways of putting the data together. Standardization aims to keep this to a minimum but it is clear that different systems often give different answers (e.g., the findings with respect to age of onset in ADHD (69), number of symptoms in antisocial diagnoses (70) or diagnostic algorithms in autism (71)).

Diagnostic validity concerns the extent to which a diagnostic construct truly reflects a syndrome that is different from others. The testing of validity, therefore, requires research that examines correlates of diagnosis with respect to basic features that are external to the behaviors that define the hypothesized diagnostic construct (72). Such correlates might include genetic influences, neuropathology, biologic indices, course, and response to specific treatments. From a measurement perspective, validity concerns the extent to which empirical measures tap the crucial features that provide the basis of the diagnostic construct—that is, the vertical connections between the top level (latent construct) and the bottom level (empirical measures) in Figure 3.2.1.4. The main measurement issue concerns the possible operation of biases in those vertical connections, expressed as Vn in Figure 3.2.1.4.

The main, possibly biasing, factor considered up to now has been the mental state of the informant (e.g., a depressed mother might overreport psychopathology in her child). To test that possibility it is necessary to determine whether maternal depression alters the pattern of associations between maternal reports of child psychopathology and teacher or child reports (73). The key statistic here relates to pattern differences and not to correlations as such. Thus, with respect to maternal depression the issue is whether a difference in child psychopathology is found on maternal reports that is not evident on reports from others. If there is, a bias is suggested. The weight of evidence from a range of studies indicates that there is some biasing effect, although not a great one. Recently, attention has broadened to consider whether depression in one parent alters the rating of the *other* parent by virtue of its influence on the overall family context (74). A comparable rating bias concern was raised with respect to possible *contrast* effects in parental ratings of twins. Thus, it was hypothesized that parents, in their ratings, might exaggerate differences between dizygotic (nonidentical) twins. Again, the test involves pattern effects in relation to the others. Such contrast effect biases have been found with respect to parental ratings of hyperactivity but, interestingly, not of other forms of disruptive behavior (75). Other examples of such possible rating biases concern the effects of a person's current social situation and mental state on their retrospective rating of negative childhood experiences (76). Findings suggest that there is a slight tendency for people who are doing well to *under* report past adversities but no tendency for people who are not doing well to *overreport* (an illustration of recall bias). Obviously, to test this possibility, it is necessary to have longitudinal data involving contemporaneous measurement of the adverse experiences. Yet another example concerns the possibility that people with a mental disorder may overreport comparable disorders in relatives (77,78). In all these examples the tests have involved some form of pattern difference that involves comparisons among different informants. Usually, the biases found have been small, but equally they have not been zero. The implication is that investigators need to use multiple informants and need to test for such possible biases, statistically correcting for them when required.

Latent Measurement Models

Historically, researchers tended to deal with these measurement problems either by choosing what seemed to be the "best" informant or alternatively by combining the ratings in some way (such as by adding them together or counting a report of a behavior if it comes from just one of a number of informants). Such composite strategies have the advantage of simplicity and, for this reason, they continue to have a worthwhile place in research. However, they fail to make use of all the data, they do not deal quantitatively with possible biases, and they do not remove random measurement error. Latent variable models were developed to deal with these issues (see Fergusson (79,80) for clear descriptions of the rationale and the assumptions involved). In brief, multivariate statistics are used to *infer* the latent construct (which can be either dimensional or categorical) that underlies the associations among a variety of behavioral measures. The focus is on the variance that is *shared* across measures—in effect putting to one side the variance component which is unique to just one measure on the ground that, whatever its intrinsic importance, it is not measuring that which is common across measures. This "special" component is not thrown away but it can be isolated and examined in its own right. Latent variable methods also take into account prior probabilities and assessments in evaluating measurement error. Applications of latent construct measures in child psychiatry include studies of the impact of maternal depression on ratings of child psychopathology (81,82), the cross-informant correlations of behavioral reports (83,84), or the adult outcomes of antisocial behavior (85).

Impairment

The importance of including impaired functioning in case definition was well shown in Bird et al.'s (26) general population epidemiologic study. The prevalence of psychiatric disorder was 50% if assessed on the basis of symptoms and diagnoses alone, without taking account of impairment, but 18% if the latter was required for case definition (26). Similar results have been found in other studies (34,38,39,86).

The need to assess functional impairment is now generally accepted but it has proved difficult to define and measure in a valid fashion. Impairment is related to concepts of role performance that reflect individual's adaptation into his social environment (87). This must be related to developmental level and sociocultural context. Typically, impairment resulting from psychopathology is assessed in four domains: interpersonal relationships, academic/work performance, social and leisure activities, and ability to enjoy and obtain satisfaction from life. These need to be evaluated with respect to functioning at home, school, and in the community.

In earlier epidemiologic surveys (88) and in most classification schemes (62,89), the assessment of impairment was left largely to a global clinical judgment by the interviewer. In the early 1980s, instruments were developed to address this issue with the development of the Children's Global Assessment Scale (90). This instrument was shown to have adequate psychometric properties but it still relied on an experienced clinician, and did not specify how impairment data should be obtained. Further developments of this scale led to a simplified nonclinician version (87,91). Another instrument, the Columbia Impairment Scale (92), was devised to be completed by both parent and adolescent respondents; it has the advantage of being brief and providing scores for specific domains. Preliminary data suggest that it is a useful measure, with the parent CIS having consistently better validity than the children's version. Other instruments exist, such as the Social Adjustment Inventory for Children and Adolescents (93) and the Child and Adolescent Functional Assessment Scale (87).

The issues to be addressed still include: (1) the differentiation between impairment and psychiatric symptoms (e.g., aggression to peers is both a symptom of conduct disorder and a reflection of impaired functioning with respect of peer relationships); (2) how to determine causal connections between symptoms and impairment (preliminary findings suggest that informants found this difficult (87) and interrater agreement was low (94)); (3) the difference between impairment and symptom severity; and (4) how to partition and attribute impairment in the case of comorbid presentations. Pickles et al. (95) found that depressive symptoms predicted later depression equally well with and without the presence of impairment; by contrast, the predictive power of conduct symptoms was increased in the presence of impairment. Angold et al. (96) found, in a community study, that over a fifth of children showed impairment even though their number of symptoms fell below specified cutoffs for diagnosis. These impaired children with subthreshold disorders were likely later to be referred to services, especially to school services in one study (39). Conversely, disorders without impairment tended to have a good outcome (97). The findings from the Ontario study tell much the same story (94).

Diagnostic interviews now include separate measures of impairment associated with disorders and symptoms (98,99). However, research is still needed on the origins of impairment; it cannot be presupposed that they will necessarily be the same as for symptoms.

CASE IDENTIFICATION AND SCREENING

Case Identification

Once a case definition has been established, case identification methods are selected. Adequate sampling techniques are required to provide unbiased estimates of rates and risk factors associated with disorders. Drawing of a sample requires the availability of a sampling frame and of sampling units covering the population of interest. In child psychiatry, surveys have often relied upon school rosters (e.g., Fombonne (11)) because, with compulsory education, they provide comprehensive sampling frames. Alternatively, households may be used as sampling units (e.g., Bird et al. (26); Ford et al. (37)). These approaches will still miss some children, such as homeless or street children (see Bird (26)) or those from families who migrate seasonally for employment reasons. Children in long-term residential facilities may also be overlooked. These losses will bias the findings if psychosocial factors associated with these unusual living circumstances are also risk factors for psychiatric disorders. Other sampling issues were discussed earlier.

Samples used in psychiatric surveys are often large, and direct interviewing of all study participants is not always convenient or possible. The two-phase design used in the Isle of Wight survey (88) has been frequently employed to deal with this difficulty. It requires a first phase of screening of all subjects with questionnaires easy to administer, followed by a diagnostic confirmation phase, more labor intensive, on a subsample of participants selected according to their results at the screening phase. The importance of understanding how screening instruments operate and how to measure their properties cannot therefore be overlooked.

Screening: Sensitivity, Specificity, Predictive Values

Dimensional measurements (whether by questionnaire or interview) lead to total scores ranging from a minimum (usually implying normality) to a maximum (mostly implying psychopathology). For both clinical and research reasons, investigators may want to transform these scores into categories (e.g., inferred normality vs. inferred disorder). Figure 3.2.1.5 depicts a fairly common situation in which scores among normal (noncases) are plotted next to those with a disorder (cases) and show a degree of overlap. Any cutoff will partition these two distributions into four groups, designated false and true positives and false and true negatives. All cutoffs (obtained by moving the vertical line C to the right or to the left in Figure 3.2.1.5) would of course result in some degree of misclassification. The measurement question concerns the determination of what score provides the best discrimination between cases and noncases and how the screening instrument performs in general. In practice, a cutoff has often been chosen before going to the field, and the results of the screening phase of an epidemiologic survey would lead to a tabular presentation as illustrated in Table 3.2.1.3. Various important indices can be used to summarize the data in this situation, including specificity, sensitivity, and positive predictive value. Sensitivity and specificity are two important proportions that are often quoted to summarize the properties of an instrument. Investigators wish both of them to be high, but as is obvious from Table 3.2.1.3 and Figure 3.2.1.5, they vary in opposite directions.

Estimating Prevalence from Screening Data

One consequence of the imperfection of our screening instruments is that the prevalence of a disorder cannot be directly

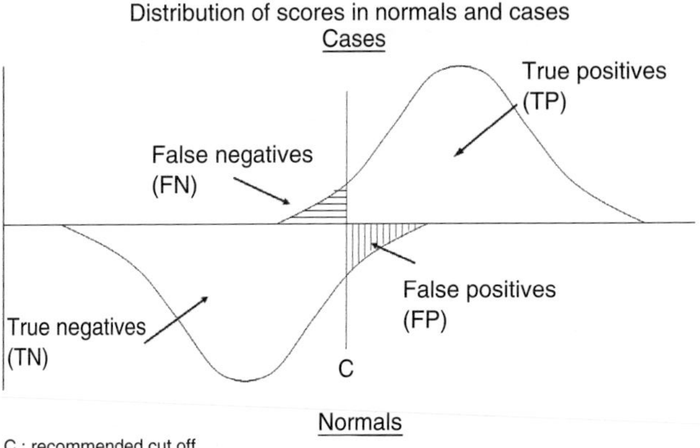

FIGURE 3.2.1.5. Distribution of scores in normals and cases.

TABLE 3.2.1.3

TYPICAL RESULTS OF A SCREENING EXERCISE

	Cases D	Normal $\bar{D}$	
Test positive: T+	a	b	a + b
Test negative: T–	c	d	c + d
	a + c	b + d	a + b + c + d = N

True positives: TP = a False negatives: FN = c D = diseased
False positives: FP = b True negatives: TN = d $\bar{D}$ = nondiseased
Sensitivity (or rate of true positives: RTP): Se = a/a + c = p(T + /D)
Specificity (or rate of true negatives: RTN): Sp = d/b + d = p(T – / $\bar{D}$)
Rate of false negatives: RFN = c/a + c = p(T – /D)
Rate of false positives: RFP = b/b + d = p(T + / $\bar{D}$)
Prevalence: P = a + c/N = p(D)
Positive predictive value: PPV = a/a + b = p(D/T+)
Negative predictive value: NPV = d/c + d = p($\bar{D}$/T–)

estimated from the screening data of a survey. Unfortunately, some authors sometimes report the "prevalence" of a condition to be equivalent to the proportion of subjects who scored above the cutoff during the screening phase (the prevalence of eating disorders or that of depression has often been reported as the proportion of subjects scoring high on eating or depression inventories). This approach is wrong as the proportion of screened positives in a survey is made of the sum of true positives and false positives (a + b/N in Table 3.2.1.3), which is very different from the prevalence rate that corresponds to the sum of true positives and false negatives (a + c/N in Table 3.2.1.3). To take a practical example, assuming that a near-perfect screening instrument is available with a sensitivity and specificity of 90%, the results of the hypothetical screening of 1,000 individuals are shown in Table 3.2.1.4 under two separate hypotheses regarding the true population prevalence rate. In both examples, the prevalence rate is different than the proportion of screened positives and, in the case of a low prevalence rate of 0.01 (Table 3.2.1.4A), the proportion of screen positives (10.8%) overestimates the prevalence by a factor greater than 10. Thus, the results of any screening test administered in a population cannot be directly interpreted in terms of prevalence, unless sensitivity and specificity are known for this survey and taken into account in a more complex estimating function.

Screening At-Risk Individuals

Another implication of the lack of perfect measurements has to do with screening particular individuals for the disorder of interest. If screening was perfect, we could infer in an individual with a positive screening score that he has the disorder; furthermore, we would expect that all individuals with the disorder would be picked up by the screening instrument. This ideal (but unrealistic) situation would correspond to a sensitivity and specificity of the screening tool of 100% (b and c would be equal to 0 in Table 3.2.1.3). As shown in the practical example of Table 3.2.1.4, the probability of detecting a disorder in a screened positive individual is in fact variable, and disappointing in the case of a low prevalence rate (Table 3.2.1.4A). This is despite using an instrument with excellent performance in terms of its sensitivity and specificity (both set at 90%). When the prevalence is low, cases in the screen-positive group remain too few in comparison to false positives, making inferences about the presence of the disorder in a screen-positive individual child too hazardous to draw. The situation is much different when the prevalence is higher (Table 3.2.1.4B). Illustrations of this issue abundant in child psychiatry. For example, in initial studies of screening questionnaires (for suicidality, eating disorders, etc.), excellent performances are often reported in differentiating cases and controls. However, the validation samples typically contain roughly equal proportions of cases and controls (which amounts to an artificial study population with a prevalence near 50%); when used later in more representative samples (where the prevalence is much lower), the questionnaire performances drop precipitously (100). A corollary message is that properties of an instrument are context-specific and *not* inherent qualities of the instrument. Sensitivity, specificity, and positive predictive value are empirical, tangible indices of the validity of a measuring instrument. The example shows that some of these properties can be affected by the context of their application (the prevalence) and that validity is not an intrinsic, absolute, instrument property. Rather, validity must be (re)evaluated according to the goals and context of a study and validity assessment is best viewed as an ongoing process.

Receiving Operating Characteristics Analysis

A scale or questionnaire is generally presented with one suggested cutoff point apparently associated with optimal performances (sensitivity and specificity). It is obvious that, as we move the cutoff point along the scale values, we would obtain different pairs of values for sensitivity and specificity. The investigator may want to vary the cutoff of an instrument to maximize sensitivity or specificity, depending on their study goals, the consequences of misclassification (sometimes, it is highly desirable to limit the false-positive rate [increase the specificity] even at the expense of sensitivity, as in some biologic or genetic studies), or on the prevalence of the disorder. The receiving operating characteristics (ROC) curve simply plots sensitivity on one axis of a graph and the false-positive rate (1 – specificity) on the other for all possible cut points on a scale (see Figure 3.2.1.6). An ROC curve close to the diagonal corresponds to a poorly discriminant instrument, whereas the discriminant power of the instrument increases the farther

TABLE 3.2.1.4

TWO SCREENING EXAMPLES

A: Prevalence of 0.01	Cases	Noncases		B: Prevalence of 0.30	Cases	Noncases	
Screen +	9	99	108	Screen +	270	70	340
Screen –	1	891	892	Screen –	30	630	660
	10	990	1,000		300	700	1,000
P = 0.01	Sp = 0.90			P = 0.30	Sp = 0.90		
Se = 0.90	PPV = 9/108 = 0.083			Se = 0.90	PPV = 270/340 = 0.794		

P, prevalence; Sp, specificity; Se, sensitivity; PPV, positive predictive value.

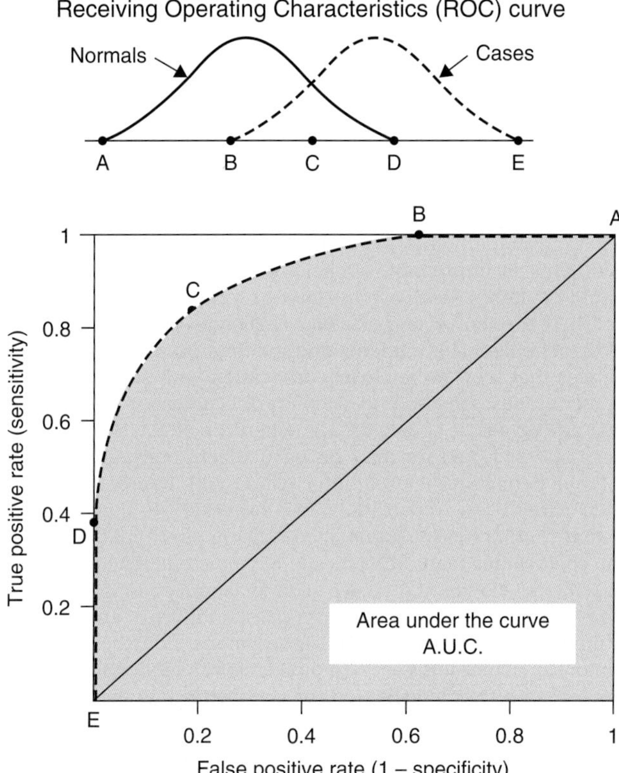

FIGURE 3.2.1.6. Receiving operating characteristics (ROC) curve.

on the upper left the ROC curve deviates from the diagonal. The area under the curve (AUC) is used as an overall summary index of the discriminant power of the scale. AUCs can be statistically compared to gauge the screening properties of different instruments, or to evaluate the gains or losses of discriminant power of a given tool when scoring instructions are changed, or items added or subtracted from the questionnaire. ROC analyses can also take into account the effect of the prevalence of the disorder on determining a best cutoff and evaluating the overall performance of an instrument, of the severity of cases under detection, and of the consequences of all types of misclassification errors (101,102). ROC analyses have been helpful in promoting a flexible use of instruments that can suit better investigators' needs in their research contexts.

Major Psychiatric Surveys

It is outside the scope of this chapter to review the substantive findings of child psychiatry epidemiologic surveys. Data on the incidence or prevalence of individual psychiatric disorders can be found in other chapters. In this section, we concentrate on current figures for overall psychiatric morbidity attributable to the most common internalizing and externalizing disorders.

Psychiatric Morbidity among Children and Adolescents. Epidemiologic surveys to assess prevalence usually rely on cross-sectional methods. Numerous prevalence surveys have now been conducted across the world (see Verhulst and Koot (40), Canino et al. (103), Bird (86), Roberts et al. (104)). Table 3.2.1.1 presents the main results of recent surveys. The overall rates of psychiatric disorders underscore the most important finding. Psychopathology in young people is common, most studies estimating the prevalence to be between 10% and 20%. Verhulst and Koot (40) reviewed 49 surveys and computed an average rate of 12.9%. Emotional disturbances and disorders of disruptive behavior are equally common (with rates of 6% to 8%). It should be noted that many of these surveys will not have included neurodevelopmental disorders such as intellectual disability, language and other specific developmental disorders or autism and may not have picked up psychotic, bipolar, or eating disorders with an onset in late adolescence.

Community samples have also shown that only a small proportion (typically between 10% and 30%) of children with a disorder have had contact with specialist mental health services (25,37,105–107). Disorders involving disruptive behavior (37,108), and those that are severe or of long duration (109) are more likely to get referred. However, contextual factors (such as parental psychopathology) and family features also influence referral (110). The findings therefore indicate the need for caution in extrapolating from clinical samples or experience. Children seen in clinics often differ in systematic ways from nonreferred children with comparable levels of psychopathology. Epidemiologic findings are needed for the development of psychopathologic models.

Age of Onset. Age of onset is a definitional feature of several disorders. In ICD-10 (and DSM-IV), enuresis cannot be diagnosed before the age of 5, ADHD symptoms must be present before age 7, and Asperger syndrome is differentiated from high-functioning autism by the absence of a significant language delay by age 3. Age of onset is usually assessed retrospectively. However, the interrater and retest reliabilities of age of onset have been found to be poor outside the last 3 months for disorders with a recent onset and outside 1 year for those with a longer duration (111). Imperfect measurement of onset and offset of disorder can therefore influence prevalence estimates that are contingent upon specific time periods.

Age of onset also indexes differential outcomes. Moffitt (112) found that conduct disorders with an adolescent onset differed from early-onset conduct problems, with the latter more likely to be associated with neuropsychological impairments and with a worse long-term outlook. Similarly, adolescent-onset depression is associated with a particularly strong risk of recurrence in adult life (113,114), whereas the course and correlates of depression beginning before puberty is rather different (115–117). The timing of onset is also crucial in order to explore the direction of causal effects in patterns of comorbidity. The demonstration that ADHD is a risk factor for later conduct disorder (but that the reverse does not apply) (118,119) and that dysthymic disorder is a gateway to major depressive disorders (120) provide examples of this issue. Retrospective assessment of age of onset is also an issue in adult studies (121), particularly as accurate assessment of this variable can influence results from familial studies (122) and from studies of secular trends (123). One way to avoid the problem of unreliability in the timing of onsets is to use lifetime prevalence estimates (e.g., Lewinsohn et al. (31)). These have the advantage of avoiding the problem of unreliability in the timing of onset and are probably the best approach for disorders present at the time of assessments. However, doubts arise over the reliability and validity of reports of past disorders that are no longer present. Such doubts probably apply less to disorders in childhood than in adult life because time spans are shorter and because multiple informants are available.

Risk Factors. A detailed review of risk factors for child psychiatric disorders identified in epidemiologic studies is out of the scope of this chapter (see chapters on individual disorders). Nevertheless, multiple risk mechanisms are now solidly established for specific disorders that have led to the development and systematic testing of treatments targeting these risk factors and to the consolidation of evidence-based practices. For example, the relationship between parenting problems, lack of maternal warmth, harsh discipline, marital discord, and the onset of antisocial symptoms in children has subsequently led to effective parent–child interventions (124). For many disorders, risk factors have been identified within the child (prenatal exposures, low birth weight, developmental delays, medical and especially brain disorders, IQ, cognitive style), in the family (parental psychopathology, marital discord, maternal sensitivity and warmth), in the school (classroom size, peer relationships, discipline practices, teaching styles), in the community (poverty, crime rates, access to drugs), and in broader societal factors (media viewing, body ideals).

There have been recent exciting developments in the systematic testing of causal mechanisms in child psychiatry epidemiology. Two are worth mentioning. First, the need is not only to identify a long collection of individual risk factors associated with psychiatric disorders but to develop models of psychopathology by examining the joint contribution of several risk factors operating in different domains (biologic *and* psychological *and* social) and in the course of individual development. Thus, the first examples of the importance of gene and environmental interactions were found in a cohort study where young adults homozygous for the short allele of the serotonin transporter gene were found to be at much increased risk of depression when (and only when) exposed to negative life events as compared to those individuals homozygous for the long allele (125). The findings clearly indicated that psychosocial risk factors operate differently in individuals according to their genetic background. The simultaneous study of risk factors is necessary to refine our understanding of child psychopathology and move beyond the frequent oversimplified explanations that are in use in clinical settings (the patient *is* depressed *because* something bad happened to her). The key point, though, is that carefully selected epidemiologic samples and measures, adequate sample sizes, and longitudinal designs are necessary to fully evaluate these complex explanatory models. Second, new techniques of analyses of complex longitudinal data (trajectory methods) have shifted the focus from classical group-based predictor–outcome relationships to the identification of patterns of individual trajectories. Predictors of trajectory membership can then be identified, such as in the studies by Tremblay et al. (126) on the persistence or desistance of aggression over time. These methods are particularly suitable to the lifespan study of psychopathology and to a focus on individual differences in the onset and offset of psychopathologic conditions.

Comorbidity. The high frequency of cooccurrence of two supposedly separate forms of psychopathology was noted in the Isle of Wight studies over 50 years ago (88). However, it is only in the last 25 years that it has received much conceptual attention and empirical study (47,51,127–130). In their thorough review of the topic, Angold et al. (47) concluded that artifacts cannot account entirely for the frequency and patterns of comorbidity and that mechanisms underlying comorbid presentations should be studied more systematically, preferably with epidemiologic samples. Several research findings show how comorbidity may carry meaning. For example, the results of a family study of depression changed once comorbidity in the probands was properly taken into account (131) and a trend emerged for a positive drug response to tricyclic antidepressants in noncomorbid depressed subjects when results from a clinical trial were stratified according to the presence or absence of comorbid conduct disorder (132).

However, in order to undertake research using comorbidity it is necessary that the epidemiologic studies' methods of measurement are adequate for dealing with the assessment of psychopathology that involves comorbid patterns.

Special Topics

Preschool Studies. Epidemiologic investigations of preschool samples have been surprisingly few (133–139, 140). Nevertheless, studies have shown that psychiatric disorders starting in the preschool years show a high degree of persistence over time and that their course is systematically associated with identifiable risk and protective factors. For example, a difficult temperament in the child interacts with characteristics of family dysfunction to increase the risk of psychopathology 5 years later (141); and a shy, inhibited style of interaction predicts later onset of anxiety disorders in childhood (142). Furthermore, evidence has accumulated that developmental disorders usually identified in the early years have short- (143) and long-term consequences (144) with respect to psychosocial disturbances and functioning. Long-term follow-up of birth cohorts have also shown continuities between preschool behavior and adult psychopathology (145). Thus, identification of preschool problems is important, especially since early intervention might be more effective in the case of some disorders (146).

There are, however, particular challenges in the assessment of preschoolers (147). Infants and toddlers present with disturbances that tend to be closely associated with somatic development. Thus, feeding and sleeping difficulties are common in this age group. It is also an age when the effects of prenatal/perinatal risk factors may be particularly marked. Second, infants' behavior is closely intertwined with interactions with their caregivers. Accordingly, it is necessary to consider the extent to which any disturbance reflects psychopathology in the child rather than difficulties in a dyadic relationship. Third, specific developmental delays such as language or social relationships are first evident in the preschool years and call for a multifaceted developmental assessment. Fourth, very few dimensional measures assessing behavioral/emotional deviance have been properly validated for children below the age of 4. Finally, current diagnostic schemes have acknowledged limitations for use with very young children (148). Scales such as the Temperament and Atypical Behavior Scale (149) and classifications such as the Zero-to-Three diagnostic classification (150) have been developed for infants and toddlers but they are based on particular conceptual frameworks and are closely linked to intervention strategies. However, downward extensions of psychiatric interviews have been recently developed and tested in preschoolers and have shown good psychometric properties (151). The use of this new generation of instruments in population-based samples of preschool children indicates that both rates and patterns of disorders and comorbidity in preschool samples are comparable to those of older children (152).

Norm-Referenced Instruments. Reference to normative data is implicit in the assessment of psychopathology. However, it was only in the late 1950s that systematic surveys of children's behaviors and emotions were undertaken on large samples of nonreferred children (22). The epidemiologic surveys of child psychiatric disorders that followed helped to promote knowledge of normative behavior at different ages with the useful development of standardized questionnaires for use with multiple informants (40,41,88,153). Increasingly, data from large representative samples of nonreferred children have been used to calibrate measures in order to provide the best identification of probable psychopathology. However, not all standardizations have used fully representative general population samples. There must be reservations about generalizability when convenience samples have been used. Second, norms are derived from particular regional or national samples and the query is whether it is justifiable to extrapolate to other regions or countries. For example, a 10- to 15-point difference in mean CBCL total scores has been reported among American, Australian (154), French (155), and Puerto Rican children (156). The question is whether these differences reflect true regional differences in psychopathology or rating tendencies that have been influenced by cultural contextual features. Both possibilities have to be considered seriously, but their differentiation requires the use of external validators of some kind. The Isle of Wight–Inner London comparison indicated that a true difference in rate of psychopathology was likely (157), whereas the United Kingdom–Hong Kong comparison with respect to hyperactivity suggested a rating difference effect (158). Investigators are well advised to be cautious about assumptions that one set of norms can be generalized to different populations.

Similar issues concern extrapolations from one large representative population to subgroups within. For example, are associations between social class and behavioral disturbance (41,42) a true reflection of valid differences or a contextual rating bias effect? The same applies to age and gender differences. An automatic assumption that subgroup norms should be used or that any differences from total population norms are necessarily valid should be resisted. As ever, external validation is essential.

Third, norms apply to one particular point in time. Evidence has accumulated that there have been secular changes in the incidence of various psychosocial disorders (159–161) and of individual behavioral problems. Thus, Achenbach and Howell (162) compared two large representative samples of American youth surveyed 13 years apart and found increased scores on 46 of 118 behavioral problems and on all scale scores (the mean total score increasing from 18 to 24.2) in the most recent birth cohorts. Periodic recalibration of instruments is necessary in child psychopathology, just as it is for other measures such as psychometric tests (163,164) or physical indices such as height, weight, head circumference, and pubertal maturation (165).

Cultural Issues. Most industrialized societies today are multicultural, multiethnic, and multilingual, a fact that has important implications for clinical practice. In addition, it has consequences for the assessment of psychopathology by means of standardized interviews or questionnaires. It would be a mistake to exaggerate the methodologic difficulties. Rating scales have usually been found to function in much the same way across cultures (166–169) with, for example, comparable gender differences (154,155,169).

Nevertheless, three issues require attention. First, there is a concern to ensure linguistic equivalence. This is usually accomplished by a series of back translations from one language to the other by independent bilingual translators who are familiar with the psychopathologic concepts. The last specification is important to ensure that the appropriate words are selected to tap the intended meaning. That is relevant, too, in relation to the need to ensure equivalence between American and British versions of instruments. The problems of going across languages are even greater and it is crucial that the translators appreciate the intended meaning in relation to psychopathology. Issues in relation to the translation of diagnostic interviews for Hispanics were described by Canino and Bravo (170) and examples of translation inaccuracies and of their effects on deviance scores were noted by Woodward et al. (171).

Second, there is the question of conceptual and perceptual equivalence. Thus, Weisz et al. (172) reported differences between Thai and American adults in their concern over particular behaviors; Lee (173) queried whether a morbid fear of fatness had the same implications for anorexia nervosa in Hong Kong as it does in Western societies; and King and Bhugra (174) posed the same question with respect to questions on dieting when used in cultures where this is part of religious practice. It cannot be claimed that there is an adequate knowledge base to show either the importance of these concerns or how they are best dealt with, but investigators need to be alert to their possible effects on measurement. They are likely to have effects because most ratings involve an explicit or implicit comparison with some norms, the behaviors being normal at a low level but abnormal at some higher level.

Third, there is the question of diagnostic equivalence. Some cultures have syndromes that appear to have no obvious equivalent in other cultures, although systematic evidence on this is largely lacking. From a measurement perspective, perhaps the key point is that when different cultures express the same disorder through differently expressed manifestations, there needs to be caution in the application of diagnostic algorithms. For example, there is evidence that cultures vary in the extent to which they express depression in reports of feelings of misery; some are more likely to report these in terms of somatic complaints (175). Similar issues arise with respect to age variations, as reflected in the different role given to irritability in the diagnosis of depression in childhood and in adult life (89). Once more, there is at least as much of a danger of wrongly assuming an age (or cultural) difference as of overlooking a real difference. The arbitration has to lie in empirical studies. Recent systematic comparisons of children's emotional and behavioral problems assessed in over 30 cultures with the same instruments indicate that cultural differences are relatively small across countries, with mean scores for most samples falling close to the omnicultural mean (176,177).

Language of Assessment. Practically, as population samples in most countries reflect a mixture of cultures and languages, it has become essential for epidemiologists but also for clinicians to have access to instruments adequately translated and validated in different languages. The common instruments used to evaluate general psychopathology in children and adolescents are available in multiple languages. For example, access to non-English versions is obtained through specific websites associated to the corresponding instruments, for example, http://www.aseba.org/ordering/translations.html for the 90 international versions of the Child Behavior Checklist and http://www.sdqinfo.com/b3.html for the 86 translations of the Strengths and Difficulties Questionnaire. Translated versions of various instruments tapping specific dimensions of child psychopathology also exist and are available either from their authors or commercial distributors. Non-English versions of various diagnostic interviews also exist in different languages, although the work is less advanced than that for general psychopathologic rating scales. It is prudent to check with the original authors of an instrument whether or not an available translation has been approved by them and properly established.

Studying Transitions to Adulthood. With a growing emphasis on lifespan perspectives on developmental psychopathology and an increasing focus on the study of continuities and discontinuities between child and adult disorders, psychiatric epidemiologists have now developed adult versions of child instruments that are suitable for longitudinal research and provide investigators with measurements that are highly consistent across age groups. For example, adolescent samples evaluated with a combination of the Child Behavior Checklist and Youth Self-Report Form can be followed as young adults with parallel adult versions of these instruments such as the Adult Self-Report and the Adult Behavior Checklist that can be used up to age 59. Versions for subjects aged 60 or older are also available (http://www.aseba.org). Similarly, adult extensions of child psychiatric interviews such as the CAPA or the DISC are being developed.

Interviewing and Computer Technology. Modern technology has allowed many assessment procedures to be computerized. For example, Berg et al. (178) compared the reliability, concurrent and criterion validity of two standard and computer-assisted procedures to collect data using two common psychopathology scales, the Rutter A2 scale and the CBCL. Psychometric properties were similar with the two procedures, suggesting that computer-assisted technologies might be used more extensively in routine practice.

There are numerous advantages to computerization: It eliminates observer bias; it ensures that all respondents receive precisely the same instructions and questions; by having a voice read the questions aloud it circumvents illiteracy problems; it allows more complex and flexible skip and branching patterns than possible with paper and pencil procedures; it makes immediate checking of the consistency and range of responses possible; and it provides error-free computation of scores with or without reference to existing norms. Data are stored readily in a format that allows for further analysis; computer storage also makes the data collection procedure less vulnerable to errors such as accidental loss of data, theft, or inadvertent disclosure of confidential materials.

Several structured diagnostic interviews already have computerized versions. The role of the computer does, however, vary considerably. Computers are sometimes used to assist interviewers in their task of conducting the interview. In this instance, the interviewer still performs a face-to-face interview and records the answers of the respondent on a laptop computer as the interview proceeds. This procedure has both the advantage and disadvantage of allowing some degree of interviewer judgment. Fully computerized diagnostic interviews tend to be highly structured, with restricted response options. Computer-aided administration is particularly useful in helping the interviewer to follow complex skip rules and to track respondent's answers that require follow-up questions in the course of the interview. The NIMH DISC-IV (98) is typical of such interviews devised for large-scale epidemiologic surveys. The DAWBA (179), used in the U.K. National Survey of Child Mental Health (37), provides another example, with the additional feature that space is allocated to record respondents' descriptions verbatim as well, so allowing a subsequent overarching clinical interpretation of all structured data and of open-ended commentaries. This procedure, however, detracts somewhat from the greater efficiency of the computerized interviews—a major selling point. In other developments, computers are used to replace interviewers fully. Some sound versions of diagnostic interviews have now been developed for full self-administration, using headphones or speakers. The Voice DISC (98) and a substance abuse module of the CAPA (99) are examples of such developments, which totally eliminate interviewer costs.

Investigator-based interviews have been, for obvious reasons, less amenable to computerization, although some attempts have been made, such as with the DICA (180). One diagnostic interview relying on displays of pictures or cartoons to elicit symptomatic data has been released in computerized form (Interactive Dominic Questionnaire (181)), but more data are still needed on its basic properties.

Computerized interviewing does not usually decrease the time needed to administer the interview, but it can lead to substantial savings in terms of interviewer time (and costs) by eliminating that used for coding and interpretation. Successful use has been achieved in recent epidemiologic surveys (37,182).

It is possible, too, that computerized interviews may be better at eliciting potentially embarrassing personal information, because it eliminates the interpersonal context. Reich et al. (183) found that children enjoyed the computerized DICA-R interview, preferred it over a person interview, and said that they would tell things to the computer that they would not tell to a person. Survey research has shown that rates of at-risk behaviors involving sexual contacts and use of addictive substances were three times higher when questions were asked via audio-computerized methods than when asked face to face (184). Similar results have been found regarding suicidal behaviors (e.g., Reich et al. (183)).

It is too early to draw firm conclusions on the merits and demerits of computerized interviews. Clearly, they have very important advantages for some purposes and there is no doubt that they will be used more in the future. However, for some purposes, their chief advantage of eliminating the need for interviewers may be a disadvantage, just because it eliminates personal contact. The structural format, too, will be limiting in relation to the eliciting of important unexpected information.

Computerized Clinical Databases. The progress made in the measurement of child psychopathology in epidemiologic research has been paralleled by similar advances in the systematic evaluation of patients referred to mental health teams. Multiaxial diagnostic formulations and use of norm-referenced general psychopathology questionnaires are now standards in most clinical centers. Yet, despite the easy access to computers and databases, the data collected are usually not made readily available for research applications to clinical researchers (be they epidemiologists or clinicians). A good example of the usefulness of such clinical data recording systems is the Item Sheet that has been in place at the Maudsley Hospital for over half a century and which records diagnoses, symptoms, demographic details, psychosocial features, test findings, details of referral, and rating of clinical outcome. This large computerized database has allowed for the study of specific problem behaviors, sampling for long-term follow-up studies, patient comparisons between centers in different countries, the investigation of trends over time in specific behavioral problems and of their causes, and the study of comorbid patterns (113,160,161,185). More streamlined data recording systems could easily achieve the same goals if a core set of variables were defined. Also, centers could decide to add on, for specific groups of patients of interest, or for defined periods of time, more exhaustive data recording procedures, because databases can easily be managed on modularity principles. Progress in information technology has made it easy and cheap to set up such databases and to exchange data when appropriate. Indeed, the need to audit services and to be accountable with regard to services activity for the health service will make such systems increasingly mandatory in most countries. Timely recognition of these needs and of the usefulness of these databases will help mental health professionals to influence these information systems in a way that might be more clinically relevant and useful for their own research and practice.

CONCLUSION

Progresses in child psychiatric epidemiology have been impressive in the last 40 years and have been made possible by the development of empirical and replicable measurement approaches to children's maladaptive behaviors and psychiatric disorders. The impact of epidemiology has been on several areas. For clinical practice, epidemiology has provided normative data on child behavior that are necessary to evaluate problems seen in clinical settings. As physiology is needed in medicine to understand disease pathology, knowledge of typically developing children acquired through epidemiologic inquiries is needed for understanding child psychopathology.

Knowledge of the clinical significance of individual symptoms, of the risk factors associated with psychiatric disorders, of their population prevalence and incidence, is required for developing appropriate models of child psychopathology. For public health, surveys have drawn the attention on the importance of global morbidity in children due to mental health problems. In addition, disorders with an onset in childhood or adolescence have strong continuities with adult disorders, thus contributing to the burden of mental illness across the lifespan. Unfortunately, and despite increasing availability of evidence-based practices with demonstrated efficacy in controlled studies, access to services is insufficient in most countries. At a time where several indicators have shown upward trends in rates of behavioral disturbances in young people, service planners and policymakers should be made aware of this discrepancy. Progress in understanding causal mechanisms underlying some disorders has been substantial. Several risk factors are now well established that could be targeted by treatment and prevention programs. More refined understanding of child psychopathology is emerging, with new studies that now incorporate a joint assessment of genetic, biologic, and psychosocial factors, and combine longitudinal and developmental approaches in genetically informative designs to test competing hypotheses on psychopathologic mechanisms.

References

1. Susser E, Neugebauer R, Hoek HW, Brown AS, Lin S, Labovitz D, Gorman JM: Schizophrenia after prenatal famine. Further evidence. *Arch Gen Psychiatry* 53(1):25–31, 1996.
2. St Clair D, Xu M, Wang P, et al.: Rates of adult schizophrenia following prenatal exposure to the Chinese famine of 1959–1961. *JAMA* 294(5):557–62, 2005.
3. Fombonne E: The importance of choosing the right type and sufficient numbers of controls in research on neurodevelopmental disorders and mental health conditions [Editorial]. *J Child Psychol Psychiatry* 57(11):1203–1204, 2016. Erratum in *J Child Psychol Psychiatry* 58(1):E1, 2017.
4. Fombonne E, Zakarian R, Bennett A, Meng L, McLean-Heywood D: Pervasive developmental disorders in Montreal, Quebec, Canada: prevalence and links with immunizations. *Pediatrics* 118(1):e139–e150, 2006.
5. Rothman KGS: *Modern Epidemiology*. Philadelphia, PA, Lippincott-Raven, 1998.
6. Dunn G, Pickles A, Tansella M, Vazquez-Barquero JL: Two-phase epidemiological surveys in psychiatric research. *Br J Psychiatry* 174:95–100, 1999.
7. Madsen KM, Hviid A, Vestergaard M, et al.: A population-based study of measles, mumps, and rubella vaccination and autism. *N Engl J Med* 347(19):1477–82, 2002.
8. Hviid A, Stellfeld M, Wohlfahrt J, Melbye M: Association between thimerosal-containing vaccine and autism. *JAMA* 290(13):1763–1766, 2003.
9. Smeeth L, Cook C, Fombonne E, et al.: MMR vaccination and pervasive developmental disorders: a case-control study. *Lancet* 364(9438):963–969, 2004.
10. Madsen KM, Lauritsen MB, Pedersen CB, et al.: Thimerosal and the occurrence of autism: negative ecological evidence from Danish population-based data. *Pediatrics* 112(3 Pt. 1):604–606, 2003.
11. Fombonne E: The Chartres study: I. Prevalence of psychiatric disorders among French school-aged children. *Br J Psychiatry* 164:69–79, 1994.
12. Boyle MH, Offord DR, Racine YA, Catlin G: Ontario Child Health Study follow-up: evaluation of sample loss. *J Am Acad Child Adolesc Psychiatry* 30(3):449–456, 1991.
13. Kalton G: *Compensating for Missing Data*. Ann Arbor, Institute for Social Research, 1983.
14. Little DR: *Statistical Analysis with Missing Data*. New York, Wiley, 1987.
15. Stott DH: Some psychosomatic aspects of casualty in reproduction. *J Psychosom Res* 3(1):42–55, 1958.
16. Hill AB: The environment and disease: association or causation? *Proc R Soc Med* 58:295–300, 1965.
17. Fombonne E, Chakrabarti S: No evidence for a new variant of measles-mumps-rubella–induced autism. *Pediatrics* 108(4):E58, 2001.
18. Lucas AR, Beard CM, O'Fallon WM, Kurland LT: 50-year trends in the incidence of anorexia nervosa in Rochester, Minn.: a population-based study. *Am J Psychiatry* 148(7):917–922, 1991.
19. Barbaresi WJ, Katusic SK, Colligan RC, Weaver AL, Jacobsen SJ: The incidence of autism in Olmsted County, Minnesota, 1976–1997: results from a population-based study. *Arch Pediatr Adolesc Med* 159(1):37–44, 2005.
20. Rutter M, Tizard J, Whitmore K: *Education, Health and Behavior*. New York, Robert E. Krieber Publishing, 1970.
21. Rutter M, Tizard J, Yule W, Graham P, Whitmore K: Research report: Isle of Wight studies, 1964–1974. *Psychol Med* 6:313–332, 1976.
22. Lapouse R, Monk M: An epidemiologic study of behavior characteristics in children. *Am J Public Health* 48:1134–1144, 1958.
23. Rutter M: Isle of Wight revisited: twenty-five years of child psychiatric epidemiology. *J Am Acad Child Adolesc Psychiatry* 28:633–653, 1989.
24. Anderson JC, Franz CP, Williams S, McGee R, Silva PA: DSM-III disorders in preadolescent children. *Arch Gen Psychiatry* 44:69–76, 1987.
25. Offord DR, Boyle MH, Szatmari P, et al.: Ontario Child Health Study. II: Six-month prevalence of disorder and rates of service utilization. *Arch Gen Psychiatry* 44(9):832–836, 1987.
26. Bird HR, Canino G, Rubio-Stipec M, et al.: Estimates of the prevalence of childhood maladjustment in a community survey in Puerto Rico. The use of combined measures [published erratum appears in Arch Gen Psychiatry 1994 May;51 (5):429]. *Arch Gen Psychiatry* 45(12):1120–1126, 1988.
27. Esser G, Schmidt MH, Woerner W: Epidemiology and course of psychiatric disorders in school-age children—results of a longitudinal study. *J Child Psychol Psychiatry* 31:243–263, 1990.
28. Morita H, Suzuki M, Kamoshita S: Screening measures for detecting psychiatric disorders in Japanese secondary school children. *J Child Psychol Psychiatry Allied Discipl* 31(4):603–617, 1990.
29. Jeffers A, Fitzgerald M: *Irish Families Under Stress*. Vol. 2. Dublin, Eastern Health Board, 1991.
30. Fergusson DM, Horwood LJ, Lynskey MT: Prevalence and comorbidity of DSM-III-R diagnoses in a birth cohort of 15 year olds. *J Am Acad Child Adolesc Psychiatry* 32(6):1127–1134, 1993.
31. Lewinsohn PM, Hops H, Roberts RE, Seeley JR, Andrews JA: Age cohort changes in the lifetime occurrence of depression and other mental disorders. *J Abnorm Psychol* 102(1):110–120, 1993.
32. Costello E, Angold A, Burns B, Erkanli A, Stangl D, Tweed D: The Great Smoky Mountains Study of Youth: functional impairment and serious emotional disturbance. *Arch Gen Psychiatry* 53:1137–1143, 1996.
33. Verhulst F, van der Ende J, Ferdinand R, Kasius M: The prevalence of DSM-111-R diagnoses in a national sample of Dutch adolescents. *Arch Gen Psychiatry* 54(4):329–336, 1997.
34. Simonoff E, Pickles A, Meyer JM, et al.: The Virginia Twin Study of Adolescent Behavioral Development. Influences of age, sex, and impairment on rates of disorder. *Arch Gen Psychiatry* 54(9):801–808, 1997.
35. Steinhausen H, Meier M, Angst J: The Zurich long-term outcome study of child and adolescent psychiatric disorders in males. *Psychol Med* 28:375–383, 1998.
36. Breton JJ, Bergeron L, Valla JP, et al.: Quebec child mental health survey: prevalence of DSM-III-R mental health disorders. *J Child Psychol Psychiatry Allied Discipl* 40(3):375–384, 1999.
37. Ford T, Goodman R, Meltzer H: The British Child and Adolescent Mental Health Survey 1999: the prevalence of DSM-IV disorders. *J Am Acad Child Adolesc Psychiatry* 42(10):1203–1211, 2003.
38. Costello EJ, Mustillo S, Erkanli A, Keeler G, Angold A: Prevalence and development of psychiatric disorders in childhood and adolescence. *ArchGen Psychiatry* 60(8):837–814, 2003.
39. Canino G, Shrout PE, Rubio-Stipec M, et al.: The DSM-IV rates of child and adolescent disorders in Puerto Rico: prevalence, correlates, service use, and the effects of impairment. *Arch Gen Psychiatry* 61(1):85–93, 2004.
40. Verhulst F, Koot H: *The Epidemiology of Child and Adolescent Psychopathology*, Oxford, UK, Oxford University Press, 1995.
41. Achenbach TM, Edelbrock CS: Behavioral problems and competencies reported by parents of normal and disturbed children aged four through sixteen. *Monogr Soc Res Child Dev* 46(1):82, 1981.
42. Fombonne E: Parent reports on behavior and competencies among 6–21-year-old French children. *Euro Child Adolesc Psychiatry* 1(4):233–243, 1992.
43. Petersen A, Compas B, Brooks-Gunn J, Stemmler M, Ey S, Grant K: Depression in adolescence. *Am Psychol* 48:155–168, 1993.
44. Fombonne E: Eating disorders: time trends and explanatory mechanisms, In: Rutter M, Smith D (eds): *Psychosocial Disorders in Young People: Time Trends and Their Causes*. Chichester, Wiley, 616–685, 1995.
45. Fombonne E: The Chartres Study: I. Prevalence of psychiatric disorders among French school-age children. *Br J Psychiatry* 164(1):69–79, 1994.
46. Achenbach TM, McConaughy SH, Howell CT: Child/adolescent behavioral and emotional problems: implications of cross-informant correlations for situational specificity. *Psychol Bull* 101(2):213–232, 1987.
47. Angold A, Costello E, Erkanli A: Comorbidity. *J Child Psychol Psychiatry* 40(1):57–87, 1999.
48. Ambrosini PJ: Historical development and present status of the schedule for affective disorders and schizophrenia for school-age children (K-SADS). *J Am Acad Child Adolesc Psychiatry* 39(1):49–58, 2000.
49. Bird HR, Gould MS, Staghezza B: Aggregating data from multiple informants in child psychiatry epidemiological research. *J Am Acad Child Adolesc Psychiatry* 31(1):78–85, 1992.
50. Achenbach TM: *Integrative guide for the 1991 CBCL/4–18, YSR and TRF profiles*. Burlington, VT, University of Vermont, Department of Psychiatry, 1991.
51. Achenbach T: "Comorbidity" in child and adolescent psychiatry: categorical and quantitative perspectives. *J Child Adolesc Psychopharmacol* 1:271–278, 1991.
52. Achenbach TM: Diagnosis, assessment, and comorbidity in psychosocial treatment research. *J Abnorm Child Psychol* 23(1):45–65, 1995.
53. Kraemer HC, Measelle JR, Ablow JC, Essex MJ, Boyce WT, Kupfer DJ: A new approach to integrating data from multiple informants in psychiatric assessment and research: mixing and matching contexts and perspectives. *Am J Psychiatry* 160(9):1566–1577, 2003.
54. Spitzer RL, Endicott J, Cohen J, Fleiss JL: Constraints on the validity of computer diagnosis. *Arch Gen Psychiatry* 31(2):197–203, 1974.
55. Bartko JJ: On various intraclass correlation reliability coefficients. *Psychol Bull* 83(5):762–765, 1976.
56. Cronbach L: Coefficient alpha and the internal structure of tests. *Psychometrika* 16:297–334, 1951.
57. Elander J, Rutter M: Use and development of the Rutter Parents' and Teachers' Scales. *Int J Meth Psychiatr Res* 5(151):1–16, 1995.
58. Achenbach TM, Edelbrock CS: The classification of child psychopathology: a review and analysis of empirical efforts. *Psychol Bull* 85(6):1275–1301, 1978.
59. Rutter M TA, Lann I (eds): *Assessment and Diagnosis in Child Psychopathology*. London, David Fulton, 1988.
60. Spitzer R, Endicott J, Robins E: Research diagnostic criteria: rationale and reliability. *Arch Gen Psychiatry* 35:773–782, 1978.
61. American PA: *Diagnostic and Statistical Manual of Mental Disorders—DSM III*, Washington, DC, American Psychiatric Association, 1980.
62. World Health Organization: *The ICD-10 Classification of Mental and Behavioural Disorders: Clinical Descriptions and Diagnostic Guidelines*. Geneva, Switzerland, World Health Organization, 1992.
63. World Health Organization: *The ICD-10 Classification of Mental and Behavioural Disorders—Diagnostic criteria for Research*. Geneva, Switzerland, World Health Organization, 1993.
64. Shaffer D, Lucas C, Richters J: *Diagnostic Assessment in Child and Adolescent Psychopathology*, New York, Guilford, 1999.

65. Piacentini J, Roper M, Jensen P, et al.: Informant-based determinants of symptom attenuation in structured child psychiatric interviews. *J Abnorm Child Psychol* 27(6):417–428, 1999.
66. Lucas CP, Fisher P, Piacentini J, et al.: Features of interviews questions associated with attenuation of symptom reports. *J Abnorm Child Psychol* 27(6):429–437, 1999.
67. Gould M, Rutter M, Shaffer D, Sturge C: UK/WHO study of ICD 9. In: Rutter M, Tuma A, Lann I (eds): *Assessment and Diagnosis in Child Psychopathology.* London, David Fulton, 1988.
68. Prendergast M, Taylor E, Rapoport JL, et al.: The diagnosis of childhood hyperactivity: a U.S.-U.K. cross-national study of DSM-III and ICD-9. *J Child Psychol Psychiatry Allied Discipl* 29(3):289–300, 1988.
69. Applegate B, Lahey BB, Hart EL, et al.: Validity of the age-of-onset criterion for ADHD: a report from the DSM-IV field trials. *J Am Acad Child Adolesc Psychiatry* 36(9):1211–1221, 1997.
70. Lahey BB, Applegate B, Barkley RA, et al.: DSM-IV field trials for oppositional defiant disorder and conduct disorder in children and adolescents. *Am J Psychiatry* 151(8):1163–1171, 1994.
71. Volkmar FR, Klin A, Siegel B, et al.: Field trial for autistic disorder in DSM-IV. *Am J Psychiatry* 151(9):1361–1367, 1994.
72. Rutter M: Diagnostic validity in child psychiatry. *Adv Biol Psychiatry* 2:2–22, 1978.
73. Chilcoat HD, Breslau N: Does psychiatric history bias mothers' reports? An application of a new analytic approach. *J Am Acad Child Adolesc Psychiatry* 36(7):971–979, 1997.
74. Borge A, Samuelsen S, Rutter M: Observer variance within families: confluence among maternal, paternal and child ratings. *Int J Meth Psychiatr Res* 10:11–21, 2001.
75. Simonoff E, Pickles A, Hervas A, Silberg JL, Rutter M, Eaves L: Genetic influences on childhood hyperactivity: contrast effects imply parental rating bias, not sibling interaction. *Psychol Med* 28(4):825–837, 1998.
76. Maughan B, Rutter M: Retrospective reporting of childhood adversity: issues in assessing long-term recall. *J Personal Disord* 11(1):19–33, 1997.
77. Kendler K, Silberg J, Neale M, Kessler R, Heath A, Eaves L: The family history method: whose psychiatric history is measured? *Am J Psychiatry* 148:1501–1504, 1991.
78. Rende R, Weissman M: Assessment of family history of psychiatric disorder. In: Shaffer D, Lucas C, Richters J (eds): *Diagnostic Assessment in Child and Adolescent Psychopathology.* New York, Guilford, 230–255, 1999.
79. Fergusson D: A brief introduction to structural equation models. In: Verhulst F, Koot H (eds): *The Epidemiology of Child and Adolescent Psychopathology.* Oxford, UK, Oxford University Press, 122–145, 1995.
80. Fergusson DM: Structural equation models in developmental research. *J Child Psychol Psychiatr Allied Discipl* 38(8):877–887, 1997.
81. Boyle MH, Pickles AR: Influence of maternal depressive symptoms on ratings of childhood behavior. *J Abnorm Child Psychol* 25(5):399–112, 1997.
82. Boyle MH, Pickles A: Maternal depressive symptoms and ratings of emotional disorder symptoms in children and adolescents. *J Child Psychol Psychiatry Allied Discipl* 38(8):981–992, 1997.
83. Fergusson D, Horwod L: The trait and method components of ratings of conduct disorder. Part 1: Maternal and teacher evaluations of conduct disorder in young children. *J Child Psychol Psychiatry* 28:249–260, 1987.
84. Fergusson DM, Horwood LJ: The trait and method components of ratings of conduct disorder—Part II. Factors related to the trait component of conduct disorder scores. *J Child Psychol Psychiatry* 28(2):261–72, 1987.
85. Zoccolillo M, Pickles A, Quinton D, Rutter M: The outcome of childhood conduct disorder: implications for defining adult personality disorder and conduct disorder. *Psycholo Med* 22(4):971–986, 1992.
86. Bird HR: Epidemiology of childhood disorders in a cross-cultural context. *J Child Psychol Psychiatry* 37(1):35–19, 1996.
87. Bird H: The assessment of functional impairment. In: Shaffer D, Lucas C, Richters J (eds): *Diagnostic Assessment in Child and Adolescent Psychopathology.* New York, Guilford Press, 1999.
88. Rutter M, Tizard J, Whitmore K: *Education, Health and Behaviour,* New York, Robert E Krieger Publishing Co, 1970.
89. American Psychiatric Association: *Diagnostic and Statistical Manual of Mental Disorders—DSM IV.* Washington, DC, American Psychiatric Association, 1994.
90. Shaffer D, Gould MS, Brasic J, et al.: A children's global assessment scale (CGAS). *Arch Gen Psychiatry* 40(11):1228–1231, 1983.
91. Bird H, Andrews H, Schwab-Stone M, et al.: Global measures of impairment for epidemiologic and clinical use with children and adolescents. *Int J Method Psychiatr Res* 6:1–13, 1996.
92. Bird H, Shaffer D, Fisher P, et al.: The Columbia Impairment Scale (CIS): pilot findings on a measure of global impairment for children and adolescents. *Int J Method Psychiatr Res* 3:167–176, 1993.
93. John K, Gammon GD, Prusoff BA, Warner V: The Social Adjustment Inventory for Children and Adolescents (SAICA): testing of a new semistructured interview. *J Am Acad Child Adolesc Psychiatry* 26(6):898–911, 1987.
94. Sanford MN, Offord DR, Boyle MH, Peace A, Racine YA: Ontario child health study: social and school impairments in children aged 6 to 16 years. *J Am Acad Child Adolesc Psychiatry* 31(1):60–67, 1992.
95. Pickles A, Rowe R, Simonoff E, Foley D, Rutter M, Silberg J: Child psychiatric symptoms and psychosocial impairment: relationship and prognostic significance. *Br J Psychiatry* 179:230–235, 2001.
96. Angold A, Costello E, Farmer E, Burners B, Erkanli A: Impaired but undiagnosed. *J Am Acad Child Adolesc Psychiatry* 38(2):129–137, 1999.
97. Costello E, Angold A, Keeler G: Adolescent outcomes of childhood disorders: the consequences of severity and impairment. *J Am Acad Child Adolesc Psychiatry* 38(2):121–128, 1999.
98. Shaffer D, Fisher P, Lucas CP, Dulcan MK, Schwab-Stone ME: NIMH Diagnostic Interview Schedule for Children Version IV (NIMH DISC-IV): description, differences from previous versions, and reliability of some common diagnoses.*J Am Acad Child Adolesc Psychiatry* 39(1):28–38, 2000.
99. Angold A, Costello EJ: The Child and Adolescent Psychiatric Assessment (CAPA). *J Am Acad Child Adolesc Psychiatry* 39(1):39–48, 2000.
100. Shaffer D, Scott M, Wilcox H, et al.: The Columbia Suicide Screen: validity and reliability of a screen for youth suicide and depression. *J Am Acad Child Adolesc Psychiatry* 43(1):71–79, 2004.
101. Fombonne E: The use of questionnaires in child psychiatry research: measuring their performance and choosing an optimal cut-off. *J Child Psychol Psychiatry Allied Discipl* 32(4):677–693, 1991.
102. Hsiao J, Bartko J, Potter W: Diagnosing diagnoses. *Arch Gen Psychiatry* 46:664–667, 1989.
103. Canino G, Bird H, Smaritza R, Bravo M: Child psychiatric epidemiology: what we have learned and what we need to learn. *Int J Method Psychiatr Res* (special issue):79–92, 1995.
104. Roberts RE, Attkisson CC, Rosenblatt A: Prevalence of psychopathology among children and adolescents. *Am J Psychiatry* 155(6):715–725, 1998.
105. Leaf PJ, Alegria M, Cohen P, et al.: Mental health service use in the community and schools: results from the four-community MECA study. Methods for the Epidemiology of Child and Adolescent Mental Disorders Study. *J Am Acad Child Adolesc Psychiatry* 35(7):889–897, 1996.
106. Costello EJ, Janiszewski S: Who gets treated? Factors associated with referral in children with psychiatric disorders. *Acta Psychiatrica Scandinavica* 81(6):523–9, 1990.
107. Zahner GE, Pawelkiewicz W, DeFrancesco JJ, Adnopoz J: Children's mental health service needs and utilization patterns in an urban community: an epidemiological assessment. *J Am Acad Child Adolesc Psychiatry* 31(5):951–960, 1992.
108. Verhulst F, Koot H: *Child Psychiatric Epidemiology: Concepts, Methods and Findings.* Newbury Park, Sage Publications, 1992.
109. Whitaker A, Johnson J, Rapoport J, et al.: Uncommon troubles in young people: prevalence estimates of selected psychiatric disorders in a nonreferred adolescent population. *Arch Gen Psychiatry* 47(5):487–496, 1990.
110. Jensen P, Bloedau L, Davis H: Children at risk. II: risk factors and clinic utilization. *J Am Acad Child Adolesc Psychiatry* 29:804–812, 1990.
111. Angold A, Erkanli A, Costello EJ, Rutter M: Precision, reliability and accuracy in the dating of symptom onsets in child and adolescent psychopathology. *J Child Psychol Psychiatry Allied Discipl* 37(6):657–664, 1996.
112. Moffitt TE: Adolescence-limited and life-course-persistent antisocial behavior: a developmental taxonomy. *Psychol Rev* 100(4):674–701, 1993.
113. Fombonne E, Wostear G, Cooper V, Harrington R, Rutter M: The Maudsley long-term follow-up study of adolescent depression: I. Adult rates of psychiatric disorders. *Br J Psychiatry* 179:210–217, 2004.
114. Weissman MM, Wolk S, Goldstein RB, et al.: Depressed adolescents grown up. *JAMA* 281(18):1707–1713, 1999.
115. Weissman M, Wolk S, Wickramaratne P, et al.: Children with prepubertal-onset major depressive disorder and anxiety grown up. *Arch Gen Psychiatry* 56:794–801, 1999.
116. Harrington R, Rutter M, Weissman M, et al.: Psychiatric disorders in the relatives of depressed probands. I. Comparison of prepubertal, adolescent and early adult onset cases. *J Affect Disord* 42(1):9–22, 1997.
117. Rende R, Weissman M, Rutter M, Wickramaratne P, Harrington R, Pickles A: Psychiatric disorders in the relatives of depressed probands. II. Familial loading for comorbid nondepressive disorders based upon proband age of onset. *J Affect Disord* 42(1):23–28, 1997.
118. Taylor E, Chadwick O, Heptinstall E, Danckaerts M: Hyperactivity and conduct problems as risk factors for adolescent development. *J Am Acad Child Adolesc Psychiatry* 35(9):1213–1226, 1996.
119. Taylor E: Developmental neuropsychopathology of attention deficit and impulsiveness. *Dev Psychopathol* 11(3):607–628, 1999.
120. Kovacs M, Akiskal H, Gatsonis C, Parrone P: Childhood onset dysthymic disorder. Clinical features and prospective naturalistic outcome. *Arch Gen Psychiatry* 51:365–374, 1994.
121. Kessler R, Mroczek D, Belli R: Retrospective adult assessment of childhood psychopathology. In: Shaffer D, Lucas C, Richters J (eds): *Diagnostic Assessment in Child and Adolescent Psychopathology.* New York, Guilford, 256–284, 1999.
122. Schurhoff F, Bellivier F, Jouvent R, et al.: Early and late onset bipolar disorders: two different forms of manic depressive illness? *J Affect Disord* 58:215–221, 2000.
123. Simon G, Von Korff M: Re-evaluation of secular trends in depression rates. *Am J Epidemiol* 135:1411–1422, 1992.
124. Webster-Stratton C, Reid MJ, Hammond M: Treating children with early-onset conduct problems: intervention outcomes for parent, child, and teacher training. *J Clin Child Adolesc Psychol* 33(1):105–124, 2004.
125. Caspi A, Sugden K, Moffitt TE, et al.: Influence of life stress on depression: moderation by a polymorphism in the 5-HTT gene. *Science* 301(5631):386–389, 2003.

126. Tremblay RE, Nagin DS, Seguin JR, et al.: Physical aggression during early childhood: trajectories and predictors. *Pediatrics* 114(1):43–50, 2004.
127. Rutter M: Comorbidity: concepts, claims and choices. *Crim Behav Ment Health* 7:265–285, 1997.
128. Caron C, Rutter M: Comorbidity in child psychopathology: concepts, issues and research strategies. *J Child Psychol Psychiatry Allied Discipl* 32(7):1063–1080, 1991.
129. Hinshaw S, Lahey B, Hart E: Issues of taxonomy and comorbidity in the development of conduct disorder. *Dev Psychopathol Special Issue* 5:310–349, 1993.
130. Nottelmann E, Jensen P: Comorbidity of disorders in children and adolescents: developmental perspectives. In: Ollendick T, Prinz R (eds): *Advances in Clinical Child Psychology*. Vol 17. New York, Plenum Press, 109–55, 1995.
131. Merikangas KR, Mehta RL, Molnar BE, et al.: Comorbidity of substance use disorders with mood and anxiety disorders: results of the International Consortium in Psychiatric Epidemiology. *Addict Behav* 23(6):893–907, 1998.
132. Hughes C, Sheldon H, Preskorn S, et al.: The effect of concomitant disorder in childhood depression on predicting treatment response. *Psychopharmacol Bull* 26:235–238, 1990.
133. Richman N, Stevenson J, Graham P: *Pre-school to School: A Behavioural Study*. London, Academic Press, 1982.
134. Earls F: Prevalence of behavior problems in 3-year-old children. *Arch Gen Psychiatry* 37:1153–1157, 1980.
135. van den Oord E, Koot H, Boomsma D, Verhulst F, Orlebeke J: A twin-singleton comparison of problem behaviour in 2–3-year-olds. *J Child Psychol Psychiatry* 36:449–458, 1995.
136. Lavigne JV, Gibbons RD, Christoffel KK, et al.: Prevalence rates and correlates of psychiatric disorders among preschool children. *J Am Acad Child Adolesc Psychiatry* 35(2):204–214, 1996.
137. Pianta R, Castaldi J: Stability of internalizing symptoms from kindergarten to first grade and factors related to instability. *Dev Psychopathol* 1:305–316, 1989.
138. Pianta R, Caldwell C: Stability of externalizing symptoms from kindergarten to first grade and factors related to instability. *Dev Psychopathol* 2:246–258, 1990.
139. Cohen S, Bromet E: Maternal predictors of behavioral disturbance in preschool children: a research note. *J Child Psychol Psychiatry Allied Discipl* 33(5):941–946, 1992.
140. Gudmundsson OO, Magnusson P, Saemundsen E, et al.: Psychiatric disorders in an urban sample of preschool children. *Child Adolesc Ment Health* 18(4):210–217, 2013.
141. Maziade M, Cote R, Boutin P, Bernier H, Thivierge J: Temperament and intellectual development: a longitudinal study from infancy to four years. *Am J Psychiatry* 144(2):144–150, 1987.
142. Kagan J, Snidman N, Arcus D: Childhood derivatives of high and low reactivity in infancy. *Child Dev* 69(6):1483–1493, 1998.
143. Stevenson J, Richman N, Graham P: Behaviour problems and language abilities at three years and behavioural deviance at eight years. *J Child Psychol Psychiatry Allied Discipl* 26(2):215–230, 1985.
144. Mawhood L, Howlin P, Rutter M: Autism and developmental receptive language disorder—a comparative follow-up in early adult life. I: Cognitive and language outcomes. *J Child Psychol Psychiatry Allied Discipl* 41(5):547–559, 2001.
145. Caspi A, Moffitt TE, Newman DL, Silva PA: Behavioral observations at age 3 years predict adult psychiatric disorders: longitudinal evidence from a birth cohort. *Arch Gen Psychiatry* 53:1033–1039, 1996.
146. Rogers S: Empirically supported comprehensive treatments for young children with autism. *J Clin Child Psychol* 27(2):168–179, 1998.
147. Mayes LC: Addressing mental health needs of infants and young children. *Child Adolesc Psychiatr Clin North Am* 8(2):209–224, 1999.
148. Emde R, Bingham R, Harmon R: Classification and the diagnostic process in infancy, In: Zeanah C (ed): *Handbook of Infant Mental Health*. New York, Guilford, 1993.
149. Bagnato S, Neisworth J, Salvia J: *Early Childhood Indicators of Developmental Dysfunction*. Baltimore, Paul H Brookes, 1999.
150. Zero to Three: Diagnostic Classification—DC:0–3: *Diagnostic Classification of Mental Health and Developmental Disorders of Infancy and Early Childhood*. Washington, DC, National Center for Clinical Infant Programs, 1994.
151. Egger HL, Erkanli A, Keeler G, Potts E, Walter BK, Angold A: Test-retest reliability of the preschool age psychiatric assessment (PAPA). *J Am Acad Child Adolesc Psychiatry* 45(5):538–549, 2006.
152. Egger HL, Angold A: Common emotional and behavioral disorders in preschool children: presentation, nosology, and epidemiology. *J Child Psychol Psychiatry* 47(3–4):313–337, 2006.
153. Bourdon KH, Goodman R, Rae DS, Simpson G, Koretz DS: The strengths and difficulties questionnaire: U.S. normative data and psychometric properties. *J Am Acad Child Adolesc Psychiatry* 44(6):557–564, 2005.
154. Achenbach TM, Hensley VR, Phares V, Grayson D: Problems and competencies reported by parents of Australian and American children. *J Child Psychol Psychiatry Allied Discipl* 31(2):265–286, 1990.
155. Stanger C, Fombonne E, Achenbach TM: Epidemiological comparisons of American and French children: parent reports of problems and competencies for ages 6–21. *Euro Child Adolesc Psychiatry* 3(1):16–28, 1994.
156. Achenbach TM, Bird HR, Canino G, Phares V, Gould MS, Rubio-Stipec M: Epidemiological comparisons of Puerto Rican and U.S. mainland children: parent, teacher, and self-reports. *J Am Acad Child Adolesc Psychiatry* 29(1):84–93, 1990.
157. Rutter MQD: Psychiatric disorder: ecological factors and concepts of causation, In: McGurk H (ed): *Ecological Factors in Human Development*. Amsterdam, North Holland, 173–187, 1977.
158. Leung PW, Luk SL, Ho TP, Taylor E, Mak FL, Bacon-Shone J: The diagnosis and prevalence of hyperactivity in Chinese schoolboys. *Br J Psychiatry* 168(4):486–496, 1996.
159. M Rutter DS (ed): *Psychosocial Disorders in Young People: Time Trends and Their Causes*, Chichester, Wiley, 1995.
160. Fombonne E: Increased rates of psychosocial disorders in youth. *Euro Arch Psychiatry Clin Neurosci* 248(1):14–21, 1998.
161. Fombonne E: Suicidal behaviours in vulnerable adolescents. Time trends and their correlates. *Br J Psychiatry* 173:154–159, 1998.
162. Achenbach TM, Howell CT: Are American children's problems getting worse? A 13-year comparison. *J Am Acad Child Adolesc Psychiatry* 32(6):1145–1154, 1993.
163. Flynn J: Massive IQ gains in 14 nations: What IQ tests really measure. *Psychol Bull* 101:171–191, 1987.
164. Fuggle PW, Tokar S, Grant DB, Smith I: Rising IQ scores in British children: recent evidence. *J Child Psychol Psychiatry Allied Discipl* 33(7):1241–1247, 1992.
165. Fredriks AM, van Buuren S, Burgmeijer RJ, et al.: Continuing positive secular growth change in The Netherlands 1955–1997. *Pediatr Res* 47(3):316–323, 2000.
166. Verhulst FC, Achenbach TM: Empirically based assessment and taxonomy of psychopathology: cross-cultural applications. A review. *Euro Child Adolesc Psychiatry* 4(2):61–76, 1995.
167. Weisz J, Eastman K: Cross-national research on child and adolescent psychopathology. In: Koot FV (ed): *The Epidemiology of Child and Adolescent Psychopathology*. Oxford, Oxford University Press, 42–65, 1995.
168. Ivanova MY, Dobrean A, Dopfner M, et al.: Testing the 8-syndrome structure of the Child Behavior Checklist in 30 societies. *J Clin Child Adolesc Psychol* 36(3):405–17, 2007.
169. Crijnen AA, Achenbach TM, Verhulst FC: Problems reported by parents of children in multiple cultures: the child behavior checklist syndrome constructs. *Am J Psychiatry* 156(4):569–574, 1999.
170. Canino G, Bravo M: The translation and adaptation of diagnostic instruments for cross-cultural use. In: Shaffer D, Lucas C, Richters J (eds): *Diagnostic Assessment in Child and Adolescent Psychopathology*. New York, Guilford Press, 1999.
171. Woodward CA, Thomas HB, Boyle MH, et al.: Methodologic note for child epidemiological surveys: the effects of instructions on estimates of behavior prevalence. *J Child Psychol Psychiatry Allied Discipl* 30(6): 919–924, 1989.
172. Weisz JR, Suwanlert S, Chaiyasit W, Weiss B, Walter BR, Anderson WW: Thai and American perspectives on over- and undercontrolled child behavior problems: exploring the threshold model among parents, teachers, and psychologists. *J Consult Clin Psychol* 56(4):601–609, 1988.
173. Lee S: Anorexia nervosa in Hong Kong: a Chinese perspective. *Psychol Med* 21:703–711, 1991.
174. King M, Bhugra D: Eating disorders: lessons from a cross-cultural study. *Psychol Med* 19:955–958, 1989.
175. Kleinman A, Good B: *Culture and Depression: Studies in the Anthropology and Cross-cultural Psychiatry of Affect and Disorder*. Berkeley, University of California, 1985.
176. Rescorla L, Achenbach M, Ivanova M, et al.: Behavioral and emotional problems reported by parents of children ages 6 to 16 in 31 societies. *J Emot Behav Disord* 15(3):130–142, 2007.
177. Ivanova M, Rescorla L, Achenbach TM, et al.: Testing the teacher's report form syndromes in 20 societies. *School Psych Rev* 36(3):468–483, 2007.
178. Berg I, Lucas C, McGuire R: Measurement of behaviour difficulties in children using standard scales administered to mothers by computer: reliability and validity. *Euro Child Adolesc Psychiatry* 1(1):14–23, 1992.
179. Goodman R, Ford T, Richards H, Gatward R, Meltzer H: The development and well-being assessment: description and initial validation of an integrated assessment of child and adolescent psychopathology. *J Child Psychol Psychiatry* 41:645–656, 2000.
180. Reich W: Diagnostic interview for children and adolescents (DICA). *J Am Acad Child Adolesc Psychiatry* 39(1):59–66, 2000.
181. Valla J, Bergeron L, Smolla N: The Dominic-R: a pictorial interview for 6- to 11-year old children. *J Am Acad Child Adolesc Psychiatry* 39(1):85–93, 2000.
182. Patton GC, Coffey C, Posterino M, Carlin JB, Wolfe R, Bowes G: A computerised screening instrument for adolescent depression: population-based validation and application to a two-phase case-control study. *Soc Psychiatry Psychiatr Epidemiol* 34(3):166–172, 1999.
183. Reich W, Cottler L, McCallum K, Corwin D, Eerdewegh V: Computerized interviews as a method of assessing psychopathology in children. *Compre Psychiatry* 36:40–45, 1995.
184. Turner C, Ku L, Rogers S, Lindberg L, Pleck J, Sonenstein F: Adolescent sexual behavior, drug use, and violence: increased reporting with computer survey technology. *Science* 280:867–873, 1998.
185. Simic M, Fombonne E: Depressive conduct disorder: symptom patterns and correlates in referred children and adolescents. *J Affect Disord* 62:175–185, 2001.

CHAPTER 3.2.2 ■ HEALTH PROMOTION AND PREVENTION IN CHILD AND ADOLESCENT PSYCHIATRY

KERRY O'LOUGHLIN, ROBERT R. ALTHOFF, AND JAMES J. HUDZIAK

The perfect storm for positioning the field of child and adolescent psychiatry to the forefront of health care reform is upon us. If we embrace the power and scope of health promotion and illness prevention, our field will become central to the care and well-being of all children and families. Child and adolescent psychiatrists are the only physicians trained to understand the emotional and behavioral correlates of the structure and function of the developing brain. No other field combines classic medical training with an understanding of brain and behavior development from birth to age 24, the age span that defines the children and families we serve. Over the past two decades multiple domains in medical research have matured to the point that child and adolescent psychiatry is perfectly positioned to execute a paradigm shift in how our field is defined and practiced.

The change agents include rapid advances in the understanding of genetics (1), epigenetics (2), and structural (3) and functional (4) neuroimaging studies of large populations of children across development (5). This research allows our field to understand the unique vulnerabilities and opportunities that occur during the epoch of brain development. Second, with the explosion of interest and evidence from the multiple Adverse Childhood Experiences (ACEs) study, it is now clear that the same factors that place children at risk for anxiety, depression, and substance abuse also contribute to similarly elevated risk for obesity, diabetes, and hypertension (and many other general medical problems) (6). These data allow our field to rightly claim a special role in addressing and preventing the factors that precede the most common and costly of all medical illnesses, not just psychiatric illness. The third major advance exists in the area of health promotion. Cardiologists would never define themselves as physicians who only care for patients' with end-stage heart disease, rather cardiology is defined as a field that also has developed heart health promotion and illness prevention programs (e.g., through diet and exercise) (7). This has led the rest of medicine to appreciate the importance of promoting cardiac health in all humans. Child and adolescent psychiatry should and can follow that same method. Modern neuroscience has positioned child and adolescent psychiatrists to design brain healthy health promotion programs from pregnancy to adulthood. Next, epidemiologic research in the fields of psychiatry and child psychiatry has moved away from dependence on categorical models of diagnoses such as embodied by the Diagnostic and Statistical Manual of Mental Disorders, 5th edition (DSM-5) (8) and into quantitative research diagnostic procedures. It has become increasingly obvious that all children (indeed all humans) experience symptoms of sadness, anxiety, inattention, risk-taking, rule-breaking behavior, and quirkiness thus redefining the target populations for child and adolescent psychiatry away from serving only children who meet criteria for largely inadequate diagnoses to all children (9). In other words, all of us carry symptoms of emotional behavioral vulnerability and a new child psychiatry can devote itself to the service of all children. Finally, the era of family-based medical care is upon us. The realization that treating a child as if she/he exists in a vacuum is no longer tenable in our field or any other field in medicine. However, we can take the lead in developing new programmatic approaches. For almost as long as our field has existed the argument for family-based care has been made, however, with new research, we now have the evidence to confidently move the argument forward that the best way to help a child or adolescent achieve wellness is to help his or her family become well.

These advances, taken together, invite child and adolescent psychiatry to operate under the following coda: the environment influences genomic health, which in turn influences the structure and function of the brain, which in turn influences a child's thoughts, feelings, and behaviors. Given that all health begins with emotional behavioral health, the path to wellness begins with creating healthy environments for all children and families.

With this in mind child psychiatry can enter the epoch of accountable care and health care reform with the following charge: we must design, test, and implement health promotion programs aimed at building healthy brains from birth to adulthood. We must design, test, and implement illness prevention programs aimed at helping those at risk for developing psychopathologies and medical morbidities (that are very difficult to treat in adulthood). When we intervene we should do so in a family-based manner with the knowledge that the best way to serve a child is to serve a child's family. If child psychiatry accepts this charge, we essentially place ourselves at the center of health care reform. Our profession already contributes to the health and well-being of children in school settings, in pediatric and community settings, as well as in our clinics and hospitals. Armed with new evidence we can contribute strategies to promote health in all children, to prevent the development of illness in many, and to intervene in a more empirical and family-based way for those who struggle with emotional behavioral illness.

In this chapter we provide child and adolescent psychiatry with the evidence for illness prevention and health promotion, and provide one model of family-based intervention that is already in place in schools, pediatric settings, and clinics in the United States and abroad (9,10).

HISTORY OF PREVENTION

Over the last 50 years, the terminology surrounding prevention has undergone a number of revisions (11). In 1964, in an effort to establish a consistent nomenclature, the field of psychiatry adopted a series of definitions to describe efforts toward prevention. In Caplan's *Principles of Prevention Psychiatry*, prevention was subdivided into three categories: primary prevention, secondary prevention, and tertiary prevention (12). Primary prevention was defined as "an intervention designed to decrease the number of new cases of a disorder or illness," secondary prevention was defined as "an intervention designed to lower the rate of established cases of a disorder or illness," and tertiary prevention was defined as "an intervention designed to decrease the amount of disability associated with an existing illness" (11).

In 1983, Gordon proposed a prevention classification system based on the costs and benefits of delivering an intervention to a targeted population (13,14). Gordon's taxonomy distinguished between universal prevention, selected prevention, and indicated prevention. In this framework, universal prevention referred to strategies for the entire population. Selective prevention referred to strategies that targeted a subpopulation deemed to be at risk for a disorder. Finally, indicated prevention referred to strategies that targeted *individuals* who were asymptomatic, but deemed, based on an individualized assessment, to be at increased risk (13).

In 1994, the Institute of Medicine (IOM) report *Reducing Risk for Mental Disorders: Frontiers for Preventive Intervention Research* established a continuum of care beginning with prevention, and including both treatment and maintenance (15). Prevention referred to interventions implemented prior to a patient receiving a diagnosis, treatment referred to interventions provided to individuals with diagnoses, and maintenance referred to long-term interventions designed to reduce rates of relapse and disability and to promote rehabilitation among individuals with chronic mental illness (11,14). Approximating the model proposed by Gordon (13), the 1994 IOM committee divided what was formally referred to as primary prevention into indicated, selective, and universal preventive interventions. In this model, distinction among indicated, selective, and universal preventive interventions was based on the population being targeted. Universal preventive interventions were designed to serve the entire population, selective preventive interventions were designed to serve individuals at heightened risk, and indicated preventative interventions were designed to serve populations manifesting early symptoms of a disorder (15). This conceptualization differed from Gordon's model as indicated preventive interventions targeted individuals with prodromal symptoms (rather than individuals who were at-risk, yet asymptomatic) (14). Within the context of such definitions, the IOM's 1994 report also proposed that as risk increased the intensity of the intervention and the costs associated with that intervention would also increase (16).

While the IOM model provides a useful framework for conceptualizing the nature and degree of risk faced by vulnerable populations, it is important to note that there is often significant overlap and interrelatedness among vulnerable populations (16). Indeed, individuals manifesting the early symptoms of psychopathology (i.e., an indicated population), are often a subset of individuals at increased risk (i.e., a selective population). As such, the distinction between selective and indicated preventive interventions is often nebulous. Beyond the broad definitions provided by the IOM in 1994, there are no explicit criteria for whether a preventive intervention be classified as selective or indicated (16).

HEALTH PROMOTION

In 2009, the National Academy of Sciences (NAS) committee largely concurred with the continuum (i.e., including prevention, treatment, and maintenance) laid out in the IOM's 1994 report (14). However, the NAS report suggested that in addition to prevention, treatment, and maintenance, the conceptualization of mental health should be broadened to include the *promotion* of mental health. Citing the World Health Organization's (1986) proclamation that health is more than merely the absence of disease, the NAS committee defined mental, emotional, and behavioral health promotion as, "efforts to enhance individuals' ability to achieve developmentally appropriate tasks (developmental competence) and a positive sense of self-esteem, mastery, well-being, and social inclusion and to strengthen their ability to cope with adversity" (14,17). In the NAS report, health promotion was characterized as focusing on well-being rather than on the prevention of illness. While drawing this distinction, however, the report also highlighted the considerable overlap between prevention and health promotion, stating that: "both (prevention and health promotion) focus on changing common influences on the development of children and adolescents in order to aid them in functioning well in meeting life's tasks and challenges and remaining free of cognitive, emotional, and behavioral problems that would impair their functioning" (14).

Established Preventive Interventions

Both the IOM and NAS have acknowledged, on a conceptual level, the importance of prevention. However, research within child and adolescent psychiatry has lagged behind such conceptual advances. To date, there are a limited number of preventive interventions, and even fewer with a strong empirical base. Therefore, selecting an evidence-based preventive intervention can prove difficult for physicians, mental health care providers, communities, schools, and parents alike.

There are, however, a number of registries which evaluate and rank preventive interventions based on the strength of their empirical evidence. One such registry is the Blueprints for Healthy Youth Development Program (18). Funded by the Annie E. Casey Foundation, the Blueprints for Healthy Youth Development Program provides a freely available registry of evidence-based preventive interventions. Since its inception, the Blueprints program has reviewed more than 1,400 preventive interventions. During this time, only 14% of programs have met the registry's minimum inclusion criteria, and less than 1% have been designated as "model" programs (18).

To be designated as a "model" program, a preventive intervention must have: (1) a minimum of either two high-quality randomized controlled trials or one high-quality randomized controlled trial and one high-quality quasiexperimental evaluation; (2) positive intervention impact sustained for 12 months after the program intervention ends; and (3) significant impact, intervention specificity, and dissemination readiness (19). To be a "model plus" program an intervention must meet the above model criteria and have undergone independent replication (19).

In the interest of providing an overview of the existent preventive interventions with the largest evidence base, each of the programs receiving the "model" or "model plus" designation from the Blueprints registry are briefly described below. Based on the definitions established in the IOM's 1994 report (15), the programs reviewed below have been categorized as: universal or selective/indicated preventive interventions.

Universal Preventive Interventions

The LifeSkills Training Program

The LifeSkills Training Program (LST) is a classroom-based program designed to prevent adolescents from engaging in alcohol use, drug use, and violent behavior (20). The LST is designed to teach students self-management skills, social skills, and drug-resistance skills, and has been associated with short- and long-term reductions in tobacco use, alcohol use, illicit substance use, polysubstance abuse, violence, and delinquency (20). In addition, at 6- and 10-year follow-up, the LST has been associated with reductions in risky driving (21), and HIV-risk behaviors (22).

The Positive Action Program

The Positive Action Program is a school-based program designed to enhance social–emotional learning and positive behavior in elementary and middle school students. The classroom component teaches self-management skills, as well as strategies to increase the use of positive social behavior (23). The Positive Action Program also includes a school-wide component designed to reinforce the classroom-level intervention (23). The Positive Action Program has been associated with reductions in suspensions and absenteeism; reductions in substance use, violence, and sexual activity; increased rates of socioemotional development; higher life satisfaction; reduced rates of depression and anxiety; reduced rates of unhealthy food consumption; as well as overall improvements in school quality (23,24).

The Promoting Alternative Thinking Strategies

The Promoting Alternative Thinking Strategies (PATHS) program is a school-based program designed to reduce aggression, and promote emotional and social competencies in children grades K-6 (25). The PATHS intervention targets five domains: self-control, emotional understanding, positive self-esteem, relationships, and interpersonal problem-solving skills (25). The PATHS intervention attempts to involve parents by incorporating home activity assignments and providing parents with information. PATHS has been associated with lower rates of conduct and externalizing behaviors, lower internalizing scores, better emotion recognition abilities, reductions in delinquency, and higher proficiency scores in reading, writing, and math (25–27).

Project Toward No Drug Abuse

Project Toward No Drug Abuse (TND) is a drug prevention program for high school students who are at risk for substance use and violent behaviors (28). Project TND is designed to enhance self-control, communication, resource acquisition, and decision-making. Project TND has been implemented as a universal preventive intervention in general populations, as well as a selective preventive intervention among high-risk students (28). Project TND has been associated with reductions in cigarette use, marijuana use, hard substance use, weapon carrying, and victimization, with reductions in hard drug use being sustained for up to 5 years post-intervention (29,30).

Selective and/or Indicated Preventive Interventions

Nurse-Family Partnership

The Nurse-Family Partnership (NFP) is a maternal health program which provides first-time low-income mothers with maternal and child health nurses (31). The intervention is designed to improve pregnancy outcomes, improve infant health, promote infant development, and improve the mother's life course trajectory (31). In particular, during pregnancy, the NFP is designed to eliminate cigarette, alcohol, and drug use and encourage rest, exercise, and sound personal hygiene habits (31,32). The NFP also aims to prepare mothers for labor, delivery, and child care (31). Among mothers, the NFP program has been associated with reductions in unintended pregnancies, domestic violence, and increased rates of employment (31,32). Among children, the NFP has been associated with reductions in hospitalization for injury and illness, accelerated language development, reduced rates of behavior problems at age 6, and reduced rates of arrests, internalizing disorders, and substance use at age 12 (33).

New Beginnings

The New Beginnings program is an intervention for divorced mothers with children ranging in age from 5 to 18 (34). The New Beginnings program is a parent-driven intervention designed to help mothers engage in effective child behavior management strategies, enhance the quality of mother–child interactions, and reduce children's exposure to interparental conflict (34). Among children, the Blueprints program has been associated with decreases in internalizing, externalizing (34,35), and aggressive behaviors (34,36). With respect to family dynamics, the New Beginnings intervention has been associated with improvements in the use of effective discipline strategies, parent–child communication, and positive routines (36).

Treatment Foster Care Oregon

Treatment Foster Care Oregon (TFCO) is a 6-month intervention for adolescents with a history of antisocial behavior, emotional disturbance, and delinquency (37). Foster families from the community are recruited and trained to provide adolescents with clear and consistent limits, appropriate consequences, and positive reinforcement for appropriate behavior (37). In so doing, the TFCO system also provides adolescents with a mentoring adult and separation from delinquent peers groups (37). The TFCO uses a behavior modification system where adolescents can accrue points for appropriate behavior, and over time gain increased levels of independence. The TFCO also includes individual and family therapy and emphasizes that adolescents develop interpersonal skills and participate in social and recreational activities (37). The TFCO program is associated with reductions in days spent incarcerated, reductions in tobacco and marijuana use, reductions in violent offenses (37), and among females, reductions in the odds of becoming pregnant (37,38).

Multisystemic Therapy

Multisystemic Therapy (MST) is a family- and community-based intervention designed to improve antisocial behavior patterns in adolescent juvenile offenders (39). MST works across multiple settings (i.e., in the home, school, and community) to increase prosocial behavior and decrease antisocial behavior. MST has been associated with decreased rates of rearrest, recidivism, incarceration, psychopathology, and substance use, as well as increased rates of community service (39,40).

Multisystemic Therapy-Problem Sexual Behavior

Similar to the broader MST intervention, the Multisystemic Therapy-Problem Sexual Behavior (MST-PSB) intervention focuses on the family, school, peer, and community systems in which an adolescent is embedded in order to reduce antisocial behavior (41). However, MST-PSB focuses specifically on the dimensions of the youth's environment that are related to problematic sexual behavior. MST-PSB strives to increase each adolescent's friendships and age-appropriate sexual experiences, and works with adolescents to increase perspective taking abilities and maladaptive beliefs and attitudes, particularly around sexual offending (41). MST-PSB is associated with reductions in rearrests for sexual and nonsexual crimes (42), parent and child psychiatric symptoms, youth behavior problems, as well as improvements in peer relationships, family functioning, and academic performance (41,43).

The Blues Program

The Blues Program is a cognitive-behavioral group depression intervention designed for adolescents with prodromal symptoms of depression (44). The program aims to provide social support and help adolescents restructure maladaptive thinking, develop plans to respond to future stressors, and participate in pleasant activities (44). The Blues Program has been associated with reductions in depressive symptoms immediately following the intervention (45), 6 months post-intervention (46), and both 1 and 2 years post-intervention (44,47). Adolescents participating in the Blues program also report reductions in substance abuse immediately following the intervention and 6 months post-intervention (44,46).

The Body Project

The Body Project is a 4-week group intervention designed for high school and college-aged females with disordered eating. The Body Project engages participants in body acceptance exercises and teaches strategies to avoid peer pressure (48). Post-intervention, the Body Project is associated with decreases in thin ideal internalization, body dissatisfaction, negative affect, risk for obesity onset, symptoms of bulimia, and disordered eating (48,49). Many of these effects are maintained for 3 years (48).

Brief Alcohol Screening and Intervention for College Students

Brief Alcohol Screening and Intervention for College Students (BASICS) is a two-session intervention designed for individuals aged 18 to 24 who are at risk for alcohol use disorders (50). BASICS strives to help college-aged students better understand the risks associated with drinking, enhance motivation to change, develop skills to moderate drinking, and ultimately make better alcohol use–related decisions (50). College-aged students who participate in BASICS demonstrate reduced rates of drinking and problem behaviors at 2- and 4-year follow-ups (50,51). Among first-year college students, BASICS has been associated with lower levels of peak blood alcohol concentration and reductions in the number of drinks consumed during the weekend (50).

Functional Family Therapy

Functional Family Therapy (FFT) is a family-based intervention for delinquent adolescents and their families (52). FFT is designed to enhance parenting skills, youth compliance, family communication and supportiveness, and decrease negativity and dysfunctional behavioral patterns (52). FFT is associated with reductions in recidivism, youth internalizing and externalizing symptoms, substance use, as well as enhanced family interactions (52,53).

Parent Management Training—Oregon Model

Parent Management Training—Oregon Model (PMTO) is a group-based parent training intervention for the parents of children ranging in age from early childhood to late adolescence (54). PMTO is designed to enhance effective family management skills and thereby reduce antisocial and problematic behavior in children (54). Research suggests that PMTO is associated with reductions in coercive parenting, noncompliance, and negative reinforcement, and increases in effective and positive parenting (54,55). Among children, PMTO is associated with reduced rates of Oppositional Defiant Disorder, aggression, internalizing disorders, and externalizing disorders (54,56,57). Nine years post-intervention, PMTO is associated with decreases in teacher-rated delinquency (54,58) and arrest rates (54,59).

A Summary of Existent Preventive Interventions

Irrespective of the population being targeted, the goal of preventive interventions is to reduce the influence of established causal risk factors, augment the availability and/or influence of known protective factors, and reduce the likelihood that children will develop (or progress toward) psychopathology.

Cutting across the many contexts (e.g., individual, peer, family, school, community) in which a given child or adolescent is embedded, and utilizing a variety of therapeutic modalities (e.g., school based, individual, group, family) the preventive interventions outlined above exert a significant influence on a variety of known risk and protective factors. Broadly speaking, these interventions can be broken down into those involving the child and those involving the family.

The child-based risk factors modified by the preventive interventions reviewed above include low school commitment, body image concerns, substance use, aggressive behavior, physical violence, poor academic performance, positive attitudes toward drug use, favorable attitudes toward antisocial behavior, and interaction with antisocial peers (60). The child-based protective factors enhanced by the interventions reviewed above include coping skills, problem-solving skills, perceived risk of drug use, social interaction skills, prosocial involvement, interaction with prosocial peers, drug refusal skills, and academic self-efficacy (60).

The family-based risk factors modified by the programs reviewed above include family violence, parental mental health difficulties, poor family management, neglectful parenting, lack of prenatal care, household adults involved in antisocial behavior, low socioeconomic status, maternal substance use during pregnancy, parental unemployment, unplanned pregnancy, and parent stress (60). The family-based protective factors modified by the programs reviewed above include: clear standards for behavior, nonviolent discipline, attachment to parents, and parental social support (60). Thus, many of the most well-supported preventive interventions alter family-level risk and protective factors and thereby prevent illness and promote health in children and adolescents.

Established and Emerging Modalities for Prevention and Health Promotion

Clearly, at both the child and family level, preventive interventions have the capacity to shore up protective factors and reduce risk factors. Given the prominence of family-level variables in the preventive interventions outlined above, and given the known genetic and environmental contributions to every developmental psychopathology that has been studied, we view parental emotional behavioral well-being and positive parenting as critical components of prevention and health promotion in children and adolescents. As such, next we will briefly review the research surrounding parental psychopathology and positive parenting. Then keeping in mind that emotional behavioral health is a key component of overall health, we present the emerging science supporting the health-promoting capacities of: music, mindfulness, nutrition, and exercise.

Established Modalities for Child and Adolescent Psychiatry

Parental Psychopathology

The presence of a parent with psychopathology serves as a nonspecific risk factor for multiple forms of offspring psychopathology including internalizing, externalizing, and substance use disorders (61–63). The risk associated with parental psychopathology is conferred via genetic and environmental mechanisms (10,64–66). Yet even when the influence of prominent environmental risk factors (e.g., childhood adversity, low socioeconomic status) are controlled for, a child who has a parent with psychopathology is still 1.5 to 8 times more likely to develop emotional behavioral illness (67,68).

Research also suggests, however, that when parental psychopathology is treated, the risk conferred to offspring is reduced. For example, children who have a parent with a depressive disorder are four times more likely to develop psychopathology (61). Yet, when maternal depression is treated, children show reduced rates of psychopathology, improved academic performance, and enhanced overall functioning (69,70). The reductions in child problem behaviors associated with the successful treatment of maternal depression are sustained at 6-month and 1- and 4-year follow-ups (69,71–73). Thus, to date research suggests that, treating parental psychopathology, can promote offspring mental health.

Parent Training

Along with parental psychopathology, the parenting practices employed within a home exert an influence on the environment in which a child's development occurs. It has been suggested that a potential mechanism through which some forms of parental psychopathology confer risk for child psychopathology is via parenting behavior. Indeed, research suggests that parental psychopathology can compromise effective parenting behavior (74), and that a reciprocal relationship exists between parenting behavior and child psychopathology (75).

Parent training programs are designed to provide parents with parenting strategies to increase their child's compliance and prosocial behavior, and reduce their child's oppositional and aggressive behavior. Some of the most well-researched behavioral parent training programs are: Helping the Noncompliant Child (76), Incredible Years (77), Parent Management Training (78), and Triple-P (79).

It is well established that parent training programs are effective treatments for children struggling with clinically significant disruptive and externalizing behavior (80). However, as PMT's designation as a model preventive intervention suggests, parent training is also effective in children and adolescents without clinically significant levels of psychopathology. Even among otherwise healthy toddlers, the preventative use of parent training has been associated with reductions in the development of externalizing and disruptive behavior over a 5-year period (81). Therefore, research suggests that effective and positive parenting can both treat and prevent the development of child psychopathology.

Emerging Modalities for Child and Adolescent Psychiatry

Beyond the established role of parental psychopathology and parent training in developmental psychopathology, there are a number of health-promoting modalities that have an emerging evidence base and are established enough, with little risk, that we believe they can begin to be implemented in standard practice. These are mindfulness training, nutrition, exercise, and music training.

Mindfulness

As it applies to modern western health care, mindfulness has been defined as the ability to disengage from one's beliefs, thoughts, and actions, and attend to moment-to-moment experience in a nonjudgmental manner (82). It has been suggested that such a state can be fostered using a variety of techniques (e.g., mindfulness meditation, mindful breathing, mindful movement, and short meditations during the course of the day) (83).

Over the last 35 years, mindfulness has been incorporated into a number of psychosocial interventions including: Dialectical Behavior Therapy (DBT) (84), Acceptance and Commitment Therapy (ACT) (85), Mindfulness-Based Stress Reduction (MBSR) (86), and Mindfulness-Based Cognitive Therapy (MBCT) (87) with research suggesting that such interventions can effectively treat a range of conditions, including: Borderline Personality Disorder (88), anxiety disorders (89), mood disorders (90), eating disorders (91), high stress levels (92), and chronic pain (83,93).

Beyond mindfulness' application to clinical populations, research also suggests that mindfulness may be a helpful strategy for individuals who do not evidence clinically significant levels of psychopathology. Among otherwise healthy adults, MBSR is associated with increases in mindfulness that temporally precede reductions in negative affect (94). Similarly, among college students without clinical levels of psychopathology, MBSR is associated with decreases in the symptoms of psychopathology (83,95).

A body of work suggests that mindfulness may be particularly beneficial for women during pregnancy. Both randomized controlled (96,97) and uncontrolled (98) studies suggest that mindfulness training for pregnant women is associated with reductions in physical pain, stress, depression, and anxiety. Maternal stress and anxiety during pregnancy have been associated with infants being born preterm and at low birth weights (99), as well as a cognitive, emotional, and developmental outcomes in infancy and childhood (97,100). Thus, some have argued that helping mothers achieve emotional behavioral wellness during pregnancy may be a means to prevent the development of negative outcomes in children (97,101).

In addition to work suggesting that mindfulness may be an effective intervention for adults, research also suggests that mindfulness may be an effective prevention and treatment strategy in children. Meta-analytic work suggests that mindfulness interventions have a small-to-moderate effect on emotional behavioral symptoms in general populations of children and adolescents, and a slightly larger effect on emotional behavioral symptoms in clinical populations (102,103). However, while mindfulness interventions may effectively promote resilience in universal populations of children and treat psychopathology in children with mental illness, more randomized controlled trials exploring the affect of mindfulness training in children are needed (104).

Nutrition

It has long been established that consuming a nutritious and well-balanced diet is a critical component of overall wellness. Research suggests that a healthy diet contributes to enhanced cardiovascular health (105), reduced rates of cancer, and longevity (106). Recently, research has begun to suggest that there is an association between nutrition and mental health.

In both children and adults, diet quality has been demonstrated to influence learning, memory, and mood (107,108). In adolescents, internalizing and externalizing disorders are positively associated with increased consumption of fast food, red meat, and sugar, and negatively associated with increased consumption of fresh fruits and vegetables (109). Prospective longitudinal work suggests that among adolescents diet quality may be causally related to mental health (110). In adults, diets of low quality are associated with increased rates of anxiety and depression, reductions in molecular substrates involved in cognitive processing, and increased risk for neurologic disorders (108).

In addition to overall diet quality, a variety of nutritional deficiencies have been associated with emotional behavioral illness. Cross-sectional work with adults suggests that low serum cholesterol is associated with antisocial, violent, and self-injurious behavior (111). Cross-sectional work with children suggests that iron and zinc deficiencies are associated with externalizing behavior and Attention-Deficit Hyperactivity Disorder (ADHD), respectively (111). Longitudinal work with children suggests that zinc, iron, and vitamin B deficiencies during early childhood are associated with externalizing disorders during adolescence (111). In children, diets low in omega-3 fatty acids have been associated with hyperactivity, learning disorders, and behavioral problems, and recent interventional work suggests that omega-3 fatty acid supplementation results in reductions in externalizing behaviors (111). It has been hypothesized that this association between nutritional deficiencies and mental health may be mediated by epigenetic changes and altered brain structure and function (111).

Exercise

Engaging in physical exercise is associated with a decreased risk for a host of general medical conditions including obesity, diabetes, and cardiovascular disease (112). It has also been suggested that physical exercise may be a viable preventive intervention and treatment for psychopathology (113).

The majority of research exploring the effects of exercise on clinically significant psychopathology in adults has explored the influence of exercise on depression and anxiety (114). Among adults with depression, meta-analytic work suggests that exercise has a moderate-to-strong effect on the symptoms of depression (115). Among adults with anxiety, results are inconsistent with some research suggesting that exercise has a minimal effect on the symptoms of anxiety (116) and others reporting a large effect (117).

Among otherwise healthy adults, correlational work suggests that individuals who are regularly physically active report fewer symptoms of anxiety and depression and have 45% lower odds of developing a depressive disorder and between 24% and 48% lower odds of developing an anxiety disorder (118). While such work does not elucidate the direction of these effects, a recent meta-meta-analysis using data from 400 randomized trials and 14,000 participants suggests that among adults with nonclinical levels of anxiety and depression, exercise results in a medium but significant reductive effect on depressive symptoms, and a small but significant reductive effect on the symptoms of anxiety (114). Such work suggests that exercise may be a viable preventive intervention among individuals with subclinical symptomatology.

Research has also explored the relationship between physical activity and psychopathology in children and adolescents. Research suggests that physical activity appears to have a small but beneficial effect on the symptoms of anxiety and depression, a large effect on self-esteem, and to be associated with improved cognitive performance, classroom behavior, and academic achievement (119). In addition, meta-analytic work suggests that in children aerobic exercise programs have a moderate-to-large effect on the symptoms of ADHD (120).

Music

Recently, there has been an explosion of interest in the neurophysiologic, cognitive, and behavioral correlates of playing music. To date, research suggests that playing a musical instrument is associated with alterations in brain structure and function, enhanced cognitive functioning, and improvements in academic performance.

A long-standing body of work with children and adults suggests that relative to amateur musicians and nonmusicians, practiced musicians evidence structural and functional differences in various regions of the brain. In adults, practiced musicians evidence structural differences in the: primary sensorimotor cortex, superior premotor cortex, superior parietal cortex, primary auditory cortex, cerebellum, inferior frontal gyrus, and lateral temporal lobe (121). Research among adult professional musicians, suggests positive associations between music training during childhood, adolescence, and adulthood and white matter tract development (122). Similarly, cross-sectional work with children suggests that relative to children who do not play musical instruments, children who play an instrument evidence increased gray matter in the sensorimotor cortex and occipital lobe, increased activation of the temporal lobe during rhythmic and melodic discrimination tasks (123), and distinct patterns of cortical thickness maturation in the dorsolateral prefrontal cortex (124).

Given the cross-sectional and correlational nature of much of the research on music, such work cannot address whether structural and functional brain differences are a consequence of increased musical practice, or rather reflect underlying neuroanatomical differences that predate exposure to music. Recently, however, research with children has begun to suggest that musical training may indeed be causally related to both changes in cognition, as well as changes in brain structure and function. Relative to a control group of children matched on age, verbal IQ, and socioeconomic status (SES), children who played an instrument for 1 year evidenced significantly greater fine motor and visual discrimination skills (123). Relative to a control group, children who engage in 15 months of musical training evidence improvements in motor and auditory skills, as well as structural changes in the right precentral gyrus, the corpus callosum, the right primary auditory region, the pericingulate, and the left middle occipital lobe (125).

In children, music training may be causally related to changes in cognition. Relative to a control group who did not receive musical instruction, 5-year-old children who received 20 minutes of twice weekly music instruction showed improvements in spatial temporal tasks after 4 months as well as after 8 months (126). Research with low-income 4 to 5 year olds also suggests that relative to a control group, children receiving a 30-week, 75-minute daily music instruction evidence improvements in visuospatial reasoning (127).

Despite such evidence, the majority of children in America do not regularly play a musical instrument. Indeed, roughly 74% of 10th graders and 86% of 12th graders "rarely or never" participate in out-of-school music lessons (124). There are, however, two emerging preventive intervention programs that use music training as a means to offset risk: El Sistema (128) and the Harmony Project (HP) (129).

El Sistema originated in Caracas, Venezuela, and is a music education program serving more than 500,000 Venezuelan children. More recently, El Sistema has been implemented in the United States, and currently more than 2 million at-risk American children partake in the El Sistema curriculum. The El Sistema program has resulted in: a 20% reduction in school dropout, a 22% increase in participation in community activities, and a 28% increase in employment among children who participate (128).

Similarly, the HP is a nonprofit organization based in the United States that provides music instruction and ensemble performance experiences for low-income youth. The HP is currently being implemented in 17 sites in Los Angeles as well as 7 other major cities across the United States. Students participating in the HP receive several hours of musical instruction per week (129). Children enrolled in the HP demonstrate significant gains in neural and auditory processing mechanisms linked with reading and language skills (130,131). In addition, participating in the HP is associated with parent-rated improvements in mood, health, grades, and behaviors. Relative to schools that do not participate in the HP, schools participating in the HP evidence improvements in high school graduation rates and college attendance (129). While music training is an integral part of the HP, the HP also utilizes a mentorship model and thereby offsets risk by capitalizing on other known protective factors (e.g., social support).

The Vermont Family-Based Approach

Examining these emerging domains of prevention and health promotion, it becomes evident that few, if any, of the evidence-based preventive interventions described above take into account the emerging literature from neuroscience, psychology, and genetics to incorporate treating family psychopathology, positive parenting, mindfulness, nutrition, music training, and exercise into one cohesive approach. With that in mind, we present here an emerging clinical and public health paradigm, The Vermont Family-Based Approach (VFBA).

The VFBA was developed by James J. Hudziak, M.D. at the Vermont Center for Children, Youth, and Families and is designed to integrate research on developmental psychopathology into a family-based therapeutic intervention. The VFBA is conceptualized as a means to both treat and prevent the development of emotional behavioral illness in children, and is based on a few central tenets: (1) emotional behavioral health is the cornerstone of all health; (2) all health is familial; (3) health promotion, prevention, and intervention should take into account the emerging science of music, mindfulness, nutrition, and exercise.

VFBA Tenet #1: *Emotional behavioral health is the foundation of all health.*

This concept arises from the emerging literature on the role of psychopathology in nearly every other medical discipline. There is nowhere that this is more evident than in the role of adverse childhood experiences on a wide range of child and adult pathologies from obesity and diabetes to sexually transmitted diseases (6). This literature demonstrates that the way that experiences are managed during childhood does not just affect later mood and behavior, but also affects other medical conditions seemingly "unrelated" to psychopathology. Further, attending to patients' emotional behavioral health allows for more adequate treatment of multiple other conditions including heart disease (132), cancer (133), and diabetes (134), again demonstrating that the cornerstone of health promotion, prevention, and intervention of medical conditions is attending to emotional behavioral health.

VFBA Tenet #2: *All health is familial.*

In the VFBA paradigm, the treatment of parental psychopathology and the utilization of parent training are viewed as means to both treat and prevent the development of child psychopathology. Given that parental psychopathology is a known risk factor for child psychopathology, the VFBA seeks to improve child and adolescent mental health by providing mental health care to both the child and his or her parents. The VFBA is based on the premise that addressing parents' clinical and subclinical mental health needs will help to prevent and facilitate the treatment of existent emotional behavioral illness in children.

Along with parental psychopathology, the parenting practices employed within a home exert an influence on the environment in which a child's development occurs. As such, in addition to addressing both children's and parents' mental health needs, the VFBA utilizes evidence-based parent training strategies to improve parent–child dynamics. Thus, within the VFBA paradigm parenting training is conceptualized as a treatment to help families who are struggling with child psychopathology, as well as a means to bolster parenting skills and prevent the development of psychopathology among children who are otherwise healthy.

VFBA Tenet #3: *Health promotion, prevention, and intervention should take into account emerging science of mindfulness, nutrition, exercise, and music.*

The VFBA promotes family wellness by encouraging the entire family to engage in health-promoting activities including: mindfulness training, healthy eating, exercise, and music training. In this way, the components of the VFBA serve as both effective treatments for children and parents with psychopathology, as well as selective, indicated, and universal preventive interventions for families who are well.

Mindfulness

Given the growing body of empirical evidence suggesting mindfulness' utility as both a treatment and a preventive intervention strategy, there is reason to be optimistic about mindfulness' role in mental health. However, while there are some randomized controlled studies on the effects of mindfulness-based interventions (e.g., MBCT) many studies on the effects of mindfulness are compromised by small sample sizes, lack of control groups, lack of randomization, and lack of data on treatment compliance (75). In particular, more well-controlled work is needed on the effect of mindfulness in children. Nonetheless, the state of the evidence is such that within the VFBA paradigm mindfulness is conceptualized as a health-promoting activity. As such, parents and children who are well, at risk, and struggling with psychopathology are encouraged to engage in mindfulness practices.

Nutrition

Given the body of research implicating overall diet quality and specific nutritional deficiencies in general medical as well as emotional behavioral disorders, the VFBA paradigm conceptualizes a healthy well-balanced diet as a treatment strategy among families who are struggling with emotional behavioral illness, as well as a preventive intervention among those who are well.

Exercise

While it cannot be concluded with certainty that the relationship between exercise and mental health is direct and causal, it seems reasonable to hypothesize that the reductive effects of physical activity on psychopathology "cannot be explained by a single mechanism acting in isolation; rather the effects are most likely due to the contribution of several mechanisms (e.g., mood, feelings of mastery, self-efficacy) and neurophysiologic (hippocampal neurogenesis, hypothalamic–pituitary–adrenal axis regulation)" (107). Given the available research, the VFBA paradigm conceptualizes exercise as a viable treatment and preventive strategy, and encourages parents and children to engage in physical activity through structured exercise programs, often using fitness coaching and positive reinforcement.

Music

Because of the large body of research suggesting that music training is associated with changes in brain structure and function, and the findings from school-based programs such as El Sistema and HP that music training is associated with improvement in cognition as well as improved academic performance, the VFBA strongly encourages a musical component for the entire family. Although a randomized controlled trial using clinical samples has yet to establish a direct relationship between music training and reductions in psychopathology, the available evidence suggesting music training's utility as a preventive strategy as well as music training's impact on neuroanatomy has led to its incorporation into the VFBA. Within the VFBA paradigm, children who are well and children who are struggling with emotional behavioral illness, along with their families, are encouraged to play a musical instrument.

Demonstrating the Effectiveness of the VFBA

While the effectiveness of each of the essential components of the VFBA has been demonstrated, the VFBA in its entirety has not been formally tested. A randomized clinical trial of the VFBA paradigm is currently underway at the University of Vermont Medical Center. This trial is projected to include 120 to 160 families with a child between the ages of 3 and 6. Families enrolled in the treatment condition will be partnered with a family wellness coach who will help them implement a health and wellness plan based on the results of a family-wide assessment. This assessment will include standardized measures of each family members' emotional behavioral health, as well as assessment of the health-promoting activities in which they engage. Each family's health and wellness plan will be tailored to their specific needs, but will rely on the fundamental principles of the VFBA: family-wide mental health care, positive parenting strategies, mindfulness, nutrition, exercise, and music training.

Summary

Child and adolescent psychiatry is now perfectly positioned to play a critical role in health promotion, illness prevention, and family-based intervention. We are the only medical professionals who understand the impact of the environment on: the genome (epigenome), the structure and function of the developing brain, and related thoughts, feelings, and behaviors (symptoms). We can prescribe wellness to all children (e.g., mindfulness, exercise, nutrition, sleep, music, etc.), regardless of whether or not they are at risk or already struggling with emotional behavioral problems. We can assist in prevention by assuring that all parents have access to parent training, and promote the idea that treating parental emotional behavioral problems is a far more powerful tool than ignoring such problems. We can become the field that recognizes the importance of prescribing social supports and education around the difficult task of raising healthy children. And, when we treat children who are in the grips of psychopathology, we should do so in a family-based manner that includes concomitant health promotion and illness prevention perscriptions. Basic developmental neuroscience and genomic evidence exist, the ACEs study provides a perfect platform for national attention, and accountable care is an invitation to fund reform that will place child and adolescent psychiatry at the center of health care reform.

References

1. Rijlaarsdam J, Stevens GW, Jansen PW, et al.: Maternal childhood maltreatment and offspring emotional and behavioral problems: maternal and paternal mechanisms of risk transmission. *Child Maltreat* 19(2):67–78, 2014.
2. Weder N, Zhang H, Jensen K, et al.: Child abuse, depression, and methylation in genes involved with stress, neural plasticity, and brain circuitry. *Am Acad Child Adolesc Psychiatry* 53(4):417–424.e415, 2014.
3. Ducharme S, Hudziak JJ, Botteron KN, et al.: Right anterior cingulate cortical thickness and bilateral striatal volume correlate with child behavior checklist aggressive behavior scores in healthy children. *Biol psychiatry* 70(3):283–290, 2011.
4. Stringaris A, Vidal-Ribas Belil P, Artiges E, et al.: The Brain's response to reward anticipation and depression in adolescence: dimensionality, specificity, and longitudinal predictions in a community-based sample. *Am J psychiatry* 172(12):1215–1223, 2015.
5. Verhulst FC, Tiemeier H: Epidemiology of child psychopathology: major milestones. *Eur Child Adolescent psychiatry* 24(6):607–617, 2015.
6. Felitti VJ, Anda RF, Nordenberg D, et al.: Relationship of childhood abuse and household dysfunction to many of the leading causes of death in adults. The Adverse Childhood Experiences (ACE) Study. *Am J Prev Med* 14(4):245–258, 1998.
7. Grace SL, Turk-Adawi KI, Contractor A, et al.: Cardiac rehabilitation delivery model for low-resource settings: an international council of cardiovascular prevention and rehabilitation consensus statement. *Prog Cardiovasc Dis* 59(3):303–322, 2016.
8. American Psychiatric Association: *Diagnostic and Statistical Manual of Mental Disorders:DSM-5.* Washington, DC: American Psychiatric Association, 2013.
9. Hudziak JJ: The Vermont family-based approach. 2010. Available at: https://www.uvm.edu/medicine/documents/CMS_Hudziak_Family_Approa h_091410.pdf. Accessed October 9, 2016.
10. Hudziak JJ, Bartels M: Genetic and environmental influences on wellness, resilience, and psychopathology a family-based approach for promotion, prevention, and intervention. In: Hudziak JJ (ed): *Developmental Psychopathology and Wellness.* Arlington, VA, American Psychiatric Publishing Inc, 267–286, 2008.
11. Mrazek DA, Mrazek PJ: Prevention of psychiatric disorders. In: Martin A, Volkmer FR (eds): *Lewis Child and Adolescent Psychiatry.* 4th ed. Philadelphia, PA, Lippincott Williams & Wilkins, 171–177, 2007.
12. Caplan G: *Principles of Prevention Psychiatry.* Oxford, England, Basic Books, 1964.
13. Gordon RS Jr: An operational classification of disease prevention. *Public Health Rep* 98:107–109, 1983.
14. National Research Council (US) and Institute of Medicine (US) Committee on the Prevention of Mental Disorders and Substance Abuse Among Children, Youth, and Young Adults: Research advances and promising interventions. In: O'Connell ME, Boat T, Warner KE (eds): *Preventing Mental, Emotional, and Behavioral Disorders Among Young People: Progress and Possibilities.* Washington, DC, National Academies Press (US), 2009.
15. Institute of Medicine: Reducing risks for mental disorders: frontiers for preventive intervention research. In: Mrazek PJ, Haggerty RJ (eds): *Committee on Prevention of Mental Disorders, Division of Biobehavorial Sciences and Mental Disorders.* Washington, DC, National Academy Press, 1994.
16. Springer F, Phillips JL: The IOM model: a tool for prevention planning and implementation. *Tactics* 8(13):1–7, 2006. Available at: http://www.cars-rp.org/publications/Prevention%20Tactics/PT8.13.06.pdf. Accessed August 28, 2016.
17. World Health Organization: *Ottawa Charter for Health Promotion.* Geneva, Switzerland: Author, 1986.
18. Blueprints for Healthy Youth Development. Available at: http://www.blueprintsprograms.com/about. Published 2012–2016. Accessed August 28, 2016.
19. Blueprints for Healthy Youth Development. Available at: http://www.blueprintsprograms.com/criteria. Published 2012–2016. Accessed August 28, 2016.
20. Blueprints for Healthy Youth Development. Available at: http://www.blueprintsprograms.com/factsheet/lifeskills-training-lst. Published 2012–2016. Accessed August 28, 2016.
21. Griffin KW, Botvin GJ, Nichols TR: Long-term follow-up effects of a school-based drug abuse prevention program on adolescent risky driving. *Prev Sci* 5:207–212, 2004.
22. Griffin KW, Botvin GJ, Nichols TR: Effects of a school-based drug abuse prevention program for adolescents on HIV risk behaviors in young adulthood. *Prev Sci* 7:103–112, 2006.
23. Blueprints for Healthy Youth Development. Available at: http://www.blueprintsprograms.com/factsheet/positive-action. Published 2012–2016. Accessed August 28, 2016.
24. Washburn IJ, Acock A, Vuchinich S, et al.: Effects of a social-emotional and character development program on the trajectory of behaviors associated with social-emotional and character development: findings from three randomized trials. *Prev Sci* 12(3):314–323, 2011.
25. Blueprints for Healthy Youth Development. Available at: http://www.blueprintsprograms.com/factsheet/promoting-alternative-thinking-strategies-paths. Published 2012–2016. Accessed August 28, 2016.
26. Riggs NR, Greenberg MT, Kusché CA, Pentz MA: The mediational role of neurocognition in the behavioral outcomes of a social-emotional prevention program in elementary school students: effects of the PATHS curriculum. *Prev Sci* 7:91–102, 2006.
27. Schonfeld DJ, Adams RE, Fredstrom BK, et al.: Cluster-randomized trial demonstrating impact on academic achievement of elementary social-emotional learning. *Sch psychol Q* 30(3):406–420, 2015.
28. Blueprints for Healthy Youth Development. Available at: http://www.blueprintsprograms.com/factsheet/project-towards-no-drug-abuse. Published 2012–2016. Accessed August 28, 2016.
29. Sussman S, Dent CW, Stacy AW: Project towards no drug abuse: a review of the findings and future directions. *Am J Health Behav* 26(5):354–365, 2002.
30. Sun W, Skara S, Sun P, Dent CW, Sussman S: Project towards no drug abuse: long-term substance use outcomes evaluation. *Prev Med* 42(3):188–192, 2006.
31. Blueprints for Healthy Youth Development. Available at: http://www.blueprintsprograms.com/factsheet/nurse-family-partnership. Published 2012–2016. Accessed August 28, 2016.
32. Olds DL, Eckenrode J, Henderson CR Jr, et al.: Long-term effects of home visitation on maternal life course and child abuse and neglect. Fifteen-year follow-up of a randomized trial. *JAMA* 278(8):637–643, 1997.
33. Olds DL, Kitzman H, Knudtson MD, Anson E, Smith JA, Cole R: Effect of home visiting by nurses on maternal and child mortality: results of a 2-decade follow-up of a randomized clinical trial. *JAMA pediatr* 168(9):800–806, 2014.

34. Blueprints for Healthy Youth Development. Available at: http://www.blueprintsprograms.com/factsheet/new-beginnings-for-children-of-divorce. Published 2012–2016. Accessed August 28, 2016.
35. Wolchik SA, West SG, Sandler IN, et al.: An experimental evaluation of theory-based mother and mother-child programs for children of divorce. *J Consult Clin Psychol* 68(5):843–856, 2000.
36. Wolchik SA, West SG, Westover S, et al.: The children of divorce parenting intervention: outcome evaluation of an empirically based program. *Am J Community Psychol* 21(3):293–231, 1993.
37. Blueprints for Healthy Youth Development. Available at: http://www.blueprintsprograms.com/factsheet/treatment-foster-care-oregon. Published 2012–2016. Accessed August 28, 2016.
38. Kerr DC, Leve LD, Chamberlain P: Pregnancy rates among juvenile justice girls in two randomized controlled trials of multidimensional treatment foster care. *J Consult Clin Psychol* 77(3):588–593, 2009.
39. Blueprints for Healthy Youth Development. Available at: http://www.blueprintsprograms.com/factsheet/multisystemic-therapy-mst. Published 2012–2016. Accessed August 28, 2016.
40. Fain T, Greathouse SM, Turner SF, Weinberg HD: Effectiveness of multisystemic therapy for minority youth: outcomes over 8 years in Los Angeles County. *J Juv Justice* 3(2):24–37, 2014.
41. Blueprints for Healthy Youth Development. Available at: http://www.blueprintsprograms.com/factsheet/multisystemic-therapy-problem-sexual-behavior-mst-psb. Published 2012–2016. Accessed August 28, 2016.
42. Borduin CM, Henggeler SW, Blaske, DM, Stein RJ: Multisystemic treatment of adolescent sexual offenders. *Int J Offender Ther Comp Criminol* 35:105–114, 1990.
43. Borduin CM, Schaeffer CM, Heiblum N: A randomized clinical trial of multisystemic therapy with juvenile sexual offenders: effects on youth social ecology and criminal activity. *J Consult Clin Psychol* 77(1):26–37, 2009.
44. Blueprints for Healthy Youth Development. Available at: http://www.blueprintsprograms.com/factsheet/blues-program. Published 2012–2016. Accessed August 28, 2016.
45. Rohde P, Stice E, Shaw H, Briere FN: Indicated cognitive behavioral group depression prevention compared to bibliotherapy and brochure control: acute effects of an effectiveness trial with adolescents. *J Consult Clin Psychol* 82(1):65–74, 2014.
46. Stice E, Rohde P, Seeley JR, Gau JM: Brief cognitive-behavioral depression prevention program for high-risk adolescents outperforms two alternative interventions: a randomized efficacy trial. *J Consult Clin Psychol* 76(4):595–606, 2008.
47. Stice E, Rohde P, Gau JM, Wade E: Efficacy trial of a brief cognitive-behavioral depression prevention program for high-risk adolescents: effects at 1- and 2-year follow-up. *J Consult Clin Psychol* 78(6):856–867, 2010.
48. Blueprints for Healthy Youth Development. Available at: http://www.blueprintsprograms.com/factsheet/body-project. Published 2012–2016. Accessed August 28, 2016.
49. Stice E, Shaw H, Burton E, Wade E: Dissonance and healthy weight eating disorder prevention programs: a randomized efficacy trial. *J Consult Clin Psychol* 74(2):263–275, 2006.
50. Blueprints for Healthy Youth Development. Available at: http://www.blueprintsprograms.com/factsheet/brief-alcohol-screening-and-intervention-for-college-students-basics. Published 2012–2016. Accessed August 28, 2016.
51. Baer JS, Kivlahan DR, Blume AW, McKnight P, Marlatt GA: Brief intervention for heavy-drinking college students: 4-year follow-up and natural history. *Am J Public Health* 91(8):1310–1316, 2001.
52. Blueprints for Healthy Youth Development. Available at: http://www.blueprintsprograms.com/factsheet/functional-family-therapy-fft. Published 2012–2016. Accessed August 28, 2016.
53. Alexander JF, Parsons BV: Short-term behavioral intervention with delinquent families: impact on family process and recidivism. *J Abnorm psychol* 81(3):219–225, 1973.
54. Blueprints for Healthy Youth. Available at: http://www.blueprintsprograms.com/factsheet/parent-management-training. Published 2012–2016. Accessed August 28, 2016.
55. Forgatch MS, DeGarmo DS: Parenting through change: an effective prevention program for single mothers. *J Consult Clin psychol* 67(5):711–724, 1999.
56. DeGarmo DS, Patterson GR, Forgatch MS: How do outcomes in a specified parent training intervention maintain or wane over time? *Prev Sci* 5(2):73–89, 2004.
57. Martinez CR Jr, Forgatch MS: Preventing problems with boys' noncompliance: effects of a parent training intervention for divorcing mothers. *J Consult Clin Psychol* 69(3):416–428, 2001.
58. Forgatch MS, Degarmo DS: Accelerating recovery from poverty: prevention effects for recently separated mothers. *J Early Intensive Behav Interv* 4(4):681–702, 2007.
59. Forgatch MS, Patterson GR, Degarmo DS, Beldavs ZG: Testing the Oregon delinquency model with 9-year follow-up of the Oregon Divorce Study. *Dev Psychopathol* 21(2):637–660, 2009.
60. Blueprints for Healthy Youth Development. Risk and protective factors. Available at: http://www.blueprintsprograms.com/programs. Published 2012–2016. Accessed August 28, 2016.
61. Beardslee WR, Versage EM, Gladstone TR: Children of affectively ill parents: a review of the past 10 years. *J Am Acad Child Adolesc Psychiatry* 37(11):1134–1141, 1998.
62. Rutter M, Quinton D: Parental psychiatric disorder: effects on children. *Psychol Med* 14(4):853–880, 1984.
63. McLaughlin KA, Gadermann AM, Hwang I, et al.: Parent psychopathology and offspring mental disorders: results from the WHO World Mental Health Surveys. *Br J Psychiatry* 200(4):290–299, 2012.
64. Althoff RR, Rettew DC, Faraone SV, Boomsma DI, Hudziak JJ: Latent class analysis shows strong heritability of the child behavior checklist-juvenile bipolar phenotype. *Biol Psychiatry* 60(9):903–911, 2006.
65. Boomsma DI, van Beijsterveldt CE, Hudziak JJ: Genetic and environmental influences on Anxious/Depression during childhood: a study from the Netherlands Twin Register. *Genes Brain Behav* 4(8):466–481, 2005.
66. Van Grootheest DS, Cath DC, Beekman AT, Boomsma DI: Genetic and environmental influences on obsessive-compulsive symptoms in adults: a population-based twin-family study. *Psychol Med* 37(11):1635–1644, 2007.
67. Wansink HJ, Drost RM, Paulus AT, et al.: Cost-effectiveness of preventive case management for parents with a mental illness: a randomized controlled trial from three economic perspectives. *BMC Health Serv Res* 16:228, 2016.
68. Bijl RV, Cuijpers P, Smit F: Psychiatric disorders in adult children of parents with a history of psychopathology. *Soc Psychiatry Psychiatr Epidemiol* 37(1):7–12, 2002.
69. Gunlicks ML, Weissman MM: Change in child psychopathology with improvement in parental depression: a systematic review. *J Am Acad Child Adolesc Psychiatry* 47(4):379–389, 2008.
70. Weissman MM, Pilowsky DJ, Wickramaratne PJ, et al.: Remissions in maternal depression and child psychopathology: a STAR*D-child report. *JAMA* 295:1389–1398, 2006.
71. Modell JD, Modell JG, Wallander J, Hodgens B, Duke L, Wisely D: Maternal ratings of child behavior improve with treatment of maternal depression. *Fam Med* 33:691–695, 2001.
72. Billings AG, Moos RH: Children of parents with unipolar depression: a controlled 1-year follow-up. *J Abnorm Chil Psychol* 14:149–166, 1986.
73. Lee CM, Gotlib IH: Maternal depression and child adjustment: a longitudinal analysis. *J Abnorm Psychol* 98:78–85, 1989.
74. Harvey E, Stoessel B, Herbert S: Psychopathology and parenting practices of parents of preschool children with behavior problems. *Parent Sci Pract* 11(4):239–263, 2011.
75. Burke JD, Pardini DA, Loeber R: Reciprocal relationships between parenting behavior and disruptive psychopathology from childhood through adolescence. *J Abnorm Child Psychol* 36(5):679–692, 2008.
76. McMahon RJ, Forehand RL: *Helping the Noncompliant Child: A Family-Based Treatment for Oppositional Behavior.* 2nd ed. New York, Guilford Press, 2015.
77. Webster-Stratton C: *The Incredible Years: A Trouble Shooting Guide for Parents of Children Age 2–8.* Seattle, WA, Incredible Years, 2006.
78. Kazdin AE: *Parent Management Training: Treatment for Oppositional, Aggressive, and Antisocial Behavior in Children and Adolescents.* New York, Oxford University Press, 2005.
79. Sanders MR, Markie-Dadds C: *Turner KMT. Practitioner's Manual for Standard Triple P.* Brisbane (Australia), Families International Publishing, 2000.
80. Maughan DR, Christiansen E, Jenson WR, et al.: Behavioral parent training as a treatment for externalizing behaviors and disruptive behavior disorders: a meta-analysis. *Sch Psychol Rev* 34(3):267–286, 2005.
81. Dishion TJ, Brennan LM, Shaw DS, McEachern AD, Wilson MN, Jo B: Prevention of problem behavior through annual family check-ups in early childhood: intervention effects from home to early elementary school. *J Abnorm Child Psychol* 42(3):343–354, 2014.
82. Ludwig DS, Kabat-Zinn J: Mindfulness in medicine. *JAMA* 300(11): 1350–1352, 2008.
83. Allen NB, Chambers R, Knight W; Melbourne Academic Mindfulness Interest Group: Mindfulness-based psychotherapies: a review of conceptual foundations, empirical evidence and practical considerations. *Aust N Z J Psychiatry* 40(4):285–294, 2006. Available at: http://search.proquest.com.ezproxy.uvm.edu/docview/621173653?accountid = 14679. Accessed August 28, 2016.
84. Linehan MM: *Cognitive-Behavioral Treatment of Borderline Personality Disorder.* New York, Guilford, 1993.
85. Hayes SC, Strosahl KD, Wilson KG: *Acceptance and Commitment Therapy: An Experiential Approach to Behavior Change.* New York, Guilford, 1999.
86. Kabat-Zinn J; University of Massachusetts Medical Center/Worcester; Stress Reduction Clinic: *Full Catastrophe Living: Using the Wisdom of Your Body and Mind to Face Stress, Pain, and Illness.* New York, Delta, 1990.
87. Segal ZV, Williams JMG, Teasdale J: *Mindfulness-Based Cognitive Therapy for Depression: A New Approach to Preventing Relapse.* New York, Guilford, 2002.
88. Linehan MM, Korslund KE, Harned MS, et al.: Dialectical behavior therapy for high suicide risk in individuals with borderline personality disorder: a randomized clinical trial and component analysis. *JAMA psychiatry* 72(5):475–482, 2015.

89. Kabat-Zinn J, Massion AO, Kristeller J, et al.: Effectiveness of a meditation-based stress reduction program in the treatment of anxiety disorders. *Am J Psychiatry* 149:936–943, 1992.
90. Teasdale JD, Segal ZV, Williams JM, Ridgeway VA, Soulsby JM, Lau MA: Prevention of relapse/recurrence in major depression by mindfulness-based cognitive therapy. *J Consult Clin Psychol* 68:615–623, 2000.
91. Kristeller JL, Hallett CB: An exploratory study of a meditation-based intervention for binge eating disorder. *J Health Psychol* 4:357–363, 1999.
92. Shapiro SL, Schwartz GE, Bonner G: Effects of mindfulness-based stress reduction on medical and premedical students. *J Behav Med* 21:581–599, 1998.
93. Kabat-Zinn J: An out-patient program in behavioral medicine for chronic pain patients based on the practice of mindfulness meditation: theoretical considerations and preliminary results. *Gen Hosp Psychiatry* 4:33–47, 1982.
94. Snippe E, Nyklicek I, Schroevers MJ, Bos EH: The temporal order of change in daily mindfulness and affect during mindfulness-based stress reduction. *J Couns Psychol* 62(2):106–114, 2015.
95. Williams KA, Kolar MM, Reger BE, Pearson JC: Evaluation of a wellness-based mindfulness stress reduction intervention: a controlled trial. *Am J Health Promot* 15:422–432, 2001.
96. Vieten C, Astin J: Effects of a mindfulness-based intervention during pregnancy on prenatal stress and mood: results of a pilot study. *Arch Women's Ment Health* 11(1):67–74, 2008.
97. Guardino CM, Dunkel Schetter C, Bower JE, Lu MC, Smalley SL: Randomized controlled pilot trial of mindfulness training for stress reduction during pregnancy. *Psychol Health* 29(3):334–349, 2014.
98. Dunn C, Hanieh E, Roberts R, Powrie R: Mindful pregnancy and childbirth: effects of a mindfulness-based intervention on women's psychological distress and well-being in the perinatal period. *Arch Women's Ment Health* 15:139–143, 2012.
99. Dunkel Schetter C: Psychological science on pregnancy: stress processes, biopsychosocial models, and emerging research issues. *Ann Rev Psychol* 62:531–558, 2011.
100. Van den Bergh BR, Mulder EJ, Mennes M, Glover V: Antenatal maternal anxiety and stress and the neurobehavioural development of the fetus and child: links and possible mechanisms. *Neurosci Biobehav Rev* 29(2):237–258, 2005.
101. Beddoe AE, Lee KA: Mind-body interventions during pregnancy. *J Obstet Gynecol Neonatal Nurs* 37(2):165–175, 2008.
102. Zoogman S, Goldberg SB, Hoyt WT, Miller L: Mindfulness interventions with youth: a meta-analysis. *Mindfulness* 6(2):290–302, 2015.
103. Zenner C, Herrnleben-Kurz S, Walach H: Mindfulness-based interventions in schools-a systematic review and meta-analysis. *Front Psychol* 5:603, 2014.
104. Greenberg MT, Harris AR: Nurturing mindfulness in children and youth: current state of the research. *Child Dev Perspect* 6(2):161–166, 2012.
105. Hooper L, Summerbell CD, Thompson R, et al.: Reduced or modified dietary fat for preventing cardiovascular disease. *Cochrane Database Syst Rev* (7):CD002137, 2011.
106. Daniel M, Tollefsbol TO: Epigenetic linkage of aging, cancer and nutrition. In: Hoppeler HH (ed): *J Exp Biol* 218(1):59–70, 2015.
107. Zainuddin MS, Thuret S: Nutrition, adult hippocampal neurogenesis and mental health. *Br Med Bull* 103(1):89–114, 2012.
108. Gomez-Pinilla F: Brain foods: the effects of nutrients on brain function. *Nat Rev Neurosci* 9:568–578, 2008.
109. Oddy WH, Robinson M, Ambrosini GL, et al.: The association between dietary patterns and mental health in early adolescence. *Prev Med* 49(1):39–44, 2009.
110. Jacka FN, Kremer PJ, Berk M, et al.: A prospective study of diet quality and mental health in adolescents. *PLoS One* 6(9):e24805, 2011.
111. Liu J, Zhao SR, Reyes T: Neurological and epigenetic implications of nutritional deficiencies on psychopathology: conceptualization and review of evidence. In: Qi L (ed): *Int J Mol Sci* 16(8):18129–18148, 2015.
112. Booth FW, Roberts CK, Laye MJ: Lack of exercise is a major cause of chronic diseases. *Compr Physiol* 2(2):1143–1211, 2012.
113. Byrne A, Byrne DG: The effect of exercise on depression, anxiety and other mood states: a review. *J Psychosom Res* 37(6):565–574, 1993.
114. Rebar AL, Stanton R, Geard D, Short C, Duncan MJ, Vandelanotte C: A meta-meta-analysis of the effect of physical activity on depression and anxiety in non-clinical adult populations. *Health Psychol Rev* 9(3):366–378, 2015.
115. Cooney GM, Dwan K, Greig CA, et al.: Exercise for depression. *Cochrane Database Syst Rev* (9):CD004366, 2013.
116. Bartley CA, Hay M, Bloch MH: Meta-analysis: aerobic exercise for the treatment of anxiety disorders. *Prog Neuropsychopharmacol Biol Psychiatry* 45:34–39, 2013.
117. Wipfli BM, Rethorst CD, Landers DM: The anxiolytic effects of exercise: a meta-analysis of randomized trials and dose-response analysis. *J Sport Exerc Psychol* 30(4):392–410, 2008.
118. Physical Activity Guidelines Advisory Committee: *Physical Activity Guidelines Advisory Committee Report.* Washington, DC, U.S. Department of Health and Human Services, 2008.
119. Biddle SJ, Asare M: Physical activity and mental health in children and adolescents: a review of reviews. *Br J Sports Med* 45(11):886–895, 2011.
120. Cerrillo-Urbina AJ, Garcia-Hermoso A, Sanchez-Lopez M, Pardo-Guijarro MJ, Santos Gomez JL, Martinez-Vizcaino V: The effects of physical exercise in children with attention deficit hyperactivity disorder: a systematic review and meta-analysis of randomized control trials. *Child Care Health Dev* 41(6):779–788, 2015.
121. Gaser C, Schlaug G: Brain structures differ between musicians and non-musicians. *J Neurosci* 23(27):9240–9245, 2003.
122. Bengtsson SL, Nagy Z, Skare S, Forsman L, Forssberg H, Ullen F: Extensive piano practicing has regionally specific effects on white matter development. *Nat Neurosci* 8(9):1148–1150, 2005.
123. Schlaug G, Norton A, Overy K, Winner E: Effects of music training on the child's brain and cognitive development. *Ann N Y Acad Sci* 1060:219–230, 2005.
124. Hudziak JJ, Albaugh MD, Ducharme S, et al.: Cortical thickness maturation and duration of music training: health-promoting activities shape brain development. *J Am Acad Child Adolesc Psychiatry* 53(11):1153–1161, 1161.e1151–1152, 2014.
125. Hyde KL, Lerch J, Norton A, et al.: The effects of musical training on structural brain development: a longitudinal study. *Ann N Y Acad Sci* 1169:182–186, 2009.
126. Rauscher FH, Zupan MA: Classroom keyboard instruction improves kindergarten children's spatial-temporal performance: a field experiment. *Early Child Res Q* 15:215–228, 2000.
127. Bilhartz TD, Bruhn RA, Olson JE: The effect of early musical training on childcognitive development. *J Applied Dev Psychol* 20:615–636, 2000.
128. Cuesta J, Antola LC, Castillo G, et al.: *Proposal for a Loan for a Program to Support the Centro de Accio n Social por la Mu sica, Phase II.* Venezuela, Inter-American Development Bank, 2007.
129. Harmony-project.org. Harmony Project. 2015. Available at: http://www.harmony-project.org. Accessed September 5, 2015.
130. Kraus N, Hornickel J, Strait D, Slater J, Thompson E: Engagement in community music classes sparks neuroplasticity and language development in children from disadvantaged backgrounds. *Front Psychol* 5, 2014.
131. Kraus N, Slater J, Thompson E, et al.: Music enrichment programs improve the neural encoding of speech in at-risk children. *J Neurosci* 34(36):11913–11918, 2014.
132. Kohlmann S, Gierk B, Murray AM, Scholl A, Lehmann M, Lowe B: Base rates of depressive symptoms in patients with coronary heart disease: an individual symptom analysis. *PLoS One* 11(5):e0156167, 2016.
133. Cheruvu VK, Oancea SC: Current depression as a potential barrier to health care utilization in adult cancer survivors. *Cancer Epidemiol* 44:132–137, 2016.
134. Meurs M, Roest AM, Wolffenbuttel BH, Stolk RP, de Jonge P, Rosmalen JG: Association of depressive and anxiety disorders with diagnosed versus undiagnosed diabetes: an epidemiological study of 90,686 participants. *Psychosom Med* 78(2):233–241, 2016.

3.3 ■ NEUROBIOLOGY AND GENETICS

CHAPTER 3.3.1 ■ FROM GENES TO BRAIN: DEVELOPMENTAL NEUROBIOLOGY

HANNA E. STEVENS, JAMES F. LECKMAN, PAUL J. LOMBROSO, AND FLORA M. VACCARINO

Human beings are complex living organisms that can be generally characterized as a species by their appearance and behavior at each point in their life cycle. Many of these characteristics are uniquely human, such as language that facilitates interpersonal communication and permits a meaningful interplay of ideas and emotions. Other characteristics, such as affection and aggression, are less distinctive and place our species as one among many that populate the earth. Scientific advances over the past 150 years clearly indicate that hereditary factors, transmitted from generation to generation, account for much of the variation among and within species. Genetic factors are essential for the general characteristics all humans share and their unfolding during development, which is orchestrated at many levels—from the higher order interplay of the environment and the individual to the microscopic interactions inside cell nuclei. Although the complexities of human existence cannot be reduced simply to the effects of genes, it is inescapable that genetic factors and their regulation over the course of development provide the biologic basis for many of our potentialities and vulnerabilities as human beings (1).

Our genetic endowment as a species is a unique collection of discrete units of heredity (genes and the regulatory regions of our genomes) that are linearly arranged on 46 chromosomes (22 pairs of homologous chromosomes and two sex chromosomes) (Figure 3.3.1.1). Analysis of the data compiled in the human genome project (2,3) has identified approximately 20,000 genes in our genome (4).

It is now clear that genes, canonically defined as those parts of DNA that code for proteins, represent only 1% of the nuclear DNA and are not the only elements that encode information in the nucleus. Until recently, the function of the vast majority of the three billion bases of the human genome outside of genes was not known and was labeled as "junk DNA." The Encyclopedia of DNA Elements (ENCODE) project, through large scale integrative analyses of many different cells types, has undertaken a systematic mapping of all DNA elements and has assigned regulatory functions to 80% of what was previously considered "junk" (5).

Our genes and other DNA elements make us both alike and different from other organisms. Although the precise genetic determinants of our interspecies similarities and differences are largely obscure, it is probable that many of the responsible genetic factors will be identified. For example, sequence differences between human and chimpanzees at specific gene enhancers drive species-specific activity in cranial neural crest cells, leading to emergence of human craniofacial traits (6). Investigators are in the midst of discovering the cascade of genes that have contributed to the remarkable neuroanatomical and functional evolution of the cerebral neocortices across different mammalian species over the past 50 million years (7–10). Intriguingly, variation of gene expression from "junk DNA," rather than variation in protein sequence, is almost certainly the dominant factor in human brain evolution (10). Such changes are thought to have led to the creation of many new combinatorial expression patterns during development and ultimately to the formation of distinct neuronal circuits (11).

Genetic factors also contribute to variations within our species. A large number of physical and psychological traits, including gender, height, and intelligence, are at least partially under genetic control. One need only examine the striking physical and psychological similarities between monozygotic (genetically identical) twins reared apart to recognize the powerful influence of genes in determining who we are (12). Some of these differences, such as gender, are due to differences in the number and type of genes present in the individual. For example, genes on the Y chromosome are present in males. Other variations are due to differences in the linear sequence of nucleotides (polymorphic alleles) of specific genes and DNA regulatory elements that are distributed within the population. While most polymorphisms are "silent" and do not change protein activity, some changes lead to new amino acids in

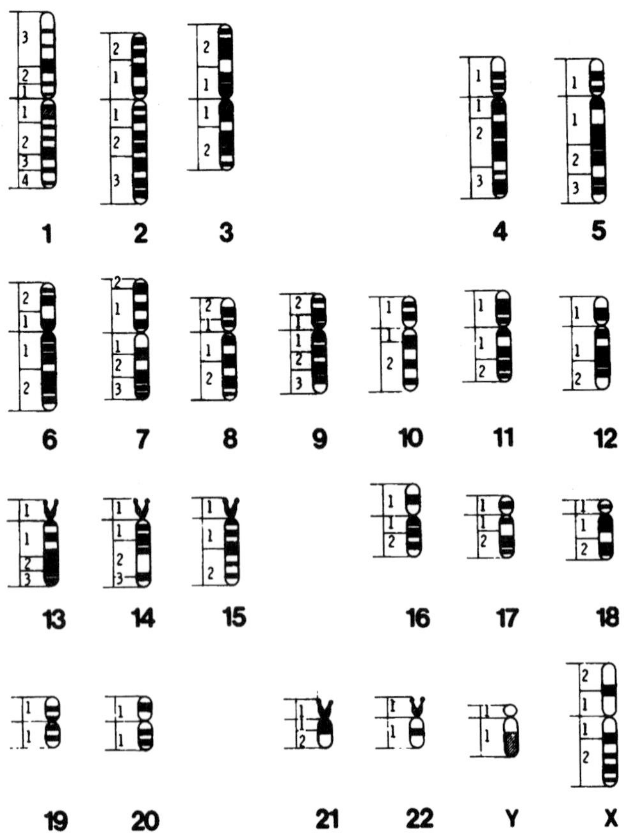

FIGURE 3.3.1.1. Depiction of high-resolution banded human chromosomes. (Adapted from *Yale-HHMI Human Gene Mapping Library Chromosome Plots*, Number 5. New Haven, CT, Howard Hughes Medical Institute, 1989.)

proteins, resulting in differences in the structure, activity, or amount of the protein and contribute to traits such as blood type, height, or eye color. In other cases, polymorphisms may render an individual more susceptible to additional factors, be they genetic or environmental that in turn lead to observable differences. These include sequence changes in gene regulatory regions effecting differential binding of transcription factors and sequence and quantity changes in regulatory RNAs.

The Human Genome Project was very important for its systematic study of allelic variation but also for its discovery of larger variations in DNA among individuals. Variation in the "dosage" or copy number of genes was discovered in all individuals studied (13). These copy number variations (CNVs) occur when a gene or portion of DNA is removed—termed deletions—or when a gene or portion of DNA is added—termed duplications. Deletions and duplication can involve just few nucleotides (called InDels) or encompass thousand to millions of base pairs spanning multiple genes (large CNVs). CNVs actually occur surprisingly frequently, accounting for about 13% of each person's DNA (14). CNVs are mostly inherited and are thought to contribute to both unique traits of our human species—such as having enough copies of a gene for the enzyme amylase to digest the food we eat—and to individual variation. On average, a typical genome varies from the reference human genome at 4 to 5 million sites, of which 99.9% are single nucleotide variants (SNVs) or InDels and about 3,000 are large CNVs (15–18). Some allelic variation and CNVs are so significant that we use the term mutation or disease-associated CNV to signify that the changes will usually lead to disease states such as Rett syndrome, Huntington disease, Marfan syndrome, or sickle cell anemia, disorders in which ameliorating factors will have little effect.

Differences in the expression of genes over the life span are critically important for the physical and cognitive functioning of individual organisms, from *Drosophila* to humans. Not all genes are active at the same time. For example, the hemoglobin genes active during fetal life are different from those that are active in adulthood. These differences are also responsible for the allocation of specific characteristics and functions to specific cells of the body (e.g., for making muscle cells different from brain cells), and are orchestrated by master developmental genes. Differences in gene expression can be also induced by the environment and by experience. However, the influence of these external factors is stronger at specific phases of development such as sensitive periods for learning and social affiliation during juvenile periods.

The next sections, Genes, and Regulation of Gene Function, present a condensed summary of some of the fundamental aspects of the structure and function of genes and gene products. Several excellent general references cover this material in greater depth (19,20).

GENES

Mendel first postulated the existence of discrete hereditary factors or genes in 1865 (21) but their importance was not appreciated until the early 1900s. Genes are arranged linearly on chromosomes that are found in the nuclei of most cells (Figure 3.3.1.2). They are composed of DNA, double helix strings of nucleotides (molecules that contain a sugar moiety, a phosphate group, and a base) that are linked together. Four nucleotides are found in DNA. Two contain purine bases (adenine and guanine) and two contain pyrimidine bases (thymine and cytosine). Hydrogen bonds between complementary base pairs (adenine binds to thymine and guanine to cytosine) (Figure 3.3.1.3) provide the basis for replication of the information, which is essential for all the cells of our body to arise from a single embryonic cell. Since each strand in the double helix is exactly complementary to the other, knowing the sequence

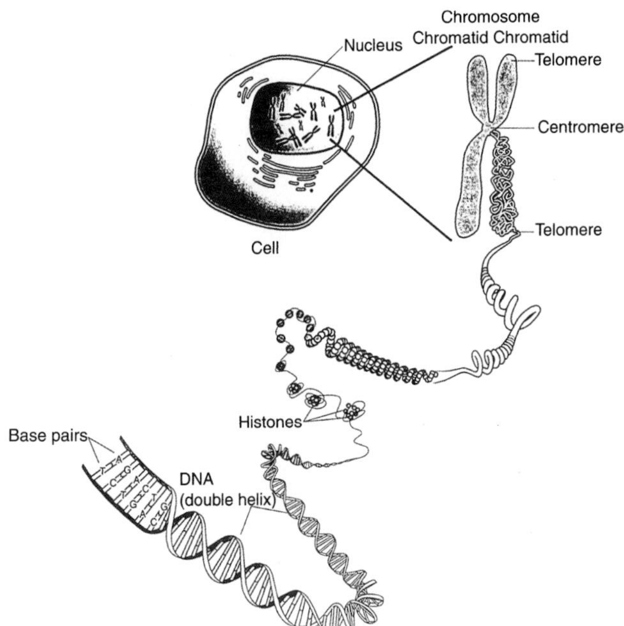

FIGURE 3.3.1.2. The structure of chromosomes. Chromosomes are thread-like packages of DNA in the nucleus of a cell. This drawing also depicts a diagram of the DNA double helix in its common form showing the orientation of the two complementary strands and the wrapping of DNA around histone cores. (Adapted from the *Glossary of Genetic Terms* and associated illustrations found on the website of the National Genome Research Institute, 2000.)

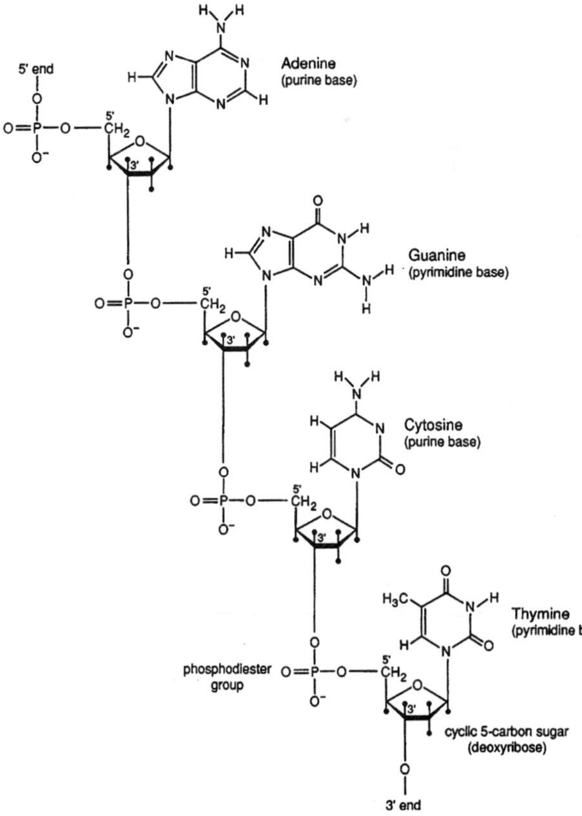

FIGURE 3.3.1.3. Chemical structure of DNA, showing the phosphodiester 3′5′ linkages that connect the nucleotides. (Adapted from Watson JD, Hopkins NH, Roberts JW, et al.: *Molecular Biology of the Cell*. Menlo Park, CA, Benjamin/Cummings, 1987.)

of one strand provides precise knowledge of the sequence of the other.

The sequence of nucleotides determines the specification and order of the amino acids in the protein encoded by the gene. As a consequence, the information contained in DNA provides the instructions for all cellular functions, including growth and cell division, regulation of gene expression, and maintenance of a diversified population of cells that are necessary for the success of a complex organism.

In order for temporary or time-sensitive expression of genes to occur, a more temporary RNA copy of the information is created. A gene is first transcribed, or complementarily copied, from one DNA strand into what is called a pre-RNA transcript. This is then processed to produce the mature messenger RNA (mRNA), typically by bringing together the sequences that actually encode for the eventual protein (exons) and removing the intervening sequences (introns) that do not contain coding sequences. Mature mRNA molecules are rapidly transported out of the nucleus, where they serve as the template for protein synthesis.

The translation of a message into a specific amino acid sequence occurs at ribosomes located either in the cytoplasm or attached to the endoplasmic reticulum. The amino acid sequence is determined by the sequence of bases, with sets of three bases constituting a codon that stands for one amino acid. At the ribosome, codons of an mRNA molecule bind to complementary anticodons of transfer RNAs (tRNAs), which then transfer specific amino acids to a growing protein chain, first proposed by Crick et al. (22).

While genes are extremely stable and precisely copied when cells divide, any mistakes that occur could disturb the normal sequence of amino acids in the encoded proteins. There are a number of proteins within the nucleus whose function is to prevent, recognize, and repair errors within the DNA sequence. Very rarely, however, mistakes go uncorrected and will result in *"de novo"* changes in the original nucleotide sequence. Any error in DNA sequence or copy number that is not repaired will result in a somatic mutation in a particular cell, mutation that will be transmitted through that cell's lineage and, if that cell is a progenitor, amplified in many generations of cell division. The majority of such changes do not affect the proteins made as they occur in regions on the DNA molecule that are not involved in encoding proteins. However, changes that occur within the sequence that encodes for protein or within regulatory portions of genes may have functional consequences. First, they may change the enzymatic function or regulation of the protein. Second, if a critical amino acid or gene regulatory region is mutated, there may be dramatic changes in the cell and, ultimately, in the organism. This capacity for change can, if occurring in germline cells and if leading to positive consequences, serve as the basis for evolution.

REGULATION OF GENE FUNCTION

According to some estimates, about 1% of the genome is expressed at a given time in higher eukaryotic cells (20). Regulation of gene function—across development, for tissue specificity or in response to the environment—can occur at any of the many steps required for gene expression (Figure 3.3.1.4). By correlating RNA abundance and processing of a specific gene with the chromatin structure and variation in nucleotide sequence of DNA, it has been demonstrated that most of the variation in gene expression can be explained by sequence or structural changes within non–protein-coding regions of DNA, which in turn change transcription factor binding at enhancers and promoters for that gene. These processes are described in the next two subsections, "transcription factors" and "epigenetic regulation."

The vast regions of DNA that are not genes themselves are one of the newest areas of discovery in genetics. This "Junk" DNA is far from useless, containing multiple different kinds of nucleotide sequences that play fundamental roles in gene regulation, cell function, and development. Furthermore, many mutations associated with psychiatric disorders through genome-wide association studies (GWAS) reside within these regions. The largest component of non–gene-encoding DNA, 62% of the genome, are sequences that are transcribed into RNA molecules of all sizes that are not translated into proteins (23). There are over 70,000 novel elements of this kind, not previously annotated, which outnumber the already known 20,000 or so protein-coding genes (24).

Some types of non–protein-coding RNA have roles that are well understood, including RNA molecules used in translation (transfer RNA and ribosomal RNA, both of which are part of the protein-making machinery). Others have regulatory functions for genes, either in the nucleus through RNA–DNA binding or in the cytoplasm, through RNA–RNA binding. Interestingly, the majority of novel RNAs, particularly those over 200 nucleotides, are cell-type specific. Conversely, less than 10% of the protein-coding genes are cell-type specific (24). Therefore, noncoding RNAs contribute more to cell-line specificity than protein-coding genes and are likely to be more involved in cell fate and cell lineage determination during development.

Still other regions of DNA regulate gene expression. Indeed, a large novel component of the genome uncovered by the ENCODE project is represented by regulatory elements, DNA regions that bind proteins to regulate the extent that a gene is transcribed. Only a small minority of such sites is active in each cell type. Almost all of these regulatory elements are located between introns or between genes (25).

As novel noncoding RNAs and regulatory elements are largely cell-type specific, it is of high interest to discover those involved in brain tissue. In this regard, the PsychENCODE project will begin exploring this landscape of transcription in the human brain, both in normal development and in neuropsychiatric disorders (10,26).

Transcription Factors

Transcription of a gene into mRNA is initiated by the binding of RNA polymerase II and a complex of regulatory proteins termed transcription factors to the regulatory region of a gene, termed the promoter. Regulatory regions are usually found immediately upstream of the transcriptional start site. Other highly conserved DNA sequences have been identified that either "enhance" or "repress" the transcription of target genes. These sequences, called "enhancers," are usually found near the regulatory promoter region or in further upstream regions of DNA. These allow the RNA polymerase II complex to bind more, or less, efficiently and thus modulate transcription of the gene. In this way, specific sets of genes are expressed while others are repressed, depending on the precise mixture of enhancers, repressors, and transcription factors present in the cell. It is now emerging that mammalian corticogenesis involves a high level of coordination in the expression of transcription factors and other regulatory elements across multiple developmental pathways (10). Mutations in nucleotide sequence that occur within the promoter and/or enhancer regions of genes could have a dramatic effect on the expression of the encoded protein by disrupting the binding sites of the transcriptional machinery. Indeed, SNVs that influence gene expression and splicing patterns have been shown to fall within regulatory elements in the genome (27).

There are several classes of DNA-binding proteins that regulate transcription. The best characterized contain conserved

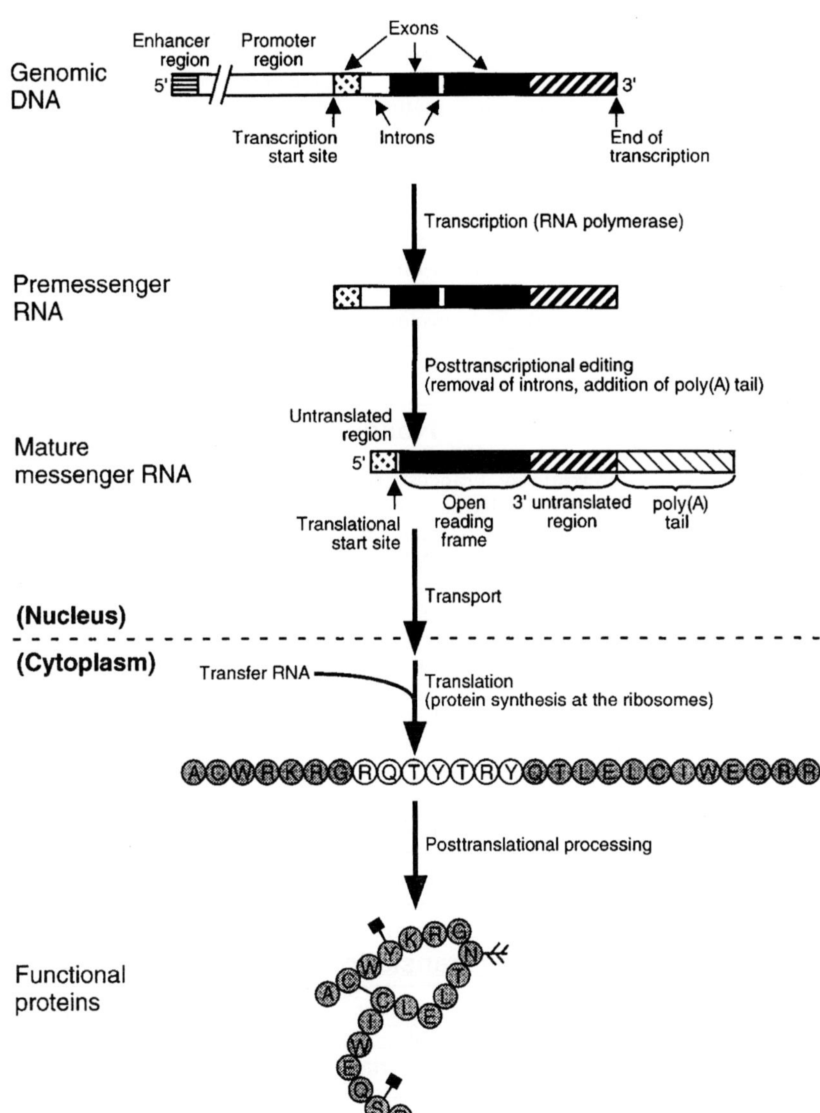

FIGURE 3.3.1.4. Sequence of events leading to gene expression. A protein-coding gene comprises a stretch of genomic DNA that contains instructions for making the protein, as well as adjacent control regions—promoters and enhancers—where the gene's trans criptional mechanism is switched on or off. The promoter region is the site at which RNA polymerase II binds and initiates transcription. Enhancer regions may be thousands of base pairs distant from the promoter. Transcription of the gene into mRNA may be either stimulated or inhibited by transcription factors that bind to promoter and enhancer regions. The mRNA formed by transcription is spliced to remove introns and processed within the cell nucleus to produce mRNAs that are exported to the cytoplasm for translation into protein. Some proteins go through post-translational modification to become biologically active. The four examples depicted include: cleavage of precursor proteins, conformational change through covalent cysteine–cysteine (C–C) bonds, phosphorylation of serine (S), threonine (T), or tyrosine (Y) (*black squares*), and glycosylation of asparagine (N, *branching motif*).

amino acid regions that bind to specific enhancer or promoter sequences. For example, *homeodomain* transcription factors have a highly conserved 60-amino acid region that binds to specific DNA sequences in the regulatory regions of multiple genes that encode for proteins required during development (28). Others known as *zinc fingers* and *leucine zippers* also bind to DNA regulatory sequences within promoters and enhancers and regulate transcription (29,30). It is interesting to note that the discovery of the structure of these endogenous molecules and other molecules in bacteria has itself led to further discovery of research tools (Zinc finger, TALEN, and CRISPR/cas nucleases) that have been used to change or disrupt gene sequences in zebrafish, rodents, and cultured human cells in order to study their function (31,32).

Epigenetic Regulation

Another major mechanism by which genes are regulated is through "epigenetic" mechanisms—literally changing structures "around" the DNA sequence. This generally means changes in the three-dimensional structure and organization of DNA, which determines the portions that are "open" to bind regulatory RNA and transcription factors, and the portions that are excluded from transcription. The epigenetic "silencing" of genes can occur through enzymes adding or removing methyl or acetyl groups from the histones around which DNA is coiled. Another silencing mechanism occurs through addition of methyl groups to DNA itself. Repression of gene expression in this manner is remarkably efficient. For example, changes in expression of globin or growth factor genes due to epigenetic regulation can result in ratios of 1:10,000,000 or more of RNAs in cells repressing these genes compared with those where these genes are actively transcribed (33,34).

Histone methylation and acetylation have a direct impact on the compactness of the DNA/histone complexes. In normal transcription, histone acetylation removes the electrical charge that attracts DNA to the histone and causes an unwinding of the DNA that permits the transcriptional machinery to access the DNA. Consequently, factors that activate histone acetylases promote gene transcription and those that activate histone deacetylases repress gene transcription. Histone methylation is a more complex mechanism that may either promote or repress gene transcription depending on exactly where the histones are methylated. Both processes are critical for the regulation of genes that play specific roles at different time points in development.

Within the promoters of most genes, DNA methylation can occur in "CpG islands" (DNA sequences rich in C + G nucleotides). Cytosine is the only nucleotide that can be replaced with a methylated version. Typically methylation of DNA in a CpG island will prevent activation of a promoter and therefore prevent transcription of a gene. Methyl-CpG–binding protein (Mecp2) binds to methylated CpG dinucleotides in the mammalian genome and recruits repressors (35,36). In addition, Mecp2 associates with DNA methyltransferases (37), which inhibit transcription via methylation of DNA. Repression of transcription via Mecp2 and associated proteins has emerged as an important factor in two neurodevelopmental disorders, Rett and fragile X syndrome (38) (see Chapter 3.3.3 for a more detailed examination of these syndromes).

Epigenetic regulation may also involve the methylation of cytosines within a gene itself. The exact role of this epigenetic modification is currently unknown but one possible role for methylation of gene exons may be to determine what exons are included and the eventual splicing of the gene transcript (39).

DNA in somatic tissue is characterized by a bimodal pattern of methylation, which is established through a series of developmental events (40). Very early in development, most DNA is unmethylated, but after implantation, a wave of *de novo* methylation modifies most of the genome, excluding the majority of CpG islands. These genomic methylation patterns are broadly maintained during the life of the organism with each replication of chromosomes during cell division. As developmental events occur, specific needs for gene silencing or activation will result in changes to the methylation of promoter regions. These developmental processes also interact with methylation change from experience and even those inherited from either parent (discussed in later section: The Role of Early Life Experience) (41,42).

Methylation can also contribute to another type of "gene dosage" control, which is a crucial process in the regulation of genes. One example is the early coordinated inactivation of one of the two X chromosomes in women. Genes may be unexpressed due to genomic *imprinting,* which means repression. Imprinting is a process that occurs normally for some classes of gene loci by which the methylation of either the maternal or the paternal locus results in only one of the two inherited copies being expressed (43,44). This process on occasion has been associated with disease when the silencing of one of an individual's alleles unmasks problems that might otherwise be compensated in the other allele. One example of this concerns two distinctively different developmental disorders, Prader–Willi and Angelman syndrome, caused by differential imprinting of the same region of the maternal or paternal chromosome 15 (see Chapter 3.3.3 for a further discussion of imprinting).

Posttranscriptional Regulation

Transcribed mRNA typically goes through a number of modifications before it leaves the nucleus. As described above, pre-RNA molecules are spliced to form a mature message containing the sequence of nucleotides that encode the amino acids that form the protein. Multiple different splice sites can be present within a pre-RNA transcript and allow for the exons of the gene to be brought together in different combinations, sometimes excluding one or more exons. This results in alternative splicing into several different mRNAs. In this way, a single gene may produce similar proteins that differ in certain critical amino acid regions, or domains. These proteins may have different enzymatic functions or binding affinities for target proteins. Alternatively spliced messages are enriched within the central nervous system (CNS), where the different exon combinations may be expressed at different developmental periods (45). For example, one version of a protein may only be expressed during embryonic development or may be targeted to the nucleus to regulate gene transcription. An alternatively spliced adult form may have a novel domain that targets it to the synapse, where it participates in specific signaling pathways.

Another gene regulatory mechanism involves the addition of long stretches of adenine nucleotides, the poly(A) tail, to the mRNA message prior to its being shuttled out of the nucleus. The stability of a mature mRNA is a critical determinant of how many copies of a protein will be synthesized by the ribosomal apparatus. Certain base sequences in the message as well as the poly(A) tail are thought to influence the stability of many mRNA molecules and their rate of degradation. Translation of mRNA to protein can also be modified through the regulation of RNA-binding proteins necessary for translation. Mutations in proteins that underlie translation can lead to a number of developmental disorders including fragile X syndrome (46).

Noncoding RNAs

Interestingly, Frances Crick et al. hypothesized 70 years ago that RNA molecules themselves would be natural regulators of other RNAs due to their biochemical structure. However, the role of noncoding RNA molecules as regulators of mRNAs was not confirmed until the early 2000s (47).

There are two main classes of noncoding RNA, the long noncoding RNA (lncRNA) described above, which are larger than 200 nucleotides and mostly act in the nucleus, and the microRNAs. The latter are complementary in sequence to mRNAs, bind to mRNAs, and prevent them from being translated into proteins. The importance of these molecules in brain development is demonstrated by one prominent example: mutations of the Dicer gene, which codes for an enzyme involved in microRNA processing. Without functional Dicer gene products, microRNAs in general cannot be produced and multiple aspects of brain development are abnormal (48).

Posttranslational Modifications

Once a protein has been formed, it often undergoes further modification that will control how it contributes to overall cell function. One important posttranslational modification is termed phosphorylation, and refers to the addition of a phosphate group to the amino acids serine, threonine, or tyrosine on target proteins. The addition of this bulky negatively charged group often leads to a conformational change in the shape of a protein, with a previously hidden domain now exposed and the activity or intracellular localization of the protein changed (e.g., translocation from the cytoplasm to the nucleus).

Another posttranslational modification is the addition of a ubiquitin peptide to specific lysine residues on a target protein. Addition of a single ubiquitin molecule (monoubiquitination) may regulate the subcellular localization of a protein or its state of activity. The addition of a string of ubiquitin molecules to a lysine residue (polyubiquitination) targets the protein for degradation by the proteasome; this can rapidly decrease the levels of a protein. For example, many proteins in the synaptic compartment need to be degraded for the development of synaptic strengthening between neurons.

There are additional posttranslational modifications that can occur. The crosslinking of sulfhydryl groups in two cysteine residues of a protein allows them to covalently bond together and stabilize the protein as it folds into a final tertiary structure. The tertiary structure of a protein often determines its activity level. Several other chemical modifications also occur, such as the glycosylation of the amino acid asparagine, the acetylation of the NH2 terminal amino acids, or the hydroxylation of proline and lysine residues. Glycosylation can change protein location, structure, and activity (20).

The removal of amino acids from a protein is another posttranslational modification. For example, neuropeptides like dynorphin are formed from the cleavage of precursor proteins at specific sites. Intriguingly, differential processing of prodynorphin, the initial dynorphin protein, in different tissues is commonplace, so that the form of dynorphin found in the anterior lobe of the pituitary is different from the form of dynorphin found in the neurointermediate lobe (49).

MICROENVIRONMENTAL INFLUENCES ON DEVELOPMENT

Growth factors are naturally occurring substances that regulate a variety of processes including cellular growth, proliferation, and differentiation (50,51). Growth factors typically act as signaling molecules between cells and have been implicated in a broad range of developmental processes in the CNS in which cell specification, growth, migration, and survival have to be coordinated across cell and tissue compartments.

For example, in early embryonic development, fibroblast growth factors (FGFs), WNT, bone morphogenetic proteins (BMPs), and sonic hedgehog (Shh), synthesized within the neural tube and/or diffusing from adjacent nonneural structures, determine the anteroposterior and dorsoventral identity of cells and subregions (52). The same factors are also critical for other aspects of brain growth. For example, basic fibroblast growth factor (FGF2) and other FGF family members, acting primarily through the FGF receptor 1 and FGFR2, are required for the growth of the hippocampus (53) and cerebral cortex (54) by regulating cell proliferation and neurogenesis (55–57). In postnatal development, different growth factor families, particularly neurotrophins which include brain-derived neurotrophic factor (BDNF), participate in the activity-dependent pruning of connections and synapses (58,59), processes underlying learning and memory (60). Thus, growth factors are required for both structural development and CNS functioning (61).

Growth factors are produced often in only minute amounts. Neurons compete for the small amounts of trophic factors present through receptors on their outer membranes. These receptors have an extracellular portion that binds to the growth factor and an intracellular domain that passes along the signal (Figure 3.3.1.5). The intracellular domains are

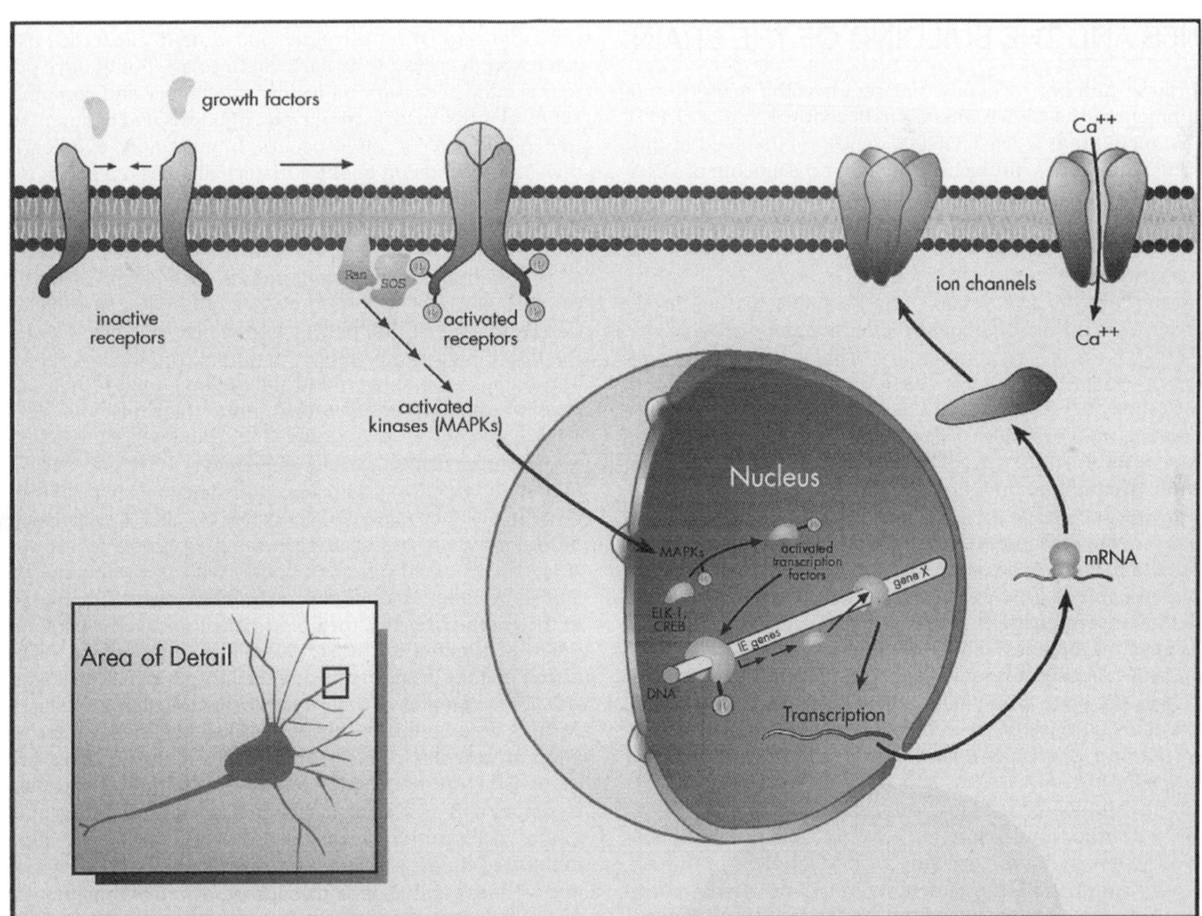

FIGURE 3.3.1.5. Signal transduction and the action of growth factors. Growth factors generate signals in a cell by binding to specific receptors on the plasma surface and initiating transcription, leading to the transcription and translation of proteins needed at that moment. Two molecules of a growth factor are shown binding to their receptor. The receptors are transmembrane tyrosine kinases receptors that associate with each other after ligand binding and phosphorylate each other at regulatory tyrosine residues. In their phosphorylated state, the receptors attract other signaling proteins, including the adapter protein SOS that activates the enzyme, Ras. The newly formed complex of proteins activates several kinase pathways, one of which is shown here (MAPKs). In this pathway, transcription factors (e.g., Elk-1, Jun) are activated by phosphorylation, often within the nucleus, and rapidly initiate the transcription of genes, some of which are themselves transcription factors (immediate early, or IE, genes). The IE transcription factors initiate transcription of additional genes, and their mRNA messages are transported out of nucleus and translated into proteins, such as the ion channels shown. In this example, an ion channel is being synthesized and leads to an increased level of the second messenger, Ca^{2+}. (Adapted from Vaccarino FM, Lombroso PJ: Growth factors. *J Am Acad Child Adol Psychiatry* 37:789–790, 1998.)

protein kinases that regulate themselves and other proteins through their phosphorylating actions. This generates a phosphorylation cascade, recruiting other proteins that are often themselves phosphorylated by the receptors, ultimately leading to the activation of transcription factors and the transcription of specific sets of genes. One of the best-studied signaling pathways is called "mitogen-activated protein kinase" (MAPK).

The cascade of signals that growth factors initiate promote the growth, differentiation, and long-term survival of cells and the synaptic plasticity underlying learning during development. It is not surprising that mutations in some of these receptor proteins disrupt normal intracellular signaling, leading to a number of developmental disorders affecting the structure and function of the CNS (62,63).

Other molecules such as hormones (i.e., thyroid hormone) and immune factors (i.e., cytokines) are present in the systemic environment and may have more distant sources than brain intrinsically produced growth factors. However, little is known about how these factors play a role in the genetic regulation of brain development and research is ongoing to determine their importance in the developing brain.

GENES AND THE BUILDING OF THE BRAIN

The precise number of genes that regulate the growth and development of the CNS is unknown. Recently, Kang et al. (11) have estimated that at least ~15,000 genes are involved in this task. This figure does not include noncoding elements of DNA or constitutively expressed genes that maintain the basic functions of cellular life, including the regulation of the cell cycle, production of subcellular organelles, and maintenance of the cellular structure.

The process of development is a heritable feature of all organisms. The unfolding of gene expression must provide virtually all of the information necessary to guide the orderly succession of events that will transform portions of the fertilized egg into a fully developed CNS. The morphogenesis of the nervous system involves at least five major genetically regulated processes: the birth of specific cell types, their migration to their final destination, their growth, the development of neural connections, and cell death (64). A fundamental understanding of these processes requires precise knowledge of: (a) the developmental information relevant to the CNS that is encoded in the human genome, (b) how this information is regulated and utilized in "morphogenetic" time and space, and (c) how the products of these genes endow the differentiating and differentiated cells of the embryonic CNS with their functional characteristics. Although we remain largely ignorant of the critical determinants of these processes, remarkable progress toward understanding them has been made during the past three decades (65).

Genetic studies of the development of the CNS in flies, worms, and other model systems have recently been complemented by new methods for studying development in human cells, confirming that fundamental processes about genes and development also occur in humans. About 8 years ago, a method for studying development in human cells not derived from embryos was introduced, namely induced pluripotent stem cells (iPSCs). The breakthrough that began this line of research was the discovery that a handful of transcription factors could "reprogram" a cell from its mature, differentiated state to an immature pluripotent state (66). This method has been now used in an explosion of research on human cellular development but more critically for an understanding of disease, using skin cells or white blood cells reprogrammed from patients. The iPSC approach provides the ability to closely examine, manipulate, and perhaps even try to rescue the cellular development that goes awry in a person with a specific disease. In the case where known mutations have led to disease, such as Huntington disease, the iPSC approach may show the precise ways cells are affected and provide a model in which molecular treatments can be tested (67). In cases where a disease has an unknown etiology, such as autism spectrum disorders, the iPSC approach may help uncover specific causes (68). For example, the study of iPSCs from patients with autism spectrum disorders with macrocephaly has demonstrated that abnormal neuronal proliferation and differentiation likely occurs in patients and involves abnormally high levels of the transcription factor FOXG1 and altered activity of the genes it regulates (69). Research efforts with iPSCs represent a large part of the fertile ground upon which gene-based discoveries with promise for developmental disorders can be explored and brought to fruition.

Spatial Differentiation and Determination of Specific Cell Lineages

The creation of specific cell types requires the production of massive numbers of cells while maintaining a blueprint of the entire CNS, all guided by genes, their transcription, translation, and regulation through biosynthetic capacities of cells. Interestingly, cells of the early embryo are not mature enough to make the necessary molecular machinery and contain thousands of mRNAs formed during oogenesis and dormant within the egg until fertilization occurs. Interestingly, even early cell division depends on enough maternally derived cyclin protein to trigger mitosis (70). In some species, the set of maternal genes constitutes the majority of all genomic loci active during ontogeny (71).

Throughout the important phases of cell division in the CNS primordium, two important classes of highly conserved genes determine the fundamental tridimensional organization of the developing brain: segmentation and homeotic genes (72). These genes are clustered in the genome where their relative chromosomal positions correspond to their relative expression throughout the body and the CNS (Figure 3.3.1.6). Acting as transcription factors, vertebrate versions of these genes such as *engrailed, wingless,* and *distalless* organize the transcription of other genes that establish distinctive cellular phenotypes of the different axes of the brain (i.e., rostral–caudal, dorsal–ventral) (73,74). This occurs in conjunction with morphogens such as FGFs and Shh. Other regulators of early developmental events in the cerebral cortex, including Notch and FGF signaling and the downstream Hes transcription factors, determine the switch of cell identity from a neuroepithelial to a radial glial stem cell (75). The evolution of the human brain to such a large size and with its large number of neurons likely depends on the generation of neurons from radial glial neural stem cells, a process regulated by transcription factors including Pax6 and the Neurogenins (76) as well as posttranslational regulation through ubiquitin ligase that degrade proteins determining stem cell identity (77). The intricate cascade of genetic and molecular events that lead to the development of the mammalian CNS is one of the most exciting stories in developmental neuroscience.

Not surprisingly, defects in the human homologues of homeodomain transcription factors and growth factor genes are being recognized with increasing frequency as a cause of cortical malformations due to aberrant neuronal proliferation and differentiation (78). Examples of this phenomenon are dystonia (79) and intellectual disability associated with schizencephaly or other disorders of cortical formation (80–82).

Finally, it is now well established that neurogenesis occurs in adults as well as in the prenatal period. New neurons have been identified that originate in the hippocampal subgranular zone and then migrate to the dentate gyrus, where they extend axons, and become functionally active (83).

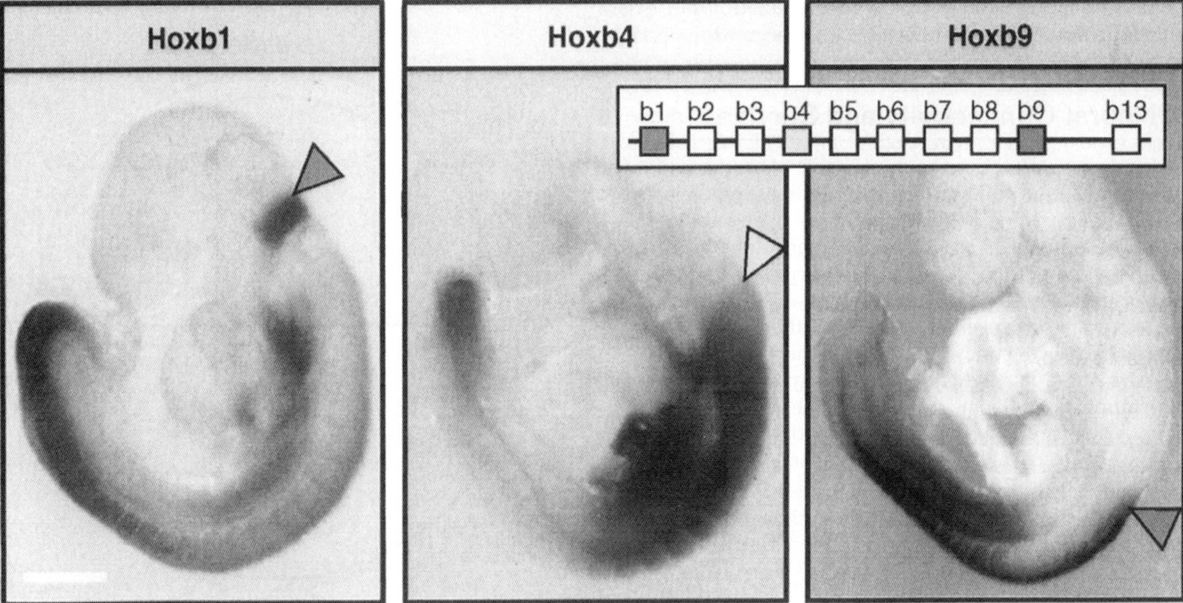

FIGURE 3.3.1.6. Homeodomain-containing genes and their expression in the neural axis. Hox gene expression in the mouse embryo. The three panels show lateral views of 9.5-day-old mouse embryos stained with antibodies specific for the protein products of *Hoxb1*, *Hoxb4*, and *Hoxb9* genes. (Adapted from Wolpert L, Beddington J, Brockes J, et al.: *Principles of Development*. Oxford, Oxford University Press, 103, 1998.)

Migration of Neurons and Microglia

The early embryonic development of the nervous system is characterized in part by the migration of populations of neurons and the immune cells of the brain, microglia. Examples of this phenomenon include the migration of neural crest cells to form elements of the peripheral nervous system (autonomic and sensory ganglia, glial cells, and adrenomedullary cells) and the migration of neurons born within the ventricular zone to their final destination within the cortical laminae. A range of factors mediate these events, and some have been identified, including proteins that contribute to inherent directional preferences, chemotaxis, and differential adhesion of cells as they migrate (84).

In the case of corticogenesis, it has been established that, as glutamatergic projection neurons are produced, they migrate along radial glial guides that stretch between the ventricular surface and outer cortical surface (85). Cytoskeletal proteins, molecular motors, and adhesion molecules are necessary for this migratory process to occur (86,87). One example is the extracellular glycoprotein reelin, which is secreted by interneurons in the outermost cortical and hippocampal marginal zone, and whose deficiency results in aberrant migratory patterns and layering of glutamate projection neurons in cerebral cortex and hippocampus (as is seen in the "reeler" mouse mutant) (88). Another example is the microtubule-binding protein doublecortin, which is selectively expressed by newly generated, migrating neurons. Cortical neurons are unable to complete their migration when doublecortin expression is decreased in mouse models (89) and in humans with doublecortin loss of function mutations. Inborn mutations in the doublecortin gene and other genes that govern neuronal migration have been implicated in a number of human disorders, including X-linked lissenencephaly, focal pachypolymicrogyria, and the "double-cortex" syndrome (90) (see Chapter 3.3.3). Isolated cortical dysplasia, which are patches of cortical neurons with abnormal layering, have been found in autism spectrum disorders (91). In many instances, the genes responsible for the abnormal migration have not yet been identified (92).

A second type of migration has been described, which is independent from radial glial cell guides, and involves the rapid "tangential" movement of GABAergic neurons from their site of origin in the medial, lateral, and caudal ganglionic eminences to the cerebral cortex, hippocampus, basal ganglia, and olfactory bulb (93,94). The gene Arx plays an important role in GABAergic progenitor migration and mutations of Arx are known to cause several different developmental brain disorders including cortical dysplasia (95). An abnormal number and location of GABAergic cells in prefrontal regions of the cortex is considered the most replicated biologic abnormality in schizophrenia (96), and an abnormal distribution of GABAergic neurons has been also found in severe cases of Tourette syndrome and possibly other hyperactivity disorders (97,98). Hence, the regulation of tangential migration, which is the focus of considerable attention in current neuroscience research, may turn out to be of fundamental importance for the pathogenesis of common neuropsychiatric disorders.

Another important component of early developing brains are microglial cells. Microglial progenitors migrate after generation from myeloid precursors in the yolk sac to the embryonic neuroepithelium (99). Although microglia are the resident macrophages of the brain that are constantly scavenging the CNS for damaged neurons, plaques, and infectious agents, they also play an important role in neural circuit formation. Indeed, they have now been shown to express and secrete immune-related signaling molecules that alter synaptic transmission and plasticity even in the absence of inflammation (100). Furthermore, throughout life the microglia have been shown to respond to immune signals from the periphery and from within the brain leading to changes in the strength of synaptic connections between neurons, even altering the activity-dependent changes that are required for learning and memory. Remarkably, PET neuroimaging studies and postmortem human brain analyses have provided clear evidence for aberrant microglial activation in a number of disorders, including Tourette syndrome (101,102), and autism (103,104). Indeed there is mounting evidence that neuroinflammation may well play an important role in a number of developmental neuropsychiatric disorders including autism and schizophrenia (105).

Neural Connectivity and Survival

Developing nerve cells have the remarkable characteristic of being able to maintain contact with literally thousands of other nerve cells by extending cellular processes over substantial distances. These contacts are of crucial importance in establishing and maintaining the functional integrity of the nervous system. These processes initially develop by way of local extension and retraction of specialized areas on the surface of the neurons called growth cones. A variety of external signals regulate the formation, maintenance, and/or degradation of these neuronal connections, including mechanical guides, differential adhesiveness including interactions with astroglial cells, the influence of electrical fields, and interaction with gradients of trophic substances (84,106,107).

Once neuronal processes reach their target field, the neurons acquire obligatory trophic dependencies. Target fields contain growth factors such as nerve growth factor (NGF) that bind to the axons projecting to that field and are retrogradely transported to the afferent cell body. A given target field, however, is able to support only a limited number of neurons, and the "extra" neurons are lost. For example, although NGF does not attract sensory nerve fibers to their target fields, it is intimately involved in the target-mediated survival of neurons. Indeed, from the first appearance of the neuronal processes in the target field, there is a marked increase in the rate of transcription of the NGF gene and the amount of NGF in the target field. There is also a rapid appearance of cell surface receptors for NGF on the sensory neurons (mediated by the transcription of the NGF receptor gene) (108).

Genetic factors are likely to play an important facilitatory role in neurite outgrowth and synaptogenesis throughout life. The dynamic equilibrium between neurite outgrowth and the formation of synapses versus neurite pruning and synapse withdrawal may well be a crucial mechanism that allows organisms to modify their behavior or "learn" as a result of experience. Although the precise genetic and molecular mechanisms that underlie these complex processes are not fully understood, one mechanism involves genes that code for molecules involved in neuronal communication. For example, in vitro and in vivo studies have indicated that neurotransmitters that are present in the early developing brain, such as GABA, in addition to their communicative function in mature neural systems, play important roles in the addition and pruning of neural processes and synapse formation (109). The ephrin family of genes is implicated in ensuring that there is accurate interconnectivity between similar topographic maps in different regions of the brain that neuronally represent the outside world (110). Microglia also monitor synaptic activity that leads to changes in neural circuits and the strength of synaptic connections. Indeed, many neurodevelopmental disorders, including Tourette syndrome and autism are associated with immature and anomalous neural circuits (111,112). A number of mouse mutants are also providing valuable insights into the genes, molecules, and mechanisms that mediate the connection of cortical neurons to other cortical and subcortical targets (113).

The Role of Early Life Experience

The development of the nervous system depends on environmental as well as genetic factors. At each level and stage of development, the micro- and macroenvironments of the organism play a crucial role, in part by modulating the epigenetic status of the cell. This means that our ability to separate out the relative contributions of genetic and epigenetic influences is difficult because the genes influence the environment through the production of various proteins and the environment, in turn, alters the expression of genes (Figure 3.3.1.7).

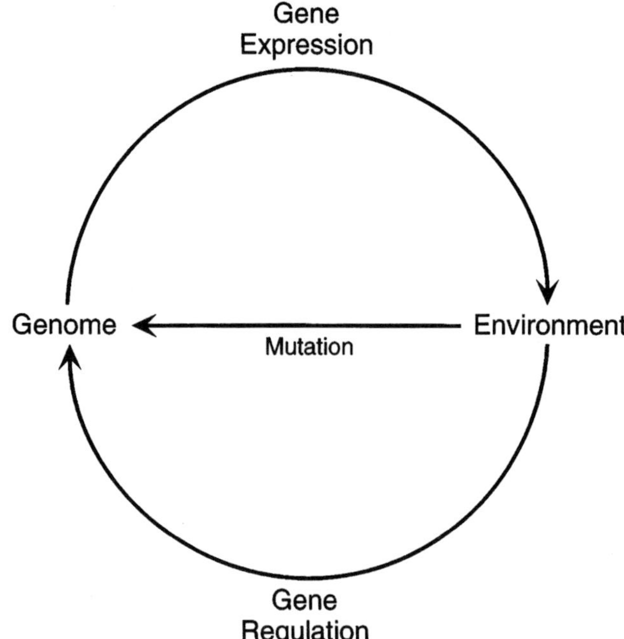

FIGURE 3.3.1.7. Gene–environment interactions. (Adapted from Purves D, Lichtrnan JW. *Principles of Neural Development*. Sunderland, MA, Sinauer, 1985.)

Environmental factors can certainly influence early developmental events. It is well established that drugs, alcohol, altered nutrition (including a lack of oxygen, or hypoxia), and infectious illnesses disrupt the orderly progression of neuronal growth during critical periods of brain development. The situation changes significantly during the latter part of gestation onward as the CNS becomes functionally active. A great deal of experimental evidence has indicated that neuronal activity, triggered by interactions of the organism with its environment, is required for the proliferation of these connections, as well as their later refinement (114,115). Hubel and Wiesel demonstrated that activity from both eyes was necessary to form the normal ocular dominance columns in visual cortex (116). Prior to and immediately following birth, inputs from the eyes make overlapping synaptic contacts in cortex. Through visual activity, there is a progressive segregation of the visual inputs from each eye into adjacent columns, a specific example of activity-dependent plasticity. Deprivation of vision from one eye during early postnatal development has been shown to result in loss of normal vision from the deprived eye, because during this "critical" period, sensory input is crucial for development of visual cortex structure and function. Vision restored later may not be sufficient for a complete "catch-up" in development, and the failure to develop properly segregated columns becomes permanent (117).

While this has traditionally held in humans who did not experience normal visual inputs during their first years of life, such as infants born with either unilateral or bilateral cataracts, some recovery of visual function has now been documented with sufficient time/experience after vision restoration (118,119). However, the importance of early sensitive periods is still clear, since adults may have cataracts for years and regain visual acuity once they are removed.

Recent research has also suggested that development begins earlier than believed, with ocular dominance columns developing before any activity is detectable in the cortex (120). Hence, it appears that experience confirms or modifies rather than establishes cortical architecture. This activity-dependent refinement occurs in many regions of the cortex involved in sensory perception such as the remodeling of cortical regions after amputation of a finger (121). The earlier this occurs, the more plastic is the cortex in remodeling. Regions that used to subserve the amputated finger regress and nearby digits expand their representations into the region. An extreme example of neural plasticity and the capacity for the brain to reorganize connections involves the artificial rewiring of visual projections to the auditory cortex that allows the animal to "see" using its auditory cortex.

A different kind of critical period with distinct types of genetic regulation was discovered in the early 2000s concerning the role of maternal stimuli and pup–mother interactions in shaping the future behavior of the progeny (122). In animal studies, the level of maternal care as measured by licking and grooming by a mother profoundly influenced her female offspring to offer high or low levels of maternal care a generation later. It also established an enduring pattern of stress response in offspring as they matured. The pups raised with more licking showed less stress in response to novel environments (123). These findings are consistent with other studies that have documented the enduring impact of maternal stress in the perinatal period (124,125). Importantly, many of these effects appear to result from environmental effects on gene expression in limbic regions of the brain. For example, the level of care by the mother regulates the DNA methylation and histone acetylation of the glucocorticoid receptor gene promoter and the entire genome in rodents, non-human primates as well as in our species (126–128). These findings demonstrate that early epigenetic alterations in these neurobiologic systems may alter an individual's vulnerability to later psychopathology, including mood and affective disorders (129). These findings also point to the daunting complexity of neural development given that the epigenetic signatures seen in the periphery are not exactly the same as those seen in the CNS (127).

Finally, it is likely that events in early family life, interactions with peers, and educational opportunities shape the course of development just as surely as the developing individual profoundly influences his or her environment. The developmental perspectives of child psychiatry echo in the study of developmental neurobiology.

FUTURE PROSPECTS

Genetics, epigenetics, and the developmental neurosciences are on the threshold of a new era in which we can study not only the sequence of the human genome but the entire sequenced genome of populations of individuals with particular disorders and even variations in genome and RNA sequences between their cells. This has been possible through astounding advances in molecular technology (130), dropping the price of sequencing a genome below $2,000 and heading still lower. We also have unprecedented tools now to manipulate genetics using silencing RNA constructs, molecular tools such as CRIPSRs and zinc finger nucleases that can produce gene knock outs without the use of transgenic technology (131), and even methods that can target the methylation to specific loci in the DNA (132). Using these tools, the genetic underpinning of neuropsychiatric syndromes can be explored (133,134), models of these diseases successfully created, and treatments based on understanding of their etiologies developed.

The human brain with its 100 billion neurons and its 100 trillion synapses is the most sophisticated computational machine known, about whose self-construction or function we know little. But one thing we do know is that events early in life matter, in part due to the complex layers of genetic and epigenetic influences upon patterns of gene expression. A deeper understanding of the impact of these mechanisms may also set the stage for preventative interventions in our field. One area worthy of pursuit is the refinement and implementation in a sustainable fashion of early childhood education and family support programs of proven value (135). It will also be important to study the mechanisms by which phenotypic traits can be inherited through male or female germlines, as this may well be unique form of adaptation that has occurred over the course of our evolutionary history (41).

Although the scientific, information management, and logistical challenges to understanding the complexity of the human genome vis-à-vis brain development are daunting, they are likely to pale in comparison to the ethical dilemmas to be faced as information about our genetic vulnerability becomes accessible. The ethical problems will multiply as even more potent pharmacologic tools are developed that can influence these developing neurobiologic systems. We also predict that this new knowledge will emphasize the importance of early life events in shaping the CNS and will point the way to the profound and enduring importance of selective early interventions for families at high risk (136,137).

References

1. Leckman JF, Mayes LC: Understanding developmental psychopathology: how useful are evolutionary accounts? *J Am Acad Child Adolesc Psychiatry* 37:1011–1021, 1998.
2. Venter JC, Adams MD, Myers EW, et al.: The sequence of the human genome. *Science* 291:1304–1351, 2001.
3. Lander ES, Linton LM, Birren B, et al.: Initial sequencing and analysis of the human genome. *Nature* 409:860–921, 2001.
4. Clamp M, Fry B, Kamal M, et al.: Distinguishing protein-coding and noncoding genes in the human genome. *Proc Natl Acad Sci U S A* 104: 19428–19433, 2007.
5. ENCODE Project Consortium: An integrated encyclopedia of DNA elements in the human genome. *Nature* 489:57–74, 2012.
6. Prescott SL, Srinivasan R, Marchetto MC, et al.: Enhancer divergence and cis-regulatory evolution in the human and chimp neural crest. *Cell* 163:68–83, 2015.
7. Hoerder-Suabedissen A, Molnar Z: Development, evolution and pathology of neocortical subplate neurons. *Nat Rev Neurosci* 16:133–146, 2015.
8. Sun T, Hevner RF: Growth and folding of the mammalian cerebral cortex: from molecules to malformations. *Nat Rev Neurosci* 15:217–232, 2014.
9. Finlay BL, Uchiyama R: Developmental mechanisms channeling cortical evolution. *Trends Neurosci* 38:69–76, 2015.
10. Reilly SK, Yin J, Ayoub AE, et al.: Evolutionary genomics. Evolutionary changes in promoter and enhancer activity during human corticogenesis. *Science* 347:1155–1159, 2015.
11. Kang HJ, Kawasawa YI, Cheng F, et al.: Spatio-temporal transcriptome of the human brain. *Nature* 478:483–489, 2011.
12. Shields J: *Monozygotic Twins, Brought Up Apart and Brought Up Together; An Investigation into the Genetic and Environmental Causes of Variation in Personality.* London, New York, Oxford University Press, 1962.
13. Feuk L, Carson AR, Scherer SW: Structural variation in the human genome. *Nat Rev Genet* 7:85–97, 2006.
14. Stankiewicz P, Lupski JR: Structural variation in the human genome and its role in disease. *Annu Rev Med* 61:437–455, 2010.
15. Perry GH, Dominy NJ, Claw KG, et al.: Diet and the evolution of human amylase gene copy number variation. *Nat Genet* 39:1256–1260, 2007.
16. Abyzov A, Mariani J, Palejev D, et al.: Somatic copy number mosaicism in human skin revealed by induced pluripotent stem cells. *Nature* 492:438–442, 2012.
17. 1000 Genomes Project Consortium, Auton A, Brooks LD, et al.: A global reference for human genetic variation. *Nature* 526:68–74, 2015.
18. Sudmant PH, Rausch T, Gardner EJ, et al.: An integrated map of structural variation in 2,504 human genomes. *Nature* 526:75–81, 2015.
19. Alberts B: *Molecular Biology of the Cell.* 6th ed. New York, Garland Science, Taylor & Francis Group, 2015.
20. Watson JD: *Molecular Biology of the Gene.* 7th ed. Boston, Pearson/CSH Press, 2014.
21. Mendel G, Tschermak E: *Versuche über Pflanzenhybriden. Zwei abhandlungen. (1865 und 1869.).* Leipzig, W. Engelmann, 1901.
22. Crick FH, Barnett L, Brenner S, Watts-Tobin RJ: General nature of the genetic code for proteins. *Nature* 192:1227–1232, 1961.
23. Guil S, Esteller M: RNA-RNA interactions in gene regulation: the coding and noncoding players. *Trends Biochem Sci* 40:248–256, 2015.
24. Djebali S, Davis CA, Merkel A, et al.: Landscape of transcription in human cells. *Nature* 489:101–108, 2012.

25. Thurman RE, Rynes E, Humbert R, et al.: The accessible chromatin landscape of the human genome. *Nature* 489:75–82, 2012.
26. PsychENCODE Consortium, Akbarian S, Liu C, et al.: The PsychENCODE project. *Nat Neurosci* 18:1707–1712, 2015.
27. GTEx Consortium: Human genomics. The Genotype-Tissue Expression (GTEx) pilot analysis: multitissue gene regulation in humans. *Science* 348:648–660, 2015.
28. McGinnis W, Levine MS, Hafen E, Kuroiwa A, Gehring WJ: A conserved DNA sequence in homoeotic genes of the Drosophila Antennapedia and bithorax complexes. *Nature* 308:428–433, 1984.
29. Landschulz WH, Johnson PF, McKnight SL: The leucine zipper: a hypothetical structure common to a new class of DNA binding proteins. *Science* 240:1759–1764, 1988.
30. Miller J, McLachlan AD, Klug A: Repetitive zinc-binding domains in the protein transcription factor IIIA from Xenopus oocytes. *EMBO J* 4:1609–1614, 1985.
31. Lin SC, Chang YY, Chan CC: Strategies for gene disruption in Drosophila. *Cell Biosci* 4:63, 2014.
32. Hendel A, Bak RO, Clark JT, et al.: Chemically modified guide RNAs enhance CRISPR-Cas genome editing in human primary cells. *Nat Biotechnol* 33:985–989, 2015.
33. Groudine M, Weintraub H: Rous sarcoma virus activates embryonic globin genes in chicken fibroblasts. *Proc Natl Acad Sci U S A* 72:4464–4468, 1975.
34. Ivarie RD, Schacter BS, O'Farrell PH: The level of expression of the rat growth hormone gene in liver tumor cells is at least eight orders of magnitude less than that in anterior pituitary cells. *Mol Cell Biol* 3:1460–1467, 1983.
35. Nan X, Ng HH, Johnson CA, et al.: Transcriptional repression by the methyl-CpG-binding protein MeCP2 involves a histone deacetylase complex. *Nature* 393:386–389, 1998.
36. Jones PL, Veenstra GJ, Wade PA, et al.: Methylated DNA and MeCP2 recruit histone deacetylase to repress transcription. *Nat Genet* 19:187–191, 1998.
37. Kimura H, Shiota K: Methyl-CpG-binding protein, MeCP2, is a target molecule for maintenance DNA methyltransferase, Dnmt1. *J Biol Chem* 278:4806–4812, 2003.
38. Amir RE, Van den Veyver IB, Wan M, Tran CQ, Francke U, Zoghbi HY: Rett syndrome is caused by mutations in X-linked MECP2, encoding methyl-CpG-binding protein 2. *Nat Genet* 23:185–188, 1999.
39. Singer M, Kosti I, Pachter L, Mandel-Gutfreund Y: A diverse epigenetic landscape at human exons with implication for expression. *Nucleic Acids Res* 43:3498–3508, 2015.
40. Greally JM, State MW: Genetics of childhood disorders: XIII. Genomic imprinting: the indelible mark of the gamete. *J Am Acad Child Adolesc Psychiatry* 39:532–535, 2000.
41. Yuan TF, Li A, Sun X, et al.: Transgenerational inheritance of paternal neurobehavioral phenotypes: stress, addiction, ageing and metabolism. *Mol Neurobiol* 53(9):6367–6376, 2015.
42. Fernandez-Twinn DS, Constancia M, Ozanne SE: Intergenerational epigenetic inheritance in models of developmental programming of adult disease. *Semin Cell Dev Biol* 43:85–95, 2015.
43. Kalsner L, Chamberlain SJ: Prader-Willi, Angelman, and 15q11-q13 duplication syndromes. *Pediatr Clin North Am* 62:587–606, 2015.
44. Sleutels F, Barlow DP: The origins of genomic imprinting in mammals. *Adv Genet* 46:119–163, 2002.
45. Revil T, Gaffney D, Dias C, Majewski J, Jerome-Majewska LA: Alternative splicing is frequent during early embryonic development in mouse. *BMC Genomics* 11:399, 2010.
46. Laggerbauer B, Ostareck D, Keidel EM, Ostareck-Lederer A, Fischer U: Evidence that fragile X mental retardation protein is a negative regulator of translation. *Hum Mol Genet* 10:329–338, 2001.
47. Cheng LC, Tavazoie M, Doetsch F: Stem cells: from epigenetics to microRNAs. *Neuron* 46:363–367, 2005.
48. Giraldez AJ, Cinalli RM, Glasner ME, et al.: MicroRNAs regulate brain morphogenesis in zebrafish. *Science* 308:833–838, 2005.
49. Molineaux CJ, Hassen AH, Rosenberger JG, Cox BM: Response of rat pituitary anterior lobe prodynorphin products to changes in gonadal steroid environment. *Endocrinology* 119:2297–2305, 1986.
50. Chao MV: Neurotrophins and their receptors: a convergence point for many signalling pathways. *Nat Rev Neurosci* 4:299–309, 2003.
51. Poon VY, Choi S, Park M: Growth factors in synaptic function. *Front Synaptic Neurosci* 5:6, 2013.
52. Wilson SW, Rubenstein JL: Induction and dorsoventral patterning of the telencephalon. *Neuron* 28:641–651, 2000.
53. Ohkubo Y, Uchida AO, Shin D, Partanen J, Vaccarino FM: Fibroblast growth factor receptor 1 is required for the proliferation of hippocampal progenitor cells and for hippocampal growth in mouse. *J Neurosci* 24:6057–6069, 2004.
54. Stevens HE, Smith KM, Maragnoli ME, et al.: Fgfr2 is required for the development of the medial prefrontal cortex and its connections with limbic circuits. *J Neurosci* 30:5590–5602, 2010.
55. Raballo R, Rhee J, Lyn-Cook R, Leckman JF, Schwartz ML, Vaccarino FM: Basic fibroblast growth factor (Fgf2) is necessary for cell proliferation and neurogenesis in the developing cerebral cortex. *J Neurosci* 20:5012–5023, 2000.
56. Vaccarino FM, Schwartz ML, Raballo R, et al.: Changes in cerebral cortex size are governed by fibroblast growth factor during embryogenesis. *Nat Neurosci* 2:848, 1999.
57. Rash BG, Lim HD, Breunig JJ, Vaccarino FM: FGF signaling expands embryonic cortical surface area by regulating Notch-dependent neurogenesis. *J Neurosci* 31:15604–15617, 2011.
58. Cabelli RJ, Shelton DL, Segal RA, Shatz CJ: Blockade of endogenous ligands of trkB inhibits formation of ocular dominance columns. *Neuron* 19:63–76, 1997.
59. Gianfranceschi L, Siciliano R, Walls J, et al.: Visual cortex is rescued from the effects of dark rearing by overexpression of BDNF. *Proc Natl Acad Sci U S A* 100:12486–12491, 2003.
60. Klintsova AY, Greenough WT: Synaptic plasticity in cortical systems. *Curr Opin Neurobiol* 9:203–208, 1999.
61. Vaccarino FM, Schwartz ML, Raballo R, Rhee J, Lyn-Cook R: Fibroblast growth factor signaling regulates growth and morphogenesis at multiple steps during brain development. *Curr Top Dev Biol* 46:179–200, 1999.
62. Sweatt JD: Mitogen-activated protein kinases in synaptic plasticity and memory. *Curr Opin Neurobiol* 14:311–317, 2004.
63. Sweatt JD, Weeber EJ, Lombroso PJ: Genetics of childhood disorders: LI. Learning and memory, Part 4: human cognitive disorders and the ras/ERK/CREB pathway. *J Am Acad Child Adolesc Psychiatry* 42:741–744, 2003.
64. Jacobson M, Rao MS: *Developmental Neurobiology*. 4th ed. New York, Kluwer Academic/Plenum, 2005.
65. Nord AS, Pattabiraman K, Visel A, Rubenstein JL: Genomic perspectives of transcriptional regulation in forebrain development. *Neuron* 85:27–47, 2015.
66. Takahashi K, Tanabe K, Ohnuki M, et al.: Induction of pluripotent stem cells from adult human fibroblasts by defined factors. *Cell* 131:861–872, 2007.
67. Zhang N, Bailus BJ, Ring KL, Ellerby LM: iPSC-based drug screening for Huntington's disease. *Brain Res* 1638(Pt A):42–56, 2016.
68. Nestor MW, Phillips AW, Artimovich E, Nestor JE, Hussman JP, Blatt GJ: Human inducible pluripotent stem cells and autism spectrum disorder: emerging technologies. *Autism Res* 9(5):513–535, 2016.
69. Mariani J, Coppola G, Zhang P, et al.: FOXG1-Dependent dysregulation of GABA/Glutamate neuron differentiation in autism spectrum disorders. *Cell* 162:375–390, 2015.
70. O'Farrell PH, Edgar BA, Lakich D, Lehner CF: Directing cell division during development. *Science* 246:635–640, 1989.
71. Watson JD: *Molecular Biology of the Gene*. 6th ed. Cold Spring Harbor, NY, CSHL Press, 2008.
72. Murtha MT, Leckman JF, Ruddle FH: Detection of homeobox genes in development and evolution. *Proc Natl Acad Sci U S A* 88:10711–10715, 1991.
73. Puelles L, Rubenstein JL: Forebrain gene expression domains and the evolving prosomeric model. *Trends Neurosci* 26:469–476, 2003.
74. Joyner AL: Engrailed, Wnt and Pax genes regulate midbrain–hindbrain development. *Trends Genet* 12:15–20, 1996.
75. Martynoga B, Drechsel D, Guillemot F: Molecular control of neurogenesis: a view from the mammalian cerebral cortex. *Cold Spring Harb Perspect Biol* 4(10):pii: a008359, 2012.
76. Nieto M, Schuurmans C, Britz O, Guillemot F: Neural bHLH genes control the neuronal versus glial fate decision in cortical progenitors. *Neuron* 29:401–413, 2001.
77. Zhao X, D' Arca D, Lim WK, et al.: The N-Myc-DLL3 cascade is suppressed by the ubiquitin ligase Huwe1 to inhibit proliferation and promote neurogenesis in the developing brain. *Dev Cell* 17:210–221, 2009.
78. Raymond AA, Fish DR, Sisodiya SM, Alsanjari N, Stevens JM, Shorvon SD: Abnormalities of gyration, heterotopias, tuberous sclerosis, focal cortical dysplasia, microdysgenesis, dysembryoplastic neuroepithelial tumour and dysgenesis of the archicortex in epilepsy. Clinical, EEG and neuroimaging features in 100 adult patients. *Brain* 118(Pt 3):629–660, 1995.
79. Pohlenz J, Dumitrescu A, Zundel D, et al.: Partial deficiency of thyroid transcription factor 1 produces predominantly neurological defects in humans and mice. *J Clin Invest* 109:469–473, 2002.
80. Kato M, Dobyns WB: X-linked lissencephaly with abnormal genitalia as a tangential migration disorder causing intractable epilepsy: proposal for a new term, "interneuronopathy". *J Child Neurol* 20:392–397, 2005.
81. Brunelli S, Faiella A, Capra V, et al.: Germline mutations in the homeobox gene EMX2 in patients with severe schizencephaly. *Nat Genet* 12:94–96, 1996.
82. Stepp ML, Cason AL, Finnis M, et al.: XLMR in MRX families 29, 32, 33 and 38 results from the dup24 mutation in the ARX (Aristaless related homeobox) gene. *BMC Med Genet* 6:16, 2005.
83. Jessberger S, Gage FH: Adult neurogenesis: bridging the gap between mice and humans. *Trends Cell Biol* 24:558–563, 2014.
84. Sanes DH, Harris WA, Reh TA: *Development of the Nervous System*. 2nd ed. Amsterdam, Boston, Elsevier, xiii, 373, 2006.
85. Rakic P: Specification of cerebral cortical areas. *Science* 241:170–176, 1988.
86. Rakic P: Defects of neuronal migration and the pathogenesis of cortical malformations. *Prog Brain Res* 73:15–37, 1988.

87. Gates MA, O'Brien TF, Faissner A, Steindler DA: Neuron-glial interactions during the in vivo and in vitro development of the nigrostriatal circuit. *J Chem Neuroanat* 6:179–189, 1993.
88. Rakic P, Sidman RL: Sequence of developmental abnormalities leading to granule cell deficit in cerebellar cortex of weaver mutant mice. *J Comp Neurol* 152:103–132, 1973.
89. Bai J, Ramos RL, Ackman JB, Thomas AM, Lee RV, LoTurco JJ: RNAi reveals doublecortin is required for radial migration in rat neocortex. *Nat Neurosci* 6:1277–1283, 2003.
90. Walsh CA, Goffinet AM: Potential mechanisms of mutations that affect neuronal migration in man and mouse. *Curr Opin Genet Dev* 10:270–274, 2000.
91. Stoner R, Chow ML, Boyle MP, et al.: Patches of disorganization in the neocortex of children with autism. *N Engl J Med* 370:1209–1219, 2014.
92. Yoshimura K, Hamada F, Tomoda T, Wakiguchi H, Kurashige T: Focal pachypolymicrogyria in three siblings. *Pediatr Neurol* 18:435–438, 1998.
93. Anderson SA, Eisenstat DD, Shi L, Rubenstein JL: Interneuron migration from basal forebrain to neocortex: dependence on Dlx genes. *Science* 278:474–476, 1997.
94. Nadarajah B, Parnavelas JG: Modes of neuronal migration in the developing cerebral cortex. *Nat Rev Neurosci* 3:423–432, 2002.
95. Kato M: Genotype-phenotype correlation in neuronal migration disorders and cortical dysplasias. *Front Neurosci* 9:181, 2015.
96. Lewis DA, Volk DW, Hashimoto T: Selective alterations in prefrontal cortical GABA neurotransmission in schizophrenia: a novel target for the treatment of working memory dysfunction. *Psychopharmacology (Berl)* 174:143–150, 2004.
97. Kleiner-Fisman G, Calingasan NY, Putt M, Chen J, Beal MF, Lang AE: Alterations of striatal neurons in benign hereditary chorea. *Mov Disord* 20:1353–1357, 2005.
98. Kalanithi PS, Zheng W, Kataoka Y, et al.: Altered parvalbumin-positive neuron distribution in basal ganglia of individuals with Tourette syndrome. *Proc Natl Acad Sci U S A* 102:13307–13312, 2005.
99. Arnold T, Betsholtz C: The importance of microglia in the development of the vasculature in the central nervous system. *Vasc Cell* 5:4, 2013.
100. Wu Y, Dissing-Olesen L, MacVicar BA, Stevens B: Microglia: dynamic mediators of synapse development and plasticity. *Trends Immunol* 36:605–613, 2015.
101. Kumar A, Williams MT, Chugani HT: Evaluation of basal ganglia and thalamic inflammation in children with pediatric autoimmune neuropsychiatric disorders associated with streptococcal infection and Tourette syndrome: a positron emission tomographic (PET) study using 11C-[R]-PK11195. *J Child Neurol* 30:749–756, 2015.
102. Lennington JB, Coppola G, Kataoka-Sasaki Y, et al.: Transcriptome analysis of the human striatum in Tourette syndrome. *Biol Psychiatry* 79(5):372–382, 2016.
103. Vargas DL, Nascimbene C, Krishnan C, Zimmerman AW, Pardo CA: Neuroglial activation and neuroinflammation in the brain of patients with autism. *Ann Neurol* 57:67–81, 2005.
104. Morgan JT, Chana G, Pardo CA, et al.: Microglial activation and increased microglial density observed in the dorsolateral prefrontal cortex in autism. *Biol Psychiatry* 68:368–376, 2010.
105. Leckman JF, Vaccarino FM: Editorial commentary: "what does immunology have to do with brain development and neuropsychiatric disorders?" *Brain Res* 1617:1–6, 2015.
106. Guan KL, Rao Y: Signalling mechanisms mediating neuronal responses to guidance cues. *Nat Rev Neurosci* 4:941–956, 2003.
107. Kalil RE, Dubin MW, Scott G, Stark LA: Elimination of action potentials blocks the structural development of retinogeniculate synapses. *Nature* 323:156–158, 1986.
108. Davies AM, Bandtlow C, Heumann R, Korsching S, Rohrer H, Thoenen H: Timing and site of nerve growth factor synthesis in developing skin in relation to innervation and expression of the receptor. *Nature* 326:353–358, 1987.
109. Lipton SA, Kater SB: Neurotransmitter regulation of neuronal outgrowth, plasticity and survival. *Trends Neurosci* 12:265–270, 1989.
110. Torii M, Rakic P, Levitt P: Role of EphA/ephrin-a signaling in the development of topographic maps in mouse corticothalamic projections. *J Comp Neurol* 521:626–637, 2013.
111. Delorme C, Salvador A, Valabregue R, et al.: Enhanced habit formation in Gilles de la Tourette syndrome. *Brain.* 2016;139(Pt 2):605–615.
112. Sahin M, Sur M: Genes, circuits, and precision therapies for autism and related neurodevelopmental disorders. *Science* 350(6263): pii: aab3897, 2015.
113. O'Leary DD, Yates PA, McLaughlin T: Molecular development of sensory maps: representing sights and smells in the brain. *Cell* 96:255–269, 1999.
114. Edelman GM: *Neural Darwinism: The Theory of Neuronal Group Selection.* New York, Basic Books, 1987.
115. Shatz CJ: Impulse activity and the patterning of connections during CNS development. *Neuron* 5:745–756, 1990.
116. Wiesel TN: Postnatal development of the visual cortex and the influence of environment. *Nature* 299:583–591, 1982.
117. Katz LC, Shatz CJ: Synaptic activity and the construction of cortical circuits. *Science* 274:1133–1138, 1996.
118. Takesian AE, Hensch TK: Balancing plasticity/stability across brain development. *Prog Brain Res* 207:3–34, 2013.
119. Ostrovsky Y, Andalman A, Sinha P: Vision following extended congenital blindness. *Psychol Sci* 17:1009–1014, 2006.
120. Crowley JC, Katz LC: Ocular dominance development revisited. *Curr Opin Neurobiol* 12:104–109, 2002.
121. Merzenich MM, Kaas JH, Wall JT, Sur M, Nelson RJ, Felleman DJ: Progression of change following median nerve section in the cortical representation of the hand in areas 3b and 1 in adult owl and squirrel monkeys. *Neuroscience* 10:639–665, 1983.
122. Francis D, Diorio J, Liu D, Meaney MJ: Nongenomic transmission across generations of maternal behavior and stress responses in the rat. *Science* 286:1155–1158, 1999.
123. Meaney MJ: Maternal care, gene expression, and the transmission of individual differences in stress reactivity across generations. *Annu Rev Neurosci* 24:1161–1192, 2001.
124. Ladd CO, Huot RL, Thrivikraman KV, Nemeroff CB, Meaney MJ, Plotsky PM: Long-term behavioral and neuroendocrine adaptations to adverse early experience. *Prog Brain Res* 122:81–103, 2001.
125. Vallee M, MacCari S, Dellu F, Simon H, Le Moal M, Mayo W: Long-term effects of prenatal stress and postnatal handling on age-related glucocorticoid secretion and cognitive performance: a longitudinal study in the rat. *Eur J Neurosci* 11:2906–2916, 1999.
126. McGowan PO, Suderman M, Sasaki A, et al.: Broad epigenetic signature of maternal care in the brain of adult rats. *PLoS One* 6:e14739, 2011.
127. Provencal N, Suderman MJ, Guillemin C, et al.: The signature of maternal rearing in the methylome in rhesus macaque prefrontal cortex and T cells. *J Neurosci* 32:15626–15642, 2012.
128. Provencal N, Suderman MJ, Guillemin C, et al.: Association of childhood chronic physical aggression with a DNA methylation signature in adult human T cells. *PLoS One* 9:e89839, 2014.
129. Maccari S, Krugers HJ, Morley-Fletcher S, Szyf M, Brunton PJ: The consequences of early-life adversity: neurobiological, behavioural and epigenetic adaptations. *J Neuroendocrinol* 26:707–723, 2014.
130. van Dijk EL, Auger H, Jaszczyszyn Y, Thermes C: Ten years of next-generation sequencing technology. *Trends Genet* 30:418–426, 2014.
131. Singh P, Schimenti JC, Bolcun-Filas E: A mouse geneticist's practical guide to CRISPR applications. *Genetics* 199:1–15, 2015.
132. Heller EA, Cates HM, Pena CJ, et al.: Locus-specific epigenetic remodeling controls addiction- and depression-related behaviors. *Nat Neurosci* 17:1720–1727, 2014.
133. Mirnics K, Levitt P, Lewis DA: Critical appraisal of DNA microarrays in psychiatric genomics. *Biol Psychiatry* 60:163–176, 2006.
134. Evans SJ, Choudary PV, Neal CR, Li JZ, Vawter MP, Tomita H, et al.: Dysregulation of the fibroblast growth factor system in major depression. *Proc Natl Acad Sci U S A* 101:15506–15511, 2004.
135. Leckman JF, Panter-Brick C, Salah R: *Pathways to Peace: The Transformative Power of Children and Families.* Cambridge, MA, MIT Press, 2014.
136. Olds DL, Kitzman H, Cole R, et al.: Effects of nurse home-visiting on maternal life course and child development: age 6 follow-up results of a randomized trial. *Pediatrics* 114:1550–1559, 2004.
137. Harris IB: *Children in Jeopardy: Can we Break the Cycle of Poverty?* New Haven, CT: Yale Child Study Center, 1996.

CHAPTER 3.3.2 ■ ASSESSING RISK: GENE DISCOVERY

THOMAS V. FERNANDEZ, ABHA R. GUPTA, AND ELLEN J. HOFFMAN

INTRODUCTION

There is indisputable evidence for the heritability of most early-onset neuropsychiatric illnesses. However, most of the genes conferring risk for these disorders remain largely unknown. Up until approximately the last decade, the process of risk gene discovery had been surprisingly slow and frustrating, especially when considering the strength of the data regarding genetic contributions to childhood disorders. This, of course, was not for lack of effort, ingenuity, or determination on the part of patients, families, and researchers. However, the tide has been changing as technologic advancements have been the main driving force accelerating risk gene discovery. The advent of affordable, high-throughput genotyping (whole-genome microarrays) and massively parallel sequencing (whole-exome and whole-genome) over the last several years has revolutionized the field and is facilitating an ever increasing pace of progress. Furthermore, an extraordinary level of involvement by private foundations, parent and advocacy groups, research consortia, and broad interdisciplinary research efforts involving clinicians, geneticists, and neuroscientists has been transformational, allowing for large collections of patient biomaterials that are shared with the broader scientific community. This synergistic convergence of technology and collaborative efforts has ushered in an era of risk gene discovery in several common childhood neuropsychiatric disorders, including autism spectrum disorder (ASD), schizophrenia, and intellectual disabilities (ID). The pace of these discoveries has been accelerating, and they are beginning to deepen our understanding of the biology of these disorders. As work on this front continues, the potential for these insights to influence clinical practice and inform new treatments is coming into clearer focus.

In this chapter, we will address the general challenges to risk gene identification that have confounded investigations of childhood neuropsychiatric disorders, outline the major research strategies and technologic advances that are helping to overcome these obstacles, and discuss the use of animal and cell models to begin translation of genetic discoveries from "bench to bedside." This discussion is intended to lay the groundwork for subsequent chapters, which will review more specific genetic findings relevant to individual disorders, describe the interplay of environment and genetics in conferring both risk and resilience, and highlight the potential contribution of genetics to research in the areas of psychopharmacology and neuroimaging.

OBSTACLES TO GENE DISCOVERY IN CHILDHOOD NEUROPSYCHIATRIC DISORDERS

Multiple Interacting Genes

Over the last four decades, the identification of disease-causing genes has become commonplace (1). These successes have largely been in the area of single gene disorders exhibiting Mendelian patterns of inheritance: that is, dominant, recessive, or X-linked (Table 3.3.2.1). In general, the inheritance of psychiatric disorders, such as schizophrenia, bipolar disorder, ASD, and Tourette disorder (TD) do not appear to fall into this category, in the sense that they cannot be accounted for by the transmission of a single gene. Rather, the commonly accepted view is that, for the most part, these disorders will be found to be the result of multiple interacting alleles, each with relatively small contributions, compared to the genetic effects observed in Mendelian disorders. For instance, in the case of ASD, analysis of linkage data, family studies, and more recent genome-wide genotyping and sequencing data has led to a hypothesis that as many as one thousand genes are likely to be involved (2).

Many psychiatric conditions are also strongly influenced by nongenetic factors. For instance, in the case of schizophrenia, the monozygotic concordance rate (Table 3.3.2.1) is approximately 50% (3,4). The observation that twins sharing all their genetic material share a diagnosis only half the time strongly suggests that influences apart from the sequence of their DNA are contributing to disease risk. These influences may be environmental in the classic sense, or may involve heritable genetic mechanisms that are not coded for in the sequence of DNA (epigenetic factors). The elaboration of the extent and nature of gene–environment interactions in developmental neuropsychiatric disorders is a vibrant area of research that has resulted in important recent insights into the etiopathology of mood, anxiety, psychotic, and attentional disorders, among others (5–7). These findings are reviewed in more detail in subsequent chapters.

An Uncertain Genetic Architecture

The combination of multigene inheritance, environmental, and epigenetic influences present significant challenges to researchers interested in gene identification. In addition, fundamental questions remain regarding the genetic architecture of nearly every childhood neuropsychiatric disorder. For instance, it is not known whether genetic variation that is common or rare in the population is likely to carry most of the risk for common childhood neuropsychiatric conditions. This issue is important for selecting appropriate research strategies to identify contributing genes as well as in interpreting the resulting findings.

Two alternatives are most commonly investigated. One is the "common disease-common variant" hypothesis, which holds that most of the risk for complex neuropsychiatric disorders will be accounted for by variations, or alleles, that are common in the population. By definition, these are genetic polymorphisms that are present in more than 1% of individuals. An often-cited early example is Alzheimer disease and the increased risk conferred by the e4 allele at the apolipoprotein E (APOE) gene locus, a variance that occurs with relatively high frequency in the general population (8,9). In the case of common disorders that begin late in life, it is widely accepted that common alleles are likely to play a major role. This is because

TABLE 3.3.2.1

GLOSSARY OF SELECTED TERMS (COURTESY OF NATIONAL HUMAN GENOME RESEARCH INSTITUTE)

Allele	One of the variant forms of a gene at a particular locus (gene location), on a particular chromosome. Different alleles may have functional significance or may be normal variants.
Association study	These studies examine the relative allele frequencies among populations with and without a phenotype of interest.
Candidate gene	A gene suspected of being involved in a disease, based on prior suggestive evidence. For example, the gene may be located within a region of a chromosome detected by linkage analysis, the gene's protein product may suggest that it could be associated with a disease, or the gene may be located near a chromosomal abnormality.
Chromosome	One of the thread-like "packages" of DNA in the nucleus of a cell. Humans normally have 23 pairs of chromosomes, with 22 pairs of autosomes and 1 pair of sex chromosomes. Each parent contributes one chromosome to each pair.
Complex disease	A disease caused by the interaction of multiple genes and environmental factors; they are also called multifactorial.
Copy number variation (CNV)	When the number of copies of a particular genetic region varies from one individual to the next. Gains and losses of genetic material.
Concordance	The presence of a given trait or phenotype in both members of a twin pair.
Deletion	A particular kind of mutation: Loss of a piece of DNA from a chromosome. Deletion of a gene or part of a gene can lead to a disease or abnormality, but can also be benign.
Dominant	A Mendelian pattern of inheritance in which a single transmitted gene variant results in a specific phenotypic characteristic, including, for example, a disease. Typically there is a strong relationship between carrying the genetic variant and having the disease. With a dominant gene, the chance of passing on the gene (and therefore the disease) to children is 50% in each pregnancy.
Duplication	An extra copy or copies of a chromosome segment.
Epigenetics	An emerging scientific field that studies heritable changes caused by the activation and deactivation of genes without any change in the underlying DNA sequence.
Exon	The region of a gene that contains the code for producing the gene's protein. Each exon codes for a specific portion of the complete protein.
FISH	Fluorescence in situ hybridization. A technique that uses fluorescent probes that attach to unique known regions of chromosomes. It is useful for determining the location and extent of chromosomal abnormalities and for gene mapping.
Gene	The basic functional and physical unit of heredity passed from parent to offspring. Genes are pieces of DNA, and most genes contain the information for making a specific protein.
Genome	The complete sequence of DNA contained in an organism or a cell, which includes all chromosomes within the nucleus and the DNA in mitochondria.
Genome-wide association studies (GWAS)	An approach to associate specific genetic variations with particular diseases. The method involves scanning the genomes from many different people and looking for genetic markers that can be used to predict the presence of a disease.
Genotype	An individual's collection of genes, or the two alleles inherited for a particular gene. The genotype is expressed when the information encoded in the genes' DNA is used to make protein and RNA molecules. The expression of the genotype contributes to the individual's observable traits, called the phenotype
Insertion	A type of chromosomal abnormality in which a DNA sequence is inserted into a gene, likely disrupting the normal structure and function of that gene.
Intron	The region of a gene containing a sequence of DNA that does not code for the gene's protein product.
Linkage	The relationship between genes and/or markers that lie near each other on a chromosome. Linked genes and markers tend to be inherited together. A marker and a phenotype are linked when they are inherited together.
Linkage analysis	Statistical examination of the likelihood that markers are linked to a particular phenotype by tracing inheritance through families. A high likelihood of linkage (expressed as a LOD score) at a locus suggests that the variation causing or contributing to disease is near the marker(s) being investigated.
Locus	The location on a chromosome where a specific gene is located.
LOD score	Logarithm of the odds. A likelihood ratio that expresses the statistical evidence in favor of linkage.
Marker	A variable segment of DNA with an identifiable physical location on a chromosome and whose inheritance can be followed. Because DNA segments that lie near each other on a chromosome tend to be inherited together, markers are often used as an indirect means of tracking the inheritance pattern of a gene that has not yet been identified.
Mutation	A permanent structural alteration in DNA. DNA changes may have no effect, may cause harm, or may improve an organism's chance of surviving and passing this alteration on to descendants.
Phenotype	The observable traits or characteristics of an organism (hair color, weight, or the presence or absence of a disease). Phenotypic traits are not necessarily genetic.
Polymorphism	A common variation in the sequence of DNA among individuals, typically defined as frequency of 1% or greater; often used as genetic markers for association studies.
Recessive	A Mendelian pattern of inheritance in which two copies of a mutant gene, one from each parent, are necessary to cause a genetic disorder.
Sequencing	Determining the exact order of the base pairs in a segment of DNA.

(*continued*)

TABLE 3.3.2.1

(CONTINUED)

SNPs	Single nucleotide polymorphisms. Variations at a single nucleotide that occur in human DNA at a frequency of approximately one every 1,000 bases. These variations can be used as markers to track inheritance in families and to analyze linkage with a phenotype. By definition an SNP with a population frequency of greater than 1% is defined as "common."
Translocation	Breakage and removal of a large segment of DNA from one chromosome, followed by the segment's attachment to a different chromosome. May be unbalanced (loss of DNA) or balanced (no loss of DNA).
Whole-exome sequencing (WES)	DNA sequencing that targets the exons (parts of genes that code for proteins) of all genes in the genome. The exome makes up about 1% of the genome.
Whole-genome sequencing (WGS)	DNA sequencing that targets the entire genome.
X-linked	A Mendelian pattern of inheritance in which a disease-gene variant is located on the X chromosome, often causing X-linked diseases to be seen preferentially in males or to have a more severe manifestation in males (due to the presence of one normal copy of the gene in females carrying two X chromosomes).

natural selection is not likely to suppress variants whose effects occur after the age at which individuals typically reproduce. Hence, deleterious alleles contributing to late-onset conditions may attain a substantial frequency in the general population.

This same logic, with minor modifications, can be applied to early-onset disorders: if one presumes that such conditions result from a conspiracy of multiple genes and that each contributing genetic variant has a relatively small effect, selection against any individual allele may be weak, allowing disease-related variations to become common in the population (10–12). In addition, it is possible that certain ancient alleles may have historically conferred some selective advantage, and only more recently contributed to disease. This is thought to be the case with respect to the identification of a common genetic variant associated with both childhood and adult-onset obesity (13). One can imagine that a gene allele predisposing to higher body mass index could have previously been advantageous during times of scarcity, and that relatively recent environmental changes would have transformed this into a genetic risk.

The common disease-common variant hypothesis is also consistent with what is known about the overall structure of the normal human genome (14). The majority of overall variation within a population is accounted for by common alleles. It would follow then that if selective pressure does not act to limit the frequency of incrementally contributing loci, common diseases would reflect this underlying structure, that is, common variation would account for common disease.

An alternate possibility is that a significant proportion of early-onset childhood neuropsychiatric disorders may be the result of rare genetic variation. This could occur via several scenarios: either through the accumulation of many different rare mutations within one or a small number of genes (allelic heterogeneity), or rare mutations in any of a large number of genes resulting in a similar or overlapping phenotype (locus heterogeneity). Moreover, these two mechanisms, locus and allelic heterogeneity, could combine within what is now considered a single psychiatric syndrome, a scenario which would present significant challenges to progress in genetic research.

The rare variant hypothesis is intuitively attractive, particularly in the case of severe early-onset illnesses. One could imagine that a genetic variation contributing to fundamental impairments in social functioning arising early in life could be subject to selective pressures, as affected individuals might be less likely to have offspring than those who are unaffected. If one looks to other areas of medicine for clues, and from what we have learned so far from the most studied psychiatric disorders, it is most likely that a combination of rare and common variants plays a role in child psychiatric illness. For instance, in the case of ASD, rare alleles carrying significant disease risks have been identified. However, these mutations do not appear to account for the majority of population risk. Nonetheless, the discovery of rare alleles has provided vitally important insights into the pathophysiology of ASD (REFS).

The question of whether childhood neuropsychiatric disorders involve common or rare genetic variation is relevant because those methods and study designs that may be most appropriate to identify the contribution of one type of risk may have less power to identify the other (Figure 3.3.2.1). However, as sequencing technologies are advancing and costs

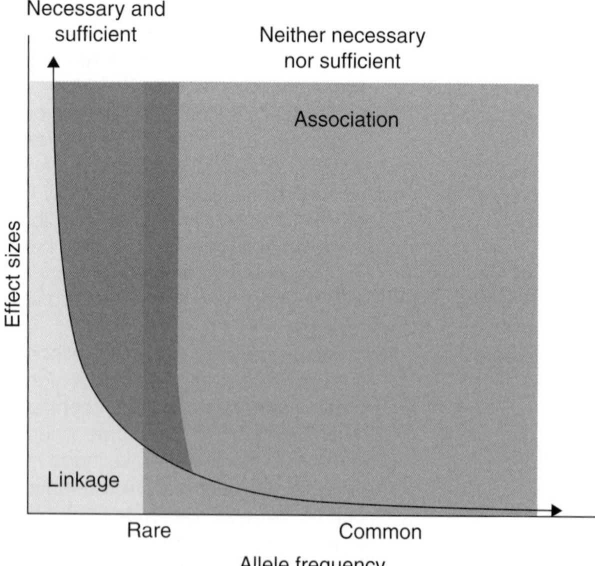

FIGURE 3.3.2.1. Allele frequency, effect size, and detection methods. (*Reproduced from State & Levitt, 2011, Nature Neuroscience 14, 1499–1506, doi:10.1038/nn.2924.*) Rare mutations have been found to carry larger effects than common variants. Linkage and association sections show typical approaches to demonstrating the role of rare versus common variation in disease. Relationships between rare alleles and a phenotype are often demonstrated using linkage analyses; common variant relationships are usually demonstrated using association (case–control) methods. The shaded area shows the approximate range of effect sizes seen for rare alleles identified in ASD.

are declining, research designs have been gradually turning toward comprehensively gathering data on both common and rare variation throughout the genome. This will be discussed further as the various approaches to gene hunting are presented below.

Phenotypic Heterogeneity

In addition to the obstacles presented by complex inheritance and an uncertain genetic architecture, diagnostic issues in childhood neuropsychiatric disorders present major challenges to geneticists. Ultimately, irrespective of the specific methodology employed, disease-gene hunting involves identifying observable clinical phenomena that bring together individuals with some degree of shared genetic risk and then uncovering the responsible or contributing variants within the genome. If one has difficulty identifying a group of affected individuals who share a proportion of their risk in common, gene identification can be quite difficult.

The absence of reliable and specific physiologic markers for childhood neuropsychiatric illnesses presents a significant challenge. Of course, one problem is that our current diagnostic approaches may have weak correlations with underlying biologic mechanisms. It is not yet possible to determine, for instance, whether similar genetic liabilities may underlie several diagnostic categories that are considered as quite separate within the boundaries imposed by current systems of classification (15). The high frequency of comorbidities and wide-ranging clinical presentations seen in childhood neuropsychiatric syndromes certainly suggest that this may be the case. New guidelines for categorizing research subjects with neuropsychiatric symptoms have recently been proposed and adopted by national research funding institutes in an attempt to alleviate this obstacle (16). In addition, while severe forms of any disorder may be quite easily recognized, more subtle manifestations may be difficult to assess and verify. The unambiguous delineation of affected versus unaffected individuals, even within an extended family, can also be complicated by clinical phenomena that change through the course of development, either through an age-dependent onset, a waxing and waning course, or symptoms that decrease markedly in adulthood.

The issue of diagnostic uncertainty in child psychiatry can also pose significant logistical problems in that it can be quite difficult to ascertain comparable samples across sites that are geographically remote. For example, in the case of hypertension, large-scale studies of individuals may be undertaken in which the diagnostic measures may involve little more than multiple readings from a blood pressure cuff. Contrast this with what is typically required for a state-of-the-art diagnosis in almost any psychiatric disorder. One can imagine that the effort and expense required to collect useful data on large numbers of patients in child psychiatry is considerably more challenging than in many other fields of medicine.

APPROACHES TO GENE DISCOVERY AND CHARACTERIZATION

Assessing Heritability and Patterns of Transmission

Most often, gene discovery efforts are preceded by epidemiologic investigations aimed at determining the general nature and extent of the genetic risk. Such studies typically seek to identify whether a particular disorder aggregates within families and, if so, whether there is an identifiable pattern of transmission. This can be useful to identify whether genes might be involved. Moreover, a comparison of this risk among different degrees of relatedness may provide a clue as to the nature of the genetic transmission (17,18).

However, such investigations typically cannot determine whether the observed familial aggregation or increased risk is the direct result of genetic influences. In this regard, both twin and adoption studies play a critical role in teasing apart the relative contribution of genetic factors versus environmental factors in disease etiology. For twin studies, the rates at which monozygotic twins (MZ) share a diagnosis are compared to the rates for dizygotic twins (DZ). An assumption is made that both types of same-sex twins will have a similar degree of shared environmental influences. Consequently, if genes "trump" environment in the etiology of a disorder, those siblings that share all of their DNA (MZ) should be more likely to share a diagnosis than twins who share the same amount of DNA as any sibling pair (DZ). Conversely, if environment predominates as a contributing factor, rates of concordance should not fundamentally differ based on the amount of shared genetic material. Adoption studies accomplish a similar goal by comparing monozygotic twins who are raised together versus those in which twins are raised apart. These types of investigations are quite powerful, but are less common in the literature than twin studies.

For ASD, MZ concordance has been found to be in the neighborhood of 60% for the full syndrome and 90% for the broad spectrum. In contrast, DZ concordance has been found to be relatively low, about 3% to 15%, depending on the diagnostic criteria employed. These data support the conclusion that the observed familial clustering is largely the result of genetic factors and translate into an estimate of heritability that places ASDs among the most strongly genetic of all neuropsychiatric conditions (2,19).

Once family, twin, and adoption studies have demonstrated that genetic factors are likely to play a role in the pathogenesis of a disorder, there are several different means to identify the specific genes involved: linkage analysis, including whole-genome screens in affected sibling pairs; gene association studies, including candidate gene studies, family-based studies of association, and genome-wide association studies (GWAS); molecular cytogenetic methods, including karyotyping, fluorescence in situ hybridization (FISH), and microarray comparative genomic hybridization (CGH); and high-throughput next-generation sequencing (NGS), including whole-exome and whole-genome sequencing. We will next examine the basic principles behind these methods, as well as advantages and pitfalls of each as they relate to the search for susceptibility genes in child psychiatric disorders.

Linkage Analysis

Linkage analysis assesses the probability that a given phenotype and a particular genetic marker (or series of markers) are transmitted together from one generation to another (Figure 3.3.2.2A). This method is based on the principle that, within affected families, genetic loci associated with a disorder are transmitted from parents to children more often than would be expected by chance (20). Results are expressed as a logarithm of the odds (LOD) score, such that, for example, an LOD score of 3 indicates the odds in favor of linkage between a marker and the disease are 1,000 (10^3):1. Indeed, this particular score is taken as the threshold for statistical significance in an investigation of the whole genome, due to the fact that multiple comparisons are conducted (one simultaneously investigates multiple markers). For a parametric analysis, in which one specifies a hypothesis about the nature of the proposed genetic transmission (e.g., that a disorder is the result of a dominantly

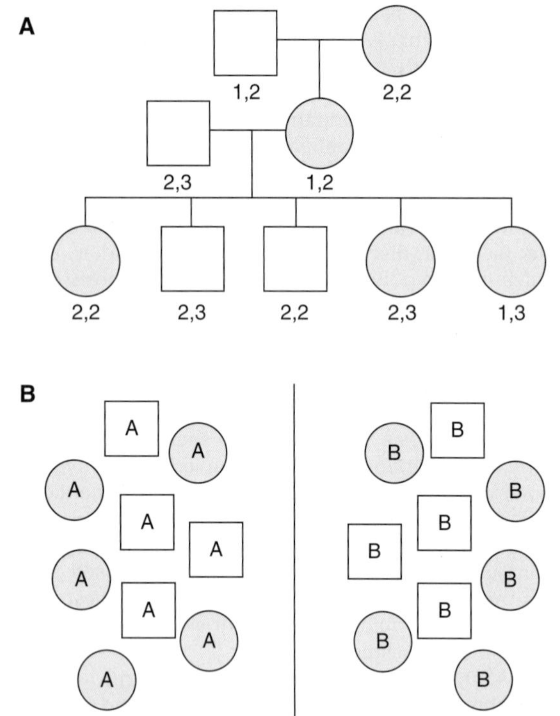

FIGURE 3.3.2.2. Schematic illustrations of linkage and association principles. **A:** Linkage analysis. A pedigree showing disease (*solid shade*) among males (*squares*) and females (*circles*) in multiple generations. The pair of numbers under each member of the pedigree represents the alleles of a DNA marker which was used to genotype the family. By analyzing the pattern of affected status within pedigrees, one may hypothesize the pattern of disease inheritance (dominant in this case) and then use a parametric linkage approach. By analyzing the frequency with which a particular genotype occurs along with disease in one or multiple families, it may be possible to conclude that a gene involved in disease phenotype is likely to lie in close proximity to a DNA marker. In this case, grandmaternal marker allele 2 appears to be linked to disease. **B:** Association studies. Individuals with a particular disorder or phenotype (*labeled A*) are compared with control subjects without the disease or phenotype (*labeled B*) to determine whether one group is more likely to carry particular allele(s) of the gene(s) being studied.

acting mutation that is rare in the population), 1,000:1 odds in favor of linkage at a marker (LOD score of 3) roughly corresponds to a genome-wide *p* value of 0.05.

There was initially great optimism in the potential of linkage analysis to uncover genes for neuropsychiatric illnesses, based on a host of dramatic discoveries, including the identification of genes for Huntington disease, hypertension, ID, and various cancers (1,21,22). However, early returns in several areas of child psychiatry were not as rewarding as anticipated. For instance, with respect to TD, when early parametric linkage studies did not identify TD-related loci, an international genetics consortium turned to nonparametric approaches. Several such studies have been reported in TD (23–27), with several "hits" approaching genome-wide statistical significance in individual studies (defined as a LOD score of 3.6). However, independent studies have not converged on any genomic region. Similarly, linkage analysis efforts in schizophrenia (28–33) and ADHD (34–39) have shown little overlap and poor replication, although several loci containing potential candidate genes have been reported for some disorders, such as dyslexia (40).

In retrospect, linkage studies have been most successful in identifying loci associated with Mendelian disorders. For genetically heterogeneous neuropsychiatric disorders, success has been limited when looking across families. Reasons for this include locus and allelic heterogeneity, differing inclusion criteria, and low statistical power, given the relatively small sample collections studied to date. Studies in other complex disorders in psychiatry and across medicine suggest that robust identification of risk alleles in nonparametric linkage analyses is likely to require cohorts of many thousands of patients (41). An alternate and perhaps more promising approach to complex disorders is linkage analysis within single pedigrees that display a clear pattern of inheritance and include multiple affected members. Such families can be difficult to identify and the risk alleles they carry may be rare, yet linkage analysis can offer unique insights into biologic mechanisms that can cause the disorder.

One example of single pedigree linkage analysis leading to a novel understanding of disease pathogenesis and a potential new treatment target can be found in TD. In 2010, Ercan-Sencicek et al. (42) described a two-generation pedigree in which a father and all eight of his children had TD, a pattern suggestive of a single dominant allele of large effect size in this family. Parametric analysis identified a single region on chromosome 15 yielding the maximum theoretically possible LOD score for the pedigree. Sequencing of the 55 genes in this region led to the identification of a nonsense point mutation (W317X) in the gene *histidine decarboxylase* (*HDC*). *HDC* encodes the enzyme required for the synthesis of histamine from histidine, and in vitro studies showed the nonsense mutation completely abolished its biosynthetic function (Figure 3.3.2.3).

This study represented the first association of disrupted histamine biosynthesis with TD (43). While this particular mutation has not been found in any other individual (affected or unaffected) to date, subsequent studies of copy number variation (CNV) in TD (44) and modeling HDC disruption in an animal system (45–47) support a role for histamine in TD biology and have led to a clinical trial of a histamine-targeting pharmaceutical, the histamine H3 receptor antagonist AZD5213 (ClinicalTrials.gov Identifier: NCT01904773). This relatively rapid progress, moving from a single index family to a new mechanism and potential new treatment, demonstrates the utility of linkage analysis in particular families as well as the more general promise of using genetic findings as an entry point into a translational science pipeline that will lead to a better understanding of disease biology and novel treatments (Figure 3.3.2.4).

Association Analysis

In contrast to linkage studies, which examine transmission within families, association studies assess gene frequencies within populations. The first association studies typically investigated one or a number of known, common genetic polymorphisms (markers) in or near predetermined candidate genes of interest. In essence, the methodology is a variation on the classic case–control design. In general, in the field of human genetics, one seeks to determine if individuals with a particular disorder or phenotype are significantly more (or less) likely than controls to carry particular allele(s) of the gene or genes being studied (Figure 3.3.2.2B).

Association methods have been shown to be more powerful than linkage methods under a number of conditions that typically prevail in complex disease. In particular, they are considered to be more powerful in detecting common susceptibility variants of relatively small effect, unlike linkage analysis, which requires relatively strong genetic effects given feasible sample sizes (15,48–50). Association studies are also popular for practical reasons. The most commonly used designs study either affected individuals versus unrelated controls, or as is often the case in pediatric disorders, affected probands and

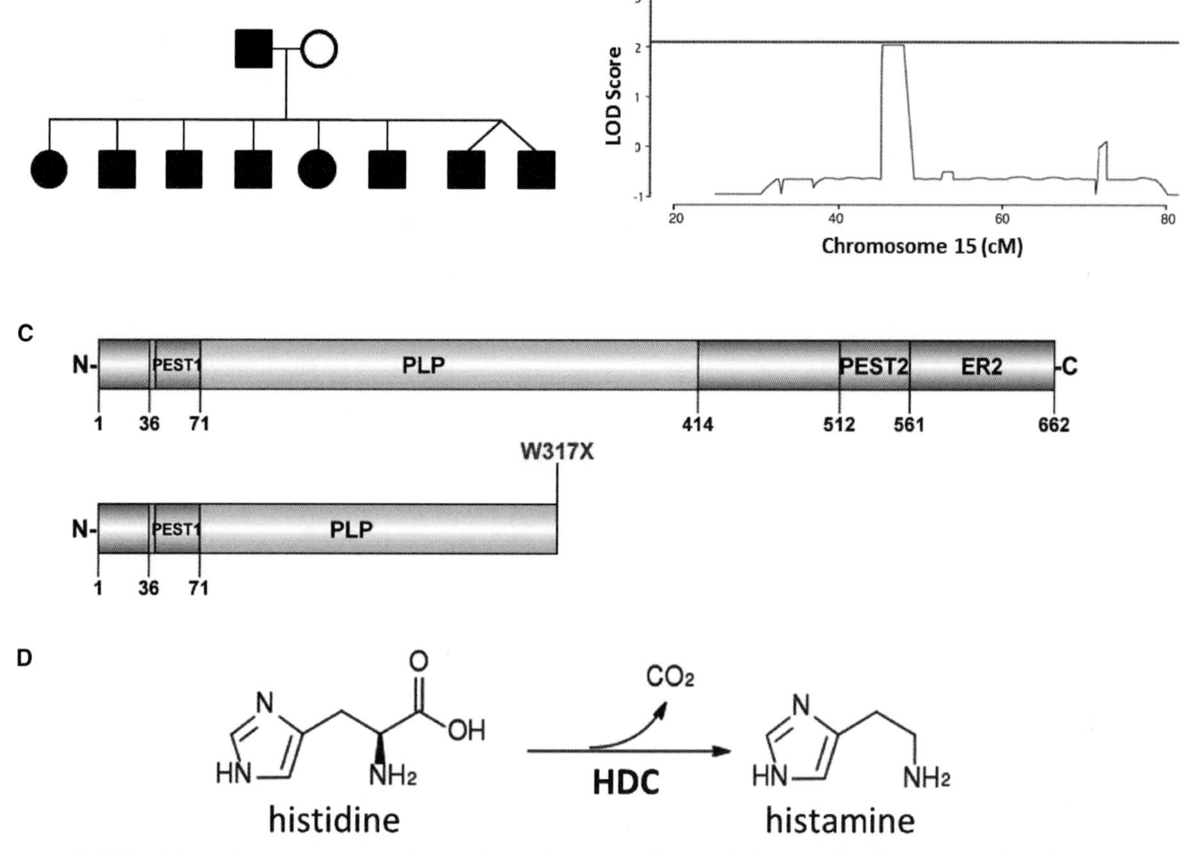

FIGURE 3.3.2.3. Linkage analysis of an outlier pedigree identifies a mutation in *HDC*. (*Reproduced from Tourette Syndrome. Davide Martino and James F. Leckman, Editors Oxford University Press.*) **A:** Two-generation pedigree with 9 TD affected individuals (*solid symbols*). **B:** Parametric linkage LOD scores along a section of chromosome 15. The horizontal line indicates the maximum theoretical LOD score (2.1) for this family. **C:** All affected family members carry a nonsense mutation affecting the *HDC* gene transcript. The wild-type HDC protein (**top**) contains 662 amino acids; the mutant HDC protein (**bottom**) is predicted to be truncated at the site of the W317X mutation. **D:** The HDC protein (L-histidine decarboxylase) is the rate-limiting enzyme in histamine biosynthesis. See (42).

their parents (where the nontransmitted parental alleles are used as the control). This contrasts with parametric linkage analyses, in which extended families must be identified and characterized, or nonparametric linkage studies that often require the identification of two affected siblings, thus excluding a significant number of patients who present to clinic. As a result, association studies make the study of large numbers of subjects reasonably practical and often allow this type of investigation to dovetail with other case–control studies being conducted simultaneously, such as pharmacologic studies.

For many years, candidate gene association studies were popular across all fields of medicine due to the ease and low cost of genotyping a small number of variants. Furthermore, the required number of statistical comparisons was low, allowing nominal statistical significance to be achieved using relatively small cohorts. However, as genomic tools have advanced and more robust approaches (reviewed below) have largely replaced candidate gene studies, several important weaknesses have come into focus, which can explain why such studies have been largely unsuccessful in yielding significant reproducible findings for complex disorders. First, the genetic markers or SNPs used in these studies are preselected based on existing pathophysiologic hypotheses; given the presence of millions of SNPs and our limited understanding of disease mechanisms, there is a very low prior probability that any selected marker will be associated with the disorder (41,51). Furthermore, even if the correct genes are selected, the specific markers interrogated may not be adequately linked to the specific variants that influence disease risk.

A second important limitation of association studies is their vulnerability to false-positive results (52). One source of this error may be population stratification. This results from variations in the frequencies of certain genetic markers among different ethnic groups. If one compares individuals with a particular phenotype to controls, and the two groups are not ethnically similar, a genetic marker that is found more frequently in the affected group will erroneously appear to be associated with the identified phenotype. In retrospect, many candidate gene association studies have failed to adequately control for population stratification, and precise matching is essential for reliable and reproducible results. Finally, based on the small effect sizes expected for common alleles contributing to most common disorders, very large cohort sizes are required for reliable gene discovery; it is clear that the candidate gene association studies reported to date for almost all neuropsychiatric disorders have employed sample sizes that are far too small.

Genome-Wide Association Studies

Due to the limitations described above, there has been a shift in methodology from candidate gene association to studies of genome-wide association, simultaneously testing hundreds of thousands to millions of common SNPs for association with

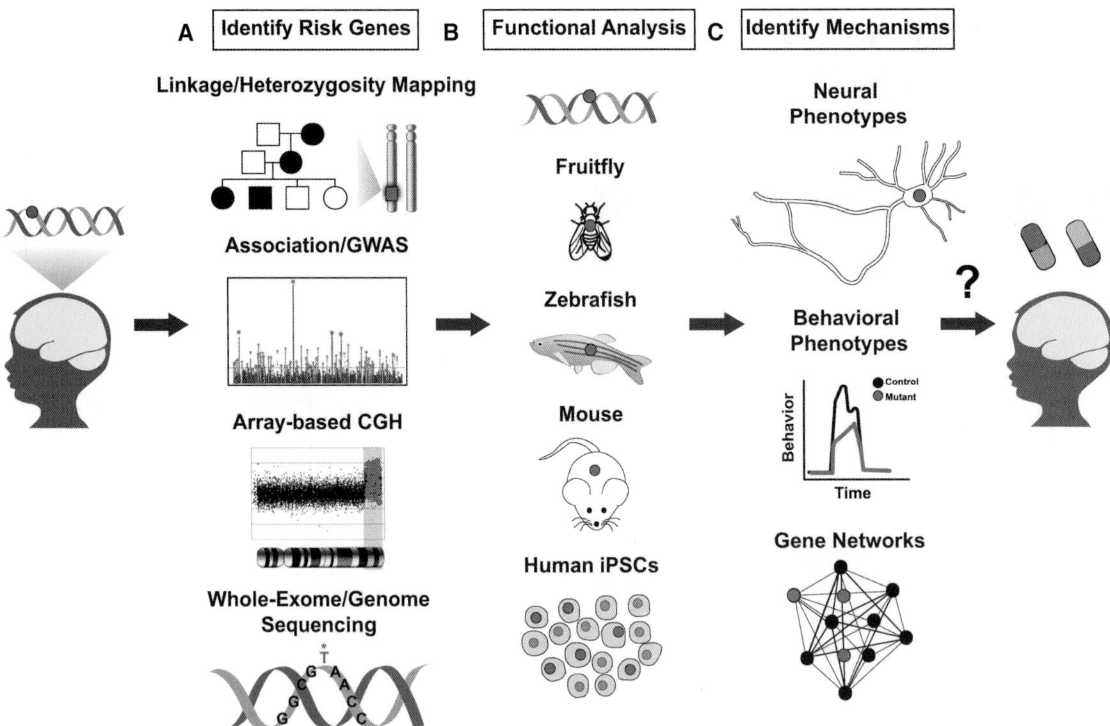

FIGURE 3.3.2.4. Schematic representation of the identification and functional analysis of risk genes in childhood neuropsychiatric disorders. **A:** Risk genes (*circle* in DNA strand) associated with childhood neuropsychiatric disorders are identified in human genetics studies using multiple methods discussed in this chapter: linkage; genome-wide association studies (GWAS); array-based comparative genomic hybridization (CGH); and whole-exome and whole-genome sequencing. (Manhattan plot adapted from www.nimh.nih.gov) **B:** Functional analysis of risk genes is conducted using in vivo and in vitro approaches. These include: nonhuman animal model systems, such as *Drosophila* (fruit fly), zebrafish, and mouse; and human induced pluripotent stem cells (iPSCs). **C:** Functional analyses using the methods shown in (**B**) are used to identify biologic mechanisms and convergent pathways by examining a range of phenotypes resulting from risk gene loss, some of which are shown here, including neuroanatomical, cellular, physiologic, behavioral, circuit-level, gene expression, and gene network phenotypes. By revealing novel mechanisms, the functional analysis of risk genes has the potential to identify novel pharmacologic targets for childhood neuropsychiatric disorders.

complex disorders. This movement toward GWAS coincided with advances in microarray technologies that delivered affordable high-density genotyping platforms. Querying genetic markers throughout the genome eliminates the need to identify candidate variants a priori and allows hypothesis-neutral investigations. This method also yields data that allows rigorous matching for ancestry between cases and controls, an aforementioned confounder in earlier association studies. The primary challenge in GWAS is the large number of independent comparisons performed, requiring a widely accepted genome-wide significance threshold of $p \leq 5 \times 10^{-8}$. Given the heterogeneity of complex disease, large sample sizes are required to achieve this level of significance. Nevertheless, this technique has led to renewed excitement in the field, with somewhat mixed results to date for complex neuropsychiatric disorders.

For example, in ASD, none of the candidate genes emerging from earlier association or linkage studies have reached the threshold for genome-wide significance using GWAS (53,54), suggesting either that these candidate genes had initial false-positive associations or that the current GWAS lacks sufficient statistical power to detect common variant association. Indeed, a GWAS study of schizophrenia from the Psychiatric Genomics Consortium (PGC) demonstrates that much larger sample sizes (>10,000 subjects) are required for the detection of variants reaching genome-wide significance (55). This study reported an association between schizophrenia risk and genetic markers across the major histocompatibility complex (MHC). More recently, data from the Schizophrenia Working Group of the PGC advanced this finding by showing that SNPs in complement component (C4) alleles are associated with schizophrenia and that these alleles lead to altered expression of C4 in the brain, leading to putative increased synapse elimination in brains of individuals with schizophrenia (56). In this way, results from GWAS can help to pinpoint susceptibility loci as well as begin to further our understanding of biologic mechanisms underlying disease.

Chromosomal Alterations

Another method for identifying risk loci contributing to complex disease in individual patients is to examine genomic regions affected by chromosomal abnormalities (e.g., deletions, duplications, translocations, inversions) in affected individuals and then identify genes in this region that may be disrupted as a result. These studies were most popular prior to the era of high resolution genome-wide investigations and involved using cytogenetic techniques such as karyotyping and FISH to map de novo chromosomal alterations. Because these types of findings derive from only one or a few patients, replication of the implicated loci is essential to establish that the findings are pathogenic.

This approach has been used successfully to identify the genes for multiple medical disorders (1) as well as a host of ID syndromes (22). For complex childhood neuropsychiatric disorders, it is assumed that genes affected by such rare gross chromosomal abnormalities are unlikely to account for any

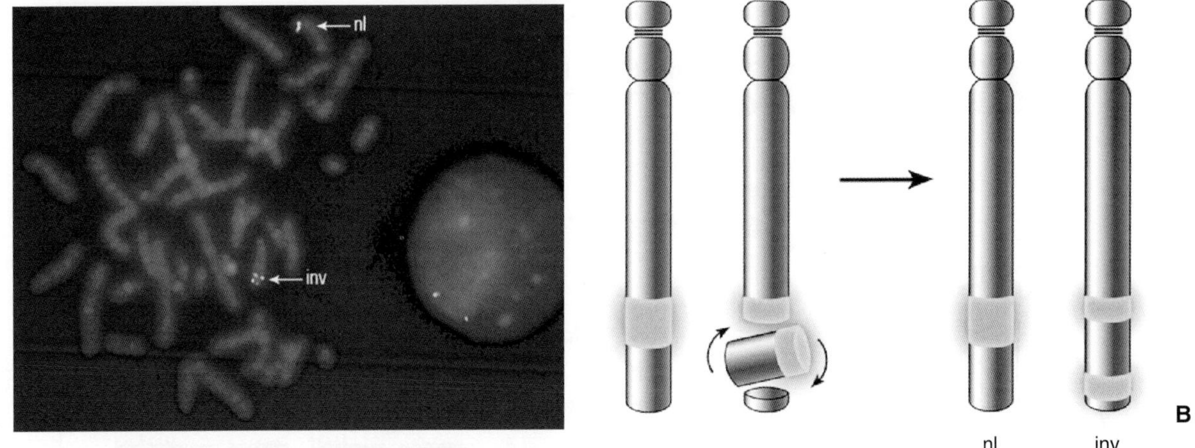

FIGURE 3.3.2.5. Using FISH to map a chromosome 13 inversion in a patient with TS. **A:** Photograph of metaphase chromosomes under 100× objective lens after hybridization with a fluorescent-labeled probe specific for a DNA sequence at 13q31.1. The experimental probe is visualized at the expected position on the normal (nl) chromosome 13. Two fluorescence signals are visible on the inverted (inv) chromosome 13, indicating that this probe spans the breakpoint. **B:** Illustration of how the chromosome 13 inversion results in two fluorescence signals when the DNA probe spans one of the inversion breakpoints. In this case, the breakpoint at 13q31.1 mapped near the gene SLITRK1 and further investigation of its sequence revealed rare mutations in three unrelated individuals affected with TS.

significant portion of susceptibility risk in most of the overall affected population. However, identifying genes involved in these rearrangements may identify loci that are mutated in affected but cytogenetically normal individuals or identify genetic pathways providing insights into the pathogenesis of more common forms of these disorders.

One illustrative example pointing to the potential value of this approach in common complex psychiatric disorders involves TD. Abelson et al. (57) studied a de novo chromosomal inversion in the only member of a family affected with TD (Figure 3.3.2.5). One of the two breakpoints identified in this child mapped near a gene known as *SLIT and Trk-Like family member 1* (*SLITRK1*). The other three genes mapping closest to the two breakpoints were thought to be less likely candidates, in part because *SLITRK1* was the only one known in the group to be expressed in brain regions thought relevant to TD and related disorders.

Given a starting hypothesis that mutations in *SLITRK1* would likely be rare among individuals with TD, the authors directly queried the entire coding and regulatory regions of *SLITRK1* among unrelated affected individuals. They identified a mutation in a second family with TD and related disorders that was predicted to lead to a truncation of the resulting protein, and which was not present in several thousand control individuals. Additional screening also demonstrated a rare variant in a regulatory region of *SLITRK1* that was present in two unrelated affected individuals and absent in several thousand unrelated controls, indicating a significant association (57).

The function of *SLITRK1* is not well understood. It is broadly expressed during development and may have a role in axon pathfinding. Expression is greatly reduced in adulthood, though it persists in cholinergic neurons of the striatum (58). In vitro, overexpression of *SLITRK1* in cortical neurons promotes dendritic growth, while the TD-associated alleles lead to dendritic regression (57). A mouse knockout of *SLITRK1* exhibits anxiety and increased noradrenergic activity that is attenuated by the alpha-2 adrenergic receptor agonist clonidine (59), recapitulating some characteristics of TD (60,61). However, no tic-like movements were documented. Mouse knockouts of a closely related gene, *SLITRK5*, were found to exhibit excessive grooming, anxiety, and altered dendritic morphology in the striatum (62).

Subsequent examinations of the association of *SLITRK1* alleles with TD have produced inconsistent results, which is to be expected in studies of rare variation in samples of modest size. Resequencing of several hundred TD probands did not identify any additional coding mutations (63–65). In trichotillomania (66) and OCD (67), on the other hand, several rare missense mutations have been identified; the functional significance of these remains unclear. Associations with common variants have been reported in a small candidate gene association study (68) and in a subsequent haplotype analysis of 376 families with a TD proband (69). However, no SNPs within or near *SLITRK1*—including those examined in these common variant studies (68,69)—emerged as even nominally significant in the first TD GWAS study (70). This does not, however, rule out the possibility that the reported mutations in *SLITRK1* are causal, but rare.

The initial work by Abelson et al. identifying *SLITRK1* mutations in TD demonstrated both the important strengths as well as the potential weaknesses of the molecular cytogenetic approach. On the positive side, the work was able to identify both a specific candidate disease gene as well as specific functional genetic changes for further investigation. The study also demonstrated the liabilities of searching for rare genetic variants in a common disease. By definition, the results are likely to affect only a small number of individuals and no single piece of evidence may be a "smoking gun." The ultimate implications of the work can only come into focus through the identification of additional rare families with clear mutations in this gene, the elaboration of a biologic pathway including other genes that may carry risk for TD, and through further study of animal and cellular models (reviewed below), which may offer more clues regarding the relationship of *SLITRK1* to TD and related disorders.

Copy Number Variation

Over the last decade, advancements in microarray technologies have permitted detection of submicroscopic structural variation. These deletions and duplications of blocks of DNA throughout the human genome—called CNV when their length is at least 1 kilobase (kb)—are common both in the clinical and the general population (71–74) (Figure 3.3.2.6). CNVs may encompass a single part of a gene, an entire gene, or multiple genes. Screening for large CNVs, both inherited and de novo, has proven an efficient strategy for detecting mutations potentially contributing to

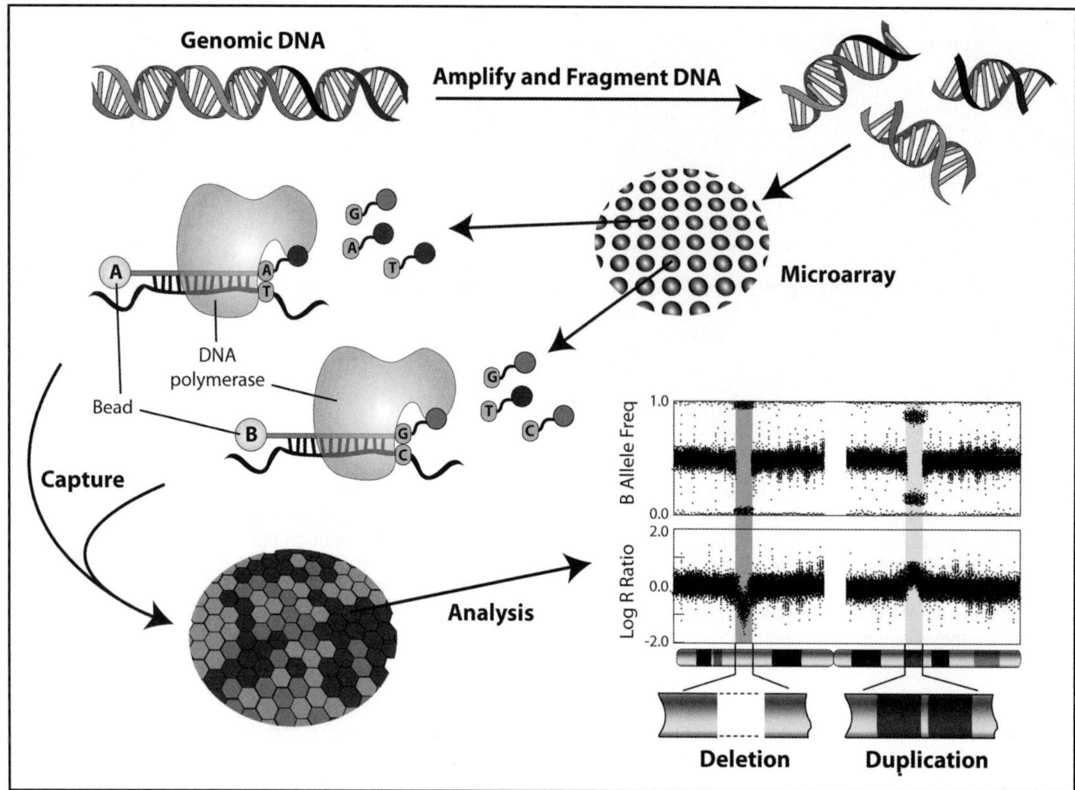

FIGURE 3.3.2.6. Schematic representation of copy number variant analysis. (*Reproduced from Hoffman EJ, State MW, J Am Acad Child Adolesc Psychiatry 49:736–751, 2010.*) One common approach to CNV analysis that can detect millions of SNPs using a microarray is shown here. First, genomic DNA is fragmented, denatured, and applied to a SNP microarray. Each microarray position contains beads (A and B) attached to a short DNA sequence found in the human genome. Genomic DNA binds to these short sequences, which end before a known SNP. A fluorescent-labeled nucleotide is added to the end of each sequence in the presence of a DNA polymerase enzyme, based on which SNP is present in that location in the particular individual. Next, an informatics-based analysis is used to identify the presence of a CNV. Specifically, the relative amount of DNA at a particular location (log R ratio) in the individual being tested compared to a control population is determined, along with a measurement of whether an individual is heterozygous or homozygous for a particular SNP (B allele frequency). For example, the B allele frequency for AA, AB, and BB genotypes are 0, 0.5, and 1, respectively. If a deletion is present, the log R ratio is negative and the region appears homozygous, such that the B allele frequency is 1 or 0. If a duplication is present, the log R ratio is positive and the B allele frequencies are between 0 and 1 (e.g., if three copies of a region are present, the possible genotypes are AAA, AAB, ABB, and BBB, and the respective B allele frequencies are 0, 0.33, 0.66, and 1). This method allows for an assessment of the presence of CNVs in an individual throughout the genome.

risk due to their rarity in the genome (75,76). Studies in schizophrenia (77–83) and ASD (84–88) have revealed an increased burden of rare CNVs, particularly genic de novo variants, in these disorders (80,84,85,89,90). For ASD, CNV detection using SNP genotyping arrays in >4,500 families has led to the identification of dozens of specific risk loci via recurrent de novo CNVs at 16p11.2, 7q11.23 (del), 15q12 (del), and 1q21.1, among other regions (84,89–93). Through integrative analyses of de novo CNV mutations in ASD, it is estimated that more than 200 risk loci are vulnerable to such mutations (90). Furthermore, when considered together, ASD-associated genes from CNV studies appear to cluster into networks enriched for neuronal synaptic function and chromatin regulation (90,93). These studies in ASD demonstrate the utility of CNVs to identify risk loci and provide further insights into the underlying biology and genomic architecture of complex disorders.

High-Throughput, Next-Generation Sequencing

In recent years, DNA sequencing technologies have advanced tremendously. In contrast to Sanger sequencing, a long-standing method of reading the individual base letters of the genetic code developed in the 1970s, next-generation sequencing (NGS, also referred to as high-throughput, massively parallel, or deep sequencing) has revolutionized genomic research. NGS allows millions of small fragments of DNA to be sequenced in parallel, then uses bioinformatic analyses to reassemble these fragments by mapping the individual reads onto the reference human genome. This methodology dramatically accelerates the sequencing process, allowing an entire human genome (~3 billion base pairs) to be sequenced in about a day, although one can also use these methods to sequence just the coding regions of the genome, referred to as the exome (~1.5% of the genome) or particular targeted regions. Furthermore, due to target amplification, fragmentation, and parallel sequencing, NGS sequences each targeted region multiple times, providing high coverage of most regions (Figure 3.3.2.7). This high (or deep) coverage allows more accurate detection of genomic variants that might otherwise be missed with fewer sequence reads. It also allows for detection of a broader spectrum of mutations (e.g., CNVs) than is possible with traditional Sanger sequencing.

Whole-exome sequencing (WES) was first used for clinical diagnosis in 2009 (94) and it is now common in clinical

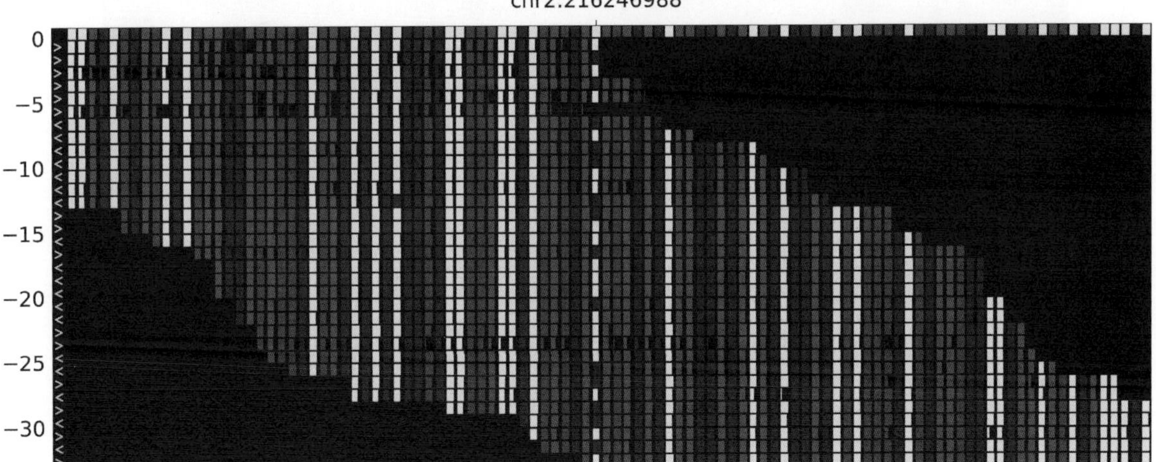

FIGURE 3.3.2.7 Alignment representation of next-generation sequencing reads. Blocks represent particular nucleotides (A, C, T, or G) at that position. The width of each block is proportional to the quality score of the base. The first row is the reference human genome sequence that is expected. Subsequent rows are the sequencing reads that have been aligned to the human genome sequence. The vertical axis represents the number of reads (or depth) at each location. In this example, a heterozygous C/T single nucleotide variant (SNV) is detected on chromosome 2 at position 216246988 (within the gene *FN1*).

use (95–97). One particularly fruitful use of sequencing data for gene discovery has been the search for protein-altering de novo SNVs and indels that occur in the same gene in more than one unrelated individual. Because de novo mutations are rare and often lead to changes with large effect size, recurrent mutations can signal high-confidence risk genes. This approach has been especially successful in the search for ASD genes (90,98,99); dozens of genes have been implicated without the need for prior hypotheses, which had been the hallmark of less successful candidate gene association studies. Furthermore, the identification of risk genes in this manner facilitates systems analyses that seek to discover the way in which these genes may coalesce within common biologic pathways and gene networks and reveal the important underlying neurobiology of disease (90,98,100).

While there are still discoveries to be made by WES, the ENCODE project has demonstrated the importance of intergenic regulatory regions (101), leading to the realization that sequencing regions outside the exome will be necessary to identify all important genetic variants. Sequencing the complete genome of individuals is more data intensive and expensive than WES, but advancements in sequencing technologies and market competition has facilitated dramatic decreases in sequencing costs over the last few years (Figure 3.3.2.8), which now makes whole-genome sequencing (WGS) a more realistic endeavor for many laboratories. Early studies of WGS in ASD are indicating that interrogation of regulatory regions outside of the exome will lead to discoveries that will help explain additional disease risk (102,103), positioning WGS as a promising tool to further our understanding of complex genetic disorders.

TRANSLATING GENE DISCOVERY FROM BENCH TO BEDSIDE

Animal Modeling

As the technology for identifying risk genes in childhood neuropsychiatric disorders continues to improve, there is an increased need to develop systems to progress from risk gene discovery to the identification of biologic mechanisms and pharmacologic targets. Given the expanding list of susceptibility genes associated with these disorders, such as ASD, the field of human genetics is approaching a bottleneck where the rate of ascertaining risk variants is beginning to exceed the ability to interpret their biologic significance. For this reason, after confirming the association of a gene with a particular disorder, a critical next step is modeling its function in a biologic system. The objective of such a system is to elucidate how disruption of a risk gene leads to the alteration of specific neuronal populations or neural circuits at defined stages of development, predisposing to behavioral dysfunction. In this way, these studies aim to illuminate the pathophysiology of childhood neuropsychiatric disorders, which remains incompletely understood, and to provide a path forward from risk gene identification to the discovery of biologic mechanisms and potential targets for pharmacologic treatments (Figure 3.3.2.4).

Model systems typically include either in vitro approaches, such as human induced pluripotent stem cells (iPSCs) (discussed in detail in the section, Stem Cell Modeling), or in vivo models, such as nonhuman animal systems, which may include a range of organisms from mouse to fish to fly. While there are benefits of in vitro methods, including the ability to study risk genes in human cells, animal models offer several key advantages. First, animal models provide a means of assessing the effect of risk gene disruption on the establishment of neural circuits in a live, behaving organism (104). In particular, the development of novel technologies for imaging neuronal activity in vivo has the potential to bridge the gap between gene and circuit function. Second, animal models are optimal for studying the role of a gene over time in an intact, developing nervous system (105), which is highly relevant to childhood neuropsychiatric disorders. Third, animal models can be used to identify novel pharmacologic targets and to conduct initial assessments of their potential to reverse structural or behavioral phenotypes resulting from risk gene loss (104). With respect to pharmacologic screens, both in vitro and in vivo methods may occur in parallel and complement each other, providing information on the effects of novel compounds on cellular and circuit-level phenotypes identified in human cell culture and animal models, respectively. In this way, both methods will play important roles in the functional analysis of susceptibility genes.

As noted, one major advantage of animal models is the ability to study the role of a risk gene in the establishment of neural circuits underlying behavioral abnormalities. To

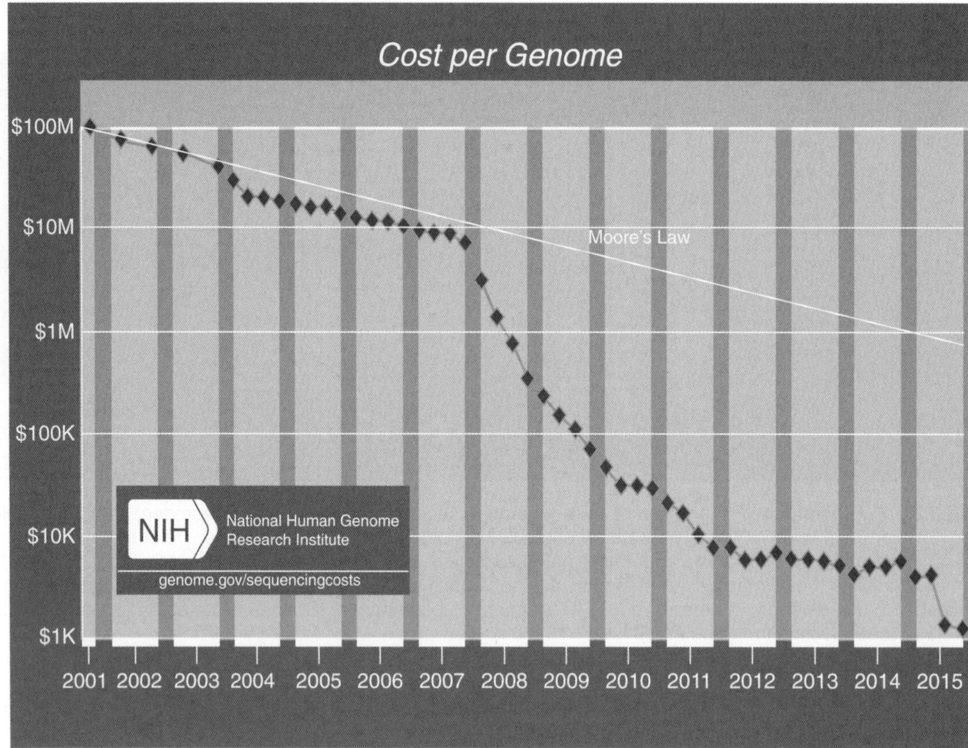

FIGURE 3.3.2.8. The cost of sequencing a human genome. The National Human Genome Research Institute (NHGRI) has tracked the costs associated with DNA sequencing performed at the sequencing centers funded by the Institute. This information has served as an important benchmark for assessing improvements in DNA sequencing technologies. To illustrate the nature of the reductions in DNA sequencing costs, the graph also shows hypothetical data reflecting Moore's Law, which describes a long-term trend in the computer hardware industry that involves the doubling of "compute power" every 2 years. Technology improvements that "keep up" with Moore's Law are widely regarded to be doing exceedingly well, making it useful for comparison. Note the logarithmic scale on the y-axis and the sudden and profound outpacing of Moore's Law beginning in January 2008; this is the time when sequencing centers transitioned from Sanger-based "next-generation" DNA sequencing technologies. (*Courtesy of the National Human Genome Research Institute.*)

accomplish this, various molecular techniques can be used to disrupt or "knockout" the function of a gene. Mouse knockout models have been instrumental in studying risk genes in multiple childhood neuropsychiatric disorders, including ASD, obsessive–compulsive disorder, and schizophrenia (106). These studies highlight the utility of using mouse knockout models to elucidate biologic mechanisms involving genes that confer risk for these disorders. For example, Fragile X syndrome (FXS) is the most common inherited cause of ID and is associated with an increased risk of ASD. Mice lacking the function of *FMR1,* the gene that causes FXS, exhibit hyperactivity and deficits in a novel spatial learning task (107). *FMR1* knockout mice also display structural abnormalities in their dendritic spines, similar to findings in individuals with FXS (108). Additional studies revealed that loss of *FMR1* in the mouse hippocampus results in increased long-term depression, a form of synaptic plasticity dependent on metabotropic glutamate receptor signaling (109). Importantly, these studies using a mouse knockout model identified a novel biologic mechanism underlying FXS and a potential pharmacologic pathway for therapeutic interventions (109).

Animal models also enable the investigation of risk gene function along a developmental trajectory, including embryonic stages (105). This is highly relevant for ASD, given that many recently identified ASD risk genes are expressed embryonically (98). Moreover, it is possible to generate animal models in which the function of a particular gene can be activated or silenced only under certain conditions, for example, in a specific cell type or at a defined developmental stage. These studies are instrumental in establishing when and where a gene is necessary for brain development. For example, mice lacking the function of *MeCP2,* which is disrupted in most cases of Rett syndrome, a neurodevelopmental disorder affecting motor coordination and language development, exhibit similar behaviors as affected humans, including the developmental onset of stereotypical forelimb movements (110). Interestingly, a recent study utilized a mouse model to demonstrate that the selective loss of *MeCP2* in inhibitory neurons leads to behavioral abnormalities, while the introduction of functional *MeCP2* in these cells is able to reverse some of these behavioral deficits (111). This study highlights the role of a risk gene in a specific neuronal population, providing insight into a biologic pathway underlying Rett syndrome.

Further, animal models can be used to assess the function of variants identified in human genetics studies. This is critically important, given that one of the current challenges in the genetics of neuropsychiatric disorders is distinguishing deleterious and neutral variation. That is, large-scale whole-exome and whole-genome sequencing projects have revealed considerable variation at the sequence and structural levels in the genomes of both affected and unaffected individuals, complicating the assignment of risk to rare transmitted missense variants or common variants in a known risk gene (112). While in silico approaches are useful for predicting the effect of a mutation on protein function, animal models provide an in vivo system to assess this. For example, it is possible to introduce or "knock-in" a gene carrying a patient-specific mutation in an animal model to test the extent to which this version of the gene can reverse or "rescue" phenotypes in a knockout animal. In this way, these studies provide a biologic readout of the function of variants identified in risk genes.

In addition, there are various emerging molecular technologies that are expanding the range of information that can be obtained from animal models both at the neuroanatomical and circuit levels. For example, a recently developed method, called CLARITY, allows for imaging intact tissue from mouse brain at high resolution without the need for sectioning (113). The application of this technology to analyze brain tissue from animal models of neuropsychiatric disorders as well as human clinical specimens has the potential to reveal subtle structural differences and to provide insight into pathophysiology (113). Also, there have been recent advances in techniques for imaging cellular activity in an awake, behaving animal, such as optogenetics, in which specific cells are engineered to express a channel that can be activated in response to light during a behavioral task, or the use of genetically encoded calcium indicators, such as GCaMP, which generate a fluorescent signal when cells are active (114,115). These techniques are beginning to illuminate the neural circuitry underlying behavior (116–118). Further, the availability of improved molecular technologies, such as the CRISPR (clustered regularly interspaced short palindromic repeats)/Cas9 system (119), which induces mutations in a gene of interest with a high degree of efficiency and flexibility, is facilitating the generation of knockout or knock-in animal models. The ability to generate animal models efficiently is critical to keep pace with the rapidly expanding list of risk genes emerging from large-scale human genetics studies.

Another advantage of animal models is the ability to conduct pharmacologic screens to identify compounds that reverse phenotypes resulting from the disruption of a specific risk gene. Here, model systems such as *Drosophila* and zebrafish are emerging as practical alternatives to mice, given the ease of genetic manipulation and the ability to conduct high-throughput drug screens in these systems at a scale that is impractical in mice, given their larger size (104). While mice offer greater conservation to humans (mice and humans share 99% of their genes), these less complex model systems share a reasonable degree of conservation to humans at the genetic level, with *Drosophila* and zebrafish sharing 75% and over 80% of their genes with humans, respectively (104). There is also evidence for conservation of neurochemical pathways (104,120,121), such that studies using these systems are translatable to neuropsychiatric disorders. For example, disruption of the fly ortholog of the *FMR1* gene resulted in abnormal courtship behavior and neuroanatomical changes that were reversed by treatment with metabotropic glutamatergic antagonists (121), similar to findings implicating this pathway in knockout mice. In addition, studies of zebrafish lacking the function of risk genes associated with ASD or epilepsy led to the identification of novel pharmacologic compounds with relevance to these disorders (122,123). While there is a "tradeoff" between the range of studies that can be conducted in less complex systems and their similarity to humans (104), it is likely that an increasing number of functional analyses of risk genes will utilize multiple animal models to harness the distinct advantages of each system.

At the same time, there are limitations to the use of animal systems for modeling neuropsychiatric disorders. First, human-specific behaviors cannot be fully recapitulated in an animal system (104–106). Face validity, or the extent to which a quantifiable behavior in an animal model represents a related behavior in humans, may be limited (106). For example, in mouse models, the time an animal spends in an open field compared to the rim of an enclosure may be used as a measure of anxiety, and repetitive grooming is considered representative of obsessive–compulsive behavior (106). While these assays cannot encompass the range of clinical symptoms associated with neuropsychiatric disorders in humans, animal models can provide critical insights into the biologic processes underlying behavior at the molecular and circuit levels. Second, pharmacologic compounds identified in animal models may not translate to humans. For example, metabotropic glutamatergic receptor antagonists reverse physiologic and behavioral abnormalities in animal models of FXS, yet these compounds have yet to be successful in clinical trials (124). Their apparent lack of efficacy may be due in part to issues in clinical trial design, such that administering the medication to younger individuals for a longer period of time or developing more precise measures to assess efficacy may improve outcomes (124). Third, it may not be possible to recapitulate some genetic abnormalities using animal models due to limits of genetic conservation. For example, CNVs are more difficult to replicate in animals than single nucleotide mutations, and animal models cannot capture the genetic diversity present in a particular individual, which may influence clinical presentation. Nonetheless, animal models play an important role in advancing from risk gene identification to the discovery of biologic mechanisms with relevance to childhood neuropsychiatric disorders.

Animal models are a key component of translating human genetics findings "from bench to bedside." Given the growing list of risk genes in neuropsychiatric disorders resulting from large-scale sequencing efforts, there is an increased need to investigate the extent to which these genes converge on common neurodevelopmental pathways using in vivo systems. With the emergence of novel technologies to examine neuronal activity in an awake, behaving animal, animal models offer considerable promise to illuminate the effect of risk gene disruption on the establishment of neural circuits underlying behavioral deficits. At the same time, the relevance of an animal model for a human disorder often relies on the strength of the evidence from human genetic studies implicating the risk gene under investigation. Therefore, continued progress in the ability to identify with confidence genes that are strongly associated with childhood neuropsychiatric disorders will be critical for elucidating the biologic mechanisms underlying these disorders and developing improved pharmacologic treatments.

Stem Cell Modeling

Another strategy for translating human genetic findings is the generation of iPSCs to model disease. In 2007, Yamanaka et al. reported in their landmark paper that adult human dermal fibroblasts could be reprogrammed into a pluripotent state using just four transcription factors, Oct3/4, Sox2, Klf4, and c-Myc (125). These iPSCs could, in turn, be differentiated into any cell type of the body, including neural cells. This development revolutionized the biologic investigation of neuropsychiatric disorders since the field is severely challenged by the unavailability of living brain tissue for cellular and molecular studies. Since then, numerous research groups have adopted this technique to reprogram a variety of mature cell types, including fibroblasts, lymphocytes (126), lymphoblastoid cell lines (127), dental pulp cells (128), and renal epithelial cells present in urine (129).

Although postmortem studies have been invaluable in revealing abnormalities of patient brain tissue, such as in cytoarchitecture (130) and gene expression (131) for disorders like ASD and schizophrenia, postmortem tissue also has limitations that can be overcome by iPSCs (130,132). Variability in parameters such as cause of death, time to collection, fixation methods, and storage conditions can confound results. Furthermore, it is difficult to determine if any findings are specific to the pathophysiology of the disorder as opposed to the lifetime accumulation of environmental effects, including treatments. The absence of living cells does not allow for functional studies, such as the electrophysiologic properties of neurons and neural circuits.

As discussed above, animal models have a long tradition of providing valuable insights into human disorders but also have limitations that can be complemented by iPSCs. Compared to iPSCs, animal breeding is more resource intensive in terms of time, space, and expense. The genome of animal models is often manipulated to recreate mutations identified in patients. Although it can be very informative to isolate the effects of a single mutation, the genetic background of the patient, which can have critical influence on disease expression, is missing (133). Also, multiple mutations within an individual and large CNVs make important contributions to the genetic architecture of complex neuropsychiatric disorders, but these are very difficult to model in animals (130). Species differences in genetics, neurobiology, and behavior mean that it is difficult to recapitulate the cognitive, affective, social, and behavioral phenotypes, which are often uniquely human. Still, no one model will completely elucidate the pathophysiology of a disorder. The multimodal approach is most likely to reveal the fullest picture. In their review, Habela et al. (130) provide the example of FXS: while postmortem studies and mouse models show increased dendritic spine density, iPSC-derived neurons show fewer and shorter spines. Further investigation will be needed to resolve these contradictory results, which may be due to possibilities such as compensatory mechanisms in the patient condition or the influence of culture conditions on iPSC-derived neurons (130).

As with any modeling technique, there are important advantages and limitations to using iPSCs. Since they can be generated from mature cells, iPSCs avoid the ethical and policy complications of using embryonic stem cells (ESCs). Source cells can be obtained by relatively simple, noninvasive, and common procedures, such as skin biopsy, blood draw, saving teeth which have been naturally shed, and urine collection. Unlike primary cell cultures, which have limited proliferative capability, iPSCs propagate indefinitely. Through specific culture conditions, which require the addition and/or withdrawal of the appropriate growth factors, iPSCs can be differentiated into any cell type of the body. Protocols have been developed to direct differentiation into electrically active glutamatergic, GABAergic, dopaminergic, and motor neurons; astrocytes; and oligodendrocytes. However, protocols need to be established for other important cell populations in the brain, such as cortical layer-specific neurons, various GABAergic neuronal subtypes, Purkinje cells, microglia, and endothelial cells (134,135). Co-culturing neuronal and nonneuronal cells would be expected to better capture disease-relevant phenotypes. The ability to produce excitatory neurons, inhibitory interneurons, and astrocytes can be very useful to probe the excitatory/inhibitory imbalance that has been identified as a feature of neuropsychiatric disorders such as ASD and schizophrenia (134).

Two popular approaches to iPSC modeling involve: (1) generating iPSCs from patient cells and (2) generating iPSCs from a healthy individual, which are then engineered to carry a patient mutation. The obvious advantage of the first approach is that it preserves the genetic background of the patient. This is especially important in complex neuropsychiatric disorders, which may result from the interaction of multiple mutations within an individual. Furthermore, iPSCs can be generated from patients for whom a genetic etiology has not been established; abnormal cellular and molecular phenotypes can still provide clues as to disease mechanism, as has been shown for idiopathic ASD (136). In those with defined genetics, genome editing techniques, such as the CRISPR/Cas9 system mentioned above (137), can be used to correct the mutation(s) to determine whether it was necessary to cause any abnormal phenotypes. By the second approach, a panel of isogenic lines can be created, each of which is engineered to carry a different disease-associated mutation. This allows for isolating and comparing the effects of each mutation without the confound of differing genetic backgrounds, and tests whether a mutation is sufficient to cause abnormal phenotypes. Combined, these approaches provide two pairs of well-matched, rigorously controlled cell lines, which can strengthen the evidence for association between any one mutation and disease (Figure 3.3.2.9), and is especially important in highly multigenic disorders.

Another advantage of iPSC modeling is that the differentiation of iPSCs to neural progenitor cells (NPCs) and mature neural cells enables the study of the full developmental process. Numerous features can be examined, including gene expression, cell proliferation, differentiation, organization, migration, morphology, synapse formation and function, etc. Neural cells can be grown in a two-dimensional monolayer culture, which facilitates cell-based assays. Neural cells can also be grown as three-dimensional organoids, which more closely, but by no means completely, recapitulate early human brain development. They may better capture cell–cell signaling and simplified network activity (134,138). iPSC modeling allows for the testing of environmental stressors on neural development and function. It is generally believed that both genetics and environmental factors contribute to many neuropsychiatric disorders; gene x environment interactions can be investigated in iPSCs and iPSC-derived neural cell lines. Through automation, iPSCs can offer a platform to screen the effects of hundreds of mutations and identify potential targets for treatment. Similarly, iPSCs can offer a high-throughput platform to screen for drugs that reverse abnormal phenotypes. The use of patient iPSCs also furthers the goal of personalized medicine.

As no one technique is expected to perfectly model neuropsychiatric disorders, it is important to be aware of the limitations of iPSCs. Despite its many advantages, it is still an in vitro

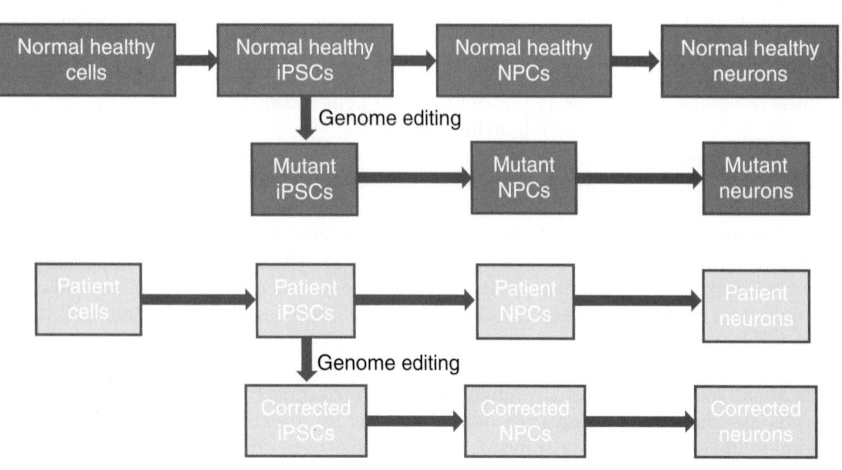

FIGURE 3.3.2.9. Two popular approaches to induced pluripotent stem cell (iPSC) modeling. Two pairs of well-matched cell lines derived from (1) a normal healthy individual in whom a mutation has been introduced and (2) a patient in whom the mutation has been corrected by genome editing. Combined, these approaches provide two pairs of well-matched, rigorously controlled cell lines, which can strengthen the evidence for association between any one mutation and disease, and is especially important in highly multigenic disorders. NPCs, neural progenitor cells.

model of complex brain organization and function. The neural cell lines produced by current differentiation methods allow for the identification of cellular and molecular phenotypes but limit the interrogation of complex neural networks. The generation of iPSCs, NPCs, and neural cells are not quick protocols. It can take a month to reprogram source cells into iPSCs, a month to differentiate iPSCs into NPCs, and 3 to 4 months for NPCs to develop into neural cells. The generation of iPSCs is labor intensive, since iPSC clones are prone to spontaneous differentiation at their periphery and require frequent "cleaning." Gene expression profiling studies have shown that the neurons tend to be immature (139), which could decrease their relevance to disease modeling. Therefore, it is important to determine the maturation status of iPSC-derived neurons. Some research groups are developing protocols to transform source cells directly into neural cells by forcing expression of lineage-specific transcription factors (133). This would greatly speed up these investigations. However, eliminating the normal developmental process may also eliminate important disease-related phenotypes, especially for neurodevelopmental disorders such as ASD.

A major concern of iPSC modeling is genetic and epigenetic variability, which has been detected between iPSC lines, between iPSC and ESC lines, between different passages of the same iPSC line, and between different populations at the same passage number of the same iPSC line (140). Concerns have been raised that the reprogramming process may introduce mutations, although a study showed that genetic mosaicism of the source cells accounted for most of what appeared to be de novo CNVs (141). Given the variability, it is critical that multiple, independent iPSC lines are generated for each mutation or patient. It is also critical to study well-matched, rigorously controlled cell lines as described earlier. The magnitude of this problem was clearly demonstrated by a study of iPSC models of Parkinson disease (PD) (142). The researchers generated iPSCs from patients with the PD-associated LRRK2 G2019S mutation and unrelated healthy controls. They used genome editing to correct the G2019S mutation in patient iPSCs and introduce this mutation into control iPSCs. Transcriptome profiling and cluster analysis of the iPSC-derived neurons revealed that some patient and control lines clustered with each other rather than with their own groups as would be expected. Only the matched patient and patient-corrected lines consistently clustered closely together.

Reprogramming, by definition, involves genome-wide epigenetic changes, including changes in DNA methylation and histone modification (143). However, there are reports of incomplete reprogramming and epigenetic alterations, including at imprinted loci and the inactivated X chromosome, during prolonged culturing (140). This raises concerns for modeling disorders of genomic imprinting and X-linked disorders. However, iPSCs generated from patients with Angelman and Prader–Willi syndromes were found to retain the appropriate DNA methylation patterns (144). In addition to studying multiple, independent, rigorously controlled cell lines, it may be advisable to assess epigenetic patterns before and after generation of iPSCs. Mutation correction experiments can also help determine if abnormal phenotypes are due to the specific mutation under study or confounded by genetic and/or epigenetic variability.

Several reviews have catalogued iPSC modeling of a variety of neuropsychiatric disorders, including genetic syndromes, ASD, schizophrenia, bipolar disorder, and depression (130,132–135,145). The growing number of studies are providing critical insights into pathophysiology, and identifying potential targets for treatment.

CONCLUSIONS

Rapidly advancing technologies in human genetics have provided significant insights into the etiology of childhood neuropsychiatric disorders, but they have only uncovered the tip of the iceberg regarding pathophysiology. Now that a growing list of genes are being strongly associated with these disorders, it is critical to determine precisely how mutations affect the structure and function of proteins and contribute to the development of disease. As discussed above, a multimodal approach, which includes the study of animal models, postmortem brain tissue, and cellular models, will yield the best information since each technique has strengths and weaknesses and, indeed, complement each other. They will help achieve the ultimate goals of elucidating pathophysiology, identifying targets for treatment, and screening therapeutic agents.

References

1. Collins FS: Positional cloning: let's not call it reverse anymore. *Nat Genet* 1(1):3–6, 1992.
2. Willsey AJ, State MW: Autism spectrum disorders: from genes to neurobiology. *Curr Opin Neurobiol* 30:92–99, 2015.
3. Kendler KS: Overview: a current perspective on twin studies of schizophrenia. *Am J Psychiatry* 140(11):1413–1425, 1983.
4. Cardno AG, Marshall EJ, Coid B, et al.: Heritability estimates for psychotic disorders: the Maudsley twin psychosis series. *Arch Gen Psychiatry* 56(2):162–168, 1999.
5. Battaglia M: Gene-environment interaction in panic disorder and posttraumatic stress disorder. *Can J Psychiatry* 58(2):69–75, 2013.
6. Lopizzo N, Bocchio Chiavetto L, Cattane N, et al.: Gene-environment interaction in major depression: focus on experience-dependent biological systems. *Front Psychiatry* 6:68, 2015.
7. Uher R: Gene-environment interactions in severe mental illness. *Front Psychiatry* 5:48, 2014.
8. Corder EH, Saunders AM, Strittmatter WJ, et al.: Gene dose of apolipoprotein E type 4 allele and the risk of Alzheimer's disease in late onset families. *Science* 261(5123):921–923, 1993.
9. Fullerton SM, Clark AG, Weiss KM, et al.: Apolipoprotein E variation at the sequence haplotype level: implications for the origin and maintenance of a major human polymorphism. *Am J Hum Genet* 67(4):881–900, 2000.
10. Reich DE, Lander ES: On the allelic spectrum of human disease. *Trends Genet* 17(9):502–510, 2001.
11. Pritchard JK, Cox NJ: The allelic architecture of human disease genes: common disease-common variant...or not? *Hum Mol Genet* 11(20):2417–2423, 2002.
12. Pritchard JK: Are rare variants responsible for susceptibility to complex diseases? *Am J Hum Genet* 69(1):124–137, 2001.
13. Herbert A, Gerry NP, McQueen MB, et al.: A common genetic variant is associated with adult and childhood obesity. *Science* 312(5771): 279–283, 2006.
14. Altshuler D, Brooks LD, Chakravarti A, et al.: A haplotype map of the human genome. *Nature* 437(7063):1299–1320, 2005.
15. Rutter M, Silberg J, O'Connor T, Simonoff E. et al.: Genetics and child psychiatry: I Advances in quantitative and molecular genetics. *J Child Psychol Psychiatry* 40(1):3–18, 1999.
16. Insel T, Cuthbert B, Garvey M, et al.: Research domain criteria (RDoC): toward a new classification framework for research on mental disorders. *Am J Psychiatry* 167(7):748–751, 2010.
17. Risch N: Linkage strategies for genetically complex traits. II. The power of affected relative pairs. *Am J Hum Genet* 46(2):229–241, 1990.
18. Risch N: Linkage strategies for genetically complex traits. I. Multilocus models. *Am J Hum Genet* 46(2):222–228, 1990.
19. Robinson EB, Neale BM, Hyman SE: Genetic research in autism spectrum disorders. *Curr Opin Pediatr* 27(6):685–691, 2015.
20. Dawn Teare M, Barrett JH: Genetic linkage studies. *Lancet* 366(9490): 1036–1044, 2005.
21. Lifton RP, Gharavi AG, Geller DS: Molecular mechanisms of human hypertension. *Cell* 104(4):545–556, 2001.
22. Ropers HH, Hamel BC: X-linked mental retardation. *Nat Rev Genet* 6(1):46–57, 2005.
23. Tourette Syndrome Association International Consortium for Genetics: A complete genome screen in sib pairs affected by Gilles de la Tourette syndrome. *Am J Hum Genet* 65(5):1428–1436, 1999.
24. Tourette Syndrome Association International Consortium for Genetics: Genome scan for Tourette disorder in affected-sibling-pair and multigenerational families. *Am J Hum Genet* 80(2):265–272, 2007.
25. Curtis D, Brett P, Dearlove AM, et al.: Genome scan of Tourette syndrome in a single large pedigree shows some support for linkage to regions of chromosomes 5, 10 and 13. *Psychiatr Genet* 14(2):83–87, 2004.
26. Paschou P, Feng Y, Pakstis AJ, et al.: Indications of linkage and association of Gilles de la Tourette syndrome in two independent family samples: 17q25 is a putative susceptibility region. *Am J Hum Genet* 75(4):545–560, 2004.

27. Zhang H, Leckman JF, Pauls DL, et al.: Genomewide scan of hoarding in sib pairs in which both sibs have Gilles de la Tourette syndrome. *Am J Hum Genet* 70(4):896–904, 2002.
28. Straub RE, MacLean CJ, O'Neill FA, et al.: A potential vulnerability locus for schizophrenia on chromosome 6p24–22: evidence for genetic heterogeneity. *Nat Genet* 11(3):287–293, 1995.
29. Lindholm E, Ekholm B, Shaw S, et al.: A schizophrenia-susceptibility locus at 6q25, in one of the world's largest reported pedigrees. *Am J Hum Genet* 69(1):96–105, 2001.
30. Lerer B, Seqman RH, Hamdan A, et al.: Genome scan of Arab Israeli families maps a schizophrenia susceptibility gene to chromosome 6q23 and supports a locus at chromosome 10q24. *Mol Psychiatry* 8(5):488–498, 2003.
31. Williams NM, Norton N, Williams H, et al.: A systematic genomewide linkage study in 353 sib pairs with schizophrenia. *Am J Hum Genet* 73(6): 1355–1367, 2003.
32. Escamilla M, Hare E, Dassori AM, et al.: A schizophrenia gene locus on chromosome 17q21 in a new set of families of Mexican and Central American ancestry: evidence from the NIMH Genetics of schizophrenia in Latino populations study. *Am J Psychiatry* 166(4):442–449, 2009.
33. Walters KA, Huang Y, Azaro M, et al.: Meta-analysis of repository data: impact of data regularization on NIMH schizophrenia linkage results. *PLoS One* 9(1):e84696, 2014.
34. Arcos-Burgos M, Castellanos FX, Pineda D, et al.: Attention-deficit/hyperactivity disorder in a population isolate: linkage to loci at 4q13.2, 5q33.3, 11q22, and 17p11. *Am J Hum Genet* 75(6):998–1014, 2004.
35. Asherson P, Zhou K, Anney RJ, et al.: A high-density SNP linkage scan with 142 combined subtype ADHD sib pairs identifies linkage regions on chromosomes 9 and 16. *Mol Psychiatry* 13(5):514–521, 2008.
36. Hebebrand J, Dempfle A, Saar K, et al.: A genome-wide scan for attention-deficit/hyperactivity disorder in 155 German sib-pairs. *Mol Psychiatry* 11(2):196–205, 2006.
37. Ogdie MN, Bakker SC, Fisher SE, et al.: Pooled genome-wide linkage data on 424 ADHD ASPs suggests genetic heterogeneity and a common risk locus at 5p13. *Mol Psychiatry* 11(1):5–8, 2006.
38. Ogdie MN, Macphie IL, Minassian SL, et al.: A genomewide scan for attention-deficit/hyperactivity disorder in an extended sample: suggestive linkage on 17p11. *Am J Hum Genet* 72(5):1268–1279, 2003.
39. Romanos M, Freitag C, Jacob C, et al.: Genome-wide linkage analysis of ADHD using high-density SNP arrays: novel loci at 5q13.1 and 14q12. *Mol Psychiatry* 13(5):522–530, 2008.
40. Peterson RL, Pennington BF: Developmental dyslexia. *Lancet* 379(9830): 1997–2007, 2012.
41. Altshuler D, Daly MJ, Lander ES. Genetic mapping in human disease. *Science* 322(5903):881–888, 2008.
42. Ercan-Sencicek AG, Stillman AA, Ghosh AK, et al.: L-histidine decarboxylase and Tourette's syndrome. *N Engl J Med* 362(20):1901–1908, 2010.
43. Bloch M, State M, Pittenger C: Recent advances in Tourette syndrome. *Curr Opin Neurol* 24(2):119–125, 2011.
44. Fernandez TV, Sanders SJ, Yurkiewicz IR, et al.: Rare copy number variants in Tourette syndrome disrupt genes in histaminergic pathways and overlap with autism. *Biol Psychiatry* 71(5):392–402, 2012.
45. Ohtsu H, Tanaka S, Terui T, et al.: Mice lacking histidine decarboxylase exhibit abnormal mast cells. *FEBS Lett* 502(1–2):53–56, 2001.
46. Castellan Baldan L, Williams KA, Gallezot JD, et al.: Histidine decarboxylase deficiency causes Tourette syndrome: parallel findings in humans and mice. *Neuron* 81(1):77–90, 2014.
47. Parmentier R, Ohtsu H, Djebbara-Hannas Z, Valatx JL, Watanabe T, Lin JS: Anatomical, physiological, and pharmacological characteristics of histidine decarboxylase knock-out mice: evidence for the role of brain histamine in behavioral and sleep-wake control. *J Neurosci* 22(17):7695–7711, 2002.
48. Sanders AR, Duan J, Gejman PV: Complexities in psychiatric genetics. *Int Rev Psychiatry* 16(4):284–293, 2004.
49. Risch N, Merikangas K: The future of genetic studies of complex human diseases. *Science* 273(5281):1516–1517, 1996.
50. Risch NJ: Searching for genetic determinants in the new millennium. *Nature* 405(6788):847–856, 2000.
51. Manolio TA, Collins FS, Cox NJ, et al.: Finding the missing heritability of complex diseases. *Nature* 461(7265):747–753, 2009.
52. Hirschhorn JN, Lohmueller K, Byrne E, Hirschhorn K: A comprehensive review of genetic association studies. *Genet Med* 4(2):45–61, 2002.
53. Anney R, Klei L, Pinto D, et al.: Individual common variants exert weak effects on the risk for autism spectrum disorders. *Hum Mol Genet* 21(21): 4781–4792, 2012.
54. Chaste P, Klei L, Sanders SJ, et al.: A genome-wide association study of autism using the Simons Simplex Collection: Does reducing phenotypic heterogeneity in autism increase genetic homogeneity? *Biol Psychiatry* 77(9):775–784, 2015.
55. Ripke S, O'Dushlaine C, Chambert K, et al.: Genome-wide association analysis identifies 13 new risk loci for schizophrenia. *Nat Genet* 45(10): 1150–1159, 2013.
56. Sekar A, Bialas AR, de Rivera H, et al.: Schizophrenia risk from complex variation of complement component 4. *Nature* 530(7589):177–183, 2016.
57. Abelson JF, Kwan KY, O'Roak BJ, et al.: Sequence variants in SLITRK1 are associated with Tourette's syndrome. *Science* 310(5746):317–320, 2005.
58. Stillman AA, Krsnik Z, Sun J, et al.: Developmentally regulated and evolutionarily conserved expression of SLITRK1 in brain circuits implicated in Tourette syndrome. *J Comp Neurol* 513(1):21–37, 2009.
59. Katayama K, Yamada K, Ornthanalai VG, et al.: Slitrk1-deficient mice display elevated anxiety-like behavior and noradrenergic abnormalities. *Mol Psychiatry* 15(2):177–184, 2010.
60. Bloch MH: Emerging treatments for Tourette's disorder. *Curr Psychiatry Rep* 10(4):323–330, 2008.
61. Leckman JF, Goodman WK, Anderson GM, et al.: Cerebrospinal fluid biogenic amines in obsessive compulsive disorder, Tourette's syndrome, and healthy controls. *Neuropsychopharmacology* 12(1):73–86, 1995.
62. Shmelkov SV, Hormigo A, Jing D, et al.: Slitrk5 deficiency impairs corticostriatal circuitry and leads to obsessive-compulsive-like behaviors in mice. *Nat Med* 16(5):598–602, 1p following 602, 2010.
63. Chou IC, Wan L, Liu SC, Tsai CH, Tsai FJ: Association of the Slit and Trk-like 1 gene in Taiwanese patients with Tourette syndrome. *Pediatr Neurol* 37(6):404–406, 2007.
64. Deng H, Le WD, Xie WJ, Jankovic J.: Examination of the SLITRK1 gene in Caucasian patients with Tourette syndrome. *Acta Neurol Scand* 114(6):400–402, 2006.
65. Zimprich A, Hatala K, Riederer F, Stogmann E, Aschauer HN, Stamenkovic M: Sequence analysis of the complete SLITRK1 gene in Austrian patients with Tourette's disorder. *Psychiatr Genet* 18(6):308–309, 2008.
66. Zuchner S, Cuccaro ML, Tran-Viet KN, et al.: SLITRK1 mutations in trichotillomania. *Mol Psychiatry* 11(10):887–889, 2006.
67. Ozomaro U, Cai G, Kajiwara Y, et al.: Characterization of SLITRK1 variation in obsessive-compulsive disorder. *PLoS One* 8(8):e70376, 2013.
68. Miranda DM, Wigg K, Kabia EM, Feng Y, Sandor P, Barr CL: Association of SLITRK1 to Gilles de la Tourette syndrome. *Am J Med Genet B Neuropsychiatr Genet* 150B(4):483–486, 2009.
69. Karagiannidis I, Rizzo R, Tarnok Z, et al.: Replication of association between a SLITRK1 haplotype and Tourette Syndrome in a large sample of families. *Mol Psychiatry* 17(7):665–668, 2012.
70. Scharf JM, Yu D, Mathews CA, et al.: Genome-wide association study of Tourette's syndrome. *Mol Psychiatry* 18(6):721–728, 2013.
71. Sebat J, Lakshmi B, Troge J, et al.: Large-scale copy number polymorphism in the human genome. *Science* 305(5683):525–528, 2004.
72. Iafrate AJ, Feuk L, Rivera MN, et al.: Detection of large-scale variation in the human genome. *Nat Genet* 36(9):949–951, 2004.
73. Conrad DF, Pinto D, Redon R, et al.: Origins and functional impact of copy number variation in the human genome. *Nature* 464(7289):704–712, 2010.
74. Redon R, Ishikawa S, Fitch KR, et al.: Global variation in copy number in the human genome. *Nature* 444(7118):444–454, 2006.
75. Itsara A, Cooper GM, Baker C, et al.: Population analysis of large copy number variants and hotspots of human genetic disease. *Am J Hum Genet* 84(2):148–161, 2009.
76. Itsara A, Wu H, Smith JD, Nickerson DA, Romieu I, London SJ, Eichler EE, et al.: De novo rates and selection of large copy number variation. *Genome Res* 20(11):1469–1481, 2010.
77. Stefansson H, Rujescu D, Cichon S, et al.: Large recurrent microdeletions associated with schizophrenia. *Nature* 455(7210):232–236, 2008.
78. Walsh T, McClellan JM, McCarthy SE, et al.: Rare structural variants disrupt multiple genes in neurodevelopmental pathways in schizophrenia. *Science* 320(5875):539–343, 2008.
79. Wilson G, Flibotte S, Chopra V, Melnyk BL, Honer WG, Holt RA: DNA copy-number analysis in bipolar disorder and schizophrenia reveals aberrations in genes involved in glutamate signaling. *Hum Mol Genet* 15(5):743–749, 2006.
80. Xu B, Roos JL, Levy S, van Rensburg EJ, Gogos JA, Karayiorgou M: Strong association of de novo copy number mutations with sporadic schizophrenia. *Nat Genet* 40(7):880–885, 2008.
81. Mulle JG, Dodd AF, McGrath JA, et al.: Microdeletions of 3q29 confer high risk for schizophrenia. *Am J Hum Genet* 87(2):229–236, 2010.
82. International Schizophrenia Consortium: Rare chromosomal deletions and duplications increase risk of schizophrenia. *Nature* 455(7210):237–241, 2008.
83. McCarthy SE, Makarov V, Kirov G, et al.: Microduplications of 16p11.2 are associated with schizophrenia. *Nat Genet* 41(11):1223–1227, 2009.
84. Marshall C, Noor A, Vincent JB, et al.: Structural variation of chromosomes in autism spectrum disorder. *Am J Hum Genet* 82(2):477–488, 2008.
85. Sebat J, Lakshmi B, Malhotra D, et al.: Strong association of de novo copy number mutations with autism. *Science* 316(5823):445–449, 2007.
86. Autism Genome Project Consortium, Szatmari P, Paterson AD, et al.: Mapping autism risk loci using genetic linkage and chromosomal rearrangements. *Nat Genet* 39(3):319–328, 2007.
87. Glessner JT, Wang K, Cai G, et al.: Autism genome-wide copy number variation reveals ubiquitin and neuronal genes. *Nature* 459(7246):569–573, 2009.
88. Pinto D, Pagnamenta AT, Klei L, et al.: Functional impact of global rare copy number variation in autism spectrum disorders. *Nature* 466(7304):368–372, 2010.
89. Sanders S, Ercan-Sencicek AG, Hus V, et al.: Multiple recurrent de novo copy number variations (CNVs), including duplications of the 7q11.23 Williams-Buren syndrome region, are strongly associated with autism. *Neuron* 70(5):863–885, 2011.

90. Sanders SJ, He X, Willsey AJ, et al.: Insights into autism spectrum disorder genomic architecture and biology from 71 risk loci. *Neuron* 87(6):1215–1233, 2015.
91. Kumar R, KaraMohamed S, Sudi J, et al.: Recurrent 16p11.2 microdeletions in autism. *Hum Mol Genet* 17(4):628–638, 2008.
92. Weiss L, Shen Y, Korn JM, et al.: Association between microdeletion and microduplication at 16p11.2 and autism. *N Engl J Med* 358(7):667–675, 2008.
93. Pinto D, Delaby E, Merico D, et al.: Convergence of genes and cellular pathways dysregulated in autism spectrum disorders. *Am J Hum Genet* 94(5):677–694, 2014.
94. Choi M, Scholl UI, Ji W, et al.: Genetic diagnosis by whole exome capture and massively parallel DNA sequencing. *Proc Natl Acad Sci U S A* 106(45):19096–19101, 2009.
95. Lee H, Deignan JL, Dorrani N, et al.: Clinical exome sequencing for genetic identification of rare Mendelian disorders. *JAMA* 312(18):1880–1887, 2014.
96. Yang Y, Muzny DM, Reid JG, et al.: Clinical whole-exome sequencing for the diagnosis of Mendelian disorders. *N Engl J Med* 369(16):1502–1511, 2013.
97. Yang Y, Muzny DM, Xia F, et al.: Molecular findings among patients referred for clinical whole-exome sequencing. *JAMA* 312(18):1870–1879, 2014.
98. Iossifov I, O'Roak BJ, Sanders SJ, et al.: The contribution of de novo coding mutations to autism spectrum disorder. *Nature* 515(7526):216–221, 2014.
99. Sanders SJ, Murtha MT, Gupta AR, et al.: De novo mutations revealed by whole-exome sequencing are strongly associated with autism. *Nature* 485(7397):237–241, 2012.
100. Willsey AJ, Sanders SJ, Li M, et al.: Coexpression networks implicate human midfetal deep cortical projection neurons in the pathogenesis of autism. *Cell* 155(5):997–1007, 2013.
101. ENCODE Project Consortium: An integrated encyclopedia of DNA elements in the human genome. *Nature* 489(7414):57–74, 2012.
102. Turner TN, Hormozdiari F, Duyzend MH, et al.: Genome sequencing of autism-affected families reveals disruption of putative noncoding regulatory DNA. *Am J Hum Genet* 98(1):58–74, 2016.
103. Yuen RK, Thiruvahindrapuram B, Merico D, et al.: Whole-genome sequencing of quartet families with autism spectrum disorder. *Nat Med* 21(2):185–191, 2015.
104. McCammon JM, Sive H: Challenges in understanding psychiatric disorders and developing therapeutics: a role for zebrafish. *Dis Model Mech* 8(7):647–656, 2015.
105. Stevens HE, Vaccarino FM: How animal models inform child and adolescent psychiatry. *J Am Acad Child Adolesc Psychiatry* 54(5):352–359, 2015.
106. Robertson HR, Feng G: Annual Research Review: transgenic mouse models of childhood-onset psychiatric disorders. *J Child Psychol Psychiatry* 52(4):442–475, 2011.
107. Fmr1 knockout mice: a model to study fragile X mental retardation. The Dutch-Belgian Fragile X Consortium. *Cell* 78(1):23–33, 1994.
108. Comery TA, Harris JB, Willems PJ, et al.: Abnormal dendritic spines in fragile X knockout mice: maturation and pruning deficits. *Proc Natl Acad Sci U S A* 94(10):5401–5404, 1997.
109. Huber KM, Gallagher SM, Warren ST, Bear MF: Altered synaptic plasticity in a mouse model of fragile X mental retardation. *Proc Natl Acad Sci U S A* 99(11):7746–7750, 2002.
110. Shahbazian M, Young J, Yuva-Paylor L, et al.: Mice with truncated MeCP2 recapitulate many Rett syndrome features and display hyperacetylation of histone H3. *Neuron* 35(2):243–254, 2002.
111. Ure K, Lu H, Wang W, et al.: Restoration of Mecp2 expression in GABA-ergic neurons is sufficient to rescue multiple disease features in a mouse model of Rett syndrome. *Elife* 5:e14198, 2016.
112. Ji W, Foo JN, O'Roak BJ, et al.: Rare independent mutations in renal salt handling genes contribute to blood pressure variation. *Nat Genet* 40(5):592–599, 2008.
113. Chung K, Wallace J, Kim SY, et al.: Structural and molecular interrogation of intact biological systems. *Nature* 497(7449):332–337, 2013.
114. Cardin JA, Carlén M, Meletis K, et al.: Targeted optogenetic stimulation and recording of neurons in vivo using cell-type-specific expression of Channelrhodopsin-2. *Nat Protoc* 5(2):247–254, 2010.
115. Akerboom J, Chen TW, Wardill TJ, et al.: Optimization of a GCaMP calcium indicator for neural activity imaging. *J Neurosci* 32(40):13819–13840, 2012.
116. Sohal VS, Zhang F, Yizhar O, Deisseroth K: Parvalbumin neurons and gamma rhythms enhance cortical circuit performance. *Nature* 459(7247):698–702, 2009.
117. Ferenczi EA, Zalocusky KA, Liston C, et al.: Prefrontal cortical regulation of brainwide circuit dynamics and reward-related behavior. *Science* 351(6268):aac9698, 2016.
118. Bianco IH, Engert F: Visuomotor transformations underlying hunting behavior in zebrafish. *Curr Biol* 25(7):831–846, 2015.
119. Jinek M, Chylinski K, Fonfara I, Hauer M, Doudna JA, Charpentier E: A programmable dual-RNA-guided DNA endonuclease in adaptive bacterial immunity. *Science* 337(6096):816–821, 2012.
120. Rihel J, Prober DA, Arvanites A, et al.: Zebrafish behavioral profiling links drugs to biological targets and rest/wake regulation. *Science* 327(5963):348–351, 2010.
121. McBride SM, Choi CH, Wang Y, et al.: Pharmacological rescue of synaptic plasticity, courtship behavior, and mushroom body defects in a Drosophila model of fragile X syndrome. *Neuron* 45(5):753–764, 2005.
122. Hoffman EJ, Turner KJ, Fernandez JM, et al.: Estrogens suppress a behavioral phenotype in zebrafish mutants of the autism risk gene, CNTNAP2. *Neuron* 89(4):725–733, 2016.
123. Baraban SC, Dinday MT, Hortopan GA: Drug screening in Scn1a zebrafish mutant identifies clemizole as a potential Dravet syndrome treatment. *Nat Commun* 4:2410, 2013.
124. Berry-Kravis E, Des Portes V, Hagerman R, et al.: Mavoglurant in fragile X syndrome: results of two randomized, double-blind, placebo-controlled trials. *Sci Transl Med* 8(321):321ra5, 2016.
125. Takahashi K, Tanabe K, Ohnuki M, et al.: Induction of pluripotent stem cells from adult human fibroblasts by defined factors. *Cell* 131(5):861–872, 2007.
126. Loh YH, Agarwal S, Park IH, et al.: Generation of induced pluripotent stem cells from human blood. *Blood* 113(22):5476–5479, 2009.
127. Rajesh D, Dickerson SJ, Yu J, Brown ME, Thomson JA, Seay NJ: Human lymphoblastoid B-cell lines reprogrammed to EBV-free induced pluripotent stem cells. *Blood* 118(7):1797–1800, 2011.
128. Beltrao-Braga PC, Pignatari GC, Maiorka PC, et al.: Feeder-free derivation of induced pluripotent stem cells from human immature dental pulp stem cells. *Cell Transplant* 20(11–12):1707–1719, 2011.
129. Zhou T, Benda C, Dunzinger S, et al.: Generation of human induced pluripotent stem cells from urine samples. *Nat Protoc* 7(12):2080–2089, 2012.
130. Habela CW, Song H, Ming GL: Modeling synaptogenesis in schizophrenia and autism using human iPSC derived neurons. *Mol Cell Neurosci* 73:52–62, 2016.
131. Voineagu I, Wang X, Johnston P, et al.: Transcriptomic analysis of autistic brain reveals convergent molecular pathology. *Nature* 474(7351): 380–384, 2011.
132. Acab A, Muotri AR: The use of induced pluripotent stem cell technology to advance autism research and treatment. *Neurotherapeutics* 12(3): 534–545, 2015.
133. Kim DS, Ross PJ, Zaslavsky K, Ellis J, et al.: Optimizing neuronal differentiation from induced pluripotent stem cells to model ASD. *Front Cell Neurosci* 8:109, 2014.
134. Nestor MW, Phillips AW, Artimovich E, Nestor JE, Hussman JP, Blatt GJ: Human inducible pluripotent stem cells and autism spectrum disorder: emerging technologies. *Autism Res* 9(5):513–535, 2016.
135. Wen Z, Christian KM, Song H, Ming GL: Modeling psychiatric disorders with patient-derived iPSCs. *Curr Opin Neurobiol* 36:118–127, 2016.
136. Mariani J, Coppola G, Zhang P, et al.: FOXG1-dependent dysregulation of GABA/glutamate neuron differentiation in autism spectrum disorders. *Cell* 162(2):375–390, 2015.
137. Cong L, Ran FA, Cox D, et al.: Multiplex genome engineering using CRISPR/Cas systems. *Science* 339(6121):819–823, 2013.
138. Ben-Reuven L, Reiner O: Modeling the autistic cell: iPSCs recapitulate developmental principles of syndromic and nonsyndromic ASD. *Dev Growth Differ* 58(5):481–491, 2016.
139. Mariani J, Simonini MV, Palejev D, et al.: Modeling human cortical development in vitro using induced pluripotent stem cells. *Proc Natl Acad Sci U S A* 109(31):12770–12775, 2012.
140. Liang G, Zhang Y: Genetic and epigenetic variations in iPSCs: potential causes and implications for application. *Cell Stem Cell* 13(2):149–159, 2013.
141. Abyzov A, Mariani J, Palejev D, et al.: Somatic copy number mosaicism in human skin revealed by induced pluripotent stem cells. *Nature* 492(7429):438–442, 2012.
142. Reinhardt P, Schmid B, Burbulla LF, et al.: Genetic correction of a LRRK2 mutation in human iPSCs links parkinsonian neurodegeneration to ERK-dependent changes in gene expression. *Cell Stem Cell* 12(3):354–367, 2013.
143. Brix J, Zhou Y, Luo Y: The epigenetic reprogramming roadmap in generation of iPSCs from somatic cells. *J Genet Genomics* 42(12):661–670, 2015.
144. Chamberlain SJ, Chen PF, Ng KY: Induced pluripotent stem cell models of the genomic imprinting disorders Angelman and Prader-Willi syndromes. *Proc Natl Acad Sci U S A* 107(41):17668–17673, 2010.
145. Beltrao-Braga PC, Muotri AR: Modeling autism spectrum disorders with human neurons. *Brain Res* pii:S0006-8993(16)30034–30038, 2016.

CHAPTER 3.3.3 ■ MOLECULAR BASIS OF SELECT CHILDHOOD PSYCHIATRIC DISORDERS

SIMONE TOMASI, JESSICA B. LENNINGTON, JAMES F. LECKMAN, AND PAUL J. LOMBROSO

The past several decades have seen remarkable progress in the application of molecular genetic strategies to the study of neurologic and neuropsychiatric disorders (1,2). The chromosomal location for many autosomal-dominant, autosomal-recessive, and X-linked disorders has been accomplished (Table 3.3.3.1). The genes mutated in a number of these illnesses have been identified and determining the function of both the normal and mutated proteins has begun. This chapter reviews some of the important accomplishments in this area. It begins with a discussion of the molecular basis of normal learning and memory and how mutations of key signaling proteins can lead to developmental disorders, and concludes with a brief consideration of the molecular basis of additional child psychiatric disorders.

LEARNING AND MEMORY

The ability to learn something new and then consolidate that information into long-term memories is part of normal development. As clinicians, we are often asked to evaluate whether a child is developing appropriately. Are specific skills emerging at the appropriate time points or are there delays? Landmarks include the ability to speak, to read, or to interact appropriately with peers. The mechanisms by which children learn to sit and crawl, walk and talk, and develop social skills have been the intensive focus of psychologists and psychiatrists over the years.

It is only in the past few decades that investigators have begun to study these questions at a molecular level (3,4). What has emerged is a fascinating story of how cells within the central nervous system (CNS) communicate with each other during learning and initiate a series of events that lead to the formation of long-lasting memories. Equally interesting is the finding that disruptions to these normal processes can contribute to developmental disorders. First we review some of the mechanisms by which normal learning develops before discussing disorders that occur when these processes are disrupted.

A central concept to emerge from research on learning and memory is that the formation of long-term memories requires both biochemical and structural modifications within neurons. The transformation of short-term, labile memories into more stable, long-term memories requires growth at specialized points of neuronal contact termed synapses. Synapses change shape as learning proceeds—new synapses are formed and old ones are strengthened. This phenomenon, termed synaptic strengthening, is found in all parts of the brain where memories are formed.

When an action potential arrives at the end of the axon, synaptic vesicles fuse with the presynaptic terminal membrane and release one or more of a variety of neurotransmitters. The transmitters diffuse across the narrow synaptic cleft and bind to receptors on the postsynaptic terminal. Neurons communicate in this way, and the subsequent processing of the incoming signal at the postsynaptic terminal results in long-lasting changes in both the shape and biochemical composition of synapses.

A tremendous amount of research has been devoted to understanding this process over the last decade (5). To summarize, a signal arrives at the surface of a neuron and induces the production of proteins required for the morphologic and biochemical changes at the synapse. This experience-induced synaptic strengthening underlies memory formation, and the molecular mechanisms by which this occurs are reviewed next.

One of several key players in these events is a member of the mitogen-activated protein kinase (MAPK) family of proteins, the extracellular signal-regulated kinases 1/2 (ERK1/2) (6–8). The arrival of a signal at the postsynaptic terminal activates a cascade of signaling proteins that leads to the activation of ERK1/2 (Figure 3.3.3.1). The ERK pathway is activated in all brain regions where synaptic plasticity occurs and is necessary for the formation of new long-term memories (5).

ERK1/2 are members of a family of enzymes termed kinases that add phosphate groups to its target substrate proteins. The addition of bulky negatively charged phosphate groups often results in a change in the three-dimensional shape of the phosphorylated protein. As an example, the conformational change may expose a previously hidden amino acid domain buried deep within the structure of the protein. The exposure of the domain now permits interactions of the protein with other proteins further downstream in a cascade. Phosphorylation and activation of ERK1/2 leads to the phosphorylation of a set of target transcription factors and these now initiate gene transcription (9). In this way, a signal originating at the surface of a neuron is communicated to the interior of the cell, and a group of proteins are produced that are necessary for the modifications at that specific spine that accompany synaptic strengthening. As a consequence, the neuron becomes more sensitive to future synaptic input; it responds with higher excitatory potentials than before. Moreover, the increase in responsiveness may last for prolonged periods of time, months, years or longer. This phenomenon, termed long-term potentiation, is thought to underlie the molecular changes that occur during the formation of stable, long-term memories (5,10).

As mentioned, ERK1/2 belong to the family of MAPK, which also includes c-Jun N-terminal kinase (JNK) and p38. JNK activation has been implicated in stress-induced associative learning in the hippocampus (11), whereas signaling through ERK1/2 is critical for long-, but not short-term memory (12–14). This role for ERK1/2 has been demonstrated by blocking the activity of ERK1/2 by injecting inhibitors of the activator of this enzyme into specific brain regions, such as the amygdala. As a consequence, the formation of memories that are normally consolidated within that structure does not occur (e.g., fear conditioning) (15,16). Similarly, if ERK1/2 activity is blocked within the hippocampus, formation of memories that require the hippocampus is prevented (e.g., visual–spatial learning) (17). In a different set of experiments, ERK1/2 signaling was shown to be a critically involved in the control

TABLE 3.3.3.1

CHROMOSOMAL LOCALIZATION AND GENE ABNORMALITIES IN SELECTED PSYCHIATRIC AND NEUROLOGIC DISORDERS

Genetic Disorder	Chromosomal Location	Genetic Mutation (Protein)
Autosomal Dominant		
Amyotrophic lateral sclerosis	21q22.1	Point mutations (superoxide dismutase)
Benign familial neonatal convulsions 1	20q13.2	Point mutations (voltage-gated potassium channel)
Benign familial neonatal convulsions 2	8q24	Point mutations (a second voltage-gated potassium channel)
Charcot–Marie–Tooth disease		
Type 1A	17p11.2	Gene duplication, deletions, point mutations (peripheral myelin protein-22, PMP22)
Type 1B	1q23.3	Point mutations (myelin protein zero protein)
Alzheimer disease		
AD1	21q21	Point mutations (amyloid precursor protein)
AD2	19q13.2	Increased frequency of apoE4 allele
AD3	14q24.3	Point mutations (presenilin-1)
AD4	1q31-q42	Point mutations (presenilin-2)
Huntington disease	4p16.3	Triplet repeat (huntingtin)
Myotonic dystrophy	19q13.2	Triplet repeat (myotonin protein kinase)
Neurofibromatosis	17q11.2	Deletions, insertions, translocations, and point mutations (neurofibromin)
Von Recklinghausen		
Acoustic neuroma	22q.12.2	Translocations, deletions, point mutations (merlin)
Parkinson disease	4q21	Point mutations (α-synuclein)
Spinocerebral ataxia	6p23	Triplet repeat (SCA1)
Imprinting Disorders		
Angelman syndrome	15q11-12	Deletion, uniparental disomy, point mutations, imprinting center mutation (UBE3A)
Prader–Willi syndrome	15q11-12	Deletion, uniparental disomy, imprinting center mutation (candidate protein: SNRNP)
Autosomal Recessive		
Ataxia telangiectasia	11q23	Translocation, deletions, point mutations (ATM)
Gaucher disease	1q21	Point mutations (glucocerebrosidase)
Lissencephaly Miller–Dieker	17q13.3	Deletions (lissencephaly 1)
Milder lissencephaly	17q13.3	Point mutations (lissencephaly 1)
Phenylketonuria	12q24	Deletions, point mutations (phenylalanine hydroxylase)
Parkinson disease	6q25.2-q27	Point mutations, deletions (parkin)
Retinoblastoma	13q14	Deletions, point mutation (retinoblastoma)
Rubinstein–Taybi syndrome	16p13.3	Translocation, deletions, point mutations (CREB-binding protein)
Schizencephaly	3q25-q26	Candidate gene (homeobox gene emx2)
Waardenburg syndrome	2q35	Deletions, point mutation (Pax-3)
Williams syndrome	7q11.23	Deletions (multiple candidate genes)
Wilson disease	13q14.21	Point mutations, deletions (copper-transporting ATPase)
Velocardiofacial syndrome	22q11	Candidate gene (UFDIL)
X-Linked Recessive		
Muscular dystrophy		
Duchenne dystrophy	Xp21.21	Large deletion (dystrophin)
Becker dystrophy	Xp21.21	Small deletion (dystrophin)
Fragile X syndrome	Xq27.3	Triplet repeat (FMR-1)
Lesch–Nyhan syndrome	Xq27	Deletions, point mutations (HGPRT)
Lissencephaly (double-cortex)	Xq22.3	Translocation, point mutations (doublecortin)
Rett syndrome	Xq28	Point mutations (MeCP2)
Spinobulbar muscular atrophy	Xp21.3	Triplet repeat (androgen receptor)
Mitochondrial Diseases with Maternal Transmission		
Leber hereditary optic atrophy	Mitochondria	Point mutations (NADH dehydrogenase)
Mitochondrial myopathy	Mitochondria	Deletion (candidate genes: Cox II and cytochrome b)

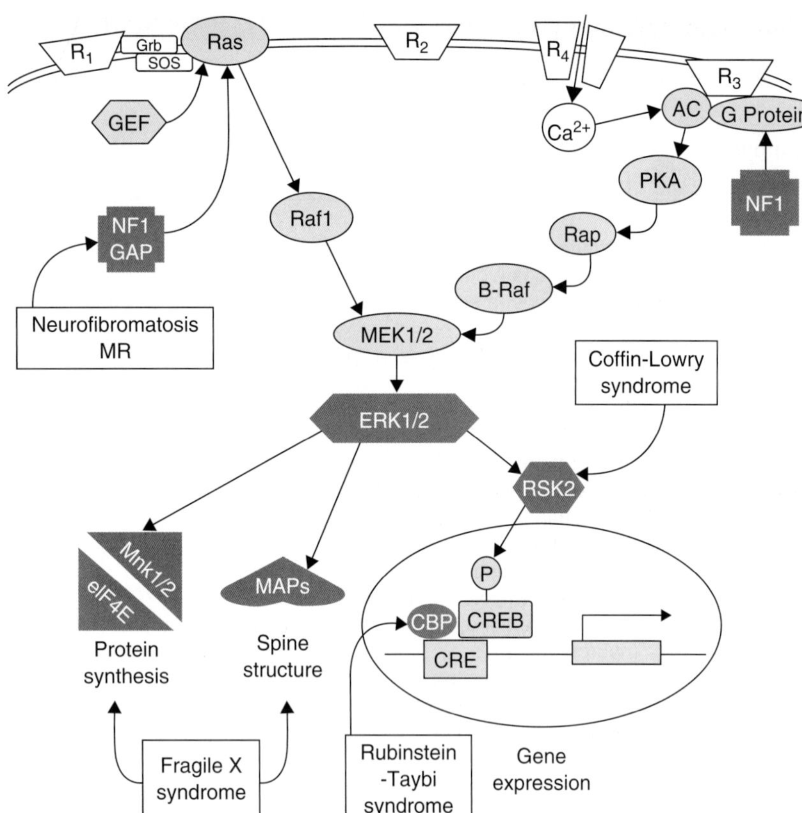

FIGURE 3.3.3.1. The ERK MAPK cascade is affected in human mental retardation syndromes. The mitogen-activated protein kinase (MAPK) family includes two important members that are involved in many different forms of learning and memory. These proteins are termed extracellular signal-regulated kinases (ERKs) to reflect the fact that they were initially characterized as kinases that became activated after growth factors bound to specific receptors at the outer surface of a cell's membrane. Upstream regulators and selected potential downstream targets of the ERK MAP kinase cascade are shown, along with known sites of derangement in human mental retardation syndromes. One current model is that MAPK plays multiple roles in memory formation: Modulating the induction of lasting synaptic changes through regulating voltage-dependent potassium channels and triggering long-lasting changes through regulating gene expression via CREB phosphorylation. Other possible sites of action are regulating local protein synthesis, regulating cytoskeletal proteins, and regulating other ion channels such as the AMPA subtype of glutamate receptor. (Adapted with permission from Sweatt JD, Weeber EJ, Lombroso PJ: Cognitive disorders and the ras/ERK/CREB pathway. *J Am Acad Child Adol Psychiatry* 42:741–744, 2003.)

of reward-seeking behavior in the nucleus accumbens (18), a region of the basal brain which receives broad glutamatergic (from prefrontal cortex, hippocampal subiculum, thalamus, and amygdala) and dopaminergic (from ventral tegmental areas) inputs and plays an important role in reward and learning, as well as in addiction. Disruption of ERK1/2 activation resulted in a decrease in reward-seeking behavior (19).

A key point in the present discussion is that a series of proteins are "upstream" of ERK1/2 and therefore necessary for its activation, while other proteins are "downstream" of activated ERK1/2 and are required for transcriptional activation. ERK1/2 signaling is activated by both glutamate (20) and dopamine signaling (21), as well as by neurotrophins such as brain-derived neurotrophic factor (BDNF) (22). Several targets have been characterized downstream of ERK1/2; among these, cyclic AMP response element binding protein (CREB) and Elk1 are two well-characterized transcription factors involved in long-term synaptic plasticity and memory in the hippocampus and other brain regions (23,24). It follows that disruption of components of this multistep pathway might disrupt the development of synaptic strengthening and contribute to developmental delays. Mutations have recently been discovered in several genes involved in this pathway and these mutations lead to the three developmental disorders that are discussed next.

Neurofibromatosis. Neurofibromatosis is an autosomal-dominant disease with clinical features that include neural-derived tumors and café-au-lait spots throughout the body. Approximately half of the affected individuals are also intellectually disabled (25). The gene that causes neurofibromatosis type I (*NF1*) was recently characterized and several mutations were identified in affected patients (26). Variability in the types of mutations (point mutations, insertions, or deletions) reflects a high level of phenotypic heterogeneity. It has been recently proposed that nongenetic, stochastic factors may contribute to the severity of symptoms, as suggested by the occurrence of loss of heterozygosity at *NF1* and "second-hit" mutations in neurofibromas, astrocytomas, malignant peripheral nerve sheath tumors, and pheochromocytomas from patients with *NF1* mutations (27).

The region of the gene that is mutated determines whether or not the child develops cognitive deficits, in addition to the characteristic benign tumors. In other words, the normal neurofibromin protein has several amino acid domains with distinct cellular functions. One of the domains regulates cellular proliferation, and mutations within this region of the gene lead to the unregulated proliferation of cells and the formation of tumors. Another portion of the protein regulates the ERK1/2 pathway, and mutations within this region interfere with the ability of neurofibromin to downregulate the ERK1/2 pathway. At least 200 mutations of another gene, *NF2*, have been reported for neurofibromatosis type II. *NF2* encodes a tumor-suppressor protein, merlin, which normally suppresses the Ras-ERK1/2 signaling pathway (28). As a consequence, the ERK1/2 pathway is overactive and does not respond appropriately to incoming neuronal signals. Normal synaptic strengthening does not occur and individuals with this type of mutation have cognitive disabilities (29).

Coffin–Lowry syndrome. A mutation in another protein in the classical ERK1/2 pathway leads to Coffin–Lowry syndrome, which is inherited in an X-linked manner (30). Several pathogenic allelic variants have been described throughout the *RSK2* gene, although their correlation with a specific phenotype has not been identified. Most variants are associated with protein truncation due to missense or nonsense mutations; intragenic deletions were observed in 21% of cases, as well as partial or full gene duplications. Interestingly, benign allelic variants have also been described, which are not associated with Coffin–Lowry syndrome (31,32). One of the downstream targets of the ERK1/2 pathway is a kinase called ribosomal S6 kinase (RSK2). RSK2 is a protein kinase that rapidly enters the nucleus upon activation and phosphorylates the transcription factor, CREB. The transcription factor CREB targets specific genes and induces their expression; in the absence of phosphorylation by RSK2, CREB remains less active. Mutations in the *RSK2* gene thus disrupt the normal cascade from the neuronal surface to the nucleus, interfere with gene transcription and the synthesis of proteins required for synaptic modifications (33). During neurite formation, nerve growth factor activates RSK2 that results in synthesis of phosphatidic acids and contributes to vesicle fusion at sites of synaptic growth (34). RSK2 has also been implicated in DNA repair and the control of genome stability (35).

Rubinstein–Taybi syndrome. A third disorder associated with mutations in the ERK1/2 pathway is Rubinstein–Taybi syndrome (RTS) (36). RTS individuals have characteristic clinical signs that include facial abnormalities, broad digits, and cognitive deficits. Recently, a mutation to the CREB-binding protein gene (*CBP*) was discovered in approximately 50% to 60% of patients with the RTS phenotype. The CBP protein is required for the normal unwinding of DNA that precedes the binding of transcription factors to promoter regions. As a result of the mutation, the transcription factor CREB cannot bind properly to the targeted DNA sequences that promote the initiation of gene transcription. Once again, synaptic strengthening is disrupted and normal learning does not develop. Pathogenic variants at the *EP300* locus have been recently described in 3% to 5% of patients with a milder cognitive impairment (37). EP300 is a histone acetyltransferase that acts as a transcriptional coactivator and tumor-suppressor protein; CBP and EP300 display high primary protein sequence similarities, but are implicated in distinct cellular functions, although the molecular alterations caused by *EP300* mutations have not been characterized yet.

FRAGILE X SYNDROME

The molecular biology of fragile X syndrome has advanced dramatically over the past few decades (38). This disorder is the second most common cause of cognitive deficits after Down syndrome and the most common form of inherited intellectual disability. Initial estimates of the prevalence of disorder were based on the detection of the Xq27.3 fragile site and reported that as many as 1 in every 1,000 to 2,600 males were affected. However, recent molecular diagnostic tests assessing the *FMR-1* gene revised the prevalence to approximately 1 in 5,000 males (39) with prevalence in females approximately one-half of this estimate.

Children with fragile X syndrome are born with mild to severe cognitive deficits and approximately 50% of them meet the diagnostic criteria for autism (40). Additional clinical symptoms include facial, testicular, and connective tissue abnormalities (41,42). Abnormal speech patterns are present in the majority of cases and include echolalia and high-pitched speech, as well as poor articulation, dysfluency, and dyspraxia. Social anxiety and gaze aversion are common among these children, as well as stereotypic behaviors, hyperactivity, and attentional difficulties. Attention-deficit hyperactivity disorder (ADHD) is often diagnosed, with a peak in disruptive behavior during preschool years and a progressive decline with age, although attentional difficulties may persist (43). Aggressive and self-injurious behaviors are prominent features in some cases (44). Although there has been some interest in identifying specific linguistic, cognitive, or behavioral deficits among affected individuals, these have not been found (45–48). This is of some interest given the recent molecular discoveries discussed below indicating a general disruption to synaptic plasticity throughout the brain.

Fragile X syndrome is transmitted from one generation to the next as an X-linked disorder. It has been known for many years that the phenotype of fragile X syndrome often cosegregates with what appears to be a "fragile" site on the

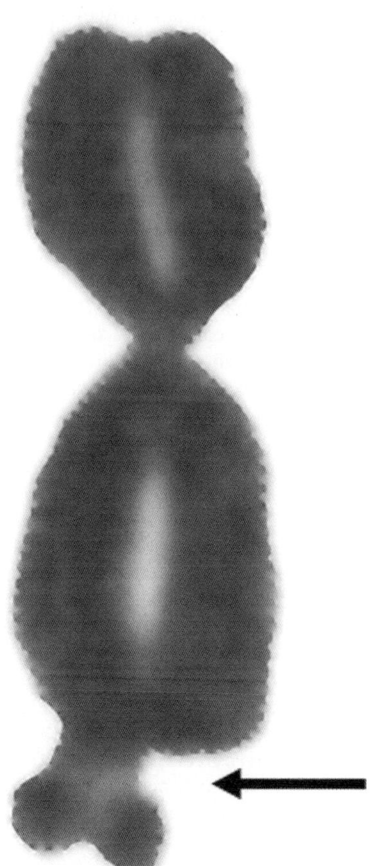

FIGURE 3.3.3.2. Fragile X site. The fragile site is shown on an affected chromosome of an individual with fragile X syndrome. (Adapted with permission from Lubs H: A marker X chromosome. *Am J Hum Gen* 21:231–244, 1969.)

X chromosome. In a certain proportion of cells grown in the absence of the nutrient, folic acid, an apparent breakpoint becomes visible on one of the X chromosomes (Figure 3.3.3.2) (49). The chromosomal region is not in fact separated but rather does not stain normally on karyotype analyses. These findings suggested that the gene or gene(s) involved in the disorder might lie near the disrupted site.

Several unusual aspects of the disorder were noted before the gene was actually cloned. Approximately 20% of the males who carry the abnormal gene are not cognitively impaired. If the gene lies on the X chromosome, why were these individuals not affected, as they have no normal copy of the gene to compensate for the mutated gene? These individuals are called "normal transmitting males," and pass the abnormal gene to their daughters, who may also be unaffected; however, their grandsons are at high risk for the full syndrome.

Several neurocognitive disorders show a progressive increase in severity over several generations, a genetic phenomenon known as anticipation. The molecular basis for anticipation is now understood, and relates to the molecular defect found in the affected *FMR-1* gene (50). A novel type of mutation was identified, termed a triplet repeat expansion. Triplet repeats refer to any three bases in the nucleotide sequence that are repeated as a unit several times. In the case of fragile X syndrome, the three repeated nucleotides are cytosine-guanine-guanine (CGG) in the 5′ untranslated region of exon 1, associated with hypermethylation, gene inactivation, and absence of the FMR protein (FMRP). Normal individuals have between 6 and 50 repeats of these bases at a specific site in their *FMR-1* gene, with 29 to 31 repeats being the most frequent (50). Affected individuals, however, have a dramatic increase in the number of repeated sequences, typically 200 to 1,000 repeats (*full mutation*). Mothers of affected probands often have numbers of CGG repeats that fall in between those seen in normal individuals and those affected with the full fragile X syndrome. Carriers thus typically have between 50 and 200 CGG repeats (50), and repeats in this range are called premutations. Expansion to a full mutation was observed in over 90% of mothers carrying 100 or more repeats (51). Mosaicism, the occurrence of two or more cell lines within the same individual with different genetic profiles, has been described in 15% to 20% of individuals with *FMR-1* mutations. This condition is associated with nearly 100% occurrence of intellectual disabilities in males, whereas a highly variable range was reported in females, from normal intellect to various degrees of cognitive impairment.

Individuals who carry the premutation of the FMR-1 gene may have mild cognitive and behavioral symptoms (52), including learning difficulties and social anxiety. Heterozygotic fragile X females perform poorly on visuospatial and/or memory subtests (53,54). Moreover, magnetic resonance imaging (MRI) and positron emission tomography (PET) analysis show that premutation female carriers have significant decreases in total brain volumes, as well as metabolic increases in the hippocampus and cerebellum (55).

Two phenotypes have been described more recently in premutation carriers. Premature ovarian failure is reported to affect 15% to 25% of female carriers (56). One-third of male premutation carriers over the age of 50 develop fragile X-associated tremor and ataxia syndrome (57,58). The molecular biology of these two distinct disorders remains unclear and does not appear directly related either to the CGG triplet repeat size or to the extent of FMRP deficit. Interestingly, a study from 2001 reported a paradoxical decrease in FMRP in permutation carriers with high levels of expression of the *FMR-1* gene (59). To explain this inconsistency, it has been hypothesized that overproduction of *FMR-1* mRNA might affect cytoplasmic translocation of other mRNAs. In this view, premature ovarian failure and fragile X-associated tremor and ataxia is interpreted as a result of RNA-mediated toxicity (60).

In addition to the 200 to 1,000 CGG repeats in affected individuals, other DNA abnormalities are present. CpG islands were discussed in the previous chapter, and are regions often found within promoter regions with high content of the two bases, cytosine and guanine. Cytosines may be chemically modified by the addition of a methyl group, and large regions of methylated nucleotides regulate whether a gene is expressed or not. The relatively small triplet repeat found in unaffected individuals is present immediately downstream of the promoter region, in a region of the message that does not encode protein (61).

The triplet repeat expansion in fragile X produces a large increase in the number of methylated CpG islands (62), and methylated cytosines lead to a very tight DNA winding. Transcription factors that must gain access to the DNA to form transcriptional complexes are unable to bind and the normal transcription of the *FMR-1* gene is disrupted. The extent of methylation over the region correlates directly with the loss of functional protein (63). The methylated region also explains the observed "fragile site," as this region of DNA is tightly wound and does not stain well on karyotype analyses and therefore appears as a broken chromosomal region. To summarize, the abnormal methylation pattern is adjacent to the promoter region, interferes with normal transcription of the gene, and ultimately leads to the absence of functional protein in most affected individuals.

In individuals with normal allelic variants, it has been proposed that the presence of an AGG repeat between the CGG repeats could represent a protective mechanism against triplet repeat expansion, as it would anchor DNA and prevent the formation of secondary structures during DNA duplication. Indeed, the presence of long, uninterrupted CGG repeats seems to confer an increased risk for expansion (51,64,65).

What is the normal function of FMRP and how does its absence lead to clinical symptoms? Soon after the gene was isolated in 1991, researchers noticed that the protein contained three domains with highly conserved amino acid patterns. These domains are homologous to a motif found in proteins that bind to ribonucleic acid (RNA) molecules. These proteins are called RNA-binding proteins and are involved at multiple steps during the processing, trafficking, or translating of mRNA transcripts within cells (66–68). Indeed, FMRP contains both nuclear localization and nuclear export signals; this, along with the RNA-binding capacity, suggested that FMRP was regulating RNA subcellular localization by acting as a nucleocytoplasmic shuttling protein (69,70). A mutation in an RNA-binding protein might impair the ability of cells to produce mature messages or translate those messages into protein.

This disruption was in fact described in a fragile X patient who did not have the expected triplet repeat expansion, but instead had a point mutation that changed a single highly conserved amino acid normally present within one of the RNA-binding motifs (68,71,72). The domain thus appeared to be critical for the proper function of FMR-1 protein, and mutations in this domain interfere with its ability to bind RNA molecules. In addition, this case indicated that although the majority of fragile X cases are caused by a triplet repeat expansion, any mutation that disrupts the functional activity of the FMR-1 protein could reasonably lead to a similar clinical syndrome. It is a good example of allelic heterogeneity, where mutations in different parts of a single gene lead to similar phenotypes.

Studies of the expression pattern of the *FMR-1* gene have identified areas of the brain that normally have high level of expression during development, including the basal forebrain and hippocampus (73). Both are involved in sequential processing of information and memory formation, and are affected in neurodegenerative disorders, such as Alzheimer disease. In addition, clinical neuroimaging studies have detected age-related volumetric changes in fragile X individuals in the cerebellar vermis, fourth ventricle, and hippocampus (74–76). Finally, the production of animal models, such as knockout mice, has been helpful in studying the underlying processes that are disrupted, as many of the clinical features seen in fragile X syndrome are present in these knockout mice (77).

A major advance in our understanding of the normal function of FMRP has come from two lines of investigation. The first has to do with the question of where proteins are translated within neurons. The older dogma was that messages produced within the nucleus were rapidly transported into the cytoplasm where they attached to ribosomes and deposit the translated proteins into the endoplasmic reticulum for further processing. This is the case for the majority of messages. However, within neurons, studies have now shown that a population of messages is actually transported throughout the dendrites and adjacent to the spines where synaptic contact is made. They remain there until an incoming signal arrives and initiates local protein synthesis at the very spines where the proteins are needed.

This new model has been helpful in solving a major difficulty with the earlier dogma. A typical neuron has up to 10,000 spines. Incoming synaptic activity arrives at perhaps a hundred of these spines. The previous model would have had the incoming signal activate a protein that would need to travel to the nucleus, initiate gene transcription and protein translation in the perinuclear region. The problem that arose was how proteins were then transported back to the hundred or so spines where the original signal arrived and where synaptic modifications were required.

The new model posits that the mRNA messages themselves are transported throughout the dendrites and deposited near spines, ready for an incoming signal to initiate translation. Evidence for this model has been extensive over the past several years, as various components of the translational machinery have been detected throughout dendrites and within the spines (77). These include the mRNAs themselves as well as ribosomes and a number of other proteins required for local protein synthesis (78).

It should be added that local protein synthesis does not preclude a signal from being sent from the activated spines back to the nucleus to initiate gene transcription. In fact, these signals must occur for long-term potentiation to be maintained and as long-term memories are consolidated. Thus, there is an initial burst of local protein synthesis that induces long-term potentiation, and a later phase during when mRNA messages are transcribed in the nucleus to maintain long-term potentiation. An interesting consequence of this process can be demonstrated by injecting transcriptional inhibitors into specific brain regions. If these inhibitors are injected into the amygdala, for example, short-term fear conditioning memories are formed, but this learning is not consolidated into long-term memories, as the maintenance of LTP requires protein synthesis.

Knowledge of the intracellular location of the FMRP protein has extended our understanding of its function. FMRP binds to ribosomes, the organelles within cells that are made from ribosomal RNA and various RNA-binding proteins, to function as factories that translate mRNA transcripts into proteins (79). FMRP has been shown to interact with several other molecules to inhibit translation of mRNA into proteins. FMRP is detected in several cellular structures, including P bodies (complexes of enzymes involved in mRNA decapping, storing and/or degradation of mRNAs), stress granules, and messenger ribonucleoproteins (mRNPs), consistent with its role in controlling translational events. In particular, FMRP is known to form homodimers and interact with a number of nuclear and cytosolic proteins, including the protein argonaute, microspherule protein, nuclear fragile X intellectual disability interacting protein, nuclear RNA export factor, dicer, and two FMRP paralogs (80).

FMRP binding to additional proteins leads to the repression of mRNA translation (81). Thus the loss of FMRP should cause an increase in protein synthesis. Control of mRNA translation by FMRP seems to be particularly important at synapses, as several crucial components of synaptic machinery are known targets of FMRP (82–85). A role in modulating mRNA stability has also been proposed for FMRP, which could either sustain or prevent mRNA decay (86). This work supports the notion that the loss of FMRP may have profound consequences on the molecular machinery controlling neuronal function.

Having solved one problem, researchers were left with another. Obviously, the messages that are transported down the neurites must not be translated until the proper synaptic input arrives. Recent work from several laboratories has suggested that inhibited translation is an important function of FMRP (38). FMRP attaches to newly synthesized mRNAs in the nucleus, accompanies these messages along the neuronal network, while inhibiting translation of the messages into proteins. When a signal arrives that normally would induce synaptic strengthening, the inhibitory actions of FMRP cease and the message is translated into proteins.

Exactly how this happens is not yet understood (85). One possibility is that the kinase ERK1/2 is involved. It is known that besides its ability to transduce signals into the nucleus as described above, another function of activated ERK1/2 is to participate in the regulation of local protein synthesis at the spine itself (87,88). Presumably, these functions of ERK1/2 work in parallel: one to initiate rapid local protein synthesis and the second to translocate into the nucleus and activate gene transcription.

Several lines of evidence suggest that mRNA translation can be fine-tuned by posttranslational modifications of FMRP. Phosphorylation of FMRP on serine 499 residue was suggested to result in its association with stalled polyribosomes and translational repression, an event mediated by mTOR-dependent activation of S6K1 (89,90). However, mTOR-independent phosphorylation of FMRP has also been proposed (91). Because nonphosphorylated FMRP is associated with actively translating polyribosomes, it is also possible that releasing the inhibited translation induced by FMRP may depend upon a yet to be described mechanism (82,92).

The messages that are transported to the spines are a subset of messages found in neurons: messages that encode proteins necessary for the biochemical and structural modifications occurring at the synapse (93,94). FMRP is probably only one of a number of proteins required for this process. Many proteins are needed to support the transport of messages, their inhibition, and providing the scaffolding for local protein translation. It is possible that mutations that affect the function of these proteins may also disrupt synaptic strengthening to varying degrees and produce cognitive deficits in affected individuals.

The model presented in the previous paragraphs leads to certain predictions. If FMRP is necessary for synaptic strengthening, then the absence of this key player might result in detectable disruptions in spine morphology. William Greenough et al. showed that this was the case by using anatomical techniques to examine spines from patients with fragile X syndrome as well as a mouse model of the syndrome (95,96). Compared to the controls, they found larger numbers of long, spindly, and immature-looking spines in the fragile X cases, and fewer numbers of short, mushroom-shaped, and mature-looking spines. Taken together, these studies suggest that FMRP is involved in spine development by regulating the shape, number, and maturity of spines, which depends on the ability of FMRP to regulate local protein synthesis.

Expansion of the *FMR-1* gene by triplet repeats was originally thought to be a genetic anomaly unique to fragile X syndrome. However, more than a dozen other triplet repeat disorders have now been identified (Figure 3.3.3.3) including Huntington chorea, Friedreich ataxia, and myotonic dystrophy (97–101). The phenomenon of anticipation was apparent in most of these disorders but early investigators dismissed it as the result of ascertainment bias: affected individuals were more likely to bring in their children as symptoms emerged. The discovery of triplet repeat expansions, however, provided a molecular explanation. The degree of anticipation can be quite remarkable (Figure 3.3.3.4). In myotonic dystrophy, for example, expansions that are just above the threshold for disease may result in cataract development late in life. Several generations later, descendants have the full expansion with long repeats and fatal congenital illness (102). Anticipation has also been described in families with schizophrenia and bipolar disorder, and some investigators believe triplet repeat expansions may account for a subset of these affected patients (103–109).

GENOMIC IMPRINTING: PRADER–WILLI AND ANGELMAN SYNDROMES

Half of our 46 chromosomes derive from our mothers and the other half from our fathers. For years, it had been assumed that genes that lay on either chromosomal pair were equivalent and that each produced the same amount of functional protein. Mutations present in one gene could often be overcome through the actions of the normal protein derived from the homologous gene.

This is an accurate description of the molecular events for the majority of genes; however, recent studies over the

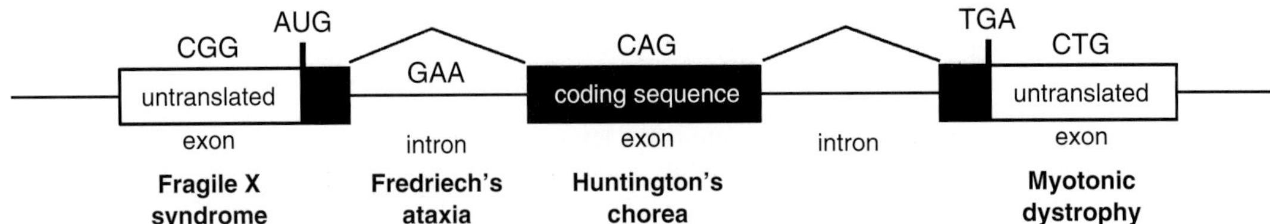

FIGURE 3.3.3.3. Triplet repeat disorders. A hypothetical gene is shown prior to the splicing together of exons and the removal of introns to produce a mature RNA message. Triplet repeat expansions have been discovered in all regions of a gene. In fragile X syndrome, the cytosine-guanine-guanine (CGG) repeat lies in the 5′ untranslated region immediately adjacent to the promoter region. The expansion to 1,000 to 2,000 repeats leads to abnormal methylation patterns and disrupts normal transcription of the gene. In myotonic dystrophy, the cytosine-adenine-guanine (CAG) repeat is found at the other end of the gene within the 3′ untranslated region. It is believed that the expansion there results in an unstable mRNA prone to degradation, as well as perhaps affecting the transcription of a second nearby homeobox gene. In Huntington chorea, the triplet repeat expansion occurs in the open reading frame of the gene and leads to the inappropriate incorporation of an amino acid, in this case glutamine, within the protein sequence. Triplet repeat expansions have also been found in introns, where they presumably interfere with the proper splicing of the message. Friedreich ataxia is an example of this type of expansion.

past decade have demonstrated that some gene pairs are not functionally equivalent. Instead, only one of the two genes is active and the other is repressed. The production of functional proteins depends on whether it is encoded by a gene on the chromosome derived from the mother or the one from the father. In some cases, the maternal gene is the gene expressed; in others cases, it is the paternal gene. This phenomenon is termed genomic imprinting.

For the majority of disorders, mutations change the specific nucleotide sequence of a gene and thereby change the amino acid sequence of the encoded protein, but for a smaller group of disorders, factors other than the underlying nucleotide sequence determine whether the DNA produces useful patterns of gene expression. These epigenetic phenomena are fundamentally different from events that have an effect on the actual nucleotide sequences. We have discussed some epigenetic factors earlier in our discussion of methylation in fragile X syndrome and will do so again when we discuss Rett syndrome. In these disorders, chromatin and DNA packaging influences gene expression rather mutated nucleotide sequences.

Approximately 100 genes have been discovered so far that are imprinted, mostly, although not exclusively, in the brain (110). Many of them influence the growth and differentiation of various tissues, and their disruption is implicated in several cancers and developmental disorders. These advances are reviewed in the following section with an emphasis on two developmental disorders caused by imprinting defects, Prader–Willi and Angelman syndromes.

Prader–Willi syndrome. Prader–Willi syndrome (PWS) is a rare disorder with a prevalence of 1 in 10,000 to 1 in 30,000 births that results in a constellation of symptoms arising shortly after birth (111). Infants are often hypotonic and fail to thrive; however, their dietary habits change within the first year or two of life, and these individuals typically become hyperphagic and obese (112). They often have mild to moderate cognitive disabilities and a number of additional behavioral problems that include temper tantrums, aggressive behaviors, and obsessive–compulsive symptoms outside of the compulsive food-related behaviors (45,113,114).

Angelman syndrome is also a relatively rare disorder with a prevalence of 1 in 12,000 to 24,000 births. Individuals with the disorder are also hypotonic as infants and develop motor delays and moderate to severe cognitive disabilities. They have a characteristic face with a large mandible with an open-mouth expression, disproportionate head circumference, abnormal gait, and puppet-like limb movements; they rarely develop speech. Affected individuals often have an abnormal electroencephalogram and develop epilepsy early in life (115).

By the mid-1980s, it was known that both disorders are caused by a deletion on chromosome 15 (15q11.2–q13) (Figure 3.3.3.5). Cytogenetic and molecular techniques showed that the same region of chromosome 15 is deleted in individuals with either syndrome. The disorders are very different, yet the identical deletion seemed to cause PWS in some cases and Angelman syndrome in others (116,117). It was then discovered that the clinical symptoms depend on which parent donates the deleted chromosome (118). The deletion derives from the father in most cases of PWS, and most individuals with Angelman syndrome have the same deletion but it is on the chromosome derived from the mother.

A further clarification of the underlying mechanism came when the region for each disorder was pinpointed to a small region on chromosome 15. The section of DNA responsible for PWS is distinct but very close to the area responsible for Angelman syndrome. Part of the puzzle was thus clarified. A large deletion often spans both regions. The child develops PWS if the deletion occurs on the paternal chromosome and Angelman syndrome if the deletion occurs on the maternal copy.

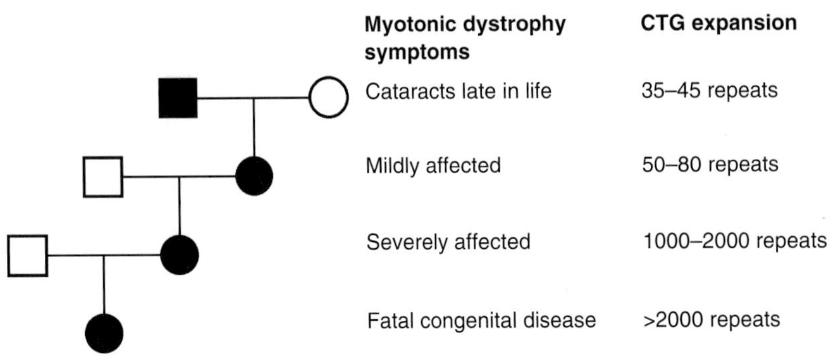

FIGURE 3.3.3.4. Anticipation. Anticipation refers to the increase in severity for a disorder over several generations. In myotonic dystrophy, for example, the increase in symptoms ranges from cataracts late in life in a great-grandfather, to milder symptoms in a grandfather and more severe muscle disorder in the father, to fatal congenital illness in the proband. A corresponding increase is found in the triplet repeat expansion for cytosine-thymidine-guanine (CTG).

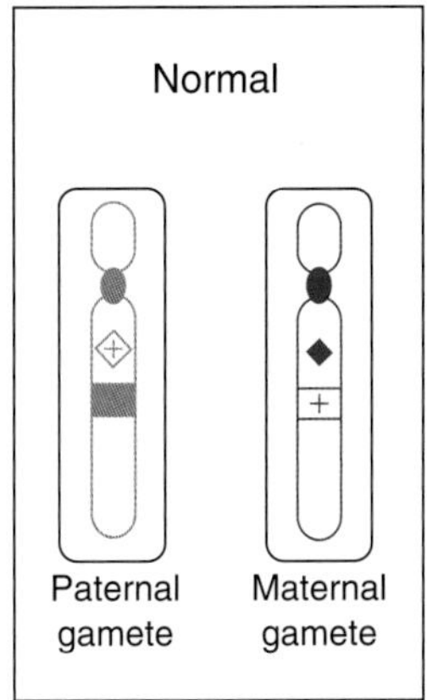

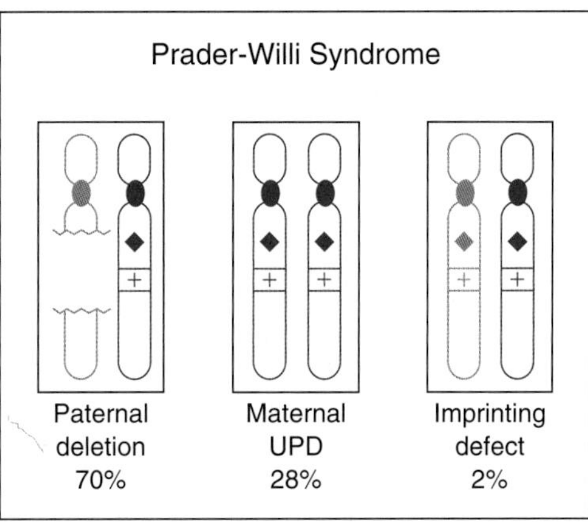

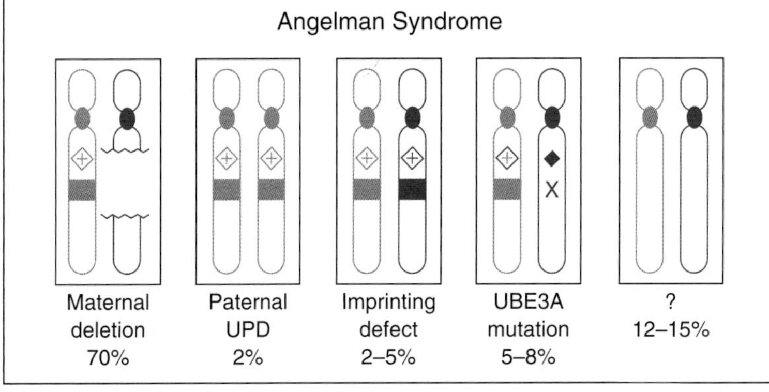

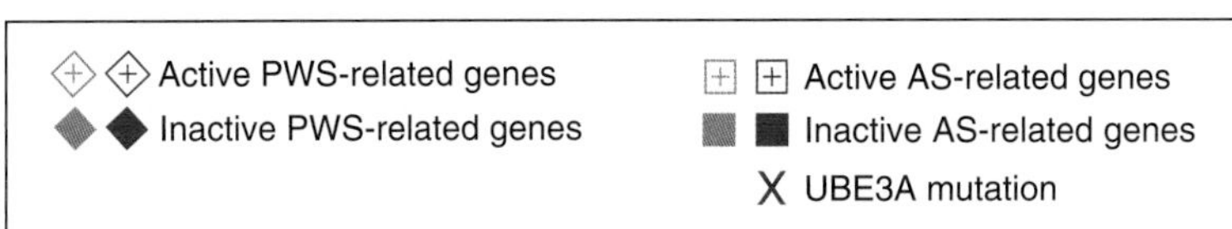

FIGURE 3.3.3.5. Imprinting in Prader–Willi and Angelman syndromes. Imprinting refers to the silencing of certain genes. It is a stable and reversible event that depends on the parental origin of the chromosome on which the gene lies and results in repression of a gene. For some genes, the paternal gene is silenced, whereas for other genes, it is the maternal gene. On chromosome 15, two adjacent regions are imprinted. In the normal situation (shown in the left, top panel), genes in the Prader–Willi syndrome (PWS) region are expressed on the paternal chromosome, whereas genes in the Angelman region are imprinted. The opposite situation exists on the maternal chromosome: genes in the PWS region are repressed, whereas genes in the Angelman region are expressed. Three mechanisms for developing PWS are shown, whereas four mechanisms have been discovered for Angelman syndrome (AS). The key at the bottom indicates genes, imprinting patterns, and mutations in both disorders. The relative proportion of each type of genetic abnormality in each syndrome is also shown. UPD, uniparental disomy. (Adapted with permission from Everman D, Cassidy S: Genomic imprinting: breaking the rules. *J Am Acad Child Adol Psychiatry* 39:386–389, 1999.)

These two nearby regions on chromosome 15 are differentially imprinted. Normally, genes within the PWS region are expressed on chromosomes that derive from the father. Immediately downstream a second set of genes lie within the Angelman critical region. These paternal-derived genes are imprinted and not expressed. The opposite expression pattern is found on the maternal chromosome. Genes within the PWS region are silenced, whereas genes within the Angelman region are expressed (Figure 3.3.3.5) (119,120). Deletions are responsible for approximately 70% of cases of both PWS and Angelman syndrome. In most cases, specific proximal and distal breakpoints have been identified that flank a portion of the chromosome and cause the approximately 5- to 6-Mb deletion (121,122).

The illnesses may also occur when children receive two copies of chromosome 15 from one of their parents (123). This unusual mechanism is called uniparental disomy (UPD). It occurs after an initial trisomy event in which two chromosomes from one parent are inappropriately passed along with one copy of the chromosome from the other parent, resulting in a total of three (rather than two) chromosomes. One chromosome is lost during gamete formation. If the initial trisomy involves two maternal and one paternal chromosome, then loss of the extra paternal copy results in two maternal chromosomes, or maternal UPD. If the initial trisomy involves two paternal and one maternal chromosome, then loss of the extra maternal copy results in paternal UPD.

Maternal UPD results in PWS (124) and it accounts for approximately 20% to 30% of cases. In this situation, the genes that lie within the PWS region are not expressed on the two maternal chromosomes and no functional proteins are produced. Paternal UPD represents the opposite situation. PWS genes are present on both paternal chromosomes and both sets are expressed. However, the genes that lie within the Angelman region are imprinted on the paternal chromosomes; therefore, even though there are two copies of all the genes, both sets are repressed and no proteins are expressed.

A third mechanism that leads to these disorders involves a region of DNA called the imprinting center. This center controls imprinting by regulating the extent of methylation and chromatin compaction for hundreds of kilobases of DNA on either side. It appears that one center determines the state of imprinting within both the PWS and Angelman critical regions. Mutations within the imprinting center have been discovered that lead to inappropriate imprinting or a lack of imprinting where it should normally occur. These types of mutations cause PWS or Angelman syndrome in about 2% to 3% of affected individuals (125). Mosaic methylation imprinting defects were recently reported in association with mild developmental impairment. This led to the hypothesis that undiagnosed groups of individuals with mild cognitive impairment could be explained on the basis of a mosaicism in the DNA imprinting center (126).

Finally, a fourth mechanism causes Angelman syndrome in approximately 10% of the cases. This is a mutation within a single gene lying within the Angelman critical region called UBE3A (127–129). The protein encoded by this gene normally regulates the lifespan of other proteins within the cell by regulating their degradation (Figure 3.3.3.6).

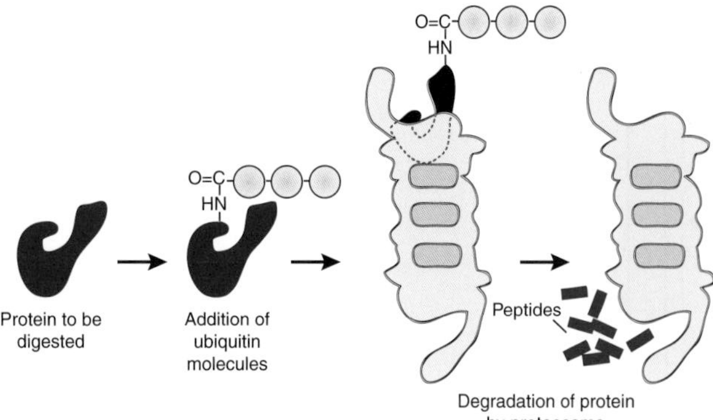

FIGURE 3.3.3.6. Angelman syndrome. It is critical to remove unwanted proteins from within cells before they disrupt cellular metabolism. Several steps are involved in this process and lead to the addition of one or more ubiquitin molecules to proteins targeted for degradation. The addition of ubiquitin to the protein serves as a signal to the proteasome, an organelle that breaks down proteins and serves as the cellular equivalent of a garbage disposal for a cell's unwanted proteins. (Adapted with permission from Lombroso PJ: Genetics of childhood disorders: XVI Angelman syndrome. *J Am Acad Child Adol Psychiatry*, 39:931–933, 2000.)

Many proteins must be quickly degraded and removed from the intracellular environment to ensure proper cell function. These include signaling proteins in which rapid turnover permits repeated signaling. It is also critical to remove certain enzymes that have become damaged before they interfere with normal intracellular signaling pathways. Several copies of a small molecule are added to proteins destined for degradation. This molecule, ubiquitin, acts as a flag to target the protein for degradation. The protein product of *UBE3A* is required in this process (32,42,107,128). It is one of several proteins that act in sequential order to attach ubiquitin molecules to targeted proteins. Intracellular organelles called proteasomes recognize ubiquitinated proteins, bind to them, and activate proteases that degrade the protein into its constitutive amino acids. When this protein is mutated and unable to function properly, an inappropriate accumulation of proteins within CNS neurons disrupts normal function. Thus, elevated peripheral BDNF levels were reported in patients with Angelman syndrome compared to neurotypical controls, which was interpreted as the consequence of deficient *UBE3A* expression (130).

The *UBE3A* gene encodes the E6-associated protein (E6AP), also known as ubiquitin-protein ligase E3A, whose function is to transfer ubiquitin from E2 ubiquitin-conjugating enzyme to its substrate, a process that eventually results in its degradation. This function is mediated by a specific domain termed the HECT domain. The silencing of the paternal allele at this locus is mediated by a nuclear localized, noncoding RNA antisense transcript (*UBE3A-ATS*) (131,132). Recently, it was reported that unsilencing of this allele by means of antisense oligonucleotides targeting the *UBE3A-ATS* transcript partially restored the expression of the UBE3A protein and ameliorated cognitive impairment in mice (133).

Several target proteins that are ubiquitinated by E6AP have been identified, including the tumor suppressor p53, MCM7 (a protein involved in DNA duplication), Arc, MecP2, and TSC2 (134–136). Alterations in a potassium channel were recently reported in the hippocampus of *UBE3A*-deficient mice with impaired synaptic strengthening and LTP (137). Disruption of activity-dependent phosphorylation of ERK1/2 has also been observed in *UBE3A*-deficient mice (138).

More than 150 pathogenic variants in *UBE3A* gene have been observed, mostly involving frameshifts (139). Interestingly, mutations that increase the activity of UBE3A lead to another developmental disorder. Thus, duplication of the region on the maternal chromosome region where *UBE3A* is found (Dup15q syndrome) is associated with developmental delays, autism, speech deficits, and epilepsy (140–142). These results indicate that the activity of UBE3A is tightly regulated within neurons. A recently reported mechanism that regulates UBE3A activity is the phosphorylation of UBE3A (142). A high rate of mutations is concentrated in a particular region within UBE3A containing a threonine residue that is phosphorylated. Phosphorylation at this residue leads to the inactivation of UBE3A within neurons that contributes to the tight regulation of UBE3A activity. Mutations that change the threonine residue result in a UBE3A mutant that is constitutively active and also leads to developmental delays and autism; in contrast, mutations that decrease UBE3A activity lead to Angelman syndrome.

Several enzymes in addition to UBE3A are required for the enzymatic reactions that result in the addition of ubiquitin molecules to proteins targeted for destruction. Mutations in these genes may lead to similar clinical problems. Such mutations would represent examples of locus heterogeneity in which mutations in distinctly different genes produce similar phenotypes. A number of laboratories are actively investigating this possibility.

On the other hand, no single gene mutation has yet been found in patients with PWS, and it remains unclear whether the absence of a single gene or the deletion of several genes within the critical PWS region is necessary for the disorder. Several genes were mapped to the region affected by the deletion, including the growth suppressor *NECDIN* and the ubiquitin ligase modulators *MAGEL2* and *MKRN3*. Truncating mutations in *MAGEL2* were recently described in four individuals with intellectual disabilities, autism spectrum disorder, and hyperphagia (143). This chromosomal region also contains a bicistronic gene that encodes two different proteins, the small ribonuclear protein SNRPN and a protein identified as SNRPN upstream reading frame (SNURF). The 5′ region of this gene has been identified as an imprinting center. The SNRPN/SNURF locus controls the expression of several small nucleolar RNAs (snoRNA), which are located in the chromosome telomeres (144). SnoRNAs are noncoding RNAs whose function has not been fully elucidated, but they may be implicated in the modification (by methylation or splicing) of other small RNAs involved in telomeres maintenance. Two snoRNAs in the PWS region of the chromosome 15 have been identified, *SNORD115* and *SNORD116*, which are present in 29 and 42 tandem repeats respectively. Specific targets of these snoRNAs have not been characterized yet, with the exception of serotonin 2C receptor for *SNORD115*, although a recent study in families carrying specific deletions and translocations allowed investigators to narrow down the PWS phenotype to *SNORD116* gene cluster (145). Additionally, mice carrying mutation at the *SNORD116* locus displayed PWS-like phenotype, including hyperphagia and growth retardation (146,147).

Two final notes should be made regarding Angelman syndrome. Recent work suggests that the maternally imprinted genes are differentially imprinted depending on the brain region where they are expressed (148). In addition, one of the genes within the region deleted in Angelman syndrome encodes a subunit of the GABAa receptor (149). The absence of this gene and a related disturbance in GABA transmission is believed to be responsible for the seizure disorders in individuals with the full deletion syndrome. As expected, individuals with a point mutation within only the UBE3A gene do not have epilepsy.

WILLIAMS SYNDROME

Deletions that span a number of adjacent genes and cause a constellation of symptoms are called contiguous gene syndromes.

Williams syndrome is one such disorder, caused by a deletion of 25 genes located on chromosome 7 (7q11.23). This developmental disorder is characterized by distinct facial features, a variable degree of cognitive disability, cardiovascular disease, and a very distinctive cognitive profile characterized by attention problems, an unusual cheerful demeanor, social disinhibition, and nonsocial anxiety (150,151). The cognitive problems consist of visual–spatial deficits. Affected children are unable to integrate the parts of a picture into a whole pattern (152). Interestingly, these children frequently exhibit strengths in other cognitive areas, such as verbal skills. Indeed, some elements of their speech are normal, such as the quality of their vocabulary, auditory memory, and social use of language. Moreover, many patients sing or play musical instruments with considerable talent. The disorder, first described by Williams in 1961 (153), has a rather low prevalence of 1 per 20,000 live births, although other estimates have suggested the prevalence is as high as 1 in 7,500 (154), and remains a topic of considerable interest because of the striking disparity in cognitive strengths and weaknesses (153,155–157). This disparity raises the possibility that the gene(s) responsible for Williams syndrome influence(s) the development of specific cortical regions and related cognitive abilities. This is in contrast to other forms of cognitive disabilities, such as fragile X syndrome, where a more uniform effect occurs across many cognitive skills.

Functional imaging studies have helped clarify some of the underlying neuropathologic mechanisms in Williams syndrome (158). Investigators of one rigorous study of the observed visuospatial difficulties identified a localized region within the dorsal pathway of the visual system around the intraparietal sulcus. Jernigan and Bellugi (159) examined MRIs of IQ- and age-matched subjects with Williams and Down syndromes. The cerebral cortices of both groups showed an overall decrease in volume. Cerebellar size, on the other hand, was normal among the Williams syndrome subjects but significantly hypoplastic among Down syndrome subjects.

Jernigan et al. extended this study by focusing in greater detail on the morphologic abnormalities in the cortices of subjects with Williams syndrome (160). The overall volume of the cerebral cortex was reduced compared to normal subjects, with relative sparing of the frontal areas and limbic structures, as well as a greater degree of hypoplasia in more posterior cortical structures. Different cortical regions are apparently affected to different degrees in Williams syndrome. MRI studies suggested the decrease in size was particularly prominent in the parietal lobule and occipital gray matter, with preserved cerebellar size; white matter decrease was estimated to be approximately 18% (161,162). Gray matter volume reductions were also documented in a cohort of high-functioning individuals with Williams syndrome in the intraparietal sulcus, the hypothalamus, and the orbitofrontal cortex. Additional morphologic changes occur in the brain of individuals with Williams syndrome, including flattening of the corpus callosum and abnormal protrusion of the cerebellum into the spinal canal (Chiari malformation), as well as increased gyrification in the parietal, temporoparietal, and occipital areas, and length reductions in the central gyrus (163–166).

Additional morphologic data comes from the autopsy of a Williams subject. Galaburda et al. (167) found abnormal organization among the neurons in posterior cortical regions (area 17), an increase in cell packing density throughout the cortex, and abnormal neuronal clustering. This result was recently confirmed by another study from the same group, where altered cell size and density were documented particularly in the primary visual cortex (168), although this single autopsy report requires additional work to clarify the underlying pathologic process.

Together, these findings suggest that abnormal, nonuniform development of the cerebral cortex may be responsible for the nonuniform cognitive findings that characterize these patients. The relatively intact cognitive skills related to affective recognition, face processing, and linguistic skills may be a consequence of the relatively normal development of limbic and frontal cortices and perhaps the relatively normal cerebellar structures. Poor functioning in visuospatial skills may be due, at least in part, to the abnormalities in the posterior cortical structures, such as the parietal and occipital cortices known to be involved in visual processing. It is reasonable to suggest that the gene or genes affected in Williams syndrome may have their greatest impact on the development or normal functioning of more posterior regions of the cerebral cortex.

Nearly all patients with Williams syndrome have a large deletion of a segment of chromosome 7, in the Williams–Beuren syndrome critical region (WBSCR) (169,170). The deletion encompasses a region of approximately 1.55 Mb in 95% of individuals with Williams syndrome. Phenotype severity correlates with the extent of the deletion; individuals with shorter deletions not including the *GTF21* locus at the telomeric breakpoint retain the peculiar cognitive profile, but without intellectual disabilities (171). A number of researchers note that cardiovascular symptoms cosegregate with a gene in the deleted region for elastin, which is a major component of skin, blood vessels, and lung tissues. The haplodeficiency caused by the deletion of elastin is likely to cause the vascular abnormalities and characteristic facies in these patients (169). Elastin, however, is not detectable in fetal or adult nervous tissue and probably does not contribute to the cognitive abnormalities (172).

Tassabehji et al. (173) were the first to report the deletion of a second gene in 20 out of 20 Williams syndrome patients. The sequence of this gene is nearly identical to a previously characterized gene called LIM kinase 1. Because it is expressed in high concentrations in the brain (174,175), mutations in this gene are possible candidates responsible for the cognitive deficits in Williams syndrome (176). LIM kinase is involved in growth cone motility in cultured neurons (173). In fact, LIM kinase knockout mice show abnormal dendritic organization, disrupted LTP, abnormalities in synaptic morphology, and deficits in learning (177). Intriguing cognitive deficits in these mice include difficulties with "unlearning." For example, once they have learned the position of a hidden platform in the Water Maze test, they are unable to learn the new location for the platform, something that normal mice can do (177).

For a brief period, it was thought that elastin and LIM kinase 1 were the only genes within the deleted region. It is now known that approximately 25 genes are present within the Williams syndrome critical region (Figure 3.3.3.7). In addition to elastin (152,168) and the LIM kinase 1 (170,171), other genes include *syntaxin 1A* (178), *Cyln2* (179), and *Frizzled 9*, a receptor for Wnt signaling (180), the gene encoding the replication factor C subunit (181), and the general transcription factors *GTF2I* and *GTF2IRD1* (182). Several laboratories are currently investigating the function of these genes (183). *Cyln2* is a protein that controls dynamic aspects of the cytoskeleton through the microtubule network; deficit of this protein is thought to be responsible for the decrease size of the corpus callum detected in individuals with Williams syndrome (184). *GFT2I* and *GFT2IRD1* are two related genes in a cluster on chromosome 7. GFTI2RD1 has strong gene repression capabilities, a DNA-binding site and plays a role in chromatin regulation (185,186). Recently, multivariate pattern classification analysis aimed at integrating morphometric brain pattern, genetics, and behavioral correlates in Williams syndrome suggested an association between (i) *GFT2I/GFT2IRD1* and visuospatial motor integration and intraparietal structures, (ii) the DNA region containing the LIM kinase gene associated with social cognition and with orbitofrontal, amygdala, and fusiform anatomy, (iii) while *syntaxin 1* and *Cyln2* was associated with overall white matter organization (187).

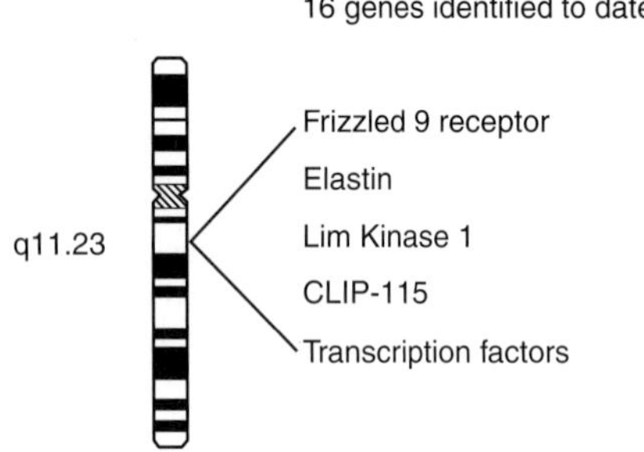

FIGURE 3.3.3.7. Williams syndrome. The deletion at 7q11.23 in patients with Williams syndrome contains at least 16 genes. Several of these genes are expressed within the central nervous system. Shown are candidate genes for the neuropsychiatric symptoms observed in subjects with Williams syndrome. When several genes contribute to the expression of a disorder through their deletion, the illness is termed a contiguous gene syndrome.

RETT SYNDROME

Rett syndrome is a disorder within the autism spectrum (188) with a prevalence of 1 in 8,500 (189). Affected children develop normally and reach developmental milestones within the first year of life and parents are unaware of any abnormalities. One of the first clinical symptoms is the loss of purposeful hand movements. Other clinical findings soon emerge, including loss of speech, growth retardation with microcephaly, ataxia, and a severe disruption of normal cognitive functioning. Clinical symptoms stabilize for the next several decades of life after this initial rapid regression (190).

One unusual feature of the disorder is that females are almost exclusively affected. An early explanation for the preponderance of affected females is that the mutated gene is located on the X chromosome. There are many examples of X-linked disorders in which males die in utero because males only have one X chromosome and only a single copy of the gene in question. Females have a second copy of the gene on their other X chromosome, and it appears that transcription of this gene in a subset of cells provides some degree of protection during fetal development and early postnatal life. However, symptoms eventually emerge because haploinsufficiency, a single functional copy of a gene, is unable to confer lasting protection.

The chromosomal location for the gene at Xq28 was facilitated by analysis of affected sisters (191). Candidate genes known to be present in this region were systematically excluded when their nucleotide sequences revealed no mutations compared to the identical sequences from normal individuals. On the other hand, a gene that is mutated in several affected individuals encodes the methyl CpG–binding protein 2 (MeCP2).

How are mutations in this gene related to clinical symptoms? As discussed in the previous chapter, many genes are expressed in certain tissues and not in others. Of the approximately 20,000 protein-coding genes on the human genome, only about one-third are expressed exclusively within the CNS. Some of these genes and their protein products are important for normal development during critical periods of brain development. Others are needed only after birth, whereas others must be expressed at all times because they are involved in normal housekeeping functions required of the cell. This functional heterogeneity illustrates how carefully gene expression must be regulated for normal development and maintenance of tissues to proceed.

The previous chapter reviewed how transcription factors and other regulatory proteins such as enhancers and repressors bind to promoter regions of genes and either initiate transcription of specific subsets of genes or maintain their stable repression. The proteins involved in these regulatory events bind to specific DNA sequences within the promoter regions that control gene expression. A protein mutated in Rett syndrome plays a critical role in this process.

The accessibility of DNA sequences depends to a large extent on the degree of methylation within the regulatory regions (192). Methylation is a chemical modification to DNA that occurs when methyl groups are added to cytosine nucleotides. It is particularly prevalent in regions of DNA that contain a high content of cytosine and guanine pairs, so-called CpG islands. Although CpG islands are present throughout the genome, they are enriched within the promoter regions of genes. In fact, one approach to identifying transcriptional start sites is to look for CpG islands because they are often found immediately upstream of the transcriptional start site.

It was originally thought that DNA methylation alone was capable of repressing gene expression. RNA polymerase II is the enzyme that transcribes most DNA into RNA. Methylation of CpG islands within promoter regions was initially believed to be sufficient to prevent this enzyme from gaining access to these regions of DNA and initiating transcription; however, what actually occurs is somewhat more complicated.

The protein implicated in Rett syndrome, MeCP2, has two functional domains. One end of the protein recognizes methylated cytosines and binds tightly to them (MBD). The second domain is then activated and functions by recruiting another set of proteins, the histone deacetylase complex, to the immediate vicinity (TRD). Histones are a family of proteins present within the nuclei of all cells. Their role in modifying the secondary structure of DNA has been recognized for some time because they provide a core of protein around which the chromosomal DNA is wrapped (193). The histone deacetylase complex that has been recruited by MeCP2 chemically modifies histones. The result is a compaction of the DNA surrounding the promoter region such that the transcriptional machinery of the nucleus is no longer able to gain efficient access to the gene, effectively silencing it.

The initial report on Rett syndrome identified six distinct mutations among the patients who had a mutation of their MeCP2 gene (194). To date, 487 pathogenic variants have been characterized, particularly in the two functional domains, MBD and TRD (Figure 3.3.3.8) (195). Most mutations are de novo and several types of mutations have been characterized, including silent, missense, nonsense, and frameshift mutations. In most cases, they result in the formation of truncated proteins that may still retain the capacity to bind to the target DNA, but are not able to recruit corepressor molecules (e.g., Sin3A) and form proper silencing complexes. Recently, it has been proposed that MeCP2 acts as a transcriptional activator as well (196), and plays a role in gene splicing and chromatin remodeling (197,198).

Missense mutations replace critical amino acids within the protein. Mutations of this type are located within the methyl-binding domain and disrupt the ability to recognize and interact with methyl groups. The remaining mutations are found in the second functional region, the domain that recruits the deacetylation complex. Two types of mutations have been found in this second domain. One is the insertion of a single nucleotide that leads to a shift in the downstream codons. A shift such as this results in the translation of a new amino acid sequence downstream of the point of mutation. The second mutation results in a novel stop codon. This type of mutation leads to the production of a truncated protein. Each of the mutations results in an impaired or nonfunctional protein (194).

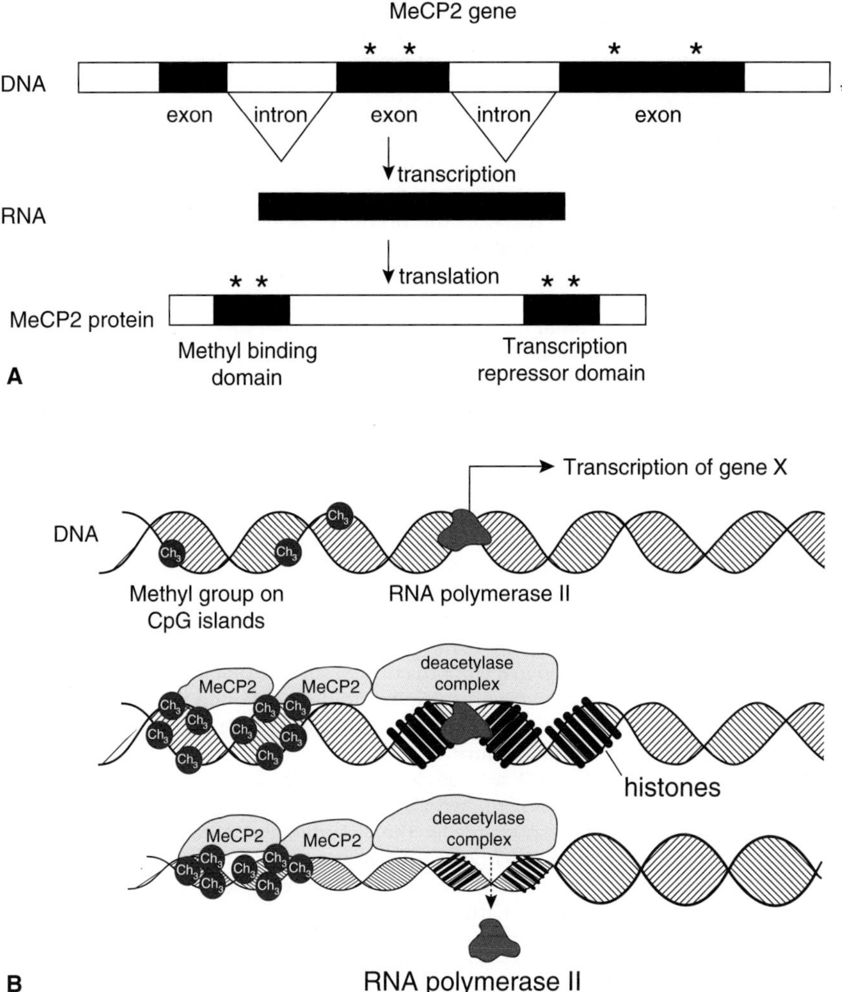

FIGURE 3.3.3.8. Rett syndrome. **A:** The MeCP2 gene consists of three exons separated by two introns. The exons are spliced together to produce a mature RNA message that is translated into MeCP2 protein. The gene has been implicated in Rett syndrome after several mutations were found within the coding regions in a number of patients. These are indicated by asterisks (*) in the nucleotide sequence and protein. Mutations to date have been found to change the amino acid sequence within two functional domains of the protein. **B:** MeCP2 protein, through one of its functional domains, binds to methylated cytosine nucleotides present in CpG islands that are enriched within regulatory regions of many genes. After binding to DNA, the second functional domain is activated and recruits a deacetylase complex that chemically modifies nearby histone molecules. The chemical modification of histones leads to a further compacting of the DNA into chromatin. The transcriptional machinery, including DNA polymerase II, no longer has easy access to the underlying DNA and is unable to initiate transcription. (Adapted with permission from Lombroso PJ: Rett syndrome. *J Am Acad Child Adol Psychiatry*, 38:671–674, 2000.)

Only certain regions of the MeCP2 gene were actually sequenced in this initial study: those that contain the open reading frame, or that portion of the gene that encodes the protein. These regions are often analyzed first because they require far fewer nucleotides to be sequenced compared to an analysis of the entire gene with its multiple introns and regulatory regions, and are therefore considerably less expensive to conduct. However, mutations in regulatory regions or in introns can also disrupt gene expression. For example, mutations at a promoter area may interfere with the initiation of transcription, whereas mutations in introns may interfere with the splicing of exons by disrupting a splice site regulatory sequence.

As mentioned earlier, allelic heterogeneity refers to the presence of different mutations within a single gene. In the majority of disease-causing mutations studied so far, the same or a very similar clinical phenotype is seen when different functional domains of a single gene are mutated. This type of allelic heterogeneity was demonstrated in the initial study on Rett syndrome (194). Six distinct mutations were found in different regions of the same gene, yet all the patients had the same disorder. It is likely that additional mutations will be found within regulatory sequences of MeCP2 that result in a similar phenotype. On the other hand, mutations to a single gene occasionally cause very different clinical presentations. For example, several mutations within the receptor for the fibroblast growth factor are responsible for a number of distinctly different skeletal and growth abnormalities (199).

By way of contrast, locus heterogeneity refers to mutations in different genes that result in a similar clinical presentation among affected individuals. This can happen, for example, when several proteins are involved in a series of related enzymatic reactions. For example, MeCP2 encodes one member of a larger family of proteins. At least two other members have been discovered that also bind to DNA and are involved in the recruitment of the histone deacetylation complex. Each of these proteins is now being examined to determine whether mutations in their genes also cause Rett syndrome. Moreover, as discussed, a number of proteins besides MeCP2 are required to repress target genes. Mutations of any of these other genes may result in a related clinical phenotype. In fact, mutations have now been documented in a second gene that results in a clinical phenotype very similar to Rett syndrome (200,201). Aside from the congenital form, several atypical variants of Rett syndrome have been recently described, including the preserved speech variant and the early-onset seizures variant. With particular regard to the latter, a mutation at the *CDKL5* locus was described. Similarly, a mutation in the repressor gene *FoxG1* was also described in a 7-year-old girl exhibiting intellectual disabilities, facial dysmorphisms, and Rett-like features (202). Autistic and Rett-like features were also recently described in an individual with a de novo heterozygous deletion in chromosome 2, with no abnormalities at the *MeCP2* locus (203).

The recent findings with Rett syndrome raise a number of interesting questions. One relates to the predominance of neurologic symptoms in the clinical examination. MeCP2 is not uniquely expressed in the brain but is found in many other tissues. Nevertheless, symptoms outside of the brain are not a predominant part of the disorder. It appears that the CNS is particularly vulnerable to disruptions of this gene. One possibility is that during brain development alternate transcripts are differentially expressed; spatial and temporal control of gene expression requires a fine balance between activating and repressing stimuli, at both the transcriptional and the epigenetic level. Moreover, the brain tissue may be more susceptible than other tissues to MeCP2 dysfunction because of the postmitotic nature of neurons (204). A similar situation occurs in Huntington chorea, where neurologic symptoms are also the central part of an illness, although the mutated gene is expressed in many tissues.

A second related question concerns the normal developmental trajectory early in life that precedes the development of symptoms. Much longer delays are seen with a number of neurodegenerative disorders where symptoms are not detected until the fourth or fifth decade of life. One explanation put forward is that toxic compounds are slowly produced over time and must accumulate before neuronal damage occurs. Free radicals are examples of toxic compounds implicated in a number of neurodegenerative disorders, including Huntington chorea. Normally, enzymes are present that detoxify free radicals within cells. If these enzymes lose their full functional activity through a mutation or are expressed in smaller amounts with age, the toxins will accumulate over time and eventually interfere with normal neuronal function.

This may be what happens in the brains of Rett syndrome patients. As discussed, the normal function of the MeCP2 protein is to repress transcription of several additional genes. These downstream target genes are only partially known, but it is reasonable to assume that mutations to MeCP2 lead to the inappropriate expression of these genes. MeCP2 has been show to silence several genes, including *BDNF, hairy2A, Dlx5, and Sgk* (197,205–207). It was recently pointed out that MeCP2 appears to play distinct roles in neuronal subclasses. Mice carrying a mutated *MeCP2* allele in the excitatory neuronal lineage developed cortical hyperexcitation and seizures, whereas removal of *MeCP2* in interneurons recapitulated several features of the Rett syndrome, including stereotyped behavior, autonomic, sensory, motor, and social dysfunction. In fact distinct behavioral phenotypes can be ascribed to *MeCP2* removal from specific interneuron subclasses. For example, particular sensorimotor and social deficits were observed when targeting parvalbumin-expressing neurons, whereas seizures and stereotypies arose in mice carrying the mutation in somatostatin-expressing lineage (202,208,209). *MeCP2* mutant mice were reported to have a genome-wide, length-dependent increase in gene expression, a finding consistent with observations in the brains of humans with Rett syndrome. Apparently long genes can be enriched for neuronal functions and appear to be selectively enriched in the brain, therefore providing some biologic explanation for why the brain is particularly affected by *MeCP2* mutations (210).

It is possible that the products of these genes are themselves toxic, or interfere with the normal signaling pathways that function during this developmental period. Neuroanatomical studies might clarify this hypothesis. The literature contains a single autopsy report (211) showing abnormalities in pyramidal neurons in layers II–III of the cerebral cortex. They had fewer dendrites than normal and many fewer dendritic arborizations.

LISSENCEPHALY

The cerebral cortex is formed of billions of cells that are born during just a few months of embryonic life from a small population of progenitor cells. The cells that are born must differentiate and migrate to reach the appropriate layer of the cortex. However, a number of disorders are caused by mutations in genes whose proteins are required for the orderly progression from neuronal birth, differentiation into appropriate neuronal subtypes, migration, and eventual elaboration of synaptic connections.

Neurogenesis occurs in a region called the ventricular zone, which lies adjacent to the lumen of the neural tube. Although neurogenesis primarily occurs during the development of the brain in utero, some degree of neurogenesis occurs throughout life (212). In the prenatal cerebral cortex, neurons must migrate past layers of earlier born cells to reach their final destinations. Those born at later periods have more complex migratory routes. Many employ a guidance system composed of radial glial cells (213). The radial glial cells are thought to send a process that spans the developing cortex and serves as scaffolding along which certain neurons migrate. Chemotaxic signals are produced that keep the neuron moving along the radial glial process. When migrating neuron reaches its final destination, other signaling molecules are produced that instruct it to stop migrating, enter the proper layer, and begin to elaborate processes (214).

Disrupted neuronal migration characterizes several human disorders. The most common of these are the lissencephalies, which consist of several distinct syndromes: isolated lissencephaly (ILS), Miller–Dieker syndrome (MDS), and X-linked lissencephaly (215). In each, disrupted neuronal migration is reflected in a smooth cortical surface that lacks the normal pattern of gyri and sulci. In addition, although the cerebral cortex normally has six layers, cortices of affected individuals have only four (Figure 3.3.3.9).

In 1993, a large deletion on chromosome 17 was identified in two patients with MDS. The search then began to clone the gene responsible for the disorder, and it was soon isolated and termed LIS-1 (216). The deletion spans this gene and genes on either side of it and is another example of a contiguous gene syndrome. Large deletions within the LIS-1 account for up to 70% of cases of MDS, and are not shared by individuals with ILS or subcortical band heterotopia (SBH), where smaller deletions are more commonly reported. The absence of several genes is believed to be responsible for the more severe MDS phenotype, which also has numerous congenital abnormalities. Smaller deletions and/or point mutations in the same LIS-1 gene were soon found in other affected individuals. These individuals had the milder form of lissencephaly (ILS).

How does a mutation in LIS-1 cause the observed cortical abnormalities? LIS-1 encodes a regulatory protein that controls the activity of a second protein, termed platelet activating factor (PAF)-acetylhydrolase (217,218). PAF acts as a signaling protein that binds to the surface of neurons. The ensuing cascade of signals is required for the normal migration of neurons (219). LIS-1 is expressed at its highest levels in the developing cortex, consistent with the protein's putative role in signaling. Exactly how mutations in LIS-1 interfere with normal migration is not well understood, although one model suggests a disruption in cytoskeletal proteins that need to rearrange themselves at the growing tip of the migrating neuron (220). Indeed, LIS-1 was shown to organize the cytoskeleton by controlling the interaction between microtubules protein (like tubulin) and the centrosome components, including dynein, dynactin, NUDE and NUDEL, and to regulate mitotic spindle assembly (221–223). Doublecortin (DCX) also interacts with LIS-1 and the two control the operation of dynein (224). In ILS, intragenic deletions and duplications *LIS-1* are present in approximately 14% of patients, along with pathogenic variants of DCX (also implicated in subcortical band heterotopia) and tubulin alpha 1A (*TUBA1A*) (225,226). The 14-3-3 family of proteins, which is involved in several cellular function including protein transport and cell migration through its binding to NUDEL, has also been correlated with the severity of cortical malformations in MDS (227–231).

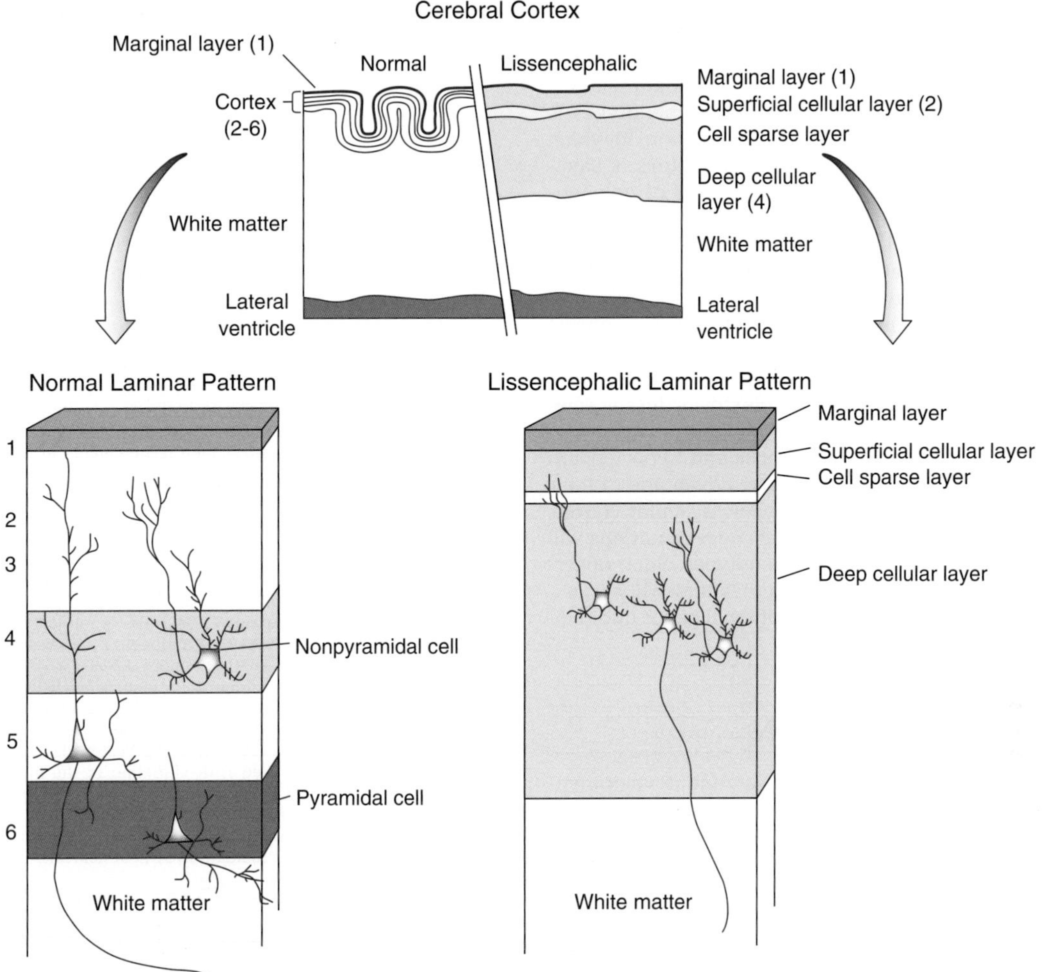

FIGURE 3.3.3.9. Lissencephaly. The normal cerebral cortex is a highly organized structure, and its six layers are shown on the left (12,13,55,73,146,192). In contrast, the lissencephalic brain lacks the normal pattern of sulci and gyri, and there are only four layers. (Adapted with permission from Reiner O, Lombroso PJ: Lissencephaly. *J Am Acad Child Adol Psychiatry* 37:231–232, 1998.)

A second disorder that affects neuronal migration also is due to SBH (232). This disorder, also known as X-linked lissencephaly or double cortex, is associated with cognitive deficits and epilepsy. The histologic findings are made of bilateral bands of gray matter consisting of disorganized neurons present in the central white matter between the cortex and ventricular wall. The degree of cognitive disabilities is directly related to the thickness of the extra neuronal tissue. The gene that causes double cortex encodes the protein DCX (233–235). Mutations in DCX sequence are most common, with very few cases of deletions or duplications reported. Somatic mosaicism in the *DCXI* has been reported recently (236).

Structurally, this protein is homologous to a family of kinases, called calcium calmodulin–dependent kinases. Although its exact role in neuronal migration remains to be clarified, recent studies indicate that it binds to and appears to stabilize cytoskeletal proteins required for the normal movement of neurons (237,238). As previously discussed, neuronal migration occurs through the establishment of specific cell–cell interactions between the migrating neuron and the radial glia cell that, besides its role in maintaining the neuronal progenitors pool in the ventricular zone, also serves as a scaffold for guidance of differentiating neurons. A radial glia–specific role in the onset of SBH has been proposed in mice, based on the observation that absence of a specific class of proteins regulating the actin and microtubule cytoskeleton, termed small Rho GTPases, led to SBH and cobblestone lissencephaly, a condition characterized by abnormal protrusion of migrating neurons beyond the pial surface (239). Interestingly, layering defects have been recently reported in other cognitive disorders that include schizophrenia and autism (240–242).

Over 20% of individuals with lissencephaly have no detectable mutation in *LIS-1*, whereas a similar number of individuals with SBH have no detectable mutation of DCX. It is possible that additional studies will detect novel mutations within these genes; however, mutations of several other genes have been recently reported for SBH (243,244).

GENETIC BASIS OF COMMON CHILD PSYCHIATRIC DISORDERS

Child psychiatry has yet to establish the molecular basis for most of its more common disorders. The reasons for this failure lie beyond the scope of this chapter, but genetic complexity is one culprit. Many of the disorders described in the preceding sections exhibit Mendelian patterns of inheritance, such as the X-linked transmission of Rett and fragile X syndromes; however, pedigree studies of most common child and adolescent mental disorders fail to show such a pattern of vertical transmission across generations. The presence of non-Mendelian patterns of transmission does not necessarily imply that genetic factors are unimportant, only that their role in the transmission and expression of disease phenotypes is complex. Examples include polygenetic transmission, in which a multiplicity of genetic and environmental factors is causative. Height and intelligence are good examples of polygenetic traits and it may be that some forms of childhood-onset anxiety disorders and ADHD will also fall into this category. Interestingly, the alleles that contribute to the vulnerability to develop these disorders may be common in the population and be seen as normal variants. However, when they act in concert with other vulnerability alleles or with adverse environments, they may lead to the syndrome in question.

Understanding the genetics of complex disorders is relevant to other fields of medicine and important progress has been made in areas such as breast cancer and hypertension (32,128,245,246). Our field is poised to take advantage of their success. If child psychiatric disorders follow a similar course, we can expect that in rare instances single gene mutations will be responsible for common disease phenotypes. Such observations will set the stage for animal studies that will serve a valuable heuristic role in elucidating additional genes and relevant neurobiologic pathways.

CONCLUSION

Advances in genomics, molecular genetics, and developmental neuroscience provide an impressive array of accomplishments as the foundation for a deeper understanding of the biologic bases of some childhood-onset neuropsychiatric disorders. Success in these areas will likely herald success in other rare diseases, such as autism and other pervasive developmental disorders. Therapeutic advances also can be anticipated as pharmaceutical agents are developed that specifically target the molecular and cellular consequences of specific genetic mutations. Perhaps even the promise of gene therapy can be realized for some of the single gene conditions. Nevertheless, the road ahead, particularly for common disorders, will not be an easy one given the complexities involved and the crucial role of the environment in shaping and reshaping the CNS within the constraints of our genetic endowment.

ACKNOWLEDGMENTS

This work was supported by the National Institute of Health grant MH01527 (PJL). Portions of this work appeared in: Lombroso P: learning and memory. *Rev Bras Psiquiatr* 26:207–210, 2004.

References

1. Kandel ER: A new intellectual framework for psychiatry. *Am J Psychiatry* 155:457–469, 1998.
2. Nestler EJ, Barrot M, DiLeone RJ, et al.: Neurobiology of depression. *Neuron* 34:13–25, 2002.
3. Squire LR, Kandel ER: *Memory: From Mind to Molecule.* New York, Scientific American Library, 85a, 1999.
4. Weeber EJ, Levenson JM, Sweatt JD: Molecular genetics of human cognition. *Mol Interv* 2:376–391, 339, 2002.
5. Sweatt JD: *Mechanisms of Memory.* New York, Elsevier Press, 2003.
6. Atkins CM, Selcher JC, Petraitis JJ, Trzaskos JM, Sweatt JD: The MAPK cascade is required for mammalian associative learning. *Nat Neurosci* 1:602–609, 1998
7. Orban PC, Chapman PF, Brambilla R: Is the Ras-MAPK signalling pathway necessary for long-term memory formation? *Trends Neurosci* 22:38–44, 1999.
8. Roberson ED, English JD, Adams JP, et al.: The mitogen-activated protein kinase cascade couples PKA and PKC to cAMP response element binding protein phosphorylation in area CA1 of hippocampus. *J Neurosci* 19:4337–1348, 1999.
9. Impey S, Obrietan K, Wong ST, et al.: Cross talk between ERK and PKA is required for Ca2+ stimulation of CREB-dependent transcription and ERK nuclear translocation. *Neuron* 21:869–883, 1998.
10. English JD, Sweatt JD: A requirement for the mitogen-activated protein kinase cascade in hippocampal long term potentiation. *J Biol Chem* 272:19103–19106, 1997.
11. Sherrin T, Blank T, Hippel C, et al.: Hippocampal c-Jun-N-terminal kinases serve as negative regulators of associative learning. *J Neurosci* 30:13348–13361, 2010.
12. Adaikkan C, Rosenblum K: The role of protein phosphorylation in the gustatory cortex and amygdala during taste learning. *Exp Neurobiol* 21:37–51, 2012.
13. Adams JP, Sweatt JD: Molecular psychology: roles for the ERK MAP kinase cascade in memory. *Annu Rev Pharmacol Toxicol* 42:135–1163, 2002.
14. Philips GT, Tzvetkova EI, Carew TJ: Transient mitogen-activated protein kinase activation is confined to a narrow temporal window required for the induction of two-trial long-term memory in Aplysia. *J Neurosci* 27:13701–13705, 2007.
15. Rodrigues SM, Schafe GE, LeDoux JE: Molecular mechanisms underlying emotional learning and memory in the lateral amygdala. *Neuron* 44:75–91, 2004.
16. Schafe GE, Atkins CM, Swank MW, et al.: Activation of ERK/MAP kinase in the amygdala is required for memory consolidation of pavlovian fear conditioning. *J Neurosci* 20:8177–8187, 2000.
17. Blum S, Moore AN, Adams F, Dash PK: A mitogen-activated protein kinase cascade in the CA1/CA2 subfield of the dorsal hippocampus is essential for long-term spatial memory. *J Neurosci* 19:3535-3544, 1999.
18. Shiflett MW, Martini RP, Mauna JC, et al.: Cue-elicited reward-seeking requires extracellular signal-regulated kinase activation in the nucleus accumbens. *J Neurosci* 28:1434–1443, 2008.
19. Kirschmann EK, Mauna JC, Willis CM, Foster RL, Chipman AM, Thiels E: Appetitive cue-evoked ERK signaling in the nucleus accumbens requires NMDA and D1 dopamine receptor activation and regulates CREB phosphorylation. *Learn Mem* 21:606–615, 1994.
20. Vincent SR, Sebben M, Dumuis A, Bockaert J: Neurotransmitter regulation of MAP kinase signaling in striatal neurons in primary culture. *Synapse* 29:29–36, 1998.
21. Valjent E, Pascoli V, Svenningsson P, et al.: Regulation of a protein phosphatase cascade allows convergent dopamine and glutamate signals to activate ERK in the striatum. *Proc Natl Acad Sci U S A* 102:491–496, 2005.
22. Kaplan DR, Miller FD: Neurotrophin signal transduction in the nervous system. *Curr Opin Neurobiol* 10:381–391, 2000.
23. Davis S, Vanhoutte P, Pages C, Caboche J, Laroche S: The MAPK/ERK cascade targets both Elk-1 and cAMP response element-binding protein to control long-term potentiation-dependent gene expression in the dentate gyrus in vivo. *J Neurosci* 20:4563–4572, 2000.
24. Impey S, Smith DM, Obrietan K, et al.: Stimulation of cAMP response element (CRE)-mediated transcription during contextual learning. *Nat Neurosci* 1:595–601, 1998.
25. Silva AJ, Elgersma Y, Costa RM: Molecular and cellular mechanisms of cognitive function: implications for psychiatric disorders. *Biol Psychiatry* 47:200–209, 2000.
26. Costa RM, Federov NB, Kogan JH, et al.: Mechanism for the learning deficits in a mouse model of neurofibromatosis type 1. *Nature* 415:526–530, 2002.
27. Upadhyaya M, Spurlock G, Thomas L, et al.: Microarray-based copy number analysis of neurofibromatosis type-1 (NF1)-associated malignant peripheral nerve sheath tumors reveals a role for Rho-GTPase pathway genes in NF1 tumorigenesis. *Hum Mutat* 33:763–776, 2012.
28. Lim JY, Kim H, Kim YH, et al.: Merlin suppresses the SRE-dependent transcription by inhibiting the activation of Ras-ERK pathway. *Biochem Biophys Res Commun* 302:238–245, 2003.
29. Weeber EJ, Sweatt JD: Molecular neurobiology of human cognition. *Neuron* 33:845–848, 2002.
30. Jacquot S, Merienne K, De Cesare D, et al.: Mutation analysis of the RSK2 gene in Coffin-Lowry patients: extensive allelic heterogeneity and a high rate of de novo mutations. *Am J Hum Genet* 63:1631–140, 1998.
31. Delaunoy J, Abidi F, Zeniou M, et al.: Mutations in the X-linked RSK2 gene (RPS6KA3) in patients with Coffin-Lowry syndrome. *Hum Mutat* 17:103–116, 2001.
32. Matsumoto A, Kuwajima M, Miyake K, et al.: An Xp22.12 microduplication including RPS6KA3 identified in a family with variably affected intellectual and behavioral disabilities. *J Hum Genet* 58:755–757, 2013.
33. Johnston MV: Clinical disorders of brain plasticity. *Brain Dev* 26:73–80, 2004.
34. Ammar MR, Reiss AL, Freund LS, Abrams MT: The Coffin-Lowry syndrome-associated protein RSK2 regulates neurite outgrowth through phosphorylation of phospholipase D1 (PLD1) and synthesis of phosphatidic acid. *J Neurosci* 33:19470–19479, 2013.
35. Lim HC, Xie L, Zhang W, et al.: Ribosomal S6 Kinase 2 (RSK2) maintains genomic stability by activating the Atm/p53-dependent DNA damage pathway. *PLoS One* 8:e74334, 2013.

36. Petrij F, Giles RH, Dauwerse HG, et al.: Rubinstein-Taybi syndrome caused by mutations in the transcriptional co-activator CBP. *Nature* 376:348–351, 1995.
37. Negri G, Milani D, Colapietro P, et al.: Clinical and molecular characterization of Rubinstein-Taybi syndrome patients carrying distinct novel mutations of the EP300 gene. *Clin Genet* 87:148–154, 1993.
38. Bagni C, Greenough WT: From mRNP trafficking to spine dysmorphogenesis: the roots of fragile X syndrome. *Nat Rev Neurosci* 6:376–387, 2005.
39. Coffee B, Keith K, Albizua I, et al.: Incidence of fragile X syndrome by newborn screening for methylated FMR1 DNA. *Am J Hum Genet* 85: 503–514, 2009.
40. Budimirovic DB, Kaufmann WE: What can we learn about autism from studying fragile X syndrome? *Dev Neurosci* 33:379–394, 2011.
41. Baumgardner TL, Reiss AL, Freund LS, Abrams MT: Specification of the neurobehavioral phenotype in males with fragile X syndrome. *Pediatrics* 95:744–752, 1995.
42. Martin JP, Bell J: A pedigree of mental defect showing sex-linkage. *J Neurol Psychiatry* 6:154–157, 1943.
43. McLennan Y, Polussa J, Tassone F, Hagerman R: Fragile x syndrome. *Curr Genomics* 12:216–224, 2011.
44. Bregman JD, Dykens E, Watson M, Ort SI, Leckman JF: Fragile-X syndrome: variability of phenotypic expression. *J Am Acad Child Adolesc Psychiatry* 26:463–471, 1987.
45. Dykens EM, Hodapp RM, Ort SI, Leckman JF, et al.: Trajectory of adaptive behavior in males with fragile X syndrome. *J Autism Dev Disord* 23:135–145, 1993.
46. Freund LS, Reiss AL, Hagerman R, Vinogradov S: Chromosome fragility and psychopathology in obligate female carriers of the fragile X chromosome. *Arch Gen Psychiatry* 49:54–60, 1992.
47. Fryns JP: The female and the fragile X. A study of 144 obligate female carriers. *Am J Med Genet* 23:157–169, 1986.
48. Hodapp RM, Leckman JF, Dykens EM, et al.: K-ABC profiles in children with fragile X syndrome, Down syndrome, and nonspecific mental retardation. *Am J Ment Retard* 97:39–46, 1992.
49. Lubs HA: A marker X chromosome. *Am J Hum Genet* 21:231–244, 1969.
50. Fu YH, Kuhl DP, Pizzuti A, et al.: Variation of the CGG repeat at the fragile X site results in genetic instability: resolution of the Sherman paradox. *Cell* 67:1047–1058, 1991.
51. Nolin SL, Glicksman A, Ding X, et al.: Fragile X analysis of 1112 prenatal samples from 1991 to 2010. *Prenat Diagn* 31:925–931, 2011.
52. Hagerman RJ, Staley LW, O'Conner R, et al.: Learning-disabled males with a fragile X CGG expansion in the upper premutation size range. *Pediatrics* 97:122–126, 2004.
53. de von Flindt R, Bybel B, Chudley AE, Lopes F, et al.: Short-term memory and cognitive variability in adult fragile X females. *Am J Med Genet* 38:488–492, 1991.
54. Kemper MB, Hagerman RJ, Ahmad RS, Mariner R: Cognitive profiles and the spectrum of clinical manifestations in heterozygous fra (X) females. *Am J Med Genet* 23:139–156, 1986.
55. Murphy DG, Mentis MJ, Pietrini P, et al.: Premutation female carriers of fragile X syndrome: a pilot study on brain anatomy and metabolism. *J Am Acad Child Adolesc Psychiatry* 38:1294–1301, 1999.
56. Allingham-Hawkins DJ, Babul-Hirji R, Chitayat D, et al.: Fragile X premutation is a significant risk factor for premature ovarian failure: the International Collaborative POF in Fragile X study–preliminary data. *Am J Med Genet* 83:322–325, 1999.
57. Hagerman PJ, Hagerman RJ: Fragile X-associated tremor/ataxia syndrome (FXTAS). *Ment Retard Dev Disabil Res Rev* 10:25–30, 2004.
58. Jacquemont S, Hagerman RJ, Leehey MA, et al.: Penetrance of the fragile X-associated tremor/ataxia syndrome in a premutation carrier population. *JAMA* 291:460–149, 2004.
59. Kenneson A, Zhang F, Hagedorn CH, Warren ST: Reduced FMRP and increased FMR1 transcription is proportionally associated with CGG repeat number in intermediate-length and premutation carriers. *Hum Mol Genet* 10:1449–1454, 2001.
60. Galloway JN, Nelson DL: Evidence for RNA-mediated toxicity in the fragile X-associated tremor/ataxia syndrome. *Future Neurol* 4:785, 2009.
61. Nelson DL: The fragile X syndromes. *Semin Cell Biol* 6:5–11, 1995.
62. Oberle I, Rousseau F, Heitz D, et al.: Instability of a 550-base pair DNA segment and abnormal methylation in fragile X syndrome. *Science* 252:1097–1102, 1991.
63. Pieretti M, Zhang FP, Fu YH, et al.: Absence of expression of the FMR-1 gene in fragile X syndrome. *Cell* 66:817–822, 1991.
64. Eichler EE, Holden JJ, Popovich BW, et al.: Length of uninterrupted CGG repeats determines instability in the FMR1 gene. *Nat Genet* 8:88–94, 1994.
65. Kunst CB, Warren ST: Cryptic and polar variation of the fragile X repeat could result in predisposing normal alleles. *Cell* 77:853–861, 1994.
66. Eichler EE, Richards S, Gibbs RA, Nelson DL: Fine structure of the human FMR1 gene. *Hum Mol Genet* 2:1147–1153, 1993.
67. Siomi H, Siomi MC, Nussbaum RL, Dreyfuss G: The protein product of the fragile X gene, FMR1, has characteristics of an RNA-binding protein. *Cell* 74:291–298, 1993.
68. Siomi H, Choi M, Siomi MC, Nussbaum RL, Dreyfuss G: Essential role for KH domains in RNA binding: impaired RNA binding by a mutation in the KH domain of FMR1 that causes fragile X syndrome. *Cell* 77:33–39, 1994.
69. Fridell RA, Benson RE, Hua J, Bogerd HP, Cullen BR: A nuclear role for the Fragile X mental retardation protein. *EMBO J* 15:5408–5414, 1996.
70. Ling SC, Fahrner PS, Greenough WT, Gelfand VI: Transport of Drosophila fragile X mental retardation protein-containing ribonucleoprotein granules by kinesin-1 and cytoplasmic dynein. *Proc Natl Acad Sci U S A* 101:17428–17433, 2004.
71. De Boulle K, Verkerk AJ, Reyniers E, et al.: A point mutation in the FMR-1 gene associated with fragile X mental retardation. *Nat Genet* 3:31–35, 1993.
72. Musco G, Stier G, Joseph C, et al.: Three-dimensional structure and stability of the KH domain: molecular insights into the fragile X syndrome. *Cell* 85:237–245, 1996.
73. Abitbol M, Menini C, Delezoide AL, Rhyner T, Vekemans M, Mallet J: Nucleus basalis magnocellularis and hippocampus are the major sites of FMR-1 expression in the human fetal brain. *Nat Genet* 4:147–153, 1993.
74. Mostofsky SH, Mazzocco MM, Aakalu G, et al.: Decreased cerebellar posterior vermis size in fragile X syndrome: correlation with neurocognitive performance. *Neurology* 50:121–130, 1998.
75. Mostofsky SH, Reiss AL, Lockhart P, Denckla MB: Evaluation of cerebellar size in attention-deficit hyperactivity disorder. *J Child Neurol* 13:434–439, 1998.
76. Reiss AL, Lee J, Freund L: Neuroanatomy of fragile X syndrome: the temporal lobe. *Neurology* 44:1317–1324, 1994.
77. Steward O, Schuman EM: Protein synthesis at synaptic sites on dendrites. *Annu Rev Neurosci* 24:299–325, 2001.
78. Ostroff LE, Fiala JC, Allwardt B, Harris KM: Polyribosomes redistribute from dendritic shafts into spines with enlarged synapses during LTP in developing rat hippocampal slices. *Neuron* 35:535–545, 2002.
79. Khandjian EW, Corbin F, Woerly S, Rousseau F: The fragile X mental retardation protein is associated with ribosomes. *Nat Genet* 12:91–93, 1994.
80. Fernandez E, Rajan N, Bagni C: The FMRP regulon: from targets to disease convergence. *Front Neurosci* 7:191, 2013.
81. Napoli I, Mercaldo V, Boyl PP, et al.: The fragile X syndrome protein represses activity-dependent translation through CYFIP1, a new 4E-BP. *Cell* 134:1042–1054, 2008.
82. Darnell JC, Jensen KB, Jin P, et al.: FMRP stalls ribosomal translocation on mRNAs linked to synaptic function and autism. *Cell* 146:247–261, 2011.
83. Darnell JC, Klann E: The translation of translational control by FMRP: therapeutic targets for FXS. *Nat Neurosci* 16:1530–1536, 2013.
84. Goebel-Goody SM, Wilson-Wallis ED, Royston S, et al.: Genetic manipulation of STEP reverses behavioral abnormalities in a fragile X syndrome mouse model. *Genes Brain Behav* 11:586–600, 2012.
85. Zalfa F, Giorgi M, Primerano B, et al.: The fragile X syndrome protein FMRP associates with BC1 RNA and regulates the translation of specific mRNAs at synapses. *Cell* 112:317–327, 2003.
86. De Rubeis S, Bagni C: Fragile X mental retardation protein control of neuronal mRNA metabolism: insights into mRNA stability. *Mol Cell Neurosci* 43:43–50, 2010.
87. Kelleher RJ 3rd, Govindarajan A, Jung HY, Kang H, Tonegawa S: Translational control by MAPK signaling in long-term synaptic plasticity and memory. *Cell* 116:467–479, 2004.
88. Kelleher RJ 3rd, Govindarajan A, Tonegawa S: Translational regulatory mechanisms in persistent forms of synaptic plasticity. *Neuron* 44:59–73, 1986.
89. Ceman S, O'Donnell WT, Reed M, Patton S, Pohl J, Warren ST: Phosphorylation influences the translation state of FMRP-associated polyribosomes. *Hum Mol Genet* 12:3295–3305, 2003.
90. Narayanan U, Nalavadi V, Nakamoto M, et al.: S6K1 phosphorylates and regulates fragile X mental retardation protein (FMRP) with the neuronal protein synthesis-dependent mammalian target of rapamycin (mTOR) signaling cascade. *J Biol Chem* 283:18478–18482, 2008.
91. Bartley CM, O'Keefe RA, Bordey A: FMRP S499 is phosphorylated independent of mTORC1-S6K1 activity. *PLoS One* 9:e96956, 2014.
92. Zhang Y, Venkitaramani DV, Gladding CM, et al.: The tyrosine phosphatase STEP mediates AMPA receptor endocytosis after metabotropic glutamate receptor stimulation. *J Neurosci* 28:10561–10566, 2008.
93. Brown V, Jin P, Ceman S, et al.: Microarray identification of FMRP-associated brain mRNAs and altered mRNA translational profiles in fragile X syndrome. *Cell* 107:477-87, 2001.
94. Darnell JC, Jensen KB, Jin P, Brown V, Warren ST, Darnell RB: Fragile X mental retardation protein targets G quartet mRNAs important for neuronal function. *Cell* 107:489–499, 2001.
95. Comery TA, Harris JB, Willems PJ, et al.: Abnormal dendritic spines in fragile X knockout mice: maturation and pruning deficits. *Proc Natl Acad Sci U S A* 94:5401–5404, 1997.
96. Irwin SA, Patel B, Idupulapati M, et al.: Abnormal dendritic spine characteristics in the temporal and visual cortices of patients with fragile-X syndrome: a quantitative examination. *Am J Med Genet* 98:161–167, 2001.
97. Caskey CT, Pizzuti A, Fu YH, Fenwick RG Jr, Nelson DL: Triplet repeat mutations in human disease. *Science* 256:784–789, 1992.
98. Hendricks AE, Latourelle JC, Lunetta KL, et al.: Estimating the probability of de novo HD cases from transmissions of expanded penetrant CAG alleles in the Huntington disease gene from male carriers of high normal alleles (27-35 CAG). *Am J Med Genet A* 149A:1375–1381, 2009.

99. Nelson DL, Warren ST: Trinucleotide repeat instability: when and where? *Nat Genet* 4:107–108, 1993.
100. Uhlmann WR, Peñaherrera MS, Robinson WP, Milunsky JM, Nicholson JM, Albin RL: Biallelic mutations in Huntington disease: a new case with just one affected parent, review of the literature and terminology. *Am J Med Genet A* 167A:1152–1160, 2015.
101. Warren ST: The expanding world of trinucleotide repeats. *Science* 271:1374–1375, 1996.
102. Fu YH, Pizzuti A, Fenwick RG Jr, et al.: An unstable triplet repeat in a gene related to myotonic muscular dystrophy. *Science* 255:1256–1258, 1992.
103. Fortune MT, Kennedy JL, Vincent JB: Anticipation and CAG*CTG repeat expansion in schizophrenia and bipolar affective disorder. *Curr Psychiatry Rep* 5:145–154, 2003.
104. Galimberti D, Reif A, Dell'osso B, et al.: C9ORF72 hexanucleotide repeat expansion is a rare cause of schizophrenia. *Neurobiol Aging* 35:1214 e7–1214 e10, 2014.
105. Jones I, Gordon-Smith K, Craddock N: Triplet repeats and bipolar disorder. *Curr Psychiatry Rep* 4:134–140, 2002.
106. Margolis RL, McInnis MG, Rosenblatt A, Ross CA: Trinucleotide repeat expansion and neuropsychiatric disease. *Arch Gen Psychiatry* 56:1019–1031, 1999.
107. McInnis MG, McMahon FJ, Chase GA, et al.: Anticipation in bipolar affective disorder. *Am J Hum Genet* 53:385–390, 1993.
108. Morris AG, Gaitonde E, McKenna PJ, Mollon JD, Hunt DM: CAG repeat expansions and schizophrenia: association with disease in females and with early age-at-onset. *Hum Mol Genet* 4:1957–1961, 1995.
109. O'Donovan MC, Guy C, Craddock N, et al.: Expanded CAG repeats in schizophrenia and bipolar disorder. *Nat Genet* 10:380–381, 1995.
110. Wilkinson LS, Davies W, Isles AR: Genomic imprinting effects on brain development and function. *Nat Rev Neurosci* 8:832–843, 2007.
111. Prader A, Labhart A, Willi H: Ein Syndrom von Adipositas, Kleinwuchs, Kryptorchismus und Oligophrenie nach Myatonieartigem Zustand im Neugeborenenalter. *Schweiz Med Wschr* 86:1260–1261, 1956.
112. Holm VA, Cassidy SB, Butler MG, et al.: Prader-Willi syndrome: consensus diagnostic criteria. *Pediatrics* 91:398–402, 1993.
113. Dykens EM, Cassidy SB: Correlates of maladaptive behavior in children and adults with Prader-Willi syndrome. *Am J Med Genet* 60:546–549, 1995.
114. State MW, Dykens EM, Rosner B, Martin A, King BH: Obsessive-compulsive symptoms in Prader-Willi and "Prader-Willi-Like" patients. *J Am Acad Child Adolesc Psychiatry* 38:329–334, 1999.
115. Angelman H: "Puppet children": A report of three cases. *Dev Med Child Neurol* 7:681–688, 1965.
116. Ledbetter DH, Riccardi VM, Airhart SD, Strobel RJ, Keenan BS, Crawford JD: Deletions of chromosome 15 as a cause of the Prader-Willi syndrome. *N Engl J Med* 304:325–329, 1981.
117. Magenis RE, Brown MG, Lacy DA, Budden S, LaFranchi S: Is Angelman syndrome an alternate result of del(15)(q11q13)? *Am J Med Genet* 28:829–838, 1987.
118. Cassidy SB, Schwartz S: Prader-Willi and Angelman syndromes. Disorders of genomic imprinting. *Medicine (Baltimore)* 77:140–151, 1998.
119. Cassidy SB: Prader-Willi syndrome. *J Med Genet* 34:917–923, 1997.
120. Nicholls RD, Saitoh S, Horsthemke B: Imprinting in Prader-Willi and Angelman syndromes. *Trends Genet* 14:194–200, 1998.
121. Castronovo C, Crippa M, Bestetti I, et al.: Complex de novo chromosomal rearrangement at 15q11-q13 involving an intrachromosomal triplication in a patient with a severe neuropsychological phenotype: clinical report and review of the literature. *Am J Med Genet A* 167A:221–230, 2015.
122. Depienne C, Moreno-De-Luca D, Heron D, et al.: Screening for genomic rearrangements and methylation abnormalities of the 15q11-q13 region in autism spectrum disorders. *Biol Psychiatry* 66:349–359, 2009.
123. Ledbetter DH, Engel E: Uniparental disomy in humans: development of an imprinting map and its implications for prenatal diagnosis. *Hum Mol Genet* 4 Spec No:1757–1764, 1995.
124. Nicholls RD, Knoll JH, Butler MG, Karam S, Lalande M: Genetic imprinting suggested by maternal heterodisomy in nondeletion Prader-Willi syndrome. *Nature* 342:281–285, 1989.
125. Ohta T, Gray TA, Rogan PK, et al.: Imprinting-mutation mechanisms in Prader-Willi syndrome. *Am J Hum Genet* 64:397–413, 1999.
126. Fairbrother LC, Cytrynbaum C, Boutis P, et al.: Mild Angelman syndrome phenotype due to a mosaic methylation imprinting defect. *Am J Med Genet A* 167:1565–1569, 2015.
127. Kishino T, Lalande M, Wagstaff J: UBE3A/E6-AP mutations cause Angelman syndrome. *Nat Genet* 15:70–73, 1994.
128. Matsuura T, Sutcliffe JS, Fang P, et al.: De novo truncating mutations in E6-AP ubiquitin-protein ligase gene (UBE3A) in Angelman syndrome. *Nat Genet* 15:74–77, 1997.
129. Nicholls RD: Strange bedfellows? Protein degradation and neurological dysfunction. *Neuron* 21:647–649, 1998.
130. Wink LK, Fitzpatrick S, Shaffer R, et al.: The neurobehavioral and molecular phenotype of Angelman Syndrome. *Am J Med Genet A* 167:2623–2628, 2015.
131. Chamberlain SJ, Brannan CI: The Prader-Willi syndrome imprinting center activates the paternally expressed murine Ube3a antisense transcript but represses paternal Ube3a. *Genomics* 73:316–322, 2001.
132. Rougeulle C, Cardoso C, Fontés M, Colleaux L, Lalande M: An imprinted antisense RNA overlaps UBE3A and a second maternally expressed transcript. *Nat Genet* 19:15–16, 1998.
133. Meng L, Ward AJ, Chun S, et al.: Towards a therapy for Angelman syndrome by targeting a long non-coding RNA. *Nature* 518:409–412, 2015.
134. Mandel-Brehm C, Salogiannis J, Dhamne SC, Rotenberg A, Greenberg ME: Seizure-like activity in a juvenile Angelman syndrome mouse model is attenuated by reducing Arc expression. *Proc Natl Acad Sci U S A* 112:5129–5134, 2015.
135. Margolis SS, Salogiannis J, Lipton DM, et al.: EphB-mediated degradation of the RhoA GEF Ephexin5 relieves a developmental brake on excitatory synapse formation. *Cell* 143:442–455, 2010.
136. Scheiffele P, Beg AA: Neuroscience: Angelman syndrome connections. *Nature* 468:907–978, 2010.
137. Sun J, Zhu G, Liu Y, et al.: UBE3A regulates synaptic plasticity and learning and memory by controlling sk2 channel endocytosis. *Cell Rep* 12:449–461, 2015.
138. Filonova I, Trotter JH, Banko JL, Weeber EJ: Activity-dependent changes in MAPK activation in the Angelman syndrome mouse model. *Learn Mem* 21:98–104, 2014.
139. Sadikovic B, Fernandes P, Zhang VW, et al.: Mutation update for UBE3A variants in Angelman syndrome. *Hum Mutat* 35:1407–1417, 2014.
140. Hogart A, Wu D, LaSalle JM, Schanen NC: The comorbidity of autism with the genomic disorders of chromosome 15q11.2-q13. *Neurobiol Dis* 38:181–191, 2010.
141. Urraca N, Cleary J, Brewer V, et al.: The interstitial duplication 15q11.2-q13 syndrome includes autism, mild facial anomalies and a characteristic EEG signature. *Autism Res* 6:268–279, 2013.
142. Yi JJ, Berrios J, Newbern JM, et al.: An autism-linked mutation disables phosphorylation control of UBE3A. *Cell* 162:795–807, 2015.
143. Schaaf CP, Gonzalez-Garay ML, Xia F, et al.: Truncating mutations of MAGEL2 cause Prader-Willi phenotypes and autism. *Nat Genet* 45:1405–1408, 2013.
144. Laufer BI, Singh SM: A macro role for imprinted clusters of microRNAs in the brain. *Microrna* 1:59–64, 2006.
145. Buiting K: Prader-Willi syndrome and Angelman syndrome. *Am J Med Genet C Semin Med Genet* 154C:365–376, 2010.
146. Ding F, Li HH, Zhang S, et al.: SnoRNA Snord116 (Pwcr1/MBII-85) deletion causes growth deficiency and hyperphagia in mice. *PLoS One* 3:e1709, 2008.
147. Skryabin BV, Gubar LV, Seeger B, et al.: Deletion of the MBII-85 snoRNA gene cluster in mice results in postnatal growth retardation. *PLoS Genet* 3:e235, 2007.
148. Albrecht U, Sutcliffe JS, Cattanach BM, et al.: Imprinted expression of the murine Angelman syndrome gene, Ube3a, in hippocampal and Purkinje neurons. *Nat Genet* 17:75–78, 1997.
149. DeLorey TM, Handforth A, Anagnostaras SG, et al.: Mice lacking the beta3 subunit of the GABAA receptor have the epilepsy phenotype and many of the behavioral characteristics of Angelman syndrome. *J Neurosci* 18:8505–8514, 1998.
150. Morris CA: The behavioral phenotype of Williams syndrome: a recognizable pattern of neurodevelopment. *Am J Med Genet C Semin Med Genet* 154C:427–431, 2010.
151. Pober BR, Dykens EM: Williams syndrome: an overview of medical, cognitive, and behavioral features. *Child Adolesc Psychiatr Clin North Am* 5:929–943, 1996.
152. Ewart AK, Morris CA, Atkinson D, et al.: Hemizygosity at the elastin locus in a developmental disorder, Williams syndrome. *Nat Genet* 5:11–16, 1993.
153. Williams JC, Barratt-Boyes BG, Lowe JB: Supravalvular aortic stenosis. *Circulation* 24:1311–1318, 1961.
154. Stromme P, Bjornstad PG, Ramstad K: Prevalence estimation of Williams syndrome. *J Child Neurol* 17:269–271, 2002.
155. Bellugi U, Bihrle A, Jernigan T, Trauner D, Doherty S: Neuropsychological, neurological, and neuroanatomical profile of Williams syndrome. *Am J Med Genet Suppl* 6:115–125, 1990.
156. Bellugi U, Lichtenberger L, Jones W, Lai Z, St George M: I. The neurocognitive profile of Williams syndrome: a complex pattern of strengths and weaknesses. *J Cogn Neurosci* 12 (Suppl 1):7–29, 2000.
157. Wang PP, Doherty S, Rourke SB, Bellugi U: Unique profile of visuo-perceptual skills in a genetic syndrome. *Brain Cogn* 29:54–65, 1995.
158. Meyer-Lindenberg A, Hariri AR, Munoz KE, et al.: Neural correlates of genetically abnormal social cognition in Williams syndrome. *Nat Neurosci* 8:991–993, 2005.
159. Jernigan TL, Bellugi U: Anomalous brain morphology on magnetic resonance images in Williams syndrome and Down syndrome. *Arch Neurol* 47:529–533, 1990.
160. Jernigan TL, Bellugi U, Sowell E, Doherty S, Hesselink JR: Cerebral morphologic distinctions between Williams and Down syndromes. *Arch Neurol* 50:186–191, 1993.
161. Eckert MA, Hu D, Eliez S, et al.: Evidence for superior parietal impairment in Williams syndrome. *Neurology* 64:152–153, 2005.
162. Reiss AL, Eckert MA, Rose FE, et al.: An experiment of nature: brain anatomy parallels cognition and behavior in Williams syndrome. *J Neurosci* 24:5009–5015, 2004.
163. Eckert MA, Galaburda AM, Karchemskiy A, et al.: Anomalous Sylvian fissure morphology in Williams syndrome. *Neuroimage* 33:39–45, 2006.

164. Mercuri E, Atkinson J, Braddick O, et al.: Chiari I malformation in asymptomatic young children with Williams syndrome: clinical and MRI study. *Eur J Paediatr Neurol* 1:177–181, 1997.
165. Meyer-Lindenberg A, Mervis CB, Berman KF: Neural mechanisms in Williams syndrome: a unique window to genetic influences on cognition and behaviour. *Nat Rev Neurosci* 7:380–393, 2006.
166. Schmitt JE, Eliez S, Warsofsky IS, Bellugi U, Reiss AL: Corpus callosum morphology of Williams syndrome: relation to genetics and behavior. *Dev Med Child Neurol* 43:155–159, 2001.
167. Galaburda AM, Wang PP, Bellugi U, Rossen M: Cytoarchitectonic anomalies in a genetically based disorder: Williams syndrome. *Neuroreport* 5:753–757, 1994.
168. Galaburda AM, Holinger DP, Bellugi U, Sherman GF: Williams syndrome: neuronal size and neuronal-packing density in primary visual cortex. *Arch Neurol* 59:1461–1467, 2002.
169. Lowery MC, Morris CA, Ewart A, et al.: Strong correlation of elastin deletions, detected by FISH, with Williams syndrome: evaluation of 235 patients. *Am J Hum Genet* 57:49–53, 1995.
170. Nickerson E, Greenberg F, Keating MT, McCaskill C, Shaffer LG: Deletions of the elastin gene at 7q11.23 occur in approximately 90% of patients with Williams syndrome. *Am J Hum Genet* 56:1156–1161, 1995.
171. Morris CA, Mervis CB, Hobart HH, et al.: GTF2I hemizygosity implicated in mental retardation in Williams syndrome: genotype-phenotype analysis of five families with deletions in the Williams syndrome region. *Am J Med Genet A* 123A:45–59, 2003.
172. Frangiskakis JM, Ewart AK, Morris CA, et al.: LIM-kinase1 hemizygosity implicated in impaired visuospatial constructive cognition. *Cell* 86:59–69, 1996.
173. Tassabehji M, Metcalfe K, Fergusson WD, et al.: LIM-kinase deleted in Williams syndrome. *Nat Genet* 13:272–273, 1996.
174. Mizuno K, Okano I, Ohashi K, et al.: Identification of a human cDNA encoding a novel protein kinase with two repeats of the LIM/double zinc finger motif. *Oncogene* 9:1605–1612, 1994.
175. Proschel C, Blouin MJ, Gutowski NJ, Ludwig R, Noble M: Limk1 is predominantly expressed in neural tissues and phosphorylates serine, threonine and tyrosine residues in vitro. *Oncogene* 11:1271–1281, 1995.
176. Hoogenraad CC, Akhmanova A, Galjart N, De Zeeuw CI: LIMK1 and CLIP-115: linking cytoskeletal defects to Williams syndrome. *Bioessays* 26:141–150, 2004.
177. Meng Y, Zhang Y, Tregoubov V, et al.: Abnormal spine morphology and enhanced LTP in LIMK-1 knockout mice. *Neuron* 35:121–133, 2002.
178. Osborne LR, Martindale D, Scherer SW, et al.: Identification of genes from a 500-kb region at 7q11.23 that is commonly deleted in Williams syndrome patients. *Genomics* 36:328–336, 1996.
179. Osborne LR, Soder S, Shi XM, et al.: Hemizygous deletion of the syntaxin 1A gene in individuals with Williams syndrome. *Am J Hum Genet* 61:449–452, 1997.
180. Wang YK, Samos CH, Peoples R, Pérez-Jurado LA, Nusse R, Francke U: A novel human homologue of the Drosophila frizzled wnt receptor gene binds wingless protein and is in the Williams syndrome deletion at 7q11.23. *Hum Mol Genet* 6:465–472, 1997.
181. Peoples R, Perez-Jurado L, Wang YK, Kaplan P, Francke U: The gene for replication factor C subunit 2 (RFC2) is within the 7q11.23 Williams syndrome deletion. *Am J Hum Genet* 58:1370–1373, 1996.
182. Jurado Perez LA, Wang YK, Peoples R, et al.: A duplicated gene in the breakpoint regions of the 7q11.23 Williams-Beuren syndrome deletion encodes the initiator binding protein TFII-I and BAP-135, a phosphorylation target of BTK. *Hum Mol Genet* 7:325–334, 1998.
183. Zhao C, Avilés C, Abel RA, Almli CR, McQuillen P, Pleasure SJ: Hippocampal and visuospatial learning defects in mice with a deletion of frizzled 9, a gene in the Williams syndrome deletion interval. *Development* 132:2917–2927, 2005.
184. van Hagen JM, van der Geest JN, van der Giessen RS, et al.: Contribution of CYLN2 and GTF2IRD1 to neurological and cognitive symptoms in Williams Syndrome. *Neurobiol Dis* 26:112–124, 2007.
185. Carmona-Mora P, Widagdo J, Tomasetig F, et al.: The nuclear localization pattern and interaction partners of GTF2IRD1 demonstrate a role in chromatin regulation. *Hum Genet* 134:1099–1115, 2015.
186. Thompson PD, Webb M, Beckett W, et al.: GTF2IRD1 regulates transcription by binding an evolutionarily conserved DNA motif 'GUCE'. *FEBS Lett* 581:1233–1242, 2007.
187. Hoeft F, Dai L, Haas BW, et al.: Mapping genetically controlled neural circuits of social behavior and visuo-motor integration by a preliminary examination of atypical deletions with Williams syndrome. *PLoS One* 9:e104088, 2014.
188. Rett A: *Über ein zerebral-atrophisches syndrome bei Hypesammonemie.* Vienna, Bruder Hollinek, 1966.
189. Laurvick CL, de Klerk N, Bower C, et al.: Rett syndrome in Australia: a review of the epidemiology. *J Pediatr* 148:347–352, 2006.
190. Naidu S: Rett syndrome: natural history and underlying disease mechanisms. *Eur Child Adolesc Psychiatry* 6 Suppl 1:14–17, 1997.
191. Webb T, Clarke A, Hanefeld F, Pereira JL, Rosenbloom L, Woods CG: Linkage analysis in Rett syndrome families suggests that there may be a critical region at Xq28. *J Med Genet* 35:997–1003, 1998.
192. Kass SU, Pruss D, Wolffe AP: How does DNA methylation repress transcription? *Trends Genet* 13:444–449, 1997.
193. Nan X, Campoy FJ, Bird A: MeCP2 is a transcriptional repressor with abundant binding sites in genomic chromatin. *Cell* 88:471–481, 1997.
194. Amir RE, Van den Veyver IB, Wan M, Tran CQ, Francke U, Zoghbi HY: Rett syndrome is caused by mutations in X-linked MECP2, encoding methyl-CpG-binding protein 2. *Nat Genet* 23:185–188, 1999.
195. Christodoulou J, Grimm A, Maher T, Bennetts B: RettBASE: The IRSA MECP2 variation database-a new mutation database in evolution. *Hum Mutat* 21:466–472, 2003.
196. Chahrour M, Jung SY, Shaw C, et al.: MeCP2, a key contributor to neurological disease, activates and represses transcription. *Science* 320:1224–1229, 2008.
197. Horike S, Cai S, Miyano M, Cheng JF, Kohwi-Shigematsu T: Loss of silent-chromatin looping and impaired imprinting of DLX5 in Rett syndrome. *Nat Genet* 37:31–40, 2005.
198. Young JI, Hong EP, Castle JC, et al.: Regulation of RNA splicing by the methylation-dependent transcriptional repressor methyl-CpG binding protein 2. *Proc Natl Acad Sci U S A* 102:17551–17558, 2005.
199. Park WJ, Meyers GA, Li X, et al.: Novel FGFR2 mutations in Crouzon and Jackson-Weiss syndromes show allelic heterogeneity and phenotypic variability. *Hum Mol Genet* 4:1229–1233, 1995.
200. Evans JC, Archer HL, Colley JP, et al.: Early onset seizures and Rett-like features associated with mutations in CDKL5. *Eur J Hum Genet* 13:1113–1120, 2005.
201. Weaving LS, Christodoulou J, Williamson SL, et al.: Mutations of CDKL5 cause a severe neurodevelopmental disorder with infantile spasms and mental retardation. *Am J Hum Genet* 75:1079–1093, 2004.
202. Papa FT, Mencarelli MA, Caselli R, et al.: A 3 Mb deletion in 14q12 causes severe mental retardation, mild facial dysmorphisms and Rett-like features. *Am J Med Genet A* 146A:1994–1948, 2008.
203. Jang DH, Chae H, Kim M: Autistic and Rett-like features associated with 2q33.3-q34 interstitial deletion. *Am J Med Genet A* 167A:2213–2218, 2015.
204. Mnatzakanian GN, Lohi H, Munteanu I, et al.: A previously unidentified MECP2 open reading frame defines a new protein isoform relevant to Rett syndrome. *Nat Genet* 36:339–341, 2004.
205. Chen WG, Chang Q, Lin Y, et al.: Derepression of BDNF transcription involves calcium-dependent phosphorylation of MeCP2. *Science* 302:885–889, 2003.
206. Nuber UA, Kriaucionis S, Roloff TC, et al.: Up-regulation of glucocorticoid-regulated genes in a mouse model of Rett syndrome. *Hum Mol Genet* 14:2247–2256, 2005.
207. Stancheva I, Collins AL, Van den Veyver IB, Zoghbi H, Meehan RR: A mutant form of MeCP2 protein associated with human Rett syndrome cannot be displaced from methylated DNA by notch in Xenopus embryos. *Mol Cell* 12:425–435, 2003.
208. Ito-Ishida A, Ure K, Chen H, Swann JW, Zoghbi HY: Loss of MeCP2 in parvalbumin-and somatostatin-expressing neurons in mice leads to distinct Rett syndrome-like phenotypes. *Neuron* 88:651–658, 2015.
209. Zhang W, Peterson M, Beyer B, Frankel WN, Zhang ZW: Loss of MeCP2 from forebrain excitatory neurons leads to cortical hyperexcitation and seizures. *J Neurosci* 34:2754–2763, 2014.
210. Gabel HW, Kinde B, Stroud H, et al.: Disruption of DNA-methylation-dependent long gene repression in Rett syndrome. *Nature* 522:89–93, 2015.
211. Belichenko PV, Oldfors A, Hagberg B, Dahlström A: Rett syndrome: 3-D confocal microscopy of cortical pyramidal dendrites and afferents. *Neuroreport* 5:1509–1513, 1994.
212. Gould E, Tanapat P: Stress and hippocampal neurogenesis. *Biol Psychiatry* 46:1472–1479, 1999.
213. Rakic P: Mode of cell migration to the superficial layers of fetal monkey neocortex. *J Comp Neurol* 145:61–83, 1972.
214. Rakic P, Cameron RS, Komuro H: Recognition, adhesion, transmembrane signaling and cell motility in guided neuronal migration. *Curr Opin Neurobiol* 4:63–69, 1994.
215. Dobyns WB, Truwit CL: Lissencephaly and other malformations of cortical development: 1995 update. *Neuropediatrics* 26:132–147, 1995.
216. Reiner O, Carrozzo R, Shen Y, et al.: Isolation of a Miller-Dieker lissencephaly gene containing G protein beta-subunit-like repeats. *Nature* 364:717–721, 1993.
217. Hattori M, Adachi H, Tsujimoto M, Arai H, Inoue K: Miller-Dieker lissencephaly gene encodes a subunit of brain platelet-activating factor acetylhydrolase [corrected]. *Nature* 370:216–128, 1994.
218. Hattori M, Adachi H, Aoki J, et al.: Cloning and expression of a cDNA encoding the beta-subunit (30-kDa subunit) of bovine brain platelet-activating factor acetylhydrolase. *J Biol Chem* 270:31345–31352, 1995.
219. Reiner O, Albrecht U, Gordon M, et al.: Lissencephaly gene (LIS1) expression in the CNS suggests a role in neuronal migration. *J Neurosci* 15:3730–3738, 1995.
220. Sapir T, Cahana A, Seger R, Nekhai S, Reiner O: LIS1 is a microtubule-associated phosphoprotein. *Eur J Biochem* 265:181–188, 1999.
221. Dix CI, Soundararajan HC, Dzhindzhev NS, et al.: Lissencephaly-1 promotes the recruitment of dynein and dynactin to transported mRNAs. *J Cell Biol* 202:479–494, 2013.
222. Huang J, Roberts AJ, Leschziner AE, Reck-Peterson SL: Lis1 acts as a "clutch" between the ATPase and microtubule-binding domains of the dynein motor. *Cell* 150:975–986, 2012.
223. Moon HM, Youn YH, Pemble H, et al.: LIS1 controls mitosis and mitotic spindle organization via the LIS1-NDEL1-dynein complex. *Hum Mol Genet* 23:449–466, 2014.

224. Tanaka T, Serneo FF, Higgins C, Gambello MJ, Wynshaw-Boris A, Gleeson JG: Lis1 and doublecortin function with dynein to mediate coupling of the nucleus to the centrosome in neuronal migration. *J Cell Biol* 165:709–721, 1996.
225. Haverfield EV, Whited AJ, Petras KS, Dobyns WB, Das S: Intragenic deletions and duplications of the LIS1 and DCX genes: a major disease-causing mechanism in lissencephaly and subcortical band heterotopia. *Eur J Hum Genet* 17:911–918, 2009.
226. Keays DA, Tian G, Poirier K, et al.: Mutations in alpha-tubulin cause abnormal neuronal migration in mice and lissencephaly in humans. *Cell* 128:45–57, 2007.
227. Cardoso C, Leventer RJ, Ward HL, et al.: Refinement of a 400-kb critical region allows genotypic differentiation between isolated lissencephaly, Miller-Dieker syndrome, and other phenotypes secondary to deletions of 17p13.3. *Am J Hum Genet* 72:918–930, 2003.
228. Hyon C, Marlin S, Chantot-Bastaraud S, et al.: A new 17p13.3 microduplication including the PAFAH1B1 and YWHAE genes resulting from an unbalanced X;17 translocation. *Eur J Med Genet* 54:287–291, 2011.
229. Mignon-Ravix C, Cacciagli P, El-Waly B, et al.: Deletion of YWHAE in a patient with periventricular heterotopias and pronounced corpus callosum hypoplasia. *J Med Genet* 47:132–136, 2010.
230. Nagamani SC, Zhang F, Shchelochkov OA, et al.: Microdeletions including YWHAE in the Miller-Dieker syndrome region on chromosome 17p13.3 result in facial dysmorphisms, growth restriction, and cognitive impairment. *J Med Genet* 46:825–833, 2009.
231. Toyo-oka K, Shionoya A, Gambello MJ, et al.: 14-3-3epsilon is important for neuronal migration by binding to NUDEL: a molecular explanation for Miller-Dieker syndrome. *Nat Genet* 34:274–285, 2003.
232. Walsh CA: Genetic malformations of the human cerebral cortex. *Neuron* 23:19–29, 1999.
233. Portes des V, Francis F, Pinard JM, et al.: Doublecortin is the major gene causing X-linked subcortical laminar heterotopia (SCLH). *Hum Mol Genet* 7:1063–1070, 1998.
234. Gleeson JG, Allen KM, Fox JW, et al.: Doublecortin, a brain-specific gene mutated in human X-linked lissencephaly and double cortex syndrome, encodes a putative signaling protein. *Cell* 92:63–72, 1998.
235. Manent JB, Wang Y, Chang Y, Paramasivam M, LoTurco JJ: Dcx reexpression reduces subcortical band heterotopia and seizure threshold in an animal model of neuronal migration disorder. *Nat Med* 15:84–90, 2009.
236. Quelin C, Saillour Y, Souville I, et al.: Mosaic DCX deletion causes subcortical band heterotopia in males. *Neurogenetics* 13:367–373, 2012.
237. Francis F, Koulakoff A, Boucher D, et al.: Doublecortin is a developmentally regulated, microtubule-associated protein expressed in migrating and differentiating neurons. *Neuron* 23:247–256, 1999.
238. Gleeson JG, Lin PT, Flanagan LA, Walsh CA: Doublecortin is a microtubule-associated protein and is expressed widely by migrating neurons. *Neuron* 23:257–271, 1999.
239. Cappello S, Böhringer CR, Bergami M, et al.: A radial glia-specific role of RhoA in double cortex formation. *Neuron* 73:911–924, 2012.
240. Beal JC: Case report: neuronal migration disorder associated with chromosome 15q13.3 duplication in a boy with autism and seizures. *J Child Neurol* 29:NP186–NP188, 2014.
241. Deutsch SI, Burket JA, Katz E: Does subtle disturbance of neuronal migration contribute to schizophrenia and other neurodevelopmental disorders? Potential genetic mechanisms with possible treatment implications. *Eur Neuropsychopharmacol* 20:281–287, 2010.
242. Muraki K, Tanigaki K: Neuronal migration abnormalities and its possible implications for schizophrenia. *Front Neurosci* 9:74, 2015.
243. Fry AE, Cushion TD, Pilz DT: The genetics of lissencephaly. *Am J Med Genet C Semin Med Genet* 166C:198–210, 2014.
244. Guerrini R, Parrini E: Neuronal migration disorders. *Neurobiol Dis* 38:154–166, 2010.
245. Lifton RP: Molecular genetics of human blood pressure variation. *Science* 272:676–680, 1996.
246. Miki Y, Swensen J, Shattuck-Eidens D, et al.: A strong candidate for the breast and ovarian cancer susceptibility gene BRCA1. *Science* 266:66–71, 1994.

SECTION IV
CLINICAL ASSESSMENT AND NOSOLOGY

CHAPTER 4.1 ■ FORMULATION AND INTEGRATION

SCHUYLER W. HENDERSON AND ANDRÉS MARTIN

A formulation distills a child's and family's nuanced life stories and experiences into a meaningful synopsis (1). Being able to formulate a case effectively is one of the key skills for clinicians working in child and adolescent mental health, but it is not an easy skill to master. A good formulation is more than just a summary: It turns a patient's narrative and all the information derived from examinations, interviews with parents and teachers, and medical and school reports into a coherent story that will help to develop a treatment plan.

THE SHAPE OF A FORMULATION

A formulation is a narrative with a clinical purpose. To achieve this purpose, it must convey relevant signs and symptoms as well as pertinent negatives, reflecting the breadth and detail of the clinical interview without reproducing the entirety of the interview. It must also provide explanatory contexts for these signs and symptoms, including familial, social, educational, and cultural contexts, so that the signs and symptoms are relevant and meaningful. When it accomplishes these tasks, the formulation can then justify diagnoses (or no diagnosis, if warranted) and point the way toward treatment options based on the diagnostic considerations.

The core components of the formulation typically follow a conventional trajectory with common signposts to guide the reader: referral source, identifying information, history of present illness, significant past psychiatric and medical histories, psychosocial contexts including family history and educational history, mental status, diagnostic considerations, and treatment planning (Table 4.1.1). Consistency in the formulation's route through these domains permits clinicians to follow a familiar path while attuned to important details and nuances.

Whether in psychoanalytic case studies or in brief presentations on ward rounds, and across systems—hospitals, clinical, juvenile justice—and countries, the overall route of the formulation usually remains the same. But as noted, the formulation has a clinical purpose, and that purpose may be different in different settings, and the formulation can be adapted: briskly oriented, for example, toward safety and risk assessments in a crisis service, or with a more leisurely exploration of family and interpersonal factors for a psychodynamic psychotherapy.

Within this broad shape, there are two common models that can organize the conceptual backbone of the formulation. These are the *biopsychosocial formulation* and the *Four Ps*.

THE BIOPSYCHOSOCIAL MODEL

As the biologic sciences became increasingly sophisticated and dominant in the 20th century, concerns were raised about the value of nonbiologic factors in the etiology, presentation, and treatment of diseases and disorders. In the face of these changes, Meyer (2) promoted the "psychobiologic" approach and Engel subsequently developed, named, and advocated for the "biopsychosocial" model, describing it as a "way of thinking that enables the physician to act rationally in areas now excluded from a rational approach" (3). Over the past three decades, the biopsychosocial model has become the most common model for formulating a case in mental health circles and has been widely adopted throughout medicine. The fundamental goal of the model is to prevent reductionism, particularly biologic reductionism, by ensuring that psychological and social factors are not excluded (see Table 4.1.2). The biopsychosocial model may appear to be a neutral mediator between the three domains but, quite specifically, it is not neutral: It is intended to oppose biomedical, psychological, and social reductionism. Regardless of anatomical lesions, clear psychological or obvious social etiologies, this model insists that all three domains be accounted for. By doing so, it has been a powerful and successful model for physicians in all fields of medicine.

The *biologic* domain circumscribes neuropsychiatric, genetic, and physiologic issues, focusing on, but not limited to, the functional operations of the brain and what might be

TABLE 4.1.1

CORE COMPONENTS INFORMING A DIAGNOSTIC FORMULATION

Component	Details Can Include:
Source	Patient, collateral information, records
Chief complaint	What brought the patient in
History of present illness	Symptoms, course, severity, triggering events, pertinent negatives
Past psychiatric history	Previous evaluations, therapies, hospitalizations, medications, and treatments; history of aggression or harm toward self or others; substance abuse history
Past medical history	Illnesses, hospitalizations, surgeries, and medications including folk and alternative medicine remedies, etc.
Family psychiatric and medical history	Pertinent positives and negatives in the family's psychiatric and medical history, especially substance abuse, suicide, and cardiac history
Social history	Family constellation, peer relations, interactions with the law and social services, and key events such as immigration
Education history	Schools, grades, report cards, special or regular education, changes in schools, suspensions
Developmental history	Mother's pregnancy and labor, delivery, milestones during infancy; stages of motor, cognitive, social, and behavioral development
Psychological testing	IQ, tests of adaptive functioning, speech and language evaluations
Mental status examination	
Assessment	Diagnoses, hypotheses of causality
Plan	Treatment goals and options, other persons or agencies to contact

directly affecting it. The *psychological* dimension includes an evaluation of the child's psychological make-up, including strengths and vulnerabilities, and offers the opportunity to include psychodynamic principles like defense structures, consciously and unconsciously driven patterns of behavior, responses to trauma and conflict, transferences and counter-transferences. The *social* dimension situates the child in their communities, exploring relationships with family and friends, as well as larger collective cultural organizations like schools, religion, socioeconomic class, and ethnicity.

Advocates for the biopsychosocial model argue convincingly that it is needed because a "broad approach [is] essential to avoid premature closure of our efforts to understand the patient's needs, tunnel vision or an overly narrow approach to treatment" (4). Furthermore, it is particularly useful for psychiatrists, who are in a unique position within medicine to address the biologic, psychological, and social dimensions of the patient (5), and therefore are responsible for being attuned to each.

Nevertheless, critics of the model, also convincingly, note that the biopsychosocial model is "silent as to how to understand those aspects under different conditions and in different circumstances" (6,7). While insisting that medical materialism or psychological and social dogmatism cannot suffice, this model does not guide the clinician how to weigh the relative contributions of each in any given patient. If a child is being bullied and has an aunt who is depressed, and has always been noted to be a worrier, the biopsychosocial model would provide slots for where each of these facts would fit, but no guidance on what needs to be addressed first, what is most important, what treatment should ensue, *etc.* An additional flaw in this regard is that because the model is agnostic about the roles of biology, psychology, and society, those who prefer one particular realm can devote their attention to it while paying lip service to the others in a few short sentences (4). In particular, the tailing "social" domain is often the least explored (8). Virchow said that "medicine is a social science" and although psychiatry has a history of collaborating with sociology (9), the academic and clinical intersections between mental health and other social sciences remain underexplored. This is especially true in regard to children, many of whom present to child and adolescent mental health workers fundamentally due to social concerns, such as impulsivity and hyperactivity in the classroom, conflict with parents, truancy and school refusal, or other externalizing disorders (10), and where the "social" component is nevertheless given short shrift.

TABLE 4.1.2

THE COMPONENTS OF THE BIOPSYCHOSOCIAL MODEL

Biologic	Psychological	Social
Family history	Emotional development	Family constellation
Genetics	Personality structure	Peer relationships
Physical development	Self-esteem	School
Constitution	Insight	Neighborhood
Intelligence	Defenses	Ethnic influences
Temperament	Patterns of behavior	Socioeconomic issues
Medical comorbidities	Patterns of cognition	Culture(s)
	Responses to stressors	Religion(s)
	Coping strategies	

The most worrying critique of the biopsychosocial model is that it does not blend or integrate the three dimensions as much as loosely knit them together through proximity in the formulation. Thus, how the social, biologic, and psychological are integrated is left unanswered (11).

The biopsychosocial model has been a step toward rethinking reductionism and an opportunity for generating hypotheses about multiply determined etiologies, which may lead to improved capacity for further synthesis and understanding (12). It is, nevertheless, not sufficient and barely good enough.

THE FOUR Ps

The Four Ps model is more sophisticated than the biopsychosocial model in that it imposes a chronology and an etiology on the formulation that suggests how and where interventions can and should take place. The Four Ps model organizes the patient's presentation into *Predisposing, Precipitating, Perpetuating,* and *Protective* factors (Table 4.1.3).

Predisposing factors are the constellation of features that render the child vulnerable to the presenting symptoms. These may include family history, genetics, medical and psychiatric

TABLE 4.1.3

EXAMPLES OF WHERE THE BIOPSYCHOSOCIAL MODEL MEETS THE FOUR Ps

The "P" Characteristic and Trigger Question	Biologic	Psychological	Social
Predisposing *Why me?*	Genetic loading	Immature defensive structure	Poverty and adversity
Precipitating *Why now?*	Iatrogenic reaction	Recent loss	School stressors
Perpetuating *Why does it continue?*	Poor response to medication	No support at school	Unable to attend therapy sessions because of parents' work schedule
Protective *What can I rely on?*	Family history of treatment response	Insightful	Community and faith as sources of support

history, and chronic social stressors. By including these factors here, the clinician is arguing that they are directly relevant to the child's current symptoms. *Precipitating* factors identify the current stressors, inciting events, and concurrent illness. *Perpetuating* factors are those that make the suffering endure, such as the severity of the condition, compliance, deficits in coping or exacerbating social circumstances, and unresolved predisposing and precipitating factors. *Protective* factors describe a patient's strengths, resilience, and supports. Although other models, including the biopsychosocial model, can include strengths and resilience, this model explicitly foregrounds it.

The Four Ps can be easily used in conjunction with other models. As a framework, it can also be used to organize a psychodynamic formulation, including *predisposing* vulnerabilities, personality structure, and family and developmental history; *precipitating* trauma or life events; *perpetuating* maladaptive behaviors and resistances; and *protective* facets of the identity. And it can easily be blended with the biopsychosocial model (see Table 4.1.3).

The Four Ps can be used with the Collaborative Problem Solving (CPS) model (13). The CPS model comprehensively assesses cognitive deficits around frustration tolerance, flexibility and problem-solving, and it exemplifies a collaborative approach to the formulation, with caregivers coming together to understand the child and then working with the child to prevent dangerous or aggressive behaviors. As the child is also involved in formulating the plan, the Four Ps provides a concrete way of organizing the different factors that lead to problematic behaviors in a manner comprehensible to staff and patients alike.

The CPS approach expands on the precipitating and perpetuating factors, especially the ones pertaining to the child's learning (including his or her social learning). It then allows the staff to formulate appropriate, testable, and patient-specific interventions based on observed behaviors and analysis of triggers (precipitating events), continued stresses (perpetuating factors), and strengths that can be tapped into (protective factors). This combination of the Four Ps formulation and the CPS model may be particularly apt on inpatient units (14).

Similarly, Havinghurst and Downey (15) propose a "Mindful Formulation." After collecting information, the Mindful Formulation uses a "patterns" worksheet where the child's affective responses, behaviors, and cognitions are collected in four domains: child functioning; parents'/carers'/siblings'/significant other's functioning; relationships with the child and among significant others; and relationships with and among the community. The goal is trying to discern patterns of strength as well as patterns of weakness and vulnerability and then to use these patterns to flesh out the Four Ps.

Biologic, psychological, and social elements can fall under each category. The limitations of the Four Ps model include the nonstandard format (one does not begin a formulation with "predisposing factors") and an uneasy overlap between categories. There is little consolidation of the many factors except as to how they affect the patient's symptomology, although strength of the model is that it is nevertheless explicit about arranging potentially etiologic factors.

TABLE 4.1.4

THE FOUR PERSPECTIVES

Perspective	Treatment	Problem/Critique	Requirement
Disease What a patient *has*	Cure	Medicines can be toxic	Compliance
Dimension What a patient *is*	Guide	Guidance can be paternalistic	Location of strength
Behavior What a patient *does*	Interrupt	Stopping can be stigmatizing	Will to change
Life story What a patient *wants*	Rescript	Interpretations can be hostile	Insight

Adapted from McHugh PR, Slavney PR: *The Perspectives of Psychiatry*. 2nd ed. Baltimore, MD, The Johns Hopkins University Press, 1998.

THE VARIETY OF FORMULATIONS

Tauber writes that in science "observations assume their meanings within a particular context, for facts are not just products of sensation or measurement, as the positivists averred, but rather they reside within a conceptual framework that places the fact into an intelligible picture of the world" (16). A formulation is not a value-neutral format containing dispassionately arranged facts. The choice as to which facts to include and which to reject and the subsequent ordering and presentation of the facts collude to produce a value-laden product. A formulation is thus a condensation of values, informed by the nature of the encounter between the clinician and the patient; practical goals; training and experience; and implicit and explicit ethics. The formulation is not a value-neutral format containing dispassionately arranged facts. Although there is a historical precedent and pragmatic use for the overall shape of the formulation, we ought not to be naive about the theoretical work a formulation performs and how values influence the shape of a formulation.

We turn now to how different types of values influence the formulation.

Location

The shape of a formulation may depend less on the patient's narrative and more on the location of the clinical encounter. As an example, on a crisis service, an excellent trainee with a longstanding interest in psychoanalysis was presenting thoughtful and rich formulations about children with a focus on developmental conflicts with family and peers; although these issues were far from irrelevant, they did not help the team decide what treatment options were required that day or what immediate services we wanted to offer the family. The trainee's formulations were, however, well suited to his long-term therapy cases. With education on how to revise the formulation for the clinical milieu, the trainee was able to provide thoughtful, psychodynamically informed formulations in concert with other observations and information that resulted in our ability to make plans for the families right then and there.

A formulation needs to reflect the imperatives of the system in which the encounter takes place and therefore mirrors clinical priorities. A formulation may focus on the severity and acuity of a patient's symptoms and needs in a crisis service; it may develop a working model of treatment trials and planning in an inpatient unit; it may narrate the gradual blossoming of relationships, defenses, and cathexes (emotional investments) cultivated and analyzed in a psychodynamic treatment. What each clinical milieu values is reflected in how the child's assessment and treatment will be formulated.

Treatment Values

One of the goals of a formulation is to drive a treatment plan (including no treatment, if warranted), and therefore the shape of a formulation will be influenced by treatment options. Depending upon the type of treatment, the clinician will select questions and areas of assessment to explore. A clinician's training, biases, and experiences will naturally influence how questions are asked and what is explored; one of the advantages of learning different types of formulation techniques and perspectives is that it allows the clinician to become aware of his or her own biases, but also allows them to be explicit about their perspective and why it leads to certain treatment options.

Etiologic Values and Pluralism

What causes mental health disorders, maladies, diseases, and problems? What factors conspire to make a child drop out of school or begin to take illicit drugs? Why is this particular child depressed, or that particular child reporting psychotic symptoms? The biopsychosocial and Four Ps models create a great deal of space in which these questions can be answered, and yet they do not *compel* an answer. They do no prognostic work themselves. There has subsequently been a push toward models that are less flimsy and wishy-washy. A goal has been to develop models that confidently assert etiologic claims (not with arrogant hubris, but based on what we know as clinicians and with respect for what we have learned from our science and our history).

Attempting to provide an alternative to the biopsychosocial and Four Ps models is the *Four Perspectives* (not to be confused with the Four Ps) (Table 4.1.4). The Four Perspectives distinguish mental health conditions based not on the conglomerative biopsychosocial model, but on etiology and treatment options (17). The concept of pluralism, defined by Havens (18) as a process of "refining methods, not mixing them" has deeply informed the Four Perspectives.

The perspectives in this model each come with a treatment paradigm:

- *Disease*, the keystone of the biomedical perspective, is a clinical entity, a pathologic condition with a specific etiology and with a likely prognosis. The treatment for disease involves prevention and cure, by interventions that directly or indirectly affect the pathologic process and/or symptom relief (which may include psychological interventions).
- *Dimensions* are based on vulnerabilities due to a person's position within ranges of psychological domains (such as intellectual disability or temperament). These vulnerabilities are not "cured" but are addressed with guidance.
- *Behaviors*, maladaptive or undesirable goal-directed activities, need to be ameliorated, stopped, or interrupted, through social, psychological, and/or medical means.
- The fourth perspective is *The Life Story*, based on the reconstruction of narratives through talk therapy. Treatment is usually sought due to emotional states of distress and proceeds through interpretation.

This model includes something rarely discussed in formulations and rarely included in psychiatric models: McHugh (19,20) points to the potential adverse effects of each intervention. All medications can be toxic; guidance can be paternalistic; stopping a behavior can be stigmatizing; and interpretations can be hostile. By making the assessment and acknowledgment of potential adverse effects a cornerstone of the formulation, mental health professionals can collaborate more fully with the patient and family in a transparent and compassionate way.

There is another potential category, "requirement," that could be included in a Four Perspectives formulation. The "requirement" is what is needed for the intervention to work. For a biomedical cure to be effective, there must be an assessment of compliance or adherence to treatment. With guidance, there must be identification of developmental potential, which the guidance can support: For example, in working with a patient with intellectual disability, intellectual, vocational, and occupational strengths must be assessed. Changing behavior requires a will to change, whether this is intuitive, as in the case of a boy who wishes to stop smoking marijuana and has moved from precontemplation into contemplation, or cultivated through a system of positive and negative reinforcement. And for interpretations to be effective, the patient's insight needs to be appraised.

A formulation based on the Four Perspectives would take as its conceptual point of origin a conviction about the patient's presentation, which would remain adaptable within the overall formulation, and which would then guide the formulation toward specific interventions. One advantage of the Four Perspectives is that they make "explicit aspects of reasoning about patients that are often left implicit or vague" (17).

The pluralistic formulation would proceed as the mental health professional ascertains which categories, perspectives, or dimensions best describe the child's condition; the formulation would then explain how the mental health professional engages in appropriate, directed treatment, having assessed the requirements and acknowledged the concerns. For example, biologic approach (the disease model) has a better fit with bipolar disorder, schizophrenia, and Rett syndrome than it does with grief. The behavioral approach, which targets known harmful behaviors, may be best for substance abuse (although, of course, medical interventions directed toward addiction as a disease can be countenanced as supplemental). The *Life Story model* is geared toward understanding and narrativizing stresses and so would be more helpful for bereavement or stagnation in life's journey.

Culture

In addition to living in a world of etiologic pluralism, we live in a world of cultural pluralism. The formulation can integrate the individual with his or her cultural contexts, without which it may not be possible to understand the patient. A cultural formulation itself has several core components: The cultural identity of the individual (including self-identified cultural affiliations, languages spoken, and levels of involvement with cultures of origin and host/local/dominant cultures); cultural explanations of illness (meanings, cultural explanations for symptoms or cause, and idioms to describe illness); cultural adaptations to the environment and stresses (such as specific stresses in the community as well as areas of support in the community, including possible sources of collaboration); and cultural areas of convergence and divergence between the clinician and the individual (21,22). Attending to this allows for culturally valid assessments on the part of the clinician, but can also be essential in formulating subsequent plans that are acceptable to the patient (23). Culture is everywhere, and children are usually exploring it with vigor. Of all the cultures children participate in, few are more important than the culture of childhood itself. A good formulation will include the child's relationship to this rich culture, including the child's interactions with peers and participation in childhood rituals, and his or her engagement with the cultural life of childhood, from television, games, and sports, to movies, books, and social media. Regarding the latter, specific adaptations of the cultural formulation for children may include a closer look at their sociocultural immersion in social media: where they spend their time, how they communicate, what they communicate, what adults do and do not know about what they are communicating, and stressors they experience in this virtual world.

A Composite Case Is Presented, Followed by a Biopsychosocial Formulation Focusing on *Risk Ractors for Depression*, and a Four Ps Formulation Focusing on *Suicidality*

A 14-year-old girl, Sara, comes to the clinic after trying to swallow a handful of lithium tablets during an argument with her father. She was stopped by her father and then threw the pills on the floor. Her chief complaint when she meets you is that she is depressed and angry. She says she was angry that her father wanted her to go back to her hometown to live with her mother. Her father had become increasingly frustrated that Sara was smoking so much marijuana and failing at school. Sara says that her depressed mood preceded coming to live with her father. She says she has had months of trouble falling asleep because she's ruminating on her day's failures, and then can't wake up because she's exhausted after a long night of tossing and turning. She says she can't concentrate in her new school, which is why she says she leaves school every day to smoke marijuana. She says it helps her focus and relax and is the one time she enjoys being her new friends. She misses being with her old friends. She says that she has no desire to die right now, but that when she gets really upset she thinks about wanting to be gone forever, particularly because her parents would be sorry and would miss her.

Her father adds that she has been irritable for about 2 months since joining him in the city and that she wasn't like this as a little girl. He says that it has been worsening recently as her school performance has worsened. He says that during arguments she has said with increasing vigor that she wishes she weren't alive. He took her to a doctor who prescribed lithium for mood lability, irritability, and depressed symptoms. Neither Sara nor her father report that she has ever had any psychotic episodes or manic symptoms, although she has been anxious at times, just like her mother was. Her father says that he has no psychiatric history but her mother was "moody" and tried to kill herself when he first said he was leaving for the city.

Biopsychosocial Formulation Focused on Risk for a Clinically Significant Depressive Disorder

Sara is a 14-year-old girl with symptoms of depression, including depressed mood and irritability, trouble sleeping, poor concentration, negative ruminations, and a recent interrupted suicide attempt. Biologic risks for a depressive disorder include a family history of mood lability; substance abuse, which may be exacerbating her depression or her performance in school; and lithium toxicity. Psychological factors include ongoing distress over her parents' separation, feeling trapped between them, and school failure. Social factors include decreased supervision now that she has moved to live with her father, distance from her old friends and family, and conflict with new friends at school.

The Four Ps for Suicidality

Sara is a 14-year-old girl with symptoms of depression and a recent suicide attempt. Predisposing factors for suicidality include her mother's history of suicide attempts; Sara's suicidal ideation, expressed as threats during arguments with her father; and having less supervision and being in a new, isolating environment. Precipitating factors include the stresses of moving to a new city, being in a new school, and a fight with her father. Perpetuating factors include insufficient treatment and worsening depressive symptoms. Protective factors include strong social relationships prior to the move, which can be developed, and a willingness to start new treatments.

THE USES OF A FORMULATION

A case formulation is hypothesis generating and iterative, and can change over time depending upon further clinical encounters, new information, and the clinician's evolving understanding of the child. So what purpose does a formulation serve?

A formulation is a way in which the clinician can understand and explain the patient. As proposed by Jaspers' understanding and explaining may be distinct ways of knowing the patient (24). The depth of our understanding of a patient's experience may not explain the etiology of a symptom in a way conducive to treatment, and likewise a model of behavior may not adequately impart the patient's experience of that behavior. Nevertheless, formulating a case allows the clinician to balance his or her understanding of the patient with his or her explanations.

Understanding a patient requires an intersubjective appreciation of the patient's experiences, hopes and concerns, and is acquired through listening, talking, and interacting with the patient (as well as his or her family and others occupying important roles in his or her world). Explanation of a patient's symptoms and conditions itself has two dimensions: the interpretative task, where psychological, sociologic, and neurobiologic theories are used, ideally in an explicit and evidence-based manner, in order to locate the contributing factors; and the explanatory task, which connects these factors with the patient's experience. Understanding and explanation work in concert.

A formulation is also a mode of communication. The question of its utility then depends upon the audience and the purpose of the communication. Formulations may need to be comprehensible to the clinicians who will treat the child next; clinicians in another discipline; the audiences for discharge summaries (which, for children, can include parents, schools, social service agencies, and, at times, the children themselves); for outside insurance company employees who review or authorize treatment for an insurance company (which frequently includes adult psychiatrists); and for legal purposes.

Consultation letters are another area where the case formulation is essential. It is widely believed that poor communication between healthcare professionals is responsible for many problems. In one worrying study, the authors reviewed 150 assessment letters from psychiatrists at a clinic in Rotherham, UK, and discovered that 94% of them did not include a case formulation (25).

Keely et al. (26) provide a useful guide for how to formulate a case in the context of a consultation letter.

Information

- Explain the purpose of the consultation at the outset.
- Explain the role the consultation letter will take (e.g., what the letter will include, such as historical information, diagnosis, and recommendations for further treatment).

Include an appropriate case formulation with diagnostic rationale and clear plans for follow-up.

As they note, the role of the formulation may be to educate, especially when the consultation is for those outside the field, and so may include references and explanations to educate the various potential audiences of the letter.

This also raises the question of what should not be included in a formulation.

Being able to discreetly convey information about sex, drugs, conflicts with family, and other potentially inflammatory topics is an important skill to develop. The broader issue is that a formulation requires communication skills that are sensitive to ethical and clinical relationships. An ethical formulation includes these values as well as the values of accuracy and veracity; it should convey clinical material in a way that is sensitive to patients, their confidentiality, and their privacy.

CHILDREN AND FORMULATIONS

The models for case formulation have typically been derived from adult psychiatry. Although child and adolescent psychiatry has offered much to adult psychiatry, and vice versa, the mantra that children are not simply "little adults" is nowhere more true than in the mental health and experience of youngsters.

How do we specifically adapt formulations for children?

1. *Jargon*: The language of the formulations needs to be precise and relevant to the child's life. This means resisting reliance on jargon, with a cautious use of terminologies that might be derived from and more epidemiologically justified in adult populations. For example, children are frequently referred for mental health evaluation, including from other mental health professionals, for "auditory hallucinations," not necessarily because they are having auditory hallucinations but because they have answered "yes" to questions that are, for them, vague and strange, that possibly approximate their experience, or that are answered concretely ("do you hear voices?"). Although the referral may warrant expert evaluation, the subsequent formulation should resist using "auditory hallucination" unless that precise term is clinically warranted, and not, for example, when the child is lying in bed, trying to go to sleep, and spooked by vivid memories of a horror film watched the night before. The language used in the formulation should therefore be effectively descriptive and the use of clinical terms should be age and developmentally appropriate.
2. *The chief complaint*: This is usually a single line or a symptom, but with children who are brought in by adults, it is worth considering assessing two chief complaints: the chief complaint of the adults and the chief complaint of the child (which, it is true, will often be "I don't know").
3. *Explicitly including family and school as separate categories*: Although this might also be good for adult patients (with a focus on employment rather than school), these realms should be explicitly and comprehensively evaluated in children and thus may merit sections of their own, rather than subsections of "social" in a formulation. Stressors in the family and school can reflect a child's symptoms, exacerbate them, or, indeed, be fundamentally etiologic. In fact, there are no situations in which a child's presentation for services does not reflect difficulties in one or both of these realms, whether the child is reacting to stressors, posing challenges to these domains with his or her behavior, or where his or her symptoms are exacerbated by what he or she is experiencing at home or at school.
4. *Development as a separate category versus inclusion of developmental factors in all categories*: Children deserve an assessment of their developmental history that is not cursory. Much of a child mental health professional's diagnosis and treatment planning is predicated on what is typical or atypical and one of the key concerns in developing a treatment plan and making recommendations is how the presenting symptoms will affect subsequent development. Putting development into its own section may seem to foreground development, but it typically permits a cursory glance at development, instead of integrating development into all aspects of the formulation. Including development explicitly in all the domains of the formulation can be helpful as a yardstick, instead of relying on a gestalt sense of whether hyperactivity or moodiness is deemed excessive, and can also be helpful in justifying interventions, because sometimes

typical behaviors coalesce to produce a constellation of symptoms that would be detrimental to a child's developmental trajectory.

5. *Models of development*: A formulation that is not book length cannot run stage by stage through, for example, Freud, Erikson, and Piaget; the formulation requires choices about which models of development are appropriate. In this regard, as well as others, children suffer from the guild frictions and antagonisms. Using or thinking through various paradigms does not necessarily imply allegiance and dogmatism. This is not to say that all models of development are equally accurate, but the capacity to invoke or countenance different models should not be based on professional competition. Although everybody changes over time, children are in a whirlwind of growth and maturation, accumulating language and skills, experimenting with their expanding world, gaining mastery over tasks while being introduced to more complicated ones on a daily basis. This process is not straightforward and may be better viewed as a punctuated evolution than as a smooth and even progression. Nevertheless, a basic appreciation of expected norms can situate the child and alert the clinician to delays and disorders. In light of this, a useful tool for the formulation can be an assessment of the child's tasks in terms of motor, cognitive, and social development, based on models including Piaget's stages of cognitive development and Erikson's tasks. Expressing the child's development in these terms in the formulation will have additional longitudinal value, documenting development just as growth charts map a child's somatic development.
6. *The individual focus of case formulations*: Formulations are typically written about an individual, not, for example, about a family or a social milieu. They therefore have an ideologic bias toward assessing children as individuals. A formulation, however, can recognize that the child may be presenting for services when the primary problem may not be the child's. Children can be the canaries in the coal mine. Profound family stressors may become manifest in the child's behavior, and it is the family stressor that needs to be addressed primarily; similarly, parents may present the healthiest member of their family to services. The formulation of the child needs to be able to accommodate this, not only to prevent the child from getting unnecessary treatment when better treatments could address the situation, but to avoid collusion in a failure to address predisposing and precipitating symptoms.

CONCLUSION

The formulation in child and adolescent psychiatry is an exciting confluence of ideas. The values of child and adolescent mental health professionals come together with the patient's experience to create a narrative about that patient leading to treatment. It is an iterative and adaptive format, able to accommodate different theories and perspectives to explain what is happening to our patients while we strive better to understand them. Despite these variables, the formulation need not be either intimidating or cumbersome. The science of the formulation is its hypothesis-generating format, modifiable with new information, in service of causal explanations. The art of the formulation is not instantaneously pinning down the right diagnosis, but rather providing a thoughtful, sympathetic portrait of a child in the world.

Disclosure: This chapter is a revision of: Henderson SW, Martin A. Case formulation and integration of information in child and adolescent mental health. In: Rey JM (ed): *IACAPAP e-Textbook of Child and Adolescent Mental Health*. International Association for Child and Adolescent Psychiatry and Allied Professions, Geneva, 2015.

ACKNOWLEDGMENT

We wish to thank Joseph Rey for his constructive editing and contributions to this chapter.

References

1. Winters NC, Hanson G, Stoyanova V: The case formulation in child and adolescent psychiatry. *Child Adolesc Psychiatr Clin N Am* 16(1):111–132, ix, 2007.
2. Meyer A: The psychobiological point of view. In: Lief A (ed): *The Commonsense Psychiatry of Dr. AdolfMeyer*. New York, McGraw Hill, 1948.
3. Engel GL: The clinical application of the biopsychosocial model. *Am J Psychiatry* 137:535–544, 1980.
4. Jellinek MS, McDermott JF: Formulation: putting the diagnosis into a therapeutic context and treatment plan. *J Am Acad Child Adolesc Psychiatry* 43(7):913–916, 2004.
5. Gabbard GO, Kay J: The fate of integrated treatment: whatever happened to the biopsychosocial psychiatrist? *Am J Psychiatry* 158(12):1956–1963, 2001.
6. Ghaemi SN: *The Concepts of Psychiatry: A Pluralistic Approach to the Mind and Mental Illness*. Baltimore, MD, The Johns Hopkins University Press, 2003.
7. Ghaemi SM: *The Rise and Fall of the Biopsychosocial Model*. Baltimore, MD, The Johns Hopkins University Press, 2009.
8. Grunebaum H: Letter to the editor. *Am J Psychiatry* 160(1):186, 2003.
9. Bloom SW. The Relevance of medical sociology to psychiatry: a historical view. *J Nerv Ment Dis* 193(2):77–84, 2005.
10. Centers for Disease Control and Prevention. Mental health in the United States: health care and wellbeing of children with chronic emotional, behavioral, or developmental problems—United States, 2001. *MMWR Morb Mortal Wkly Rep* 54(39):985–989, 2005.
11. McLaren N: A critical review of the biopsychosocial model. *Aust N Z J Psychiatry* 32:86–92, 1998.
12. Freedman AM: The biopsychosocial paradigm and the future of psychiatry. *Compr Psychiatry* 36(6):397–406, 1995.
13. Greene RW, Ablon JS: *Treating Explosive Kids: The Collaborative Problem Solving Approach*. New York, Guilford Press, 2005.
14. Greene RW, Ablon JS, Martin A: Use of collaborative problem solving to reduce seclusion and restraint in child and adolescent inpatient units. *Psychiatric Services*, 57(5):610–612, 2006.
15. Havighurst SS, Downey L: Clinical reasoning for child and adolescent mental health practitioners: the mindful formulation. *Clin Child Psychol Psychiatry* 14(2):251–271, 2009.
16. Tauber AA: Medicine and the call for a moral epistemology. *Perspect Biol Med* 48(1):42–53, 2005.
17. McHugh PR, Slavney PR: *The Perspectives of Psychiatry*. 2nd ed. Baltimore, MD, The Johns Hopkins University Press, 1998.
18. Havens L: *Psychiatric Movements: From Sects to Science*. New Brunswick, NJ, Transaction Publishers, 2005.
19. McHugh PR: Striving for coherence: psychiatry's efforts over classification. *J Am Med Assoc* 293:2526–2528, 2005.
20. McHugh PR: *The Mind Has Mountains*. Baltimore, MD, The Johns Hopkins University Press, 2005.
21. American Psychiatric Association: *Diagnostic and Statistical Manual of Mental Disorders, Fourth Edition (DSM-IV)*. Washington, DC, APA, 1994.
22. Pumariega AJ, Rothe E, Mian A, et al.: Practice parameter for cultural competence in child and adolescent psychiatric practice. *J Am Acad Child Adolesc Psychiatry* 52(10):1101–1115, 2013.
23. Lewis-Fernández R, Díaz N: The cultural formulation: a method for assessing cultural factors affecting the clinical encounter. *Psychiatr Q* 73(4):271–295, 2002 Winter.
24. Jaspers K: *General Psychopathology*, Vol 1. Translated: Hoenig J, Hamilton MW (eds): Baltimore, MD, The Johns Hopkins University Press, 1997.
25. Abbas MJ, Premkumar L, Goodarzi A, Walton R: Lost in documentation: a study of case-formulation documentation in letters after outpatient assessment. *Academic Psychiatry* 37:336–338, 2013.
26. Keely E, Dojeiji S, Myers K: Writing effective consultation letters: 12 tips for teachers. *Med Teach* 24(6):585–589, 2002.

CHAPTER 4.2 ■ CLINICAL ASSESSMENT OF INFANTS AND TODDLERS

WALTER S. GILLIAM, LINDA C. MAYES, AND AMALIA LONDONO TOBON

Why perform infant assessments? It is perhaps easier to state definitively what infant assessments cannot provide. They do not provide a measure of fixed or immutable intelligence, a trajectory for future development, or a window on future adjustment, nor can they typically partial out the various potential causal factors. Results are descriptive, with only limited application for etiologic understanding or detailed prognosticating. Questions such as "How much of this infant's delay comes from his environment, versus how much from his prematurity?" or "What will be the eventual extent of this child's developmental disability?" are not definitively answerable by a developmental assessment. Developmental assessments, however complete and skillfully done, cannot provide sure predictions of long-term outcome or parcel out the complex contributions of endowment, experience, and maturational forces.

Despite the above caveats, assessment of infant development can be highly useful, and in many cases essential to proper clinical treatment. Skillfully done, these assessments can help create a picture of the child's current developmental level and environmental context that can be invaluable to sound clinical decision-making and treatment planning. Essentially, developmental assessment results help provide a lens through which we might be better able to perceive the world from the child's perspective. Indeed, Bagnato and Neisworth (1) have pointed out that the word *assidere* (the Greek origin of *assessment*) literally means "to sit beside," and hence to get to know someone.

Clinical assessment of infants and toddlers is a subspecialty area of clinical practice. Not all psychiatrists, psychologists, pediatricians, and other professionals will possess the training and degree of closely supervised practice necessary to competently and independently conduct such evaluations. Those professionals who do possess these specialized skills typically have acquired them through formal subspecialization near the end of their professional training.

A BRIEF HISTORY OF INFANT DEVELOPMENTAL ASSESSMENT

A brief discussion of the history of infant assessment may provide an illustration of the evolving aims and technologic advances in this field. (A more complete history is provided by Brooks & Weinraub (2) and Wyly (3).)

In the late 19th century, the European scientific community was consumed with a fervor and creativity best characterized by the studies of evolution, theories about the unconscious mind, and a growing concern for persons with mental illness and intellectual challenges. The science of child development was dominated by single-child case studies—often the children of the scientists. By the early 20th century, a concept of measuring infant capacities grew out of the concern of scientists of the time to find a metric for human intelligence that would permit the creation of criteria for schools for children with intellectual deficiencies (4,5). By the 1920s to 1940s, two basic approaches were used in exploring intellectual development in infants. One approach, the infant IQ model, sought to extend downward the IQ assessment model to children younger than school age, eventually including infants. Overall, "infant IQ tests" were found to be inadequate at meaningfully extending the IQ assessment model into infancy and are now all but extinct in use. A second approach, the gesellian model, sought to create a new model of assessment that began with the newborn and extended upward.

Several aspects of Gesell's work distinguish it from those of his predecessors and contemporaries. First, whereas the infant IQ tradition grew from an interest in identifying deviant patterns of development, Gesell's interest was mostly in documenting normal developmental trends. Second, Gesell's model supported the conceptualization of development occurring simultaneously in many distinct but interrelated domains (6), as opposed to a singular factor of intellectual ability. Third, Gesell's model of developmental maturation supported an understanding of the effects of the child's environment in altering the course of development, as opposed to viewing IQ as a stable and static trait, opening the way for the more transactional and dynamic understanding of developmental processes that would later prevail. Gesell's work was far-reaching, and subsequent researchers, such as Nancy Bayley, relied heavily on the developmental tasks and techniques he pioneered. Bayley applied testing concepts more familiar to the infant IQ model to the assessment techniques developed by Gesell, resulting in two scales of infant development that would later revolutionize and dominate the field of infant assessment.

In the 1940s and 1950s, the science of infant developmental assessment gained greater international attention, through the publishing of the *Griffiths Mental Development Scale* (7) in London. American developmentalists first began to consider seriously the stage theory of Jean Piaget, which clearly favored the view of qualitative, rather than simply quantitative, differences in the abilities of children of various ages. The 1960s and 1970s were breakthrough decades that brought a new wave of infant development tests, more rigorously standardized on larger numbers of infants, with careful testing of interobserver agreement and test–retest reliability. The *Bayley Scales of Infant Development* (BSID) (8) consolidated Bayley's original two scales into one assessment instrument with norms based on a nationally representative sample of infants. The BSID set a new and enduring standard of sophistication for the development and standardization of infant developmental assessment tools. Concomitant interest in newborn capacities and the rapidly emerging field of newborn sensory perception also led to the development of a number of scales to measure competency in newborns.

The last three decades have led to further psychometric improvements, a renewed interest in diagnostic functionality, and the application of information-processing theory to the study of infant development. Federal mandates for the special education of young children created the need for an arsenal of assessment tools that encompassed all of the qualifying areas of delay, utilized information from both direct assessment of the child and parent report, and facilitated early intervention treatment planning and program accountability. The federal early childhood special education laws also instantiated the notion of a five-factor model of development (Motor [gross and fine], Communication [receptive and expressive], Cognitive, Adaptive or Self-Help, and Personal–Social or Social–Emotional) that has since been replicated in nearly all currently existing developmental measure. Also, a plethora of brief developmental screening instruments also were developed for use by professionals with relatively little training in formal assessment.

INTERVIEWING, OBSERVING, AND SYTNTHESIZING INFORMATION

The developmental assessment of infants involves more than the simple administration of a set of developmental test protocols. Assessments performed in the first 3 years of life require the clinician to function simultaneously as a generalist and a specialist, to blend quiet observation with active probing, to synthesize information from caregivers with that gathered through direct observation of the child, and to be involved in a curious blend of searching for specifically defined responses from a child with inferences based on behavior. This set of skills is indeed important for adequate clinical assessment of children of all ages. However, the need is even greatest for those providing clinical services to these youngest of patients, since development during the early years is the most rapid, context dependent, and intersystemic. (See Table 4.2.1 for a summary of some of the information obtained during an infant assessment.) While interviewing, observation, and synthesis are the skills of medical diagnosis in general, there are unique aspects to each in the process of assessing infants.

Interviewing

Skillful interviewing is central to a complete developmental assessment, since much of the data about infants' daily functioning and their relationships with others come from interviews with the caregivers. Skillful interviewing techniques include letting caregivers begin their story wherever they choose; using directed, information-gathering questions in such a way as to clarify but not disrupt the parents' account; and listening for affect as much as content. Importantly, nearly every step of the assessment process requires an alliance between clinician and caregiver, since infants usually perform better when they are in the company of familiar adults, and the initial interview between clinician and family is crucial in setting the tone for such an alliance. Moreover, establishing an alliance is central to evaluating infants' interactions with the adults in their world. Indeed, infant assessments are quite compromised when there are no familiar adults available to meet with the clinician and be with the infant. Parenthetically, it is often in cases involving the most severe environmental disturbance that clinicians do not have access to caregivers that are able to describe the infant's history.

Addressing Caregiver Fears Regarding the Assessment

When parents, foster parents, or other caregivers are available, skillful interviewing is also critical in helping parents follow through with the assessment process. Coming for a developmental evaluation or participating in one while their infant is hospitalized is enormously stressful and often frightening for caregivers. Clinicians working with infants and their families need to understand that, regardless of what caregivers have been told about the assessment, caregivers' fears and fantasies about the process are as potent as the facts of the presenting problem. Not uncommonly, caregivers have begun to see the infant as damaged or defective in some way and are afraid and guilty about the effect of their own behavior on the infant. Their fears of what the infant's problems signify may

TABLE 4.2.1

SOME OF THE INFORMATION OBTAINED DURING AN INFANT ASSESSMENT

Caregiver Interview	Observation or Formal Evaluation of Child
• Family history • Genetic influences • History of pregnancy, delivery, perinatal period • Developmental history (developmental milestones, previous assessments) • Medical history • Child care and extended family arrangements • Child's psychological role in family • Caregiver perceptions and expectations of child • Stability of home/family environment • Family social support systems • Family functioning, stress, and coping (alcohol and drug abuse, domestic violence, etc.) **Observation of Caregiver and Infant** • Infant's use of caregiver for support and reassurance • Caregiver's attunement and responsiveness to child's affective state • Elicitation and receipt of positive interactions • Security of attachment between caregiver and infant • Caregiver affective response to child's efforts during assessment	• Physical health, appearance, and growth parameters • Sensory development (vision, hearing, tactile, etc.) • Gross motor development • Fine motor development • Communication development • Receptive communication • Expressive communication • Speech clarity and fluency • Cognitive problem-solving • Developing sense of self • Social relatedness and interest in environment • Capacity for affect regulation and coping skills • Emerging mastery motivation • Capacity for symbolic representation and play

be expressed in many ways. They may anticipate that their infant has a serious developmental disability, such as autism or intellectual disability, or that the infant will have serious emotional difficulties in school, or that they themselves will be, or already are, inadequate caregivers. It is a vulnerable time for caregivers, and clinicians should keep in mind that what seem inconsequential moments and statements to them may be memorable and powerful for many caregivers. Furthermore, the stress of coming for an assessment affects the caregivers' abilities to report about the infant's development. Often, the "facts" start to change as the alliance between caregivers and clinician develops.

Active Listening

When first interviewed, caregivers may be reluctant to be candid or may not themselves be fully aware of their own perceptions and beliefs about the infant. Open-ended questions, allowing caregivers to begin their story wherever they feel most comfortable, and conveying a nonjudgmental attitude are crucial beginning points in establishing the working alliance. Also, at the risk of stating the obvious, such "interviews" involve considerably more listening than active questioning. Indeed, the type of active listening involved in this type of interview requires the clinician to do much more than passively collect and record requested information, it involves forming numerous connections between "factual" information, observational information (the reactions of the caregivers and their affective responses), and an appreciation of the context of the relationship between the caregiver and the clinician.

Content of the Interview

The important areas to cover in terms of the infant's development are the medical history and major developmental milestones; the history of the mother's pregnancy, delivery, and immediate perinatal period; the number, ages, and health of family members; and how the infant fits in the family's daily life (9). The meaning of the individual child for all caregivers is an important window on the infant's place in the family. Many infants and toddlers attend child care or early intervention programs, and the perception of those teachers, as well as their relationship with the infant's primary caregivers at home, is also important.

More specifically, the interviewer should try to get a picture of the caregivers' perceptions of the infant's level of functioning in several areas. These include motor development and activity level, speech and communication, problem-solving and play, self-regulation (ease of comforting, need for routines), relationships with others, and level of social responsiveness. Questions about whether or not the pregnancy was planned or came at a good time for the family and what expectations the parents had for the infant provide important information about perceptions, disappointments, and stresses. Similarly, asking the caregivers of whom the infant reminds them or what traits in their infant they like best and least may be useful avenues for learning about how the parents view both the infant's problem and his or her place within their family.

Techniques of Organizing Information

Provence (10) has suggested that a productive method of gathering developmental and family data is to ask the caregivers to describe a day in the life of their child. Provence outlines how this question can be the framework for learning about daily activities, how the infant and caregivers interact throughout the day, and about interactions around mealtime, bedtime, or times of distress. When all major caregivers are present for the interview, this question provides a time for each of them to present descriptions of his or her time with, and perceptions of, the child. Additionally, clinicians may use structured interviews, such as the *Vineland Adaptive Behavior Scales* (11) currently under revision, in order to collect both quantitative developmental data and provide an opportunity to open new areas of clinical discussion. Also, the *Infant-Toddler Developmental Assessment* (IDA) (12), appropriate for infants from birth to 36 months, is particularly useful in providing a schemata for organizing important information from caregiver interviews, medical/developmental records, and behavioral observations.

Implicit in this overview of interviewing is the assumption that such assessments require several sessions. Minimally, one meeting with caregivers, two or more with the child and caregivers together, and another to present the results to the caregivers are necessary. The sessions with the infant also provide an opportunity to gather more interview information, as other questions will occur in the context of the child's behavior and performance. For example, asking whether the child's response to a particular situation within the evaluation context is usual for him or her may open up another area of information from the caregivers. As is likely clear from these suggestions, infant assessment is a process of constantly gathering information, revising impressions, and testing hypotheses—and that requires time.

Observing

Observation is the fundamental skill needed for measuring infants' development. After all, most diagnostic evaluations are based on observation of physical signs and/or behavioral responses. However, what distinguishes the observational skill necessary for developmental assessment is that it occurs on many levels simultaneously and is perhaps the area in which the developmentalist's dual role as both generalist and specialist is most evident. Moreover, the observational skills inherent in assessments of infants require a blend of free-floating attention bounded by a structure. In other words, while the clinician must be comfortable enough in the setting to attend to whatever occurs, he or she must also have a mental framework by which to organize the observations collected during the session. Such a framework entails at least four broad areas: (a) predominant affective tone of the participants, (b) involvement in the situation (curiosity and interest), (c) use of others (child's use of the caregivers or examiner), and (d) reactions to transitions (initial meetings, end of sessions, and changes in amount of structure).

What to Observe

Clinical observation begins from the very first contact with the caregivers and infant, including the caregiver interview addressed above. Many important observations of the infant and infant–caregiver and familial interactions can be obtained during the course of formal developmental assessment. Benham (13) has provided an elaborated framework for structuring observations of infants and toddlers based on the familiar psychiatric mental status examination. In many cases, however, the formal developmental evaluation alone may not provide sufficient opportunity to observe all of the important behaviors of the infant and caregiver. Infants may behave differently with different caregivers and in varying contexts. For this reason, both naturalistic and structured analog procedures, where the examiner attempts to recreate specific "home-like" scenarios (e.g., a parent requesting the child to clean up the toys), can often be used to gather additional observational data that can be useful for both clinical and research purposes (14). Play-based assessment allows the clinician the opportunity to observe the infant and caregivers in a less structured format than provided by the formal developmental assessment. Also, play observations can be very useful in gaining additional information about the infant's cognitive, symbolic/linguistic, social, and motor development, as well as in assessing internal emotional states and conflicts and the infant's internal dynamic representations of the world (15).

Levels of Observing

Within the four broad areas of observation described earlier, the clinician makes observations continuously on at least three levels. Perhaps the most obvious level is the observations of how the child responds to the structured assessment items administered during formal testing. As already stated above, observations during formal testing should not be confined to whether or not the child passes or fails a given item, but to how the child approaches the task. The second level of observation during an infant assessment is how the child reacts to the situation apart from the formal testing structure. Does the child approach toys, initiate interactions, refer to the examiner or his caregivers? How does the child react in the beginning of the evaluation versus later, when the situation and the examiner are more familiar? The third observational level is a specific focus on the interactions between caregivers (and other adults) and infant.

The clinician makes these observations throughout the evaluation process and revises hypotheses as both caregivers and infant become familiar with the process. How to interpret the behaviors one observes between caregivers and child in terms of their ongoing relationship is learned partially by experience and requires time to gather many observational points. However, several general areas may provide important descriptive clues. Does the child refer to the caregivers for both help and reassurance? Similarly, does the child show his successes to the caregivers, and do the caregivers respond?

Another important observation for toddlers is whether or not the child leaves his caregivers' immediate company to work with items or explore. For infants, how caregivers hold, feed, and comfort their baby may be windows in the emerging dyadic and familial relationships. A caregiver participates with his or her child during such sessions in varying ways, and the clinician continuously will be assessing qualitative aspects of that participation—how intrusively involved, withdrawn, or comfortably facilitative the caregivers are.

One of the most important lessons when learning how to observe interactions between infants and caregivers is that clinical observations, even when based in a naturalistic setting, may or may not be an adequate reflection of what is typical for that particular family. Adults may appear very different as individuals in their own right, compared to when they are interacting with their children. Also, the assessment context where one's child (and by implication, one's self as a person and as a caregiver) is observed by another is anxiety provoking in varying degrees for all parents, and may profoundly alter their parenting style. Also, it is important that the assessor realize that he or she is also an integral component of the assessment. How does the infant respond to the evaluator? How does the infant use her familiar caregiver to navigate the introduction of the stranger (evaluator) and manage her stranger anxieties? How does the infant warm to the stranger over time? And, how does the evaluator observe her own internal feelings or countertransference regarding the infant, the caregiver, and their relationship?

For very young children, assessing development involves elaborating a more complex view of the child and his or her environment, and at this age, every developmental evaluation must include descriptions of behavior and the qualitative aspects of the child's behavior in the structured setting. For example, *when* the infant first turned to a voice or successfully retrieved a toy in a manner appropriate for age may be less important than *how* he or she responded to these tasks (with excitement, positive affect, and energy versus slowly, deliberately, and with little affective response). Such qualitative observations are often the best descriptors of those capacities for which we have few standardized assessment techniques but that are absolutely fundamental to fueling the development of motor, language, and problem-solving skills. Through observing how infants do what they do, the clinician gains information about how infants cope with frustration and how they engage the adult world, as well as about their emotional expressiveness, their capacity for persistence and sustained attention, and the level of investment and psychological energy given to their activities.

Synthesizing

Synthesizing the large amount of data obtained from a comprehensive clinical infant assessment can be quite daunting. The clinician must draw upon and synthesize knowledge from child psychiatry, pediatrics, neurology, developmental psychology, speech/language therapy, physical and occupational therapy, and often genetics and endocrinology (16). Increasingly, clinicians evaluating young children need also know about early childhood education programs and early intervention, as well as laws regarding child abuse, neglect, and domestic violence. Knowledge from these diverse fields allows a clinician to place the results of a developmental assessment in a meaningful context for the individual child and leads to a better conceptualization of treatment options. For example, understanding the physiologic effects of prolonged malnutrition and episodic starvation in infancy (17,18) helps the clinician evaluate the relatively greater gross motor delays of a child with failure to thrive who has no other neurologic signs. Similarly, understanding the effects of a parent's affective disorder on a child's responsiveness to the external world (19) adds another dimension to understanding the infant's muted or absent social interactiveness, babbling, and smiling.

Finally, it is often during the synthesis process that the therapeutic effect for caregivers participating in the assessment is most evident. At the very least, caregivers often change their perceptions of their infant's capacities. They may see strengths in their infant they had not previously recognized or become deeply and painfully aware of weaknesses and vulnerabilities that they may or may not have feared before the assessment. Any of these changes in perceptions may affect the caregivers' view of themselves and of their role as caregivers. Also, infants often change during the assessment process, as their caregivers become more involved in the alliance with the clinician, and they experience, at least temporarily, another adult's concern and interest in their family. Emphasizing the potentially therapeutic value of an assessment underscores that the synthesis process is not simply wrapping up the assessment and conveying information, but is also a time to explore with the caregivers the meaning of the process for them and their infant.

SELECTING AN INFANT ASSESSMENT TOOL

Below are some basic guidelines for choosing an infant developmental test that best meets the clinician's specific needs. These guidelines also help provide a framework for evaluating the usefulness of some of the various tests currently in use. Four areas of consideration are presented: purpose, sources of data, standardization, and psychometric properties.

Purpose

A developmental test may be useful for one or more of several different purposes: diagnosis, screening, and early intervention planning. Tests designed for these three purposes are quite different, and selecting the correct tests to match the stated purpose is essential. First, *diagnostic tests* are used to provide information necessary for either clinically or eligibility-oriented diagnoses. Second, *screening tests* are used when it is desirable to use a relatively brief instrument to identify infants who may be "at risk" for delayed development and would benefit from further diagnostic testing. Third, *intervention-planning tests* are used to plan an individualized early intervention program once children have been diagnosed and are used almost exclusively in early intervention and educational settings.

Sources of Data

Developmental tests for infants use one or more of at least three different types of data: direct assessment, incidental observation, and caregiver report. Direct assessment has the strength of potentially being standard in its presentation, so that an infant's performance may be directly compared to other infants with the assumption that the material was presented in a similar standard method. The limitation of direct assessment, however, is that it represents only a small sample of the infant's developmental repertoire and is influenced greatly by current issues regarding the infant's motivation, mood, comfort, and responsiveness to the examiner and the evaluative process. Caregiver report surveys are a useful addition to formal assessment, in particular to document behaviors that occur too infrequently to be observed in a clinical evaluation or to assess the caregivers' individual perspectives of their infant. However, caregiver reports should not be the sole measure of the infant's development, since they are highly subject to rater bias (20). Given the strengths and limitations of each of these sources of data, a comprehensive assessment should utilize multiple sources of data across multiple contexts.

Standardization

Test standardization involves the process of developing a consistent method of administration and collecting normative data regarding children's typical performance on the test. It is by this normative data that evaluators determine a specific infant's standing relative to the normative group. It is the responsibility of the test user, however, to decide whether a given test's standardization and normative samples are representative of the type of infants the test user plans to assess. Some tests are normed on very specific populations of children, such as children from a specific city or state or a particular economic status. The use of standard scores derived from these tests with infants from other localities or economic backgrounds, without specific empirical evidence to justify their generalization, is generally not recommended. Furthermore, in order to yield reliable results, tests (and their normative data) should be no more than about a decade old in order to keep pace with intergenerational escalation in test performance (21). Grossly outdated norms often yield inflated scores that may lead to erroneously disqualifying infants for needed services.

Psychometric Properties

The soundness of a psychometric test is judged based on its reliability (the ability to produce similar results under differing conditions) and validity (the collection of evidence that suggests that the test measures what it is supposed to measure). Several forms of reliability exist, such as test–retest (reliability over time), interrater (reliability between assessors), and internal consistency (reliability between items on the test). As a guideline, reliability coefficients of at least 0.90 for diagnostic tests and 0.80 for screening tests are recommended in each of these three areas of reliability (22). *Validity* is even more multifaceted. There is no single or preferred way to establish a test's validity. Rather, validity represents an accumulation of evidence that together builds a case that the test measures what it is supposed to measure. Specifically, infant developmental tests are expected to correlate significantly with other similar tests, to reflect developmental changes that result from expected maturation, and to be sensitive to the presence of diagnosable disorders with clear developmental manifestations.

REVIEW OF SELECTED DEVELOPMENTAL TESTS

A few of the more widely used developmental tests are presented in Table 4.2.2, and some of the most common examples are further described below, organized under three basic headings: neonatal, infant/toddler development, and screening.

Neonatal Assessment Tests

Brazelton Neonatal Behavioral Assessment Scale, Fourth Edition (NBAS-4)

The NBAS-4 (24) dominates the field of neonatal assessment and is intended to assess the neonate's current level of neurobehavioral organization, capacity to respond to the stress of labor and delivery, and adjustment to the ex utero environment. It is designed for use with neonates of 37 to 44 weeks' gestational age who do not currently need mechanical supports or supplemental oxygen. Though it is recommended that neonates be at least 3 days old before testing, it has been used on neonates during the first day of life. It takes about 20 to 30 minutes to administer, followed by about 15 minutes to record and score the neonate's performance. Although the NBAS was originally designed for use with full-term healthy newborns, it has been used extensively with premature and otherwise medically fragile newborns.

The NBAS is used to describe the range of behavioral responses to social and nonsocial stimuli, as the neonate moves from sleeping to alert states. Items assess the neonate's neurologic intactness, behavioral organization (state regulation and autonomic reactivity), and interactiveness and responsiveness with both animate and inanimate stimuli on the basis of 28 behavioral items and 18 reflexes. Lester et al. (40) have summarized the behavioral items as six factors (habituation, orientation, motor, range of states of alertness, regulation of state, and autonomic regulation) and use neurologic reflex behaviors to define a seventh factor. Each of the seven factors can be used to yield a numerical score describing the infant's performance in that area.

With training, interrater reliability for the behavioral items has been shown to be adequate, although a considerable degree of judgment is required of the examiner for assigning a rating to the neonate's responses, and temporal stability is poor for most items (41,42). The NBAS has been shown to be an effective intervention tool for increasing the maternal involvement and responsiveness of low-income and adolescent mothers (43) and has been shown to predict infant–parent attachment and subsequent infant development. Unfortunately, research

TABLE 4.2.2

SELECTED FORMAL TESTS OF INFANT/TODDLER DEVELOPMENT

	Age	Domains[a]	Norm Sample	Reliability/Validity	Comments
Neonatal Assessment Tests					
Graham/Rosenblith Behavioral Test for Neonates (23)		M, TA, V, A, MT	Not applicable	Encouraging early findings	Seldom used
Brazelton Neonatal Behavioral Assessment Scale-4 (24)	37–44 weeks GA	NI, B, PS	Not applicable	High interrater reliability, weak test–retest, poor predictor beyond first year	Most widely used neonatal test
Infant/Toddler Development Tests					
Bayley Scales of Infant Development-III (25)	1–42 mo	Ad, Cg, EC, RC, FM, GM, PS	Large, representative	Excellent for cognitive and language, adequate for adaptive behavior and socioemotional	Most widely used and validated infant test, used as gold standard
Mullen Scales of Early Learning (26)	0–68 mo	GM, FM, VR, RC, EC	Large, representative	Adequate to exceptional	Mostly useful for toddlers and preschoolers
Battelle Developmental Inventory-2 (27)	0–95 mo	PS, Ad; GM; FM; EC; RC; Cg (and subdomains)	Large, representative	Excellent reliability, adequate validity	Used considerably
Griffiths Mental Development Scales—Revised: Birth to 2 years (7)	0–24 mo	Lm, PS, RC, EC, EH, P	Medium, all from UK	Mixed results	Mostly used in Europe
Uzgiris–Hunt Infant Psychological Development Scales (28)	NA	See text	Not applicable	Adequate to exceptional reliability	Most popular Piagetian infant test
Screening Tests					
Battelle Developmental Inventory Screening Test (27)	6–95 mo	PS, Ad; GM; FM; EC; RC; Cg	Large, representative	Strong correlation with full BDI	
Bayley Infant Neurodevelopmental Screen (29)	3–24 mo	N; RC; EC/M; Cg	Large; representative	Excellent reliability; promising validity	
Birth to Three Developmental Scale (30)	0–36 mo	EC/RC; Cg; PS; M	Small; questionable representation	Strong interrater reliability, but little evidence of validity	
Child Development Inventory (31)	15–72 mo	GM; FM; EC; RC; Ad; PS; L; N	Small; from St. Paul, MN	Little evidence of reliability and validity	300 parent report items
Denver Developmental Screening Test-II (32)	0–72 mo	GM; FM/Cg; PS; EC/RC	Large, all from Denver area	See text	See text
Developmental Activities Screening Inventory-II (33)	0–60 mo	15 sensory and problem-solving	>200 disabled children	Little evidence of reliability; valid for severely delayed	Can be used with linguistically and visually impaired children
Developmental Indicators for the Assessment of Learning-4 (34)	30–71 mo	M; EC/RC; B; PS; AS	Large; representative	Acceptable reliability and validity	One of better screeners for age level
Diagnostic Inventory for Screening Children—fifth edition (35)	0–60 mo	FM; GM; RC; EC; AM; VM; Ad; PS	Small; all from southwest Ontario	Excellent reliability; limited validity	
Developmental Observation Checklist System (36)	0–72 mo	Cg; EC/RC; PS; FM/GM; Adj; PS&S	Adequate; representative	Sound reliability and concurrent validity	Parent report only
Developmental Profile-III (37)	0–155 mo	M; Ad; PS; AS; EC/RC	Large	Adequate reliability and validity	Parent report only

TABLE 4.2.2

(CONTINUED)

	Age	Domains[a]	Norm Sample	Reliability/Validity	Comments
Early Screening Profile (38)	24–72 mo	Cg; EC/RC; M; Ad/PS; Ar	Adequate; representative	Good reliability; exceptional validity	One of better screeners for age level
Kent Infant Development Scales (39)	0–12 mo	Cg; M; EC/RC; Ad; PS	All from Northeast Ohio	Adequate reliability and validity	Primarily parent report

[a]A, auditory responsiveness; Adj, adjustment; Ad, adaptive, self-help or daily living; AM, auditory attention and memory; Ar, articulation; AS, academic or preacademic skills; B, behavior; Cg, cognitive or problem-solving; EC, expressive communication/language; EH, eye–hand coordination; FM, fine motor; GM, gross motor; L, letters; Lm, locomotor; M, motor or physical; MT, muscle tone; N, numbers; NI, neurologic intactness; P, performance; PS, personal–social; PS&S, parental stress and support; RC, receptive communication/language; TA, tactile adaptive; V, visual responsiveness; VM, visual attention and memory; VR, visual reception. A slash mark (/) indicates that multiple domains are assessed in the same scale or subtest.

not consistently shown the NBAS to be a good predictor of infant development much beyond the first year of life (44,45).

Infant/Toddler Development Tests

Bayley Scales of Infant and Toddler Development-III (BSID-3)

The BSID-3 (25) is the most widely used measure of the development of infants and toddlers in both clinical and research settings. The BSID's extensive history of test development and validation makes it the most psychometrically sophisticated infant test on the market. The BSID is applicable to children from 1 to 42 months of age. Administration time is about 25 to 35 minutes for infants under 15 months and up to 60 to 90 minutes for children over 15 months.

The BSID is subdivided into five components following the five domains covered by federal early intervention law: Cognition, Language, Motor, Social-Emotional, and Adaptive Behaviors. The Cognition portion provides information on the child's problem-solving and cognitive abilities, the Language portion assesses the child's expressive and receptive communication, while the Motor component assesses the child's fine and gross motor skills. The new Social-Emotional scale (self-regulation and relationship formation) and Adaptive Behavior scales (adaptive and coping skills) are mainly based on parental report.

Normative samples are large and nationally representative, reliability is acceptable to high. It is important to note that Bayley did not intend BSID scores to be interpreted as intelligence quotients. For the most part, performance on the BSID does not consistently predict later cognitive measures, particularly when socioeconomic status and level of functioning are controlled (46).

Mullen Scales of Early Learning

A relatively recent addition is the Mullen Scales of Early Learning (MSEL) (26). This revision of the original Mullen scales combined earlier versions of the test designed for infants and preschoolers into one test with continuous norms from birth to 68 months. The MSEL takes about 15 to 60 minutes to administer, depending on the age of the child (15 minutes at 1 year old, 30 minutes at 3 years, and 60 minutes at 5 years). The MSEL assesses child development in five separate domains: gross motor, visual reception (primarily visual discrimination and memory), fine motor, receptive language, and expressive language. The gross motor scale is only applicable to children birth through 33 months old and does not contribute to the overall early learning composite score. The normative sample is large, but somewhat overrepresentative of children from the Northeast. Reliability is acceptable to high. However, with normative data over two decades old, the MSEL is in dire need of renorming and may therefore overestimate scores.

Griffiths Mental Development Scales

Although the Griffiths Mental Development Scales (GMDS) is seldom used in America, it warrants a brief description due to its continued use in Europe and early influence on extending infant developmental testing internationally. The GMDS consists of two tests: *Griffiths Mental Development Scales—Revised: Birth to 2 years (GMDS 0-2)* (7), designed for infants birth to 24 months, and *Griffiths Mental Development Scales—Extended Revised: 2 to 8 years (GMDS-ER 2-8)* (47), for children 24 months to 8 years. The GMDS 0-2 scale consists of five domains: locomotor, personal and social, language, eye and hand coordination, and performance. The GMDS-ER 2-8 has the same five subdomains but also incorporates a practical reason subscale. The test is administered in about 1 hour, however, extensive training is required, and scales are only supplied to pediatricians or health care professionals. The GMDS 0-2 is normed on 665 UK children ages 0 to 2 from 1996. The GMDS-ER 2-8 is normed on 1,026 UK children ages 2 through 8 and is stratified according to 1997 UK Office of National Statistics data. The GMDS remains rather popular in Europe, Quebec, and South Africa, with some evidence of cross-cultural validity (48). However, the normative data are quite old and in need of updating.

Infant/Toddler Screening Tests

Denver Developmental Screening Test-II

The Denver Developmental Screening Test-II (DDST-2) (32) is one of the most popular developmental screening tests, especially in medical settings. This may be due at least in part to its brevity, as it can be administered in as little as 15 to 20 minutes. It is applicable for children from birth to 6 years. Items are scored based on a combination of caregiver report, direct assessment of the child, and observation. The DDST-2 produces one overall score, placing children in one of four descriptive categories: pass, questionable, abnormal, or untestable. Since the Denver-II was normed exclusively on children living in Colorado, caution should be used when employing this screener in other localities. The original edition of the DDST (49) had been criticized for not being sensitive enough, missing as many as 80% of children with delays or disabilities (50). Although the

DDST-2 is a clear improvement over the original DDST, there is evidence that it now significantly over-identifies as many as 72% of children (51).

Early Screening Profiles

The Early Screening Profiles (ESP) (38) is applicable for children 2 through 6 years. It screens for cognitive, language, speech, physical, and social disabilities or delays that may interfere with a child's learning and warrant further diagnostic assessment. Children complete three different subtests: cognitive/language (assessing children's visual discrimination, logical reasoning, verbal concepts, basic school readiness skills), motor (assessing both fine and gross motor skills), and speech articulation. Total testing time per child is only 15 to 30 minutes, depending on the child's age. Additionally, the person who administers the test completes a 2- to 3-minute Behavior Survey documenting the child's behaviors during the assessment (e.g., activity level, attention span, cooperativeness, independence). Caregivers, or sometimes teachers, complete three different rating forms: the self-help/social profile (which provides a rating of the child's adaptive behaviors), the home survey (regarding the caregiver's perception of the child's home environment and caregiver–child interaction), and the health history survey (which provides information regarding immunizations, health problems, and prenatal health and delivery). Each of these rating forms can be completed in about 5 minutes. The ESP provides a wide variety of scores for all domains and subdomains, including age equivalents, standard scores, percentile ranks, and easy-to-use six-point screening categories. Screener cut-points can be set at several different levels in order to manipulate the false-positive to false-negative ratio. The primary drawback of the ESP is that it has no Spanish version. Psychometrically, the ESP is quite sound and represents one of the very best screening tests on the market.

CONCLUSIONS

Infant assessments are clinical explorations involving a fair amount of uncertainty and inference. While the medical diagnostic process always involves some element of uncertainty, the assessments made in infancy require of the clinician a particular comfort with uncertainty and the unknown. Though the latter half of the last century brought a veritable explosion of knowledge about infancy and the neonatal period, the more we learn, the greater we understand how inexplicably woven are the forces of development. As emphasized throughout this chapter, infant assessment involves far more than the infant and is as much a measure of the infant's environment as it is of his or her functional status. Thus, clinicians assessing infants are always dealing more with what they cannot know than with what they can, ever exploring the limits of predictive capabilities and constantly mindful of those limitations.

References

1. Bagnato SJ, Neisworth JT: Collaboration and teamwork in assessment for early intervention. *Child Adolesc Psychiatr Clin N Am* 8:347–363, 1999.
2. Brooks J, Weinraub J: A history of infant intelligence testing. In: Lewis M (ed): *Origins of Intelligence: Infancy and Early Childhood.* New York, Plenum, 19–58, 1976.
3. Wyly MV: *Infant Assessment.* Boulder, CO, Westview Press, 1997.
4. Esquirol JD: *Des Maladies Mentales Considerees Sous Les Rapports Medical, Hygienique, and Medicolegal.* Paris, Bailliere, 1938.
5. Terman LM: *The Measurement of Intelligence.* Boston, MA, Houghton-Mifflin, 1916.
6. Gesell A: *The First Five Years of Life: A Guide to the Study of the Preschool Child.* New York, Harper, 1940.
7. Griffiths R: *Griffiths Mental Development Scales—Revised: Birth to 2 years (GMDS 0-2).* Oxford, Hogrefe, 1996.
8. Bayley N: *Bayley Scales of Infant Development.* New York, Psychological Corporation, 1969.
9. Cox CE: Obtaining and formulating a developmental history. *Child Adolesc Psychiatr Clin N Am* 8:271–279, 1999.
10. Provence S: Developmental assessment. In: Green M, Haggarty R (eds): *Ambulatory Pediatrics.* Philadelphia, PA, Saunders, 374–383, 1977.
11. Sparrow SS, Balla DA, Chicchetti DV: *Vineland Adaptive Behavior Scales.* Circle Pines, American Guidance Service, 1984.
12. Provence S, Erikson J, Vater S, Palmeri S: *Infant-Toddler Developmental Assessment.* Chicago, Riverside Publishing, 1995.
13. Benham AL: The observation and assessment of young children including use of the Infant-Toddler Mental Status Exam. In: Zeanah CH (ed): *Handbook of Infant Mental Health.* New York, Guilford Press, 249–265, 2000.
14. Zeanah CH, Boris NW, Heller SS, et al.: Relationship assessment in infant mental health. *Infant Ment Health J* 18:182–197, 1997.
15. Close N: Diagnostic play interview: its role in comprehensive psychiatric evaluation. *Child Adolesc Psychiatr Clin N Am* 8:239–255, 1999.
16. Mayes LC, Gilliam WS (eds): *Comprehensive Psychiatric Assessment of Young Children. Child and Adolescent Psychiatric Clinics of North America.* Philadelphia, PA, Saunders, 1999.
17. Dickerson JWT: Nutrition, brain growth and development. In: Connolly KJ, Prechtl HR (eds): *Maturation and Development: Biological and Psychological Perspectives.* Philadelphia, PA, JB Lippincott, 110–130, 1981.
18. Shonkoff JP, Marshall PC: Biological bases of developmental dysfunction. In: Meisels SJ, Shonkoff JP (eds): *Handbook of Early Childhood Intervention.* New York, Cambridge University Press, 35–52, 1990.
19. Seifer R, Dickstein S: Parental mental illness and infant development. In: Zeanah CH (ed): *Handbook of Infant Mental Health.* New York, Guilford Press, 145–160, 2000.
20. Meisels SJ Waskik BA: Who should be served? identifying children in need of early intervention. In: Meisels SJ, Shonkoff JP (eds): *Handbook of Early Childhood Intervention.* New York, Cambridge University Press, 605–632, 1990.
21. Flynn JR: The mean IQ of Americans: massive gains 1932 to 1978. *Psychol Bull* 95:29–51, 1984.
22. Salvia J, Ysseldyke JE: *Assessment.* 5th ed. Boston, MA, Houghton Mifflin, 1991.
23. Rosenblith JF: The Graham/Rosenblith behavioral examination for newborns: Prognostic value and procedural issues. In: Osofsky J (ed): *Handbook of Infant Development.* New York, Wiley, 1979.
24. Brazelton TB, Nugent JK: *Neonatal Behavioral Assessment Scale.* 4th ed. London, Mac Keith Press, 2011.
25. Bayley N: *Bayley Scales of Infant and Toddler Development.* 3rd ed. San Antonio, TX, Harcourt, 2006.
26. Mullen EM: *Mullen Scales of Early Learning: AGS Edition.* Circle Pines, American Guidance Service, 1995.
27. Newborg J: *Battelle Developmental Inventory.* 2nd ed. Itasca, IL, Riverside Publishing, 2005.
28. Uzgiris I, Hunt JM: *Assessment in Infancy: Toward Ordinal Scales of Psychological Development in Infancy.* Champaign-Urbana, University of Illinois Press, 1975.
29. Aylward GP: *Bayley Infant Neurodevelopmental Screener.* San Antonio, TX, Psychological Corporation, 1995.
30. Bangs TE, Dodson S: *Birth to Three Developmental Scale.* Allen, TX, DLM Teaching Resources, 1979.
31. Ireton H: *Child Development Inventory.* Minneapolis, Behavior Science Systems, 1992.
32. Frankenburg WK, Dodds J, Archer P, et al.: *Denver II: Technical Manual.* Denver, Denver Developmental Materials, 1990.
33. Fewell RR, Langley MB: *Developmental Activities Screening Inventory-II.* Austin, Pro-Ed, 1984.
34. Mardell-Czudnowski CD, Goldenberg D: *DIAL-4 (Developmental Indicators for the Assessment of Learning-Fourth Edition).* San Antonio, TX, Pearson Clinical Assessment, 2011.
35. Amdur JR, Mainland JK, Parker KCH: *Diagnostic Inventory for Screening Children (DISC) Manual.* 5th ed. Kitchner, ON, Kitchner-Waterloo Hospital, 1999.
36. Hrescko WP, Miguel SA, Sherbenou RJ, et al.: *Developmental Observation Checklist System.* Austin, TX, Pro-Ed, 1994.
37. Alpern GD: *Developmental Profile-III.* San Antonio, TX, Western Psychological Services, 2007.
38. Harrison PL: *Early Screening Profiles (ESP): Manual.* Circle Pines, American Guidance Service, 1990.
39. Reuter J, Bickett L: *Kent Infant Development Scale (KIDS).* Kent, Developmental Metrics, 1985.
40. Lester B, Als H, Brazelton TB: Regional obstetric anesthesia and newborn behavior: a reanalysis toward synergistic effects. *Child Dev* 53:687–692, 1982.
41. Lancione E, Horowitz FD, Sullivan JW: The NBAS-K 1: a study of its stability and structure over the first month of life. *Infant Behav Dev* 3:341–359, 1980.
42. Sameroff AJ: Organization and stability of newborn behavior: a commentary on the Brazelton Neonatal Behavioral Assessment Scale. *Monogr Soc Res Child Dev* 43:76, 1978.
43. Worobey J, Brazelton TB: Newborn assessment and support for parenting. In: Gibbs ED, Teti DM (eds): *Interdisciplinary Assessment of Infants:*

A Guide for Early Intervention Professionals. Baltimore, MD, Brookes, 1990.
44. Horowitz FD, Linn LP: The Neonatal Behavioral Assessment Scale. In: Wolraich M, Routh DK (eds): *Advances in Developmental Pediatrics, 3*. Greenwich, CT, JAI, 223–256, 1982.
45. Vaughn BE, Taraldson B, Crichton L, Egeland B: Relationships between neonatal behavioral organization and infant behavior during the first year of life. *Infant Behav Dev* 3:47–66, 1980.
46. Rubin RA, Balow B: Measures of infant development and socio-economic status as predictors of later intelligence and school achievement. *Dev Psychol* 15:225–227, 1979.
47. Luiz D, Barnard A, Knoesen N, et al.: *Griffiths Mental Development Scales, Extended Revised: GMDS-ER; 2 to 8 years*. Oxford, Hogrefe, 2006.
48. Luiz DM, Foxcroft CD, Stewart R: The construct validity of the Griffiths Scales of Mental Development. *Child Care Health Dev* 27:73–83, 2001.
49. Frankenburg WK, Dodds J, Fandal A: *Denver Developmental Screening Test*. Denver, LADOCA, 1975.
50. Greer S, Bauchner H, Zuckerman B: The Denver Developmental Screening Test: how good is its predictive validity? *Dev Med Child Neurol* 31:774–781, 1989.
51. Glascoe FP, Byrne KE: The accuracy of three developmental screening tests. *J Early Interv* 17:368–379, 1993.

CHAPTER 4.3 ■ CLINICAL ASSESSMENT OF CHILDREN AND ADOLESCENTS: CONTENT AND STRUCTURE

JEFF Q. BOSTIC, MONA P. POTTER, AND ROBERT A. KING

The most common purposes of psychiatric assessment are (a) to determine if psychopathology is present, and if so, to establish target symptom priorities; (b) to determine what treatments/interventions might address the target symptoms and evaluate with the family and patient the relative benefits and risks of any proposed treatments; and (c) to gain understanding and build rapport that encourages patient and family engagement (1). The child (except as noted in identified sections, "child" will refer to "child and adolescent") is evaluated in the context of his or her functioning in the family, the school, extracurricular activities, and with peers, with sensitivity to cultural and community influences. The clinical assessment seeks to detect any developmental aberrations and maladaptive patterns, while casting a wide net to identify the patient's symptoms, as well as protective/resilience factors and relevant environmental variables and resources that may affect treatment outcomes. Many symptom constellations will respond to established treatments, so the clinician must prioritize intervention targets to devise a treatment plan that will address multiple problems, including comorbid disorders (2).

DISTINCTIVE ASPECTS OF THE PSYCHIATRIC ASSESSMENT OF CHILDREN

The psychiatric assessment of the child differs from the assessment of adults in several respects.

First, children rarely initiate psychiatric assessment or treatments themselves; rather, in most cases their parents or other adults provide the impetus for seeking treatment for the child. The child's behavior may cause greater distress to these adults than it does to the child. In some situations, the adult's expectations for the child may exceed the child's abilities, or the adult's own parenting or teaching style may be a poor fit with this child, yet these adults may seek means to alter the child to remedy this poor fit. On the other hand, children may not recognize their behaviors as problematic for others, or may not be receptive to changing these behaviors. Often these misbehaviors have "worked" by getting parents or teachers to avoid requesting the child to complete chores or tasks, or have culminated in others giving in to the child's requests. Children also may attribute problems to others and be unable or unwilling to accept their personal contribution to an identified problem. The psychiatric assessment of children thus requires consideration of both adult and child contributions to the distressing behaviors for which evaluation is being sought. In addition, the assessment requires explicit attention to the child's perceptions of the problems and what the child desires to change (e.g., a child with severe anxiety might feel complacent with limiting activities and remaining in the comfort and safety of home versus pushing to tackle anxiety by engaging in anxiety-provoking situations).

Second, the child and the clinician are at different developmental levels, such that they may essentially speak different languages. The school-age child may lack the maturity to abstract "patterns" from isolated events, while the adolescent may perceive the clinician's questions as another inquisition resembling that of parents or school staff. Moreover, phase-specific developmental features may further impede communication. For example, young children may not trust unfamiliar adults, while adolescents may feel reluctant to express vulnerabilities they are experiencing (3).

Third, the child may function differently in different settings. The child may function relatively well in multiple domains (with family, at school or work, with peers), function poorly in only one domain, or may function poorly across multiple domains. This underlines the necessity of multiple informants (4), not only to discern accurately the child's overall functioning, but also to identify the child's areas of strength on which the clinician can build and to identify others (peers or adults) effective with the child and potentially able to introduce or reinforce more adaptive skills or behaviors.

Fourth, the child's presenting problems must be examined in a developmental context. The child may have a delay in skill development, such as delay in speaking or in areas of self-care, such as toileting. The child may not yet possess the social skills necessary to interact appropriately with age-similar peers, and thus will require interventions to introduce skills not yet present. The child's problems may also emanate from an inability to select appropriate coping/emotion regulation skills from an existing repertoire. For example, an anxious child may overgeneralize that "everyone" is negatively judging him and therefore feel unable to go to school and challenge those faulty cognitions, or an adolescent may understand that isolating worsens her depression, but still feel unable to get out of bed and reach out to friends. Finally, the child's problems may follow the loss of previously attained skills, often consequent to serious medical and psychiatric disorders, loss, or trauma. For example, a medically hospitalized school-age child may transiently regress with immature behaviors or loss of bowel or bladder control; adolescents developing schizophrenia may lose previously effective interaction and cognitive skills.

Further complicating this developmental context is developmental differences in presentation of mental illnesses. Many DSM diagnoses were primarily defined among adult samples. Although some disorders, such as obsessive–compulsive disorder, look quite similar in children and adults, other disorders, such as major depression or PTSD, can present notably differently in younger patients as compared to adults (Chapter 5.4.2). For example, in major depression, some school-age children may be less likely than adults to manifest dysthymic, self-accusatory feelings and more likely to manifest irritability or somatic symptoms (e.g., headaches, stomachaches, body pain). Discerning "categories" of mental disorders in children can be difficult, since symptoms overlap across diagnostic categories; more importantly, numbers of symptoms in children predict psychosocial function more so than the diagnostic category where a child appears to best fit (5). A dimensional approach can, therefore, provide additional formulation insights; efforts to consider common underlying tendencies (e.g., difficulty tolerating emotions) and determining where a particular child fits on the depressed mood axis, the inattention spectrum, and the impulsive axis, for example, may ultimately prove fruitful for prioritizing intervention targets.

Finally, an underestimated but critical facet of the psychiatric assessment of children is the necessity for forming alliances with the multiple parties, including among the clinician and the child, the parent, the school, and any additional outside agencies. A breach or rupture in any of these relationships can markedly impair treatment efforts. It is during the assessment phase that efforts must begin to identify and align the agendas of these various treatment "partners" to enhance any intervention efforts. Parental permission should be obtained to contact and elicit information and collaboration from the various relevant parties who may have important information or who play an important role in the child's progress; such contacts include step- and noncustodial parents, teachers (by phone, via school records, and/or requested rating scales), and primary medical care providers. Following the initial evaluation, follow-up contacts with parents living apart from the child, school staff, and other health providers can often help clarify obstacles to treatment and can help invest others in the child's improvement.

CONTENT OF THE CLINICAL INTERVIEW

Core contents of the clinical assessment of children and adolescents are common across purposes; these components are summarized in Table 4.3.1. The core components are similar to the adult psychiatric assessment, though with added emphasis on developmental and environmental (e.g., family, school, peer, media) factors and contributions. They illuminate the need for a consistent, thorough assessment of the multiple variables that may contribute to the child's presentation, and the importance of synthesizing the input from multiple informants to derive an accurate picture of each child's unique predicament.

Depending on the complexity of the problem(s), the initial assessment might need to be completed over more than one session; priorities of the initial evaluation include safety assessment, rapport and empathy building (so that they are willing to come back), clear understanding of what the acute problem is and how it is affecting the child and system (family, school, peers), barriers to seeking/engaging in treatment as well as strengths and motivating factors, and list of invested others with whom to collaborate and seek additional information.

TABLE 4.3.1

CONTENT COMPONENTS OF THE PSYCHIATRIC ASSESSMENT OF CHILDREN AND ADOLESCENTS

Content Component	Primary Informant	Additional Resources
Reason for referral	Usually parents/guardian, sometimes school or legal agency	Letter from school or other agency seeking evaluation
History of present illness/problems(s)	Child and parents	Referral source, pediatrician/primary care provider
Past problems	Child and parents	Structured interviews, rating scales
Safety assessment	Child and parents	School
Comorbid symptoms	Child and parents	Structured interviews, rating scales
Substance use	Child and parents	Toxicology screening (as relevant)
Previous assessment/treatment(s)	Child, parents, clinicians	Mental health records
Developmental history (motor, cognitive, interpersonal, emotional, moral), trauma	Parents, school staff	School records, including Special Education Evaluations, home videos (as relevant)
Family history	Parents	Genogram
Medical history	Parents, health care provider(s)	Review of symptoms checklist, laboratory tests (as relevant)
Child's strengths	Parents, child, teachers, coaches, peers	Activity video (sports, music); cognitive, school, neuropsychological testing
Environmental supports	Parents, child, adults familiar to child	Activity schedules (scouting, teams), afterschool/summer programs, mentorships/Big Brother or Sister relationships
Child's media diet	Parents, child, caregivers, siblings	Media diary, Apps on phone
Mental status examination	Child, Clinician (observations during interview)	

Reason for Referral (Chief Complaint)

Clarity about who actually initiated the referral, their motivations, and what changes they seek is essential to the success of any evaluation. While parents may schedule an evaluation, opening questions about who suggested it, who recognized a need for an evaluation, or who is most uncomfortable with the child's behavior may all help clarify the impetus for the evaluation. More importantly, clarifying the circumstances and concerned individuals driving the evaluation request may reveal the expectations of relevant parties and their willingness to implement treatment recommendations. For example, a parent may indicate the school or a grandparent identified distressing behaviors in the child. The parent may be required to obtain an evaluation for the child to return to school. The expectations of these various parties may in fact be in conflict and must be reconciled if effective treatments are to be implemented and for adherence to occur. For example, the school may seek to have parents manage the child differently or consider medication treatments, while the parents may wish for the evaluation to validate their current parenting efforts or provide diagnoses and recommendations that would yield additional school services. Similarly, grandparents may wish for different parenting approaches, while the parents may seek confirmation that their current approach is appropriate.

History of Present Illness

Current Problem(s)

Narrative. The evolution of the child's problem should be elicited by the clinician mindful of the pain most parents encounter while recounting the deterioration or anguish of their child. To minimize this distress, and to obtain a full description, clinicians should provide parents some opportunity to chronicle this history in their own words. Parents diverge widely in terms of their own experience with and views of psychiatry, how they understand people's behaviors, and in their acceptance of alternatives to their current responses. Attention throughout the interview to these parent variables allows the clinician to explain behaviors and select interventions in terms acceptable to these particular parents. The more treatment recommendations can be framed within the parents' own description and understanding, by using the parents' words or concepts, the greater the probability parents will feel heard and collaborate in treatment.

As the parents describe the history of the problem, the clinician attends to the context in which the behavior emerged and occurs, changes in frequency and intensity of the behaviors, and the current progression of the problem. The clinician ultimately needs also to inquire directly about specific instances of the child's problematic behaviors, parental responses to these behaviors, and the child's response to current parental interventions.

Functional Assessment of Problem Behaviors. Since any given symptom or behavior (anxiety, inattention, arguing, theft, hallucinations) may have quite different meanings, functions, and clinical implications in different children, it is important not to jump immediately from symptom to diagnosis. The clinician may need to inquire directly about the *functions* of the problem behavior, including any secondary gains for the behavior (tantrums diminish parental expectations of chore completion, complaining of headaches every morning decreases time spent in a painful school class, running away causes parents to unite in efforts to find the child). Identifying specific antecedents and precipitants of the problem behavior and its consequences, both for the child and for others (including the family or classroom), may provide valuable insights into the functions of the problem behavior. In addition, the clinician should clarify the impact of the problem on the patient's quality of life, with particular attention as to whether the problem is specific to one functional domain or whether the behavior pervades multiple or all areas of the child's functioning, such as home, school, extracurricular activities, and with peers.

Problem behaviors may reflect an underlying disorder within the child, but may also reveal a problem within the child's environment (6). For example, a particular teacher, peer, or adult may contribute to the child's distress, although it is the child's symptom that is being labeled as the problem behavior. The *fit* between the child and a particular teacher, peer, or adult may culminate in expression or exacerbation of the child's symptoms. Accordingly, even when the child's symptoms occur pervasively across multiple domains of life (home, school/work, peers), attention to changes in school circumstances and peer and adult/parent networks may clarify forces fueling the symptoms.

Daily Routine. Given the impact a breech in basic functioning can have on exacerbating and perpetuating symptoms, it is helpful to inquire about a child's current functioning in everyday essentials such as sleeping, eating, physical activity, and self-care (developmentally appropriate tasks, e.g., brushing teeth, showering). Asking parents and child to map out a typical weekday and weekend day (morning to next morning) for the child can paint a picture and provide insight into how much time is being spent on various activities and with what level of ease/distress (e.g., getting ready for school, doing homework, extracurricular activities, social media/video games, sleep), as well as offer opportunities for interventions (e.g., sleep hygiene/bedtime routine for a child with poor sleep, behavioral activation for a sedentary and isolated child).

Past Problems

Significant past problems that have impaired the child should be identified, as this provides a historical context for understanding the current problem. It is especially important to understand whether a problem has been persistent since early childhood, is intermittent, or represents a deterioration from a previously better level of functioning. (If the latter, the inquiry naturally leads to the questions of what events and circumstances have accompanied this deterioration.) Identification of significant past problems that have interfered substantially with functioning at home, school, or with peers can also be facilitated through the use of screening instruments (see Chapter 4.6).

Inquiring about past episodes of harmful comments or acts may reveal important developmental progressions or patterns that warrant intervention. Headbanging or self-injurious behaviors may reveal underlying sensory disturbances, sometimes seen in developmental disorders; thoughts or comments about death may reveal suicidality; and self-harmful acts such as burning or cutting may reveal primitive coping mechanisms (7).

Safety Assessment. A safety assessment, both through direct and indirect questioning, may reveal need for close monitoring to preserve safety while diagnostic or treatment interventions occur. For example, directly asking a child if thoughts of death or not wanting to be alive have occurred will give a clinician a sense of how stuck and hopeless the child feels. Indirectly paying attention to how much or little the child talks about future-oriented events and meaningful connections, such as looking forward to an upcoming concert with friends, can help the clinician gauge how engaged and connected the child feels, thus providing insight into protective factors. Typical parts of the core safety evaluation include:

- Current suicidal ideation, intent, plan, means (e.g. access to pills if plan is to overdose)
- Past suicidal ideation, intent, plan

- Past suicide attempt(s), including method of the attempt, result of the attempt (e.g., hospitalized?), perception about outcome (i.e., how the child feels about the attempt being unsuccessful)
- Past and current nonsuicidal self-injury (NSSI) (e.g., cutting, burning), purpose of this behavior, does it fulfill that purpose (feelings before/during/after), desire to continue/stop, need for stitches/medical attention
- Current conflict(s); thoughts, plan, intent to harm anyone
- Past aggression/violence toward others

Additional acute safety issues important to investigate include substance abuse, impulsivity, risky behaviors, restrictive eating, agitation/aggression, and access to guns/weapons. This information should be put in context of information gained through the entire psychiatric interview to help determine level of risk.

Comorbid Problems

As parents describe the symptoms that appear most prominently in their child, the clinician begins thinking implicitly about what diagnostic categories (or other means of conceptualizing the symptoms) might apply. Symptom constellations may be described by a parent in such a way as to suggest one particular diagnostic category, particularly when parents have heard from other parents, books, or Internet resources about potential diagnoses. However, it is important to recall that psychiatric symptoms often overlap between various disorders, so consideration of disorders that may share similar symptoms should be considered. For example, inattention may occur in children with attention deficit hyperactivity disorder (ADHD), but also among children with bipolar disorder, posttraumatic stress disorder, anxiety disorders, or autism spectrum disorders, as well as in children who may be preoccupied with obsessions that distract them from focusing on what others are discussing.

Comorbidity is common in childhood psychiatric disorders and can complicate the course of treatment. For example, a child presenting with depression might also struggle with severe anxiety; the child will therefore require interventions not only to address mood symptoms, but also to tackle fear and avoidance (that also worsens the depression). Conducting a Psychiatric Review of Systems by asking screening questions about core DSM-5 diagnostic categories will help inform the clinician about possible comorbidities requiring further investigation. In addition, Section III of DSM-5 provides a Cross-Cutting Symptom Measure for Children ages 6 to 17, which assesses 12 domains of functioning across psychiatric diagnostic categories (i.e., somatic symptoms, sleep problems, inattention, depression, anger, irritability, mania, anxiety, psychosis, repetitive thoughts and behaviors, substance use, and suicidal ideation/suicide attempts). Screening instruments can also be useful to provide comprehensive information about less conspicuous conditions. This may be particularly important in detecting *internalizing* disorders, such as anxiety or mood disorders, which may be difficult for children to articulate, or which may be less troublesome or apparent to adults than disruptive *externalizing* disorders.

Substance Use History

Some symptom patterns, such as substance use, are particularly worrisome, both in terms of the direct hazards they pose to the child's development and as markers for a broader constellation of risk behaviors (8). Hence, it is particularly important to inquire regarding the child's exposure to and use of substances, including tobacco, alcohol, synthetic, and illicit substances, and how they may contribute to current symptoms. Asking about substance use in the child's peer group, views of use (e.g., "is it ok to occasionally drink socially?"), and perceived risk of use (e.g., "how harmful is it to smoke marijuana?") might provide insight into factors increasing likelihood of use. Previous exposures (including prenatal), contexts surrounding use, and effects of substances may impact treatment. Some children identify specific reasons for taking certain substances, while others proceed through many substances with diverse motives for taking or continuing use of these agents. For example, some children perceive that substances temporarily alleviate some of their symptoms (anxiety, depression) and so "self-medicate." In such cases, clarifying what impact these substances have on symptoms can clarify symptom priorities of the child, as well as possible intervention points more likely to be embraced by the child.

Previous Testing and Treatment(s)

Previous evaluations, including educational and neuropsychological testing, as well as past treatments, including medications, therapy, hospitalizations, and alternative treatments, may provide useful information about the evolution of a child's problems. Chronologic assessment of past treatment efforts may reveal seasonal patterns or escalation of a disorder. In addition, past treatment history may suggest which treatment modalities have been tolerable and effective (or not) for this patient (and family), signaling adherence issues or approaches that will be important in this case.

Developmental History

The developmental history is a detailed account of the child's development from birth forward. This history includes bodily/basic function regulation, motor development, language development, cognitive growth, social development, emotional regulation, moral development, and exposure to trauma. Parents vary widely in their recollection of precise timing of developmental milestones. Comparisons with other siblings or children, comparative recollections by different adults, and review of earlier videotapes of the child by the parents may improve the reliability and completeness of parent reports.

Bodily/basic functions include sleeping, eating, and toileting (including inquiries into bedwetting and soiling). Challenges in achieving milestones in these areas may result from or exacerbate episodes of difficulty. Similarly, previously attained skills may suddenly be lost, sometimes signaling the importance of emotional events at particular times. Eating behavior has become complicated as the availability of various types of food and times to eat have increased. While hunger remains a risk factor for psychopathology (9), obesity has become more common among younger people and markedly increases risk for both physical and mental illness (10,11).

Motor development includes milestones such as standing, walking, throwing, running, hopping, skipping, and playing sports or musical instruments. Fine motor and gross motor skills may not be congruent and therefore require specific inquiry into possible areas needing intervention or accommodation. Inquiry as to how the child enjoys or fares at activities such as sports and/or music may suggest treatment options through nonverbal modalities. In addition, history from parents may clarify periods when the child could not employ skills or became frustrated in attempting activities requiring motor coordination.

Cognitive development usually begins with the child's verbal and attentional skills. Assessment of the child's academic progression in preschool and school can reveal cognitive weaknesses that may contribute to the current problem, or potential strengths to be harnessed to ameliorate the current problem. Specific inquiry concerning learning disorders—e.g., reading, writing, and math skill progression—may reveal global difficulties or uneven skills in development (12). Evaluation of executive functioning skills, particularly at times of transition to middle and high school, can uncover underlying skills deficits that manifest through emotional and behavioral challenges. It is important to bear in mind that adequate progress in school requires more than adequate innate cognitive abilities; it also reflects factors such as the child's motivation, freedom from distraction, attitudes toward authority, capacity for peer relations, tolerance for frustration and delayed gratification, and degree of parental support for learning.

Interpersonal development assesses how the child interacts with others, particularly family members, other children, and adults. Early interactions, especially with parents, provide important information about this child's comfort around others and the environment. For example, early aloofness, disinterest in others, absence of interactive play with parents or attention to objects pointed out by parents may be early markers of autism spectrum disorder. The child's (and parents') reactions to significant changes in the social environment of the home can be important precipitants for the child's symptoms, particularly births/deaths of family members, marital changes (separations or conflicts, divorce, remarriages), and changes in caretaking arrangements (parent returning to work, or custody/visitation changes).

The child's interactions with peers and adults outside the family are also important. Interactions with other children and preferences in play activities and friends (gender, age, interests) are important data for assessing the child's social skills and interest in relating to others. Stability of relationships, numbers of friends, types of activities shared, and expectations of peers ("plays with me when I want," "plays what I want to play," "helps me out if I need it," etc.) can reveal strengths, sources of difficulty, or persistent maladaptive clashes where only the names of the antagonists change.

Emotional development and *temperament* is a key component in the evaluation of every child. A child's capacity to recognize his or her own mood state and to self-soothe or regulate negative affect should be investigated. Prevailing moods can be described by parents, as well as past suicidality, irritability, specific fears and anxieties, and conditions associated with the child's happiness and pleasure. Whether the child can recognize when a mood is mild or severe, and what steps the child will take when anxious, sad, or when encountering change, boredom, or disappointment provide insight into vital coping mechanisms. Circumstances which provoke aggression or anger and the child's responses and capacity to accept input or direction from others may clarify intervention options such as parenting or behavioral treatments. These traits commonly exist along a spectrum, so that bullying, for example, may have started as assertiveness and progressed to exploitation or intimidation of others.

Assessment of the child's *moral development* provides an important gauge of whether the child's conscience or moral values are too lax, too harsh, overly focused on particular areas, or uneven and out of proportion to daily events. The child's religious, cultural, and ethical views and practices and how those fit with those of the family also provide helpful information guiding potential treatment interventions. Similarly, the child's ability to recognize the plight of others, to recognize impacts of decisions on others, to reconcile principles with mistakes the child makes, and to acknowledge and correct mistakes often provides clarity about the child's strengths and limitations.

Trauma experienced at any stage of the child's development can substantially impact or even arrest development. Investigation of not only actual events (such as documented physical or sexual abuse), but also of events perceived traumatic by the child and the vicissitudes of these events for the child and family shed important light on the child's behaviors and patterns of relating to others. Identifying episodes of trauma, the events surrounding the trauma, the child's role in disclosing such trauma to others, and the reactions of adults to such disclosures are important for the clinician to recognize and address. It is also essential to ensure current safety of the child, such that any risk of re-traumatization is minimized.

Family History

Parental variables may impact the child's problems and warrant examination. First, family conflict, or differences in parenting style, may culminate in the child manifesting symptoms; however, the converse is equally true, in that disturbed behavior by a child may stress otherwise adequate parental coping skills or provoke conflict between parents (13). Parents may have grown up themselves with different parenting practices in their families of origin that they wish to employ, or avoid, and these influences are important to understand in assessing the consistencies and discrepancies within and between each parent's style. In the face of a child's distressing behaviors, parents may attempt a wide variety of approaches, some uncharacteristic of their usual parenting style, poorly conceived, and enacted at inopportune times (e.g., unenforceable threats during a tantrum); such responses may not improve the problem but do increase parental guilt and hopelessness. Accordingly, the clinician must be mindful that the approach parents ordinarily employ may not be described if it does not work with this child. Clarifying the evolution of the approaches parents have attempted for this child's problems, and how these approaches may have differed from approaches employed with their other children, may help the clinician disentangle child and parent contributions to the current problem. In addition, exploring the child's compliance with family rules and expectations, the consequences for noncompliance, and the child's reaction to parental interventions in response to noncompliance often provide opportunities for behavioral interventions to diminish symptom expression. It is important to identify parents' style of limit setting in a variety of areas. For school-age children, these concern hygiene; sleep; diet; television, Internet, and video game use; and the expression of aggression. For adolescents, it is additionally important to know what sort of expectations parents do or do not set regarding curfew, dress, leisure activities, and choice of friends. Effective parental monitoring of an adolescent's activities, whereabouts, and peers is an important aspect of problem behaviors and usually reflects not only parents' efforts at active, close surveillance, but also a close parent–child relationship that encourages open communication and child disclosure (14).

Second, parents may have problems with the child at particular developmental periods. Certain developmental stages may have particularly challenged the parent's skills or coping responses, or may have reminded the parent of a painful time in his or her own childhood. Discussion with parents about how they navigated past difficulties with this child, their rationales for certain parenting practices, and their expectations (and fears) during this given developmental phase of the child often provide clues about potential parental contributions to the problem. Similarly, information about parents' cultural, educational, occupational, and religious background may reveal not only sources of adversity or conflict between parents or family members, but also sources of pride and resilience that inform interventions to enhance treatment adherence among parents and children.

Third, parental genetic contributions remain an important variable to consider, particularly since some parents perceive that the child's psychopathology may be attributed to one or the other parent based on that parent's personal or family history. Few if any common psychiatric disorders appear exclusively through genetic transmission alone, although increased vulnerabilities to various disorders are likely. In addition, growing up with a parent who has struggled with a psychiatric disorder such as depression, anxiety, psychosis, or substance abuse is likely to have an impact on the child, over and above any genetically transmitted vulnerability. Tactful but thorough investigation into psychopathology in each parent and among the extended family may suggest which disorders or general conditions (mood, anxiety) may be more probable. Patterns can also be visualized by constructing a genogram, particularly in complex families with multiple psychopathologies. Although unspoken during psychiatric evaluations, many parents fear that their other children may be destined to suffer psychopathology when one sibling manifests a disorder, so clarification of genetic contributions to expression of disorders can often be helpful in reducing unwarranted fear, guilt, and distress among parents.

Divorce, separation, and single-parent family circumstances may stress all family members, including the children. Even when parents part amicably, children may have difficulty with change from what has been familiar. Similarly, even in circumstances where parents and children experience reduced conflict after parents separate, children sometimes exhibit symptoms which coincide with marital changes. The child's symptoms may reveal overwhelming stress or fear, but also may reveal efforts to reunite family members. In addition, children may exhibit symptoms months or years after separations as difficulty adjusting to new roles or environments occurs or as they enter a new developmental phase (15). Therefore, the clinician should be attuned to how the divorce/separation is affecting each member of the family, e.g., what is the child's understanding of circumstances leading to divorce? How does communication between parents occur (e.g., routinely and amicably vs. angrily and only via child as messenger)? Are parents reasonably consistent in their approach to parenting (vs. one parent being "the mean/difficult parent" while the other becomes the "fun/easy parent")?

Adoption is usually a positive event for the child and for the adoptive parents. The circumstances of the adoption warrant tactful attention by the clinician, including age of the child and biologic parents, the degree of ongoing contact with or interest in biologic parents, the child's understanding of the adoption and attitudes about the biologic and the adoptive parents, and how the adoption is discussed at home. In addition, adoptive parent expectations and feelings about the adoption, particularly as their child now undergoes a psychiatric evaluation, may reveal underlying parental fears, guilt, or disappointments. However, the family system is currently configured, the clinician should inquire about how the family system functions, with whom the child spends time, and the nature of the relationships between the various household members and the child. Boundaries and alliances, conflicts, and the child's affinities or resentments of other family members should be determined. Family communication and problem solving, including how issues of disagreement are handled, should be assessed. The emotional tone of families vary widely from constricted to overly expressive and dramatic, and should be examined both by observation of family interactions during the interview, as well as by direct inquiry. Clarification of family stressors that are chronic family stressors (family member illness or disability) or acute (sudden illness, job loss/change, financial or legal difficulties) may identify determinants of the child's current problems as well as potential targets for intervention.

Medical History

Obtaining consent to contact the patient's pediatrician allows for collaboration across health care providers. Checking into compliance with well-child visits and pediatrician recommendations (e.g., vaccinations), and pediatrician's involvement in ongoing care can provide helpful information related to resources and follow-through.

Medical conditions experienced by the child should be identified beginning with conception (including any difficulties the mother had in conceiving or the use of assisted reproductive technologies). Pregnancy complications, birth difficulties, extended hospital stays, and medical illnesses requiring recurrent or ongoing treatments (e.g., asthma, diabetes) should be investigated, since these appear to increase the child's risk for psychopathology (16). In addition, inquiry into hospitalizations, emergency room visits, or surgeries can help shed light on severity of illness as well as the child's fears or parental over/underprotectiveness.

Age of menarche and stage of pubertal development should be inquired about when relevant. If the child's weight and/or stature is out of the normal range for age (as plotted on a standard growth chart), a detailed review of the child's growth history and eating habits should be made in consultation with the child's pediatrician.

Accidents or illnesses with a potential for central nervous system impact, such as lead exposure, seizures, head trauma, and loss of consciousness, deserve specific inquiry.

Medications and Allergies

A list of all medications (including over-the-counter and naturopathic agents), indication for the medication, length of treatment (or dates taken if known), max doses, benefits, side effects, compliance, and reason for discontinuation should be obtained for all current and past medications. Additional attention to patient and family attitudes to use and effects of medication can provide opportunity to address potential sensitivities and barriers to treatment.

Allergies, particularly to medications, also should be elicited and documented.

School and Educational History

As noted earlier, putting the child in context of family, school, and the broader environment is essential in gaining a full understanding of the presenting problem and possible interventions. Creating a timeline by grade level provides opportunity evaluate connections between academic progress (e.g., report card grades, standardized testing, evaluation of learning disabilities), behavioral challenges (e.g., disruptive classroom behaviors, tardies/early dismissals, absences/school refusal), social stressors (e.g., bullying, social exclusion, or isolation), environmental events (e.g., death of beloved family member), and interventions (retentions, accommodations/modifications [504 plan/IEPs], treatment) to evaluate areas in need of particular attention. Focusing on notable years/grades that went particularly well or poorly can shed light on the impact of classroom/teacher fit, social experiences—including bullying (17,18), and learning challenges/disabilities on progression of symptoms. Understanding the culture of the school and classroom, the system's approach to bullying and social/emotional support, and the most trusted allies/adults at school can provide additional insights and opportunities for interventions.

In addition, gaining an understanding of how the child views himself as a student (e.g., "I'm really smart, but my emotions get in the way" versus "The work is just too hard for me." versus "My teacher doesn't know how to teach so that I can understand") and what the child's priorities are as a student (e.g., valuing education and progressing through high school to college vs. wanting to drop out as soon as possible) can provide insight into self-esteem and self-efficacy and possible need for additional school-related interventions.

Child Strengths and Supports

In addition to clarifying the child's problems, the evaluation simultaneously elicits the child's areas of strength so that interventions can build on these existing assets rather than focusing exclusively on areas of weakness. It often can be helpful to start an assessment by asking parents what the like about their child, or what their child does particularly well. In addition, finding out what the child takes pride in or values offers an opportunity to help boost the child's sense of efficacy; this can be a nice balance given that children presenting for evaluation often experience an emphasis on negative behaviors and events.

Interests, hobbies, and talents of the child should be obtained from both the child and the parents, since these accounts may not match or may even be in conflict. Parents may have aspirations for their children that the child does not share, or the child may have fantasies beyond apparent abilities. In most cases, though, the child will have some identifiable interests or abilities that serve as potential points of connection with peers and adults (including the therapist) and may serve to facilitate therapy. Exploration of the child's interests, including newly emerging ones, may allow the interviewer to anchor recommendations or treatment metaphors to language or subjects familiar to or valued by the patient. Similarly, the child's and parents' accounts of time spent in an activity (10 years of ballet and modern dance) or perceived fruits of the child's labor ("I won trophies twice," vs. "I've lost most games I've played in") illuminate what effect the activity has had on the child, including pride or disappointment, as well as the parents' and the child's own expectations.

Although many children must contend with moves or changes in the family constellation, other *environmental supports and buffers* often provide stability and even sanctuary and warrant investigation. Adults other than the parents (such as grandparents and other relatives, coaches, teachers) may play significant, ongoing roles in the lives of children, while community involvements, such as church groups, athletic team participation, outdoor clubs, musical ensembles, or even preferred places to convene, may provide opportunities for intervention or support in natural settings on a regular basis.

The Child's Media Diet

In an information-processing society, children are exposed to immense doses of media, including television, music, videos, electronic games, cell phones, e-mail, and social media platforms and apps. These media, which may provide exposure of the child to violent and sexually provocative material, can have positive or negative effects. It is important to clarify which media the child uses, how much time each day is spent with these various media, how the child decides what personal information to post and share publically, and what consequences these media have on the child (e.g., in response to watching action television shows the child becomes more violent vs. has developed interest in Asian food through watching cooking programs, or listening to music at school serves to distract the child from classroom instruction vs. helps the child calm down on the bus or ignore other disruptions) (19). Social media can be used to multiple ends, which may be adaptive (maintaining friendships with camp friends), problematic (bullying, harassment, or dangerous exhibitionism), or both (permitting a socially anxious child to maintain a modicum of electronic social contacts, but at the cost of face-to-face relationships) (20). As with other aspects of parental monitoring, the degree of parental awareness and appropriate limit setting regarding television, video games, and social media is important to determine, in part as an indicator of parental structure and expectations. As with other of the child's interests, preferred television show, favorite movies, favored musicians, or bands provide a common language to examine topics, as well as clues about the child's aspirations and behavioral self-expectations ("[Music idol] swears at adults all the time, so why can't I?") (21). Asking a child to describe an episode of a favorite TV show or movie also provides a convenient picture of the quality of the child's social language and grasp of others' motives and feelings.

Mental Status Examination

The mental status examination is an essential part of any psychiatric interview, as it provides direct information about how the child presents and interacts with the clinician. The mental status examination includes a clinical description of the child's appearance, engagement, behaviors, mood and affect, sensorium, apparent cognitive functioning, and thought content and process. Although often conceptualized as a separate component that is distinct from the history-taking interview, in reality much of the mental status examination takes place implicitly as the clinician interacts with and observes the child during the child and family interviews. Although some components of the examination will require specific inquiry or examination (such as orientation, memory, fund of knowledge, and mental contents), most will be noted as the clinician organizes his or her ongoing observations of the child according to the elements of the mental status examination. A format for the child mental status examination is provided in Table 4.3.2.

In addition, the mental status examination provides an opportunity for further screening of organic or neurologic contributions to the child's symptoms. A mini-mental status examination (MMSE) (Table 4.3.3) can provide more detailed assessment of an older child's higher-order mental functions, including orientation, attention, memory, language, and constructional ability (22). This MMSE contains items appropriate for older children, although some modified versions provide questions for younger patients (23). More reliable and detailed assessment of a child's speech, language, intellectual, academic achievement, attention and executive functioning, memory, and complex thinking requires standardized psychometric testing (Chapters 4.4 and 4.5).

STRUCTURE OF THE CLINICAL INTERVIEW

While the steps in the process of the psychiatric assessment of the child may unfold in multiple ways, a stepwise approach, individualized by the clinician for the requirements of each specific case, helps ensure thoroughness. More importantly, the quality of the information obtained from which all diagnoses and treatment planning will follow is contingent on the approach the clinician employs, and how well this approach fits the particular patient. A sample checklist for the preparatory stage of the psychiatric assessment of children is summarized in Figure 4.3.1. The clinician or staff may begin completing such a checklist during the initial phone contact with the child's family, although the entire checklist may not be completed until after the assessment.

Preparatory Phase of the Child Interview

Preparation is paramount in child psychiatry interviews. Families are often unfamiliar with what occurs during such an assessment, and concern by the child or the parent that they

TABLE 4.3.2

THE MENTAL STATUS EXAMINATION IN CHILDREN

Appearance	Appears stated age, notable physical attributes, clothing, hygiene and grooming
Orientation and alertness	Self (name), place (location), time (awareness of morning, day of week, month, etc., varies by age), situation (why here)
Manner of relating to clinician and parents	Ease of separating from parents, quick or slow to warm up, level of engagement, eye contact, eagerness to please, defiance
Activity level	Psychomotor agitation or slowing, fidgeting, goal-oriented or erratic movements, coordination, unusual postures or motor patterns (e.g., tics, stereotypies, akathisia, dystonia, tremors), compulsions
Speech	Spontaneous or forced, fluency (including stuttering, speech impediments), rate, volume, prosody, latency
Mood	As described by child, e.g., "happy," "sad," "mad"
Affect	Congruent with mood? Examples: anxious, blunted/restricted, dysthymic, euphoric, euthymic, flat, full range, irritable, inappropriate/odd, labile
Thought process	Logic, linear, goal-directed, perseverative, circumstantial, disorganized, tangential (consider age-appropriateness), looseness of associations, word salad (incoherent, clanging, neologisms) Poverty of thought (latency, blocking) Racing thoughts, flight of ideas Abstract vs. concrete: Proverbs (e.g., what does "Grass is always greener in somebody else's yard" mean?)
Thought content and perceptions	[note: ego-syntonic or dystonic] Thoughts to harm self or others (plan, intent) Obsessions, delusions, ideas of reference, paranoia Depersonalization, derealization, hallucinations
Attention, calculation, working memory	Need for redirection/repeating, length of time sustained in activity, degree to which child shifts from activity to activity, distractibility (e.g., to outside noises) Serial Sevens (start from 100, subtract 7) or Digit Span (repeat 2–5 digit strings forward and backwards), spell "WORLD" backwards
Memory	Immediate (repeat words) Short-term (recall three words at 2 and 2 min) Long-term (recall events from past week, month, etc.)
Intelligence/fund of knowledge	Age-appropriate recognition of letters, vocabulary, reading, counting, computational skills Age-appropriate knowledge of geography, history, culture (e.g., celebrities, sports, movies) Ability to classify and categorize
Insight	Ability to see alternative explanations, others' points of view, locus of control (internal vs. external), defense mechanisms
Judgment	Sample questions: What would you do if. "you found a stamped envelope next to a mailbox" "a fire started in a theater" "you saw a man with big feet"

will be "judged" is almost universal. Unlike routine well-child visits with a pediatrician, a child psychiatry interview is rarely perceived by parents as a mental health checkup for their child, but rather as potentially indicative of their failures as parents. Invocation of a psychiatric diagnosis may help exonerate some parents from feelings of guilty (but sometimes spurious) responsibility for the child's presenting difficulties and, indeed, some parents may seek evidence of a "chemical imbalance" outside their control as responsible for the child's symptoms. Others, however, might view a psychiatric diagnosis as stigmatizing for their child (and themselves). Accordingly, interactions prior to the actual interview can help clarify parental fears and expectations. For example, parents may report, "I did toilet training wrong, and now my child—..." as they search for the root of the child's current problems. Similarly, parent anxieties often emerge, as some parents report, "My child only acts badly toward me—I bring out the worst in my child," fearing they uniquely cause the child's symptoms. The parent interview also provides clues as to what difficulties may be encountered in trying to change parental behavior, such as how overwhelmed a parent may become when even basic interventions are suggested for them to enact (e.g., in response to questions such as "What would happen if you were to simply turn the television off and tell him it is bedtime?"). At the other extreme, some parents may have hopes or expectations that the clinician cannot fulfill, for example, "You [the child psychiatrist] need to tell him how good he has it at home" or "Tell him if he is gay I will disown him and throw him out of the house." Such expectations may require clarifying what expectations the child psychiatrist can or cannot fulfill. Parents may come with other preconceived agendas, such as that their child is bipolar or that they are determined that under no condition will their child ever receive any medication. Preparing parents for what to expect during the assessment diminishes parent and child anxieties, and initiates a process for shared goals and appropriate parent and child expectations. Sample letters clarifying the assessment are provided in Appendices 4.3.1 and 4.3.2.

Children also usually have little idea of what occurs in a psychiatric assessment, and may fear being hospitalized, or otherwise punished, especially if their difficulties have been a source of recrimination in the family. A child who harbors a family secret or concerns about a parent's behavior may fear punishment, relocation, or loss of contact with that parent if he or she speaks openly. Other children only know they are being expected to articulate explanations for behaviors that may not make sense to them, let alone to adults.

TABLE 4.3.3

MINI-MENTAL STATUS EXAMINATION

		Score	Points
Orientation			
1. What is the	Year?	___	1
	Season?	___	1
	Date?	___	1
	Day?	___	1
	Month?	___	1
2. Where are we?	Country	___	1
	State or territory	___	1
	Town or city?	___	1
	Hospital or suburb?	___	1
	Floor or address?	___	1
Registration			
3. Name three objects, taking 1 s to say each. Then ask the patient all three after you have said them. (Tree, clock, boat, or body parts for children <7 yrs.) Give one point for each correct answer. Repeat the answers until patient learns all three.		___	3
Attention and Calculation			
4. Serial sevens. Give one point for each correct answer. Stop after five answers. For children <age 7, have them repeat 2–5 digit strings (e.g., "4–7," then 3–5–8," and score one point for each digit string repeated forward correctly).		___	5
5. Spell "world" backwards. For children <7, have them repeat 2–4 digit strings backwards (e.g., examiner says "5–2" and child repeats back "2–5," etc.).		___	5
Recall			
6. Ask for names of three objects learned in 3 above. Give one point for each correct answer.		___	3
Language			
7. Point to a pencil and a watch or to body parts. Have the patient name them as you point.		___	2
8. Have the patient repeat, "No ifs, ands, or buts."		___	1
9. Have the patient follow a three-stage command. "Take a piece of paper in your right hand. Fold the paper in half. Put the paper on the floor."		___	3
10. Have the patient read and obey the following: "CLOSE YOUR EYES." (Write it in large letters.) For children <7, have them read their name.		___	1
11. Have the patient write a sentence of his or her choice. (The sentence should contain a subject and an object and should make sense. Ignore spelling errors when scoring.) For children <7, have them write their name.		___	1
12. Have the patient copy the design printed below. (Give one point if all sides and angles are preserved and if the intersecting sides form a diamond shape.) For children under age 7, have drawn a circle or oval.		___	1
TOTAL:		___	(24)

(From Ouvrier RA, Goldsmith RF, Ouvrier S, Williams IC: The value of the mini-mental state examination in childhood: a preliminary study. *J Child Neurol* 8:145–148, 1993, and Jain M, Passi GR: Assessment of a modified mini-mental scale for cognitive functions in children. *Indian Peds* 42: 907–912, 2005, both with permission.)

Similarly, interested others (such as school staff or other health care providers) may have diverse (or unrealistic) expectations of what a psychiatric assessment can provide or how it might be implemented (such as a month-long inpatient observation).

In order to diminish unreasonable fears and to encourage more honest, accurate reporting, the clinician will seek, even prior to the first interview, to cultivate a partnership with the parents and interested others to support the child. A brief (under 15 minutes) initial phone call can help clarify how parents and teachers perceive the identified problem and introduce potential areas of exploration (e.g., specific patient strengths or interests) that may facilitate the family's and child's functioning and comfort with the assessment. If such calls are not possible or feasible, trained office staff may make these initial inquiries or request that the family completes a pre-intake survey prior to the initial appointment.

During this same initial phone contact, clarification of preferred contact numbers where the parents can be reached without embarrassment, billing information, and consent to speak with others familiar with the child can often be accomplished in advance of the actual interview. Some parents are reluctant to consent to contact between the clinician and others (such as the school) until they feel more comfortable with the clinician. Parental preferences for e-mail correspondence can also be discussed before the actual interview, so that efficient methods for data acquisition from others can be determined. Finally, special needs of the child (e.g., visual difficulties) can be discussed in a less embarrassing context than in front of the patient. Similarly, ideas from the parents for making the

_____ 1. Child's Name: ______________________________ Preferred Name: ______________________________

_____ 2. Parents/Guardians: ____

_____ 3. Contact Information:

Home Phone: ______________________________ Cell Phone: ______________________________

Billing Address: ____

____

_____ E-mail: ____

_____ E-mail parameters including privacy caveats, discussed/acceptable to family: YES NO

_____ 4. Reasons for Referral: ____

____

____

_____ 5. Expectations from This Assessment: ______________________________________

____

____

_____ 6. Consents Given to Speak with:

_____ Family _____ School _____ Other Providers

Names/Contact Numbers: ______________________________

____

____

____

_____ 7. Taping/Video/Recording: ______________________________

_____ 8. Special Needs: _____ Language _____ Audiovisual

(Does the family have videotapes of the child's early years? If yes, reviewing these with attention to when the child walked, talked, played with other children, showed any concerning behaviors or mannerism, maybe helpful during discussions of the child's developmental history.)

_____ 9. Parent Preparation of Child for Clinical Interview

_____ 10. Making Comfortable at Office:

_____ Preferred Toys/Games/Activities: ______________________________________

_____ Interests (Sports, Music, Extracurricular): ______________________________

_____ 11. Condentiality (HIPAA, e-mail) Discussed: ______________________________________

FIGURE 4.3.1. Preparatory checklist for clinical assessment.

assessment flow more comfortably, such as allowing the child to bring and demonstrate favored toys or electronics, or preferred discussion topics for teenagers, enhance the initial alliance, crucial in any later treatment efforts.

Initial Meeting

While circumstances may call for an alternative initial interview structure, it can be helpful to first meet together with parents and child, then separately with the child and the parents, and then bring everyone back together to wrap-up the meeting. When first meeting, depending on the reason for presentation, it may be helpful to start by eliciting strengths and future goals of the child. This can help build rapport and frame the interview toward a positive experience for the child and family (25).

Meeting with Child and Parents Together

The child and parents are often seen together at the beginning of the child psychiatric interview; this allows the clinician to make introductions, describe the purpose and structure of the assessment, begin to establish rapport and level of comfort, and discuss confidentiality so that parents and child understand what information will and will not be shared. Allowing the child to become sufficiently comfortable before parents depart can cultivate an environment where the child is less guarded. Children can often indicate an acceptable point for the parents to leave the room, usually within a matter of minutes, and transitional objects (from blankets to handheld computer game devices) may ease these transitions.

Confidentiality is one of the most challenging issues surrounding child psychiatric interviews, especially with adolescents who may be particularly concerned about who might hear what from the clinician. Parents and children should be informed of the confidential nature of the doctor–patient relationship so that the clinician is not seen as a parental spy. However, findings such as diagnoses often must be reported to parents, to insurance companies (for reimbursement), and to schools for classroom or curricular modifications to occur. Describing to the adolescent what will be told to specific others is usually sufficient, as well as what information will not be revealed. Parents and child should be told explicitly that confidentiality does *not* extend to situations that pose a clear danger to the child or others. In cases where this emerges (e.g., the child describes hoarding pills in a drawer to commit suicide or obtaining bullets to threaten a student at school), the clinician should clarify with the child how they will tell appropriate others, and ideally how the child will participate in the disclosure to others. State laws vary and change regarding what information must be shared or kept confidential between clinicians and patients, even minors, about substance use, pregnancy/abortion, and weapons possession, so clinicians should remain familiar with local legal standards of confidentiality. While treatment may not be possible with some children unless certain information remains confidential, confidentiality should not become collusion.

The Parent Interview

In the initial face-to-face parent interview, the clinician seeks to understand the parents' perspective on the problems leading to the referral. The clinician endeavors to identify the "why now?" reasons that this evaluation is occurring, how parents understand the evolution of their child's symptoms, what current priorities each parent or other party (such as the school or court) describes for this evaluation, what impact the child's difficulties now have on the family, and how the child's symptoms impact his or her functioning with peers and at school or beyond (e.g., work, extracurricular activities). As noted earlier, throughout each component of the interview, the clinician remains alert to the potential functions or benefits the current symptoms carry for the child, the apparent attunement of the parents to the child's needs, and available resources; these resources include special skills or talents the child may possess and the presence of other individuals who exert a positive influence on this child. The clinician will also be attentive to any relevant cultural factors that may affect the child's symptoms. The goal is to obtain as full a picture as possible of the child's current developmental trajectory. Sample questions for eliciting each component of this interview are provided in Table 4.3.4.

The parent interview can be complicated by multiple factors, including parental ambivalence about having a child evaluated by a psychiatrist, by divergent perceptions among parents and adults about the origin of the child's problems, fears of loss of control or criticism, or parental shame or embarrassment about perceived parenting faults or personal past history. Just as the child's level of development will impact the content of the interview, so too do adults vary in their sophistication about parenting techniques or understanding their child's developmental needs. To understand parents' descriptions about the child in their proper context, the clinician will remain attentive throughout the interview to the parents' own vulnerabilities and concerns about parenting. Parents may have their own past experiences rekindled when they see their child in distress, and may seek to prevent outcomes they experienced (26). Clinicians may detect reflexive inclinations in some parents to revert, when stressed, to doing what their parents did to them, and clinicians may detect distressing parental recollections about their own childhood adversities brought back through their child's problems. Multiple techniques may be required for the clinician to help parents overcome such obstacles during the course of the interview.

The Child Interview

Inquiring what the child has been told or understands about the purpose of the interview often provides initial information on the child's experience of presenting to the clinic, the communication style between the child and parent(s), and the child's understanding of the circumstances. The child's description of what he or she has been told regarding the evaluation may further reveal the child's priorities for intervention.

In addition to the purpose of this evaluation generally, the clinician should inquire about what the child believes parents, teachers, or other adults want to be different as a result of this interview. While the child may not know what others seek, this approach helps elucidate what the child recognizes about others' perspectives, and also facilitates the child projecting thoughts or fantasies about this evaluation.

The interviewer then focuses attention on gathering additional history from the child's point of view, paying particular attention to how the child attributes meaning to things. Although the reliability of information from the child on any given point will vary with the topic and with the individual child, the clinical information derived from direct observation of and interaction with the child is essential (27). The child's description of feelings, moods, levels of distress, and significant events contribute to a complete understanding of the child, and to matching and framing viable treatments with the individual child. In addition, symptoms such as compulsions, urges, obsessive or suicidal thoughts, hallucinations, tics, or a thought disorder may not be recognized or acknowledged by the adults in the child's life, and children are often more reliable reporters of internalizing symptoms such as anxiety (28). Similarly, the child may be the only informant with knowledge of traumatic events (e.g., sexual abuse of the child, bullying), delinquent acts, or the child's idiosyncratic interpretation of certain events.

TABLE 4.3.4

INTERVIEW: SAMPLE CLINICIAN QUESTIONS

Component	Description	Sample Questions for Caregiver	Sample Questions for Child
Reason for referral	Chief complaint/primary reason for presenting for evaluation	What are the primary concerns bringing you in today? Whose idea was it that [child] might need this evaluation? Who is most concerned about [child's] behavior? Has anyone else, such as other family members, school staff, or other agencies, encouraged this evaluation? What do you/they hope this evaluation will accomplish?	What is your understanding of why you are here today? [What did your parent(s) tell you about coming here today?] Who wanted you to meet with me today? Why do you think they want us to meet? What do you think they are worried about? What do you think/feel about being here?
History of problems/ present illness	Why now: narrative about events leading to current presentation [open ended questions]	When did you first notice concerns about [child]? How did the problem develop over time? Have there been times when things have gotten much better or worse?	What is not going so well for you? What do you wish would be different? When was the last time you remember things going pretty well? What do you think is making it such a hard time?
	Functional assessment of problem behaviors	How do you understand [child's] behavior? When/Where does the problem occur most often? How does the problem impact [child] at home? At school? With peers? Is the problem behavior worse in one of these places? What usually occurs right before [problem behavior]? What happens after [child] does [problem behavior]? Does anything make the behavior worse/ better?	When/Where do you notice having a hard time? [triggers] What happens when you [exhibit symptoms]? How does your [parent, teacher, friend] respond when you [exhibit symptom]? How do you feel after you [exhibit symptom]?
	Daily routine	Please walk through what an average day looks like for [child], starting from waking up in the morning and going through waking up the next morning? How about over the weekend?	Let's walk through a typical day for you. What time do you normally wake up...
	Past problems	Has [child] experienced problems in the past that have caused concern? Have things escalated to this point in the past?	Do you remember ever feeling this badly when you were younger? Was there anything you can remember that helped make things feel better?
	Comorbid symptoms (Psychiatric review of systems): Basic functioning: Sleeping Eating Physical activity Self-care DSM-5 diagnostic criteria screening [Substance abuse and trauma assessed separately]	Does [child] have any other symptoms that are concerning and/or interfere at home, school, or with friends? Basic functioning: Let's talk about some of the essentials for staying healthy: How does [child] sleep at night? Does [child] take naps during the day? How has [child's] appetite been? Has [child] ever been under/overweight? How often does [child] get physical activity? How much prompting does [child] require to take care of everyday tasks such as brushing teeth, showering, getting dressed? DSM-5 diagnostic criteria e.g., ADHD, Anxiety Disorders, OCD, Depression, Bipolar disorder, Psychosis, Eating disorder, Conduct Disorder, Oppositional Defiant Disorder, Anger/Aggression	Is there anything else going on that you wish were different? Is there anything else that is bothering you? Basic functioning: Do you have any trouble falling asleep? Staying asleep? What are your favorite foods to eat? Are you usually hungry for breakfast, lunch, and dinner? Snacks? Do you feel like you have enough energy during the day or do you usually feel tired? How much exercise are you getting? Is it pretty easy or hard to get active?

TABLE 4.3.4

(CONTINUED)

Component	Description	Sample Questions for Caregiver	Sample Questions for Child
	Substance use	How is drug/alcohol use discussed in the family? Has [child] done anything to suggest use of alcohol and/or drugs? Have you detected [child] to be drunk/high? Have you seen or found any drug paraphernalia that might be [child's]? Has [child] spoken about drinking, smoking, or drug use? How about his/her friends?	Have you ever been around any drugs or alcohol? How harmful (or not) do you think it is to drink, smoke marijuana, use drugs, etc.? Have you ever tried cigarettes? Alcohol? Drugs? How often do your friends drink/use? Have you ever been high/drunk? Has that ever led to problems for you? [If positive use] What do you notice when you use [substance used]? It is helpful in any way?
Safety assessment	Suicidal ideation, prior suicide attempts, future orientation Homicidal ideation, agitation, aggression Access to guns, history of stealing/legal involvement, running away, fire setting Risky behaviors (e.g., promiscuity, restrictive eating, substance use)	Has [child] ever talked about wanting to die? Has [child] ever talked about hurting himself? Others? Has [child] ever done things to hurt himself? To hurt other people or animals? Has [child] ever been involved with school officials or police because of threats or harm toward others? Does [child] tend to be on the more cautious or risk-taking end of the spectrum? Have you noticed that [child] tends to be impulsive?	Have you ever thought about not wanting to be alive anymore? Have you ever thought about hurting yourself? Others? Have you ever done something to hurt yourself? What was the purpose? How did you feel after you did _____? Have you ever hurt anyone else on purpose? How did you feel about that? How do you feel about that now?
Previous testing and treatments	Prior diagnoses Prior treatments and efficacy (including outpatient, ER visit, and inpatient hospitalizations) Independent neuropsychological testing, academic or SPED testing via school, etc.	Has [child] received any diagnoses or treatment(s) in the past for emotional or behavioral concerns? Has [child] undergone any testing through school or independent entities?	
Develop-mental history	Bodily/basic function	How did toilet training progress with [child]? Has [child] had periods of wetting or soiling?	
	Motor development	When did [child] start walking? Have concerns been raised about [child's] handwriting? In what sports/activities has [child] participated? Which ones have gone well? Not so well?	Which sports do you like to do? Which ones are harder? Do you have any problems playing games/sports/ music /dancing?
	Cognitive development	When did [child] begin preschool/school? How did that go? How does [child] do with reading? Math? Writing? In which subjects does [child] do particularly well? Which subjects are more difficult?	

(*continued*)

TABLE 4.3.4

(CONTINUED)

Component	Description	Sample Questions for Caregiver	Sample Questions for Child
	Interpersonal development	How did [child] relate to you as an infant/toddler? As a toddler, did [child] show interest in things you pointed to? Did [child] point things out to you? How did [child] respond to your requests or directions? When did [child] start interacting with other children? How did that go? Did [child] have any significant attachments or relationships to others that ended? What kind of friends does [child] have at this point? How does [child] get along with these children? Does [child] get invited to play dates, birthday parties, sleepovers?	How do you get along with the other kids in your class? With your teacher? Who are some of your good friends now (when/where met, what do together, how often)? How often do you and play together? How long do you stay at [friend's house]? Do you spend the night at [friend's house]? How does that go (What do you do?) Any rough spots between you and other kids? How come? Have you lost any good friends (because of moves, misunderstandings)?
	Emotional development	Does [child] recognize when he or she is sad, happy, etc.? How does [child] soothe him/herself when unhappy or in a bad mood? What is the child's prevailing/most common mood? How does the child respond to unexpected changes? Disappointments? Frustrations? Worries?	How often do you feel sad? Mad? Worried? Happy? Does anything in particular make you sad/mad/worried? What do you do when you are feeling that way? How do you calm yourself down when you're upset?
	Moral development	Does [child] recognize right from wrong? Does [child] describe any "principles" that guide his/her actions? How does [child] contend with mistakes or when confronted about doing something wrong? Has [child] ever deliberately hurt any animals or other kids? Bullied or been bullied by other kids? Does [child] show remorse after hurting someone? Does [child] consider consequences of decisions on others? Is [child] either too perfectionistic or morally rigid?	Do you ever do things that you wish you hadn't? Do you ever hurt others? Even if it's not on purpose? What do you wish will happen when you [hit other, say something really mean, break/steal someone's toy]? What does happen when you do something that hurts or upsets [someone else]? Can you keep yourself from hitting/getting back at someone if you want to?
Trauma history		Has [child] ever been hurt/injured? Has [child] ever witnessed anything really bad or frightening or been traumatized? Has [child] described frightening dreams/nightmares? Have you [parent] had any traumatic experiences that remind you of what [child] is going through?	Have you ever been hurt? Injured? Have you ever seen anything really bad? Frightening? Have you ever seen anyone get hurt badly? Do you ever have scary dreams or nightmares? Do you ever see or hear something that reminds you of something really scary? Who did/would you tell if someone tried to hurt you?
Family history	Family conflict, differences in parenting style	Do [parents] agree on how to respond to [child]? Is there anything [one parent] does quite differently from [other parent], or from your own parents?	Do your parents tend to agree on how to help you? Punishment and discipline? How have your symptoms affected your family?

TABLE 4.3.4

(CONTINUED)

Component	Description	Sample Questions for Caregiver	Sample Questions for Child
	Developmentally sensitive parenting challenges	Do you treat [child] differently from how you were treated by your parents? Did [parents] grow up in similar type families?	
	Familial/genetic contributions: Mental illness Learning disabilities Notable medical illness Completed suicide Response to medications Anyone who presented similar to child?	Has anyone on father's (mother's) side of the family had depression, anxiety, . . . ? Has anyone in the family had serious medical problems? Has anyone in the family ever been psychiatrically or medically hospitalized? Incarcerated? [If relevant] what was that like for [the child]? What do you think [child] has inherited from [all parents, biologic, and adoptive] ?	Are you like anyone else in your family? Do you know if anyone in your family has ever felt like you do?
	Family constellation	What were the circumstances surrounding the conception and pregnancy with [child]? Have there been any times when [child's parents] were separated/together? Have any changes in the family [loss/addition of parent, loss/addition of sibling or other in the home] contributed to [child's] symptoms? What kind of contact does [child] have with [parents, grandparents, primary caregiving relatives]? What does [child] say about [other parent, caregivers?]	Who lives at home? How does everyone at home get along? How do your parents understand you? Have either of your parents ever been away very long? Doe you miss anyone from your family? With whom do you get along best in your home? With whom do you have the hardest time? Why?
Medical history	Name and contact of pediatrician Most recent physical exam, blood work/labs, imaging Active medical problems Past medical problems, including history of head injuries, loss of consciousness, seizures, medical work-ups Prior medical hospitalizations, surgeries	Has [child] ever had any medical illnesses or serious injuries? Been hospitalized? Had any operations? Was [child] physically ill before these symptoms started? Has [child] had any physical symptoms that occur with/since the emotional symptoms?	Have you ever been really sick? Have you ever had to go to the hospital (what happened?) Have you ever had any surgeries (what was that like)? Have you been physically sick since you have had problems with_____?
Medications and allergies	Include efficacy, tolerability, and compliance: Current Past Allergies or adverse reactions	[Walk through medication treatment history] How is [child] with taking medications? Do you have any concerns about the medications? What is your sense of how helpful (or not) the current regimen is? Has [child] ever been allergic to anything?	What's your understanding of why you're taking medications? Have they been helpful? Have you had any side effects?
Educational history	School functioning, including type of school, grade, attendance, accommodations, social connection, strongest and weakest classes, etc. Extracurricular activities and level of mastery and engagement Future orientation (e.g., what do you want to be when you grow up?)	How did [child] do each year in school? Did [child] ever receive any special educational services? Has [child] ever been suspended, expelled, or asked to leave as school? Did [child] ever have any periods of excessive absences? Did [child] ever fail in subjects or grades? Has [child] even had any summer school or after-school tutoring? Is there anything [child] particularly enjoys or does well at in school?	Which subjects do you like best at school? Is the academic work at school reasonable, or too hard or fast? Is there anything you have trouble understanding at school? Has anyone ever helped you with school work? What do they do? Is there anything that would make being in class easier? Who do you sit with at lunch? What do you do at recess?

(continued)

TABLE 4.3.4

(CONTINUED)

Component	Description	Sample Questions for Caregiver	Sample Questions for Child
Strengths and supports	Areas of strength and interest	What is [child] good at? What does [child] do for fun? What does [child] do during the day? What does [child] want to do/wish he could do?	What do you most like to do? What are you really good at? What do your friends/other students think you are really good at? What would you like to be better at? Do you feel special in any way? What do you want to do when you grow up?
	Community and environmental supports	What is your neighborhood like? Do kids play outside much in your neighborhood? Any neighborhood problems or tensions? Is a language other than English spoken at home? If so, by whom, and does [child] also speak/understand that language? [If family is of recent immigrant origins], does [the child] still have close relatives there? Does [child] visit there often? What is the family's religious tradition? Does [the child] attend services regularly or have strong religious identifications? What activities does [child] participate in? Are there others who work with [child]? Do you have any help/support managing these problems with [child]? How do your family members view [child's problems]? Does [child] benefit from interactions/ participation with neighbors/scouting/ hobbies/shared interests with others?	Outside of your home, where are you most happy? Are there any other adults who are special to you/work with you? Can you tell me about your best friends? Are there any kids that bother you or make you uncomfortable? Is there a group you feel a part of? Who do you "hang out" with? Is there a group you would rather be a part of? Are there particular others you'd like to hang out with? Is there any place you really like to go to feel better?
Media diet		What does [child] watch/read/listen to? How much time does [child] spend on social media? Video games? Watching television/movies? Listening to music? Reading? How does media (e.g., social media, television) influence [child]? What effects do you think [child's] musical choices have on him?	How much time do you spend on electronics every day—social media, video games, TV, listening to music? What about [TV show, music, magazine] most appeals to you? How do you feel after watching/ listening/reading ____? Do you ever get into trouble after watching/listening/reading ____? Which apps do you use? What appeals to you about them? What are your go-to social media platforms, and how often are you on them? How do you decide what you post on social media?

For the psychiatric interview of the child to yield accurate, clinically useful information, the interview process and wording of questions must be tailored to fit with the child's understanding (29). The child may simply not understand what the interviewer is seeking, or comprehend terms necessary to answer the questions accurately. In addition, the interviewer must be attuned to the child's efforts with current developmental tasks. The child may provide misleading answers to shield other family members, to protect self-esteem against acknowledging some perceived failing, or to avoid changes even in painful circumstances if the child fears it will entail unwanted change. The adolescent may not trust the interviewer and may provide evasive or misleading answers for fear that the clinician will see him or her as "weird" or "crazy" or might collude with the parents against the teen.

The Adolescent Interview

Adolescents sometimes require additional modifications for this interview (30). First, adolescents sometimes fear parents will skew the interview by getting to tell their "version" first, and the clinician, as an adult, will side with the parents against the adolescent. To prevent this, the clinician may want to speak over the phone initially with the parent about their concerns and about any information they consider important for the clinician to know prior to meeting with the adolescent. This also affords an opportunity for parents to identify information they have not yet shared with the adolescent (e.g., finding drug paraphernalia in the adolescent's room, previous marriages of parents). Meeting briefly for a few minutes with the parent and adolescent to clarify objectives and the format of the evaluation, and then meeting with the adolescent alone at length is more likely to enhance an alliance with an adolescent. Clarifying during this initial segment that the clinician and the parents will later meet alone to review birth history, developmental milestones, and family history usually is acceptable to adolescents.

Adolescents may articulate that they do not want to participate in this evaluation or may resist answering questions. In such situations, the clinician may first validate the adolescent's reluctance to talk about personal matters with an unknown individual and then attempt to encourage the adolescent's cooperation by trying to identify goals the adolescent may wish to be advanced by the assessment and siding with those. For example, the adolescent may respond to clinician efforts to help identify what the adolescent needs to do to satisfy parents so that the adolescent no longer needs to see a psychiatrist. In addition, clinicians can decrease resistance by beginning the history taking by inquiring first about the adolescent's interests, strengths, and musical/athletic preferences, rather than a too-exclusive focus on "problems." Adolescents are often exquisitely sensitive to feeling that they are being perceived or judged as vulnerable, "weird," or "different" from peers; hence it is generally best to begin with strengths before introducing areas of difficulty. In the same spirit, it is best to try to use lay terms, rather than technical terms or those laden with implications of pathology or transgression.

DEVELOPMENTALLY SENSITIVE TECHNIQUES FOR THE PSYCHIATRIC INTERVIEW

The choice of developmentally appropriate techniques to elicit information from children and adolescents is not strictly dictated by chronologic age. As part of their presenting difficulties, some children may have delayed or aberrant development in some realms that impact the conduct of the interview, such as social language. For other children, regression in the face of stress or anxiety may lead to refusal to speak, oppositionality, tantrums, or retreating to other immature behaviors, either in the context of the interview or as an aspect of the child's more general functioning. Distressing content may similarly require interviewer techniques (drawing, puppets, or play) ordinarily used for younger patients. With some children, once they are at ease with the interview situation, more explicit discussion may be able to take the place of play. The optimal combination of techniques most likely to place the child at ease and to obtain useful information will depend on where a given child is on the developmental (cognitive, emotional, interpersonal) spectrum. The choice and timing of techniques further depend on the emotional valence or difficulty of the issue being addressed, and the fluctuations in the rapport between the child and the clinician. In child psychiatric interviews, the clinician continuously monitors the usefulness of a technique at a particular moment and shifts between techniques as the interview unfolds, according to the waxing or waning of the child's anxiety, trust, and engagement.

Four categories of techniques are generally employed in the child psychiatric interview. First, *engagement* techniques are often required to help put the child at ease and elicit the child's willingness to actively participate in the psychiatric interview so that the child will provide accurate and meaningful clinical information. Second, *projective* techniques are used to allow the child to reveal underlying themes or issues which the child may be unable to verbalize directly and to assess the child's unique ways of thinking and responding to stimuli. Third, *direct questioning* techniques are required to clarify particular points or elicit specific information needed to distinguish disorders, contributions to the child's problems, and intervention options. Fourth, *interactive* techniques are needed to clarify how the child relates to, as well as accepts or integrates input from, others. Throughout the psychiatric interview, opportunities for the child to express content in his or her own way must be balanced with the clinician retaining enough control of the interview to ensure sufficient information is obtained to allow effective clinical assessments and treatment planning.

Techniques to Engage the Child

Engaging the child can be challenging, particularly since the child is in an unfamiliar setting with unfamiliar adults involved in an unfamiliar task. Accordingly, making the setting and tasks more familiar often helps put the child at ease and accelerates engagement. To make the setting more attractive, many child psychiatri sts will provide toys in both the waiting room and clinical office. In addition, child-friendly art or even movie posters may simultaneously make the setting more appealing and provide a stimulus for the child to describe reactions to the poster, characters, or movie preferences that may provide important information about the child's underlying concerns or perceptions. Similarly, toy figures, puppets, and similar relationship-oriented toys may ease the child into the interview. Generic toy figures are usually preferable, since they are more likely to evoke the child's specific themes and concerns rather than the prefabricated scripts associated with specific toy characters based on TV shows or movies. Tasks that are framed as games or that involve activities (drawing a house or family) familiar to the child often help the child transition into the psychiatric interview.

In addition to making the child feel comfortable, engagement techniques facilitate the child's presentation of information. Imaginative play with puppets, toys, or the interviewer provides useful inferential material about the child's concerns, perceptions, and characteristic modes of regulating affect, impulses, and transitions. By allowing the child to direct the content, the interviewer can follow the sequence of the child's concerns, note themes that emerge, and observe the points at which a child backs away from the story line, shifts to a new activity or topic, or falls into a repetitive loop. The form of the child's play further provides mental status information about the child's coordination and motor skills, speech and language development, attention span, readiness to engage the interviewer, capacity for complex thought, and affective state. Absence of imaginative play or concrete, repetitive, noninteractive play, for example, may suggest autism spectrum disorder.

Adolescents can be difficult to engage. Efforts to indicate familiarity with contemporary adolescent tastes (music, movies, terms) can be perceived as disingenuous by the adolescent. Instead, clinicians may engage the adolescent by inquiring about current interests, musical preferences, and adherence to current adolescent values, but from a curious, "just help me understand it" perspective, rather than from one of "trying to be hip." Adolescents often are ambivalent about the talking relationship, so fidget toys (squeeze balls, modeling clay, finger cuffs, cards) allow a socially acceptable option for keeping their hands busy during the interview and make the interview feel less like an interrogation. Complex games, such as chess or video games, require such focus that the interview may become subordinate to the game itself, impeding the clinical interview.

Concern about judgment can limit how vulnerable a child is willing to be with a clinician. It can be helpful for the clinician to maintain a goal of figuring out what is compelling/likeable about the child to help create a genuine interest in and connection with the child. Sometimes, the clinician is in the position of holding hope until the child can regain hope that things can get better, so finding ways to genuinely portray interest can improve patient engagement and alliance.

Projective Techniques

In addition to imaginative play, projective techniques may help the child express concerns indirectly, so that anxiety about significant fears, telling family secrets, or betraying loyalties is minimized. Among the most common projective techniques is picture drawing. Commonly, the child is asked to draw a picture of him/herself or family doing something. By complimenting the picture close to its completion and expressing curiosity about what is happening in the drawing, the clinician can help ensure that the content of the picture, rather than its artistic quality, remains the focus of the interview. For pictures of the child, body details including sizes of appendages or body parts (e.g., fingers, toes), relative size of the figure to the page, and frequent erasures can all reveal underlying issues of anxiety, perceived agency to address difficulties, or needs to control the environment. Depictions of the self as nonhuman, grotesque, imbued with super powers, or of the opposite gender may provide clues about the child's self-image and underlying wishes. The relative size and placement or omission of family members in a family drawing may illuminate the child's feelings about family relationships. Aggressive or sexual themes may be revealed more readily in drawings than in words.

Verbal projective techniques can similarly yield important information. Asking what animal or character (TV/movie star, cartoon, superhero) the child would most like to be, or whom the child would take along to a deserted island, or asking what the child would do with three magic wishes often allow underlying issues to emerge. For example, children may describe wishes to be dominant predator animals to avoid being harmed, or to be gentle animals so that their rage might become less of a problem. Wishes may reveal basic needs, such as food or a safe place to live, or longings for parents to reunite or for the return of a departed friend. Wishes sometimes reveal specific desires, such as "not to have tics anymore," or "never to get teased." Very general or altruistic wishes, such as "world peace" or "to live in a big house with lots of money" warrant further exploration, such as "Are there particular fights you would especially like to stop?" or "Who else would live there?" and "What would you do first with lots of money?"

Open-ended interactive techniques require the child to respond to changes introduced by the clinician. The squiggle game described by Winnicott (31) consists of the clinician drawing a "squiggle," or curvy line, and asking the child to turn it into a picture of something. The resulting picture can then be described and discussed between the child and clinician. The child may also produce a squiggle for the clinician to develop, and the clinician can draw pictures of subjects or topics suspected significant to the child. In addition, incomplete, affectively evocative beginnings of stories or fables can be described to the child, who then elaborates or completes the story (1).

Projective techniques may help adolescents to reveal and share emotionally significant concerns with the clinician despite the developmentally expectable suppression of fantasy in favor of more realistic discourse and reluctance to reveal vulnerabilities or anxieties to adults. Inquiries into favorite, or most disliked, movies, television characters, political or historical figures, musicians or artists, or sports figures all allow elaboration of the teenager's ideas (and ideals) in displacement. The more the adolescent resists direct discussion of his or her own concerns, the greater the displacement that may be required between the projective figure and the adolescent's real life. For example, adolescents less distrustful of the clinician may readily speak about their own social longings or anxieties regarding friends at school, while those adolescents more suspicious of the clinician's motives or wary of self-revelation may be more likely to reveal personal concerns or feelings as projected on or embodied in celebrities or other characters distant from the adolescent's real life. Adolescent resistances are often revealed by reluctance to divulge names of friends, or even questions about why the clinician needs to know this information. If resistance is detected, questions about what the adolescent most admires about a character, or what the adolescent imagines this character would do in given situations, may reveal the adolescent's perceptions or repertoire of response options through projection onto the character.

Since one of the developmental tasks of the adolescent is to find a place among peers, the vicissitudes of joining, rejecting, or being rebuffed by various groups of peers is an essential part of the adolescent's process of social self-definition. Amidst this preoccupation with ingrouping/outgrouping, adolescents are very sensitive to being included or excluded, and issues of fairness, justice, and revenge arise. Asking the adolescent about the different cliques or groups at school and his or her relationship to them provides useful information about the teen's self-image. Similarly, questions about what the adolescent sees as fair or not fair and what he or she would most like to change about his or her school or the world often reveals underlying concerns and issues.

Older adolescents may be able to respond to second-order or circular questions about what others think someone else's motives or thoughts were. For example, the clinician might ask what the adolescent thinks his best friend was thinking when the friend skipped school. Again, if the adolescent finds a topic too emotionally charged or fears betraying a peer, the clinician may need to ask about those more distant. For example, the clinician might ask what the adolescent thought a celebrity or movie character was thinking or trying to accomplish (motive) when the movie star made certain comments or engaged in certain behaviors.

Additional projective techniques are appropriate for all age levels and provide another vehicle to elicit significant information unique to that child. Asking the child or adolescent about favorite books, magazines, music, television shows, movies, or video games may provide important information and help cultivate bonds of common interest between the child and clinician. Particularly if the evaluation is to extend over multiple sessions, or if treatment with the clinician is anticipated, the clinician's exploration of the child's preferred media may help convey interest in the child's world, as well as help illuminate important concerns on the child's part. While the clinician has to be careful not to impose ideas or judgments of characters important to the child, such figures often provide a vehicle or mechanism for discussing difficult content.

Direct Questioning

The goal of direct questioning is to clarify the presence or chronology of symptoms or events, to explore how the child sees the world and functions within it, and to follow up on themes suggested by the history or through play and other interactions with the clinician. Direct questioning can help fill in gaps not revealed by the child, and may help focus attention if responses become circumstantial or tangential. Direct questions may seem to benefit clinician needs more than the concerns of the child, so children may resist answering direct questions, particularly if the child imputes a critical or intrusive intent to the question or an effort to label him or her in some way as crazy, weird, or otherwise deviant. Tact, timing, and the phrasing of the question; appreciation of the child's cognitive and linguistic development; and regard for the impact of the question on the child's self-esteem all influence the effort the child will make to respond to a direct question. In addition, the structure of the question will markedly affect the quality of the child's response.

Questions that allow the child control of the depth of the response are usually preferred early in the interview, and more focused questions can be employed later as needed. Asking the child to describe friends ("Tell me about your best friend"), siblings, or parents, is preferable to "Do you get along with your brother?" which may invite only a "yes" or "no" response. Open-ended questions such as "What sorts of things make you mad/afraid/happy?" and "What do you daydream about?" are similarly preferable to "Do you get mad?" or "Do you ever daydream?" Early in the interview, less anxiety-provoking questions are preferred ("What is your school like?"), as momentum can be generated for the more difficult questions about family relationships or why others are distressed by the child's symptoms or behaviors.

For younger children, anchoring direct questions chronologically to major events may help children provide more accurate answers. For example, "Did that happen before or after your birthday?" or "How has that (problem) been since school ended?" allow greater precision by the respondent. At the same time, direct questions should continue to elicit feelings rather than "just the facts," since the child's affective narrative history is usually more important than the actual chronicle of events.

Similarly, direct questioning in adolescents may require particular tact and attention to positives or strengths before questions about the adolescent's negative behaviors can be addressed. For example, inquiries into the adolescent's best school subjects or what avocations the adolescent is good at may need to occur before inquiries about troublesome school subjects, or the adolescent's current problems. "No fault" phrasing of sensitive questions can help diffuse defensiveness on teens' parts. For example, "Are there ever any rough spots between you and other kids?" is a preferable starting point for inquiring about social difficulties rather than "Do you ever have trouble getting along with other kids?" Asking about future aspirations ("What would you like to do once you've finished with school?") also often provides a useful window into the adolescent's ideals, interests, quality of self-appraisal, and degree of identification with his or her family's values.

Substance abuse, sexuality, and risky behaviors are, by necessity, often assessed through direct questions. However, more general questions initially may make these topics more comfortable and thus the information obtained more accurate. The clinician can often use a simple question, such as "What's your take on drugs and alcohol?" that allow substantial latitude, and then focus in further, contingent on the child's responses. For example, the clinician may hear "No, I don't do any of that anymore," which could then be followed by "What led to that decision?" and then proceed backward to when and what substances were used. Similarly, sexuality can be assessed by gentle direct questions such as "Have you ever had romantic feelings toward another (or liked someone as more than a friend)? How did that go?" (instead of "Have you had a boyfriend yet?"). Children and adolescents are often very cautious about discussing sexual urges, even more so if they fear the interviewer will be disapproving; hence, non-gender-specific grammar is useful initially ("romantic feelings toward anyone" rather "Are there any girls you like?") (1) to indicate, at least implicitly, that one is open to hearing about homoerotic, as well as heterosexual, attractions. Finally, direct inquiries into risky behaviors (stealing, vandalism, assaults, gambling) often require general questions such as "Have you done anything that you now look back on and think 'that was pretty dangerous'?" "Have you ever done anything that would have gotten you in trouble if your parents or other grownups knew about it?" before proceeding to specific questions ("Have you ever stolen anything? Have you ever been beat up? Beat up someone else?"). Suicidal risk behaviors may be minimized or trivialized, particularly in adolescents, so additional questions to examine the adolescent's historical "genogram" of connections to others, fantasies about impacts of the suicide on family and friends, and value contradictions may be needed to clarify suicidality risks (32).

Interactive Techniques

During the interview, the clinician is uniquely positioned to observe firsthand how the child relates to another person and what feelings or reactions this elicits. How the child initially reacts to a new person, how the child sustains interaction throughout the interview, and how the child terminates the interview often reveal patterns important in the child's larger social life. Social rules of conduct, forced transitions, and game playing all allow the clinician to evaluate the child's ways of relating to others. The clinician can employ normal social conventions such as smiling, bending down to the child's level to obtain eye contact, and offering to shake hands to discern the child's initial reactions to unfamiliar others. The clinician can assess how the child negotiates social situations even in small interactions such as determining who will sit in which chair. The clinician can evaluate more complex social interactions during transitions ("It's time to put these toys up in the box.") and during games. Short games (tic tac toe) are useful since the clinician can quickly detect how the child responds to winning, tying, and losing.

Adolescents rely on more complex patterns of relating, often specific to a subgroup to which they now belong. For example, dress or language may be imbued with special meaning within adolescent subgroups, so clarifying what clothing symbols represent, idiosyncratic meanings of confusing terms, and values espoused by any identified subgroup the adolescent appears to embrace can all clarify the adolescent's patterns of relating and values. For example, an adolescent may wear a shirt with Bob Marley's picture on it, and inquiry may reveal the adolescent's commitment to equality. Similarly, the child may describe being "Goth," "punk," "straight-edge," "hip-hop," or other terms. Rather than attempting to be "with it" or assuming one knows what these imply to the patient, it is helpful to inquire what that term or ethos means to this adolescent. In addition, the adolescent may employ gestures or language ordinarily offensive or off-putting to the clinician. The clinician should observe whether these appear to be efforts to provoke the clinician, to titrate space between the clinician and the adolescent, or to be the adolescent's customary idiom, which the adolescent may not realize alienates others.

CONCLUDING THE INTERVIEW

Allowing the interview to end in a collaborative fashion increases the likelihood that the child will feel positive about the interview and any subsequent encounters with clinicians, including other evaluations or treatments. The clinician may wind up the interview by empowering the child with some degree of ownership of this interview. Questions which turn the interview topics over to the child such as "Are there other things that would be important for me to know about you or how things have been for you?" or "What else have I not asked about that is important?" facilitate this process. Similarly, questions such as "I've asked you lots of questions—do you have any questions for me?" demonstrate respect for the child.

The child may be curious about what the clinician thinks about the child and with whom the clinician will share findings. Most often, the clinical interview is but one piece of a larger evaluation, so the clinician may need to clarify that additional laboratory or paper–pencil testing, conversations with teachers or family members, or additional meetings may be needed for the clinician to have a fuller or more accurate impression. Discussing findings (including treatment recommendations) with parents first before discussing them with the child is usually advisable so that additional conflict is not generated if parents should disagree with the clinician's conclusions or resist certain suggested interventions (medication, individual therapy, changes in school placement).

LABORATORY EVALUATION IN THE CHILD PSYCHIATRIC EVALUATION

New techniques of molecular genetics, neurobiology, functional and structural imaging, and neuroendocrinology are deepening our understanding about the pathogenesis and biologic underpinnings of developmental psychopathology. Still, at this time, few, if any, definitive clinical tests exist to identify specific child psychiatric disorders. In the child psychiatry evaluation, laboratory testing remains a vehicle to identify a small number of specific etiologies of certain psychiatric symptoms, as suggested by history or physical findings that warrant such testing, rather than a widely applicable method of screening for specific psychiatric disorders.

Pediatric Collaboration in the Laboratory Evaluation

Close collaboration with the child's pediatrician or primary care provider remains important throughout the child psychiatry evaluation. These providers are familiar with the child's medical and developmental trajectory, as well as family background, and are often positioned to provide essential input on the emergence or progression of a child's symptoms. In addition, the pediatrician or other primary care provider may serve as an invaluable collaborator in the child's ongoing care.

The pediatric examination is a useful complement to the child psychiatric evaluation. The pediatric review of systems may clarify physical changes important in the evolution of the child's symptoms. In addition, growth charts may reveal changes in head circumference relevant to autism spectrum disorder, abnormalities in weight suggestive of an eating disorder or failure to thrive, or changes in stature relevant to hormonal changes. Similarly, the pediatric physical examination may identify visual or hearing problems that explain learning, language, social, attentional, or oppositional problems, as well as pubertal precocity or delays which have important psychosocial consequences. The pediatric examination may also reveal emerging complications associated with treatment (such as weight gain or metabolic dysregulation associated with atypical antipsychotic use). The pediatrician may also identify congenital anomalies or other developmental physical features suggestive of specific developmental disorders or other medical disorders accompanied by psychiatric symptoms.

Collaboration with the primary pediatric care provider may help guide decisions about possible further medical consultations (e.g., audiometric, genetic, neurologic, speech) or other diagnostic tests (e.g., blood tests, electroencephalograms, neuroimaging, sleep studies).

Testing in Specific Childhood Disorders

Laboratory evaluation is warranted when other history or physical findings suggest a particular potential medical diagnosis, such as hyperthyroidism. Routine use of laboratory testing yields findings which alter the working diagnosis in approximately 1% of cases, and the yield for laboratory abnormalities, without the presence of other supportive signs or symptoms, remains less than 5% (33). Laboratory tests commonly considered in key forms of child psychopathology, particularly when other symptoms accompany the psychiatric symptoms, are summarized in Table 4.3.5; the interested reader is also referred to the related chapters elsewhere in this

TABLE 4.3.5

LABORATORY TESTING TO CONSIDER FOR PSYCHIATRIC DISORDERS

Disorder	Testing
ADHD	• Consider lead level if reason for concern
Anxiety disorder	• Consider thyroid function test (TFT), complete blood count (CBC), basic metabolic profile (BMP)
Autism spectrum disorder	• Consider workup to identify comorbid conditions important for treatment or genetic counseling, e.g., Fragile X, Angelman syndrome, and tuberous sclerosis complex • Consider EEG to detect possible comorbid seizures
Depression/Mood disorder (24)	• Consider CBC, BMP, TFT, vitamin B12, vitamin D, folate, urinalysis, toxicology screen • Also consider infectious etiology per clinical history, e.g., mononucleosis, Lyme, HIV
Anorexia	• Comprehensive metabolic profile (CMP), calcium, magnesium, phosphorous, CBC including differential (anemia, leukopenia, thrombocytopenia), TFT, vitamin B12, vitamin D, internationalized normalized ratio (INR) • Urinalysis for specific gravity (hydration status) • EKG +/– fuller cardiac evaluation as indicated • Consider bone density test
Bulimia	• CMP, calcium, magnesium, phosphorous, CBC, urinalysis • Consider EKG

OCD and related disorders (34)	If abrupt, dramatic onset of symptoms consider: PANS (pediatric acute-onset neuropsychiatric syndrome) or PANDAS (pediatric autoimmune neuropsychiatric disorders associated with strep infections)
	• CBC with manual differential, CMP, erythrocyte sedimentation rate (ESR) and C-reactive protein (CRP)
	• Urinalysis; clean-catch urine culture for those with pyuria
	• (PANDAS) Confirm group A beta-hemolytic streptococcal bacteria (GAS) infection via
	  • throat or skin culture or rapid antigen detection test for GAS at the beginning of a PANDAS exacerbation (follow-up culture if the test is negative) or
	  • clinically significant rise in antistreptococcal antibody (anti-DNase B (ADB) and antistreptolysin O (ASO)) between the onset of symptoms and 4–8 wks later.

Psychosis (35)	• CBC, CMP, calcium and phosphorus, TFT, ESR, antinuclear antibodies, ceruloplasmin, HIV screening, FTA-Abs for syphilis (strongly recommended. *RPR not sufficient*), vitamin B12 • Urinalysis, urine drug screen • MRI to rule out demyelinating disease, brain tumor (e.g. meningioma) • EEG to rule out a seizure disorder

APPENDIX 4.3.1

SAMPLE LETTER FOR PARENTS DESCRIBING THE CHILD PSYCHIATRIC ASSESSMENT

Dear [Parent],

We look forward to seeing [child's name] on [date]. This assessment will last approximately [time allotted]. Unless your child is very young, or uncomfortable separating from you, usually [clinician's name] will meet briefly with the parent or adults alone to understand their primary concerns, to obtain relevant medical and family history, and to review any sensitive information important to the assessment, but which may not have been discussed with your child. Bringing toys or activities (books, mazes) to occupy your child during this part of the assessment can be helpful in making him or her comfortable. Report cards, reports from school, prior clinicians, or others involved in the child's care (daycare, courts), or educational or psychological testing reports can be very helpful, so we encourage you to bring these.

[Clinician's name] will usually then meet with your child alone for [allocated time], as well as, perhaps, with all of you together. This interview will include questions about how he or she interacts with friends, parents, and teachers; your child does not need to prepare for this interview. [Clinician's name] may measure your child's height, weight, and pulse and blood pressure, but the child will not need to change clothes or to expect to be examined like during a pediatric visit. No needles or shots are given during psychiatric interviews.

After interviews with you, and with your child, [clinician's name] will finish up the meeting by discussing "next steps" with you, and depending on the recommendations, with your child present as well. Commonly, additional input from teachers or other adults familiar with your child may be needed, so your giving consent to speak/interact with them may be discussed. In some situations, [clinician's name] may recommend certain types of treatment and discuss options, including risks and benefits of these treatments. In some cases, rating scales may be provided for you and others to describe or rate symptoms, or to measure changes as interventions are implemented.

At all times, please feel encouraged to clarify any concerns or advance any questions you may have about any part of this assessment or proposed treatment. We are eager to collaborate with you throughout this process.

Sincerely,

[Clinician's name]

APPENDIX 4.3.2

SAMPLE LETTER FOR PARENTS DESCRIBING THE ADOLESCENT PSYCHIATRIC ASSESSMENT

Dear [Parent],

We look forward to seeing [adolescent's name] on [date]. This assessment will last approximately [time allotted]. Usually [clinician's name] will meet briefly with both you and your adolescent to clarify the purpose of this assessment, and then meet for [allocated time] with your adolescent. This interview will include questions about how your teenager interacts with friends, parents, and teachers; he or she does not need to prepare for this interview. [Clinician's name] may measure your adolescent's height, weight, and pulse and blood pressure, but the adolescent will not need to change clothes or to expect to be examined like a regular medical visit. There will not be any needles or shots.

[Clinician's name] usually will then meet with the parent or guardian to review primary concerns, to obtain relevant medical and family history, and to review any sensitive information important to the assessment, but which may not have been discussed with the adolescent. Report cards, reports from school, prior clinicians, or others (daycare, courts), or educational or psychological testing reports can be very helpful, so bringing these is encouraged.

After interviews with you and with your adolescent, [clinician's name] will conclude the meeting by discussing "next steps" with the adults, and depending on the recommendations, with your teenager present as well. Commonly, additional input from teachers or other adults familiar with the adolescent may be needed, so consents to speak/interact with them may be discussed.

Confidentiality can be very important to adolescents, and issues of safety or danger are usually the only circumstances where confidentiality cannot be preserved. Often, however, sensitive subjects may warrant discussion with either the adolescent or parents/guardians alone, so our normal approach is to discuss and decide with adolescents how any sensitive information will be discussed with parents.

In some situations, following this initial evaluation, [clinician's name] may recommend certain types of treatment, and discuss options, including risks and benefits of these treatments. Rating scales may be provided for you and others to describe symptoms, or to measure changes as interventions are implemented.

At all times, please feel encouraged to clarify any concerns or advance any questions you may have about any part of this assessment or proposed treatment. We are eager to collaborate with you throughout this process.

Sincerely,

[Clinician's name]

volume for additional details. More specialized technologies, such as positron emission tomography (PET), single-photon emission computerized tomography (SPECT), functional MRI (fMRI), and brain electrical activity mapping (BEAM) remain attractive research tools, but currently have no routine clinical or diagnostic usefulness in child and adolescent psychiatric populations.

CONCLUSION

The goal of assessment is to determine the presence of psychopathology, assess contributing factors to the presenting problem(s), and determine appropriate treatment interventions. A clinician can gain vital information through a developmentally sensitive interview with a child and parents; simultaneously, clinicians can benefit greatly from collaboration with pediatricians, schools, and other interested adults who can offer additional insights into predisposing, precipitating, perpetuating, and even protective factors. Emphasis on rapport building, empathy for the child and parents, clear understanding of the problem(s) and function of behaviors(s), hopes and expectations of interested parties, as well as strengths and resilience factors can help facilitate accurate information gathering and successful treatment planning. Being flexible in approach and technique during the interview, genuinely listening, and taking parent and child feedback (verbal and nonverbal) into consideration can help put the family at ease and allow for more fluid sharing of information.

References

1. King RA, AACAP Work Group on Quality Issues: Practice parameters for the psychiatric assessment of children and adolescents. American Academy of Child and Adolescent Psychiatry. *J Am Acad Child Adolesc Psychiatry* 36(10 Suppl):4S–20S, 1997.
2. Bostic JQ, Rho Y: Target-symptom psychopharmacology: between the forest and the trees. *Child Adolesc Psychiatr Clin N Am* 15(1):289–302, 2006.
3. Hong DS: Here/in this issue and there/abstract thinking: the secret lives of adolescents: are we asking the right questions? *J Am Acad Child Adolesc Psychiatry* 54(9):697–698, 2015.
4. Ferdinand RF, Hoogerheide KN, van der Ende J, et al.: The role of the clinician: three-year predictive value of parents', teachers' and clinicians' judgment of childhood psychopathology. *J Child Psychol Psychiatry* 44(6):867–876, 2003.
5. Pickles A, Rowe R, Simonoff E, Foley D, Rutter M, Silberg J: Child psychiatric symptoms and psychosocial impairment: relationship and prognostic significance. *Br J Psychiatry* 179:230–235, 2001.
6. Johnson JG, Cohen P, Gould MS, Kasen S, Brown J, Brook JS: Childhood adversities, interpersonal difficulties, and risk for suicide attempts during late adolescence and early adulthood. *Arch Gen Psychiatry* 59(8):741–749, 2002.
7. King RA, Ruchkin VV, Schwab-Stone M: Suicide and the "continuum of adolescent self-destructiveness": is there a connection? In: King RA, Apter A (eds): *Suicide in Children and Adolescents.* Cambridge: Cambridge University Press, 41–62, 2003.
8. King RA, Schwab-Stone M, Flisher AJ, et al.: Psychosocial and risk behavior correlates of youth suicide attempts and suicidal ideation. *J Am Acad Child Adolesc Psychiatry* 40(7):837–846, 2001.
9. Weinreb L, Wehler C, Perloff J, et al.: Hunger: its impact on children's health and mental health. *Pediatrics* 110(4):e41, 2002.
10. Vila G, Zipper E, Dabbas M, et al.: Mental disorders in obese children and adolescents. *Psychosom Med* 66(3):387–394, 2004.
11. Erermis S, Cetin N, Tamar M, Bukusoglu N, Akdeniz F, Goksen D: Is obesity a risk factor for psychopathology among adolescents? *Pediatr Int* 46(3):296–301, 2004.
12. Maehler C, Schuchardt K: The importance of working memory for school achievement in primary school children with intellectual or learning disabilities. *Res Dev Disabil* 58:1-8, 2016.
13. Yeh MT, Chen P, Raine A, Baker LA, Jacobson KC: Child psychopathic traits moderate relationships between parental affect and child aggression. *J Am Acad Child Adolesc Psychiatry* 50(10):1054–1064, 2011.
14. Stattin H, Kerr M: Parental monitoring: a reinterpretation. *Child Dev* 71(4):1072–1085, 2000.
15. Wallerstein JS, Blakeslee S: *The Unexpected Legacy of Divorce: A 25 Year Landmark Study.* New York, Hyperion, 2000.
16. Indredavik MS, Vik T, Heyerdahl S, Kulseng S, Fayers P, Brubakk AM. Psychiatric symptoms and disorders in adolescents with low birth weight. *Arch Dis Child Fetal Neonatal Ed* 89(5):F445–F450, 2004.
17. Silberg JL, Copeland W, Linker J, Moore AA, Roberson-Nay R, York TP: Psychiatric outcomes of bullying victimization: a study of discordant monozygotic twins. *Psychol Med* 46(9):1875–1883, 2016.
18. Bowes L, Joinson C, Wolke D, Lewis G: Peer victimization during adolescence and its impact on depression in early adulthood: prospective cohort study in the United Kingdom. *BMJ* 350:h2469, 2015.
19. Pataki C, Bostic JQ, Schlozman S: The functional assessment of media in child and adolescent psychiatric treatment. *Child Adolesc Psychiatr Clin N Am* 14(3):555–570, 2005.
20. Daley ML, Becker DF, Flaherty LT, et al.: Case study: the internet as a developmental tool in an adolescent boy with psychosis. *J Am Acad Child Adolesc Psychiatry* 44(2):187–190, 2005.
21. Bostic JQ, Schlozman S, Pataki C, Ristuccia C, Beresin EV, Martin A: From Alice Cooper to Marilyn Manson: the significance of adolescent antiheroes. *Acad Psychiatry* 27(1):54–62, Spring 2003.
22. Ouvrier RA, Goldsmith RF, Ouvrier S, Williams IC: The value of the mini-mental state examination in childhood: a preliminary study. *J Child Neurol* 8(2):145–148, 1993.
23. Jain M, Passi GR: Assessment of a modified mini-mental state scale for cognitive functions in children. *Indian Pediatr* 42:907–912, 2005.
24. Pan LA, Martin P, Zimmer T, et al.: Neurometabolic disorders: potentially treatable abnormalities in patients with treatment-refractory depression and suicidal behavior. *Am J Psychiatry* 174(1):42–50, 2016.
25. O'Brien KH, Schlechter A: Is talking about what's wrong necessarily right: a positive perspective on the diagnostic interview. *J Am Acad Child Adolesc Psychiatry* 55(4):262–264, 2016.
26. Shemesh E, Newcorn JH, Rockmore L, et al.: Comparison of parent and child reports of emotional trauma symptoms in pediatric outpatient settings. *Pediatrics* 115(5):e582–e589, 2005.
27. Close N: Diagnostic play interview: its role in comprehensive psychiatric evaluation. *Child Adolesc Psychiatr Clin N Am* 8(2):239–255, 1999.
28. Wren FJ, Bridge JA, Birmaher B: Screening for childhood anxiety symptoms in primary care: integrating child and parent reports. *J Am Acad Child Adolesc Psychiatry* 43(11):1364–1371, 2004.
29. Lewis M (ed): Psychiatric assessment of infants, children, and adolescents. In: Lewis M (ed): *Child and Adolescent Psychiatry: A Comprehensive Textbook.* Baltimore, MD: Williams and Wilkins, 561–572, 1991.
30. King RA, Schowalter JE: The clinical interview of the adolescent. In: Wiener JA, Dulcan MK (eds): *Textbook of Child and Adolescent Psychiatry.* 3rd ed. Washington, DC: American Psychiatric Publishing, 113–116, 2004.
31. Winnicott DW: *Therapeutic Consultations in Child Psychiatry.* London, Hogarth Press, 1971.
32. Galvin MR, Fletcher J, Stilwell BM: Assessing the meaning of suicidal risk behavior in adolescents: three exercises for clinicians. *J Am Acad Child Adolesc Psychiatry* 45(6):745–748, 2006.
33. Challman TD, Barbaresi WJ, Katusic SK, Weaver A: The yield of the medical evaluation of children with pervasive developmental disorders. *J Autism Dev Disord* 33(2):187–192, 2003.
34. Chang K, Frankovich J, Cooperstock M, et al: Clinical evaluation of youth with pediatric acute onset neuropsychiatric syndrome (pans): recommendations from the 2013 pans consensus conference. *J Child Adolesc Psychopharmacol* 1–11, 2014.
35. Freudenreich O: Chapter 5: secondary schizophrenia. *Practical Guides in Psychiatry: Psychotic Disorders.* Philadelphia, PA: Lippincott Williams & Wilkins, 36–44, 2008.

CHAPTER 4.4 ■ PSYCHOLOGICAL AND NEUROPSYCHOLOGICAL ASSESSMENT OF CHILDREN

KATHERINE D. TSATSANIS, LESLEY HART, AND KELLY K. POWELL

NATURE AND USE OF PSYCHOLOGICAL AND NEUROPSYCHOLOGICAL ASSESSMENT

The broad aims of a psychological and/or neuropsychological assessment are threefold: (i) to provide a more complete description and understanding of a child's behavioral, emotional, and cognitive functioning; (ii) to assist with diagnosis; and (iii) to inform strategies for intervention. This is accomplished in part through the use of psychological tests that offer an objective and standardized measure of a sample of behavior, one that allows performance to be evaluated on the basis of empirical data (1). However, it must be emphasized that psychological or neuropsychological tests and resulting test scores are but one part of the assessment process. Test selection and administration are important factors as is, above all, test interpretation. The final analysis is formed from multiple lines of converging evidence and takes into consideration the developmental and environmental context.

Psychological Assessment

Psychological tests were developed as a means to measure individual differences. Although diverse with regard to content, such measures shared a common use, which was to categorize and classify individuals based on observations of their behavior under uniform conditions (1). At the outset such measures were applied toward educational, personnel, and military classification. Differential diagnosis was also identified as a concern in the context of changes taking place in the 19th century in institutional care, and as test development was intended to aid in the educational placement of children, specifically in the study and instruction of children with intellectual disabilities. Experimental psychology was concerned with universal descriptions of human behavior, particularly in the physiology of sensory responses at this time; however, the general emphasis on the need for controlled conditions when making observations has remained at the heart of the standardization of procedures (uniform conditions) in psychological testing (1).

Early interest in educational testing led to the development of more sophisticated principles and measurement techniques that are now used to assess a wide variety of domains of functioning, including social, emotional, neuropsychological, and adaptive behavior. However, it is intellectual assessment that holds a place of notoriety in the history of psychology. Two of the more fundamental issues that have beset intelligence testing are the definition of intelligence, and the use and interpretation of measures of intelligence. As illustrated in Table 4.4.1, theories of intelligence abound. More than this, each theorist posits multiple components or abilities as part of his account of intelligence. As such, it is worth keeping in mind that intelligence is a construct that is neither unitary nor fixed. Additionally, there is a distinction to be made between theories of intelligence and psychometric intelligence. Whereas the former provides conceptualizations of the nature of intelligence, the latter represents the measurement of general mental ability using standardized tests. The global scores yielded from these measures are usually stable and have general predictive value for educational, social, and job outcome. The instruments are limited to what they are measuring, and their interpretation is contingent on valid use, and they are of course subject to misuse.

The use and interpretation of IQ scores is an important matter and a lengthy subject. In brief, from a psychometric perspective, early approaches to psychometric intelligence focused on quantifying a general level of intelligence as represented by a single number (the IQ score) and assignment to a descriptive classification (e.g., "dull" or "very bright"). Subsequent methods have involved profile analysis or a consideration of individual areas of strength and weakness. This approach may be most powerful when integrated with theories of cognitive abilities (13). Indeed, the cross-battery assessment approach (14,15) that has emerged of late in the arena of psychological assessment emphasizes the usefulness of identifying cognitive processes versus, for example, reporting cognitive functioning in the context of a single IQ number. This represents a shift in thinking of cognitive activity in terms of a single function—intelligence—to a multifaceted entity.

Psychological Assessment Goals

The fundamental first step toward treatment planning is gaining a more complete understanding of the individual child. As noted, the psychological/neuropsychological examination is considered to be an integral part of this process. The psychologist/neuropsychologist is in a unique position to consider the influence of the child's cognitive functioning on academic and social emotional functioning (and vice versa). One purpose for seeking an assessment is that of diagnosis and/or differential diagnosis. The referral question may focus on a diagnostic ambiguity or the question may be one of levels of functioning or the development of a specific skill. The second major purpose for an evaluation is to gain information about a child's cognitive and academic profile and/or an augmented understanding of his/her behavioral and emotional functioning. Diagnosis is often emphasized, but what may be needed to design educational as well as treatment objectives is a more detailed assessment of the child's strengths and weaknesses in several areas. For example, language deficits may interfere with the child's ability to form a personal narrative; memory deficits may account for challenges in learning or treatment gains; a child's learning strengths/difficulties may inform the

TABLE 4.4.1

FACTOR ANALYTIC THEORIES OF INTELLIGENCE

Thurstone's Primary Mental Abilities
Thurstone (2) identified 13 factors of which a subset was considered to represent primary mental abilities. These included spatial visualization, perceptual speed, numerical facility, verbal meaning, word fluency, memory, and inductive reasoning.

Cattell–Horn Theory of Cognitive Abilities
Cattell (3,4) proposed two distinct general factors: fluid and crystallized intelligence. Fluid intelligence refers to reasoning ability that is not dependent on prior experience, whereas crystallized intelligence represents learned or stored information. Hence, a distinction is made between those abilities needed in novel problem-solving conditions vs. rote or familiar learning strategies. Horn (5,6) modified this theory to include nine abilities: crystallized ability, fluid ability, visual and auditory processing, short-term and long-term memory, processing speed, decision speed, and quantitative knowledge.

Guilford's Structure of Intellect Model
The three dimensions of this model are operations, contents, and products. Content refers to the kind of information that is being processed (figural, symbolic, semantic, and behavioral). Guilford (7) also identifies five types of mental operations or procedures (evaluation, convergent production, divergent production, memory, and cognition), and six products (units, classes, relations, systems, transformations, implications).

Sternberg's Triarchic Theory of Intelligence
Sternberg (8) proposes a systems approach or integrative theory in which different aspects of intelligence are interrelated. The three main parts of the triarchic theory are componential, experiential, and contextual. In more recent accounts, Sternberg (9) expands his theory and examines the relationship between intelligence and the internal world, experience, and external world of the individual.

Gardner's Multiple Intelligence Theory
Gardner (10) proposes multiple types of intelligence or competencies, including linguistic, musical, logical–mathematical, spatial, bodily kinesthetic, intrapersonal, interpersonal, and naturalist. Although not easily supported, each of the intelligence is viewed as unrelated or separate in their determination.

Carroll's Three-Stratum Factor Analytic Theory of Cognitive Abilities
Carroll's (11) account of intelligence is based on an impressive meta-analysis of test-based research datasets. From this factor analysis of the data, three levels were identified: narrow (65 ability areas), broad (8 factors), and general (a single general factor, g). The second broad stratum includes fluid intelligence, crystallized intelligence, general memory and learning, broad visual perception, broad auditory perception, broad retrieval ability, broad cognitive speediness, and processing speed (reaction time/decision speed).

Das, Naglieri, and Kirby's Planning-Attention-Simultaneous-Successive Processing Model of Intelligence (PASS)
The PASS theory (12) is based on the seminal work of A.R. Luria in neuropsychology, but is also consistent with information processing models of more recent development. Three fundamental and related functional units of the brain are considered to represent four basic psychological processes of attention and arousal, simultaneous processing (organization of information into a coherent whole), successive processing (sequential processing or processing of information in a specific order), and planning (developing the plans or strategies to arrive at a solution or complete tasks).

best modality for presenting information. Third, clinically and in research, assessment measures may be used for pre- and postcomparisons (e.g., in the case of brain trauma, in the evaluation of medication or a treatment program). Measurement through well-constructed tests further serves an important function in research toward the identification of environmental and biologic factors associated with behavioral differences (e.g., gene–brain–behavior relationships).

Neuropsychological Assessment

The traditional neuropsychological assessment is distinguished by its emphasis on producing a description and understanding of the relationship between brain and behavior. A fundamental approach to neuropsychological assessment is measurement of multiple ability domains sufficient to (i) represent the principal areas of functioning thought to be mediated by the brain and (ii) gather the information needed to address the clinical problems presented by the child (16). The assessment is typically quite comprehensive, as it is designed to sample a broad range of skills and abilities in the child. Given the emphasis on brain and behavior, it has been the longstanding practice of neuropsychologists to consider cognitive functioning as multidimensional. In describing the brain–behavior relationship, there is an implicit recognition that cognition as an operation of the brain is complex and any inferences that are made about behavior conceptualized in terms of cognition should reflect this complexity (17).

The basic neuropsychological framework for understanding dimensions of behavior reflects the functional systems of the brain. These divisions may be represented broadly as cognitive, emotional, and control processes, and as connected systems in the brain they can be thought to have reciprocal influence. The domains for assessment include (i) alertness/arousal; (ii) sensory perception; (iii) motor activity; (iv) attention; (v) memory or the encoding, storage, and retrieval of information; (vi) information processing, such as analysis and synthesis of information, problem solving, concept formation, etc.; and (vii) intentional or goal-directed activity, i.e., the organizational programs of behavior, sometimes referred to as executive functions (EFs). Alterations in motivation and emotional capacity are also evidenced in brain injury or disease and should be considered for their impact on these other systems.

A neuropsychological assessment specifically may be sought to (i) ascertain the likelihood that the child's problems in adaptation are the result of compromised brain functioning (versus, for example, the result of a psychiatric disturbance); (ii) enhance understanding of the child's psychosocial behavior by examining cognitive and control processes, such as how information is received, processed, and expressed by the child; and ultimately (iii) identify the pattern or constellation of neuropsychological assets and deficits displayed by the child toward developing strategies for behavioral or educational intervention.

THE ASSESSMENT PROCESS

The psychological/neuropsychological assessment involves (i) clarifying the referral question, (ii) selection and administration of psychological tests, (iii) observation, (iv) interpretation, and (v) diagnostic formulation and recommendations.

Referral Question and Background History

The referral question(s) are initially identified by the parents and/or referring professional involved in the child's care. They are further refined by obtaining information from multiple sources, including interviews with key people in the child's life (parents, teachers, and other professionals), a review of past records (school reports, previous testing, and medical information), thorough history-taking, and talking with the child.

Selection and Administration of Psychological Tests

The types of assessment methods used and the breadth of the battery formed are key to test selection. Typically, a comprehensive evaluation will make use of a variety of assessment methods and assess a range of domains of functioning. One reason for sampling a range of functions lies in the fact that most psychological measures are not "pure"—that is, they do not assess one ability domain alone. It is important to discern whether, for example, on a timed task in which the child is asked to copy figures, poor performance is related to a motor, visual perceptual, attentional, and/or speed of processing issue. Difficulty on a measure of math skills may reflect limits in understanding numerical concepts, remembering math facts, understanding the *language* of mathematics (symbol use), knowing which operations to apply when sequencing (e.g., performing the correct steps in the correct order), copying errors, and/or attending to meaningful visual details (operational sign, place, columns of numbers). Test selection is guided by evaluation of the test itself and related constructs such as norm groups, reliability, and validity (see Table 4.4.2 and discussion below).

Test administration variables include the environmental setting (e.g., quiet, well-lit room, free of interruptions), establishing rapport with the child, and engaging the child in a manner so as to obtain the best possible performance. The rationale for creating optimal performance conditions is related to the purpose of the evaluation; that is, to determine if the child has the component cognitive skills or abilities necessary to function adequately (or more than adequately) at home, at school, or with others. Standardization, which refers to the uniformity of procedure in administering and scoring a test, is also a key concept in test administration. The examiner must know and adhere to the test procedures, including presentation of directions, use of materials, response to queries, etc. In all, the assessment must be conducted effectively to obtain information regarding the level of performance that the child is capable of but also in a standardized manner to ensure comparability of the scores obtained.

TABLE 4.4.2

CRITICAL VARIABLES IN TEST SELECTION

Evidence of reliability
Evidence of validity
Representativeness of standardization group
Up-to-date norms
Ample sample (size) of normative group
Difficulty gradients (3 raw score points or more per standard deviation [SD])
Floors and ceilings (the test is sensitive enough to discriminate the lowest and highest scorers)
Clear presentation of instructions, administration, and scoring
Cost and administration time

Observation of Test Behavior

In addition to obtaining test data, the examiner makes qualitative observations of the child's presentation and performance during the test sessions. Clinical observation is an essential aspect of test interpretation. Test scores represent how a child performs on a particular test at a particular time. Qualitative observations must be integrated with the quantitative information or test scores to provide a more complete understanding of the results and conditions under which they were obtained. This includes variables such as attention, motivation, persistence, fatigue, illness, and rapport, as well as observations regarding how the child approached the tasks (e.g., use of verbal mediation, trial and error, slow but accurate style).

Interpretation of Results

Test interpretation typically involves an analysis of levels and patterns of test performance. The clinician engages in a dynamic process of hypothesis testing and information gathering, reasoning deductively and inductively from the data collected. Interpretation of test results also requires taking into consideration the behavior observed during testing and other relevant behavioral data (e.g., suspicions of a primary visual or hearing impairment) and case history information (cultural, economic, family variables).

Summary and Recommendations

Assessment conclusions and recommendations should be based on all sources of information. The comprehensive assessment is designed to identify the child's assets and deficits in a variety of domains of functioning. This approach promotes an understanding of the challenges the child faces and why, but also the strengths he/she possesses and how these can be used to help remediate areas of weakness. Inferences are derived from these data to determine the services and strategies that will facilitate the child's social, emotional, and academic functioning.

PRINCIPLES OF ASSESSMENT

The psychometric principles of assessment influence test selection, administration, and interpretation. These measurement issues are outlined below to familiarize the reader with the basic constructs and related issues.

Standardization Sampling/ Developmental Norms

The raw scores obtained from tests are for practical purposes meaningless without a basis of comparison. As such, the data obtained from psychological tests are interpreted with reference to a norm group. This aspect of test development and use is fundamental as it permits that evaluation of a child's behavior need not rely on subjective interpretation alone. Rather, such norm-referenced tests offer (1) quantification of the child's level of performance with reference to his/her peer group, (2) an ipsative ("of the self") comparison or analysis of the child's performance across different measures to determine areas of personal asset and deficit, and (3) longitudinal comparison or assessment of gains/loss over time.

Norms are developed empirically on the basis of the performance of the normative sample, also sometimes referred to as the standardization sample. Standardization sampling represents the procedure used; the normative data are obtained under standard conditions with regard to consistency of item content, administration procedures, and scoring criteria. The norm group should be evaluated for representativeness, size, and relevance (18). The norm group should be a representative group of the child's peers and large enough to ensure stability of the test scores. Sattler (18) recommends at least 100 subjects for each age group in the normative sample. In most cases, test developers will draw from U.S. Census Bureau data to determine the composition of this sample based on stratification variables such as age, gender, socioeconomic level, race, geographic region, etc. Many instruments will also offer normative data obtained from special populations to permit comparisons of the child to other children with the same disorder (a peer group as well).

Reliability

The reliability of a test refers to the consistency of measurement; as such, it also speaks to the degree to which test scores are free from random fluctuations of measurement (19). The example of a scale used to measure weight vividly illustrates the importance of the stability of test scores as concerns accuracy or dependability of measurement. Let us say that on one day when you step on the scale it shows a weight of 150 pounds, 100 pounds on the next day, and then 175 pounds the following day. The scale could not be considered a meaningful or accurate measure of your weight. The same could be said for a psychological test that is not reliable. Test results are not interpretable if the test is not reliable, making reliability a fundamental factor in test selection and interpretation.

There are different types of reliability, each of which reflects a different aspect of how a test score is reproducible (Table 4.4.3). The reliability coefficient, symbolized by the letter *r* with two identical subscripts, is used to express the degree of consistency of test scores. It is a particular kind of correlation coefficient with a range of .00 (indicating no association or consistency between scores) to 1.00 (perfect reliability). No assessment measure is 100% reliable, and as such, some error of measurement is to be expected. The reliability coefficient can be used to determine the degree of error variance or random or unsystematic variation in the measurement instrument (1). The error variance of a test is calculated by subtracting the reliability coefficient from 1.00, where 1.00 indicates perfect reliability. Thus, a reliability coefficient of .80 indicates 80% reliability and 20% error variance. Typically, a minimum acceptable level of reliability is .80 (18).

The reliability coefficient is an important number as a measure of consistency, but also as a source of the amount of reliable variance associated with the test. As such, it is used in the calculation of the standard error of measurement (SEM) of a test score and in turn the confidence interval. Scores for a psychological test (e.g., an IQ score) are often reported as falling within a specific range of scores, or within a confidence interval. The psychometric properties of a test are such that although they may aim to quantify level of functioning in a real way, the obtained test score is actually composed of a true score (hypothetical) and an error score (1). The confidence interval represents the range of scores surrounding the obtained score within which the true score is likely to lie. For example, if a child obtains an IQ score of 90, we can state at the 95% confidence level (the usual reported level) that her IQ score on any single administration of the test will lie between 84 and 96. That is, 95 times out of 100, her IQ score will fall within this band of values. The confidence interval is determined by the SEM for the instrument, which in turn is computed from the reliability coefficient.

The major point to underscore here is that the obtained test score is not precise or definitive, as each test inherently contains measurement error that should be taken into consideration

TABLE 4.4.3

OVERVIEW OF TYPES OF RELIABILITY

Types of Reliability	Description
Test–retest reliability	A measure of temporal stability. The reliability coefficient is expressed as r_{tt} and is the correlation between scores obtained by the same persons taking the same test on two different occasions.
Alternate-form reliability	Consistency of test scores when alternate forms of a test are given to the same person. The tests may be given at different times or on the same occasion. As such, this method may be used to minimize practice effects and also to examine whether two different forms (items and item composition) of the test give the same result.
Split-half reliability	A measure of internal consistency or consistency of the content of the test. This type of reliability is measured from a single administration of a single test form, splitting the test in half (e.g., odd and even items of the test) and comparing the two half-scores, usually by means of the Spearman-Brown formula.
Inter-item reliability	Another measure of internal consistency using a single test form and a single administration. In this case, however, reliability is measured based on performance on *each* item relative to the other items of the test and thus gives some indication of the homogeneity of the measure. The usual formula used is Kuder Richardson (when items are scored 0 or 1) or Cronbach's alpha coefficient (for items not scored as right or wrong).
Interrater reliability	Apart from temporal, content, and examinee variables, variance in test scores can arise from examiner factors, such as differences in scoring. Interrater reliability provides a measure of consistency of scores obtained when the same test is scored by two different examiners. This is an especially critical variable when evaluating test forms that leave judgment open to the scorer.

TABLE 4.4.4

OVERVIEW OF TYPES OF VALIDITY

Types of Validity	Description
Construct validity	Examines the extent to which a test measures what it purports to measure, such as a psychological construct or trait. Two constituents of construct validity are *convergent* (measures of related constructs should correlate) and *divergent* (measures of unrelated constructs should not correlate) validity.
Content validity	Refers to the degree to which a test covers the behavior or skill or subject matter being measured. A discussion of the content validity of a test should help to answer whether the test offers representative coverage of the domain assessed, and whether there is influence from other variables.
Face validity	As the name suggests, face validity refers to whether on the surface of things the test appears to be appropriate for its intended use.
Concurrent validity	A form of criterion-related validation in which the current measure is compared to a criterion or outcome to which it is related (e.g., ratings or other test scores).
Predictive validity	Another form of criterion-related validation that examines the degree to which the measure predicts some other criterion in the future (e.g., IQ and later academic success).
Treatment validity	Refers to the clinical utility of an instrument as it relates to the impact of the test results on the examinee's behavior.

when decisions are being made based on a single score (e.g., IQ score for qualification of services). The second and related point is that measurement error must be accounted for when reported scores are compared over time or across instruments. The difference between two test scores may be due to chance factors or the error variance associated with each test. Correspondingly, the reliability coefficient for each test is taken into consideration in the calculation of discrepancy scores.

Validity

Test validity is a term used to represent the meaning or relevance of a test, specifically, whether it measures what it is purported to measure (1). It is a fundamental psychometric concept that can be approached in several ways, as detailed in Table 4.4.4. The validity of a test is relevant when assessing what is being measured and how completely, as well as how to use a test appropriately. Validity coefficients are a type of correlation coefficient and accordingly are impacted by the range of attributes being measured (the narrower the range, the lower the value of the validity coefficient). Examinee variables also can impact validity; if an examinee presents with severe test-taking anxiety, extreme fatigue or illness, a hearing or vision impairment (and, for example, forgets to wear her glasses), or fails to understand the instructions, these factors are likely to render the test scores invalid, as the test is no longer measuring the characteristic it is intended to measure. As such, psychological reports include a section on observations of test behavior and a description of any presenting factors that are a threat to validity. Extrinsic or environmental factors such as socioeconomic status, access to quality teaching or textbooks, or cultural experiences can similarly impact validity and are addressed in the interpretation of test scores.

INTERPRETATION OF TEST SCORES

Derived Scores

A basic feature of interpretation of test scores is the comparison of scores to some standard or norm. As mentioned above, raw test scores, whether the number of points earned, items successfully completed, or symptoms endorsed, are meaningless on their own. Rather, the raw test score is evaluated relative to the test performance of the standardization sample. The question that is answered in this process is where this particular child's score falls relative to the distribution of scores produced by the standardization sample, where the mean represents the average and the standard deviation (SD) represents the variability. There are a variety of derived scores or ways in which this comparison can be reported.

Standard Scores

Standard scores are the most typical and often the most suitable kind of score to report. Standard scores are particularly useful for making comparisons across tests, as the mean and SD are set and there are equal units along the scale (19). For all standard scores, a score falling 1 SD below the mean (below the average range) or a score falling 2 SD above the mean (well above average) occupies the same position relative to the group apart from the instrument used. Comparability of scores in this manner is achieved through a transformation of the raw data. The usual types of reported scores are standard scores, scaled scores, and T-scores (Table 4.4.5). The typical standard score has a mean set at 100 and an SD of 15. Most major cognitive and achievement assessment batteries report global scores in this format. Individual subtest scores, however, may be represented as scaled scores with a mean of 10 and an SD of 3. Some tests and many behavior checklists yield T-scores, which have a mean of 50 and an SD of 10.

Percentile Scores

Percentile scores are a popular means for reporting test performance as they are easy to understand; a percentile rank is a way of positioning the child's performance relative to the norm group in familiar terms (18). For example, a percentile rank of 84 indicates that the child scored as well as or better than 84%

TABLE 4.4.5

Z-SCORES AND DERIVED SCORE EQUIVALENTS

Z-Score	Standard Score	T-Score	Scaled Score	Percentile Rank
−3	55	20	1	1
−2	70	30	4	2
−1	85	40	7	16
0	100	50	10	50
+1	115	60	13	84
+2	130	70	16	98
+3	145	80	19	>99

of the norm group. There are some caveats. Naïve consumers of these test scores may confuse percentile ranks with percent of items passed (such as an 84% on a test). A major concern also with regard to percentile ranks (vs. standard scores) is that the units are unequal. The numbers can be deceptive and may overemphasize or underemphasize differences between standard scores. For example, note that scores between the 25th and 75th percentile are all within the average range.

Age and Grade Equivalent Scores

Test scores in some cases are also reported in terms of age and grade equivalents. An age equivalent score is determined based on the performance of each age group in the norm sample. If the average raw score of the 8 year olds in the sample is 14, then a raw score of 14 yields an age equivalent of 8 years. Age equivalent scores thus describe the raw score obtained and do not necessarily correspond to the child's level of functioning, nor do they represent equal units.

Grade equivalents are similar in that grade norms are computed from the mean raw score obtained by children in each grade in the standardization sample. Again, if the average raw score on a reading test for single words corresponds to 25 for fourth graders, then a raw score of 25 corresponds to a grade equivalent of 4. Grade units are unequal and do not represent the variability between subject areas at different levels. It is also important to recognize that when a fourth-grade child obtains a grade equivalent score of 6.5 on an arithmetic test, it does not necessarily indicate that the child is capable of grade 6 arithmetical processes or should be placed in the seventh-grade curriculum (1). Rather, the child's total raw score may reflect superior performance on fourth-grade arithmetic. The point is that psychological tests are typically constructed to provide a range of scores. If we consider the standardization sample of children in the fourth grade, there will be a distribution of scores for this group of children; an average raw score for this group will represent the average score on the test at the fourth-grade level. The children who perform well above average within this distribution will produce a well-above average score on the test for their comparison group and may in turn share a total raw score with the average sixth grader. Additionally, the same raw score yielding the same age or grade equivalent could be obtained in a very different way relative to the individual items of the test and thus have a different meaning. Although appealing, age and grade equivalent scores are easily subject to misinterpretation; they do not necessarily reflect a particular level of knowledge but are rather another means of indicating where a child falls relative to a particular kind of reference group (19). On the other hand, the advantage of reporting scores in this format is that they are easily understandable and place performance within a familiar developmental context. In this case, correct interpretation is paramount.

Descriptive Levels

In addition to a quantitative representation of performance, classification of ability levels is applied to standard scores, based on whether the score corresponds to the average performance of the normative group or, for example, the upper or lower extreme end of the distribution. These descriptions of performance are widely used to represent how far a child's score deviates above or below the mean. The qualitative descriptors provided vary from instrument to instrument. Two examples are detailed in Table 4.4.6. In the event that a child's file contains several different reports, one should keep in mind that derived scores can be converted to a uniform metric for comparison. Knowing the child's test score, the mean and SD of the test, and assuming that the scores on the test fit to a normal distribution (which would be true of most major assessment instruments), then it is easy to determine where the child's scores fall relative to the mean. This would be achieved by taking the child's test score, subtracting the mean, and dividing by the SD. Thus, if a child obtained an IQ score of 115 on a test that has a mean of 100 and SD of 15, his or her score would be 1 SD above the mean. Similarly, if the same child obtained a T-score of 60 on a different measure (with a mean of 50 and SD of 10), his or her score would also be 1 SD above the mean. If percentile scores are reported on a given test, these too can represent the child's position relative to the standardization sample (see Table 4.4.5). A special note about IQ scores: The traditional means of obtaining an IQ score (or intelligence *quotient*) was to take the ratio of mental age (MA) divided by chronologic age (CA) and multiply by 100. The problem with

TABLE 4.4.6

CLASSIFICATION OF ABILITY LEVELS

Standard Score	Percentile Rank	Descriptive Classification[a]
69 and below	<2	Extremely low
70–79	2–8	Very low
80–89	9–23	Low average
90–109	25–73	Average
110–119	75–90	High average
120–129	91–97	Very high
130 and above	98–99.99	Extremely high

Standard Score	Descriptive Classification (10-Point Scale)[b]	Standard Score	Descriptive Classification (15-Point Scale)[b]
69 and below	Very low	40–54	Very low
70–79	Low	55–69	Low
80–89	Below average	70–84	Below average
90–109	Average	85–115	Average
110–119	Above average	116–130	Above average
120–129	High	131–145	High
130 and above	Very high	146–160	Very high

[a]Widely used WISC-V (20) descriptive classifications.
[b]KTEA-3 (21) descriptive classifications.

this procedure is that ratio IQ scores at different ages are not comparable and thus not psychometrically sound in practice. Although the term IQ has been retained, current measures of IQ do not derive scores based on the above formula; rather, these so-called deviation IQs are a type of standard score and as described above fit to a distribution with a mean of 100 and an SD of 15. However, knowledge of the ratio IQ is handy when there is limited information and a need to make a *rough* approximation of the child's ability level.

Significant Difference

Derived scores and classification of ability levels provide a means to compare a child's performance relative to his or her peers as defined by the norm group. However, test interpretation also involves a comparison of the child's different ability levels across domains of functioning and in some cases across time. For example, we may want to know whether Sam is more able on verbal versus visual spatial tasks, whether Alice's reading skills are consistent with expectations given her overall IQ, or whether ratings of Justin's behavior at home and school are significantly different. There are two considerations to keep in mind when comparing whether two scores are different or not: (a) statistical significance and (b) unusualness or abnormality of difference. The first, statistical significance, answers whether the results differ from what would be expected based on chance alone (18). The usual p-value for this calculation is .05, meaning that, if the difference between two scores is significant (not due to chance factors), we accept a 5 out of 100 chances of being wrong. Test publishers will report domain and subtest score differences in their manuals or computerized printouts. When making comparisons between two different tests, either of the following two calculations can be made, which take into account the error variance of each test:

$$SE_{diff} = \sqrt{(SEM_1)^2 + (SEM_2)^2}$$

$$SE_{diff} = SD\sqrt{2 - r_{11} - r_{22}}$$

The standard error of the difference (SE_{diff}) is then multiplied by 1.96 to determine how large a score difference could be obtained by chance at the .05 level (1).

In addition to answering whether two scores are significantly different in statistical terms, the second part of interpretation lies in determining whether the difference is clinically significant. One way to address this particular question is to examine base rate frequency; that is, to ask how unusual it is to find this difference in scores. Test publishers of cognitive and achievement test batteries will typically provide this information in supplementary tables. A difference of scores that is found in only 5% of the norm sample can be considered unusual and highly unusual when present in only 1% of the sample.

Sometimes standard scores in a domain of functioning may decline over time. This finding does not necessarily represent a deterioration or regression, but rather, may reflect a failure to make age-appropriate gains (rate of gain slower than rate of change in chronologic age). If standard scores on the *same* test are found to be significantly different across time, it would be important to look at the raw scores and pattern of scores obtained on each test before assuming there has been a loss of skill. Additionally, of course, it will be important to consider other variables that might have affected the test performance (such as fatigue, illness, compliance). Table 4.4.7 lists several other factors to consider when test scores for the same child on (ostensibly) the same kind of test differ (the child scores in

TABLE 4.4.7

SOME REASONS WHY TEST SCORES MAY DIFFER

Norms	A difference in the age of the norms could impact test scores. The Flynn effect refers to a finding by J.R. Flynn (22) that there is a continued rise in IQ test performance. The average rate of rise seems to be around three IQ points per decade. The composition of the normative sample used to develop the test scores is different and may represent a less or more able group.
Test Units	The scores are reported in different units of measurement. For example, a score of 115 on one test and a score of 60 on another may in fact represent the same level of performance if in the case of the former the mean is 100 with an SD of 15 and in the case of the latter the mean is 50 with an SD of 10. Alternatively, two tests could both have a mean of 100 but different SDs.
Floor and Ceiling Effects	Floor effects occur when the test lacks enough easy items to discriminate between low scorers, and ceiling effects refer to when the measure lacks enough hard items to adequately assess upper levels of ability. A raw score of 0 on one test may produce an IQ score of 40 but an IQ of 70 on another test as a result of differences in the lower limits of the test items. If the referral includes a question of MR, test selection is paramount to ensure adequate range at the lower levels to make this discrimination.
Correlations Between Tests	Two tests may yield score differences because the tests are not correlated or only moderately related.
Reliability	Test scores for children 5 yrs of age and under are typically less reliable than those obtained in school-age children. Test length can also affect reliability. To determine how large a difference is needed for statistical significance (to be confident that the discrepancy between scores is not due to chance factors alone), a calculation is made that takes into account the reliability of each test.
Item Content Differences	Tests intended to measure the same domain may diverge in content and response despite sharing a similar name. For example, IQ measures may differ in terms of the level of language, memory, and/or speed of processing demands that factor into the overall score. A reading comprehension test may involve reading a sentence or a passage, aloud or silently. Additionally, the response required may be dissimilar between tests, ranging from filling in a missing word, enacting what is read, or responding to oral questions about what was read.
Practice Effects	Scores may improve because of familiarity with the test or test items or prior exposure. Practice effects appear to be most pronounced on nonverbal vs. verbal tasks, perhaps because of their novelty. Most tests should not be re-administered until after a period of time has passed (typically, 1 yr) in order to minimize such effects.
Other Factors	Differences related to variables such as fatigue, illness, medication, motivation. Actual gain, loss, or discrepancy in skill level can be noted.

the intellectually disabled range on one cognitive test but not another). These factors are important to consider, particularly in the interpretation of IQ scores, as they impact diagnosis and the procurement of services.

Levels of Analysis

Interpretation involves the analysis and synthesis of all of the data obtained as part of the assessment. To assure ecologically valid conclusions regarding adaptive behavior, it is necessary to sample a wide variety of abilities and skills that interact for successful accomplishment (16). Test performance is examined for statistically significant discrepancies between observed and expected levels. Expected levels of performance may be based on earlier known levels of functioning, age norms, and/or other abilities. It is also generally expected that test scores will converge around the same level, and when functions are not proportionate, one should consider factors such as uneven brain development or brain disturbance, socialization, educational experience, emotional disturbance, physical illness/fatigue, economics, or primary sensory impairments to account for discontinuities in the child's profile (17). Base rates and contextual factors must be taken into account for those discrepancies that are commonly found in the normal population or those measures that are differentially sensitive to cultural, economic, and educational background (e.g., vocabulary level). The test results are further examined for particular patterns of performance. Comparisons may be made along the following lines as examples: domain of functioning (language, visual spatial, memory, problem-solving skills), modality (visual, auditory, tactile), level of task difficulty (simple or complex), speed of processing (speeded versus no time limit), closed or open response structure (forced choice versus generative, recognition versus recall), laterality (right vs. left performances), and so on. Strengths and weaknesses in the child's information processing are thus examined according to how the information is represented and processed, as well as the nature of the response that is required.

DOMAINS OF ASSESSMENT

The domains of functioning assessed and the methods used in psychological/neuropsychological testing are far reaching in their scope, with an overview presented in this section. Individual tests are selected relative to the clinical or research need and developmental capacities of the child or adolescent initially based on an understanding of the child developed from prior assessment and clinical history, and updated with additional tests and subtests to evaluate diagnostic hypotheses based on performance during assessment. Many commonly used assessment instruments organized according to the functional domain assessed are presented in Tables 4.4.8 and 4.4.9. Computer-assisted assessment and scoring is also available for many of these instruments. For more detailed information, key resources on psychological assessment as well as test selection and acquisition are identified in Table 4.4.10.

Psychological Assessment

General Ability and Intelligence

Broad measures of cognitive ability and intelligence provide an estimate of a child's general ability level at a particular point in time in relation to the given age norms (1). Although most cognitive or intelligence tests yield a single IQ or ability score, this should not be interpreted to suggest that intelligence is a single unitary construct. Rather, such measures are typically composed of a variety of subtests measuring a range of functions. Careful interpretation involves an analysis of domain and subtest scores for areas of normative and relative strength and weakness. It is also worth noting that such tests are developed based on different theories of intelligence. Thus, in spite of assessing a shared construct, intelligence tests may differ greatly in terms of content, including emphasis on verbal versus visual information, extent to which speed of processing is emphasized, the type of response format, and so on. In general, tests of cognitive ability and intelligence assess the extent to which a child has acquired information and is able to think abstractly. IQ scores are generally stable in children 5 years of age and older and are predictive of academic abilities in school-aged children. IQ and cognitive assessments may provide useful information with regard to how the child takes in, processes, and responds to information, useful toward treatment planning and provision of differentiated instruction.

Achievement

Achievement tests measure educationally relevant skills or acquired knowledge in subject areas such as reading, spelling, mathematics, written expression, science, social studies, and humanities. Such tests provide a means of identifying strengths or weaknesses in the acquisition of basic academic skills and knowledge in core subject areas. In the past, learning disability (LD) service eligibility had been determined on the basis of IQ-achievement discrepancy scores. There were a host of problems with this approach, both theoretically and practically, including for example that the magnitude of the difference (typically greater than 1 SD) could vary between school districts. The Individuals with Disabilities Education Act (IDEA), revised in 2004, does not allow the use of a discrepancy definition of LD, but instead recommends the use of a procedure for assessing students' response to scientific, research-based intervention. This Response to Intervention (RTI) approach uses a tiered approach in which students receive mainstream education at Tier 1, additional instruction in small groups at Tiers 2 and 3, and only after they have failed to meet benchmarks with this additional instruction, evaluates for special educational services and LD. Thus, children receive services before they are allowed to experience school failure to a point at which they are significantly behind their peers, a requirement of the discrepancy definition of LD. See Fletcher et al. (109) and Fuchs and Vaughn (110) for more information. IDEA also recognizes the importance of examining various cognitive processes and their impact on school learning (111). For example, phonologic awareness, familiarity with words, and ability to retrieve words rapidly are relevant components of reading and spelling competence, and these and other cognitive abilities such as nonverbal reasoning have been found to predict reading ability as much as 5 years later (112). Deficits in working memory are likely to impact math learning, and planning and organization problems can affect written expression. Of note, achievement tests differ widely in content, presentation, and response format. Reading comprehension, for example, may be assessed using written words, sentences, or passages, with responses to oral questions or by filling in the blank. Decoding may be measured using real words, in which vocabulary and sight word recognition can drive scores, or using pseudowords, a more "pure" measure of decoding. Math questions may be presented orally or as a written calculation, with or without visual support, and timed or untimed. Therefore, in interpreting achievement scores, it is also important to understand how the subject matter was assessed.

Behavioral, Social, and Emotional

As a complement to direct behavioral observation and clinical interviewing, behavior rating scales and personality inventories offer a psychometric approach to assessing social emotional problems in children and adolescents (104,113,114).

TABLE 4.4.8

COMMONLY USED CHILD AND ADOLESCENT ASSESSMENT INSTRUMENTS

Tests	For Ages (yrs)
General Ability/Intelligence Tests	
Differential Ability Scales, 2nd edition (DAS-II) (23)	2:6–17:11
Kaufman Assessment Battery for Children, 2nd edition (KABC-2) (24)	3:0–18:11
Stanford-Binet, Fifth Edition (SB-5) (25)	2:0–89:11
Wechsler Preschool and Primary Scale of Intelligence, 4th edition (WPPSI-III) (26)	2:6–7:7
Wechsler Intelligence Scale for Children, 5th edition (WISC-V) (20)	6:0–16:11
Wechsler Adult Intelligence Scale, 4th edition (WAIS-IV) (27)	16:0–90:11
Woodcock Johnson Tests of Cognitive Abilities, 4th edition (WJ-IV) (28)	2–90+ yrs
Abbreviated Intelligence Test Batteries	
Kaufman Brief Intelligence Test, 2nd edition (KBIT-2) (29)	4:0–90:0
Wechsler Abbreviated Scale of Intelligence™ (WASI) (30)	6:0–89:11
Wide Range Intelligence Test (WRIT) (31)	4:0–85:0
Achievement Test Batteries	
Kaufman Test of Educational Achievement, 3rd edition (KTEA-3) (21)	4:6–25;11
Wechsler Individual Achievement Test, 3rd edition (WIAT-III) (32)	4:0–50:11
Wide Range Achievement Test 4 (WRAT4) (33)	5–94 yrs
Woodcock Johnson Tests of Achievement, 4th edition (WJ-IV) (34)	2–90+ yrs
Neuropsychological Test Batteries	
Delis–Kaplan Executive Function System (DKEFS) (35)	8–89 yrs
Halstead–Reitan Neuropsychological Test Batteries (36)	5–8, 9–14, 15+ yrs
Luria–Nebraska Neuropsychological Battery—Children's Revision (37)	8–12 yrs
Luria–Nebraska Neuropsychological Battery (LNNB) (38)	15+ yrs
NEPSY-II: A developmental neuropsychological assessment (39)	3–16 yrs
Reitan–Indiana Neuropsychological Test Battery (40)	5–8 yrs
Nonverbal Tests[a]	
Comprehensive Test of Nonverbal Intelligence, 2nd edition (C-TONI-2) (41)	6:0–89:11
Leiter International Performance Scale, 3rd edition (Leiter-3) (42)	3:0–75+ yrs
Naglieri Nonverbal Ability Test, 3rd edition (NNAT-3) (43)	5–18 yrs (Grades K-12)
Test of Nonverbal Intelligence, 4th edition (TONI-4) (44)	6:0–89:11 yrs
Universal Nonverbal Intelligence Test, 2nd edition (UNIT-2) (45)	5;0–21;11
Wechsler Nonverbal Scale of Ability (46)	4:0–21:11
Adaptive Behavior	
AAMR Adaptive Behavior Scale-School, 2nd edition (ABS-S2) (47)	3–21 yrs
Adaptive Behavior Assessment System, 3rd edition (ABAS-3) (48)	0–89 yrs
Scales of Independent Behavior-Revised (SIB-R) (49)	Infancy–80+ yrs
Vineland Adaptive Behavior Scales, 3rd edition (50)	0–90 yrs
Vineland Social-Emotional Early Childhood Scales (SEEC) (51)	0–5:11
Diagnostic Instruments	
Child and Adolescent Psychiatric Assessment (CAPA) (52)	8–17
Children's Interview for Psychiatric Symptoms (ChIPS) (53)	6–18
Diagnostic Interview for Children and Adolescents (DICA) (54,55)	6–18
Diagnostic Interview Schedule for Children (DISC-IV) (56)	6–17
Schedule for Affective Disorders and Schizophrenia for School-Aged Children (K-SADS) (57)	6–18
Structured Clinical Interview for DSM-IV Childhood Diagnoses (KID-SCID) (58)	7–17

[a]The KABC-2, DAS-II, and SB5 also yield nonverbal composite scores.

General-purpose rating scales provide information about multiple areas of psychopathology as well as attitudes and interpersonal relationships whereas single domain syndrome measures typically assess specific areas such as depression or anxiety according to DSM criteria. Personality tests or inventories are intended to assess relatively stable characteristics of the individual, but in children usually cover a range of psychological and adjustment problems. Social competence measures focus on the assessment of social skills as well as peer relationships; most behavioral scales and personality inventories include these domains but not to the same extent. Behavioral summaries are based on checklists that use dichotomous ratings and an additive scale; the symptom is rated as present or absent and the number of checked items is summed. Rating scales, on the other hand, permit an indication as to whether a symptom is present or not and also the degree to which it is present in terms of frequency (never, sometimes, usually).

TABLE 4.4.9

COMMONLY USED CHILD AND ADOLESCENT BEHAVIORAL, SOCIAL, EMOTIONAL MEASURES

	Behavior Rating Scales				
	Self	**Parent**	**Teacher**	**Clinician**	**Ages (yrs)**
Broad Measures					
Adolescent Psychopathology Scale (59)	x				12–19
Behavior Assessment System for Children, 3rd Edition (BASC3) (60)	x	x	x	x	2:0–21:11 (self 6; 0–college)
Achenbach System of Empirically Based Assessment, Child Behavior Checklist (CBCL) (61)		x			1.5–18
Achenbach System of Empirically Based Assessment, Youth Self Report (YSR) (61)	x				11–18
Achenbach System of Empirically Based Assessment, Teacher Report Form (TRF) (61)			x		6–18
Minnesota Multiphasic Personality Inventory for Adolescents (MMPI-A) (62,63) and Restructured Form (MMPI-A-RF) (64)	x				14–18
Personality Inventory for Children, 2nd Edition (PIC-2) (65)		x			5–19
Personality Inventory for Youth (PIY) (66)	x				9–19
Specialized Measures					
Attention					
ADHD Rating Scale-5 (67)		x	x		5–17
Conners 3rd Edition Rating Scales (Conners-3) (68)	x	x	x		6–18 (self 8–18)
Conners Early Childhood (Conners EC) (69)		x	x		2–6
Swanson, Nolan, and Pelham (SNAP)-IV Rating Scale (70)		x	x		6–18
Strengths and Weaknesses of ADHD symptoms and Normal behavior (SWAN) Rating Scale (71)		x	x		6–18
Anxiety					
Revised Children's Manifest Anxiety Scale, 2nd edition (RCMAS-2) (72)	x				6–19
State-Trait Anxiety Inventory for Children (STAIC) (73)	x				9–12
Beck Anxiety Inventory for Youth (74), Beck Anxiety Inventory (75)	x				7–18; 18+
Multidimensional Anxiety Scale for Children, 2nd edition (MASC-2) (76)	x	x			8+
Screen for Childhood Anxiety Related Disorders (SCARED) (77)	x	x			8+
Depression					
Beck Depression Inventory for Youth (BDI-Y) (74), Beck Depression Inventory-II (BDI-II) (78)	x				7–18; 13–80
Children's Depression Inventory, 2nd edition (CDI-2) (79)	x	x	x		7–17
Reynolds Child Depression Scale (RCDS) (80)	x				7–13
Reynolds Adolescent Depression Scale, 2nd edition (RADS-2) (81)	x				11–20
Children's Depression Rating Scale-Revised (CDRS-R) (82)				x	6–12
Executive Function					
Behavior Rating Inventory for Executive Function (BRIEF) (83)		x	x		5–18
BRIEF—Preschool Version (BRIEF–P) (84)		x	x		2:0–5:11
BRIEF—Self-Report Version (BRIEF–SR) (85)	x				11–18
Learning					
Academic Competence Evaluation Scales (ACES) (86)	x		x		Gr K-12 (teacher), Gr 6–college (self)
Learning And Study Strategies Inventory-High School (87) and Learning And Study Strategies Inventory, 3rd edition (88)	x				High School College
Self Concept					
Beck Youth Inventories™ Self Concept Inventory (74)	x				7–18
Self-Esteem Index (SEI) (89)	x				7–18
Projective Tests:					
Children's Apperception Test (90)					3–10
Draw-a-Person Technique (91,92)					5–17
Kinetic Drawing System for Family and School (93)					5–20
Rorschach Inkblot Test (94)					5–adult
Roberts Apperception Technique for Children (Roberts-2) (95)					6–18
Sentence Completion Techniques e.g., Hart Sentence Completion Test for Children (96), Rotter Incomplete Sentence Blank (97)					Children, adolescent–adult
Thematic Apperception Test (98)					6–adult

TABLE 4.4.10

SOURCES OF INFORMATION ON ASSESSMENT AND ASSESSMENT INSTRUMENTS

Websites

American Psychological Association Testing and Assessment http://www.apa.org/science/testing.html

Resource for guidelines and standards for testing, information about psychological tests, as well as links to other testing websites.

Test Publishers

Publishers provide a description of published tests, age range, administration time, user qualifications, types of scores yielded, cost of purchasing, etc.

Pearson Assessments www.pearsonassessments.com

Pro-Ed www.proedinc.com

Psychological Assessment Resources www.parinc.com

Riverside Publishing www.riverpub.com

Stoelting Company www.stoeltingco.com

Western Psychological Services www.wpspublish.com

Major Test Reviews

The *Mental Measurements Yearbook* (99) and *Tests in Print* (100), from the Buros Institute, contain the most recent descriptive information and critical reviews of new and revised tests. Typically available in the reference section/online at most college/university libraries, they can also be accessed for a fee at http://www.unl.edu/buros/. *Tests: A Comprehensive Reference for Assessments in Psychology, Education, and Business* (101) and *Test Critiques* (102) also a major source for test descriptions and critical review.

Sample Assessment Texts

Assessment of Children: Cognitive Foundations (5th edition) (18)

Essentials of Cross-battery Assessment (3rd edition) (15)

Foundations of Behavioral, Social, and Clinical Assessment of Children (6th edition) (103)

Clinical Assessment of Child and Adolescent Intelligence (2nd edition) (19)

Clinical Assessment of Child and Adolescent Personality and Behavior (3rd edition) (104)

Compendium of Neuropsychological Tests: Administration, Norms, and Commentary (105)

Handbook of Nonverbal Assessment (106)

Handbook of Psychological Assessment (107)

Practice of Child-Clinical Neuropsychology: An Introduction (16)

Neuropsychological Assessment (5th edition) (17)

The Neuropsychological Evaluation of the Child (108)

Through the assessment of behavioral, social, and emotional functioning, information is obtained in a systematic and standardized format, producing quantified data, relative to normative developmental reference groups. In addition, rating scales make use of the judgments and observations of others who are familiar with the child, including the child him/herself, parents, or teachers. In some instances, it is possible (and useful) to compare results between reporters and settings. As with other types of measures, scale names may be similar across behavioral instruments, but item content may differ; also, scales of different names may share content (e.g., when hyperactive behaviors are subsumed under the conduct domain) (103,114). Although objective in the sense that information is collected under standard conditions, rating scales are subject to respondent variables. Most behavioral measures include scales to assess the response style of the informant, such as whether the individual is reporting in a manner to create a favorable impression ("faking good"), an unfavorable impression ("faking bad"), a more/less socially acceptable picture, as well as to evaluate consistency of response. It is important to interpret these scales first in order to determine whether the results as a whole are valid.

Projective techniques are another method for accessing the "inner life" of the child or adolescent. This assessment method may in fact be particularly useful for children and adolescents. Tasks such as drawing, completing sentences, and providing narratives to pictures may be more engaging and less confrontational than direct questioning. (See Frick et al. (104) for a discussion.) The projective techniques are based upon the premise that responses to and interpretations of ambiguous stimuli provide insight into the examinee's unconscious mental processes, such as needs, motives, and conflicts. Most projective tasks have been in longstanding use and continue to be widely employed; several have an extensive research literature (such as the Rorschach Inkblot Test and Thematic Apperception Test). Although an understanding of projective techniques is typically embedded in psychodynamic theory, these measures can also be viewed as an additional means of capturing how the child processes and organizes novel, ambiguous, or unstructured information.

Adaptive Behavior

Adaptive behavior scales measure domains related to personal independence and social competence. These are the day-to-day activities necessary to take care of oneself and get along with others, as defined by age and cultural standards. The usual domains assessed include independent living skills (eating, toileting, simple household chores), functional communication and academic skills, fine and gross motor skills, as well as social behavior such as relations with others, participation in leisure activity, and awareness of community rules. An assessment of adaptive behavior enhances the clinical picture of a child or adolescent by providing information about what the individual *actually* does, as opposed to what he or she is capable of doing in the home, school, or community. It is especially valuable when working with children with developmental disabilities toward treatment planning and toward intellectual disability classification. As with other measures, interpretation of the results requires a consideration of the variables that are likely to impact performance, including motivation, family expectations, cultural values, and level of cognitive functioning.

Diagnostic Interviews

The unstructured clinical interview is commonly used in psychology, as in psychiatry. However, several instruments are available for use that offer a more structured and uniform approach to the diagnostic interview, which is of particular relevance in research but is becoming increasingly used in the clinical setting (115). These interviews are tied to DSM criteria and provide a set of questions and explicit guidelines for how responses are to be scored. They offer the following advantages when compared to behavior scales: They provide information about symptom duration and onset, intensity and level of impairment, and are tied to diagnostic criteria. The explicit interview format may also be helpful for the interviewer in training. Disadvantages include the use of these instruments requires more time (60 to 90 minutes), they are not norm-referenced, and they are subject to the biases of the reporter, which are not captured in any systematic way (104). There are four other factors to keep in mind when evaluating diagnostic interviews relative to one's research or clinical needs. First, there are usually multiple versions of the same instrument (as they are being constantly updated as DSM criteria change). Second, although the interviews are structured, they vary in their degree of explicit instruction (e.g., the Schedule for Affective Disorders and Schizophrenia for School-aged Children (57) provides questions to guide the examiner, whereas the Diagnostic Interview Schedule for Children (56) requires the questions to be read as written). Third, most interview responses are scored in a dichotomous fashion (present or absent), although some instruments permit a rating of severity for each symptom, allowing for assessment of subclinical presentations. The last point to be made is that the time frame used to assess symptomatology differs among instruments, for example, in terms of how "present episode" is defined, and also whether lifetime diagnosis information is collected. (See Frick et al. (104) for a further discussion.)

Neuropsychological Assessment

A comprehensive neuropsychological assessment will include measures in one or more of the domains above. The basic test battery will also evaluate cognitive behavior in depth by including measures in each of the following domains and then selecting tests to emphasize one area or another according to initial results of the child's particular pattern of assets and deficits.

Sensory Perception

Measures of tactile, visual, and auditory perception are fundamental to the neuropsychological assessment battery. At a basic level, the individual will be evaluated for evidence of sensory imperception and suppression in each sensory domain, and on each side of the body. Higher-level perceptual abilities also are evaluated in each domain. A comparison of performance on the two sides of the body is significant for evidence of lateral or bilateral brain impairment. Each sensory system is also subserved by different regions of the brain and thus yields initial information about areas that are likely to be maximally involved (16). This aspect of the assessment is also relevant to particular types of brain impairment, such as the agnosia. From a developmental perspective, information about the child's sensory and perceptual processes is essential to understanding how the child takes in and assembles information in each of these domains and evaluating the impact on more complex or higher-order information processing.

Motor Skills

Motor ability is assessed for basic skills such as force, speed, steadiness, and dexterity; it may also be evaluated in the context of more complex skills such as visual motor coordination, visual motor integration, and constructional abilities. If a deficit in one of these multisystem tasks is obtained, then an analysis of each of the individual component processes is important. Motor function is examined both for overall level as well as laterality. It is relevant to the performance of activities of daily living, play, leisure involvement, classroom tasks, drawing, and handwriting. Assessment of motor and visual motor function is relevant to the question of apraxia.

Attention

Attention is a core capacity that is central to the processes of information reduction, response selection, and preparation for eventual action. The widespread use of the phrase "pay attention," illustrates that attentional resources come at some cost and require effort (we have to "concentrate hard"). Further, there is an implicit notion that attention is selective (we pay attention to one aspect of a complex environment to the exclusion of another). New information arrives in the form of a continuous flow of both internal and external stimuli. Children develop an increasing capacity to override the impulse to attend to what is most striking or novel or desired in order to anticipate, direct, or guide attention, based on prior knowledge and internal goals. Components of attention are distinguished in terms of modality (e.g., tactile, auditory, visual) and process (e.g., focusing or sustaining attention and shifting or dividing attention) assessed. Intact attention is relevant for focused behavior as well as mental tracking (such as following a sequence of ideas or steps in one's head) (17).

Memory

It is important to understand the role of memory, as very few aspects of higher cognitive function and learning could operate successfully without some memory contribution. Memory is often treated as a unitary construct but should be recognized as comprising multiple interrelated systems. Performance may be modality (verbal or visual), task (recall versus recognition), or system (immediate vs. long term; semantic vs. episodic; implicit vs. explicit) specific. Organization has a role in memory, as do other executive control processes. Working memory tasks require the ability simultaneously to attend to, recall, and act upon information held in an online state. This aspect of memory function is often considered in the domain of EF and is fundamental to most aspects of problem solving.

Language

Language is typically assessed for the intactness of the child's ability to discriminate and produce speech sounds, repeat words and phrases, retrieve words rapidly, appreciate word meanings, make verbal associations, and express him/herself, as well as comprehend more complex utterances (16), understand and use nonliteral language, and understand and use language in social contexts. The significance of assessing language abilities is understandable, with regard to the functional lateralization of this system (e.g., left cerebral dominance), evaluation of the aphasias, as well as the importance of language development with regard to reading, spelling, and written expression, concept formation, and the regulation of behavior.

Problem Solving, Concept Formation, and Reasoning

Measures of problem-solving ability, concept formation, and reasoning have in common an emphasis on abstract reasoning ability; the task demands are typically complex and require higher-order problem-solving strategies. The stimuli may be verbal, visual, or tactile in nature, although the child may restructure the task such that a visual task is verbally mediated or a verbal reasoning measure is guided by visual imagery (16). Conceptual and reasoning tasks are likely to represent the integrity of brain functioning, given the need for recruitment of multiple systems in the performance of such tasks. Such tasks provide insights into how the examinee thinks, for example, revealing concreteness and/or mental inflexibility to form concepts and logic relationships.

Executive Functions

EF is a term generally used to capture several higher-order cognitive functions. It refers to the ability to maintain an appropriate problem solving set to guide future goal-directed behavior, and is composed of a set of abilities including (1) inhibition, (2) set shifting, (3) planning, (4) working memory, and (5) self-monitoring. Most cognitive or intelligence test batteries do not comprehensively assess this domain. Adequate assessment of these areas is relevant to evaluating the child's ability to formulate plans of action, test hypotheses, benefit from feedback, and work toward an end goal. The child who presents with problem solving (as above) and/or EF deficits is likely to require a greater deal of structure and contingent feedback in his or her treatment or educational program.

COGNITIVE AND LEARNING CHALLENGES IN PSYCHIATRIC AND NEURODEVELOPMENTAL DISORDERS

There is consistent evidence that psychiatric and neurodevelopmental disorders of childhood are associated with cognitive and learning challenges, although the pattern is neither uniform (there is considerable heterogeneity within disorders versus a single core deficit) nor diagnostic (specificity is often lacking and process deficits are being identified that are shared across disorders). (See Coghill (116) for a discussion.) The constellation of behavioral deficits that encompasses attention-deficit hyperactivity disorder (ADHD) is typically identified relative to day-to-day behaviors in real-world settings. It would be reasonable to consider that performance-based measures of EF deficits would also be consistently associated with ADHD; however, the evidence suggests that the degree and nature of involvement varies in children with ADHD and the presence of EF deficits does not necessarily lead to a higher level of ADHD symptoms but rather potentially represents a notable subtype (e.g., 117,118). Different diagnostic groups may be distinguished based on profiles of everyday EF problems; for example, children with Tourette syndrome (TS) showed elevations in the domain of emotional control relative to elevated concerns for inhibitory control for children with ADHD-C, planning/organization for children with ADHD-I, and cognitive flexibility for children with ASD (119). Indeed, conceptual flexibility versus perceptual or attentional flexibility (or simple inhibitory control) appears to be the predominant deficit in higher-functioning individuals with autism (120–123). Sustained attention for simple repetitive visual information is generally intact in individuals with autism compared to developmentally matched controls, as measured by continuous performance tasks (124–128). TS is associated with problems with attention, fine motor coordination, and visual motor integration, where fine motor skill deficits may be a predictor of future tic severity and global psychosocial function in children with TS (129). In addition, although the disorder is defined by the presence of tics, it is the co-occurring disorders such as behavioral disinhibition, hypersensitivity to sensory stimuli, problems with visual motor integration, ADHD, obsessive–compulsive disorder, depression, and anxiety that may be especially impairing and thus important to assess (130). Anxiety and depression may impact attention, memory, and learning. Bipolar disorder has been linked to impairments in sustained attention, working memory, and processing speed after controlling for ADHD (131). Neuropsychological studies of childhood onset schizophrenia have revealed deficits in attentional capacities and the processing of information (132–136). Premorbid neuropsychological deficits are also reported in a large proportion of children who later develop schizophrenia, and less so in bipolar disorder, suggesting neurodevelopment underlying cognition in children prior to the onset of schizophrenia may be especially impaired (137).

Several disorders clearly necessitate a psychological or neuropsychological evaluation, such as suspicion of an LD or intellectual disability. One specific type of LD, nonverbal learning disability (NLD), is defined by a profile of neuropsychological strengths and weaknesses. The NLD syndrome is so named because the clinical presentation is thought to arise from deficits that are primarily nonverbal in nature (138). These primary deficiencies, which include visual, tactile, and motor functioning, also impact apprehension and use of nonverbal aspects of communication, such as facial expressions, gestures, and general body language. Academically, these children show better reading and spelling skills relative to arithmetic. At present, there is no formal provision for NLD in the DSM-5, although rules for classification have been developed (139,140). For the purposes of obtaining services, the needs of these children may be partially captured by diagnostic labels such as specific learning disorder with impairment in mathematics or written expression.

SUMMARY: INTEGRATED APPROACH

The psychological and neuropsychological assessment represents a systematic process for arriving at a more complete understanding of the child. The determinants of human behavior are many and varied; accordingly, when presented with problem behaviors, thought must be given to factors both intrinsic and extrinsic to the child. Intrinsic factors include (a) cognition and learning, which can be thought of as the information processing aspect of behavior; (b) emotional status, including feelings, motivation, regulation; and (c) EFs or execution of purposeful behavior (17). An overly simplistic approach is eschewed in favor of considering the relative contributions of each of the domains, the processes within them, and most interestingly, their interaction (e.g., the impact of a child's cognitive style on his/her affect, how a child's emotional state impacts information processing). In the final analysis, this information is integrated with extrinsic factors, including past experiences, current environmental demands, and the availability of resources toward guiding future treatment planning.

References

1. Anastasi A: *Psychological Testing*. 7th ed. New York, Pearson, 1997.
2. Thurstone LL: *Primary Mental Abilities: Psychometric Monographs No. 1*. Chicago, IL, University of Chicago Press, 1938.
3. Cattell RB: Theory of fluid and crystallized intelligence: a critical experiment. *J Educ Psychol* 54:1–22, 1963.
4. Cattell RB: *Intelligence: Its Structure, Growth, and Action*. New York, North-Holland, 1987.
5. Horn JL: Organization of abilities and the development of intelligence. *Psychol Rev* 75:242–259, 1968.
6. Horn JL: The theory of fluid and crystallized intelligence. In: Sternberg RJ (ed): *The Encyclopedia of Intelligence*. New York, Macmillan, 443–451, 1994.
7. Guilford JP: *The Nature of Human Intelligence*. New York, McGraw-Hill, 1967.
8. Sternberg RJ: *The Triarchic Mind: A New Theory of Human Intelligence*. New York, Viking, 1988.

9. Sternberg RJ: The triarchic theory of successful intelligence. In: Flanagan DP, Harrison PL (eds): *Contemporary Intellectual Assessment: Theories, Tests, and Issues.* New York, Guilford Press, 103–119, 2004.
10. Gardner H: *Frames of Mind: The Theory of Multiple Intelligences.* New York, Basic Books, 1993.
11. Carroll JB: *Human Cognitive Abilities: A Survey of Factor Analytic Studies.* New York, Cambridge University Press, 1993.
12. Das JP, Naglieri JA, Kirby JR: *Assessment of Cognitive Processes: The PASS Theory of Intelligence.* Needham Heights, MA, Allyn & Bacon, 1994.
13. Kamphaus RW, Winsor AP, Rowe EW, Kim S: A history of intelligence test interpretation. In: Flanagan DP, Harrison PL (eds): *Contemporary Intellectual Assessment: Theories, Tests, and Issues.* New York, Guilford Press, 23–38, 2004.
14. Flanagan DP, Ortiz S: *Essentials of Cross-Battery Assessment.* New York, Wiley, 2001.
15. Flanagan DP, Ortiz SO, Alfonso VC. *Essentials of Cross-battery Assessment.* Hoboken, NJ, Wiley Press, 2013.
16. Rourke BP, van der Vlugt H, Rourke SB: *Practice of Child-Clinical Neuropsychology: An Introduction.* Lisse, Swets & Zeitlinger, 2002.
17. Lezak M, Howieson DB, Bigler ED, Tranel D: *Neuropsychological Assessment.* 5th ed. Oxford, Oxford University Press, 2012.
18. Sattler J: *Assessment of Children: Cognitive Foundations.* 5th ed. San Diego, CA, Jerome M. Sattler, Publisher, Inc., 2008.
19. Kamphaus RW: *Clinical Assessment of Child and Adolescent Intelligence.* 2nd ed. New York, Springer, 2005.
20. Wechsler D: *Wechsler Intelligence Scale for Children.*5th ed. San Antonio, TX, Psychological Corporation, 2014.
21. Kaufman AS, Kaufman NL: *Kaufman Test of Educational Achievement.* 3rd ed. San Antonio, TX, Pearson, 2014.
22. Flynn JR: Massive gains in 14 nations: What IQ tests really measure. *Psychol Bull* 101:171–191, 1987.
23. Elliott CD: *Differential Ability Scales.* 2nd ed. San Antonio, TX, Harcourt Assessment, Inc, 2006.
24. Kaufman AS, Kaufman NL: *Kaufman Assessment Battery for Children.* 2nd ed. Circle Pines, MN, AGS Publishing, 2004.
25. Roid GH: *Stanford-Binet Intelligence Scales.* 5th ed. Itasca, IL: Riverside Publishing, 2003.
26. Wechsler D: *Wechsler Preschool and Primary Scale of Intelligence.* 4th ed. San Antonio, TX, Psychological Corporation, 2012.
27. Wechsler D: *Wechsler Adult Intelligence Scale.* 4th ed. San Antonio, TX, Psychological Corporation, 2008.
28. Schrank FA, McGrew KS, Mather N: *Woodcock Johnson-IV Tests of Cognitive Abilities.* Rolling Meadows, IL, Riverside, 2014.
29. Kaufman AS, Kaufman NL: *Kaufman Brief Intelligence Test, Second Edition (KBIT-2).* San Antonio, TX, Pearson, 2004.
30. Wechsler D: *Wechsler Abbreviated Scale of Intelligence.* San Antonio, TX, The Psychological Corporation/A brand of Harcourt Assessment Inc, 1999.
31. Glutting J, Adams W, Sheslow D. *Wide Range Intelligence Test (WRIT).* San Antonio, TX, Pearson, 1999.
32. *Wechsler Individual Achievement Test.* 3rd ed. San Antonio, TX, NCS Pearson, 2009.
33. Wilkinson GS, Robertson GJ: *Wide Range Achievement Test 4.* Lutz, FL, Psychological Assessment Resources, Inc., 2006.
34. Schrank FA, Mather N, McGrew KS: *Woodcock Johnson Tests of Achievement.* 4th ed. Rolling Meadows, IL, Riverside, 2014.
35. Delis DC, Kaplan E, Kramer JH: *Delis-Kaplan Executive Function System.* San Antonio, TX, PsychCorp, A brand of Harcourt Assessment, Inc, 2001.
36. Reitan RM, Wolfson D: *Halstead-Reitan Neuropsychological Test Battery: Theory and Clinical Interpretation.* Tucson, Arizona, Reitan Neuropsychology, 1985.
37. Golden CJ: *Luria-Nebraska Neuropsychological Battery, Children's Revision.* Los Angeles, CA, Western Psychological Services, 1987.
38. Golden CJ, Purisch AD, Hammeke TA: *Luria-Nebraska Neuropsychological Battery: Forms I and II.* Los Angeles, CA, Western Psychological Services, 1985.
39. Korkman M, Kirk U, Kemp S: *NEPSY-Second Edition (NEPSY II).* San Antonio, TX, Harcourt Assessment, 2007.
40. Reitan RM: *Reitan-Indiana Neuropsychological Test Battery.* Tucson, AZ, Reitan Neuropsychology Laboratory/Press, 1981.
41. Hammill DD, Pearson NA, Wiederholt JL: *Comprehensive Test of Nonverbal Intelligence.* 2nd ed. Austin, TX, PRO-ED, Inc., 2009.
42. Roid GH, Miller LJ, Pomplun M, Koch C: *Leiter International Performance Scale.* 3rd ed. Lutz, FL, PAR, 2013.
43. Naglieri JA: *Naglieri Nonverbal Ability Test.* 3rd ed. San Antonio, TX, Pearson, 2015.
44. Brown L, Sherbenou RJ, Johnson SK: *Test of Nonverbal Intelligence,* 4th ed. Austin, TX, PRO-ED, Inc., 2010.
45. Bracken BA, McCallum RS: *Universal Nonverbal Intelligence Test.* 2nd ed. Torrance, CA, WPS, 2016.
46. Wechsler D, Naglieri JA: *Wechsler Nonverbal Scale of Ability.* San Antonio, TX, Harcourt Assessment Inc., 2006.
47. Lambert N, Nihira K, Leland H: *AAMR Adaptive Behavior Scale-School.* 2nd ed. Austin, TX, PRO-ED, Inc., 1993.
48. Harrison PL, Oakland T: *Adaptive Behavior Assessment System.* 3rd ed. San Antonio, TX, Pearson, 2015.
49. Bruininks RH, Woodcock RW, Weatherman RF, Hill BK: *Scales of Independent Behavior, Revised.* Itasca, IL, Riverside Publishing, 1997.
50. Sparrow SS, Cicchetti DV, Saulnier, C: *Vineland Adaptive Behavior Scales.* 3rd ed. Minneapolis, MN, Pearson Assessments, a business of Pearson Education, 2016.
51. Sparrow SS, Balla DA, Cicchetti DV: *Vineland Social Emotional Early Childhood Scales.* Circle Pines, MN: AGS, Inc., 1998.
52. Angold A, Costello EJ: The child and adolescent psychiatric assessment (CAPA). *J Am Acad Child Adolesc Psychiatry* 39:39–48, 2000.
53. Weller EB, Weller RA, Fristad MA, Rooney MT: *ChIPS—Children's Interview for Psychiatric Syndromes.* Arlington, VA, American Psychiatric Publishing, Inc., 1999.
54. Reich W: Diagnostic interview for children and adolescents (DICA). *J Am Acad Child Adolesc Psychiatry* 39:59–66, 2000.
55. Reich W, Welner Z, Herjanic B: *Diagnostic Interview for Children and Adolescents-IV (DICA-IV).* North Tonawanda, NY, Multi-Health Systems, Inc., 1997.
56. Shaffer D, Fisher P, Lucas CP, Dulcan MK, Schwab-Stone ME: NIMH Diagnostic Interview Schedule for Children Version IV (NIMH DISCIV): description, differences from previous versions, and reliability of some common diagnoses. *J Am Acad Child Adolesc Psychiatry* 39:28–38, 2000.
57. Ambrosini PJ. Historical developments and present status of the schedule for affective disorders and schizophrenia for school age children (K-SADS). *J Am Acad Child Adolesc Psychiatry* 39:49–58, 2000.
58. Matzner F, Silva R, Silvan M, Chowdhury M, Nastasi L: *Preliminary Test-retest Reliability of the KID-SCID,* Scientific Proceedings, American Psychiatric Association Meeting, 1997.
59. Reynolds WM: *Adolescent Psychopathology Scale.* Odessa, FL: Psychological Assessment Resources, Inc., 1998.
60. Reynolds WM, Kamphaus RW: *BASC3: Behavior Assessment System for Children.* 3rd ed. Minneapolis, MN, Pearson Assessments, a business of Pearson Education, 2015.
61. Achenbach TM, Rescorla LA, McConaughey S, et al.: *Achenbach System of Empirically Based Assessment.* Burlington, VT, ASEBA, 2006.
62. Butcher JN, Williams CL, Graham JR, et al.: *MMPI-A (Minnesota Multiphasic Personality Inventory—Adolescent): Manual for Administration, Scoring, and Interpretation.* Minneapolis, MN, University of Minnesota Press, 1992.
63. Butcher JN, Williams CL, Graham JR, et al.: *MMPI-A (Minnesota Multiphasic Personality Inventory—Adolescent): Manual for Administration, Scoring, and Interpretation, Manual Supplement.* Minneapolis, MN, University of Minnesota Press, 2006.
64. Archer RP, Handel RW, Ben-Porath YS, Tellegen A: *MMPI-A-RF (Minnesota Multiphasic Personality Inventory—Adolescent-Restructured Form): Manual for Administration, Scoring, and Interpretation.* Minneapolis, MN, University of Minnesota Press, 2016.
65. Wirt RD, Lachar D, Seat PD, Broen WE Jr: *Personality Inventory for Children.* 2nd ed. Los Angeles, CA, Western Psychological Services, 2001.
66. Lachar D, Gruber CP: *Personality Inventory for Youth (PIY) Manual: Administration and Interpretation Guide.* Los Angeles, CA, Western Psychological Services, 1995.
67. DuPaul GJ, Power TJ, Anastopulos AD, Reid R: *ADHD Rating Scale-IV: Checklists, Norms, and Clinical Interpretation.* New York, Guilford Press, 1998.
68. Conners CK: *CRS-R: Conners' Rating Scales Revised.* Minneapolis, MN, Pearson Assessments, 2000.
69. Conners CK: *Conners Early Childhood.* Torrance, CA, WPS, 2009.
70. Swanson JM: The SNAP-IV teacher and parent rating scale. In: Fine A, Kotkin R (eds): *Therapists Guide to Learning and Attention Disorders.* San Diego, CA, Elsevier Science, pp. 487–500, 2003.
71. Swanson JM: The SWAN rating form. In: Fine A, Kotkin R (eds): *Therapist's Guide to Learning and Attention Disorders.* San Diego, CA, Elsevier Science, 501–502, 2003.
72. Reynolds CR, Richmond BO: *Revised Children's Manifest Anxiety Scale.* Los Angeles, CA, Western Psychological Services, 1985.
73. Spielberger CD: *State-Trait Anxiety Inventory for Children.* Palo Alto, CA, Consulting Psychologists Press, 1973.
74. Beck JS, Beck AT, Jolly J, Steer R: *Beck Youth Inventories™, Second Edition for Children and Adolescents (BYI-II).* San Antonio, TX, Harcourt Assessment, Inc, 2005.
75. Beck AT, Steer RA: *Beck Anxiety Inventory.* San Antonio, TX, PsychCorp, A brand of Harcourt Assessment, Inc, 1993.
76. March JS: *Multidimensional Anxiety Scale for Children.* 2nd Ed. San Antonio, TX, Pearson Assessment, 2012.
77. Birmaher B, Khetarpal S, Cully M, Brent D, McKenzie S: *Screen for Child Anxiety Related Disorders (SCARED).* Pittsburgh, PA: Western Psychiatric Institute and Clinic, University of Pittsburgh, 1995.
78. Beck AT, Steer RA, Brown GK: *Beck Depression Inventory—II.* San Antonio, TX, PsychCorp, A brand of Harcourt Assessment, Inc, 1996.
79. Kovacs M: *Children's Depression Inventory.* Minneapolis, MN, Pearson Assessments, 1992.
80. Reynolds WM: *Reynolds Child Depression Scale.* Odessa, FL, Psychological Assessment Resources, Inc., 1989.

81. Reynolds WM: *Reynolds Adolescent Depressive Scale.* 2nd ed. Lutz, FL, Psychological Assessment Resources, Inc., 2002.
82. Poznanski E, Mokros HB: *Children's Depression Rating Scale, Revised.* Los Angeles, CA, Western Psychological Services, 1996.
83. Gioia GA, Isquith PK, Guy SC, Kenworthy L: *Behavior Rating Inventory of Executive Function.* Odessa, FL, Psychological Assessment Resources, Inc., 2000.
84. Gioia GA, Espy KA, Isquith PK: *Behavior Rating Inventory of Executive Function—Preschool Version.* Odessa, FL, Psychological Assessment Resources, Inc., 2003.
85. Guy SC, Isquith PK, Gioia GA: *Behavior Rating Inventory of Executive Function—Self-Report Version.* Lutz, FL, Psychological Assessment Resources, Inc., 2004.
86. DiPerna J, Elliott JN: *Academic Competence Evaluation Scales.* San Antonio, TX, Pearson Assessments, 2000.
87. Weinstein CE, Palmer DR: *Learning and Study Strategies Inventory—High School Version.* Clearwater, FL, H&H Publishing Company, Inc., 1990.
88. Weinstein CE, Palmer DR, Acee TW: *Learning and Study Strategies Inventory.* 3rd ed. Clearwater, FL, H&H Publishing Company, Inc., 2016.
89. Brown L, Alexander J: *Self-Esteem Index.* Austin, TX: Pro-Ed, 1991.
90. Bellak L, Bellak SS: *Children's Apperception Test (1991 Revision).* Larchmont, NY, C.P.S., Inc., 1991.
91. Koppitz EM: *Psychological Evaluation of Children's Human Figure Drawings.* New York, Grune & Stratton, 1968.
92. Naglieri JA: *Draw A Person: A quantitative Scoring System.* San Antonio, TX, PsychCorp, A brand of Harcourt Assessment, Inc, 1988.
93. Knoff HM, Prout HT: *Kinetic Drawing System for Family and School: A Handbook.* Los Angeles, CA, Western Psychological Services, 1985.
94. Weiner IB: *Principles of Rorschach® Interpretation* 2nd ed. Odessa, FL, Psychological Assessment Resources, Inc., 2003.
95. Roberts GE, McArthur DS: *Roberts Apperception Test for Children.* 2nd ed. Odessa, FL, Psychological Assessment Resources, Inc., 2005.
96. Hart DH: *The Hart Sentence Completion Test for Children.* Salt Lake City, UT, Educational Support Systems, 1972.
97. Rotter JB, Lah MI, Rafferty JE: *Rotter Incomplete Sentences Blank.* 2nd ed. San Antonio, TX, PsychCorp, A brand of Harcourt Assessment, Inc, 1992.
98. Murray HA: *Thematic Apperception Test.* Cambridge, MA, Harvard University Press, 1943.
99. Carlson JF, Geisinger KF, Jonson JL (eds): *The Nineteenth Mental Measurements Yearbook.* Lincoln, NE, Buros Center for Testing, 2014.
100. Buros Center: In: Anderson N, Schlueter JE, Carlson JF, Geisinger KF (eds): *Tests in Print IX: An Index to Tests, Test Reviews, and the Literature on Specific Tests.* Lincoln, NB, University of Nebraska Press, 2016.
101. Maddox T (ed): *Tests: A Comprehensive Reference for Assessments in Psychology, Education, and Business.* 6th ed. Austin, TX: Pro-Ed, 2008.
102. Keyser DJ, Sweetland RC (eds): *Test Critiques.* Kansas City, MO, Test Corporation of America, 1994.
103. Sattler J: *Foundations of Behavioral, Social, and Clinical Assessment of Children.* 6th ed. San Diego, CA, Jerome M. Sattler, Publisher, Inc., 2014.
104. Frick PJ, Barry C, Kamphaus RW: *Clinical Assessment of Child and Adolescent Personality and Behavior.* 3rd ed. New York, Springer, 2009.
105. Strauss E, Sherman EMS, Spreen O: *A Compendium of Neuropsychological Tests: Administration, Norms, and Commentary.* 3rd ed. New York, Oxford University Press, 2006.
106. McCallum RS: *Handbook of Nonverbal Assessment.* New York, Kluwer Academic/Plenum Publishers, 2003.
107. Groth-Marnat G, Wright AJ: *Handbook of Psychological Assessment.* 6th ed. Hoboken, NJ, Wiley, 2016.
108. Baron IS: *Neuropsychological Evaluation of the Child.* New York, Oxford University Press, 2004.
109. Fletcher JM, Coulter WA, Reschly DJ, Vaughn S. Alternative approaches to the definition and identification of learning disabilities: some questions and answers. *Ann Dyslexia* 54:304–331, 2004.
110. Fuchs LS, Vaughn S: Responsiveness-to-intervention a decade later. *J Learn Disabil* 45:195–203, 2012.
111. Mather N, Wendling BJ: Linking cognitive assessment result to academic interventions for students with learning disabilities. In: Flanagan DP, Harrison PL (eds): *Contemporary Intellectual Assessment: Theories, Tests, and Issues.* New York, Guilford Press, 269–294, 2004.
112. Fuchs D, Compton DL, Fuchs LS, Bryant J, Hamlett C, Lambert W: First-grade cognitive abilities as long-term predictors of reading comprehension and disability status. *J Learn Disabil* 45:217–231, 2012.
113. Merrell KW: *Behavioral, Social, and Emotional Assessment of Children and Adolescents.* 2nd ed. Mahwah, NJ, Lawrence Erlbaum Associates, 2002.
114. Sattler J: *Assessment of Children: Behavioral and Clinical Applications.* 4th ed. San Diego, CA, Jerome M. Sattler, Publisher, Inc., 2002.
115. Jensen Doss A: Evidence-based diagnosis: incorporating diagnostic instruments into clinical practice. *J Am Acad Child Adolesc Psychiatry* 44:947–952, 2005.
116. Coghill D: Editorial: Acknowledging complexity and heterogeneity in causality—implications of recent insights into neuropsychology of childhood disorders for clinical practice. *J Child Psychol Psychiatry* 55:737–740, 2014.
117. Willcutt EG, Doyle AE, Nigg JT, Faraone SV, Pennington BF: Validity of the executive function theory of attention-deficit/hyperactivity disorder: a meta-analytic review. *Biol Psychiatry* 57:1336–1346, 2005.
118. Lambek R, Tannock R, Dalsgaard S, Trillingsgaard A, Damm D, Thomsen PH: Validating neuropsychological subtypes of ADHD: how do children with and without an executive function deficit differ? *J Child Psychol Psychiatry* 51:895–904, 2010.
119. Hovik KT, Egeland J, Isquith PK, et al.: Distinct patterns of everyday executive function problems distinguish children with Tourette syndrome from children with ADHD or autism spectrum disorders. *J Atten Disord* 1–13, 2014.
120. Goldstein G, Johnson CR, Minshew NJ: Attentional processes in autism. *J Autism Dev Disord* 31:433–440, 2001.
121. Minshew NJ, Meyer J, Goldstein G: Abstract reasoning in autism: a dissociation between concept formation and concept identification. *Neuropsychology* 16:327–334, 2002.
122. Ozonoff S, Cook I, Coon H, et al.: Performance on Cambridge Neuropsychological Test Automated Battery subtests sensitive to frontal lobe function in people with autistic disorder: evidence from the Collaborative Programs of Excellence in Autism Network. *J Autism Dev Disord* 34:139–150, 2004.
123. Ozonoff S, McEvoy RE: A longitudinal study of executive function and theory of mind development in autism. *Dev Psychopathol* 6:415–431, 1994.
124. Buchsbaum MS, Siegel BV Jr, Wu JC, et al.: Brief report: attention performance in autism and regional brain metabolic rate assessed by positron emission tomography. *J Autism Dev Disord* 22:115–125, 1992.
125. Casey BJ, Gordon CT, Mannheim GB, Rumsey JM: Dysfunctional attention in autistic savants. *J Clin Exp Neuropsychol* 15:933–946, 1993.
126. Garretson HB, Fein D, Waterhouse L: Sustained attention in children with autism. *J Autism Dev Disord* 20:101–114, 1990.
127. Minshew NJ, Goldstein G, Siegel DJ: Neuropsychological functioning in autism: profile of a complex information processing disorder. *J Int Neuropsychol Soc* 3:303–316, 1997.
128. Pascualvaca DM, Fantie BD, Papageorgiou M, Mirsky AF: Attentional capacities in children with autism: is there a general deficit in shifting focus? *J Autism Dev Disord* 28:467–478, 1998.
129. Bloch MH, Sukhodolsky DG, Leckman JF, Schultz RT: Fine-motor skill deficits in childhood predict adulthood tic severity and global psychosocial functioning in Tourette's syndrome. *J Child Psychol Psychiatry* 47:551–559, 2006.
130. Leckman JF, King RA, Bloch MH. Clinical features of Tourette syndrome and tic disorders. *J Obsessive Compuls Relat Disord* 3:372–379, 2014.
131. Doyle AE, Wilens TE, Kwon A, et al.: Neuropsychological functioning in youth with bipolar disorder. *Biol Psychiatry* 58:540–548, 2005.
132. Asarnow RF, Asamen J, Granholm E, Sherman T, Watkins JM, Williams ME: Cognitive/neuropsychological studies of children with a schizophrenic disorder. *Schizophr Bull* 20:647–669, 1994.
133. Asarnow RF, Brown W, Strandburg R: Children with a schizophrenic disorder: neurobehavioral studies. *Eur Arch Psychiatry Clin Neurosci* 245:70–79, 1995.
134. Karatekin C, Asarnow RF: Working memory in childhood-onset schizophrenia and attention-deficit/hyperactivity disorder. *Psychiatry Res* 80:165–176, 1998.
135. Karatekin C, Asarnow RF: Components of visual search in childhood onset schizophrenia and attention-deficit/hyperactivity disorder. *J Abnorm Child Psychol* 26:367–380, 1998.
136. Karatekin C, Asarnow RF: Exploratory eye movements to pictures in childhood-onset schizophrenia and attention-deficit/hyperactivity disorder. *J Abnorm Child Psychol* 27:35–49, 1999.
137. Seidman LJ, Cherkerzian S, Goldstein JM, Agnew-Blais J, Tsuang MT, Buka SL: Neuropsychological performance and family history in children at age 7 who develop adult schizophrenia or bipolar psychosis in the New England Family Studies. *Psychol Med* 43:119–131, 2013.
138. Rourke BP: *Nonverbal Learning Disabilities: The Syndrome and the Model.* New York, Guilford Press, 1989.
139. Drummond CR, Ahmad SA, Rourke BP: Rules for the classification of younger children with nonverbal learning disabilities and basic phonological processing disabilities. *Arch Clin Neuropsychol* 20:171–182, 2005.
140. Pelletier PM, Ahmad SA, Rourke BP: Classification rules for basic phonological processing disabilities and nonverbal learning disabilities: formulation and external validity. *Child Neuropsychol* 7:84–98, 2001.

CHAPTER 4.5 ■ ASSESSING COMMUNICATION

RHEA PAUL AND MEGAN C. LYONS

This chapter provides a brief outline of the process involved in assessing how children use speech and language for communication. We describe clinical assessment as a process that involves screening, evaluation—the process of establishing the degree of disability and diagnosis that best fits based on evidence from the child's history and performance and/or to establish continuing eligibility for services—and assessment, the ongoing process of gathering information to monitor the child's progress, strengths and needs and to make educational decisions (1). Evaluation, ideally, is conducted by a team of professionals from multiple disciplines who contribute their expertise in identifying the child's disorder and needs. For very young children (birth to 3 years), the evaluation team may include family members, a service coordinator, and persons conducting the evaluations and typically takes place in natural environments (e.g., home or daycare setting). For school-age children, The Individuals with Disabilities Education Act (1) regulations identify members of the team as: parents; regular education teacher; special education teacher; representative of the public agency, and at the discretion of the parent or agency, other individuals who have expertise regarding the child. Older children may also be included in the team. A speech-language pathologist (SLP) is the member of the team who specializes in the assessment and treatment of disorders of communication, including speech, language, and hearing. Qualified SLPs are certified by the American Speech-Language-Hearing Association (ASHA), and usually licensed by the state, as well.

Assessment of communication typically includes the evaluation of:

- Articulation: the pronunciation of the sounds of speech. Errors of articulation can be confined to the distorted production of a few sounds, such as a lisp. Alternatively, a speaker may substitute a range of sounds for others (saying /dot/ for *goat* or /to/ for *sew*), or may omit sounds in words ('pay' for *play;* 'so' for *soap*). Some articulation errors may make speech sound childish or immature; more frequent errors can lead to difficulty in understanding what the speaker says.
- Language Comprehension: the understanding of words and sentences. Difficulties in comprehending what others say can result in a failure to follow directions, to provide appropriate responses to questions, and to understand both spoken and written material.
- Language Production: the ability to use words and sentences to express meanings. These disorders can result in difficulties in both social interactions and academic and vocational activities.
- Pragmatic Communication: Children with disorders in this area may have large vocabularies and use complex sentence types, but may have difficulty following the rules of conversation, such as taking turns appropriately, maintaining conversational topics introduced by others, and giving the appropriate amount of information (not too much, not too little) based on the conversational partner's needs and interests. These deficits can result in rejection by peers and attributions of "rudeness" by others.

Screening involves the collection of data to decide whether there is a strong likelihood that an individual has a problem that will require a more in-depth assessment. An appropriate speech-language screening measure is one that meets high levels of psychometric criteria, including well-established reliability, validity, sensitivity, and specificity, as well as assessing relevant areas of communication. A well-designed screening measure will look beyond a single area of concern; for example, it will examine both the child's expressive ability, as well as the understanding of language. Failure to achieve a criterion level on a screening measure should result in a child's referral for evaluation and more in-depth assessment. Some examples of language screening measures appear in Table 4.5.1.

EVALUATION

Review of existing and/or historical data is typically the first step of the evaluation process. Information can be gathered from parent interviews, teacher report, clinical observations, previous testing, and/or data kept on intervention progress from either internal (e.g., school; Birth to Three services) or external sources (e.g., medical records). When gathering this information, the team must determine what is known about the child versus what needs to be learned in the current evaluation to establish risk factors, the presence and type of disorder, and to contribute to the development of a treatment plan. The following are examples of basic questions to consider when gathering this initial information regarding a child's communication:

1. Reason for referral (e.g., who referred the child; what are the concerns regarding the child's current speech, language, and communication skills; when did the problem begin; impact of problem across settings)
2. Speech and language development (babbling by 10 months; first words by 18 months; two-word combinations and following simple directions by 24 months; sentences by 3 years); moreover, for those children who already received early intervention services, questions regarding their current mode of communication are asked: Are they using gestures, signs, communication devices or demonstrating pretend play skills?
3. Feeding (solid food by 6 months; using a cup by 18 months; drinking from a straw by 30 months)
4. Therapy (prior language evaluation/s; current and/or past intervention services)
5. Education (daycare; school; special education)
6. Birth/medical history (e.g., cleft lip; cleft palate; ear infections; PE tubes; prematurity)
7. Significant family history (e.g., hearing; articulation; learning disabilities)
8. What does the family see as the child's most important problem in communication?
9. When did the problem begin?

TABLE 4.5.1

EXAMPLES OF SPEECH-LANGUAGE SCREENING MEASURES

Screening (Name/Author(s)/Date/Publisher)	Developmental Range
Battelle Development Inventory—2nd ed. Screening Test Newborg J (2005). Itasca, IL: Riverside Publishing	Birth–7:11 yrs
Clinical Evaluation of Language Fundamentals—5th ed. Screening Test Wiig EH, Secord WA, Semel E (2013). Bloomington, MN: Pearson	5–21:11 yrs
Developmental Indicators for the Assessment of Learning—4th ed. Mardell C, Goldenberg DS (2011). Bloomington, MN: Pearson	2:6–5:11 yrs
Diagnostic Evaluation of Language Variation—Screening Test Seymour HN, Roeper TW, deVilliers J, deVilliers PA (2003). Bloomington, MN: Pearson	4–9 yrs
Early Screening Profiles Harrison P, Kaufman A, Kaufman N, et al. (1990). Bloomington, MN: Pearson	2–6:11 yrs
Hodson Assessment of Phonological Patterns-Preschool Phonological Screening—3rd ed. Hodson BW (2004). Austin, TX: Pro-Ed	Preschool
Fluharty Preschool Speech and Language Screening Test—2nd ed. Fluharty NB (2000). Austin, TX: Prod-Ed	3–6:11 yrs
Joliet 3-Minute Speech and Language Screen (Revised) Kinzler MC, Johnson CC (1992). Tucson, AZ: Communication Skill Builders	K, 2nd and 5th grades
Kindergarten Language Screening Test—2nd ed. Gauthier SV, Madison CL (1998). Austin, TX: Pro-Ed	3:6–6:11 yrs
Screening Test for Developmental Apraxia of Speech: Examiner's Manual—2nd ed. Blakely RW (2001). Austin, TX: Pro-Ed	4–12 yrs
Adolescent Language Screening Test Morgan DL, Guilford AM (1984). Austin, TX: Pro-Ed	11–17 yrs

10. Does this problem vary in terms of its severity or occurrence?
11. Can the child's speech be understood by people outside the family?
12. Can the child follow verbal directions at home or at school?
13. How does this problem influence the child's social communication across various environments, including school and within social settings?

A common method for gathering this case history information is to ask families to fill out a questionnaire with queries like the above, prior to the evaluation session, and to conduct an interview with the parent at the time of the assessment to clarify and supplement the written information. *Caregiver information* gained through questionnaire and interview procedures can supplement results gathered from direct interaction between the clinician and child. Caregivers can provide information about the child's communicative functioning among a variety of contexts, including home, school, and with peers. Caregivers can describe their own concerns by outlining the child's communication performance across these natural contexts. Parent report can give the clinician a better sense of the child's everyday communication challenges and areas of weakness. Sachse and Von Suchodoletz (2) support the validity of parent report measures in comparison to direct language measures (e.g., spontaneous language samples) when it comes to their young child's language skills and identifying potential delays. The advantages of parent report include the tendency for young children to be reluctant to interact with a clinician or in an unfamiliar environment. Allowing a child to play or converse with a parent, for example, provides a way for the clinician to observe the child's communication and interaction style indirectly, and may put the child and parent at ease. Additionally, parents may be reluctant or anxious to raise certain of their concerns or reveal specific information in direct conversation with an unfamiliar clinician. In order to decrease both caregiver and child stress, to minimize additional testing sessions, and to obtain a representative sample of the child's skills, gathering information from parents and caregivers as they both describe and interact with their child, can increase the efficiency of an assessment, as well as decrease the stress induced by long testing sessions. Some examples of parent report instruments appear in Table 4.5.2.

Once sufficient information about the history and the problem has been gathered, the team will determine the child's general developmental level to begin the evaluation process. Assessment of general developmental level, usually through psychological testing of cognitive and motor function, will help to establish the level of communication skills that might be expected, and help to select instruments that will target skills at the appropriate level. It will also be important to consider cultural and linguistic variables when planning the evaluation. Cultural variables to be considered may include child-rearing practices, ethnicity, rules of interaction, gender identity and socioeconomic status as well as linguistic variables such as oral, written, and manual languages used by the child and family.

A communication evaluation will usually include a battery of standardized assessments that provide an answer to the question of whether this child is significantly different from a sample of age-matched children whom the measure was normed in terms of the ability to speak, understand language, and use of speech and language to communicate with family, teachers, and peers. For this purpose, again, tests with strong psychometric properties must be chosen in order to answer the question in a fair and valid way. Some examples of tests often used for evaluation at various stages of development are listed in Table 4.5.3.

If testing confirms the observations of parents and teachers and corroborates the screening results that the child is showing difficulty with communication skills relative to others at his/her developmental level, the child can be identified as having a disorder in this area. However, not every child who tests low on a standardized test will be able to receive services for a communication deficit. Eligibility criteria are based on local, state, and federal regulations determining the requisite level of impairment for services based on norm-referenced measures, observational assessment, whether the language impairment

TABLE 4.5.2

EXAMPLES OF PARENT REPORT INSTRUMENTS FOR COMMUNICATION

Parent Report Instrument (Name/Author(s)/Date/Publisher)	Developmental Level
Autism Diagnostic Interview—Revised Rutter M, LeCouteur A, Lord C (2003). Los Angeles, CA: Western Psychological Services	2–21 yrs
Communication and Symbolic Behavior Scales—Normed Edition: Record Forms and Caregiver Questionnaires Wetherby AM, Prizant BM (2002). Baltimore, MD: Paul H. Brookes Publishing Co., Inc.	6–24 mo
Children's Communication Checklist—2nd ed. Bishop DVM (2003). Austin, TX: Harcourt Assessment	4–16:11 yrs
The Language Development Survey: A Screening Tool for Delayed Language in Toddlers Rescorla L (1989)	18–35 mo
Manual for the ASEBA Preschool Forms & Profiles Achenbach TM, Rescorla LA (2000). Burlington, VT: University of Vermont, Research Center for Children, Youth, & Families	
The MacArthur-Bates Communicative Development Inventories—User's Guide and Technical Manual—2nd ed. Fenson L, Marchman VA, Thal DJ, Dale PS, Reznick JS, Bates E (2006). Baltimore, MD: Paul H. Brookes Publishing Co., Inc.	8–37 mo
The Vineland Adaptive Behavior Scales—2nd ed. Sparrow SS, Cicchetti DV, Balla DA (2005). Bloomington, MN: Pearson, Inc.	Birth–90 yrs

interferes with spoken language or primary mode of communication and whether the impairment affects the child's educational, social, or emotional development. Thus, one outcome of evaluation will be a determination as to whether a child's disability is severe or pervasive enough to qualify for publicly funded services. Clinicians need to be aware of local requirements for eligibility. If a child fails to meet eligibility criteria, parents may opt to obtain services privately.

In addition to establishing eligibility for services, the evaluation process is aimed at integrating data from the various professionals on the team in order to arrive at a diagnostic label that best describes the child's conditions. Communication disorders are very frequently associated with a variety of conditions, as Chapter 5.2.4 explains. So although failure to talk or poor speech development is frequently a child's presenting problem, it is often the case that evaluation uncovers deficits in other areas

TABLE 4.5.3

EXAMPLES OF COMMONLY USED GENERAL LANGUAGE TEST BATTERIES

Test Name, Author(s)/Date, Publisher	Developmental Level
Clinical Evaluation of Language Fundamentals—Preschool—2nd ed. Semel E, Wiig EH, Secord WA (2004). San Antonio, TX: Pearson	3–0–6:11 yrs
Clinical Evaluation of Language Fundamentals—5th ed. Wiig EH, Semel E, Secord WA (2013). San Antonio, TX: Pearson	5–0–21:11 yrs
Comprehensive Assessment of Spoken Language Carrow-Woolfolk E (1999). Bloomington, MN: Pearson	3–0–21–0 yrs
Detroit Tests of Learning Aptitude-Primary—3rd ed. Hammill DD, Bryant BR (2005). Austin, TX: Pro-Ed	3–9:11 yrs
Oral and Written Language Scales—2nd ed. Carrow-Woolfolk E (2012). Austin, TX: Pro-Ed	3–21:11 yrs
Preschool Language Scales—5th ed. Zimmerman IL, Steiner VG, Pond RE (2011).Bloomington, MN: Pearson	Birth–7:11 yrs
Sequenced Inventory of Communication Development—Revised Hedrick DL, Prather EM, Tobin AR (1984). Seattle: University of Washington Press	4 mo–4 yrs
Test of Adolescent and Adult Language—4th ed. Hammill DD, Brown VL, Larsen SC, Wiederholt JL (2007). Austin, TX: Pro-Ed	12–24:11 yrs
Test of Early Language Development—3rd ed. Hresko WP, Reid DK, Hammill DD (1999). Austin, TX: Pro-Ed	2–7:11 yrs
Test of Language Development Primary—4th ed. Newcomer PL, Hammill DD (2008). Austin, TX: Pro-Ed	4–8:11 yrs
Test of Language Development Intermediate—4th ed. Newcomer PL, Hammill DD (2008). Austin, TX: Pro-Ed	8:6–12:11 yrs
Test of Early Written Language—3rd ed. Hresko WP, Herron SR, Peak PR, Hicks DL (2012). Austin, TX: Pro-Ed	4–11:11 yrs
Utah Test of Language Development—4th ed. Mecham MJ (2003). Australia: Pro-Ed	3–9:11 yrs
Woodcock Language Proficiency Battery—Revised. Woodcock RW (1991). Chicago, IL: Riverside Publishing	2–95 yrs

of development, such as cognition, hearing, motor or social skills that contribute to the choice of diagnostic label. When this happens, the child may receive a primary diagnosis of intellectual disability, autism, or hearing impairment, with language described as a secondary or comorbid condition. The conferring of a primary diagnosis other than language disorder, however, does not mean that the child's need for communication assessment and intervention diminishes. Even when a child's primary diagnosis is something other than a specific speech or language disorder, assessment of communication strengths and needs remains important in order to develop an intervention program that will address all of the child's developmental concerns.

One additional issue explored by the evaluation team concerns the nonverbal child. Children may fail to acquire expressive language function for a variety of reasons, primarily because of neuromotor deficits that affect vocal function, such as cerebral palsy. However, some children without diagnosable neuromotor disorders may also fail to begin speaking during early childhood; children with Down syndrome and autism can sometimes show this pattern, for example. When this is the case, the SLP will be charged with deciding whether the child should be taught to use an alternative or augmentative communication (AAC) modality, such as sign language, picture exchange communication system, assistive communication application (e.g., such as those for iOS platform) or a designated speech generating device (SGD). Although the considerations that go into this decision are beyond the scope of this discussion (see (3) for further discussion), in general, SLPs will attempt to ensure that the child has some way to communicate with others if speech is not an accessible modality for the child (3). AAC may be provided on a short-term basis, until more usable speech emerges, or may be part of the child's long-term communication program. The SLP will attempt, in investigating AAC usage for a particular child, to identify the best match of a system to a child's developmental level and communication needs. This investigation may be expanded as part of the assessment portion of the team's activities.

ASSESSMENT

Once it has been determined that the child has a disorder that includes communication deficits, a detailed assessment of the child's functioning is undertaken. This process has three main goals: to establish the child's baseline level of communicative function, to identify goals for intervention, and to monitor progress within the therapy program. To achieve these aims, SLPs typically use a range of methods that include not only standardized tests, but criterion-referenced, observational, and dynamic procedures. Norm-referenced tests, or standardized instruments, are, as we have discussed, used to compare a child's skills to those of other children of similar age and background. These formal instruments have specific statistical properties that allow meaningful comparisons among children to determine if their functioning is significantly different from typical performance. Standardized tests are particularly useful in determining the existence of a communication disorder, and for establishing eligibility for speech and language services. That said, norm-referenced assessments are not designed to identify the specific behaviors that constitute the child's deficits; only whether or not the child's performance differs from developmental norms. Criterion-referenced assessments, on the other hand, do not provide statistical comparisons to other children's abilities, but rather determine whether the child can perform particular tasks deemed to be important for communication. Criterion-referenced assessments may examine specific forms of speech and language in more informal ways or in naturalistic contexts, without standardized rules and methods. Instead, the clinician can establish criteria and learn whether the child meets these particular milestones. Criterion-referenced assessments allow the clinician to individualize the assessment to examine targeted communication behaviors and are ideal for evaluating whether intervention methods have been successful or to monitor progress in a course of therapy. These methods can be developed by the clinician to answer particular questions, such as whether a child understands past tense forms, whether a child can understand vocabulary related to a school curricular unit, or whether a child can participate in language arts assignments given by a particular teacher (4).

The assessment of communication, of necessity, involves some observation of what a child's communication is like in natural situations. It is important to supplement standardized tests with real-life measures for a reliable index of the child's communication in everyday interactions. Observational, or *authentic*, assessment allows for a closer look at a child's communication, by examining the child's spontaneous language use and understanding in contextualized settings pertinent to the child and provides a record of the child's growth in skills over time. McCauley (5) argued for the importance of supplementing standardized measures with authentic assessment due to the fact that norm-referenced testing, even when high sensitivity and specificity were present, nonetheless was inconsistent in identifying actual errors made in a child's spontaneous speech. Thus, to get a realistic perspective of a child's expressive functioning, and to determine appropriate goals for expressive language use, sampling spontaneous communication is an important part of assessment. A range of methods of analyzing spontaneous speech in children at all stages of language development are available, using both paper and pencil as well as automated methods making use of software packages that apply to samples transcribed with codes to indicate various semantic, phonologic, and syntactic features. Examples of these methods can be found in Paul and Norbury (4), McCauley (5), MacWhinney (6), and Miller and Iglesias (7).

Dynamic assessment, an additional nonstandardized form of authentic assessment, is specifically designed to take a closer look at what factors, supports, or modifications enhance the child's communication performance. Dynamic assessment is used to manipulate the linguistic context through the use of prompts, cues, or various scaffolds to determine what best supports positive changes in communication. In turn, dynamic assessment provides important initial information about what techniques or teaching styles may be appropriate for treatment. Moreover, dynamic assessment measures have been found to reduce test bias for children learning English as a second language (8). With emphasis on the learning process (test-teach-test) rather than what has already been learned, dynamic assessment is especially helpful in determining whether real communicative impairments are present in bilingual school-age children who may appear to show deficits due to their lack of experience in English, rather than due to inherent language learning problems (9).

Another form of dynamic assessment is use of the *Response to Intervention* (RTI) model of classroom instruction. RTI is aimed at determining whether a child's poor performance is due to limited previous exposure to the concept or skill rather than inherent learning problems. This is accomplished by carefully monitoring each child's progress within a course of regular classroom instruction in language and literacy, identifying children who perform poorly on these ongoing assessments, and providing them with supplemental small group instruction to determine whether their response to this additional input allows them to catch up to classmates and go on to perform at grade level. Children who respond to this level of intervention are spared the experience of evaluation for, and possibly mistaken placement in special education. Those who do not respond to the initial intervention may be provided with some additional one-to-one instruction, before being referred for an evaluation for special educational needs. SLPs working in school districts using the RTI model may be called upon to collaborate and consult with classroom teachers in the development of progress monitoring and initial intervention, before determining whether a child meets criteria for services in language and special education (10).

Having examined the range of methods available for assessing communication skills, we can now discuss the three major aims of the assessment process: establishing baseline function, identifying goals for intervention, and monitoring progress in therapy.

Establishing Baseline Function

The purpose of this phase of assessment is not merely to show that the child scores below other children on tests, but to document in detail the child's communicative strengths and weaknesses and whether there is a difference in how the child communicates across various contexts. Typically, a thorough assessment will include measures of both understanding and production of sounds, words, sentence structures, conversation, and storytelling. Profiles of relative strengths and weaknesses among these communicative skills will be used to decide on the child's overall level of communication, which will determine the goal level for areas that are less well developed. When determining the child's baseline level of communicative functioning, standardized tests can, again, be useful, especially those that focus on specific areas of function, rather than those in Table 4.5.3, which assess general receptive versus expressive skills more broadly. Some examples of these focused tests appear in Table 4.5.4.

In addition to testing, though, SLPs often employ more observational methods to round out their picture of the child's ability to communicate in real settings. Frequently, they collect a sample of the child's communication as he/she engages in play or other age-appropriate activities with family or peers. These observations are aimed at discovering how the child uses the communication skills available to him/her to interact socially. Some children with very limited language can show strengths in using gesture, facial expression, and tone of voice to convey a range of meanings, while others at the same level of language show few of these abilities. Conversely, some children with nearly age-appropriate vocabulary and sentence structures who score well on standardized tests are nonetheless severely lacking in social communication skills, and this deficit would not be documented unless data from natural observation were collected. To that end, SLPs often collect samples of spontaneous communication in dyadic conversation. They may also sample the child's ability to construct a coherent narrative about a set of pictures or by discussing a personal experience or retelling a favorite story or video plot. Narrative tasks are known to be highly related to success in school (11), and have been documented to represent weaknesses in children with various kinds of language problems (12). Thus, assessment of narrative skill is often an aspect of the communication assessment for language comprehension and production for school-age children. A range of methods are available in the literature for analyzing various aspects of children's narrative production (4,9,11–14).

As noted earlier, assessment for baseline functioning can also involve answering questions such as, does this child communicate better with adults than peers? in structured or

TABLE 4.5.4

EXAMPLES OF STANDARDIZED TESTS FOR FOCUSED LANGUAGE ASSESSMENT

Test	Developmental Level
Boehm Test of Basic Concepts—3rd ed. Boehm AE (2000). San Antonio, TX: Pearson	K–2nd grade
Expressive Vocabulary Test—2nd ed. Williams KT (2007). San Antonio, TX: Pearson	2:6–adulthood
Expressive One-Word Picture Vocabulary Test—4th ed. Martin NA, Brownell R (2010). Austin, TX: Pro-Ed	2–adulthood
Lindamood Auditory Conceptualization Test—3rd ed. Lindamood PC, Lindamood P (2004). San Antonio, TX: Pearson	5–18:11 yrs
Peabody Picture Vocabulary Test—4th ed. Dunn LM, Dunn DM (2007). Minneapolis, MN: Pearson	2:6 yrs–adulthood
Receptive One-Word Picture Vocabulary Test—4th ed. Martin NA, Brownell R (2010). San Antonio, TX: Pearson	2:11–adulthood
Structured Photographic Expressive Language Test—3rd ed. Dawson JI, Stout CE, Eyer JA (2003). Austin, TX: Pro-Ed	4–9:11 yrs
Test of Adolescent/Adult Word Finding—2nd ed. German DJ (2015). Austin, TX: Pro-Ed	12–adulthood
Test for Auditory Comprehension of Language—4th ed. Carrow-Woolfolk E (1999). Austin, TX: Pro-Ed	3–12:11 yrs
Test of Narrative Language. Gillam RB, Pearson, NA (2004). Austin, TX: Pro-Ed	5–11:11 yrs
Test of Pragmatic Language—2nd ed. Phelps-Terasaki D, Phelps-Gunn, T (2007). Austin, TX: Pro-Ed	6–18:11 yrs
Elementary: Test of Problem Solving—3rd ed. Bowers L, Barrett M, Huisingh R, Orman J, LoGiudice C (2005). Austin, TX: LinguiSystems	6–12 yrs
Test of Word Finding—3rd ed. German DJ (2014). Austin, TX: Pro-Ed	4:6–12:11 yrs
Test of Word Knowledge. Wiig EH, Secord W (1992). San Antonio, TX: Pearson	5–17:0 yrs
Test of Written Language—4th ed. Hammill DD, Larsen SC (2009). Austin, TX: Pro-Ed	9–17:11 yrs

informal settings? in familiar environments? To answer these questions, a child's communication may be observed in several settings and among different partners. The SLP may, for example, collect language samples of the preschool child playing with a parent and then with a peer, of a toddler playing with a parent and then with a clinician, or of a school-age child having a conversation with a clinician and then telling him/her a story. By taking several observations in varying contexts, a fuller picture of the child's relative strengths and needs can be drawn.

Identifying Goals for Intervention

The completion of a comprehensive communication assessment leads to the identification of appropriate targets for a child's intervention program. Criterion-referenced, dynamic, and observational assessments are central to this aim. The SLP uses these methods to determine where a particular child is in the developmental sequence of communication acquisition, what skills are next in the developmental sequence of language acquisition, and what components and subcomponents of the language system the child has mastered, is using inconsistently, or is not using at all. Observation and language sampling will be used to identify aspects of communication that are most troublesome in preventing the child from effectively communicating with parents, teachers, and peers. Criterion-referenced assessment will be used to fill out the picture of strengths and needs. Dynamic assessment or RTI will help to determine what kinds of supports, cues, prompts, and materials will be most facilitating for the acquisition of new forms. The end result of this phase of the assessment will be a set of long-term goals that state the desired changes in communication to be targeted over the next 1- to 3-year period (depending on the child's current age). Typically measurable annual goals are based on the child's needs and present level of performance and align along a developmental continuum or with grade-level curriculum. Based on the identified speech or language impairment, goals are created to address identified impairment with speech production (e.g., articulation, phonology, fluency) or language: form (phonology, morphology, syntax), content (semantics), and/or use (social communication). Each long-term goal will be broken down into a sequence of short-term objectives, which state the steps the child will be led through in order to attain the long-term goal. Short-term objectives typically follow a three-part format:

1. "Do" statement: What the child will do to demonstrate achievement of the goal (James will produce sentences with "I want" and an object ["cookies"])
2. A context: Under what circumstances the child will be able to perform the behavior at this phase of the therapy (when shown a desired object and prompted with "Tell me what you want")
3. A criterion: How frequently the child must perform the activity correctly in order to move on to the next step in the sequence (in 90% of trials).

Monitoring Change in Intervention

Once the basic plan of the intervention program has been designed, the SLP proceeds through each of the short-term objectives. In order to move on to the next step, however, the SLP must show that the child has achieved the criterion level stated in the short-term objective. Further, the SLP will need to document when the long-term goal has been achieved and therefore no longer needs to be addressed in therapy. These require tracking the degree to which the client is producing correct responses within and outside therapy sessions.

The child's intervention plans—the Individualized Family Service Plan (IFSP) intended for families of children from birth to three years of age or the Individualized Education Program (IEP) for school-age children—will specify how the child's progress on goals will be measured (e.g., given the category 'animals,' the child will name 4-5 animals, after exposure to animal names and pictures in picture books presented by the clinician). SLPs routinely record and analyze client responses to therapy activities in order to document these changes. Monitoring change in intervention, however, not only requires that SLPs show their clients can get, for example, 90% correct responses in a treatment activity; they also need to show that these changes generalize to real conversation and interaction. To demonstrate these broader changes, SLPs often use criterion-referenced assessments, as well as language sampling. These assessment methods allow the demonstration of change not only in structured activities, but also in the real-world situations that determine a child's communicative competence.

SUMMARY

The assessment of communication is part of the larger process of diagnostic evaluation and educational planning that goes into determining the strengths and needs of children with disabilities. In conducting these assessments, professionals from a variety of disciplines collaborate to determine a child's diagnostic classification and eligibility for publicly funded services, to describe in detail the child's needs in all areas of functioning, to identify the most appropriate goals for an intervention program, and to monitor the program as it proceeds to ensure it is efficient and effective. SLPs typically function as members of an assessment team whose primary responsibility is to evaluate the child's use of communication. They use a variety of methods to achieve these goals, including standardized tests, criterion-referenced assessments, observations of authentic communication, and dynamic methods to identify effective supports for learning.

References

1. Individuals with Disabilities Education Act (IDEA), Part C: Early Intervention for Infants and Toddlers with Disabilities, 20 U.S.C., Part C § 303.321, 2004.
2. Sachse S, Von Suchodoletz W: Early identification of language delay by direct language assessment or parent report? *J Dev Behav Pediatr* 29:34–41, 2008.
3. Beukelman DR, Mirenda P: *Augmentative and Alternative Communication: Supporting Children and Adults with Complex Communication Needs.* 4th ed. Baltimore, MD, Paul H. Brookes Publishing Co., Inc., 2013.
4. Paul R, Norbury C: *Language Disorders From Infancy Through Adolescence.* St. Louis, MO, Elsevier, 2012.
5. McCauley RJ: *Assessment of Language Disorders in Children.* New York, Psychology Press, 2013.
6. MacWhinney B: *The CHILDES Project: Tools for Analyzing Talk–Electronic Edition Part 1: The CHAT Transcription Format.* 2012.
7. Miller J, Iglesias A: *SALT: Systematic Analysis of Language Transcripts. Software for the Analysis of Oral Language.* Middleton, WI, SALT Software LLC, 2012.
8. Patterson JL, Rodriguez BL, Dale PS: Response to dynamic language tasks among typically developing Latino preschool children with bilingual experience. *Am J Speech Lang Pathol* 22:103–112, 2013.
9. Peña ED, Gillam RB, Malek M, et al.: Dynamic assessment of school-age children's narrative ability: an experimental investigation of classification accuracy. *J Speech Lang Hear Res* 49:1037–1057, 2006.
10. Wixson KK, Valencia SW: Assessment in RTI: what teachers and specialists need to know. *The Reading Teacher* 64:466–469, 2011.
11. Petersen DB, Gillam SL, Spencer T, Gillam RB: The effects of literate narrative intervention on children with neurologically based language impairments: an early stage study. *J Speech Lang Hear Res* 53:961–981, 2010.
12. Petersen D, Spencer T: The narrative language measures: tools for language screening, progress monitoring, and intervention planning. *Perspect Lang Learn Educ* 19:119–129, 2012.
13. Liles BZ: Cohesion in the narratives of normal and language-disordered children. *J Speech Hear Res* 28:123–133, 1985.
14. Norbury CF, Bishop DV: Narrative skills of children with communication impairments. *Int J Lang Commun Disord* 38:287–313, 2003.

CHAPTER 4.6 ■ STRUCTURED INTERVIEWING

ADRIAN ANGOLD, ELIZABETH JANE COSTELLO, AND HELEN EGGER

INTRODUCTION

Interviews are necessary tools for all forms of clinical medical diagnosis, and they have a singularly prominent position in psychiatry because of the lack of other "tests" for psychiatric disorders. All structured interviews used in psychiatry have their roots in the phenomenologic clinical interview, although different interviews take rather different routes in the standardization of the collection of phenomenologic data relevant to diagnosis. The questioning strategies involved now represent a mature technology, and the sometimes acrimonious methodologic debates that once characterized the field have been replaced by the recognition that each approach has advantages and disadvantages that must be weighed in selecting a structured interview for each individual application.

The Limitations of Unstructured Diagnostic Interviews

It has been known for a long time that clinical training is sufficiently varied that colleagues of the same discipline, working in the same establishment, are often unable to agree about an individual's diagnosis, even when presented with exactly the same information (1–4). An apparent difference in rates of schizophrenia between New York and London proved to be almost entirely due to differences in diagnostic criteria applied to observed phenomenology (5). Observations such as these motivated the development of the formalized sets of diagnostic criteria familiar to us today from the DSM-IV and ICD-10.

The literature on medical decision-making had already shown that clinicians suffer from a number of information collection biases: (1) They tend to come to diagnostic determinations before they have collected all the relevant information; (2) they tend then to focus on collecting information to *confirm* that diagnosis (confirmatory bias); (3) they tend to ignore disconfirmatory information; (4) they combine information in idiosyncratic ways; and (5) they tend to make judgments based on the most readily available cognitive patterns (the availability heuristic). Further problems arise because of a tendency to see correlations where none exist (illusory correlation), and to miss real correlations (6).

Added to all these problems is the fact that, even today, standard diagnostic manuals do not provide very detailed descriptions of how to assess psychopathology at the symptom level. All of the criteria for oppositional defiant disorder, for instance, begin with the word "often." But "how often is often?" There is a great deal of room for clinicians to adopt very different decision rules about when to regard such symptoms as being present.

In the face of all these difficulties it became apparent that methods were required to standardize the collection, quantification, and combination of diagnostic information. As a result, all structured interviews aim to:

1. Structure information coverage, so that all interviewers will have collected all relevant information (both confirmatory and disconfirmatory) from all subjects.
2. Define the ways in which relevant information is to be collected.
3. Structure the process by which relevant confirmatory and disconfirmatory information is combined to produce a final diagnosis.

Early Structured Diagnostic Interviews

In the early days of structured interviews, it was supposed that *clinicians* would be using them, because it was felt that only they had the necessary training and experience to be able to decide about the presence or absence of symptoms, even when quite detailed definitions were provided. The interview schedule served as a tool to guide the clinician interviewer in determining whether symptoms were present, but the interviewer made the decisions, on the basis of information provided by the child or adult. Interviews of this sort, like the Present State Examination (7) and the Reynard (8) for adults, and the Isle of Wight interview for children (9,10), were the first to be developed, since they sprang naturally from clinical practice. They were called *semi*-structured because the interviewer was allowed latitude in the specific form of the questions used.

Although the PSE and Isle of Wight interviews were used extensively in community surveys, it was clear that the use of clinician interviewers created both logistic and budgetary problems. Large-scale epidemiologic studies, such as the Epidemiologic Catchment Area (ECA) studies (11) mandated the use of nonclinician ("lay") interviewers. Some felt that such interviewers would be incapable of making the judgments about symptoms; so, following methodologies used by political and marketing surveys, interviews were developed that required only that the interviewer asks a set of fixed questions in a preset order, and collects the simple answers to those questions. In such interviews, it is the *questions* put to the subject which are structured, and the interviewer makes no decisions about the presence of symptoms. Hence they came to be called *highly* or *fully* structured. The Diagnostic Interview Schedule (DIS) was the paradigmatic example of this sort of interview in adult psychiatry (12), while the original Diagnostic Interview Schedule for Children and Adolescents (DICA) was the first child-oriented example (13,14).

Emergence of the Diagnostic Interview with the Child

Until the late 1960s, interviews and questionnaires directed to a parent or teacher about a child's behavior and *observation* of the child's behavior were the predominant methods of assessment in child and adolescent psychiatry. Verbal information from the child was typically regarded as being only supplemental, or material for psychodynamic interpretation (15).

More attention was paid to playing with the child than to the collection of information through direct questioning. In 1968, a key transitional paper reported on the reliability and validity of the Isle of Wight interview with the child (9). Here the behavior of the child in a face-to-face interview was examined directly, but little was made of the factual content of the child's reports. In 1975, Herjanic and her colleagues (16) asked: "are children reliable reporters" of factual information, and presented evidence that they are. Since then, a great deal of work has confirmed the importance of children's self-reports as a source of factual information, with the result that fact-finding (as opposed to interpretative) interviews with both parents and children are now regarded as being of equal weight in the diagnostic process, at least from late childhood (prior to about age 9, children are incapable of completing such "adult-style" interviews). The one exception is in the evaluation of attention-deficit hyperactivity disorder (ADHD) symptoms, where child reports have been found to be of little help (17,18). Even here, however, the recent growth of interest in ADHD in adolescence and adulthood has led to the development of new measures in this area (e.g., 19).

Disagreement among Informants and Its Implications

Until the 1980s, agreement between child and parent reports of symptomatology was widely regarded as being a test of the *validity* of *child* reports (9,14). However, it soon became apparent that only low levels of agreement among informants (correlation coefficients around 0.3 for agreement among children, parents and teachers) could be expected (20,21). It is now considered that low levels of agreement among different informants about the child's clinical state are to be expected and do not invalidate the reports of any of them. Rather, each key informant presents a particular view of the child's problems. Indeed, it is precisely because agreement among informants is low that multiple informants are needed. Were agreement very high, taking the history from more than one informant would be redundant.

The problem is that disagreement among informants means that one has to decide how to weight the information from each informant in arriving at a diagnosis. Since it is uncommon for informants to invent fictitious symptoms, the simple rule of regarding a symptom as being present if any informant reports it usually suffices. When symptoms are combined to make diagnoses, the usual procedure is to ignore the source, and to add up all positive symptoms from any source. Thus, a diagnosis of a major depressive episode (which requires the presence of at least five symptoms) might be made on the basis of three relevant symptoms being reported by the child (say depressed mood, anhedonia, and excessive guilt), with two other relevant symptoms (perhaps sleep and appetite disturbances) being reported by another informant (typically a parent and/or teacher). Although some interview developers have recommended "reconciliation" discussions involving the interviewer, the parent, and the child to clear up discrepancies between their reports (22), such a discussion is problematic. Reconciliation requires one informant to modify his or her story, but that means admitting being wrong, or at least uninformed. The knowledge that such a discussion will occur could cause informants (e.g., drug-using adolescents) to withhold important information that they did not wish other informants (such as their parents) to hear about. Finally, in most research applications, one wishes to assure informants that what they say will not be revealed to anyone else, in which case a reconciliation interview is ruled out.

The remainder of this chapter is concerned with the description of key points relating to general psychiatric diagnostic interviews, that is, those that cover a broad range of the common disorders of childhood and adolescence. A number of interviews and observational systems exist for more specialized tasks (for instance, the Autism Diagnostic Interview and the Autism Diagnostic Observation Schedule (23,24)), but such instruments will not be considered further here.

A TYPOLOGY OF INTERVIEWS

As we have already seen, a distinction between semi-structured and highly structured interviews has found its way into the description and discussion of diagnostic interviewing techniques. However, these terms are not very helpful for two reasons. First, they imply that the key difference between different types of interview concerns the *amount* of structure they impose. The problem is that the real issue is not one of amount of structure, but rather who makes the final decision as to whether a symptom is present.

Respondent-Based Interviews

In interviews where the questions are absolutely prespecified, it is the respondent who makes the final decision (typically by answering yes or no to each question). The interviewer makes no such decisions, but merely reads the questions. Since the decisions as to the presence or absence of psychopathology lie with the respondent in such interviews, we refer to them as being *respondent-based*. The Diagnostic Interview Schedule for Children (DISC (25)) and the computer-assisted version of the DICA (26), and the Dominic-R (27) are the three representatives of this approach.

Interviewer-Based Interviews and Glossary-Based Interviews

We call interviews that require the interviewer to make an informed decision based on what the respondent says *interviewer-based*. The interviewer is expected to question until s/he can decide whether a symptom meeting the definitions provided by the interview (or known to them from their training) is present. This group of interviews includes the Anxiety Disorders Interview Schedule (ADIS (28)), the Child and Adolescent Psychiatric Assessment (CAPA (29)), the Child Assessment Schedule (CAS (30,31)), the paper and pencil (not the computerized) versions of the DICA (26) and its close relative the Missouri Assessment of Genetics Interview for Children (MAGIC), the Interview Schedule for Children and Adolescents (ISCA (32)), the various versions of the Kiddie Schedule for Affective Disorders and Schizophrenia (K-SADS (33)), and the Pictorial Instrument for Children and Adolescents (PICA-IIIR (34)). Three of these interviewer-based interviews (the K-SADS-P IVR, the DICA, and the CAPA) provide extensive sets of definitions of symptoms and/or detailed guidance on the conduct of the interview, and we call these *glossary-based*. Such glossaries are particularly important when an interviewer-based interview is to be used by nonclinician interviewers because they provide detailed guidance as to what the interviewer is supposed to be looking for in making symptom ratings. Nonclinician interviewers have been shown to be able to make such "clinical" judgments with high reliability when they have received adequate training with such glossaries (35).

The distinction between interviewer- and respondent-based interviews is not hard and fast in actual practice, because there has been considerable cross-fertilization between these approaches. For instance, the CAPA, which has its roots in the interviewer-based tradition, includes a subset of questions that are to be asked verbatim of all subjects, as in a respondent-based interview, but then allows further questioning for clarification. On the other hand, the DICA, which had previously been a respondent-based interview, now requires interviewers to question much more flexibly, and is now an interviewer-based instrument (26). Though the distinction between interviewer- and respondent-based interviews provides a useful rough-and-ready typology, it is really better to consider interviews as lying at various locations along three dimensions: (1) degree of specification of questions, (2) degree of definition of symptom concepts, and (3) degree of flexibility in questioning permitted to the interviewers. Interviews that provide extensive definitions and require interviewers to make judgments lie in the interviewer-based region of that three-dimensional space, while those that specify every question and allow no interviewer deviation from those questions lie in the respondent-based region.

PICTORIAL INTERVIEWS

More recently, respondent-based child self-report interviews that add *pictorial* cues have been added to the assessment armamentarium. The most developed pictorial interview at this time is the Dominic-R (27,36,37) which is intended for use with 6 to 11 year olds. Pictures representing psychopathology relevant to seven diagnoses are shown to the child, and questions about whether each symptom is present are read at the same time. Because no frequency, duration, or onset data are collected, it is not yet clear how such information should be combined with diagnostic information from other sources. This is, however, a general problem for interviews with younger children, because before the age of 8 or 9, they simply cannot provide all the frequency, dating, and timing information that full diagnostic interviews require. Although diagnostic test–retest reliabilities cannot be reported for the Dominic-R, its item reliabilities are respectable in comparison with those reported from studies of older children with other interviews.

The PICA-IIIR, for children aged 6 to 16, adopts a somewhat similar approach, but the questions to be asked with the pictures are more loosely specified, and it is intended to be used by clinicians. It covers a broader range of diagnoses than the Dominic-R, but no test–retest reliability data are yet available (34).

Parent-Only Interviews for Younger Children

Standard practice in adult psychiatry is to rely upon a single key informant for structured diagnostic interviews. The person who is the subject of the interview alone is interviewed. Parent and teacher interviews are added in child and adolescent psychiatry because the child him/herself is regarded as being a limited informant. The point is that, at any age, interviews need to be conducted with whoever is needed to provide adequate reliable information coverage. We have already noted that younger children cannot provide all the information necessary for making DSM-style diagnoses, but there is no reason why the child's lack of capacity in this regard should invalidate the use of the available best informants (parents and sometimes teachers) for diagnostic purposes. After all, in clinical practice diagnosis for young children is very largely based on parent reports of the child's behavior supplemented by office observations and teacher reports. Following this logic, several groups have modified interviews originally developed for use with parents of older children to allow structured diagnostic assessments down to age 2 (38–40). A test–retest study of one of these (the Preschool Age Psychiatric Assessment [PAPA]) suggests that preschoolers' diagnoses assessed in this way are just reliable as those of older children (38).

Screened Interviews

The Children's Interview for Psychiatric Syndromes (ChIPS (41)) was designed as a *screening* tool covering 20 DSM-IV Axis 1 disorders. "Cardinal questions" concerning symptoms most often seen in children with a particular disorder are asked at the beginning of each section. If the answers to these screening questions are in the negative, then the rest of that section is skipped. No test–retest reliability data are yet available for the ChIPS. A similarly screened version of the CAPA is also available, but in practice, it has been found to save only about 10 minutes of interview time, so the loss of information resulting from not asking about all symptoms may not really be worth the time saving.

Computerized Interviews

Computer-*assisted* psychiatric interviews (CAPI) employ an interviewer to read questions from the screen and enter the appropriate codes into the computer as the interview progresses. The machine takes the interviewer to the appropriate stem questions, and stores the responses in a database. There is no need for bulky interview schedules to be copied and carried around, and data entry is completed during the interview (or during coding of the interview later in the office with some interviews). Furthermore, the computer will not accidentally skip parts of the interview, or accidentally vary the order of its presentation. On the other hand, computerized interviews can be programmed to vary the order in which sections are presented deliberately, so as to reduce the order of presentation effects observed when respondents learn that saying no tends to shorten the interview. However, interviews for use with children do not currently incorporate this potential feature. Recent advances in programming technology for structured interviews mean that even the most "interviewer-based" interviews can now be produced in CAPI formats. For instance, the CAPI version of the PAPA allows interviewers to write and store text notes with a stylus on a tablet PC; similar versions of the CAPA and YAPA are also available. When some interview schedules run to over 300 pages, the costs of buying computers can soon be offset against savings on schedule reproduction and data entry. The DISC has become progressively more complex over the last 20 years (largely because of the ever-increasing complexity of the DSMs), and, except as discussed below, the DISC-IV is now supposed always to be completed in its CAPI format, because it is really too difficult to administer it effectively in a paper-and-pencil format. There is also a CAPI version of the DICA, but this differs from the paper-and-pencil version of the interview in being fully respondent-based (42). Given the advantages of CAPI administration, we predict that paper and pencil will soon disappear as a means of interview administration.

The next level of computerization is referred to as *audio computer-administered* survey interviewing (ACASI). Here no interviewer is used at all. Rather, digitized audio recordings of the questions (sometimes even with digitized video of an interviewer) are played back by the computer as the written form of the question is displayed. The respondent enters a response to the question, which is saved to the database. Obviously, such an approach can only be adopted with a respondent-based interview, and the DISC provides the paradigmatic example of this approach (43).

INTRODUCTION TO THE INTERVIEWS

Here we present a brief introduction to each of the diagnostic interviews, with a focus on their characteristic *response formats.*

The Schedule for Affective Disorders and Schizophrenia for School-Age Children (Kiddie-SADS, K-SADS)

The K-SADS "family" of interviews consists of a group of very diverse assessments. Indeed, the only features that all of the current versions of the K-SADS share in common are the name, the ability to make DSM-IV diagnoses, and the fact that all were designed to be administered *by clinicians*. The original version of the K-SADS (the K-SADS-P (44)) was a downward extension of the adult Schedule for Affective Disorders and Schizophrenia (SADS) and focused on the Research Diagnostic Criteria (45). Note that the "P" in its title stands for *present* (not parent). It was designed for use with children aged 6 to 17, but covered only a relatively limited range of symptoms and diagnoses. It was revised to cover DSM-IIIR (46) and DSM-IV.

K-SADS-P IVR

The version of the K-SADS-P most recently developed by Ambrosini and colleagues (46) is called the K-SADS-P IVR. This version is closest conceptually to the original K-SADS-P in including quite detailed definitions of severity codings for each symptom. The modal form for these symptom codings is a six-point scale, involving judgments about various combinations of intensity, duration, frequency, environmental responsiveness, psychosocial impairment, and observed behavior.

K-SADS-E

The K-SADS-E (47) (E for epidemiologic) collects ratings of the present episode of any disorder *and* the *worst* past episode. This interview was never even remotely similar in format to the K-SADS-P, because it rated only the presence or absence of symptoms, rather than employing the carefully defined severity codings of the K-SADS-P. The latest edition is DSM-IV compatible, and allows the current *episode* (not individual symptoms) to be rated as mild, moderate or severe.

K-SADS-PL

A group in Pittsburgh has developed the K-SADS-PL (present and lifetime), as a sort of cross between the K-SADS-P and the K-SADS-E (48,49). Symptom ratings have been reduced to three-point scales (typically not at all, subthreshold, threshold), and fairly minimal anchoring definitions of each point are provided. An initial 82-item screen interview, which allows skipping of substantial symptom areas, is also available.

WASH-U-KSADS

Rather brief definitions of symptoms are given, and level of severity is coded, but the severity codings are idiosyncratic, and bear little relation to those in other versions of the K-SADS.

COLUMBIA K-SADS

The symptom "definitions" provided are often simply restatements of the DSM-IV criteria. Sometimes (particularly in relation to depression) a little more guidance is given. Symptom severity is typically rated on what appears to be a six-point scale like the K-SADS-P and K-SADS-P IVR, but closer inspection reveals that two of the points are usually defined only as being intermediate between two other points. Thus, only four points (one being symptom absence) are really defined.

Although K-SADS interviews were developed for use by clinicians, some have also been used with lay interviewers (31).

The K-SADS family differs from most interviews (but not the ISCA) in directing that the parent should be interviewed first and then the child should be seen by the same interviewer, who is then expected to resolve any discrepancies between the child's reports and those of the parent. The interviewer then completes a record representing his/her summation of the two interviews. This procedure is highly dependent on clinical judgment, and means that the process of combining the information is not structured. It also seems likely to bias the results of the interview in favor of the parental reports, and some workers have instead scored the interviews with the parent and the child separately (50).

The Child and Adolescent Psychiatric Assessment (CAPA) and Its Congeners

The CAPA is one of an integrated group of instruments developed to assess a variety of risk factors for, manifestations of, and outcomes of child and adolescent psychiatric disorders. In addition to the usual symptom and impairment assessments, it also includes extensive ratings of the family environment and relationships, family psychosocial problems, and life events (including traumatic events and physical and sexual abuse). A separate module called the Child and Adolescent Impact Assessment (CAIA (51)) measures the impact of the child's problems on the family, while the Child and Adolescent Services Assessment (CASA (52,53)) covers service use for mental health problems in multiple sectors and settings. Psychosocial impairment in 17 domains of functioning is measured at both the syndromic level and overall. In the interview with the child, 62 items reflecting the child's observed behavior during the interview are also coded. In order to facilitate completion of the interview by nonclinicians, the CAPA provides a more molecular approach to symptom codings. Extensive symptom definitions are given in a glossary and on the schedule, and rules are specified to allow nonclinicians make separate codings of the intensity, frequency, duration, date of onset of symptoms, and psychosocial impairment resulting from them. The CAPA emphasizes getting descriptions and examples of possible pathology to ensure that codings are not based on the informant's misunderstanding of what was being asked about (35,54,55).

A version of the CAPA has been developed for use with *young adults* (the Young Adult Psychiatric Assessment, YAPA), and a substantially modified version is now available for use with the parents of preschool children (PAPA (38)). The latter includes assessment of a number of areas of particular relevance to preschoolers that are not included in any other diagnostic interview. In addition, a version of the CAPA with empirically derived screen items is available, which allows sections to be skipped if screen symptoms are absent. A streamlined version of the CAPA for collecting data for twin studies has also been developed (56).

Diagnostic Interview for Children and Adolescents

The DICA started out as a respondent-based interview over 20 years ago (16,42,57,58). Since then it has been progressively modified so that its paper and pencil version is now an interviewer-based interview (26,59,60). However, there is also a computer-based version of the DICA that remains fully respondent-based (26,60). In addition, the group responsible for the development of the DICA has produced a modification called the Missouri Assessment for Genetics Interview for Children (MAGIC). The major difference between the DICA and the MAGIC is that the MAGIC has a specifications manual, which includes a great deal of guidance on how to elicit key features of symptoms, and a variety of clarifications of coding instructions (26).

The DICA and the MAGIC provide alternate versions for self-reports from children aged 6 (or 7) to 12 and 13 to 17, which have differently worded questions. The DICA has also been used with even younger children, but special training is required for its administration in those under 6 or 7, and the instructions to interviewers essentially tell them to ignore the usual questioning format laid out in the schedule and use their own questions.

Symptoms are typically coded on a three-point scale (no, sometimes/somewhat, yes) for items about emotional symptoms, and a two-point scale (no, yes) for disruptive behaviors with additional information on frequency sometimes being added. Impairment is measured at the syndrome level by three items asking about symptoms making it hard to "get along" with the family, friends, and at school, rated on four-point scales (not at all, not too much, somewhat, quite a bit).

CHILD ASSESSMENT SCHEDULE

The CAS is organized around thematic topics and provides ratings of many items that are not required if all one wants to do is make ratings of the DSM criteria for disorders (31,61–64). The CAS now exists in child (7–12), adolescent, and parent report versions. Although originally developed for use by experienced clinicians, the CAS has now been used by lay interviewers in several studies. Symptoms are scored on a four-point scale (yes; no; ambiguous; not scored). This is followed by questioning about the onset and duration of positive symptoms. The items to be coded are defined in brief sentences which outline each symptom concept. The interviewer is expected to make a judgment about the coding based on the answer to the questions on the schedule (plus any additional questions that may be thought necessary).

The CAS also has a 56-item section for recording observations of the child's behavior during the interview. Diagnoses can be generated manually by interviewers using algorithms provided by the developer of the interview, but computerized scoring is recommended. The algorithms also generate symptom scales pertaining to a number of areas of psychopathology.

Psychosocial impairment is measured using a separate measure, the Child and Adolescent Functional Assessment Scale (CAFAS), which can also be used alone or with another diagnostic interview (65–67).

The Anxiety Disorders Interview Schedule

Notwithstanding its title, the ADIS also provides brief ratings of symptoms pertinent to other disorders, but its coverage of the anxiety disorders is more thorough (68–73). The interview is designed for clinician use, and was derived from the adult ADIS (74). Questions that *should* be asked are provided, and guidance is given about when to use additional questions. Most symptoms are scored on a simple three-point scale (yes, no, other). However, in the anxiety section a good deal of use is also made of nine-point scales (represented by a thermometer) ranging from not at all to very, very much. Similar scales are used to rate "interference," which is the ADIS term for psychosocial impairment resulting from disorders. Skip structures are frequently employed, so many individuals will not be asked about all symptoms.

The Interview Schedule for Children and Adolescents

The ISCA mandates administration by experienced clinicians with extensive structured interviewing training, and full understanding of the principles of diagnosis and its application to children with psychopathology. Interviewers must be able to combine the symptom information from both parent and child into diagnoses themselves, since formal algorithms for this process (other than the official diagnostic manual itself) do not appear to be available (32). Questions are clearly specified, but much additional clarification is expected of interviewers, who are not expected slavishly to stick to the written questions. Sixty-nine "major" symptoms plus 10 "mental status" items are covered, and typically coded on a nine-point severity scale that incorporates judgments about associated distress, functional impairment, and the amount of effort required to counteract symptoms. "Subsidiary information" about many symptoms is also collected, typically in a yes/no format. In addition, 17 intra-interview behavioral observation items are assessed.

A version of the interview for use with young adults (the Follow-up Interview Schedule for Adults, FISA) has also been developed.

The Diagnostic Interview Schedule for Children (DISC)

As already indicated, the questions on a respondent-based instrument are designed in a fixed, ordered sequence, and require very simple responses (typically yes/no, or picking one from a set of multiple choices for frequencies and durations of symptoms). Symptom severity is defined by similar yes/no answers on subsidiary questions (asked only if a positive response was obtained to a superordinate question) and forced choices from short sets of frequency ranges. All data combination is performed by computerized algorithms. The DISC covers a wide range of childhood and adolescent disorders and is suitable for use with 9 to 18 year olds (75). A version for use with the parents of preschoolers is currently under development. CAPI and ACASI versions are available.

INTERVIEW TIME FRAMES

The K-SADS interviews, the ADIS, the CAS, the Dominic, the PICA-IIIR, and the ISCA all focus on the child's current status or the current episode of disorder, though the definition of "current" is largely unspecified, except in the case of the ISCA, where the assessment period is specified (e.g., 2 weeks for irritability). The Columbia K-SADS adds a past 2-week time frame to the current frame. The K-SADS-PL, the Columbia K-SADS, and K-SADS-E also explore lifetime histories of "worst" episodes, while the ISCA also provides for assessment of lifetime disorder, and an interim version provides an assessment of current status plus the child's status in the interim between the current assessment and the last assessment for use in follow-up studies. The DICA and MAGIC focus on the whole lifetime, but for some disorders an additional shorter time frame is also included. For instance, in the depression section, the MAGIC asks about the past month as well as whether the child has "ever" had symptoms. The CAPA covers a "primary period" of 3 months, but also notes whether certain uncommon symptoms (such as suicide attempts) have ever occurred, and a version that provides lifetime coverage of major episodes of certain syndromes is also available (56). The full DISC-IV can be used to assess either the last month or the last year, and also offers a module to determine whether certain syndromes that did not occur during the preceding year had occurred at any point since the age of five.

SPECIFICATION OF QUESTIONS, INTERVIEWER FLEXIBILITY, AND DEFINITION OF SYMPTOMS

In a fully respondent-based interview like the DISC, or the computerized version of the DICA, all questions are completely specified and no others may be used. There is no interviewer flexibility, and no need to provide definitions of symptoms. All variability in these features concerns the interviewer-based interviews.

The ADIS, CAPA, DICA, and MAGIC all contain questions that, under most circumstances, should be asked as written in the schedule. Additional questions are then asked as necessary to allow the interviewer to determine exactly whether the symptom is present. Many such questions are provided on the schedule of the CAPA, a smaller number is provided by the CAS schedule (but it is not clear to what extent the "set" questions of the CAS are mandated for use). Most guidance on this process for the DICA and MAGIC is provided in the MAGIC's specifications manual. All these interviews provide at least some additional instructions about when to probe further. The K-SADS group of interviews provides a range of suggested questions, but no formal rules about when they are to be used or skipped. Interviewers are also expected to ask any additional follow-up questions that may be necessary to clarify responses.

By interviewer flexibility, we mean the degree to which the interviewer is expected or encouraged to use judgment in asking additional clarifying questions. In this respect, the K-SADS and ISCA (and perhaps the ADIS) interviews may be seen as providing most flexibility because they demand that judgments based on clinical experience be made, and in the case of the K-SADS do not mandate the use of any particular questions. The problem question is "flexible to do what?" The answer is relatively clear in the case of the K-SADS-P IV and the CAPA, where detailed coding rules are provided for each symptom. The task of the interviewer is to determine whether those coding criteria are met. With the other interviewer-based instruments it often seems that the interviewer's job is to get the answer *to the original question*. Variable amounts of guidance on how to do so are provided; in considerable detail in the MAGIC specifications manual, with brief symptom definitions in the CAS, but little or no guidance in the K-SADS-E or ADIS.

The K-SADS-P IV and the CAPA provide detailed *definitional* glossaries covering each symptom, which means that the task of the interviewer is quite clearly specified at the level of the definition of symptoms. The CAPA glossary also contains many procedural instructions relating both to questioning in general and questioning about specific symptoms; but these are presented as being secondary to the definitional issues. The MAGIC specifications manual can also be seen as being a glossary, but it is, first and foremost, a *procedural* manual. It is primarily about how to collect the information. In the course of this discussion of procedure, it also includes a good deal of definitional material, but does not provide formal definitions of items in the way that the K-SADS-P IV or CAPA do.

RELIABILITY OF STRUCTURED DIAGNOSTIC INTERVIEWS

A difficulty with the literature on "reliability" is that the term is applied to several very different sorts of design and statistical approaches. Three of these are commonly seen in the literature on structured interviews, but only one presents a useful test of what one ultimately requires in a diagnostic interview. For instance, one often sees reports of *interrater* reliabilities in the interview literature. However, interrater reliability is not a very useful index of interview performance. With respondent-based interviews it tests nothing but whether one interviewer can read aloud adequately while another codes a schedule. With such interviews, if interrater reliability is not in the high 0.9s, one should retrain or fire one's interviewers! In an interviewer-based interview, the questions are not fixed, and so different interviewers could use different questions to elicit the same information. Since the interrater reliability paradigm uses multiple raters to score the same interview, this major source of potential unreliability is eliminated, with the result that the interrater reliability is likely to substantially overestimate the reliability of the interview in actual use. However, if interrater reliabilities fall below about 0.8, that is an indication that something is either wrong with interviewer training, or that the interview needs to be revised to provide greater clarity about what is supposed to be rated. The point is that, if very high interrater reliability coefficients cannot be obtained, we can be certain that test–retest reliability will be poor.

"Internal reliability" is sometimes reported for scales resulting from diagnostic interviews. Typically the statistic given is Cronbach's alpha. This statistic provides a measure of the degree to which the items in the scale are correlated with one another. There are two problems with the use of such a statistic here. First, it has nothing to do with whether *raters* are coding items "reliably"; it concerns the degree to which the items in a scale are all measuring the same thing. Second, a perfectly good diagnosis could be associated with low correlations among the symptoms that signal the presence of that diagnosis. Most medical (and psychiatric) diagnoses are more concerned with pattern recognition than with scalar values. For instance, in the general population it is unlikely that dry eyes, dry mouth, and arthritis are very highly correlated with one another, but that does not mean that Sjorgren's syndrome is a bad diagnosis. Of course, if the task is to develop a scalar measure of some construct, then the scale's alpha is important information. However, from the perspective of a diagnostic interview, low alphas are not necessarily a bad thing, nor are high alphas necessarily a good thing. It is entirely possible to have a perfect measure of a diagnostic entity where Cronbach's alpha for the symptoms constituting that entity was close to zero.

Table 4.6.1 shows the results of studies of the *test–retest* reliabilities (Kappas) of diagnoses measured by the instruments considered in this chapter. Test–retest reliability is what is needed in judging an instrument. In the absence of reasonable test–retest reliability, all other reliabilities are moot. It can be seen that all the interviews that have been tested do a reasonably good job, and that there is not much to choose between them. These reliability coefficients are similar to those reported for psychiatric interviews with adults.

Reliabilities for scale scores derived from the interviews are typically rather higher than they are for diagnosis, but that is nearly always true of comparisons between scale score reliabilities and the reliabilities of categories generated by imposing cut points on the same scales. It is also important to remember that some of the unreliability of diagnostic measures is the product of the diagnostic system itself, thanks to its requirement that numerous unmemorable details about past psychopathology be considered. Particular problems have been identified with the reliability of responses concerning the duration of symptoms and the dates of their onsets (76,77).

Despite enormous efforts on the part of interview developers, it cannot be said that the reliability of diagnostic

TABLE 4.6.1

DIAGNOSTIC TEST–RETEST RELIABILITIES (KAPPAS) OF INSTRUMENTS

	MDD[a]	Dysthy/ Minor D	Any Depress	GAD/ OAD	Sep Anx	Specific Phobia	Social Phobia	Any Anx	PTSD	ADHD	CD	ODD	SA/D
K-SADS-P	0.54	0.70						0.24					
K-SADS-P IIIR	0.77	0.89						0.72		0.91		0.46	
K-SADS-PL current	0.90			0.78				0.80	0.67	0.63		0.74	
K-SADS-PL lifetime	1.0			0.78				0.60	0.60	0.55	0.83	0.77	
CAS	1.0	0.85	0.83	0.38				0.72		0.43			
DICA			0.90					0.76		1.0		0.61	
CAPA child only	0.90	0.85	0.82	0.79				0.64	0.64		0.55		1.0
PAPA			0.72	0.39	0.60	0.36	0.54	0.49	0.73	0.74	0.60	0.57	
ISCA child only				0.82	0.81								
ADIS—combined P & C. DSM-IIIR				0.64		0.84	0.73	0.75					
ADIS—combined P & C. DSM-IV. Clinic sample				0.80	0.84	0.81	0.92			1.0		0.62	
DISC-IV—combined P & C. Clinic sample.	0.65			0.58	0.51	0.86	0.48			0.62	.55	0.59	
DISC-IV—combined P & C. Clinic sample. Chinese	0.61				0.53					0.75		0.56	
DISC 2.3—combined P & C. Community sample	0.45			0.52	0.49		0.44	0.47		0.48	0.66	0.59	

[a]MDD, major depressive disorder/episode; Dysthy, dysthymia; Minor, minor depression; Any Anx, any anxiety disorder; PTSD, spot traumatic stress disorder; ODD, oppositional defiant disorder; SA/D, substance abuse or minor depression; GAD, generalized anxiety disorder, OAD, over-anxious disorder; Sep, separation anxiety disorder; ADHD, attention-deficit hyperactivity disorder; CD, conduct dependence.

interviews has increased much over the years. We now have a fairly mature interview technology which has been repeatedly refined in the hope of increasing the reliability of assessments. The current arsenal of diagnostic interviews probably offers as good reliability as can be achieved until quite different means of arriving at psychiatric diagnoses appear.

A problem with the test–retest assessment of reliability is that it requires that the interview be repeated within a short period of time. With both questionnaires and interviews one typically finds that fewer symptoms are endorsed at the second interview than at the first (78,79). There are many possible explanations for this effect (80), but some evidence suggests that the results of the first interview are probably the most accurate representation of reality. The usual interpretation of test–retest reliability statistics such as Cohen's Kappa for categorical data (such as diagnoses) and the intraclass correlation coefficient (ICC) for continuous data (such as scale scores) involves the supposition that the relationship between scores at the first interview and those at the second involves two components, agreement and random error. The presence of a *consistent difference* between first interviews and second interviews indicates that such statistics underestimate the "true" (and ultimately unmeasurable) reliability of both interviews and psychopathology scales.

VALIDITY OF STRUCTURED DIAGNOSTIC INTERVIEWS

The problem with trying to assess the validity of psychiatric interviews is that there is no noninterview test for most psychiatric disorders. The structured interview itself is now the closest approximation we have to a gold standard. So how are we to validate the diagnoses obtained from such interviews? This is a version of a problem that psychologists have been grappling with for decades, one that led to the concept of *construct validity*. The central idea here is that the validity of an instrument for the measurement of a psychological construct inheres not in some single agreement coefficient with one external standard, but in the instrument's performance within the *nomologic net* of theory and data concerning the construct or constructs that the instrument purports to measure (81–89). As Gulliksen (84) pointedly remarked over half a century ago, "at some point in the advance of psychology it would seem appropriate for the psychologist to lead the way in establishing good criterion measures, instead of just attempting to construct imperfect tests for attributes that are presumed to be assessed more accurately and more validly by the judgment of experts." Structured interviews were developed because of the dismal psychometric properties of unaided clinical diagnosis, so comparisons with unstructured clinical judgment (as might be found for instance in chart diagnoses) are hopelessly flawed tests of diagnostic interview validity. That has been obvious to interview developers for a long time, so "validity" studies have sometimes provided the clinicians with all the information from the interviews to be validated, in addition to allowing them to collect further information should they wish to. In such a circumstance it will often be the case that *most* of the information available to the clinician comes from the interview under test. It will hardly be surprising, then, if there is good agreement between clinician and interview, but no real test will have been done.

In considering the validity of any interview we should take a construct validation approach, and describe what we currently know about it in relation to the nomologic net pertaining to child and adolescent psychiatric diagnosis. So far, only the developers of the CAPA have explicitly laid out the evidence for the validity of the CAPA using this approach, but most of the interviews considered here can point to similar chains of evidence. To give a flavor of the sort of evidence relevant to construct validation, the following findings have been adduced as construct validators of the CAPA (29):

1. Diagnostic rates and age and gender patterns of disorder given by the CAPA are consistent with those found using other interviews.
2. Patterns of diagnostic comorbidity are consistent with those found by other interviews.
3. Symptomatic diagnoses are associated with psychosocial impairment.
4. Parent and child reports of psychopathology on the CAPA are related to parent and teacher reports of problems on well-established scales for detecting psychopathology.
5. Children with CAPA-identified disorders use more mental health services than children without diagnoses.
6. CAPA-diagnosed children tend to come from families with a history of mental illness.
7. There is genetic loading for a number of CAPA scales scores and diagnoses.
8. CAPA diagnoses show consistency over time.
9. CAPA diagnoses predict negative life outcomes.
10. Different CAPA diagnoses are differentially related to the physiologic changes of puberty.

There is, of course, a big drawback to this approach. No new interview will be able to point to such chains of evidence until it has been in use for quite a time. How then is any new instrument ever to be developed? The answer lies in the application of common sense and well-established assessment principles. When a new assessment is needed, it is perfectly proper to use the best available information about the nature of the phenomena to be measured to design what seems, on the face of it, to be an adequate measure. Attention needs to be given to keeping questions short, and focused on single constructs; to defining the task of the interviewer clearly; and to providing good definitions of the constructs to be studied in the case of interviewer-based interviews. If initial test–retest reliability is adequate, then in general, it is unlikely that the interview will prove to be completely "invalid." Since it is very unusual to be trying to assess a construct that has been utterly unmeasured before, or about which nothing whatever is known, it will also usually be possible to include in the test–retest study other measures that will give some indication of the concurrent, predictive, or divergent validity of the new instrument.

ADVANTAGES AND DISADVANTAGES OF INTERVIEWER- AND RESPONDENT-BASED INTERVIEWS

Neither interviewer- nor respondent-based interviews are ideal tools, and there is simply no answer to the question "Which type is best?" In this section, we list the general advantages of each type of interview, and the lack of each advantage can be regarded as a disadvantage of the other type. However, it is worth noting here that it has sometimes been said that respondent-based interviews are more appropriate for general population studies. Since it has now been shown that lay interviewers can provide reliable and valid ratings using interviewer-based interviews, this position is no longer tenable. Indeed a number of larger-scale longitudinal general population studies have used (and are still using) interviewer-based interviews (for instance) (90,91).

Advantages of Interviewer-Based Interviews

Interviewer-based interviews have four theoretical and practical advantages: (1) If the interview has been conducted and coded properly, the meaning of the ratings is precisely known; (2) they provide opportunities to cross-check discrepant or confusing information; (3) they enable the use of efficient open-ended questioning strategies, and allow the use of redundant questioning, which has been shown in adults to improve the quality of responses; and (4) they appear to be less prone to overdiagnosis on the basis of symptom reports, so arbitrary impairment scale cutoffs do not have to be employed to produce reasonable diagnostic rates in unselected community samples.

What Do the Codings Mean?

In an interviewer-based interview, a positive coding for a symptom means that it has been determined that the symptom as defined in the schedule is present. In a respondent-based interview, one knows only that a child or parent responded positively to a particular question. One does not know exactly what the child or parent understood the question to mean. This problem has been documented with unusual symptoms that most children never experience, such as obsessive–compulsive or psychotic symptoms. Such symptoms were greatly overreported using early versions of the DISC (92). When clinicians reviewed what the children said, it was obvious that what was being reported was not obsessive–compulsive disorder or psychosis. However, if an unstructured clinician review is added to the diagnostic process, one no longer knows exactly what factors went into the final rating, and one great advantage of the respondent-based interview is lost.

Cross-Checking Information

It is common in clinical practice to find that certain answers appear to contradict previously given information, or lead to uncertainty about whether a symptom is present. In an interviewer-based interview, one simply attempts to clarify the contradiction or confusion. The respondent-based approach provides no mechanism for resolving such difficulties, since interviewers are not allowed to exercise their judgment about such matters.

Use of Open-Ended and Redundant Questions

The distinction between open and closed questions is not absolute, but open questions are those that offer the chance to provide a wide range of answers or free-recall descriptions of phenomena, while closed questions call for one of a limited set of responses. For example, an open question in response to being told by a child that he had received a bad school report might be "How did you feel about your bad grades?," whereas "Did your bad grades make you feel unhappy?" would be a closed question. If a child had just admitted to stealing, responding with "Tell me more about that" involves an open question, whereas "What did you steal?" is a closed question. Basically, closed questions call for a yes/no answer or a date, frequency, duration, or other quite specific piece of information, while open questions give the opportunity for the child to provide a description of his feelings, which might or might not involve sadness or hostility. The work of Rutter and Cox and their colleagues offers some direct guidance on the best ways to use these different sorts of questions with adults, and in the light of the literature on children's memory, there is little reason not to use a similar approach with children (93–97). They concluded that, in general, most factual information was collected when a systematic approach that relied heavily on open questions was used. This approach was also conducive to parental expressions of emotion, since it involved less talking on the part of the interviewer and gave more time for parents to discuss their concerns. On the other hand, a noninterventionist approach resulted in the provision of less relevant information, while challenging interpretations and a confrontational style proved less effective in eliciting emotions. Thus, open questions can be effective in collecting information efficiently, but, of necessity, respondent-based interviews must rely on closed questions. On the other hand, closed questions are necessary to elicit information that is otherwise not forthcoming, and respondent-based interviews have been a substantial help to the developers of interviewer-based interviews in establishing well thought-out logic structures for series of closed questions.

A redundant question is one that is asked more than once in different ways; that is, questions that contain two presentations of the same item, as in "Have you been more irritable than usual?," followed by "or made angry more easily?" The adult survey literature (98) suggests that such redundancy is actually helpful in providing both additional time for thought and a second chance to pick up symptoms. If the answer to one question is positive and the other negative, then that is no problem for an interviewer-based interview, where follow-up questions can be used to clarify the situation. However, this cannot be done in a respondent-based interview, where specific chains of questions in response to initially discrepant information would be required. Collapsing the two questions into one is no help because this generates a "multiple question" which requires the respondent to remember and process the two parts of the question simultaneously.

Reasonable Rates of Disorder

Rates of diagnosis based only on symptom reports were found to be unreasonably high with early versions of the DISC. To correct this tendency, it is now usual to require that a diagnosis only be allocated when the score on the Child Global Assessment Scale (CGAS) is less than 60 (or sometimes 70; i.e., when notable psychosocial impairment is present). However, in most cases, the DSM-IV requires that *either* impairment *or* distress be present, not that significant impairment always be present. Furthermore, the typical impairment cutpoint of 60 was established because it generated what appeared to be sensible rates of diagnosis, not because anyone with a score over 60 is necessarily unimpaired. Since the K-SADS-P and the CAPA employ exacting definitions at the individual symptom level, community studies using these instruments do not need to apply additional rules about impairment to generate sensible rates of diagnosis.

Advantages of Respondent-Based Interviews

We can also identify three advantages of respondent-based interviews: (1) Less intensive training need be provided to interviewers, (2) a lesser degree of quality control is required, and (3) computer-administered (ACASI) interviews offer the prospect of providing a "preclinical" screening for use in clinical settings.

Intensity of Training

There is no doubt that an interviewer-based interview makes greater demands on an interviewer than does a respondent-based interview. For instance, training on the full CAPA package takes a month, compared with a few days for the DISC.

Quality Control

"Interviewer drift" occurs with respondent-based interviews, necessitating continuing quality control throughout a study, but it is unarguable that there is much more to check with an interviewer-based interview. Care must be taken, not only that the interview is being conducted and coded properly, but mechanisms must also be in place to ensure that interviewers continue to interpret the responses of interviewees correctly. Whether this additional burden is worth the effort depends on the situation in which the interview is being used.

Preclinical Screening

We have reached the point where it is feasible to have parents and children complete a computer-administered diagnostic interview like the DISC-IV before they see a clinician at all. The possible output from the DISC-IV is almost infinitely flexible, and requires only programming to allow the production of reports tailored to particular clinical needs that can be generated as soon as the interview is finished. Equipped with such a report, a clinician familiar with one of the interviewer-based interviews would then be starting with a very respectable initial diagnostic formulation to guide further elucidation of the clinical status of the child. For instance, the ACASI version of the DISC has also been found suitable for use in juvenile justice settings where staff are rarely available to conduct diagnostic interviews.

SELECTING A STRUCTURED INTERVIEW

As we have already seen, reliability and validity quotients are little help in selecting the "best" interview, because there is little to choose between interviews in this regard. Similarly, all the interviews considered here take quite a long time to complete, and their length is proportional to the amount of symptomatology manifested by a child. None has been shown to be notably shorter than any other in practice, and so reported mean interview durations are also no help in selecting and interview for any particular application. Rather, the key to selecting an interview is to be very clear about what that application demands. This means having thought through what the ideal interview for that application would be like, so that the characteristics of each can be matched against those criteria. It is also worthwhile to prioritize these demand characteristics in advance. It may not be possible to have everything, so it is a big help to have thought through the relative impact of different tradeoffs. In the following sections, we consider some questions that prospective interview users should ask themselves as part of the process of selecting an interview.

1. *What content areas need to be covered?* All interviews do not cover all diagnoses (indeed, none covers all possibly relevant diagnoses). It is essential in the first instance to decide what areas must be covered, and what additional areas would be nice to have, but not essential.
2. *What assessment time frame is needed?* The addition of a lifetime frame involves either compromises in the assessment of current or recent symptomatology (as with the

K-SADS-PL) or combining a short time-frame interview with a separate lifetime interview, which results in a very long assessment. If one is conducting a 3-month follow-up assessment following treatment, an interview that focuses on diagnostic status over the last year will not be very helpful.

3. *What sort of interviewers will be available?* In general, clinicians are not enthusiastic about using a respondent-based interview because they have to follow a fixed schedule of questions, and it provides no means to collect more detailed information that may be relevant to a variety of treatment decisions. So it makes sense for them to use one of the interviewer-based interviews. Such interviews can also be very useful clinical training tools, since they provide excellent models for the clinical interviewing process.

   If lay interviewers are to be used, then the K-SADS family of interviews may not be the best choice because these interviews have all been developed for use by clinicians and provide less guidance for the training of lay interviewers. No reliability data on their use with lay interviewers are available. On the other hand, the CAS, CAPA, DICA, and ADIS were all developed for use with trained lay interviewers and have been shown to have acceptable reliability in their hands; all of these interviews are also acceptable to clinicians.

4. *What is the age and developmental level of the children to be assessed?* It is clear that "adult-style" diagnostic interviews (all of the interviews considered in this chapter fall into this category) with preschool children are a waste of time, because they are cognitively incapable of providing all the information required by the DSM-IV or ICD-10 diagnostic criteria. Several groups are working on this problem at present, but none of the instruments reviewed here is of any use for interviewing very young children directly. The K-SADS and DICA are said to be suitable for face-to-face use with children down to the age of 6, but others doubt that a *full* diagnostic interview really works with children under the age of 8 or 9, unless the interviewer simply "goes off interview" to get a relatively impressionistic view of the child's symptomatology. Even the interview with the parent requires substantial modification for preschoolers. We would not recommend the use of any of these instruments in face-to-face interviews with children under the age of 8 or 9. Picture-enhanced interviews like the Dominic-R may be suitable down to the age of 6, but even here, reliability appears to be somewhat lower with younger children, and such interviews do not generate full diagnoses. The same problem applies to older individuals with substantial intellectual deficits. When an individual's IQ is much below 70, it becomes very difficult to complete a full diagnostic interview. Interviews with parents and teachers may still be conducted, but we know little about their performance characteristics in such circumstances.

   At the other end of the juvenile age range (late adolescence and early adulthood), the researcher or clinician has the choice of shifting to an adult measure, or using an age-appropriate modification of a child interview (such as the YAPA).

5. *How much can I afford to spend on training and quality control?* "Spend" here refers to both time and money. If less than a week is available, then none of the interviewer-based interviews is suitable, because good training for them demands a greater time investment. However, DISC training can be provided in as short a time as this, because the DISC requires far less of interviewers. On the other hand, when amortized over the life of a study or clinical program, initial costs for training usually turn out to be only a small percentage of total costs, so training on an interviewer-based interview may constitute a good investment.

6. Once each interview is completed, the DICA and CAPA both expect that it will be reviewed for appropriateness of codings. In addition, regular (both recommend weekly) continuing training sessions for interviewers are required to prevent interviewer drift. Are funds and personnel available to support such continuing quality control and training procedures? The CAS and K-SADS interviews do not appear to have standard recommendations for quality control and continuing training, but there is no reason to suppose that data quality and consistency are any easier to maintain with these instruments. Since the DISC-IV is computerized, and the DISC interviewer's task is much less arduous than that required of interviewers using any of the interviews considered in this chapter, it demands less effort to control interviewer drift. However, interviewer monitoring is still necessary to ensure that interviewers are following the questioning rules exactly, and to ensure that they are actually conducting interviews and not simply falsifying them (yes, this does happen!).

7. *What needs and resources do I have for data entry and manipulation of the data?* The K-SADS family of interviews produces diagnoses through the medium of score sheets completed by the interviewer and scored by that person to produce diagnoses. The CAS provides formal algorithms for making diagnoses that can be implemented either by the interviewer or a computer. The CAPA offers only computerized algorithms because its developers (like those of the DISC) believe that the process of producing a final diagnosis from a large array of symptom data is of such complexity that errors are bound to occur if humans do it unaided. These different approaches to producing a final diagnostic formulation have very different implications for data entry and manipulation. If the computer is to make the diagnoses, then all the symptom information must be entered (this task easily runs to hundreds or thousands of variables per case), and diagnostic algorithms must be available. If the clinician makes the final diagnosis, then one could simply enter only that information (or not computerize any data at all in a clinical setting where the interview is being used just as a clinical assessment whose results appear only in the medical record). CAPI interviews reduce the need to budget for data entry per se, but consideration still has to be given to data management over the course of an interviewing project.

Once these demand characteristics have been determined, one can begin the task of actually selecting an interview:

1. *Review the available instruments and make a shortlist.* It may seem surprising that we place a review of available measures so late in the process. There are two reasons for doing this. First, the choice of measure should be dependent on the nature of the application, not the other way around, so until the application has been well defined, the issue of instrumentation is moot. Second, once one has answered questions 1 to 6, a brief review of instruments may indicate that only one is even remotely suitable. To put it another way, it is more efficient to decide which interview to use relatively late in the process, because one may be able to save a lot of time that would otherwise have been spent in considering instruments that cannot meet the needs of the study. If there seem to be several possibilities at hand, one has at least reduced the number of instruments that need to be considered to a shortlist for further evaluation.

2. *Get copies of the instruments on the shortlist and conduct a detailed evaluation.* Unfortunately, there is absolutely no substitute for getting copies of the instruments still left on the shortlist and reviewing them in detail. The manifold differences between instruments make it impossible to provide more than a flavor of what an interview is like in a review chapter such as this. It is worth remembering that you will be asking the interview developers to send several hundred pages of schedules, glossaries, instruction manuals, and the like, and that these will need to be paid for. At this stage, it should be possible to make a final choice, but if there are still questions that have not been answered in all these materials, a telephone call to someone in the relevant interview development group can be very helpful. If the "homework" outlined above has been done, it is also likely to be well received.
3. *Plan training well ahead of time.* It is not unknown for an interview developer to receive a request like the following: "Hello, I put the... in a grant proposal, and the funding has just come through. I need you to train my interviewers next month." Interview developers have busy research and clinical lives, and they cannot provide training programs at a moment's notice. The time to be setting a hopeful date for training is *before the grant proposal is submitted,* not after it has been reviewed and funded.

FUTURE DIRECTIONS

A great deal of work has gone into producing the interviews we have today, and there is little sign that recent efforts to further "improve" such measures have had much effect on their reliability. Of course, as we learn more about psychopathology we will need to modify our measures' content to reflect what we need to measure, but the basic principles used to design new or revised modules will not change in the foreseeable future (and will work just as well or poorly as they do today). What is needed now is to extend the range of structured assessments down to younger ages. There is astonishingly little research on preschool psychopathology, for instance, and it was only in 2000 that the first structured parent-report diagnostic interview specifically designed for use with this age group became available. It remains to be seen how information from the child and caretakers other than parents can usefully be integrated into diagnostic assessments, but work has begun in this area. Newer "self-report" assessments of the mental status of the child that do not tie themselves rigidly to current diagnostic criteria show great promise for the future. For instance, with the MacArthur Story-Stem Battery (99–101) the interviewer uses toys to act out the beginnings of stories which the child is then asked to complete. The videotapes of these interactions are then scored to provide indices of a variety of internal states. The Berkeley Puppet Interview (102) employs two puppets to express two moods/states, and the child indicates the puppet most like him- or herself, thereby providing self-report assessments of perceived academic functioning, social relationships, depression, anxiety, and aggression/hostility. Some simpler "questionnaires with pictures" have also shown promise with preschoolers in relation to the assessment of depression and anxiety (103,104). Observational assessments, such as the Disruptive Behaviors Diagnostic Observational Schedule (DB-DOS), a structured observational measure to identify clinically significant disruptive behaviors in preschoolers (105), will also likely play a role in the diagnosis of preschool psychiatric symptoms and impairment in the future.

Now that many diagnostic measures are available, it is likely that they will move progressively into ordinary clinical practice. It seems strange that the unstructured clinical interview has been almost entirely supplanted for research purposes because of its well-documented inadequacies as a diagnostic procedure, but continues to be the main assessment tool in clinical practice, where good phenomenologic assessment is surely of the greatest importance. All clinicians dealing with psychopathology can benefit from training on an interviewer-based structured interview (particularly one of the glossary-based interviews), and it is to be hoped that such training will soon become part of all training programs for psychiatric clinicians. However, it must be admitted that the time to conduct a full psychiatric assessment is not always available, and when that is the case it would be helpful to have shorter interviews available to serve as screening tools. Here, a good start has been made with the DISC predictive scales (106), which have been shown to have good screening properties in relation to DSM-IIIR diagnoses. The idea here is not to force slavish dependence on any particular structured interview on clinicians, but to use the strengths of standardized interviews to underpin their explorations of the nature and meaning of psychopathology. Our understanding of psychopathology and its measurement has have come a long way, and it is time to bring the benefits of what are still typically regarded as being research assessment methods to all of our patients and clients.

References

1. Cantwell DP: DSM-III studies. In: Rutter M, Tuma A, Lann IS (eds): *Assessment and Diagnosis in Child Psychopathology.* New York, Guilford Press, 3–36, 1988.
2. Gould MS, Shaffer D, Rutter M, Sturge C: UK/WHO study of ICD-9. In: Rutter ME, Tuma ALann IS (eds.): *Assessment and Diagnosis in Child Psychopathology.* New York, Guilford Press, 37–65, 1988.
3. Remschmidt H: German study of ICD-9. In: Rutter M, Tuma AHLann IS (eds): *Assessment and Diagnosis in Child Psychopathology.* London: Guilford Press, 66–83, 1988.
4. Prendergast M, Taylor E, Rapoport JL, et al.: The diagnosis of childhood hyperactivity a U.S.-U.K. Cross-national study of DSM-III and ICD-9. *J Child Psychol Psychiatry* 29:289–300, 1988.
5. Cooper JE, Kendell RE, Gurland BJ, Sharpe L, Copeland JRM: *Psychiatric Diagnosis in New York and London: A Comparative Study of Mental Hospital Admissions.* 20th ed. London, Oxford University Press, 1972.
6. Achenbach TM: *Assessment and Taxonomy of Child and Adolescent Psychopathology.* Beverly Hills, CA, Sage Publications, 1985.
7. Wing JK: *Measurement and Classification of Psychiatric Symptoms.* Oxford, Oxford University Press, 1974.
8. Guze SB, Goodwin DW, Crane JB: Criminality and psychiatric disorders. *Arch Gen Psychiatry* 20:583–591, 1969.
9. Graham P, Rutter M: The reliability and validity of the psychiatric assessment of the child: II. Interview with the parent. *Br J Psychiatry* 114:581–592, 1968.
10. Rutter M, Graham P: The reliability and validity of the psychiatric assessment of the child: I. Interview with the child. *Br J Psychiatry* 114:563–579, 1968.
11. Regier DA, Myers JK, Kramer M, et al.: The NIMH Epidemiological Catchment Area Program: historical context, major objectives, and study population characteristics. *Arch Gen Psychiatry* 41(10):934–941, 1984.
12. Robins LN, Helzer J, Croughan J, Williams JBW, Spitzer RL: The NIMH Diagnostic Interview Schedule (DIS): version II. *National Institutes of Mental Health* 1979.
13. Herjanic B, Campbell W: Differentiating psychiatrically disturbed children on the basis of a structured interview. *J Abnorm Child Psychol* 5:127–134, 1977.
14. Herjanic B, Herjanic M, Brown F, Wheatt T: Are children reliable reporters? *J Abnorm Child Psychol* 3(1):41–48, 1975.
15. Lapouse R: The epidemiology of behavior disorders in children. *Am J Dysfunctional Children* 111:594–599, 1966.
16. Herjanic B, Reich W: Development of a structured psychiatric interview for children: agreement between child and parent on individual symptoms. *J Abnorm Child Psychol* 10(3):307–324, 1982.
17. Loeber R, Green SM, Lahey BB, Stouthamer-Loeber, M: Differences and similarities between children, mothers, and teachers as informants on disruptive child behavior. *J Abnorm Child Psychol* 19(1):75–95, 1991.
18. Lahey BB: *Validity of Informants and Combinations of Informants in Assessing Childhood Psychopathology,* 1990.
19. Conners CK: *Conners' Rating Scales revised: Instruments for Use with Children and Adolescents,* North Tonawanda, NY, Multi-Health Systems, Inc, 1997.
20. Reich W, Herjanic B, Welner Z, Gandhy PR: Development of a structured psychiatric interview for children: agreement on diagnosis

comparing child and parent interviews. *J Abnorm Child Psychol* 10:325–336, 1982.

21. Stanger C, Lewis M: Agreement among parents, teachers, and children on internalizing and externalizing behavior problems. *J Clin Child Psychol* 22(1):107–115, 1993.
22. Chambers WJ, Puig-Antich J, Hirsch M, et al.: The assessment of affective disorders in children and adolescents by semistructured interview: test-retest reliability of the schedule for affective disorders and schizophrenia for school-age children, present episode version. *Arch Gen Psychiatry* 42:696–702, 1985.
23. Lord C, Rutter M, Goode S, et al.: Autism diagnostic observation schedule. A standardized observation of communicative and social behavior. *J Autism Dev Disord* 19(2):185–212, 1989.
24. Lord C, Rutter M, LeCouteur A: Autism diagnostic interview—revised: a revised version of a diagnostic interview for caregivers of individuals with possible pervasive developmental disorders. *J Autism Dev Disord* 24(5):659–685, 1994.
25. Shaffer D, Fisher P, Lucas CP, Dulcan MK, Schwab-Stone ME: NIMH diagnostic interview schedule for children version IV (NIMH DISC-IV): description, differences from previous versions, and reliability of some common diagnoses. *J Am Acad Child Adolesc Psychiatry* 39:28–38, 2000.
26. Reich W: Diagnostic interview for children and adolescents (DICA). *J Am Acad Child Adolesc Psychiatry* 59–66, 2000.
27. Valla JP, Bergeron L, Smolla N: The Dominic-R: a pictorial interview for 6- to 11-year-old children. *J Am Acad Child Adolesc Psychiatry* 39:85–93, 2000.
28. Silverman WK, Rabian B: Test-retest reliability of the DSM-III-R childhood anxiety disorders symptoms using the anxiety disorders interview schedule for children. *J Anxiety Disord* 9(2):139–150, 1995.
29. Angold A, Costello EJ: The Child and Adolescent Psychiatric Assessment (CAPA). *J Am Acad Child Adolesc Psychiatry* 39:39–48, 2000.
30. Hodges K: Structured interviews for assessing children. *J Child Psychol Psychiatry* 34(1):49–68, 1993.
31. Hodges K, McKnew D, Cytryn L, Stern L, Kline J: The Child Assessment Schedule (CAS) diagnostic interview: a report on reliability and validity. *J Am Acad Child Psychiatry* 21(5):468–473, 1982.
32. Sherrill JT, Kovacs M: Interview schedule for children and adolescents (ISCA). *J Am Acad Child Adolesc Psychiatry* 39:67–75, 2000.
33. Ambrosini PJ: Historical development and present status of the schedule for affective disorders and schizophrenia for school-age children (K-SADS). *J Am Acad Child Adolesc Psychiatry* 39:49–58, 2000.
34. Ernst M, Cookus BA, Moravec BC: Pictorial instrument for children and adolescents (PICA-III-R). *J Am Acad Child Adolesc Psychiatry* 39:94–99, 2000.
35. Angold A, Costello EJ: A test-retest reliability study of child-reported psychiatric symptoms and diagnoses using the Child and Adolescent Psychiatric Assessment (CAPA-C). *Psychol Med* 25:755–762, 1995.
36. Murphy DA, Cantwell C, Jordan DD, Lee MB, Cooley-Quille MR, Lahey BB: Test-retest reliability of Dominic anxiety and depression items among young children. *J Psychopathol Behav Assess* 22:257–270, 2000.
37. Valla JP, Kovess V, Chan Chee C, et al.: A French study of the Dominic interactive. *Soc Psychiatry Psychiatr Epidemiol* 37(9):441–448, 2002.
38. Egger HL, Erkanli A, Keeler G, Potts E, Walter B, Angold A: The test-retest reliability of the preschool age psychiatric assessment. *J Am Acad Child Adolesc Psychiatry* 45(5):538–549, 2006.
39. Luby J, Heffelfinger AK, Mrakotsky C, et al.: The clinical picture of depression in preschool children. *J Am Acad Child Adolesc Psychiatry* 42:340–348, 2003.
40. Wakschlag LS, Keenan K: Clinical significance and correlates of disruptive behavior in environmentally at-risk preschoolers. *J Clin Child Psychol* 30(1):262–275, 2001.
41. Weller EB, Weller RA, Fristad MA, Rooney MT, Schecter J: Children's interview for psychiatric syndromes (ChIPS). *J Am Acad Child Adolesc Psychiatry* 39:76–84, 2000.
42. Reich W, Cottler L, McCallum K, Corwin D, VanEerdewegh M: Computerized interviews as a method of assessing psychopathology in children. *Compr Psychiatry* 36(1):40–45, 1995.
43. Wasserman GA, McReynolds LS, Ko SJ, Katz LM, Carpenter JR. Gender differences in psychiatric disorders at juvenile probation intake. *Am J Public Health* 95:131–137, 2005.
44. Joan K, Birmaher B, Brent D, et al.: Schedule for affective disorders and schizophrenia for school-age children-present and lifetime version (K-SADS-PL): initial reliability and validity data. *Am Acad Child Adolesc Psychiatry* 36(7):980–988, 1997.
45. Spitzer RL, Endicott J, Robins E: Research diagnostic criteria: rationale and reliability. *Arch Gen Psychiatry* 35:773–782, 1978.
46. Ambrosini P, Metz C, Prabucki K, Lee J-C: Videotape reliability of the third revised edition of the K-SADS. *J Am Acad Child Adolesc Psychiatry* 28:723–728, 1990.
47. Orvaschel H, Puig-Antich J, Chambers W, Tabrizi MA, Johnson R: Retrospective assessment of prepubertal major depression with the Kiddie-SADS-e. *J Am Acad Child Psychiatry* 21:392–397, 1982.
48. Kaufman J, Birmaher B, Brent D, et al.: Schedule for affective disorders and schizophrenia for school-age children—present and lifetime version (K-SADS-PL): initial reliability and validity data. *J Am Acad Child Adolesc Psychiatry* 36(7):980–988, 1997.
49. Shanee N, Apter A, Weizman A. Psychometric properties of the K-SADS-PL in an Israeli adolescent clinical population. *Isr J Psychiatry Relat Sci* 34(3):179–186, 1997.
50. Weissman MM, Wickramaratne P, Warner V, et al.: Assessing psychiatric disorders in children: discrepancies between mothers' and children's reports. *Arch Gen Psychiatry* 44:747–753, 1987.
51. Messer SC, Angold A, Costello EJ, Burns BJ: The Child and Adolescent Burden Assessment (CABA): measuring the family impact of emotional and behavioral problems. *Int J Methods Psychiatric Res* 6:261–284, 1996.
52. Ascher BH, Farmer EM, Burns BJ, Angold A: The Child and Adolescent Services Assessment (CASA): description and psychometrics. *J Emot Behav Disord* 4:12–20, 1996.
53. Farmer EMZ, Angold A, Burns BJ, Costello EJ: Reliability of self-reported service use: test-retest consistency of children's responses to the Child and Adolescent Services Assessment (CASA). *J Child and Fam Stud* 3(3):307–325, 1994.
54. Angold A, Prendergast M, Cox A, Harrington R, Simonoff E, Rutter M: The Child and Adolescent Psychiatric Assessment (CAPA). *Psychol Med* 25:739–753, 1995.
55. Costello EJ, Angold A, March J, Fairbank J: Life events and post-traumatic 79. stress: the development of a new measure for children and adolescents. *Psychol Med* 28:1275–1288, 1998.
56. Simonoff E, Pickles A, Meyer JM, et al.: The Virginia Twin Study of adolescent behavioral development: influences of age, sex and impairment on rates of disorder. *Arch Gen Psychiatry* 54:801–808, 1997.
57. Welner Z, Reich W, Herjanic B, Jung KG, Amado H: Reliability, validity, and parent–child agreement studies of the Diagnostic Interview for Children and Adolescents (DICA). *J Am Acad Child Adolesc Psychiatry* 26:649–653, 1987.
58. Reich W, Earls F. Rules of making psychiatric diagnoses in children on the basis of multiple sources of information: preliminary strategies. *J Abnorm Child Psychol* 15:601–616, 1987.
59. de la Osa N, Ezpeleta L, Domenech JM, Navarro JB, Losilla JM: 83. Convergent and discriminant validity of the structured diagnostic interview for children and adolescents (DICA-R). *Psychology in Spain* 1(1):37–44, 84. 1997.
60. Ezpeleta L, de la Osa N, Domenech JM, Navarro JB, Losilla JM, Judez J: 85. Diagnostic agreement between clinician and the Diagnostic Interview for 86 Children and Adolescents—DICA-R in an outpatient sample. *J Child Psychol Psychiatry Allied Discip* 38(4):431–440, 87, 1997.
61. Hodges K, Cools J, McKnew D: Test-retest reliability of a clinical 88 research interview for children: the child assessment schedule. *J Consult Clin Psychol* 1(4):317–322, 1989.
62. Hodges K, Kline J, Stern L, Cytryn L, McKnew D: The development 89. of a child assessment interview for research and clinical use. *J Abnorm Child Psychol* 10:173–189, 1982.
63. Hodges K, Saunders W: Internal consistency of a diagnostic interview 91 for children: the child assessment schedule. *J Abnormal Child Psychology* 17:691–701, 1989.
64. Hodges K, Saunders WB, Kashani J, Hamlett K, Thompson RJ Jr: Internal 93 consistency of DSM-III diagnoses using the symptom scales of the child assessment schedule. *J Am Acad Child Adolesc Psychiatry* 29:635–641, 1990.
65. Hodges K, Wong MM: Psychometric characteristics of a multidimensional 94 measure to assess impairment: the child and adolescent functional assessment scale. *J Child Fam Stud* 5(4):445–467, 1996.
66. Hodges K, Wong MM: Use of the child and adolescent functional assessment scale to predict service utilization and cost. *J Ment Health Adm* 24(3):278–290, 1997.
67. Hodges K, Wong MM, Latessa M: Use of the child and adolescent functional assessment scale (CAFAS) as an outcome measure in clinical settings. *J Behav Health Serv Res* 25(3):325–336, 1998.
68. Grills A, Ollendick TH: Multiple informant agreement and the anxiety disorders interview schedule for parents and children. *J Am Acad Child Adolesc Psychiatry* 42(1):30–40, 2003.
69. Silverman W, Saavedra LM, Pina AA: Test-retest reliability of anxiety symptoms and diagnoses with the anxiety disorders interview schedule for 99 DSM-IV: child and parent versions. *J Am Acad Child Adolesc Psychiatry* 40(8):937–944, 2001.
70. Silverman WK: Diagnostic reliability of anxiety disorders in children using 100 structured interviews. *J Anxiety Disorders* 5:105–124, 1991.
71. Silverman WK, Eisen AR: Age differences in the reliability of parent and child reports of child anxious symptomatology using a structured 101 interview. *J Am Acad Child Adolesc Psychiatry* 31:117–124, 1992.
72. Silverman WK, Nelles WB: The anxiety disorders interview schedule for children. *J Am Acad Child Adolesc Psychiatry* 27(6):772–778, 1988.
73. Wood J, Piacentini JC, Bergman RL, McCracken J, Barrios V: Concurrent validity of the anxiety disorders section of the anxiety disorders interview schedule for DSM-IV: child and parent versions. *J Clin Child Adolesc Psychol* 31(3):335–342, 2002.
74. Di Nardo PA, Moras K, Barlow DH, Rapee RM, Brown TA: Reliability of DSM-III-R anxiety disorder categories: using the anxiety disorders interview schedule—revised (ADIS-R). *Arch Gen Psychiatry* 50(4):251–256, 1993.
75. Ho TP, Leung PW, Lee CC, et al.: Test-retest reliability of the Chinese version of the Diagnostic Interview Schedule for Children-Version 4 (DISC-IV). *J Child Psychol Psychiatry* 46(10):1135–1138, 2005.

76. Angold A, Erkanli A, Costello EJ, Rutter M: Precision, reliability and accuracy in the dating of symptom onsets in child and adolescent psychopathology. *J Child Psycholo Psychiatry* 37:657–664, 1996.
77. Breton JJ, Bergeron L, Valla JP, Lepine S, Houde L, Gaudet N: Do children aged 9 to 11 years understand the DISC version 2.25 questions? *J Am Acad Child Adolesc Psychiatry* 34:946–956, 1995.
78. Angold A, Erkanli A, Loeber R, Costello EJ, Van Kammen W, Stouthamer-Loeber M: Disappearing depression in a population sample of boys. *J Emot Behav Disord* 4:95–104, 1996.
79. Piacentini J, Roper M, Jensen P, et al.: Informant-based determinants of symptom attenuation in structured child psychiatric interviews. *J Abnorm Child Psychol* 27:417–428, 1999.
80. Jensen PS, Shaffer D, Rae D, et al.: *Attenuation of the Diagnostic Interview Schedule for Children (Disc 2.1): Sex, Age and IQ Relationships.* Paper presented at the 39th Annual Meeting of the AACAP, Washington, DC, 1992.
81. Anastasi A: The concept of validity in the interpretation of test scores. *J Psychol Educ Measures* 10:67–78, 1950.
82. Anastasi A: Evolving concepts of test validation. *Annu Rev Psycholo* 37:1–15, 1986.
83. Cronbach LJ, Meehl PE: Construct validity in psychological tests. *Psychol Bull* 52(4):281–302, 1955.
84. Gulliksen H: Intrinsic validity. *Am Psychol* 5:511–517, 1950.
85. Jenkins JG: Validity for what? *J Consult Clin Psychol* 10:93–98, 1946.
86. Novick MR: *Standards for Educational and Psychological Testing.* Washington, DC: American Psychological Association, 1985.
87. Peak H: Problems of objective observation. In: Festinger L, Katz D (eds): *Research Methods in the Behavioral Sciences.* New York, Dryden Press, 243–300, 1953.
88. Wallace SR: Criteria for what? *Am Psychol* 20:411–417, 1965.
89. Weitz J: Criteria for criteria. *Am Psychol* 16:228–231, 1961.
90. Costello EJ, Mustillo S, Erkanli A, Keeler G, Angold A: Prevalence and development of psychiatric disorders in childhood and adolescence. *Arch Gen Psychiatry* 60:837–844, 2003.
91. Lewinsohn PM, Hops H, Roberts RE, Seeley JR, Andrews JA: Adolescent psychopathology: I. Prevalence and incidence of depression and other DSM-III-R disorders in high school students. *J Abnorm Psychol* 102:133–144, 1993.
92. Breslau N: Inquiring about the bizarre: false positives in Diagnostic Interview Schedule for Children (DISC) ascertainment of obsessions, compulsions, and psychotic symptoms. *J Am Acad Child Adolesc Psychiatry* 26:639–644, 1987.
93. Cox A, Holbrook D, Rutter M: Psychiatric interviewing techniques: VI. Experimental study: eliciting feelings. *Br J Psychiatry* 139:144–152, 1981.
94. Cox A, Hopkinson K, Rutter M: Psychiatric interviewing techniques: II. Naturalistic study—eliciting factual information. *Br J Psychiatry* 138:283–291, 1981.
95. Cox A, Rutter M, Holbrook D: Psychiatric interviewing techniques: V. Experimental Study—eliciting factual information. *Br J Psychiatry* 139:27–37, 1981.
96. Rutter M, Cox A: Psychiatric interviewing techniques: I. Methods and measures. *Br J Psychiatry* 138:273–282, 1981.
97. Rutter M, Cox A, Egert S, Holbrook D, Everitt B: Psychiatric interviewing techniques: IV. Experimental study—four contrasting styles. *Br J Psychiatry* 138:456–465, 1981.
98. Cannell CF, Marquis KH, Laurent A: A summary of studies of interviewing methodology: 1959–1970. *Vital Health Stat 2* 26:1–78, 1977.
99. Emde R, Wolfe DP, Oppenheim D: *Revealing the Inner Worlds of Young Children: The MacArthur Story Stem Battery and Parent–Child Narratives.* New York, Oxford University Press, 2003.
100. Warren SL, Emde RN, Sroufe A: Internal representations: predicting anxiety from children's play narratives. *J Am Acad Child Adolesc Psychiatry* 39:100–107, 2000.
101. Warren SL, Oppenheim D, Emde RN: Can emotions and themes in children's play predict behavior problems? *J Am Acad Child Adolesc Psychiatry* 35:1331–1337, 1996.
102. Measelle JR, Ablow JC, Cowan PA, Cowan CP: Assessing young children's views of their academic, social, and emotional lives: an evaluation of the self-perception scales of the Berkeley Puppet Interview. *Child Dev* 69:1556–1576, 1998.
103. Ialongo N, Edelsohn G, Werthamer-Larsson L, Crockett L, Kellam S: Are self-reported depressive symptoms in first-grade children developmentally transient phenomena? A further look. *Dev Psychopathol* 5:433–457, 1993.
104. Martini DR, Strayhorn JM, Puig-Antich J: A symptom self-report measure for preschool children. *J Am Acad Child Adolesc Psychiatry* 29:594–600, 1990.
105. Wakschlag LS, Leventhal B, Briggs-Gowan MJ, et al.: Defining the "disruptive" in preschool behavior: what diagnostic observation can teach us. *Clin Child Fam Psychol Rev* 8(3):183–201, 2005.
106. Lucas CP, Zhang H, Fisher PW, et al.: The DISC Predictive Scales (DPS): efficiently screening for diagnoses. *J Am Acad Child Adolesc Psychiatry* 40:443–449, 2001.

CHAPTER 4.7 ■ DIAGNOSTIC CLASSIFICATION

FRED R. VOLKMAR, DENIS G. SUKHODOLSKY, MARY SCHWAB-STONE, AND MICHAEL B. FIRST

PRINCIPLES OF CLASSIFICATION

The ability and the urge to classify are unique aspects of human experience. They provide us with the capacity to observe, to order our observations, and to formulate general principles and hypotheses. Classification enables us to make use of information for purposes of communication, prediction, and explanation. At the present time in child and adolescent psychiatry, classification systems have their greatest role in facilitating communication for both clinical and research purposes; their role in prediction is somewhat more limited, and their explanatory value is often quite limited although the process of being assigned a diagnostic label may itself be associated with some sense of relief on the part of the patient or the patient's parents (1). Sometimes this reflects the misconception that having a label implies having an explanation (2). Like all human constructions, classification schemes can be abused or ill-used (3). This chapter provides an overview of classification in child and adolescent psychiatry and an overview of the current official systems, that is, the 10th edition of the *International Classification of Diseases* (ICD-10) (4) and the 5th edition of the *Diagnostic and Statistical Manual Mental Disorders* (DSM-5) (5). (Definitions for each disorder are discussed in detail in the respective chapters.)

Various authors (2,6–11) discuss criteria for psychiatric classification systems. There is no single "right" way to classify disorders in childhood. Classification systems vary, depending on the purpose of classification and what is being classified. As described later, "official" diagnostic systems have tended to adopt, on the whole, a categorical approach, but a dimensional approach would be equally as applicable, if perhaps less useful for clinical purposes.

The goals of classification include facilitating communication among professionals, providing information about given disorders that is relevant to treatment or to prevention, and providing information useful for research aimed at understanding the pathogenesis of disorders. To achieve these goals, classification schemes must be readily and reliably used by clinicians and researchers; hence the need for systems that are readily comprehensible. The disorders should be described, so they can be differentiated from one another. Disorders should differ in important ways, such as associated features and course. The classification system must be applicable over the range of development and must be comprehensive and logically consistent (12). A classification of disorders implies that some clinically significant patterns of symptoms, behaviors, and signs are observed and comprise a source of significant distress or impairment (5). Deviant behavior itself does not necessarily constitute a disorder unless it is a manifestation of dysfunction within the individual person (e.g., conflicts over political beliefs do not constitute a mental disorder). Although it is often assumed that mental disorders must have a biologic basis, this need not be the case; for example, maladaptive, enduring personality patterns can readily be classified as disorders (13).

Development of a general classification system for psychiatric disorders inevitably involves various tradeoffs. General classification systems must cover the entire range of disorders in a logically consistent fashion; classification systems developed for a highly specific purpose or setting do not share this concern. The need for reasonable parsimony must be balanced with the need for adequate coverage (1,9). The needs for a clinically relevant system differ somewhat from those for a research system; for example, highly detailed criteria may be useful for research purposes but are cumbersome in clinical practice. Different diagnostic systems address these issues in different ways. Thus, the DSM-IV (5) was intended to be useful for *both* clinical work and research, whereas the ICD-10 (4) system provides *separate* clinical and research descriptions.

ISSUES IN CLASSIFICATION

Developmental Aspects

Developmental considerations assume major importance in the provision of a classification scheme for children and adolescents, and, indeed, for adults as well (14). Some disorders such as autism have their origin in a specific developmental period, whereas others are frequently associated with developmental problems, for example, Tourette syndrome may be associated with attentional or learning difficulties. At other times, the child's overall level of development may have a major impact on the ways in which various disorders can be expressed (the child with intellectual disability who also exhibits conduct problems). Classification systems must be able to encompass such issues without simultaneously making the disorder so developmentally specific that the utility of the category is compromised.

The developmental approach to classification is used whenever disorders are viewed in the context of the unfolding of basic developmental processes. The use of standard, developmentally based assessment instruments such as tests of intelligence or communication skills exemplifies this approach. In contrast, many categorical and dimensional classification systems rely on assessment of deviant behavior. The use of such an approach is often complicated because issues of how deviant behavior is to be evaluated and how instruments are to be "normed" become quite important, and reliability among examiners can be low. Both the ICD-10 and the DSM-5 systems include some categories in which the definition is fundamentally developmental (intellectual disabiltiy, articulation disorders), whereas in others the "deviant" nature of the disorder predominates (autism, schizophrenia of childhood onset).

Role of Theory

Theoretical models of psychological disturbance have developed from diverse historical traditions and have considerable value for the individual clinician in understanding and treating children with emotional and behavioral problems. For example, Anna Freud (15) proposed a developmental profile based on and applicable to psychoanalytic assessment of children. More phenomenologically based classification systems can be traced to Kraeplin's delineation of schizophrenia and bipolar disorder (16). In the early "official" classifications (e.g., DSM-I and DSM-II), theoretical concerns were reflected in terms such as "schizophrenic reaction of childhood" or "obsessional neurosis." Classification schemes that are driven by theory are limited because, by their nature, they are based on a set of assumptions and hypotheses not usually generally shared and may give rise to different terms used to describe the same clinical phenomena; for example, a learning theorist may invoke principles of conditioning to explain a child's phobia, whereas a psychoanalytically oriented clinician may be more concerned with the child's level of psychosexual organization. Particularly following the work on development of research diagnostic criteria (17), starting with DSM-III in 1980, the phenomenologic approach to classification has predominated in the various "official" diagnostic systems. The more robust diagnostic concepts have typically emerged from clinical experience rather than from theory (18). In some instances, a theory has been invoked to account for a given set of phenomena, but it is the set of phenomena rather than the theory that has endured. For example, Langdon Down provided a complex theoretical explanation for children with the condition now known as Down syndrome. His theory, based on obsolete racial stereotypes (mongolism), was incorrect, but his observation of some element of commonality among a large group of children with intellectual disability has proved enduring.

For clinicians with pronounced theoretical views, the more phenomenon-based approach can be a source of frustration. It is sometimes incorrectly assumed that in such an approach matters as history, course, and outcome, and, for that matter, etiology and theory are irrelevant to classification. Information on course and outcome may provide important data relative to external validation of diagnostic categories, and information on the development of the disorder may be highly relevant to differential diagnosis regardless of how similar, at one point, two different disorders may appear to be. For example, the syndrome of childhood disintegrative disorder clearly appears to resemble autistic disorder once it is established; however, patterns of early development and outcome differ in these conditions (19). Theoretical views of conditions and mechanisms remain highly relevant for both clinical work and research because they are more likely to generate truly testable hypotheses.

Etiology and Classification

It is often assumed that classification systems are developed to approximate some ideal diagnostic system in which the etiology could be directly related to clinical condition. This is not, in fact, the case, in that no single ideal system is waiting to be discovered and that etiology need not be included in classification systems (12). Similarly, classification need not reflect a "disease" model (12). Different etiologic factors may result in rather similar clinical presentations and the same etiologic factor may be associated with a range of quite different clinical presentations. Aspects of intervention may be more directly related to the clinical presentation than to the cause. Remedial services for children with intellectual disability are, for example, much more likely to be oriented around aspects of developmental level than around the precise etiologic origin of the intellectual disability. With a few exceptions (reactive attachment or posttraumatic stress disorders), etiologic factors are not generally included in official diagnostic systems.

Contextual Factors

In certain situations and populations, contextual variables such as family, school, or cultural setting pose major complications to diagnosis. The attentional problems of a child whose difficulties arise only as a result of an inappropriate school placement would not, for example, merit a diagnosis of attention-deficit disorder. Contextual variables are particularly problematic in disorders of infancy and early childhood in which the infant exerts effects on the parents, who, in turn, exert effects on the child; attributions of causality in such situations may be particularly difficult to make (20). A few of the traditional categorical disorders can be readily observed in infants and young children (e.g., autism), but generally clinical complaints in this age group are centered around problems that encompass the infant in the context of the family, the individual's age or developmental level, or life situation. These issues are particularly relevant for diagnosis of disorders in infancy—an area that remains somewhat controversial so that, for example, a diagnosis of autism can often be made in very young children (21), although in some cases not all features are exhibited until around age 3 (22). Although research on disorders of infancy is limited (23), it is clear that infants exhibit a tremendous ability to react, even over relatively short periods, to their environment, and change, rather than stability, is often the rule (24). Clinical problems often relate more to issues of *goodness of fit* between parents and the infant than to a disorder in the infant (25). As children become slightly older, traditional diagnostic groupings become more readily applicable (26). Issues of developmental level also become important in specifying inclusion and exclusion criteria for diagnostic categories; for example, a diagnosis of Pica may be appropriate for a 12-year-old child with profound intellectual disability but is less appropriate for a normally developing 10-month-old infant. These are important issues for DSM-5 and for the new ICD-11.

Cultural differences may also affect diagnostic concepts and practice (27). Clearly, certain sociocultural factors are associated with certain types of problems (e.g., economic disadvantage is associated with conduct and attentional problems), but the meanings of such relationships often remain unclear (28).

What Is Classified?

It is particularly important that clinicians and researchers alike bear in mind that disorders, rather than children, are classified. This is a source of considerable confusion. Concerns have been raised about the possible effects of labeling children (3), and to some extent these concerns are valid. It is, of course, also the case that having an adequate label for a child's disorder may be helpful, for example, in securing needed services. Thus, a diagnosis of intellectual disability or specific learning disorder may be associated with social stigma or other untoward effects, or it may be associated with more realistic expectations on the part of parents and teachers and provision of potentially more appropriate services. These tensions are also exemplified in the debate between those who advocate broad and encompassing definitions (to maximize clinical and educational service provision) and those who advocate narrow definitions (by defining more homogenous groups of research subjects).

Similar debates arise about aspects of social stigma related to mental illness and behavioral and developmental problems. In this regard, it is always important to refer to the child's disorder, *not to the child as the disorder* (e.g., "child with a diagnosis of schizophrenia" rather than "schizophrenic child"). The term *diagnosis* refers both to the notion of assigning a label to a given problem and to the act of evaluation. In important respects, it is the diagnostic process (29) that is the most important of the two. Although diagnostic labels have considerable value, they do not provide information specifically about the individual person, who is unique and uniquely related to intervention.

VALIDATION AND STATISTICAL ISSUES

As official classification systems have become more complex and sophisticated, issues of reliability and validity have assumed increasing importance. For example, both the DSM-IV and the ICD-10 used results of large national or international field trials in providing definitions of disorders. Categorical and dimensional approaches to classification share certain statistical concerns (6).

Validity

Validity is the extent to which a classification system does what it purports to do in terms of facilitating communication, intervention, and research. Various types of validity have been identified, for example, *face validity* (a judgment about whether the description of a category appears to represent the diagnostic construct reasonably), *predictive validity* (whether some aspect of subsequent course or response to treatment is predicted), and *construct validity* (whether the category has meaning in terms of what it purports to assess). Generally, such concepts are most useful in measuring the validity of psychometric assessment instruments; their applicability to classification systems is somewhat different. In general, childhood psychiatric disorders have face validity but not necessarily predictive or construct validity (11). The validity of a given diagnostic category can be established on the basis of its association with various features other than those incorporated in the definition (response to treatment, natural history in the absence of treatment, family pattern, biologic correlates, and developmental correlates such as age at onset and intelligence quotient).

The sensitivity and specificity of a given categorical diagnostic instrument can be assessed relative to the true presence or absence of a specific disorder. However, a general problem for both categorical and dimensional classification systems is the nature of the standard against which a given category or criteria set is to be judged. Given the usual absence of an unequivocal diagnostic marker for the various conditions, clinical judgment is often used as the standard against which new instruments or definitions are assessed. The issues of "caseness" and diagnostic thresholds are particularly important in the derivation and validation of diagnostic systems (30,31). These issues can be complex, for example, if impairment is a necessary feature of a condition like Tourette's disorder what is the best approach given the strong genetic component of the condition, that is, a father might have mild and nonimpairing tics but have a son who is quite disabled.

Reliability

In addition to validity, classification systems should exhibit *reliability;* that is, users in different locations seeing rather similar disorders should be able to agree on the applicability of a specific category or criterion (32). Various kinds of reliability have been identified: interrater, test–retest, and internal consistency. If a given category is not used reliably, it has little value for purposes of communication. Some disorders, almost by definition, have limited test–retest reliability over a relatively short time period (adjustment disorder), whereas other highly stable disorders tend to have better test–retest reliability (profound intellectual disability). Sources of unreliability in psychiatric diagnosis include differences in the kinds of information clinicians collect, theoretical biases in the clinician, and differences in internalized diagnostic thresholds, as well as, of course, the true differences that persons with disorders will exhibit at various points over the course of their condition.

High reliability does not guarantee validity. It is possible for a disorder to be reliably defined but have little or no validity. Conversely, a disorder may have validity, but criteria and diagnostic instruments designed to detect its presence may have little or no reliability. In providing diagnostic criteria and descriptions, there is often a tradeoff between the level of detail of a definition and its reliability. What appear to be relatively minor changes in the wording of a criterion can produce major changes in the way in which a diagnosis or diagnostic criterion is applied.

Statistical Analyses

Various *statistical techniques* have been applied to data derived from assessment methods (8,33,34). These techniques are theoretically of great interest in that they can provide more rational and empirical approaches to the derivation of diagnostic schemes. The fundamental assumption of such techniques is that the variables of interest lie along some dimension of function and dysfunction that all persons exhibit to some degree. For many types of problems, this assumption is probably justified, such as relative to anxiety or depression. However, the usefulness of such techniques is limited in important ways (12). In the first place, these methods are highly dependent on both the sample and the type of data entered in the analysis. For example, *factor analysis* of an instrument designed to detect conduct problems would not likely produce a factor related to eating disturbance. Similarly, cluster analysis of even a very large normative sample would not likely produce a cluster that corresponded to autism, given the low base rate of this disorder in the population. For rare disorders, other statistical approaches may be useful. Other relevant statistical procedures include *signal detection analysis* (35), which can be used to establish which symptoms and symptom combinations are more strongly related to a particular diagnosis. Similarly, *latent trait analysis* and *latent class analysis* (36,37) provide other approaches.

MODELS OF CLASSIFICATION

Werry (1) delineated three general approaches to classification of disorders: categorical, dimensional, and ideographic. The *categorical approach,* sometimes referred to as the medical model of classification, views disorders as either present or absent (the patient does or does not have appendicitis). This approach assumes that patients exhibiting a given disorder display certain similarities, that these similarities outweigh differences, and that this knowledge has certain implications for understanding pathophysiology, course, treatment, and so on. Unlike the categorical approach, which views disorders as dichotomous, the *dimensional approach* to classification relies on assessment of dimensions of function or dysfunction by reducing phenomena to various dimensions along which a child can be placed. Various sources of data can be used for this approach, such as behavioral ratings, parental reports, sums of yes–no criteria, developmentally based test scores, and the like. Although the dimensional approach is more commonly used in nonmedical settings, many medical phenomena also exhibit continuous (dimensional) characteristics (stature, blood pressure). For some purposes, categorical diagnoses (levels of intellectual disability) are derived from what is essentially a continuous variable, whereas some dimensional assessment instruments can similarly be used to generate categorical diagnoses. *Ideographic classifications* reject simple labels and focus on the total context of the individual person; this approach may be theory-driven (by psychoanalytic or behavioral theories) or may be used eclectically. Ideographic approaches are commonly used in clinical work; that is, the child or adolescent is viewed in the totality of life circumstance, and various disorders, problems, and psychosocial situations may be viewed as worthy of notation and treatment.

Categorical Approaches

The most widely used "official" systems are those developed by the World Health Organization (WHO) (ICD-10) (4) and the American Psychiatric Association (DSM-5) (5). There systems have their historical origins in medicine in the 19th and 20th centuries as advances in diagnosis and public health concerns necessitated more systematic approaches to record-keeping (Table 4.7.1). During the 19th century, many advances in the taxonomy of adult psychiatric disorders were made, and this led Kraepelin to attempt a comprehensive classification system (38). By the mid-20th century, certain psychiatric disorders were generally recognized. The second edition of the DSM (DSM-II) (39) includes only a handful of diagnostic categories specific to children: intellectual disability, childhood schizophrenia, adjustment, and other "reactions" (hyperkinetic, withdrawing, overanxious, runaway, unsocialized aggressive, group delinquent, and "other"). By the time the DSM-III appeared (40), the number of disorders first evidenced in infancy, childhood, or adolescence had increased more than fourfold to include the following major classes of disorder, each of which included some specific diagnostic categories: intellectual disability, specific developmental disorders, attention-deficit disorder, conduct disturbance, eating disorders, stereotyped movement disorders, pervasive developmental

TABLE 4.7.1

LANDMARKS IN THE DEVELOPMENT OF PSYCHIATRIC TAXONOMIES[a]

Kraepelin (1883): Proposal for a comprehensive classification system
ICD-6 (1948): Psychiatric disorders included
DSM-I (1952): First US official classification system
Group for the Advancement of Psychiatry (1966): Diagnostic system for children
DSM-II (1968): Some child disorders, emphasis on theory and Meyer's concept of reaction types
DSM-III (1980): Fourfold increase in child psychiatric disorders, greater diagnostic precision, multiaxial
DSM-III-R (1987): Refinements in criteria, categories
ICD-10 (1992): Separation of research diagnostic criteria from clinical descriptions
DSM-IV (1994): More emphasis on data based modifications in categories and criteria
DSM-IV-TR (2000): Generally minor revisions in text (not criteria)
DSM-5
(2013): Major revision, drops subthreshold concept
(2002): Research agenda and white papers
(2012): Anticipated publication date

[a]DSM, Diagnostic and Statistical Manual of Mental Disorders; ICD, International Classification of Diseases.

disorders, other disorders with physical manifestations, and other disorders of infancy, childhood, or adolescence (16). Similar, although not precisely corresponding, changes occurred in the revision of the ICD 10 (4). In the DSM-III, for example, disorders generally specific to childhood were grouped together, and there were many more DSM-III subcategories (40). The DSM-III and its successor, the DSM-III-R (41), differ from the ICD-9 in terms of their greater diagnostic reliance on explicit (if not always truly operationalized) diagnostic criteria (42,43). Both the DSM and the ICD incorporate multiaxial framework, although the specific systems adopted differ from each other in some respects. Both systems were hierarchically organized, although the DSM-III and the DSM-III-R encourage multiple diagnoses. Changes in the DSM-III-R and DSM-IV are generally less dramatic than in the DSM-III (44). Work on the DSM-IV began in 1988 (45), stimulated, in part, the desirability of harmonizing DSM-IV with ICD-10, which was also undergoing revision at that time. As part of the process of producing the DSM-IV, steps were undertaken to ensure that changes made were based on solid empirical data and thorough documentation (45). This task was somewhat facilitated because it was clear that the DSM-III and III-R had stimulated considerable research of relevance to the DSM-IV (46). Other issues for the DSM-IV relate to clinical utility and compatibility with ICD-10. As part of the revision process, extensive literature reviews were conducted, datasets were aggregated and analyzed or reanalyzed, and working groups of experts convened to evaluate the available data and, in some cases, to generate new data. For the child disorders section, field trials were conducted for disruptive behavior disorders (47) and for autism and related conditions (48).

The *International Classification of Causes of Death* was adopted by the International Statistical Institute in 1893 (49). By the 1960s, the ICD had been revised six times, and the deficiencies of the ICD-7 for psychiatric disorders (10) were particularly clear. Many changes were made in the eighth edition of the ICD in 1968. Even when this edition was adopted, however, it was clear that further revision would be needed, and a process was instituted for further revision. An important part of this work was the development of a multiaxial classification system for child disorders (10).

The ICD-9 was published in 1977, and work on its revision began shortly thereafter (50–52). As part of the extensive revision process, the number of categories increased substantially (53), and a decision was made to have several versions of the system—one for primary health care providers, another for specialty-based researchers, and one for psychiatric practitioners. The ICD-10 had good clinical utility and good, although variable, reliability (the latter being less optimal for disorders with more subtle symptoms such as personality disorders) (51,54,55); it also included a handful of mixed categories (e.g., depressive conduct disorder) for the more frequent co-occuring disorders in childhood (56).

DSM-5

DSM-5 (5) was published in 2013 and marked the first major DSM revision in nearly two decades (57,58). Prior to starting formal work on DSM-5, a research planning effort was initiated with the goal of stimulating research in advance of starting the revision process. The first phase of the effort produced a series of white papers, which were published in 2002 in *A research agenda for DSM-V* (59). One of the white papers (60) reviewed advances in the developmental sciences and proposed a research agenda for the next decade focusing on six areas of research that have the potential to refine the classification of developmental psychopathology. These included (1) developmental neuroscience and genetics, such as studies in animals to determine associations between maternal behavior and hypothalamic–pituitary–adrenal axis regulation; (2) prevention, including studies of early intervention for children and adolescents; (3) improved diagnostic classification of disorders of infancy and early childhood; (4) improvements in the multiaxial system; (5) approaches to psychiatric assessment: integration of information from different assessment approaches; and (6) developmental epidemiology, entailing large-scale population-based samples of children studied from birth, or even earlier, through adulthood.

The final version of DSM-5 was released in May of 2013 and sought to address both the challenges in diagnosing mental disease and the advances that have been made in the 20 years since the last version (58,59,61). Significant changes to the overall structure, including the elimination of the section for Disorders Usually First Diagnosed in Infancy, Childhood, or Adolescence and the decision to rely, as much as possible (59), on standardized diagnostic instruments and neuropsychiatric findings for the source of defining the included disorders, were made. The overall approach to childhood-onset disorders, that is, in general (apart from those disorders with strong developmental components), to move descriptions to overarching categories, for example, anxiety disorders, rather than have a section of the manual focused on childhood-onset conditions. The NOS categories were replaced with "Other Specified Disorder" and "Unspecified Disorder" categories.

Also, it was noteworthy that the previous multiaxial system was eliminated with a list of all disorders on a single axis along with the potential for listing psychosocial and contextual features and the potential for using the WHO disability assessment schedule (rather than the previous axis V).

At the level of disorders included decisions were made to drop a number of categories, for example, Asperger's syndrome. Newly recognized conditions were relevant to social communication disorder (a communication disorder with a strong social component). Gender identity disorder was renamed as gender dysphoria. A new category of disruptive mood dysregulation disorder was included specifically for children and adolescents with chronic irritability punctuated by frequent temper outbursts, which is intended to be used instead of juvenile bipolar disorder. The name for mental retardation was replaced with intellectual disability. The DSM-IV categories of phonologic disorder and stuttering were renamed speech–sound disorder and childhood-onset fluency disorder, respectively. Similarly, a new category of motor disorder includes tic disorder, coordination, and stereotyped mood disorders. For some disorders, for example, enuresis, no major changes were made from the DSM-IV approach. Clarifications were made in some cases, for example, for Pica, to indicate that the behavior could be observed at any age. Newly recognized diagnosis included binge eating disorder and changes were made in criteria for both bulimia nervosa and anorexia nervosa. The rarely used DSM-IV category of feeding disorder was reconceptualized as avoidant/restrictive food intake disorder with a new set of criteria. Changes were made in the DSM-IV approach to oppositional and conduct disorder.

Criticisms of the new approaches included the inclusion of new disorders with little or no empirical support (e.g., social communication disorder) and, low inter-rater reliability (e.g., disruptive mood dysregulation disorder). For childhood-onset disorders, concern was raised regarding changes in the autism section—the name change for the overall category (from pervasive developmental disorders) to autism spectrum disorder (ASD) was applauded although a substantial body of work (62) suggests paradoxically that the definition for ASD is much more appropriate to more "classic" autism (as typified by Kanner's original cases). As a result, the final autistic disorder definition "grandfathered" in previous "well-established" diagnoses like Asperger's and PDD–NOS effectively maintaining the DSM-IV approach.

ICD-11

The 11th revision of the *International Classification of Diseases* (ICD-11) is currently being developed by the WHO and is expected to be approved by the World Health Assembly in 2018 with implementation by WHO member countries in subsequent years. Given that the neuroscience and genetics evidence that has accumulated over the past 20 years does not support major changes for individual conditions or provide definitive support for specific structure, the primary focus of the revision of the Mental and Behavioural Disorders chapter is to improve the clinical utility of the classification. A significant change in ICD-11 as compared to ICD-10 is the use of a standardized template for the presentation of the clinical descriptions and diagnostic guidelines (63). At present, it appears that, on balance, ICD-11 will be more similar to DSM-5 than different but important details remain to be decided. A draft version of ICD-11 clinical descriptions and diagnostic guidelines is available (63). Moreover, extensive Internet-based case vignette studies and clinic-based diagnostic agreement studies are underway (64).

Dimensional Approaches

In contrast to the more clinically oriented (categorical) approach, multivariate (dimensional) approaches to diagnosis offer several potential advantages in that various behaviors and dimensions of behavior are assessed, rather than single, presumably pathognomonic, features (8,33,34). Similarly, the dimensional approach can encompass symptom coding in other than a dichotomous fashion; for example, "never," "sometimes," and "always" could be coded, rather than simply presence or absence, to rate specific diagnostic features. Various rating scales, checklists, and so forth can be used for multivariate classification schemes based on self, parent, or teacher report or on direct observation; many such instruments are described in subsequent chapters. As noted previously, various statistical techniques such as factor and cluster analysis may be used to derive relevant clinician patterns or profiles. These patterns may, in turn, be used to derive categorical diagnoses. Given the inherent problems in sample selection and instrument development, issues of replication are particularly important (12).

Early work focused on examination of patterns of relationships (correlations) between variables to derive syndrome groupings (65). A large series of case records was studied, and the presence or absence of specific behaviors was noted in each case. Clusters of deviant behavior were noted, and broad patterns of disturbance (socialized delinquent, overinhibited, unsocialized aggressive) were identified. Subsequently, more sophisticated methods have been applied to a range of children using a variety of assessment instruments (33). Studies done using this approach generally identify several factors with relative consistency; factors identified have included conduct disturbance, overactivity, and emotional disturbance (12,66). Not surprisingly, the stability of more narrowly defined factors is less robust. Similarly, as would be expected, such techniques have limited usefulness in detecting children with disorders of very low prevalence.

Reliability of dimensions derived from multivariate studies has been assessed and is generally satisfactory (8). Stability of dimensions or profiles is somewhat more complex to assess, in that some change is, of course, expected, but short-term stability appears to be within acceptable limits (8). The use of dimensional assessment instruments clearly avoids certain of the pitfalls inherent in the categorical approach, for example, in terms of the loss of information inherent in the application of dichotomous categories, in increasing reliability, and in issues of "caseness." These issues are relevant to medicine in general and not just to psychiatry.

For some purposes, dimensional assessment instruments are particularly valuable. For such assessments to be clinically useful, their validity must be demonstrated, for example, in terms of some associated features, such as familial pattern or course. The assumption that characteristics have the same meaning throughout their distribution is often questionable (e.g., severe intellectual disability differs in a host of ways from normal intelligence) (55). Certain disorders clearly do *not* shade off into normality. At the same time, it is important to note effects of biologic development on syndrome expression (67).

RELATIONSHIP OF CATEGORICAL AND DIMENSIONAL APPROACHES

There are major areas of agreement between both the categorical and dimensional approaches; this is particularly true for the more common disorders. Analysis of data from dimensional assessment instruments has proved useful in the development of categorical systems, for example, in supporting division of conduct disorder into various types. Probably the greatest drawback to the use of such assessments in clinical practice arises from the difficulty in using such instruments in a simple way for purposes of communication; for clinical purposes, it is more helpful to know that a child has attention-deficit hyperactivity disorder and learning problems than to know his or her factor or profile scores on a dimensional assessment instrument. Dimensional and categorical approaches need not be used in mutually exclusive ways; the multiaxial classification used in the DSM-III-R, for example, employs both approaches in that although disorders are categorically defined, assessments of severity of psychosocial stressors and global assessment of functioning are dimensional.

IDEOGRAPHIC APPROACHES

Ideographic approaches (1) to diagnosis are common in clinical practice. In the broader sense of diagnosis (as diagnostic process) (29), most clinicians target certain problems or issues for intervention that relate only in part to categorical or even dimensional diagnosis. In some ways, such approaches are more practical in certain situations (family therapy), although again they can be used in conjunction with categorical approaches. They are less useful for certain purposes (in considering pharmacologic intervention) (1). Past the level of the individual cases, the utility of ideographic approaches is limited. Such approaches make it very difficult to communicate information for clinical and research purposes in a concise and readily understood fashion. Chapter 4.1 suggests efficient ways of incorporating the various classification systems into a meaningful understanding of the patient, in order to institute a balanced and informed treatment plan.

RDoC

The Research Domain Criteria (RDoC) project is a framework for conducting research that has been launched by the NIMH in order to gather empirical data to ultimately develop a new classification of psychopathology based on the dimensions of neurobiology and behavior that cut across traditional categories of mental disorders (68). In contrast to the DSM and ICD classification systems which are intended for clinical use, the RDoC approach is not a classification system per se but is intended for researchers to provide a working model to stimulate research on the core dimensions (or constructs) of psychopathology. First, in 2009, an NIMH workgroup devised a proposal for a new system and outlined five major domains of functioning such as cognition and emotions, and units of analysis ranging from genes to neural circuits to behavior. Then, five groups of experts in basic and behavioral sciences representing each of the domains were convened for a series of workshops and asked to determine and define specific dimensions to be included in each domain. In order to be included, the domains (e.g., "fear") had to reflect validated behavioral functions and show evidence for a neural circuit or system responsible for implementing this function.

The ensuing RDoC constructs are organized in a two-dimensional matrix of five domains that include constituent constructs in the rows and seven units of analysis as the columns (69). The *units of analysis* include genes, molecules, cells, circuits, physiology, behavior, and self-report, reflecting a range of methodologic approaches from genetics to psychology. The first three levels of analysis pertain to neurobiologic mechanism of circuitry essential to each construct. In turn, neural circuits is a central unit that can be studied with neuroimaging methods such as functional magnetic resonance imaging or indices of circuit activity such as fear-potentiated startle. Physiology refers to variables such as event-related potentials or heart rate variability that can be validated as indirect measures of neural circuits. Measures of observable behavior and performance on laboratory task are grouped under the unit of analysis termed "behavior." Lastly, self-report category is reserved for interviews, rating scales, and other psychometric instruments of various aspects of the construct of interest that represent signs and symptoms of psychopathology. This emphasis on the multifaceted characterization of constructs is part of the RDoC's aim to incorporate methods of genetics, neuroscience, and cognitive science into the future classification scheme of mental disorders.

The RDoC constructs are grouped into domains of functioning that reflect key aspects of emotion, motivation, cognition, social behavior, and regulatory systems (70). The first domain, *negative valence systems,* includes constructs defined by responses to acute threat ("fear"), potential threat ("anxiety"), sustained threat, loss, and frustration. The second domain, *positive valence system,* contains constructs defined by reward learning and habit formation. For example, approach motivation construct encompasses goal pursuit behaviors subserved by the mesolimbic dopamine system. A dysfunction of this system can lead to abnormally low (e.g., avolition) or high (e.g., addition) goal-directed behaviors. Another construct within this domain called "habit" is viewed as a manifestation of reinforcement learning where repetitive motor or cognitive behaviors occur and manifest without serving an adaptive goal. The *cognitive systems domain* encompasses six broad constructs: attention, perception, declarative memory, language, cognitive control, and working memory. The *social processes domain* includes constructs that bridge social behavior with neural circuits of attachment, social dominance and perception, and understanding of self and others. For example, facial communication may include receptive aspects of facial affect recognition and productive aspects of eye contact and gaze following. The neural underpinnings of these behaviors have been studied with an array of neuroimaging and electrophysiologic methods in order to established biomarkers of psychiatric disorders such as ASD and schizophrenia. The fifth domain includes *arousal and regulatory systems* that subserve many of the other domains and are central in sleep and wakefulness.

The RDoC framework is based on three core assumptions: (1) mental illnesses are presumed to be disorders of brain circuits, (2) neuroscience tools can identify the pathophysiology, and (3) the discovery of biosignatures will supplement diagnoses based on clinical signs and symptoms and direct assessment and treatment of mental illness (71). These assumptions have been critiqued for overly biologizing mental illness and their relative lack of emphasis on developmental and environmental influences on mental health and illness, as these variables are missing in the RDoC matrix (72). However, since its inception, the RDoC approach has stimulated an increasing body of research on developing and validating the proposed constructs along the lines that are outlined in the RDoC matrix. In addition, RDoC offers a new perspective to study co-occurring disorders. For example, autism commonly co-occurs with anxiety, but when using symptom-based criteria, it is hard to know whether anxiety is a true comorbidity or a feature of autism. However, measures that have been validated to test relevant functions within anxiety/fear circuitry and social brain networks can provide an alternative way for characterizing anxiety in autism (73). Treatment studies can also benefit from the RDoC approach by focusing on brain/behavior associations as the primary outcome variables. For example, randomized control studies can test whether reduction of behavior (e.g., aggression) is associated with changes in socio-emotional circuitry (e.g., connectivity of the amygdala with ventromedial prefrontal cortex), thus testing the constructs of the RDoC matrix (e.g., frustrative nonreward) (74).

SUMMARY

Classification in child and adolescent psychiatry has multiple meanings and functions. Complications for classification of child and adolescent disorders are myriad: The child is often not the person complaining; different kinds of data may be used in making a diagnosis; developmental factors may have a major impact on the expression of disorders; and certain features (e.g., beliefs in fantasy figures) are normative at certain ages but not at others. Additional complications are posed by the unintended, but no less real, uses to which diagnostic concepts are put, such as their inclusion in legislation and their use as mandates for services in educational programs or for purposes of insurance reimbursement for services. Different kinds and levels of classification are needed for different purposes.

The past 20 years witnessed tremendous advances in the area of diagnosis and classification of child and adolescent psychopathology. These advances are particularly welcome because work in this area had lagged behind that in the adult psychiatric disorders. Various approaches to classification have been employed; each has its advantages and limitations. Issues of reliability and validity remain to be addressed for many categories and classification systems; the attempt to address these issues through examining empirical data rather than theorizing is perhaps the greatest accomplishment of these efforts.

Tensions between clinical and research utility will continue to exist. As classification systems become more complex, they are less readily used; conversely, simplistic systems fail to capture important aspects of clinical experience. The likely ability, over the next decade, to identify more clearly the role of genetic factors for at least a few conditions and the growing sophistication of statistical approaches to aspects of classification and diagnosis represent important areas for future work.

A classification scheme is best used by persons with considerable training who take the task of diagnosis (in its broadest sense) seriously. Although categorical systems increasingly use diagnostic criteria, these are often not truly operationalized, although they are often abstracted and reified for specific purposes (development of interview schedules administered by lay interviewers, or the use of simple frequency counts or symptom duration that obscures the more central aspects of the underlying clinical construct). Although the various "official" systems present areas of disagreement, the areas of agreement are even more noteworthy. Certain issues, such as classification of combination categories versus the use of multiple diagnoses, remain to be resolved. Specific issues arise with respect to inclusionary and exclusionary rules and aspects of comorbidity. Although much has been accomplished, considerable work remains to be done.

References

1. Werry JS: ICD 9 and DSM III classification for the clinician. *J Child Psychol Psychiatry* 26:1–6, 1985.
2. Jaspers K: *General Psychopathology.* Hoenig J, Hamilton M (trans, eds). Manchester, University Press, 1962.
3. Hobbs N (ed): *Issues in the Classification of Children.* San Francisco, CA, JosseyBass, 1975.
4. World Health Organization: Mental and behavioral disorders, clinical descriptions and diagnostic guidelines. In: *International Classification of Diseases,* 10th ed. Geneva, World Health Organization, 1992.
5. American Psychiatric Association: *Diagnostic and Statistical Manual of Mental Disorders,* 5th ed. Washington, DC, American Psychiatric Association, 2013.
6. Blashfield RG, Draguns JG: Evaluative criteria for psychiatric classification. *J Abnorm Psychol* 85:140–150, 1976.
7. Hempel CG: Problems of taxonomy. In: Zubin J (ed.): *Field Studies in the Mental Disorders.* London, Grune & Stratton, 3–22 1961.
8. Quay HC: Classification. In: Quay HC, Werry JS (eds.): *Psychopathological disorders of childhood,* 3rd ed. New York, Wiley, 1–34, 1986.
9. Rutter M: Classification and categorization in child psychiatry. *J Child Psychol Psychiatry* 6:71–83, 1965.
10. Rutter M, Shaffer D, Shepherd M: A multiaxial classification of child psychiatric disorders. Geneva, World Health Organization, 1975.
11. Spitzer RL, Cantwell DP: The DSM-III classification of the psychiatric disorders of infancy, childhood, and adolescence. *J Am Acad Child Psychiatry* 19:356–370, 1980.
12. Rutter M, Gould M: Classification. In: Rutter M, Hersov L (eds): *Child and Adolescent Psychiatry: Modern Approaches,* 2nd ed. Oxford, Blackwell Scientific, 304–321, 1985.
13. Morey LC: Personality disorders in DSM-III and DSM-III-R: convergence, coverage, and internal consistency. *Am J Psychiatry* 145:573–577, 1988.
14. Zigler E, Glick M: *A Developmental Approach to Psychopathology.* New York, Wiley, 1986.
15. Freud A: *Normality and Pathology in Childhood.* New York, International Universities Press, 1965.
16. Mattison RE, Hooper SR: The history of modern classification of child and adolescent psychiatric disorders: an overview. In: Hooper SR, Hynd GW, Mattison RE (eds): *Assessment and Diagnosis of Child and Adolescent Psychiatric Disorders. Vol. 1: Psychiatric Disorders.* Hillsdale, NJ, Erlbaum, 1992.
17. Feighner J, Robbins E, Guze DB, Woodruff RA, Winokur G, Munoz R: Diagnostic criteria for use in psychiatric research. *Arch Gen Psychiatry* 26:57–63, 1972.
18. Weber AC, Scharfetter C: The syndrome concept: history and statistical operationalizations. *Psychol Med* 14:315–325, 1984.
19. Volkmar FR, Cohen DJ: Disintegrative disorder or "late onset" autism. *J Child Psychol Psychiatry* 30:717–724, 1989.
20. Bell RQ, Harper LV: *Child Effects on Adults.* Hillsdale, NJ, Erlbaum, 1977.
21. Klin A, Chawarska K, Paul R, Rubin E, Morgan T, Wiesner L, Volkmar F: Autism in a 15-month-old child. *Am J Psychiatry* 161(11):1981–1988, 2004.
22. Lord C: Follow-up of two-year-olds referred for possible autism. *J Child Psychol Psychiatry* 36(8):1365–1382, 1995.
23. Zeanah C (ed): *Handbook of Infant Mental Health.* New York, Guilford, 236–249, 1993.
24. Kagan J: *Change and Continuity in Infancy.* New York, Wiley, 1971.
25. Chess S, Thomas A: *Temperament in Clinical Practice.* New York, Guilford, 1986.
26. Earls FR: Application of DSM-III in an epidemiological study of preschool children. *Am J Psychiatry* 139:242–243, 1982.
27. Mezzich JE, von Cranach M: *International Classification in Psychiatry: Unity and Diversity.* Cambridge, Cambridge University Press, 1988.
28. Ozonoff S, Rogers SJ, Hendren RL (eds): Autism spectrum disorders: a research review for practitioners. Washington, DC, American Psychiatric Publishing, Inc, 2003.
29. Cohen DJ, Leckman JF, Volkmar FR: The diagnostic process and classification in child psychiatry: issues and prospects. In: Mezzich JE, von Vranach M (eds.): *International Classification in Psychiatry: Unity and Diversity.* Cambridge, Cambridge University Press, 284–297, 1988.
30. Swets JA: Measuring the accuracy of diagnostic systems. *Science* 240:1285–1292, 1988.
31. Valliant GE, Schnurr P: What is a case? *Arch Gen Psychiatry* 45:313–319, 1988.
32. Grove WM, Andreasen NC, McDonald-Scott P, Keller MB, Shapiro RW: Group for the advancement of psychiatry, 1966. Reliability studies of psychiatric diagnosis: theory and practice. *Arch Gen Psychiatry* 38:408–413, 1981.
33. Achenbach TM: Integrating assessment and taxonomy. In: Rutter M, Tuma H, Lann IS (eds): *Assessment and Diagnosis in Child Psychopathology.* New York, Guilford, 300–339, 1988.
34. Achenbach TM, Edelbrock CS: The classification of child psychopathology: a review and analysis of empirical efforts. *Psychol Bull* 85:1275–1301, 1978.
35. Kraemer HC: Assessment of 2×2 associations: generalization of signal detection methodology. *Am Statist* 42:37–49, 1988.
36. Szatmari P, Volkmar F, Walter S: Latent class models and the evaluation of diagnostic criteria for autism. *J Am Acad Child Adolesc Psychiatry* 34:216–222, 1995.
37. Zoccolillo M, Pickes A, Quinton D, et al.: The outcome of conduct disorder: implications for defining adult personality disorder and conduct disorder. *Psychol Med* 22:971–986, 1992.
38. Kraepelin E: *Compendium der Psychiatrie.* Leipzig, Abel, 1883.
39. American Psychiatric Association: *Diagnostic and Statistical Manual of Mental Disorders,* 2nd ed. Washington, DC, American Psychiatric Association, 1968.
40. American Psychiatric Association: *Diagnostic and Statistical Manual of Mental Disorders,* 3rd ed. Washington, DC, American Psychiatric Association, 1980.
41. American Psychiatric Association: *Diagnostic and Statistical Manual of Mental Disorders,* 3rd ed., rev. Washington, DC, American Psychiatric Association, 1987.
42. Puig-Antich J: The use of RDC criteria for major depressive disorder in children and adolescents. *J Am Acad Child Psychiatry* 21:291–293, 1982.
43. Spitzer RL, Endicott JE, Robins E: Research diagnostic criteria. *Arch Gen Psychiatry* 35:773–782, 1978.
44. Schwab-Stone M, Towbin KE, Tarnoff GM: Systems of classification: ICD-10, DSM-III-R, and DSM-IV. In: Lewis M (ed.): *Child and Adolescent Psychiatry: A Comprehensive Textbook.* Baltimore, MD, Williams & Wilkins, 422–434, 1991.
45. Frances AJ, Widiger TA, Pincus HA: The development of DSM-IV. *Arch Gen Psychiatry* 46:373–375, 1989.
46. Widiger TA, Frances AJ, Pincus HA, et al.: Toward an empirical classification for the DSM-IV. *J Abnorm Psychol* 100:280–288, 1991.
47. Lahey BB, Applegate B, McBurnett K, et al.: DSM-IV field trials for attention deficit hyperactivity disorder in children and adolescents. *Am J Psychiatry* 151:1673–1685, 1994.
48. Volkmar FR, Klin A, Siegel B, et al.: Field trial for autistic disorder in DSM-IV. *Am J Psychiatry* 151:1361–1367, 1994.
49. Kramer M: The history of the efforts to agree on an international classification of mental disorders. In: *Diagnostic and Statistical Manual of Mental Disorders,* 2nd ed. Washington, DC, American Psychiatric Association, xi–xx, 1968.
50. Brämer G: Tenth revision of the international classification of diseases: in progress. *Br J Psychiatry* 152[Suppl]:29–32, 1988.
51. Sartorius N: International perspectives of psychiatric classification. *Br J Psychiatry* 152[Suppl]:9–14, 1988.
52. World Health Organization: *International Classification of Diseases,* 9th ed. Geneva, World Health Organization, 1977.
53. Cooper JE: The structure and presentation of contemporary psychiatric classifications with special reference to ICD-9 and 10. *Br J Psychiatry* 152[Suppl]:21–28, 1988.
54. Rutter M: Annotation: child psychiatric disorders in ICD-10. *J Child Psychol Psychiatry* 30:499–513, 1989.
55. Rutter M, Tuma AN: Diagnosis and classification: some outstanding issues. In: Rutter M, Tuma H, Lann IS (eds): *Assessment and Diagnosis in Child Psychopathology.* New York, Guilford, 437–445, 1988.
56. Volkmar FR, Woolston JL: Comorbidity of psychiatric disorders in children and adolescents. In: Wexler S (ed.): *Comorbidity in Psychiatry.* New York, Wiley, 307–322, 1997.
57. American Psychiatric Association: Diagnostic and statistical manual of mental disorders, 4th ed, text rev. Washington, DC, American Psychiatric Association, 2000.
58. First MB, Pincus HA: The DSM-IV text revision: rationale and potential impact on clinical practice. *Psychiatr Serv* 53(3):288–92, 2002.
59. Kupfer DA, First MB, Regier DA: A research agenda for DSM-V. Washington, DC, American Psychiatric Publishing, 2002.
60. Pine DS, Alegria M, Cook EH, et al.: Advances in developmental science and DSM-V. In: Kupfer DA, First MB, Regier DA (eds). *A research agenda for DSM-V.* Washington, DC, American Psychiatric Publishing, 85–122, 2002.
61. Rutter, M, Uher R: Classification issues and challenges in child and adolescent psychopathology. *Int Rev Psychiatry* 24(6):514–529, 2012.
62. Smith IC, Reichow B, Volkmar FR. The effects of DSM-5 criteria on number of individuals diagnosed with autism spectrum disorder: a systematic review. *J Autism Dev Disord* 45(8):2541–2552, 2015.
63. Reed GM, First MB, Elena Medina-Mora M, Gureje O, Pike KM, Saxena S. Draft diagnostic guidelines for ICD-11 mental and behavioural disorders available for review and comment. *World Psychiatry* 15(2):112–113, 2016.

64. Keeley JW, Reed GM, Roberts MC, et al. Developing a science of clinical utility in diagnostic classification systems field study strategies for ICD-11 mental and behavioral disorders. *Am Psychol* 2016;71(1):3–16.
65. Hewitt LE, Jenkins RL: *Fundamental Patterns of Maladjustment: The Dynamics of Their Origin.* Springfield, IL, State of Illinois, 1946.
66. Achenbach TM, Conners CK, Quay HC, et al.: Replication of empirically derived syndromes as a basis for taxonomy of child/adolescent psychopathology. *J Abnorm Child Psychol* 17:299–323, 1989.
67. Angold A, Rutter M: Effects of age and pubertal status on depression in a large clinical sample. *Dev Psychopathol* 4:5–28, 1992.
68. Insel T, Cuthbert B, Garvey M, et al.: Research Domain Criteria (RDoC): toward a new classification framework for research on mental disorders. *Am J Psychiatry* 167(7):748–751, 2010.
69. Cuthbert BN: The RDoC framework: facilitating transition from ICD/DSM to dimensional approaches that integrate neuroscience and psychopathology. *World Psychiatry* 13(1):28–35, 2014.
70. National Institute of Mental Health: *Research Domain Criteria Matrix.* Retrieved November 9, 2015, from http://www.nimh.nih.gov/research-priorities/rdoc/research-domain-criteria-matrix.shtml
71. Cuthbert BN: Research Domain Criteria: toward future psychiatric nosologies. *Dialogues Clin Neurosci* 17(1):89–97, 2015.
72. Lilienfeld SO: The Research Domain Criteria (RDoC): an analysis of methodological and conceptual challenges. *Behav Res Ther* 62:129–139, 2014.
73. Sukhodolsky DG, Scahill L, Gadow KD, et al.: Parent-rated anxiety symptoms in children with pervasive developmental disorders: frequency and association with demographic and clinical characteristics. *J Abnorm Child Psychol* 36:117–128, 2008.
74. Sukhodolsky DG, Vander Wyk BC, Eilbott JA, et al.: Neural mechanisms of cognitive-behavioral therapy for aggression in children: design of a randomized controlled trail within the RDoC construct of frustrative non-reward. *J Child Adolesc Psychopharmacol* 26:38–48, 2016.

SECTION V
SPECIFIC DISORDERS AND SYNDROMES

5.1 ■ ATTENTION AND DISRUPTIVE DISORDERS

CHAPTER 5.1.1 ■ ATTENTION-DEFICIT HYPERACTIVITY DISORDER

LACRAMIOARA SPETIE AND EUGENE L. ARNOLD

DEFINITION

Attention-deficit hyperactivity disorder (ADHD) is a syndrome of inattention, distractibility, restless overactivity, impulsiveness, and other deficits of executive function. It involves impairment of the ability to "plan your work and work your plan." DSM-5 diagnosis of ADHD requires either six of nine inattentive symptoms (e.g., carelessness about details, easy distraction, not listening when spoken to, easily losing focus, failure to complete tasks, avoiding tasks that require sustained attention, forgetfulness, and easily losing things) or six of nine hyperactive-impulsive symptoms (e.g., often fidgeting, squirming, or leaving seat when expected to remain in place, running, climbing or talking excessively, unable to be still or quiet for extended reasonable time, often having a hard time waiting their turn, often intruding or interrupting others) present for at least 6 months, dating from before age 12, not better explained by another disorder, and causing impairment in at least two settings academically, socially, or in daily living function. Six inattentive symptoms qualify for a diagnosis of inattentive presentation; six hyperactive/impulsive symptoms qualify as hyperactive/impulsive presentation; and six of each qualify as combined presentation. For patients age 17 and older, five symptoms from a list are sufficient.

It can be full expression (combined type—DSM-IV (1) or combined presentation—DSM-5, with six symptoms from each list of nine) (2) or partial expression (inattentive or hyperactive-impulsive types or presentations, with six symptoms from one of the lists). It is not necessary to have all the symptoms to qualify for the diagnosis. It is possible for two patients to meet diagnostic criteria with no symptoms in common and it is even possible to have the same presentation with only half the symptoms in common. This leads to wide variability in presenting problems and severity, which is further complicated by common associated symptoms such as irritability, boredom, and impaired social skills, and by psychiatric comorbid diagnoses.

There has been controversy in the literature as to whether the diagnosis of ADHD should be regarded as a category or as a dimension. Recent findings from genome-wide association studies question the basis of current classifications and the extent to which disorder categories reflect overlapping or distinct neuropathologic entities. The categorical view proposes that ADHD is qualitatively different from any variation of normal. The dimensional view proposes ADHD symptoms are on a continuum with variations on a spectrum of severity and only differ from normal in degree (3).

THE ATTENTION-DEFICIT HYPERACTIVITY DISORDER CONCEPT AND TERMINOLOGY

As early as the mid-19th century, the problems of inattentiveness and overactivity in children were recognized by Heinrich Hoffman (4) in the moralistic children's book *Slovenly Peter*, which featured the characters Fidgety Phil and Harry Who Looks in the Air. In the early 20th century, Still's disease was recognized as the behavioral sequelae of viral encephalitis. The behavioral constellation, particularly the overactivity and impulsiveness, were therefore considered "minimal brain damage," which morphed over time into "minimal brain dysfunction" as diagnosticians realized it was not possible to find evidence of actual brain damage in most cases (at least not with the technology available through the 1970s). Other descriptive terms used by the second half of the 20th century included hyperkinesis, hyperkinetic syndrome, hyperactivity, hyperactive-impulse disorder, psychoneurologic integration deficit, and pseudoneurosis.

The first diagnosis to describe children with symptoms of ADHD was the diagnosis of Hyperkinetic Impulse Disorder introduced by Laufer et al in 1957 (5a). In 1970 the second

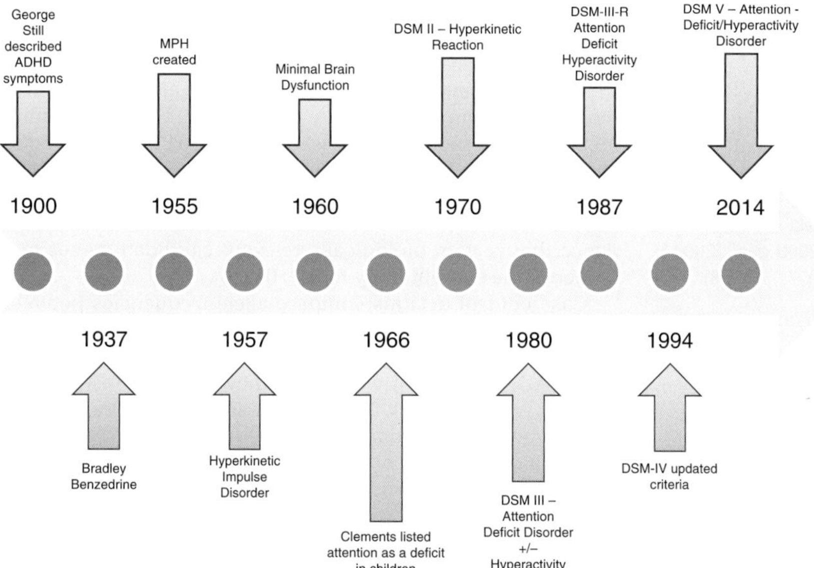

FIGURE 5.1.1.1. Timeline of names from industry set. (Courtesy of Novartis Pharmaceuticals.)

edition of the Diagnostic and statistical Manual (5b) identified the syndrome as "hyperkinetic reaction" based on the then-prevailing psychodynamic philosophy that mental disorders were always reactions to some stressor. The term "hyperkinetic disorder" (HD) is still used in the current International Code of Diseases (6). Recognizing that the cause of most mental disorders is more complex than a reaction to stress, the DSM-III (7) changed in 1980 to descriptive phenomenologic terms without causal implication. By that time the importance of inattentive symptoms had been recognized, leading to the appellation "attention deficit disorder," which could be diagnosed either without (ADD) or with hyperactivity (ADDH). The term ADD is still used by many to refer to the inattentive subpresentation, and is preserved in the names of such support/advocacy groups as Attention-Deficit Disorder Association (ADDA) (8) and Children and Adults with ADD (ChADD) (9). DSM-III-R (10) added overactivity back to the name of the disorder via the term "attention-deficit/hyperactivity disorder (ADHD)." This name was retained by DSM-IV although the symptom list changed somewhat, being expanded from 14 to 18 symptoms and being split into two lists of 9 each (Figure 5.1.1.1). The age requirement for symptom onset was changed to age 12 in DSM-5 (rather than age 7 in DSM-IV), but the name of the disorder was preserved as in DSM-III-R.

The ICD-10 criteria for HD (11) are more restrictive than the DSM-IV criteria in that all three symptom clusters of inattention, hyperactivity and impulsivity should be present and pervasive across settings and that the presence of anxiety or mood disorder is in itself an exclusion criterion. ICD 10 also includes the diagnosis of hyperkinetic conduct disorder (HKD), which would be roughly the same as the DSM equivalent of ADHD combined presentation with comorbid conduct disorder.

EPIDEMIOLOGY

ADHD is one of the most common childhood-onset psychiatric disorders, affecting 5% to 12% of children worldwide. ADHD is a costly public health concern (12) since it can cause significant impairment in functioning that interferes with normal development and all areas of functioning in patients of all ages.

Epidemiologic studies of ADHD addressing issues of frequency, distribution, determinants, comorbidity, long-term outcome, and impact of treatment have been complicated by several problems. The first is integrating the different types of information from various sources required to make the diagnosis. A related problem is how to correct for the subjective nature of the information provided by the informants. The diagnosis could be easily overestimated if the information obtained does not include the level of impairment caused by the symptoms reported (13). Another problem is the difficulty integrating epidemiologic information obtained over time due to the ongoing refinement in the diagnostic criteria for ADHD. The current DSM-5 criteria allow the inclusion of more females, preschoolers, and adults presenting with significant impairment but who would have been otherwise excluded (14). The definition of ADHD may continue to flux over time, as experts consider age-specific thresholds for symptom counts.

Further, there are differences between the DSM-5 criteria used to make the diagnosis in the United States and the ICD-10 criteria used to make the diagnosis in Europe and other parts of the world, although many investigators worldwide use the DSM system. Because of the difference in stringency of definition, DSM-5 ADHD is more prevalent than ICD HKD, a finding that could be easily misinterpreted to show that ADHD is more common in countries using DSM criteria than in countries using ICD-10 criteria (15). The reanalysis of the data of the National Institute of Mental Health (NIMH) Multimodal Treatment Study of children with ADHD (the MTA) found that only 145 of the 579 children who had DSM-IV combined type ADHD also met criteria for ICD-10 HKD (16). A further complication is whether all the inattentive presentation cases are detected in a given study.

Results of various prevalence studies in the United States and worldwide are similar: conservatively 5% in children and 2.5% in adults. The male:female ratio is about 2:1 in epidemiologically discerned samples, in contrast to 3 to 5:1 and even up to 9:1 in mental health clinic samples. Girls present more often with less disruptive symptoms, more attention problems and more internalizing problems such as depression and anxiety (17), while boys present with more disruptive behavior leading to clinical referral. Male sex, low socioeconomic status, and young age are associated with a higher prevalence of ADHD.

In preschoolers the hyperactive presentation is more common and the prevalence may vary from a low of 2% in the primary care setting to a high of 59% in a child psychiatry clinic (18). The symptoms of hyperactivity tend to decrease with age. In elementary school-age children, the combined type/presentation has been more frequently diagnosed, while the inattentive type was more common in middle and high school. As many as 60% of the childhood cases continue to have some symptoms as adults (19). Emotional symptoms are likely to persist and cause impairment in adults with ADHD (20–22).

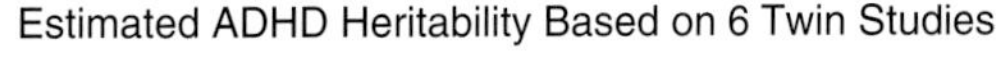

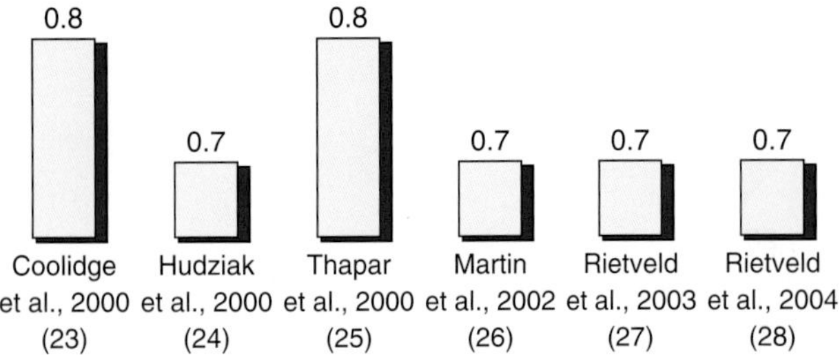

FIGURE 5.1.1.2. Estimated ADHD heritability based on six studies.

ETIOLOGY

The etiology of ADHD is complex and most likely includes genetic and environmental factors.

Genetics

Studies have shown that ADHD is a phenotypically complex diagnosis that is strongly genetically influenced and is transmitted in families. In the past twin and adoption studies yielded an estimated heritability of about 75% (Figure 5.1.1.2) (23–28). A more recent analysis by Faraone et al (28a) found that genetic factors accounted for 60% of the heritability, with the rest being split between environmental influences and child specific environmental influences.

Recent genetic studies have been using endophenotypes as tools to detect the effects of individual genes. Endophenotypes are phenotypes that are assumed to be less complex in presentation and etiology than signs and symptoms of the clinical disorder but are still influenced by one or more of the same susceptibility genes as the disorder. Neuropsychological measures of inhibitory control and impairments in state regulation and delay aversion are considered potential candidates for ADHD endophenotypes (29–32). Other methods focus on distinct components or clusters of symptoms of the complex phenotypes that may be heritable and may characterize phenotypically homogenous groups of individuals.

There are several different chromosomal regions shared more often than expected by chance among ADHD family members. These regions have included 5p12, 10q26, 12q23, and 16p13 (33); 15q15, 7p13, and 9q33 (34); and 8q12, 11q23, 4q13, 17p11, 12q23, and 8p23 (35).

Association studies of candidate genes have looked for evidence that certain biologically relevant candidate genes may influence the susceptibility to ADHD (36).

Case control designs compare allele frequencies between patients with ADHD and non-ADHD control subjects, while family-based designs compare the alleles that parents transmit to ADHD children with those they do not transmit. If an allele increases the risk for ADHD, it should be more common among the transmitted alleles than the nontransmitted alleles. The data obtained in both study designs can be analyzed to derive odds ratio (OR) or relative risk (RR) statistics that assess the magnitude of the association between the risk alleles and the diagnosis of ADHD. An OR or RR of 1.0 indicates no association, greater than 1.0 indicates that the allele increases the risk for ADHD, and those less than 1.0 indicate that the allele decreases the risk for ADHD. The most studied candidate genes for ADHD are listed in Table 5.1.1.1 (37–123).

STRUCTURAL, FUNCTIONAL, AND ELECTROPHYSIOLOGIC FINDINGS IN THE BRAIN

Structural Findings in ADHD

Similarities between the symptoms of ADHD and symptoms observed in certain neurologic patients following damage to the prefrontal cortex (126) have prompted researchers to theorize that brain structural abnormalities may be at the root of ADHD symptomatology.

TABLE 5.1.1.1

CANDIDATE GENES FOR ADHD

Gene	Reference	Summary Findings
Dopamine Transporter Gene (DAT; SLC6A3)	Cook et al. (37); Waldman et al. (38); Dougherty et al. (39); Krause et al. (40); Todd et al. (41); Payton et al. (42); Muglia et al. (43); van Dyck et al. (44); Chen et al. (45); Smith et al. (46) Meta-analysis: Curran et al. (47); Gizer IR et al. (48); Azeredo LA et al. (49)	Pooled OR = 1.13
D2 Dopamine Receptor Gene (DRD2)	Case-control studies: Comings (50); Comings (51) Family-based studies: Rowe et al. (52); Kirley et al. (53); Huang et al. (54)	Pooled OR = 1.16 No conclusive results
D4 Dopamine Receptor Gene (DRD4–7)	Faraone et al. (55)—meta-analysis of case studies (CS) and family-based studies (FB)	Found a significant association between 7-repeat allele CR studies—pooled OR = 1.9 FB studies—pooled OR = 1.4
	Other positive case control studies: Payton et al. (42) Meta-analysis: Gizer et al. (48) Other positive family-based studies: Holmes et al. (56); Grady et al. (57); Arcos Burgos et al. (21) Negative case control studies: Qian et al. (58) Negative family-based studies: Mill et al. (59); Manor et al. (60); Kustanovich et al. (61); Smith et al. (46)	
Other DRD4 polymorphisms (120 bp repeat 1.2 kb; 240 allele FspI-521 C to T and Ava-II—616 C to G; 5'120-bp repeat)	McCracken et al. (62); Todd et al. (63); Barr et al. (64); Rowe et al. (65); Kustanovich et al. (61); Kustanovich et al. (66); Arcos Burgos et al. (21); Barkley et al. (18)	No conclusive results

TABLE 5.1.1.1

(CONTINUED)

Gene	Reference	Summary Findings
D5 Dopamine Receptor Gene (DRD5)	Case control studies: Comings et al. (67) Family-based studies: Daly et al. (68); Barr et al. (69); Tahir et al. (70); Payton et al. (42); Kustanovich et al. (61); Kustanovich et al. (66); Mill et al. (71); Lasky-Su, Biederman et al. (72); Meta-analysis: Gizer et al. (48)	Probable association; results need independent replication
	Meta-analysis of family-based studies: Maher et al. (73); Lowe et al. (74); Manor et al. (75)	Significant association: pooled OR 1.2
D3 Dopamine Receptor gene (DRD3)	Barr et al. (76); Payton et al. (42); Muglia et al. (77); Coming et al. (67); Retz et al. (78)	Pooled OR = 1.2
Serotonin Transporter Gene (5-HTT; SLC6A4)	Case control studies: Retz et al. (79); Seeger et al. (80); Zoroglu et al. (81); Beitchman et al. (82) Family studies: Manor et al. (83); Kent et al. (84); Cadoret et al. (85) Meta-analysis: Gizer IR et al. (48)	Pooled OR = 1.31
Serotonin Receptor Genes (5HT2A)	Ribases M, Ramos-Quirgoa et al. (86)	Found evidence of association only with the combined ADHD subtype in adults (OR = 1.63) and children (OR = 1.49)
Aromatic L-amino acid decarboxylase (DDC)	Ribases M, Ramos-Quirgoa, et al. (86)	Strongly associated with adulthood (OR = 2.17) and childhood (OR = 1.90) ADHD
Norepinephrine Receptor Gene (SLC6A2, ADRA2A)	Case report studies: Comings et al. (67) Family-based studies: Barr et al. (87); McEvoy et al. (88); DeLuca et al. (89)	No conclusive results
	Yang L, Qian Q, Li H, et al. (90)	One study suggests DNA variants of SLC6A2 and ADRA2A might alter the response to atomoxetine (results need further replication)
Dopamine Beta Hydroxylase Gene (DBH)	Case-control studies: Smith, 2003 (91) Family studies: Daly et al. (68); Payton et al. (42); Roman et al. (92); Wigg et al. (93); Hawi et al. (94); Barkley et al. (18)	Pooled OR = 1.33
Synaptosomal Associated Protein 25 Gene (SNAP 25)	Family-based studies: Hess et al. (95); Hess et al. (96); Barr et al. (97); Brophy et al. (98); Kustanovich et al. (61); Mill et al. (99); Kirley (100) Meta-analysis: Gizer et al. (48)	Pooled OR = 1.19
Tyrosine Hydroxylase Gene (TH)	Case control: Comings et al. (101) Family studies: Barr et al. (97); Payton et al. (42)	All studies negative
Catechol O COMT, Val108Met)	Family studies: Syvanen et al. (102); Barr et al. (103); Hawi et al. (104); Manor et al. (105); Tahir et al. (106); Payton et al. (42); Qian et al. (107); Beijsterveldt (108)	No significant association (pooled OR = 1.0)
Monoamine Oxidase A (MAO-A)	Case control: Manor et al. (109) Family studies: Payton et al. (42); Manor et al. (109); Lawson et al. (110)	All studies but one (Payton et al., 2001) found a significant association
Monoamine Oxidase B (MAO-B)	Ribases, Ramos-Quirgoa, et al. (86)	Specifically associated in the adult ADHD sample (OR = 1.90)
Noradrenergic Receptors ADRA2A	Comings et al. (111); Xu et al. (112); Comings et al. (113); Barr, Wigg (114) Roman et al. (115)	No conclusive results
ADRA1C and ADRA2C	Comings et al. (111); Barr et al. (114); De Luca et al. (89)	No conclusive results
Serotonin Receptors HTR1B (G861C SNP)	Family studies: Hawi et al. (116); Quist et al. (117)	Pooled OR = 1.44
HTR2A (T102C; G1438A; His438Tyr)	Case control: Zoroglu et al. (81) Family studies: Quist et al. (117); Hawi et al. (116); Beijsterveldt et al. (108)	No significant association (pooled OR = 1.1)
Tryptophan Hydroxylase (TPH-SNP's A218C; 6526G)	Family studies: Tang et al. (124); Li et al. (125); Beijsterveldt et al. (108)	No conclusive results
Acetylcholine Receptors CHRNA4 and CHRNA7	Case control: Comings et al. (67) Family studies: Kent et al. (120); Todd et al. (121)	No conclusive results
Glutamate Receptors GRIN2A	Family studies: Turic et al. (122); Adams et al. (123)	Contradicting results

TABLE 5.1.1.2

STRUCTURAL BRAIN ABNORMALITIES IN ADHD

Brain Region	Reference	Summary Findings
Prefrontal Cortex	Castellanos et al. (127); Filipek et al. (128); Overmeyer et al. (129); Castellanos et al. (123); Mostofsky et al. (130); Hill et al. (131); Durston et al. (132)	General findings in ADHD compared to healthy controls: smaller volumes in various areas, especially in the dorsolateral prefrontal and orbitofrontal regions and anterior cingulate
Caudate	Hynd et al. (133); Semrud-Clickeman et al. (134); Castellanos et al. (135); Castellanos et al. (127); Filipek et al. (128); Mataro et al. (136); Castellanos et al. (137); Castellanos et al. (123); Pineda et al. (138); Bussing et al. (139); Hill et al. (131); Castellanos et al. (140)	General findings in ADHD compared to healthy controls: smaller total caudate volume and/or smaller caudate head, but difference from normal lost with age
Pallidum	Aylward et al. (141); Castellanos et al. (127); Overmeyer et al. (142); Castellanos et al. (137)	General findings in ADHD compared to healthy controls: smaller pallidum volume
Corpus Callosum	Hynd et al. (143); Hynd et al. (144); Semrud-Clickeman et al. (145); Giedd et al. (146); Baumgardner et al. (147); Lyoo et al. (148); Castellanos et al. (149); Mostofsky et al. (150); Kates et al. (151); Hill et al. (152)	General findings in ADHD compared to healthy controls: smaller volumes especially in the posterior regions linked to temporal and parietal cortices
Cerebellum	Castellanos et al. (153); Filipek et al. (154); Berquin et al. (155); Mostofsky et al. (156); Castellanos et al. (149); Bussing et al. (157); Hill et al. (152)	General findings in ADHD compared to healthy controls: smaller volumes in various regions, including vermis

The most consistent structural brain imaging findings in children with ADHD have been significantly smaller volumes in the dorsolateral prefrontal cortex, caudate, pallidum, corpus callosum, and cerebellum (Table 5.1.1.2).

Neurocognitive studies of patients with ADHD also identified patterns of executive dysfunction in patients with ADHD (158,159) that are thought to reflect abnormalities in the functioning of the prefrontal cortex, therefore, supporting the hypothesis of an alteration of the prefrontal cortex neuroanatomy in ADHD. The robust symptom response to psychostimulant drugs that target the dopaminergic system, very well represented in the prefrontal cortex, further support this theory (160). With the introduction of totally automated imaging methods it has been possible to identify more widespread volumetric and cortical changes.

One of the most comprehensive longitudinal case control imaging studies was of 152 children and adolescents with ADHD (age range 5 to 18 years) and 139 age- and sex-matched controls (age range 4.5 to 19 years) completed at the National Institute of Mental Health (NIMH) from 1991 to 2001. The patients with ADHD had significantly smaller brain volumes on the initial scan in all regions (total cerebrum; cerebellum; gray and white matter for the four major lobes: frontal–temporal, parietal and occipital; unmedicated children with ADHD had significantly smaller total cerebral volumes and significantly smaller total white matter (161); the volumetric abnormalities persisted with age in total and regional cerebral measures and in the cerebellum except for the caudate nucleus volumes, which were initially abnormal in patients with ADHD but lost the diagnostic difference from controls during adolescence; developmental trajectories for all structures except the caudate remained roughly parallel for patients and controls during childhood and adolescence and are unrelated to stimulant treatment (162).

Prospective longitudinal case control brain MRI studies also identified abnormalities in the brain developmental trajectory in ADHD such as delayed prefrontal cortical development in children with ADHD compared to typical individuals (163–165). A prospective longitudinal study that followed ADHD patients into adulthood (166) found that fixed cortical thinning in the prefrontal cortex correlated with the persistence of the diagnosis in adulthood (167). Prefrontal cortical thinning and slowing of cortical development were also associated with inattention symptoms in healthy children in another study (168) and cortical thinning of the attention and executive function networks in adults was associated with ADHD in adults (169).

Twin studies using structural neuroimaging suggest that the volume of brain regions relevant to ADHD (subcortical and cortical volumes, left and right neocortex, variation of cerebellar volume) is under significant genetic control and might be used to define neuroimaging ADHD endophenotypes (170).

Brain Functional Abnormalities

New brain imaging techniques, including single-photon emission computed tomography (SPECT); positron emission tomography (PET); functional MRI (fMRI), and proton magnetic resonance spectroscopy (PMRS), have made it possible to obtain dynamic measures of brain metabolism at rest and during certain cognitive tasks. Most studies have found abnormalities in cerebral activation in ADHD, with a hypoperfusion of frontal and possibly striatal areas (Table 5.1.1.3). The studies looking at brain function during tasks that challenge the brain inhibitory control also show deficits in the activation of the brain inhibitory control area in the frontal and striatal regions. Because of the important role dopamine (DA) and the dopamine transporter (DAT) seem to have in the pathophysiology and response to treatment in ADHD, several imaging studies using ligands highly selective for the dopamine transporter sites have studied their density in ADHD subjects compared to controls. These studies consistently found an increase in the DAT binding in the striatum of ADHD subjects compared to controls. Several studies also showed a normalization of this brain function following treatment with methylphenidate.

Such functional investigative tools have opened a window on the dynamic nature of ADHD and started to elucidate the flexible and multidirectional causal relationship among brain structure, its neurochemistry, and brain function. Several recent studies found that stimulants prescribed for ADHD improved function and normalized neuroanatomy (215–217). Possible explanations for such findings are that either the stimulant itself directs the brain toward more typical development or the drug enhances function-driven normalization.

Multiple lines of evidence support the role of dopamine in the etiology and the response to treatment (Figure 5.1.1.3). The dopamine circuits are influenced by inputs from multiple areas

TABLE 5.1.1.3

FUNCTIONAL NEUROIMAGING STUDIES OF ADHD

Imaging Technique	Reference	Summary Findings
SPECT Studies	Lou et al. (171–174); Sieg et al. (175); Amen et al. (176); Gustaffson et al. (51); Langleben et al. (177,178); Spalletta et al. (179); Kim et al. (180,181)	General findings in ADHD compared to healthy controls: hypoperfusion in various cortical areas, especially in the frontal and prefrontal cortex, striatum and cerebellum
fMRI Studies	Sunshine et al. (182); Vaidya et al. (183); Bush et al. (184); Rubia et al. (185); Teicher et al. (186); Anderson et al. (187); Durston et al. (188); Schulz et al. (189); Tamm et al. (190)	General findings in ADHD compared to healthy controls: decreased cerebral blood flow to the frontal, prefrontal, and the basal ganglia; decreased activation of frontal/prefrontal regions and basal ganglia during certain cognitive tasks; atypical increase in activity in other brain areas possibly to compensate for hypoactivation; normalization of cerebral blood flow to frontal/prefrontal areas following administration of methylphenidate
PET Studies	Zametkin et al. (191,192); Matochik et al. (193,194); Ernst et al. (195–198); Schweitzer et al. (199–201)	General findings in ADHD compared to healthy controls: decreased glucose metabolism in prefrontal/frontal and other cortical areas and reduced metabolic rate in same areas during cognitive tasks
Positive DAT Binding SPECT Studies	Dougherty et al. (202); Dresel et al. (203); Cheon et al. (204)	Elevated DAT binding in ADHD compared to healthy controls compared to controls
Negative DAT Binding SPECT Studies	Van Dyke et al. (205)	No difference in striatum binding in ADHD compared to healthy controls compared with controls
Positive DAT Binding PET Studies	Spencer et al. (206,207)	Elevated binding in striatum in ADHD compared to healthy controls compared to controls
Negative DAT Binding PET Studies	Jucaite et al. (208)	No difference in DAT binding or D2 receptor binding in the striatum and decreased DAT binding in the midbrain between ADHD subjects and controls
		Significant correlation between DAT and D2 binding in the striatum and measures of hyperactivity
	Pedro Rosa-Neto et al. (209)	Estimated binding potential for D2/3 receptors in the striatum in ADHD within range of estimates obtained in healthy subjects; significant correlation between binding in the right striatum and severity of inattention and impulsivity; significant decrease in binding potential following administration of methylphenidate
PMRS Studies	Jin et al. (210)	Low *N*-acetyl aspartate/creatine ratio in globus pallidus in ADHD
	MacMaster et al. (211)	Elevated glutamate in the right prefrontal cortex and left striatum
	Yeo et al. (212)	Lower *N*-acetyl aspartate levels in girls with ADHD
	Courvoisie et al. (213)	Significantly higher ratios of *N*-acetyl aspartate; glutamate and choline/creatine in the frontal lobes of ADHD subjects
	Moore et al. (214)	Glutamatergic dysfunction in the anterior cingulated cortex in ADHD subjects compared to healthy controls and subjects with bipolar disorder

of the brain involving other neurotransmitter systems, including norepinephrine and serotonin.

Table 5.1.1.4 presents one of the theories explaining the abnormal dopamine transporter density in ADHD subjects and the response to methylphenidate.

Electrophysiologic Studies

Electroencephalograms (EEGs) provide information about the background electrical activity of the brain with good temporal resolution but poor spatial resolution. EEG studies of patients with ADHD were first done as early as 1938 (218) when they included mostly qualitative EEG studies that used visual evaluation of paper recordings of the EEG. Most studies consistently found elevated levels of slow-wave activity in comparison to normal children, with the most reliable measure being the relative theta power and reduced amounts of relative alpha and beta waves.

Several studies have looked at EEG as a diagnostic tool and reported that the theta/beta ratio could discriminate ADHD subjects from control subjects with sensitivity and specificity (219–222). However, more recent studies have noted attenuation of the difference in theta/beta ratio over time due to the theta/beta ratio of normal controls approaching that of individuals with ADHD, possibly as a result of sleep deprivation (223). Several models of ADHD and ADHD presentations have been proposed based on EEG studies: the Maturational Lag Model; the Developmental Deviation Model; and the Hypoarousal Model (Table 5.1.1.5). All models fail to account for the complex clinical presentation in ADHD.

Event-Related Potentials

Event-related potentials (ERPs) provide information about the brain electrical activity underlying sensory and cognitive brain processes in response to stimuli. The small subject

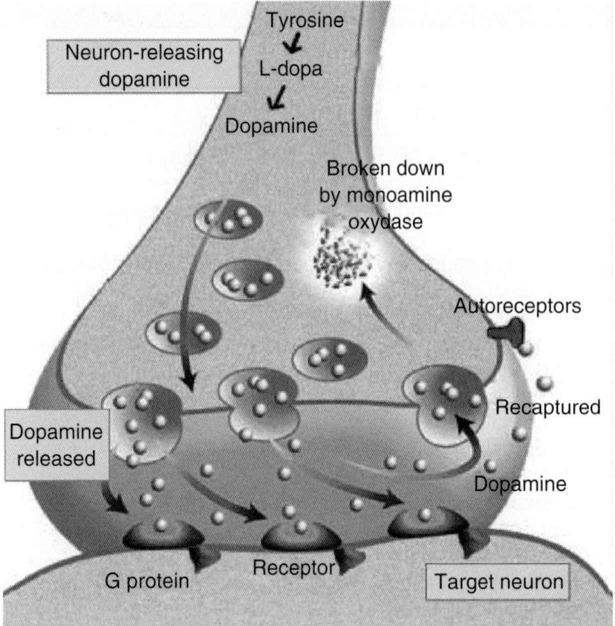

FIGURE 5.1.1.3. Dopamine synapse. Genetic studies indicate that patients with ADHD have a higher rate of certain polymorphisms for the dopamine and other receptors and for the dopamine transporter, resulting in either lower sensitivity of the receptor or faster reuptake of dopamine molecules. Stimulant drugs inhibit reuptake, keeping each dopamine molecule longer in the synaptic cleft so that it is available to stimulate the receptors longer. Similar considerations apply also to norepinephrine, another neurotransmitter believed to be involved in ADHD.

numbers, the use of different types of task performance indicators and reward systems, and other methodologic flows have made the results of most of the studies to date difficult to interpret (241).

TABLE 5.1.1.4

THE DOPAMINE TRANSPORTER AND ADHD

Theory	Rationale
Abnormal DAT binding as a "trait"	"Hypertrophy" of the dopaminergic neurons as a result of inadequate pruning during neurodevelopment genetic abnormalities
Abnormal DAT binding as a "state"	Result of processes compensating for abnormal (increased or decreased) dopamine transmission an attempt to increase efficiency of dopamine clearing resulting from abnormalities at the dopamine synapse level (excess dopamine production and/or release; decreased vesicular storage; increased activity of D1–D5 receptors; abnormal receptor–effector coupling)

With the development of molecular genetics, attempts have been made to identify electrophysiologic endophenotypes of ADHD. A meta-analytic review of twin studies of electrophysiologic measures indicates that genetic factors contribute significantly to both EEG and ERP measures, with significant heritability scores for the EEG alpha power and alpha peak frequency and ERP P3 amplitude (242). More studies are needed to refine such endophenotypes (243).

Special Etiologic Subgroups

Because ADHD is a phenomenologic diagnosis rather than etiologic, there can be various causes manifested through the same symptom constellations. Genetic predisposition, of course, is a major cause, but genes can exert their influence only through

TABLE 5.1.1.5

EEG-BASED MODELS OF ATTENTION-DEFICIT HYPERACTIVITY DISORDER

Model	Rationale	EEG Characteristics	Reference
Maturational Lag	1. ADHD results from a developmental lag in central nervous system functioning. 2. EEG measures in the ADHD subject would be considered normal in a younger child and EEG findings mature in a normal fashion.	Increased centroposterior relative delta; increased relative theta across the scalp; decreased frontocentral relative beta; decreased relative alpha across the scalp; greater levels of theta and deficiencies of alpha and beta in comparison to the control group	Kinsbourne et al. (224); Satterfield et al. (225); Matsuura et al. (226); John et al. (227); Clarke et al. (228); Lazzaro et al. (229)
Developmental Deviation	1. ADHD results from an abnormality in central nervous system functioning. 2. Beta levels in the ADHD combined group were greater than mean values for control group; the theta levels were greater than control groups; less relative alpha compared to control group		Klinkerfuss et al. (230); Wikler et al. (231); John et al. (232); Clarke et al. (233,234)
Hypoarousal	1. ADHD results from cortical hypoarousal. 2. EEG measures in the ADHD subject indicate lower levels of beta activity during cognitive tasks. 3. EEG findings of hypoarousal in the ADHD subject should correlate with other functional measures of the brain activity showing decreased cortical activation.	Reduced suppression of alpha waves; increased frontal relative theta; decreased relative beta suppression across the scalp;	Satterfield and Cantwell (235); Satterfield et al. (236,237); Grunewald-Zuberbier et al. (238); Ackerman et al. (239); Lubar et al. (240)
Overaroused		Excess beta activity	

interaction with the environment and other genes. The pathogenetic mechanisms for expression of various genes in interaction with various environments—physical, chemical, nutritional, familial, social—can vary widely from one individual to another. The multiple-allele polymorphisms described above allow for multiple environmental sensitivities or special environmental needs, and there are probably further polymorphisms not yet discovered. For example, there appears to be a subgroup of children with ADHD who have some kind of food or food additive sensitivity demonstrated in placebo-controlled studies (124,125,244,245). Another very small subgroup has thyroid abnormality intimately linked to ADHD symptoms (246,247). Heavy metal poisoning can cause ADHD symptoms, and at least one study suggested that in cases of lead toxicity, ADHD symptoms improve as much (or more) with deleading as with a stimulant drug (248). It is possible that because of genetic differences in enzymes and other metabolic features, some individuals may be more sensitive to heavy metal poisoning than others. Some anticonvulsants can make ADHD symptoms worse.

Recent studies have found some evidence that tryptophan depletion and vitamin D deficiency may be linked to ADHD (249–251). Many authors believe that thresholds of vitamin and mineral requirements vary from person to person, so that some may be more susceptible to borderline deficiency symptoms.

DIAGNOSIS AND CLINICAL FEATURES

Importance of History

ADHD is a diagnosis primarily made by history: by caregiver report (or in the case of some adolescents and adults, by self-report) of a chronic pattern of inattentiveness, overactivity, and/or impulsiveness. Rarely is a short sampling of behavior in an office visit adequate to detect the symptoms, and even then the diagnostician needs caregiver confirmation of their chronicity and pervasiveness. Often a child with ADHD can appear calm and attentive in a novel setting with an adult one-on-one, especially a strange adult. Therefore, careful collection of the observations of parents, teachers, and other caregivers (bus drivers, coaches, sitters) is the most essential diagnostic strategy.

Parent and Teacher Rating Scales

An excellent way to collect caregiver observations is by using one of the many standardized rating scales. Probably the best ones are those that use the actual DSM-IV symptoms rated on a standard metric, usually 0 to 3, from no symptom to severe. Examples include the ADHD Rating Scale (252) and the SNAP (Swanson, Nolan, & Pelham, adhd.net), which have only DSM symptoms, and the Conners 3 long forms (253) which have the DSM symptoms embedded in a longer scale. When counting symptoms, a rating of 2 or 3 on the 0 to 3 scales is usually considered as the presence of the symptom. Numerous other scales are also useful and have been used in research and clinical practice.

Family History

Additional diagnostic information can come from family history, both positive and negative. For example, relatives with ADHD help to confirm the diagnosis. On the other hand, the absence of relatives with ADHD, coupled with either history of traumatic stress or family history of bipolar disorder, thyroid disorder, or severe anxiety may alert the diagnostician to the possibility that the patient's symptoms may be another disorder mimicking ADHD and point the direction for further investigation.

Mental Status Examination

The main value of mental status examination is to rule out other mental disorders that might better explain the symptoms (Criterion E of DSM-5). These include psychosis, bipolar disorder, depression, autism, and severe anxiety—especially posttraumatic stress disorder—as well as intellectual disability. A reasonable mental status examination for this purpose would include appearance/demeanor, orientation, alertness, speech clarity and content, affect, ability to develop rapport, relevance and logic of thought processes, some estimate of cognitive ability, queries about depressive or other mood symptoms, worries, fears, obsessions, compulsions, hallucinations, and traumatic events, and some projective elicitation such as drawing, three wishes, or fable completion.

Physical Examination and Medical History

Although there are no diagnostic physical signs in ADHD (when abnormalities occur, they usually reflect a comorbid disorder such as intellectual disability, cerebral palsy, or genetic syndromes), a physical examination and medical history can be useful in ruling out other mimicking disorders and in discovering or confirming the common comorbidity of developmental coordination disorder. Also, the presence of soft neurologic signs and/or minor physical anomalies may somewhat increase confidence in the ADHD diagnosis, even though there is no 1:1 link. Soft neurologic signs are nonfocal motor deficits that include deficits in balance, motor planning and control, and sensory integration (254,255) (Table 5.1.1.6). Gustaffson et al. also found a significant correlation between the soft neurologic signs and decreased cerebral blood flow measures in the frontal lobes bilaterally in children with ADHD. At this time, functional imaging is not a part of the routine workup of ADHD. Physical examination would note hyperdynamics or hypodynamics, abnormal deep tendon reflexes, fine or coarse skin or hair, and any other signs of endocrine disorder, as well as allergic stigmata (swollen eyes, darkened lids, nasal congestion, and allergic salute) and pallor of nail beds or conjunctivae. Positive findings should, of course, prompt appropriate laboratory tests. The diagnostician should inquire about things like food sensitivities (especially in younger children), dietary imbalance, cardiac problems, and heat or cold intolerance. Prominent allergic signs suggest a possible etiologic or exacerbating condition (e.g., food intolerance, atopy).

TABLE 5.1.1.6

SOFT NEUROLOGIC SIGNS IN ADHD

Clinical Finding	Putative Explanation
Difficulties performing repetitive motor tasks (such as hand flipping; foot rocking; serial thumb to finger opposition)	Impaired ability to use cognitive control to alternately inhibit and excite motor activity to maintain a regular cadence
Difficulties performing sequential timed tasks (such as foot rocking; hand flipping; serial finger)	Impaired ability to use cognitive control to adjust motor performance) flexibly in a multistep task
Difficulties maintaining gait and balance (sustained motor stance; tandem balance)	Difficulties maintaining balance; integrating proprioceptor input/body position sense; abnormal vestibular function; etc.

Presentations

The distinction among presentations (types) is more dimensional than categorical. For example, a child with six inattentive symptoms and five hyperactive-impulsive symptoms would have predominantly inattentive presentation, while someone with six symptoms of each kind would have combined presentation ADHD. Further, the presentation/type does not even firmly predict the ratio of the two kinds of symptoms. For example, six inattentive and five hyperactive-impulsive would make inattentive presentation, but nine inattentive and six hyperactive-impulsive symptoms would make combined presentation despite having a greater excess of inattentive symptoms than the first symptom profile. Despite this threshold-definition problem, some experts believe that a substantial proportion of inattentive presentation, those who are sluggishly hypoactive, may actually constitute a distinct disorder with different etiology. In any event, the inattentive presentation tends to be referred less often for treatment and tends to be missed diagnostically more often, especially if of high enough intelligence to get by in school without using full potential.

Comorbidity

ADHD has a high rate of comorbid psychiatric disorders. Half of clinical samples have oppositional defiant disorder (ODD) or conduct disorder (CD), 25% to 30% have anxiety disorder, and 20% to 25% have a learning disorder (256,257). There is increased risk for mood disorders (which may develop later). Although the rate of comorbid Tourette's is low (about 2%), it is much higher than in the random population or in other psychiatric disorders. Comorbidity can introduce some diagnostic challenges because the comorbid disorders can mimic ADHD, with overlapping symptoms, so the diagnostician must differentiate between comorbidity and primary diagnosis. Table 5.1.1.7 presents some comparisons and differences.

TABLE 5.1.1.7

SOME MENTAL DISORDERS THAT CAN MIMIC ADHD: THEIR OVERLAPPING OR SIMILAR SIGNS/SYMPTOMS

ADHD Symptoms	Depression	Bipolar (Manic)	Anxiety, Including PTSD	Psychosis	Autism/PDD
Inattentiveness, distractibility, forgetfulness, losing things, careless mistakes	Impairment of concentration and memory; preoccupation with mood	Flight of ideas, thought racing, distraction by delusions or grandiosity	Preoccupation with worry; intrusive memories; flashbacks, psychic numbing, hypervigilance	Withdrawal from reality, preoccupation, loose association, "distraction" by hallucinations As above; abrupt change of activity	Disregard of people, decreased responsiveness to attempted communication
Failure to finish tasks or activities; reluctance to start if needs sustained mental effort	Fatigue, anergia, loss of interest	Flight of ideas/ activities; grandiosely above common tasks	Fear-induced paralysis of function; afraid to try, expecting failure; avoiding of reminders		Abrupt change of activity, resistance to instructed activity, adherence to preferred activity
Difficulty organizing	Anergia, cognitive impairment	Flightiness		Psychotic fragmentation	
Hyperactivity, fidgeting/squirming restlessness, always on the go	Agitation	Hyperactivity, driven quality	Panic, agitation, anxiety-driven restlessness, "nervousness"	Psychotic agitation, response to hallucinations	Hyperactivity, twirling, pacing, flapping
Excessive talking	Agitated complaining	Pressured speech	Anxious verbosity, obsessions, verbal rituals Anxious eagerness; reenactments	Talking to hallucinations	Compulsive stereotyped repetitions
Impulsive blurting of answers, interrupting, intruding	Preoccupied complaining (pain, worry)	Pressured speech, flight of ideas, impulsive poor judgment		Responding to hallucinations	Obliviousness of personal space of others
Impatience, easy frustration, difficulty waiting	Easy frustration	Pressured hyperactivity and impulsiveness	Intolerance of delay that builds suspense or reminds of trauma	Lack of social orientation	Easy frustration
Irritability	Irritability	Irritability	Anger when rituals frustrated	Paranoid irritability	Irritability, tantrum when rituals or routine interrupted
Restless sleep, lability, instability (emotional and physiologic)	Insomnia	Insomnia Labile affect	Insomnia or nightmares Physiologic instability, nervousness	Nocturnal agitation Psychotic unpredictability	Insomnia, lability, unpredictability
Distinguishing from ADHD	Depressed mood, anorexia, weight loss, suicidal ideation, guilt feelings, psychomotor slowing, mutism, fatigue	F.H. of mood disorder; extreme driven quality; sometimes episodic; prominent mood: irritable, grandiose; possible appetite change, weight change	Phobias, worries, stress-induced onset, obsessions, compulsions, perfectionism, tremor, physiologic symptoms (palpitations, SOB, sweating), posttraumatic play	Delusions, poverty of thought, disorientation, command hallucinations, inappropriate affect	Impaired nonverbal/verbal communication, lack of social relatedness, fantasy, or social or imaginative play

Adapted with permission from Arnold LE: *Contemporary Diagnosis and Management of ADHD*. Newtown, PA: Handbooks in Health Care, 2004.

TABLE 5.1.1.8

NEUROPSYCHOLOGICAL TESTS OF EXECUTIVE FUNCTIONING

Test Stop Signal Reaction Time (SSRT)	Executive Function Assessed Response Inhibition
Continuous performance test commission errors	Response inhibition
Continuous performance test omission errors and hit reaction time variability	Vigilance
Wisconsin card sorting test	Set shifting
Trail-making test, Part B	Set shifting
Tower of Hanoi/London	Planning ability
Porteus Mazes	Planning ability
Rey–Osterreith complex figure test	Planning/organization
Working memory sentence span test	Working verbal memory
Digits backward test	Working verbal memory
Self-ordered pointing test	Spatial working memory
CANTAB spatial working memory test	Spatial working memory

NEUROPSYCHOLOGICAL TEST RESULTS

A great deal of research done within the past 30 years supports the view that ADHD is a heterogeneous disorder related to multiple neuropsychological deficits (31). Executive functions are neurocognitive processes that maintain an appropriate problem solving set to attain a future goal (258). Executive function tasks include response inhibition and execution; working memory and updating; set shifting and task switching; interference control; planning and organization; vigilance; visuospatial orienting; and verbal and spatial working memory. Children with ADHD, for example, exhibit significant working memory deficits compared to typically developing children (259). Executive functions employ multiple neural networks that involve the thalamus, basal ganglia, and prefrontal cortex. The most common neuropsychological test results measuring different aspects of executive functioning in ADHD are listed in Table 5.1.1.8.

Several theories have been developed based on the neuropsychological profile of children with ADHD.

1. The deficit in inhibitory control theory suggests that the general pattern of executive impairment is caused by developmental abnormalities in inhibitory control processes (260). A meta-analysis of neuropsychological studies in adults found a somewhat different profile of neurocognitive deficits compared to children and adolescents, with deficits related mostly to impairment in measures of verbal memory, focused attention, sustained attention, and abstract verbal problem solving with working memory. Simple alertness tasks were less impaired than more complex attention tasks (261).
2. The delay aversion theory posits a biologically based impairment in the ability to tolerate delay and its consequences on behavior and cognitive style. A test used to measure ability to tolerate delay is the Choice Delay Task (262,263).
3. In the cognitive energetic model (264), neurocognitive performance deficits in ADHD are determined by information processing abnormalities at the computational (encoding, search, decision, and motor organization) and state levels (effort, arousal, and activation). The model proposes the existence of three energetic pools: effort (necessary energy to meet the demands of the task); arousal (time locked to stimulus processing) and activation (tonic changes in physiologic activity in significant brain areas, including the basal ganglia and corpus striatum), and the existence of a management or evaluation mechanism associated with planning, monitoring, detection, and correction of errors that overlaps with the concept of executive functions in other theories.
4. The sluggish cognitive tempo theory proposes that inattention presents differently in ADHD without hyperactivity compared with combined presentation (265), the main features including slow retrieval and information processing; low levels of alertness; and mild problems with memory and orientation. Further studies are needed to answer the question of whether the group of sluggish cognitive tempo children may represent a distinct category of ADHD with a different pathophysiology or may even represent a different disorder altogether.
5. The multiple pathway model emphasizes the parallels between the core deficits in ADHD as defined by major theories of ADHD and relevant temperament and personality domains, in particular effortful control and regulation (266,267).

COURSE AND PROGNOSIS

Up to 60% of childhood cases continue symptomatic into adulthood (268,269). The ratio of males to females in adult samples approximates 2:1 or even close to 1:1, much more equal than in childhood, where it is more likely 4 or 5 to 1 in clinical samples. The change in sex ratio of clinical cases in adulthood may partly reflect a sex difference in willingness to seek help, or possibly girls who had not shown enough problems in school to be identified, finally realizing deficits as grown women. ADHD can seriously impair the quality of life of children with ADHD (270,271) and have co-occurring aggressive and depressive symptoms.

The manifestations of ADHD change over the course of life (Figure 5.1.1.4). Just as normal children develop better impulse

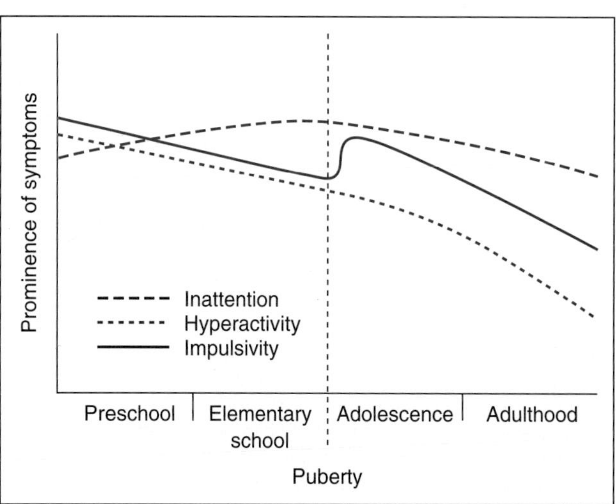

FIGURE 5.1.1.4. Course of different ADHD symptoms over the life span. Hyperactivity tends to wane with maturity, being replaced by a feeling of restlessness. Impulsivity also tends to wane except for a possible blip in adolescence under the influence of "raging hormones." The most persistent cluster of symptoms is inattentiveness, with the main adult manifestations being disorganization, difficulty managing money, keeping schedules, and sticking with a relationship or job. (Reproduced with permission from Arnold LE: *Contemporary Diagnosis and Management of ADHD.* Newtown, PA: Handbooks in Health Care, 2004.)

control, attentional focus, other executive function, and ability to remain calm as they mature, so do those with ADHD, just at a slower pace, lagging behind their age mates. Childhood ADHD severity and childhood treatment significantly predicted the persistence of ADHD in adulthood in the National Comorbidity Survey Replication Study (272). ADHD symptoms in adults are more heterogeneous and subtle, leading some researchers to suggest the need for different diagnostic criteria in adults.

Hyperactivity is the most likely symptom to be outgrown. Adolescents and adults with ADHD, even those who started with combined presentation, may have only an inner feeling of restlessness. The most persistent symptom cluster involves inattention, distractibility, disorganization, and failure to finish things. Males with a childhood history of significant hyperactivity, impulsivity, and disruptive behavior disorder comorbidity are more likely to develop polysubstance abuse and adult antisocial behavior. Adults with ADHD may struggle with frequent job changes, frequent partner changes, divorce, difficulty with schedules and money management, and driving accidents. Girls and women with ADHD have a higher rate of unwed pregnancy than those who do not have ADHD. Adults with ADHD may present with significant self-esteem issues and feelings of hopelessness and helplessness related to ongoing difficulties in managing everyday life. Several follow-up studies have found a high rate of major depression in adult patients with ADHD. Effective treatment significantly improves quality of life. Ambivalence about the existence of an adult ADHD diagnosis and concerns over prescribing psychostimulants with a high potential for abuse have made it difficult for adults with ADHD to receive treatment. Minority status, female sex, and low income were found in several studies to predict failure to be diagnosed and treated (153,273).

TREATMENT

Because ADHD is a chronic and pervasive disorder, affecting all areas of function, the treatment plan must be farsighted, comprehensive, and flexibly adapted over time to changing needs. The commitment of patient and family to the plan must be cultivated. This implies that treatment must be not only effective, but also feasible, palatable, and affordable for the particular patient. Therefore, treatment planning has to be individualized, with consideration for family preferences. From the beginning, the child, as star of the therapeutic team, should be involved in planning, with an eye toward the day when he or she has to assume responsibility for his or her own treatment as an adult. Other members of the team—physician, teacher, psychologist, and other professional—can come and go; even parents are eventually outgrown; but the patient is permanently involved.

The necessary gradual assumption of personal responsibility for managing the disorder should be discussed periodically with the child and adolescent. For the younger child, this can involve parents. For example, for a 10-year old, lay out the fact that in 8 years, the child will have to assume responsibility for self and discuss how parents can coach and support in gradual assumption of responsibility. A 14-year old can be seen alone briefly and reminded that he or she has only 4 years to prepare for personal responsibility; it may be useful to inquire if the idea scares them before asking how they plan gradually to take more responsibility. Attention to such psychosocial and psychodynamic aspects of management is important especially for patients who are treated mainly with medication. See also Psychoeducation below.

Established Treatments

Two treatment modalities have been endorsed by both the American Academy of Child and Adolescent Psychiatry (154) and American Academy of Pediatrics (150,152,274). They are behavioral treatment and the FDA-approved agents (amphetamine, methylphenidate, atomoxetine, guanfacine, and clonidine). Additional drugs are expected to be added to the list of agents with an approved indication for ADHD. The flow chart of evaluation and treatment recommendations published by the American Academy of Pediatrics is reproduced in Figure 5.1.1.5. In acute and medium-length studies (up to 2 years) medication generally outperforms behavioral treatment for symptom suppression, but three-fourth of children with ADHD can be managed with intensive behavioral treatment alone, and the combination offers several advantages, including equal or better results with a lower medication dose, saving side effects (245,275,276).

For some comorbid subgroups, such as ADHD combined with both anxiety and ODD/CD, the combination is impressively more effective (145,277). Behavioral treatment appears especially effective in the presence of comorbid anxiety.

Behavioral Treatment

Behavioral treatments are based on social learning theory. Behaviors that are reinforced increase in frequency and those that are not reinforced in some way (or are punished) tend to extinguish. A number of practical behavioral treatments can be implemented from the first contact. These include star charts for target behaviors, clear house rules, written or pictorial instructions making use of the visual channels if auditory instructions seem unattended to, and contingencies for doing various things. With more time and effort, more refined interventions can be set up, such as a home token economy or a daily report card to tie school behavior to home reinforcement. There are several programs for providing parent training in behavioral management, now called parent management training (PMT). For younger children and milder cases, these may provide sufficient intervention, but once diagnosed, a case should be monitored over time. Sometimes additional need for treatment emerges as the child progresses to more challenging academic stresses.

Pharmacologic Treatment

Most psychiatric drugs have some evidence of benefit in ADHD (notable exceptions being the selective serotonin reuptake inhibitors), but only a few have a Food and Drug Administration (FDA)-approved indication (Table 5.1.1.9A). The evidence for many of the others, such as tricyclic antidepressants, bupropion, monoamine oxidase inhibitors, and modafinil, is nevertheless rather good, with multiple placebo-controlled trials (Table 5.1.1.9B). However, some have only open trials or a single-controlled trial. Tables 5.1.1–5.1.9 show approximate relative effect sizes (the number of standard deviations by which active drug differs from placebo).

With any of the drugs, it is important to start low and titrate, preferably weekly, to individual optimal effect. Generally for school-age children, the smallest size stimulant dosage marketed is a good place to start. Because of wide individual variability in sensitivity, the size of the patient is only a rough guide to dose: One 30-kg child may require and tolerate 30 mg/day of amphetamine while another 30-kg child has an optimal response to 5 mg/day, with severe side effects above 10 mg. Clinical art is required to optimize the benefit and minimize side effects by size of dose, timing, and management of time–action effects such as "evening rebound" with stimulants. Generally, the new extended-release preparations yield a smoother effect with fewer ups and downs. They also avoid the necessity of taking pills at school, which some children find stigmatizing. For such reasons, extended-release formulations of stimulants are preferred, and titration can be initiated directly with one of them without any need to first establish dose with immediate-release tablets.

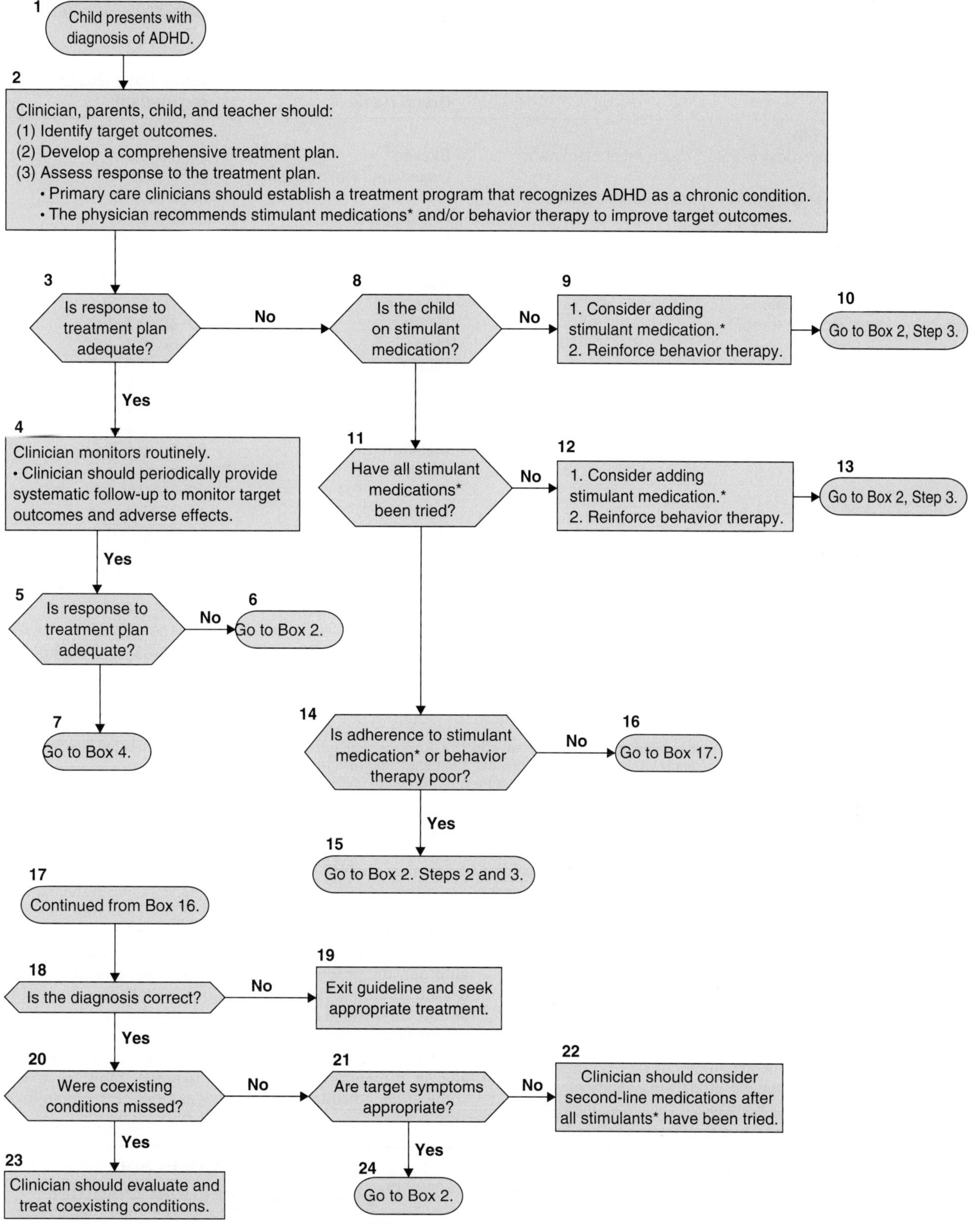

* Excluding pemoline. Another FDA-approved option is atomoxetine (Strattera©), approved since the guideline was published. Used with the permission of the Academy of Pediatrics. From Clinical practice guideline: treatment of the school-aged child with attention deficit/hyperactivity disorder. *Pediatrics* 108:1033–1044, 2001.

FIGURE 5.1.1.5. Clinical guidelines by American Academy of Pediatrics, which were written before availability of atomoxetine, which, as an FDA-approved treatment for ADHD, should be considered after a stimulant before resorting to off-label drugs. (From American Academy of Pediatrics: Clinical practice guideline for the school-age child with ADHD. *Pediatrics* 108:1033–1048, 2001.)

TABLE 5.1.1.9A

DRUGS WITH FDA APPROVAL FOR ADHD

Generic Name	Brand Name	Usual Daily Dose[c] mg (mg/kg)
Stimulants (ES 0.7–1.8)		
Amphetamine, racemic (dextro–levo)[a] dextroamphetamine[a,b]	Evekeo®	10–40 (0.3–1)
	Dexedrine® DextroStat®	5–30 (0.2–0.7)
mixture 3/4 d-, 1/4 L-amphetamine[a,b] mixed amphetamine salts (MAS)	Adderall®	5–40 (0.2–1)
	Adderall® XR	5–40 (0.2–1)
methamphetamine[b,d]	Desoxyn®	5–25 (0.2–0.7)
	Adzenys XR	6.3–12.5 (0.2–0.5)
	Dyanavel XR	2.5–20 (0.1–0.8)
lisdexamfetamine dimesylate	Vyvanse	20–70
Methylphenidate, racemic threo[a,b]	Ritalin®,	10–60 (0.3–1.5)
	Methylin®	10–60 (0.3–1.5)
	Ritalin® LA	20–60 (0.6–1.5)
	Metadate®	10–60 (0.3–1.5)
	Metadate® CD	20–60 (0.6–1.5)
	Aptensio XR	10–60 (0.3–1.5)
	Metadate ER	20–60 (0.6–1.5)
	Quillivant XR	20–60 (0.6–1.5)
	QuilliChew ER	20–60 (0.6–1.5)
osmotic release[a,b]	Concerta®	18–72 (0.4–1.8)
Transdermal release	Daytrana patch	10–30 (0.3–0.7)
dextro-threomethylphenidate[a,b]	Focalin™	5–30 (0.2–0.7)
	Focalin XR™	5–30 (0.2–0.7)
Nonstimulants with FDA-Approved Indication (ES 0.5–1.4)		
Atomoxetine[a,b]	Strattera®	18–100 (0.7–1.4)
Guanfacine XR[a,b]	Intuniv	1–4 (0.05–0.12 mg/kg/day)
Clonidine XR[a,b]	Kapvay	0.1–0.4 mg

[a]Supported by controlled studies.
[b]FDA-approved indication for ADHD.
[c]Usual daily dose should not be interpreted as either a cap or a minimal effective dose if a higher or lower dose is clinically indicated in individual cases. Actual patient doses must be individually titrated using direct teacher and parent information.
[d]Although it carries an FDA-approved indication for ADHD, methamphetamine, in contrast to other forms of amphetamine, is not favored by many experts because of suspected neurotoxicity in animal data.
ΔBecause only 5/6 of the MPH in the osmotic-release form is released, 72 mg = 60 mg of other MPH preparations.
ES, effect size, the number of standard deviations different from placebo or from pre-drug measure. It is a measure of clinical significance. An ES of 1 is considered large, 0.5 medium.
Reproduced with permission from Arnold LE, *Contemporary Diagnosis and Management of ADHD.* Newtown, PA: Handbooks in Health Care, 2004.

Labeled and Off-Label Drugs

The drugs with currently approved FDA indications for ADHD are the stimulants, atomoxetine, guanfacine, and clonidine, with others being developed for that indication. Some antipsychotics also have an indication for "childhood hyperactivity" grandfathered from previous use in the 1970s, and there is no doubt that antipsychotics have a moderate benefit for hyperactive symptoms. However, because of their greater risk and less impressive benefit, they would usually be a last resort, logically used mainly when a stimulant worsens the symptoms. Some off-label drugs with good evidence would be preferred to antipsychotics early in the search for an effective medication. Antidepressants other than selective serotonin reuptake inhibitors (SSRIs) have many placebo-controlled studies supporting their use. These include tricyclics, monoamine oxidase inhibitors (MAOIs), and bupropion. For children the effect is not on average as good as for stimulants, but some individuals may respond better, and comorbid depression or anxiety might point toward considering one of them. The danger of interaction with food amines would limit the feasibility of MAOIs for children. Another class with reasonable evidence is the alpha-agonists; of these, guanfacine has the advantages over clonidine of longer half-life and less sedation. They may be good for severely overaroused agitation and comorbid aggression. Clonidine is often used at bedtime alone to promote sleep, although the practice has been questioned on safety grounds if used in conjunction with daytime stimulants. Diphenhydramine, an antihistamine with some dopamine effect, was an arcane treatment before more modern drug development; for a few patients, especially those whose behavior fluctuates with allergy, it may have considerable benefits. Table 5.1.1.10 lists some of the advantages and disadvantages of the main drugs.

Educational Plan and Psychoeducation about Disorder

Education is important in two ways in ADHD: as a problem area that needs to be addressed and as a treatment modality. Most children with diagnosed ADHD have some problem with academic performance; in fact, that is often what brings them to clinical attention. Although most are able to function in a regular classroom with appropriate treatment and support, some will need an individual educational plan (IEP) or even a special class or resource room. This is particularly so for the 20% to 25% with comorbid learning disorders. Parents may need some coaching in obtaining appropriate educational

TABLE 5.1.1.9B

OTHER DRUGS USED FOR ADHD

Generic Name	Brand Name	Usual Daily Dose[b] mg (mg/kg)
Not all of the following drugs have been documented as effective by well-controlled studies, let alone approved by the FDA for ADHD.		
Antidepressants (ES 0.5–1.5)[c]		
Imipramine (TCA)[a]	Tofranil®	20–100 (0.7–3)
Desipramine (TCA)[a]	Norpramin®, Pertofrane®	20–100 (0.7–3)
Amitriptyline (TCA)[a]	Elavil®, Endep®	20–100 (0.7–3)
Nortriptyline (TCA)	Pamelor®	10–50 (0.4–2)
Bupropion[a]	Wellbutrin®	75–300 (3–6)
Clomipramine (TCA)[a]	Anafranil®	25–100
Tranylcypromine (MAOI A + B)[c]	Parnate®	5–15
Clorgyline (MAOI A)[a]		5–20
Pargyline (MAOI)	Eutonyl®	
Venlafaxine[d]	Effexor®	25–100 (1.4)
SSRIs (e.g., fluoxetine[d])	Prozac®	5–40
Miscellaneous (ES variable)		
Buspirone (ES < 1)	BuSpar®	5–30 (0.2–0.6)
Diphenhydramine	Benadryl®	75–150
Nicotine (adults only, ES > 1)[a]	(lower dose for nonsmokers)	7–21 mg patch
Modafinil (ES ~ 1)[a]	Provigil®	50–400
Anticonvulsants (ES up to 1.0)		
Carbamazepine[a]	Tegretol®	50–800, serum level
Valproate	Depakote®, Depakene®	serum level
Phenytoin	Dilantin®	50–300
Antipsychotics (ES usually about half of stimulants)[f]		
Thioridazine[a]	Mellaril®	25–150 (1–6)
Haloperidol[a,e]	Haldol®	0.5–5.0 (0.03–0.075)
Chlorpromazine[a,c]	Thorazine®	25–150 (1–6)
Risperidone	Risperdal®	0.25–2.0 (0.01–0.1)
Precursors (ES < 0.6, short term)[g]		
Deanol (possible precursor of acetylcholine)	Deaner®	>500
Tryptophan (precursor of serotonin)		(70–100)
Tyrosine (precursor of dopamine and norepinephrine)		(100–140)
Phenylalanine (precursor of dopamine and norepinephrine)		(100–140)
Levo–DOPA (precursor of dopamine and norepinephrine)	Carbidopa	
Others		
β-blockers (e.g., propranolol)	Inderal®	10–300
Caffeine		100–450

[a]Supported by controlled studies.
[b]Usual daily dose should not be interpreted as either a cap or a minimal effective dose if a higher or lower dose is clinically indicated in individual cases. Actual patient doses must be individually titrated, using direct teacher and parent information.
[c]No antidepressants are FDA approved for ADHD, despite well-controlled studies demonstrating efficacy for many of them. In fact, some (but not all) studies show imipramine, desipramine, amitriptyline, and tranylcypromine equal to stimulants, although with worse side effects. For adults, they may equal stimulants despite not seeming to benefit attention as much as behavior.
[d]Despite a report of a positive open trial of fluoxetine, most experts do not consider selective serotonin reuptake inhibitors (SSRIs) generally effective for ADHD core symptoms, in contrast with the documented effectiveness of other antidepressant classes. The newer antidepressants, with both serotonin and catecholamine action (such as venlafaxine, mirtazapine, and nefazodone) are expected to be effective. The number of standard deviations different from placebo or from pre-drug measure. It is a measure of clinical significance. An ES of 1 is considered large, 0.5 medium.
[e]FDA-approved for short-term treatment of hyperactive children.
[f]Although haloperidol and chlorpromazine have FDA-approved indications for short-term treatment of hyperactive children; antipsychotics should be a last resort because of the risk of tardive dyskinesia. Newer ones, such as risperidone, olanzapine, and quetiapine, may carry less risk.
[g]The precursors of neurotransmitters are nutrients found in the normal diet. They are included because they are used like drugs in supplemental dosage. Deanol (dimethylaminoethanol [DMAE]) was formerly marketed as Deaner®, but initial FDA approval was withdrawn as "possibly effective."
Not ordinarily used: most minor tranquilizers, benzodiazepines Contraindicated: barbiturates (aggravate hyperactivity; can even cause it)
TCA, tricyclic antidepressant; MAOI, monoamine oxidase inhibitor; SSRI, selective serotonin reuptake inhibitor; ES, effect size, the number of standard déviations different from placebo or from pre-drug measure. It is a measure of clinical significance. An ES of 1 is considered large, 0.5 medium.
Arnold LE, Jensen PS: Attention-deficit hyperactivity disorder. In: Kaplan H, Sadock B (eds): *Comprehensive Textbook of Psychiatry*. Baltimore, MD: Williams and Wilkins, 2295–2311, 1995. Adapted with permission.
Adapted from Arnold LE, Jensen PS: Attention-deficit hyperactivity disorder. In: Kaplan H, Sadock B (eds): *Comprehensive Textbook of Psychiatry.* Baltimore, MD: Williams and Wilkins, 2295–2311, 1995 and Arnold LE, *Contemporary Diagnosis and Management of ADHD.* Newtown, PA: Handbooks in Health Care, 2004.

TABLE 5.1.1.10

RELATIVE ADVANTAGES AND DISADVANTAGES/SIDE EFFECTS OF ADHD DRUG CLASSES

Drug Class	Advantages	Side Effects, Disadvantages
Stimulants (FDA indication)	Specifically treat ADHD core symptoms of inattention, overactivity, and impulsiveness Largest and most rapid effect on ADHD of any drug class, especially for children Significant benefit in 85–90% of ADHD if two or more tried in succession and titrated carefully Calms comorbid aggression and oppositional defiant behavior Results of given dose seen immediately; relatively easy titration	Appetite, weight loss Sleep disturbance (if taken late in day) Cramps (first few wks) Headaches Mild BP and pulse increase Evening crash "Zombie" appearance (amphetamine look): constricted affect and spontaneity, emotional blunting Depression Tics Hallucinations (skin crawling, visions) Mild growth slowing first 2 yrs (31) Dose for behavior may not be optimal for attention Nuisance of schedule II Rx
Atomoxetine (Strattera®) (FDA indication)	Specifically treats ADHD core symptoms of inattention, overactivity, and impulsiveness FDA indication for ADHD, like stimulants, but not Schedule II Refills by phone Nearly as effective as stimulants (slower onset), better for some; may help stimulant failures Continuous duration of effect Little or no insomniac side effect Can be given any time of day No tic side effect (good choice with comorbid tics) Some benefit for comorbid oppositional defiant symptoms May help comorbid depression Smooth action over time (long pharmacodynamic half-life), cumulative benefit	Appetite, weight loss Gastrointestinal Sx (nausea, vomiting, diarrhea, constipation) Fatigue, dizziness Probable mild growth slowing Allergic reactions In adults: dry mouth, urinary retention, sexual dysfunction Irritating to skin if capsules opened Possibly longer time than stimulants to flush out if adverse effect Slower attainment of full effect than stimulants
Antidepressants Tricyclics, bupropion (Wellbutrin), MAOIs (32), probably newer antidepressants with both serotonin action and dopamine	Treat both ADHD and comorbid depression and anxiety Helps some stimulant nonresponders Third most effective drug class for ADHD (except for SSRIs, which are not very effective) Some patients/families who are prejudiced against stimulants will accept antidepressants May equal stimulant effectiveness for adults	Sedation BP changes (down or up) Dizziness (especially on standing) Dry mouth Cardiac conduction block: TCAs require ECG monitoring in children Constipation, urinary retention (rare in children) Headache (deserves evaluation) Overdose lethal, and sudden deaths at therapeutic dose (DMI) Response delayed, especially bupropion Dietary restrictions for MAOIs Not as good as stimulants for attention
α_2-Agonists	Treat both hyperactivity impulsiveness and comorbid tic disorder or comorbid aggression Helps some nonresponders to stimulants and antidepressants Good for those overaroused, possibly with comorbid anxiety May be especially good with comorbid autism	Response delayed Sedation Hypotensive dizziness (especially postural) Dry mouth Rare hallucinations Hypertensive rebound if dose missed Sudden deaths (when used with stimulant) Not as helpful for attention as stimulants
Buspirone	Good for comorbid anxiety and aggression, possibly depression Relatively safe (similar to stimulants) Smooth effect Relatively free of side effects	Possible paradoxical excitation Several weeks needed to see full effect of a given dose; therefore, hard/slow to titrate
Antihistamines (older)	Safe, cheap, over the counter Especially good in patients with possible allergic etiology (but not restricted to those)	Sedation Risk of seizures in high doses Not as effective as stimulants, atomoxetine, or antidepressants: unsatisfactory in many patients

TABLE 5.1.1.10

(CONTINUED)

Drug Class	Advantages	Side Effects, Disadvantages
Antipsychotics*	May work when stimulant or atomoxetine does not, especially if stimulant makes worse Good for comorbid anxiety, aggression, tic disorder, or bipolar disorder	Sedation Extrapyramidal side effects Endocrine effects Tardive dyskinesia Paradoxical agitation (akathisia) Weight gain Not specific, generally less effective than stimulants or atomoxetine Riskiest drug, last resort
Anticonvulsants	Good for comorbid mood disorder, aggression, explosiveness, impulsiveness May work when stimulant, atomoxetine, or antidepressant does not	Blood tests for levels and safety monitoring Liver toxicity Blood dyscrasia Sedation or agitation Ataxia

*Although some antipsychotics (haloperidol and chlorpromazine) have an FDA-approved indication, they should not be preferred to unapproved drugs higher on the list unless for a specific reason, such as comorbid bipolar disorder.
TCA, tricyclic antidepressant; MAOI, monoamine oxidase inhibitor; DMI, desipramine; SSRIs, selective serotonin reuptake inhibitors.
Reproduced with permission from Arnold LE: *Contemporary Diagnosis and Management of ADHD.* Newtown, PA: Handbooks in Health Care, 2004.

services for the child, such as is required by PL 94–142 (Education for All Handicapped Act), IDEA (Individuals with Disabilities Education Act), or section 504 of the Civil Rights Act. Children with learning disorders are likely to be covered by the first two mandates, and those without a specific learning disorder are usually covered by section 504, which provides for "other health impaired."

This brings us to the other side of educational considerations: the education of patient and family (and other caregivers) about ADHD, its symptoms, course, chronicity, treatments, and services available. Some "talking points" for this are listed in Table 5.1.1.11. Referral to a support/advocacy organization, such as ChADD or ADDA for further peer education may also be useful. There are also numerous explanatory books written for both children and adults, such as *A Family Guide to ADHD* (278). The local support group may have a lending library of these. Such psychoeducation is important in cementing a commitment to enduring treatment for a chronic disorder.

Other Treatments

Treatments other than medication, behavioral treatment, psychoeducation, and special educational services are often called "alternative." The term "alternative" implies substitution for

TABLE 5.1.1.11

POINTS FOR EXPLANATION AND CLARIFICATION TO PATIENT AND FAMILY

Talking Point	Reason
Acknowledge what they already know.	Shows respect and attention to their story. Imparts feeling of cognitive familiarity, a base on which to hook the new information.
Give them the current name of the disorder, indicating there are numerous other names.	Defines and clarifies the disorder.
ADHD has many symptoms, and not every patient with ADHD has all of them. Some have partial expressions of the syndrome.	Prevents confusion from having symptoms that are different from those of an acquaintance with ADHD.
Three main symptoms are inattention, hyperactivity, and impulsivity.	Focuses the targets of treatment. Prevents assumption the patient needs to be aggressive.
Other symptoms are frequent and often disabling, though not important for the diagnosis.	Puts all symptoms in perspective.
Symptoms are just excess amounts of normal behavior.	Implies need to control symptoms, not eliminate them.
Symptoms are not the patient's fault, but the patient can improve with help.	Breaks up the blame game, prevents giving up. Promotes teamwork in fighting ADHD.
ADHD lasts a long time, perhaps a lifetime, although it tends to get better with age.	Prepares for long-term treatment.
Important not to give up or neglect treatment.	Giving up allows secondary problems, dropping farther behind.
Treatment helps prevent secondary problems.	So they don't just wait for things to get better.
Many different treatments are available, relative advantages/disadvantages, and scientific basis of each.	So they'll know the options, be involved in choice of treatment, and, therefore, commit to it.

Reproduced with permission from Arnold LE: *Contemporary Diagnosis and Management of ADHD.* Newtown, PA: Handbooks in Health Care, 2004.

TABLE 5.1.1.12

SCIENTIFIC STATUS OF TREATMENT ALTERNATIVES FOR ATTENTION DEFICIT HYPERACTIVITY DISORDER (ADHD)

Treatment	Etiology or Mechanism	Type of Data	Effect Size d and/or p	Rating[a] (0–6); Recommendation and/or Need	Risks, Discomforts, Disadvantages
Sympathomimetic meds: stimulants, atomoxetine	Catecholamine, esp. dopamine	>100 placebo XOs and RCTs in 1000s	ES 0.5–1.8 *p*. 01–0.0001	6; Use if no cause found	Side effects; doubt neurotoxic
Antidepressants, other psychotropic medications	Catecholamine? serotonin	Multiple placebo-controlled RCTs	ES 0.5–1.5 *p*. 05–0.005	6; When stimulants fail	Cardiotoxicity, other side effects
Behavioral Tx: BM, contingency	Social learning theory, shaping	ABAB, random waitlist controls	ES 0.5–1.2 *p*. 05–0.005	6; Selective use (severe, or comorbid anxiety)	Nuisance, time
Few foods diet (oligoantigenic)	Food or additive sensitivity	Controlled trial; placebo challenges	ES 0.5–1.0 *p*. 05–0.001	5; Define subgroup (profile; % ADHD)	Nuisance, expense, nutrition balance
Enzyme-potentiated desensitization	Food or additive sensitivity	Controlled comparison to placebo injections	*p*. 001	4; Replication Define subgroup	Injection
Elimination of sugar alone	Sugar malaise	Placebo-controlled challenges	$p > 0.1$	0; Take FH of diabetes	Delay standard Tx
Amino acid supplementation	Precursors of neurotransmitters	Placebo-controlled comparisons	ES up to 0.6, *p*. 01	0; Despite short-lived effect of little utility	Eosinophilia, neurotoxicity
Essential fatty acid supplement	Prostaglandins neural membrane	Serum level in controls 10 placebo-controlled trials	ES 0.5, *p*. 0.1	3; Trials of specific n-3 or n-6 by serum profile	Upsetting balance
L-carnitine	Promotes EFA anabolism	1 published placebo trial ADHD	ES ~ 0.5, $p < 0.05$; only in inattentive type	2; Better placebo trial	Upsetting balance
Dimethylaminoethanol (DMAE)	Acetylcholine precursor?	Many open and DB trials	ES 0.1–0.6; 0.1 > *p*. > 0.05	3; Rigorous PBO trial in ADHD	Modest effect, SE, expense
Vitamins	Deficiency vs. idiopathic need for higher dose	Placebo-controlled trial multivitamin/mineral in adults with ADHD	ES ~ 0.05	4; Trials in children	GI upset
Iron supplementation	Co-factor make catecholamine	Open trial; ferritin levels cf. controls; r ferritin and p rating	ES 1.0 $p < 0.05$–0.001, r = −0.34	3[b]; Controlled trials	Hemochromatosis from excess
Zinc supplementation	Co-factor for many enzymes	2 DB RCT, flawed, high dose	ES~1, $p < 0.002$ in mid-east studies; 0 in American study	3[b]; Better trials	WBC aplasia from excess
Magnesium supplementation	Deficiency cf. to controls	Open trial with control group	ES 1.2–1.4, $p < 0.05$	3[b]; Placebo trials	Aggression from excess
Chinese herbals	Clinical experience	Open trials, one w. MPH control	$p < 0.05$; no diff. MPH	3; Placebo trials	Delay of other Tx
Other herbals	Clinical experience	French maritime pine bark small RCT	Significant	3; Pilot trials	Delay Tx
Homeopathic prep	Clinical experience	3 studies	Equivocal but generally positive	3; Better trials	Delay Tx

Laser acupuncture	Stimulate foci for calming	Open trial	ES 1.0	2; Controlled trial	Burn
EEG biofeedback	Suppress theta, increase beta	Open and randomized nonblind controlled trials	ES > 0.5, $p < 0.05$	3; Sham-controlled trial	Expense, time
EMG biofeedback, relaxation, hypnosis	Lower arousal, muscle tone	Randomized trials with controls	ES 1.0–1.3, $p < 0.01$	0 for hypnosis; 4 for EMG/ relaxation; cf. med	Delay other Tx
Meditation	Autonomic effect focused attention	cf. relaxation, wait list ctrl, med	$p < 0.05$	3; Rigorous replication, sham ctrl	Delay other Tx
Mirror feedback	Improve deficiency in self-focus	Randomized crossover w. and w/o cf. controls	ES 0.5, $p < 0.05$	3; Replication,	May impair non-ADHD children
Channel-specific perceptual training	Basic readiness skills, focus	Randomized trial with 2 control groups	ES 0.9, $p < 0.01$	3; Controlled Tx trials	Delay other Tx
Vestibular stimulation	Modulate behavior, attention, perception	Open and single-blind trials rotary stimulation	ES 0.4–1.2, p ns–0.001	3; Randomized sham-controlled trials	Nausea, accident
Cerebellar training	Patterning of behavior, organization of perceptions	Open trials, not well diagnosed, one with waitlist control	$p < 0.05$	1; Controlled trials with comparison Tx of equal duration and intensity	Nuisance, expense, And delay of other Tx
Massage	Vagal tone, 5HT, soothing	Single-blind comparison to relaxation	ES med-large $p < 0.05$	3; Replication, better assessments	Bruising if too hard
Antifungal Tx	GI yeast toxin; breach mucosa	No data in ADHD; other placebo trials	(ES 1.1–3; $p < 0.003$)	1; Trials in ADHD	Medium risk
Thyroid Tx	Thyroid function affects ADHD Sx	Placebo trial: 5/8 GRTH, 1/9 other	ns. If thyroid function not abnormal	0, if thyroid normal; 6, if thyroid abnormal	Thyroid toxicity
Deleading	Lead toxicity causes ADHD Sx	Placebo-controlled trial of chelation (= MPH)	ES 0.7–1.6, p. 05–0.001	4, if blood Pb > 20; 2 if Pb < 20; ctrl trial	Toxicity of chelator
Comprehensive vitamin/mineral supplementation	Correct dietary insufficiency; meet genetic special needs	RCT in adults	ES 0.69, $p = 0.002$	3; Compatible with other treatments; may reduce optimal dose of medication Needs replication	Expense, nuisance, GI upset

[a]Ratings: 0 = not worth considering further (despite, in the case of amino acids, some evidence of short-lived effect); 1 = credible hypothesis or collateral support or wide clinical experience, needs pilot data; 2 = promising systematic data, but not prospective trial; 3 = promising prospective data (perhaps with random assignment to control or objective/blind measures) lacking some important control or controlled trial(s) with trends suggesting further exploration; 4 = one significant double-blind controlled trial needing replication or multiple positive controlled trials in a treatment not easily blinded; 5 = convincing double-blind controlled evidence but needs further refinement (e.g., define target subgroup) for clinical application; 6 = should be considered established Tx for the appropriate subgroup.

[b]The rating would be 6 for patients showing frank deficiency of vitamins, iron, zinc, or other nutrients.

ES, effect size, Cohen's d (number of standard deviations difference between means): small ES < 0.3; moderate ES = 0.5; large ES = 1.0; p, probability; DB, double-blind; DO, dropout rate; MPH, methylphenidate; RCT, randomized clinical trial; RDI, recommended dietary intake; Sx, symptoms; Tx, treatment; XO, cross-over trial.

Adapted with permission from Arnold, LE: *Contemporary Diagnosis and Management of ADHD.* 3rd ed. Newtown, PA: Handbooks in Health Care Co., 2004.

proven standard treatment. A better name for most alternative treatments would be complementary treatments because they can theoretically be used in combination with standard treatments (analogous to combining two standard treatments such as medication and behavioral treatment), either to enhance benefit of the standard treatment or to address a problem not covered by the standard treatment. For example, mirror feedback might be used to ease evening homework angst at a time when the daytime stimulant is wearing off.

Unfortunately, the evidence base for most such treatments is rather thin. For example, the mirror feedback mentioned has only one published small randomized controlled trial, which showed a medium effect compared to the control condition. Some other treatments (149,157,279–281) are supported only by open trials or clinical observation. The reported improvement for some is likely due to nonspecific effects (placebo, maturation, history, regression to the mean). However, others have multiple placebo-controlled trials showing medium to large effects, often for only a small subgroup. Objective assessment of the evidence is complicated by unsubstantiated claims and assumptions made by some advocates of such treatments. The task of understanding them is discouraging enough to induce many busy practitioners to discard the lot as not worth the effort. Nevertheless, impatient rejection of such treatments without examining the evidence is as unscientific as uncritical acceptance. Most important, surveys indicate that a high proportion of patients use such treatments on their own, without professional guidance. Therefore, it behooves the practitioner to know enough about them and their varying evidence bases to advise and guide the families about likelihood of benefit, possible risks, and risk–benefit ratio. (Summaries of evidence for various treatments may be found in the references for Table 5.1.1.12.)

The following points may be useful in guiding families:

1. The easier, cheaper, and safer a treatment is, the less evidence is needed to justify an individual trial, especially if it can be done along with a proven standard treatment. Risky treatments need controlled convincing evidence. Difficult or expensive treatments risk diverting family emotional and financial resources from better proven treatments.
2. Look for controlled trials in well-characterized samples, not anecdotes or testimonials. A major flaw in many published alternative/complementary treatment studies is lack of diagnostic rigor, second only to lack of controls.
3. Herbs are crude drugs (if they work) and can have interactions with other drugs, either prescription or over the counter. Most families do not realize this because herbs are peddled as "nutritional" and "natural" or "dietary supplements," which most people mistakenly interpret as perfectly safe. Some herbs, with further research, may indeed be found useful for treatment of ADHD, and may contain psychoactive chemicals, such as nicotine from tobacco leaf, that can be refined into useful drugs. For now, the unknown risk appears to exceed any proven benefit. To prevent herb–drug interactions, physicians should inquire about herbs or "dietary" supplements containing herbs before prescribing, and explain the risk.
4. Remember that delay of proven treatment is a risk, varying in seriousness with the urgency of the presenting clinical picture. This is a consideration where the family wishes to substitute an alternative they have heard about for standard treatment.
5. Rather than merely advising against an unproven treatment, it is more useful to discuss what is known about it and help the family reach a considered decision. If the treatment is easy, cheap, and safe, there would seem little harm in accepting a trial and providing some guidance about how to monitor the results (baseline and follow-up measures, log of observed behavior), and the clinician's open-mindedness may help the family accept the recommended standard treatment.
6. When any treatment (including standard treatments) is tried, it is important to document the effect. Some rating scale or behavior count at baseline can be repeated periodically to see if there is reasonable progress. If there is, a trial of stopping the treatment can test whether the benefit was nonspecific (e.g., placebo benefit) or specific to the treatment. Lack of progress after a reasonable trial would seem prima facie evidence that it is not working for this patient.

Each family must find its own palatable and effective combination of treatment with professional guidance. The 36-month results of the Multimodal Treatment Study of children with ADHD (282) demonstrated that with treatment, symptoms abate significantly by the end of a year for most patients, and at 3 years continue to be significantly better than baseline, even though a substantial minority were able to terminate treatment by that time.

References

1. *Diagnostic and Statistical Manual of Mental Disorders, Fifth Edition (DSM IV)* Washington, DC, APA (American Psychiatric Association), c2013.
2. *Diagnostic and Statistical Manual of Mental Disorders, Fourth Edition (DSM-V).* Washington DC, APA (American Psychiatric Association, c2004.
3. Salum GA, Sonuga-Barke E, Sergeant J, et al.: Mechanisms underpinning inattention and hyperactivity: neurocognitive support for ADHD dimensionality. *Psychol Med* 44:3189–3201, 2014.
4. Struwwel P: *Fearful Stories and Vile Pictures to Instruct Good Little Folks/Stories by Heinrich Hoffman.* Venice, CA, Feral House, 1999.

5a. Laufer MW, Denhoff E, Solomons G: Hyperkinetic impulse disorder in children's behavior problems. *Psychosom Med* 19(1):38–49, 1957.

5b. *Diagnostic and Statistical Manual of Mental Disorders, Second Edition (DSM II).* Washington, DC, APA (American Psychiatric Association), c1970.

6. The ICD 10 Classification of Mental and Behavioural Disorders: *Diagnostic Criteria for Research.* Geneva, World Health Organization (WHO), 1993.
7. *Diagnostic and Statistical Manual of Mental Disorders, Third Edition (DSM III).* Washington, DC, APA (American Psychiatric Association), c1980.
8. Attention Deficit Disorder Association (ADDA). Available at: https://add.org. Accessed June 1, 2017.
9. *Children and Adults with Attention Deficit Hyperactivity Disorder.* Available at: www.chadd.org.
10. *Diagnostic and Statistical Manual of Mental Disorders, Third Edition—Revised (DSM III R).* Washington, DC, APA (American Psychiatric Association), c1987.
11. Taylor E, Dopfner M, Sergeant J, et al: European clinical guidelines for hyperkinetic disorder- first upgrade. *Eur Child Adolesc Psychiatry* 13 (Suppl 1): I/7-I/30, 2004.
12. Rowland AS, Lesesne CA, Abramowitz AJ: The epidemiology of ADHD—a public health view. *Ment Retard Dev Disabil Res Rev* 8:162–170, 2002.
13. Faraone SV, Biederman J, Zimmerman BA: Correspondence of parent and teacher reports in medication trials. *Eur J Child Adolesc Psychiatr* 14:20–27, 2005.
14. Faraone SV, Sergeant J, Gillberg C, Biederman J: The worldwide prevalence of ADHD—is it an American condition? *World Psych* 2:104–113, 2003.
15. Lahey BB, Applegate B, McBurnett K, et al.: DSM IV field trials for ADHD in children and adolescents. *Am J Psychiatry* 151:1673–1685, 1994.
16. Santosh P, Taylor E, Swanson J, et al.: Refining the diagnoses of inattention and overactivity syndromes: a reanalysis of the multimodal treatment study of attention deficit hyperactivity disorder (ADHD) based on ICD-10 criteria for hyperkinetic disorder. *J Clin Neurosci Res* 5–6: 307–314, 2005.
17. Biederman J, Monuteaux MC, Mick E, et al.: Adolescent outcome of females with ADHD: a controlled 5 year prospective study of girls into adolescence. Presented at the NIMH Pediatric Bipolar Conference, Coral Gables, FL, April 2005.
18. Preschool ADHD: A review of prevalence, diagnosis, neurobiology and stimulant treatment. *Dev Behav Pediatr* 23(1 Suppl):S1–S9, 2002.
19. Asherson P: ADHD across the lifespan. *Medicine* 40(11):623–627.
20. Morestedt B, Corbisiero S, Bitto H, Stieglitz RD: Emotional symptoms and their contribution to functional impairment in adults with attention

deficit/hyperactivity disorder. *Atten Defic Hyperact Disord* 8(1):21–33, 2016.

21. Skirrow C, Asherson P: Emotional lability, comorbidity and impairment in adults with attention deficit hyperactivity disorder. *J Affect Disord* 147:80–86, 2013.
22. Childress AC, Sallee FR: emotional lability in patients with attention deficit/hyperactivity disorder: impact of pharmacotherapy. *CNS Drugs* 29(8):683–693, 2015.
23. Coolidge F, Thede L, Young S: Heritability and the comorbidity of attention deficit hyperactivity disorder with behavioral disorders and executive function deficits: a preliminary investigation. *Dev Neuropsychology* 17(3):273–287, 2000.
24. Hudziak JJ, Rudiger LP, Neale MC, Heath AC, Todd RD: A twin study of inattentive, aggressive, and anxious/depressed behaviors. *J Am Acad Child Adolesc Psychiatry* 39:469–476, 2000.
25. Thapar A, Harrington R: Does the definition of ADHD affect heritability? *J Am Acad Child Adolesc Psychiatry* 39(12):1528–1536, 2000. (9p, 5 charts 1 diagram.)
26. Martin N, Scourfield J, McGuffin P: Observer effects and heritability of childhood attention-deficit hyperactivity disorder symptoms. *Br J Psychiatry* 180:260–265, 2002.
27. Rietveld MJ, Hudziak JJ, Bartels M, Van Beijsterveldt CE, Boomsma DI: Heritability of attention problems in children: I. cross-sectional results from a study of twins, age 3–12 years. *Am J Med Genet B Neuropsychiatry Genet* 117:102–113, 2003.
28. Rietveld M, Hudziak J, Bartels M, Van Beijsterveldt C, Boomsma D: Heritability of attention problems in children: longitudinal results from a study of twins, age 3 to 12. *J Child Psychol Psychiatry* 45(3):577–588, 2004.

28a. Faraone SV, Perlis RH, Doyle AE et al.: Molecular genetics of attention-deficit/hyperactivity disorder. *Biol Psychiatry* 57:1313–1323, 2005.

29. Kebir O, Joober R: Neuropsychological endophenotypes in attention deficit/hyperactivity disorder: a review of genetic association studies. *Eur Arch Psychiatry Clin Neurosci* 261:583–594, 2011.
30. Sonuga-Barke JS, Coghill D: Introduction: The foundations of next generation attention deficit/hyperactivity disorder neuropsychology: building on progress during the last 30 years. *J Child Psychol and Psychiatry* 55(12): e1-e5, 2014.
31. Sjwwall D, Roth L, Lindqvist S, Thorell LB: Multiple deficits in ADHD: executive dysfunction, delay aversion, reaction time variability, and emotional deficits. *J Child Psychol and Psychiatry* 54(6):619–627, 2013.
32. Doyle AE, Seidman LJ, Biederman J, Chourinard VA, Silva J, Faraone SV: Attention deficit hyperactivity disorder endophenotypes. *Biol Psychiatry* 57:1313–1323, 2005.
33. Fisher SE, Francks C, McCracken JT, et al.: A genomewide scan for loci involved in ADHD. *Am J Hum Gen* 70:1183–1196, 2002.
34. Bakker SC, Van der Maulen EM, Buitelaar JK, et al.: A whole genome scan in 164 Dutch sib pairs with ADHD: suggestive evidence for linkage on chromosome 7p and 15q. *Am J Hum Genet* 72:1251–1260, 2003.
35. Arcos Burgos M, Castellanos FX, Konecki D, et al.: Pedigree disequilibrium test (PDT) replicates association and linkage between DRD4 and ADHD in multigenerational and extended pedigrees from a genetic isolate. *Mol Psychiatry* 9:252–259, 2004.
36. Li Z, Chang S, Zhang L, Wang J: Molecular genetic studies of ADHD and its candidate genes: a review. *Psychiatry Res* 219:10–24, 2014.
37. Cook EH, Stein MA, Krasowski MD, et al.: Association of ADHD and the dopamine transporter gene. *Am J Hum Genet* 56:993–998, 1995.
38. Waldman ID, Rowe DC, Abramowitz A, Kozel ST, Mohr JH, Sherman, SL: Association and linkage of the dopamine transporter gene and attention deficit hyperactivity disorder in children: Heterogeneity owing to diagnostic subtype and severity. *Am J Hum Genet* 63:1767–1776, 1998.
39. Dougherty DD, Bonab AA, Spencer TJ, Rausch SL, Madras BK, Fischman AJ: Dopamine transporter density is elevated in patients with ADHD. *Lancet* 354:2132–2133, 1999.
40. Krause K, Dresel SH, Krause J, Kung HF, Tatsch K: Increased striatal dopamine transporter in adult patients with ADHD: effects of methylphenidate as measured by single photon emission computed tomography. *Neurosci Lett* 285:107–110, 2000.
41. Todd RD, Jong YG, Lobos EA, Reich W, Heath AC, Neumann RJ: No association of the dopamine transporter gene 3; VNTR polymorphism with ADHD subtypes in a population sample of twins. *Am J Med Genet* 105:745–748, 2001.
42. Payton A, Holmes J, Barrett JH, et al.: Examining for association between candidate gene polymorphisms in the dopamine pathways and ADHD: a family based study. *Am J Med Genet* 105:464–470, 2001.
43. Muglia P, Jain U, Iukster B, Kennedy JL: A quantitative trait locus analysis of the dopamine transporter gene in adults with ADHD. *Neuropsychopharmacology* 27:655–662, 2002.
44. VanDyck CH, Quinlan DM, Cretella LM, Staley JK, Malison RT, Baldwin RM: Unaltered dopamine transporter availability in adult attention deficit hyperactivity disorder. *Am J Psychiatry* 159:309–312, 2002.
45. Chen CK, Chen SL, Mill J, et al.: The dopamine transporter gene is associated with ADHD in a Taiwanese sample. *Mol Psychiatry* 8:393–396, 2003.
46. Smith KM, Daly M, Fischer M, et al.: Association of the dopamine beta Hydroxylase gene with attention deficit hyperactivity disorder: genetic analysis of the Milwaukee longitudinal study. *Am J Genet* 119:77–85, 2003.
47. Curran S, Mill J, Tahir E, et al.: Association study of a dopamine transporter polymorphism and ADHD in UK and Turkish samples. *Mol Psychiatry* 6:425–428, 2001.
48. Gizer IR, Ficks C, Waldman ID: Candidate gene studies of ADHD: a meta-analytic review. *Hum Genet* 126:51–90, 2009.
49. Azeredo LA, Rovaris DL, Mota NR, Polia ER, et al.: Further evidence for the association between a polymorphism in the promoter region of SLC6A3/DAT1 and ADHD: findings from a sample of adults. *Eur Arch Psychiatry Clin Neurosci* 264:401–408, 2014.
50. Comings DE, Comings BG, Muhleman D, et al.: The dopamine D2 receptor locus as a modifying gene in neuropsychiatric disorders. *JAMA* 266:1793–1800, 1991.
51. Comings DE, Wu H, Chiu C, et al.: Polygenic inheritance of Tourette syndrome, stuttering, ADHD, conduct and oppositional defiant disorder: the additive and subtractive effect of the three dopamine genes—DRD2, DBH and DAT1. *Am J Genet* 67:264–288, 1996.
52. Rowe DC, den Oord EJ, Stever C, et al.: The DRD2 Taq1 polymorphism and symptoms of ADHD. *Mol Psychiatry* 4:580–586, 1999.
53. Kirley A, Hawi Z, Daly G, et al.: Dopaminergic system genes in ADHD: Toward a biological hypothesis. *Neuropsychopharmacology* 27:607–619, 2002.
54. Huang YS, Lin SK, Wu YY, Chao CC, Chen CK: A family based association study of ADHD and dopamine D2 receptor Taq1A alleles. *Chang Gung Med J* 26:897–903, 2003.
55. Faraone SV, Doyle AE, Mick E, Biederman J: Metaanalysis of the association between the 7-repeat allele of the dopamine D4 receptor gene and ADHD. *Am J Psychiatry* 158:1052–1057, 2001.
56. Holmes J, Payton A, Barrett J, et al.: Association of DRD4 in children with ADHD and comorbid conduct problems. *Am J Med Genet* 114:150–153, 2002.
57. Grady DL, Chi HC, Ding YC, et al.: High prevalence of rare dopamine D4 alleles in children diagnosed with ADHD. *Mol Psychiatry* 8:536–545, 2003.
58. Qian Q, Wang Y, Zhou R: Association studies of dopamine D4 receptor gene and dopamine transporter gene polymorphisms in Han Chinese patients with ADHD. *Beijing Da Xue Xue Bao* 35:412–418, 2003.
59. Mill J, Curran S, Kent L, et al.: ADHD and the dopamine D4 receptor gene: Evidence of association but no linkage in a UK sample. *Mol Psychiatry* 6:440–444, 2001.
60. Manor I, Tyano S, Mel E, Eisenberg J, et al.: Family based and association studies of MAO-A and attention deficit hyperactivity disorder: preferential transmission of the long-promoter region repeat and its and its association with impaired performance on a continuous performance test (TOVA). *Mol Psychiatry* 7:626–632, 2002.
61. Kustanovich V, Ishii J, Crawford L, et al.: Transmission disequilibrium testing of dopamine-related candidate gene polymorphisms in ADHD: confirmation of association of ADHD with DRD4 and DRD5. *Mol Psychiatry* 9:711–717, 2003.
62. McCracken JT, Smalley SL, McGough JJ, et al.: Evidence for linkage of a tandem duplication polymorphism upstream of the dopamine D4 receptor gene (DRD4) with attention deficit hyperactivity disorder (ADHD). *Mol Psychiatry* 119(5):531–536, 2000.
63. Todd RD, Neuman RJ, Lobos EA, Jong YJ, Reich W, Heath AC: Lack of association of dopamine D4 receptor gene polymorphisms with ADHD subtypes in a population sample of twins. *Am J Med Genet* 105:432–438, 120, 2001.
64. Barr CL, Wigg KG, Bloom S, et al.: Further evidence from haplotype analysis for linkage of the dopamine D4 receptor gene and attention-deficit hyperactivity disorder. *Am J Med Genet* 96:244–250, 2000.
65. Rowe DC, Stever C, Chase D, Sherman S, Abramowitz A, Waldman ID: Two dopamine genes related to reports of childhood retrospective inattention and conduct disorder symptoms. *Mol Psychiatry* 6:429–433, 2001.
66. Kustanovich V, Ishii J, Crawford L, et al.: Transmission disequilibrium testing of dopamine – related candidate gene polymorphisms in ADHD: confirmation of association of ADHD with DRD4 and DRD5. *Mol Psychiatry* 9(7):711–717, 2004.
67. Comings David E, Gade-Andavolu R, Gonzalez N, et al.: Comparison of the role of dopamine, serotonin, and noradrenaline genes in ADHD, ODD and conduct disorder: multivariate regression analysis of 20 genes. *Clin Genet* 57(3):178–196, 2000.
68. Daly G, Hawi Z, Fitzgerald M, Gill M: Mapping susceptibility loci in ADHD: Preferential transmission of parental alleles of DAT1; DBH; and DRD5 to affected children. *Mol Psychiatry* 4:192–196, 1999.
69. Barr CL, Wigg KG, Feng Y, et al.: Attention-deficit hyperactivity disorder and the gene for the dopamine D5 receptor. *Mol Psychiatry* 5:548–551, 2000.
70. Tahir E, Yazgan Y, Cirakoglu OF, Waldman I, Asherson PJ: Association and linkage of DRD4 and DRD5 with attention deficit hyperactivity disorder. *Mol Psychiatry* 5:396–404, 2000.
71. Mill J, Richards S, Knight J, Curran S, Taylor E, Asherson P: Haplotype analysis of SNAP 25 suggests a role in the aetiology of ADHD. *Mol Psychiatry* 9:801–810, 2004.
72. Lasky-Su J, Biederman J, Laird N, et al.: Evidence for an association of the dopamine D5 receptor gene on age at onset of attention deficit hyperactivity disorder. *Ann Hum Genet* 71:648–659, 2007.
73. Maher BS, Marazita ML, Ferrell RE, Vanuykov MM: Dopamine system genes and ADHD: A meta-analysis. *Psychiatr Genet* 12:207–215, 2002.

74. Lowe N, Kirley A, Hawi Z, et al.: Joint analysis of DRD5 marker concludes association with ADHD confined to the predominantly inattentive and combined types. *Am J Hum Genet* 74:348–356, 2004.
75. Manor I, Corbex M, Eisenberg J, et al.: Association of the dopamine D5 receptor with attention deficit hyperactivity disorder (ADHD) and scores on a continuous performance test (TOVA). *Am J Med Genet* 127B:73–77, 2004.
76. Barr CL, Wigg KG, Wu J, et al.: Linkage study of two polymorphisms at the dopamine D3 receptor gene and attention-deficit hyperactivity disorder. *Am J Med Genet* 96:114–117, 2000.
77. Muglia P, Jain U, Kennedy JL: A transmission disequilibrium test of the Ser 9/Gly dopamine D3 receptor gene polymorphism in adult attention deficit hyperactivity disorder. *Behav Brain Res* 130:91–95, 2002.
78. Retz W, Rosler M, Supprian T, Retz-Junginger P, Thome J: Dopamine D3 receptor polymorphism and violent behavior: relation to impulsiveness and ADHD related psychopathology. *J Neural Transm* 110:561–572, 2003.
79. Retz W, Thome J, Blocker D, Baaden M, Rosler M: Association of ADHD related psychopathology and personality traits with the serotonin transporter promoter region polymorphism. *Neurosci Lett* 319:133–136, 2002.
80. Seeger G, Schloss P, Schmidt MH: Functional polymorphism within the promoter of the serotonin transporter gene is associated with severe hyperkinetic disorders. *Mol Psychiatry* 6:235–238, 2001.
81. Zoroglu SS, Erdal ME, Alasehirli Erdal N, et al.: Significance of serotonin transporter gene 5-HTTLPR and variable number of tandem repeat polymorphism in attention deficit hyperactivity disorder. *Neuropsychobiology* 45:176–181, 2002.
82. Beitchman JH, Davidge KM, Kennedy JL, et al.: The serotonin transporter gene in aggressive children with and without ADHD and nonaggressive matched controls. *Ann N Y Acad Sci* 1008:248–251, 2003.
83. Manor I, Eisenberg J, Tyano S, et al.: Family based association study of the serotonin transporter promoter region polymorphism (5-HTTLPR) in ADHD. *Am J Med Genet* 105:91–95, 2001.
84. Kent L, Doerry U, Hardy E, et al.: Evidence that variation at the serotonin transporter gene influences susceptibility to ADHD: analysis and pooled analysis. *Mol Psychiatry* 7:908–912, 2002.
85. Cadoret RJ, Langbehn D, Caspers K, et al.: Association of the serotonin transporter promoter polymorphism with aggressivity, attention deficit, and conduct disorder in an adoptee population. *Compr Psychiatry* 44:88–101, 2003.
86. Ribases M, Ramos-Quiroga JA, Hervas A, et al: Exploration of 19 serotnergic candidate genes in adults and children with attention deficit/hyperactivity disorder identifies association for 5HT2A, DDC and MAOB. *Mol Psychiatry* 14:71–85, 2009.
87. Barr CL, Kroft J, Feng Y, et al.: The norepinephrine transporter gene and attention-deficit hyperactivity disorder. *Am J Med Genet* 114:255–259, 2002.
88. McEvoy B, Hawi Z, Fitzgerald M, Gill M: No evidence of linkage or association between the norepinephrine transporter (NET) gene polymorphisms and ADHD in the Irish population. *Am J Med Genet* 114:665–666, 2002.
89. De Luca V, Muglia P, Vincent J, Lanktree M, Jain U, Kennedy JL: Adrenergic alpha 2C receptor genomic organization: association study in adult ADHD. *Am J Med Genet* 127:65–67, 2004.
90. Yang L, Qian Q, Liu L, Li H, Faraone SV, Wang Y: Adrenergic neurotransmitter system transporter and receptor genes associated with atomoxetine response in attention deficit hyperactivity disorder. *J Neural Transm* 120:1127–1133, 2013.
91. Smith KM, Daly M, Fischer M, et al.: Association of the dopamine beta Hydroxylase gene with attention deficit hyperactivity disorder: genetic analysis of the Milwaukee longitudinal study. *Am J Genet* 119:77–85, 2003.
92. Roman T, Schmitz M, Polanczyk G, Eizirik M, Rohde LA, Hutz MH: Further evidence for the association between attention deficit hyperactivity disorder and the dopamine beta hydroxylase gene. *Am J Med Genet* 114:154–158, 2002.
93. Wigg K, Zai G, Schachar R, et al.: Attention deficit hyperactivity disorder and the gene for dopamine beta hydroxylase. *Am J Psychiatry* 159:1046–1048, 2002.
94. Hawi Z, Lowe N, Kirley A, et al.: Linkage disequilibrium mapping at DAT1, DRD5, and DBH narrows the search for ADHD susceptibility alleles at these loci. *Mol Psychiatry* 8:299–308, 2003.
95. Hess EJ, Jinnah HA, Kozac CA, Wilson MC: Spontaneous locomotor hyperactivity in a mouse mutant with a deletion including the SNAP gene on chromosome 2 *J Neurosci* 12:2865–2874, 1992.
96. Hess EJ, Rogan PK, Domoto M, Tinker DE, Ladda RL, Ramer JC: Absence of linkage of apparently single gene mediated ADHD with the human synterric region of the mouse mutant coloboma. *Am J Med Genet* 60:573–579, 1995.
97. Barr CL, Feng Y, Wigg K, et al.: Identification of DNA variants in the SNAP-25 gene and linkage study of these polymorphisms and attention-deficit hyperactivity disorder. *Mol Psychiatry* 5:405–409, 2000.
98. Brophy K, Hawi Z, Kirley A, Fitzgerald M, Gill M: Synaptosomal-associated protein 25 (SNAP-25) and attention deficit hyperactivity disorder (ADHD): evidence of linkage and association in the Irish population. *Mol Psychiatry* 7:913–917, 2002.
99. Mill J, Curran S, Kent L, et al.: Association study of a SNAP-25 microsatellite and attention deficit hyperactivity disorder. *Am J Med Genet* 114:269–271, 2002.
100. Kirley A, Brophy K, Hawi Z, Fitzgerald M, Gill M: Synaptosomal-associated protein 25 (SNAP 25) and ADHD: evidence of linkage and association in the Irish population. *Mol Psychiatry* 7:913–917, 2002.
101. Comings D, Gade R, Muhleman D, Sverd J: No association of a tyrosine Hydroxylase gene tetranucleotide polymorphism in autism, Tourette syndrome, or ADHD. *Biol Psychiatry* 37:484–486, 1995.
102. Syvanen AC, Tilgmann C, Rinne J, Ulmanen I: Genetic polymorphism of COMT; correlation of genotype with individual variation of S-COMT activity and comparison of the allele frequencies in the normal population and parkinsonian patients in Finland. *Pharmacogenetics* 7:65–71, 1997.
103. Barr CL, Wigg K, Malone M, et al.: Linkage study of COMT and attention deficit hyperactivity disorder. *Am J Med Genet* 88:710–713, 1999.
104. Hawi Z, Millar N, Daly G, Fitzgerald M, Gill M: No association between COMT gene polymorphism and ADHD in an Irish sample. *Am J Med Genet* 96:241–243, 2000.
105. Manor I, Kotler M, Sever Y, Eisenberg J, Cohen H, Ebstein RP: Failure to replicate an association between the COMT polymorphism and attention deficit hyperactivity disorder in a second, independently recruited Israeli cohort. *Am J Med Genet* 96:858–860, 2000.
106. Tahir E, Curran S, Yazgan Y, Ozbay F, Cirakoglu Asherson PJ: No association between low and high activity COMT and attention deficit hyperactivity disorder in a sample of Turkish children. *Am J Med Genet* 96:285–288, 2000.
107. Qian Q, Wang Y, Zhou R, et al.: Family based and case control association studies of COMT in attention deficit hyperactivity disorder suggest genetic sexual dimorphism. *Am J Med Genet* 118:103–109, 2003.
108. Beijsterveldt CE, Middeldorp CM, Slof-Op't Landt M, et al.: Influence of Candidate genes on attention problems in children: a longitudinal study. *Behav Genet* 41:155–164, 2011.
109. Manor I, Tyano S, Mel E, et al.: Family based and association studies of MAO-A and attention deficit hyperactivity disorder: preferential transmission of the long-promoter region repeat and its and its association with impaired performance on a continuous performance test (TOVA). *Mol Psychiatry* 7:626–632, 2002.
110. Lawson DC, Turic D, Langley K, et al.: Association analysis of monoamine oxidase A and attention deficit hyperactivity disorder. *Am J Med Genet* 116:84–89, 2003.
111. Comings D, Gade-Andavolu R, Gonzales N, Blake H, MacMurray J: Additive effect of three noradrenergic genes (ADRA2A, ADRA2C, DBH) on attention deficit hyperactivity disorder and learning disabilities in Tourette syndrome subjects. *Clin Genet* 55:160–172, 1999.
112. Xu C, Schachar R, Tannock R, et al.: Linkage study of the alpha2A adrenergic receptor in attention deficit hyperactivity disorder families. *Am J Med Genet* 105:159–162, 2001.
113. Comings DE, Gonzales NS, Cheng Li SC, MacMurray J: A line item approach to the identification of genes involved in polygenic behavioral disorders: the adrenergic alpha2A (ADRA2A) gene. *Am J Med Genet* 118:110–114, 2003.
114. Barr CL, Wigg K, Zai G, et al.: Attention deficit hyperactivity disorder and the adrenergic receptors alpha1C and alpha2C. *Mol Psychiatry* 6:334–337, 2001.
115. Roman T, Schmitz M, Polanczyk GV, Eizirik M, Rohde LA, Hutz MH: Is the alpha-2A adrenergic receptor gene (ADRA2A) associated with attention deficit hyperactivity disorder? *Am J Med Genet* 120:116–120, 2003.
116. Hawi Z, Dring M, Kirley A, et al.: Serotonergic system and attention deficit hyperactivity disorder (ADHD): a potential susceptibility locus at the 5-HT (1B) receptor gene in 273 nuclear families from a multi-center sample. *Mol Psychiatry* 7:718–725, 2002.
117. Quist JF, Barr CL, Schachar R, et al.: Evidence for the serotonin 5-HTR2A receptor gene as a susceptibility factor in attention deficit hyperactivity disorder (ADHD). *Mol Psychiatry* 5:537–541, 2000.
118. Tang G, Ren D, Xin R, Qian Y, Wang D, Jiang S: Lack of association between the tryptophan hydroxylase gene A218C polymorphism and attention deficit hyperactivity disorder in Chinese Han population. *Am J Med Genet* 105:485–488, 2001.
119. Li J, Wang YF, Zhou RL, Yang L, Zhang HB, Wang B: Association between the tryptophan hydroxylase gene polymorphisms and attention deficit hyperactivity disorder with or without learning disorder. *Zhong-hua Yi Xue Za Zhi* 83:2114–2118, 2003.
120. Kent L, Middle F, Hawi Z, et al.: Nicotinic acetylcholine receptor alpha4 subunit gene polymorphism and attention deficit hyperactivity disorder. *Psychiatr Genet* 11:37–40, 2001.
121. Todd RD, Lobos EA, Sun LW, Neumann RJ: Mutational analysis of the nicotinic acetylcholine receptor alpha 4 subunit gene in attention deficit hyperactivity disorder: evidence for association of an intronic polymorphism with attention problems. *Mol Psychiatry* 8:103–108, 2003.
122. Turic D, Langley K, Mills S, et al.: Follow up of genetic linkage findings on chromosome 16p13: evidence of association of N-methyl-D-aspartate glutamate receptor 2A gene polymorphism with ADHD. *Mol Psychiatry* 9:169–173, 2004.

123. Adams J, Crosbie J, Wigg K, et al.: Glutamate receptor, ionotropic, N-methyl D-aspartate 2A (GRIN2A) gene as a positional candidate for attention deficit hyperactivity disorder in the 16p13 region. *Mol Psychiatry* 9:494–499, 2004.
124. Wu Z, Yang L, Wang Y: Applying imaging genetics to ADHD: the promises and the challenges. *Mol Neurobiol* 50:449–462, 2014.
125. Arnold LE: Treatment alternatives for attention-deficit/hyperactivity disorder (ADHD). *J Attention Disord* 3:30–48, 1999.
126. Mattes JA: The role of frontal lobe dysfunction in childhood hyperkinesis. *Compr Psychiatry* 21:358–369, 1980.
127. Castellanos FX, Giedd JN, Marsh WL, et al.: Quantitative brain magnetic resonance imaging in attention deficit hyperactivity disorder. *Arch Gen Psychiatry* 53:607–616, 1996.
128. Filipek PA, Semrud-Clickeman M, Steingard R, Kennedy D, Biederman J: Volumetric MRI analysis: comparing subjects having attention deficit hyperactivity disorder with normal controls. *Neurology* 48:589–601, 1997.
129. Overmeyer S, Bullmore ET, Suckling J, et al.: Distributed gray and white matter deficits in hyperkinetic disorder: MRI evidence for anatomical abnormality in an attentional network. *Psychol Med* 31:1425–1435, 2001.
130. Mostofsky S, Cooper K, Kates W, Denckla M, Kaufmann W: Smaller prefrontal and premotor volumes in boys with attention deficit hyperactivity disorder. *Biol Psychiatry* 52:785–794, 2002.
131. Hill DE, Yeo RA, Campbell RA, Hart B, Vigil J, Brooks W: Magnetic resonance imaging correlates of attention deficit hyperactivity disorder in children. *Neuropsychology* 17:496–506, 2003.
132. Durston S, Hulshoff Pol HE, Schnack HG, et al.: Magnetic resonance imaging of boys with attention deficit hyperactivity disorder and their unaffected siblings. *J Am Acad Child Adolesc Psychiatry* 43:332–340, 2004.
133. Hynd GW, Hern KL, Novey ES, et al.: Attention deficit hyperactivity disorder and asymmetry of the caudate nucleus. *J Child Neurol* 8:339–347, 1993.
134. Semrud-Clickeman MS, Filipek PA, Biederman J, et al.: Attention deficit hyperactivity disorder: Magnetic resonance imaging morphometric analysis of the corpus callosum. *J Am Acad Child Adolesc Psychiatry* 33:875–881, 1994.
135. Castellanos FX, Giedd JN, Eckburg P, et al.: Quantitative morphology of the caudate nucleus in attention deficit hyperactivity disorder. *Am J Psychiatry* 151:1791–1796, 1994.
136. Mataro M, Garcia-Sanchez C, Junque C, Estevez-Gonzales A, Pujol J: Magnetic resonance imaging measurement of the caudate nucleus in adolescents with attention deficit hyperactivity disorder and its relationship with neuropsychological and behavioural measures. *Arch Neurol* 54:963–968, 1997.
137. Castellanos FX, Giedd JN, Berquin PC, et al.: Quantitative brain magnetic resonance imaging in girls with attention-deficit/hyperactivity disorder. *Arch Gen Psychiatry* 58:289–295, 2001.
138. Pineda DA, Restrepo A, Sarmiento RJ, et al.: Statistical analyses of structural magnetic resonance imaging of the head of the caudate nucleus in Colombian children with attention deficit hyperactivity disorder. *J Child Neurol* 17:97–105, 2002.
139. Bussing R, Grudnick J, Mason D, Wasiak M, Leonard C: ADHD and conduct disorder: an MRI study in a community sample. *World J Biol Psychiatry* 3:216–220, 2002.
140. Castellanos FX, Sharp WS, Gottesman RF, Greenstein DK, Giedd JN, Rapoport JL: Anatomic brain abnormalities in monozygotic twins discordant for attention deficit disorder. *Am J Psychiatry* 160:1693–1696, 2003.
141. Aylward EH, Reiss AL, Reader MJ, Singer HS, Brown JE, Denckla MB: Basal ganglia volumes in children with attention deficit hyperactivity disorder. *J Child Neurol* 11:112–115, 1996.
142. Overmeyer S, Simmons A, Santosh J, et al.: Corpus callosum may be similar in children with ADHD and siblings of children with ADHD. *Dev Med Child Neurol* 42:8–13, 2000.
143. Hynd GW, Semrud-Clickeman MS, Lorys AR, Novey ES, Eliopulos D: Brain morphology in developmental dyslexia and attention deficit hyperactivity disorder. *Arch Neurol* 47:919–926, 1990.
144. Hynd GW, Semrud-Clickeman MS, Lorys AR, Novey ES, Eliopulos D, Lytinen H: Corpus callosum morphology in attention deficit hyperactivity disorder: morphometric analysis of MRI. *J Learn Disabilities* 24:141–146, 1991.
145. Swanson JM, Kraemer HC, Hinshaw SP, et al.: Clinical relevance of the primary findings of the MTA: success rates based on severity of ADHD and ODD symptoms at the end of treatment. *J Am Acad Child Adolesc Psychiatry* 40:168–179, 2001.
146. Giedd JN, Castellanos FX, Casey BJ, et al.: Quantitative morphology of the corpus callosum in attention deficit hyperactivity disorder. *Am J Psychiatry* 151:665–669, 1994.
147. Baumgardner TL, Singer HS, Denckla MB, et al.: Corpus callosum morphology in children with Tourette syndrome and attention deficit hyperactivity disorder. *Neurology* 47:1–6, 1996.
148. Lyoo I, Noam G, Lee H, Kennedy B, Renshaw P: The corpus callosum and lateral ventricles in children with attention deficit hyperactivity disorder: a brain magnetic resonance imaging study. *Biol Psychiatry* 40:1060–1063, 1996.
149. Arnold LE, Robert MD, DiSilvestro RA, et al.: Zinc for attention-deficit/hyperactivity disorder: placebo-controlled double-blind pilot trial alone and combined with amphetamine. *J Child Adolesc Psychopharmacol* 21(1) 1–19, 2011.
150. American Academy of Pediatrics Subcommittee on Attention Deficit/Hyperactivity Disorder, Steering Committee on Quality Improvement and Management: Implementing the key action statements: an algorithm and explanation for process of care for the evaluation, diagnosis, treatment, and monitoring of ADHD in *Child Adolesc Pediatri* 128(5): S11–S121, 2011.
151. Kates WR, Frederikse M, Mostofsky SH, et al.: MRI parcellation of the frontal lobe in boys with attention deficit hyperactivity disorder or Tourette syndrome. *Psychiatry Res* 116:63–81, 2002.
152. The MTA Cooperative Group: A 14-month randomized clinical trial of treatment strategies for attention-deficit/hyperactivity disorder. *Arch Gen Psychiatry* 56:1073–1086, 1999.
153. Pastor P, Reuben C: Racial and ethnic differences in ADHD and learning disorders in young school age children: parental reports in the National Health Interview Survey. *Public Health Rep*120:383–392, 2005.
154. American Academy of Child and Adolescent Psychiatry: Practice parameters for the assessment and treatment of children and adolescents with attention deficit/hyperactivity disorder. *J Am Acad Child Adolesc Psychiatry* 46(7): 894–921, 2007.
155. Berquin PC, Giedd JN, Jacobsen LK, et al.: Cerebellum in attention deficit hyperactivity disorder: a morphometric MRI study. *Neurology* 50:1087–1093, 1998.
156. Mostofsky SH, Reiss AL, Lockhart P, Denckla MB: Evaluation of the cerebellar size in attention deficit hyperactivity disorder. *J Child Neurol* 13:434–439, 1998.
157. Rucklidge JJ, Frampton CM, Gorman B, Boggis A: Vitamin- mineral treatment of attention-deficit hyperactivity disorder in adults: double-blind randomized placebo-controlled trial. *Br J Psychiatry* 207(3):1–10, 2014.
158. Pennington BF, Ozonoff S: Executive functions and developmental psychopathology. *J Child Psychol Psychiatry* 37:51–87, 1996.
159. Barkley RA: Behavioral inhibition, sustained attention, and executive function: constructing a unified theory of ADHD. *Psychol Bull* 121:65–94, 51. 1997.
160. Seidman LJ, Doyle A, Fried R, Valera E, Crum K, Matthews L: Neuropsychological function in adults with attention deficit hyperactivity disorder. *Psychiatr Clin North Am* 27:261–282, 2004.
161. Volkow ND, Fowler JS, Wang GJ, Ding YS, Gatley SJ: Role of dopamine in the therapeutic and reinforcing effects of methylphenidate in humans: results from imaging studies. *Eur Neuropsychopharmacol* 12:557–566, 2002.
162. Greven C, Bralten J, Mennes M, et al.: Developmentally stable whole brain volume reductions and developmentally sensitive caudate and putamen volume alterations in those with attention deficit/hyperactivity disorder and their unaffected siblings. *JAMA Psychiatry* 72(5):490–499, 2015.
163. Castellanos FX, Lee PP, Sharp W, et al.: Developmental trajectories of brain volume abnormalities in children and adolescents with attention deficit hyperactivity disorder. *JAMA* 288:1740–1748, 2002.
164. Shaw P, Malek M, Watson B, Sharp W, Evans A, Greenstein D: Development of cortical surface area and gyrification in attention deficit/hyperactivity disorder. *Biol Psychiatry* 72:191–197, 2012.
165. Shaw P, Eckstrand K, Sharp W, et al.: Attention deficit/hyperactivity disorder is characterized by a delay in cortical maturation. *PNAS* 104(49): 19649–19654, 2007.
166. Sripada CS, Kessler D, Angstadt M: Lag in maturation of the brain's intrinsic functional architecture in attention deficit/hyperactivity disorder. *PNAS* 111(39):14259–14264, 2014.
167. Giedd JN, Raznahan A, Alexander-Bloch A, Schmitt E, Gogtay N, Rapoport J: Child Psychiatry Branch of the National Institute of Mental Health Longitudinal Structural Magnetic Resonance Imaging Study of Human Brain Development. *Neuropsychopharmacology* 40:43–49, 2015.
168. Shaw P, Malek M, Watson B, Greenstein D, de Rossi P, Sharp W: Trajectories of cerebral cortical development in childhood and adolescence and adult attention deficit/hyperactivity disorder. *Br J Psychiatry* 194:123–129, 2009.
169. Ducharme S, Hudziak JJ, Botteron KN, et al.: Decreased regional cortical thickness and thinning rate are associated with inattention symptoms in healthy children. *J Am Acad Child Adolesc Psychiatry* 51(1):18–27.
170. Makris N, Biederman J, Valera EM, et al.: Cortical thinning of the attention and executive function networks in adults with attention deficit/hyperactivity disorder. *Cereb Cortex* 17:1364–1375, 2007.
171. Lou HC, Henricksen L, Bruhn P: Focal cerebral hypoperfusion in children with dysphasia and/or attention deficit hyperactivity disorder. *Arch Neurol* 41(8):825–829, 1984.
172. Lou HC, Henricksen L, Borner H, Nielsen JB: Striatal dysfunction in attention deficit and hyperkinetic disorder. *Arch Neurol* 46(1):48–52, 1989.
173. Lou HC, Henricksen L, Bruhn P: Focal cerebral dysfunction in developmental learning disabilities. *Lancet* 335(8680):8–11, 1990.
174. Lou HC, Andresen J, Steinberg B, McLaughlin T, Friberg L: The striatum in a putative cerebral network activated by verbal awareness in normals and in ADHD children. *Eur J Neurol* 5(1):67–74, 1998.
175. Sieg KG, Gaffney GR, Preston DF, Hellings JA: SPECT brain abnormalities in attention deficit hyperactivity disorder. *Clin Nucl Med* 20(1):55–60, 1995.

176. Amen DG, Carmichael BD: High resolution brain SPECT imaging in ADHD. *Ann Clin Psychiatry* 9(2):81–86, 1997.
177. Langleben DD, Austin G, Krikorian G, Ridlehuber HW, Goris ML, Strauss HW: Interhemispheric asymmetry of regional cerebral blood flow in prepubescent boys with attention deficit hyperactivity disorder. *Nucl Med Commun* 22(12):1333–1340, 2001.
178. Langleben DD, Acton PD, Austin G, et al.: Effects of methylphenidate discontinuation on cerebral blood flow in prepubescent boys with attention deficit hyperactivity disorder. *J Nucl Med* 43(12), 2002.
179. Spalletta G, Pasini A, Pau F, Guido G, Menghini L, Caltagirone C: Prefrontal blood flow dysregulation in drug naïve ADHD children without structural abnormalities. *J Neurol Transm* 108(10):1203–1216, 2001.
180. Kim BN, Lee JS, Cho SC, Lee DS: Methylphenidate increased regional cerebral blood flow in subjects with attention deficit hyperactivity disorder. *Yonsei Med J* 42(1):19–29, 2001.
181. Kim BN, Lee JS, Shin MS, Cho SC, Lee DS: Regional cerebral perfusion abnormalities in attention deficit hyperactivity disorder: statistical parametric mapping analysis. *Eur Arch Psychiatry Clin Neurosci* 252(5):219–225, 2002.
182. Sunshine JL, Lewis JS, Wu DH, et al.: Functional MR to localize sustained visual activation in patients with attention deficit hyperactivity disorder: a pilot study. *AJNR Am J Neuroradiol* 18(4):633–637, 1997.
183. Vaidya CJ, Austin G, Kirkorian G, et al.: Selective effects of methyl-phenidate in attention deficit hyperactivity disorder: a functional magnetic resonance study. *Proc Natl Acad Sci USA* 95(24):14494–14499, 1998.
184. Bush G, Frazier JA, Rauch SL, et al.: Anterior cingulated cortex dysfunction in attention deficit hyperactivity disorder revealed by fMRI and the Counting Stroop. *Biol Psychiatry* 45(12):1542–1552, 1999.
185. Rubia K, Overmeyer S, Taylor E, et al.: Hypofrontality in attention deficit hyperactivity disorder during higher-order motor control: a study with functional MRI. *Am J Psychiatry* 156(6):891–896, 1999.
186. Teicher MH, Anderson CM, Polcari A, Glod CA, Maas LC, Renshaw PF: Functional deficits in basal ganglia of children with attention deficit hyperactivity disorder shown with functional magnetic resonance imaging relaxometry. *Nat Med* 6(4):470–473, 2000.
187. Anderson CM, Polcari A, Lowen SB, Renshaw PF, Teicher MH: Effects of methylphenidate on functional magnetic resonance relaxometry of the cerebellar vermis in boys with ADHD. *Am J Psychiatry* 159:1322–1328, 2002.
188. Durston S: A review of the biological bases of ADHD: what have we learned from imaging studies? *Ment Retard Dev Disabil Res Rev* 9:184–195, 2003.
189. Schulz KP, Fan J, Tang CY, et al.: Response inhibition in adolescents diagnosed with attention deficit hyperactivity disorder during childhood: an event-related FMRI study. *Am J Psychiatry* 161:1650–1657, 2004.
190. Tamm L, Menon V, Ringel J, Reiss AL: Event-related FMRI evidence of frontotemporal involvement in aberrant response inhibition and task switching in attention-deficit/hyperactivity disorder. *J Am Acad Child Adolesc Psychiatry* 43:1430–1440, 2004.
191. Zametkin AJ, Nordahl TE, Gross M, et al.: Cerebral glucose metabolism in adults with hyperactivity of childhood onset. *N Engl J Med* 323:1361–1366, 1990.
192. Zametkin AJ, Liebenauer LL, Fitzgerald GA, et al.: Brain metabolism in teenagers with attention-deficit hyperactivity disorder. *Arch Gen Psychiatry* 50:333–340, 1993.
193. Matochik JA, Nordahl TE, Gross M, et al.: Effects of acute stimulant medication on cerebral metabolism in adults with hyperactivity. *Neuropsychopharmacology* 8:377–386, 1993.
194. Matochik JA, Liebenauer LL, King AC, Szymanski HV, Cohen RM, Zametkin A: Cerebral glucose metabolism in adults with attention deficit hyperactivity disorder after chronic stimulant treatment. *Am J Psychiatry* 151:658–664, 1994.
195. Ernst M, Liebenauer LL, King AC, Fitzgerald GA, Cohen RM, Zametkin A: Reduced brain metabolism in hyperactive girls. *J Am Acad Child Adolesc Psychiatry* 33:858–868, 1994a.
196. Ernst M, Zametkin AJ, Matochik JA, Liebenauer L, Fitzgerald GA, Cohen RM: Effects of intravenous dextroamphetamine on brain metabolism in adults with attention-deficit hyperactivity disorder (ADHD): preliminary findings. *Psychopharmacol Bull* 30:219–225, 1994b.
197. Ernst M, Zametkin AJ, Phillips RL, Cohen RM: Age-related changes in brain glucose metabolism in adults with attention-deficit/hyperactivity disorder and control subjects. *J Neuropsychiatry Clin Neurosci* 10:168–177, 1998.
198. Ernst M, Kimes AS, London ED, et al.: Neural substrates of decision making in adults with attention deficit hyperactivity disorder. *Am J Psychiatry* 160:1061–1070, 2003.
199. Schweitzer JB, Faber TL, Grafton ST, Tune LE, Hoffman JM, Kilts CD: Alterations in the functional anatomy of working memory in adult attention deficit hyperactivity disorder. *Am J Psychiatry* 157:278–280, 2000.
200. Schweitzer JB, Lee DO, Hanford RB, et al.: Positron emission tomography study of methylphenidate in adults with ADHD: alterations in resting blood flow and predicting treatment response. *Neuropsychopharmacology* 28:967–973, 2003.
201. Schweitzer JB, Lee DO, Hanford RB, et al.: Effect of methylphenidate on executive functioning in adults with attention-deficit/hyperactivity disorder: normalization of behavior but not related brain activity. *Biol Psychiatry* 56:597–606, 2004.
202. Dougherty DD, Bonab AA, Spencer TJ, Rauch SL, Madras BK, Fischman AJ: Dopamine transporter density in patients with attention deficit hyperactivity disorder. *Lancet* 354:2132–2133, 1999.
203. Dresel S, Krause J, Krause KH, et al.: Attention deficit hyperactivity disorder: Binding of [99mTc] TRODAT-1 to the dopamine transporter before and after methylphenidate treatment. *Eur J Nucl Med* 27:1518–1524, 2000.
204. Cheon KA, Ryu YH, Kim YK, Namkoong K, Kim CH, Lee JD: Dopamine transporter density in the basal ganglia assessed with [123I] IPT SPECT in children with attention deficit hyperactivity disorder. *Eur J Nucl Med Mol Imaging* 30:306–311, 2003.
205. van Dyke CH, Quinlan DM, Cretella LM, et al.: Unaltered dopamine transporter availability in adult attention deficit hyperactivity disorder. *Am J Psychiatry* 159:309–312, 2002.
206. Spencer T: In vivo neuroreceptor imaging of attention-deficit/hyperactivity disorder: a focus on the dopamine transporter. *Biol Psychiatry* 57:1293–1300, 2005.
207. Spencer TJ, Biederman J, Ciccone PE, et al.: PET study examining pharmacokinetics, detection and likeability, and dopamine transporter receptor occupancy of short-and long-acting oral methylphenidate. *Am J Psychiatry* 163(3):387–395, 2006.
208. Jucaite A, Fernell E, Halldin C, Forssberg H, Farde L: Reduced midbrain dopamine transporter binding in male adolescents with attention-deficit/hyperactivity disorder: association between striatal dopamine markers and motor hyperactivity. *Biol Psychiatry* 57:229–238, 2005.
209. Rosa-Neto P, Lou H, Cumming P, et al.: Methylphenidate evoked changes in striatal dopamine correlate with inattention and impulsivity in adolescents with attention deficit hyperactivity disorder. *NeuroImage* 25:868–876, 2005.
210. Jin Z, Zang YF, Zeng YW, Zhang L, Wang YF: Striatal neuronal loss or dysfunction and choline rise in children with attention-deficit hyperactivity disorder: a 1H-magnetic resonance spectroscopy study. *Neurosci Lett* 315:45–48, 2001.
211. MacMaster FP, Carrey N, Sparkes S, Kusumakar V: Proton spectroscopy in medication free pediatric attention deficit hyperactivity disorder. *Biol Psychiatry* 53:184–187, 2003.
212. Yeo RA, Hill DE, Campbell RA, et al.: Proton magnetic resonance spectroscopy investigation of the right frontal lobe in children with attention-deficit/hyperactivity disorder. *J Am Acad Child Adolesc Psychiatry* 42:303–310, 2003.
213. Courvoisie H, Hooper SR, Fine C, Kwock L, Castillo M: Neurometabolic functioning and neuropsychological correlates in children with ADHD-H: Preliminary findings. *J Neuropsychiatry Clin Neurosci* 16:63–69, 2004.
214. Moore CM, Biederman J, Wozniak J, et al.: Differences in brain chemistry in children and adolescents with attention deficit hyperactivity disorder with and without comorbid bipolar disorder: a proton magnetic resonance spectroscopy study. *Am J Psychiatry* 163:316–318, 2006.
215. Doyle AE, Seidman LJ, Biederman J, Chourinard VA, Silva J, Faraone SV: Attention deficit hyperactivity disorder endophenotypes. *Biol Psychiatry* 57:1313–1323, 2005.
216. Bledsoe J, Semrud-Clikeman M, Pliszka SR: A magnetic resonance imaging study of the cerebellar vermis in chronically treated and treatment-naïve children with attention deficit/hyperactivity disorder combined type. *Biol Psychiatry* 65:620–624, 2009.
217. Pliszka SR, Lancaster J, Liotti M, Semrud-Clikeman M: Volumetric MRI differences in treatment-naïve vs chronically treated children with ADHD. *Neurology* 67:1023–1027, 2006.
218. Rubia K, Alegria AA, Cubillo AI, Smith AB, Brammer MJ, Radua J: Effects of stimulants on brain function in attention deficit/hyperactivity disorder: a systematic review and meta-analysis. *Biol Psychiatry* 76:616–628, 2014.
219. Jasper H, Solomon P, Bradley C: Electroencephalographic analyses of behaviour problem children. *Am J Psychiatry* 95:641–658, 1938.
220. Mann C, Lubar J, Zimmerman A, Miller C, Muenchen R: Quantitative analysis of EEG in boys with attention deficit hyperactivity disorder—controlled study with clinical implications. *Pediatr Neurol* 8:30–36, 1992.
221. Chabot R, Merkin H, Wood L, Davenport T, Serfontein G: Sensitivity and specificity of QEEG in children with attention deficit hyperactivity disorder or specific developmental learning disorders. *Clin Electroencephalogr* 27:26–34, 1996.
222. Monastra V, Lubar J, Linden M, et al.: Assessing attention deficit hyperactivity disorder via quantitative electroencephalography: an initial validation study. *Neuropsychology* 13:424–433, 1999.
223. Arns M, Conners CK, Kraemer HC: A Decade of EEG Theta/Beta Ratio Research in ADHD: A Meta-Analysis. *J Attention Disord* 17(5):374–383, 2011.
224. Kinsbourne M: Minimal brain dysfunction as a neurodevelopmental lag. *Ann NY Acad Sci* 205:268–273, 1973.
225. Satterfield J, Lesser M, Saul R, Cantwell D: EEG aspects in the diagnosis and treatment of minimal brain dysfunction. *Ann N Y Acad Sci* 205:274–282, 1973.
226. Matsuura M, Ojubo Y, Toru M, et al.: A cross national EEG study of children with emotional and behavioural problems: a WHO collaborative study in the Western Pacific region. *Biol Psychiatry* 34:52–58, 1993.
227. John E, Princhep L, Easton P: Normative data banks and neurometrics: basic concepts, method and results of norm construction. In: Gevins A, Remond A (eds.): *Handbook of Electroencephalography and Clinical Neurophysiology 1*. Amsterdam, Elsevier, 919–923, 1987.

228. Clarke A, Barry R, McCarthy R, Selikowitz M: EEG analysis in attention deficit hyperactivity disorder: a comparative study of two subtypes. *Psychiatry Res* 81:19–29, 1998.
229. Lazzaro I, Gordon E, Whitmont S, et al.: Quantitative EEG activity in adolescent attention deficit hyperactivity disorder. *Clin Electroencephalogr* 29:37–42, 1998.
230. Klinkerfuss G, Lange P, Weinberg W, O'Leary J: Electroencephalo-graphic abnormalities of children with hyperkinetic behaviour. *Neurology* 15:883–891, 1965.
231. Wikler A, Dixon J, Parker J: Brain function in children and controls: Psychometric, neurological and electroencephalographic comparisons. *Am J Psychiatry* 127:634–645, 1970.
232. John E, Princhep L, Ahn H, Easton P, Fridman J, Kaye H: Neurometric evaluation of cognitive dysfunctions and neurological disorders in children. *Prog Neurobiol* 21:239–290, 1983.
233. Clarke A, Barry R, McCarthy R, Selikowitz M: EEG differences in two subtypes of attention deficit hyperactivity disorder. *Psychophysiology* 38:212–221, 2001.
234. Clarke A, Barry R, McCarthy R, Selikowitz M: EEG defined subtypes of children with attention deficit hyperactivity disorder. *Clin Neurophysiol* 112:2098–2105, 2001.
235. Satterfield J, Cantwell D: CNS function and response to methylphenidate in hyperactive children. *Psychopharmacol Bull* 10:36–37, 1974.
236. Satterfield J, Cantwell D, Saul R, Lesser M, Podsin R: Response to stimulant drug treatment in hyperactive children: predictions from EEG and neurological findings. *J Autism Child Schizophr* 3:36–48, 1973.
237. Satterfield J, Cantwell D, Satterfield B: Pathophysiology of the hyperactive child syndrome. *Arch Gen Psychiatry* 31:839–844, 1974.
238. Grunewald-Zuberbier E, Grunewald G, Rasche A: Hyperactive behaviour and EEG arousal reactions in children. *Electroenceph Clin Neurophysiol* 38:149–159, 1975.
239. Ackerman P, Dykman R, Oglesby D, Newton J: EEG power spectra of children with dyslexia, slow learners, and normally reading children with ADD during verbal processing. *J Learn Disabil* 27:619–630, 1994.
240. Lubar J, Swartwood J, O'Donnell P: Evaluation of the effectiveness of EEG neurofeedback training for ADHD in a clinical setting as measured by changes in T.O.V.A. scores, behavioral ratings, and WISC-R performance. *Biofeedback Self Regul* 20:83–99, 1995.
241. Kovatchev B, Cox D, Hill R, Reeve R, Robeva R, Loboschefski T: A psychophysiological marker of attention deficit hyperactivity disorder—defining the EEG consistency index. *Appl Psychophysiol Biofeedback* 26:127–140, 2001.
242. Barry R, Johnstone SJ, Clarke AR: A review of electrophysiology in attention deficit hyperactivity disorder—event related potentials. *Clin Neurophysiol* 114:184–198, 2003.
243. van Beijsterveldt CE, van Baal GC: Twin and family studies of the human electroencephalogram: a review and a meta-analysis. *Biol Psychol* 61:111–138, 2002.
244. Arnold LE: Treatment alternatives for attention-deficit/hyperactivity disorder. In: Jensen PS, Cooper J (eds.): *Attention Deficit Hyperactivity Disorder: State of the Science; Best Practices.* Kingston, NJ: Civic Research Institute, 2002.
245. Rojas NL, Chan E: Old and new controversies in the alternative treatment of attention-deficit/hyperactivity disorder. *Mental Retard Dev Disabil Res Rev* 11:116–130, 2005.
246. Rovet J, Alvarez M: Thyroid hormone and attention in school-age children with congenital hypothyroidism. *J Child Psychol Psychiatry* 37:579–585, 1996.
247. Hauser P, Soler R, Brucker-Davis F, Weintraub BD: Thyroid hormones correlate with symptoms of hyperactivity but not inattention in ADHD. *Psychoneuroendocrinology* 22:107–114, 1997.
248. David OJ, Hoffman SP, Clark J, Grad G, Sverd J: The relationship of hyperactivity to moderately elevated lead levels. *Arch Environ Health* 38:341-B 346, 1983.
249. Mette C, Zimmermann M, Grabemann M et al: The impact of acute tryptophan depletion on attentional performance in adult patients with ADHD. *Acta Psychiatr Scand* 128: 124–132, 2013.
250. Kotting WF, Bubenzer S, Helmbold K, Eisert A et al: Effects of tryptophan depletion on reactive aggression and aggressive decision-making in young people with ADHD. *Acta Psychiatr Scand* 128: 114–123, 2013.
251. Goksugur SB, Tufan AE, Semiz M, Gunes C, et al: Vitamin D status in children with attention-deficit-hyperactivity disorder. *Pediatr Int* 56: 515–519, 2014.
252. DuPaul GJ, Power TJ, Anastopoulos AD, Reid R: *ADHD Rating Scale-IV: Checklists, Norms, and Clinical Interpretations.* New York, Guilford Press, 1998.
253. Conners, CK: *Manual for Conners' Rating Scales.* 3rd ed. Pearson's Clinical Assessment Group: Pearson PsychCorp, 2008.
254. Gustaffson P, Thernlund G, Ryding E, Rosen I, Cederblad, M. Associations between cerebral blood-flow measured by single photon computed tomography (SPECT), electro-encephalogram (EEG), behaviour symptoms, cognition and neurological soft signs in children with attention deficit hyperactivity disorder. *Acta Paediatr* 89(7):830–835, 2000.
255. Dickstein DP, Garvey M, Pradella AG, et al.: Neurologic examination abnormalities in children with attention deficit hyperactivity disorder. *Biol Psychiatry* 58:517–524, 2005.
256. The MTA Cooperative Group: A 14-month randomized clinical trial of treatment strategies for attention-deficit/hyperactivity disorder. *Arch Gen Psychiatry* 56:1073–1086, 1999a.
257. Hechtman L, Etcovitch J, Platt R, et al.: Does multimodal treatment of ADHD decrease other diagnoses? *Clin Neurosci Res* 5(5/6), 273–282, 2005.
258. Welsh MC, Pennington BF: Assessing frontal lobe functioning in children: views from developmental psychology. *Dev Neuropsychol* 4:199–230, 1988.
259. Kasper LJ, Alderson RM, Hudec KL: Moderators of working memory deficits in children with attention deficit /hyperactivity disorder (ADHD): a meta-analytic review. *Clin Psychol Rev* 32:605–617, 2012.
260. Schoechlin C, Engel RR: Neuropsychological performance in adult attention deficit hyperactivity disorder: meta-analysis of empirical data. *Arch Clin Neuropsychol* 20:727–744, 2005.
261. Sonuga-Barke EJS: On dysfunction and function in psychological accounts of childhood disorder. *J Child Psychol Psychiat* 35:801–815, 1994.
262. Ployelis Y, Asherson P, Kuntsi J: Are ADHD symptoms associated with delay aversion or choice impulsivity? A general population study. *J Am Acad Child Adolesc Psychiatry* 48(8):837–846, 2009.
263. Killeen PR: Models of ADHD: five ways smaller sooner is better. *J Neurosci Methods* 252:2–13, 2015.
264. Sergeant J: The cognitive energetic model: an empirical approach to attention deficit hyperactivity disorder. *Neurosci Biobehav Rev* 24:7–12, 2000.
265. McBurnett K, Pfiffner LJ, Frick PJ: Symptom properties as a function of ADHD type: an argument for continued study of sluggish cognitive tempo. *J Abnorm Child Psychol* 29:207–213, 2001.
266. Nigg JT, Goldsmith HH, Sachek J: Temperament and attention deficit hyperactivity disorder: the development of a multiple pathway model. *J Clin Child Adolesc Psychol* 33, 1:42–53, 2004.
267. Gomez R, Corr PJ: ADHD and personality: a meta-analytic review. *Clin Psychol Rev* 34: 376–388, 2014.
268. Biederman J, Mick E, Faraone SV: Age dependent decline of symptoms of attention deficit hyperactivity disorder: impact of remission definition and symptom type. *Am J Psychiatry* 157:816–818, 2000.
269. Kessler RC, Lenard AA, Barkley R, et al.: Patterns and predictors of attention deficit hyperactivity disorder persistence in adulthood: results from the National Comorbidity Survey Replication. *Biol Psychiatry* 57:1442–1451, 2005.
270. Danckaerts M, Sonuga-Barke EJ, Banschewski T, Buitelaar J, et al.: The quality of life of children with attention deficit/hyperactivity disorder: a systematic review. *Eur Child Adolesc Psychiatry* 19:83–105, 2010.
271. Jiang Y, Johnston C: Co-occurring aggressive and depressive symptoms as related to overestimations of competence in children with attention deficit/hyperactivity disorder. *Clin Child Fam Psychol Review* 17:157–172, 2014.
272. Kessler RC, Lenard AA, Barkley R, et al.: Patterns and predictors of attention deficit hyperactivity disorder persistence in adulthood: results from the National Comorbidity Survey Replication. *Biol Psychiatry* 57:1442–1451, 2005.
273. Brownell MD, Yogendran MS: Attention deficit hyperactivity disorder in manitoba children: medical diagnosis and psychostimulant treatment rates. *Can J Psychiatry* 46:264–272, 2001.
274. American Academy of Pediatrics Subcommittee on Attention Deficit/Hyperactivity Disorder, Steering Committee on Quality Improvement and Management: ADHD: clinical practice guideline for the diagnosis, evaluation, and treatment of attention deficit/hyperactivity disorder in children and adolescents. *Pediatrics* 128(5):1007–1022, 2011.
275. Conners CK, Epstein JN, March JS, et al.: Multimodal treatment of ADHD in the MTA: an alternative outcome analysis. *J Amer Acad Child & Adolesc Psychiatry* 40:159–167, 2001.
276. Farmer C, Brown NV, Gadow KD, Arnold LE, et al: Comorbid symptomatology moderates response to risperidone, stimulant, and parent training in children with severe aggression, disruptive behavior disorder, and attention deficit/hyperactivity disorder. *J Child Adolesc Psychopharmacology* 25(3):213–224, 2015.
277. Jensen PS, Hinshaw SP, Kraemer HC, et al.: ADHD comorbidity findings from the MTA study: comparing comorbid subgroups. *J Amer Acad Child & Adolesc Psychiatry* 40:147–158, 2001.
278. Arnold LE: *A Family Guide to ADHD.* Newtown, PA: Handbooks in Health Care Co., 2004.
279. Arnold LE, Lofthouse N, Hersch S, et al.: EEG neurofeedback for ADHD: double-blind-sham-controlled randomized pilot feasibility trial. *J Attention Disord* 17(5):410–419, 2013.
280. Lofthouse N, Hurt E, Arnold LE: Complementary and alternative treatments for pediatric and adult ADHD. In: Adler L, Spencer TJ, and Wilens TE (eds): *Attention Deficit Hyperactivity Disorder in Adults and Children,* Chapter 24. University Printing House, Cambridge CB2 8BS United Kingdom: Cambridge University Press, 2014.
281. Hurt E, Arnold LE: Dietary management of ADHD in attention-deficit hyperactivity disorder. In: Barkley RA (ed): *A Handbook for Diagnosis and Treatment,* 4th ed., Chapter 25. Guilford Press, 2014.
282. 36-month MTA follow-up and other new insights into ADHD treatment. Symposium at 51st Annual Meeting American Academy of Child and Adolescent Psychiatry, October 19–24, Washington, DC, 2004.

CHAPTER 5.1.2 ■ OPPOSITIONAL DEFIANT AND CONDUCT DISORDERS

JOSEPH M. REY, GARRY WALTER, AND CESAR A. SOUTULLO

Children and adolescent who are sullen, argumentative, uncooperative, miss school, and lie about their whereabouts, refuse to adhere to curfews, steal money from home, etc. represent one of the largest group of patients seen in child and adolescent mental health settings; they are usually labeled as suffering from oppositional defiant disorder (ODD), conduct disorder (CD), or disruptive behavior disorder (DBD). The last term was often used to include also children with attention-deficit hyperactivity disorder (ADHD). However, in this chapter, the term DBD refers only to young people with ODD or CD. The cost of DBDs to the individuals themselves, their families, and society is high (1,2).

Individuals with ODD and CD share many characteristics. For example, their conduct is socially unacceptable, they cause disruption or distress to others more than to themselves (i.e., they "externalize" their problems), and they are more likely to be male and to find it difficult to learn from experience. Yet, they also differ widely from one another: they may be aggressive or not, break the law or not, feel guilt and empathy or not, may be sensation-seeking or not. Although ODD and CD represent well-characterized, reliable behavioral syndromes, they do not fit easily into a traditional "illness" model because children with these problems are heterogeneous in relation to etiology, natural history, response to treatment, and outcome. This is similar to what happens with heart disease, where multiple factors contribute to the pathology and other illness characteristics, but the construct has heuristic value. Because of their heterogeneity, the usefulness of a diagnosis of ODD or CD for treatment planning is limited. For example, "an 8-year old child who initiates fights, bullies others, and hurts animals and a 16-year-old adolescent who sets fires, steals from others' homes and is truant from school would both receive a diagnosis of CD" despite having a very different picture and probably requiring a different management (3). An emphasis on identifying each child's problems and modifying the individual risk factors is likely to be the best way of managing these disorders, as is the case with heart disease.

ODD and CD are described together here to highlight their similarities and differences and to avoid unnecessary repetitions. The content of this chapter overlaps and should be read in conjunction with topics discussed in other parts of the book.

CLASSIFICATION

DSM-5 and ICD-11

DSM-5 (4) incorporated only minor modifications to the DBDs—criteria for diagnosis remaining the same as in DSM-IV—but are grouped differently. In DSM-5, ODD and CD have been placed in the chapter "Disruptive, Impulse-Control, and Conduct Disorders" together with conditions such as intermittent explosive disorder, pyromania, kleptomania, and antisocial personality disorder (ASPD). This grouping seems to assume that these conditions—involving problems with self-control that impinge on others—are part of a continuum with ODD at one end and ASPD at the other. In the provisional draft of ICD-11 (5), impulse control disorders other than ODD and CD are listed in a separate chapter (see Table 5.1.2.1). At this stage, ICD-11 is not expected to provide diagnostic criteria but model descriptions of the disorders.

While criteria for ODD have not been changed, in DSM-5 symptoms are grouped into three types: angry/irritable mood, argumentative/defiant behavior, and vindictiveness—highlighting the emotional and behavioral aspects of the syndrome (Table 5.1.2.2). In DSM-IV, a diagnosis of CD pre-empted a diagnosis of ODD; this exclusion has been removed in DSM-5. That is, individuals can be diagnosed as suffering from both ODD and CD concurrently. Criteria for CD remain the same as in DSM-IV (6) but the specifier "with limited prosocial emotions" has been added in DSM-5. This specifier applies to young people with CD who show a callous and unemotional interpersonal style across multiple settings and relationships (see below).

The clustering of ODD symptoms in DSM-5 in a subgroup of anger/irritability and another of argumentativeness/defiance is supported by studies showing that these behaviors tend to occur together and predicted, respectively, internalizing and externalizing behavior later on (7,8).

DSM-III (9) divided CD into four subgroups according to whether children are socialized or undersocialized, and aggressive or nonaggressive (e.g., socialized/aggressive; socialized/nonaggressive). This was changed in DSM-III-R to "solitary type" and "group type." DSM-IV classified CD according to age of onset (childhood- or adolescent-onset type, depending on whether there were symptoms prior to the age of 10 years). DSM-5 retains the same two types and adds the further specifier of "with limited prosocial emotions."

In recent years, there has been a resurgence in interest on the traditionally described as "psychopathic" traits, in the case of young people often referred to with the term "callous–unemotional." These youth are described in DSM-5 as "with limited prosocial emotions." This label defines children and adolescents who show lack of remorse and guilt after doing something wrong, do not care about the negative consequences of their actions, appear cold and uncaring, show no concern for the feelings of others, are undaunted by their poor performance at school, and their emotions appear shallow or insincere. These young people respond poorly to punishment, show lower cortisol levels, seek novel, exciting, and dangerous activities, are prone to boredom, and have lower trait anxiety than other youth with the same level of conduct problems (4,10).

ICD-10 (11) describes three subtypes of CD: confined to the family context, unsocialized, and socialized. It is not clear what subtypes, if any, will be included in ICD-11.

TABLE 5.1.2.1

COMPARISON BETWEEN DSM-5 AND ICD-11[a] CLASSIFICATION AND DESCRIPTION OF DISRUPTIVE BEHAVIOUR DISORDERS

	DSM-5	ICD-11[a]
Chapter	Disruptive, impulse control and conduct disorders	Disruptive behavior and dissocial disorders
Disorders included	• Oppositional defiant disorder • Conduct disorder • Intermittent explosive disorder • Pyromania • Kleptomania • Antisocial personality disorder • Other specified disruptive, impulse control and conduct disorder	• Oppositional defiant disorder • Conduct–dissocial disorder • Other specified disruptive behavior and dissocial disorders
ODD	• A pattern lasting more than 6 mo of angry or irritable mood, argumentative and defiant behavior, or vindictiveness and exhibited at least with one individual who is not a sibling as manifested by the presence of at least 4 of 9 behaviors in the previous 6 mo (see Table 5.1.2.2) • Associated with distress in the individual or others or results in significant impairment in in functioning	• A pattern lasting more than 6 mo of markedly defiant, disobedient, provocative or spiteful behavior that occurs more frequently than is typically observed in individuals of comparable age and developmental level and that is not restricted to interaction with siblings • Of sufficient severity to result in significant impairment.

CD	• A repetitive and persistent pattern of behavior in which the basic rights of others or major age-appropriate societal norms or rules are violated, as manifested by the presence of at least 3 of 15 behaviors in the previous 12 mo (see Table 5.1.2.2).
	• These behaviors results in significant impairment in personal, family, social, or academic functioning
	• Specifiers:
	  • Of childhood- or adolescent-onset
	  • With limited prosocial emotions
		• A repetitive and persistent pattern of behavior in which the basic rights of others or major age-appropriate societal norms, rules, or laws are violated
		• The behavior pattern must be enduring over a significant period of time (e.g., 6 mo or more). Isolated dissocial or criminal acts are not in themselves grounds for the diagnosis.

[a]Beta draft (5). The ICD-11 working definitions are not final, are subject to change, and have not been approved by the WHO.
ODD, oppositional defiant disorder; CD, conduct disorder.

TABLE 5.1.2.2

BEHAVIORS[a] SUGGESTIVE OF OPPOSITIONAL DEFIANT DISORDER (ODD) AND CONDUCT DISORDER (CD) ACCORDING TO DSM-5[b]

Oppositional Defiant Disorder	Conduct Disorder
Anger/Irritability 1. Losing temper 2. Touchy or easily annoyed 3. Angry and resentful **Argumentativeness/Defiance** 4. Arguing with adults 5. Defying or refusing to comply with adults' requests or rules 6. Deliberately annoying people 7. Blaming others for their mistakes or misbehavior **Vindictiveness** 8. Spiteful and vindictive	**Aggressiveness** 1. Bullying, threatening or intimidating others 2. Initiating physical fights 3. Has used a weapon 4. Physically cruel to people 5. Physically cruel to animals 6. Stealing while confronting a victim 7. Forcing someone into sexual activity **Destruction of Property** 8. Setting fires 9. Destroying others' property **Deceitfulness or Theft** 10. Breaking into someone's house, building or car 11. Lying to obtain goods or favors or to avoid obligations 12. Stealing without confronting a victim **Serious Violations of Rules** 13. Staying out at night before age 13 despite parental prohibitions 14. Running away from home overnight 15. Truanting from school before age 13

[a]Wording is summarized.
[b]ICD-11 does not envisage including criteria for diagnosis; it plans to provide diagnostic descriptions instead.

Some researchers have emphasized the importance for outcome of overt (characterized by confrontation and fighting) and covert (typified by deception, such as stealing and lying) symptoms (12), which overlaps with the aggressive–nonaggressive distinction. There are data showing that two different types of covert antisocial behavior may exist: property violations (e.g., stealing) and status offenses (truancy, running away). Other scholars suggest that life-course persistent (beginning during childhood and persisting past adolescence) and adolescence limited is a prognostically useful distinction (13), and this has been incorporated in DSM-5.

Comorbidity

The vexatious issue of comorbidity is highly relevant for ODD and CD since both often co-occur with other diagnoses. The most frequent comorbidities are with ADHD (about 10 times more often than expected (14)), major depression (about seven times (14)), and substance abuse (in adolescents, about four times (15)). According to ICD-10, CD is not diagnosed if ADHD is present (it would warrant a diagnosis of hyperkinetic CD), or if CD is associated with emotional disorders (mixed disorder of conduct and emotions). It is not clear yet how ICD-11 will deal with this issue. In similar circumstances, DSM-5 allows multiple diagnoses to be made (e.g., ODD *and* CD, ODD *and* ADHD, CD *and* major depression). However, a diagnosis of ODD or CD should not be made if symptoms occur exclusively during the course of a psychotic, substance use, depressive, or bipolar disorder, and the young person does not meet criteria for disruptive mood dysregulation disorder.

Reliability

The diagnoses of ODD and CD have acceptable interrater and test–retest reliability, comparable to or better than the reliability of most psychiatric diagnoses in young people (16,17). Agreement varies according to the informant and age of the child, being usually higher when parent or teacher reports or multiple informants are used, for aggressive than nonaggressive behaviors, and in older children or adolescents. Reliability is also higher in clinic than in community samples due to base rate issues. For example, test–retest agreement of CD using the NIMH Diagnostic Interview Schedule for Children Version IV in a clinic sample was $K = 0.70$ for parents as informants, 0.86 for children, and 0.71 when using data from both. The parallel results in a community sample were 0.56, 0.64, and 0.66 (17). Reliability of ODD is lower, in the range of $K = 0.4–0.6$ (16,17).

Validity

Developmental Considerations

Children's prosocial impulses already become apparent in the first year of life, for example, through cooperative interactions and sharing. Learning how to deal with and tolerate frustration are important aspects of the socialization process. A degree of defiance and noncompliance is normal in toddlers, probably reflecting the child's assertiveness and search for autonomy or ignorance of what parents are prepared to tolerate. Notwithstanding this, toddlers' behavior may already be indicative of problems when it is too intense, persistent, or pervasive. However, there are considerable individual variations and distinguishing behaviors that are within the normal range from problematic defiance or noncompliance is difficult at that age. Prosocial behaviors usually increase up to the age of 3 years; a temporary decline then begins to emerge. Defiance and noncompliance, particularly in boys, may also increase about the age of 2 or 3 years.

Males report greater involvement in physical fights (58% of grade 9 students in the United States) than females (43%). Among US students, physical fighting generally decreases with age, from 43% among grade 9 females to 25% in grade 12; the corresponding figures for males being 58% and 42%. There has also been a reduction in reports of involvement in physical fights from 1991 to 2013: a decrease of 43% in grade 9 males and 46% among females (18).

ODD symptoms appear earlier than CD symptoms. Aggressive behavior (hitting, biting, smashing objects) is common in 4 to 8 year olds and decreases with age, although severely aggressive acts typically start after puberty. Covert antisocial actions such as property and status violations (stealing, truancy, running away) increase as children become older, being more prevalent during adolescence. Early adolescence is often associated with an increase in rebellious behavior. Teachers' reports indicate that most oppositional symptoms, such as arguing, screaming, disobedience, and defiance, peak between 8 and 11 years and then decline in frequency.

Stability and Change

Disruptive behaviors are quite prevalent in children but often extinguish as they grow older. However, many data show that CD symptoms are more enduring than changeable (19). Callous–unemotional traits can be identified as early as 2 years of age and are present in about half of the children who meet criteria for CD. It is possible that callus–unemotional traits are largely responsible for the stability of CD, although they can change from childhood to adulthood (they remain in about 20% to 30% of youth) (20,21).

ODD and CD

The relationship between ODD and CD is complex. In some children, ODD symptoms begin in infancy, persist during childhood, and evolve into CD, often after puberty. Other young people show noncompliance and defiance for short periods or do not progress to CD; this may occur more often in females than in males (22). Oppositional behavior is present only at home in some children, while symptoms occur in most settings in others. ODD often starts in the family context and generalizes to other settings over time. Taken together, these and other findings already mentioned suggest that ODD and CD are best considered as distinguishable if highly correlated dimensions of psychopathology at the phenotypic level (23).

Adult Outcomes

The continuity between childhood CD and adult ASPD has long been known (24), so much so that DSM-5 requires evidence of CD symptoms prior to the age of 15 to make a diagnosis of ASPD—implying that ODD, CD, and ASPD are part of a dimension of psychopathology.

Data are mounting showing that childhood DBDs are associated not only with ASPD but with a wide range of other psychiatric disorders in adulthood (e.g., substance abuse, major depression, psychosis), as well as with many adverse outcomes such as suicidal behavior, delinquency, educational difficulties, unemployment, and teenage pregnancy (25–28). For example, in a cohort studied prospectively, 25% to 60% of adults with any psychiatric diagnosis had a history of CD or ODD (25). The association, which applies equally to males and females (26), reflects not only the already noted stability of disruptive behaviors, but also the fact that childhood DBDs often trigger a chain of events that increase the likelihood of such unfavorable outcomes (e.g., early defiance may lead to harsh parental discipline, aggressiveness, and peer rejection, which may in turn be followed by association with deviant peers, antisocial acts, substance use, conflict with the law, and mental illness). Studies by and large show a dose–response relationship: The higher the number and variety of disruptive behaviors, the worse the adult outcomes. This said, most adolescents with CD do not develop ASPD in adulthood. A large decline in delinquent and antisocial activities is a commonly reported phenomenon in early adulthood (29). It is not clear if this parallels a reduction in DBDs or if their manifestations change with age (e.g., whether behaviors extinguish, mutate into other psychiatric problems, or delinquent acts become more covert). This decline may reflect the existence of a *desisting* adolescent-limited CD—as opposite to a life-course *persistent* (13). Early onset (displaying mostly ODD symptoms), severity, and exposure to risk factors would predict the latter group (29).

Most epidemiologic studies in adults have neglected to examine the prevalence of the so-called childhood-onset disorders. A survey of people older than 18 years in the United States reported a 12-month prevalence of 1% each for ODD and CD (30). Thus, ODD symptoms can persist into adulthood and significantly interfere with functioning, particularly in social or interpersonal contexts (31). Symptoms consistent with ODD can, therefore, be found in adults although it is not clear whether they appear *de novo* or—more likely—are a continuation of childhood problems.

There is less information about what happens to children with ODD who do not develop CD when they grow up. Some data suggest heterotypic continuity between symptoms of irritability (losing temper, being touchy or easily annoyed, angry and resentful) and later internalizing problems, particularly depression, which is not gender specific (32). Chronic irritability during the preschool years is associated with a variety of anxiety, depressive and DBD symptoms, functional impairment, and service use 6 years later (33).

In relation to criminality, individuals with high levels of psychopathic traits are more likely to engage in criminal behavior but individuals engaging in criminal activities do not necessarily have high levels of psychopathic traits. Nevertheless, adolescents with callous–unemotional traits are at a higher risk of violent reoffending earlier than their young offender peers and appear to be more chronic in their adolescent offending (21).

EPIDEMIOLOGY

Prevalence

Estimates of the prevalence of ODD and CD vary depending on the population, diagnostic criteria, instrument used, period considered (point or lifetime), and informant. Recent surveys (mostly using DSM-IV criteria) in several countries have produced reasonably consistent results, summarized in Table 5.1.2.3. Overall, about 3% of children aged 6 to 18 years met criteria for ODD or CD in the previous 3 or 6 months, slightly lower rates than those reported in earlier studies using DSM-III or DSM-III-R criteria (34).

An examination of questionnaire data of 6 to 17 year olds from nine cultures showed that cultural differences had a small effect on delinquent behavior (1%) and aggressive behavior (5%) syndromes (35). ODD and CD are two to three times more prevalent in males than females, though this may vary according to age. Earlier studies suggested that ODD was more prevalent in children (this was incorporated in ICD-10, where diagnosis of ODD is discouraged after the age of 10 years), while CD was more prevalent in adolescents. Epidemiologic data is inconsistent with this view; prevalence across studies is similar in both age groups.

TABLE 5.1.2.3

PREVALENCE (PERCENT) OF OPPOSITIONAL DEFIANT DISORDER (ODD) AND CONDUCT DISORDER (CD) IN SELECTED EPIDEMIOLOGIC STUDIES

	ODD					CD				
Sample	Male	Female	Children	Adolescents	Total	Male	Female	Children	Adolescents	Total
3,171 Australian children aged 6–17 yrs (95)						4.4	1.6	4.4	2.4	3.0
1,420 children from North Carolina aged 9–13 yrs (96)	3.1	2.1	2.0	3.0	2.7	4.2	1.2	2.4	2.7	2.7
10,438 British 5–15 yr olds (97)	3.2	1.4	2.6	1.4	2.3	2.1	0.8	0.9	3.3	1.5
1,886 children aged 4–17 yrs from Puerto Rico (98)					2.0					5.5
1,251 children aged 7–14 yrs attending school in Brazil (99)					3.2					2.2
541 students in Hong Kong (100)	6.9	6.8		6.8		1.9	1.4		1.7	
6,150 children aged 7–9 yrs in Norway (101)	4.0	1.3	2.7		2.7					
10,148 US adolescents aged 13–17 yrs (102)				8.3					5.4	
1,049 school students aged 6–16 in Spain (103)	6.8	4.3			5.6					

Secular Changes

It has been suggested that children, particularly females, born later in the 20th century show higher rates of antisocial behavior than those born earlier (36). Conversely, changes in diagnostic criteria may have led to a progressive "masculinization" of the disorder over time because aggressive girls use verbal abuse more often than physical fighting (37). This is difficult to verify given the limitations of epidemiologic surveys (e.g., changes in diagnostic criteria over time). Indirect approaches, such as variations in juvenile delinquency rates or arrests, are also hazardous because of legal and law enforcement changes over time.

ETIOLOGY

The literature on etiologic and risk factors for DBDs is voluminous and compelling but rather nonspecific; it makes reference to ODD, CD, aggression, juvenile offending, and disruptive behaviors defined in a variety of ways (e.g., (38–43)). Data specific to ODD are scarce. This is not necessarily a major issue given the nature and heterogeneity of the DBDs. Dodge and Pettit (44) note that the model used to study and treat or prevent heart disease is applicable to disruptive behavior problems. Both are vaguely defined, heterogeneous constructs but with easily identifiable outcomes, such as a myocardial infarction or, in the case of disruptive behaviors, truancy. While the traditional goal in medicine is to identify a cluster of symptoms and then to seek a single causal agent, this is not appropriate for heart disease or DBDs, where a single causal agent does not exist. Multiple risk factors or vulnerabilities contribute to the development of heart disease and DBDs, and their recognition has allowed the implementation of successful preventive interventions.

Inheritance

Heritability of antisocial behavior has been estimated at about 50%, though it is not diagnosis specific (45). It appears that what might be transmitted is a general liability to externalizing disorders although there are also disorder-specific liabilities (e.g., for ADHD). Shared environment may specifically influence CD, highlighting the importance of examining shared environmental variables as processes underlying the comorbidity among ODD and CD (46). Although it needs further corroboration, a study showed that an allele of the neurotransmitter-metabolizing enzyme monoamine oxidase A gene increased the risk for adult antisocial behavior among individuals who had experienced childhood adversity (47).

Risk Factors

Well-known risk factors are listed in Table 5.1.2.4. It is important to emphasize that a large component of the association between risk factors, DBDs, and poor outcomes is probably noncausal. Risk factors include, among others, socioeconomic disadvantage, exposure to family violence and dysfunction, lower IQ, and attentional difficulties (e.g., (26,38–47)).

Interactions between risk factors are complex. First, the accumulation of risk may not only act additively, but also multiplicatively. For example, impulsivity may convey a small risk for a child developing CD, but in combination with other factors (e.g., poor socializing experiences, harsh discipline), the risk for antisocial outcomes becomes quite high. Second, while genes are important, they interact with, and are modified by environmental variables in complex ways (48). Thus, it has been shown that genetic influences are stronger in children from poor families than in those from affluent backgrounds (49), and that heritability of problem behavior is significantly lower in children with very low birth weight in relation to gestational age than in those with a normal birth weight (50). Third, genetic factors influence individuals' choices and shaping of their own environment (48). In this line, active children tend to participate in sports and energetic activities; antisocial individuals are more likely to find problematic partners (assortative mating). Fourth, the same risk factor may have different consequences depending on other circumstances. For example, while parental separation increases the risk of DBDs in the children, it may actually reduce that risk if separation means losing contact with an antisocial father (40).

It is firmly established that CD is more prevalent among disadvantaged families, though this applies to relative deprivation; the risk seems to flow from being worse off than other people in the child's community rather than from the absolute level of poverty (51). An ingenious natural experiment in North Carolina confirmed this but also showed that reducing poverty among native American families resulted in a reduction in behavior problems in their children (52). The mechanisms by which this occurred do not seem directly monetary, rather higher incomes resulted in more parents working, fewer single parents, fewer demands on parents' time, and ultimately better parental supervision, which probably led to the change.

Neuropsychological Aspects

Low resting heart rate, probably reflecting autonomic underarousal, is the best replicated biologic correlate of antisocial behavior in children and adolescents, although its meaning is still poorly understood (53). Studies using a range of imaging techniques have enabled speculation about the brain regions that may be involved in ODD and CD. The frontal lobe has been a focus of attention. Thus, it has been suggested that atypical frontal lobe activation, as detected on EEG, is a basis for negative affective style in children with ODD (54). Positron emission tomography has shown violence to be associated with decreased glucose metabolism in the prefrontal cortex (55), and orbitofrontal lobe damage has been linked to impulsive aggression (56). Research has also focused on the role of various neurotransmitters, with serotonin having received most attention; there is a suggested link between aggression and low levels of serotonin in the CNS (e.g., (57)).

"What is striking to people who come into contact with these children (...) are the repeated poor choices that they make. Children with DBDs often act impulsively, with apparently little ability to compute the consequences of their poor behavioral choices. Many of these children desperately want to make better choices but become upset when they find themselves yet again in trouble that they did not see coming. Others may pursue selfish goals but with overly optimistic predictions of the likely outcome of their actions and experience frustrated aggression when things do not work out" (58,59). Interest in the neuropsychological processes in children suffering from DBDs is growing. A better understanding of the information processing abnormalities that characterize their decision-making is needed to devise more effective interventions (58). For example, young people with CD, especially if they are aggressive, tend to misperceive other people's intentions as hostile and threatening more often than their peers, thus responding in an unnecessarily aggressive manner, which they feel is justified (4).

As already highlighted, there is considerable evidence that development of CD is negatively associated with IQ, particularly with the verbal components of psychometric tests, compared with their performance as a whole. Children with ODD and CD appear to have a lower sensitivity to punishment, which may reduce their ability to associate inappropriate behaviors and consequences (the result of impaired fear conditioning,

TABLE 5.1.2.4

SUMMARY OF FACTORS ASSOCIATED WITH THE DEVELOPMENT OF DISRUPTIVE BEHAVIOR DISORDERS AND OPPORTUNITIES FOR PREVENTION

Risk Factor	Potential Prevention Interventions
Biologic	
• Genetic • Low birth weight • Antenatal, and perinatal complications • Brain injury, brain disease • Male sex	• Improved antenatal, prenatal, and obstetric care. • Quit smoking and drug treatment programs targeted to intending parents • Programs to reduce domestic violence
Individual	
• Below average IQ • Difficult temperament • Aggressiveness • Impulsivity and hyperactivity • Attentional problems • Language impairment • Reading problems	• Early identification, adequate support and services for families and individuals with intellectual disability • Quality home visiting programs which aim to facilitate attachment and enhance parenting skills • Parent management training programs • Head start-type programs • Early speech and reading remediation programs
Family	
• Parental antisocial behavior or substance use • Domestic violence • Single parent, divorce • Harsh discipline, maltreatment, or neglect • Parent–child conflict • Lack of parental supervision • Excessive parental control • Maternal depression and anxiety • Early motherhood	• Quality home visitation programs • Parent management training programs • Programs to reduce domestic violence • Drug-treatment programs • Child protection initiatives • Early identification and treatment of maternal depression • Prevention of teenage pregnancy • Support programs for teenage mothers
Social and School	
• Poverty • Association with deviant peers/siblings • Rejection by peers • History of victimization or of being bullied • Disorganized, disadvantaged, or high-crime neighborhoods • Dysfunctional or disorganized schools • Intense exposure to media violence	• Measures to reduce poverty and provide a social safety net • Enhance the quality of schools • School programs to reduce bullying and prevent behavior problems • Initiatives to reduce access to firearms, and gang activities • Programs to reduce school truancy • Initiatives to enhance neighborhood cohesion • Law enforcement initiatives to reduce crime targeted to high-crime areas • Public campaigns to reduce media violence and education about how to monitor and prevent children's exposure to it

reduced cortisol reactivity to stress, amygdala hyporeactivity to negative stimuli, and altered serotonin and noradrenaline neurotransmission). They also show hyposensitivity to reward, which is mediated by sympathetic nervous system hyporeactivity to incentives, low basal heart rate, orbitofrontal cortex hyporeactivity to reward, and altered dopamine function. The emotional state associated with these changes may make these young people prone to break rules, delinquency, and substance abuse—risk-taking, sensation-seeking behavior—while impairment in executive functions suggests poorer control of emotions and decision-making (60).

DIAGNOSIS

Diagnostic Assessment

An evaluation performed by an experienced clinician based on information from multiple sources and supplemented by questionnaire data should allow making a diagnosis of ODD or CD quite reliably. Given the range of problems shown by children with DBDs, it is important to clarify to all concerned the purpose of the evaluation from the outset. Assessment may be requested by parents, schools, courts, children's lawyers, or social services. The purpose will influence how the assessment is conducted and the tone of the interviews. This may also pose limitations to confidentiality, which should be explained to the relevant parties. Building rapport with and achieving cooperation from these children is often problematic because of their difficulty accepting ownership of their actions and hostility to authority figures. Often they do not see a distinction between mental health professionals, parents, teachers, and police. Thus, noncooperation and resistance to disclose information are to be expected. Because referral is often triggered by a disciplinary or legal crisis after months or, more often, years of discord, clinicians are usually confronted with stressed, angry families who are unable to see anything positive in one another.

Reports from children, parents, or teachers may disagree but these sets of information often complement each other. Since sexual abuse, inconsistent parenting, maternal depression, and parental drug use are not uncommon in these children's backgrounds, these areas need to be explored carefully. Learning as much as possible about the parenting style, parent–child interactions, and the child's strengths and relationships with peers will be valuable when planning and delivering treatment.

Boundaries of the Disorder

The developmental issues noted raise the question of the boundaries between disorder and extremes of normal behavior. ICD-10 states that judgments concerning the presence of ODD/CD should take into account the child's developmental level. Temper tantrums, for example, are a normal part of a 3 year old's development and mere presence would not be grounds for diagnosis. While there is much evidence that children who display symptoms of ODD or CD persistently and intensely are significantly impaired (e.g., (61)), it is also clear that a continuum of symptoms exist and that children with a subsyndromal level of diagnostic criteria can be impaired (62).

Gender and Age

Rather than physical attack, females are more prone to use indirect, verbal, and relational violence such as ostracism and character defamation (63). These behaviors can be difficult to document, are not clearly described as CD symptoms, and may result in underdiagnosis of CD in girls (34).

The lowest age at which a valid diagnosis of ODD or CD can be made is unresolved. For example, ICD-10 states that a violation of other people's civic rights (such as by violent crime) is not within the capacity of most 7 year olds and so it is not a necessary diagnostic criterion for that age group. In most cases, symptoms of ODD begin to appear during the preschool years and a valid diagnosis of ODD or CD may be made in preschoolers (64,65). Conversely, the ICD-10 statement warning about diagnosing ODD after the age of 10 years is without foundation since as many young people qualify for ODD in adolescence as in childhood. Further, even some adults may meet criteria for ODD or CD (30).

Social and Cultural Context

DSM-5 highlights that a diagnosis of CD should be made only when the behavior in question is symptomatic of an underlying dysfunction within the individual and not simply a reaction to the immediate social or cultural context. This is to circumvent concerns that a diagnosis of CD may at times be misapplied to individuals in particular settings (threatening, impoverished, high crime, war) where patterns of undesirable behavior could be protective. This does not necessarily imply an absence of CD in those settings, it only means that the context in which symptoms occur needs to be taken into consideration. Although the difference appears theoretically difficult, clinicians seem able to make such a distinction in practice (66).

Comorbidity and Differential Diagnosis

Assessment must cover all symptom domains to ensure that comorbid disorders are not overlooked. It is common for parents, teachers, and clinicians to focus on the more obvious and annoying behaviors and neglect mentioning or inquiring about less conspicuous symptoms and disorders, which nevertheless may be important for treatment and prognosis. As noted, the most frequent are ADHD, mood disorders, and in adolescents, substance misuse. Conditions such as anxiety disorders, tic disorders, specific developmental and learning disorders, autism spectrum disorders, and intellectual disability ought to be considered also. Antisocial behavior is not uncommon in the prodromal stage of schizophrenia (67).

It has been suggested that some children with severe impulsivity, hyperactivity, unstable mood, irritability, defiance, and conduct problems may suffer from bipolar disorder, resulting in a higher prevalence of bipolar disorder in this age group. The association between DBDs and bipolar disorder in prepubertal children—important for its therapeutic implications—has received much attention and created controversy at the turn of the 21st century, leading to the introduction in DSM-5 of a new diagnosis—*disruptive mood dysregulation disorder*—to describe primary school-age children with severe and chronic negative mood and temper outbursts. There is considerable symptom overlap between ODD and disruptive mood dysregulation disorder but, according to DSM-5, the latter and not ODD should be diagnosed when symptoms are particularly severe and negative mood predominates. The validity of this condition is still questioned; it may represent an extreme form of ODD (68).

A diagnosis of ODD should not be made when defiance, grouchiness, and noncompliance occur only in the course of *major depression* or if ODD symptoms appear when parents try to force anxious children, for example, with a phobia, to confront their fears. Ignoring ODD symptoms when making a diagnosis of depression or ADHD may also occur. ODD may be present if the child has shown symptoms of defiance, temper tantrums, etc. prior to the onset of the other disorder or if oppositionality persists after symptoms of the comorbid condition have lessened.

The possibility of *intermittent explosive disorder* should be considered also. This condition is characterized by impulsive, unpremeditated outbursts of anger and aggression. Such aggressive episodes are uncommon in ODD, while they differ from those in CD in that children with explosive disorder do not seek an ulterior benefit and nonaggressive symptoms of CD (e.g., lying, truancy) are absent.

The existence of intellectual disability creates significant problems when diagnosing DBDs. A diagnosis of ODD is made in individuals with developmental disability only if oppositionality is markedly greater than that observed in youth with similar IQ. Aggressive behavior in intellectually disabled young people is common and often results in placement in residential programs. When present, CD behaviors tend to persist over time, particularly in males, and a comorbid diagnosis of CD would be justified in these cases.

Clinical Assessment

Questionnaires and checklists provide quantifiable data, reliably supplement information obtained at interview, and are useful to measure progress and outcome. Besides general questionnaires such as the Child Behavior Checklist (69), a variety of specific rating scales are available (70), including the Eyberg Child Behavior Inventory (71), the New York Teacher Rating Scale for Disruptive and Antisocial Behavior (72), and the Home and School Situations Questionnaire (73). A comprehensive list of instruments to assist in the diagnosis of ODD can be found here (74).

Psychometric and educational assessment is often useful as part of the initial evaluation; it should be performed when children show difficulties at school or if learning problems are suspected. A careful medical history and review of systems is mandatory in all cases. Routine biochemical, EEG, or radiologic investigations are unnecessary, with the exception of urine drug screen in adolescents (75). Laboratory investigations should be conducted when the clinician uncovers symptoms suggestive of a physical illness (e.g., epilepsy), or for sexually transmitted diseases when sexual abuse has occurred, or there is suspicion of unprotected sexual activity.

TREATMENT

In practice, children with DBDs are treated with a variety of psychological, behavioral, or pharmacologic approaches, alone or in combination, targeting the child and/or the family. Professionals largely believe that therapy is of limited effectiveness in the patients with CD typically seen in mental health settings (more chronic, more disturbed, and usually with comorbid conditions). While there have been considerable advances in the last 25 years, effective treatments are few and no great breakthroughs have occurred. Moreover, treatment research, though vast, is hampered by poor definition of target symptoms, mixed populations, small sample sizes, and poor randomization and blinding, among other limitations. Few trials specifically focus on participants with ODD or CD and it is often difficult to translate findings to the complex circumstances of individual patients. This is compounded by psychosocial treatments being less efficacious when delivered in the average clinic than in academic research settings.

General principles to keep in mind when treating these disorders are (74,76,77):

- DBDs tend to be chronic conditions, more similar to heart disease than pneumonia, and treatment should be tailored accordingly.
- Most guidelines concur that structured psychosocial and behavioral interventions should be the first line of treatment for ODD and CD, and should be continued even if medications are subsequently initiated.
- Treatment is more likely to be effective when administered early in the course of the disorder. Typically, maladaptive behaviors are continually reinforced; over time, negative perceptions, emotions, and patterns of relating become deeper and more entrenched. Once CD is established, it becomes more resistant to intervention.
- Treatment should involve the parents. In almost all instances, improving parenting skills and parent–child interactions are core goals.
- Comorbid conditions (ADHD, depression) ought to be identified and, if appropriate, treated.
- Parental depression, psychosis, or substance abuse should also be noted and treated.
- It is very useful to ascertain children's and families' strengths and build on them in addition to focusing on their problems.
- Dealing with the stress, anger, and hopelessness that many of these families experience and achieving some calm and control is often a necessary initial step.
- The goals of treatment need to be realistic and modified as progress occurs. For example, preventing or minimizing drug use or involvement in delinquent activities in adolescents with CD may be a more appropriate initial step than seeking symptom resolution.
- Because these young people usually show disturbance in a variety of settings (e.g., school, home) and impairment in several aspects of functioning, addressing their multiple needs in the various domains is likely to increase effectiveness (multimodal treatment).
- Association with deviant peers is a well-established factor that increases the likelihood of conduct problems, delinquency, and drug use, particularly in adolescence. A goal should be to enhance participation in activities with well-functioning peers.
- In the case of ODD, the main goal of treatment is to increase compliance and reduce conflict. Therefore, the treatment plan should include ways of helping the young person become more cooperative, less argumentative, and be better accepted by peers, often in a family therapy context.
- Medication should not be offered for the routine management of ODD or CD. In cases of severe aggressive behavior that has not responded to psychosocial interventions, the use of risperidone can be considered in the short term and with the appropriate precautions (e.g., metabolic syndrome monitoring).

Emergencies

Presentation of young people with DBDs to emergency services is not uncommon. For example, 16% of all the child and adolescent presentations to a psychiatric emergency service in Albany, NY, between 1990 and 1995 were due to DBDs (78). Emergencies usually occur following conflict, legal, or disciplinary crises that result in the child losing control and becoming aggressive toward the self, others, or property. Differentiating DBDs from other psychiatric problems in the emergency room is reasonably straightforward, but establishing whether ODD or CD is the more appropriate diagnosis is harder because a comprehensive evaluation is often difficult in that context. Children with DBDs who present to emergency services tend to have more severe disorders, more aggression, more comorbid conditions, and fewer family and social supports than those without DBDs. Police or mobile psychiatric services involvement is often required. Some of the management principles to be followed in these cases are (79):

- Crisis intervention strategies should be employed before resorting to the use of medication to control behavior.
- Physical and mechanical restraints and locked seclusion should be used only as a last resort, when all other approaches have failed.
- The choice to use emergency ("stat" or "p.r.n.") pharmacologic management should correspond to the risk for potential injury.
- Emergency staff should be aware of the risks and side effects of acute sedation and follow the appropriate protocols.
- When antipsychotic "p.r.n." or "stat" medications are used several times per day to manage agitation or aggression, clinicians should re-evaluate the diagnosis and the adequacy of behavioral and environmental interventions and then readjust the treatment plan and medication regimen. In most cases, physicians should consider using standing antipsychotic medications rather than frequent "stat" medications.

Acute situations similar to the ones seen in emergency settings also occur during inpatient treatment or in institutions. In these settings, crises usually build up over days or hours and can often be predicted. While their management follows the principles listed above, clinicians working in these services need to be skilled in detecting the early symptoms of loss of control and preventing the crisis.

Psychosocial Treatments

Psychosocial interventions that include a parent component, either alone or in combination with other treatments, are likely to be more effective at reducing disruptive behaviors than those that include only a child component (77).

Parent Management Training

Parent management training (PMT) is based on the principles of operant conditioning and social learning theory. In PMT, parents are encouraged to use positive reinforcement, to adopt more effective discipline strategies, and to learn how to negotiate with their children (for a review, see Chapter "6.2.4" in this textbook and (80)).

PMT has been the most extensively researched therapy in this field. It has the potential to produce improvements in child behavior to within the nonclinical range at home and, sometimes, at school. Further, these effects can be maintained, together with indirect improvement in other areas such as sibling behavior, maternal psychopathology, marital satisfaction, and family cohesion (81). Key limitations of PMT include the substantial number of parents who do not complete the program, their frequent ineffectiveness in the most dysfunctional families, and that it has been targeted to younger children.

Multimodal Interventions

Given the variety of symptom and impairment domains, it is thought that multimodal interventions may optimize the chances of success. For example, PMT alone often does not generalize to the school context, and antisocial behavior at school is a predictor of poor outcomes. Also, PMT does not necessarily influence the child's capacity to make friends, when having well-functioning friends is a protective factor. Hence, adding to PMT a component that addresses the child's problem-solving abilities or a teacher-training element may enhance efficacy (82). This multimodal approach has been shown to produce better results than PMT alone (83). Examples of multimodal programs are Multisystemic Therapy (MST) and Families and Schools Together (FAST Track). The former predominantly targets adolescents with severe conduct problems and delinquency, while the latter focuses on conduct disordered children starting school.

MST (see Chapter "6.2.7") also draws on a range of interventions, is home-based, goal-oriented and intensive—it provides therapy 7 days a week for about 4 months (84). A meta-analysis reported that MST is moderately effective in reducing offending, but this appears to be very dependent on the skills of the treatment team (effect sizes ranging from 0.26 to 0.81) (85). MST is resource intensive and there are doubts about its cost-effectiveness (86).

Therapeutic foster care is another multimodal approach in which adolescents are placed with specially trained, intensely supervised foster parents who are supported by a team. There is some evidence this reduces these youths' criminal activities (82).

Evidence for the effectiveness of wilderness programs, boot camps, and other residential treatments is conflicting and studies are of poor quality. A concern about these interventions is that they provide opportunities to associate and identify with deviant peers, and that gains may not generalize outside the treatment setting.

Individual Interventions

Problem-solving skills training is the best studied and it results in a clinically significant improvement (87). In this therapy, children are taught to understand interpersonal problems and find adaptive solutions using various techniques including games, structured activities, stories, modeling, role play, and reinforcement. Studies have also demonstrated at least modest benefits for other individual interventions. A review of 82 controlled trials found that individual assertiveness training, anger control/stress inoculation, and rational emotive therapy were "probably efficacious" (at least two studies showed the treatment to be better than a control condition) (87). Child CBT-based interventions showed a small-to-moderate effect in decreasing antisocial behavior (88).

Pharmacotherapy

Medication is *not* a mainstay of treatment of ODD and CD, and research in this area suffers from most of the shortcomings already noted (77). Psychotropic drugs may be used for the treatment of ODD or CD symptoms if psychosocial and educational interventions have failed and as a part of a comprehensive management plan, although medication is often used for those individuals who have coexisting conditions, such as ADHD, and in emergency situations.

Some principles should be followed when prescribing medication for DBDs besides those already highlighted in the section on emergencies, including (79):

- The dosing strategy of "start low, go slow, taper slowly" should be followed, particularly when using antipsychotic drugs.
- Caution and careful monitoring should be exercised when prescribing stimulants to adolescents with CD, given the high rate of substance misuse in this population.
- Adherence, side effects, and drug interactions should be monitored routinely and systematically. In particular, it is important to ascertain whether patients are concurrently using psychoactive substances or complementary therapies that may interact with prescribed drugs.
- Before switching, augmenting, combining, or discontinuing medications because of a lack of response, it should be ensured that patients have received an adequate trial (dose and duration) as well as psychosocial interventions.
- Polypharmacy should be avoided whenever possible.

Psychostimulants are effective in children with ADHD with significant symptoms of oppositional behavior, conduct problems, or aggression. Treatment with atomoxetine, guanfacine, and clonidine may also provide some lesser symptom relief (89). There is evidence to support the efficacy of risperidone for the treatment of aggressive behavior (90).

Antipsychotic drugs have often been prescribed to manage disruptive behavior in individuals with intellectual disability. Controlled trials suggest these medications, particularly risperidone, are beneficial in this population, at least in the short term (91).

PREVENTION

There is no reason to believe the incidence of DBDs cannot be reduced, since that has been achieved with other scourges such as heart disease, but doing so will require a concerted effort and substantial resources. Child and adolescent mental health professionals have a critical role in educating the community and political leaders on the advantages of prevention over treatment and retribution, notwithstanding that treatment and law enforcement are important also. Reducing DBDs is one of the challenges for child mental health in the 21st century. Yet simply addressing conduct problems without tackling the social, family, and individual factors associated with these conditions will lead to disappointment. Little may be achieved in communities that fail to protect the disadvantaged and to ensure that all its citizens, particularly women and families with children, are treated with dignity and afforded access to a minimum of resources and life opportunities, as well as having developmental difficulties such as attention and learning problems addressed. Schools can play a key role in this endeavor (92).

Table 5.1.2.3 lists some of the opportunities for prevention and the range of potential interventions. Many prevention programs already exist (93), often implemented *ad hoc* and without much data about their effectiveness; finding that evidence should be a priority for research. Home visitation is one of the most widespread, though with many variations. Evaluations show that home visitation is no silver bullet, but results of the better programs are encouraging. Participation can improve children's cognitive, social, and linguistic development, and reduce child maltreatment and behavioral problems (94).

Most of the therapies used to treat DBDs can be adapted for prevention purposes. For example, there are packages based on PMT principles, such as Triple-P (80), designed for use at several levels: (i) in broad community education (e.g., through media campaigns); (ii) for children at risk in a group format; (iii) for children with a full-blown syndrome in group or individual format. There is limited data on the effectiveness of these programs outside preschool or early primary school-age children.

References

1. Foster, EM, Jones, DE: The high costs of aggression: public expenditures resulting from conduct disorder. *Am J Public Health* 95:1767–1772, 2005.
2. Scott S, Knapp M, Henderson J, Maughan B: Financial cost of social exclusion: follow up study of antisocial children into adulthood. *BMJ* 323:191–194, 2001.
3. Quay HC: Classification of the disruptive behaviour disorders. In: Quay HC, Hohgan AE (eds): *Handbook of Disruptive Behavior Disorders.* New York, Springer, 1999.
4. American Psychiatric Association: *Diagnostic and Statistical Manual of Mental Disorders.* 5th ed. Washington, DC, American Psychiatric Press, 2013.
5. Beta draft. Available at: http://apps.who.int/classifications/icd11/browse/l-m/en#/http%3a%2f%2fid.who.int%2ficd%2fentity%2f310393530. Accessed 02/28/2017.
6. American Psychiatric Association: *Diagnostic and Statistical Manual of Mental Disorders,* 4th ed. Washington, DC, American Psychiatric Association, 1994.
7. Burke JD, Hipwell AE, Loeber R: Dimensions of oppositional defiant disorder as predictors of depression and conduct disorder in preadolescent girls. *J Am Acad Child Adoles Psychiatry* 49:484–492, 2010.
8. Herzhoff K, Tackett JL: Subfactors of oppositional defiant disorder: converging evidence from structural and latent class analyses. *J Child Psychol Psychiatry* 57:18–29, 2016.
9. American Psychiatric Association: *Diagnostic and Statistical Manual of Mental Disorders,* 3rd ed. Washington, DC, American Psychiatric Association, 1980.
10. Kimonis ER, Frick PJ: Oppositional defiant disorder and conduct disorder grown-up. *J Dev Behav Pediatr* 31:244–254, 2010.
11. World Health Organisation. *The ICD-10 Classification of Mental and Behavioural Disorders: Diagnostic Criteria for Research.* Geneva, World Health Organization, 1993.
12. Frick PJ, Lahey BB, Loeber R, et al.: Oppositional defiant disorder and conduct disorder: a meta-analytic review of factor analyses and cross validation in a clinical sample. *Clin Psychol Rev* 13:319–340, 1993.
13. Moffitt TE: Adolescence-limited and life-course-persistent antisocial behavior: a developmental taxonomy. *Psychol Rev* 100:674–701, 1993
14. Angold A, Costello EJ, Erkanli A: Comorbidity. *J Child Psychol Psychiatry* 40:57–87, 1999.
15. Armstrong TD, Costello EJ: Community studies on adolescent substance use, abuse, or dependence and psychiatric comorbidity. *J Consult Clin Psychol* 70:1224–1239, 2002.
16. Rey JM, Plapp JM, Stewart GW: Reliability of psychiatric diagnosis in referred adolescents. *J Child Psychol Psychiatry* 30:879–888, 1989.
17. Shaffer D, Fisher P, Lucas CP, et al.: NIMH Diagnostic Interview Schedule for Children Version IV (NIMH DISC-IV): description, differences from previous versions, and reliability of some common diagnoses. *J Am Acad Child Adolesc Psychiatry* 39:28–38, 2000.
18. Centres for Disease Control and Prevantion: *1991–2013 High School Youth Risk Behavior Survey Data.* Available at https://nccd.cdc.gov/youthonline/App/Default.aspx Accessed 13/01/2016.
19. Fergusson DM: Stability and change in externalising behaviors. *Eur Arch Psychiatry Clin Neurosci* 248:4–13, 1998.
20. Kimonis ER, Frick PJ: Oppositional defiant disorder and conduct disorder grown-up. *J Dev Behav Pediat* 31:244–254, 2010.
21. Piquero AR, Farrington DP, Fontaine NG, et al.: Childhood risk, offending trajectories, and psychopathy at age 48 years in the Cambridge study in delinquent development. *Psychol Public Policy Law* 18:577–598, 2012.
22. Rowe R, Maughan B, Pickles A, Costello EJ, Angold A: The relationship between DSM-IV oppositional defiant disorder and conduct disorder: findings from the Great Smoky Mountains Study. *J Child Psychol Psychiatry* 43:365–373, 2002.
23. Lahey BB, Waldman ID: Phenotypic and causal structure of conduct disorder in the broader context of prevalent forms of psychopathology. *J Child Psychol Psychiatry* 53:536–557, 2012.
24. Helgeland MI, Kjelsberg E, Torgersen S: Continuities between emotional and disruptive behavior disorders in adolescence and personality disorders in adulthood. *Am J Psychiatry* 2005;162:1941–1947.
25. Kim-Cohen J, Caspi A. Moffitt TE, Harrington H, Milne BJ, Poulton R: Prior juvenile diagnoses in adults with mental disorder: developmental follow-back of a prospective-longitudinal cohort. *Arch Gen Psychiatry* 60:709–717, 2003.
26. Fergusson DM, Horwood LJ, Ridder EM: Show me the child at seven: the consequences of conduct problems in childhood for psychosocial functioning in adulthood. *J Child Psychol Psychiatry* 46:837–849, 2005.
27. Caspi A, Wright BRE, Moffitt TE, Silva PA: Early failure in the labor market: childhood and adolescent predictors of unemployment in the transition to adulthood. *Am Sociol Rev* 3:424–451, 1998.
28. Fergusson DM, Lynskey MT: Conduct problems in childhood and psychosocial outcomes in young adulthood: a prospective study. *J Emot Behav Disord* 6:2–18, 1998.
29. Stouthamer-Loeber M, Wei E, Loeber R, Mastenb AS: Desistance from persistent serious delinquency in the transition to adulthood. *Dev Psychopathol* 16:897–918, 2004.
30. Kessler RC, Chiu WT, Demler O, Merikangas KR, Walters EE: Prevalence, severity, and comorbidity of 12-month DSM-IV disorders in the national comorbidity survey replication. *Arch Gen Psychiatry* 62:617–627, 2005.
31. Burke JD, Rowe R, Boylan K: Functional outcomes of child and adolescent oppositional defiant disorder symptoms in young adult men. *J Child Psychol Psychiatry* 55:264–272, 2014.
32. Leadbeater BJ, Homel J: Irritable and defiant sub-dimensions of ODD: their stability and prediction of internalizing symptoms and conduct problems from adolescence to young adulthood. *J Abnorm Child Psychol* 43:407–421, 2015.
33. Dougherty LR, Smith VC, Bufferd SJ, Kessel E, Carlson GA, Klein DN: Preschool irritability predicts child psychopathology, functional impairment, and service use at age nine. *J Child Psychol Psychiatry* 56:999–1007, 2015.
34. Loeber R, Burke JD, Lahey BB, Winters A, Zera M: Oppositional defiant and conduct disorder: a review of the past 10 years, part I. *J Am Acad Child Adolesc Psychiatry* 39:1468–1484, 2000.
35. Crijnen A, Achenbach TM, Verhulst FC: Problems reported by parents of children in multiple cultures: The Child Behavior Checklist syndrome constructs. *Am J Psychiatry* 156:569–574, 1999.
36. Rutter M, Smith DJ: *Psychosocial Disorders in Young People: Time Trends and Their Causes.* Chichester, Wiley, 1995.
37. Robins L N: A 70-year history of conduct disorder: variations in definition, prevalence, and correlates. In: Cohen P, Slomkowski C, Robins LN (eds): *Historical and Geographical Influences in Psychopathology.* Mahwah, NJ, Lawrence Erlbaum, 32–49, 1999.
38. Fergusson D, Swain-Campbell N, Horwood J: How does childhood economic disadvantage lead to crime? *J Child Psychol Psychiatry* 45:956–966, 2004.
39. Hack M, Taylor G, Drotar D, et al.: Chronic conditions, functional limitations, and special health care needs of school-aged children born with extremely low birth-weight in the 1990s. *JAMA* 294:318–325, 2005.
40. Jaffee SR, Moffitt TE, Caspi A, Taylor A: Life with (or without) father: the benefits of living with two biological parents depend on the father's antisocial behavior. *Child Dev* 74:109–126, 2003.
41. Kim-Cohen J, Moffitt TE, Taylor A, et al.: Maternal depression and children's antisocial behavior. *Arch Gen Psychiatry* 62:173–181, 2005.
42. Lansford JE, Dodge KA, Pettit GS, Bates JE, Crozier J, Kaplow J: A 12 year prospective study of the long-term effects of early child physical maltreatment on psychological, behavioral and academic problems in adolescence. *Arch Pediatr Adolesc Med* 156:824–830.
43. Maughan B, Pickels A, Hagell A, Rutter M, Yule W: Reading problems and antisocial behaviour: developmental Trends in Comorbidity. *J Child Psychol Psychiatry* 37:405–418, 1996.
44. Dodge KA, Pettit GS: A biopsychosocial model of the development of chronic conduct problems in adolescence. *Dev Psychol* 39:349–371, 2003.
45. Moffitt TE: The new look of behavioral genetics in developmental psychopathology: gene-environment interplay in antisocial behaviors. *Psychol Bull* 131:533–544, 2005.
46. Bornovalova MA, Hicks BM, Iacono WG McGue M: Familial transmission and heritability of childhood disruptive disorders. *Am J Psychiatry* 167:1066–1074, 2010.
47. Caspi A, Mcclay J, Moffitt TE, et al.: Role of genotype in the cycle of violence in maltreated children. *Science* 297:851–854, 2002.
48. Rutter M, Moffitt TE, Caspi A: Gene-environment interplay and psychopathology: multiple varieties but real effects. *J Child Psychol Psychiatry* 47:226–261, 2006.
49. Tuvblad C, Grann M, Lichtenstein P: Heritability for adolescent antisocial behavior differs with socioeconomic status: gene-environment interaction. *J Child Psychol Psychiatry* 47:734–743, 2006.
50. Wichers M, Purcell S, Danckaerts, et al.: Prenatal life and post-natal psychopathology: evidence for negative gene-birth weight interaction. *Psychol Med* 32:1165–1174, 2002.
51. Wilkinson R, Marmot M: *Social Determinants of Health: The Solid Facts,* 2nd ed. Copenhagen, WHO, 2003.

52. Costello EJ, Compton SN, Keeler G, Angold A: Relationships between poverty and psychopathology: a natural experiment. *JAMA* 290:2023–2029, 2003.
53. Ortiz J, Raine A: Heart rate level and antisocial behavior in children and adolescents: a meta-analysis. *J Am Acad Child Adolesc Psychiatry* 43:154–162, 2004.
54. Baving L, Laucht M, Schmidt MH: Oppositional children differ from healthy children in frontal brain activation. *J Abnorm Child Psychol* 28:267–275, 2000.
55. Pliszka SR: The psychobiology of oppositional defiant disorder and conduct disorder. In: QuayHC, Hogan AE (eds): *Handbook of Disruptive Behavior Disorders*. New York, Kluwer Academic/Plenum, 1999.
56. Brower MC, Price BH: Neuropsychiatry of frontal lobe dysfunction in violence and criminal behavior: a critical review. *J Neurol Neurosurg Psychiatry* 71:720–726, 2001.
57. Kruesi MJP, Keller S, Wagner MW: Neurobiology of aggression. In: Martin A, Scahill L, Charney D, Leckman JF (eds): *Pediatric Psychopharmacology. Principles and Practice*. New York: Oxford University Press, 210–223, 2003.
58. Viding S, Seara-Cardoso A. Why do children with disruptive behavior disorders keep making bad choices? *Am J Psychiatry* 170:253–255, 2013.
59. White SF, Pope K, Sinclair S, et al.: Disrupted expected value and prediction error signaling in youths with disruptive behavior disorders during a passive avoidance task. *Am J Psychiatry* 70:315–323, 2013.
60. Matthys W, Vanderschuren LJ, Schutter DJ: The neurobiology of oppositional defiant disorder and conduct disorder: altered functioning in three mental domains. *Dev Psychopathol* 25:193–207, 2013.
61. Vostanis P, Meltzer H, Goodman R, Ford T: Service utilization by children with conduct disorders—findings from the GB national study. *Eur Child Adolesc Psychiatry* 12:231–128, 2003.
62. Rowe R, Maughan B, Costello EJ, et al.: Defining oppositional defiant disorder. *J Child Psychol Psychiatry* 46:309–1316, 2005.
63. Crick NR, Grotpeter JK: Relational aggression, gender, and social psychological adjustment. *Child Dev* 199 66:710–722, 1995.
64. Keenan K, Wakschlag LS: Can a valid diagnosis of disruptive behavior disorder be made in preschool children? *Am J Psychiatry* 159:351–358. 2002.
65. Kim-Cohen J, Arseneault L, Caspi A, Tomás MP, Taylor A, Moffitt TE: Validity of DSM-IV conduct disorder in 41/2–5-year-old children: a longitudinal epidemiological study. *Am J Psychiatry* 162:1108–1117, 2005.
66. Wakefield JC, Pottick KJ, Kirk SA: Should the DSM-IV diagnostic criteria for conduct disorder consider social context? *Am J Psychiatry* 159:380–386, 2002.
67. Gosden NP, Kramp P, Gabrielsen G, Andersen TF, Sestoft D: Violence of young criminals predicts schizophrenia: a 9-year register-based follow-up of 15- to 19- year-old criminals. *Schizophrenia Bull* 31:759–768, 2005.
68. Axelson D: Taking disruptive mood dysregulation disorder out for a test drive. *Am J Psychiatry* 170:136–139, 2013.
69. Achenbach TM: *The Achenbach System of Empirically Based Assessment (ASEBA): Development, Findings, Theory, and Applications*. Burlington, VT: University of Vermont, Research Center for Children, Youth, and Families, 2009.
70. Collett BR, Ohan JL, Myers K: Ten-year review of rating scales. VI: scales assessing externalizing behaviors. *J Am Acad Child Adolesc Psychiatry* 42:1143–1170, 2003.
71. Eyberg SM, Pincus D: *Eyeberg Child Behavior Inventory and Sutter-Eyberg Student Behavior Inventory-Revised, Professional Manual*. Odessa, FL, Psychological Assessment Resources, 1999.
72. Miller LS, Klein RG, Piacentini J, et al.: The New York teacher rating scale for disruptive and antisocial behavior. *J Am Acad Child Adolesc Psychiatry* 34:359–370, 1995.
73. Barkley RA: *Defiant Children: A Clinician's Manual for Assessment and Parent Training*, 2nd ed. New York, Guilford, 1997.
74. American Academy of Child and Adolescent Psychiatry: Practice parameter for the assessment and treatment of children and adolescents with oppositional defiant disorder. *J Am Acad Child Adolesc Psychiatry* 46:126–141, 2007.
75. Zametkin AJ, Ernst M, Silver R: Laboratory and diagnostic testing in child and adolescent psychiatry: a review of the past 10 years. *J Am Acad Child Adolesc Psychiatry* 37:464–472, 1998.
76. The National Institute for Health and Care Excellence (NICE): *Antisocial Behaviour and Conduct Disorders in Children and Young People: Recognition And Management*. NICE guidelines CG158. March 2013. Available at http://www.nice.org.uk/guidance/cg158 Accessed January 19, 2016.
77. Epstein R, Fonnesbeck C, Williamson E, et al.: *Psychosocial and Pharmacologic Interventions for Disruptive Behavior in Children and Adolescents*. Comparative Effectiveness Review No. 154. AHRQ Comparative Effectiveness Review No. 154. AHRQ Publication No. 15(16)-EHC019-EF. Available at http://effectivehealthcare.ahrq.gov/ehc/products/555/2133/disruptive-behavior-disorder-report-151201.pdf. Accessed January 25, 2016.
78. Breslow RE, Klinger BI, Erickson BJ: The disruptive behavior disorders in the psychiatric emergency service. *Gen Hosp Psychiatry* 21:214–219, 1999.
79. Pappadopulos E, Macintyre LiI JC, Crismon ML, et al.: Treatment recommendations for the use of antipsychotics for aggressive youth (TRAAY). Part II. *J Am Acad Child Adolesc Psychiatry* 42:145–161, 2003.
80. Haslam D, Mejia A, Sanders MR, et al.: Parenting programs. In: Rey JM (ed): *IACAPAP e-Textbook of Child and Adolescent Mental Health*. Geneva: International Association for Child and Adolescent Psychiatry and Allied Professions 2016. Available at: http://iacapap.org/iacapap-textbook-of-child-and-adolescent-mental-health. Accessed 1/20/2016.
81. Scott S: Do parenting programs for severe child antisocial behavior work over the longer term, and for whom? One year follow-up of a multi-centre controlled trial. *Behav Cogn Psychother* 33:403–421, 2005.
82. Woolgar M, Scott S: Evidence-based management of conduct disorders. *Curr Opin Psychiatry* 18:392–396, 2005.
83. Webster-Stratton C, Reid M, Hammond M: Treating children with early-onset conduct problems: intervention outcomes for parent, child, and teacher training. *J Clin Child Adolesc Psychol* 33:105–124, 2004.
84. Henggeler SW, Scoenwald SK, Borduin CM, et al.: *Multisystems Treatment of Antisocial Behavior in Children and Adolescents*. New York, Guilford Press, 1998.
85. Curtis NM, Ronan KR, Borduin CM: Multisystemic treatment: a meta-analysis of outcome studies. *J Fam Psychol* 18:411–419, 2004.
86. Olsson TM: MST with conduct disordered youth in Sweden: costs and benefits after 2 years. *Res Social Work Prac* 20:561–571, 2010.
87. Brestan EV, Eyberg SM: Effective psychosocial treatment of conduct disordered children and adolescents: 29 years, 82 studies and 5272 kids. *J Clin Child Psychol* 27:180–189, 1998.
88. Bennett DS, Gibbons TA: Efficacy of child cognitive behavior interventions for antisocial behaviour: a meta-analysis. *Child Fam Behav Ther* 22:1–15, 2000.
89. Pringsheim T, Hirsch L, Gardner D, Gorman DA: The pharmacological management of oppositional behaviour, conduct problems, and aggression in children and adolescents with attention-deficit hyperactivity disorder, oppositional defiant disorder, and conduct disorder: a systematic review and meta-analysis. Part 1: psychostimulants, alpha-2 agonists, and atomoxetine. *Can J Psychiatry* 60:42–51, 2015.
90. Pringsheim T, Hirsch L, Gardner DM, et al.: The pharmacological management of oppositional behaviour, conduct problems, and aggression in children and adolescents with attention-deficit hyperactivity disorder, oppositional defiant disorder, and conduct disorder: a systematic review and meta-analysis. Part 2: antipsychotics and traditional mood stabilizers. *Can J Psychiatry* 60:52–61, 2015.
91. Aman MG, De Smedt G, Derivan A, Lyons B, Findling RL: Risperidone Disruptive Behavior Study Group: Double-blind, placebo-controlled study of risperidone for the treatment of disruptive behaviors in children with subaverage intelligence. *Am J Psychiatry* 159:1337–1346, 2002.
92. van Lier PAC, Vuijk P, Crijnen AAM: Understanding mechanisms of change in the development of antisocial behavior: the impact of a universal intervention. *J Abnorm Child Psychol* 33:521–553, 2005.
93. Bor W: Prevention and treatment of childhood and adolescent aggression and antisocial behavior: a selective review. *Aust N Z J Psychiatry* 38:373–380, 2004.
94. Lyons-Ruth K, Melnick S: Dose–response effect of mother-infant clinical home visiting on aggressive behavior problems in kindergarten. *J Am Acad Chil Adolesc Psychiatry* 43:699–707, 2004.
95. Sawyer M, Arney F, Baghurst P, et al.: The mental health of young people in Australia: key findings from the child and adolescent component of the national survey of mental health and well-being. *Aust NZ J Psychiatry* 35:806–814, 2001.
96. Costello EJ, Mustillo S, Erkanli A, Keeler G, Angold A: Prevalence and development of psychiatric disorders in childhood and adolescence. *Arch Gen Psychiatry* 60:837–844, 2003.
97. Ford T, Goodman R, Meltzer H: The British child and adolescent mental health survey 1999: the prevalence of DSM-IV disorders. *J Am Acad Child Adolesc Psychiatry* 42:1203–1211, 2003.
98. Canino G, Shrout PE, Rubio-Stipec M, et al.: The DSM-IV rates of child and adolescent disorders in Puerto Rico: prevalence, correlates, service use, and the effects of impairment. *Arch Gen Psychiatry* 61:85–93, 2004.
99. Fleitlich-Bilyk B, Goodman R: Prevalence of child and adolescent psychiatric disorders in Southeast Brazil. *J Am Acad Child Adolesc Psychiatry* 43:727–734, 2004.
100. Leung PWL, Hung S-F, Ho T-p, et al.: Prevalence of DSM-IV disorders in Chinese adolescents and the effects of an impairment criterion: a pilot community study in Hong Kong. *Eur Child Adolesc Psychiatry* 17:452–461, 2008.
101. Munkvold LH, Lundervold AJ, Manger T: Oppositional defiant disorder—gender differences in co-occurring symptoms of mental health problems in a general population of children. *J Abnorm Child Psychol* 39:577–587, 2011.
102. Kessler RC, Avenevoli S, Costello EJ, et al.: Prevalence, persistence, and sociodemographic correlates of DSM-IV disorders in the National Comorbidity Survey Replication Adolescent Supplement. *Arch Gen Psychiatry* 69:372–380, 2012.
103. López-Villalobos JA, Andrés-De Llano JM, Rodríguez-Molinero L, et al.: Prevalence of oppositional defiant disorder in Spain. *Rev Psiquiatr Salud Ment* 7:80–87, 2014.

CHAPTER 5.1.3 ■ AGGRESSION IN CHILDREN: AN INTEGRATIVE APPROACH

JOSEPH C. BLADER AND DANIEL F. CONNOR

INTRODUCTION

Aggressive and Prosocial Behavior

A central goal of every human community is the mitigation of aggression between its members. From the earliest writings, most reflections on human interactions suggest an intrinsic capacity for aggression and brutality (1). Natural drives to acquire resources, to protect those resources and personal safety, and to enhance and defend one's status cause antagonisms that humans, like other animals, resolve through force. Social order demands less destructive alternatives to violence, and moral development and social organization strive to suppress such behavior. Thomas Hobbes (1588–1679) memorably summarized this viewpoint by showing how human communities would not advance very much if we lived in fear of one another (2):

> ...In such condition there is no place for Industry because the fruit thereof is uncertain...no commodious Building;... no Arts; no Letters; no Society; and which is worst of all, continuall feare, and danger of violent death; And the life of man, solitary, poore, nasty, brutish, and short.

When Charles Darwin considered these issues within a biologic framework some 200 years later, these predecessors who depicted life as a struggle for existence influenced his work (3). Natural selection involves competition for the resources that are essential to survival and successful reproduction. Scarcity of these resources means that some creatures inevitably deprive others within their species of access to them, often through aggressive behavior. However, Darwin also devoted much attention to the adaptive benefits of the "social instincts," such as sympathy, cooperation, altruism, and the desire to maintain the approval of one's group, which exert an equally natural countervailing force on intraspecific aggression. After all, when danger is at hand humans tend to seek safety in one another's company. Potential procreative partners may also favor these characteristics, accelerating their proliferation through the process of sexual selection (4).

As man is a social animal, it is almost certain that he would inherit a tendency to be faithful to his comrades, and obedient to the leader of his tribe; for these qualities are common to most social animals. He would consequently possess some capacity for self-command. He would from an inherited tendency be willing to defend, in concert with others, his fellow men; and would be ready to aid them in any way, which did not too greatly interfere with his own welfare or his own strong desires (5).

Since then, behavioral research has supported the overall view that a combination of affective, cognitive, and social factors inhibits the majority of people from harming others most of the time (6,7). We also know a fair amount about when social factors could lose their potency to inhibit aggressive behavior, even in the absence of psychopathology. For instance, aggressive behavior becomes more likely when a potential target belongs to a different social grouping; when one perceives another person as threatening; when one believes that others will approve of or encourage aggressive acts; or, when one believes that the benefits of aggression will exceed its probable cost.

Because many psychiatric disorders have the potential to disrupt cognitive, affective, and behavioral processes that ordinarily inhibit aggressive and other harmful behaviors, these behaviors often arise as a highly disconcerting complication. High negative emotionality may predispose to a low threshold for anger or frustration, so that one reacts forcefully to situations others would find only mildly bothersome. Distorted cognitive processes may lead to unwarranted alarm about environmental threats, to feeling impelled by some force to hurt others, or to erroneous beliefs about entitlement to impose one's will on others. High anxiety may trigger avoidance or escape behaviors that can injure others who get in the way. Inadequate impulse control can disrupt response selection so that aggression has precedence over alternatives. Abnormal development may impair the acquisition of coping behaviors and self-regulatory capabilities that ordinarily suppress dyscontrolled outbursts. A diminished capacity for empathy removes an important restraining factor whereby cues that show the distress of others can reverberate uncomfortably within ourselves.

Certain experiential factors can contribute to persistent aggression and therefore have psychiatric significance. Early severe maltreatment may disrupt the development of empathy. Socialization that promotes violence and threats as vehicles for self-preservation may lead to aggression that persists even in new social contexts that disapprove of such behavior.

Aggressive behavior is therefore an important concern for all mental health professions. Because persistent aggressive behavior most often originates in childhood, and is in itself a frequent reason for which youth obtain psychiatric care, it is especially significant for the practice of child and adolescent psychiatry. Aggressive behavior among school-age children confers high risk for unfavorable outcomes not only during youth but also throughout later life, including early mortality (8–12).

AGGRESSION AND VICTIMIZATION AMONG YOUTH

Community- and Clinic-Based Estimates

Physically aggressive behavior among preschoolers is common but diminishes upon school entry and during the elementary school years. Tremblay et al. (13) found that only a minority (28%) of 3 year olds were said to display little or no aggression. Parent reports indicate that 27% of 3-year-old boys hit, push, or trip others. The comparable rate for girls is 19%. Parents reported "modest aggression" for 58% with equal gender representation (13). Parents reported quite high aggressive behavior among 14%, of whom 57% were male.

In elementary school samples, larger gender differences emerge for "starts fights," with parent reports indicate that fighting is present among about 12% of boys and 6% of girls (14). However, the prevalence of "bullies, threatens, or intimidates" is relatively similar between genders (boys 13%, girls 10%).

Several longitudinal studies have tracked teacher-reported conduct problems through elementary school. Some also had initial assessments from infancy and some had follow-ups through young adulthood. Data from six of these studies found that 8% of boys consistently obtain the highest physical aggression ratings (15). Stability in teachers' ratings of aggressive behavior across many school years is even more striking than the continuity of parent report, because teachers and classmates change annually for most children.

Aggressive behavior is among the most prevalent chief complaints for youth seen in inpatient, outpatient, and residential treatment services. Among preadolescents, aggressive dyscontrol may be the most frequent reason for treatment in specialty mental health services. By adolescence, rising prevalence of mood disorders and self-injurious behavior, particularly among females, eclipses aggressive behavior as a chief complaint. However, new-onset aggressive behavior among girls in early to middle adolescence seems rather frequent, and in clinical samples may be an associated feature of depressive disorders (16). Therefore, despite a shift from "externalizing" to "internalizing" diagnoses with age, aggression may remain a formidable concern.

The majority of youngsters who fight seem to do so in some settings and not others. Aggressive behavior at home only is especially common: about half of boys who fight show physical aggression within the family exclusively. Only 20% were reported to display physical aggression at both home and school (17).

CHARACTERIZING AND SUBTYPING AGGRESSION

The prevailing approach to distinguishing types of aggressive behavior focuses on whether its motivation is mainly (a) to repel a perceived threat or source of frustration, or (b) to acquire something desirable. The former defines *reactive, affective, frustrative, impulsive,* or *defensive* aggression. The latter is associated with terms like *proactive* or *instrumental aggression.* In general, psychometric and psychobiologic evidence supports such a distinction between these behaviors (18–20). As an approach to categorizing *people,* rather than behaviors, it may have some shortcomings, since many individuals display aggressive behaviors characteristic of both types at various times, and the correlations between them are high (21–25).

Impulsive, Affective, or Reactive Aggression

Affective or impulsive aggression refers to dyscontrolled reactions, which have the potential or the intent to hurt others or oneself, occur upon exposure to events perceived as noxious. The provocations are usually things that one might agree are annoyances, but within a level of intensity that most other children handle with composure. Triggers may appear quite trivial, such as not getting the right cereal for breakfast. Directions to comply with an adult request or the need to end a preferred activity to transition to something else are very frequent antecedents to full-blown rage episodes. Hitting, kicking, destruction of property, and self-abusive behavior are common. A verbal onslaught of screaming, vulgarity, threats, and hurtful insults are themselves very disturbing, even without physical contact. Since the behavior is most often reactive and nearly instantaneous, it tends to be overt and unplanned. These events can also show a self-defeating character. Youngsters in their explosive rage may end up hurting themselves by, for instance, punching walls or glass, damaging their own possessions, or escalating when it should be obvious, that doing so only makes matters worse. They may attack people much larger and stronger than themselves. A few children calm down when placated, but it is also common for these outbursts, once kindled, to have to run their course before the child regains control.

Children with these difficulties typically meet criteria for oppositional defiant disorder (ODD), since its symptoms include frequent loss of temper, anger, susceptibility to slight provocation, and argumentativeness. This pattern of behavior can also contribute to diagnosis of conduct disorder, usually with childhood onset, when it includes threats, fighting, and destruction of property.

Rageful outbursts are the cardinal symptom of disruptive mood dysregulation disorder (DMDD). DSM-5 introduced DMDD as a mood disorder to designate persistent irritability, and better distinguish it from other disorders in which irritability can be prominent but that is typically episodic (e.g., bipolar disorder, major depressive disorder). The DMDD diagnosis therefore requires that one's prevailing mood in between rageful outbursts is irritable or angry. However, only a minority of youth with significant reactive aggression also show abnormalities of mood when they are not acutely distressed (26,27).

Proactive, Instrumental, or Appetitive Aggression

Proactive or instrumental aggression includes assaultive or coercive behavior purposefully used to achieve a goal such as material goods or social status. Willful property destruction is also included by some. Descriptions of proactive/instrumental aggression sometimes liken it to hunting, but for many species predation and intraspecific aggression have different underpinnings and phenomenology (28). A few features of proactive aggression make plain that the actor is in control. For instance, proactive aggression stops once the goal is achieved or when it becomes clear that it has become unobtainable. Victims are chosen to make success likely. The aggressor may take protective measures to avoid getting hurt and evasive action to avoid apprehension. While planning and premeditation are certainly consistent with proactive aggressive behavior, it is probably not a requirement. A number of "acquisitive" violent acts, such as certain robberies and sexual assaults, are often opportunistic and not necessarily performed with much forethought.

Among youth whose aggressive behavior is principally of the proactive/instrumental type, we can also discriminate two important subgroups.

Adolescent-Onset, Peer-Facilitated Proactive Aggression

First, a group of proactively aggressive youth show adolescent onset of antisocial behavior. Aggressive acts in this context are on the whole less violent, rely on peer encouragement, and seem likely to diminish by adulthood (29–31). However, the boundary between obnoxious pranks and major violations that cause serious injury or damage is fortified by common sense and restraint. The group dynamics of adolescents behaving recklessly do not promote these qualities, often with tragic results. In these situations, a young person may become ensnared by the consequences of delinquent participation. School expulsion, increased wariness of other peers, and involvement with law enforcement or correctional facilities can promote further identification and involvement with delinquent peers, and deflect what had hitherto been a pathway of overall positive adjustment.

Callous–Unemotional ("Psychopathic") Proactive Aggression

Another important subgroup of proactively aggressive youth is profoundly indifferent to the consequences that their misbehavior has upon others. Displays of genuine remorse are rare, and a current descriptor for this group's salient personality features, "callous–unemotional traits," is highly evocative of their lack of empathy, self-centeredness, and shallowness (32). In this respect, they resemble adults with *psychopathic* or *sociopathic* personality traits. When these features are present, the DSM-5 diagnosis of conduct disorder can be accompanied by the specifier, "with limited prosocial emotions." These youth are responsible for a large number of violent offenses, their aggressive behavior is often persistent and development of these characteristics may be early in childhood (33,34).

Many individuals exhibit *both* the angry overreactivity of affective/impulsive aggression and the deliberate, calculated injury to others characteristic of psychopathy. Indeed, some definitions of psychopathy include both impulsive "hotheadedness" along with the capacity to trample calmly upon the rights of others when it suits one's purpose.

INFLUENCES ON AGGRESSIVE BEHAVIOR: PSYCHOPATHOLOGY AND PROCESSES

In keeping with the view that diverse forms of psychopathology and unfavorable experiences can lead to aggressive behavior, this section offers a framework that links them (Figure 5.1.3.1). Four broad categories of specific deficits and experiential factors that we distinguish are: impulse control deficits, affective instability, sensory and cognitive abnormalities, and environments that can promote antisocial behavior. Linkages on the left acknowledge the frequent co-occurrence and interdependence of these factors. To the right are several psychiatric disorders and psychosocial processes to which these factors often integral, and that in turn constitute the "psychopathologic context" for aggressive behavior problems in youth. Finally, severely disruptive behavior itself has sequelae that can abate (e.g., interventions) or increase (e.g., social marginalization) persistence and impairments; some of these "impact outcomes" appear on the far right.

Impulse Control Deficits

Generalized problems with situational awareness and self-control are strongly associated with aggressive behavior (35–37). These problems are "generalized" because affected children often show undercontrol of many functions in numerous settings. These include weak self-restraint of conduct and activity level that often biases action toward disproportionately physical and disruptive responses to

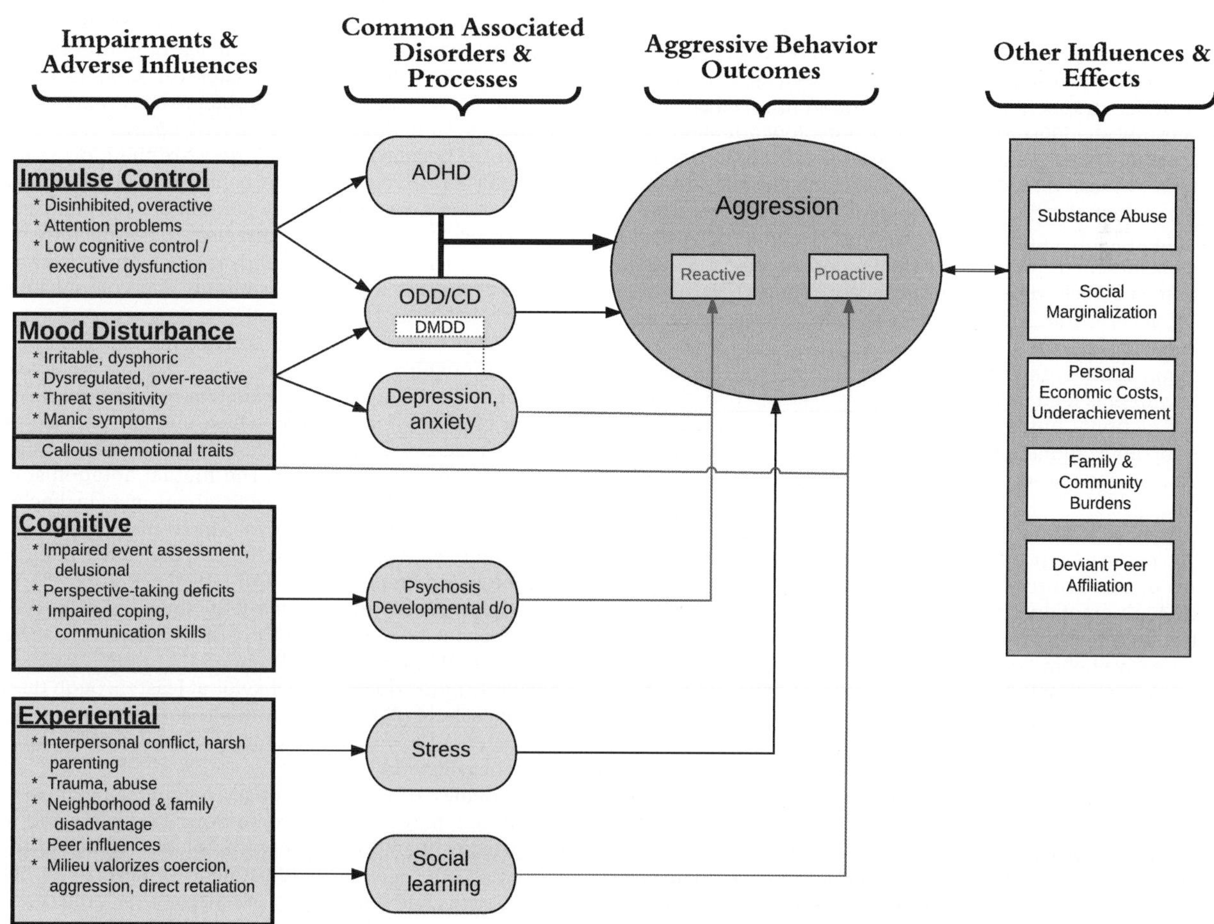

FIGURE 5.1.3.1. Influences on the development of aggressive behavior. ADHD, attention-deficit/hyperactivity disorder; ODD, oppositional defiant disorder; CD, conduct disorder; DMDD, disruptive mood dysregulation disorder.

minimal provocation, and low effortful cognitive control over one's behavior (e.g., sustaining attention, problem-solving, verbal mediation of conflicts, perspective taking), that make willful selection of alternative responses problematic. Dimensional measures of impulsivity correlate with aggression and self-harming behavior (38,39). Early hyperactivity predicts subsequent aggression (40,41) and, in tandem with early aggressive conduct problems, strongly predisposes to persistent antisocial behavior (42).

These predisposing factors toward behavioral volatility and aggression are prominent in youth diagnosed with attention-deficit/hyperactivity disorder (ADHD). Self-regulation of affect, while not currently part of ADHD's criteria, is often regarded as practically intrinsic to at least some presentations of ADHD (43,44), and ADHD is ubiquitous among youth with high negative emotional reactivity (45–47).

Although we emphasize ADHD because of its prevalence among aggressive youth, problems with impulsiveness that develop later in life, can also contribute to the onset of aggressive behavior. Impaired self-control can occur in several psychiatric disorders discussed below that often develop in adolescence (such as bipolar disorder, psychosis, and chronic substance abuse), as well as traumatic brain injury (48,49).

Impairments of Mood, Affect Reactivity, and Anxiety

Negative Affect, Mood Disorders

Evidence from several sources implicates affect disturbances in aggression and other early-onset disruptive behaviors. The correlation between negative affective features (e.g., irritability, lability, anger, dysphoria, frustrability) and disruptive behavior is well established (50–52). Unconsolability, low adaptability, and irritability predict subsequent aggression (53,54). Parental reactions to these difficult characteristics may moderate the ultimate impact of difficult temperament (55,56). From a diagnostic standpoint, longitudinal studies indicate that early ODD confers heightened risk for adolescent mood disorders (57,58). This outcome likely reflects the presence among ODD symptoms of several that highlight negative affect (anger, easily annoyed, etc.) (59,60).

Among youth with conduct problems, those with negative affect symptoms tend to be more aggressive and to experience worse functional outcomes. Unfavorable outcomes include more hospitalizations, police contacts, impaired social relations, substance abuse, and less improvement with treatment (61–65).

Emotion regulation can be disturbed episodically, with or without persistent problems in prevailing mood (26,66,67). Aspects of emotion regulation that are relevant to aggression include high emotional reactivity, poor emotion modulation, lability, and slow recovery from upset (68–71).

Aggressive behavior may also arise in the context of major depression and bipolar disorder. Heightened irritability and anger are frequent aspects of both disorders, so a lowered threshold for lashing out is not surprising, and the risk for self-directed harm among affected individuals is of course high. Among adults, comorbid substance abuse significantly raises risk of violent and suicidal behavior (72,73). Bipolar disorder may confer a higher lifetime risk for aggression than unipolar depression (74). Clinician-rated aggressive behavior may be less frequent among inpatient adolescents than adults with bipolar disorder (75), but there may be sample biases wherein adults are more likely to be hospitalized for dangerousness than youth.

Anxiety

With the reclassification or trauma-related disorders in DSM-5, the remaining anxiety disorders by themselves seldom increase the liability for aggressive behavior. The situation changes, though, when comorbid conditions enter the picture (76). Anxious children with ADHD and ODD are more likely to become behaviorally agitated, perhaps by virtue of impulse control problems making it more difficult for them to tolerate anxious discomfort. For instance, efforts to interrupt compulsive rituals for a child with obsessive–compulsive disorder or to enforce school attendance with a child who has separation anxiety can at times provoke reactive aggression.

Coldheartedness

Besides these "hot" affective features, callousness and *under*-emotionality may, as mentioned earlier, influence aggressive behavior used for instrumental goals (77,78). These individuals appear to display rather blunted emotional reactivity to the distress of others, a stimulus that is thought to inhibit gratuitous violence in most people (79). Similarly, the disapproval of others appears to carry little significance for them and it seems they are more interested in asserting control and gaining advantage over others than in companionship.

Environmental Influences

Interpersonal Conflict, Trauma, and Stress

Diminished Positive Parental Interactions; Harsh and Inconsistent Discipline. Child-rearing practices probably affect the development of children's aggressive behavior though both stress-related and social learning processes, and the next section will focus on the latter. It is obvious that children with early-onset conduct problems often make difficult housemates, and those with frequent aggressive behavior still more so because family members are the most common targets (80–83). Even when the behavior is not particularly harmful, many aspects of family life that are normally almost effortless are fraught with the prospect that a meltdown or a "scene" will disrupt otherwise enjoyable activities, draw attention and resources away from siblings, and complicate relations with schools.

The compound effects are to corrode the quality of parent–child relationships, particularly when parents believe misbehavior to be volitional (84). Family stress and discord and frequent repercussions (85–88), which may further degrade a parent's capacity to apply measured discipline consistently and with composure (56,87,89–91). The mutual antagonism that results, and the child's own unpredictability, may incline a parent toward disengagement or involvement that depends on the parent's own energy and mood, than on the child's behavior.

Parental psychopathology and substance abuse can also lead to suboptimal interactions with their children (92–94). Low maternal education and hostile/ineffective parenting behaviors both increase the likelihood that toddlers will show persistently high aggressive behavior at least through the start of middle school (95). However, this risk was reduced among preschoolers of low-education mothers who received nonmaternally provided day care (96).

Poor quality of a child's primary relationships, however it comes about, may predict a worse overall outcome and treatment prospects among those with behavioral volatility and aggression, after statistical adjustment for severity of behavioral problems and disciplinary practices (97,98). Interestingly, it has been suggested that among children with callous–unemotional traits, quality of parenting may play a *smaller* role in the development of their conduct problems (99), a finding that is consistent with the apparent indifference of psychopathic individuals to others' feelings.

Trauma, Abuse, Frequent Endangerment. Maltreatment and other direct trauma during childhood significantly increase one's liability for lifetime psychopathology. The largest effect size of child abuse for both genders is the increase in antisocial behavior (100). A connection between living helplessly with frequent, random infliction of pain and development of defensive hyperreactivity to even minimal threat is both intuitive and supported by recent studies indicating abnormalities in the structures and processes that subserve fear and affect regulation (101,102). Early maltreatment correlates equally well with measures of reactive and proactive aggression (103), and abuse was slightly more prevalent among youth categorized as proactively aggressive than reactively aggressive (104).

Peers and siblings can also inflict torment and fear that heighten threat sensitivity leading to self-regulatory problems and aggression. Bullying and other victimization experiences have recently gained overdue recognition as sources of distress that can culminate in harmful behavior toward others or oneself (105–107).

Community Factors. Studies focused on disadvantaged communities indicate that children's exposure to neighborhood violence is associated with both aggressive behavior and post-traumatic stress disorder (108). Exposure effects on development of aggressive behavior seem especially strong for highly stressed families with conflictual relationships (108).

Besides exposure-related risk, neighborhood socioeconomic disadvantage augments the risk for aggressive behavior in children, but the effect may be largest for children in single-parent households (109). It has also been suggested that the proportion of single-adult-led households may be a community-level risk factor (110). While single-parent homes are not inherently pathogenic, communities where they predominate have fewer adults providing supervision and those present are more likely to be busy with the burdens of raising children with fewer resources than would be typical in child-rearing homes with at least two adults.

Social Learning

Benefits for One's Own Aggressive Behavior. If aggressive behavior has a payoff, basic learning theory would predict that it will be more likely in the future. Therefore, if a conflict involving the child's aggression ends with the child prevailing in getting his or her way, escaping from an undesirable situation, or gaining some other reward, aggressive behavior is in effect reinforced.

Likewise, victim acquiescence to one's aggressive behavior offers further incentive to attack or intimidate others. Some bullies may also attain high status among peers at least for brief periods (29). In addition, peer encouragement can also provide powerful inducement toward antisocial behavior that outweighs adult-imposed consequences for it. Vicarious enjoyment of a peer's antisocial conduct, and reinforcement for the performer, may be related to the findings that outpatient group treatments for youth with severe conduct problems may do more harm than good (111). A similar process may also occur by which a youth with severe conduct problems may enlist the collusion of sibling to erode the authority structure within the home (112).

Modeling, Observed Benefits for Aggression. The phenomenon of learning by observing the consequences that accompany behaviors modeled by *others* is called social or vicarious learning (113). The weight of the current evidence seems to indicate that high exposure to depictions of violence in mass media may contribute to the risk of aggressive behavior, particularly among young children (114). Similar effects have been shown for violent video games, but interestingly video games that involve cooperation have been linked to increased prosocial behavior.

Cognitive or Sensory Impairments

Several psychiatric and developmental disorders may have aggression as a complication because they distort one's information processing or the capacity to communicate and handle distress.

Aggressive behavior frequently accompanies schizophrenia among adolescents and adults (115,116). The few children who develop the disorder are more typically terrified, withdrawn and perplexed, rather than belligerent or agitated. Several factors that seem to augment the risk of violence include severity of positive symptoms, paranoid delusions, male gender, and premorbid history of aggressive behavior. Following stabilization of acute psychotic symptoms, violence does not seem especially characteristic of residual phase schizophrenia among adults, and indeed increased belligerence, suspiciousness, and lashing out often signify risk of relapse, drug or alcohol use, or effects of other nonpsychotic disturbances (116).

Aggressive behavior is more prevalent in certain developmental major disorders than others. Aggressive behavior frequently occurs among those with autism spectrum disorders (ASD), and may be more severe than among those with other significant developmental disabilities (117,118). By contrast, it is less of a complication in Down or Williams syndrome (119). Within any given syndrome, as well as idiopathic intellectual disability in general, severity of aggression seems a function of lower IQ and male gender.

Self-injurious behavior is an aspect of several developmental syndromes. Difficulties communicating the nature and cause of discomfort, and a limited repertoire of behaviors to gain the attention of others, mandate careful assessment to identify the triggers for aggressive outbursts and consider environmental changes to reduce their impact.

Behavioral Pharmacotoxicity

Prescription Drugs: Complications of Therapeutic Use, Overdose

Medication regimens for many aggressive children currently involve coadministration of multiple agents (120–122). Pharmacotherapy may contribute to irritability and behavioral dyscontrol in idiosyncratic ways. Agitation or "activation" that accompanies selective serotonin reuptake inhibitor (SSRI) treatment seems more prevalent among children than adolescents (123). Stimulant medications may also worsen irritability among some youth (124), but this is often a dose-dependent effect. Compounds used mainly for nonpsychiatric reasons also warrant review when behavior changes. For instance higher doses of corticosteroids can precipitate aggressive behavior (125).

Drugs of Abuse

It is difficult to attribute any specific amount of aggressive behavior to the effects of alcohol and other substances, because the risk factors for substance use resemble many of those for aggression. Because chronic aggressive behavior in youth often originates before exposure to illicit drugs, we show substance abuse in Figure 5.1.3.1 as a sequela of conduct problems that in turn further impairs functioning. Adolescent-onset aggressive behavior, though, may coincide with drug and alcohol use. Drug use by adolescents, including cannabinoids, cocaine, and hallucinogens, may aggravate psychiatric illness among psychosis-prone individuals.

TREATMENT

Treatment Planning

Psychopathology and Context

This chapter emphasizes the significance of specific "underlying" psychopathology and other influences in the emergence of aggressive behavior, in large part because successful treatment of the primary disorder ameliorates aggression. An alternate view is that aggression, regardless of specific disorder, might be amenable to some antiaggressive treatment. Current practice and guidelines combine these approaches, especially in regard to pharmacotherapy (126–128). Generally, the primary psychiatric disorder should be the target of initial interventions. Then, if aggressive behavior does not subside adequately, other medications are often prescribed on the basis of their antiaggression effects. As a practical matter, the most common scenario, especially for preadolescents, involves initiating pharmacotherapy targeting ADHD symptoms among the large group of youngsters whose aggressive behavior develops in the context of ADHD plus a disruptive disorder or DMDD. Another large patient group shows aggressive volatility and agitation that accompany depression, usually among adolescents, which often raises concerns about bipolar disorder risk.

Clinicians therefore often face a decisional dilemma of how long and to what doses should one persist in trying to optimize first-line treatments (such as stimulants for ADHD) versus initiating an adjunctive medication (often antipsychotics that incur higher adverse effect risks) to achieve behavioral stability in troubling situations. There is only limited research to guide these choices.

Multiple Impairments in Several Settings Are Common

It is common for a child to exhibit aggressive behavior in one setting and other problems in other venues. For example, loss of control may be most prominent at home, but school problems can include academic frustration, low achievement, and social problems. Aggressive behavior at home may relate to these other stresses, and managing these triggers may be the key to reducing volatility at home.

Prioritizing and Sequencing Treatments

When psychosocial treatments should precede medications or vice versa, is a common issue. Family preference is a pivotal factor, and the pros and cons of each approach should be discussed openly along with an agreement about how to monitor the outcome and when to change course. Productive shared decision-making, however, requires well-informed partners. Many families would prefer to give nonpharmacologic treatments a chance, in which case it is worthwhile to find discuss their expectations for therapy. Most evidence-based psychosocial treatments for youth conduct problems involve significant parental effort to change interaction patterns with the child, and to manage behavioral upsets in a firm but calm manner. When impulsivity and inattention are significant problems, behavioral therapies stand a greater chance of gaining traction when self-control and focus have improved somewhat, and medications for ADHD remain the most effective means to that outcome.

In any case, severe conduct problems that include aggression often have had a corrosive impact on family life, and relationships become fraught with negative expectations, resentment, or guilt. Whether or not formal psychosocial treatment is part of the plan, assuming it is even available, the child psychiatrist has to be mindful of these stresses and try to foster opportunities for family members to enjoy one another's company, and warmly recognize and support any progress toward handling troubling situations with greater composure.

Pharmacotherapy

A common view is that medication affects only reactive or impulsive aggression (129,130). However, trials involving impulsive youth indicate that proactive aggressive behavior often decreases alongside improvements in reactive aggression, and parent ratings of callous–unemotional features also decline (20,131–133). Nevertheless, among proactively aggressive individuals without contributing psychopathology (such as impulsivity, mood disturbances, etc.), pharmacotherapy currently lacks justification.

Stimulant and Nonstimulant Treatments When ADHD Is Present

Most controlled trials of stimulant medications for ADHD show treatment-related reductions in aggression and other conduct problems (35,131,134–137). However, very few of these trials involve patients selected for high aggressive behavior that is the primary outcome. Instead, ratings of conduct problems are most often secondary outcomes for patients with ADHD and no prespecified level of aggression. Some trials involve patients with a broad spectrum of disruptive behavior, not aggression per se (131,135,138).

More recent trials examining treatment strategies for children with significant aggressive behavior who have ADHD, though, indicate large effects following stimulant monotherapy on reducing aggression or a composite of disruptive behavior symptoms, as well as mood symptoms (20,26,133,139–141). These trials employed either extended or brief stimulant optimization, along with behavioral therapy, before starting adjunctive treatment risperidone, divalproex sodium (DVPX), or placebo. Across two trials using extended stimulant monotherapy optimization, 50% and 62% of children, all of whom had prior stimulant treatment before enrollment, showed remission of aggression that obviated the need for adjunctive treatments. A trial using a briefer period of stimulant monotherapy before starting adjunctive risperidone or placebo, showed significant continued improvement for those randomized to placebo with no difference in overall responder rates, but an advantage on mean disruptive behavior ratings for those receiving adjunctive risperidone.

Two nonstimulant medications with affinity for noradrenergic α_2 receptors, the antihypertensive agents guanfacine and clonidine, have long been used to treat ADHD, and as add-on to stimulant targeting conduct problems including aggression. Long-acting preparations of these agents have made their use in this context more attractive, especially with their smaller adverse effect liability relative to antipsychotic treatment. They do seem to provide additional benefit to stimulant monotherapy for disruptive behavior symptoms when added to stimulants (142), but it is unclear from the relevant trials how often stimulant medication was optimized, nor was high aggressive behavior usually their focus. However, one small trial comparing methylphenidate and clonidine monotherapies with these drugs combined among aggressive youth with ADHD indicated that all three treatment approaches had comparable effects in reducing aggression (143).

Other approved nonstimulant treatments for childhood ADHD, bupropion and atomoxetine, have not yet been shown to affect aggressive behavior.

In the context of other primary disorders, the benefits of stimulant treatment on aggressive behavior are less well studied. Youngsters with major developmental disorders, autism in particular, have more variable responses to stimulant therapy, which at times may worsen aggression and irritability (144,145).

Antipsychotics and Antimanic/Mood Stabilizers

Antipsychotics. Antipsychotics have long held a prominent place in treating aggression in nonpsychotic individuals. Their broad spectrum of effects includes antimanic effects. Early studies suggested the efficacy of antipsychotic medications among nonpsychotic aggressive youth (146,147), but concerns about their potential to produce adverse extrapyramidal symptoms (EPS) and other unfavorable effects restrained their use. The advent of nonclozapine "second-generation" antipsychotic medications led to their wide use for nonpsychotic youth partly because they have overall lower risk for neuromotor adverse effects, at least among adults. Consequently, the past 15 years or so have witnessed a tremendous increase in the use of second-generation antipsychotics (SGAs) to treat severe behavioral disturbances in children (121,148–151). However, obesity, insulin resistance, type II diabetes, hypertension, and indices of atherosclerosis risk, known collectively as cardiometabolic adverse effects, are elevated among SGA-treated youth relative to non-SGA-treated youth (152,153). Children treated with these agents also remain more susceptible to EPS than adults with these agents (154,155).

Risperidone currently has the most extensive data from controlled trials supporting its efficacy as monotherapy among children with aggressive behavior (156,157). It has FDA approval for the treatment of irritability in autism. These studies show marked reductions relative to placebo in parent or clinician ratings of aggression and in some instances improvements in the asociality associated with autism spectrum disorders. Trials of risperidone added on to stimulant medication for aggressive children with ADHD (and without ASD or other developmental handicap) also show some advantage over placebo, but of smaller magnitude than risperidone monotherapy trials (133,158). Weight gain and hyperprolactinemia are frequently reported.

Aripiprazole also has an indication for irritability and aggression for 6 to 17 year olds with autistic disorder. Despite widespread clinical use for aggression outside of psychosis or autism, controlled trials for other populations are pending.

Two other SGAs marketed in the United States have adverse effect profiles that make them generally inappropriate for youth without psychotic illness: olanzapine's weight gain risk is very high, and ziprasidone has the highest risk for QTc prolongation (159). Lurasidone seems to have lower weight gain liability among adults relative to SGAs currently prescribed to youth, but was no more effective than placebo for irritability in autism (160) and EPS risk is higher than other SGAs (159).

Mood Stabilizer Agents. The use of lithium and anticonvulsant medications that have indications for mania (often referred to collectively as "mood stabilizers") for aggressive behavior among youth has been largely overtaken by SGAs. For some patient groups, however, the adverse effect profile of these treatments may be more favorable than SGAs.

Supportive data for lithium came from a few inpatient studies, and there are to date no outpatient trials that have shown its efficacy (130,146,161). A recent outpatient trial involving children and adolescents with bipolar I disorder showed improvement on symptom severity ratings compared with placebo, which may spur renewed interest on potential antiaggressive benefit for a subgroup of patients with primary mood disturbances (162).

A trial of adjunctive DVPX for children with ADHD whose aggressive behavior was refractory to optimized stimulant monotherapy showed higher rates of remission than those who received adjunctive placebo (140). A study using a similar stepped treatment approach but stimulant-refractory randomizing patients to adjunctive DVPX, risperidone, or placebo also showed advantages for DVPX over placebo on aggression and other measures of conduct disturbance. However, the magnitude of improvement for children who had stimulant plus either DVPX or risperidone cotherapy was substantially less than for the 64% of children whose aggression remitted after the stimulant monotherapy protocol.

Trials of DVPX monotherapy in more patients with more heterogeneous conduct or mood problems also showed greater improvement relative to placebo (163–165). For youth with bipolar disorder, reductions in aggressive behavior accompanied DVPX treatment and were comparable to quetiapine (166), though among 10 to 17 year olds with bipolar I disorder extended-release DVPX was not more advantageous than placebo (167).

Carbamazepine treatment was associated with reduced aggression among hospitalized preadolescents with conduct disorder (168), however a randomized controlled trial at the same facility showed no benefit over placebo (169).

Antidepressants, Anxiolytics, Micronutrients

Despite the general principle that encourages choosing initial pharmacotherapy for aggressive or volatile patients based on his or her primary psychiatric disorder, there are practically no data on this approach for young people with major depression. Reluctance to include rage-prone adolescents in clinical trials is understandable, because the risk for harms is greater than among those who are less behaviorally activated or experiencing psychomotor retardation. Concern that such a symptom picture portends conversion to bipolar disorder also often dissuades clinicians from antidepressant monotherapy, even though data are lacking on the true magnitude of such risk compared to the risk of "overtreatment" with antipsychotic medications.

In clinical practice, adjunctive treatment with SSRIs for irritable youth with comorbid ADHD is not uncommon, but there are no data to support or denigrate this strategy. Trials of stimulant and adjunctive SSRI treatment for youth with DMDD are in progress.

Benzodiazepines may increase disinhibition and aggression (170) and are disfavored for treating childhood aggression outside acute management for agitation associated with psychosis.

One intriguing double-blind controlled trial conducted in a British penitentiary showed marked reductions in violent incidents among inmates randomized to receive a combination of vitamins, and omega-3 fatty acid pills compared to those who received matching placebo pills (171). The fact that this study effectively standardized all other aspects of environment and diet appears to strengthen the potential significance of micronutrients in violence-prone populations.

A recent trial with 11 and 12 year olds evaluated micronutrients, including three common omega-3 fatty acids, crossed with cognitive behavioral treatment (CBT) emphasizing anger control and reappraisal strategies (172). Child self-reports of reactive aggression showed larger reductions among those who had CBT plus nutrient supplementation than CBT and control groups. However, parent reports of externalizing behaviors showed no treatment effect.

Psychosocial Treatments

Overview

Interventions to reduce aggressive behavior alter the environmental context that promotes it, help individuals develop

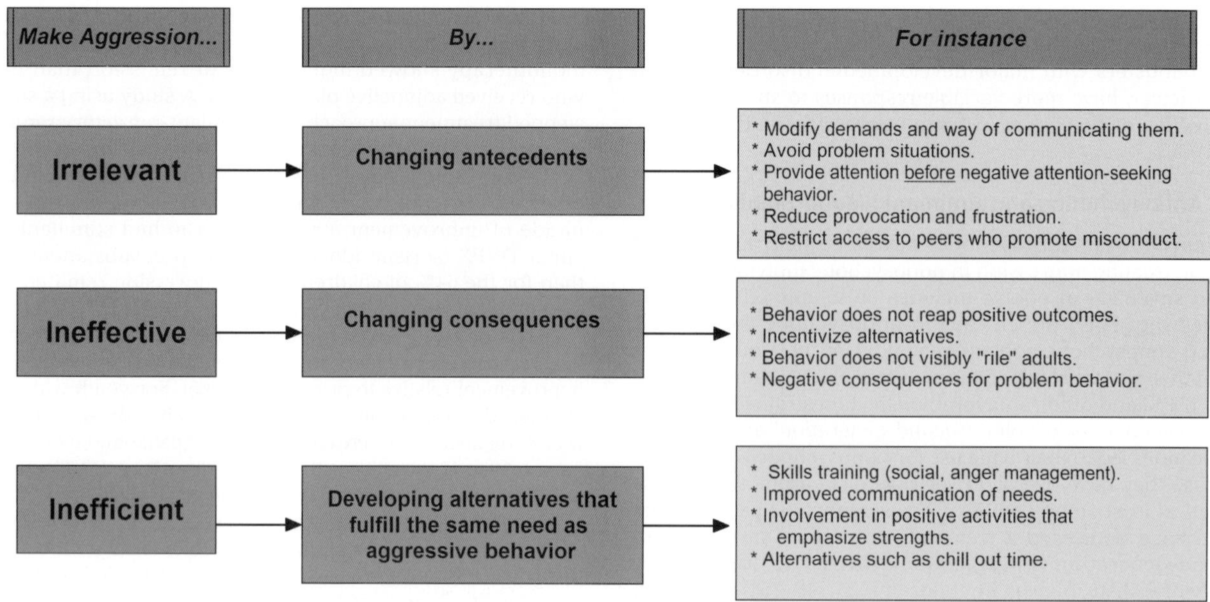

FIGURE 5.1.3.2. Goals and approaches of psychosocial treatment.

alternatives to aggression that meet their goals more adaptively. Other chapters contain descriptions of specific therapies for these purposes (consequence-based approaches, anger control, multisystemic therapy, etc.). This section offers a framework to appreciate at a more general level the avenues through which treatments may reduce aggressive behavior. Borrowing from the framework of functional behavior assessment we organize the discussion to show how psychosocial interventions try to make aggressive behavior *irrelevant, ineffective,* or *inefficient* (Figure 5.1.3.2) (173).

Make Aggression Irrelevant

Aggressive behavior is generally not a random event. Situations, or antecedents, usually trigger problem behaviors, these antecedents affect patients to differing degrees. One approach is to reduce exposure to these precipitants. From a functional viewpoint, if aggression is the child's "solution" to that situation, minimizing exposure to that situation makes aggression irrelevant. If a child frequently fights with a sibling when they're both in their shared bedroom together in the morning, then it seems sensible to have child eat breakfast while the other is getting dressed, then switch. A reminder to get homework finished might precipitate arguments, escalation, and finally an explosion. Enrolling the youngster in an after-school program that includes homework may help. The same idea also applies to reducing exposure to situations that actively encourage problematic behavior. Curtailing a youth's exposure to behaviorally deviant peers is one example (174).

Besides avoiding situations that provoke aggressive responses, increasing exposure to situations that already lead to cooperative behavior is another way in which altering antecedents can make aggression irrelevant. After reaching high rates of cooperation and exposure by asking the child to do only things he or she would want to do anyway, one then moves on to requests that the child had hesitated to do before (175).

Make Aggression Ineffective

How other people react to aggressive behavior might maintain or reinforce it. If outbursts lead others to acquiesce, or, alternatively, remove the child from a situation he or she wanted to escape, then problem behaviors are essentially rewarded. Changing consequences of aggressive behavior would therefore make it ineffective in achieving the goal that sustains it. Contingency management approaches (reward systems, time out, and the like), or ignoring milder misbehavior altogether, makes aggressive behavior less effective by diminishing the "payoff" that previously reinforced it.

Similarly, bullying and intimidation become ineffective if the social milieu expresses intolerance for the behavior, rather than fear and subservience. This often means supporting victims who come forward as the real "heroes" so that a community undermines the secrecy and fear on which such behavior thrives.

Make Aggression Inefficient

If the purpose that aggressive behavior seemed to serve can be achieved with behavior that is easier to perform, then aggression becomes relatively inefficient, and should reduce in favor of the alternative. Many skills training interventions (anger management, social skills training, problem-solving, etc.) develop proficiency in alternatives that enable a child to cope with otherwise aggression-provoking situations more adaptively. However, one has to take care that these alternatives really are easier for a given child, and make sure that the alternative has the desired result. One can teach a child to ask to borrow something, but if limited verbal skills make it harder rather than easier relative to grabbing, altercation can follow. Likewise, if the other child does not willingly share then "asking behavior" may not be reinforced. "Bridging" can help smooth the process, where the child can easily signal to an adult that he or she wants something from another child and the adult facilitates the exchange, and reward the child for handling a rebuff with composure. At the other end of the age range, if an adolescent had obtained some social esteem by being antisocial, consider exploiting his or her prosocial talents and interests as a vehicle to gaining prestige.

Selected Trials of Psychosocial Interventions for Aggressive Behavior

A range of psychosocial interventions exists for children and adolescents with various conduct and oppositional defiant behaviors, often including aggression. Treatment studies targeting aggression per se have been somewhat less common.

Nonetheless, various psychosocial treatment strategies have yielded significant reductions in aggressive behaviors, both in prevention trials and clinical treatment settings (176–180). Thus, parent management training (PMT) is an efficacious strategy for treating aggression and related conduct problems (176,179,181,182). Some evidence suggest that PMT may yield durable improvements in behavioral problems across various settings (183). Parent–child interaction training (PCIT) has also been found to reduce aggressive symptoms among young children, in large part through making parental attention and positive engagement a scheduled an enjoyable time to reduce child reliance on negative behavior for attention (184). Individual and some group-based cognitive-behavioral treatments, including anger management training and problem-solving skills training, have also had some success in improving aggressive behavior (177,178,181,185–187).

CONCLUSIONS

Nevertheless, aggressive behavior still eludes consistently effective intervention. The combined force of troubling outcomes, adverse community impact, high prevalence, and uncertain treatment prospects propels childhood-onset aggression to the forefront of challenges in mental health today. Timely and thoughtful assessment and intervention may save a child from a spiral of chronic conflict, social maladjustment, and marginalization. The child psychiatrist has an especially privileged position because the complications that arise from chronic antisocial behavior cause their own hardships, lifestyle problems, and impairments that make successful treatment far less likely.

References

1. Pinker S: *The Better Angels of Our Nature: Why Violence has Declined.* New York, Viking, 2011.
2. Hobbes T: *Leviathan; or The Matter, Forme, and Power of a Commonwealth Ecclesiaticall and Civil.* (Oakeshott M, editor). Oxford, UK, Blackwell, 1960. Original work published 1651.
3. Malthus TR: *An Essay on the Principle of Population.* (Gilbert G, editor). New York, Oxford University Press, 1993. Original work published 1798.
4. Miller G: *The Mating Mind: How Sexual Choice Shaped the Evolution of Human Nature.* London, Heineman, 2000.
5. Darwin C: *The Descent of Man, and Selection in Relation to Sex.* Princeton, NJ, Princeton University Press (Originally published 1871), 1981.
6. de Waal F: *Good Natured: The Origins of Right and Wrong in Humans and Other Animals.* Cambridge, MA, Harvard University Press, 1996.
7. Ridley M: *The Origins of Virtue: Human Instincts and the Evolution of Cooperation.* New York, Viking, 1996.
8. Moffitt TE, Caspi A, Rutter M, et al.: *Sex Differences in Antisocial Behaviour: Conduct Disorder, Delinquency, and Violence in the Dunedin Longitudinal Study.* New York, Cambridge University Press, 2001.
9. Lahey BB, Loeber R, Burke JD, Applegate B: Predicting future antisocial personality disorder in males from a clinical assessment in childhood. *J Consult Clin Psychol* 73:389–399, 2005.
10. Tremblay RE: Why socialization fails: the case of chronic physical aggression. In: Lahey BB, Moffitt TE, Caspi A (eds): *Causes of Conduct Disorder and Juvenile Delinquency.* New York, Guilford Press, 182–224, 2003.
11. Jokela M, Ferrie J, Kivimaki M: Childhood problem behaviors and death by midlife: the British national child development study. *J Am Acad Child Adolesc Psychiatry* 48:19–24, 2009.
12. Temcheff CE, Serbin LA, Martin-Storey A, et al.: Childhood aggression, withdrawal and likeability, and the use of health care later: a longitudinal study. *Can Med Assoc J* 183:2095–2101, 2011.
13. Tremblay RE, Nagin DS, Seguin JR, et al.: Physical aggression during early childhood: trajectories and predictors. *Pediatrics* 114:e43–e50, 2004.
14. Gadow KD, Sprafkin J: *Child Symptom Inventory 4: Screening and Norms Manual.* Stony Brook, NY, Checkmate, 2002.
15. Broidy LM, Nagin DS, Tremblay RE, et al.: Developmental trajectories of childhood disruptive behaviors and adolescent delinquency: a six-site, cross-national study. *Dev Psychol* 39:222–245, 2003.
16. Keenan K, Loeber R, Green S: Conduct disorder in girls: a review of the literature. *Clin Child Fam Psychol Rev* 2:3–19, 1999.
17. Loeber R, Stouthamer-Loeber M: Juvenile aggression at home and at school. In: Elliott DS, Hamburg BA, Williams KR (eds): *Violence in American Schools.* New York, Cambridge University Press, 94–126, 1998.
18. Scarpa A, Haden SC, Tanaka A: Being hot-tempered: autonomic, emotional, and behavioral distinctions between childhood reactive and proactive aggression. *Biol Psychol* 84:488–496, 2010.
19. Fite PJ, Colder CR, Lochman JE, Wells KC: Developmental trajectories of proactive and reactive aggression from fifth to ninth grade. *J Clin Child Adolesc Psychol* 37:412–421, 2008.
20. Blader JC, Pliszka SR, Kafantaris V, et al.: Callous-unemotional traits, proactive aggression, and treatment outcomes of aggressive children with attention-deficit/hyperactivity disorder. *J Am Acad Child Adolesc Psychiatry* 52:1281–1293, 2013.
21. Waschbusch DA, Willoughby MT, Pelham WE Jr: Criterion validity and the utility of reactive and proactive aggression: comparisons to attention deficit hyperactivity disorder, oppositional defiant disorder, conduct disorder, and other measures of functioning. *J Clin Child Psychol* 27:396–405, 1998.
22. Raine A, Dodge K, Loeber R, et al.: The reactive–proactive aggression questionnaire: differential correlates of reactive and proactive aggression in adolescent boys. *Aggress Behav* 32:159–171, 2006.
23. Atkins MS, Stoff DM: Instrumental and hostile aggression in childhood disruptive behavior disorders. *J Abnorm Child Psychol* 21:165–178, 1993.
24. Davidson RJ, Putnam KM, Larson CL: Dysfunction in the neural circuitry of emotion regulation—a possible prelude to violence. *Science* 289:591–594, 2000.
25. Barker ED, Tremblay RE, Nagin DS, Vitaro F, Lacourse E: Development of male proactive and reactive physical aggression during adolescence. *J Child Psychol Psychiatry* 47:783–790, 2006.
26. Blader JC, Pliszka SR, Kafantaris V, et al.: Prevalence and treatment outcomes of persistent negative mood among children with attention-deficit/hyperactivity disorder and aggressive behavior. *J Child Adolesc Psychopharmacol* 26:164–173, 2016.
27. Roy AK, Lopes V, Klein RG: Disruptive mood dysregulation disorder: a new diagnostic approach to chronic irritability in youth. *Am J Psychiatry* 171:918–924, 2014.
28. Gendreau PL, Archer J: Subtypes of aggression. In: Tremblay RE, Hartup WW, Archer J (eds): *Developmental Origins of Aggression.* New York, Guilford, 25–46, 2005.
29. Moffitt TE: Adolescence-limited and life-course persistent antisocial behavior: a developmental taxonomy. *Psychol Rev* 100:674–701, 1993.
30. Loeber R, Green SM, Lahey BB, Kalb L: Physical fighting in childhood as a risk factor for later mental health problems. *J Am Acad Child Adolesc Psychiatry* 39:421–428, 2000.
31. Moffitt TE: Life-course-persistent versus adolescence-limited antisocial behavior. In: Cicchetti D, Cohen DJ (eds): *Developmental Psychopathology.* 2nd ed. Hoboken, NJ, John Wiley & Sons, 570–598, 2015.
32. Frick PJ, Ellis M: Callous-unemotional traits and subtypes of conduct disorder. *Clin Child Fam Psychol Rev* 2:149–168, 1999.
33. Frick PJ, White SF: Research review: the importance of callous-unemotional traits for developmental models of aggressive and antisocial behavior. *J Child Psychol Psychiatry* 49:359–375, 2008.
34. Steiner H, Cauffman E, Duxbury E: Personality traits in juvenile delinquents: relation to criminal behavior and recidivism. *J Am Acad Child Adolesc Psychiatry* 38:256–262, 2000.
35. Saylor KE, Amann BH: Impulsive aggression as a comorbidity of attention-deficit/hyperactivity disorder in children and adolescents. *J Child Adolesc Psychopharmacol* 26:19–25, 2016.
36. King S, Waschbusch DA: Aggression in children with attention-deficit/hyperactivity disorder. *Expert Rev Neurother* 10:1581–1594, 2010.
37. Connor DF, Chartier KG, Preen EC, Kaplan RF: Impulsive aggression in attention-deficit/hyperactivity disorder: symptom severity, co-morbidity, and attention-deficit/hyperactivity disorder subtype. *J Child Adolesc Psychopharmacol* 20:119–126, 2010.
38. Barratt ES, Stanford MS, Dowdy L, Liebman MJ, Kent TA: Impulsive and premeditated aggression: a factor analysis of self-reported acts. *Psychiatry Res* 86:163–173, 1999.
39. Mann JJ, Waternaux C, Haas GL, Malone KM: Toward a clinical model of suicidal behavior in psychiatric patients. *Am J Psychiatry* 156:181–189, 1999.
40. Campbell SB: Hard-to-manage preschool boys: externalizing behavior, social competence, and family context at two-year followup. *J Abnorm Child Psychol* 22:147–166, 1994.
41. Tremblay RE, Pihl RO, Vitaro F, Dobkin PL: Predicting early onset of male antisocial behavior from preschool behavior. A test of two personality theories. *Arch Gen Psychiatry* 51:732–738, 1994.
42. Simonoff E, Elander J, Holmshaw J, Pickles A, Murray R, Rutter M: Predictors of antisocial personality. Continuities from childhood to adult life. *Br J Psychiatry* 184:118–127, 2004.
43. Karalunas SL, Fair D, Musser ED, Aykes K, Iyer SP, Nigg JT: Subtyping attention-deficit/hyperactivity disorder using temperament dimensions: toward biologically based nosologic criteria. *JAMA Psychiatry* 71:1015–1024, 2014.
44. Barkley RA: Emotional dysregulation is a core component of ADHD. In: Barkley RA (ed): *Attention-Deficit Hyperactivity Disorder: A Handbook for Diagnosis and Treatment.* 4th ed. New York, Guilford Press, 81–115, 2015.

45. Axelson D, Findling RL, Fristad MA, et al.: Examining the proposed disruptive mood dysregulation disorder diagnosis in children in the longitudinal assessment of manic symptoms study. *J Clin Psychiatry* 73:1342–1350, 2012.
46. Leibenluft E: Severe mood dysregulation, irritability, and the diagnostic boundaries of bipolar disorder in youths. *Am J Psychiatry* 168:129–142, 2011.
47. Althoff RR, Kuny-Slock AV, Verhulst FC, Hudziak JJ, van der Ende J: Classes of oppositional-defiant behavior: concurrent and predictive validity. *J Child Psychol Psychiatry* 55:1162–1171, 2014.
48. Geraldina P, Mariarosaria L, Annarita A, et al.: Neuropsychiatric sequelae in TBI: a comparison across different age groups. *Brain Inj* 17:835–846, 2003.
49. Max JE, Robertson BA, Lansing AE: The phenomenology of personality change due to traumatic brain injury in children and adolescents. *J Neuropsychiatry Clin Neurosci* 13:161–170, 2001.
50. Lahey BB, Applegate B, Barkley RA, et al.: DSM-IV field trials for oppositional defiant disorder and conduct disorder in children and adolescents. *Am J Psychiatry* 151:1163–1171, 1994.
51. Frick PJ, Lahey BB, Loeber R, et al.: Oppositional defiant disorder and conduct disorder: a meta-analytic review of factor analyses and cross-validation in a clinic sample. *Clin Psychol Rev* 13:319–340, 1993.
52. Okado Y, Bierman KL: Differential risk for late adolescent conduct problems and mood dysregulation among children with early externalizing behavior problems. *J Abnorm Child Psychol* 43:735–747, 2015.
53. Sanson A, Smart D, Prior M, Oberklaid F: Precursors of hyperactivity and aggression. *J Am Acad Child Adolesc Psychiatry* 32:1207–1216, 1993.
54. Eisenberg N, Fabes RA, Guthrie IK, Reiser M: Dispositional emotionality and regulation: their role in predicting quality of social functioning. *J Pers Soc Psychol* 78:136–157, 2000.
55. Lytton H: Child and parent effects in boys' conduct disorder: a reinterpretation. *Dev Psychol* 26:683–697, 1990.
56. Stoolmiller M: Synergistic interaction of child manageability problems and parent-discipline tactics in predicting future growth in externalizing behavior for boys. *Dev Psychol* 37:814–825, 2001.
57. Burke JD: An affective dimension within oppositional defiant disorder symptoms among boys: personality and psychopathology outcomes into early adulthood. *J Child Psychol Psychiatry* 53:1176–1183, 2012.
58. Burke JD, Boylan K, Rowe R, et al.: Identifying the irritability dimension of ODD: application of a modified bifactor model across five large community samples of children. *J Abnorm Psychol* 123:841–851, 2014.
59. Stringaris A, Goodman R: Three dimensions of oppositionality in youth. *J Child Psychol Psychiatry* 50:216–223, 2009.
60. Stringaris A, Cohen P, Pine DS, Leibenluft E: Adult outcomes of youth irritability: a 20-year prospective community-based study. *Am J Psychiatry* 166:1048–1054, 2009.
61. Biederman J, Faraone SV, Hatch M, Mennin D, Taylor A, George P: Conduct disorder with and without mania in a referred sample of ADHD children. *J Affect Disord* 44:177–188, 1997.
62. Biederman J, Mick E, Bostic JQ, et al.: The naturalistic course of pharmacologic treatment of children with maniclike symptoms: a systematic chart review. *J Clin Psychiatry* 59:628–637, 1998.
63. Carlson GA, Kelly KL: Manic symptoms in psychiatrically hospitalized children—what do they mean? *J Affect Disord* 51:123–135, 1998.
64. Wozniak J, Biederman J, Kiely K, et al.: Mania-like symptoms suggestive of childhood-onset bipolar disorder in clinically referred children. *J Am Acad Child Adolesc Psychiatry* 34:867–876, 1995.
65. Wu P, Hoven CW, Bird HR, et al.: Depressive and disruptive disorders and mental health service utilization in children and adolescents. *J Am Acad Child Adolesc Psychiatry* 38:1081–1090; discussion 1090–1092, 1999.
66. Gross JJ: Emotion regulation: past, present, future. *Cogn Emot* 13:551–573, 1999.
67. Thompson RA: Emotion and self-regulation. In: Thompson RA (ed): *Nebraska Symposium on Motivation. 36 [1988]*. Lincoln, NE, University of Nebraska Press, 1990.
68. Cole PM, Zahn-Waxler C, Fox NA, Usher BA, Welsh JD: Individual differences in emotion regulation and behavior problems in preschool children. *J Abnorm Psychol* 105:518–529, 1996.
69. Sanson A, Prior M: Temperament and behavioral precursors to oppositional defiant disorder and conduct disorder. In: Quay HC, Hogan AE (eds): *Handbook of Disruptive Behavior Disorders*. New York, Kluwer Academic/Plenum Publishers, 397–417, 1999.
70. Shields A, Cicchetti D: Emotion regulation among school-age children: the development and validation of a new criterion Q-sort scale. *Dev Psychol* 33:906–916, 1997.
71. Wakschlag LS, Estabrook R, Petitclerc A, et al.: Clinical implications of a dimensional approach: the normal:abnormal spectrum of early irritability. *J Am Acad Child Adolesc Psychiatry* 54:626–634, 2015.
72. Sher L, Oquendo MA, Galfalvy HC, et al.: The relationship of aggression to suicidal behavior in depressed patients with a history of alcoholism. *Addict Behav* 30:1144–1153, 2005.
73. Elizabeth Sublette M, Carballo JJ, Moreno C, et al.: Substance use disorders and suicide attempts in bipolar subtypes. *J Psychiatr Res* 43:230–238, 2009.
74. Corrigan PW, Watson AC: Findings from the National Comorbidity Survey on the frequency of violent behavior in individuals with psychiatric disorders. *Psychiatry Res* 136:153–162, 2005.
75. McElroy SL, Strakowski SM, West SA, Keck PE Jr, McConville BJ: Phenomenology of adolescent and adult mania in hospitalized patients with bipolar disorder. *Am J Psychiatry* 154:44–49, 1997.
76. Bubier JL, Drabick DA: Co-occurring anxiety and disruptive behavior disorders: the roles of anxious symptoms, reactive aggression, and shared risk processes. *Clin Psychol Rev* 29:658–669, 2009.
77. Christian RE, Frick PJ, Hill NL, Tyler L, Frazer DR: Psychopathy and conduct problems in children: II. Implications for subtyping children with conduct problems. *J Am Acad Child Adolesc Psychiatry* 36:233–241, 1997.
78. Viding E: Annotation: understanding the development of psychopathy. *J Child Psychol Psychiatry* 45:1329–1337, 2004.
79. Blair RJR: Responsiveness to distress cues in the child with psychopathic tendencies. *Pers Individ Dif* 27:135–145, 1997.
80. Glaser BA, Kronsnoble KM, Forkner CBW: Parents and teachers as raters of children's problem behaviors. *Child Fam Behav Ther* 19:1–13, 1997.
81. MacLeod RJ, McNamee JE, Boyle MH, Offord DR, Friedrich M: Identification of childhood psychiatric disorder by informant: comparisons of clinic and community samples. *Can J Psychiatry* 44:144–150, 1999.
82. Nock MK, Kazdin AE: Parent-directed physical aggression by clinic-referred youths. *J Clin Child Adolesc Psychol* 31:193–205, 2002.
83. Baillargeon RH, Boulerice B, Tremblay RE, Zoccolillo M, Vitaro F, Kohen DE: Modeling interinformant agreement in the absence of a "gold standard." *J Child Psychol Psychiatry* 42:463–473, 2001.
84. Johnston C, Ohan JL: The importance of parental attributions in families of children with attention deficit/hyperactivity and disruptive behavior disorders. *Clin Child Fam Psychol Rev* 8:167–182, 2005.
85. Angold A, Messer SC, Stangl D, Farmer EM, Costello EJ, Burns BJ: Perceived parental burden and service use for child and adolescent psychiatric disorders. *Am J Public Health* 88:75–80, 1998.
86. Burt SA, McGue M, Krueger RF, Iacono WG: How are parent-child conflict and childhood externalizing symptoms related over time? Results from a genetically informative cross-lagged study. *Dev Psychopathol* 17:145–165, 2005.
87. Barry TD, Dunlap ST, Cotten SJ, Lochman JE, Wells KC: The influence of maternal stress and distress on disruptive behavior problems in boys. *J Am Acad Child Adolesc Psychiatry* 44:265–273, 2005.
88. Stormshak EA, Speltz ML, DeKlyen M, Greenberg MT: Observed family interaction during clinical interviews: a comparison of families containing preschool boys with and without disruptive behavior. *J Abnorm Child Psychol* 25:345–357, 1997.
89. Baker BL, Heller TL, Henker B: Expressed emotion, parenting stress, and adjustment in mothers of young children with behavior problems. *J Child Psychol Psychiatry* 41:907–915, 2000.
90. Crouch JL, Behl LE: Relationships among parental beliefs in corporal punishment, reported stress, and physical child abuse potential. *Child Abuse Negl* 25:413–419, 2001.
91. Rodriguez CM, Green AJ: Parenting stress and anger expression as predictors of child abuse potential. *Child Abuse Negl* 21:367–377, 1997.
92. Stanger C, Dumenci L, Kamon J, Burstein M: Parenting and children's externalizing problems in substance-abusing families. *J Clin Child Adolesc Psychol* 33:590–600, 2004.
93. Cassidy B, Zoccolillo M, Hughes S: Psychopathology in adolescent mothers and its effects on mother-infant interactions: a pilot study. *Can J Psychiatry* 41:379–384, 1996.
94. Frick PJ, Lahey BB, Loeber R, Stouthamer-Loeber M, Christ MA, Hanson K: Familial risk factors to oppositional defiant disorder and conduct disorder: parental psychopathology and maternal parenting. *J Consult Clin Psychol* 60:49–55, 1992.
95. Côté SM, Vaillancourt T, LeBlanc JC, Nagin DS, Tremblay RE: The development of physical aggression from toddlerhood to pre-adolescence: a nation wide longitudinal study of Canadian children. *J Abnorm Child Psychol* 34:71–85, 2006.
96. Côté SM, Boivin M, Nagin DS, et al.: The role of maternal education and nonmaternal care services in the prevention of children's physical aggression problems. *Arch Gen Psychiatry* 64:1305–1312, 2007.
97. Blader JC: Which family factors predict children's externalizing behaviors following discharge from psychiatric inpatient treatment? *J Child Psychol Psychiatry* 47:1133–1142, 2006.
98. Blader JC: Symptom, family, and service predictors of children's psychiatric rehospitalization within one year of discharge. *J Am Acad Child Adolesc Psychiatry* 43:440–451, 2004.
99. Wootton JM, Frick PJ, Shelton KK, Silverthorn P: Ineffective parenting and childhood conduct problems: the moderating role of callous-unemotional traits. *J Consult Clin Psychol* 65:292–300, 1997.
100. MacMillan HL, Fleming JE, Streiner DL, et al.: Childhood abuse and lifetime psychopathology in a community sample. *Am J Psychiatry* 158:1878–1883, 2001.
101. Teicher MH, Andersen SL, Polcari A, Anderson CM, Navalta CP, Kim DM: The neurobiological consequences of early stress and childhood maltreatment. *Neurosci Biobehav Rev* 27:33–44, 2003.
102. Gerson R, Rappaport N: Traumatic stress and posttraumatic stress disorder in youth: recent research findings on clinical impact, assessment, and treatment. *J Adolesc Health* 52:137–143, 2013.
103. Connor DF, Steingard RJ, Cunningham JA, Anderson JJ, Melloni RH Jr: Proactive and reactive aggression in referred children and adolescents. *Am J Orthopsychiatry* 74:129–136, 2004.

104. Dodge KA, Pettit GS, Bates JE: How the experience of early physical abuse leads children to become chronically aggressive. In: Cicchetti D, Toth SL (eds): *Rochester Symposium on Developmental Psychology. 8, Developmental perspectives on trauma: Theory, Research, and Intervention.* Rochester, NY, University of Rochester Press, 263–288, 1997.
105. Klomek AB, Sourander A, Niemelä S, et al.: Childhood bullying behaviors as a risk for suicide attempts and completed suicides: a population-based birth cohort study. *J Am Acad Child Adolesc Psychiatry* 48:254–261, 2009.
106. Veenstra R, Lindenberg S, Oldehinkel AJ, De Winter AF, Verhulst FC, Ormel J: Bullying and victimization in elementary schools: a comparison of bullies, victims, bully/victims, and uninvolved preadolescents. *Dev Psychol* 41:672–682, 2005.
107. Kim Y, Leventhal BL, Koh YJ, Hubbard A, Boyce WT: School bullying and youth violence: causes or consequences of psychopathologic behavior? *Arch Gen Psychiatry* 63:1035–1041, 2006.
108. Gorman-Smith D, Henry DB, Tolan PH: Exposure to community violence and violence perpetration: the protective effects of family functioning. *J Clin Child Adolesc Psychol* 33:439–449, 2004.
109. Kupersmidt JB, Griesler PC, DeRosier ME, Patterson CJ, Davis PW: Childhood aggression and peer relations in the context of family and neighborhood factors. *Child Dev* 66:360–375, 1995.
110. Laub JH, Lauritsen JL: The interdependence of school violence with neighborhood and family conditions. In: Elliott DS, Hamburg BA, Williams KR (eds): *Violence in American Schools.* New York, Cambridge University Press, 127–155, 1998.
111. Dishion TJ, McCord J, Poulin F: When interventions harm. Peer groups and problem behavior. *Am Psychol* 54:755–764, 1999.
112. Bullock BM, Dishion TJ: Sibling collusion and problem behavior in early adolescence: toward a process model for family mutuality. *J Abnorm Child Psychol* 30:143–153, 2002.
113. Masia CL, Chase PN: Vicarious learning revisited: a contemporary behavior analytic interpretation. *J Behav Ther Exp Psychiatry* 28:41–51, 1997.
114. Browne KD, Hamilton-Giachritsis C: The influence of violent media on children and adolescents: a public-health approach. *Lancet* 365:702–710, 2005.
115. Swanson JW, Swartz MS, Van Dorn RA, et al.: A national study of violent behavior in persons with schizophrenia. *Arch Gen Psychiatry* 63:490–499, 2006.
116. Volavka J, Citrome L: Pathways to aggression in schizophrenia affect results of treatment. *Schizophr Bull* 37:921–929, 2011.
117. Mayes SD, Calhoun SL, Aggarwal R, et al.: Explosive, oppositional, and aggressive behavior in children with autism compared to other clinical disorders and typical children. *Res Autism Spectr Disord* 6:1–10, 2012.
118. Farmer CA, Aman MG: Aggressive behavior in a sample of children with autism spectrum disorders. *Res Autism Spectr Disord* 5:317–323, 2011.
119. Graham JM Jr, Rosner B, Dykens E, Visootsak J: Behavioral features of CHARGE syndrome (Hall-Hittner syndrome) comparison with down syndrome, Prader-Willi syndrome, and Williams syndrome. *Am J Hum Genet* 133A:240–247, 2005.
120. Kreider AR, Matone M, Bellonci C, et al.: Growth in the concurrent use of antipsychotics with other psychotropic medications in medicaid-enrolled children. *J Am Acad Child Adolesc Psychiatry* 53:960–970.e2, 2014.
121. Blader JC: Pharmacotherapy and postdischarge outcomes of child inpatients admitted for aggressive behavior. *J Clin Psychopharmacol* 26:419–425, 2006.
122. Martin A, Van Hoof T, Stubbe D, Sherwin T, Scahill L: Multiple psychotropic pharmacotherapy among child and adolescent enrollees in Connecticut Medicaid managed care. *Psychiatr Serv* 54:72–77, 2003.
123. Safer DJ, Zito JM: Treatment-emergent adverse events from selective serotonin reuptake inhibitors by age group: children versus adolescents. *J Child Adolesc Psychopharmacol* 16:159–169, 2006.
124. Posner J, Kass E, Hulvershorn L: Using stimulants to treat ADHD-related emotional lability. *Curr Psychiatry Rep* 16:478, 2014.
125. Kayani S, Shannon DC: Adverse behavioral effects of treatment for acute exacerbation of asthma in children: a comparison of two doses of oral steroids. *Chest* 122:624–628, 2002.
126. Pappadopulos E, Macintyre li JC, Crismon ML, et al.: Treatment recommendations for the use of antipsychotics for aggressive youth (TRAAY). Part II. *J Am Acad Child Adolesc Psychiatry* 42:145–161, 2003.
127. Schur SB, Sikich L, Findling RL, et al.: Treatment recommendations for the use of antipsychotics for aggressive youth (TRAAY). Part I: a review. *J Am Acad Child Adolesc Psychiatry* 42:132–144, 2003.
128. Pliszka SR, Crismon ML, Hughes CW, et al; Texas Consensus Conference Panel on Pharmacotherapy of Childhood Attention Deficit Hyperactivity Disorder: The Texas Children's Medication Algorithm Project: revision of the algorithm for pharmacotherapy of attention-deficit/hyperactivity disorder (ADHD). *J Am Acad Child Adolesc Psychiatry* 45:642–657, 2006.
129. Campbell M, Kafantaris V, Cueva JE: An update on the use of lithium carbonate in aggressive children and adolescents with conduct disorder. *Psychopharmacol Bull* 31:93–102, 1995.
130. Campbell M, Adams PB, Small AM, et al.: Lithium in hospitalized aggressive children with conduct disorder: a double-blind and placebo-controlled study. *J Am Acad Child Adolesc Psychiatry* 34:445–453, 1995.
131. Klein RG, Abikoff H, Klass E, Ganeles D, Seese LM, Pollack S: Clinical efficacy of methylphenidate in conduct disorder with and without attention deficit hyperactivity disorder. *Arch Gen Psychiatry* 54:1073–1080, 1997.
132. Hinshaw SP, Heller T, McHale JP: Covert antisocial behavior in boys with attention-deficit hyperactivity disorder: external validation and effects of methylphenidate. *J Consult Clin Psychol* 60:274–281, 1992.
133. Aman MG, Bukstein OG, Gadow KD, et al.: What does risperidone add to parent training and stimulant for severe aggression in child attention-deficit/hyperactivity disorder? *J Am Acad Child Adolesc Psychiatry* 53: 47–60.e1, 2014.
134. Pringsheim T, Hirsch L, Gardner D, Gorman DA: The pharmacological management of oppositional behaviour, conduct problems, and aggression in children and adolescents with attention-deficit hyperactivity disorder, oppositional defiant disorder, and conduct disorder: a systematic review and meta-analysis. Part 1: psychostimulants, alpha-2 agonists, and atomoxetine. *Can J Psychiatry* 60:42–51, 2015.
135. Connor DF, Glatt SJ, Lopez ID, Jackson D, Melloni RH Jr: Psychopharmacology and aggression. I: a meta-analysis of stimulant effects on overt/covert aggression-related behaviors in ADHD. *J Am Acad Child Adolesc Psychiatry* 41:253–261, 2002.
136. MTA Cooperative Group: A 14-month randomized clinical trial of treatment strategies for attention-deficit/hyperactivity disorder. The MTA Cooperative Group. Multimodal Treatment Study of Children with ADHD. *Arch Gen Psychiatry* 56:1073–1086, 1999.
137. Pappadopulos E, Woolston S, Chait A, Perkins M, Connor DF, Jensen PS: Pharmacotherapy of aggression in children and adolescents: efficacy and effect size. *J Can Acad Child Adolesc Psychiatry* 15:27–39, 2006.
138. Hinshaw SP, Lee SS: Ritalin effects on aggression and antisocial behavior. In: Greenhill LL, Osman BB (eds): *Ritalin: Theory and Practice.* 2nd ed. Larchmont, NY, Mary Ann Liebert, 237–251, 2000.
139. Blader JC, Pliszka SR, Jensen PS, Schooler NR, Kafantaris V: Stimulant-responsive and stimulant-refractory aggressive behavior among children with ADHD. *Pediatrics* 126:e796–e806, 2010.
140. Blader JC, Schooler NR, Jensen PS, Pliszka SR, Kafantaris V: Adjunctive divalproex versus placebo for children with ADHD and aggression refractory to stimulant monotherapy. *Am J Psychiatry* 166:1392–1401, 2009.
141. Gadow KD, Arnold LE, Molina BS, et al.: Risperidone added to parent training and stimulant medication: effects on attention-deficit/hyperactivity disorder, oppositional defiant disorder, conduct disorder, and peer aggression. *J Am Acad Child Adolesc Psychiatry* 53:948–959.e1, 2014.
142. Hirota T, Schwartz S, Correll CU: Alpha-2 agonists for attention-deficit/hyperactivity disorder in youth: a systematic review and meta-analysis of monotherapy and add-on trials to stimulant therapy. *J Am Acad Child Adolesc Psychiatry* 53:153–173, 2014.
143. Connor DF, Barkley RA, Davis HT: A pilot study of methylphenidate, clonidine, or the combination in ADHD comorbid with aggressive oppositional defiant or conduct disorder. *Clin Pediatr (Phila)* 39:15–25, 2000.
144. Stigler KA, Desmond LA, Posey DJ, Wiegand RE, McDougle CJ: A naturalistic retrospective analysis of psychostimulants in pervasive developmental disorders. *J Child Adolesc Psychopharmacol* 14:49–56, 2004.
145. Handen BL, Johnson CR, Lubetsky M: Efficacy of methylphenidate among children with autism and symptoms of attention-deficit hyperactivity disorder. *J Autism Dev Disord* 30:245–255, 2000.
146. Campbell M, Small AM, Green WH, et al.: Behavioral efficacy of haloperidol and lithium carbonate: a comparison in hospitalized aggressive children with conduct disorder. *Arch Gen Psychiatry* 41:650–656, 1984.
147. Greenhill LL, Solomon M, Pleak R, Ambrosini P: Molindone hydrochloride treatment of hospitalized children with conduct disorder. *J Clin Psychiatry* 46:20–25, 1985.
148. Patel NC, Crismon ML, Hoagwood K, et al.: Trends in the use of typical and atypical antipsychotics in children and adolescents. *J Am Acad Child Adolesc Psychiatry* 44:548–556, 2005.
149. Zito JM, Safer DJ, DosReis S, et al.: Psychotropic practice patterns for youth: a 10-year perspective. *Arch Pediatr Adol Med* 157:17–25, 2003.
150. Olfson M, King M, Schoenbaum M: Treatment of young people with antipsychotic medications in the United States. *JAMA Psychiatry* 72:867–874, 2015.
151. Birnbaum ML, Saito E, Gerhard T, et al.: Pharmacoepidemiology of antipsychotic use in youth with ADHD: trends and clinical implications. *Curr Psychiatry Rep* 15:382, 2013.
152. Correll CU, Blader JC: Antipsychotic use in youth without psychosis: a double-edged sword. *JAMA Psychiatry* 72:859–860, 2015.
153. Correll CU, Manu P, Olshanskiy V, Napolitano B, Kane JM, Malhotra AK: Cardiometabolic risk of second-generation antipsychotic medications during first-time use in children and adolescents. *JAMA* 302:1765–1773, 2009.
154. Correll CU: Antipsychotic use in children and adolescents: minimizing adverse effects to maximize outcomes. *J Am Acad Child Adolesc Psychiatry* 47:9–20, 2008.
155. Pringsheim T, Lam D, Ching H, Patten S: Metabolic and neurological complications of second-generation antipsychotic use in children: a systematic review and meta-analysis of randomized controlled trials. *Drug Saf* 34:651–668, 2011.
156. Loy JH, Merry SN, Hetrick SE, Stasiak K: Atypical antipsychotics for disruptive behaviour disorders in children and youths. *Cochrane Database Syst Rev* 9:CD008559, 2012.

157. Pringsheim T, Hirsch L, Gardner D, Gorman DA: The pharmacological management of oppositional behaviour, conduct problems, and aggression in children and adolescents with attention-deficit hyperactivity disorder, oppositional defiant disorder, and conduct disorder: a systematic review and meta-analysis. Part 2: antipsychotics and traditional mood stabilizers. *Can J Psychiatry* 60:52–61, 2015.
158. Blader JC, Pliszka SR, Kafantaris V: *Stepped treatment for attention-deficit/hyperactivity disorder and aggressive behavior: a randomized trial of risperidone, valproate, and placebo after optimized stimulant monotherapy.* Presented at the 63rd Annual Meeting of the American Academy of Child and Adolescent Psychiatry; New York, 2016.
159. Leucht S, Cipriani A, Spineli L, et al.: Comparative efficacy and tolerability of 15 antipsychotic drugs in schizophrenia: a multiple-treatments meta-analysis. *Lancet* 382:951–962, 2013.
160. Loebel A, Brams M, Goldman RS, et al.: Lurasidone for the treatment of irritability associated with autistic disorder. *J Autism Dev Disord* 46:1153–1163, 2016.
161. Malone RP, Delaney MA, Leubbert JF, Cater J, Campbell M: A double-blind placebo-controlled study of lithium in hospitalized aggressive children and adolescents with conduct disorder. *Arch Gen Psychiatry* 57:649–654, 2000.
162. Findling RL, Robb A, McNamara NK, et al.: Lithium in the acute treatment of bipolar I disorder: a double-blind, placebo-controlled study. *Pediatrics* 136:885–894, 2015.
163. Donovan SJ, Susser ES, Nunes EV, Stewart JW, Quitkin FM, Klein DF: Divalproex treatment of disruptive adolescents: a report of 10 cases. *J Clin Psychiatry* 58:12–15, 1997.
164. Donovan SJ, Stewart JW, Nunes EV, et al.: Divalproex treatment for youth with explosive temper and mood lability: a double-blind, placebo-controlled crossover design. *Am J Psychiatry* 157:818–820, 2000.
165. Steiner H, Petersen ML, Saxena K, Ford S, Matthews Z: Divalproex sodium for the treatment of conduct disorder: a randomized controlled clinical trial. *J Clin Psychiatry* 64:1183–1191, 2003.
166. Barzman DH, DelBello MP, Adler CM, Stanford KE, Strakowski SM: The efficacy and tolerability of quetiapine versus divalproex for the treatment of impulsivity and reactive aggression in adolescents with co-occurring bipolar disorder and disruptive behavior disorder(s). *J Child Adolesc Psychopharmacol* 16:665–670, 2006.
167. Wagner KD, Redden L, Kowatch RA, et al.: A double-blind, randomized, placebo-controlled trial of divalproex extended-release in the treatment of bipolar disorder in children and adolescents. *J Am Acad Child Adolesc Psychiatry* 48:519–532, 2009.
168. Kafantaris V, Campbell M, Padron-Gayol MV, Small AM, Locascio JJ, Rosenberg CR: Carbamazepine in hospitalized aggressive conduct disorder children: an open pilot study. *Psychopharmacol Bull* 28:193–199, 1992.
169. Cueva JE, Overall JE, Small AM, Armenteros JL, Perry R, Campbell M: Carbamazepine in aggressive children with conduct disorder: a double-blind and placebo-controlled study. *J Am Acad Child Adolesc Psychiatry* 35:480–490, 1996.
170. Bond AJ: Pharmacological manipulation of aggressiveness and impulsiveness in healthy volunteers. *Prog Neuropsychopharmacol Biol Psychiatry* 16:1–7, 1992.
171. Gesch CB, Hammond SM, Hampson SE, Eves A, Crowder MJ: Influence of supplementary vitamins, minerals and essential fatty acids on the antisocial behaviour of young adult prisoners. Randomised, placebo-controlled trial. *Br J Psychiatry* 181:22–28, 2002.
172. Raine A, Cheney RA, Ho R, et al.: Nutritional supplementation to reduce child aggression: a randomized, stratified, single-blind, factorial trial. *J Child Psychol Psychiatry* 57:1038–1046, 2016 .
173. O'Neill RE, Horner RH, Albin RW, et al.: *Functional Assessment and Program Development for Problem Behavior: A Practical Handbook.* 2nd ed. Pacific Grove, CA, Brooks/Cole Publishing, 1997.
174. Henggeler SW, Schoenwald SK, Borduin CM, et al.: *Multisystemic Treatment of Antisocial Behavior in Children and Adolescents.* New York, Guilford Press, 1998.
175. Ducharme JM, Atkinson L, Poulton L: Success-based, noncoercive treatment of oppositional behavior in children from violent homes. *J Am Acad Child Adolesc Psychiatry* 39:995–1004, 2000.
176. Kazdin AE, Bass D, Siegel T, Thomas C: Cognitive-behavioral therapy and relationship therapy in the treatment of children referred for antisocial behavior. *J Consult Clin Psychol* 57:522–535, 1989.
177. Lochman JE, Curry JF: Effects of social problem-solving training and self-instruction training with aggressive boys. *J Clin Child Psychol* 15:159–164, 1986.
178. Lochman JE, Lampron LB: Cognitive-behavioral interventions for aggressive boys: 7-month follow-up effects. *J Child Adolesc Psychotherapy* 5:15–23, 1988.
179. Kazdin AE, Siegel T, Bass D: Cognitive problem-solving skills training and parent management training in the treatment of antisocial behavior in children. *J Consult Clin Psychol* 60:733–747, 1992.
180. Kellam SG, Ling X, Merisca R, Brown CH, Ialongo N: The effect of the level of aggression in the first grade classroom on the course and malleability of aggressive behavior into middle school. *Dev Psychopathol* 10:165–185, 1998.
181. Brestan EV, Eyberg SM: Effective psychosocial treatments of conduct-disordered children and adolescents: 29 years, 82 studies, and 5,272 kids. *J Clin Child Psychol* 27:180–189, 1998.
182. Burke JD, Loeber R, Birmaher B: Oppositional defiant disorder and conduct disorder: a review of the past 10 years, part II. *J Am Acad Child Adolesc Psychiatry* 41:1275–1293, 2002.
183. Kazdin AE: Practitioner review: psychosocial treatments for conduct disorder in children. *J Child Psychol Psychiatry* 38:161–178, 1997.
184. Schuhmann EM, Foote RC, Eyberg SM, Boggs SR, Algina J: Efficacy of parent-child interaction therapy: interim report of a randomized trial with short-term maintenance. *J Clin Child Psychol* 27:34–45, 1998.
185. Newcomer AR, Roth KB, Kellam SG, et al.: Higher childhood peer reports of social preference mediates the impact of the good behavior game on suicide attempt. *Prev Sci* 17:145–156, 2016.
186. Sukhodolsky DG, Kassinove H, Gorman BS: Cognitive-behavioral therapy for anger in children and adolescents: a meta-analysis. *Aggress Violent Behav* 9:247–269, 2004.
187. Sukhodolsky DG, Smith SD, McCauley SA, Ibrahim K, Piasecka JB: Behavioral interventions for anger, irritability, and aggression in children and adolescents. *J Child Adolesc Psychopharmacol* 26:58–64, 2016.

CHAPTER 5.1.4 ■ FIRE BEHAVIOR IN CHILDREN AND ADOLESCENTS

STEVEN J. BARRETO, JOHN R. BOEKAMP, ELIZABETH L. REICHERT, KAREN R. HEBERT, AND MARGARET PACCIONE-DYSZLEWSKI

INTRODUCTION

All children will naturally be exposed to fire during the early years of life. It is part of the normal course of development that they acquire knowledge that is linked both to mastery over fire and its potential for destruction and harm. In contrast to the development of fire interest, the emergence of fire behavior in children and adolescents carries with it the potential for death, injury, and property loss of striking proportions. Children who become involved with fire early in life, and those who use fire in an unsafe and destructive manner, are at risk, not only for continued involvement with fire, but for psychopathology and behavioral problems. The challenge for clinicians is meeting the need for early identification of children at risk, in order to help parents and caregivers curb maladaptive forms of fire activity that may lead a child down a maladaptive developmental pathway.

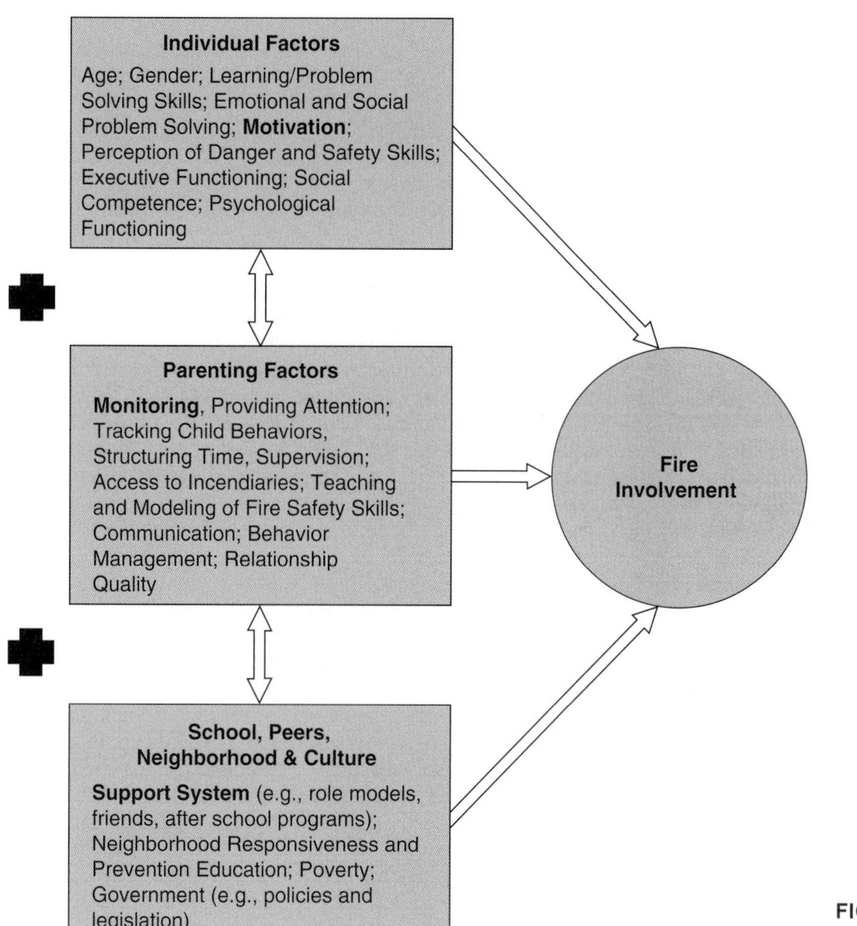

FIGURE 5.1.4.1. The ecologic–transactional model of juvenile firesetting.

In this chapter, we summarize the literature on juvenile fire behavior, presenting a foundation for assessment and intervention. In this review, we will define the phrase juvenile fire behavior as including both intentional firesetting and unintentional and unsupervised match and lighter play. The term juvenile fire-setting will be used to refer to intentional fire-starting. The term fire involvement will be used to refer to the widest range of fire behaviors including pulling of smoke/fire alarms, hiding matches/lighters, or bomb-making. Occasionally, we will identify where the term fire involvement is defined in a more restrictive manner by an instrument or specific study. In child psychiatric settings, the behavioral health clinician occupies a critical role in adequately identifying children at risk, and offering treatment options that decrease the likelihood of maladaptive developmental outcomes. We will present an ecologic–transactional model (Fig. 5.1.4.1) of the development of fire behavior that can serve as a foundation for research, but also a heuristic for clinical practice. We view this model as more accurately capturing the complexity of the developmental nature of fire behavior when compared with dominant motivational typology models. The ecologic model will suggest characteristics of both maladaptive and adaptive pathways of fire behavior. Throughout the chapter, we will stress that fire behavior carries both short- and long-term risks, ranging from more immediate concerns including property damage, risk for human injury, behavioral problems, and psychopathology to more destructive forms of fire play potentially emerging at a later point in development. We will review important considerations in the clinical evaluation of fire behavior and follow with a contemporary selection of the empirically supported educational and psychosocial interventions.

PREVALENCE, RISK, AND DANGER

Youth who engage in unsupervised fire behavior pose a significant threat to the health and safety of every community throughout the United States. Annually, fire behavior among children accounts for thousands of uncontrolled fires, millions of dollars in property damage, as well as injury and death (1–5). The number of incidents of injury and death is cause for concern. From 2004 to 2008, there were 57,700 fires attributed to youth associated with over 100 civilian deaths and over 900 civilian injuries and $286 million in direct losses (6). Arson is the charge most likely to bring a child under 10 in contact with the legal system, as children aged 10 and under are arrested for arson more than for any other crime (7). Of the individuals arrested for arson in 2009 in the United States, 45% were under the age of 18 (8).

Although prevalence rates vary considerably, it is clear that juvenile firesetting remains an issue of significant clinical concern. Among child and adolescent psychiatric samples, incidence of firesetting has ranged from 2.3% to 15% for outpatients, and 14.3% to 34.7% for inpatients (2,3). Statistics from community samples have been somewhat more variable, with estimates ranging from as low as 3% (4), as high as 45% (5), and with over 80% of males noted to be interested in fire and fire play. As these data suggest, firesetting is a problem affecting boys more frequently than girls (6). In a review of 22 descriptive studies, Kolko (9) found that 82% of identified firesetters were male and the age of these children was on average 10 years, with older children having more extensive firesetting histories. Although prevalence estimates have focused primarily on US samples, juvenile firesetting is a problem in other countries as well (10).

Two recent community sample studies found nearly a third of adolescents reported engaging in firesetting within the past year (11,12). According to the data collected from the Melbourne (Australia) Metropolitan Fire Brigade, nearly 20% of all reported fires are started by children (2). Further complicating the problem are the high recidivism rates among youth, with up to 59% engaging in recidivistic behavior (4,13,14).

These statistics are alarming and underscore the seriousness of juvenile firesetting. Among children, fires started by children annually number in the thousands, leading to millions of dollars in property damage, severe injury, and even death (1–5). In fact, fires and burns have been documented as the fourth most common cause of unintentional injury-related death, resulting in more than 4,000 deaths each year (1,15). In 1997, statistics documented that 8% of deaths from residential fires occurred as a result of children's fire behavior, most often the result of the unsupervised use of lighters and matches. Furthermore, a survey conducted by the National Association of Fire Marshals determined that children were responsible for nearly 100,000 fires annually causing more than $250 million in property damage (5). This research clearly highlights the substantial role that children play in fire-related damages, injuries, and deaths. The damages resulting from fires set by children are likely much larger than these estimates suggest; as many fires set by children are never reported to fire departments. One study indicates that as few as 10% of all fires set by children are ever reported to the appropriate authorities (2,16).

ETIOLOGY AND DEVELOPMENTAL PATHWAYS

Although most descriptive studies have focused on dangers immediate to juvenile fire behavior (e.g., property loss, injury, death), enduring developmental outcomes associated with early fire experimentation are of integral importance to correction and prevention efforts. Interest in and attraction to fire is a common feature of childhood (14,17–22). Early fire curiosity and activity that are ignored or dismissed by supervising adults can lead a child down several possible maladaptive pathways. In a study of males aged 5 through 9 years, researchers found that interest in fire was almost universal across the sample, with one-half of the boys actually engaging in fire behavior, often in the form of match or lighter play (23). Some children become involved in early fire activity that leads to continued experimentation and heightened interest and fascination in later childhood and adolescence. Other children remain interested in fire but cease to engage in fire behavior. Still others remain interested and engage in planned and deliberate fire behavior with the intention of causing damage or harm. The present section will serve to explore the etiology and developmental pathways associated with early fire play and eventual firesetting behavior. Recognizing risk may be the first step for parents and supervising adults in altering maladaptive developmental outcomes.

We present an ecologic–transactional model that integrates theory and empirical findings (Fig. 5.1.4.1). This model describes the individual, family, social, and ecologic factors associated with the onset and perpetuation of juvenile fire activity. Elements of these factors may combine to place a child on one of several pathways associated with dangerous fire behavior. As children mature, their cognitive and emotional development may place them at risk, or protect them against, engagement in destructive or dangerous fire behavior. Broadly, risk factors include the child's individual characteristics and motivational repertoire, parental and family features, as well as peer group factors, and school and community characteristics (24). It is important for clinicians to identify early distinguishing characteristics of juvenile firesetters so that intervention efforts can build upon strengths, target problem behaviors, and broaden the child and family's problem-solving repertoire, to protect against deviant developmental pathways and long-term maladaptive outcomes (25,26). In the present discussion, a focus will be placed on elements of the model that may contribute to the development of fire competency in children, despite exposure to conditions of adversity or the experience of failures at early points in development.

As the ecologic–transactional model highlights, individual risk factors include age, gender, cognitive ability, fire safety knowledge, social competence, executive functioning, as well as overt and covert delinquent behavior (27–29). Males, particularly those in the elementary and middle school years, are at high risk for fire experimentation. Furthermore, even younger children (ages 3 to 8) are at risk for fire behavior that may be associated with higher base rates of inattention and impulsive behavior, as well as a limited understanding of the consequences of fire behavior (30). Others have found juvenile fire behavior samples to be socially immature, isolated, and overall socially incompetent (9). Children who have firesetting histories have also exhibited a higher incidence of other emotional and behavioral disturbances (18,31). In one pathway, limited social competence and diminished learning capacities can be associated with noncompliance, impulsivity, hyperactivity, emotional dysregulation, and reactive–aggressive behavior, creating a constellation of elements placing the child at risk of firesetting behavior. In another pathway, individual factors may combine to place a child at risk of overt and covert conduct problems and delinquent behavior including the destruction of property, stealing, lying, running away, and truancy. The presence of these behaviors may increase the child's risk for engaging in firesetting behavior (9). In a study of 3,965 adolescents of grades 7 to 12, 27% reported firesetting in the last year, with over 13% reporting 3 or more episodes. Teens who persisted in fire behavior were more likely to report psychiatric distress, binge drinking, cannabis use, and sensation-seeking behaviors. This study highlights the association of psychopathology and substance use among adolescent firesetters (12). More generally, externalizing problems are thought to be developmental antecedents to fire behavior by some researchers (27), with others suggesting that firesetting behavior is an extreme form of conduct disorder (32).

In addition to the learning capacities and the frequency and intensity of disruptive behaviors, the child's emotion regulation skills play a significant role in early fire behavior. This construct has been subsumed under the domain of motivation (33); however, we think it is important to examine self-regulation skills separately to clarify a child's capacity for self-soothing, self-control, responsiveness to emotional stimuli, and the capacity for self-monitoring emotional status. We have suggested elsewhere that curiosity and anger may be emotional triggers for firesetting behavior (16). Curiosity has demonstrated strong associations to parent reports of internalizing and externalizing behavior problems in clinical samples of children who have engaged in fire behavior. Some children who display excessive curiosity may be more emotionally dysregulated and display more frequent, earlier, or more significant forms of fire involvement (34). Compared to firesetting children scoring high on curiosity or interest, children reporting elevated anger have lower levels of psychopathology by parent report, and may engage in more deliberate and destructive involvement with fire (34). These findings highlight the possibility that difficulties regulating intense emotion (e.g., curiosity, fascination, or anger) influence the child's development of maladaptive strategies or skills that lead to potentially more destructive forms of fire play. It will be fruitful for future studies to examine more closely the effects of emotional dysregulation and its relationship to juvenile firesetting.

The child's individual characteristics need to be considered in his/her environmental context to clarify risk of firesetting when evaluating developmental pathways toward firesetting. Cognitive behavioral models emphasize how children's behavioral repertoires develop through observation, modeling, and conditioning processes. Researchers have noted that early fire experiences, access to incendiary materials, family members who smoke, and siblings and peers who have had a history of firesetting all contribute to the child's development of maladaptive strategies which may increase the risk of firesetting (16,18,19,24). In an early study, juvenile firesetting was found to be more frequent among boys whose fathers' occupations directly or indirectly involved the use of fire when compared with those children whose fathers' occupations were unrelated to fire (35). Furthermore, child and adolescent firesetters have reported more frequent observation of friends and family members who smoke and use fire regularly (28). Kolko and Kazdin (24) report that access to firesetting materials alone can provide the conditions sufficient for children to become involved in fire-related activities (a child who uses a candle to light paper on a stove). Accessibility may be facilitated by peers or adults who model smoking or other fire-related behaviors or who carelessly leave materials accessible to children. Observation and modeling appear to be an important mechanism in the development of fire behavior.

Fire-related learning, impulse control, and emotional dysregulation are influenced by the family context. Familial risk factors for trajectories leading toward firesetting behaviors include parental psychopathology, emotional distance and communication, harsh disciplinary strategies, limited supervision, and stressful life events (28,34,36). For example, parents of juvenile firesetters have been found to demonstrate a significantly greater incidence of psychological disturbance including schizophrenia, other psychotic disorders, depression, and substance abuse. Parents of juvenile firesetters have also been found to be less nurturing, unresponsive, and at times rejecting (27,34). These relationships have been described as conflict laden and unaffectionate (34) and frequently involve limited communication between parent and child. A prospective study found a link between marital violence, paternal abuse of animals, paternal alcohol use, and children's firesetting behavior (37). Additional work has documented a significant relationship between parental disciplinary strategies and fire behavior. In particular, research suggests that juvenile firesetters tend to come from families who either use unduly harsh punishment practices (38), or mild, less-effective, forms of discipline (28). Related to this finding, researchers report that prolonged absence and insufficient supervision from parental figures can also lead to engagement in antisocial behavior (34). Left to their own, children are more likely to participate in covert behaviors and may even act out in an effort to engage otherwise inattentive parents. Moreover, stressful events such as a death in the family, divorce, or the introduction of a new step-parent may also be associated with firesetting among children and adolescents (27). Taken together, these findings suggest that ineffective parenting patterns are both directly and indirectly linked to firesetting.

As the ecologic–transactional model suggests, children's developmental pathways are also linked to other social and ecologic factors including peers, school, neighborhood, and culture. The presence or absence of a support system, the community's response to fire behavior, and government policies and regulations are all factors that can contribute to a child's risk of continued fire involvement. For example, exposure to peers who smoke or engage in fire activity themselves may contribute to a child's risk for early fire experimentation. Moreover, peer support and attention can serve as significant reinforcers for juvenile firesetters (39), particularly because these children tend to grapple with social skill deficits and often are not accepted by the peer group. However influential the peer group, community response to a child's early fire behavior can have significant impact on continued involvement with fire as well. For example, educational intervention and awareness programs provided by fire departments and other community organizations may be effective in reducing the frequency and severity of children's firesetting behavior (2,15). Over the past several years, major insurance companies have sponsored training opportunities for parents and providers working with juvenile firesetters and associated intervention coalitions (40). The juvenile justice system plays a role in the diversion of youth who are charged with arson (41) and, in many cases, coordinates or provides behavioral health treatment (42). Delinquent youth may be at risk of firesetting but charged with other crimes. The continued allocation of public and private resources in support of interagency collaborations and networks that support fire-specific intervention efforts is crucial.

The influence of cultural values regarding fire use and the level of assimilation of families is an unexplored, but potentially significant, factor in firesetting behavior. Less industrialized societies expose children more regularly to fire use for instrumental purposes (cooking, heating, agriculture/crop maintenance). In one case anecdote, a child referred for fire-starting, whose family had recently immigrated from the Dominican Republic, was receiving inconsistent messages regarding fire safety from his mother and grandfather. While his mother emphasized the importance of never using fire without proper supervision and responded with firm prohibition and consequences for this behavior, his grandfather disregarded this approach to home fire safety, noting that in their country of origin, he would be encouraged to use fire without supervision at an early age to meet developmental expectations.

PSYCHOPATHOLOGY AND FIRE BEHAVIOR

As our discussion of risk factors implies, the pathways to juvenile firesetting are multiple and interactive. For example, there is no clear evidence that early fire experimentation and activity causes later fire behavior. Some of the complex factors that influence an early fire-starter's later fire behavior include (1) the individual child's developmental maturation, together with impulse control and behavioral inhibition, emotion regulation skills particularly pertaining to fire fascination/curiosity, anger, and loneliness, and the development of social competence; (2) parenting practices including warmth, attention, monitoring, behavior control and discipline, communication, and modeling of safe behavior in the presence of fire; (3) the influence of peer modeling expectations; and (4) the constructive response of the neighborhood as well as the availability of ongoing prevention and intervention collaborative efforts in the community through fire service, juvenile justice, and behavioral health networks. Studies of juvenile firesetting have focused on the association of psychopathology to early fire experimentation and activity that are related to individual risk factors. Although over the years an emphasis has been placed on externalizing symptoms, likely because these features are more observable and intrusive to adults, research has also shown internalizing problems to be significantly related to early fire activity.

Externalizing problems including aggression and covert behavior such as lying and stealing are the most frequently cited correlates of early firesetting (17,29,33). A great deal of empirical work has associated firesetting diagnostically with conduct disorder (32,36,43–45) and firesetting is one of the symptoms of conduct disorder in the DSM-5. For example, when compared to a group of children who had committed murder, firesetters aged 10 through 17 were found to have higher rates of previous violent offenses, and they also were more likely than the homicidal group to carry a diagnosis of conduct disorder (43). Among clinical populations, several authors have noted that the primary reason for referral among firesetters was not for fire activity per se, but rather other externalizing symptomology (e.g., hyperactivity, truancy, running away, destructiveness, aggression) (24,27). As noted previously, some theorists suggest a developmental framework for understanding firesetting amid other kinds of disruptive behavior. Specifically, early fire activity is conceptualized as part of a deviant pathway characterized by stealing, lying, and other kinds of antisocial behaviors, only eventually ending in fire activity or arson (27). Alternatively, some have suggested that fire behavior signifies an extreme form of conduct disorder (32). A recent prospective study of six 12-year-old children found that reports of firesetting increased the likelihood of delinquent behavior within the following 10 years by as much as 2- to 10-fold (37).

We do not view firesetting as isomorphic with antisocial behavior, as there is clearly a much larger and heterogeneous group of children at risk of firesetting. For example, in several comparative studies of firesetting, delinquency, and other kinds of violent offenders, juvenile firesetters with and without histories of delinquent behavior did not differ across multiple domains (36,46,47). These authors determined that firesetters tended to demonstrate the same kinds of behavioral problems as children who had no previous history of fire experimentation, but who were classified as delinquent for other reasons. However, recent research has suggested that even when a fire safety education (FSE) intervention is administered, juvenile firesetting behavior may be a marker for significantly increased risk of future antisocial or criminal behavior in an important and large subgroup of youth (48).

Although externalizing behaviors tend to be the most widely cited and observed correlates of early fire activity, internalizing problems should not be overlooked. Researchers have found some significant associations between fire behavior and the presence of depressive and anxious characteristics. For example, in an investigation of the personality profiles of adolescent firesetters, investigators found that these teens scored significantly higher than non-firesetters on scales of depression, alienation, and on symptoms such as fear, worry, and withdrawal (49). In the prospective study mentioned earlier, firesetting and cruelty to animals were shown to be related to depression as well as conduct disorder, ADHD, and ODD (37). Furthermore, it has been noted that juvenile arsonists tend to have heightened suicidal thinking and an increased risk of suicide attempts (50). These children frequently have been involved in recent stressful life events including separations, divorces, and deaths in the family (17,27), all of which tend to heighten internalizing symptomology such as anxiety and depression. In an investigation of female firesetters, depression and low self-esteem were cited as significant antecedents to fire activity (51). Nevertheless, depression and anxiety are reviewed much less often in the firesetting literature than aggression and conduct behaviors. Studies that rely on parent report may be more likely to document associations between externalizing symptom and juvenile firesetting because externalizing behaviors are more easily observed, compared to internalizing symptoms which are more reliably endorsed through child self-report. As such, while the majority of research suggests firesetting is mostly associated with disruptive behaviors, anxious and depressive symptomology should remain a clinical consideration. Of particular interest are children with a mixed constellation of externalizing and internalizing psychopathology. These are children who may have multiple diagnoses over their lifetime (e.g., ADHD, ODD, mood or anxiety disorder) who are at risk for a variety of behavioral problems (e.g., impulsivity, irritability, emotion dysregulation, defiance, noncompliance, self-injury, or reactive aggression toward others). Such children may not be as likely to endorse anger as a primary motivation for firesetting and they may struggle with family environments lacking in critical parenting practices of monitoring, structured and responsive behavior management, warmth, and attention.

Two additional clinical considerations are social skill deficits, briefly reviewed in our discussion of etiology and developmental pathways, and substance abuse. Both are strongly associated with psychopathology as well as firesetting among children and adolescents. Kolko, Kazdin, and Meyer (29) conducted a comparative study of firesetters and non-firesetters, and found that firesetters demonstrated significantly lower social ability than their counterparts. In a follow-up work, this same finding has been consistently reported (24,33,51). Some have suggested that firesetters are averse to social interaction, and therefore are less likely to develop solutions to problems via socially acceptable routes (33). This aversion may lead to acting out aggressively, and indirectly, in the form of fire play, when a child's limited problem-solving repertoire leads to the aversion of assertive social confrontation and the expression of aggression through covert fire behavior. Another maladaptive pathway is through fire experimentation as a method by which to gain the attention and, potentially, admiration of peers, by children who are unable to do so by more skillful methods.

In addition to social skill deficits, substance abuse has also been implicated in the constellation of psychiatric difficulties observed among adolescent firesetters. Specifically, this population is noted to have difficulties including alcohol dependence (52) and inhalant abuse (50). We view substance abuse as likely linked to increased impulsivity through disinhibition contributing to poor decision making in critical areas of fire competence (e.g., fire safety knowledge and reasoning). The combination of social skill deficits and substance abuse may be associated with deviant peer socialization that may place a child at greater risk of engaging in firesetting behavior and other serious rule-violating behaviors.

FIRESETTING TYPOLOGIES AND CATEGORIZATIONS

Over the last half century, clinical theorists have attempted to identify a typology of firesetters in which different motivations (such as curiosity or anger) are thought to influence recidivism or severity of fire behavior (33). It has been suggested that children's motivation for becoming involved in fire play is predictive of continued involvement with fire as well as other forms of antisocial behavior (33). Several taxonomies have been suggested (39,53–55). For purposes of integrating these categories and typologies into the ecologic–transactional model, we organize these into four domains: fire curiosity/excitement, family dysfunction and parenting practices, and delinquency and conduct disorder, and serious psychopathology (such as psychosis or the diagnosis of pyromania).

Fire Curiosity/Excitement

By far, the most well-known category is that of the child who is motivated by curiosity (17,50). Retrospective studies of incidents reported to fire departments over the span of several years have demonstrated that a clear majority of fires and fire play were the result of curiosity (56,57). In retrospective incident report studies, the term curious refers to a child who has few to no behavioral difficulties and is in the early stages of fire experimentation (54). These studies, and the broader definition of curiosity, continue to influence strongly the firefighter literature that has driven much of the continuing education and training, particularly among fire education specialists. This literature describes children in the curious category as unlikely to set fires again after receiving FSE, with less-intensive intervention assumed to be warranted. In the past, research reported the curious firesetter to be less pathologic, younger, and generally only involved in one serious fire incident across the life span (17).

The curious firesetter categorization, however, is evolving and has been expanded by more recent empirical findings. Specifically, Kolko and Kazdin (33) found that children motivated to set fires by curiosity were also found to demonstrate elevations on measures of psychopathology including internalizing and externalizing dysfunction, overt and covert antisocial behaviors, expressed hostility and social skill deficits. These children also had more early experiences with fire and reported to be more interested in, exposed to, and in contact with fire over the previous year. This was in contrast to children scoring high on anger, who did not show more psychopathology than those low in anger, but had greater exposure to models of fire interest, elicited more community complaints about fire behavior, and were more frequently hiding matches or incendiary materials. These findings suggest that curiosity, when compared with anger among firesetters, is more strongly associated with a different constellation of risk factors that combine into distinct maladaptive pathways. The findings also suggest that the broader type of curiosity, associated with one-time fire experimentation, and thought to be developmentally common in children, may be distinct from fire curiosity/ excitement as identified in studies using the Firesetting Risk Interview (FRI) or the Children's Firesetting Inventory (CFI) (18,19). The comparatively smaller group of children described by these measures may show more psychopathology, hostility, social skill deficits, and engage in more disruptive behaviors than those children in the more broadly curious category. High levels of curiosity, as measured by the FRI/CFI, may be associated with heightened risk for repeat fire play and/or intentional firesetting behavior. Fire interest/excitement and antisocial behavior have also been linked to more severe and persistent firesetting (14,22). Similar to some children with high levels of anger, some children with high levels of fire curiosity and excitement may set fires with a specific intention to harm (33).

Family Dysfunction and Parenting Practices

Children may also set fires as an individual expression of family dysfunction or a response to overwhelming life or family stress. This stress may be related to deficits in family functioning such as parental modeling around fire, communication, monitoring, behavior control, or parental psychiatric illness. In this category, children are thought to be inadvertently using fire as way of calling out for help (17). Several researchers have indeed found firesetting to be intimately tied to family and life stressors (17,27,36). We term this second category family dysfunction and parenting practices. This family dysfunction and parenting practice group includes families where there is an association between child maltreatment and juvenile firesetting. In a review of 4,155 youth in the child welfare system, results suggested that children were three times more likely to engage in firesetting behavior (58). A study of 205 juvenile firesetting youth (ages 4 to 17) showed 48% to have a history of maltreatment. Among this group, firesetters had an increased likelihood of family stress as a motivating factor, used more versatile ignition sources and targets, and showed higher rates of recidivism (59).

Delinquency/Conduct Disorder

The third category refers to children who become involved with fire as part of the development of a pervasive pattern of antisocial behavior. This category (17) may represent a distinctive maladaptive pathway (32). This category may also include many children scoring high in anger and thought to be engaging in firesetting that is more purposive or deliberate than children in the family functioning and parenting practices category. However, this relationship has yet to be tested. This group may also include those youth who are at risk for reoffending through delinquent behaviors other than firesetting, even after firesetting educational intervention has been received. A 10-year follow-up study of offending behaviors among 182 child and adolescent firesetters in New Zealand showed that while arson recidivism was only 2% for this sample, rates of other offending behavior were high with 59% of the sample reoffending during the follow-up period (12.8% imprisoned, 40% rated as moderate, and 4% rated as minor offenses). Offending behavior was predicted by the experience of abuse. Involvement in family violence was associated with more severe offending behavior. Living in a two-parent home was associated with decreased likelihood of offending behavior. Results suggested that repeat firesetting (in this study, defined by more than one incident and representing more than the half of the sample) significantly predicted the risk of later offending behavior (48).

It has been speculated that enuresis, cruelty to animals, and firesetting are not only highly correlated to one another, but also predictive of violent crimes later in adulthood (17,27). Two studies have failed to identify a relationship between firesetting and enuresis (47,60). However, juveniles reported to be cruel to animals have been shown to be more likely to engage in repeat firesetting when compared with children not cruel to animals (60). It is possible that the behavior of cruelty to animals when combined with firesetting will increase the likelihood of subsequent delinquent behaviors (37), thus signifying a distinctive maladaptive antisocial pathway that may be included in the category of delinquency.

Serious Psychopathology

The fourth category of children and adolescents accounts for a very small portion of child and adolescent fire behavior. This category includes children who set fires as a result of extreme psychopathology including compulsive behaviors and/or psychotic ideation that may be specifically related to the firesetting (17,61). The DSM-IV diagnosis of pyromania represents another dimension of this category that is also extremely rare in children. Pyromania describes fire behavior that is deliberate, purposeful, involving an obsession with fire, with children showing tension or affective excitement before the act, and pleasure or gratification during the act (62).

Fire-Specific Variables

The modest body of empirical research over the last 30 years has converged to emphasize the critical role of fire-specific variables in the classification of firesetters. A treatment outcome study from 2006 examined recidivism at one-year follow-up among 48 juvenile firesetters. Findings supported the view that children who persist in lighting fires show a wider range of fire involvement and more intense fascination with fire at the start of treatment. Recidivists had a higher frequency of match play and more firesetting incidents including a greater involvement in fire-related acts such as hiding matches or lighters and pulling fire alarms. Repeat firesetters also demonstrated heightened curiosity, personal interest in fire, and fire attraction, as well as more externalizing behaviors (22).

A more recent analysis of firesetters 4 to 17 has yielded 3 clusters which combine multiple factors from the ecologic model with a focus on fire-specific variables. The three clusters are termed as conventional limited (CL), home instability (HI), moderate and multi-problem (MP) risk. Firesetting behavior in the conventional limited category is distinguished by a relatively low fire interest or curiosity, but combined with: (1) a relatively low number of firesetting incidences, (2) a relatively late age of firesetting onset and child mental health contact, (3) the least varied range of ignition sources and target, (4) the highest percentage expressing remorse, and (5) the lowest percentage endorsing antisocial motivation. These children also had the most contact with their biologic parents.

In contrast, the home instability–moderate cluster is characterized by relatively larger number of firesetting incidents, greater fire interest and curiosity, and more varied ignition sources and targets when compared with conventional limited firesetters. There was a higher proportion of antisocial motivation and less expressed remorse in this group. This group was also characterized by less parental involvement, the highest percentage of abuse exposure, and the greatest number of children in care of a children's welfare agency, as well as more difficulties (when compared with CL) for social relationships, attention and externalizing behaviors. Of note, the abuse exposures were the highest in this group when compared with all other categories.

Finally, the multi-problem risk group engaged in the overall highest number of firesetting incidents and had the youngest firesetting onset. They demonstrated high levels of fire interest and curiosity and had, among all groups, the most varied number of ignition sources and targets. In addition, this cluster was distinguished from the other two groups by the highest levels of social skill deficits, attentional difficulties, and externalizing behaviors. Interestingly, none of these youth were placed in care of a child welfare agency (although many had been referred) and, as noted above, this category had a lower level of abuse than the home instability group, but higher levels than the conventional limited group. Like the home instability group, the multi-risk group included few youth expressing remorse and greater number of youth with antisocial motivation (63).

ASSESSMENT

Prior to any evaluation of children's fire behavior it must be determined whether the purpose is to assess for treatment or to evaluate the risk of recidivism. There is currently little empirical support for the predictive validity of risk categories as they primarily rely upon the clinical expertise of individual practitioners (16,50,62). The ecologic model and the expertise of experienced practitioners, when combined with training in a thorough assessment protocol, are currently considered the standard of practice for juvenile firesetter risk assessment. A good example of a thorough protocol would be the FRAT-Y Firesetting Risk Assessment Tool for Youth (64). In some states, risk assessments are requested by the courts to inform placement decisions. Such assessments can provide useful information that can guide treatment decisions and should be obtained prior to beginning treatment. In this section, we will restrict our discussion to treatment assessment using the ecologic–transactional model (65).

Information from referral sources and other outside agencies should be obtained prior to the assessment. Many referrals of children who have set fires are initially screened through the fire department or juvenile diversion programs. This interdisciplinary involvement has influenced the development of standardized screening measures, which in some states are widely used, but have yet to be validated (66). Examples of screenings/assessments are the Oregon Screening Tool, Maine Screening Tool, and the Federal Emergency Management Tool (66). The evaluating clinician can identify whether any screening measures are being administered in their region and follow up by requesting a copy of the measure prior to interviewing the child and the family. These screenings provide a basis for further inquiry into the nature of the firesetting incident and the existence of other behavior problems or delinquent activities at home or school. In addition, there may be a written report summarizing the fire investigation that rests with the fire department or a law enforcement agency. Reviewing this "cause and origin" or fire/arson investigation report (55,67) from the fire department can be particularly helpful with preteens and adolescents, who may be less inclined to be truthful regarding the nature of the incident. The report can provide a foundation for confronting the child with inconsistencies in their narrative and promote accountability as well as provide a basis for assessment of the complexity of the fire behavior (e.g., the use of accelerants, covert hiding of materials, deliberation). Finally, prior to the assessment, older children, adolescents, and parents must be informed about the limits of confidentiality and protections of disclosure within the larger community or juvenile justice system, particularly whether or not disclosure of firesetting may lead to criminal justice involvement.

Once these initial steps are taken, child assessment should proceed with a thorough understanding of firesetting behavior both past and present. Recognizing when fire behavior deviates from normative development requires an understanding of the child's behaviors, cognitions, and emotions surrounding the firesetting incident, including what was used to start the fire, the location, if others were present, the child's response to the event and how the fire was extinguished (27,61,67). Several preliminary questions may precede more structured assessment methods. For example, children are generally asked if they have ever played with matches or lighters and if they have ever "set a fire," or "set a fire in order to burn something" (see Wilcox and Kolko (67) for a more thorough discussion of unstructured interview techniques).

Prior to the assessment, the evaluator should consider modifying the interview format to match the developmental level of the child. In general, preschool-aged children will require visual stimuli (e.g., "Play Safe; Be Safe" drawings, empty match boxes) (68) and an emphasis on obtaining a simple narrative of the sequence of events around the fire incident, with minimal focus on motivational states as these are difficult for most preschool-aged children to report. Elementary school–aged children, particularly those with learning disabilities and attentional/concentration difficulties can benefit from these methods and techniques as well. Wilcox and Kolko (67) noted several questions that capture important nuances of the child's degree of planning and learning from the experience that may be particularly helpful for elementary school–aged children ("How did you get the idea to start the fire?" "What did you think would happen when you actually started the fire?" "Did the fire act the way you thought it would?" "Did you learn anything from what happened?"). The latter questions can be helpful in linking assessment to educational or psychosocial interventions. With adolescents, the interviewer may need to confront denial or avoidance directly by using collateral reports and discussion of the context and purpose of the interview in the larger system (69). Self-monitoring techniques have been popular among evaluators in helping children to report accurately on thoughts, feelings, and behavior related to the firesetting incident; however, they may be beneficial in the interview process as well (70). One study has simplified this method using vignettes to introduce the relationship among thoughts, feelings, and actions (16), which can help children become acquainted with the concepts before applying them to their own firesetting incidents. One area that has received very little attention is the assessment of fire behavior among developmentally disabled populations. As with younger children, the interview will likely focus less on more complex motivation and more on curiosity or fascination, use more visual cues and prompts, and include more inquiry on fire safety skills awareness, as well as family and ecologic factors that may be contributing to lapses in supervision or monitoring.

Multi-source (parent, child, and teacher report) and multi-method assessment protocols are recommended across at least two settings (e.g., home and school environments) to identify the scope and intensity of firesetting or associated behavioral disturbance. Some instruments have been validated in general clinical populations, but clinical utility in firesetting populations is less well established. Other fire-specific instruments have been developed for research purposes, but have not been as well examined in clinical populations.

Both structured interviews and behavioral rating scales have been developed for use with juvenile firesetters. These tools include questions about how materials were obtained, the site of fire, type of property damage, fire competence, exposure to fire models, fire involvement (hiding of matches/lighters), and curiosity/fascination with fire (19). The domain of learning and exposure relates to how the child acquired exposure and knowledge of fire in his/her family. Attempts should be made to identify (1) the current and past adult, sibling, or peer models of fire behavior, (2) the age of exposure to fire and to models of fire safety, (3) the nature of the exposure (whether unsupervised, supervised, or guided with developmentally appropriate explanations), (4) the consistency of the caregiver or peer modeling, and caregiver supervision, and (5) child fire competence (knowledge) and fire safety skill (both child report and parental perception).

One important domain is that of fire competence, skill, and understanding. Firesetters (6 to 13 years old), when compared with non-firesetters with similar behavioral health profiles, have been shown to be more knowledgeable about types of things that burn, more curious, less fire competent (lacking in both fire safety skills awareness and an understanding of the properties of fire). In addition, exposure to fire activities in the home and community should also be assessed (e.g., individuals in home who smoke or have been burned, fires in neighborhood, or friends who smoke) (18).

Assessment of problems in family functioning is the next important domain for assessment. This may include an evaluation of the quality of the parent–child relationship/communication, the degree of parental involvement, warmth and nurturance, disciplinary practices, as well as parental psychiatric distress and exposure to stressful life events. Generally, the parenting process can be organized into three dimensions: (1) motivation (parental belief systems including norms, values, and parent goals), (2) parental monitoring, or the tracking and structuring of the child's activities, social ecology or environments, and (3) behavior management (the parent's active attempt to shape positive outcomes by using incentives, reinforcement, limit-setting, and negotiation). Parental monitoring is thought to be the common denominator within this process and is associated strongly with both parenting practices and measures of the parenting relationship/communication. In this way, parental monitoring may act as a protective factor for children living in high-risk settings and can provide a foundation for brief interventions for child and adolescent problem behavior and child injury prevention (71). Future research should examine the application of these dimensions of parenting as they pertain specifically to fire behavior.

The FRI contains sections assessing parenting regarding both fire-specific issues and more general concerns. Fire-specific domains in the FRI include parental fire awareness (parental safety instruction in the home, fire safety instruction in the home, practicing fire-escape drills), as well as general parenting practices (use of mild vs. harsh punishment, parental supervision). In Table 5.1.4.1, we list several measures of family functioning and stressful life events that are used in the assessment of disruptive behavior disorders and may be useful in the assessment of family functioning among juvenile firesetters specifically (18). Assessment may also include parental psychiatric history/distress, as this is more commonly found among firesetters when compared with non-firesetters (24).

TABLE 5.1.4.1

ASSESSMENT TOOLS FOR USE IN EVALUATION OF JUVENILE FIRESETTING[a]

Name of Measure	Brief Description	Reporter
The Firesetting Incident Analysis—Parent and Child Version[b] (FIA-P, FIA-C) (60)	Structured interview that obtains information regarding specific fire incidents	Parent and Child Report
The Firesetting Risk Interview[b] (FRI) (14)	Structured interview used to assess several domains related to fire involvement	Parent Report
Children's Firesetting Inventory[b] (CFI) (15)	Structured interview used to assess several domains related to fire involvement, administered to children	Child Report
Fire Interest Questionnaire[b] (63)	Structured interview used to assess several domains related to fire involvement, administered to children	Parent and Child Report
Child Behavior Checklist (CBCL) (61)	Rating scale used to assess several dimensions of children's emotional and behavioral functioning	Parent Report (Teacher Report Form also available)
IOWA/Conners (IOWA/C) (62)	Rating scale used to determine the presence of hyperactivity, impulsivity, and inattention in children	Parent Report
Children's Hostility Inventory (CHI) (63) and Children's Inventory of Anger (CHIA) (64)	Questionnaires used to assess aggression and hostility among children	Parent or Child Report
Children's Depression Inventory (CDI) (65)	Brief rating scale used to measure children's level of depressive symptoms	Child Report
Trauma Symptom Checklist for Children (TSCC) (66)	Rating scale measuring psychological distress and related symptomology	Child Report
The Parent–Child Conflict Tactics Scales (CTSPC) (67)	Assesses parental disciplinary strategies during child conflicts (nonviolent discipline, psychological aggression, physical assault)	Parent Report
Parent–Child Relationship Inventory (PCRI) (68)	Assesses parent–child communication strategies	Parent Report

[a]This table is not an exhaustive battery, but reflects an array of tools that have been clinically useful and often incorporated into empirical investigations of juvenile firesetting. For a more extensive review of measures, see Kolko DJ, Swenson CC: *Assessing and Treating Physically Abused Children and Their Families*. Thousand Oaks, CA, Sage Publications, 2002.
[b]These instruments can be solicited from the first author upon request.

Finally, the evaluator should be sure to obtain information regarding the range of delinquent behaviors that may be associated with firesetting behavior. In particular, cruelty to animals, violence toward others or property, truancy, running away, breaking and entering, and court involvement may increase risk for future delinquency and firesetting. A history of exposure to domestic violence and early modeling of paternal cruelty toward animals are also activities (37) that may be associated with a higher risk of maladaptive outcomes (e.g., delinquency and court involvement).

TREATMENT

A thorough assessment of fire behavior guided by the ecologic–transactional model yields information that corresponds with skill-based, multimodal approaches that can stand alone or be used to supplement ongoing treatment interventions such as fire safety skills training (FSST), self-monitoring, parent–child communication, parental psychoeducation, promoting emotion regulation and alternative coping strategies, and restitution for damages (2,16,72,73). Treatment outcome studies for juvenile firesetting are few and yield limited, if promising, results. Samples are heterogeneous, making it difficult to identify whether subgroups based on severity or breadth of dysfunction would benefit from a specific element of treatment (e.g., children vs. adolescents; match players vs. repeat firesetters). Treatment protocols are also varied, making it difficult to identify specific elements of treatment that are more or less effective. There is a relative lack of randomized controlled studies when compared with other areas of child behavioral health (e.g., depression, aggression). Reductions in recidivism may reflect change over time following treatment, additional behavioral health treatment for other problems, or change due to a nonspecific factor in fire treatment. Yet there is accumulating evidence that FSST and cognitive behavioral therapy (CBT) are promising interventions, particularly when combined or delivered in a collaborative format (2,3). FSST has been shown to be more effective than a general discussion of the fire incident with inpatient children aged 4 to 8 years (33). Another study compared one-time fire safety discussion/pamphlet with a combined educational and home-based psychosocial intervention delivered by fire educators (satiation, response cost, self-monitoring/graphing of antecedents, and associated emotions and cognitions). Of the children, 67% demonstrated improved fire behavior, with 42% setting no fires in the 12 months following the intervention. Thirty percent of the families were not assessed because they could not be located. In this study, even the very brief fire safety intervention had an impact on reducing recidivism, with a one-time pamphlet shown to effectively reduce repeated fire activity (2).

FSE remains a core component of most interventions for juvenile firesetters. One-classroom-style FSE program included live tours of a burn unit, a curriculum on fire knowledge and safety awareness, and lectures from returning veterans of the program. There are innovative programs being developed that involve collaboration with fire departments (74) and more standard group treatment models for disruptive behaviors. In fact, there appears to be a variety of fire-specific psychosocial interventions and/or safety education/skills training that can reduce recidivism from 6 months up to 2-year follow-up (2,33). Given findings that a significant percentage of firesetters will repeat if untreated (19), it seems imperative that intervention efforts be early and swift.

The most rigorous outcome study to date shows that when FSST and brief cognitive behavioral treatment (average number of sessions was 5.5) are administered in a highly standardized format, they can be superior to a one-time pamphlet and safety contract (75), although not superior to each other. This study set the standard for multimodal and collaborative treatment of juvenile firesetters by integrating self-monitoring techniques (identifying the personal and environmental context of the firesetting) into a treatment including relaxation, cognitive restructuring, assertion skills training, problem solving, and parental skills training (selective attention, reinforcement, contingency management) (3).

A subsequent small outcome study of firesetting treatment outcome of 48 youth compared FSE, CBT and FHV (a single-informational firefighter home visit). This study suggested that FHV may be less effective for families with heightened dysfunction. Interestingly, FSE appeared more effective with children who had greater fire safety knowledge. These exploratory findings suggest the potential benefit of systematically examining the characteristics of youth who respond to treatment, to better match firesetting youth with a potentially successful treatment (22).

Influenced by Kolko's work, other innovative and cost-effective fire-specific interventions for parents and families have been developed that include clearly defined treatment objectives that can lead to standardization of administration and some evaluation of recidivism. One intervention effort has offered classes to 247 families of firesetters from 2000 to 2005 through the Washington County Fire Academy (57), with estimates of 3% to 6% recidivism. These classes meet two times per week for 6 weeks with parents and children attending concordant programs. Children receive FSE with their peers, while parents meet with one another and identify the ecologic factors contributing to their child's firesetting (Oregon "Cycles" Model) (57), learn myths and facts about firesetting behavior, are instructed in contingency management, positive praise techniques and response–cost techniques, and identify areas of psychopathology that may need attention (e.g., untreated ADHD, parental conflict, or other family stressors).

Similarly, in a treatment study through Bradley Hospital in Rhode Island, families of firesetters receive 4 weeks of 1.5-hour concordant sessions. Children meet with their peers prior to working directly with their parents in Multiple Family Group Intervention (MFGT). This model focuses on improving the quality of family communication about fire and uses group and individual exercises (e.g., affect identification, self-monitoring) to facilitate children's experience of mastery over fire behavior. Children learned to identify and monitor both emotions and thoughts associated with fire behavior and identify coping strategies through four exercises: group discussion designed to destigmatize fire communication, vignette and game activities, review of firesetting incidents, and coping strategy contracts. These strategies were then refined with children and parents in an MFGT session. Parents received psychoeducation about the ecologic model and cyclical nature of firesetting (57) combined with experiential discussion related to fire communication in the family (e.g., how parents first learned about the fire behavior, the quality of the family communication around fire behavior/safety, the parent's history of modeling safe fire behavior, and development of a home fire safety checklist and escape plan).

In a third example developed in Ontario, Canada, and operating for over 20 years, fire safety education and parent–child intervention are delivered simultaneously by a trained local behavioral health clinician (76). The content of the protocol is described in a detailed manual with fire-specific exercises and worksheets for caregivers and children. The protocol is conducted in five sessions (total of 7.5 hours) and includes modules on fire safety (attitudes, high-risk situations, and behaviors) in and out of the home, rewarding fire safety behavior, parental supervision and monitoring access to ignition materials, understanding antecedents to fire involvement, and teaching a systematic approach to consequences of future fire involvement. Follow-up of over 200 families receiving the intervention indicate that approximately 75% had no further fire involvement over 1 to 2 years (77). Interestingly, this is the only program to evaluate the adoption and implementation of the protocol through a survey of approximately 700 community professionals trained over 8 years. Findings indicated that although 89% of the clinicians made a commitment to use the protocol, only 29% implemented the protocol on a routine basis. Factors such as the compatibility of the protocol with existing practice, ease of use, and adopter self-efficacy may have influenced implementation (78).

Remarkably, there has been little empirical evaluation of the specific treatment needs of preschool or adolescent firesetters, given that preschool fire behavior may be associated with some of the greatest danger for loss of life and adolescent fire behavior can lead to the most costly treatments (i.e., residential and juvenile justice incarceration). Existing FSE program curriculums that are directed toward preschoolers can be incorporated into daycare programming for children (68,74). Parental participation is critical to any systematic approach to treatment of preschoolers and two of the four psychosocial interventions previously described have been used with preschoolers (72,79).

Many adolescents come to the attention of behavioral health providers through the criminal justice system, and may be engaging in a broad range of delinquent behaviors. Some may be charged with arson and then referred to intervention programs that specialize in working with delinquent adolescents engaging in fire behavior. Several models have been developed, ranging from those offering individually supervised restitution or community service activities to more structured fire safety and CBT skill-based group interventions (42). These court diversion intervention programs designed specifically for children convicted of arson have yet to be evaluated using more rigorous experimental designs, although some conform to best practice guidelines for youth offender programs established by the Office of Juvenile Justice and Delinquency Prevention programs (42). Multisystemic therapy has also shown some promise in the treatment of serious juvenile offenders, some of which included those teens 13.7 years old charged with arson (80). However, many of the studies and treatment models previously reviewed in this chapter included children referred by the court system and may have been influential in reducing or eliminating dangerous fire behavior among these court-referred youth. For group or residential treatments, there is a potential for negative impact for modestly deviant or delinquent adolescents, if these teens are exposed to deviant older youth. Such deviant peer exposure effects may detract from the overall positive impact of the intervention and are in need of rigorous evaluation (81).

There have been calls for clearer standards of care in residential settings for evaluation and placement of firesetters (74). Recently, one study comparing 17 adolescent firesetters in residential treatment with 30 adolescents with first-time fire histories demonstrated no differences in psychopathology, delinquent personality characteristics, and surprisingly, fire-specific characteristics (e.g., number of fires set, use of accelerants, location of the fire, injuries caused by the fire). Instead, a greater proportion of residential teens came from single-parent homes and had higher scores of aggression (82), suggesting that lack of safety, supervision, and monitoring in the home environment, coupled with aggressive behavior, may be the primary factors leading to out-of-home placement. There has been a call for better integration of fire-specific treatment with residential facilities, making FSST a treatment objective that is actively monitored in clinical care meetings throughout placement along with coordination of resources outside of the residential program as necessary to provide FSST (83).

The treatment of specific populations, such as children diagnosed with mental retardation or significant learning and communication limitations (e.g., autism, impaired attention/concentration, reading and writing challenges, limited reasoning capacities) has received little attention. There is need for specialized delivery of FSST or CBT techniques for these groups. One case study describes the use of a multicomponent behavioral treatment approach with a hospitalized 6-year-old boy with developmentally disabilities. Treatment included negative practice with correction from his mother, token reinforcement, and routine discipline instruction (84). Another study used a virtual reality computer game to teach fire safety skills to children diagnosed with fetal alcohol syndrome. The games were administered without direct assistance from parents or observers (85). We have found the use of educational videotapes and testimonials useful for children with limited cognitive abilities who are resistant to FSST. We have adapted and simplified techniques by avoiding discussions of motivations of firesetting or past experiences (beyond the initial assessment) and adapting workbooks and curriculum available online to create structured learning sequences. The sequences maintain a focus on understanding "how things work" and reinforce a sense of mastery and competence with fire for these youngsters.

Children repeatedly lighting matches to satiate interest under the supervision of an adult is one of the earliest behavioral interventions reported to be effective in decreasing a child's interest in fire and firesetting behaviors (86). This practice, however, is rarely encouraged, due to the risks of the potential negative effects of modeling fire behavior and reports of the large number of sessions required to be effective. Given the prominent association of curiosity or fascination and psychopathology, further development of behavioral interventions that target fire fascination is warranted, perhaps through the specification of overt or covert sensitization techniques (i.e., use of stories, narratives, testimonials, or visual stimuli to discourage contact with fire). If such programs were systematically evaluated and included measures related to specific treatment components, we may better understand the cognitive and behavioral change processes that make both FSE and psychosocial treatment effective.

As noted earlier, FSE delivered in a classroom, combined with experiential format, has been shown to reduce recidivism significantly (87), and FSST delivered to children individually has been shown to be as effective as CBT (88). The modality of delivering of FSE, however, may differ considerably between local communities and service providers. Guidelines for FSE are broad, and the availability of FSE intervention will depend upon community resources. Thus, it is incumbent upon the behavioral health clinician to have some knowledge of exactly what is being delivered in the community to facilitate clinical treatment objectives, to avoid duplication of services, and to assess and monitor the child's generalization of fire safety skills. FSE can include the following topics: fire facts (e.g., fuel, how fire grows/spreads and how is it extinguished/controlled, smoke inhalation dangers), fire safety awareness (i.e., "matches are tools and not toys," safe distance, home fire safety "projects" such as identifying common fire safety hazards in the home or collecting information regarding the causes and consequences of fire in the community), fire survival (e.g., smoke detectors, home fire escape plan and strategies, "stop, drop, and roll"), fire consequences (potential criminal justice involvement, burns, damages to community both direct and indirect) (15,28).

Fire behavior crosses over the boundaries of several disciplines (fire service, juvenile justice, behavioral health, pediatric injury prevention, and child protection), with many of these disciplines using public health prevention education techniques (89). Basic FSE principles (stop, drop, and roll; use of 911; and match/lighter safety slogans) are delivered in many elementary school classrooms around the country. Unfortunately, the efficacy of these education programs has yet to be established. For example, many children do not effectively generalize simple fire safety instruction following a single classroom exposure. Two examples of preschool prevention programs are the "Learn Not to Burn Program" and the "Play Safe; Be Safe" curricula. A middle school curriculum has been designed (72). Many of the tools and exercises in these prevention education curricula can be adapted for use in clinical therapies with individuals, families, or groups.

Psychopharmacologic techniques for treatment of juvenile firesetting populations have largely been neglected in the empirical literature. To date, no specific medications are used to treat firesetting behavior per se. Instead, juvenile firesetters are treated for associated difficulties such as disruptive behavior problems, ADHD, or internalizing distress. In many cases, and as suggested by the ecologic–transactional model, risk for future firesetting will decrease secondary to the improvement of associated psychological and behavioral difficulties, as these factors increase vulnerability for repeated fire activity. Improvement in these areas, in turn, provides opportunity for more adaptive developmental outcomes.

As noted earlier, juvenile arson is not merely a clinical concern, but a public health and safety problem of large proportions. Inter-agency collaborative relationships among city departments, community-based organizations, city residents, and state law enforcement and fire prevention agencies are needed to develop multilayered community prevention programs (90). In Detroit (a metropolitan area of over 500,000), one such collaborative effort successfully reduced the incidence of fires set in the community on Halloween night from record numbers of fires set in 1984 (810 fires over a 3-day period) to levels consistent with incidence at other times of the year. Many of these fires were suspected to be set by youth; the intervention included after-school and evening programs as well as a curfew to monitor more effectively children's whereabouts and limit access to dumpsters and abandoned buildings. Moreover, the intervention included the deployment of public safety personnel, the elimination of arson targets through community cleanup, volunteer mobilization and training, public media and communications campaigns, and prohibitions on the safe use of fuel (90).

CONCLUSION

Fire behavior in children and adolescents is a problem of surprising scope, carrying with it the potential for death, injury, and property loss of striking proportions. The problem spans all ages, is particularly prevalent among children in psychiatric settings, and often is not identified unless the clinician specifically asks about experiences with firesetting and fire play. The complexity of the development of juvenile firesetting behavior is best captured by an ecologic–transactional model that includes factors related to individual functioning, parental processes, peer socialization, neighborhood and school safety, and cultural socialization. Assessment should be fire specific, but correspond with the best practices in the assessment and treatment of disruptive behavior disorders (multimodel, parent and child report, developmentally sensitive methods), internalizing disorders, and mixed internalizing/externalizing disorders. When child and adolescent fire behavior is associated with externalizing and internalizing disorders, families may benefit from promising collaborative treatment programs combining FSE with cognitive–behavioral treatment and/or parent–child treatments. While children without associated emotional disorders will likely benefit from FSE alone, some children with behavioral disorders may also see a reduction in repeat fire behavior, without any additional psychosocial treatment.

ACKNOWLEDGMENT

This research was supported through grants from the Providence Mutual Fire Insurance Agency and the Shriner's Foundation. The authors are grateful to the contributions of Kristen Durbin, Lauren Mernick, Beth Hollander, James Leverone, LCMHC; Julie Lucier, Psy.D.; and Peter Gillen, Psy.D.

References

1. American Academy of Pediatrics, Committee on Injury and Poison Prevention: Reducing the number of deaths and injuries from residential fires. *Pediatrics* 105:1355–1357, 2000.
2. Adler R, Nunn R, Northam E, Lebnan V, Ross R: Secondary prevention of childhood firesetting. *J Am Acad Child Adolesc Psychiatry* 33:1194–1202, 1994.
3. Kolko DJ: Efficacy of cognitive-behavioral treatment and fire safety education for children who have set fires: initial and follow-up outcomes. *J Child Psychol Psychiatry* 42:359–369, 2001.
4. Kolko DJ, Kazdin AE: The emergence and recurrence of child firesetting: a one-year prospective study. *J Abnorm Child Psychol* 20:17–37, 1992.
5. National Association of State Fire Marshals: *Juvenile Firesetter Intervention Research Project: Final Report.* Washington, DC, Office of Juvenile Justice and Delinquency Prevention, 2001. Available at: www.firemarshalsarchive.org. Accessed 03/05/2017.
6. Hall JR: *Children Playing with Fire.* Quincy, MA: Fire Analysis and Research Division, National Fire Protection Association, 2010.
7. Hall JR: *Intentional Fires and Arson.* Quincy, MA: National Fire Protection Association, 2007.
8. U.S. Department of Justice—Federal Bureau of Justice. Crime in the United States, 2009. Table 36: current year over previous year arrest trends, 2010. Available at: http://www2.fbi.gov/ucr/cius2009/data/table_36.html.
9. Kolko DJ: Juvenile firesetting: a review and methodological critique. *Clin Psychol Rev* 5:345–376, 1985.
10. Juvenile firesetting intervention practices, National Association of State Fire Marshals International Conference, January 24–25, 2003.
11. Del Bove G, Caprara GV, Pastorelli C, Paciello M: Juvenile firesetting in Italy: relationship to aggression, psychopathology, personality, self-efficacy, and school functioning. *Eur Child Adolesc Psychiatry* 17:235–244, 2008.
12. MacKay S, Paglia-Boak A, Henderson J, Marton P, Adlaf E: Epidemiology of firesetting in adolescents: mental health and substance use correlates. *J Child Psychol Psychiatry* 50:1282–1290, 2009.
13. Kolko DJ, Day BT, Bridge JA, Kazdin AE: Two-year prediction of children's firesetting in clinically referred and nonreferred samples. *J Child Psychol Psychiatry* 42:371–380, 2001.
14. MacKay S, Henderson J, Del Bove G, Marton P, Warling D, Root C: Fire interest and antisociality as risk factors in the severity and persistence of juvenile firesetting. *J Am Acad Child Adolesc Psychiatry* 45:1077–1084, 2006.
15. Pinsonneault IL: Fire safety education and skills training. In: Kolko DJ (ed): *Handbook on Firesetting in Children and Youth.* San Diego, CA, Academic Press, 219–260, 2002.
16. Barreto SJ, Boekamp JR, Armstrong LM, Gillen P: Community-based interventions for juvenile firestarters: a brief family-centered model. *Psychol Serv* 1:158–168, 2004.
17. Cole R, Grolnick W, Schwartzman P: Firesetting. In: Ammerman R, Hersen M, Last C (eds): *Prescriptive Treatment for Children and Adolescents.* Boston, MA, Allyn & Bacon, 293–307, 1999.
18. Kolko DJ, Kazdin AE: Assessment of dimensions of childhood firesetting among patients and nonpatients: the Firesetting Risk Interview. *J Abnorm Child Psychol* 17:157–176, 1989.
19. Kolko DJ, Kazdin AE: The Children's firesetting interview with psychiatrically referred and nonreferred children. *J Abnorm Child Psychol* 17:609–624, 1989.
20. Simonsen B, Bullis M: *Fire Interest Survey: Final Report.* Salem, Oregon Office of the State Fire Marshal, 2001.
21. Cotterall A, McPhee B, Plecas D: *Fireplay Report—A Survey of School-Aged Youth in Grades 1 to 12.* Abbotsford, University College of the Fraser Valley, 1999.
22. Kolko DJ, Herschell AD, Scharf DM: Education and treatment for boys who set fires: specificity, moderators, and predictors of recidivism. *J Emot Behav Disord* 14(4), 227–239, 2006.
23. Kafry D: Playing with matches: children and fire. In: Canter D (ed): *Fires and Human Behavior.* New York, Wiley and Sons, 47–62, 1980.
24. Kolko DJ, Kazdin AE: A conceptualization of firesetting in children and adolescents. *J Abnorm Child Psychol* 14:49–61, 1986.
25. Rutter M, Sroufe LA: Developmental psychopathology: concepts and challenges. *Dev Psychopathol* 12:265–296, 2000.
26. Sroufe LA: Psychopathology as an outcome of development. *Dev Psychopathol* 9:251–268, 1997.
27. Fineman KR: Firesetting in childhood and adolescence. *Psychiatr Clin North Am* 3:483–500, 1980.

28. Kolko DJ: Education and counseling for child firesetters: a comparison of skills training programs with standard practice. In: Hibbs ED, Jensen PS (eds): *Psychosocial Treatments for Child and Adolescent Disorders: Empirically Based Strategies for Clinical Practice.* Washington, DC, American Psychological Association, 187–206, 1996.
29. Kolko DJ, Kazdin AE, Meyer EC: Aggression and psychopathology in childhood firesetters: parent and child reports. *J Consult Clin Psychol* 53:377–385, 1985.
30. Mackay S, Ruttle EM, Ward AK. *The Developmental Aspects of Firesetting. Firesetting and Mental Health: Theory, Research, and Practice.* London: RCPsych, 84–101, 2012.
31. Stickle TR, Blechman EA: Aggression and fire: antisocial behavior in firesetting and nonfiresetting juvenile offenders. *J Psychopathol Behav* 24:177–193, 2002.
32. Forehand R, Wierson M, Frame CL, Kemptom T, Armistead L: Juvenile firesetting: a unique syndrome or an advanced level of antisocial behavior? *Behav Res Therapy* 29:125–128, 1991.
33. Kolko DJ, Kazdin AE: Motives of child firesetters: firesetting characteristics and psychological correlates. *J Child Psychol Psychiatry* 32:535–550, 1991.
34. Kolko DJ, Kazdin AE: Matchplay and firesetting in children: relationship to parent, marital, and family dysfunction. *J Clin Child Psychol* 19:229–238, 1990.
35. Macht LB, Mack JE: The firesetter syndrome. *Psychiatry* 31:277–288, 1968.
36. Stewart MA, Culver KW: Children who set fires: the clinical picture and a follow-up. *Br J Psychiatry* 140:357–363, 1982.
37. Becker K, Stuewig J, Herrera V, McCloskey L: A study of firesetting and animal cruelty in children: family influences and adolescent outcomes. *J Am Acad Child Adolesc Psychiatry* 43:905–912, 2004.
38. Sakheim GA, Vigdor MG, Gordon M, Helprin LM: A psychological profile of juvenile firesetters in residential treatment. *Child Welfare* 64:453–476, 1985.
39. Fineman KR: A model for the qualitative analysis of child and adult fire deviant behavior. *Am J Forensic Psychol* 13:31–61, 1995.
40. Doherty J: Parent and community fire education: integrating awareness in public education programs. In: Kolko DJ (ed): *Handbook on Firesetting in Children and Youth.* San Diego, CA, Academic Press, 283–303, 2002.
41. Schwartzman P, Stambaugh H, Kimball J: *Arson and Juveniles: Responding to the Violence.* Emmitsburg, MD: United States Fire Administration, 1998.
42. Elliott EJ: Juvenile justice diversion and intervention. In Kolko DJ (ed): *Handbook on Firesetting in Children and Youth.* San Diego, CA, Academic Press, 383–394, 2002.
43. Bailey S, Smith C, Dolan M: The social background and nature of "children" who perpetrate violent crimes: a UK perspective. *J Community Psychol* 29:305–317, 2001.
44. Heath GA, Hardesty VA, Goldfine PE, Walker AM: Diagnosis and childhood firesetting. *J Clin Psychol* 41:571–575, 1985.
45. Sakheim GA, Osborn E: A psychological profile of juvenile firesetters in residential treatment: a replication study. *Child Welfare* 65:495–503, 1986.
46. Hanson M, Mackay-Soroka S, Staley S, Poulton L: Delinquent firesetters: a comparative study of delinquency and firesetting histories. *Can J Psychiatry* 39:230–232, 1994.
47. Ritvo E, Shanok SS, Lewis DO: Firesetting and nonfiresetting delinquents: a comparison of neuropsychiatric, psychoeducational, experiential, and behavior characteristics. *Child Psychiatry Hum Dev.* 13:259–267, 1983.
48. Lambie I, Ioane J, Randell I, and Seymour F. Offending behaviors of child and adolescent firesetters over a 10-year follow-up. *J Child Psychol Psychiatry* 54(12), 1295–1307, 2013.
49. Moore JM Jr, Thompson-Pope SK, Whited RM: MMPI—a profile of adolescent boys with a history of firesetting. *J Pers Assess* 67:116–126, 1996.
50. Kolko DJ: Research studies on the problem. In: Kolko DJ (ed): *Handbook on Firesetting in Children and Youth.* San Diego, CA, Academic Press, 33–52, 2002.
51. Stewart LA: Profile of female firesetters: implications for treatment. *Br J Psychiatry* 163:248–256, 1993.
52. Repo E, Virkkunen M: Young arsonists: history of conduct disorder, psychiatric diagnoses and criminal recidivism. *J Forens Psychiatry* 8:311–320, 1997.
53. Sakheim GA, Osborn E: *Firesetting Child: Risk, Assessment, and Treatment.* Washington, DC, Child Welfare League of America, 1994.
54. Wooden WS, Berkey ML: *Children and Arson.* New York, Plenum Press, 1984.
55. Gaynor J, Hatcher C: *The Psychology of Child Firesetting: Detection and Intervention.* New York, Brunnel/Mazel, 1987.
56. Cole R, Grolnick W, Laurenitis L, McAndrews M, Matkowski K, Schwartzman P: *Children and Fire: Rochester Fire-Related Youth Project Progress Report.* Rochester, NY: University of Rochester, 1986.
57. Porth D: *Juvenile Firesetting: A Four Year Perspective.* Portland, OR: SOS Fire Youth Intervention Program, 1997.
58. Lyons JS, McClelland G, Jordan N: Fire setting behavior in a child welfare system: Prevalence, characteristics and co-occurring needs. *J Child Fam Stud* 19(6):720–727, 2010.
59. Root C, Mackay S, Henderson J, Del Bove G, Warling D: The link between maltreatment and juvenile fire setting: correlates and underlying mechanisms. *Child Abuse Neg* 32(2):161–176, 2008.
60. Slavkin ML: Enuresis, firesetting, and cruelty to animals: does the ego triad show predictive validity? *Adolescence* 36:461–466, 2001.
61. Stadolnik RF: *Drawn to the Flame: Assessment and Treatment of Juvenile Firesetting Behavior.* Sarasota, FL, Professional Resource Press, 2000.
62. American Psychiatric Association: *Diagnostic and Statistical Manual of Mental Disorders.* 4th ed. Arlington, VA, American Psychiatric Association, 2000.
63. Del Bove G, Mackay S. An empirically derived classification system for juvenile firesetters. *Crim Justice Behav* 38:796–817, 2011.
64. Stadolnik R. *FRAT-Y: Firesetting Risk Assessment Tool for Youth, Professional Manual.* Norwood, MA, FirePsych, Inc., 2010.
65. Kolko DJ, Nishi-Strattner L, Wilcox DK, Kopet T: Clinical assessment of juvenile firesetters and their families: tools and tips. In: Kolko DJ (ed): *Handbook on Firesetting in Children and Youth.* San Diego, CA, Academic Press, 177–212, 2002.
66. DiMillo J: Screening and triage tools. In Kolko DJ (ed): *Handbook on Firesetting in Children and Youth.* San Diego, CA, Academic Press, 141–159, 2002.
67. Wilcox DK, Kolko DJ: Assessing recent firesetting behavior and taking a firesetting history. In Kolko DJ (ed): *Handbook on Firesetting in Children and Youth.* San Diego, CA, Academic Press, 161–175, 2002.
68. Bic Corporation: *Play safe! Be safe! Teacher's Manual and Resource Book for Children's Fire Safety Education Program, Ages 3–5.* Milford, CT, Author, 1994.
69. Slavkin ML, Fineman K: What every professional who works with adolescents should know about firesetters. *Adolescence* 35:759–774, 2000.
70. Kolko DJ: Child, parent, and family treatment: cognitive-behavioral interventions. In Kolko DJ (ed): *Handbook on Firesetting in Children and Youth.* San Diego, CA, Academic Press, 305–336, 2002.
71. Dishion TJ, McMahon RJ: Parental monitoring and the prevention of child adolescent problem behavior: a conceptual and empirical formulation. *Clin Child Fam Psychol Rev* 1:61–75, 1998.
72. Nishi-Strattner L: Are first-time firesetters different from repeat firesetters? *Hot Issues.* Winter:1–4, 2005.
73. Bumpass ER, Brix RJ, Preston D: A community-based program for juvenile firesetters. *Hosp Commun Psychiatry* 36:529–533, 1985.
74. Massachusetts Coalition for Juvenile Firesetter Intervention Programs. *Expanding the Circles of Care.* Fall River, MA, Author, 2002.
75. Kolko DJ: ed. *Handbook on Firesetting in Children and Youth.* San Diego, CA, Academic Press, 2002.
76. MacKay S, Hanson M, Dickens S, Henderson J: *Fire Involvement Interview (FII): TAPP-C.* Toronto, Arson Prevention Program for Children, 1999.
77. MacKay S, Henderson J, Root C, Warling D, Gilbert KB, Johnstone J: *TAPP-C: Clinician's Manual for Preventing and Treating Juvenile Fire Involvement, Version 1.0.* Toronto, Centre for Addiction and Mental Health, 2004.
78. Henderson JL, MacKay S, Peterson-Badali M: Closing the research-practice gap: factors affecting adoption and implementation of a children's mental health program. *J Clin Child Adolesc Psychol* 35:2–12, 2006.
79. Hanson M, MacKay S, Atkinson L, Staley S, Pignatiello A: Firesetting during the preschool period—assessment and intervention issues. *Can J Psychiatry* 40:299–303, 1995.
80. Klietz SJ, Borduin CM, Schaeffer CM: Cost-benefit analysis of multisystemic therapy with serious and violent juvenile offenders. *J Fam Psychol* 24(5):657–666, 2010.
81. Dodge KA, Dishion TJ, Lansford JE: Deviant peer influences in intervention and public policy for youth. *Social Policy Report* XX:1–19, 2006.
82. Pollinger J, Samuels L, Stadolnik R: A comparative study of the behavioral, personality, and fire history characteristics of residential and outpatient adolescents (ages 12–17) with firesetting behaviors. *Adolescence* 40:345–353, 2005.
83. Richardson JP: Secure residential treatment for adolescent firesetters. In Kolko DJ (ed): *Handbook on Firesetting in Children and Youth.* San Diego, CA, Academic Press, 353–381, 2002.
84. Kolko DJ: Multicomponent parental treatment of firesetting in a six-year-old boy. *J Behav Ther Exp Psychiatry* 56:628–630, 1983.
85. Padgett LS, Strickland D, Coles CD: Case study: using a virtual reality computer game to teach fire safety skills to children diagnosed with fetal alcohol syndrome. *J Pediatr Psychol* 31:65–70, 2006.
86. Wolff R: Satiation in the treatment of inappropriate fire setting. *J Behav Ther Exp Psychiatry* 15:337–340, 1984.
87. Franklin GA, Pucci PS, Arbabi S, Brandt M, Wahl WL, Taheri PA: Decreased juvenile arson and firesetting recidivism after implementation of a multidisciplinary prevention program. *J Trauma* 53:260–266, 2002.
88. Kolko DJ, Swenson CC: *Assessing and Treating Physically Abused Children and Their Families.* Thousand Oaks, CA, Sage Publications, 2002.
89. Pinsonneault IL, Richardson JP Jr, Pinsonneault J. Three models of educational interventions for child and adolescent firesetters. In Kolko DJ (ed): *Handbook on Firesetting in Children and Youth.* San Diego, CA, Academic Press, 261–282, 2002.
90. Maciak BJ, Moore MT, Leviton LC, Guinan ME: Preventing Halloween arson in an urban setting: a model for multisectoral planning and community participation. *Health Educ Behav* 25:194–211, 1998.

5.2 DEVELOPMENTAL DISORDERS

CHAPTER 5.2.1 ■ AUTISM SPECTRUM DISORDER

FRED R. VOLKMAR, GERRIT I. VAN SCHALKWYK, AND BRENT VAN DER WYK

DEFINITION

In Kanner's original (1) description of autism he felt that two features were essential for the diagnosis: autism and "resistance to change"—the latter category including literal troubles with change but also an "insistence on sameness" and the stereotyped mannerism and behaviors so frequently associated with autism in children. Various attempts were made to provide more formal guidelines and to clarify the early confusions, for example, about whether autism was a form of schizophrenia. By 1980, a sufficient body of work had accumulated to suggest that autism was a disorder in its own right and it was included as an official diagnosis for the first time in the ground-breaking Diagnostic and Statisical Manual (DSM)-III (2). That definition focused more on "infantile" autism, in so far as it did not really encompass an understanding of developmental change. Subsequent editions of DSM attempted to cope with this problem. DSM-III coined a new term "pervasive developmental disorder" for the class of conditions to which autism was assigned. The DSM-IV approach provided considerable flexibility in terms of coverage of the broad range of autism (over both age and developmental level) and also converged with the International Classification of Diseases (ICD)-10 approach (3). This convergence facilitated research and clinical work. In both DSM-IV and ICD-10 other disorders were recognized within the broader pervasive developmental disorder (PDD) category, for example, Asperger disorder and a subthreshold concept for individuals with some but not all features of autism or other formal diagnosis (4). These two approaches continued for nearly two decades. However, major changes were undertaken in DSM-5.

A number of overall changes were made in DSM-5, for example, relative to multiaxial classification and a move toward modifiers and specifications of severity as well as an emphasis on the use of existing diagnostic instruments to develop criteria (see Chapter 4.1). The term pervasive developmental disorder (as the overall term for the class of disorders) was replaced by autism spectrum disorder. A new disorder (social communication disorder [SCD]) was added. Asperger's, Rett's and other types recognized in DSM-IV were not identified. In contrast to the traditional grouping (as in DSM-IV) of criteria into social, communication, and behavioral problems (such as resistance to change), the social communication criteria were reduced in number and placed in a single category, with the requirement that all features should be met for the diagnosis to be made. The restricted and repetitive behaviors domain criteria were reduced in number (although a new feature related to hypo/hypersensitivity was added) and for this group two of the four diagnostic features were required. The marked change in approach from DSM-IV was based on analysis of a large body of standardized data (5). The previous social and communication category is now monothetic (i.e., all features must be met) while the restricted behavior category remains polythetic, requiring evidence of symptoms in two of four symptom groupings; the respective and restricted behavior domain also includes a new (to DSM) symptom cluster reflecting sensory difficulties. A specification that symptoms must be present in early development enacted a universal onset criterion, with the caveat that problems may not manifest until social demands exceed limited capacities. Other innovations of the DSM-5 approach included the specification of modifiers (e.g., with catatonia) and levels of severity. A new diagnostic category, SCD, defined by difficulties in the social use of language was introduced.

Despite some clear advances (e.g., the change of name to autism spectrum disorder), other aspects of the DSM-5 approach have proven controversial (4). The rationale for the new SCD remains unclear with a miniscule body of supporting research (6). Probably most importantly, as the draft DSM-5 criteria began to appear, a series of studies (7) have fairly consistently shown problems with the DSM-5 approach particularly relative to higher cognitively functioning individuals (8) and very young children (9). This result has potentially serious implications for service eligibility and as a result, a final decision was made to add the criterion to the new DSM-5 approach that allows individuals with previously well-established diagnoses (under DSM-IV and ICD-10) to keep them. Effectively, this creates two approaches—continuing the old one and adding a new one that appears to be more restricted for newly diagnosed cases. In addition, the implications of the Research Domain Criteria (R-DOC) approach and ICD-11 remain unclear (see Chapter 4.7). The various approaches to diagnosis of autism/autism spectrum disorder (ASD) are summarized in Table 5.2.1.1.

HISTORY

Following Kraepelin's description of dementia praecox in adolescents, the concept was extended to children and the terms childhood schizophrenia and/or childhood psychosis became blanket terms for all apparent severe psychiatric disturbance in children (apart from what was then recognized as intellectual disability) (see Chapter 5.2.2). These early assumptions of continuity with adult-onset psychotic disorder began to describe unique constellations of difficulty of childhood onset. Kanner's classic description of the syndrome of early infantile autism exemplifies this approach (1). His presentation of 11 cases of "inborn disturbance of affective contact" was a landmark in the field. He emphasized two core features for diagnosis: (1) autism (a marked lack of interest in others) and (2) insistence on sameness/resistance to change (this included both literal insistence on rigid adherence to routines and difficulties with change as well as the motor mannerisms and stereotyped behaviors). Kanner believed these problems were of early onset—from the beginning of life or in the first year or two of life. Kanner noted many of the clinical features that continue to be recognized in classic autism, for example, mutism or echolalia, marked communication problems, and so forth. One year after Kanner's description Hans Asperger (10) also reported a small series of cases—all boys who had marked social difficulties along with unusual circumscribed interests but relatively good verbal abilities. Asperger disorder was officially recognized in DSM-IV and ICD-10 for the first time and work on it increased dramatically (11) with various lines of research suggesting the validity of this concept as distinct from autism (12). In important ways, the

TABLE 5.2.1.1

ICD-10 CRITERIA FOR CHILDHOOD AUTISM (F84.0)

A. Abnormal or impaired development is evident before the age of 3 years in at least one of the following areas:
   1. Receptive or expressive language as used in social communication
   2. The development of selective social attachments or of reciprocal social interaction; functional or symbolic play

B. A total of at least six symptoms from (1), (2), and (3) must be present, with at least two from (1) and at least one from each of (2) and (3).
   1. Qualitative impairments in social interaction, as manifested by at least two of the following areas:
      a. Failure adequately to use eye-to-eye gaze/facial expression, body postures, and gestures to regulate social interaction
      b. Failure to develop (in a manner appropriate to mental age, and despite ample opportunities) peer relationships that involve a mutual sharing of interests, activities, and emotions
      c. Lack of socioemotional reciprocity as shown by an impaired or deviant response to other people's emotions; or lack of modulation of behavior according to social context; or a weak integration of social, emotional, and communicative behaviors
      d. Lack of spontaneous seeking to share enjoyment, interests, or achievements with other people (e.g., a lack of showing, bringing, or pointing out to other people objects of interest to the individual)
   2. Qualitative abnormalities in communication, as manifested by at least one of the following areas:
      a. Delay in, or total lack of, development of spoken language that is not accompanied by an attempt to compensate through the use of gestures or mime as an alternative mode of communication (often preceded by a lack of communicative babbling)
      b. Relative failure to initiate or sustain conversational interchange (at whatever level of language skill is present), in which there is reciprocal responsiveness to the communications of the other person
      c. Stereotyped and repetitive use of language or idiosyncratic use of words or phrases
      d. Lack of varied spontaneous make-believe play or (when young) social imitative play
   3. Restricted, repetitive, and stereotyped patterns of behavior, interests, and activities, as manifested by at least one of the following:
      a. An encompassing preoccupation with one or more stereotyped and restricted patterns of interest that are abnormal in content or focus; or one or more interests that are abnormal in their intensity and circumscribed nature, though not in their content or focus
      b. Apparently compulsive adherence to specific, nonfunctional routines or rituals
      c. Stereotyped and repetitive motor mannerisms that involve either hand or finger snapping, or twisting or complex whole-body movements
      d. Preoccupations with part objects or nonfunctional elements of play materials (such as their odor, the feel of their surface, or the noise or vibration they generate)

C. The clinical picture is not attributable to the other varieties of pervasive developmental disorders; specific development disorder of receptive language (F80.2) with secondary socioemotional problems, reactive attachment disorder (F94.1), or disinhibited attachment disorder (F94.2); intellectual disability (F70–F72) with some associated emotional or behavioral disorders; schizophrenia (F20) of unusually early onset; and Rett syndrome (F84.12).

issues of making discriminations among various forms of social disability remain an open topic for research, particularly given the genetic work suggesting involvement of a number of genes and a growing awareness of the potentially broader spectrum of heritable social vulnerabilities (Table 5.2.1.2).

EPIDEMIOLOGY

It is now the case that hundreds of studies of the epidemiology of ASD/autism have been completed around the world—as summarized elsewhere (Table 5.2.1.3) (13). Several issues complicate the interrelation of results obtained and comparisons across studies. These include differences in diagnosis approach (e.g., school vs. clinical data), methods of ascertainment, potential problems of undersamplings relative to specific populations, and so forth. The problem of diagnostic substitution is significant (14), for example, in the United States in particular a single label is typically used for identifying students for service eligibility and, as awareness of autism has increased, schools and parents may be more likely to use this label for service eligibility thus inflating estimates compared if such data, rather than direct child assessment, are used to establish "caseness." Conversely there are also data suggesting that in some populations, for example, with impoverished students in inner cities, underdiagnosis may be common (15). Overall, however, it appears that for ASD an estimate of 6.6 children per 1,000 is reasonable (13). What is often assumed to be a real secular increase over time most likely reflects changes in diagnostic concepts, increased awareness of the range of ASD, and availability of services. It does appear that boys are three to four times more likely to have ASD than girls, although females can have subtler social difficulties (16).

ETIOLOGY

In the years following Kanner's initial description considerable debate centered on the pathogenesis of autism. Kanner's observation of high levels of occupational success in parents led some to assume a role of psychological factors in the etiology of the condition. Additional complexity arose given the early confusion of autism with childhood schizophrenia (17). During the 1970s it became clear that autism was a distinct disorder in its own right. Longitudinal studies suggested a high risk for onset of epilepsy particularly in adolescence (18) as well as a very strong role of genetic factors given the higher concordance of autism in identical, as compared to same-sex fraternal twins (19). By 1980, when infantile autism was first recognized as an official diagnosis (2) considerable evidence suggested that it was a highly genetic and strongly brain-based disorder.

In the decades subsequent to its official recognition, research on ASD had expanded dramatically. Much work has centered on understanding the neurobiologic basis of the disorder as well as potential genetic contributions; increasing efforts have been made to understand the core "autism" aspect, that is, the marked social learning problems that characterize autism. Different approaches have been used to understand the social brain in autism.

In 1990, Brothers (20) published a seminal article arguing that a small set of regions comprised the "social brain" dedicated to processing socially relevant information about

TABLE 5.2.1.2

EVOLUTION OF DIAGNOSITC CONCEPTS

Source/Term	Summary	Comment/Critique
DeSanctis (1906) Dementia praecox	Childhood schizophrenia, rapid extension of Kraepelin's original concept	Childhood psychosis became a blanket term; in reality, schizophrenia onset before adolescence is rare
Heller (1906) Dementia infantilis	Late-onset autism with marked regression in previously normal child	Recognized in DSM-IV and ICD-10 as childhood disintegrative disorder
Kanner (1943) Early infantile autism	The classic description of autism. "Autism" and "resistance to change" cardinal features	Concept has evolved over time. Early work began to show strong brain and genetic basis and need for structured treatment
Asperger (1944) Autistic psychopathy/autistic personality disorder	Marked social difficulties and motor problems but good verbal skills, marked circumscribed interests	Included in DSM-IV and ICD-10 but definition controversial, not included in DSM-5, often associated with unusual IQ profiles (better verbal than nonverbal skills)
DSM-III (1980) Infantile autism development	First official recognition, included in new class of disorder "pervasive developmental disorders"	Definition more appropriate to younger and more impaired case
DSM-III-R (1987) Autistic disorder	More developmentally oriented definition, polythetic criteria grouped in three categories	Definition probably overly broad, attempt to have developmental orientation a plus
DSM-IV/ICD-10 (1994/1993) Autistic disorder	Definition finalized in large field trial that brought convergence of DSM and ICD definitions, included another disorder such as Asperger's	Inclusion of new categories somewhat controversial Two decades of diagnostic stability and consistency of the two major definitions advanced research, polythetic with continued use of three categories of disturbance, many (<2,000) combinations of criteria could produce diagnosis, social items more heavily weighed
DSM-5 (2014) Autism spectrum disorder	Better term for condition, based on data from structured diagnostic instruments	Limited field trial data, definition more focused on "classic" cases with higher cognitive functioning individuals and very young less likely to get label. Social communication criteria (all must be met) and at least 2 of 4 resistance to change criteria. Potential for specification of severity and use of some modifiers, for example, autism with catatonia

conspecifics (21). These regions included the amygdala, the orbitofrontal cortex, and the ventral and lateral temporal cortex (see Table 5.2.1.4). The theory was supported by evidence from nonhuman primate electrophysiology and human neuropsychology (20). This theory was highly influential in guiding early human studies in the emerging discipline of neuroimaging. Paralleling the growth of neuroimaging, there was an increasing appreciation of ASD as both a brain disorder and as a disorder of social cognition (22). Thus, it was natural that many early neuroimaging studies in ASD focused on the neural correlates of social cognition (23–25). Indeed, although ASD research has broadened substantially, the study of the neural correlates of social function continues to be the dominant topic and has centered on several areas.

Face processing has high face validity in tapping into the core social cognition deficits associated with autism (26) and can readily be studied using different approaches. Face processing as a developmental phenomenon in normative development has been extensively studied and has become one of the best studied areas in the cognitive neuroscience of ASD. Neuroimaging approaches rely heavily on the *method of difference, that is, a contrast must be made relative to some* control process to serve as the contrast. This question is a key component of study design and often a source of methodologic variability between

TABLE 5.2.1.3

SELECTED EPIDEMIOLOGIC STUDIES OF AUTISM

Study	Location	Diagnostic Criteria	Prevalence/10,000	Gender Ratio (M:F)
Lotter (1966)	UK	Rating scale	4.1	2.6
Bohman et al. (1983)	Sweden	Rutter criteria	5.6	1.6
Ritvo et al. (1989)	US	DSM-III	2.47	3.73
Gillberg et al. (1991)	Sweden	DSM-III-R	9.5	2.7
Baird et al. (2000)	UK	ICD-10	30.8	15.7
Chakrabarti and Fombonne (2005)	UK	ICD-10 DSM-IV	22.0	3.8
Fombonne et al. (2006)	Canada	DSM-IV	5.7	21.6
Parner et al. (2011)	Australia	DSM-IV/TR	4.4	39.3
Isakesn et al. (2011)	Norway	ICD-10 + ADI + ADOS	3.2	14
Kcocovscka et al. (2012)	Faroe Island	ICD-10 + DSM-IV	2	21
Parner et al. (2012)	Denmark	ICD-8, 9, 10	4.4	18.65

Data adapted from Hill AP, Zuckerman KE, Fombonne E: Epidemiology of autism spectrum disorders. In: Volkmar F, Rogers S, Paul R, Pelphery K (eds): *Handbook of Autism and Developmental Disorders*, Vol 1. 3rd ed. Hoboken, NJ, John Wiley & Sons, Inc., 63–66, 2005.

TABLE 5.2.1.4

BRAIN REGIONS POTENTIALLY INVOLVED IN AUTISM

Neural System	Areas	Comment/Function
Social perception system		Evolutionarily conserved and shared with other primates, refers to the initial stages in social information processing
	Superior temporal sulcus (STS)	Decoding of nonverbal social signals such as gaze direction and facial expression
	The fusiform gyrus (FFG)	Face processing
	Extrastriate body area (EBA) in lateral occipitotemporal cortex	Visual perception and recognition of the human body
	The amygdala and limbic system	Perception of emotional states and salient emotional experiences
	The orbitofrontal cortex (OFC) and ventrolateral prefrontal cortex (VLPFC)	Social reward and reinforcement
Mirror neuron system	The inferior frontal gyrus and the inferior parietal lobe (IPL)	An evolutionarily conserved system, plays an important role in action perception, understanding, and prediction
The mental state reasoning system		Probably unique to humans
	The medial prefrontal cortex (MPFC) and temporoparietal junction (TPJ)	Responsible for reasoning about others' thoughts

studies and labs. For example, some studies consider face processing relative to the processing of nonface stimuli such as complex objects or scrambled faces. One early study that used a simple contrast between faces and objects found hypoactivation in the fusiform gyrus in individuals with ASD relative to typical controls (25); this area is thought to be a key component of the face-processing network in typically developing individuals (27). These results supported the idea that social cognition problems in ASD may be due to poor activation of this key region. This finding has been generally confirmed by further work (for a review, see (28)), but the dysfunction may not reflect a general processing deficit, rather some combination of task complexity and attention (29). Table 5.2.1.4 summarizes some of the regions of interest relative to the social brain in autism.

Other studies considered subtler aspects of face processing and processing of affective dimensions relative to nonaffective dimensions, operationalized as a contrast between emotional and neutral faces. An early finding along these lines identified lower activation in the limbic areas (23) in support of an amygdala theory of ASD (30). However, a finding of amygdala hypoactivation is not as consistently replicated in face-processing studies as other effects (28).

Other approaches have also been employed, using electroencephalogram EEG (31) as well as eye tracking (32). Differences in processing both faces and dynamic faces have been noted. Individuals with ASD also show slower event-related face processing (31). Similarly, differences in dynamic face processing using eye tracking have been observed with the earliest studies highlighting a tendency to focus on the lower versus upper part of the face (32). Thus, differences in brain activation may not be due to inherent processing differences but instead due to differences in stimulus intake (see Fig. 5.2.1.1) (33). Subsequent work has made it clear that these issues are complex but generally speaking there does appear to be important differences in the ways faces are processed in autism (34,35). Similar findings arise with respect to perception of biologic motion (36), affect perception, and so forth. This work has important limitations given variations in methods, samples, etc. but does suggest important areas for future work. The results have already been extended to use in high-risk samples (i.e., infant siblings) with interesting differences observed as early as 6 months (37).

Genetic studies of ASD have similarly increased dramatically—in scope, sophistication and complexity. A range of methods has been used since the earliest studies of twins suggested high heritability of the condition (38). Several findings are of note. Although in the past it was suggested that autism was associated with a host of medical conditions, this literature rested largely on case reports (where positive associations are much more likely to be published). It became clear that, apart from epilepsy, the strongest association of autism with medical conditions related to two strong genetic conditions—fragile X and tuberous sclerosis (39).

It has become increasingly clear that genetic influences are complex but important in the pathogenesis of autism. One interesting development has been the recognition that the "broader spectrum" of social vulnerability (NOT qualifying for an ASD diagnosis as such) may reflect the operation of some of these factors. There clearly is the potential impact of some environmental factor or factors in this complex process (40), although to date it is the genetic factors that appear to be most robustly elucidated. Many genes potentially involved have now been identified and these often appear to have an important role in the central nervous system. In perhaps 10% of cases, some associated genetic syndrome associated with autism can be identified, that is, in the majority of cases this is not the case. An interesting related issue is the frequent association of autism with other conditions, for example, anxiety problems, attention difficulties, that themselves may have strong genetic components.

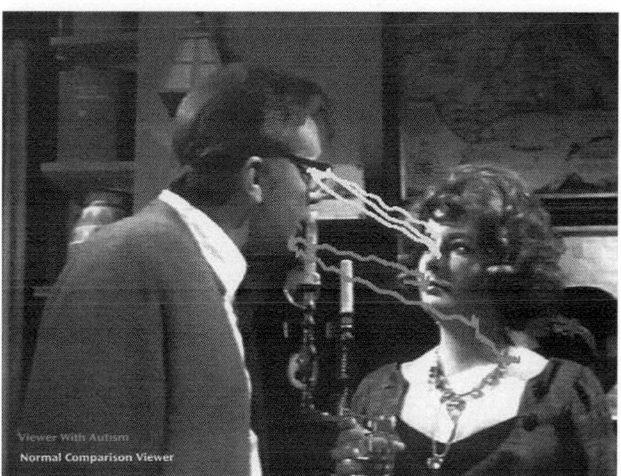

FIGURE 5.2.1.1. Differences in eye tracking in an individual with high functioning autism (*bottom line*) and a typically developing person (*top line*) watching an intensely social scene; the individual with autism focuses on the mouth losing much of the social-affective information conveyed in the top part of the face.

Social Features

Kanner emphasized the centrality of "autism" as one of the two defining features of the condition in his initial description of the syndrome; subsequent research has consistently shown him to be correct, in that the social difficulties observed appear to be a (if not the) hallmark of the condition (41,42). The social problems are not simply due to cognitive disability, and if anything they probably lead to the latter (43). Social difficulties can be most profound in the youngest individuals but, over time, may progress to the point where the child passively accepts interaction or develops a one-sided and eccentric interactive style (44). Social and adaptive skills are among the more powerful predictors of ultimate outcome (45). Even for individuals with "optimal outcome," some social eccentricity may remain (46).

Communicative Features

In the past a majority of individuals were mute or had very limited communicative speech but with earlier and more intensive intervention, this appears to be changing (47). It is, however, common for parents to become concerned because of the delayed development of speech (48). Communicative difficulties are a central aspect of the condition. For the individual who does talk, speech is often remarkable in various respects. The child may repeat sentences or phrases (echolalia) either one just heard or remembers from the past; this may be functional in some sense and also reflects the unusual "gestalt" learning style typical of ASD. Problems with pronoun use are frequent (49). Deficits in the development of expressive language are one of the more frequent sources of initial concern for parents of children later diagnosed with autism. Often prosody is unusual (monotonic or poorly inflected with a loud voice volume) and idiosyncratic language may be observed (and is often only understood by parents or family members). Even for the most able individual, problems with pragmatic language are frequent, for example, in understanding figurative language, humor, sarcasm, irony, and so forth (49).

Behavioral Features

In addition to emphasizing social problems, Kanner also emphasized the presence of unusual difficulties with change—"insistence on sameness"—in the cases he described. Often the contrast between a child's lack of social interest stands in stark contrast to his sensitivity to environmental change or interest in aspects of the nonsocial world, for example, early interest in fans, letters, iconic images. Occasionally the child is attached to an unusual object (differing from transitional objects, in that this is usually hard rather than soft and the category of object is more important than the specific object). Although parents are sometimes worried that children may be deaf, the child may actually respond with great alarm to some sounds. Younger children often are more interested in the taste, texture, and smell of objects than their function. Unusual sensory interests often antedate the development of more "classic" stereotyped mannerisms.

Cognitive Functioning

It took investigators and clinicians many years to realize that autism/ASD could be, and at that point usually was, associated with intellectual deficiency. The child's ability to cooperate with some parts of IQ tests (e.g., puzzles) was in stark contrast to the child's verbal ability but these deficits were "written off" as due to poor testability or negativism. It gradually became clear that unusual cognitive profiles are common in individuals with social learning problems and are powerful predictors of outcome. Scatter on cognitive testing is common often in children with more classic autism exhibiting better nonverbal than verbal abilities. The reverse profile may be seen in individuals with Asperger disorder (11).

In a minority of cases, individuals may exhibit remarkable abilities, for example, in drawing, calculating dates, or memory. These "savant skills" sometimes stand in stark contrast to the individual's overall ability and may offer insight into unusual approaches to solving problems (50). Sometimes these skills diminish with age, although not always. Typically one skill is exhibited. Similarly in Asperger's, intense special interests are usual and often interfere with the individual's learning and family functioning although, on occasion, these can be turned into potentially valuable vocational skills (51); unfortunately, they can sometimes lead to legal issues (52).

ONSET

Kanner initially thought that autism was congenital and while this seems often to be true, it is the case that in a small number of cases (perhaps 1 in 5) parents will report a loss of skills. In the majority of cases, warning signs of autism are evidence in the first year of life (see Table 5.2.1.5) and these warning signs are used in screening for the condition (53). Early concerns may have to do with the concern that the child is deaf or that speech is delayed; sometimes, unusual interests or preoccupations may be resorted.

The issue of "regressive" autism is a complex one. Sometimes parents report regression but also report earlier delayed milestones or sometimes it is less a regression than a failure to progress (54). However, in a small number of cases there is a clear, marked, and dramatic regression with loss of words, deterioration of social skills, and loss of adaptive skills. DSM-IV and ICD-10 included the concept of childhood disintegrative disorder to accent for these cases which, unfortunately, appear to have a much worse prognosis (55).

PHYSICAL CHARACTERISTICS, PATHOLOGY, AND LABORATORY EXAMINATION

Kanner's initial report noted the absence of obvious physical dysmorphology. Subsequently, autism has been noted to be associated with several genetic conditions—notably, fragile X and tuberous sclerosis; and physical signs may be associated with the condition in these cases (39). As noted previously, the risk for onset of epilepsy is markedly increased with peaks on onset early in life and again in adolescence (39). In some cases macrocephaly develops in toddlerhood (56). A small number of neuropathologic studies have been conducted that suggest issues in the organization of the cortex (57). As noted previously, a considerable body of work on brain mechanisms has now emerged from studies using EEG and functional magnetic resonance imaging (fMRI). Laboratory studies are guided by history and physical examination; the American College of Medical Genetics and Genomics periodically updates its recommendations for genetic studies (58).

DIFFERENTIAL DIAGNOSIS AND ASSESSMENT

Autism must be differentiated from intellectual deficiency, communication disorders, severe deprivation, and sensory impairment (particularly deafness). In intellectual deficiency without autism, social skills are usually on par with cognitive development. In the communication disorders (apart from the new "SCD"), social skills are generally well preserved, even

TABLE 5.2.1.5

SYMPTOMS OF AUTISM IN THE FIRST 3 YEARS OF LIFE

	0–12 Months	12–36 Months
Social	Limited ability to anticipate being picked up Low frequency of looking at people Limited interest in interactional games Limited affection toward familiar people Content to be left alone Limited range of facial expression	Abnormal eye contact Limited social referencing Limited interest in other children Limited social smile Low frequency of looking at people Limited sharing of affect/enjoyment
Play	Little interest in interactive games	Limited functional play No pretend play Limited motor imitation
Communication	Poor response to name (does not respond to call) Does not frequently look at objects held by others	Low frequency of verbal or nonverbal communication Failure to share interests (e.g., through pointing, sharing, giving, showing) Poor response to name Failure to respond to communicative gestures (pointing, giving, showing) Use of others' body as a tool (pulls hand to desired object without making eye contact, as if *hand* rather than person obtains object)
Restricted interests/ behaviors	Mouths objects excessively Does not like to be touched	Unusual sensory behaviors Hyper/hyposensitivity to sounds, texture, tastes, visual stimuli Hand or finger mannerisms Inappropriate use of objects Repetitive interest/play

Reprinted with permission from Volkmar F, Chawarska K, Klin A: Autism in infancy and early childhood. *Annu Rev Psychol* 56:315–336, 2005.

in the face of major language vulnerabilities. For individuals with Asperger disorder, the differential diagnosis may include personality problems and occasionally psychotic disorders are considered—the intense circumscribed interests and marked social impairments are usually indicative of Asperger's but in some cases differentiation can be difficult (11).

It is typical for individuals with autism to have problems in multiple areas of functioning, with areas of strength and weakness. It is important to understand these profiles as they may indicate approaches to treatment (using strengths to address weaknesses) (11). It is also important to keep in mind the broad range of syndrome expression. It is usual for intellectual testing to reveal significant scatter with social and language-based skills, lower than would be expected, given the child's nonverbal abilities (the opposite profile may be seen in Asperger's). It is often the case that various specialists are involved, for example, psychologists, speech pathologists, special and regular education teachers, occupational and physical therapists. A wide range of normative assessment instruments can be used to assess intellectual level, communicative skills, academic achievement, and other domains (59); given the unusual and often rigid patterns of learning in ASD assessment should address the issue of adaptive skills—that is, the child's capacity to generalize skills to "real-world" settings (59).

A number of screening instruments for preschool and school-age children (53), as well as diagnostic instruments (60), have been developed. Of the former, probably the most widely used is the M-Char (61). A number of good diagnostic instruments have been developed and include the Autism Diagnostic Interview-Revised (an interview for parents) (62) as well as the Autism Diagnostic Observation Schedule (ADOS) (63) (both instruments require relatively extensive training). The Childhood Autism Rating Scale—second edition (64) is frequently used in schools. It is important to realize that the diagnostic instruments presently available have, for the most part, focused on school-age children with borderline to mild intellectual disability, that is, their use may be more complex in older or younger or lower or higher cognitively functioning individuals.

Initial examination should include a physical and careful history with referral to neurology or genetics as indicated for additional assessment. Hearing and vision should be evaluated. As part of the examination of the child observation in both structured and unstructured settings is helpful. A number of rating scales and diagnostic instruments have been developed (60); these can be based on parent report and/or child assessment. It is important to keep in mind that the traditional rating scales and checklists often work best in children of school age with borderline to mild intellectual disability, that is, older individuals and the very young may present diagnostic challenges as do the more intellectually gifted and more intellectually impaired. Assessment procedures are summarized in Table 5.2.1.6.

The strongest associations of autism are with a handful of medical conditions. Probably the strongest connection is with epilepsy that develops in about 20% of cases of individuals with strictly diagnosed autism. Autism is also observed at higher than expected rates in connection with two strongly genetic conditions—fragile X syndrome and tuberous sclerosis. Brain size appears to be increased in toddlers with autism, although this difference becomes less pronounced over time. Medical assessment should include a careful medical and family history. Testing for fragile X and of hearing is typically indicated. More extensive genetic testing is indicated by physical examination or family history. Signs of possible seizures should prompt EEG and neurologic examination. Neuroimaging studies may be indicated by examination or history.

COURSE AND PROGNOSIS

As noted previously, parents are typically worried about their child's development in the first year of life—typical concerns centering on language delay or possible deafness. However, the first screening instruments (at present) only begin to be useful around 18 months so that delay in diagnosis is relatively common. In addition, some children seem to develop normally for a time and then lose skills. Sometimes children at ages 1 or 2 will exhibit the more typical social communication

TABLE 5.2.1.6

EVALUATION PROCEDURES: AUTISM AND PERVASIVE DEVELOPMENTAL DISORDERS

1. Historical information
   - Early development and characteristics of development
   - Age and nature of onset
   - Medical and family history
2. Developmental and psychological assessment
   - Intellectual level and profile of learning
   - Communicative assessment (receptive and expressive language skills, use of nonverbal communication, pragmatic use of language)
   - Adaptive behavior (ability to generalize skills to real-world settings)
   - Occupational/physical therapy assessments as appropriate
3. Psychiatric examination
   - Nature of social relatedness (eye contact, attachment behaviors, reciprocity, insight)
   - Behavioral features (stereotypy/self-stimulation, resistance to change, unusual sensitivities to the environment)
   - Language/communication difficulties (echolalia, presence of communicative speech, etc.)
   - Play skills (nonfunctional use of play materials, symbolic play, and imagination)
4. Medical evaluations
   - Search for associated medical conditions, genetic abnormalities, presence of seizures
   - With additional tests as needed
   - Hearing/vision test
   - Additional consultation (neurologic/pediatric/genetic) as indicated by history and current presentation (see reference 58 for current genetic testing recommendations)
   - Examination (e.g., EEG, CT/MRI scan, chromosome analysis)

Reprinted with permission from Volkmar FR, Lord C, Bailey A, Schultz RT, Klin A: Autism and pervasive developmental disorders. In: Martin A, Volkmar FR, Lewis M (eds): *Lewis's Child and Adolescent Psychiatry: A Comprehensive Textbook*. 4th ed. Philadelphia, PA, Wolters Kluwer, 391, 2007.

problems but not yet all the unusual behaviors (although sometimes exhibiting precursors to these behaviors, for example, staring at fans or fixating on some object more than on parents and family members). However, by age 3 the vast majority of children with ASD will exhibit the diagnosis (65) and often intervention has started even before that time due to language delay (66). Early diagnosis is increasingly common and schools are mandated to provide services after the age of 3.

Young children with autism may exhibit an aloof social style, although sometimes the more cognitively able are more passively accepting of social interaction or somewhat one sided and eccentric as they mature (44). Behavioral difficulties often increase during childhood and may further increase in adolescence before diminishing in young adulthood. Although the DSM-5 definition of ASD is somewhat restricting in the broader sense of the autistic spectrum, it is very clear that a tremendous range of features and symptoms are exhibited. See Box 5.2.1.1 for an illustrative case.

Over time, the prognosis of autism appears to have improved substantially. In the 1980s, about 90% of children with classic autism were functioning in the intellectually impaired range. At that time, only perhaps 50% of individuals with autism would ever speak. Perhaps two-thirds of cases were institutionalized as adults with only a small fraction living independently. As time has gone on, there appear to have been major changes in outcome, for example, perhaps only 20% or so now remain mute, many individuals are now functioning in the normal cognitive range and often are going to college, perhaps 30% or so (at least) are independent and self-sufficient as adults (67). Indeed some individuals become sufficiently capable that they "lose" their diagnosis (although often retaining some social vulnerability) (46). The change in outcome reflects several factors including, to some extent, changes in diagnostic practice but probably more importantly, providing of early and more effective intervention.

Associated clinical problems include the increased risk for epilepsy (often of adolescent onset) as well as several psychiatric problems. These include attention problems in middle childhood and, particularly in the more cognitively able, anxiety and depression in adolescence and young adulthood. There may be an increased risk for other problems as well.

BOX 5.2.1.1

CASE REPORT—AUTISTIC DISORDER

John was the second of two children born to middle-class parents after normal pregnancy, labor, and delivery. As an infant, John appeared undemanding and relatively placid; motor development proceeded appropriately, but language development was delayed. Although his parents indicated that they were first concerned about his development when he was 18 months of age and still not speaking, in retrospect they noted that, in comparison to their previous child, he had seemed relatively uninterested in social interaction and the social games of infancy. Stranger anxiety had never really developed, and John did not exhibit differential attachment behaviors toward his parents. Their pediatrician initially reassured John's parents that he was a "late talker," but they continued to be concerned. Although John seemed to respond to some unusual sounds, the pediatrician obtained a hearing test when John was 24 months old. Levels of hearing appeared adequate for development of speech, and John was referred for developmental evaluation. At 24 months, motor skills were age appropriate and John exhibited some nonverbal problem-solving skills close to age level. His language and social development, however, were severely delayed, and he was noted to be resistant to changes in routine and unusually sensitive to aspects of the inanimate environment. His play skills were quite limited and he used play materials in unusual and idiosyncratic ways. His older sister had a history of some learning difficulties, but the family history was otherwise negative. A comprehensive medical evaluation revealed a normal EEG and CT scan; genetic screening and chromosome analysis were normal as well.

John was enrolled in a special education program, where he gradually began to speak. His speech was characterized by echolalia, extreme literalness, a monotonic voice quality, and pronoun reversal. He rarely used language in interaction and remained quite isolated. By school age, John had developed some evidence of differential attachments to family members; he also had developed a number of self-stimulatory behaviors and engaged in occasional periods of head banging. Extreme sensitivity to change continued. Intelligence testing revealed marked scatter, with a full-scale IQ in the moderately retarded range. As an adolescent, John's behavioral functioning deteriorated, and he developed a seizure disorder. Now an adult, he lives in a group home and attends a sheltered workshop. He has a rather passive interactional style but exhibits occasional outbursts of aggression and self-abuse.

Comment: With earlier intervention, more children with autism are doing better. Unfortunately in this case, although the child developed speech, his overall outcome has not been as good as might have been hoped.

Adapted from Volkmar FR, Lord C, Klin A, Cook E: Autism and the pervasive developmental disorders. In: Lewis M (ed): *Lewis's Child and Adolescent Psychiatry: A Comprehensive Textbook*. Philadelphia, PA, Lippincott, 595, 2002.

Unfortunately, information on aging in autism is severely limited with most outcome studies stopping in early adulthood (68).

TREATMENTS

After autism was first identified, the only available treatments were psychotherapy—which had little impact. During the 1960s, the first school for children with autism was founded and during the 1970s, the first studies appeared suggesting that structured educational interventions were more effective than psychopathy (69). The passage of public law 94-142 mandated schools to provide educational service for all children and this mandate increased services and research. Over time, more treatments have been extensively researched so that many individual intervention procedures as well as some model programs and drug treatments can now be regarded as having some, or extensive, basis in evidence (70). Areas of intervention typically address the core diagnostic features of autism—deficits with social interaction and communication—but also include other issues including problems in learning (47). As a result of the growing body of work on assessment and intervention, practice guidelines have also now appeared (71,72).

Educational and Behavioral Treatments

Beginning in the 1970s, a number of research-based methods have been used to enhance effective learning. Behavioral techniques were among the first to be developed based on principles of learning derived from psychology and principles of learning theory. These techniques have a strong research basis (73) and have been used in a range of settings and for a range of problems. These also have been integrated into model treatment programs and serve as the basis for programs using applied behavior analysis (ABA) (73). Social skills are another area for support and a range of methods have been used to teach social skills (74)—ranging from use of peers to teach preschoolers, to social skills groups in children and adolescents. Peer-based approaches have, by far, the strongest base in the research literature and tend to revolve around integration of preschoolers and young school-age children in mainstream educational settings (75). Similarly, various approaches can be used to foster communication (in the broader sense) as well as spoken language (49). For children who don't speak, augmentative approaches (76) can be used to increase functional communicative abilities. For the more cognitively able and verbal individuals, work may center on social language use. Finally, it is important to note that organizational issues can be significantly helped with supportive technology—methods range from low-to-high tech. These can include simple things like visual schedule, timers, and so forth to organizational software and apps designed specifically to help individuals with ASD (77).

In addition to evidence-based intervention techniques several evidence-based model treatment programs have been developed. These share many similarities and some differences (70). Model programs for intervention fall into four general types. Probably the most widely known are behaviorally based/focused programs or ABA programs which employ principles from behavioral psychology to teach and can be very effective for younger and more impaired individuals; discrete trial teaching is one of the more frequently used methods in these programs (78). In contrast, more developmentally oriented programs (79) build on the child's interest using developmentally oriented and focused intervention. Pivotal response training (PRT) is a third approach that uses behavioral techniques within a more developmentally oriented framework (80). Eclectic approaches exist, such as a program used statewide in North Carolina (81). Autism-oriented curricula have also been developed, and many techniques and methods from model programs and empirically validated interventions are employed within public school settings (82). It is important to emphasize that in the United States, children with ASD are entitled to school programs beginning at age 3 years (and preschool services before that); this likely has contributed to the improved outcome that is now more frequently seen.

Pharmacologic Treatments

At present no specific drug treatments exist for the core social disability of autism (although efforts are underway to examine potential treatments). Effective drug treatments are available to help with the "irritability" often seen in inidividuals with ASD. In addition, a host of medications (and some behavioral techniques) can be used to treat attention difficulties, anxiety, and depression (83). It is important to be judicious in the use of drug treatments and avoid overmedication. It is important as well to keep in mind the special issues posed in each case, for example, abrupt behavioral deterioration associated with face slapping or head banging in a more cognitively impaired individual should prompt a search for any associated ear infection, erupting wisdom teeth, etc. (39). Similarly, it is important to realize that a bad educational program cannot be medicated. The clinician should be alert to any features that are unusual, for example, learning that a behavioral problem occurs only in one situation or context should prompt careful review. Finally, it is important to note that having behavioral data can greatly help monitor medication effects (as long as only the medication is being adjusted). Despite extensive research over the last two decades, there are no drug treatments that are broadly considered to be effective for the core symptoms of ASD. A large number of drugs have been studied in ASD, none to a greater extent than the digestive hormone secretin, which has consistently been found to be ineffective (84–86). Other agents have been successful in treating behavioral symptoms of ASD and associated psychiatric comorbidity. The drug risperidone has also been demonstrated to reduce symptoms of repetitive behaviors, but without impact on social deficits (87). Drug treatment is not routinely indicated in all individuals with ASD and should be considered only to target problematic symptoms. In this section we consider the evidence base for the use of medications to manage behavioral symptoms of ASD. In addition, we will explore treatments for comorbid symptom dimensions. For the purpose of this section, we will leave aside the issue of distinguishing between a true comorbidity and a set of symptoms that is in fact part of an underlying ASD. Rather we will employ a pragmatic lens toward understanding how the literature can inform the use of medication in individuals who may experience a range of symptoms in the context of an ASD diagnosis.

It is not standard care to use medication in all individuals with ASD. There is insufficient evidence to support the use of medication for core ASD symptoms. By contrast, early behavioral and educational interventions are safe and effective, and these should be emphasized in treatment planning.

Medication may be particularly useful for managing irritability and aggressive behavior, and in this regard, risperidone and aripiprazole are significantly superior to other agents in terms of the extent of their evidence base. Both are however associated with significant adverse metabolic effects, potentially limiting their use and necessitating careful monitoring. Similarly, pharmacotherapy for either inattention or repetitive behaviors is inconsistently helpful and with greater potential for adverse effects, and in each case a decision to initiate drug treatment should involve a thoughtful discussion with a patient and their family, setting appropriate expectations and highlighting relevant risks. A number of medications are prescribed in ASD which have not been subjected to rigorous study, despite evidence that medication tolerance and response rates may differ substantially in these individuals. This highlights both the need for a cautious clinical approach and ongoing research. As noted previously, a growing body of evidence-based treatments are available and it is incumbent on the practitioner to review this small but growing body of evidence (83,88).

AGGRESSION AND IRRITABILITY

Aggression is a problematic behavior with consequences for the individual and the family system. Aggressive behavior is more common in individuals with ASD (89), and an important predictor for engagement with crisis management services and medication utilization (90). A number of atypical antipsychotic medications have been studied for this intervention, including several randomized controlled trials.

Risperidone

Risperidone was the first antipsychotic medication shown to be effective for serious problem behaviors in ASD, including aggression, tantrums, and self-injurious behavior (91). In addition to behavioral improvements, measures of irritability were also substantially improved. Improvements were noted in around two-thirds of participants. These findings have since been replicated (92). In both these studies the dose was lower than typically used for the treatment of psychosis. However, in both studies, risperidone was associated with around 4 lb greater weight gain than placebo over an 8-week period. The potential benefits may not always outweigh the significant morbidity resulting from this degree of weight gain, and the choice to use this medication should include a clear discussion with the patient and family about this and other adverse effects.

Aripiprazole

More recent study supports the use of aripiprazole as a similarly effect agent for irritability and associated behaviors (93,94). The degree of weight gain appears to be less than for risperidone, but remains a significant adverse effect. Extrapyramidal symptoms, sedation and presyncope, were also reported as potentially significant side effects. Longer-term open-label study suggests that weight gain on aripiprazole may eventually plateau, but may be associated with metabolic abnormalities in a significant subset of patients (95).

Haloperidol

The earliest evidence from randomized controlled trials for behavioral symptoms of ASD supported the use of haloperidol (96). Although effective for a number of maladaptive symptoms, including stereotypies, labile and angry affect, its use was associated with significant side effects of sedation, and a 25% incidence of acute dystonia. Concern regarding the latter side effect is likely the primary reason why haloperidol is less often used for ongoing treatment of aggression in ASD. There is little recent study of haloperidol for this indication, despite concerns related to the metabolic side effects of newer agents.

Other Antipsychotics

There is very limited robust evidence supporting the use of other antipsychotics in ASD. One small randomized controlled trial of olanzapine did not demonstrate improvement on measures of irritability (97), and an open-label study of quetiapine found no clear evidence of benefit, with significant adverse effects (98). In clinical practice, it appears common for patients with ASD to be prescribed a broader range of antipsychotics. This is not an evidence-based approach. It should be noted that not all patients with ASD will respond to medication, or may experience only a partial improvement. This should serve as an impetus to explore potential exacerbating or sustaining factors for these symptoms and to explore additional behavioral treatments and does not justify the use of unproven treatments with significant potential for side effects.

Antiepileptic Drugs

Sodium valproate has been found to be an effective treatment for aggression in ASD in one randomized controlled trial (99). The effect size reported in this study was moderate. Side effects including weight gain were uncommon. Additional study could support the use of valproate as a more tolerable treatment option. Of the other antiepileptics, levetiracetam and lamotrigine have been studied in a randomized fashion and found to be ineffective (100,101). Owing to the high comorbidity between ASD and epilepsy, a broader range of antiepileptics have been used in ASD—however, this does not support their utility for managing behavioral symptoms, and they should not be considered a first line for this indication.

REPETITIVE BEHAVIOR

Selective Serotonin Reuptake Inhibitors (SSRIs)

Repetitive behavior, including self-injury, is a treatment-refractory symptom. An early trial was promising in reporting a moderate to large effect size for the use of fluoxetine in reducing repetitive behaviors in ASD (102). However, a subsequent study using citalopram was negative (103), and a recent Cochrane review found no evidence supporting the use of SSRIs in children with ASD (104).

Atypical Antipsychotics

Studies of risperidone and aripiprazole, in addition to detecting improvements in irritability and aggression, also found improvement in the symptom dimension of repetitive behavior. However, these effects were quantified using the Aberrant Behavior Checklist stereotypy subscale, whereas most of the SSRIs made use of the Children's Yale-Brown Obsessive Compulsive Scale. The aberrant behavior checklist stereotypy (ABC-S) captures a broad range of movements which may include purposeful behaviors (such as waving or shaking extremities) that may improve in the context of decreased irritability or anxiety—these behaviors are phenomenologically distinct from the more distinct subtype of stereotyped behavior which is considered a core dimension of ASD (105). It is therefore unclear whether atypical antipsychotics truly alter a core symptom dimension of ASD, or whether this apparent effect is attributable to improvements in irritability that are being captured by the instruments used in these studies.

Other Agents

A number of studies have examined the utility of tricyclic antidepressants; clomipramine in particular has demonstrated efficacy in a randomized controlled trial (106). In practice, its use is limited by concerns regarding side effects, including severe urinary retention and worsening aggression (107).

INATTENTION AND ATTENTION DEFICIT HYPERACTIVITY DISORDER (ADHD)

Stimulants

Comorbid difficulties with attention are common in ASD and there is much argument about whether or not this represents a true comorbid diagnosis or an expected symptom dimension in ASD. The answer to this question is less relevant in the context of evidence that supports the use of stimulants in individuals with ASD who have significant ADHD symptom. A randomized controlled trial of methylphenidate in children (N = 72) with ASD and ADHD symptoms found a response rate of 49% (108). This is lower than rates reported for children with ADHD who do not have ASD. In addition, effect sizes reported were smaller, and side effects were more frequent. Given these findings, stimulant treatment remains appropriate in some cases, but the threshold may be higher given the greater potential for adverse effects and lower likelihood for a positive outcome.

Other Agents

In clinical practice, the alpha-2 agonists guanfacine and clonidine are frequently used for both ADHD symptoms and irritability in children with ASD. Their efficacy is well established in larger trials of children without ASD, and there is a small body of evidence specific to ADHD symptoms in ASD (109). A trial of atomoxetine reported moderate improvement in ADHD in children with ASD compared to placebo, with adverse effects comparable to studies in non-ASD populations (110).

Social Deficits

There are no medications which have consistently been shown to be effective for the social deficits which characterize ASD. The neurohormone oxytocin remains a focus of study, with recent meta-analysis suggesting that current data are potentially promising, but that additional, rigorous research is required (111). A subsequent clinical trial reported that oxytocin enhanced orientation to social information in specific subgroups of individuals with ASD only (112).

A recent study of the glutamatergic agent memantine showed good tolerance but no statistically significant improvement in core ASD symptoms, including social domains.

ALTERNATIVE TREATMENTS

Nonestablished (i.e., alternative and complementary) treatments are frequently used by parents. These include a range of interventions from special diets or megavitamins to correction-presumed nutritional problems, chelation to rid the body of presumed toxic meals, to somatic treatments. By definition, evidence is either lacking or, less commonly, multiple negative studies are taken to strongly suggest the treatment doesn't work (the use of secretin and facilitated communication are examples of this). Complementary treatments are used along with evidence-based treatments and alterative treatment instead of such treatments. Probably between 50% and 75% of families will use such treatment at some point (113).

As a practical matter, it is important to elicit information from parents about all treatments they are using and engage in a supportive and understanding way with them regarding complementary interventions. When negative evidence is available it can be pointed out, and when treatments carry some risk (e.g., chelation) this should also be discussed. The risk of alternative treatments displacing evidenced-based interventions should also be highlighted. Helping parents secure quality sources of information is important.

SUMMARY AND DIRECTIONS FOR FUTURE RESEARCH

Over the past decades, considerable progress has been made: we now understand that autism is a strongly brain-based disorder, is also strongly genetic, and that it responds best to structured treatment approaches. A major focus of research has been on understanding the social brain processes involved in autism and it is clear that there are fundamental differences in such processes such as face processing, monitoring ongoing social interaction, perception of biologic movement, and so forth. Although a number of findings have proved robust, others have not. One complexity is the tendency for investigators to employ slight variations in replication studies, for example, differences in sample, methods, materials, techniques, can lead to differences in results which must, in turn be sorted out. With this caveat, it is exciting that genetic research and work on brain mechanisms is starting to converge.

Findings from more recent large scale genetics research are informing new approaches to development of pharmacotherapy—such as the targeting of glutamate receptors and, perhaps, processes more fundamentally connected with social cognition and learning.

Translation of promising preclinical research into positive results in human studies remains a prominent challenge. Oxytocin treatment continues to offer promise, although recent mixed results highlight the need for further study (114). Currently available agents warrant further study for behavioral symptoms—in particular, newer atypical antipsychotics like ziprasidone offer a promise of improved side-effect burden and appear to be effective in clinical practice. Nicotinic agents appear to be a promising area for further investigation, with some early reports of positive effects for both cognition and behavioral symptoms (115).

References

1. Kanner L: Autistic disturbances of affective contact. *Nervous Child* 2:217–250, 1943.
2. American Psychiatric Association: *Diagnostic and Statistical Manual*. Washington, DC, APA Press, 1980.
3. World Health Organization: *International Classification of Diseases (Draft Version: Diagnostic Criteria for Research)*. 10th ed. Geneva, WHO, 1990.
4. Volkmar FR, McPartland JC: From Kanner to DSM-5: autism as an evolving diagnostic concept. *Ann Rev Clin Psychol* 10:193–212, 2014.
5. Huerta M, Bishop SL, Duncan A, Hus V, Lord C: Application of DSM-5 criteria for autism spectrum disorder to three samples of children with DSM-IV diagnoses of pervasive developmental disorders. *Am J Psychiatry* 169(10):1056–1064, 2012.
6. Miller M, Young GS, Hutman T, Johnson S, Schwichtenberg AJ, Ozonoff S: Early pragmatic language difficulties in siblings of children with autism: implications for DSM-5 social communication disorder? *J Child Psychol Psychiatry* 56(7):774–781, 2014.
7. Smith IC, Reichow B, Volkmar FR: The effects of DSM-5 criteria on number of individuals diagnosed with autism spectrum disorder: a systematic review. *J Autism Dev Disord* 45(8):2541–2552, 2015.
8. McPartland JC, Reichow B, Volkmar FR: Sensitivity and specificity of proposed DSM-5 diagnostic criteria for autism spectrum disorder. *J Am Acad Child Adolesc Psychiatry* 51(4):368–383, 2012.
9. Barton ML, Robins DL, Jashar D, Brennan L, Fein D: Sensitivity and specificity of proposed DSM-5 criteria for autism spectrum disorder in toddlers. *J Autism Dev Disord* 43(5):1184–1195, 2013.
10. Asperger H: Die "autistischen psychopathen" im kindesalter. *Archiv für psychiatrie und Nervenkrankheiten* 117:76–136, 1944.
11. Volkmar FR, Klin A, McPartland JC: Asperger syndrome: an overview. In: *Asperger Syndrome: Assessing and Treating High-Functioning*

Autism Spectrum Disorders. 2nd ed. New York, Guilford Press, 1–42, 2014.
12. Chiang HM, Tsai LY, Cheung YK, Brown A, Li H: A meta-analysis of differences in IQ profiles between individuals with Asperger's disorder and high-functioning autism. *J Autism Dev Disord* 44(7):1577–1596, 2014.
13. Hill AP, Zuckerman KE, Fombonne E: Epidemiology of autism spectrum disorders. In: *Handbook of Autism and Pervasive Developmental Disorders, Volume 1: Diagnosis, Development, and Brain Mechanisms.* 4th ed. Hoboken, NJ, John Wiley & Sons, Inc., 57–96, 2014.
14. Shattuck PT: The contribution of diagnostic substitution to the growing administrative prevalence of autism in US special education. *Pediatrics* 117(4):1028–1037, 2006.
15. Mandell DS, Wiggins LD, Carpenter LA, et al.: Racial/ethnic disparities in the identification of children with autism spectrum disorders. *Am J Public Health* 99(3):493–498, 2009.
16. Dworzynski K, Ronald A, Bolton P, Happé F: How different are girls and boys above and below the diagnostic threshold for autism spectrum disorders? *J Am Acad Child Adolesc Psychiatry* 51(8):788–797, 2012.
17. Rutter M: Childhood schizophrenia reconsidered. *J Autism Childhood Schizophr* 2(4):315–337, 1972.
18. Volkmar FR, Nelson DS: Seizure disorders in autism. *J Am Acad Child Adolesc Psychiatry* 29(1):127–129, 1990.
19. Folstein S, Rutter M: Infantile autism: a genetic study of 21 twin pairs. *J Child Psychol Psychiatry* 18(4):297–321, 1977.
20. Brothers L: The neural basis of primate social communication. *Motiv Emot* 14(2):81–91, 1990.
21. Brothers L, Ring B: A neuroethological framework for the representation of minds. *J Cogn Neurosci* 4(2):107–118, 1992.
22. Piven J: The biological basis of autism. *Curr Opin Neurobiol* 7(5):708–712, 1997.
23. Critchley HD, Daly EM, Bullmore ET, et al.: The functional neuroanatomy of social behaviour: changes in cerebral blood flow when people with autistic disorder process facial expressions. *Brain* 123(Pt 11):2203–2212, 2000.
24. Ring HA, Baron-Cohen S, Wheelwright S, et al.: Cerebral correlates of preserved cognitive skills in autism: a functional MRI study of embedded figures task performance. *Brain* 122(Pt 7):1305–1315, 1999.
25. Schultz RT, Gauthier I, Klin A, et al.: Abnormal ventral temporal cortical activity during face discrimination among individuals with autism and asperger syndrome. *Arch Gen Psychiatry* 57(4):331–340, 2000.
26. Volkmar F, Chawarska K, Klin A: Autism in infancy and early childhood. *Annu Rev Psychol* 56:315–336, 2005.
27. Kanwisher N, McDermott J, Chun MM: The fusiform face area: a module in human extrastriate cortex specialized for face perception. *J Neurosci* 17(11):4302–4311, 1997.
28. Philip RC, Dauvermann MR, Whalley HC, Baynham K, Lawrie SM, Stanfield AC: A systematic review and meta-analysis of the fMRI investigation of autism spectrum disorders. *Neurosci Biobehav Rev* 36(2):901–942, 2012.
29. Hadjikhani N, Chabris CF, Joseph RM, et al.: Early visual cortex organization in autism: an fMRI study. *Neuroreport* 15(2):267–270, 2004.
30. Baron-Cohen S, Ring HA, Bullmore ET, Wheelwright S, Ashwin C, Williams SC: The amygdala theory of autism. *Neurosci Biobehav Rev* 24(3):355–364, 2000.
31. McPartland J, Dawson G, Webb SJ, Panagiotides H, Carver LJ: Event-related brain potentials reveal anomalies in temporal processing of faces in autism spectrum disorder. *J Child Psychol Psychiatry* 45(7):1235–1245, 2004.
32. Klin A, Jones W, Schultz R, Volkmar F, Cohen D: Visual fixation patterns during viewing of naturalistic social situations as predictors of social competence in individuals with autism. *Arch Gen Psychiatry* 59(9):809–816, 2002.
33. Dalton KM, Nacewicz BM, Johnstone T, et al.: Gaze fixation and the neural circuitry of face processing in autism. *Nat Neurosci* 8(4):519–526, 2005.
34. Apicella F, Sicca F, Federico RR, Campatelli G, Muratori F: Fusiform gyrus responses to neutral and emotional faces in children with autism spectrum disorders: a high density ERP study. *Behav Brain Res* 251:155–162, 2013.
35. Lozier LM, Vanmeter JW, Marsh AA: Impairments in facial affect recognition associated with autism spectrum disorders: a meta-analysis. *Dev Psychopathol* 26(4 Pt 1):933–945, 2014.
36. Pelphrey KA, Morris JP, Michelich CR, Allison T, McCarthy G: Functional anatomy of biological motion perception in posterior temporal cortex: an FMRI study of eye, mouth and hand movements. *Cereb Cortex* 15(12):1866–1876, 2005.
37. Chawarska K, Macari S, Shic F: Decreased spontaneous attention to social scenes in 6-month-old infants later diagnosed with autism spectrum disorders. *Biol Psychiatry* 74(3):195–203, 2013.
38. Rutter M, Thapar A: Genetics of autism spectrum disorders. In: *Handbook of Autism and Pervasive Developmental Disorders, Volume 1: Diagnosis, Development, and Brain Mechanisms.* 4th ed. Hoboken, NJ, John Wiley & Sons, Inc., 411–423, 2014.
39. Volkmar FR, Rowberry J, Vinck-Baroody OD, et al.: Medical care in autism and related conditions. In: *Handbook of Autism and Pervasive Developmental Disorders, Volume 1: Diagnosis, Development, and Brain Mechanisms.* 4th ed. Hoboken, NJ, John Wiley & Sons, Inc., 2014.
40. Hertz-Picciotti I, Lyall L, Schmidt R: Environmental factors in ASD. In: Volkmar FR, Paul R, Rogers SJ, Pelphrey KA (eds): *Handbook of Autism and Pervasive Developmental Disorders.* 4th ed. Hoboken, NJ, John Wiley & Sons, Inc., 2014.
41. Siegel B, Vukicevic J, Spitzer RL: Using signal detection methodology to revise DSM-III-R: re-analysis of the DSM-III-R national field trials for autistic disorder. *J Psychiatr Res* 24(4):293–311, 1990.
42. Davis NO, Carter AS: Social development in autism. In: *Handbook of Autism and Pervasive Developmental Disorders, Volume 1: Diagnosis, Development, and Brain Mechanisms.* 4th ed. Hoboken, NJ, John Wiley & Sons, Inc., 212–229, 2014.
43. Mundy P, Burnette C: Joint attention and neurodevelopmental models of autism. In: Volkmar FR, Rogers SJ, Paul R, Pelphrey KA (eds): *Handbook of Autism and Pervasive Developmental Disorders.* Vol 1. 3rd ed. Hoboken, NJ, John Wiley & Sons, Inc., 650–681, 2014.
44. Wing L, Gould J: Severe impairments of social interaction and associated abnormalities in children: epidemiology and classification. *J Autism Dev Disord* 9(1):11–29, 1979.
45. Howlin P, Moss P, Savage S, Rutter M: Social outcomes in mid- to later adulthood among individuals diagnosed with autism and average nonverbal IQ as children. *J Am Acad Child Adolesc Psychiatry* 52(6):572–581, 2013.
46. Fein D, Barton M, Eigsti IM, et al.: Optimal outcome in individuals with a history of autism. *J Child Psychol Psychiatry* 54(2):195–205, 2013.
47. National Research Council: *Educating Young Children with Autism.* Washington, DC, National Academy Press, 307, 2001.
48. Chawarska K, Macari SL, Volkmar FR, Kim SH, Shic F: ASD in infants and toddlers. In: *Handbook of Autism and Pervasive Developmental Disorders, Volume 1: Diagnosis, Development, and Brain Mechanisms.* 4th ed. Hoboken, NJ, John Wiley & Sons, Inc., 121–147, 2014.
49. Tager-Flusberg H, Paul R, Lord C: Language and communication in autism. In: Volkmar FR, Rogers SJ, Paul R, Pelphrey KA (eds): *Handbook of Autism and Pervasive Developmental Disorders.* 4th ed. Hoboken, NJ, John Wiley & Sons, Inc., 335–364, 2014.
50. Hermelin B: *Bright Splinters of the Mind: A Personal Story of Research With Autistic Savants.* London, Jessica Kingsley Publishers Ltd, 176, 2001.
51. Attwood T: Understanding and managing circumscribed interests. In: *Learning and Behavior Problems in Asperger Syndrome.* New York, Guilford Press, 126–147, 2003.
52. Woodbury-Smith MR, Clare ICH, Holland AJ, et al.: Circumscribed interests and 'offenders' with autism spectrum disorders: a case-control study. *J Forens Psychiatry Psychol* 21(3):366–377, 2010.
53. Ibañez LV, Stone WL, Coonrod EE: Screening for autism in young children. In: *Handbook of Autism and Pervasive Developmental Disorders.* 4th ed. Hoboken, NJ, John Wiley & Sons, Inc., 2014.
54. Siperstein R, Volkmar F: Brief report: parental reporting of regression in children with pervasive developmental disorders. *J Autism Dev Disord* 34(6):731–734, 2004.
55. Westphal AR: The place of childhood disintegrative disorder on the autism spectrum. Dissertation Abstracts International: Section B: The Sciences and Engineering. 75(5-B(E)), 2014.
56. Klein S, Sharifi-Hannauer P, Martinez-Agosto JA: Macrocephaly as a clinical indicator of genetic subtypes in autism. *Autism Res* 6(1):51–56, 2013.
57. Casanova MF: The neuropathology of autism. In: *Handbook of Autism and Pervasive Developmental Disorders.* 4th ed. Hoboken, NJ, John Wiley & Sons, Inc., 2014.
58. Schaefer GB, Mendelsohn NJ; Professional Practice and Guidelines Committee: Clinical genetics evaluation in identifying the etiology of autism spectrum disorders: 2013 guideline revisions. *Genet Med* 15(5):399–407, 2013.
59. Volkmar FR, Booth LL, McPartland JC, Wiesner L: Clinical evaluation in multidisciplinary settings. In: *Handbook of Autism and Pervasive Developmental Disorders, Volume 2: Assessment, Interventions, and Policy.* 4th ed. Hoboken, NJ, John Wiley & Sons, Inc., 661–672, 2014.
60. Lord C, Corsello C, Grzadzinski R: Diagnostic instruments in autistic spectrum disorders. In: *Handbook of Autism and Pervasive Developmental Disorders.* Vol 2. 4th ed. John Wiley & Sons, Inc., 609–660, 2014.
61. Robins DL, Casagrande K, Barton M, Chen CM, Dumont-Mathieu T, Fein D: Validation of the modified checklist for autism in toddlers, revised with follow-up (M-CHAT-R/F). *Pediatrics* 133(1):37–45, 2014.
62. Mildenberger K, Sitter S, Noterdaeme M, Amorosa H: The use of the ADI-R as a diagnostic tool in the differential diagnosis of children with infantile autism and children with a receptive language disorder. *Eur Child Adolesc Psychiatry* 10(4):248–255, 2001.
63. Gotham K, Risi S, Dawson G, et al.: A replication of the Autism Diagnostic Observation Schedule (ADOS) revised algorithms. *J Am Acad Child Adolesc Psychiatry* 47(6):642–651, 2008.
64. Schopler E, Van Bourgondien ME: *Childhood Autism Rating Scale™, Second Edition (CARS™-2).* Los Angeles, CA, Western Psychological Services, 2010.
65. Lord C: Follow-up of two-year-olds referred for possible autism. *J Child Psychol Psychiatry* 36(8):1065–1076, 1996.
66. Volkmar FR, Wiesner LA: *A Practical Guide to Autism: What Every Parent, Family Member, and Teacher Needs to Know.* Hoboken, NJ, John Wiley & Sons, Inc., 2009.

67. Howlin P: Outcomes in adults with autism spectrum disorders. In: *Handbook of Autism and Pervasive Developmental Disorders.* 4th ed. Hoboken, NJ, John Wiley & Sons, Inc., 2014.
68. Volkmar FR, Reichow B, McPartland JC (eds): *Adolescents and Adults with Autism Spectrum Disorders.* New York, Springer Science+Business Media, p. 337, 2014.
69. Rutter M, Bartak L: Special educational treatment of autistic children: a comparative study. II. Follow-up findings and implications for services. *J Child Psychol Psychiatry* 14(4):241–270, 1973.
70. Reichow B, Barton EE: Evidence-based psychosocial interventions for individuals with autism spectrum disorders. In: *Handbook of Autism and Pervasive Developmental Disorders.* Vol 2. 4th ed. John Wiley & Sons, Inc., 2014.
71. Volkmar F, Siegel M, Woodbury-Smith M, King B, McCracken J, State M; American Academy of Child and Adolescent Psychiatry (AACAP) Committee on Quality Issues (CQI): Practice parameter for the assessment and treatment of children and adolescents with autism spectrum disorder. *J Am Acad Child Adolesc Psychiatry* 53(2):237–257, 2014.
72. Wilson EC, Roberts G, Gillan N, Ohlsen C, Robertson D, Zinkstok J: The NICE guideline on recognition, referral, diagnosis and management of adults on the autism spectrum. *Adv Ment Health Intellect Disabil* 8(1):3–14, 2014.
73. Powers MD, Palmieri MJ, Egan SM, Rohrer JL, Nulty EC, Forte S: Behavioral assessment of individuals with autism: current practice and future directions. In: *Handbook of Autism and Pervasive Developmental Disorders, Volume 2: Assessment, Interventions, and Policy.* 4th ed. Hoboken, NJ, John Wiley & Sons, Inc., 695–736, 2014.
74. Laugeson EA, Ellingsen R: Social skills training for adolescents and adults with autism spectrum disorder. In: *Adolescents and Adults With Autism Spectrum Disorders.* New York, Springer Science+Business Media, 61–85, 2014.
75. Kohler FW, Strain PS, Goldstein H: Learning experiences…an alternative program for preschoolers and parents: peer-mediated interventions for young children with autism. In: Hibbs ED, Jensen PS (eds): *Psychosocial Treatments for Child and Adolescent Disorders: Empirically Based Strategies for Clinical Practice.* 2nd ed. Washington, DC, American Psychological Association, 659–687, 2005.
76. Mirenda P: Augmentative and alternative communication. In: *Handbook of Autism and Pervasive Developmental Disorders, Volume 2: Assessment, Interventions, and Policy.* 4th ed. Hoboken, NJ, John Wiley & Sons, Inc., 813–825, 2014.
77. Ozonoff S, South M, Provencal S: Executive functions. In: Volkmar FR, Rogers SJ, Paul R, Pelphrey KA (eds): *Handbook of Autism and Pervasive Developmental Disorders.* Hoboken, NJ, John Wiley & Sons, Inc., 606–627, 2014.
78. Odom SL, Boyd BA, Hall LJ, Hume KA: Comprehensive treatment models for children and youth with autism spectrum disorders. In: *Handbook of Autism and Pervasive Developmental Disorders, Volume 2: Assessment, Interventions, and Policy.* 4th ed. Hoboken, NJ, John Wiley & Sons, Inc., 770–787, 2014.
79. Rogers SJ, Dawson G, Vismara LA: *An Early Start for Your Child with Autism: Using Everyday Activities to Help Kids Connect, Communicate, and Learn.* New York, Guilford Press, 2012.
80. Koegel RL, Koegel LK (eds): *Pivotal Response Treatments for Autism: Communication, Social, and Academic Development.* Baltimore, MD, Paul H. Brookes Publishing Co., Inc., 2006.
81. Schopler E: Implementation of TEACCH philosophy. In: Cohen DJ, Volkmar FR (eds): *Handbook of Autism and Pervasive Developmental Disorders.* New York, John Wiley & Sons, Inc., 767–795, 1997.
82. Olley JG: Curriculum and classroom structure. In: Volkmar FR, Paul R, Klin A, Cohen D (eds): *Handbook of Autism and Pervasive Developmental Disorders.* Vol 2. 3rd ed. Hoboken, NJ, John Wiley & Sons, Inc., 863–881, 2005.
83. Scahill L, Tillberg CS, Martin A: Psychopharmacology. In: *Handbook of Autism and Pervasive Developmental Disorders.* 4th ed. Hoboken, NJ, John Wiley & Sons, Inc., 2014.
84. Carey T, Ratliff-Schaub K, Funk J, Weinle C, Myers M, Jenks J: (2002). Double-blind placebo-controlled trial of secretin: effects on aberrant behavior in children with autism. *J Autism Dev Disord* 32(3):161–167, 2002.
85. Levy SE, Souders MC, Wray J, et al.: Children with autistic spectrum disorders. I: comparison of placebo and single dose of human synthetic secretin. *Arch Dis Child* 88(8), 731–736, 2003.
86. Owley T, McMahon W, Cook EH, et al.: Multisite, double-blind, placebo-controlled trial of porcine secretin in autism. *J Am Acad Child Adolesc Psychiatry* 40(11):1293–1299, 2001.
87. McDougle CJ, Scahill L, Aman MG, et al.: Risperidone for the core symptom domains of autism: results from the study by the autism network of the research units on pediatric psychopharmacology. *Am J psychiatry* 162(6):1142–1148, 2005.
88. Reichow B, Doehring P, Cicchetti DV, Volkmar FR (eds): *Evidence-Based Practices and Treatments for Children with Autism.* New York, Springer Science+Business Media, p. 408, 2011.
89. Hartley SL, Sikora DM, McCoy R: Prevalence and risk factors of maladaptive behaviour in young children with autistic disorder. *J Intellect Disabil Res* 52(10):819–829, 2008.
90. Kanne SM, Mazurek MO: Aggression in children and adolescents with ASD: prevalence and risk factors. *J Autism Dev Disord* 41(7):926–937, 2011.
91. McCracken JT, McGough J, Shah B, et al.: Risperidone in children with autism and serious behavioral problems. *New Engl J Med* 347(5):314–321, 2002.
92. Shea S: Risperidone in the treatment of disruptive behavioral symptoms in children with autistic and other pervasive developmental disorders. *Pediatrics* 114(5):e634–e641, 2004.
93. Marcus RN, Owen R, Kamen L, et al.: A placebo-controlled, fixed-dose study of aripiprazole in children and adolescents with irritability associated with autistic disorder. *J Am Acad Child Adolesc Psychiatry* 48(11):1110–1119, 2009.
94. Owen R, Sikich L, Marcus RN, et al.: Aripiprazole in the treatment of irritability in children and adolescents with autistic disorder. *Pediatrics* 124(6):1533–1540, 2009.
95. Marcus RN, Owen R, Manos G, et al.: Safety and tolerability of aripiprazole for irritability in pediatric patients with autistic disorder: a 52-week, open-label, multicenter study. *J Clin Psychiatry* 72(9):1270–1276, 2011.
96. Anderson LT, Campbell M, Grega DM, Perry R, Small A, Green W: Haloperidol in the treatment of infantile autism: effects on learning and behavioral symptoms. *Am J Psychiatry* 141(10):1195–1202, 1984.
97. Hollander E, Wasserman S, Swanson EN, et al.: A double-blind placebo-controlled pilot study of olanzapine in childhood/adolescent pervasive developmental disorder. *J Child Adolesc Psychopharmacol* 16(5):541–548, 2006.
98. Martin A, Koenig K, Scahill L, Bregman J: Open-label quetiapine in the treatment of children and adolescents with autistic disorder. *J Child Adolesc Psychopharmacol* 9(2), 99–107, 1999.
99. Hollander E, Chaplin W, Soorya L, et al.: Divalproex sodium vs placebo for the treatment of irritability in children and adolescents with autism spectrum disorders. *Neuropsychopharmacology* 35(4):990–998, 2010.
100. Belsito KM, Law PA, Kirk KS, Landa RJ, Zimmerman AW: Lamotrigine therapy for autistic disorder: a randomized, double-blind, placebo-controlled trial. *J Autism Dev Disord* 31(2):175–181, 2001.
101. Wasserman, Stacey, Rupa Iyengar, et al.: "Levetiracetam versus placebo in childhood and adolescent autism: a double-blind placebo-controlled study." *International clinical psychopharmacology* 21(6):363–367, 2006.
102. Hollander E, Phillips A, Chaplin W, et al.: A placebo controlled crossover trial of liquid fluoxetine on repetitive behaviors in childhood and adolescent autism. *Neuropsychopharmacology* 30(3): 582–589, 2005.
103. King BH, Hollander E, Sikich L, et al.: Lack of efficacy of citalopram in children with autism spectrum disorders and high levels of repetitive behavior: citalopram ineffective in children with autism. *Arch Gen Psychiatry* 66(6):583–590, 2009.
104. Williams K, Brignell A, Randall M, Silove N, Hazell P: Selective serotonin reuptake inhibitors (SSRIs) for autism spectrum disorders (ASD). *Cochrane Database Syst Rev* 8:CD004677, 2013.
105. Accordino RE, Kidd C, Politte LC, Henry CA, McDougle CJ: Psychopharmacological interventions in autism spectrum disorder. *Expert Opin Pharmacother* 17(7):937–952, 2016.
106. Gordon CT, State RC, Nelson JE, Hamburger SD, Rapoport JL: A double-blind comparison of clomipramine, desipramine, and placebo in the treatment of autistic disorder. *Arch Gen Psychiatry* 50(6):441–447, 1993.
107. Brasić JR, Barnett JY, Sheitman BB, Tsaltas MO: Adverse effects of clomipramine. *J Am Acad Child Adolesc Psychiatry* 36(9):1165–1166, 1997.
108. Research Units on Pediatric Psychopharmacology Autism Network: Randomized, controlled, crossover trial of methylphenidate in pervasive developmental disorders with hyperactivity. *Arch Gen Psychiatry* 62(11): 1266–1274, 2005.
109. Fankhauser MP, Karumanchi VC, German ML, Yates A, Karumanchi SD: A double-blind, placebo-controlled study of the efficacy of transdermal clonidine in autism. *J Clin Psychiatry* 53(3):77–82, 1992.
110. Harfterkamp M, van de Loo-Neus G, Minderaa RB, et al. A randomized double-blind study of atomoxetine versus placebo for attention-deficit/hyperactivity disorder symptoms in children with autism spectrum disorder. *J Am Acad Child Adolesc Psychiatry* 51(7):733–741, 2012.
111. Preti A, Melis M, Siddi S, Vellante M, Doneddu G, Fadda R: Oxytocin and autism: a systematic review of randomized controlled trials. *J Child Adolesc Psychopharmacol* 24(2):54–68, 2014.
112. Althaus M, Groen Y, Wijers AA, Noltes H, Tucha O, Hoekstra PJ: Oxytocin enhances orienting to social information in a selective group of high-functioning male adults with autism spectrum disorder. *Neuropsychologia* 79(Pt A):53–69, 2015.
113. Smith T, Oakes L, Selver K: Alternative treatments. In: *Handbook of Autism and Pervasive Developmental Disorders, Volume 2: Assessment, Interventions, and Policy.* 4th ed. Hoboken, NJ, John Wiley & Sons, Inc., 1051–1069, 2014.
114. Accordino RE, Kidd C, Politte LC, Henry CA, McDougle CJ: Psychopharmacological interventions in autism spectrum disorder. *Expert Opin Pharmacother* 17(7):937–952, 2016.
115. Van Schalkwyk GI, Lewis AS, Qayyum Z, Koslosky K, Picciotto MR, Volkmar FR: Reduction of aggressive episodes after repeated transdermal nicotine administration in a hospitalized adolescent with autism spectrum disorder. *J Autism Dev Disord* 45(9):3061–3066, 2015.

CHAPTER 5.2.2 ■ INTELLECTUAL DISABILITY

FRED R. VOLKMAR, ELISABETH M. DYKENS, AND ROBERT M. HODAPP

DEFINITION

Traditionally intellectual disability (ID) (previously termed mental retardation) has been defined based on three key features: subnormal intellectual functioning, commensurate deficits in adaptive functioning, and onset before 18 years. Of these three criteria, the first two are most often discussed. Subnormal intellectual functioning is characterized by an intelligence quotient (IQ) lower than 70, based in most cases on the administration of an appropriate standardized assessment of intelligence. Deficits in adaptive skills, which involve one's social and personal sufficiency and independence, are generally measured on instruments such as the recently rerevised Vineland Adaptive Behavior Scales (1). Various levels of ID were specified in the DSM-IV and ICD-10: mild (IQ 50 to 70), moderate (IQ 35 to 49), severe (IQ 20 to 34), and profound (IQ <20). The overall diagnostic approach to ID in DSM-IV and ICD-10 is summarized in Table 5.2.2.1.

The DSM-5 (2) approach is largely consistent with this approach albeit with a few changes. Most importantly the name of the condition has been changed to ID. Cognitive intellectual functioning should be two or more standard deviations below the mean (with some potential for flexibility in the "borderline" range). In addition to the name change the condition is now grouped as one of the neurodevelopmental disorders (these include ASD, communication disorders, and so forth); this was part of a broader effort to avoid having a childhood disorders section of the manual. ID is defined based on three features: deficits in intellectual functioning (as defined by both clinical observation and standardized assessments of intelligence), deficits in adaptive functioning (the capacity to cope with real world situations—again assessed both clinically and by standard tests), and onset in the developmental period. Specifiers can be used to note severity, associations with specific medical problems, and so forth. Accordingly this generally is in consistent with the approach in DSM-IV and ICD-10. It is important to note that the validity of specifiers (e.g., severe vs. profound levels) remains the topic of debate, the precise age of the "developmental period" is left unclear, and, rather oddly, it is suggested that deficits in adaptive function must be "directly related" to the cognitive deficits. On the latter score this might be complicated in the case of an individual with ASD and ID since the ASD may be an even greater factor impacting delayed adaptive skills. Other issues (see Chapter 4.7) arise with the overarching DSM-5 move away from multiaxial classification which was particularly important in noting comorbid conditions associated with ID.

Most persons with ID in childhood are those with mild ID (about 85% of cases); the remainder of cases are comprised of those with moderate (about 10%), severe (about 4%), and profound (1% to 2%) ID (Fig. 5.2.2.1). In the past, the distinction was made between educable (IQ 50 to 70) and trainable (IQ <50). Although no longer commonly used, this distinction is important. Persons with mild ID often have psychiatric difficulties that are fundamentally similar (if generally more frequent) to those seen in the general population; this is not true for more severely impaired persons. Similarly, specific medical conditions associated with ID are more likely in the group with an IQ lower than 50, whereas poverty and lower socioeconomic status are more frequent in the group with mild ID (3). The proportion of persons with severe and profound ID is higher than would be expected given the normal curve, reflecting the impact of genetic disorders and severe medical problems on development (4).

The tests chosen for assessment of intellectual functioning should be appropriate to the patient, have reasonable reliability and validity, and be administered in a standardized way by

TABLE 5.2.2.1

OVERALL DIAGNOSTIC APPROACH TO INTELLECTUAL DISABILITY IN ICD-10 AND DSM-IV

1. Cognitive ability (as assessed by an appropriate standardized test) in the significantly subaverage range (IQ below 70)
2. Adaptive skills (also as assessed by an appropriate standardized test) also below 70
3. Onset in the developmental period

Levels of intellectual deficiency
- Mild (IQ 50–69) (ultimate adult cognitive level or mental age 9–12 yrs)
- Moderate (IQ 35–49) (ultimate adult cognitive level or mental age 6–9 yrs)
- Severe (IQ 20–34) (ultimate adult cognitive level or mental age 3–6 yrs)
- Profound (IQ <20) (ultimate adult cognitive level or mental age <3-yr level)

Note: Clinical sensitivity is needed, especially in situations where cultural, language, or others issues complicate usual assessment.

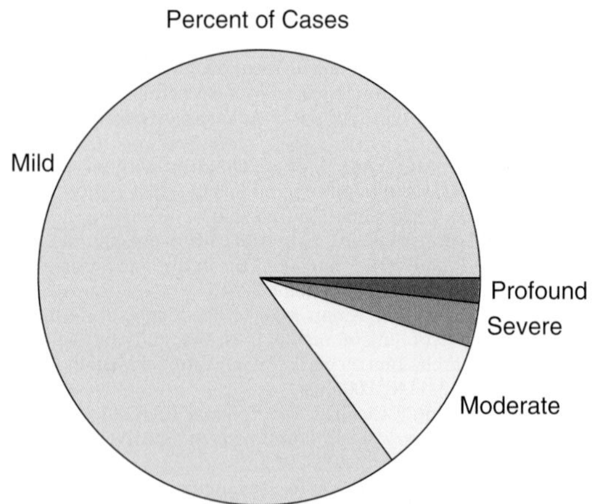

FIGURE 5.2.2.1. Levels of intellectual disability.

appropriately trained examiners (see Chapter 4.4, for a discussion of psychological assessment). Unfortunately, in some situations, the selection of an appropriate test can be difficult, such as for a very low functioning person. Other aspects of assessment can also be problematic, such as when some modification must be made in terms of administration given the specific circumstance. Such modifications may limit the validity of the results obtained. The examiner must then make an informed decision depending on the nature of the issue at hand, for example, determination of eligibility for services versus information on levels of functioning that can guide remediation. Particularly in terms of eligibility for services, it is critical that the examiner administer the test in exactly the standardized fashion. Measures of adaptive skills are generally based on parent or caregiver report, although, in some cases, the person may be interviewed directly. In essence, the conceptual notion is that the term *adaptive skills* refer to the performance of day-to-day activities required for personal or social self-sufficiency.

The inclusion of adaptive skills in the definition of ID rests on the observation that some persons with IQ scores below 70 may, as adolescents or adults, have learned sufficient adaptive skills, so that they are able to function totally or largely independently. Technically, then, such individuals would not meet criteria for ID. This situation is more typical of persons who, as children, score in the mildly retarded range (5).

The approach to the definition of ID is fundamentally the same in the 10th edition of the *International Classification of Diseases* (ICD-10) (6). However, the definition of ID promulgated by the American Association of Mental Retardation (AAMR)—first in its 1992 manual (7) and later (in revised form) in its 2002 manual (8)—discards the use of IQ levels in favor of a "needs-based" nosology that identifies the intensity of supports that persons require to function best within multiple adaptive domains. This definition also gives the clinician leeway to extend the upper IQ bound to 75; this seemingly small increase would actually considerably broaden the diagnostic concept of ID, potentially doubling the total number of cases (9). The AAID definition was much criticized and has had very little empirical support. Partly as a result, the AAID definition (particularly its 1992 version) has not been widely used either in research (10) or in state guidelines (11).

HISTORICAL NOTE

Interest in ID can be traced to antiquity (12,13). Modern interest in ID began at the time of the enlightenment and increased greatly during the 19th century; this emphasis occurred at the time of great social upheaval and as infant and child mortality began to decline. There was increased interest in children, in education, and in the role of experience (nurture) versus endowment (nature). The interest in the "nature–nurture problem" is exemplified in Itard's work with Victor, a child who was thought to be wild or "feral" but who may have had autism (14,15).

Subsequently, educators such as Seguin began to develop specific educational methods for stimulating children's development. By the latter half of the 19th century, many facilities had been developed for the care of persons with ID. Although the initial goal of such facilities was to provide a period of treatment before the child was returned to the family, these institutions gradually became places for custodial care (12). This problem has led to a strong counterreaction in recent years and to a renewed emphasis of caring for persons with ID in their homes and communities (16).

During the 19th century attempts were made to distinguish between levels of ID by using what now would be seen as rather pejorative terms (imbecile, cretin, idiot). Originally, the etiologic basis of any such distinctions was quite limited. On one hand, there was little systematic information on intellectual functioning that could be used for purposes of categorization. On the other, there were few known etiologic causes of ID.

Toward the end of the 19th and the beginning of the 20th centuries, both these limitations began to be addressed. Binet developed the first test of intelligence, which was translated into English and adapted in the United States by Terman (17,18). As a model psychometric assessment instrument for many years, the Stanford–Binet test allowed much more precise characterization of levels of ID. In addition, Terman had the brilliant notion of taking the mental age, dividing it by the child's chronologic age, and multiplying this quotient by 100. The resulting IQ score allowed for comparisons across children of different ages. Although Binet had originally developed his scale to identify children who were delayed in order to help them, the IQ score quickly became the object of much study.

Faith in the IQ as a predictor variable led to several unfortunate practices. First, developmental testing began to be performed on infants and young children (19). Second, proponents of the new tests believed that, when the test was properly administered, the resulting score from an IQ test was fixed and reflected a person's genetic endowment. This proved incorrect. In a classic study, Skeels and Dye (20) demonstrated this practically by transferring infants and young children from an orphanage to a home for the "feeble minded" to make the children normal. This fantastic plan had been prompted by clinical observation that children in the home for the feeble minded received considerably more stimulation than those in the orphanage. Skeels (21) later reported major differences in outcomes for these better-cared-for children, both in childhood and in later adult life. By the 1940s and 1950s, there was increased awareness that the IQ score was indeed the product of both experience and endowment, and therapeutic optimism again increased for improving the functioning of children with ID.

In addition to the focus on intellectual functioning, it also became apparent that the person's capacity to engage in appropriate self-care or "adaptive" skills was a major aspect of ID. In the 1930s, the psychologist Edgar Doll developed the Vineland Social Maturity Scale in an attempt to quantify such skills. Originally revised two decades ago (22), the Vineland Adaptive Behavior Scales have recently been rerevised (1). The Vineland Scales, now published in several versions, continue to serve as an important tool in the assessment of children with ID. Along with lower IQs, deficits in adaptive skills are now required as part of the diagnosis of ID. In contrast to IQ, however, adaptive skills can be readily taught.

Another major line of work centers on the origin of ID syndromes. In the 19th century, Dr. Langdon Down reported on a syndrome (which now bears his name) that is currently recognized as being the result of a trisomy of chromosome 21. At the time of his report, Dr. Down, of course, had no notion of chromosomes. Indeed, though his theoretical understanding was fundamentally flawed, Down's clinical observation has been remarkably robust. As time went on, more and more syndromes of ID were identified. It became clear that ID could result from a range of risk factors, including problems related to the developing fetus, and ranging from genetic factors (Down syndrome) to exposure to toxins in utero (fetal alcoholism) to maternal infections (congenital rubella). As noted subsequently, advances in genetics have led to an explosion in the recognition of such syndromes, often with a very precise understanding of their cause (3,23).

In recent years, several developments have substantially changed the approach to treatment and prevention of ID in the United States. Beginning in the 1960s, there has been increased emphasis on the care of persons in their homes and communities. The trend toward deinstitutionalization reflects various concerns about the effects of prolonged institutionalization and has led to creation of many community services.

This movement has been further stimulated by the mandate of the U.S. federal government that schools provide appropriate education for all children with disabilities, within integrated settings when possible. In the United States, many students with ID are largely or entirely integrated into classrooms with typically developing age mates, although there are marked state-to-state variations (24), and the benefits of mainstreaming are the focus of some debate (25). It is clear that students with more severe disabilities are most likely to spend their school time in more restricted settings.

One unfortunate aspect of current practice has been the often complete separation of services for those who are mentally ill from those who are mentally retarded. Although administratively useful, this approach has made provision of high-quality psychiatric care even more difficult to obtain for many persons with ID. With renewed interest in the field of "dual diagnosis" of ID and psychiatric disorders (26), we can only hope that this separation will soon be ending.

PREVALENCE AND EPIDEMIOLOGY

The use of both subnormal intellectual functioning and deficits in adaptive behavior in the definition of ID has important implications for epidemiology. If only the IQ criterion is used, the expectation, based on the normal curve, would be that about 2.3% of the population should exhibit the condition. This number is significantly decreased, particularly in adulthood, if the adaptive criterion is included. For example, in the Isle of Wight study, Rutter et al. (27) noted that, in 9- to 11-year-old children, about 2.5% would be classified as mentally retarded if IQ were the sole criterion. But if the prevalence were based only on those receiving services, this rate would be cut almost in half (1.3%) (Fig. 5.2.2.2). The drop in cases based on inclusion of IQ and adaptive skills is more common among those with mild ID (28,29); these children (and adults) may, however, need services and support at times of stress (30,31). As children, such persons are more likely to have academic and behavioral problems (27).

Additional findings have also recently been reported from large-scale epidemiologic studies (32). For individuals with severe ID, prevalence levels mostly converge on 3 to 4 children per 1,000; for mild ID, rates range wildly from 5.4 to 10.6 children per 1,000 (29,30). Studies also examine correlates of ID as gender, age, and social economic status (SES). More boys than girls have ID, and rates of ID are generally low in the early years, peak at around 10 to 14 years, and decrease slightly in the late-school years and markedly during adulthood. Individuals of lower SES and of ethnic minority groups (in several cultures) (13) also show higher-than-expected rates of ID.

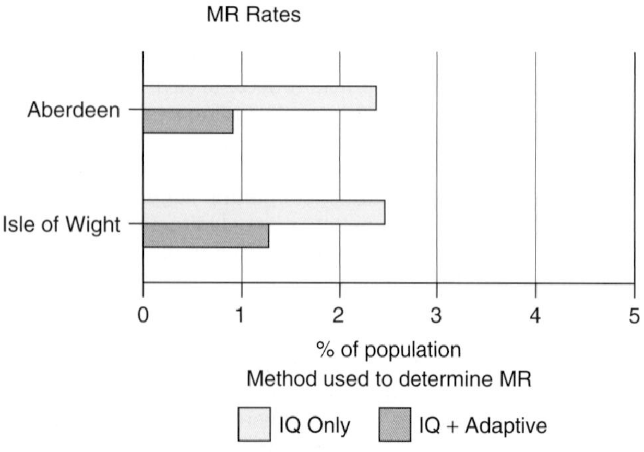

FIGURE 5.2.2.2. Isle of Wight study.

CLINICAL DESCRIPTION

Clinical Features

Associated clinical features vary depending on several factors, most importantly the cognitive level. Persons with severe and profound ID come to diagnosis at a younger age, more often exhibit related medical conditions, may exhibit dysmorphic features, and have a range of behavioral and psychiatric disturbances. In contrast, persons with mild ID often come to diagnosis much later (typically when academic demands become more prominent in school), are less likely to have medical conditions that could account for the ID, and usually are of normal appearance without dysmorphic features. In this latter group, although rates of psychopathology are increased relative to nondisabled populations, the range and nature of problems seen are fundamentally similar to those in normative samples (3). Persons with moderate levels of ID are intermediate between these two extremes. It is well recognized that the nature of associated psychiatric and behavioral disorders undergoes a marked shift between the mild and more severe levels of ID (33). Chapters 3.2.2 and 3.3.3 discuss some aspects of genetic contributions to intellectual disabilities.

ASSOCIATED PSYCHIATRIC AND BEHAVIORAL PROBLEMS

A growing body of work focuses on psychiatric and behavioral difficulties relative to specific genetic causes (34,35). Features have been identified that are highly frequent to specific syndromes, such as hyperphagia and compulsivity in Prader–Willi syndrome (36), attentional and social problems in fragile X syndrome (37), inappropriate laughter in Angelman syndrome (38), the unusual cry in 5p– syndrome (39), and the self-hug in Smith–Magenis syndrome (40). In some instances, aspects of syndrome expression have even been related to the genetic features of the syndrome, such as the severity of ID in fragile X syndrome (41,42) and the type and severity of maladaptive behaviors in Prader–Willi syndrome (43–45). Furthermore, some of these connections between genetic disorder and behavioral outcome appear unique to a single syndrome, whereas others are "shared" among two or more syndromes (46–48). Thus, in some instances, features are relatively syndrome specific, such as the unusual hand-washing stereotypies of Rett syndrome (49), or the extreme hyperphagia in Prader–Willi syndrome (50). More often, however, features are shared in two or more conditions. Thus, attentional problems are frequent in fragile X, Williams, and 5p– syndromes (51,52).

Somewhat paradoxically, for many years the diagnosis of ID tended to cause clinicians and researchers to overlook the presence of associated psychiatric and behavioral problems; such difficulties, when noted at all, were assumed to be a function of the ID. This "diagnostic overshadowing" (53) remains a problem in clinical practice (54). Although more clinicians and researchers are being specifically trained to work with this population, the separation of ID and mental health services in most states is a further obstacle to appropriate identification and treatment of mental disorders.

Although rates vary, as many as 25% of persons with ID may have significant psychiatric problems; these rates are much higher if persons with salient behavior disorders are included (55). Problems are invariably seen in children who present clinically (56), whereas rates are lower, from 10% to 15%, in more population-based studies, including two large-scale medical record surveys of all clients served in New York and California (57,58). Rates that fall between these two extremes, from 30% to 40%, are found in other studies based on informant checklists of behavior problems of children or adults in nonreferred samples (59).

Persons with ID experience the same range of psychiatric problems as seen in the general population (60), but prevalence rates for specific disorders vary widely. Some of this variability may be associated with different methods for determining "caseness," with common approaches including record reviews, behavioral checklists, and, to a lesser extent, direct interviews (61–64). An additional concern is that although some researchers assess DSM- or ICD-based diagnoses, others identify maladaptive features commonly seen in the general population (e.g., inattention or sadness), whereas still others focus on a narrow range of behaviors seen primarily in persons with ID (e.g., stereotypies or self-injury) (47).

For example, rates of schizophrenia or psychosis in persons with ID range from 1% to 9% among nonreferred samples and 2.8% to 24% in referred samples. Although variable, these rates are much higher than the 0.5% to 1% of the general population with schizophrenia (1). Rates for depression vary from 1.1% to 11% across nonreferred and clinic samples of persons with ID, and rates of attention deficit hyperactivity disorder range from 7% to 15% in children with ID, a finding that contrasts with the 3% to 5% estimate among children in general (1). Patterns of psychopathology also differ across persons with or without ID. Relative to the general population, for example, people with ID are more likely to show psychosis, autism, and behavior disorders and are less apt to be diagnosed with substance abuse and affective disorders (35,36).

ASSESSMENT OF PSYCHIATRIC DISORDERS

As researchers increasingly began to appreciate the scope of problems in persons with ID, they also developed various ways of assessing these problems. Some work has been devoted to the development of specialized rating scales and surveys; most of these measures are geared specifically for persons with ID and have well-developed psychometric properties (65). Among the more widely used are the Aberrant Behavior Checklist (66), Reiss Screen (67), and Developmental Behaviour Checklist (62). A tradeoff in using these scales is that, although they are sensitive to the unique concerns of those with ID, they are not necessarily compatible with DSM or ICD psychiatric diagnoses. Further, because each scale has a different set of items and factor structures, these differences may ultimately contribute to inconsistent findings across studies (61).

At the same time, other researchers have taken issue with the applicability of traditional DSM or ICD diagnoses for persons with ID (33). Many of these concerns relate to the psychiatric interview itself, including acquiescence bias, and the limited abilities of many persons with ID to answer questions about the onset, duration, frequency, and severity of symptoms (36). In response to these challenges, several groups have adapted traditional DSM or ICD criteria for persons with developmental delay (3,60), whereas others have designed interview schedules specifically for those with ID, including the Psychiatric Assessment Schedule for Adults with Developmental Disability (68). Direct interviews with both respondents and informants result in fewer cases of missed diagnoses (69). Still others advocate a more functional analysis of challenging behavior (70).

CAUSES OF INCREASED PSYCHOPATHOLOGY

Although the field has done well with assessment and diagnostic issues, less progress has been made in advancing theories on why persons with ID are at heightened risk of psychopathology in the first place. Many reasons have been discussed over the years and most fall within the "biopsychosocial" spectrum. Yet a comprehensive model of "dual diagnosis" is lacking, in part because researchers cannot simply apply existing risk factors for psychopathology in the general population to the unique characteristics of those with ID (71). In addition, the causal direction of most risk factors is unclear. Poor peer or social relations, for example, may be a precursor of psychopathology or a consequence of disruptive behavior.

Even so, some advances have been made, and heightened psychopathology in persons with ID has now been linked to specific biopsychosocial problems. Biologically, these include increased rates of seizure disorders (72,73), abnormal neurologic functioning that in most cases is undetected (74,75), high rates of sensory or motor impairments among persons with ID (76), biochemical or neurologic anomalies associated with unusual behaviors such as severe self-injury (77), and genetic causes that carry higher than usual risks of certain maladaptive or psychiatric vulnerabilities (78).

Psychological risk factors include the following: aberrant personality styles, including an outer-directed orientation and being too wary or disinhibited with others (79,80); atypical motivational styles or abnormal levels of sensitivity to basic human drives such as the need for attention or acceptance (81); increased risk of failure experiences, which may lead to learned helplessness, low expectancies for success, and depression (81,80); more global and less differentiated self-concepts that may lead to more sweeping negative evaluations of the entire self instead of not liking just one aspect of one's self (82); and reinforcement of negative behaviors, leading to more entrenched maladaptive behavior or interactions (83).

Finally, specific social risk factors include the following: poor communication or assertiveness skills, which may lead to increased frustration and acting-out behavior (84); social strain or stressful social interactions, more strongly correlated with psychopathology than low levels of social support (85); social stigma, with a subsequent negative impact on daily living, adjustment, and esteem (30); peer rejection and ostracism and, among children, atypical patterns of friendship with typically developing children (86); compromised "social intelligence," or inappropriate responses to social cues, that may exacerbate stigma and isolation from others (87); heightened risks of exploitation and abuse, which may worsen behavioral or emotional problems (88,89); and family stress, including low levels of emotional, service, or financial support to families (90).

GENETIC RISK AND PSYCHOPATHOLOGY

As previously noted, a comprehensive model has yet to be developed that identifies the relative importance of these many risk factors. To date, research aimed at doing so has generally relied on heterogeneous groups with ID. Yet each of the factors listed earlier can just as easily apply to those with a genetic diagnosis, and syndrome-specific studies may shed new light on genetic or other mechanisms associated with certain psychopathologic conditions (47,63). The latter are of particular interest as they offer the potential for new treatments.

ETIOLOGY AND PATHOGENESIS

Historically, researchers have used two broad categories to classify persons with ID (13,91). One group has organic causes of their ID and consists of people with known prenatal, perinatal, and postnatal insults. Estimates suggest that approximately one-half of people with ID have known "organic" causes (92). The second group has no clearly identifiable organic cause

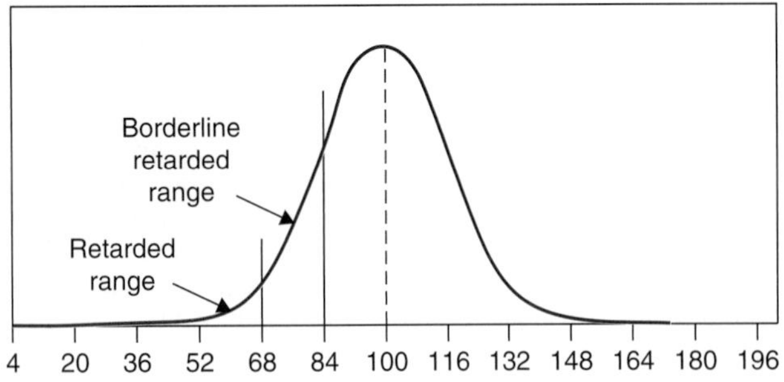

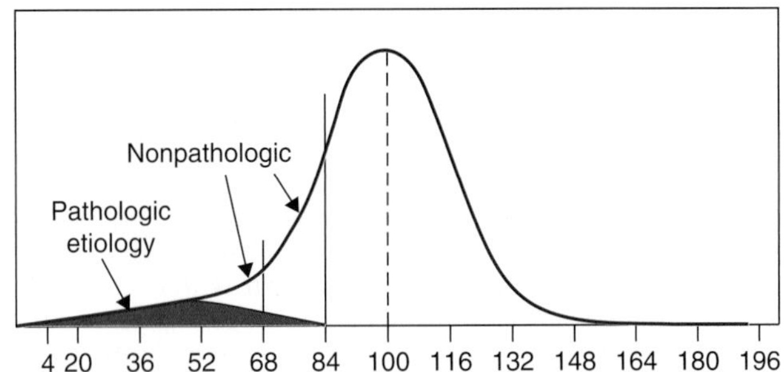

FIGURE 5.2.2.3. **A:** Distribution of Stanford–Binet IQ expected from the normal curve. **B:** Approximate distribution of IQs actually found, with persons having signs of pathologic origin separated from those not having signs of pathologic origin. (From Achenbach T: *Developmental Psychopathology*. 2nd ed. New York, Wiley, 1974, with permission.)

and is postulated to account for most persons with mild ID. In years past, the terms "sociocultural" or "cultural-familial" retardation reflected the view that nonorganic ID stemmed from environmental deprivation. Although impoverished, chaotic environments may indeed be implicated in a few cases, this theory has generally fallen out of favor as an explanation for the population as a whole. Even so, a complicating factor is that disproportionately more persons with sociocultural ID are poor, from minority backgrounds, and of low IQ parents (92).

With increased diagnostic precision and with the discovery of new genetic disorders, many workers speculate that more persons with nonspecific delay will receive specific genetic diagnoses in the years ahead. The complex interplay of organic and genetic (including polygenic) factors with sociocultural and environmental factors has been increasingly recognized (93). Progress has been slower in identifying clear neurologic causes in persons with unspecified ID, because most neuroimaging research is conducted with persons with known genetic or other causes (75). However, some persons with nonorganic causes may simply represent the lower end of the normal, Gaussian distribution of intelligence (94,95). Assuming that nonorganic ID is the extreme end of the normal IQ distribution, then some persons will always belong to this group, even as progress is made in uncovering genetic or neurologic causes for other persons at the same IQ levels (Fig. 5.2.2.3).

In the organic group as well, many unresolved issues remain. Early researchers grouped people together who had different types of organic causes and often compared these heterogeneous groups with those with familial or nonspecific ID. Even today, mixed or heterogeneous groups, consisting of those with known and unknown causes for their delay, predominate in behavioral ID research (23). Yet with the remarkable progress in molecular genetics, and improved diagnostic accuracy, researchers are now much better positioned to examine people with specific genetic causes. Indeed, there are now nearly 1,000 known genetic causes of ID (96), and as many as one-third of all persons with ID have already been diagnosed with a known genetic disorder (97). Further, although genetic and other organic causes are typically seen in persons with severe and profound delay, high functioning persons with Down syndrome, fragile X syndrome, Prader–Willi, Williams, and other syndromes may comprise 10% to 50% of persons with mild ID (93).

With these advances, research on so-called behavioral phenotypes is gaining momentum, including both between-syndrome and within-syndrome designs (23,34,94). Between-group studies help to identify possible unique syndromic behaviors that may accelerate our understanding of gene or brain function. Further, and as shown in Table 5.2.2.2, some syndromes feature unique psychiatric vulnerabilities, including increased rates of obsessive–compulsive symptoms in Prader–Willi syndrome (43), as well as anxiety, fears, and phobias in Williams syndrome (95). Groups without these syndromes can also have these vulnerabilities, albeit much less often. As such, studies on these syndromes hold much promise for differentiating genetic from other pathways to these psychiatric endpoints.

Cognitively as well, some syndromes show distinctive profiles of relative strength or weakness that are not typically seen in studies of persons with mixed or nonspecific causes of ID. As summarized in Table 5.2.2.2, persons with Williams, Prader–Willi, Down, and other syndromes often show distinctive patterns of cognitive strength or weakness. Many people with Williams syndrome, for example, show relative strengths in specific aspects of expressive language, along with pronounced deficits in visual–spatial functioning. Despite visual–spatial deficits, however, many persons with Williams syndrome have a remarkable sparing of facial recognition and memory. Many, although not all, persons with Prader–Willi syndrome show remarkable skills solving jigsaw puzzles, with performances that exceed those of their chronologic age mates (96).

TABLE 5.2.2.2

EXAMPLES OF COGNITIVE AND BEHAVIORAL PROFILES IN SELECTED INTELLECTUAL DISABILITY SYNDROMES

Syndrome	Cognitive Weakness	Cognitive Strengths	Behavioral Profiles
Fragile X	Sequential processing, auditory STM, planning	Verbal LTM-acquired information	Social anxiety, shyness, gaze aversion, inattention, hyperactivity, autism/PDD
Prader–Willi	Sequential processing	Verbal LTM, visual-spatial processing	Hyperphagia, nonfood obsessive-compulsive symptoms, skin picking, tantrums
Williams	Spatial organization, visual motor coordination	Facial recognition, auditory STM, expressive language	Social disinhibition, anxiety, fears, inattention, hyperactivity, hyperacusis
Down	Auditory processing	Visual-spatial processing, expressive language	Noncompliance, stubbornness, inattention, depression and dementia in adults

LTM, long-term memory; PDD, pervasive developmental disorder; STM, short-term memory.

However, most syndromic behaviors appear to be "partially specific" or shared across one or more conditions (46). For example, persons with both fragile X and Prader–Willi syndromes appear to have relative weaknesses in certain short-term memory and sequential processing tasks (50), and inattention and hyperactivity are seen in Williams, fragile X, and 5p– syndromes (51,52,62). These disorders, however, show qualitative differences in symptoms. Inattention in Williams syndrome, for example, may be associated with heightened anxiety and social disinhibition, whereas in fragile X syndrome, these difficulties may be related to hyperarousal and anomalies in the size of the posterior cerebellar vermis and caudate nucleus (98).

Although between-group studies help to identify distinctive syndromic behaviors, within-syndrome studies help to explain individual variation in these behaviors. Researchers now need to identify the genetic, environmental, developmental, and psychosocial factors that help to explain individual behavioral differences in people with the same genetic disorder. For example, the level of cognitive delay in fragile X syndrome is associated with both age and molecular genetic status (42). Similarly, in Prader–Willi syndrome, the frequency and severity of maladaptive behaviors such as skin picking appear to vary across genetic subtypes of this disorder (36).

Whereas research on heterogeneous groups is still necessary, both between-syndrome and within-syndrome studies offer many advantages (35,47). In the long term, work on behavioral phenotypes facilitates the search for gene–brain–behavior relationships, as well as contributing toward a more precise science of ID. In the short term, phenotypic data refine intervention and treatment (99,100). Although many syndrome-specific recommendations for interventions have now been made, the efficacy of these approaches needs to be evaluated, including how they fare relative to more generic interventions.

DIFFERENTIAL DIAGNOSIS

The diagnosis of ID is based on the appropriate assessment of cognitive abilities and adaptive skills; clinical assessment also includes a careful developmental and family history, physical examination, and laboratory studies as appropriate. The clinician should be alert to any medical or environmental conditions that may be associated with developmental disability. For example, a strong family history or certain dysmorphic features in the child should raise the possibility of an inherited condition; a history of significant birth trauma, exposure to environmental toxins, and exposure to marked psychosocial adversity are some of the factors that should be considered.

As noted, the age of diagnosis often varies depending on the severity of the disability, so persons with more severe ID present for clinical assessment earlier than those with mild, or borderline, ID. Careful psychological assessment of the child (Chapter 4.4) is obviously critical. Various other developmental difficulties, notably language and other specific developmental disorders and autism and related conditions, may be associated with some degree of mental disability or may be confused with it. Diagnosis can be complicated because persons with ID can exhibit other developmental problems that can complicate the task of both diagnosis and assessment. For example, children with a marked expressive language disorder often do poorly on a test of intelligence test that is highly verbal. In autism and related disorders, social abilities tend to be the area of greatest weakness (see Chapter 5.2.1). Potential genetic and toxic environmental contributions should also be considered particularly in children with greater degrees of intellectual impairment (see Chapters 3.2.2 and 3.3.3).

TREATMENT

In most developed countries, the treatment of ID has undergone a marked shift over the past few decades. More persons with ID now reside with their families and in their communities. More children now receive services within regular educational settings, and more services are available to support them and their families. At the same time, it is clear that placement in the community is not sufficient in and of itself, and the provision of adequate and appropriate support is critical. This is particularly important for the growing numbers of older persons with ID, many of whom still reside with their aging parents.

In general, treatment planning begins with a consideration of the underlying cause, if one is known, of the ID. In many instances, knowing the cause can guide both medical and psychosocial interventions; indeed, many syndrome-specific parent and professional organizations have published "best practice" guidelines across the lifespan (e.g., Prader–Willi, Williams, and Down syndromes). However, for disorders that are more rare, such data are lacking.

Medical Treatment

Medically, laboratory studies should be based on the results of a careful history (including family history) and evaluation. Physical examination should include assessment of growth and developmental status as well as observation for facial features or other physical findings that could suggest a specific medical condition. It is sometimes the case that the evolution of the condition provides important clues to its cause, such as in Rett syndrome. Depending on the clinical circumstance, hearing or visual testing may be indicated as are, at times, specific metabolic studies, chromosome analysis (including fragile X testing), neuroimaging or neurologic assessment, skeletal radiography, screening for organic acidurias, associated genetic conditions, and so forth (101,102).

Persons with ID may be at increased risk for certain medical conditions (103). In their review of the Aberdeen cohort of cases, Goulden et al. (104) noted that at least 15% of patients developed epilepsy by adulthood; the risk was increased when associated disabilities were present or when there was a history of postnatal injury.

To some extent, associated medical conditions vary depending on the cause of the ID. Consider Down syndrome, the most common genetic (i.e., chromosomal) cause of ID. Although the median age of death among individuals with Down syndrome has increased from 25 to 49 years over the period from 1983 to 1997 (105), specific medical problems persist for these individuals throughout their lifetimes. Congenital heart defects occur in approximately 50% of newborns with Down syndrome (106,107), and the large majority of these children are hospitalized for heart or other problems (mostly pneumonia, bronchitis, or other respiratory problems), often within the first few months of life (108). Later, children with Down syndrome are more likely than other children to have leukemia, and, by age 40, the plaques and tangles of Alzheimer disease strike virtually all adults with the syndrome (109). Other genetic disorders, notably Prader–Willi syndrome, also show particularly high rates of etiology-related health problems and higher death rates in the young adult and middle-aged years (110).

Cognitive and Adaptive Intervention

Regardless of the origin of ID, accurate assessment of each person's intellectual and adaptive strengths and weaknesses is essential, because specific recommendations for intervention depend on the overall level and profiles of cognitive functioning. Although there are many different models of intelligence (111), investigators generally agree about such basic features of intelligence as the ability to use conceptual thinking in solving problems and in acquiring knowledge (112). Various IQ tests are now available, and they differ in certain dimensions, such as the degree to which they emphasize language-based problem-solving or short-term memory. Tests differ in other ways as well: some tests include timed tasks, whereas others provide the opportunity for demonstration of tasks by the examiner. As part of the standard administration of test items, the examiner is also able to collect considerable amounts of qualitative information that may be particularly important for treatment.

Some special considerations are involved in assessing persons with ID. To the extent possible, tests should be appropriate for the person's chronologic age as well as her or his levels of receptive and expressive language. In some cases, cultural and other factors also need to be considered. The behavioral problems sometimes associated with ID may pose special problems; particularly if they arise around times of change or frustration.

Assessment of adaptive functioning has the goal of providing a representative picture of the person's typical abilities in home, school, and community environments. In this regard, the goal is somewhat different from that of the intellectual assessment, in which the aim is to obtain optimal performance in a structured and standardized situation. Large discrepancies between intellectual level and adaptive skills suggest that the treatment should include a major focus on acquisition and generalization of adaptive skills.

Various measures of adaptive functioning have been proposed. The most widely used instrument is the Vineland Adaptive Behavior Scales (2), which assess capacities for self-sufficiency in various domains of functioning, including communication (receptive, expressive, and written language), daily living skills (personal, domestic, and community skills), socialization (interpersonal relationships, play and leisure time, and coping skills), and motor skills (gross and fine). The Vineland scales are available as a survey interview, an expanded interview for use in more detailed program planning, an informant-administered rating form, and a teacher rating form.

Psychiatric Treatment

As previously described, persons with ID are at increased risk of psychiatric problems, and these are often a major source of distress to the individual and family and may severely limit opportunities for self-sufficiency and independence (102). Yet these mental and physical health problems are frequently overlooked. Ryan and Sunada (103) report that up to 75% of persons with ID who are referred for psychiatric assessment have undiagnosed or undertreated medical conditions, and nearly 50% receive no psychotropic medications that could have behavioral side effects.

Even though associated psychiatric problems can severely limit personal and social sufficiency, there is often a tendency to neglect or overlook the mental health needs of this population (59). Although some of the many rating scales, checklists, and other instruments for assessment of psychopathology in the general population are applicable, other instruments have been developed that are specific for persons with ID. Psychiatric assessment may entail some modification in usual procedures, particularly for persons with more severe ID, in whom the psychiatric assessment must be comprehensive and multifocal. The presence of associated difficulties (seizures, motor impairments, sensory problems) may further complicate accurate psychiatric diagnosis.

Other Psychosocial Treatment

General quality-of-life issues are receiving renewed attention in the ID field, with particular emphasis on improving how people with ID live, work, and play in inclusive, community-based settings. Most persons with ID benefit from employment or from structured programs that emphasize vocational, adaptive, or socialization skills, long after formal schooling. Indeed, the transition from school to work is a vulnerable point for many persons and their families. Unlike the school years, when special education and related services (e.g., occupational, physical, and speech and language therapies) are typically provided at school under one roof, the services for adults risk being more fragmented. These young adults may particularly benefit from *case coordination,* to avoid becoming isolated or lost between various cracks in services (113).

A particularly troublesome outgrowth of adult service needs concerns residential placements. As individuals with ID live longer lives, our society increasingly needs to deal with who will take care of these individuals when aging parents can no longer do so. Currently in the United States, 526,000 individuals with disabilities are 60 years and over; by the year 2030, that number is expected to triple, to 1.5 million (114). Since over 60% of these individuals live in their parents' home, who will take care of these aging individuals? Such concerns have recently led to a call from more research on adult siblings of individuals with ID (115), as these adult siblings (116) are likely to become tomorrow's caregivers for aging brothers and sisters with disabilities.

OUTCOME AND FOLLOW-UP DATA

As expected, the course and outcome of ID vary considerably, depending on various factors. These include the level of severity of the ID, associated biologic or other vulnerabilities, and aspects of the individual's psychological functioning, family support, and other factors (3). Levels of ability to cope with the demands of daily life (i.e., adaptive skills) are critical in determining adult outcome. It is also clear that the expectations of caregivers and the provision of intervention services and environmental supports are also important. For persons with known medical causes of ID, certain risks may be present, such as the risk of early development of Alzheimer dementia in persons with Down syndrome (117). Conversely, even when the specific biomedical cause is known, there may be a wide range in ultimate outcome. To simplify the discussion of outcome, we focus the discussion on levels of ID but again emphasize that the outcome in a given individual patient varies considerably, depending on a host of factors.

In mild ID, many children with the condition go on, as adolescents and adults, to make major gains in adaptive functioning and thus may "lose" the diagnosis as they become older. Such persons may be self-supporting, may marry, and may raise families. At the same time, such persons are not without difficulties, because several studies (27,31) show that persons with intellectual deficits who have not required special services in school have higher rates of educational and behavioral problems. In their follow-up study of the Aberdeen cohort of children first seen at 9 to 11 years of age and then followed up at the age of 22 years, Richardson and Koller (118) report that more than 75% no longer require services as adults, although only about 25% of the entire group are judged to be functioning adequately in all areas. Mild ID is likely to be diagnosed only at the time of school entry, that is, when academic demands increase. As discussed previously, persons from backgrounds of social disadvantage or adversity and from certain minority groups are more likely to be represented in these cases.

As adults, persons with moderate levels of ID (IQ 40 to 55) typically have more serious impairment. It is common for such persons to need services as adults. At this, and lower, levels of cognitive functioning, specific medical causes are more likely to be identified, and minority group membership and psychosocial adversity in the family are less frequent. The prognosis for adult self-sufficiency is more guarded, although many persons can live semiindependently or with partial support (119).

For persons with severe or profound retardation, case identification may occur in infancy or early childhood. Generally, high levels of supervision and support are required during the person's life. Goals for these patients include facilitating self-care and other skills as far as possible. Associated medical problems and behavioral difficulties are frequent. Communication skills may be impaired and are a further source of disability.

Legislation, legal decisions, and some important social policy changes have markedly changed the provision of remedial programs. The provision of early diagnosis and intervention and the availability of community-based resources and educational interventions within public schools have dramatically improved the care of persons with ID as well as overall outcome.

PREVENTION

Estimates of recurrence risk vary depending on the situation, ranging from instances in which a clear genetic origin can be identified (e.g., fragile X syndrome) to those in which the difficulties appear to be of nongenetic origin (e.g., congenital rubella). When no specific cause is identified, estimates of recurrence risk vary considerably, such as between 3.5% and 14% for the siblings of a boy with ID (120). For some disorders, such as autism, there has been a growing appreciation of genetic factors, and it now appears that, for parents who have one child with autism, the risk of having a second child with autism is between 2% and 10% (121). Siblings of children with ID who are not themselves affected may be at increased risk of other difficulties, due to increased family and personal stress, although data are sorely needed on the range of both positive and negative outcomes in these siblings (122). Support for siblings, and for their parents, is an important element of long-term treatment planning (3).

RESEARCH DIRECTIONS

Several issues will likely dominate the research agenda for the coming decade. They include the interplay between genetic and environmental (including psychosocial) risk factors in the origin of ID as well as the study of basic neural mechanisms (94). Understanding of basic processes that underlie phenotypic expression, including various forms of psychopathology, offers the opportunity to advance knowledge more generally about mechanisms of disorder. Although many advances in the care and treatment of persons with intellectual deficiency have been made, studies of treatment methods remain an important priority. Identification of genetic contributions (particularly for single gene disorders) and specific mechanisms likely will hasten development of more targeted treatments approaches; this is already happening in some conditions like fragile X and, in turn, these may have implications for other disorders as well (123).

References

1. Sparrow S, Balla D, Cicchetti D: *Vineland Adaptive Behavior Scales.* Circle Pines, MN, American Guidance Service, 2005.
2. American Psychiatric Association: *Diagnostic and Statistical Manual of Mental Disorders.* 5th ed. Washington, DC, American Psychiatric Association, 2013.
3. Szymanski L, King BH: Practice parameters for the assessment and treatment of children, adolescents, and adults with mental retardation and comorbid mental disorders: American Academy of Child and Adolescent Psychiatry Working Group on Quality Issues. *J Am Acad Child Adolesc Psychiatry* 38(Suppl):5S–31S, 1999.
4. Dingman HG, Tarjan G: Mental retardation and the normal distribution. *Am J Ment Defic* 64:991–994, 1960.
5. Edgerton RB, Bollinger M, Herr B: The cloak of competence: after two decades. *Am J Ment Defic* 88:345–351, 1984.
6. World Health Organization: Mental and behavioral disorders, clinical descriptions and diagnostic guidelines. In: *International Classification of Diseases.* 10th ed. Geneva, World Health Organization, 1992.
7. American Association on Mental Retardation (AAMR): *Mental Retardation: Definition, Classification, and Systems of Support.* 9th ed. Washington, DC, AAMR, 1992.
8. American Association on Mental Retardation. *Mental Retardation: Definition, Classification, and Systems of Supports.* 10th ed. Washington, DC: Author, 2002.
9. MacMillan DL, Gresham FM, Siperstein GN: Heightened concerns over the 1992 AAID definition: advocacy vs. precision. *Am J Ment Retar* 100:87–95,1995.
10. Polloway EA, Smith JD, Chamberlain J, Denning CB, Smith TE: Levels of deficits or supports in the classification of mental retardation: implementation practices. *Edu Train Mental Retard* 34:200–206, 1999.
11. Denning CB, Chamberlain JA, Polloway EA: An evaluation of state guidelines for mental retardation: focus on definition and classification practices. *Edu Train Mental Retard* 35:226–232, 2000.
12. Trent JW: *Inventing the Feeble Mind: A History of Mental Retardation in the United States.* Berkeley, CA, University of California Press, 1994.
13. Zigler E, Hodapp R: *Understanding Mental Retardation.* New York, Cambridge University Press, 1986.
14. Candland DK: *Feral Children and Clever Animals: Reflections on Human Nature.* Oxford, Oxford University Press, 1993.
15. Simon N: Kaspar Hauser's recovery and autopsy: a perspective on neurological and sociological requirements for language development. *J Autism Child Schizophr* 8:209–217, 1978.
16. Anderson LL, Lakin KC, Mangan TW, Prouty RW: State institutions: thirty years of depopulation and closure. *Mental Retard* 36:431–443, 1998
17. Binet A, Simon T: *The Development of Intelligence in Children. [E.S. Kit, trans.]* Baltimore, MA, Williams & Wilkins, 1916.
18. Terman LM: The Binet-Simon Scale for measuring intelligence: impressions gained by its application. *Psychol Clin* 5:199–206, 1911.
19. Bayley N: Consistency and variability in the growth of intelligence from birth to eighteen years. *J of Gen Psychology* 75:165–196, 1949.
20. Skeels A, Dye HB: A study of the effects of differential stimulation on mentally retarded children. *Proc Am Assoc Mental Def* 44:114–136, 1939.
21. Skeels HM: Adult status of children with contrasting early life experiences. *Monogr Soc Res Child Dev* 31:1–56, 1966.
22. Sparrow S, Balla D, Cicchetti D: *Vineland Adaptive Behavior Scales.* Circle Pines, MN, American Guidance Service, 1984.
23. Dykens EM, Hodapp RM, Finucance BM: *Genetics and Mental Retardation Syndromes: A New Look at Behavior and Interventions.* Baltimore, MA, Paul H. Brookes Pub. Co., 2000.
24. Hallahan DP, Kauffman JM: *Exceptional Children: Introduction to Special Education.* 10th ed. Boston, MA, Allyn & Bacon, 2006.
25. Burack JA, Kurtz L, Derevensky JL: Services for persons with mental retardation: a debate for all seasons. *McGill J Educ* 27:275–278, 1992.
26. Bouras N, Holt G (eds): *Psychiatric and Behavioural Disorders in Developmental Disabilities.* 2nd ed. Cambridge, Cambridge University Press, 2006.
27. Rutter M, Tizard J, Yule W, Graham P, Whitmore K: Research report: Isle of Wight studies, 1964–1974. *Psychol Med* 6:313–332, 1976.
28. McLaren J, Bryson SE: Review of recent epidemiological studies of mental retardation: prevalence, associated disorders, and etiology. *Am J Ment Retard* 92(3):243–254, 1987.
29. Leonard H, Wen X: The epidemiology of mental retardation: challenges and opportunities in the new millennium. *Ment Retard Dev Dis Res Rev* 8:117–134, 2002.
30. Roeleveld N, Zielhus GA, Gabreels F: The prevalence of mental retardation: a critical review of recent literature. *Dev Med Child Neurol* 39:125–132, 1997.
31. Granat K, Granat S: Adjustment of intellectually below-average men not identified as mentally retarded. *Scand J Psychol* 19:41–51, 1978.
32. Yeargin-Allsopp M, Boyle C: Overview: the epidemiology of neurodevelopmental disorders. Special issue on "The Epidemiology of Neurodevelopmental Disorders" (M. Yeargin-Allsopp & C. Boyle, Eds.). *Ment Retard Dev Dis Res Rev* 8(3):113–116, 2002.
33. Sovner R: Limiting factors in the use of DSM-III with mentally ill/mentally retarded persons. *Psychopharmacol Bull* 22:1055–1059, 1986.
34. Hodapp RM, Dykens EM: Strengthening behavioral research on genetic mental retardation syndromes. *Am J Ment Retard* 160:4–15, 2001.
35. Hodapp RM, Dykens EM: Measuring behavior in genetic disorders of mental retardation. *Ment Retard Dev Dis Res Rev* 11:340–346, 2005.
36. Dykens EM, Cassidy SB: Prader–Willi syndrome. In: Goldstein S, Reynolds CR (eds): *Handbook of Neurodevelopmental and Genetic Disorders in Children.* New York, Guilford Press, 525–554, 1999.

37. Hagerman RJ, Jackson AW, Levitas A, Rimland B, Braden M: An analysis of autism in 50 males with the fragile X syndrome. *Am J Med Genet* 23:359–374, 1986.
38. Williams CA, Zori RT, Hendrickson J, et al.: Angelman syndrome. *Curr Probl Pediatr* 25:216–231, 1995.
39. Gersh M, Goodard SA, Pasztor LM, Harris DJ, Weiss L, Overhauser J: Evidence for a distinct region causing a cat-cry in patients with 5p deletions. *Am J Hum Gen* 56:1404–1410, 1995.
40. Finucane BM, Konar D, Haas-Givler B, Kurtz MB, Scott CI Jr: The spasmodic upper body squeeze: a characteristic behavior in Smith-Magenis syndrome. *Dev Med Child Neurol* 36:78–83, 1994.
41. Dykens EM, Hodapp RM, Leckman JF: *Behavior and Development in Fragile X Syndrome.* Thousand Oaks, CA, Sage, 1994.
42. Tassone FI, Hagerman RJ, Ikle D, Dyer PN, Lampe M: FMRP expression as a potential prognostic indicator in fragile X syndrome. *Am J Med Genet* 84:250–261, 1999.
43. Dykens EM, Leckman JF, Cassidy SB: Obsessions and compulsions in Prader–Willi syndrome. *J Child Psychol Psychiatry* 37:995–1002, 1996.
44. Verhoeven WM, Tuinier S, Curfs L: Prader-Willi syndrome: cycloid psychosis in a genetic subtype? *Acta Neuropsychiatrica* 15:32–37, 2003.
45. Vogels A, De Hert M, Descheemaeker MJ, et al.: Psychotic disorders in Prader-Willi syndrome. *Am J of Med Gen* 127:238–243, 2004.
46. Hodapp RM: Direct and indirect behavioral effects of different genetic disorders of mental retardation. *Am J Ment Retard* 102:67–79, 1997.
47. Dykens EM: Measuring behavioral phenotypes: provocations from the new genetics. *Am J Ment Retard* 99:522–532, 1995.
48. Dykens EM: Direct effects of genetic mental retardation syndromes: maladaptive behavior and psychopathology. *Int Rev Res Ment Retard* 22:1–26, 1999.
49. VanAcker R: Rett's Syndrome. In: Cohen DJ, Volkmar FR (eds): *Handbook of Autism and Pervasive Developmental Disorders.* 2nd ed. New York, Wiley, 60–93, 1997.
50. Dykens EM, Cassidy SB, King BH: Maladaptive behavior differences in Prader–Willi syndrome due to paternal deletion versus maternal uniparental disomy. *Am J Ment Retard* 104:67–77, 1999.
51. Baumgardner TL, Reiss AL, Freund LS, Abrams MT: Specification of the neurobehavioral phenotype in males with fragile X syndrome. *Pediatrics* 95:744–752, 1995.
52. Dykens EM, Clarke DJ: Correlates of maladaptive behavior in individuals with 5p- (cri du chat) syndrome. *Dev Med Child Neurol* 39:752–756, 1997.
53. Reiss S, Levitan GW, Szyszko J: Emotional disturbance and mental retardation: diagnostic overshadowing. *Am J Ment Retard* 86:567–574, 1982.
54. White MJ, Nichols CN, Cook RS, Spengler PM, Walker BS, Look KK: Diagnostic overshadowing and mental retardation: a meta-analysis. *Am J Ment Retard* 100:293–298, 1995.
55. Jacobson JW: Dual diagnosis services: history, progress and perspectives. In: Bouras N (ed): *Psychiatric and Behavioural Disorders in Developmental Disabilities and Mental Retardation.* Cambridge, Cambridge University Press, 329–358, 1999.
56. Philips I, Williams N: Psychopathology and mental retardation: a study of 100 mentally retarded children I: psychopathology. *Am J Psychiatry* 132:1265–1271, 1975.
57. Borthwick–Duffy SA, Eyman RK: Who are the dually diagnosed? *Am J Ment Retard* 94:586–595, 1990.
58. Jacobson JW: Problem behavior and psychiatric impairment within a developmentally delayed population. I. Behavioral frequency. *Appl Res Ment Retard* 3:121–139, 1982.
59. Einfeld SL, Tonge BJ: Population prevalence of psychopathology in children and adolescents with intellectual disability. II. Epidemiological findings. *J Intellect Disabil Res* 40:99–109, 1996.
60. King BH, DeAntonia C, McCracken JT, Forness SR, Ackerland V: Psychiatric consultation in severe and profound mental retardation. *Am J Psychiatry* 151:1802–1808, 1994.
61. Dykens EM: Psychopathology in children with intellectual disabilities. *J Child Psychol Psychiatry* 41:407–417, 2000.
62. Einfeld SL, Tonge BJ: *Manual for the Developmental Behavioural Checklist: Primary Carer Version.* Sydney, Australia, School of Psychiatry, University of New South Wales, 1992.
63. Holland AJ, Koot HM: Conference report: mental health and intellectual disabilities. *J Intellect Disabil Res* 42:505–512, 1998.
64. Moss SC: Assessment: conceptual issues. In: Bouras N (ed): *Psychiatric and Behavioural Disorders in Developmental Disabilities and Mental Retardation.* Cambridge, Cambridge University Press, 18–37, 1999.
65. Aman MG: *Assessing Psychopathology and Behavior Problems in Persons with Mental Retardation: A Review of Available Instruments.* Rockville, MD, U.S. Department of Health and Human Services, 1991.
66. Aman MG, Singh NN: *Aberrant Behavior Checklist: Community Supplementary Manual.* East Aurora, NY, Slosson Educational Publications, 1994.
67. Reiss S: *The Reiss Screen for Maladaptive Behavior.* Worthington, OH, IDS Publishing, 1988.
68. Moss SC, Ibbotson B, Prosser H, Goldberg D, Patel P, Simpson N: Validity of the PAS-ADD for detecting psychiatric symptoms in adults with learning disability. *Soc Psychiatric Epidemiol* 32:344–354, 1997.
69. Moss SC, Prossner H, Ibbotson B, Goldberg D: Respondent and informant accounts of psychiatric symptoms in a sample of patients with learning disability. *J Intellect Disabil Res* 40:457–465, 1996.
70. Sturmey P: Classification: concepts, progress, and future. In: Bouras N (ed): *Psychiatric and Behavioural Disorders in Developmental Disabilities and Mental Retardation.* Cambridge, Cambridge University Press, 3–17, 1999.
71. Reiss S: Prevalence of dual diagnosis in community-based day programs in the Chicago metropolitan area. *Am J Ment Retard* 94:578–588, 1990.
72. Bird J: Epilepsy and learning disabilities. In: Russell O (ed): *Seminars in the Psychiatry of Learning Disabilities.* London, Gaskell, 223–244, 1997.
73. Caplan R, Arbelle S, Magharious W, et al.: Psychopathology in pediatric complex partial and primary generalized epilepsy. *Dev Med Child Neurol* 40:805–811, 1998.
74. Peterson BS: Neuroimaging in child and adolescent neuropsychiatric disorders. *J Am Acad Child Adolesc Psychiatry* 34:1560–1576, 1995.
75. Robertson D, Murphy D: Brain imaging and behavior. In: Bouras N (ed): *Psychiatric and Behavioural Disorders in Developmental Disabilities and Mental Retardation.* Cambridge, Cambridge University Press, 49–70, 1999.
76. Hodapp RM: *Development and Disabilities: Intellectual, Sensory and Motor Impairments.* New York, Cambridge University Press, 1998.
77. King BH: Self-injury by people with mental retardation: a compulsive behavior hypothesis. *Am J Ment Retard* 98:93–112, 1993.
78. Dykens EM: Personality-motivation: new ties to psychopathology, etiology, and intervention. In: Zigler E, Bennett-Gates D (eds): *Personality Development in Individuals with Mental Retardation.* New York, Cambridge University Press, 249–270, 1999.
79. Bybee J, Zigler E: Outerdirectedness in individuals with mental retardation: a review. In: Burack J, Hodapp RM, Zigler E (eds): *Handbook of Mental Retardation and Development.* New York, Cambridge University Press, 434–461, 1998.
80. Zigler E, Bennett–Gates D (eds): *Personality Development in Individuals with Mental Retardation.* New York, Cambridge University Press, 1999.
81. Reiss S, Havercamp SH: Toward a comprehensive assessment of functional motivation: factor structure of the Reiss profiles. *Psychol Assess* 10:97–106, 1998.
82. Evans DW: Development of the self-concept in children with mental retardation: organismic and contextual factors. In: Burack J, Hodapp RM, Zigler E (eds): *Handbook of Mental Retardation and Development.* New York, Cambridge University Press, 462–480, 1998.
83. Reiss S, Havercamp SH: The sensitivity theory of motivation: why functional analysis is not enough. *Am J Ment Retard* 101:553–566, 1997.
84. Nezu CM, Nezu AM: Outpatient psychotherapy for adults with mental retardation and concomitant psychopathology: research and clinical imperatives. *J Consult Clin Psychol* 62:34–42, 1994.
85. Lunsky Y, Havercamp SM: Distinguishing low level of social support and social strain: implications for dual diagnosis. *Am J Ment Retard* 104:200–204, 1999.
86. Siperstein GH, Leffert JS, Wenz–Gross M: The quality of friendships between children with and without learning problems. *Am J Ment Retard* 102:111–125, 1997.
87. Greenspan S, Granfield JM: Reconsidering the construct of mental retardation: implications of a model of social competence. *Am J Ment Retard* 96:442–453, 1992.
88. Ammerman RT, Hersen M, Van Hasselt VB, Lubstsky MJ, Sieck WR: Maltreatment in psychiatrically hospitalized children and adolescents with developmental disabilities: prevalence and correlates. *J Am Acad Child Adolesc Psychiatry* 33:567–576, 1994.
89. Sullivan PM, Knutson JF: Maltreatment and disabilities: a population-based epidemiological study. *Child Abuse & Neglect* 24:1257–1273, 2000.
90. Minnes P: Mental retardation: the impact on the family. In: Burack JA, Hodapp RM, Zigler E (eds): *Handbook of Mental Retardation and Development.* New York, Cambridge University Press, 693–712, 1998.
91. Zigler E: Developmental versus difference theories of retardation and the problem of motivation. *Am J Ment Defic* 73:536–556, 1969.
92. Hodapp RM: Cultural-familial mental retardation. In: Sternberg R (ed): *Encyclopedia of Intelligence.* New York, Macmillan, 711–717, 1994.
93. Rutter M, Simonoff E, Plomin R: Genetic influences on mild mental retardation: concepts, findings, and research implications. *J Biosoc Sci* 28:509–526, 1996.
94. Simonoff E, Bolton P, Rutter M: Mental retardation: genetic findings, clinical implications, and research agenda. *J Child Psychol Psychiatry* 37:259–280, 1996.
95. Zigler E: Familial mental retardation: a continuing dilemma. *Science* 155:292–298, 1967.
96. Opitz JM: Vision and insight in the search for gene mutations causing nonsyndromal mental deficiency. *Neurol* 55:335–340, 2000.
97. Matalainen R, Aiaksinen E, Mononen T, Launiala K, Kaariainen R: A population-based study on the causes of severe and profound mental retardation. *Acta Pediatr* 84:261–266, 1995.
98. Mostofsky SH, Mazzocco MM, Aakalu G, Warsofsky IS, Denckla MB, Reiss AL: Decreased cerebellar posterior vermis size in fragile X syndrome: correlation with neurocognitive performance. *Neurology* 50:121–130, 1998.
99. Dykens EM, Hodapp RM: Treatment issues in genetic mental retardation syndromes. *Profess Psychol Res Pract* 28:263–270, 1997.
100. Hodapp RM, Fidler DJ: Special education and genetics: connections for the 21st century. *J of Special Ed* 33:130–137, 1999.

101. Curry CJ, Stevenson RE, Aughton D, Byrne JC: Evaluation of mental retardation: recommendations of a consensus conference: American College of Medical Genetics. *Am J Med Genet* 72:468–477, 1997.
102. Szymanski LS, King BH, Goldberg B, et al.: Diagnosis of mental disorders in people with mental retardation. In: Reiss S, Aman MG (eds): *Psychotropic Medications and Developmental Disabilities: The International Consensus Handbook.* Columbus, OH, Ohio State University Press, 3–17, 1998.
103. Ryan R, Sunada K: Medical evaluation of persons with mental retardation referred for psychiatric assessment. *Gen Hosp Psychiatry* 19:274–280, 1997.
104. Goulden KK, Shinnnar S, Koller K, Katz M, Richardson SA: Epilepsy in children with mental retardation: a cohort study. *Epilepsia* 32:690–697, 1991.
105. Yang Q, Rasmussen SA, Friedman JM: Mortality associated with Down's syndrome in the USA from 1983 to 1997: a population-based study. *Lancet* 359:1019–1025, 2002.
106. Cohen WI (ed): Health care guidelines for individuals with Down syndrome (Down syndrome preventive medical check list). *Down Syn Quaterly* 1(2), 1996.
107. Roizen NJ: The early interventionist and the medical problems of the child with Down syndrome. *Infant Young Child* 16:88–95, 2003.
108. So SA, Urbano RC, Hodapp RM: Hospitalizations for infants and young children with Down syndrome: evidence from person-records from a statewide administrative database. *J Intellect Disabil Res* 51(Pt 12):1030–1038, 2007.
109. Zigman WB, Silverman W, Wisniewski HM: Aging and Alzheimer's disease in Down syndrome: clinical and pathological changes. *Ment Retard Dev Dis Res Rev* 2:73–79, 1996.
110. Whittington JE, Holland AJ, Webb T, Butler J, Clarke D, Boer H: Population prevalence and estimated birth incidence and mortality rate for people with Prader-Willi syndrome in one UK Health Region. *J Med Genet* 38(11):792–798, 2001.
111. Sternberg RJ (ed): *Handbook of Intelligence.* Cambridge, Cambridge University Press, 2000.
112. Sparrow SS, Davis SM: Recent advances in the assessment of intelligence and cognition. *J Child Psychol Psychiatry* 41:117–131, 2000.
113. Rusch FR, Chadsey JG (eds): *Beyond High School: Transition From School to Work.* Boston, MD, Allyn & Bacon, 1998.
114. National Center for Family Support: *Aging Family Caregivers: Needs and Policy Concerns.* Family support policy brief #3. National Center for Family Support @ HSRI, Winter, 2000.
115. Hodapp RM, Glidden LM, Kaiser AP: Siblings of persons with disabilities: toward a research agenda. *Ment Retard* 43:334–338, 2005.
116. Orsmond GI, Seltzer MM: Brothers and sisters of adults with mental retardation: gendered nature of the sibling relationship. *Am J on Ment Retard* 105:486–508, 2000.
117. Aylward EH, Burt DB, Thorpe LV, Lai F, Dalton A: Diagnosis of dementia in individuals with intellectual disability. *J Intellect Disabil Res* 41:152–164, 1997.
118. Richardson S, Koller H: Vulnerability and resilience of adults who were classified as mildly mentally handicapped in childhood. In: Tizard B, Varma V (eds): *Vulnerability and Resilience in Human Development.* London, Jessica Kingsley, 102–119, 1992.
119. Ross TT, Begab MK, Dondis EH, Giampiccolo JS, Meyers CE: *Lives of the Mentally Retarded: A Forty-Year Follow-Up Study.* Stanford, CA, Stanford University Press, 1985.
120. Crow YJ, Tolmie JL: Recurrence risks in mental retardation. *J Med Genet* 35:177–182, 1998.
121. Fombonne E, Bolton P, Prior J, et al.: A family study of autism: cognitive patterns and levels in parents and siblings. *J Child Psychol Psychiatry* 38:667–683, 1997.
122. Hodapp RM, Glidden LM, Kaiser AP: Siblings of persons with disabilities: toward a research agenda. *Ment Retard* 43:334–338, 2005.
123. Wang LW, Berry-Kravis E, Hagerman RJ. Fragile X: leading the way for targeted treatments in autism. *Neurotherapeutics* 7(3):264–274, 2010.

CHAPTER 5.2.3 ■ LEARNING DISABILITIES

ELENA L. GRIGORENKO

Fundamentally, the concept of learning disabilities (LD) enabled society to identify and serve children demonstrating unexplained school failure in a way that was not possible before the LD category was introduced in 1968 and legally recognized in 1969. The LD category replaced a variety of loose qualifiers such as "slow," "backward," and "feeble-minded" learner, among others. This public law, which ensures that students with LD are provided with Free Appropriate Public Education (FAPE) that is tailored to their individual needs has undergone a number of editions; its current version is known as the "Individuals with Disabilities Education Improvement Act" (IDEIA or IDEA,[1] used interchangeably, or Public Law 108–446 signed in 2004). It has included the category of LD in all of its editions, yet the identification of LD has been surrounded by controversy since the inception of this diagnostic category (1–3). This controversy, in many ways, is still a mark of the field.

In current practice, the LD label typically assumes the following. Under typical circumstances, LD are not diagnosable prior to the child's engagement with schooling and the opportunity to master key academic competencies. It is presumed that in school, a child is assigned tasks that are grade appropriate. These tasks suppose some degree of variability in children's performance; these assumptions constrain the definitions of acceptable and worrisome variability in performance. When the child's performance consistently falls out of the acceptable range in one or more academic subjects, then the child becomes the focus of intense observation and documentation and is referred for evaluation to appropriate professionals (e.g., educational psychologists, school counselors, clinical psychologists, neurologists, pediatricians, and psychiatrists). An important qualifier here is that such observation, documentation, and evaluation are considered only for children whose performance is below that expected based on their general capacity to learn; thus, the concept of "unexpected" school failure is central to the definition of LD. If something is "unexpected," then it could not have been predicted (or, at the minimum, predicted accurately). There are important safeguards that are used to minimize the risk of missing such unexpected events. First, although a diagnosable manifestation of LD can be unexpected, there are numerous risk factors that forewarn the relevant professionals about a possible onset of LD. These risk factors may be assessed and monitored as early as 3 years of age and are typically defined through various psychological processes that have to be recruited into the construction of a new academic skill. Second, public laws have special provisions—the Child Find Section of the IDEA (Child Find), Section 504 of the Rehabilitation Act of 1973, as amended (Section 504), and Title II of the Americans with Disabilities Act of 1990 (Title II)—that require local education

[1]The previous version of this law, Public Law 105–17 (signed in 1997), was called Individuals with Disabilities Education Act, IDEA.

agencies to identify and serve children with such "unexpected" difficulties in the acquisition of academic skills while in school.

When reports on the child's performance in the classroom, testing results, and clinical evaluations are compiled, the child and his or her family are referred to a committee (Planning and Placement Team), which determines the child's eligibility for individualized special education services. If eligibility is established, an individualized education program (IEP) is created for that child. The IEP refers to a specific diagnostic label carried by the child and cites the proper category of public laws that guarantees services for an individual with such a diagnosis.

DEFINITION

The definition that currently drives federal regulations was produced by the National Advisory Committee on Handicapped Children in 1968 and subsequently adopted by the U.S. Office of Education in 1977 (4). This definition has remained virtually unchanged in the IDEA (Title I, Part A, Sec. 602, §30). According to this definition, "*specific learning disability* means a disorder in one or more of the basic psychological processes involved in understanding or in using language, spoken or written, which may manifest itself in an imperfect ability to listen, think, speak, read, write, spell, or to do mathematical calculations. The term includes conditions such as perceptual handicaps, brain injury, minimal brain dysfunction, dyslexia, and developmental aphasia. The term does not include learning problems which are primarily the result of visual, hearing, or motor disabilities, of intellectual disability, or emotional disturbance, or of environmental, cultural, or economic disadvantage" (5).

The *Diagnostic and Statistical Manual of Mental Disorders*, fifth edition (DSM-5 (6)) does not use the term learning disabilities, but makes a reference to the term learning disorders. According to the DSM-5, "specific learning disorder can only be diagnosed after formal education starts but can be diagnosed at any point afterward in children, adolescents, or adults, providing there is evidence of onset during the years of formal schooling (i.e., the developmental period). No single data source is sufficient for a diagnosis of specific learning disorder. Rather, specific learning disorder is a clinical diagnosis based on a synthesis of the individual's medical, developmental, educational, and family history; the history of the learning difficulty, including its previous and current manifestation; the impact of the difficulty on academic, occupational, or social functioning; previous or current school reports; portfolios of work requiring academic skills; curriculum-based assessments; and previous or current scores from individual standardized tests of academic achievement" (p. 70). Of interest here is that this is one of the very few categories of the DSM-5 where a reference is made explicitly to psychological tests, although, as stated, DSM-5 does not provide specific guidelines as to what "substantially below" means. Thus, DSM-5 implicitly refers to evidence-based practices as they exist in the field. The problem, of course, is that there are multiple interpretations of these best practices (see discussion following). Yet, assuming there are consistent and coherent guidelines in place for establishing the diagnosis of LD, the DSM-5 classifies types of LD by referencing the primary academic areas of difficulty. The classification includes three specific categories: specific learning disorder with impairment in reading (315.00, F81.0), written expression (315.2, F81.81), and mathematics (315.1, F81.2). A common practice in the field is to view a diagnosis of a learning disorder as established by DSM-IV as an equivalent to "specific learning disability," which qualifies a child for special services under federal regulations. Of particular importance is the recognition that LD are lifelong disorders; however, reassessments are needed at meaningful intervals to trace the developmental transformations of LD.

HISTORY

The introduction of the concept of LD is typically credited to Samuel Kirk (then a professor of special education at the University of Illinois), who, while presenting at a conference in Chicago on April 6, 1963, proposed the term *learning disability* to refer to children who have disorders in development of language, speech, reading, and associated communication skills. The category was well received and promoted shortly thereafter by an established parent advocacy group known as the Association for Children with Learning Disabilities. Prior to the formal introduction of this concept, the literature had accumulated numerous descriptions of isolated cases and group analyses of children with specific deficits in isolated domains of academic performance (e.g., reading and mathematics) whose profiles were later reinterpreted as those of individuals with specific LD (e.g., specific reading and math disabilities). It is those examples in the literature and the experiences of many distressed parents desperate to find adequate educational support for their struggling children that, in part, resulted in the creation of the field of LD as a social reality and professional practice (7). The subsequent accumulation of research evidence and experiential pressure led to the formulation of legislation protecting the rights of children with LD.

Congress enacted the *Education for All Handicapped Children Act* (Public Law 94–142) in 1975 to support states and educational institutions in protecting the rights of, meeting the individual needs of, and improving the results of schooling for infants, toddlers, children, and youth with disabilities, and their families. This landmark law is currently enacted as the IDEA, as amended in 2004. In its 2004 version, the law was tightly associated with the No Child Left Behind (NCLB) Act. As NCLB was replaced in 2015 by the Every Student Succeeds Act (ESSA), major changes are expected in IDEA as well, as it is due for reauthorization. The importance of this law is difficult to overstate given that, prior to its enactment, in 1970, US schools provided education to only one in five children with disabilities (8). By the school year 2013–14, the number of children served under IDEA was 6.5 million, or 13% of the total public school enrollment. Approximately 35% of these students were classified as LD (9).

In its 2004 amendment, IDEA recognizes 13 categories under which a child can be identified as having a disability: autism; deaf-blindness; deafness; emotional disturbance; hearing impairment; intellectual disability; multiple disabilities; orthopedic impairment; other health impairment; specific learning disability; speech or language impairment; traumatic brain injury; and visual impairment, including blindness. Notably, LD as described above in IDEA are referred to as "specific learning disabilities" (SLD, hereafter, LD) to emphasize the difference between children with SLD and those with general learning difficulties (GLD) characteristic of other IDEA categories (e.g., autism and intellectual disability). The consensus in the field is that children with LD possess average to above-average levels of intelligence across general domains of functioning, but demonstrate specific deficits within a narrow range of academic skills. Finally, as stated above, exclusionary factors have been central to diagnoses of LD (10); a child cannot be diagnosed with an LD unless other factors such as other disorders or lack of exposure to high-quality age-, language-, and culture-appropriate educational environments have been ruled out. To rule out the lack of exposure to high-quality environments as an exclusionary factor, the 2004 amendment of IDEA introduced the concept of Response to Treatment Intervention (RTI)—"individual, comprehensive student-centered assessment models that apply a problem-solving framework to identify and address a student's learning difficulties" (11) (p. 483).

EPIDEMIOLOGY

There are two main sources for obtaining estimates for prevalence rates of LD. The first and most obvious one is linked to the number of children served under this category of IDEA. Figure 5.2.3.1 provides relevant data. When these data are mapped on the total number of children in the United States, although the number fluctuates from year to year, the average estimates of prevalence rates for LD are around 5% to 6% of the total school-age population.

Yet it is important to note that prevalence rates vary substantially from district to district and from state to state. For example, in 2011, of all students receiving special education services, those who received them under the category of LD comprise 14.1% in Kentucky compared with 60.4% in Iowa. Thus, based on these numbers, the prevalence rates of LD in Iowa are about 4.2 times as high as in Kentucky, two states not very far apart geographically! This observation stresses the mosaic-like situation of LD diagnosis: there is no unified approach to these diagnoses across different local education agencies in the United States.

When IDEA-related prevalence rates are considered, LD are diagnosed more frequently in boys than in girls (in 2013, these numbers were 9% and 6% for boys and girls aged 6 to 17, respectively). Of interest is that, in 2013, there were no significant differences in the rate of LD by race or Hispanic origin, although such differences (12) (i.e., LD was diagnosed more frequently in underrepresented minority groups than in Asian American or White) were often observed prior to the 2004 reauthorization.

The second source for these rates is research studies. Per results from these studies, it is assumed that although up to 10% to 12% of school-age children show specific deficits in selected academic domains, high-quality classroom instruction and supplemental intensive small-group activities can reduce this number to approximately 6% of children. It is assumed that these 6% will meet strict criteria for LD and will need special education intervention.

It is important to note that most of the research in the field of LD is disproportionally conducted with reading and, correspondingly, specific reading disability (SRD). Although there has been an exponential growth of the literature on mathematics (and specific math disability [SMD]) and writing (and specific writing disability [SWD]), the research on reading and SRD is where the frontiers of LD science currently are.

To illustrate, according to the results of current research on early reading acquisition, 2% to 6% of children do not show expected progress even in the context of the highest-quality evidence-based reading instructions. Based on US national data, the risk for reading problems as defined through failure to reach age- and grade-adequate milestones ranges from 20% to 80%. Specifically, data from the National Assessment of Educational Progress (http://www.nationsreportcard.gov/) 2015 show that only 36% of 4th, 34% of 8th, and 37% of 12th graders perform at or above a proficient level in reading, that is, possess the adequate reading skills required for the completion of grade-appropriate educational tasks. Similarly, only 40% of 4th, 33% of 8th, and 25% of 12th graders perform at or above a proficient level in math. The numbers for writing are available only for 2011 and only for 8th and 12th graders and they are 27% and 27%, respectively. However, it is clear that far from all of the children who perform below the proficiency level have SRD, SMD, or SWD. The majority of these children underachieve, most likely because of inadequate educational experiences or causes other than SRD.

Some changes in the 2004 version of IDEA were invoked directly because of concerns regarding the overidentification of students as having LD. The category of LD has often been the largest single category of children served under IDEA. The reality of everyday practices in school districts was such that most diagnoses prior to the 2004 reauthorization were based on so-called aptitude–achievement discrepancy criteria (AADC), which required a severe discrepancy between IQ and achievement scores (e.g., two standard deviations, 2 years of age equivalence), although IDEA had never specifically required a discrepancy formula. Correspondingly, it has been argued that these discrepancy-based approaches are flawed and might have led to overidentification, especially among minority youth (13). In light of this hypothesis, IDEA 2004 emphasizes that there is *no* explicit ability-achievement discrepancy requirement for the diagnosis of LD. As a possible alternative approach for identification and diagnosis, IDEA 2004 states that local educational agencies may use a child's RTI in lieu of the classification processes. A local educational agency (e.g., a school) may choose to administer to the child in question an evidence-based intervention program and, depending on the child's response to this program, determine his or her eligibility for special education services under IDEA.

Specifically, the statutory language of the IDEA 2004 states:

> *(6) Specific Learning Disabilities.*
> (A) In general.
> Notwithstanding section 607(b), when determining whether a child has a specific learning disability as defined in section 602, a local educational agency shall not be required to take

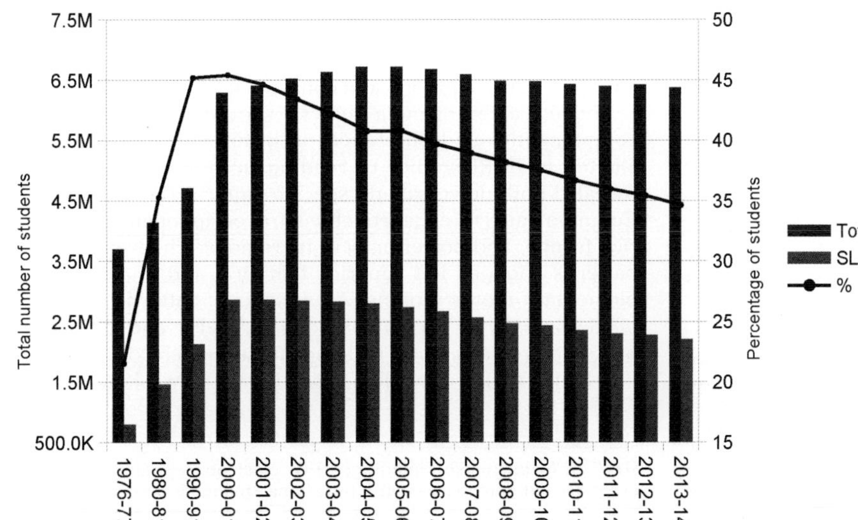

FIGURE 5.2.3.1. The absolute numbers (*left axis*, shown in *bars*) and percentage of children (*right axis*) diagnosed with SLD, out of the total number of children in special education in the United States, from 1976 to 2014.

into consideration whether a child has a severe discrepancy between achievement and intellectual ability in oral expression, listening comprehension, written expression, basic reading skill, reading comprehension, mathematical calculation, or mathematical reasoning.
(B) Additional authority.
In determining whether a child has a specific learning disability, a local educational agency may use a process that determines if the child responds to scientific, research-based intervention as a part of the evaluation procedures described in paragraphs (2) and (3). [§614(b)(6)].

As a consequence of this language, although AADC has been and continues to remain the common, although not required, practice for local educational agencies, there is a new "entry point" for RTI.[2] Moreover, as the IDEA language is rather ambiguous and alternative (to RTI) research-based approaches to the identification of LD are permitted, such approaches have been developed since 2004. One such approach is the Pattern of Strengths and Weaknesses (PSW) (14), which attempts to identify a core cognitive processing deficit (or a combination of deficits) as a source of LD. Yet, although present in the literature, this approach is considerably underresearched, compared to either discrepancy criteria or RTI.

Needless to say, these changes are of great theoretical and practical importance. A recent review of LD regulations and guidelines utilized in 2013 by all 50 of the United States and the District of Columbia (3) revealed a quilt-like variability of the interpretation of the IDEA across the United States. Specifically, with regard to the AADC, 67% of states allow and 20% of states explicitly prohibit its use. Approximately 16% of states require the sole use of RTI models and there are considerable differences in how this requirement is implemented. About 50% of states do not allow the use of PSW models, and most states allowing these models provide little information regarding ideal identification practices.

The implementation of RTI since the introduction of IDEA 2004 has generated much data. These data and their analyses have led to a number of observations. Specifically, although the field readily recognizes that the overall intentions and goals of RTI are laudable, (1) the empirical data for evidence-based intervention are rather inconsistent (again, it is more so for mathematics and writing, than reading); (2) the implementation of the RTI model is complex at best, driven in part by nonoverlap of different identification models and, in part, by inadequate teacher training; and (3) evidence of the power of RTI to prevent LD or introduce early identification is weak. It is because of these complexities that the concept of RTI was not included in the DSM-5. The DSM-5's requirement for "6-month persistence, despite targeted intervention" is there as an exclusionary criterion (i.e., to rule out the influence of inadequate instruction and to broadly view targeted intervention as any type of instruction, at home, school, or specialized services), not as a reference to RTI (15).

ETIOLOGY

There is a consensus in the field that LD arise from intrinsic factors and have neurobiologic bases, specifically atypicalities

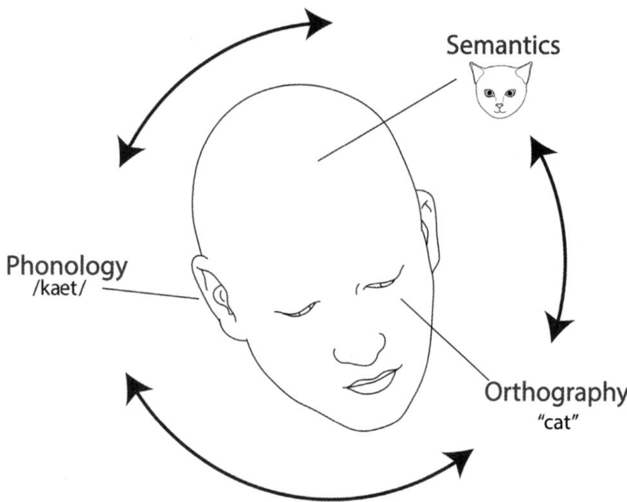

FIGURE 5.2.3.2. The componential view of reading.

of brain maturation and function that are rooted in the genome. There is a substantial body of literature convincingly supporting this consensus and pointing to genetic factors as major etiologic factors of LD. The working assumption is that these genetic factors affect the development, maturation, and functional structure of the brain, which in turn, influences cognitive processes associated with LD. Yet, the field is acutely aware that a number of external risk factors, such as poverty and lack of educational opportunities, affect patterns of brain development and function and, correspondingly, might worsen the prognosis for biologic predisposition for LD or act as a trigger in LD manifestation.

Although this model, in main strokes, appears to be relevant to all LD, far more research on relevant genes and brain structure and function is available for children with SRD (16) than for any other LD. Thus, here illustrative findings are presented from SRD; there are comprehensive reviews reflecting the state of the field for SMD (17) and SWD (18).

Multiple methodologic techniques (e.g., DTI, EEG, ERP, (f) MRI, MEG, PET, TMS, to name a few[3]) have been used to elicit brain-reading relationships. When data from multiple sources are combined, it appears that a developed, automatized skill of reading engages a wide, bilateral (but predominantly left hemispheric) network of brain areas passing activation from occipitotemporal, through temporal (posterior), toward frontal (precentral and inferior frontal gyri) lobes. The process of reading is multifaceted and involves the evocation of orthographical, phonologic, and semantic representations (Figure 5.2.3.2) that, in turn, call for the activation of brain networks participating in visual, auditory, and conceptual processing.

Indeed, a recent meta-analysis synthesizing age-related commonalities and differences in brain activation patterns elicited in fMRI studies of reading in children and adults revealed both universal and specific patterns (Figure 5.2.3.3). Common patterns engaged left ventral occipitotemporal, inferior frontal, and posterior parietal regions. Children-specific patterns engaged left superior temporal and bilateral supplementary motor regions. Adult-specific patterns engaged bilateral posterior occipitotemporal/cerebellar and left dorsal precentral regions. Thus, imaging studies underscore both the distributed nature of reading-related brain networks as well as

[2]It is important to note that RTI might appear counterintuitive at first: How can a disorder be defined through treatment if treatment is prescribed for a particular disorder? This "circularity" of RTI, however, is only superficial. An implicit assumption behind RTI is that teaching is inadequate and that is why schools "produce" such a high level of LD. A closer analogy would not be with treatment, but with prevention with vitamins; if vitamins were delivered properly, then many deficiencies could be avoided. Thus, if all children get preventive extensive instruction, the frequencies of LD will diminish.

[3]DTI, diffusion tensor imaging; EEG, electroencephalogram; ERP, event-related potentials; (f)MRI, (functional) magnetic resonance imaging; MEG, magnetoencephalography; PET, positron emission tomography; TMS, transcranial magnetic stimulation.

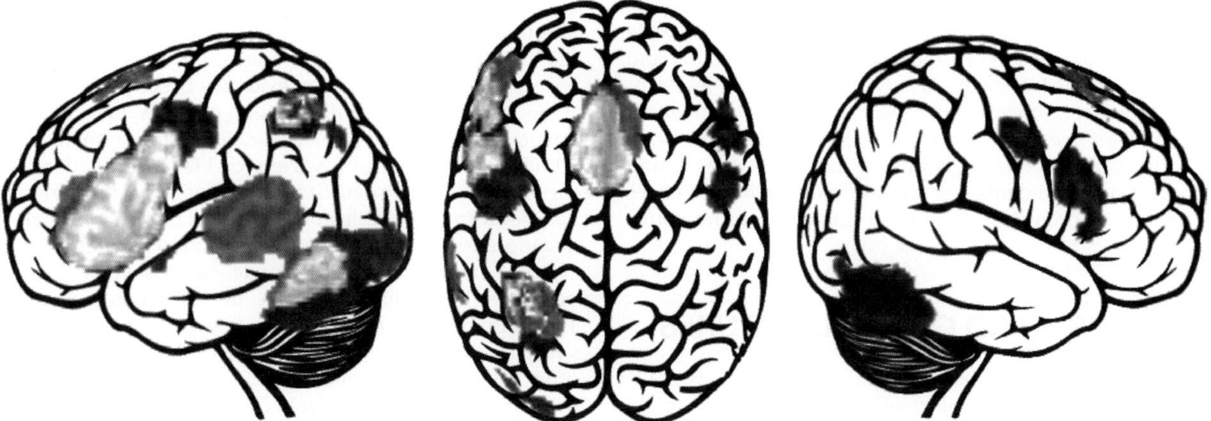

FIGURE 5.2.3.3. Surface renderings of maps of the brain circuitry for reading. Light gray indicates the overlapping areas of activation, medium gray—the areas specific to children, and dark gray—the areas specific to adults.

their malleability attributable to the maturation and automatization of reading-related skills. Globally speaking, the mastery of reading is marked by progressive, behaviorally modulated development of the left and progressive disengagement of the right hemisphere. In addition, there appears to be a shift of regional activation preferences: The frontal regions are used by fluent more than by beginning readers, and readers with difficulties activate the parietal and occipital regions more than the frontal regions.

In an attempt to understand the mechanism of the "deficient" pattern of brain activation while engaged in reading, researchers are looking for genes that might be responsible, at least partially, for these observed differences in functional brain patterns. This search is supported by a set of convergent lines of evidence (19–21). First, SRD has been considered a familial disorder since the late 19th century. This consideration is grounded in years of research into the familiality of SRD (similarity in the skill of reading among relatives of different degrees), characterized by studies that have engaged multiple genetic methodologies, specifically twin, family, sib-pair, and case-control designs. Although each of these methodologies has its own resolution power with regard to obtaining corresponding estimates of relative contributions of genes and environments, all methodologies have produced data that unanimously point to the genome as the main source of individual differences in reading and of the manifestation of SRD.

Today, it is assumed that multiple genes contribute to the biologic risk factor that forms the foundation for the development of SRD (Figure 5.2.3.4). Specifically, nine candidate regions of the human genome have been implicated. These regions are recognized as SRD candidate regions; they are abbreviated as DYX1–9 (DYX for dyslexia, a term often used to refer to SRD) and refer to the regions on chromosomes 15q, 6p, 2p, 6q, 3cen, 18p, 11p, 1p, and Xq, respectively. Each of these regions harbors dozens of genes, and some of them have been named as risk genes for SRD. These genes are: two for the 15q region, *DYX1C1* and *SEMA6D;* two for the 6p region, *KIAA0319* and *DCDC2;* two for the 2p region, *C2Orf3* and *MRPL19;* and one for the 3cen region, *ROBO1.* Although the field has not yet converged on "firm" candidates, it is remarkable and of scientific interest that of the current candidate genes for SRD, five genes (*DYX1C1, SEMA6D, KIAA0319, DCDC2,* and *ROBO1*) are involved in biologic functions of neuronal migration and axonal crossing. Thus, all these genes are plausible candidates

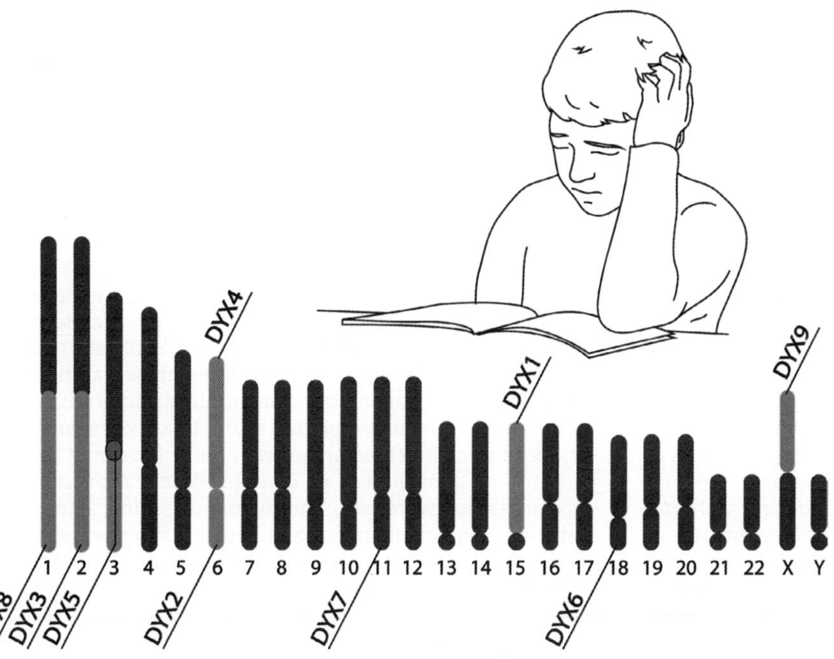

FIGURE 5.2.3.4. Genomic regions of interest for specific reading disability (SRD).

for understanding the pattern of brain functioning in SRD. Yet, there are caveats. Specifically, until now, three genome-wide association studies (GWAS) (22–24) have been carried out and none have identified, in an unbiased manner, any of these candidates. Moreover, other genes known to be associated with a variety of cognitive processes, have been shown to be associated with reading and other cognitive functions, questioning the specificity of the genetic sources of individual differences for variation in reading as well as in related brain functions (25,26).

DIAGNOSIS AND CLINICAL FEATURES

As stated earlier, it is crucially important in a diagnosis of LD to establish the "typical" intellectual performance of the child and to document that the child's performance in the area of difficulty (i.e., reading, writing, or mathematics) does not correspond to what would be expected given average ability level. Although this general principle is relatively easy to grasp, the field of LD has, since its inception in the early 1960s, struggled with establishing specific steps that prescriptively should lead to the establishment of the diagnosis.

As mentioned earlier, prior to the 2004 reauthorization of IDEA, the most common way of establishing an LD diagnosis was the AADC. Historically, the introduction of the discrepancy between ability and achievement as a criterion for LD in the 1977 law was not based on empirical research, but rather driven by a need for a more objective approach to the diagnosis than those commonly used and largely discredited at the time (27). Two decades of research and practical explorations of the discrepancy model have resulted in it being discredited from points of view of theory, reliability of diagnosis and classification, robustness of implementation, and treatment validity. In response to the overwhelming amount of evidence for the inadequacy of the discrepancy model, however realized (through psychometric indices, age equivalences, regression approaches, or expert opinions), a number of alternative models have been proposed. The major dividing line between these new models and previous discrepancy-based models is in their theoretical orientation. Previous diagnostic models attempted to identify children diagnosable with LD by looking for characteristic cognitive deficits, so that an intervention could be delivered to children with such deficits, whereas modern models argue for the need to deliver the best pedagogical practices to all children and then best remediation-intervention approaches to those children who do not respond well to good teaching.

In its most general form, the RTI model has a number of features. First, the performance of the student in question is compared with the performance of his/her immediate peers on academic tasks. Specifically, RTI assumes tracking the academic performance and the rate of growth for all students within a given class, with a goal of identifying those students in a class whose performance differs from that of their peers both in absolute (level) and relative (rate of growth) terms. Second, the model is structured primarily by intervention, so that students identified by these means are offered individualized accommodations and interventions with a goal of maximizing the effectiveness of the learning environment for a given student in need. Third, the model is multilayered, so that each layer offers an opportunity for the further differentiation and individualization of education for students who need it. Typically, three layers are recommended. The first tier covers the regular classroom environment; the second tier is characterized as "supplemental" to tier 1; and tier 3 is "intensive," "individualized," and "strategic." Fourth, only when these multilayered attempts to modify the regular classroom pedagogical environment have proved unsuccessful is the prospect of establishing an LD diagnosis considered. In summary, a child could be identified as having an LD if he or she consistently fails to perform at a level and rate of progress comparable with the child's peers in general education, after having experienced and participated in an evidence-based intervention.

As per the 2004 reauthorization of IDEA, local educational agencies have some choice in selecting diagnostic models, which has resulted in a variety of LD identification models throughout the United States. Specifically, the federal law has permitted the utilization of an RTI approach for over a decade and some states have mandated it. Similarly, some states opened up to the PSW model. So, has either RTI or PSW proven to be better than AADC for the identification of LD? The bottom line is that opinions (and data) vary. Specifically, some researchers assert that an RTI approach does indeed offer a superior approach to LD identification, because, in part, this identification is embedded in the educational process and is instructive, if nothing else, for providing accommodations and services (1). Congruently, there is an argument that the focus on both assessing and remediating specific cognitive processes, as proposed by the PSW model, does not pan out to be advantageous (28). Yet, there are also multiple criticisms of RTI and suggestions that the true solution lies in combining elements of RTI and PSW approaches (29), as they inform identification differentially and have different roles in answering questions of the *why* LD and *how* to remediate it.

RELEVANT THEORETICAL MODELS AND CONSIDERATIONS

As mentioned earlier, the literature on LD is uneven, with the vast majority of it relating to SRD, although within the last few years much progress has been made with regard to SMD and SWD. Although psychological models of other LD have been developed, here only those for SRD are exemplified for illustration purposes.

So far, there have been only generic references to the disruption of both the acquisition and mastery of reading skills that constitutes the texture of SRD. When this generic reference is closely considered, another massive body of literature materializes: (1) cognitive psychology literature (30) on the types of representation of information involved in reading (reading involves the translation of meaningful symbolic visual codes [orthographical representation] into pronounceable and distinguishable sounds of language [phonologic representation] so that a meaning [semantic representation] can be derived); (2) developmental psychology literature on when these representations develop and what might cause the development of a dysfunctional representational system (31); and (3) educational psychology literature on how the formation of functional representations can be aided or corrected when at risk for malfunctioning (32). One of the major theoretical frameworks for reading (30) is shown in Figure 5.2.3.2.

Here only brief commentaries relevant to these literatures are offered. Today, given the predominance of the phonology-based connectionist accounts of SRD, the behavioral manifestation of SRD is captured through a collection of correlated psychological traits. Although different researchers use different terms for specific traits, these can be loosely structured into groups aimed at capturing different types of information representation, for example: (1) performance on orthographic choice or homonym choice judgment tasks for quantifying parameters of orthographical representation; (2) phonemic awareness, phonologic decoding, and phonologic memory for quantifying phonologic representation; and (3) vocabulary and indices of comprehension at different levels of linguistic processing for quantifying semantic representation. Correspondingly, in studies of the etiology, development, and educational malleability of SRD, the quantification of the disorder is carried out through these various traits (or components of SRD). Thus, many studies attempt to subdivide SRD into its components and explore their etiologic bases, developmental trajectories, and susceptibility to pedagogical interventions separately as well as jointly.

DIFFERENTIAL DIAGNOSIS

The majority of students with LD are identified in middle and high school; this occurrence can be explained by the fact that early years of schooling might simply be insufficient for exposing and making evident a deficit in a particular academic domain. As mentioned, the core conceptual piece of the LD definition is that the deficit could have not been predicted reliably prior to the child's school entry because a child with LD demonstrates otherwise typical levels of cognitive functioning. Yet, there are known risk factors, the major cluster of which implicates atypicalities in early language development (33).

Previously, when the discrepancy criteria were applied, the diagnosis of LD was different from other forms of learning difficulties because of its stress on the specificity of the deficit (i.e., a discrepancy was expected not in *all* academic domains, but in a *specific* academic domain). The introduction of RTI-based approaches to diagnosis makes the question of differential diagnosis somewhat difficult to address. In fact, students with intellectual disability, emotional or behavior disorders, attention deficit hyperactivity disorder (ADHD), and other childhood and adolescent disorders might also exhibit low responsiveness to intervention. Yet their nonresponsiveness will occur for reasons very different from those experienced by students with LD. In other words, if RTI cannot differentiate LD from other diagnoses where learning difficulties are present but nonspecific, can RTI even be considered a classification/diagnostic instrument (34)?

Although this question has been raised, it has not yet been answered. The pre-2004 conceptualization of LD assumed that the texture of LD was in deficient (or different, atypical) psychological processing of information. In other words, the field was driven by the assumption that LD were likely to represent a dysfunction in one or more basic psychological processes (phonologic processing, sustained attention, different types of memory, executive functioning). These deficient processes, in turn, could slow down or inhibit mastery of a particular academic domain (reading or mathematics). Under this assumption, intensive academic instruction could improve performance in specific academic domains, but could not treat the disorder. Even if reading improves as a result of intervention, in this paradigm, the disorder might remanifest as a deficiency in a bordering domain (writing). In other words, although reading skills might be enhanced, the deficient psychological skills might impede some other academic domain of functioning.

Throughout the existence of the category of LD, there has been a consistent and strong demand from parents, researchers, and educators for the differentiation of these disorders from GLD. In its current iteration, RTI does not differentiate nonspecific and specific learning difficulties, because nonresponsiveness to intervention can occur with a variety of developmental disorders. In sum, because IDEA preserved the category of SLD, there is a new demand to differentiate SLD and GLD by means of RTI and possibly other methods in the field.

One of these "other" methods has to do, of course, with psychological testing. Many researchers argue for the necessity of maintaining the role of psychoeducational and neuropsychologic tests on a variety of indicators, including IQ, in establishing an LD diagnosis (35). And this is exactly why the PSW model was introduced, although, at this point, there is not enough evidence to argue for its advantages.

COURSE AND PROGNOSIS

There is an accepted understanding in the field that LD are typically lifelong disorders, although their manifestations might and often do vary depending on the developmental stage and the demands of the environment (school, work, retirement) imposed on an individual at a particular time. This understanding assumes that LD do not manifest themselves exclusively in academic settings. In fact, the assumption here is that, although it might be successfully remediated during years of schooling, a particular LD might need further assistance and remediation in later years of functioning (as a part of the workforce). Although the literature on adults with LD is still somewhat limited, there is an accumulation of evidence that LD constitute a serious public health problem even after the schooling years. Such evidence is particularly rich in the field of studies of SRD.

LD are comorbid with a number of other disorders typically diagnosed in childhood or adolescence, especially attention deficit (36) and disruptive behavior disorders (37). LD also often co-occur with anxiety and depression (38). Correspondingly, individuals with LD are at higher risk for developing other mental health problems.

Yet the main drawback for individuals with LD has to do with their educational achievement. On average, only approximately 50% of students aged 14 and older diagnosed with LD graduate with regular high school diplomas. Correspondingly, the dropout rate among these students is very high (approximately 45%), and even higher for underrepresented minority students. The employment prospects of these students are also troubling—only about 60% of students aged 14 and older diagnosed with LD have paid jobs outside the home.

Thus, it is important to realize that the impact of LD is not limited to any one academic domain (reading or mathematics); these are lifetime disorders with wide-ranging consequences.

TREATMENT

Currently, there are no approved medical treatments for children with LD. There is a consensus in the field that children with LD should be provided special education and related services upon establishing their eligibility and determining the necessity, content, duration, and desired outcomes of such education and services.

Yet, in much of the literature, many educators have expressed concern with the possible presence of faulty identification procedures in states and districts across the country, which has resulted in the possible abuse of the classification and service systems. In response to this concern, the 2004 reauthorization of IDEA makes reference to a set of prevention mechanisms intended to establish a better classification strategy for identifying children with LD. By law, schools need to implement systemic models of prevention that address (1) primary prevention: the provision of high-quality education for all children; (2) secondary prevention: targeted, scientifically based interventions for children who are not responding to primary prevention; and (3) tertiary prevention: the provision of intensive individualized services and interventions for those children who have not responded to high-quality instruction or subsequent intervention efforts. Per new regulations, it is assumed that this third group of children, those children who have failed to respond to age-, language-, and culture-appropriate, evidence-based, domain-specific instruction (in reading or mathematical cognition), can be identified as eligible for special education services. Of importance here is that these prevention mechanisms are also assumed to be used as diagnostic mechanisms (see the earlier discussion of RTI).

This circular system of an outcome of intervention being also an entry point to diagnosis is currently creating significant turmoil in the literature and in practice.

In general, RTI approaches are conceived as a twofold simultaneous realization of high-quality, domain-specific instruction and continuous formative evaluation of students' performance and learning (39,40). In other words, RTI refers to ongoing assessment of students' response to evidence-based pedagogical interventions in particular academic domains. Thus, it is assumed that LD can be identified *only* when underachievement related to poor instruction is ruled out (6). Although present in a number of alternative forms, RTI includes eight central features and six common attributes. Among the central features linking all forms of RTI are: (1) high-quality classroom instruction; (2) research-based instruction; (3) classroom performance measures; (4) universal screening; (5) continuous progress monitoring; (6) research-based intervention; (7) progress monitoring during intervention; and (8) fidelity measures. Among common attributes of different RTI models, there are concepts of (1) multiple tiers; (2) transition from instruction for all to increasingly intense interventions; (3) implementation of differentiated curricula; (4) instruction delivered by staff other than the classroom teacher; (5) varied duration, time, and frequency of intervention; and (6) categorical or noncategorical placement decisions (41). Clearly, the concept of RTI is centered on the field's consensus of what high-quality, research-validated instruction is. It is important to note that, although there is growing consensus with regard to critical elements for effective reading instruction, other domains of teaching for academic competencies are still not consensus driven.

There are numerous examples of RTI-based treatment of LD; two oft-cited ones are the Minneapolis Public School's Problem Solving Model, which has been in action since 1994 (42), and the Heartland (Iowa) Area Education Association's (AEA) Model, implemented in 1986 (43). The Minneapolis model is a three-tier intervention model where the referral to special education is made only after consecutive failures to benefit from instruction throughout all three tiers of pedagogical efforts. The Iowa model originally included four tiers, where the third tier was subdivided into two related steps, but then collapsed into one tier, similar to the Minneapolis model. Unfortunately, neither model has published empirical data on its effectiveness. Yet, years of implementations have resulted in appreciation from the communities they serve in a stable, relatively low special education population.

Currently, the concept of RTI is under careful examination by researchers supported by both the U.S. Department of Education and the National Institute of Child Health and Development. The future of RTI and its role in diagnosing and treating LD is dependent on answers to critical questions: (1) whether an RTI model can be implemented on a large scale; (2) how an RTI model can be used for LD eligibility determination; (3) whether RTI is an effective prevention system; and (4) whether RTI enhances LD determination and minimizes the number of false positives. As the field is getting ready for the reauthorization of the IDEA, answers to these questions become essential for how the federal law, in its next iteration, will define LD.

CONCLUSION

Currently, students with LD constitute about one-third of all students served under IDEA. Effective identification of such students and their efficacious and efficient remediation are crucial steps to addressing their individual educational needs and providing them with adequate and equitable life opportunities.

Given changes in IDEA 2004, it is of no surprise that RTI is central to current discourse on LD. RTI is central to professional discussions of educators, diagnosticians, and policymakers because of its promise to alleviate many long-standing concerns with the AADC predominant in the field of LD for the last 30 years. At this point, however, RTI has yet to deliver on its promise and PSW has yet to be thoroughly researched. The next year or two, as the reauthorization of IDEA gets underway, will be key, once again, for revisiting the criteria for the identification of LD.

AUTHOR NOTE

Preparation of this chapter was supported by grants R305H140050 from the Institute for Educational Sciences, Department of Education, and P50 HD052120 from the National Institutes of Health. Grantees undertaking such projects are encouraged to express freely their professional judgment. This article, therefore, does not necessarily represent the position or policies of the IES or the NIH, and no official endorsement should be inferred. The author expresses sincere gratitude to Ms. Mei Tan for her editorial assistance and Ms. Natalie Banker for preparing the figures.

References

1. Reschly DJ: Response to intervention and the identification of specific learning disabilities. *Top Lang Disord* 34:39–58, 2014.
2. Zumeta RO, Zirkel PA, Danielson L: Identifying specific learning disabilities legislation, regulation, and court decisions. *Top Lang Disord* 34:8–24, 2014.
3. Maki KE, Floyd RG, Roberson T: State learning disability eligibility criteria: a comprehensive review. *Sch Psychol Q* 30:457–469, 2015.
4. Mercer CD, Jordan L, Allsopp DH, Mercer AR: Learning disabilities definitions and criteria used by state education departments. *Learn Disabil Q* 19:217–232, 1996.
5. U.S. Department of Education: *Building the Legacy: IDEA 2004*. Vol 20162006. Washington, DC, U.S. Department of Education.
6. APA: *Diagnostic and Statistical Manual of Mental Disorders*. 5th ed. Washington, DC, American Psychiatric Association, 2013.
7. Hallahan DP, Mock DR: A brief history of the field of learning disabilities. In: Swanson HL, Harris KR, Graham S (eds): *Handbook of Learning Disabilities*. New York, Guilford Press, 16–29, 2003.
8. OSEP: *History: Twenty-Five Years of Progress in Educating Children With Disabilities Through IDEA*. Washington, DC, US Department of Education, Office of Special Education Programs, 2000.
9. Kena G, Hussar W, McFarland J, et al.: The Condition of Education 2016. *NCES 2016-144*. Washington, DC, National Center for Education Statistics, U.S. Department of Education, 2016.
10. Fletcher JM, Lyon GR, Fuchs LS, Barnes MA: *Learning Disabilities: From Identification to Intervention*. 2nd ed. New York, Guilford Press, 2016.
11. Deshler DD, Mellard DF, Tollefson JM, Byrd SE: Research topics in responsiveness to intervention: introduction to the special series. *J Learn Disabil* 38:483–484, 2005.
12. Pane NE: *How are students with disabilities performing in school?* Bethesda, MD, Child Trends, 2015. Available at: https://www.childtrends.org/how-are-students-with-disabilities-performing-in-school/.
13. Cavendish W: Identification of learning disabilities: implications of proposed DSM-5 criteria for school-based assessment. *J Learn Disabil* 46:52–57, 2013.
14. Hale JB, Kaufman A, Naglieri JA, Kavale KA: Implementation of IDEA: integrating response to intervention and cognitive assessment methods. *Psychol Sch* 43:753–770, 2006.
15. Tannock R: Provision of evidence-based intervention is not part of the DSM-5 diagnostic criteria for specific learning disorder. *Eur Child Adolesc Psychiatry* 25:209–210, 2016.
16. Elliott JG, Grigorenko EL: *The Dyslexia Debate*. New York, Cambridge, 2014.
17. Geary DC: Consequences, characteristics, and causes of mathematical learning disabilities and persistent low achievement in mathematics. *J Dev Behav Pediatr* 32:250–263, 2011.
18. Grigorenko EL, Mambrino E, Preiss D: *Writing: A Mosaic of Perspectives*. New York, Psychology Press, 2012.
19. Kere J: The molecular genetics and neurobiology of developmental dyslexia as model of a complex phenotype. *Biochem Biophys Res Commun* 452:236–243, 2014.
20. Peterson RL, Pennington BF: Developmental dyslexia. *Annu Rev Clin Psychol* 11:283–307, 2015.
21. Bishop DV: The interface between genetics and psychology: lessons from developmental dyslexia. *Proc Biol sci* 282:20143139, 2015.
22. Gialluisi A, Newbury DF, Wilcutt EG, et al.: Genome-wide screening for DNA variants associated with reading and language traits. *Genes Brain Behav* 13:686–701, 2014.

23. Luciano M, Evans DM, Hansell NK, et al.: A genome-wide association study for reading and language abilities in two population cohorts. *Genes Brain Behav* 12:645–652, 2013.
24. Eicher JD, Powers NR, Miller LL, et al.; Pediatric Imaging, Neurocognition, and Genetics Study: Genome-wide association study of shared components of reading disability and language impairment. *Genes Brain Behav* 12:792–801, 2013.
25. Landi N, Frost S, Mencl EW, et al.: COMT Val/Met polymorphism is associated with reading-related skills and consistent patterns of functional neural activation. *Dev Sci* 16(1):13–23, 2012.
26. Jasińska KK, Molfese PJ, Kornilov SA, et al.: The BDNF Val66Met polymorphism influences reading ability and patterns of neural activation in children. *PLoS One* 11:e0157449, 2016.
27. Gresham FM, Reschly DJ, Tilly WD, et al.: Comprehensive evaluation of learning disabilities: a response to intervention perspective. *The School Psychologist* 59:26–29, 2004.
28. Fletcher JM, Stuebing KK, Barth AE, Miciak J, Francis DJ, Denton CA: Agreement and coverage of indicators of response to intervention: a multi-method comparison and simulation. *Top Lang Disord* 34:74–89, 2014.
29. Johnson ES: Understanding why a child is struggling to learn the role of cognitive processing evaluation in learning disability identification. *Top Lang Disord* 34:59–73, 2014.
30. Harm MW, Seidenberg MS: Computing the meanings of words in reading: cooperative division of labor between visual and phonological processes. *Psychol Rev* 111:662–720, 2004.
31. Karmiloff-Smith A: Development itself is the key to understanding developmental disorders. *Trends Cogn Sci* 2:389–398, 1998.
32. Blachman BA, Schatschneider C, Fletcher JM, et al.: Effects of intensive reading remediation for second and third graders and a 1-year follow-up. *J Educ Psychol* 96:444–461, 2004.
33. Sun L, Wallach GP: Language disorders are learning disabilities: challenges on the divergent and diverse paths to LLD. *Top Lang Disord* 34:25–38, 2014.
34. Mastropieri MA, Scruggs TE: Feasibility and consequences of response to intervention: examination of the issues and scientific evidence as a model for the identification of individuals with learning disabilities. *J Learn Disabil* 38:525–531, 2005.
35. Semrud-Clikeman M: Neuropsychological aspects for evaluating learning disabilities. *J Learn Disabil* 38:563–568, 2005.
36. Semrud-Clikeman M, Biederman J, Sprich-Buckminster S, Lehman BK, Faraone SV, Norman D: Comorbidity between ADDH and learning disability: a review and report in a clinically referred sample. *J Am Acad Child Adolesc Psychiatry* 31:439–448, 1992.
37. Grigorenko EL: Learning disabilities in juvenile offenders. *Child Adolesc Psychiatr Clin N Am* 15:353–371, 2006.
38. Martinez RS, Semrud-Clikeman M: Emotional adjustment and school functioning of young adolescents with multiple versus single learning disabilities. *J Learn Disabil* 37:411–420, 2004.
39. Mellard DF, Deshler DD, Barth A: LD identification: it's not simply a matter of building a better mousetrap. *Learn Disabil Q* 27:229–242, 2004.
40. Mellard DF, Byrd SE, Johnson E, Tollefson JM, Boesche L: Foundations and research on identifying model Responsiveness-to-Intervention sites. *Learn Disabil Q* 27:243–256, 2004.
41. Graner PS, Faggetta-Luby MN, Fritschmann NS: An overview of responsiveness to intervention: what practitioners ought to know. *Top Lang Disord* 25:93–105, 2005.
42. Marston D, Muyskens P, Lau M, Canter A: Problem-solving model for decision making with high-incidence disabilities: the minneapolis experience. *Learn Disabil Res Prac* 18:187–200, 2003.
43. Ikeda MJ, Gustafson JK: *Heartland AEA 11' Problem Solving Process: Impact on Issues Related to Special Education.* Johnston, IA, Heartland Area Educational Agency 11, 2002.

CHAPTER 5.2.4 ■ DISORDERS OF COMMUNICATION

ELIZABETH SCHOEN SIMMONS AND RHEA PAUL

Language, a unique and characteristic capacity of the human mind, is also one of its most vulnerable faculties. Virtually any disruption in cognitive function, particularly during early development, can affect language acquisition. For this reason, disorders of language development typically accompany a variety of conditions but they can occur in relative isolation as well. It is also true that language is just one form of communication. The term *communication* refers to all forms of sending and receiving messages, not only with spoken language, but in other ways, such as with gestures or facial expressions. Within the realm of communication, *language* represents one specific type, which involves generating a potentially infinite set of never-before conveyed messages through the combination of symbols in rule-governed ways that allow the formation of sentences to express meaning to others. Language, like communication, can be conveyed in a variety of forms including written expression or manual signs seen in American Sign Language (ASL). *Speech,* on the other hand, is a particular modality of language, its expression through the use of sounds produced by oral movements (Figure 5.2.4.1).

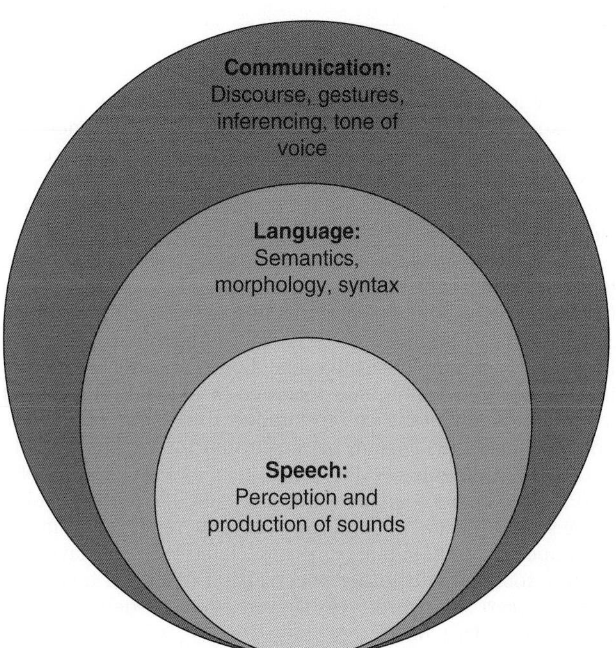

FIGURE 5.2.4.1. Relationship among speech, language, and communication and their components.

DEFINITIONS

The American Speech-Language-Hearing Association (ASHA) has defined *language disorder* as an impairment in "comprehension and/or use of a spoken, written, and/or other symbol system. The disorder may involve (1) the form of language (phonologic, morphologic, and syntactic systems), (2) the content of language (semantic system), and/or (3) the function of language in communication (pragmatic system), in any combination" (1, p. 40). This definition means that a language disorder can be seen as a disruption in any aspect of verbal communication, whether oral or written. It is important to note that this impairment is not necessarily defined only in relation to cognitive level or mental age. Current practice (2) dictates that any child whose language is inadequate for communication can be diagnosed as having a language disorder, even a child who is intellectually disabled with a mental age commensurate with his current level of language function.

Speech disorders are more limited difficulties that refer to problems with the production of spoken language, although comprehension may be intact. Speech disorders can affect the fluency of speech (e.g., stuttering), the perceived quality of production (e.g., voice disorders), or the pronunciation of particular sounds (e.g., articulation disorders).

EPIDEMIOLOGY

Accurate estimates of prevalence of specific language disorders are difficult to come by because of methodologic differences across studies (e.g., in the subclassifications and definitions; in the cutoffs and inclusionary criteria; and in the age, sex, and other characteristics of the children sampled). However, delays in language development are the most common presenting symptom in preschool children (3). The most recent NIH estimates prevalence for speech/language disorders at 11% for children 3 to 5 years old and 9% for those 6 to 8 years old (4,5). The prevalence estimate is 8% for boys and 6% for girls (6).

In post-primary school age, the prevalence of primary language disorders is thought to be between 4% and 7% (7), although there is overlap with related disorders, because some preschoolers with language disorders "grow into" school-age learning disabilities and dyslexia (8). Specific language disorders and learning disabilities combined are some of the most prevalent disorders of school-age children (9).

ETIOLOGY

Again, etiologic discussions are complicated by the fact that language disorders can exist as circumscribed syndromes, but also accompany a range of other developmental disorders. For this reason, we will restrict our discussion of etiology to specific language impairment (SLI). Neurobiologic factors are clearly implicated in the disorder as evidenced by genetic factors in SLI (10), including higher concordance in monozygotic than dizygotic twins (11) and higher than normal risk in family members for language and learning problems if a child has SLI (12–14). Additionally, there is emerging evidence that has identified candidate genes that may be responsible for behavioral phenotypes commonly observed in SLI (15). The results of these linkage investigations suggest that single nucleotide polymorphisms (SNPs) may be responsible for language ability and disability. While specific genes, such as FOXP2 and CNTNAP2 (16,17) have been identified as candidate genes in SLI in some studies, these findings have yet to be replicated. Finally, it is important to note that genes associated with SLI have also been associated with other psychiatric conditions including autism spectrum disorder (ASD) and attention-deficit hyperactivity disorder (18).

Just how specific are specific language disorders? Children with SLI are at greatly increased risk for attention and activity problems (19,20). Other "soft" neurologic signs are also frequently present in children with SLI (21). A variety of nonverbal cognitive skills have also been implicated in SLI (22,23). These findings have led to the hypothesis that children with SLI may have not just a language problem, but a general representational deficit, affecting a variety of kinds of symbolic functioning (24), deficits in aspects of cognition, primarily memory (25,26).

Imaging studies have demonstrated some differences in brain function between children with and without specific language disorders. Typically, individuals have asymmetrical brains; language structures (such as the planum temporale) tend to be bigger in the left hemisphere. However, children with SLI have generally smaller and more symmetrical brain hemispheres (27). Studies of adults with language difficulties have revealed that they were more likely than individuals with no history of language impairment to have an extra sulcus in Broca's area, in either brain hemisphere (28). Studies that employ functional imaging techniques have revealed less activation within the gray matter during auditory tasks (29). A recent review of neuroimaging studies in language disorders (30) reports both functional and structural anomalies associated with language disorders, primarily in the finding of greater activity and volume relative to controls. Cortical and subcortical atypicalities in the language network have been reported, with little consistency across studies, except in the superior temporal gyri. It is important to realize that no single patten of brain architecture has been shown consistently in all individuals with language impairment. Instead, these structural differences appear to act as risk factors for language difficulty.

In summary, there is evidence for a genetic component in specific speech and language disorder. However, there are few agreed upon biologic markers of SLI. Although neurobiologic methods have demonstrated differences in the neural structure and auditory functioning of children with SLI, reliable clinical markers have not yet emerged.

SYNDROMES INVOLVING COMMUNICATION DISORDERS

Intellectual Disability

Limitation in communicative skill is often one of the first signs of intellectual disability (ID). Children with ID are often first recognized because of their failure to begin talking at the normal time. The sequence of language acquisition in children with this disability follows, in general, the sequence of normal acquisition, although some differences can be identified (31). Many children with ID show communicative skills that are commensurate with their developmental level, but more than half have language skills that are less than what would be expected for mental age (32). Phonologic errors are prevalent in children with ID. These children make similar errors to those seen in normal development, but errors are more frequent (33). Pragmatic skills are usually similar to those seen in children at similar developmental levels (34). The two most prevalent syndromes of ID, Down syndrome (DS) and fragile X syndrome, are both very frequently associated with various problems in language development (35,36). About a third of children with fragile X also exhibit symptoms of autism (37). Social communication skills in many children with DS tend to be relatively preserved, although 8% to 14% of this population, too, is reported to show symptoms of autism (38). Other syndromes, such as Prader–Willi, also exhibit language deficits (31). Even in Williams syndrome, in which it was previously thought that language was an unexpected strength, research has shown that language is preserved relative to nonverbal skills, but does not typically exceed developmental level (39).

Hearing Impairment

Children with impaired hearing are vulnerable to language disorders because of their lack of access to the linguistic information from the auditory signal. Still, children with hearing impairments (HIs) vary greatly in their oral language ability. With hearing aids, children can be moved from greater to lesser levels of severity of hearing loss. Cochlear implants and tactile aids are also used to provide auditory information to children who would otherwise be considered deaf (40). In recent years, cochlear implants are being used more routinely at earlier ages to facilitate language development in children born with severe hearing loses, and research (41–43) suggests this results in very good outcomes in terms of speech and understanding language.

Use of language for communication is not a major problem area for children with HI. Rather, most of their difficulties lie in acquiring the conventional verbal forms of communication. Reading and writing present particular problems, primarily because of the language basis necessary for acquiring these skills. Average reading comprehension level for adolescents with HI without cochlear implants is third to fourth grade (44–46). Language and reading outcomes for children who receive cochlear implants are generally higher (42,47).

Some children with HI, especially those who come from families in which one or more parent is deaf, can be taught to bypass the auditory channel through the use of manual Sign language. Using this method, children can develop fluency and eloquence in sign that would never be available to them through the modality of speech. There is controversy within the community of the hearing impaired as to the role of Sign language versus oral language instruction for children with severe hearing loss. In general, nonimplanted deaf children taught sign develop higher-level language skills than those taught speech, although their communication may be limited to those in the deaf community who use sign as their mode of communication.

Psychiatric Disorders

There is a very high comorbidity between sociobehavioral and communicative disorders (47,48). Benner et al. (50) found, in a meta-analysis, that over 70% of children diagnosed with emotional–behavioral disorders (EBD) had clinically significant language deficits. The deficits were broad-based and included expressive, receptive, and pragmatic aspects of language. This finding has been confirmed in studies of bilingual children as well (51). In addition, over 50% of children diagnosed with language deficits also had diagnosable EBD. Further, the number of children who have both communicative and behavioral–socioemotional disorders increases as children with language disorders get older (52). It may be impossible to know the source of this connection. Some writers (53) hold that a communication problem leads to frustration, creating behavioral or emotional disorders. It may, alternatively, be the case that a behavioral–socioemotional problem leads to decreased motivation to communicate or an inability to "tune in" to learn the rules of communication or use language for self- and other-regulation (54) or perhaps diagnostic overlap between disorders (55). Studies of genetics may help us understand diagnostic comorbidity, especially when two disorders arise from similar genetic underpinnings (56). Whatever the answer to these questions, children with language problems are vulnerable to socioemotional difficulties, and children with psychiatric diagnoses show a higher than normal prevalence of language disorders.

Selective Mutism

The psychiatric problems that most commonly co-occur with language disorders include attention-deficit hyperactivity disorders, conduct disorders, and anxiety disorders. One particular form of anxiety disorder, selective mutism, has the most obvious communicative concomitants. DSM-5 (57) defines selective mutism as a persistent refusal to talk in one or more major social situations, including school, despite the ability to comprehend and use spoken language (58). High levels of social anxiety are often also present (58). The problem has been recognized for at least a century (60) and is relatively rare, with prevalence rates of 0.3 to 0.8 per 1,000 (57). Selective mutism is most often seen in school settings, where the child refuses to speak despite being verbal at home. Cultural and linguistic differences (CLDs) can exacerbate the problem, especially when the child has limited English proficiency (LEP) and feels uncomfortable using the language of the classroom (61). The condition shows a 2:1 ratio in favor of girls (62). In spite of the fact that the diagnostic criteria require the child to have the ability to use language in some situations, a high incidence of speech and language difficulties has been reported in this population. Seventy-five percent of children with selective mutism have been found to have articulation disorders and expressive language problems; 60% show significant deficits in receptive language (63,64). Speech-language pathologists often work in collaboration with mental health professionals to address the needs of the selectively mute child. Recent reviews (65,66) report evidence that behavioral intervention was the most effective approach. These techniques include contingency management (positive reinforcement of verbalizations and nonreinforcement for nonverbal responses), stimulus fading (gradually extending the number of people with whom and environments wherein verbalization is rewarded), shaping (rewarding gradual approximations to speech, such as mouthing and whispering), and response cost procedures (losing money or tokens for not speaking) (67,68). Multimodal interventions that combine behavioral or cognitive-behavioral approaches with psychodynamic approaches, family involvement, and other therapies such as music or dance also showed some degree of efficacy (69). Pharmacologic intervention produced no recovery when used alone, but use of selective serotonin reuptake inhibitors (SSRIs) appears to have an ancillary role in the treatment of selective mutism when combined with other approaches (70). Music therapy also showed emerging evidence of efficacy (71).

Autism Spectrum Disorder

The psychiatric disorder most consistently associated with communication deficits is ASD. Communication problems—including severe delays in language, inability to communicate nonverbally, inability to sustain conversation, stereotyped and repetitive use of idiosyncratic language, and abnormal ability to use language for social communication—are included in the diagnostic criteria for ASD (72). Virtually all children with autism have some form of communication disorder that presents as part of their syndrome. What differentiates autism from a more circumscribed language disorder is the global nature of the child's communication problem. Not only is language affected, but also the ability and motivation to send messages by any means, either verbal or nonverbal, is severely impaired.

From early in development, children with ASD show differences in intentional communication. Major differences seen in 1 year olds later diagnosed with ASD include a lack of joint attentional behavior and an abnormal response to human faces and voices. These babies use gestures to show and point less often than language-matched controls, although they do use gestures to request, protest, and regulate others' behavior (73). In general, they do not communicate in order to share focus as normal infants do, but only to express wants and needs (74). Some children with ASD do not develop speech, approximately 30% depending on study; although the proportion who do not is declining as earlier identification and intervention is being implemented (75–77). When speech is absent, it is not spontaneously replaced by communicative gestures, as it is in children with HI, for example. Furthermore, children with ASD may develop maladaptive means for expressing requests and protests. They may begin head-banging, for example, to express rejection of an activity. In children with ASD who do develop speech, some expansion of communicative intentions occurs, along with an elaboration of more socially acceptable means of communicating (78).

Children with ASD who do talk begin speaking late and develop speech at a significantly slower rate than other children (78). About 25% of children with ASD appear to acquire a few words by 12 or 18 months, and then lose them or fail to acquire more (79). When children with ASD begin talking, aspects of language form, including phonology, syntax, and morphology, are relatively spared. These children generally show skills in language form that are at or close to those of mental-age mates (78), although a subgroup of children with ASD show deficits in language form that are similar to those of children with SLI (74). Vocabulary skills also are usually on par with developmental level. Meaning and pragmatic aspects are disproportionately impaired, though (80). For individuals with ASD who develop spoken language, verbal output may lack spontaneity and remain somewhat sparse. They generally have trouble adapting what they say to the needs and status of the listener, distinguishing given from new information, following politeness rules, making relevant comments, maintaining topics outside their own obsessive interests, and giving listeners their fair share of conversational turns (78).

A classic characteristic of autistic language is *echolalia*, either immediate or delayed (81,82). Although echolalia was long thought to be a dysfunctional language behavior, investigators such as Fay (83) and Prizant and Duchan (84) have shown that children with ASD often use echolalia for communicative purposes. Echolalia in ASD is selective, as it is in normal development (85). Children with ASD who echo tend to do so when they do not understand what has been said to them or when they lack the language skills to generate an original reply (86). Although echolalia is a "classic" symptom of autistic disorders, not all verbal children with ASD use it. Fay (87) estimated that it appears, at least briefly, in about 75% of autistic children who speak. Also, echolalia is used by children with other syndromes, such as blindness and fragile X syndrome. As language skill in children with ASD improves, echolalia decreases, as it does in typical development.

Paralinguistic aspects of communication also are affected in verbal children with ASD. Intonation is often monotonous and machinelike, and stress, vocal quality, rate, rhythm, prosody, and loudness deviances also have been reported for approximately half of higher-functioning speakers with ASD (88,89). The reasons for these paralinguistic differences are not known. Paralinguistic aspects of communication do, though, carry some of the pragmatic and emotional information in the message. The deficits in affective development seen in children with ASD may, then, form some part of the explanation.

Social (Pragmatic) Communication Disorder

This new diagnostic classification is identified in DSM-5 (57). Those diagnosed with this disorder demonstrate a primary deficit in the social use of language, specifically pragmatics, but fail to display the restricted and repetitive behaviors (RRBs) seen in ASDs. Children who are diagnosed with social communication disorder (SCD) may demonstrate difficulties initiating and maintaining conversation, adapting their communication style to accommodate various listeners or show problems in comprehending higher-level language needed for social exchanges (e.g., inferences). Children with SCD have intact formal language skills; that is, vocabulary, morphology, and syntax, are roughly in the average range; they show no history of RRBs (90). This new diagnostic classification may be useful in better quantifying the social language impairments observed in other psychiatric conditions (91), but there is limited evidence of its diagnostic validity (92).

ACQUIRED DISORDERS OF COMMUNICATIVE FUNCTION

Language disorders acquired during the developmental period can be broadly categorized as those related to focal lesions (93,94); and those in which more widespread damage is sustained, usually in association with seizure disorders (95,96) or traumatic brain injury. These disorders and their remediation are described in Paul and Norbury (97).

Disorders with Environmental Components

Fetal Alcohol Syndrome

Fetal alcohol syndrome (FAS) is the most impairing form of fetal alcohol spectrum disorder, which is a continuum of impairments as a result of exposure to alcohol in utero (98). Communication disabilities are almost universal in those with FAS (99) and are related to the level of intellectual impairment. These disorders include delayed development, poor receptive vocabulary and comprehension, and pragmatic difficulties. Perseveration and echolalia are often present in children with more severe impairments (100).

Drug Exposure

Although prenatal drug exposure is a developmental risk, fewer than half of children exposed to drugs prenatally experience low birth weight, prematurity, intrauterine growth retardation, or small head circumference (100,101). Sparks (101) reported that drug-exposed newborns are often irritable and stiff and show arousal and attention problems, but these traits do not appear to last past the first year. In general, cognition is not impaired, except when reduced head size is present. Still, catch-up head growth is a marker of good prognosis for long-term development (100). Several studies (102–105) have found that children with a history of cocaine exposure show delays in language acquisition, particularly in the area of expressive language, with exposure to higher-doses prenatally resulting in higher levels of impairment. However, these studies also find that effects are modified by an enriched environment; children placed in foster or adoptive homes show higher levels of communicative skill than those who remain with biologic mothers.

Child Abuse and Neglect

Children with communicative and other developmental disorders are, as Knutson and Sullivan (106) pointed out, more likely than normally developing children to experience maltreatment. Similar findings were reported in a meta-analysis of 17 studies examining the prevalence of abuse and neglect in children with developmental disorders, including communication impairments (107). Fox et al. (108) suggested that a child with a communication disorder might be less satisfying for a parent to care for and provide less rewarding interactions. These difficulties might predispose a child to abuse.

Maltreatment itself also constitutes a risk for language disorder. Culp et al. (109) argued that language development is particularly vulnerable in the maltreatment situation, because of the disruption in social interaction it entails. Preschool children who were maltreated are more likely to exhibit language delay compared to other developmental issues, such as motor or cognitive impairments (110). Coster et al. (111) showed that maltreated toddlers used shorter sentences and more limited vocabularies during play with their mothers than peers from nonabusing homes. Both Allen and Oliver (112) and Eigsti and Cicchetti (113) found that preschoolers with a history of maltreatment had significantly lower language scores than peers of similar socioeconomic level, with impairments in both vocabulary and sentence production. Lynch and Roberts (114) showed that these children scored significantly lower on verbal IQ relative to nonverbal scores. Fox et al. (108) found that maltreated children had receptive language deficits, with neglected children suffering greater lags than those shown by children who were abused. Moreover, there are cascading effects on development for children who have been maltreated, including altered cognitive functioning in adulthood and increased risk of psychiatric disorders (115).

SPECIFIC SPEECH AND LANGUAGE DISORDERS

Communication disorders can be associated with a variety of conditions but they can also occur in relative isolation. These more specific disorders of speech and language development can still have broad effects on a child's ability to succeed in social and academic pursuits because communication is so central to human interaction and the development of the intellect. We will examine the types of specific speech and language disorders discussed in the DSM-5 (57): Childhood-onset fluency disorder (stuttering), speech sound disorder, and language disorder.

Specific Speech Disorders

Stuttering

This syndrome involves abnormal and persistent dysfluencies that result in deviations in the continuity, smoothness, rhythm, and/or effort with which phonologic, lexical, morphologic, and/or syntactic language units are spoken (116); these are often accompanied by affective and behavioral reactions. Several types of speech dysfluencies also may be involved, including blocking of sounds, hesitations, and tense pauses. Incidence of childhood stuttering is highest between a child's second and fourth birthdays, ultimately affecting 4% to 5% of the population. Although many children go through periods of dysfluency during the developmental period, these "normal dysfluencies" tend to occur in the larger linguistic units (word, phrases, and sentences). For children who tend to persist in stuttering over time, dysfluencies are more likely to occur in repetitions of syllables ("vi-vi-vi-vi-video") and sounds ("g-g-g-g-ot"). Other "red flags" for persistent stuttering include sound prolongations ("WWWWWait!"), silent blocks in which the child attempts to speak but no sound comes out, and visible struggle behaviors during speech, such as blinks or grimaces (8). If dysfluencies continue to be relatively effortless, there is a good chance of recovery. In addition, Yairi et al. (117) reported that children who recover from stuttering begin to show reductions in their number of dysfluencies within the first year, whereas those who persist in stuttering are relatively stable in their rate of dysfluency.

When recovery occurs, it usually does so by adolescence, often around the time of puberty. For individuals with chronic stuttering, the severity of the disturbance varies from situation to situation and is more severe when there is pressure to communicate. Stress or anxiety has been shown to exacerbate stuttering, but is not thought to play a role in the etiology; however, in a study of adolescents, those who stutter have a higher rates of social and trait anxiety compared to nonstuttering controls (118). Reducing stress during speaking can reduce stuttering episodes (119), but general treatments for anxiety, including the use of tranquilizing medication, have not been found to be effective for the stuttering itself (120). In general, speech therapy is used both to shape fluent speech and help the patient to stutter with less tension, avoidance, and interruption of the flow of communication (121,122). Psychotherapy alone has not been shown to be an effective treatment for stuttering, but counseling is often helpful for overcoming the secondary effects of stuttering on self-concept, thoughts, and feelings (123). Today, stuttering is believed by most researchers to have a complex multiplicity of causes that include biologic vulnerability, environmental demands and expectations, and temperamental characteristics of the speaker (124).

Speech Sound Disorders

These difficulties with speech articulation are characterized by impaired production of developmentally expected speech sounds. To diagnose a speech sound disorder, it is necessary to ascertain that the problem is not attributable to deficits or abnormalities in intelligence, hearing, or the structure and physiology of the speech mechanism. So a speech sound disorder is one in which, although there is no organic reason for the disability, the child's speech is marked by developmentally inappropriate misarticulations, including distortions of sounds (e.g., /s/ is produced with a lisp), omissions of sounds (e.g., *up* is pronounced "uh," *play* is pronounced "pay"), and incorrect substitutions of one sound for another (e.g., *cat* is pronounced "dat"). Many of these misarticulations represent processes that are typical in the speech of young typical children (e.g., deletions of final consonants, simplifications of consonant clusters), but in speech sound disorders more of them are used, they are used more often, and their use persists beyond the normal developmental period. There may also be idiosyncratic preferences for and/or avoidances of certain sounds or sound simplification processes (125–127), and/or reversals or misordering of sounds in words (128). Speech sound disorders are the most prevalent type of communication problem. Edwards (129) reported that 80% of speech clinic referrals were for articulation disorder. Six percent of school-age children have phonologic disorders. The prevalence is higher for preschoolers, with estimates ranging from 10% to 15% (4).

Speech sound disorders can, of course, occur with many of the syndromes discussed in the preceding. They can also occur in isolation, and are commonly associated with specific language disorders. Shriberg and Kwiatkowski (130) found that over 50% of children with speech sound disorders have delays in expressive language, and 10% to 40% have delays in language comprehension. Shriberg and Kwiatkowski (130) reported that a significant minority of these children, with either speech-only or speech/language delays as preschoolers, required continuing special services throughout their elementary school years.

Childhood Apraxia of Speech

A subset of children with severe, persistent speech disorders accompanied by certain language and behavioral features are sometimes said to have a *childhood apraxia of speech (CAS)* (131–134). Although there is not a well-established set of diagnostic criteria, characteristics most commonly attributed to this syndrome (131–136) include:

- Limited repertoires of speech sounds
- Predominant use of simple syllable shapes
- Frequent sound omission errors

- Slow rate of speech
- Difficulties with imitating sounds and speech
- Production in single words is better than in connected speech
- Stress and pausing may be unusually equal across words, with loss of normal intonation quality

Davis (137) and Shriberg (138) discussed some of the controversies surrounding this disorder. First, some degree of connected speech is necessary to make the diagnosis. Children who are not speaking at all cannot technically be diagnosed with CAS for this reason, although nonverbal children do often receive this diagnosis erroneously. Second, CAS was originally defined as an analog to an adult-acquired neurologic disorder: apraxia of speech, or a neurologically based difficulty in programming speech movements, thought to take place at a prearticulatory motor planning level. Intensive investigation, however, has not been able to document any consistent neuropathology in children who show this speech pattern, even with sophisticated new techniques. Partly as a result of this failure to identify a neurologic lesion similar to the one that causes apraxia in adults, and the fact that the behavioral symptomatology associated with CAS overlaps extensively with other conditions, such as developmental phonologic disorders and expressive language delays, accurate and reliable diagnosis is difficult. In general, it is best to be conservative about the diagnosis of CAS, and to reserve it for children who have demonstrated some connected speech production but fail to make progress in articulation after an intensive trial of traditional speech therapy.

Specific Language Impairment

Some kinds of language disorders have no known concomitants. These disorders have been traditionally defined by exclusion, that is, by the absence of the other factors—ID, sensory disorders, neurologic damage, emotional problems, or environmental deprivation.

Rescorla and Lee (139) have argued on the basis of recent evidence regarding the development of very young children with delayed speech (140,141) that it is not appropriate to make the diagnosis of SLI until age 4. Research suggests that younger children with delayed language have a good chance of "outgrowing" their slow start, although their language functioning may seem very similar to children with SLI at earlier ages (142) and they frequently retain subtle weaknesses when compared to matched social-economic peers (143–147).

Children with SLI are frequently late to begin talking. When they do begin to talk, they add new words slowly. They may continue to use single word or telegraphic utterances into their third year. In general, communication patterns of children with SLI are similar to those of younger children at comparable levels of language development. While this pattern holds true when looking at one specific feature of development at a time, Leonard (148) pointed out that children may be 1 year below age level in one set of features, 1½ years below in another, 6 months below in a third, and so on. The result will be that the overall profile of language skills in a child with SLI may not resemble that of a child with normal language function at any point in development. This does not mean that language development is deviant, but rather that it is in some ways asynchronous (31).

Early lexical usage in children with SLI is very much like that of normally developing children at similar language levels but is acquired at a slower pace. Vocabulary sizes of normally developing 2 year olds are more than 200 words, whereas those of children with SLI are in the range of 20 words (141–151). Moreover, children with SLI talk and communicate less often than same-age peers (139). While these children acquire sounds and make speech errors that are similar to those of peers, their repertoires of consonant sounds are smaller, and they take longer to acquire basic word forms (152–155).

Although vocabulary deficits are the first sign of language delay, these typically resolve by ages 3 to 4 (150,151). Use of early semantic relations appears similar to that of language-matched peers (148). Vocabulary in school-aged children with SLI lags behind that of peers (156,157), perhaps because of reduced experience through reading (which is often problematic for these children) (158).

Delays in syntax emerge between 18 to 24 months of age in children with SLI as evidenced by a failure to spontaneously (141,149,159,160). Follow-up studies indicate that these children continue to lag behind in syntactic development through the preschool period (142,161). They appear to acquire grammatical structures in roughly the same order as normally speaking children do, although they make more errors for longer periods and use higher rates of ungrammatical sentences (139,160). Some recent electrophysiologic evidence suggests reduced sensitivity to cues within sentences to the grammar of subject–verb agreement (162), although there are several alternative theories to explain this widespread observation in English-speaking children with SLI.

Pragmatic skills are generally better than skills in language form, and this is one of the characteristics that differentiates SLI from ASD (163). While children with SLI have been reported to be less interactive than age-matched peers, they are often similar to younger language-matched children (139), and pragmatic deficits seen are usually in the mild range (30). Still, Marton et al. (164) report finding significant deficits in social knowledge in children with SLI and others have reported subthreshold autism symptomatology (165).

For children with chronic mild to moderate language disorders, problems in the school years tend to narrow in their focus and to be concentrated in subtle difficulties of language organization and efficiency, rather than frank errors (143,144). Word retrieval or "word finding" difficulties, are common. A child with SLI may substitute an incorrect word of related meaning (e.g., "table"); or use functional descriptors (e.g., "thing to sit on"), vague or general terms (e.g., "thing"). Storytelling and discourse problems often persist and affect both oral and written modes of expression (149,166). There may be tangential or inappropriate responses to questions, a limited range of communicative functions (e.g., requests, imperatives, questions) expressed, difficulty maintaining and/or changing topics, and difficulty initiating interactions (167). Academic problems tend to involve primarily reading and writing. Despite their persistent problems, however, most of these children do finish high school, some go on to college, and most live independent lives (144,145,168).

DIFFERENTIAL DIAGNOSIS

When seeing children suspected of having specific speech and language disorders, the main diagnostic task is to rule out other syndromes with which speech and language problems are frequently associated. These syndromes include the ones discussed in the early section of this chapter; that is, deafness or significant hearing loss, ID, ASD, psychiatric disorder, organically based communication disorders (e.g., cleft palate, apraxia, cerebral palsy, or childhood-acquired aphasia), or a disorder associated with maternal substance abuse or maltreatment.

The absence of significant HI must be established by audiometric testing by a certified audiologist. Because subtle deficits in hearing can affect language acquisition, it is important to get complete and accurate results in order to assure that hearing deficits do not play a role in the disorder. Although chronic middle ear pathology is sometimes associated with speech and language problems, research (169,170), suggests that chronic otitis media alone does not significantly increase the risk of language disorder in otherwise normal children.

ID must be diagnosed by means of an individually administered, standardized test of intelligence, as well as by a standardized measure of adaptive behavior. For children suspected of language disorders, it is necessary to use nonverbal intelligence tests to assess intellectual ability, so as not to penalize the child for the language deficit and to obtain an estimate of intelligence unbiased by language performance. It should be noted, though, that even in nonverbal measures, children with SLI tend to score lower (though within the normal range) than average (171). It is not necessary to show that a child has language skills that are lower than expected for IQ in order for the child to receive communication services through the public schools. According to Individuals with Disabilities Education Act (IDEA) Part B, Children with ID can qualify for these school-based services if their communication skills significantly impact their access to social and academic opportunities.

Organic disorders that can affect the speech mechanism, such as dyspraxia, dysarthria, and motor deficits associated with cerebral palsy, can be ruled out by physical and functional assessment of the speech mechanism. A speech-language pathologist (SLP) typically examines the morphology, symmetry, and alignment of the facial features. The functional integrity of the larynx, lips, tongue, and velopharyngeal structures, as well as the respiratory support for speech are also assessed. The quality of oral volitional movements also may be examined if an apraxia is suspected. If physical limitations to speech production are identified, an alternative system of communication—such as a picture board or electronic communicative device—may be indicated (172,173). However, it is important to note that difficulties in imitation and cognition can affect a child's ability to participate in these assessments. Finding typical speech motor performance can rule out neuromotor involvement, but a finding of poor performance is more difficult to interpret, especially in developmentally young children.

Psychiatric/behavioral assessment can rule out ASD and other psychiatric disorders. Features associated with ASD include lack of (nonverbal) social interactions, absence of imaginative activity, stereotypic behaviors, self-injurious behaviors, odd responses to sensory input, and mood abnormalities. Formal measures, such as the Autism Diagnostic Interview (ADI; 174) and the Autism Diagnostic Observation Schedule (ADOS; 175), as well as checklists such as the Childhood Autism Rating Scale (CARS; 176) can assist in differential diagnosis.

The differential diagnosis among stuttering, speech sound disorder, language disorder, and selective mutism requires comprehensive speech/language testing. To diagnose stuttering, a clinician should ascertain, by means of standardized testing, that other language skills are age appropriate. If dysfluency coexists with other speech and language disorders, it may be appropriate to delay making a diagnosis of stuttering until some of the other problems resolve, then reevaluate to determine whether the dysfluency has persisted. For young children, too, dysfluency may be transient. If the preschool dysfluent child is not showing any signs of struggle or self-consciousness about speech, it may be wise to "watch and see," and re-evaluate the child in 6 months before initiating a course of speech therapy.

Speech sound disorders are diagnosed by means of standardized testing of sound production, usually using procedures that ask children to name pictures or objects and transcribing the child's rendition of the target word for comparison with adult production standards. Because these disorders typically coexist with other language disorders, it is acceptable to confer a concurrent diagnosis of speech sound disorder even if other language disorders are present. However, it is necessary to rule out HI, ID, and speech mechanism limitations before diagnosing a specific speech disorder.

To diagnose a specific a language disorder, it is necessary to demonstrate—by means of individually administered, standardized tests—that expressive and/or receptive language skills are below the expected level of function. Again, because speech sound disorders so frequently coexist with language deficits, especially expressive language impairments, both conditions can be diagnosed concurrently.

TREATMENT OF SPEECH AND LANGUAGE DISORDERS

It is important to make a careful differential diagnosis of any communication disorder in order to decide whether the problem is specific to speech and language or is part of a larger syndrome. In the case of communication disorders associated with syndromes such as HI, ID, and autism, treatment must address all aspects of the child's problem, not just those of speech and language.

The treatment of choice for all the disorders discussed here, except selective mutism, is individual or small group therapy administered by a certified SLP. Because associated educational and/or psychiatric problems are common with these disorders, educational tutoring, social skills training, and/or psychiatric intervention also may be indicated, even if the disorder is specific to communication.

Methods of intervention are essentially behavioral and educational. Some clinicians use strict operant procedures, whereas others favor more child-centered approaches such as indirect language stimulation, which involves a rich communicative environment with opportunities for incidental learning. Many SLPs take a middle ground between these extremes, using structured play opportunities and focused stimulation to provide examples of desired forms and elicit language targets. Although all these methods have been shown to be effective in small studies (97,177,178), much more research is needed on the efficacy and effectiveness of particular approaches to intervention and variables that can be used to best match the method to the child.

Caution should be exerted when treatments make claims of dramatic improvement, particularly when the improvement is claimed for a broad range of disorders. Clinicians who work with families of children with communication disorders need to maintain a healthy skepticism regarding these programs that make extravagant claims. Any intervention, whether familiar or innovative, must be shown to meet the particular needs of the patient receiving it. Communicative interventions need to be evaluated with the same kind of rigor that would be used to evaluate the efficacy of a medical or surgical treatment. Although double-blind, placebo-controlled, randomized assignment trials are difficult to design for behavioral interventions, clinicians must strive to achieve some degree of objective evaluation before deciding that a treatment is appropriate for a given individual.

ACKNOWLEDGMENTS

Preparation of this chapter was supported by Research Grant P01-03008 funded by the National Institute of Mental Health (NIMH); by the Studies to Advance Autism Research and Treatment (STAART) Center grant U54 MH66494 funded by the National Institute on Deafness and Other Communication Disorders (NIDCD), the National Institute of Environmental Health Sciences (NIEHS), the National Institute of Child Health and Human Development (NICHD), the National Institute of Neurological

Disorders and Stroke (NINDS); by a MidCareer Development grant to Dr. Paul, K24 HD045576 funded by NIDCD; the National Alliance for Autism Research; as well as the Integrative Graduate Education and Research Traineeship Program (IGERT) Grant 1144399 funded by the National Science Foundation (NSF).

References

1. American Speech-Language-Hearing Association: Guidelines for caseload size and speech-language service delivery in the schools. *ASHA Suppl* 35:33–39, 1993.
2. Bishop DVM, Snowling MJ, Thompson PA, Greenhalgh T, CATALISE consortium: CATALISE: A Multinational and Multidisciplinary Delphi Consensus Study. Identifying Language Impairments in Children. *PLoS ONE* 11(7):e0158753, 2016. doi:10.1371/journal.pone.0158753
3. Van Dyke DC, Holte L: Communication disorders in children. *Pediatric Ann* 32:436–437, 2003.
4. Hoffman H, Li C, Bainbridge K, Losonczy K, Chiu M, Rice M: *Voice, Speech, and Language Problems in the U.S. Pediatric Population: The 2012 National Health Interview Survey (NHIS).* Anchorage, AK, Poster # 3852 presented at the IEA 20th World Congress of Epidemiology, 2014.
5. NIDCD: Statistics and human communication [Internet]: *National Institute on Deafness and Other Communication Disorders*; c2010 [cited 2015 December 7]. Available at: http://www.nidcd.nih.gov/health/statistics/pages/vsl.aspx.
6. Tomblin JB, Records NL, Buckwalter P, Zhang X, Smith E, O'Brien M: Prevalence of specific language impairments in kindergarten children. *J Speech Lang Hear Res* 40:1245–1260, 1997.
7. Bartlett CW, Flax JF, Logue MW, et al.: A major susceptibility locus for special language impairment is located on 13q21. *Am J Hum Genet* 71(1):45–55, 2002.
8. Plante E, Beeson P: *Communication and Communication Disorders.* Boston, Allyn & Bacon, 1999.
9. Pore SG, Reed KL: *Quick Reference to Speech-Language Pathology.* Gaithersburg, MD, Aspen, 1999.
10. Bishop DV, Adams C, Norbury CF: Distinct genetic influences on grammar and phonological short-term memory: evidence from 6-year-old twins. *Genes Brain Behav* 5:158–169, 2006.
11. Bishop DV, North T, Donlan C: Genetic basis of specific language impairment: evidence from a twin study. *Dev Med Child Neurol* 37:56–71, 1995.
12. Tallal P, Ross R, Curtiss S: Familial aggregation in specific language impairment. *J Speech Hear Disord* 54:167–173, 1989.
13. Tomblin JB: Familial concentration of developmental language impairment. *J Speech Hear Disord* 54:287–295, 1989.
14. Viding E, Spinath FM, Price TS, Bishop DV, Dale PS, Plomin R: Genetic and environmental influence on language impairment in 4-year-old same-sex and opposite-sex twins. *J Child Psychol Psychiatry* 45:315–325, 2004.
15. Reader R, Covill L, Nudel R, Newbury D: Genome-wide studies of specific language impairment. *Curr Behav Neurosci Rep* 1(4):242–250, 2014.
16. Lai CS, Fisher SE, Hurst JA, Vargha-Khadem F, Monaco AP: A forkhead-domain gene is mutated in a severe speech and language disorder. *Nature* 413:519–523, 2001.
17. Vernes SC, Newbury DF, Abrahams BS, et al.: A functional genetic link between distinct developmental language disorders. *N Engl J Med* 359:2337–2345, 2008.
18. Bartlett CW, Hou L, Flax JF, et al.: A genome scan for loci shared by autism spectrum disorder and language impairment. *Am J Psychiatry* 171:72–81, 2014.
19. Wittke K, Spaulding TJ, Schechtman CJ: Specific language impairment and executive functioning: parent and teacher ratings of behavior. *Am J Speech Lang Pathol* 22:161–172, 2013.
20. Henry LA, Messer DJ, Nash G: Executive functioning in children with specific language impairment. *J Child Psychol Psychiatry* 53:37–45, 2012.
21. Eisenson J: *Aphasia in Children.* New York, Harper & Row, 1972.
22. Ullman MT, Pierpont EI: Specific language impairment is not specific to language: the procedural deficit hypothesis. *Cortex* 41:399–433, 2005.
23. Conti-Ramsden G, St. Clair MC, Pickles A, Durkin K: Developmental trajectories of verbal and non-verbal skills in individuals with a history of SLI: From childhood to adolescence. *J Speech Lang Hear Res* 55:1716–1735, 2012.
24. Rakhlin N, Kornilov SA, Grigorenko EL: Gender and agreement processing in children with developmental language disorder. *J Child Lang* 41:241–274, 2014.
25. Lum JA, Conti-Ramsden G, Page D, Ullman MT: Working, declarative and procedural memory in specific language impairment. *Cortex* 48: 1138–1154, 2012.
26. Hutchinson E, Bavin E, Efron D, Sciberras E: A comparison of working memory profiles in school-aged children with specific language impairment, attention deficit/hyperactivity disorder, comorbid SLI and ADHD and their typically developing peers. *Child Neuropsychol* 18:190–207, 2012.
27. Leonard CM, Lombardino LJ, Walsh K, et al.: Anatomical risk factors that distinguish dyslexia from SLI predict reading skill in normal children. *J Commun Disord* 35:501–531, 2002.
28. Clark MM, Plante E: Morphology of the inferior frontal gyrus in developmentally language-disordered adults. *Brain Lang* 61:288–303, 1998.
29. Badcock NA, Bishop DV, Hardiman MJ, Barry JG, Watkins KE: Co-localisation of abnormal brain structure and function in specific language impairment. *Brain Lang* 120:310–320, 2012.
30. Liegeois R, Mayes A, Morgan A: Neural correlates of developmental speech and language disorders: evidence from neuroimaging. *Curt Dev Disord Rep* 1:215–227, 2014.
31. Rice ML, Warren SF, Betz SK: Language symptoms of developmental language disorders: an overview of autism, Down syndrome, fragile X, specific language impairment, and Williams syndrome. *Applied Psycholing* 26:7–27, 2005.
32. Abbeduto L, Boudreau D: Theoretical influences in research on language development and intervention in individuals with mental retardation. *Mentl Retard Dev Disabil Res Rev* 10:184–192, 2004.
33. Shriberg LD, Widder CJ: Speech and prosody characteristics of adults with mental retardation. *J Speech Hear Res* 33:627–653, 1990.
34. Lahey M: *Language Disorders and Language Development.* New York, Macmillan, 1988.
35. Dykens E, Hodapp R, Leckman J: *Behavior and Development in Fragile X Syndrome.* London, Sage Publications, 1994.
36. Abbeduto L, Murphy MM: Language, social cognition, maladaptive behavior and communication in Down syndrome and fragile X syndrome. In: Rice ME, Warren S (eds): *Developmental Language Disorders: From Phenotypes to Etiology.* Mahwah, NJ, Erlbaum, 77–96, 2004.
37. Hall SS, Lightbody AA, Hirt M, Rezvani A, Reiss AL: Autism in fragile X syndrome: a category mistake? *J Am Acad Child Adolesc Psychiatry* 49:921–933, 2010.
38. Moss J, Richards C, Nelson L, Oliver C: Prevalence of autism spectrum disorder symptomatology and related behavioural characteristics in individuals with Down syndrome. *Autism* 17:390–404, 2013.
39. Laws G, Bishop D: Pragmatic language impairment and social deficits in Williams syndrome: a comparison with Down's syndrome and specific language impairment. *Int J Lang Commun Disord* 39:45–64, 2004.
40. Roeser R: Cochlear implants and tactile aids for the profoundly deaf student. In: Roeser RJ, Downs MP (eds): *Auditory Disorders in School Children.* New York, Thieme Medical Publishers, 260–280, 1988.
41. Peng SC, Spencer LJ, Tomblin JB: Speech intelligibility of pediatric cochlear implant recipients with 7 years of device experience. *J Speech Lang Hear Res* 47:1227–1236, 2004.
42. Colletti L, Mandalà M, Zoccante L, Shannon RV, Colletti V: Infants versus older children fitted with cochlear implants: performance over 10 years. *Int J Pediatr Otorhinolaryngol* 75:504–509, 2011.
43. Colletti L, Mandalà M, Colletti V: Cochlear implants in children younger than 6 months. *Otolaryngol Head Neck Surg* 147:139–146, 2012.
44. Paul P, Quigley S: *Language and Deafness.* San Diego, Singular Publishing Group, 1994.
45. King C, Quigley S: *Reading and Deafness.* San Diego, College-Hill Press, 1985.
46. Trybus R, Karchmer M: School achievement scores of hearing impaired children: national data on achievement status and growth patterns. *Am Ann Deaf* 122:62–69, 1977.
47. Tomblin JB, Spencer L, Flock S, Tyler R, Gantz B: A comparison of language achievement in children with cochlear implants and children using hearing aids. *J Speech Lang Hear Res* 42:497–509, 1999.
48. Giddan JJ, Milling L: Comorbidity of psychiatric and communication disorders in children. *Child Adolesc Psychiatr Clin N Am* 8:19–36, 1999.
49. Helland WA, Helland T, Heimann M: Language profiles and mental health problems in children with specific language impairment and children with ADHD. *J Atten Disord* 18:226–235, 2014.
50. Benner G, Nelson J, Epstein M: Language skills of children with EBD: a literature review. *J Emot Behav Disord* 10:43–57, 2002.
51. Toppelberg CO, Medrano L, Peña Morgens L, Nieto-Castañon A: Bilingual children referred for psychiatric services: associations of language disorders, language skills, and psychopathology. *J Am Acad Child Adolesc Psychiatry* 41:712–722, 2002.
52. Baltaxe C: Emotional, behavioral, and other psychiatric disorders of childhood associated with communication disorders. In: Layton T, Crais E, Watson W (eds): *Handbook of Early Language Impairment in Children: Nature.* Albany, NY, Delmar Publishers, 63–125, 2001.
53. Redmond SM, Rice ML: The socioemotional behaviors of children with SLI: social adaption or social deviance? *J Speech Hear Res* 41:688–700, 1998.
54. Paul R, Cohen D, Klin A, Volkmar F: Multiplex developmental disorders. The role of communication in the construction of a self. *Child Adolesc Psychiatr Clin N Am* 8:189–202, 1999.
55. First MB: Mutually exclusive versus co-occurring diagnostic categories: the challenge of diagnostic comorbidity. *Psychopathology* 38:206–210, 2005.
56. Tomblin JB, Mueller KL: How can the comorbidity with ADHD aid understanding of language and speech disorders? *Top Lang Disord* 32:198–206, 2012.
57. American Psychiatric Association. *Diagnostic and Statistical Manual of Mental Disorders (DSM-V).* Arlington, American Psychiatric Publishing, 2013.

58. McInnes A, Manassis K: When silence is not golden: an integrated approach to selective mutism. *Semin Speech Lang* 26:201–210, 2005.
59. Viana AG, Beidel DC, Rabian B: Selective mutism: a review and integration of the last 15 years. *Clin Psychol Rev* 29:57–67, 2009.
61. Kussmaul A: *Die Stoerungen der Sprache. [Disturbances in linguistic function.]* Basel, Germany, Benno Schwabe, 211, 1877.
60. Elizur Y, Perednik R: Prevalence and description of selective mutism in immigrant and native families: a controlled study. *J Am Acad Child Adolesc Psychiatry* 42:1451–1459, 2003.
62. McInnes A, Fung D, Manassis K, Fiksenbaum L, Tannock R: Narrative skills in children with selective mutism: an exploratory study. *Am J of Speech Lang Pathol* 13:304–315, 2004.
63. Giddan J, Ross G, Sechler L, Becker B: Selective mutism in elementary school: multidisciplinary interventions. *Lang Speech Hear Serv Sch* 28:127–133, 1997.
64. Kristensen H: Selective mutism and comorbidity with developmental disorder/delay, anxiety disorder, and elimination disorder. *J Am Acad Child Adolesc Psychiatry* 39:249–256, 2000.
65. Sutherland L: *Treatment Approaches to Selective Mutism; Types, Professional Involvement, Motivation and Effectiveness: A Systematic Literature Review (1990–2011) [other thesis].* Edinburgh, Queen Margaret University, 2012.
66. Bergman RL: *Treatment for Children with Selective Mutism: An Integrated Approach.* New York, Oxford University Press, 2012.
67. Labbe EL, Williamson D: Behavioral treatment of elective mutism: a review of the literature. *Clin Psychol Rev* 4:273–292, 1984.
68. Viana AG, Beidel DC, Rabian B: Selective mutism: a review and integration of the last 15 years. *Clin Psychol Rev* 29:57–67, 2009.
69. Muris P, Ollendick TH: Children who are anxious in silence: a review on selective mutism, the new anxiety disorder in DSM-5. *Clin Child Fam Psychol Rev* 18:151–169, 2015.
70. Carlson JS, Mitchell AD, Segool N: The current state of empirical support for the pharmacological treatment of selective mutism. *Sch Psychol Q* 23:354–372, 2008.
71. Amir D: Re-finding the voice: music therapy with a girl who has selective mutism *Nor J Music Ther* 14:67–77, 2005.
72. Volkmar F, Reichow B, Westphal A, Mandell D: Autism and the autism spectrum. In: Volkmar F, Rogers S, Paul R, Pelphrey K (eds): *Handbook of Autism and Pervasive Developmental Disorders.* 4th ed. New York, Wiley, 3–27, 2014.
73. Chawarska K, Macari S, Volkmar F, Kim S, Shic F: ASD in infants and toddlers. In: Volkmar F, Rogers S, Paul R, Pelphrey K (eds): *Handbook of Autism and Pervasive Developmental Disorders.* 4th ed. New York, Wiley, 121–147, 2014.
74. Tager-Flusberg H, Joseph R: Identifying neurocognitive phenotypes in autism. *Philos Trans R Soc Lond B Biol Sci* 358:303–314, 2004.
75. Paul R, Chawarska K, Klin A, Volkmar F: Dissociations in communication development in children with ASD. In: Paul R (ed): *Language Disorders From a Developmental Perspective: Essays in Honor of Robin Chapman.* Mahwah, NJ, Erlbaum, 163–194, 2006.
76. Rogers S: Evidence-based intervention for language development in young children with autism. In: Charman T, Stone W (eds): *Social and Communication Development in Autism Spectrum Disorders: Early Identification, Diagnosis, and Intervention.* New York, Guilford, 143–179, 2006.
77. Tager-Flusberg H, Kasari C: Minimally verbal school-aged children with autism spectrum disorder: the neglected end of the spectrum. *Autism Res,* 6:468–478, 2013.
78. Kim S, Paul R, Tager-Flusberg H, Lord C: Language and communication is autism. In: Volkmar F, Rogers S, Paul R, Pelphrey K (eds): *Handbook of Autism and Pervasive Developmental Disorders.* 4th ed. New York, Wiley, 230–262, 2014.
79. Lord C, Shulman C, DiLavore P: Regression and word loss in autistic spectrum disorders. *J Child Psychol Psychiatry* 45:936–955, 2004.
80. Simmons ES, Paul R, Volkmar F: Assessing pragmatic language in autism spectrum disorder: the Yale in vivo Pragmatic Protocol. *J Speech Lang Hear Res* 57:2162–2173, 2014.
81. Kanner L: Autistic disturbances of affective contact. *Nervous Child* 2:416–426, 1943.
82. Tager-Flusberg H: Dissociations in form and function in the acquisition of language in autistic children. In: Tager-Flusberg H (ed): *Constraints on Language Acquisition: Studies of Atypical Children.* Hillsdale, NJ, Erlbaum, 175–194, 1995.
83. Fay W: On the basis of autistic echolalia. *J Commun Disord* 2:38–47, 1969.
84. Prizant B, Duchan J: The functions of immediate echolalia in autistic children. *J Speech Hear Disord* 46:241–249, 1981.
85. Carr E, Schriebman I, Lovaas O: Control of echolalic speech in psychotic children. *J Abnorm Child Psychol* 3:331–351, 1975.
86. Prizant B: Communication, language, social, and emotional development. *J Autism Dev Disord* 26:173–178, 1996.
87. Fay W: Infantile autism. In: Bishop D, Mogford K (eds): *Language Development in Exceptional Circumstances.* Hillsdale, NJ, Erlbaum, 190–202, 1992.
88. Shriberg LD, Paul R, McSweeney JL, Klin AM, Cohen DJ, Volkmar FR: Speech and prosody characteristics of adolescents and adults with high functioning autism and Asperger syndrome. *J Speech Lang Hear Res* 44:1097–1115, 2001.
89. Lyons M, Simmons ES, Paul R: Prosodic development in middle childhood and adolescence in high-functioning autism. *Autism Res* 7:181–196, 2014.
90. Reisinger LM, Cornish KM, Fombonne E: Diagnostic differentiation of autism spectrum disorders and pragmatic language impairment. *J Autism Dev Disord* 41:1694–1704, 2011.
91. Cohen NJ, Farnia F, Im-Bolter N: Higher order language competence and adolescent mental health. *J Child Psychol Psychiatry* 54:733–744, 2013.
92. Norbury CF: Practitioner review: social (pragmatic) communication disorder conceptualization, evidence and clinical implications. *J Child Psychol Psychiatry* 55:204–216, 2014.
93. Trauner DA, Eshagh K, Ballantyne AO, Bates E: Early language development after peri-natal stroke. *Brain Lang* 127:399–403, 2013.
94. Reilly JS, Wasserman S, Appelbaum M: Later language development in narratives in children with perinatal stroke. *Dev Sci* 16:67–83, 2013.
95. Caraballo RH, Cejas N, Chamorro N, Kaltenmeier MC, Fortini S, Soprano AM: Landau–Kleffner syndrome: a study of 29 patients. *Seizure* 23:98–104, 2014.
96. Landi N, Montoya J, Kober H, et al.: Maternal neural responses to infant cries and faces: relationships with substance use. *Front Psychiatry* 2:32, 2011.
97. Paul R, Norbury C: *Language Disorders from Infancy through Adolescence: Listening, Speaking, Reading, Writing, and Communicating.* New York, Elsevier Health Sciences, 2012.
98. Riley EP, Infante MA, Warren KR: Fetal alcohol spectrum disorders: an overview. *Neuropsychol Rev* 21:73–80, 2011.
99. Mattson SN, Riley EP: A review of the neurobehavioral deficits in children with fetal alcohol syndrome or prenatal exposure to alcohol. *Alcohol Clin Exp Res* 22:279–294, 1998.
100. Sparks S: Prenatal substance use and its impact on young children. In: Layton T, Crais E, Watson L (eds): *Handbook of Early Language Impairment in Children: Nature.* Albany, NY, Delmar Publishers, 451–487, 2001.
101. Sparks S: *Children of Prenatal Substance Abuse.* San Diego, Singular Publishing Group, 1993.
102. Bandstra ES, Morrow CE, Accornero VH, Mansoor E, Xue L, Anthony JC: Estimated effects of in utero cocaine exposure on language development through early adolescence. *Neurotoxicol Teratol* 33:25–35, 2011.
103. Cone-Wesson B: Prenatal alcohol and cocaine exposure: influences on cognition, speech, language, and hearing. *J Commun Disord* 38:279–302, 2005.
104. Morrow C, Vogel A, Anthony J, Ofir A, Dausa A, Bandstra E: Expressive and receptive language functioning in preschool children with prenatal cocaine exposure. *J Pediatr Psychol* 29:543–554, 2004.
105. Lewis BA, Minnes S, Short EJ, et al.: The effects of prenatal cocaine on language development at 10 years of age. *Neurotoxicol Teratol* 33:17–24, 2011.
106. Knutson J, Sullivan P: Communicative disorders as a risk factor in abuse. *Top Lang Disord* 13:1–14, 1993.
107. Jones L, Bellis MA, Wood S, et al.: Prevalence and risk of violence against children with disabilities: a systematic review and meta-analysis of observational studies. *Lancet* 380:899–907, 2012.
108. Fox L, Long SH, Anglois A: Patterns of language comprehension deficit in abused and neglected children. *J Speech Hear Disord* 53:239–244, 1988.
109. Culp R, Watkins R, Lawrence H, Letts D, Kelly D, Rice M: Maltreated children's language and speech development: abused, neglected, and abused and neglected. *First Lang* 11:377–390, 1991.
110. McDonald JL, Milne S, Knight J, Webster V: Developmental and behavioural characteristics of children enrolled in a child protection pre-school. *J Paediatr Child Health* 49:E142–E146, 2013.
111. Coster W, Gersten M, Beeghly, M, Cicchetti D: Communicative functioning in maltreated toddlers. *Devl Psychol* 25:1020–1029, 1989.
112. Allen RE, Oliver JM: The effects of child maltreatment on language development. *Child Abuse Negl* 6:299–305, 1982.
113. Eigsti IM, Cicchetti D: The impact of child maltreatment on expressive syntax at 60 months. *Dev Sci* 7:88–102, 2004.
114. Lynch M, Roberts J: *The Consequences of Child Abuse.* NY, Academic Press, 1982.
115. Gould F, Clarke J, Heim C, Harvey PD, Majer M, Nemeroff CB: The effects of child abuse and neglect on cognitive functioning in adulthood. *J Psychiatr Res* 46:500–506, 2012.
116. American Speech-Language-Hearing Association. *Incidence and Prevalence of Communication Disorders and Hearing Loss in Children.* Rockville, MD, Author, 2006.
117. Yairi E, Ambrose N, Cox N: Genetics of stuttering: a critical review. *J Speech Hear Res* 40:49–58, 1996.
118. Mulcahy K, Hennessey N, Beilby J, Byrnes M: Social anxiety and the severity and typography of stuttering in adolescents. *J Fluency Disord* 33:306–319, 2008.
119. Van Riper C: *The Treatment of Stuttering.* Englewood Cliffs, NJ, Prentice-Hall, 1973.
120. Ham R: *Therapy of Stuttering: Preschool through Adolescence.* Englewood Cliffs, NJ, Prentice-Hall, 1990.
121. Guitar B, McCauley R: *Treatment of Stuttering: Established and Emerging Interventions.* Baltimore, MD, Lippicott Williams & Wilkins, 2010.

122. Guitar B: *Stuttering: An Integrated approach to its Nature and Treatment.* Baltimore, MD, Lippincott Williams & Wilkins, 2013
123. Cooper EB, Cooper CS: Treating fluency disordered adolescents. *J Comm Disord* 28:125–142, 1995.
124. Packman A: Theory and therapy in stuttering: a complex relationship. *J Fluency Disord* 37:225–233, 2012.
125. Dunn C, Davis B: Phonological process occurrence in phonologically disordered children. *App Psycholing* 4:187–207, 1983.
126. Ingram D: *Phonologic Disability in Children.* New York, Elsevier, 1976.
127. Weiner F: Systematic sound preference as a characteristic of phonologic disability. *J Speech Hear Disord* 46:281–286, 1981.
128. Trantham C, Pedersen J: *Normal Language Development: The Key to Diagnosis and Therapy for Language Disordered Children.* Baltimore, MD, Williams & Wilkins, 1976.
129. Edwards M: Speech disability in children: some general considerations. *Int Rehabil Med* 6:114–116, 1984.
130. Shriberg LD, Kwiatkowski J: Developmental phonologic disorders. I: a clinical profile. *J Speech Hear Res* 37:1100–1126, 1994.
131. American Speech-Language-Hearing Association. Childhood apraxia of speech [Technical Report]. 2007. Available at www.asha.org/policy Accessed February 17, 2017.
132. Shriberg LD, Kwiatkowski J: A follow-up study of children with phonologic disorders of unknown origin. *J Speech Hear Disord* 53:144–155, 1988.
133. Rosenbek J, Wertz R: A review of 50 cases of developmental apraxia of speech. *Lang Speech Hear Serv Sch* 3:23–33, 1972.
134. Yoss KA, Darley FL: Developmental apraxia of speech in children with defective articulation. *J Speech Hear Res* 7:399–416, 1974.
135. Shriberg LD, Campbell TF, Karlsson HB, Brown RL, McSweeny JL, Nadler CJ: A diagnostic marker for childhood apraxia of speech: the lexical stress ratio. *Clin Linguist Phon* 17:549–574, 2003.
136. Davis B, Velleman S: Differential diagnosis and treatment of developmental apraxia of speech in infants and toddlers. *Infant-Toddler Interven Trans J* 10:177–192, 2000.
137. Davis B, Jakielski K, Marquardt T: Differential diagnosis of developmental apraxia of speech: determiners of deferential diagnosis. *Clin Linguist Phon* 12:25–45, 1998.
138. Shriberg LD: A neurodevelopmental framework for research in childhood apraxia of speech. In: Maassen B, van Lieshout P (eds): *Speech Motor Control: New Developments in Basic and Applied Research.* Oxford, Oxford University Press, 259–270, 2010b.
139. Rescorla L, Lee E: Language impairment in young children. In: Layton T, Crais E, Watson L (eds): *Handbook of Early Language Impairment in Children: Nature.* Albany, New York, Delmar Publishers, 1–55, 2001.
140. Paul R: Ethical implications of the natural history of slow expressive language development. In: Bishop D, Leonard L (eds): *Proceedings of the Third International Symposium for Aphasic and Speech Impaired Children.* London, Psychology Press, 2000.
141. Rescorla L, Roberts J, Dahlsgaard K: Late talkers at 2: outcome at age 3. *J Speech Lang Hear Res* 40:556–566, 1997.
142. Bishop DV, Price TS, Dale PS, Plomin R: Outcomes of early language delay: II. Etiology of transient and persistent language difficulties. *J Speech Lang Hear Res* 46:561–575, 2003.
143. Rescorla L: Language and reading outcomes to age 9 in late-talking toddlers. *J Speech Lang Hear Res* 45:360–371, 2002.
144. Rescorla L: Age 13 language and reading outcomes in late-talking toddlers. *J Speech Lang Hear Res* 48:459–472, 2005.
145. Snowling MJ, Adams JW, Bishop DV, Stothard SE: Educational attainments of school leavers with a preschool history of speech-language impairments. *Int J Lang Commun Disord* 36:173–183, 2001.
146. Weismer S, Evans JL: The role of processing limitations in early identification of specific language impairment. *Top Lang Disord* 22:15–29, 2002.
147. Rescorla L: Age 17 language and reading outcomes in late-talking toddlers: support for a dimensional perspective on language delay. *J Speech Lang Hear Res* 52:16–30, 2009.
148. Leonard L: *Children with Specific Language Impairment.* Cambridge, MA, MIT press, 2014.
149. Paul R: Clinical implications of slow expressive language development. *Am J Speech Lang Pathol* 5:5–21, 1996.
150. Rescorla L, Alley A: Validation of the language development survey (LDS): a parent report tool for identifying language delay in toddlers. *J Speech Lang Hear Res* 44:434–445, 2001.
151. Rescorla L, Mirak J, Singh L: Vocabulary growth in late talkers: lexical development from 2;0 to 3;0. *J Child Lang* 27:293–311, 2000.
152. Paul R, Jennings P: Phonological behavior in toddlers with slow expressive language development. *J Speech Lang Hear Res* 35:99–107, 1992.
153. Pharr A, Ratner N, Rescorla L: Syllable structure development of toddlers with expressive specific language impairment. *App Psycholing* 21:429–449, 2000.
154. Rescorla L, Ratner NB: Phonetic profiles of typically developing and language-delayed toddlers. *J Speech Hear Res* 39:153–165, 1996.
155. Roberts J, Rescorla L, Giroux J, Stevens L: Phonological skills of children with specific expressive language impairment (SLI-E): outcome at age 3. *J Speech Lang Hear Res* 41:374–384, 1998.
156. Rice ML, Hoffman L: Predicting vocabulary growth in children with and without specific language impairment: a longitudinal study from 2;6 to 21 years of age. *J Speech Lang Hear Res* 58:345–359, 2015.
157. Rice ML, Redmond SM, Hoffman L: Mean length of utterance in children with specific language impairment and in younger control children shows concurrent validity and stable and parallel growth trajectories. *J Speech Lang Hear Res* 49:793–808, 2006.
158. St. Clair MC, Durkin K, Conti-Ramsden G, Pickles A: Growth of reading skills in children with a history of specific language impairment (SLI): the role of autistic symptomatology and language related abilities. *Br J Dev Psychol* 28:109–131, 2010.
159. Rescorla L, Dahlsgaard K, Roberts J: Late-talking toddlers: MLU and IPSyn outcomes at 3;0 and 4;0. *J Child Lang* 27:643–664, 2000.
160. Rescorla L, Roberts J: Nominal versus verbal morpheme use in late talkers at ages 3 and 4. *J Speech Lang Hear Res* 45:1219–1231, 2002.
161. Rescorla L, Mirren L: Communicative intent in late-talking toddlers. *App Psycholing* 19:393–411, 1998.
162. Purdy JD, Leonard LB, Weber-Fox C, Kagnovich N: Decreased sensitivity to long-distance dependencies in children with a history of specific language impairment: electrophysiological evidence. *J Speech Lang Hear Res* 57:1040–1059, 2014.
163. Caparulo B, Cohen D: Developmental language studies in the neuropsychiatric disorders of children. In: Nelson KE (ed): *Children's Language.* Hillsdale, NJ, Erlbaum, 423–463, 1983.
164. Marton K, Abramoff B, Rosenzweig S: Social cognition and language in children with specific language impairment (SLI). *J Comm Disord* 38:143–162, 2005.
165. Conti-Ramdsden G, Simkin Z, Btting N: The prevalence of autistic spectrum disorders in adolescents with a history of specific language impairment (SLI). *J Child Psychol Psychiatry* 47:621–628, 2006.
166. Reilly J, Losh M, Bellugi U, Wulfeck B: "Frog, where are you?" Narratives in children with specific language impairment, early focal brain injury, and Williams syndrome. *Brain Lang* 88:229–247, 2004.
167. Kuder J: *Teaching Students with Language and Communication Disabilities.* Boston, Allyn & Bacon, 1997.
168. Hall PK, Tomblin JB: A follow-up study of children with articulation and language disorders. *J Speech Hear Disor* 43:227–241, 1978.
169. Roberts J, Wallace I, Henderson F: *Otitis Media in Young Children.* Baltimore, MD, Paul H. Brookes Publishing, 1997.
170. Roberts JE, Rosenfeld RM, Zeisel SA: Otitis media and speech and language: a meta-analysis of prospective studies. *Pediatrics* 113:238–248, 2004.
171. Gallianat E, Spaulding TJ: Differences in the performance of children with specific language impairment and their typically developing peers on nonverbal cognitive tests: a meta-analysis. *J Speech Lang Hear Res* 57:1363–1382, 2014.
172. Beukelman D, Mirenda P: *Augmentative and Alternative Communication: Supporting Children and Adults with Complex Communication Needs.* 4th ed. Baltimore, MD, Paul H. Brookes Publishing, 2012.
173. Glennen S, DeCoste D: *Handbook of Augmentative and Alternative Communication.* San Diego, Singular Publishing Group, 1997.
174. Rutter M, Le Couteur A, Lord C: *Autism Diagnostic Interview—Revised.* Los Angeles, CA, Western Psychological Services, 2003.
175. Lord C, Rutter M, DiLavore P, Risi S, Gotham K, Bishop S: *The Autism Diagnostic Observation Schedule.* 2nd ed. Los Angeles, CA, Western Psychological Services, 2012.
176. Schopler E, Van Bourgondien M: *Childhood Autism Rating Scale.* 2nd ed. Los Angeles, CA, Western Psychological Services, 2010.
177. Fey M, Windsor J, Warren S: *Language Intervention: Preschool Through Elementary Years.* Baltimore, MD, Paul H. Brookes Publishing, 1995.
178. McCauley R, Fey M: *Treatment of Language Disorders in Children.* Baltimore, MD, Paul H. Brookes Publishing, 2006.

5.3 ■ PSYCHOTIC DISORDERS

CHAPTER 5.3 ■ CHILDHOOD-ONSET SCHIZOPHRENIA AND OTHER EARLY-ONSET PSYCHOTIC DISORDERS

ANNA E. ORDÓÑEZ AND NITIN GOGTAY

BACKGROUND

Psychotic disorders are rare in children although transient psychotic experiences are more common in otherwise healthy children than generally recognized (1–3). As is often the case with other very early-onset illnesses, psychotic disorders in children are usually more severe than their adult counterparts (4), and the disruption of cognitive and social development as well as the burden to the family can be devastating. Systematic research in this area was initially limited by diagnostic uncertainty and the general lack of knowledge about the psychotic processes in children (5).

History of Childhood-Onset Psychoses

Although the existence of childhood schizophrenia was recognized early in the twentieth century (6), the term psychosis was used so broadly in children that a spectrum of behavioral disorders and autism were grouped together under the category of childhood schizophrenia (7). The landmark studies of Kolvin (8) first established the clinical distinction between autism and other psychotic disorders of childhood. However, even today high rates of initial misdiagnosis remain due to symptom overlap, particularly for mood disorders (9–11), and the presence of transient hallucinations and delusions in nonpsychotic pediatric patients (3,12,13). Overall, hallucinations and delusions appear more prevalent in children and early adolescents than in older adolescents (14,15), with a recent meta-analysis of population studies reporting median prevalence of psychotic symptoms among children ages 9 to 12 years of 17%, and among adolescents 13 to 18 years of 7.5%.

Nonetheless, while the occurrence of psychotic-like experiences in many children and early adolescents will have short-term discontinuation, older age (14), greater severity, and frequency (12) appear associated to persistence of symptoms. Furthermore, psychotic symptoms in adolescents can be important indicators of risk for a range of psychotic (13) and nonpsychotic mental disorders (14–16) as well as conferring greater risk of poorer outcomes (17). In summary, while prevalent and usually transient in nonclinical populations particularly at earlier ages, psychotic symptoms in childhood and adolescents can be predictive of psychopathology later in life (16,18), suggesting that these symptoms probably exist as a continuous phenotype rather than an all-or-none phenomenon (19).

Childhood-Onset Schizophrenia—Diagnosis, Clinical Presentation, and Differential Diagnoses

Given the relatively high rate of hallucinations in children, with prevalence estimates in large population studies of 8% (20), and reports as high as 21.3% in some community samples (21), the distinction of pathologic psychotic symptoms in childhood is very important. For instance, 28% to 65% of children between the ages of 5 and 12 years of age report experiencing imaginary friends (22) which could be inappropriately misinterpreted as pathologic. Similarly, hallucinations associated with the periods of transition from wakefulness to sleep (hypnagogic) or from sleep to wakefulness (hypnopompic), are frequent in childhood and decline with age (23). It is noteworthy that some cases of sleep-associated hallucinations can be indicative of sleep disorders such as narcolepsy (24).

Although rare, with an incidence in the National Institute of Mental Health (NIMH) cohort of less than 0.04% (25), Kolvin's work established that children can be diagnosed with unmodified criteria for schizophrenia (8,25). Childhood-onset schizophrenia (COS) shows a pattern similar to that of poor-outcome adult cases, and the psychosis of COS can usually be distinguished by its severe and pervasive nature and its nonepisodic, unremitting course (25). Additionally, these children show poorer premorbid functioning in social, motor, and language domains, learning disabilities, and disruptive behavior disorders (26–28), and although not reported in studies of the premorbid history of adult-onset schizophrenia (AOS) (29,30), transient autistic symptoms such as hand flapping and echolalia in toddler years are common (26), probably reflecting more compromised early brain development.

Because COS is rare, it must be distinguished from several childhood conditions that can manifest with psychotic symptoms and/or deterioration in function:

1. Affective disorders: Hallucinations are relatively common in pediatric bipolar disorder and major depression (9,17,31,32). However, the psychotic symptoms in these conditions tend to be mood congruent (33) and follow-up studies on this population generally suggest a less disabling long-term course in a large number of cases (34,35).
2. Psychosis due to medical conditions such as migraine (36), inborn errors of metabolism (37), and substance abuse disorders (38) should be carefully ruled out.
3. Autism spectrum disorders and childhood disintegrative disorder can often be mistaken for psychosis, as they show severe impairment in reciprocal communication, social interactions, and odd stereotyped behaviors (39,40).
4. Conduct disorder and various other behavioral disturbances can be associated with hallucinations (41,42).
5. Atypical psychosis is an important differential diagnosis and is described in detail below.

Atypical Psychosis

A sizeable, heterogeneous group of children referred to the NIMH COS study over the past 20 years had transient psychotic symptoms and multiple developmental abnormalities, but were not adequately characterized by existing DSM-IV categories and were given a provisional diagnosis of "multidimensionally impaired (MDI)" (43–45). In the DSM nosology, these patients might be considered as having either psychosis NOS or mood disorder NOS.

The MDI group, although showing similarities with COS, has distinct features which were used as the operational diagnostic criteria by the NIMH group (43,44) including:

1. Brief, transient episodes of psychosis and perceptual disturbance, typically in response to stress (as opposed to the pervasive hallucinations/delusions in COS)
2. Nearly daily periods of emotional lability disproportionate to precipitants
3. Impaired interpersonal skills despite the desire to initiate peer friendships (distinction from COS)
4. Cognitive deficits as indicated by multiple deficits in information processing
5. No clear thought disorder (although this can be difficult to define clinically, particularly in the presence of a communication disorder)
6. Comorbid ADHD

The MDI children resemble syndromes such as the borderline syndrome of children, or the multiple complex developmental disorder (MCDD) (45–48). However, these syndromes have more predominant symptoms of autism spectrum disorders; greater evidence of a formal thought disorder; and onset before age 5 (as opposed to about age 8 for the MDI group) (44,45,49,50).

Initially, the neuropsychologic test profiles, smooth pursuit eye movement (SPEM) abnormalities, and familial risk factors suggested that some of the MDI children fell within the schizophrenia *spectrum* (44), but the MDI cohort appears to have a distinct long-term clinical course, and none have progressed to schizophrenia (51).

THE NIMH COS EXPERIENCE

The NIMH COS study has been ongoing since 1990. Inclusion criteria for the study are as follows: onset of psychosis before 13, premorbid IQ of 70 or above, and absence of significant neurologic disorder. In the last 24 years, over 2,000 charts have been reviewed, of which 80% are declined from further consideration as they fail to meet criteria for COS. About 400 children have been screened in person, of whom about 60% receive other psychiatric diagnoses, such as affective disorders, anxiety, or behavioral disorders. About 250 children who appeared likely to meet criteria for COS have been admitted to the research unit and undergone a complete medication washout followed by 1 to 3 weeks' drug-free inpatient observation. An additional 40% did not meet criteria for COS, most frequently because a diagnosis of affective disorder was made (5,43,52). A 4- to 6-year follow-up study of 33 of the ruled-out cases indicated good stability of the alternative diagnoses and confirmed the absence of schizophrenia (53).

PHENOMENOLOGY AND NEUROBIOLOGY OF COS

Premorbid Development

A striking phenomenologic feature of COS relative to AOS appears to be the higher rates of early language, social, and motor developmental abnormalities, possibly reflecting greater impairment in early brain development. In the NIMH COS sample, premorbid development (defined as development prior to 1 year before psychosis onset and assessed using the Cannon-Spoor Premorbid Adjustment Scale (PAS) (54) and the Hollis premorbid development scale (27) and social, speech and language impairments were clearly impaired (55,56), as has been previously observed by other independent research centers (27,28,57,58).

Risk Factors

Since COS represents a more severe phenotype of schizophrenia than AOS, our initial hypothesis was that most risk factors identified in adult studies would be more striking in our very early-onset cases.

Parental Age and Obstetric Complications

AOS studies suggest associations of the illness with advanced paternal age (59–63), raising the possibility of increased de novo mutations in the paternal germ cells, and also increased rates of maternal/fetal obstetric complications (64–66). The NIMH COS cohort showed no correlation with maternal or paternal age (67). In our cohort, we compared the obstetric records of 60 children with COS and 48 healthy siblings using the Columbia Obstetrics Complication Scale (68), a comprehensive measurement scale consisting of 37 variables. Contrary to our hypothesis, the incidence of obstetric complications in COS patients did not differ from that for the healthy sibling control group (69).

Eye Tracking

SPEM abnormalities have been reported in 25% to 40% of first-degree relatives of schizophrenia patients (70). Other studies have suggested more striking abnormalities in COS than in AOS, with a bilineal pattern of inheritance (71). Our group compared 70 COS parents, 64 AOS parents, and 20 COS siblings to separate matched control groups and found that the effect sizes for SPEM abnormalities were higher for COS than for AOS relatives, indicating that genetic factors underlying eye-tracking dysfunction may be more salient for COS (72).

Familial Schizophrenia Spectrum Disorders

Schizophrenia spectrum disorders consist of schizophrenia and schizoaffective disorders on axis I, and schizotypal, paranoid, and schizoid personality disorders on axis II (73). A prior study by Asarnow et al. (74) showed higher rates of schizophrenia spectrum diagnoses for COS relatives than for relatives of patients with attention-deficit hyperactivity disorder (ADHD) or community controls. Similarly, our analyses of 97 parents of COS patients, 97 parents of AOS patients and matched community controls, found a higher rate of familial schizophrenia spectrum disorders in COS than AOS, with the lowest rate in community controls. This observation further supported the continuity between COS and AOS, and the salience of familial/genetic risk in COS (75).

Familial Neurocognitive Functioning

It is well documented that subtle cognitive deficits, including abnormalities of attention (76,77), executive functioning (78,79), spatial working memory (80), and verbal memory (81,82) are seen in healthy relatives of patients with AOS (83–85). Deficits in auditory attention, verbal memory, and executive functioning are generally considered consistent (86,87), although it is unclear whether these represent an underlying global cognitive deficit or each deficit represents a discrete endophenotype transmitted in families of patients with schizophrenia (78,86). When we compared neuropsychologic deficits in 67 parents and 24 full siblings of COS patients to matched community controls in the Trail Making Tests A and B and the Wechsler Intelligence Scale-Revised Digit Span and Vocabulary, COS siblings had significantly poorer performance than community controls, although the rates of neuropsychologic abnormalities for COS were not significantly higher than for AOS (88).

Pervasive Developmental Disorder and COS

The diagnosis of autism or pervasive developmental disorder (PDD) has been raised early in the development in our cases (n = 28 of 97, 28%) (26) and several studies have claimed that autism per se might be a risk factor for later psychosis (89–92). Premorbid PDD may be a nonspecific manifestation of impaired neurodevelopment, and also may provide an independent additive risk factor for COS. We ascertained the premorbid diagnosis of past or current autism or PDD in 97 COS probands in whom the diagnosis of PDD was made according to DSM-IV criteria (American Psychiatric Association, 1994) based on early chart reviews and clinical interviews of patients and parents. The diagnoses of PDD was made in cases in which there was a clear clinical history of symptoms of autistic/PDD spectrum prior to the onset of psychosis that were still observable at the time of the NIH evaluation.

Twenty-eight (29%) of our COS patients had a lifetime diagnosis of PDD: 3 met criteria for autism, 1 for Asperger disorder, and 24 for PDD NOS (26). Premorbid social impairment was the most common feature for COS-PDD subjects; the PDD group did not differ significantly from the rest of the COS sample with respect to SES, age of onset, IQ, or severity as measured by the Global Assessment of Severity (GAS). However, similar to demographic characteristics seen in the literature for children with PDD, the COS patients with PDD were predominantly male (p = 0.04) and non-African American (p = 0.02) (26). In an earlier study, our group also failed to find any differences in baseline or 2- to 6-year clinical outcome measures, parental SES, response to medications, and rate of familial schizotypy (56). Furthermore, there was no difference between PDD and non-PDD groups with respect to initial brain magnetic resonance imaging (MRI) measures after controlling for gender, although the rate of gray matter (GM) loss appeared to be greater for PDD (n = 12) than for the non-PDD (n = 27) subgroup (−19.5 ± 11.3 mL/yr vs. −9.6 ± 15.3 mL/yr; p = 0.05) (56). These results may indicate that PDD in COS may be a nonspecific marker of more severe early abnormal neurodevelopment. However, siblings of the PDD-COS patients had significantly higher scores on the autism screening questionnaires, and 2 of 12 (17%) siblings of PDD patients were diagnosed with autism, a total rate similar to that seen for sibling of autistic patients (4.9%) (93), which may still imply a familial–genetic connection between COS and autism.

Neurocognitive Functioning in COS Patients

Neuropsychologic function in COS outpatients has been studied by Asarnow et al. (94–96). While rote language skills and simple perceptual processing are not impaired, these children perform poorly on tasks involving fine motor coordination, attention, short-term and working memory (97). Evoked potential studies show diminished amplitude of brain electrical activity during these tasks, suggesting that allocation of necessary attentional resources is deficient, which is also shared by adults with schizophrenia (96). It is generally established for adult schizophrenia that cognitive function deteriorates at onset of psychosis but remains stable afterward (98–100). Our earlier study had shown that children with COS (n = 27) as well as those with MDI (n = 24) share similar deficits in attention, learning, and abstraction, resembling the pattern in adult patients with schizophrenia (101). A subsequent analyses of 71 COS patients where preadmission IQ data were also available from medical and school records for a subgroup (n = 27), pre- and postpsychosis decline in IQ was noted as for adults, but postpsychotic cognitive function for up to 8+ years did not show continued decline (Fig. 5.3.1). Thus, in spite of greater severity and generally poor clinical outcome, there was no evidence for a longer-term degenerative cognitive process in COS, at least through early adulthood (102).

Comorbid Disorders

Comorbid psychiatric disorders, particularly DSM defined mood, anxiety, and substance abuse disorders, often coexist with schizophrenia and can significantly alter the presentation, clinical course, or prognosis of the illness (103–106). As the symptom manifestations of these disorders can also be part of (or masked by) the symptoms of the primary illness, the diagnoses of independent axis I conditions are often ignored (107–109). Furthermore, medical comorbidities in schizophrenia are also frequent (110), including cardiovascular disease (due to tobacco, diabetes, obesity, and increased lipids), HIV, and infectious hepatitis (111). We analyzed the rate of coexistent axis I diagnoses for 76 COS cases at the time of first NIMH admission, and correlated the comorbid diagnoses with age of onset, ratings of illness severity, familiarity, and premorbid development.

As seen with AOS, the most frequent comorbid diagnosis at NIMH screening was depression (54%), followed by

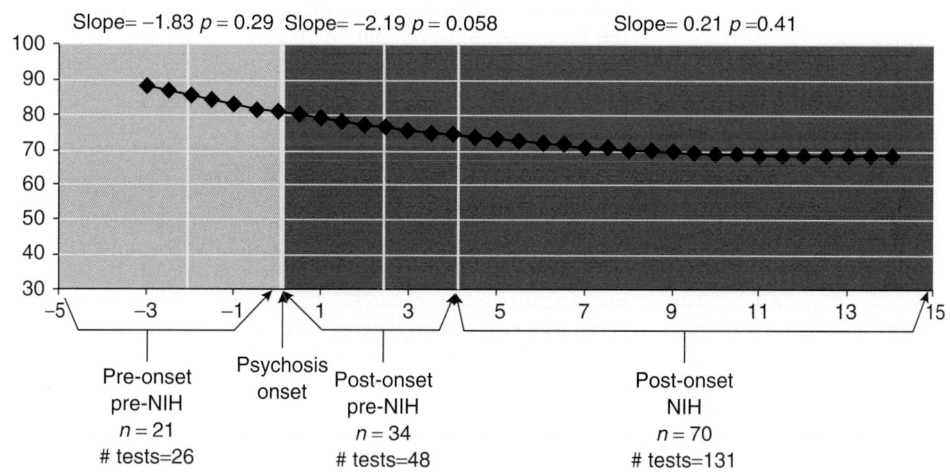

FIGURE 5.3.1. Full scale IQ measures for 70 COS children plotted before (n = 21) and after (n = 70) the onset of psychosis, and also before (n = 56; obtained from prior charts) and after (n = 70) the children were admitted to the NIMH study. Although the children show significant decline in full scale IQ after the onset of psychosis, there is no significant long-term decline over next 14 years.

obsessive-compulsive disorder ([OCD] 21%), generalized anxiety disorder ([GAD] 15%), and ADHD (15%). The rate of "any" anxiety disorder (GAD, OCD, separation anxiety, PTSD, and panic disorder combined) at screening was 42%. In general, comorbid diagnoses were independent of other illness indices, but comorbid depression correlated with poorer GAS scores ($p = 0.01$), and presence of an anxiety disorder only predicted anxiety at 4-year follow-up ($p = 0.05$). No other psychiatric diagnoses showed correlations with any clinical measures, and there were no significant associations between comorbid diagnoses and IQ, familiarity, medication status, premorbid functioning, or age of onset at psychosis. Interestingly, no "current" comorbid depression was seen at the 4-year follow-up for a subgroup of 28 subjects for whom there was complete diagnostic information available, possibly due to our high use of antidepressant treatment (45%). In contrast, anxiety disorders remained highly comorbid despite adjuvant anxiety medication use, suggesting either the refractory nature of these conditions, or a close association with core schizophrenia pathology.

BRAIN IMAGING: STRUCTURAL, FUNCTIONAL, AND POSITRON EMISSION TOMOGRAPHY

The majority of the imaging studies of COS come from the NIMH sample, with more recent contributions from other groups (112–115). Using both cross-sectional and longitudinal data, and rapidly developing state-of-the-art brain mapping methods, neuroimaging in COS has addressed some broad questions about brain development in COS and schizophrenia in general.

Structural Neuroimaging

A fundamental question in brain imaging studies of any illness is whether there are overall differences in brain size. Studies in AOS have documented decreased intracranial volume (116,117), longitudinal reduction in total cerebral volume (118), and ventricular enlargement (119). It is also predicted that brain growth in AOS is stunted even before the onset of illness (116). Similarly, in COS patients, overall brain volume at initial scan is smaller and is followed by a progressive decline in volume during adolescence (120). Patients with COS have also been found to have larger ventricular volume (121) as well as greater progressive increase in ventricular size compared to healthy controls (120,122). Understanding how these brain changes are meaningfully related to clinical features remains an important unanswered question, but collective research points toward the significance of key findings, which are highlighted in the following sections.

Cortical Gray Matter Thickness

Progressive cortical GM loss in COS was first described by Thompson et al. in 2001 (123). This study demonstrated a dynamic wave of GM loss, which started in the parietal and motor cortices and advanced into the superior frontal, dorsolateral prefrontal, and temporal cortices (including the superior temporal gyri). While temporal and dorsolateral prefrontal cortex deficits were among the most severe, they began in late adolescence and were observed only after the onset of psychotic symptoms. The progressive deterioration in GM also correlated with overall deterioration in global functioning. Seeking to determine whether psychosis itself was associated with GM loss, the study included a comparison group of participants with atypical (nonschizophrenic) psychosis, matched for IQ and medications, in addition to healthy volunteers. This atypical psychosis group showed subtle but significantly greater GM loss than healthy volunteers, pointing to a successively increasing rate of GM loss, with COS patients experiencing the greatest loss. In 2004, prompted by the Thompson study, using a similar analysis we evaluated cortical maturation in typically developing children for prospective cortical changes between the ages of 4 to 21 years (124). This study highlighted the timelines of cortical maturation, and importantly, it suggested that COS neurodevelopment appeared to be an exaggeration of normal GM loss and maturation patterns, possibly indicating a loss of inhibitory regulation of the development process (Fig. 5.3.2).

These initial observations generated an important question: Does the GM loss persist into early adulthood and if so, does it continue at the same rate? A longitudinal study addressed this question by following COS patients and controls into adulthood (125). This study found a 7.5% difference in mean cortical thickness (MCT) ($p = 0.001$) between COS patients ($n = 70$, ages 7 to 26) and age-matched healthy controls ($n = 72$), as well as progressive cortical thinning in the parietal, frontal, and temporal regions, although the parietal thinning normalized by early adulthood (125). These results are continuous with findings from AOS patients, which demonstrate cortical thinning in the frontal and temporal cortices only (126,127). Together, these findings established that the profound GM thinning in adolescence appears to slow down as the children mature. Whether this lessening rate is part of the natural course of the disease, a resilience process, or due to medical treatment remains difficult to conclude.

It has also been established that COS patients do not differ from healthy controls with regard to sex differences in cortical thickness (128), or cross-sectional or longitudinal developmental changes in asymmetry (129). Cortical thickness deficits in COS are also largely uninfluenced by clozapine versus olanzapine intake, aside from a small area of the right prefrontal cortex (130). These findings are consistent with AOS, in which age, dose, or type of antipsychotic medication is not significantly linked to changes in cortical thickness (127).

Subcortical Structures

Hippocampus. Critical in learning and memory, the hippocampus has been a structure of significant interest in schizophrenia, where cognitive deficits remain a primary feature of the disease. Deficits in hippocampal volume are well documented in AOS bilaterally (131) and is suggested in COS (120,132).

Prospective studies (133,134) have demonstrated fixed longitudinal volumetric deficits in COS patients compared to controls. Of these, the study with the largest sample (134) (89 COS patients, 78 siblings, and 79 controls) corroborated prior findings (120,133) that suggest that the hippocampal deficits in COS are significant but do not vary over time. These findings are consistent with the animal model of schizophrenia suggested by Lipska et al. in 1993 (135), in which an early fixed deficit in the hippocampus, which is relatively quiescent during the first years of development, manifests later during periods of increased stress or with exposure to particular substances.

Anatomically, subregional shape abnormalities of hippocampus have also been described in AOS (136,137) and COS (138). Bilateral inward deformations of the anterior hippocampus have been found in COS (138), and greater differences have been associated with increased symptom severity. The affected hippocampal regions are commonly associated with hippocampal CA1 pyramidal neurons, whose migration is disrupted by genetic differences associated with schizophrenia (e.g., disruption of the Disc1 gene) (139). The CA1 neurons serve as a connection between the hippocampus and the prefrontal cortex, which is also widely implicated in schizophrenia (140). While the exact involvement of hippocampal abnormalities in COS is unclear, it is possible that abnormal neurodevelopment in these interconnected regions holds further information regarding symptom development.

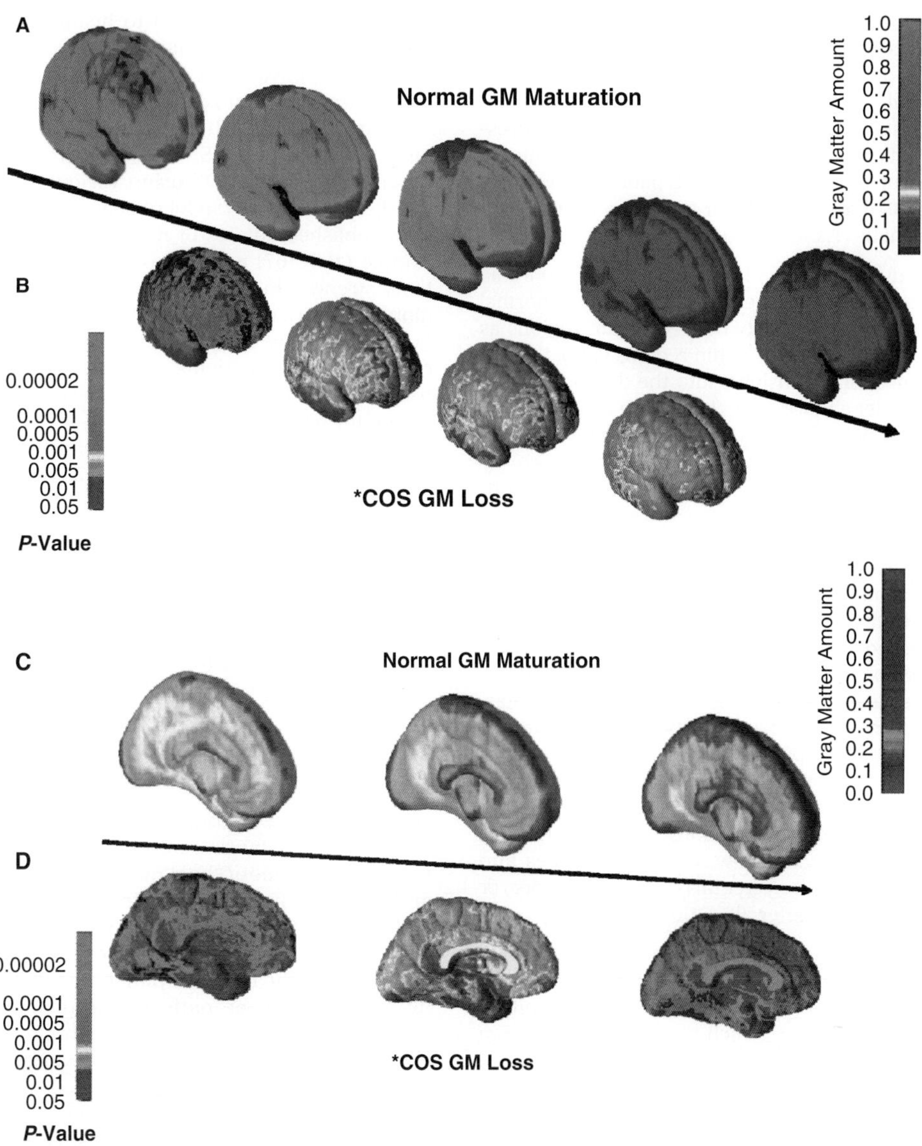

FIGURE 5.3.2. Comparison of the patterns of cortical GM loss in COS (between ages 12 and 16) to that seen in normal cortical maturation (between ages 4 and 22). (**A,C**) Lateral and medial views of the dynamic sequences of cortical GM maturation in healthy children between ages 4 and 22 ($n = 13$; 54 scans) rescanned every 2 years. Scale bar shows GM amount at each of the 65,536 cortical points across the entire cortex represented using a color scale (red to pink—more GM; blue—GM loss). Cortical GM maturation appears to progress in a back to front (parietotemporal) manner on the lateral surface and in a top-down fashion on the medial surface. (**B,D**) Lateral and medial views of the dynamic sequence of cortical GM maturation in COS between ages 12 and 16 compared with age- and sex-matched healthy controls ($n = 12$; 36 scans in each group), where children are rescanned every 2 years. Dynamic maps represent *p*-values for the difference in GM amount between COS and controls at each of the 65,536 cortical points, and *p*-values are represented using a color scale (e.g., pink $p < 0.00002$) which can be observed in color in the original paper or in the online figure. Cortical GM loss in COS also appears to follow in a back to front direction on the lateral surface and in top-down direction on medial surface, thus suggesting that the COS pattern is an exaggeration of the normal GM maturation. (Adapted from Gogtay N, Giedd JN, Lusk L, et al.: Dynamic mapping of human cortical development during childhood through early adulthood. *Proc Natl Acad Sci USA* 101(21):8174–8179, 2004; Thompson PM, Vidal C, Giedd JN, et al.: Mapping adolescent brain change reveals dynamic wave of accelerated gray matter loss in very early-onset schizophrenia. *Proc Natl Acad Sci USA* 98(20):11650–11655, 2001.)

Cerebellum. The cerebellum has a highly heritable development (141), may contribute to higher cognitive functions (142), and it is a potential key site of dysregulated circuitry in schizophrenia (143). In line with this, cerebellar deficits have been linked to COS (144). An early cross-sectional study of COS patients between the ages of 9 and 18 demonstrated decreased cerebellar volume relative to controls in the vermis (11.7% smaller), midsagittal inferior posterior lobe area (10.9% smaller), and midsagittal inferior posterior lobe (8.9% smaller) (145). Studies of AOS have reported a progressive decline in cerebellar volume (146), or a smaller cerebellar volume during the first episode in AOS (147).

In a prospective study of COS patients ($n = 94$) ages 6 to 29 and their nonpsychotic siblings ($n = 80$), COS subjects had smaller bilateral anterior lobes and anterior and total vermis volumes compared to controls (148). Siblings did not differ from healthy controls initially, but demonstrated decreased cerebellar volume over time in the total and right cerebellum, left inferior posterior, left superior posterior, and superior vermis (148). The presence of cerebellar deficits in healthy siblings of COS patients, as well as the presence of abnormalities in AOS patients during the first episode, suggests that the cerebellar trajectory described is likely related to a genetic risk for schizophrenia.

White Matter. The dysconnectivity hypothesis of schizophrenia first proposed that aspects of the illness could be due to abnormal (increased or decreased) connectivity between brain regions as opposed to localized abnormalities within regions (149). Studies of white matter provide initial insights into the dysconnectivity hypothesis. White matter abnormalities have been demonstrated in both AOS and COS patients. Using tensor-based morphometry, we demonstrated that teenage COS patients have a slower rate of white matter growth per year, particularly in the right hemisphere, and that growth deficits are associated with lower functioning in terms of the GAS (150). AOS patients show similar white matter deficits longitudinally (117).

Diffusion tensor imaging (DTI), which examines directional diffusion of water in the brain to infer the structural integrity of neural fibers, has led to less conclusive results. In the largest study of DTI in COS to date, examining eleven regions of interest, we found decreased white matter integrity in the bilateral cuneus, a portion of the occipital lobe (151). In another DTI study, COS patients exhibited a decrease in white matter integrity in relation to their level of linguistic impairment (152). Overall though, DTI research in COS is limited, and inconsistent with the frontal abnormalities demonstrated by AOS DTI research (153); more observations with larger samples and better image resolution are likely required to provide clearer insight into potential white matter alterations in COS.

Corpus Callosum. The majority of patients with schizophrenia manifest neurologic soft signs that include errors in sensory integration, motor coordination, and inhibition (154). These processing deficits, which may arise partly from decreased interhemispheric neural communication, have been associated with irregularities in the corpus callosum (155) and meta-analyses have generally established a reduced midsagittal cross-sectional area in the corpus callosum (156,157). First episode patients showed decreased corpus callosum areas, while chronic patients were more likely to demonstrate an increase in the area (156). The only longitudinal study of the corpus callosum in AOS schizophrenia patients demonstrated progressive decline in callosal size, with poor-outcome patients showing more pronounced decline (158).

The largest to-date longitudinal study in COS (159) (n = 98), their siblings (n = 71), and healthy controls (n = 100) found no differences in total corpus callosum or in the area of any subregion cross-sectionally or in developmental trajectories of any measurement of corpus callosum area or volume (159). Similarly, a study examining healthy siblings of COS patients found no significant differences in corpus callosum area (159). These data suggest that the behavioral deficits in sensorimotor integration in COS may originate not in callosal connections but in the interaction of multiple networks, possibly reflecting a dysfunction in predictive processing (160–162).

Functional Magnetic Resonance Imaging

Functional imaging studies are difficult to conduct in the COS due to illness severity, which make it difficult for patients to perform tasks in the scanner and often introduce behavioral confounds. In a unique fMRI study of language processing in COS, Borofsky et al. (163) found that COS patients have overall reduced activity compared to healthy controls during both semantic and syntactic language processing tasks. The differences in activation were not related to performance on the task, as there were no group differences in success rate.

Resting state fMRI (R-fMRI) studies have been relatively more feasible in COS. R-fMRI has been used to examine dysconnectivity in AOS using various methods, and support the dysconnectivity model of schizophrenia (164). To date, the four published studies of R-fMRI in COS are from the NIMH sample (165–167) and demonstrate decreased local connectivity strength in COS that is partially balanced by increased global network efficiency relative to healthy controls (166,167). Furthermore, we found widespread decreased functional correlations in COS patients compared to healthy volunteers, in brain regions that organized into a social-cognitive and a sensorimotor processing network. These findings emphasized the role of dysfunctional integration of these two major systems, and importantly, found that resting state alterations were linked to behavioral symptoms. Specifically, decreases in functional connectivity across these two networks in COS were related to the severity of positive symptoms, while connectivity decreases within the social-cognitive network related to the severity of negative symptoms (165). These results are consistent with the proposal that dysfunctional network interactions play a crucial role in the disease, particularly with respect to sensorimotor integration and predictive processing.

Healthy Siblings

Studying nonsymptomatic or healthy siblings of patients with heritable illnesses improves understanding of the contribution of genetic background to an illness state versus an illness predisposition or trait. Nonpsychotic biologic full siblings of COS patients, share about 50% of their genetic material and can add valuable context to neuroimaging findings (168). In the most simplified form, consistent phenotypic differences between patients and their healthy biologic full siblings suggest that the patient phenotype is related to the expression of symptoms (disease state), assuming that the healthy sibling group and unrelated healthy control group do not differ. On the other hand, similarities between healthy and ill siblings, despite the difference in their health status, can relate phenotypes to genetic vulnerability that may not contribute directly to symptoms (disease trait). Due to the early-onset nature of COS, siblings of COS patients enter studies at early ages and thus provide a unique opportunity to address questions of state versus trait within a neurodevelopmental window.

State Markers

State markers are characteristics unique to the expression of symptoms that do not occur in unrelated healthy controls or healthy siblings of patients despite their predisposition for the illness. Because these differences occur despite similarities in genetic background between patients and their unaffected siblings, they are assumed to be associated with the development of the disease, for example, psychosis in the case of schizophrenia. The brain area most consistently identified as a state marker for schizophrenia through COS studies is the hippocampus, which demonstrates volumetric deficits, that are fixed over time, in patients but not their nonpsychotic siblings (134).

Trait Markers

Trait markers are defined as phenotypes that may be related to predisposition for the illness, but may not be directly related to the disease. Nonpsychotic siblings of COS patients

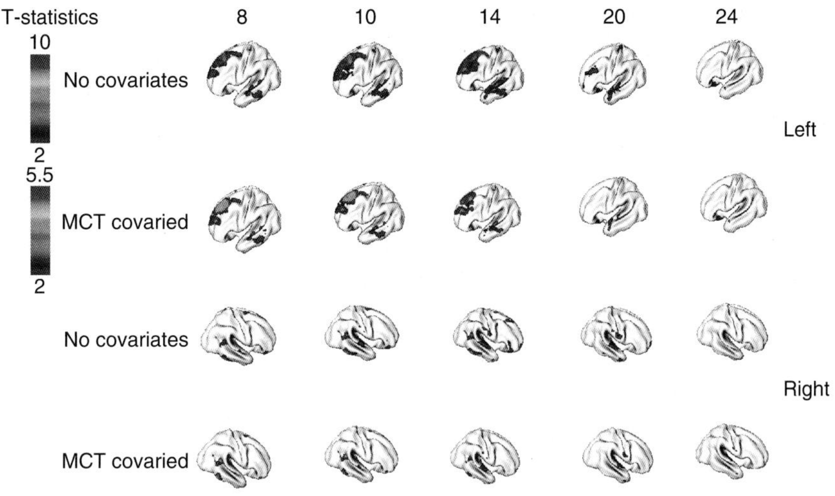

FIGURE 5.3.3. Cortical GM development in healthy COS siblings (n = 56; 100 scans) compared with age- and sex-matched normal volunteers (n = 56; 100 scans) between 6 and 30 years. Analyses were done using automated cortical thickness measure across 40,000 cortical points over the entire cortex using mixed-effect regression model analyses which allowed using cross-sectional as well as longitudinal scans. Color bars, which can be observed in color in the original paper or in the online figure, represent t-statistics where $t > 2$ (adjusted for multiple comparisons, using false discovery rate at $t = 2$) indicates significant loss of GM in healthy siblings compared to controls at that cortical point. GM differences at various ages were obtained by age recentering the data at that age. Healthy siblings showed GM loss in prefrontal and temporal cortices in early ages, but the GM differences were normalized by age 24 years. Images are shown both with and without adjusting for mean cortical thickness (MCT). (From Gogtay N, Greenstein D, Lenane M, et al.: Cortical brain development in nonpsychotic siblings of patients with childhood-onset schizophrenia. *Arch Gen Psychiatry* 64(7):772–780, 2007.)

share a number of characteristic abnormalities with their affected relatives, including differences in cerebral volume, GM thickness, and white matter growth (169–171). Two nonoverlapping studies of unaffected siblings (n = 52; ages 8 to 28 and n = 43, ages 5 to 26 years) versus healthy controls (n = 52 and n = 86) demonstrated no significant difference in MCT between the two groups, however the sibling group had a pattern of early restricted GM loss (171,172). Both studies examined cortical thickness in siblings by region, revealing GM deficits in prefrontal, temporal, and parietal areas during early life. Each of these deficits, though initially similar to those seen in young COS patients, were undetectable by adulthood (171,172) (Fig. 5.3.3). This deficit "normalization," which is likely to be an age-specific trait marker, may also help explain inconsistent results from studies of cortical thickness in healthy siblings of AOS patients (173) where the average age of sibling sample is much older and past the developmental window. Furthermore, siblings of COS patients have also been shown to exhibit deficits in white matter growth during adolescence at early stages in life, however the growth rate normalizes by adulthood in healthy siblings, suggesting that white matter growth may also represent a trait marker (170).

To date, a single task-based fMRI study has been reported in a COS sibling population which demonstrated that healthy siblings of COS patients showed aberrant frontal and striatal activation relative to healthy controls during a cognitive skill learning task (174). If feasible, it would be interesting to conduct a similar study in COS patients, in order to understand to what extent these findings may represent a functional endophenotype.

To our knowledge, no R-fMRI studies have been published describing functional connectivity in healthy siblings of COS patients although preliminary findings from our unpublished data suggest they are intermediate, similar to that seen for structural abnormalities, suggesting a potential functional trait marker.

GENETIC STUDIES

Schizophrenia is a complex disorder with a heterogeneous phenotype in which most likely numerous genetic and environmental exposures are involved (175). While inheritance patterns vary, a strong genetic inheritance is supported by twin, family, and adoption studies (175,176). Observations across pediatrics and medicine suggest that early-onset cases may have more salient genetic causes (4,177,178), and as with breast cancer (179), Alzheimer disease (180), and type II diabetes (181), the familial risk for schizophrenia spectrum disorders appears higher for COS than in AOS contrast groups (74,75).

In genetic studies of complex disease there are currently two salient working hypotheses, the common disease–common allele model, which proposes that combinations of common genetic variations (i.e., polymorphisms in >1% of the population) contribute a modest effect to disease cause or susceptibility (182). Alternatively, the common disease–rare allele hypothesis proposes that some individually rare mutations (<1% of the population, which a single individual or family may have) with high penetrance contribute to disease cause or susceptibility (183).

Common Variant Alleles

While now considered generally inadequate, earlier studies of common variants focused on candidate genes, which utilized existing biologic knowledge to identify single-nucleotide polymorphisms (SNPs) as markers to map and trace transmission of regions of the chromosome (182). One of the key issues about this approach is that many disease genes have been unanticipated based on what was previously known. Notwithstanding, using the hypothesis that there may be more detrimental/penetrant mutations in known schizophrenia susceptibility genes in COS, several genes previously implicated in AOS samples showed significant association with COS including G72 (now DAOA) (184), neuregulin 1 (NRG1) (185), GAD1 (186), and dysbindin

(DTNBP1) (187). In addition to supporting the genetic continuity between COS and AOS, these data suggested that the very early-onset COS population, with more pronounced neurobiologic abnormalities and a more homogeneous phenotype, might turn out to be a relatively efficient population to target for the identification of genetic risk of schizophrenia more generally.

With the technologic advances in microarray analyses, genome-wide association studies (GWASs) have opened a new window into the genome at a submicroscopic level by systematically assessing a broad array of SNPs independent of prior scientific knowledge (188). Because GWASs require stringent corrections for multiple comparisons, studies must have very large numbers of participants/samples in order to be adequately powered. This encouraged international collaborative efforts such as the Psychiatric Genomic Consortium (PGC) in order to pool samples. Despite these efforts, samples for rare diseases such as COS remain small with pooled numbers of less than 300 which cannot compare to AOS studies of over 16,000 patients (189). Results from large GWAS studies in AOS have included the association of the major histocompatibility complex and the intron 4 transcription factor (TCF4) involved in neurogenesis and brain development (190). GWAS results have also supported polygenicity, with multiple small genetic variations conferring risk for AOS, genetic overlap with other mental illnesses, and difficulties replicating findings from prior candidate gene studies (191–193). To overcome the issue of small sample size, the NIMH team created polygenic risk scores for 130 COS participants and their healthy sibling controls, using 80 genomic variants associated to schizophrenia PGC GWAS. Despite the small sample size, COS participants had higher risk scores than their healthy siblings ($p < 0.05$). Although only with the most liberal significance threshold, the study also described overlap between polygenic risk for autisms and COS (194).

Rare Variant Alleles

Studies of rare variant alleles have focused primarily on structural variations in stretches of DNA known as copy number variations (CNVs). Essential to these studies is that these types of variations are common in human populations and, while they may denote disease risk, they may also represent standard genetic variation. One of the initial seminal studies of CNVs in schizophrenia found a progressive increase in novel CNVs with earlier age of onset of schizophrenia. While only 5% of the controls had any CNVs >100 kb, 15% of AOS cases and 20% of young onset (< age 18) had CNVs. An independent replication in the same study found that 28% of COS patients had CNVs compared to 13% in their control sample of COS parents. A large number of the CNVs affected genes in brain development and regulation pathways (183). This study was followed by numerous additional findings of CNVs in schizophrenia (195–200). Using whole genome sequencing, the NIMH team assessed CNVs in 126 COS patients and 69 of their healthy full siblings. Focusing on a group of 46 CNVs associated to risk for AOS, autism, intellectual disabilities, and seizures, the study found that COS patients had not only significantly higher rates of disease-related CNVs compared to their healthy sibling controls ($p = 00.17$), but also than that reported in AOS ($p < 0.0001$) (201).

Cytogenetic Abnormalities

High-resolution banding karyotype and fluorescent in situ hybridization (FISH) analyses are done routinely on all COS participants to look for fragile X, 22q11 deletions, Smith–Magenis (17p11.2del), and 15q11–q13 deletions/duplications. Almost 10% of the NIMH COS participants show chromosomal abnormalities. The 22q11 deletion syndrome (22q11DS), manifest as velocardiofacial syndrome (VCFS), is estimated to occur 1 in 4,000 live births (202), and is a known risk factor for schizophrenia (203,204). Five out of 126 (4.0%) of the NIMH COS patients have VCFS with spontaneous 22q11.2 deletion, a rate significantly higher than reported in healthy controls (0.2%) ($p < 0.0001$) (205), AOS patients (0.3% to 1%) (206–208) ($p < 0.0001$), or any clinical population at present. Despite the association between autism and the 22q.11.2 deletion (209,210), and the presence of prepsychotic autism spectrum disorders in 20% of our sample, none of the individuals with the 22q11.2 deletion had prepsychotic autism symptoms (201). Similarly, 7 out of 133 have large chromosomal abnormalities such as Turner syndrome, XYY, trisomy X, or either translocations or frameshift mutations (211,212).

TREATMENT STUDIES IN CHILDHOOD PSYCHOSES

Although rare, COS is a devastating disorder, frequently resistant to treatment, and with an unfortunately narrow evidence base to guide treatment, particularly as there are few trials comparing atypical antipsychotics, which have become the mainstay of current treatment (213). Two prior randomized controlled trials established the superiority of typical antipsychotics over placebo in COS (214,215). A single trial in a small group of treatment refractory COS patients had demonstrated the efficacy of clozapine over the typical antipsychotic haloperidol (216). However, as there was no placebo arm in the study, it is hard to assess the true effect size for clozapine. A later double-blind randomized controlled trial of comparing clozapine ($n = 12$) with olanzapine ($n = 13$) showed a significant advantage for clozapine in the alleviation of negative symptoms of schizophrenia, which was not correlated with improvement in mood or extrapyramidal side effects. As anticipated, clozapine was associated with more overall side effects, including enuresis, tachycardia, hypertension, and significant weight gain by 2 years (217). The results of the NIMH cohort and studies in AOS patients (218,219) show that clozapine has the greatest antipsychotic efficacy, particularly in a pediatric population, with our recent study finding over 70% of the 120 children available at follow-up adhering to clozapine treatment for more than 2 years, despite its side effects and need for close monitoring (220).

Adverse Effects of Clozapine

In spite of its unique efficacy for some COS patients, clozapine is associated with several side effects, in particular agranulocytosis, weight gain, cardiovascular changes such as postural hypotension and tachycardia, and incontinence. The NIMH study has started addressing the questions of how to manage these side effects so that these children can continue to stay on clozapine.

Neutropenia and Akathisia

Children and adolescents treated with clozapine have increased susceptibility to neutropenia, particularly in male children with African American decent (221). This can be successfully managed by addition of lithium (222). Similarly, akathisia, seen only rarely in adults on clozapine, appears more common in children and can frequently manifest as worsening of psychotic symptoms or agitation in children, which frequently results in dosage increment. This side effect is responsive to adjunctive propranolol treatment (223).

Weight Gain

Weight gain is a significant effect of atypical antipsychotics and appears more pronounced in pediatric patients (224,225). Clozapine particularly has been noted to cause significant weight gain during childhood (226). Although the mechanism of weight gain in poorly understood, genetic risks (polymorphism in beta 3 and alpha-1A adrenergic, 5HT-2C, TNF-alpha, and histamine receptors) and a number of biochemical correlates (e.g., leptin, prolactin, triglyceride, and HDL levels) of weight gain have been reported in the literature (227). In our group, an analysis of 23 COS patients treated with clozapine and 21 matched healthy controls showed increases in BMI ($p < 0.001$) and leptin levels ($p = 0.003$) after 6 weeks of treatment. For COS patients, BMI at baseline and week 6 correlated with insulin level ($r = 0.5$, $p = 0.004$) and BMI was positively correlated with clinical improvement in CGI, SAPS, and SANS rating scales ($p < 0.05$) (228). Based on these correlations, we have used the antidiabetic medication metformin (which improves peripheral insulin sensitivity) with some success although no formal trial was done.

References

1. Schreier HA: Hallucinations in nonpsychotic children: more common than we think? *J Am Acad Child Adolesc Psychiatry* 38(5):623–625, 1999.
2. McGee R, Williams S, Poulton R: Hallucinations in nonpsychotic children. *J Am Acad Child Adolesc Psychiatry* 39(1):12–13, 2000.
3. Kelleher I, Connor D, Clarke MC, Devlin N, Harley M, Cannon M: Prevalence of psychotic symptoms in childhood and adolescence: a systematic review and meta-analysis of population-based studies. *Psychol Med* 42(9):1857–1863, 2012.
4. Childs B, Scriver CR: Age at onset and causes of disease. *Perspect Biol Med* 29(3 Pt 1):437–460, 1986.
5. Nicolson R, Rapoport JL: Childhood-onset schizophrenia: rare but worth studying. *Biol Psychiatry* 46(10):1418–1428, 1999.
6. Kraepelin E: *Dementia Praecox and Paraphrenia.* Huntington, NY, Robert E Krieger, 1919.
7. Volkmar FR: Childhood and adolescent psychosis: a review of the past 10 years. *J Am Acad Child Adolesc Psychiatry* 35(7):843–851, 1996.
8. Kolvin I: Studies in the childhood psychoses. I. Diagnostic criteria and classification. *Br J Psychiatry* 118(545):381–384, 1971.
9. Ulloa RE, Birmaher B, Axelson D, et al.: Psychosis in a pediatric mood and anxiety disorders clinic: phenomenology and correlates. *J Am Acad Child Adolesc Psychiatry* 39(3):337–345, 2000.
10. Edelsohn GA, Rabinovich H, Portnoy R: Hallucinations in nonpsychotic children: findings from a psychiatric emergency service. *Ann NY Acad Sci* 1008:261–264, 2003.
11. Yung AR, Buckby JA, Cosgrave EM, et al.: Association between psychotic experiences and depression in a clinical sample over 6 months. *Schizophr Res* 91(1–3):246–253, 2007.
12. Escher S, Romme M, Buiks A, Delespaul P, van Os J: Independent course of childhood auditory hallucinations: a sequential 3-year follow-up study. *Br J Psychiatry Suppl* 43:s10–s18, 2002.
13. Rubio JM, Sanjuan J, Florez-Salamanca L, Cuesta MJ: Examining the course of hallucinatory experiences in children and adolescents: a systematic review. *Schizophr Res* 138(2-3):248–254, 2012.
14. Kelleher I, Keeley H, Corcoran P, et al.: Clinicopathological significance of psychotic experiences in non-psychotic young people: evidence from four population-based studies. *Br J Psychiatry* 201(1):26–32, 2012.
15. Calkins ME, Moore TM, Merikangas KR, et al.: The psychosis spectrum in a young U.S. community sample: findings from the Philadelphia Neurodevelopmental Cohort. *World Psychiatry* 13(3):296–305, 2014.
16. Dhossche D, Ferdinand R, Van der Ende J, Hofstra MB, Verhulst F: Diagnostic outcome of self-reported hallucinations in a community sample of adolescents. *Psychol Med* 32(4):619–627, 2002.
17. De Loore E, Gunther N, Drukker M, et al.: Persistence and outcome of auditory hallucinations in adolescence: a longitudinal general population study of 1800 individuals. *Schizophr Res* 127(1–3):252–256, 2011.
18. Poulton R, Caspi A, Moffitt TE, Cannon M, Murray R, Harrington H: Children's self-reported psychotic symptoms and adult schizophreniform disorder: a 15-year longitudinal study. *Arch Gen Psychiatry* 57(11): 1053–1058, 2000.
19. van Os J, Linscott RJ, Myin-Germeys I, Delespaul P, Krabbendam L: A systematic review and meta-analysis of the psychosis continuum: evidence for a psychosis proneness-persistence-impairment model of psychotic disorder. *Psychol Med* 39(2):179–195, 2009.
20. Laurens KR, Hobbs MJ, Sunderland M, Green MJ, Mould GL: Psychotic-like experiences in a community sample of 8000 children aged 9 to 11 years: an item response theory analysis. *Psychol Med* 42(7): 1495–1506, 2012.
21. Yoshizumi T, Murase S, Honjo S, Kaneko H, Murakami T: Hallucinatory experiences in a community sample of Japanese children. *J Am Acad Child Adolesc Psychiatry* 43(8):1030–1036, 2004.
22. Pearson D, Burrow A, FitzGerald C, Green K, Lee G, Wise N: Auditory hallucinations in normal child populations. *Pers Individ Differ* 31(3): 401–407, 2001.
23. Ohayon MM: Prevalence of hallucinations and their pathological associations in the general population. *Psychiatry Res* 97(2–3):153–164, 2000.
24. Nevsimalova S: Narcolepsy in childhood. *Sleep Med Rev* 13(2):169–180, 2009.
25. Driver DI, Gogtay N, Rapoport JL: Childhood onset schizophrenia and early onset schizophrenia spectrum disorders. *Child Adolesc Psychiatr Clin N Am* 22(4):539–555, 2013.
26. Rapoport J, Chavez A, Greenstein D, Addington A, Gogtay N: Autism spectrum disorders and childhood-onset schizophrenia: clinical and biological contributions to a relation revisited. *J Am Acad Child Adolesc Psychiatry* 48(1):10–18, 2009.
27. Hollis C: Child and adolescent (juvenile onset) schizophrenia. A case control study of premorbid developmental impairments. *Br J Psychiatry* 166(4):489–495, 1995.
28. Alaghband-Rad J, McKenna K, Gordon CT, et al.: Childhood-onset schizophrenia: the severity of premorbid course. *J Am Acad Child Adolesc Psychiatry* 34(10):1273–1283, 1995.
29. Laurens KR, Luo L, Matheson SL, et al.: Common or distinct pathways to psychosis? A systematic review of evidence from prospective studies for developmental risk factors and antecedents of the schizophrenia spectrum disorders and affective psychoses. *BMC Psychiatry* 15:205, 2015.
30. Bucci P, Mucci A, Piegari G, et al.: Characterization of premorbid functioning during childhood in patients with deficit vs. non-deficit schizophrenia and in their healthy siblings. *Schizophr Res* 2016.
31. Tillman R, Geller B, Klages T, Corrigan M, Bolhofner K, Zimerman B: Psychotic phenomena in 257 young children and adolescents with bipolar I disorder: delusions and hallucinations (benign and pathological). *Bipolar Disord* 10(1):45–55, 2008.
32. Niarchou M, Zammit S, Lewis G: The Avon Longitudinal Study of Parents and Children (ALSPAC) birth cohort as a resource for studying psychopathology in childhood and adolescence: a summary of findings for depression and psychosis. *Socl Psychiatr Psychiatr Epidemiol* 50(7):1017–1027, 2015.
33. Pavuluri MN, Herbener ES, Sweeney JA: Psychotic symptoms in pediatric bipolar disorder. *J Affect Disord* 80(1):19–28, 2004.
34. Geller B, Tillman R, Bolhofner K, Zimerman B: Child bipolar I disorder: prospective continuity with adult bipolar I disorder; characteristics of second and third episodes; predictors of 8-year outcome. *Arch Gen Psychiatry* 65(10):1125–1133, 2008.
35. Birmaher B, Gill MK, Axelson DA, et al.: Longitudinal trajectories and associated baseline predictors in youths with bipolar spectrum disorders. *Am J Psychiatry* 171(9):990–999, 2014.
36. Smith RA, Wright B, Bennett S: Hallucinations and illusions in migraine in children and the Alice in Wonderland Syndrome. *Arch Dis Child* 100(3):296–298, 2015.
37. Sedel F, Baumann N, Turpin JC, Lyon-Caen O, Saudubray JM, Cohen D: Psychiatric manifestations revealing inborn errors of metabolism in adolescents and adults. *J Inherit Metabol Dis* 30(5):631–641, 2007.
38. Linscott RJ, van Os J: An updated and conservative systematic review and meta-analysis of epidemiological evidence on psychotic experiences in children and adults: on the pathway from proneness to persistence to dimensional expression across mental disorders. *Psychol Med* 43(6):1133–1149, 2013.
39. Cochran DM, Dvir Y, Frazier JA: "Autism-plus" spectrum disorders: intersection with psychosis and the schizophrenia spectrum. *Child Adolesc Psychiatr Clin N Am* 22(4):609–627, 2013.
40. Rosman NP, Bergia BM: Childhood disintegrative disorder: distinction from autistic disorder and predictors of outcome. *J Child Neurol* 28(12):1587–1598, 2013.
41. Garralda ME: Hallucinations in children with conduct and emotional disorders: II. The follow-up study. *Psychol Med* 14(3):597–604, 1984.
42. Garralda ME: Hallucinations in children with conduct and emotional disorders: I. The clinical phenomena. *Psychol Med* 14(3):589–596, 1984.
43. McKenna K, Gordon CT, Lenane M, Kaysen D, Fahey K, Rapoport JL: Looking for childhood-onset schizophrenia: the first 71 cases screened. *J Am Acad Child Adolesc Psychiatry* 33(5):636–644, 1994.
44. Kumra S, Jacobsen LK, Lenane M, et al.: "Multidimensionally impaired disorder": is it a variant of very early-onset schizophrenia? *J Am Acad Child Adolesc Psychiatry* 37(1):91–99, 1998.
45. Towbin KE, Dykens EM, Pearson GS, Cohen DJ: Conceptualizing "borderline syndrome of childhood" and "childhood schizophrenia" as a developmental disorder. *J Am Acad Child Adolesc Psychiatry* 32(4):775–782, 1993.
46. Dahl EK, Cohen DJ, Provence S: Clinical and multivariate approaches to the nosology of pervasive developmental disorders. *J Am Acad Child Psychiatry* 25(2):170–180, 1986.
47. Petti TA, Vela RM: Borderline disorders of childhood: an overview. *J Am Acad Child Adolesc Psychiatry* 29(3):327–337, 1990.
48. Van der Gaag RJ, Buitelaar J, Van den Ban E, Bezemer M, Njio L, Van Engeland H: A controlled multivariate chart review of multiple complex developmental disorder. *J Am Acad Child Adolesc Psychiatry* 34(8): 1096–1106, 1995.
49. Cohen DJ, Paul R, Volkmar FR: Issues in the classification of pervasive and other developmental disorders: toward DSM-IV. *J Am Acad Child Psychiatry* 25(2):213–220, 1986.
50. Ad-Dab'bagh Y, Greenfield B: Multiple complex developmental disorder: the "multiple and complex" evolution of the "childhood borderline

syndrome" construct. *J Am Acad Child Adolesc Psychiatry* 40(8):954–964, 2001.
51. Nicolson R, Lenane M, Brookner F, et al.: Children and adolescents with psychotic disorder not otherwise specified: a 2- to 8-year follow-up study. *Compr Psychiatry* 42(4):319–325, 2001.
52. Kumra S, Briguglio C, Lenane M, et al. Including children and adolescents with schizophrenia in medication-free research. *Am J Psychiatry* 156(7):1065–1068, 1999.
53. Calderoni D, Wudarsky M, Bhangoo R, et al.: Differentiating childhood-onset schizophrenia from psychotic mood disorders. *J Am Acad Child Adolesc Psychiatry* 40(10):1190–1196, 2001.
54. Cannon-Spoor HE, Potkin SG, Wyatt RJ: Measurement of premorbid adjustment in chronic schizophrenia. *Schizophr Bull* 8(3):470–484, 1982.
55. Nicolson R, Lenane M, Singaracharlu S, et al.: Premorbid speech and language impairments in childhood-onset schizophrenia: association with risk factors. *Am J Psychiatry* 157(5):794–800, 2000.
56. Sporn AL, Addington AM, Gogtay N, et al.: Pervasive developmental disorder and childhood-onset schizophrenia: comorbid disorder or a phenotypic variant of a very early onset illness? *Biol Psychiatry* 55(10):989–994, 2004.
57. Schaeffer JL, Ross RG: Childhood-onset schizophrenia: premorbid and prodromal diagnostic and treatment histories. *J Am Acad Child Adolesc Psychiatry* 41(5):538–545, 2002.
58. Green WH, Padron-Gayol M, Hardesty AS, Bassiri M: Schizophrenia with childhood onset: a phenomenological study of 38 cases. *J Am Acad Child Adolesc Psychiatry* 31(5):968–976, 1992.
59. Tsuchiya KJ, Takagai S, Kawai M, et al.: Advanced paternal age associated with an elevated risk for schizophrenia in offspring in a Japanese population. *Schizophr Res* 76(2–3):337–342, 2005.
60. Frans EM, McGrath JJ, Sandin S, et al.: Advanced paternal and grandpaternal age and schizophrenia: a three-generation perspective. *Schizophr Res* 133(1–3):120–124, 2011.
61. Torrey EF, Buka S, Cannon TD, et al.: Paternal age as a risk factor for schizophrenia: how important is it? *Schizophr Res* 114(1–3):1–5, 2009.
62. Lehrer DS, Pato MT, Nahhas RW, et al.: Paternal age effect: Replication in schizophrenia with intriguing dissociation between bipolar with and without psychosis. *Am J Med Genet B Neuropsychiatr Genet* 171(4):495–505, 2015.
63. Malaspina D, Harlap S, Fennig S, et al.: Advancing paternal age and the risk of schizophrenia. *Arch Gen Psychiatry* 58(4):361–367, 2001.
64. Lewis SW, Murray RM: Obstetric complications, neurodevelopmental deviance, and risk of schizophrenia. *J Psychiatr Res* 21(4):413–421, 1987.
65. Cannon M, Jones PB, Murray RM: Obstetric complications and schizophrenia: historical and meta-analytic review. *Am J Psychiatry* 159(7):1080–1092, 2002.
66. Clarke MC, Harley M, Cannon M: The role of obstetric events in schizophrenia. *Schizophr Bull* 32(1):3–8, 2006.
67. Nicolson R, Malaspina D, Giedd JN, et al.: Obstetrical complications and childhood-onset schizophrenia. *Am J Psychiatry* 156(10):1650–1652, 1999.
68. Malaspina D: *Columbia Obstetrics Complication Scale, Diagnostic Center for Schizophrenia Linkage Studies.* New York, New York State Psychiatric Institute, 2003.
69. Ordonez AE, Bobb A, Greenstein D, et al.: Lack of evidence for elevated obstetric complications in childhood onset schizophrenia. *Biol Psychiatry* 58(1):10–15, 2005.
70. Holzman PS: Eye movements and the search for the essence of schizophrenia. *Brain Res Brain Res Rev* 31(2-3):350–356, 2000.
71. Ross RG, Olincy A, Harris JG, et al.: Evidence for bilineal inheritance of physiological indicators of risk in childhood-onset schizophrenia. *Am J Med Genet* 88(2):188–199, 1999.
72. Sporn A, Greenstein D, Gogtay N, et al.: Childhood-onset schizophrenia: smooth pursuit eye-tracking dysfunction in family members. *Schizophr Res* 73(2–3):243–252, 2005.
73. Asarnow JR, Ben-Meir S: Children with schizophrenia spectrum and depressive disorders: a comparative study of premorbid adjustment, onset pattern and severity of impairment. *J Child Psychol Psychiatr Allied Discipl* 29(4):477–488, 1988.
74. Asarnow RF, Nuechterlein KH, Fogelson D, et al.: Schizophrenia and schizophrenia-spectrum personality disorders in the first-degree relatives of children with schizophrenia: the UCLA family study. *Arch Gen Psychiatry* 58(6):581–588, 2001.
75. Nicolson R, Brookner FB, Lenane M, et al.: Parental schizophrenia spectrum disorders in childhood-onset and adult-onset schizophrenia. *Am J Psychiatry* 160(3):490–495, 2003.
76. Chen WJ, Faraone SV: Sustained attention deficits as markers of genetic susceptibility to schizophrenia. *Am J Med Genet* 97(1):52–57, 2000.
77. Harris JG, Adler LE, Young DA, et al.: Neuropsychological dysfunction in parents of schizophrenics. *Schizophr Res* 20(3):253–260, 1996.
78. Schulze-Rauschenbach S, Lennertz L, Ruhrmann S, et al.: Neurocognitive functioning in parents of schizophrenia patients: attentional and executive performance vary with genetic loading. *Psychiatry Res* 230(3):885–891, 2015.
79. Faraone SV, Seidman LJ, Kremen WS, Toomey R, Pepple JR, Tsuang MT: Neuropsychological functioning among the nonpsychotic relatives of schizophrenic patients: a 4-year follow-up study. *J Abnorm Psychol* 108(1):176–181, 1999.
80. Park S, Holzman PS, Goldman-Rakic PS: Spatial working memory deficits in the relatives of schizophrenic patients. *Arch Gen Psychiatry* 52(10):821–828, 1995.
81. Skelley SL, Goldberg TE, Egan MF, Weinberger DR, Gold JM: Verbal and visual memory: characterizing the clinical and intermediate phenotype in schizophrenia. *Schizophr Res* 105(1–3):78–85, 2008.
82. Gold JM, Blaxton TA, Hermann BP, et al.: Memory and intelligence in lateralized temporal lobe epilepsy and schizophrenia. *Schizophr Res* 17(1):59–65, 1995.
83. Egan MF, Hyde TM, Bonomo JB, et al.: Relative risk of neurological signs in siblings of patients with schizophrenia. *Am J Psychiatry* 158(11):1827–1834, 2001.
84. Sitskoorn MM, Aleman A, Ebisch SJ, Appels MC, Kahn RS: Cognitive deficits in relatives of patients with schizophrenia: a meta-analysis. *Schizophr Res* 71(2–3):285–295, 2004.
85. Snitz BE, Macdonald AW 3rd, Carter CS: Cognitive deficits in unaffected first-degree relatives of schizophrenia patients: a meta-analytic review of putative endophenotypes. *Schizophr Bull* 32(1):179–194, 2006.
86. Krabbendam L, Marcelis M, Delespaul P, Jolles J, van Os J: Single or multiple familial cognitive risk factors in schizophrenia? *Am J Med Genet* 105(2):183–188, 2001.
87. Faraone SV, Seidman LJ, Kremen WS, Toomey R, Pepple JR, Tsuang MT: Neuropsychologic functioning among the nonpsychotic relatives of schizophrenic patients: the effect of genetic loading. *Biol Psychiatry* 48(2):120–126, 2000.
88. Gochman PA, Greenstein D, Sporn A, et al.: Childhood onset schizophrenia: familial neurocognitive measures. *Schizophr Res* 71(1):43–47, 2004.
89. Sullivan S, Rai D, Golding J, Zammit S, Steer C: The association between autism spectrum disorder and psychotic experiences in the Avon longitudinal study of parents and children (ALSPAC) birth cohort. *J Am Acad Child Adolesc Psychiatry* 52(8):806–814.e802, 2013.
90. Selten JP, Lundberg M, Rai D, Magnusson C: Risks for nonaffective psychotic disorder and bipolar disorder in young people with autism spectrum disorder: a population-based study. *JAMA Psychiatry* 72(5): 483–489, 2015.
91. Chisholm K, Lin A, Abu-Akel A, Wood SJ: The association between autism and schizophrenia spectrum disorders: A review of eight alternate models of co-occurrence. *Neurosci Biobehav Rev* 55:173–183, 2015.
92. Joshi G, Wozniak J, Petty C, et al.: Psychiatric comorbidity and functioning in a clinically referred population of adults with autism spectrum disorders: a comparative study. *J Autism Dev Disord* 43(6):1314–1325, 2013.
93. Jorde LB, Hasstedt SJ, Ritvo ER, et al.: Complex segregation analysis of autism. *Am J Hum Genet* 49(5):932–938, 1991.
94. Asarnow RF: Neurocognitive impairments in schizophrenia: a piece of the epigenetic puzzle. *Euro Child Adolesc Psychiatry* 8(Suppl 1):I5–I8, 1999.
95. Asarnow RF, Asamen J, Granholm E, Sherman T, Watkins JM, Williams ME: Cognitive/neuropsychological studies of children with a schizophrenic disorder. *Schizophr Bull* 20(4):647–669, 1994.
96. Asarnow RF, Brown W, Strandburg R: Children with a schizophrenic disorder: neurobehavioral studies. *Eur Arch Psychiatry Clin Neurosci* 245(2):70–79, 1995.
97. Karatekin C, Asarnow RF: Working memory in childhood-onset schizophrenia and attention-deficit/hyperactivity disorder. *Psychiatry Res* 80(2):165–176, 1998.
98. Goldberg TE, Hyde TM, Kleinman JE, Weinberger DR: Course of schizophrenia: neuropsychological evidence for a static encephalopathy. *Schizophr Bull* 19(4):797–804, 1993.
99. Russell AJ, Munro JC, Jones PB, Hemsley DR, Murray RM: Schizophrenia and the myth of intellectual decline. *Am J Psychiatry* 154(5):635–639, 1997.
100. Mesholam-Gately RI, Giuliano AJ, Goff KP, Faraone SV, Seidman LJ: Neurocognition in first-episode schizophrenia: a meta-analytic review. *Neuropsychology* 23(3):315–336, 2009.
101. Kumra S, Wiggs E, Bedwell J, et al.: Neuropsychological deficits in pediatric patients with childhood-onset schizophrenia and psychotic disorder not otherwise specified. *Schizophr Res* 42(2):135–144, 2000.
102. Gochman PA, Greenstein D, Sporn A, et al.: IQ stabilization in childhood-onset schizophrenia. *Schizophr Res* 77(2–3):271–277, 2005.
103. Buckley PF, Miller BJ, Lehrer DS, Castle DJ: Psychiatric comorbidities and schizophrenia. *Schizophr Bull* 35(2):383–402, 2009.
104. Fenton WS: Comorbid conditions in schizophrenia. *Curr Opin Psychiatry* 14:17–23, 2001.
105. Fenton WS, McGlashan TH: The prognostic significance of obsessive-compulsive symptoms in schizophrenia. *Am J Psychiatry* 143(4):437–441, 1986.
106. Huppert JD, Weiss KA, Lim R, Pratt S, Smith TE: Quality of life in schizophrenia: contributions of anxiety and depression. *Schizophr Res* 51(2–3):171–180, 2001.
107. Bermanzohn PC, Porto L, Arlow PB, Pollack S, Stronger R, Siris SG: Hierarchical diagnosis in chronic schizophrenia: a clinical study of co-occurring syndromes. *Schizophr Bull* 26(3):517–525, 2000.
108. Green AI, Canuso CM, Brenner MJ, Wojcik JD: Detection and management of comorbidity in patients with schizophrenia. *Psychiatr Clin North Am* 26(1):115–139, 2003.
109. Huppert JD, Smith TE: Anxiety and schizophrenia: the interaction of subtypes of anxiety and psychotic symptoms. *CNS Spectr* 10(9):721–731, 2005.

110. Lambert TJ, Velakoulis D, Pantelis C: Medical comorbidity in schizophrenia. *Med J Australia* 178(Suppl):S67–S70, 2003.
111. Goff DC, Cather C, Evins AE, et al.: Medical morbidity and mortality in schizophrenia: guidelines for psychiatrists. *J Clin Psychiatry* 66(2): 183–194; 147, 273–184, 2005.
112. Matsumoto H, Simmons A, Williams S, Pipe R, Murray R, Frangou S: Structural magnetic imaging of the hippocampus in early onset schizophrenia. *Biol Psychiatry* 49(10):824–831, 2001.
113. Sowell ER, Toga AW, Asarnow R: Brain abnormalities observed in childhood-onset schizophrenia: a review of the structural magnetic resonance imaging literature. *Ment Retard Dev Disabil Res Rev* 6(3):180–185, 2000.
114. Sowell ER, Levitt J, Thompson PM, et al.: Brain abnormalities in early-onset schizophrenia spectrum disorder observed with statistical parametric mapping of structural magnetic resonance images. *Am J Psychiatry* 157(9):1475–1484, 2000.
115. Matsumoto H, Simmons A, Williams S, et al.: Superior temporal gyrus abnormalities in early-onset schizophrenia: similarities and differences with adult-onset schizophrenia. *Am J Psychiatry* 158(8):1299–1304, 2001.
116. Haijma SV, Van Haren N, Cahn W, Koolschijn PCMP, Hulshoff Pol HE, Kahn RS: Brain volumes in schizophrenia: a meta-analysis in over 18000 subjects. *Schizophr Bull* 39(5):1129–1138, 2013.
117. Kahn RS, Sommer IE: The neurobiology and treatment of first-episode schizophrenia. *Mol Psychiatry* 20(1):84–97, 2015.
118. Veijola J, Guo JY, Moilanen JS, et al.: Longitudinal changes in total brain volume in schizophrenia: relation to symptom severity, cognition and antipsychotic medication. *PLoS One* 9(7):e101689, 2014.
119. Sayo A, Jennings RG, Van Horn JD: Study factors influencing ventricular enlargement in schizophrenia: a 20 year follow-up meta-analysis. *Neuroimage* 59(1):154–167, 2012.
120. Giedd JN, Jeffries NO, Blumenthal J, et al.: Childhood-onset schizophrenia: progressive brain changes during adolescence. *Biol Psychiatry* 46(7):892–898, 1999.
121. Alaghband-Rad J, Hamburger SD, Giedd JN, Frazier JA, Rapoport JL: Childhood-onset schizophrenia: biological markers in relation to clinical characteristics. *Am J Psychiatry* 154(1):64–68, 1997.
122. Rapoport JL, Giedd J, Kumra S, et al.: Childhood-onset schizophrenia. Progressive ventricular change during adolescence. *Arch Gen Psychiatry* 54(10):897–903, 1997.
123. Thompson PM, Vidal C, Giedd JN, et al.: Mapping adolescent brain change reveals dynamic wave of accelerated gray matter loss in very early-onset schizophrenia. *Proc Natl Acad Sci U S A* 98(20):11650–11655, 2001.
124. Gogtay N, Giedd JN, Lusk L, et al.: Dynamic mapping of human cortical development during childhood through early adulthood. *Proc Natl Acad Sci U S A* 101(21):8174–8179, 2004.
125. Greenstein D, Lerch J, Shaw P, et al.: Childhood onset schizophrenia: cortical brain abnormalities as young adults. *J Child Psychol Psychiatry* 47(10):1003–1012, 2006.
126. Gutiérrez-Galve L, Chu EM, Leeson VC, et al.: A longitudinal study of cortical changes and their cognitive correlates in patients followed up after first-episode psychosis. *Psychol Med* 45(1):205–216, 2015.
127. Nesvag R, Lawyer G, Varnas K, et al.: Regional thinning of the cerebral cortex in schizophrenia: effects of diagnosis, age and antipsychotic medication. *Schizophr Res* 98(1–3):16–28, 2008.
128. Weisinger B, Greenstein D, Mattai A, et al.: Lack of gender influence on cortical and subcortical gray matter development in childhood-onset schizophrenia. *Schizophr Bull* 39(1):52–58, 2013.
129. Bakalar JL, Greenstein DK, Clasen L, et al.: General absence of abnormal cortical asymmetry in childhood-onset schizophrenia: a longitudinal study. *Schizophr Res* 115(1):12–16, 2009.
130. Mattai A, Chavez A, Greenstein D, et al.: Effects of clozapine and olanzapine on cortical thickness in childhood-onset schizophrenia. *Schizophr Res* 116(1):44–48, 2010.
131. Adriano F, Caltagirone C, Spalletta G: Hippocampal volume reduction in first-episode and chronic schizophrenia: a review and meta-analysis. *Neuroscientist* 18(2):180–200, 2012.
132. Jacobsen LK, Giedd JN, Castellanos FX, et al.: Progressive reduction of temporal lobe structures in childhood-onset schizophrenia. *Am J Psychiatry* 155(5):678–685, 1998.
133. Nugent TF 3rd, Herman DH, Ordonez A, et al.: Dynamic mapping of hippocampal development in childhood onset schizophrenia. *Schizophr Res* 90(1–3):62–70, 2007.
134. Mattai A, Hosanagar A, Weisinger B, et al.: Hippocampal volume development in healthy siblings of childhood-onset schizophrenia patients. *Am J Psychiatry* 168(4):427–435, 2011.
135. Lipska BK, Jaskiw GE, Weinberger DR: Postpubertal emergence of hyperresponsiveness to stress and to amphetamine after neonatal excitotoxic hippocampal damage: a potential animal model of schizophrenia. *Neuropsychopharmacology* 9(1):67–75, 1993.
136. Narr KL, Thompson PM, Szeszko P, et al.: Regional specificity of hippocampal volume reductions in first-episode schizophrenia. *Neuroimage* 21(4):1563–1575, 2004.
137. Csernansky JG, Wang L, Jones D, et al.: Hippocampal deformities in schizophrenia characterized by high dimensional brain mapping. *Am J Psychiatry* 159(12):2000–2006, 2002.
138. Johnson SL, Wang L, Alpert KI, et al.: Hippocampal shape abnormalities of patients with childhood-onset schizophrenia and their unaffected siblings. *J Am Acad Child Adolesc Psychiatry* 52(5):527–536.e522, 2013.
139. Booth CA, Brown JT, Randall AD: Neurophysiological modification of CA1 pyramidal neurons in a transgenic mouse expressing a truncated form of disrupted-in-schizophrenia 1. *Euro J Neurosci* 39(7):1074–1090, 2014.
140. Godsil BP, Kiss JP, Spedding M, Jay TM: The hippocampal-prefrontal pathway: the weak link in psychiatric disorders? *Euro Neuropsychopharmacol* 23(10):1165–1181, 2013.
141. Wallace GL, Eric Schmitt J, Lenroot R, et al.: A pediatric twin study of brain morphometry. *J Child Psychol Psychiatr Allied Discipl* 47(10):987–993, 2006.
142. Middleton FA, Strick PL: Cerebellar output: motor and cognitive channels. *Trends Cogn Sci* 2(9):348–354, 1998.
143. Andreasen NC, Pierson R: The role of the cerebellum in schizophrenia. *Biol Psychiatry* 64(2):81–88, 2008.
144. Keller A, Castellanos FX, Vaituzis AC, Jeffries NO, Giedd JN, Rapoport JL: Progressive loss of cerebellar volume in childhood-onset schizophrenia. *Am J Psychiatry* 160(1):128–133, 2003.
145. Jacobsen LK, Giedd JN, Berquin PC, et al.: Quantitative morphology of the cerebellum and fourth ventricle in childhood-onset schizophrenia. *Am J Psychiatry* 154(12):1663–1669, 1997.
146. Kong L, Bachmann S, Thomann PA, Essig M, Schröder J: Neurological soft signs and gray matter changes: A longitudinal analysis in first-episode schizophrenia. *Schizophr Res* 134(1):27–32, 2012.
147. Bottmer C, Bachmann S, Pantel J, et al.: Reduced cerebellar volume and neurological soft signs in first-episode schizophrenia. *Psychiatry Res* 140(3):239–250, 2005.
148. Greenstein D, Lenroot R, Clausen L, et al.: Cerebellar development in childhood onset schizophrenia and non-psychotic siblings. *Psychiatry Res* 193(3):131–137, 2011.
149. Pettersson-Yeo W, Allen P, Benetti S, McGuire P, Mechelli A: Dysconnectivity in schizophrenia: where are we now? *Neurosci Biobehav Rev* 35(5):1110–1124, 2011.
150. Gogtay N, Lu A, Leow AD, et al.: Three-dimensional brain growth abnormalities in childhood-onset schizophrenia visualized by using tensor-based morphometry. *Proc Natl Acad Sci U S A* 105(41):15979–15984, 2008.
151. Moran ME, Luscher ZI, McAdams H, et al.: Comparing fractional anisotropy in patients with childhood-onset schizophrenia, their healthy siblings, and normal volunteers through DTI. *Schizophr Bull* 41(1):66–73, 2015.
152. Clark K, Narr KL, O'Neill J, et al.: White matter integrity, language, and childhood onset schizophrenia. *Schizophr Res* 138(2–3):150–156, 2012.
153. Samartzis L, Dima D, Fusar-Poli P, Kyriakopoulos M: White matter alterations in early stages of schizophrenia: a systematic review of diffusion tensor imaging studies. *J Neuroimaging* 24(2):101–110, 2014.
154. Chan RC, Xu T, Heinrichs RW, Yu Y, Wang Y: Neurological soft signs in schizophrenia: a meta-analysis. *Schizophr Bull* 36(6):1089–1104, 2010.
155. Bersani G, Quartini A, Paolemili M, et al.: Neurological soft signs and corpus callosum morphology in schizophrenia. *Neurosci Lett* 499(3):170–174, 2011.
156. Arnone D, McIntosh AM, Tan GM, Ebmeier KP: Meta-analysis of magnetic resonance imaging studies of the corpus callosum in schizophrenia. *Schizophr Res* 101(1–3):124–132, 2008.
157. Woodruff PW, McManus IC, David AS: Meta-analysis of corpus callosum size in schizophrenia. *J Neurol Neurosurg Psychiatry* 58(4):457–461, 1995.
158. Mitelman SA, Nikiforova YK, Canfield EL, et al.: A longitudinal study of the corpus callosum in chronic schizophrenia. *Schizophr Res* 114(1–3): 144–153, 2009.
159. Johnson SL, Greenstein D, Clasen L, et al.: Absence of anatomic corpus callosal abnormalities in childhood-onset schizophrenia patients and healthy siblings. *Psychiatry Res* 211(1):11–16, 2013.
160. Frith CD, Blakemore S, Wolpert DM: Explaining the symptoms of schizophrenia: abnormalities in the awareness of action. *Brain Res Brain Res Rev* 31(2-3):357–363, 2000.
161. Ford JM, Mathalon DH: Anticipating the future: automatic prediction failures in schizophrenia. *Int J Psychophysiol* 83(2):232–239, 2012.
162. Picard F, Friston K: Predictions, perception, and a sense of self. *Neurology* 83(12):1112–1118, 2014.
163. Borofsky LA, McNealy K, Siddarth P, Wu KN, Dapretto M, Caplan R: Semantic processing and thought disorder in childhood-onset schizophrenia: insights from fMRI. *J Neurolinguist* 23(3):204–222, 2010.
164. Yu Q, Allen E, Sui J, Arbabshirani M, Pearlson G, Calhoun V: Brain connectivity networks in schizophrenia underlying resting state functional magnetic resonance imaging. *Curr Top Med Chem* 12(21):2415–2425, 2012.
165. Berman RA, Gotts SJ, McAdams HM, et al.: Disrupted sensorimotor and social-cognitive networks underlie symptoms in childhood-onset schizophrenia. *Brain* 139(Pt 1):276–291, 2016.
166. Alexander-Bloch AF, Gogtay N, Meunier D, et al.: Disrupted modularity and local connectivity of brain functional networks in childhood-onset schizophrenia. *Front Syst Neurosci* 4:147, 2010.
167. Alexander-Bloch AF, Vertes PE, Stidd R, et al.: The anatomical distance of functional connections predicts brain network topology in health and schizophrenia. *Cerebral Cortex* 23(1):127–138, 2013.
168. Moran ME, Hulshoff Pol H, Gogtay N: A family affair: brain abnormalities in siblings of patients with schizophrenia. *Brain* 136(Pt 11):3215–3226, 2013.

169. Gogtay N, Sporn A, Clasen LS, et al.: Structural brain MRI abnormalities in healthy siblings of patients with childhood-onset schizophrenia. *Am J Psychiatry* 160(3):569–571, 2003.
170. Gogtay N, Hua X, Stidd R: Delayed white matter growth trajectory in young nonpsychotic siblings of patients with childhood-onset schizophrenia. *Arch Gen Psychiatry* 69(9):875–884, 2012.
171. Gogtay N, Greenstein D, Lenane M, et al.: Cortical brain development in nonpsychotic siblings of patients with childhood-onset schizophrenia. *Arch Gen Psychiatry* 64(7):772–780, 2007.
172. Mattai AA, Weisinger B, Greenstein D, et al.: Normalization of cortical gray matter deficits in nonpsychotic siblings of patients with childhood-onset schizophrenia. *J Am Acad Child Adolesc Psychiatry* 50(7):697–704, 2011.
173. Boos HB, Cahn W, van Haren NE, et al.: Focal and global brain measurements in siblings of patients with schizophrenia. *Schizophr Bull* 38(4):814–825, 2012.
174. Wagshal D, Knowlton BJ, Suthana NA, et al.: Evidence for corticostriatal dysfunction during cognitive skill learning in adolescent siblings of patients with childhood-onset schizophrenia. *Schizophr Bull* 40(5):1030–1039, 2014.
175. Harrison PJ, Weinberger DR: Schizophrenia genes, gene expression, and neuropathology: on the matter of their convergence. *Mol Psychiatry* 10(1):40–68, 2005; image 5.
176. Kendler KS, Diehl SR: The genetics of schizophrenia: a current, genetic-epidemiologic perspective. *Schizophr Bull* 19(2):261–285, 1993.
177. St George-Hyslop PH: Genetic factors in the genesis of Alzheimer's disease. *Ann NY Acad Sci* 924:1–7, 2000.
178. Bishop DT: BRCA1 and BRCA2 and breast cancer incidence: a review. *Ann Oncol* 10(Suppl 6):113–119, 1999.
179. Hall JM, Lee MK, Newman B, et al.: Linkage of early-onset familial breast cancer to chromosome 17q21. *Science* 250(4988):1684–1689, 1990.
180. Murrell J, Farlow M, Ghetti B, Benson MD: A mutation in the amyloid precursor protein associated with hereditary Alzheimer's disease. *Science* 254(5028):97–99, 1991.
181. Fajans SS, Bell GI, Polonsky KS: Molecular mechanisms and clinical pathophysiology of maturity-onset diabetes of the young. *New Engl J Med* 345(13):971–980, 2001.
182. Altshuler D, Daly MJ, Lander ES: Genetic mapping in human disease. *Science* 322(5903):881–888, 2008.
183. Walsh T, McClellan JM, McCarthy SE, et al.: Rare structural variants disrupt multiple genes in neurodevelopmental pathways in schizophrenia. *Science* 320(5875):539–543, 2008.
184. Addington AM, Gornick M, Sporn AL, et al.: Polymorphisms in the 13q33.2 gene G72/G30 are associated with childhood-onset schizophrenia and psychosis not otherwise specified. *Biol Psychiatry* 55(10):976–980, 2004.
185. Addington AM, Gornick MC, Shaw P, et al.: Neuregulin 1 (8p12) and childhood-onset schizophrenia: susceptibility haplotypes for diagnosis and brain developmental trajectories. *Mol Psychiatry* 12(2):195–205, 2007.
186. Addington AM, Gornick M, Duckworth J, et al.: GAD1 (2q31.1), which encodes glutamic acid decarboxylase (GAD67), is associated with childhood-onset schizophrenia and cortical gray matter volume loss. *Mol Psychiatry* 10(6):581–588, 2005.
187. Gornick MC, Addington AM, Sporn A, et al.: Dysbindin (DTNBP1, 6p22.3) is associated with childhood-onset psychosis and endophenotypes measured by the Premorbid Adjustment Scale (PAS). *J Autism Dev Disord* 35(6):831–838, 2005.
188. Price AL, Patterson NJ, Plenge RM, Weinblatt ME, Shadick NA, Reich D: Principal components analysis corrects for stratification in genome-wide association studies. *Nat Genet* 38(8):904–909, 2006.
189. Gejman PV, Sanders AR, Kendler KS: Genetics of schizophrenia: new findings and challenges. *Annu Rev Genomics Hum Genet* 12:121–144, 2011.
190. Stefansson H, Ophoff RA, Steinberg S, et al.: Common variants conferring risk of schizophrenia. *Nature* 460(7256):744–747, 2009.
191. Neale BM, Sklar P: Genetic analysis of schizophrenia and bipolar disorder reveals polygenicity but also suggests new directions for molecular interrogation. *Curr Opin Neurobiol* 30:131–138, 2015.
192. Loh PR, Bhatia G, Gusev A, et al.: Contrasting genetic architectures of schizophrenia and other complex diseases using fast variance-components analysis. *Nature Genet* 47(12):1385–1392, 2015.
193. Asarnow RF, Forsyth JK: Genetics of childhood-onset schizophrenia. *Child Adolesc Psychiatr Clin N Am* 22(4):675–687, 2013.
194. Ahn K, An SS, Shugart YY, Rapoport JL: Common polygenic variation and risk for childhood-onset schizophrenia. *Mol Psychiatry* 21(1):94–96, 2016.
195. International Schizophrenia Consortium: Rare chromosomal deletions and duplications increase risk of schizophrenia. *Nature* 455(7210):237–241, 2008.
196. Kirov G, Grozeva D, Norton N, et al.: Support for the involvement of large copy number variants in the pathogenesis of schizophrenia. *Hum Mol Genet* 18(8):1497–1503, 2009.
197. McCarthy SE, Makarov V, Kirov G, et al.: Microduplications of 16p11.2 are associated with schizophrenia. *Nat Genet* 41(11):1223–1227, 2009.
198. Rujescu D, Ingason A, Cichon S, et al.: Disruption of the neurexin 1 gene is associated with schizophrenia. *Hum Mol Genet* 18(5):988–996, 2009.
199. Stefansson H, Rujescu D, Cichon S, et al.: Large recurrent microdeletions associated with schizophrenia. *Nature* 455(7210):232–236, 2008.
200. Ingason A, Rujescu D, Cichon S, et al.: Copy number variations of chromosome 16p13.1 region associated with schizophrenia. *Mol Psychiatry* 16(1):17–25, 2011.
201. Ahn K, Gotay N, Andersen TM, et al.: High rate of disease-related copy number variations in childhood onset schizophrenia. *Mol Psychiatry* 19(5):568–572, 2014.
202. Papolos DF, Faedda GL, Veit S, et al.: Bipolar spectrum disorders in patients diagnosed with velo-cardio-facial syndrome: does a hemizygous deletion of chromosome 22q11 result in bipolar affective disorder? *Am J Psychiatry* 153(12):1541–1547, 1996.
203. Pulver AE, Nestadt G, Goldberg R, et al.: Psychotic illness in patients diagnosed with velo-cardio-facial syndrome and their relatives. *J Nerv Ment Dis* 182(8):476–478, 1994.
204. Murphy KC, Jones LA, Owen MJ: High rates of schizophrenia in adults with velo-cardio-facial syndrome. *Arch Gen Psychiatry* 56(10):940–945, 1999.
205. Goodship J, Cross I, LiLing J, Wren C: A population study of chromosome 22q11 deletions in infancy. *Arch Dis Child* 79(4):348–351, 1998.
206. Need AC, Ge D, Weale ME, et al.: A genome-wide investigation of SNPs and CNVs in schizophrenia. *PLoS Genet* 5(2):e1000373, 2009.
207. Grozeva D, Conrad DF, Barnes CP, et al.: Independent estimation of the frequency of rare CNVs in the UK population confirms their role in schizophrenia. *Schizophr Res* 135(1–3):1–7, 2012.
208. Hoogendoorn ML, Vorstman JA, Jalali GR, et al.: Prevalence of 22q11.2 deletions in 311 Dutch patients with schizophrenia. *Schizophr Res* 98(1–3):84–88, 2008.
209. Niklasson L, Rasmussen P, Oskarsdottir S, Gillberg C: Autism, ADHD, mental retardation and behavior problems in 100 individuals with 22q11 deletion syndrome. *Res Dev Disabil* 30(4):763–773, 2009.
210. Vorstman JA, Morcus ME, Duijff SN, et al.: The 22q11.2 deletion in children: high rate of autistic disorders and early onset of psychotic symptoms. *J Am Acad Child Adolesc Psychiatry* 45(9):1104–1113, 2006.
211. Addington AM, Rapoport JL: The genetics of childhood-onset schizophrenia: when madness strikes the prepubescent. *Curr Psychiatr Rep* 11(2):156–161, 2009.
212. Addington AM, Gauthier J, Piton A, et al.: A novel frameshift mutation in UPF3B identified in brothers affected with childhood onset schizophrenia and autism spectrum disorders. *Mol Psychiatry* 16(3):238–239, 2011.
213. Campbell M, Young PI, Bateman DN, Smith JM, Thomas SH: The use of atypical antipsychotics in the management of schizophrenia. *Br J Clin Pharmacol* 47(1):13–22, 1999.
214. Pool D, Bloom W, Mielke DH, Roniger JJ, Gallant DM: A controlled evaluation of loxitane in seventy-five adolescent schizophrenic patients. *Curr Ther Res Clin Exp* 19(1):99–104, 1976.
215. Spencer EK, Campbell M: Children with schizophrenia: diagnosis, phenomenology, and pharmacotherapy. *Schizophr Bull* 20(4):713–725, 1994.
216. Kumra S, Frazier JA, Jacobsen LK, et al.: Childhood-onset schizophrenia. A double-blind clozapine-haloperidol comparison. *Arch Gen Psychiatry* 53(12):1090–1097, 1996.
217. Shaw P, Sporn A, Gogtay N, et al: Childhood-onset schizophrenia: A double-blind, randomized clozapine-olanzapine comparison. *Arch Gen Psychiatry* 63(7):721–730, 2006.
218. Davis JM, Chen N, Glick ID: A meta-analysis of the efficacy of second-generation antipsychotics. *Arch Gen Psychiatry* 60(6):553–564, 2003.
219. Moncrieff J: Clozapine v. conventional antipsychotic drugs for treatment-resistant schizophrenia: a re-examination. *Br J Psychiatry* 183:161–166, 2003.
220. Kasoff LI, Ahn K, Gochman P, Broadnax DD, Rapoport JL: Strong treatment response and high maintenance rates of clozapine in childhood-onset schizophrenia. *J Child Adolesc Psychopharmacol* 26(5):428–35, 2016.
221. Maher KN, Tan M, Tossell JW, et al: Risk factors for neutropenia in clozapine-treated children and adolescents with childhood-onset schizophrenia. *J Child Adolesc Psychopharmacol* 23(2):110–116, 2013.
222. Sporn A, Gogtay N, Ortiz-Aguayo R, et al.: Clozapine-induced neutropenia in children: management with lithium carbonate. *J Child Adolesc Psychopharmacol* 13(3):401–404, 2003.
223. Gogtay N, Sporn A, Alfaro CL, Mulqueen A, Rapoport JL: Clozapine-induced akathisia in children with schizophrenia. *J Child Adolesc Psychopharmacol* 12(4):347–349, 2002.
224. Ratzoni G, Gothelf D, Brand-Gothelf A, et al.: Weight gain associated with olanzapine and risperidone in adolescent patients: a comparative prospective study. *J Am Acad Child Adolesc Psychiatry* 41(3):337–343, 2002.
225. Sikich L, Hamer RM, Bashford RA, Sheitman BB, Lieberman JA: A pilot study of risperidone, olanzapine, and haloperidol in psychotic youth: a double-blind, randomized, 8-week trial. *Neuropsychopharmacology* 29(1):133–145, 2004.
226. Taylor DM, McAskill R: Atypical antipsychotics and weight gain—a systematic review. *Acta Psychiatr Scand* 101(6):416–432, 2000.
227. Basile VS, Masellis M, McIntyre RS, Meltzer HY, Lieberman JA, Kennedy JL: Genetic dissection of atypical antipsychotic-induced weight gain: novel preliminary data on the pharmacogenetic puzzle. *J Clin Psychiatry* 62(Suppl 23):45–66, 2001.
228. Sporn AL, Bobb AJ, Gogtay N, et al.: Hormonal correlates of clozapine-induced weight gain in psychotic children: an exploratory study. *J Am Acad Child Adolesc Psychiatry* 44(9):925–933, 2005.

5.4 ■ MOOD DISORDERS

CHAPTER 5.4.1 ■ DEPRESSIVE DISORDERS

DAVID A. BRENT

In this chapter, we describe the nosology and epidemiology of unipolar depressive disorders in youth, risk factors for depression onset and recurrence, and the evidence base for psychosocial and pharmacologic treatments. We conclude with suggested areas for future inquiry.

CLINICAL PICTURE

Depressive disorders in childhood and adolescence are characterized by core persistent and pervasive sadness, anhedonia, boredom or irritability that is functionally impairing, and relatively unresponsive to usual experiences that might usually bring relief, such as pleasurable activities and interactions and attention from other people. The single most important distinction between depression as an illness and the "normal ups and downs" of childhood and adolescence is that depression is associated with functional impairment, mediated through the intensity, duration, and lack of responsiveness of depressed mood and associated symptoms.

Depressive disorders exist on a continuum, and are classified on the basis of severity, pervasiveness, and presence or absence of mania (1). At the mildest end of the spectrum are adjustment disorders with depressed mood, which are mild, self-limited, and occur in response to a clear stressor. Other specified depression, which has sufficient duration (at least 2 weeks) and impairment, but fewer symptoms than major depression, also referred to as "minor" or sub-syndromal depression, and is diagnosed in the presence of depressed mood, anhedonia, or irritability, and up to three symptoms of major depression (2). Persistent depressive disorder, which in DSM-5 replaces dysthymic disorder, is a chronic depressive condition with fewer symptoms than major depression, but lasts a minimum of 1 year. Major depression requires the greatest number of symptoms, with either sad or irritable mood, or anhedonia, along with at least five other symptoms, such as social withdrawal, worthlessness, guilt, suicidal thoughts or behavior, increased or decreased sleep, decreased motivation and/or concentration, and increased or decreased appetite. Rarely, young patients with major depression also have psychotic symptoms such as auditory hallucinations or delusions, usually with self-derogatory, paranoid, or depressive content. Depression may be seasonal in onset, typically beginning in the fall when exposure to sunlight decreases.

There is one new mood-related condition in DSM-5, termed disruptive mood dysregulation disorder (DMDD), which is characterized by severe, persistent irritability, namely, at least three temper outbursts weekly, and has its onset in youth aged 6 and no older than age 10. According to DSM-5, if the symptoms of DMDD are present, one cannot make a diagnosis of oppositional defiant disorder (ODD). However, if hierarchical diagnostic procedures are not applied, DMDD shows extremely high diagnostic overlap with ODD and mood disorders, and in the National Comorbidity Survey, Adolescent Supplement (NCS-A), its 12-month prevalence shrinks from 5.2% to 0.12% (3,4).

Comorbidity is the rule rather than the exception in depressed children and adolescents, especially in clinical samples (5). Anxiety is frequently a precursor of mood disorder and may also occur simultaneously with depression (6). The relationship between behavioral disorders, such as ADHD and conduct disorder is in part mediated by their comorbidity with ODD, which is a strong predictor of eventual depression (6). Alcohol, tobacco, and cannabis use and abuse are highly comorbid with depression, but longitudinal analyses suggest that alcohol and substance use are more likely to precede and lead to depression, than vice versa (7–9).

DESCRIPTIVE EPIDEMIOLOGY

Estimates of Population Prevalence

The point prevalence of depressive disorders is 1% to 2% for prepubertal children and in the National Comorbidity Survey, Adolescent Supplement, the lifetime and 12-month prevalence for adolescent depression were 11.0% and 7.5%, respectively (10,11).

Gender Distribution and the Onset of Puberty

The 3:1 female predominance in mood disorders first emerges in adolescence (10). The higher female-to-male rate of depression after the onset of puberty may be due to higher rates of anxiety disorder and a tendency to rumination in females, and greater sensitivity to interpersonal stressors in females, all of which predispose to depression (12). Early onset of puberty increases the risk of depression in girls (13). Other peripubertal developmental factors that may contribute to an increased risk of depression after puberty include changes in prefrontal and limbic circuitry involved in emotion regulation, social attribution, and reward, as well as a greater incidence of sleep deficit and experimentation with drugs and alcohol (7,8,14,15).

Age and Developmental Factors

Most typically, prepubertal depression has a set of risk factors and course similar to conduct disorder, characterized by family discord, parental criminality, and parental substance abuse, and increased risk of antisocial disorder, but not depression in adult life (16). Less commonly, prepubertal depression is highly familial, with multigenerational loading for depression, with high rates of anxiety and bipolar disorder, and recurrences of mood disorder in adolescence and adulthood (17). Adolescent-onset depression is more likely to result in recurrent episodes in adult life (16,17). Depressive disorders have been reported in preschool children, with evidence of strong family loading for depression, and continuity of depressive disorders into later childhood (18).

RISK FACTORS FOR DEPRESSION ONSET AND RECURRENCE

Genetic

Twin studies demonstrate that depressive symptoms have a heritability of around 40% to 65%, with higher estimates of heritability in adolescent versus prepubertal children (19). Both "bottom-up" and "top-down" family studies have shown a two- to fourfold increased risk of depression in first-degree relatives (20). Greater family loading, either due to both parents having depressive disorders, or having an affected parent and an affected grandparent further increase the likelihood of depression in offspring (20).

Possible intermediate phenotypes that might account for the familial transmission of depression include traits of fearfulness, cognitive bias toward sad emotional stimuli, difficulty with mood repair, decreased heart rate variability, and increased awakening cortisol levels (19–23).

Identification of loci linked to depression has been elusive. Meta-analyses have found genetic linkage to neuroticism, a trait related to the onset of depression, and other studies have suggested linkage to genes involving glutamatergic neurotransmission, the hypothalamic–pituitary–adrenal (HPA) axis, and neural structure (24).

The most commonly reported candidate gene associated with depression is the less functional, short allele of the serotonin transporter gene, which has been reported to interact with stressful life events to result in an increased risk for depression (25). The consistency of this finding has been questioned (26), although it has been linked to a number of potential intermediate phenotypes for depression, such as hypersecretion of cortisol in response to a social stressor (27), increased amygdala reactivity to emotional faces (28), and negative cognitive bias (22).

Familial/Environmental Risk and Protective Factors

Twin studies show that the effect of shared environment is nearly as potent as are heritable factors (19). In the ROOTS study conducted in the United Kingdom, parent–child interactions characterized either by maltreatment or discord were most consistently associated with increased risk for depression (12). Parental depression, particularly if chronic, may exert its deleterious effect on child mood disorder not only through genetic mechanisms, but also via modeling of cognitive distortions, and through either passive and withdrawn, or discordant parent–child interactions (29–32). Longitudinal studies show reciprocal interrelationships between maternal and child interpersonal difficulties, child behavior symptoms, cognitive distortions, and depressive outcome (29–32). Treatment of maternal depression results in prevention of onset, and reduction in child symptomatology (33).

Neglect and child maltreatment not only increases the risk for depression, but also for comorbid conditions (e.g., substance abuse), an earlier age of onset, more chronic and persistent depression, and greater likelihood of treatment nonresponse (34–36). The impact of maltreatment may be mediated through its impact on the inflammatory system, and via alterations in brain structure and brain function related to emotion regulation and reward response (37,38).

Bereavement due to the loss of a sibling, parent, or close friend is associated with an increased risk for depression (39,40). The negative impact of parental bereavement on youth depression is mediated by the functioning of the surviving parent and the adaptiveness of the child's coping style and may be more deleterious in the case of maternal loss (40). Bereavement is no longer an exclusion for the diagnosis of depression, consistent with findings that the risk factors, phenomenology, and course of depression are similar regardless of bereavement history (41).

Those who are bullied, as well as the bulliers show an increased risk for depression, possibly mediated by increases in negative cognitions about self, as well as an exaggerated cortisol response to social stress (42–44). Sexual minority youth have about a threefold increased risk for depression, explained in part by contributions due to parent–child conflict, parental rejection, peer victimization, and maltreatment (45,46).

Connection to family, friends, and to school, parental behavioral and academic expectations, and nondeviant peer group are all protective against depression, as well as health-risk behaviors (47,48).

Cognitive Bias

Depressed individuals have been shown to have a negative view of self, future, and the world, and these biases predict the onset and growth of depressive symptoms, particularly in the face of stressful life events (29,30,49). Both the presence and growth of depressive symptoms are associated with performance-based tasks that show evidence of cognitive bias, including bias toward negative emotional stimuli, cognitive disruption in the face of emotional stimuli, and difficulty with inhibition of negative affect (22,50–53). Rumination, a cognitive style that involves preoccupation with emotionally upsetting thoughts and events, is a predictor of the onset and growth of depressive symptomatology, particularly in girls (30).

Mood Repair

Mood repair, or emotion regulation, is the ability to moderate extremes in emotional responses, and is posited to be a core ingredient in vulnerability to depression (54,55). Laboratory assessment of mood repair, including assessment of persistence in the face of frustration, and altered heart rate variability and respiratory sinus arrhythmia, has been shown to be related to the onset and growth of depressive symptomatology (54,55). Moreover, those with atypical respiratory sinus arrhythmia show greater difficulty in learning how to repair mood in a laboratory setting (55).

Sleep

Subjective sleep complaints are a very prominent component of early-onset depression, although subjective complaints and objective observations of sleep in a sleep laboratory are not closely correlated (56). The most consistent sleep laboratory finding associated with depressive onset, persistence, and recurrence is increased sleep latency (57). Insomnia has been found to have a stronger relationship with onset and growth of depressive symptoms than vice versa (58), perhaps explained by the impact of insomnia on attention to negative emotional stimuli, mood lability, and response to reward (59–61).

Anxiety

Behavioral inhibition and anxiety disorders pose an increased risk for depression, in part due to a shared genetic diathesis (19,62,63). The link between behavioral inhibition and latter depression may be mediated through the development of social anxiety (62). Consistent with this, cognitive bias *away* from negative emotional stimuli (e.g., avoidance) has been shown to predict growth of depressive symptomatology in anxious youth (64).

Externalizing Disorders and Irritability

Depression is a frequent outcome in youth with ADHD, perhaps due to peer and adult criticism and social rejection, and in part due to poor emotional regulation (65). ODD and conduct disorders are also associated with an increased risk of depression, mediated by negative affect and lability in ODD (66) and via irritability in those with conduct disorder, respectively (67).

Medical Illness

Illnesses that involve the central nervous system (e.g., epilepsy, migraine) or that involve systemic inflammation (e.g., asthma, inflammatory bowel disease) as well some of the treatments for chronic illness (e.g., steroids, interferon) increase the risk for depression in youth (68–71). In addition to systemic effects of chronic illness, medical illness may predispose to depression by interfering with the youth's ability to engage in behaviors that promote positive mood.

Cortisol

A *blunted* response to social threat and low waking cortisol have found to be associated with depression in prepubertal samples (72,73), while *increased* morning cortisol has been associated with depression onset in postpubertal samples (72). High morning cortisol has been reported to be predictive of onset of depression in boys, but not girls, and in other studies, this relationship is qualified by past adversity, and current stressful life events (74–76).

Inflammation

There is growing evidence of involvement of inflammatory processes in youth depression, although the relationship between levels of inflammatory cytokines and depressive symptoms in some cases has been reported to be bidirectional (77). Inflammatory processes may partially mediate the relationship between adversity and depression (78), and may play a role in depression via its potential neurotoxicity and interference with central serotonin metabolism (37,77).

Neuroimaging Studies

Structural and functional neuroimaging studies are consistent with self-report and performance task studies of youth at risk for depression as well as those with depressive disorders, with alterations in structures and circuits that result in deploying greater attention to negative emotional cues, decreased ability to use prefrontal cortical mechanisms to inhibit subcortical activation to negative emotional cues, and impaired ability to anticipate, and experience positive affect and reward (79,80). Structural imaging studies of adult subjects with early onset, familial depression as well as in adolescents with depression have found reduced volume of the left subgenual prefrontal cortex and orbital prefrontal cortex (OFC) (81–83). Smaller hippocampal volume has been posited to be a risk for early-onset depression, particularly if there is a history of maltreatment (84).

Functional magnetic resonance imaging (fMRI) studies find that depressed youth show greater activation in the amygdala, dorsal anterior cingulate, and insula in response to negative emotional stimuli, with *decreased* reactivity in the dorsolateral prefrontal cortex (DLPFC) on these same tasks (79,80). Studies of resting-state connectivity are consistent with these findings, showing *decreased* connectivity between the amygdala and DLPFC (79). Diffusion tensor imaging (DTI) studies have found decreased fractional anisotropy in the uncinate fasciculus, which connects the subgenual anterior cingulate cortex (ACC) and the ventromedial PFC (85,86).

Low positive affect is a risk factor for early-onset depression (87). Depressed adolescents and those at high risk for depression show a blunted response in the striatum, caudate, ACC, and orbitofrontal cortex during reward anticipation and receipt (80,88,89). The above-noted neural correlates of reward anticipation and response in adolescents at high risk for depression appear to be moderated by parent–child warmth, parental depression, parent–child conflict, and exposure to early adversity (87,90).

COURSE AND OUTCOME

Episode Length and Recovery

The duration for depressive episodes ranges between 3 and 6 months for community samples, and between 5 and 8 months for clinically referred samples (91). Factors associated with a longer episode duration include previous chronicity, comorbidity with anxiety disorder or substance abuse, greater initial severity of the depressive condition, current or past suicidal ideation or behavior, chronicity and number of episodes of parental depression, and family discord (91). In both clinical and community samples, around 20% of adolescents have a persistent depression of 2 or more years' duration (91).

Risk for Recurrence

In one study of the course of depressive disorder in children aged 8 to 13 years, the risk of recurrence was 40% in 2 years, and 72% in 5 years (91). Other longitudinal studies in treated samples have shown that the risk for relapse or recurrent depression in adolescent depression is between 30% and 70% in 1 to 2 years of follow-up (91–93). Risk factors for persistence and recurrence include parental depression, family discord, history of maltreatment, and comorbidity (36,91).

Risk for Bipolar Disorder

The risk for bipolar disorder in early-onset depression is estimated to be around 10% to 20%, and is higher in patients who present with a history of antidepressant-induced or spontaneous hypomania, psychotic features, hypersomnia, and a family history of bipolar disorder (94). Depressed children and younger adolescents exposed to antidepressants may be at particularly high risk for manic switch (95).

Other Sequelae

Depressed youth are at increased risk for suicidal behavior, impairments in interpersonal, educational, and occupational functioning, as well as increased risk for obesity and cardiovascular disease (96–99). Poor functioning can be a sequelae of depression as well as an indicator of incomplete recovery (99), but comorbidity with alcohol, tobacco, and cannabis use is more likely to be due to the impact of substance use on mood than vice versa (7–9).

CLINICAL MANAGEMENT

There are currently three well-established evidence-based treatments for adolescent depression, namely, antidepressant treatment, cognitive behavior therapy (CBT), and interpersonal therapy (IPT) (100). There has been considerably less research on treatment of prepubertal children with depression, although there is some support for the efficacy of antidepressants. Each of these three approaches will be discussed, followed by a recommendation for current "best practice" treatment of youth depression.

Antidepressant Medication

Evidence of Efficacy

Both the single largest placebo-controlled comparison study of tricyclic antidepressants (TCAs) and placebo, and a subsequent meta-analysis showed no difference between TCAs and placebo (101,102), while several studies have demonstrated efficacy with selective serotonin reuptake inhibitor (SSRI) antidepressants (103). A meta-analysis of both published and unpublished available clinical trials, shows that SSRIs are superior to placebo, with the average response rate for antidepressant versus placebo of 60% versus 49%, for an overall Number Need to Treat (NNT) of 9 (103). A higher risk difference between drug and placebo was found in studies with fewer sites, and those that selected participants with greater global severity (104).

Fluoxetine is the best-studied antidepressant with the strongest efficacy data, and consequently is the only antidepressant to receive FDA and MHRA approval for use for the treatment of depression in both children and adolescents, with an NNT = 5 (103). In the Treatment of Adolescent Depression Study (TADS), fluoxetine was more efficacious than placebo after 12 weeks of treatment (proportion "much or very much" improved, 61% vs. 35%, respectively) (105). The impact of escitalopram, sertraline, and venlafaxine on pediatric depression is more modest, with stronger effects in adolescents (103,106,107). Paroxetine is not superior to placebo for adolescent depression, and so this agent is not recommended in this age group (103,108).

Adverse Events in Antidepressant Treatment

The FDA conducted a meta-analysis that found a higher rate of suicide-related, spontaneously reported adverse events on drug than on placebo (4% vs. 2%) (109). There were relatively few suicide attempts and no completions. A more recent meta-analysis that included additional studies and using random rather than fixed effects models reported a risk difference for suicidal adverse events between drug and placebo of 0.9% (103). Between 4.5 and 11 times more youth will respond to an antidepressant than will experience a suicidal event (103,108). Suicidal events are most common in the first 4 weeks of treatment and are more likely to occur in those who enter clinical trials with suicidal ideation, a history of nonsuicidal self-injury, substance use, family conflict, and who do not respond to antidepressant treatment (110).

Meta-analyses have also found that antidepressant-treated youth have about twice the incidence of hostility and aggression and a much higher incidence of mania compared to those treated with placebo (for the latter, 10% vs. 0.5%) (111,112), with the risk greatest of mania in those under the age of 14 (95). In addition, antidepressants are associated with increased incidence of sleep disruption, vivid dreams, nausea and gastrointestinal distress, agitation, akathisia, anxiety, headache, serotonin syndrome (particularly in combination with other serotonergic agents) and bruising (due to a prolongation of clotting time) (113). The latter side effect is usually not clinically significant, but can become so in patients with intrinsic coagulation disorders or who are undergoing surgery.

Predictors of Antidepressant Response

Clinical severity, comorbidity, insomnia, and family conflict predict a poorer response to antidepressants (114–116). Lower drug concentration, nonadherence, anhedonia, and subsyndromal manic symptoms have also been reported to be associated with antidepressant nonresponse (117–120).

Cognitive Behavior Therapy

Theory and Techniques

CBT is predicated on the observation that depressed individuals show biases in their thinking and information processing, preferentially attending to negative emotional stimuli that reinforce a depressed mood (29), especially during times of stress (49). CBT treatments for depression focus on interrupting this cycle of negative thinking, mood, and maladaptive action, through a variety of cognitive techniques and behavioral skill-building exercises. Central to the treatment model is *cognitive restructuring*—an effort to make the patient aware of negative distortions and to teach the individual how to counteract them, thus relieving depression as a result. The cognitive theory of depression has been supported by studies of performance-based tasks and fMRI studies. fMRI studies show impaired top-down cognitive control of emotion response, and CBT aims to strengthen the ability of the patient to deploy prefrontal cortical resources through cognitive restructuring (80,121).

Also key to the application of CBT is the use of *behavioral activation* (BA) techniques, that is, encouraging patients to normalize their routine and engage in rewarding activities, even if they do not feel like it at the time. BA is based on the observation that depressed individuals tend to withdraw from activities that are potentially reinforcing, but that if coaxed to participate, can experience those activities as rewarding. Preliminary evidence shows that BA approaches can increase activation in reward-related circuitry and that this change appears to mediate improvement in depressive symptoms (122).

While these two techniques appear to be core to the theory and practice of CBT, the content of CBT treatment manuals tested in clinical trials varies greatly in the emphasis on each of these techniques and the inclusion of other, adjunctive skill-building elements (e.g., problem solving, relaxation, emotion regulation, assertiveness training). In addition, CBT approaches are heterogeneous with regard to the overall number of sessions, the number of sessions devoted to each CBT technique, degree of structure, and therapy format (group or individual), differences that make it difficult to interpret the varying effects of CBT reported across clinical trials.

In Acute Treatment, Efficacy of CBT

CBT has been shown to be more efficacious than supportive, relaxation, and one form of family therapy. However in longer-term follow-up, the outcomes of CBT and these other types of therapy converged (123,124). CBT has been shown to be more efficacious than other forms of treatment in reducing cognitive distortions, and also appears to work by improvement in problem-solving ability (125,126). Internet versions of CBT has been shown to be efficacious for adolescents and young adults, including one version of game-based CBT (NNT = 3) (127,128).

The most comprehensive clinical efficacy trial in adolescent depression is the TADS study (105), which compared CBT, fluoxetine, their combination, and placebo in 439 depressed adolescent patients. After 12 weeks of treatment, CBT (43% significantly improved) was not superior to placebo (35%), and whereas both fluoxetine monotherapy (61%) and the combination of fluoxetine and CBT (71%) were superior to placebo (105). By 18 weeks, CBT has similar outcomes to the other two active treatments (129). CBT may not have shown as vigorous a response in the TADS trial as in other studies because the manual contained many different techniques that were all offered to patients at a low "dose" (130).

Predictors of Outcome

Naturalistic data suggest that an adequate response requires at least nine sessions, and that active ingredients include social skills training and problem solving (131). CBT, either alone, or in combination with medication appears to be particularly efficacious for those with high levels of cognitive distortions and comorbidity, whereas in the presence of parental depression or history of maltreatment, CBT is not better, and sometimes worse than alternative treatments (115,116,132). When CBT management of insomnia was added to CBT treatment for depression, the long-term outcome for remission of depression was superior to that achieved by CBT for depression alone (133).

Combined CBT and Medication

In the TADS study, the combination of CBT and fluoxetine was similar to fluoxetine alone with regard to initial response rates, but combination had a higher remission rate, showed superior adaptive functioning, and evoked faster declines in self-reported depression and suicidal ideation (105,134). In TADS, fewer suicidal events were found in those treated with combination relative to fluoxetine alone (129), although other studies of combined CBT and antidepressant medication did not find a protective benefit on suicidal outcomes compared to medication monotherapy (135,136). Clarke et al. (137) studied the addition of CBT to antidepressant management in primary care. This combined treatment resulted in some modest improvement in quality of life, but improvement in depressive symptoms never reached statistical significance; moreover, patients in the combined treatment were more likely to stop their antidepressants or receive a reduced dose. A second study, the Adolescent Depression Antidepressant and Psychotherapy Trial (ADAPT), conducted an open run-in of brief supportive therapy and randomized nonresponders to this brief intervention to either fluoxetine monotherapy, or the combination of CBT and fluoxetine (135). CBT did not add to medication alone with regard to global functioning, quality of life, or depressive symptomatology, although this sample was probably the most severe and complex of any of the large clinical trials.

INTERPERSONAL THERAPY

Theory and Techniques

IPT for adolescents (IPT-A) is an adaptation of IPT, a well-established, efficacious treatment for adult unipolar depression (138). In this treatment, depression is conceptualized as occurring within an interpersonal matrix and IPT-A targets resolution of interpersonal stress that seems to be associated with the adolescent's depression. IPT-A begins by taking an interpersonal inventory of important relationships in order to determine appropriate treatment targets. The types of problems typically targeted by IPT-A are loss, role disputes, role transitions, interpersonal skills deficits, or adjustment to a single-parent family. The goal of treatment is to replace conflictual, unfulfilling relationships with those that are more meaningful, rewarding, and less conflictual.

The IPT formulation and set of techniques are not fundamentally incompatible with the cognitive view of depression. In fact, there are several similarities, including education about depression as an illness, encouragement of the individual to resume normal activities, problem solving, and skill building. However, IPT tends to look from the outside in, whereas, CBT tends to look at inner experience and how it relates to the interpersonal. IPT-A is a very developmentally appropriate treatment, since adolescence is a time of role changes, conflicts with parents, and the investment of more emotional capital in peer relationships.

Evidence of IPT Efficacy

Mufson et al. (138) conducted the first efficacy trial of IPT-A in a patient population of depressed adolescents. Forty-eight adolescents were randomized to either IPT-A or monthly clinical management. A much higher proportion of adolescents met recovery criteria (Hamilton Depression Scale-Depression ≤6) in the IPT-A group (75% vs. 46%, NNT = 4). Analyses of dimensional measures of depressive symptomatology, functional status, and social adaptiveness also favored IPT-A. Two clinical trials compared CBT and IPT for depressed Puerto Rican adolescents, with one study finding IPT superior to CBT, and other finding CBT superior to IPT (139,140). In one of the few clinical psychotherapy trials for prepubertal depressed youth, an adaptation of IPT, termed family-based IPT (FB-IPT) was tested against supportive psychotherapy (141). FB-IPT was superior to supportive therapy in achievement of remission (66% vs. 31%), and in the reduction in social impairment, with the latter mediating FB-IPT's impact on depressive symptoms (141).

Predictors and Moderators of Response

IPT-A is particularly efficacious in youth with greater depressive severity, comorbid anxiety, poorer interpersonal functioning, high levels of conflict with parents, and a greater cortisol response to a lab-based assessment of parent–child conflict (138,142–144).

TREATMENT, PREVENTION, AND EFFICACY

Treatment-Resistant Depression

Treatment-resistant depression is defined as the persistence of depression after having received adequate quality and dose of an evidence-based treatment. The Treatment of SSRI-Resistant Depression in Adolescents (TORDIA) study was designed to determine what clinicians should do next after a patient does not respond to an adequate trial with an SSRI (107). In TORDIA, 334 adolescents were randomized to a switch to another SSRI, switch to venlafaxine, switch to another SSRI plus CBT, or switch to venlafaxine plus CBT. After 12 weeks, the addition of CBT to either medication strategy resulted in a superior outcome to medication monotherapy, and the effects of the SSRI and venlafaxine interventions were similar, except that venlafaxine resulted in more side effects.

Prevention of Relapse

In depressed adolescents who have responded to fluoxetine treatment, continued treatment with fluoxetine is much superior to placebo in preventing depressive relapses (92). The addition of 12 sessions of a wellness-based CBT to continuation pharmacotherapy decreased the relapse rate even further (93).

Effectiveness

In one test of the effectiveness of evidence-based CBT treatment, community therapists were randomized to training and supervision in CBT versus usual care for adolescent depression (145). CBT was not superior to usual care, but accomplished its results in significantly fewer sessions and involved fewer other services, resulting in a lower net cost for similar therapeutic outcomes. Another approach designed to make evidence-based treatments more effective is modular treatment, which employs an algorithm for prioritizing and sequencing different types of evidence-based treatments, whereas "regular" evidence-based care allowed for clinician discretion in the selection, prioritization, and sequencing of manual-based treatments. In one clinical trial that treated several conditions, including depression, modular treatment was superior to manualized care and usual care, and manualized care and usual care were not different from one another (146). Mufson et al. (147) tested the effectiveness of IPT-A versus usual care in school-based mental health clinics. School social workers delivered both interventions, after a brief training in IPT-A and weekly supervision. IPT-A was superior to usual care on dimensional measures of depression, global function, social adjustment, and global clinical status (50% vs. 33% symptomatically improved). Studies have examined the transportability of CBT and antidepressant treatment into primary care settings, and shown that evidence-based primary care interventions are dramatically superior to usual care, both for depression and other conditions as well (148,149).

Prevention

The impact of Coping with Depression for Adolescents (CWD-A) on the prevention of depressive onset or recurrence in youth who are the offspring of depressed parents was tested in a 4-site study. CWD-A significantly reduced the onset of depressive disorders relative to treatment as usual at 9 months after the intervention (depression onset of 21.4% vs. 32.7%, NNT = 9) (150). If one of the parents was currently depressed during the intervention, the CWD-A was no better than usual care (150). The positive effects of the program on depression outcomes and adult functioning were present 75 months after the intervention, with the effects of the intervention on adult functioning mediated by the number of depression-free days, illustrating the importance of relief of depression at this critical stage of development (151). Both universal and indicated preventive interventions have been shown to be efficacious, although indicated interventions have larger effects (152). A family CBT intervention has been found to be efficacious in the reduction of depressive onsets in the offspring of depressed parents, with the effects mediated by changes in youth coping, and parenting behavior (153,154). A modification of IPT-A delivered in a group format that included adolescent skills training (IPT-AST) was compared to supportive counseling in a school setting, and IPT-AST showed a greater decrease in levels of depressive symptomatology and improvement in functioning (155). One study compared IPT-AST, CBT, and a no-treatment group, and found that both active conditions were superior to no-treatment on reduction in depression, with stronger effects in those with higher levels of depressive symptomatology (156).

Other Available Interventions

One promising treatment that is currently being evaluated in a large clinical trial, attachment-based family therapy (ABFT), has been found to be superior to clinical management in the reduction of depression and suicidal ideation in two clinical trials of largely impoverished and minority youth (157,158). With regard to somatic treatments, 1 hour of light therapy in the morning has been shown to be beneficial for pediatric seasonal affective disorder, and may be beneficial for treatment of mild depression and as an augmentation of pharmacotherapy of depression (159–161).

Recommendations for Current Best Practice Treatment

Since there is a relatively high response rate to placebo or brief supportive treatment and education in many of the published treatment studies, the first approach for mild depression should be family education, supportive counseling, case management, and problem solving. For more persistent, moderate depression, one of the three empirically validated treatments, SSRI medication, CBT, or IPT, is indicated. Initial treatment with any of the three treatments for moderate depression is reasonable, with the choice informed primarily by patient preference and the availability of local expertise. If the patient does not show any improvement after 6 to 8 weeks, consideration should be given to a change of treatment (e.g., psychotherapy to medication or vice versa), or augmentation (adding psychotherapy to medication or vice versa). In many communities, there is a paucity of clinicians trained in CBT or IPT-A, and the evidence suggests that more generic psychotherapies practiced in the community may not be helpful in the treatment of youth depression (123,162). In the absence of available specialized psychotherapy, or in the face of a patient's disinclination to engage in psychotherapy, use of an antidepressant as a first-line intervention is indicated. Patients should be seen or evaluated by phone weekly for the first 4 weeks of antidepressant treatment or after a dose adjustment in order to monitor for adverse effects of antidepressants such as suicidality, hostility, and mania.

For more severely depressed adolescents, particularly those with difficulties with motivation, concentration, sleep, and appetite, medication should be a first-line treatment. The combination of CBT and antidepressant results in a more rapid improvement, and is more effective than medication monotherapy for first onset, and for chronic, treatment-resistant depression (105,107). Relative contraindications for use of antidepressant medication are a history of mania or hypomania, for whom mood stabilization should be undertaken prior to the use of antidepressants, and for those with a strong family history of bipolar disorder, for whom it may be safer to begin with psychotherapy for the same reason.

Given that the most and strongest evidence for efficacy exists for fluoxetine, this should be the first-line medication. For those who have failed to respond to fluoxetine, cannot tolerate it, or for some reason do not wish to take it, use of one of the other SSRIs for which there is some evidence of efficacy is warranted, such escitalopram or sertraline. Current clinical recommendations are to begin with half the usual initial target dose (e.g., the equivalent of 10 mg fluoxetine) for 1 week, to determine if the patient can tolerate the medication, and then increase to 20 mg for the next 3 weeks. If the patient does not respond to 20 mg and is tolerating the medication, it is reasonable to increase the dosage to 40 mg, in light of previous studies (120). Further dose increases would be indicated if there is evidence of rapid metabolism, or if the patient has comorbid obsessive compulsive disorder or anxiety disorders, for which higher doses of SSRIs may be useful (163). If a patient fails to respond to a fluoxetine at an adequate dose and duration then, based on the TORDIA study, patients should be switched to another SSRI and in addition should receive CBT (107). However, it is important to rule out reasons for continued depression such as rapid drug metabolism, nonadherence, presence of undiagnosed medical or psychiatric comorbidity (e.g., insomnia, psychosis, cannabis abuse, bipolar disorder), or environment stressors, such as family conflict, parental depression, peer victimization, or same-sex attraction. Expert consensus recommends that if a patient shows partial response to an agent, then augmentation should be considered, and while empirical studies in youth are lacking, adult studies support augmentation with lithium, bupropion, and antipsychotics among other agents (100). After nonresponse to a second SSRI, one should consider switching to an antidepressant of a different class. If the patient has prominent anxiety, then a selective norepinephrine/serotonin reuptake inhibitor is a logical next step. If a patient has low motivation and fatigue, or comorbid ADHD, then bupropion might be a logical next step. After treatment nonresponse to three antidepressants, patients should be considered for ECT, with naturalistic studies indicating best outcomes in those with psychosis or mania, and less favorable outcomes in those with personality disorder (164).

Treatment should focus on achievement of remission, because residual symptoms of depression can increase the likelihood of depressive relapse (2). Moreover, if a patient has achieved symptomatic remission, he or she should continue on the same regimen for at least 6 months before considering withdrawal of medication (92). Addition of CBT to continuation medication treatment can increase the likelihood of staying well (93). Patients with more severe and chronic disorder, or who are about to embark on potentially stressful transition, for example, a year abroad, should receive continuation treatment for longer periods of time.

FUTURE CHALLENGES

1. *Improving access to care for child and adolescents with depression.* Since the black box warning about the risk of suicidal events associated with use of antidepressants in adolescents and young adults, there has been a decline in the use of antidepressants in adolescents and even a decline in the rendering of a depressive diagnosis in adolescents (165). Collaborative care, that is the colocation of mental health specialists in pediatric and family medicine primary care, has been shown to improve access to care and outcome in depression, and in overall mental health issues (148,149). The dissemination of evidence-based treatments that can be delivered with less intense clinician involvement, such as via the Internet can also help to improve access to evidence-based care (166).
2. *Deconstruction of depressive disorders into dimensions that can be reliably assessed and can be linked to neural mechanisms that can be targeted with effective treatments.* The Research Diagnostic Criteria (RDoC) initiative aims to deconstruct current nosologically heterogeneous entities such as depression into biologically coherent sub-groups that then frame appropriate treatment targets and mechanisms (167). For example, anhedonia is a dimension associated with depression as well as with other psychiatric conditions that has a unique neurocircuitry and may respond to specific types of interventions such as BA, as compared to cognitive therapy (122).
3. *Improved understanding of the contribution of early and current adversity to the pathogenesis of early onset and treatment.* Maltreatment accounts for a very high proportion of the population attributable risk of early-onset depression, and also greatly increases the likelihood of nonresponse to treatment (36). Research is indicated to identify the neurobiologic basis of the more extreme clinical phenotype of depression associated with early and current adversity, and the translation of those findings into interventions that are more effective than our current interventions for this important sub-population of depressed individuals (38).
4. *Translation of the explosion in our understanding of the neurocircuitry of depressive disorders into improvements in interventions.* Currently, our ability to identify neural abnormalities associated with depression greatly outstrip our ability to translate those findings into viable interventions. Novel approaches that target neural circuitry may be useful as research probes and therapeutic interventions (168).
5. *Metabolomic approaches to treatment-resistant depression may help shed light in improving outcome in youth and adults with chronic, treatment-resistant depression.* Promising research into the etiology and treatment of chronic, resistant depression has identified that a surprisingly high proportion of treatment-resistant depressed patients may have one or more metabolic abnormalities, such as cerebral folate deficiency, that may in turn respond to replacement treatment (e.g., folinic acid) (169).
6. *Prevention of cardio-metabolic disorders in depressed youth.* Depressed youth have greatly increased risk of cardio-metabolic disease (170), and share risk factors for these physical conditions such as inflammation and reduced heart rate variability (21,77). Interventions to target these shared risk factors might greatly improve mortality and morbidity in depressed youth.

References

1. DSM-5 American Psychiatric Association: *Diagnostic and Statistical Manual of Mental Disorders*. Arlington, American Psychiatric Publishing, 2013.
2. Wesselhoeft R, Sorensen MJ, Heiervang ER, et al.: Subthreshold depression in children and adolescents—a systematic review. *J Affect Disord* 151(1):7–22, 2013.
3. Althoff RR, Crehan ET, He JP, et al.: Disruptive mood dysregulation disorder at ages 13-18: Results from the National Comorbidity Survey-Adolescent Supplement. *J Child Adolesc Psychopharmacol* 26(2): 107–113, 2016.
4. Copeland WE, Angold A, Costello EJ, et al.: Prevalence, comorbidity, and correlates of DSM-5 proposed disruptive mood dysregulation disorder. *Am J Psychiatry* 170(2):173–179, 2013.
5. Copeland WE, Shanahan L, Erkanli A, et al.: Indirect comorbidity in childhood and adolescence. *Front Psychiatry* 4:144, 2013.
6. Copeland WE, Adair CE, Smetanin P, et al.: Diagnostic transitions from childhood to adolescence to early adulthood. *J Child Psychol Psychiatry* 54(7):791–799, 2013.
7. Lev-Ran S, Roerecke M, Le Foll B, et al.: The association between cannabis use and depression: a systematic review and meta-analysis of longitudinal studies. *Psychol Med* 44(4):797–810, 2014.
8. Boden JM, Fergusson DM: Alcohol and depression. *Addiction* 106(5): 906–914, 2011.
9. Boden JM, Fergusson DM, Horwood LJ: Cigarette smoking and depression: tests of causal linkages using a longitudinal birth cohort. *Br J Psychiatry* 196(6):440–446, 2010.
10. Costello EJ, Mustillo S, Erkanli A, et al.: Prevalence and development of psychiatric disorders in childhood and adolescence. *Arch Gen Psychiatry* 60(8):837–844, 2003.
11. Avenevoli S, Swendsen J, He JP, et al.: Major depression in the National Comorbidity Survey-Adolescent Supplement: prevalence, correlates, and treatment. *J Am Acad Child Adolesc Psychiatry* 54(1):37–44 e32, 2015.
12. Lewis G, Jones PB, Goodyer IM: The ROOTS study: a 10-year review of findings on adolescent depression, and recommendations for future longitudinal research. *Soc Psychiatry Psychiatr Epidemiol* 51(2):161–170, 2016.
13. Graber JA, Seeley JR, Brooks-Gunn J, et al.: Is pubertal timing associated with psychopathology in young adulthood. *J Am Acad Child Adolesc Psychiatry* 43(6):718–726, 2004.
14. Dahl RE: Regulation of sleep and arousal: comments on part VII. *Ann N Y Acad Sci* 1021:292–293, 2004.
15. Casey B, Jones RM, Somerville LH: Braking and accelerating of the adolescent brain. *J Res Adolesc* 21(1):21–33, 2011.
16. Shanahan L, Copeland WE, Costello EJ, et al.: Child-, adolescent- and young adult-onset depressions: differential risk factors in development? *Psychol Med* 41(11):2265–2274, 2011.
17. Harrington R, Rutter M, Weissman M, et al.: Psychiatric disorders in the relatives of depressed probands. I. Comparison of prepubertal, adolescent and early adult onset cases. *J Affect Disord* 42(1):9–22, 1997.

18. Luby JL, Gaffrey MS, Tillman R, et al.: Trajectories of preschool disorders to full DSM depression at school age and early adolescence: continuity of preschool depression. *Am J Psychiatry* 171(7):768–776, 2014.
19. Thapar A, Rice F: Twin studies in pediatric depression. *Child Adolesc Psychiatr Clin N Am* 15(4):869–881, 2006.
20. Weissman MM, Wickramaratne P, Gameroff MJ, et al.: Offspring of depressed parents: 30 years later. *Am J Psychiatry* 173(10):1024–1032, 2016.
21. Su S, Lampert R, Lee F, et al.: Common genes contribute to depressive symptoms and heart rate variability: The Twins Heart Study. *Twin Res Hum Genet* 13(1):1–9, 2010.
22. Owens M, Goodyer IM, Wilkinson P, et al.: 5-HTTLPR and early childhood adversities moderate cognitive and emotional processing in adolescence. *PLoS One* 7(11):e48482, 2012.
23. LeMoult J, Chen MC, Foland-Ross LC, et al.: Concordance of mother-daughter diurnal cortisol production: understanding the intergenerational transmission of risk for depression. *Biol Psychol* 108:98–104, 2015.
24. Smith DJ, Escott-Price V, Davies G, et al.: Genome-wide analysis of over 106 000 individuals identifies 9 neuroticism-associated loci. *Mol Psychiatry* 21(6):749–757, 2016.
25. Caspi A, Hariri AR, Holmes A, et al.: Genetic sensitivity to the environment: the case of the serotonin transporter gene and its implications for studying complex diseases and traits. *Am J Psychiatry* 167(5):509–527, 2010.
26. Risch N, Herrell R, Lehner T, et al.: Interaction between the serotonin transporter gene (5-HTTLPR), stressful life events, and risk of depression: a meta-analysis. *JAMA* 301(23):2462–2471, 2009.
27. Gotlib IH, Joormann J, Minor KL, et al.: HPA axis reactivity: a mechanism underlying the associations among 5-HTTLPR, stress, and depression. *Biol Psychiatry* 63(9):847–851, 2008.
28. Hariri AR, Tessitore A, Mattay VS, et al.: The amygdala response to emotional stimuli: a comparison of faces and scenes. *Neuroimage* 17(1):317–323, 2002.
29. Gotlib IH, Joormann J: Cognition and depression: current status and future directions. *Annu Rev Clin Psychol* 6:285–312, 2010.
30. Hankin BL: Future directions in vulnerability to depression among youth: integrating risk factors and processes across multiple levels of analysis. *J Clin Child Adolesc Psychol* 41(5):695–718, 2012.
31. Hayden EP, Olino TM, Mackrell SV, et al.: Cognitive vulnerability to depression during middle childhood: stability and associations with maternal affective styles and parental depression. *Pers Individ Dif* 55(8):892–897, 2013.
32. Olino TM, McMakin DL, Nicely TA, et al.: Maternal depression, parenting, and youth depressive symptoms: mediation and moderation in a short-term longitudinal study. *J Clin Child Adolesc Psychol* 45(3):279–290, 2016.
33. Cuijpers P, Weitz E, Karyotaki E, et al.: The effects of psychological treatment of maternal depression on children and parental functioning: a meta-analysis. *Eur Child Adolesc Psychiatry* 24(2):237–245, 2015.
34. Infurna MR, Reichl C, Parzer P, et al.: Associations between depression and specific childhood experiences of abuse and neglect: a meta-analysis. *J Affect Disord* 190:47–55, 2016.
35. Brown J, Cohen P, Johnson JG, et al.: Childhood abuse and neglect: specificity of effects on adolescent and young adult depression and suicidality. *J Am Acad Child Adolesc Psychiatry* 38(12):1490–1496, 1999.
36. Nanni V, Uher R, Danese A: Childhood maltreatment predicts unfavorable course of illness and treatment outcome in depression: a meta-analysis. *Am J Psychiatry* 169(2):141–151, 2012.
37. Nusslock R, Miller GE: Early-life adversity and physical and emotional health across the lifespan: a neuroimmune network hypothesis. *Biol Psychiatry* 80(1):23–32, 2015.
38. Teicher MH, Samson JA: Childhood maltreatment and psychopathology: a case for ecophenotypic variants as clinically and neurobiologically distinct subtypes. *Am J Psychiatry* 170(10):1114–1133, 2013.
39. Brent DA, Moritz G, Bridge J, et al.: Long-term impact of exposure to suicide: a three-year controlled follow-up. *J Am Acad Child Adolesc Psychiatry* 35(5):646–653, 1996.
40. Brent D, Melhem N, Donohoe MB, et al.: The incidence and course of depression in bereaved youth 21 months after the loss of a parent to suicide, accident, or sudden natural death. *Am J Psychiatry* 166(7):786–794, 2009.
41. Hamdan S, Melhem NM, Porta G, et al.: The phenomenology and course of depression in parentally bereaved and non-bereaved youth. *J Am Acad Child Adolesc Psychiatry* 51(5):528–536, 2012.
42. Rudolph KD, Troop-Gordon W, Granger DA: Individual differences in biological stress responses moderate the contribution of early peer victimization to subsequent depressive symptoms. *Psychopharmacology (Berl)* 214(1):209–219, 2011.
43. Sinclair KR, Cole DA, Dukewich T, et al.: Impact of physical and relational peer victimization on depressive cognitions in children and adolescents. *J Clin Child Adolesc Psychol* 41(5):570–583, 2012.
44. Zwierzynska K, Wolke D, Lereya TS: Peer victimization in childhood and internalizing problems in adolescence: a prospective longitudinal study. *J Abnorm Child Psychol* 41(2):309–323, 2013.
45. Marshal MP, Dietz LJ, Friedman MS, et al.: Suicidality and depression disparities between sexual minority and heterosexual youth: a meta-analytic review. *J Adolesc Health* 49(2):115–123, 2011.
46. Friedman MS, Marshal MP, Guadamuz TE, et al.: A meta-analysis of disparities in childhood sexual abuse, parental physical abuse, and peer victimization among sexual minority and sexual nonminority individuals. *Am J Public Health* 101(8):1481–1494, 2011.
47. van Harmelen AL, Gibson JL, St Clair MC, et al.: Friendships and family support reduce subsequent depressive symptoms in at-risk adolescents. *PLoS One* 11(5):e0153715, 2016.
48. Resnick MD, Bearman PS, Blum RW, et al.: Protecting adolescents from harm. Findings from the National Longitudinal Study on Adolescent Health. *JAMA* 278(10):823–832, 1997.
49. Carter JS, Garber J: Predictors of the first onset of a major depressive episode and changes in depressive symptoms across adolescence: stress and negative cognitions. *J Abnorm Psychol* 120(4):779–796, 2011.
50. Kyte ZA, Goodyer IM, Sahakian BJ: Selected executive skills in adolescents with recent first episode major depression. *J Child Psychol Psychiatry* 46(9):995–1005, 2005.
51. Park RJ, Goodyer IM, Teasdale JD: Effects of induced rumination and distraction on mood and overgeneral autobiographical memory in adolescent major depressive disorder and controls. *J Child Psychol Psychiatry* 45(5):996–1006, 2004.
52. Ladouceur CD, Dahl RE, Williamson DE, et al.: Altered emotional processing in pediatric anxiety, depression, and comorbid anxiety-depression. *J Abnorm Child Psychol* 33(2):165–177, 2005.
53. Ladouceur CD, Dahl RE, Williamson DE, et al.: Processing emotional facial expressions influences performance on a Go/NoGo task in pediatric anxiety and depression. *J Child Psychol Psychiatry* 47(11):1107–1115, 2006.
54. Kovacs M, Lopez-Duran N: Prodromal symptoms and atypical affectivity as predictors of major depression in juveniles: implications for prevention. *J Child Psychol Psychiatry* 51(4):472–496, 2010.
55. Yaroslavsky I, Rottenberg J, Bylsma LM, et al.: Parasympathetic nervous system activity predicts mood repair use and its effectiveness among adolescents with and without histories of major depression. *J Abnorm Psychol* 125(3):323–336, 2016.
56. Forbes EE, Bertocci MA, Gregory AM, et al.: Objective sleep in pediatric anxiety disorders and major depressive disorder. *J Am Acad Child Adolesc Psychiatry* 47(2):148–155, 2008.
57. Augustinavicius JL, Zanjani A, Zakzanis KK, et al.: Polysomnographic features of early-onset depression: a meta-analysis. *J Affect Disord* 158:11–18, 2014.
58. Gregory AM, Rijsdijk FV, Lau JY, et al.: The direction of longitudinal associations between sleep problems and depression symptoms: a study of twins aged 8 and 10 years. *Sleep* 32(2):189–199, 2009.
59. Soffer-Dudek N, Sadeh A, Dahl RE, et al.: Poor sleep quality predicts deficient emotion information processing over time in early adolescence. *Sleep* 34(11):1499–1508, 2011.
60. Dagys N, McGlinchey EL, Talbot LS, et al.: Double trouble? The effects of sleep deprivation and chronotype on adolescent affect. *J Child Psychol Psychiatry* 53(6):660–667, 2012.
61. Casement MD, Keenan KE, Hipwell AE, et al.: Neural reward processing mediates the relationship between insomnia symptoms and depression in adolescence. *Sleep* 39(2):439–447, 2016.
62. Gladstone GL, Parker GB: Is behavioral inhibition a risk factor for depression? *J Affect Disord* 95(1–3):85–94, 2006.
63. Waszczuk MA, Zavos HM, Gregory AM, et al.: The phenotypic and genetic structure of depression and anxiety disorder symptoms in childhood, adolescence, and young adulthood. *JAMA Psychiatry* 71(8):905–916, 2014.
64. Price RB, Rosen D, Siegle GJ, et al.: From anxious youth to depressed adolescents: prospective prediction of 2-year depression symptoms via attentional bias measures. *J Abnorm Psychol* 125(2):267–278, 2016.
65. Seymour KE, Chronis-Tuscano A, Halldorsdottir T, et al.: Emotion regulation mediates the relationship between ADHD and depressive symptoms in youth. *J Abnorm Child Psychol* 40(4):595–606, 2012.
66. Burke JD: An affective dimension within oppositional defiant disorder symptoms among boys: personality and psychopathology outcomes into early adulthood. *J Child Psychol Psychiatry* 53(11):1176–1183, 2012.
67. Stringaris A, Lewis G, Maughan B: Developmental pathways from childhood conduct problems to early adult depression: findings from the ALSPAC cohort. *Br J Psychiatry* 205(1):17–23, 2014.
68. Szigethy E, McLafferty L, Goyal A: Inflammatory bowel disease. *Child Adolesc Psychiatr Clin N Am* 19(2):301–318, ix, 2010.
69. Hoppe C, Elger CE: Depression in epilepsy: a critical review from a clinical perspective. *Nat Rev Neurol* 7(8):462–472, 2011.
70. Bruti G, Magnotti MC, Iannetti G: Migraine and depression: bidirectional co-morbidities? *Neurol Sci* 33(Suppl 1):S107–S109, 2012.
71. Goodwin RD, Bandiera FC, Steinberg D, et al.: Asthma and mental health among youth: etiology, current knowledge and future directions. *Expert Rev Respir Med* 6(4):397–406, 2012.
72. Colich NL, Kircanski K, Foland-Ross LC, et al.: HPA-axis reactivity interacts with stage of pubertal development to predict the onset of depression. *Psychoneuroendocrinology* 55:94–101, 2015.

73. Suzuki H, Belden AC, Spitznagel E, et al.: Blunted stress cortisol reactivity and failure to acclimate to familiar stress in depressed and sub-syndromal children. *Psychiatry Res* 210(2):575–583, 2013.
74. Owens M, Herbert J, Jones PB, et al.: Elevated morning cortisol is a stratified population-level biomarker for major depression in boys only with high depressive symptoms. *Proc Natl Acad Sci U S A* 111(9):3638–3643, 2014.
75. LeMoult J, Ordaz SJ, Kircanski K, et al.: Predicting first onset of depression in young girls: interaction of diurnal cortisol and negative life events. *J Abnorm Psychol* 124(4):850–859, 2015.
76. Rao U, Morris MC: Cortisol responses to psychosocial stress: the role of childhood maltreatment and depression. *Int J Public Ment Health Neurosci* 2(1), 2015, pii: 0018.
77. Kim JW, Szigethy EM, Melhem NM, et al.: Inflammatory markers and the pathogenesis of pediatric depression and suicide: a systematic review of the literature. *J Clin Psychiatry* 75(11):1242–1253, 2014.
78. Miller GE, Cole SW: Clustering of depression and inflammation in adolescents previously exposed to childhood adversity. *Biol Psychiatry* 72(1):34–40, 2012.
79. Hulvershorn LA, Cullen K, Anand A: Toward dysfunctional connectivity: a review of neuroimaging findings in pediatric major depressive disorder. *Brain Imaging Behav* 5(4):307–328, 2011.
80. Miller CH, Hamilton JP, Sacchet MD, et al.: Meta-analysis of functional neuroimaging of major depressive disorder in youth. *JAMA Psychiatry* 72(10):1045–1053, 2015.
81. Schmaal L, Veltman DJ, van Erp TG, et al.: Subcortical brain alterations in major depressive disorder: findings from the ENIGMA Major Depressive Disorder working group. *Mol Psychiatry* 21(6):806–812, 2015.
82. Schmaal L, Hibar DP, Samann PG, et al.: Cortical abnormalities in adults and adolescents with major depression based on brain scans from 20 cohorts worldwide in the ENIGMA Major Depressive Disorder Working Group. *Mol Psychiatry* 2016. doi: 10.1038/mp.2016.60.
83. Arnone D, Job D, Selvaraj S, et al.: Computational meta-analysis of statistical parametric maps in major depression. *Hum Brain Mapp* 37(4):1393–1404, 2016.
84. Rao U, Chen LA, Bidesi AS, et al.: Hippocampal changes associated with early-life adversity and vulnerability to depression. *Biol Psychiatry* 67(4):357–364, 2010.
85. Cullen KR, Klimes-Dougan B, Muetzel R, et al.: Altered white matter microstructure in adolescents with major depression: a preliminary study. *J Am Acad Child Adolesc Psychiatry* 49(2):173–183.e1, 2010.
86. Huang H, Fan X, Williamson DE, et al.: White matter changes in healthy adolescents at familial risk for unipolar depression: a diffusion tensor imaging study. *Neuropsychopharmacology* 36(3):684–691, 2011.
87. Morgan JK, Olino TM, McMakin DL, et al.: Neural response to reward as a predictor of increases in depressive symptoms in adolescence. *Neurobiol Dis* 52:66–74, 2013.
88. Forbes EE, Dahl RE: Research Review: Altered reward function in adolescent depression: what, when and how? *J Child Psychol Psychiatry* 53(1):3–15, 2012.
89. Olino TM, McMakin DL, Morgan JK, et al.: Reduced reward anticipation in youth at high-risk for unipolar depression: a preliminary study. *Dev Cogn Neurosci* 8:55–64, 2014.
90. Morgan JK, Shaw DS, Olino TM, et al.: History of depression and frontostriatal connectivity during reward processing in late adolescent boys. *J Clin Child Adolesc Psychol* 45(1):59–68, 2016.
91. Birmaher B, Arbelaez C, Brent D: Course and outcome of child and adolescent major depressive disorder. *Child Adolesc Psychiatr Clin N Am* 11(3):619–637, 2002.
92. Emslie GJ, Kennard BD, Mayes TL, et al.: Fluoxetine versus placebo in preventing relapse of major depression in children and adolescents. *Am J Psychiatry* 165(4):459–467, 2008.
93. Kennard BD, Emslie GJ, Mayes TL, et al.: Sequential treatment with fluoxetine and relapse–prevention CBT to improve outcomes in pediatric depression. *Am J Psychiatry* 171(10):1083–1090, 2014.
94. Geller B, Zimerman B, Williams M, et al.: Bipolar disorder at prospective follow-up of adults who had prepubertal major depressive disorder. *Am J Psychiatry* 158(1):125–127, 2001.
95. Martin A, Young C, Leckman JF, et al.: Age effects on antidepressant-induced manic conversion. *Arch Pediatr Adolesc Med* 158(8):773–780, 2004.
96. Fergusson DM, Woodward LJ: Mental health, educational, and social role outcomes of adolescents with depression. *Arch Gen Psychiatry* 59(3):225–231, 2002.
97. Pine DS, Goldstein RB, Wolk S, et al.: The association between childhood depression and adulthood body mass index. *Pediatrics* 107(5):1049–1056, 2001.
98. Rottenberg J, Yaroslavsky I, Carney RM, et al.: The association between major depressive disorder in childhood and risk factors for cardiovascular disease in adolescence. *Psychosom Med* 76(2):122–127, 2014.
99. Lewinsohn PM, Rohde P, Seeley JR, et al.: Psychosocial functioning of young adults who have experienced and recovered from major depressive disorder during adolescence. *J Abnorm Psychol* 112(3):353–363, 2003.
100. Birmaher B, Brent D, Bernet W, et al.: Practice parameter for the assessment and treatment of children and adolescents with depressive disorders. *J Am Acad Child Adolesc Psychiatry* 46(11):1503–1526, 2007.
101. Hazell P, O'Connell D, Heathcote D, et al.: Efficacy of tricyclic drugs in treating child and adolescent depression: a meta-analysis. *BMJ* 310(6984):897–901, 1995.
102. Keller MB, Ryan ND, Strober M, et al.: Efficacy of paroxetine in the treatment of adolescent major depression: a randomized, controlled trial. *J Am Acad Child Adolesc Psychiatry* 40(7):762–772, 2001.
103. Bridge JA, Iyengar S, Salary CB, et al.: Clinical response and risk for reported suicidal ideation and suicide attempts in pediatric antidepressant treatment: a meta-analysis of randomized controlled trials. *JAMA* 297(15):1683–1696, 2007.
104. Bridge JA, Birmaher B, Iyengar S, et al.: Placebo response in randomized controlled trials of antidepressants for pediatric major depressive disorder. *Am J Psychiatry* 166(1):42–49, 2009.
105. March J, Silva S, Petrycki S, et al.: Fluoxetine, cognitive-behavioral therapy, and their combination for adolescents with depression: Treatment for Adolescents With Depression Study (TADS) randomized controlled trial. *JAMA* 292(7):807–820, 2004.
106. Emslie GJ, Findling RL, Yeung PP, et al.: Venlafaxine ER for the treatment of pediatric subjects with depression: results of two placebo-controlled trials. *J Am Acad Child Adolesc Psychiatry* 46(4):479–488, 2007.
107. Brent D, Emslie G, Clarke G, et al.: Switching to another SSRI or to venlafaxine with or without cognitive behavioral therapy for adolescents with SSRI-resistant depression: The TORDIA randomized controlled trial. *JAMA* 299(8):901–913, 2008.
108. Hetrick SE, McKenzie JE, Cox GR, et al.: Newer generation antidepressants for depressive disorders in children and adolescents. *Cochrane Database Syst Rev* 11:CD004851, 2012.
109. Hammad TA, Laughren T, Racoosin J: Suicidality in pediatric patients treated with antidepressant drugs. *Arch Gen Psychiatry* 63(3):332–339, 2006.
110. Wilkinson P, Kelvin R, Roberts C, et al.: Clinical and psychosocial predictors of suicide attempts and nonsuicidal self-injury in the Adolescent Depression Antidepressants and Psychotherapy Trial (ADAPT). *Am J Psychiatry* 168(5):495–501, 2011.
111. Offidani E, Fava GA, Tomba E, et al.: Excessive mood elevation and behavioral activation with antidepressant treatment of juvenile depressive and anxiety disorders: a systematic review. *Psychother Psychosom* 82(3):132–141, 2013.
112. Sharma T, Guski LS, Freund N, et al.: Suicidality and aggression during antidepressant treatment: systematic review and meta-analyses based on clinical study reports. *BMJ* 352:i65, 2016.
113. Goldstein BJ, Goodnick PJ: Selective serotonin reuptake inhibitors in the treatment of affective disorders–III. Tolerability, safety and pharmacoeconomics. *J Psychopharmacol* 12(3 Suppl B):S55–S87, 1998.
114. Emslie GJ, Kennard BD, Mayes TL, et al.: Insomnia moderates outcome of serotonin-selective reuptake inhibitor treatment in depressed youth. *J Child Adolesc Psychopharmacol* 22(1):21–28, 2012.
115. Curry J, Rohde P, Simons A, et al.: Predictors and moderators of acute outcome in the Treatment for Adolescents with Depression Study (TADS). *J Am Acad Child Adolesc Psychiatry* 45(12):1427–1439, 2006.
116. Asarnow JR, Emslie G, Clarke G, et al.: Treatment of selective serotonin reuptake inhibitor-resistant depression in adolescents: predictors and moderators of treatment response. *J Am Acad Child Adolesc Psychiatry* 48(3):330–339, 2009.
117. McMakin DL, Olino TM, Porta G, et al.: Anhedonia predicts poorer recovery among youth with selective serotonin reuptake inhibitor treatment-resistant depression. *J Am Acad Child Adolesc Psychiatry* 51(4):404–411, 2012.
118. Maalouf FT, Porta G, Vitiello B, et al.: Do sub-syndromal manic symptoms influence outcome in treatment resistant depression in adolescents? A latent class analysis from the TORDIA study. *J Affect Disord* 138(1–2):86–95, 2012.
119. Woldu H, Porta G, Goldstein T, et al.: Pharmacokinetically and clinician-determined adherence to an antidepressant regimen and clinical outcome in the TORDIA trial. *J Am Acad Child Adolesc Psychiatry* 50(5):490–498, 2011.
120. Sakolsky DJ, Perel JM, Emslie GJ, et al.: Antidepressant exposure as a predictor of clinical outcomes in the Treatment of Resistant Depression in Adolescents (TORDIA) study. *J Clin Psychopharmacol* 31(1):92–97, 2011.
121. DeRubeis RJ, Siegle GJ, Hollon SD: Cognitive therapy versus medication for depression: treatment outcomes and neural mechanisms. *Nat Rev Neurosci* 9(10):788–796, 2008.
122. Mori A, Okamoto Y, Okada G, et al.: Behavioral activation can normalize neural hypoactivation in subthreshold depression during a monetary incentive delay task. *J Affect Disord* 189:254–262, 2016.
123. Brent DA, Holder D, Kolko D, et al.: A clinical psychotherapy trial for adolescent depression comparing cognitive, family, and supportive therapy. *Arch Gen Psychiatry* 54(9):877–885, 1997.
124. Wood A, Harrington R, Moore A: Controlled trial of a brief cognitive-behavioural intervention in adolescent patients with depressive disorders. *J Child Psychol Psychiatry* 37(6):737–746, 1996.

125. Kolko DJ, Brent DA, Baugher M, et al.: Cognitive and family therapies for adolescent depression: treatment specificity, mediation, and moderation. *J Consult Clin Psychol* 68(4):603–614, 2000.
126. Dietz LJ, Marshal MP, Burton CM, et al.: Social problem solving among depressed adolescents is enhanced by structured psychotherapies. *J Consult Clin Psychol* 82(2):202–211, 2014.
127. van der Zanden R, Kramer J, Gerrits R, et al.: Effectiveness of an online group course for depression in adolescents and young adults: a randomized trial. *J Med Internet Res* 14(3):e86, 2012.
128. Fleming T, Dixon R, Frampton C, et al.: A pragmatic randomized controlled trial of computerized CBT (SPARX) for symptoms of depression among adolescents excluded from mainstream education. *Behav Cogn Psychother* 40(5):529–541, 2012.
129. March JS, Silva S, Petrycki S, et al.: The Treatment for Adolescents With Depression Study (TADS): long-term effectiveness and safety outcomes. *Arch Gen Psychiatry* 64(10):1132–1143, 2007.
130. Hollon SD, Garber J, Shelton RC: Treatment of depression in adolescents with cognitive behavior therapy and medications: a commentary on the TADS project. *Cogn Behav Pract* 12(2):149–155, 2005.
131. Kennard BD, Clarke GN, Weersing VR, et al.: Effective components of TORDIA cognitive-behavioral therapy for adolescent depression: preliminary findings. *J Consult Clin Psychol* 77(6):1033–1041, 2009.
132. Brent DA, Kolko DJ, Birmaher B, et al.: Predictors of treatment efficacy in a clinical trial of three psychosocial treatments for adolescent depression. *J Am Acad Child Adolesc Psychiatry* 37(9):906–914, 1998.
133. Clarke G, McGlinchey EL, Hein K, et al.: Cognitive-behavioral treatment of insomnia and depression in adolescents: a pilot randomized trial. *Behav Res Ther* 69:111–118, 2015.
134. Kennard B, Silva S, Vitiello B, et al.: Remission and residual symptoms after short-term treatment in the Treatment of Adolescents with Depression Study (TADS). *J Am Acad Child Adolesc Psychiatry* 45(12):1404–1411, 2006.
135. Goodyer I, Dubicka B, Wilkinson P, et al.: Selective serotonin reuptake inhibitors (SSRIs) and routine specialist care with and without cognitive behaviour therapy in adolescents with major depression: randomised controlled trial. *BMJ* 335(7611):142, 2007.
136. Brent DA, Emslie GJ, Clarke GN, et al.: Predictors of spontaneous and systematically assessed suicidal adverse events in the treatment of SSRI-resistant depression in adolescents (TORDIA) study. *Am J Psychiatry* 166(4):418–426, 2009.
137. Clarke G, Debar L, Lynch F, et al.: A randomized effectiveness trial of brief cognitive-behavioral therapy for depressed adolescents receiving antidepressant medication. *J Am Acad Child Adolesc Psychiatry* 44(9):888–898, 2005.
138. Mufson L, Weissman MM, Moreau D, et al.: Efficacy of interpersonal psychotherapy for depressed adolescents. *Arch Gen Psychiatry* 56(6): 573–579, 1999.
139. Rossello J, Bernal G: The efficacy of cognitive-behavioral and interpersonal treatments for depression in Puerto Rican adolescents. *J Consult Clin Psychol* 67(5):734–745, 1999.
140. Rossello J, Bernal G, Rivera-Medina C: Individual and group CBT and IPT for Puerto Rican adolescents with depressive symptoms. *Cultur Divers Ethnic Minor Psychol* 14(3):234–245, 2008.
141. Dietz LJ, Weinberg RJ, Brent DA, et al.: Family-based interpersonal psychotherapy for depressed preadolescents: examining efficacy and potential treatment mechanisms. *J Am Acad Child Adolesc Psychiatry* 54(3):191–199, 2015.
142. Gunlicks-Stoessel M, Mufson L, Cullen KR, et al. A pilot study of depressed adolescents' cortisol patterns during parent-adolescent conflict and response to interpersonal psychotherapy (IPT-A). *J Affect Disord* 150(3):1125–1128, 2013.
143. Young JF, Gallop R, Mufson L: Mother-child conflict and its moderating effects on depression outcomes in a preventive intervention for adolescent depression. *J Clin Child Adolesc Psychol* 38(5):696–704, 2009.
144. Gunlicks-Stoessel M, Mufson L, Jekal A, et al.: The impact of perceived interpersonal functioning on treatment for adolescent depression: IPT-A versus treatment as usual in school-based health clinics. *J Consult Clin Psychol* 78(2):260–267, 2010.
145. Weisz JR, Southam-Gerow MA, Gordis EB, et al.: Cognitive-behavioral therapy versus usual clinical care for youth depression: an initial test of transportability to community clinics and clinicians. *J Consult Clin Psychol* 77(3):383–396, 2009.
146. Weisz JR, Chorpita BF, Palinkas LA, et al.: Testing standard and modular designs for psychotherapy treating depression, anxiety, and conduct problems in youth: a randomized effectiveness trial. *Arch Gen Psychiatry* 69(3):274–282, 2012.
147. Mufson L, Dorta KP, Wickramaratne P, et al.: A randomized effectiveness trial of interpersonal psychotherapy for depressed adolescents. *Arch Gen Psychiatry* 61(6):577–584, 2004.
148. Richardson LP, Ludman E, McCauley E, et al.: Collaborative care for adolescents with depression in primary care: a randomized clinical trial. *JAMA* 312(8):809–816, 2014.
149. Asarnow JR, Rozenman M, Wiblin J, et al.: Integrated medical-behavioral care compared with usual primary care for child and adolescent behavioral health: a meta-analysis. *JAMA Pediatr* 169(10):929–937, 2015.
150. Garber J, Clarke GN, Weersing VR, et al.: Prevention of depression in at-risk adolescents: a randomized controlled trial. *JAMA* 301(21):2215–2224, 2009.
151. Brent DA, Brunwasser SM, Hollon SD, et al.: Effect of a cognitive-behavioral prevention program on depression 6 years after implementation among at-risk adolescents: a randomized clinical trial. *JAMA Psychiatry* 72(11):1110–1118, 2015.
152. Merry SN, Hetrick SE, Cox GR, et al.: Psychological and educational interventions for preventing depression in children and adolescents. *Cochrane Database Syst Rev* (12):CD003380, 2011.
153. Compas BE, Champion JE, Forehand R, et al.: Coping and parenting: mediators of 12-month outcomes of a family group cognitive-behavioral preventive intervention with families of depressed parents. *J Consult Clin Psychol* 78(5):623–634, 2010.
154. Compas BE, Forehand R, Thigpen JC, et al.: Family group cognitive-behavioral preventive intervention for families of depressed parents: 18- and 24-month outcomes. *J Consult Clin Psychol* 79(4):488–499, 2011.
155. Young JF, Benas JS, Schueler CM, et al.: A randomized depression prevention trial comparing interpersonal psychotherapy-adolescent skills training to group counseling in schools. *Prev Sci* 17(3):314–324, 2016.
156. Horowitz JL, Garber J, Ciesla JA, et al.: Prevention of depressive symptoms in adolescents: a randomized trial of cognitive-behavioral and interpersonal prevention programs. *J Consult Clin Psychol* 75(5): 693–706, 2007.
157. Diamond GS, Reis BF, Diamond GM, et al.: Attachment-based family therapy for depressed adolescents: a treatment development study. *J Am Acad Child Adolesc Psychiatry* 41(10):1190–1196, 2002.
158. Diamond GS, Wintersteen MB, Brown GK, et al.: Attachment-based family therapy for adolescents with suicidal ideation: a randomized controlled trial. *J Am Acad Child Adolesc Psychiatry* 49(2):122–131, 2010.
159. Swedo SE, Allen AJ, Glod CA, et al.: A controlled trial of light therapy for the treatment of pediatric seasonal affective disorder. *J Am Acad Child Adolesc Psychiatry* 36(6):816–821, 1997.
160. Niederhofer H, von Klitzing K: Bright light treatment as add-on therapy for depression in 28 adolescents: a randomized trial. *Prim Care Companion CNS Disord* 13(6), 2011, pii: PCC.11m01194.
161. Niederhofer H, von Klitzing K: Bright light treatment as mono-therapy of non-seasonal depression for 28 adolescents. *Int J Psychiatry Clin Pract* 16(3):233–237, 2012.
162. Weersing VR, Weisz JR: Community clinic treatment of depressed youth: benchmarking usual care against CBT clinical trials. *J Consult Clin Psychol* 70(2):299–310, 2002.
163. Bloch MH, McGuire J, Landeros-Weisenberger A, et al.: meta-analysis of the dose-response relationship of SSRI in obsessive-compulsive disorder. *Mol Psychiatry* 15(8):850–855, 2010.
164. Walter G, Rey JM: Has the practice and outcome of ECT in adolescents changed? Findings from a whole-population study. *J ECT* 19(2):84–87, 2003.
165. Libby AM, Orton HD, Valuck RJ: Persisting decline in depression treatment after FDA warnings. *Arch Gen Psychiatry* 66(6):633–639, 2009.
166. Stasiak K, Fleming T, Lucassen MF, et al.: Computer-based and online therapy for depression and anxiety in children and adolescents. *J Child Adolesc Psychopharmacol* 26(3):235–245, 2016.
167. Garvey M, Avenevoli S, Anderson K: The National Institute of Mental Health research domain criteria and clinical research in child and adolescent psychiatry. *J Am Acad Child Adolesc Psychiatry* 55(2):93–98, 2016.
168. Camprodon JA, Pascual-Leone A: Multimodal Applications of Transcranial Magnetic Stimulation for Circuit-Based Psychiatry. *JAMA Psychiatry* 73(4):407–408, 2016.
169. Pan L, Martin P, Zimmer T, et al.: Neurometabolic disorders: potentially treatable abnormalities in patients with treatment refractory depression and suicidal behavior. *Am J Psychiatry* 174(1):42–50, 2017.
170. Goldstein BI, Carnethon MR, Matthews KA, et al.: Major depressive disorder and bipolar disorder predispose youth to accelerated atherosclerosis and early cardiovascular disease: a scientific statement from the American Heart Association. *Circulation* 132(10):965–986, 2015.

CHAPTER 5.4.2 ■ BIPOLAR SPECTRUM DISORDERS

BORIS BIRMAHER, TINA GOLDSTEIN, DAVID A. AXELSON, AND MANI PAVULURI

INTRODUCTION

Consistent with Kraepelin's early descriptions (1921) (1), it is now recognized that bipolar disorder (BP) occurs in children and adolescents. This disorder severely affects the normal development and psychosocial functioning of the child and is associated with increased risk for suicide, psychosis, sexual risk behaviors, substance abuse, as well as for behavioral, academic, social, and legal problems. However, many youth do not receive treatment, and of those who do, many receive treatment for comorbid conditions rather than for their mood condition (2). Moreover, it takes an average of 10 years to identify and begin treatment of BP (3), and the longer it takes to start appropriate treatment, the worse the adult outcomes.

The goal of this chapter is to review the clinical picture, epidemiology, differential diagnosis, course and prognosis, risk factors, and pharmacologic and psychosocial treatment of pediatric BP. For the purposes of this chapter, the word *youth,* unless specified, denotes children and adolescents. To date, all studies in pediatric BP employed Diagnostic and Statistical Manual of Mental Disorders-IV (DSM-IV) criteria (4). However, with some exceptions (e.g., adding increased goal-directed activity or high energy to elevated or irritable mood to the criterion A and modification of "mixed" from episode to specifier), the DSM-5 (5) diagnostic criteria for mania and hypomania are similar to the DSM-IV (for the DSM-5 criteria, see Tables 5.4.2.1 and 5.4.2.2).

TABLE 5.4.2.1

DSM-5 CRITERIA FOR A MANIC EPISODE

A. A distinct period of abnormally and persistently elevated, expansive, or irritable mood and persistent increase in goal-directed activity or energy for at least 1 wk and present most of the day, nearly every day (or any duration if hospitalization is necessary).
B. During the period of mood disturbance and increased energy or activity, three (or more) of the following symptoms (four if the mood is only irritable) are present to a significant degree and represent noticeable change from usual behavior:
   1) Inflated self-esteem or grandiosity
   2) Decreased need for sleep (e.g., feels rested after only 3 hrs of sleep)
   3) More talkative than usual or pressure to keep talking
   4) Flight of ideas or subjective experience that thoughts are racing
   5) Distractibility (i.e., attention too easily drawn to unimportant or irrelevant external stimuli)
   6) Increase in goal-directed activity (either socially, at work or school, or sexually) or psychomotor agitation (e.g., purposeless nongoal-directed activity)
   7) Excessive involvement in pleasurable activities that have a high potential for painful consequences (engaging in unrestrained buying sprees, sexual indiscretions)
C. The mood disturbance is sufficiently severe to cause marked impairment in occupational functioning or in usual social activities or relationships with others, or to necessitate hospitalization to prevent harm to self or others, or there are psychotic features.
D. The symptoms are not due to the direct physiological effects of a substance (a drug of abuse, a medication, or other treatment) or to another medical condition.

Note: A full manic episode that emerges during antidepressant treatment (medication, electroconvulsive therapy, light therapy), but persists at a fully syndromal level; beyond the physiological effect of that treatment is sufficient evidence for a manic episode and therefore, a bipolar I diagnosis.
Criteria A to D constitute a manic episode. At least one lifetime manic episode is required for the diagnosis of bipolar I disorder.

CLINICAL CHARACTERISTICS

Most clinicians acknowledge that pediatric BP exists, and that the symptoms of pediatric BP are similar to those in adults when accounting for the effects of psychosocial development. However, there is debate on the following issues regarding the phenomenology of pediatric BP: (1) the necessity of cardinal or

TABLE 5.4.2.2

DSM-5 CRITERIA FOR A HYPOMANIC EPISODE

A. A distinct period of persistently elevated, expansive, or irritable mood and persistent increase in goal-directed activity or energy lasting at least 4 consecutive days and present most of the day, nearly every day.
B. Same as B criterion for manic episode.
C. The episode is associated with an unequivocal change in functioning that is uncharacteristic of the person when not symptomatic.
D. The disturbance in mood and the change in functioning are observable by others.
E. The episode is not severe enough to cause marked impairment in social or occupational functioning, or to necessitate hospitalization, and there are no psychotic features.
F. The episode is not attributable to the physiological effects of a substance (a drug of abuse, a medication, or other treatment) or a medical condition.

Note: A full hypomanic episode that emerges during antidepressant treatment (medication, electroconvulsive therapy, light therapy), but persists at a fully syndromal level; beyond the physiological effect of that treatment is sufficient evidence for a hypomanic episode. However, *caution is indicated so that one or two symptoms (particularly increased irritability, edginess, or agitation following antidepressant use) are not taken as sufficient for the diagnosis of a hypomanic episode, nor necessarily indicative of a bipolar diathesis.*
Criteria A to D constitute a hypomanic episode. Hypomanic episodes are common in bipolar I disorder but are not required for the diagnosis of bipolar I disorder.

key symptoms (e.g., elated mood and/or grandiosity) for a BP diagnosis; (2) the role of irritable mood in pediatric BP; (3) the requirement of clearly demarcated mood episodes; (4) the temporal relation between manic and depressive symptoms and mood cycling patterns; (5) the validity and importance of manic symptoms that do not meet the DSM symptom requirements or duration thresholds for a manic, hypomanic, or mixed episode; and (6) the best way to attribute potential symptoms of mania that also commonly present in other pediatric psychiatric disorders. Though the issue of diagnostic features of BP in youth has provoked considerable controversy, it is important to note that many of these issues similarly remain unclear in the adult BP literature. Thus, the conceptualization of BP will continue to evolve as more research becomes available.

Applying the DSM Criteria

It is clear from the work of several groups that some youth meet the full DSM-IV criteria for BP, despite the fact that the criteria were not specifically developed for use in the pediatric population (1,6–9). When examining the DSM criteria for a manic or hypomanic episode, it is obvious that normal youth can exhibit some manic or hypomanic symptoms to some degree, especially in certain situations or environments. Thus, it is of utmost importance to evaluate whether the mood and symptoms are abnormal, clearly different from the youth's usual mood and behavior, above and beyond the youth's developmental level and the context where the symptoms occur, and the extent to which the symptoms affect the functioning of the youth. For instance, elevated mood, high activity level, and rapid speech would not be considered evidence of mania in a 7-year-old at a birthday party or among a group of adolescents at an amusement park.

Consideration of how manic symptoms may manifest differently across development can facilitate accurate diagnosis. For instance, in contrast with an adult who is in a manic episode, a school-age child is not likely to exhibit behaviors such as engaging in risky business ventures, driving recklessly, going on spending sprees, or having sexual relations with multiple partners. However, they can exhibit inappropriate sexual behavior (touching others inappropriately, frequent public masturbation, or drawing sexually provocative pictures) or engage in uncharacteristically dangerous, risk-taking play such as jumping from high places or performing frequent and exaggerated daredevil stunts on a bicycle (6,8).

The distinction between a manic and hypomanic episode can be challenging, but also must be taken in a developmental context. Beyond the differences in minimum duration, manic episodes require marked impairment, which should be measured against the expected level of functioning for a youth given his/her chronologic age and intellectual capabilities. Functioning should be examined across the psychosocial domains that are relevant to youth (school, family, peers). A hypomanic episode also requires impairment, but some youth may function better while hypomanic. For any type of episode, there must be an unequivocal positive or negative change from usual functioning, and the mood and functional changes must be observable by others. Given that lack of insight can be associated with mania or hypomania and that the diagnosis of pediatric BP is more accurate when parents are the reporters (see Assessment section below), it is imperative to obtain information from caregivers or other significant adults in the youth's life in order to accurately assess symptoms and potential change in functioning.

Symptoms of Mania

A recent meta-analysis of 20 published studies (N = 2,226) evaluated the weighted rates of manic symptoms in youth (average age: 11.5 years old, 64% male, mainly Caucasian) with BP-I and BP not otherwise specified (BP-NOS) (7). As shown in Table 5.4.2.3, the most common symptoms across BP subtypes included increased energy, irritability and mood lability, distractibility, and goal-directed activity (all approximately 75%), while hypersexuality, hallucinations, and delusions were the least frequent (all approximately 26%). Grandiosity and hypersexuality were the most specific symptoms, but they were less common (57% and 32%, respectively). As expected, youth with BP-I had more severe and greater number of symptoms than those with BP-NOS. As depicted in Figure 5.4.2.1, there was significant variability in the rates of many symptoms, particularly in youth with BP-NOS, and with few exceptions, the variability was not accounted for by the year of data collection, age, sex, study quality, and methodologic approach utilized in the study (e.g., informant, diagnostic instrument). Other variables not measured, such as the timing of data collection with respect to the time of the acute episode, and how

TABLE 5.4.2.3

WEIGHTED AVERAGE PREVALENCE RATES FOR MANIC SYMPTOMS FOR YOUTH WITH BIPOLAR SPECTRUM DISORDERS (BP-I, BP-II, AND BP-NOS)

Symptom	Prevalence, %	95% Confidence Interval
Increased energy	79	61–93%
Irritability	77	71–92%
Mood lability	76	61–85%
Distractibility	74	69–90%
Irritability	81	55–94%
Grandiosity	78	67–85%
Racing thoughts	74	51–88%
Decreased need for sleep	72	53–86%
Euphoria/elation	70	45–87%
Poor judgment	69	38–89%
Flight of ideas	56	46–66%
Hypersexuality	38	31–45%

From Van Meter AR, Burke C, Kowatch RA, Findling RL, Youngstrom EA: Ten-year update meta-analysis of the clinical characteristics of pediatric mania and hypomania. *Bipolar Disord* 18(1):19–32, 2016.

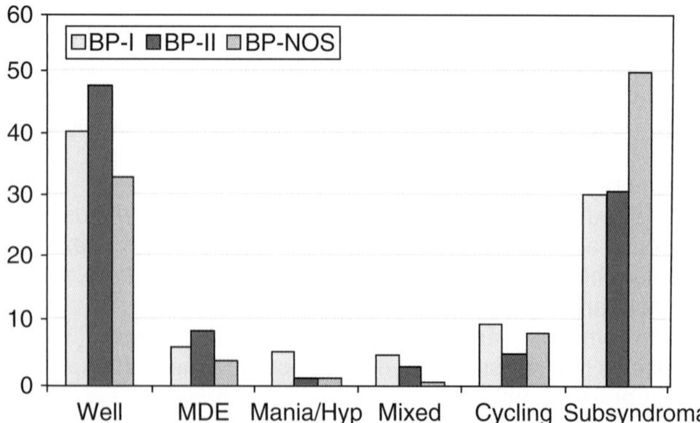

FIGURE 5.4.2.1. Comparison of weekly symptom status (the percentage of follow-up weeks spent asymptomatic or symptomatic in different mood categories during a 2-year prospective follow-up) between youth with BP-I, II and NOS. BP, bipolar disorder; NOS, not otherwise specified. (From Birmaher B, Axelson D, Strober M, et al.: Clinical course of children and adolescents with bipolar spectrum disorders. *Arch Gen Psychiatry* 63:175–183, 2006.)

the studies measured and conceptualized symptoms (e.g., "double-counting" symptoms that are diagnostic for both mania and attention deficit hyperactivity disorder [ADHD]) may also have contributed to the variability. Though it is not a symptom of mania per se, psychosis frequently occurs in BP youth. In the meta-analyses, perhaps due to the complexity assessing psychosis in youth (particularly in children), the weighted rates of psychosis were unexpectedly high (31% hallucinations and 24% delusions), although there was significant heterogeneity among the studies.

One factor that may contribute to the difficulty diagnosing BP in youth is that the most common symptoms of pediatric mania identified in the meta-analysis are also frequently present in other pediatric psychiatric disorders. A recent study comparing the phenomenology of BP and ADHD found that there were no significant differences between the BP and the ADHD subjects in rates of irritability (98% BP vs. 72% ADHD), accelerated speech (97% vs. 82%), distractibility (94% vs. 96%), or unusual energy (100% vs. 95%) (10). Thus, the lack of specificity makes it problematic to diagnose mania by simply counting the presence or absence of symptoms.

Cardinal Symptoms

The overlap of manic symptoms with features of other psychiatric illnesses emphasizes the diagnostic importance of symptoms more specific to mania. Some authors have advocated that two of these manic symptoms, elated/elevated mood and grandiosity, are core features of the manic syndrome, so they should be considered cardinal or hallmark symptoms (8–11). As shown in the meta-analysis noted above, these two symptoms are present in 64% and 57%, respectively, but there is considerable heterogeneity among studies.

Irritability in Pediatric Bipolar Disorder

Irritability has been defined as "...an emotional state characterized by having a low threshold for experiencing anger in response to negative emotional events" (12). Irritability can encompass multiple temporal features of abnormal emotional reactivity, including a lower threshold to anger, a faster increase in anger, a higher "peak" level of anger, and a longer duration of anger.

As noted above, irritability is present in nearly all manic children and adolescents, so it is a sensitive marker for pediatric BP. However it is also part of the DSM-IV diagnostic criteria for disorders such as disruptive, major depressive, generalized anxiety, and posttraumatic stress. In addition, it is frequently present in youth with other psychiatric diagnoses (e.g., ADHD, autism spectrum disorders [ASD]). Therefore irritability has low specificity for BP. The DSM-IV and the DSM-5 criteria for a manic episode explicitly allow for the presence of irritable mood alone to satisfy the "A" criterion, though it is qualified by the requirement of an additional symptom criterion. Some reports have prompted substantial controversy by stating that chronic presentations of irritability alone, particularly when the irritability is severe and accompanied by aggression and volatility, is the primary mood disturbance in BP youth and that elevated or expansive mood is uncommon (13–15). However, the high prevalence of elated/expansive mood in most cross-sectional pediatric BP samples stands in contrast to these reports. Moreover, a recent large study showed that only 10% of youth with BP had irritability or elation alone, whereas most of the sample had both symptoms at intake and during the follow-up (16,17).

Due to the controversy regarding irritability as a key symptom for the diagnosis of pediatric BP, the DSM-5 included a new disorder in the category of mood disorders entitled Disruptive Mood Dysregulation Disorder (DMDD). This disorder is characterized by frequent, severe, recurrent temper outbursts and chronically irritable and/or angry mood, both of which must be present for at least a year and cannot be accounted by other mood disorders. Since the key symptom for DMDD is irritability and this disorder is highly comorbid and sometimes indistinguishable from ODD, the same issues discussed above for irritability apply to DMDD (18–20).

Episodic Versus Chronic Mania

The DSM criteria for manic or hypomanic episode require a distinct period of abnormal mood and accompanying symptoms, and most authors have advocated that an episodic course is a key feature for a definitive diagnosis of BP (6,9,11). Nevertheless, some groups assert that BP youth present with chronic manic symptoms, and have reported mean durations of 3 to 4 years for manic or mixed episodes (21,22). As noted below, BP youth have high rates of comorbid disorders, particularly ODD and ADHD, which manifest with nonepisodic and nonspecific symptoms of mania such as irritability, rapid speech, psychomotor agitation, and distractibility. This fact together with the rapid mood fluctuations and complex admixtures of manic and depressive symptoms found in BP youth can make it difficult to identify distinct episodes that are embedded in this "miscellaneous" presentation. However, a large prospective study of BP youth showed that close longitudinal clinical observation demonstrated that pediatric BP indeed is an episodic illness (23,24).

Depression

Depressive symptoms are noted to be prominent features in most phenomenologic studies of BP youth, and BP adults frequently recall having significant depressive symptoms in childhood or adolescence (3,6,25,26). BP youth can have clear periods of depression that meet the full criteria for a major depressive episode (MDE) and recurrent subsyndromal depressive symptoms (see Chapter 5.4.1 for the DSM criteria for MDE) (23). As described in the differential diagnosis section following, major depression may precede the onset of mania, so that some youth who appear to have unipolar depression may actually have BP with depression as their initial presentation. Mild or transient manic symptomatology that does not meet the diagnostic threshold for mania or hypomania may also precede an MDE, although the presentation of full DSM-IV/5 criteria for BP-II (MDE plus at least one hypomanic episode) does not appear to be common in youth with BP (6,23). All of these factors highlight the need to carefully probe for a history of threshold or subthreshold manic symptoms in youth presenting with depression.

Temporal Relation of Manic and Depressive Symptoms

Many researchers have reported that BP youth often present with mixed states and complex cycling patterns between depression and mania (23). Some groups have reported chronic mixed states lasting years in duration and rapid cycling between mania and depression as frequently as several times per day (13,27). However, it seems that these cycles do not represent new episodes, but mood fluctuations within the same episode. Moreover, the issue is complicated by the fact that there are no clear boundaries that delineate a mixed state from an actual switch in episode polarity, or from mood lability and/or transient dysphoria occurring in the midst of mania. The DSM-IV criteria for a mixed episode require that the criteria for both a manic/hypomanic episode and an MDE be met; the DSM-5 criteria require depression with three manic symptoms or mania plus three depressive symptoms. This could be satisfied by an episode consisting of: (1) an amalgamation of manic and depressive symptoms that present concurrently (expansive, irritable, and depressed mood; high energy; racing thoughts; rapid speech; hopelessness; guilt; and suicidality); (2) cycling between distinct short periods of predominantly manic symptoms and predominantly depressive symptoms; or (3) some combination of both types of presentations. Overlapping criteria and features plus the symptoms of other comorbid psychiatric disorders can make it difficult to determine whether symptoms should be attributed to depression or mania. For example, irritability, racing thoughts, and psychomotor agitation can occur in both mood states and it can be challenging to differentiate decreased need for sleep from insomnia occurring in an agitated depression. Published studies have used patients' retrospective recall over long time intervals which limits reliable evaluation of symptom patterns. It is not clear whether the reports of multiple mood cycles in a day represent periods when the child switches from meeting the full criteria of the manic syndrome to periods when they are completely depressed, or whether they are manifestations of mood lability within the manic state. However, the evidence does indicate that the majority of BP youth have symptoms of depression interspersed in some manner with manic symptoms.

Subthreshold Presentations and Cyclothymic Disorder

Some children and adolescents present in clinical and research settings with what appears to be significant manic symptomatology, but do not meet full DSM-IV/5 criteria for BP-I or BP-II (6,28). These youth are frequently assigned the DSM-IV diagnosis of BP-NOS (in the DSM-5 "other specified or unspecified bipolar and other related disorders") (6,28). The main reason these youth are diagnosed with BP-NOS is because the manic symptoms are not present for sufficient time to meet the DSM duration criteria for a manic, hypomanic, or mixed episode; and/or they do not have enough symptoms. One large study comparing the presentation of youth with an operationalized diagnosis of BP-NOS with those who met full criteria for BP-I found that BP-NOS subjects differed from those with BP-I primarily on duration and severity of manic symptomatology, but not on the fundamental phenomenology of manic symptoms, comorbid disorders, or family psychiatric history (6,23). The majority of BP-NOS youth fulfilled the mood and symptom criteria for mania and/or hypomania, but did not meet the 4-day duration criteria for a hypomanic episode or the 7-day duration criteria for a manic/mixed episode. BP-NOS youth are younger, have more chronic course, irritability, mixed presentations with less euphoric mania than BP-I, but otherwise phenomenologically in continuum with BP-I (23,28,29). Moreover, BP-NOS youth have as much impairment, risk for suicidality and substance abuse, presence of comorbid disorders and family history of mania as youth with BP-I, and about 50% progress to meet the DSM-IV criteria for BP-I or BP-II disorders (28–32).

Youth can also be diagnosed with cyclothymic disorder, a condition manifested by at least 1 year of several episodes with hypomanic symptoms and episodes with depressive symptoms that do not fulfill the criteria for a hypomanic episode or an MDE (33). Youth with these symptoms are difficult to differentiate from BP-NOS.

Attributing Symptoms to Bipolar Disorder Versus Other Psychiatric Disorders

As described later in more detail under Differential Diagnosis, clinicians must be cautious about attributing symptoms to mania or hypomania unless they show a clear temporal association with the abnormally elevated, expansive, and/or irritable mood. The manic syndrome exists as a collection of concurrent symptoms and mood abnormalities, not a list of symptoms that occur in temporal isolation. Chronic symptoms such as hyperactivity or distractibility generally should not be considered evidence of mania unless they clearly intensify with the onset of abnormal mood. Prolonged presentations of nonspecific manic-like symptoms that do not change in overall intensity and appear episodically should raise the possibility of an alternative psychiatric diagnosis.

EPIDEMIOLOGY

Retrospective studies in adults with BP have consistently reported that up to 60% experienced onset of their mood symptoms before age 20 (25,26). However, due to the difficulties and controversies regarding the diagnosis of pediatric BP, it is not clear what the real prevalence of this disorder is in youth.

Over the last several years, the "administrative" prevalence (the number of children diagnosed with "BP" in clinical settings) of BP in youth has significantly increased, particularly in the United States (34). This increase may be accounted for by factors such as increased awareness, referral biases, and misdiagnosing youth with BP. However, due to the fact that pediatric BP was rarely diagnosed in the past, any small increment in the rate of diagnosis will produce a large increment of the administrative prevalence of this condition. In contrast to the above results, a recent meta-analysis showed that the "true prevalence" of pediatric BP-I and II does not differ among countries, with rates of 1% to 2% that increase during late adolescence (35,36). Dissimilarly, the prevalence of BP-NOS or "soft" subsyndromal symptoms varies among studies, with a prevalence as high as 6% in the United States (36).

COMORBIDITY

Pediatric BP is usually accompanied by other psychiatric disorders. A recent meta-analysis reported that the average weighted rates were as follows: ADHD 53%, ODD 42%, conduct disorder 27%, and anxiety disorders 23% (7). As expected, given the relatively young mean age of the sample, substance abuse was present in 9%. However, substance use disorders (SUD) progressively increases with age (32,37). To a lesser degree, other psychiatric disorders, such as obsessive–compulsive disorder as well as medical conditions, can accompany BP. However, the results are heterogeneous and depend on factors such as the setting where the data were collected, instruments used, clinical experience of the interviewer, and methods to interpret the data. In any case, the presence of these disorders affects the youth's response to treatment and prognosis, indicating the need to identify and treat them effectively.

DIFFERENTIAL DIAGNOSIS

As noted above, it is difficult to diagnose pediatric BP because of variability in the clinical presentation (severity, subtype of BP disorder, phase of the illness), high comorbidity and overlap in symptom presentation with other psychiatric disorders, effects of development on symptom expression, children's difficulties describing their symptoms, the environmental context in which the BP is developing (e.g., high family conflict, abuse), and potential effects of any psychotropic medications prescribed (9,38,39).

The main psychiatric conditions that can be challenging to differentiate from pediatric BP are ADHD, disruptive behavior disorders (ODD and conduct disorder), DMDD (and its predecessor severe mood dysregulation [SMD]), unipolar depression, ASD, schizophrenia and other psychotic disorders, substance abuse disorders, and in adolescents, borderline personality disorder. Medical and neurologic illnesses (head trauma, brain tumors, hyperthyroidism), and side effects of medications (corticosteroids, antidepressants, and stimulants) may also be accompanied by mood fluctuations that may mimic BP. Additionally, normal mood variability sometimes may be misinterpreted as symptoms of hypomania. In daily practice, severe disruptive behavior disorders and ADHD are the most frequent conditions that may be confused with BP (Tables 5.4.2.4 and 5.4.2.5). There are some symptoms that mainly occur in BP youth and may help to differentiate between BP and these disorders, such as clinically relevant euphoria, grandiosity, decreased need for sleep, hypersexuality (without history of sexual abuse or exposure to sex), and hallucinations (6,10,11,38,39). Some of the symptoms shared between BP, ADHD, and behaviorally disordered children, such as increased energy, irritability, and aggression, can be much more severe in BP youth. The course of the symptoms over time, the presence of family history of BP, and other issues described in Tables 5.4.2.4 and 5.4.2.5 also may help distinguish between BP and these disorders.

Most depressed youth seen at psychiatric clinics are experiencing their first episode of depression (23,39). Some of these youth may develop BP, but so far it is almost impossible to know at the time of first assessment who will go on to develop BP. Thus, a careful assessment for history of syndromal and subsyndromal manic or hypomanic symptoms is indicated. Also, the presence of psychosis, family history of BP, and pharmacologically induced mania/hypomania may indicate susceptibility to develop BP (40–44).

DMDD (and SMD) is characterized by impairing, chronic irritability that can be misdiagnosed as BP, but this disorder does not have distinct manic episodes (45). Moreover, perhaps with the exception of severely irritable youth with positive family history of mania, longitudinal data indicate that youth with SMD are not at high risk to develop BD as they age (45).

Schizophrenia is rare in children and sometimes BP may manifest with psychosis and bizarre behaviors. Therefore, mood disorders need to be ruled out in any child with psychosis. Substance abuse may also induce severe mood changes that may be difficult to differentiate from BP. In these cases, if the symptoms of mania continue after the youth is no longer using substances, there is an increased likelihood of a BP diagnosis. Moreover, youth with mood disorders are at higher risk for using illicit drugs or alcohol as a way to deal with their mood and stressors (32,38). Finally, although there is controversy about the validity of borderline personality disorder in youth, some BP teens, particularly those with BP-II, may be misdiagnosed as having this condition (and vice-versa).

The use of medications such as antidepressants may unmask or trigger a manic or hypomanic episode in a susceptible individual (46). However, not every child who becomes agitated or giddy and excited with these or other medications has BP. Family history, the severity, length, and quality of manic symptomatology may help to differentiate between BP and agitation induced by these or other medications (47).

TABLE 5.4.2.4

BIPOLAR DISORDER VERSUS ATTENTION DEFICIT HYPERACTIVE DISORDER (ADHD)[a]

Suspect the presence of bipolar disorder in a child with ADHD if:

- The ADHD symptoms appeared later in life (e.g., at age 10 yrs old or older).
- The symptoms of ADHD appeared abruptly in an otherwise healthy child.
- The ADHD symptoms were responding to stimulants and now are not.
- The ADHD symptoms come and go and tend to occur with mood changes.
- A child with ADHD begins to have periods of exaggerated elation, grandiosity, depression, no need for sleep, inappropriate sexual behaviors.
- A child with ADHD has recurrent severe mood swings, temper outbursts, or rages.
- A child with ADHD has hallucinations and/or delusions.
- A child with ADHD has a strong family history of bipolar disorder in his or her family, particularly if the child is not responding to appropriate ADHD treatments.

[a]A child may have both ADHD and BP. Moreover, the noted clinical situations may also be due to other psychiatric disorders (unipolar depression, substance abuse), medical problems (thyroid problems, seizures, tumors), use of medications (prednisone), and environmental stressors (family conflict, chaotic environment, sexual or physical abuse) that may coexist with ADHD.

Reprinted from Birmaher B: *New Hope for Children and Adolescents with BP Disorders.* New York, Three Rivers Press, a division of Random House, Inc., 2004, with permission.

TABLE 5.4.2.5

BIPOLAR DISORDER VERSUS DISRUPTIVE BEHAVIOR DISORDER

- If the behavior problems *only* occur while the child is in the midst of an episode of mania or depression, and the behavior problems disappear when the mood symptoms improve, the diagnoses of oppositional or conduct disorder should not be made.
- If a child has "off and on" oppositional or conduct symptoms or these symptoms only appear when the child has mood problems, the diagnosis of BP (or other disorders such as recurrent unipolar depression or substance abuse) should be considered.
- If the child had oppositional behaviors before the onset of the mood disorders, both diagnoses may be given.
- If a child has severe behavior problems that are not responding to treatment, consider the possibility of a mood disorder (bipolar and nonbipolar depressions), other psychiatric disorder (ADHD, substance abuse), and/or exposure to stressors.
- If a child has behavior problems and a family history of BP disorder, consider the possibility that the child has a mood disorder (unipolar major depression or BP disorder).
- If a child has behavior problems and is having hallucinations and delusions consider the possibility of BP disorder. Also consider the possibility of schizophrenia, use of illicit drugs/alcohol, or medical/neurologic conditions.

Reprinted from Birmaher B: *New Hope for Children and Adolescents with BP Disorders*. New York, Three Rivers Press, a division of Random House, Inc., 2004, with permission.

COURSE AND OUTCOME

Although there are methodologic differences among the current pediatric prospective naturalistic studies, they have consistently shown that 70% to 100% of children and adolescents with BP will eventually recover (i.e., no significant symptoms for at least 2 months) from their index episode (23,39,48,49). However, of those who recover, up to 80% will experience one or more recurrences in a period of 2 to 5 years. BP youth have high rates of hospitalizations and health service utilization, and they are at risk for psychosis, suicidality, substance abuse, unemployment, legal problems, abuse, and poor academic and psychosocial functioning (22,23,30–32). The ongoing BP symptoms may also have a negative impact on the family, marital, and sibling relationships, as well as on family finances. The considerable impairment in psychosocial functioning reported in these studies is not only due to the fact that most of them were carried out in clinical samples, but also similar findings have been reported in BP adolescents never referred for treatment (50,51).

Recent studies show that BP is not only manifested by punctuated recovery and recurrences, but by ongoing fluctuating syndromal and subsyndromal symptomatology (23). In fact, in a recent 4-year follow-up study, for approximately 60% of the observation time, BP youth experienced syndromal and subsyndromal BP symptoms, particularly depressive and mixed symptoms (Fig. 5.4.2.1) (23). In addition, pediatric BP frequently manifests with repeated changes in symptom polarity (22–24,39). These rapid fluctuations in mood appear to be more accentuated than in adults with BP and may explain, at least in part, the difficulties encountered in diagnosing and treating BP symptoms in youth (Fig. 5.4.2.2) (23,29,52). Youth diagnosed with BP-NOS are at high risk to convert to BP-I/II, with rates of conversion as high as 45% (28). To date, the main risk factor found to be associated with conversion into BP-I is family history of mania.

The above noted studies evaluated the course and outcome of BP as a group. A recent study evaluated more individualized course during a 9-year period using latent growth class analyses (48). Four longitudinal mood trajectories were found: (1) "predominantly euthymic" course (24.0%); (2) "moderately euthymic" course (34.6%), "ill with improving course" (19.1%), and "predominantly ill" course (22.3%). Within each group, youths were euthymic on average 84.4%, 47.3%, 42.8%, and 11.5% of the follow-up time, respectively. The fact that a substantial group of youth have good course gives youth and their families hope that BP disorder does not necessarily convey poor prognosis. Nonetheless, continued syndromal and subsyndromal mood symptoms in all four classes underscore the need to optimize treatment.

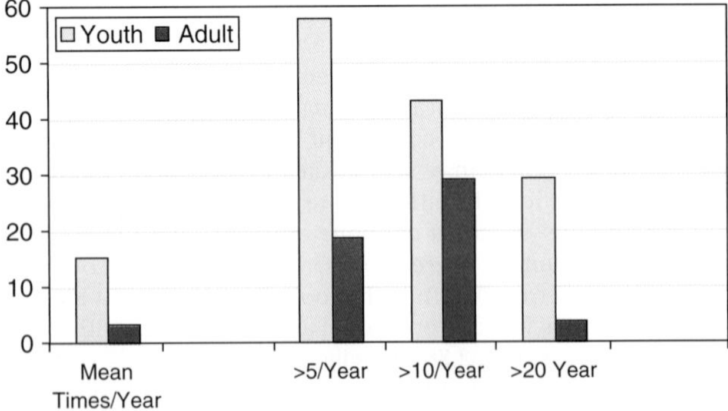

FIGURE 5.4.2.2. Change in polarity: Switch between depression and mania/hypomania or vice versa with or without intervening weeks at the asymptomatic status. Comparison between youth with BP-I versus adults with BP-I. All comparisons are significant at $p < 0.001$. (Data from Birmaher B, Axelson D, Strober M, et al.: Clinical course of children and adolescents with bipolar spectrum disorders. *Arch Gen Psychiatry* 63:175–183, 2006; and Judd LL, Akiskal HS, Schettler PJ, et al.: The long-term natural history of the weekly symptomatic status of bipolar I disorder. *Arch Gen Psychiatry* 59:530–537, 2002.)

Overall, across the extant studies the following factors have been associated with worse course and outcome: early age of onset, long duration, mixed or rapid cycling episodes, psychosis, presence of subsyndromal mood symptoms, comorbid disorders, exposure to negative life events (e.g., abuse), and family psychopathology (mood disorders and substance abuse) and low socioeconomic status (22,23,48,49).

RISK FACTORS

Twin, Adoption, and Family Studies

Twin and adoption studies have demonstrated that BP runs in families (39,53–56). The prevalence of BP in first-degree relatives of adults with BP is increased 8- to 10-fold over the expected prevalence of BP in community samples of adults, making BP one of the most familial psychiatric disorders (39,54,57–60). However, the rates of BP in relatives of BP subjects may be underestimated because most BP high-risk studies included only offspring of BP parents older than 18 years (54) without considering that many adults with BP experienced their first symptoms of BP early in life (3,25,26,39,61).

A large prospective high-risk BP study (mean follow-up 7 years), the Pittsburgh Bipolar Offspring Study (BIOS), that included offspring of parents with BP and control offspring of healthy parents and parents with non-BP psychiatric disorders (with raters blind to parental diagnosis) showed that after adjusting for confounding factors, in comparison with offspring of community controls, offspring of BP parents had significantly higher rates of BP spectrum disorders (23% vs. 3%, respectively) (57,58,61), high rates of BP-I (13% and 1.5%, respectively), and anxiety disorders. The presence of subthreshold manic or hypomanic episodes, MDEs, and disruptive behavior disorders was associated with subsequent manic, mixed, or hypomanic episodes. However, only subthreshold manic or hypomanic episodes were associated when analyses were restricted to prospective data.

The above study analyzed categorical disorders. A more recent analyses of the dimensional symptoms preceding the onset of BP showed that offspring with mood lability, depression/anxiety, and particularly those with subsyndromal manic symptoms and whose parents had early-onset BP were at 50% risk to develop BP (61).

In addition to the above high-risk family investigations, "bottom-up" studies also provide further evidence of the familial nature of BP (39,59). These studies have shown increased risk for BP and depression in first-degree relatives of youth with BP when compared with relatives of adolescents with other disorders. Further, the first-degree relatives of youth whose BP started early in life, adolescents with subsyndromal symptoms of BP, and BP children with comorbid ADHD, showed a significantly increased risk for mood disorders when compared with youth without these factors.

Genetic Studies

Extant literature has demonstrated a genetic etiology for BP with an estimated heritability at over 80% (53,54,56,62,63). Current literature suggests that multiple (interacting) loci and epigenetic factors may contribute to BP liability, but the effect of each gene is small (63,64). Moreover, variation in ascertainment, phenotype definition, control selection, limited power, and possible confounding by population substructure has led to inconsistent results.

Spectroscopy Studies

The most common spectroscopic imaging method used in BP research is ^{1}H-MR spectroscopy. Glutamatergic ^{1}H-MR spectroscopy metabolites include Glu, Gln, γ-aminobutyric acid (GABA) and *N*-acetyl aspartylglutamate (65). These compounds seem to be affected in the frontostriatal region, cingulate cortex, dorsolateral prefrontal cortex (DLPFC), and other areas of the brain in BP youth and offspring of BP parents (66–70). A recent review concluded that the predictive value of MR spectroscopy neuroimaging may relate to a disturbance in either glutamine or GABA, or in the homeostatic equilibrium of Glu and glutamine, providing further support for the exploration of the Gln/Glu ratio as a potential biomarker in pediatric BP (71). BP youth in a manic or mixed episode were treated with valproic acid and performed ^{1}H-MR spectroscopy at baseline, day 7, and day 28 (70). In subjects who achieved clinical remission with valproic acid, the investigators found a decreased baseline glutamate and a correlation between a change in the Young Mania Rating Scale (YMRS) scores and decreased Glu in the left ventrolateral prefrontal cortex. Furthermore, overall, mitochondrial studies of MR spectroscopy revealed reduced intracellular pH and that adenosine diphosphate is one of the principal controllers of oxidative metabolism (71).

Neuroimaging Studies

A recent meta-analyses showed that in contrast to BP adults, emotional dysfunction is associated with hyperactivation of the amygdala, prefrontal, and visual system and cognitive deficits with hypoactivation of the anterior cingulate cortex (72–75). Studies in BP youth also demonstrate abnormally decreased amygdala volumes, decreased OFC and anterior cingulate cortex (ACC) gray matter; abnormally reduced fractional anisotropy (FA) in white matter tracts connecting prefrontal and subcortical region; and altered resting state in prefrontal cortical circuitry and large scale networks (73–80).

Neuroimaging findings in BP youth thus may be conceptualized as parallel dysfunction in bilateral prefrontal cortical (especially vlPFC)–hippocampal–amygdala emotion processing and emotion regulation neural circuitries, together with an "overactive" left-sided ventral striatal–vlPFC–OFC reward processing circuitry, that results in characteristic behavioral abnormalities associated with BP: emotional dysregulation, heightened reward sensitivity, and predisposition to mania (73). A potential structural basis for these functional abnormalities is decrease in white matter tracts connecting prefrontal and subcortical regions that may suggest abnormal myelination or abnormal orientation of axons in these tracts, and gray matter decreases in prefrontal and temporal cortices, amygdala, and hippocampus. Resting state connectivity studies are beginning to provide evidence in support of intrinsic functional abnormalities in these neural circuitries in adults with BD.

A limitation of the current literature is the inadequate information of the impact of previous clinical mood and nonmood symptoms course and treatment upon neural functioning and structure. Prospective longitudinal follow-up studies are also critically needed to elucidate the extent to which measures of neural functioning and structure predict future course. Regarding the effects of treatment, imaging findings in BP have preliminarily reported that prefrontal cortical regions improve in function with some pharmacologic agents, while amygdala in the subcortical region does not reach normality until after longer-term treatment (15,81). Also, various medications differentially engage different brain circuitry regions, suggesting the possibility that combined therapy may be required based on severity and/or presentation.

Regarding the effects of nonmood symptomatology, preliminary evidence from studies that contrasted BD and ADHD suggests that the neural systems involved in impulsivity, reward systems, and executive function were engaged differently in the two illnesses. In BP, "emotional impulsivity" is predominantly emotionally driven, and stems from ventral frontostriatal-limbic circuitry dysfunction. In contrast, in ADHD "cognitive impulsivity" is predominantly cognitively driven, and stems from dorsal frontostriatal dysfunction (82).

Neurocognitive Function

The neurocognitive studies have limitations similar to those described under neuroimaging studies above. Extant literature has found that in comparison with healthy controls and youth with other disorders, BP youth show cognitive impairment in attention, set-shifting, working memory, and in particular, cognitive flexibility (adaptation in response to changing rewards and punishments) (83–85). These findings have also been observed in BP youth during periods of euthymia (86). Similar results have been reported in BP adults (87). There is also widespread agreement that cognitive functioning independently and robustly predicts later functional outcomes in BP (88). However, the trajectory of cognitive functioning into adulthood in young BP patients remains largely unknown. Some data support a neuroprogressive model of worsening cognitive function over the course of illness (86–90), while other reports dispute this (91–93). The neurocognitive studies have limitations similar to those described under neuroimaging studies above. However, some studies, but not all (75,81) suggest that impairment in cognitive functioning (e.g., flexibility) in BP youth may be independent of mood state and treatment exposure (83–85).

Psychosocial Factors

Very few studies have evaluated the effects of psychosocial factors on the onset and maintenance of BP in youth. These studies have suggested that low socioeconomic status (SES), exposure to negative events (e.g., abuse), and stressful family environments (i.e., high "expressed emotion" [EE]) are associated with poor prognosis (22,23,39,93). In BP adults, high EE, negative events, poor sleep hygiene, and irregular daily routines have been associated with increased risk for recurrences (64,95).

ASSESSMENT

This section briefly describes instruments and rating scales used to assess BP symptoms in youth. For further information regarding these scales and for the description of instruments related to the assessment of depressive, suicidal, and other psychiatric conditions, see Chapter 4.3 and the parameters for the psychiatric assessment of children and adolescents (96).

Psychiatric Interviews

There are several structured and semistructured interviews that can be used for the diagnosis of BP and for the evaluation of subtype and the frequency, intensity, number, and duration of each episode. The most widely used interviews in BP studies are two similar instruments: the Kiddie Schedule for Affective Disorders and Schizophrenia for School Age Children—Present and Lifetime version (K-SADSPL) (97) and the Washington University KSADS (WASH-U-KSADS) (98). However, these interviews are lengthy, and thus mainly used for research purposes. Symptom checklists based on the DSM criteria for BP as well as depressive disorders are also useful in clinical settings.

Clinician-Based Rating Scales

Two clinician-based rating scales are currently used for the assessment of manic symptoms in youth, the YMRS (99) and the KSADS Mania Rating Scale that was derived from the KSADS-P mania module (KSADS-MRS) (100). However, a recent study found that the YMRS is not a valid instrument for BP disorder in youth (101).

Youth, Parent, and Teacher Rating Scales

The above noted meta-analysis reported that in general, existing scales help to screen youth with BP from youth with other disorders (101). However, scales that include manic symptoms outperformed those with general symptom checklists. Among the scales that include manic symptoms, the General Behavior Inventory (GBI) (102), the Child Mania Rating Scale (CMRS) (103), and the Mood Disorders Questionnaire (104) have been validated in many studies and appear to be the most helpful in clinical practice. Caregiver reports are more effective in identifying mania than youth or teacher reports. Nevertheless, multiple informants and directly interviewing the youth increase the validity of the diagnosis.

Of note, studies using a scale that includes general symptoms of psychopathology, the Child Behavior Checklist (CBCL), found a consistent pattern of elevated scores on subscales assessing aggressive behavior, attention problems, delinquent behavior, and anxious/depressed domains in BP youth (105–107). However, more recent studies have demonstrated that the above symptoms are a proxy for severe psychopathology and not specific for BP (101,108).

Mood Timelines or Diaries

Mood timelines or diaries using school years, birthdays, and holidays as anchors are very helpful in the assessment of the onset and course of mood disorders. These instruments use colors or numeric ratings (e.g., from 0 to 10) to chart daily changes in mood along with any corresponding stressors, illnesses, and treatments. These instruments can help children, parents, and clinicians to visualize the course of their mood, and identify events that may have triggered the depression, hypomania/mania, or irritability and examine the relationship between treatment and response. Several electronic mood charts (e.g., websites, mobile applications) exist to evaluate daily mood fluctuations, but they vary widely in quality and usefulness.

Other Assessments

Clinicians should always evaluate for psychosocial functioning, family psychopathology, ongoing negative life events (family conflicts, abuse), functioning in several areas (peer relationships, school functioning, work), and for the presence of psychiatric and medical conditions and suicidal and homicidal ideation (for instruments to evaluate these domains, see the respective chapters). If the youth has learning difficulties before the onset of the mood disorders or these difficulties continue when the mood is stable, neuropsychologic testing is warranted (Chapter 4.4). Also, the clinician together with the child and parents should evaluate the appropriate intensity and restrictiveness of care (hospitalization). The decision for the level of care will depend on factors such as the severity of mood symptoms, presence of suicidal and/or homicidal symptoms, psychosis, substance dependence, agitation, child's and parents' adherence to treatment, parental psychopathology, and family environment.

At the present time, no biologic or imaging tests are clinically available for the diagnosis of BP.

TREATMENT

Phases of Treatment

The treatment of BP is usually divided into acute, continuation, and maintenance phases. The main goal of the acute treatment phase is to control or ameliorate the acute BP symptoms that are affecting the child's psychosocial functioning and well-being or endangering the child's life. Continuation treatment is required to consolidate the response during the acute phase and avoid relapses, and maintenance treatment is designed to avoid recurrences. Pharmacologic and psychosocial treatment strategies for each one of these three treatment phases are discussed below. In general, the choice of treatment depends on the severity, phase of illness, subtype of BP, chronicity, comorbid disorders, subject's age, family and patient preference and expectations, availability of services, family and environmental circumstances, and family psychopathology.

During each of the three treatment phases noted above, if a child does not respond to treatment, factors associated with nonresponse need to be considered, such as misdiagnosis, poor adherence to treatment, presence of comorbid psychiatric and medical conditions, and ongoing exposure to negative events (family conflict, abuse).

Support, Psychoeducation, and Case Management

At any phase of treatment, basic elements of support are indicated, including active listening. Provision of hope is critical, particularly in the face of demoralization that may occur for the youth and his/her parents both in the early phases of diagnosis and treatment, and during periods of relapse.

Psychoeducation is a common component of most manualized psychosocial treatments for pediatric BP, and data suggest its provision is associated with improved treatment adherence and reduced mood symptoms (109–111). It is important to provide psychoeducation to both the patient and family members about the causes, symptoms, course, and different treatments of BP and the possible risks and benefits associated with these treatments (and with no treatment at all). Attention should be given to helping the youth and family understand the genetic, biologic, and psychosocial influences associated with onset of mood disorders. Additionally, providers should prepare the youth and family for what may be a recurrent and chronic illness with frequent fluctuations in mood and functioning. Often, it is hard for parents and youth to accept the illness, and therefore, to adhere to treatment. A discussion highlighting the import of adherence to both medication and psychosocial treatment is therefore critical, and optimally includes identification and problem-solving potential barriers to adherence in any individual case (e.g., irregular schedules, side effects, etc.). Furthermore, psychosocial treatment should involve helping youth and parents recognize symptoms of both depression and hypomania/mania, and distinguish symptoms associated with BP (e.g., negative thinking and mood swings) from normal developmental processes (e.g., individuation in adolescence) and also from symptoms of other psychiatric disorders (e.g., oppositionality in behavioral disorders, impulsivity in ADHD). Sleep hygiene and routine are important, especially in view of sleep deprivation leading to worsening of symptoms. Ensuring a stable circadian rhythm has a positive effect on physiology and daily functioning. To further assist with psychoeducation in clinical practice, websites and books are available (112,113).

Case management is frequently an important component of treatment for BP youth and their families. This often involves coordination and ongoing contact with school personnel, who may need education to help understand the disease model of BP. Alongside parents, providers must help advocate for adequate accommodations (e.g., schedule, workload) to help the child succeed academically. Additionally, providers may need to help negotiate with parents and/or other organizations regarding reasonable expectations for the child based on his/her current symptoms, with the recognition that needs will likely change over time (113–115).

Acute Treatment

In this chapter, the term mood stabilizer refers to lithium and anticonvulsants such as valproate, carbamazepine, and lamotrigine. However, the extant literature seems to indicate that the atypical antipsychotics may also operate as mood stabilizers.

In general, and until further studies are available, doses of mood stabilizers and atypical antipsychotics and blood levels of mood stabilizers are similar to those used in BP adults (116–119). It appears that the pharmacokinetics of these medications is similar across age (120). However, a small study that deserves replication showed that youth demonstrate lower brain-to-serum lithium concentration ratios than adults, suggesting that youth may need higher serum lithium concentrations (121).

In any case, to avoid unnecessarily high dosages and decrease the risk of side effects and poor adherence to treatment, unless the youth is too agitated, it is recommended to start at low dosages and increase slowly according to response and side effects.

PHARMACOTHERAPY

Mania/Mixed Episodes

Current studies suggest that the most efficacious and fastest way to yield response for acute manic/mixed episodes is with the atypical antipsychotics (122–125). The mood stabilizers are less efficacious, but most studies only lasted 8 weeks—possibly insufficient time to observe the true response to these medications (125–129). Also, there is variability in response to mood stabilizers depending on the site of the study and the sample size. A recent multicenter study, the Treatment of Early-Age Mania (TEAM), randomly administered risperidone (average dose 3 mg), lithium (average blood levels 1.1), or valproate (average blood levels 114) to 279 youth (ages 6 to 15 years old) with BP-I (130). The treatment was open, but the assessments were blind to treatment assignment. After 8 weeks of treatment, roughly 70% of the youth responded to risperidone, 30% to lithium, and 20% to valproate. The response to risperidone was similar across sites, but in some sites, the response to lithium was higher (128). An analysis of the benefits of either an add-on or a switch of antimanic medications for an 8-week period in partial and nonresponders, respectively, showed better response to risperidone than lithium or valproate (131). A small 6-week study comparing valproate versus risperidone versus placebo for preschool BP also showed that risperidone was efficacious, but not valproate (129). These studies have also suggested that the combination of two mood stabilizers such as lithium and valproate or a mood stabilizer with an atypical antipsychotic appears to be superior to mood stabilizer monotherapy, with responses ranging from 60% to 90% (132–136). Open treatment with carbamazepine indicates that this medication appears to be effective and safe for BP youth, but randomized control trials (RCTs) are needed to confirm this (137). A RTC for oxycarbamazepine was negative (138).

Although there are no studies, for youth who require prompt response (e.g., agitation, psychosis), it is possible to start treatment with a mood stabilizer and antipsychotic, and once the youth is stable consider tapering the antipsychotic. However, atypical antipsychotic monotherapy may serve as an alternative choice. For adolescents with severe illnesses that are resistant to these treatments, electroconvulsive therapy (ECT) should be considered (139).

Hypomania, BP-NOS, and Cyclothymia

Despite the increased morbidity associated with these disorders, there are very few open studies that specifically address the treatment of youth with these conditions. Therefore, until research is available, for those youth with significant impairment, similar psychosocial and pharmacologic treatments to those described for mania are recommended.

Depression

BP youth spend substantial amounts of time with syndromal or subsyndromal depressive symptoms that significantly impair their psychosocial functioning and increase their risk for suicide (9,23,30). However, the very few studies for depressed BP youth are pharmacologic RCTs with small samples and open-label studies.

In adults, monotherapy with lithium, valproate, some of the atypical antipsychotics, and the combination of these medications are indicated for the acute treatment of depression (117,140). Although controversial, the judicial use of the serotonin reuptake inhibitors (SSRIs) or bupropion in combination with mood stabilizers, and/or the typical antipsychotic, may also be beneficial for some youth with BP depression (117,140). SSRIs or other antidepressants may trigger mania, hypomania, mixed episodes or rapid cycling, or agitation, particularly when used without concomitant mood stabilizer treatment. A recent 8-week RCT comparing quetiapine versus placebo for a small sample of BP-depressed youth was negative (141). Finally, a secondary analysis of the TEAM study showed that depressive symptoms, present in the acutely manic/mixed phase of BP, equally improved with risperidone, lithium, and valproate (142). However, risperidone yielded more rapid improvement than the other two medications.

Until more studies become available, and taking into account the limitations of extrapolating from the adult literature, it is recommended to use lithium, valproate, or the atypical antipsychotics as first-line medications for BP depression. For partial or nonresponders, combinations of these medications with atypical antipsychotics, SSRIs, or bupropion are indicated.

As described below, specific psychosocial treatments designed for BP youth appear to be efficacious for the treatment of BP symptoms, particularly depression. These treatments should also be considered as the first line of treatment, especially for youth with mild-to-moderate depression. For subjects with recurrent seasonal depression, light therapy should be considered (143). For adolescents with severe and treatment-resistant disorders, electroconvulsive treatment (ECT) may be indicated (139). Other treatments such as transcranial magnetic therapy (TMS) or augmentation with omega-3 fatty acids (144,145) appear promising, but they need to be further evaluated.

Rapid Cycling

There are no specific studies for the treatment of rapid cycling in youth. Until these studies become available, the same treatments as for mania or mixed episodes are recommended (116).

Adjunctive Medications

Almost all studies use short-term adjuvant medications or rescue paradigms during the acute phase of treatment with monotherapy or combination regimes. This strategy, in fact, becomes inevitable in managing breakthrough symptoms of mania in BP disorder. Lorazepam and clonazepam or short administration of antipsychotics sometimes may be temporarily used for the management of acute agitation or insomnia (39,116).

Psychosocial Treatments

In addition to supportive psychotherapy, specific psychosocial treatment packages for youth with BP are at various stages of investigation that target acute affective symptoms and prevention or delay of recurrences, improvement of adherence to treatment, and management of comorbid conditions. A central feature of all psychosocial treatment models for pediatric BP includes psychoeducation, problem-solving, and coping skills. Parents are closely engaged in their children's therapy and referred to treatment if they have clinically significant symptoms themselves.

To date, five distinct psychosocial approaches have been developed and are at various stages of evaluation, each with a specified target age group and method of delivery (e.g., group vs. individual treatment). First, child- and family-focused cognitive behavior therapy (CFF-CBT) was specifically designed for 8 to 12 year olds with BP (146). This approach integrates core principles of CBT with those of family-focused therapy (FFT; see below) in a 12-session intervention designed to be largely delivered jointly with parents and children. Data from open studies and an RCT suggest CFF-CBT is associated with improvement in functioning, mood symptoms, and treatment adherence (146,147). Second, Fristad et al. (110,111) employed an 8-session multiple-family group treatment for youths aged 8 to 12 years with bipolar and depressive spectrum disorders. This approach includes an emphasis on psychoeducation around the role of medications, and coping skills including problem-solving and communication skills. Studies show that multi-family psycho-education group therapy (MFPG) (vs. control condition) is associated with greater mood improvement, enhanced family interactions, subsequent treatment engagement, and greater knowledge around mood disorder (110,111,114). Third, Miklowitz et al. (2004) (115), developed a 9-month (21 session) manualized version of FFT specifically for adolescents with BP and their parents that includes psychoeducation geared toward illness management, skills to solve problems, and building communication skills to decrease stress and conflict in the family environment. A preliminary study using FFT for BP adolescents showed symptomatic improvement in mania, depression, and behavior problems at the end of 1 year of follow-up (115). A subsequent randomized trial showed less severe depressive symptoms and faster recovery from depression among adolescents receiving FFT as compared with a brief educational intervention (148). However, a more recent randomized trial failed to replicate these findings (148,149). Next, Goldstein et al. (2007) (149) developed a 1-year adaptation of Dialectical Behavior Therapy (DBT) (151) for adolescents (age 12 to 18) with BP and their family members. This approach includes both individual and family skills training sessions to provide psychoeducation, and also teach and ensure generalization of skills targeting mindfulness, emotion dysregulation, distress tolerance, interpersonal effectiveness, and parent–child conflict (150). A recent randomized trial showed adolescents receiving DBT (as compared with psychosocial treatment as usual) demonstrated less severe depressive symptoms and greater likelihood of improvement in suicidal ideation (151). Finally, Hlastala and Frank (2006) (152) adapted Interpersonal and Social Rhythm Therapy for BP adolescents ages 12 to 18 years old. This intervention highlights the connection between difficulties in relationships and mood, alongside regularizing sleep and daily rhythms as a means of preventing and improving mood symptoms in BP. This 16-session adaptation is primarily conducted with the adolescent, but family involvement is recommended. In one open study, Hlastala et al. (2010) (153) showed improvement from pre- to posttreatment in mood symptoms with interpersonal and social rhythm therapy (IPSRT). With respect to psychosocial treatment of common comorbid conditions (e.g., oppositional behaviors, substance abuse, anxiety disorder), efficacious psychosocial treatments are indicated (see respective chapters). In sum, additional research is needed to establish efficacy and determine fit between the psychosocial approaches and the individual patient most likely to respond. Nonetheless, these developmental adaptations, with significant consensus on core shared principles (e.g., psychoeducation, problem-solving, skill building), offer promise as adjunctive treatment.

Recent studies have also begun to explore the potential for early psychosocial intervention to ameliorate, delay, or even prevent the onset and/or progression of BP among youth at high risk for the disorder. Goldstein et al. (2013) (154) developed a modification of IPSRT for the adolescent offspring of parents with BP who themselves have not yet developed BP. An open pilot study demonstrated the feasibility and acceptability of the intervention for this group, and identified pre- to posttreatment improvement in sleep and circadian patterns that may contribute to increased risk for illness onset. Results from a recently completed RCT will further inform the field regarding efficacy. Additionally, given the risk for youth with mood disturbance and a positive BP family history to develop BP and progress to BP-I/II over time, Miklowitz et al. (155,156) examined whether FFT-A could be a beneficial early intervention for mood-disordered adolescents (i.e., those with BP-NOS, cyclothymia, depression) with a family history of BP. An initial pilot study demonstrated feasibility and improvement pre- to posttreatment in depression, hypomania, and functioning (155). A subsequent RCT showed more rapid recovery from mood symptoms, more weeks symptom free, and lesser manic symptoms over 1 year among high-risk youth receiving FFT-A as compared with those receiving a single-session family educational intervention; effects were more pronounced among high EE families (116). Clearly, further study of the role of early intervention for at-risk youth is warranted to determine timing and selection of those most likely to benefit.

CONTINUATION AND MAINTENANCE TREATMENTS

Randomized controlled trials in adults have suggested the use of valproate, lithium, lamotrigine (only for depression), and atypical antipsychotics for prevention of new mood episodes in stable BP adults (118). In any case, the first-line maintenance treatment is the same regimen that successfully treated the manic episode (118). The literature examining ongoing treatment for BP youth is limited and most studies have been open. An 18-month naturalistic follow-up study of BP adolescents who were stable on lithium therapy found a relapse rate of 92% in adolescents who stopped lithium treatment, compared to 38% to those who continued with lithium (157). Two controlled studies have been published examining how BP youth who remitted from acute manic symptoms while taking combination treatment responded to a switch to monotherapy. In the first, 6 out of 14 BP adolescents who were stabilized from an acute psychotic manic episode after 4 weeks of treatment with lithium and an antipsychotic relapsed within 1 week of discontinuation of the antipsychotic (135). In the second, subjects stabilized on lithium and valproate combination therapy were switched to either drug alone (134). There was no difference between the two drugs, and the majority of subjects had relapsed within 4 months of switching to monotherapy. An extended follow-up phase of this study found that approximately 90% of the subjects who had a mood relapse responded to restarting the combination treatment (158). A recent RCT showed that aripiprazole 10 mg/day or 30 mg/day were superior to placebo and generally well tolerated in BP-I youth up to 30 weeks. However, completion rates were very low in all treatment arms (122,159).

The duration of the maintenance treatment depends on many factors such as the duration of the illness, lifetime number of episodes, severity and history of hospitalizations, psychosis, and suicidality. In general, BP youth with clear BP may require many years of treatment and some lifelong. However, some BP youth, particularly those with late onset, less severe mood episodes, less comorbid disorders, high SES, less history of sexual abuse, and less family history of mood and substance use disorders may have long mostly euthymic course (23,48), careful medication taper may be considered once remission has been maintained for 12 to 24 months. Also, it may be reasonable to consider shorter treatment in cases when the diagnosis is not clearly established or the illness has been relatively mild. Conversely, severe and recurrent illness may merit more prolonged maintenance pharmacotherapy. The optimal duration of psychosocial treatments for pediatric BP has not been established. Given that BP may be best viewed as a chronic disease, it is reasonable to provide some level of ongoing psychosocial support, crisis management, and formal therapy booster sessions when appropriate.

ACUTE AND LONG-TERM PHARMACOTHERAPY SIDE EFFECTS

For a comprehensive review refer to Chapter 6.1.1. In this section we highlight practical aspects of the pharmacologic management of BP.

Lithium

The most serious problem associated with acute and long-term lithium therapy is that of toxicity due to elevated lithium blood levels. Lithium has a low therapeutic index, and severe lithium toxicity can cause permanent renal and neurologic damage, as well as death. Though initial signs and symptoms of toxicity usually do not manifest until blood levels are above 1.5 mEq/L, tolerability varies among patients and some individuals will be symptomatic at lower blood levels. The risk of lithium toxicity can be reduced by a number of basic steps. Patients and family members must be aware of the signs of lithium toxicity: dizziness, clumsiness, unsteady gait, slurred speech, coarse tremors, abdominal pain, vomiting, sedation, confusion, and blurry vision. Basically, the subject intoxicated with lithium looks and acts like a "drunk" person and in these cases a stat lithium level is indicated. If a patient has difficulty with taking fluids or has excessive fluid loss (nausea, vomiting, diarrhea, febrile illness), lithium doses should be reduced or temporarily held until regular fluid intake is maintained. If other symptoms of lithium toxicity occur in addition to gastrointestinal distress, referral for immediate evaluation is necessary.

The dose escalation of lithium should be conservative, especially in outpatient settings, and blood levels should be obtained as early as 6 to 7 days after each dose increase, if the mood symptoms are recurring (e.g., check adherence), and immediately if clinical symptoms of toxicity occur. Patients should be counseled to maintain adequate hydration during vigorous exercise or on hot days, and avoid major changes in salt, caffeine, or fluid intake. In addition, they must notify physicians and pharmacists that they are taking lithium, and do not take substances that interact with lithium. Common conditions and nonprescription drugs and substances that can elevate lithium levels include dehydration, diuretics, most nonsteroidal anti-inflammatory drugs (not acetaminophen), and alcohol. Caffeine tends to lower lithium levels. The list of prescription drugs that interact with lithium is long and should be checked prior to prescribing any new medication.

Lithium has a number of different potential side effects associated with short- and long-term treatment, which may be particularly bothersome to youth (acne, increased weight, tiredness, polyuria, poor concentration and "dullness," and rarely hair loss) (see Table 5.4.2.6). Patients have a wide range of tolerability to lithium, with some having minimal or manageable side effects while others will have significant problems. Sometimes side effects can be ameliorated by dose reduction or by switching between extended release and immediate release preparations and/or dividing the dose during the day.

Two issues that require ongoing monitoring are the potential for kidney damage and hypothyroidism. Lithium inhibits the renal tubular response to antidiuretic hormone, which decreases the ability to concentrate urine and leads to polyuria. Evidence from biopsy studies in adults indicates that in some cases lithium can lead to chronic interstitial nephritis (119,160–162). However, selection bias and the fact that similar changes have been found in adult psychiatric patients who have not been treated with lithium make it difficult to determine how much lithium treatment elevates the risk of kidney damage (160). Studies of the effects of lithium on glomerular function have generally showed minimal to mild reductions associated with long-term treatment. These data have made it difficult to know how to monitor for the undetermined but likely low risk of developing

TABLE 5.4.2.6

LITHIUM SIDE EFFECTS

Common	Polyuria, polydipsia, tremor, weight gain, nausea, diarrhea, hypothyroidism, cognitive dulling, sedation, leukocytosis
Uncommon	New onset or exacerbation of acne or psoriasis, bradycardia, hair loss, ECG changes (T-wave flattening)
Rare	Kidney, brain damage and death (due to acute toxicity), decreased renal function, pseudotumor cerebri, extrapyramidal symptoms, movement abnormalities, nystagmus, seizure, hyperparathyroidism, sinus node dysfunction, arrhythmias

TABLE 5.4.2.7

ROUTINE LABORATORY MONITORING BEFORE AND DURING PHARMACOTHERAPY

Medication	Baseline Tests	Follow-up	Test Frequency[a]	Comments
Lithium	BUN, creatinine, TSH, free T4, urinalysis, CBC, electrolytes, calcium, albumin, height, weight, BMI	Lithium level BUN, creatinine, TSH, free T4, urinalysis, calcium, albumin, height, weight, BMI	Each dose change and q3–6mo q3–6mo	24-hr urine for protein and creatinine clearance if marked polyuria, proteinuria, or change in serum creatinine
Valproate	CBC with differential and platelet count, AST, ALT, lipase, height, weight, BMI menstrual history	Valproate level and platelet count, AST, ALT Height, weight, BMI, menstrual history	q2wk × 2, then q month × 2, then q3–6mo and with each dose change Each appointment	Risk of hepatic failure is highest in first 6 mo of treatment. Repeat lipase if pancreatitis suspected
Carbamazepine	CBC with differential and platelet count, AST, ALT, sodium	Carbamazepine level, CBC with differential and platelet count, AST, ALT, sodium	1 and 3–4 wks after dose change and then q3–6mo	Check labs if unexplained fever, sore throat, lymphadenopathy, or severe fatigue
Antipsychotics	Glucose, triglycerides, total cholesterol, HDL, LDL, AIMS, height, weight, BMI For ziprasidone EKG	Glucose, triglycerides, total cholesterol, HDL, LDL AIMS Height, weight, BMI EKG as necessary	3 mo after start, then q6–12mo q3–6mo Every appointment	Check metabolic status if substantial weight gain

Note: A pregnancy test should be performed in all postmenarchal females at baseline and whenever pregnancy is a possibility over follow-up.
[a]Follow-up tests should be performed whenever clinical symptoms of serious side effects occur.
BMI, body mass index; BUN, blood urea nitrogen; TSH, thyroid-stimulating hormone; AST, aspartate aminotransferase; ALT, alanine aminotransferase; CBC, complete blood count; HDL, high-density lipoprotein; LDL, low-density lipoprotein; AIMS, Abnormal Involuntary Movement Scale; EKG, electrocardiogram.

clinically significant kidney damage. A conservative monitoring approach is noted in Table 5.4.2.7. The decision to refer for renal consultation and/or discontinue lithium treatment remains one of clinical judgment, though a significant change in serum creatinine should trigger a thorough evaluation.

Lithium inhibits the effect of thyroid-stimulating hormone (TSH) in the thyroid gland. As a consequence, approximately 25% of youth develop elevated TSH levels within 3 months of initiating lithium treatment (163). The long-term effects on the thyroid have not been determined in a pediatric population, and TSH levels can be just transiently elevated in BP adults initiating lithium treatment (162). Given the developmental implications, clear hypothyroidism induced by lithium in youth will require intervention. Whether to treat or discontinue lithium in patients with subclinical hypothyroidism is less clear. However, if lithium is clearly helping the individual, thyroid replacement treatment is indicated.

Preliminary evidence of greater mood instability and depression in BP adults with lower levels of free T4 or higher levels of TSH at baseline or during treatment with lithium indicates that adding thyroid hormone may be reasonable (162,164,165). Although not well studied, lithium can also cause hyperparathyroidism and as a consequence abnormalities in calcium, phosphorus, and magnesium blood levels.

Finally, lithium has been associated with cardiac abnormalities in the fetus when administered during the first trimester of pregnancy. Therefore, the continuation of lithium during this period of pregnancy needs to be balanced against the possibility of a manic recurrence with the deleterious consequences for the mother and the fetus.

Valproate

Valproate has gastrointestinal, neurologic, hematologic, and cognitive side effects that usually can be minimized by careful titration or dose reduction (Table 5.4.2.8). Periodic blood tests are often performed in order to monitor for the rare but serious side effects (hepatic failure, pancreatitis, thrombocytopenia) (Table 5.4.2.7) (116). It is very important that patients and family members are aware of the initial symptomatic presentations of these side effects and know to obtain an urgent assessment if they occur. For instance, hepatotoxicity can present with symptoms of vomiting, nausea, anorexia, lethargy, drowsiness, and facial edema. Mild elevations of serum transaminases do occur during treatment and are of questionable clinical significance unless they are more than three times the normal level. The risk of hepatic failure is most elevated in children under the age of 3, in those who have metabolic or neurologic disorders, and those who are taking multiple anticonvulsants.

Although uncertain, valproate has been associated with polycystic ovarian syndrome. Thus, baseline menstrual history and a gynecologic consultation of any female who develops significant changes in her menstrual cycle and/or hirsutism while on this medication are warranted. Valproate has been associated with spina bifida in fetuses exposed to this medication during the first trimester of pregnancy. As with lithium, the clinician needs to consider the benefits and risks of

TABLE 5.4.2.8

VALPROATE SIDE EFFECTS

Common	Weight gain, tremor, nausea, diarrhea, cognitive dulling, sedation, fatigue, ataxia, dizziness
Uncommon	Serum transaminase elevations, alopecia, elevated testosterone, polycystic ovarian syndrome, rash, hair loss
Rare	Hepatic failure, thrombocytopenia, pancreatitis, severe dermatologic reactions, myelosuppression, anticonvulsant hypersensitivity syndrome

TABLE 5.4.2.9

CARBAMAZEPINE SIDE EFFECTS

Common	Nausea, vomiting, clumsiness, dizziness, nystagmus, sedation, blurred vision, diplopia, cognitive dulling, ataxia, photosensitivity CYP450 enzyme induction (increased clearance of drugs metabolized by hepatic cytochrome system, including oral contraceptives)
Uncommon	Hyponatremia, rash, confusion, leukopenia
Rare	Serious dermatologic reactions, agranulocytosis, aplastic anemia, atrioventricular block, arrhythmias, hepatitis, renal dysfunction, anticonvulsant hypersensitivity syndrome

continuing valproate during the pregnancy. If valproate is going to be continued, some advocate for the use of folic acid as preventative against neurologic problems in the fetus.

Carbamazepine

As with valproate, carbamazepine has neurologic, cognitive, and gastrointestinal side effects that can usually be managed by dose adjustment, as well as rare serious side effects that are difficult to prevent via routine blood monitoring (Tables 5.4.2.7 and 5.4.2.9) (116). Decreases in platelet and white blood cell counts are not uncommon during carbamazepine treatment, but they do not necessarily predict subsequent development of aplastic anemia or agranulocytosis. Carbamazepine does induce its own metabolism, as well as other drugs that are metabolized by the hepatic cytochrome P450 1A2 and 3A4 isoenzymes. Therefore, blood levels must be repeated several weeks after dose changes and care must be taken when other medications are coadministered (such as oral contraceptives), as they may not reach therapeutic levels. A metabolite of carbamazepine, oxycarbamazepine, does not have the hematologic side effects associated with the parental compound. However, it seems that this medication is not efficacious for the treatment of BP (138).

Lamotrigine

The neurologic and cognitive side effects of lamotrigine seem similar to other anticonvulsants, and are usually managed by dose adjustment (see Table 5.4.2.10). Lamotrigine can induce rash in about 1/2,500 youth. This rash is reversible if lamotrigine is discontinued, but in some cases it may progress to a serious dermatologic reaction such as Stevens–Johnson syndrome (SJS) or toxic epidermal necrolysis (TEN). Though rare, these reactions are more common in youth than adults, and it is difficult to predict whether a rash will progress to SJS or TEN.

TABLE 5.4.2.10

LAMOTRIGINE SIDE EFFECTS

Common	Dizziness, ataxia, headache, tremor, blurred vision, diplopia
Uncommon	Rash, nausea, vomiting, ataxia, cognitive dulling, confusion
Rare	Serious dermatologic reactions, anemia, anticonvulsant hypersensitivity syndrome

TABLE 5.4.2.11

ATYPICAL ANTIPSYCHOTIC SIDE EFFECTS

Common	Weight gain,[a] postural hypotension, extrapyramidal symptoms,[a] dizziness, sedation[a]
Uncommon	Hyperglycemia, diabetes, hypercholesterolemia, increased triglycerides, hyperprolactinemia,[a] rash, photosensitivity, nausea, diarrhea, dyspepsia, constipation, elevated serum transaminases, urinary difficulties, sexual dysfunction, cognitive dulling
Rare	Tardive dyskinesia, neuroleptic malignant syndrome, seizure, hepatic failure

[a]Rate of side effect may vary substantially among the different atypical antipsychotics.

Therefore, unless a new rash is clearly attributable to something other than lamotrigine, treatment should be suspended. The rate of serious dermatologic reactions may be reduced by current dosing recommendations that prescribe small and gradual dose escalation, in particular with the concomitant use of valproate.

Atypical Antipsychotics

The atypical antipsychotics have some differences in side effect profiles, though there are some side effects that are common to all of them in varying degrees (Table 5.4.2.11). In general, there has been increasing concern about the metabolic effects (e.g., increased weight, glucose, and lipids) of some of these medications, which are of substantial concern when these agents are used in children and adolescents over extended periods of time (125,166–168). Routine monitoring parameters have not been established, but it is recommended to measure the child's body mass index (BMI) and fasting glucose and lipids before and routinely (every 6 months and whenever clinical symptoms indicate) while taking these medications (Table 5.4.2.7). If a patient exhibits significant weight gain, it should prompt a more thorough investigation of metabolic status and a reevaluation of the risk–benefit ratio of continuing the current atypical antipsychotic.

Although much less often than the typical antipsychotics, the atypical antipsychotics may cause extrapyramidal symptoms, tardive dyskinesia, and neuroleptic malignant syndrome; thus, it is necessary to evaluate the child at baseline and routinely over follow-up for abnormal movements. Finally, the long-term side effects including chronic hyperprolactinemia associated with the atypicals, particularly risperidol, have not been well studied.

MONITORING PHARMACOTHERAPY

Although the medications that are used to treat bipolar disorder have the potential for significant side effects, there is no evidence whether routine laboratory monitoring reduces the risk of adverse events. Table 5.4.2.8 gives general monitoring guidelines based on recommendations from Federal Drug Administration (FDA) package inserts and typical practice from our BP research centers. It does not have empirical support and is not a substitute for clinical judgment. In many cases, the benefits of treatment outweigh potential risks even if regular laboratory monitoring is not feasible for a patient. Laboratory tests are not a replacement for clinical evaluation, and it is important to review signs and symptoms of potential adverse events with patients and their families as well as emphasize the need to contact the prescribing physician if these symptoms occur.

MANAGEMENT OF COMORBID DISORDERS

It is crucial to treat accompanying comorbid disorders, because they may worsen the prognosis of BP (23,169,170). However, most of the existing literature regarding the treatment of comorbid disorders in BP youth is anecdotal or from open-label studies. For ADHD, few RCTs with small samples have suggested that adding stimulants is beneficial and safe (171,172).

In general, it is recommended to use the best available medications and/or psychosocial treatments for each specific comorbid disorder (see respective chapters in this book). It is important to begin treatment for each comorbid disorder sequentially. Also, since some medications may cause mood dysregulation, if appropriate, psychosocial treatments should be tried before adding new medications (e.g., CBT for anxiety disorders). For BP youth with certain comorbid psychiatric or medical conditions, sometimes the use of medications for BP may also target the other disorder (valproate for BP and seizures).

For youth with dubious diagnosis of BP, it is better to treat first the other disorder and reevaluate for the presence of mood symptoms. In particular, this is relevant to ADHD because of the stimulants' rapid action. However, for youth with clear BP, before treating the comorbid disorder(s), it is recommended first to stabilize the symptoms of BP. Likewise, if the child's "comorbid" symptoms (hyperactivity, behavior problems) appear to be secondary to the mood disorder (mania, depression, or both), it is also recommended first to treat the BP. If the symptoms of BP improve and the other symptoms persist, treatment for both the BP and the comorbid conditions is indicated.

SUMMARY AND FUTURE DIRECTIONS

BP is a recurrent familial disorder that frequently emerges early in life and is associated with significant morbidity and sometimes mortality due to suicide. Pediatric BP usually follows an ongoing changeable and sinuous course, with patients having a wide spectrum of mood symptoms that can range from mild to severe depression, mania, and/or hypomania. These results explain, at least in part, the difficulties encountered when treating youth with BP spectrum disorders. Furthermore, it is likely that the very rapid fluctuation in mood symptoms, combined with the developmental issues influencing the clinical picture of BP youth, the difficulties children and adolescents have verbalizing their emotions, and the high rates of comorbid disorders, account for the complexity and current controversies in diagnosing BP youth.

As reviewed in this chapter, it is clear that youth may manifest classical symptoms of BP. However, many youth do not fulfill the current DSM BP-I or II criteria for the diagnoses mainly because they lack the required duration of symptoms. Moreover, many youth referred for evaluation for BP have severe mood lability, "affective storms," irritability, verbal and/or physical aggression, and ODD- and ADHD-like symptoms. These youth may have BP, but careful longitudinal follow-up is mandatory to ascertain whether these symptoms are indeed manifestations of BP, prodromal symptoms for more classical manifestations of BP, the symptoms of non-BP disorders (e.g., MDD, DBD, anxiety), reactions to ongoing environmental factors (e.g., bullying, abuse, family conflicts), or indicate that these youth have other difficulties regulating their mood.

The enduring and rapid changeability of symptoms of BP in youth from very early in life and at crucial life stages deprive them of the opportunity for normal, emotional, cognitive, and social development. Moreover, this illness can negatively affect relationships with parents and siblings, and family finances. Thus, early recognition and acute and maintenance treatment of BP in children and adolescents are of utmost importance to ameliorate ongoing syndromal and subsyndromal symptomatology and to reduce or prevent the serious psychosocial morbidity that can accompany this illness.

The existent pharmacologic studies suggest that the atypical antipsychotics followed by the mood stabilizers, and their combination are helpful for the acute treatment of manic/mixed symptoms. However, studies of longer duration are warranted. Also, further pharmacologic and psychosocial acute and maintenance RCTs to reduce the risk of relapse and recurrences as well as examine the effects of development, comorbid disorders, family environment, and parental psychopathology on treatment response, and the long-term side effects of pharmacologic treatments in youth are urgently needed.

Future studies evaluating possible preventative strategies for youth at high risk for BP, especially offspring at very high risk to develop BP are indicated. Also, studies to evaluate and analyze the contributions of risk and protective factors (e.g., cognitive development, social and coping skills, environmental factors to outcome are warranted. Regarding the environmental factors, important issues such as parental lifetime and current psychopathology, support, exposure to negative events (abuse, poor school or neighborhoods, and ongoing family conflicts) should be considered.

Finally, genetic and other biologic studies including pharmacogenetic and further studies correlating the effects of treatment and biochemical changes on the brain are warranted.

ACKNOWLEDGMENTS

This work was supported in part by NIMH grants MH59929, MH60952, and MH100056. The authors would like to thank Rita Scholle for her assistance with manuscript preparation and Andrès Martin for carefully reviewing the manuscript.

References

1. Kraepelin E: *Manic Depressive Insanity and Paranoia.* London, E & S Livingstone, 1921.
2. Khazanov GK, Cui L, Merikangas KR, Angst J: Treatment patterns of youth with bipolar disorder: results from the National Comorbidity Survey-Adolescent Supplement (NCS-A). *J Abnorm Child Psychol* 43(2):391–400, 2015.
3. Egeland JA, Shaw JA, Endicott J, et al.: Prospective study of prodromal features for bipolarity in well Amish children. *J Am Acad Child Adolesc Psychiatry* 42:786–796, 2003.
4. American Psychiatric Association. *Diagnostic and Statistical Manual of Mental Disorders.* 4th ed. Washington, DC, American Psychiatric Association, 1994.
5. American Psychiatric Association. *Diagnostic and Statistical Manual of Mental Disorders.* 5th ed. Washington, DC, American Psychiatric Association, 2013.
6. Axelson D, Birmaher B, Strober M, et al.: Phenomenology of children and adolescents with bipolar spectrum disorders. *Arch Gen Psychiatry* 63:1139–1148, 2006.
7. Van Meter AR, Burke C, Kowatch RA, Findling RL, Youngstrom EA: Ten-year update meta-analysis of the clinical characteristics of pediatric mania and hypomania. *Bipolar Disord* 18(1):19–32, 2016.
8. Geller B, Zimerman B, Williams M, Delbello MP, Frazier J, Beringer L: Phenomenology of prepubertal and early adolescent bipolar disorder: examples of elated mood, grandiose behaviors, decreased need for sleep, racing thoughts and hypersexuality. *J Child Adolesc Psychopharmacol* 12:3–9, 2002.
9. Birmaher B: Pediatric bipolar disorder: epidemiology, pathogenesis, clinical manifestations and course. *UpToDate,* 2016.
10. Geller B, Zimerman B, Williams M, et al.: DSM-IV mania symptoms in a prepubertal and early adolescent bipolar disorder phenotype compared

to attention-deficit hyperactive and normal controls. *J Child Adolesc Psychopharmacol* 12:11–25, 2002.
11. Leibenluft E, Charney DS, Towbin KE, Bhangoo RK, Pine DS: Defining clinical phenotypes of juvenile mania. *Am J Psychiatry* 160:430–437, 2003.
12. Leibenluft E, Blair RJ, Charney DS, Pine DS: Irritability in pediatric mania and other childhood psychopathology. *Ann N Y Acad Sci* 1008:201–218, 2003.
13. Biederman J, Faraone SV, Wozniak J, Mick E, Kwon A, Aleardi M: Further evidence of unique developmental phenotypic correlates of pediatric bipolar disorder: findings from a large sample of clinically referred preadolescent children assessed over the last 7 years. *J Affect Disord* 82S:S45–S58, 2004.
14. Mick E, Spencer T, Wozniak J, Biederman J: Heterogeneity of irritability in attention-deficit hyperactivity disorder subjects with and without mood disorders. *Biol Psychiatry* 58:576–582, 2005.
15. Wozniak J, Biederman J, Kiely K, et al.: Mania-like symptoms suggestive of childhood-onset bipolar disorder in clinically referred children. *J Am Acad Child Adolesc Psychiatry* 34:867–876, 1995.
16. Hunt J, Birmaher B, Leonard H, et al.: Irritability without elation in a large bipolar youth sample: frequency and clinical description. *J Am Acad Child Adolesc Psychiatry* 48(7):730–739, 2009.
17. Hunt J, Case B, Birmaher B, et al.: Irritability and elation in a large bipolar youth sample: relative symptom severity and clinical outcomes over four years. *J Clin Psychiatry* 74(1):110–117, 2013.
18. Axelson D, Findling RL, Fristad MA, et al.: Examining the proposed disruptive mood dysregulation disorder diagnosis in children in the longitudinal assessment of manic symptoms study. *J Clin Psychiatry* 73(10):1342–1350, 2012.
19. Althoff RR, Crehan ET, He JP, Burstein M, Hudziak JJ, Merikangas KR: Disruptive mood dysregulation disorder at ages 13–18: results from the national comorbidity survey-adolescent supplement. *J Child Adolesc Psychopharmacol* 26(2):107–113, 2016.
20. Birmaher B: The risks of persistent irritability. *J Am Acad Child Adolesc Psychiatry* 55(7):538–539, 2016.
21. Biederman J, Faraone SV, Chu MP, Wozniak J: Further evidence of a bidirectional overlap between juvenile mania and conduct disorder in children. *J Am Acad Child Adolesc Psychiatry* 38:468–476, 1999.
22. Geller B, Tillman R, Craney JL, Bolhofner K: Four-year prospective outcome and natural history of mania in children with a prepubertal and early adolescent bipolar disorder phenotype. *Arch Gen Psychiatry* 61:459–467, 2004.
23. Birmaher B, Axelson D, Goldstein B, et al.: Four-year longitudinal course of children and adolescents with bipolar spectrum disorders: the Course and Outcome of Bipolar Youth (COBY) study. *Am J Psychiatry* 166(7):798–804, 2009.
24. Findling RL, Gracious BL, McNamara NK, et al.: Rapid, continuous cycling and psychiatric co-morbidity in pediatric bipolar I disorder. *Bipolar Disord* 3:202–210, 2001.
25. Chengappa KN, Kupfer DJ, Frank E, et al.: Relationship of birth cohort and early age at onset of illness in a bipolar disorder case registry. *Am J Psychiatry* 160:1636–1642, 2003.
26. Perlis RH, Dennehy EB, Miklowitz DJ, et al.: Retrospective age at onset of bipolar disorder and outcome during two-year follow-up: results from the STEP-BD study. *Bipolar Disord* 11(4):391–400, 2009.
27. Geller B, Williams M, Zimerman B, Frazier J, Beringer L, Warner KL: Prepubertal and early adolescent bipolarity differentiate from ADHD by manic symptoms: grandiose delusions; ultra-rapid or ultradian cycling. *J Affect Disord* 51:81–91, 1998.
28. Axelson DA, Birmaher B, Strober MA, et al.: Course of subthreshold bipolar disorder in youth: diagnostic progression from bipolar disorder not otherwise specified. *J Am Acad Child Adolesc Psychiatry* 50(10):1001–1016, 2011.
29. Hirneth SJ, Hazell PL, Hanstock TL, Lewin TJ: Bipolar disorder subtypes in children and adolescents: demographic and clinical characteristics from an Australian sample. *J Affect Disord* 175:98–107, 2015.
30. Goldstein T, Ha W, Axelson DA, et al.: Predictors of prospectively examined suicide attempts among youth with bipolar disorder. *Arch Gen Psychiatry* 69(11):1113–1122, 2012.
31. Goldstein TR, Birmaher B, Axelson D, et al.: Psychosocial functioning among bipolar youth. *J Affect Disord* 114(1–3):174–183, 2009.
32. Goldstein BI, Strober M, Axelson D, et al.: Predictors of first-onset substance use disorders during the prospective course of bipolar spectrum disorders in adolescents. *J Am Acad Child Adolesc Psychiatry* 52(10):1026–1037, 2013.
33. Van Meter A, Youngstrom E, Demeter C, Findling RL: Examining the validity of cyclothymic disorder in a youth sample: replication and extension. *J Abnorm Child Psychol* 41(3):367–378, 2013.
34. Stringaris A, Youngstrom E: Unpacking the differences in US/UK rates of clinical diagnoses of early-onset bipolar disorder. *J Am Acad Child Adolesc Psychiatry* 53(6):609–611, 2014.
35. Merikangas KR, Cui L, Kattan G, Carlson GA, Youngstrom EA, Angst J: Mania with and without depression in a community sample of US adolescents. *Arch Gen Psychiatry* 69(9):943–951, 2012.
36. Van Meter AR, Moreira AL, Youngstrom EA: Meta-analysis of epidemiologic studies of pediatric bipolar disorder. *J Clin Psychiatry* 72(9):1250–1256, 2011.
37. Wilens TE, Biederman J, Millstein RB, Wozniak J, Hahesy AL, Spencer TJ: Risk for substance use disorders in youths with child- and adolescent-onset bipolar disorder. *J Am Acad Child Adolesc Psychiatry* 38:680–685, 1999.
38. Birmaher B: Bipolar disorder in children and adolescents: assessment and diagnosis. *UpToDate,* 2016.
39. Pavuluri MN, Birmaher B, Naylor M: Pediatric bipolar disorder: ten year review. *J Am Acad Child Adolesc Psychiatry* 44:846–871, 2005.
40. Geller B, Zimerman B, Williams M, Bolhofner K, Craney JL: Bipolar disorder at prospective follow-up of adults who had prepubertal major depressive disorder. *Am J Psychiatry* 158:125–127, 2001.
41. Kovacs M: Presentation and course of major depressive disorder during childhood and later years of the life span. *J Am Acad Child Adolesc Psychiatry* 35:705–715, 1996.
42. Strober M, Carlson G: Bipolar illness in adolescents with major depression. *Arch Gen Psychiatry* 39:549–555, 1982.
43. Weissman MM, Wolk S, Goldstein RB, et al.: Depressed adolescents grown up. *JAMA* 281:1707–1713, 1999.
44. Uchida M, Serra G, Zayas L, Kenworthy T, Faraone SV, Biederman J: Can unipolar and bipolar pediatric major depression be differentiated from each other? A systematic review of cross-sectional studies examining differences in unipolar and bipolar depression. *J Affect Disord* 176:1–7, 2015.
45. Towbin K, Axelson D, Leibenluft E, Birmaher B: Differentiating bipolar disorder-not otherwise specified and severe mood dysregulation. *J Am Acad Child Adolesc Psychiatry* 52(5):466–481, 2013.
46. Martin A, Young C, Leckman JF, Mukonoweshuro C, Rosenheck R, Leslie D: Age effects on antidepressant-induced manic conversion. *Arch Pediatr Adolesc Med* 158:773–780, 2004.
47. Wilens TE, Wyatt D, Spencer TJ: Disentangling disinhibition. *J Am Acad Child Adolesc Psychiatry* 37:1225–1227, 1998.
48. Birmaher B, Gill MK, Axelson D, et al.: Longitudinal trajectories and associated baseline predictors in youth with bipolar spectrum disorders. *Am J Psychiatry* 171(9):990–999, 2014.
49. DelBello MP, Hanseman D, Adler CM, Fleck DE, Strakowski SM: Twelve-month outcome of adolescents with bipolar disorder following first hospitalization for a manic or mixed episode. *Am J Psychiatry* 164:582–590, 2007.
50. Lewinsohn PM, Klein DN, Seeley JR: Bipolar disorder during adolescence and young adulthood in a community sample. *Bipolar Disord* 2:281–293, 2000.
51. Lewinsohn P, Klein D, Seeley J: Bipolar disorders in a community sample of older adolescents: prevalence, phenomenology, comorbidity, and course. *J Am Acad Child Adolesc Psychiatry* 34:454–463, 1995.
52. Holtzman JN, Miller S, Hooshmand F, et al.: Childhood-compared to adolescent-onset bipolar disorder has more statistically significant clinical correlates. *J Affect Disord* 179:114–120, 2015.
53. Althoff RR, Faraone SV, Rettew DC, Morley CP, Hudziak JJ: Family, twin, adoption, and molecular genetic studies of juvenile bipolar disorder. *Bipolar Disord* 7:598–609, 2005.
54. Goodwin F, Jamison K: *Manic Depressive Illness.* New York, Oxford University Press, 1990.
55. Neuman RJ, Geller B, Rice JP, Todd RD: Increased prevalence and earlier onset of mood disorders among relatives of prepubertal versus adult probands. *J Am Acad Child Adolesc Psychiatry* 36:466–473, 1997.
56. Tsuang MT, Faraone SV: *The Genetics of Mood Disorders.* Baltimore, Johns Hopkins University Press, 1990.
57. Birmaher B, Axelson D, Monk K, et al.: Lifetime psychiatric disorders in school-aged offspring of parents with bipolar disorder: the Pittsburgh Bipolar Offspring study. *Arch Gen Psychiatry* 66(3):287–296,2009.
58. Axelson D, Goldstein B, Goldstein T, et al.: Diagnostic precursors to bipolar disorder in offspring of parents with bipolar disorder: a longitudinal study. *Am J Psychiatry* 172(7):638–646, 2015.
59. Wozniak J, Faraone SV, Martelon M, McKillop HN, Biederman J: Further evidence for robust familiality of pediatric bipolar I disorder: results from a very large controlled family study of pediatric bipolar I disorder and a meta-analysis. *J Clin Psychiatry* 73(10):1328–1334, 2012.
60. Strober M, Morrell W, Burroughs J, Lampert C, Danforth H, Freeman R: A family study of bipolar I disorder in adolescence. Early onset of symptoms linked to increased familial loading and lithium resistance. *J Affect Disord* 15:255–268, 1988.
61. Hafeman DM, Merranko J, Axelson D, et al.: Toward the definition of a bipolar prodrome: dimensional predictors of bipolar spectrum disorders in at-risk youths. *Am J Psychiatry* 173(7):695–704, 2016.
62. McGuffin P, Rijsdijk F, Andrew M, Sham P, Katz R, Cardno A: The heritability of bipolar affective disorder and the genetic relationship to unipolar depression. *Arch Gen Psychiatry* 60:497–502, 2003.
63. Segurado R, Detera-Wadleigh SD, Levinson DF, et al.: Genome scan metaanalysis of schizophrenia and bipolar disorder. Part III: bipolar disorder. *Am J Hum Genet* 73:49–62, 2003.
64. Stovall J: Bipolar disorder in adults: epidemiology and pathogenesis. *UpToDate,* 2016.
65. Agarwal N, Renshaw PF, Proton MR: Spectroscopy-detectable major neurotransmitters of the brain: biology and possible clinical applications. *Am J Neuroradiol* 33:595–602, 2012.
66. Cecil KM, DelBello MP, Sellars MC, Strakowski SM: Proton magnetic resonance spectroscopy of the frontal lobe and cerebellar vermis in

children with a mood disorder and a familial risk for bipolar disorders. *J Child Adolesc Psychopharmacol* 13:545–555, 2003.
67. Davanzo P, Yue K, Thomas MA, et al.: Proton magnetic resonance spectroscopy of bipolar disorder versus intermittent explosive disorder in children and adolescents. *Am J Psychiatry* 160:1442–1452, 2003.
68. Sassi RB, Stanley JA, Axelson D, et al.: Reduced NAA levels in the dorsolateral prefrontal cortex of young bipolar patients. *Am J Psychiatry* 162:2109–2115, 2005.
69. Chang K, Adleman N, Dienes K, Barnea-Goraly N, Reiss A, Ketter T: Decreased N-acetylaspartate in children with familial bipolar disorder. *Biol Psychiatry* 53:1059–1065, 2003.
70. Strawn JR, Patel NC, Chu WJ, et al.: Glutamatergic effects of divalproex in adolescents with mania: a proton magnetic resonance spectroscopy study. *J Am Acad Child Adolesc Psychiatry* 51:642–651, 2012.
71. Kondo DG, Hellem TL, Shi XF, et al.: A review of MR spectroscopy studies of pediatric bipolar disorder. *AJNR Am J Neuroradiol* 35(6 Suppl): S64–S80, 2014.
72. Wegbreit E, Cushman GK, Puzia ME, et al.: Developmental meta-analyses of the functional neural correlates of bipolar disorder. *JAMA Psychiatry* 71:926, 2014.
73. Phillips ML, Swartz HA: A critical appraisal of neuroimaging studies of bipolar disorder: toward a new conceptualization of underlying neural circuitry and a road map for future research. *Am J Psychiatry* 171(8):829–843, 2014.
74. Pfeifer JC, Welge J, Strakowski SM, Adler CM, DelBello MP: Meta-analysis of amygdala volumes in children and adolescents with bipolar disorder. *J Am Acad Child Adolesc Psychiatry* 47(11):1289–1298, 2008.
75. Pavuluri MN: Neuroscience-based formulation and treatment for early-onset bipolar disorder: a paradigm shift. *Current Treatment Options in Psychiatry* 2(3):229–251, 2015.
76. Kalmar JH, Wang F, Chepenik LG, et al.: Relation between amygdala structure and function in adolescents with bipolar disorder. *J Am Acad Child Adolesc Psychiatry* 48(6):636–642, 2009.
77. Bitter SM, Mills NP, Adler CM, Strakowski SM, DelBello MP: Progression of amygdala volumetric abnormalities in adolescents after their first manic episode. *J Am Acad Child Adolesc Psychiatry* 50(10):1017–1026, 2011.
78. Lu LH, Zhou XJ, Fitzgerald J, et al.: Microstructural abnormalities of white matter differentiate pediatric and adult-onset bipolar disorder. *Bipolar Disord* 14(6):597–606, 2012.
79. Dickstein DP, Gorrostieta C, Ombao H, et al.: Fronto-temporal spontaneous resting state functional connectivity in pediatric bipolar disorder. *Biol Psychiatry* 68(9):839–846, 2010.
80. Wu M, Lu LH, Passarotti AM, Wegbreit E, Fitzgerald J, Pavuluri MN: Altered affective, executive and sensorimotor resting state networks in patients with pediatric mania. *J Psychiatry Neurosci* 38(4):232–240, 2013.
81. Hafeman DM, Bebko G, Bertocci MA, et al.: Abnormal deactivation of the inferior frontal gyrus during implicit emotion processing in youth with bipolar disorder: attenuated by medication. *J Psychiatr Res* 58:129–139, 2014.
82. Passarotti AM, Pavuluri MN: Brain functional domains inform therapeutic interventions in attention-deficit/hyperactivity disorder and pediatric bipolar disorder. *Expert Rev Neurother* 11(6):897–914, 2011.
83. Dickstein DP, Nelson EE, McClure EB, et al.: Cognitive flexibility in phenotypes of pediatric bipolar disorder. *J Am Acad Child Adolesc Psychiatry* 46(3):341–355, 2007.
84. Dickstein DP, Brazel AC, Goldberg LD, Hunt JI: Affect regulation in pediatric bipolar disorder. *Child Adolesc Psychiatr Clin N Am* 18(2): 405–420, 2009.
85. Dickstein DP, Axelson D, Weissman AB, et al.: Cognitive flexibility and performance in children and adolescents with threshold and sub-threshold bipolar disorder. *Eur Child Adolesc Psychiatry* 25(6):625–638, 2015.
86. Pavuluri MN, Passarotti AM, Harral EM, Sweeney JA: An fMRI study of the neural correlates of incidental versus directed emotion processing in pediatric bipolar disorder. *J Am Acad Child Adolesc Psychiatry* 48(3):308–319, 2009.
87. Malhi GS, Ivanovski B, Hadzi-Pavlovic D, Mitchell PB, Vieta E, Sachdev P: Neuropsychological deficits and functional impairment in bipolar depression, hypomania and euthymia. *Bipolar Disord* 9(1–2):114–125, 2007.
88. Lee J, Altshuler L, Glahn DC, Miklowitz DJ, Ochsner K, Green MF: Social and nonsocial cognition in bipolar disorder and schizophrenia: relative levels of impairment. *Am J Psychiatry* 170(3):334–341, 2013.
89. Berk M, Kapczinski F, Andreazza AC, et al.: Pathways underlying neuroprogression in bipolar disorder: focus on inflammation, oxidative stress and neurotrophic factors. *Neurosci Biobehav Rev* 35(3):804–817, 2011.
90. Torrent C, Martinez-Arán A, del Mar Bonnin C, et al.: Long-term outcome of cognitive impairment in bipolar disorder. *J Clin Psychiatry* 73(7):e899–e905, 2012.
91. Depp CA, Savla GN, Moore DJ, et al.: Short-term course of neuropsychological abilities in middle-aged and older adults with bipolar disorder. *Bipolar Disord* 10(6):684–690, 2008.
92. Gualtieri CT, Morgan DW: The frequency of cognitive impairment in patients with anxiety, depression, and bipolar disorder: an unaccounted source of variance in clinical trials. *J Clin Psychiatry* 69(7):1122–1130, 2008.
93. Gerber AJ, Posner J, Gorman D, et al.: An affective circumplex model of neural systems subserving valence, arousal, and cognitive overlay during the appraisal of emotional faces. *Neuropsychologia* 46(8):2129–2139, 2008.
94. Miklowitz DJ, Goldstein MJ, Nuechterlein KH, Snyder KS, Mintz J: Family factors and the course of bipolar affective disorder. *Arch Gen Psychiatry* 45:225–231, 1988.
95. Hlastala SA, Frank E, Kowalski J, et al.: Stressful life events, bipolar disorder, and the "kindling model". *J Abnorm Psychol* 109:777–786, 2000.
96. King RA, The Work Group on Quality Issues: Practice parameter for the psychiatric assessment of children and adolescents. American Academy of Child and Adolescent Psychiatry. *J Am Acad Child Adolesc Psychiatry* 36(10 Suppl):4S–20S, 1997.
97. Kaufman J, Birmaher B, Brent D, et al.: Schedule for affective disorders and schizophrenia for school-age children—present and lifetime version (K-SADS-PL): initial reliability and validity data. *J Am Acad Child Adolesc Psychiatry* 36:980–988, 1997.
98. Geller B, Warner K, Williams M, Zimerman B: Prepubertal and young adolescent bipolarity versus ADHD: assessment and validity using the WASH-U-KSADS, CBCL, and TRF. *J Affect Disord* 51:93–100, 1998.
99. Fristad MA, Weller EB, Weller RA: The Mania Rating Scale: can it be used in children? A preliminary report. *J Am Acad Child Adolesc Psychiatry* 31:252–257, 1992.
100. Axelson D, Birmaher B, Brent D, et al.: A preliminary study of the kiddie schedule for affective disorders and schizophrenia for school-age children mania rating scale for children and adolescents. *J Child Adolesc Psychopharmacol* 13:463–470, 2004.
101. Youngstrom EA, Egerton GA, Van Meter AR. Multivariate meta-analysis of the discriminative validity of caregiver, youth and teacher rating scales for pediatric bipolar disorder: mother knows best about mania. *Arch Scien Psychology* 3:112–137, 2015.
102. Findling R, Youngstrom E, Danielson C, et al.: Clinical decision-making using the general behavior inventory in juvenile bipolarity. *Bipolar Disord* 4:34–42, 2002.
103. Pavuluri MN, Henry D, Devineni B, Carbray JA, Birmaher B: Child Mania Rating Scale: development, reliability and validity. *J Am Acad Child Adolesc Psychiatry* 45:550–560, 2006.
104. Wagner KD, Hirschfeld RM, Emslie GJ, Findling RL, Gracious BL, Reed ML: Validation of the mood disorders questionnaire for bipolar disorders in adolescents. *J Clin Psychiatry* 67:827–830, 2006.
105. Biederman J, Wozniak J, Kiely K, et al.: CBCL clinical scales discriminate prepubertal children with structured interview-derived diagnosis of mania from those with ADHD. *J Am Acad Child Adolesc Psychiatry* 34:464–471, 1995.
106. Dienes K, Chang K, Blasey C, Adleman NE, Steiner H: Characterization of children of bipolar parents by parent report CBCL. *J Psychiatr Res* 36:337–345, 2002.
107. Hazell PL, Lewin TJ, Carr VJ: Confirmation that child behavior checklist clinical scales discriminate juvenile mania from attention deficit hyperactivity disorder. *J Paediatr Child Health* 35:199–203, 1999.
108. Diler RS, Birmaher B, Axelson D, et al.: The Child Behavior Checklist (CBCL) and the CBCL-bipolar phenotype are not useful in diagnosing pediatric bipolar disorder. *J Child Adolesc Psychopharmacol* 19(1):23–30, 2009.
109. Brent DA, Poling K, McKain B, Baugher M: A psychoeducational program for families of affectively ill children and adolescents. *J Am Acad Child Adolesc Psychiatry* 32:770–774, 1993.
110. Fristad MA, Gavazzi SM, Mackinaw-Koons B: Family psychoeducation: an adjunctive intervention for children with bipolar disorder. *Biol Psychiatry* 53:1000–1008, 2003.
111. Fristad MA, Goldberg-Arnold JS, Gavazzi SM: Multi-family psychoeducation groups in the treatment of children with mood disorders. *Marital Fam Ther* 29:491–504, 2003.
112. Birmaher B: *New Hope for the Treatment of Children and Teens with Bipolar Disorder.* New York, Three Rivers Press, 2004.
113. Fristad MA, Goldberg JS: *Raising a Moody Child: How to Cope with Depression and Bipolar Disorder.* New York, Guilford, 2003.
114. Colom F, Vieta E: A perspective on the use of psychoeducation, cognitive-behavioral therapy and interpersonal therapy for bipolar patients. *Bipolar Disord* 6:480–486, 2004.
115. Miklowitz DJ, George EL, Axelson DA, et al.: Family-focused treatment for adolescents with bipolar disorder. *J Affect Disord* 82:113–128, 2004.
116. Stovall J: Bipolar disorder in adults: pharmacotherapy for acute mania and hypomania. *UpToDate*, 2016.
117. Stovall J: Bipolar disorder in adults: pharmacotherapy for acute depression. *UpToDate*, 2016.
118. Post RM: Bipolar disorder in adults: choosing maintenance treatment. *UpToDate*, 2016.
119. Janicak P: Bipolar disorder in adults and lithium: pharmacology, administration, and side effects. *UpToDate*, 2015.
120. Dutta S, Zhang Y, Conway JM, et al.: Divalproex-ER pharmacokinetics in older children and adolescents. *Pediatr Neurol* 30:330–337, 2004.
121. Moore CM, Demopulos CM, Henry ME, et al.: Brain-to-serum lithium ratio and age: an in vivo magnetic resonance spectroscopy study. *Am J Psychiatry* 159:1240–1242, 2002.
122. Meduri M, Gregoraci G, Baglivo V, Balestrieri M, Isola M, Brambilla P: A meta-analysis of efficacy and safety of aripiprazole in adults and pediatric bipolar disorder in randomized controlled trials and observational studies. *J Affect Disord* 191:187–208, 2016.

123. Fraguas D, Correll CU, Merchán-Naranjo J, et al.: Efficacy and safety of second-generation antipsychotics in children and adolescents with psychotic and bipolar spectrum disorders: comprehensive review of prospective head-to-head and placebo-controlled comparisons. *Eur Neuropsychopharmacol* 21(8):621–645, 2011.
124. Findling RL, Landbloom RL, Szegedi A, et al.: Asenapine for the acute treatment of pediatric manic or mixed episode of bipolar I disorder. *J Am Acad Child Adolesc Psychiatry* 54(12):1032–1041, 2015.
125. Correll CU, Sheridan EM, DelBello MP: Antipsychotic and mood stabilizer efficacy and tolerability in pediatric and adult patients with bipolar I mania: a comparative analysis of acute, randomized, placebo-controlled trials. *Bipolar Disord* 12(2):116–141, 2010.
126. Findling RL, Robb A, McNamara NK, et al.: Lithium in the acute treatment of bipolar I disorder: a double-blind, placebo-controlled study. *Pediatrics* 136(5):885–894, 2015.
127. Kowatch RA, Suppes T, Carmody TJ, et al.: Effect size of lithium, divalproex sodium, and carbamazepine in children and adolescents with bipolar disorder. *J Am Acad Child Adolesc Psychiatry* 39:713–720, 2000.
128. Vitiello B, Riddle MA, Yenokyan G, et al.: Treatment moderators and predictors of outcome in the treatment of early age mania (TEAM) study. *J Am Acad Child Adolesc Psychiatry* 51(9):867–878, 2012.
129. Kowatch RA, Scheffer RE, Monroe E, Delgado S, Altaye M, Lagory D: Placebo-controlled trial of valproic acid versus risperidone in children 3–7 years of age with bipolar I disorder. *J Child Adolesc Psychopharmacol* 25(4):306–313, 2015.
130. Geller B, Luby JL, Joshi P, et al.: A randomized controlled trial of risperidone, lithium, or divalproex sodium for initial treatment of bipolar I disorder, manic or mixed phase, in children and adolescents. *Arch Gen Psychiatry* 69(5):515–528, 2012.
131. Walkup JT, Wagner KD, Miller L, et al.: Treatment of early-age mania: outcomes for partial and nonresponders to initial treatment. *J Am Acad Child Adolesc Psychiatry* 54(12):1008–1019, 2015.
132. DelBello MP, Schwiers ML, Rosenberg HL, Strakowski SM: A double-blind, randomized, placebo-controlled study of quetiapine as adjunctive treatment for adolescent mania. *J Am Acad Child Adolesc Psychiatry* 41:1216–1223, 2002.
133. Findling RL, McNamara NK, Gracious BL, et al.: Combination lithium and divalproex sodium in pediatric bipolarity. *J Am Acad Child Adolesc Psychiatry* 42:895–901, 2003.
134. Findling RL, McNamara NK, Youngstrom EA, et al.: Double-blind 18-month trial of lithium versus divalproex maintenance treatment in pediatric bipolar disorder. *J Am Acad Child Adolesc Psychiatry* 44:409–417, 2005.
135. Kafantaris V, Coletti DJ, Dicker R, Padula G, Kane JM: Adjunctive antipsychotic treatment of adolescents with bipolar psychosis. *J Am Acad Child Adolesc Psychiatry* 40:1448–1456, 2001.
136. Pavuluri MN, Henry D, Carbray JA, Sampson G, Naylor MW, Janicak PG: One-label prospective trial of risperidone in combination with lithium or divalproex sodium in pediatric mania. *J Affect Disord* 82(Suppl 1): 103–111, 2004.
137. Findling RL, Ginsberg LD: The safety and effectiveness of open-label extended release carbamazepine in the treatment of children and adolescents with bipolar I disorder suffering from a manic or mixed episode. *Neuropsychiatr Dis Treat* 10:1589–1597, 2014.
138. Wagner KD, Kowatch RA, Emslie GJ, et al.: A double-blind, randomized, placebo-controlled trial of oxcarbazepine in the treatment of bipolar disorder in children and adolescents. *Am J Psychiatry* 163(7):1179–1186, 2006.
139. Ghaziuddin N, Kutcher SP, Knapp P, et al.: Work Group on Quality Issues: Practice parameter for the use of ECT with adolescents. *J Am Acad Child Adolesc Psychiatry* 43:1521–1539, 2004.
140. Gijsman HK, Geddes JR, Rendell JM, Nolen WA, Goodwin GM: Antidepressants for bipolar depression: a systematic review of randomized, controlled trials. *Am J Psychiatry* 161(9):1537–1547, 2004.
141. Findling RL, Pathak S, Earley WR, Liu S, DelBello MP: Efficacy and safety of extended-release quetiapine fumarate in youth with bipolar depression: an 8 week, double-blind, placebo-controlled trial. *J Child Adolesc Psychopharmacol* 24(6):325–335, 2014.
142. Salpekar JA, Joshi PT, Axelson DA, et al.: Depression and suicidality outcomes in the treatment of early age mania study. *J Am Acad Child Adolesc Psychiatry* 54(12):999–1007, 2015.
143. Swedo SE, Allen AJ, Glod CA, et al.: A controlled trial of light therapy for the treatment of pediatric seasonal affective disorder. *J Am Acad Child Adolesc Psychiatry* 36:816–821, 1997.
144. Wozniak J, Faraone SV, Chan J, et al.: A randomized clinical trial of high eicosapentaenoic acid omega-3 fatty acids and inositol as monotherapy and in combination in the treatment of pediatric bipolar spectrum disorders: a pilot study. *J Clin Psychiatry* 76(11):1548–1555, 2015.
145. Fristad MA, Young AS, Vesco AT, et al.: A randomized controlled trial of individual family psychoeducational psychotherapy and omega-3 fatty acids in youth with subsyndromal bipolar disorder. *J Child Adolesc Psychopharmacol* 25(10):764–774, 2015.
146. West AE, Weinstein SM, Peters AT, et al.: Child and family-focused cognitive-behavioral therapy for pediatric bipolar disorder: a randomized clinical trial. *J Am Acad Child Adolesc Psychiatry* 53:1168–1178, 2014.
147. Weinstein SM, Henry DB, Katz AC, Peters AT, West AE: Treatment moderators of child- and family-focused cognitive-behavioral therapy for pediatric bipolar disorder. *J Am Acad Child Adolesc Psychiatry* 54(2):116–125, 2015.
148. Miklowitz DJ, Schneck C, George EA, et al.: Pharmacotherapy and family-focused treatment for adolescents with bipolar I and II disorders: a 2-year randomized trial. *Am J Psychiatry* 171:658–667, 2014.
149. Miklowitz DJ, Axelson DA, Birmaher B, et al.: Family-focused treatment for adolescents with bipolar disorder: results of a two-year randomized trial. *Arch Gen Psychiatry* 65:1053–1061, 2008.
150. Goldstein TR, Axelson DA, Birmaher B, Brent DA: Dialectic behavior therapy for adolescents with bipolar disorder: a one-ear open trial. *J Am Acad Child Adolesc Psychiatry* 46(7):820–830, 2007.
151. Goldstein TR, Fersch-Podrat RK, Rivera M, et al.: Dialectical Behavior Therapy (DBT) for adolescents with bipolar disorder: results from a pilot randomized trial. *J Child Adolesc Psychopharmacol* 25(2):140–149, 2015.
152. Hlastala SA, Frank E: Adapting interpersonal and social rhythm therapy to the developmental needs of adolescents with bipolar disorder. *Dev Psychopathol* 18:1267–1288, 2006.
153. Hlastala S, Kotler J, McClellan J, McCauley EA: Interpersonal and social rhythm therapy for adolescents with bipolar disorder: treatment development and results from an open trial. *Depress Anxiety* 27:457–464, 2010.
154. Goldstein TR, Fersch RK, Axelson DA, et al.: Early intervention for adolescents at high risk for the development of bipolar disorder: pilot study of Interpersonal and Social Rhythm Therapy (IPSRT). *Psychotherapy* 51(1):180–189, 2014.
155. Miklowitz D, Chang K, Taylor D, et al.: Early psychosocial intervention for youth at risk for bipolar I or II disorder: a one-year treatment development trial. *Bipolar Disord* 13:67–75, 2011.
156. Miklowitz DJ, Schneck C, Singh M, et al.: Early intervention for symptomatic youth at risk for bipolar disorder: a randomized trial of family-focused therapy. *J Am Acad Child Adolesc Psychiatry* 52(2):121–131, 2013.
157. Strober M, Morrell W, Lampert C, Burroughs J: Relapse following discontinuation of lithium maintenance therapy in adolescents with bipolar I illness: a naturalistic study. *Am J Psychiatry* 147:457–461, 1990.
158. Findling RL, McNamara NK, Stansbrey R, et al.: Combination lithium and divalproex sodium in pediatric bipolar symptom restabilization. *J Am Acad Child Adolesc Psychiatry* 45:142–148, 2006.
159. Findling RL, Youngstrom EA, McNamara NK, et al.: Double-blind, randomized, placebo-controlled long-term maintenance study of aripiprazole in children with bipolar disorder. *J Clin Psychiatry* 73(1):57–63, 2012.
160. Gitlin M: Lithium and the kidney: an updated review. *Drug Safety* 20:231–243, 1999.
161. Goodwin GM. The safety of lithium. *JAMA* 72(12):1167–1169, 2015.
162. Kleiner J, Altshuler LL, Hendrik V, Hershman JM: Lithium-induced subclinical hypothyroidism: review of the literature and guidelines for treatment. *J Clin Psychiatry* 60:249–255, 1999.
163. Gracious BL, Findling RL, Seman C, Youngstrom EA, Demeter CA, Calabrese JR: Elevated thyrotropin in bipolar youths prescribed both lithium and divalproex sodium. *J Am Acad Child Adolesc Psychiatry* 43:215–220, 2004.
164. Cole DP, Thase ME, Mallinger AG, et al.: Slower treatment response in bipolar depression predicted by lower pretreatment thyroid function. *Am J Psychiatry* 159:116–121, 2002.
165. Frye MA, Denicoff KD, Bryan AL, et al.: Association between lower serum free T_4 and greater mood instability and depression in lithium-maintained bipolar patients. *Am J Psychiatry* 156:1909–1914, 1999.
166. Mitchell AJ, Delaffon V, Vancampfort D, Correll CU, De Hert M: Guideline concordant monitoring of metabolic risk in people treated with antipsychotic medication: systematic review and meta-analysis of screening practices. *Psychol Med* 42(1):125–147, 2012.
167. Nielsen RE, Laursen MF, Vernal DL, et al.: Risk of diabetes in children and adolescents exposed to antipsychotics: a nationwide 12-year case control study. *J Am Acad Child Adolesc Psychiatry* 53(9):971–979, 2014.
168. Bobo WV, Cooper WO, Stein CM, et al.: Antipsychotics and the risk of type 2 diabetes mellitus in children and youth. *JAMA Psychiatry* 70(10):1067–1075, 2013.
169. Sala R, Strober M, Axelson D, et al.: Effects of comorbid anxiety disorders on the longitudinal course of pediatric bipolar illness. *J Am Acad Child Adolesc Psychiatry* 53(1):72–81, 2014.
170. Yen S, Stout R, Hower H, et al.: The influence of comorbid disorders on the episodicity of bipolar disorder in youth. *Acta Psychiatr Scand* 133(4):324–334, 2016.
171. Scheffer RE, Kowatch RA, Carmody T, Rush AJ: Randomized, placebo-controlled trial of mixed amphetamine salts for symptoms of comorbid ADHD in pediatric bipolar disorder after mood stabilization with divalproex sodium. *Am J Psychiatry* 162:58–64, 2005.
172. Miller S, Chang KD, Ketter TA: Bipolar disorder and attention-deficit/hyperactivity disorder comorbidity in children and adolescents: evidence based approach to diagnosis and treatment. *J Clin Psychiatry* 74(6):628–629, 2013.

CHAPTER 5.4.3 ■ CHILD AND ADOLESCENT SUICIDAL BEHAVIOR

CYNTHIA R. PFEFFER

INTRODUCTION

Recent research with diverse methods expanded knowledge of child and adolescent suicide risk, treatment and prevention; but suicidal ideation and attempts among these populations continue to increase. DSM-5 described suicidal behavior and nonsuicidal self-injury as "Conditions for Further Study," indicating that "future research is encouraged" (p. 783) (1). The 2012 National Strategy for Suicide Prevention outlined comprehensive suicide prevention strategies (2). This chapter, based primarily on empirical investigations, presents an overview of suicidal behavior to assist clinicians and US public policy developers to prevent suicidal morbidities and fatalities among young populations.

EPIDEMIOLOGY

The 2014 US suicide data highlight suicide as a public health problem, particularly for adolescents, youth, and middle age adults (3). Suicide, 10th leading cause of US deaths, occurred among 42,773 people indicating a 13.0 per 100,000 population death rate, accounting for 1.6% of all deaths and a 24% higher rate than in 1999 (10.5 per 100,000). Unintentional deaths are the leading cause of death for ages 1 to 44 years. Suicide is the second leading cause of death for ages 10 to 24 years. Suicide occurred among 425 children, aged 10 to 14 years, accounting for a 2.1 per 100,000 death rate and 14.7% of all deaths in this age group. Suicide occurred among 5,079 adolescents and young adults, aged 15 to 24 years, accounting for a 11.6 per 100,000 death rate and 17.6% of all deaths in this age group. Homicide is the third leading cause of death for ages 1 to 4 and 15 to 24 years, fourth for ages 5 to 9 years, and fifth for ages 10 to 14 years.

Number of suicide deaths and percent of all deaths were higher for males, aged 10 to 14 years (males: 275, 15.5%; females 150, 13.4%) and 15 to 24 years (males: 4,089, 19.4%; females: 990, 12.9%). Female suicide rates for ages 10 to 14 years, compared to other ages, had the highest increase (200%), tripling from 0.5 in 1999 to 1.5 per 100,000 in 2014.

Suicide was the second leading cause of death among Whites and American Indians/Alaskan Natives, aged 10 to 14 accounting for 347 (16.8%) and 12 (2.8%) deaths, respectively, and for ages 15 to 24 years accounting for 4,177 (20.1%) and 129 (2.5%) deaths, respectively. It is the third leading cause of death among Hispanics aged 10 to 14 and 15 to 24 years, accounting for 66 (11.3%) and 719 (14.7%) deaths, respectively. Suicide among Blacks aged 15 to 24 years and 10 to 14 years is the third and the fourth leading cause of death, respectively, accounting for 544 (8.2%) and 56 (8.4%) suicides, respectively.

Use of firearms was the most common suicide method followed by suffocation for individuals older than 14 years. Suicide method rates for ages 15 to 24 years were firearms (44.7%), suffocation (39.6%), poisoning (7.1%), fall (3.3%), other classifiable (2.4%), and drowning, fire, transportation, unspecified (1.0%). Suicide method rates for ages 10 to 14 years were suffocation (52.9%), firearms (40.9%), poisoning (4.2%), and other classifiable and fall, transportation unspecified (1.0%).

Figure 5.4.3.1 shows annual US suicide rates per 100,000 population for both sexes and all races from 1999 through 2014 for specific age groups (3).

Suicide rates increased almost each year beginning at rate 13.9 in 1999 for ages 45 to 54 years, in 2005 at rate 13.7 for ages 55 to 64 years, and in 2005 at rate 11.0 for all ages. Suicide increased for younger ages almost yearly in 2007 at rate 9.6 for ages 15 to 24 years, in 2009 at rate 13.1 for ages 25 to 34 years, and in 2011 at rate 0.7 for ages 5 to 14 years. Notably, annual suicide rates for ages 45 to 54 years since 2007 surpassed those for all age groups and are attributed to White non-Hispanic men and women, lower educational level, declined mental and physical health, inability to work and conduct daily activities, chronic pain, and economic insecurity due to job and income loss, but not to a simple cohort effect (4). These suicide rates may have implications for increasing suicide among children, adolescents and young adults, who suffered adverse childhood experiences.

The National Youth Risk Behavior Survey (YRBS), completed during springtime every 2 years since 1991 by a US representative sample of 9th through 12th graders in public and private high schools, documented that during the 12 months before the 2015 survey 17.7% adolescents seriously considered attempting suicide, 14.6% developed a suicide attempt plan, 8.6% attempted suicide, and 2.8% attempted suicide resulting in injury, poisoning, or overdose that necessitated treatment (5). Figure 5.4.3.2 indicates YRBS suicidal ideation and attempt rates from 1991 through 2015. From 1991 through 2009, significant decreases occurred for suicidal ideation rates and significant increases occurred after 2009 through 2015; no significant suicide attempt rate changes occurred from 2009 through 2015.

YRBS documented firearm accessibility: 5.3% adolescents reported carrying a gun at least 1 day during the 30 days before the 2015 survey, accounting for a significant decrease since 1997 (7.9%) (4). Rates were higher for males (8.7%) than females (1.6%) and for White (9.6%), Black (9.6%), and Hispanic males (6.5%) than White (1.4%), Black (1.7%), and Hispanic females (1.9%).

CLINICAL DESCRIPTION

DSM-5 criteria provide "a common language for researchers and clinicians who are interested in studying these disorders" but "the proposed criteria are not intended for clinical use" (p. 783) (1). Suicidal behavior disorder criteria include "within the last 24 months, the individual has made a suicide attempt... set of actions would lead to his or her own death... does not meet criteria for nonsuicidal self-injury... not applied to suicidal ideation... not initiated during a state of

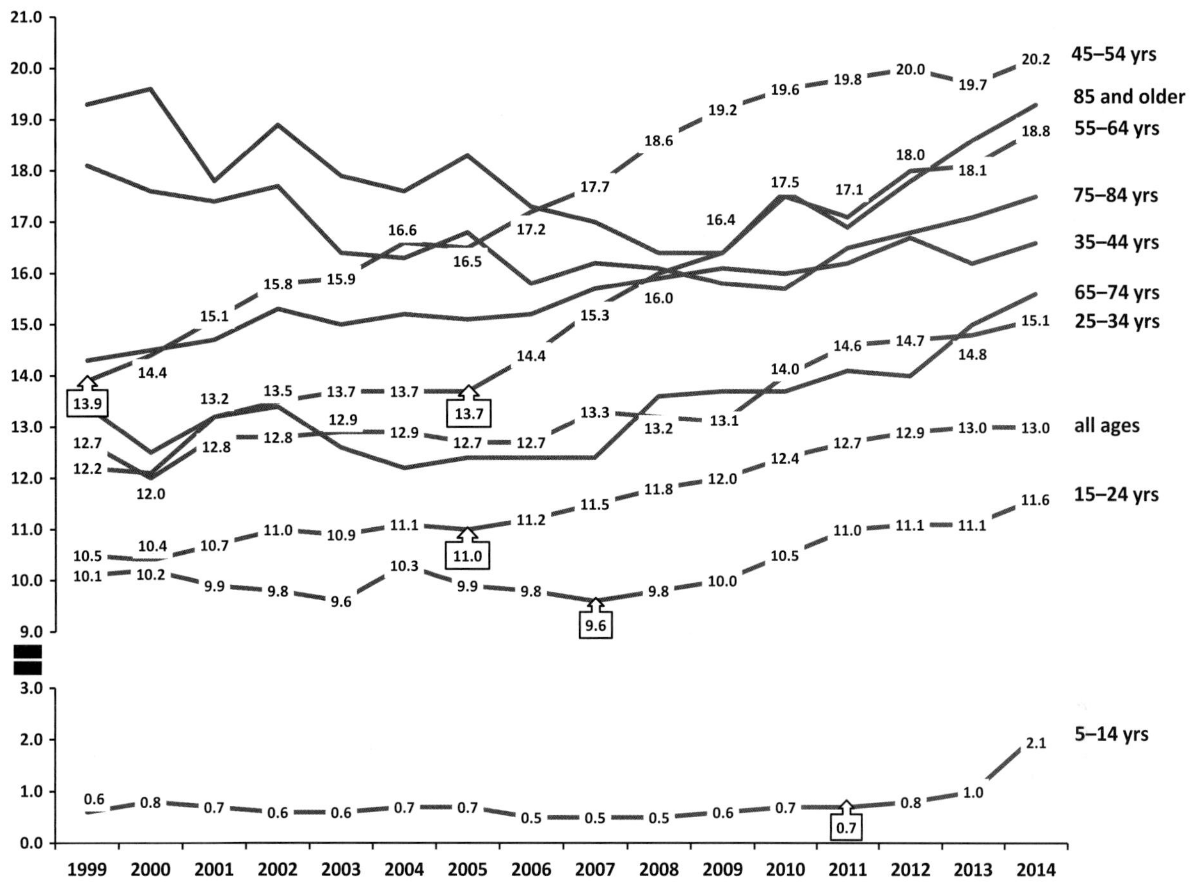

FIGURE 5.4.3.1. US suicide rates per 100,000 population from 1999 through 2014 for specific age groups.

delirium or confusion...not undertaken solely for a political or religious objective" (p. 801) (1). Nonsuicidal self-injury criteria include "in the last year, the individual has, on 5 or more days, engaged in intentional self-inflicted damage to the surface of his or her body of a sort likely to induce bleeding, bruising, or pain...expectation that the injury will lead to only minor or moderate physical harm...to obtain relief from a negative feeling or cognitive state, to resolve an interpersonal difficulty, to induce a positive feeling...preoccupation with the intended behavior that is difficult to control, thinking about self-injury that occurs frequently...behavior is not socially sanctioned...causes clinically significant distress...does not occur exclusively during psychotic episodes, delirium, substance intoxication or substance withdrawal...not part of a pattern of repetitive stereotypies, not better explained by another mental disorder or medical condition" (p. 803) (1).

Child and adolescent suicidal conditions comprise a continuum from self-harm ideas with intent to die, ideas to plan suicide, suicide attempt, and suicide (6).

RISK FACTORS FOR SUICIDAL IDEATION AND ACTS

Primary Psychiatric Disorders among Youth Suicide Victims

Psychological autopsy studies utilize information from coroner reports and direct interviews of suicide victims' relatives to identify psychosocial suicide risk factors. First child and adolescent psychological autopsy study involved all suicides in England and Wales in 1962–1068 (30 children: 21 males, 9 females), aged 12 to 14 years (7). Most common suicide method was carbon monoxide (43%). Forty-six percent reported prior suicidal ideation or acts, 57% had mixed antisocial, affective symptoms, 36% experienced recent disciplinary crisis, and 55% parents suffered emotional symptoms requiring treatment. Subsequent child and adolescent psychological autopsy studies indicated approximately 90% had a psychiatric disorder and 70% had comorbid psychiatric disorders at time of suicide (8,9). Prior suicide attempt increased suicide risk 51- to 89-fold (8,9). Majority (61% to 76%) of youth suicide victims suffered from mood disorders increasing suicide risk 8- to 13-fold. Major depressive disorder (MDD) prevalence ranged from 32% to 54%, increasing suicide risk 27-fold. Current substance abuse disorder, occurring in 27% to 62%, increased suicide risk 8.5-fold. Other disorders were bipolar disorder (20%), increasing suicide risk 9-fold, and anxiety disorders (27%), eating disorders (4%), and schizophrenia (4%) (8). Suicide victims without psychiatric disorders had high prior suicide ideation or attempt rates, low suicide intent, easy access to firearms, and disciplinary problems (10).

Suicide Ideation and Attempts, Nonsuicidal Self-Injury, and Psychopathology

Predicting risk for transitions between suicidal states is an important suicide prevention strategy. National Comorbidity Survey Replication Adolescent Supplement reported 33% suicide ideators developed a suicide plan, 60.8% with a plan and 20.4% without a plan attempted suicide; indicating that 60% of first suicide attempts are planned (11). Transitions

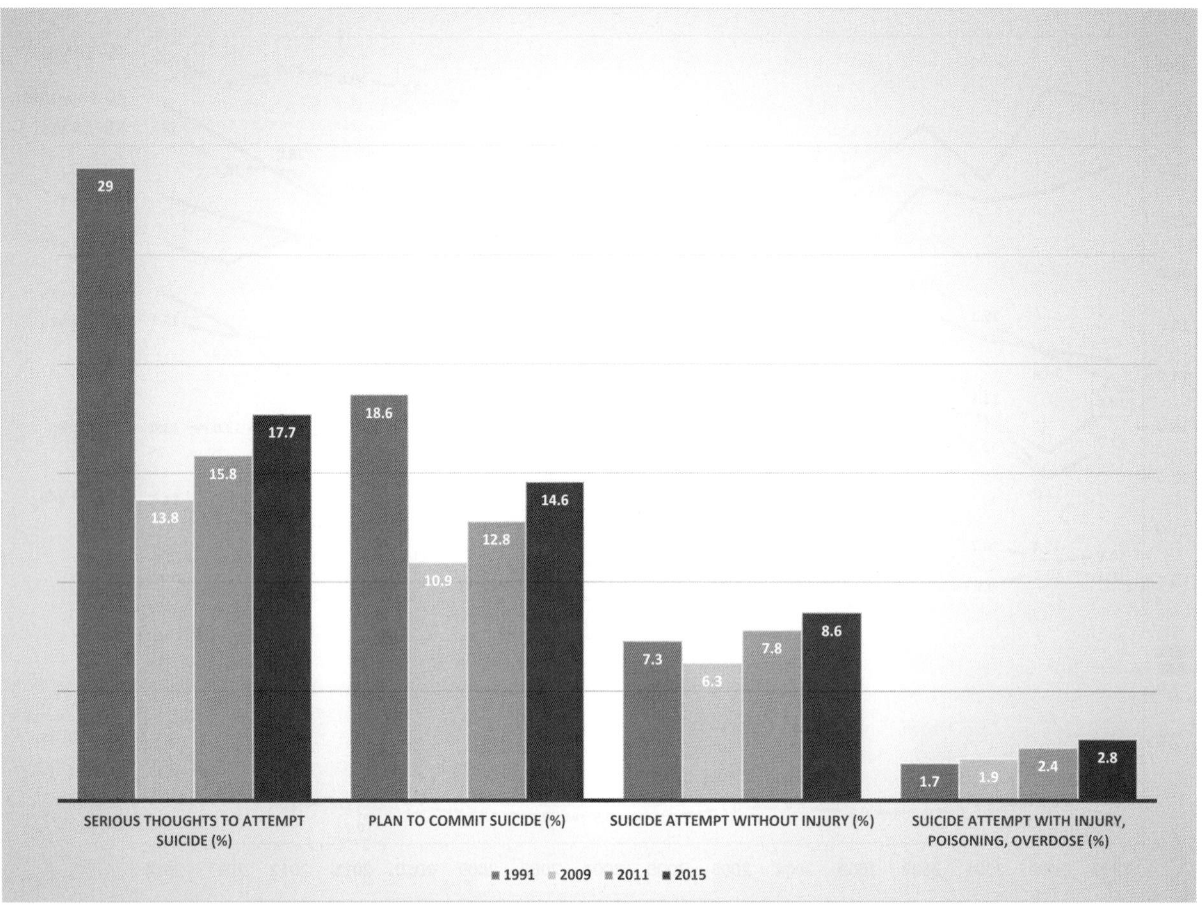

FIGURE 5.4.3.2. High school student suicidal ideation and suicide attempt rates from 1991, 2009, 2011, 2015.

from suicide ideation to plan (63.1%) and ideation to attempt (86.1%) occurred in first year of suicidal ideation onset. Only MDD predicted a suicide plan among those with suicidal ideation. Transitions from ideation to attempt were associated with MDD, eating disorder, attention-deficit hyperactivity disorder, conduct disorder, and intermittent explosive disorders.

A prospective study of 506 adolescents participating in a school-based suicide screening program identified that adolescents, who had serious repeated suicidal ideation, attempted suicide during 4- to 6-year follow-up (12). Earlier attempts were predicted by proximal suicidal ideation lasting greater than 1 hour. Other prospective research suggested developmental transitions affect suicidal risk; child psychiatric inpatients with suicidal ideation were at 4-fold and those who attempted suicide were at 6-fold increased suicide attempt risk in adolescence (13). Highest risk period was first year after discharge. Strongest predictor of adolescent suicide attempt was number of prior suicide attempts rather than a mood disorder alone; mood disorder with suicide attempt history predicted future attempts (14). Psychomotor agitation and alcohol and substance abuse increase suicide attempt lethality (15).

Inability to make decisions that provide rewarding experiences may be a cognitive suicide attempt risk factor among adolescents with MDD (16). A study of depressed adolescents suggested that suicide attempters versus suicide ideators, had more severe anhedonia and were less likely to pursue rewards during an experimental computer task, when outcomes were uncertain (17). These results imply that intense adverse emotions impair cognitive decision-making processes to integrate prior rewarding experiences when making present decisions.

Chronic nonsuicidal self-injury is among the strongest predictors for suicide (18) and suicide attempts (19) and stronger than depression, anxiety, borderline personality disorder, and impulsivity (19,20). The Avon Longitudinal Study of Parents and Children, utilizing 4,855 adolescents, identified that self-injuring adolescents with suicidal intent compared to without suicidal intent had 3.5-fold higher risk for depressive and anxiety disorders (21).

Adolescent nonsuicidal self-injury risk was associated with family dysfunction, poor parental mental health, insecure attachment, and temperamental characteristics that diminish emotion regulation, self-confidence, and problem-solving skills (22). An experimental study identified that self-injuring adolescents, compared to healthy controls, showed poorer inhibition to images depicting negative emotional content; implying that nonsuicidal self-injuring adolescents have more difficulty maintaining cognitive behavioral control when faced with negative emotional stimuli (23).

Bipolar disorder is among the most lethal diagnoses. A longitudinal study of 405 children and adolescents with bipolar disorder I, II, and NOS found 33% had history of a suicide attempt (24). Prevalent suicide attempt predictors were mixed bipolar episodes, severe depression, psychosis, self-injury, Panic and substance use disorders, psychiatric hospitalization, and family history of depression.

Psychosis is a prominent risk factor for suicide attempts. A prospective study of 110 children and adolescents with first-episode psychosis indicated suicide attempt prevalence was 12.4% at 24-month reevaluation (25). Two independent case-controlled studies of 212 adolescents, aged 11 to 13 years, and 211 adolescents, aged 13 to 15 years, attending school suggested psychotic symptoms were associated with 10-fold increased risk of suicidal ideation, plans or acts; but risk increased to 14-fold when adolescents were also depressed (26). Adolescents with suicidal ideation with, compared to without, psychotic symptoms had a 20-fold increased risk of suicide plans and attempts. Evaluating psychotic symptoms is essential during suicide risk assessment.

A consistent research finding is that comorbid anxiety and depression significantly increases risk for proximal suicidal attempts in children and adolescents (27). Posttraumatic stress disorder (PTSD) comorbid with MDD mediated the link between traumatic events and suicidal ideation and acts (28). This study suggested rates of suicidal ideation (30% to 80%) and suicide attempts (15% to 50%) in adolescents with PTSD were similar to rates in depressive disorders and schizophrenia. A longitudinal study of 613 children recruited in first grade and followed up in 10th grade suggested a predictor of 10th grader suicidal ideation involved interaction between 10th grader depressive symptoms and first grader anxiety sensitivity to cognitive concerns (i.e., fears of experiencing anxiety or panic from onset of cognitive concerns, such as depersonalization, racing thoughts, lack of concentration) (29). This study suggested a process that early-onset anxiety sensitivity amplified depression distress to promote risk for suicidal ideation.

Few studies examined relations between suicidal ideation and specific anxiety disorders. A study of 54 child and adolescent outpatients with obsessive compulsive disorder (OCD) found 13% had suicidal ideation, which was associated with OCD-specific symptoms, such as symmetry/ordering, sexuality/religiosity, need to tell, confess, or ask, and depressive and anxiety symptoms, age, and functional impairment (30). A longitudinal study of 144 female (72%) adolescent psychiatric inpatients suggested significant direct relationship between social anxiety disorder at hospitalization and suicidal ideation at 18-month follow-up, and significant indirect effect on suicidal ideation at 18-month follow-up through loneliness at 9-month follow-up (31). The study highlighted loneliness related to social anxiety as risk factor for adolescent suicidal ideation.

Personality Disorders and Traits

Psychological autopsy studies suggested 33% youth suicide victims suffered from a personality disorder, especially borderline and antisocial personality disorders (32) and narcissistic and schizoid traits (33). Among 366 adolescents with repeated self-harm, 60% suffered from a personality disorder and over 1-year follow-up had severe self-harm, suicide attempts, depressive symptoms, and functional impairment (34). Other studies suggested personality traits, such as extreme self-reliance for solving problems or high sensation-seeking behavior, were associated with suicidal ideation and attempts (35,36). Identifying adolescent personality traits is important to suicide prevention.

MINORITY SEXUAL ORIENTATION AND SUICIDAL IDEATION AND ACTS

The National Longitudinal Study of Adolescent Health reported adolescents with minority sexual orientation, compared to other adolescents, had higher risk for suicidal ideation and attempts, depression, hopelessness, alcohol abuse, victimization, and recent family or peer suicide attempts (37). The New Zealand Birth Cohort Study documented that by age 21 years, 2.8% of 1,007 participants were classified as gay, lesbian, or bisexual and exhibited more suicidal ideation and attempts, major depressive, generalized anxiety, and conduct disorders (38).

ADVERSE CHILDHOOD EXPERIENCES

Children and adolescents with history of suicidal ideation, attempts, or suicide often experienced cumulative adverse experiences (39,40). A longitudinal study of a national sample of 1,186 children and adolescents suggested suicide ideation risk was greater among those experiencing recent peer victimization (2.4-fold), sexual assault (3.4-fold), and parental maltreatment (4.4-fold); but exposure to seven or more recent types of victimization increased likelihood for suicidal ideation (6-fold) (41). A case-control longitudinal study using Danish register data of 403,321 children and adolescents of whom 0.8% (3,465 individuals) attempted suicide described a multiplicative dose–response relationship between risk of suicide attempts and number of exposures to parental adverse events including low family income, parental psychiatric illness, suicide attempt, and suicide (42). Another longitudinal Danish register study of 3,465 suicide attempters, aged 10 to 22 years, and 75,300 matched controls described a significantly higher suicide attempt rate for those bereaved by a biologic parental death, but it doubled with a second biologic parental death (43).

Family history of suicide imparts for adolescent girls and boys, a 3- and 5-fold greater suicide risk, respectively, than those in the community (44). Risk for youth suicide is transmitted in families independent of psychiatric disorders and mediated by the transmission of impulsive aggression (45). A prospective study suggested parental suicide attempts had a direct predictive effect on adolescent offspring suicide attempt in addition to risk effects of offspring mood disorder and impulsive aggression (46). Evaluating youth after family suicidal behavior is an important suicide prevention strategy.

Youth suicides and nonfatal suicide attempts sometimes occur in the context of time-space clusters stimulated by mechanisms of imitation of suicidal peers and exposure to suicide presentations on news, fictional or social media (47,48). Cultural affiliation problems related to migration and changing social supports among Black, American Indian, Alaska Native, and Native Hawaiian adolescents significantly predicted adolescent suicide attempts (49–51). Community education about suicide prevention is essential when a child or adolescent commits suicide or feels socially isolated.

Physical problems near time of birth, including respiratory distress for more than an hour after birth, no antenatal care before 20 weeks of pregnancy, chronic maternal physical disease and chronic childhood medical illnesses, such as diabetes and epilepsy, are associated with increased risk for suicidal behavior (52–54). Inquiry about medical problems is essential for youth suicide risk assessment.

Neurobiologic Factors

Serotonin neurotransmitter system dysregulation, manifest as low levels of whole blood tryptophan (55) or affected by interactions between early environmental stress and the short(s) allele of the serotonin transporter gene (56,57), increase risk for child and adolescent suicidal attempts and nonsuicidal self-injury. Suicide risk may involve more complex interactions between a specific genotype and environmental adverse event exposure during a critical window of brain development (58).

Early-life adversity was associated with HPA axis dysregulation caused by epigenetic effects involving DNA methylation that affects expression of hippocampal glucocorticoid receptor variants in adult suicide victims (59). HPA axis dysregulation was reported as elevated blood post dexamethasone cortisol levels among child suicide attempters and elevated baseline blood cortisol levels before sleep onset of adolescent suicide attempters (60,61). A differential pattern of higher cortisol secretion in response to a serotonergic agonist, meta-chlorophenylpiperazine (mCPP), was shown for adolescent depressed male suicide attempters compared to suicidal and nonsuicidal depressed females (62). A prospective study of 138 adolescent females, at risk for suicidal behavior and exposed at baseline to a psychosocial stress task, assessed salivary cortisol levels and suicidal ideation obtained pre- and post-stressor (63). HPA axis hyperresponsive females, compared to normal or hyporesponsive females, were more likely to report lifetime history of suicidal ideation at baseline and more likely to have suicidal ideation 3 months after baseline, compared to normal females. Adolescents with nonsuicidal self-injury, compared to healthy controls, and exposed to an experimental cold pain reported greater pain threshold, pain tolerance, and lower pain intensity, which was associated with heightened reactivity of the HPA axis and autonomic nervous system (64).

Extensive adolescent brain maturation highlights the importance of studying brain structure and functioning and relates these to adolescent suicidal behavior. Magnetic resonance imaging (MRI) identified that adolescents with MDD and suicide attempt history had elevated brain white matter hyperintensities (65). Functional brain magnetic resonance imaging (fMRI) of depressed adolescents with and without suicide attempt history suggested adolescent suicide attempters had elevated activity in attention control circuitry and reduced anterior cingulate–insula functional connectivity when responding to 50% intensity angry faces but no evident differences when emotional stimuli were absent (66). This study suggested markers of past suicide attempt may be abnormal functioning in the salience and attention neural circuitry when processing emotional stimuli but normal network functioning in the absence of emotional stimuli. Functional neuroimaging with cold as a pain stimulus was studied among adolescents with, compared to those without, nonsuicidal self-injury (67). Those with nonsuicidal self-injury had greater blood oxygenation level–dependent (BOLD) response in right midbrain/pons, culmen, amygdala, and parahippocampal, inferior frontal and superior temporal gyri, and orbital frontal cortex. These brain regions are associated with reward and pain processing in dopamine and opiate systems. The results suggested associations between pain and reward among nonsuicidal self-injuring adolescents.

Sleep disturbances including insomnia, shortened sleep duration, hypersomnia, nightmares, and sleep-related serotonergic functioning and growth hormone secretion may predict adolescent suicidal ideation, suicide attempts, and suicide (61,68,69). Immediate effects of sleep deprivation include mood instability, negative affect, and impulsivity in response to negative stimuli. Such symptoms increase risk for imminent suicidal ideation and attempts, especially for children and adolescents with mood and substance use disorders and psychosocial stresses. Sleep disturbances should be part of clinical suicide risk assessment.

RISK ASSESSMENT

Assessment of children and adolescents also involves parents to identify suicidal risk factors and plan for safety. Clinical interviews may be augmented with reliable and valid suicide risk rating scales, such as the Columbia-Suicide Severity Rating Scale measuring severity and intensity of suicidal ideation and lethality of suicide attempts and nonsuicidal self-injury (70). Self-report rating scales include Harkavy–Asnis Suicide Scale (71), Scale for Suicidal Ideation, Suicidal Intent Scale, Beck Depression Inventory, and Hopelessness Scale (72). Child Adolescent Suicide Potential Index (CASPI) measures risk related to recent suicidal ideation and attempts, psychiatric symptoms, and adverse childhood events (73). Implicit Association Test for Suicide Attempts or Nonsuicidal Self-Injury involves computerized measurement of adolescent reaction time to stimuli related to self and suicide or self-injury to predict future suicidal states (74).

TREATMENT

Acute Intervention

Review of randomized clinical trials to reduce child and adolescent suicidal ideation or attempts or self-injury suggested efficacy was strongest for interventions focusing on family interactions, other support, greatest number of sessions, motivational interviewing to enhance treatment compliance, and promotion of positive affect, sobriety, and healthy sleep (75). During psychiatric emergency intervention, a patient is not discharged until there is a safety plan derived from explicit discussion of suicidal intent, methods for maintaining safety, and no access to lethal suicidal methods (76). A randomized controlled emergency department intervention for adolescents at risk for suicidal behavior suggested motivational discussion and barrier-reduction to mental health services, compared to standard referral, significantly improved linkage to outpatient mental health services (77). A 12-week SAFETY cognitive behavioral family intervention integrated with emergency services focused on practicing skills to prevent repeated adolescent suicide attempts and increasing safety (78). It demonstrated significant decreased adolescent suicidal behavior, hopelessness, and parent depression 6 months after program entry.

Psychiatric hospitalization is recommended when safety is unpredictable and provides acute interventions and removal from a stressful environment. Outpatient and partial hospitalization treatments are utilized if low likelihood for imminent suicidal acts and presence of family support exist. A randomized controlled study comparing intervention as usual with an experimental collaborative care intervention including assessment of adolescent depression at initial meeting and during 12-month follow-up found significantly greater reduction in depressive symptoms for those in collaborative care; a program that increased patient motivation and reduced barriers for treatment (79).

Psychotherapy

Meta-analysis of 19 randomized controlled psychotherapeutic trials to reduce suicidal and nonsuicidal self-harm in 2,176 adolescents suggested lower self-injury rate for those in treatment (28%) compared to controls (33%) (80). Largest effects were for dialectical behavior therapy (DBT), cognitive behavioral therapy (CBT), and mentalization-based therapy (MBT). Another meta-analysis of 29 studies of child and adolescent cognitive behavioral, family, interpersonal, and psychodynamic interventions to reduce suicidal and nonsuicidal self-injury behaviors highlighted elements of efficacious treatments as family skills training to improve communication and problem solving, parent education in monitoring and managing, and child and adolescent skills training to regulate emotions and solve problems (81). Controlled treatment trials of DBT suggest total number of sessions is a partial mediator between treatment and changes in severity of suicidal ideation (82). DBT is an effective adjunct therapy for suicidal adolescents with bipolar disorder (83). Other effective therapies to reduce adolescent self-harm include attachment-based family therapy (ABFT) focusing on strengthening parent–adolescent attachment to create a protective and secure base for adolescent development, emotion regulation, and family cohesion (84) and MBT to improve self-awareness and reduced attachment avoidance (85).

Psychopharmacology

Many research methods are utilized to assess effects of psychopharmacological interventions for suicide risk. One method links large aggregated prescription data with suicide data from similar populations. Studies suggested that increased antidepressant prescription rates especially for selective serotonin reuptake inhibitors (SSRIs) were associated with lower suicide rates (86,87) and longer antidepressant drug treatment (180 vs. 55 days) reduced likelihood of suicide attempt (88).

Outcomes of depressed children and adolescents at risk for suicide were studied in randomized, double-blind, placebo-controlled medication treatment studies. Treatment of Adolescent Depression Study (TADS), sponsored by NIMH, was a 36-week pharmacologic and psychotherapeutic treatment trial including 439 adolescents, aged 12 to 17 years, with MDD without high suicide risk (89). Initial acute 12-week randomized, double-blind, placebo-controlled phase compared efficacy of fluoxetine alone, CBT alone, combined CBT and fluoxetine, and placebo. After acute phase, all treatments were unblinded and nonresponders were discontinued from study, referred to community providers, but continued with study assessments to end of 36 weeks. Six-week consolidation phase involved acute phase responders beginning maintenance treatment in their assigned treatment and partial responders receiving 6 weeks in their assigned treatment with additional CBT or higher fluoxetine dose or both in the combined group. Eighteen-week continuation phase was long-term maintenance treatment. Final phase was a 1-year open community follow-up.

During 12-week acute phase, depression symptoms decreased in 71.0% with combined treatment, 60.6% with fluoxetine alone, 43.2% with CBT alone, and 34.8% with placebo (90). Suicidal ideation and attempts were rated by adolescents and study clinicians and reassessed by expert raters using the Columbia Classification Algorithm for Suicidal Assessment (91). At baseline, 29% reported suicidal ideation, which improved with each treatment but was greatest for combined CBT and fluoxetine treatment. Suicide-related events (suicidal ideation or attempts) during 12-week study included 10 (9.2%) adolescents in fluoxetine treatment, 5 (4.6%) in combined treatment, 5 (4.6%)in CBT, and 3 (2.7%) in placebo group. Only fluoxetine, compared to placebo, had significantly greater (2-fold) suicide-related events. A 1.6% suicide attempt rate involved two in combined treatment, two in fluoxetine treatment, one in CBT, and no suicides. As depression symptoms improved, suicidal ideation decreased. Combined CBT and fluoxetine had a more favorable safety profile than fluoxetine alone.

During the 36-week study, 44 participants (10.0%) had at least 1 suicidal event (23 episodes of suicidal ideation and 21 suicide attempts) (92). These occurred between 0.4 and 31.1 weeks with mean time of 12 weeks after study onset. Adolescents receiving fluoxetine alone had a significantly higher suicide event rate (14.7%) than those receiving CBT alone (6.3%). Combined treatment suicide event rate (8.4%) was not different from fluoxetine alone or CBT alone. Suicidal events were predicted by pretreatment severity of suicidal ideation and depressive symptoms.

Open 1-year community follow-up indicated gains at end of 36-week phase were maintained 1 year later (93). Need for improved long-term treatment of adolescent depression was suggested by 6% to 33% loss of benefit at follow-up, which represented substantial deterioration.

Treatment of Adolescent Suicide Attempters (TASA) study, developed by NIMH and five academic medical centers, was a combined psychosocial and pharmacologic 6-month clinical trial including 124 depressed adolescent suicide attempters to evaluate intervention and predictors and mediators of recurrent suicide attempts (94). It identified low 6-month risks for suicidal ideation and reattempts, suggesting this intervention be studied with controlled methodology.

Treatment of SSRI-Resistant Depression in Adolescents (TORDIA) study, sponsored by NIMH as a multicenter study, involved 12-week acute and 12-week continuation phases to evaluate treatment, after adolescents with MDD did not respond adequately to usual treatment with an SSRI drug (95–97). The 334 treatment-resistant adolescents with MDD and high risk for suicidal ideation or attempts or nonsuicidal self-injury included 70% females, 82% Whites, 60% with suicidal ideation, 50% with MDD for at least 2 years, and 52% with comorbid psychiatric disorders. At study baseline, 47% reported history of self-injurious behavior (23.9% nonsuicidal self-injury only, and 14% suicide attempts and nonsuicidal self-injury, and 9.5% suicide attempts only).

Participants had prior lack of response to SSRI before beginning TORDIA when prior SSRI treatment involved at least 8 weeks and in the last 4 weeks, SSRI dose was equivalent to 40 mg fluoxetine. In first 2 weeks of TORDIA, the failed SSRI was gradually decreased and discontinued while study medication was gradually added. Adolescents were randomized to one of four treatment groups including switch to a second SSRI (either citalopram, fluoxetine, or paroxetine at doses of 20 to 40 mg orally daily), switch to venlafaxine at doses of 150 to 225 mg orally daily, switch to a different SSRI plus CBT, or switch to venlafaxine plus CBT. TORDIA used weekly CBT, similar to that in TADS.

Acute phase results indicated greater decrease of depression with CBT plus switch to another medication (54.8%) than a medication switch alone (40.5%); but no difference in response between a second SSRI (47.0%) and venlafaxine (56.0%). No differences in response occurred for the four treatments regarding suicidal ideation or attempts or self-harm behavior. Suicide attempts occurred in 11.3% (18 suicide attempts among 17 participants and no suicide). Median time to suicidal event was 3 weeks after intake. New-onset suicide attempt rate was 5% and nonsuicidal self-injury was 9%. Venlafaxine was associated with more suicidal events and nonsuicidal self-injury for those with high baseline suicidal ideation. Strongest predictors of suicidal events were high baseline suicidal ideation, self-reported parent–child conflict, and drug and alcohol use. Those with suicidal events at study baseline continued to report high levels of depression and suicidal ideation, and were less likely to respond to treatment.

Adolescents with nonsuicidal self-injury plus suicide attempts had highest 24-week incidence of suicide attempts (7%), nonsuicidal self-injury (11%), and depressive symptoms, hopelessness, family conflict, and histories of physical and/or sexual abuse. Nonsuicidal self-injury history predicted suicide attempts as well as nonsuicidal self-injury and was a stronger predictor of future suicide attempts than prior suicide attempts. Time to incident suicide attempts was predicted by baseline nonsuicidal self-injury and hopelessness. Time to nonsuicidal self-injury was predicted by history of nonsuicidal self-injury and physical and/or sexual abuse.

Depression Antidepressants and Psychotherapy Trial (ADAPT) was a 12-week acute and subsequent 16-week maintenance phase study conducted in England with 164 adolescents with MDD (98). Adolescents, assigned to SSRI medication plus CBT or SSRI medication alone, were assessed at baseline, and subsequent 6, 12, and 28 weeks. Results suggested no difference in outcomes of the two treatments; 20% did not respond. Predictors of suicide attempts were baseline serious suicidal ideation or acts, nonsuicidal self-injury, and poor family functioning. Predictors of nonsuicidal self-injury were baseline nonsuicidal self-injury, hopelessness, anxiety disorder, being younger and female. This study, like TORDIA, highlighted persistent suicidal and nonsuicidal self-injury in depressed adolescents.

Extensive discussion about safety of antidepressant drug treatment for children and adolescents began when United Kingdom Medicines and Healthcare Products Regulatory Agency (June 10, 2003) and U.S. Food and Drug Administration (FDA) (June 19, 2003) issued advisories recommending paroxetine not be prescribed to children and adolescents. FDA requested pharmaceutical companies submit their antidepressant clinical trials data about child and adolescent suicidal ideation and acts. Wyeth Pharmaceutical Company (August 2003) voluntarily changed labeling for pediatric use of venlafaxine and issued a letter to health providers indicating higher rates of suicidal ideation and acts and hostility in children and adolescents treated with venlafaxine in their clinical trials. After initial review of child and adolescent antidepressant treatment clinical trials, FDA issued an advisory (October 27, 2003) indicating association between antidepressants and suicidal ideation and acts. Additional FDA reviews resulted in a public advisory (March 22, 2004) indicating need for close observation of children, adolescents, and adults treated with antidepressants.

FDA conducted statistical analyses of randomized, double-blind, placebo-controlled pharmaceutical industry–sponsored child and adolescent studies of antidepressant drug treatment comparing incidence of suicidal ideation and acts for antidepressant drug treatment versus placebo (99). Manufacturers submitted to FDA data identifying suicidal ideation and acts, as adverse events in 22 industry-sponsored studies of various clinical indications involving 9 antidepressant drugs and a total of 2,298 children and adolescents treated with an antidepressant drug and 1,952 children and adolescents receiving placebo. Incidence of suicidal events was combined across clinical trials to yield risk estimates of suicidal ideation and attempts for those on antidepressant drugs compared to placebo. Risk estimate for serious suicidal adverse events was 1.89 (95% confidence interval: 1.18 to 3.04). FDA concluded treatment with antidepressant drugs was associated with suicidal events double the placebo rate.

FDA reanalysis on data from 23 clinical trials, involving 9 sponsored by pharmaceutical companies and the TADS study, evaluated whether antidepressant drugs used to treat 4,582 children and adolescents increased suicidal acts risk (100). Study drugs were bupropion, citalopram, fluoxetine, fluvoxamine, mirtazapine, nefazodone, paroxetine, sertraline, and venlafaxine. Psychiatric disorders included MDD (16 trials), OCD (4 trials), generalized anxiety disorder (2 trials), attention-deficit hyperactivity disorder (1 trial), and social anxiety disorder (1 trial). Four trials not reporting suicidal ideation or acts were dropped. Analysis from 20 studies focused on suicidal risk for each drug, for SSRIs in depression trials, and for all trials combined. TADS, using fluoxetine as antidepressant drug, was the only clinical trial with statistically significant risk ratio involving drug versus placebo (4.62, 95% confidence interval: 1.02 to 20.92). No child or adolescent in these studies committed suicide. Risk ratio for SSRIs in depression studies was 1.66 (95% confidence interval: 1.02 to 2.68) and for all drugs for all psychiatric indications was 1.95 (95% confidence interval: 1.28 to 2.98). Investigators concluded antidepressant drugs to treat children and adolescents were associated with increased suicidal ideation or acts risk. FDA mandated (October 15, 2004) pharmaceutical companies add a black box labeling for all antidepressants used for children and adolescents.

The FDA black box warning stimulated controversy about its validity and implications for clinical care of children and adolescents (101). Some suggested importance of the FDA black box warning was to remind prescribers and consumers of need for close monitoring for adverse behavioral effects during initiation or changes in antidepressant therapy (102). Others noted "rather than being a threat, the judicious clinical use of antidepressants actually does serve to effectively treat and indeed protect depressed patients from suicidal outcome" (103). Others believed that different outcome results may have been identified if other statistical analyses were used (104).

Study of large aggregate data indicated that national rates of diagnosing new-onset MDD in children and adolescents increased from 1999 to late 2003 but declined after the FDA advisory (October 27, 2003) through 2007 among primary care physicians, were unchanged among pediatricians, and increased among psychiatrists and rate of antidepressant prescription fills declined (105). A study of antidepressant prescribing for children and adolescents with depression, anxiety, or attention-deficit hyperactivity disorders indicated that compared to the period preceding the 2004 FDA boxed warning (2001 to 2003), a significant decline in antidepressant prescribing was detected in the immediate post-FDA boxed warning period (2006 to 2007) but increased in 2008 to 2009 (106). Another study, evaluating antidepressant dispensing and psychotropic drug poisonings as proxy for suicide attempts and suicides, reported decreased antidepressant use in 2005 among adolescents, young adults, and adults and significant increases in psychotropic drug poisonings for adolescents, young adults but not adults (107). Associations between rates of antidepressant prescribing for children and adolescents and rates of suicide and nonfatal suicidal acts after 2009 have not been studied.

SUICIDE PREVENTION STRATEGIES

The increasing child and adolescent suicide rates in recent years suggest need for new suicide prevention strategies. Educating children and adolescents through school and family programs to cope with stress, develop effective emotional and behavioral self-regulation, and avoid substance use/abuse are important primary suicide prevention issues. Identifying early-life experiences that may interact with developmental vulnerability periods to increase suicidal risk need to be targets for primary prevention. New access prevention laws and educating parents about risks for guns or firearms at home are needed to restrict availability of guns and firearms (108,109). Enhancing accessibility to mental health care by reducing barriers for receiving help and improving collaborative care among health care providers are essential for reducing suicide risk.

Other suicide prevention efforts include development of valid universal screening and monitoring methods with excellent predictive capacity to identify combinations of proximal suicide risk factors. Effective real-time monitoring methods using mobile technology to identify transitions in suicidal states may enhance provision of immediate acute intervention. Recently, NIH announced sponsorship of a multisite study to identify biomarkers for suicide risk identification. Such studies may suggest strategies for precise treatment methods to reduce suicide risk. Greater understanding of sociocultural risk factors, such as use of social media, and development of primary prevention strategies to reduce youth risk are necessary. Public health education for the general public and health care professionals may reduce stigma and improve treatment-seeking for suicidal children and adolescents and when suicide occurs in families.

References

1. American Psychiatric Association: *Diagnostic and Statistical Manual of Mental Disorders.* 5th ed. Arlington, Virginia, American Psychiatric Association, 2013.
2. U.S. Department of Health and Human Services (HHS) Office of the Surgeon General and National Action Alliance for Suicide Prevention.

2012 National Strategy for Suicide Prevention: Goals and Objectives for Action. Washington, DC, HHS, 2012.

3. Murphy SL, Kochanek KD, Xu JQ, et al.: *Mortality in the United States, 2014. NCHS Data Brief No. 229*. Hyattsville, MD, National Center for Health Statistics, 2015.
4. Case A, Deaton A: Rising morbidity and mortality in midlife among white non-Hispanic Americans in the 21st century. *Proc Natl Acad Sci U S A* 112(49):15078–15083, 2015.
5. Centers for Disease Control and Prevention Morbidity and Mortality Weekly Report—Youth Risk Behavior Surveillance—United States, 2015. 2016;65(6).
6. Pfeffer CR: *The Suicidal Child*. New York, Guilford Press, 1986.
7. Shaffer D: Suicide in childhood and early adolescents. *J Child Psychol Psychiat* 15:275–291, 1974.
8. Shaffer D, Gould MS, Fisher P, et al.: Psychiatric diagnosis in child and adolescent suicide. *Arch Gen Psychiatry* 53:339–348, 1996.
9. Brent DA, Baugher M, Bridge J, Chen T, Chiappetta L: Age- and sex-related risk factors for adolescent suicide. *J Am Acad Child Adolesc Psychiatry* 38:1497–1505, 1999.
10. Brent DA, Perper J, Moritz G, Baugher M, Allman C: Suicide in adolescents with no apparent psychopathology. *J Am Acad Child Adolesc Psychiatry* 32:494–500, 1993.
11. Nock MK, Greif JG, Hwang I, et al.: Prevalence, correlates, and treatment of lifetime suicidal behavior among adolescents: results from the national comorbidity survey replication adolescent supplement. *JAMA Psychiatry* 70(3):300–310, 2013.
12. Miranda R, Ortin A, Scott M, Shaffer D: Characteristics of suicidal ideation that predict the transition to future suicide attempts in adolescents. *J Child Psychol Psychiatry* 55(11):1288–1296, 2014.
13. Pfeffer CR, Klerman GL, Hurt SW, Kakuma T, Peskin JR, Siefker CA: Suicidal children grow up: rates and psychosocial risk factors for suicide attempts during follow-up. *J Am Acad Child Adolesc Psychiatry* 32:106–113, 1993.
14. Goldston DB, Daniel SS, Reboussin DM, Reboussin BA, Frazier PH, Kelley AE: Suicide attempts among formerly hospitalized adolescents: a prospective naturalistic study of risk during the first 5 years after discharge. *J Am Acad Child Adolesc Psychiatry* 38:660–671, 1999.
15. Barbe RP, Williamson DE, Bridge JA, et al.: Clinical differences between suicidal and nonsuicidal depressed children and adolescents. *J Clin Psychiatry* 66:492–498, 2005.
16. Bridge JA, McBee-Strayer SM, Cannon EA, et al.: Impaired decision-making in adolescent suicide attempters. *J Am Acad Child Adolesc Psychiatry* 51(4):394–403, 2012.
17. Auerbach RP, Millner AJ, Stewart JG, Esposito EC: Identifying differences between depressed adolescent suicide ideators and attempters. *J Affect Disord* 186:127–133, 2015.
18. Hawton K, Zahl D, Weatherall R: Suicide following deliberate self-harm: long-term follow-up of patients who presented to a general hospital. *Brit J Psychiatry* 182:537–542, 2003.
19. Nock MK, Joiner TE Jr, Gordon KH, Lloyd-Richardson E, Prinstein MJ: Non-suicidal self-injury among adolescents: diagnostic correlates and relation to suicide attempts. *Psychiatry Res* 144:65–72, 2006.
20. Klonsky ED, May AM, Glenn CR: The relationship between nonsuicidal self-injury and attempted suicide: converging evidence from four samples. *J Abnorm Psychol* 122(1):231–237, 2013.
21. Mars B, Heron J, Crane C, et al.: Differences in risk factors for self-harm with and without suicidal intent: findings from the ALSPAC cohort. *J Affect Disord* 168:407–414, 2014.
22. Glazebrook K, Townsend E, Sayal K: The role of attachment style in predicting repetition of adolescent self-harm: a longitudinal study. *Sui Life Threat Behavior* 45(6):664–678, 2015.
23. Allen KJ, Hooley JM: Inhibitory control in people who self-injure: evidence for impairment and enhancement. *Psychiatry Res* 225(3):631–637, 2015.
24. Goldstein TR, Ha W, Axelson DA, et al.: Predictors of prospectively examined suicide attempts among youth with bipolar disorder. *Arch Gen Psychiatry* 69(11):1113–1122, 2012.
25. Sanchez-Gistau V, Baeza I, Arango C, et al.: Predictors of suicide attempt in early-onset, first-episode psychosis: a longitudinal 24-month follow-up study. *J Clin Psychiatry* 74(1):59–66, 2013.
26. Kelleher K, Lynch F, Harley M, et al.: Psychotic symptoms in adolescence index risk for suicidal behavior: findings from 2 population-based case-control clinical interview studies. *Arch Gen Psychiatry* 69(12): 1277–1283, 2012.
27. Foley DL, Goldston DB, Costello EJ, Angold A: Proximal psychiatric risk factors for suicidality in youth: the Great Smoky Mountains Study. *Arch Gen Psychiatry* 63(9):1017–1024, 2006.
28. Panagioti M, Gooding PA, Triantafyllou K, Tarrier N: Suicidality and posttraumatic stress disorder (PTSD) in adolescents: a systematic review and meta-analysis. *Soc Psychiatry Psychiatr Epidemiol* 50:525–537, 2015.
29. Capron DW, Allan NP, Ialongo NS, Leen-Feldner E, Schmidt NB: The depression distress amplification model in adolescents: a longitudinal examination of anxiety sensitivity cognitive concerns, depression, and suicidal ideation. *J Adolesc* 41:17–24, 2015.
30. Storch EA, Bussing R, Jacob ML, et al.: Frequency and correlates of suicidal ideation in pediatric obsessive-compulsive disorder. *Child Psychiatry Hum Dev* 46:75–83, 2015.
31. Gallagher M, Prinstein MJ, Simon V, Spirito A: Social anxiety symptoms and suicidal ideation in a clinical sample of early adolescents: examining loneliness and social support as longitudinal mediators. *J Abnorm Child Psychology* 42(6):871–883, 2014.
32. Rich CL, Runeson BS: Similarities in diagnostic comorbidity between suicide among young people in Sweden and the United States. *Acta Psychiatr Scand* 86:335–339, 1992.
33. Apter A, Bleich A, King RA, et al.: Death without warning? A clinical postmortem study of suicide in 43 Israeli adolescent males. *Arch Gen Psychiatry* 50:138–142, 1993.
34. Ayodeji E, Green J, Roberts C, et al.: The influence of personality disorder on outcome in adolescent self-harm. *Br J Psychiatry* 207(4):313–319, 2015.
35. Labouliere CD, Kleinman M, Gould MS: When self-reliance is not safe: associations between reduced help-seeking and subsequent mental health symptoms in suicidal adolescents. *Int J Environ Res Public Health* 12(4):3741–3755, 2015.
36. Ortin A, Lake AM, Kleinman M, Gould MS: Sensation seeking as risk factor for suicidal ideation and suicide attempts in adolescence. *J Affect Disord* 143(1–3):214–222, 2012.
37. Fergusson DM, Horwood LJ, Beautrais AL: Is sexual orientation related to mental health problems and suicidality in young people? *Arch Gen Psychiatry* 56:876–880, 1999.
38. Russell ST, Joyner K: Adolescent sexual orientation and suicide risk: evidence from a national study. *Am J Public Health* 91(8):1276–1281, 2001.
39. Gould MS, Fisher P, Parides M, Flory M, Shaffer D: Psychosocial risk factors of child and adolescent completed suicide. *Arch Gen Psychiatry* 53(12):1155–1162, 1996.
40. Pfeffer CR, Normandin L, Kakuma T: Suicidal children grow up: relations between family psychopathology and adolescents' lifetime suicidal behavior. *J Nerv Ment Dis* 186:269–275, 1998.
41. Turner HA, Finkelhor D, Shattuck A, Hamby S: Recent victimization exposure and suicidal ideation in adolescents. *Arch Pediatr Adolesc Med* 166(12):1149–1154, 2012.
42. Christiansen D, Goldney RD, Beautrais AL, Agerbo E: Youth suicide attempts and the dose-response relationship to parental risk factors: a population-based study. *Psychol Med* 41(2):313–319, 2011.
43. Jakobsen IS, Christiansen E: Young people's risk of suicide attempts in relation to parental death: a population-based register study. *J Child Psychol Psychiatry* 52(2):176–183, 2011.
44. Shaffer D: The epidemiology of teen suicide: an examination of risk factors. *J Clin Psychiatry* 49:36–41, 1988.
45. Brent DA, Oquendo M, Birmaher B, et al.: Peripubertal suicide attempts in offspring of suicide attempters with siblings concordant for suicidal behavior. *Am J Psychiatry* 160:1486–1493, 2003.
46. Brent DA, Melhem NM, Oquendo M, et al.: Familial pathways to early-onset suicide attempt: a 5.6-year prospective study. *JAMA Psychiatry* 72(2):160–168, 2015.
47. Gould MS, Petrie K, Kleinman MH, Wallenstein S: Clustering of attempted suicide: New Zealand national data. *Int J Epidemiol* 23:1185–1189, 1994.
48. Gould MS: Suicide and media. *Ann N Y Acad Sci* 932:200–221; discussion 221–224, 2001.
49. Shaffer D, Gould M, Hicks RC: Worsening suicide rate in black teenagers. *Am J Psychiatry* 151:1810–1802, 1994.
50. Borowsky IW, Resnick MD, Ireland M, Blum RW: Suicide attempts among American Indian and Alaska Native youth: risk and protective factors. *Arch Ped Adol Medicine* 153:573–580, 1999.
51. Yuen NC, Nahulu LB, Hishinuma ES, Miyamoto RH: Cultural identification and attempted suicide in native Hawaiian adolescents. *J Am Acad Child Adolesc Psychiatry* 39:360–367, 2000.
52. Salk L, Lipsitt LP, Surner WQ, Reilly BM, Levat RH: Relationship of maternal and perinatal conditions to eventual adolescent suicide. *Lancet* 1(8429):624–627, 1985.
53. Goldston DB, Kovacs M, Ho VY, Parrone PL, Stiffler L: Suicidal ideation and suicide attempts among youth with insulin-dependent diabetes mellitus. *J Am Acad Child Adolesc Psychiatry* 33:240–246, 1994.
54. Brent DA: Overrepresentation of epileptics in a consecutive series of suicide attempters seen at a children's hospital, 1978–1983. *J Am Acad Child Psychiatry* 25:242–246, 1986.
55. Pfeffer CR, McBride PA, Anderson GM, Kakuma T, Fensterheim L, Khait V: Peripheral serotonin measures in prepubertal psychiatric inpatients and normal children: associations with suicidal behavior and its risk factors. *Biol Psychiatry* 44:568–577, 1998.
56. Caspi A, Sugden K, Moffitt TE, et al.: Influence of life stress on depression: moderation by a polymorphism in the 5-HTT gene. *Science* 301(5631):386–389, 2003.
57. Hankin BL, Barrocas AL, Young JF, Haberstick B, Smolen A: 5-HTTLPR x interpersonal stress interaction and nonsuicidal self-injury in general community sample of youth. *Psychiatry Res* 225(3):609–612, 2015.
58. Zalsman G: Timing is critical: gene, environment and timing interactions in genetics of suicide in children and adolescents. *Eur Psychiatry* 25:284–286, 2010.

59. Labonte B, Yerko V, Gross J, et al.: Differential glucocorticoid receptor exon 1(B), 1(C), and 1(H) expression and methylation in suicide completers with a history of childhood abuse. *Biol Psychiatry* 72(1):41–48, 2012.
60. Pfeffer CR, Stokes P, Shindledecker R: Suicidal behavior and hypothalamic-pituitary-adrenocortical axis indices in child psychiatric inpatients. *Biol Psychiatry* 29:909–917, 1991.
61. Dahl RE, Puig-Antich J, Ryan ND, et al.: EEG sleep in adolescents with major depression: the role of suicidality and inpatient status. *J Affect Disord* 19:63–75, 1990.
62. Ghaziuddin N, King CA, Welch K, Ghaziuddin M: Depressed suicidal adolescent males have an altered cortisol response to a pharmacological challenge. *Asian J Psychiatry* 7(1):28–33, 2014.
63. Giletta M, Calhoun CD, Hastings PD, Rudolph KD, Nock MK, Prinstein MJ: Multi-level risk factors for suicidal ideation among at-risk adolescent females: the role of hypothalamic-pituitary-adrenal axis responses to stress. *J Abnorm Child Psychology* 43(5):807–820, 2015.
64. Koenig J, Rinnewitz L, Warth M, Kaess M: Autonomic nervous system and hypothalamic-pituitary-adrenal axis response to experimentally induced cold pain in adolescent non-suicidal self-injury: study protocol. *BMC Psychiatry* 15:150, 2015.
65. Ehrlich S, Noam GG, Lyoo IK, Kwon BJ, Clark MA, Renshaw PF: White matter hyperintensities and their associations with suicidality in psychiatrically hospitalized children and adolescents. *J Am Acad Child Adolesc Psychiatry* 43:770–776, 2004.
66. Pan LA, Hassel S, Segreti AM, Nau SA, Brent DA, Phillips ML: Differential patterns of activity and functional connectivity in emotion processing neural circuitry to angry and happy faces in adolescents with and without suicide attempt. *Psychol Med* 43(10):2129–2142, 2013.
67. Osuch E, Ford K, Wrath A, Bartha R, Neufeld R: Functional MRI of pain application in youth who engaged in repetitive nonsuicidal self-injury vs. psychiatric controls. *Psychiatry Res* 223(2):104–112, 2013.
68. Bernert RA, Joiner TE: Sleep disturbance and suicide risk: a review of the literature. *Neuropsychiatr Dis Treat* 3(6):735–743, 2007.
69. Goldstein TR, Bridge JA, Brent DA: Sleep and suicidal behavior in adolescents. *J Consult Clin Psychol* 76(1):84–91, 2008.
70. Posner K, Brown GK, Stanley B, et al.: The Columbia-Suicide Severity Rating Scale: initial validity and internal consistency findings from three multisite studies with adolescents and adults. *Am J Psychiatry* 168:1266–1277, 2011.
71. Asarnow J, McArthur D, Hughes J, Barbery V, Berk M: Suicide attempt risk in youths: utility of the Harkavy-Asnis Suicide Scale for monitoring risk levels. *Suicide Life Threat Behav* 42(6):684–698, 2012.
72. Steer RA, Beck A: Use of the beck depression inventory, hopelessness scale, scale for suicidal ideation, and the suicidal intent scale with adolescents. *Adv Adolesc Mental Health* 3:219–231, 1988.
73. Pfeffer CR, Jiang H, Kakuma T: Child-Adolescent Suicidal Potential Index (CASPI): a screen for risk for early onset suicidal behavior. *Psychol Assess* 12:304–318, 2000.
74. Nock MK, Park JM, Finn CT, Deliberto TL, Dour HJ, Banaji MR: Measuring the "suicidal mind": implicit cognition predicts suicidal behavior. *Psychol Sci* 21:511–517, 2010.
75. Brent DA, McMakin DL, Kennard BD, Goldstein TR, Mayes TL, Douaihy AB: Protecting adolescents from self-harm: a critical review of intervention studies. *J Am Acad Child Adolesc Psychiatry* 52(12):1260–1271, 2013.
76. Rogers SC, DiVietro S, Borrup K, Brinkley A, Kaminer Y, Lapidus G: Restricting youth suicide: behavioral health patients in an urban pediatric emergency department. *J Trauma Acute Care Surg* 77(3 Suppl 1): S23–S28, 2014.
77. Grupp-Phelan J, McGuire L, Husky MM, Olfson M: A randomized controlled trial to engage in care of adolescent emergency department patients with mental health problems that increase suicide risk. *Pediatr Emerg Care* 28(12):1263–1268, 2012.
78. Asarnow JR, Berk M, Hughes JL, Anderson NL: The SAFETY Program: a treatment-development trial of a cognitive-behavioral family treatment for adolescent suicide attempters. *J Clin Child Adolesc Psychol* 44(1):194–203, 2015.
79. Richardson LP, Ludman E, McCauley E, et al.: Collaborative care for adolescents with depression in primary care: a randomized clinical trial. *JAMA* 312(8):809–816, 2014.
80. Ougrin D, Tranah R, Stahl D, Moran P, Asarnow JR: Therapeutic interventions for suicide attempts and self-harm in adolescents: systematic review and meta-analysis. *J Am Acad Child Adolesc Psychiatry* 54(2):97–107, 2015.
81. Glenn CR, Franklin JC, Nock MK: Evidence-based psychosocial treatments for self-injurious thoughts and behaviors in youth. *J Clin Child Adolesc Psychol* 44(1):1–29, 2015.
82. Mehlum L, Tørmoen AJ, Ramberg M, et al.: Dialectical behavior therapy for adolescents with repeated suicidal and self-harming behavior: A randomized trial. *J Am Acad Child Adolesc Psychiatry* 53(10):1082–1091, 2014.
83. Goldstein TR, Fersch-Podrat RK, Rivera M, et al.: Dialectical behavior therapy for adolescents with bipolar disorder: results from a pilot randomized trial. *J Child Adolesc Psychopharmacol* 25(2):140–149, 2015.
84. Diamond GS, Wintersteen MB, Brown GK, et al.: Attachment-based family therapy for adolescents with suicidal ideation: a randomized controlled trial. *J Am Acad Child Adol Psychiatry* 49: 122–131, 2010.
85. Rossouw TI, Fonagy P: Mentalization-based treatment for self-harm in adolescents: a randomized controlled trial. *J Am Acad Child Adolesc Psychiatry* 51:1304–1313, 2012.
86. Olfson M, Shaffer D, Marcus SC, Greenberg T: Relationship between antidepressant medication treatment and suicide in adolescents. *Arch Gen Psychiatry* 60(10):978–982, 2003.
87. Gibbons RD, Hur K, Bhaumik DK, Mann JJ: The relationship between antidepressant prescription rates and rate of early adolescent suicide. *Am J Psychiatry* 163(11):1898–1904, 2006.
88. Valuck RJ, Libby AM, Sills MR, Giese AA, Allen RR: Antidepressant treatment and risk of suicide attempt by adolescents with major depressive disorder: a propensity-adjusted retrospective cohort study. *CNS Drugs* 18(15):1119–1132, 2004.
89. The Treatment for Adolescents with Depression Study Team: Treatment for Adolescents with Depression Study (TADS): rationale, design, and methods. *J Am Acad Child Adolesc Psychiatry* 42(5):531–542, 2003.
90. Emslie G, Kratochvil C, Vitiello B, et al.: Treatment of Adolescents with Depression Study (TADS). *J Am Acad Child Adolesc Psychiatry* 45(12):1440–1455, 2006.
91. Posner K, Oquendo MA, Gould M, Stanley B, Davies M: Columbia Classification Algorithm of Suicidal Assessment (C-CASA): classification of suicidal events in the FDA's pediatric suicidal risk analysis of antidepressants. *Am J Psychiatry* 164:1035–1043, 2007.
92. Vitiello B, Silva SG, Rohde P, et al.: Suicidal events in the Treatment for Adolescents with Depression Study (TADS). *J Clin Psychiatry* 70(5):741–747, 2009.
93. Treatment for Adolescents with Depression Study (TADS) Team: The treatment for adolescents with depression study: outcomes over 1 year of naturalistic follow-up. *Am J Psychiatry* 166(10):1141–1149, 2009.
94. Brent D, Greenhill LL, Compton S, et al.: The Treatment of Adolescent Suicide Attempters (TASA) Study: predictors of suicidal events in an open trial. *J Am Acad Child Adolesc Psychiatry* 48(10):987–996, 2009.
95. Brent D, Emslie G, Clarke G, et al.: Switching to another SSRI or to venlafaxine with or without cognitive behavioral therapy for adolescents with SSRI-resistant depression: the TORDIA randomized controlled trial. *JAMA* 299(8):901–913, 2008.
96. Brent DA, Emslie GJ, Clarke GN, et al.: Predictors of spontaneous and systematically assessed suicidal adverse events in the treatment of SSRI-resistant depression in adolescents (TORDIA) study. *Am J Psychiatry* 166(4):418–426, 2009.
97. Asarnow JR, Porta G, Spirito A, et al.: Suicide attempts and nonsuicidal self-injury in the treatment of resistant depression in adolescents: findings from the TORDIA Study. *J Am Acad Child Adol Psychiatry* 50(8):772–781, 2011.
98. Wilkinson P, Kevin R, Roberts C, Dubicka B, Goodyer I: Clinical and psychosocial predictors of suicide attempts and nonsuicidal self-injury in the Adolescent Depression Antidepressants and Psychotherapy Trial (ADAPT). *Am J Psychiatry* 168:495–501, 2011.
99. Mosholder AD, Willy M: Suicidal adverse events in pediatric randomized, controlled clinical trials of antidepressant drugs are associated with active drug treatment: a meta-analysis. *J Child Adolesc Psychopharmacol* 16(1–2):25–32, 2006.
100. Hammad TA, Laughren T, Racoosin J: Suicidality in pediatric patients treated with antidepressant drugs. *Arch Gen Psychiatry* 63(3):332–339, 2006.
101. Pfeffer CR: The FDA pediatric advisories and changes in diagnosis and treatment of pediatric depression. *Am J Psychiatry* 164(6):843–846, 2007.
102. Goodman WK, Murphy TK, Storch EA: Risk of adverse behavioral effects with pediatric use of antidepressants. *Psychopharmacology (Berl)* 191(1):87–96, 2007.
103. Rihmer Z, Akiskal H: Do antidepressants t(h)reat(en) depressives? Toward a clinically judicious formulation of the antidepressant-suicidality FDA advisory in light of declining national suicide statistics from many countries. *J Affect Disord* 94(1–3):3–13, 2006.
104. Kaizar EE, Greenhouse JB, Seltman H, Kelleher K: Do antidepressants cause suicidality in children? A Bayesian meta-analysis. *Clin Trials* 3(2):73–90; discussion 91–98, 2006.
105. Libby AM, Orton HD, Valuck RJ: Persisting decline in depression treatment after FDA warnings. *Arch Gen Psychiatry* 66(6):633–639, 2009.
106. Mittal M, Harrison DL, Miller MJ, Brahm NC: National antidepressant prescribing in children and adolescents with mental health disorders after an FDA boxed warning. *Res Social Adm Pharm* 10(5):781–790, 2014.
107. Lu CY, Zhang F, Lakoma MD, et al.: Changes in antidepressant use by young people and suicidal behavior after FDA warnings and media coverage: quasi-experimental study. *BMJ* 348:g3596, 2014.
108. Grossman DC, Mueller BA, Riedy C, et al.: Gun storage practices and risk of youth suicide and unintentional firearm injuries. *JAMA* 293:707–714, 2005.
109. Webster DW, Vernick JS, Zeoli AM, Manganello JA: Association between youth-focused firearms laws and youth suicides. *JAMA* 292:594–601, 2004.

5.5 ■ ANXIETY DISORDERS

CHAPTER 5.5.1 ■ ANXIETY DISORDERS

JEROME H. TAYLOR, ELI R. LEBOWITZ, AND WENDY K. SILVERMAN

INTRODUCTION

Anxiety disorders are the most common psychiatric disorders in childhood (1–3) and are associated with poor quality of life, depression (4), and significant societal costs (5). Pediatric anxiety is also associated with poorer obesity intervention outcomes (6). Anxiety is the emotional, cognitive, and physiologic reaction related to real or imagined threat that may occur in the future. Fear is the reaction that occurs when confronted with an actual threat, like seeing a snake or while flying. Anxiety and fear are emotions that can be adaptive. Adaptive anxiety, for instance, can foster appropriate preparedness for possible challenges in the future. Anxiety is viewed as a "clinical disorder" when the anxious reaction becomes so intense that it causes psychic distress or interferes with functioning (e.g., academic performance, family/peer relationships). Many childhood anxieties are developmentally appropriate, highlighting the importance in considering the child's age as well as sociocultural context. For instance, an increase in separation anxiety distress and stranger anxiety are developmentally appropriate around age 8 months, with symptoms usually resolved by age 2 years. Similarly, preschoolers are often afraid of the dark and monsters, and it is common for youngsters in elementary school to be afraid during storms. Developmentally appropriate worries fade with time and do not interfere with functioning, making them distinguishable from anxiety disorders.

The tripartite view of anxiety postulates that individuals' anxious responses consist of three components: behavioral or motoric, cognitive or subjective, and physiologic (7). The behavioral or motoric components involve avoidance of the situations in which the negative stimulus may be encountered. The cognitive or subjective components involve apprehension and distress about an event in the future and often relates to difficulties with control of situations. Cognitions often also involve worst-case scenarios that are unlikely to occur but viewed likely by the child. Physiologically, anxiety involves autonomic arousal that can include elevated heart rate, hyperventilation, sweating, flushing, and other somatic symptoms. The settings that evoke children's anxiety distinguish the specific anxiety disorders from one another, though these three response components are generally present across all anxiety disorders (8,9). In this chapter we use "children" for youths under 18 years old unless referring to a specific developmental period.

EPIDEMIOLOGY

In this chapter, we review separation anxiety disorder (SAD), selective mutism (SM), specific phobia (SP), social anxiety disorder (also referred to as social phobia, SoP), panic disorder (PD), agoraphobia, and generalized anxiety disorder (GAD) in children and adolescents (Table 5.5.1.1). The age of onset of anxiety disorders is often determined by retrospective methods, and large prospective studies are lacking (10–12). The best estimates for prevalence in the United States are derived from the National Comorbidity Survey Replication Adolescent Supplement (NCSA) (3). The study surveyed a nationally representative cohort of 10,148 children 13 to 17 years old for DSM-IV diagnoses with structured in-person interviews. The prevalence and age of onset estimates were based on recall. Anxiety disorders were the most common mental health disorder with a 25% 12-month prevalence and 32% lifetime prevalence (posttraumatic stress disorder [PTSD] was included as an anxiety disorder and had a 4% 12-month prevalence and 5% lifetime prevalence with or without another comorbid anxiety disorder). Twelve-month and lifetime prevalence among adolescents for specific anxiety disorders were: SP—16%, 20%; SoP—8%, 9%; SAD—2%, 8%; agoraphobia—2%, 3%; PD—2%, 2%; and GAD—1%, 2% (3,13). SM was not included in NCSA, as this disorder was included as an anxiety disorder only in the 5th edition of the Diagnostic and Statistical Manual (14). In a study of 2,256 children in kindergarten to second grade, the point prevalence of SM was 0.7% (15,16). In NCSA, anxiety was less likely in adolescents whose parents were married or college graduates (2). In NCSA, girls were more likely than boys to have an anxiety disorder (2,3). However, study results have been mixed with regard to prevalence differences between boys and girls for pediatric anxiety disorders (10). For instance, a longitudinal study that followed children from latency to young adulthood found females were more likely than males to have an anxiety disorder in midadolescence and early adulthood but not overall (5).

The National Comorbidity Survey-Replication (NCSR) is the adult companion to the NCSA and the pediatric anxiety rates are based on retrospective reports. The median age of onset for anxiety disorders in the NCSR was 11 years (11). In NCSR, SoP, SP, and SAD began before adulthood in most cases; agoraphobia, PD, and GAD did not emerge in most cases until late adolescence or adulthood (11,13). In NCSR SAD was diagnosed based on DSM-IV criteria, which required onset of separation anxiety before age 18 years. DSM-5 removed the childhood-onset criterion for SAD, and thus NCSR likely underestimates the median age of onset for SAD. Silove et al. examined data from the World Mental Health Survey and found SAD onset can occur across the lifespan. The median age of SAD onset was in late adolescence in higher-income countries and in the mid-20s in lower-income countries (17). National studies on SM are lacking, though most studies suggest age of onset is usually before age 5 years (16).

SPECIFIC ANXIETY DISORDERS

In this section, we describe the DSM-5 anxiety disorders: SP, SAD, SoP, SM, PD, agoraphobia, and GAD (14). Illness anxiety disorder, which is based on the DSM-IV diagnosis hypochondriasis, was classified as a disorder related to somatic disorders in DSM-5 and is therefore not covered (14).

Specific Phobia

SP is an excessive fear of a specific object or situation. Exposure to the object or situation consistently results in immediate

TABLE 5.5.1.1

KEY FEATURES OF ANXIETY DISORDERS

DSM-5 Anxiety Disorder	Key Points
Separation anxiety disorder (SAD)	Excessive worry about being separated from caregiver Duration: >4 wks in children, 6 mo in adults
Selective mutism (SM)	Lack of speech in particular situations (e.g., school) despite talking in other settings Duration: >4 wks, not limited to the first month of school
Specific phobia (SP)	Excessive fear of a particular object or situation Duration: >6 mo
Social anxiety disorder (social phobia, SoP)	Excessive fear of social situations or being observed. Fear of negative evaluation. "Performance-only" specifier if symptoms only occur around performances Duration: >6 mo
Panic disorder (PD)	Multiple panic attacks without identifiable trigger. Persistent apprehension about having a panic attack and/or excessive behavioral changes to avoid having panic attack Duration: >4 wks *Note:* Panic attacks can occur with any anxiety disorder. Panic attacks peak within minutes and often include physical sensations and discomfort, dissociative experiences, and fear of dying or losing one's mind. A medical work-up is often indicated
Agoraphobia	Avoidance of two of the following situations: public transportation, open spaces, enclosed spaces, crowds, and being outside of the home. The avoidance is due to unrealistic fears of being trapped or inability to get help if panic-like or embarrassing symptoms arise, or in children fear of getting lost. PD not required Duration: >6 mo
Generalized anxiety disorder (GAD)	Intense worry about multiple everyday tasks or situations. In children, only one additional symptom (e.g., poor sleep, fatigue, poor concentration, restlessness, muscle tension) is needed. Duration >6 mo with symptoms on most days

excessive and irrational fear that may manifest as hiding, clinging, freezing, crying, screaming, vasovagal fainting (especially in blood and needle phobias), or autonomic arousal. Symptoms must last for 6 months and cause significant avoidant behavior and/or distress, as well as functional impairment. Phobias are divided into five categories: animals, natural environment (e.g., lightning, heights, darkness), blood-injection-injury (including other medical procedures), situational (e.g., flying, driving, bridges), and other (e.g., loud noises, choking, clowns). Research indicates that only 17% of children with SP have a single phobia, and most children have multiple phobias (18). After traumatic and frightening experiences, SP or PTSD may develop; SP is only diagnosed when the criteria for PTSD are not met.

Separation Anxiety Disorder

SAD is developmentally inappropriate anxiety or distress relating to separation from a major attachment figure or caretaker. Children with SAD may worry about being kidnapped or lost and/or that separation may result in death or injury to their parents, and they will be unable to see their caretakers again. SAD frequently presents after parental loss, a significant illness in the family or child, death of a pet, or other stressful events (19). SAD may present with children's refusal to sleep alone or be away from home and nightmares about separation. It is not uncommon for SAD to be associated with somatic symptoms such as headaches, stomachaches, muscle cramps, or dizziness. If somatic symptoms occur only when children are separated from attachment figures or when faced with separation (e.g., no somatic symptoms on weekends when there is no school), anxiety is likely rather than other medical etiologies. Young children with SAD may report seeing shadows of monsters when left alone, and are more likely to cling to their parents, follow them from room to room, and/or insist parental presence at all times (e.g., bathing). SAD may result in school refusal and can prevent playing with friends outside of the home, going to sleep overs, or participating in overnight camps. Symptoms of separation anxiety must have a duration of at least 4 weeks in children, and 6 months duration in adults.

Social Phobia (SoP)

SoP is also known as Social Anxiety Disorder. It is an excessive and impairing fear of being negatively evaluated by others. SoP must be accompanied by either avoidance of social situations or severe discomfort while enduring social situations. In children, the anxiety cannot be limited to discomfort in social situations with adults. Children with SoP are unlikely to approach peers and often feel like others are watching them. Children with SoP may worry others will think they are weird, ugly, stupid, or clumsy. If forced to attend social gatherings, children with SoP may throw a tantrum prior to the event, and younger children may cry, freeze, or cling to adults in social settings. Eye contact is often uncomfortable for children with SoP, posture may be overly rigid, and speech may be abnormally soft. Avoidance may involve retreating to one's room when company is present, eating lunch in a teacher's room instead of with other children, refusal to frequent public places such as malls or public restrooms (paruresis), and in severe cases almost complete self-isolation in the child's room, often accompanied by a reversal of diurnal cycles (20). Socially anxious children may worry about being judged by others who might notice physical symptoms of anxiety like blushing, sweating, or trembling voice. Most children and adolescents with SoP fear a variety of social situations, but when social anxiety is circumscribed to performing (e.g., sports, concerts, presentations), the diagnosis is "performance-only" SoP (14).

Before SoP is diagnosed, symptoms need to be present for 6 months and almost always occur in the feared social situation. Impairment helps distinguish between normative shyness and SoP. Examples of impairment include difficulties making or keeping friends, limited romantic relationships, school refusal, not participating in extracurricular activities, and significant child distress. Adolescents may abuse drugs prior to and/or during social situations in attempts to self-medicate. Family life also is often disrupted as the child's avoidance and impairment often constrains families' engagement in fun activities. The differential diagnosis includes avoidant personality disorder, which is sometimes conceptualized as a severe variant of SoP (21). Autism spectrum disorder is on the differential for SoP because social skills deficits from limited social interactions can mimic the social difficulties seen in autism spectrum disorder; however, children with SoP often have friends their own age and demonstrate improved social skills in established relationships. In many cases of autism spectrum disorder, a comorbid diagnosis of SoP is warranted.

Selective Mutism

SM is refusal to speak in particular settings. Children may speak at home but not school or in front of unfamiliar people. They may communicate by nodding, writing, or making sounds in lieu of speaking. Many children with SM rely on friends and parents to speak for them in social settings. Impairments due to SM include reduced class participation, academic underachievement, and isolation from peers. Symptoms must persist for 1 month and cannot be limited to the first month of school. The failure to speak cannot be due to a physical inability to speak. Children with SM are often shy and usually have comorbid social phobia (16); however, some enjoy participating in social activities that do not require speaking. Communication and developmental disorders are frequently comorbid with SM (22), and children with SM, communication, and developmental disorders all present with a lack of speech. What distinguishes children with SM from children with communication and developmental disorders is that the former have an ability to speak in certain social contexts but not in others (22).

Panic Disorder

PD is defined by having panic attacks, at least some of which *do not* have identifiable precipitants. A panic attack is a set of distressing symptoms that classically peak within 10 to 15 minutes. Physical symptoms include trembling, dizziness, palpitations, difficulties breathing, nausea, and vomiting. Derealization (i.e., out-of-body experiences) and fear of dying and/or losing one's mind may also occur. Ruling out medical etiologies is required before diagnosing panic attacks. Medical causes for panic-like symptoms include cardiac arrhythmias, hyperthyroidism, hyperparathyroidism, seizures, vestibular disorders, asthma, and neuroendocrine tumors like pheochromocytoma. In collaboration with the pediatrician, a medical evaluation including physical examination, laboratory tests, and an EKG (especially in the case of cardiac symptoms) should be considered. Cardiology consultation should also be considered. Once medical causes are ruled out, it is important to determine whether the panic attacks are evoked by stimuli associated with other disorders (e.g., panic in social evaluative settings may suggest a diagnosis of Social Anxiety with Panic Attacks). When panic attacks occur solely in response to particular situations, PD is not diagnosed. Children with PD have panic attacks without an identifiable cause and may have additional panic attacks that are associated with exposure to specific situations. Nocturnal panic attacks, which awaken an individual from sleep, are usually pathognomonic for PD.

Key to PD diagnosis is the presence of worry about having a panic attack or behavioral changes in attempts to avoid an attack or reduce possible harm due to an attack. Children with PD may not take stairs or participate in sports because of beliefs that increased heart rate might trigger a panic attack. They may only go outside with others who could help if an attack occurs. The worry or behavioral changes must be present for at least 1 month. Increased anxiety sensitivity, or the fear of anxiety-related sensations (e.g., increased heart rate, dizziness, or derealization) due to beliefs that these sensations have harmful physical, psychological, or social consequences is particularly common in PD, though anxiety sensitivity is experienced by children with other anxiety disorders as well (23,24). Somatic symptom disorder is similar to PD in that troubling somatic symptoms are often prominent. However, in PD, somatic symptoms usually present in relatively brief and intense episodes in contrast to the persistently present symptoms of somatic symptom disorder (14).

Agoraphobia

Agoraphobia is a fear of being unable to escape or get help in the event of overwhelming or embarrassing symptoms (e.g., panic symptoms). Avoidance must occur in at least two types of setting categories. The five categories of avoided situations are (1) public transportation, (2) open spaces (e.g., bridges, parking lots), (3) enclosed spaces (e.g., stores, basements, elevators), (4) crowded areas, and (5) anywhere outside of the home alone. In agoraphobic children a prominent fear is getting lost. Symptoms often begin following parental loss, life-threatening situations, or other scary situations that may produce feelings of helplessness. Agoraphobia can occur with or without PD (e.g., if fear of fainting leads to the avoidance, PD is not diagnosed). Symptoms usually last at least 6 months before a diagnosis is made. As in agoraphobia, children with SAD may fear getting lost and/or leaving home. In SAD, however, the fear relates to separation from the caretaker and not seeing the caretaker again. In agoraphobia the fear is about encountering a dire situation in which help is needed but unavailable. Further, unlike the commonly early onset for SAD, agoraphobia does not typically have an onset until late adolescence and early adulthood.

Generalized Anxiety Disorder

GAD is characterized by impairing worry about multiple situations for at least 6 months. Children with GAD express worry about potentially negative occurrences on most days, and the focus of the worry may shift from topic to topic. The anxiety in GAD is often difficult to control and interferes with completing tasks or enjoying activities, which helps to distinguish pathologic from normal anxiety. Children with GAD may have difficulties falling or staying asleep, fatigue, trouble focusing, muscle tension, or irritability, and worry must be accompanied by one of these symptoms in childhood GAD (note, diagnosis of GAD in adults requires worry be accompanied by three of these symptoms). Anxieties in GAD often involve everyday matters like completing assignments, being on time, getting good grades, and performance in sports. Worry about anticipated changes and dangerous situations like storms, home invasion, or a family member getting sick is also common. The worries can sometimes be fantastical (e.g., monsters in the basement) or extreme (e.g., terrorist attacks). Children with GAD may seek reassurance about their performance or safety frequently. GAD may also present as perfectionism, indecision for fear of making a poor choice, and a tendency to magnify minor mistakes. Somatic symptoms also often manifest including headaches and stomachaches. There is significant overlap between depressive and GAD symptoms, including sleep changes, low energy, difficulties concentrating, psychomotor changes, and irritability (particularly common in adolescent depression). In addition to symptom overlap, there is significant overlap in the age prevalence curves of GAD and depression (5): they both are relatively uncommon in younger children and increase throughout adolescence and young adulthood.

COMORBIDITY

The various anxiety disorders have many overlapping symptoms and somatic manifestations. Anxiety disorders are highly comorbid with each other and other disorders. GAD is the anxiety disorder most likely to be comorbid with another anxiety or mood disorders. In NCSA, children with GAD had a 66% lifetime comorbidity rate with other anxiety disorders: 41% with SP; 21% with SAD; and 20% with SoP (25). Children with GAD had a 59% lifetime comorbidity rate with mood disorders (e.g., major depression, dysthymia, and bipolar). In the large prospective Great Smoky Mountain Study (GSMS), described in detail in the "course of illness" section below, GAD increased the odds of having every other anxiety disorder, except agoraphobia (but there was a trend that linked GAD and agoraphobia, $p = 0.06$) (5). Still, GAD was more closely associated with depression than any other individual anxiety disorder. The converse was also true—depression had a stronger association with GAD than the other individual anxiety disorders. GAD also increased the odds of having a behavioral disorder, which included conduct disorder, oppositional defiant disorder (ODD), attention-deficit hyperactivity disorder (ADHD), and substance disorders.

SoP was associated with drug-use disorders but not alcohol-use disorders in NCSA (26). In GSMS, SoP was most tightly associated with SP with over one-half of patients with SoP meeting criteria for SP during the course of the study (5). SoP was also associated with GAD, depression, and agoraphobia. For SP, the more types of SPs that adolescents in NCSA had, the more likely they were to have mood disorders and ADHD (18). The blood-injection-injury SP subtype was specifically associated with ADHD and children with situational-type SPs (e.g., flying, bridges) were more likely to be diagnosed with conduct disorder. Adolescents with anxiety disorders in NCSA had higher lifetime prevalence of intermittent explosive disorder (23%) compared to adolescents without a history of anxiety (8% intermittent explosive disorder prevalence), and the association was particularly robust between intermittent explosive disorder and SoP and PD (27). Interestingly, although PD and agoraphobia commonly co-occur, PD was more strongly associated with GAD, depression, and SAD in childhood through young adulthood in GSMS relative to agoraphobia (5). SoP and developmental disorders are frequently comorbid with SM (16,28). In a sample of children 3 to 17 years old with SM, 68% had SoP, 43% had a phonologic disorder, 32% had an elimination disorder, 17% had a developmental coordination disorder, and 17% had mixed expressive–receptive language disorder (22).

COURSE OF ILLNESS

A tendency toward negative affectivity (i.e., experiencing fear, shame, anger, sadness, and low self-esteem) is widely observed in children before they develop anxiety disorders (29). Many children with SoP displayed patterns of behavioral inhibition (avoidance of novel experiences) in the first few years of life (30). Once childhood anxiety disorders develop, they tend to be chronic (3,31). SAD is the anxiety disorder least likely to be chronic (17). In NCSA 79% of teenagers who were previously diagnosed with SAD no longer met criteria during the previous 12 months, and in NCSR 64% of childhood SAD cases resolved by adulthood (3,32). SAD with comorbid ODD and severe ADHD is more likely to persist into adulthood (33). Rates of partial or full remission in NCSA for the previous year were 9% in SoP, 18% in SP, 18% in PD, 25% in agoraphobia, 49% in GAD, and 79% in SAD (partial or full remission defined as no longer meeting full diagnostic criteria during the past year) (2,3). Children whose social phobia persists into adulthood are less likely to achieve full occupational potential and have fulfilling social relationships (34). Studies with small samples have found most but not all children with SM improve by young adulthood, with more severe cases having poorer outcomes (35). Larger longitudinal studies of SM are needed.

Prospective longitudinal studies are best suited to track the course of illness. The Great Smokey Mountain Study (GSMS) was a prospective longitudinal study designed to examine the course of mental illness from childhood to early adulthood (36). The study began in the 1992 and has followed the cohort for nearly 25 years (37). GSMS had 1,420 participants from predominantly rural communities in North Carolina, United States. Participants were 9 to 13 years old at enrollment. Copeland et al. (2014) examined the course of anxiety from age 9 years to 26 years (36). GSMS found childhood anxiety disorders were associated with poorer outcomes in young adulthood. Specifically, childhood SAD was associated with poorer self-reported medical health (e.g., smoking, obesity, chronic illnesses) in young adulthood. Childhood SoP was associated with poorer self-reported interpersonal outcomes (quality of relationship with friends and loved ones) in young adulthood. Childhood GAD was associated with poorer self-reported health and financial outcomes (poverty, debt level) as a young adult (5). Moreover, children with GAD are at increased risk for developing depression, and the temporal association is bidirectional—that is, having GAD as a child increases the risk for adulthood depression and having major depression as a child increases the risk for adult-onset GAD (38).

A study examining GSMS data of children aged 9 to 16 years found a trend toward an association between anxiety and subsequent suicidality (defined as intrusive thoughts of wanting to die, kill oneself, or a suicide attempt) (odds ratio = 2.5, $p = 0.07$ after adjusting for comorbid disorders and demographic characteristics) (39). The analysis found a significant association between depression and subsequent suicidality (adjusted odds ratio = 21.7, $p < 0.05$). Risk for suicidality was greatest for those with comorbid depression and GAD (39).

ETIOLOGY

Learning is viewed as key in the etiology and maintenance of phobias and anxiety disorders (40). Rachman theorized three pathways (41). First, children may learn to fear stimuli verbally—that is, from others saying certain stimuli are dangerous. Second, children may learn vicariously by observing others experience distress when confronted with certain stimuli. Third, children may learn to avoid certain stimuli based on their own direct traumatic experiences. There are two types of learning processes involved in etiology and maintenance: classical conditioning and operant conditioning. Classical conditioning, also known as Pavlovian conditioning, occurs when a neutral stimulus is paired with an aversive stimulus (e.g., an electric shock) repeatedly such that the neutral stimulus becomes associated with distress. The automatic and associative learning in classical conditioning is thought to play a role in the development of phobias and anxiety disorders (e.g., a child develops a water phobia after a near-drowning experience) (42). The other learning process is operant conditioning, which occurs when an individual makes a choice based on desired outcomes (reinforcements) and/or displeasing consequences (punishments) that have resulted from the choice previously. For instance, after a child is humiliated in front of a peer group, operant conditioning may motivate the child to voluntarily avoid social interactions. Volitional avoidance of threatening stimuli contributes to the disability associated with anxiety disorders. While learning may contribute to the development of anxiety disorders, other mechanisms are also implicated.

Risk factors for developing anxiety disorders include physical or sexual abuse, parental loss, early-life stressors, parental overprotectiveness, and overcontrolling parental behaviors (43,44). A meta-analysis that included data on 8,907 children found insecure attachment, particularly ambivalent attachment, was associated with anxiety disorder development (45). Early-life stressors can affect brain development (46). Gee et al. used functional magnetic resonance imaging to examine the amygdala–medial prefrontal cortex connectivity of 41 healthy children 6 to 17 years old who had been institutionalized in orphanages in various other countries for an average of 22 months before age 8 and compared these previously institutionalized scans to the scans of 48 never-institutionalized youths. At the time of the study, the previously institutionalized children were living with high-income adoptive families in the United States. The study found that children with a history of being institutionalized had more mature amygdala–medial prefrontal cortex connectivity relative to children without histories of institutionalization (47). The changes were mediated by cortisol, intimating the changes in connectivity were related to stress and hypothalamic–pituitary–adrenal axis activity. The connections between the prefrontal cortex and amygdala are often described as the "fear circuit" (48–50), and it is possible that the impact of early-life stress on this circuit partially explains the link between early childhood adversity and anxiety disorders. In addition to the amygdala and prefrontal cortex, the hippocampus and cingulate gyrus are thought to be involved in the neurocircuitry of anxiety (48,51,52).

Anxiety disorders are caused by both genetic and environmental factors. Heritability is the proportion of the illness likely due to genetics and ranges from 0% to 100%. Estimates of anxiety disorder heritability have ranged from 20% to 50% in twin studies (53–55). Several studies have investigated the role of the serotonin transporter gene promoter (5-HTTLPR) in anxiety, though the findings are equivocal. However, a meta-analysis in 2013 found that the short allele of 5-HTTLPR had a small but statistically significant effect on amygdala reactivity (56). Similarly, a 2013 meta-analysis found the 5-HTTLPR genotype was associated with cortisol stress reactivity (57). Amygdala response to potential threats and cortisol stress reactivity have been implicated in anxiety disorder etiology (47,48). Further research is needed to clarify whether 5-HTTLPR plays a role in anxiety.

Anxiety disorders run in families, and children of anxious parents are more likely to exhibit clinical levels of anxiety than children of nonanxious parents, a consistent finding that has been confirmed in large-scale population studies (58,59). Although this is explained in part by shared genetics, nongenetic factors also contribute to the heritability of anxiety disorders. Anxious caregivers may promote more avoidance in the child by providing higher levels of family accommodation, or changes to their own behavior aimed at helping the child avoid or alleviate distress related to the anxiety (60,61). More anxious parents may also directly model fearful and avoidant behavior, providing the child with more opportunities for vicarious fear learning and with less modeling of nonavoidant coping skills (62).

While anxiety disorders share many risk factors, presumably there are etiologic distinctions underlying each disorder. For instance, one hypothesis posits that PD may be due to high anxiety sensitivity or oversensitivity to physiologic arousal (23,24). The cycle of recognizing benign physical variance in breathing and heart rate results in worry, which in turn increases physical arousal, self-perpetuating the spiral toward a panic attack. Evidence also points toward an oversensitivity to carbon dioxide (CO_2) as a cause for PD (i.e., suffocation model) (63). Both SAD and PD patients are likely to experience panic-like symptoms when exposed to CO_2-enriched air (64). Of note, SAD is a risk factor for subsequently developing PD (65,66). Studies have found genetic factors common to SAD and PD likely influence sensitivity to CO_2 (19,48). Also, it is theorized that many SPs have an evolutionary basis because exaggerated fears of dangerous animals or natural environments may have conferred a survival advantage earlier in human history (67). In addition to genetic predisposition, many phobias have an identifiable traumatic or frightening experience that resulted in the development of SP. Recent research has implicated the oxytocinergic system in childhood anxiety disorders, in particular in the anxious children's reliance on parents for proximity and family accommodation. Children with SAD were found to have lower levels of peripheral oxytocin compared to anxious children with other anxiety disorders, and the oxytocin levels were significantly linked to the degree of family accommodation reported by the mothers (68). Furthermore, a follow-up study found that the differences in oxytocin levels were no longer apparent after the children were allowed to interact with their mothers for a few minutes (69).

ASSESSMENT

The gold standard for assessing childhood anxiety in research studies is the Anxiety Disorders Interview Schedule—Child and Parents (70). Whether in research or clinical settings, a multisource, multimethod assessment approach is useful for accurate and valid assessment of childhood anxiety. There is moderate agreement on anxiety levels between parent and child reports of anxiety, and child–parent agreement is usually higher for children older than 12 years (71). Becker et al. (72) found child–parent agreement was higher on overt behavioral symptoms of SAD and school refusal compared with the less overt symptoms in SoP and GAD. Clinical assessment tools include rating scales for anxiety disorder screening, diagnosis, and monitoring treatment effects, and most include parent and child versions (see Byrne et al., 2017 for review) (73,74). The Screen for Child Anxiety Related Disorders (SCARED) is a scale commonly used to screen for anxiety with child self-rating and parent-rating versions (75). The Multidimensional Anxiety Scale for Children 2 (MASC2) is another commonly used scale with child self-rating and parent-rating versions (76). The Pediatric Anxiety Rating Scale (PARS) has questions for the child and parent, and the final score is based on clinician ratings of frequency, severity, and impairment due to symptoms (77). The Family Accommodation Scale—Anxiety (FASA) (60,78) is the most widely used scale for assessing family accommodation, or the degree to which parents change their own behavior to help their child avoid feeling anxious. There are both parent and child report versions of FASA and the total accommodation score is based on the ratings of frequency of various forms of accommodation (e.g., providing reassurance to the child).

In children presenting with anxiety, it is important to rule out substance/medication-induced anxiety. Medications that can cause anxiety include albuterol, oral steroids, pseudoephedrine, stimulants, and bupropion. Importantly, although stimulants may provoke anxiety, a 2015 meta-analysis found that in children with ADHD, stimulant treatment had a lower risk of anxiety as a side effect compared to placebo (79). Many antidepressants including selective serotonin reuptake inhibitors (SSRIs) and serotonin norepinephrine reuptake inhibitors (SNRIs) can cause anxiety, particularly at initiation. Fenfluramine/phentermine and other diet supplements are often anxiogens. Withdrawal from short-acting benzodiazepines can also present with anxiety symptoms. A wide array of illicit substances including marijuana, cocaine, anabolic steroids (e.g., testosterone), hallucinogens, and phencyclidine can result in anxiety. Use and withdrawal from nicotine and caffeine can produce anxiety. Environmental etiologies of anxiety include exposure to organophosphates and ingestion of lead in paint chips, arsenic in soil, and other toxic metals.

TREATMENT

A primary goal of treatment is for children to learn how to manage and cope with their excessive and impairing anxiety. Given the high comorbidity of the anxiety disorders, it is common to target the most impairing anxiety disorder first. In this way, success can be attained and the child comes to understand that the anxiety is manageable, and that the skills learned can be applied to the comorbid problems. Treatment of anxiety disorders affecting sleep should also be prioritized (80). First-line interventions for childhood anxiety disorders are cognitive behavioral therapy (CBT) (81) and treatment with SSRI (82–84).

PSYCHOTHERAPY

CBT is a first-line treatment for pediatric anxiety (85–87). CBT for anxiety usually includes psychoeducation about anxiety, self-monitoring of emotions and somatic manifestations of anxiety, relaxation techniques (e.g., deep breathing and progressive muscle relaxation), tracking behavioral patterns contributing to anxiety, graded exposure to feared stimuli, identification of thoughts (e.g., negative self-talk) that influence feelings, cognitive restructuring, problem-solving skills, reward systems, and relapse prevention. Practicing skills between sessions is a key element of CBT. Parents receive psychoeducation and help execute the behavioral reward system (88). CBT is usually comprised of 50- to 60-minute individual sessions every week for 12 to 20 weeks. Variations on CBT include Panic Control Treatment for Adolescents (PCTA), which includes traditional CBT elements and adds exposure to feared bodily sensations like hyperventilation or tachycardia (i.e., interoceptive exposure) in order to treat PD (89). For SP, a randomized controlled trial (RCT) found that one 3-hour CBT session was efficacious (90). Group CBT with concurrent child groups and parent groups are also effective in treating childhood anxiety (91), and have outcomes similar to individual CBT (92). It is possible that an exception is for children with SoP, who may benefit more from individual CBT relative to group CBT, but more research is needed (93). Web-based CBT with minimal therapist support is also efficacious (94).

Silk et al. found CBT was more effective than supportive therapy in pediatric anxiety. In an RCT comparing individual CBT with child-centered supportive therapy, remission rates (i.e., no longer meeting diagnostic criteria for SoP, GAD, or SAD) were higher for children randomized to CBT (67%) relative to supportive therapy (47%), and CBT superiority was maintained at 1-year follow-up (95). However, another study found that CBT and usual care in an urban mental health clinic had similar primary anxiety disorder remission rates—58% in usual care and 50% in CBT (96). Less robust findings in effectiveness trials (as opposed to efficacy trials) highlight the need for more community studies beyond the more carefully protocolized RCTs (92). Recent work has begun to pool the findings of studies that have been conducted (86,87). A 2012 meta-analysis found that among psychotherapeutic interventions for anxious youth, CBT has the most evidence with a small to medium effect size relative to active treatment controls (97).

Social effectiveness training is an evidence-based treatment for SoP that combines social skills training and behavioral therapy. A 12-week RCT of children with SoP found social effectiveness training was more effective than fluoxetine (98). In social effectiveness training, children had two sessions per week—one group session and one individual session. Social skills training was conducted in group format and included lessons on initiating and maintaining conversation, joining groups of peers, and nonverbal skills like eye contact. Immediately after social skills training, the group practiced the social skills during social outings (e.g., bowling, visiting museums, or going out to eat) aimed at "peer generalization" of the skills. Individual sessions included exposures based on the unique social fears of the child. After 12 weeks, remission rates were 53% with social effectiveness training, 21% with fluoxetine, and 3% with placebo. The treatment gains from social effectiveness training are especially notable because children with SoP generally have poorer treatment outcomes compared to children with other anxiety disorders (99,100). Furthermore, a prior study found that children with SoP who received only CBT had poorer outcomes than children who received SSRI (101).

Bergman et al. conducted an RCT in which 21 children (age 4 to 8 years) with SM were randomized to a waitlist control group or a 24-week behavioral intervention. The behavioral intervention included graded exposure to speech, a reward system, parent and teacher involvement, and some cognitive restructuring when developmentally appropriate. The intervention had a 75% treatment response rate, while the waitlisted group did not significantly improve (101). An RCT by Oerbeck et al. with 24 children (3 to 9 years old) with SM found a 3-month intervention with a behavioral reward system, an in-home component, and an in-school component involving teachers and peers was efficacious, while children on the waitlist did not improve (102). Younger children with SM had better outcomes in both studies. A pilot study by Ooi et al. randomized 21 Singaporean children (age 6 to 12 years) to a therapist-guided web-based CBT program for 14 weeks or the control group in which children played computer games while interacting with the therapist. Children in both groups improved and there were no between-group differences (103). Unlike prior studies, the web-based CBT was compared to an active control instead of a waitlist control. Furthermore, unlike other randomized trials with behavioral intervention components, in this web-based intervention the parent and teacher components were supplementary and not included in the pilot study. In summary, there is evidence for behavior interventions in children with SM when parents and teachers are active participants in the treatment program. Effective behavioral interventions for SM included psychoeducation, behavioral reward systems, and graded exposure. SM treatment should focus on social and academic functioning. Finally, once the child begins to speak, overzealous celebration can result in regression.

Limited evidence supports the use of psychodynamic psychotherapy for pediatric anxiety. In psychodynamic terms, anxiety can be viewed in the context of unacceptable desires and defense mechanisms used to respond to the desires. Failings of defense mechanisms can cause anxiety that interferes with function (104). Gottken et al. (2014) used short-term manualized psychoanalytic child therapy (PaCT) in weekly sessions for 6 months in 30 children (4 to 10 years old) with any DSM-IV anxiety disorder (the most common anxiety disorders were SP and GAD). PaCT included 5 to 6 parent sessions, which focused on improving the parent–child relationship, mentalizing capacity, and parental reflective functioning. Three children (10%)

dropped out. Eighteen children (60%) achieved remission with PaCT and no children achieved remission on the waitlist. Remission was defined as no longer meeting criteria for any anxiety disorder (105).

Children with histories of autism spectrum disorder, bipolar, and psychosis have been excluded from many large RCT examining interventions in pediatric anxiety (85,106). However, multiple studies have demonstrated that CBT is effective in reducing anxiety in children with autism spectrum disorder and comorbid anxiety (107–111). Studies examining effective treatments for anxiety in children with histories of bipolar disorders and psychotic disorders are needed.

PHARMACOLOGIC

SSRIs are effective treatments in pediatric anxiety (83,85,106,112). Serotonin and norepinephrine reuptake inhibitors (SNRIs) are also effective in pediatric anxiety; however, there is substantially more evidence supporting the efficacy and tolerability of SSRI. A 2015 meta-analysis of RCTs investigating the efficacy of SSRIs and SNRIs found a medium effect size (Cohen's $d = 0.62$) relative to placebo in SAD, SoP, and GAD. Medications with more serotonergic specificity had a greater effect size in post hoc analyses—sertraline and fluvoxamine had effect sizes >1.4 and paroxetine, fluoxetine, venlafaxine, and duloxetine had effect sizes <0.7 (84). The meta-analysis did not find evidence of increased risk for suicidality with antidepressants; however, there was a strong trend toward activation (odds ratio = 1.86, $p = 0.054$).

There are few pharmacologic RCTs conducted on SM, and most are limited by very small samples. One of the largest pharmacologic trials was conducted by Black and Uhde in which 15 children 6 to 12 years old with SM were randomized to double-blind treatment with either fluoxetine or placebo for 12 weeks. There were no significant differences in clinician- and teacher-ratings between the two groups at the end of the study, though parents rated significant improvements in SM symptoms in children who were randomized to fluoxetine. Most children in both groups continued to have considerable impairment due to SM (113). Fluoxetine was well tolerated, and there was no significant difference in side effects between the fluoxetine and placebo group. In short, SSRIs may reduce symptoms in SM, though more research is needed (114).

There is a dearth of evidence for other medications in childhood anxiety. An 8-week small open-label study investigating the efficacy of mirtazapine in 18 children 8 to 17 years old with SoP had a 56% response rate, and 22% discontinued due to adverse effects; mirtazapine also caused significant weight gain (3.3 kg) (115). Geller et al. found atomoxetine, which selectively inhibits norepinephrine reuptake, improved anxiety and ADHD symptoms in children with both disorders (116). RCTs examining the efficacy of benzodiazepines in pediatric anxiety have been negative, but the studies may have been underpowered (117,118). An unpublished Bristol-Meyers Squibb 2010 RCT with 559 children found buspirone (15 to 60 mg/day in divided doses) for 6 weeks was not significantly more effective than placebo in reducing pediatric anxiety (83). Evidence for the use of tricyclic acids is lacking. Given the substantial evidence for SSRIs relative to other agents, multiple SSRIs should be tried prior to trials of other psychotropic agents in pediatric anxiety.

CHILD/ADOLESCENT ANXIETY MULTIMODAL STUDY

The Child/Adolescent Anxiety Multimodal Study (CAMS) is the largest RCT investigating treatments for anxious youth. CAMS randomized 488 children aged 7 to 17 years who met DSM-IV criteria for GAD, SoP, or SAD to 12 weeks of treatment with sertraline (SSRI), CBT, combined sertraline and CBT, or pill placebo (85,119,120). Combined treatment was most efficacious, there were no significant differences between sertraline and CBT, and placebo had the poorest outcomes. Remission rates, or no longer meeting diagnostic criteria at week 12, were 68% with combined treatment, 46% with sertraline, 46% with CBT, and 24% with placebo (100). Response rates (i.e., "much improved" or "very much improved" on the Clinician Global Impression-Improvement scale) at week 12 were 81% for children in combined treatment, 61% for CBT, 55% for sertraline, and 24% in placebo (85). In severe anxiety, combined treatment is usually needed to achieve symptom remission (121,122). In milder anxiety, given the high response rates to monotherapy with CBT, CBT should be considered before medications.

A predictor and moderator analysis of the CAMS study by Compton et al. found patients with SoP had superior outcomes when sertraline was included in the treatment regimen and that patients with GAD had greater reductions in anxiety if CBT was included in the regimen (100). Superior outcomes with medication in SoP may be due to youth who may be too socially anxious to fully engage in psychotherapy. Children with SAD particularly benefitted from combined treatment relative to children with other anxiety disorders. Older age, minority status (i.e., either non-White race or Hispanic ethnicity), more severe baseline anxiety, having comorbid depression or additional anxiety disorders, and the presence of SoP were associated with a lower likelihood of symptom remission (99).

There was no significant difference in spontaneously reported physical or psychiatric side effects in youth who received sertraline (dosed 25 to 200 mg) or placebo in CAMS (123). Children aged 12 years and younger reported more adverse events than older children with sertraline (4% in adolescents vs. 16% in children 12 years old and under). Children who received sertraline were most likely to report increased trouble with sleeping on the Physical Symptom Checklist (28% in sertraline, 16% CBT, 15% combined, 13% placebo). There were no suicide attempts in any treatment condition in CAMS.

The acute responders, or those whose symptoms improved at week 12, in CAMS were followed for 6 additional months (119). Children who received CBT were given monthly booster sessions and children prescribed sertraline received monthly medication appointments. Children were allowed to have additional treatment from providers outside of the study during the 6 months of follow-up. At 6 months, combined treatment demonstrated slight superiority over monotherapy, and CBT and sertraline continued to have similar outcomes at 6 months (119). In a naturalistic study, 288 of the children in CAMS were followed for a mean of 6 years in Child/Adolescent Anxiety Multimodal Extended Long-term Study (CAMELS) (124). Nearly half (47%) of the children in CAMELS were in remission. A greater percentage of acute responders were in remission than nonresponders (52% remission in acute responders and 38% in acute nonresponders). Male sex and better baseline family functioning were predictors of remission at 6 years.

OTHER INTERVENTIONS

CAMS provided support for the use of CBT and SSRIs as first-line treatments in childhood anxiety. However, many children do not respond to first-line treatments. Attention bias modification, which aims to reduce anxious children's unconscious predilection to pay over-attention to threatening stimuli has demonstrated success in RCTs (125–127). Parent-based programs aimed at reducing family accommodation by parents such as Supportive Parenting for Anxious Childhood Emotions (SPACE) are also showing promise (128).

CONCLUSION

In summary, pediatric anxiety disorders are common, and diagnosis requires functional impairment or substantial distress. Further evidence is needed to determine the precise etiology of anxiety disorders; however, the evidence suggests that both genetic and environmental factors play a role in the development of anxiety disorders. During the last decade, several studies have confirmed the efficacy of SSRIs and CBT. Future research is needed to identify effective interventions for children whose anxiety does not remit with SSRIs or CBT. Finally, future studies should examine how psychiatric comorbidities like bipolar spectrum disorders affect treatment efficacy.

References

1. Merikangas KR, Nakamura EF, Kessler RC: Epidemiology of mental disorders in children and adolescents. *Dialogues Clin Neurosci* 11(1):7–20, 2009.
2. Merikangas KR, He J-p, Burstein M, et al.: Lifetime prevalence of mental disorders in US adolescents: results from the National Comorbidity Survey Replication–Adolescent Supplement (NCS-A). *J Am Acad Child Adolesc Psychiatry* 49(10):980–989, 2010.
3. Kessler RC, Avenevoli S, Costello EJ, et al.: Prevalence, persistence, and sociodemographic correlates of DSM-IV disorders in the National Comorbidity Survey Replication Adolescent Supplement. *Arch Gen Psychiatry* 69(4):372–380, 2012.
4. Avenevoli S, Swendsen J, He J-P, Burstein M, Merikangas KR: Major depression in the National Comorbidity Survey–Adolescent Supplement: prevalence, correlates, and treatment. *J Am Acad Child Adolesc Psychiatry* 54(1):37–44. e32, 2015.
5. Copeland WE, Angold A, Shanahan L, Costello EJ: Longitudinal patterns of anxiety from childhood to adulthood: the Great Smoky Mountains Study. *J Am Acad Child Adolesc Psychiatry* 53(1):21–33, 2014.
6. Taylor J, Xu Y, Li F, et al.: Psychosocial predictors and moderators of weight management programme outcomes in ethnically diverse obese youth. *Pediatr Obes* 2016.
7. Lang PJ: *Fear Reduction and Fear Behavior: Problems in Treating a Construct. Paper Presented at: Research in Psychotherapy Conference, 3rd, May-Jun, 1966,* Chicago, IL, US 1968.
8. Rachman S: Human fears: a three systems analysis. *Cogn Behav Ther* 7(4):237–245, 1978.
9. Chorpita BF: The tripartite model and dimensions of anxiety and depression: an examination of structure in a large school sample. *J Abnorm Child Psychol* 30(2):177–190, 2002.
10. Perou R, Bitsko RH, Blumberg SJ, et al.: Mental health surveillance among children—United States, 2005–2011. *MMWR Surveill Summ* 62(Suppl 2):1–35, 2013.
11. Kessler RC, Berglund P, Demler O, Jin R, Merikangas KR, Walters EE: Lifetime prevalence and age-of-onset distributions of DSM-IV disorders in the National Comorbidity Survey Replication. *Arch Gen Psychiatry* 62(6):593–602, 2005.
12. Costello EJ, Egger HL, Copeland W, Erkanli A, Angold A: The developmental epidemiology of anxiety disorders: phenomenology, prevalence, and comorbidity. *Anxiety Disord Child Adolesc Res Assess Intervent* 2:56–75, 2011.
13. Kessler RC, Petukhova M, Sampson NA, Zaslavsky AM, Wittchen HU: Twelve month and lifetime prevalence and lifetime morbid risk of anxiety and mood disorders in the United States. *Int J Methods Psychiatr Res* 21(3):169–184, 2012.
14. American Psychiatric Association: *Diagnostic and Statistical Manual of Mental Disorders.* 5th ed. 2013.
15. Bergman RL, Piacentini J, McCracken JT: Prevalence and description of selective mutism in a school-based sample. *J Am Acad Child Adolesc Psychiatry* 41(8):938–946, 2002.
16. Viana AG, Beidel DC, Rabian B: Selective mutism: a review and integration of the last 15 years. *Clin Psychol Rev* 29(1):57–67, 2009.
17. Silove D, Alonso J, Bromet E, et al.: Pediatric-onset and adult-onset separation anxiety disorder across countries in the World Mental Health Survey. *Am J Psychiatry* 172(7):647–656, 2015.
18. Burstein M, Georgiades K, He JP, et al.: Specific phobia among US adolescents: phenomenology and typology. *Depress Anxiety* 29(12):1072–1082, 2012.
19. Battaglia M, Pesenti-Gritti P, Medland SE, Ogliari A, Tambs K, Spatola CA: A genetically informed study of the association between childhood separation anxiety, sensitivity to CO2, panic disorder, and the effect of childhood parental loss. *Arch Gen Psychiatry* 66(1):64–71, 2009.
20. Lebowitz ER, King RA, Silverman WK: Anxiety disorders of childhood and adolescence. In: Ebert M, Leckman JF, Petrakis I (eds): *Current Diagnosis and Treatment Psychiatry (Lange Current Series).* 3rd ed. McGraw-Hill Education; 2017.
21. Bögels SM, Alden L, Beidel DC, et al.: Social anxiety disorder: questions and answers for the DSM-V. *Depress Anxiety* 27(2):168–189, 2010.
22. Kristensen H: Selective mutism and comorbidity with developmental disorder/delay, anxiety disorder, and elimination disorder. *J Am Acad Child Adolesc Psychiatry* 39(2):249–256, 2000.
23. Reiss S: Expectancy model of fear, anxiety, and panic. *Clin Psychol Rev* 11(2):141–153, 1991.
24. Silverman WK, Goedhart AW, Barrett P, Turner C: The facets of anxiety sensitivity represented in the Childhood Anxiety Sensitivity Index: confirmatory analyses of factor models from past studies. *J Abnorm Psychol* 112(3):364, 2003.
25. Burstein M, Beesdo-Baum K, He J-P, Merikangas K: Threshold and subthreshold generalized anxiety disorder among US adolescents: prevalence, sociodemographic, and clinical characteristics. *Psychol Med* 44(11):2351–2362, 2014.
26. Burstein M, He J-P, Kattan G, Albano AM, Avenevoli S, Merikangas KR: Social phobia and subtypes in the National Comorbidity Survey–Adolescent Supplement: prevalence, correlates, and comorbidity. *J Am Acad Child Adolesc Psychiatry* 50(9):870–880, 2011.
27. Keyes KM, McLaughlin KA, Vo T, Galbraith T, Heimberg RG: Anxious and aggressive: the co-occurrence of IED with anxiety disorders. *Depress Anxiety* 33(2):101–111, 2016.
28. Black B, Uhde TW: Psychiatric characteristics of children with selective mutism: a pilot study. *J Am Acad Child Adolesc Psychiatry* 34(7):847–856, 1995.
29. Watson D, Clark LA, Carey G: Positive and negative affectivity and their relation to anxiety and depressive disorders. *J Abnorm Psychol* 97(3):346, 1988.
30. Clauss JA, Blackford JU: Behavioral inhibition and risk for developing social anxiety disorder: a meta-analytic study. *J Am Acad Child Adolesc Psychiatry* 51(10):1066–1075. e1061, 2012.
31. Taylor JH, Jakubovski E, Bloch MH: Predictors of anxiety recurrence in the Coordinated Anxiety Learning and Management (CALM) trial. *J Psychiatr Res* 65:154–165, 2015.
32. Shear K, Jin R, Ruscio AM, Walters EE, Kessler RC: Prevalence and correlates of estimated DSM-IV child and adult separation anxiety disorder in the National Comorbidity Survey Replication. *Am J Psychiatry* 163(6):1074–1083, 2006.
33. Foley DL, Pickles A, Maes HM, Silberg JL, Eaves LJ: Course and short-term outcomes of separation anxiety disorder in a community sample of twins. *J Am Acad Child Adolesc Psychiatry* 43(9):1107–1114, 2004.
34. Kessler R: The impairments caused by social phobia in the general population: implications for intervention. *Acta Psychiatr Scand* 108(s417):19–27, 2003.
35. Steinhausen HC, Wachter M, Laimböck K, Metzke CW: A long-term outcome study of selective mutism in childhood. *J Child Psychol Psychiatry* 47(7):751–756, 2006.
36. Costello EJ, Angold A, Burns BJ, et al.: The Great Smoky Mountains Study of Youth: goals, design, methods, and the prevalence of DSM-III-R disorders. *Arch Gen Psychiatry* 53(12):1129–1136, 1996.
37. Costello EJ, Copeland W, Angold A: The Great Smoky Mountains Study: developmental epidemiology in the southeastern United States. *Soc Psychiatry Psychiatr Epidemiol* 51(5):639–646, 2016.
38. Copeland WE, Shanahan L, Costello EJ, Angold A: Childhood and adolescent psychiatric disorders as predictors of young adult disorders. *Arch Gen Psychiatry* 66(7):764–772, 2009.
39. Foley DL, Goldston DB, Costello EJ, Angold A: Proximal psychiatric risk factors for suicidality in youth: the Great Smoky Mountains Study. *Arch Gen Psychiatry* 63(9):1017–1024, 2006.
40. Field AP, Purkis HM: The role of learning in the etiology of child and adolescent fear and anxiety. *Anxiety Disord Child Adolesc Res Assess Interv* 227–256, 2011.
41. Rachman S: The conditioning theory of fear acquisition: a critical examination. *Behav Res Ther* 15(5):375–387, 1977.
42. Field AP: Is conditioning a useful framework for understanding the development and treatment of phobias? *Clin Psychol Rev* 26(7):857–875, 2006.
43. Green JG, McLaughlin KA, Berglund PA, et al.: Childhood adversities and adult psychiatric disorders in the national comorbidity survey replication I: associations with first onset of DSM-IV disorders. *Arch Gen Psychiatry* 67(2):113–123, 2010.
44. McLaughlin KA, Green JG, Gruber MJ, Sampson NA, Zaslavsky AM, Kessler RC: Childhood adversities and adult psychiatric disorders in the national comorbidity survey replication II: associations with persistence of DSM-IV disorders. *Arch Gen Psychiatry* 67(2):124–132, 2010.
45. Colonnesi C, Draijer EM, Jan JM, et al.: The relation between insecure attachment and child anxiety: a meta-analytic review. *J Clin Child Adolesc Psychol* 40(4):630–645, 2011.
46. Tottenham N, Hare T, Millner A, Gilhooly T, Zevin J, Casey B: Elevated amygdala response to faces following early deprivation. *Dev Sci* 14(2):190–204, 2011.
47. Gee D, Gabard-Durnam L, Flannery J, et al.: Early developmental emergence of mature human Amygdala-prefrontal phenotype following

maternal deprivation: evidence of stress-induced acceleration. *Proc Nat Acad Sci* 110:15638–15643, 2013.
48. Pine DS: Research review: a neuroscience framework for pediatric anxiety disorders. *J Child Psychol Psychiatry* 48(7):631–648, 2007.
49. Strawn JR, Hamm L, Fitzgerald DA, Fitzgerald KD, Monk CS, Phan KL: Neurostructural abnormalities in pediatric anxiety disorders. *J Anxiety Disord* 32:81–88, 2015.
50. Strawn JR, Dominick KC, Patino LR, Doyle CD, Picard LS, Phan KL: Neurobiology of pediatric anxiety disorders. *Curr Behav Neurosci Rep* 1(3):154–160, 2014.
51. Pine DS: Developmental biology related to emotion and anxiety. *Anxiety Disord* 69, 2015.
52. Pine DS: The brain and behavior in childhood and adolescent anxiety disorders. *Anxiety Disord Child Adolesc* 179–197, 2011.
53. Ask H, Waaktaar T, Seglem KB, Torgersen S: Common etiological sources of anxiety, depression, and somatic complaints in adolescents: a multiple rater twin study. *J Abnorm Child Psychol* 44(1):101–114, 2016.
54. McGrath LM, Weill S, Robinson EB, Macrae R, Smoller JW: Bringing a developmental perspective to anxiety genetics. *Dev Psychopathol* 24(04):1179–1193, 2012.
55. Smoller JW, Cerrato FE, Weatherall SL: The genetics of anxiety disorders. *Anxiety Disord* 47, 2015.
56. Murphy S, Norbury R, Godlewska B, et al.: The effect of the serotonin transporter polymorphism (5-HTTLPR) on amygdala function: a meta-analysis. *Mol Psychiatry* 18(4):512–520, 2013.
57. Miller R, Wankerl M, Stalder T, Kirschbaum C, Alexander N: The serotonin transporter gene-linked polymorphic region (5-HTTLPR) and cortisol stress reactivity: a meta-analysis. *Mol Psychiatry* 18(9):1018–1024, 2013.
58. Li X, Sundquist J, Sundquist K: Age-specific familial risks of anxiety. A nation-wide epidemiological study from Sweden. *Eur Arch Psychiatry Clin Neurosci* 258(7):441–445, 2008.
59. Steinhausen H-C, Foldager L, Perto G, Munk-Jorgensen P: Family aggregation of mental disorders in the nationwide Danish three generation study. *Eur Arch Psychiatry Clin Neurosci* 259(5):270–277, 2009.
60. Lebowitz ER, Woolston J, Bar-Haim Y, et al.: Family accommodation in pediatric anxiety disorders. *Depress Anxiety* 30(1), 2013.
61. Lebowitz ER, Panza KE, Bloch MH: Family accommodation in obsessive-compulsive and anxiety disorders: a five-year update. *Expert Rev Neurother* 16(1), 2016.
62. Askew C, Field AP: Vicarious learning and the development of fears in childhood. *Behav Res Ther* 45(11):2616–2627, 2007.
63. Klein DF: False suffocation alarms, spontaneous panics, and related conditions: an integrative hypothesis. *Arch Gen Psychiatry* 50(4):306–317, 1993.
64. Roberson-Nay R, Klein DF, Klein RG, et al.: Carbon dioxide hypersensitivity in separation-anxious offspring of parents with panic disorder. *Biol Psychiatry* 67(12):1171–1177, 2010.
65. Roberson-Nay R, Eaves LJ, Hettema JM, Kendler KS, Silberg JL: Childhood separation anxiety disorder and adult onset panic attacks share a common genetic diathesis. *Depress Anxiety* 29(4):320–327, 2012.
66. Kossowsky J, Pfaltz MC, Schneider S, Taeymans J, Locher C, Gaab J: The separation anxiety hypothesis of panic disorder revisited: a meta-analysis. *Am J Psychiatry* 2013.
67. Poulton R, Menzies RG: Non-associative fear acquisition: a review of the evidence from retrospective and longitudinal research. *Behav Res Ther* 40(2):127–149, 2002.
68. Lebowitz ER, Leckman JF, Feldman R, Zagoory-Sharon O, McDonald N, Silverman WK: Salivary oxytocin in clinically anxious youth: associations with separation anxiety and family accommodation. *Psychoneuroendocrinology* 65, 2016.
69. Lebowitz ER, Silverman WK, Martino A, Zagoory-Sharon O, Feldman R, Leckman JF: Oxytocin response to youth-mother interactions in clinically anxious youth is associated with separation anxiety and dyadic behavior. *Depress Anxiety* 34(2):127–136, 2017.
70. Silverman WK, Nelles WB: The anxiety disorders interview schedule for children. *J Am Acad Child Adolesc Psychiatry* 27(6):772–778, 1988.
71. Silverman WK, Eisen AR: Age differences in the reliability of parent and child reports of child anxious symptomatology using a structured interview. *J Am Acad Child Adolesc Psychiatry* 31(1):117–124, 1992.
72. Becker EM, Jensen-Doss A, Kendall PC, Birmaher B, Ginsburg GS: All anxiety is not created equal: correlates of parent/youth agreement vary across subtypes of anxiety. *J Psychopathol Behav Assess* 1–10, 2016.
73. Byrne SB, Lebowitz EL, Ollendick TH, Silverman WK: Child and adolescent anxiety disorders. In: Hunsley J, Mash E (eds): *A Guide to Assessments That Work.* 2nd ed. New York: Oxford University Press, 2017.
74. Silverman WK, Ollendick TH: Evidence-based assessment of anxiety and its disorders in children and adolescents. *J Clin Child Adolesc Psychol* 34(3):380–411, 2005.
75. Birmaher B, Khetarpal S, Brent D, et al.: The Screen for Child Anxiety Related Emotional Disorders (SCARED): scale construction and psychometric characteristics. *J Am Acad Child Adolesc Psychiatry* 36(4):545–553, 1997.
76. March JS, Parker JD, Sullivan K, Stallings P, Conners CK: The Multidimensional Anxiety Scale for Children (MASC): factor structure, reliability, and validity. *J Am Acad Child Adolesc Psychiatry* 36(4):554–565, 1997.
77. Group RUoPPAS: The pediatric anxiety rating scale (PARS): development and psychometric properties. *J Am Acad Child Adolesc Psychiatry* 41(9):1061–1069, 2002.
78. Lebowitz ER, Scharfstein L, Jones J: Child-report of family accommodation in pediatric anxiety disorders: comparison and integration with mother-report. *Child Psychiatry Hum Dev* 46(4), 2015.
79. Coughlin CG, Cohen SC, Mulqueen JM, Ferracioli-Oda E, Stuckelman ZD, Bloch MH: Meta-analysis: reduced risk of anxiety with psychostimulant treatment in children with attention-deficit/hyperactivity disorder. *J Child Adolesc Psychopharmacol* 25(8):611–617, 2015.
80. Cassiday KL. Involving the family in treatment. *Anxiety Disord* 95, 2015.
81. Silverman WK, Pina AA, Viswesvaran C: Evidence-based psychosocial treatments for phobic and anxiety disorders in children and adolescents. *J Clin Child Adolesc Psychol* 37(1):105–130, 2008.
82. Strawn JR, Prakash A, Zhang Q, et al.: A randomized, placebo-controlled study of duloxetine for the treatment of children and adolescents with generalized anxiety disorder. *J Am Acad Child Adolesc Psychiatry* 54(4):283–293, 2015.
83. Wehry AM, Beesdo-Baum K, Hennelly MM, Connolly SD, Strawn JR: Assessment and treatment of anxiety disorders in children and adolescents. *Curr Psychiatry Rep* 17(7):1–11, 2015.
84. Strawn JR, Welge JA, Wehry AM, Keeshin B, Rynn MA: Efficacy and tolerability of antidepressants in pediatric anxiety disorders: a systematic review and meta-analysis. *Depress Anxiety* 32(3):149–157, 2015.
85. Walkup JT, Albano AM, Piacentini J, et al.: Cognitive behavioral therapy, sertraline, or a combination in childhood anxiety. *N Engl J Med* 359(26):2753–2766, 2008.
86. Hudson JL, Keers R, Roberts S, et al.: Clinical predictors of response to cognitive-behavioral therapy in pediatric anxiety disorders: the Genes for Treatment (GxT) study. *J Am Acad Child Adolesc Psychiatry* 54(6):454–463, 2015.
87. Bennett K, Manassis K, Walter SD, et al.: Cognitive behavioral therapy age effects in child and adolescent anxiety: an individual patient data metaanalysis. *Depress Anxiety* 30(9):829–841, 2013.
88. Manassis K, Lee TC, Bennett K, et al.: Types of parental involvement in CBT with anxious youth: a preliminary meta-analysis. *J Consult Clin Psychol* 82(6):1163, 2014.
89. Pincus DB, May JE, Whitton SW, Mattis SG, Barlow DH: Cognitive-behavioral treatment of panic disorder in adolescence. *J Clin Child Adolesc Psychol* 39(5):638–649, 2010.
90. Ollendick TH, Halldorsdottir T, Fraire MG, et al.: Specific phobias in youth: a randomized controlled trial comparing one-session treatment to a parent-augmented one-session treatment. *Behav Ther* 46(2):141–155, 2015.
91. Silverman WK, Kurtines WM, Ginsburg GS, Weems CF, Lumpkin PW, Carmichael DH: Treating anxiety disorders in children with group cognitive-behavioral therapy: a randomized clinical trial. *J Consult Clin Psychol* 67(6):995, 1999.
92. Wergeland GJ, Fjermestad KW, Marin CE, et al.: An effectiveness study of individual vs. group cognitive behavioral therapy for anxiety disorders in youth. *Behav Res Ther* 57:1–12, 2014.
93. Manassis K, Mendlowitz SL, Scapillato D, et al.: Group and individual cognitive-behavioral therapy for childhood anxiety disorders: a randomized trial. *J Am Acad Child Adolesc Psychiatry* 41(12):1423–1430, 2002.
94. Spence SH, Donovan CL, March S, et al.: A randomized controlled trial of online versus clinic-based CBT for adolescent anxiety. *J Consult Clin Psychol* 79(5):629, 2011.
95. Silk JS, Tan PZ, Ladouceur CD, et al.: A randomized clinical trial comparing individual cognitive behavioral therapy and child-centered therapy for child anxiety disorders. *J Clin Child Adolesc Psychol* 1–13, 2016.
96. Southam-Gerow MA, Weisz JR, Chu BC, McLeod BD, Gordis EB, Connor-Smith JK: Does cognitive behavioral therapy for youth anxiety outperform usual care in community clinics? An initial effectiveness test. *J Am Acad Child Adolesc Psychiatry* 49(10):1043–1052, 2010.
97. Reynolds S, Wilson C, Austin J, Hooper L: Effects of psychotherapy for anxiety in children and adolescents: a meta-analytic review. *Clin Psychol Rev* 2012;32(4):251–262, 2010.
98. Beidel DC, Turner SM, Sallee FR, Ammerman RT, Crosby LA, Pathak S: SET-C versus fluoxetine in the treatment of childhood social phobia. *J Am Acad Child Adolesc Psychiatry* 46(12):1622–1632, 2007.
99. Ginsburg GS, Kendall PC, Sakolsky D, et al.: Remission after acute treatment in children and adolescents with anxiety disorders: findings from the CAMS. *J Consult Clin Psychol* 79(6):806–813, 2011.
100. Compton SN, Peris TS, Almirall D, et al.: Predictors and moderators of treatment response in childhood anxiety disorders: results from the CAMS trial. *J Consult Clin Psychol* 82(2):212–224, 2014.
101. Bergman RL, Gonzalez A, Piacentini J, Keller ML: Integrated behavior therapy for selective mutism: a randomized controlled pilot study. *Behav Res Ther* 51(10):680–689, 2013.
102. Oerbeck B, Stein MB, Wentzel-Larsen T, Langsrud Ø, Kristensen H: A randomized controlled trial of a home and school-based intervention for selective mutism–defocused communication and behavioural techniques. *Child Adolesc Ment Health* 19(3):192–198, 2014.
103. Ooi YP, Sung SC, Raja M, Kwan CH, Koh JB, Fung DS: Web-based CBT for the treatment of selective mutism: results from a pilot randomized controlled trial in Singapore. *J Speech Pathol Ther* 2016, 2016.

104. Silver G, Shapiro T, Milrod B: Treatment of anxiety in children and adolescents: using child and adolescent anxiety psychodynamic psychotherapy. *Child Adolesc Psychiatr Clin N Am* 22(1):83–96, 2013.
105. Göttken T, White LO, Klein AM, von Klitzing K: Short-term psychoanalytic child therapy for anxious children: a pilot study. *Psychotherapy* 51(1):148, 2014.
106. Walkup JT, Labellarte MJ, Riddle MA, et al.: Fluvoxamine for the treatment of anxiety disorders in children and adolescents. *N Engl J Med* 344(17):1279–1285, 2001.
107. Sukhodolsky DG, Bloch MH, Panza KE, Reichow B: Cognitive-behavioral therapy for anxiety in children with high-functioning autism: a meta-analysis. *Pediatrics* 132(5):e1341–e1350, 2013.
108. Reaven J, Blakeley-Smith A, Culhane-Shelburne K, Hepburn S: Group cognitive behavior therapy for children with high-functioning autism spectrum disorders and anxiety: a randomized trial. *J Child Psychol Psychiatry* 53(4):410–419, 2012.
109. Storch EA, Arnold EB, Lewin AB, et al.: The effect of cognitive-behavioral therapy versus treatment as usual for anxiety in children with autism spectrum disorders: a randomized, controlled trial. *J Am Acad Child Adolesc Psychiatry* 52(2):132–142. e132, 2013.
110. Wood JJ, Drahota A, Sze K, Har K, Chiu A, Langer DA: Cognitive behavioral therapy for anxiety in children with autism spectrum disorders: a randomized, controlled trial. *J Child Psychol Psychiatry* 50(3):224–234, 2009.
111. Wood JJ, Piacentini JC, Southam-Gerow M, Chu BC, Sigman M: Family cognitive behavioral therapy for child anxiety disorders. *J Am Acad Child Adolesc Psychiatry* 45(3):314–321, 2006.
112. Birmaher B, Axelson DA, Monk K, et al.: Fluoxetine for the treatment of childhood anxiety disorders. *J Am Acad Child Adolesc Psychiatry* 42(4):415–423, 2003.
113. Black B, Uhde TW: Treatment of elective mutism with fluoxetine: a double-blind, placebo-controlled study. *J Am Acad Child Adolesc Psychiatry* 33(7):1000–1006, 1994.
114. Manassis K, Oerbeck B, Overgaard KR: The use of medication in selective mutism: a systematic review. *Eur Child Adolesc Psychiatry* 1–8, 2016.
115. Mrakotsky C, Masek B, Biederman J, et al.: Prospective open-label pilot trial of mirtazapine in children and adolescents with social phobia. *J Anxiety Disord* 22(1):88–97, 2008.
116. Geller D, Donnelly C, Lopez F, et al.: Atomoxetine treatment for pediatric patients with attention-deficit/hyperactivity disorder with comorbid anxiety disorder. *J Am Acad Child Adolesc Psychiatry* 46(9):1119–1127, 2007.
117. Simeon JG, Ferguson HB, Knott V, et al.: Clinical, cognitive, and neurophysiological effects of alprazolam in children and adolescents with overanxious and avoidant disorders. *J Am Acad Child Adolesc Psychiatry* 31(1):29–33, 1992.
118. Graae F, Milner J, Rizzotto L, Klein RG: Clonazepam in childhood anxiety disorders. *J Am Acad Child Adolesc Psychiatry* 33(3):372–376, 1994.
119. Piacentini J, Bennett S, Compton SN, et al.: 24- and 36-week outcomes for the Child/Adolescent Anxiety Multimodal Study (CAMS). *J Am Acad Child Adolesc Psychiatry* 53(3):297–310, 2014.
120. Caporino NE, Brodman DM, Kendall PC, et al.: Defining treatment response and remission in child anxiety: signal detection analysis using the pediatric anxiety rating scale. *J Am Acad Child Adolesc Psychiatry* 52(1):57–67, 2013.
121. Connolly SD, Bernstein GA, Work Group on Quality I. Practice parameter for the assessment and treatment of children and adolescents with anxiety disorders. *J Am Acad Child Adolesc Psychiatry* 46(2):267–283, 2007.
122. Rapee R: Anxiety disorders in children and adolescents: nature, development, treatment and prevention. In: Rey JM (ed): *IACAPAP e-Textbook of Child and Adolescent Mental Health. Geneva: International Association for Child and Adolescent Psychiatry and Allied Professions.* 2012.
123. Rynn MA, Walkup JT, Compton SN, et al.: Child/Adolescent anxiety multimodal study: evaluating safety. *J Am Acad Child Adolesc Psychiatry* 54(3):180–190, 2015.
124. Ginsburg GS, Becker EM, Keeton CP, et al.: Naturalistic follow-up of youths treated for pediatric anxiety disorders. *JAMA Psychiatry* 71(3):310–318, 2014.
125. Dudeney J, Sharpe L, Hunt C: Attentional bias towards threatening stimuli in children with anxiety: a meta-analysis. *Clin Psychol Rev* 40:66–75, 2015.
126. Eldar S, Apter A, Lotan D, et al.: Attention bias modification treatment for pediatric anxiety disorders: a randomized controlled trial. *Am J Psychiatry* 169(2):213–230, 2012.
127. Linetzky M, Pergamin-Hight L, Pine DS, Bar-Haim Y: Quantitative evaluation of the clinical efficacy of attention bias modification treatment for anxiety disorders. *Depress Anxiety* 32(6):383–391, 2015.
128. Lebowitz ER, Omer H, Hermes H, Scahill L: Parent training for childhood anxiety disorders: the SPACE program. *Cogn Behav Pract* 21(4), 2014.

CHAPTER 5.5.2 ■ OBSESSIVE-COMPULSIVE DISORDER

KENNETH E. TOWBIN AND MARK A. RIDDLE

INTRODUCTION

Detailed descriptions of obsessions and compulsions are found among the oldest records of mental illness known. Classic obsessions and compulsions, depicted as possession by the devil, date back in 1467 in *Malleus Maleficarum* (1) and are described in the "Obsessi" of Paracelsus in the 16th century. In the 1600s, pious texts tell of extremes of religious doubting and "scrupulosity," or excessive devotion (2). Pioneers of psychiatry such as Esquirol (3), Maudsley (4), Freud (5), and Janet (6) took up these intriguing symptoms, and their writings reflect the prevailing views on the nature of thought, motivation, and free will.

DEFINITIONS

Obsessions are unwanted thoughts, images, or impulses that are recognized as senseless or unnecessary, intrude into consciousness involuntarily, and cause functional impairment and distress. Despite this lack of control, a person with obsessions is aware that these thoughts originate in his or her own mental activity. Since they arise in the mind, obsessions can take the form of any mental event—simple repetitive words, thoughts, fears, memories, pictures, or elaborate dramatic scenes.

Compulsions are repetitive actions that are responses to obsessions or perceived internal obligations to follow certain rituals or rules. They are distressing and cause functional impairment. Compulsions may follow directly from obsessions or indirectly as efforts to ward off certain thoughts, impulses, or fears. Children often report that their compulsions do not have a preceding mental component. Like obsessions, compulsions are often viewed as being unnecessary, excessive, senseless, involuntary, or forced. Individuals suffering from compulsions will often elaborate a variety of precise rules for the chronology, rate, order, duration, and number of repetitions of their acts.

These definitions reflect three critical concepts that are relevant to the differential diagnosis—unwanted/distressing, senseless/excessive, and impairing. An essential criterion is that symptoms produce functional impairment. The other two follow classic definitions (4,7). While most patients view their compulsions as unnecessary and their obsessions as senseless, for some, such awareness ("insight") may be absent or intermittent (8). Although the capacity for insight falls along a continuum (9), DSM-5 offers three categories (absent, poor, fair/good) (10). Patients with insight see their actions as senseless or excessive, those with poor insight think their actions are "probably necessary" (10), and those without insight are nearly delusional, entirely convinced that their actions are necessary.

Few studies differentiate between participants with childhood- and adolescent-onset obsessive-compulsive disorder (OCD). Therefore, in this chapter, "child," "childhood," or "children" will be used to signify children *and adolescents*. When studies are drawn solely on adolescent participants, the more restrictive term will be employed.

PREVALENCE AND EPIDEMIOLOGY

The prevalence of OCD in childhood should be understood in the context of the high prevalence of *subclinical* obsessions or compulsions and of developmentally appropriate magical thinking in children. In children less than 6, urges to make things "just right" and preoccupations with symmetry and rules are very common and typically decline after age 6 (11). A majority of fourth graders experience preoccupations with guilt about lying and engaging in checking behaviors and 50% report contamination and germ fears (12). By eighth grade, rates for these concerns declined to 40%, but 60% of eighth graders reported worries about cleanliness and 50% noted intrusive rude thoughts (12). However, even in this older population, rates of these behaviors and thoughts declined over time. Prevalence and incidence rates are heavily influenced by which diagnostic criteria are applied (13–16) and how diagnoses are made (such as using structured interviews by nonclinician interviewers or computers) (14–17).

Given the methodologic shortcomings of most epidemiologic studies, there is no consensus on the lifetime prevalence and incidence of OCD. Overall, the lifetime prevalence of OCD is probably greater than that reported in the 1950s (0.05%), but less than 1.3% to 3.3% reported in the ECA (18). At this point the best one can say is that, the lifetime prevalence in adults is probably between 0.5% and 2% (13,14,19–21).

Methodologically more reliable studies suggest that OCD shows an equal sex distribution. Compared to females, males with OCD appear to have an earlier age of onset (20,22–24), and a longer duration of illness prior to seeking treatment (24). Delays in diagnosis are common. One study reported an average of 7 to 8 years before patients reached clinical attention (25).

CLINICAL DESCRIPTION

The variety of obsessions and compulsions reflect the unlimited capacity of the human mind and body. Typically, patients experience both obsessions and compulsions and most patients experience multiple concurrent obsessions or compulsions. In the minority of patients who have only one or the other (22,26) having only obsessions may be more common (27). The content of obsessions can show a wide range, but some themes are more frequent and influenced by the individual's level of development. Adolescents' obsessions typically focus on dirt and germs, fears of an ill fate befalling loved ones, exactness or symmetry, and religious scrupulousness (22). Bodily functions, lucky numbers, sexual or aggressive preoccupations, and fear of harm to oneself are less common. In adults, these remain frequent, but aggressive and sexual obsessions are more common (23,28,29).

Although any action can become a compulsion, some actions are more common. An adolescent clinical cohort (22) displayed (in descending order of frequency) cleaning rituals, repeating actions (doing and undoing), and checking rituals most commonly. Many fewer subjects reported rituals to protect themselves from illness or injury, ordering maneuvers, and counting behaviors. In adults, the most common compulsions are checking and cleaning (23,29,30). Slowness (29), counting (23), or doing things by numbers (30) each have been reported as third most common.

Several investigators (31–33) suggest that obsessions and compulsions should no longer be viewed as separate entities. These investigators used factor analysis to reconfigure Children's Yale–Brown Obsessive Compulsive Scale (CY–BOCS) symptom categories and found a four-factor model that they believed was more meaningful (34). Rather than just one homogeneous entity or as "two factors" (obsessions or compulsions), there are strong reasons to consider that OCD might be better viewed as composed of four or more subtypes. A number of investigators have now identified four-factor subtypes: (1) aggressive, sexual, religious, and somatic obsessions with checking compulsions; (2) symmetry obsessions with counting, arranging, ordering, and repeating compulsions; (3) contamination obsessions with cleaning and washing; and (4) hoarding obsessions with hoarding and collection compulsions (31–38). Mataix-Cols et al. (35) found a five-factor model that has been replicated as well: (1) aggressive checking; (2) symmetry ordering; (3) contamination cleaning; (4) sexual and religious obsessions; and (5) hoarding. These solutions are close to one another and it is not yet clear which will be the most predictive. Largely building on this work, the DSM-5 committee created a separate diagnostic entity of hoarding disorder with the OC and Related Disorder section (10).

Subsequent research, using factor analyses of symptoms without starting with Y-BOCS categories, argues for a yet more useful, "multidimensional" way of grouping symptoms and thinking about OCD symptom patterns and subtypes (39). Using latent class analysis of symptoms, Mataix-Cols et al. (39) and Nestadt et al. (40,41) identified symptom groupings that were more meaningful when placed in the context of age of onset and comorbid diagnoses. From this work there is evidence for factors 1 and 2 (above) that are associated with early-onset OCD, and a factor 4 (hoarding) that does not associate with other disorders. Furthermore, these factors show some association with comorbid disorders. Factor 2, described above, has been associated with earlier age of onset and tic disorders (32,35,42). Hoarding was more associated with axis II psychopathology (particularly obsessive-compulsive personality disorder [OCPD] (43)), social disability and social anxiety disorder (39). Subsequent work looking more closely at comorbid diagnoses also relying on latent class analysis suggests greater likelihood of comorbid diagnostic groupings, such that OCD occurs with recurrent major depression and generalized anxiety (40,42), and another that associates OCD with agoraphobia, panic disorder, and tic disorders (40).

Also, these factors correlate with treatment response (35), neuroimaging results (39,44), neuropsychologic function (45), and genetics (46,47). The course, genetic risk, neuropathology, and treatment may be different among these subgroups. For example, Alsobrook et al. (48) found that a major gene locus model was more strongly supported in families ascertained where the probands had symmetry+ordering symptoms (factor grouping II), than in probands with other symptom groupings. Alonso et al. (43) found that those scoring highly on the religious–sexual obsessions dimension fared more poorly over 2 years. Nevertheless, a serotonin reuptake inhibitor (SRI) treatment study failed to support differences in response among three of these five subtypes (35). Several other caveats were suggested by Summerfeldt et al. (33), including the possibility that "more-than-four" factor models might also be viable, that a variety of items have been excluded in the analyses performed to date that use categories from the YBOCS, and problems with using "lifetime" ratings as these are subject to recall bias.

Longitudinal studies find that symptoms often change over time and individuals' symptoms are likely to change over the course of their illness (49). However, studies of adults reveal that, while symptoms changed, they remained within the same symptom groupings identified by latent class analysis (50). When adults with OCD were followed over 2 years, symptoms typically remained within the same symptom group (35,50). This change in symptoms with stability within symptom groupings has also been reported in children with OCD (51).

One might say that children with OCD are more *selectively* impaired than children with other psychiatric disorders. Academic and extracurricular functioning are often preserved, although the quality of peer relating may be variable (52). Studies with adults report significant impairment in social and role function (53). Koran et al. (53) noted that moderate to severe illness showed a linear correlation with social impairment. Data from clinical settings show that children with OCD have average intellectual abilities, although ascertainment bias is a factor in these reports.

On the surface, a child with OCD may appear to function well and seem relatively adapted to his or her life, but severe symptoms may be concealed while they are enveloping the patient and family completely (53,54). It is common to learn that washing rituals consume 4 hours of scrubbing daily, dissolve an entire bar of soap at a time, leave the patient's hands worn raw and macerated, and generate huge water bills. Counting or ordering compulsions can consume half a day and virtually obstruct functioning. Repetitive rituals from night to early morning may reduce sleep to a few hours. Checking or cleansing rituals result in physical injury such as skin lacerations, ulcers, and chemical burns.

The family's reaction to the patient's symptoms is crucial. Several common response patterns may delay evaluation and treatment of OCD. Although patients are embarrassed and secretive about the content of their symptoms and the limitations they impose, serious impairment rarely eludes family members. Parents may delay seeking treatment out a false hope that symptoms will fade if everyone acquiesces or aids in performing the activities. Parent may fear stigmatization (54,55). This kind of family assistance relieves the child's symptoms only momentarily. Many times, parents cannot extricate themselves once they become involved in the rituals. Their children demand their assistance or implore them to continue. Over time, the child and parent may become pathologically entangled in rituals. When a child has sturdy development in other domains, parents find it hard to believe that he or she suffers from a serious disorder. In addition, the child's claims that the thoughts or acts are ridiculous or unnecessary can instill false security, leading parents to think that "it's just a phase." Parents with subclinical-obsessive or compulsion-like behaviors may be unable to recognize symptoms in their child and unwittingly minimize the child's impairment. Reassurance from clinicians and pediatricians who are unfamiliar with OCD may lead to mistaking severe symptoms for "normal" reactions. It is a frightening and painful moment when parents recognize that their child is ill and has lost control of his or her thoughts and actions.

ETIOLOGY AND PATHOGENESIS

Genetic Studies

Over 50 years ago, a small twin study showed that heredity plays an important role in susceptibility to OCD (56). Since then, several family studies have found a higher rate of OCD in first-degree relatives of probands with OCD versus controls (57–60). Family studies of child and adolescent probands have found even greater differences in prevalence of OCD in relatives of case (OCD) versus control probands (61,62). These findings are consistent with previous results of increased familial loading in adult probands with early age of onset (59,60). Family studies have also identified other disorders that are associated with OCD (expanded phenotype), including chronic tic disorders, obsessive-compulsive personality, hoarding, some anxiety disorders, trichotillomania, skin picking, and body dysmorphic disorder (63).

Family studies can be used to determine "recurrence risk," a clinical proxy for genetic risk for a disorder. For six available studies, the estimates of recurrence risk range somewhat with most being in the 10% to 20% range (57–62). All recurrence risk estimates for OCD are considerably higher than the estimated lifetime prevalence of OCD in the general population of 0.7% to 3.0% (16,20,64).

Heritability is the proportion of observed variation in a particular trait (e.g., obsessions) that can be attributed to inherited genetic factors in contrast to nongenetic ones. Heritability ranges from zero (no observed variation in a particular trait attributed to inherited genetic factors) to one (all observed variation attributed to inherited genetic factors). Six large twin studies of OCD diagnosis or symptoms, comparing concordance rates in monozygotic and dizygotic twins, found heritability of about 0.50, with no significant contribution from shared environment (65–70).

Recently, methods have been developed to estimate disease heritability from genome-wide genotyping data (71,72) using a statistical package genome-wide complex trait analysis (GCTA) that can estimate the lower bound of true heritability explained by additive genetic factors. A recent study of OCD using data from a genome-wide association study (GWAS) and GCTA estimated lower bound of heritability at 0.37 (73). A large proportion of heritability in OCD was present on chromosome 15. The remaining genetic variation was distributed across the rest of the genome, with almost no heritability associated with minor allele frequency of <0.05. These results, although exciting and provocative, need to be verified in independent samples of individuals with and without OCD.

Genetic linkage is the tendency of alleles that are located close together on a chromosome to be inherited together during the meiosis phase of sexual reproduction. Genetic linkage studies of OCD have identified suggestive linkage peaks (74–76), but none reached the level of genome-wide significance. Many candidate gene association studies of OCD have been conducted of genes involved in neurotransmission (e.g., serotonergic, glutaminergic) and neurodevelopment (77–80). Some of these studies have found positive associations of interest in OCD, most convincingly the neuronal and epithelial glutamate transporter gene (SLC1A1) located on chromosome 9p24, but none have consistently, or in a meta-analysis, reached experiment-wise significance (81).

Two GWASs, which compare DNA markers across the genome (the complete genetic material in a person) in people with a disease or trait to people without the disease or trait, have been reported for OCD. The International OCD Foundation Genetic Collaborative reported on 1,465 cases and 5,557 ancestry-matched controls, as well as 400 complete trios, from 22 sites (82). Although there were some interesting findings in separate case-control and trio analyses, the findings in the combined sample did not reach genome-wide significance. Of considerable interest, in the combined sample, significant enrichment of methylation quantitative trait loci and frontal lobe expression quantitative trait loci were found within top-ranked single nucleotide polymorphisms (SNPs), possibly related to a broader role of gene expression in the brain, and the etiology of OCD.

The OCD Collaborative Genetic Association Study (OCGAS) reported on a second GWAS of 1,065 families, 1,406 patients with OCD and a population-based sample for a total of 5,061 individuals (83). Again, although there were some interesting findings, none reached genome-wide significance.

In summary, OCD is a highly heritable disorder with additive genetic factors that have yet to be identified. Future research can be expected to identify specific genes, epigenetic factors, and environmental risk. Successful genetic research will likely need larger samples of carefully selected cases and controls and improved assessment methodologies.

Imaging Studies

The aim of magnetic resonance imaging (MRI), functional magnetic resonance imaging (fMRI), and positron emission tomography (PET) studies of OCD is to integrate imaging of brain morphology or function with neuropsychology in the hope of improving treatment. Brain imaging during performance of neuropsychologic tasks may provide a clearer functional "map" of impairments in OCD. At this point, the map strongly implicates impairments in neuropsychologic functions related to: (a) key "executive functions," such as cognitive flexibility (e.g., the capacity to perceive multiple/alternate perspectives or assimilate and apply changing concepts) planning, and response inhibition (e.g., refraining from applying a learned "prepotent" response); (b) "evaluative functions," such as error and conflict monitoring, assessing risk and uncertainty; and (c) working memory. While imaging studies of those with OCD generally support the hypothesis of impairments in cortico-striato-thalamo-cortical (CSTC) circuitry (see below), employing diverse methods to study brain circuitry reveals a more intricate picture. Taken together, the data suggest that the CSTC circuit remains important, but the model for OCD points to impairments that go beyond this single network. Structures outside the CSTC circuit, such as parietal and dorsolateral prefrontal cortex, amygdala, hippocampus, insula, corpus callosum, and cerebellum appear to play key roles, too (84–89).

Structural Imaging Studies

Morphometric studies of adults with OCD have used region of interest (ROI) and voxel-based morphometry (VBM) designs (90). Generally they point to differences in the volume in frontal regions (cingulate gyrus) and decreased volumes in striatal regions (especially globus pallidus) and increased volumes in thalamic regions (84,91,92). However, findings using different methods do not replicate one another (93).

Meta-analyses suggest those with OCD have increased gray matter volume in the dorsomedial frontal gyrus, anterior cingulate, and bilateral lenticular nuclei and putamen (93,94) and that decreased volumes in lenticular nuclei and putamen may be specific to OCD (94) compared to other anxiety disorders. Another meta-analysis noted that, compared to healthy volunteers, those with OCD displayed decreased inferior frontal cortex and anterior insula volumes (93). This same pattern in the caudate, putamen, and globus pallidus was observed in children with OCD compared to age-matched healthy volunteers (95).

The application of the ROI method in MRI morphometry has declined in the last decade because it demands a priori hypotheses when selecting which regions will be studied (90,96). A meta-analysis (96) suggests reduced volume in the left anterior cingulate cortex (ACC) and the left and right orbitofrontal cortex (OFC) and significant increases bilaterally in thalamic volumes. No differences were noted in whole brain, ventricles, or prefrontal cortex in this analysis (96). The most robust finding was a positive correlation between increased thalamic volume and OCD symptom severity (96).

Functional Imaging Studies

Positron Emission Tomography

PET highlights specific dopamine and serotonin transporter proteins and the brain regions in which they are active and can be a powerful tool to learn about brain function. Since it is generally regarded as unethical to expose children to radioactivity exclusively for research that has no direct benefit to the participant, all these findings are from adults. When adults with OCD are compared to healthy volunteers, PET studies have replicated findings of increased activity in orbital-frontal cortex (OFC) and caudate nuclei (97–103) and increased activity in the anterior cingulate gyrus and thalamus (103).

By stratifying groups into dimensional subtypes by phenotype and employing provocation tasks, PET studies gained more specificity (104,105). Exposing OCD patients to feared stimuli during PET scanning showed increased activation in the right caudate, orbital, thalamic, and anterior cingulate gyrus (104). Unique, large differences between those with OCD plus hoarding and OCD without hoarding were noted in the dorsal anterior cingulate (105). Increased metabolism in premotor and mid-frontal regions was reported in patients with obsessional slowness (106).

Changes have also been observed in PET scans in response to treatment or spontaneous recovery. Medication responders displayed decreased right caudate nucleus glucose metabolism while no changes appeared in treatment nonresponders (107). Compared to nonresponders, responders to behavioral treatment showed increased OFC glucose metabolism (108).

Functional Magnetic Resonance Imaging

The relative safety of fMRI permits investigators to gather data from children as well as adults. Thus, comparisons can be made across development, across time (longitudinal changes), and between earlier- versus later-onset cohorts. At this point, fMRI studies of OCD point to: (1) executive function deficits implicating the dorsolateral prefrontal cortex and circuitry connecting the cingulate, frontal, orbitofrontal regions, and basal ganglia (86,87,103); (2) deficits in evaluative functions such as error monitoring, performance monitoring, and decision making pointing to deficits in the ACC, OFC, nucleus accumbens, and medial prefrontal cortex (mPFC) (88,109); and (3) deficits in hippocampal activation during specific learning tasks (110).

The anterior cingulate cortex (ACC) may play a pivotal role in OCD. The ACC is activated during conflict monitoring—the response to incoming streams of information that conflict with other information or in response to errors (111–113). Although behavioral data show *performance* on error monitoring tasks among participants with OCD to be the same as healthy controls, those with OCD show substantially increased ACC activation (112,114) and these increases in ACC activation correlate with OCD severity (112). The ACC also may be important in the distortion of appraisal functions leading to doubt and repetition (115–117) and in those who resist OCD symptoms compared to those who do not (114). In those with OCD, the anterior cingulate also showed significantly higher activation during "n-back" working memory tasks (118).

Pairing symptom profiles to fMRI scanning, Mataix-Cols et al. (44,45) presented highly specific aversive experiences to patients in an fMRI environment. The phenotypic profiles were derived from factor analytic studies and these fMRI study results showed significant symptom-specific activation in different brain regions based on clinical phenotype (44,45). Had the study omitted differentiating the groups, no differences in activation would have been observed. Such findings lend support to OCD being multiple conditions with separate, overlapping abnormalities in neuropsychologic function (39).

Diffusion Tensor Imaging

Diffusion tensor imaging (DTI) uses MRI and principles of water diffusion through brain tissue in order to observe connections between white matter regions (119). DTI studies of OCD, suggest there are abnormalities in fiber tracts in the anterior cingulate gyri and corpus callosum (119). Studies of children with OCD have raised the possibility of premature myelination in frontal regions (119) and "hyperconnectivity" in tracts that connect the thalamus and prefrontal cortex (95,120) and those that connect temporal structures such as the hippocampus and amygdala with the OFC (95). Illness severity may correlate with hyperconnectivity between the thalamus and prefrontal cortex (95,120) and have raised the hypothesis that OCD is related to delays in, or excessively drawn out development of those white matter tracts (120).

Magnetic Resonance Spectroscopy

Magnetic resonance spectroscopy (MRS) can show metabolic activity of the brain by measuring the density and activity of glutamate, N-acetylaspartate (NAA) (a signal of neuronal destruction or injury) and glycerophosphocholine plus phosphocholine (Cho) (a signal of membrane phospholipid metabolism). Studies of drug-naïve children with OCD suggest increased cells or abnormal myelination in medial thalamus and right prefrontal cortex (121). Positive correlations between OCD severity scores and NAA levels in the right prefrontal region were also observed (121). MRS studies of glutamate showed decreased levels in the ACC (122). In one study, elevated glutamate levels in the caudate nucleus, measured by MRS, normalized after responding to treatment with paroxetine (123).

Abrupt-Onset OCD

There are cases of children having a dramatic, abrupt onset of obsessive-compulsive symptoms. While this presentation was once thought to be tightly associated with group A beta-hemolytic streptococcal (GABS) infection, a series of studies now cast doubt over this relationship (124). Abrupt onset can be seen following traumatic brain injury (125).

Swedo et al. (126) termed the specific GABS-related syndrome PANDAS and proposed that it, like Sydenham chorea, arose from an autoimmune cross-reaction of streptococcal bacteria and basal ganglia structures. Subsequent work raised such serious doubts about PANDAS criteria (127) and theory behind it (124,128) that it has now been supplanted by another syndrome termed PANS (127) or CANS (129) that emphasizes abrupt onset, additional symptoms that arise concurrently, and the absence of medical conditions known to cause OCD (127,130). Therefore, caution is in order when considering clinical intervention for a child who might have abrupt-onset OCD. Children or parents of children with OCD, commonly report abrupt onset or exacerbation of symptoms with infection. Since viral and GABS infections are so common in the pediatric population, one might expect a frequent overlap in children with OCD. Several reviews provide details on the differential diagnosis and evaluation of PANS (127,129,130). Considering an autoimmune mechanism is only relevant for the highly specific pattern of acute-onset and concurrent-onset additional symptoms (130). In addition, there is insufficient evidence to support use of antibiotic prophylaxis, immunoglobulins, or plasmapheresis as a standard treatment for patients with PANS or abrupt onset of OCD (129–132) and, at this time, recommended treatments for abrupt-onset patients are the same as for all OCDs (132).

The Cortico-Striato-Thalamo-Cortical Circuit

Neuroscience and clinical psychiatry are closely intertwined. Explorations of the pathophysiology of serious mental disorders has increased our understanding of networks operating in the central nervous system, and the study of these circuits and networks reciprocally increases our understanding of pathophysiology of psychiatric disorders. From the study of disorders we learn about the development and functional interconnections of the central nervous system. New knowledge about the brain extends our understanding of the pathophysiology of brain disorders, our ability to treat symptoms, and our understanding of the relationship between disorders. OCD is among the best paradigms of this reciprocal process. Once it was shown that medication could improve OCD (133), the way was opened to identifying biologic mechanisms that predispose to it, precipitate it, and maintain it. In turn, this has advanced our general understanding of neural networks.

The conceptual model of OCD integrates neuropsychologic, anatomical, neurochemical, and electrophysiologic findings (107,134–138). It proposes somatotopically organized connections and circuits between brain structures as CSTC circuits that subserve planning, execution, and termination of voluntary movements (84,91,139).

This "basic model" (84,89,91,134,135) proposes that frontal cortical and limbic structures have excitatory effects on striatal structures via glutamatergic efferents. These striatal structures, including the caudate nucleus, putamen, nucleus accumbens, and olfactory tubercle, project to the internal and external globus pallidus. From the internal globus pallidus, inhibitory efferents using gamma-aminobutyric acid (GABA) have tonic activity at the thalamus. Consequently, *increased* striatal activity *decreases* inhibitory activity (or creates disinhibition) at the thalamus. Increased activation of thalamic nuclei produces excitatory transmission to cortical structures and then movement.

However, this basic model has required modification in three ways. The first modification introduces separate "direct" and "indirect" pathways between the striatum and the thalamus. The direct pathway is so termed because efferents pass directly from the striatum to the thalamus, exerting a disinhibiting (activating) effect. Conversely, the indirect pathway sends a variety of efferents to subthalamic nuclei, which in turn send efferents to both the globus pallidus externa and globus pallidus interna. The indirect pathway moderates activity in the thalamus (134,135,137).

The second modification proposes two parallel systems from the striatum, one related to the dorsolateral region and the other the ventromedial region. Input to the ventromedial region is largely from limbic structures, whereas dorsolateral regions receive input from the dorsal cortex. From the striatum, both direct and indirect systems send information to the thalamus. Activation of the dorsolateral system can produce either disinhibition or inhibition of the dorsal thalamus via the direct or indirect system, respectively. Activation of the ventromedial pathway only results in inhibition of the dorsal thalamus (134,137). Balance in the activity between the dorsolateral and ventromedial striatal systems is crucial in maintaining control (89). In OCD, increased tone in the pathway from limbic cortex to ventromedial striatum excessively activates the direct pathway, decreasing inhibition, and producing symptoms (overactivation) (134,137). SRIs attenuate afferents to the ventromedial pathway at the level of the striatum. Direct pathway tone decreases relative to the dorsolateral system and equilibrium is restored. Baxter (137) has hypothesized that behavioral treatment works by increasing tone in the dorsolateral system relative to the ventromedial system. Increasing tone in dorsolateral system restores the balance.

The third modification is to understand the influence of structures outside the CSTC circuit, including parietal and dorsolateral prefrontal cortex, amygdala, hippocampus, insula, corpus callosum, and cerebellum (84–89) that clearly play either a direct role in symptoms or an influential role in the functions of the CSTC circuit.

This model is compatible with the variety of neurochemical findings. First, it accounts for the efficacy of SRIs. Serotonin selectively activates GABA and reduces glutamatergic output from limbic efferents to the ventromedial caudate. Consequently, serotonergic augmentation substantially reduces activation in the ventromedial system.

Another dimension is the relationship between serotonin and dopamine. Dopaminergic inputs distributed throughout the caudate nucleus have downstream effects on the thalamus (134,135,137). There is a gradient of D1 and D2 receptors across the caudate. Higher concentrations of D2 receptors are observed in the dorsolateral caudate and decrease as one moves toward the ventromedial region. Conversely, a lower concentration of D1 receptors in the dorsolateral caudate increases as one moves toward the ventromedial region. Blockade of D2 receptors would have a greater effect on dorsolateral circuitry and produce a decrease in both direct and indirect pathway activity. This too would change the balance in activity between the dorsolateral and ventromedial regions.

EVALUATION

Clinical Evaluation

The treatment of children with OCD must begin with a thorough evaluation by a mental health clinician who is experienced in the assessment, differential diagnosis, and treatment of this condition. Children usually feel embarrassed about their symptoms and minimize impairment and underreport their symptoms to their parents (140). Frequently, children fear that their symptoms are bizarre and "crazy." They are most likely to describe symptoms to a clinician who resists confrontation, conveys acceptance, and respects privacy; it takes time for the patient to reveal his or her fears fully. Consequently, assessment usually cannot be completed in one meeting (132).

An adequate evaluation of OCD samples multiple sources. It is desirable to gather history from the patient alone, from his or her parents alone, and from the family together. Helpful information can be obtained from teachers on academic performance, peer relationships, areas of impairment, and tasks presenting special challenges. Siblings may provide valuable information on family responses to the patient.

The objectives of individual meetings are to ascertain the patient's developmental level, extent of impairment, and associated diagnoses and symptoms. The clinician should discover the patient's strengths and weaknesses, fears and aspirations, achievements and disappointments. Symptoms often ruin life at home, school, and work. They damage peer relations and self-image. Therefore each of these domains should be assessed. When asked directly, patients may also talk about OCD symptoms that are exhibited by others at home.

Thinking about the long-term relationship with the patient is important from the start. A clinician may feel pressure to overpower denial, root out secrets, and unmask obsessions but doing so could sacrifice the patient's trust and confidence. A clinician can become so entangled in an aggressive pursuit to unearth symptoms and penetrate concealment that he or she loses the relationship.

Information from family members can allow one to learn the extent to which symptoms interfere with the patient's life and if there are ways the family is unwittingly facilitating symptoms (54,55). The family evaluation should yield information about family dynamics and how the patient's illness influences the family. It is helpful to learn the significance of the patient's symptoms to the parents, how the parents understand their child, and what the family's responses to the patient's behaviors have been. These aims are most readily accomplished by direct observation and interaction with the family. A critical question is whether concomitant family treatment may be needed to change patterns of communication, patterns of interaction, and other sources of conflict. It is valuable for parents to obtain treatment when their psychopathology is exacerbating the patient's condition.

Meeting with parents alone is pivotal for gathering sensitive information and educating them about OCD. Personal information about each parent and their marriage, medical and psychiatric history, disappointments, concerns, and frustrations, and confidential information about the history in extended family members should be obtained without the patient. Meeting with parents alone is important for teaching and reassuring them about their child's illness. A parent may fear that their child is psychotic or untreatable, feel guilty that they have caused their child's condition, fear that the clinician is going to blame them for their child's difficulties or compete with them for their child's affection (55). Parent-only meetings are opportunities to reassure and solidify a collaborative relationship.

Although a comforting atmosphere fosters discussion of symptoms and stresses and assists in monitoring progress, it may not yield a thorough overview of strengths and difficulties. Standardized instruments do not convey the quality of difficulties or the impact of symptoms on the patient and others, but they are more effective for general assessment and screening. They also permit the clinician to assess severity in comparison with clinical populations. Two instruments have been used with children and may assist a general clinician in this way: the Leyton Obsessional Inventory—Children's Version (LOI-CV) (141,142) and the Children's Yale–Brown Obsessive Compulsive Scale (CY–BOCS) (143–145).

Differential Diagnosis

Table 5.5.2.1 offers a partial list of disorders in which obsessions or compulsions are seen. Often with chronic OCD one sees comorbid major depression or at least symptoms of fatigue, helplessness, and hopelessness. Though rare, OCD can arise as a consequence of specific brain disorders ("organic brain syndromes") (146).

When there are disorders comorbid with OCD, DSM-5 requires that the content of the obsessions not be restricted to any comorbid disorder or better explained by another disorder. Although this eliminates some difficulties, it creates others. It can be difficult to discern how related or unrelated a symptom may be. Therefore, clinicians are obligated to conduct thorough diagnostic assessments in order to detect all active comorbid conditions (147). Neglecting to do so will lead one to miss findings that are relevant to treatment and prognosis (148). Similarly, if research studies are to be generalizable and valid, investigators are obligated to provide comprehensive descriptions of their sample subjects (147). Care should be taken not to equate subclinical obsessions or compulsions with threshold OCD, especially in adolescents. Subclinical phenomena appear to be stable features that do not interfere with development and functioning (25) and are seen in as much as 80% of the population (149).

One might mistake OCPD for OCD. Most children with OCD do not have OCPD, although there is some suggestion they may

TABLE 5.5.2.1

DISORDERS MANIFESTING OBSESSIONS AND/OR COMPULSIONS

Anorexia nervosa
Autism spectrum disorder
Body dysmorphic disorder
Delusional disorder (all types)
Depression
Hypochondriasis
Obsessive-compulsive personality disorder
Organic mental disorder[a]
Panic disorder
Phobias
Posttraumatic stress disorder
Schizophrenia
Schizotypal personality
Somatization disorder
Somatoform disorders
Trichotillomania
Tourette disorder

[a]Specifically arising from CNS trauma, tumors, toxins.

be at higher risk than others for developing OCPD in adulthood. In OCD and OCPD, patients may have rigid routines, needs for orderliness, hoarding behaviors (that are subthreshold for hoarding disorder), and indecisiveness that fluctuate in severity and escalate under stress. However in those with OCPD, these behaviors typically do not cause anxiety or subjective distress. The impairment in OCPD is a product of patterns of interpersonal interactions and a detached, inflexible behavior toward others, rather than circumscribed, internally distressing experiences and symptoms that characterize OCD.

Conversely, patients with OCD generally are not emotionally cold, unexpressive, stingy, or especially rigid about moral or ethical matters. Furthermore, list making and rigidity about schedules or time are uncommon among compulsions reported by patients with OCD (23).

In relation to OCD, insight means the ability to understand that urges and/or obsessions originate in the patient's mind and are not imposed by external sources, or that fears are excessive and senseless. When insight is compromised, it can be difficult to differentiate psychosis from overvalued ideas. Some patients with OCD balance precariously between delusional conviction and insight. At some moments their compulsive behaviors seem logical and necessary to carry out and, at others, these same behaviors are viewed as senselessness, excessive, or grossly distorted (9). DSM-5 permits the diagnosis of OCD when schizophrenia or delusional disorders are present. Comorbid combinations like these can further complicate specifying the patient's level of insight. Clinicians should be mindful of comorbid diagnoses when patients have little or no insight since lack of insight in OCD is associated with a poorer prognosis and should influence treatment strategies (114).

Laboratory Studies

There are no pathognomonic laboratory findings in OCD. Appropriate laboratory evaluation follows from the findings of the history, physical, mental status, and psychological examination. An electrocardiogram, complete blood count with differential and baseline blood chemistries, including electrolytes, as well as liver function tests, blood urea nitrogen, and creatinine may be necessary before commencing somatic treatment. Measures of serum copper for Wilson disease are unnecessary in the absence of psychotic symptoms or physical findings of tics or chorea. CT or MRI scanning is warranted only when focal neurologic findings are discovered. Electroencephalography is indicated only when other features suggest a seizure disorder.

If there are concerns about a child's cognitive abilities, standardized Intelligence tests, such as the Wechsler Intelligence Scales for Children edition IV or V (WISC-IV or WISC-V) or the Differential Abilities Scale (DAS) are appropriate.

Severity measures of obsessions and compulsions are discussed below. In addition, the parent-on-child version of the Child Behavior Checklist (CBCL) (150) or the Behavior Assessment System for Children (151) may help discover other maladaptive behaviors.

TREATMENT

Although diverse treatments have been used to help children with OCD, only cognitive-behavioral therapy (CBT) and medications have been systematically studied. CBT is widely regarded as first-line treatment (132,152,153). Adjunctive family treatment is often necessary (132,152,153). In rare circumstances, inpatient hospitalization may be necessary.

Family Support and Illness Education

Whichever modalities will be used, the clinician's relationships with the patient and parent(s) are paramount. First, most children with OCD are apprehensive and secretive. In many cases they are embarrassed or anxious about what others will think of their symptoms and have mixed feelings about receiving treatment. The relationship with their treating clinician offers reassurance, reduces anxiety, promotes discussion, and furthers the treatment. Second, many patients are uneasy discussing their thoughts or rituals because the content may be scatologic or sexual. Clinicians should strive to foster a relationship in which patients feel that the clinician will not "judge them," will understand the distress they experience and can be trusted with the "unacceptable" content of their symptoms. Third, when treatments require time to take effect or produce significant anxiety, the strength of the relationship with the clinician is what sustains the work. Fourth, treatment may not lead to complete remission; many patients will have a chronic, though hopefully substantially less severe, course. Thus, the treatment relationship with the clinician may need to be maintained over years.

After the diagnosis is established, it is critical to review the causes, nature, and course of illness with the patient and his or her parents. The clinician should explain the relevance of comorbid features for interventions and prognosis. This may need to be reiterated during the course of treatment. It is helpful to the family and patient to understand that the course of OCD may be chronic. In light of this, the objectives of treatment are to reduce the interference in the patient's life caused by symptoms and to support the child's optimal development. It might be unrealistic to expect that symptoms will vanish. Furthermore, part of the evaluation is to explain how the family can best support the patient and to find the support they need to sustain themselves for a potentially lengthy treatment. Seeking risk factors for family accommodation that might compromise treatment is also critical at this early stage (154,155). While it is possible that symptoms will linger, clinicians have every reason to be encouraging and optimistic that treatment will lead to a significant reduction in impairment.

Cognitive-Behavioral Therapy

CBT is the first line of intervention for most children with mild to severe symptoms (132,152,156–159). CBT has been systematically investigated for children with OCD (152,157–159) (employing multiple rigorous tests) (161). There is ample support for the efficacy of CBT (157,158,160–163).

The most investigated type of CBT for OCD is graduated exposure with response prevention (ExRP), a less aversive version of "flooding with response prevention" (164,165). March et al. (164) studied CBT using ExRP with 15 children; 9 (60%) achieved at least a 50% reduction in symptoms that was sustained for 18 months.

Expanding on this work, the Pediatric OCD Treatment Study (POTS) (163), compared the efficacy of ExRP with sertraline treatment. POTS emphasized an adequately sized treatment cohort, standardized assessments, random assignment, control groups, and strict fidelity to treatment techniques (163). The response rates to sertraline-alone and CBT-alone were the same, roughly 40% (163). This was a significantly lower response rate to ExPR than that reported in less rigorous studies (163). Importantly, there were substantial site-specific effects in POTS. CBT-alone at the University of Pennsylvania (UPenn) yielded superior results to CBT-alone at Duke, while sertraline-alone at Duke was superior to sertraline-alone at UPenn. However, combined CBT-plus-sertraline and placebo-alone showed no between-site differences. de Haan et al. (161) also compared ExRP to medication (clomipramine), though on a much smaller scale, and found these treatments equally effective.

POTS II compared the efficacy of combined treatment using ExRP + medication, with medication-alone (166), and explored what part of ExRP treatment might be pivotal. In order to perform a more rigorous test of the importance of therapist-assisted exposure, 124 children were randomly assigned to 12 weeks of an SSRI-alone (mostly fluoxetine or sertraline), full-CBT + SSRI, or CBT-instruction + SSRI, which had no exposure sessions. The rate of responders to full-CBT + SSRI was 68% compared to the 30% to 34% in the other arms. SSRI-alone did not differ from CBT-instruction + SSRI.

Since CBT can have many different elements such as "psychoeducation, socialization to a theoretical model, parent training, anxiety management techniques," Bolton and Perrin also explored whether ExRP was a critical element (167). They studied 20 patients, randomizing them to waitlist or a modified ExRP that had minimal cognitive or psychoeducational components. Though a smaller study, ExRP was significantly more effective than the waitlist condition. Conversely, Williams et al. (168) explored an approach that, rather than using exposure techniques, draws on cognitive interventions that encourage patients to take responsibility for their thoughts, and to think about and use strategies to manage them. A pilot study of older children using this method found a large effect size although response or remission rates in this small cohort (*n*=21) were not reported (168).

The scarcity of well-trained expert therapists and the intensiveness of the treatment using ExRP have led investigators to explore modifications in the technique to boost the efficiency of this modality without compromising efficacy. Storch et al. (169) compared the efficacy of a shorter-term, intensive treatment ("90-minute psychotherapy sessions held 5 days/week for 3 weeks") for children, to conventional, 14-session weekly CBT treatment. There was no difference between the groups in the rate of remission immediately following and 3 months after treatment (169). Asbahr et al. (170) compared a 12-week group therapy ExRP to treatment with sertraline. The treatments were equally effective with a 75% response rate, but the rate of relapse 9 months after treatment was significantly lower in the group-CBT recipients. The method used to analyze the data limits the validity of these findings. The trial of sertraline was short and the majority of those in group-ExRP were not fully compliant with treatment.

When treating younger or more developmentally immature children, ExRP may be intimidating and outstrip their cognitive abilities for abstract reasoning and self-observation. In addition, for children with OCD, there appears to be a direct correlation between the extent to which their parents make accommodations (such as assisting their child with carrying out rituals or facilitating avoidance of situations that evoke anxiety) and greater functional impairment and treatment resistance (155,171). Recognizing that such children rely on their parents so much, investigators explored including parents directly in the ExRP treatment. Several studies have demonstrated efficacy of ExRP for children when modified in this way (162,172–174). Treatment conducted with this modification shows improvement in roughly 60% of participants with roughly 40% in remittance (173).

Storch et al. (175) explored the efficacy of web camera–delivered family-based ExRP treatment using random assignment to active treatment or a waitlist control. Significant differences were seen in active treatment and gains were sustained after 3 months; a large effect size was observed.

In a third POTS study, termed POTS Jr (176) 127 children, 5 to 8 years of age, were randomly assigned to 14 weeks of family-based ExRP (akin to what was used in POTS II, above, but with much greater emphasis on psychoeducation and parent-based skills plus simpler behavioral tasks) or an active control of family-based relaxation training. Family-based ExRP was superior to the control condition; rate of remission was 72% for those in FB-CBT and 41% for the group with relaxation training (176).

A review of the research and the treatment guidelines on CBT for OCD highlights two characteristics that strongly influence treatment efficacy. CBT must closely adhere to an established manual that includes ExRP elements. Also, efficacy is correlated with clinicians' depth of training in CBT for OCD and their experience with it.

Pharmacologic Treatment

It is widely known that a variety of agents that inhibit serotonin reuptake appear to be useful in the treatment of OCD. The claims for efficacy that are ubiquitous in advertisements and media may mislead patients to conclude that anyone with OCD will achieve remission by taking medication. It is helpful to inform patients at the outset that reliable studies have shown 40% to 50% of drug-naïve patients experience a reduction of 25% to 40% severity in symptoms. This is important when obtaining consent prior to treatment and in helping patients understand why they may continue to experience symptoms after a course of treatment.

The clinician also should be mindful of comorbid psychopathology when choosing medications. Coexisting panic disorder, psychotic or schizotypal features, depression, or Tourette disorder might steer toward classes of drugs and specific agents with demonstrated efficacy in these conditions and with OCD.

Determining whether a patient has responded to a medication requires that sufficient doses be given for a sufficient duration. This is separate from the time needed to gradually increment to the maximum tolerated dose. A majority of studies suggest that an adequate trial has been offered when the patient receives either the maximum allowable dose or the maximum dose that the patient can tolerate for at least 4 weeks. An important consideration in weighing efficacy is adherence to the prescription. Family accommodation affects adherence to both psychological and pharmacologic treatments and commonly results in missed doses or to taking an improper dose (155,177). Gradual dose reductions are necessary to avert withdrawal reactions when discontinuing those medications with shorter half-lives such as fluvoxamine and sertraline.

The most studied medications in the treatment of OCD are potent SRIs. While we refer to these drugs as SRIs, it should be kept in mind that all of them affect other neurotransmitter systems, too and, as a result, have different side-effect profiles. Controlled, blinded studies in children have used clomipramine (178,179), fluoxetine (180,181), fluvoxamine (182), sertraline (163,183,184), paroxetine (185), and citalopram (186,187). Of these, neither paroxetine nor citalopram has FDA indications for OCD.

Mataix-Col et al. (35) attempted to predict the outcome to placebo or active agents by stratifying the cohort according to factor-analyzed subgroups (see above). Their results suggested that the hoarding group was less likely than other subtypes to respond to SRIs. The other factor groups were not different from one another in their responsiveness to SRIs.

A meta-analysis of 12 studies of pediatric OCD employing SSRIs or clomipramine concluded that response rates among the SRRIs were comparable, and clomipramine was superior by a significant margin (188). Nevertheless, the side-effect profile and tolerance for clomipramine continue to place it outside consideration as the first-line pharmacologic treatment for pediatric OCD (189).

Augmentation Strategies

Between 40% and 50% of individuals with OCD do not respond to adequate trials of SRIs (163,190,191). The failure of response to one SRI agent does not predict failure of response to another, and side effects from one agent do not predict side effects on another. For this reason, it is important to offer adequate doses for a sufficient period of at least two and even three agents before moving on to augmentation strategies.

While the use of polypharmacy is generally to be avoided, an augmentation strategy may become necessary. There are randomized, double-blind placebo-controlled trials (RBDPCT) in adults suggesting that augmentation with haloperidol, risperidone, and aripiprazole may be useful (192,193); studies do not show benefits with olanzapine or quetiapine (192,193). A trial comparing aripiprazole versus risperidone added to existing medication for children with tic-related OCD showed both drugs were equally beneficial (194).

Use of atypical antipsychotic augmentation remains controversial (192); adding CBT to SRI was more effective than risperidone or pill placebo in a study of adults (195). Furthermore, in children who had not benefitted from an initial course of CBT, a randomized trial that extended CBT or added sertraline showed equal, and significant benefit (196). N-acetylcysteine is metabolized in the body into cysteine, a precursor to glutathione. The effects of NAC are diverse and yet to be understood but are likely to influence glutamate function (197). In adults (198) a small RBDPCT add-on study suggested NAC may be useful but no studies have been done in children with OCD.

Along the same lines, riluzole, a glutamate modulator, was assessed in an RBDPCT in children and failed to demonstrate a difference from placebo (199).

Partial Hospital and Inpatient Treatment

Hospitalizing patients to evaluate their symptoms is rarely feasible nowadays unless it can be justified by compelling concerns about safety. However, acute hospital care may be necessary and useful when patients or families are in crisis. Hospitalization may help when symptoms are severe and spiral out control, the family's capacity to support the patient is thoroughly depleted, compulsions are dangerous, or there is ongoing severe impairment despite a sufficient course of treatment. While clinicians are likely to feel pressed to initiate additional interventions in a crisis, in OCD such crises typically are the aggregation of chronic stressors that also are important to understand for the ongoing treatment.

In a crisis, partial (or day treatment) hospitalization can be a constructive alternative to inpatient care or dramatic changes in outpatient treatment. Furthermore, should partial hospital treatment fail, inpatient treatment may be more acceptable. Partial or inpatient hospitalization can reduce the pressure on parents and the patient to contain symptoms that are out of control. Also, it may provide rapid, objective assessment of the severity of the patient's impairment outside the home, facilitate integration of psychological, family, and pharmacologic treatments, and reduce stresses and anxiety of school or home.

COURSE AND OUTCOME

The mean age of onset of OCD is 19.5 years and the average duration of illness is 9 years (20,21). Skoog and Skoog (200) studied the natural history of 251 adult patients over 30 years. In this cohort, 29% had onset before age 20, 40% between ages 20 and 29 years, and 32% after age 30. Yet others report that 40% onset before age 20, and an average age of onset in the early 20s (201). In the ECA, the mean onset was 20.9 to 25.4 years of age (18). Others note that age of onset of OCD is almost exclusively before age 18 (59).

Outcome from an episode of OCD can range from complete, permanent remission to continuous decline. Points along this continuum include complete remission with discrete recurrent episodes, partial remission (chronic low to moderate symptoms), and partial remission punctuated by severe flare-ups (202).

Generalizing conclusions about outcome to all patient groups based on data derived from self-referred patients is unreliable and obtaining reliable outcome data from community samples is very challenging. Thus one study of adults reported "continuous" illness with fluctuating severity was the most common (84%) and a deteriorating course in 15% (23). Yet others (29) reported 2-year spontaneous remission rates of 65%, and another reported greater than 80% improved on all measures (203). Outcome based on hospitalized patients gives a rate of only 30% who were "greatly improved" (30,202).

Skoog and Skoog's (200) study of adults reported that intermittent illness (periods of OCD interspersed with completely symptom-free periods) occurred in 56% of their cohort, followed by chronic illness (continuous, unremitting severity lasting over 5 years) in 27%, and an episodic course (one episode of illness lasting <5 years) in 17%. In this 40-year longitudinal study, 83% of patients improved, 48% improved clinically, and 20% recovered completely (200).

A prospective study of a nonclinical public high school adolescent cohort resampled them 2 years after they were first identified with either OCD ($n = 16$) or "subclinical" obsessions or compulsions ($n = 10$) (204). Those with "subclinical" obsessions and compulsions did not worsen; only 1 of 10 developed OCD. Only 5 of 16 (31%) initially diagnosed with OCD met criteria 2 years later. Furthermore, a measure of impairment of those diagnosed with OCD diminished by 30%, beneath the cutoff for clinically significant impairment. The authors wondered if this reflected actual improvement or methodologic unreliability. The most likely predictors of an OCD diagnosis were previous diagnosis of OCD and presence of another psychiatric diagnosis with OC features. This could reflect the concept of OCD as a heterogeneous disorder with waxing and waning symptoms, and a relatively more benign, nondeteriorating course. The 69% recovery rate approaches the spontaneous adult remission rate reported by others (29,202).

Taken together for pediatric OCD, the general prognosis that emerges is of a less severe disorder than was reported in studies before 1990 (205–207). Sixty percent of children will improve to a level that they no longer meet criteria for the disorder and roughly two-thirds of those will recover (40% overall). Although this is certainly encouraging for the majority, those with co-occurring disorders, earlier onset, longer duration of symptoms, and poor psychosocial functioning are not as likely to recover. Poor response to medication, presence of tics, and parental psychopathology also predict a poorer outcome (208).

FUTURE CHALLENGES AND RESEARCH

On the treatment front, interest in OCD has produced well-informed clinicians with greater diagnostic and treatment skills. Self-help organizations, such as the International OCD Foundation (https://kids.iocdf.org; info@iocdf.org; International OCD Foundation, Inc., P.O. Box 961029 Boston, MA 02196), have informed the public and are bringing down the isolation and embarrassment experienced by persons with OCD. As organizations and clinicians educate the public, those who fear treatment or have been disappointed in previous efforts are now receiving more effective treatment and achieving some relief. A majority of seriously ill patients will improve if they receive specific CBTs or family cognitive-behavioral treatments, and, to a smaller extent, medications. Nevertheless, there is still a need to improve treatments. Current treatments produce limited success in 30% to 40% of patients (209). Hoarding remains the most refractory symptom and disorder (210).

Too many persons with OCD continue to suffer in secrecy. Epidemiologic studies remind us that the majority of persons with OCD do not obtain consultation or treatment. Too few clinicians are schooled CBT techniques (152,211). Vigorous effort to inform the public and assist primary care clinicians in recognition of OCD is still needed. Training clinicians in effective treatments, extending treatment and neuroscience research, and improving outreach and public education are the greatest challenges now.

On the research front, imaging techniques may yet illuminate structural relationships and link neuropsychologic and anatomical findings in ways that will advance more successful treatments. OCD also continues to hold out opportunities to learn about links between genetic endowment and environmental experience (212).

References

1. Kramer H, Sprenger J: *Malleus Maleficarum.* London, Pushkin Press, 1928.
2. Hunter R, Macalpine I: *Three Hundred Years of Psychiatry.* London, Oxford University Press, 1963.
3. Esquirol JED: *Des Maladies Mentales.* Paris, Ballière, 1845.
4. Maudsley H: *The Pathology of the Mind.* London, Macmillan, 1895.
5. Freud S: Notes upon a case of obsessional neurosis (1909). *Standard Edition.* London, Hogarth Press, 10:155–318, 1955.
6. Pitman RK: Pierre Janet on obsessive-compulsive disorder (1903). Review and commentary. *Arch Gen Psychiatry* 44(3):226–232, 1987.
7. Jaspers K: *General Psychopathology.* Chicago, University of Chicago Press, 1963.
8. Insel TR, Akiskal HS: Obsessive-compulsive disorder with psychotic features: a phenomenologic analysis. *Am J Psychiatry* 143(12):1527–1533, 1986.
9. Kozak MJ, Foa EB: Obsessions, overvalued ideas, and delusions in obsessive-compulsive disorder. *Behav Res Ther* 32(3):343–353, 1994.
10. American Psychiatric Association: *Diagnostic and Statistical Manual of Mental Disorders (5th ed): DSM-5.* Arlington, VA, American Psychiatric Publishing, 2013.
11. Evans DW, Leckman JF, Carter A, et al.: Ritual, habit, and perfectionism: the prevalence and development of compulsive-like behavior in normal young children. *Child Dev* 68(1):58–68, 1997.
12. Zohar AH, Bruno R: Normative and pathological obsessive-compulsive behavior and ideation in childhood: a question of timing. *J Child Psychol Psychiatry* 38(8):993–999, 1997.
13. Stein MB, Forde DR, Anderson G, Walker JR: Obsessive-compulsive disorder in the community: an epidemiologic survey with clinical reappraisal. *Am J Psychiatry* 154(8):1120–1126, 1997.
14. Crino R, Slade T, Andrews G: The changing prevalence and severity of obsessive-compulsive disorder criteria from DSM-III to DSM-IV. *Am J Psychiatry* 162(5):876–882, 2005.
15. Nestadt G, Bienvenu OJ, Cai G, Samuels J, Eaton WW: Incidence of obsessive-compulsive disorder in adults. *J Nerv Ment Dis* 186(7):401–406, 1998.
16. Fontenelle LF, Mendlowicz MV, Versiani M: The descriptive epidemiology of obsessive-compulsive disorder. *Prog Neuropsychopharmacol Biol Psychiatry* 30(3):327–337, 2006.
17. Nelson E, Rice J: Stability of diagnosis of obsessive-compulsive disorder in the epidemiologic catchment area study. *Am J Psychiatry* 154(6): 826–831, 1997.
18. Karno M, Golding JM, Sorenson SB, Burnam MA: The epidemiology of obsessive-compulsive disorder in five U.S. communities. *Arch Gen Psychiatry* 45(12):1094–1099, 1988.
19. Bebbington PE: Epidemiology of obsessive-compulsive disorder. *Br J Psychiatry Suppl* 35:2–6, 1998.
20. Ruscio AM, Stein DJ, Chiu WT, Kessler RC: The epidemiology of obsessive-compulsive disorder in the National comorbidity survey replication. *Mol Psychiatry* 15(1):53–63, 2010.
21. Koran LM, Hanna GL, Hollander E, Nestadt G, Simpson HB; American Psychiatric Association: Practice guideline for the treatment of patients with obsessive-compulsive disorder. *Am J Psychiatry* 164(7 Suppl):5–53, 2007.
22. Swedo SE, Rapoport JL, Leonard H, Lenane M, Cheslow D: Obsessive-compulsive disorder in children and adolescents: clinical phenomenology of 70 consecutive cases. *Arch Gen Psychiatry* 46(4):335–341, 1989.
23. Rasmussen SA, Tsuang MT: Clinical characteristics and family history in DSM-III obsessive-compulsive disorder. *Am J Psychiatry* 143(3):317–322, 1986.
24. Noshirvani HF, Kasvikis Y, Marks IM, Tsakiris F, Monteiro WO: Gender-divergent aetiological factors in obsessive-compulsive disorder. *Br J Psychiatry* 158:260–263, 1991.
25. Flament MF, Whitaker A, Rapoport JL, et al.: Obsessive compulsive disorder in adolescence: an epidemiological study. *J Am Acad Child Adolesc Psychiatry* 27(6):764–771, 1988.
26. Riddle MA, Scahill L, King R, et al.: Obsessive compulsive disorder in children and adolescents: phenomenology and family history. *J Am Acad Child Adolesc Psychiatry* 29(5):766–772, 1990.
27. Zohar AH, Ratzoni G, Pauls DL, et al.: An epidemiological study of obsessive-compulsive disorder and related disorders in Israeli adolescents. *J Am Acad Child Adolesc Psychiatry* 31(6):1057–1061, 1992.
28. Dowson JH: The phenomenology of severe obsessive-compulsive neurosis. *Br J Psychiatry* 131:75–78, 1977.
29. Rachman SL, Hodgson RJ: *Obsessions and Compulsions.* Englewood Cliffs, NJ, Prentice Hall Inc, 1980.
30. Welner A, Reich T, Robins E, Fishman R, Van Doren T: Obsessive-compulsive neurosis: record, follow-up, and family studies: I. inpatient record study. *Compr Psychiatry* 17(4):527–539, 1976.
31. Baer L: Factor analysis of symptom subtypes of obsessive compulsive disorder and their relation to personality and tic disorders. *J Clin Psychiatry* 55 Suppl:18–23, 1994.
32. Leckman JF, Grice DE, Boardman J, et al.: Symptoms of obsessive-compulsive disorder. *Am J Psychiatry* 154(7):911–917, 1997.
33. Summerfeldt LJ, Richter MA, Antony MM, Swinson RP: Symptom structure in obsessive-compulsive disorder: a confirmatory factor-analytic study. *Behav Res Ther* 37(4):297–311, 1999.
34. Leckman JF, Zhang H, Alsobrook JP, Pauls DL: Symptom dimensions in obsessive-compulsive disorder: toward quantitative phenotypes. *Am J Med Genet* 105(1):28–30, 2001.
35. Mataix-Cols D, Rauch SL, Manzo PA, Jenike MA, Baer L: Use of factor-analyzed symptom dimensions to predict outcome with serotonin reuptake inhibitors and placebo in the treatment of obsessive-compulsive disorder. *Am J Psychiatry* 156(9):1409–1416, 1999.
36. Mataix-Cols D, Marks IM, Greist JH, Kobak KA, Baer L: Obsessive-compulsive symptom dimensions as predictors of compliance with and response to behaviour therapy: results from a controlled trial. *Psychother Psychosom* 71(5):255–262, 2002.
37. Foa EB, Huppert JD, Leiberg S, et al.: The obsessive-compulsive inventory: development and validation of a short version. *Psychol Assess* 14(4):485–496, 2002.
38. Feinstein SB, Fallon BA, Petkova E, Liebowitz MR: Item-by-item factor analysis of the Yale-Brown Obsessive Compulsive Scale Symptom Checklist. *J Neuropsychiatry Clin Neurosci* 15(2):187–193, 2003.
39. Mataix-Cols D, Rosario-Campos MC, Leckman JF: A multidimensional model of obsessive-compulsive disorder. *Am J Psychiatry* 162(2):228–238, 2005.
40. Nestadt G, Addington A, Samuels J, et al.: The identification of OCD-related subgroups based on comorbidity. *Biol Psychiatry* 53(10):914–920, 2003.
41. Nestadt G, Samuels JF, Riddle MA, et al.: Obsessive-compulsive disorder: defining the phenotype. *J Clin Psychiatry* 63(Suppl 6):5–7, 2002.

42. Hasler G, LaSalle-Ricci VH, Ronquillo JG, et al.: Obsessive-compulsive disorder symptom dimensions show specific relationships to psychiatric comorbidity. *Psychiatry Res* 135(2):121–132, 2005.
43. Alonso P, Menchon JM, Pifarre J, et al.: Long-term follow-up and predictors of clinical outcome in obsessive-compulsive patients treated with serotonin reuptake inhibitors and behavioral therapy. *J Clin Psychiatry* 62(7):535–540, 2001.
44. Mataix-Cols D, Wooderson S, Lawrence N, Brammer MJ, Speckens A, Phillips ML: Distinct neural correlates of washing, checking, and hoarding symptom dimensions in obsessive-compulsive disorder. *Arch Gen Psychiatry* 61(6):564–576, 2004.
45. Phillips ML, Mataix-Cols D: Patterns of neural response to emotive stimuli distinguish the different symptom dimensions of obsessive-compulsive disorder. *CNS Spectr* 9(4):275–283, 2004.
46. Cavallini MC, Albertazzi M, Bianchi L, Bellodi L: Anticipation of age at onset of obsessive-compulsive spectrum disorders in patients with obsessive-compulsive disorder. *Psychiatry Res* 111(1):1–9, 2002.
47. Miguel EC, Leckman JF, Rauch S, et al.: Obsessive-compulsive disorder phenotypes: implications for genetic studies. *Mol Psychiatry* 10(3):258–275, 2005.
48. Alsobrook II JP, Leckman JF, Goodman WK, Rasmussen SA, Pauls DL: Segregation analysis of obsessive-compulsive disorder using symptom-based factor scores. *Am J Med Genet* 88(6):669–675, 1999.
49. Rettew DC, Swedo SE, Leonard HL, Lenane MC, Rapoport JL: Obsessions and compulsions across time in 79 children and adolescents with obsessive-compulsive disorder. *J Am Acad Child Adolesc Psychiatry* 31(6):1050–1056, 1992.
50. Mataix-Cols D, Rauch SL, Baer L, et al.: Symptom stability in adult obsessive-compulsive disorder: data from a naturalistic two-year follow-up study. *Am J Psychiatry* 159(2):263–268, 2002.
51. Fernández de la Cruz L, Micali N, Roberts S, et al.: Are the symptoms of obsessive-compulsive disorder temporally stable in children/adolescents? A prospective naturalistic study. *Psychiatry Res* 209(2):196–201, 2013.
52. Riddle MA, Hardin MT, King R, Scahill L, Woolston JL: Fluoxetine treatment of children and adolescents with Tourette's and obsessive compulsive disorders: preliminary clinical experience. *J Am Acad Child Adolesc Psychiatry* 29(1):45–48, 1990.
53. Koran LM, Thienemann ML, Davenport R: Quality of life for patients with obsessive-compulsive disorder. *Am J Psychiatry* 1996;153(6): 783–788.
54. Stengler-Wenzke K, Trosbach J, Dietrich S, Angermeyer MC: Coping strategies used by the relatives of people with obsessive-compulsive disorder. *J Adv Nurs* 48(1):35–42, 2004.
55. Stengler-Wenzke K, Trosbach J, Dietrich S, Angermeyer MC: Experience of stigmatization by relatives of patients with obsessive compulsive disorder. *Arch Psychiatr Nurs* 18(3):88–96, 2004.
56. Inouye E: Similar and dissimilar manifestations of obsessive-compulsive neuroses in monozygotic twins. *Am J Psychiatry* 121:1171–1175, 1965.
57. Fyer AJ, Lipsitz JD, Mannuzza S, Aronowitz B, Chapman TF: A direct interview family study of obsessive-compulsive disorder. I. *Psychol Med* 35(11):1611–1621, 2005.
58. Grabe HJ, Ruhrmann S, Ettelt S, et al.: Familiality of obsessive-compulsive disorder in nonclinical and clinical subjects. *Am J Psychiatry* 163(11):1986–1992, 2006.
59. Nestadt G, Samuels J, Riddle M, et al.: A family study of obsessive-compulsive disorder. *Arch Gen Psychiatry* 57(4):358–363, 2000.
60. Pauls DL, Alsobrook JP 2nd, Goodman W, Rasmussen S, Leckman JF: A family study of obsessive-compulsive disorder. *Am J Psychiatry* 152(1):76–84, 1995.
61. do Rosario-Campos MC, Leckman JF, Curi M, et al.: A family study of early-onset obsessive-compulsive disorder. *Am J Med Genet B Neuropsychiatr Genet* 136B(1):92–97, 2005.
62. Hanna GL, Himle JA, Curtis GC, Gillespie, BW: A family study of obsessive-compulsive disorder with pediatric probands. *Am J Med Genet B Neuropsychiatr Genet* 134B(1):13–19, 2005.
63. Browne HA, Gair SL, Scharf JM, Grice DE: Genetics of obsessive-compulsive disorder and related disorders. *Psychiatr Clin North Am* 37(3):319–335, 2014.
64. Karno M, Golding JM. Obsessive-compulsive disorder. In: Robins LN, Regier DA (eds): *Psychiatric Disorders in America.* New York, NY, The Free Press, 204–219, 1991.
65. Eley TC, Bolton D, O'Connor TG, Perrin S, Smith P, Plomin R: A twin study of anxiety-related behaviours in pre-school children. *J Child Psychol Psychiatry* 44(7):945–960, 2003.
66. Hudziak JJ, Van Beijsterveldt CE, Althoff RR, et al.: Genetic and environmental contributions to the child behavior checklist obsessive-compulsive scale: a cross-cultural twin study. *Arch Gen Psychiatry* 61(6):608–616, 2004.
67. Iervolino AC, Rijsdijk FV, Cherkas L, Fullana MA, Mataix-Cols D: A multivariate twin study of obsessive-compulsive symptom dimensions. *Arch Gen Psychiatry* 68(6):637–644, 2011.
68. Mataix-Cols D, Boman M, Monzani B, et al.: Population-based, multi-generational family clustering study of obsessive-compulsive disorder. *JAMA Psychiatry* 70(7):709–717, 2013.
69. Monzani B, Rijsdijk F, Cherkas L, Harris J, Keuthen N, Mataix-Cols D: Prevalence and heritability of skin picking in an adult community sample: a twin study. *Am J Med Genet B Neuropsychiatr Genet* 159B(5):605–610, 2012.
70. Monzani B, Rijsdijk F, Harris J, Mataix-Cols D: The structure of genetic and environmental risk factors for dimensional representations of DSM-5 obsessive-compulsive spectrum disorders. *JAMA Psychiatry* 71(2):182–189, 2014.
71. Lee SH, Wray NR, Goddard ME, Visscher PM: Estimating missing heritability for disease from genome-wide association studies. *Am J Human Genet* 88(3):294–305, 2011.
72. Yang J, Manolio TA, Pasquale LR, et al.: Genome partitioning of genetic variation for complex traits using common SNPs. *Nat Genet* 43(6):519–525, 2011.
73. Davis LK, Yu D, Keenan CL, et al.: Partitioning the heritability of Tourette syndrome and obsessive compulsive disorder reveals differences in genetic architecture. *PLoS Genet* 9(10):e1003864, 2013.
74. Hanna GL, Veenstra-VanderWeele J, Cox NJ, et al.: Genome-wide linkage analysis of families with obsessive-compulsive disorder ascertained through pediatric probands. *Am J Med Genet* 114(5):541–552, 2002.
75. Shugart YY, Samuels J, Willour VL, et al.: Genomewide linkage scan for obsessive-compulsive disorder: evidence for susceptibility loci on chromosomes 3q, 7p, 1q, 15q, and 6q. *Mol Psychiatry,* 11(8):763–770, 2006.
76. Willour VL, Yao Shugart Y, Samuels J, et al.: Replication study supports evidence for linkage to 9p24 in obsessive-compulsive disorder. *Am J Human Genet* 75(3):508–513, 2004.
77. Nestadt G, Grados M, Samuels JF: Genetics of obsessive-compulsive disorder. *Psychiatr Clin North Am* 33(1):141–158, 2010.
78. Bloch MH, Pittenger C: The genetics of obsessive-compulsive disorder. *Curr Psychiatry Rev* 6(2):91–103, 2010.
79. Hemmings SM, Stein DJ: The current status of association studies in obsessive-compulsive disorder. *Psychiatr Clin North Am* 29(2):411–444, 2006.
80. Samuels J. Grados MA, Planalp E, Bienvenu OJ: Genetic understanding of OCD and spectrum disorders. In: Steketee G (ed): *In the Oxford Handbook of Obsessive Compulsive and Spectrum Disorders.* New York, NY, Oxford University Press, 111–125, 2012.
81. Stewart SE, Mayerfeld C, Arnold PD, et al.: Meta-analysis of association between obsessive-compulsive disorder and the 3′ region of neuronal glutamate transporter gene SLC1A1. *Am J Med Genet B Neuropsychiatr Genet* 162B(4):367–379, 2013.
82. Stewart SE, Yu D, Scharf JM, et al.: Genome-wide association study of obsessive-compulsive disorder. *Mol Psychiatry* 18(7):788–798, 2013.
83. Mattheisen M, Samuels JF, Wang Y, et al.: Genome-wide association study in obsessive-compulsive disorder: results from the OCGAS. *Mol Psychiatry* 20(3):337–344, 2015.
84. Menzies L, Chamberlain SR, Laird AR, Thelen SM, Sahakian BJ, Bullmore ET: Integrating evidence from neuroimaging and neuropsychological studies of obsessive-compulsive disorder: the orbitofronto-striatal model revisited. *Neurosci Biobehav Rev* 32(3):525–549, 2008.
85. Huyser C, Veltman DJ, de Haan E, Boer F: Paediatric obsessive-compulsive disorder, a neurodevelopmental disorder? Evidence from neuroimaging. *Neurosci Biobehav Rev* 33(6):818–830, 2009.
86. Eng GK, Sim K, Chen SH: Meta-analytic investigations of structural grey matter, executive domain-related functional activations, and white matter diffusivity in obsessive compulsive disorder: an integrative review. *Neurosci Biobehav Rev* 52:233–257, 2015.
87. Abramovitch A, Abramowitz JS, Mittelman A, Stark A, Ramsey K, Geller DA: Research review: neuropsychological test performance in pediatric obsessive-compulsive disorder—a meta-analysis. *J Child Psychol Psychiatry* 56(8):837–847, 2015.
88. Stern ER, Taylor SF: Cognitive neuroscience of obsessive-compulsive disorder. *Psychiatr Clin North Am* 37(3):337–352, 2014.
89. Milad MR, Rauch SL: Obsessive-compulsive disorder: beyond segregated cortico-striatal pathways. *Trends Cogn Sci* 16(1):43–51, 2012.
90. Nakao T, Okada K, Kanba S: Neurobiological model of obsessive-compulsive disorder: evidence from recent neuropsychological and neuroimaging findings. *Psychiatry Clin Neurosci* 68(8):587–605, 2014.
91. Saxena S, Rauch SL: Functional neuroimaging and the neuroanatomy of obsessive-compulsive disorder. *Psychiatr Clin North Am* 23(3):563–586, 2000.
92. Friedlander L, Desrocher M: Neuroimaging studies of obsessive-compulsive disorder in adults and children. *Clin Psychol Rev* 26(1):32–49, 2006.
93. de Wit SJ, Alonso P, Schweren L, et al.: Multicenter voxel-based morphometry mega-analysis of structural brain scans in obsessive compulsive disorder. *Am J Psychiatry* 171(3):340–349, 2014.
94. Radua J, van den Heuvel OA, Surguladze S, Mataix-Cols D: Meta-analytical comparison of voxel-based morphometry studies in obsessive-compulsive disorder vs other anxiety disorders. *Arch Gen Psychiatry* 67(7):701–711, 2010.
95. Zarei M, Mataix-Cols D, Heyman I, et al.: Changes in gray matter volume and white matter microstructure in adolescents with obsessive-compulsive disorder. *Biol Psychiatry* 70(11):1083–1090, 2011.

96. Rotge JY, Guehl D, Dilharreguy B, et al.: Meta-analysis of brain volume changes in obsessive-compulsive disorder. *Biol Psychiatry* 65(1):75–83, 2009.
97. Baxter LR Jr, Phelps ME, Mazziotta JC, Guze BH, Schwartz JM, Selin CE: Local cerebral glucose metabolic rates in obsessive-compulsive disorder: a comparison with rates in unipolar depression and in normal controls. *Arch Gen Psychiatry* 44(3):211–218, 1987.
98. Baxter LR Jr, Schwartz JM, Mazziotta JC, et al.: Cerebral glucose metabolic rates in nondepressed patients with obsessive-compulsive disorder. *Am J Psychiatry* 145(12):1560–1563, 1988.
99. Nordahl TE, Benkelfat C, Semple WE, Gross M, King AC, Cohen RM: Cerebral glucose metabolic rates in obsessive compulsive disorder. *Neuropsychopharmacology* 2(1):23–28, 1989.
100. Swedo SE, Schapiro MB, Grady CL, et al.: Cerebral glucose metabolism in childhood-onset obsessive-compulsive disorder. *Arch Gen Psychiatry* 46(6):518–523, 1989.
101. Martinot JL, Allilaire JF, Mazoyer BM, et al.: Obsessive-compulsive disorder: a clinical, neuropsychological and positron emission tomography study. *Acta Psychiatr Scand* 82(3):233–242, 1990.
102. Perani D, Colombo C, Bressi S, et al.: [18F]FDG PET study in obsessive-compulsive disorder: a clinical/metabolic correlation study after treatment. *Br J Psychiatry* 166(2):244–250, 1995.
103. Whiteside SP, Port JD, Abramowitz JS: A meta-analysis of functional neuroimaging in obsessive-compulsive disorder. *Psychiatry Res* 132(1): 69–79, 2004.
104. Rauch SL, Jenike MA, Alpert NM, et al.: Regional cerebral blood flow measured during symptom provocation in obsessive-compulsive disorder using oxygen 15-labeled carbon dioxide and positron emission tomography. *Arch Gen Psychiatry* 51(1):62–70, 1994.
105. Saxena S, Brody AL, Maidment KM, et al.: Cerebral glucose metabolism in obsessive-compulsive hoarding. *Am J Psychiatry* 161(6):1038–1048, 2004.
106. Sawle GV, Hymas NF, Lees AJ, Frackowiak RS: Obsessional slowness. Functional studies with positron emission tomography. *Brain* 114(Pt 5): 2191–2202, 1991.
107. Baxter LR Jr, Schwartz JM, Bergman KS, et al.: Caudate glucose metabolic rate changes with both drug and behavior therapy for obsessive-compulsive disorder. *Arch Gen Psychiatry* 49(9):681–689, 1992.
108. Brody AL, Saxena S, Schwartz JM, et al.: FDG-PET predictors of response to behavioral therapy and pharmacotherapy in obsessive compulsive disorder. *Psychiatry Res* 84(1):1–6, 1998.
109. Endrass T, Ullsperger M: Specificity of performance monitoring changes in obsessive-compulsive disorder. *Neurosci Biobehav Rev* 46 (Pt 1):124–138, 2014.
110. Rauch SL, Wedig MM, Wright CI, et al.: Functional magnetic resonance imaging study of regional brain activation during implicit sequence learning in obsessive-compulsive disorder. *Biol Psychiatry* 61(3):330–336, 2007.
111. van Veen V, Carter CS: The anterior cingulate as a conflict monitor: fMRI and ERP studies. *Physiol Behav* 77(4–5):477–482, 2002.
112. Ursu S, Stenger VA, Shear MK, Jones MR, Carter CS: Overactive action monitoring in obsessive-compulsive disorder: evidence from functional magnetic resonance imaging. *Psychol Sci* 14(4):347–353, 2003.
113. Bush G, Luu P, Posner MI: Cognitive and emotional influences in anterior cingulate cortex. *Trends Cogn Sci* 4(6):215–222, 2000.
114. Viard A, Flament MF, Artiges E, et al.: Cognitive control in childhood-onset obsessive-compulsive disorder: a functional MRI study. *Psychol Med* 35(7):1007–1017, 2005.
115. Carter CS, Macdonald AM, Botvinick M, et al.: Parsing executive processes: strategic vs. evaluative functions of the anterior cingulate cortex. *Proc Natl Acad Sci U S A* 97(4):1944–1948, 2000.
116. Macdonald AW 3rd, Cohen JD, Stenger VA, Carter CS: Dissociating the role of the dorsolateral prefrontal and anterior cingulate cortex in cognitive control. *Science* 288(5472):1835–1838, 2000.
117. Botvinick M, Nystrom LE, Fissell K, Carter CS, Cohen JD: Conflict monitoring versus selection-for-action in anterior cingulate cortex. *Nature* 402(6758):179–181, 1999.
118. van der Wee NJ, Ramsey NF, Jansma JM, et al.: Spatial working memory deficits in obsessive compulsive disorder are associated with excessive engagement of the medial frontal cortex. *Neuroimage* 20(4):2271–2280, 2003.
119. Koch K, Reess TJ, Rus OG, Zimmer C, Zaudig M: Diffusion tensor imaging (DTI) studies in patients with obsessive-compulsive disorder (OCD): a review. *J. Psychiatr Res* 54:26–35, 2014.
120. Fitzgerald KD, Liu Y, Reamer EN, Taylor SF, Welsh RC: Atypical fronto-striatal-thalamic circuit white matter development in pediatric obsessive-compulsive disorder. *J Am Acad Child Adolesc Psychiatry* 53(11):1225–1233, 2014.
121. Weber AM, Soreni N, Stanley JA, et al.: Proton magnetic resonance spectroscopy of prefrontal white matter in psychotropic naïve children and adolescents with obsessive-compulsive disorder. *Psychiatry Res* 222(1–2):67–74, 2014.
122. Rosenberg DR, Mirza Y, Russell A, et al.: Reduced anterior cingulate glutamatergic concentrations in childhood OCD and major depression versus healthy controls. *J Am Acad Child Adolesc Psychiatry* 43(9):1146–1153, 2004.
123. Rosenberg DR, MacMaster FP, Keshavan MS, Fitzgerald KD, Stewart CM, Moore GJ: Decrease in caudate glutamatergic concentrations in pediatric obsessive-compulsive disorder patients taking paroxetine. *J Am Acad Child Adolesc Psychiatry* 39(9):1096–1103, 2000.
124. Leckman JF, King RA, Gilbert DL, et al.: Streptococcal upper respiratory tract infections and exacerbations of tic and obsessive-compulsive symptoms: a prospective longitudinal study. *J Am Acad Child Adolesc Psychiatry* 50(2):108–118, 2011.
125. Grados MA, Vasa RA, Riddle MA, et al.: New onset obsessive-compulsive symptoms in children and adolescents with severe traumatic brain injury. *Depress Anxiety* 25(5):398–407, 2008.
126. Swedo SE, Leonard HL, Garvey M, et al.: Pediatric autoimmune neuropsychiatric disorders associated with streptococcal infections: clinical description of the first 50 cases. *Am J Psychiatry* 155(2):264–271, 1998.
127. Chang K, Frankovich J, Cooperstock M, et al; PANS Collaborative Consortium: Clinical evaluation of youth with pediatric acute-onset neuropsychiatric syndrome (PANS): recommendations from the 2013 PANS Consensus Conference. *J Child Adolesc Psychopharmacol* 25(1):3–13, 2015.
128. Lougee L, Perlmutter SJ, Nicolson R, Garvey MA, Swedo SE: Psychiatric disorders in first-degree relatives of children with pediatric autoimmune neuropsychiatric disorders associated with streptococcal infections (PANDAS). *J Am Acad Child Adolesc Psychiatry* 39(9):1120–1126, 2000.
129. Singer HS, Gilbert DL, Wolf DS, Mink JW, Kurlan R: Moving from PANDAS to CANS. *J Pediatr* 160(5):725–731, 2012.
130. Murphy TK, Gerardi DM, Leckman JF: Pediatric acute-onset neuropsychiatric syndrome. *Psychiatr Clin North Am* 37(3):353–374, 2014.
131. Nicolson R, Swedo SE, Lenane M, et al.: An open trial of plasma exchange in childhood-onset obsessive-compulsive disorder without poststreptococcal exacerbations. *J Am Acad Child Adolesc Psychiatry* 39(10):1313–1315, 2000.
132. Practice parameter for the assessment and treatment of children and adolescents with obsessive-compulsive disorder. *J Am Acad Child Adolesc Psychiatry* 51(1):98–113, 2012.
133. Thoren P, Asberg M, Cronholm B, Jornestedt L, Traskman L: Clomipramine treatment of obsessive-compulsive disorder. I. A controlled clinical trial. *Arch Gen Psychiatry* 37(11):1281–1285, 1980
134. Parent A, Hazrati LN: Functional anatomy of the basal ganglia: I. The cortico-basal ganglia-thalamo-cortical loop. *Brain Res Brain Res Rev* 20(1):91–127, 1995.
135. Parent A, Hazrati LN: Functional anatomy of the basal ganglia. II. The place of subthalamic nucleus and external pallidum in basal ganglia circuitry. *Brain Res Brain Res Rev* 20(1):128–154, 1995.
136. Modell JG, Mountz JM, Curtis GC, Greden JF: Neurophysiologic dysfunction in basal ganglia/limbic striatal and thalamocortical circuits as a pathogenetic mechanism of obsessive-compulsive disorder. *J Neuropsychiatry Clin Neurosci* 1(1):27–36, 1989.
137. Baxter L: Functional imaging of brain systems mediating obsessive compulsive disorder. In: Charney DL, Nessler E, Bunney B (eds): *Neurobiology of Mental Illness*. London, Oxford Press, 534–547, 1999.
138. Insel TR, Winslow JT: Neurobiology of obsessive compulsive disorder. *Psychiatr Clin North Am* 15(4):813–824, 1992.
139. Alexander GE, Crutcher MD, DeLong MR: Basal ganglia-thalamocortical circuits: parallel substrates for motor, oculomotor, "prefrontal" and "limbic" functions. *Prog Brain Res* 85:119–146, 1990.
140. Rapoport JL, Inoff-Germain G: Treatment of obsessive-compulsive disorder in children and adolescents. *J Child Psychol Psychiatry* 41(4): 419–431, 2000.
141. Berg CJ, Rapoport JL, Flament M: The Leyton obsessional inventory-child version. *J Am Acad Child Psychiatry* 25(1):84–91, 1986.
142. Cooper J: The Leyton obsessional inventory. *Psychol Med* 1:48–64, 1970.
143. Goodman WK, Price LH, Rasmussen SA, et al.: The Yale–Brown obsessive compulsive scale. I. Development, use, and reliability. *Arch Gen Psychiatry* 46(11):1006–1011, 1989.
144. Goodman WK, Price LH, Rasmussen SA, et al.: The Yale–Brown obsessive compulsive scale: II. Validity. *Arch Gen Psychiatry* 46(11):1012–1016, 1989.
145. Scahill L, Riddle MA, McSwiggin-Hardin M, et al.: Children's Yale–Brown obsessive compulsive scale: reliability and validity. *J Am Acad Child Adolesc Psychiatry* 36(6):844–852, 1997.
146. Coetzer BR: Obsessive-compulsive disorder following brain injury: a review. *Int J Psychiatry Med* 34(4):363–377, 2004.
147. Towbin KE, Leckman JF, Cohen DJ: Drug treatment of obsessive-compulsive disorder: a review of findings in the light of diagnostic and metric limitations. *Psychiatr Dev* 5(1):25–50, 1987.
148. Samuels J, Bienvenu OJ 3rd, Riddle MA, et al.: Hoarding in obsessive compulsive disorder: results from a case-control study. *Behav Res Ther* 40(5):517–528, 2002.
149. Salkovskis PM, Harrison J: Abnormal and normal obsessions—a replication. *Behav Res Ther* 22(5):549–552, 1984.
150. Achenbach TM: *Manual for the Child Behavior Checklist and Revised Child Behavior Profile*. Burlington, VT, Thomas M. Achenbach, 1983.

151. Reynolds CR, Kamphaus RW. *BASC-2: Behavior Assessment System for Children*. 2nd ed. Circle Pines, MN, AGS Publishing, 2004.
152. National Institute for Health and Care Excellence (NICE): Obsessive-compulsive disorder and body dysmorphic disorder: treatment NICE guidelines CG31 [Internet] London. NICE Nov. 2005. Clinical guideline CG31 [Cited 08 April, 2016]. Available at: www.nice.org.uk/CG31
153. Sookman D, Fineberg NA; Accreditation Task Force of The Canadian Institute for Obsessive Compulsive Disorders: Specialized psychological and pharmacological treatments for obsessive-compulsive disorder throughout the lifespan: a special series by the Accreditation Task Force (ATF) of The Canadian Institute for Obsessive Compulsive Disorders (CIOCD, www.ciocd.ca). *Psychiatry Res* 227(1):74–77, 2015.
154. Flessner CA, Freeman JB, Sapyta J, et al.: Predictors of parental accommodation in pediatric obsessive-compulsive disorder: findings from the POTS trial. *J Am Acad Child Adolesc Psychiatry* 50(7):716–725, 2011.
155. Lebowitz ER, Panza KE, Su J, Bloch MH: Family accommodation in obsessive-compulsive disorder. *Expert Rev Neurother* 12(2):229–238, 2012.
156. March JS: Cognitive-behavioral psychotherapy for children and adolescents with OCD: a review and recommendations for treatment. *J Am Acad Child Adolesc Psychiatry* 34(1):7–18, 1995.
157. Franklin ME, Foa EB: Treatment of obsessive compulsive disorder. *Annu Rev Clin Psychol* 7:229–243, 2011.
158. O'Kearney RT, Anstey K, von Sanden C, Hunt A: Behavioural and cognitive behavioural therapy for obsessive compulsive disorder in children and adolescents. *Cochrane Database Syst Rev* 18(4):CD004856, 2006.
159. McKay D, Sookman D, Neziroglu F, et al; Accreditation Task Force of The Canadian Institute for Obsessive Compulsive Disorders: Efficacy of cognitive-behavioral therapy for obsessive-compulsive disorder. *Psychiatry Res* 227(1):104–113, 2015.
160. Franklin ME, Kratz HE, Freeman JB, et al; Accreditation Task Force of The Canadian Institute for Obsessive Compulsive Disorders: Cognitive-behavioral therapy for pediatric obsessive-compulsive disorder: empirical review and clinical recommendations. *Psychiatry Res* 227(1):78–92, 2015.
161. de Haan E, Hoogduin KA, Buitelaar JK, Keijsers GP: Behavior therapy versus clomipramine for the treatment of obsessive-compulsive disorder in children and adolescents. *J Am Acad Child Adolesc Psychiatry* 37(10):1022–1029, 1998.
162. Barrett P, Healy-Farrell L, March JS: Cognitive-behavioral family treatment of childhood obsessive-compulsive disorder: a controlled trial. *J Am Acad Child Adolesc Psychiatry* 43(1):46–62, 2004.
163. March JS; Pediatric Obsessive-Compulsive Treatment Study Group: Cognitive-behavior therapy, sertraline, and their combination for children and adolescents with obsessive-compulsive disorder: The Pediatric OCD Treatment Study (POTS) randomized controlled trial. *JAMA* 292(16):1969–1976, 2004.
164. March JS, Mulle K, Herbel B: Behavioral psychotherapy for children and adolescents with obsessive-compulsive disorder: an open trial of a new protocol-driven treatment package. *J Am Acad Child Adolesc Psychiatry* 33(3):333–341, 1994.
165. March JS, Frances A, Kahn D, Carpenter D: The expert consensus guidelines series: treatment of obsessive-compulsive disorder. *J Clin Psychiatry* 58(Suppl 4):1–72, 1997.
166. Franklin ME, Sapyta J, Freeman JB, et al.: Cognitive behavior therapy augmentation of pharmacotherapy in pediatric obsessive-compulsive disorder: the pediatric OCD treatment study II (POTS II) randomized controlled trial. *JAMA* 306:1224–1232, 2011.
167. Bolton D, Perrin S: Evaluation of exposure with response-prevention for obsessive compulsive disorder in childhood and adolescence. *J Behav Ther Exp Psychiatry* 39(1):11–22, 2008.
168. Williams TI, Salkovskis PM, Forrester L, Turner S, White H, Allsopp MA: A randomised controlled trial of cognitive behavioural treatment for obsessive compulsive disorder in children and adolescents. *Eur Child Adolesc Psychiatry* 19(5):449–456, 2010.
169. Storch EA, Geffken GR, Merlo LJ, et al.: Family-based cognitive-behavioral therapy for pediatric obsessive-compulsive disorder: comparison of intensive and weekly approaches. *J Am Acad Child Adolesc Psychiatry* 46:469–478, 2007.
170. Asbahr FR, Castillo AR, Ito LM, Latorre MR, Moreira MN, Lotufo-Neto F: Group cognitive-behavioral therapy versus sertraline for the treatment of children and adolescents with obsessive-compulsive disorder. *J Am Acad Child Adolesc Psychiatry* 44(11):1128–1136, 2005.
171. Anderson LM, Freeman JB, Franklin ME, Sapyta JJ: Family-based treatment of pediatric obsessive-compulsive disorder: clinical considerations and application. *Child Adolesc Psychiatr Clin N Am* 24(3):535–555, 2015.
172. Freeman JB, Garcia AM, Coyne L, et al.: Early childhood OCD: preliminary findings from a family-based cognitive-behavioral approach. *J Am Acad Child Adolesc Psychiatry* 47:593–602, 2008.
173. Piacentini J, Bergman RL, Chang S, et al.: Controlled comparison of family cognitive behavioral therapy and psychoeducation/relaxation training for child obsessive-compulsive disorder. *J Am Acad Child Adolesc Psychiatry* 50(11):1149–1161, 2011.
174. Merlo LJ, Storch EA, Lehmkuhl HD, et al.: Cognitive behavioral therapy plus motivational interviewing improves outcome for pediatric obsessive-compulsive disorder: a preliminary study. *Cogn Behav Ther* 39(1):24–27, 2010.
175. Storch EA, Caporino NE, Morgan JR, et al.: Preliminary investigation of web-camera delivered cognitive-behavioral therapy for youth with obsessive-compulsive disorder. *Psychiatry Res* 189(3):407–412, 2011.
176. Freeman J, Sapyta J, Garcia A, et al.: Family-based treatment of early childhood obsessive-compulsive disorder: the pediatric obsessive-compulsive disorder treatment study for young children (POTS Jr)—a randomized clinical trial. *JAMA Psychiatry* 71(6):689–698, 2014.
177. Murphy YE, Flessner CA: Family functioning in paediatric obsessive compulsive and related disorders. *Br J Clin Psychol* 54(4):414–434, 2015.
178. Flament MF, Rapoport JL, Berg CJ, et al.: Clomipramine treatment of childhood obsessive-compulsive disorder. A double-blind controlled study. *Arch Gen Psychiatry* 42(10):977–983, 1985.
179. DeVeaugh-Geiss J, Moroz G, Biederman J, et al.: Clomipramine hydrochloride in childhood and adolescent obsessive-compulsive disorder–a multicenter trial. *J Am Acad Child Adolesc Psychiatry* 31(1):45–49, 1992.
180. Fontaine R, Chouinard G: Fluoxetine in the treatment of obsessive compulsive disorder. *Prog Neuropsychopharmacol Biol Psychiatry* 9(5–6):605–608, 1985.
181. Geller DA, Hoog SL, Heiligenstein JH, et al.: Fluoxetine treatment for obsessive-compulsive disorder in children and adolescents: a placebo-controlled clinical trial. *J Am Acad Child Adolesc Psychiatry* 40(7):773–779, 2001.
182. Riddle MA, Reeve EA, Yaryura-Tobias JA, et al.: Fluvoxamine for children and adolescents with obsessive-compulsive disorder: a randomized, controlled, multicenter trial. *J Am Acad Child Adolesc Psychiatry* 40(2):222–229, 2001.
183. March JS, Biederman J, Wolkow R, et al.: Sertraline in children and adolescents with obsessive-compulsive disorder: a multicenter randomized controlled trial. *JAMA* 280(20):1752–1756, 1998.
184. Alderman J: Sertraline treatment of children and adolescents with obsessive-compulsive disorder or depression: pharmacokinetics, tolerability, and efficacy. *J Am Acad Child Adolesc Psychiatry* 37(4):386–394, 1998.
185. Geller DA, Wagner KD, Emslie G, et al.: Paroxetine treatment in children and adolescents with obsessive-compulsive disorder: a randomized, multicenter, double-blind, placebo-controlled trial. *J Am Acad Child Adolesc Psychiatry* 43(11):1387–1396, 2004.
186. Mukaddes NM, Abali O, Kaynak N: Citalopram treatment of children and adolescents with obsessive-compulsive disorder: a preliminary report. *Psychiatry Clin Neurosci* 57(4):405–408, 2003.
187. Alaghband-Rad J, Hakimshooshtary M: A randomized controlled clinical trial of citalopram versus fluoxetine in children and adolescents with obsessive-compulsive disorder (OCD). *Eur Child Adolesc Psychiatry* 18(3):131–135, 2009.
188. Geller DA, Biederman J, Stewart SE, et al.: Which SSRI? A meta-analysis of pharmacotherapy trials in pediatric obsessive-compulsive disorder. *Am J Psychiatry* 160(11):1919–1928, 2003.
189. March JS: Review: clomipramine is more effective than SSRIs for paediatric obsessive compulsive disorder. *Evid Based Ment Health* 7(2):50, 2004.
190. Chouinard G, Goodman W, Greist J, et al.: Results of a double-blind placebo controlled trial of a new serotonin uptake inhibitor, sertraline, in the treatment of obsessive-compulsive disorder. *Psychopharmacol Bull* 26(3):279–284, 1990.
191. Bloch MH, Storch EA: Assessment and management of treatment-refractory obsessive-compulsive disorder in children. *J Am Acad Child Adolesc Psychiatry* 54(4):251–262, 2015.
192. Veale D, Miles S, Smallcombe N, Ghezai H, Goldacre B, Hodsoll J: Atypical antipsychotic augmentation in SSRI treatment refractory obsessive-compulsive disorder: a systematic review and meta-analysis. *BMC Psychiatry* 29(14):317, 2014.
193. Dold M, Aigner M, Lanzenberger R, Kasper S: Antipsychotic augmentation of serotonin reuptake inhibitors in treatment-resistant obsessive-compulsive disorder: an update meta-analysis of double-blind, randomized, placebo-controlled trials. *Int J Neuropsychopharmacol* 18(9):pii: pyv047, 2015.
194. Masi G, Pfanner C, Brovedani P: Antipsychotic augmentation of selective serotonin reuptake inhibitors in resistant tic-related obsessive-compulsive disorder in children and adolescents: a naturalistic comparative study. *J Psychiatr Res* 47(8):1007–1012, 2013.
195. Simpson HB, Foa EB, Liebowitz MR, et al.: A randomized, controlled trial of cognitive-behavioral therapy for augmenting pharmacotherapy in obsessive-compulsive disorder. *Am J Psychiatry* 165(5):621–630, 2008.
196. Skarphedinsson G, Weidle B, Thomsen PH, et al.: Continued cognitive-behavior therapy versus sertraline for children and adolescents with obsessive-compulsive disorder that were non-responders to cognitive-behavior therapy: a randomized controlled trial. *Eur Child Adolesc Psychiatry* 24(5):591–602, 2015.
197. Dean O, Giorlando F, Berk M: N-acetylcysteine in psychiatry: current therapeutic evidence and potential mechanisms of action. *J Psychiatry Neurosci* 36(2):78–86, 2011.
198. Afshar H, Roohafza H, Mohammad-Beigi H, et al.: N-acetylcysteine add-on treatment in refractory obsessive-compulsive disorder: a

randomized, double-blind, placebo-controlled trial. *J Clin Psychopharmacol* 32(6):797–803, 2012.
199. Grant PJ, Joseph LA, Farmer CA, et al.: 12-week, placebo-controlled trial of add-on riluzole in the treatment of childhood-onset obsessive-compulsive disorder. *Neuropsychopharmacology* 39(6):1453–1459, 2014.
200. Skoog G, Skoog I: A 40-year follow-up of patients with obsessive-compulsive disorder. *Arch Gen Psychiatry* 56(2):121–127, 1999.
201. Black A: The natural history of obsessional neurosis. In: Beech HR (ed): *Obsessional States*. London, Metheun, 1–23, 1974.
202. Goodwin DW, Guze SB, Robins E: Follow-up studies in obsessional neurosis. *Arch Gen Psychiatry* 20(2):182–187, 1969.
203. Mawson D, Marks IM, Ramm L: Clomipramine and exposure for chronic obsessive-compulsive rituals: III. Two year follow-up and further findings. *Br J Psychiatry* 140:11–18, 1982.
204. Berg CZ, Rapoport JL, Whitaker A, et al.: Childhood obsessive compulsive disorder: a two-year prospective follow-up of a community sample. *J Am Acad Child Adolesc Psychiatry* 28(4):528–533, 1989.
205. Leonard HL, Swedo SE, Lenane MC, et al.: A 2- to 7-year follow-up study of 54 obsessive-compulsive children and adolescents. *Arch Gen Psychiatry* 50(6):429–439, 1993.
206. Wewetzer C, Jans T, Muller B, et al.: Long-term outcome and prognosis of obsessive-compulsive disorder with onset in childhood or adolescence. *Eur Child Adolesc Psychiatry* 10(1):37–46, 2001.
207. Stewart SE, Geller DA, Jenike M, et al.: Long-term outcome of pediatric obsessive-compulsive disorder: a meta-analysis and qualitative review of the literature. *Acta Psychiatr Scand* 110(1):4–13, 2004.
208. Leonard HL, Lenane MC, Swedo SE, Rettew DC, Gershon ES, Rapoport JL: Tics and Tourette's disorder: a 2- to 7-year follow-up of 54 obsessive-compulsive children. *Am J Psychiatry* 149(9):1244–1251, 1992.
209. Fisher PL, Wells A: How effective are cognitive and behavioral treatments for obsessive-compulsive disorder? A clinical significance analysis. *Behav Res Ther* 43(12):1543–1558, 2005.
210. Abramowitz JS, Khandker M, Nelson CA, Deacon BJ, Rygwall R: The role of cognitive factors in the pathogenesis of obsessive-compulsive symptoms: a prospective study. *Behav Res Ther* 44(9):1361–1374, 2006.
211. Lewin AB, Storch EA, Adkins J, Murphy TK, Geffken GR: Current directions in pediatric obsessive-compulsive disorder. *Pediatr Ann* 34(2):128–134, 2005.
212. Hyman SE: The millennium of mind, brain, and behavior. *Arch Gen Psychiatry* 57(1):88–89, 2000.

CHAPTER 5.5.3 ■ TRICHOTILLOMANIA AND EXCORIATION DISORDER

KENNETH E. TOWBIN

François Henri Hallopeau coined trichotillomania (TTM) from the Greek words for "hair + pulling + madness" in 1889 (1). TTM, excoriation disorder (ED), and obsessive-compulsive disorder (OCD) share a feature of repetitive behavior yet there may be more than this visible similarity between them (2,3). With publication of DSM-5, all three are part of a larger group of obsessive-compulsive and related disorders (OCRDs) (4). The DSM-5 concept of this obsessive-compulsive spectrum draws on shared characteristics of impulsive and repetitive behaviors and includes OCD, body dysmorphic disorder, hoarding disorder, TTM, and ED. The decision to place these together is controversial, particularly for TTM and ED (5,6). The rationale for encompassing them into a larger group of OCRDs grew from data suggesting (1) increased rates of hair pulling (HP) and ED among those with OCD, and of OCD among those with TTM or ED, (2) the shared phenotypic similarity of repetitive (compulsive) behaviors, preceded by urges, and followed by temporary relief, and (3) increased rates of these disorders among first-degree relatives of those with OCD and TTM (7–9). Furthermore, there are reports that childhood-onset OCD is a risk factor for TTM (10,11) and that TTM often has its onset in childhood and adolescence (8–11). Some have suggested that TTM and ED are alternative manifestations of the same genetic predisposition (3).

The DSM-5 diagnostic criteria for TTM and EM are essentially the same (4). Both require a behavioral component—recurrent HP (or skin picking) to the point of hair loss (or skin lesions), *and* a psychological component—repeated attempts to decrease or stop this behavior. In addition, there are the usual provisos that the problem must lead to distress or impairment in domains of social, occupational, or other areas of function in the person's life, not be attributable to a medical condition, and not be better explained by another condition (DSM-5, APA). Some investigators view these criteria as excessively restrictive (12–14).

TRICHOTILLOMANIA

The prevalence of HP without psychological components is 4% to 6% in the general population (13–15), compared to the 0.6% to 1% prevalence reported for TTM (13–15). Females are more common in some clinical samples while others report an equal distribution by gender (15). The age of incident peaks in early childhood and adolescence (13–15). Forty-five to 55% of TTM/HP patients report a childhood (before age 18) onset (16).

Data showing that HP and TTM have a similar course, prognosis, genetic risk, and treatment response would provide more convincing biologic evidence of a close relationship. TTM and HP are often comorbid with OCD (16–18). Four to 35% of patients with OCD report lifetime histories of TTM/HP (18–22), and 13% to 16% of those with TTM/HP report lifetime histories of OCD (16,23,24). Also, TTM and HP both are commonly associated with tic disorders (10,12,18,20,21,25). As with tics, TTM/HP appears to be particularly associated with early-onset OCD (12,18,20). TTM/HP is also associated with hoarding (26). Most studies have relied exclusively on clinical populations at risk, producing an erroneous, biased association (27). However, two studies drawing on nonreferred, community samples suggest an association may exist (13,14).

There is evidence that TTM/HP may show genetic associations with OCD (12,21) though the data are mixed. The first studies drew data from small and relatively unrepresentative samples (12,13). Bienvenu et al. (21) conducted a controlled family study of 88 adults with rigorously diagnosed OCD and their first-degree relatives. There were few individuals with TTM in the entire cohort. Comparing patient probands to healthy controls, rates of TTM were not statistically greater. Comparing first-degree relatives of probands to first-degree relatives of healthy volunteers (HVs), the rates of TTM were not significantly different. The study also ascertained rates for other "pathologic grooming behaviors" such as pathologic skin picking and nail biting. Only skin picking was statistically significantly greater among OCD probands compared to HVs. The rates for all grooming behaviors were not elevated in first-degree relatives of OCD patients compared to relatives of healthy controls (21). However, a replication study drawing on a larger number of patients and of first-degree relatives showed that, compared to a healthy control population and their relatives, the rate of TTM in those with OCD was greater both among patients and among their relatives (28).

There are preliminary, but few, neuropsychological data on TTM and there are many fewer data from pediatric patients. Compared to adults with OCD, adults with TTM display some overlapping but not entirely congruent patterns of neuropsychological impairments (29–31). One study (29) examining age- and IQ-matched adults with OCD, TTM, and HVs reported no differences between groups on measures of attention, memory, organization (verbal and nonverbal), visual–spatial abilities, and concept learning (29). The only differences were that those with TTM showed increased perseveration errors, suggesting cognitive inflexibility, compared to those with OCD and HVs, while compared to the other groups, patients with OCD showed impaired learning from feedback based on the Wisconsin Card Sort (29). Chamberlain et al. (31) examined a purported endophenotype for OCD related to "strategy implementation," which integrates cognitive functions and motor inhibition (30) and are, in turn, closely tied to the orbitofrontal striatal circuitry described for OCD (Chapter 5.5.2). Using the Stop Signal Task, to measure capacity to suppress impulsivity, these investigators (31) compared patients with only OCD to those with only TTM and HVs. They found that adults with TTM displayed abilities in strategy implementation equal to HVs (31), and significant deficits in motor inhibition compared to patients with OCD and HVs (30). In contrast, a study with pediatric patients (32) found that, after controlling for both age and symptoms of attention-deficit hyperactivity disorder, compared to HVs, children with TTM had *greater* inhibitory control.

Morphometric MRI studies have studied only a small number of patients (33–35). Taken together they suggest that compared to HVs, women with TTM have decreased volumes in the left frontal cortex. Interestingly, in contrast to reports on patients with OCD, there are no differences in the caudate or in white matter structures. A diffusion tensor imaging (DTI) study (36) of TTM showed reduced connectivity between white matter tracts that connect the orbital frontal cortex and anterior cingulate cortex, the left presupplemental motor area, and the left temporal lobe.

The relative rarity of TTM has hampers how much we know of its course and treatment. As with many uncommon disorders, the patients who come to clinical attention can be an inaccurate reflection of the entire range of the disorder, are likely to be severely impaired and to suffer from comorbid conditions such as depression or anxiety disorders. The best evidence suggests that TTM has a chronic waxing and waning course. One study (37) followed the course of only 14 participants after CBT; 12 of 14 individuals were considered responders at the end of treatment. However, at an average of 3 years 9 months follow-up, only 4 of 13 were still considered responders. When compared to the group of 10 individuals who initially refused treatment, there was no difference in overall response rates between treated and untreated groups (37). Another study (38) followed the course of 63 individuals who had participated in a "state-of-the-art" treatment study. After a mean of 42 months, 51% were still in treatment and 27% were not. Thirty-three (52%) participants considered themselves treatment responders while 16 (25%) improved with CBT alone. The investigators reported that higher rates of depression correlated with better outcome (38). However, in a subsequent follow-up of the same cohort (39) some 30 months later, 61% were still in active treatment for TTM and only 37% considered themselves treatment responders. While the first follow-up point reported improvement in self-esteem, depression, and anxiety, this progress had virtually disappeared at the second follow-up despite improvements in HP (39).

Pharmacotherapy offers modest improvement for TTM. Among all agents, serotonin reuptake inhibitors have been the most studied (38,40–44). Few randomized controlled studies have been conducted and rates of improvement have been disappointing. While open-label studies report rates of improvement of 30% to 60%, two placebo-controlled trials showed no significant difference from placebo (41,43). Generally, the response to SSRIs appears to be lower in TTM than what treatment trials report for patients with OCD (44).

Two small studies employing randomized assignment demonstrated superiority of CBT to medication (one study using clomipramine, the other fluoxetine) (42,45,46). In order to explore whether these gains could be maintained, Keijsers et al. (45) performed a 3-month and then a 2-year follow-up on 28 participants, some of whom were previously in the CBT versus fluoxetine study, while others were simply assigned to cognitive-behavioral treatment subsequently. Initial treatment effects, again showing large effect sizes, rivaled those observed in the original CBT versus fluoxetine study (46) but the benefits deteriorated at 3 months and at 2 years (45). Pretreatment depression was a significant predictor of poor outcome, and the ability to cease HP by the end of behavioral treatment was associated with a greater likelihood of improvement (45). Both of these studies present a risk of being underpowered since they randomized less than 20 individuals per treatment group.

Data suggesting that modulation of glutamatergic pathways might benefit repetitive behavior disorders led to a randomized double-blind placebo-controlled add-on study of *N*-acetyl cysteine (NAC) for TTM in adults (47). NAC showed significant benefits, with 56% responding to drug versus 16% to placebo and clinically significant change in 44% of those on NAC compared to 4% given placebo. There were few ill effects (47). However, when the study was replicated in children (48) there were no differences between drug and placebo, emphasizing that caution should be used when generalizing adult study data to children (48).

Overall, manualized CBT or habit reversal training (HRT) appears to be superior to pharmacologic treatment for TTM (49,50). However, at best the initial gains made in CBT are difficult to maintain and comorbid depression makes them even harder to sustain. At this point there are no specific indicators to suggest which patients will be more likely to respond to CBT/HRT or medication and there are no augmentation strategies that have been studied with sufficient rigor to permit one to recommend them.

Many more questions remain to be answered before we will understand the genetics, neurobiology, course, and treatment of TTM. Although the last decade has seen very significant gains, particularly in understanding the cognitive underpinnings of TTM, it is likely that the larger majority of children with TTM remain to be identified and offered treatment. Clearly without treatment the majority of patients with TTM have very severe impairment in function (49,51). Some individuals develop severe gastrointestinal complications from trichobezoars (52–54). Treatment can improve TTM but there is a gap to be closed on how to sustain those gains. Fifty to 66% of those who receive CBT find their symptoms improve, but of those for whom treatment was successful, only about 50% maintained those gains over 2 years, and the majority required ongoing treatment for many years.

EXCORIATION DISORDER

While the data on TTM are scanty, those on ED, particularly with children and youth, are more meager yet. Thus, assertions about the prevalence, pathophysiology, treatment, and course of this disorder in children are almost entirely the product of downward extrapolations of adult studies and require confirmation by pediatric-focused research.

The only community-based prevalence study of pathologic skin picking, though flawed, gives a general population estimate of 5% (55) which is close to the 4% rate reported in university students (56,57). Limitations in ascertainment and diagnostic measurement affect the reliability of all of these reports. A community-based (nonclinical) twin study reported a life-time prevalence of 1.2% (58).

The sole genetic study of ED relative to other OCRDs (3) used factor analysis in an adult cohort to explore the relationships among all the conditions in the DSM-5 OCRD chapter. The data suggest a general factor of moderate heritability for all the OCRDs, and an additional factor of moderate heritability for TTM and ED. There were no factors that differentiated genetic risk for TTM from ED, or were unique to ED (3). This is further supported by the twin study, above (58), which found 40% of the variance in the sample could be explained by genetic factors.

So far, there appears to be no unique pathophysiologic features that separate ED from TTM. Like those with TTM (30), individuals with ED show impairments in inhibitory control (59,60), which suggests impairments in the circuit linking the inferior frontal gyrus and anterior cingulate cortex. One neuroimaging study, using DTI, showed that, compared to HVs, those with ED displayed diminished connectivity between cingulate cortex and other regions (61). Of note, the same research consortium reported a similar finding using DTI in those with TTM (36). An fMRI study of females comparing those with ED to those with TTM and to HVs (62) reported greater volumes in the accumbens and thinner cortex in the inferior frontal gyrus and orbitofrontal regions, and thicker cortex in the cuneus bilaterally in the ED cohort; there were no differences in these regions between those with TTM and HVs. The investigators noted the relevance of the involvement of these frontostriatal regions in stimulus-response habit formation.

There are no pediatric treatment data available. In adults, two double-blind, placebo-controlled trials (DBPCT) using SSRIs, one with fluoxetine (63) and the other with citalopram (64), offered mixed results. The fluoxetine study showed benefits on only one of the three primary outcome measures, and in the citalopram study there was no improvement on the primary outcome measure. A DBRCT of lamotrigine showed no difference between drug and placebo (65). A DBPCT of NAC (66) for ED reported statistically significant reductions in severity although the study is marred by a 30% drop out rate among those in the placebo arm, no difference on self-reported changes in picking, and a *clinically* dubious difference of just 0.5 on the CGI-severity scale at 12 weeks. Response rates were 47% in the NAC group compared to 19% of *completers* in placebo (66).

There is only one randomized controlled study of CBT for ED (67); all participants were college students. Participants were randomly assigned to either four sessions of CBT or a waitlist group, a design with significant limitations. There were significant differences in the primary measures and positive effects were sustained at a 2-month follow-up.

Needless to say, a great deal remains to be learned about ED, particularly in pediatric populations. Nevertheless, growing awareness among clinicians and investigators opens the way to improving our understanding of its course, pathophysiology, assessment, and treatment.

References

1. Hallopeau M: Alopécia par grattage (trichomanie ou trichotillomanie). *Ann Dermatol Venereol* 10:440–441, 1889.
2. Stein DJ, Kogan CS, Atmaca M, et al.: The classification of obsessive-compulsive and related disorders in the ICD-11. *J Affect Disord* 190:663–674, 2016.
3. Monzani B, Rijsdijk F, Harris J, Mataix-Cols D: The structure of genetic and environmental risk factors for dimensional representations of DSM-5 obsessive-compulsive spectrum disorders. *JAMA Psychiatry* 71(2):182–189, 2014.
4. American Psychiatric Association: *Diagnostic and Statistical Manual of Mental Disorders*. 5th ed. Arlington, VA: American Psychiatric Publishing, 2013.
5. Mataix-Cols D, Pertusa A, Leckman JF: Issues for DSM-V: how should obsessive-compulsive and related disorders be classified? *Am J Psychiatry* 164(9):1313–1314, 2007.
6. Abramowitz JS, Jacoby RJ: Obsessive-compulsive and related disorders: a critical review of the new diagnostic class. *Annu Rev Clin Psychol* 11:165–186, 2015.
7. Flessner CA, Knopik VS, McGeary J: Hair pulling disorder (trichotillomania): genes, neurobiology, and a model for understanding impulsivity and compulsivity. *Psychiatry Res* 199(3):151–158, 2012.
8. Stein DJ, Grant JE, Franklin ME, et al.: Trichotillomania (hair pulling disorder), skin picking disorder, and stereotypic movement disorder: toward DSM-V. *Depress Anxiety* 27(6):611–626, 2010.
9. Snorrason I, Belleau EL, Woods DW: How related are hair pulling disorder (trichotillomania) and skin picking disorder? A review of evidence for comorbidity, similarities and shared etiology. *Clin Psychol Rev* 32(7):618–629, 2012.
10. Diniz JB, Rosario-Campos MC, Shavitt RG, et al.: Impact of age at onset and duration of illness on the expression of comorbidities in obsessive-compulsive disorder. *J Clin Psychiatry* 65(1):22–27, 2004.
11. Hanna GL: Trichotillomania and related disorders in children and adolescents. *Child Psychiatry Hum Dev* 27(4):255–268, 1997.
12. King RA, Scahill L, Vitulano LA, Schwab-Stone M, Tercyak KP Jr, Riddle MA: Childhood trichotillomania: clinical phenomenology, comorbidity, and family genetics. *J Am Acad Child Adolesc Psychiatry* 34(11):1451–1459, 1995.
13. Christenson GA, Pyle RL, Mitchell JE: Estimated lifetime prevalence of trichotillomania in college students. *J Clin Psychiatry* 52(10):415–417, 1991.
14. King RA, Zohar AH, Ratzoni G, et al.: An epidemiological study of trichotillomania in Israeli adolescents. *J Am Acad Child Adolesc Psychiatry* 34(9):1212–1215, 1995.
15. Duke DC, Bodzin DK, Tavares P, Geffken GR, Storch EA: The phenomenology of hairpulling in a community sample. *J Anxiety Disord* 23(8):1118–1125, 2009.
16. Christenson GA, Mackenzie TB, Mitchell JE: Characteristics of 60 adult chronic hair pullers. *Am J Psychiatry* 148(3):365–370, 1991.
17. Fontenelle LF, Mendlowicz MV, Versiani M: Impulse control disorders in patients with obsessive-compulsive disorder. *Psychiatry Clin Neurosci* 59(1):30–37, 2005.
18. Jaisoorya TS, Reddy YC, Srinath S: The relationship of obsessive-compulsive disorder to putative spectrum disorders: results from an Indian study. *Compr Psychiatry* 44(4):317–323, 2003.
19. Richter MA, Summerfeldt LJ, Antony MM, Swinson RP: Obsessive-compulsive spectrum conditions in obsessive-compulsive disorder and other anxiety disorders. *Depress Anxiety* 18(3):118–127, 2003.
20. Stewart SE, Jenike MA, Keuthen NJ: Severe obsessive-compulsive disorder with and without comorbid hair pulling: comparisons and clinical implications. *J Clin Psychiatry* 66(7):864–869, 2005.
21. Bienvenu OJ, Samuels JF, Riddle MA, et al.: The relationship of obsessive-compulsive disorder to possible spectrum disorders: results from a family study. *Biol Psychiatry* 48(4):287–293, 2000.
22. du Toit PL, van Kradenburg J, Niehaus DJ, Stein DJ: Characteristics and phenomenology of hair-pulling: an exploration of subtypes. *Compr Psychiatry* 42(3):247–256, 2001.
23. Cohen LJ, Stein DJ, Simeon D, et al.: Clinical profile, comorbidity, and treatment history in 123 hair pullers: a survey study. *J Clin Psychiatry* 56(7):319–326, 1995.
24. Swedo SE, Leonard HL: Trichotillomania. An obsessive compulsive spectrum disorder? *Psychiatr Clin North Am* 15(4):777–790, 1992.
25. Hemmings SM, Kinnear CJ, Lochner C, et al.: Early-versus late-onset obsessive-compulsive disorder: investigating genetic and clinical correlates. *Psychiatry Res* 128(2):175–182, 2004.
26. Samuels J, Bienvenu OJ 3rd, Riddle MA, et al.: Hoarding in obsessive compulsive disorder: results from a case-control study. *Behav Res Ther* 40(5):517–528, 2002.
27. Cohen P, Cohen J: The clinician's illusion. *Arch Gen Psychiatry* 41(12):1178–1182, 1984.
28. Bienvenu OJ, Samuels JF, Wuyek LA, et al.: Is obsessive-compulsive disorder an anxiety disorder, and what, if any, are spectrum conditions? A family study perspective. *Psychol Med* 42(1):1–13, 2012.
29. Bohne A, Savage CR, Deckersbach T, et al.: Visuospatial abilities, memory, and executive functioning in trichotillomania and obsessive-compulsive disorder. *J Clin Exp Neuropsychol* 27(4):385–399, 2005.
30. Chamberlain SR, Fineberg NA, Blackwell AD, Robbins TW, Sahakian BJ: Motor inhibition and cognitive flexibility in obsessive-compulsive disorder and trichotillomania. *Am J Psychiatry* 163(7):1282–1284, 2006.
31. Chamberlain SR, Blackwell AD, Fineberg NA, Robbins TW, Sahakian BJ: Strategy implementation in obsessive-compulsive disorder and trichotillomania. *Psychol Med* 36(1):91–97, 2006.

32. Brennan E, Francazio S, Gunstad J, Flessner C: Inhibitory control in pediatric trichotillomania (hair pulling disorder): the importance of controlling for age and symptoms of inattention and hyperactivity. *Child Psychiatry Hum Dev* 47(2):173–182, 2016.
33. Stein DJ, Coetzer R, Lee M, Davids B, Bouwer C: Magnetic resonance brain imaging in women with obsessive-compulsive disorder and trichotillomania. *Psychiatry Res* 74(3):177–182, 1997.
34. O'Sullivan RL, Rauch SL, Breiter HC, et al.: Reduced basal ganglia volumes in trichotillomania measured via morphometric magnetic resonance imaging. *Biol Psychiatry* 42(1):39–45, 1997.
35. Grachev ID: MRI-based morphometric topographic parcellation of human neocortex in trichotillomania. *Psychiatry Clin Neurosci* 51(5): 315–321, 1997.
36. Chamberlain SR, Hampshire A, Menzies LA, et al.: Reduced brain white matter integrity in trichotillomania: a diffusion tensor imaging study. *Arch Gen Psychiatry* 67(9):965–971, 2010.
37. Lerner J: Effectiveness of a cognitive behavioral treatment program for trichotillomania: an uncontrolled evaluation. *Behavior Therapy* 29(1): 157–171, 1998.
38. Keuthen NJ, O'Sullivan RL, Goodchild P, Rodriguez D, Jenike MA, Baer L: Retrospective review of treatment outcome for 63 patients with trichotillomania. *Am J Psychiatry* 155(4):560–561, 1998.
39. Keuthen NJ, Fraim C, Deckersbach T, Dougherty DD, Baer L, Jenike MA: Longitudinal follow-up of naturalistic treatment outcome in patients with trichotillomania. *J Clin Psychiatry* 62(2):101–107, 2001.
40. Streichenwein SM, Thornby JI: A long-term, double-blind, placebo-controlled crossover trial of the efficacy of fluoxetine for trichotillomania. *Am J Psychiatry* 152(8):1192–1196, 1995.
41. Christenson GA, Mackenzie TB, Mitchell JE, Callies AL: A placebo-controlled, double-blind crossover study of fluoxetine in trichotillomania. *Am J Psychiatry* 148(11):1566–1571, 1991.
42. Ninan PT, Rothbaum BO, Marsteller FA, Knight BT, Eccard MB: A placebo-controlled trial of cognitive-behavioral therapy and clomipramine in trichotillomania. *J Clin Psychiatry* 61(1):47–50, 2000.
43. Swedo SE, Leonard HL, Rapoport JL, Lenane MC, Goldberger EL, Cheslow DL: A double-blind comparison of clomipramine and desipramine in the treatment of trichotillomania (hair pulling). *N Engl J Med* 321(8):497–501, 1989.
44. Walsh KH, McDougle CJ: Pharmacological strategies for trichotillomania. *Expert Opin Pharmacother* 6(6):975–984, 2005.
45. Keijsers GP, van Minnen A, Hoogduin CA, Klaassen BN, Hendriks MJ, Tanis-Jacobs J: Behavioural treatment of trichotillomania: two-year follow-up results. *Behav Res Ther* 44(3):359–370, 2006.
46. van Minnen A, Hoogduin KA, Keijsers GP, Hellenbrand I, Hendriks GJ: Treatment of trichotillomania with behavioral therapy or fluoxetine: a randomized, waiting-list controlled study. *Arch Gen Psychiatry* 60(5): 517–522, 2003.
47. Grant JE, Odlaug BL, Kim SW: N-acetylcysteine, a glutamate modulator, in the treatment of trichotillomania: a double-blind, placebo-controlled study. *Arch Gen Psychiatry* 66:756–763, 2009.
48. Bloch MH, Panza KE, Grant JE, et al.: N-Acetylcysteine in the treatment of pediatric trichotillomania: a randomized, double-blind, placebo-controlled add-on trial. *J Am Acad Child Adolesc Psychiatry* 52:231–240, 2013.
49. Duke DC, Keeley ML, Geffken GR, Storch EA: Trichotillomania: a current review. *Clin Psychol Rev* 30(2):181–193, 2010.
50. Bloch MH, Landeros-Weisenberger A, Dombrowski P, et al.: Systematic review: pharmacological and behavioral treatment for trichotillomania. *Biol Psychiatry* 62(8):839–846, 2007.
51. Diefenbach GJ, Tolin DF, Hannan S, Crocetto J, Worhunsky P: Trichotillomania: impact on psychosocial functioning and quality of life. *Behav Res Ther* 43(7):869–884, 2005.
52. Ciampa A, Moore BE, Listerud RG, Kydd D, Kim RD: Giant trichophy-tobezoar in a pediatric patient with trichotillomania. *Pediatr Radiol* 33(3):219–220, 2003.
53. Frey AS, McKee M, King RA, Martin A: Hair apparent: Rapunzel syndrome. *Am J Psychiatry* 162(2):242–248, 2005.
54. Lynch KA, Feola PG, Guenther E: Gastric trichobezoar: an important cause of abdominal pain presenting to the pediatric emergency department. *Pediatr Emerg Care* 19(5):343–347, 2003.
55. Hayes SL, Storch EA, Berlanga L: Skin picking behaviors: an examination of the prevalence and severity in a community sample. *J Anxiety Disord* 23(3):314–319, 2009.
56. Keuthen NJ, Deckersbach T, Wilhelm S, et al.: Repetitive skin-picking in a student population and comparison with a sample of self-injurious skin-pickers. *Psychosomatics* 41(3):210–215, 2000.
57. Leibovici V, Murad S, Cooper-Kazaz R, et al.: Excoriation (skin picking) disorder in Israeli University students: prevalence and associated mental health correlates. *Gen Hosp Psychiatry* 36(6):686–689, 2014.
58. Monzani B, Rijsdijk F, Cherkas L, Harris J, Keuthen N, Mataix-Cols D: Prevalence and heritability of skin picking in an adult community sample: a twin study. *Am J Med Genet B Neuropsychiatr Genet* 159B(5):605–610, 2012.
59. Odlaug BL, Chamberlain SR, Grant JE: Motor inhibition and cognitive flexibility in pathologic skin picking. *Prog Neuropsychopharmacol Biol Psychiatry* 34(1):208–211, 2010.
60. Grant JE, Odlaug BL, Chamberlain SR: A cognitive comparison of pathological skin picking and trichotillomania. *J Psychiatr Res* 45(12): 1634–1638, 2011.
61. Grant JE, Odlaug BL, Hampshire A, Schreiber LR, Chamberlain SR: White matter abnormalities in skin picking disorder: a diffusion tensor imaging study. *Neuropsychopharmacology* 38(5):763–769, 2013.
62. Roos A, Grant JE, Fouche JP, Stein DJ, Lochner C: A comparison of brain volume and cortical thickness in excoriation (skin picking) disorder and trichotillomania (hair pulling disorder) in women. *Behav Brain Res* 279:255–258, 2015.
63. Simeon D, Stein DJ, Gross S, Islam N, Schmeidler J, Hollander E: A double-blind trial of fluoxetine in pathologic skin picking. *J Clin Psychiatry* 58(8): 341–347, 1997.
64. Arbabi M, Farnia V, Balighi K, et al.: Efficacy of citalopram in treatment of pathological skin picking, a randomized double blind placebo controlled trial. *Acta Medica Iranica* 46:367–372, 2008.
65. Grant JE, Odlaug BL, Chamberlain SR, Kim SW: A double-blind, placebo-controlled trial of lamotrigine for pathological skin picking: treatment efficacy and neurocognitive predictors of response. *J Clin Psychopharmacol* 30(4):396–403, 2010.
66. Grant JE, Chamberlain SR, Redden SA, Leppink EW, Odlaug BL, Kim SW: N-Acetylcysteine in the treatment of excoriation disorder: a randomized clinical trial. *JAMA Psychiatry* 73(5):490–496, 2016.
67. Schuck K, Keijsers GP, Rinck M: The effects of brief cognitive-behaviour therapy for pathological skin picking: A randomized comparison to wait-list control. *Behav Res Ther* 49(1):11–17, 2011.

5.6 ■ TIC AND MOTOR DISORDERS

CHAPTER 5.6 ■ TIC DISORDERS

MICHAEL H. BLOCH AND JAMES F. LECKMAN

Tic disorders are transient or chronic conditions associated with difficulties in self-esteem, family life, social acceptance, or school or job performance that are directly related to the presence of motor and/or phonic tics. Tic disorders have been noted since antiquity. The first identified case of Tourette syndrome (TS) in historical literature was recounted in *Malleus Maleficarum* (*The Witches' Hammer*), a 1482 treatise on recognizing and curing demonic possession. Sprenger and Kraemer, the authors of *Malleus Maleficarum*, provide a detailed description of a young priest with motor and vocal tics, who is saved from a fiery death at the stake only by successful treatment with exorcism (1). In later French historical archives, there is a chilling account of one Prince de Conde, a 17th century French nobleman in the court of Louis XIV, who resorted to stuffing objects in his mouth to prevent an involuntary bark when in the presence of his royal highness (2).

Although reported since antiquity, recognition of TS as a distinct neuropsychiatric syndrome, and systematic study of individuals with tic disorders, began only with the reports of French neurologists Itard (1825) and Gilles de la Tourette (1885) in the 19th century. Gilles de la Tourette, in his classic study of 1885, described nine cases characterized by motor "incoordinations" or tics, "inarticulate shouts accompanied by articulated words with echolalia and coprolalia" (3). In addition to identifying the cardinal features of severe tic disorders, his report noted an association between tic disorders and obsessive-compulsive (OC) symptoms, as well as the hereditary nature of the syndrome in some families.

Since the case series presented by Gilles de la Tourette, we have learned that TS typically has a much more benign course than initially suggested in his account. We have also developed some effective pharmacologic, psychological, and now, even surgical, treatments for individuals with TS. With increasing longitudinal assessment of children with tic disorders we have learned that many present or develop a broad array of behavioral difficulties, including disinhibited speech or conduct, impulsivity, distractibility, motoric hyperactivity, and OC symptoms (4). In this chapter, a presentation of the phenomenology and classification of tic disorders precedes a review of the epidemiology, clinical course, neurobiologic substrates, assessment and management of tic disorders, and their associated comorbidities.

DEFINITION

Tics are sudden, repetitive movements, gestures, or phonic productions that typically mimic some aspect of normal behavior. Usually of brief duration, individual tics rarely last more than a second. Many tics tend to occur in bouts, with brief inter-tic intervals of less than 1 second (5). Individual tics can occur singly or together in an orchestrated pattern. They vary in their intensity or forcefulness. Motor tics, which can be viewed as disinhibited fragments of normal movement, can vary from simple, abrupt movements such as eye blinking, nose twitching, head or arm jerks, or shoulder shrugs to more complex movements that appear to have a purpose, such as facial or hand gestures or sustained looks. These two phenotypic extremes of motor tics are classified as simple and complex motor tics, respectively. Similarly, phonic tics can be classified into simple and complex categories. Simple vocal tics are sudden, meaningless sounds such as throat clearing, coughing, sniffing, spitting, or grunting. Complex phonic tics are more protracted, meaningful utterances, which vary from prolonged throat clearing to syllables, words or phrases, to even more complex behaviors such as repeating one's own words (palilalia) or those of others (echolalia) and, in rare cases, the utterance of obscenities (coprolalia) (6). Clinicians typically characterize tics by their anatomical location, number, frequency, duration, forcefulness, and complexity as outlined above. Each of these elements has been incorporated into clinician rating scales that have proven to be useful in monitoring tic severity (7).

Many individuals with tics, especially those above the age of 10, are aware of premonitory urges that may either be experienced as a focal perception in a particular body region where the tic is about to occur (like an itch or a tickling *sensation*) or as a mental awareness (8,9). A majority of patients also report a fleeting sense of relief after a bout of tics has occurred, and most individuals are able to suppress their tics for short intervals of time (9,10).

DIAGNOSTIC CLASSIFICATION

The currently accepted diagnostic criteria for TS as defined in the International Classification of Disease (ICD)-10 include: (1) presence of multiple motor tics, (2) presence of one or more vocal tics, (3) onset before age 18, (4) tics that may appear many times a day, either everyday or intermittently, (5) presence of tics for a period longer than 1 year, (6) change in anatomic location and character of tics over time, and (7) occurrence of tics not attributable to CNS disease (Huntington disease or postviral encephalopathies) or psychoactive medication or substance usage. Table 5.6.1 depicts the current diagnostic criteria for tic disorders in ICD-10. Diagnostic criteria for tic disorders between ICD-10 and *Diagnostic and Statistical Manual of Mental Disorders Text-Revision (DSM-IV-TR)* are nearly identical.

Tics that appear in childhood are often ephemeral. When a patient exhibits motor and/or vocal tics for less than a year, a diagnosis of a transient tic disorder is made according to DSM-IV-TR and ICD-10, regardless of tic frequency or severity. In DSM-5, children are diagnosed with a transient tic disorder if and only if their tics have subsided within a year's time. A new category of Provisional Tic Disorder (rather than

TABLE 5.6.1

ICD-10 TIC DISORDER CLASSIFICATION

Diagnostic criteria for F95.2 Combined vocal and multiple motor tic disorder (de la Tourette syndrome)

A. Multiple motor tics and one or more vocal tics have been present at some time during the disorder, but not necessarily concurrently.
B. The frequency of tics must be many times a day, nearly every day, for more than 1 year, with no period of remission during that year lasting longer than 2 months.
C. Onset is before the age of 18 years.

Diagnostic criteria for F95.1 Chronic motor or vocal tic disorder

A. Motor or vocal tics, but not both, occur many times per day, on most days, over a period of at least 12 months.
B. No period of remission during that year lasts longer than 2 months.
C. There is no history of Tourette syndrome, and the disorder is not the result of physical conditions or side effects of medication.
D. Onset is before the age of 18 years.

Diagnostic criteria for F95.0 Transient tic disorder

A. Single or multiple motor vocal tic(s) or both occur many times a day, on most days, over a period of at least 4 weeks.
B. Duration of the disorder is 12 months or less.
C. There is no history of Tourette syndrome, and the disorder is not the result of physical conditions or side effects of medications.
D. Onset is before the age of 18 years.

From the World Health Organization used in Skin Diseases: *ICD-10 Classification of Mental and Behavioural Disorders: Diagnostic Criteria for Research*. Albany, CH, 1993.

transient tic disorder) was established for children who are currently having tics but have not had them for a full year. The additional Provisional Tic Disorder category was introduced in DSM-5 because of the recognition that some of these children may go on to develop TS (e.g., their tic disorder is in fact not transient). If either motor or phonic tics (but not both) are present for a year or more, then a diagnosis of chronic motor or phonic tic disorder, respectively, can be made, according to DSM-5 or ICD-10. Chronic tics are viewed by experts as a milder phenotypic expression of TS, while transient tic disorders are generally viewed as a separate entity (4).

CLINICAL COURSE OF TS

The onset of TS is usually characterized by the appearance of simple, transient motor tics that affect the face (typically eye blinking) around the age of 5 to 7 (11). Over time these simple motor tics generally progress in a rostrocaudal direction affecting other areas of the face, followed by the head, neck, arms and last and less frequently, the lower extremities (12). Phonic tics usually appear several years after the onset of motor tic symptoms, at 8 to 15 years of age. Phonic tics seldom appear in isolation without the prior onset of motor tics—fewer than 5% of all patients with tic disorders have isolated phonic tic disorder, whereas the vast majority of children afflicted with tic disorders have isolated motor symptomatology (10). Tic complexity, also, generally evolves with age. During the first years of TS onset there is a steady unfolding of symptoms with single, rapid motor tics evolving into stereotyped, complex movements and nonsense sounds developing into elaborate words and phrases. The character of these complex phonations and movements are highly unique to the individual. Due to the rapid progression of symptoms during childhood, the vast majority of TS cases are diagnosed by age 11 (10).

Typically, as they grow older, children with TS gain an increasing ability to recognize when tics will ultimately strike and gain control over them. The first transient motor tics TS patients experience in the latency years are usually sudden, involuntary, unconscious movements. Often the afflicted individual is only made aware of the presence of these movements through the reactions of others around him. By the age of 10 or 11, however, many children report premonitory urges: feelings of tightness, tension, or itching that are accompanied by a mounting sense of discomfort or anxiety that can be relieved only by the performance of a tic (9). These premonitory urges are similar to the sensation preceding a sneeze or an itch. Premonitory urges cause many TS patients to suffer from an endless cycle of rising tension and tic performance because the relief provided by tic performance is ephemeral. Thus, soon after tic performance the tension of the premonitory urge again rises to a crescendo (13).

With increasing awareness of premonitory urges, TS patients begin to exhibit a variable degree of voluntary control over tic performance. Ninety-two percent of TS subjects in one study reported that the tics they exhibited were either partially or totally voluntary (9). However, this voluntary control should be likened to that governing control of eye blinking. Eye blinking and tics can both be inhibited voluntarily, but only for a limited period of time and only with mounting discomfort. Thus, some adult TS patients are able to demonstrate nearly complete control over the situation when expression of their tics will occur. However, when complete or near complete control of tics is present, resistance to the mounting tension of premonitory urges can produce mental and physical exhaustion even more impairing and distracting than the tics themselves (12). However, little evidence exists from experimental studies that the active suppression of tics leads to any noticeable effect on future tic frequency and severity (e.g., there is little evidence for any rebound phenomenon due to active tic suppression) (14,15).

The severity of tics in TS waxes and wanes throughout the course of the disorder. The tics of TS and other tic disorders are highly variable from minute to minute, hour to hour, day to day, week to week, month to month, and even year to year (5). Tic episodes occur in bouts, which in turn also tend to cluster. Tic symptoms, however, can be exacerbated by stress, fatigue, extremes of temperature and external stimuli (in echolalia tics) (16). Intentional movements attenuate tic occurrence over the affected area and intense involvement and concentration in activities tends to dissipate tic symptoms. The power of this effect in many patients with TS is illustrated beautifully in Oliver Sacks' short story, *A Surgeon's Life.* As Sacks writes:

> *And, indeed, whenever the stream of attention and interest was interrupted, Bennett's (the surgeon) tics and iterations immediately reasserted themselves—in particular, obsessive touchings of his mustache and glasses. His mustache had constantly to be smoothed and checked for symmetry, his glasses had to be "balanced"—up and down, side to side, diagonally, in and out—with sudden, ticcy touchings of the fingers, until these, too, were exactly "centered." There were also occasional reachings and lungings with his right arm; sudden, compulsive touchings of the windshield with both forefingers ("the touching has to be symmetrical," he commented); sudden repositionings of the knees, or the steering wheel ("I have to have the knees symmetrical in relation to the steering wheel. They have to be exactly centered"); and sudden, highpitched vocalizations, in a voice completely unlike his own, that sounded like "Hi, Patty," "Hi, there," and, on a couple occasions, "Hideous!"*

Sacks keenly observes that Dr. Bennett's tics and tic-related compulsive behavior are noticeably absent in two situations: (1) in the morning when he is conducting preparatory reading for his later surgeries while simultaneously riding an exercise bike and (2) when performing surgery (17).

Tic severity, however, typically dissipates with the onset of adolescence. TS symptoms generally peak in severity between the ages of 8 and 12 (11,18). Reduction in TS severity generally ends by the early 20s. Although a small minority of TS patients do experience catastrophic outcomes in adulthood, on the whole, individuals rarely experience either a sustained worsening or improvement of their symptoms after the third decade of life. One-half to two-thirds of individuals with TS experience a marked reduction of symptoms by their late teens and early 20s, with one-third to one-half becoming virtually asymptomatic in adulthood (11,19). Figure 5.6.1 diagrams the general course of tic severity of TS patients through the first two decades of their illness (11,18).

PREVALENCE

Transient tic behaviors are commonplace among children. Studies have estimated that 4% to 24% of school-age children experience tics (20–23). The upper end of this estimate was based on a study by Snider et al. (21) that assessed a community sample of 553 children aged 5 to 12 years in a suburban elementary school (21). Assessment was obtained by direct observations by trained observers on each child over multiple occasions over an 8-month period. Snider et al. estimated that 18% of the children ($n = 101$) experienced a single tic or transient tics. A much smaller portion ($n = 34$), 6%, had multiple or persistent tics. A similar study by Khalifa and von Knorring examined the prevalence of tic disorders in an epidemiologic sample of 4,479 Swedish children ages 7 to 15 using a three-stage evaluation procedure including screening, parental interview, and clinical assessment. This study estimated the prevalence of chronic motor tics at 0.7% and transient

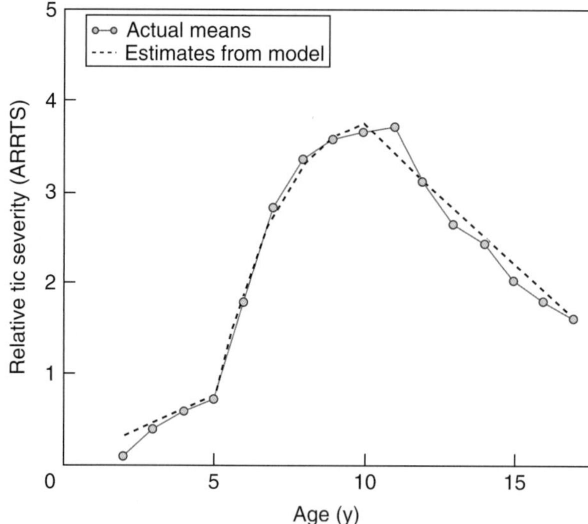

FIGURE 5.6.1. Plot of mean tic severity, ages 2 to 18 years. The *solid line* connecting the small *circles* plots the means of the annual rating of relative tic severity scores (ARRTS) recorded by the parents. The *dashed line* represents a mathematical model designed best to fit the clinical data. Two inflection points are evident that correspond to the age of tic onset and the age at worst-ever tic severity, respectively. (Adapted from Leckman JF, Zhang H, Vitale A, et al.: Course of tic severity in Tourette syndrome: the first two decades. *Pediatrics* 102(1 Pt 1):14–19, 1998.)

tics at 4.5% in this sample (22). The difference in prevalence measurements of transient and persistent motor tic disorders reported in these studies is likely due to their different ascertainment methods (parent interview vs. direct observation). Nonetheless, the relative commonness of transient tics in the school-age population is evident in both these studies and the difference in prevalence between transient and multiple tic disorders is relatively conserved across studies.

Although boys are more commonly affected with tic behaviors than girls, the male–female ratio in most community surveys is less than 2 to 1. For example, in the Isle of Wight study of 10 to 11 year olds, approximately 6% of boys and 3% of girls were reported by their parents to have "twitches, mannerisms, tics of face or body" (20). Similar estimates have been reported from Quebec and from North Carolina (24,25).

There exists drastic variation in estimates of prevalence of TS in the published medical literature. Once thought to be rare, current estimates vary 100-fold, from 2.9 per 10,000 to 299 per 10,000 (26,27). There are three main reasons for this variation in the measurement of the estimation of TS prevalence: (1) The prevalence and severity of tic disorders vary drastically as a function of age (with highest prevalence and greatest severity taking place late in the first decade and early in the second decade of life, and decreasing roughly with the onset of puberty), (2) assessment method of individual studies has varied (patient registries, parent interview, direct observation vs. clinically ascertained cases), and (3) the diagnostic criteria of TS has changed with time—specifically, whether the diagnosis of TS requires an impairment criteria. DSM-III included a requirement that tic symptoms need to "cause marked distress of significant impairment in social, occupational or other important areas of functioning" in order to qualify as TS. By contrast, the impairment criteria were removed in DSM-IV-TR and ICD-10. Estimates of TS prevalence since 1990 among school-age children have estimated a prevalence somewhere between 10 and 100 per 10,000 (22,28–32). Studies incorporating the older DSM-III definition of TS have estimated the prevalence of TS around the lower end of this range, while studies relying on the newer DSM-IV definition of TS not incorporating an impairment criteria have estimated TS prevalence toward its higher end. Estimates of older teenagers and adults with TS are considerably lower, at approximately 4.5 per 10,000 and this result is not surprising since many cases of TS improve drastically or remit completely during the course of adolescence (33).

COEXISTING CONDITIONS

Tics, which are the most prominent feature of TS, are often neither the first nor the most impairing psychological disturbance endured by patients. It has become apparent that children with TS have higher rates of obsessive-compulsive disorder (OCD), attention-deficit hyperactivity disorder (ADHD), and disinhibited speech and behavior compared to individuals in the general population. In one study, 65% of TS patients in late adolescence regarded their behavioral problems (including ADHD and OCD) and learning difficulties to have had an equal or greater impact on their life function than did the tics themselves (34). In the natural course of comorbid psychiatric illness in TS, ADHD symptoms, when they occur, typically precede the onset of tic symptoms by a couple of years, whereas OC symptoms typically present around the ages of 12 to 13 after tics have reached their peak severity (11,18) (Figure 5.6.2).

Attention-Deficit Hyperactivity Disorder

Clinical and epidemiologic studies sharply differ on rates of ADHD seen among individuals with TS (35). Clinical studies vary according to setting and established referral patterns, but it is not uncommon to see reports of 50% or more of referred children with TS diagnosed with comorbid ADHD. In contrast, epidemiologic studies typically indicate a much lower rate of comorbidity (33). Although the etiologic relationship between TS and ADHD is in dispute, it is clear that those individuals with both TS and ADHD are at a much greater risk for a variety of untoward outcomes (36). Uninformed peers frequently tease individuals with TS and ADHD. They are often regarded as less likeable, more aggressive, and more withdrawn than their classmates (37). These social difficulties are amplified in a child with TS who also has ADHD (38). In such cases, their level of social skill is often several years behind their peers (39).

Negative appraisal by peers in childhood is a strong predictor of global indices of psychopathology (40). This appears to be particularly true for children with TS and ADHD. Children with TS and comorbid ADHD are at much greater risk for disruptive behavior disorders and functional impairment

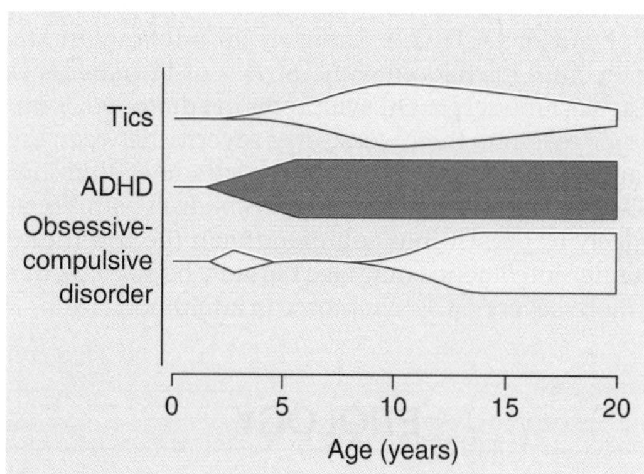

FIGURE 5.6.2. Age at which tics and coexisting disorders affect patients with TS. Width of bars shows schematically the amount the disorder affects a patient at a particular age. (Adapted from Leckman JF: Tourette's syndrome. *Lancet* 360(9345):1577–1586, 2002.)

from psychiatric illness than children with TS alone (41). Longitudinal studies confirm that these individuals are at high risk for anxiety and mood disorders, oppositional defiant disorder, and conduct disorder (36,42). Much of this negative impact appears to be due to the ADHD, as children who only have TS tend to fare better (36,41,43). Surprisingly, levels of tic severity are less predictive of peer acceptance than is the presence of ADHD (38). Furthermore, the rates of subsequent psychiatric morbidity seen in TS plus ADHD subjects are nearly identical to those seen in prior cross-sectional and longitudinal studies of ADHD subjects who do not have tics (44,45).

Obsessive-Compulsive Symptoms

Clinical and epidemiologic studies indicate that more than 40% of individuals with TS experience recurrent OC symptoms (18,46,47). Genetic, neurobiologic, and treatment response studies suggest that there may be qualitative differences between tic-related forms of OCD and cases of OCD in which there is no personal or family history of tics. Tic-related OCD tends to have an earlier age of onset, prior to the ages of 12 to 13, compared to non–tic-related OCD, which usually appears during late adolescence or early adulthood. Patients with OCD and comorbid tics have a significantly higher rate of intrusive violent or aggressive thoughts and images; sexual and religious preoccupations; concerns with symmetry and exactness; hoarding and counting rituals; and touching and tapping compulsions compared to patients with non-tic OCD, who often suffer primarily from contamination worries and cleaning compulsions (46,48). Compulsions designed to eliminate a perceptually tinged mental feeling of unease, coined in the literature as "Just Right" perceptions, are particularly typical of patients with OCD and comorbid tics (47). In addition to global rating scales for OCD, there exist both clinician-rated and self-report instruments to assess the dimensional nature of OCD symptoms. The Dimensional Yale–Brown Obsessive-Compulsive Scale (DY–BOCS), was a clinician-rated and self-report instrument designed to measure the presence and severity of OCD symptoms within six thematically related dimensions and should aid in further discriminating the OCD experienced by patients with TS compared to those with comorbid tics (49,50). Also the Dimensional Obsessive-Compulsive Scale (DOCS) was designed to measure symptom severity in the four most consistently derived symptom dimensions in OCD (51,52). In addition, tic-related OCD is significantly less responsive to pharmacologic therapy with SRIs than non–tic-related OCD and appears to be more responsive to augmentation with antipsychotic agents (53–56).

In a previous prospective longitudinal study the presence of tics in childhood and early adolescence predicted the future development of OCD (32). Similarly, in a follow-up study of adult outcomes in children with TS, 41% of TS patients experienced at least moderate OC symptoms in adulthood, with these symptoms reaching their worst-ever severity between the ages of 12 and 13 years, an average of 2 years later than tics (18). Also, OC symptoms, when present in children with TS, appear more likely to persist into adulthood than the tics themselves (18). Higher intelligence may also herald a higher risk of developing more severe OCD symptoms in adulthood (18).

ETIOLOGY

Genetic Factors

TS and other closely related disorders clearly have a strong genetic component. The overall risk of an offspring of a parent with TS developing TS is approximately 10% to 15%; the risk of their offspring developing a tic disorder (20% to 29%) or OCD (12% to 32%) is slightly higher (57–60). The risk of developing tic disorders in male offspring is higher, while the risk of developing OCD is less. Twin and family studies provide evidence that genetic factors are involved in the vertical transmission within families of a vulnerability to TS and related disorders (61). The concordance rate for TS among monozygotic twin pairs is greater than 50%, while the concordance of dizygotic twin pairs is about 10% (62,63). If co-twins with chronic motor tic disorder are included, these concordance figures increase to 77% for monozygotic and 30% for dizygotic twin pairs. Differences in the concordance of monozygotic and dizygotic twin pairs indicate that genetic factors play an important role in the etiology of TS and related conditions. These figures also suggest that nongenetic factors are critical in determining the nature and severity of the clinical syndrome.

Several studies involving segregation analysis of large multigenerational families have implicated the possible importance of single gene(s) inherited with an autosomal dominant pattern in the pathogenesis of TS (59,61,64). Unfortunately, genetic linkage studies that have screened the entire genome have eliminated the possibility of a single gene being responsible for TS (65). Despite the well-established large hereditary component of TS, establishing any definitive TS genes has proven difficult. Numerous genome wide–linkage studies in TS failed to produce any consistent results. In a recently completed genome-wide association study (GWAS), no loci achieved genome-wide significance. However, in the largest GWAS in TS involving 1,286 cases and 4,986 controls, a couple of SNPs were strongly implicated (66). The single nucleotide polymorphisms (SNP) rs7868992 on chromosome 9q32 within the gene *COL27A1* ($p = 1.9 \times 10^{-6}$) was strongly associated with a diagnosis of TS (66). This SNP was replicated in a secondary cohort of 211 cases and 285 controls from two Latin American population isolates from Costa Rica and Colombia. *COL27A1* is a fibrillar collagen primarily expressed in cartilage, although it is also expressed in cerebellum development (67). The role of COL27A1 in the development of the nervous system in unknown (68). The SNP rs6539267 on chromosome 12q23 within an intron of *POLR3B* was also strongly associated with TS in the GWAS sample ($p = 7.4 \times 10^{-6}$) (69). *POLR3B* encodes for a subunit of RNA polymerase III (70). Recessive mutations in POLR3B can cause hypomyelinating leukodystrophy. RNA polymerase III–related hypomyelinating leukodystrophy typically present between early childhood to adolescence and are associated with ataxia, motor regression with upper motor neuron signs, and some mild cognitive dysfunction or regression (71).

Recent analysis of genome-wide common variant data from the same TS GWAS study has estimated that 21% of the heritability in TS is due to inheritance of rare variant alleles (genes with minor allele frequency less than 5%) (72).

Increasingly candidate gene approaches which identify chromosomal anomalies in patients with TS have been successful in helping us better understand the pathophysiology of the disorder. This sib-pair approach is suited for diseases with an unclear mode of inheritance and has been used successfully in studies of other complex disorders such as diabetes mellitus and essential hypertension. Abelson et al. (73) identified and mapped a de novo chromosome 13 inversion in a patient with TS. The gene SLITRK1 was identified as a brain-expressed candidate gene mapping approximately 350 kilobases from the 13q31 breakpoint (73). Mutation screening of 174 patients with TS was undertaken, with the resulting identification of a truncating frame-shift mutation in a second family affected with TS. In addition, two examples of a rare variant were identified in a highly conserved region of the 3′ untranslated region of the gene corresponding to a brain-expressed micro-RNA–binding domain. None of these anomalies were demonstrated in 3,600 controls. In vitro studies showed that both the frameshift and the micro-RNA-binding site variant had functional potential and were consistent with a loss-of-function mechanism. Studies of both SLITRK1 and the micro-RNA predicted to bind in the variant-containing 3′ region showed expression in multiple neuroanatomical areas implicated in TS neuropathology, including the cortical plate, striatum, globus pallidus, thalamus, and subthalamic nucleus.

More recently, another strong candidate gene in TS was established through linkage analysis of a two-generation pedigree in a densely affected family where a father and eight of his children had TS (74). A rare functional mutation was identified in the *HDC* gene, which encodes for L-histidine decarboxylase, the rate limiting step in histamine biosynthesis. The histamine 3 receptor in the brain acts as a presynaptic autoreceptor on histaminergic projection neurons that regulate a variety of neurotransmitters including serotonin and dopamine. HDC knockout mice show decreased brain histamine and increased sensitivity to stereotypies induced by dopamine agonists (75).

Perinatal Factors

The search for nongenetic factors that mediate the expression of a genetic vulnerability to TS and related disorders has also focused on the role of adverse perinatal events. This interest dates from the report of Pasamanick and Kawi, who found that mothers of children with tics were 1.5 times more likely to have experienced a complication during pregnancy than the mothers of children without tics (76). Other investigations have reported that among monozygotic twins discordant for TS, the index twins with TS had lower birth weights than their unaffected co-twins (63,77). Severity of maternal life stress during pregnancy, severe nausea and/or vomiting during the first trimester have also emerged as potential risk factors in the development of tic disorders (78). In 1997, Whitaker and coworkers reported that premature and low birth weight children are at increased risk of developing tic disorders and ADHD. This appears to be especially true of children who had ischemic parenchymal brain lesions. Burd et al. (79) presented the results of a case-control study in which low Apgar scores at 5 minutes and *more* prenatal visits were associated with a higher risk of TS (79). Finally, there exists increasing evidence that maternal smoking during pregnancy may be associated with an increased risk of developing TS (80). Investigations into the effects of perinatal complications into the later development of TS are severely hampered by (1) the possibility that recall bias likely influences results in the retrospective case-control studies addressing this question and (2) multiple hypothesis testing without appropriate statistical correction. However, a recent prospective cohort study from the Danish National Birth Cohort examining over 73,000 singleton pregnancies demonstrated a significant association between maternal smoking during pregnancy and increased risk of development of TS or chronic tic disorders (hazard ratio = 1.66) (81). There was also some evidence of a dosing effect within this study such that children born to heavy smoking mothers during pregnancy had an even further elevated risk of TS or chronic tic disorders (81).

Neuroanatomical Factors

Strong evidence implicates the basal ganglia and corticostriatal thalamocortical (CSTC) abnormalities as central to the pathogenesis of tics. Indirect evidence for the involvement of the basal ganglia in the pathogenesis of TS comes from the association of other movement disorders, such as Huntington disease, hemiballismus, and Parkinson disease, with basal ganglia pathology. Direct evidence supporting CSTC abnormalities in TS comes from neuroimaging, neuropathologic, and neurosurgical studies.

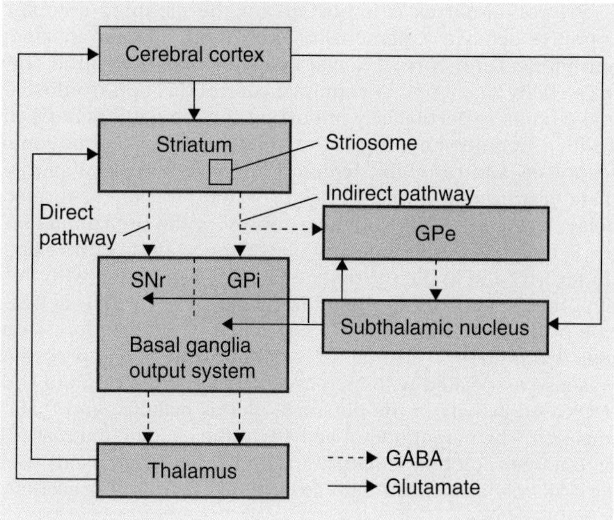

FIGURE 5.6.3. Schematic diagram of the major connections of the basal ganglia. GPe, globus pallidus, pars externa; GPi, globus pallidus, pars interna; SNr, substantia nigra, pars reticulata. (Adapted from Leckman JF: Tourette's syndrome. *Lancet* 360(9345):1577–1586, 2002.)

Dysfunction of frontostriatal circuits is hypothesized to be central to the pathogenesis of TS as well as several other major psychiatric disorders such OCD, TTM, ADHD, and eating disorders (82). Frontostriatal circuits are best known for the execution of planned movements but are also crucial for the performance of many aspects of goal-directed behavior such as elements that drive action such as cognition, emotion, and reward (82). Frontostriatal circuits are multiple, parallel but interacting neuronal circuits which project information from cortical areas to the striatum (caudate, putamen, nucleus accumbens), and back to the cortex via the thalamus (Figure 5.6.3). Frontostriatal circuits are synaptotopically and hierarchically organized. Abnormalities in two frontostriatal circuits are central to the pathogenesis of TS that initiated from and projecting to (1) premotor and motor cortex and (2) prefrontal cortex (dorsal prefrontal and orbitofrontal cortex) (82).

Premotor cortex is important for the driving, planning, initiation, and execution of voluntary movements. Electrical stimulation of the supplementary motor area can produce (1) synergistic, complex, coordinated movements involving cooperation across multiple joints—movements quite similar to the complex tics seen in TS and sensations involving the "urge" to move—analogous to the premonitory urges experienced by many patients with TS (83). Thus, in TS the frontostriatal circuits projecting from the premotor and motor cortex are hypothesized to be trait deficits of TS that are important in the pathogenesis of tic generation and the premonitory urges of TS. Supporting this hypothesis, functional MRI studies have demonstrated activation of the supplementary motor cortex just prior to tic generation (84,85). Structural neuroimaging examining 25 children with TS and 35 age-matched controls demonstrated thinning of the sensorimotor cortex of children with TS compared to healthy controls (86). Among children with TS, tic severity was associated with degree of thinning of the sensorimotor area (especially dorsal regions) (86). Furthermore, severity of facial tic symptoms was associated with degree of thinning in the ventral sensorimotor cortex (86). The ventral portions of the sensorimotor cortex control the facial, orolingual, and laryngeal musculature.

Prefrontal cortex is important for the planning complex cognitive behaviors, personality expression, decision making, and moderating correct social behavior. The prefrontal cortex's ability to engage in cognitive control through frontostriatal circuits is particularly important for the pathogenesis of TS (87). Cognitive control is the ability to regulate emotional responses and to inhibit temptations or impulses for immediate gratification in the service of waiting for longer-termed delayed rewards (88). Cognitive control of the prefrontal cortex is hypothesized to be particularly important in controlling tic severity and in the pathogenesis of TS. Consistent with this hypothesis, an fMRI study of 22 adults with TS, that activation of the frontal cortex was associated with tic suppression (89). Magnitude of frontal activation during tic suppression was also associated with increased activity in the caudate and decreased activity in the putamen, globus pallidus, and thalamus (89). The magnitude of activity in the caudate (increased) or putamen, globus pallidus, and thalamus (decreased) was significantly associated with severity of tics in the preceding month.

Anatomical neuroimaging studies have consistently demonstrated prefrontal cortex abnormalities compared to healthy controls. The largest neuroimaging on TS to date, involving 155 TS subjects and 131 controls, demonstrated larger dorsolateral prefrontal cortex volumes in children with TS and smaller dorsal prefrontal cortex in adults with active TS (90). Larger dorsal prefrontal volumes in children were associated with decreased tic severity. These data suggest that prefrontal cortex hypertrophy may represent a compensatory or adaptive process that attenuates tics. Subsequent structural neuroimaging findings have confirmed the association between prefrontal cortex hypertrophy and tic severity—demonstrating a correlation of increased dorsal prefrontal cortex thickness with decreased tic severity in children with TS (86).

The most consistent structural neuroimaging finding in TS is a reduction in caudate nucleus volumes compared to healthy controls. Large cross-sectional neuroimaging studies have demonstrated a small, but significant 5% reduction in the caudate nucleus in TS subjects compared to controls (91). Studies of monozygotic twins discordant for tic severity have demonstrated reduced caudate volumes in the more severely affected twin (92). These reduction in caudate volumes in children with TS have been further associated with the persistence of tic symptoms into adulthood (93). Postmortem neurostereologic studies assessing neuronal density and numbers in five adults with severe, intractable TS and five healthy controls have suggested a possible mechanism for this caudate volume reduction (94,95). TS subjects demonstrated reduced overall number of two types of interneurons in the striatum (94,95). Parvalbumin positive interneurons and cholinergic interneurons were both reduced by over 50% in the caudate and putamen of TS patients (94,95). Furthermore, adult TS patients showed the greatest decrease in cholinergic neurons in the anterior caudate, the area of prefrontal projections (95). Cholinergic neurons were reduced to a lesser extent than in projection areas from the sensorimotor cortex (95). The most posterior limbic projection areas demonstrated similar density of cholinergic interneurons between TS subjects and controls (95). These recent findings strongly implicate prefrontal and sensorimotor projection areas of the basal ganglia in the pathogenesis of TS. These focused loss of interneurons provide a mechanism by which TS patients have impairment of cognitive control or require increasing frontal activation to achieve normal levels of cognitive controls. This loss of interneurons in sensorimotor projection areas also suggests a possible mechanism of tic generation—abnormal firing of striatal projection neurons due to impaired inhibition.

If striatal neurons became overactive in discrete, repeated episodes, the result would be multiple, stereotyped movements—tics (96,97).

Support for this hypothesis of tic generation comes from experiments conducted by Anderson et al. (98), which demonstrated that microstimulation at numerous sites of the putamen produced tic-like stereotyped movements in awake monkeys (98). Furthermore, microstimulation of discrete striatal zones produced characteristic stereotyped movements of individual body parts and, stunningly, even stereotyped movements of multiple body parts reminiscent of complex tics (99).

Human postmortem specimens have fairly consistently demonstrated abnormalities in basal ganglia development or function in the pathogenesis of TS. A postmortem study of three adult patients with severe TS, a markedly higher total neuron number was found in the globus pallidus pars interna (GPi) of TS. In contrast, a lower neuron number and density was observed in adults with TS in the globus pallidus pars externa and in the caudate nucleus. An increased number and proportion of the GPi neurons were positive for the calcium-binding protein parvalbumin in tissue from TS subjects, whereas lower densities of parvalbumin-positive interneurons were observed in both the caudate and putamen of TS subjects. This loss of parvalbumin-positive fast-spiking interneurons in the striatum has been hypothesized to cause somatotopically arranged clusters of medium-spiny interneurons to become disengaged from their normal high-voltage spindle activity. The result could be a disturbance in discrete CSTC loops through thalamocortical dysrhythmia (a disturbance in the normal rhythmic τ-band activity by the thalamus, in conjunction with ectopic γ-band activity thought to be due to hyperpolarization of thalamic cells), resulting in the premonitory urges and tics characteristic of TS (100). Earlier postmortem studies of TS patients have also reliably demonstrated an association between abnormalities in basal ganglia anatomy, development, and function, and TS (101,102). Abnormalities of the dopaminergic system within the CSTC loops have also been demonstrated in previous postmortem studies. For example, a postmortem study of four adults with intractable TS revealed (1) an increased number of presynaptic dopamine uptake sites in their striatum, (2) increased striatal dopamine levels compared to controls, and (3) similar D2 receptor affinity between TS subjects and controls (101,103).

Neuropharmacologic support for the involvement of CSTC and basal ganglia abnormalities in TS comes from the effectiveness of dopamine-depleting agents (tetrabenazine and alpha-methyl-para-tyrosine) and dopaminergic receptor antagonists (pimozide, haloperidol) in the suppression of tics and from the exacerbation of tics caused by administration of dopamine agonists (L-DOPA) and cocaine (104). Additionally, the application of stimulants directly to specific regions of the basal ganglia of animal models can produce tic-like stereotypic movements (105).

Despite the extensive and diverse neuroimaging studies conducted in TS, it is still a matter of substantial debate whether caudate, thalamic, or cortical dysfunction is primary to the pathogenesis of this disorder. Prospective, longitudinal neuroimaging studies of children with TS are necessary to determine whether the functional and structural abnormalities observed in patients with TS are causes or consequences of the disorder.

Psychological Factors

Tic disorders have long been identified as "stress-sensitive" conditions (106,107). Typically, symptom exacerbations follow in the wake of stressful life events. Children with TS on average experience higher levels of psychosocial stress compared to matched controls (16). As noted by Shapiro et al. (108), these events need not be adverse in character (108). Clinical experience suggests that in some unfortunate instances a vicious cycle can be initiated in which tic symptoms are misunderstood by the family and teachers, leading to active attempts to suppress the symptoms by punishment and humiliation. These efforts can lead to a further exacerbation of symptoms and further increase in stress in the child's interpersonal environment. Unchecked, this vicious cycle can lead to the most severe manifestations of TS and dysthymia, as well as maladaptive characterologic traits. Although psychological factors are insufficient to cause TS, the intimate association of the content and timing of tic behaviors and dynamically important events in the lives of children make it difficult to overlook their contribution to the intramorbid course of these disorders (36,42). The interaction of TS symptom exacerbation and comorbid depressive symptoms is an area that warrants further investigation. Short-term symptom exacerbation in TS is also influenced by sleeplessness and fatigue, so proper sleep hygiene is also advisable in children with TS.

DIAGNOSTIC ASSESSMENT

Differential Diagnosis

The differential diagnosis of simple motor tics includes a variety of hyperkinetic movements: myoclonus, tremors, chorea, athetosis, dystonias, akathitic movements, paroxysmal dyskinesias, and ballistic movements (109). These movements may be associated with genetic conditions such as Huntington chorea or Wilson disease; structural lesions, as in hemiballismus (associated with lesions to the contralateral subthalamic nucleus); infectious processes as in Sydenham chorea; idiopathic functional instability of neuronal circuits, as in myoclonic epilepsy; and pharmacologic treatments such as acute akathisia and dystonias associated with the use of neuroleptic agents. Differentiation between these conditions and tic disorders is usually accomplished on clinical grounds and is based on the presentation of the disorder and its natural history. For example, although aspects of tics such as their abruptness, their paroxysmal timing, or their suppressible nature may be similar to symptoms seen in other conditions, it is rare for all of these features to be combined in the absence of a *bona fide* tic disorder. Occasionally diagnostic tests are needed to exclude alternative diagnoses.

Complex motor tics can be confused with other complex repetitive behaviors such as stereotypies or compulsive rituals. Differentiation among these behaviors may be difficult, particularly among retarded individuals with limited verbal skills. Stereotypies, as opposed to tics, tend to have an earlier age of onset (2 to 3 as opposed to 6), tend to be bilateral rather than unilateral in nature, the individual movements stay more consistent over time in stereotypies, and stereotypies usually do not have a waxing and waning course (110). In other settings where these symptoms are closely intertwined, as in individuals with both TS and OCD, efforts to distinguish between complex motor tics and compulsive behaviors may be futile. In cases of a tic disorder, it is unusual to see complex motor tics in the absence of simple tics. Involuntary vocal utterances are uncommon neurologic signs in the absence of a tic disorder. Examples include sniffing and brief sounds in Huntington disease and involuntary moaning in Parkinson disease, particularly as a result of L-dopa toxicity. Complex phonic tics characterized by articulate speech typically can be distinguished from other conditions, including voluntary coprolalia. Because of their rarity in other syndromes, phonic tics can play an important role in differential diagnosis.

Clinical history, family history, observation, and neurologic examination are usually sufficient to establish the diagnosis of a tic disorder. There are no confirmatory diagnostic tests. Neuroimaging studies, EEG-based studies, and laboratory tests are usually noncontributory except in atypical cases.

Assessment

Once the diagnosis has been established, care should be taken to focus on the overall course of an individual's development, not simply on tic symptoms. This may be a particular problem in the case of TS, where the symptoms can be dramatic and there is the temptation to organize all of an individual's behavioral and emotional difficulties under a single, all-encompassing rubric.

The principal goal of an initial assessment is to determine the individual's overall level of adaptive functioning and to identify areas of impairment and distress (4). Close attention to the strengths and weaknesses of the individual and the family is crucial. Relevant dimensions include the presence of comorbid mental, behavioral, developmental, or physical disorders; family history of psychiatric and/or neurologic disease; relationships with family and peers; school and/or occupational performance; and the history of important life events. Medication history is important, particularly if the disorder is longstanding or if medications have been prescribed for physical disorders. It may be necessary to evaluate the adequacy of the prior trials with pharmacologic agents used to treat tic disorders. Table 5.6.2 demonstrates all the components that are important in the initial evaluation of a patient suspected of having TS (111).

Inventories such as the *Yale Child Study Center: TS Obsessive-Compulsive Disorder Symptom Questionnaire* (4) completed by the family prior to their initial consultation can be valuable ancillary tools to gain a long-term perspective of the child's developmental course and the natural history of the tic disorder. In addition, valid and reliable clinical rating instruments that have been developed to inventory and quantify recent tic symptoms, such as the Yale Global Tic Severity Scale, are particularly useful in judging an individual's current level of tic severity and monitoring changes in tic severity over time (7).

The Yale Global Tic Severity Scale (YGTSS) is a clinician-rated, semi-structured scale that begins with a systematic inventory of tic symptoms that the clinician rates as present or absent over the past week. Current motor and phonic tics are then rated separately according to number, frequency, intensity, complexity, and interference on a 6-point ordinal scale (0 = absent; 1 through 5 for severity) yielding three scores: total motor, total phonic, and total tic score. The scale concludes with an overall impairment rating. The YGTSS has shown excellent inter-rater agreement as well as other desirable psychometric properties (7). Because the YGTSS permits the clinician to incorporate direct observation with historical information, it requires both training with the instrument and clinical experience with tic disorders. At present most investigators consider the YGTSS to be the state of the art with regard to clinician ratings of tic severity.

Direct observational methods include videotaped tic counting procedures (112,113) or in vivo evaluation of tic symptoms (114). These direct observational methods would appear to be the most objective measure of tic severity; however, the frequency of tics varies according to setting and activity. In addition, many individuals with TS can suppress their symptoms for brief periods of time. In practice, videotaped tic counting appears to be most useful for acute research procedures that take place over several hours. Clinically, videotaping can be quite valuable when the diagnosis is in doubt or when tics are not observed in the consultation room.

TREATMENT

Tic disorders are frequently chronic, if not lifelong, conditions. Continuity of care is desirable and should be considered before embarking on a course of treatment. Usual clinical practice focuses initially on the educational and supportive

TABLE 5.6.2

CLINICAL EVALUATION OF TIC DISORDERS AND CLOSELY RELATED CONDITIONS

1. Tics

Anatomic location and symmetry, number, frequency, intensity, complexity, degree of interference (family and clinician ratings of current and worst-ever severity).

Onset—Age, characteristics (sudden, gradual, associated with stressful life events, infections—particularly recurrent streptococcal infections).

Course—Bout-like occurrence, waxing or waning course, and changing repertoire (most occurring in the eyes, face, head, and shoulders); tic complexity likely to increase with increasing age; momentary suppressibility, reduction during fine motor or vocal tasks that require mental effort, marked diminution during sleep, and usual improvement during the second-half of the second decade of life; intramorbid factors associated with worsening or improvement (stress, fatigue, recent infections); current treatment regimen; history of response to medications (efficacy, side effects, adequacy of trials); history of other interventions.

Associated Perceptual Phenomena and Disinhibited Behavior—Premonitory sensory urges, mental tics, site sensitization, trigger stimuli; socially inappropriate urges or behaviors (calling out in libraries or other quiet public places, urges to do prohibited actions).

Comorbidity—Obsessive-compulsive symptoms; attention-deficit hyperactivity disorder; mood and anxiety disorders.

Impairment—Impact on self-esteem, family function, social acceptance, educational or job performance; risk of physical injury to self or others.

2. Obsessive-Compulsive Symptoms and Behaviors

Range of obsessive worries and thoughts with aggressive, sexual, or religious content, need for symmetry or exactness, a need for things to look, feel or sound "just right," contamination fears, thoughts about saving or hoarding; simple compulsive rituals ("evening-up," ordering behaviors); full-fledged obsessive-compulsive disorder (time-consuming ego-dystonic obsessive thoughts and compulsive rituals that are "resisted" and interfere with normal cognitive function); pathologic doubting; family and clinician ratings of current and worse-ever severity and assessment of obsessive-compulsive symptom dimensions.

Onset—Age, characteristics (associated with recurrent streptococcal infections or the onset of puberty, recent moves, separations, or losses).

Course—Time spent and types of obsessions and compulsions, level of autonomic arousal and anxiety; level of control and resistance; perceived distress if prevented from performing compulsions; role of environmental cues and avoidance behaviors; progression from ego-neutral to ego-dystonic compulsions; changing repertoire of obsessions and compulsions; intramorbid factors associated with worsening or improvement (stress, fatigue, recent infections); current treatment regimen; history of response to cognitive behavioral interventions, medications (efficacy, side effects, adequacy of trials); history of other interventions.

Comorbidity—Depression and other mood and anxiety disorders; obsessive-compulsive personality; schizophrenia; developmental disorders (autism, Prader–Willi syndrome).

Impairment—Impact on self-esteem; subjective distress; pervasive slowness and getting stuck in routine behaviors; impact on family function (level of involvement of the family in the performance of compulsions); effect on social adaptation, educational or job performance; risk of physical injury to self or others.

3. Attention-Deficit Hyperactivity Disorder

Distractibility and impulsive behavior; poor sustained attention, motoric hyperactivity and fidgetiness; associated disruptive behaviors; need for multiple sources of information, especially teachers and other school personnel.

Onset—Age, timing (before or after onset of tic syndrome).

Course—Context dependence: settings where these difficulties are less apparent versus settings of greatest difficulty; history of tutoring and other special educational services; current treatment regimen; history of response to stimulants (efficacy, side effects, adequacy of trials); history of other nonsomatic interventions.

Comorbidity—Oppositional and defiant disorder, conduct disorder, and substance abuse disorders; specific learning disabilities; depression and other mood and anxiety disorders; developmental disorders (fragile X syndrome and other intellectual disability syndromes).

Impairment—Impact on self-esteem; impact on family function especially difficulties with siblings; effect on peer relationships; school underachievement; job performance.

4. Comorbid Developmental, Behavioral, Emotional, Personality, or Substance Abuse Problems

Presence of pervasive developmental disorders (autism, Asperger syndrome, and pervasive development disorder [PDD] not otherwise specified), specific developmental disorders, mood liability and increased irritability, major depression, bipolar disorder, and anxiety disorders (panic disorder, phobias including social and agoraphobia, generalized anxiety disorders), perfectionism and other obsessive-compulsive personality traits, other personality disorders as well as any history of substance abuse.

5. Prenatal and Birth History

Prenatal events (severe nausea and vomiting, maternal emotional stress during pregnancy, history of smoking and alcohol use, other drug and hormonal exposures); birth history (hypoxic episodes, prolonged labor, use of forceps).

6. Developmental, Neurologic, and Pediatric Histories

Developmental delays; exposure to toxins (lead); medication exposures; infectious diseases (streptococcal pharyngitis and other infections such as varicella), rheumatic fever, rheumatic carditis, or Sydenham chorea; head injuries; seizures; asthma; allergies; migraine; disorders of arousal (night terrors, sleep walking).

7. Family and Social Environment, Stress and Adaptive Function, Awareness of Advocacy Organizations

Premorbid history; family environment—stability of family life, coping skills and social supports; relationship of life events (major losses or moves, changes in family circumstances) to onset and exacerbations of symptoms; current adjustment (patient's general knowledge and attitude toward tics, obsessive-compulsive symptoms, and problems with impulsivity and attention, willingness to teach others about symptoms, and the level of understanding and acceptance of the symptoms by close family members); existence of close and lasting friendships; marital status. How aware is the patient and family of the existence of national and local advocacy organizations such as the TS Association (TSA), Obsessive Compulsive Foundation (OCF), and the Children and Adults with Attention Deficit Disorder (CHADD)?

TABLE 5.6.2

(CONTINUED)

8. School Status
Cognitive level, special talents or gifts, specific learning problems, adequacy of placement, level of understanding and acceptance of the symptoms by school personnel and classmates.
9. Employment Status
Current occupation, job difficulties associated with tic behaviors or related phenomena, adequacy of placement given patient's native abilities, level of understanding and acceptance of the symptoms by employer and coworkers.
10. Family History of Developmental, Autoimmune, Behavioral, and Emotional Disorders
Review of family pedigree with regard to tics, Sydenham chorea, other movement disorders; rheumatic fever; attentional problems and hyperactivity; learning problems; developmental disorders; obsessive-compulsive behaviors; personality disorders; major depression and other mood and anxiety disorders; schizophrenia; alcoholism and other substance abuse disorders.
11. Neuropsychological Assessment
Estimate of cognitive ability, visual motor integration.
12. Physical and Neurologic Evaluations
Health history; evidence of recent physical examinations; throat culture and titers for antistreptolysin O and anti-DNAse B (if requested); presence of soft, nonlocalizing neurologic signs; consider more extensive workup (EEG and structural MRI scan) in atypical cases (negative family history, positive seizure history, history of severe hypoxia, head trauma, marked symptom severity, atypical pattern of response to medication).

Adapted from Leckman JF, Zhang H, Vitale A, et al.: Course of tic severity in Tourette syndrome: the first two decades. *Pediatrics* 102(1 Pt 1): 14–19,1998.

interventions. Pharmacologic treatments are typically held in reserve. Given the waxing and waning course of the disorders, it is likely that whatever is done (or not done) will lead in the short term to some improvement in tic severity. The decision to employ psychoactive medications is usually made after the educational and supportive interventions have been in place for a period of months, and it is clear that the tic symptoms are persistently severe and are themselves a source of impairment in terms of self-esteem, relationships with the family or peers, or the child's ability to perform at school.

Educational and Supportive Interventions

Educational activities are among the most important interventions available to the clinician. They should be undertaken first, not only with patients with severe TS, but with patients with milder presentations. Although the efficacy of these educational and supportive interventions has not been rigorously assessed, they appear to have positive effects by reshaping familial expectations and relationships (115). This is particularly true when the family and others have misconstrued the tic symptoms as being intentionally provocative. Families also find descriptions of the natural history comforting in that the disorders tend not to be relentlessly progressive and usually improve during adulthood. This information often contradicts the impressions gained from the available lay literature on TS that typically focuses on the most extreme cases. Armed with this knowledge, patients and family members and others can begin to understand why waiting before beginning medical treatment makes good sense. If a patient is in the midst of a bad period of tics, it is likely that whether or not a new medication is prescribed, the tics will probably get significantly better in the near future. This insight will also help patients and their families realize why at times in the past their medications have suddenly stopped working. These dialogues can be relieving and can interrupt a vicious cycle of recrimination that leads to further tic exacerbation, and it can help aggravated parents shift the focus from blame to problem solving.

For children, contact with their teachers can be enormously valuable. By educating the educators, clinicians can make significant progress toward securing for the child a positive and supportive environment in the classroom. If possible, teachers need to respond to outbursts of tics with grace and understanding. Repeatedly scolding a child for his tics can be counterproductive. The child may develop a negative attitude toward authority figures and may be reluctant to attend school; classmates may feel freer to tease the child. If tics interfere with a student's ability to receive information in the classroom, it is imperative to find alternative ways to present the material. By helping the student find a way to function even during periods of severe tics, teachers model problem-solving skills that will foster future self-esteem. It is also important for teachers to know that unstructured settings such as the cafeteria, gym, playground, and school bus tend to be very difficult. In these situations, peers who tease or taunt tend to take advantage of the lack of adult supervision. The assignment of a paraprofessional aide to accompany the student can be remarkably beneficial—particularly in situations where there is a history of teasing. Other useful strategies that teachers may consider include: providing short breaks out of the classroom to let the tics out in private, allowing students with severe tics to take tests in private so that a child does not have the pressure to suppress tics during the test period, and being flexible with regard to the scheduling of oral presentations so that the child is not expected to make an oral presentation at a point when his tics are severe (116). A useful compendium of educational accommodations is available at http://www.tourettesyndrome.net/.

Educated peers are equally important. Many clinicians actively encourage patients, families, and teachers to help educate peers and classmates about TS. It is remarkable what can be tolerated in the classroom and on the playground when teachers and peers simply know what the problem is and learn to disregard it.

Finally, it is important for clinicians to determine the family's awareness and potential interest in advocacy organizations such as the TS Association, Obsessive Compulsive Foundation, and the Children and Adults with Attention Deficit Disorder. In the United States, these organizations have made a positive contribution to the lives of many patients and their families by providing support and information. They can also be a valuable outlet for families, to advance research and raise the general level of awareness among health care professionals, educators, and the public at large. Readers are referred to their respective websites for additional information: Tourette Association of America: www.tourette.org; the International OCD

Foundation: www.iocdf.org; and Child and Adults with Attention Deficit: www.chadd.org.

Psychological Interventions

Habit reversal training (HRT) is the first behavioral intervention that has shown promise in reducing tic severity in patients with TS (117). HRT consists of two main focuses: (1) awareness training and (2) competing response practice. Awareness training consists of four components designed to increase an individual's awareness of his or her own tics. These components include: (1) response description, in which an individual learns how to describe tic movements and reenacts them into a mirror; (2) response detection, in which the therapist aids the patient in tic detection by pointing out each tic immediately after it occurs in the session; (3) early warning procedure, in which an individual learns how to identify the earliest signs of tic occurrence; and (4) situational awareness training, in which an analysis is conducted to identify the high-risk situations where tics are most likely to occur. Competing response practice involves teaching individuals to produce an incompatible physical response (isometric contraction of tic-opposing muscles) contingent upon the urge to perform a tic (118).

HRT in its current form, originally developed by Azrin and Nunn (119), and refined by many others over the intervening years, has been demonstrated to significantly reduce tic symptoms in adults with TS, as compared to supportive therapy in randomized controlled clinical trials (120,121). Similar randomized, controlled trials in children with TS have shown similar efficacy. Effect sizes observed for HRT in controlled trials (ES ≈ 0.6 to 0.7) are similar in magnitude to those observed for the most effective pharmacologic treatments for tics (122–124). Further studies are needed to replicate these current findings at other, less experienced sites with TS. The next challenge is to effectively disseminate this behavioral therapy available only at a few academic institutions to more therapists out in the community. The Tourette Association of America holds several weekend training sessions annually with available off-site supervision in order to help expand the supply of trained therapists.

Pharmacologic Interventions

The decision to begin medication is based on the level of symptoms and the clinical presentation of the individual case. Given the waxing and waning of tic symptoms, it is best to withhold psychotropic medications until the tics, even at their best, are a significant source of impairment. Many cases of TS can be successfully managed without medication. When patients present with coexisting ADHD, OCD, depression, or bipolar illness, it is often better to treat these comorbid conditions first, as successful treatment of these disorders often will diminish tic severity.

A variety of therapeutic agents are now available to treat tics (125). Each medication should be selected on the basis of expected efficacy and potential side effects. Dopamine D2 receptor antagonists remain the most predictably effective tic-suppressing agents in the short term. Documentation of haloperidol's effectiveness in the early 1960s was a landmark in the history of TS, as it called into question the prevailing view that tics were psychogenic in nature (126). The most widely used typical D2 receptor antagonists are haloperidol, pimozide, fluphenazine, and tiapride (not presently available in the United States). Favorable data from double-blind clinical trials are available for haloperidol, pimozide, and tiapride (127–130). The U.S. Food and Drug Administration has approved TS as an indication for haloperidol and pimozide use. Long-term experience has been less favorable, and the "reflexive" use of these agents should be avoided (131,132). Typically, treatment is initiated with a low dose (0.5 mg of haloperidol or 1 mg of pimozide) given before sleep. Further increments (0.5 mg of haloperidol or 1 mg of pimozide) may be added at 7-day intervals if the tic behaviors remain severe. In most instances, 0.5 to 6.0 mg per day of haloperidol or 1.0 to 10.0 mg per day of pimozide administered over a period of 4 to 8 weeks is sufficient to achieve adequate control of tic symptoms. Common potential side effects include tardive dyskinesia, acute dystonic reactions, sedation, depression, school and social phobias, and/or weight gain. In many instances, by starting at low doses and adjusting the dosage upward slowly clinicians can avoid these side effects. The goal should be to use as little of these medications as possible to render the tics "tolerable." Efforts to stop the tics completely often risk overmedication.

Due to the extrapyramidal side effects associated with typical neuroleptics, atypical neuroleptics, such as risperidone, aripiprazole, and ziprasidone have been used to treat tic symptoms. These agents have potent 5-HT2 blocking effects as well as more modest blocking effects on dopamine D2. Initial favorable double-blind clinical trials have now been reported for risperidone (124), olanzapine (133), and ziprasidone (134). Risperidone and olanzapine use is often associated with weight gain and sedation. Ziprasidone use can be associated with QT prolongation in children so serial monitoring with electrocardiograms may be necessary (135). Recent controlled trials suggest similar efficacy of aripiprazole to other antipsychotic agents (136).

Despite being the most effective pharmacologic agent for the treatment of tics, antipsychotic agents are not generally utilized as a first-line treatment for TS because of their unfavorable side-effect profile. Meta-analysis demonstrated a significant, medium-to-large treatment effect of antipsychotic agents in improving tic symptoms compared to placebo (ES = 0.61 (95% confidence interval [CI]: 0.36 to 0.86), $z = 4.80$, $p = 0.00001$) (137). Further stratified subgroup analysis comparing effect sizes of different antipsychotics (compared to placebo and in head-to-head antipsychotic trials) failed to demonstrate that any particular antipsychotic agent was more effective than any other for the treatment of tic disorders (137). Meta-regression also suggests that there is no association between maximum dose of antipsychotics used in trials and their measured efficacy (137). Therefore, it is advisable to keep antipsychotic doses lower in TS than those typically used for the treatment of psychotic disorders (138).

Clonidine and guanfacine are potent α2-receptor agonists that are thought to reduce central noradrenergic activity. Initial open-label studies of clonidine were favorable, subsequent double-blind clinical trials have had mixed results (138,139). Clinical trials indicate that subjects can expect on average a 25% to 35% reduction in their symptoms over an 8- to 12-week period. Motor tics may show greater improvement than phonic symptoms. The usual starting dose is 0.05 mg on arising. Further 0.05-mg increments at 3- to 4-hour intervals are added weekly until a dosage of 5 mcg per kg is reached, or the total daily dose exceeds 0.25 mg. Although clonidine is clearly less effective than haloperidol and pimozide for immediate tic suppression, it is considerably safer. The principal side effect associated with its use is sedation, which occurs in 10% to 20% of subjects and which usually abates with continued use. Other side effects include dry mouth, transient hypotension, and rare episodes of worsening behavior. Clonidine should be tapered and not withdrawn abruptly, to reduce the likelihood of symptom or blood pressure rebound (140). Guanfacine is another α2-receptor agonist that has been demonstrated in double-blind studies to be effective in the treatment of TS and TS with comorbid ADHD (141). Guanfacine is generally preferred to clonidine because it is less sedating and not associated with rebound hypertension following withdrawal. Guanfacine is generally started at a dose of 0.5 mg at night and then gradually increased by 0.5 mg roughly weekly to TID dosing, with a maximum dose of 4 mg daily (141).

Meta-analysis of randomized, placebo-controlled trials has demonstrated that α2 agonists have a small-to-medium-sized treatment effect in improving tic symptoms compared to placebo (standardized mean difference [SMD] = 0.31 [95% CI: 0.15 to 0.48], $z = 3.64$, $p < 0.001$) (137). Furthermore, comorbid ADHD appeared to have a significant moderating effect on the efficacy of α2 agonists in treating tic symptoms. Trials that only enrolled subjects with comorbid ADHD demonstrated a medium-to-large effect of α2 agonists in reducing tics (SMD = 0.68 [95% CI: 0.36 to 1.01], $z = 4.10$, $p < 0.001$). Trials that excluded subjects with ADHD demonstrated a small, nonsignificant benefit (SMD = 0.15 [95% CI: 0.06 to 0.36], $z = 1.40$, $p = 0.16$) (137). Meta-regression similarly demonstrated a strong positive association between proportion of subjects enrolled in α2 agonist trials and their measured efficacy in treating tic disorders ($\beta = 0.0053$ [95% CI: 0.0015 to 0.0091], $z = -2.72$, $p = 0.006$) (137).

Pharmacotherapy of Coexisting ADHD

The stimulants methylphenidate, d-amphetamine, and Adderall are first-line agents for the medical management of ADHD (141). However, the use of stimulants in ADHD associated with a tic disorder is controversial (143). While many patients with both ADHD and a pre-existing tic disorder will do well on stimulants, data from clinical case reports and controlled studies indicate that some children with ADHD will exhibit tics de novo when exposed to a stimulant. Based on this case report level data most psychostimulant medications carry a warning that they are contraindicated in children with tic disorders or having a family history of TS.

Pharmacotherapy of Coexisting OCD

Cognitive behavioral therapies, particularly exposure and response prevention alone or in combination with serotonin reuptake inhibitors (SRIs), are the standard interventions for OCD (144). Unfortunately, many patients with OCD and a coexisting tic disorder respond less well to first-line pharmacologic interventions such as SSRIs (145). Investigators in controlled clinical trials have found that addition of small doses of the neuroleptic haloperidol, or the atypical neuroleptic risperidone, increases the response to SRIs (55,56). OCD patients with comorbid tics seem to be particularly responsive to SRI augmentation with traditional or atypical neuroleptics (55,56). Since OCD patients with comorbid tics seem to respond slightly less well to SSRI monotherapy, it seems to be increasingly important that these children receive access to evidence-based psychotherapy for OCD (e.g., CBT) early in the treatment course especially before being exposed to the significant side-effect burden of antipsychotic medications.

Other Interventions for Tourette Syndrome Typically Reserved for Adult Patients

Botulinum toxin injections are a treatment reserved for adults with severely debilitating tics involving focal muscle groups. Vocal tics (e.g., coprolalia) or motor tics involving the upper face and neck are considered to be the best targets for treatment. These injections should be performed only by an experienced clinician. A single randomized controlled trial of 20 adolescents and adults with TS has demonstrated that botulinum toxin injection was more effective than placebo in reducing tic symptoms (146). However, weakness of the affected muscles is a side effect of treatment which commonly can cause ptosis, dysphagia, hypophonia, and loss of facial expression depending on the muscles injected.

Neurosurgical interventions for TS have been appropriately reserved for adults with intractable tics that severely affect social functioning. Many neurosurgical sites have been targeted for tics in previous lesioning studies—the frontal cortex (147), limbic cortex (148,149), thalamus (150), infrathalamic area (151,152), and cerebellum (153). Increasingly, with the successful use of deep brain stimulation—a relatively reversible, stereotactic technique to treat other movement disorders—DBS has been looked to as the preferred method of neurosurgical treatment for medically intractable tics. The original electrode placement for DBS surgery was placed in the medial part of the thalamus, based on the results of previous lesioning studies. All four patients, who received bilateral medial thalamic DBS surgery, experienced a substantial improvement in tic severity following the procedure (154,155). Two subsequent case reports demonstrated comparable efficacy in bilateral palladial stimulation compared with bilateral medial thalamic stimulation (155). Likewise, the joint activation of both pairs of electrodes did not lead to a further reduction in tic severity (155). DBS has several advantages over previous neurosurgical lesioning procedures in that it lacks many of the permanent complications typically associated with lesioning procedures (the electrodes can be removed), lends access to many surgically inaccessible sites, and allows for bilateral stimulation and thus holds great promise for adult patients with intractable tics (153). However, currently in DBS for tics, neither the appropriate site of electrode placement nor the electrode stimulation parameters have been examined in carefully controlled clinical studies and differ markedly in the few sites willing to engage in this procedure. Therefore DBS is currently not advisable for all but the most severely affected adults with TS (as children with tics will likely get better with time) and even those most severely affected with TS will likely benefit more from the procedure as the protocol is refined over the upcoming years. Any patient considering this intervention should be very discerning regarding the neurosurgical team, especially regarding experience in this area, as no one has much, and should exhaust every possible medical option to treat tics beforehand and conclude that the tics are unbearable despite these interventions. Any DBS team attempting such surgeries should minimally consist of a neurosurgeon specialized in the stereotactic technique, a neurologist and a psychiatrist trained in movement disorders and their comorbidities, and a specially trained nursing staff (96). The utmost caution is warranted from everyone when engaging in this intervention, especially until the surgical method is improved and this refined method bears the test of more rigorous scientific testing.

FUTURE DIRECTIONS

Recent research efforts have uncovered the first gene, SLTRK1, associated with TS. HRT is the first psychotherapeutic invention proven effective in double-blind studies for TS. DBS, although in its infancy, as applied to TS seems to show some promise in helping the most medically refractory adult patients with TS. Although significant advances in TS treatment have been made, our major challenge over the next few years remains to perfect them and disseminate them to the general public effectively. Despite these advances, our current best available therapies are far from optimum in treating this disorder. Only with an improved understanding of TS will future treatment advances come.

References

1. Sprenger J, Kraemer H: *Malleus Maleficarum (1489)*. London, Pushkin Press, 1948.
2. Stevens H: Gilles de la Tourette and his syndrome by serendipity. *Am J Psychiatry* 128:489–492, 1971.
3. Gilles de la Tourette G: E'tude sur une affection nerveuse caracte'rise'e par de l'incoordination motrice accompagne'e d'echolalie et de copralalie. *Archive Neurologie* 9:19–42, 158–200, 1885.
4. Leckman JF, King RA, Scahill L, Findley D, Ort S, Cohen DJ: Yale approach to assessment and treatment. In: Leckman JF, Cohen DJ (eds): *Tourette's Syndrome Tics, Obsessions, Compulsions - Developmental Psychopathology and Clinical Care*. New York, John Wiley & Sons, 285–309, 1998.
5. Peterson BS, Leckman JF: The temporal dynamics of tics in Gilles de la Tourette syndrome. *Biol Psychiatry* 44(12):1337–1348, 1998.
6. Leckman JF, Cohen DJ: Evolving models of pathogenesis. In: Leckman JF, Cohen DJ (eds): *Tourette's Syndrome—Tics, Obsessions, Compulsions—Developmental Psychopathology and Clinical Care*. New York, John Wiley & Sons, 156–175, 1999.
7. Leckman JF, Riddle MA, Hardin MT, et al.: The Yale Global Tic Severity Scale: initial testing of a clinician-rated scale of tic severity. *J Am Acad Child Adolesc Psychiatry* 28(4):566–573, 1989.
8. Lang A: Patient perception of tics and other movement disorders. *Neurology* 41(2 (Pt 1)):223–228, 1991.
9. Leckman JF, Walker DE, Cohen DJ: Premonitory urges in Tourette's syndrome. *Am J Psychiatry* 150(1):98–102, 1993.
10. Robertson MM: The Gilles de la Tourette syndrome: the current status. *Br J Psych* 154:147–169, 1989.
11. Leckman JF, Zhang H, Vitale A, et al.: Course of tic severity in Tourette syndrome: the first two decades. *Pediatrics* 102(1 Pt 1):14–19, 1998.
12. Peterson BS, Leckman JF, Cohen DJ: TS: A genetically predisposed and an environmentally specified developmental psychopathology. In: Cichetti D, Cohen DJ (eds): *Developmental Psychopathology: Vol. 2. Risk, Disorder and Adaption*. New York, Wiley, 213–241, 1985.
13. Bliss J: Sensory experiences of Gilles de la Tourette syndrome. *Arch Gen Psychiatry* 37:1343–1347, 1980.
14. Conelea CA, Woods DW: Examining the impact of distraction on tic suppression in children and adolescents with Tourette syndrome. *Behav Res Ther* 46(11):1193–1200, 2008.
15. Conelea CA, Woods DW: The influence of contextual factors on tic expression in Tourette's syndrome: a review. *J Psychosom Res* 65(5): 487–496, 2008.
16. Findley DB, Leckman JF, Katsovich L, et al.: Development of the Yale Children's Global Stress Index (YCGSI) and its application in children and adolescents with Tourette's syndrome and obsessive-compulsive disorder. *J Am Acad Child Adolesc Psychiatry* 42(4):450–457, 2003.
17. Sacks O: A surgeon's life. In: *An Anthropologist on Mars: Seven Paradoxical Tales*. New York, Random House, 77–107, 1995.
18. Bloch MH, Peterson BS, Scahill L, et al.: Adulthood outcome of tic and obsessive-compulsive symptom severity in children with Tourette syndrome. *Arch Pediatr Adolesc Med* 160(1):65–69, 2006.
19. Pappert EJ, Goetz CG, Louis ED, Blasucci L, Leurgans S: Objective assessments of longitudinal outcome in Gilles de la Tourette's syndrome. *Neurology* 61(7):936–940, 2003.
20. Rutter M, Tizard J, Whitmore K: *Education, Health, and Behaviour*. London, Longman, 1970.
21. Snider LA, Seligman LD, Ketchen BR, et al.: Tics and problem behaviors in schoolchildren: prevalence, characterization, and associations. *Pediatrics* 110(2 Pt 1):331–336, 2002.
22. Khalifa N, von Knorring AL: Prevalence of tic disorders and Tourette syndrome in a Swedish school population. *Dev Med Child Neurol* 45(5), 315–319, 2003.
23. Gadow KD, Nolan EE, Sprafkin J, Schwartz J: Tics and psychiatric comorbidity in children and adolescents. *Dev Med Child Neurol* 44(5):330–338, 2002.
24. Costello EJ, Angold A, Burns BJ, et al.: The Great Smoky Mountains Study of Youth. goals, design, methods, and the prevalence of DSM-III-R disorders. *Arch Gen Psychiatry* 53(12):1129–1136, 1996.
25. Breton JJ, Bergeron L, Valla JP, et al.: Quebec child mental health survey: prevalence of DSM-III-R mental health disorders. *J Child Psychol Psychiatry* 40(3):375–384, 1999.
26. Caine ED, McBride MC, Chiverton P, Bamford KA, Rediess S, Shiao J: Tourette's syndrome in Monroe County school children. *Neurology* 38(3):472–475, 1988.
27. Mason A, Banerjee S, Eapen V, Zeitlin H, Robertson MM: The prevalence of Tourette syndrome in a mainstream school population. *Dev Med Child Neurol* 40(5):292–296, 1998.
28. Comings DE, MacMurray J, Johnson P, Dietz G, Muhleman D: Dopamine D2 receptor gene (DRD2) haplotypes and the defense style questionnaire in substance abuse, Tourette syndrome, and controls. *Biological Psychiatry* 37(11):798–805, 1995.
29. Kadesjo B, Gillberg C: Tourette's disorder: epidemiology and comorbidity in primary school children. *J Am Acad Child Adolesc Psychiatry* 39(5):548–555, 2000.
30. Kurlan R, McDermott MP, Deeley C, et al.: Prevalence of tics in schoolchildren and association with placement in special education. *Neurology* 57(8):1383–1388, 2001.
31. Landgren M, Pettersson R, Kjellman B, Gillberg C: ADHD, DAMP and other neurodevelopmental/psychiatric disorders in 6-year-old children: epidemiology and co-morbidity. *Dev Med Child Neurol* 38(10):891–906, 1996.
32. Peterson BS, Pine DS, Cohen P, Brook JS: Prospective, longitudinal study of tic, obsessive-compulsive, and attention-deficit/hyperactivity disorders in an epidemiological sample. *J Am Acad Child Adolesc Psychiatry* 40(6):685–695, 2001.
33. Apter A: An epidemiologic study of Gilles de la Tourette's syndrome in Israel. *Arch Gen Psychiatry* 50(9):734, 1993.
34. Erenberg G, Cruse RP, David Rothner A: The natural history of Tourette syndrome: a follow-up study. *Annals of Neurology* 22(3):383–385, 1987.
35. Walkup JT, Khan S, Schuerholz L, Paik Y-S, Leckman JF, Schultz RT: Phenomenology and natural history of tic-related ADHD and learning disabilities. In: Leckman JF, Cohen DJ (eds): *Tourette's Syndrome Tics, Obsessions, Compulsions - Developmental Psychopathology and Clinical Care*. New York, John Wiley & Sons, 63–79, 1998.
36. Carter AS, O'Donnell DA, Schultz RT, Scahill L, Leckman JF, Pauls DL: Social and emotional adjustment in children affected with Gilles de la Tourette's syndrome: associations with ADHD and family functioning. Attention deficit hyperactivity disorder. *J Child Psychol Psychiatry* 41(2):215–223, 2000.
37. Stokes A, Bawden HN, Camfield PR, Backman JE, Dooley JM: Peer problems in Tourette's disorder. *Pediatrics* 87(6):936–942, 1991.
38. Bawden HN, Stokes A, Camfield CS, Camfield PR, Salisbury S: Peer relationship problems in children with Tourette's disorder or diabetes mellitus. *J Child Psychol Psychiatry* 39(5):663–668, 1998.
39. Dykens E, Leckman J, Riddle M, Hardin M, Schwartz S, Cohen D: Intellectual, academic, and adaptive functioning of Tourette syndrome children with and without attention deficit disorder. *J Abnorm Child Psychol* 18(6):607–615, 1990.
40. Hinshaw S: *Attention Deficits and Hyperactivity in Children*: SAGE Publications; 1994.
41. Sukhodolsky DG, Scahill L, Zhang H, et al.: Disruptive behavior in children with Tourette's syndrome: association with ADHD comorbidity, tic severity, and functional impairment. *J Am Acad Child Adolesc Psychiatry* 42(1):98–105, 2003.
42. Carter AS, Pauls DL, Leckman JF, Cohen DJ: A prospective longitudinal study of Gilles de la Tourette's syndrome. *J Am Acad Child Adolesc Psychiatry* 33(3):377–385, 1994.
43. Spencer T, Biederman J, Harding M, et al.: Disentangling the overlap between Tourette's disorder and ADHD. *J Child Psychol Psychiatry* 39(7): 1037–1044, 1998.
44. Greene RW, Biederman J, Faraone SV, Sienna M, Garcia-Jetton J: Adolescent outcome of boys with attention-deficit/hyperactivity disorder and social disability: results from a 4-year longitudinal follow-up study. *J Consult Clin Psychol* 65(5):758–767.
45. Mannuzza S, Klein RG, Bessler A, Malloy P, LaPadula M: Adult psychiatric status of hyperactive boys grown up. *Am J Psychiatry* 155(4):493–498, 1998.
46. Leckman JF, Grice DE, Boardman J, et al.: Symptoms of obsessive-compulsive disorder. *Am J Psychiatry* 154(7):911–917, 1997.
47. Leckman JF, Walker DE, Goodman WK, Pauls DL, Cohen DJ: "Just right" perceptions associated with compulsive behavior in Tourette's syndrome. *Am J Psychiatry* 151(5):675–680, 1994.
48. Baer L: Factor analysis of symptom subtypes of obsessive compulsive disorder and their relation to personality and tic disorders. *J Clin Psychiatry* 55 Suppl:18–23, 1994.
49. Rosario-Campos MC, Miguel EC, Quatrano S, et al.: The Dimensional Yale-Brown Obsessive-Compulsive Scale (DY-BOCS): an instrument for assessing obsessive-compulsive symptom dimensions. *Mol Psychiatry* 11(5):495–504, 2006.
50. Mataix-Cols D, do Rosario-Campos MC, Leckman JF: A multidimensional model of obsessive-compulsive disorder. *Am J Psychiatry* 162(2):228–238, 2005.
51. Bloch MH, Landeros-Weisenberger A, Rosario MC, Pittenger C, Leckman JF: Meta-analysis of the symptom structure of obsessive-compulsive disorder. *Am J Psychiatry* 165(12):1532–1542, 2008.
52. Abramowitz JS, Deacon BJ, Olatunji BO, et al.: Assessment of obsessive-compulsive symptom dimensions: development and evaluation of the Dimensional Obsessive-Compulsive Scale. *Psychol Assess* 22(1):180–198, 2010.
53. Geller DA, Biederman J, Stewart SE, et al.: Impact of comorbidity on treatment response to paroxetine in pediatric obsessive-compulsive disorder: is the use of exclusion criteria empirically supported in randomized clinical trials? *J Child Adolesc Psychopharmacol* 13 Suppl 1:S19–29, 2003.
54. March JS, Franklin ME, Leonard H, et al.: Tics moderate treatment outcome with sertraline but not cognitive-behavior therapy in pediatric obsessive-compulsive disorder. *Biol Psychiatry* 61(3):344–347, 2007.
55. McDougle CJ, Goodman WK, Leckman JF, Lee NC, Heninger GR, Price LH: Haloperidol addition in fluvoxamine-refractory obsessive-compulsive disorder. A double-blind, placebo-controlled study in patients with and without tics. *Arch Gen Psychiatry* 51(4):302–308, 1994.

56. Bloch MH, Landeros-Weisenberger A, Kelmendi B, Coric V, Bracken MB, Leckman JF: A systematic review: antipsychotic augmentation with treatment refractory obsessive-compulsive disorder. *Mol Psychiatry* 11:622–632, 2006.
57. Hebebrand J, Klug B, Fimmers R, et al.: Rates for tic disorders and obsessive compulsive symptomatology in families of children and adolescents with Gilles de la Tourette syndrome. *J Psychiatr Res* 31(5): 519–530, 1997.
58. McMahon WM, Carter AS, Fredine N, Pauls DL: Children at familial risk for Tourette's disorder: child and parent diagnoses. *Am J Med Genet B Neuropsychiatr Genet* 121(1):105–111, 2003.
59. Pauls DL, Raymond CL, Stevenson JM, Leckman JF: A family study of Gilles de la Tourette syndrome. *Am J Hum Genet* 48(1):154–163, 1991.
60. Walkup JT, LaBuda MC, Singer HS, Brown J, Riddle MA, Hurko O: Family study and segregation analysis of Tourette syndrome: evidence for a mixed model of inheritance. *Am J Hum Genet* 59(3):684–693, 1996.
61. Pauls DL, Leckman JF: The inheritance of Gilles de la Tourette's syndrome and associated behaviors. Evidence for autosomal dominant transmission. *N Engl J Med* 315(16):993–997, 1986.
62. Price RA: A twin study of Tourette syndrome. *Arch Gen Psychiatry* 42(8):815, 1985.
63. Hyde TM, Aaronson BA, Randolph C, Rickler KC, Weinberger DR: Relationship of birth weight to the phenotypic expression of Gilles de la Tourette's syndrome in monozygotic twins. *Neurology* 42(3 Pt 1):652–658, 1992.
64. Hasstedt SJ, Leppert M, Filloux F, van de Wetering BJ, McMahon WM: Intermediate inheritance of Tourette syndrome, assuming assortative mating. *Am J Hum Genet* 57(3):682–689, 1995.
65. Barr CL, Sandor P: Current status of genetic studies of Gilles de la Tourette syndrome. *Can J Psychiatry* 43(4):351–357, 1998.
66. Schultz RT, Carter AS, Gladstone M, et al.: Visual-motor integration functioning in children with Tourette syndrome. *Neuropsychology* 12(1):134–145, 1998.
67. Pace JM, Corrado M, Missero C, Byers PH: Identification, characterization and expression analysis of a new fibrillar collagen gene, COL27A1. *Matrix Biol* 22(1):3–14, 2003.
68. Fox MA: Novel roles for collagens in wiring the vertebrate nervous system. *Curr Opin Cell Biol* 20(5):508–513, 2008.
69. Scharf JM, Yu D, Mathews CA, et al.: Genome-wide association study of Tourette's syndrome. *Mol Psychiatry* 18(6):721–728, 2013.
70. Dieci G, Fiorino G, Castelnuovo M, Teichmann M, Pagano A: The expanding RNA polymerase III transcriptome. *Trends Genet* 23(12):614–622, 2007.
71. Daoud H, Tetreault M, Gibson W, et al.: Mutations in POLR3A and POLR3B are a major cause of hypomyelinating leukodystrophies with or without dental abnormalities and/or hypogonadotropic hypogonadism. *J Med Genet* 50(3):194–197, 2013.
72. Davis LK, Yu D, Keenan CL, et al.: Partitioning the heritability of Tourette syndrome and obsessive compulsive disorder reveals differences in genetic architecture. *PLoS Genet* 9(10):e1003864, 2013.
73. Abelson JF. Sequence variants in SLITRK1 are associated with Tourette's syndrome. *Science* 310(5746):317–320, 2005.
74. Ercan-Sencicek AG, Stillman AA, Ghosh AK, et al.: L-histidine decarboxylase and Tourette's syndrome. *N Engl J Med* 362(20):1901–1908, 2010.
75. Castellan Baldan L, Williams KA, Gallezot JD, et al.: Histidine decarboxylase deficiency causes Tourette syndrome: parallel findings in humans and mice. *Neuron* 81(1):77–90, 2014.
76. Pasamanick B, Kawi A: A study of the association of prenatal and paranatal factors with the development of tics in children; a preliminary investigation. *J Pediatr* 48(5):596–601, 1956.
77. Leckman JF, Price RA, Walkup JT, Ort S, Pauls DL, Cohen DJ: Nongenetic factors in Gilles de la Tourette's syndrome. *Arch Gen Psychiatry* 44(1):100, 1987.
78. Leckman JF, Dolnansky ES, Hardin MT, et al.: Perinatal factors in the expression of Tourette's syndrome: an exploratory study. *J Am Acad Child Adolesc Psychiatry* 29(2):220–226, 1990.
79. Burd L, Severud R, Klug MG, Kerbeshian J: Prenatal and perinatal risk factors for Tourette disorder. *J Perinat Med* 27(4):295–302, 1999.
80. Santangelo SL, Pauls DL, Goldstein JM, Faraone SV, Tsuang MT, Leckman JF: Tourette's syndrome: what are the influences of gender and comorbid obsessive-compulsive disorder? *J Am Acad Child Adolesc Psychiatry* 33(6):795–804, 1994.
81. Browne HA, Modabbernia A, Buxbaum JD, et al.: Prenatal maternal smoking and increased risk for Tourette syndrome and chronic tic disorders. *J Am Acad Child Adolesc Psychiatry* 55(9):784–791, 2016.
82. Marsh R, Maia TV, Peterson BS: Functional disturbances within frontostriatal circuits across multiple childhood psychopathologies. *Am J Psychiatry* 166(6):664–674, 2009.
83. Fried I, Katz A, McCarthy G, et al.: Functional organization of human supplementary motor cortex studied by electrical stimulation. *J Neurosci* 11(11):3656–3666, 1991.
84. Bohlhalter S, Goldfine A, Matteson S, et al.: Neural correlates of tic generation in Tourette syndrome: an event-related functional MRI study. *Brain* 2006.
85. Hampson M, Tokoglu F, King RA, Constable RT, Leckman JF: Brain areas coactivating with motor cortex during chronic motor tics and intentional movements. *Biol Psychiatry* 65(7):594–599, 2009.
86. Sowell ER, Kan E, Yoshii J, et al.: Thinning of sensorimotor cortices in children with Tourette syndrome. *Nat Neurosci* 11(6):637–639, 2008.
87. Marsh R, Zhu H, Wang Z, Skudlarski P, Peterson BS: A developmental fMRI study of self-regulatory control in Tourette's syndrome. *Am J Psychiatry* 164(6):955–966, 2007.
88. Mischel W, Shoda Y, Rodriguez MI: Delay of gratification in children. *Science* 244(4907):933–938, 1989.
89. Peterson BS, Skudlarski P, Anderson AW, et al.: A functional magnetic resonance imaging study of tic suppression in Tourette syndrome. *Arch Gen Psychiatry* 55(4):326–333, 1998.
90. Peterson BS, Staib L, Scahill L, et al.: Regional brain and ventricular volumes in Tourette syndrome. *Arch Gen Psychiatry* 58(5):427–440, 2001.
91. Peterson BS, Thomas P, Kane MJ, et al.: Basal ganglia volumes in patients with Gilles de la Tourette syndrome. *Arch Gen Psychiatry* 60(4):415–424, 2003.
92. Hyde TM, Stacey ME, Coppola R, Handel SF, Rickler KC, Weinberger DR: Cerebral morphometric abnormalities in Tourette's syndrome: a quantitative MRI study of monozygotic twins. *Neurology* 45(6):1176–1182, 1995.
93. Bloch MH, Leckman JF, Zhu H, Peterson BS: Caudate volumes in childhood predict symptom severity in adults with Tourette syndrome. *Neurology* 65(8):1253–1258, 2005.
94. Kalanithi PS, Zheng W, Kataoka Y, et al.: Altered parvalbumin-positive neuron distribution in basal ganglia of individuals with Tourette syndrome. *Proc Natl Acad Sci U S A* 102(37):13307–13312, 2005.
95. Kataoka Y, Kalanithi PS, Grantz H, et al.: Decreased number of parvalbumin and cholinergic interneurons in the striatum of individuals with Tourette Syndrome. *J Comparative Neurology* 518:277–291, 2010.
96. Schrock LE, Mink JW, Woods DW, et al;Tourette Syndrome Association International Deep Brain Stimulation (DBS) Database and Registry Study Group: Tourette syndrome deep brain stimulation: a review and updated recommendations. *Mov Disord* 30(4):448–471, 2015.
97. Mink JW. The basal ganglia and involuntary movements. *Arch Neurol* 60(10):1365, 2003.
98. Anderson GM, Polack ES, Chatterjee D, Leckman JF, Riddle MA, Cohen DJ: Postmortem analysis of subcortical monoamines and amonoacids in Tourette syndrome. In: Chase TN, Friedhoff AJ, Cohen DJ (eds): *Tourette Syndrome: Genetics, Neurobiology, and Treatment.* New York, Raven Press, Ltd., 253–262, 1992.
99. Alexander GE, DeLong MR: Microstimulation of the primate neostriatum. II. Somatotopic organization of striatal microexcitable zones and their relation to neuronal response properties. *J Neurophysiol* 53(6):1417–1430, 1985.
100. Leckman JF, Vaccarino FM, Kalanithi PS, Rothenberger A: Annotation: Tourette syndrome: a relentless drumbeat–driven by misguided brain oscillations. *J Child Psychol Psychiatry* 47(6):537–550, 2006.
101. Singer HS: Neurochemical analysis of postmortem cortical and striatal brain tissue in patients with Tourette syndrome. *Adv Neurol* 58:135–144, 1992.
102. Richardson EP: Neuropathological Studies of TS. In: Friedhoff AJ, Chase TN (eds): *Advances in Neurology Vol. 35: Gilles de la TS.* New York, Raven Press, 83–87, 1982.
103. Haber SN: The primate basal ganglia: parallel and integrative networks. *J Chem Neuroanat* 26(4):317–330, 2003.
104. Peterson BS: Neuroanatomical Circuitry. In: Leckman JF, Cohen DJ (eds): *TS – Tics, Obsessions, Compulsions: Developmental Psychopathology and Clinical Care.* New York, Wiley, 230–260, 1999.
105. Kelley A, Lang C, Gauthier A: Induction of oral stereotypy following amphetamine microinjection into a discrete subregion of the striatum. *Psychopharmacology* 95(4), 1988.
106. Silva RR, Munoz DM, Barickman J, Friedhoff AJ: Environmental factors and related fluctuation of symptoms in children and adolescents with Tourette's disorder. *J Child Psychol Psychiatry* 36(2):305–312, 1995.
107. Jagger J, Prusoff BA, Cohen DJ, Kidd KK, Carbonari CM, John K: The epidemiology of Tourette's syndrome: a pilot study. *Schizophr Bull* 8(2):267–278, 1982.
108. Shapiro AK, Shapiro ES, Young JG, Freinberg TE: *Gilles de la Tourette Syndrome.* 2nd ed. New York, Raven Press, 1988.
109. Towbin KE, Peterson BS, Cohen DJ, Leckman JF: Differential diagnosis. In: Leckman JF, Cohen DJ (eds): *Tourette's Syndrome Tics, Obsessions, Compulsions—Developmental Psychopathology and Clinical Care.* New York, John Wiley & Sons: 118–139, 1998.
110. Mahone EM, Bridges D, Prahme C, Singer HS: Repetitive arm and hand movements (complex motor stereotypies) in children. *J Pediatr* 145(3):391–395, 2004.
111. Leckman JF: Tourette's syndrome. *Lancet* 360(9345):1577–1586, 2002.
112. Chappell PB, McSwiggan-Hardin MT, Scahill L, et al.: Videotape tic counts in the assessment of Tourette's syndrome: stability, reliability, and validity. *J Am Acad Child Adolesc Psychiatry* 33(3):386–393, 1994.
113. Goetz CG, Pappert EJ, Louis ED, Raman R, Leurgans S: Advantages of a modified scoring method for the Rush Video-Based Tic Rating Scale. *Mov Disord* 14(3):502–506, 1999.
114. Nolan EE, Gadow KD, Sverd J: Observations and ratings of tics in school settings. *J Abnorm Child Psychol* 22(5):579–593, 1994.
115. Cohen DJ, Ort SI, Leckman JF, Riddle MA, Hardin MT: Family functioning and Tourette's syndrome. In: Cohen DJ, Bruun RD, Leckman JF (eds): *Tourette's Syndrome and Tic Disorders.* New York: John Wiley & Sons, 179, 1988.

116. Bronheim S: An educator's guide to Tourette syndrome. *J Learn Disabil* 24(1):17–22, 1991.
117. Woods DW, Twohig MP, Flessner CA, Roloff TJ: Treatment of vocal tics in children with Tourette syndrome: investigating the efficacy of habit reversal. *J Appl Behav Anal* 36(1):109–112, Spring 2003.
118. Piacentini JC, Chang SW: Behavioral treatments for tic suppression: habit reversal training. *Adv Neurol* 99:227–233, 2006.
119. Azrin HG, Nunn RG: Habit-reversal: a method of eliminating nervous habits and tics. *Behav Res Ther* 11(4):619–628, 1973.
120. Deckersbach T, Rauch S, Buhlmann U, Wilhelm S: Habit reversal versus supportive psychotherapy in Tourette's disorder: a randomized controlled trial and predictors of treatment response. *Behav Res Ther* 2005.
121. Wilhelm S, Deckersbach T, Coffey BJ, Bohne A, Peterson AL, Baer L: Habit reversal versus supportive psychotherapy for Tourette's disorder: a randomized controlled trial. *Am J Psychiatry* 160(6):1175–1177, 2003.
122. McGuire JF, Piacentini J, Brennan EA, et al.: A meta-analysis of behavior therapy for Tourette syndrome. *J Psychiatr Res* 50:106–112, 2014.
123. Piacentini J, Woods DW, Scahill L, et al.: Behavior therapy for children with Tourette disorder: a randomized controlled trial. *JAMA* 303(19):1929–1937, 2010.
124. Bruggeman R, van der Linden C, Buitelaar JK, Gericke GS, Hawkridge SM, Temlett JA: Risperidone versus pimozide in Tourette's disorder: A comparative double-blind parallel-group study. *J Clin Psychiatry* 62(1):50–56,2001.
125. Scahill L, Erenberg G, Berlin CM, Jr., et al.: Contemporary assessment and pharmacotherapy of Tourette syndrome. *NeuroRx* 3(2):192–206, 2006.
126. Kushner HI: *A Cursing Brain? The Histories of Tourette Syndrome.* Cambridge, MA, Harvard University Press, 1999.
127. Eggers C, Rothenberger A, Berghaus U: Clinical and neurobiological findings in children suffering from tic disease following treatment with tiapride. *Eur Arch Psychiatry Neurol Sci* 237(4):223–229, 1988.
128. Sallee FR, Nesbitt L, Jackson C, Sine L, Sethuraman G: Relative efficacy of haloperidol and pimozide in children and adolescents with Tourette's disorder. *Am J Psychiatry* 154(8):1057–1062, 1997.
129. Shapiro E: Controlled study of haloperidol, pimozide, and placebo for the treatment of Gilles de la Tourette's syndrome. *Arch Gen Psychiatry* 46(8):722, 1989.
130. Tourette_Syndrome_Study_Group: Short-term versus longer-term pimozide therapy in Tourette's syndrome: a preliminary study. *Neurology* 52:874–877, 1999.
131. Kurlan R: Treatment of tics. *Neurologic Clinics* 15:403–409, 1997.
132. Silva RR, Munoz DM, Daniel W, Barickman J, Friedhoff AJ: Causes of haloperidol discontinuation in patients with Tourette's disorder: management and alternatives. *J Clin Psychiatry* 57(3):129–135, 1996.
133. Stephens RJ, Bassel C, Sandor P: Olanzapine in the treatment of aggression and tics in children with Tourette's syndrome–a pilot study. *J Child Adolesc Psychopharmacol* 14(2):255–266, Summer 2004.
134. Sallee FR, Kurlan R, Goetz CG, et al.: Ziprasidone treatment of children and adolescents with Tourette's syndrome: a pilot study. *J Am Acad Child Adolesc Psychiatry* 39(3):292–299, 2000.
135. Blair J, Scahill L, State M, Martin A: Electrocardiographic changes in children and adolescents treated with ziprasidone: a prospective study. *J Am Acad Child Adolesc Psychiatry* 44(1):73–79, 2005.
136. Yang CS, Huang H, Zhang LL, Zhu CR, Guo Q: Aripiprazole for the treatment of tic disorders in children: a systematic review and meta-analysis. *BMC Psychiatry* 15:179, 2015.
137. Weisman H, Qureshi IA, Leckman JF, Scahill L, Bloch MH: Systematic review: pharmacological treatment of tic disorders—efficacy of antipsychotic and alpha-2 adrenergic agonist agents. *Neurosci Biobehav Rev* 37(6):1162–1171, 2013.
138. Murphy TK, Lewin AB, Storch EA, Stock S, American Academy of C, Adolescent Psychiatry Committee on Quality I. Practice parameter for the assessment and treatment of children and adolescents with tic disorders. *J Am Acad Child Adolesc Psychiatry* 52(12):1341–1359, 2013.
139. Goetz CG, Tanner CM, Wilson RS, Carroll VS, Como PG, Shannon KM: Clonidine and Gilles de la Tourette's syndrome: double-blind study using objective rating methods. *Ann Neurol* 21(3):307–310, 1987.
140. Leckman JF. Clonidine treatment of Gilles de la Tourette's syndrome. *Arch Gen Psychiatry* 48(4):324, 1991.
141. Scahill L, Chappell PB, Kim YS, et al.: A placebo-controlled study of guanfacine in the treatment of children with tic disorders and attention deficit hyperactivity disorder. *Am J Psychiatry* 158(7):1067–1074, 2001.
142. Dulcan M: Practice parameters for the assessment and treatment of children, adolescents, and adults with attention-deficit/hyperactivity disorder. American Academy of Child and Adolescent Psychiatry. *J Am Acad Child Adolesc Psychiatry* 36(10 Suppl):85S–121S, 1997.
143. Castellanos FX: Stimulants and tic disorders: from dogma to data. *Arch Gen Psychiatry* 56(4):337–338, 1999.
144. Practice parameter for the assessment and treatment of children and adolescents with obsessive-compulsive disorder. *J Am Acad Child Adolesc Psychiatry* 51(1):98–113, 2012.
145. McDougle CJ, Goodman WK, Leckman JF, Barr LC, Heninger GR, Price LH: The efficacy of fluvoxamine in obsessive-compulsive disorder: effects of comorbid chronic tic disorder. *J Clin Psychopharmacol* 13(5):354–358, 1993.
146. Marras C, Andrews D, Sime E, Lang AE: Botulinum toxin for simple motor tics: a randomized, double-blind, controlled clinical trial. *Neurology* 56(5):605–610, 2001.
147. Baker EFW: Gilles de la TS treated by medial frontal leucotomy. *Can Med Assoc J* 86:746–747, 1962.
148. Kurlan R, Kersun J, Ballantine HT, Jr., Caine ED: Neurosurgical treatment of severe obsessive-compulsive disorder associated with Tourette's syndrome. *Mov Disord* 5(2):152–155, 1990.
149. Sawle GV, Lees AJ, Hymas NF, Brooks DJ, Frackowiak RS: The metabolic effects of limbic leucotomy in Gilles de la Tourette syndrome. *J Neurol Neurosurg Psychiatry* 56(9):1016–1019, 1993.
150. Hassler R, Dieckmann G: Relief of obsessive-compulsive disorders, phobias and tics by stereotactic coagulations of the rostral intralaminar and medial-thalamic nuclei. In: Laitinen L, Livingston K (eds): *Surgical Approaches in Psychiatry: Proceedings of the Third International Congress of Psychosurgery.* Cambridge, Garden City Press, 206–212, 1973.
151. Leckman JF, de Lotbiniere AJ, Marek K, Gracco C, Scahill L, Cohen DJ: Severe disturbances in speech, swallowing, and gait following stereotactic infrathalamic lesions in Gilles de la Tourette's syndrome. *Neurology* 43(5):890–894, 1993.
152. Babel TB: Immediate and long term outcome after infrathalamic and thalamic lesioning for intractable Tourette's syndrome. *J Neurol, Neurosurg Psychiatry* 70(5):666–671, 2001.
153. Singer HS. Tourette's syndrome: from behaviour to biology. *Lancet Neurol* 4(3):149–159, 2005.
154. Visser-Vandewalle V, Temel Y, Boon P, et al.: Chronic bilateral thalamic stimulation: a new therapeutic approach in intractable Tourette syndrome. Report of three cases. *J Neurosurg* 99(6):1094–1100, 2003.
155. Ackermans L, Temel Y, Cath D, et al.: Deep brain stimulation in Tourette's syndrome: two targets? *Mov Disord* 21(5):709–713, 2006.

5.7 ■ EATING DISORDERS

CHAPTER 5.7.1 ■ ANOREXIA NERVOSA, BULIMIA NERVOSA, AND BINGE EATING DISORDER

KATHERINE A. HALMI

DEFINITION

Anorexia nervosa (AN) and bulimia nervosa (BN) for many years were regarded as the two major eating disorders. They are complex syndromes with considerable psychiatric and medical comorbidities. After years of obtaining sufficient data and evidence, binge eating disorder (BED) has become a primary diagnosis in the DSM-5. Current abbreviated diagnostic criteria for AN, BN, and BED from DSM-5 (1) are shown in Tables 5.7.1.1, 5.7.1.2, and 5.7.1.3. For those patients who have serious problems with eating behavior but do not fall into the above primary diagnostic categories, the DSM-5 has

TABLE 5.7.1.1

DIAGNOSTIC CRITERIA FOR ANOREXIA NERVOSA

A. Restriction of energy intake leading to low body weight in the context of age, sex, developmental trajectory, and physical health. Significant low weight for children and adults is less than minimally expected.
B. Intense fear of gaining weight or becoming fat or persistent behavior that interferes with weight gain.
C. Disturbance in experiencing body weight or shape, undue influence of the latter on self-regard or persistent lack of recognition or the seriousness of low body weight.

Subtype—Restricting or Binge Eating/Purging

Condensed from the American Psychiatric Association: *Diagnostic and Statistical Manual of Mental Disorders*. 5th ed. Washington, DC, American Psychiatric Association, 2013.

TABLE 5.7.1.3

DIAGNOSTIC CRITERIA FOR BINGE EATING DISORDER

A. Recurrent episodes of binge eating
B. More episodes of eating: more rapidly than normal, until uncomfortably full, large amounts when not physically hungry, alone due to embarrassment, and feeling disgusted, depressed or guilty afterward
C. Marked distress over binge eating
D. Binge eating on average at least once a week for 3 months
E. Binge eating does not occur with inappropriate compensatory behaviors and does not occur exclusively in the course of anorexia or bulimia nervosa occur exclusively in the course of anorexia or bulimia nervosa

Condensed from American Psychiatric Association: *Diagnostic and Statistical Manual of Mental Disorders*. 5th ed. Washington, DC, American Psychiatric Association, 2013.

designated a category of "Other Specified Feeding or Eating Disorder." Most cases of eating disorders have an onset during adolescence.

There are three major criteria which define AN. The first criterion is a guideline for defining weight loss, recommending considering age, sex developmental trajectory, and physical health. For children up to the age of 18, pediatric growth charts should be used. Some children may not have weight loss but still weigh less than expected weight because they have failed to make weight gains during a growth in height.

There is no consensus on how weight loss should be calculated, especially with adolescent patients. Some clinicians calculate weight loss below a normal weight for age and height and others figure the amount loss from an original baseline. Body mass index (BMI) is weight in kilograms divided by height in meters squared. This measure is a standard score that somewhat corrects for height and different body build. This index has the advantage of not being subjected to cultural influences. The World Health Organization (WHO) regards a BMI of 18.5 kg/m^2 as the lower limit of normal body weight for adults. The Center for Disease Control and Prevention (CDC) recommends their BMI for age percentile calculator for children and adolescents and suggests below the 5th percentile as underweight, a BMI between 25 and 30 is considered overweight, and over 30 is labeled obesity.

The second criterion, "intense fear of gaining weight," is present even during emaciated states. Anorectic patients often deny this fear since they are resistant to treatment and thus, their fear of gaining weight must often be inferred by reports of their behavior which reveal rigorous attempts to prevent weight gain such as severe food restriction and exercising.

TABLE 5.7.1.2

DIAGNOSTIC CRITERIA FOR BULIMIA NERVOSA

A. Recurrent episodes of binge eating.
B. Recurrent inappropriate behaviors to prevent weight gain; e.g., self-induced vomiting; laxative, diuretic or other medicine misuse; fasting; excessive exercise.
C. Binge eating and inappropriate compensatory behaviors occur, on average, once a week for 3 months.
D. Self-evaluation is unduly influenced by body shape and weight.
E. Above symptoms do not occur exclusively during episodes of anorexia nervosa.

Condensed from American Psychiatric Association: *Diagnostic and Statistical Manual of Mental Disorders*. 5th ed. Washington, DC, American Psychiatric Association, 2013.

The third criterion, concerning conception of body shape and weight, has evolved into a more complex concept. The significance of body weight and shape are greatly distorted in these individuals. Some feel globally overweight and others realize they are thin but feel certain parts of their body, especially the abdomen and thighs, are too fat. The distorted significance of body weight and shape is related to feelings of insecurity and ineffectiveness. Losing weight and being thin is one area in which these individuals can be effective and in control. The latter undoubtedly influences their denial of the serious medical complications of their malnourished state.

There are two subtypes of AN: the restricting type and the binge–purge type. Studies have consistently demonstrated that impulsive behaviors including stealing, drug abuse, suicide attempts, self-mutilation, and promiscuity are more prevalent in anorectic binge/purgers compared with anorectic restrictors. Those with anorexia binge–purge type also have a higher prevalence of premorbid obesity, familial obesity, debilitating personality traits, and specific medical complications compared with the anorexia restrictive type (3–5).

The criteria for BN are more arbitrary and less specific than the criteria for AN. In the first criterion for BN in DSM-5, binge eating is defined as eating more food than most people eat in similar circumstances and in a similar period of time. The sense of losing control is a significant subjective aspect that needs to be present. The second criterion, which is the recurrent use of inappropriate compensatory behaviors to avoid weight gain, usually means self-induced vomiting. However, bulimic patients often use cathartics for weight control and have an eating pattern of alternate binges and long fasting periods. The third criterion designed to address chronicity and frequency was changed from twice to once a week for 3 months in DSM-5 in response to clinician-based data that once per week was associated with significant impairment of function. The fourth criterion acknowledges that BN patients are also concerned about their body shape and weight and tend to place excessive estimation of their worth in terms of appearance. The fifth criterion of BN differentiates the latter from the binge–purge subtype of AN.

The first criterion for BED is the same as that for BN, defining binge eating and emphasizing the sense of lack of control. The second criterion provides descriptive criteria surrounding a binge eating episode. Binge eating in BED is associated with significant distress which constitutes the third criterion. The fourth criterion of frequency and chronicity is the same as that for BN, once a week for 3 months. Exclusion of evidence of BN and AN comprise the fifth criterion.

In DSM-5 for the three primary eating disorders specifications are required for partial or full remission and the level of current severity. There are several changes in diagnostic criteria from DSM-IV (2) to DSM-5 for AN, BN, and "not otherwise specified" category. For AN, the most significant change is the deletion of the amenorrhea criterion which did not apply to prepubescent girls, males, or females on contraceptives. Also accurate menstrual history data was often difficult to obtain and comparison between those who were and who were not menstruating revealed no consistent differences. The subtyping of AN into restricting type and binge eating/purging type has changed from current episode to a duration of at least 3 months. Terms implying deliberateness of AN patients; for example, refusal and denial are changed to restriction of energy intake and persistent lack of recognition of the seriousness of current low body weight. Persistent behavior that interferes with weight gain is added to the intense fear of gaining weight since many patients do not admit to the latter. The term "significantly low body weight" remains wisely broad in consideration of age, sex, and developmental trajectory.

For BN, the only major change in DSM-IV criteria is the frequency of binge eating and compensatory behaviors from twice to once/weekly for 3 months.

BED received an official classification in DSM-5 after years of extensive data collection to demonstrate that this diagnosis had sufficient validity and clinical usefulness (24). Although less common in children and adolescents compared to adults, an association was found between binge eating and being overweight.

Eating disorders not otherwise specified (EDNOS) have been replaced with other specified feeding or eating disorder (OSFED). This category includes the three major eating disorders without meeting full criteria but having presence of significant distress or impairment. Also in this category is purging disorder—recurrent purging in the absence of binge eating, and night eating syndrome—recurrent eating after awakening from sleep or excessive eating after the evening meal.

Unspecified feeding or eating disorder is a category for which eating-related symptoms are causing significant distress but criteria are not met for the DSM-5 designated eating disorder diagnoses.

HISTORICAL CONTEXT

Disturbances of eating behavior were described in the Middle Ages. Well-documented case reports of AN are found in the literature describing early Christian saints. Monastery documents record the severe starving behavior and binging episodes of Saint Catherine of Siena, along with the kind of reed she used to induce vomiting and the herbal cathartics she used for purging (3). Another example of this irreversible self-starvation in a fasting female saint is Princes Margaret of Hungary, who lived from 1240 to 1271 (4). She was the daughter of a king and was raised in a Dominican convent where she excelled in all of her studies and in the undesirable chores of the monastery. It is likely that biologic vulnerability factors are similar in those dieting for sainthood during the Middle Ages and those dieting for thinness (attractiveness) in the 20th century. In the 17th century both John Reynolds (5) and Richard Morton (6) described cases of typical AN symptomatology and distinguished them from consumption. In the 19th century Marcé (7), Sir William Gull (8), and Laséque (9) described additional cases of AN and recommended treatment. In the 20th century the first major publication on AN was a book by Bliss and Branch (10) that presented endocrine studies as well as psychological descriptions of the disorder. A decade later, Hilda Bruch (11) further articulated the psychology of AN in her phrase "the relentless pursuit of thinness" and "the paralyzing sense of ineffectiveness, which pervades all thinking and activities." In 1979, Russell identified BN as a separate entity from AN (12). Subsequently it became apparent that there were young women who had the full syndrome of BN without a history of AN.

After DSM-III-R (13) was published in 1987, clinical evidence was accumulating for a condition in which binge eating was not followed by compensatory weight reducing behavior. Controlled studies to investigate this condition were strongly encouraged by Robert Spitzer, MD, Chair of the DSM-III-R work group. By 1994, when DSM-IV was published, sufficient studies justified placing BED in the EDNOS section with research criteria. The difficulty in identifying BED as a specific disorder was distinguishing it from BN—nonpurging type and obesity with overeating and defining compensatory behavior. By 2013, BED which qualified as a prime specific diagnosis was presented as such in DSM-5.

EPIDEMIOLOGY, DEMOGRAPHIC CHARACTERISTICS, AND OUTCOME

Most of the studies of incidence and prevalence of eating disorders have been conducted on limited populations such as primary care clinics or medical records with self-report questionnaires. Thus, the true incidence and prevalence of AN, BN, and BED within various countries is not likely truly accurate. The incidence rate, the number of new cases of a disorder in a population over a specific period, is usually expressed for eating disorders as per 100,000 persons per year. Adequate incidence studies are costly and require large samples. Most published data for eating disorders reflect data collection from at least a decade ago using DSM-IV criteria.

Since 1980 until 2000 the incidence of AN in Europe has remained relatively stable. For example, in the United Kingdom new cases in 1988–1993 were 4.2 per 100,000 and in 1994–2000 were 4.7 per 100,000 (14). In the Netherlands, in 1985–1989 there were 7.4 per 100,000 new cases of AN and in 1995–1999 there were 7.7 per 100,000 (15). The incidence of AN in the Netherlands was highest for females aged 15 to 19 and comprised 40% of all cases; 56.4 per 100,000 in 1985 and 109.2 per 100,000 in 1995–1999 (15). Incidence of males was less than 1 per 100,000 in both countries. In the United States, the overall age adjusted incidence in Minnesota for females was 14.6 per 100,000 and 1.8 for males from 1935 to 1989 (16). Among 10- to 19-year-old girls, the incidence rates increased substantially from 1950 to 1984.

Published prevalence studies of eating disorders are more abundant and often conducted on limited populations with varying sensitivity of assessments. Prevalence is usually expressed as point prevalence, occurring at a specific point in time, or lifetime prevalence, proportion of persons that had the disorder at any time in their life.

In the United States, an 8-year prospective study of adolescent girls had a lifetime prevalence by age 20 of AN to be 0.6% with DSM-IV criteria and 2.0% for atypical AN (17). Lifetime prevalence of AN in the United States was assessed in two other large sample studies revealing a lifetime prevalence of 0.3% in 13- to 18-year-old females and males (18) and 0.9% among adult females and 0.3% in males (19). A population-based study in six European countries (20) had a 0.9% AN lifetime prevalence in females and none in males. More recently over 2,000 children were assessed from age 11 in 2001 to ages 19 to 20 in 2010 in a Dutch community sample. At ages 19 to 20 there was a 1.7% lifetime prevalence of DSM-5 AN in women and 0.1% in men (21).

Mortality rates in AN are high. A 20-year follow-up study had 6.5% deaths with a standardized mortality rate (SMR) of 4.37 for lifetime AN. Duration of illness effected the SMR; 0 to

15 years had a 3.25 SMR and 15 to 30 years had a 6.6 SMR (22). A meta-analysis of 36 studies had an SMR of 5.86 for AN. One in five persons who died committed suicide (23).

A younger age at detection and treatment of AN predicted recovery in a Dutch study. Those 19 years and younger had an odds ratio of recovery of 4.3 compared to those 20 years and older (24). An analysis of 119 studies of outcome found less than half of AN patients had full recovery, 33% improved, and 20% developed a chronic course (25).

BN has few incidence but many prevalence studies. An incidence of 438 per 100,000 person years was found in 15 to 18 Finnish females with BN including those who lacked one criteria for BN (26). In a nation-wide primary care study in the Netherlands the incidence BN rate was 8.6 per 100,000 person years in 1985–1989 and decreased to 6.1 per 100,000 person years in 1995–1999 (15). Likewise, the incidence of BN in the United Kingdom decreased from 12.2 per 100,000 person years in 1993 to 6.6 in 2000. In women aged 10 to 19, the incidence rate of BN remained stable around 40 per 100,000 person years in 1993 and 2000 (14).

Soundy et al. (27) found that the community-based incidence of BN rose sharply from 1980 to 1983 and then remained relatively constant through 1990. The incidence rates of Rochester, MN during that decade were 26.5 per 100,000 per year for females and 0.8 per 100,000 per year for males. The mean age of onset for females is 23 years. Among 15- through 24-year-old adolescent girls and young women, it had become at least twice as common as AN.

Lifetime prevalence of BN in a six European country study was 0.88% in females and 0.12% in males (25). In the United States, a lifetime prevalence of 1.6% for BN was found at age 20 in adolescent females followed for 8 years (17). A point prevalence of 0.6% was reported in 14-year-old Australian adolescents (28). The point prevalence of BN among university women decreased from 4.2% in 1982 to 1.3% in 1992 to 1.7% in 2002 (29). Initially, high rates for BN found in the 1980s were based on DSM-III criteria (30). DSM-IV BN criteria (2) were more restrictive and DSM-5 BN criteria (1) are again less restrictive. Thus increases in BN prevalence may be anticipated with DSM-5 criteria.

There is some evidence that the age of onset of BN is decreasing. Italian BN patients born in 1970–1972 had a mean age onset of 18.5 years compared to 17.1 years in those born between 1979 and 1981 (31). A Dutch high-risk group of BN changed from 25- to 29-year-old females in 1985–1989 to 15- to 24-year-old females in 1995–1999 (15).

A longitudinal assessment of mortality over 8 to 25 years in 906 BN clinic outpatients produced a crude mortality rate of 3.9% and an SMR of 1.57. The elevated risk for suicide 0.9% was significant and accounted for 23% of the deaths (32). Inconsistent findings are present in outcome studies of BN and vary from recovery in 48% (33) to 70% (34) to 77% (35). Likewise, studies of the effect of various comorbidities on outcome of BN are inconsistent. The most replicable unfavorable outcome factor has been the presence of borderline personality symptoms (36).

BED lifetime prevalence assessed with DSM-IV criteria in the United States found 3.5% women and 2.0% men were effected (19). With DSM-5 criteria applied to this sample BED lifetime, prevalence increased to 3.6% in women and 2.1% in men (37). In a nationally representative sample of US adolescents aged 13 to 18 years the lifetime prevalence of BED was 2.3% in females and 0.8% in males (18). In the six European country study the lifetime prevalence of BED was 1.9% for women and 0.3% for men (20). There were no published incidence studies of BED at the time of this article preparation.

Mortality and outcome studies of BED have been embedded in the EDNOS DSM-IV criteria. However, a German 12-year follow-up of 68 BED inpatients revealed that 2 had died giving a crude mortality rate of 2.9% and a nonsignificant SMR of 2.29 (38). A high comorbidity, 42%, of obesity with BED was present in a large population-based study (19,24).

CLINICAL DESCRIPTION

Two hallmark characteristics of patients with AN are denial of the seriousness of their illness and resistance to treatment, both of which make obtaining an accurate history and producing an effective treatment result a challenge. Anorectic individuals demonstrate their intense fear of gaining weight by their intense preoccupation with thoughts of food and irrational worries about fatness. They frequently look in mirrors to make sure they are thin and incessantly express concern about their appearance. They will take a great deal of time cutting up food into small pieces and rearranging food on their plates in order to eat less. An overwhelming feeling of inadequacy and ineffectiveness is a core symptom of all anorectics. Their success at losing weight is an impressive accomplishment and boosts their self-confidence. Obsessive-compulsive behaviors often develop or become worse as their AN becomes more severe. Obsessions with cleanliness and an increase in cleaning activities and compulsive studying are commonly observed. Perfectionistic traits are common in the restricting type of AN patient.

Many adolescent anorectics have delayed psychosocial development and adults often have a markedly decreased interest in sex with the onset of AN.

There are important physiologic differences between the two subtypes of anorectic patients. Most of the physiologic and metabolic changes in AN are secondary to the starvation state or to purging behavior. These changes revert to normal with nutritional rehabilitation and the cessation of purging behavior.

In patients with AN who engage in self-induced vomiting or abuse laxatives and diuretics, hypokalemic alkalosis may develop (Table 5.7.1.4). These electrolyte disturbances are associated with physical symptoms of weakness, lethargy, and at times cardiac arrhythmias. The latter condition may result in sudden cardiac arrest, a cause of death in patients who purge. Mild elevation of serum liver enzymes may occur both in the emaciated anorectic phase and during refeeding. This reflects some fatty degeneration of the liver. Elevated serum cholesterol levels tend to occur more frequently in younger patients and return to normal with weight gain. Other common laboratory findings in emaciated AN patients are listed in Table 5.7.1.5. Laboratory findings present with bingeing and purging behavior are listed in Table 5.7.1.6.

Patients with BN should not be below 15% of the normal weight range. If they are, in most circumstances the correct diagnosis will be AN binge–purge (AN-BP) subtype.

TABLE 5.7.1.4

COMPLICATIONS OF BINGEING AND PURGING BEHAVIOR

1. Dental enamel erosion and caries
2. Perioral dermatitis
3. Periodontitis
4. Subconjunctival hemorrhage
5. Esophageal or gastric rupture
6. Metabolic alkalosis with hypokalemia
7. Cardiac arrhythmias
8. Cardiomyopathy and cardiac failure secondary to ipecac abuse
9. Renal failure
10. Seizures

TABLE 5.7.1.5

COMMON LABORATORY FINDINGS IN EMACIATED ANOREXIA NERVOSA

1. Hematologic
   - Anemia
   - Leukopenia with relative lymphocytosis
2. Serum and plasma
   - Hypercarotenemia
   - Hypoproteinemia
   - Hypercholesterolemia
3. Endocrine
   - Decreased estrogens
   - Decreased testosterone (in males)
   - Immature secretion pattern of luteinizing hormone
   - Decreased or blunted luteinizing hormone-releasing hormone
   - Decreased triiodothyronine
   - Increased corticotropin-releasing hormone
   - Increased fasting and impaired growth hormone secretion responses
   - Blunted diurnal cortisol levels
   - Uncoupled vasopressin secretion from osmotic challenge
   - Low basal metabolic rate
   - Reduced bone density

BN patients can be overweight. The sense of losing control of eating is a significant subjective aspect that occurs during binge eating. Abdominal pain or discomfort, self-induced vomiting, sleep, or social interruption usually terminate the bulimic episode, which is followed by feelings of guilt, depression, or self-disgust. Bulimic patients have a fear of not being able to stop eating voluntarily. Thus, ironically they may fast for long periods of time, lose control because of severe hunger, and then binge eat. Thus, they completely forgo a normal eating pattern and establish a routine of alternate binges and fasts. The food consumed during a binge usually has a high dense caloric content and a texture that facilitates rapid eating. Frequent weight fluctuations occur in BN but without the severity of weight loss present in AN. Most bulimic patients have difficulty feeling satiety at the end of a normal meal. They usually prefer to eat alone and at their homes. About one-fourth to one-third of these patients will have had a previous history of AN.

Majority of BN patients have depressive signs and symptoms. They have problems with interpersonal relationships, self-concept, impulsive behaviors, and also show high levels of anxiety and compulsivity. Alcohol abuse and other drug dependency are not uncommon in this disorder. Bulimics will abuse amphetamines to reduce their appetite and lose weight. As is present in the binge–purge type anorectic patient, BN patients can have severe erosion of the enamel of their teeth, pathologic pulp exposures, loss of integrity of dental arches, diminished masticatory ability, and an obvious unaesthetic appearance of their teeth.

Parotid gland enlargement is associated with elevated serum amylase in bulimics who binge and vomit. Other complications of bingeing and purging behavior are listed in Table 5.7.1.5. Severe abdominal pain in the bulimic patients should alert the physician to a diagnosis of gastric dilatation and a need for nasal gastric suction, x-rays, or surgical consultation.

TABLE 5.7.1.6

COMMON LABORATORY FINDINGS WITH BINGEING AND PURGING BEHAVIOR

- Hypokalemia
- Hypochloremic alkalosis
- Elevated serum amylase
- Electrocardiogram—QT- and T-wave changes
- Photon absorptiometry—reduced bone density

Cardiac failure may be caused by a cardiomyopathy from ipecac abuse. This is a medical emergency that usually results in death. Symptoms of pericardial pain, dyspnea, and generalized muscle weakness associated with hypotension, tachycardia, and electrocardiogram abnormalities should alert one to possible ipecac intoxication (39).

BED patients are similar to those with BN in that they engage in binge eating and feel a loss of control over eating. Also in common with many BN patients, those with BED feel disgusted, depressed, or guilty after a binge. However, the difference is those with BED do not engage in behaviors such as vomiting, laxative abuse, or exercise to lose the calories gained in a binge. Shame and embarrassment about their eating behavior makes it difficult for BED persons to seek treatment and be forthcoming about their problem. The majority have functional impairments in work, school, social, or family domains. Comorbid psychiatric disorders such as mood, anxiety, impulse control, or substance use are common (40).

ETIOLOGY AND PATHOGENESIS

The development of AN and BN is best conceptualized within the framework of a multidimensional model, which states that these disorders begin with dieting behavior. Antecedent conditions such as social and cultural influences, family environment, psychological or personality characteristics, and biologic vulnerabilities impact on the dieting behavior to produce the full-blown disorders of AN and BN. As fasting behavior, weight loss, and binge/purge behavior continue, significant psychological and physiologic changes occur. Some of these changes are strong secondary reinforcers that allow the process of fasting, weight loss, and binge/purge behavior to continue.

Secondary psychological reinforcement occurs when the young women initially receive compliments for their weight loss and later realize this is one area of their life in which they can be extremely effective and in control. Binge eating patients soon achieve a relief of anxiety during their binge eating even though that is followed by unpleasant feelings of guilt and depression. The physiologic reinforcements are less precisely defined. For example, with the period of only 8 hours of fasting, there is an increased secretion of corticotrophin-releasing hormone (CRH), which is a potent anorectic agent. This may be effective in assisting some anorectics to continue their decreased calorie intake. Exercising causes a release of norepinephrine and endogenous opioids, which may also reinforce a feeling of exhilaration. Dopamine is released during vomiting and this may reinforce purging behavior. Some chronic BN patients have described receiving a high after self-induced vomiting.

SOCIAL AND CULTURAL INFLUENCES

Data obtained in the 21st compared to the 20th century show epidemiologic and demographic changes have occurred in eating disorders most likely due to social and cultural influences. Whereas in Western Europe and North America in the past decade the incidence of AN has been relatively stable with BN decreasing in Caucasian women (14,15,29), eating disorders are increasing in minority groups as well as increasing in Asian and Arab countries along with industrialization, urbanization, and globalization (41). There is evidence that eating disorders and disturbed eating behaviors are increasing in

China, Singapore, South Korea, Egypt, Pakistan, United Arab Emirates, Oman, Lebanon, Kuwait, Iran, and Jordan (41).

Conceptualization of the emergence of eating disorders has consistently included social and cultural influences. The latter has been investigated within ethnic groups in the United States as well as globally. Most of the recent studies in the United States were conducted on college students with questionnaire surveys rather than structured interviews.

Data from the NIMH Collaborative Psychiatric Epidemiological Studies (CPES) found no significant differences in prevalence for AN and BED in the United States across Latinos, Asians, African Americans, and non-Latino Whites (42,43). BN was more prevalent among Latinos and African Americans than non-Latino Whites (43). Utilization of mental health services was lower in all ethnic minority groups compared to non-Latino Whites (43). Other differences were present among ethnic groups. For African American women, perceived levels of peer attitudes toward weight and shape were positively associated with levels of body dissatisfaction. For white women, body dissatisfaction remained constant across low and high perceived levels of peer attitudes on weight and shape (44). For those presenting for BED treatment, blacks had a higher BMI and binge eating frequency than whites and lower depression than white and Hispanic groups (45). A survey of female college students found black women compared to white, Asian, and Hispanic women had greater self-esteem, were less likely to compare their body to those in the media, and felt less pressure to attain the media set physical appearance (46).

Another study has emphasized a small proportion of Latinos reporting distress with eating disorders seek treatment. Factors contributing to this are lack of health insurance, lack of affordable and accessible treatment services, and beliefs about seeking treatment (47). A study of Mexican American women suggests those who are less acculturated are more satisfied with their bodies (48). A survey of American college students found Arab Americans reported the highest prevalence, 10%, of binge eating (49). Despite some of the ethnic differences in eating disorders found in the United States, it is of interest to note that a prevention program was similarly effective for Asian, African, European, and Hispanic American female college students (50).

The development of eating disorders has also been found to be associated with various social factors. It is possible that the social and economic disadvantages present in non-Caucasian girls may sensitize them toward the culturally dominant body ideals and thus instill a risk factor for developing eating disorders. For example, a study of AN in Curacao found cases in only mixed ethnicity women who reported that thinness allowed them greater acceptance in the more affluent white community (51).

Feminist theories emphasize that women are indoctrinated into a belief system that overvalues feminine beauty, and in particular thinness. Women cannot achieve satisfactory self-esteem without attaining ideals that are impossible to fulfill. Eating disorders then become the adaptive response to the stress of demands that women conform to an impossible and oppressive social expectation. Some support for this hypothesis comes from a study done in Japan, which suggested eating pathology there may be linked to a conflict between traditional and modernizing roles for women (52).

Peer groups that tout slimness contribute to the risk for the development of eating disorders. In a study of 9- to 11-year-old girls, Wardell and Watters (53) found that greater exposure to older peers in school was associated with increased weight concern, dieting, and thinner size ideals. In another study, sorority women were found to maintain a more rigorous dietary control than nonsorority women (54). Peer groups transmit and reinforce social values that perpetuate risk for body dissatisfaction and eating disorders (55). Higher rates of eating disorders are reported in sport activities in which leanness is valued, such as dance, gymnastics, and among jockeys (56). A study in England showed that girls from a higher social economic status environment reported greater exposure to weight loss and dieting by family and friends and the higher SES girls indicated a greater awareness of ideals of thinness (57).

Several studies have found an adverse effect of the media on body image, eating attitudes, and behaviors. In one study, magazine exposure to thin body images found the resulting body dissatisfaction was mediated by internalization of thin ideals (58). In another study of college women, Low et al. (59) found internalization of the thin ideal was associated with increased eating and weight concerns. An increased desire to emulate unrealistic body standards was found in grade school girls and boys who were exposed to pictures of "ideal men and women" (60). Adolescent girls exposed to commercials depicting thin, attractive models reported feeling more dissatisfied with their bodies and expressed a greater drive for thinness 2 years later in a study by Hargreaves and Tiggeman (61).

STRESSFUL LIFE EVENTS

Childhood trauma which consists of either emotional abuse, physical abuse, sexual abuse, emotional neglect, physical neglect, or any combination of the above has been the most frequently investigated stressful life event related to eating disorders. Most studies of childhood trauma have been conducted with retrospective questionnaires. A meta-analysis of sexual abuse studies found an increased risk of a lifetime diagnosis of multiple psychiatric disorders including eating disorders (62). One study found childhood physical abuse and childhood sexual abuse contributed independently to increased risk of eating disorders among women (63). However, sexual abuse rarely occurs in isolation since physical and emotional abuse are often present. Another study found that emotional abuse was the only abuse type that consistently related to eating disorder symptoms (64). In this study, emotional dysregulation mediated the effect of emotional abuse on eating disorder symptoms. In girls, negative/depressive affect mediated the relationship between childhood maltreatment and eating disorder psychopathology in a study of adolescent psychiatric inpatients (65).

Additional personality characteristics or traits were found to interact with child sexual abuse and eating disorders. Avoidant personality disorder and child sexual abuse interacted in predicting poor outcome in chronic eating disorder patients (66). Another study found those with eating disorders and childhood abuse had elevations of a dysregulated or impulsive psychopathology (67). Emotional dysregulation explained the relationship between childhood emotional abuse and AN symptom severity in patients from an intensive treatment facility (68).

Binge eating behavior has been especially associated with childhood abuse. Higher rates of the latter were found in AN with binge–purge behavior than AN restricting type (69). Women with BED reported rates of childhood maltreatment much higher than those in community samples (70). Childhood onset in comparison to adult onset of binge eating was associated with higher rates of lifetime BN, greater severity of BN symptoms, and higher rates of abuse (71).

There is some evidence that childhood abuse in genetically susceptible persons may lower modulation of stress reactions and thus increase the likelihood of developing an eating disorder. For example, an association was found between BN and the low function variant of the Bcll polymorphism (low glucocorticoid receptor sensitivity) and prior abuse (72). Another study found genes within the dopamine system (DRD2 and

COMT) were interacting with childhood abuse and bulimic behaviors (73). The effect of adverse life events on binge eating was moderated by the 5-HTTLPR serotonin transporter promotor polymorphism (74).

For clinicians it is important to inquire into the full range of childhood traumatic experience including physical abuse, emotional abuse and neglect as well as sexual abuse.

In the premorbid vulnerable individual, normative developmental events such as the onset of puberty, leaving home, beginning school, and the start of new relationships have been precipitating events for the onset of an eating disorder (75). Adverse life events such as the death of a close relative, the breakup of a relationship, or an illness have also been related as precipitant of eating disorder problems.

BIOLOGIC FACTORS

Genetic Factors

A genetic vulnerability may be direct, through the inheritance of genes that are directly associated with the development of AN or BN. An indirect genetic predisposition on the other hand could become manifest with genetic vulnerability under adverse conditions such as inappropriate dieting or emotional stress. These predispositions could be a particular personality type, a tendency to susceptibility to psychiatric instability (especially affective or anxiety disorders), or a neurocircuitry dysfunction.

Behavioral genetics including family, twin, and adoption studies have provided evidence for a genetic influence on a liability to eating disorders (76,77). Family studies found an increased risk of both AN and BN in relatives of AN and BN probands and more BED in first-degree relatives of those with BED. Twin studies comparing identical with fraternal twins have reported heritability estimates ranging from 33% to 84% for AN, 28% to 83% for BN, and 41% to 57% for BED with the remaining variance attributable to unique environmental factors (78,79). Twin studies have also identified possible endophenotypes (measurable markers observable in the affected proband in both well and ill states). For example, puberty and age seem to moderate genetic influence on eating disorder traits (80,81). Adoption studies comparing biologic and adopted female sibling pairs found heritability estimates for disordered eating symptoms ranged from 59% to 82% (82).

Molecular genetic studies have rapidly increased in the past decade. Those involving eating disorders have used either a linkage, case association method, or genome-wide association analysis. In linkage analyses, variation in the paternal and the maternal contribution to the genome of the offspring is used to localize genes that influence a trait. In the association study, cases that display a trait of interest are compared to controls who do not have the trait. Candidate genes are genotyped and the allele and genotype frequencies are compared in cases versus controls. An association study can also be done in an affected individual and both biologic parents. This is called a transmission disequilibrium test (TDT). In the TDT approach, the transmission versus nontransmission of marker alleles to affected offspring is compared.

Linkage analyses identify genomic regions that may harbor risk or protective loci by identifying genetic markers that are coinherited with the eating disorder phenotype. A multisite found significant peak linkage for AN on chromosome 1 and for BN on chromosome 10 (83,84). Genotyping single nucleotide polymorphisms (SNPs) in the peak linkage area on chromosome 1 revealed possible candidate gene variants at the delta opioid receptor (OPRD1) and the serotonin 1 D receptor (HTR1D) (85). These associations were confirmed by an independent study (86).

Genetic case association compares variants that are hypothesized to be involved in the pathophysiology of eating disorders in those with eating disorders and controls. In the past decade many of these analyses conducted resulted in contradictory or nonreplicable findings. These investigations focused on SNPs in genes involved in the regulation of neurotransmitters, serotonin, dopamine, and norepinephrine or neuronal function and growth brain-derived neurotropic factor (BDNF) or the regulation of hormones, leptin, ghrelin, and adrenocorticotropin. The BDNF polymorphism, Met 66 variant was associated with the restricting type of AN and confirmed with both a case control design and a TDT approach (87).

Genome-wide association studies (GWAS) compares over 500,000 loci (SNPs) in each case and control. Extremely conservative significance thresholds are necessary for these multiple comparisons usually requiring sample sizes of more than 5,000 cases to detect significance. One GWAS with 1,033 cases of AN and 3,773 controls was negative for SNPs meeting genome-wide significance (88).

Epigenetics, the study of mechanisms that regulate gene expression independently of DNA sequence, most frequently examine DNA methylation. Methylation changes are usually examined in the blood and if present may not be in other tissues such as the brain. A methylation study of AN women found global DNA hypomethylation and hypermethylation of the DRD2 promotor (89). BN women had hypermethylation of the atrial natriuretic peptide (ANP) gene promotor region and down regulation of ANP in RNA (90). DRD2 is associated with dopamine regulation and ANP inhibits CRH which may have an anxiolytic effect (91).

Genetic studies at this date have had limited success in identifying gene variants associated with eating disorders. However, epigenetic mechanisms have produced gene x environment interactions which future research may discover highly relevant to the development of eating disorders.

Neuroendocrine and Neurocircuitry Factors

Ingestive behavior which is disturbed in eating disorders is controlled and influenced by many biologic factors. In the past two decades biologic investigations have focused on neurotransmitters and peptide hormones.

Under stress, such as severe dieting, vulnerability for destabilization of some of the endocrine and metabolic mechanisms affecting eating behavior may influence the development of a full-blown eating disorder. Most of the neuroendocrine changes in the eating disorders are directly related to dieting behaviors, weight loss, and reduced caloric intake. These changes revert to normal with resumption of normal eating behavior and nutritional rehabilitation. For example, increased CRH secretion occurs in underweight anorectic patients and in normal weight dieting individuals but returns to normal with weight restoration. However, CRH is a potent anorectic hormone and may have a role in maintaining anorectic behaviors and initiating a relapse.

It is well established that pituitary cells producing luteinizing hormone are understimulated in patients with AN because of hyposecretion of GnRH by the hypothalamus. A dysfunction may be present in the neurotransmitter systems that influence GnRH release and secretion. The considerable difference in patterns of severe dieting and fasting in BN patients probably explains the variability in the function of the hypothalamic–pituitary–ovarian axis as measured in various studies of BN patients. Some anorectic women remain amenorrheic for long periods of time (several years) after weight restoration. Studies have shown these women to be more psychologically disturbed compared to those who have a rapid resumption of menses (92).

Serum levels of leptin, a product of an obesity gene, were shown to correlate significantly with BMI and the amount of adipose tissue in AN patients. Thus, emaciated anorectics have extremely low levels of leptin, which increase as the patients gain weight (93). Baseline serum leptin levels in BN patients compared with controls have shown variable results (94). A compounding factor is that leptin levels decreased during short periods of caloric deficit. It is unlikely that leptin is a causal agent for producing eating disorders. Adiponectin is another adipokine protein that is released from adipose tissue and has an effect of enhancing insulin sensitivity. An inverse correlation between adiponectin and BMI is consistent with the increased adiponectin levels found in AN and variable findings in BN (95).

Ghrelin is a peptide released from endocrine cells in the stomach which acts in the hypothalamus to increase meal size (96). Fasting baseline plasma ghrelin levels were not different in BN patients compared with controls (97). However, the ghrelin response to standardize meals was significantly attenuated in patients with BN compared to controls (98). This suggests an impairment of postingestive satiety in BN with abnormal ghrelin regulation possibly contributing to the binge eating episodes. In AN patients' plasma ghrelin levels are elevated in comparison to healthy controls, and these levels decrease toward normal values as patients regain their weight (99). The relationship of these peptide levels to various clinical symptom patterns needs to be clarified.

More recently, neuroimaging paradigms have provided much information on serotonin and dopamine circuitry in the processing of food, reward, fear, and cognitive stimuli. In studying eating disorders it is important to document state-related factors such as electrolyte and metabolic conditions. The neurotransmitters, serotonin and dopamine, have been conceptualized within anxiety and reward circuitries. Serotonin which is associated with anxiety is also inhibitory to feeding, exploratory and sexual behaviors, all of which are inhibited in AN. Positron emission tomography (PET) studies showed 5HT2A binding was reduced in recovered restricting AN (AN-R) in the insula, cingulate, mesial, temporal, and occipital cortex. In AN-BP recovered women 5HT2A binding was reduced in the cingulate, parietal, and occipital cortex. In both AN subtypes 5HT2A binding was positively related to harm avoidance, an anxious trait (100). These findings may influence connections between the affected cortical areas and the amygdala and thus produce impairment in cognitive and emotional pathways.

In recovered BN reduced orbital-frontal 5HT2A receptor binding could be related to impulsiveness and emotional dysregulation (100). 5HT1A from two PET studies showed increased activity across frontal, temporal, and parietal cortex areas as well as in the dorsal raphe in recovered AN (101,102). This activity was also positively correlated with harm avoidance. BN persons showed increased 5HT1A receptor binding in the prefrontal, cingulate, and parietal cortical areas, also implicating anxiety features (100). No differences were found in serotonin transporter (5HT-T) availability between AN individuals and controls (100). However a single-photon emission computerized tomography (SPECT) study showed reduced 5HT-T binding in the thalamus and hypothalamus in ill BN persons and varying binding results in different brain areas after recovery (103). 5 HT-T regulates serotonin levels in the synapses. Low serotonin synaptic levels may explain higher dosages of serotonin reuptake inhibitors needed to reduce binge eating.

Food image studies with functional magnetic resonance imaging (fMRI) provoked anxiety and increased activation in the anterior cingulate and medial prefrontal cortex in both ill and recovered AN persons compared to controls, suggesting a possible trait marker for AN (104,105). Similar responses were present in BN persons (105).

Changes in brain dopamine and reward functioning have been demonstrated in AN. PET studies in recovered AN women revealed increased D2/3 receptor availability in the ventral striatum (106). AN women had a greater response in the striatum during fMRI to images of thin bodies compared to controls (107). Recovered AN women had a reduced functional brain response with fMRI to repeated applications of taste in the insula and ventral and dorsal striata (108). Those with AN did not distinguish between win and loss in the ventral striatum in response to monetary reward stimuli (109). These findings may indicate altered brain dopamine reward circuitry in AN. There are few studies of dopamine reward circuitry in BN. One fMRI study found reduced response in the ventral putamen, insula, and prefrontal cortex in BN persons to a dopamine-related reward paradigm (110).

More recently, the technique of diffusion tensor imaging was used to demonstrate larger anteroventral gray and white matter volume in adolescents with AN compared to controls. Also present was lower white matter integrity in posterior frontal and parietal regions. The authors implied this finding may indicate developmental factors such as gray matter pruning and white matter growth could contribute to brain alterations in AN (111). Another study using diffusion imaging processing in adult recovered AN women found white matter integrity was reduced across large frontal regions and in the cerebellum. The authors suggested this abnormality could result in less efficient information processing and interfere with the neurocircuitry of food–reward processing. These findings may reflect a premorbid trait or a remodeling after an underweight state (112). It is not clear how these findings suggesting impairments in brain neurocircuitry involving anxiety and reward-related brain pathways, especially in the insular and cingulate cortex and basal ganglia, may specifically effect eating behavior.

PSYCHOLOGICAL FACTORS

Psychological factors may be conceptualized as predating the onset of eating disorders, occurring in the acute phase of illness and persisting after recovery. Perfectionism is a psychological feature initially identified with AN. A multisite genetic study found higher perfectionism scores on the Frost Multidimensional Perfection Scale in AN persons compared to healthy persons. In those with AN greater perfectionism was associated with lower body weight, greater eating preoccupations and rituals, and diminished motivation to change (113). Also perfectionism was most severe in those with obsessional compulsive personality disorder (OCPD) or the combination of OCPD and obsessive-compulsive disorder (OCD) (114). Trait anxiety, which is a common feature of AN, predicted a lower likelihood of recovery in a multisite study of 680 AN women (115).

A meta-analysis of the Temperament and Character Inventory (TCI) in 14 studies found persistence and harm avoidance was significantly higher in AN persons compared to BN, BED persons, and controls. Recovered AN persons had significantly lower harm avoidance and higher reward dependence compared to those acutely ill with AN. Novelty seeking was significantly elevated only in those with BN (116). Other studies found BN, compared to controls, to have greater impulsivity and low self-directedness (117). These psychological features may represent enduring temperament traits that contribute to eating disorder pathogenesis.

In a community sample personality features associated with BED included high novelty seeking, higher harm avoidance and low self-directedness (118). The authors suggested two types of BED; an impulsive novelty seeking type and another with harm avoidance and mood dysregulation.

Current research suggests high harm avoidance, low self-directedness, perfectionism, and anxiety traits are risk factors for developing and maintaining an eating disorder.

Negative affect which includes depression, anxiety, anger, fear, hostility, and guilt was positively associated with binge-ing, laxative use, vomiting, and exercising in both AN and BN (119). Negative affect in women with BN had a positive correlation on fMRI with activity in the putamen, caudate, and pallidum measured during anticipated intake of a palatable food (120). The authors suggested negative affect may increase the reward value of food in BN or be a conditioned cue due to binge eating in a negative mood.

Set shifting, which involves various cognitive functions, was impaired in 22.9% AN-R, 45.5% AN-BP, 36.7% BN, 16.7% recovered AN, and 9% controls (121). Those with impaired versus those with intact set shifting were twice as likely to have a longer duration of illness, a higher Yale-Brown-Cornell Eating Disorder Scale (YBC-EDS) rituals score, and a diagnosis of social phobia. Two studies have demonstrated the set-shifting deficits do not exist in AN adolescents in contrast to AN adults (122,123). This may be due to not fully developed brain circuits in adolescents.

All eating disorders were found to be sensitive to punishment compared to controls. However, AN-R were least sensitive to reward and had higher levels of behavioral inhibition whereas bulimic types were more sensitive to reward and had higher levels of behavioral activation (124,125). Impaired behavioral response shifting in AN measured by fMRI revealed hypoactivation in the ventral anterior cingulate–striatal–thalamic loop (126). Dopamine and norepinephrine modulate the functioning of the striatal–cortical loops. Since dopamine is active in the ventral–striatal–cortical loop for set shifting and norepinephrine is active in response inhibition and sustained attention, it is reasonable to suggest these monoamines may be involved in initiating and maintaining core eating disorder symptomatology.

Psychiatric disorders comorbid with eating disorders are predominantly in four categories: affective, anxiety, substance use, and personality disorders. According to the National Comorbidity Survey Replication any mood disorder was present in 42.1% of AN, 70% of BN, and 46.4% of BED persons. Any anxiety disorder was present in 47.9% AN, 80.6% BN and 65.1% of BED persons. Any substance use disorder was present in 27% of AN, 36.8% of BN, and 23.3% of BED persons (19). The above figures represent a general pattern and will vary according to the sample studied. In the same survey Impulse Control Disorder was found in 30.8% AN which included both types of AN. Fernandez-Aranda et al. (127) found only 1.7% of restricting AN had this disorder. Impulse control disorder is highly associated with binge eating and is present in 63.3% of BN and 43.3% BED persons (19). Likewise, oppositional and conduct disorders are more prevalent in disorders with binge eating (19). Cluster B, the impulsive personality disorders are almost exclusively associated with binge eating (128).

Comorbid psychological features and psychiatric diagnoses are common in eating disorders and must be incorporated in comprehensive treatment strategies.

FAMILY FACTORS

Family factors influencing the development and maintenance of eating disorders can be parental psychiatric diagnoses, parental practices, and family interaction characteristics. Information of these factors may be obtained by interviews, self-questionnaires, or observed behavior.

Analyses from the Stockholm Youth Cohort revealed a diagnosis in one or both parents of bipolar affective disorder, anxiety and depression disorders, or a personality disorder was a risk factor for eating disorders in their offspring (129). One study found girls of AN women were more likely to have emotional, conduct, and hyperactive disorders and boys to have emotional disorders compared to offspring of healthy women. In the same study girls of BN women were more likely to show hyperactivity and boys to show emotional and conduct disorders compared to controls (130).

Adolescent self-report on the Family Assessment Device (FAD) found parental psychological control moderated the protective relationship between family functioning and disordered eating behaviors in adolescent girls. Parent psychological control was associated with greater odds of engaging in dieting and disordered eating behaviors while parents knowledge of the child's whereabouts was associated with lower odds of dieting and having disordered eating behavior (131). A study of adolescents in the United Kingdom found for both girls and boys lower perceived parental responsibility for food was significantly related to greater eating psychopathology. For girls pressure to eat and for boys parental restriction of food led to unhealthy eating-related attitudes (132).

A multicenter European project found perceived abusive parenting was related to the development of AN-BP and BN but not AN-R (133). Other studies found perceived family influences such as negative attitudes about weight and shape, promoting dieting, and parental weight loss practices to be associated with disordered eating behavior (134,135). Mothers eating and exercising attitudes predicted their activity-related parenting practices with daughters (more controlling) and sons (136).

A study using the FAD self-report measure found half of AN families experience some impairment of family function. Adolescent's perspective on family function reflected greater family dysfunction compared to parental ratings. Adolescent but not parent ratings of global family function were associated with more severe eating disorder symptoms, greater depression, lower self-efficacy and self-esteem, and more functional impairment. The authors suggested that the adolescent's view of family functioning was more clinically relevant (137).

A direct effect of marital conflict occurring during a child's kindergarten year was found on adolescent disordered eating and was mediated through the child's emotional insecurity about the marital relationship (138). Another study found adolescent reports of the level of family cohesion were more accurate than parent reports in predicting changes in adolescent mental health (139). In a study of BN adolescents, low patient/low parent expressed emotion showed greater reduction in purging overtreatment with high patient/low parent expressed emotion showing smallest reduction in purging (140).

Patients with BED perceived their mothers as high expressed emotion and reported significantly higher levels of perceived maternal criticism, emotional overinvolvement, and lower levels of perceived warmth than did controls (141). Parental perception of family functioning is affected by both the presence of binge eating/purging behavior and nonsuicidal self-injuring behaviors with worse family functioning occurring in the latter group (142).

DIFFERENTIAL DIAGNOSIS

In making a diagnosis of AN it is important to be certain the patient has no medical illness that can account for weight loss. Occasionally, a patient may have both AN and a medical illness contributing to weight loss. In this situation the diagnosis of AN is made by the positive criteria for the disorder, and both the underlying medical condition and the AN are diagnosed and treated as such. Weight loss frequently occurs in depressive disorders. However, in the latter the patient usually has a decreased appetite, whereas an anorectic patient denies the existence of an appetite. The hyperactivity seen in AN differs from the agitated activity seen in depressive disorders in that the anorectic's activity is planned and ritualistic, such as exercising programs of jogging and cycling. The preoccupation with the calorie content of food, collecting recipes, and preparing meals for others is typical of the anorectic patient but not present in those with a depressive disorder. The latter do not have a fear of becoming fat or a disturbance in their body image, as is characteristic in AN.

Delusions about food in schizophrenia are rarely concerned with the calorie content of food. A fear of becoming obese and hyperactivity is also uncommon in the schizophrenic but is typical of the anorectic patient.

Chronic medical illnesses frequently associated with weight loss are Crohn disease, hyperthyroidism, Addison disease, and diabetes mellitus. Overeating episodes may occur in the Kluver–Bucy syndrome, which consists of visual agnosia, compulsive licking and biting, inability to ignore any stimulus, and hypersexuality. Another uncommon syndrome associated with hyperphasia is the Kleine–Levin syndrome, which is characterized by periodic hypersomnia lasting for several weeks.

TREATMENT

Anorexia Nervosa

The British National Institute for Clinical Excellence (NICE) developed a grading scheme for which all treatment was classified according to an accepted hierarchy of evidence (143). A summary of the NICE guidelines for AN is as follows: (1) Patients should be managed on an outpatient basis whenever possible with psychological treatment given by an experienced and competent service that also assesses physical risks. (2) Inpatient treatment should be in an experienced setting that can implement refeeding with careful physical monitoring and give psychosocial intervention. (3) Family intervention that directly addresses the eating disorder should be offered to children and adolescents.

The above recommendations for treating AN continue to be valid. However, in the past decade more specific evidence-based data have emerged. Meeting the criteria for the highest level of "well established" is family therapy with a behavioral focus often referred to as family-based treatment. This approach which has a manualized published version (144) promotes parental management of weight restoration through education and support by focusing on eating disorder symptoms in the early phase of treatment and emphasizing general family interactions after weight gain is well underway.

Probably, efficacious criteria are applied to family systems therapy and insight-oriented individual psychotherapy referred to as adolescent-focused therapy or ego-oriented individual therapy. Family systems therapy focuses on general systematic and interactive concerns in the family. The therapist adopts a neutral stance, explores family patterns of beliefs and behaviors and seeks ways to enable the family to generate solutions (145). The adolescent-focused therapy, also manualized (146), is based in self-psychology and cognitive individual therapy that targets self-esteem, self-efficacy, and autonomy. Randomized controlled trials (RCTs) have shown family-based (behavioral) therapy to be superior to adolescent-focused therapy (147) and family systems therapy (145). Family behavioral therapy resulted in a faster weight gain, greater recovery rates, and fewer days of hospitalizations during treatment.

Additional analyses of the above studies revealed information moderating treatment. Patients with higher levels of obsessive-compulsive features and those from single parent families had greater improvement with a high dose of therapy. Intact families and those with AN-R adolescents had higher rates of remission regardless of treatment. Adolescents with greater obsessive-compulsive features gained more weight with systems family therapy compared to behavioral family therapy. Other studies have shown that the use of hospitalization solely for the purpose of weight gain may not be useful for most AN adolescents (148).

Exploratory studies are examining the utility of multifamily therapy in both adults and adolescents with eating disorders (149,150).

Family therapy for AN has been predominantly applied to children and adolescents. Other forms of AN individual therapy receiving an experimental level designate and studied mainly in adults are beginning to be tested in adolescents. Cognitive therapy which addresses cognitive inflexibility is considered an adjunctive treatment (151) with the purpose of enhancing quality of life in social, work and health domains (152). Dialectical behavioral therapy (DBT) is another experimental treatment that targets emotion regulation and is most often used in patients with bingeing and purging behaviors (153).

Weight restoration and nutritional rehabilitation are extremely important since the state of being underweight is associated with depression, difficulty concentrating, irritability, and preoccupation with food. Also, cognitive impairment is present during this state of calorie restriction. In order to accomplish necessary changes with psychotherapy the patient must be in a condition where she can actually concentrate on the issues of psychotherapy. Monitoring is an important part of CBT. In an outpatient setting the patient is taught to record not only her food intake but stressful circumstances during the day and her emotional responses to them. Cognitive restructuring is a method in which patients are taught to identify their disturbing cognitions and challenge their core beliefs. In this process they become aware of specific negative thoughts and present arguments and evidence both to support their validity and to cast doubt on their validity. From this they try to form a reasoned conclusion based on the evidence. Problem solving is another method whereby patients learn to reason through difficult food-related and/or interpersonal situations. Adolescents from age 12 onward are fully capable of participating in this type of therapy.

A family analysis should be done on all anorectic patients who are living with their families. From this analysis a clinical judgement should be made as to what type of family therapy or counseling is clinically advisable. There will be some cases in which family therapy is not possible, and in those instances family relationships can be addressed in individual therapy. In other situations brief counseling sessions with the immediate family members may be the best manner of dealing with family issues. A controlled family therapy study (154) has shown that anorectic patients under the age of 18 benefited from this whereas patients over age 18 did worse in family therapy compared with the control therapy. In another randomized controlled treatment trial 40 adolescent patients with AN were randomly assigned to conjoint family therapy or to separated family therapy with one therapist conducting both forms of treatment. On a global measure of outcome, the two forms of therapy had equivalent end of treatment results. For those patients with high levels of maternal criticism toward the patient the separated family therapy was shown to be superior to the conjoint family therapy (155). In actual practice, many clinicians provide individual therapy and some sort of family counseling in managing AN.

Medication should only be considered as adjunct therapy for AN patients with severe or resistant symptoms. RCTs have been severely compromised with small samples and lack of actual serum drug levels making meta-analyses meaningless. AN individuals are extremely reluctant to take medication even after agreeing to participate in a drug trial. RCTs of typical antipsychotics in AN did not reveal significant results (156). Treatment studies of atypical antipsychotics in AN have produced vaying results. The one study measuring actual serum levels of olanzapine showed an effect for weight gain over placebo (157). Other RCTs have shown a modest effect on improved AN psychopathology (156). Atypical antipsychotics such as risperidone, quetiapine, amisulpride, and aripiprazole have had little effect on improving core AN symptoms (157).

Antidepressants have not been effective for improving core AN psychopathology and may not effect depression symptoms until AN patients are medically stable with adequate weight gain (158).

Although there is conflicting evidence for zinc promoting weight gain, both the WFSBP and APA recommend zinc supplementation may be useful since it is an essential micronutrient (156).

Using estrogen compounds for treating decreased bone density in adolescents remains controversial. NICE guidelines do not recommend it since estrogen replacement may lead to premature fusion of the epiphyses. One study using physiologic estrogen replacement (159) and another using a combination of dehydroepiandrosterone (DHEA) with estradiol and levonorgestrel (160) found increasing bone density and cortical thickness with these compounds in adolescents and young adults. Early detection of illness and weight restoration with nutritional rehabilitation remain the primary treatment of osteopenia in AN.

There have been several double-blind studies to show that cyproheptadine—especially in high doses, up to 24 mg/day—is effective in facilitating weight gain and reducing depressive symptomatology. This drug has the advantage of very few side effects, which make it attractive for use in emaciated anorectic patients (161).

In the exploratory status of AN treatment are intranasal oxytocin, D-cycloserine facilitation of exposure therapy, repetitive transcranial magnetic stimulation, internet-based interventions (computer or mobile), and for adults with severe intractable AN, deep brain stimulation and stereotactic surgery to inactivate the nucleus accumbens.

Medical management, a necessary part of the treatment of AN patients, is based on the experience of clinicians and not RCTs. Nutritional rehabilitation programs should establish healthy target weights with a weight gain of 2 to 3 lb per week for inpatient and 1 lb per week for outpatient treatment programs. Patients must be monitored for discarding food, vomiting, or exercising frequently. Medical monitoring during refeeding includes assessment of vital signs, food, and fluid intake and output, assessment of electrolytes (including phosphorous), observation for edema, rapid weight gain with fluid overload, congestive heart failure, constipation, and bloating. Physical activity should be adapted to the food intake and energy expenditure of the patient. Liquid food supplements may be very helpful in the initial stages of treatment. Forceful intervention should be considered only when patients are unwilling to cooperate with oral feedings and their physical safety is in danger. Nasal gastric feedings may be required in life-threatening circumstances. During hospitalization the use of liquid formula in the early stages of weight gain with gradual exposure to food and gradual increase in activity can be very effective for inducing weight gain (162). Specialized eating disorder units yield better outcome than general psychiatric units because of the specific nursing expertise and more effective protocols (163). A study by Watson et al. (163) showed that short-term outcomes for involuntarily hospitalized patients are similar to those voluntarily admitted.

Early detection and treatment of adolescents before adulthood is the best prevention of chronic AN. Family therapy is the first recommended treatment with attention to multifaceted needs such as weight restoration, nutritional rehabilitation, and medical stabilization.

Bulimia Nervosa

CBT is the first-line treatment for (BN). It has been found to be the most effective treatment in over 35 controlled studies. In these studies the treatment program was usually 16 to 20 weeks, after which 40% to 50% of the patients were abstinent from both bingeing and purging. A reduction of bingeing and purging occurred in 70% to 95% of patients. Another 30% of those who did not show improvement immediately after treatment did show improvement to full recovery 1 year after treatment. In BN, CBT interrupts the self-maintaining cycle of bingeing and purging and alters the individual's dysfunctional cognitions and beliefs about food, weight, body image, and overall self-concept. It should be noted that in order for therapists to be effective in using CBT for the treatment of BN, they need to be trained in these specific manuals available for this purpose. Wilson and Fairburn (164) have written an excellent review of these studies.

In the past decade cognitive behavior therapy (CBT) has been modified in recognition that more than half of BN patients receiving CBT do not recover. Enhancements to address perfectionism, mood, interpersonal problems, and low self-esteem were added to the tested CBT and this is referred to as CBT enhanced (CBT-E) (165). Few RCTs exist for treatment of BN in adolescents. CBT adapted for children (CBT-A) and family-based therapy for BN (FBT-BN) were found to be effective for treating adolescent BN (166,167). These therapies have a designated level of possibly efficacious. A more recent RCT found FBT-BN was more efficacious in promoting abstinence from binge eating and purging than CBT-A in adolescent BN at end of treatment and 6 months but no difference was present at the 12-month follow-up (168).

Multifamily therapy for adolescent BN is in the developmental stage (169).

Interpersonal therapy (ITP) which targets specific interpersonal problems associated with eating disorder symptoms is an effective treatment for adults with BN but produces results slower than CBT (170) and has not been studies in BN adolescents. Other treatment strategies being tested for BN include the use of the internet to support self-help and phone messages for behavioral monitoring.

Although group therapy has not been adequately studied in a controlled manner, in practice many clinicians are conducting group CBT for patients with BN. This seems to be especially effective and popular with college students and young adults. Furthermore, it is a cost-effective treatment modality for both patients and therapists.

Over a dozen double-blind, placebo-controlled trials of antidepressants, including desipramine, imipramine, amitriptyline, nortriptyline, phenelzine, and fluoxetine, have been conducted in normal-weight outpatients with BN. The dosage of antidepressant medication used was similar to that used for the treatment of depression. In all trials, antidepressants were significantly more effective than placebo in reducing binge eating. These medications also improved mood and reduced eating disorder symptoms such as preoccupation with shape and weight. However, the abstinence rate from bingeing and purging on the average was only 22%. An excellent review of these studies is available in Mitchell and DeZwaan (171). There is some indication that combining antidepressant medication with CBT is helpful in some individuals (172).

More recently topiramate, an antiepileptic drug associated with appetite suppression and weight loss, was investigated as a treatment for BN in a randomized control trial involving 69 patients treated for 10 weeks. The median dose was 100 mg daily (range 25 to 400 mg daily). Topiramate was more effective than placebo in its effects on binge eating and purging and on measures of psychosocial impairment (173,174).

An analysis from two large fluoxetine trials found BN patients who failed to report a greater than 60% decrease in the frequency of binge eating or vomiting by week 3 of treatment were unlikely to respond to this drug (175). This is a helpful indication to guide clinical management in BN.

Binge Eating Disorder

A large number of RCTs provide evidence that CBT is the most well-established psychological treatment of adults with BED (176,177). CBT produces substantial reduction in binge eating and related symptomatology that is maintained for a long time (178). ITP has also been demonstrated in RCTs to be effective in treating BED (153). Fewer RCTs suggest that DBT and group therapy are promising for treating BED (179).

For adolescents with BED only pilot preliminary RCTs exist. CBT compared with a delayed treatment control was efficacious in producing abstinence from binge eating over a 3-month follow-up in 12- to 18-year-old adolescents (180). An internet-based CBT program reduced binge eating and shape and weight concerns and facilitated weight loss in overweight adolescents over a 5-month follow-up (181). Another RCT of 12- to 17-year-old girls showed group ITP reduced binge eating at 3-month follow-up compared to a standard health education group (182).

Although 25 placebo-controlled drug trials and 13 trials comparing two or more active treatments with drugs have been conducted, there is no FDA approved drug for the treatment of BED. Of the selective serotonin reuptake inhibitors (SSRIs) studied, only citalopram (183), escitalopram (184), and sertraline (185) were associated with a greater reduction of binge frequency reduction and symptom severity. The tricyclic antidepressants, desipramine and imipramine, were greater than placebo for reducing binge eating, weight, and depression in those with BED (186).

The antiepileptics, topiramate and zonisamide, have been the most effective drugs for reducing binge eating frequency and weight (187,188). The selective norepinephrine reuptake inhibitor, atomoxetine, reduced binge frequency and weight more than placebo in one study (189). Several trials of lisdexamfetamine dimesylate, a drug used to treat ADHD, provided evidence that this drug was also effective for reducing binge frequency and weight (190). Orlistat, an anti-obesity drug, when combined with CBT was more effective than CBT for reducing binge eating (191). Acamprosate, a mixed GABA agonist/glutamate antagonist, had a greater reduction in binge days per week compared with placebo (192) but no difference in achieving abstinence.

At present evidence-based data indicate cognitive behavioral therapy should be the first-line treatment for BED. Most drug studies for BED have had limited follow-up periods and have not reported on remission of binge eating.

RESEARCH DIRECTIONS

Many questions need to be answered in order to create effective prevention and treatment programs for eating disorders. It is necessary to learn how an individual's genotype and environment interact to create, maintain, and recover from an eating disorder. Advancing techniques in genetics and neuroimaging are producing information on normal brain developmental changes in adolescence, the time period most eating disorders develop. Knowledge is needed on the role of genetic, environmental factors (life stress), weight loss, food restriction (starvation), and other core eating disorder behaviors (purging) in mediating the effects of brain developmental trajectories. Probing how patterns of neuropsychological assets and deficits (perfectionism, anxiety, negative mood states) may influence the development of an eating disorder can be conducted via various neuroimaging techniques. Although the above personality traits may influence susceptibility to cultural messages, peer influences, and internalization of the thin ideal, the mechanism in the brain by which this is accomplished is unknown.

Information on how dysregulation within and/or between limbic and executive corticostriatal circuitry may contribute to inhibition and self-control would be useful for treatment interventions in anorexia and BN. Neuroimaging studies of alterations of structural and functional connectivity are needed to identify specific brain circuits involved in the core eating disorder symptomatology.

Prospective longitudinal studies are needed to observe how brain alterations are related to risk, causing, maintaining, or the consequence of an eating disorder. Current research indicates eating disorders will have a polygenic etiology. Genes identified by epigenetic studies are likely to have a significant influence in the development of eating disorders and need more extensive investigation.

Improving treatment strategies will come about with the integration of emerging data from multiple sources. Problems of high treatment dropout rates, motivation for treatment, individualized treatment, insurance coverage, early diagnosis to facilitate early treatment, dissemination of effective treatment knowledge, and support for innovative treatment approaches and innovative research will continue to be a challenge in the next decade.

References

1. American Psychiatric Association: *Diagnostic and Statistical Manual of Mental Disorders.* 5th ed. Washington, DC, American Psychiatric Association, 2013.
2. American Psychiatric Association: *Diagnostic and Statistical Manual of Mental Disorders.* 4th ed. Washington, DC, American Psychiatric Association, 1994.
3. Bell RM: *Holy Anorexia.* Chicago, IL, University of Chicago Press, 1985.
4. Halmi KA: Images in psychiatry. *Am J Psychiatry* 151:1216, 1994.
5. Reynolds JA: *Discourse by the 12 Months Fasting of Martha Taylor, the Famed Derbyshire Damosell.* London, RW, 1669.
6. Morton R: *Phthisiologia Seu Exercitationes de Phtisi.* London, S. Smith.
7. Marcé LV: On a form of hypochondriacal delirium occurring consecutive to dyspepsia and characterized by refusal of food. *J Psychol Med Ment Pathol* 13:264–266, 1860.
8. Gull W: Anorexia nervosa. *Lancet* 1:516–517, 47, 1888.
9. Laséque EC: On hysterical anorexia. *Med Times Gazette* 2:265–266, 1873.
10. Bliss EL, Branch CH: *Anorexia Nervosa: Its History, Psychology and Biology.* New York, Hoeber, 1960.
11. Bruch AH: *Eating Disorders: Obesity, Anorexia Nervosa, and the Person Within.* New York, Basic Books, 1973.
12. Russell GFM: Bulimia nervosa: an ominous variant of anorexia nervosa. *Psychol Med* 9:492–448, 1979.
13. American Psychiatric Association: *Diagnostic and Statistical Manual of Mental Disorders,* 3rd ed-Revised. Washington, DC, American Psychiatric Association, 1987.
14. Currin L, Schmidt U, Treasure J, Jick H: Time trends in eating disorder incidence. *Br J Psychiatry* 186:132–135, 2005.
15. van Son GE, van Furth EF, Barteld AI, van Furth EF, Hoek HW: Time trends in the incidence of eating disorders: a primary care study in the Netherlands. *Int J Eat Disord* 39:565–569, 2006.
16. Lucas AR, Beerd CM, O'Fallon WN, Kurland LT: 50 year trend in the incidence of anorexia nervosa in Rochester Minn: a population based study. *Am J. Psychiatry* 148:917–922, 1991.
17. Stice E, Marti C, Shaw HC, et al.: An 8 year longitudinal study of the natural history of threshold, subthreshold, and partial eating disorders from a community sample of adolescents. *J Abnorm Psychol* 118:587–597, 2009.
18. Swanson SA, Crow SJ, Le Grange D, Swendsen J, Merikangas KR: Prevalence and correlates of eating disorders in adolescents—results from the national comorbidity survey replication adolescent supplement. *Arch Gen Psychiatry* 68:714–723, 2011.
19. Hudson JI, Hiripi E, Pope HG Jr, Kessler RC: The prevalence and correlates of eating disorders in the national comorbidity survey replication. *Biol Psychiatry* 61:348–358, 2007.

20. Preti A, Girolamo GD, Vilagut G, et al.: The epidemiology of eating disorders in six European countries: results of the ESE-MeD-WMH project. *J Psychiatr Res* 43:1125–1132, 2009.
21. Smink FR, van Hoeken D, Oldehinkel AJ, Hoek HW: Prevalence and severity of DSM V eating disorders in a community cohort of adolescents. *Int J Eat Disord* 47:610–619, 2014.
22. Franko DL, Keskaiah A, Eddy KT, et al.: A longitudinal investigation of mortality in anorexia nervosa and bulimia nervosa. *Am J Psychiatry* 170:917–925, 2013.
23. Arcelus J, Mitchell AJ, Wales J, Nielsen S: Mortality rates in patients with anorexia nervosa and other eating disorders. *Arch Gen Psychiatry* 68:724–731, 2011.
24. van Son G, Hoeken D, Furth E: Course and outcome of eating disorders in a primary care based cohort. *Int J Eat Disord* 43:130–138, 2010.
25. Steinhausen HC: The outcome of anorexia nervosa in the 20th century. *Am J Psychiatry* 159:1284–1293, 2002.
26. Isomaa R, Isomaa A, Marttunen M, Kaltiala-Heino R, Björkqvist K: The prevalence, incidence and development of eating disorders in Finnish adolescents: a two-step 3 year follow-up study. *Eur Eat Disord Rev* 17:199–207, 2009.
27. Soundy TJ, Lucas AR, Suman VJ, Melton LJ 3rd: Bulimia nervosa in Rochester Minnesota, 1980–1990. *Psychol Med* 25:1065–1071, 1995.
28. Allen KL, Byrne SM, Forbes D, Oddy WH: Risk factors for full- and partial-syndrome early adolescent eating disorders: a population-based pregnancy cohort study. *J Abnorm Psychol* 118:587–597, 2009.
29. Keel PK, Heatherton TF, Dorer DJ, Joiner TE, Zalta AK: Point prevalence of bulimia nervosa in 1982, 1992, and 2002. *Psychol Med* 36:119–127, 2006.
30. American Psychiatric Association: *Diagnostic and Statistical Manual of Mental Disorders*. 3rd ed. Washington, DC, American Psychiatric Association, 1980.
31. Favaro A, Caregaro L, Tenconi E, Bosello R, Santonastaso P: Time trends in age at onset of anorexia nervosa and bulimia nervosa. *J Clin Psychiatry* 70:1715–1721, 2009.
32. Crow SJ, Peterson CB, Swanson SA, et al.: Increased mortality in bulimia nervosa and other eating disorders. *Am J Psychiatry* 166:1342–1346, 2009.
33. Fairburn CG, Cooper Z, Doll HA, Norman P, O'Connor M: The natural course of bulimia nervosa and binge eating disorder in young women. *Arch Gen Psychiatry* 57:659–665, 2000.
34. Fichter MM, Quadflieg W: Twelve year course and outcome of bulimia nervosa. *Psychol Med* 34:1396–1406, 2004.
35. Ben-Tovim D, Walker K, Gilchrist F, Freeman R, Kalucy R, Esterman A: Outcome in patients with eating disorders: a five year study. *Lancet* 357:1254–1257, 2001.
36. Steinhausen HC: Outcome of rating disorders. *Child Adol psychiatry Clin N Am* 18:225–242, 2008.
37. Hudson JI, Coit CE, Lalonde JK, Pope HG Jr: By how much will the proposed new DSM 5 criteria increase the prevalence of binge eating disorder? *Int J Eat Disord* 45:139–141, 2012.
38. Fichter MM, Quadflieg W, Hedlund S: Long term course of binge eating disorder and bulimia nervosa; relevance for nosology and diagnostic criteria. *Int J Eat Disord* 41:577–586, 2008.
39. Halmi KA: Eating disorders. In: Hales RE, Yudofsky SC, Gabbard GO (eds): *Essentials of Psychiatry*. 3rd ed. Washington, DC, APPI, pp. 429–453, 2011.
40. Mitchell JE, Devlin M, de Zwann M, et al.: *Binge Eating Disorder : Clinical Foundations and Treatment*. New York, Guilford Press, 2008.
41. Pike KM, Hoek HW, Dunne PE: Cultural trends and eating disorders. *Cur Opinion* 27:436–442, 2014.
42. National Institute of Mental Health [NIMH]: *Data Set: Collaborative Psychiatric Epidemiology Survey Program [CPES]: Integrated Weights and Sampling Error Codes for Design-based Analysis*. 2007.
43. Marques L, Alegria M, Becker AE, et al.: Comparative prevalence, correlates of impairment and service utilization for eating disorders across US ethnic groups: implications for reducing ethnic disparities in health care access for eating disorders. *Int J Eat Disord* 44:412–420, 2011.
44. Javier SJ, Moore MP, Belgrave FZ: Racial comparisons in perceptions of maternal and peer attitudes, body dissatisfaction and eating disorders among African American and White women. *Women Health* 56(6):615–633, 2015.
45. Lydecker JA, Grilo CM: Different yet similar: examining race and ethnicity in treatment-seeking adults with binge eating disorder. *J Consult Clin Psychol* 84:88–94, 2016.
46. Quick VM, Byrd-Bredbenner C: Disordered eating, socio-cultural media influences, body image and psychological factors among a racially/ethnically diverse population of college women. *Eat Behav* 15:37–41, 2014.
47. Cachelin FM, Gil-Rivas V, Vela A: Understanding eating disorders among Latinas. *Adv Eat Disord* 2(2):204–208, 2014.
48. Stein KF, Corte C, Ronis DL: Personal identities and disordered eating behaviors in Mexican American women. *Eat Behav* 11:197–200, 2010.
49. Reslan S, Saules KK: Assessing the prevalence of and factors associated with overweight, obesity and binge eating as a function of ethnicity. *Eat Weight Disord* 18:209–219, 2013.
50. Stice E, Marti CN, Cheng ZH: Effectiveness of a dissonance-based eating disorder prevention program for ethnic groups in two randomized controlled trials. *Behav Res Ther* 55:54–64, 2014.
51. Katzman MA, Hermans KME, Van Koeken D, Hoek HW: Not your typical island woman: anorexia nervosa is reported only in subcultures in Curacão. *Cult Med Psychiatry* 28:463–492, 2004.
52. Pike KM, Borovoy A: The rise of eating disorders in Japan: issues of culture and limitations of the model of westernization. *Cult Med Psychiatry* 28:493–531, 2004.
53. Wardle J, Watters R: Sociocultural influences on attitudes on weight and eating: results of a natural experiment. *Int J Eat Disord* 35:589–596, 2004.
54. Allison KC, Park CL: A prospective study of disordered eating among sorority and non-sorority women. *Int J Eat Disord* 35:354–358, 2004.
55. Presnell K, Bearman SK, Stice E: Risk factors for body dissatisfaction in adolescent boys and girls: a prospective study. *Int J Eat Disord* 36:389–401, 2004.
56. Thompson SH, Digsby S: A preliminary survey of dieting, body dissatisfaction, and eating problems among high school cheerleaders. *J Sch Health* 74:85–90, 2004.
57. Wardel J, Robb KA, Johnson F, et al.: Social economic variation and attitudes to eating and weight in female adolescence. *Health Psychol* 23:275–282, 2004.
58. Tiggeman NM: Media exposure, body dissatisfaction and disordered eating: television and magazines are not the same. *Eur Eat Dis Rev* 11:418–430, 2003.
59. Low KA, Charanasomeoon S, Brown C, et al.: Internalization of the thin deal, weight and body image concerns. *Soc Behav Pers* 31:81–90, 2003.
60. Murnen SK, Smolak L, Mills JA, Good L: Thin, sexy women and strong, muscular men: grade school children's responses to objectified images of women and men. *Sex Roles* 49:427–437, 2003.
61. Hargreaves D, Tiggeman M: Younger-term implications of responsiveness to thin-ideal television: support for a cumulative hypothesis of body image disturbance. *Eur Eat Dis Rev* 11:465–477, 2003.
62. Chen LP, Murad MH, Paras ML, et al.: Sexual abuse and lifetime diagnosis of psychiatric disorders: systematic review and meta-analysis. *Mayo Clin Proc* 85:618–629, 2010.
63. Gentile K, Raghavan C, Rajah V, Gates K: It doesn't happen here; eating disorders in an ethnically diverse sample of economically disadvantaged urban college students. *Eat Disord* 15:405–425, 2007.
64. Burns EE, Fischer S, Jackson JL, Harding HG: Deficits in emotion regulation mediate the relationship between childhood abuse and later eating disorder symptoms. *Child Abuse Negl* 36:32–39, 2012.
65. Hopwood CJ, Ansell GB, Fehon DC, et al.: The mediational significance of negative/depressive affect in the relationship of childhood maltreatment and eating disorder features in adolescent psychiatric inpatients. *Eat Weight Disord* 16:e9–e16, 2011.
66. Urabel KR, Hoffart A, Ro O, Martinsen EW, Rosenvinge JH: Co-occurrence of avoidant personality disorder and child sexual abuse predicts poor outcome in long-standing eating disorder. *J Abn Psychol* 119:623–629, 2010.
67. Steiger H, Richardson J, Schmitz N, Israel M, Bruce KR, Gauvin L: Trait-defined eating-disorder subtypes and history of childhood abuse. *Int J Eat Disord* 43:428–432, 2010.
68. Racine SE, Wildes JE: Emotion dysregulation and anorexia nervosa: an exploration of the role of childhood abuse. *Int J Eat Disord* 48:55–58, 2015.
69. Jaite C, Schneider N, Hilbert A, Pfeiffer E, Lehmkuhl U, Salbach-Andrae H: Etiological role of childhood emotional trauma and neglect in adolescent anorexia nervosa: a cross-sectional questionnaire analysis. *Psychopathology* 45:61–66, 2012.
70. Becker DF, Grilo CM: Childhood maltreatment in women with binge-eating disorder: association with psychiatric comorbidity, physiological function and eating pathology. *Eat weight Disord* 16:e113–e120, 2011.
71. Brewerton TD, Rance SJ, Damsky BS, O'Neil PM, Kilpatrick DG: A comparison of women with child-adolescent versus adult onset binge eating: results from the National Women's Study. *Int J Eat Disord* 47:836–843, 2014.
72. Steiger H, Bruce K, Gauvin L, et al.: Contributions of the glucocorticoid receptor polymorphism [BclI] and childhood abuse to risk of bulimia nervosa. *Psychiatry Res* 187:193–197, 2011.
73. Groleau P, Steiger H, Joober R, et al.: Dopamine-system genes, childhood abuse and clinical manifestations in women with bulimia-spectrum disorders. *J Psychiatr Res* 46:1139–1145, 2012.
74. Akkermann K, Kaasik K, Kiive E Nordquist N, Oreland L, Harro J: The impact of adverse life events and the serotonin transporter gene promotor polymorphism on the development of eating disorder symptoms. *J Psychiatr Res* 46:38–43, 2012.
75. Cooper Z: The development and maintenance of eating disorders. In: Brownell KD, Fairburn CG (eds): *Eating Disorders and Obesity: A Comprehensive Handbook*. New York and London, Guilford Press, pp. 199–206, 1995.
76. Strober M, Freeman R, Lampert C, Diamond J, Kaye W: Controlled family study of anorexia nervosa and bulimia nervosa: evidence of shared liability and transmission of partial syndromes. *Am J Psychiatry* 157:393–401, 2000.
77. Bulik CM, Sullivan PF, Tozzi F, Furberg H, Lichtenstein P, Pedersen NL: Prevalence, heritability and prospective risk factors for anorexia nervosa. *Arch Gen Psychiatry* 631:305–312, 2006.

78. Javaras KW, Laird NM, Reichborn-Kjennerud T, Bulik CM, Pope HG Jr, Hudson JI: Familiality and heritability of binge eating disorder: results of a case-control family study and a twin study. *Int J Eat Disord* 41:174–179, 2008.
79. Thrornton LM, Mazzeo SE, Bulik CM: The heritability of eating disorders: methods and current findings. *Curr Top Behav Neurosci* 6:141–156, 2011.
80. Baker JH, Maes HH, Lissner L, Aggen SH, Lichtenstein P, Kendler KS: Genetic risk factors for disordered eating in adolescent males and females. *J Abnorm Psychol* 118:576–586, 2009.
81. Klump KL, Burt SA, Spanos A, McGue M, Iacono WG, Wade TD, et al.: Age differences in genetic and environmental influences on weight and shape concerns. *Int J Eat Disord* 43:679–688, 2010.
82. Klump KL, Suisman H, Burt SA, McGue M, Iacono WG: Genetic and environmental influences on disordered eating: an adoption study. *J Abnorm Psychol* 118:797–805, 2009.
83. Devlin B, Jones B, Bacanu SA, Roeder K: Mixture and linear models for linkage analysis of affected sibling pairs with covariates. *Gebet Epidemiol* 22:52–65, 2002.
84. Bulik CM, Devlin B, Bacanu SA, et al.: Significant linkage on chromosome 10p in families with bulimia nervosa. *Am J Hum Genet* 72:200–207, 2003.
85. Bergen AM, van den Bree MB, Yeager M, et al.: Candidate genes for anorexia nervosa in the 1p33-36 linkage region: serotonin 1 D and delete opioid receptor loci exhibited significant association with anorexia nervosa. *Mol Psychiatry* 81:397–406, 2003.
86. Brown KM, Bujar SR, Marn ET, Campbell DA, Stubbins MJ, Blundell JE: Further evidence of association of ORD1 and HTR1D polymorphisms with susceptibility to anorexia nervosa. *Biol Psychiatry* 61:367–373, 2006.
87. Ribases M, Gratacos M, Armengol L, et al.: Met66 in the brain-derived neurotrophic factor (BDNF) precursor is associated with anorexia nervosa restrictive type. *Mol Psychiatry* 8:745–751, 2003.
88. Wang K, Zhang H, Bloss CS, et al; Price Foundation Collaborative Group. A genome-wide association study on common SNPs and rare CNVs in anorexia nervosa. *Mol Psychiatry* 16:949–959, 2011.
89. Frieling H, Romer KD, Scholz S, et al.: Epigenetic dysregulation of dopaminergic genes in eating disorders. *Int J Eat Disord* 43:577–583, 2010.
90. Frieling H, Bleich S, Otten J, et al.: Epigenetic downregulation of atrial natriuretic peptide but not vasopressin mRNA expression in females with eating disorders related to impulsivity. *Neuropsychopharmacology* 33:2605–2609, 2008.
91. Strohe A, Kellner M, Holsboer F, Wiedemann K: Anxiolytic activity of atrial natriuretic peptide in patients with panic disorder. *Am J Psychiatry* 158:1514–1516, 2001.
92. Halmi KA, Falk JR: Behavioral and dietary discriminators of menstrual function in anorexia nervosa. In: Darby, Garner, Garfinkel (eds): *Anorexia Nervosa: Recent Development*. New York, Allen R. Liss, pp. 323–329, 1983.
93. Eckert E, Pomeroy C, Raymond N, Kohler PF, Thuras P, Bowers CY: Leptin in anorexia nervosa. *J Clin Endocrinol Metab* 83:791–795, 1998.
94. Monteleone P, Di Lieto A, Castaldo E, Maj M: Leptin functioning in eating disorders. *CNS Spectr* 9:523–529, 2004.
95. Monteleone P, Fabrazzo M, Martiadis Z., et al.: Opposite changes in circulating adiponectin in women with bulimia nervosa or binge eating disorder. *J Clin Endocrinol Metab* 88:5387–5391, 2003.
96. Chen HA, Trumbauer ME, Chen AS, et al.: Orexigenic action of peripheral ghrelin is mediated by neuropeptide Y and agouti-related protein. *Endocrinology* 145:2607–2612, 2004.
97. Monteleone P, Fabrazzo M, Tortorella A, Martiadis V, Serritella C, Maj M: Circulating ghrelin is decreased in non-obese and obese women with binge eating disorder was well as in obese non-binge eating women, but not in patients with bulimia nervosa. *Psychoneuroendocrinology* 30:243–250, 2005.
98. Monteleone P, Martiadis V, Fabrazzo M, Serritella C, Maj M: Ghrelin and leptin responses to food ingestion in bulimia nervosa: implications for binge eating and compensatory behaviors. *Psychol Med* 33:1387–1394, 2003.
99. Otto B, Cuntz U, Fruhauf E, et al.: Weight gain decreased elevated plasma ghrelin concentrations of patients with anorexia nervosa. *Eur J Endocrinol* 145:669–673, 2001.
100. Bailer UF, Kaye WH: Serotonin: imaging findings in eating disorders. *Curr Top Behav Neurosci* 6:59–79, 2011.
101. Bailer UF, Frank GK, Henry SE, et al.: Altered brain serotonin 5-HT1A receptor binding after recovery from AN measured by PET and carbonyl 11 C WAY-1000635. *Arch Gen Psychiatry* 62:1032–1041, 2005.
102. Galusca B, Costea N, Zito NG, et al.: Organic background of restrictive-type anorexia nervosa suggested by increased serotonin 1 A receptor binding in right frontotemporal cortex of both lean and recovered patients: [18F]MPPF PET scan study. *Biol Psychiatry* 64:1009–1013, 2008.
103. Tauscher J, Pirker W, Willeit M, et al.: I^{123} B-CIT and single photon emission computed tomography reveal reduce brain serotonin transporter availability in bulimia nervosa. *Biol Psychiatry* 49:326–332, 2001.
104. Joos AA, Saum B, van Elst LT, et al.: Amygdala hyperreactivity in restrictive anorexia nervosa. *Psychiatry Res* 191:189–195, 2011.
105. Uher R, Murphy T, Brammer MJ, et al.: Medial prefrontal cortex activity associated with symptom provocation in eating Disorders. *Am J Psychiat* 161:1238–1246, 2004.
106. Frank GK, Bailer UF, Henry SE, et al.: Increased dopamine D2/D3 receptor binding after recovery from anorexia nervosa measured by positron emission tomography and [11c]raclopride. *Biol Psychiatry* 58:908–912, 2005.
107. Fladung AK, Gron G, Grammer K, et al.: A neural signature of anorexia nervosa in the ventral striatal reward system. *Am J Psychiatry* 167:206–212, 2010.
108. Wagner A, Aizenstein H, Mazurkewicz L, et al.: Altered insula response to taste stimuli in individuals recovered from restricting-type anorexia nervosa. *Neuropsychopharmacology* 33:513–523, 2008.
109. Wagner A, Aizenstein H, Venkatraman VK, et al.: Altered reward processing in women recovered from anorexia nervosa. *Am J Psychiatry* 164:1842–1849, 2007.
110. Frank GK, Reynold JR, Shott ME, O'Reilly RC: Altered temporal difference learning in bulimia nervosa. *Biol Psychiatry* 70:728–735, 2011.
111. Frank GK, Shott ME, Hagman JO, Yang TT: Localized brain volume and white matter integrity alteration in adolescent anorexia nervosa. *J Am Acad Child Adolesc Psychiatry* 52:1066–1075.e5, 2013.
112. Shott ME, Pryor TL, Yang TT, Frank GKW: Greater insula white matter fiber connectivity in women recovered from anorexia nervosa. *Neuropsychopharmacology* 41, 498–507, 2015.
113. Halmi KA, Sunday SR, Strober M, et al.: Perfectionism in anorexia nervosa: variation by clinical subtype, obsessionality, and pathological eating behavior. *Am J Psychiatry* 1157:1799–1805, 2000.
114. Halmi KA, Tozzi F, Thornton L, et al.: The relation among perfectionism, obsessive compulsive personality disorder and obsessive compulsive disorder in individuals with eating disorders. *Int J Eat Disord* 38:371–374, 2005.
115. Zerwas A, Lund BC, Von Holle A, et al.: Factors associated with recovery from anorexia nervosa. *J Psychiatr Res* 47:972–979, 2013.
116. Atiye M, Mietunen J, Raevuori-Helkamaa A: A meta-analysis of temperament in eating disorders. *Eur Eat Dis Rev* 23:89–99, 2015.
117. Rotella F, Fioravanti G, Godini L, Mannucci E, Faravelli C, Ricca V: Temperament and emotional eating: a crucial relationship in eating disorders. *Psychiatry Res* 225:452–457, 2015.
118. Grucza R, Przybeck TR, Cloninger CR: Prevalence and correlates of binge eating disorder in a community sample. *Compr Psychiatry* 48:124–131, 2007.
119. Wonderlich JA, Lavender JM, Wonderlich SA, et al.: Examining convergence of retrospective and ecological momentary assessment measures of negative affect and eating disorder behaviors. *Int J Eat Disord* 48:305–311, 2015.
120. Bohon C, Stice E: Negative affect and neural response to palatable food intake in bulimia nervosa. *Appetite* 58:964–970, 2013.
121. Roberts M, Tchanturia K, Treasure JL: Exploring the neurocognitive signature of poor set-shifting in anorexia and bulimia nervosa. *J Psychiatr Res* 44:964–970, 2010.
122. Shott ME, Filotes JV, Bhatnager K, et al.: Cognitive set-shifting in anorexia nervosa. *Eur Eat Disord Rev* 20:343–349, 2012.
123. Buhren K, Mainz V, Herpertz-Dahlmann B, et al.: Cognitive flexibility in juvenile anorexia patients before and after weight recovery. *J Neural Transm (Vienna)* 119:1047–1057, 2012.
124. Jappe LM, Frank G, Shott ME, et al.: Heightened sensitivity to reward and punishment in anorexia nervosa. *Int J Eat Disord* 44:317–324, 2011.
125. Harrison A, O'Brien N, Lopez C, Treasure J: Sensitivity to reward and punishment in eating disorders. *Psych Res* 117:1–11, 2010.
126. Zastrow A, Kaiser S, Stippich C, et al.: Neural correlates of impaired cognitive-behavioral flexibility in anorexia nervosa. *Am J Psychiatry* 166:608–616, 2009.
127. Fernandez-Aranda F, Pinheiro AP, Thornton LM, et al.: Impulse control disorders in women with eating disorders. *Psychiatry Res* 157:147–157, 2008.
128. Braun DL, Sunday SR, Halmi KA: Psychiatric comorbidity in patients with eating disorders. *Psychol Med* 24:859–867, 1994.
129. Bould H, Koupil I, Dalman C, DeStavola B, Lewis G, Magnusson C: Parental mental illness and eating disorders in offspring. *Int J Eat Disord* 48:383–391, 2015.
130. Micali N, Stahl D, Treasure J, Simonoff E: Childhood psychopathology in children of women with eating disorders: understanding risk mechanisms. *J Child Psychol Psychiatry* 55:124–134, 2014.
131. Berge J, Wall M, Larson N, Eisenberg ME, Loth KA, Neumark-Sztainer D: The unique and additive association of family functioning and parenting practices with disordered eating behaviors in diverse adolescents. *J Behav Med* 37:205–217, 2014.
132. Haycraft E, Godwin H, Meyer C: Adolescents level of eating psychopathology in relation to perceptions of their parents current feeding practices. *J Adolesc Health* 54:204–208, 2014.
133. Krug I, Fuller-Tyszkiewicz M, Anderhul M, et al.: A new social-family model for eating disorders: a European multicenter project using a case-control design. *Appetite* 95:544–553, 2015.
134. Kluck AS: Family influence on disordered eating: the role of body image dissatisfaction. *Body Image* 7:8–14, 2010.
135. Palfreyman Z, Haycraft E, Meyer C: Parental modelling of eating behavior: observational validation of the Parental Modelling of Eating Behaviours scale (PARM). *Appetite* 86:31–37, 2015.
136. Haycraft E, Powell F, Meyer C: Activity-related parenting practices: development of the Parenting Related to Activity Measure (PRAM) and

links with mother's eating psychopathology and compulsive exercise beliefs. *Eur Eat Disord Rev* 23:51–61, 2015.
137. Ciao A, Accurso E, Fitzsimmons E, Lock J, Le Grange D: Family functioning in two treatments for adolescent anorexia nervosa. *Int J Eat Disord* 48:81–90, 2015.
138. George MW, Fairchild AJ, Mark Cummings E, Davies PT: Marital conflict in early childhood and adolescent disordered eating: emotional insecurity about the marital relationship as an explanatory mechanism. *Eat Behav* 15:532–539, 2014.
139. White J, Shelton KH, Elgar FJ: Prospective association between family environment, family cohesion and psychiatric symptoms among adolescent girls. *Child Psychiatry Hum Dev* 45:544–554, 2014.
140. Hoste R, Lebow J, Le Grange D: A bidirectional examination of expressed emotion among families of adolescents with bulimia nervosa. *Int J Eat Disord* 48:249–252, 2015.
141. Schmidt R, Tetzloff A, Hilbert A: Perceived expressed emotion in adolescents with binge-eating disorder. *J Abnorm Child Psychol* 43:1369–1377, 2015.
142. Depestele L, Claes L, Dierckx E: The role of non-suicidal self-injury and binge-eating/purging behavior in family functioning in eating disorders. *Eur Eat Disord Rev* 23:413–416, 2015
143. NICE (National Institute for Clinical Excellence): *Core Interventions in the Treatment and Management of Anorexia Nervosa, Bulimia nervosa and Related Eating Disorders.* London, Clinical Guidelines 9 2004, pp. 1–55.
144. Lock J, Le Grange D: *Treatment Manual for Anorexia Nervosa: A Family-Based Approach.* 2nd ed. New York, Guilford, 2013.
145. Agras W, Lock J, Brandt H, et al.: Comparison of 2 family therapies for adolescent anorexia nervosa: a randomized parallel trial. *JAMA Psychiatry* 72:1279–1286, 2014.
146. Fitzpatrick KK, Moye A, Hoste R, Lock J, Le Grange D: Adolescent focused therapy for adolescent anorexia nervosa. *J Cont Psychother* 40:31–39, 2010.
147. Lock J, Le Grange D, Agras W, Moye A, Bryson SW, Jo B: Randomized clinical trial comparing family-based treatment with adolescent-focused individual therapy for adolescents with anorexia nervosa. *Arch Gen Psychiatry* 67:1025–1032, 2010.
148. Madden S, Miskovic-Wheatley J, Wallis A, et al.: A randomized controlled trial of inpatient treatment for anorexia nervosa in medically unstable adolescents. *Psychol Med* 45:415–427, 2015.
149. Dimitropoulos G, Farquhar J, Freeman V, Colton PA, Olmsted MP: Pilot study comparing multi-family therapy to single family therapy for adults with anorexia nervosa in an intensive eating disorder program. *Eur Eat Disord Rev* 23:294–303, 2015.
150. Gelin Z, Fuso S, Hendricks S, Cook-Darzens S, Simon Y: The effects of a multiple family therapy on adolescents with eating disorders: an outcome study. *Fam Process* 54:160–172, 2015.
151. Whitney J, Easter A, Tchanturia A: Service users feedback on cognitive training in the treatment of anorexia nervosa: a qualitative study. *Int J Eat Disord* 41:542–550, 2008.
152. Dingemans AE, Danner UN, Donker JM, et al.: The effectiveness of cognitive remediation in patients with a severe eating disorder: a randomized controlled trial. *Psychother Psychosom* 83:29–36, 2013.
153. Safer D, Robinson A, Jo B: Outcome from a randomized controlled trial of group therapy for binge eating disorder: comparing dialectical behavior therapy adapted for binge eating to an active comparison group therapy. *Behav Ther* 41:106–120, 2010.
154. Russell GF, Szmukler GI, Dare C, Eisler I: An evaluation of family therapy and anorexia and bulimia nervosa. *Arch Gen Psychiatry* 44:1047–1056, 1987.
155. Eisler I, Dare C, Hodes M, Russell G, Dodge E, Le Grange D: Family therapy for adolescent anorexia nervosa ; the result of a control comparison of two-family interventions. *J Child Psychol Psychiatry* 41:727–736, 2000.
156. Aigner M, Treasure J, Kaye W, Kasper S; WFSBP Task Force On Eating Disorders. World Federation of Societies of Biological Psychiatry [WFSBP] guidelines for the pharmacological treatment of eating disorders. *World J Biol Psychiatry* 12:400–443, 2011.
157. Attia E, Kaplan AS, Walsh BT, et al.: Olanzapine versus placebo for outpatients with anorexia nervosa. *Psychol Med* 41:2177–2182, 2011.
158. Flament MF, Bissada H, Spettigue W: Evidence based pharmacotherapy of eating disorders. *Int J Neuropsychopharmacol* 15:189–297, 2012.
159. Misra M, Katzman D, Miller KK, et al.: Physiologic estrogen replacement increases bone density in adolescent girls with anorexia nervosa. *J Bone Mineral Res* 26:2430–2438, 2011.
160. DiVasta AD, Feldman HA, Beck TJ, LeBoff MS, Gordon CM: Does hormone replacement normalize bone geometry in adolescents with anorexia nervosa? *J Bone Miner Res* 29:151–157, 2014.
161. Okamoto A, Yamachita T, Nagoshi Y: A behavior therapy program combined with liquid nutrition designed for anorexia nervosa. *Psychiatry Clin Neurosci* 56:515–520, 2002.
162. Wolfe BE, Gimby LB: Caring for the hospitalized patient with an eating disorder. *Nurs Clin North Am* 38:75–99, 2003.
163. Watson TL, Bowers WA, Anderson AE: Involuntary treatment of eating disorders. *Am J Psychiatry* 157:1806–1810, 2000.
164. Wilson GT, Fairburn CG: Cognitive treatments for treating eating disorders. *J Consult Clin Psychol* 61:261–269, 1993.
165. Fairburn C, Cooper Z, Shafron R: Enhanced cognitive behavioral therapy for eating disorders [CBT-E]. In: Fairburn CG (ed): *Cognitive Behavioral Therapy and Eating Disorders.* New York, Guilford, pp 23–34, 2008.
166. Scmidt U, Lee S, Beecham J, et al.: A randomized controlled trial of family therapy and cognitive guided self-care for adolescents with bulimia nervosa and related disorders. *Am J Psychiatry* 164:591–598, 2007.
167. Le Grange D, Crosby RD, Rathauz PJ, Leventhal BL, et al.: A randomized controlled comparison of family-based treatment and cognitive behavioral therapy for adolescent bulimia nervosa. *Arch Gen Psychiatry* 64:1049–1056, 2007.
168. Le Grange D, Loch J, Agras S, Bryson SW, Jo B: Randomized clinical trial of family-based treatment and cognitive behavioral therapy for adolescent bulimia nervosa. *J Am Acad Child Adol Psychiatry* 54:886–894, 2015.
169. Stewart C, Voulgari S, Eisler I, Hunt K, Simic M: Multi-family therapy for bulimia nervosa in adolescence. *Eat Disord* 23:345–355, 2015.
170. Wilson GT, Fairburn CC, Agras WS, Walsh BT, Kraemer H: Cognitive behavioral therapy for bulimia nervosa: time course and mechanisms of change. *J Consult Clin Psychol* 70:267–274, 2002.
171. Mitchell JE, DeZwaan M: Pharmacological treatments of binge eating. In: Fairburn CG, Wilson GT (eds): *Binge Eating: Nature, Assessment and Treatment.* New York, Guilford Press, 1993.
172. Agras WS, Rossiter EM, Arnow B, et al.: Pharmacologic and cognitive behavioral treatment for bulimia nervosa: a control comparison. *Am J Psychiatry* 149:82–87, 1992.
173. Hedges DW, Reimherr FW, Hoopes SP, et al.: Treatment of bulimia nervosa with Topiramate in a randomized double-blind, placebo-controlled trial, part 2: improvements in psychiatric measures. *J Clin Psychiatry* 64:1449–1454, 2003.
174. Hoopes SP, Riemherr FW, Hedges DW, et al.: Treatment of bulimia nervosa with Topiramate in a randomized-double-blind placebo-controlled trial, part 1: improvement in binge and purge measures. *J Clin Psychiatry* 64:1335–1341, 2003.
175. Sysko R, Sha N, Wang N, Duan N, Walsh BT: Early response to antidepressant treatment in bulimia nervosa. *Psychol Med* 40:999–1005, 2010.
176. Brownley KA, Berkman ND, Sedway JA, Lohr KN, Bulik CM: Binge eating disorder treatment: a systematic review of randomized controlled trials. *Int J Eat Disord* 40:337–348, 2007.
177. Fischer S, Meyer A, Dremmel D, Schlup B, Munsch S: Short term cognitive behavioral therapy for binge eating disorder: long term efficacy and predictors of long term success. *Behav Res Ther* 58:36–42, 2014.
178. Hilbert A, Bishop ME, Stein RI, et al.: Long term efficacy of psychological treatment for binge eating disorder. *Br J Psychiatry* 200:232–237, 2012.
179. Wilson GT, Wilfley DE, Agras WS, Bryson SW, et al.: Psychological treatment of binge eating disorder. *Arch Gen Psychiatry* 67:94–101, 2010.
180. Debar LL, Wilson GT, Yarborough BJ, et al.: Cognitive behavioral treatment for recurrent binge eating in adolescent girls: a pilot trial. *Cogn Behav Pract* 20:147–161, 2013.
181. Jones M, Luce KK, Osborne MI, et al.: Randomized controlled trial of an internet-facilitated intervention for reducing binge eating and overweight in adolescents. *Pediatrics* 121:453–462, 2008.
182. Tanofsky-Kraff M, Wilfrey DE, Young JF, et al.: A pilot study of interpersonal psychotherapy for preventing excess weight gain in adolescent girls at-risk for obesity. *Int J Eat Disord* 43:701–706, 2010.
183. McElroy SL, Hudson JI, Malhotra S, et al.: Citalopram in the treatment of binge-eating disorder: a placebo-controlled trial. *Int J Clin Psychiatry* 64:807–813, 2003.
184. Guerdjikova AI, McElroy SL, Kotwal R, et al.: High dose escitalopram in the treatment of binge-eating disorder with obesity: a placebo-controlled monotherapy trial. *Hum Psychopharmacol* 23:1–11, 2008.
185. McElroy S, Casuto L, Nelson E, et al.: Placebo-controlled trial of sertraline in the treatment of binge eating disorder. *AM J Psychiatry* 157:1004–1006, 2000.
186. McCann UD, Agras WS: Successful treatment of nonpurging bulimia nervosa with desipramine: a double-blind, placebo-controlled study. *Am J Psychiatry* 149:1509–1513, 1990.
187. McElroy S, Hudson JI, Capece JA, et al.: Topiramate for the treatment of binge eating disorder associated with obesity: a placebo-controlled study. *Biol Psychiatry* 61:1039–1048, 2007.
188. McElroy SL, Kotwal R, Guerdjikova AI, et al.: Zonisamide in the treatment of binge eating disorder with obesity: a randomized controlled trial. *J Clin Psychiatry* 67:1897–1906, 2006.
189. McRoy S, Guerdjikova A, Kotwal R, et al.: Atomoxetine in the treatment of binge-eating disorder: a randomized placebo-controlled trial. *J Clin Psychiatry* 68:390–398, 2007.
190. McRoy S: SPD489 in adults aged 18-55 years with moderate to severe BED. *ClinicalTrials.gov Identifier: NCT01718483.* U.S. National Institutes of Health. Accessed November 20, 2014.
191. Grilo C, Masheb R, Salant S: CBT guided self-help and Orlistat for treatment of BED. *Int J Eat Disord* 44:81–90, 2011.
192. McElroy S, Guerdjikova AI, Winstanley EL, et al.: Acamprosate in the treatment of binge eating disorder: a placebo-controlled trial. *Int J Eat Disord* 44:81–90, 2011.

CHAPTER 5.7.2 ■ PICA, RUMINATION DISORDER, AND AVOIDANT/RESTRICTIVE FOOD INTAKE DISORDER

KATHRYN A. CONIGLIO AND JENNIFER J. THOMAS

INTRODUCTION

Although anorexia nervosa (AN), bulimia nervosa (BN), and binge eating disorder (BED) get considerable attention in research and clinical practice, other lesser known feeding and eating disorders exist. *The Diagnostic and Statistical Manual*, fifth edition (DSM-5) also describes pica, rumination disorder (RD), and avoidant/restrictive food intake disorder (ARFID). Earlier descriptions of both pica and RD were included in DSM-IV. ARFID, however, is a revised version of DSM-IV feeding disorder of infancy and early childhood, meant to capture inadequate volume or variety of food intake throughout the lifespan. While none of these disorders are characterized by the distorted body image and overvaluation of shape and weight that characterize AN and BN, all three can cause significant medical and psychological impairment. Although less is known about these disorders, clinicians should be familiar with their presentations to aid in detection, and their more prominent placement in DSM-5 has inspired new research on their optimal assessment and treatment.

PICA

Clinical Definition

Four diagnostic criteria characterize pica (1). The first and *sine qua non* is persistent consumption of nonfood, nonnutritive substances for 1 month or more. Unlike individuals with AN or BN, those with pica do not show aversion to food in general and may consume food in addition to nonfood substances. Pica substances include chalk, coal, ash, clay, dirt, laundry starch, other powdery substances such as talcum powder or makeup, and feces (2). Previous versions of DSM did not include "nonfood" as a qualifier for substances consumed; this term was added in DSM-5 to exclude individuals who consume items—such as ice, raw pasta, or artificial sweetener—that, despite having minimal nutritional value, are still considered food (3).

The second criterion describes the consumption of nonfood, nonnutritive substances as inappropriate given the individual's developmental level (1). For example, a teething infant who eats or sucks on nonnutritive substances should not be diagnosed with pica. For this reason, an age of 2 years is the suggested minimum for a pica diagnosis.

The third criterion for pica is that the consumption of nonfood substances is not attributable to a socially or culturally normative behavior (1). In some cultures, dirt, clay, or other nonfood, nonnutritive substances are consumed for their believed medicinal or spiritual benefits (2). For example, geophagia, or the consumption of earth, has been documented as early as 460 BC in ancient Greece and Rome (4). Geophagia has since been observed, primarily among women from communities in sub-Saharan Africa, for believed benefits of skin softening and increased fertility (5). Thus, among communities where geophagia or similar practices are culturally accepted, a diagnosis of pica would not be warranted.

The fourth criterion for pica states that, in the presence of other comorbid medical complications, pica should only be diagnosed if the consumption of nonfood, nonnutritive substances is serious enough to warrant additional clinical attention (1). Likewise, a diagnosis of pica is not warranted when a person consumes nonfood, nonnutritive substances for perceived appetite suppression effects, as a method of nonsuicidal self-injury, or because the person feels compelled to do so as a result of a psychotic disorder, like schizophrenia.

Of note, pregnancy is included as an exemptive medical condition in DSM-5, unless the consumption of nonfood substances is severe enough to warrant additional clinical attention (1). This is partly because pica-like ingestion of nonfood, nonnutritive substances has been associated with iron and zinc deficiencies, which can be present in pregnant women (6). Micronutrients such as iron and zinc are commonly found in soil, clay, and other earthen materials that people who have pica may consume. Available data provide conflicting evidence as to whether pica is correlated with micronutrient deficiencies (7,8). Further studies are needed to examine the strength of this relationship and its implications for the etiology and treatment of pica.

Prevalence of pica are largely unknown and vary widely. A recent study by Delaney et al. (9) found that pica prevalence was 1.3% among adolescent and young adult females in residential eating disorder treatment in the United States, whereas another study found a 74.4% prevalence in a sample of mixed sex schoolchildren in Lusaka, Zambia (10). Prevalence estimates for pica vary widely due in part to differing definitions across studies (e.g., inclusion vs. exclusion of ice as a pica substance) and changing definitions of pica from DSM-IV to DSM-5. For example, a recent review of four prevalence studies of pica among "institutionalized individuals with intellectual disability" (p. 206) found that prevalence ranged from 9.2% to 25.8% (11). However, the latter figure came from a study that used a broader definition of pica that included some potentially nutritive substances (e.g., coffee grounds, excessive water consumption) (12) that would not meet the first DSM-5 criterion.

Pica is often associated with intellectual developmental disorders and developmental disabilities (1). Pica also often co-occurs with obsessive-compulsive spectrum disorders such as trichotillomania, in which individuals may consume the hair they have pulled. Case studies also indicate that individuals with OCD may engage in consuming nonfood, nonnutritive substances, such as cigarettes or paint chips, as part of compulsion rituals (13).

Medical Complications

Individuals with pica can experience from potentially fatal medical consequences, depending on the level of toxicity of the substance ingested. Complications of pica can include injuries to the mouth and gastrointestinal (GI) tract, intestinal blockages, lead poisoning, constipation, parasites, and infections (2,14). In a retrospective medical record review of 35 individuals with pica described as "mentally handicapped" (p. 552) and undergoing surgery to remove foreign bodies from the GI tract in an inpatient community hospital, 11% eventually died from surgical complications directly related to pica (15).

Iron-deficiency anemia (IDA) is often associated with pica, although it is unclear whether IDA is a consequence or a cause. Some research has suggested that clay and dirt can block absorption of iron in the bloodstream, thus leading to iron deficiency (7), while others have suggested that individuals may crave iron-containing substances (e.g., dirt or soil) in order to correct a pre-existing iron deficiency (2).

Pica can impair psychosocial functioning as well. Many people with pica do not seek treatment, citing embarrassment and shame as primary deterrents (9,16). Purchasing and consuming nonfood substances are typically done in secret. One case report documented that an individual with pica often resisted the urge to engage in the eating behavior, only to find that the urge did not relent until she consumed her preferred pica substance (16).

Etiology

Although DSM-IV categorized pica under Disorders Usually First Diagnosed in Infancy, Childhood, or Adolescence; DSM-5 recategorized pica under Feeding and Eating Disorders in recognition that pica can occur across the lifespan. However, pica typically onsets in childhood (17). Multiple theories of pica etiology have been posited, from both anthropologic and behavioral standpoints. Young (2) suggested three main etiologic theories: pica is an adaptive response during times of food shortage/famine; pica represents a pre-existing micronutrient deficiency; and pica acts as a natural protection against toxins and illness. While these theories may hold true for some individuals with pica, they do not represent a comprehensive etiologic framework, and are largely unsupported by empirical work. In contrast, behavioral theorists hypothesize that pica may be the result of a learned behavior from environments with little social interaction (18). Indeed, in children, pica has specifically been associated with environments of parental neglect (19). The link between diminished or inappropriate social interaction, be it a cause or consequence of pica, has inspired behavioral techniques to target pica behaviors (20,23).

Assessment

Pica is underreported in clinical settings, likely due to individuals not spontaneously volunteering symptoms, and clinicians not inquiring (9). Individuals with pica may conceal their consumption of nonfood items for fear of being viewed as financially poor or intellectually disabled (2,9). Indeed, historically, pica was more heavily documented among people with low socioeconomic status (e.g., enslaved and/or indigenous populations) or intellectual disability (2). For these reasons, individuals with pica may initially present with physical ailments such as stomach cramping or injuries to the GI tract. Thorough physical examinations (including x-ray or MRI if needed), blood tests, and nutritional consultation may be helpful to rule out medical complications in instances where pica is suspected (17).

Clinically, the individual should be questioned about the types of items that he or she consumes that aren't "normal food." This can be done through unstructured clinical interviewing based upon DSM-5 criteria, or by using a standardized assessment. The Eating Disorder Assessment for DSM-5 (EDA-5) (21) is a brief "app"-based interview with good psychometric properties that clinicians or researchers can implement to ascertain the presence or absence of DSM-5 feeding and eating disorders including pica. For a more detailed assessment, the Pica, ARFID, and Rumination Disorder Interview (PARDI) is a semi-structured interview that can be used clinically to diagnose pica and assess severity and related impairment among individuals ages 2 and older (22). For respondents under age 13, a parent/carer version of the interview can be implemented to obtain collateral information to supplement self-report. The PARDI is the only standardized clinical assessment tool that provides a continuous measure of pica severity, and is currently undergoing pilot testing in a multisite validation trial.

Treatment

At present, no evidence-based treatment protocol exists for pica specifically. However, case reports have described behavioral techniques that have been effective in reducing the severity and overall occurrence of pica behaviors. Functional analyses are useful prior to starting treatment, as the function that pica behaviors serve likely vary by individual (23). Common to most individuals, however, is that pica is a stimulating behavior that is maintained through positive automatic reinforcement. Applied Behavioral Analysis (ABA) has been effective in treating pica, specifically among children with developmental disorders. In a qualitative review of pica treatment techniques, Matson et al. (24) found that successful components of ABA to treat pica include both "punishment procedures" (p. 2565) and "positive procedures" (p. 2568). Punishment procedures can include incorporating taste aversion techniques (such as pairing lemon juice or aromatic ammonia [e.g., smelling salts] with the pica substance), and overcorrection following the behavior (i.e., encouraging an individual who eats cigarettes to thoroughly wash his or her teeth and clean up trash around him or her following the behavior). Positive procedures can include offering appropriate and preferred food substances and introducing novel and enriching elements to the environment (e.g., new types of play) to increase engagement in replacement behaviors (24).

RUMINATION DISORDER

Clinical Definition

RD is characterized in DSM-5 by persistent regurgitation of food for 1 month or more (1). Regurgitated food can be rechewed, reswallowed, or spit out. DSM-5 describes that this behavior typically occurs several times per week—often daily—though this is not a formal diagnostic criterion (1). In a study of clinical features in a pediatric sample of individuals with RD, 100% of the sample endorsed daily rumination, after almost every meal (25). It is important to note that rumination is different from vomiting; individuals with RD typically do not retch or feel nauseous when food is regurgitated, and often, the food is not acidic. For instance, a person with gastroesophageal reflux disease (GERD) who experiences frequent regurgitation as a result of reflux cannot be diagnosed with RD unless he or she also engages in persistent regurgitation outside of reflux episodes (1). Rather, rumination behaviors must occur independent of a medical condition that is better able to account for the behavior.

RD must also occur independently of other eating disorders, such as AN, BN, BED, or ARFID (1). While previous studies have shown that rumination behavior can co-occur with other eating disorders, a formal diagnosis of RD is inappropriate in these cases, according to DSM-5 (9). In cases of intellectual disability or other mental disorders, however, RD can be a comorbid diagnosis if the behaviors are severe enough to warrant additional clinical attention (1).

Prevalence of RD in the general population are unknown. One study in a residential eating disorder facility in the United States indicated that 7.4% of the (all-female) participants endorsed rumination behavior, but none received a formal diagnosis of RD due to DSM-5 trumping rules, which specify that RD cannot co-occur with another eating disorder (9). Just as with pica, RD is no longer a Feeding Disorder of Infancy or Early Childhood; adults are able to receive this diagnosis under DSM-5 and adult cases have been documented in the literature (26,27). A recent prevalence study among male and female school-aged children (ages 10 to 16 years) in Sri Lanka found that 5.1% met criteria for rumination syndrome (RS) using Rome III criteria (28). Similar to DSM-5, Rome III criteria state that a diagnosis of RS should involve repeated, painless regurgitation of food. This regurgitation should occur shortly after a meal, not occur during sleep, and not involve retching (29). Unlike DSM-5, however, Rome III criteria need only be present once per week for 2 months. While DSM-5 does not include a definitive behavior frequency in RD criteria, it suggests this behavior will occur many times per week, perhaps even daily. Although methodologic differences make prevalence difficult to compare across studies, available data suggest that, like pica, RD is relatively rare in the general population.

Medical Complications

Although different from vomiting, the regurgitation of food in RD can yield medical consequences that are similar to those found in patients who frequently purge through vomiting. These can vary depending on severity and length of illness, and some can be quite serious. Electrolyte imbalances, dehydration, dental erosions, and weight loss are among the most clinically impairing complications (30).

RD can have a negative impact on social activities as well. Among pediatric patients with RD, 73% endorsed missing school or work due to associated symptoms of RD, such as abdominal pain or constipation (25). Some people with RD may attempt to conceal this behavior in social settings, due to shame or embarrassment (27).

Etiology

The etiology of RD is largely unknown, though it appears that rumination may function in infants and those with developmental disabilities as a self-soothing behavior (14). Clinically, patients endorse varying degrees of self-control over rumination behavior (31), yet behavioral theory posits that the physiologic mechanisms that allow one to ruminate are voluntary (32). Among individuals with RD, rumination may serve as a learned habit in response to external cues, including starting or ending a meal, or feelings of fullness while eating. Individuals may habitually, yet subconsciously, initiate rumination by contracting the abdominal wall and ruminating in a controlled fashion (32). Individuals with RD may be unaware that this behavior is a learned response. In such cases, developing insight into the individual's own role in maintaining the regurgitation behavior is often a key component of RD treatment.

Assessment

Patients with RD may not volunteer information to family, friends, or healthcare workers without prompting (27,30). To assess symptoms of RD, clinicians can use the EDA-5 (21) as a brief diagnostic measure, or the PARDI (22) to confer a diagnosis and also assess RD severity and associated clinical impairment. The clinician should be sure to differentiate the rumination behavior from food coming back up into the mouth due to vomiting or acid reflux. For the latter, the clinician can inquire if acid reflux medication helped to alleviate the rumination, as certain medications that are helpful to alleviate symptoms of GERD (i.e., reducing gastric secretion volume and acidity using proton pump inhibitors) (33) have not been studied for use with RD, and may exacerbate the problem.

Treatment

At present, no randomized controlled trials have identified preferred treatments for RD. However, several case reports have documented success in symptom alleviation using diaphragmatic breathing (26,34). Diaphragmatic breathing is a technique designed to relax the abdominal muscle contractions thought to initiate rumination behavior. Clinicians can demonstrate this technique during a routine medical visit or therapy session, as follows:

1. The therapist instructs the patient to place one hand on his or her chest and the other on his or her abdomen, and to inhale deeply. Typically, the patient will inhale through the chest, noticing the hand on his or her chest rise, while the hand on his or her abdomen barely moves.
2. The therapist then instructs the patient to inhale deeply through the abdomen only, attempting to keep the hand on his or her chest motionless. Breaths should be slow and last at least 3 seconds to inhale and 3 seconds to exhale. It may be appropriate, given the developmental level of the patient, to use imagery (e.g., a balloon being inflated and deflated) to help the patient achieve slow and deliberate breaths.
3. The therapist encourages the patient to practice diaphragmatic breathing during times when rumination behavior typically occurs. For some, this may occur partway through the meal, while for others it may occur post-prandially. Ultimately, with practice, the patient should engage in diaphragmatic breathing automatically during high-risk times, thus preventing the muscle contractions necessary to trigger regurgitation behavior.

AVOIDANT/RESTRICTIVE FOOD INTAKE DISORDER

Clinical Definition

ARFID is a revised and expanded DSM-5 version (1) of the disorder formerly known as DSM-IV Feeding or Eating Disorder of Infancy or Early Childhood (3). Specifically, DSM-5 includes ARFID to offer a specific diagnosis for individuals who obtain inadequate nutrition due to limiting the variety or volume of food consumed, whereas DSM-IV grouped these individuals heterogeneously along with other types of feeding and eating problems in youth. In addition, while DSM-IV stipulated that the disorder must onset before age 6, DSM-5 acknowledges that these presentations may onset later in life.

ARFID has four main DSM-5 diagnostic criteria, all of which must be fully met for diagnosis (1). The first is an eating disturbance that leads to significant weight loss, nutritional deficiency, dependence on a gastronomy (G) or nasogastric (NG) tube, and/or psychosocial impairment. Typically the individual eats a limited volume or variety of food due to (a) apparent lack of interest in eating or food, (b) avoidance based on the sensory characteristics of food, or (c) concern about aversive consequences of eating (e.g., vomiting or choking), but this is not an exhaustive list. Second, this disturbance in eating cannot be accounted for by lack of food availability. Third, the eating disturbance cannot occur solely during the course of AN or BN. Unlike individuals with AN or BN, those with ARFID do not restrict their food intake to influence their shape or weight, or to avoid an episode of overeating. Rather, restrictive eating is a consequence of lack of interest, sensory sensitivity, fear of aversive consequences, or another reason unrelated to shape or weight, as stated in the first criterion. Finally, the eating disturbance cannot be better explained by the presence of another physical or mental disorder, including food allergies and intolerances, GI disease, and neuromuscular disorders that may affect swallowing.

It is important to note that the inclusion of ARFID in DSM-5 is not meant to over-pathologize picky eating or to ascribe psychological dysfunction to individuals with medical problems that limit their diets. While selective eating patterns are relatively normative among young children, a study of over 2,000 pediatric patients ages 8 to 18 years seeking treatment for GI issues found that only 1.5% met criteria for ARFID (35). As outlined in criterion one, the eating disturbance must be accompanied by medical or psychosocial impairment that warrants additional clinical attention.

Medical Complications

Individuals with ARFID and related presentations can experience serious medical consequences. Those with avoidant/restrictive eating—especially those who present with the sensory phenotype—are less likely to eat fruits, vegetables, meats, or fish than nonselective eaters, citing bitter taste and aversive textures as key deterrents (36,37). Additionally, some individuals with selective eating rely as dietary staples on high-carbohydrate foods that are not nutrient dense (38). This limited diet can lead to nutritional deficiencies that must be corrected either through supplementation, or in more extreme cases, enteral feeding (39). A recent case report of ARFID in an adolescent boy documented multiple nutritional deficiencies including low levels of vitamins A, D, E, K, B_{12}, and folate (40), resulting in macrocytic anemia, osteoporosis, and subacute combined degeneration (SCD) of the spinal cord.

In cases of extreme food restriction, the patient may be underweight. Indeed, in one retrospective study of outpatients receiving an initial evaluation at an eating disorder clinic, there was no significant difference in BMI between youth with ARFID versus those with AN (41). Approximately one-third of ARFID patients in an outpatient eating disorder clinic required medical hospital admission due to extreme low weight or unstable vital signs (41). In the same study, bone mineral density (BMD) scores were significantly lower among ARFID patients than among AN patients ($p < 0.001$), with 25% of ARFID patients showing scores in the osteoporotic range.

Comorbidity

ARFID is common among people with ASD; estimates of picky or selective eating are as high as 89% among children with ASD, though the rates of the full ARFID phenotype are unknown. In an eating disorder day treatment program, patients with ARFID showed significantly higher rates of comorbid anxiety disorders compared to those with AN (42). However, another study that also highlighted high rates of psychiatric comorbidity among individuals with ARFID found that, in contrast, those with ARFID were less likely than patients with AN to initiate psychopharmacological interventions (41). Therefore, it is important for clinicians to assess for any comorbid mood disorders and consider appropriate interventions.

Etiology

Multiple etiologies have been proposed for ARFID, though most are speculative, as ARFID is a burgeoning area of research. Behavioral theory, which has focused mainly on child presentations, posits that implicit associations form between the child's behaviors around declining to eat (i.e., arguing, spitting out food) and the desired outcome (i.e., not having to eat the nonpreferred food). That this behavior is reinforced over time makes it difficult to extinguish. For traumatic experiences like vomiting or choking, implicit associations can be formed between the food and the aversive outcome. In extreme cases, this may be difficult to extinguish without clinical attention. In one study of 5,294 children ages 10 to 11 years, children who were identified by their mothers as being "choosy eaters" were more likely to be "supertasters" (or, were more likely to have heightened taste sensitivity and experience taste sensation with more intensity than nonsupertasters) than children who did not self-identify as being choosy eaters (43), highlighting the possibility that biologic differences in taste preferences contribute to ARFID etiology.

Assessment

Compared to those with AN and BN, individuals with ARFID are more likely to be younger and male (44). Three classic phenotypes are associated with ARFID; these correspond to the three examples provided by DSM-5 as follows:

(a) *ARFID with apparent lack of interest in eating or food*: Amit is an 11-year-old boy who often forgets to eat and requires prompting from his parents at mealtimes. When he does eat, he only tolerates small amounts before losing interest, often preferring to engage in other activities (e.g., talking, watching television) during mealtimes. He presents for treatment at the request of his pediatric gastroenterologist, who suggests the use of a feeding tube to ensure adequate caloric intake in the short-term.

(b) *ARFID with avoidance based on the sensory characteristics of food*: Shoshannah is a 28-year-old woman whose intense anxiety and panic around eating results in her eating the same foods every day (e.g., a specific brand and flavor of yogurt for breakfast, plain pasta without sauce for lunch, etc.). She often goes through phases in which she only eats one food (e.g., a specific type of chocolate bar) for several days, and then becomes surfeited of that food, selecting a new preferred food and reinitiating the cycle.

(c) *ARFID with concern about the aversive consequences of eating*: Sarah is a 6-year-old girl who choked on a piece of chicken, developed an intense fear of choking, and subsequently has eaten nothing at all for 6 consecutive days. Due to the extreme weight loss following the food restriction, Sarah requires a brief medical hospitalization for rehydration.

It is important to note that these phenotypes are neither mutually exclusive nor exhaustive. Patients may, and often do, exhibit features from more than one phenotype. At present, ARFID diagnoses do not require a phenotypic specifier in the way that a clinician may characterize AN with a restricting or binge/purge subtype. However, classification is important to assess in a clinical setting, as phenotypic presentations inform treatment modalities.

The PARDI can be used to diagnose ARFID and assess severity and clinical impairment (22). The PARDI includes subscales to establish the degree of similarity with each of the three classic ARFID presentations. Patients receive a score for each subscale, and can be matched with multiple phenotypes if applicable, which is consistent with the nature of ARFID presentations in a clinical setting. ARFID can also be assessed using the EDA-5 (21). As with pica and RD, the EDA-5 assesses diagnostic criteria, but does not assess severity or impairment.

In clinical practice, it is important to ascertain the patient's current food intake on a typical day, including both the range of foods consumed as well as amounts, to fully assess the degree of potential nutritional deficiency (45). Individuals whose diets are quite limited in variety may benefit from blood tests to screen for nutritional deficiency, and those who are underweight may benefit from BMD scans. The clinician should also assess the patient's current weight and height, and, among children, whether there has been a recent drop in BMI centile. Failure to grow as expected for age is a potentially telling sign of inadequate nutrition (38).

Treatment

At present, there is no evidence-based treatment for ARFID, and available data on the effectiveness of specific interventions have focused largely on very young children. In clinical practice, approaches vary widely by discipline. In the absence of evidence for any specific treatment, we suggest that the intensity of any intervention be informed by the severity of nutritional compromise. For example, individuals who are very underweight may require inpatient hospitalization for refeeding, while those who are not underweight may benefit from outpatient care alone. Similarly, those with nutritional deficiencies may benefit from close medical monitoring and vitamin supplementation while they are working to expand their diets. In contrast, we suggest that within any given level of treatment intensity, specific therapeutic interventions be informed by the clinician's assessment of the presenting ARFID phenotype(s):

ARFID with apparent lack of interest in eating or food: Individuals who have diminished appetite or little interest in eating, like Amit, may present at low weight and require interventions designed to increase calorie intake. It is unclear whether evidence-based interventions for adolescent AN (e.g., family-based treatment in which parents take control of renourishing their child) will generalize to ARFID. The potential role of medication is also unknown. Although in clinical practice an appetite stimulant called cyproheptadine (CY) is sometimes used, a recent no-randomized case record review from a pediatric feeding clinic found that patients who took CY gained significant weight over a 6.5-month period, but remained in the underweight range at the end of the study and did not surpass weight gain in an unmedicated control group (46).

ARFID with avoidance based on the sensory characteristics of food: Individuals with heightened sensitivity to the taste or texture of novel foods, like Shoshannah, may present for treatment with a very limited diet and a desire to increase food variety. Motivation for increased food variety can range from counteracting the effects of poor nutrition, to enhancing self-esteem, to increasing opportunities to participate in food-related social activities (45). Techniques for increasing food variety include operant conditioning (a reward-based intervention style) and systematic desensitization (modeling and hierarchical exposures) (47). A recent randomized controlled trial comparing operant conditioning to systematic desensitization for 2 to 6 year olds with selective eating found that, although both groups successfully added 7.9 and 4.7 new foods, respectively, compared to baseline, the two therapies did not differ significantly in terms of efficacy (48). Additionally, a recent case report described an adaptation of FBT in which parents supported their 11-year-old child in increasing the variety of foods consumed through family-oriented food exposure techniques (49).

ARFID with concern about the aversive consequences of eating: Individuals like Sarah who have had a traumatic experience with eating (e.g., choking or vomiting) may present to treatment having omitted foods that are similar to those that led to the aversive experience, or declining to eat altogether. Case reports of treatment for similar presentations have conceptualized this type of avoidance as a phobia and consequently utilized exposure techniques to reintroduce avoided foods (50,51). For example, one case report described the treatment of a 4-year-old boy who limited his intake to oatmeal, soft baby food, water, and protein drinks following a choking incident on partially solid food. He was able to successfully reincorporate solid foods (such as crackers and meats) via graduated exposure to increasingly feared categories of food using both office and in-home visits in order to generalize desired eating behavior across contexts (i.e., home, school, etc.) (52).

CONCLUSION

Although lesser known than other eating disorders, pica, RD, and ARFID can have serious physical and psychosocial consequences that impair both physical health and quality of life for many individuals. At present, there are no tested treatment manuals for any of these disorders, but each is an area of active research inquiry. Meanwhile, a comprehensive assessment is critical, and techniques already familiar to clinicians to treat classical eating disorders, anxiety disorders, low weight, and GI disorders may have heuristic value.

References

1. American Psychiatric Association: *Diagnostic and Statistical Manual of Mental Disorders: DSM-5*. Washington, DC, American Psychiatric Association, 2013.
2. Young S: *Craving Earth: Understanding Pica – The Urge to Eat Clay, Starch, Ice, and Chalk*. New York, Columbia University Press, 2011.
3. American Psychiatric Association: *Diagnostic and Statistical Manual of Mental Disorders: DSM-IV*. Washington, DC, American Psychiatric Association, 1994.
4. Woywodt A, Kiss A: Geophagia: the history of earth-eating. *J R Soc Med* 95:143–146, 2002.
5. Parry-Jones B, Parry-Jones WL: Pica: symptom or eating disorder? A historical assessment. *B J Psych* 160:341–354, 1992.
6. Mills M: Craving more than food: the implications of pica in pregnancy. *Nurs Womens Health* 11:268–273, 2007.
7. Singhi S, Ravishanker R, Singhi P, Nath R: Low plasma zinc and iron in pica. *Indian J Pediatr* 70:139–143, 2003.
8. Khan Y, Tisman G: Pica in iron deficiency: a case series. *J Med Case Rep* 4:86, 2010.
9. Delaney CB, Eddy KT, Hartmann AS, Becker AE, Murray HB, Thomas JJ: The prevalence of pica and rumination behavior among individuals seeking treatment for eating disorders and obesity. *Int J Eat Disord* 48:238–248, 2015.
10. Nchito M, Geissler PW, Mubila L, Friis H, Olsen A: Effects of iron and multimicronutrient supplementation on geophagy: a two-by-two factorial study among Zambian schoolchildren in Lusaka. *Trans R Soc Trop Med Hyg* 98:218–227, 2004.
11. Ali Z: Pica in people with intellectual disability: a literature review of aetiology, epidemiology and complications. *J Intellect Dev Disabil* 26:205–215, 2001.
12. Danford DE, Huber AM: Pica among mentally retarded adults. *Am J Ment Defic* 87:141–146, 1982.
13. Gundogar D, Demir SB, Eren I: Is pica in the spectrum of obsessive-compulsive disorders? *General Hosp Psych* 7:293–294, 2003.
14. Hartmann AS, Becker AE, Hampton C, Bryant-Waugh R: Pica and rumination disorder in DSM-5. *Psychiatr Ann* 42:426–430, 2012.
15. Decker CJ: Pica in the mentally handicapped: a 15-year surgical perspective. *Can J Surg* 36:551–554, 1993.
16. Hartmann AS, Jurilj V: Pica. In: de Vries S, Goldstein S (eds): *Handbook of DSM-5 Childhood Disorders*. Heidelberg, Springer (in press).
17. Rose EA, Porcerelli JH, Neale AV: Pica: common but commonly missed. *J Am Board Fam Pract* 13:353–358, 2000.

18. Mace FC, Knight D: Functional analysis and treatment of severe pica. *J Appl Behav Anal* 19:411, 1986.
19. Singhi S, Singhi P, Adwani GB: Role of psychosocial stress in the cause of pica. *Clin Ped* 20:783–785, 1981.
20. Wasano LC, Borrero JC, Kohn CS: Brief report: a comparison of indirect versus experimental strategies for the assessment of pica. *J Autism Dev Disord* 39:1582–1586, 2009.
21. Sysko R, Glasofer DR, Hildebrandt T, et al.: The eating disorder assessment for DSM-5 (EDA-5): development and validation of a structured interview for feeding and eating disorders. *Int J Eat Disord* 48:452–463, 2015.
22. Bryant-Waugh R, Thomas JJ, Eddy KT, Micali N, Melhuish L, Cresswell L: The development of the Pica, ARFID, and Rumination Disorder Interview (PARDI). Poster presentation at the annual Eating Disorders Research Society conference, New York, NY; 2016.
23. Piazza CC, Fisher WW, Hanley GP, et al.: Treatment of pica through multiple analyses of its reinforcing functions. *J Appl Behav Anal* 31:165–189, 1998.
24. Matson JL, Hattier MA, Belva B, Matson ML: Pica in persons with developmental disabilities: approaches to treatment. *Res Dev Disabil* 34:2564–2571, 2013.
25. Chial HJ, Camilleri M, Williams DE, Litzinger K, Perrault J: Rumination syndrome in children and adolescents: diagnosis, treatment, and prognosis. *Pediatrics* 111:158, 2003.
26. Thomas JJ, Murray HB: Cognitive-behavioral treatment of adult rumination disorder in the setting of disordered eating: a single case experimental design. *Int J Eat Disord* 49(10):967–972, 2016.
27. Tamburrino M, Campbell NB, Franco KN, Evans CL: Rumination in adults: two case histories. *Int J Eat Disord* 17:101–104, 1994.
28. Rajindrajith S, Devanarayana NM, Perera BJ: Rumination syndrome in children and adolescents: a school survey assessing prevalence and symptomatology. *BMC Gastroenterology* 12:1, 2012.
29. Drossman DA, Corazziari E, Delvaux M, et al.: *Rome III: The Functional Gastrointestinal Disorders*. 3rd ed. McLean, VA, Degnon Associates, 2006, pp. 885–893.
30. Fredericks DW, Carr JE, Williams WL: Overview of the treatment of rumination disorder for adults in a residential setting. *J Behav Ther Exp Psy* 29:31–40, 1998.
31. Eckern M, Stevens W, Mitchell J: The relationship between rumination and eating disorders. *Int J Eat Disord* 26:414–419, 1998.
32. Chitkara DK, Van Tilburg M, Whitehead WE, Talley NJ: Teaching diaphragmatic breathing for rumination syndrome. *Am J Gastroenterol* 101:2449–2452, 2006.
33. Steingoetter A, Sauter M, Curcic J, et al.: Volume, distribution and acidity of gastric secretion on and off proton pump inhibitor treatment: a randomized double-blind controlled study in patients with gastro-esophageal reflux disease (GERD) and healthy subjects. *BMC Gastroenterology* 15(1):111, 2015.
34. Wagaman JR, Williams DE, Camilleri M: Behavioral intervention for the treatment of rumination. *J Pediatr Gastroenterol Nutr* 27:596–598, 1998.
35. Eddy K, Thomas JJ, Hastings E, et al.: Prevalence of DSM-5 avoidant/restrictive food intake disorder in a pediatric gastroenterology healthcare network. *Int J Eat Disord* 48(5):464–470, 2014.
36. Galloway AT, Lee Y, Birch LL: Predictors and consequences of food neophobia and pickiness in young girls. *J Am Diet Assoc* 103:692–698, 2003.
37. Dubois L, Farmer AP, Girard M, Peterson K: Preschool children's eating behaviours are related to dietary adequacy and body weight. *Euro J Clin Nutr* 7:846–855, 2006.
38. Carruth BR, Ziegler PJ, Gordon A, Barr SI: Prevalence of 'picky/eaters among infants and toddlers and their caregivers' decision about offering new food. *J Am Diet Assoc* 104:S57–S64, 2004.
39. Williams KE, Hendy HM, Field DG, Belousov Y, Riegel K, Harclerode W: Implications of avoidant/restrictive food intake disorder (ARFID) on children with feeding problems. *Children's Health Care* 44:307–321, 2014.
40. Chandran JJ, Anderson G, Kennedy A, Kohn M, Clarke S: Subacute combined degeneration of the spinal cord in an adolescent male with avoidant/restrictive food intake disorder: a clinical case report. *Int J Eat Disord* 48:1176–1179, 2015.
41. Norris ML, Robinson A, Obeid N, Harrison M, Spettigue W, Henderson K: Exploring avoidant/restrictive food intake disorder in eating disordered patients: a descriptive study. *Int J Eat Disord* 47:495–499, 2014.
42. Nicely TA, Lane-Loney S, Masciulli E, Hollenbeak CS, Ornstein RM: Prevalence of avoidant/restrictive food intake disorder in a cohort of young patients in day treatment for eating disorders. *IntJ Eat Disord* 2:21, 2014.
43. Golding J, Steer C, Emmett P, Bartoshuk LM, Horwood J, Smith GD: Associations between the ability to detect bitter taste, dietary behavior, and growth: a preliminary report. *Ann N Y Acad Sci* 1170:553–557, 2009.
44. Fisher MM, Rosen DS, Ornstein RM, et al.: Avoidant/restrictive food intake disorder: a proposed diagnosis in DSM-5. *J Adol Health* 52:S9, 2013.
45. Bryant-Waugh R: Avoidant restrictive food intake disorder: an illustrative case example. *Int J Eat Disord* 46:420–423, 2013.
46. Sant'Anna A, Hammes PS, Porporino M, Martel C, Zygmuntowicz C, Ramsay M: Use of cyproheptadine in young children with feeding difficulties and poor growth in a pediatric feeding program. *J Pediatr Gastroenterol Nutr* 59:674–678, 2014.
47. Toomey KA: *SOS Basic Training Workshop*. Little Rock, AR, Sponsored by the Sensory Processing Disorder Foundation, December 4–7, 2014.
48. Marshall J, Hill RJ, Ware RS, Ziviani J, Dodrill P: Multidisciplinary intervention for childhood feeding difficulties: a randomized clinical trial. *J Pediatr Gastroenterol Nutr* 60:680–687, 2015.
49. Fitzpatrick KK, Forsberg SE, Colborn D: Family-based therapy for avoidant restrictive food intake disorder: families facing food neophobias. In: Loeb KL, LeGrange D, Lock J (eds): *Family Therapy for Adolescent Eating and Weight Disorders: New Applications (256–276)*. New York, Routledge.
50. Moran DJ, Obrien RM: Competence imagery: a case study treating emetophobia. *Psychol Rep* 96:635–636, 2005.
51. Boschen MJ: Reconceptualizing emetophobia: a cognitive-behavioral formulation and research agenda. *J Anxiety Disord* 21:407–419, 2007.
52. Nock MK: A multiple-baseline evaluation of the treatment of food phobia in a young boy. *J Behav Ther Exp Psychiatry* 33:217–225, 2002.

5.8 ■ SUBSTANCE USE DISORDERS

CHAPTER 5.8 ■ SUBSTANCE USE DISORDERS

CHRISTIAN HOPFER, JESSE D. HINCKLEY, AND PAULA RIGGS

DEFINITION

Substance-related disorders encompass two major categories in *DSM-5*: substance use disorders (SUDs) and substance-induced disorders (SIDs) (1). Substances are divided into 10 classes, including alcohol; caffeine; cannabis; hallucinogens; inhalants; opioids; sedatives, hypnotics, or anxiolytics; stimulants; tobacco; and other or unknown. SUD is defined by cognitive, behavioral, and physiologic symptoms due to continued use of a substance despite significant substance use–related problems. Diagnostic criteria are divided into four central categories: impaired control over substance use (criteria 1 to 4), social impairment due to substance use (criteria 5 to 7), risky use of the substance (criteria 8 to 9), and pharmacologic criteria of tolerance and withdrawal (criteria 10 and 11, respectively). SUD can further be classified by severity based on the number of symptoms endorsed and by course specifiers. SID includes intoxication and withdrawal states, as well as other substance-induced mental disorders, related to each specific substance. Intoxication is defined as a constellation of reversible symptoms that develop during or shortly after recent ingestion of a substance and that are attributable to physiologic effects of the substance on the central nervous system (CNS). Intoxication only applies when symptoms of use result in problematic behavior. Withdrawal is defined as physiologic and cognitive symptoms due to reduction in or cessation of use of a substance that result in problematic behavioral change. In comparison

TABLE 5.8.1

CRITERIA FOR SUBSTANCE USE DISORDER, INTOXICATION, AND WITHDRAWAL

Substance Use Disorder: Two or more within a 12-mo period

Impaired Control
1. Taken in larger amounts or over a longer period than intended
2. Persistent desire or unsuccessful effort to cut down or control use
3. Great deal of time spent to obtain, use, or recover from substance
4. Craving, or strong desire or urge to use

Social Impairment
5. Failure to fulfill major role obligations
6. Continued use despite social or interpersonal problems
7. Reduction in important social, occupational, or recreational activities

Risky Use
8. Recurrent use in physically hazardous situations
9. Continued use despite knowledge of physical or psychological problem

Pharmacologic Effect
10. Tolerance (need for increased amount or diminished effect)
11. Withdrawal (withdrawal syndrome or use to relieve/avoid withdrawal)

Intoxication
A. Recent ingestion
B. Problematic behavior or psychological changes
C. One or more sign or symptom attributable to the substance
D. Not attributable to another medical condition, mental disorder, or substance

Withdrawal
A. Cessation or reduction in heavy, prolonged use
B. Two or more signs or symptoms attributable to cessation or reduction in use
C. Clinically significant distress or impairment in important areas of functioning
D. Not attributable to another medical condition, mental disorder, or substance

to *DSM-IV* "abuse" and "dependence" are enfolded into the diagnostic criteria of SUD. Furthermore, the diagnosis of SID does not require nor preclude the diagnosis of SUD. The criteria for these diagnoses are described in Table 5.8.1.

HISTORY

Use and abuse of substances have been documented throughout history and date back to ancient times. The active ingredients in substances of abuse were initially identified and extracted during the 19th century, leading to an increase in the purity of substances available for consumption as more concentrated formulations were made. Initially, when substances such as opiates or cocaine were first identified, they were either freely available or prescribed widely by physicians and made available through many tonics. The liability of certain substances to result in "addiction" was recognized in the late 19th and early 20th centuries, when laws regulating substances of abuse were introduced. The 1914 Harrison Narcotic Act, which forbade the sale of cocaine or opiates except by licensed physicians or pharmacists, was one of the first laws introduced to regulate substances seen as having a liability for abuse. Also, the widespread perception that alcohol created societal problems led to the Prohibition Amendment of 1919 to the American Constitution, which made alcohol an illegal substance. This amendment, however, was overturned in 1933.

With the creation of the U.S. Federal Bureau of Narcotics (now the Drug Enforcement Administration) in 1930, the federal government took a more active role in regulating drugs and also defining which drugs could be legally purchased, could be available only by prescription, or would be completely banned. Throughout the latter half of the 20th century, major societal changes occurred in the acceptance and use of various substances—including marijuana, tobacco, cocaine, amphetamines, and "designer" drugs such as Ecstasy.

Along with changes in societal views and consumption of various substances came an increased scientific understanding of the mechanisms of actions of most addictive compounds, including the realization that these were binding to specific brain receptor sites. Animal models of addiction established the neurobiologic basis for understanding addiction as a psychiatric illness (2).

EPIDEMIOLOGY

Annual surveys of US adolescents' drug use are conducted by the Monitoring the Future Survey (MTF) (3). Overall, American adolescents over the past decade have been using fewer substances, although there are some exceptions. Alcohol continues to be the most widely used substance among adolescents, with up to two-thirds of students having consumed "more than a few sips" of alcohol by the end of high school. Overall alcohol consumption has declined since the 1980s and is currently at the lowest level since the 1970s. However, lifetime prevalence of having been drunk in 2014 remains 11% among 8th grade and 50% among 12th grade students. Tobacco use has also continued to decline over the past decade and is currently at the lowest level since the 1970s. Thirty-day prevalence of cigarette smoking peaked in 1996–1997, and has fallen by 81%, 77%, and 63% since among 8th, 10th, and 12th grade students, respectively. In 2014, the estimated lifetime prevalence of cigarette use was 14% in 8th grade, 23% in 10th grade, and 34% in 12th grade. Increases in taxes on tobacco products may help explain the further decline in prevalence as perceived risk has remained level over the past decade.

The annual prevalence of using any illicit drug continued to decrease slightly, with the largest decrease among 10th and 12th grade students. Much of this decrease is likely due to a decrease in the annual prevalence of marijuana use over the past decade, though perceived risk of regular marijuana use is also declining. Marijuana remains the most widely used illicit drug among adolescents. While experimentation with alcohol and tobacco declined somewhat, marijuana experimentation increased from 35% in 1991 to a peak of 50% in 1997, and then drifted down again to approximately 45% in 2004. Over the past decade marijuana use prevalence again increased, peaking in 2010 to 2012. Overall roughly a third of twelfth graders reported lifetime experimentation with an illicit substance besides marijuana.

Opioid use is arguably the greatest adolescent and young adult substance use epidemic of the past decade. Illicit use of prescription opioids among 12th grade students nearly tripled from an annual prevalence of 3.3% in 1992 to a peak of 9.4% in 2004, declining to 5.4% in 2015. The annual prevalence of heroin use fell sharply in the latter half of the 1970s and remained steady through 1994. Heroin use again increased in the 1990s,

TABLE 5.8.2

PRIMARY ADMITTING SUBSTANCE OF ABUSE (% OF TOTAL ADMISSIONS), BY AGE, FROM THE TREATMENT EPISODE DATA SET

Substance	Age 12–14 (%)	Age 15–17 (%)	Age 18–19 (%)	Age 20–24 (%)
Other/none	5.9	2.7	2.5	1.9
Alcohol only	6.9	4.3	9.0	11.1
Alcohol + secondary drug	6.4	8.3	11.7	12.3
Opioids, heroin	0.3	2.0	15.3	25.9
Opioids, other	0.8	1.7	6.9	12.1
Cocaine, smoked	0.2	0.2	0.6	1.0
Cocaine, other route	0.2	0.4	0.9	1.3
Marijuana	77.0	75.5	44.2	24.4
Methamphetamine/ amphetamine	1.4	3.7	7.1	8.3
Tranquilizers	0.3	0.5	1.0	1.0
Sedatives	0.1	0.1	0.2	0.1
Hallucinogens	0.2	0.4	0.5	0.2
PCP	<0.05	<0.05	0.1	0.2
Inhalants	0.4	0.1	0.1	0.1
Total percent	100	100	100	100
(Total, *N*)	(17,842)	(83,823)	(54,509)	(244,893)

(From TEDS. *Treatment Episode Data Set: 2003 Highlights. National Admissions to Substance Abuse Treatment Services, DASIS Series: S-27.* Rockville, MD; Services DoHaH (ed); 2005. DHHS Publication No. SMA 05–4043, with permission.)

along with increased use of most drugs, peaking in 2000 among 12th grade students at 1.5%. Prevalence again declined over 2005–2010, with slowing rates of decline in 2011, and have remained level since 2013 at 0.6% among 12th graders. Injection heroin use has also remained relatively stable among adolescents (3). Although the MTF study has found some decline in opiate use from peak levels in high school surveys, a number of other studies demonstrate the depth of the adolescent opiate epidemic. Thus, in 2014 an estimated 467,000 adolescents were using opiates for pain relief, with approximately a third of these having an opiate use disorder. Another estimated 28,000 adolescents used heroin in the past year, and an estimated 18,000 adolescents had a heroin use disorder in 2014 (4).

The most commonly abused substances resulting referral of adolescents to publicly funded substance abuse treatment programs in the United States, by age group, are shown in Table 5.8.2 (5). For the youngest age group (12 to 14), marijuana constitutes the most frequently cited primary admitting substance of abuse. For the older (18 to 20) age group, marijuana and alcohol continue to represent a large portion of treatment admissions, but other illicit substances such as cocaine, methamphetamine, and heroin are more commonly cited as reasons for admission compared with younger adolescents.

While adolescents only represent 6% of the total patient population that accesses substance abuse treatment, 64.6% of all patients report first use of primary substance by 18 years old (5). The vast majority of patients entering treatment for alcohol, alcohol with a secondary drug, or marijuana use endorsed first use in adolescence (78.2%, 87.6%, and 92.1%, respectively). Over half of patients whose primary drug is methamphetamines/amphetamines, hallucinogens, PCP, or inhalants also began use as teenagers, as well as 35.9% of heroin users and 35% users of other opiates. Although initiation and progression to SUD is common during adolescence, only an estimated 10% to 15% of adolescents who could benefit from substance treatment receive it. These findings strongly suggest the importance of improving drug and alcohol screening and developing earlier interventions for substance-involved adolescents and underscores the critical need to increase access and availability of substance treatment for youth and families.

General population surveys of adolescent SUDs indicate clear marked age trends. The prevalence of substance use and SUDs increases almost linearly from early to late adolescence (6). Approximately one in four older adolescents meets criteria for DSM-IV abuse for at least one substance, and one in five meets criteria for DSM-IV dependence (7). Nearly one in three adolescents reports daily smoking and 8.6% meet criteria for tobacco dependence by age 18. Although alcohol is the most commonly abused substance (10%), a slightly larger proportion of adolescents meet criteria for dependence on marijuana (4.3%) than alcohol (3.5%) (6). Additionally, there are gender differences, as males report more substance use than females, and more frequently meet criteria for dependence on alcohol and marijuana in late adolescence, while females are more often nicotine dependent (6). In clinical populations, rates of comorbidity are even higher. Approximately 60% of adolescents in juvenile justice settings and 40% in mental health treatment settings have co-occurring SUD (8) and as many as three-quarters of adolescents with SUD have other nonsubstance psychiatric disorders. The most frequent of these are externalizing disorders, but internalizing disorders are also more prevalent than in the general population. The Methods for the Epidemiology of Child and Adolescent Mental Disorders (MECA) study found past 6-month prevalence for comorbid psychiatric disorders with an adolescent SUD sample to be 76% for any comorbid disorder, 68% for any disruptive behavior disorder, 32% for any mood disorder, and 20% for any anxiety disorder (9).

ETIOLOGY

SUDs can only develop if substances are available for experimentation to occur. However, despite widespread availability of many substances, only a portion of youth experiment, and only a smaller percentage of those who do experiment go on to become regular users or to develop SUDs. Thus, the etiology of SUDs lies in those factors that predispose an individual to experiment with substances, and among experimenters, factors that predict progression to SUD. Although a comprehensive review of these substance-related risk factors is beyond the scope of this chapter, major theories about the etiology of adolescent SUDs are discussed below.

Genetic and Environmental Influences

Twin and adoption studies have demonstrated that considerable shared environmental influences exist for the initiation of substance use, with genetic influences becoming more apparent when environments allow for their expression (10). Thus, for example, Koopmans et al. (11) demonstrated that there were no genetic influences on the liability to initiate alcohol use when adolescents were raised in a religious household, but that 40% of the variation in initiation could be explained by genetic factors when adolescents were raised in a nonreligious household. Genetic influences on the development of adolescent SUDs may act through a direct effect on psychophysiological reactions or subjective effects (12) to substances or their metabolism, or indirectly through genetic effects on personality traits such as behavioral disinhibition, which leads to substance experimentation (13). Thus, genetic factors influence individual risk, but do not account for population-wide shifts in patterns of substance use.

Externalizing Disorders

Externalizing disorders have been shown to be major risk factors predicting the initiation of substance use and the development of abuse and dependence (14–17). Many of the risk factors associated with the development of externalizing disorders similarly predispose to the development of SUDs. Conduct disorder has consistently been shown to be a predictor of substance use initiation (18) and progression toward SUDs (19). Attention-deficit hyperactivity disorder (ADHD) appears to increase risk for developing SUDs somewhat, although there is controversy about the magnitude of the effect of ADHD due to its comorbidity with CD (20). Externalizing disorders and SUDs can also be thought of as influenced by one or more common antecedent risk factors (21).

Stage Theory and the "Gateway" Theory

Stage theory posits that there is a temporal ordering of substance experimentation in which lower-order substances, which are more commonly used, precede the use of higher-order substances. Thus, typically a licit substance, such as alcohol or cigarettes, is used first in a sequence, followed by marijuana, which is usually the first illicit substance before progressing on to use of other illicit substances (22). Related to stage theory is the gateway hypothesis as it relates to marijuana. This posits that the use of marijuana facilitates the entry into other illicit substance use.

A review of the available literature about the effect of marijuana use on other drug use concluded that there is a relationship between marijuana use and progression to other drugs. This effect can be explained by: (1) the selective recruitment to heavy cannabis use of persons with pre-existing traits that predispose to the use of a variety of different drugs (i.e., that marijuana use is a marker for a tendency to use multiple drugs); (2) the affiliation of cannabis users with drug-using peers in settings that provide more opportunities to use other illicit drugs at an earlier age; and (3) that marijuana use results in socialization into an illicit drug subculture which creates favorable attitudes toward the use of other illicit drugs (23). Whether these relationships derived from past studies generalize to an environment where marijuana is legal for adult use is unclear however (24).

Early Onset of Use

Early onset of substance use has been shown to be a strong predictor for the development of SUDs over the lifetime (25). Whether this is due to early use being a marker for other risk factors that predict substance involvement or whether it has a causal effect is unknown. Animal work has suggested that the adolescent brain may be particularly vulnerable to the effects of drug sensitization, providing a possible neurobiologic explanation for the increased incidence of SUDs among those who begin drug use early (26).

Family and Peer Effects

SUDs tend to aggregate in families. This may be in part due to some common genetic influences within families; however, there is substantial evidence of environmental mediation. Parental drug use, as well as drug use by older siblings, is a significant risk factor for the development of adolescent substance use. However, the mechanism of transmission is complex, with individual personality dimensions mediating the effect of sibling and parent influences (27,28). Association with delinquent peers has been one of the hallmarks of the development of adolescent SUDs. However, while the common notion has been that peers create "peer pressure" to consume substances, most studies support the notion that there exists a complex process by which individuals select peer groups, and then in turn influence these, as well as are influenced by them (29).

Biologic Mechanisms in the Etiology of Substance Use Disorders

A large body of animal work has shown that repeated exposure to substances leads to neural adaptations altering the hedonic "tone" of individuals. This tone is reset by substance use so that it is lower over time, resulting in dysphoria and craving when not using, and driving the substance dependence cycle (30). This animal work has been key in demonstrating that all substances of abuse, although acting at different receptors, create a common downstream pathway resulting in neural adaptations that perpetuate the addictive cycle.

Substance-Specific Risks

Although all substances of abuse share common neurologic pathways that are involved in the development of SUDs, there are differences between substances in terms of their addictive potential. The time course toward the development of dependence varies by individual, by substance, and by route of administration. Some substances, such as cocaine, are characterized by a rapid onset of the development of dependence, as for example, 6% of cocaine users develop dependence within one year of experimenting with cocaine (31). In a longitudinal study, Wagner and Anthony (32), for example, demonstrated that whereas some 15% to 16% of cocaine users had developed cocaine dependence within 10 years of first use, the corresponding values were about 8% for marijuana users, and 12% to 13% for alcohol users. There is growing evidence that adolescents may be more vulnerable to addiction compared to adults (26,33). For example, 1/6 adolescents who experiment with marijuana progress to dependence compared to about 1/11 adults (34).

DIAGNOSIS AND CLINICAL FEATURES

The diagnosis of SUD is made primarily through the clinical interview with the adolescent, as well as through obtaining collateral information from parents and teachers. Adolescents are likely to be in a "precontemplative" stage of change and may thus minimize the extent of their substance involvement (35). Establishing rapport with the adolescent is critical in order to increase the chance of self-disclosure of drug use. Early strong therapeutic alliance is facilitated by use of motivational interviewing (MI) style which is characterized by a nonjudgmental, collaborative approach (36).

Of primary clinical concern is the extent or severity of substance involvement, the specific substances that the patient is abusing or dependent on, and the length of time that the pattern has persisted. When an MI approach is taken and the limits of confidentiality are carefully explained to adolescents and parent/guardians, clinicians are much more likely to get an honest history of substance severity along with other behavioral problems.

When conducting an initial assessment with an adolescent for SUDs, the parents or caretakers should ideally be present during the initial interview, including discussion of the parameters and limits of confidentiality, and to obtain relevant developmental and family history. The interview with the parents or caretakers can also be used to obtain a history of the presenting complaint, early development history, and assess family dynamics. However, it is recommended that the substance use history be obtained in a private interview with the adolescent because adolescents' self-reports of drug use have been shown to be more reliable when confidentiality is assured (37). The interviewing technique should be empathic, nonjudgmental, and supportive, using a MI approach to foster development of a strong therapeutic alliance (see http://www.motivationalinterview.org) (36). In general, the substance use history should be obtained with a similar style and sensitivity to obtaining medical/clinical information for any other disorder or evaluation of a medical review of systems. For substances that the adolescent reports using more than five times in his/her lifetime, clinicians should inquire about age of first use or experimentation, age of progression to regular use; peak use, current use (past month); and last use.

Following that, DSM-5 diagnostic criteria for SUD should be assessed to establish which SUDs should be targeted in treatment. Calendar-based timeline follow-back procedures (38) are often used at baseline/intake to better understand the current pattern and severity of substance use prior to treatment initiation. Other important information includes triggers for craving and use; context of use (e.g., with particular peers, or at or before school); perceived motivation for using; positive and negative consequences of use; and current motivation and goals for treatment (39).

Adolescents with SUD commonly meet diagnostic criteria for other psychiatric disorders. Thus, is quite important to obtain a longitudinal development history that enables the clinician to evaluate the temporal relationship between the onset and progression of psychiatric symptoms and the onset and progression of substance use. Use of a lifetime timeline to anchor this information is useful in consideration of differential diagnosis.

SPECIFIC LABORATORY TESTING OF SUBSTANCES—UPDATED

Detection of substances is a key component of SUD diagnosis and treatment. While the technologies to detect specific substances are changing, urinalysis remains the most commonly used method (for the detection of substances). Most commercial laboratories offer standard "panels" that may include the "NIDA 5." These are commonly abused substances that are detected by urinalysis. The NIDA 5 includes marijuana, cocaine, methamphetamine, heroin, and PCP, which were considered the most important substances to detect following passage of the Drug-Free Workplace Act of 1988. Table 5.8.3 shows the detection time of commonly tested substances by urinalysis.

There are a number of substances where urinalysis is ineffective or inefficient: Detection of alcohol use by urinalysis is limited by the quick elimination time of alcohol; similarly, detection of inhalants by urinalysis is ineffective. Detection of alcohol is usually done via breathalyzer. If inhalant abuse is suspected, a commercial product is a Toxtrap that will detect the presence of residual volatile organic compounds. If there is a clinical suspicion of the abuse of hallucinogens, 3,4-methylenedioxymethamphetamine (MDMA), or GHB, usually specific laboratory tests for these must be ordered. Though commonplace, urinalysis of drugs of abuse is further limited in an evolving drug market of synthetic and designer drugs. Many synthetic cannabinoids, opioids, and amphetamines that are now widespread are not detectable by routine analysis (40). Many commonly used medications may result in false-positive detection of amphetamines, including pseudoephedrine, ephedrine, phenylephrine, and beta blockers propranolol and atenolol. Furthermore, doxylamine and dextromethorphan may result in false-positive detection of PCP. Ingestion of poppy seeds or hemp-containing food products may cause false-positive results for opioids and cannabinoids, respectively. Urinalysis may also be subverted by consuming free water (41,42); ingestion of "masking agents," though the concept is controversial (43); and adding adulterants to urine, including common household products ammonia, bleach, hydrogen peroxide, iodine, liquid soap, papain, and vinegar (43–46).

TABLE 5.8.3

URINE SUBSTANCE DETECTION PERIODS (TYPICAL)

Substance	Urine Detection Time
Alcohol	After absorption, decreases by −0.02 g%/hr
Amphetamine	24–72 hrs
Barbiturates	1–2 days
Benzodiazepines	3 days for therapeutic dose
Cannabis (single use)	1–3 days
Cannabis (moderate use)	3–5 days
Cannabis (heavy use)	10 days
Cocaine	24–96 hrs
Codeine/morphine	24–72 hrs
Heroin	24–72 hrs
Methamphetamine	24–72 hrs
PCP	14–30 days
LSD	1.5–5 days

Though urinalyses using immunoassays are considered specific and sensitive, urinalysis for drugs of abuse is less reproducible and may be unreliable when performed using on-site or point-of-care assays (47–49). Furthermore, proper training of personnel performing screening tests may significantly impact outcomes (50). If laboratory testing is going to be used in a legal proceeding, the laboratory must meet certain standards defined in federal law as the Clinical Laboratory Improvement Amendments (CLIA). In addition, for youth with chronic Δ-9 tetrahydrocannabinol (THC) use, a quantitative test is available that will show a decline in use over time, and thus can distinguish current from past use (51).

SUBSTANCE-SPECIFIC CLINICAL FEATURES

While all SUDs have common features that are characterized by the criteria for abuse and dependence, there are substance-specific issues of clinical relevance.

Alcohol

Alcohol is one of the first substances that adolescents usually experiment with, and alcohol use disorders constitute a major proportion of adolescent SUDs (4). The acute effects of alcohol intoxication include sedation, loss of balance, restlessness, slurred speech, decreased heart rate, and lowered blood pressure. Tolerance to alcohol develops with repeated ingestion, and withdrawal symptoms, although rare in adolescents, can be observed. These may include increased heart rate, elevated blood pressure, elevated temperature, vomiting and diarrhea, sweating, and possibly confusion, seizures, delirium, or psychosis. Withdrawal from alcohol can be medically life threatening and may need to be managed in a medically supervised setting. Detection of alcohol use is usually accomplished via breathalyzer, as its detection time in a urinalysis is limited.

Tobacco

The addictive ingredient in tobacco is nicotine, which has been shown to produce dependence in a substantial proportion of users (52). The primary concern with tobacco dependence is the long-term medical sequelae of use, as well as evidence that consumption of tobacco may facilitate the use of other substances. Nicotine is rapidly absorbed through either smoking or chewing and results in CNS stimulation, followed by withdrawal symptoms. It binds to the nicotinic acetylcholine receptors. Blood and brain levels of nicotine increase with each puff of a cigarette, and nicotine accumulates throughout the day. The half-life of nicotine is usually about 2 hours. Withdrawal symptoms from nicotine typically include craving, irritability, difficulty concentrating, and possibly anxiety and depressed mood.

Marijuana

Marijuana use disorders accounts for the largest proportion of adolescent SUDs (4) and recent changes in state-by-state marijuana policies have multiple implications for adolescents (24). There is mixed evidence regarding the effect of medical marijuana laws on adolescent marijuana use, with some evidence that states that enacted laws already had more liberal attitudes toward marijuana consumption (53–55). However, commercialization allowing operation of dispensaries is associated with increased use and decreased perceived risk among adolescents and young adults (56). Laws legalizing and regulating the marijuana industry also do not provide guidelines for potency or set limits on maximum potency of marijuana products (57). Thus, commercialized marijuana products have higher potency based on strain and can be further concentrated in edibles or other products than marijuana purchased on the black market. Medical marijuana is also diverted to adolescents (58,59). Treatment-seeking teens who reported diversion of marijuana were also more likely to report easy availability, no friend disapproval of regular marijuana use, increased use, and more substance use problems (58).

There is a paucity of data on the impact of state laws legalizing recreational marijuana in the United States. Two approaches to decriminalize marijuana possession have been implemented regionally in Europe and elsewhere: depenalization and legalization (60). Legalization of recreational marijuana provides a path to commercialize marijuana sales, which subsequently is associated with decreased risk perception and increased access and use similar to medical marijuana commercialization. Among US high school seniors, 10% of non–marijuana-using students and 18% of lifetime marijuana-using students report intent to initiate or increase use of marijuana, respectively, if recreational marijuana was legalized. Thus, policies decriminalizing recreational marijuana use in the United States are likely to have varying effect determined by approach, limitations, and implementation.

As marijuana policies have evolved over the last decade, much has been learned about marijuana's effect on the brain and development. The active ingredient in marijuana is A-9 tetrahydrocannabinol (THC). THC binds to the cannabinoid receptor (CNR1), which is broadly distributed throughout the CNS. The endogenous cannabinoid system is an important neurotransmitter system involved in memory formation, appetite regulation, and coordinated movement. Brain development continues through adolescents, with increases in white matter volume and development of functional connectivity underlying tasks such as executive function (61,62). Analysis of the Dunedin Study (prospective cohort of 1,037 individuals followed from birth to 38 years old) showed that persistent marijuana use in adolescence was associated with a decline in intelligence quotient (IQ) among multiple domains (63). IQ did not fully recover after cessation, which is consistent with previous research demonstrating persistent neuropsychological deficits in executive function and psychomotor speed tests during prolonged periods of abstinence (64–66). Longitudinal functional MRI (fMRI) analysis of treatment-seeking adolescents and healthy controls demonstrated a dose-related decrease in functional connectivity of cortices essential for executive functioning over time (67). High amounts of marijuana use was also associated with lower IQ and slower cognitive function.

Marijuana has a range of effects on the user, consistent with the widespread distribution of the CNR1 receptor. It may have sedative, analgesic, hallucinogenic, appetite-enhancing, and anxiolytic properties for the user. It usually results in a relatively short-lived intoxication state, often characterized as euphoria. THC intoxication impairs cognitive and psychomotor performance, although it is unclear currently if these effects persist after abstinence. There is also increasing evidence that marijuana use may be a causal factor in the development of other psychiatric disorders. In particular, evidence points to marijuana use increasing the risk for developing psychosis, as well as other psychiatric disorders (34). It remains unclear how higher-potency marijuana products will affect prevalence and severity of cannabis-induced psychiatric disorders. Cannabis withdrawal syndrome, which is now recognized in *DSM-5* consists of including irritability, anger, aggression, anxiety, sleep disturbance, restlessness, and depressed mood (1,68).

Opiates

Heroin use and abuse of prescription opiates has risen during the past two decades. Adolescents are commonly exposed to prescription opioids, with an estimated one in four high school seniors in the United States endorsing use of these drugs either medically or nonmedically between 2007 and 2009 (69). In a recent epidemiologic study, 12.9% of high school seniors report nonmedical use of prescription opioids, of whom over half were given the drugs for free by friends or relatives (69). Another survey of 14- to 20-year-old patients at university-affiliated emergency departments found that 8.7% report nonprescription opioid use (70). Furthermore, ambulatory opioid prescriptions for adolescents and young adults nearly doubled between 1994 and 2007, including for noninjury encounters (71).

Regional studies from across the United States estimate 39% to 86% of young adults used nonmedical opioids prior to transitioning to heroin (72–77). As shown in analysis of 2011–2013 national data, frequent nonmedical opioid use is the most significant risk factor for heroin use (odds ratio 40, 95% CI 24.6–65.3) (78). However, the conversion rate to heroin has remained low overall. The price of heroin has decreased ($465 in 2012 per gram compared to $2,690 per gram in 1982) and more readily available (78–80). The increasing purity of heroin has made it possible to smoke or snort it, and this has led to an increase in its use over the past decade among adolescents. Heroin dependence in adolescents is typically associated with a rapid psychosocial decline, school failure, criminal behaviors, and family problems (81). The intense pleasurable effects of heroin are largely responsible for the addictive potential of heroin and tolerance may develop rapidly.

Unintentional death due to opioid overdose has been on the rise over the past 30 years, with the most dramatic increases in over the past decade (82). This rise in opioid deaths contributed significantly to unintentional overdose becoming the second most common cause of accidental death in the United States by 2007. Designer opioid drugs are up to 1,000 times more potent than heroin, with frequent changes in formulation (83,84). Furthermore, heroin is often adulterated with various agents, including prescription drugs, resulting in compounds that differ in final concentration by up to 20-fold (85). Thus, opioid use is more likely to result in unintentional overdose than abuse of other substances.

Opioid ingestion affects multiple organ systems and can result in a life-threatening toxidrome. Intoxication may produce analgesia, euphoria, or dysphoria. Physical symptoms often include miosis, flushing, nausea, emesis, and constipation. Co-ingestion of contaminants such as cocaine or anticholinergics may cause mydriasis or normal pupils confusing the clinical picture. Opioids cause both CNS and respiratory depression, ranging from altered mental status and bradypnea or hypopnea to coma, apnea, and noncardiogenic pulmonary edema. Patients may also have bradycardia, hypotension, cardiac arrhythmias, or seizures. Arrhythmias are caused by opioid effects on ion channels within the heart or contaminants mixed with opioids. Early stages of opioid withdrawal manifest as anxiety, insomnia, restlessness, diaphoresis, abdominal discomfort, and rhinorrhea. Symptoms of fevers, chills, emesis, diarrhea, muscle spasms, and tremors may persist for 3 days after last ingestion. Other clinical signs of withdrawal include tachycardia, hypertension, and tachypnea.

Cocaine

Physical effects of cocaine use include constricted blood vessels, dilated pupils, increased temperature, heart rate, and blood pressure. The duration of cocaine's euphoric effects, which include hyperstimulation, reduced fatigue, and mental clarity, depends on the route of administration. The faster the absorption, the more intense the high and the shorter the duration. The high from snorting may last 15 to 30 minutes, while that from smoking may last 5 to 10 minutes.

Amphetamines

Methamphetamine is known by a variety of street names including ice, speed, crystal, glass, and crank. It is an addictive stimulant that can be smoked, injected, or inhaled. Its use is associated with major health consequences, including memory loss, aggression, violence and psychotic behavior, and neuropsychological deficits (86). Similar to cocaine, dependence can develop quickly and be associated with rapid psychosocial decline. The physical effects of acute intoxication include increased wakefulness, increased physical activity, decreased appetite, increased respiration, hyperthermia, and euphoria. Convulsions and seizures may occur.

MDMA

Past year use of MDMA, or ecstasy, surged in the early 2000s to its highest prevalence, subsiding by 2004. Over the past decade MDMA past year prevalence peaked again in 2010, subsequently declining to 0.9%, 2.3%, and 3.6% of 8th, 10th, and 12th grade students in 2014 (3). This represents all-time lows among adolescents less than 16 years old. MDMA is a synthetic drug with both psychedelic and stimulant effects. In the past, some therapists in the United States used the drug to facilitate psychotherapy. In 1988, however, MDMA became a Schedule I substance under the Controlled Substances Act. MDMA is a stimulant usually taken orally in pill form and whose psychedelic effects can last between 4 and 6 hours. The psychological effects of MDMA include confusion, depression, anxiety, sleeplessness, and paranoia. Physical effects may include muscle tension, involuntary teeth clenching, nausea, blurred vision, feeling faint, tremors, rapid eye movement, and sweating or chills. In rare cases, severe hyperthermia may develop. The epidemiologic evidence suggests that most users do not develop dependence upon MDMA and that its use spontaneously remits in the early 20s. However, a minority of users, primarily those who meet dependence symptoms, will continue to use MDMA (87).

GHB

Approximately 2% of US high school seniors reported using gamma hydroxy butyrate (GHB) within the past year (8). GHB is known by such street names such as "grievous bodily harm," "G," or "liquid ecstasy." It is a CNS depressant originally sold in health food stores as a muscle growth agent. The effects of GHB have been described as being similar to those of alcohol, except that periods of unconsciousness appear to be more frequent and unpredictable. Effects usually last about 4 hours. Some users report developing dependence upon GHB and experience rebound symptoms, with features similar to benzodiazepine withdrawal.

Inhalants

Approximately 5% of US high school students reports having tried inhalants at least once in the past year (3); however, rates of inhalant abuse or dependence are much lower, as only 0.1% of adolescents report abuse or dependence upon inhalants (88). Inhalants are volatile organic compounds that include many gases and fumes that are deliberately taken in order to achieve intoxication. Their abuse is more common among young adolescents, since these are some of the first substances available to them. Inhalants may be taken by directly spraying them into the mouth, "huffed"—meaning that the substance is held in a cloth and several breaths are taken, or "bagged"—meaning that the vapors are inhaled from a bag. The acute effects of inhalant intoxication resemble alcohol intoxication in that the youth often experiences acute euphoria and disorientation, which may be followed by a period of drowsiness, as inhalants are CNS depressants. Because inhalants encompass a wide range of possible compounds, it is not possible to cover all aspects of their presentation. However, inhalant use may quickly result in neurologic sequelae and persistent use has been associated with white matter changes and loss of cognitive performance. Due to the neurotoxicity of inhalants, any use must be taken seriously.

Steroids

Approximately 0.6% to 2.0% of male US high school students report having used anabolic steroids within the past year, which is down by approximately half among younger adolescents over the past decade (3). Steroids are used generally not in order to achieve an immediate pleasurable effect, but in order to increase muscle mass, and thereby body image. Thus, the abuse of steroids differs from abuse of other substances, which are usually taken because of their immediate, rewarding effects. Steroids are typically taken in order to achieve a long-term goal: improved body image or physical performance.

Anabolic steroids are usually taken in "cycles" and typically combined with weight-lifting regimens. There are numerous medical consequences of administering exogenous steroids, including premature growth stoppage and either shrinking testicles for men or the development of male sexual characteristics for women. In addition, mood swings or psychotic episodes may result from steroid abuse. Details of the medical and psychiatric sequelae are described by Brown (89).

COURSE AND PROGNOSIS

The course and prognosis of SUDs is varied. Earlier onset, more severe substance use, and comorbid conditions predict a more severe course and outcome. In general, substance disorder implies a chronic, relapsing condition.

Treatment

Treatment for adolescent SUDs involves recognizing that these are chronic relapsing conditions. Patients may need multiple episodes of treatment over time. Treatment typically involves initial attempts to create abstinence or markedly reduced drug use, a period of addressing the biopsychosocial aspects of SUDs, and a maintenance or "relapse prevention" phase. Adolescents usually do not self-refer for treatment, but are often pressured into treatment by family, school, or court. They often present as defiant, or minimizing of their drug use. The primary initial goals of treatment are to engage the adolescent and the family in processes that interrupt drug-seeking and drug-using behaviors and to replace these with prosocial behaviors. A variety of evidence-based approaches have been shown to be successful. Typically, effective treatments are multimodal and address individual, family, peer, and other social environment domains simultaneously. Pharmacotherapy may be an important component for certain SUDs, as well as comorbid conditions.

Specific Therapeutic Approaches

Motivational Interviewing

Motivational enhancement techniques have been demonstrated to promote treatment engagement and can be used to establish a strong treatment alliance and to elicit patient-generated treatment goals (90). This approach increases the patient's motivation to change by increasing the frequency and strength of "change talk," which in turn is positively correlated with making behavioral changes. Adolescents are generally resistant to more directive, confrontational approaches and are often ambivalent and relatively unmotivated for treatment, making motivational approaches critical. MI principles can be effectively used in conjunction with cognitive-behavioral or family-based treatment (91,92).

Cognitive-Behavioral Therapy

Cognitive-behavioral therapy (CBT), based on learning theory, also has been shown to be effective in treating adolescent SUDs (93). Treatment manuals have been developed for courses of weekly CBT treatment ranging from 5 to 16 weeks. Both group and individual format CBT have been shown to reduce adolescent SA and improve related behavior problems (94). However, individual CBT has more consistently been associated with sustained or even emerging treatment effect size (92). CBT typically relies on a "functional analysis" that identifies reinforcers of substance use as well as competing behaviors, skills deficits, and specific cognitive distortions associated with substance use. An important feature of CBT is its emphasis on skills training used to enhance coping strategies to deal effectively with drug cravings, regulate negative mood states, avoid high-risk situations; and strengthen problem solving and communication skills (95).

Family and Multisystemic Therapies

A range of family-based therapies have been shown to be successful in treating adolescent SUDs. Family and multisystemic therapies all treat adolescents within the context of their environment, and try to modify multiple environmental factors contributing to SUDs (96). These approaches have been widely studied and shown to be effective for adolescent SUDs. Multisystemic therapy is an approach that addresses social and family influences of drug use and associated antisocial behaviors. Therapists make frequent home visits and are available on a full-time basis to families. Henggeler et al. (97) demonstrated that over 98% of youth receiving MST remained in treatment, compared to very few youth in a control group accessing treatment. Other approaches include brief strategic family therapy, which is a less intensive approach and can be delivered through weekly office visits. Other family therapies include multidimensional family therapy (98), which has also reported positive outcomes in controlled, randomized trials.

Community Reinforcement and Behavioral Approaches

Community reinforcement therapy is a skills-based approach to treatment that focuses largely on changing environmental factors in the community in order that nonusing behaviors be rewarded. A manual has been developed for the treatment of adolescent cannabis use (the most common presentation for adolescents with SUDs), and is available from the Substance Abuse and Mental Health Services Administration. This approach, and similar ones that focus on altering environmental rewards for drug use and non–drug-using behaviors, has been shown to be superior to a supportive model (99). The primary goal of these approaches is to promote abstinence by altering the conditions that promote substance use. Typically, therapists conduct a functional analysis of substance use that identifies antecedents to drug use, actual behaviors, and positive and negative consequences of substance use. Therapists aim to promote positive social activities that are not compatible with drug use and improve relationships with family members. The primary goal with parents is to motivate them to participate in the community reinforcement process and to teach the family members skills to promote abstinence and discourage drug use. Furthermore, other systems such as school or probation may be engaged in order to affect their behavior to promote adolescent abstinence. Waldron et al. (91) demonstrated that it was possible to engage 71% of treatment-resistant youth in treatment using a community-reinforcement family therapy model. Both parents and youth showed significant improvements in multiple domains of functioning and significant reduction in drug use for the youth who participated in treatment.

Contingency Management

Contingency management (CM) is based on well-established principles of behavioral reinforcement. The use of CM in the treatment of addiction has shifted away from negative reinforcement approaches (e.g., confrontation, punishment) and toward more positive reinforcement approaches. For example, abstinence is often reinforced by providing tangible rewards (vouchers or opportunities to draw for prizes) for urine drug screens. Numerous studies in adults and an increasing number of adolescent studies show higher rates of abstinence when CM is added to other psychosocial substance treatment interventions (100–102). For example, most adolescent psychosocial substance treatment interventions report that 10% to 30% achieve abstinence during treatment compared to approximately 50% with the addition of CM/abstinence-based incentives (101,103). The addition of contingencies can help retain adolescents in treatment as well as improve outcomes (104,105).

Pharmacotherapies

For many SUDs, there are no effective pharmacotherapies. However, for the abuse of alcohol, nicotine, and opioids, there are effective pharmacotherapies. In addition, comorbid conditions may often be the target of pharmacotherapy. These are described in Tables 5.8.4 and 5.8.5.

Integrated Mental Health and Addiction Treatment Principles

Taken together, current research indicates that most adolescents with SUD have other nonsubstance psychiatric disorders and poorer substance treatment outcomes compared to noncomorbid youth with SUD. There is also considerable consensus among both researchers and clinicians that treatment for co-occurring disorders should be integrated or concurrent treatment. Despite practice parameters recommending integrated treatment (116), existing evidence-based substance treatment interventions and most adolescent substance treatment programs do not systematically assess or concurrently treat co-occurring substance and other psychiatric disorders. Progress toward integrated mental health and substance treatment has been impeded by the lack of dually trained clinicians, systemic and economic barriers, and limited research to guide integrated treatment approaches.

TABLE 5.8.4

COMMON COMORBID DISORDERS PHARMACOTHERAPY FOR ADOLESCENTS WITH A SUBSTANCE USE DISORDER

Comorbid Disorder	Effective Treatment for Adolescents without SUD	Impact of Treatment on Adolescents with SUD
Attention-deficit hyperactivity disorder (ADHD)	• First line: pharmacotherapy (generally; psychostimulants) • Medication options with low abuse potential: pemoline, bupropion, atomoxetine	**One controlled trial of pemoline (Riggs et al., 2004 (106); *N* = 69) suggests:** • Efficacy for ADHD despite nonabstinence • Good safety profile in 12-wk trial; potential for hepatotoxicity, relative contraindication for pemoline • No decrease (or increase) in drug use in the absence of specific behavioral intervention for SUD • Potential for hepatoxicity relative contraindication for pemoline given other current options • Clonidine relatively contraindicated
Bipolar disorder	• First line: pharmacotherapy • Mood stabilizers (lithium, valproic acid, carbamazepine)	**One randomized controlled trial of lithium in adolescents with SUD and comorbid bipolar (Geller et al., 1998 (107); *N* = 25) suggests:** • Efficacy and reasonable safety for bipolar disorder despite nonabstinence • Not adequate as an effective treatment for SUD in the absence of specific behavioral treatment for SUD
Depression	• First line: combined pharmacotherapy and psychotherapy • Pharmacotherapy: SSRIs (> support, fluoxetine) in adolescents without SUD • Psychotherapy: cognitive-behavioral therapy (CBT) and interpersonal psychotherapy, combined with medication for severe depression fluoxetine + CBT > efficacy than either alone (TADS study March/TADS team 2004, *JAMA*) (108)	**One randomized controlled trial of fluoxetine in adolescents with SUD and comorbid MDD + CBT for SUD (Riggs et al. (109); *N* = 126) suggests:** • Efficacy for depression despite nonabstinence (16-wk trial) • Good safety profile. • High rate of depression remission in both fluoxetine and placebo-treated subjects suggests that CBT also + impact on depression despite focus on drug abuse, not depression • Remission of depression, regardless of medication assignment, was a more important predictor of decreased drug use than fluoxetine vs. placebo • Remitters drug use decreased significantly; nonremitters had no change in drug use • Tricyclics relatively contraindicated in adolescents with SUD (e.g., arrhythmias; anticholinergic adverse effects)
Anxiety disorder (often comorbid with depressive disorders)	• First line: combined psychotherapy (CBT) and pharmacotherapy (> evidence, SSRIs)	**40% of adolescents in aforementioned controlled trial of fluoxetine for MDD in adolescents with SUD (Riggs et al., 109) suggests:** • Fluoxetine efficacy and safety in reducing symptoms of anxiety in depressed, substance-dependent adolescents with significant anxiety symptoms and/or anxiety disorders (GAD, SAD, PTSD) • No difference in depression and drug use outcomes comparing those with and without anxiety disorders

TABLE 5.8.5

PHARMACOTHERAPIES FOR ADOLESCENT SUBSTANCE USE DISORDER

Substance	Medication	Dose	Comments
Alcohol	Disulfiram	250 mg po qd or 500 mg po qod	FDA approved for alcohol dependence in adults Carroll et al. (110) showed that, in adults, it was also effective for cocaine dependence when alcohol involved
	Acamprosate	1–4 g per day given in a tid dosing schedule	FDA approved for alcohol dependence in adults. One study (Niederhofer and Steffan (111); *N* = 26) suggests similar efficacy in adolescents as for adults
	Naltrexone	50 mg po qd, also available in injection form	FDA approved for alcohol dependence in adults. Deas et al. (112) showed in open-label trial (*N* = 5) that it was safe and well tolerated
	Topiramate	25–300 mg po qd	Not FDA approved yet. Review by Johnson (113) indicates effectiveness for adults
Nicotine	Bupropion	100–300 mg po qd	FDA approved for smoking cessation in adults
	Nicotine patch	Varies depending upon product	
Opiates	Methadone	Varies	Adolescents under 18 must have two documented failures at drug-free detoxification. Needs to be prescribed at a certified clinic. See Hopfer et al. (114).
	Buprenorphine	8–32 mg	Marsch et al. (115) showed effectiveness for adolescent detoxification in randomized controlled trial. However, consider maintenance therapy.
	Naltrexone	50 mg po qd	Low compliance without monitoring. Injectable form has been approved and is available (Vivitrol).

However, in the context of national healthcare reform (e.g., Affordable Care Act, 2010; Mental Health and Addiction Parity Act, 2008) there are early signs of progress toward greater integration of mental health and addiction treatment and behavioral health integration within mainstream medical care. There has also been progress in research that informs the development of integrated treatment models, including a handful of controlled pharmacotherapy and behavioral treatment trials of adolescents with SUD and other psychiatric comorbidities. Taken together, results of these studies, summarized below, provide an important foundation from which research-based principles for integrated treatment can be derived.

Only a handful of controlled pharmacotherapy and behavioral intervention trials have been conducted in adolescents with co-occurring substance and nonsubstance psychiatric disorders. The strikingly similar results of three similarly designed studies are particularly informative and relevant to integrated treatment principles. In the first study, 126 adolescents (ages 13 to 17) meeting DSM-IV diagnostic criteria for major depressive disorder (MDD), lifetime conduct disorder (CD), and at least one nontobacco SUD were randomized to 20 mg daily dose of fluoxetine or matching placebo. Participants in both groups received weekly, individual MET/CBT as outpatient substance treatment throughout the 16-week medication trial. Fluoxetine showed greater efficacy compared to placebo on reductions in Childhood Depression Rating Scale-Revised (CDRS-R) scores (primary outcome measure). Reductions in substance use were clinically and statistically significant in both groups but not different between groups (109).

Rates of depression remission (defined as final CDRS-R raw score ≤28) were unexpectedly high in both the fluoxetine (70%) and placebo (52%) treatment groups. This led investigators to speculate that CBT (targeting substance abuse), received by participants in both groups, may have contributed to depression treatment response despite its primary focus on substance abuse. Similar findings have been reported in adult studies including a meta-analysis of controlled antidepressant medication trials (mostly serotonin reuptake inhibitors/SSRIs) in adults with co-occurring depression and SUD. The authors concluded that mixed findings across studies were due to an unusually high "placebo response rate" especially in the studies in which participants concurrently received individual CBT as outpatient substance treatment (40,41).

Two similarly designed controlled trials of pharmacotherapy for ADHD in adolescents with SUD reported similar results. The first was a multi-site placebo-controlled trial of Osmotic-Release Methylphenidate (OROS-MPH) conducted in the NIDA Clinical Trials Network (CTN). In this study, 303 adolescents (ages 13 to 17) meeting DSM-IV diagnostic criteria for ADHD and SUD were randomized to OROS-MPH or matching placebo across 11 participating sites. Adolescent participants assigned to both groups received individual, manual-standardized MET/CBT as outpatient substance treatment throughout the 16-week medication trial. Results showed significant reductions in ADHD symptom severity and substance use in both groups but no difference between groups on either the primary ADHD (ADHD-RS) or primary substance (change in days of past 28-day substance use) outcome measures. Some secondary outcome measures suggested "added benefit" with OROS-MPH compared to placebo treatment. Specifically, participants treated with OROS-MPH reported greater improvement in their problem-solving and coping skills related to substance use and had more negative urine drug screens compared to participants in the placebo group (43).

A similarly designed randomized controlled trial of atomoxetine versus placebo in 70 adolescents (ages 13 to 18) with ADHD and SUD reported similar findings. Participants in both groups received individual MET/CBT as outpatient substance treatment throughout the 12-week medication trial. Both groups showed significant and comparable reductions in ADHD symptom severity (ADHD-RS) and substance use (days of past 28-day substance use) but no difference between groups on either primary outcome measure (44).

The higher than expected placebo response rates in both of these adolescent studies led authors to speculate about the potential contribution of CBT to ADHD symptom reduction. Similar findings have been reported in adult studies. For example, in a 12-week, 3-arm trial comparing methylphenidate (MPH), bupropion, or placebo for ADHD in adults receiving concurrent CBT (outpatient SUD treatment), all groups showed significant reductions in ADHD symptoms but no difference between active medication and placebo groups (45).

Two other placebo-controlled trials of MPH for ADHD in cocaine-dependent adults also reported no greater improvement in ADHD with MPH treatment compared to placebo in the context of concurrent weekly CBT (outpatient substance treatment) (46,47). This is in contrast to two randomized placebo-controlled trials of pemoline (adolescent study) and atomoxetine (adult study) reporting moderately greater efficacy for active medication compared to placebo for ADHD in participants who did not receive concurrent CBT or other psychosocial substance treatment during these trials (48,49).

Implications for Integrated Mental Health/Substance Treatment

Taken together, results of these studies have important implications for clinical practice and provide a foundation for deriving research-based principles for integrating the treatment of SUD and other co-occurring psychiatric disorders:

1. Each of these studies utilized a standardized and comprehensive semi-structured diagnostic interview to determine substance and other psychiatric diagnoses at baseline.
2. Based on psychiatric diagnosis (e.g., MDD/CDRS-R; ADHD/ADHD-RS) psychometrically valid and clinically informative measures of psychiatric symptom severity were administered at baseline and repeated at least monthly throughout treatment to monitor changes in psychiatric symptom severity in response to treatment.
3. Changes in substance use was assessed at baseline and throughout treatment using standard TLFB procedures based on self-reports. Urine drug screens were also obtained at baseline and weekly during treatment as a biologic measure of substance use.
4. The medications used in the aforementioned trials (i.e., fluoxetine, OROS-MPH, atomoxetine) demonstrated relatively good safety profiles, despite nonabstinence in most participants, in the context of concurrent participation in substance treatment and regular safety monitoring. This suggests that these medications may be considered to treat co-occurring depression or ADHD if psychiatric symptoms are not significantly improving during the first month of substance treatment, even in patients who have not yet achieved abstinence.

Finally, the consistency of findings across adolescent and adult studies showing significant reductions in psychiatric symptom severity or high "placebo response rates" in the context of substance treatment with individual CBT warrants additional research and studies specifically designed to determine the separate and combined contribution of CBT (targeting SUD) to treatment response for other (nonsubstance) co-occurring psychiatric disorders.

CONCLUSION

Adolescent substance use present in a myriad number of ways in clinical settings. Often the use of substances may complicate the assessment or treatment of another psychiatric conditions and the primary clinical task is to establish whether a use disorder exists. In other contexts, the substance use disorder is primary and potentially life threatening. Placement criteria developed by the American Society of Addiction Medicine are commonly used to determine level of care (117). While the mainstay of treatment consists of multimodal psychosocial treatments, pharmacotherapy has an important role in the management of co-occurring psychiatric disorders, nicotine and alcohol use disorders, as well as for opiate use disorders, where pharmacotherapy (either agonist or antagonist) is the standard of care.

References

1. Association AP: *Diagnostic and Statistical Manual of Mental Disorders, Fifth Edition.* Arlington, VA, American Psychiatric Publishing, 2013.
2. Volkow ND, Koob GF, McLellan AT: Neurobiologic advances from the brain disease model of addiction. *N Engl J Med* 374(4):363–371, 2016.
3. Johnston LD, O'Malley PM, Miech RA, Bachman JG, Schulenberg JE: *Monitoring the Future National Survey Results on Drug Use: 1975–2015: Overview, Key Findings on Adolescent Drug Use.* Ann Arbor, The University of Michigan, 2016.
4. SAMHSA: *Behavioral Health Trends in the United States: Results from the 2014 National Survey on Drug Use and Health.* 2015. Available at: http://www.samhsa.gov/data/sites/default/files/NSDUH-FRR1-2014/NSDUH-FRR1-2014.pdf. Accessed January 11, 2016.
5. Substance Abuse and Mental Health Services Administration CfBHSaQ: *Treatment Episode Data Set (TEDS): 2003–2013. National Admissions to Substance Abuse Treatment Services.* Rockville, MD: Substance Abuse and Mental Health Services Administration; 2015.
6. Young SE, Corley RP, Stallings MC, Rhee SH, Crowley TJ, Hewitt JK: Substance use, abuse and dependence in adolescence: prevalence, symptom profiles and correlates. *Drug Alcohol Depend* 68(3):309–322, 2002.
7. Harrison PA, Fulkerson JA, Beebe TJ: DSM-IV substance use disorder criteria for adolescents: a critical examination based on a statewide school survey. *Am J Psychiatry* 155(4):486–492, 1998.
8. Aarons GA, Brown SA, Hough RL, Garland AF, Wood PA: Prevalence of adolescent substance use disorders across five sectors of care. *J Am Acad Child Adolesc Psychiatry* 40(4):419–426, 2001.
9. Kandel DB, Johnson JG, Bird HR, et al.: Psychiatric comorbidity among adolescents with substance use disorders: findings from the MECA Study. *J Am Acad Child Adolesc Psychiatry* 38(6):693–699, 1999.
10. Hopfer CJ, Crowley TJ, Hewitt JK: Review of twin and adoption studies of adolescent substance use. *J Am Acad Child Adolesc Psychiatry* 42(6):710–719, 2003.
11. Koopmans JR, Slutske WS, van Baal GC, Boomsma DI: The influence of religion on alcohol use initiation: evidence for genotype X environment interaction. *Behav Genet* 29(6):445–453, 1999.
12. Haberstick BC, Zeiger JS, Corley RP, et al.: Common and drug-specific genetic influences on subjective effects to alcohol, tobacco and marijuana use. *Addiction* 106(1):215–224, 2011.
13. McGue M, Iacono WG: The adolescent origins of substance use disorders. *Int J Methods Psychiatr Res* 17 Suppl 1:S30–S38, 2008.
14. Iacono WG, Malone SM, McGue M: Substance use disorders, externalizing psychopathology, and P300 event-related potential amplitude. *Int J Psychophysiol* 48(2):147–178, 2003.
15. Kirisci L, Tarter R, Ridenour T, Reynolds M, Horner M, Vanyukov M: Externalizing behavior and emotion dysregulation are indicators of transmissible risk for substance use disorder. *Addict Behav* 42:57–62, 2015.
16. Magallon-Neri E, Diaz R, Forns M, Goti J, Castro-Fornieles J: Personality psychopathology, drug use and psychological symptoms in adolescents with substance use disorders and community controls. *Peer J* 3:e992, 2015.
17. Salom CL, Betts KS, Williams GM, Najman JM, Alati R: Predictors of comorbid polysubstance use and mental health disorders in young adults—a latent class analysis. *Addiction* 111(1):156–164, 2016.
18. Hopfer C, Salomonsen-Sautel S, Mikulich-Gilbertson S, et al.: Conduct disorder and initiation of substance use: a prospective longitudinal study. *J Am Acad Child Adolesc Psychiatry* 52(5):511–518.e514, 2013.
19. Brook DW, Brook JS, Zhang C, Koppel J: Association between attention-deficit/hyperactivity disorder in adolescence and substance use disorders in adulthood. *Arch Pediatr Adolesc Med* 164(10):930–934, 2010.
20. Disney ER, Elkins IJ, McGue M, Iacono WG: Effects of ADHD, conduct disorder, and gender on substance use and abuse in adolescence. *Am J Psychiatry* 156(10):1515–1521, 1999.
21. McGue M, Iacono WG, Legrand LN, Malone S, Elkins I: Origins and consequences of age at first drink. I. Associations with substance-use disorders, disinhibitory behavior and psychopathology, and P3 amplitude. *Alcohol Clin Exp Res* 25(8):1156–1165, 2001.
22. Kandel DB, Yamaguchi K, Chen K: Stages of progression in drug involvement from adolescence to adulthood: further evidence for the gateway theory. *J Stud Alcohol* 53(5):447–457, 1992.
23. Hall WD, Lynskey M: Is cannabis a gateway drug? Testing hypotheses about the relationship between cannabis use and the use of other illicit drugs. *Drug Alcohol Rev* 24(1):39–48, 2005.
24. Hopfer C: Implications of marijuana legalization for adolescent substance use. *Subst Abus* 35(4):331–335, 2014.

25. Grant BF, Dawson DA: Age at onset of alcohol use and its association with DSM-IV alcohol abuse and dependence: results from the National Longitudinal Alcohol Epidemiologic Survey. *J Subst Abuse* 9:103–110, 1997.
26. Chambers RA, Taylor JR, Potenza MN: Developmental neurocircuitry of motivation in adolescence: a critical period of addiction vulnerability. *Am J Psychiatry* 160(6):1041–1052, 2003.
27. Brook DW, Brook JS, Rubenstone E, Zhang C, Singer M, Duke MR: Alcohol use in adolescents whose fathers abuse drugs. *J Addict Dis* 22(1):11–34, 2003.
28. Brook JS, Whiteman M, Brook DW, Gordon AS: Sibling influences on adolescent drug use: older brothers on younger brothers. *J Am Acad Child Adolesc Psychiatry* 30(6):958–966, 1991.
29. Schulenberg JE, Maggs JL: A developmental perspective on alcohol use and heavy drinking during adolescence and the transition to young adulthood. *J Stud Alcohol Suppl* (14):54–70, 2002.
30. Koob GF. Neurocircuitry of alcohol addiction: synthesis from animal models. *Handb Clin Neurol* 125:33–54, 2014.
31. O'Brien MS, Anthony JC: Risk of becoming cocaine dependent: epidemiological estimates for the United States, 2000–2001. *Neuropsychopharmacology* 30(5):1006–1018, 2005.
32. Wagner FA, Anthony JC: From first drug use to drug dependence; developmental periods of risk for dependence upon marijuana, cocaine, and alcohol. *Neuropsychopharmacology* 26(4):479–488, 2002.
33. Crews F, He J, Hodge C: Adolescent cortical development: a critical period of vulnerability for addiction. *Pharmacol Biochem Behav* 86(2): 189–199, 2007.
34. Volkow ND, Baler RD, Compton WM, Weiss SR: Adverse health effects of marijuana use. *N Engl J Med* 370(23):2219–2227, 2014.
35. Prochaska JO, DiClemente CC, Norcross JC: In search of how people change. Applications to addictive behaviors. *Am Psychol* 47(9):1102–1114, 1992.
36. Miller WR, Rose GS: Toward a theory of motivational interviewing. *Am Psychol* 64(6):527–537, 2009.
37. Winters KC, Stinchfield RD, Henly GA, Schwartz RH: Validity of adolescent self-report of alcohol and other drug involvement. *Int J Addict* 25(11A):1379–1395, 1990.
38. Robinson SM, Sobell LC, Sobell MB, Leo GI: Reliability of the timeline followback for cocaine, cannabis, and cigarette use. *Psychol Addict Behav* 28(1):154–162, 2014.
39. Riggs PD, Davies RD: A clinical approach to integrating treatment for adolescent depression and substance abuse. *J Am Acad Child Adolesc Psychiatry* 41(10):1253–1255, 2002.
40. Melanson SE, Baskin L, Magnani B, Kwong TC, Dizon A, Wu AH: Interpretation and utility of drug of abuse immunoassays: lessons from laboratory drug testing surveys. *Arch Pathol Lab Med* 134(5): 735–739, 2010.
41. Cone EJ, Lange R, Darwin WD: In vivo adulteration: excess fluid ingestion causes false-negative marijuana and cocaine urine test results. *J Anal Toxicol* 22(6):460–473, 1998.
42. Price JW: Dilution of urine drug tests: is it random? *J Addict Med* 7(6):405–409, 2013.
43. Mittal MK, Florin T, Perrone J, Delgado JH, Osterhoudt KC: Toxicity from the use of niacin to beat urine drug screening. *Ann Emerg Med* 50(5):587–590, 2007.
44. Cody JT, Valtier S: Effects of Stealth adulterant on immunoassay testing for drugs of abuse. *J Anal Toxicol* 25(6):466–470, 2001.
45. Paul BD, Jacobs A: Spectrophotometric detection of iodide and chromic (III) in urine after oxidation to iodine and chromate (VI). *J Anal Toxicol* 29(7):658–663, 2005.
46. Larson SJ, Holler JM, Magluilo J, Jr, Dunkley CS, Jacobs A: Papain adulteration in 11-nor-delta9-tetrahydrocannabinol- 9-carboxylic acid-positive urine samples. *J Anal Toxicol* 32(6):438–443, 2008.
47. Taylor EH, Oertli EH, Wolfgang JW, Mueller E: Accuracy of five on-site immunoassay drugs-of-abuse testing devices. *J Anal Toxicol* 23(2):119–124, 1999.
48. George S, Braithwaite RA: Use of on-site testing for drugs of abuse. *Clin Chem* 48(10):1639–1646, 2002.
49. Attema-de Jonge ME, Peeters SY, Franssen EJ: Performance of three point-of-care urinalysis test devices for drugs of abuse and therapeutic drugs applied in the emergency department. *J Emerg Med* 42(6):682–691, 2012.
50. Bush DM: The U.S. Mandatory Guidelines for Federal Workplace Drug Testing Programs: current status and future considerations. *Forensic Sci Int* 174(2–3):111–119, 2008.
51. Huestis MA, Scheidweiler KB, Saito T, et al.: Excretion of Delta9-tetrahydrocannabinol in sweat. *Forensic Sci Int* 174(2–3):173–177, 2008.
52. Apelberg BJ, Corey CG, Hoffman AC, et al.: Symptoms of tobacco dependence among middle and high school tobacco users: results from the 2012 National Youth Tobacco Survey. *Am J Prev Med* 47(2 Suppl 1): S4–S14, 2014.
53. Cerda M, Wall M, Keyes KM, Galea S, Hasin D: Medical marijuana laws in 50 states: investigating the relationship between state legalization of medical marijuana and marijuana use, abuse and dependence. *Drug Alcohol Depend* 120(1-3):22–27, 2012.
54. Lynne-Landsman SD, Livingston MD, Wagenaar AC: Effects of state medical marijuana laws on adolescent marijuana use. *Am J Public Health* 103(8):1500–1506, 2013.
55. Choo EK, Benz M, Zaller N, Warren O, Rising KL, McConnell KJ: The impact of state medical marijuana legislation on adolescent marijuana use. *J Adolesc Health* 55(2):160–166, 2014.
56. Schuermeyer J, Salomonsen-Sautel S, Price RK, et al.: Temporal trends in marijuana attitudes, availability and use in Colorado compared to non-medical marijuana states: 2003–11. *Drug Alcohol Depend* 140:145–155, 2014.
57. Sevigny EL, Pacula RL, Heaton P: The effects of medical marijuana laws on potency. *Int J Drug Policy* 25(2):308–319, 2014.
58. Thurstone C, Lieberman SA, Schmiege SJ: Medical marijuana diversion and associated problems in adolescent substance treatment. *Drug Alcohol Depend* 118(2–3):489–492, 2011.
59. Salomonsen-Sautel S, Sakai JT, Thurstone C, Corley R, Hopfer C: Medical marijuana use among adolescents in substance abuse treatment. *J Am Acad Child Adolesc Psychiatry* 51(7):694–702, 2012.
60. MacCoun R, Reuter P: Evaluating alternative cannabis regimes. *Br J Psychiatry* 178:123–128, 2001.
61. Lenroot RK, Giedd JN. Brain development in children and adolescents: insights from anatomical magnetic resonance imaging. *Neurosci Biobehav Rev* 30(6):718–729, 2006.
62. Kelly AM, Di Martino A, Uddin LQ, et al.: Development of anterior cingulate functional connectivity from late childhood to early adulthood. *Cereb Cortex* 19(3):640–657, 2009.
63. Meier MH, Caspi A, Ambler A, et al.: Persistent cannabis users show neuropsychological decline from childhood to midlife. *Proc Natl Acad Sci U S A* 109(40):E2657–E2664, 2012.
64. Bolla KI, Brown K, Eldreth D, Tate K, Cadet JL: Dose-related neurocognitive effects of marijuana use. *Neurology* 59(9):1337–1343, 2002.
65. Lane SD, Cherek DR, Tcheremissine OV, Steinberg JL, Sharon JL: Response perseveration and adaptation in heavy marijuana-smoking adolescents. *Addict Behav* 32(5):977–990, 2007.
66. Schweinsburg AD, Brown SA, Tapert SF: The influence of marijuana use on neurocognitive functioning in adolescents. *Curr Drug Abuse Rev* 1(1):99–111, 2008.
67. Camchong J, Lim KO, Kumra S: Adverse effects of cannabis on adolescent brain development: a longitudinal study [published online ahead of print February 8, 2016]. *Cereb Cortex*. doi 10.1093/cercor/bhw015.
68. Crowley TJ, Macdonald MJ, Whitmore EA, Mikulich SK: Cannabis dependence, withdrawal, and reinforcing effects among adolescents with conduct symptoms and substance use disorders. *Drug Alcohol Depend* 50(1):27–37, 1998.
69. McCabe SE, West BT, Teter CJ, Boyd CJ: Medical and nonmedical use of prescription opioids among high school seniors in the United States. *Arch Pediatr Adolesc Med* 166(9):797–802, 2012.
70. Whiteside LK, Walton MA, Bohnert AS, et al.: Nonmedical prescription opioid and sedative use among adolescents in the emergency department. *Pediatrics* 132(5):825–832, 2013.
71. Fortuna RJ, Robbins BW, Caiola E, Joynt M, Halterman JS: Prescribing of controlled medications to adolescents and young adults in the United States. *Pediatrics* 126(6):1108–1116, 2010.
72. Siegal HA, Carlson RG, Kenne DR, Swora MG: Probable relationship between opioid abuse and heroin use. *Am Fam Physician* 67(5):942, 945, 2003.
73. Pollini RA, Banta-Green CJ, Cuevas-Mota J, Metzner M, Teshale E, Garfein RS: Problematic use of prescription-type opioids prior to heroin use among young heroin injectors. *Subst Abuse Rehabil* 2(1):173–180, 2011.
74. Lankenau SE, Teti M, Silva K, Jackson Bloom J, Harocopos A, Treese M: Initiation into prescription opioid misuse amongst young injection drug users. *Int J Drug Policy* 23(1):37–44, 2012.
75. Peavy KM, Banta-Green CJ, Kingston S, Hanrahan M, Merrill JO, Coffin PO: "Hooked on" prescription-type opiates prior to using heroin: results from a survey of syringe exchange clients. *J Psychoactive Drugs* 44(3):259–265, 2012.
76. Kallupi M, Vendruscolo LF, Carmichael CY, George O, Koob GF, Gilpin NW: Neuropeptide YY(2)R blockade in the central amygdala reduces anxiety-like behavior but not alcohol drinking in alcohol-dependent rats. *Addict Biol* 19(5):755–757, 2014.
77. Mateu-Gelabert P, Guarino H, Jessell L, Teper A: Injection and sexual HIV/HCV risk behaviors associated with nonmedical use of prescription opioids among young adults in New York City. *J Subst Abuse Treat* 48(1):13–20, 2015.
78. Compton WM, Jones CM, Baldwin GT: Relationship between nonmedical prescription-opioid use and heroin use. *N Engl J Med* 374(2):154–163, 2016.
79. Mars SG, Fessel JN, Bourgois P, Montero F, Karandinos G, Ciccarone D: Heroin-related overdose: the unexplored influences of markets, marketing and source-types in the United States. *Soc Sci Med* 140:44–53.
80. Unick G, Rosenblum D, Mars S, Ciccarone D: The relationship between US heroin market dynamics and heroin-related overdose, 1992–2008. *Addiction* 109(11):1889–1898, 2014.
81. Hopfer CJ, Khuri E, Crowley TJ, Hooks S: Adolescent heroin use: a review of the descriptive and treatment literature. *J Subst Abuse Treat* 23(3):231–237, 2002.
82. Okie S: A flood of opioids, a rising tide of deaths. *N Engl J Med* 363(21): 1981–1985, 2010.
83. Brittain JL: China white: the bogus drug. *J Toxicol Clin Toxicol* 19(10): 1123–1126, 1982.

84. Hibbs J, Perper J, Winek CL: An outbreak of designer drug-related deaths in Pennsylvania. *JAMA* 265(8):1011–1013, 1991.
85. Schwartz RH: Adolescent heroin use: a review. *Pediatrics* 102(6):1461–1466, 1998.
86. Monterosso JR, Aron AR, Cordova X, Xu J, London ED: Deficits in response inhibition associated with chronic methamphetamine abuse. *Drug Alcohol Depend* 79(2):273–277, 2005.
87. von Sydow K, Lieb R, Pfister H, Hofler M, Wittchen HU: Use, abuse and dependence of ecstasy and related drugs in adolescents and young adults—a transient phenomenon? Results from a longitudinal community study. *Drug Alcohol Depend* 66(2):147–159, 2002.
88. Sakai JT, Hall SK, Mikulich-Gilbertson SK, Crowley TJ: Inhalant use, abuse, and dependence among adolescent patients: commonly comorbid problems. *J Am Acad Child Adolesc Psychiatry* 43(9):1080–1088, 2004.
89. Brown JT: Anabolic steroids: what should the emergency physician know? *Emerg Med Clin North Am* 23(3):815–826, ix–x, 2005.
90. Brown RA, Abrantes AM, Minami H, et al.: Motivational interviewing to reduce substance use in adolescents with psychiatric comorbidity. *J Subst Abuse Treat* 59:20–29, 2015.
91. Waldron HB, Kern-Jones S, Turner CW, Peterson TR, Ozechowski TJ: Engaging resistant adolescents in drug abuse treatment. *J Subst Abuse Treat* 32(2):133–142, 2007.
92. Waldron HB, Turner CW: Evidence-based psychosocial treatments for adolescent substance abuse. *J Clin Child Adolesc Psychol* 37(1):238–261, 2008.
93. Kaminer Y, Burleson JA, Goldberger R: Cognitive-behavioral coping skills and psychoeducation therapies for adolescent substance abuse. *J Nerv Ment Dis* 190(11):737–745, 2002.
94. Kaminer Y: Adolescent substance abuse treatment: evidence-based practice in outpatient services. *Curr Psychiatry Rep* 4(5):397–401, 2002.
95. Wagner EF, Brown SA, Monti PM, Myers MG, Waldron HB: Innovations in adolescent substance abuse intervention. *Alcohol Clin Exp Res* 23(2):236–249, 1999.
96. Sheidow AJ, Henggeler SW: [Multisystemic therapy with substance using adolescents: a clinical and research overview]. *Prax Kinderpsychol Kinderpsychiatr* 57(5):401–419, 2008.
97. Henggeler SW, Pickrel SG, Brondino MJ, Crouch JL: Eliminating (almost) treatment dropout of substance abusing or dependent delinquents through home-based multisystemic therapy. *Am J Psychiatry* 153(3):427–428, 1996.
98. Robbins MS, Bachrach K, Szapocznik J: Bridging the research-practice gap in adolescent substance abuse treatment: the case of brief strategic family therapy. *J Subst Abuse Treat* 23(2):123–132, 2002.
99. Azrin NH, McMahon PT, Donohue B, et al.: Behavior therapy for drug abuse: a controlled treatment outcome study. *Behav Res Ther* 32(8):857–866, 1994.
100. Budney AJ, Higgins ST, Radonovich KJ, Novy PL: Adding voucher-based incentives to coping skills and motivational enhancement improves outcomes during treatment for marijuana dependence. *J Consult Clin Psychol* 68(6):1051–1061, 2000.
101. Stanger C, Budney AJ, Kamon JL, Thostensen J: A randomized trial of contingency management for adolescent marijuana abuse and dependence. *Drug Alcohol Depend* 105(3):240–247, 2009.
102. Stanger C, Ryan SR, Scherer EA, Norton GE, Budney AJ: Clinic- and home-based contingency management plus parent training for adolescent cannabis use disorders. *J Am Acad Child Adolesc Psychiatry* 54(6):445–453 e442, 2015.
103. Riggs P: Want change? Try honey instead of vinegar. *J Am Acad Child Adolesc Psychiatry* 54(6):440–441, 2015.
104. Kamon J, Budney A, Stanger C: A contingency management intervention for adolescent marijuana abuse and conduct problems. *J Am Acad Child Adolesc Psychiatry* 44(6):513–521, 2005.
105. Lash SJ, Burden JL, Parker JD, et al.: Contracting, prompting and reinforcing substance use disorder continuing care. *J Subst Abuse Treat* 44(4):449–456, 2013.
106. Riggs PD, Hall SK, Mikulich-Gilbertson SK, Lohman M, Kayser A: A randomized controlled trial of pemoline for attention-deficit/hyperactivity disorder in substance-abusing adolescents. *J Am Acad Child Adolesc Psychiatry* 43(4):420–429, 2004.
107. Geller B, Cooper TB, Sun K, et al.: Double-blind and placebo-controlled study of lithium for adolescent bipolar disorders with secondary substance dependency. *J Am Acad Child Adolesc Psychiatry* 37(2):171–178, 1998.
108. Treatment for Adolescents With Depression Study (TADS) Team: Fluoxetine, cognitive-behavioral therapy, and Their Combination for Adolescents with depression. *JAMA* 292:807–820, 2004.
109. Riggs PD, Mikulich-Gilbertson SK, Davies RD, Lohman M, Klein C, Stover SK: A randomized controlled trial of fluoxetine and cognitive behavioral therapy in adolescents with major depression, behavior problems, and substance use disorders. *Arch Pediatr Adolesc Med* 161(11):1026–1034, 2007.
110. Carroll KM, Nich C, Ball SA, McCance E, Frankforter TL, Rounsaville BJ: One-year follow-up of disulfiram and psychotherapy for cocaine-alcohol users: sustained effects of treatment. *Addiction* 95(9):1335–1349, 2000.
111. Niederhofer H, Staffen W: Acamprosate and its efficacy in treating alcohol dependent adolescents. *Eur Child Adolesc Psychiatry* 12(3):144–148, 2003.
112. Deas D, May MP, Randall C, Johnson N, Anton R: Naltrexone treatment of adolescent alcoholics: an open-label pilot study. *J Child Adolesc Psychopharmacol* 15(5):723–728, 2005.
113. Johnson BA: Recent advances in the development of treatments for alcohol and cocaine dependence: focus on topiramate and other modulators of GABA or glutamate function. *CNS Drugs* 19(10):873–896, 2005.
114. Hopfer CJ, Khuri E, Crowley TJ: Treating adolescent heroin use. *J Am Acad Child Adolesc Psychiatry* 42(5):609–611, 2003.
115. Marsch LA, Moore SK, Borodovsky JT, et al.: A randomized controlled trial of buprenorphine taper duration among opioid-dependent adolescents and young adults. *Addiction* 111:1406–1415, 2016.
116. Bukstein OG, Bernet W, Arnold V, et al.: Practice parameter for the assessment and treatment of children and adolescents with substance use disorder. *J Am Acad Child Adolesc Psychiatry* 44(6):609–621, 2005.
117. ASAM. The ASAM criteria: treatment criteria for addictive, substance-related, and co-occurring conditions. 2016. Available at: http://www.asam.org/quality-practice/guidelines-and-consensus-documents/the-asam-criteria/text. Accessed March 3, 2016.

5.9 ■ SLEEP DISORDERS

CHAPTER 5.9 ■ SLEEP DISORDERS

ARGELINDA BARONI AND THOMAS F. ANDERS

INTRODUCTION

Sleep is crucial for emotional, cognitive, and physical well-being. Most psychiatric conditions are associated with sleep disorders (1); additionally, sleep disturbances are risk factors for the development of mood, anxiety, and substance use disorders and suicidal behaviors (1,2). Insufficient or disrupted sleep in children and adolescents is also associated with sport and motor vehicle accidents and metabolic disorders, including increased obesity and insulin resistance (2,3).

Sleep complaints are common among both typically developing children and children with psychiatric and developmental disorders (4). Moreover, population-wide studies have found a high prevalence of children getting inadequate sleep (5). Unfortunately, most medical and mental health professionals receive insufficient training in sleep medicine and parental knowledge on sleep is limited (4,6,7). For these reasons, sleep disorders are vastly underdiagnosed and undertreated, despite strong evidence for effective interventions (8). This chapter begins with a brief overview of normal sleep physiology, sleep assessment, and prevention across development and

TABLE 5.9.1

FEATURES OF NREM SLEEP AND REM SLEEP

NREM Sleep	REM Sleep
EEG: synchronized, slower frequencies and higher voltages than wakefulness and REM	EEG: desynchronized, mixed, low amplitude fast frequencies, similar to wakefulness
Reduced metabolic activity	Increased metabolic activity
Autonomic slowing	Autonomic activation
Maintained thermoregulation	Altered thermoregulation: poikilothermia
Episodic, involuntary movements	Skeletal muscle atonia
Slow rolling eye movements	Rapid eye movements
Few penile erections or little vaginal lubrication	Partial or full penile erections or significant vaginal lubrication
Limited mentation/dreaming	Dreaming
Defined as quiet sleep in infants	Defined as active sleep in infants
Sleepwalking and sleep terrors arise from NREM sleep	Nightmares arise from REM sleep

concludes with an overview of common pediatric sleep disorders. For simplicity, we will refer to children and adolescents as children throughout, except when referring specifically to adolescents.

SLEEP PHYSIOLOGY

Behaviorally, sleep can be defined as perceptual disengagement from the environment that is easily reversed with intense stimulation and is accompanied by specific physiologic concomitants. These include variations in brain and cardiovascular activity, muscle tone, breathing pattern, and body temperature. Physiologic systems are routinely recorded via polysomnography (PSG) in the sleep laboratory or, increasingly, at home. Eye movement, muscle tone, and electroencephalographic (EEG) patterns are the primary parameters used to score the two major sleep states, non–rapid eye movement (NREM) and rapid eye movement (REM) sleep. These states alternate cyclically throughout the night. NREM sleep is further divided into N1, N2, N3 "stages" based on EEG characteristics. N1 is the lightest sleep stage, characterized by limited sensory disconnection, while N3, also called "deep sleep," is characterized by slow-wave activity, disengagement from the environment, and a high arousal threshold. See Table 5.9.1 for differences between REM and NREM sleep. Patterns of abnormal breathing, heart rate irregularity, and episodic behaviors, including limb movements, can be observed during PSG and are associated features useful in diagnosing specific sleep disorders. PSG can also be used to assess quantitatively the amount of excessive daytime sleepiness that patients with disorders of hypersomnolence experience, with the Multiple Sleep Latency Test (MSLT) protocol (9). The test is done in a sleep laboratory and uses PSG to measure the amount of sleep obtained during five 20-minute trials, from mid-morning to early evening, usually after a nocturnal PSG. At each 20-minute period, the subject tries to fall asleep, and the latency to sleep onset for each attempted nap represents how sleepy the individual is. The test, standardized for use with adults and for adolescents, is a sensitive indicator of sleepiness and is significantly correlated with the performance decrement associated with sleepiness.

SLEEP–WAKE STATE ORGANIZATION ACROSS DEVELOPMENT

The characteristics of the electrophysiologic patterns and the proportions of sleep–wake states change markedly across development as a function of multiple processes, including myelination, cortical synaptic density, and circadian system maturation. Adult sleep organization is achieved by early adolescence. Neonates and infants have shorter sleep cycles (~50 minutes) compared to older children, adolescents, and adults (90 to 120 minutes) (10). Moreover, their sleep cycles are characterized by sleep-onset REM (active) sleep and higher proportion of REM sleep (50%). REM sleep declines to 25% in toddlers and children, close to adult proportions. Slow-wave sleep (SWS, N3) also emerges in the first 2 years of life and accounts for approximately 30% of total sleep time in toddlers and preschoolers. SWS declines to 20% or less in older adolescents and young adults. The proportion of NREM–REM sleep per cycle also changes across development. The proportions of REM–NREM do not differ appreciably from early- to late-sleep periods in infants, whereas the length of REM periods increases during each cycle as the night progresses in older children and adults. See Table 5.9.2 for differences between infants and adults sleep.

Sleep cycles are also characterized by multiple, brief arousals throughout the night usually at points of REM/NREM transitions. These physiologic arousals are normative, but can lead to night awakenings when children are unable to return to sleep on their own. Finally, circadian rhythms, responsible for daily variations of alertness, core body temperature, and melatonin secretion, emerge within the first 4 weeks but become more soundly synchronized to day–night cycles by 2 to 6 months (11,12).

Finally, sleep duration decreases with maturation of the central nervous system. See Table 5.9.3 for average sleep durations in children and adolescents (13).

TABLE 5.9.2

DIFFERENCES BETWEEN SLEEP IN INFANTS AND ADULTS

	Infants	Adults
NREM/REM %	50/50	80/20
Ultradian cycle length	50–60 min	90 min
Circadian cycle	Polyphasic	Diurnal
Temporal distribution of NREM/REM during the night	Equi-distributed	First third/last third
Sleep stages	Quiet Sleep (NREM) Active Sleep (REM)	NREM (N1–N2–N3) REM

TABLE 5.9.3

SLEEP DURATIONS IN CHILDHOOD AND ADOLESCENCE

	Mean Nighttime Sleep Duration (hours)	Mean Daytime Sleep Duration (hours)
6 mos old	14.2	3.4
3 yrs old	12.5	1.7
6 yrs old	11	—
10 yrs old	9.9	—
12 yrs old	9.3	—
15 yrs old	8.5	—

SLEEP REGULATION

The sleep–wake cycle is regulated by two core processes, as postulated by Borbely et al. (12). One, defined as process S, is sleep-dependent, homeostatic, and contingent on the amount of time spent awake preceding sleep time plus the accumulated sleep debt; process S increases with wakefulness and decreases with sleep. The second component, process C, is regulated by circadian rhythms, self-sustained rhythms of approximately 24 hours. Process C is responsible for circadian variations in alertness, activity, and physiologic systems. It is regulated by a combination of internal and external factors. Internal factors include the activity of the suprachiasmatic nucleus (SCN), the body's master clock, and its effects on melatonin secretion, among others. The SCN rhythm is slightly longer than 24 hours in most individuals and must be entrained into a 24-hour pattern by environmental cues, the most powerful of which is the light–dark cycle. Activity and feeding also help maintain circadian stability. The S and C processes operate simultaneously, determining the level of alertness in individuals. While process S progressively increases with time, process C produces two periods of increased alertness, one at the end of the morning, and one in the evening, prior to sleep onset. This latter increase in alertness is responsible for "the second wind," or the sense of increased energy and vigilance most individuals experience in the last part of the day. The relationship between process C and shared social time determines the circadian preference, that is, whether a child or an adolescent is a lark (morningness preference) or an owl (eveningness preference).

ASSESSMENT

Clinicians can assess normal and pathologic sleep subjectively using clinical interviews, questionnaires, and sleep diaries. Objective methods such as actigraphy and PSG can be useful in assessing specific sleep disorders, as shown in Tables 5.9.4 and 5.9.5 (9,14).

CLINICAL INTERVIEW

The use of screening tools increases the detection of sleep disorders and should be included in any evaluation of children even in the absence of sleep complaints (15). The BEARS acronym is a validated screening tool for reminding primary care clinicians to assess the following domains: (1) Bedtime Issues (including insomnia or bedtime refusal), (2) Excessive Daytime Sleepiness, (3) Awakenings/Abnormal Behaviors During Sleep, (4) Regularity or Duration of Sleep, and (5) Snoring (15,16). Routine use of a screening method such as BEARS leads to significant increase in detection of sleep disorders. The BEARS can also be administered as a form; see

TABLE 5.9.4

COMMON RESPIRATORY INDICATIONS FOR POLYSOMNOGRAPHY IN CHILDREN

Suspicion of obstructive sleep apnea (OSA)	Presence of respiratory symptoms (e.g., habitual snoring, witnessed apneas) and associated symptoms (e.g., hyperactivity, enuresis) Any of the above symptoms plus obesity → low threshold for PSG
Low threshold in neurodevelopmental syndromes (high prevalence of sleep-disordered breathing)	For example, Down syndrome, Prader–Willi, Chiari malformation
Low threshold in craniofacial abnormalities, neuromuscular disorders or abnormal chest wall syndromes	For example, Duchenne muscular dystrophy, achondroplasia, craniofacial dysostosis
Post-tonsillectomy in case of:	Moderate to severe OSA at baseline, obesity, craniofacial anomalies, neurodevelopmental disorders
Suspicion of sleep-related breathing disorder in infants who have experienced an apparent life-threatening event (ALTE)	

Table 5.9.5 (7). If sleep problems are reported, a more detailed sleep and medical history should be gathered, along with current medications and a physical examination including a calculation of body mass index (BMI) and an examination of the tonsils. See Table 5.9.6 for content and examples of probing questions for a sleep interview.

MONITORING SLEEP AND WAKING BEHAVIOR

Sleep diaries are useful tools for sleep assessment and treatment monitoring and show good reliability with actigraphy for actual sleep start and end (17). The parents and the child should compile a sleep diary daily for 1 to 2 weeks, ideally prior to assessment. In the sleep diary the informants can mark the occurrence of a sleep problem (e.g., sleepwalking or nightmare events) but also indicate multiple sleep behaviors such as sleep duration, sleep-onset latency, nap duration and timing, sleep–wake regularity, and circadian preference. Sleep diaries can be downloaded from the American Academy of Pediatrics (https://www2.aap.org/sections/dbpeds/pdf/sleeplog.pdf). Parental report measures include the Child Sleep Habits Questionnaire (CSHQ) (18) and the Pediatric Sleep Questionnaire (PSQ) (19), both of which are dimensional scales of problem sleep behaviors (bedtime problems, sleep-disordered breathing, etc.). These questionnaires have demonstrated reliability and validity with respect to identifying both behaviorally based and medically based sleep disorders in children aged 2 to 18 years (19) and 2 to 10 years (18,20). Circadian preference can be assessed with the Children's Chronotype Questionnaire (CCTQ), along with a sleep diary (21).

TABLE 5.9.5

BEARS FORM
CIRCLE OR HIGHLIGHT ANY QUESTION YOU WOULD ANSWER YES

	Toddler/Preschool (3–5 yrs)	School-aged (6–12 yrs)	Adolescent (13–18 yrs)
1. Bedtime problems	Does your child have any problems going to bed? Falling asleep?	Does your child have any problems at bedtime (fights, complaints, fears)? Does your child have difficulties falling asleep?	Does your teenager have any problems falling asleep at bedtime?
2. Excessive daytime sleepiness	Does your child seem overtired or sleepy a lot during the day? Does he/she still take naps?	Does your child have difficulty waking in the morning, or seem sleepy during the day or take naps during the day?	Does your teenager have difficulty waking in the morning, seem sleepy during the day or take naps during the day? More than average?
3. Awakenings during the night	Does your child wake up a lot at night? Night terrors? Sleep walking?	Does your child seem to wake up a lot at night? Any sleepwalking or nightmares? Bedwetting?	Does your teenager wake up a lot at night? Does your teenager have trouble getting back to sleep in the middle of the night? Any sleepwalking or nightmares?
4. Regularity and duration of sleep	Does your child have difficulties maintaining a regular bedtime and wake time? (Falling asleep/ waking up at different times)	Does your child have difficulties maintaining a regular bedtime and wake time during school days? During weekends? Do you think he/ she is not getting enough sleep?	Does your teenager have difficulties maintaining a regular bedtime and wake time during school days? During weekends?
5. Snoring	Does your child snore a lot or have difficulty breathing at night?	Does your child have loud or nightly snoring or any breathing difficulties at night?	Does your teenager snore loudly or nightly? Does your teenager ever stop breathing during the night?

Sleepiness can be assessed using a modified version of the Epworth Sleepiness Scale, the Pediatric Daytime Sleepiness Scale, or the Cleveland Adolescent Sleepiness Questionnaire (22).

PREVENTION AND PARENT EDUCATION

Parents and children should be regularly educated on how to maintain or improve sleep using healthy sleep practices, referred to as sleep hygiene, starting in infancy (7,16,23). Good sleep hygiene practices have been found to be associated with good sleep in children from birth to age 10 (1,23). In order to stabilize circadian rhythms (process C) and regulate sleep drive (process S), children should, as best as possible: (1) maintain a regular sleep–wake schedule both on weekdays and weekends; (2) keep a regular daily schedule, including meals and physical activity; (3) avoid bright light and screen use, including e-readers, for at least 1 hour prior to the target bedtime (to avoid melatonin suppression secondary to light); (4) be exposed to natural bright light in the morning (blinds open at wake-up time, walking to school if possible) to stabilize circadian rhythms; and (5) schedule age-appropriate or strategic naps when indicated. Consistency of wake-up time is more relevant than bedtime for circadian entrainment and parents should enforce wake-up time within 2 hours on weekends compared to weekdays. Clinicians should also educate parents and children regarding appropriate sleep need requirements by age and suggest that an age-appropriate amount of sleep should be scheduled in the child's day, as for any other fundamental activity. This is increasingly challenging, as most adults engage in poor sleep hygiene.

Positive sleep associations can be promoted by: (1) encouraging an age-appropriate and consistent bedtime routine; (2) avoiding sleep-incompatible or arousing activities in bed during the day and at bedtime, including watching TV, computer use, doing homework or drinking of caffeinated beverages; and (3) limiting parental interaction with the child prior to sleep onset. A soothing and enjoyable bedtime routine creates positive associations with sleep-time and sets the tone for both body and mind to prepare for sleep. Similarly, avoiding stimulating or unpleasant activities in bed eliminates the association between bed and arousing activities. For this reason, ideally, the bedroom should not be routinely used for timeout or other negative consequences in pre-school age children and toddlers. Suitable bedtime routines change according to the child's age and can include bathing, cuddling, or reading a story. Ideally, bedtime routines should be consistent, repeating in the same order and lasting no longer than 30 minutes. Independent sleep onset should be encouraged as early as possible, and is achieved by limiting or removing parental interaction with the child prior to sleep (see insomnia). The use of a transitional object (a blanket, a stuffed animal) can be used to redirect sleep associations in children after 6 months of age, when the child does not require night feedings.

Use of caffeine or any other sleep-impacting substances, including nicotine, marijuana or other illicit drugs, should be assessed, as their effects on sleep are usually underestimated by parents and children. Caffeine use has been understudied in adolescents but appears to be associated with chronic sleep loss, worse academic functioning, nicotine use, and higher risk of other substance use (2).

CLASSIFICATION OF SLEEP DISORDERS IN CHILDHOOD

Sleep disorders are differently represented at different ages. During infancy, difficulties falling asleep independently and night

TABLE 5.9.6

SLEEP INTERVIEW

History of Sleep Problems		Example Probing Questions	Comments
	Onset, timing and course	What is the frequency of the symptom in terms of events per week or per night? What has been its course (stable, worsening, improving)?	
Functioning	Excessive daytime sleepiness	Does the child fall asleep in class or watching TV? Does the child struggle to wake up?	Excessive daytime sleepiness is always pathologic in children
	Social and family dysfunction	Is the child embarrassed to sleep at a friend's house because of the sleep problem? Is the child's sleep problem negatively affecting parents?	Child sleep problems are associated with high degree of parental stress
Sleep–Wake Schedule	Bedtime and wake-up time sleep duration	What is the usual bedtime and rise time?	Sometimes parental expectations do not match developmental sleep needs
	Time and circumstances needed to fall asleep	Does the child fall asleep easily or need parental intervention or presence?	
	Awakenings: How frequent? How long?	Does the child signal to parents? Or is she able to self-soothe if she wakes up at night? What is the parents' response?	
	Naps and their duration		Naps are developmentally appropriate until ages 4–5. Naps after this age may indicate excessive daytime sleepiness
	Regular schedule on schooldays vs. vacation days	What is the sleep–wake schedule on school days and vacation days?	More than 2 hrs difference can indicate sleep deprivation and/or circadian rhythm disorder
Bedtime Routine		Does the child have a regular bedtime routine? Is it soothing? Is there screen use within 1–2 hrs of sleep time? Are bedtime rituals present?	Regular bedtime routine is associated with better sleep; screen use within 1 hour of sleep onset can worsen sleep and decrease melatonin secretion
Bedtime Environment	Consistent? Dark? Quiet? Co-sleeping? TV or computer in the room? Cellphone use overnight?	What are the sleeping arrangements? With whom does the child share a room or bed? Does the child fall asleep in his bed? Is co-sleeping a choice or a consequence of inability to set limits?	TV in the bedroom is associated with worse sleep in children. White noise machine, earplugs, blinds or eye-masks should be considered if sleep environment is inadequate
Sleep Review of System	Snoring/gasping; excessive movements during sleep; restless legs syndrome; abnormal behaviors; enuresis; nightmares; teeth clenching	Is snoring prominent, habitual, even in absence of a cold? Are pauses in breathing audible? Is the child restless during sleep? Have the parents noted abnormal behaviors or movement during sleep? Sleepwalking? Does the child endorse "funny" "strange" feelings in her legs before sleep time? Does she say that her legs need to kick at night?	

awakenings are the most common problems. By contrast, toddlers and children also present sleepwalking, obstructive sleep apnea (OSA) and nightmares, while adolescents tend to display insufficient sleep hygiene and circadian rhythm disorders.

Whereas there was only partial agreement for the criteria of sleep disorders among different classification systems in the past, recent revisions have strived to harmonize diagnostic criteria. Currently, there is fair concordance in sleep disorder classifications and criteria between *The International Classification of Sleep Disorders*, 3rd Edition (ICSD-3) (24) and the *Diagnostic and Statistical Manual of Mental Disorders* (DSM-5) (25), even if the ICSD-3 contains a greater level of detail, because it is geared toward sleep specialists. The major classification changes in DSM-5 and ICSD-3 are related to the collapse of different insomnia diagnoses into a single entity, defined as chronic insomnia, and the adoption of unique criteria for both adults and children, with age-appropriate specifiers. This has led to the possibility of diagnosing DSM-5 insomnia in children and the elimination of the "behavioral insomnia of childhood" diagnosis from ICSD-3.

Currently, both nosologies include sections on (1) insomnia, (2) sleep-related breathing disorders, (3) hypersomnias, (4) circadian rhythms disorders, (5) parasomnias, (6) sleep-related movement disorders; see Table 5.9.7. The other clinically relevant change in DSM-5 is that sleep disorders and psychiatric disorders can be diagnosed concurrently. For example, the diagnoses of depression and insomnia can both be assigned if the insomnia does not appear to be simply secondary to the depression. This change in DSM-5 reflects the awareness that sleep disorders have an impact on the course and severity of psychiatric conditions and that they warrant their own attention and treatment.

For younger children, the Diagnostic Classification: Zero to Three, Revised (DC 0–3R) (26) can also be used. DC 0–3R is a multiaxial nosology of mental disorders developed specifically for use in infancy and early childhood. DC 0–3R provides several opportunities to classify sleep problems, either as a primary entity or as a symptom of another Axis 1 disorder such as traumatic stress disorder, adjustment disorder, regulatory disorder, anxiety disorder, or mood disorder. This classification is currently being revised.

TABLE 5.9.7

MAIN CATEGORIES OF SLEEP DISORDERS IN DSM-5 AND ICSD-3

Category	Description
Insomnia	• Persistent difficulties sleeping • Adequate opportunity for sleep • Daytime impairment (e.g., chronic insomnia)
Sleep-related breathing disorders	• Irregular breathing during sleep, possibly accompanied by sleep disruption (e.g., obstructive sleep apnea)
Hypersomnolence disorder and narcolepsy	• Excessive daytime sleepiness, in spite of adequate sleep (e.g., narcolepsy, hypersomnolence disorder)
Circadian rhythms disorders	• Misalignment of circadian rhythms and social requirement (e.g., delayed sleep phase)
Parasomnias	• Abnormal physical and emotional experiences during sleep or sleep–wake transitions (e.g., sleepwalking, nightmares)
Sleep-related movement disorders	• Presence of movements that delay sleep onset or disrupt sleep (e.g., restless legs syndrome)

Insomnia

General Features

Bedtime resistance, night awakenings, difficulties falling asleep or remaining asleep are the main symptoms of insomnia in childhood. Difficulty falling asleep without caregiver intervention, for example, a parent sitting or lying next to the child, is also considered a feature of pediatric insomnia. This was defined as sleep-onset association type insomnia in prior classifications (16). Bedtime resistance and bedtime "stalling" (calling out, getting out of bed, fighting bedtime routines) was previously described as limit-setting type insomnia (16). Other than nighttime problems, children with insomnia can display behavioral and cognitive problems, including sleepiness, tiredness, irritability, aggression, hyperactivity and social withdrawal (22). Pediatric insomnia is common and can begin at any age, although it is not usually diagnosed before 6 months of age, as nocturnal feedings and irregular sleep patterns are typical in infants (22) (ICSD-3). In community samples of infants, toddlers and preschoolers, the prevalence rates of insomnia are 20% to 30% (16). In older children, insomnia prevalence ranges between 10% and 30%, depending on criteria stringency. In European and American adolescents the prevalence of insomnia ranges between 6% and 11% (22). In children with psychiatric disorders or developmental delays, the prevalence of insomnia can be substantially higher, for example, 80% among children with autistic spectrum disorder have some difficulties sleeping (4,27).

The pathophysiology of insomnia remains unclear, but current models support a combination of behavioral, developmental, familial, and temperamental risk factors. Behavioral aspects include parental handling, especially for younger children. Sleep-related hypervigilance or hyperarousal, along with negative sleep associations are common elements of insomnia across the lifespan. The process of decreasing vigilance and/or extinguishing negative associations through relaxation, predictability of positive bedtime routines, and extinction of dysfunctional associations (such as parental presence) are common treatment strategies (22).

Insomnia needs to be distinguished from other sleep or psychiatric disorders. Delayed sleep phase, OSA, restless legs syndrome, and primary mood or anxiety disorders should be considered in the differential diagnosis when assessing for insomnia (5). For adolescents, along with delayed sleep phase disorder, volitional sleep restriction should also be considered.

Behavioral strategies are the first line of treatment for pediatric insomnia. However, most of the literature has focused on infants and preschoolers, and there is a lack of well-established treatments for older children, adolescents, and children with special needs (22,28). Use of medications should be considered only as an add-on after an appropriate behavioral plan has been implemented (29). In younger typically developing children, behavioral treatments are highly effective; 80% of children have a clinically significant positive response in terms of sleep latency and night awakenings that is maintained for up to 6 months (23) with large within-subject effect sizes (28). Unmodified extinction (ignoring all negative behaviors after lights out until a set time in the morning, unless the child is in danger or ill), graduated extinction (brief parental checks with decreased frequencies after lights out, accompanied by ignoring all negative behavior) and prevention/parent education are considered established and effective treatments for young children. Extinction strategies can be emotionally challenging for parents who typically resist implementing them. Parents should be reassured that these behavioral interventions have not been associated with negative outcomes (28). While there are limited studies on cognitive-behavioral interventions for older children and adolescents, it seems plausible to use them as well, pending controlled studies (28). Stimulus control is considered standard of care for insomnia in adults and targets the associations between bed and negative feelings and behaviors associated with insomnia. It involves going to bed only when sleepy, and leaving the bedroom when unable to sleep for extended times (20 to 30 minutes), engaging only in boring activities in dim light, for example, reading a boring book. Additionally, the bed should be only used for sleep. As the child or adolescent engages in stimulus control, she starts associating her bed with feeling sleepy, rather than with frustration or the arousal secondary to sleep-incompatible behaviors, such as watching TV or texting. Both the patient's understanding of these principles and parental support and monitoring are crucial for success. Often, phone and computer removal from the bedroom is necessary for effective implementation. Relaxation is also considered standard of care and includes classic progressive muscle relaxation and diaphragmatic breathing that should be mastered by the child during the day, prior to nighttime use. Other components of cognitive-behavioral therapy for insomnia that can be implemented are sleep restriction/bedtime fading and cognitive restructuring, when clinically and developmentally appropriate (22,30).

The U.S. Federal Drug Administration has not approved any medications for the treatment of pediatric insomnia and most of the guidelines for pediatric insomnia are based on expert consensus rather than randomized controlled trials (31). Indications for pharmacotherapy include acute stressors or medical illness, and lack of response to or parental inability to conduct behavioral intervention. Contraindications include potential negative interactions, for example, presence of other sedating medications, alcohol or illicit drug use. Other sleep disorders such as OSA and restless legs syndrome should be ruled out, as medication might exacerbate and/or mask the primary condition. The choice of medication should be based on clinical characteristics (e.g., age, sleep-onset vs. maintenance insomnia, comorbidities, other medications used) and should minimize side effects. Parents should be educated on goals, side effects (e.g., possible "paradoxical" effects such as stimulation and disinhibition, tolerance), optimal duration and possible modifications (nightly vs. intermittent use) of medication treatment. Attempts to discontinue the agent should be made regularly. Gradual taper is preferred to decrease recrudescence and symptomatic rebound. Melatonin is often considered a first-line agent for pediatric insomnia, given its efficacy and relatively benign short-term side-effect profile both in neurotypical children and children with psychiatric conditions. Melatonin doses range between 1 and 3 mg, with even lower doses recommended for treatment of delayed sleep phase (32). Alpha-2 agonists such as clonidine or guanfacine are also widely used by pediatricians and child psychiatrists and can have a role in treating insomnia in children with attention-deficit/hyperactivity disorder (ADHD) given their indications for this condition (31). Risk of rebound hypertension on abrupt discontinuation, narrow therapeutic index, and possible onset of tolerance for sedating effects should be considered, especially for clonidine (31). Antihistamines such as diphenhydramine are the most commonly used sedatives in pediatric practice, but their chronic use for insomnia is not supported by empirical data, secondary to lack of demonstrated efficacy, rapid tolerance with consequent dose escalation and anticholinergic, histaminergic, and adrenergic side effects (31). Other agents might be specifically indicated for insomnia with specific comorbidities, for example, long-acting benzodiazepines such as clonazepam for comorbid anxiety disorders or disorders of arousal (31).

Sleep-Related Breathing Disorders

The physiology of the respiratory system and ventilatory control changes dramatically during sleep. This determines the occurrence of specific breathing disorders during sleep, such as sleep-related hypoventilation or central sleep apnea. Since these potentially fatal disorders are usually diagnosed and treated by sleep specialists or pulmonologists, only OSA will be presented, given its high prevalence and impact on children and adolescents.

Obstructive Sleep Apnea

OSA is a well-known but still under recognized sleep disorder and should be suspected in any child who snores. The prevalence of OSA is 1% to 5% in the general pediatric population but likely much higher in obese children and children with medical or neurodevelopmental conditions and habitual snoring (33). However, as parents get used to their children snoring, they tend not to report it, unless specifically probed. Notably, primary snoring, even in the absence of OSA, is associated with symptoms and consequences similar to OSA (34).

Clinically, symptoms of OSA include chronic snoring, labored breathing, gasping, or choking during sleep, apneas (breathing pauses) witnessed by parents and/or frequent arousals in a child with chronic snoring. Nocturnal enuresis often accompanies pediatric OSA. Excessive daytime sleepiness is less prominent in children than in adults, but children with OSA are prone to develop psychiatric symptoms mimicking ADHD, irritability, and behavioral problems (7,33). OSA requires PSG for definitive diagnosis and assessment of severity. Polysomnographycally, it is identified by the presence of apneas, hypopneas and brief cortical arousals during sleep, secondary to intermittent upper-respiratory obstructions. In children and adolescents, the upper airway obstruction is often secondary to enlarged tonsils and adenoids, but obesity, craniofacial and muscular abnormalities can also determine or worsen OSA. Chronic snoring and OSA should be routinely screened in children with ADHD; PSG is indicated for detection of OSA in typical children in the presence of clinical symptoms. Clinicians should have a low threshold for requesting a PSG whenever sleep-disordered breathing is suspected or when evaluating children with neurodevelopmental conditions such as Down syndrome, Prader–Willi, or neuromuscular diseases. See Table 5.9.4 for respiratory indications for PSG.

Consequences of untreated OSA include cardiovascular, growth, cognitive, and behavioral abnormalities (33). Cognitive deficits associated with OSA include lower scores on objective and subjective measures of general intelligence, attention, memory, and executive function (33).

Adenotonsillectomy is the primary treatment for OSA in children. Successful treatment of OSA typically results in improvements in behavioral problems and cognitive functions, though residual OSA after adenotonsillectomy is common. Post-adenotonsillectomy OSA is found in up to a third in low-risk populations and up to two-thirds in obese children (33). Nasal steroids can be considered for mild cases.

Parasomnias

Parasomnias are disorders characterized by the recurrence of undesirable behaviors or emotions during sleep or at sleep transitions. Parasomnias are classified as NREM parasomnias, REM parasomnias, or other parasomnias. Examples of NREM parasomnias or disorders of arousal are sleepwalking and sleep terrors. Examples of REM-related parasomnias are nightmare disorder, REM behavior disorder, and recurrent sleep paralysis; enuresis is considered an "other parasomnia" (24). The concomitant presence of features of wakefulness and sleep at the same time, such as locomotory behavior during sleep, is a key feature of parasomnias. This section covers disorders of arousals (NREM parasomnias) and nightmare disorders, given their high prevalence in children. Enuresis is covered in Chapter 5.12.

Disorders of Arousal, NREM Parasomnias

The two most common, and clinically relevant, NREM parasomnias in childhood are sleep terrors and sleepwalking. Essential features are presence of arousal and motor behaviors and/or significant autonomic activation while the person is still asleep or only partially aroused (35). Complete amnesia is usual, unless the individual wakes up during the event. They are associated with risk for serious injury (36).

During sleepwalking episodes, the child leaves the bed and wanders and can engage in potentially dangerous activity such as leaving the house or cooking. The child appears confused, with limited response to verbal or physical stimulation and emits no or reduced verbal responses (usually basic words). Occasionally, the family becomes aware of sleepwalking behaviors when the child wakes up in the morning, not in bed. Episodes usually last a few minutes but can occasionally last up to half an hour.

Night terrors are characterized by a sudden arousal, accompanied by loud screaming, possible simple vocalizations, and autonomic activation with tachypnea, tachycardia, and diaphoresis. The child may appear glassy-eyed, staring without seeing, and unresponsive to visual or verbal cues. Sleep terrors are usually briefer, lasting from 30 seconds to 5 minutes, but they occasionally can be longer. Frequency of episodes ranges from a few episodes a year to daily. Episode frequency tends to decrease with age.

NREM parasomnias are common. The prevalence of sleep terrors has been reported in up to 34% in children below age 2, and lifetime episodes of sleepwalking have been reported in up to 29% in older children with a peak between ages 6 and 12 (35,36). These disorders persist in 3% to 4% of adults (35). Boys and girls are equally affected (35,36). Familial aggregation has been consistently reported. Pathophysiologic overlap among disorders of arousal is suggested by the emergence of later sleepwalking in up to a third of young children with sleep terrors (36). Both kinds of episodes are triggered by the same factors, including sleep deprivation, noise, fever, medications, and sleep disruptions in general, including sleep-related breathing disorders (36).

Electroencephalographically, sleep terrors and sleepwalking arise from SWS (N3), and during the events, the individual is cortically asleep, despite motor or vocal behavior and apparent distress. This explains the amnesia and lack of mentation (no dreaming content) if awakened, inconsolability, and the temporal distribution (emergence in the first third of the night when N3 is maximally represented).

The differential diagnosis of NREM parasomnias includes nightmares and seizure disorders, specifically nocturnal frontal lobe epilepsy. Nightmares are more frequent in the last part of the night and are associated with vivid dream imagery, a fully alert, frightened and oriented youngster, and recollection of the episode in the morning. Nocturnal seizures are usually briefer than parasomnias, lasting often less than 2 minutes, can present multiple times per night, do not cluster in the first third of the sleep time, and behaviors are often highly stereotyped (35). A PSG is indicated when nocturnal epilepsy is suspected, or when episodes are extremely frequent, atypical or violent or might be associated to OSA. See Table 5.9.8 for nonrespiratory indications for PSG.

TABLE 5.9.8

COMMON NONRESPIRATORY INDICATIONS FOR POLYSOMNOGRAPHY AND MULTIPLE SLEEP LATENCY TEST IN CHILDREN

Evaluation of hypersomnolence and narcolepsy	Unexplained excessive daytime sleepiness should be assessed with PSG followed by multiple sleep latency test (MSLT)
Parasomnias	In presence of frequent or potentially injurious parasomnias, to differentiate parasomnia from nocturnal epilepsy, in case of enuresis, or if there is suspicion for parasomnia comorbid with sleep-disordered breathing or periodic limb movement disorder
Suspicion for periodic limb movement disorder and possibly for supportive data for restless leg syndrome (RLS)	For children with RLS who also complains of poor sleep or those symptoms suggestive of periodic limb movement disorder

The basic treatment for parasomnias includes child and family reassurance, education, and safety measures. The family should be informed that episodes are usually transient, not serious, and in most cases require no specific pharmacologic intervention. Since sleep deprivation and/or irregular schedules might trigger episodes in predisposed children, parents should be advised of the importance of strict sleep hygiene and sufficient amounts of sleep for the child's age. An after-school nap may be suggested to reduce night N3 intensity and reduce propensity for episodes. Sleep terrors and sleepwalking have a potential for injuries and safety should be addressed. See Table 5.9.9 for safety measures for NREM parasomnias. A possible behavioral approach to frequent episodes of parasomnias is to establish scheduled awakenings. Parents are instructed to monitor the time of the episodes through a sleep diary and to briefly awaken the child approximately half an hour prior to the expected episode. While often successful, this technique might also trigger more events. When the episodes do not respond to sleep hygiene, are frequent or severe with concern for dangerous activities, a low dose of long half-life benzodiazepine, for example, clonazepam, can be used at bedtime for 2 to 3 months and then tapered slowly, monitoring for reoccurrence upon discontinuation.

Nightmares

Dreams are normally reported by children after age 3 (37) and nightmares shortly thereafter. Whereas a standard definition is still lacking, nightmares can be broadly defined as dreams characterized by intense negative emotions such as fear, but also anger, disgust, or sadness, which awaken the individual from sleep (38). Disturbing dreams or "bad dreams" are similar to nightmares but do not interrupt sleep. There is a phenomenologic and likely qualitative continuity between nightmares and disturbing dreams. Clinically, both require

TABLE 5.9.9

SAFETY MEASURES FOR SLEEP TERRORS AND SLEEPWALKING

Assess for injuries or dangerous behaviors	Injuring self or others? Falling? Leaving the house? Using the stove? Inappropriate ingestion of food or medications? Aggressive behaviors?
Establish safety	Parent notification measures, e.g., bells/alarm on the door Secure front door Remove sharp objects Cover sharp obstacles Barricade and/or cover windows Lock firearms and medications Mattress on the floor if indicated Manage sleepovers and college living arrangement (ideally first floor dorm room for frequent episodes)

attention if they are associated with waking emotional distress. Nightmares mostly occur during REM sleep and thus are considered an REM parasomnia. After waking up from a nightmare, the child is often scared but awake, oriented and able to recount the dream content. This helps differentiate them from sleep terrors. Because REM sleep occurs most commonly in the latter third of the night, nightmares generally are noted in the early morning hours, after 2:00 AM. For preschool children, nightmares often include images of monsters and frightening animals; for older school-age children, nightmares typically include more usual human imagery including being injured, lost, or abandoned. If nightmares are frequent, they can be a source of bedtime resistance. Nightmares and disturbing dreams are associated with both acute and posttraumatic stress disorders, anxiety disorders, and suicidal ideation, even when controlling for depression in children and adolescents (39). They are also associated with sleep disorders including sleep deprivation and other parasomnias (38,39). Nightmares and disturbing dreams are common in children and adolescents, up to three to four times the rates reported for adults (38). At ages 3 to 5, 10% to 50% of children report having experienced disturbing dreams. Prevalence rises with age and peaks at ages 10 to 12, with frequent nightmares reported by up 44% (38,39). Disturbed dreams are approximately equally present in boys and girls but toward early adolescence, they become more common in girls and less common in boys (38,39).

Although treatment of nightmares in adults has progressed (40), limited interventions address this condition in children (39). If nightmares are frequent or distressing, the presence of possibly undisclosed trauma and/or other concurrent anxiety symptoms, including separation anxiety should be explored. Imagery rehearsal therapy appears to be the most promising treatment both in children and adolescents (39). During treatment, the child is invited to modify the content of his most recent nightmare to something not distressing, and then visualize and rehearse (cognitive intervention and exposure) the new imagined version while in a state of relaxation (behavioral intervention) (41). The child can also use drawings rather than mental imagery, if developmentally appropriate (39). Although some research has been done on the treatment of nightmares using pharmacologic agents, insufficient evidence supports such treatments for children (39).

Hypersomnolence Disorders and Narcolepsy

Hypersomnolence (excessive daytime sleepiness) is the main characteristic of several sleep disorders. DSM-5 classifies syndromes with primary hypersomnolence into two groups: (1) hypersomnolence disorder and (2) narcolepsy. ICSD-3 differentiates narcolepsy into two subtypes. ICSD-3 "narcolepsy type 1" requires demonstration of orexin/hypocretin deficiency or presence of cataplexy. Hypersomnolence accompanied by objective measures of sleepiness via MSLT and/or presence of sleep-onset REM periods is defined as "narcolepsy type 2." In the ICSD-3, other conditions characterized by hypersomnolence are classified as other disorders. These include idiopathic hypersomnia and hypersomnia associated with a mental disorder. This section follows the DSM-5 classification.

Hypersomnolence Disorder

Historically, hypersomnolence was a key feature of narcolepsy, but starting from the late 1970s, the diagnosis of idiopathic hypersomnia became attached to excessive sleepiness not associated to narcolepsy (42).

The main feature of hypersomnolence disorder is excessive daytime sleepiness, in the absence of substantial sleep deprivation. Clinically, patients usually complain of excessively long night sleep, restorative sleep, and need for frequent naps or dozing off. They can also struggle with awakening in the morning, or present prolonged confusion upon awakening (i.e., sleep drunkenness or sleep inertia). Associated features can be manifestations of autonomic dysfunction such as headache, cold extremities, temperature dysregulation, digestive problems, and cognitive symptoms such as attention and memory problems and mental fatigability (42). Pathophysiologic, genetic, traumatic or immunologic hypotheses have been proposed but mechanisms of the disorder remains unclear (42). Prevalence is between 0.5% and 1% in the general population (25,42) with onset generally beginning in adolescence or young adulthood and usually a stable course (42). Psychiatrically, hypersomnolence disorder often accompanies affective illnesses, especially depressive episodes including unipolar and bipolar types; the presence of a mental disorder can be specified in DSM-5. The diagnostic process is complex and patients should be referred to a sleep specialist for a conclusive diagnostic workup including actigraphy, PSG and MSLT, and for treatment. Differential diagnoses include insufficient sleep syndrome, narcolepsy, OSA, delayed sleep phase disorder, or medical conditions such as hypothyroidism (42).

Narcolepsy

Clinically, narcolepsy is characterized by severe and chronic hypersomnolence and brief intrusions of REM sleep–like states during wakefulness. These REM sleep intrusions are responsible for most of the symptoms of narcolepsy, namely cataplexy, sleep paralysis, and hypnagogic hallucinations. Cataplexy is pathognomic for narcolepsy and presents as a sudden loss of peripheral muscle tone, usually provoked by strong affect, often positive, such as laughter. The face and neck are often involved and cataplexy can present as slurred speech. Cataplexy reflects the muscle atonia of REM sleep. In children, cataplexy can also present as long-lasting periods of decreased muscle tone, unsteady gait, grimacing, and tongue protrusions (43). Cataplectic attacks are brief, rarely lasting more than 1 to 2 minutes, with immediate and complete recovery. Attacks may occur only a few times a year or as frequently as many times a day. Consciousness and memory remain intact, if the child remains awake. Sleep paralysis is characterized by inability to move at sleep–wake transitions. The paralysis lasts for seconds to a few minutes and is another manifestation of REM sleep atonia incursion into wakefulness. Similarly, REM-related mentation (dreaming) can intrude during wakefulness at sleep–wake transitions as hypnagogic or hypnopompic hallucinations. They often present as complex hallucinations (visual and auditory), rarely lasting longer than 1 to 2 minutes. Fragmentation of nocturnal sleep is also common but brief naps are usually refreshing. Obesity and depression are also often associated features of narcolepsy (43).

Narcolepsy affects about 1 in 2,000 people in the general population. Onset is usually in the second decade, although onset can be earlier. The diagnosis is often delayed 5 to 15 years and approximately half of all individuals with narcolepsy remain undiagnosed (43). The diagnosis is established objectively with PSG and MSLT. The form of narcolepsy associated with low cerebrospinal fluid level of orexin/hypocretin is often accompanied by cataplexy and generally has more severe symptoms (43). Other forms of narcolepsy present with PSG and MSLT abnormalities diagnostic of narcolepsy, without cataplexy and/or low orexin/hypocretin levels. These forms may be phenotypically similar disorders with different etiologies and pathogeneses (43). Low levels of orexin/hypocretin and cataplexy are usually associated with loss of orexin-producing neurons. Genetic factors play a role in this degenerative process; more than 98% of individuals with low orexin/hypocretin and/or cataplexy are positive for the human leukocyte antigen (HLA)DQB1*06:02, which is present in 12% to 30% of the general population (43). Polymorphisms of other genes affecting immune function have also been associated to this form of narcolepsy. Autoimmune processes, secondary to infections but also to vaccinations, have been proposed as mechanism of neuronal destruction (43). The pathogenesis of forms of narcolepsy not associated with low orexin/hypocretin is unknown (43).

The treatment of narcolepsy is based on a combination of behavioral and pharmacologic approaches. A regular sleep–wake schedule is strongly advised for children and adolescents with narcolepsy. Regular meal times and physical activity should also be encouraged at an early stage to avoid weight gain, which can be severe. Additionally, routine naps of 20 to 30 minutes are generally recommended to increase daytime wakefulness and psychomotor performances. This can be difficult during school hours, but the gym or infirmary can be used. The adolescent naps for 20- to 40-minute periods, awakening refreshed. The cycle is repeated again within 2 to 3 hours. This refreshed feeling contrasts with the disorientation and persistent fatigue associated with hypersomnolence disorder secondary to other causes.

Pharmacologically, stimulant medications are used most commonly for treating excessive daytime sleepiness, and venlafaxine and tricyclic antidepressant medications for cataplexy. Sodium oxybate (sodium salt of gamma-hydroxybutyrate) is effective for both hypersomnolence and cataplexy and in prepubertal children with orexin/hypocretin deficiency can improve obesity, normalize sleep, wake, and cataplexy by itself (44). Sodium oxybate can only be prescribed by sleep specialists because of the risk of diversion and is usually reserved for severe cases.

Patients with narcolepsy usually adjust poorly to their disorder. They exhibit problems in school and in social relationships, thus behavioral management, emotional and psychosocial support, and counseling are essential components of treatment.

Circadian Rhythm Sleep Disorder, Delayed Sleep Phase Type

As mentioned in the section on sleep regulation, circadian rhythms are one of main physiologic systems which regulate sleep–wake cycles. When individuals fall asleep and wake up naturally roughly at the socially expected times, they are considered to have a normal sleep phase. When the sleep and wake-up times occur earlier than socially expected, for example, 7 PM to 3 AM, the sleep phase is defined as "advanced." Conversely, when sleep and wake-up times occur later than socially expected, for example, 3 AM to 11 AM, the sleep phase is "delayed." At times, this misalignment between endogenous rhythms and expected sleep–wake schedule causes social or academic problems, becoming a circadian rhythm disorder.

Development and social demands both affect circadian rhythms and melatonin secretion timing, and most adolescents naturally experience a sleep phase delay, that is , they tend to fall asleep and wake up later than during childhood and often later than expected or required. Clinically, the adolescent complains of being unable to fall asleep and struggles to awake in the morning. Absences and tardiness or dozing off in class are common associated features. As the adolescent stays up late and arises early for school, he tends to accumulate sleep debt and, as a consequence, he often "sleeps in" or does "sleep marathons" on weekends to catch up. This lack of regularity reinforces and worsens the problem, causing a perpetual social jetlag.

Delayed sleep phase disorder prevalence is estimated to be greater than 7% in adolescents (25). Pathogenesis is multifactorial. Delayed sleep phase has been associated with polymorphisms of genes regulating circadian rhythms such as *Per3*, inappropriately timed light exposure, abnormal light sensitivity and social gains, such as unsupervised time for adolescents (7,24).

Differential diagnoses include narcolepsy, given the excessive daytime sleepiness, and insomnia. However, while individuals with insomnia struggle to fall asleep in most circumstances, adolescents with delayed sleep phase report no difficulties in their sleep patterns when allowed to follow their natural schedule. This can be clarified by asking about their sleep during vacations, sleep during weekends, and asking about circadian variation (do they consider themselves night owls?). Questionnaires, such as the CCTQ, show eveningness preference and a 2-week sleep diary often shows the delayed sleep-onset and extremely delayed wake-up times on weekends. Once a phase delay syndrome is chronic and persistent, phase advance methods of resetting the biologic clock may be necessary. Behavioral methods include strict adherence to sleep hygiene, avoidance of light emitting devices for at least 2 hours prior to scheduled sleep time (as this can cause further phase delay), and avoiding more than 2 hours discrepancy in wake-up time between weekdays and weekends. Ideally, phones and other electronic devices use should be restricted at night. Bright light exposure after natural awakening and low-dose melatonin (0.5 to 1 mg 6 to 4 hours prior to bedtime) are commonly used as chronotherapeutic agents (6,45).

Restless Legs Syndrome/ Willis–Ekbom Disease

RLS is a neurologic disorder presenting with sensory-motor symptoms, usually creepy or crawling sensations in the extremities and an urge to move the legs usually relieved by movement. The sensations and the urge to move are more prominent or only present in the evening and are exacerbated by immobility, thus interfering with sleep initiation and maintenance. While the sensory component often accompanies the syndrome, only the urge to move the legs and the other associated features are required. Difficulty falling asleep is a major consequence of RLS along with fatigue, inattentiveness, or sleepiness. Simple questions such as "Do your legs want to kick at night?" and "Do your legs bother you at night?" can be good screening probes for the disorder. The pediatric prevalence of

RLS is 2% to 4% in the United States, United Kingdom, and Turkey; moderate to severe RLS was found in 0.5% to 1% of children (24). Childhood RLS is often misdiagnosed as growing pains, limiting access to appropriate treatment. On PSG, during sleep, patients with RLS often show periodic, stereotyped jerks, which are defined as periodic limb movements and can be associated with further sleep disruption. RLS is highly familial, with recent adult studies showing familial rates up to 77% in early-onset cases (46); multiple gene variants have been associated with the disorder in genome-wide studies (47). The pathophysiology of RLS is still unclear but likely related to iron and dopamine metabolism. Iron is a cofactor for tyrosine hydroxylase, which is essential for dopamine synthesis. Thus, ferritin, a measure of iron storage, should be routinely assessed in children with RLS. Oral iron supplementation should be considered for ferritin below <50 mcg/L (47). Adult RLS responds to dopaminergic agents and an abnormal dopaminergic system may be responsible for the association between RLS and ADHD; approximately one-quarter of individuals with RLS have attention problems and conversely, 13% to 35% of individuals with ADHD meet criteria for RLS (46). For children, iron supplementation and nonpharmacologic treatments are indicated for mild cases. Moderate to severe cases should be referred for medication trials in the setting of long-term specialty care (46).

Disordered Sleep in Psychiatric Conditions

Less information about sleep disorders in children and adolescents with medical and psychiatric conditions is available than for adults. However, the last decade has seen long overdue surge of interest in pediatric sleep disorders. It is becoming evident that sleep disturbances in childhood are common, associated with a wide range of psychopathologies, and represent a risk factor for the development of future psychiatric disorders (1).

Children who live in institutions are reported to have short sleep periods, repeated nighttime awakenings, and phase delay disorders. Children with neurodevelopmental disorders such as autism experience shorter sleep duration, frequent night awakenings and difficulties falling asleep, possibly secondary to melatonin secretion abnormalities (1). Extensive research has demonstrated the association between ADHD and sleep disturbances, although the mechanisms for this association remain unclear (1,48). Children with ADHD often struggle with difficulties falling asleep, RLS, OSA, and periodic limb movements. Objectively, they are more likely to have lower efficiency, more stage shifts, and higher number of apneas or hypopneas, and they tend to have variable sleep–wake schedules (48).

Sleep disturbances, including insomnia, hypersomnia, and nightmares may be important indicators of depression severity and suicidality in children and adolescents (49). Polysomnographycally, youth with depression also display short REM latency, a biologic marker for depression in adults. However, other indicators of disturbed sleep present in adults with depression, including disruptions of sleep-related endocrine regulation, have not been found consistently in children and adolescents (50,51). Sleep extension and circadian manipulation (phase advance) have been considered possible adjunctive treatments for juvenile depression.

So far, limited research has focused on sleep in children and adolescents with psychotic disorders, although difficulties sleeping may predict psychosis onset in high-risk adolescents/young adults. Additionally, the extent of sleep problems was found to correlate with decreased thalamic volume (1), a key brain region involved in sleep. An association between psychotic symptoms at puberty and nightmares and sleep terrors during childhood has also been found (1).

Sleep disturbances have been consistently connected with anxiety disorders in youth, and often interpreted as secondary to anxiety. Conversely, longitudinal studies have shown that sleep disturbances are often more predictive of later anxiety than vice versa (1).

Finally, poor sleep is associated with increased substance use and risk-taking behaviors; specifically, sleep deprivation can compromise self-regulation and reward-related behaviors, and most substances, including alcohol, exert deleterious effects on sleep–wake cycles and sleep architecture, potentially leading to a vicious cycle. Finally, most psychotropic medications, including serotonin reuptake inhibitors and stimulants, negatively affect sleep or circadian rhythm and require close monitoring.

In closing, more research continues to be needed to better understand the associations and interactions of sleep disturbances with psychopathology. Delineating the underlying mechanisms of these associations will inform causal influences which may have direct implications for therapeutics across a wide spectrum of disorders and functioning.

References

1. Gregory AM, Sadeh A: Annual Research Review: sleep problems in childhood psychiatric disorders—a review of the latest science. *J Child Psychol Psychiatry* 57:296–317, 2015.
2. Owens J. Insufficient sleep in adolescents and young adults: an update on causes and consequences. *Pediatrics* 134(3):e921–e932, 2014.
3. Sadeh A, Tikotzky L, Kahn M: Sleep in infancy and childhood: implications for emotional and behavioral difficulties in adolescence and beyond. *Curr Opin Psychiatry* 27(6):453–459, 2014.
4. Schreck KA, Richdale AL: Knowledge of childhood sleep: a possible variable in under or misdiagnosis of childhood sleep problems. *J Sleep Res* 20(4):589–597, 2011.
5. Lipton J, Becker RE, Kothare SV: Insomnia of childhood. *Curr Opin Pediatr* 20(6):641–649, 2008.
6. Kotagal S, Chopra A: Pediatric sleep-wake disorders. *Neurol Clin* 30(4):1193–1212, 2012.
7. Mindell JA, Owens JA: *A Clinical Guide to Pediatric Sleep: Diagnosis and Management of Sleep Problems*. Philadelphia, PA, Lippincott Williams & Wilkins, 2015.
8. Boerner KE, Coulombe JA, Corkum P: Barriers and facilitators of evidence-based practice in pediatric behavioral sleep care: qualitative analysis of the perspectives of health professionals. *Behav Sleep Med* 13(1):36–51, 2015.
9. Aurora RN, Lamm CI, Zak RS, et al.: Practice parameters for the non-respiratory indications for polysomnography and multiple sleep latency testing for children. *Sleep* 35(11):1467–1473, 2012.
10. Roffwarg HP, Muzio JN, Dement WC: Ontogenetic development of the human sleep-dream cycle. *Science* 152(3722):604–619, 1966.
11. Mirmiran M, Maas YG, Ariagno RL: Development of fetal and neonatal sleep and circadian rhythms. *Sleep Med Rev* 7(4):321–334, 2003.
12. Borbely AA, Daan S, Wirz-Justice A, Deboer T: The two-process model of sleep regulation: a reappraisal. *J Sleep Res* 25(2):131–143, 2016.
13. Iglowstein I, Jenni OG, Molinari L, Largo RH: Sleep duration from infancy to adolescence: reference values and generational trends. *Pediatrics* 111(2):302–307, 2003.
14. Aurora RN, Zak RS, Karippot A, et al.: Practice parameters for the respiratory indications for polysomnography in children. *Sleep* 34(3):379–388, 2011.
15. Owens JA, Dalzell V: Use of the 'BEARS' sleep screening tool in a pediatric residents' continuity clinic: a pilot study. *Sleep Med* 6(1):63–69, 2005.
16. Honaker SM, Meltzer LJ: Bedtime problems and night wakings in young children: an update of the evidence. *Paediatr Respir Rev* 15(4):333–339, 2014.
17. Werner H, Molinari L, Guyer C, Jenni OG: Agreement rates between actigraphy, diary, and questionnaire for children's sleep patterns. *Arch Pediatr Adolesc Med* 162(4):350–358, 2008.
18. Owens JA, Spirito A, McGuinn M: The Children's Sleep Habits Questionnaire (CSHQ): psychometric properties of a survey instrument for school-aged children. *Sleep* 23(8):1043–1051, 2000.
19. Chervin RD, Hedger K, Dillon JE, Pituch KJ: Pediatric sleep questionnaire (PSQ): validity and reliability of scales for sleep-disordered breathing, snoring, sleepiness, and behavioral problems. *Sleep Med* 1(1):21–32, 2000.
20. Goodlin-Jones BL, Sitnick SL, Tang K, Liu J, Anders TF: The Children's Sleep Habits Questionnaire in toddlers and preschool children. *J Dev Behav Pediatr* 29(2):82–88, 2008.
21. Werner H, Lebourgeois MK, Geiger A, Jenni OG. Assessment of chronotype in four- to eleven-year-old children: reliability and validity of the Children's Chronotype Questionnaire (CCTQ). *Chronobiol Int* 26(5):992–1014, 2009.

22. Reid GJ, Huntley ED, Lewin DS: Insomnias of childhood and adolescence. *Child Adolesc Psychiatr Clin N Am* 18(4):979–1000, 2009.
23. Mindell JA, Kuhn B, Lewin DS, Meltzer LJ, Sadeh A; American Academy of Sleep Medicine: Behavioral treatment of bedtime problems and night wakings in infants and young children. *Sleep* 29(10):1263–1276, 2006.
24. Medicine, A.A.o.S.: *International Classification of Sleep Disorders*. Darien, IL, American Academy of Sleep Medicine, 2014.
25. Association A.P.: *Diagnostic and Statistical Manual of Mental Disorders : DSM-5*. Washington, DC, American Psychiatric Association, 2013.
26. Three ZT: *Diagnostic Classification of Mental Health and Developmental Disorders of Infancy and Early Childhood: Revised Edition (DC: 0-3R)*. Washington, DC, Zero To Three Press, 2005, .
27. Cortesi F, Giannotti F, Ivanenko A, Johnson K: Sleep in children with autistic spectrum disorder. *Sleep Med* 11(7):659–664, 2010.
28. Meltzer LJ, Mindell JA. Systematic review and meta-analysis of behavioral interventions for pediatric insomnia. *J Pediatr Psychol* 39(8):932–948, 2014.
29. Owens JA, Babcock D, Blumer J, et al.: The use of pharmacotherapy in the treatment of pediatric insomnia in primary care: rational approaches. A consensus meeting summary. *J Clin Sleep Med* 1(1):49–59, 2005.
30. Taylor DJ, Roane BM: Treatment of insomnia in adults and children: a practice-friendly review of research. *J Clin Psychol* 66(11):1137–1147, 2010.
31. Owens JA, Moturi S: Pharmacologic treatment of pediatric insomnia. *Child Adolesc Psychiatr Clin N Am* 18(4):1001–1016, 2009.
32. Bruni O, Alonso-Alconada D, Besag F, et al.: Current role of melatonin in pediatric neurology: clinical recommendations. *Eur J Paediatr Neurol* 19(2):122–133, 2015.
33. Marcus CL, Brooks LJ, Draper KA, et al.: Diagnosis and management of childhood obstructive sleep apnea syndrome. *Pediatrics* 130(3):e714–e755, 2012.
34. Brockmann PE, Urschitz MS, Schlaud M, Poets CF: Primary snoring in school children: prevalence and neurocognitive impairments. *Sleep Breath* 16(1):23–29, 2012.
35. Avidan AY, Kaplish N: The parasomnias: epidemiology, clinical features, and diagnostic approach. *Clin Chest Med* 31(2):353–370, 2010.
36. Petit D, Pennestri MH, Paquet J, et al.: Childhood sleepwalking and sleep terrors: a longitudinal study of prevalence and familial aggregation. *JAMA Pediatr* 169(7):653–658, 2015.
37. Foulkes D: A cognitive-psychological model of REM dream production. *Sleep* 5(2):169–187, 1982.
38. Levin R, Nielsen TA: Disturbed dreaming, posttraumatic stress disorder, and affect distress: a review and neurocognitive model. *Psychol Bull* 133(3):482–528, 2007.
39. Gauchat A, Seguin JR, Zadra A: Prevalence and correlates of disturbed dreaming in children. *Pathol Biol (Paris)* 62(5):311–318, 2014.
40. Seda G, Sanchez-Ortuno MM, Welsh CH, Halbower AC, Edinger JD: Comparative meta-analysis of prazosin and imagery rehearsal therapy for nightmare frequency, sleep quality, and posttraumatic stress. *J Clin Sleep Med* 11(1):11–22, 2015.
41. St-Onge M, Mercier P, De Koninck J: Imagery rehearsal therapy for frequent nightmares in children. *Behav Sleep Med* 7(2):81–98, 2009.
42. Billiard M, Sonka K: Idiopathic hypersomnia. *Sleep Med Rev* 29:23–33, 2015.
43. Scammell TE: Narcolepsy. *N Engl J Med* 373(27):2654–2662, 2015.
44. Mignot EJ: A practical guide to the therapy of narcolepsy and hypersomnia syndromes. *Neurotherapeutics* 9(4):739–752, 2012.
45. Morgenthaler TI, Lee-Chiong T, Alessi C, et al.: Practice parameters for the clinical evaluation and treatment of circadian rhythm sleep disorders. An American Academy of Sleep Medicine report. *Sleep* 30(11):1445–1459, 2007.
46. Picchietti DL, Bruni O, de Weerd A, et al.: Pediatric restless legs syndrome diagnostic criteria: an update by the International Restless Legs Syndrome Study Group. *Sleep Med* 14(12):1253–1259, 2013.
47. Picchietti MA, Picchietti DL: Advances in pediatric restless legs syndrome: iron, genetics, diagnosis and treatment. *Sleep Med* 11(7):643–651.
48. Cortese S, Brown TE, Corkum P, et al.: Assessment and management of sleep problems in youths with attention-deficit/hyperactivity disorder. *J Am Acad Child Adolesc Psychiatry* 52(8):784–796, 2013.
49. Pigeon WR, Pinquart M, Conner K: Meta-analysis of sleep disturbance and suicidal thoughts and behaviors. *J Clin Psychiatry* 73(9):e1160–e1167, 2012.
50. Waterman GS, Dahl RE, Birmaher B, et al.: The 24-hour pattern of prolactin secretion in depressed and normal adolescents. *Biol Psychiatry* 35(7):440–445, 1994.
51. Dahl RE, Ryan ND, Williamson DE, et al.: Regulation of sleep and growth hormone in adolescent depression. *J Am Acad Child Adolesc Psychiatry* 31(4):615–621, 1992.

5.10 ■ SOMATIZATION IN CHILDREN AND ADOLESCENTS

CHAPTER 5.10 ■ FUNCTIONAL SOMATIC SYMPTOMS AND DISORDERS

JOHN V. CAMPO, MARY LYNN DELL, AND GREGORY K. FRITZ

INTRODUCTION

The biomedical model, a central tenet of Western medicine, maintains that the subjective suffering of patients, most commonly described as *illness*, is best understood as a consequence of demonstrable biophysical or biochemical abnormalities at the intracellular, intercellular, organ, organ system, and/or gross anatomical levels known as *disease*. Nevertheless, patients in general and specialty care settings commonly present with physical symptoms and associated disabilities absent explanatory disease in the traditional biomedical sense. "Unexplained" physical symptoms have traditionally been conceptualized as "mental" or "psychological" in nature, and a psychological model of illness causation with its own analogous terminology (psychopathology vs. pathology) and separate system of reimbursement and service delivery (mental health care vs. health care) developed alongside the biomedical model. Despite contemporary understanding that physical and mental health are inextricably linked and that health is a unitary construct, a practical dualism continues to influence our conceptualizations, attitudes, behaviors, and the structure of modern health care.

Illness and disease are associated with cultural expectations. "Sickness" implies individual suffering, lack of responsibility for the illness, and willingness to seek competent medical help (1). The sick are exempted from usual duties and obligations (e.g., school attendance) after a physician has evaluated, diagnosed, and legitimized the illness. While illness associated with disease is readily accepted as "legitimate," the very same symptoms and sufferings in the absence of explanatory disease may be stigmatized as somehow "illegitimate" due to individual weakness, duplicity, or sociomoral failure.

The term somatization has been used descriptively to refer to the experience of physical symptoms where standard medical evaluation reveals no disease or biophysical process sufficient to explain the symptoms or their impact, and such symptoms have commonly been referred to as functional somatic symptoms (FSS) (2,3). A variety of related descriptive terms have been applied to medically unexplained symptoms in the past. For example, the term "neurosis" was initially applied to patients with "nervous symptoms" unassociated with explanatory pathology in the brain or nervous system. Other descriptors such as "psychogenic," "nonorganic," and "hysterical" have typically fallen out of favor after acquiring an inappropriately dualistic and pejorative connotation.

FSS and disorders in children and adolescents are of relevance not simply because they are common. Affected children do suffer and are viewed by parents as being in poorer health than unaffected peers (4,5). Pediatric FSS are associated with considerable functional impairment, most notably school absenteeism and poor school performance (5–10). Pediatric FSS are also well-known risk markers for current and future anxiety and depressive disorders (11–13) and may predict suicide attempts and completion later in life (14). Children and adolescents with FSS use more health services than unaffected peers (4,5,15), and are at risk to fall between the cracks of a polarized health care system that triages care based on whether a problem is considered to be "physical or mental." They are also at risk for unnecessary medical investigations and treatments that not only put the child at risk for iatrogenic (i.e., physician caused) suffering and harm (16), but also may have the unintended consequence of increasing the family's conviction that the child is "sickly" and that serious disease is being overlooked (6). Patients with FSS and their families may feel profoundly misunderstood or even dismissed after hearing that "nothing is physically wrong." Conversely, efforts to explain away the pain simply as a manifestation of a mental disorder can generate confusion and be perceived as an empathic failure.

This chapter builds upon several previous reviews and will address the clinical challenges posed by children and adolescents presenting for evaluation and management of FSS and associated disorders, describe current attempts at diagnostic classification, and outline a practical approach to management (6–8,17).

NOSOLOGY

Efforts to classify the problems suffered by patients with medically unexplained or FSS diverge depending on whether they were initiated from the general medicine perspective, where the approach has been to develop descriptive diagnostic criteria for functional somatic syndromes based on the organ system of interest, or from the mental health perspective, where FSS have been addressed in the existing classification system for mental disorders.

The way clinicians currently conceptualize FSS and disorders has been influenced heavily by the somatoform disorders classification set forth in American Psychiatric Association's *Diagnostic and Statistical Manual of Mental Disorders*, fourth edition (DSM-IV) in 1994 and the DSM-IV-TR in 2000. Somatoform disorders were introduced to account for physically ill patients who did not suffer from an explanatory general medical condition or disease and where the symptoms did not appear to be deliberately produced by the patient or perceived to be under the patient's voluntary control (18,19). The somatoform disorders included somatization disorder, undifferentiated somatoform disorder, conversion disorder, pain disorder, hypochondriasis, body dysmorphic disorder, and somatoform disorder not otherwise specified. However helpful these versions of the DSM might have been, clinicians and researchers alike struggled with the somatoform disorder classification, and some argued that the category should be eliminated entirely, based in part on concerns that the category unintentionally reinforced mind–body dualism by requiring clear-cut distinctions between presumably psychological and physiologic causes for symptoms (20).

Distinguishing somatoform disorders from malingering and factitious disorders often proved difficult, as determining whether a symptom intentionally produced is often based on subjective judgment. Critics also pointed out that common somatic symptoms and concerns presented by patients in ambulatory, nonpsychiatric settings did not receive enough attention (21–25). Finally, children and adolescents were largely excluded in the development of diagnostic criteria and studies of diagnostic validity and reliability.

The DSM-5 groups the entities historically known as somatoform disorders into a section entitled "Somatic Symptom and Related Disorders" (26). The primary diagnoses include somatic symptom disorder, illness anxiety disorder, conversion disorder (functional neurologic symptoms disorder), psychological factors affecting other medical conditions, and factitious disorder, including factitious disorder imposed on self and factitious disorder imposed on others. The two diagnoses of other specified somatic symptom and related disorder, and unspecified somatic symptom and related disorder, capture clinical instances that may not totally qualify for the other diagnoses in this DSM-5 category, but the seriousness and degree of impairment are worthy of diagnosis and treatment focus. The work group charged with updating and reorganizing the DSM-IV somatoform diagnostic category strove to improve diagnostic relevance and utility for primary care and general medical settings. Secondly, somatoform disorders were essentially diagnoses of exclusion, made only after structural or cellular pathologies and/or toxic, metabolic, or chemical insults had been ruled out as etiologies for the presenting symptoms. In other words, the medically unexplained symptoms themselves were the largest focus within the diagnostic schemas. The DSM-5 classification attempts to shift diagnostic attention to the presence of positive, or affirmative, signs and symptoms, such as the association of somatic distress and impairment with abnormal or maladaptive thoughts, feelings, actions, and patterns of behavior (26–32).

Somatic symptom disorder is the diagnosis designed to describe many, if not most, instances in which one or more somatic symptoms cause serious distress or significant disruption in daily living. The individual presents with excessive thoughts, feelings, or behaviors related to the somatic symptoms or associated health concerns as manifested by persistent and disproportionate thoughts about the gravity of the symptoms, a high level of anxiety about health or the symptoms, and/or the devotion of excessive amounts of time and energy to the symptoms and health concerns. This maladaptive preoccupation usually is present for longer than 6 months, though the somatic symptoms themselves may vary and do not need to be present the entire time. Specifiers include mild, moderate, and severe for symptom number and intensity, and persistent if symptoms are severe with marked impairment and last longer than 6 months. A final specifier is "with predominant pain," which both captures this disabling subtype and brings the DSM-IV-TR pain disorder into the folds of the new DSM-5 somatic symptom disorder (26).

Illness anxiety disorder is new to DSM-5. It is diagnosed in the presence of a significant preoccupation with having or acquiring a serious illness when there are no somatic symptoms or when existing symptoms are only mild in intensity. If a comorbid medical condition is also present or if the patient is at risk for such a condition, the preoccupation with somatic symptoms is extreme or out of proportion to what would reasonably be expected. There is high anxiety about health, the patient is easily upset by health-related matters, and these behaviors cannot be explained satisfactorily as a manifestation of another psychiatric disorder such as delusional disorder, obsessive–compulsive disorder, or others of the somatic symptom and related disorders group of diagnoses. Specifiers include *care-seeking type* for those who demonstrate either excessive health-related behaviors such as professional appointments, tests, and procedures; and *care-avoidant type*, for individuals whose illness anxiety leads them to complete avoidance of medical professionals and settings. A 6-month period of symptoms is required for diagnosis, though the feared illnesses may change over time. Individuals previously diagnosed with hypochondriasis in DSM-IV-TR will qualify for either somatic symptom disorder or illness anxiety disorder in DSM-5 (26,33–35).

Conversion disorder is an important consideration in child and adolescent medical and psychiatric care. DSM-5 criteria include one or more symptoms of altered sensory or voluntary motor functioning with clinical findings inconsistent or not compatible with known or recognized medical and neurologic conditions. The symptom(s) cannot be explained better by other medical or psychiatric disorders, and cause distress or impairment in social, occupational, or other important domains of functioning and/or require medical evaluation. DSM-5 recognizes the multiple ways symptoms may be expressed, and incorporates ICD-10-CM codes to signify symptom subtypes. Subtypes noted include with weakness or paralysis, abnormal movement, swallowing symptoms, attacks or seizures, anesthesia or sensory loss, special sensory symptom, and mixed symptoms. Other specifiers include acute or persistent episode, and with or without psychological stressors (26,36).

The diagnosis of *psychological factors affecting other medical conditions* is often used by psychiatrists and other clinicians caring for children and adolescents in whom a medical symptom or condition is indisputably present. Psychological or behavioral elements may affect the medical condition adversely by influencing the onset, course, or recovery from the medical condition, or interfere with the proper treatment of the condition. These factors may influence the underlying pathophysiology of the condition, thus affecting the timing of and severity of symptoms and the need for medical attention or care. These factors present a demonstrable health risk for the individual, and cannot be better explained by the presence of another psychiatric disorder. Specifiers include mild, moderate, severe, and extreme. There is no time length or duration of symptoms specified for this diagnosis, which may also take into account the common scenario of poor or absent treatment adherence (26).

The DSM-5 *factitious disorder* includes two subtypes, *factitious disorder imposed on self* and *factitious disorder imposed on another*. The latter replaces DSM-IV-TR factitious disorder by proxy, commonly known as Munchausen syndrome by proxy. In both types, whether the symptoms are falsified by the patient or others, physical or psychological signs or symptoms are created and there is deception regarding the origin of those signs and symptoms. There are no obvious external rewards for the deceptive behaviors, and the presentation cannot be explained better or more appropriately by another mental disorder. Specifiers denote whether the occurrence is a single episode or recurrent (26).

Other specified somatic symptom and related disorder permits diagnosis of presentations that may fall short of meeting full criteria for another disorder in this category but are nevertheless clinically significant. Examples include pseudocyesis, or the false belief one is pregnant, accompanied by signs and reported symptoms of pregnancy, and brief somatic symptom and illness anxiety disorders of durations less than 6 months (26).

Current discussion and literature both support and applaud the nosologic changes to somatoform disorders in DSM-5, as well as point out shortcomings and areas for future clarification and updates (25,27–37). Minimal literature exists at this time regarding the utility of the DSM-5 diagnostic classifications in the child and adolescent population (38). Therefore, the discussions of epidemiology, assessment, and management that follow remain just as important, if not more so, for contemporary clinical practice.

EPIDEMIOLOGY

Prevalence

FSS and complaints are exceptionally common in children and adolescents, yet most available studies are not comprehensive, relying on self- or parent-report checklists, focusing on some physical symptoms but not others, and failing to include independent medical assessments to determine if the reported symptoms are truly "medically unexplained" (6–9). With rare exception (39), most available studies have focused on the prevalence of specific somatic symptoms rather than the prevalence of specific mental disorders, and standardized research interviews have not typically assessed for the presence of somatoform or somatic symptom disorders as currently categorized in the DSM-5 (26). With these caveats aside, all manner of FSS have been reported by children and adolescents in clinical- and community-based studies, with approximately half of preschool and school-age children reporting at least one somatic complaint in the previous 2 weeks, and approximately 15% endorsing four or more symptoms (10,40,41).

Although individuals typically focus on a single symptom when presenting for medical evaluation, it has been consistently shown that the presence of one FSS predicts another (42). Children and adolescents with one type of somatic complaint are at significantly greater risk of experiencing other types of FSS, both cross-sectionally and longitudinally (12). Empirical support for a "somatic complaints syndrome" is provided by principal components analysis of parent ratings for over 8,000 youth referred for mental health services (43). Recurrent somatic symptoms were reported by 11% of girls and 4% of boys ages 12 to 16 years in the Ontario Child Health Study (44), and other studies report multiple and frequent somatic complaints in 10% to 15% of adolescents (45). Population-based studies have also found that reports of somatic symptoms tend to cluster, with examples of common symptom clusters including pain/weakness, gastrointestinal (GI), conversion/pseudoneurologic, and cardiovascular (41).

Pain is defined as an unpleasant sensory and emotional experience that is associated with tissue damage or perceived as representative of such damage (46). Although typically considered to signal tissue damage, pain and nociception are not identical, which means that pain can be experienced in the absence of nociceptor activity or can be minimal or absent in the presence of great nociceptor activation. Pain is essentially subjective and must be assessed by self-report. Recurrent complaints of pain are particularly common in children and adolescents. Just over one-third of the children and adolescents assessed in the Great Smoky Mountains Study for headaches, stomach aches, and musculoskeletal pain at multiple time points between the ages of 9 and 16 reported at least one somatic complaint that occurred weekly over 3 months prior to the interview assessment (12). Headaches were the most common complaint (24.7%), followed by stomach aches (9.6%) and muscle aches (8.4%). Perquin et al. (47) found a 3-month prevalence of 25% for painful somatic symptoms, with over half of affected children taking medication and over 40% seeking medical help for the pain.

Headache is the most common type of pain reported by school-age children and adolescents, with 10% to 30% endorsing "frequent" headaches, or headaches at least on a weekly basis (10,12,48–51). Headache is cited as the reason for 1% to 2% of pediatric ambulatory visits (52). The classification system currently in use for headaches is descriptive in nature, since most headaches are considered "primary" and not attributable to an underlying physical disease (53). The primary headaches of greatest relevance are migraine and tension-type headache (TTH). Migraine may be diagnosed when a child or adolescent presents with a history of at least five headache attacks where the headache lasts 1 to 72 hours (4 to 72 hours in adults); the headache has at least two of the following characteristics—unilateral location, pulsating quality, moderate to severe pain intensity, and/or is aggravated by routine physical activity; and the headache is accompanied by nausea and/or vomiting or photophobia and phonophobia. Migraine may be accompanied by aura, defined as focal neurologic features that may precede or accompany the headache such as visual scintillating scotoma, sensory symptoms such as numbness, tingling, or paresthesias, and motor symptoms such as motor weakness or dysphasia. TTH may be episodic or chronic, with the main features being bilateral location, nonpulsatile quality, mild to moderate intensity, and lack of aggravation by routine physical activity. Dizziness is another common symptom reported by up to 15% of children in surveys (41,49) that may at times be related to migraine.

Functional abdominal pain (FAP) is quite common, with a prevalence of 7% to 25% in school-age youth (54,55), and is responsible for 2% to 4% of pediatric visits (52). It is the most common somatic symptom reported by preschool children (40). Most cases of pediatric abdominal pain prove to be representative of FAP, particularly in the absence of clues to unrecognized disease such as involuntary weight loss, bleeding, fever, other systemic symptoms, or laboratory abnormalities (56). GI symptoms such as nausea, vomiting, and bowel-related complaints are also common, often in association with FAP, and are commonly associated with headaches as well, particularly with migraine (57,58). Gastroenterologists have developed symptom-based diagnostic criteria for functional gastrointestinal disorders (FGIDs), with the most recent iteration (Rome IV) creating three broad categories of pediatric FGIDs: functional abdominal pain disorders (FAPD), functional nausea and vomiting disorders, and functional defecation disorders (56). A recent review reported the worldwide-pooled prevalence of FAPD to be 13.5% (54). Irritable bowel syndrome (IBS) is diagnosed when FAP is related to defecation and/or changes in the frequency or character of bowel movements, and is the most commonly reported FAPD in the pediatric population with an estimated prevalence of 8.8%. Notable among the functional nausea and vomiting disorders is cyclical vomiting syndrome (CVS). CVS has a community prevalence of 1% or less, and is characterized by recurrent and stereotyped episodes of intense, unexplained nausea and paroxysmal vomiting (56). CVS has been associated with migraine (59).

Chest pain is reported by approximately 10% of school-age children and adolescents (6,41), and is a frequent presentation in pediatric emergency rooms and in pediatric cardiology (60,61). Other common pains include musculoskeletal pains such as limb pain and back pain (6,12). Approximately one-third of Finnish youth reported musculoskeletal pain at least once per week in a community study, with 7.5% endorsing widespread musculoskeletal pains in a number of sites and approximately 1% meeting criteria for fibromyalgia (62). Fibromyalgia is characterized by at least 3 months of multiple musculoskeletal aches and pains, most often in association with fatigue, sleep difficulties, anxiety and depressive symptoms, and pain to palpation on physical examination in so-called "tender points" (63). Other varieties of musculoskeletal complaints may present in pediatric settings, including complex regional pain syndrome type I, or reflex sympathetic dystrophy, which typically develops after immobilization or injury to the limb (64). Clinical features include pain disproportionate to any inciting event such as allodynia (i.e., pain from innocuous tactile stimulation) and/or hyperalgesia (i.e., an exaggerated response to painful stimulation), as well as swelling, changes in skin blood flow, changes in skin temperature, and limitation of functioning. Fatigue is among the most common physical symptoms reported by youth, with up to one-half of adolescents complaining of at least weekly fatigue and 15% reporting daily fatigue (45,65). Chronic fatigue syndrome (CFS), sometimes referred to as myalgic encephalitis (ME) in the United Kingdom, more specifically refers to a condition characterized by severe, disabling fatigue of at least 6 months' duration where alternative medical and psychiatric explanations (e.g., hypothyroidism, malignancy, hepatitis, narcolepsy, obstructive sleep apnea, medication side effects, major mood disorder, schizophrenia, or eating disorder) have been excluded (66). The Centers for Disease Control and Prevention (CDC) definition requires four additional symptoms from a list that includes sleep disturbance, cognitive difficulties such as self-reported limitations in concentration and short-term memory, postexertional malaise, headaches, and musculoskeletal aches and pains. Prevalence of CFS in adolescents is estimated to be between 0.5% and 2%, and the condition is less common in younger children (66). Using data from the Avon Longitudinal Study of Parents and Children, chronic disabling fatigue of at least 6 months' duration was identified in 1.3% of 13 year olds and 1.86% of 16 year olds (67). Onset typically follows an acute febrile illness in approximately two-thirds of cases, with Epstein–Barr virus (EBV) being the best known virus associated with CFS (66).

A variety of functional respiratory symptoms have been reported in children and adolescents, including complaints of cough characterized as somatic cough syndrome and tic cough (68), and shortness of breath or dyspnea (69). Vocal cord dysfunction (VCD) is an often unrecognized condition in which presumed vocal cord spasm leads to symptoms that can mimic acute asthma (70). Affected youth may present with a history of "asthma" unresponsive to aggressive medical management. VCD may be differentiated from asthma by the absence of nocturnal symptoms, localization of wheezing to the upper chest and throat, normal blood gases despite extreme symptoms, and significant adduction of the vocal cords when visualized on laryngoscopy.

Conversion symptoms are symptoms that suggest a neurologic illness in the absence of explanatory neurologic disease. Although these symptoms have generated considerable interest in the psychiatric literature, epidemiologic data are relatively sparse and conversion symptoms appear to be unusual in community samples of Western youth (6,71–74). An Australian population-based study reported an incidence of 2.3 to 4.2 per 100,000 children under 16 years (72) and a more recent UK study found an incidence of 1.3 per 100,000 children between the ages of 7 and 15 (71). Motor abnormalities are the most common presentation at the population level. Presentations with conversion symptoms become increasingly common in tertiary referral centers and pediatric neurology services, where nonepileptic seizures, unresponsiveness, faints, falls, and abnormalities of gait or sensation are the most commonly reported symptoms (75–80). Nonepileptic seizures, in the past sometimes described as "pseudoseizures," resemble epileptic seizures but are not associated with the electroencephalographic abnormalities or clinical course characteristic of true epilepsy, though affected individuals may also suffer from concomitant epilepsy. Relatively little definitive is known about course, though the outcome is favorable in the majority of cases (81), with most resolving within 3 months of diagnosis (82). Though past clinical teaching has emphasized that symptoms considered to be representative of conversion disorder are commonly found to be caused by unrecognized physical disease (83), a systematic review found that the rate of misdiagnosis of conversion symptoms averaged 4% across studies since 1970 (84).

Although hypochondriacal fears and beliefs have not been well studied in childhood and adolescence and the diagnosis of hypochondriasis is quite unusual in younger populations (39), clinical experience and some epidemiologic data suggest that health-related anxiety and fear of suffering from a serious physical disease can be experienced prior to adulthood (15,85). Such illness fears or disease convictions may be rooted in misinterpretation or exaggeration of the threat associated with one or multiple physical sensations, a process sometimes referred to as somatosensory amplification (86). Just over 15% of a sample of Italian adolescents screened positive on a screen for hypochondriacal symptoms and preoccupations (85), and health anxiety has been noted in preadolescents as well, with hypochondriacal fears being associated with FSS, emotional disorders, and increased health expenditures (15). Perhaps counterintuitively, higher levels of illness fears were associated with less health behaviors such as smoking, illicit substance use, poor sleep habits, and physical inactivity. Health anxiety has also been noted in younger children (15).

A prospective epidemiologic study that applied past diagnostic criteria for somatoform disorders in a sample of 3,021 German youth aged 14 to 24 years found the lifetime prevalence of any specific somatoform disorder to be 3% at baseline, and clinically meaningful somatoform illness that did not meet diagnostic criteria for a specific somatoform disorder was reported by an additional 10% of the sample (39). Complaints of pain were most common, but no specific cases of somatization disorder or hypochondriasis were identified in children and adolescents, and the lifetime prevalence of conversion disorder was 0.3%.

Individual and Sociocultural Factors

Reporting of FSS appears to increase with increasing age into adolescence (6,50). Although headache is the most common complaint of pain across childhood and adolescence, FAP is likely the most common complaint in early childhood, with headache prevalence peaking at approximately age 12 (40,50). Polysymptomatic presentations become more common in adolescence (44,87,88). Conversion disorder is especially rare in very young children, and clinicians should be skeptical of presumed conversion symptoms in children younger than age 6 years (6,75,76,89).

In general, FSS such as recurrent complaints of pain occur equally in boys and girls until late childhood and puberty, after which female symptom reporting predominates (6,8). Chronic fatigue (66) and hypochondriacal fears (85) are more common in females, and conversion symptoms are more common among girls than boys across all age groups (77–79). Girls tend to use health services for FSS more than boys (47) and are more consistent in symptom reporting across time (6). Female gender predicts the persistence of FSS and related disorders in adolescents, along with depression and poor self-rated health (39,90).

Low socioeconomic status and lower levels of parental education have been associated with somatic symptom reporting in childhood and adolescence in some studies (4,39,91), as well as with symptom stability (39), but not in others (88). Though often considered a disorder of the upper strata, CFS appears to be more common in children exposed to social deprivation (66). The impact of race/ethnicity and the role of social and cultural factors have been inadequately studied, but culture does appear to be influential. For example, conversion symptoms are reported to be common presentations of psychiatric disorder in non-Western clinical settings, including Turkey and India, and cultural differences in pain expression and behavior have been suggested (6). Unfortunately, existing studies may confound ethnicity, socioeconomic status, and acculturation.

Lack of exercise, sedentary behavior, and low levels of physical fitness have been associated with a variety of FSS in children and adolescents (90) and specifically with CFS (92).

Psychopathology and Temperament

FSS are consistently associated with anxiety and depressive symptoms and disorders in children and adolescents both cross-sectionally and longitudinally, and the likelihood of concurrent anxiety or depression increases with the number of FSS reported (11). Children and adolescents with FSS in the methodologically strong Great Smoky Mountains Study experienced higher rates of anxiety, depression, and behavioral disorders than peers, and were significantly more likely in adulthood to suffer from depression, generalized anxiety, and "combined distress disorders" of mixed depression and anxiety, suggesting a specific relationship between pediatric FSS and later depression and generalized anxiety (12). Persistent FSS across developmental periods were particularly strong predictors of later emotional disorders, and FSS in childhood also predicted suicidality in later life in bivariate analysis, but the finding attenuated in multivariate regression. In a large Finnish sample, FSS at age 8 predicted antidepressant use in young adulthood, and childhood abdominal pain predicted later suicide attempts and completions in boys, but not in girls (14,93).

High rates of psychiatric symptoms and disorders have been consistently observed in studies comparing children and adolescents with FSS to unaffected controls, with particularly high rates of anxiety and/or depressive symptoms and disorders reported in association with FAP, headache, musculoskeletal pain, and chest pain (8,11,12,94). An anxiety disorder can be diagnosed in approximately three-quarters of youth with FAP presenting in primary care (95) and specialty care (96,97). Youth suffering from CFS also report higher levels of anxiety and depressive symptoms and disorders than healthy controls (66,92). Comorbid emotional disorder likely contributes to the functional impairment experienced by youth with FSS (98).

Just as internalizing psychiatric symptoms and disorders appear to be overrepresented in children and adolescents with FSS and disorders, children with internalizing disorders are more likely to suffer from FSS such as FAP and headache (99). A systematic review of the relationship between FSS, anxiety, and depression concluded that childhood anxiety and depression predicted FSS later in life (11), and depressive symptoms appear to be a predictor of the persistence of FSS (90). A longitudinal study of somatoform disorders in adolescents and young adults found pre-existing anxiety, depressive, and substance use disorders to be associated with the new onset of somatoform disorders, and also reported that depression and substance abuse were associated with persistence of FSS (39). Children with autism spectrum disorder also appear to suffer higher rates of functional GI symptoms such as abdominal pain and bowel complaints than controls (100).

Temperamental traits such as behavioral inhibition, harm avoidance, neuroticism, and negative affect have been consistently associated with FSS, anxiety, and depression (95,101), and trait neuroticism prospectively predicts headaches and stomach aches in adolescents (102). These traits share associations with pessimistic worry, fear of uncertainty, and a tendency to respond to environmental challenge at lower thresholds (103,104). Children and adolescents with conversion disorder showed significantly faster reaction times to sad faces than did healthy controls in a study that examined reaction times to facial expressions of emotion, suggesting greater vigilance to expressions of negative emotion and interpersonal threat (105). Physiologic responses of youth with FAP to a social stressor also appear more akin to those of anxiety-disordered youth than of healthy controls (106). Anxiety sensitivity, a tendency to fear bodily sensations associated with anxious arousal based on the belief that they signal real harm, has also been associated with FSS.

Taken together, it is plausible that youth with FSS, anxiety, and depression may share a common tendency to respond to perceived threat with some combination of somatic and cognitive emotional distress (11). It has also been suggested that children with FSS may be "hypersensitive" to pain or "pain prone," responding to painful stimuli at lower thresholds that controls (107). Given existing evidence for a shared neural system that mediates both physical discomfort and social distress, it is plausible that individuals at risk for FSS may indeed be more vulnerable to the impact of both physical pain and social adversity (108).

Life Events and Trauma

A variety of negative experiences and stressors have been associated with FSS in childhood and adolescence, including maltreatment (6,8). A recent study found that the combined severity of negative life events predicted FSS in adolescents even when adjusted for pre-event levels of FSS and anxiety and depression (109). Although most children with FSS have not been maltreated, sexual abuse predicts FSS in children and adolescents (39,110,111). Exposure to parental neglect and the experience of poor care in childhood have also been associated with FSS later in life (112,113). Persistence of FSS has also been associated with exposure to traumatic events (39), and youth with posttraumatic stress disorder appear to be at increased risk of FSS and somatoform disorders (114).

Family and Genetic Factors

The experience of FSS can be familial, and youth with FSS are more likely to have parents and family members who experience higher levels of FSS and report negative health perceptions than unaffected peers (6–8,50,80,87,88,115–120). Recurrent pain such as FAP and headache is more likely to be reported by the family members of affected youth than by those of controls, raising questions regarding so-called "pain-prone" families (108). CFS tends to cluster in the families of affected children, and twin studies suggest a heritable component (65,66,92). Children of parents with somatization disorder have also been found to endorse higher levels of FSS than children of controls (116). Anxiety and depressive symptoms and disorders are associated with FSS within families and across generations (11).

Exposure to illness in a parent has been associated with later FSS, and offspring of adults with FSS are more likely to suffer from health anxieties and higher levels of health service use for FSS than those of controls (117). Parents may influence the experience of FSS in children and adolescents via a number of psychological mechanisms, most notably by reinforcement of illness behaviors and social learning through modeling (121). Selective attention to the expression of FSS and limiting the child's activities and responsibilities can reinforce illness behavior and increase disability associated with the symptoms (118,121). Parents of youth with FSS have been described as overprotective and prone to view their children as particularly vulnerable, which may increase the degree to which the child's symptoms are viewed as threatening. Clinical observers often note that there is a family "model" for an ill child's FSS, suggesting that family members may model maladaptive illness behaviors and methods of coping with FSS, emotional distress, and adversity.

Family systems theorists have sometimes understood pediatric FSS as serving a specific function within the family system, with the child's symptoms potentially allowing the family to avoid conflict, most notably parental–marital conflict, and thus preserving family homeostasis (122,123). Families of youth with FSS are more likely than those of peers to be described as low in perceived support, and affected children are more likely to come from nonintact families and those characterized by parental–marital conflict (5,120). Some observers have also called attention to how a particular child's somatic symptoms may serve a communicative function in the family on the order of "body language" or a "plea for help" (124,125).

Genetic and environmental factors play an interactive role in the development of FSS and related disorders, but some evidence suggests a prominent heritable component (118,126–130). A functional polymorphism in the promoter region of the serotonin transporter gene has been associated with FSS (131,132), as well as trait neuroticism and anxiety (133,134). Other polymorphisms in genes important to the metabolism of specific neurotransmitters have been related to susceptibility for FSS, including association of a polymorphism in catecholamine-*O*-methyltransferase (COMT) with pain sensitivity (135) and in the gene coding for tryptophan hydroxylase, the rate-limiting enzyme in the biosynthesis of serotonin, with somatic anxiety (136), but subsequent studies of potential associations with FSS have been unrevealing (137,138).

Coping

Vulnerability to FSS may be understood as being derivative of individual differences in stress reactivity, stress exposure, threat appraisal, distress tolerance, and coping skills (139,140). Coping refers to voluntary efforts to regulate emotion, thought, behavior, and/or environment in response to challenge or adversity. Several coping styles have been described, and some appear to be more adaptive than others with regard to the management of FSS and emotional distress. Active coping applies problem-focused strategies to resolve the FSS and make the discomfort "go away." In addition to problem solving, active coping strategies may sometimes include emotional expression and emotional regulation. Accommodative coping is characterized by efforts to accept and adjust to adversity, generally by regulating attention or thought patterns via strategies such as acceptance, distraction/ignoring, self-encouragement, and cognitive restructuring. Accommodative strategies are consistently associated with lower levels of FSS and emotional distress in youth. Passive coping reflects strategies that avoid confronting pain such as avoidance, denial, and wishful thinking, and is considered maladaptive given strong associations with worsening levels of pain and emotional distress in children (141,142). Existing research highlights the importance of exaggerated threat appraisal in magnifying and sustaining FSS, and how beliefs about the nature of the illness may influence choice of coping strategy (65,143). Unchecked fears that the child's illness represents a serious threat to the child and family can provoke maladaptive responses that may be active, such as frenetic efforts to "make it just go away," or passive, such as despair and a wish to "give up," rather than more adaptive accommodative responses (143).

Persistence

Somatic symptom reporting early in life predicts FSS later in life. Predictors of persistent FSS include female gender, poor self-rated health, and depression (144). Children who complain of stomach aches at the age of 4 are three times more likely to have similar complaints on follow-up at age 10 than peers (145). Early follow-up studies reported persistence of FAP into adulthood for one-third to one-half of affected children

(16,146–148). Young adults with a childhood history of FAP not only are more likely to report more FSS than controls with no history of childhood pain, but are also much more likely to experience psychiatric symptoms and disorders in adulthood, particularly anxiety and depressive disorders (12,13,119,149). Adults with multiple FSS are more likely to have experienced physical illness before age 17 than other ill adults (112).

ASSESSMENT AND DIAGNOSIS

Approach to the Patient and Family

Assessment establishes the foundation for successful intervention, and both content and process are critically important (17). Empathic acknowledgment of the patient's suffering and the family's very real fears and concerns can aid in establishing a working partnership, and it is both unproductive and presumptuous to challenge the subjective reality of the child's symptoms. Clinicians managing patients with FSS do well to remember that empathic failure by professionals can generate embarrassment, anger, and even a perceived sense of entitlement on the part of patients and family members. Patients and especially parents may fear that the child's symptoms indicate the presence of a life-threatening disease, yet may also be concerned that the child's presentation might be perceived as feigned, imaginary, or an indication of personal weakness or family dysfunction. Youth presenting with FSS have often visited a variety of health care professionals prior to referral for consultation with a psychiatrist or other mental health professional, making it important to explore patient and family experiences with previous providers. For example, families may have had experiences that generated mistrust of medical professionals and the health care system in general, and it is not uncommon for patients and families to believe that the child's FSS have not been taken seriously or have been "dismissed" by previous providers. Patients and families may bristle if they believe they are being told that "nothing is wrong" after weeks or months of worrisome physical symptoms and distress—not to mention several hours in a waiting room.

Patients and families may misinterpret psychiatric referral as an indication that the child's symptoms have not and will not be taken seriously. Conversely, mental health professionals risk a loss of credibility if the child's physical suffering is approached narrowly as being purely "psychological" or as a consequence of "stress," without exploring other possible explanations and the beliefs of the patient and family. Concerns related to stigma can interfere with the willingness of patients and families to engage with mental health professionals and even motivate patients, families, and clinicians to push for potentially dangerous and unnecessary medical investigations and procedures. Ideally, psychiatric assessment will take place within the context of a relationship with a collaborating primary care physician or specialist.

Multiple sources of information are helpful, with important resources beyond the patient including parents, other professionals, teachers, and school nurses. Useful questionnaires with child and parent self-report versions include the Children's Somatization Inventory (CSI), a measure of the presence and intensity of a variety of somatic symptoms (150) and the Functional Disability Inventory (FDI), an assessment of impairment associated with FSS (151). It is important to explore a particular symptom's timing, context, and characteristics, as well as to examine associated social reinforcements and other potential benefits associated with the child assuming the sick role. Parents may inadvertently encourage sick role behaviors by responding to complaints of pain with attention, rewards, or opportunities to avoid unpleasant activities or school (121,152). Identifying any school difficulties can be especially relevant, since learning problems or peer problems such as bullying can reinforce absenteeism. The child's FSS may become part of a self-handicapping strategy by becoming a ready "explanation" for the child not performing up to expectations (152).

Differential Diagnosis

The specific components necessary to a competent assessment of the youthful patient with presumably "medically unexplained" physical symptoms are best determined on a case-by-case basis and dictated by clinical judgment and experience, but should be informed by the development of a differential diagnosis at the outset. Thoughtful clinicians will remain alert to the possibility of unrecognized physical disease, conduct the assessment with an open mind, and communicate an unwillingness to prejudge the etiology of the symptom. Previous records should be carefully reviewed, and there should be no reluctance to initiate additional medical evaluation if the assessment generates new concerns about physical disease or if the clinical picture appears to be changing over time. A balanced approach that avoids excessive testing is nevertheless of great importance, since unnecessary medical tests and treatments carry the risk of iatrogenic disease, as well as of miscommunicating physician uncertainty, which can help maintain or worsen FSS and related disorders (8,17).

There is no simple answer to the question as to when the medical workup is complete, since it may be impossible definitively to rule out unrecognized disease, but unless the treating professionals are reasonably comfortable that serious physical disease has not been missed and are able to communicate this conviction to the patient and family, it is difficult to adequately build a solid foundation for intervention. A given symptom may prove functional despite the presence of a coexisting physical disease, as the simple presence of disease (e.g., epilepsy) does not exclude the possibility of a functional disorder (nonepileptic seizure) and FSS are commonly observed to develop following an acute physical illness or accident (6–8). Beyond unrecognized physical disease, medically unexplained symptoms in a child or adolescent most often are considered functional or FSS, meaning that they are quite real and subjectively outside the patient's sense of voluntary control. From the mental disorder perspective, FSS and syndromes are generally classified as being representative of a somatic symptom disorder or understood as a component of an anxiety or depressive disorder. In addition, "psychological factors affecting medical condition" may be the diagnosis if the FSS is codified by the diagnostician as a general medical condition where emotional or psychological factors are impacting on the illness. As noted previously, the many decision points requiring a clinician to judge "physical versus mental" certainly complicate the diagnostic process and can affect diagnostic reliability. So-called positive findings or clues to a symptom being considered functional go beyond simply eliminating or ruling out physical disease. Such clues include contiguity of the symptom with a psychosocial stressor or stressors; the presence of another diagnosable psychiatric disorder; the association of a symptom with some interpersonal, familial, or social gain for the patient (secondary gain), or even a presumed intrapsychic gain (primary gain); existence of a model for the symptom within the child's immediate environment; a communicative or symbolic meaning for the symptom within the family or immediate social milieu; the violation of known anatomic or physiologic patterns by the symptom; and the response of the symptom to placebo, suggestion, or psychological treatment. Clearly, these clues should not be considered to be definitive in any way, since virtually all could be found in association with physical disease (e.g., asthmatic bronchoconstriction that responds to placebo or suggestion). However, a constellation of such clues taken together is most persuasive (6–8,17). For example, while *"la belle indifférence"* (an apparent lack of concern in relation to the symptom) has often been considered to be suggestive of conversion disorder, it hardly constitutes proof that a given symptom is functional (153).

In circumstances where the child's physical symptoms are judged to be intentionally produced or feigned, FSS and disorders are distinguished from factitious disorders and malingering (26). In factitious disorder, physical symptoms are deliberately feigned or self-inflicted by the patient, with the patient's goal appearing to be an internal one in the form of the psychological gain presumably associated with the sick role. In factitious disorder by proxy, a parent or caretaker feigns, simulates, or causes disease in a child with the motivation being an internal one for the caretaker. Malingering is the deliberate feigning, simulation, or production of physical symptoms in pursuit of an external incentive, such as the avoidance of a particular responsibility or punishment, or the pursuit of financial gain. Inconsistencies or apparent fabrications in the history should raise concerns about these uncommon but real problems. Medical or psychiatric records hand-carried by a parent are certainly not uncommon, yet should provoke at least mild suspicion given that record tampering has been reported in some cases of factitious disorder by proxy.

Careful assessment of the social and family environment is similarly critical. Family history of psychiatric disorder, functional somatic syndromes, chronic physical illness, and disability should be explored, with attention to known risk factors. Because pediatric FSS are commonly associated with separation fears, consideration should be given to experiences which may have led to the family perceiving the child to be especially vulnerable from a physical or emotional perspective (154). Other relevant areas include possible marital conflict and parent–child relational problems, as well as other negative life events. Perhaps the most critical environmental issue to consider is that of maltreatment, which is particularly relevant in youth suffering from conversion symptoms, genitourinary complaints, and chronic polysymptomatic somatization.

Diagnosis and Psychoeducation

The diagnostic impression should be developed carefully, often in consultation with the referring provider, and discussed in the context of a collaborative relationship with the patient and the family. It is generally wise for the clinician first to review and gather consensus with regard to the number and types of physical, emotional, and behavioral symptoms noted during the assessment, as well as the time course and context of the symptoms with the patient and family prior to arriving at and discussing the diagnosis formulation. In circumstances where there is confidence in the diagnostic formulation, the diagnosis should be discussed clearly, frankly, and directly with the patient and family together (8,17). Once a diagnosis has been made with reasonable confidence, additional medical workup should be avoided in the absence of new information, a change in clinical status, or a strong conviction that a relatively low-risk investigation is needed to reassure the patient and family in order for treatment to proceed. When the diagnosis is presumptive or uncertain, truthful acknowledgment of uncertainty is superior to feigned certainty or avoidance. Humility is essential since presumably "medically unexplained" symptoms are sometimes just that—truly unexplained. Said differently, there may be occasions where the consensus of evidence suggests that a particular physical symptom is best considered simply unexplained in the usual sense.

Competent education of the patient and family provides a solid foundation for treatment, challenges stigma, and instills hope and positive expectations. The clinician should avoid communicating any sense of unease or embarrassment about the diagnosis, since this might contribute to treatment resistance and a wish to perpetuate the search for unrecognized disease. Patients and families can be educated about how physical symptoms of distress in the absence of serious disease are common and considered to be quite real by physicians and other health care professionals, and should be reassured that although our knowledge base is limited, much practical help is still available. Examples of common psychophysiologic reactions, such as cold or sweating hands associated with nervousness or heart racing in response to excitement, may be useful. Discussing the relationship between mind and body and the false dichotomy implied by separate systems of care for "physical" and "mental" disorders can also be useful. Efforts to explain FSS purely as reactions to adversity or stress may sometimes prove unproductive, since the patient may not recognize the presence of stress, may believe that illness in response to stress implies personal weakness, or may jump to the potentially maladaptive conclusion that avoidance of all life stress is the solution.

Education about the nature of painful FSS may be helpful to patients and families. Pain is typically perceived as a signal of threat to organismal integrity and accompanied by a wish to avoid additional discomfort and physical harm. Patients with FSS may benefit from knowing that some individuals may be especially vulnerable to experiencing bodily sensations as painful and a special threat to health. For example, youth with FAP may be especially sensitive to gut sensations or discomfort (155,156). Like fear, pain can serve a defensive neurobehavioral function, steering the organism away from perceived threats and motivating adaptive behaviors. Functional pain is essentially pain in the absence of demonstrable tissue damage, and is analogous to psychopathologic anxiety, which may be understood as fear inappropriate to context. The pain sensitivity observed in youth with FAP creates conditions for abdominal pain inappropriate to context (i.e., pain in the absence of tissue damage). The analogy of an overly sensitive car alarm that is triggered by simply walking past the car rather than a real attempt to enter or damage the vehicle can sometimes be helpful in educating patients and families about the sort of vulnerability to experience bodily sensations as painful and threatening often exhibited by youth with FSS.

The collaborative nature of the treatment process should be discussed early and often, and the importance of a therapeutic partnership—the foundation for therapeutic success emphasized. Patient, family, and professional roles and responsibilities should be delineated, with an emphasis on solid communication and the importance of working together. Determining shared functional goals for the patient, family, and treating professionals is an important task, as it deemphasizes unequivocal "cure" and encourages the rehabilitative mindset that typically serves as the successful foundation for treatment.

MANAGEMENT

Children and adolescents presenting with one type of FSS commonly experience other FSS, and FSS and disorders are often comorbid with anxiety and depressive symptoms and disorders, suggesting a common pathophysiology (11). The management model presented below builds upon common approaches and a few core principles distilled from the available pediatric and adult treatment literature. It should nevertheless be understood that successful interventions for one type of FSS or disorder may not prove effective for other FSS and disorders and that well-designed trials of specific interventions are a requirement of evidence-based medicine.

Therapeutic approaches to FSS and disorders often share common features, but care for individual patients is best individualized (17,157). Randomized controlled trials of interventions for youth with FSS are relatively sparse, so much of what follows is a synthesis of available evidence and accepted practice. Child and adolescent psychiatrists and other behavioral health professionals may be helpful as formal or informal consultants to primary care physicians and general medicine specialists, who are most often "out front" in managing children with FSS, but youth with FSS and their families may resist psychiatric referral, either actively or passively. Communication and coordination between the consultant and the referring physician are critical in maintaining the referring physician–patient alliance and avoiding unnecessary "doctor shopping."

Reassurance

Reassurance that a life-threatening or serious physical disease is not present is often a necessary step in the treatment process. It is usually essential for the patient and family to view the presenting symptoms as less threatening, as it is often difficult to proceed with intervention until fears related to the FSS have decreased. Parents must understand that the child's quite real subjective distress does not appear to be associated with actual tissue damage. If it is suspected that the parents fear that a serious diagnosis such as cancer has been missed, the feared diagnosis and the rationale for eliminating it from serious consideration should be specifically discussed. Excessive reassurance may nevertheless prove counterproductive in cases where obsessional illness worry and hypochondriacal fears are prominent. In such cases, the illness worry should be addressed directly and framed as a problem to be solved rather than attempting to overcome it by reassurance alone.

Rehabilitative Approach

Many authors have discussed the advantages of a rehabilitative approach to pediatric FSS (8,17,157). By encouraging the patient to return to usual activities and responsibilities prior to definitive symptomatic relief and by discouraging illness-related behaviors, the rehabilitative approach directs the patient and family focus away from finding a "cure" to instead finding a way to cope with and overcome a distressing physical problem. This approach challenges the notion that symptom resolution is necessary for the child to return to normal functioning, and can empower the patient and family by shifting the burden of responsibility for therapeutic success to the patient in the context of professional support and encouragement. The metacommunication of a rehabilitative approach is that the child will not be harmed by activity and effort, which can help neutralize concerns about FSS and foster health-promoting behaviors for both child and parents. Achievement of functional goals is understood and acknowledged as a personal success due to individual courage and hard work, and rightly treated as an accomplishment of which the patient can be proud of. The rehabilitative approach has been applied with some success in CFS, producing superior results to energy management strategies such as "pacing" that involve accepting the limitations associated with the illness and resting based on subjective need (158). Indeed, there is little evidence that rest alone is helpful in CFS, and may in fact exacerbate the condition (65). In keeping with a rehabilitative model, the use of physical therapy has sometimes been advocated, including in the management of conversion disorder (159).

Cognitive factors such as expectations and beliefs that the child's symptoms signal the threat of tissue damage appear to be important in youth with FSS, and addressing such concerns has been associated with response to psychotherapy (160). The rehabilitative approach challenges misperceptions about the child's health and capabilities, and serves as the linchpin of a cognitive-behavioral strategy by emphasizing the child's fundamental health, strength, and adaptability. Success largely depends on the clinician's ability to address patient and family anxiety about the child's illness and to successfully challenge patient- and family-distorted health beliefs. Parents and caretakers must understand that rehabilitative expectations in the face of the child's real distress are not cruel. Instead, a discussion of how kindness demands a firm approach is often indicated. Clinician speech and behavior should communicate that the child is fundamentally strong, competent, and capable of overcoming the challenge presented by the illness. To expect less may actually be countertherapeutic and representative of "misplaced kindness." Specifically, school attendance and performance should be emphasized as critical indicators of developmentally appropriate functioning. Homebound instruction is sometimes sought by youth with somatoform illness and/or their parents, but should almost always be avoided or challenged by treatment professionals. Respect for the importance of school should be communicated by attempting to schedule follow-up visits outside of regular school hours whenever possible.

Psychotherapeutic Interventions

Recent systematic reviews found psychological therapies to be beneficial in reducing pain intensity for children and adolescents with headache and other recurrent pains when delivered face to face (161,162) or remotely via the internet, computer program, audiotape, smartphone, or telephone (163). Cognitive-behavioral therapy (CBT) addresses attitudes, cognitions, and behaviors that may generate or maintain FSS, and has been reported to be helpful, often as part of a multimodal intervention, in the treatment of headache (164), FAP (165–167), fibromyalgia (168), and CFS (158,169). Interpersonal and expressive psychotherapies have not been systematically studied in the treatment of pediatric FSS, but case reports suggest they may be useful, particularly in the presence of psychological trauma (170).

Behavioral and operant interventions are common to most successful interventions, with core features being the reward of health-promoting behaviors and the discouragement of illness behaviors and disability. Most behavioral interventions emphasize positive reinforcement for functional improvement, as well as *extinction* or withdrawal of reinforcement for illness-promoting behaviors (17). The use of punishment per se is not advisable. Negative reinforcement, which produces an increase in the frequency of a desired response by removing an aversive event immediately after the desired response, has typically been applied by lifting restrictions theoretically imposed by illness contingent upon functional improvement (17,171). For example, discharge from the hospital might be allowed only if the patient demonstrates convincing clinical improvement, or persistent bed rest might be imposed with removal contingent on the patient returning to premorbid functioning and responsibilities such as school attendance. Implementing behavioral interventions typically requires a strong therapeutic alliance with the family, as parents may have difficulty cooperating unless their illness-related fears and concerns have been addressed.

Encouraging results have been reported with the use of self-management strategies, including self-monitoring, training in coping and relaxation, guided imagery, hypnotherapy, and biofeedback (162,172). Such strategies not only offer symptomatic relief, but may also encourage more active coping strategies, which may help improve functional status.

Family therapy and family-based interventions have been advocated (122,123) and a family focus has often been included as a component of CBT-based interventions (166,167). Since children with FSS are more likely as a group to be viewed as health impaired and have sick role behaviors inadvertently encouraged by parents, it is important to respectfully challenge the perceived physical vulnerability of the child and any familial encouragement of illness behavior (160,167). Group psychotherapy has not been systematically evaluated in the management of pediatric FSS.

In summary, psychotherapeutic approaches to FSS in children and adolescents seek to help child and family: (1) diminish the perceived threat associated with the FSS; (2) modulate affective and physiologic reactivity to relevant environmental or physical triggers; (3) promote healthy coping by encouraging accommodative coping strategies such as acceptance, distraction, self-encouragement, and cognitive restructuring, while discouraging passive strategies such as avoidance, denial, and wishful thinking; (4) optimize social reinforcement by using positive reinforcement for healthy behaviors and withdrawal of reinforcement for illness behaviors; and (5) strengthen the child's perceived competence and self-worth.

Suggestion and Placebo

Though sometimes tempting, particularly to generalists, the use of placebo and/or sham interventions is discouraged for both ethical and practical reasons. Such efforts may inadvertently contribute to patient and family convictions that the symptom is caused by physical disease, and if suggestion or placebo prove unsuccessful, the clinician is then forced to perpetuate new deceptions or must backtrack and attempt to convince the patient that serious physical disease is absent and that symptom removal is not really necessary for functional improvement to take place.

Psychopharmacologic Treatment

Pharmacologic management has the advantage of relative simplicity and acceptability within general medical settings, and is in keeping with traditional office practice. Unfortunately, large randomized controlled trials of psychoactive medications in the treatment of pediatric FSS and disorders are relatively lacking, so psychopharmacologic treatment of youth with FSS has largely been presumptive and based on experience with adults. Psychopharmacologic interventions are nevertheless worthy of consideration in the treatment of refractory and/or painful FSS, GI symptoms, or fatigue, particularly in the presence of psychiatric comorbidity or when psychotherapeutic interventions have not been entirely successful. Antidepressant medications have been reported to be of benefit in the treatment of a number of somatoform disorders and FSS in adults, including somatoform pain, IBS, and a variety of other FSS and syndromes such as fibromyalgia, FGIDs, and headache (173). Because pediatric FSS are commonly associated with comorbid internalizing symptoms and disorders (11) attention to comorbid psychopathology is very much indicated and clinical experience suggests that active intervention for comorbid anxiety and depression can ameliorate the functional impact of associated FSS. In the clinical setting, medications such as SSRIs, selective serotonin–norepinephrine reuptake inhibitors (SNRIs) such as duloxetine and venlafaxine, other novel antidepressants such as mirtazapine and milnacipran, benzodiazepines, and antipsychotics have been used anecdotally in pediatric patients struggling with FSS, but randomized controlled trials have been lacking in general. Although medications used for FSS that are not typically considered to be psychoactive are not within the scope of this chapter, they may be worthy of exploration in the care of individual patients.

The literature on the psychopharmacologic treatment of pediatric FAP has been judged to be inconclusive and inadequate (174,175). Although an open trial of citalopram for pediatric FAP reported positive response in 21 of 25 (84%) treated youth (176), subsequent randomized controlled trials have produced mixed results. An Iranian study that randomized 115 school-age children and adolescents to citalopram 20 mg daily or placebo in a 4-week trial failed to demonstrate statistically significant between-group differences on intent-to-treat (ITT) analysis, but completer analysis revealed statistically significant reductions in pain and the clinical global severity for the citalopram group (177). Another as yet unpublished double-blind, placebo-controlled trial that randomized 81 subjects ages 7 to 18 years to citalopram or placebo for 8 weeks failed to demonstrate the superiority of citalopram versus placebo on ITT analysis of clinical global improvement and abdominal pain using a mixed effects model, but citalopram was superior in reducing global illness burden relative to placebo ($p = 0.037$). Endpoint analysis for the ITT sample revealed a trend favoring citalopram with 52.5% of citalopram-treated subjects rated "much" or "very much" improved relative to 31.7% of placebo-treated subjects ($p = 0.058$), but no between-group differences in reported abdominal pain. Endpoint analysis for completers classified 60.0% of citalopram-treated subjects as responders compared to 29.7% of those taking placebo ($p = 0.010$). Citalopram was well tolerated relative to placebo in both controlled studies, and there were no serious adverse events (178).

Though pediatric gastroenterologists have often favored the use of tricyclic antidepressants in youth with FAP based in part on adult experience, controlled trials have failed to demonstrate efficacy (174,175,179). It is thus difficult to advocate their use, particularly given the potential for toxicity in households with young children, past reports of sudden death, and the lack of proven efficacy in pediatric emotional disorders.

With regard to pediatric headache, both acetaminophen and ibuprofen have been shown to be effective in the acute treatment of pediatric migraine, as has sumatriptan nasal spray (180). Antipsychotic medications such as chlorpromazine, prochlorperazine, and haloperidol have been used effectively in the acute management of adult migraine with effects comparable to sumatriptan, though pediatric experience is limited (181). Antidepressant medications such as amitriptyline and trazodone, anticonvulsants such as topiramate, beta-adrenergic blockers such as propranol, and cyproheptadine have been applied to the management of pediatric headache, but data remain insufficient to draw firm conclusions about efficacy (162,182,183). The alpha-adrenergic agonist clonidine has not demonstrated efficacy and is most likely ineffective. Serotonergic antimigraine drugs such as sumatriptan have been used in combination with serotonergic antidepressants (184), but caution is suggested given the U.S. Food and Drug Administration (FDA) warning about the risk of serotonin syndrome issued in 2006 and the relative paucity of research (185).

The use of low-dose clonidine in adolescent CFS had a negative effect on physical activity relative to placebo, and was not clinically useful despite reductions in markers of sympathetic outflow and inflammation (186). Given the common association of anxiety and depressive disorders with the symptom profile in CFS, consideration might be given to the use of antidepressant medications, including more activating antidepressants such as bupropion, though such approaches cannot be recommended as standard practice and deserve careful study.

Clinical experience suggests that some patients who experience physical symptoms associated with emotional arousal and anxiety may benefit from a short course of a benzodiazepine such as clonazepam or lorazepam, which can sometimes produce rapid symptomatic relief, help reassure the patient and family, and demonstrate the potential contribution of emotional activation to somatic distress (8,17). For youth with refractory symptoms of nausea or vomiting in the presence of symptoms suggesting acute migraine, the brief use of an antipsychotic medication or antiemetic such as ondansetron may be worthy of consideration.

Coordination of Care

Successful communication and collaboration with other professionals involved in the child's care, including teachers and school nurses, can prove critical to success over time. Because FSS commonly present in general medical settings, a close working relationship with the primary care physician or referring specialist is essential. As integrated care models of health care delivery become more widespread, effective communication between medical and mental health providers becomes easier. Poor communication is the most frequent complaint made by pediatricians about child and adolescent psychiatrists (187), and increases the risk that treatment efforts will be misapplied, diluted, or overlooked. A simple consultation letter outlining a general approach to adult somatization disorder patients from a consulting psychiatrist to primary care physicians was shown to be effective in improving patient satisfaction and reducing disability and health care expenditures (188). Because absenteeism from school is common in youth with FSS, communication and collaboration with school officials can prove instrumental in developing a rehabilitative plan. The clinician can serve as a bridge to help bring together the school and the patient's family. A retrospective excuse for past school absences can be negotiated with the family and school as being contingent upon the child's commitment to a forward-looking management plan which will treat subsequent absenteeism for known FSS as inexcusable. It is thus useful to define what constitutes a legitimate, medically excused absence for the child, family, and school, and the physician who will be responsible for legitimizing medical excuses should be specified beforehand in order to prevent doctor shopping in search of medical excuses. Absence from school without the approval of the treatment team can then be legitimately viewed as truancy, allowing the school to leverage attendance and benefit overall treatment efforts.

Ideally, coordination of the child's medical care should be consolidated with a single physician or clinician. Regularly scheduled medical visits can prove useful in reassuring the patient and family that their concerns have not been dismissed (188). The primary physician may serve as a powerful attachment figure for patients and families. Regularly scheduled visits allow the patient and family to see the physician without the requirement that the child be sick.

CONCLUSION

The study and management of pediatric FSS and associated disorders remain handicapped by problems of conceptualization and classification. Clinicians often feel confused and intimidated by these patients, their distressed and sometimes demanding families, and the general medical colleagues who call on us for help. New ways of conceptualizing and managing the problems posed by patients with swill require additional epidemiologic, mechanistic, and treatment studies. Future studies should examine not only the efficacy of tested interventions, but whether symptomatic and functional improvements are independent of changes in comorbid anxiety and depressive symptoms. The need to develop relatively potent, tiered interventions applicable to primary care and other general medical settings is clear given the prevalence and impact of FSS in children and adolescents across the lifespan.

References

1. Parsons T: *Social Structure and Personality*. New York, The Free Press, 1964.
2. Kellner R: *Somatization and Hypochondriasis*. New York, Praeger, 1986.
3. Lipowski ZJ: Somatization: the concept and its clinical application. *Am J Psychiatry* 145(11):1358–1368, 1988.
4. Campo JV, Jansen-McWilliams L, Comer DM, Kelleher KJ: Somatization in pediatric primary care: association with psychopathology, functional impairment, and use of services. *J Am Acad Child Adolesc Psychiatry* 38(9):1093–1101, 1999.
5. Campo JV, Comer DM, Jansen-McWilliams L, Gardner W, Kelleher KJ: Recurrent pain, emotional distress, and health service use in childhood. *J Pediatr* 141:76–83, 2002.
6. Campo JV, Fritsch SL: Somatization in children and adolescents. *J Am Acad Child Adolesc Psychiatry* 33(9):1223–1235, 1994.
7. Fritz GK, Fritsch S, Hagino O: Somatoform disorders in children and adolescents: a review of the past 10 years. *J Am Acad Child Adolesc Psychiatry* 36(10):1329–1338, 1997.
8. Dell ML, Campo JV: Somatoform disorders in children and adolescents. *Psychiatr Clin North Am* 34(3):643–660, 2011.
9. Garralda ME: A selective review of child psychiatric syndromes with a somatic presentation. *Br J Psychiatry* 161:759–773, 1992.
10. Fichtel A, Larsson B: Psychosocial impact of headache and comorbidity with other pains among Swedish school adolescents. *Headache* 42:766–775, 2002.
11. Campo JV: Annual research review: functional somatic symptoms and associated anxiety and depression–developmental psychopathology in pediatric practice. *J Child Psychol Psychiatry* 53(5):575–592, 2012.
12. Shanahan L, Zucker N, Copeland WE, Bondy CL, Egger HL, Costello EJ: Childhood somatic complaints predict generalized anxiety and depressive disorders during young adulthood in a community sample. *Psychol Med* 45(8):1721–1730, 2015.
13. Shelby GD, Shirkey KC, Sherman AL, et al.: Functional abdominal pain in childhood and long-term vulnerability to anxiety disorders. *Pediatrics* 132(3):475–482, 2013.
14. Luntamo T, Sourander A, Gyllenberg D, et al.: Do headache and abdominal pain in childhood predict suicides and severe suicide attempts? Finnish nationwide 1981 birth cohort study. *Child Psychiatry Hum Dev* 45(1):110–118, 2014.
15. Rask CU, Munkholm A, Clemmensen L, et al.: Health anxiety in pre-adolescence–associated health problems, healthcare expenditure, and continuity in childhood. *J Abnorm Child Psychol* 44(4):823–832, 2016.
16. Stickler GB, Murphy DB: Recurrent abdominal pain. *Am J Dis Child* 133:486–489, 1979.
17. Campo JV, Fritz G: A management model for pediatric somatization. *Psychosomatics* 42:467–476, 2001.
18. American Psychiatric Association: *Diagnostic and Statistical Manual of Mental Disorders*. 4th ed. Arlington, VA, American Psychiatric Association, 1994.
19. American Psychiatric Association: *Diagnostic and Statistical Manual of Mental Disorders-TR*. 4th ed. Washington, DC, American Psychiatric Association, 2000.
20. Mayou R, Kirmayer LJ, Simon G, Kroenke K, Sharpe M: Somatoform disorders: time for a new approach in DSM-V. *Am J Psychiatry* 162:847–855, 2005.
21. Fink P, Rosendal M, Olesen F: Classification of somatization and functional somatic symptoms in primary care. *Aust N Z J Psychiatry* 39:772–781, 2005.
22. Kirmayer LJ, Young A: Culture and somatization: clinical, epidemiological, and ethnographic perspectives. *Psychosom Med* 60:420–430, 1998.
23. Kroenke K, Sharpe M, Sykes R: Revising the classification of somatoform disorders: key questions and preliminary recommendations. *Psychosomatics* 48:277–285, 2007.
24. Oken D: Evolution of psychosomatic diagnosis in DSM. *Psychosom Med* 69:830–831, 2007.
25. Abbey SE, Wulsin L, Levenson JL: Somatization and somatoform disorders. In: Levenson JL (ed): *Textbook of Psychosomatic Medicine: Psychiatric Care of the Medically Ill*. 2nd ed. Arlington, VA, American Psychiatric Publishing, Inc., 2011, 261–289.
26. American Psychiatric Association: *Diagnostic and Statistical Manual of Mental Disorders*. 5th ed. Arlington, VA, American Psychiatric Association, 2013.
27. Barsky AJ: Assessing the new DSM-5 diagnosis of somatic symptom disorder. *Psychosom Med* 78:2–4, 2016.
28. Dimsdale JE, Creed F, Escobar J, et al.: Somatic symptom disorder: an important change in DSM. *J Psychosom Res* 75:223–228, 2013.
29. van Dessel NC, van der Wouden JC, Dekker J, van der Horst HE: Clinical value of DSM IV and DSM 5 criteria for diagnosing the most prevalent somatoform disorders in patients with medically unexplained physical symptoms (MUPS). *J Psychosom Res* 82:4–10, 2016.

30. Rosic T, Kalra S, Samaan Z: Somatic symptom disorder, a new DSM-5 diagnosis of an old clinical challenge. *BMJ Case Rep* 2016, 2016.
31. Voigt K, Nagel A, Meyer B, Langs G, Braukhaus C, Löwe B: Towards positive diagnostic criteria: a systematic review of somatoform disorder diagnoses and suggestions for future classification. *J Psychosom Res* 68:403–414, 2010.
32. Voigt K, Wollburg E, Weinmann N, et al.: Predictive validity and clinical utility of DSM-5 somatic symptom disorder—comparison with DSM-IV somatoform disorders and additional criteria for consideration. *J Psychosom Res* 73:345–350, 2012.
33. Bailer J, Kerstner T, Witthöft M, Diener C, Mier D, Rist F: Health anxiety and hypochondriasis in the light of DSM-5. *Anxiety Stress Coping* 29:219–239, 2016.
34. Brakoulias V: DSM-5 bids farewell to hypochondriasis and welcomes somatic symptom disorder and illness anxiety disorder. *Aust N Z J of Psychiatry* 48:688, 2014.
35. Scarella TM, Laferton JA, Ahern DK, Fallon BA, Barsky A: The relationship of hypochondriasis to anxiety, depressive, and somatoform disorders. *Psychosomatics* 57:200–207, 2016.
36. Stone J, LaFrance WC Jr, Brown R, Spiegel D, Levenson JL, Sharpe M: Conversion disorder: current problems and potential solutions for DSM-5. *J Psychosom Res* 71:369–376, 2011.
37. Mayou R: Is the DSM-5 chapter on somatic symptom disorder any better than DSM-IV somatoform disorder? *Br J Psychiatry* 204:418–419, 2014.
38. van Geelen SM, Rydelius PA, Hagquist C: Somatic symptoms and psychological concerns in a general adolescent population: exploring the relevance of DSM-5 somatic symptom disorder. *J Psychosom Res* 79:251–258, 2015.
39. Lieb R, Zimmermann P, Friis RH, Höfler M, Tholen S, Wittchen HU: The natural course of DSM-IV somatoform disorders and syndromes among adolescents and young adults: a prospective-longitudinal community study. *Eur Psychiatry* 17:321–331, 2002.
40. Domènech-Llaberia E, Jané C, Canals J, Ballespí S, Esparó G, Garralda E: Parental reports of somatic symptoms in preschool children: prevalence and associations in a Spanish sample. *J Am Acad Child Adolesc Psychiatry* 43:598–604, 2004.
41. Garber J, Walker L, Zeman J: Somatization symptoms in a community sample of children and adolescents: further validation of the Children's Somatization Inventory. *Psychol Assessment* 3:588–595, 1991.
42. Alfvén G: The covariation of common psychosomatic symptoms among children from socio-economically differing residential areas. An epidemiological study. *Acta Paediatr* 82:484–487, 1993.
43. Achenbach TM, Conners CK, Quay HC, Verhulst FC, Howell CT: Replication of empirically derived syndromes as a basis for taxonomy of child/adolescent psychopathology. *J Abnorm Child Psychol* 17:299–323, 1989.
44. Offord DR, Boyle MH, Szatmari P, et al.: Ontario Child Health Study. II. Six-month prevalence of disorder and rates of service utilization. *Arch Gen Psychiatry* 44(9):832–836, 1987.
45. Belmaker E, Espinoza R, Pogrund R: Use of medical services by adolescents with non-specific somatic symptoms. *Int J Adolesc Med Health* 1:149–156, 1985.
46. Basbaum AI, Jessell T: *The Perception of Pain*. New York, McGraw-Hill, 2000.
47. Perquin CW, Hazebroek-Kampschreur AA, Hunfeld JA, et al.: Pain in children and adolescents: a common experience. *Pain* 87(1):51–58, 2000.
48. Aro H: Life stress and psychosomatic symptoms among 14 to 16-year old Finnish adolescents. *Psychol Med* 17(1):191–201, 1987.
49. Larsson BS: Somatic complaints and their relationship to depressive symptoms in Swedish adolescents. *J Child Psychol Psychiatry* 32:821–832, 1991.
50. Oster J: Recurrent abdominal pain, headache and limb pains in children and adolescents. *Pediatrics* 50:429–436, 1972.
51. Rutter M, Tizard J, Whitmore K: *Education, Health and Behavior*. London, Longman Group Limited, 1970.
52. Starfield B, Gross E, Wood M, et al.: Psychosocial and psychosomatic diagnoses in primary care of children. *Pediatrics* 66:159–167, 1980.
53. Caviness V, Ebinger F: Headache in pediatric practice. *Handb Clin Neurol* 112:827–838, 2013.
54. Korterink JJ, Diederen K, Benninga MA, Tabbers MM: Epidemiology of pediatric functional abdominal pain disorders: a meta-analysis. *PLoS One* 10(5):e0126982, 2015.
55. Apley J, Naish N: Recurrent abdominal pains: a field survey of 1,000 school children. *Arch Dis Child* 33:165–170, 1958.
56. Hyams JS, Di Lorenzo C, Saps M, Shulman RJ, Staiano A, van Tilburg M: Functional disorders: children and adolescents. *Gastroenterology* pii: S0016-5085(16)00181-5, 2016.
57. Abu-Arafeh I, Russell G: Prevalence and clinical features of abdominal migraine compared with those of migraine headache. *Arch Dis Child* 72(5):413–417, 1995.
58. Mortimer MJ, Kay J, Jaron A: Clinical epidemiology of childhood migraine in an urban general practice. *Dev Med Child Neurol* 35:243–248, 1993.
59. Fleisher D: Cyclic vomiting syndrome and migraine. *J Pediatr* 134:533–535, 1999.
60. Lipsitz JD, Masia-Warner C, Apfel H, et al.: Anxiety and depressive symptoms and anxiety sensitivity in youngsters with noncardiac chest pain and benign heart murmurs. *J Pediatr Psychol* 29:607–612, 2004.
61. Selbst SM, Ruddy RM, Clark BJ, Henretig FM, Santulli T Jr: Pediatric chest pain: prospective study. *Pediatrics* 82:319–323, 1988.
62. Mikkelsson M, Sourander A, Piha J, Salminen JJ: Psychiatric symptoms in preadolescents with musculoskeletal pain and fibromyalgia. *Pediatrics* 100:220–227, 1997.
63. Kashikar-Zuck S, King C, Ting TV, Arnold LM: Juvenile fibromyalgia: different from the adult chronic pain syndrome? *Curr Rheumatol Rep* 18(4):19, 2016.
64. Weissmann R, Uziel Y: Pediatric complex regional pain syndrome: a review. *Pediatr Rheumatol Online J* 14(1):29, 2016.
65. Garralda ME, Chalder T: Practitioner review: chronic fatigue syndrome in childhood. *J Child Psychol Psychiatry* 46:1143–1151, 2005.
66. Crawley E: The epidemiology of chronic fatigue syndrome/myalgic encephalitis in children. *Arch Dis Child* 99(2):171–174, 2014.
67. Collin SM, Norris T, Nuevo R, et al.: Chronic fatigue syndrome at age 16 years. *Pediatrics* 137(2):e20153434, 2016.
68. Vertigan AE, Murad MH, Pringsheim T, et al; CHEST Expert Cough Panel: Somatic cough syndrome (previously referred to as psychogenic cough) and tic cough (previously referred to as habit cough) in adults and children: CHEST guideline and expert panel report. *Chest* 148(1):24–31, 2015.
69. Goodwin RD, Lewinsohn PM, Seeley JR: Respiratory symptoms and mental disorders among youth: results form a prospective, longitudinal study. *Psychosom Med* 66(6):943–949, 2004.
70. McQuaid EL, Spieth LE, Spirito A: The pediatric psychologist's role in differential diagnosis: vocal-cord dysfunction presenting as asthma. *J Pediatr Psychol* 22:739–748, 1997.
71. Ani C, Reading R, Lynn R, Forlee S, Garralda E: Incidence and 12-month outcome of non-transient childhood conversion disorder in the U.K. and Ireland. *Br J Psychiatry* 202:413–418, 2013.
72. Kozlowska K, Nunn KP, Rose D, Morris A, Ouvrier RA, Varghese J: Conversion disorder in Australian pediatric practice. *J Am Acad Child Adolesc Psychiatry* 46(1):68–75, 2007.
73. Stefánsson JG, Messina JA, Meyerowitz S: Hysterical neurosis, conversion type: clinical and epidemiological considerations. *Acta Psychiatr Scand* 53:119–138, 1976.
74. Tomasson K, Kent D, Coryell W: Somatization and conversion disorders: comorbidity and demographics at presentation. *Acta Psychiatr Scand* 84:288–293, 1991.
75. Grattan-Smith P, Fairley M, Procopis P: Clinical features of conversion disorder. *Arch Dis Child* 63:408–414, 1988.
76. Leslie SA: Diagnosis and treatment of hysterical conversion reactions. *Arch Dis Child* 63:506–511, 1988.
77. Goodyer IM, Mitchell C: Somatic emotional disorders in childhood and adolescence. *J Psychosom Res* 33:681–688, 1989.
78. Spierings C, Poels PJ, Sijben N, Gabreëls FJ, Renier WO: Conversion disorders in childhood: a retrospective follow-up study of 84 inpatients. *Dev Med Child Neurol* 32:865–871, 1990.
79. Steinhausen HC, von Aster M, Pfeiffer E, Göbel D: Comparative studies of conversion disorders in childhood and adolescence. *J Child Psychol Psychiatry* 30:615–621, 1989.
80. Volkmar F R, Poll J, Lewis M: Conversion reactions in childhood and adolescents. *J Am Acad Child Adolesc Psychiatry* 23:424–430, 1984.
81. Pehlivantürk B, Unal F: Conversion disorder in children and adolescents: a 4-year follow-up study. *J Psychosom Res* 52:187–191, 2002.
82. Turgay A: Treatment outcome for children and adolescents with conversion disorder. *Can J Psychiatry* 35:585–589, 1990.
83. Rivinus TM, Jamison DL, Graham PJ: Childhood organic neurological disease presenting as psychiatric disorder. *Arch Dis Child* 50:115–119, 1975.
84. Stone J, Smyth R, Carson A, et al.: Systematic review of misdiagnosis of conversion symptoms and "hysteria." *BMJ* 331(7523):989, 2005.
85. Sirri L, Ricci Garotti MG, Grandi S, Tossani E: Adolescents' hypochondriacal fears and beliefs: relationship with demographic features, psychological distress, well-being and health-related behaviors. *J Psychosom Res* 79(4):259–264, 2015.
86. Barsky AJ, Goodson JD, Lane RS, Cleary PD: The amplification of somatic symptoms. *Psychosom Med* 50:510–519, 1988.
87. Walker LS, Greene JW: Children with recurrent abdominal pain and their parents: more somatic complaints, anxiety, and depression than other patient families? *J Pediatr Psychol* 14(2):231–243, 1989.
88. Walker LS, Garber J, Greene JW: Somatization symptoms in pediatric abdominal pain patients: relation to chronicity of abdominal pain and parent somatization. *J Abnorm Child Psychol* 19(4):379–394, 1991.
89. Lehmkuhl G, Blanz B, Lehmkuhl U, Braun-Scharm H: Conversion disorder (DSM-III 300.11): symptomatology and course in childhood and adolescence. *Eur Arch Psychiatry Neurol Sci* 238:155–160, 1989.
90. Janssens KA, Oldehinkel AJ, Bonvanie IJ, Rosmalen JG: An inactive lifestyle and low physical fitness are associated with functional somatic symptoms in adolescents. The TRAILS study. *J Psychosom Res* 76(6):454–457, 2014.
91. Aro H, Paronen O, Aro S: Psychosomatic symptoms among 14–16 year old Finnish adolescents. *Soc Psychiatry* 22(3):171–176, 1987.

92. Lievesley K, Rimes KA, Chalder T: A review of the predisposing, precipitating and perpetuating factors in chronic fatigue syndrome in children and adolescents. *Clin Psychol Rev* 34(3):233–248, 2014.
93. Luntamo T, Sourander A, Sillanmäki L, et al.: Pain at age eight as a predictor of antidepressant medication use by age 24: findings from the Finnish nationwide 1981 birth cohort study. *J Affect Disord* 138 (1–2):153–159, 2012.
94. Egger HL, Costello EJ, Erkanli A, Angold A: Somatic complaints and psychopathology in children and adolescents: stomach aches, musculoskeletal pains, and headaches. *J Am Acad Child Adolesc Psychiatry* 38: 852–860, 1999.
95. Campo JV, Bridge J, Ehmann M, et al.: Recurrent abdominal pain, anxiety, and depression in primary care. *Pediatrics* 113(4):817–824, 2004.
96. Garber J, Zeman J, Walker LS: Recurrent abdominal pain in children: psychiatric diagnoses and parental psychopathology. *J Am Acad Child Adolesc Psychiatry* 29(4):648–656, 1990.
97. Liakopoulou-Kairis M, Alifieraki T, Protagora D, et al.: Recurrent abdominal pain and headache: psychopathology, life events and family functioning. *Eur Child Adolesc Psychiatry* 11:115–122, 2002.
98. Peterson CC, Palermo TM: Parental reinforcement of recurrent pain: the moderating impact of child depression and anxiety on functional disability. *J Pediatr Psychol* 29:331–341, 2004.
99. Yacob D, Di Lorenzo C, Bridge JA, et al.: Prevalence of pain-predominant functional gastrointestinal disorders and somatic symptoms in patients with anxiety or depressive disorders. *J Pediatr* 163(3):767–770, 2013.
100. McElhanon BO, McCracken C, Karpen S, Sharp WG: Gastrointestinal symptoms in autism spectrum disorder: a meta-analysis. *Pediatrics* 133(5):872–883, 2014.
101. Watson D, Pennebaker JW: Health complaints, stress, and distress: exploring the central role of negative affectivity. *Psychol Rev* 96:234–254, 1989.
102. Wilner JG, Vranceanu AM, Blashill AJ: Neuroticism prospectively predicts pain among adolescents: results from a nationally representative sample. *J Psychosom Res* 77(6):474–476, 2014.
103. Boyce WT, Barr RG, Zeltzer LK: Temperament and the psychobiology of childhood stress. *Pediatrics* 90:483–486, 1992.
104. Kagan J, Reznick JS, Snidman N: Biological bases of childhood shyness. *Science* 40:167–171, 1988.
105. Kozlowska K, Brown KJ, Palmer DM, Williams LM: Specific biases for identifying facial expression of emotion in children and adolescents with conversion disorders. *Psychosom Med* 75(3):272–280, 2013.
106. Dorn LD, Campo JC, Thato S, et al.: Psychological comorbidity and stress reactivity in children and adolescents with recurrent abdominal pain and anxiety disorders. *J Am Acad Child Adolesc Psychiatry* 42(1):66–75, 2003.
107. Winger A, Kvarstein G, Wyller VB, et al.: Pain and pressure pain thresholds in adolescents with chronic fatigue syndrome and healthy controls: a cross-sectional study. *BMJ Open* 4(9):e005920, 2014.
108. Landa A, Peterson BS, Fallon BA: Somatoform pain: a developmental theory and translational research review. *Psychosom Med* 74(7):717–727, 2012.
109. Bonvanie IJ, Janssens KA, Rosmalen JG, Oldehinkel AJ: Life events and functional somatic symptoms: a population study in older adolescents. *Br J Psychol* 2016.
110. Bonvanie IJ, van Gils A, Janssens KA, Rosmalen JG: Sexual abuse predicts functional somatic symptoms: an adolescent population study. *Child Abuse Negl* 46:1–7, 2015.
111. Livingston R, Taylor JL, Crawford SL: A study of somatic complaints and psychiatric diagnosis in children. *J Am Acad Child Adolesc Psychiatry* 27(2):185–187, 1988.
112. Craig TK, Boardman AP, Mills K, Daly-Jones O, Drake H: The South London Somatisation Study. I: longitudinal course and the influence of early life experiences. *Br J Psychiatry* 163:579–588, 1993.
113. Craig TK, Drake H, Mills K, Boardman AP: The South London Somatisation Study. II. Influence of stressful life events and secondary gain. *Br J Psychiatry* 165:248–258, 1994.
114. Perkonigg A, Pfister H, Stein MB, et al.: Longitudinal course of posttraumatic stress disorder and posttraumatic stress disorder symptoms in a community sample of adolescents and young adults. *Am J Psychiatry* 162:1320–1327, 2005.
115. Kriechman AM: Siblings with somatoform disorders in childhood and adolescence. *J Am Acad Child Adolesc Psychiatry* 26:226–231, 1987.
116. Livingston R: Children of people with somatization disorder. *J Am Acad Child Adolesc Psychiatry* 32:536–544, 1993.
117. Craig TK, Cox AD, Klein K: Intergenerational transmission of somatization behavior: a study of chronic somatizers and their children. *Psychol Med* 32:805–816, 2002.
118. Levy RL, Jones KR, Whitehead WE, Feld SI, Talley NJ, Corey LA: Irritable bowel syndrome in twins: heredity and social learning both contribute to etiology. *Gastroenterology* 121(4):799–804, 2001.
119. Campo JV, Di Lorenzo C, Chiappetta L, et al.: Adult outcomes of pediatric recurrent abdominal pain: do they just grow out of it? *Pediatrics* 108:E1, 2001.
120. Campo JV, Bridge J, Lucas A, et al.: Physical and emotional health of mothers of youth with functional abdominal pain. *Arch Pediatr Adolesc Med* 161(2):131–137, 2007.
121. van Tilburg MA, Levy RL, Walker LS, et al.: Psychosocial mechanisms for the transmission of somatic symptoms from parents to children. *World J Gastroenterol* 21(18):5532–5541, 2015.
122. Mullins LL, Olson RA: Familial factors in the etiology, maintenance, and treatment of somatoform disorders in children. *Family Systems Medicine* 8:159–175, 1990.
123. Wood BL: Physically manifested illness in children and adolescents: a biobehavioral family approach. *Child Adolesc Psychiatr Clin N Am* 10:543–562, 2001.
124. Goodyer I, Taylor DC: Hysteria. *Arch Dis Child* 60:680–681, 1985.
125. Maisami M, Freeman JM: Conversion reactions in children as body language: a combined child psychiatry/neurology team approach to the management of functional neurologic disorders in children. *Pediatrics* 80:46–52, 1987.
126. Kendler KS, Walters EE, Truett KR, et al.: A twin-family study of self-report symptoms of panic-phobia and somatization. *Behav Genet* 25:499–515, 1995.
127. Gillespie NA, Zhu G, Heath AC, Hickie IB, Martin NG: The genetic aetiology of somatic distress. *Psychol Med* 30:1051–1061, 2000.
128. Morris-Yates A, Talley NJ, Boyce PM, Nandurkar S, Andrews G: Evidence of a genetic contribution to functional bowel disorder. *Am J Gastroenterol* 93(8):1311–1317, 1998.
129. Ask H, Waaktaar T, Seglem KB, Torgersen S. Common etiological sources of anxiety, depression, and somatic complaints in adolescents: a multiple rater twin study. *J Abnorm Child Psychol* 44(1):101–114, 2016.
130. Torgersen S: Genetics of somatoform disorders. *Arch Gen Psychiatry* 43:502–505, 1986.
131. Camilleri M, Atanasova E, Carlson P, et al.: Serotonin-transporter polymorphism pharmacogenetics in diarrhea-predominant irritable bowel syndrome. *Gastroenterology* 123(2):425–432, 2002.
132. Hennings A, Zill P, Rief W: Serotonin transporter gene promoter polymorphism and somatoform symptoms. *J Clin Psychiatry* 70(11):1536–1539, 2009.
133. Greenberg BD, Li Q, Lucas FR, et al.: Association between the serotonin transporter promoter polymorphism and personality traits in a primarily female population sample. *Am J Med Genet* 96:202–216, 2000.
134. Lesch KP, Bengel D, Heils A, et al.: Association of anxiety-related traits with a polymorphism in the serotonin transporter gene regulatory region. *Science* 274:1527–1531, 1996.
135. Diatchenko L, Slade GD, Nackley AG, et al.: Genetic basis for individual variations in pain perception and the development of a chronic pain condition. *Hum Mol Genet* 14:135–143, 2005.
136. Du L, Bakish D, Hrdina PD: Tryptophan hydroxylase gene 218A/C polymorphism is associated with somatic anxiety in major depressive disorder. *J Affect Disord* 65:37–44, 2001.
137. Jakobi J, Bernateck M, Tran AT, et al.: Catechol-O-methyltransferase gene polymorphisms are not associated with multisomatoform disorder in a group of German multisomatoform disorder patients and healthy controls. *Genet Test Mol Biomarkers* 14(3):293–297, 2010.
138. Koh KB, Choi EH, Lee YJ, Han M: Serotonin-related gene pathways associated with undifferentiated somatoform disorder. *Psychiatry Res* 189(2):246–250, 2011.
139. Compas BE, Thomsen AH: Coping and responses to stress among children with recurrent abdominal pain. *J Dev Behav Pediatr* 20(5):323–324, 1999.
140. Thomsen AH, Compas BE, Colletti RB, Stanger C, Boyer MC, Konik BS: Parent reports of coping and stress responses in children with recurrent abdominal pain. *J Pediatr Psychol* 27(3):215–226, 2002.
141. Walker LS, Smith CA, Garber J, et al.: Development and validation of the Pain Response Inventory for children. *Psychological Assessment* 9(4):392–405, 1997.
142. Lavigne JV, Saps M, Bryant FB: Models of anxiety, depression, somatization, and coping as predictors of abdominal pain in a community sample of school-age children. *J Pediatr Psychol* 39(1):9–22, 2014.
143. Walker LS, Smith CA, Garber J, Claar RL: Testing a model of pain appraisal and coping in children with chronic abdominal pain. *Health Psychol* 24(4):364–374, 2005.
144. Janssens KA, Klis S, Kingma EM, Oldehinkel AJ, Rosmalen JG: Predictors for persistence of functional somatic symptoms in adolescents. *J Pediatr* 164(4):900–905.e2, 2014.
145. Borge AI, Nordhagen R, Moe B, Botten G, Bakketeig LS: Prevalence and persistence of stomach ache and headache among children. Follow-up of a cohort of Norwegian children from 4 to 10 years of age. *Acta Paediatr* 83:433–437, 1994.
146. Apley J, Hale B: Children with recurrent abdominal pain: how do they grow up? *Br Med J* 3:7–9, 1973.
147. Christensen MF, Mortensen O: Long-term prognosis in children with recurrent abdominal pain. *Arch Dis Child* 50:110–114, 1975.
148. Horst S, Shelby G, Anderson J, et al.: Predicting persistence of functional abdominal pain from childhood into young adulthood. *Clin Gastroenterol Hepatol* 12(12):2026–2032, 2014.
149. Hotopf M, Carr S, Mayou R, Wadsworth M, Wessely S: Why do children have chronic abdominal pain, and what happens to them when they grow up? Population based cohort study. *BMJ* 316:1196–1200, 1998.
150. Walker LS, Beck JE, Garber J, Lambert W: Children's Somatization Inventory: psychometric properties of the revised form (CSI-24). *J Pediatr Psychol* 34(4):430–440, 2009.

151. Walker LS, Greene JW: The Functional Disability Inventory: measuring a neglected dimension of child health status. *J Pediatr Psychol* 16:39–58, 1991.
152. Walker LS, Garber J, Van Slyke DA: Do parents excuse the misbehavior of children with physical or emotional symptoms? An investigation of the pediatric sick role. *J Pediatr Psychol* 20:329–345, 1995.
153. Dubowitz V, Hersov L: Management of children with non-organic (hysterical) disorders of motor function. *Dev Med Child Neurol* 18:358–368, 1976.
154. Green M, Solnit AJ: Reactions to the threatened loss of a child: a vulnerable child syndrome. Pediatric management of the dying child, part III. *Pediatrics* 34:58–66, 1964.
155. Di Lorenzo C, Youssef NN, Sigurdsson L, Scharff L, Griffiths J, Wald A: Visceral hyperalgesia in children with functional abdominal pain. *J Pediatr* 139:838–843, 2001.
156. Van Ginkel R, Voskuijl WP, Benninga MA, Taminiau JA, Boeckxstaens GE: Alterations in rectal sensitivity and motility in childhood irritable bowel syndrome. *Gastroenterology* 120:31–38, 2001.
157. Garralda ME: Practitioner review: assessment and management of somatization in childhood and adolescence: a practical perspective. *J Child Psychol Psychiatry* 40:1159–1167, 1999.
158. Knight SJ, Scheinberg A, Harvey AR: Interventions in pediatric chronic fatigue syndrome/myalgic encephalomyelitis: a systematic review. *J Adolesc Health* 53(2):154–165, 2013.
159. FitzGerald TL, Southby AK, Haines TP, Hough JP, Skinner EH: Is physiotherapy effective in the management of child and adolescent conversion disorder? A systematic review. *J Paediatr Child Health* 51(2):159–167, 2015.
160. Levy RL, Langer SL, Romano JM, et al.: Cognitive mediators of treatment outcomes in pediatric functional abdominal pain. *Clin J Pain* 30(12): 1033–1043, 2014.
161. Eccleston C, Palermo TM, Williams AC, et al.: Psychological therapies for the management of chronic and recurrent pain in children and adolescents. *Cochrane Database Syst Rev* (5):CD003968, 2014.
162. Rutten JM, Korterink JJ, Venmans LM, Benninga MA, Tabbers MM: Nonpharmacologic treatment of functional abdominal pain disorders: a systematic review. *Pediatrics* 135(3):522–535, 2015.
163. Fisher E, Law E, Palermo TM, Eccleston C: Psychological therapies (remotely delivered) for the management of chronic and recurrent pain in children and adolescents. *Cochrane Database Syst Rev* (3):CD011118, 2015.
164. Powers SW, Kashikar-Zuck SM, Allen JR, et al.: Cognitive behavioral therapy plus amitriptyline for chronic migraine in children and adolescents: a randomized clinical trial. *JAMA* 310(24):2622–2630, 2013.
165. Sanders MR, Rebgetz M, Morrison M, et al.: Cognitive-behavioral treatment of recurrent nonspecific abdominal pain in children: an analysis of generalization, maintenance, and side effects. *J Consult Clin Psychol* 57(2):294–300, 1989.
166. Sanders MR, Shepherd RW, Cleghorn G, Woolford H: The treatment of recurrent abdominal pain in children: a controlled comparison of cognitive-behavioral family intervention and standard pediatric care. *J Consult Clin Psychol* 62(2):306–314, 1994.
167. Levy RL, Langer SL, Walker LS, et al.: Cognitive-behavioral therapy for children with functional abdominal pain and their parents decreases pain and other symptoms. *Am J Gastroenterol* 105(4):946–956, 2010.
168. Kashikar-Zuck S, Swain NF, Jones BA, Graham TB: Efficacy of cognitive-behavioral intervention for juvenile primary fibromyalgia syndrome. *J Rheumatol* 32:1594–1602, 2005.
169. Nijhof SL, Bleijenberg G, Uiterwaal CS, Kimpen JL, van de Putte EM: Effectiveness of internet-based cognitive behavioural treatment for adolescents with chronic fatigue syndrome (FITNET): a randomised controlled trial. *Lancet* 379(9824):1412–1418, 2012.
170. Pennebaker JW, Susman JR: Disclosure of traumas and psychosomatic processes. *Soc Sci Med* 26:327–332, 1988.
171. Campo JV, Negrini BJ: Case study: negative reinforcement and behavioral management of conversion disorder. *J Am Acad Child Adolesc Psychiatry* 39:787–790, 2000.
172. Palsson OS, van Tilburg M: Hypnosis and guided imagery treatment for gastrointestinal disorders: experience with scripted protocols developed at the University of North Carolina. *Am J Clin Hypn* 58(1):5–21, 2015.
173. Kleinstäuber M, Witthöft M, Steffanowski A, van Marwijk H, Hiller W, Lambert MJ: Pharmacological interventions for somatoform disorders in adults. *Cochrane Database Syst Rev* (11):CD010628, 2014.
174. Korterink JJ, Rutten JM, Venmans L, Benninga MA, Tabbers MM: Pharmacologic treatment in pediatric functional abdominal pain disorders: a systematic review. *J Pediatr* 166(2):424–431.e6, 2015.
175. Saps M, Biring HS, Pusatcioglu CK, Mintjens S, Rzeznikiewiz D: A comprehensive review of randomized placebo-controlled pharmacological clinical trials in children with functional abdominal pain disorders. *J Pediatr Gastroenterol Nutr* 60(5):645–653, 2015.
176. Campo JV, Perel J, Lucas A, et al.: Citalopram treatment of pediatric recurrent abdominal pain and comorbid internalizing disorders: an exploratory study. *J Am Acad Child Adolesc Psychiatry* 43(10):1234–1242, 2004.
177. Roohafza H, Pourmoghaddas Z, Saneian H, Gholamrezaei A: Citalopram for pediatric functional abdominal pain: a randomized, placebo-controlled trial. *Neurogastroenterol Motil* 26(11):1642–1650, 2014.
178. Campo JV, Bridge J, Fontanella CA, et al.: *Citalopram for Functional Abdominal Pain: A Randomized Controlled Trial. Poster Presented at the 60th Annual Meeting of the American Academy of Child and Adolescent Psychiatry*. Orlando, FL, October 24, 2013.
179. Saps M, Youssef N, Miranda A, et al.: Multicenter, randomized, placebo-controlled trial of amitriptyline in children with functional gastrointestinal disorders. *Gastroenterology* 137(4):1261–1269, 2009.
180. Lewis D, Ashwal S, Hershey A, Hirtz D, Yonker M, Silberstein S; American Academy of Neurology Quality Standards Subcommittee; Practice Committee of the Child Neurology Society: Practice parameter: pharmacological treatment of migraine headache in children and adolescents: report of the American Academy of Neurology Quality Standards Subcommittee and the Practice Committee of the Child Neurology Society. *Neurology* 63:2215–2224, 2004.
181. Kabbouche MA, Vockell AL, LeCates SL, Powers SW, Hershey AD: Tolerability and effectiveness of prochlorperazine for intractable migraine in children. *Pediatrics* 107(4):E62, 2001.
182. Battistella PA, Ruffilli R, Cernetti R, et al.: A placebo-controlled crossover trial using trazodone in pediatric migraine. *Headache* 33:36–39, 1993.
183. El-Chammas K, Keyes J, Thompson N, Vijayakumar J, Becher D, Jackson JL: Pharmacologic treatment of pediatric headaches: a meta-analysis. *JAMA Pediatr* 167(3):250–258, 2013.
184. Putnam GP, O'Quinn S, Bolden-Watson CP, Davis RL, Gutterman DL, Fox AW: Migraine polypharmacy and the tolerability of sumatriptan: a large-scale, prospective study. *Cephalalgia* 19:668–675, 1999.
185. Napoletano F, Lionetto L, Martelletti P: Sumatriptan in clinical practice: effectiveness in migraine and the problem of psychiatric comorbidity. *Expert Opin Pharmacother* 15(3):303–305, 2014.
186. Sulheim D, Fagermoen E, Winger A, et al.: Disease mechanisms and clonidine treatment in adolescent chronic fatigue syndrome: a combined cross-sectional and randomized clinical trial. *JAMA Pediatr* 168(4):351–360, 2014.
187. Fritz GK, Bergman AS: Child psychiatrists seen through pediatricians' eyes: results of a national survey. *J Am Acad Child Psychiatry* 24:81–86, 1985.
188. Smith GR Jr, Monson RA, Ray DC: Psychiatric consultation in somatization disorder. A randomized controlled study. *N Engl J Med* 314: 1407–1413, 1986.

CHAPTER 5.11 ■ DELIRIUM AND CATATONIA

DANIEL T. WILLIAMS

With a growing level of sophistication in recent years, we have come to appreciate important neurophysiologic substrates of central nervous system (CNS) dysfunction inherent in many traditional psychiatric disorders. By virtue of functional neuroimaging studies clarifying that every behavior and subjective experience has a neurophysiologic correlate, it is now well recognized that the organic versus psychiatric distinction is ultimately a semantic one, determined by our current level of neurophysiologic sophistication or lack thereof.

Perturbations of consciousness and motor function that are a byproduct of a significant change in the functional integrity of the CNS from its baseline state merit specific clinical consideration by both neurologists and psychiatrists. Two such patterns of perturbation, delirium, and catatonia, are classic neuropsychiatric syndromes. We will address here the phenomenology, evaluation, and treatment of these disorders in children and adolescents.

DELIRIUM

Delirium may be defined as a transient and usually reversible dysfunction in cerebral activity that has an acute or subacute onset and is manifest clinically by a wide array of neuropsychiatric abnormalities, including impairment of consciousness or cognition, which causes a "confusional state" (1–3). Associated symptoms may include perceptual disturbances, delusions, affective lability, disordered thought processes, sleep disturbances, and psychomotor symptoms. If there is a progression of functional derangement of consciousness from normal alertness through delirium to further impairment, the patient can decline into a state of stupor, coma, and eventually death.

Insofar as there are a variety of underlying causes of delirium in different patients, it is reasonable to consider it as a syndrome rather than a single disorder. Although the term has been used with differing connotations over the years and has many synonyms in the neurologic and psychiatric literature, it seems best for current purposes to define delirium as outlined in DSM-IV-TR (Table 5.11.1).

Predisposing Factors

Children and the elderly reportedly are at higher risk to the development of delirium under circumstances of physiologic stress (4–6). While the elderly are thought to be more vulnerable because of diminished cholinergic reserve, children are thought to be more vulnerable because of immature and evolving structural and biochemical brain development. Intrinsic predisposing patient vulnerabilities in addition to age would include a previous delirium episode, pre-existing cognitive impairment, a CNS disorder, and increased blood–brain barrier permeability. Environmental risk factors include social isolation, sensory extremes, visual or hearing deficits, immobility, as well as environmental novelty or stress. Other risk factors include medical illness, surgery, and pharmacologic influences. Clearly, during hospitalization, there is often a confluence of these predisposing and precipitating factors.

Some of the above risk factors may be modifiable and consequently present opportunities for preventive intervention. Closer observation of patients at high risk for delirium could allow for earlier detection of emergent delirium and allow for attenuation of modifiable risk factors. Probably the most readily modifiable is medication exposure, particularly of anticholinergic medications (7). Because of the general acceptance of a tendency for children to regress under stressful circumstances, milder forms of delirium may be mistaken for simply regressive or provocative behavior. As with adults, however, undetected delirium may proceed to the point of self-injury or serious interference with medical treatment.

Paradoxically, children may have a reduced risk of postcardiotomy delirium compared to adults. Kornfeld et al. (8) reported on a sample of 119 unselected open heart patients that included 20 children who had surgical procedures for repair of congenital lesions. Only one of the children developed delirium, whereas 30% of the adults operated on for congenital repairs did. It is noteworthy that preoperative psychiatric interviews may reduce postoperative delirium and psychosis by 50% (9). Others have also reported the benefit of using preoperative psychological interventions to reduce anxiety and improve perioperative management in children (10). A clinical consensus suggests that as the severity of pathophysiologic strain increases, so does the probability of developing a delirium (11). This is particularly true for burn patients, as well as for postoperative patients. Additional factors that are considered to foster the development of delirium include sleep deprivation, sensory deprivation, and sensory overload. Thiamine deficiency can be a risk factor for delirium in pediatric intensive care and oncology patients (12). Low serum albumin is another factor, resulting in a greater bio availability of drugs that are transmitted in the bloodstream, potentially contributing to delirium (13).

TABLE 5.11.1

DIAGNOSTIC CRITERIA FOR DELIRIUM DUE TO . . .* (1–5)

A. Disturbance of consciousness (reduced clarity of awareness of the environment) with reduced ability to focus, sustain, or shift attention.
B. A change in cognition (such as memory deficit, disorientation, language disturbance) or the development of a perceptual disturbance that is not better accounted for by a pre-existing, established, or evolving dementia.
C. The disturbance develops over a short period of time (usually hours to days) and tends to fluctuate during the course of the day.
D. There is evidence from the history, physical examination, or laboratory findings that the disturbance is caused by the direct physiologic consequences of . . .* (1–5)
   *(1) . . . a general medical condition.
   *(2) . . . substance intoxication.
   *(3) . . . substance withdrawal.
   *(4) . . . multiple etiologies.
   *(5) . . . not otherwise specified.

Adapted from American Psychiatric Association: *Diagnostic and Statistical Manual of Mental Disorders*. 4th ed. Text Revision. Washington, DC, American Psychiatric Association, 2000.

Clinical Features

Given that there is a wide variety of etiologies for delirium, it may be most useful to conceptualize delirium as a final common neural pathway that leads to its characteristic symptoms (4). These symptoms often fluctuate in intensity over a 24-hour period and may be associated with shifts between hypoactive and hyperactive states or with disruption of the sleep–wake cycle. Table 5.11.2 outlines symptoms generally associated with delirium that may be variably represented in different patients. Review of studies of delirium in adults with a variety of underlying etiologies shows that some symptoms are reported more often and more consistently than others, suggesting that there may be some core symptoms, irrespective of etiology. Postulated core symptoms include attentional deficits, memory impairment, disorientation, sleep–wake cycle disturbance, thought process abnormalities, motoric alterations, and language disturbances. Associated or noncore symptoms would include perceptual disturbances (illusions, hallucinations), delusions, and affective changes (14). The associated symptoms might reflect the impact of either specific etiologic influences or individual differences in brain circuitry and vulnerability.

TABLE 5.11.2

SIGNS AND SYMPTOMS OF DELIRIUM ("PLASTRD")

***P*sychosis**
Perceptual disturbances (especially visual), including illusions, hallucinations, metamorphopsias
Delusions (usually paranoid and poorly formed)
Thought disorder (tangentiality, circumstantiality, loose associations)
***L*anguage Impairment**
Word-finding difficulty/dysnomia/paraphasia
Dysgraphia
Altered semantic content
Severe forms can mimic expressive or receptive aphasia
***A*ltered or Labile Affect**
Any mood can occur, usually incongruent to context
Anger or increased irritability common
Hypoactive delirium often mislabeled as depression
Lability (rapid shifts) common
Unrelated to mood preceding delirium
***S*leep–Wake Disturbance**
Fragmented throughout 24-hour period
Reversal of normal cycle
Sleeplessness
***T*emporal Course**
Acute/abrupt onset
Fluctuating severity of symptoms over 24-hour period
Usually reversible
Subclinical syndrome may precede and/or follow the episode
***R*eactivity Altered**
Hyperactive
Hypoactive
Mixed
***D*iffuse Cognitive Deficits**
Attention
Orientation (time, place, person)
Memory (short- and long-term; verbal and visual)
Visuoconstructional ability
Executive functions

Adapted from Trzepacz PT, Meagher DF, Wise M: Neuropsychiatric aspects of delirium. In: Yudofsky SC, Hales RE (eds): *The American Psychiatric Publishing Textbook of Neuropsychiatry and Clinical Neurosciences*. 4th ed. Washington, DC, American Psychiatric Publishing, 525–564, 2002.

Some studies suggest that the motoric profile in delirium is influenced by etiology. Thus, delirium due to drug and alcohol related causes is more commonly hyperactive, whereas delirium due to metabolic disturbances, including hypoxia, is more frequently hypoactive (15,16). As yet, however, available studies have not provided clear evidence that gross motoric subtypes have discernible neurobiologic mechanisms.

Mortality rates during a hospitalization involving delirium for adults have ranged from 1.5% to 65% in different case series (17). Turkel and Tavare (18) retrospectively reviewed 84 children and adolescents with delirium, among 1,027 consecutive inpatient psychiatric consultations during a 4-year period. They found a mortality rate of 20% and a prolonged length of stay when delirium was documented. It is clear therefore that the diagnosis of delirium constitutes a matter of severe medical urgency. Since some of the medical conditions contributing to delirium are potentially reversible, early clarification of diagnosis and aggressive initiation of treatment are clinically imperative.

Etiology

When a diagnosis of delirium is established, a thorough search for causes must be pursued, insofar as correction or amelioration of specific underlying causes is important in reversing the condition. However, this process of investigation should not unduly delay prompt treatment of the delirium itself, since such treatment can reduce symptoms even before the underlying medical causes have been reversed. As noted above, from a DSM-IV-TR perspective, delirium is broadly categorized according to etiology into five groups. These include delirium due to a general medical condition, due to substance use or withdrawal, due to multiple causes, and due to no apparent cause that can be identified. It is probably useful to spell out in more detail a list of the wide variety of etiologies that may pertain, either individually or in combination. These are listed in Table 5.11.3.

Delirium in children and adolescents involves the same categories of etiologies as adults, though the relative frequency of specific etiologies differs. Thus, delirium related to illicit drugs is more common in the child and adolescent age group, as is the incidence of delirium from hypoxia due to foreign-body inhalation, drowning, and asthma, as well as delirium related to head trauma.

Differential Diagnosis

Delirium frequently goes undetected in a variety of therapeutic settings by a variety of medical specialists, including neurologists and psychiatrists (19). Failure of detection may derive from insidious onset and fluctuating course involving multiple symptom constellations that can generate much clinical variability. Thus an agitated, hyperactive delirium, that is more likely to be recognized, contrasts with the more common, mixed or hypoactive symptom pattern that may be more readily overlooked. This is particularly true in a hospital setting, with multiple shift changes of staff, where subtle and gradual changes of mental status may not be discerned. Diagnosis can be improved by routinely assessing cognitive function, by improving staff awareness of the varied presentations of delirium, and by using one of the screening instruments for delirium currently available (4).

Differential diagnosis includes depression, psychosis, anxiety, somatoform disorders, dementia (more commonly in the elderly and particularly in children), behavioral disturbance. Because of the general tendency for children to regress under stressful circumstances, milder forms of delirium may be mistaken for simply regressive or provocative behavior. As with adults, however, undetected delirium may proceed to the point

TABLE 5.11.3

ETIOLOGIES OF DELIRIUM

Drug intoxication	Intracranial infection
Drug withdrawal	Systemic infection
Metabolic/endocrine disturbances	Cerebrovascular disorder
Traumatic brain injury	Organ insufficiency
Seizures	Other CNS etiologies
Neoplastic disease	Other systemic etiologies

Adapted from Hales RE, Yudofsky SC: *The American Psychiatric Publishing Textbook of Neuropsychiatry and Clinical Neurosciences*. 3rd ed. Washington, DC, American Psychiatric Press, 2002.

of self-injury or serious interference with medical treatment. Effective diagnosis requires close attention to symptom pattern, temporal sequence, and objective clinical test results (laboratory, cognitive, electroencephalographic). Since delirium is often the first indication of serious medical deterioration, any patient manifesting an abrupt decline in attentional or cognitive function should be evaluated for possible delirium.

Assessment

To allow more accurate diagnosis and monitoring, more than 10 different assessment instruments suitable for adults have been developed (20). One of these, the delirium rating scale, has been systematically evaluated retrospectively with 84 children and adolescents diagnosed with delirium (age range 6 months to 19 years) (21). The delirium rating scale is composed of 10 items: two items ascertain the temporal onset of symptoms and their relationship to a physical disorder; eight other items evaluate major symptoms of delirium. These eight items rate perceptual disturbances, hallucinations, delusions, changes in psychomotor behavior, diffuse cognitive dysfunction, disturbances of sleep–wake cycle, lability of mood, and variability of symptoms. The cognitive dysfunction item includes impairment of attention, concentration, and memory. The results of the Turkel et al. study (21) suggest that the delirium rating scale can be used effectively to evaluate delirium in the pediatric population.

In most cases, electroencephalograms (EEGs) are not needed to make a clinical diagnosis of delirium, but are used when seizures are suspected or when differential diagnosis is difficult. The degree of slowing on EEGs recorded serially over time in children and adolescents correlates with the severity of, and recovery from, delirium (22).

The psychiatrist will clearly not be primarily responsible for diagnosing and managing the underlying medical condition contributing to the delirium. However, supportively maintaining the morale and involvement of family members who can be invaluable observers and informers to the medical staff regarding the patient's mental status can be a vital part of the consulting psychiatrist's function. This, of course, is supplementary to the psychiatrist's own longitudinal assessments of the patient, which should be documented systematically.

Treatment

Prompt treatment is vital because of the substantial morbidity and mortality associated with delirium. Symptomatic treatments include medication, environmental manipulation, as well as patient and family psychosocial support (11). These should be initiated concomitant with the attempts to identify and reverse underlying causes of the delirium.

Pharmacologic treatment with a neuroleptic, most commonly haloperidol, is the most commonly reported medical intervention for delirium, despite the absence of double-blind, placebo-controlled trials documenting efficacy. Haloperidol can be given orally, intramuscularly, or intravenously, although haloperidol is not approved by the U.S. Food and Drug Administration for intravenous use. Clinical experience with haloperidol in pediatric delirium supports its beneficial effects, although purely based on uncontrolled case reports (23). Based on such existing clinical experience, one suggested dosage regimen for children younger than 4 years of age starts with 0.25 mg slowly intravenously over 30 to 45 minutes as a loading dose, and 0.05 to 0.5 mg/kg/24 hr intravenously as a continuing dose. When using higher doses of IV haloperidol (e.g., >20 mg/day), electrocardiographic tracking of QTc interval prolongation and other relevant parameters should be done daily, as well as monitoring and correction of magnesium, phosphate, and other electrolytes in order to minimize the risks of cardiotoxicity (up to torsade de pointes and other tachyarrhythmias). The oral dose of haloperidol is twice the intravenous dose. Although no fixed dosing schedule based on controlled studies is available for either children or adults, a protocol for haloperidol use in agitated delirium in adults has been proposed (11). Intravenous administration of haloperidol is reportedly associated with fewer extrapyramidal symptoms compared with oral administration (24). The rationale for this neuroleptic treatment intervention is based on clinical evidence suggesting a low cholinergic, excess dopaminergic state as the final common neural pathway for delirium (4).

Benzodiazepines are generally reserved for delirium due to alcohol or sedative–hypnotic withdrawal. Occasionally, lorazepam may be used as an adjunct with haloperidol in cases of delirium where agitation and insomnia persist. Caution is needed, however, to avoid over-sedation or paradoxical disinhibition.

Environmental interventions for delirium are often helpful but are not by themselves adequate treatment. Family members and nurses can help reorient the patient with a clock, calendar, and familiar objects. A room with a window can help with diurnal cues and adequate lighting at night can diminish frightening visual misperceptions. Encouraging a stable parent to stay overnight, with appropriate explanation to the parent about the phenomenon of delirium and about the merits of supportive measures for the patient, can be quite reassuring.

Psychiatrists are often called to evaluate the fluctuating, confusing, and bizarre behaviors that may characterize delirium. Insofar as significant morbidity and mortality can be associated with this condition, it is important for the psychiatrist to help organize a systematic differential diagnosis, collaborate with the primary care physician in identifying the underlying cause(s), and help formulate a plan for monitoring and treating the associated agitation as well as related psychiatric symptomatology in both the patient and family.

CATATONIA

In contrast to delirium, which is defined primarily by alterations in level of consciousness as reflected by attention and cognition, with occasionally accompanying psychomotor symptoms, catatonia is defined by a cluster of motor symptoms, including a rigid posture, mutism, fixed staring, stereotypic movements, hyperkinetic movements, or stupor. Implicit in this varied constellation of motor symptoms, however, is the presumption of an underlying neuropsychiatric derangement which presents the clinician with a differential diagnostic and treatment challenge of comparable complexity to that posed by delirium. Like delirium, catatonia is best understood as a syndrome that may be associated with a wide array of psychiatric and medical disorders that lead to the final common path of these motor manifestations. In some patients, the differential diagnostic challenge will include differentiating between delirium and catatonia.

In the current diagnostic classification nomenclature of the American Psychiatric Association, there are three domains in which catatonia is represented and these are represented in Tables 5.11.4 to 5.11.6. This diverse representation speaks to the multifactorial contributants to this syndrome from diverse etiologies.

Predisposing Factors

By definition in the existing psychiatric nomenclature, predisposing factors to catatonia include the three clinical domains

TABLE 5.11.4

DSM-IV-TR CRITERIA FOR CATATONIC DISORDER DUE TO . . . [INDICATE THE GENERAL MEDICAL CONDITION]

A. ***Cat**atonia is manifested by motoric immobility, excessive motor activity (that is apparently purposeless and not influenced by external stimuli), extreme negativism or mutism, peculiarities of voluntary movement, or echolalia or echopraxia.
B. ***Med:*** There is evidence from the history, physical examination, or laboratory findings that the disturbance is the direct physiologic consequence of a general medical condition.
C. ***Not Ment:*** The disturbance is not better accounted for by another mental disorder (e.g., a manic episode).
D. ***Not Del:*** The disturbance does not occur exclusively during the course of a delirium.

Adapted from American Psychiatric Association: *Diagnostic and Statistical Manual of Mental Disorders*. 4th ed., Text Revision. Washington, DC, American Psychiatric Association, 2000.

referred to above, namely a variety of medical conditions, a variety of mood disorders, and a particular type of schizophrenia. Although the occurrence of catatonia in children and adolescents is well documented in the clinical literature (25), there are no epidemiologic studies that indicate a relative difference in incidence associated with age (26). It appears that the range of primary diagnoses with which catatonia is associated in youngsters broadly overlaps that reported in adults. In addition, there are a significant number of reports of catatonia associated with autism, the Prader–Willi syndrome, and intellectual disability (27,28). As with delirium, catatonia in youngsters may be more difficult to diagnose because of the more limited expressive capacity of children and adolescents, as well as the tendency of observers to ascribe symptomatic behavior to willful regression of an oppositional nature.

TABLE 5.11.5

DSM-IV-TR CRITERIA FOR CATATONIC FEATURES SPECIFIER OF A MOOD DISORDER

Specify if:
With Catatonic Features (can be applied to the current or most recent major depressive episode, manic episode, or mixed episode in major depressive disorder, bipolar I disorder, or bipolar II disorder)
The clinical picture is dominated by at least two of the following characteristics (***MUMEE***)
(1) ***M**otoric immobility as evidenced by catalepsy (including waxy flexibility) or stupor
(2) ***U**tmost negativism (an apparently motiveless resistance to all instructions or maintenance of a rigid posture against attempts to be moved) or mutism
(3) ***M**otor hyperactivity (i.e., apparently purposeless and not influenced by external stimuli)
(4) ***E**ccentricities of voluntary movement as evidenced by posturing (voluntary assumption of inappropriate or bizarre postures), stereotyped movements, prominent mannerisms, or prominent grimacing
(5) ***E**cholalia or echopraxia

Adapted from American Psychiatric Association: *Diagnostic and Statistical Manual of Mental Disorders*. 4th ed. Text Revision. Washington, DC, American Psychiatric Association, 2000.

TABLE 5.11.6

CATATONIC TYPE OF SCHIZOPHRENIA

A type of schizophrenia in which the clinical picture is dominated by at least two of the following characteristics (***MUMEE***):
(1) ***M**otoric immobility as evidenced by catalepsy (including waxy flexibility) or stupor
(2) ***U**tmost negativism (an apparently motiveless resistance to all instructions or maintenance of a rigid posture against attempts to be moved) or mutism
(3) ***M**otor hyperactivity (i.e., apparently purposeless and not influenced by external stimuli)
(4) ***E**ccentricities of voluntary movement as evidenced by posturing (voluntary assumption of inappropriate or bizarre postures), stereotyped movements, prominent mannerisms, or prominent grimacing
(5) ***E**cholalia or echopraxia

Clinical Features

The principal motor signs associated with catatonia are mutism, immobility, negativism, posturing, stereotypy, and echophenomena. Although DSM-IV-TR defines a requirement for two of these to be present in cases of mood disorder or schizophrenia, it does not specify a duration. Some clinicians advocate that these signs be present for at least an hour or be reproducible on at least two occasions (29). Prolonged immobility may generate malnutrition, dehydration, weight loss, muscle wasting, contractures, and bedsores. Death may ensue from venous thrombosis and pulmonary emboli. A summary description of clinical features frequently associated with catatonia is presented in Table 5.11.7.

Etiology

As with delirium, there have been efforts to define a final common neurophysiologic pathway, whereby many different pathophysiologic conditions may contribute to the clinical features of catatonia. Recent views implicate frontal lobe circuitry dysfunction (29). Disruption of connections from perceptual-integrating brain systems because of thalamic or parietal lobe lesions as well as limbic interference (as occurs in certain mood states) have been postulated to play etiologic roles. The neurotransmitters dopamine and GABA have been implicated and this has therapeutic relevance.

As previously noted, conditions in which catatonia is expressed include mood disorders, psychosis, and a variety of medical conditions, including neurologic disorders, metabolic disorders, as well as drug intoxication and withdrawal.

Catatonia has been reported in about 15% of manic episodes in adult patients with bipolar mood disorders, with one series of 99 manic patients finding as high as a 27% incidence (30). Bipolar mood disorder is the most common cause of catatonia. Depression is the second most common condition underlying catatonia in adults. Catatonia in depressed patients is often manifest as profound psychomotor retardation, sometimes progressing to stupor or pseudodementia. Delay in diagnostics and treatment intervention for treating catatonia in mood disorder patients clearly can increase morbidity and mortality.

Schizophrenia accounts for about 10% of adult patients with catatonia (31). Catatonic features more commonly encountered in these patients include catalepsy, mannerisms, posturing, and mutism. Historically, this diagnosis has been invoked more frequently than that of mood disorder in patients

TABLE 5.11.7

PRINCIPAL FEATURES OF CATATONIA

Feature	Description
Mutism	Verbal unresponsiveness, not always associated with immobility.
Stupor	Unresponsiveness, hypoactivity, and reduced or altered arousal during which the patient fails to respond to queries; when severe, the patient is mute, immobile, and does not withdraw from painful stimuli.
Negativism (Gegenhalten)	Patient resists examiner's manipulations, whether light or vigorous, with strength equal to that applied, as if bound to the stimulus of the examiner's actions.
Posturing (catalepsy)	Maintains postures for long periods. Includes facial postures, such as grimacing or *Schnauzkrampf* (lips in an exaggerated pucker). Body postures, such as *psychological pillow* (patient lying in bed with his head elevated as if on a pillow), lying in a jackknifed position, sitting with upper and lower portions of body twisted at right angles, holding arms above the head or raised in prayer-like manner, and holding fingers and hands in odd positions.
Waxy flexibility	Offers initial resistance to an induced movement before gradually allowing himself to be postured, similar to bending a candle.
Stereotypy	Non–goal-directed, repetitive motor behavior. The repetition of phrases and sentences in an automatic fashion, similar to a scratched record, termed *verbigeration*, is a verbal stereotypy. The neurologic term for similar behavior is *palilalia*, during which the patient repeats the sentence just uttered, usually with increasing speed.
Automatic obedience	Despite instructions to the contrary, the patient permits the examiner's light pressure to move his limbs into a new position (posture), which may then be maintained by the patient despite instructions to the contrary.
Ambitendency	The patient appears "stuck" in an indecisive, hesitant movement, resulting from the examiner verbally contradicting his own strong nonverbal signal, such as offering his hand as if to shake hands with stating, "Don't shake my hand; I don't want you to shake it."
Echophenomena	Includes *echolalia*, in which the patient repeats the examiner's utterances, and *echopraxia*, in which the patient spontaneously copies the examiner's movements or is unable to refrain from copying the examiner's test movements, despite instruction to the contrary.
Mannerisms	Odd, purposeful movements, such as holding hands as if they were handguns, saluting passerby, or exaggerations or stilted caricatures of mundane movements.

Reprinted from Fink M, Taylor MA: *Catatonia. A Clinician's Guide to Diagnosis and Treatment*. New York, Cambridge University Press, 2003, with permission.

with catatonia, which is a disservice if it leads to premature or exclusive reliance on neuroleptic medication, with associated increased risks of disabling side effects. (These side effects can include neuroleptic malignant syndrome [NMS], an admittedly rare complication that can initially be difficult to differentiate from catatonic schizophrenia.)

Many general medical conditions can manifest with catatonia, including many of the same conditions that are associated with delirium. These include a variety of neurologic syndromes, metabolic, autoimmune, and endocrine disorders, infections, burns, and drug-induced states. The latter may include both recreational and prescribed drugs, including NMS. Neurologic conditions and metabolic disorders associated with catatonia are outlined in Tables 5.11.8 and 5.11.9.

A review of the literature regarding catatonia in children and adolescents suggests that signs of catatonia in youngsters are similar to those in adults (29). It appears that catatonia is sufficiently frequent in this age group that children and adolescents with otherwise unexplained motor symptoms should be formally assessed for it.

Differential Diagnosis

The first task in diagnosis is recognizing the constellation of motor symptoms that constitute catatonia. If, after initial evaluation, there is no clear etiology, it is often diagnostically helpful to administer an intravenous infusion of lorazepam in a medically supervised setting. Because of the possibility of respiratory depression, facilities for assisted respiration should be available. In either adolescents or adults, intravenous infusion of lorazepam, 0.1 mg/kg, with a maximum dose of 1 to 2 mg, can be infused over 2 minutes. This is often helpful in alleviating mutism, posturing, and rigidity. The infusion should be accompanied by supportive communication to the patient of the prospect of benefit of this intervention. A positive response, including relaxation of posture, improvement or restoration of speech, diminished mannerisms, and responsiveness to commands would confirm the diagnosis of catatonia (29). There is insufficient data to allow for an advisory on dosage of diagnostic intravenous infusion in children with catatonia, although one may be influenced in this regard by the dose range indicated for treatment of status epilepticus (maximum pediatric dose of 0.32 mg/kg/day, as specified by the Physician's Desk Reference).

When catatonia is ascertained in a child or adolescent, the differential diagnosis regarding underlying etiology in order of decreasing frequency is mood disorder, seizure disorder, pervasive developmental disorder, and schizophrenia, followed by other neurologic and metabolic disorders, including the effects of psychoactive substances (29). Although some underlying etiologies can be clarified by laboratory tests, catatonia secondary to a mood disorder or a schizophreniform disorder has no pathognomonic laboratory correlate. In those cases, personal and family history, most often with input from parents or other informants, is crucial in establishing the psychiatric diagnosis.

EEGs can be diagnostic if an epileptiform disorder is presenting as catatonia. The EEG will be diagnostic in these cases if obtained during the symptomatic episode, but not necessarily if administered interictally. Clearly, if there are indications that there may be nonpsychiatric contributants to the catatonia, it is imperative that a neurologist and often other primary care physicians become involved in the medical workup seeking to define the underlying etiology.

TABLE 5.11.8

NEUROLOGIC CONDITIONS ASSOCIATED WITH CATATONIA

Encephalitis
Postencephalitic states
Parkinsonism
Subacute sclerosing panencephalitis
Bilateral lesions of the globus pallidus
Bilateral infarction of the parietal lobes
Temporal lobe infarction
Thalamic lesions
Periventricular diffuse pinealoma
Anterior cerebral and anterior communicating artery aneurysms and hemorrhagic infarcts
Frontal lobe traumatic contusions, arteriovenous malformations, neoplasms
Primary frontal lobe degeneration
Traumatic hemorrhage in the region of the third ventricle
Subdural hematoma
General paresis
Tuberous sclerosis
Paraneoplastic encephalopathy
Multiple sclerosis
Pediatric autoimmune neuropsychiatric disorder associated with streptococcal infections (PANDAS)
Familial cerebellar-pontine atrophy
Epilepsy (particularly psychosensory)
Creutzfeldt–Jakob disease
Alcohol degeneration and Wernicke encephalopathy
AIDS-related dementia and other white matter dementias
Narcolepsy

Adapted from Fink M, Taylor MA: *Catatonia. A Clinician's Guide to Diagnosis and Treatment*. New York, Cambridge University Press, 2003.

TABLE 5.11.9

METABOLIC DISORDERS ASSOCIATED WITH CATATONIA

Diabetic ketoacidosis
Hyperthyroidism
Hypercalcemia from a parathyroid adenoma
Pellagra, vitamin B_{12} deficiency
Acute intermittent porphyria
Endocrinopathies: Addison disease, Cushing disease
Syndrome of inappropriate antidiuretic hormone secretion
Hereditary coproporphyria, porphyria
Homocystinuria, uremia, glomerulonephritis
Hepatic dysfunction or encephalopathy
Thrombocytopenic purpura
Lupus erythematosus or other causes of arteritis
Infectious mononucleosis
Bacterial infections: tuberculosis, typhoid, malaria
Langerhans carcinoma
Toxic states secondary to mescaline, amphetamine, phencyclidine, cortisone, disulfiram, aspirin, antipsychoticagents, illuminating gas, organic fluorides

Adapted from Fink M, Taylor MA: *Catatonia. A Clinician's Guide to Diagnosis and Treatment*. New York, Cambridge University Press, 2003, with permission.

Conditions that can be mistaken for catatonia include elective mutism, involving conscious and volitional withholding of speech. However, elective mutism is generally not accompanied by any of the motor signs needed for the diagnosis of catatonia. Juvenile Parkinson disease (PD) can present in childhood or adolescence with bradykinesia (slowing of movement) and bradyphrenia (slowing of cognition). However, PD will often include tremor, pill-rolling finger movements, a shuffling gait, and does not present with bizarre posturing or mutism. Torsion dystonia may present with seemingly bizarre posturing and indeed is often initially misdiagnosed as a psychiatric disorder, but is generally not associated with mutism and will be readily diagnosable by a neurologist familiar with this movement disorder. Somatoform disorder should also be considered in the differential diagnosis, with a different personal and family history pattern, as well as atypical physical presentations often being helpful in the differential (32).

Delirium and its devolution to stupor will often present with reduced CNS arousal that is also a hallmark of catatonia. Indeed, as noted above, some of the neurologic and metabolic conditions that can generate either delirium or catatonia can also generate the other. The diagnostic distinction between these two syndromes is at this point primarily phenomenologic. Delirium is defined by the primary presenting deficits in the areas of consciousness, attention, and cognition, while variable alterations in motor function, generally considered to be associated phenomena, are not necessarily present. Catatonia is defined by the primary presenting deficits in motor function, often with preservation of awareness and memory, as demonstrable on resolution of the catatonic state, when patients can often reproduce conversations and observations that occurred during the catatonic state. Undoubtedly there are some patients in which these syndromes may coexist, though the frequency of this is not clearly documented in the clinical literature. The clinician's primary task, after defining and documenting the presenting phenomenology, is to actively search for the underlying etiology in an effort to delineate routes of treatment intervention and symptomatic resolution.

Assessment

Rating scales have value both for enhancing precision in documenting clinical symptoms as well as for teaching and clinical research purposes. There are several rating scales available for catatonia with good reported interrater reliability (33–35). The Stony Brook scale (33) has a reported interrater reliability of 0.9 and is easy to administer in a simpler version for screening purposes as well as in a more detailed version for rating severity.

Treatment

As with any serious medical condition, early diagnosis and prompt, effective treatment diminishes morbidity and mortality. The clinical literature documents that there have often been unfortunate delays in both of these domains. Insofar as patients with catatonia need protection, intensive treatment, and close monitoring, this is usually best administered in a hospital setting. The number and pattern of catatonic symptoms do not predict response to treatment, but clinical data suggest that most patients respond well to treatment, with prognosis strongly influenced by that of the underlying etiology.

Different treatment algorithms have been outlined for different varieties of catatonia (29). Patients with "retarded catatonia" often present in a stuporous state or with rigid posture. They may become dehydrated and nutrition may be compromised. If untreated for extended periods, bedsores and contractures may develop. Supportively explaining to family members the diagnosis and need for prompt treatment is a

TABLE 5.11.10

MANAGEMENT FOR MALIGNANT CATATONIA/NEUROLEPTIC MALIGNANT SYNDROME

Goal	Measures to Take
Reverse hyperthermia	Aspirin or acetaminophen suppositories; place patient under cooling blankets or give alcohol bath; gastric lavage with ice water.
Reverse dehydration	Intravenous normal or half normal saline. Ringer lactate is avoided as it may increase acidosis. Glucose loads may precipitate a Wernicke encephalopathy in a chronic alcoholic or other persons with chronically low thiamine levels.
Maintain stable blood pressure and cardiac rhythm	Blood pressure and pulse rate are monitored. Hyperkalemia from muscle breakdown is prevented or resolved. Hypertension is controlled with labetalol or esmolol; hypotension by increasing blood volume, and giving vasopressors.
Ensure adequate oxygenation	Continuously monitor oxygen saturation. Maintain airway artificially if rigidity blocks air exchange. Use 100% oxygen if oximetry shows blood saturation less than 95%.
Avoid complications of immobility: thrombosis, embolism, aspirationpneumonia, bedsores	Critical care nursing, moving of limbs, changing of position, skin care.
Avoid renal failure	Frequent monitoring of serum creatinine phosphokinase (as an indicator of muscle necrosis), creatine, and urea nitrogen. Check urine for myoglobinuria to monitor renal function. Dialysis may be required if the syndrome is not promptly and fully resolved.

Reprinted from Fink M, Taylor MA: *Catatonia. A Clinician's Guide to Diagnosis and Treatment*. New York, Cambridge University Press, 2003, with permission.

top priority. Restoration and maintenance of hydration with intravenous fluid and electrolytes is often necessary, with appropriate EKG monitoring. If antipsychotic drugs have been previously in place without benefit, they are best discontinued to avoid precipitating or perpetuating a neurotoxic effect. If a specific etiology is identified, its treatment takes priority (e.g., nonconvulsive status epilepticus). If no such cause is identified, treatment is started with a benzodiazepine, most often lorazepam, and most often initially by the intravenous route (36,37). As noted earlier, an intravenous infusion of lorazepam, 0.1 mg/kg, with a maximum dose of 1 to 2 mg, can be infused over 2 minutes with adolescents or adults. If there is a positive response with symptom attenuation, one shifts to a maintenance dose geared to sustain and enhance improvement, with a maximum pediatric dose of 0.32 mg/kg/day specified by the Physician's Desk Reference (the dose indicated for treatment of status epilepticus). For adolescents, one will often start with a daily dose of 3 to 4 mg. If improvement is only partial, the dose can be titrated within a few days to 8 to 16 mg/day (38). If clinical status stabilizes and improves on this benzodiazepine regimen, one addresses further the issues of nutrition, physical rehabilitation, and treatment of the underlying etiologic influences. If, however, response remains inadequate after a few days, ECT becomes the treatment of choice (29).

Patients with "excited catatonia," including patients with "delirious mania," are a potential danger both to themselves and to others, frequently requiring not only hospitalization but physical restraints and isolation. If no specific treatable etiology can be identified, aggressive treatment with a benzodiazepine is recommended. A common protocol with adolescents or adults is 1 to 2 mg of lorazepam IV every 20 to 30 minutes, up to 10 mg within a few hours (38). If this intervention is not rapidly effective, daily or twice-daily ECT for several days may be needed to achieve stabilization.

"Malignant catatonia" is a life-threatening condition with many features of catatonia plus fever and autonomic instability. Some consider NMS to be a variant and the most common current presenting manifestation of malignant catatonia, precipitated by neuroleptics (29). The first treatment interventions for malignant catatonia/NMS should be the stopping of neuroleptics, the physical protection of the patient when agitated, control of temperature and hydration, as well as close medical monitoring of vital signs in a hospital setting (Table 5.11.10). Two alternative treatment approaches have evolved for management of this disorder. The dopaminergic-muscle relaxant approach considers NMS to be an idiosyncratic response to the dopamine blockade that is generated by neuroleptics. This formulation led to a treatment strategy using the presynaptic dopamine agonist amantadine; the postsynaptic dopamine receptor agonist bromocriptine; and the muscle relaxant dantrolene (39). An alternate strategy involves the benzodiazepine/ECT approach which is a variant of that described above in the treatment of excited catatonia (29,40). Finally, conservative management consisting of stopping potentially offending agents and hydrating vigorously has also been endorsed by some. Controlled studies are needed to clarify the preferred management strategy for NMS.

Once a patient has recovered from an acute episode of catatonia, current advisories call for a maintenance dose of benzodiazepine for at least 6 months. Recurrence of catatonia requires dose augmentation and the possible use of ECT (29). This maintenance recommendation is a supplement to the designated treatment strategy addressed to the patient's underlying clinical condition.

CONCLUSIONS

Delirium and catatonia are neuropsychiatric conditions representing perturbations of consciousness and motor function that are byproducts of significant changes in the functional integrity of the CNS. It is vital that child and adolescent psychiatrists be familiar with the phenomenology, assessment, differential diagnosis, and treatment of these syndromes, insofar as early diagnosis and treatment intervention can have significant impact on the patient's survival and prognosis for future functioning.

References

1. Stewart JT: Behavioral and emotional complications of neurological disorders. In: Noseworthy JH (ed): *Neurological Therapeutics: Principles and Practices*. London, Martin Dunitz, pp. 2855–2870, 2003.
2. Taylor DA, Ashwal S: Impairment of consciousness and coma. In: Swaiman KF, Ashwal S, Ferriero DM (eds): *Pediatric Neurology: Principles and Practice*. 4th ed. Philadelphia, Mosby/Elsevier, pp. 1377–1400, 2006.

3. American Psychiatric Association: *Diagnostic and Statistical Manual of Mental Disorders*. Text Revision. 4th ed. Washington, DC, American Psychiatric Association, 2000.
4. Trzepacz PT, Meagher DF, Wise M: Neuropsychiatric aspects of delirium. In: Yudofsky SC, Hales RE (eds): *The American Psychiatric Publishing Textbook of Neuropsychiatry and Clinical Neurosciences*. 4th ed. Washington, DC, American Psychiatric Publishing, pp. 525–564, 2002.
5. Inouye SK, Charpentier PA: Precipitating factors for delirium in hospitalized elderly patients: predictive model and interrelationships with baseline vulnerability. *JAMA* 275:852–857, 1996.
6. O'Keefe S, Lavan J: The prognostic significance of delirium in older hospital patients. *J Am Geriatr Soc* 45:174–178, 1997.
7. Inouye SK, Bogardus ST Jr, Charpentier PA, et al.: A multicomponent intervention to prevent delirium in hospitalized older patients. *New Engl J Med* 340:669–676, 1999.
8. Kornfeld DS, Zimberg S, Malm J: Psychiatric complications of open-heart surgery. *New Engl J Med* 273:287–292, 1965.
9. Kornfeld DS, Heller SS, Frank KA, Moskowitz R: Personality and psychological factors in postcardiotomy delirium. *Arch Gen Psychiatry* 31:249–253, 1974.
10. Stoddard FJ, Wilens TE: Delirium. In: Jellinek MS, Herzog DB (eds): *Psychiatric Aspects of General Hospital Pediatrics*. Chicago, Yearbook Medical Publishers, pp. 254–259, 1995.
11. Wise MG, Hilty DM, Cerda GM: Delirium due to a general medical condition, delirium due to multiple etiologies, and delirium not otherwise specified. In: Gabbard GO (ed): *Treatment of Psychiatric Disorders*. 3rd ed. Washington, DC, American Psychiatric Publishing, pp. 387–412, 2001.
12. Seear M, Lockitch G, Jacobson B, Quigley G, MacNab A: Thiamine, riboflavin and pyridoxine deficiency in a population of critically ill children. *J Pediatrics* 121:533–538, 1992.
13. Dickson LR: Hypoalbuminemia in delirium. *Psychosomatics* 32:317–323, 1991.
14. Trzepacz PT: Update on the neuropathogenesis of delirium. *Dement Geriatr Cogn Disord* 10:330–334, 1999.
15. Meagher DJ, O'Hanlon D, O'Mahony E, Casey PR: Use of environmental strategies and psychotropic medication in the management of delirium. *Br J Psychiatry* 168:512–515, 1996.
16. O'Keeffe ST, Lavan J: Clinical significance of delirium subtypes in older people. *Age Ageing* 28:115–119, 1999.
17. Oloffseon SM, Weitzner MA, Valentine AD, Baile WF, Meyers CA: A retrospective study of the psychiatric management and outcome of delirium in the cancer patient. *Support Care Cancer* 4:351–357, 1996.
18. Turkel SB, Tavare CJ: Delirium in children and adolescents. *J Neuropsychiatry Clinical Neuroscience* 15:431–435, 2003.
19. Johnson JC, Kerse NM, Gottlieb G, Wanich C, Sullivan E, Chen K: Prospective versus retrospective methods of identifying patients with delirium. *J Am Geriatrics Society* 40:316–319, 1992.
20. Trzepacz PT: A review of delirium assessment instruments. *General Hospital Psychiatry* 16:394–405, 1994.
21. Turkel SB, Brazlow K, Tavare CJ, Trzepacz PT: The delirium rating scale in children and adolescents. *Psychosomatics* 44:126–129, 2003.
22. Montgomery EA, Fenton GW, McClelland RJ, MacFlynn G, Rutherford WH: Psychobiology of minor head injury. *Psychosomatic Med* 21:375–384, 1991.
23. Schieveld JN, Leentjens AF: Delirium in severely ill young children in the pediatric intensive care unit. *J Am Acad Child & Adolescent Psychiatry* 44:392–394, 2005.
24. Menza MA, Murray GB, Holmes VF, Rafuls WA: Decreased extrapyramidal symptoms with intravenous haloperidol. *J Clinical Psychiatry* 48:278–280, 1987.
25. Fink M, Taylor MA: The many varieties of catatonia. *Eur Arch Psychiatry Clin Neurosci* 251(Suppl 1): 8–13, 2001.
26. Thakur A, Jagadheesan K, Dutta S, Sinna VK: Incidence of catatonia in children and adolescents in a paediatric psychiatric clinic. *Aust N Z J Psychiatry* 37:200–203, 2003.
27. Wing L, Shah A: Catatonia in autistic spectrum disorders. *Br J Psychiatry* 176:357–362, 2000.
28. Cohen D: Towards a valid nosography and psychopathology of catatonia in children and adolescents. *Int Rev Neurobiol* 72:131–47, 2006.
29. Fink M, Taylor MA: *Catatonia. A Clinician's Guide to Diagnosis and Treatment*. New York, Cambridge University Press, 2003.
30. Braunig P, Kruger S, Shugar G: Prevalence and clinical significance of catatonic symptoms in mania. *Compr Psychiatry* 39:35–46, 1998.
31. Kruger S, Braunig P: Catatonia in affective disorder: new findings and a review of the literature. *CNS Spectrums* 5:48–53, 2000.
32. Williams DT: Somatoform disorders. In: Rowland LP (ed): *Merritt's Neurology*. 11th ed. Philadelphia, PA, Lippincott Williams & Wilkins, pp. 1140–1145, 2005.
33. Bush G, Fink M, Petrides G, Dowling F, Francis A: Catatonia: I: rating scale and standardized examination. *Acta Psychiatr Scand* 93:129–136, 1996.
34. Braunig P, Kruger S, Shugar G, Hoffler J, Borner I: The catatonia rating scale I: development, reliability and use. *Compr Psychiatry* 41:147–158, 2000.
35. Northoff G, Kock A, Wenke J, et al.: Catatonia as a psychomotor syndrome: a rating scale and extrapyramidal motor symptoms. *Mov Disord* 14:404–416, 1999.
36. Bush G, Fink M, Petrides G, Dowling F, Francis A: Catatonia: II: treatment with lorazepam and electroconvulsive therapy. *Acta Psychiatr Scand* 93:137–143, 1996.
37. Ungvari GS, Kau LS, Wai-Kwong T, Shing NF: The pharmacological treatment of catatonia: an overview. *Eur Arch Psychiatry Clin Neurosci* 251(Suppl 1):31–34, 2001.
38. Ungvari GS, Chiu HFK, Chow LY, Lau BST, Tang WK: Lorazepam for chronic catatonia: a randomized, double-blind, placebo-controlled crossover study. *Psychopharmacology* 142:393–398, 1999.
39. Davis JM, Caroff SN, Mann SC: Treatment of neuroleptic malignant syndrome. *Psychiatr Ann* 30:325–331, 2000.
40. Slooter AJ, Balk FJ, van Nieuwenhuizen O, van der Hoeven J: Electroconvulsive therapy for malignant catatonia in childhood. *Pediatr Neurol* 32:190–192, 2005.

5.12 ■ ELIMINATION DISORDERS

CHAPTER 5.12 ■ ELIMINATION DISORDERS: ENURESIS AND ENCOPRESIS

EDWIN J. MIKKELSEN

ENURESIS

Definition and Historical Note

Enuresis is divided into two subtypes: primary and secondary. Primary enuresis encompasses children who have never achieved continence, whereas secondary enuresis refers to those children who maintain continence for at least 1 year, only to lose it at some point after that. The term itself is derived from the Greek word *enourein,* "to void urine," and has come to imply nocturnal events, although that connotation is not inherent in the derivation of the word itself. There is a rich literature concerning enuresis and its treatment over the centuries. In retrospect, many of these treatment approaches now appear to have been quite sadistic. This history has been summarized in an excellent review by Glicklich (1), which covers material dating back to the Ebers Papyrus of 1550 BC.

There has been substantial progress in the treatment of enuresis, which in turn has contributed to a greater understanding of the fundamental pathophysiologic processes involved. These advances are reviewed in this chapter.

Prevalence and Epidemiology

Statistics concerning the prevalence of enuresis also must take into account the severity of the disorder. For example, in the Isle of Wight Study, Rutter and colleagues (2) found that 15.2% of boys were wet less often than once a week, whereas only 6.7% wet at least once a week. The corresponding figures for girls were 12.2% and 3.3%, respectively. By the age of 14 years, only 1.9% of boys were wet less often than once a week, and 1.1% were wetting at least once a week, with the corresponding figures for girls being 1.2% and 0.5%, respectively (3). Longitudinal data from the Isle of Wight Study have illustrated that wetting develops in many children between the ages of 5 and 7 years. Enuresis also was found in greater frequency in children undergoing psychosocial stress and in those living in socially disadvantaged circumstances (2).

A Scandinavian study of 3,206 7-year-old children found an overall prevalence of 9.8%; 6.4% of this group was accounted for by children with night wetting, 1.8% by day wetters, and 1.6% by those with mixed day and night wetting. This study also showed a strong genetic influence in that the risk of a child having enuresis was 7.1 times greater if the father manifested enuresis after 4 years of age, and 5.2 times greater if the mother did (4).

An 8-year longitudinal study in New Zealand found a prevalence of 7.4% for nocturnal enuresis in 8 year olds. This figure was accounted for by 3.3% with primary enuresis and 4.1% with secondary enuresis (5).

More recent studies have found remarkably similar results. In a group of 392 7-year-old children from Sweden, Wille (6) reported a prevalence of 7.3% for monosymptomatic primary enuresis. A questionnaire study involving a large cohort of Australian children in the 5- to 12-year-old range reported an overall incidence of 5.1% for nocturnal enuresis of at least weekly frequency and 1.4% for daytime wetting of similar frequency (7). In a population-based questionnaire study, Soderstrom et al. (8) reported bedwetting at a frequency of at least once per month in 7.1% of first-graders, and 2.7% of fourth-graders.

Clinical Description

As noted, the term enuresis itself denotes only the voiding of urine, but over the years, it has acquired both a pathologic and a nocturnal connotation. Daytime wetting is correctly referred to as diurnal enuresis, whereas nighttime wetting is referred to as nocturnal enuresis.

In the fifth edition of the *Diagnostic and Statistical Manual of Mental Disorders* (DSM-5*)*, the American Psychiatric Association (2013) defines primary enuresis as "repeated voiding of urine during the day or at night into bed or clothes, whether involuntarily or intentionally." The DSM-5 goes on to specify that "the behavior is clinically significant as manifested by either a frequency of at least twice per week for at least three consecutive months or impairment in social, academic (occupational) or other important areas of functioning." The child must also have reached an age at which continence could reasonably be expected. The criteria require a chronologic age of 5 years as a cutoff or a mental age of 5 years for those children with developmental delays. The DSM-5 also stipulates that the wetting not be the result of "the physiological effects of a substance (e.g., a diuretic, an antipsychotic agent) or a general medical condition (e.g., diabetes, spina bifida, a seizure disorder)." Three subtypes of enuresis are defined: nocturnal only (nighttime wetting), diurnal only (daytime wetting), and nocturnal and diurnal (mixed day and night wetting). A distinction also is made between primary and secondary enuresis. Primary enuresis refers to those children who have never achieved urinary continence, whereas secondary enuresis refers to those children who have achieved continence and then lost it. The period of continence necessary to differentiate between primary and secondary enuresis had variously been proposed to be 6 months to 1 year. The criteria do not specify a precise period of time for the distinction, but instead makes reference to "a secondary type in which the disturbance develops after a period of established urinary continence." A child is not considered to have primary functional enuresis until 5 years of age. Secondary enuresis can begin at any time, once the criterion of initial continence has been fulfilled, but the usual onset is between 5 and 7 years of age (2). These criteria are essentially unchanged from the prior edition of the DSM. It is unfortunate that the inclusion of the term "involuntarily or intentionally" has been continued, as the number of children whose incontinence is involuntary or intentional is quite small.

Etiology and Pathogenesis

The physiologic manifestations of this disorder have led to a wide range of etiologic theories. A primary focus of these studies has naturally been the anatomy of the bladder and urinary tract. A study that investigated bladder capacity in children with primary nocturnal enuresis, former enuretic patients, and control subjects, failed to find any significant difference in bladder capacity between the groups (9). It also has been demonstrated that fluid loading can produce enuretic events in children who do not have a history of enuresis (10,11). Children with enuresis were found to have developmental delays twice as often as those without in a large longitudinal population study (12) and Touchette et al. (13) have reported an association between bedwetting and related developmental milestones. An investigation of event-related potentials and brainstem auditory-evoked responses found longer latencies in children with enuresis, as compared to controls, which the authors interpreted as evidence of a maturational delay (14).

There is an obvious relationship between enuresis and bladder infection (15); thus, an infection of the urogenital tract should be ruled out before a diagnosis of functional enuresis is made. This is especially important for girls, who are more prone to urinary tract infections (16). The possibility of urinary tract obstruction as a widespread cause of enuresis has been reported (17) but has been criticized because such a hypothesis can lead to unnecessary surgery (18). After extensively reviewing the literature on this subject, Shaffer (19) concluded: "There is no evidence that urethral dilatation or bladder neck repair is an effective treatment for enuresis." The only exception to this would be if there were very specific pathophysiologic findings.

Other investigations into the role of urodynamic abnormalities in the pathogenesis of primary enuresis support Schaffer's conclusion (20). In a large study, Kawauchi et al. (21) found an incidence of urologic abnormalities of 1.8% on intravenous pyelography (n = 940), 7.1% on voiding cystourethrography (n = 695), 11.5% on cystometry (n = 487), and no abnormalities on renal ultrasonography (n = 58). Of those who did manifest reflux on voiding cystourethrography, the degree of reflux was assessed as mild in 92.1%.

Yeung et al. (22) utilized noninvasive ultrasound techniques to assess physiologic bladder parameters in 514 children with primary enuresis (age 5 to 18 years; mean age 11.2 years), and 339 age-matched controls. Analysis of the data from the entire study group yielded three subtypes: small-capacity bladder with thick wall; normal-capacity bladder with normal wall thickness; and large-capacity bladder with thin wall. There was also a 4-week period of treatment with desmopressin acetate (DDAVP) for the children with enuresis. The authors found that "poor response to treatment was significantly associated with pathological bladder conditions, that is, small-capacity bladder with thick bladder wall or large-capacity bladder with thin bladder wall."

The nature of the enuretic phenomenon has naturally led to speculation concerning a psychodynamic etiology. These hypotheses have in general evolved from case reports or have been derived from theoretical considerations. There has been one rigorous attempt to define the generalizations derived from the literature regarding enuresis and encopresis and then to determine with what frequency these generalizations were borne out by an analysis of the clinical material. This elegant study by Achenbach and Lewis (23) revealed that "only two of the twenty-four generalizations derived from the literature regarding encopresis and enuresis received support at the conventional level (probability = 0.05) of statistical significance."

Epidemiologic studies have, however, shown a correlation between psychological disturbance and enuresis, which is more pronounced in older children (2). This observation then raises the question of the nature of the relationship: Is it a causal, incidental, or secondary relationship? The aforementioned link between enuresis and developmental delays, which are also linked to psychopathology, would suggest that there is a common underlying maturational factor that predisposes vulnerable children to manifest both behavioral disturbances and enuresis. In further support of this hypothesis are the observations that the nature of the behavioral disturbance in children with enuresis is nonspecific (24) and that no physiologic marker can be found that reliably differentiates psychologically disturbed from nondisturbed children with enuresis (25). Biederman et al. (26) have evaluated the possible linkage between enuresis and attention-deficit hyperactivity disorder (ADHD). Their findings indicated that enuresis did not increase the risk for psychopathology in children with or without ADHD but was associated with increased risk for learning disability in normal control children, but not in those with ADHD. Baeyens et al. (27) investigated the prevalence of ADHD in 120 children (age 6 to 12 years) with primary enuresis, utilizing parent and teacher questionnaires as well as diagnostic interviews. Their results indicated that 15% met the criteria for ADHD, and a further 22.5% met the criteria for ADHD-inattentive type. A 2-year follow-up study of the same cohort indicated that 73% of those diagnosed with ADHD had the diagnosis reconfirmed at the follow-up (28). The authors also noted that the odds of a child with ADHD still having episodes of nocturnal enuresis at 2-year follow-up were 3.2 times higher than those for a child who did not have comorbid ADHD. The association with behavioral disturbance has been reported as being greater for secondary enuresis (29,30) and for enuresis persisting into adolescence (31). One study that specifically evaluated risk factors for the development of secondary enuresis found that delayed attainment of initial nocturnal continence and exposure to four or more stressful life events in a year were significantly related to the development of secondary enuresis (32). Similar results with regard to the relationship between psychosocial stress and secondary enuresis have been reported by von Gontard et al. (33). However, at least one large study in the Netherlands found no difference in psychopathology between children with primary and secondary enuresis (34). Of interest is an investigation by Van Hoecke et al. (35) that compared the results of the Child Behavior Checklist and the Disruptive Behavior Disorder Rating Scale in 154 children with enuresis and 153 controls. The results indicated that although the children with enuresis scored significantly higher on both scales, when the socioeconomic status of the children was controlled for the relationship was no longer present.

The occurrence of the enuretic episodes during sleep naturally led to a series of studies investigating the relationship between sleep states and the occurrence of enuretic events. The earliest of these studies suggested that the enuretic events occurred in "deep" sleep and led to a theory that enuretic events were dream equivalents (36). This theory was subsequently supplanted by Broughton's (37,38) view that enuresis was a disorder of arousal. This research suggested that enuretic episodes were preceded by arousal signals and originated in delta sleep. A further elaboration of this theory held that psychiatrically disturbed children with enuresis received normal arousal signals but did not respond to them, whereas those without psychiatric disturbance did not generate arousal signals (39). The largest and most convincing sleep studies indicate that enuretic episodes occur in each sleep stage in proportion to the time spent in that stage, when time of night also is considered (24,40,41). There have been three studies that suggested children with primary enuresis may be more difficult to arouse from sleep than control subjects, although the methodology is somewhat subjective with regard to defining arousability (6,42,43). Other research in this area has focused on combining sleep studies with cystometry (44), and may eventually lead to the identification of subtypes of children with enuresis (45,46).

The development of DDAVP as a treatment for enuresis (described later) has led to the observation that some children with enuresis do not have the ability to concentrate the urine they produce during the night and reduce urine volume (47). In a further investigation of this hypothesis, Rittig et al. (48) compared the circadian variation of plasma atrial natriuretic peptide (ANP) with the clearance of creatinine and the excretion of sodium and potassium. Subjects in the study consisted of 15 children with nocturnal enuresis and 11 control subjects matched for age, sex, and weight. The children with enuresis did not differ from control subjects with regard to ANP, but during the first hours of sleep, they did manifest significantly more polyuria, natriuresis, and kaliuresis despite normal levels of ANP. The authors concluded that children with enuresis display abnormal diurnal rhythmicity in the urinary excretion of potassium and sodium that is not correlated with plasma levels of ANP. They speculated that the abnormalities in sodium and potassium may be related to abnormal tubular handling. This hypothesis has been further supported by subsequent research (49–51) that used radioimmunoassay to evaluate the circadian rhythmicity of plasma arginine vasopressin (AVP) in 55 children with enuresis and 15 control subjects. The AVP levels were measured under conditions of controlled water intake 3 times per day for 72 hours. Only 14 of the 55 children with enuresis had a significant decrease in AVP compared with control subjects. Nine of these 14 AVP-deficient children subsequently were found to be totally dry with DDAVP treatment.

The circadian rhythmicity of AVP has continued to be a focus of investigation because it theoretically could explain both the pathophysiology of enuresis and its response to DDAVP. Accordingly, researchers have been particularly interested in any differences that could be detected between DDAVP responders and nonresponders. One study has reported significant differences in morning values of AVP between normal control subjects ($n = 7$) and children whose enuresis responded to DDAVP ($n = 6$), as well as between the responders ($n = 6$) and nonresponders to DDAVP ($n = 5$). Thus, the morning AVP levels were able to differentiate the children with enuresis from the control subjects, and the responders from the nonresponders (52). However, further complicating this line of research has been the finding that AVP is secreted in a "pulsatile pattern," requiring frequent sampling of plasma levels to be meaningful (53). Studies using frequent measurements of AVP have produced mixed results. Two studies that used more frequent AVP measurements (53,54) found no differences between responders and nonresponders to DDAVP. Aikawa et al. (55,56) addressed this question in a series of studies that measured AVP secretion on an hourly basis for 24 hours. The first set of these studies looked at AVP secretion profiles in children with enuresis ($n = 9$) and control subjects ($n = 8$). The results did establish that the plasma AVP level was significantly lower in the children with enuresis in the 11 PM to 4 AM time period. They then looked at the secretion dynamics in two phenomenologic subgroups of children with enuresis: those with low urinary osmotic pressure and large nocturnal urine output, as opposed to a group with normal urinary osmotic pressure and small nocturnal urine output. The results showed that the mean nocturnal AVP levels were significantly lower in the first (large nocturnal output) group and that treatment with DDAVP did produce a significant increase in AVP for this group as a whole, but not for every child.

The effect of fluid restriction on AVP levels and urine osmolality also has been investigated. These studies indicate that AVP levels are increased in both control subjects and in children with enuresis in response to fluid restriction, and that the degree of AVP secretion is related to plasma osmolality (57). When DDAVP responders and nonresponders are compared with control subjects, all three groups manifest an increase in AVP, but the DDAVP responders showed a smaller increase than the other groups (58). Studies involving adolescents and adults with refractory enuresis also have suggested that the primary pathophysiologic mechanism may be an abnormal tubular processing of sodium related to a relative insensitivity to AVP (59,60) that is corrected to some degree by DDAVP. Similar research in children led Eggert and Kuhn (61) to hypothesize that the primary difference between children with enuresis and control subjects may be at the distal tubular AVP receptor level.

One of the newest areas of research has been the exploration of genetic linkages. It has long been known that enuresis tends to run in families, and that a positive family history can be related to positive treatment outcome (62). In general, genetic studies involve large numbers of families with multigenerational transmission of primary nocturnal enuresis. The chromosomes that have been identified to date include 13q, 12q, 8, and 22 (63–65). In some families, an autosomal dominant mode of transmission with penetrance above 90% has been identified (66).

Loeys et al. (67) studied 32 families with extensive histories of nocturnal enuresis, which ranged from two to four generations. Linkage to an area on chromosome 22q11 was noted in nine families, to 13q13–14 in six, and to 12q in four. Evidence of linkage to chromosome 8q could not be established. Thus, the findings were heterogeneous with regard to the chromosome sites involved. A genetic investigation of a large, four-generation family with a history of both nocturnal and diurnal enuresis indicated an autosomal dominant pattern with high penetrance. The author concluded that, "The most likely genetical model in this kindred seems to be a gene located on chromosome 4p16.1 causing primary nocturnal enuresis." However, involvement of chromosome 12q24.3 could not be excluded (68).

The results of this line of research to date would support the view of von Gontard et al. (66) that "Nocturnal enuresis is a common, genetic, and heterogeneous disorder. The association between genotype and phenotype are complex and are susceptible to environmental influences."

Laboratory Studies

The fact that urinary tract infections can precipitate enuretic events in children means that a urinalysis should be performed to rule out this readily treatable cause of enuresis.

The use of more invasive and painful studies remains controversial. Although it is certainly possible that altered bladder physiology may lead to primary enuresis, the yield from these studies does not appear to be of sufficient magnitude to warrant subjecting all children with enuresis to them. A thorough review of this subject by Cohen (69) found the incidence of obstructive lesions in children with enuresis to be 3.7% in a primary care pediatric setting. Accordingly, he suggested that, "contrast studies are indicated only when there is significant evidence of anatomical or functional pathology by history or exam." Subsequent studies have supported this general position (23,24), while suggesting that those children with daytime wetting and overt symptoms of voiding disturbance are more apt to have urinary tract abnormalities than those who wet solely at night (70). As discussed above, ultrasound bladder measurements may prove useful in the future, but currently this is viewed as a technique utilized in research only (25).

Differential Diagnosis

The differential diagnosis includes the possibility of urinary tract infection and altered bladder physiology. There are scattered case reports of enuresis being secondary to other primary medical problems, such as hyperthyroidism (71), constipation (72), and central hormonal abnormalities (73). Although such reports are infrequent, the clinician should do a thorough physical examination and consider the possibility of underlying organic illness—particularly readily treatable constipation. Brooks and Topol (74) have reported an association between obstructive sleep apnea in children and nocturnal enuresis. They hypothesize that this could be related to the effects of sleep apnea on arousal patterns, and bladder dynamics on urinary hormone production.

There are reports of nocturnal enuresis occurring as a side effect of treatment with selective serotonin reuptake inhibitor antidepressants (SSRIs). Given the frequency with which these agents are prescribed to children, this should be considered. The chronologic correlation between the initiation of treatment with an SSRI and the onset of enuretic episodes would tend to substantiate the diagnosis (75–78). This side effect has also been reported with risperidone (79). Psychological testing in conjunction with structured interviews may provide further insight into the coexistence of psychopathology. However, the studies reviewed previously suggest that any coexisting psychological disorder should be viewed as an accompanying finding rather than as a causal effect.

The distinction between primary and secondary enuresis can be made by history.

Treatment

Although psychotherapy may be helpful for managing the behavioral disorders that accompany enuresis, it appears to have little effect on primary enuresis itself, with studies showing a success rate of 20%, which may largely be accounted for by spontaneous remission (69). Psychotherapy may be more useful for those children with secondary enuresis, especially those whose episodes begin after a traumatic event or parental divorce, or in those cases where a specific parent–child conflict appears to be contributing to the continuation of the enuresis (Table 5.12.1) (80).

It has been shown that having nocturnal enuresis has a negative impact on self-esteem, which can be normalized by effective treatment (81–83). The factors related to negative self-image were male gender, primary enuresis, and a greater frequency of wet nights.

The two primary means of treating children with enuresis fall into the categories of behavioral and psychopharmacologic methods.

Behavioral Methods

Behavioral treatment should be attempted first because it is usually more innocuous than pharmacologic intervention.

TABLE 5.12.1

FACTORS TO CONSIDER WHEN CONSTRUCTING A TREATMENT ALGORITHM FOR PRIMARY NOCTURNAL ENURESIS

Age of child
Medical cause has been ruled out
Rate of spontaneous remission (approximately 14–16% per year)
Behavioral conditioning with bell and pad or similar methodology
Equally effective as pharmacologic treatment
Lower rate of relapse than with pharmacologic treatment
Safer than pharmacologic treatment
Most commonly used pharmacologic intervention is desmopressin acetate (DDAVP)
Most serious side effect (rare) is hyponatremia, leading to seizures
Imipramine is no longer first-line choice for pharmacologic treatment, but can be used for refractory individuals
Combination of behavioral and pharmacologic treatment can be considered for refractory enuresis

The underlying assumption of the behavioral strategy is that it is helping children with enuresis and their families master an affliction rather than tacitly implying that the children are either consciously or unconsciously causing the wetting themselves. One unfortunate consequence of various reward–punishment strategies is that they can subtly imply to children and their families that the disorder is quasi-volitional. The bell and pad method of conditioning is a reasonable first approach. A review of this treatment modality indicated that it was first reported in 1904 and has been in routine use since the 1930s (84). In reviewing the results of several studies involving over 1,000 children, Werry (85) found a success rate of 75%, and subsequent studies have been consistent with this (86). Glazener et al. (87) noted that approximately two-thirds of children treated with the alarm achieved nocturnal continence during treatment and nearly half who complete this form of treatment remained dry after the termination of treatment. In a similar study, Butler and Gasson (88) reviewed 38 studies involving at least 10 children, and found that the success rate ranged from 30% to 87%. However, there were considerable methodologic differences, including the definition of success. When they narrowed the review to 20 relatively homogeneous studies, they found an overall 65% success rate and a relapse rate of 42%. There appear to be two subgroups of responders: those who sleep through the night after treatment without wetting, and those who wake up spontaneously to go to the bathroom (89). A psychiatric disorder in the child and family stress appear to be negative prognostic factors when predicting outcome with this modality (86).

Butler and Robinson (90) found low functional bladder capacity and inability to be aroused by the alarm to correlate with lack of success, and a higher pretreatment frequency of enuretic events has been found to correlate with increased success with this form of treatment (91,92).

Bladder capacity also has been investigated with regard to changes occurring during treatment. Oredsson and Jorgensen (93) measured bladder capacity in 18 children with severe nocturnal enuresis before beginning a 6-week period of treatment with the bell and pad and again after treatment. Ten of the 18 children ceased wetting, but overall, there was a significant increase in bladder capacity for the entire group that did not correlate with outcome. Subsequent investigations have also reported an increase in bladder capacity following treatment with the alarm method (94,95). This may explain why one study found that children whose nocturnal enuresis responded to the alarm also had significant improvement in daytime wetting (96). Behavioral treatment continues to evolve. In a study involving 125 children, an attempt was made to replace the bell and pad mechanism with a simple alarm clock that was either set to go off at a time when the bladder might be expected to be reaching maximal capacity (group I) or after 2 to 3 hours of sleep (group II). The results were comparable with previously published figures for the bell and pad, with success noted in 77.1% of group I and 61.8% of group II, and respective 6-month relapse rates of 24.1% and 14.7% (97).

Another innovation involves replacing the pad that signals the enuretic event with a small ultrasonic monitor mounted to an elastic abdominal belt that signals the alarm when bladder capacity is reaching a predetermined threshold (98). Results of a clinical trial of this methodology were comparable with those obtained with the traditional bell and pad technique, and increases in nighttime bladder capacity also were noted (99).

An approach using bladder biofeedback has been developed for children with enuresis who are refractory to other forms of treatment, have small bladder capacities, and have evidence of an unstable detrusor (100). A subsequent report by the same group (101) also reported an increase in bladder capacity with biofeedback treatment. As noted earlier, the presence of behavioral or family functioning problems can have a negative impact on the outcome of behavioral treatment. A successful intervention in refractory children with severe wetting who have these issues has been to combine traditional alarm therapy with treatment with DDAVP (102,103).

Glazener and Evans (104) performed a review of studies involving simple behavioral interventions for enuresis. The procedures involved included reward systems, such as star charts, nighttime awakening to urinate, retention-control training, and fluid restriction. They noted that many of the studies were small and poorly controlled, which precluded a meta-analysis. There was some suggestion that star charts and nighttime awakening achieved better outcome than no treatment. A similar review was completed for the more complex behavioral and educational interventions of dry bed training and full-spectrum home training (105). Again, there were methodologic issues that compromised many of the studies. These modalities were found to be superior to no treatment, but as stand-alone treatments were not as effective as alarm treatment. However, there was some indication that combining dry bed treatment with the alarm might provide better results than the alarm alone in some children. Bennett (106) has developed a protocol that utilizes educational and simple behavioral interventions as a prelude to treatment with the bell and pad. He reports a success rate of 85%, and a relapse rate of 15% (many of whom become dry with a repeat of the program) with this methodology. Bennett's book also contains a very useful chapter that describes the advantages and disadvantages of each of the various subtypes of the bell and pad form of treatment that are commercially available.

Psychopharmacologic Methods

The Australian psychiatrist MacLean (107) first described the efficacy of imipramine for nocturnal enuresis in 1960. Since then, there have been over 40 double-blind studies confirming the efficacy of imipramine for nocturnal enuresis. Lack of response to imipramine often can be traced to the reluctance of primary care physicians to exceed dosages of 25 to 50 mg. Nevertheless, it is reasonable to begin at a dose of 25 mg and to titrate up slowly because some children respond to the lower dosages. Allowing 4 to 7 days between dosage increments makes it possible to detect these low-dose responders. Most children respond in the 75- to 125-mg range. The upper range of dosage is determined by the child's weight, with the standard upper limit being 5 mg/kg/d. A baseline electrocardiogram should be obtained before instituting treatment with imipramine, and monitoring is advised above 3.5 mg/kg (24).

The relatively high rate of spontaneous remission in enuresis mitigates against keeping children on medication for long periods. A practical approach is to taper slowly and discontinue the imipramine every 3 months. If wetting resumes as the dosage is tapered or after it is discontinued, then the dosage can simply be titrated back up to the effective dose for another 3-month period.

There have been tragic reports of children who reasoned that if three pills would stop the wetting for a night, then taking the whole bottle should stop it permanently. Thus, it is important to warn parents about the magical thinking of children in this regard and the importance of controlling the medication. Younger siblings also are at risk of overdosing with the medication if it is not controlled. In cases of mild-to-moderate overdose, supportive measures, including the symptomatic management of seizures and cardiac arrhythmias, may be sufficient.

There have been five studies investigating the relationship between blood level of imipramine and clinical response. One study found no correlation between improvement in enuresis and the blood level of imipramine either alone or in conjunction with its metabolites (108). However, three studies have now demonstrated a significant correlation between the diminution of enuretic events and the steady-state concentrations of imipramine plus its metabolite desipramine (109–112). One of these studies found an optimal effect when the combined steady-state imipramine plus desipramine concentrations were above 60 ng/mL (111), and another reported favorable outcomes when steady-state combined levels were greater than 80 ng/mL (109). An investigation into the role of dosage response (113) evaluated the blood level–efficacy equation in 18 children who, after baseline and placebo, received increasing dosages of imipramine at 2-week intervals. The specific dosages used were 1, 1.5, 2, and 2.5 mg/kg/d. They found that efficacy was "moderately but significantly" related to increasing dose. However, there was wide variation (sevenfold) in serum levels between the individual children at every dosage level. There is a good correlation between side effects and blood level, especially dry mouth (122). This may prove clinically useful in monitoring children who are phobic about having their blood drawn. As might be expected, the advent of treatment with DDAVP has led to a marked decline in new research concerning imipramine.

Gepertz and Neveus (114) utilized imipramine in the treatment of 49 children who had been refractory to treatment with DDAVP, the alarm, and anticholinergic treatment. They reported that 31 children (64.6%) achieved a 50% reduction in the frequency of enuresis and 22 of these realized complete cessation of the enuresis. It was also noted that seven children with comorbid attention deficit showed improvement in those symptoms as well. Thus, the authors concluded that it was reasonable to consider imipramine for children who had not responded well to other modalities.

Despite the efficacy of behavioral interventions, survey studies tend to indicate that in clinical practice medication is more apt to be used than behavioral interventions (115). A large population-based study found that only 38% of children with enuresis had seen a physician. Over one-third of this physician-treated group had been prescribed some form of pharmacotherapy, and only 3% had been advised to use the bell and pad conditioning technique (116). This may be changing, as a subsequent study reported 80% of physicians recommended the bell and pad (117). Boulis and Long (118) have reported that family practitioners are more likely to recommend DDAVP as a first treatment for enuresis than are pediatricians.

The newest research into pharmacotherapy for enuresis involves the use of DDAVP. Moffatt et al. (119) reviewed all of the then-existing controlled studies concerning the use of DDAVP for enuresis. In the process, they located 18 randomized controlled trials (11 crossover and 7 parallel), which included a total of 689 subjects, most of whom had been refractory to prior treatment. The decreased frequency of enuretic events in the study ranged from 10% to 91%. In general, wetting resumes once the medication is discontinued. Those studies that reported long-term follow-up indicated that 5.7% remained dry after stopping the medication. The most common side effects were nasal stuffiness, headache, epistaxis, and mild abdominal pain. Positive prognostic factors appear to be fewer initial (pretreatment) wet nights and age greater than 9 years. Hogg and Husmann (62) and Terho (120) particularly looked at the efficacy of DDVAP for children who had been refractory to conditioning treatment and imipramine, using a randomized, double-blind, placebo-controlled crossover study. Of the 52 children studied (age range 5 to 13 years), 53% had a complete cessation of wetting, 19% were partial responders, and 28% had no or minimal response. The dosages used ranged from 20 to 40 μg (intranasal) and response did not persist after termination of treatment. In a 5-year retrospective review of 59 children, Key et al. (121) suggested that lower doses may be just as effective. In their series, 5 μg at bedtime was the initial starting dose, and 81% improved on less than 10 μg.

A study investigating the differential response of children with enuresis to DDAVP and the bell and pad method of conditioning found that 70% improved with the DDAVP and 86% improved with the alarm method, yielding no significant differences (122). A similar experiment that compared the therapeutic benefits of DDAVP in combination with the bell and pad to placebo found that the combination of DDAVP and the alarm resulted in significantly more dry nights (123). Leebeek-Groenewegen et al. (124) found that the combination of the alarm with DDAVP provided a more rapid response than monotherapy with the alarm, but the long-term success rates were comparable. However, Naitoh et al. (125) found that neither combination treatment with the alarm and imipramine nor the alarm and DDAVP were superior to the alarm alone. There have been reports of hyponatremia (126) and hyponatremic seizures (127–129) with intranasal use of DDAVP. A case report and literature review documented 14 cases in the English language literature with symptomatic hyponatremia involving seizures or mental status changes (130). A similar review noted that excess fluid intake was identified in 6 of 11 case reports, leading the authors to recommend that patients receiving DDAVP for nocturnal enuresis should not ingest more than 8 ounces of fluid on the nights when DDAVP is administered (131). The most comprehensive review of this subject identified a total of 93 instances of symptomatic hyponatremia in children treated with DDAVP (132). Younger children appeared to be more susceptible and the risk was greater at the beginning stages of treatment. This increasing literature, which included some fatalities, led the U.S. Food and Drug Administration (FDA) to warn clinicians that the intranasal form of DDAVP for the treatment of primary nocturnal enuresis should be discontinued. In addition, the warning indicated that the treatment with the oral form should be discontinued during acute illnesses that might disrupt the fluid/electrolyte balance.

The formulation of oral DDAVP has made it significantly easier and safer to administer (133,134). In an early open 6-week trial involving 33 children with primary nocturnal enuresis, 5 children responded to 200 μg/d and 17 to 400 μg/d, whereas 7 showed no response, and 4 dropped out. A multicenter, randomized study compared 200- and 400-μg doses of the oral preparation, as well as a 20-μg dose of the spray. No significant differences were found between any of the treatment conditions. However, there tended to be fewer wet nights when the children who initially received 200 μg of the oral preparation were increased to 400 μg (135). Similar positive results with oral DDAVP have been reported by Schulman et al. (136).

The dose response of oral DDAVP was explored in a randomized, placebo-controlled study that used 200-, 400-, and 600-μg daily doses. The 400- and 600-μg doses were significantly more effective than placebo, and there also was a significant linear trend for decreases in wet nights with increasing dosage (137).

An early oral DDAVP study with adolescents (138) has also provided long-term follow-up data (139). The initial study included two 12-week treatment periods with most of the patients receiving 400 μg/d. The initial studies showed that oral DDAVP was significantly more effective than placebo. The long-term, 7-year follow-up indicated that the "cure rate" at both the 2-year and 7-year follow-ups was greater than would be expected by data on the rate of spontaneous remission.

A large Canadian study found that long-term administration of oral DDAVP was safe and well tolerated (140). Consistent findings related to predictors of successful treatment are older age, larger bladder capacity, and fewer pretreatment numbers of wet nights (141–147).

Outcome and Follow-up

The natural history of primary enuresis must be taken into account in any treatment plan, whether it is primarily behavioral or pharmacologic. There is a high rate of spontaneous remission between the ages of 5 and 7 and again after the age of 12 years. Accordingly, the clinician might want to wait until after the age 7 of years before instituting pharmacologic treatment, unless other factors indicate otherwise. Similarly, the strong possibility of spontaneous remission should be considered in any positive treatment response after 10 or 11 years of age. In general, the rate of spontaneous remission from year to year is in the range of 14% to 16% (89,112). There has been one large follow-up study that compared observation, imipramine, DDAVP, and the alarm system. Patients were weaned from therapy after 6 months. Continence was assessed at the 3-, 6-, 9-, and 12-month points of the protocol, so that the 12-month assessment would be 6 months after treatment ceased. Among the observation group ($n = 50$), only 6% were continent at 6 months and 16% at 12 months. Of the imipramine group ($n = 44$), 36% were continent at 6 months while still on medication, but this decreased to 16% at the 12-month assessment. The corresponding figures for DDAVP ($n = 88$) were 68% continent at 6 months, but only 10% at 12 months. The alarm system showed the best long-term effects, with 63% continent at 6 months, and 56% at 12 months (148). A systematic review of the literature with regard to treatment with the alarm, imipramine, and DDAVP indicated that there is less risk of relapse with the alarm (149). The data with regard to treatment outcomes clearly indicate that behavioral interventions should constitute the first line of treatment, as they do not possess the side-effect potential of pharmacologic interventions (150). The bell and pad method of conditioning is the most thoroughly researched form of behavioral treatment. The relapse rate after termination of this treatment is also substantially less than that seen with either DDAVP or imipramine. For children who do not respond to the bell and pad, treatment with DDAVP is a reasonable alternative. Treatment with imipramine is now usually reserved for children who have been refractory to other interventions.

Following the introduction of DDAVP, there were significant cost differentials related to the different forms of treatment, as treatment with DDAVP was significantly more expensive than treatment with either the bell and pad or imipramine (151). However, DDAVP is now available in generic form, so the large cost differentials no longer exist.

Areas for Future Research

As indicated by the new research reviewed previously, there has been a dramatic increase in research into the etiology and treatment of enuresis. Much of this has been stimulated by the recognition that DDAVP is an effective treatment for the disorder. Despite this new research, a definitive explanation that would link DDAVP efficacy with the pathophysiology of the disorder has yet to be proven, and there is no consistently reliable way to differentiate DDAVP responders from nonresponders, either retrospectively or prospectively.

This and other findings related to bladder physiology and anatomy suggest that we might ultimately be able to differentiate distinct phenomenologic subgroups that relate to treatment outcome. Of particular interest in this regard are the studies involving changes in bladder capacity that result from treatment and correlate with outcome.

The longstanding observation that enuresis has a hereditary basis has been advanced by the elucidation of genetic linkages in some large, multigenerational pedigrees. This research will likely continue to advance and, when coupled with physiologic variables that predispose to enuresis, may ultimately provide important information on clinical subtypes. Thus, while it appears increasingly likely that a single etiology for all children with enuresis will not be identified, it may be possible to identify clinically relevant subtypes.

ENCOPRESIS

Definition

Encopresis is defined by DSM-5 (American Psychiatric Association, 2013) as the "repeated passage of feces into inappropriate places." There is a notation that the soiling is usually involuntary, but may be intentional in some cases. The manual goes on to note that the soiling must occur at least once a month for at least 3 months and that the mental or chronologic age of the child must be at least 4 years. Physical disorders must, of course, be ruled out. If there has been a period of fecal continence preceding the recurrence of soiling, it is classified as secondary encopresis.

The DSM-5 also denotes two subtypes of encopresis, which it labels as "with constipation and overflow incontinence" and "without constipation and overflow incontinence." The former category roughly corresponds to what has been referred to in the literature as retentive encopresis, whereas the latter corresponds to what has been known as nonretentive encopresis.

Prevalence and Epidemiology

A study involving 8,863 children found a prevalence of 1.5% among children between 7 and 8 years of age, with a male-to-female ratio of over 3:1 (152). In the Isle of Wight Study, Rutter and colleagues (2) found that 1.3% of boys between the ages of 10 and 12 years soiled at least once a month, with the corresponding figure for girls being 0.3%. That study also found a significant relationship between enuresis and encopresis (153). A more recent, large population-based study in the Netherlands investigated the prevalence in a sample of 13,111 5- to 6-year-old children, and 9,780 11- to 12-year-old children. The authors report a prevalence of 4.1% in the 5- to 6- year age group. The corresponding frequency for the older age (11 to 12 years) group was 1.6%. Of interest is the finding that 37.7%

of the younger age group children and 27.4% of the older age group had not been taken to a physician for evaluation (154). A large population-based questionnaire study reported episodes of fecal incontinence in 9.8% of first-graders, and 5.6% of fourth-graders (8). Of interest was a positive correlation between daytime urinary incontinence and fecal soiling.

Clinical Description

Encopresis has been classified in different ways. As noted, DSM-5 made a distinction between primary and secondary encopresis and has added subtypes that denote the distinction between retentive and nonretentive encopresis. Retentive encopresis is characterized by a cycle of several days of retention, a painful expulsion, and another period of retention. While the fecal mass is growing, there may be leakage around the mass. The category of nonretentive encopresis applies to those children who simply do not control the expulsion of feces on a psychological, physiologic, or combined basis.

Hersov (155) has proposed three categories: (a) children who have adequate bowel control and volitionally deposit feces in inappropriate places; (b) children who either are unaware that they are soiling or are aware but unable to control the process; and (c) situations where the soiling is due to excessive fluid, which may be caused by diarrhea, anxiety, or the retentive overflow process described previously. The last mechanism is responsible for approximately 75% of this category.

The importance of constipation to the development of retentive encopresis has led to the formulation of proposed criteria for functional fecal retention (FFR), which include a history greater than 12 weeks with passage of large diameter stools that are sufficiently large to obstruct the toilet, abdominal pain that is relieved by laxatives or enemas, and fecal soiling (156).

Etiology and Pathogenesis

There have been extensive investigations into the physiologic basis for encopresis. Loening-Baucke (157) found that 56% of children with retentive encopresis were unable to defecate rectal balloons, and most of these children had abnormal contractions of the external anal sphincter. This study also had prognostic significance in that only 14% of those who were unable to defecate the rectal balloons had responded to treatment after 1 year, whereas 64% of those who could defecate the balloons recovered after 1 year. Similarly, only 13% of patients who were unable to relax the anal sphincter at initial evaluation were improved 1 year later, whereas the corresponding figure for those who could relax the sphincter was 70%. Interestingly, none of the patients who presented with an abdominal fecal mass at the time of the initial evaluation showed improvement 1 year later, regardless of the ability to defecate the rectal balloons. Constipated children subsequently were compared with control subjects on a wide range of physiologic measures during the act of bearing down (158). These studies revealed that the act of bearing down led to decreased anal sphincter activity in 100% of control children, 58% of constipated children who were able to defecate a rectal balloon, and 7% of those constipated children who were unable to defecate the balloon. The latter group was significantly less likely to respond to conventional laxative treatment, and the authors concluded that the increased external sphincter activity could relate to their chronic fecal retention and encopresis. A companion study (159) investigated the social competence and behavioral profiles of 38 children with encopresis and correlated physiologic variables of anorectal manometric and electromyographic evaluations to treatment outcome. The study found that social competence and behavioral rating scores were not significantly different between those boys who were or were not able to defecate the balloons. The behavioral problem ratings also were similar in both physiologic subgroups of girls. The social competence score of the girls who could not defecate the balloons was lower than that of those who could. The follow-up data indicated that the behavioral and social competence scores did not correlate with successful outcome at 6-month and 1-year follow-ups, but there was a significant negative correlation between positive outcome in the inability to defecate the balloon and the inability to relax the sphincter. Thus, the physiologic variables were predictive of outcome, and the psychological variables were not. A subsequent study by the same group with a similar design continued to demonstrate some predictive value of the balloon test, in that children with functional constipation and encopresis who were able to defecate the balloon were twice as likely to have recovered at 12-month follow-up. However, the author concluded that even though these results were statistically significant, the calculation of predictive value indicated that the defecation test could not, in and of itself, reliably predict recovery (160).

A similar study at a different center concluded that a significant number of boys with encopresis have abnormalities of anorectal expulsion dynamics, but the researchers could not find abnormalities of anorectal sensory or motor function (161,162). They specifically investigated pudendal nerve terminal motor latency in 23 children with encopresis, compared with 23 control subjects, and could find no significant difference. However, anal electromyography did indicate nonrelaxation of the external anal sphincter in 75% of the encopretic children, as opposed to 13% of the control subjects, as well as lower pressures at rest and with squeezing. Complementary abnormalities of anal sphincter function have been reported by others (163,164).

Another approach has been to investigate potential involvement of hormones that affect gastrointestinal motility. Stern et al. (165) measured plasma levels of gastrin, pancreatic polypeptide, cholecystokinin, motilin, thyroxin, estrogen, and insulin at several intervals after the administration of a standardized meal to 10 children with encopresis and the same number of matched control subjects. The authors reported significant differences for postprandial levels of pancreatic polypeptide, which peaked earlier and remained higher in children with encopresis, as well as a lower motilin response. However, the authors could not entirely rule out that their findings were not the result of chronic constipation, rather than the cause (165).

Environmental factors have been noted for some time and include the observations of Freud and Burlingham (166), who noted a high frequency of soiling and wetting in children separated from their parents during World War II.

At least three studies that revealed no correlation between social class and soiling (153,167,168) specifically looked at associated psychopathology in boys with primary encopresis, compared with those with secondary encopresis. They found that the children with primary encopresis were more likely to have experienced developmental delays and to have associated enuresis, whereas those with secondary encopresis had experienced more psychosocial stressors and had higher rates of associated conduct disorder. A study involving 86 children with encopresis and 62 control children found that children with encopresis had more symptoms of anxiety and depression, more attentional difficulties, more disruptive behavior, and poorer school performance. However, the differences only reached significant levels for a minority of the children with encopresis (169). Mellon et al. (170) have reported higher rates of fecal soiling in children who have been sexually abused.

Klages et al. (171) reported higher rates of both enuresis and encopresis in children with a prepubertal and early adolescent bipolar disorder phenotype as compared to controls. An investigation utilizing the Child Behavior Checklist identified significantly more behavioral difficulties in children with functional nonretentive fecal soiling when compared to a Dutch normative sample. Von Gontard and Hollmann (172) have reported elevated Child Behavior Checklist scores and comorbid psychiatric disorders in children who present with both enuresis and encopresis. Large epidemiologic studies have suggested higher rates of psychological disturbance in children with encopresis (173,174).

Laboratory Studies

The physiologic studies described previously must be considered research investigations and not the representation of a usual and customary workup. However, they do suggest that a more detailed physiologic investigation than usually is done may be warranted. Usually, once the more obvious physiologic problems, such as Hirschsprung disease, are ruled out, the problem is considered to be psychogenic.

The plain abdominal x-ray reveals evidence of fecal retention. In general, a positive rectal examination is sufficient to determine fecal retention, but a negative rectal examination does not rule it out, and in those cases, the abdominal x-ray can be helpful in establishing the diagnosis (175).

One of the most important investigations may well be a thorough history that documents the frequency, nature, and circumstances of the soiling events in great detail. This history should be elicited both from the parents and from the child.

Psychological testing and evaluation are important in providing a thorough picture of the child, but it remains difficult to know if concomitant psychological problems are associated, causal, or secondary.

Differential Diagnosis

The differential diagnosis of encopresis must take into account that the soiling can be either a symptom of another problem or the primary problem itself. For example, historically, encopresis and enuresis have been reported to occur under stress in normal children and to remit when the stressor is removed. Similarly, in children who have significant developmental delays, the encopresis may be only one expression of the primary problem. Children who are impulsive and hyperactive may have occasional episodes of encopresis simply because they do not attend to the stimuli until it is too late. Thus, the symptom of encopresis must be viewed in the context of the child's larger psychological and environmental profile. Strictly medical causes, such as Hirschsprung disease, stenosis of the rectum or anus, smooth muscle disease, and endocrine abnormalities, also should be ruled out.

Treatment

The most widely accepted first line of treatment is one that encompasses educational, psychological, and behavioral approaches. As outlined by Levine (176), this approach entails an initial meeting that is designed to educate both the parents and child about bowel function and to diffuse the psychological tension that may have developed in the family around the encopresis. This educational and psychological intervention is then followed by an initial bowel catharsis, after which the child receives daily doses of laxatives or mineral oil. There also is a behavioral component to the treatment, which consists of daily timed intervals on the toilet with rewards for success. A 78% success rate has been reported for this approach, without symptom substitution (177–179). The addition of a behavior management component to the intensive medical treatment provides some additional benefit (Table 5.12.2).

TABLE 5.12.2

FACTORS TO CONSIDER WHEN CONSTRUCTING A TREATMENT ALGORITHM FOR ENCOPRESIS

- Subtypes of encopresis
  - Retentive (most common)
  - Nonretentive
  - Volitional (least frequent)
- A thorough history is essential that documents frequency, nature, and circumstances of event
- First line of treatment for retentive subtype usually includes:
  - Education about bowel functioning with both parents and child
  - Physiologic treatment with laxatives or mineral oil
- Behavioral component with time intervals on toilet and positive reinforcement
- Extensive research into biofeedback
  - Not proven to be more effective than traditional interventions
  - May be a consideration in refractory cases
- Case reports of imipramine in the treatment of nonretentive encopresis
- Psychodynamic assessment for those with volitional encopresis

Stark et al. (180) have replicated earlier work reporting the efficacy of group treatment with an educational and behavioral focus in conjunction with medical management for children who had not responded to medical management alone.

The adjunctive use of oral laxatives and conditional rectal cathartics also has been investigated (181). Specifically, the authors compared the results obtained with children who were all treated with a high-fiber diet, initial bowel evacuation, behavior modification program, and random assignment to either oral laxatives ($n = 24$) or conditioning rectal cathartics ($n = 37$). Only 61 of 136 patients evaluated completed treatment, and thus there was a high dropout rate. No significant outcome difference was found between the two groups, and 87% continued in remission at 6- to 12-month follow-up. Nolan et al. (182) used a random allocation design to compare combined treatment with laxatives and behavior modification ($n = 83$) to behavior modification alone ($n = 86$). At 12-month follow-up, 51% of the combined therapy group had at least one 4-week period without an encopretic episode, compared with 36% of the behavior modification group. After the authors excluded children with poor compliance, there was no statistical difference between groups, although the authors maintained that from a clinical perspective, the use of laxatives combined with behavior modification was superior to behavior modification alone. Laxative therapy is an important component of treatment for children who have encopresis related to chronic constipation. A number of studies have reported success with polyethylene glycol (PEG) 3350 for this group (183–186).

Loening-Baucke (187) has expanded on the pathophysiologic studies described earlier by exploring the utility of biofeedback training in children with abnormal defecation dynamics. Specifically, patients (ages 5 to 16 years) were randomly assigned to traditional medical treatment alone ($n = 19$) or conventional treatment plus up to six biofeedback sessions. Eighty-six percent of the biofeedback group had learned normal defecation dynamics at the conclusion of biofeedback treatment. At 7-month follow-up, 77% of the biofeedback group had normal defecation dynamics, as opposed to only 13% of the conventionally treated. The improvement in defecation dynamics was correlated with clinical improvement at 12 months (16% with conventional treatment and 50% with biofeedback). Similar successful results were reported in a European study (188).

A longer follow-up study (4.1 ± 1.5 years) compared the long-term outcome in 129 children with constipation and encopresis, as well as abnormal defecation dynamics, who were treated with conventional treatment, with 63 children who received additional biofeedback training that was directed toward normalizing the defecation dynamics. The results indicated that both groups showed similar rates of improvement (86% of the conventionally treated and 87% of the biofeedback group). At long-term follow-up, complete recovery was documented in 62% of the conventionally treated, 50% of those who had achieved success with the biofeedback treatment, and 23% of those who had not responded to biofeedback treatment. The length of time at follow-up was significantly related to recovery for the group as a whole, suggesting that the natural history of the disorder is to move toward continence. The author concluded that biofeedback treatment cannot be demonstrated to be statistically superior to conventional treatment (189).

A subsequent study by another group with a somewhat similar design reached the same conclusion (190), and two large literature reviews also failed to demonstrate any benefit from biofeedback as compared to the standard medical treatment (191,192). However, research into biofeedback treatment continues using a newly developed portable apparatus (193), and as an adjunctive treatment in combination with other behavioral strategies and laxative therapy (194,195), have reported a significant decrease in soiling frequency and laxative use in a group of 36 patients treated with biofeedback who had a history of constipation and encopresis, and who had not responded to 6 months of conventional treatment.

Pharmacologic treatment with imipramine also has been reported as useful for encopresis. There have been 15 reported cases of children with encopresis responding to imipramine, which have been described in six papers (196–201). All but three of the reported subjects are male. In general, the therapeutic effect occurred within a few days to 2 weeks. The doses of imipramine reported are relatively low, in the 25- to 75-mg range. There also is a similar positive case report involving amitriptyline treatment of a 6 year old (202). There is one double-blind study demonstrating the effectiveness of the prokinetic agent cisapride (Propulside) for encopresis related to constipation (203). However, this agent has been removed from the market in the United States by the FDA, due to serious side effects.

Outcome and Follow-up Data

The 78% success rate described by Levine suggests that most children will respond to a relatively innocuous approach that involves educational, behavioral, and physiologic components, as do the follow-up data of Loening-Baucke (189). In general, the longer-term follow-up studies consistently indicate that the passage of time is an important contributor to remission of the disorder (189,204). The epidemiologic data also indicate that the effects of maturation will provide a significant number of spontaneous remissions from year to year. The evaluation of any long-term intervention such as psychotherapy should take this factor into account. All but a few children will have either responded to treatment or spontaneously remitted by age 16 years, and persistence beyond that age is quite unusual (205).

Areas for Future Research

This review suggests that encopresis is an excellent paradigm for assessing the relative impacts of biologic, psychological, and social factors. For example, do the physiologic findings described previously represent a constitutional vulnerability, or are they the result of the effects of chronic constipation on the bowel? The symptom of encopresis in its various presentations can be a fruitful area of research for those interested in elucidating the interrelation of mind, body, and culture in children.

APPENDIX: ANTIENURETIC AGENTS

Desmopressin, Oxybutynin, and Tolterodine

Table 5.12.3 depicts the pharmacologic characteristics of medications used for enuresis. Desmopressin (DDAVP) is a synthetic antidiuretic hormone (ADH), a powerful inhibitor of the production of urine. It can be administered orally or via intranasal spray. One review suggested that desmopressin helps approximately 25% of children who use it, with minimal risk of adverse effects. Although desmopressin is usually well tolerated, the beneficial effects often do not endure over time. The most effective treatment for enuresis is the use of behavioral interventions, such as a "pad and buzzer" or a "moisture alarm." However, DDAVP can be a useful short-term adjunct, as in the facilitation of sleepovers or overnight camp stays. For longer-term pharmacologic management of enuresis, usually in cases unresponsive or only partially responsive to behavioral interventions, antimuscarinic agents can occasionally be useful. Alternatives to the time-tested use of low (25 to 50 mg hs) or regular dose imipramine include oxybutynin (Ditropan) or the less sedating tolterodine (Detrol). As is the case of other pharmacologic interventions for enuresis, beneficial effects usually disappear rapidly upon drug discontinuation (Table 5.12.3).

TABLE 5.12.3

CLINICAL GUIDANCE ON ANTIENURETIC AGENTS USED IN PEDIATRIC PRACTICE

Drug	Mechanism of Action	Main Indications and Clinical Uses	Dosage (mg/day)	Schedule	Adverse Effects
Desmopressin[a]	Antidiuretic hormone analog	Enuresis	0.1–0.6	qhs/bid	Headache Nausea Hyponatremia and water intoxication at toxic doses
Oxybutynin	Antimuscarinic agents		5.0–15	bid/tid	Anticholinergic side effects
Tolterodine			1–2	bid	Less anticholinergic effects, less sedation

[a]Can be useful for acute situations (e.g., sleepaways).

ACKNOWLEDGMENT

The author wishes to thank Ms. Patsy Kuropatkin for her invaluable assistance in the preparation of this manuscript.

References

1. Glicklich LB: A historical account of enuresis. *Pediatrics* 8:859–876, 1951.
2. Rutter M: Isle of Wight revisited: twenty-five years of child psychiatric epidemiology. *J Am Acad Child Adolesc Psychiatry* 28:633–653, 1989.
3. Rutter ML, Yule W, Graham PJ: Enuresis and behavioural deviance: some epidemiological considerations. *Clin Dev Med* 48(49):137–147, 1973.
4. Jarvelin MR, Vikevainen-Tervonen L, Moilanen I, Huttunen NP: Enuresis in seven-year-old children. *Acta Paediatr Scand* 77:148–153, 1988.
5. Fergusson DM, Horwood LJ, Shannon FT: Factors related to the age of attainment of nocturnal bladder control: an 8-year longitudinal study. *Pediatrics* 78:884–890, 1986.
6. Wille S: Primary nocturnal enuresis in children: background and treatment. *Scand J Urol Nephrol* 156:1–48, 1994c.
7. Bower WF, Moore KH, Shepherd RB, Adams RD: The epidemiology of childhood enuresis in Australia. *Br J Urol* 78:602–606, 1996.
8. Söderstrom U, Hoelcke M, Alenius L, Söderling AC, Hjern A: Urinary and faecal incontinence: a population-based study. *Acta Paediatr* 93(3):386–389, 2004.
9. Wille S: Functional bladder capacity and calcium-creatinine quota in enuretic patients, former enuretic and non-enuretic controls. *Scand J Urol Nephrol* 28:353–357, 1994a.
10. Kirk J, Rasmussen PV, Rittig S, Djurhuus JC: Provoked enuresis-like episodes in healthy children 7 to 12 years old. *J Urol* 156:210–213, 1996.
11. Rasmussen PV, Kirk J, Rittig S, Djurhuus JC: The enuretic episode: a complete micturition from a bladder with normal capacity? A critical reappraisal of the definition. *Scand J Urol Nephrol* 183:23–24, 1997.
12. Essen J, Peckham C. Nocturnal enuresis in childhood. *Dev Med Child Neurol* 18:577–589, 1976.
13. Touchette E, Petit D, Paquet J, Tremblay RE, Boivin M, Montplaisir JY: Bed-wetting and its association with developmental milestones in early childhood. *Arch Pediatr Adolesc Med* 159(12):1129–1134, 2005.
14. Iscan A, Ozkul Y, Unal D, et al: Abnormalities in event-related potential and brainstem auditory evoked response in children with nocturnal enuresis. *Brain Dev* 24(7):681–687, 2002.
15. Hansson S: Urinary incontinence in children and associated problems. *Scand J Urol Nephrol* 141:47–55, 1992.
16. Hjalmas K: Functional daytime incontinence: definitions and epidemiology. *Scand J Urol Nephrol* 141:39–44, 1992.
17. Mahony DT: Studies of enuresis: I. The incidence of obstructive lesions and pathophysiology of enuresis. *J Urol* 106:951–958, 1971.
18. Smith DR: Critique on the concept of vesical neck obstruction in children. *JAMA* 207:1686–1692, 1969.
19. Shaffer D: Enuresis. In: Rutter M, Hersov L (eds): *Child and Adolescent Psychiatry: Modern Approaches,* 2nd ed. London, Blackwell Scientific, 465–481, 1985.
20. McDermott VG, Merrick MV: Isotope renography in childhood enuresis. *Clin Radiol* 49:705–707, 1994.
21. Kawauchi A, Kitamori T, Imada N, Tanaka Y, Watanabe H. Urological abnormalities in 1,328 patients with nocturnal enuresis. *Eur Urol* 29:231–234, 1996a.
22. Yeung CK, Sreedhar B, Leung VT, Metreweli C: Ultrasound bladder measurements in patients with primary nocturnal enuresis: a urodynamic and treatment outcome correlation. *J Urol* 171(6 Pt 2):2589–2594, 2004.
23. Achenbach TM, Lewis M: A proposed model for clinical research and its application to encopresis and enuresis. *J Am Acad Child Psychiatry* 10:535–554, 1971.
24. Mikkelsen EJ, Rapoport JL, Nee L, Gruenau C, Mendelson W, Gillin JC: Childhood enuresis: I. Sleep patterns and psychopathology. *Arch Gen Psychiatry* 37:1139–1144, 1980.
25. Mikkelsen EJ, Rapoport JL: Enuresis: psychopathology, sleep stage, and drug response. *Urol Clin North Am* 7:361–377, 1980.
26. Biederman J, Santangelo SL, Faraone SV: Clinical correlates of enuresis in ADHD and non-ADHD children. *J Child Psychol Psychiatry* 36:865–877, 1995.
27. Baeyens D, Roeyers H, Hoebeke P, Verté S, Van Hoecke E, Walle JV: Attention deficit/hyperactivity disorder in children with nocturnal enuresis. *J Urol* 171(6 Pt 2):2576–2579, 2004.
28. Baeyens D, Roeyers H, Demeyere I, Verté S, Hoebeke P, Vande Walle J: Attention-deficit/hyperactivity disorder (ADHD) as a risk factor for persistent nocturnal enuresis in children: a two-year follow up study. *Acta Paediatr* 94(11):1619–1625, 2005.
29. Feehan M, McGee R, Stanton W, Silva PA: A six-year follow-up of childhood enuresis: prevalence in adolescence and consequences for mental health. *J Paediatr Child Health* 26(2):75–79, 1990.
30. von Gontard A, Mauer-Mucke K, Pluck J, Berner W, Lehmkuhl G: Clinical behavioral problems in day- and night-wetting children. *Pediatr Nephrol* 13:662–667, 1999b.
31. Fergusson DM, Horwood LJ: Nocturnal enuresis and behavioral problems in adolescence: a 15-year longitudinal study. *Pediatrics* 95:662–668, 1994.
32. Fergusson DM, Horwood LJ, Shannon FT: Secondary enuresis in a birth cohort of New Zealand children. *Paediatr Perinat Epidemiol* 4:53–63, 1990.
33. von Gontard A, Hollmann E, Eiberg H, Benden B, Rittig S, Lehmkuhl G: Clinical enuresis phenotypes in familial nocturnal enuresis. *Scand J Urol Nephrol* 183:11–16, 1997.
34. Hirasing RA, Van Leerdam FJ, Bolk-Bennink LB, Bosch JD: Bedwetting and behavioural and/or emotional problems. *Acta Paediatr* 86:1131–1134, 1997.
35. Van Hoeck E, Baeyens D, Vande Walle J, Hoebeke P, Roeyers H: Socioeconomic status as a common factor underlying the association between enuresis and psychopathology. *J Dev Behav Pediatr* 24(2):109–114, 2003.
36. Pierce CM, Whitman RM, Mass JW, Gay ML: Enuresis and dreaming: experimental studies. *Arch Gen Psychiatry* 166–170, 1961.
37. Broughton RF: Sleep disorders: disorders of arousal? *Science* 159:1070–1078, 1968.
38. Gastaut H, Broughton R: A clinical and polygraphic study of episodic phenomena during sleep. In: Wortis J (ed): *Recent Advances in Biological Psychiatry.* New York, Plenum, 196–221, 1964.
39. Ritvo ER, Ornitz EM, Gottlieb F, et al.: Arousal and nonarousal enuretic events. *Am J Psychiatry* 126(1):77–84, 1969.
40. Kales A, Kales JD, Jacobson A, Humphrey FJ 2nd, Soldatos CR: Effects of imipramine on enuretic frequency and sleep stages. *Pediatrics* 1977;60:431–436.
41. Robert M, Averous M, Besset A, et al.: Sleep polygraphic studies using cystomanometry in twenty patients with enuresis. *Eur Urol* 24(1) 97–102, 1993.
42. Neveus T, Hetta J, Cnattingius S, et al.: Depth of sleep and sleep habits among enuretic and incontinent children and incontinent children. *Acta Paediatr* 88(7):748–752, 1999a.
43. Wolfish N: Sleep arousal function in enuretic males. *Scand J Urol Nephrol* 202:24–26, 1999.
44. Norgaard JP, Hansen JH, Wildschiotz G, Sørensen S, Rittig S, Djurhuus JC: Sleep cystometries in children with nocturnal enuresis. *J Urol* 141:1156–1159, 1989.
45. Imada N, Kawauchi A, Tanaka Y, Yamao Y, Watanabe H, Takeuchi Y: Classification based on overnight simultaneous monitoring by electroencephalography and cystometry. *Eur Urol* 33(3):45–48, 1998.
46. Watanabe H, Kawauchi A, Kitamori T, Azuma Y: Treatment system for nocturnal enuresis according to an original classification system. *Eur Urol* 25:43–50, 1994.
47. Miller K, Atkin B, Moody ML: Drug therapy for nocturnal enuresis: current treatment recommendations. *Drugs* 44:47–56, 1992.
48. Rittig S, Knudsen UB, Norgaard JP, Gregersen H, Pedersen EB, Djurhuus JC: Diurnal variation of plasma atrial natriuretic peptide in normals and patients with enuresis nocturna. *Scand J Clin Lab Invest* 51:209–217, 1991.
49. Natochin YV, Kuznetsova AA: Defect of osmoregulatory renal function in nocturnal enuresis. *Scand J Urol Nephrol* 202:40–43, 1999.
50. Vurgun N, Gumus BH, Ece A, Ari Z, Tarhan S, Yeter M: Renal functions of enuretic and nonenuretic children: hypernatriuria and kaliuresis as causes of nocturnal enuresis. *Eur Urol* 32:85–90, 1997.
51. Steffens J, Netzer M, Isenberg E, Alloussi S, Ziegler M: Vasopressin deficiency in primary nocturnal enuresis: results of a controlled prospective study. *Eur Urol* 24:366–370, 1993.
52. Medel R, Dieguez S, Brindo M, et al.: Monosymptomatic primary enuresis: differences between patients responding or not responding to oral desmopressin. *Br J Urol* 3:46–49, 1998.
53. Wood CM, Butler RJ, Penny MD, Holland PC: Pulsatile release of arginine vasopressin (AVP) and its effect on response to desmopressin in enuresis. *Scand J Urol Nephrol* 163:93–101, 1994.
54. Lackgren G, Neveus T, Stenberg A: Diurnal plasma vasopressin and urinary output in adolescents with monosymptomatic nocturnal enuresis. *Acta Paediatr* 86:385–390, 1997.
55. Aikawa T, Kashara T, Uchiyama M: The arginine-vasopressin secretion profile of children with primary nocturnal enuresis. *Eur Urol* 33(3):41–44, 1998.
56. Aikawa T, Kashara T, Uchiyama M: Circadian variation of plasma arginine vasopressin concentration, or arginine vasopressin in enuresis. *Scand J Urol Nephrol* 202:47–49, 1999.
57. Eggert P, Muller-Schluter K, Muller D: Regulation of arginine vasopressin in enuretic children under fluid restriction. *Pediatrics* 103:452–455, 1999.
58. Hunsballe JM, Rittig S, Pedersen EB, Djurhuus JC: Fluid deprivation in enuresis: effect on urine output and plasma arginine vasopressin. *Scand J Urol Nephrol* 1999;202:50–51.
59. Hunsballe JM, Hansen TK, Rittig S, Pedersen EB, Djurhuus JC: The efficacy of DDAVP is related to the circadian rhythm of urine output in patients with persisting nocturnal enuresis. *Clin Endocrinol* 49:793–801, 1998.

60. Robertson G, Rittig S, Kovacs L, Gaskill MB, Zee P, Nanninga J: Pathophysiology and treatment of enuresis in adults. *Scand J Urol Nephrol* 202:36–38, 1999.
61. Eggert P, Kuhn B: Antidiuretic hormone regulation in patients with primary nocturnal enuresis. *Arch Dis Child* 73:508–511, 1995.
62. Hogg RJ, Husmann D: The role of family history in predicting response to desmopressin in nocturnal enuresis. *J Urol* 150:444–445, 1993.
63. Arnell H, Hjalmas K, Jagervall M, et al.: The genetics of primary nocturnal enuresis: inheritance and suggestion of a second major gene on chromosome 12q. *J Med Genet* 34:360–365, 1997.
64. Eiberg H, Berendt I, Mohr J: Assignment of dominant inherited nocturnal enuresis (ENUR1) to chromosome 13q. *Nat Genet* 10:354–356, 1995.
65. von Gontard A, Eiberg H, Hollmann E, Rittig S, Lehmkuhl G: Molecular genetics of nocturnal enuresis: linkage to a locus on chromosome 22. *Scand J Urol Nephrol* 202:76–80, 1999a.
66. von Gontard A, Schaumburg H, Hollmann E, Eiberg H, Rittig S: The genetics of enuresis: a review. *J Urol* 166(6):2438–2443, 2001.
67. Loeys B, Hoebeke P, Raes A, Messiaen L, De Paepe A, Vande Walle J: Does monosymptomatic enuresis exist? A molecular genetic exploration of 32 families with enuresis/incontinence. *BJU Int* 90(1):76–83, 2002.
68. Eiberg H, Shaumburg HL, von Gontard A, Rittig S: Linkage study of a large Danish four-generation family with urge incontinence and nocturnal enuresis. *J Urol* 166(6):2401–2403, 2001.
69. Cohen M: Enuresis. *Pediatr Clin North Am* 22:545–560, 1975.
70. Jarvelin MR, Huttunen NP, Seppanen J, Seppänen U, Moilanen I: Screening of urinary tract abnormalities among day and nightwetting children. *Scand J Urol Nephrol* 24:181–189, 1990.
71. Stoffer SS: Loss of bladder control in hyperthyroidism. *Postgrad Med* 84:117–118, 1988.
72. O'Regan S, Yazbeck S, Hamberger B, Schick E: Constipation a commonly unrecognized cause of enuresis. *Am J Dis Child* 140(3):260–261, 2010.
73. Kikuchi K, Fujisawa I, Ohie T, et al.: Ectopic posterior lobe of the pituitary gland and intractable nocturnal enuresis in a case with pituitary dwarfism. *Acta Paediatr Scand* 78(3):479–481, 1989.
74. Brooks LJ, Topol HI: Enuresis in children with sleep apnea. *J Pediatr* 142(5):515–518, 2003.
75. Monji A, Yanagimoto K, Yoshida I, et al.: SSRI-induced enuresis: a case report. *J Clin Psychopharmacol* 24(5):564–565, 2004.
76. Kandil ST, Aksu HB, Ozyavuz R: Reversible nocturnal enuresis in children receiving SSRI with or without risperidone: presentation of five cases. *Isr J Psychiatry Relat Sci* 41(3):218–221, 2004.
77. Ramadan MI, Khan AY, Weston WE: Response to SSRI-induced enuresis: a case report. *J Clin Psychopharmacology* 26(1):99–100, 2006.
78. Hergüner S, Kilingaslan A, Gürker I, Tüzün U: Serotonin-selective reuptake inhibitor-induced enuresis in three pediatric cases. *J Child Adolesc Psychopharmacol* 17(3):367, 2007.
79. Hergüner S, Mukaddes NM: Risperidone-induced enuresis in two children with autistic disorder. *J Child Adolesc Psychopharmacol* 17(4):527, 2007.
80. Fritz G, Rockney R, Bernet W, et al.: Practice parameter for the assessment and treatment of children and adolescents with enuresis. *J Am Acad Child Adolesc Psychiatry* 1540–1550, 2004.
81. Hagglof B, Andren O, Bergstrom E, Marklund L, Wendelius M: Self-esteem in children with nocturnal enuresis and urinary incontinence: improvement of self-esteem after treatment. *Eur Urol* 33(3):16–19, 1998.
82. Moffatt ME, Kato C, Pless IB: Improvements in self-concept after treatment of nocturnal enuresis: randomized controlled trial. *J Pediatr* 110:647–652, 1987.
83. Collier J, Butler RJ, Redsell SA, Evans JH: An investigation of the impact of nocturnal enuresis on children's self-concept. *Scand J Urol Nephrol* 36(3):204–208, 2002.
84. Rappaport L: Prognostic factors for alarm treatment. *Scand J Urol Nephrol* 183:55–57, 1997.
85. Werry J: The conditioning treatment of enuresis. *Am J Psychiatry* 123:226–229, 1996.
86. Devlin JB, O'Cathain C: Predicting treatment outcome in nocturnal enuresis. *Arch Dis Child* 65:1158–1161, 1990.
87. Glazener CM, Evans JH, Peto RE: Alarm interventions for nocturnal enuresis in children. *Cochrane Database Syst Rev* (2):CD002911, 2003. Update in *Cochrane Database Syst Rev* (2):CD002911, 2005.
88. Butler RJ, Gasson SL: Enuresis alarm treatment. *Scand J Urol Nephrol* 39(5):349–357, 2005.
89. Bonde HV, Andersen JP, Rosenkilde P: Nocturnal enuresis: change of nocturnal voiding pattern during alarm treatment. *Scand J Urol Nephrol* 28:349–352, 1994.
90. Butler RJ, Robinson JC: Alarm treatment for childhood nocturnal enuresis: an investigation of within-treatment variables. *Scand J Urol Nephrol* 36(4):268–272, 2002.
91. Jensen N, Kristensen G: Frequency of nightly wetting and the efficiency of alarm treatment of nocturnal enuresis. *Scand J Urol Nephrol* 35(5):357–363, 2001.
92. Butler RJ, Holland P, Basson S, Norfolk S, Houghton L: Exploring potential mechanisms in alarm treatment for primary nocturnal enuresis. *Scand J Urol Nephrol* 41(5):407, 2007.
93. Oredsson AF, Jorgensen TM: Changes in nocturnal bladder capacity during treatment with the bell and pad for normosymptomatic nocturnal enuresis. *J Urol* 160:166–169, 1998.
94. Hvistendahl GM, Kamperis K, Rawashdeh YF, Rittig S, Djurhuus JC: The effect of alarm treatment on the functional bladder capacity in children with monosymptomatic nocturnal enuresis. *J Urol* 171(6 Pt 2): 2611–2614, 2004.
95. Taneli C, Ertan P, Taneli F, et al.: Effect of alarm treatment on bladder storage capacities in monosymptomatic nocturnal enuresis. *Scand J Urol Nephrol* 38(3):207–210, 2004.
96. Van Leerdam FJ, Blankespoor MN, van der Heijden AJ, et al.: Alarm treatment is successful in children with day- and night-time wetting. *Scand J Urol Nephrol* 38(3):211–215, 2004. Erratum in: *Scand J Urol Nephrol* 38(4):350. Hiraing, RA [corrected to Hirasing, Remy A].
97. El-Anany FG, Maghraby HA, Shaker SE, Abdel-Moneim AM: Primary nocturnal enuresis: a new approach to conditioning treatment. *Urology* 53:405–408, 1999.
98. Petrican P, Sawan MA: Design of a miniaturized ultrasonic bladder volume monitor and subsequent preliminary evaluation on 41 enuretic patients. *IEEE Trans Rehabil Eng* 6:66–74, 1998.
99. Pretlow RA: Treatment of nocturnal enuresis with an ultrasound bladder volume controlled alarm device. *J Urol* 162:1224–1228, 1999.
100. Hoekx L, Wyndaele JJ, Vermandel A: The role of bladder biofeedback in the treatment of children with refractory nocturnal enuresis associated with idiopathic detrusor. *J Urol* 160:858–860, 1998.
101. Hoekx L, Vermandel A, Wyndaele JJ: Functional bladder capacity after bladder biofeedback predicts long-term outcome in children with nocturnal enuresis. *Scand J Urol Nephrol* 37(2):120–123, 2003.
102. Bradbury M: Combination therapy for nocturnal enuresis with desmopressin and an alarm device. *Scand J Urol Nephrol* 183:61–63, 1997.
103. Bradbury MG, Meadow SR: Combined treatment with enuresis alarm and esmopressin for nocturnal enuresis. *Acta Paediatr* 84:1014–1018, 1995.
104. Glazener CM, Evans JH: Simple behavioural and physical interventions for nocturnal enuresis in children. *Cochrane Database Syst Rev* (2):CD003637, 2004.
105. Glazener CM, Evans JH, Peto RE: Complex behavioural and educational interventions for nocturnal enuresis in children. *Cochrane Database Sys Rev* (1):CD004668, 2004.
106. Bennett HJ: *Waking Up Dry: A Guide to Help Children Overcome Bedwetting*. Vol. 241. Illinois, IL, American Academy of Pediatrics, 2005.
107. MacLean RE: Imipramine hydrochloride (Tofranil) and enuresis. *Am J Psychiatry* 117:551, 1960.
108. Devane CL, Walker RD 3rd, Sawyer WP, Wilson JA: Concentrations of imipramine and its metabolites during enuresis therapy. *Pediatr Pharmacol* 4:245–251, 1984.
109. de Gatta MF, Garcia MJ, Acosta A, Rey F, Gutierrez JR, Dominguez-Gil A: Monitoring of serum levels of imipramine and desipramine and individualization of dose in enuretic children. *Ther Drug Monit* 1984;6:438–443.
110. Fernandez de Gatta MM, Galindo P, Rey F, et al.: The influence of clinical and pharmacological factors on enuresis treatment with imipramine. *Br J Clin Pharmacol* 30:693–698, 1990.
111. Jorgensen OS, Lober M, Christiansen J, Gram LF: Plasma concentration and clinical effect in imipramine treatment of childhood enuresis. *Clin Pharmacokinet* 5:386–393, 1980.
112. Rapoport JL, Mikkelsen EJ, Zavadil A, et al.: Childhood enuresis: II. Psychopathology, tricyclic concentration in plasma, and antienuretic effect. *Arch Gen Psychiatry* 37:1146–1152, 1980.
113. Fritz GK, Rockney RM, Yeung AS: Plasma levels and efficacy of imipramine treatment for enuresis. *J Am Acad Child Adolesc Psychiatry* 33:60–64, 1994.
114. Gepertz S, Neveus T: Imipramine for therapy resistant enuresis: a retrospective evaluation. *J Urol* 171(6 Pt 2):2607–2610, 2004.
115. Devlin JB: Prevalence and risk factors for childhood nocturnal enuresis. *Ir Med J* 84:118–120, 1991.
116. Foxman B, Valdez RB, Brook RH: Childhood enuresis: prevalence, perceived impact, and prescribed treatments. *Pediatrics* 77:482–487, 1986.
117. Vogel W, Young M, Primack W: A survey of physician use of treatment methods for functional enuresis. *J Dev Behav Pediatr* 17:90–93, 1996.
118. Boulis AK, Long J: Variation in the treatment of children by primary care physician specialty. *Arch Pediatr Adolesc Med* 156(12):1210–1215, 2002.
119. Moffatt ME, Harlos S, Kirshen AJ, Burd L: Desmopressin acetate and nocturnal enuresis: how much do we know? *Pediatrics* 92:420–425, 1993.
120. Terho P: Desmopressin in nocturnal enuresis. *J Urol* 145:818–820, 1991.
121. Key DW, Bloom DA, Sanvordenker J: Low-dose DDAVP in nocturnal enuresis. *Clin Pediatr* 31:299–301, 1992.
122. Wille S: Comparison of desmopressin and enuresis alarm for nocturnal enuresis. *Arch Dis Child* 61:30–33, 1986.
123. Sukhai RN, Mol J, Harris AS: Combined therapy of enuresis alarm and desmopressin in the treatment of nocturnal enuresis. *Eur J Paediatr* 148:465–467, 1989.
124. Leebeek-Groenewegen A, Blom J, Sukhai R, Van Der Heijden B: Efficacy of desmopressin combined with alarm therapy for monosymptomatic nocturnal enuresis. *J Urol* 166(6):2456–2458, 2001.

125. Naitoh Y, Kawauchi A, Yamao Y, et al.: Combination therapy with alarm and drugs for monosymptomatic nocturnal enuresis not superior to alarm monotherapy. *Urology* 66(3):632–635, 2005.
126. Kallio J, Rautava P, Huupponen R, Korvenranta H: Severe hyponatremia caused by intranasal desmopressin for nocturnal enuresis. *Acta Paediatr* 82:881–882, 1993.
127. Beach PS, Beach RE, Smith LR: Hyponatremic seizures in a child treated with desmopressin to control enuresis: a rational approach to fluid intake. *Clin Pediatr* 31:566–569, 1992.
128. Schwab M, Wenzel D, Ruder H: Hyponatraemia and cerebral convulsion due to short-term DDAVP therapy for control of enuresis nocturna. *Eur J Pediatr* 155:46–48, 1996.
129. Yaouyanc G, Jonville AP, Yaouyanc-Lapalle H: Seizure with hyponatremia in a child prescribed desmopressin for nocturnal enuresis. *J Toxicol* 30:637–641, 1992.
130. Bernstein SA, Williford SL: Intranasal desmopressin-associated hyponatremia: a case report and literature review. *J Fam Pract* 44:203–208, 1997.
131. Robson WL, Norgaard JP, Leung AK: Hyponatremia in patients with nocturnal enuresis treated with DDAVP. *Eur J Pediatr* 155:959–962,1996.
132. Thumfart J, Roehr CC, Kapelari K, Querfeld U, Eggert P, Müller D: Desmopressin associated symptomatic hyponatremic hypervolemia in children. Are there predictive factors? *J Urol* 174(1):294–298, 2005.
133. Lottmann H, Froeling F, Alloussi S, et al.: A randomized comparison of oral desmopressin in lyophilisate (MELT) and tablet formulations in children and adolescents with primary nocturnal enuresis. *Int J Clin Pract* 61(9):1454–1460, 2007.
134. Robson WL, Leung AK, Norgaard JP: The comparative safety of oral versus intranasal desmopressin for the treatment of children with nocturnal enuresis. *J Urol* 78(1):24, 2007.
135. Janknegt RA, Zweers HM, Delaere KP, Kloet AG, Khoe SG, Arendsen HJ: Oral desmopressin as a new treatment modality for primary nocturnal enuresis in adolescents and adults: a double-blind, randomized, multicenter study. Dutch Enuresis Study Group. *J Urol* 157:513–517, 1997.
136. Schulman SL, Stokes A, Salzman PM: The efficacy and safety of oral desmopressin in children with primary nocturnal enuresis. *J Urol* 166(6):2427–2431, 2001.
137. Skoog SJ, Stokes A, Turner KL: Oral desmopressin: a randomized double-blind placebo controlled study of effectiveness in children with primary nocturnal enuresis. *J Urol* 158:1035–1040, 1997.
138. Stenberg A, Lackgren G: Desmopressin tablets in the treatment of severe nocturnal enuresis in adolescents. *Pediatrics* 94:841–846, 1994.
139. Lackgren G, Lilja B, Neveus T, Stenberg A: Desmopressin in the treatment of severe nocturnal enuresis in adolescents: a 7-year follow-up study. *Br J Urol* 81(3):17–23, 1998.
140. Wolfish NM, Barkin J, Gorodzinsky F, Schwarz R: The Canadian enuresis study and evaluation—short- and long-term safety and efficacy of an oral desmopressin preparation. *Scand J Urol Nephrol* 37(1):22–27, 2003.
141. Butler R, Holland P, Devitt H, Hiley E, Roberts G, Redfern E: The effectiveness of desmopressin in the treatment of childhood nocturnal enuresis: predicting response using pretreatment variables. *Br J Urol* 81(3):29–36, 1998.
142. Eller DA, Homsy YL, Austin PF, Tanguay S, Cantor A: Spot urine osmolality, age and bladder capacity as predictors of response to desmopressin in nocturnal enuresis. *Scand J Urol Nephrol* 183:41–45, 1997.
143. Eller DA, Austin PF, Tanguay S, Homsy YL: Daytime functional bladder capacity as a predictor of response to desmopressin in monosymptomatic nocturnal enuresis. *Eur Urol* 1998;33(3):25–29.
144. Folwell AJ, Macdiarmid SA, Crowder HJ, Lord AD, Arnold EP: Desmopressin for nocturnal enuresis: urinary osmolality and response. *Br J Urol* 80(3):480–484, 1997.
145. Neveus T, Lackgren G, Tuvemo T, Stenberg A: Osmoregulation and desmopressin pharmacokinetics in enuretic children. *Pediatrics* 103:65–70, 1999b.
146. Rushton HG, Belman AB, Zaontz MR, Skoog SJ, Sihelnik S: The influence of small functional bladder capacity and other predictors on the response to desmopressin in the management of monosymptomatic nocturnal enuresis. *J Urol* 156:651–655, 1996.
147. Kruse S, Hellstrom AL, Hanson E, et al.: Swedish Enuresis Trial (SWEET) Group: treatment of primary monosymptomatic nocturnal enuresis with desmopressin: predictive factors. *BJU Int* 88(6):572–576, 2001.
148. Monda JM, Husmann DA: Primary nocturnal enuresis: a comparison among observation, imipramine, desmopressin acetate and bed-wetting alarm systems. *J Urol* 154:745–748, 1995.
149. Glazener CM, Evans JH: Desmopressin for nocturnal enuresis in children. *Cochrane Database Syst Rev* (3):CD002112, 2002.
150. Önol FF, Guzel R, Tahra A, et al.: Comparison of long-term efficacy of desmopressin lyophilisate and enuretic alarm for monosymptomatic enuresis and assessment of predictive factors for success: a randomized prospective trial. *J Urol* 193(2):665–661, 2015.
151. Mikkelsen EJ: Enuresis and encopresis: ten years of progress. *Am Acad Child and Adol Psychiatry* 40(10):1146–1158, 2001.
152. Bellman M: Studies on encopresis. *Acta Paediatr Scand* 170:1+, 1966.
153. Rutter M, Tizard J, Whitmore K, eds.: *Education, Health and Behavior.* New York, Krieger, Huntington, 1981.
154. van der Wal MF, Benninga MA, Hirasing RA: The prevalence of encopresis in a multicultural population. *J Pediatr Gastroenterol Nutr* 40(suppl 3): 345–348, 2005.
155. Hersov L: Faecal soiling. In: Rutter M, Sersov L, eds.: *Child and Adolescent Psychiatry: Modern Approaches.* 2nd ed. London, Blackwell Scientific, 482–489, 1985.
156. Loening-Baucke V: Functional fecal retention with encopresis in childhood. *J Pediatr Gastroenterol Nutr* 38(suppl 1):79–84, 2004.
157. Loening-Baucke VA: Factors responsible for persistence of childhood constipation. *J Pediatr Gastroenterol Nutr* 6:915–922, 1987.
158. Loening-Baucke VA, Cruikshank BM: Abnormal defecation dynamics in chronically constipated children with encopresis. *J Pediatr* 108:562–566, 1986.
159. Loening-Baucke V, Cruikshank B, Savage C: Defecation dynamics and behavior profiles in encopretic children. *Pediatrics* 80:672–679, 1987.
160. Loening-Baucke V: Balloon defecation as a predictor of outcome in children with functional constipation and encopresis. *J Pediatr* 128:336–340, 1996.
161. Wald A, Chandra R, Chiponis D, Gabel S: Anorectal function and continence mechanisms in childhood encopresis. *J Pediatr Gastroenterol Nutr* 5:346–351, 1986.
162. Sentovich SM, Kaufman SS, Cali RL: Pudendal nerve function in normal and encopretic children. *J Pediatr Gastroenterol Nutr* 26:70–72, 1998.
163. Catto-Smith AG, Nolan TM, Coffey CM: Clinical significance of anismus in encopresis. *J Gastroenterol Hepatol* 13:955–960, 1998.
164. Sutphen J, Borowitz S, Ling W, Cox DJ, Kovatchev B: Anorectal manometric examination in encopretic-constipated children. *Dis Colon Rectum* 40:1051–1055, 1997.
165. Stern HP, Stroh SE, Fiedorek SC, et al.: Increased plasma levels of pancreatic polypeptide and decreased plasma levels of motilin in encopretic children. *Pediatrics* 96:111–117, 1995.
166. Freud A, Burlingham DT: *War and Children.* New York, Medical War Books, 1943.
167. Stein Z, Susser M: Social factors in the development of sphincter control. *Dev Med Child Neurol* 9:692–706, 1967.
168. Foreman DM, Thambirajah MS: Conduct disorder, enuresis and specific developmental delays in two types of encopresis: a case-note study of 63 boys. *Eur Child Adolesc Psychiatry* 5:33–37, 1996.
169. Cox DJ, Morris JB Jr, Borowitz SM, Sutphen JL: Psychological differences between children with and without chronic encopresis. *J Pediatr Psychol* 27(suppl 7):585–591, 2002.
170. Mellon MW, Whiteside SP, Friedrich WN: The relevance of fecal soiling as an indicator of child sexual abuse: a preliminary analysis. *J Dev Behav Pediatr* 27(1):25, 2006.
171. Klages T, Geller B, Tillman R, Bolhofner K, Zimerman B: Controlled study of encopresis and enuresis in children with a prepubertal and early adolescent bipolar-I disorder phenotype. *J Am Acad Child Adolesc Psychiatry* 44(suppl 10):1050–1057, 2005.
172. von Gontard A, Hollmann E: Comorbidity of functional urinary incontinence and encopresis: somatic and behavioral associations. *J Urol* 71(suppl 6 Pt 2):2644–2647, 2004.
173. Joinson C, Heron J, Butler R, von Gontard A; Avon Longitudinal Study of Parents and Children Study Team: Psychological differences between children with and without soiling problems. Avon longitudinal study of parents and children study team. *Pediatrics* 117(5):1575–1584, 2006.
174. Joinson C, Heron J, Butler R, et al.: A United Kingdom population-based study of intellectual capacities in children with and without soiling, daytime wetting, and bedwetting. *Pediatrics* 120(2):308, 2007.
175. Rockney RM, McQuade WH, Days AL: The plain abdominal roentgenogram in the management of encopresis. *Arch Pediatr Adolesc Med* 149:623–627, 1995.
176. Levine MD: Encopresis: its potentiation, evaluation and alleviation. *Pediatr Clin North Am* 29:315–330, 1982.
177. Levine MD, Bakow H: Children with encopresis: a study of treatment outcome. *Pediatrics* 58:845–852, 1976.
178. Levine MD, Mazonson P, Bakow H: Behavioral symptom substitution in children cured of encopresis. *Am J Dis Child* 134:663–667, 1980.
179. Borowitz SM, Cox DJ, Sutphen JL, Kovatchev B: Treatment of childhood encopresis: a randomized trial comparing three treatment protocols. *J Pediatr Gastroenterol Nutr* 34(suppl 4):378–384, 2002.
180. Stark LJ, Opipari LC, Donaldson DL, Danovsky MB, Rasile DA, DelSanto AF: Evaluation of a standard protocol for retentive encopresis: a replication. *J Pediatr Psychol* 22:619–633, 1997.
181. Sprague-McRae JM, Lamb W, Homer D: Encopresis: a study of treatment alternatives and historical and behavioral characteristics. *Nurse Pract* 18(suppl 10):52–53,56–63, 1993.
182. Nolan T, Debelle G, Oberkland F, Coffey C: Randomized trial of laxatives in treatment of childhood encopresis. *Lancet* 31:523–527, 1991.
183. Pashankar DS, Bishop WP: Efficacy and optimal dose of daily polyethylene glycol 3350 for treatment of constipation and encopresis in children. *J Pediatr* 139(suppl 3):428–432, 2001.
184. Loening-Baucke V. Polyethylene glycol without electrolytes for children with constipation and encopresis. *J Pediatr Gastroenterol Nutr* 4(suppl 4): 372–377, 2002.
185. Pashankar DS, Bishop WP, Loening-Baucke V: Long-term efficacy of polyethylene glycol 3350 for the treatment of chronic constipation in children with and without encopresis. *Clin Pediatr* 42(suppl 9):815–819, 2003.

186. Voskuijl W, de Lorijn F, Verwijs W, et al.: PEG 3350 (Transipeg) versus lactulose in the treatment of childhood functional constipation: a double-blind, randomized, controlled, multicentre trial. *Gut* 53(11):1590–1594, 2004.
187. Loening-Baucke V: Modulation of abnormal defecation dynamics by biofeedback treatment in chronically constipated children with encopresis. *J Pediatr* 116:214–222, 1990.
188. Benninga MA, Buller HA, Iaminiau JA: Biofeedback training in chronic constipation. *Arch Dis Child* 68:126–129, 1993.
189. Loening-Baucke V: Biofeedback treatment for chronic constipation and encopresis in childhood: long-term outcome. *Pediatrics* 96:105–110, 1995.
190. Nolan T, Catto-Smith T, Coffey C, Wells J: Randomised controlled trial of biofeedback training in persistent encopresis with anismus. *Arch Dis Child* 1998;79:131–135.
191. Brooks RC, Copen RM, Cox DJ, Morris J, Borowitz S, Sutphen J: Review of the treatment literature for encopresis, functional constipation, and stool-toileting refusal. *Ann Behav Med* 2(suppl 3):260–267, 2000.
192. Brazzelli M, Griffiths P: Behavioural and cognitive interventions with or without other treatments for defecation disorders in children. *Cochrane Database Syst Rev* (4):CD002240, 2001.
193. Griffiths P, Dunn S, Evans A, Smith D, Bradnam M: Portable biofeedback apparatus for treatment of anal sphincter dystonia in childhood soiling and constipation. *J Med Eng Tech* 23(suppl 3):96–101, 1999.
194. Cox DJ, Sutphen J, Borowitz S, Kovatchev B, Ling W: Contribution of behavior therapy and biofeedback to laxative therapy in the treatment of pediatric encopresis. *Ann Behav Med* 20:70–76, 1998.
195. Croffie JM, Ammar MS, Pfefferkorn MD, et al.: Assessment of the effectiveness of biofeedback in children with dyssynergic defecation and recalcitrant constipation/encopresis: does home biofeedback improve long-term outcomes? *Clin Pediatr* 44(suppl 1):63–71, 2005.
196. Abrahams D: Treatment of encopresis with imipramine. *Am J Psychiatry* 119:891–892, 1963.
197. Connell HM: The practical management of encopresis. *Aust Paediatr J* 8:279–281, 1972.
198. Gavanski M: Treatment of non-retentive secondary encopresis with imipramine and psychotherapy. *CMAJ* 104:46–48, 1971.
199. Geormaneanu M, Voiculescu VP: Treatment of encopresis with imipramine. *Rev Roum Med Neurol Psychiatr* 18:209–210, 1980.
200. Siomopoulos V: Psychogenic encopresis treated with imipramine. *JAMA* 235:1842, 1976.
201. White JH: *Pediatric Psychopharmacology*. Baltimore, MD: Williams & Wilkins, 109–114, 1977.
202. Dossetor D, Stiefel I, Gomes L: A case of predominantly nocturnal soiling treated with amitriptyline. *Eur Child Adolesc Psychiatry* 7:114–118, 1998.
203. Nurko S, Garcia-Aranda JA, Worona LB, Zlochisty O: Cisapride for the treatment of constipation in children: a double-blind study. *J Pediatr* 136:135–140, 2000.
204. Rockney RM, McQuade WH, Days AL, Linn HE, Alario AJ: Encopresis treatment outcome: long-term follow-up of 45 cases. *J Dev Behav Pediatr* 17:380–385, 1996.
205. Rex DK, Fitzgerald JF, Goulet RJ: Chronic constipation with encopresis persisting beyond 15 years of age. *Dis Colon Rectum* 35:242–244, 1992.

5.13 ■ PERSONALITY DISORDERS

CHAPTER 5.13 ■ PERSONALITY DISORDERS IN CHILDREN AND ADOLESCENTS: A FOCUS ON BORDERLINE PERSONALITY DISORDER

EFRAIN BLEIBERG AND CARLA SHARP

The study of personality disorders (PD) is fraught with more controversies than any other area of psychopathology, as Millon and Davis noted. The controversies have been particularly pronounced regarding the child and adolescent antecedents of the PD of adulthood. Until recently, there has been considerable reluctance to diagnose PD in children and adolescents, a reluctance that is still present among many mental health professions (1,2).

Such reluctance is based on concerns about stigma—a significant issue particularly in regard to diagnosis such as psychopathy, and antisocial, borderline, or narcissistic personality disorder (3), which evoke rather intense negative responses in others, including mental health professionals, the difficulty of distinguishing the "normal" turmoil of adolescence from PD; and the incompleteness and fluidity of children and adolescent's development. This fluidity accounts for constant chances in every aspect of children and adolescent's bodies and personalities, which in turn, affects their self-image and their patterns of coping, thinking, feeling, and relating.

This chapter will focus on borderline personality disorder (BPD) in adolescence, which has been the subject of the largest body of empirical investigation among the PD in children and adolescents over the last two decades. BPD is illustrative of the processes by which biologic and psychosocial risk and protective factors interact to shape, organize, and reinforce the developmental trajectories leading to the PD that emerge in adolescence. This review will seek to establish whether there is sufficient data to justify a valid and reliable diagnosis of BPD in adolescence with a definable clinical presentation, developmental trajectory, course and outcome, including continuities and discontinuities between adolescent and adult BPD. Furthermore, this chapter also examines the literature on evidence-based psychosocial and biologic treatment, including promising treatment currently under development or undergoing testing of effectiveness.

DEFINITION AND PHENOMENOLOGY OF BORDERLINE PERSONALITY DISORDERS IN ADOLESCENCE

DSM-5 (4) section II lists nine criteria, of which at least five must be present to qualify for a diagnosis of BPD. These are:

1. A pattern of unstable intense relationships
2. Inappropriate, intense anger
3. Frantic efforts to avoid abandonment affective instability
4. Affective instability
5. Impulsive actions
6. Recurrent self-harm and suicidality
7. Chronic feelings of emptiness or boredom (dysphoria)
8. Transient, stress-related paranoid thoughts
9. Identity disturbance and severe dissociative symptoms

DSM-5 includes also a section III that indicates that more research is needed to validate a model of PD that is not based on categorical symptoms (3), but on impairments in self and interpersonal function (criterion A) and pathologic personality traits (criterion B). This alternative model of diagnosing PD reflects a growing consensus that PD should be understood as *dimensional* disorders in which individuals present varying degrees of pathologic personality traits that impair functioning.

This dimensional model of PD is consistent with the model proposed in this chapter. The aspects of impairment proposed in DSM-5's alternative model are particularly relevant to this chapter's proposed description of core dysfunctions in adolescent BPD.

They include:

1. *Identity:* Referring to the degree of difficulty experiencing the self as a distinct and coherent entity with a sense of continuity over time.
2. *Self-direction:* Involving the extent of impairment in experiencing oneself as an *agent,* the originator and "owner" of one's behavior, capable of setting and pursuing short- and long-term goals.
3. *Empathy:* Describing the extent of impairment in the capacity to understand the experience and intentions of others, appreciate and tolerate other people's perspective, and understand the impact one has on others and others have on us.
4. *Intimacy:* Assessing the impairment in the capacity for closeness, trust, and reciprocity in relations.

These impairments are highly consistent with an emerging consensus (5) that the core dimensional impairments characterizing BPD are *affective dysregulation, impulsivity,* pervasive *social dysfunction,* and *impairments in identity.*

Despite long-standing agreement that PD, in general, and BPD, in particular, are rooted in childhood and adolescent—and that youngsters are unlikely to wake up after their 18th birthday to discover that they have become borderline overnight—there is much debate about the validity and stability of the BPD diagnosis in adolescence over time.

Two decades of research (6–9), however, provide evidence that the reliability and validity of the BPD diagnosis in mid-to-late adolescence are comparable to that of adults.

DSM-5 provides criteria for BPD unmodified by developmental considerations but suggests that BPD—as well as other PD—can be diagnosed in children and adolescents when maladaptive traits have been present for at least 1 year and the traits are pervasive, persistent, and unlikely to be limited to a particular developmental stage. In both adolescent and adults, BPD is broadly defined by affect dysregulation, marked impulsivity, including self-injurious behavior, and a pervasive pattern of instability of interpersonal relationships and self-image. At a psychological level, the core features of adolescent and adult clinical presentations are high sensitivity and anxious expectation of rejection, abandonment or loss, difficulties with trust and cooperation, proneness to shame, negative perception of self and body, and explosive rage and intermittent hostility (10). Several studies (11–13), however, show relatively low stability of categorical symptoms (if a symptom present or not) as part of a polythetic criterion (e.g., a set of five of nine categorical features) for the adolescent BPD diagnosis.

Greater stability and accuracy of diagnosis can be achieved when considering the core dysfunctions of affect dysregulation, impulsivity and pervasive disturbances in interpersonal relations, and self-image in a *dimensional* approach. Diagnosing BPD with a dimensional, rather than a categorical approach is particularly relevant in adolescence, as a dimensional approach can account for the developmental variability during adolescence and in the transition to adulthood, identifying a population of adolescents with current psychopathology and psychosocial dysfunction (4); very high comorbidity with other psychiatric disorders (14) such as eating disorders, depression and anxiety disorders, and substance use disorders; and poor outcomes in longitudinal studies (15).

Differences between adolescents and adults indeed suggest a developmental trajectory of consistent and continuing impairment but with changing clinical features. Compared to adults with BPD, adolescents with BPD present with more acute and dramatic symptoms, such as self-harm and suicidality (see section on Diagnosis and Clinical Features), explosive rage, and other impulsive and self-damaging behaviors. By contrast, unstable relationships and identity disturbance are more often diagnosed in adults with BPD.

Fear and anticipation of rejection and abandonment appear to be a specific inclusion criterion in adolescents, with patients endorsing this symptom meeting full diagnostic criteria in 85% of cases (16). Westen et al. (8) conclude that feelings of emptiness, dramatic fluctuations in self-image, and dependence on the presence and responsiveness of others to maintain a sense of identity are the most distinctive features associated with the diagnosis of BPD in adolescents. These findings were confirmed in recent work utilizing modern latent trait approaches (17).

Assessing the dimensional features of personality pathology emerging in adolescence and the more pervasive and persistent dysfunctions in the core dimensions that characterize BPD in adolescents are critical in order to differentiate BPD in adolescents from the acute or episodic manifestations of other psychiatric disorders or developmental crisis, which can occur comorbidly with BPD. Of particular note are the diagnostic entities of nonsuicidal self-injury (NSSI) and suicidal behavior disorder, which have been included in section III of DSM-5 (4). NSSI is common in adolescence and suicide attempts can be associated with a range of conditions or developmental crisis, including major depression and substance abuse. However, repetitive NSSI, in which self-harm becomes a device to achieve emotion regulation, relieve feelings of emptiness, and a response to perceived or anticipated rejection or abandonment are highly associated with BPD (18). Moreover, BPD is much more likely in adolescents who present both NSSI *and* suicide attempt than in those adolescents who present one or the other.

According to Ha et al. (19), a confluence of internalizing (mood and anxiety disorders, including obsessive-compulsive disorder (OCD), posttraumatic stress disorder (PTSD), and separation anxiety disorder) and externalizing disorders (attention-deficit hyperactivity disorder [ADHD], oppositional disorder, conduct disorder, and substance use disorders) is predictive of a BPD diagnosis. Thus, clinicians should use the presence of this complex suggestive of a BPD diagnosis.

History

Clinical descriptions of BPD in childhood, beginning in the late 1940s, formulated these children's symptoms within a psychoanalytic framework (2). Margaret Mahler et al. (20) suggested the term "borderline psychosis" to refer to children at the milder end of a proposed continuum that extended to the most severe psychotic conditions of childhood. Ekstein and Wallerstein (21) used the term "borderline" to describe children who were not mildly or incipiently psychotic but presented, instead, a stable condition, paradoxically defined by its persistent instability, and characterized by rapid and ongoing shifts in levels of ego functioning, including reality testing, relationships with others, and defense mechanisms. Such formulations defined borderline children as less severely disturbed than psychotic children but more seriously impaired than neurotic children. In a similar vein, Kernberg (22) characterized "borderline" as a level of development and organization underlying several PD. This developmental pattern, according to Kernberg, included limitations in the capacity to differentiate self from others, reliance in primitive defenses, and attainment of reality testing, without the achievement of object constancy and identity integration.

Such formulations of borderline pathology in children used diverse clinical criteria, and likely described a heterogeneous population (23), but laid the foundation for the development of formal criteria for BPD in children and adolescents.

Goldman et al. (24) were the first to adapt standardized adult DSM criteria for BPD in children and adolescents, thus allowing for the comparison of findings from different studies and the application of adult assessment tools to child and adolescent samples.

Epidemiology

Recent reviews of epidemiologic studies suggest that the prevalence of BPD in adolescence is similar or higher than in adults, affecting 3% to almost 6% in community samples (25), 11% of those seeking outpatient services (26,27), and almost 50% of those admitted to inpatient treatment. For example, Grilo et al. (28) demonstrated similar rates of BPD in inpatient settings for adolescents (49%) and young adults (43%) using the same measures for both samples.

Etiology

Models are emerging seeking to integrate biologic and psychosocial interaction factors interacting with one other to generate, organize, and reinforce a developmental trajectory leading to the emergence of BPD in adolescence with core dimensional features of affect dysregulation, impulsivity, and a pervasive pattern of impairment in relationships and self-image (29). Existing research, as section III of DSM-5 points out, does not yet support a comprehensive developmental–etiologic interactional model of BPD. In this section, we discuss growing understanding BPD as emerging from biologic vulnerabilities interacting with specific psychosocial factors.

A selective review of investigations of genetic, biologic, and psychosocial factors in the etiology of BPD will be followed by an examination of these emerging interactional models.

Genetic Factors

Studies investigating genetic factors associated with BPD have included family, adoption, and twin studies.

Twin studies suggest that BPD features in adults have heritability between 40% and 50% (30–32). Two studies show that children aged 9 to 15 who carried the S allele of the serotonin transporter gene promoter region (5-HTTLPR) presented with the highest degree of BPD features (33). This finding is suggestive that the genetic diathesis driving the core features of BPD development is a *high sensitivity* and *reactivity to stress* and thus, a heightened sensitivity to the adequacy or inadequacy of the child's attachment context to regulate and modulate stress.

Evidence of this interaction between genetic diathesis and attachment context is provided by a large study of a birth cohort of over 1,100 families with twins. In this study, Belsky et al. (34) found that the likelihood of extreme dimensional features of BPD, assessed at age 12, more than doubled (8% vs. 3%) in children with a family history of psychiatric disorder, as an index of genetic vulnerability. The likelihood of extreme dimensional features of BPD also more than doubled (7% vs. 3%) in children with a history of maltreatment. However, in those with *both* a genetic vulnerability *and* maltreatment, the extreme dimensional features of BPD were present in 40%.

Neurobiologic Factors

Studies of adults with BPD suggest dysfunctions in 5-HT, dopamine, monoamine oxidase, and vasopressin are likely associated with impulsivity, aggression, and self-injury in BPD. On the other hand affective dysregulation, a core dimension of BPD, may be associated with dysfunctions in the acetylcholine and noradrenaline systems (35).

Neuroimaging studies in adults with BPD identify reduced volumes of the amygdala; hippocampus, orbitofrontal cortex (OFC) and anterior cingulate cortex (ACC), brain areas that play key roles in emotion regulation and in the processing of social and social–emotional information (36). In response to affective stimuli, BPD patients show bilateral increases in activation of the amygdala, suggesting an increased reactivity to emotionally relevant stimuli (37), further supporting the notion of deficient processing of affective stimuli in BPD.

Taken together, studies of the neurobiologic correlates of BPD converge in pointing to a dysfunctional frontolimbic network that may account for both symptoms of impulsive aggression and affective dysregulation and the characteristic hyperreactivity of BPD individuals to loss, rejection of frustration.

Reduced volumes in left ACC and right orbitofrontal cortex (OFC) have been identified in adolescent patients with BPD and correlate with impulsivity and NSSI (38,39). However, contradictory findings have also been reported (40).

Diffusion tensor imaging studies show decreased fractional anisotropy in the fornix of adolescents with BPD (41). New et al. (42) report decreased fractional anisotropy in the inferior longitudinal fasciculus and other areas, which appear to be present in adolescents but not in adults with BPD.

These findings, and the overall inconsistency in neuroimaging studies of BPD on adolescence, suggest neurodevelopmental differences between adolescents and adults with BPD, that highlight that during adolescence there are increased deficits in connectivity between the medial prefrontal cortex and the orbitofrontal cortex, on the one hand, and the amygdala, hippocampus, posterior cingulate and insular cortex, on the other hand (42). These findings correlate with at least one FMRI study documenting hyperresponsiveness of the amygdala in adolescents with repetitive NSSI.

These findings are associated with the characteristic neurodevelopmental features of adolescence involving synaptogenesis (increase in the number of synaptic connections) followed by synaptic pruning and axonal myelination. The brain areas involved in this structural reorganization are particularly the prefrontal cortex, the anterior cingulate, and the superior temporal cortex, areas that, as discussed below, are involved in social cognition, mentalizing, and social cognition–mediated ("top-down") affect regulation (43).

While this reorganization will eventually lead to more efficient brain networks and neural transmission in early adulthood, while it is taking place, it significantly impairs social cognition, mentalizing, and affect regulation in adolescence, arguably creating a critical vulnerability to the emergence of BPD in predisposed adolescents.

Psychosocial and Psychological Factors

A large body of research, including longitudinal studies, offers robust evidence that a range of adverse and traumatic childhood experiences (in particular experiences of emotional neglect and abuse and broader problems in family environment [including parental conflict, separation, and loss and parental psychopathology]) and low socioeconomic status are associated with the key features of BPD (43–46).

The children in the community study (47), for example, found that childhood maltreatment prospectively predicted a high risk for BPD in young adulthood even after controlling for other PD, parental education, and psychiatric disorders in the parents in this same study. Early separations from the mother and the family's low socioeconomic status also predicted BPD symptomatology in adolescence and were largely independent from other predictive factors such as maltreatment.

Lyons-Ruth et al. (48) identified maternal withdrawal at age 18 months as a predictor of BPD symptoms in adolescence. Carlson et al. (49) identified a strong relationship between early exposure to maltreatment and parental hostility and attachment disorganization (see section Interactional-Integrating Models), which, in turn, is prospectively predictive of BPD symptoms in middle childhood, adolescence, and adulthood.

Association between the broader psychosocial context and BPD symptomatology is suggested by Wilkinson and Pickett (50) who find a substantial correlation between countries' levels of income inequality and levels of mental health problems such as substance abuse and teen parenthood associated with BPD.

Arguably, income inequality is a marker of social cohesiveness and social reciprocity versus lack of cohesion and social exclusion.

Psychological research has illuminated the relationship between patterns of social interaction and emotional–interpersonal problems. The domains of sensitivity to social rejection and abandonment, aggression in interpersonal relationships, and difficulties forming trusting and cooperative relationship appear particularly relevant to BPD symptomatology (51).

These studies offer a bridge to integrating perspectives that focus on the interactive development of genetically prepared mechanisms to appraise and regulate self, affect and relationships, and the psychosocial and attachment contexts in which these mechanisms are shaped, organized, and reinforced in ways that lead to developmental trajectories marked by adaptive or maladaptive patterns of relationships, coping, and experiencing.

INTERACTIONAL-INTEGRATING MODELS

Attachment theory has been proposed by a number of authors as a particularly useful framework for conceptualizing the relationship of psychosocial adversity, such as maltreatment and loss, and BPD symptomatology (52). A review of attachment studies in BPD shows an inverse relationship between adult BPD and insecure or disorganized attachment (53,54).

Fonagy et al. (52) suggest that security of attachment is, in turn, linked to the caregiver's mentalizing capacity. Mentalizing refers to the genetically prepared capacity to understand the self and others in terms of intentional mental states, such as thoughts, feelings, needs, desires, and goals. These authors propose that mentalizing is a fundamental maturational achievement underpinning personality development, particularly the capacity for self-agency and the construction of an autobiographical narrative; the ability for social reciprocity and empathy; the capacity for self-regulation and affect modulation; and the capacity to represent experience and symbolize.

Functional neuroimaging studies provide compelling evidence of brain systems mediating mentalization, particularly a neural network including the superior temporal sulcus, the medial prefrontal cortex (including the ACC) and, to a lesser extent, the amygdala and the orbitofrontal cortex associated with BPD (55).

Secure attachment appears to be the optimal and perhaps the necessary developmental context for the unfolding of the psychobiologic capacity to mentalize. At the root of the core symptomatology of BPD appears to lie a diminished capacity to mentalize in the context of attachment relationships (56).

Neurodevelopmental models of BPD have attempted to examine the reciprocal relationship between biologic and psychosocial factors underlying the developmental disruptions postulated to account for BPD.

An example of such models is proposed by Fonagy and Bateman, and Bleiberg (56,57), who advanced the hypothesis that the developmental trajectory leading to BPD comprises the following elements in various combinations: (1) infants with an exceptional disposition to mentalization (hypersensitivity to social cues); (2) a disposition to increased arousal or affective dysregulation associated to neuropsychiatric vulnerabilities, such as mood disorders (58) or ADHD (59); (3) parents who share similar genetic, neuropsychiatric vulnerabilities or histories of maltreatment; (4) a parental disposition to respond to their children's hyperarousal and signals of distress with hyperarousal and distress of their own and inhibition of their capacity to mentalize, interfering with the capacity to accurately match the children's internal state (60); (5) a corresponding impairment in children's capacity to maintain a stable, mentalized representation of affect and intentionality in self and others in the context of close attachments (56); (6) children's adaptation to stress and relationship trauma with an inhibition of their capacity to deal with mental states, relying instead on prementalistic, coercive maneuvers aiming at achieving self-stability and a sense of attachment; and (7) a reinforcement of this psychological and psychosocial adaptation by changes in neural mechanisms of arousal that lead to a low threshold for the triggering of the arousal system with a concurrent inhibition of the frontal and prefrontal structures involved in mentalizing in response to relatively mild emotional stimuli (61). The prototype of such adaptation appears to be the disorganized pattern of attachment.

Such a model may help explain one of the paradoxes of borderline psychopathology of an uncanny sensitivity and reactivity to other people's mental states, accounting for their exquisite capacity to know what are the right buttons to push in order to evoke responses from others, and the dramatic intensity of their responses to interpersonal events, incongruously coexisting with remarkable self-centeredness and utter disregard for other people's feelings.

Diagnosis and Clinical Features

Beginning in the early 1980s, a number of authors reported on a substantial consensus among clinicians on the diagnostic criteria for borderline children. These clinical criteria closely parallel the adult criteria for BPD.

Petti and Vela (23) described the confusion in the clinical literature between children with borderline personality or borderline spectrum disorders and children who, although often referred to as borderline, are more appropriately described as falling within the schizotypal personality or schizophrenia spectrum disorders. Both groups of children present transient psychotic episodes, idiosyncratic fantasies, and magical thinking. Yet only schizotypal children have a family history of schizophrenia spectrum disorder or present constricted, flat, or inappropriate affect; oddness of speech; and discomfort in social situations, these features contrast with the intense, dramatic affect and hunger for social response of borderline youths. This differentiation is supported by genetic, epidemiologic, and follow-up studies of adult BPD that discriminate BPD from the schizophrenia-schizotypal spectrum.

Clinical Evaluation

Early manifestations of developmental difficulties are apparent in children who subsequently develop BPD, including a difficult temperament, high activity levels, poor adaptability, negative mood, and problems settling into rhythmic patterns of sleep–wakefulness and feeding. Cranky and hard to soothe, these infants frequently challenge and burden their caretakers.

Hyperactivity and temper tantrums are common in the preschool years of many children on the path to BPD, whereas others are more notable for their clinginess and vulnerability to separations. By school age, these children almost invariably meet diagnostic criteria for an axis I diagnosis, more commonly ADHD, conduct disorder, separation anxiety disorder, or mood disorder.

Many of these youngsters appear anxious, moody, irritable, and explosive. Minor upsets or frustrations trigger intense affective storms—episodes of uncontrolled emotion wholly out of proportion to the apparent precipitant. The lability of their affect mirrors the kaleidoscopic quality of their sense of self and others. One moment they feel elated and expansive, blissfully connected in perfect love and harmony to an idealized partner. Next, they plunge into bitter disappointment and rage coupled with self-loathing and despair.

On clinical examination, school-age borderline children may appear helpless and vulnerable, provocative and suspicious, or eager to comply and ingratiate themselves with the examiner. These youngsters quickly attempt to establish highly coercive, controlling relationships with their examiners (62). Some show surprisingly little anxiety about meeting alone with the clinician and proceed to take over the office as if they owned it. Even those who seem vulnerable and anxious try vigorously to set the agenda for the meeting. They become anxious and even more desperate and arbitrary when the examiner does not comply with their demands or when they feel that their control is threatened. A distorted sense of reality is a distinctive and puzzling feature of borderline children, as they create a vivid fantasy world in which they become intensely absorbed. They then attempt to coerce others to assume certain roles that fit their particular fantasy. While they can generally recognize the arbitrariness with which they treat reality, they behave as if they must believe their own falsification of reality. When others do not match the prescribed roles, borderline children become desperate, enraged, and transiently psychotic.

Psychological testing reveals rigid and tenuous repressive defenses coexisting with primitive defenses; a highly egocentric, arbitrary interpretation of reality; transitory disturbances in reality testing and impairments in formal thought processes in unstructured tests; constant or recurrent disturbances in ego functions, such as frustration tolerance, attention, and goal directedness; primitive, unmodulated experience of affects and drives; and marked disturbances in interpersonal relationships and in the experiences of self and others (62).

The developmental and psychosocial pressures of adolescence typically trigger the onset of the full range of borderline psychopathology and allow for greater diagnostic certainty. Adolescence may be the point at which the coping mechanisms, relationship patterns, and modes of organizing experience acquire self-perpetuating rigidity and the capacity to coercively evoke responses from others that maintain and reinforce these youngsters' maladjustment.

Unstable relationships with peers become prominent as transient idealization and clingy overdependence alternate with rage, devaluation, and feelings of abandonment and betrayal. Regardless of whether idealization or anger predominates, all of their interpersonal exchanges have an intense, dramatic quality. Promiscuity is more common in borderline girls, particularly in sexually abused girls, for whom aggressive seductiveness affords the opportunity to turn around and gain control of the helplessness associated with being abused.

Borderline boys are often burdened with intense shyness and fears of rejection. Manipulative efforts to secure attention and prevent abandonment become prominent interpersonal strategies for both boys and girls. Bulimic binges or drugs are relied on for soothing and comfort and become essential regulators of well-being and self-esteem (63,64). Yet, the transient nurturance derived from food binges, drug abuse, or promiscuous sex only leads to shame, guilt, and a dreaded feeling of inner deadness or emptiness. Self-mutilation and suicidal gestures result from a wish to "feel something" and relieve the emptiness, an effort to escape unbearable feelings of anxiety and depression, a desire to punish a previously idealized partner, and a manipulative attempt to evoke guilt and involvement. Dissociative episodes appear more commonly in sexually abused borderline adolescents.

A central feature of BPD—and all PD—is the construction of a rigid set of beliefs, mental representations, and coping mechanisms. As Zanarini et al. (65) remark, individuals with BPD believe that people cannot be loved comfortably or left gracefully and transform anxiety, sorrow, and rage into indirect, dramatic, reproachful attempts to evoke attention. They anticipate experiencing subjective dyscontrol and fragmentation, so they actively provoke these very experiences, thus gaining an illusion of control over themselves and others. Borderline children's rigid and desperate insistence on inducing interpersonal responses that support and validate their own mental representations and expectations turns into one of the most daunting therapeutic challenges facing child and adolescent clinicians.

The use of well-established interview tools to support clinical assessment is recommended for a reliable diagnosis in adolescents. Structured interviews such as the structured clinical interview for PD is an interview-based assessment that shows good reliability (66) and validity. The Personality Disorder Examination (PDE) a child version of the Diagnostic Interview for Borderline patients (C-DIB) for adolescents (67) and the borderline personality features scale (SCID-II), also show reliability and validity.

For children (BPFS-C) (10) shows good psychometric properties. The BPFS-C includes age-appropriate items adapted from the original scale for adults to reflect the domains of affective instability (e.g., "My feelings are very strong. For instance, when I get mad, I get really, really mad. When I get happy, I get really, really happy"); identity problems (e.g., "I feel that there is something important missing about me, but I don't know what it is"); negative relationships (e.g., "I've picked friends who have treated me badly"); and self-harm (e.g., "I get into trouble because I do things without thinking"). A newly developed parent report (BPFS-P) has been validated and shows good psychometric properties. An 11-item version has recently been developed for use in large-scale epidemiologic studies or outcomes studies where shorter measures are required (68).

Differential Diagnosis

Adult BPD is often comorbid with other disorders, including major depression, substance misuse, posttraumatic stress disorder, other anxiety disorders, and eating disorders. Evidence is now accumulating of a similar cooccurrence of diagnosis of other PD. The strongest comorbidity demonstrated for BPD is with externalizing disorder (69,70). In one study (71), conduct disorder was the only axis I disorder significantly more prevalent in adolescents with BPD than in those without.

Physical and sexual abuse and early losses are common features in BPD and conduct disorders. ADHD uncomplicated by BPD does not include the array of problems with self-destructiveness, unstable relationships, and fragile sense of reality. Conduct disorders can also be associated with other PD—for example, narcissistic personality disorder—as well as with depression and learning disorders such as dyslexia.

Equally complex is the differentiation between BPD and mood disorders. A vulnerability to affective dysregulation and a proneness to excessive rage may be significant predisposing factors to BPD. Children of bipolar parents present a range of psychiatric difficulties, including conduct disorders, substance abuse, and dysthymia. Clinical descriptions of childhood presentations of bipolar or dysthymic disorders portray moody, irritable, and affectively labile children with a low tolerance for frustration and explosive anger. More definite mood changes in late school-age years or adolescence should point to a diagnosis of mood disorder, particularly exuberant affect, loud giggling, increased activity, disturbed sleep, recent onset of angry outbursts, and decreased attention. Manic adolescents may do poorly in school because of poor concentration or high-flown thinking or end relationships because of irritability or impulsivity. The acute onset of a depressive episode characterized by hypersomnia, psychomotor retardation, and psychosis in a child or adolescent with a family history of two or more generations with mood disorders is predictive of a bipolar course.

A history of trauma, particularly sexual abuse, is common in BPD. PTSD follows exposure to an identifiable, overwhelming stressor. Repeated traumatization can result in a response of reenactment, avoidance, dissociation, and hyperarousal that becomes woven into the child's or adolescent's habitual and pervasive patterns of coping, relating, and experiencing and can contribute to the development of BPD.

Eating disorders, particularly bulimia nervosa, are often part of the clinical picture of BPD. In younger children, separation anxiety disorder should be differentiated from the clinginess and distress following separations characteristic of borderline youths. Children with an uncomplicated anxiety disorder do not exhibit the impulsivity, rage, self-destructiveness, and impaired sense of reality typical of borderline psychopathology.

The cross-sectional presentation of mood disorders and externalizing disorders (including ADHD and conduct disorder) may mimic BPD. Thus, adequate treatment of the comorbid disorder and a longitudinal perspective is needed before arriving at a dual diagnosis.

Another group of disorders that must be ruled out is schizophrenia spectrum disorders. Transient psychotic episodes, suspiciousness, and a disturbed sense of reality are typical features of BPD, but delusions, hallucinations, and loose associations are not. A family history of schizophrenia spectrum disorders is suggestive of these disorders.

The most common disorders cooccurring with adult BPD include avoidant, dependent, narcissistic, antisocial, and paranoid personality disorders. The child clinical literature often confuses BPD and schizotypal personality disorder. Schizotypal children present magical thinking, unusual perceptual experiences, idiosyncratic fantasies, and paranoid ideation, all common in borderline children. Schizotypal children, however, have a family history of schizophrenia spectrum disorders and present constricted or inappropriate affect, oddness of speech and behavior, and extreme discomfort in social situations, which contrast with the intense and dramatic affect and hunger for social response of borderline youths.

Children with a schizoid disorder of childhood may become intensely absorbed in a world of fantasy of their own making but are not distressed by their social isolation and do not attempt to coerce caretakers and peers to play roles prescribed by their idiosyncratic fantasies or play themes.

Children in the process of developing narcissistic personality or histrionic personality disorders present significant clinical overlap with children with BPD. Narcissistic or histrionic children are self-centered and self-absorbed, need constant attention, respond with rage to rejection or indifference, alternate between idealization and devaluation, are seductive and manipulative, express affect with undue intensity and drama, and, in the case of narcissistic youngsters, are preoccupied with fantasies of power and control. Borderline children, however, display much greater impulsivity, self-destructiveness, affective instability, disturbances in the sense of reality, and transient psychotic episodes.

Course and Prognosis

The few prospective longitudinal studies conducted to assess the course and prognosis of juvenile BPD have shown inconsistent findings. Some studies provide limited evidence of developmental continuity of BPD symptoms from adolescence into adulthood. But most support a developmental trajectory that begins with childhood externalizing disorder mixed with internalizing disorders leading to adolescent BPD and developing into adult BPD. For example, Crawford et al. (11) examined the developmental link between personality disorder symptoms (borderline, histrionic, and narcissistic) and comorbid internalizing and externalizing symptoms in a community sample of 407 adolescents. Cross-lagged longitudinal models tested the hypothesis that symptoms reflect primary disturbances that give rise to cooccurring internalizing and externalizing symptoms, versus the alternative hypothesis that these axis I symptom clusters reflect primary problems that interfere with normal personality development and lead to dysfunctional patterns of coping and relating. Instead of clearly supporting one hypothesis over the other, longitudinal models suggested gender-specific developmental effects that were partially consistent with both hypotheses.

Current evidence supports the conclusion that adolescence and young adulthood of BPD patients are marked by dramatic crises of affective dyscontrol, interpersonal storms, and impulsive and self-destructive behavior, which often require extensive use of health and mental health resources. Family dysfunction and occupational impairment associated with suicide risk and substance abuse are most notable during the late adolescent and young adult years and tend to decrease in intensity during middle age, a time when a significant percentage of patients with BPD "mellow" and are able to gain greater stability in their relationships.

Treatment

Psychopharmacotherapy

The use of medications can powerfully support the parents' competence and the alliance between parents and treaters. Randomized controlled trials (RCTs) of pharmacologic interventions with BPD children and adolescents are very limited and thus, pharmacotherapy is largely based on clinical studies and research with adults. Pharmacotherapy is also grounded in clinical experience with these youths and in studies documenting the effectiveness of medications in a range of related or comorbid child and adolescent problems. The role of pharmacotherapy in the treatment of children and adolescents with BPD is to target dysregulations of arousal, cognition, affect, and impulse.

Pharmacotherapy targets both the symptoms that emerge during episodes of acute psychobiologic decompensation and the trait vulnerabilities that represent an enduring diathesis to dysfunction. No one-to-one correspondence has been identified between specific neurobiologic vulnerabilities and types of PD. Thus, given the current level of knowledge, pharmacotherapy targets personality dimensions, such as affective dysregulation and impulsive-behavior dysregulation, and axis I disorders, such as depression, anxiety disorders, ADHD, and mood disorders. By impacting the neurobiologic underpinnings of arousal, cognition, affect, and impulse, pharmacotherapy creates optimal conditions for psychotherapy and family treatment.

Psychosocial Interventions

Children and adolescents can more readily become engaged in treatment when they are not buffeted by subjective distress, anxiety, or hyperarousal, or when their depressed energy level and reduced capacity for concentration have improved. Parents' position as provider of containment and support is enhanced when they collaborate with the treaters in administering medication effectively.

While BPD is not regularly evaluated or treated in routine clinical practice (72), its assessment and treatment has been identified as an important public health priority. This priority reflects the reality that evidence-based psychosocial treatment for BPD in adolescents is available (10). Prominent in this regard are mentalization-based treatment for adolescents (MBT-A) (63), dialectical behavior therapy (DBT) (73), and cognitive analytic therapy (CAT) (74) for which RCTs have been conducted (63). While these therapeutic modalities share some features, they can be distinguished by the mechanism of change they each assume. MBT assumes that the development of BPD in adolescence is grounded in a phase-specific compromise in the capacity to mentalize that occurs during adolescence. DBT synthesizes a change orientation from behavior therapy with an acceptance orientation from Zen philosophy specifically to target the emotional dysregulation, distress tolerance, and interpersonal difficulties associated with BPD. CAT integrates elements of psychoanalytic object relations theory and cognitive psychology and identifies procedural sequences or chains of events that may include thoughts, emotions, and motivations to explain how a target problem (e.g., interpersonal aggression) is established and maintained.

Recently, focus in BPD intervention has shifted to indicate prevention. This notion is promoted by Chanen et al. who suggest that neither stand-alone universal, nor selective prevention of BPD is currently practical, and argue for indicated prevention that targets adolescents with subthreshold (two or three) symptoms of BPD. Data have begun to emerge to suggest indicated prevention to be a viable option for early intervention in BPD (75).

References

1. Millon T, Davis AD: *Disorders of Personality: DSM-IV and Beyond.* New York, Wiley, 1996.
2. Bleiberg E: Borderline disorders in children and adolescents: the concept, the diagnosis and the controversies. *Bull Menninger Clin* 58(2): 169–196, 1994.
3. Griffiths M: Validity, utility and acceptability of borderline personality disorder diagnosis in childhood and adolescence: survey of psychiatrists. *Psychiatrist* 35:19–22, 2011.
4. American Psychiatric Association: *Diagnostic and Statistical Manual of Mental Disorders, Fifth Edition (DSM-5).* Arlington, TX, American Psychiatric Publishing, 2013.
5. Fonagy P, Speranza M, Luyten P, Kaess M, Hessels C, Bohus M: ESCAP expert article: borderline personality disorder in adolescence: an expert research review with implications for clinical practice. *Eur Child Adolesc Psychiatry* 24:1307–1320, 2015.
6. Miller AL, Muehlenkamp JJ, Jacobson CM: Fact or fiction: diagnosing borderline personality disorder in adolescents. *Clin Psychol Rev* 28:969–981, 2008.
7. Chanen AM, Jovev M, McCutchion LK, Jackson HJ, McGorry PD: Borderline personality disorder in young people and the prospects for prevention and early intervention. *Curr Psychiatry Rev* 4:48–57, 2008.
8. Westen D, DeFife JA, Malne JC, DiLallo J: An empirically derived classification of adolescent personality disorders. *J Am Acad Child Adolesc Psychiatry* 53:528–549, 2014.
9. Sharp C: Bridging the gap: the assessment and treatment of adolescent personality disorder in routine clinical care. *Arch Dis Child* 102(1):103–108, 2017.
10. Sharp C, Fonagy P: Practitioner review: borderline personality disorder in adolescence—recent conceptualization, intervention, and implications for clinical practice. *J Child Psychol Psychiatry* 56(12):1266–1288, 2015.
11. Crawford TN, Cohen P, Brook JS: Dramatic-erratic personality disorder symptoms: II. Developmental pathways from early adolescence to adulthood. *J Pers Disord* 15:336–350, 2001.
12. Mattanah JJ, Becker DF, Levy KN, Edell WS, McGlashan TH: Diagnostic stability in adolescents followed up 2 years after hospitalization. *Am J Psychiatry* 152:889–894, 1995.
13. Crawford TN, Cohen P, Brook JS: Dramatic-erratic personality disorder symptoms: I. Continuity from early adolescence into adulthood. *J Pers Disord* 15:319–335, 2001.
14. Kaess M, Brunner R, Chanen A: Borderline personality disorder in adolescence. *Pediatrics* 134:782–793, 2014.
15. Zanarini MC, Frankenberg FR, Hennen J, Silk KR: The longitudinal course of borderline psychopathology: 6-year prospective follow-up of the phenomenology of borderline personality disorder. *Am J Psychiatry* 160:274–283, 2003.
16. Becker DF, Grilo CM, Edell WS, McGlashan TH: Diagnostic efficiency of borderline personality disorder criteria in hospitalized adolescents: comparison with hospitalized adults. *Am J Psychiatry* 159:2042–2047, 2002.
17. Michonski JD, Sharp C, Steinberg L, Zanarini MC: An item response theory analysis of the DSM-IV borderline personality disorder criteria in a population-based sample of 11- to 12-year-old children. *Personal Disord* 4(1):15–22, 2013.
18. Nock MK, Joiner TE Jr, Gordon KH, Lloyd-Richardson E, Prinstein MJ: Non-suicidal self-injury among adolescents: diagnostic correlates and relation to suicide attempts. *Psychiatry Res* 144:65–72, 2006.
19. Ha C, Balderas JC, Zanarini MC, Oldham J, Sharp C: Psychiatric comorbidity in hospitalized adolescents with borderline personality disorder. *J Clin Psychiatry* 75:e457–e464, 2014.
20. Mahler MS, Ross JR Jr, de Friess Z: Clinical studies in benign and malignant cases of childhood psychosis (schizophrenia-like). *Am J Orthopsychiatry* 19:295–305, 1949.
21. Ekstein R, Wallerstien J: Observations on the psychology of borderline and psychotic children. *Psychoanal Study Child* 19:344–372, 1954.
22. Kernberg O: Borderline personality organization. *J Am Psycholoanal Assoc* 15:641–685, 1967.
23. Petti TA, Vela RM: Borderline disorders of childhood: an overview. *J Am Acad Child Adolesc Psychiatry* 29(3):327–337, 1990.
24. Goldman SJ, D'Angelo EJ, DeMaso DR, Mezzacappa E: Physical and sexual abuse histories among children with borderline personality disorder. *Am J Psychiatry* 149(12):1723–1726, 1992.
25. Bernstein DP, Cohen P, Velez CN, Schwab-Stone M, Siever LJ, Shinsato L: Prevalence and stability of the DSM-III-R personality disorders in a community-based survey of adolescents. *Am J Psychiatry* 150:1237–1243, 1993.
26. Chanen AM, Jackson HJ, McGorry PD, Allot KA, Clarkson V, Yuen HP: Two-year stability of personality disorder in older adolescent outpatients. *J Pers Disord* 18:526–541, 2004.
27. Chanen AM, McCutchion LK, Jovev M, Jackson HJ, McCorry PD: Prevention and early intervention for borderline personality disorder. *Med J Aust* 187(7 Suppl):S18–S21, 2007.
28. Grilo CM, McGlashan TH, Quinlan DM, Walker ML, Greenfeld D, Edell WS: Frequency of personality disorders in two age cohorts of psychiatric inpatients. *Am J Psychiatry* 155(1):140–142, 1998.
29. Fonagy P, Lyten P: A multilevel perspective on the development of borderline personality disorder In: Cicchetti D (ed): *Development and Psychopathology.* New York, Wiley, 2015.
30. Bornavalova MA, Hicks BM, Iacono WG, McGue M: Stability, change, and heritability of borderline personality disorder traits from adolescence to adulthood: a longitudinal twin study. *Dev Psychopathol* 21:1335–1353, 2009 Fall.
31. Distel MA, Trull TJ, Derom CA, et al.: Heritability of borderline personality disorder features is similar across three countries. *Psychol Med* 38:1219–1229, 2008.
32. Kenler KS, Aggen SH, Czajkosski N, et al.: The structure of genetic and environmental risk factors for DSM-IV personality disorders: a multivariate twin study. *Arch Gen Psychiatry* 65:1438–1446, 2008.
33. Hankin BL, Barrocas AL, Jenness J, et al.: Association between 5-HTTLPR and borderline personality traits among youth. *Front Psychiatry* 2:6, 2011.
34. Belsky DW, Caspi A, Arseneault L, et al.: Etiological features of borderline personality related characteristics in a birth cohort of 12-year-old children. *Dev Psychopathol* 24:251–265, 2012.
35. Skodol AE, Siever LJ, Livesley WJ, Gunderson JG, Pfohl B, Widiger TA: The borderline diagnosis II: biology, genetics and clinical course. *Biol Psychiatry* 51:951–963, 2002.
36. Rocco AC, Amirthavasagam S, Zukzanis KK: Amygdala and hippocampal volume reductions as candidate endophenotypes for borderline personality disorder: a meta-analysis of magnetic resonance imaging studies. *Psychiatry Res* 201:245–252, 2012.
37. Herpetz SC, Dietrich TM, Wenning B, et al.: Evidence of abnormal amygdala functioning in borderline personality disorder: a functional MRI study. *Biol psychiatry* 50:292–298, 2001.
38. Whittle S, Chanen AM, Fornito A, McGorry PD, Pantelis C, Yucel M: Anterior cingulate volume in adolescents with first-presentation borderline personality disorder. *Psychiatry Res* 172:155–160, 2009.
39. Brunner R, Henze R, Parzer P, et al.: Reduced prefrontal and orbitofrontal gray matter in female adolescents with borderline personality disorder: is it disorder specific? *Neuroimage* 49:114–120, 2010.
40. Chanen AM, Velakoulis D, Carison K, et al.: Orbitofrontal, amygdala and hippocampal volumes in teenagers with first-presentation borderline personality disorder. *Psychiatry Res* 163:116–125, 2008.

41. New AS, Carpenter DM, Perez-Rodriquez MM, et al.: Developmental differences in diffusion tensor imaging parameters in borderline personality disorder. *J Psychiatry Res* 47:1101–1109, 2013.
42. New AS, Goodman M, Triebwasser J, Siever LJ: Recent advances in the biological study of personality disorders. *Psychiatr Clin North Am* 31(3):441–461, 2008.
43. Sebastian C, Viding E, Williams KD, Blakemore SJ: Social brain development and the affective consequences of ostracism in adolescence. *Brain Cogn* 72:134–145, 2010.
44. Chanen AM, Kaess M: Developmental pathways to borderline personality disorder. *Curr Psychiatry Rep* 14:45–53, 2012.
45. Crawford TN, Cohen PR, Chen H, Anglin DM, Ehrensaft M: Early maternal separation and the trajectory of borderline personality disorder symptoms. *Dev Psychopathol* 21:1013–1030, 2009 Summer.
46. Cohen P, Chen H, Gordon K, Johnson J, Brook J, Kasen S: Socioeconomic background and the developmental course of schizotypal and borderline personality disorder symptoms. *Dev Psychopathol* 20:633–650, 2008 Spring.
47. Johnson JG, Cohen P, Brown J, Smailes EM, Bernstein DP: Childhood maltreatment increases risk for personality disorders during early adulthood. *Arch Gen Psychiatry* 56:600–606, 2008.
48. Lyons-Ruth K, Bureau JF, Holmes B, Easterbooks A, Brooks NH: Borderline symptoms and suicidality/self-injury in late adolescence: prospectively observed relationship correlates in infancy and childhood. *Psychiatry Res* 206(2–3):273–281, 2013.
49. Carlson EA, Egeland B, Sroufe LA: A prospective investigation of the development of borderline personality disorder: a review of recent findings and methodological challenges. *Dev Psychopathol* 21:1311–1334, 2009.
50. Wilkinson R, Pickett K: *The Spirit Level: Why Equality is Better for Everyone*. London, Penguin Books, 2009.
51. Lis S, Bohus M: Social interaction in borderline personality disorder. *Curr Psychiatry Rep* 15:338, 2013.
52. Fonagy P, Gergely G, Jurist E, Target M: *Affect Regulation, Mentalization and the Development of the Self*. New York, Other Press, 2002.
53. Agrawal HR, Gunderson J, Bjarne M, Holmes BM, Lyons-Ruth K: Attachment studies with borderline patients: a review. *Harv Rev Psychiatry* 12(2):94–104, 2004.
54. Fonagy P, Leigh T, Steele M, et al.: The relation of attachment status, psychiatric classification, and response to psychotherapy. *J Consult Clin Psychol* 64:22–31, 1996.
55. Brendel GR, Stern E, Silbersweig DA: Defining the neurocircuitry of borderline personality disorder: functional neuroimaging approaches. *Dev Psychopathol* 17(4):1197–1206, 2005 Fall.
56. Bateman A, Fonagy P: *Mentalization-Based Treatment for Personality Disorders*. Oxford, Oxford University Press, 2016.
57. Bleiberg E: *Treating Personality Disorders in Children and Adolescents: A Relational Approach*. New York, Guilford Press, 2001.
58. Posner MI, Rothbart MK, Vizueta N, et al.: Attentional mechanisms of borderline personality disorder. *Proc Natl Acad Sci U S A* 99(25):16366–16370, 2002.
59. Kutcher SP, Marton P, Korenblum M: Adolescent bipolar illness and personality disorder. *J Am Acad Child Adolesc Psychiatry* 29(3):355–358, 1990.
60. Carndell LE, Patrick MP, Hobson RP: 'Still-face' interactions between mothers with borderline personality disorder and their 2-month-old infants. *Br J Psychiatry* 183:239–247, 2003.
61. Arnsten RF: The biology of being frazzled. *Science* 280:1711–1712, 1998.
62. Leichtman M, Nathan S: A clinical approach to the psychological testing of borderline children. In: Robson KS (ed): *The Borderline Child: Approaches to Etiology, Diagnosis, and Treatment*. New York, McGraw-Hill, 1983.
63. Rossouw TI, Fonagy P: Mentalization-based treatment for self-harm in adolescents: a randomized controlled trial. *J Am Acad Child Adolesc Psychiatry* 51:1304–1313, 2012.
64. Kaes M, Von Ceumern-Lindenstjerna IA, Parzer P, et al.: Axis I and II comorbidity and psychosocial functioning in female adolescents with borderline personality disorder. *Psychopathology* 46:55–62, 2013.
65. Zanarini MC, Williams AA, Lewis RE: Reported pathological childhood experiences associated with the development of borderline personality disorder. *A M J Psychiatry* 154(8):1101–1106, 1997.
66. First MB, Gibbon M, Spitzer RL, Williams JB, Benjamin LS: *User's Guide for the Structured Clinical Interview for DSM-IV Axis II Personality Disorders (SCID-II)*. Washington, DC, American Psychiatric Press, 1997.
67. Chanen AM, Jovev M, Djaja D, et al.: Screening for borderline personality disorder in outpatient youth. *J Pers Disord* 22:353–364, 2008.
68. Sharp C, Steinberg L, Temple J, Newlin E: An 11-item measure to assess borderline traits in adolescents: refinement of the BPFSC using IRT. *Personal Disord* 5(1):70–78, 2014.
69. Eppright TD, Kashani JH, Robison BD, Reid JC: Comorbidity of conduct disorder and personality disorders in an incarcerated juvenile population. *Am J Psychiatry* 150(8):1233–1236, 1993.
70. Myers WC, Burket RC, Otto TA: Conduct disorder and personality disorders in hospitalized adolescents. *J Clin Psychiatry* 54(1):21–26, 1993.
71. Guzder J, Paris J, Zelkowitz P, Feldman R: Psychological risk factors for borderline pathology in school-age children. *J Am Acad Child Adolesc Psychiatry* 38(2):206–212, 1999.
72. Chanen A, Sharp C, Hoffman P, and the Global Alliance for Prevention and Early Intervention for Borderline Personality Disorder: Prevention and early intervention for borderline personality disorder: a public health priority. *World Psychiatry* 16(2):215–216, 2017.
73. Mehlum L, Tørmoen AJ, Ramberg M, et al.: Dialectical behavior therapy for adolescents with repeated suicidal and self-harming behavior: a randomized trial. *J Am Acad Child Adolesc Psychiatry* 53(10):1082–1091, 2014.
74. Chanen AM, Jackson HJ, McCutcheon LK, et al.: Early intervention for adolescents with borderline personality disorder using cognitive analytic therapy: randomised controlled trial. *Br J Psychiatry* 193(6):477–484, 2008.
75. Chanen AM, McCutcheon L: Prevention and early intervention for borderline personality disorder: current status and recent evidence. *Br J Psychiatry Suppl* 54:S24–S29, 2013.

5.14 ■ GENDER VARIANCE AND GENDER DYSPHORIA

CHAPTER 5.14 ■ GENDER DYSPHORIA AND GENDER INCONGRUENCE

JACK L. TURBAN III, ANNELOU L. C. DE VRIES, AND KENNETH J. ZUCKER

INTRODUCTION

Transgender (gender incongruent) youth include children and adolescents who experience a marked incongruence between their gender assigned at birth and their gender identity (1). Since the last edition of this volume, which was published 10 years ago (2), there has been a remarkable increase in attention to transgender issues across the life span. Television has begun to highlight transgender individuals from childhood to adulthood (3,4). News outlets from *The New York Times Magazine* to *Le Monde* have explored the life experiences of transgender youth (5–7). Legislative bodies have examined transgender rights through restroom access, hate crime legislation, insurance regulations, and antidiscrimination policies, with physicians playing key roles in these discussions (8). Parallel to this growing attention, there has been a marked increase in the establishment of specialized gender identity clinics for children and adolescents in North America and in Europe (9), which likely reflects the marked increase in referrals that has been noted internationally (10–12). At the same time, the scientific literature on gender incongruence has expanded as well,

TABLE 5.14.1

TERMINOLOGY

Term	Definition
Gender assigned at birth/natal sex/ birth sex	Gender assigned to an infant at birth, generally based on physical characteristics (genitalia, etc.)
Experienced gender/gender identity	An individual's psychological understanding of one's own gender
Affirmed gender	An individual's psychological understanding of one's own gender, typically referring to one who lives socially as that understood gender
Sexuality/sexual orientation	Refers to the types of individuals toward whom one is romantically and/or sexually attracted
Transgender	Refers to an individual whose gender identity is incongruent with that of one's gender assigned at birth. Sometimes also used as a term for an individual whose gender identity is binary opposite one's gender assigned at birth.
Gender dysphoria	Refers to psychological distress in relationship to one's experienced gender; is also the classification used in the DSM 5 (requiring fulfillment of certain clinical criteria)
Cisgender	Refers to an individual whose experienced gender matches that of one's gender assigned at birth
Gender non-conforming/gender variant	Refers to variation from developmental norms in gender role behavior that may be considered as nongender stereotypical. This may include identifying as both genders or identifying with neither gender, among others.
Transsexual	Typically used to refer to individuals who desire medical interventions to align their physiologies with the gender identities. This term is used synonymously with transgender by some and has largely fallen out of favor (though it was used commonly in the past).

with a flux of new studies on co-occurring psychological functioning, long-term follow-up studies, biologic correlates, and outcomes of medical interventions. Practicing child and adolescent psychiatrists should be familiar with the basics of this field to appropriately assess and treat these patients.

TERMINOLOGY AND DEFINITIONS

Terminology in this specialized area is continuously evolving. This section describes terms and definitions that are in most common usage at this time, but different regions, cultures, and families may have their own preferred terminology (Table 5.14.1).

The term *gender assigned at birth* refers to a newborn's gender (boy, girl, indeterminate), as generally declared by a medical professional. Other relevant terms include *natal sex* and *birth sex*. The term *biologic sex* is somewhat vague, as it is unclear whether it would be based on karyotyping of the sex chromosomes, internal reproductive structures, the configuration of the external genitalia, etc. The vast majority of newborns are assigned the gender of boy or girl through prenatal diagnostics or, at birth, based on genital anatomy. A small number of newborns may be classified as having a "disorder of sex development" (DSD), or what others have called "differences of sex development" (13), congenital conditions in which biologic parameters of sex (e.g., the sex chromosomes, the gonads or the configuration of the external genitalia, etc.) are incongruent with one another. These conditions include complete or partial androgen insensitivity syndrome, mixed gonadal dysgenesis, 5-alpha-reductase deficiency, penile agenesis, and congenital adrenal hyperplasia (CAH), among others. Such patients may experience gender identity issues that can be unique from those experienced by those without a DSD (14).

Experienced gender refers to one's gendered sense of self as a boy, as a girl, or some alternative gender that is different from the traditional boy–girl dichotomy (e.g., "gender fluid," "agender," or "nonbinary"). Other terms include *affirmed gender* (typically used for individuals who have transitioned socially to living as the desired gender). For the majority of individuals, experienced gender matches the gender assigned at birth. These individuals are referred to as *cisgender*. For some patients, experienced gender is opposite from the gender assigned at birth, and these individuals are referred to as *transgender*.

Transgender, gender variant, and *gender nonconforming* are sometimes used as terms for individuals whose experienced gender does not strictly match that of their gender assigned at birth. One who experiences psychological distress in relation to one's gender identity may be referred to as *gender dysphoric*. Gender dysphoria is the diagnostic term that has been adopted in the DSM-5 (see below) (1).

Sexual attraction or *sexual orientation* is a separate concept from gender identity. Sexual orientation refers to the types of individuals toward whom one is romantically or sexually attracted. Terms such as androphilia (attraction to males), gynephilia (attraction to females), biphilia (attraction to males and females), and aphilia (attraction to neither males nor females) are used more commonly nowadays, slowly replacing older terms such as heterosexual, bisexual, homosexual, and asexual. In the scientific literature, the sexual orientation of individuals who identify as transgender can be described in relation to their experienced gender or their gender assigned at birth. For example, an adolescent female who identifies as male and is sexually attracted to females can be described as "heterosexual" in relation to experienced gender but as "homosexual" in relation to birth sex (15). From either a clinical or research perspective, it is critical to identify the referent in describing a patient's sexual orientation. Most individuals who identify as transgender will describe their sexual orientation in relation to their gender identity, not their gender assigned at birth (e.g., a transgender woman who is attracted to men would likely consider herself to be heterosexual).

The "genderbread person" has been developed as an educational tool to clarify the distinctions among *gender assigned at birth, experienced gender,* and *sexual orientation* (Figure 5.14.1). Note that as a published educational instrument, this graphic diverges somewhat from the contemporary terminology we described above. Nonetheless, this tool has proven useful for introducing this terminology to families and students new to the topics of gender and sexuality.

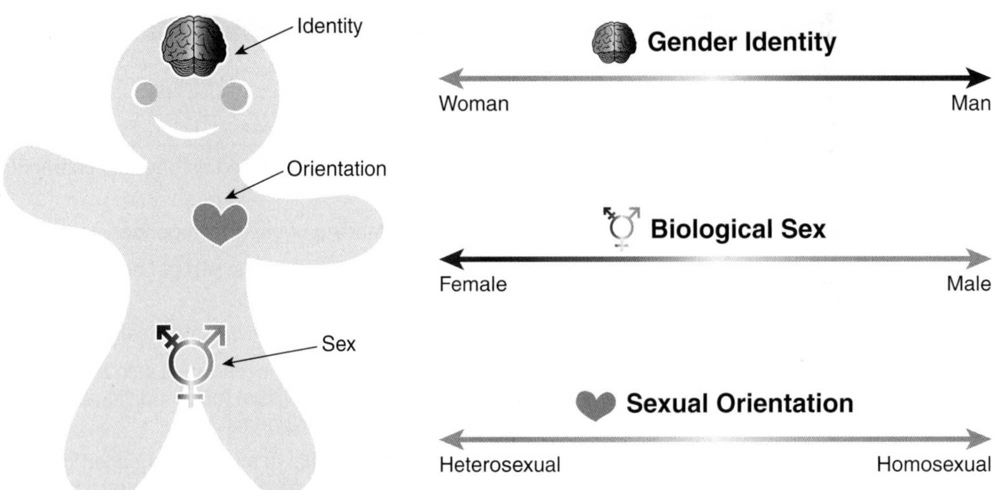

FIGURE 5.14.1. The Genderbread Person. The genderbread person is an educational tool used to explain the distinctions between experienced gender (termed gender identity here), gender assigned at birth (termed biological sex here), and sexual or romantic orientation. This educational tool may be useful for students new to the field and when explaining these phenomena to families with gender incongruent and gender dysphoric children. These terms are further described in Table 5.14.1. (Modified from Killermann S. (2016). *The Genderbread Person.* Available at: itspronouncedmetrosexual.com)

HISTORY OF GENDER IDENTITY AND MEDICINE

John Money (1921–2006) was a psychologist and sexologist whose empirical and theoretical contributions regarding gender identity, gender role, and gender development were innovative and of great influence, beginning in the 1950s. Money originally proposed a theory of "gender neutrality," suggesting that gender identity was predominantly determined by social factors, including the gender assigned at birth and subsequent socialization processes (16). Money proposed that, for individuals with a DSD, early surgical interventions to correct genital ambiguity were often needed so that a child could then be supported with rearing in the gender assigned at birth.

Over the past few decades, Money's original theory of gender neutrality at birth has been challenged by various lines of evidence suggesting the importance of biologic factors, particularly patterns of prenatal hormone exposure, in also contributing to gender identity formation and differentiation. For example, chromosomal females with CAH, assigned female at birth are exposed to elevated levels of prenatal testosterone and many of these girls are behaviorally masculinized and a higher percentage than the general population develop gender dysphoria and transition from male to female (17,18).

Perhaps the most widely cited case pertains to a biologically "normal" male (one of a pair of identical twins) who, after a circumcision accident at the age of 7 months led to penile ablation, underwent a vaginoplasty and was socially reassigned to female at the age of 17 months (19,20).

Although this patient was described by Money (21) as a "tomboy" during childhood, subsequent follow-up revealed that the patient rejected estrogen therapy at the time of puberty and subsequently transitioned back to living as a male (19,20). Tragically, this patient committed suicide at the age of 38 (22). The "John–Joan" case, as it was called, has been used as evidence of the importance of biologic factors in contributing to a person's sense of gender identity. A subsequent summary of seven similar such patients reared as female after traumatic loss of the penis have shown both male and female gender identities in adolescence and adulthood, further complicating the picture (23).

In the 1960s, research into the developmental histories of adults with "transsexualism" suggested that childhood cross-gender identification was common in these individuals (24). This work was then followed by research with children who showed patterns of gender-related behavior similar to the recalled patterns of transsexual adults (24). During this period, there was much less attention given to adolescents with a marked history of cross-gender identification.

By the late 1990s, however, more attention was given to adolescents with a DSM diagnosis of gender identity disorder, including the possibility of treatments with gonadotropin-releasing hormone analogs (GnRHa), as reported by a research team in the Netherlands (25). This approach, described below, was ultimately outlined in the 2009 Endocrine Society Guidelines for the Treatment of Transsexual Persons (26) and in the periodically updated Standards of Care by the World Professional Association for Transgender Health (27). Research into these hormonal interventions has since garnered significant attention, including increased NIH funding to study the long-term benefits and risks of these endocrine treatments (28).

DIAGNOSIS AND ASSESSMENT

Gender identity diagnoses first entered the DSM in its third edition with three diagnoses: transsexualism, gender identity disorder of childhood, and atypical gender identity disorder. The essential feature of these three diagnoses was "an incongruence between anatomic sex and gender identity" (29). Revisions in the DSM-III-R were modest, though in this edition, exclusion of individuals with schizophrenia or a DSD was removed, noting that individuals with either of these diagnoses could also have a gender identity disorder (30).

In the DSM-IV, the three diagnoses from DSM-III were collapsed into the overarching diagnosis "gender identity disorder" with distinct criteria sets for children versus adolescents and adults. This edition also added a criterion stating "The disturbance causes clinically significant distress or impairment in social, occupational, or other important areas of functioning" (31).

The DSM-5 renamed "gender identity disorder" as "gender dysphoria," aiming to decrease stigma associated with the diagnosis while maintaining a diagnosis that could be used to secure access to care for those who needed it (32). The DSM-5 removed sexual orientation subtyping, but noted in the text its relevance in understanding variations in developmental trajectories and for research on biologic factors and long-term outcomes (1). The DSM-5 also made an effort to make the childhood diagnosis stricter, requiring more than just gender nonconforming behavior. The new criteria required that a child expresses an actual desire or insistence of being the other gender. The adolescent and adult criteria simultaneously became more inclusive, allowing for nonbinary gender identities that would allow for gender variant, but not strictly binary, transgender adolescents and adults to receive the diagnosis and subsequently access to care.

Current DSM-5 criteria for gender dysphoria in children require a marked incongruence between one's experienced/expressed gender and assigned gender, of at least 6 months' duration, as evidenced by at least six of eight criteria, one of which must be a strong desire to be of the other gender or an insistence that one is the other gender (or some alternative gender different from one's assigned gender) (1). Additionally, the patient must experience clinically significant distress or impairment in social, school, or other important areas of functioning as introduced in the DSM-IV (Table 5.14.2). DSM-5 criteria for gender dysphoria in adolescents and adults are similar, though with different requirements for the manifestation of gender dysphoria. This diagnosis requires at least two of six manifestations (Table 5.14.3). For a summary and rationale for the DSM-5 changes, see Zucker et al. (33).

Some have argued for use of the term "gender incongruence," including the Working Group on Sexual Disorders and Sexual Health for the forthcoming 11th edition of the

TABLE 5.14.2

DSM-5 CRITERIA FOR GENDER DYSPHORIA IN CHILDREN AND IN ADOLESCENTS AND ADULTS

Diagnostic Criteria
Gender Dysphoria in Children
302.6 (F64.2)

A. A marked incongruence between one's experienced/expressed gender and assigned gender, of at least 6 months' duration, as manifested by at least six of the following (one of which must be Criterion A1):
   1. A strong desire to be of the other gender or an insistence that one is the other gender (or some alternative gender different from one's assigned gender).
   2. In boys (assigned gender), a strong preference for cross-dressing or simulating female attire; or in girls (assigned gender), a strong preference for wearing only typical masculine clothing and a strong resistance to the wearing of typical feminine clothing.
   3. A strong preference for cross-gender roles in make-believe play or fantasy play.
   4. A strong preference for the toys, games, or activities stereotypically used or engaged in by the other gender.
   5. A strong preference for playmates of the other gender.
   6. In boys (assigned gender), a strong rejection of typically masculine toys, games, and activities and a strong avoidance of rough-and-tumble play; or in girls (assigned gender), a strong rejection of typically feminine toys, games, and activities.
   7. A strong dislike of one's sexual anatomy.
   8. A strong desire for the primary and/or secondary sex characteristics that match one's experienced gender.

B. The condition is associated with clinically significant distress or impairment in social, school, or other important areas of functioning.

Specify if:

- With a disorder of sex development (e.g., a congenital adrenogenital disorder such as 255.2 [E25.0] congenital adrenal hyperplasia or 259.50 [E34.50] androgen insensitivity syndrome).
- Coding note: Code the disorder of sex development as well as gender dysphoria.

Gender Dysphoria in Adolescents and Adults
302.85 (F64.1)

A. A marked incongruence between one's experienced/expressed gender and assigned gender, of at least 6 mo duration, as manifested by at least two of the following:
   1. A marked incongruence between one's experienced/expressed gender and primary and/or secondary sex characteristics (or in young adolescents, the anticipated secondary sex characteristics).
   2. A strong desire to be rid of one's primary and/or secondary sex characteristics because of a marked incongruence with one's experienced/expressed gender (or in young adolescents, a desire to prevent the development of the anticipated secondary sex characteristics).
   3. A strong desire for the primary and/or secondary sex characteristics of the other gender.
   4. A strong desire to be of the other gender (or some alternative gender different from one's assigned gender).
   5. A strong desire to be treated as the other gender (or some alternative gender different from one's assigned gender).
   6. A strong conviction that one has the typical feelings and reactions of the other gender (or some alternative gender different from one's assigned gender).

B. The condition is associated with clinically significant distress or impairment in social, occupational, or other important areas of functioning.

Specify if:

- **With a disorder of sex development** (e.g., a congenital adrenogenital disorder such as 255.2 [E25.0] congenital adrenal hyperplasia or 259.50 [E34.50] androgen insensitivity syndrome).
- **Coding note:** Code the disorder of sex development as well as gender dysphoria.

Specify if:

- **Posttransition:** The individual has transitioned to full-time living in the desired gender (with or without legalization of gender change) and has undergone (or is preparing to have) at least one cross-sex medical procedure or treatment regimen—namely regular cross-sex hormone treatment or gender reassignment surgery confirming the desired gender (e.g., penectomy, vaginoplasty in a natal male; mastectomy or phalloplasty in a natal female).

TABLE 5.14.3

TREATMENT OF TRANSGENDER YOUTH

Timing	Intervention
Prepubertal	No endocrine intervention recommended. Patient should have regular psychotherapy to discuss gender identity and assess possible future need for hormonal intervention.
Early signs of puberty	Pubertal blockade with gonadotropin-releasing hormone analogs to prevent the development of secondary sex characteristics and provide additional time for psychotherapy and consideration regarding partially reversible interventions.
Age 14+ or 16+, depending on the center	Cross-sex hormonal therapy with estrogen or testosterone. Less frequently with other endocrine-acting medications that have less favorable side effect profiles.
Age 18 for most centers	Gender-affirming surgeries may be considered. Note that some surgeries may be performed earlier for select patients (generally mastectomies for transgender males).

International Classification of Diseases. This group suggested that the term gender incongruence highlights that not all transgender individuals experience dysphoria. The group noted that the term gender dysphoria might increase inappropriate stigmatization and pathologization. Only for the practical purpose of preserving access to medical care did the group recognize the necessity of classification. The group additionally argued that the diagnosis be moved out of the chapter on mental health and behavioral disorders and into another section, provisionally termed Conditions Related to Sexual Health (34).

EPIDEMIOLOGY OF GENDER DYSPHORIA AND GENDER NONCONFORMITY

A range of methodologic challenges, including but not limited to shifting terminology and stigma associated with self-identification, have made it difficult to establish the true prevalence of gender dysphoria or gender incongruence.

Prevalence in Adults

In adults, most studies have used the numbers of individuals that seek out clinical care for gender-affirming treatment as a proxy for determining prevalence in a certain country or catchment area. A recent meta-analysis based on 21 studies that applied this method concluded that the prevalence of transsexualism (the definition used in most of these studies) was 6.8 transwomen in 100,000 gender at birth-assigned males (1:14,705) and 2.6 transmen in 100,000 gender at birth-assigned females (1:38,461) (35). A time trend was also found, with recent studies reporting higher prevalence rates. These studies are, of course, limited by the fact that they do not include transgender individuals who do not seek medical care. Indeed, much higher prevalence rates, ranging from 4.2% having an ambivalent gender identity to around 0.5% identifying as transgender and considering medical interventions, are suggested by recent studies that have used broader definitions and probability samples (36–38). A recent population-based survey in the United States found that 0.6% of adults self-identified as transgender, with rates ranging from 0.3% to 0.8% in the states for which data were available. Compared to the older age groups, young adults between 18 and 24 years old were most likely to identify as transgender (39).

Prevalence in Children and Adolescents

Although formal epidemiologic studies of gender dysphoria in children and adolescents have not been conducted, looser or more liberal definitions of "caseness" in children and adolescents have been examined in several recent studies. In a random sample of 2,730 grade 6 to 8 students from San Francisco, Shields et al. (40) found that 1.3% self-identified as "transgender" in response to the question "What is your gender?," with the other response options being female or male. In a random sample of 8,166 high school students from New Zealand, Clark et al. (41) found that 1.2% self-identified as transgender and 2.5% reported that they were not sure about their gender, in response to the question "Do you think you are a transgender?" which was followed by a definition of the term. Interestingly, another 1.7% reported that they did not understand the question.

In the 1999 standardization sample of the Child Behavior Checklist (CBCL) for children aged 6 to 18 years and the Youth Self-Report (YSR) form, aged 11 to 18 years, there is one item pertaining to gender identity ("Wishes to be of opposite sex") (42). On the CBCL (total $N = 3{,}210$), less than 1% of parents of nonreferred boys and 1.2% of nonreferred girls endorsed this item as either somewhat or sometimes true or very true or often true. The percentages were higher for referred boys and girls (2.8% and 5.4%, respectively). On the YSR, about 10% of nonreferred girls and 2% of nonreferred boys endorsed this item compared to about 18% of referred girls and 3% of referred boys. In the prior 1991 CBCL standardization sample, two age groups were reported (4 to 11 and 12 to 18). For the 4 to 11 year olds, 1% of parents of nonreferred boys and girls endorsed this item compared to 3% and 5% of referred boys and girls. For the 12 to 18 year olds, none of the parents endorsed this item for nonreferred boys and girls compared to 2% and 5% of referred boys and girls. Consistent with the original CBCL and YSR standardization studies, two consistent findings emerge: the item is endorsed more often for girls than for boys and it is endorsed more often for referred than for nonreferred children and adolescents.

Gender Assigned at Birth Ratio

Of prepubertal children referred to gender identity clinics, the majority has a male gender assigned at birth. Among 577 Canadian children referred to a gender identity clinic between 1976 and 2011, the male-to-female ratio was 4.49:1 (12). This was significantly higher than the 2.02:1 ratio in the Netherlands (12). These differences are theorized, in part, to be a reflection of increased parental anxiety regarding gender-variant behavior in males compared to females, particularly in North America. For adolescents with gender dysphoria, the gender ratio is much closer to 1:1 and appears to be more consistent across nations (10). Of note, however, there has been a recent temporal shift from more birth-assigned males (prior to 2006) to more birth-assigned females (2006 to 2013), though the ratio remains closer to 2:1 in either direction (10).

BIOLOGIC AND PSYCHOSOCIAL DETERMINANTS

The etiology of cross-gender identification and behavior continues to be elusive. While psychological and social factors were once the focus of study, especially in normative gender development, attention has shifted to biologic mechanisms more recently. At present, the evidence suggests that both psychosocial and biologic elements are involved. A monocausal mechanism is unlikely and gender dysphoria most likely results from a complex interaction between these factors (43).

Biologic Factors

Twin studies suggest a strong heritable component with additional environmental contributors. In a large-scale CBCL study of Dutch twins (N = 23,393) ages 7 and 10 (44), monozygotic (MZ) and dizygotic (DZ) twins were compared and estimated genetic factors contributed to 70% of cross-gender behavior (as assessed via the two CBCL gender items). Another study of 314 MZ and DZ twins (mean ages 9.4 and 10.1 years, respectively) roughly replicated this finding, with genetic factors contributing to 62% of the variance on a DSM-IV-based gender dysphoria scale (45). In a third study of 3,337 Japanese MZ and DZ twins ranging in age from 3 to 26 years (46), there was also strong evidence for genetic factors for females, but much less so for males.

Many studies, both in animals and humans, have shown that differences in brain anatomy and function in cis-gender males and females underlie the sex differences in their behavioral (47). Sex hormones play an important role in these differences. The *organizational* effect, predominantly prenatally but also during puberty, leads to the sex differences in brain structures. On average, males have larger brain volumes, more white matter, gray matter, and cerebrospinal fluid than females, although when corrected for total volume, females have more gray matter and a larger volume of the cortex (48–50).

The sexual differentiation hypothesis suggests that transgender individuals may have brain structures and brain functioning more closely aligned with their experienced gender (51). Postmortem studies have suggested a sex reversal in several hypothalamic nuclei in transgender adults (52,53). More recent neuroimaging techniques have allowed the in vivo study of brain morphology and functioning of larger numbers of adolescents and adults with gender incongruent feelings (50,54). Findings of these studies are more mixed. Before they received any medical gender affirmative treatment, brain anatomy with regard to volume, gray and white matter, and cerebrospinal fluid did not differ compared to their birth-assigned sex (50). Differences are, however, found with regard to the white matter microstructure, with results of transgender individuals in between males and females (50). In the realm of functional neuroimaging, task-related imaging studies show that transgender people may have either similar reactions as their experienced gender (e.g., smelling odorous steroids (55)) or activity different from their assigned gender as well as their experienced gender (e.g., mental rotation (56)), or not different from their assigned gender (e.g., verbal fluency (57)). The results so far show that we are still far away from a situation where imaging or other medical testing may serve as a diagnostic tool.

In animal studies, where prenatal hormones can be manipulated, the strong effect of prenatal testosterone on gender role behavior is clear (47). The effects on gender identity, however, can only be studied in humans. Individuals with DSD may be exposed to high levels of prenatal testosterone, and XX individuals with CAH (58) indeed have higher rates of gender dysphoria and cross-gender identification (18). The majority of female-raised individuals with CAH (~95%), however, appear to develop a female gender identity (17). Other evidence for the importance of prenatal testosterone comes from studies in XY individuals with complete androgen insensitivity syndrome (CAIS) who lack the receptors necessary to respond to endogenous testosterone. The vast majority of these patients develop a female gender identity, suggesting that downstream testosterone signaling may be important for the development of a male gender identity (59). Others have noted that these patients are reared unambiguously as females and that social factors may play a strong role in their female identity formation (60). Some studies have shown that those with CAIS have lower scores on tests of female identity scales (61) and there have been some case reports of gender dysphoria ultimately leading to gender-affirming surgeries (62). This notably could be secondary to the psychological stress of learning about the diagnosis, as well as the possibility of undetected functional androgen receptors (43). Overall, studies of gender identity in individuals with DSD, while implicating androgens in the development of gender identity, have yet to show a simple direct relationship.

Psychosocial Factors

Past literature has investigated the potential role of parental characteristics on the development of gender dysphoria (maternal wish for a child of the opposite gender, paternal absence, and parental psychological functioning, among others). None of these hypotheses have been validated (43). Mothers of gender dysphoric boys have been noted to have higher scores on the Beck Depression Inventory and the Diagnostic Interview for Borderlines (63), but these higher scores might be due to external pressures placed on these parents by unaccepting social environments and such studies cannot determine the direction of causation. One study noted that gender dysphoric boys were rated as more feminine and "beautiful" by blinded college students (64) while another study of gender dysphoric girls showed that these girls were rated as less "cute" (65), raising the question of whether perceived physical appearance and resultant social treatment may contribute to gender incongruence. An alternative interpretation of this data is that those with a more male gender identity might alter their appearances to appear more "masculine" (e.g., culturally masculine haircuts) while those with a more female gender identity alter their appearances to appear more "feminine" (66). Some have suggested that a lack of parental limit-setting, particularly around cross-gender behavior, is associated with gender dysphoria (67), though this again does not prove causation, as more insistence on cross-gender behavior (i.e., transgender identity or stronger cross-gender behavior preferences) may make this limit-setting more difficult. Overall, there have been no proven causative psychosocial factors in the development of gender incongruence. Since studies on normative gender identity development show that cognitive psychological factors and social environment play a role, this may also be the case for gender nonconforming development.

CLINICAL COURSE

Persistence of Gender Dysphoria from Childhood to Adolescence

The natural history of gender identity for children who express gender nonconforming or transgender identities is an area of active research (68). To date, the long-term follow-up studies of clinic-referred children have been based on samples that have included children who were either threshold or subthreshold for the gender identity diagnosis in DSM-III, III-R, or IV and some of the earliest studies began prior to the availability of formal diagnostic criteria.

These follow-up studies have classified participants as either "persisters" or "desisters" with regard to their cross-gender identification, using various metrics (semi-structured interviews based on DSM criteria for gender identity disorder, dimensional scores on standardized questionnaires, etc.). Ristori and Steensma (69) have provided the most recent summary of 10 follow-up studies, in which the percentage of participants classified as persisters ranged from 2% to 39% (collapsed across natal boys and girls). In one study (70), the percentage of natal girls who were persisters appeared to be substantially higher than the percentage of natal boys (50% vs. 12%), but in two other studies from the same clinic, the percentage was similar across natal sex (71,72).

One criticism of these studies is that either formal diagnostic criteria were not used (because they were not available at the time of the study) or that subthreshold cases were included. Some studies have found that threshold cases were more likely to be classified as persisters (73), but other studies have not (72). It has also been suggested that more recent cohorts (after the year 2000) have found higher rates of persistence (12% to 39% (61,64–66)) than older cohorts (2% to 9% prior to 2000 (74,75)); however, it is not clear if such differences are related to variations in sampling procedures or something more substantive. Comparisons of persisters with desisters have found that the intensity of gender dysphoria (using dimensional metrics), older age at the time of assessment in childhood, a lower social class background, and having a female gender assigned at birth are associated with higher rates of persistence (72,73). Despite this work, it remains difficult to predict, for an individual child, the likelihood of cross-gender identification persistence from childhood into adolescence (73).

Persistence of Gender Dysphoria from Adolescence to Adulthood

In contrast to the low rates of persistence from childhood into adolescence, it appears that the vast majority of transgender adolescents persist in their transgender identity (76).

Childhood Gender-Variant Behavior and Sexual Orientation

Childhood gender-variant behavior has been found to be a strong predictor of a same-sex sexual orientation (using gender assigned at birth as a reference point) in adults. In a study of 879 Dutch boys and girls, gender-variant behavior was assessed using the CBCL and sexual orientation was assessed 24 years later (77). It was found that the prevalence of a same-sex sexual orientation was, depending on the domain (attraction, fantasy, behavior, and identity), between 8.4 and 15.8 times higher in the gender-variant subgroup as compared to the nongender-variant subgroup. In summary, the current literature, though limited as described above, suggests that the majority of gender incongruent prepubescent children will grow up to identify as cisgender individuals with either a bisexual or a same-sex sexual orientation (70,72,74).

ASSOCIATED COEXISTING PSYCHIATRIC CONDITIONS AND BEHAVIORS

Children and adolescents with gender incongruence exhibit higher internalizing and externalizing psychopathology as compared to nonreferred controls, with internalizing psychopathology being more common, particularly in natal boys (78–84). One hypothesis is that this problem behavior is a result of minority stress and dysphoria toward their gender assigned at birth. These individuals are also subjected to rates of peer bullying as high as 80% (85). Poor peer relations is one of the strongest investigated predictors for behavioral and emotional problems in gender incongruent youth (79). In a study of 105 gender dysphoric Dutch adolescents whose parents completed the Diagnostic Interview Schedule for Children (DISC), 32.4% had one or more psychiatric disorders, with 21% suffering from anxiety, 12.4% from mood disorders, and 11.4% from disruptive disorders (85). A study with the same DISC measure in prepubertal children revealed higher percentages, with 52% having one or more psychiatric disorders other than GD (80).

Chart review studies of gender incongruent youth presenting to specialized gender identity clinics have shown similarly high or even higher rates of psychiatric conditions: mood (12.4% to 64%), anxiety (16.3% to 55%), and disruptive disorders (9% to 11.4%) (82,83,86–88). The prevalence range across studies may be secondary to cultural differences, differing diagnostic criteria, and differing ages of clinical populations. These psychiatric conditions appear to become more common in gender incongruent individuals with increasing age. Some studies have shown that older transgender youth suffer a greater burden of co-occurring psychiatric conditions (82), and that gender incongruent adults suffer a greater burden of co-occurring psychiatric conditions as compared to adolescents (89).

Self-harming Behavior and Suicidality

Self-harming behavior and suicide attempts are prevalent among gender incongruent youth. Gender clinics have reported high rates of past suicide attempts by patients presenting for care: Boston (9.3%, mean age 14.8 (87)), London (10%, mean age 13.5 (82)), Los Angeles (30%, mean age 19.2 (86)). Rates of self-harm and suicidality appear to increase with age within this population (90).

Autism Spectrum Disorder

A number of studies have shown autism spectrum disorder (ASD) symptoms to be over-represented among transgender individuals. Clinical level rates of ASD symptomatology in transgender adults have been reported in the range of approximately 5% to 20% (91–93). A single study of 204 children and adolescents referred for gender dysphoria reported an ASD prevalence of 7.8% as measured by the Diagnostic Interview for Social and Communication Disorders (94). This compares to rates of ASD in the general population of around 1% (95). Two studies found increased gender variance (5.4%, 11.3%), defined by a positive response to "wishes to be of opposite sex" sometimes or often on the CBCL or YSR) in referred children, adolescents, and adults with ASD compared to nonreferred controls (96,97). However, the same was true for an ADHD-referred control sample (97), raising the issue that a higher probability of gender variance is characteristic of clinic-referred samples in general. Several hypotheses for shared underlying etiology that explains the link between these two conditions have been suggested (98–100).

Clinically, the co-occurrence of gender dysphoria and ASD may complicate transgender care, as diagnosing gender dysphoria can be difficult (e.g., in the context of the rigid thinking that is characteristic of ASD). Case reports have described instances cross-gender identification represented a transient preoccupation in youth with ASD (101). Additionally, language difficulties can make expression of gender dysphoria difficult for patients with ASD. Nonetheless, a comprehensive narrative review of the literature has shown a role for transition with pubertal blockade and cross-sex hormonal therapy in these patients following an extended diagnostic process (99). By use of a Delphi method, a group of experts on the ASD-gender dysphoria co-occurrence developed initial clinical guidelines assessment and treatment for adolescent transgender care (98). Careful diagnosis of both conditions by specific specialists, collaboration of clinicians from both fields, an extended diagnostic phase, and risk assessment and safety issues are part of the suggested management protocol.

THERAPEUTICS

Treatment of Prepubescent Children

Over the past 10 years, best practice treatment for children with gender dysphoria has been the subject of intense controversy (102). As noted below, there are now three broad approaches that have been delineated in the literature: (1) the oldest one—characterized by Dreger (103) as the "therapeutic model"—consists of efforts, either directly (e.g., via specific suggestions that parents can implement in the day-to-day environment) or indirectly (e.g., psychodynamically informed approaches that treat the putative underlying "causes" of the gender dysphoria) and actively attempt to reduce cross-gender identification (104); (2) an intermediate approach, which some have characterized as "watchful waiting" (105), in which no direct efforts are made to "prohibit" a child's gender-variant behavior, but one that also advises parents to keep options open about the child's long-term gender identity and to avoid early social transition; (3) and, more recently, an approach characterized by Ehrensaft (106) as the "affirmative model" that considers all outcomes of gender identity to be equally valid and desirable and allows children who express a desire to socially transition to do so after careful counseling. These approaches have been discussed in great detail in three Task Force reports (107–109), in a special volume of the *Journal of Homosexuality* (102), and various other essays and case reports, the references for which can be found in these major reviews.

For the nonspecialist, there are several key issues to keep in mind when appraising this literature: (1) Some of these approaches may be influenced by particular theoretical formulations regarding the determinants of gender dysphoria and these formulations guide or influence recommended treatment plans; (2) there are no randomized controlled trials that have compared the effects of these treatments with regard to both short-term and long-term outcomes. Indeed, Byne et al. (109) noted that, by and large, "the highest level of evidence…can best be characterized as expert opinion" (p. 762); (3) with some rare exceptions (110), there are no manualized or even semi-manualized treatments that a clinician can follow in developing a therapeutic plan. Thus, the clinician needs to self-educate by reading about the therapeutic model that one intends to follow and tailor it on a case-by-case basis. Below, we provide relatively brief summaries of these three treatment approaches.

Promoting Identification with the Gender Assigned at Birth

This first approach aims, through psychosocial interventions, to reduce the child's cross-gender identification and gender dysphoria. These treatments (which have been described in the literature since the 1960s) have, however, been quite varied. They include classical behavior therapy, psychodynamic therapy (including psychoanalysis and dynamically informed play psychotherapy), parental counseling, and parent-guided interventions in the naturalistic environment (e.g., encouragement of peer relations of the same natal sex) (110,111).

Perhaps the underlying assumption of all of these approaches rests on the view that gender identity is not yet fixed in childhood and may be malleable through psychosocial treatments. There is also an implicit assumption or value judgment that might be inferred from this approach, namely that all things considered a child's long-term adaptation might be easier if he or she could come to feel content with a gender identity that matches their natal sex and to avoid the necessity of a lifelong regimen of cross-sex hormonal treatment and sex-reassignment surgery (or what nowadays is also called gender-affirming surgery).

Critics of this approach have argued that there is nothing inherently "wrong" with a cross-gender identity and have challenged the view that trying to change such an identity is warranted. Indeed, there are now several US states and one province in Canada that have passed legislation stating that it is inappropriate to try and change a minor's gender identity when the minor is unable to consent to the treatment, but exempt from this directive is "identity exploration" (112). Critics have also rightly noted that some of the earliest proponents of this treatment held the belief that it might also reduce the odds of the child's later development of a same-sex sexual orientation (113), although other proponents of this treatment rejected this as an ethically defensible treatment goal (111). Another expressed concern has been that this type of treatment might cause a child to feel shame or other negative and maladaptive feelings (108).

Watchful Waiting

The second approach takes an intermediate therapeutic position. On the one hand, it does not recommend an early gender social transition on the grounds that the extant follow-up studies have shown that the majority of children with gender dysphoria desist for one reason or another. On the other hand, it does not explicitly recommend any type of limit-setting on the child's gender-variant behavior, with the exception that in certain environments it might be risky or dangerous to display such behavior, which Hill et al. (114) described as the "only at home" rule.

This approach also does not privilege one type of long-term outcome over another, noting that it is difficult to predict outcome for an individual child and that the more important focus should be on the child's general psychosocial adjustment and well-being. This approach does, however, include recommendations to parents that they try to encourage in their child a variety of gender-related interests and social affiliation with children of both genders. In some respects, the "watchful waiting" label is a bit of a misnomer because clinical protocols appear to include information provided to the parents that is more than "wait-and-see." As noted by de Vries and Cohen-Kettenis (115), appropriate limit-setting with good explanation of why the limits are set to their child may be helpful so that the child will learn "that not all desires will be met," which is important because "someone's deepest desire or fantasy to have been born in the body of the other gender will never be completely fulfilled." Although social transition according to this approach is not recommended at a very young age, an increasing number of children have already socially transitioned when they come to gender identity clinics (115). Some of these children may have no clear memories of a time that they were socially living in the birth-assigned gender and have stopped talking about being born different from their experienced gender. In these cases, it is encouraged that parents create an open situation where the child has the possibility of returning to the birth-assigned gender. It is discussed with the child that when gender identity feelings change, it is nothing to be ashamed of, that nobody will be angry, that the child may speak out, and that it is good to have tried. A form of psychotherapy that helps the child to verbalize his or her feelings may be advised so that, by the time the child may come back for GnRHa, the child is able to talk about his or her feelings and can give informed consent.

Affirmative Approach

The affirmative approach theorizes that clinician and parental attempts to push children with gender incongruence toward conforming to their gender assigned at birth might produce shame and stigma that can ultimately lead to internalizing psychopathology (108). The approach considers all outcomes of gender identity to be equally desirable and affirms any gender identity the child expresses.

Though similar to the watchful waiting approach, an important departure is in its approach regarding early social transition. In the affirmative model, prepubertal children who ultimately express a desire to socially transition and live full time in their experienced gender (i.e., using cross-gender pronouns, a cross-gender name, cross-gender clothing, etc.) are allowed to do so. The approach to social transition must be carefully individualized with a nuanced understanding of the child's gender identification and the level of support within the child's community; there must also be an open discussion with the child highlighting that despite the social transition that the patient is free to transition back at any time (115).

Some have noted cases where this transition back to living as one's birth gender can be particularly difficult mostly due to fear of peer judgment (116), though this must be weighed against the potential negative consequences of refusing to affirm a child's identity and desire to transition socially. The affirmative model predicts that this lack of affirmation might lead to shame and consequent internalizing psychopathology (117). The therapeutic relationship in these cases could also be negatively affected if the clinician strongly discourages an early transition for a patient who ultimately persists in cross-gender identification.

Critics of social transitions in prepubertal children have raised the question of whether early social transition increases the rates of gender incongruence persistence from childhood into adolescence. Indeed, a multivariate regression analysis revealed that early social transition was associated with persistence (73). However, the direction of this association cannot be determined by this study. While some believe that prepubertal social transition makes children more likely to persist, the alternative interpretation is that those likely to persist are also more likely to undergo early social transition, due to currently unidentified factors. This additionally raises the ethical question of whether persistence should be considered an undesirable outcome. The affirmative model suggests that all outcomes of gender identity are equally desirable.

Separate from the question of persistence is the question of mental health outcomes following social transition. There is a relative paucity of literature studying the effect of prepubertal social transition. One study examined 73 American prepubertal children who were transgender in a binary fashion and allowed to socially transition. Parents of these children completed short forms for anxiety and depression at an unspecified time following the transition (118). Data from these scales revealed that these children had notably lower rates of internalizing psychopathology than previously reported children who did not transition. Furthermore, socially transitioned children in this study showed developmentally normal levels of depression and only minimally elevated (subclinical) levels of anxiety. It is important to note that families in this study had a relatively high median income, raising the question of whether this cohort is representative of a broader sociodemographic cohort (119). Though this early work suggests that socially transitioned children have better mental health metrics than previously reported children who did not socially transition, future research is needed to fully understand the dynamic and long-term effects of social transition in a broader population (119).

Treatment of Adolescents

Once children have reached puberty, transgender identity persists in the vast majority of cases, and medical intervention is often considered. At present, the effectiveness of an approach that includes puberty suppression and is followed by cross-hormones and surgeries has been evaluated in two studies on the same cohort of Dutch adolescents. The first study evaluated gender dysphoria and psychological functioning at two time points; first, when the 70 adolescents entered the clinic (mean age, 13.65 years), and second, just before they started cross-hormones (mean age, 16.64 years). Of interest, while adolescents improved with regard to psychological functioning on several domains, gender dysphoria did not improve and all adolescents went on with the next step of gender-affirming hormones (120). The second study added a third assessment, around one year after gender affirmative surgeries, when the first 55 adolescents who had been in this treatment protocol had reached young adulthood (mean age, 20.70 years). This time, gender dysphoria was resolved and psychological functioning measures had even further improved with scores that were comparable to normative samples. The same accounted for quality of life, subjective happiness, and satisfaction with life scores (121). These positive results are promising and give trust that starting treatment at a relatively young age is possible. However, the results come from only one clinic and concern a highly selected sample that received support from their parents and often their further school and social environment that started the treatment only after extensive assessment and received further mental health counseling during the years of treatment. Whether the same positive results can be expected for the larger number of adolescents that are treated at clinics that strongly vary in their approach to gender-variant adolescents has yet to be determined.

Assessing Eligibility

According to Endocrine Society Guidelines, hormonally based medical intervention may be initiated at the earliest signs of puberty (i.e., Tanner 2 or 3) (26). Other eligibility criteria include meeting criteria for gender dysphoria (termed gender identity disorder in the 2009 guidelines), experiencing dysphoria toward early pubertal changes, having adequate psychological and social support for treatment, understanding the risks and benefits of treatment, and not suffering from a psychiatric comorbidity that would interfere with treatment (26). To assess eligibility, most clinics offer an assessment by a mental health professional that sees the adolescent and his or her family over a longer period of time before decisions regarding medical interventions are made. This time is used to prepare for the long period of medical treatment with lifelong consequences that is likely to follow and weigh the pros and cons of treatment so that an informed decision can be made. Although many adolescents come with a clear wish for medical treatment, some are not sure yet and want to explore their gender dysphoric feelings more broadly. Sometimes co-occurring psychiatric difficulties like ASD with rigid thinking, severe depression with acute suicidality or anxiety with worrisome avoidance and school refusal, complicate this diagnostic work and make coming to regular medical checkups and taking medication impossible. Treatment of these psychiatric disorders may then be necessary before endocrine intervention. The importance of parental support for the psychological well-being of adolescents is widely acknowledged (122). The time that is used for assessment may also be helpful in addressing parents' concerns and improving the adolescent–parent relationship. The time that is needed before medical intervention is provided may vary for each individual case, but tends to be longer when psychosocial comorbidities occur (115,123).

Fully Reversible Interventions (Pubertal Blockade)

The first such intervention (implemented at Tanner 2 or 3 of puberty) is pubertal blockade with GnRHa. Gonadotropin-releasing hormone is produced by neurons in hypothalamus. In prepubertal children, this hormone is secreted at very low levels. At the initiation of puberty, release of gonadotropin-releasing hormone becomes cyclical. This cyclical release of hormone results in release of follicle-stimulating hormone (FSH) and luteinizing hormone (LH) from the anterior pituitary. These hormones then enter the peripheral circulation, where they initiate the production of sex hormones (estrogen in natal women and testosterone in natal men). These hormones then initiate the irreversible development of secondary sex characteristics.

GnRHa (either implants, depot injections, or regular injections) maintain high levels of gonadotropin-releasing hormone in the circulation. Without physiologic cyclical fluctuations in GnRH levels, FSH and LH are not released and all downstream signaling is prevented. This allows the patient to remain in a prepubertal state (124).

Pubertal blockade prevents the development of irreversible secondary sex characteristics (voice deepening, breast development, etc.) and provides additional time for gender dysphoric children to decide if they wish to fully transition physically into the body of the opposite sex. Therefore, it does not need to be considered actual gender affirmative medical treatment, but rather may function as an extended diagnostic phase. If the GnRHa implant is removed or the injections discontinued, the effects of the medication are reversible. With removal or discontinuation of the GnRHa, the patient will undergo natal puberty. Follow-up studies into young adulthood on the first cohort of puberty-suppressed adolescents are reassuring with regard to side effects. Although there was some deprived bone density, there were no concerns regarding liver and kidney functioning and lipid profile (125,126). Some advise clinicians to evaluate bone age for these patients every 3 months (26) and have regular blood monitoring to ensure that the central axis of puberty is sufficiently suppressed (26).

Partially Reversible Interventions (Cross-sex Hormonal Therapy)

Around the age of 16, patients may choose to move onto the next intervention of cross-sex hormonal therapy with estrogen or testosterone, according to Endocrine Society guidelines. Some groups have noted that cross-sex hormones can be instituted earlier, as delaying puberty outside the developmentally appropriate age may cause social problems for these youth (127). Additional criteria for cross-sex hormonal therapy are identical to those for GnRHa in the Endocrine Society guidelines.

Cross-sex hormones will initiate the development of secondary sex characteristics of the desired puberty. These interventions are mostly irreversible and carry a more significant side-effect profile. The most prominent side effect of estrogen therapy is hypercoagulability, though clinicians prescribing these medications should be aware of the full spectrum of side effects. Of note, this hypercoagulability can be particularly problematic for patients undergoing high-risk surgery such as vaginoplasty. Patients on these medications should be regularly monitored for serum hormone concentrations and maintained within normal testosterone and estrogen serum concentrations for their desired gender. Spironolactone has been used for its antiandrogenic properties in select cases but is generally not considered a first-line treatment given its unfavorable side-effect profile as a diuretic (26).

Irreversible Interventions (Gender-Affirming Surgeries)

At the legal age of adulthood, patients may choose to undergo a variety of surgical interventions, including vaginoplasty, phalloplasty, scrotoplasty, breast augmentation, facial reconstruction, hysterectomy, reduction thyroid chondroplasty, among others. Patients should be carefully counseled on the risks and benefits of surgery. Specific surgical interventions are many and are out of scope for the purpose of this review. Of note, some surgical interventions may be considered earlier in the course of treatment. In the WPATH's Standards of Care, mastectomies are being considered earlier than age 18 (27).

Fertility Considerations

There is a paucity of research on the effects of pubertal blockade and cross-sex hormonal therapy on future fertility. Interested patients should be counseled on fertility preservation options early in treatment. Include LGBT Health study showing that most transgender youth do not desire fertility preservation, however most adults which they had. More longitudinal research needed (128).

SUMMARY

Gender incongruent and gender dysphoric youth represent a vulnerable demographic with high rates of co-occurring psychiatric conditions and suicidal behavior, likely secondary to minority stress and dysphoria related to living in a body that does not match one's experienced gender. Prepubescent children with gender-variant behavior or identification are best supported with psychotherapy. For those children who continue to have strong cross-sex identification in adolescence, pubertal blockade, and cross-sex hormone therapy to align patients' bodies with their identities have been shown to improve mental health outcomes.

References

1. American Psychiatric Association: *Diagnostic and Statistical Manual of Mental Disorders*, 5th ed. Arlington, VA, American Psychiatric Press, 2013.
2. Zucker KJ: Gender identity disorder. In: Martin A, Volkmar FR (eds): *Lewis's Child and Adolescent Psychiatry: A Comprehensive Textbook*, 4th ed. Baltimore, MD, Lippincott Williams & Wilkins, 669–680, 2007.
3. Morrison EG: Transgender as ingroup or outgroup? Lesbian, gay, and bisexual viewers respond to a transgender character in daytime television. *J Homosex* 57:650–665, 2010.
4. Vrouenraets LJ, Fredriks AM, Hannema SE, Cohen-Kettenis PT, de Vries MC: Perceptions of sex, gender, and puberty suppression: a qualitative analysis of transgender youth. *Arch Sex Behav* 45:1697–1703, 2016, doi:10.1007/s10508-016-0764-9
5. Padawer R: Boygirl. *The New York Times Magazine*, 18–23, 36, 46, 12 August 2012.
6. Rosin H: A boy's life. *The Atlantic* 302(4):56–59, 62, 64, 66–68, 70–71, 2008.
7. Chayet S: *Moi, Nikki, 13 ans, née Niko*. Le Monde, 2014. Available at: http://www.lemonde.fr/m-actu/article/2014/12/10/moi-nikki-13-ans-nee-niko_4534297_4497186.html. Accessed 10 December 2014.
8. Schuster MA, Reisner SL, Onorato SE: Beyond bathrooms—meeting the health needs of transgender people. *N Engl J Med* 375:101–103, 2016.
9. Hsieh S, Leininger J: Resource list: clinical care programs for gender-nonconforming children and adolescents. *Pediatr Ann* 43:238–244, 2014.
10. Aitken M, Steensma TD, Blanchard R, et al.: Evidence for an altered sex ratio in clinic-referred adolescents with gender dysphoria. *J Sex Med* 12:756–763, 2015.
11. Chen M, Fuqua J, Eugster EA: Characteristics of referrals for gender dysphoria over a 13-year period. *J Adolesc Health* 58:369–371, 2016.
12. Wood H, Sasaki S, Bradley SJ, et al.: Patterns of referral to a gender identity service for children and adolescents (1976–2011): age, sex ratio, and sexual orientation [Letter to the Editor]. *J Sex Marital Ther* 39:1–6, 2013.
13. Hughes IA, Houk C, Ahmed SF, et al.: Consensus statement on management of intersex disorders. *Arch Dis Child* 91:554–563, 2006.

14. Meyer-Bahlburg HF, Baratz Dalke K, Berenbaum SA, Cohen-Kettenis PT, Hines M, Schober JM: Gender assignment, reassignment and outcome in disorders of sex development: update of the 2005 consensus conference. *Horm Res Paediatr* 85:112–118, 2016.
15. Lawrence AA: Sexual orientation versus age of onset as bases for typologies (subtypes) for gender identity disorder in adolescents and adults. *Arch Sex Behav* 39:514–545, 2010.
16. Money J, Hampson JG, Hampson JL: Imprinting and the establishment of gender role. *Arch Neurol Psychiatry* 77:333–336, 1957.
17. Dessens AB, Slijper FM, Drop SL: Gender dysphoria and gender change in chromosomal females with congenital adrenal hyperplasia. *Arch Sex Behav* 34:389–397, 2005.
18. Pasterski V, Zucker KJ, Hindmarsh PC, et al.: Increased cross-gender identification independent of gender role behavior in girls with congenital adrenal hyperplasia: results from a standardized assessment of 4- to 11-year-old children. *Arch Sex Behav* 44:1363–1375, 2015.
19. Colapinto J: *As Nature Made Him: The Boy Who Was Raised as a Girl.* New York, Harper Collins Publishers, 2000.
20. Diamond M, Sigmundson HK: Sex reassignment at birth: long-term review and clinical implications. *Arch Pediatr Adolesc Med* 151:298–304, 1997.
21. Money J: Ablatio penis: normal male infant sex-reassigned as a girl.*Arch Sex Behav* 4:65–71, 1975.
22. The Associated Press. *David Reimer, 38, Subject of the John/Joan Case.* 2004. Available at: http://www.nytimes.com/2004/05/12/us/david-reimer-38-subject-of-the-john-joan-case.html?_r=0. Accessed 12 May 2004.
23. Meyer-Bahlburg HFL: Gender identity outcome in female-raised 46,XY persons with penile agenesis, cloacal exstrophy of the bladder, or penile ablation. *Arch Sex Behav* 34:423–438, 2005.
24. Green R: *Sexual Identity Conflict in Children and Adults.* New York, Basic Books, 1974.
25. Cohen-Kettenis PT, van Goozen SH: Pubertal delay as an aid in diagnosis and treatment of a transsexual adolescent. *Eur Child Adolesc Psychiatry* 7:246–248, 1998.
26. Wylie CH, Cohen-Kettenis PT, Delemarre-van de Waal H, et al.: Endocrine treatment of transsexual persons: an Endocrine Society Clinical Practice Guideline. *J Clin Endocrinol Metab* 94:3132–3154, 2009.
27. Coleman E, Bockting W, Botzer M, et al.: Standards of care for the health of transsexual, transgender and gender non-conforming people, version 7. *Int J Transgenderism* 13:165–232, 2011.
28. Reardon S: Largest ever study of transgender teenagers set to kick off. *Nature* 531:560, 2016.
29. American Psychiatric Association: *Diagnostic and Statistical Manual of Mental Disorders,* 3rd ed. Washington, DC, Author, 1980.
30. American Psychiatric Association: *Diagnostic and Statistical Manual of Mental Disorders,* 3rd ed., rev. Washington, DC, Author, 1987.
31. American Psychiatric Association: *Diagnostic and Statistical Manual of Mental Disorders,* 4th ed.Washington, DC, Author, 1994.
32. Vance SR, Cohen-Kettenis PT, Drescher J, et al.: Opinions about the DSM gender identity disorder diagnosis: results from an international survey administered to organizations concerned with the welfare of transgender people. *Int J Transgenderism* 12:1–14, 2010.
33. Zucker KJ, Cohen-Kettenis PT, Drescher J, Meyer-Bahlburg HF, Pfäfflin F, Womack WM: Memo outlining evidence for change for gender identity disorder in the DSM-5. *Arch Sex Behav* 42:901–914, 2013.
34. Drescher J, Cohen-Kettenis PT, Reed GM: Gender incongruence of childhood in the ICD-11: controversies, proposal, and rationale. *Lancet Psychiatry* 3:297–304, 2016.
35. Arcelus J, Bouman WP, Van Den Noortgate W, Claes L, Witcomb G, Fernandez-Aranda F: Systematic review and meta-analysis of prevalence studies in transsexualism. *Eur Psychiatry* 30:807–815, 2015.
36. Conron KJ, Scott G, Stowell GS, Landers SJ: Transgender health in Massachusetts: results from a household probability sample of adults. *Am J Public Health* 102:118–122, 2012.
37. Kuyper L, Wijsen C: Gender identities and gender dysphoria in the Netherlands. *Arch Sex Behav* 43:377–385, 2014.
38. Van Caenegem E, Wierckx K, Elaut E, et al.: Prevalence of gender nonconformity in Flanders, Belgium. *Arch Sex Behav* 44:1281–1287, 2015.
39. Andres R, Flores JL, Gates GJ, et al.: *How Many Adults Identify as Transgender in the United States?* Los Angeles, CA, The Wiliams Institute, 2016.
40. Shields JP, Cohen R, Glassman JR, Whitaker K, Franks H, Bertolini I: Estimating population size and demographic characteristics of lesbian, gay, bisexual, and transgender youth in middle school. *J Adolesc Health* 52:248–250, 2013.
41. Clark TC, Lucassen MF, Bullen P, et al.: The health and well-being of transgender high school students: results from the New Zealand adolescent health survey (Youth'12). *J Adolesc Health* 55:93–99, 2014.
42. Achenbach TM, Rescorla LA: *Manual for the ASEBA School-Age Forms & Profiles: An Integrated System of Multi-informant Assessment.* Burlington, VT, University of Vermont, Research Center for Children, Youth, & Families, 2001.
43. Steensma TD, Kreukels BP, de Vries AL, Cohen-Kettenis PT: Gender identity development in adolescence. *Horm Behav* 64:288–297, 2013.
44. van Beijsterveldt CE, Hudziak JJ, Boomsma DI: Genetic and environmental influences on cross-gender behavior and relation to behavior problems: a study of Dutch twins at ages 7 and 10 years. *Arch Sex Behav* 35:647–658, 2006.
45. Coolidge FL, Thede LL, Young SE: The heritability of gender identity disorder in a child and adolescent twin sample. *Behav Genet* 32:251–257, 2002.
46. Sasaki S, Ozaki K, Yamagata S, et al.: Genetic and environmental influences on traits of gender identity disorder: a study of Japanese twins across developmental stages. *Arch Sex Behav* 45:1681–1695, 2016.
47. Hines M: Gender development and the human brain. *Annu Rev Neurosci* 34:69–88, 2011.
48. Ruigrok AN, Salimi-Khorshidi G, Lai MC, et al.: A meta-analysis of sex differences in human brain structure. *Neurosci Biobehav Rev* 39:34–50, 2014.
49. Giedd JN, Raznahan A, Mills KL, Lenroot RK: Magnetic resonance imaging of male/female differences in human adolescent brain anatomy. *Biol Sex Differ* 3(1): 2012, doi:10.1186/2042–6410–3–19.
50. Guillamon A, Junque C, Gomez-Gil E: A review of the status of brain structure research in transsexualism. *Arch Sex Behav* 45:1615–1648, 2016.
51. Swaab DF, Garcia-Falgueras A: Sexual differentiation of the human brain in relation to gender identity and sexual orientation. *Funct Neurol* 24:17–28, 2009.
52. Kruijver FP, Zhou JN, Pool CW, Hofman MA, Gooren LJ, Swaab DF: Male-to-female transsexuals have female neuron numbers in a limbic nucleus. *J Clin Endocrinol Metab* 85:2034–2041, 2000.
53. Zhou JN, Hofman MA, Gooren LJ, et al.: A sex difference in the human brain and its relation to transsexuality. *Nature* 378:68–70, 1995.
54. Kreukels BP, Guillamon A. Neuroimaging studies in people with gender incongruence. *Int Rev Psychiatry* 28:120–128, 2016.
55. Berglund H, Lindstrom P, Dhejne-Helmy C, Savic I: Male-to-female transsexuals show sex-atypical hypothalamus activation when smelling odorous steroids. *Cereb Cortex* 18:1900–1908, 2008.
56. Schoning S, Engelien A, Bauer C, et al.: Neuroimaging differences in spatial cognition between men and male-to-female transsexuals before and during hormone therapy. *J Sex Med* 7:1858–1867, 2010.
57. Soleman RS, Schagen SE, Veltman DJ, et al.: Sex differences in verbal fluency during adolescence: a functional magnetic resonance imaging study in gender dysphoric and control boys and girls. *J Sex Med* 10:1969–1977, 2013.
58. Merke DP, Bornstein SR: Congenital adrenal hyperplasia. *Lancet* 365:2125–2136, 2005.
59. Mazur T: Gender dysphoria and gender change in androgen insensitivity or micropenis. *Arch Sex Behav* 34:411–421, 2005.
60. Hines M. Gonadal hormones and sexual differentiation of human brain and behavior. In: Pfaff DW, Arnold AP, Etgen AM, et al.: (eds.). *Hormones, Brain and Behavior,* 2nd ed. San Diego, CA, Academic Press, 1869–1910, 2009.
61. Richter-Appelt H, Discher C, Gedrose B: Gender identity and recalled gender related childhood play-behaviour in adult individuals with different forms of intersexuality. *Anthropol Anz* 63:241–256, 2005.
62. T'Sjoen G, De Cuypere G, Monstrey S, et al.: Male gender identity in complete androgen insensitivity syndrome. *Arch Sex Behav* 40:635–638, 2011.
63. Marantz S, Coates S: Mothers of boys with gender identity disorder: a comparison of matched controls. *J Am Acad Child Psychiatry* 30:310–315, 1991.
64. Zucker KJ, Wild J, Bradley SJ, Lowry CB: Physical attractiveness of boys with gender identity disorder. *Arch Sex Behav* 22:23–36, 1993.
65. Fridell SR, Zucker KJ, Bradley SJ, Maing DM: Physical attractiveness of girls with gender identity disorder. *Arch Sex Behav* 25:17–31, 1996.
66. McDermid SA, Zucker KJ, Bradley SJ, Maing DM: Effects of physical appearance on masculine trait ratings of boys and girls with gender identity disorder. *Arch Sex Behav* 27:253–267, 1998.
67. Zucker KJ, Bradley, SJ: *Gender Identity Disorder and Psychosexual Problems in Children and Adolescents.* New York, Guilford Press, 1995.
68. Olson KR: Prepubescent transgender children: what we do and do not know. *J Am Acad Child Adolesc Psychiatry* 55:155–156, 2016.
69. Ristori J, Steensma TD: Gender dysphoria in childhood. *Int Rev Psychiatry* 28:13–20, 2016.
70. Wallien MS, Cohen-Kettenis PT: Psychosexual outcome of gender-dysphoric children. *J Am Acad Child Adolesc Psychiatry* 47:1413–1423, 2008.
71. Drummond KD, Bradley SJ, Peterson-Badali M, Zucker KJ: A follow-up study of girls with gender identity disorder. *Dev Psychol* 44:34–45, 2008.
72. Singh D: *A Follow-up Study of Boys with Gender Identity Disorder.* Unpublished doctoral dissertation. University of Toronto, 2012.
73. Steensma TD, McGuire JK, Kreukels BPC, et al.: Factors associated with desistence and persistence of childhood gender dysphoria: a quantitative follow-up study. *J Am Acad Child Adolesc Psychiatry* 52:582–590, 2013.
74. Green R: *The "Sissy Boy Syndrome" and the Development of Homosexuality.* New Haven, CT, Yale University Press, 1987.

75. Zuger B: Early effeminate behavior in boys: outcome and significance for homosexuality. *J Nerv Ment Dis* 172:90–97, 1984.
76. Cohen-Kettenis PT, Pfäfflin F: *Transgenderism and Intersexuality in Childhood and Adolescence: Making Choices.* London, Sage, 2003.
77. Steensma TD, van der Ende J, Verhulst FC, Cohen-Kettenis PT: Gender variance in childhood and sexual orientation in adulthood: a prospective study. *J Sex Med* 10:2723–2733, 2013.
78. Cohen-Kettenis PT, Owen A, Kaijser VG, Bradley SJ, Zucker KJ: Demographic characteristics, social competence, and behavior problems in children with gender identity disorder: a cross-national, cross-clinic comparative analysis. *J Abnorm Child Psychol* 31:41–53, 2003.
79. Steensma TD, Zucker KJ, Kreukels BP, et al.: Behavioral and emotional problems on the Teacher's Report Form: a cross-national, cross-clinic comparative analysis of gender dysphoric children and adolescents. *J Abnorm Child Psychol* 42:635–647, 2014.
80. de Vries AL, Steensma TD, Cohen-Kettenis PT, VanderLaan DP, Zucker KJ: Poor peer relations predict parent- and self-reported behavioral and emotional problems of adolescents with gender dysphoria: a cross-national, cross-clinic comparative analysis. *Eur Child Adolesc Psychiatry* 25:579–588, 2016.
81. Wallien MS, Swaab H, Cohen-Kettenis PT: Psychiatric comorbidity among children with gender identity disorder. *J Am Acad Child Adolesc Psychiatry* 46:1307–1314, 2007.
82. Skagerberg E, Carmichael P: Internalizing and externalizing behaviors in a group of young people with gender dysphoria. *Int J Transgenderism* 14:105–112, 2013.
83. Holt V, Skagerberg E, Dunsford M: Young people with features of gender dysphoria: demographics and associated difficulties. *Clin Child Psychol Psychiatry* 21:108–118, 2016.
84. Kaltiala-Heino R, Sumia M, Tyolajarvi M, Lindberg N: Two years of gender identity service for minors: overrepresentation of natal girls with severe problems in adolescent development. *Child Adolesc Psychiatry Ment Health* 9: 2015, doi:10.1186/s13034-015-0042-y.
85. McGuire JK, Anderson CR, Toomey RB, Russell ST: School climate for transgender youth: a mixed method investigation of student experiences and school responses. *J Youth Adolesc* 39:1175–1188, 2010.
86. Olson J, Schrager SM, Belzer M, Simons LK, Clark LF: Baseline physiologic and psychosocial characteristics of transgender youth seeking care for gender dysphoria. *J Adolesc Health* 57:374–380, 2015.
87. Spack NP, Edwards-Leeper L, Feldman HA, et al.: Children and adolescents with gender identity disorder referred to a pediatric medical center. *Pediatrics* 129:418–425, 2012.
88. Khatchadourian K, Amed S, Metzger DL: Clinical management of youth with gender dysphoria in Vancouver. *J Pediatr* 164:906–911, 2014.
89. de Vries ALC, Kreukels BPC, Steensma TD, Doreleijers TA, Cohen-Kettenis PT: Comparing adult and adolescent transsexuals: an MMPI-2 and MMPI-A study. *Psychiatry Res* 186:414–418, 2011.
90. Aitken M, VanderLaan DP, Wasserman L, Stojanovski S, Zucker KJ: Self-harm and suicidality in children referred for gender dysphoria. *J Am Acad Child Adolesc Psychiatry* 55:513–520, 2016.
91. Jones RM, Wheelwright S, Farrell K, et al.: Female-to-male transsexual people and autistic traits. *J Autism Dev Disord* 42:301–306, 2012.
92. Pasterski V, Gilligan L, Curtis R: Traits of autism spectrum disorders in adults with gender dysphoria. *Arch Sex Behav* 43:387–393, 2014.
93. Pohl A, Cassidy S, Auyeung B, Baron-Cohen S: Uncovering steroidopathy in women with autism: a latent class analysis. *Mol Autism* 5:27, 2014.
94. de Vries AL, Noens IL, Cohen-Kettenis PT, van Berckelaer-Onnes IA, Doreleijers TA: Autism spectrum disorders in gender dysphoric children and adolescents. *J Autism Dev Disord* 40:930–936, 2010.
95. Lai MC, Lombardo MV, Baron-Cohen S: Autism. *Lancet* 383:896–910, 2014.
96. Strang JF, Kenworthy L, Dominska A, et al.: Increased gender variance in autism spectrum disorders and attention deficit hyperactivity disorder. *Arch Sex Behav* 43:1525–1533, 2014.
97. van der Miesen AI, Hurley H, Bal A, et al. Gender variance and autism spectrum disorder. Manuscript submitted for publication, 2016.
98. Strang JF, Meagher H, Kenworthy L, et al.: Initial clinical guidelines for co-occurring autism spectrum disorder and gender dysphoria in adolescents. *J Clin Child Adolesc Psychol* 2016. doi:10.1080/15374416.2016.1228462.
99. van der Miesen AI, Hurley H, de Vries AL: Gender dysphoria and autism spectrum disorder: a narrative review. *Int Rev Psychiatry* 28:70–80, 2016.
100. VanderLaan DP, Leef JH, Wood H, Hughes SK, Zucker KJ: Autism spectrum disorder risk factors and autistic traits in gender dysphoric children. *J Autism Dev Disord* 45:1742–1750, 2015.
101. Parkinson J: Gender dysphoria in Asperger's syndrome: a caution. *Australas Psychiatry* 22:84–85, 2014.
102. Drescher J, Byne W: Introduction to the special issue on "The Treatment of Gender Dysphoric/Gender Variant Children and Adolescents." *J Homosex* 59:295–300, 2012.
103. Dreger A: Gender identity disorder in childhood: inconclusive advice to parents. *Hastings Cent Rep* 39:26–29, 2009.
104. Zucker KJ, Wood H, Singh D, Bradley SJ: A developmental, biopsychosocial model for the treatment of children with gender identity disorder. *J Homosex* 59:369–397, 2012.
105. Zucker KJ: On the "natural history" of gender identity disorder in children [Editorial]. *J Am Acad Child Adolesc Psychiatry* 47:1361–1363, 2008.
106. Ehrensaft D: From gender identity disorder to gender identity creativity: true gender self child therapy. *J Homosex* 59:337–356, 2012.
107. American Psychological Association: Guidelines for psychological practice with transgender and gender nonconforming people. *Am Psychol* 70:832–864, 2015.
108. Adelson SL: Practice parameter on gay, lesbian, or bisexual sexual orientation, gender nonconformity, and gender discordance in children and adolescents. *J Am Acad Child Adolesc Psychiatry* 51:957–974, 2012.
109. Byne W, Bradley SJ, Coleman E, et al.: Report of the American Psychiatric Association Task Force on Treatment of Gender Identity Disorder. *Arch Sex Behav* 41:759–796, 2012.
110. Meyer-Bahlburg HF: Gender identity disorder in young boys: a parent-and peer-based treatment protocol. *Clin Child Psychol Psychiatry* 7:360–376, 2002.
111. Zucker KJ: Treatment of gender identity disorders in children. In: Blanchard R, Steiner BW (eds). *Clinical Management of Gender Identity Disorders in Children and Adults.* Washington, DC, American Psychiatric Press, 25–47, 1990
112. Green R: Banning therapy to change sexual orientation or gender identity in patients under 18 [Editorial]. *Am Acad Psychiatry Law* 45:7–11, 2017.
113. Pleak R. Ethical issues in diagnosing and treating gender-dysphoric children and adolescents. In: Rottnek M (ed.): *Sissies & Tomboys: Gender Nonconformity & Homosexual Childhood.* New York, New York University Press, 44–51, 1999.
114. Hill DB, Menvielle E: "You have to give them a place where they feel protected and safe and loved": the views of parents who have gender-variant children and adolescents. *J LGBT Youth* 6:243–271, 2009.
115. de Vries AL, Cohen-Kettenis PT: Clinical management of gender dysphoria in children and adolescents: the Dutch approach. *J Homosex* 59:301–320, 2012.
116. Steensma TD, Cohen-Kettenis PT: Gender transitioning before puberty? [Letter to the Editor]. *Arch Sex Behav* 40:649–650, 2011.
117. Edwards-Leeper L, Leibowitz S, Sangganjanavanich VF: Affirmative practice with transgender and gender nonconforming youth: expanding the model. *Psychol Sexual Orientat Gender Diversity* 3:165–172, 2016.
118. Olson KR, Durwood L, DeMeules M, McLaughlin KA: Mental health of transgender children who are supported in their identities. *Pediatrics* 137(3), 2016. doi:10.1542/peds.2015-3223.
119. Olson KR, Durwood L, DeMeules M, et al.: Author response to McKean, Vande Voort, and Croarkin (2016). *Pediatrics* 130(1), 2016. doi:10.1542/peds.2016-1203B.
120. de Vries AL, Steensma TD, Doreleijers TA, Cohen-Kettenis PT: Puberty suppression in adolescents with gender identity disorder: a prospective follow-up study.*J Sex Med* 8:2276–2283, 2011.
121. de Vries AL, McGuire JK, Steensma TD, Wagenaar EC, Doreleijers TA, Cohen-Kettenis PT: Young adult psychological outcome after puberty suppression and gender reassignment. *Pediatrics* 134:696–704, 2014.
122. Simons L, Schrager SM, Clark LF, Belzer M, Olson f: Parental support and mental health among transgender adolescents. *J Adolesc Health* 53:791–793, 2013.
123. de Vries AL, Doreleijers TA, Steensma TD, Cohen-Kettenis PT: Psychiatric comorbidity in gender dysphoric adolescents. *J Child Psychol Psychiatry* 52:1195–1202, 2011.
124. Costa R, Dunsford M, Skagerberg E, Holt V, Carmichael P, Colizzi M: Psychological support, puberty suppression, and psychosocial functioning in adolescents with gender dysphoria. *J Sex Med* 12:2206–2214, 2015.
125. Klink D, Caris M, Heijboer A, van Trotsenburg M, Rotteveel J: Bone mass in young adulthood following gonadotropin-releasing hormone analog treatment and cross-sex hormone treatment in adolescents with gender dysphoria. *J Clin Endocrinol Metab* 100:E270-E275, 2015, doi: 10.1210/jc.2014-2439.
126. Schagen SE, Cohen-Kettenis PT, Delemarre-van de Waal HA, Hannema SE: Efficacy and safety of gonadotropin-releasing hormone agonist treatment to suppress puberty in gender dysphoric adolescents. *J Sex Med* 13:1125–1132, 2016.
127. Rosenthal SM: Approach to the patient: Transgender youth: Endocrine considerations. *J Clin Endocrinol Metab* 99:4379–4389, 2014.
128. Nahata et al. 2017 Journal of Adolescent Health

5.15 ■ NEGLECT, ABUSE, AND TRAUMA-RELATED CONDITIONS

CHAPTER 5.15.1 ■ CHILD ABUSE AND NEGLECT

JOAN KAUFMAN AND DANIEL HOOVER

INTRODUCTION

If you work in mental health, you work with maltreated children. The best available data suggest that approximately 30% of child and adolescent outpatients (1), and as many as 55% of child and adolescent psychiatric inpatients have a lifetime history of abuse or neglect (2). While not all abused children go on to develop psychiatric problems, a history of abuse is a highly significant risk factor for the development of a number of different psychiatric disorders (3,4), as well as a notable risk factor for a host of medical health problems later in life (5).

This chapter reviews definitions and prevalence of child abuse and neglect. It also discusses developmental, clinical, and neurobiological sequelae of child maltreatment, and findings from the fields of genetics, epigenetics, and neuroscience relevant for understanding risk, resilience, and recovery. A number of treatment interventions are also reviewed.

DEFINITIONS

Each state has its own definitions of child abuse and neglect that are based on minimal standards set by federal law. Definitions of the various maltreatment categories have also been drafted by the American Academy of Child and Adolescent Psychiatry (6). Federal legislation defines child abuse and neglect as (7):

> *Any recent act or failure to act on the part of a parent or caretaker which results in death, serious physical or emotional harm, sexual abuse or exploitation; or an act or failure to act, which presents an imminent risk of serious harm.*

Most states have laws pertaining to the four major types of maltreatment: physical abuse, sexual abuse, psychological maltreatment, and neglect. While physical abuse, the nonaccidental injury of children is unlawful nationwide, corporal punishment is allowed in the home of birth families in every state. It is not allowed in most out-of-home placement settings though. As of June 2014, 40 states prohibited the use of corporal punishment in foster homes or institutions (8). Given the state-by-state variation in legal standards, clinicians should familiarize themselves with the maltreatment criteria and corporal punishment laws specific to the state where they practice.

PREVALENCE

The federal government has been analyzing annual data on child abuse and neglect since 1990 (9). Between 1990 and 1994, the number of annual cases of child abuse and neglect that were substantiated rose from 861,000 to 1,032,000 (10). Since 1994, the rates of substantiated cases of maltreatment have declined, with only 679,000 confirmed cases of maltreatment reported in the most recent recorded year (9). These 679,000 cases were from 3.5 million referrals of families for suspected maltreatment involving approximately 6.4 million children.

The decline in rates of child maltreatment is believed to be "real," and has been attributed to prevention efforts, more aggressive criminal prosecution of perpetrators, and increased dissemination of psychiatric medications targeting behaviors that increase risk for abuse (11). It is likely, however, that some of the drop in substantiation rates is an artifact of changing practices and standards for responding to allegations of maltreatment (12), as there have been no corresponding decreases in rates of referrals for suspected maltreatment, or rates of child abuse–related fatalities during this same time period (13). Specifically, 1994, the year rates of substantiated reports of maltreatment began to drop, is the same year states began to implement differential response programs (14). Differential response programs, also referred to as alternative responses or family assessment programs are part of a two-tier response to allegations of abuse and neglect that have been implemented in most states. The most severe maltreatment allegations involving injury or imminent risk still involve forensic evaluations and determination of whether or not maltreatment occurred, but moderate- to low-risk cases are referred for family assessments instead. The goal of the contact is no longer a formal determination of whether abuse or neglect occurred, but rather an evaluation of whether or not services are needed to strengthen families.

Preliminary data from research conducted on differential response programs suggest child safety is better served by this alternative approach to responding to child maltreatment allegations. Families who receive differential response family assessments have fewer subsequent maltreatment reports, a longer period of time between re-reports, and less severe new reports than families receiving traditional protective services forensic investigative interventions. Differential response interventions are also associated with greater family satisfaction, and most importantly, greater involvement with community services (15).

While the true rate of abuse and neglect will likely never be known (16), a synthesis of self-report studies suggests official documented rates of abuse and neglect grossly underestimate the true prevalence of these experiences (17). There are many reported cases of actual abuse that are not verified (18), and countless other cases which never come to the attention of authorities (19).

ASSESSING CHILD ABUSE, NEGLECT, AND OTHER TRAUMA EXPERIENCES

Given the high prevalence of maltreatment experiences in child psychiatric populations (1,2), psychiatric assessment of children should routinely include screening for abuse, neglect, and other traumatic experiences (20). It is best to assess children's trauma experiences utilizing information from multiple informants (e.g., parent, children, child protective service workers) (21–23). Rating scales to facilitate assessment of child abuse, neglect, and other traumatic experiences are reviewed in the Chapter 5.15.2 of this text.

NEW DISCLOSURES OF CHILD MALTREATMENT

Mental health providers are mandated reporters. They are required by law to report suspected abuse and neglect. Unfortunately, there is no systematic research on optimal procedures for handling mandated reporting requirements. In our clinical experience, it is usually best to inform the parent or guardian of one's intention to file a report, and to suggest that the parent or guardian call in the information and report the concerns as well. The parent's response to this fact will provide valuable information in evaluating the parent's capacity to support and protect the child, and determine the safety of the child staying in the immediate custody of the parent. It also gives the parent a sense of control at a very stressful time, and in truth, protective service workers look favorably upon a parent who calls to report the problem independently. Regardless of whether the parent agrees to call in the alleged maltreatment or not, the mental health professional is obligated to make the report.

As the process of case investigation can be idiosyncratic (24), it is recommended that detailed information about the alleged abuse and known risk (e.g., prior reports of maltreatment, parental substance abuse, domestic violence, number of birth to 3-year-old children living in the home) and protective (e.g., parent engaged in treatment, extended positive family supports) factors be included in suspected child maltreatment reports. Clinicians should not attempt to conduct forensic evaluations in the context of clinical assessments though, as specific guidelines must be followed for forensic evaluations (20,25).

RISK FACTORS FOR CHILD MALTREATMENT

Child abuse most often occurs in the context of other risk factors. Child abuse can and does occur across all socioeconomic classes, but is most prevalent among the poor (26). While most poor families do not maltreat their children, poverty is a significant risk factor for child abuse and neglect, with more than half of the families participating in a large-scale representative sample of protective services cases falling below the federal poverty line (27).

Substance abuse and domestic violence are two other problems that frequently co-occur in association with child maltreatment. It is estimated that 60% of cases involved with protective services have histories of severe domestic violence (27), and 60% to 70% of parents with substantiated child welfare cases, and more than 80% of parents who lose custody of their children have a substance use disorder (28). These co-occurring problems significantly complicate the management of child maltreatment cases.

SEQUELAE

Indices of Adaptive Functioning

A history of maltreatment is associated with deficits on numerous indices of adaptation across the lifecycle. When compared to community controls, maltreated children have significantly more disturbances in attachment relations in infancy, delays in autonomous functioning and deficits in frustration tolerance in toddlerhood, and problems with self-esteem and peer relations in later childhood (29). Problems in language development and school performance have also been reported, including below average standardized achievement test scores, frequent repeated grades, low cumulative grade point averages, and significant social and behavior problems in the school setting (30). In studies examining resiliency in maltreated children (31,32), a quarter or fewer children could be classified resilient when multiple domains of functioning were considered.

Sexual Behavior Problems

Sexual behavior problems are frequently utilized as indicators of child sexual abuse. While inappropriate sexual behaviors are strongly related to experiences of sexual abuse, they are also associated with histories of physical abuse, witnessing domestic violence, inappropriate exposure to family sexuality, and child psychiatric illness (33). Table 5.15.1.1 delineates behaviors that are highly suggestive of a possible sexual abuse history, behaviors that are relatively prevalent in abuse victims and psychiatric controls with no history of abuse, and behaviors that are frequently observed in these high-risk groups and normal controls (33,34).

Intergenerational Transmission of Abuse

Victims of child maltreatment are more likely than controls to be involved in intimate partner violence in adolescence (35) and adulthood (36). They are also more likely to experience teen parenthood (37), and have difficulties parenting their own children. While approximately 80% to 90% of abusive parents have a history of child maltreatment, and being abused puts one at risk of experiencing parenting problems, retrospective (38) and prospective longitudinal (39) studies estimate that only

TABLE 5.15.1.1

DISTINCTIVENESS OF SEXUALIZED BEHAVIORS IN INDICATING ABUSE HISTORY

Moderately Prevalent in Sexually Abused Children, Exceedingly Rare in Psychiatric and Normal Controls	Moderately Prevalent in Sexually Abused Children *and* Psychiatric Controls, Uncommon in Normal Controls	Moderately Prevalent in Sexually Abused Children, Psychiatric Controls, *and* Normal Controls
Puts mouth on sex parts	Stands too close to others	Talks flirtatiously
Asks to engage in sexual acts	Hugs adults they do not know well	Masturbates with hand
Masturbates with an object	Talks about sexual acts	Touches sex parts at home
Inserts objects in vagina or anus	Wants to watch movies that show nudity	Tries to look at nude pictures/undressing people
	Knows more about sex than other children their age	

one in three individuals who were abused as children repeat the cycle in the next generation. Most break the cycle—or there would be exponential increases in rates of abuse with each generation.

Psychiatric Diagnoses and Symptomatology

Child maltreatment is a nonspecific risk factor for multiple forms of psychopathology (4,40,41). Compared to community controls, maltreated children have elevated externalizing and internalizing behavior problems according to parent and teacher reports (42). They also have increased rates of posttraumatic stress disorder (PTSD) (43); depression diagnoses (44,45); reactive attachment disorder and disinhibited social engagement disorder (46); dissociative symptoms (47); suicidality, self-destructive behavior, and borderline traits (48); drug and alcohol problems (4,49); eating disorders (50); oppositional defiant disorder (51); and conduct disorder and sociopathy later in life (51).

GENETIC PREDICTORS OF PSYCHIATRIC PROBLEMS IN MALTREATED CHILDREN

Genetic factors, in part, appear to explain why some maltreated children go on to develop certain psychiatric problems, and others do not. Caspi et al. were the first to show that risk for antisocial behavior in individuals maltreated as children was moderated by genotype—in particular, variation in the neurotransmitter-metabolizing enzyme monoamine oxidase A (*MAOA*) gene (52). Since this seminal study, there have been over a hundred studies published that examined gene by environment (GxE) interactions and the moderating effects of various candidate genes on a range of mental health outcomes among individuals with a history of abuse (41). Consistent with other data in the field showing that genetic markers do not map on to distinct DSM diagnoses, but rather individual genetic markers are associated with a range of psychiatric disorders (53), results of the GxE candidate gene studies with maltreated cohorts demonstrate pleiotropy in the genetics of stress-related psychiatric disorders, with each candidate gene examined associated with a variety psychiatric disorders.

As reviewed elsewhere (41), the greatest number of studies in the field have examined genetic variation in the serotonin transporter (*5-HTTLPR*) gene, and replicated reports have found variation in *5-HTTLPR* predicts a range of outcomes. Specifically, among individuals with a history of child abuse and neglect, genetic variation in *5-HTTLPR* has been found to predict risk for depression, PTSD and other anxiety disorders, substance use problems, and antisocial behavior in children and adolescents and aggressive behavior in adults. While not as many studies have been conducted examining the moderating effect of other candidate genes, there is also evidence for pleiotropy in studies examining genetic variation in *MAOA*, the catechol-O-methyltransferase (*COMT*) gene, brain-derived neurotropic factor (*BDNF*) gene, corticotropin-releasing hormone receptor (*CRHR1*) gene, and the FK506 binding protein 5 (*FKBP5*) gene (41).

Genome-wide association studies (GWAS) that have examined predictors of PTSD have also identified genetic markers that interact with trauma history that show evidence of pleiotropy (41). For example, the first PTSD GWAS conducted reported an association between PTSD and the retinoid-related orphan receptor alpha (*RORA*) gene (54), a gene which has also been associated with multiple other psychiatric disorders including depression, bipolar disorder, attention-deficit hyperactivity disorder (55), and autism (41).

Pleiotropy may be due to overlapping symptoms across diagnoses (56,57), or the high rates of comorbidity among disorders (58), which is true even among disorders that share no common symptoms (59). Alternatively, a central tenet of the National Institute of Mental Health Research Domain Criteria (RDoC) initiative is that pleiotropy and comorbidity occur because the various DSM diagnoses are associated with abnormalities in interlocking brain circuits (60). Using an RDoC framework that incorporates dimensional assessments of behaviors that map onto discrete brain circuits, would likely help to advance research on the genetics of stress-related psychopathologies (61).

Advancing the genetics of stress-related psychiatric outcomes will also likely require incorporating emerging understandings of the various mechanisms of gene regulation that affect disease risk. As reviewed elsewhere (41), three of the five other published PTSD GWAS identified unique markers in intergenic nonprotein coding regions of the DNA that predicted risk for PTSD in individuals with a history of abuse or other lifetime traumatic experiences. Many intergenic regions are enriched for factor-binding sites and are involved in the three-dimensional organization of the genome and gene regulation (62). Transcription factor-binding sites and chromatin insulators within intergenic regions are believed to mediate intra- and interchromosomal interactions, affecting gene expression at both proximal and distal locations (62). Epigenetic modifications in intergenic regions have been implicated in other neuropsychiatric diseases as well (63). As less than 2% of the over three billion DNA base pairs in the human genome code for proteins, it is not surprising that a role in gene regulation and disease risk is emerging for intergenic regions of DNA.

CHILD ABUSE AND EPIGENETIC MECHANISMS OF DISEASE RISK

There is an emerging appreciation of the role of epigenetic mechanisms in understanding how experiences of abuse can confer risk for deleterious outcomes later in life (64,65). Epigenetic processes do not result in genetic mutations, but rather chemical modifications to the DNA that alter gene expression. While some epigenetic modifications are hardwired and responsible for producing cell-specific phenotypic differences, emerging research suggests that the genome is highly sensitive to environmental influences that can promote epigenetic changes. DNA methylation, histone modifications, and posttranslational regulation of gene expression via noncoding RNA species are three different epigenetic mechanisms by which adverse experience such as childhood trauma can alter gene expression, with the most available data examining the role of early adversity on epigenetic changes via DNA methylation (64).

Research by Weaver, Meaney, and colleagues provided the first evidence that variations in early maternal care could produce stable alterations of DNA methylation, providing a mechanism for the long-term effects of early adversity (66). Utilizing a rat model of neglect, operationalized as decreased maternal pup licking and grooming and arched-back nursing, Meaney et al. found offspring of "neglectful" mothers had increased DNA methylation of the glucocorticoid receptor gene in the hippocampus when compared to offspring of "non-neglectful" mothers. The glucocorticoid receptor in the hippocampus is key for putting the brakes on the stress response, and DNA methylation of this gene leads to fewer available glucocorticoid receptors, which is associated with greater stress reactivity and anxiety- and depressive-like behaviors in the rat pups. These behavioral differences emerge early in life and persist into adulthood, and through a series of elegant experiments epigenetic changes programmed by early experience were shown to be causally related to the negative outcomes (66). This was the first series of studies to show that deviations in early experience could alter gene expression that mediated long-term negative physiological and behavioral outcomes.

Over the past decade there have been at least 40 preclinical and human studies published examining the impact of early adversity on methylation in the glucocorticoid receptor gene (67), and numerous other studies examining the impact of early adversity on expression of a wide variety of genes across multiple brain regions and in the periphery (e.g., blood and saliva DNA) (41). It is now well established that experience can alter gene expression. Results of these preclinical and clinical studies suggest adverse experiences early in life are associated with changes in gene expression of multiple known candidate genes, genes involved in DNA transcription and translation, and genes necessary for brain circuitry development, with changes in gene expression reported in key brain structures implicated in the pathophysiology of psychiatric and substance use disorders (41).

NEUROIMAGING STUDIES IN ABUSED AND NEGLECTED CHILDREN

While there are inconsistencies in the literature, as recently reviewed by Bick and Nelson (68) and Teicher and Samson (69), experiences of child abuse and neglect are associated with structural and functional brain changes across multiple brain regions and circuits that mediate a wide variety of social, emotional, and cognitive processes. Hippocampal volume deficits are one of the best replicated findings in adults with maltreatment-related PTSD; although these deficits have been less consistently observed in pediatric cohorts (68,69). One of the best replicated findings in pediatric cohorts is atrophy of the medial and/or posterior portions of the corpus callosum, with reduced integrity of white matter tracts in this region also reported (69). Relatively consistent findings are also emerging which suggest maltreatment-related changes in corticolimbic circuitry involving enhanced amygdala activation in response to threat stimuli (69), with changes in threat processing circuitry in maltreated cohorts observed in association with depressive, anxiety, and PTSD symptoms, and independent of psychopathology. Several studies have also reported maltreated individuals have a blunted response in the striatal regions in response to anticipated reward in the monetary incentive delay task (69), with reduced activity in the striatal region during this reward task associated with the later development of alcohol problems (70). Preliminary data suggest structural and functional brain changes associated with child maltreatment may vary as a function of family loading for psychopathology (71), genetic variation (72), the age when the experiences occurred (73), and the presence or absence of positive social supports (74).

REVERSIBILITY OF BRAIN CHANGES ASSOCIATED WITH CHILD MALTREATMENT

While brain changes associated with early adversity can be long-lasting, there are emerging data that they can be reversed (75). The notion that early deviant experience can lead to permanent changes in brain development and behavior stems partly from the groundbreaking experiments on monocular deprivation in cats by Wiesel and Hubel (76). The development of central visual pathways in several mammalian species, like many other brain systems, is known to be experience-dependent. Wiesel and Hubel deprived kittens of vision in one eye for different lengths of time and at different ages. They found that after suturing one lid during the first 3 months of life, there was no vision in that eye later in development after the sutures were removed, and the visual cortex did not develop normally. The effects of visual deprivation on subsequent brain development and visual processing was evident only in kittens, not in adult cats, which led to the conclusion that vision development in kittens has a "critical period," and if the eyes are not exposed to the required stimuli during that period, vision would be lost and associated brain structures altered permanently.

Emerging findings, however, are challenging previous understandings of the impact of early experience on brain function and development (75). Further studies revisiting the initial experiments of Wiesel and Hubel have shown that the brain alterations associated with monocular deprivation are due to epigenetic changes, and the effects can be reversed with pharmacologic interventions and environmental enrichment (75). What was previously deemed to be permanent brain damage secondary to adverse early experiences during formative periods of development has now been shown to be amenable to treatment, allowing complete function to be restored.

There are emerging data that some of the brain changes associated with a history of child maltreatment can also be remediated with therapeutic foster care interventions (77–79), and preliminary data that the availability of positive social supports can diminish risk for alterations in key brain circuits affected by experiences of child maltreatment (74). In addition, in a study with adults with PTSD secondary to military trauma, exposure therapy was associated with normalization of fear circuitry functioning in the amygdala and other key brain regions (80). Comparable pre- and posttreatment imaging studies have yet to be conducted in child cohorts, but the findings are promising.

PROMOTING RESILIENCE AND RECOVERY IN MALTREATED CHILDREN

Promoting resilience and recovery in maltreated children is facilitated by: (1) promoting the development and maintenance of positive attachment relationships; (2) providing enrichment opportunities; and (3) child and birth parent–focused clinical interventions. Data related to each of these are discussed briefly in the following sections.

Attachment

In our work and the work of others, the availability of positive stable social supports has emerged as one of the most important factors in promoting resilience in maltreated children. In our studies with maltreated cohorts, the availability of a positive stable attachment figure has been found to decrease risk for the development of depressive disorders (44), minimize hypothalamic–pituitary–adrenal (HPA) stress axis abnormalities (44), ameliorate the negative effect of genes associated with risk for psychopathology (81), and reduce the negative impact of abuse and neglect on brain structure and function (74,82).

Dozier et al. have developed an attachment-based intervention to facilitate the establishment of secure attachments for infants and toddlers who enter the child welfare system (83). As maltreated infants who enter the system frequently have a history of insecure attachments and multiple disruptions in parenting, these infants may not elicit caregiver support and may actually initially avoid or reject their foster parents' attempt to provide comfort. The intervention, called the Attachment Biobehavioral Catch-up (ABC) intervention, is designed to help caregivers provide nurturance even when children do not elicit it, and even when it does not come naturally to them. The ABC intervention is associated with improvements evaluated into the preschool years in attachment relations (84), measures of affect regulation (85), cognitive flexibility (86), and HPA stress axis indices (87).

Attachment and the availability of stable caring adult caregivers are important across the lifecycle (88). Despite federal legislation passed in 1997 to promote adoptions and permanency for children involved with the child welfare system (89), approximately 25,000 children "age-out" of the foster care system each year without consistent or stable adults in their lives, with approximately 25% of these youth age 12 or younger when they entered care, and more than 30% of them with histories of having experienced eight or more placements before aging out of the system (90). As clinicians working with these youth, helping youth to identify and maintain positive stable supports is an important component of the treatment planning process.

Enrichment

Environmental enrichment in early adolescence has been found to ameliorate the negative effects associated with maternal separation and low licking and grooming "neglectful" rearing in rodents studies (91). In a study of matched samples of foster care alumni (92), alumni from the enhanced foster care program had significantly fewer psychiatric problems as young adults than alumni from public sector foster care programs. The enhanced foster care program provided a greater number of enrichment opportunities for youth, like participation in summer day camp programs, music lessons, and involvement in sports. While the two foster care programs differed in numerous other significant ways, involvement in enriching extracurricular activities provides youth an opportunity to develop positive self-esteem and establish supportive relationships with coaches and other adults who can become meaningful resources for the youth. In addition, there are emerging data that exercise (93) and music training (94) can promote positive brain changes via neuroplasticity. While more data are needed to demonstrate that enrichment experiences can positively impact the outcome of maltreated children, in our clinical experience these types of experiences appear invaluable in tipping the scale in favor of positive outcomes.

Child and Birth Parent Clinical Interventions

Trauma Informed Systems of Care

While it has been acknowledged for decades that parents involved with the child welfare system have high rates of childhood trauma, it is only within the past 5 to 10 that this knowledge has started to shape practice. Emerging data now suggest when mental health and child welfare systems do not appropriately assess, identify, and address underlying trauma issues, services are often more expensive and less effective (95). For further information, the interested reader is referred to the Child Traumatic Stress Network website for state-of-the-art updates on trauma-informed practices (http://www.nctsnet.org).

Posttraumatic Stress Disorder Treatments

PTSD treatment interventions are discussed in greater detail in the Chapter 5.15.2 of this text. Briefly, trauma-focused cognitive-behavioral therapy (TF-CBT) is the intervention with the strongest evidence base for the treatment of PTSD and other trauma-related psychopathology in children (96). In one study that provided TF-CBT to children in foster care (97), compared to children who received treatment as usual, children who received TF-CBT had significantly greater reduction in PTSD and other emotional and behavioral symptomatology, and were half as likely to disrupt from their current foster care placement. Providing trauma-informed care and involving foster parents in children's clinical interventions appear to be essential in promoting continuity of care and facilitating recovery (98).

Interventions That Target Physically Abusive Parenting Behaviors

Parent–child interaction therapy (PCIT) is the therapeutic intervention with the strongest results in reducing physically abusive parenting behaviors (99,100). PCIT is a model of intervention which was originally developed for young children with externalizing behavior problems that combines concrete teaching and "bug-in-the-ear" coaching to help caregivers interact more effectively with their 2- to 7-year-old children (101). PCIT has shown strong evidence of effectiveness in terms of improving child behavior, and reducing self-reported parental stress, harsh parenting behaviors, child welfare referrals, and recurrence of physical abuse (99,100). Perhaps the main drawback of PCIT is the high dropout rate, especially in families with the most severe child behavior problems, maltreatment, and court-mandated participation (99). Home-based PCIT (102) or utilizing initial motivational sessions prior to implementing PCIT (103) have been shown to enhance treatment completion.

Psychopharmacology

A number of papers have been published raising concerns about the rate of psychotropic drug use among children in the foster care system (104–107). In a large sample of over 15,000 births to 19-year-old children with Medicaid insurance, 30% of the children and adolescents in the sample who were living in foster care were reported to be prescribed psychotropic medications, a rate nearly double the rate of psychotropic drug use among youth receiving supplemental security income (SSI) for diagnosed disabilities, and 15 times the rate of youngsters receiving welfare (105). Another study reported that 41% of the foster care children on psychotropic drugs were prescribed three or more different types of medications (e.g., stimulant, antidepressant, antipsychotic), with atypical antipsychotic drugs used at very high rates (107). In another report, comparably high rates of psychotropic drug use and polypharmacy were documented among youth aging out of the system, however, 41% of the adolescents diagnosed with ADHD and 19% of the youth with a history of mania were not on any medications (108). This raised doubts about the overall appropriateness of medication use in children within the child welfare system, with concerns about both overuse and underuse.

This growing body of research was the impetus for federal legislation requiring states to track and monitor psychotropic drug use among children in the child welfare system (109,110). States were required to develop protocols, not just for the monitoring of psychotropic medications, but for their appropriate uses as well. As recently as 2007, only three states maintained databases to monitor the use of psychotropic medications of children in state custody (111); finding out what drugs children were prescribed required workers in most states to hunt and peck through random case notes.

In a recent survey of key informants from child welfare and affiliated agencies in 47 states and the District of Columbia (112), two-thirds of states adopted at least one "red flag" marker signaling a need for heightened scrutiny. The most commonly used red flags were use of psychotropic medications in young children (defined variously as 3 to 6 years old), endorsed by nearly one-half of the states; use of multiple concurrent psychotropic medications (defined variously as three to five medications), endorsed by two-fifths of the states; and use of multiple medications within the same class for longer than 30 days, endorsed by two-fifths of the states. Dosage exceeding maximum recommendations (e.g., manufacturer, professional, federal, or state) and medications inconsistent with current recommendations (e.g., professional or state guidelines) were endorsed as red flags by more than one-fourth of the states.

At the time of the survey, most states had or were developing a written policy on the appropriate use of psychotropic medication for youth in the child welfare system (112). But what is the appropriate use of psychotropic medications for youth in state custody due to abuse and neglect? Meta-analyses of adolescent and adult treatment studies have found, compared to individuals who meet criteria for the diagnosis of major depression without a history of child abuse, individuals with a history of child abuse who meet criteria for depression are less likely to remit following standard evidence-based pharmacological (e.g., selective serotonin reuptake inhibitor medications) interventions (45). Individuals with a history of child maltreatment also appear to have a poorer treatment response across a range of diagnoses (113). The database steering the existing guidelines is limited, and will be discussed further in Chapter 5.15.2 of this text. The bottom line is the drugs are being used without a truly adequate research database in maltreated cohorts to guide clinical practice.

Parent-Focused Interventions

As noted earlier in this chapter, an estimated that 60% to 70% of parents with substantiated child welfare cases, and 80% or more of parents whose children are placed in foster care, meet criteria for a substance use disorder (28). Among child welfare cases, parental substance abuse is associated with higher rates of child revictimization, greater likelihood of out-of-home placement, longer stays in care, and higher rates of termination of parental rights and child adoption (28). As reviewed elsewhere (28), over the past decade there has been a burgeoning of research aimed at improving the effectiveness of substance abuse interventions for parents involved in the child welfare system, and addressing parental substance abuse is key to promoting positive outcomes in youth.

CONCLUDING REMARKS

A history of maltreatment puts children at risk for a host of negative outcomes. Over the past decade there have been remarkable advances in the field in terms of dissemination of evidence-based practices to treat trauma-related psychopathology, and insights regarding the mechanisms by which experiences of abuse confer risk for a broad range of psychiatric and medical health problems. Data to guide best practices in terms of pharmacological treatments are sorely lacking, and an absence of services to address child and parent problems leaves far too many children lost in the child welfare system.

Child maltreatment cases are frequently quite challenging, presenting with high rates of diagnostic comorbidity and co-occurring family and social problems. As discussed previously, recent data suggest that as many as 25,000 children "age-out" of the foster care system each year without consistent or stable adults in their lives, with approximately 25% of these youth age 12 or younger when they entered care, and more than 30% of them with histories of eight or more placements. Through multidisciplinary research efforts with foci that span from neurobiology to social policy, we can, and must do better.

References

1. Lanktree C, Briere J, Zaidi L: Incidence and impact of sexual abuse in a child outpatient sample: the role of direct inquiry. *Child Abuse Negl* 15:447–453, 1991.
2. McClellan J, Adams J, Douglas D, McCurry C, Storck M: Clinical characteristics related to severity of sexual abuse: a study of seriously mentally ill youth. *Child Abuse Negl* 19:1245–1254, 1995.
3. McLaughlin KA, Green JG, Gruber MJ, Sampson NA, Zaslavsky AM, Kessler RC: Childhood adversities and adult psychiatric disorders in the national comorbidity survey replication II: associations with persistence of DSM-IV disorders. *Arch Gen Psychiatry* 67:124–132, 2010.
4. Molnar BE, Buka SL, Kessler RC: Child sexual abuse and subsequent psychopathology: results from the National Comorbidity Survey. *Am J Public Health* 91:753–760, 2001.
5. Felitti VJ, Anda RF, Nordenberg D, et al.: Relationship of childhood abuse and household dysfunction to many of the leading causes of death in adults. The Adverse Childhood Experiences (ACE) Study. *Am J Prev Medicine* 14:245–258, 1998.
6. Lawson L, Chaffin M: False negatives in sexual abuse interviews: incidence and influence of caretaker's belief in abuse in cases of accidental abuse discovery by diagnosis of STD. *J Interpers Violence* 7:532–542, 1992.
7. Child Abuse Prevention and Treatment Act (CAPTA) as amended by P.L. 111–320, the CAPTA Reauthorization Act of 2010, in PL 111–320, 2010. Available at: http://www.acf.hhs.gov/sites/default/files/cb/capta2010.pdf Accessed May 13, 2015.
8. EACPC: Corporal Punishment of Children in the USA. *Global Initiative to End All Corporal Punishment of Children*, 2014.
9. ACYF: Child Maltreatment 2013. Edited by U.S. Department of Health and Human Services Administration for Children and Families Administration on Children YaFCsB 2015.
10. Child_Trends_Databank: Child Maltreatment: Indicators on Children and Youth, 2015.
11. Jones LM, Finkelhor D, Halter S: Child maltreatment trends in the 1990s: why does neglect differ from sexual and physical abuse? *Child Maltreat* 11:107–120, 2006.
12. Janczewski CE: The influence of differential response on decision-making in child protective service agencies. *Child Abuse Negl* 39:50–60, 2015.
13. ACYF: *Child Abuse and Neglect Fatalities 2013: Statistics and Interventions. in Child Welfare Information Gateway.* Washington, DC, Children's Bureau, Administration of Children Youth and Families; 2015.
14. Siegel GL: Lessons from the Beginning of Differential Response: Why it Works and When it Doesn't. In: *A Monograph of the Institute of Applied Research.* St. Louis, MO, 2012.
15. Kyte A, Trocme N, Chamberland C: Evaluating where we're at with differential response. *Child Abuse Negl* 37:125–132, 2013.
16. Fallon B, Trocme N, Fluke J, MacLaurin B, Tonmyr L, Yuan YY: Methodological challenges in measuring child maltreatment. *Child Abuse Negl* 34:70–79, 2010.
17. Vizard E: Practitioner review: the victims and juvenile perpetrators of child sexual abuse–assessment and intervention. *J Child Psychol Psychiatry* 54:503–515, 2013.
18. Kaufman J, Zigler E: Child abuse and social policy. In: Zigler E, Kagan S, Hall N (eds): *Children, Families and Government: Preparing for the Twenty-first Century.* New York, Cambridge University Press; 1996, pp. 233–255.
19. Wolfner GD, Gelles RJ: A profile of violence toward children: a national study. *Child Abuse Negl* 17:197–212, 1993.
20. Cohen JA, Bukstein O, Walter H, et al.: Practice parameter for the assessment and treatment of children and adolescents with posttraumatic stress disorder. *J Am Acad Child Adolesc Psychiatry* 49:414–430, 2010.
21. Grasso D, Boonsiri J, Lipschitz D, et al.: Posttraumatic stress disorder: the missed diagnosis. *Child Welfare* 88:157–176, 2009.
22. Shaffer A, Huston L, Egeland B: Identification of child maltreatment using prospective and self-report methodologies: a comparison of maltreatment incidence and relation to later psychopathology. *Child Abuse Negl* 32:682–692, 2008.
23. Hambrick EP, Tunno AM, Gabrielli J, Jackson Y, Belz C: Using multiple informants to assess child maltreatment: concordance between case file and youth self-report. *J Aggress Maltreat Trauma* 23:751–771, 2014.
24. Drake B, Jonson-Reid M, Way I, Chung S: Substantiation and recidivism. *Child Maltreat* 8:248–260, 2003.
25. Kraus LJ, Thomas CR, Bukstein OG, et al.: Practice parameter for child and adolescent forensic evaluations. *J Am Acad Child Adolesc Psychiatry* 50:1299–1312, 2011.
26. DHHS: *Third National Incidence Study of Child Abuse and Neglect (NIS-3).* Edited by Department of Health and Human Services AfCNCoCAaN, Washington, DC, 1996.
27. Connelly CD, Hazen AL, Coben JH, Kelleher KJ, Barth RP, Landsverk JA: Persistence of intimate partner violence among families referred to child welfare. *J Interpers Violence* 21:774–797, 2006.
28. Oliveros A, Kaufman J: Addressing substance abuse treatment needs of parents involved with the child welfare system. *Child Welfare.* 2011;90:25–41.
29. Myers J, Berliner L, Briere J, Hendrix CT, Jenny C, Reid TA: *The APSAC Handbook on Child Maltreatment.* 2nd ed. Thousand Oaks, CA, Sage Publications, Inc.; 2002.
30. Stahmer AC, Leslie LK, Hurlburt M, et al.: Developmental and behavioral needs and service use for young children in child welfare. *Pediatrics* 116:891–900, 2005.
31. Kaufman J, Cooke A, Arny L, Jones B, Pittinsky T: Problems defining resiliency: illustrations from the study of maltreated children. *Develop and Psychopathol* 6:215–229, 1994.

32. Walsh WA, Dawson J, Mattingly MJ: How are we measuring resilience following childhood maltreatment? Is the research adequate and consistent? What is the impact on research, practice, and policy? *Trauma Violence Abuse* 11:27–41, 2010.
33. Friedrich WN, Fisher JL, Dittner CA, et al.: Child Sexual Behavior Inventory: normative, psychiatric, and sexual abuse comparisons. *Child Maltreat* 6:37–49, 2001.
34. Friedrich WN, Grambsch P, Damon L, et al.: Child Sexual Behavior Inventory: normative and clinical comparisons. *Psychol Assessm* 4: 303–311, 1992.
35. Wolfe DA, Wekerle C, Scott K, Straatman AL, Grasley C: Predicting abuse in adolescent dating relationships over 1 year: the role of child maltreatment and trauma. *J Abnorm Psychol* 113:406–415, 2004.
36. Noll JG, Horowitz LA, Bonanno GA, Trickett PK, Putnam FW: Revictimization and self-harm in females who experienced childhood sexual abuse: results from a prospective study. *J Interpers Violence* 18:1452–1471, 2003.
37. Noll JG, Trickett PK, Putnam FW: A prospective investigation of the impact of childhood sexual abuse on the development of sexuality. *J Consult Clin Psychol* 71:575–586, 2003.
38. Kaufman J, Zigler E: Do abused children become abusive parents? *Am J Orthopsychiatry* 57:186–192, 1987.
39. Widom CS, Czaja SJ, DuMont KA: Intergenerational transmission of child abuse and neglect: real or detection bias? *Science* 347:1480–1485, 2015.
40. Kendler KS, Bulik CM, Silberg J, Hettema JM, Myers J, Prescott CA: Childhood sexual abuse and adult psychiatric and substance use disorders in women: an epidemiological and cotwin control analysis. *Arch Gen Psychiatry* 57:953–959, 2000.
41. Montalvo-Ortiz JL, Gelernter J, Hudziak J, Kaufman J: RDoC and translational perspectives on the genetics of trauma-related psychiatric disorders. *Am J Med Genet B Neuropsychiatr Genet* 171:81–91, 2016.
42. Vachon DD, Krueger RF, Rogosch FA, Cicchetti D: Assessment of the harmful psychiatric and behavioral effects of different forms of child maltreatment. *JAMA Psychiatry* 72:1135–1142, 2015.
43. Ruggiero K, McLeer S, Dixon J: Sexual abuse characteristics associated with survivor psychopathology. *Child Abuse Negl.* 24:951–964, 2000.
44. Kaufman J: Depressive disorders in maltreated children. *J Am Acad Child Adolesc Psychiatry* 30:257–265, 1991.
45. Nanni V, Uher R, Danese A: Childhood maltreatment predicts unfavorable course of illness and treatment outcome in depression: a meta-analysis. *Am J Psychiatry* 169:141–151, 2012.
46. Zeanah CH, Gleason MM: Annual research review: attachment disorders in early childhood–clinical presentation, causes, correlates, and treatment. *J Child Psychol Psychiatry* 56:207–222, 2015.
47. Putnam FW, Helmers K, Horowitz LA, Trickett PK: Hypnotizability and dissociativity in sexually abused girls. *Child Abuse Negl* 19:645–655, 1995.
48. Fergusson DM, Horwood LJ, Miller AL, Kennedy MA: Life stress, 5-HTTLPR and mental disorder: findings from a 30-year longitudinal study. *Br J Psychiatry* 198:129–135, 2011.
49. Afifi TO, Henriksen CA, Asmundson GJ, Sareen J: Childhood maltreatment and substance use disorders among men and women in a nationally representative sample. *Can J Psychiatry* 57:677–686, 2012.
50. Ackard DM, Neumark-Sztainer D: Multiple sexual victimizations among adolescent boys and girls: prevalence and associations with eating behaviors and psychological health. *J Child Sex Abus* 12:17–37, 2003.
51. Garland A, Hough R, McCabe K, Yeh M, Wood P, Aarons G: Prevalence of psychiatric disorders in youths across five sectors of care. *J Am Acad Child Adolesc Psychiatry* 40:409–418, 2001.
52. Caspi A, McClay J, Moffitt TE, et al.: Role of genotype in the cycle of violence in maltreated children. *Science* 297:851–854, 2002.
53. Cross-Disorder_Group_of_the_Psychiatric_Genomics_Consortium: Genetic relationship between five psychiatric disorders estimated from genome-wide SNPs. *Nat Genet* 45:984–994, 2013.
54. Logue MW, Baldwin C, Guffanti G, et al.: A genome-wide association study of post-traumatic stress disorder identifies the retinoid-related orphan receptor alpha (RORA) gene as a significant risk locus. *Mol Psychiatry* 18:937–942, 2013.
55. Neale BM, Lasky-Su J, Anney R, et al.: Genome-wide association scan of attention deficit hyperactivity disorder. *Am J Med Genet B Neuropsychiatr Genet* 147B:1337–1344, 2008.
56. APA: *Diagnostic and Statistical Manual of Mental Disorders.* 4th ed. Washington, DC, American Psychiatric Association, 2000.
57. APA: *Diagnostic and Statistical Manual of Mental Disorders: DSM-5.* 5th ed. Washington, DC, American Psychiatric Association, 2013.
58. Kessler RC, Avenevoli S, McLaughlin KA, et al.: Lifetime co-morbidity of DSM-IV disorders in the US National Comorbidity Survey Replication Adolescent Supplement (NCS-A). *Psychol Med* 42:1997–2010, 2012.
59. Kessler RC, Crum RM, Warner LA, Nelson CB, Schulenberg J, Anthony JC: Lifetime co-occurrence of DSM-III-R alcohol abuse and dependence with other psychiatric disorders in the National Comorbidity Survey. *Arch Gen Psychiatry* 54:313–321, 1997.
60. Etkin A, Cuthbert B: Beyond the DSM: development of a transdiagnostic psychiatric neuroscience course. *Acad Psychiatry* 38:145–150, 2014.
61. Cuthbert BN: The RDoC framework: facilitating transition from ICD/DSM to dimensional approaches that integrate neuroscience and psychopathology. *World Psychiatry* 13:28–35, 2014.
62. Yang J, Corces VG: Chromatin insulators: a role in nuclear organization and gene expression. *Adv Cancer Res* 110:43–76, 2011.
63. Qureshi IA, Mattick JS, Mehler MF: Long non-coding RNAs in nervous system function and disease. *Brain Res* 1338:20–35, 2010.
64. Turecki G, Ota V, Belangero S, Jackowski A, Kaufman J: Early life adversity, genomic plasticity, and psychopathology. *Lancet Psychiatry* 1:461–466, 2014.
65. Yang B-Z, Zhang H, Ge W, et al.: Child abuse and epigenetic mechanisms of disease risk. *Am J Prevent Med* 44:101–107, 2013.
66. Weaver IC, Cervoni N, Champagne FA, et al.: Epigenetic programming by maternal behavior. *Nat Neurosci* 7:847–854, 2004.
67. Turecki G, Meaney MJ: Effects of the social environment and stress on glucocorticoid receptor gene methylation: a systematic review. *Biol Psychiatry* 022:2014.
68. Bick J, Nelson CA: Early adverse experiences and the developing brain. *Neuropsychopharmacol* 41:177–196, 2016.
69. Teicher MH, Samson JA: Annual Research Review: enduring neurobiological effects of childhood abuse and neglect. *J Child Psychol Psychiatry* 57:241–266, 2016.
70. Nees F, Tzschoppe J, Patrick CJ, et al.: Determinants of early alcohol use in healthy adolescents: the differential contribution of neuroimaging and psychological factors. *Neuropsychopharmacol* 37:986–995, 2012.
71. Carballedo A, Lisiecka D, Fagan A, et al.: Early life adversity is associated with brain changes in subjects at family risk for depression. *World J Biol Psychiatry* 13:569–578, 2012.
72. Almli LM, Srivastava A, Fani N, et al.: Follow-up and extension of a prior genome-wide association study of posttraumatic stress disorder: gene x environment associations and structural magnetic resonance imaging in a highly traumatized African-American civilian population. *Biol Psychiatry* 76:e3–e4, 2014.
73. Pechtel P, Lyons-Ruth K, Anderson CM, Teicher MH: Sensitive periods of amygdala development: the role of maltreatment in preadolescence. *Neuroimage* 97:236–44, 2014.
74. Orr CA, Hudziak J, Albaugh MD, et al.: *Relations between childhood adversity, post-traumatic symptoms, and neural activity.* Paper presented at the Annual meeting of the society for research in child development. Philadelphia, PA, 2015.
75. Weder N, Kaufman J: Critical periods revisited: implications for intervention with traumatized children. *J Am Acad Child Adolesc Psychiatry* 50:1087–1089, 2011.
76. Wiesel TN, Hubel DH: Effects of visual deprivation on morphology and physiology of cells in the cats lateral geniculate body. *J Neurophysiol* 26:978–993, 1963.
77. Bick J, Fox N, Zeanah C, Nelson CA: Early deprivation, atypical brain development, and internalizing symptoms in late childhood. *Neuroscience* 026, 2015.
78. Bruce J, McDermott JM, Fisher PA, Fox NA: Using behavioral and electrophysiological measures to assess the effects of a preventive intervention: a preliminary study with preschool-aged foster children. *Prev Sci* 10:129–140, 2009.
79. McDermott JM, Troller-Renfree S, Vanderwert R, Nelson CA, Zeanah CH, Fox NA: Psychosocial deprivation, executive functions, and the emergence of socio-emotional behavior problems. *Front Hum Neurosci* 7:167, 2013.
80. Roy MJ, Costanzo ME, Blair JR, Rizzo AA: Compelling evidence that exposure therapy for PTSD normalizes brain function. *Stud Health Technol Inform* 199:61–65, 2014.
81. Kaufman J, Yang BZ, Douglas-Palumberi H, et al.: Social supports and serotonin transporter gene moderate depression in maltreated children. *Proc Natl Acad Sci U S A* 101:17316–17321, 2004.
82. Sheridan MA, Fox NA, Zeanah CH, McLaughlin KA, Nelson CA, 3rd: Variation in neural development as a result of exposure to institutionalization early in childhood. *Proc Natl Acad Sci U S A* 109:12927–12932, 2012.
83. Dozier M, Peloso E, Lewis E, Laurenceau JP, Levine S: Effects of an attachment-based intervention on the cortisol production of infants and toddlers in foster care. *Dev Psychopathol* 20:845–859, 2008.
84. Bernard K, Dozier M, Bick J, Lewis-Morrarty E, Lindhiem O, Carlson E: Enhancing attachment organization among maltreated children: results of a randomized clinical trial. *Child Dev* 83:623–636, 2012.
85. Lind T, Bernard K, Ross E, Dozier M: Intervention effects on negative affect of CPS-referred children: results of a randomized clinical trial. *Child Abuse Negl* 38:1459–1467, 2014.
86. Lewis-Morrarty E, Dozier M, Bernard K, Terracciano SM, Moore SV: Cognitive flexibility and theory of mind outcomes among foster children: preschool follow-up results of a randomized clinical trial. *J Adolesc Health* 51:S17–S22.
87. Bernard K, Hostinar CE, Dozier M: Intervention effects on diurnal cortisol rhythms of Child Protective Services-Referred infants in early childhood: preschool follow-up results of a randomized clinical trial. *JAMA Pediatrics* 169:112–119, 2015.
88. Dozier M, Kaufman J, Kobak R, et al.: Consensus Statement on Group Care. In: Annie E (ed): *Applying Research in Child and Adolescent Development to Child Welfare Placement Practices Meeting Participants.* New York, Casey Foundation YLC, 2012.
89. PL105-89: Adoption and Safe Families Act in PL 105-89, 1997.

90. DHHS: The AFCARS Report. In: *Adoption and Foster Care Analysis and Reporting System (AFCARS) FY 2013 data, U.S. Department of Health and Human Services, Administration for Children and Families, Administration on Children, Youth and Families,* Children's Bureau, Available at http://www.acf.hhs.gov/programs/cb, 2014.
91. Bredy TW, Humpartzoomian RA, Cain DP, et al.: Partial reversal of the effect of maternal care on cognitive function through environmental enrichment. *Eur J Neurosci* 18:571–576, 2003.
92. Kessler RC, Pecora PJ, Williams J, et al.: Effects of enhanced foster care on the long-term physical and mental health of foster care alumni. *Arch Gen Psychiatry* 65:625–633, 2008.
93. Davidson RJ, McEwen BS: Social influences on neuroplasticity: stress and interventions to promote well-being. *Nat Neurosci* 15:689–695, 2012.
94. Hudziak JJ, Albaugh MD, Ducharme S, et al.: Cortical thickness maturation and duration of music training: health-promoting activities shape brain development. *J Am Acad Child Adolesc Psychiatry* 53:1153–1161, e1152, 2014.
95. Harris M, Fallot RD: Using trauma theory to design service systems. In: Lamb HR (ed): *New Directions for Mental Health Services.* San-Francisco, CA, Jossey-Bass, 2001.
96. Cohen JA, Mannarino AP: Trauma-focused cognitive behavior therapy for traumatized children and families. *Child Adolesc Psychiatr Clin N America* 24:557–570, 2015.
97. Cohen J: Providing comprehensive care for traumatized children. In: *American Academy of Child and Adolescent Psychiatry.* New York, 2010.
98. Barth RP, Greeson JK, Zlotnik SR, Chintapalli LK: Evidence-based practice for youth in supervised out-of-home care: a framework for development, definition, and evaluation. *J Evid Based Soc Work* 8:501–528, 2011.
99. Batzer S, Berg T, Godinet MT, Stotzer RL: Efficacy or chaos? Parent-child interaction therapy in maltreating populations: a review of research. *Trauma Violence Abuse.* 2015, pii: 1524838015620819.
100. Kennedy SC, Kim JS, Tripodi SJ, Brown SM, Gowdy G: Does parent-child interaction therapy reduce future physical abuse? A meta-analysis. *Research on Social Work Practice* 26:147–156, 2016.
101. Urquiza AJ, McNeil CB: Parent–child interaction therapy: an intensive dyadic intervention for physically abusive families. *Child Maltreatment* 1:134–144, 1996.
102. Lanier P, Kohl PL, Benz J, Swinger D, Drake B: Preventing maltreatment with a community-based implementation of parent-child interaction therapy. *J Child Fam Stud* 23:449–460, 2014.
103. Chaffin M, Funderburk B, Bard D, Valle LA, Gurwitch R: A combined motivation and parent-child interaction therapy package reduces child welfare recidivism in a randomized dismantling field trial. *J Consult Clin Psychol* 79:84–95, 2011.
104. Zima BT, Bussing R, Crecelius GM, Kaufman A, Belin TR: Psychotropic medication treatment patterns among school-aged children in foster care. *J Child Adolesc Psychopharmacol* 9:135–147, 1999.
105. dosReis S, Zito JM, Safer DJ, Soeken KL: Mental health services for youths in foster care and disabled youths. *Am J Public Health* 91:1094–1099, 2001.
106. THHSC: Use of psychoactive medication in Texas foster children, state fiscal year 2005. Edited by Commission. THaHS2006.
107. Zito JM, Safer DJ, Sai D, et al.: Psychotropic medication patterns among youth in foster care. *Pediatrics* 121:e157–163, 2008.
108. Raghavan R, McMillen JC: Use of multiple psychotropic medications among adolescents aging out of foster care. *Psychiatr Serv* 59:1052–1055, 2008.
109. P.L.110–351: The Fostering Connections to Success and Increasing Adoptions Act of 2008.
110. P.L.112–34. The Child and Family Services Improvement and Innovation Act, 2011.
111. Naylor MW, Davidson CV, Ortega-Piron DJ, Bass A, Gutierrez A, Hall A: Psychotropic medication management for youth in state care: consent, oversight, and policy considerations. *Child Welfare* 86:175–192, 2007.
112. Leslie LK, Mackie T, Dawson EH, et al.: Multi-state study on psychotropic medication oversight in foster care. Edited by Institute TCaTS. Boston, MA, 2010.
113. Teicher MH, Samson JA: Childhood maltreatment and psychopathology: a case for ecophenotypic variants as clinically and neurobiologically distinct subtypes. *Am J Psychiatry* 170:1114–1133, 2013.

CHAPTER 5.15.2 ■ POSTTRAUMATIC STRESS DISORDER

DANIEL HOOVER AND JOAN KAUFMAN

Deshawn is a 9-year-old African-American boy who resides in his maternal great-grandmother's care along with his younger brother, James, in an urban neighborhood. The brothers were placed with relatives 8 months ago, after witnessing an altercation between their mother and her boyfriend, which ended in their mother's death. The boys' father has been incarcerated for several years and they have had no contact with him since his arrest. While James is making a relatively positive adjustment following his mother's death, Deshawn initially refused to talk about it, then showed increasing irritability, withdrawal, and angry blow-ups at home and school. He has been getting into fights with other children, has trouble concentrating on schoolwork, and has difficulty going to sleep at night. During a diagnostic interview, Deshawn reported having frequent nightmares since his mother's death, some specific to traumatic memories, and some nonspecific. Deshawn has also had illusory experiences of "hearing noises" in the house and worries that someone is trying to break in. He thinks that his misbehavior was the cause of the fight that led to his mother's death.

Deshawn is displaying a constellation of symptoms characteristic of posttraumatic stress disorder (PTSD). His irritability, explosiveness, and nightmares are common features of PTSD. His self-blame, concentration difficulties, and concerns related to safety are symptoms that are also frequently observed in children with PTSD. The difference between his and his brother's adaptation following his mother's traumatic death is also not atypical. As will be discussed later in this chapter, there are many factors that make some children more prone than others to develop PTSD following traumatic events.

This chapter reviews the diagnosis, assessment, and treatment of PTSD in children and adolescents. Data on the genetics, epigenetics, and neurobiology of PTSD and other stress-related disorders are reviewed in the Child Abuse chapter of this text.

ACUTE STRESS DISORDER AND POSTTRAUMATIC STRESS DISORDER DIAGNOSTIC CRITERIA

The DSM-5 places trauma- and stressor-related disorders in their own category (1); previously acute stress disorder (ASD) and PTSD were included with the anxiety disorders.

The diagnoses contained in the trauma- and stressor-related disorders section of the DSM include: PTSD, ASD, reactive attachment disorder, disinhibited social engagement disorder, the adjustment disorders and other unspecified trauma-related disorders. These diagnoses are distinct from other disorders in the DSM in that they require exposure to overt stressors or potentially traumatic events (PTEs) to attain the diagnoses, and the etiology of the diagnoses is specifically linked to the adverse life experiences. The diagnostic criteria for ASD and PTSD are delineated in Table 5.15.2.1.

Exposure to Traumatic Events

As noted above, the diagnoses of ASD and PTSD require exposure to a PTE. In the DSM-5 this is defined as "actual or threatened death, serious injury, or sexual violence." This may be through direct experiencing; witnessing the event(s) in person; learning that the traumatic event(s) happened to a close friend or family member; or "repeated or extreme exposure" to aversive details of the traumatic event(s), like that experienced by first responders. Television or other electronic media exposure

TABLE 5.15.2.1

DSM-5 CRITERIA

Acute Stress Disorder	Posttraumatic Stress Disorder
A. Exposure to actual or threatened death, serious injury, or sexual violence in one or more of the following ways: 1. Directly experiencing the traumatic event(s). 2. Witnessing, in person, the event(s) as it occurred to others. 3. Learning that the traumatic event(s) occurred to a close family member or close friend. In cases of actual or threatened death of a family member or friend, the event(s) must have been violent or accidental. 4. Experiencing repeated or extreme exposure to aversive details of the traumatic event(s) (e.g., first responders collecting human remains; police officers repeatedly exposed to details of child abuse). *Note:* Criterion A4 does not apply to exposure through electronic media, television, movies, or pictures, unless this exposure is work related. B. Presence of nine (or more) of the following symptoms: Intrusion Symptoms: 1. Recurrent, involuntary, and intrusive distressing memories of the traumatic event(s). *Note:* In children, repetitive play may occur in which themes or aspects of the traumatic event(s) are expressed. Also, in children less than six, spontaneous and intrusive memories may not appear distressing. 2. Recurrent distressing dreams in which the content and/or affect of the dream are related to the traumatic event(s). *Note:* In children, there may be frightening dreams without recognizable content. 3. Dissociative reactions (e.g., flashbacks) in which the individual feels or acts as if the traumatic event(s) were recurring. (Such reactions may occur on a continuum, with the most extreme expression being a complete loss of awareness of present surroundings.) *Note:* In children, trauma-specific reenactment may occur in play. 4. Intense or prolonged psychological distress or marked physiologic reactions at exposure to internal or external cues that symbolize or resemble an aspect of the traumatic event(s). Avoidance Symptoms: 5. Efforts to avoid distressing memories, thoughts, or feelings about or closely associated with the traumatic event(s). 6. Efforts to avoid external reminders (people, places, conversations, activities, objects, situations) that arouse distressing memories, thoughts, or feelings about or closely associated with the traumatic event(s).	A. Exposure to actual or threatened death, serious injury, or sexual violence in one or more of the following ways: 1. Directly experiencing the traumatic event(s). 2. Witnessing, in person, the event(s) as it occurred to others. 3. Learning that the traumatic event(s) occurred to a close family member or close friend. In cases of actual or threatened death of a family member or friend, the event(s) must have been violent or accidental. 4. Experiencing repeated or extreme exposure to aversive details of the traumatic event(s) (e.g., first responders collecting human remains; police officers repeatedly exposed to details of child abuse). 5. *Note:* Criterion A4 does not apply to exposure through electronic media, television, movies, or pictures, unless this exposure is work related. B. Presence of one (or more) of the following intrusion symptoms associated with the traumatic event(s), beginning after the traumatic event(s) occurred: 1. Recurrent, involuntary, and intrusive distressing memories of the traumatic event(s). *Note:* In children, repetitive play may occur in which themes or aspects of the traumatic event(s) are expressed. Also, in children less than six, spontaneous and intrusive memories may not appear distressing. 2. Recurrent distressing dreams in which the content and/or affect of the dream are related to the traumatic event(s). *Note:* In children, there may be frightening dreams without recognizable content. 3. Dissociative reactions (e.g., flashbacks) in which the individual feels or acts as if the traumatic event(s) were recurring. (Such reactions may occur on a continuum, with the most extreme expression being a complete loss of awareness of present surroundings.) *Note:* In children, trauma-specific reenactment may occur in play. 4. Intense or prolonged psychological distress at exposure to internal or external cues that symbolize or resemble an aspect of the traumatic event(s). 5. Marked physiologic reactions to internal or external cues that symbolize or resemble an aspect of the traumatic event(s). C. Persistent avoidance of stimuli associated with the traumatic event(s), beginning after the traumatic event(s) occurred, as evidenced by one or both of the following: 1. Avoidance of or efforts to avoid distressing memories, thoughts, or feelings about or closely associated with the traumatic event(s). 2. Avoidance of or efforts to avoid external reminders (people, places, conversations, activities, objects, situations) that arouse distressing memories, thoughts, or feelings about or closely associated with the traumatic event(s).

TABLE 5.15.2.1

(CONTINUED)

Acute Stress Disorder	Posttraumatic Stress Disorder
Negative Mood and Dissociative Symptoms: 7. Persistent inability to experience positive emotions (e.g., inability to experience happiness, satisfaction, or loving feelings). 8. Inability to remember an important aspect of the traumatic event(s) (typically due to dissociative amnesia and not to other factors such as head injury, alcohol, or drugs). 9. An altered sense of the reality of one's surroundings or oneself (e.g., seeing oneself from another's perspective, being in a daze, time slowing).	D. Negative alterations in cognitions and mood associated with the traumatic event(s), beginning or worsening after the traumatic event(s) occurred, as evidenced by two (or more) of the following: 1. Persistent inability to experience positive emotions (e.g., inability to experience happiness, satisfaction, or loving feelings). 2. Inability to remember an important aspect of the traumatic event(s) (typically due to dissociative amnesia and not to other factors such as head injury, alcohol, or drugs). This item is not included in the criteria for children six and below. 3. Persistent and exaggerated negative beliefs or expectations about oneself, others, or the world (e.g., "I am bad," "No one can be trusted," "The world is completely dangerous," "My whole nervous system is permanently ruined"). This item is not included in the criteria for children six and below. 4. Persistent, distorted cognitions about the cause or consequences of the traumatic event(s) that lead the individual to blame himself/herself or others. This item is not included in the criteria for children six and below. 5. Persistent negative emotional state (e.g., fear, horror, anger, guilt, or shame). 6. Markedly diminished interest or participation in significant activities. 7. Feelings of detachment or estrangement from others. This item is behaviorally anchored as "socially withdrawn" for children six and below. *Note:* For children six and below, only one symptom is required from the combined set of items included in criterion C and criterion D.
Arousal Symptoms: 10. Irritable behavior and angry outbursts (with little or no provocation) typically expressed as verbal or physical aggression toward people or objects. 11. Hypervigilance. 12. Exaggerated startle response. 13. Problems with concentration. 14. Sleep disturbance (e.g., difficulty falling or staying asleep or restless sleep).	E. Marked alterations in arousal and reactivity associated with the traumatic event(s), beginning or worsening after the traumatic event(s) occurred, as evidenced by two (or more) of the following: 1. Irritable behavior and angry outbursts (with little or no provocation) typically expressed as verbal or physical aggression toward people or objects. 2. Reckless or self-destructive behavior. This item is not included in the criteria for children six and below. 3. Hypervigilance. 4. Exaggerated startle response. 5. Problems with concentration. 6. Sleep disturbance (e.g., difficulty falling or staying asleep or restless sleep).
C. The duration of the disturbance (symptoms in criterion B) is 3 days to 1 mo after trauma exposure.	F. Duration of the disturbance (criteria B, C, D, and E) is more than 1 mo.

to traumatic events does not qualify for the diagnoses of ASD or PTSD.

Symptom Clusters

In addition to exposure to a traumatic event, the diagnosis of PTSD requires the presence of symptoms from four categories: reexperiencing, avoidance, negative alteration of cognition and mood, and hyperarousal symptoms. The negative alteration of cognition and mood symptom cluster is new with the DSM-5, as is the reckless and the self-destructive behavior item in the hyperarousal symptom cluster. The diagnosis in children over age 6 and adults requires at least one reexperiencing, one avoidance, two negative alteration of cognition and mood, and two hyperarousal symptoms. The diagnosis of PTSD also has two subtype specifiers, one based on the presence of predominant dissociative symptoms and the other based on the timing of PTSD onset (e.g., acute vs. delayed onset).

Acute Stress Disorder

The diagnosis of ASD utilizes many of the same symptoms required for the diagnosis of PTSD. Nine symptoms are required for the diagnosis of ASD, however, they can be derived from any of the symptom clusters. ASD symptoms typically begin immediately after the trauma, but persistence for at least 3 days and up to a month is needed to meet ASD criteria. If the symptoms persist beyond 1 month, a diagnosis of PTSD is indicated.

Diagnostic Criteria for PTSD for Children Ages 6 and Younger

Specific modifications are delineated for diagnosing children of age 6 and younger with PTSD. The exposure and reexperiencing criteria are essentially unchanged from the adult and older child criteria. The diagnosis of PTSD in young children, however only requires one symptom from a combined set of items including the two avoidance symptoms included in the adult and older child criteria, and four of the seven symptoms included in the adult and older child negative alteration of cognition and mood symptom items. The first three items in this section of the adult and older child criteria are omitted from the young child criteria (e.g., inability to remember events, exaggerated negative beliefs, distorted cognitions), given limitations in young children's ability to describe internal thoughts, and the feelings of detachment item were behaviorally anchored (e.g., socially withdrawn) to enhance the appropriateness of this symptom with young children. Like with adults and older children, two hyperarousal symptoms are required for the diagnosis of PTSD in children of age 6 and younger, although the reckless and self-destructive behavior item is omitted from the hyperarousal set of criteria developed for young child. Adopting these changes in diagnostic criteria for young children results in greater temporal stability of diagnosis (2) and a higher, but likely more accurate, prevalence rate of PTSD in young children (3,4).

PREVALENCE

Exposure to PTEs and Rates of PTSD among Adolescents

A recent national survey of US adolescents (5,6) estimates that 61.8% of youth in the United States are exposed to at least one PTE by age 17. This rate of trauma exposure is similar to that found in other previous samples (7). Lifetime prevalence of PTSD among adolescents is considerably lower than rates of trauma exposure and estimated at 4.7%, with significantly higher rates of PTSD observed among females (7.3%) than males (2.2%) (8). The most common PTEs for children and adolescents are the unexpected death of a loved one (28.2%) and man-made or natural disasters (14.8%), with these PTEs associated with the lowest rates of subsequent PTSD. Only 10.3% of youth exposed to the unexpected death of a loved one, and 6.5% of youth exposed to man-made or natural disasters go on to develop PTSD. It is the least common PTEs, kidnapping (0.6%), physical abuse by a caregiver (2.0%), physical assault by a romantic partner (1.3%), sexual abuse (3.8%), and rape (2.5%) that are associated with the highest rates of PTSD (range: 25.2% to 39.3%).

RISK FACTORS FOR THE DEVELOPMENT OF PTSD

Genetic Factors

As reviewed in the child abuse chapter in this text, genetic factors, in part, explain why some traumatized children go on to develop PTSD, and others do not. The genetic risk factors associated with PTSD, however, are not unique to PTSD. Nearly all genetic markers that have been reported to increase risk for PTSD following experiences of child abuse or other traumatic events have been associated with risk for a range of different psychiatric problems, as well as risk for the development of substance use disorders (9).

Trauma Characteristics

Trauma factors are among the best replicated predictors of PTSD onset, severity, and persistence. As noted above, type of trauma predicts risk for PTSD, with risk for PTSD greatest after experiences of kidnapping, physical abuse by a caregiver, physical assault by a romantic partner, sexual abuse, and rape (8). In addition, the greater the severity of the sexual (10) and physical assaults (11), the greater the likelihood of PTSD developing. Increased risk for PTSD is also associated with traumatic events that are unexpected (12) and chronic (13,14), and when the victim is in close emotional and physical proximity to the event (15). Polyvictimization is another factor that adds to the severity and complexity of trauma symptoms (16).

Posttrauma Factors

Factors in the posttrauma environment contribute most in determining the likelihood of PTSD becoming chronic. The absence of social supports and exposure to ongoing psychosocial adversity are the most potent predictors of PTSD chronicity (15,17,18). Low parental support and a hostile and coercive parenting style, as perceived by children, are also potent predictors of PTSD severity (19). Enhancing the caregiver response and capacity to support the child posttrauma, is therefore an important component of prevention and treatment interventions following traumatic experiences.

ASSESSMENT OF TRAUMA EXPERIENCES

It is best to assess children's trauma experiences utilizing information from multiple informants (e.g., parent, children, child protective service workers) (20–22). As reviewed elsewhere (23), several rating scales have been developed to assess abuse, neglect, and other traumatic experiences in children and adolescents. The Childhood Trauma Questionnaire (24) provides an excellent self-report assessment of a range of maltreatment experiences and can be utilized with children of age 12 and above. The UCLA Posttraumatic Stress Disorder Reaction Index (UCLA-PTSD-RI) is one of the most widely used trauma symptom assessment scales and includes a survey of maltreatment- and nonmaltreatment-related traumatic events (25). The PTSD-RI can be downloaded at no cost with administration and scoring instructions from the National Child Traumatic Stress Network (NCTSN) website (http://www.nctsn.org/nctsn_assets/pdfs/mediasite/ptsd-training.pdf). The Structured Trauma-Related Experiences and Symptoms Screener (STRESS) is a relatively new computer-administered measure with excellent psychometric properties (26).

TRAUMA SYMPTOM ASSESSMENT

In our clinical and research practice, we aim to have trauma history data from multiple informants prior to assessing psychiatric symptomatology in children. We then query them about various trauma experiences. If children deny a trauma we know they have experienced via other sources, we consider that evidence of "avoidance." We then let them know what we learned about from the other source, let them know that we are not going to ask them too much about those experiences at the time of the evaluation, and just want to know if they have any problems that many other children experience who have been through the type of things they experienced. We then query them regarding the presence of PTSD symptoms. If children are particularly reticent to talk, we begin by asking the more benign hyperarousal items (sleep difficulties, concentration problems, and irritability), progress to ask about the negative cognition and mood and avoidance symptoms, and then query about the more stressful reexperiencing items.

If children are living in foster care or with other guardians who do not know them well, obtaining adjunctive information from birth parents and/or school teachers can be enormously helpful. In addition, parents and caretakers are notoriously poor at identifying internalizing (depression, anxiety) symptoms. Children are the best informants of these symptoms. Children are also frequently the best to ask about nightmares and sleeping difficulties. As traumatized children frequently have not received comfort when distressed, many do not seek adult reassurance when they wake up from a nightmare. Rather, they stay in their beds alone, terrified. Their guardians have no idea they are not sleeping through the night.

There are several well-validated trauma symptom rating scales (23), including: the UCLA PTSD-RI (27) discussed previously, Trauma Symptom Checklist for Young Children (28), Trauma Symptom Checklist for Children (29), Child Dissociative Checklist (30), Adolescent Dissociative Experiences Scale (31), and Child Sexual Behavior Inventory (32). There are also several story-based/cartoon measures available, including the Darryl (33), Andy/Angie Cartoon Trauma Scales (34), and the Levonn Cartoon-Based Interview for Assessing Children's Distress (35). Trauma-related symptomatology is also well assessed using semistructured diagnostic interviews for young (36) and school-age children (37).

PSYCHIATRIC COMORBIDITY AND DIFFERENTIAL DIAGNOSIS

Approximately three-quarters of individuals with PTSD experience one or more comorbid lifetime diagnoses, and 37% to 48% report a lifetime history of major depression (38–40). In one-half to three-quarters of all cases, the onset of PTSD is primary. The risk for major depressive disorder (MDD) following PTSD is about the same as the risk of MDD following any other anxiety disorder, and 30% to 40% more likely in individuals with a history of a pre-existing anxiety disorder. PTSD is also highly comorbid with alcohol and substance abuse disorders in adolescents and adults (41–43), highlighting the importance of routine screening for substance use disorders in youth with significant trauma histories.

The diagnosis of PTSD has numerous symptoms in common with multiple other childhood psychiatric diagnoses. In the DSM-5, PTSD and MDD have five symptoms in common. Concentration difficulties associated with PTSD are frequently misattributed to attention deficit hyperactivity disorder (ADHD) (44), and extreme irritability reported in PTSD is sometimes misattributed to mania or oppositional defiant disorder (ODD).

Determining the presence of PTSD and potential comorbid diagnoses requires careful assessment of the developmental timing of the onset of symptoms, evaluating the pattern of problem behaviors, the severity of difficulties across different settings, and the association of problem behaviors with trauma triggers. For the diagnosis of PTSD to be given, there must be at least one reexperiencing symptom, a cardinal feature of the disorder. For comorbid MDD to be diagnosed, beyond symptoms that overlap with the diagnosis of PTSD, there should ideally be at least one symptom that is uniquely associated with MDD (appetite disturbance, low self-esteem, and suicidality). For concentration problems to be attributed to ADHD, they should have been evident before the trauma, be relatively chronic, and generally worse in a school setting. If they emerged after the trauma and are worse in the home setting or when the child is exposed to trauma triggers, they are likely not related to ADHD. Irritability is a totally nonspecific symptom associated with many of the major childhood psychiatric diagnoses. Most symptoms of ODD involve some expression of irritability, but for a comorbid ODD diagnosis to be given there should be evidence of marked and persistent defiance, disrespect, or vindictiveness. In PTSD, irritability is frequently worse when the child is exposed to trauma triggers and less evident in nonemotionally charged environments. Sleep disturbance is another symptom shared by several child diagnoses. While both PTSD and mania are associated with sleep disturbances, decreased need for sleep is the cardinal feature of mania, and nightmares and insomnia—wanting to sleep, but not being able to—are the sine qua non of PTSD.

When psychotic-like symptoms are present, differentiating between PTSD, mood disorders with psychotic features, or a primary psychotic disorder has extremely important treatment implications. A number of distinctive features of psychotic-like symptoms in traumatized children facilitate this differential diagnosis. For example, hallucinations in maltreated children are frequently trauma related, such as hearing the perpetrator's voice, or as depicted in the case example at the beginning of this chapter, are frequently illusory experiences related to safety. They are also often nocturnal (30), and frequently resolve with psychotherapeutic intervention, cessation of the trauma, and safety reassurances (45). In addition, the presence of hallucinations in traumatized children is not typically associated with other psychotic symptoms that would suggest schizophrenia or another primary psychotic diagnosis. They are less likely to be associated with negative symptoms (withdrawn behavior, blunted affect) or abnormal early development as would be typical in childhood-onset schizophrenia (46). Hallucinations in traumatized children tend to be associated with impulsive, aggressive, and self-injurious behavior, nightmares, and trance-like states, and less likely to be associated with evidence of formal thought disorder (47).

COURSE AND TRAJECTORY

Bonanno et al. (13) describe four typical trajectories that have been found in a variety of studies among individuals with different types of traumatic experiences: resilient, delayed, recovered, and chronic. The majority of individuals who experience trauma, from 35% to 65% of those exposed, tend to be in the resilient category, showing healthy functioning even shortly after the traumatic event that is maintained over time. The delayed course, comprising approximately 0% to 15% of cases, appears to show subclinical adjustment problems that increase in severity over time. Those who can be termed recovered, making up roughly 15% to 25% of cases, show significant symptoms early on, which resolve to a large degree over time and with treatment. Those in the chronic distress category, estimated at 5% to 30% of exposed individuals, show serious symptoms and functional limitations that are resistant to treatment.

PREVENTION

There is no clear evidence supporting the use of psychological debriefing approaches posttrauma (48,49). Traditionally conceived, psychological debriefing is delivered in the early aftermath of an event in a single group session in which survivors share their experiences and reactions and reconstruct the event. Methodologic limitations restrict the conclusions that can be drawn from the available empirical evidence, but most studies show no clear benefit with debriefing interventions, and some studies in adults reported worse outcomes among individuals participating in the debriefing intervention.

The NCTSN developed a trauma-informed modular approach to psychological first aid (PFA) for use by mental health responders in diverse settings under diverse conditions which is available on the NCTSN website (http://www.nctsn.org/content/psychological-first-aid). The PFA intervention involves providing for the basic safety and comfort of survivors, connecting survivors with social supports and practical assistance, psychoeducation about typical trauma responses, tips for helping children cope, and teaching basic relaxation techniques. The PFA intervention, however, has yet to undergo rigorous evaluation (49,50).

The Child and Family Traumatic Stress Intervention (CFTSI) is a four-session prevention protocol developed for children within 30 days of a PTE (51). The central goals are to increase parent–child communication about feelings, symptoms, and behaviors related to the PTE, and to provide behavioral coping skills to the child and caregiver. The child and caregiver are separately provided psychoeducation about trauma and coping and then brought together in the final session to facilitate mutual communication and use of the skills imparted in the intervention. In an initial randomized controlled trial comparing the effectiveness of this preventive intervention to four nondirective support sessions, 3 months posttreatment CFTSI was associated with significantly lower rates of PTSD diagnoses and fewer PTSD and other trauma symptoms in the children (51).

There are currently no strongly supported pharmacologic approaches to prevent the development of PTSD posttrauma exposure. An early pilot study supported the use of propranolol (52), but a meta-analyses of studies conducted in adults suggest propranolol treatment after a traumatic event does not alter the incidence of PTSD (53). Consistent with the results of the meta-analysis of adult studies, a randomized controlled trial with 29 youth likewise failed to show an advantage of propranolol over placebo in preventing the onset of PTSD posttrauma exposure (54). For child burn victims, there is some suggestion that enhanced pain management with morphine treatment is associated with lower rates of PTSD (55), and one small open treatment trial of three physically abused preschool-age children diagnosed with ASD secondary to serious burns that reported significant improvement in symptoms with risperidone treatment (56).

PSYCHOSOCIAL TREATMENTS

Since its inception in 2000, the NCTSN has had a far-reaching impact on extending understanding and treatment of childhood trauma in the United States. The mission of the NCTSN is to raise the standard of care and increase access to evidence-based trauma-informed interventions. Clinicians, families, and other interested parties can access a wealth of information through the website www.nctsn.org. NCTSN provides education to a wide range of audiences, from children and families to clinicians, educators, first responders, and others. Continuing education about various types of trauma, their effects, special populations, evidence-based treatments, and assessment tools is available both on the website and through webinars and in-person venues.

Trauma-Focused Cognitive Behavior Therapy (TF-CBT) is the psychotherapeutic intervention with the strongest empirical support for PTSD and other trauma-related symptoms in children and adolescents (25,57–59). TF-CBT is a 12-to-16-session intervention that was designed for children aged 3 to 18 years to reduce PTSD symptoms and other behavioral and emotional problems associated with child trauma exposure. The central components of TF-CBT are represented by the PRACTICE acronym. The "P" stands for psychoeducation (e.g., educating children and parents about the prevalence of the type of traumatic event the child experienced and common trauma reactions) and parenting skills training (parent management principles). "R" stands for relaxation skills; "A" for affective modulation skills (e.g., feeling identification; self-regulation skills); "C" for cognitive coping and processing (e.g., recognizing relations among thoughts, feelings, and behaviors); "T" for the trauma narrative (creating a narrative of the child's traumatic experiences); "I" for in vivo mastery of trauma reminders; "C" for conjoint child–parent sessions (joint sessions in which the child shares the trauma narrative with parents and other family issues are addressed); and "E" for enhancing future safety and development (25).

TF-CBT training can be obtained via attending workshops conducted by certified trainers, reviewing published treatment manuals (58,60,61), and completing a web-based training available at www.musc.edu/tfcbt. Extant data suggest the model is implemented with the strongest fidelity when the web-based training and two-day in-person workshop are completed and augmented with follow-up consultation (62).

As reviewed elsewhere (25,59), the efficacy of TF-CBT has been demonstrated in over a dozen randomized controlled trials and has been deemed "supported and efficacious" based on current standards. Among the currently available evidence-based child trauma treatments, TF-CBT alone has been evaluated across the child and adolescent developmental spectrum (3 to 18 years), for multiple index traumas (e.g., sexual abuse, commercial sexual exploitation, domestic violence, disaster, war, traumatic grief, and multiple and complex trauma), in different settings (e.g., clinics, foster care, community domestic violence center, refugee nongovernmental organization, juvenile detention centers, human immunodeficiency virus treatment centers), in group- and individual-administered formats, in multiple countries and cultures (e.g., United States, Native American, Africa, Europe, Australia), and with both mental health and nonmental health providers (59). In all of these studies, TF-CBT has been found to be superior to the comparison conditions for improving PTSD symptoms and diagnosis, as well as other related outcomes including, depression, internalizing symptoms, externalizing problems, anxiety ratings, sexualized behaviors, relationship difficulties, and adaptive functioning (59). Moreover, the therapeutic effects of TF-CBT have been shown to be maintained over 6, 12, and 24 months following treatment (63,64).

Child–Parent Psychotherapy (65) and the Attachment Biobehavioral Catch-up intervention (66,67) represent two trauma-focused treatment models that have been developed for working with infants, toddlers, and preschoolers. For an updated list of empirically supported treatments and promising practices the interested reader is referred to the NCTSN website (http://www.nctsnet.org/resources/audiences/parents-caregivers/treatments-that-work) and a recent review by Barth et al. (68).

PSYCHOPHARMACOLOGY

Trauma-focused psychotherapies are considered the first line of treatment for PTSD in children and adolescents (25), and as of the writing of this book, there were no Federal Drug Administration (FDA) approved pharmacologic treatments for youth with PTSD. While studies of pharmacologic treatment of PTSD have demonstrated the efficacy of selective serotonin reuptake inhibitors (SSRI's) in adults (69), support for SSRIs in children and adolescents with PTSD is lacking (70). Two randomized controlled studies examined the use of sertraline to treat childhood PTSD and both reported no advantage for SSRI medications over placebo (71,72).

Overall there is a paucity of data to guide the pharmacologic treatment of youth with PTSD. In small-scale open treatment trials with samples ranging in size from 3 to 19 youth, benefits in treating PTSD have been suggested with quetiapine (73), clonidine (74), and guanfacine (75). In a B-A-B off-on-off design, propranolol was also shown to reduce reexperiencing and hyperarousal symptoms in a study with 11 youth (76), and in secondary analyses of data from 12 youth with comorbid PTSD who were part of a double-blind, randomized controlled trial of two doses of divalproex sodium treatment in boys with conduct disorder, those assigned to the high-dose condition of divalproex sodium had a greater reduction in PTSD symptoms than youth assigned the lower dose (77).

Glutamate N-methyl-d-aspartic acid (NMDA) receptors have been shown to be involved in fear extinction, and although the findings have been mixed, there are data showing that D-cycloserine (DCS), a partial NMDA agonist, can enhance fear extinction and the efficacy of cognitive behavioral and exposure-based therapies for PTSD in adults and a range of anxiety disorders in children, adolescents, and adults (78). In the one DCS trial completed with youth with PTSD, 57 children and adolescents were randomized to DCS or placebo plus CBT exposure-based treatment. The authors reported a trend toward DCS speeding PTSD symptom recovery during the exposure-based sessions, and evidence that the CBT and DCS group better maintained clinical gains 3 months after treatment than the CBT plus placebo group (79).

While trauma-focused psychotherapies are considered the first line of treatment for PTSD in children and adolescents (25), it is estimated that approximately 20% of youth who complete a course of TF-CBT will still meet diagnostic criteria for PTSD posttreatment (80). Further research is needed to identify pharmacologic agents effective in the treatment of PTSD, and the augmentation of evidence-based psychotherapies. Preclinical and early clinical studies in adults suggest the utility of several potential novel agents, including nabilone, norbinaltorphimine, 7,8-dihydroxyflavone, and oxytocin (OT) to target cannabinoids, opioids, brain-derived neurotrophic factor, and the OT receptor systems, respectively (81). To date, pharmacologic treatment choice for children with PTSD is best guided by the comorbid diagnostic profile of the child, and ideally used to augment evidence-based psychotherapy approaches.

CONCLUSIONS

The child trauma field has made considerable advances in recent years, promoted in large part by the efforts of the NCTSN. Trauma exposure among children and adolescents is a common phenomenon that leads to PTSD and other mental health symptoms in a significant proportion of cases. While most children show a degree of resilience in response to traumatic events, those exposed to interpersonal violence and polytraumatization are at greatest risk for ongoing distress and compromised functioning. Good trauma-informed care requires an understanding of the factors that modify outcome, thorough multi-informant assessment, and evidence-based therapy in combination with psychopharmacologic treatment when clinically indicated.

References

1. APA: *Diagnostic and Statistical Manual of Mental Disorders: DSM-5*. 5th ed. Washington, DC, American Psychiatric Association, 2013.
2. Meiser-Stedman R, Smith P, Glucksman E, Yule W, Dalgleish T: The posttraumatic stress disorder diagnosis in preschool- and elementary school-age children exposed to motor vehicle accidents. *Am J Psychiatry* 165:1326–1337, 2008.
3. Scheeringa MS, Wright MJ, Hunt JP, Zeanah CH: Factors affecting the diagnosis and prediction of PTSD symptomatology in children and adolescents. *Am J Psychiatry* 163:644–651, 2006.
4. DeYoung CG, Cicchetti D, Rogosch FA: Moderation of the association between childhood maltreatment and neuroticism by the corticotropin-releasing hormone receptor 1 gene. *J Child Psychol Psychiatry* 52:898–906, 2011.
5. Kessler RC, Avenevoli S, Costello EJ, et al.: Design and field procedures in the US National Comorbidity Survey Replication Adolescent Supplement (NCS-A). *Int J Methods Psychiatr Res* 18:69–83, 2009.
6. Kessler RC, Avenevoli S, McLaughlin KA, et al.: Lifetime co-morbidity of DSM-IV disorders in the US National Comorbidity Survey Replication Adolescent Supplement (NCS-A). *Psychol Med* 42:1997–2010, 2012.
7. Copeland WE, Keeler G, Angold A, Costello EJ: Traumatic events and posttraumatic stress in childhood. *Arch Gen Psychiatry* 64:577–584, 2007.
8. McLaughlin KA, Koenen KC, Hill ED, et al.: Trauma exposure and posttraumatic stress disorder in a national sample of adolescents. *J Am Acad Child Adolesc Psychiatry* 52:815–830.e14, 2013.
9. Montalvo-Ortiz JL, Gelernter J, Hudziak J, Kaufman J: RDoC and translational perspectives on the genetics of trauma-related psychiatric disorders. *Am J Med Genet B Neuropsychiatr Genet* 171:81–91, 2016.
10. Lynskey MT, Fergusson DM: Factors protecting against the development of adjustment difficulties in young adults exposed to childhood sexual abuse. *Child Abuse Negl* 21:1177–1190, 1997.
11. Boney-McCoy S, Finkelhor D: Psychosocial sequelae of violent victimization in a national youth sample. *J Consult Clin Psychol* 63:726–736, 1995.
12. Lobb EA, Kristjanson LJ, Aoun SM, Monterosso L, Halkett GK, Davies A: Predictors of complicated grief: a systematic review of empirical studies. *Death Stud* 34:673–698, 2010.
13. Bonanno GA, Westphal M, Mancini AD: Resilience to loss and potential trauma. *Annu Rev Clin Psychol* 7:511–535, 2011.
14. McCart MR, Smith DW, Saunders BE, Kilpatrick DG, Resnick H, Ruggiero KJ: Do urban adolescents become desensitized to community violence? Data from a national survey. *Am J Orthopsychiatry* 77:434–442, 2007.
15. Brewin CR, Andrews B, Valentine JD: Meta-analysis of risk factors for posttraumatic stress disorder in trauma-exposed adults. *J Consult Clin Psychol* 68:748–766, 2000.
16. Clark DB, Lesnick L, Hegedus AM: Traumas and other adverse life events in adolescents with alcohol abuse and dependence. *J Am Acad Child Adolesc Psychiatry* 36:1744–1751, 1997.
17. Charuvastra A, Cloitre M: Social bonds and posttraumatic stress disorder. *Annu Rev Psychol* 59:301–328, 2008.
18. Pynoos RS, Steinberg AM, Piacentini JC: A developmental psychopathology model of childhood traumatic stress and intersection with anxiety disorders. *Biol Psychiatry* 46:1542–1554, 1999.
19. Valentino K, Berkowitz S, Stover CS: Parenting behaviors and posttraumatic symptoms in relation to children's symptomatology following a traumatic event. *J Trauma Stress* 23:403–407, 2010.
20. Grasso D, Boonsiri J, Lipschitz D, et al.: Posttraumatic stress disorder: the missed diagnosis. *Child Welfare* 88:157–176, 2009.
21. Shaffer A, Huston L, Egeland B: Identification of child maltreatment using prospective and self-report methodologies: a comparison of maltreatment incidence and relation to later psychopathology. *Child Abuse Negl* 32:682–692, 2008.
22. Hambrick EP, Tunno AM, Gabrielli J, Jackson Y, Belz C: Using multiple informants to assess child maltreatment: concordance between case file and youth self-report. *J Aggress Maltreat Trauma* 23:751–771, 2014.
23. Stover CS, Berkowitz S: Assessing violence exposure and trauma symptoms in young children: a critical review of measures. *J Trauma Stress* 18:707–717, 2005.
24. Bernstein D, Ahluvalia T, Pogge D, Handelsman L: Validity of the childhood trauma questionnaire in an adolescent psychiatric population. *J Am Acad Child Adolesc Psychiatry* 36:340–348, 1997.
25. Cohen JA, Bukstein O, Walter H, et al.: Practice parameter for the assessment and treatment of children and adolescents with posttraumatic stress disorder. *J Am Acad Child Adolesc Psychiatry* 49:414–430, 2010.
26. Grasso DJ, Felton JW, Reid-Quinones K: The Structured Trauma-Related Experiences and Symptoms Screener (STRESS): development and preliminary psychometrics. *Child Maltreat* 20:214–220, 2015.
27. Pynoos R, Steinberg AM: *UCLA PTSD Reaction Index for Children and Adolescents--DSM-5 Version*. Los Angeles, University of California, 2013.
28. Briere J, Johnson K, Bissada A, et al.: The Trauma Symptom Checklist for Young Children (TSCYC): reliability and association with abuse exposure in a multi-site study. *Child Abuse Negl* 25:1001–1014, 2001.
29. Briere J: *Trauma Symptom Checklist for Children (TSCC) Professional Manual*. Odessa, FL, Psychological Assessment Resources, 1996.
30. Putnam FW, Helmers K, Trickett PK: Development, reliability, and validity of a child dissociation scale. *Child Abuse Negl* 17:731–741, 1993.
31. Armstrong JG, Putnam FW, Carlson EB, Libero DZ, Smith SR: Development and validation of a measure of adolescent dissociation: the adolescent dissociative experiences scale. *J Nerv Ment Dis* 185:491–497, 1997.
32. Friedrich WN, Grambsch P, Damon L, et al.: Child sexual behavior inventory: normative and clinical comparisons. *Psychol Assess* 4:303–311, 1992.

33. Geller PA, Neugebauer R, Possemato AK, Walter P, Dummit ES, Silva RR: Psychometric properties of Darryl, a cartoon based measure to assess community violence-related PTSD in children. *Psychiatr Q* 78:157–168, 2007.
34. Praver F, DiGiuseppe R, Pelcovitz D, Mandel FS, Gaines R: A preliminary study of a cartoon measure for children's reactions to chronic trauma. *Child Maltreat* 5(3):273–285, 2000.
35. Richters J, Martinez P, Valla J: *Levonn: A Cartoon Based Interview for Assessing Children's Distress Symptoms*. Washington, DC, National Institute of Mental Health, 1990.
36. Scheeringa MS, Haslett N: The reliability and criterion validity of the diagnostic infant and preschool assessment: a new diagnostic instrument for young children. *Child Psychiatry Hum Dev* 41:299–312, 2010.
37. Kaufman J, Birmaher B, Brent D, Rao U: Schedule for Affective Disorders and Schizophrenia for School-Age Children-Present and Lifetime version (K-SADS-PL): initial reliability and validity data. *J Am Acad Child Adolesc Psychiatry* 36:980–988, 1997.
38. Breslau N, Davis GC, Andreski P, Peterson E: Traumatic events and posttraumatic stress disorder in an urban population of young adults. *Arch Gen Psychiatry* 48:216–222, 1991.
39. Breslau N, Davis GC, Andreski P, Peterson EL, Schultz LR: Sex differences in posttraumatic stress disorder. *Arch Gen Psychiatry* 54:1044–1048, 1997.
40. Kessler R, Sonnega A, Bromet E, Hughes M, Nelson C: Posttraumatic stress disorder in the National Comorbidity Survey. *Arch Gen Psychiatry* 52:1048–1060, 1995.
41. Kendler KS, Kessler RC, Walters EE, et al.: Stressful life events, genetic liability, and onset of an episode of major depression in women. *Am J Psychiatry* 152:833–842, 1995.
42. Clark DB, Pollock N, Bukstein OG, Mezzich AC, Bromberger JT, Donovan JE: Gender and comorbid psychopathology in adolescents with alcohol dependence. *J Am Acad Child Adolesc Psychiatry* 36:1195–1203, 1997.
43. Adams ZW, Danielson CK, Sumner JA, McCauley JL, Cohen JR, Ruggiero KJ: Comorbidity of PTSD, major depression, and substance use disorder among adolescent victims of the spring 2011 Tornadoes in Alabama and Joplin, Missouri. *Psychiatry* 78:170–185, 2015.
44. Weinstein D, Staffelbach D, Biaggio M: Attention-deficit hyperactivity disorder and posttraumatic stress disorder: differential diagnosis in childhood sexual abuse. *Clin Psychol Rev* 20:359–378, 2000.
45. Putnam FW, Hornstein N, Peterson G: Clinical phenomenology of child and adolescent dissociative disorders: gender and age effects. *Child Adolesc Psychiatr Clin N Am* 5:351–360, 1996.
46. Nurcombe B, Mitchell W, Begtrup R, Tramontana M, LaBarbera J, Pruitt J: Dissociative hallucinosis and allied conditions. In: Volkmar FR, Volkmar FR (eds): Arlington, VA, US, American Psychiatric Association, 107–128, 1996.
47. Kaufman J, Birmaher B, Clayton S, Retano A, Wongchaowart B: Case study: trauma-related hallucinations. *J Am Acad Child Adolesc Psychiatry* 36(11):1602–1605, 1997.
48. Pfefferbaum B, Jacobs AK, Nitiema P, Everly GS Jr: Child debriefing: a review of the evidence base. *Prehosp Disaster Med* 30:306–315, 2015.
49. Pfefferbaum B, Shaw JA: Practice parameter on disaster preparedness. *J Am Acad Child Adolesc Psychiatry* 52:1224–1238, 2013.
50. Allen B, Brymer MJ, Steinberg AM, et al.: Perceptions of psychological first aid among providers responding to Hurricanes Gustav and Ike. *J Trauma Stress* 23:509–513, 2010.
51. Berkowitz SJ, Stover CS, Marans SR: The child and family traumatic stress intervention: secondary prevention for youth at risk of developing PTSD. *J Child Psychol Psychiatry* 52:676–685, 2011.
52. Pitman RK, Sanders KM, Zusman RM, et al.: Pilot study of secondary prevention of posttraumatic stress disorder with propranolol. *Biol Psychiatry* 51:189–192, 2002.
53. Argolo FC, Cavalcanti-Ribeiro P, Netto LR, Quarantini LC: Prevention of posttraumatic stress disorder with propranolol: a meta-analytic review. *J Psychosom Res* 79:89–93, 2015.
54. Nugent NR, Christopher NC, Crow JP, Browne L, Ostrowski S, Delahanty DL: The efficacy of early propranolol administration at reducing PTSD symptoms in pediatric injury patients: a pilot study. *J Trauma Stress* 23:282–287, 2010.
55. Saxe G, Stoddard F, Courtney D, et al.: Relationship between acute morphine and the course of PTSD in children with burns. *J Am Acad Child Adolesc Psychiatry* 40:915–921, 2001.
56. Meighen KG, Hines LA, Lagges AM: Risperidone treatment of preschool children with thermal burns and acute stress disorder. *J Child Adolesc Psychopharmacol* 17:223–232, 2007.
57. Cohen JA, Mannarino AP, Deblinger E: *Treating Trauma and Traumatic Grief in Children and Adolescents*. New York, Guilford Press, 2006.
58. Cohen JA, Mannarino A: *Trauma-Focused CBT for Children and Adolescents: Treatment Applications*. New York, Guilford Press, 2012.
59. Cohen JA, Mannarino AP: Trauma-focused cognitive behavior therapy for traumatized children and families. *Child Adolesc Psychiatr Clin N Am* 24:557–570, 2015.
60. Cohen JA, Deblinger E, Mannarino AP: Trauma-focused cognitive-behavioral therapy for sexually abused children. In: Hibbs ED, Jensen PS (eds): *Psychosocial Treatments for Child and Adolescent Disorders, Empirically Based Strategies for Clinical Practice*. 2nd ed. Washington, DC, American Psychological Association, 2005.
61. Scheeringa M: *Treating PTSD in Preschoolers: A Clinical Guide*. New York, Guilford Press, 2015.
62. Cohen JA, Mannarino AP, Jankowski K, Rosenberg S, Kodya S, Wolford GL 2nd: A randomized implementation study of trauma-focused cognitive behavioral therapy for adjudicated teens in residential treatment facilities. *Child Maltreat* 21:156–167, 2016.
63. Deblinger E, Mannarino AP, Cohen JA, Steer RA: A follow-up study of a multisite, randomized, controlled trial for children with sexual abuse-related PTSD symptoms. *J Am Acad Child Adolesc Psychiatry* 45:1474–1484, 2006.
64. Deblinger E, Steer RA, Lippmann J: Two-year follow-up study of cognitive behavioral therapy for sexually abused children suffering post-traumatic stress symptoms. *Child Abuse Negl* 23:1371–1378, 1999.
65. Lieberman AF, Van Horn P: *"Don't hit my mommy!": A Manual for Child-Parent Psychotherapy with Young Witnesses of Family Violence*. Washington, DC, Zero to Three Press, 2005.
66. Bernard K, Hostinar CE, Dozier M: Intervention effects on diurnal cortisol rhythms of child protective services-referred infants in early childhood: preschool follow-up results of a randomized clinical trial. *JAMA pediatrics* 169:112–119, 2015.
67. Dozier M, Peloso E, Lewis E, Laurenceau JP, Levine S: Effects of an attachment-based intervention on the cortisol production of infants and toddlers in foster care. *Dev Psychopathol* 20:845–859, 2008.
68. Barth RP, Greeson JK, Zlotnik SR, Chintapalli LK: Evidence-based practice for youth in supervised out-of-home care: a framework for development, definition, and evaluation. *J Evid Based Soc Work* 8:501–528, 2011.
69. Hoskins M, Pearce J, Bethell A, et al.: Pharmacotherapy for post-traumatic stress disorder: systematic review and meta-analysis. *Br J Psychiatry* 206:93–100, 2015.
70. Cohen JA, Bukstein O, Walter H, et al.: Practice parameter for the assessment and treatment of children and adolescent with posttraumatic stress disorder. *J Am Acad Child Adolesc Psychiatry* 49:414–430, 2010.
71. Cohen JA, Mannarino AP, Perel JM, Staron V: A pilot randomized controlled trial of combined trauma-focused CBT and sertraline for childhood PTSD symptoms. *J Am Acad Child Adolesc Psychiatry* 46:811–819, 2007.
72. Robb AS, Cueva JE, Sporn J, Yang R, Vanderburg DG: Sertraline treatment of children and adolescents with posttraumatic stress disorder: a double-blind, placebo-controlled trial. *J Child Adolesc Psychopharmacol* 20:463–471, 2010.
73. Stathis S, Martin G, McKenna JG: A preliminary case series on the use of quetiapine for posttraumatic stress disorder in juveniles within a youth detention center. *J Clin Psychopharmacol* 25:539–544, 2005.
74. Harmon RJ, Riggs PD: Clonidine for posttraumatic stress disorder in preschool children. *J Am Acad Child Adolesc Psychiatry* 35:1247–1249, 1996.
75. Connor DF, Grasso DJ, Slivinsky MD, Pearson GS, Banga A: An open-label study of guanfacine extended release for traumatic stress related symptoms in children and adolescents. *J Child Adolesc Psychopharmacol* 23:244–251, 2013.
76. Famularo R, Kinscherff R, Fenton T: Propranolol treatment for childhood posttraumatic stress disorder, acute type. A pilot study. *Am J Dis Child* 142:1244–1247, 1988.
77. Steiner H, Saxena KS, Carrion V, Khanzode LA, Silverman M, Chang K: Divalproex sodium for the treatment of PTSD and conduct disordered youth: a pilot randomized controlled clinical trial. *Child Psychiatry Hum Dev* 38:183–193, 2007.
78. Ori R, Amos T, Bergman H, Soares-Weiser K, Ipser JC, Stein DJ: Augmentation of cognitive and behavioural therapies (CBT) with d-cycloserine for anxiety and related disorders. *Cochrane Database Syst Rev* 5:CD007803, 2015.
79. Scheeringa MS, Weems CF: Randomized placebo-controlled D-cycloserine with cognitive behavior therapy for pediatric posttraumatic stress. *J Child Adolesc Psychopharmacol* 24:69–77, 2014.
80. Cohen JA, Deblinger E, Mannarino AP, Steer RA: A multisite, randomized controlled trial for children with sexual abuse-related PTSD symptoms. *J Am Acad Child Adolesc Psychiatry* 43:393–402, 2004.
81. Ragen BJ, Seidel J, Chollak C, Pietrzak RH, Neumeister A: Investigational drugs under development for the treatment of PTSD. *Expert Opin Investig Drugs* 24:659–672, 2015.

CHAPTER 5.15.3 ■ REACTIVE ATTACHMENT DISORDER AND DISINHIBITED SOCIAL ENGAGEMENT DISORDER

MARY MARGARET GLEASON AND CHARLES H. ZEANAH

INTRODUCTION

Since the mid-20th century, psychiatric literature has included descriptions of the negative impact of severe emotional deprivation (1). Descriptive studies of young children raised in institutions have consistently described abnormalities in social and emotional development in children raised in extreme caregiving adversity. Although disorders of attachment were not described in formal nosologies until the DSM-III (2), attachment theory has been the focus of active investigation for decades beginning with Bowlby (3,4). Bowlby proposed that infants are born with a biologic predisposition to develop an attachment relationship with a small number of caregiving adults from whom the child seeks comfort, nurturance, support, and protection (Table 5.15.3.1).

DEVELOPMENTAL STAGES OF THE ATTACHMENT RELATIONSHIP

In the first 2 months of life, infants preferentially orient to people's movement, faces, sounds, although they do not discriminate among people, except in very subtle ways. From ages 2 to 7 months, children become more socially interactive and appear to respond differentially to their caregivers, although they continue to socially engage with unfamiliar adults as well. Focused attachment behavior, characterized by proximity seeking in times of stress, appears around 7 to 9 months of age, heralded by the onset of separation protest and stranger anxiety. According to attachment theory, the attachment system works in conjunction with a number of other biologically driven systems, most prominently the exploration system. An equilibrium develops between the attachment and exploration systems. The parent serves as a secure base from which the child can explore the world when the exploration system is more highly activated, and a safe haven to whom she/he can return in times of stress when the attachment behaviors are more prominent.

Interactions of Attachment, Exploration, and Social Systems

In human infants, attachment formation appears to be an example of experience-expectant neural development, by which infants are hardwired to form selective attachments to caregiving adults. Environmental and relationship factors play a strong role in the type of attachment relationship that the child develops. Ainsworth demonstrated a relationship between early patterns of parental, sensitivity, and infant responsiveness, and the development of a secure attachment relationship at age 12 months (5,6).

Patterns of attachment serve as risk and protective factors for subsequent psychosocial adaptation. Children with insecure attachment patterns are at higher risk for subsequent psychiatric disorders and impairment from emotional and behavioral symptoms than securely attached infants (7,8).

TABLE 5.15.3.1

DEVELOPMENT OF ATTACHMENT

	0–2 Months	2–7 Months	7–18 Months	18–26 Months
Bowlby's characterization	• Orientation and signals without discrimination	• Orientation and signals directed toward >1 or more discriminated figures	• Maintenance of proximity to a discriminated figure	• Formation of a reciprocal relationship
Social interaction Patterns	• Physical and social attributes attract adults for social interactions • Recognition of maternal face • Olfactory/auditory recognition • Spontaneous smile	• Able to engage adults in reciprocal social interactions • Evidence of differential responses to adults	• Focused attachment • Separation protest • Stranger reactions • Intersubjectivity evident • Social referencing	• Develop negotiating abilities with caregivers ("goal-corrected partnership") • Increased interest in peers; move toward interactive play and exploration
Communication/ methods of cueing adults to needs	• Crying, cooing	• Eye contact • Social smile • Responsive cooing, babbling	• Intentional communication with gestures and then words	• Able to express needs • Rapid vocabulary expansion

Disorders of Attachment

Definitions of the categorical disorders related to attachment patterns have evolved over the last decades, with different nomenclature, but with fairly consistent core features. For the first time in the DSM-III-R, the two subtypes of "inhibited" and "disinhibited" reactive attachment disorder were introduced; these distinctions remain in all extant nosologies.

The ICD-10, which preceded the DSM-5 and is used primarily in Europe, similarly describes two separate disorders, both with an emphasis on social relatedness. The first is simply "reactive attachment disorder of childhood" and describes children with inhibited emotional responsiveness and contradictory social responses. In the ICD-10 nosology, "disinhibited attachment disorder of childhood" describes children with diffuse attachments and indiscriminate behaviors (9).

For the purposes of this chapter, the DSM-5 classifications will be used. The DSM-5, published in 2013, also describes two distinct disorders in place of what was previously called reactive attachment disorder (RAD) (10). In the DSM-5, the disorders are called RAD and disinhibited social engagement disorder (DSED). These two disorders are explicitly linked to observable patterns of attachment-related behaviors and to a child's lack of adaptive use of the primary attachment figure. Both require "insufficient care" and provide specific examples that may increase the risk of the disorders, highlighting the importance that social and emotional neglect play in the development of both disorders (11).

In the DSM-5, both sets of criteria require a developmental age of at least 9 months to ensure that the child has the potential to have developed a focused attachment relationship. Both disorders also require pervasive, rather than relationship-specific patterns. However, beyond these commonalities, the two disorders have distinct clinical presentations as well as different patterns of associated features, different trajectories, and strikingly different responses to intervention (12,13).

Phenomenology of RAD and DSED

Reactive Attachment Disorder

In RAD, children show restriction of affect and behavior in situations that would normally activate the attachment system. In a healthy attachment behavioral system, stressors activate the attachment system and a child seeks comfort from his or her attachment figure. Children with RAD demonstrate a consistent pattern of inhibition or emotional withdrawal around adult caregivers as well as significant negative emotional regulation and limited reciprocity. Specifically, children with RAD do not seek comfort from an attachment figure when distressed and are not calmed when comfort is offered. The difficulties in social or affective interactions may present with minimal social or emotional responsiveness to other people, a lack of positive affect and periods of sadness, distress, or irritability that does not seem to be related to typical triggers. Although some of these features may be seen in children with other disorders, it is their presentation in the context of a lack of attachment patterns that makes the criteria specific and the disorder distinguishable from other disorders (14).

Disinhibited Social Engagement Disorder

In DSED, children exhibit pervasive social disinhibition. In novel situations, these children are overly familiar with strangers. They do not demonstrate social reticence when meeting new adults, they tend not to check back with a caregiver in new situations, and caregivers report the child might go off with a stranger (10). Preschool children may exhibit verbal in addition to physical intrusiveness, by asking overly personal questions with unfamiliar adults. These behaviors are often experienced by others as intrusive and excessive rather than social or friendly (15).

Other Areas of Clinical Concern

Comorbid RAD and DSED. The DSM-5 does not preclude concurrent RAD and DSED. A number of studies of maltreated and institutionalized children, have revealed modest intercorrelations between signs of RAD and DSED, but no association among categorical diagnoses in children with a history of institutional care (12,14,16). However, in a large study of children ages 26 to 89 months in the Netherlands, 15% of children in therapeutic foster care and 3% of children in typical foster care met criteria for both inhibited RAD and DSED (17). Importantly, the mixed pattern was associated with more internalizing and externalizing problems than the single diagnosis, suggesting distinct groups or a higher level of severity. However, the clinical presentation of these children is not clear and it is possible that they present with apparent indiscriminate behaviors because of passivity of RAD rather than pervasive disinhibition.

Relationship Disorders. Although RAD and DSED occur within the context of insufficient caregiving, they do not indicate a relationship specific disorder. Some parent–child relationships may not function in a way that supports a child's development adequately, resulting in problems in the relationship between a caregiver and a child, rather than the patterns specific to the child. Disorders of relationships may present as severely disordered attachment behavior within the context of a relationship, revealed by the child's distorted use of the caregiver as an emotional secure base (18,19). Four major types of these disorders were described: role-reversed behaviors, provocative self-endangering behaviors, excessive clinginess and restriction in exploration, and excessive vigilance and hypercompliance. These relationship classifications have been shown to be associated with less adaptive relationship qualities and have proven interrater reliability (19). Moreover, they have not been well studied and have limited established validity. The *DC: 0–5* includes a categorical disorder, "Relationship Specific Disorder of Early Childhood," that would subsume the previously described attachment relationship disorders (20).

Associated Clinical Features

The particular risks and contexts that give rise to RAD and DSED also have been associated with other clinical conditions. The differences in these clinical correlates support the distinction of RAD and DSED as separate disorders.

Clinical Correlates of RAD. RAD has been shown to be associated with atypical patterns and incomplete development of attachment, developmental delays, depressive symptoms, and a quasiautistic clinical presentation. Attachment classifications and security are consistently associated with RAD. In the Bucharest Early Intervention Project (BEIP), a randomized controlled trial of foster care as an intervention for children exposed to institutional care, both attachment and RAD were examined concurrently (21). In this study, the signs of RAD were inversely associated with the degree of attachment formed, with the highest level of RAD in children classified as unclassifiable (22). In longitudinal follow-up, the association between low attachment security and signs of RAD was evident throughout the preschool years (14).

Developmental delays are modestly associated with signs of RAD (14). This association likely stems from the shared risk factor of caregiving adversity, rather than a causal association between RAD and developmental delays.

Signs of RAD are associated with signs of depression, which shares a presentation of limited positive affect and negative emotionality. However, in the BEIP, fewer than half of children with RAD met full criteria for major depressive disorder at 54-month follow-up, suggesting that the disorders themselves are distinct (14).

Rutter et al. (23,24) described a small subgroup of previously institutionalized children who presented with "quasi-autistic" features, including limited social reciprocity, poor observance of social boundaries, and poor social awareness. These children, who represented 9.2% of previously institutionalized children, demonstrated several features that distinguished them from typically described autism, including a normal or small head circumference, association of quasiautistic feature severity with duration of institutionalization, and a reduction in quasiautistic features over a course of 2 years following adoption.

Clinical Correlates of DSED. The association between DSED and attachment is less clear than that of RAD. In a study of high-risk infants, Lyons-Ruth (25) demonstrated a higher level of indiscriminate behaviors associated with disorganized attachment (compared to organized) patterns and with insecure (compared with secure) attachment patterns in the strange situation. In the English and Romanian Adoption Study (ERA), Rutter et al. (26) also reported that children adopted from Romania to the United Kingdom between 6 and 42 months with no signs of disinhibition had higher rates of secure attachment (79%) compared to those who had some disinhibition (53.4%). On the other hand, the association between signs of DSED and attachment has been examined in diverse samples, with most studies indicating a modest inverse association with attachment security. Consistently, a few children exhibit both secure attachments and signs of DSED (26–29). Some have argued that if children with DSED can have a secure attachment relationship, that the disorder does not represent a core deficit of an attachment problem (11) whereas others suggest that the associations with attachment indicate that attachment theory provides a parsimonious way of understanding the outcomes related to signs of DSED (30). Because of the centrality of child-caregiving relationships in early life, there is certainly no question that attachment plays an important part in most areas of development in children exposed to adversity.

Others have explored other possible core deficits to explain socially indiscriminate behavior in children exposed to adversity. In the BEIP, cognitive impulsivity (inhibitory control deficits) as measured by the Bear Dragon task (a research variant of "Simon Says") was only modestly associated with levels of signs of DSED, suggesting that cognitive inhibitory control also does not fully explain DSED. Others have explored whether DSED is associated with a deficit in theory of mind or an exaggerated hostile attribution bias, neither of which explained the variability in signs of DSED (31).

Biologic underpinnings of DSED have also been explored. In a study of 4 to 17 year olds with a history of institutional care compared with noninstitutionalized children, higher levels of indiscriminate social behaviors were associated with lesser differentiation in amygdala activation on functional MRI between mother and stranger faces in institutionalized compared to noninstitutionalized children (32). The finding suggests that indiscriminate behavior is associated with a neurodevelopmental lack of discrimination, although caution is warranted in extrapolating from studies of school-age children to younger children. Similarly, indiscriminate social behaviors have also been linked to abnormal cortisol secretion patterns in children with the most severe growth restriction after institutional care (33). Lastly, Drury et al. who studied functional polymorphisms in brain-derived neurotrophic factor (BDNF) and the serotonin transporter (5httlpr) on levels of indiscriminate behavior over time in the BEIP sample. They found that those children who were short/short 5-httlpr or the met 66 BDNF allele carriers—thought to be most associated with responsivity to environment—demonstrated the lowest levels of indiscriminate behavior in children in foster care and the highest levels in the care as usual group (34). These findings highlight the complex interactions between genes and susceptibility to adverse or advantageous environments with respect to indiscriminate social behaviors.

Indiscriminate behavior has also been noted to be accompanied by hyperactivity and inattention. While these symptoms are not part of DSED, some have suggested that the inattention and overactivity seen in children with a history of institutionalization and attachment disturbances may reflect an "institutional deprivation syndrome" (12). Rather than invoking traditional attention deficit hyperactivity disorder (ADHD), these investigators suggest this syndrome is directly related to institutional experience, citing correlations between hyperactivity and attachment disturbances and duration of institutional care. In the BEIP, there was no association between caregiver-reported signs of DSED at 24, 30, or 42 months and activity, but a strong association at 54 months with signs of ADHD (14). However, discriminant validity was demonstrated as only 25% of the children who met criteria for DSED also met DSM-IV criteria for ADHD.

Epidemiology

Although believed by most to be a rare disorder, RAD has not been included in population-based studies, and the actual prevalence is unknown. Interpretation of estimates in other groups must be limited because of varying application of diagnostic criteria. Nevertheless, experts agree that the disorder is rare in the general population (22).

Rates of RAD in high-risk samples have been studied slightly more extensively, but some of the studies used outdated diagnostic criteria and combined the inhibited and disinhibited forms. Taken together, rates range from 1% to 20%, in a range of settings (19,35,36). These differences likely reflect differences in referral patterns and method of diagnosis. In a large cohort study that applied rigorous diagnostic classifications, 1% of children met ICD-10 criteria for RAD (37). In a study of 10- to 47-month-old maltreated children in US foster care, 35% of children met criteria for RAD, with an additional 17% who met criteria both for RAD and DAD (the ICD-10 disorder that parallels DSED) (38). In the BEIP, rates of RAD in the longitudinal sample of children with a history of institutional care were under 5% at four time points from mean age of 22 months baseline to 54 months, with rates higher among children randomized to care as usual rather than those randomized to foster care (14).

Rates of DSED are higher than RAD. In the US maltreated toddlers, 22% met criteria for the ICD-10 diagnosis that parallels DSED, with an additional 17% who met criteria for both forms of the disorders (38). In the BEIP, rates of DSED in the longitudinal sample of children with a history of institutional care were 31.8%, 17.9%, 18.0%, and 17.6% at baseline before randomization (mean age 22 months), 30, 42, and 54 months, respectively (14).

Etiology

Insufficient care is required as a criterion in the diagnoses of RAD and DSED in the DSM-5 and strongly recommended in ICD-10 for the parallel disorders. This caregiving may include social neglect or deprivation, changes in caregivers that limit opportunities to form stable attachments, such as multiple caregiving disruptions in foster placements, or atypical caregiving environments such as institutions, that provide structural impediments to forming selective attachments (10). The DSM-5 criteria further state that the care is thought to contribute to the behaviors noted in both RAD and DSED.

Although it can be difficult to confirm early adversity if a child's early experiences are not known, this criterion ensures that children with either social inhibition or social disinhibition without a known history of caregiving adversity are not diagnosed with either disorder. This is particularly important because children who have experienced excellent caregiving but a microdeletion on chromosome 7 (i.e., Williams syndrome) show indiscriminate behavior that is similar to the patterns in DSED (39). To date, no studies have examined the phenomenology of indiscriminate behavior in the two conditions to determine if they are clinically distinguishable.

There is evidence to support a dose-dependent effect of insufficient care on attachment behavior disturbances. Romanian toddlers on a pilot institution unit with a higher staff ratio and staffing schedules more conducive to the development of attachment relationships had lower rates of indiscriminate behaviors than those in the traditional unit, and higher rates than children who had never been institutionalized (40). Within standard institutional care, children who received higher-quality caregiving also were more likely to have lower rates of disturbed attachment behaviors (22). After adoption, the same dose-dependent relationship has been documented, with length of institutionalization correlating closely with the severity of indiscriminant attachment disorder behaviors (15,41). In the United States, rates of RAD parallel the environmental or family risk of adverse caregiving. Children in foster care had the highest rates of RAD, followed by homeless children and then children in Head Start (42). A number of studies have demonstrated an association between length of institutional care and level of indiscriminate behavior in children adopted internationally. Rutter et al. (26) reported that 8.9% children who had been adopted before age 6 months showed marked disinhibition, compared with 26% of those adopted between 6 months and 42 months showed the same level of disinhibition. The association between social disinhibition and duration of institutional exposure persisted at follow-up at age 11.

It should be emphasized that most children exposed to maltreatment or institutionalization do not develop DSED (26). While the protective mechanisms are not yet sufficiently understood, being considered a "favorite child" may be one factor favoring a resilient outcome to young children in institutions (22). It is likely that dose of exposure to institutional care, quality of care within that institution, and a child's biologic and genetic make-up influence the development and persistence of signs of DSED. Very early life experiences, which are almost impossible to measure systematically in children who are placed in institutional or other adverse care, likely also contribute to the outcomes. For example, in the BEIP, the sole independent predictor of signs of DSED at 54 months was the degree of disorganization of attachment behaviors in the strange situation at the baseline data point (mean of 22 months), suggesting that very early caregiving may put a child at risk for persistent signs of DSED (14).

Diagnosis

Clinical History and Interview

As with all other psychiatric disorders in young children, evaluation of a child who may have RAD is a multimodal process that should involve more than one appointment, ideally in more than one setting. Interviews with caregivers as well as child–caregiver observations provide the central core of the diagnostic evaluation. An interview reviewing RAD and DSED should address a child's attachment behavior with the primary caregiver, including the presence of a focused attachment relationship, inhibited or indiscriminate patterns, as well as patterns of secure base distortions.

First, the presence of a focused attachment relationship should be explored. Specifically, an interviewer should assess whether the child has one adult (or more) from whom he or she seeks comfort, reassurance and nurturing, particularly in times of distress. In addition, patterns of inhibited attachment behaviors (not using attachment figure for comfort), and indiscriminate attachment behaviors should be identified. It is also useful to assess the child's use of caregiver as a secure emotional base and to explore distortions of this secure base (43). Relationship-specific patterns of behaviors and interaction patterns are also important to establish. The use of a semi-structured interview, such as the Disturbances of Attachment Interview (44), may be helpful to assess these categories of RAD and DSED behaviors in a systematic manner.

The context of the child's attachment behaviors and relationships must be investigated during the interview, including details of a child's caregiving. To meet criteria for RAD and DSED, insufficient caregiving must be established. Details of the caregiving history, with attention to neglect, changes in caregiving relationships, significant losses, or institutional care should be investigated during the interview. It should be noted that for some children who have experienced adversity, the information about past caregiving is not available or that elements of current adversity may not be disclosed in early assessments. Thus, a low threshold for considering these disorders should be maintained when a clinician notes the clinical syndromes.

Because of the high rates of other psychiatric disorders in children with high-risk family or environmental backgrounds, reviewing other areas of disturbance is an essential part of the history. Disruptive behavior disorders, mood disorders, and anxiety disorders are seen at higher rates in maltreated populations. With any child, but particularly one whose history includes a deprived caregiving context, assessment of both developmental and cognitive status is important. In particular, a child who is not developmentally 9 months of age should not be diagnosed with RAD because he or she may not have the developmental capacity for an attachment relationship and therefore cannot have a disorder of such.

Clinical Observations

Clinical practice settings provide opportunities to observe and stimulate attachment behaviors (45). Observing children in the beginning of the assessment when first meeting the interviewer (a stranger) can provide information about how a child references and/or seeks comfort from a caregiver in the context of a new person and setting. In addition, creating a brief separation can activate the child's attachment system and provide valuable information about how a child uses the parent upon reunion. A single observation is rarely sufficient to make a diagnosis of RAD, and serial observations are recommended (45). Throughout the assessment, it is valuable to compare the child's interactions with a caregiver and the stranger. In addition, observations of a child with all important caregivers can help to distinguish between child-specific behaviors and relationship-specific behaviors (46).

Standardized observations of attachment behaviors have primarily been studied for assessment of attachment classification, a qualitatively different categorization of attachment.

However, one clinical assessment of attachment involving a stranger, separations and reunions and the introduction of a robot as a mildly distressing stimulus have also been used reliably to diagnose attachment disorders in a clinical context (42). Another structured interaction procedure, the Crowell, has been used for relationship assessments, although not necessarily diagnoses, in multiple clinical settings. The procedure includes opportunities for unstructured play interactions, joy sharing with bubbles, structured tasks of increasing difficulty, and a separation and reunion procedure. The use of standardized procedure provides the clinician the opportunity to observe patterns of children's attachment behaviors in a consistent manner in repeated episodes and potentially with different caregivers, reducing the influence of other variables.

Differential Diagnosis and Comorbid Disorders

Institutionalized and maltreated children are at risk for other diagnoses related to their early experiences, and both RAD and DSED must be distinguished from these disorders. Most prominent among them are disruptive behavior disorders, anxiety disorders, particularly posttraumatic stress disorder, and mood disorders (47–49).

The differential diagnosis of RAD is broad and includes developmental concerns as well as externalizing and internalizing problems, and neurodevelopmental concerns. A child with developmental delays who is not yet 9 months developmental age will not show the usual patterns of healthy attachment but will also have other findings consistent with developmental delay. RAD must be distinguished from oppositional defiant patterns. While both share negativistic affect and both may include noncompliance, the pattern in RAD is a passive noncompliance rather than an outright defiance seen in ODD. Children with anxiety disorders may present with an inhibited affect, but in RAD, the presentation is pervasive, whereas the inhibition related to anxiety tends to dissipate in comfortable situations. Depression should be evaluated in children with signs of RAD, as the signs of both show moderate–strong correlations as early as 22 months. Posttraumatic stress disorder shares an etiology of adversity with RAD but shows limited overlap in the clinical presentation, with the exception that dissociative patterns will cause a lack of reciprocity and both can present with negativistic emotions.

The differentiation between quasiautism described by Rutter et al., which shares some traits with RAD, and an autism spectrum disorder may be hard to assess when a child is first evaluated and this differentiation should be considered in any child with a history of caregiving adversity who is diagnosed with autism as well. In longitudinal follow-up, they will improve in a safe caregiving environment, although this differentiation is not useful when a patient is first presenting for care. While children with quasiautistic features present with behaviors similar to those of children with autism, they may be distinguished by (1) normal or small (not large) head circumference, (2) frequent (though socially inappropriate) approaches to others and even indiscriminate behavior, and (3) more use of language (24). Stereotypies can occur in children with a history of institutional care as well as those with autism spectrum disorders, so may not serve as a differentiating factor.

For children for whom DSED is considered, a range of disorders must be considered as well. Externalizing symptoms have been associated with signs of DSED, especially as children move into the later preschool and school-age years (14,50). ADHD is common among children with history of adversity, and may be associated with DSED, but the hyperactive-impulsive form can be distinguished by the pervasiveness of the impulsivity, which is not confined to social interactions. Aggressive behaviors are not associated with signs of DSED in toddlerhood and early preschool years, although there is a moderate association between disruptive behavior patterns beginning at 54 months (14,40). Mood and anxiety disorders should be considered in any child with a history of caregiving adversity. There is little phenotypical overlap between DSED and depressive disorders or anxiety disorders or of posttraumatic stress disorder, although the shared risk factor of adversity means a full assessment of these possibly comorbid conditions is warranted.

Course and Prognosis

In a small study of young children in foster care, nearly all of the dyads showed a distinct pattern of attachment behaviors, most within days of placement, although those patterns were vulnerable to external disruptions like respite placement (51). While this study did not address a clinical diagnosis of RAD, it highlights the rapidity with which infants can develop new attachment relationships, particularly when placed in favorable caregiving settings.

At this time, prospective longitudinal studies of RAD follow children through the school-age years. The challenges of diagnosing RAD in infants and preschoolers are magnified in older children; measures of normal attachment exist but there is no gold standard as there is in early childhood. The application of the infant and preschool definitions of a disorder is likely inappropriate (45). In a study in the United Kingdom, using a single diagnosis that included both inhibited and disinhibited forms of the DSM-IV diagnosis of RAD generated by the Child Age Psychiatric Assessment interview, the diagnosis was associated with lower rates of security based on the McMaster Child Attachment Story Task (52). As in younger children, the diagnosis did not preclude a secure attachment classification, especially in girls. This study may be the beginning of more rigorous study of the constructs of RAD and DSED in older children, but unfortunately the merged diagnostic category limits its contribution. Other studies of attachment disorders in older children have used a broadly defined syndrome (called "RAD") that includes criteria included in both the inhibited syndrome of RAD and disinhibited DSED as well as sometimes signs of disruptive behavior patterns and moral deficits (53–55). To date, it is unclear how this construct relates to RAD and DSED as well as whether it describes children not currently well described in existing nosologies.

Treatment

Data related to specific interventions for RAD are limited. A commonality on which most infant mental health interventions are based, is the inclusion of both child and primary caregiver as participants in the intervention and the promotion of sensitive, responsive caregiving relationships.

Foster Care Placement

While the need to remove a child from pathologic care or the extremes of deprivation seems to be an obvious intervention for RAD, only one study has examined the effect of this process on children's attachment disorder behaviors. The BEIP, the only randomized controlled trial of foster care for children with a history of institutional care, includes baseline data about the children before their placement into foster care. After randomization to care as usual or foster care at a mean age of 22 months, children randomized to foster care and their families received regular visits and support from social workers who were supervised by experts in infant mental health and foster care (56). At follow-up at 30, 42, 54 months and 8 years, signs of RAD in children placed in foster care were indistinguishable from community controls (13). The rate of resolution in signs of RAD is striking.

Signs of DSED decreased far more slowly than signs of RAD. Signs of DSED were higher in the care as usual group than in community controls, with children in foster care showing an intermediate level. Importantly, early placement in foster care was associated with a greater reduction in signs of DSED. These results suggest that placement in a safe, family environment is an effective intervention for inhibited attachment disorder behaviors, but is not sufficient to eliminate signs of indiscriminate attachment disorder. The relative persistence of DSED after removal from institutional care and placement in family care has been documented in other populations as well, with follow-up after intervention into adolescence (12,41,57). Clearly, more effective interventions for DSED are needed, although prevention and early intervention for maltreatment or adversity will be the most powerful approaches to reduce the impact of DSED in high-risk populations.

Attachment-based Therapies

Attachment-focused therapies have not been studied as interventions for RAD, but the enhanced foster care of the BEIP, which influenced both RAD and DSED albeit at different magnitudes, was strongly influenced by attachment theory. Given the lack of other specific treatments for RAD or DSED, there is reason to consider attachment-based interventions in this discussion. Attachment-based therapies seek, through various mechanisms and points of entry, to strengthen the primary caregiving relationship.

A number of caveats must be identified when considering attachment-based therapies in the context of RAD (58). While these attachment-based therapies assume a focused attachment relationship (albeit usually an unsatisfying one) not all children with RAD or DSED have a focused attachment relationship. It is not known whether attachment-based interventions can stimulate development of an attachment relationship where none exists.

For RAD, there is a theoretical basis for believing that interventions that strengthen the attachment relationship may create an environment in which a child's negative internal representations can be modified and which can interrupt the perpetuation of RAD, which is thought to be closely tied to attachment security (57). Particularly important may be helping the child's caregiver reinterpret the child's behaviors in order to function as a more effective secure base (59).

Given the different correlates and responsivity to family-based living, it seems likely that RAD and DSED might require different interventions, and that DSED might be less likely to respond to an attachment-based treatment. In spite of these caveats, the BEIP findings suggest that promotion of a healthy parent–child relationship and family environment through an attachment-focused supports may have a place in a treatment plan for DSED as well as RAD.

Infant–Parent Psychotherapy. Infant–Parent Psychotherapy (IPP) and Child–Parent Psychotherapy (CPP) are therapies which draw on psychoanalytic and attachment theory to provide corrective attachment experiences to the parent and infant. In keeping with its psychodynamic roots, the development of parental insight into her use of the child as a negative transference object is defined as one target of treatment. In addition, through the therapeutic relationship and interventions, IPP provides the dyad with corrective attachment experiences that model and emphasize nurturing, support, protection, and reciprocity. The third mutative factor is described as the power of mutually satisfying interactions. IPP and CPP sessions are flexibly structured, and access a parent's current and past experiences to increase awareness and insight into the relationship. The therapist provides a nurturing, and supportive experience for both partners in the dyad. CPP shares the same foundation, but uses play as the modality through which the child and parent together can create joint meaning in their interactions (60).

IPP and CPP have been used and studied extensively with sustained positive effects on security of attachment, child trauma-related symptom and behavioral difficulties, cognitive functioning, parent trauma-related symptoms, as well as regulating cortisol release patterns (61–63).

Attachment and Biobehavioral Catch-up. Attachment and Biobehavioral Catch-Up (ABC) was developed for foster caregivers to support them in developing sensitive, nurturing, nonfrightening parenting behaviors (64). In ABC, dyadic interactions provide opportunities for psychoeducation and support in understanding the needs of infants and young children as well as caregiver state of mind. In randomized controlled trials, ABC has been associated with decreased rates of disorganized attachment status and with increased caregiver sensitivity and, notably, normalized diurnal cortisol patterns in toddlers (65–67). With the intense focus on the developing caregiver–child relationship, this model may have promise for RAD and to a lesser extent with DSED.

Circle of Security. The Circle of Security (COS) is an intervention designed to enhance attachment relationships between young children and their caregivers through psychoeducation, video review, and insight-oriented psychotherapy (68). Originally, it was disseminated as a manualized, time-limited group psychotherapy using video feedback. This intervention has since been adapted for dyadic therapy. More recently, parenting DVDs based on the model have been created; these combine education about attachment with an opportunity for caregivers to reflect on their child's needs and the challenges each faces in meeting those needs (69). For the video therapy approach, an observational procedure including the standard SSP and the COS Interview is completed at baseline for treatment planning (70). The intervention emphasizes the sophisticated capabilities of young children and draws caregivers' attention to the meaning of subtle behaviors. It also teaches parents to recognize their own maladaptive responses and how to override them (71).

Video-based Intervention to Promote Positive Parenting. Video-based intervention to promote positive parenting (VIPP) is a brief, manualized attachment intervention delivered in four home visits to parents of infants less than 1 year of age (72). VIPP was drawn explicitly from attachment research and attempts to promote mothers' sensitive interactions with their infants. Interveners' present written materials and review videotaped infant–parent interactions during home visits. An expanded version, VIPP-R, provides an additional 3-hour home visit that focuses on the parent's childhood attachment experiences. Research has documented enhancement of sensitive and nurturing parenting behaviors, attachment disorganization, and externalizing behavior problems during preschool (73,74).

Parent Management Training Models. No intervention other than foster care has been explicitly studied as a treatment for DSED. In part, as the core deficit of this disorder is not as well understood, designing a focused treatment may be more difficult. DSED has some overlapping presentation with disruptive behavior patterns, especially in the older preschool ages, although there is no suggestion that it shares a common etiology with these problems. Parent–Child Interaction

Therapy (PCIT), a parent management training approach, has been shown to reduce child disruptive behaviors as well as child internalizing problems, executive functioning, and emotional recognition skills (75–77). In maltreating families, PCIT was associated with improvement in a number of aspects of observable parent–child interactions, including more praise and use of verbal positive reinforcement as well as parental sensitivity on the Emotional Availability Scale in these high-risk families (78). Despite limitations in generalizing from this sample, a parent management training approach that increases parental sensitivity and reduces types of impulsivity may also have some promise in reducing impairment associated with DSED.

Treatments not Recommended. Perhaps because of the high intensity clinical needs of children who have experienced severe deprivation or maltreatment, alternative treatments for emotional and behavioral problems in adopted children have proliferated. Coercive treatments including holding and rebirthing have been associated with fatalities, are not supported empirically, and have been condemned by the American Academy of Child and Adolescent Psychiatry (AACAP) (45,79–82).

Summary and Future Directions

The empirical support for RAD and DSED has grown substantially in recent decades. RAD is strongly associated with incompletely developed attachment and resolves quickly after removal from adversity and placement into adequate caregiving environment. DSED, on the other hand, appears to derive from the persistence of behavioral adaptations to very early experiences rather than concurrent caregiving experiences. Despite the substantial progress in characterizing the disorders, a number of questions persist. First, we must identify the factors and interactions that put some children at risk of developing RAD or DSED or confer protection against either of these disorders. Additionally, better understanding the core deficits of each disorder will provide opportunities for focused interventions. Most importantly, prevention of both disorders can be achieved through advocacy for healthy caregiving environments for all children, especially those whose families cannot protect them. First-line intervention must include removal from an adverse caregiving environment and placement in a safe, sensitive environment. After placement in a safe caregiving environment, current treatment recommendations focus on enhancing positive caregiver interactions, although the specific modalities have not been established.

References

1. Spitz R: Hospitalism: an inquiry into the genesis of psychiatric conditions in early childhood. *Psychoanal Study Child* 1:53–74, 1945.
2. American Psychiatric Association: *Diagnostic and Statistical Manual of Mental Disorders III*. Washington, DC, American Psychiatric Press, 1980.
3. Bowlby J: *Attachment and Loss: Attachment*. New York, Basic Books, 1962.
4. Ainsworth MD: Object relations, dependency and attachment: a theoretical review of the infant-mother relationship. *Child Dev* 40:969–1025, 1969.
5. Bretherton I: The origins of attachment theory: John Bowlby and Mary Ainsworth. *Dev Psychol* 28:759–775, 1992.
6. Bell SM, Ainsworth MD: Infant crying and maternal responsiveness. *Child Dev* 43:1171–1190, 1972.
7. Main M, Cassidy J: Categories of response to reunion with the parent at age 6: predictable from infant attachment classifications and stable over a 1-month period. *Dev Psychopathol* 24:1–12, 1998.
8. Van Ijzendoorn M, Schuengel C, Bakermans-Kraneburg MJ: Disorganized attachment in early childhood: meta-analysis of precursors, concomitants, and sequelae. *Dev Psychopathol* 11(02):225–250, 1999.
9. WHO: *The IDC-10 Classification of Mental and Behavioral Disorders: Clinical Descriptions and Diagnostic Guidelines*. 10th ed. Geneva, Switzerland, World Health Organization, 1992.
10. APA: *Diagnostic and Statistical Manual of Mental Disorders 5*. Washington, DC, American Psychiatric Press, 2013.
11. Zeanah CH, Gleason MM: Annual research review: attachment disorders in early childhood—clinical presentation, causes, correlates, and treatment. *J Child Psychol Psychiatry* 56(3):207–222, 2015.
12. Rutter M, Kreppner J, Sonuga-Barke E: Emanuel Miller lecture: attachment insecurity, disinhibited attachment, and attachment disorders: where do research findings leave the concepts? *J Child Psychol Psychiatry* 50(5):529–543, 2009.
13. Smyke AT, Zeanah CH, Gleason MM, et al.: A randomized controlled trial comparing foster care and institutional care for children with signs of reactive attachment disorder. *Am J Psychiatry* 5(169):508–514, 2012.
14. Gleason MM, Fox NA, Drury S, et al.: Validity of evidence-derived criteria for reactive attachment disorder: indiscriminately social/disinhibited and emotionally withdrawn/inhibited types. *J Am Acad Child Adolesc Psychiatry* 50(3):216–231, 2011.
15. O'Connor TG, Bredenkamp D, Rutter M: Attachment disturbances and disorders in children exposed to early severe deprivation. *Infant Ment Health J* 20(1):10–29, 1999.
16. Kreppner JM, O'Connor TG, Rutter M; English and Romanian Adoptees Study Team: Can inattention/hyperactivity be an institutional deprivation syndrome? *J Abnorm Child Psychol* 29:513–528, 2001.
17. Jonkman CS, Oosterman M, Schuengel C, Bolle EA, Boer F, Lindauer RJ: Disturbances in attachment: inhibited and disinhibited symptoms in foster children. *Child Adolesc Psychiatry Ment Health* 8(1):21, 2014.
18. Zeanah CH, Smyke AT: Attachment disorders in family and social context. *Infant Ment Health J* 29(3):219–233, 2008.
19. Boris NW, Zeanah CH, Larrieu JA, Scheeringa MS, Heller SS: Attachment disorders in infancy and early childhood: a preliminary investigation of diagnostic criteria. *Am J Psychiatry* 155:295–297, 1998.
20. Zero to Three. *DC: 0-5; Diagnostic Classification of Mental Health and Developmental Disorders in Infancy and Early Childhood*. Washington, DC, Zero to Three Press, 2016.
21. Zeanah C, Nelson C, Fox N, et al.: Designing research to study the effects of institutionalization on brain and behavioral development: the Bucharest early intervention project. *Dev Psychopathol* 15:885–907, 2003.
22. Zeanah CH, Smyke AT, Koga SF, Carlson E: Attachment in institutionalized and community children in Romania. *Child Dev* 76(5):1015–1028, 2005.
23. Rutter M, Kreppner J, Croft C, et al.: Early adolescent outcomes of institutionally deprived and non-deprived adoptees. III. Quasi-autism. *J Child Psychol Psychiatry* 48(12):1200–1207, 2007.
24. Rutter M, Andersen-Wood L, Beckett C, et al.: Quasi-autistic patterns following severe early global privation. *J Child Psychol Psychiatry* 40(4): 537–549, 1999.
25. Lyons-Ruth K, Bureau J, Riley C, Atlas-Corbett A: Socially indiscriminate attachment behavior in the strange situation: convergent and discriminant validity in relation to caregiving risk, later behavior problems, and attachment insecurity. *Dev Psychopathol* 21:355–372, 2009.
26. Rutter M, Colvert E, Kreppner J, et al.: Early adolescent outcomes for institutionally-deprived and non-deprived adoptees. I: disinhibited attachment. *J Child Psychol Psychiatry* 48(1):17–30, 2007.
27. Bruce J, Tarullo AR, Gunnar MR: Disinhibited social behavior among internationally adopted children. *Dev Psychopathol* 21(1):157–171, 2009.
28. Soares I, Belsky J, Oliveira P, et al.: Does early family risk and current quality of care predict indiscriminate social behavior in institutionalized Portuguese children? *Attach Hum Dev* 1–12, 2014.
29. Oosterman M, Schuengel C: Attachment in foster children associated with caregivers' sensitivity and behavioral problems. *Infant Men Health J* 29(6):609–623, 2008.
30. Lyons-Ruth K, Zeanah CH, Gleason MM: Commentary: should we move away from an attachment framework for understanding disinhibited social engagement disorder (DSED)? A commentary on Zeanah and Gleason (2015). *J Child Psychol Psychiatry* 56(3):223–227, 2015.
31. Kay CL, Green JM: Social cognitive deficits and biases in maltreated adolescents in UK out-of-home care: relation to disinhibited attachment disorder and psychopathology. *Dev Psychopathol* 28(1):73–83, 2016.
32. Olsavsky AK, Telzer EH, Shapiro M, et al.: Indiscriminate amygdala esponse to mothers and strangers after early maternal deprivation. *Biol Psychiatry* 74(11):853–860, 2013.
33. Johnson AE, Bruce J, Tarullo AR, Gunnar MR: Growth delay as an index of allostatic load in young children: predictions to disinhibited social approach and diurnal cortisol activity. *Dev Psychopathol* 23(3):859–871, 2011.
34. Drury S, Gleason MM, Theall KP, et al.: Genetic sensitivity to the caregiving context: the influence of 5httlpr and BDNF val66met on indiscriminate social behavior. *Physiol Behav* 106(5):728–735, 2012.
35. Dunitz M, Scheer PJ, Kvas E, Macari S: Psychiatric diagnoses in infancy: a comparison. *Infant Ment Health J* 17(1):12–23, 1996.
36. Frankel KA, Boyum LA, Harmon RJ: Diagnoses and presenting symptoms in an infant psychiatry clinic: comparison of two diagnostic systems. *J Am Acad Child Adolesc Psychiatry* 43(5):578–587, 2004.
37. Skovgaard AM, Houmann T, Christiansen E, et al.: The prevalence of mental health problems in children 1 1/2 years of age—the Copenhagen Child Cohort 2000. *J Child Psychol Psychiatry* 48(1):62–70, 2007.

38. Zeanah CH, Scheeringa M, Boris NW, Heller SS, Smyke AT, Trapani J: Reactive attachment disorder in maltreated toddlers. *Child Abuse Negl* 28(8):877–878, 2004.
39. Tager-Flusberg H, Plesa-Skwerer D: Social engagement in Williams syndrome. In: Marshall PJ, Fox NA (eds). *The Development of Social Engagement: Neurobiological Perspectives.* New York, Oxford University Press, 2005.
40. Zeanah CH, Smyke AT, Dumitrescu A: Attachment disturbances in young children. II: indiscriminate behavior and institutional care. *J Am Acad Child Adolesc Psychiatry* 41(8):983–989, 2002.
41. Tizard B, Rees J: The effect of early institutional rearing on the behavior problems and affectional relationships of four-year-old children. *J Child Psychol Psychiatry* 27:61–73, 1975.
42. Boris NW, Hinshaw-Fuselier SS, Smyke AT, Scheeringa MS, Heller SS, Zeanah CH: Comparing criteria for attachment disorders: establishing reliability and validity in high-risk samples. *J Am Acad Child Adolesc Psychiatry* 43(5):568–577, 2004.
43. Gleason MM: Relationship assessment in clinical practice. *Child Adolesc Psychiatr Clin North Am* 18(3):581–591, 2009.
44. Smyke AT, Zeanah CH: *Disturbances of Attachment Manual.* New Orleans, Tulane University Health Sciences Center, 1999.
45. Boris NW, Zeanah CH: Practice parameter for the assessment and treatment of children and adolescents with reactive attachment disorder of infancy and early childhood. *J Am Acad Child Adolesc Psychiatry* 44(11):1206–1219, 2005.
46. Zeanah CH, Larrieu JA, Valliere J, et al.: Infant-parent relationship assessment. In: Zeanah CH (ed). *Handbook of Infant Mental Health.* New York, Guilford, 222–235, 2000.
47. Scheeringa MS, Zeanah CH: Reconsideration of harm's way: onsets and comorbidity patterns of disorders in preschool children and their caregivers following Hurricane Katrina. *J Clin Child Adolesc Psychol* 37(3):508–518, 2008.
48. Chemtob CM, Nomura Y, Abramovitz RA: Impact of conjoined exposure to the world trade center attacks and to other traumatic events on the behavioral problems of preschool children. *Arch Pediatr Adolesc Med* 162(2):126–133, 2008.
49. Reams R: Children birth to three entering the state's custody. *Infant Ment Health J* 20(2):166–174, 1999.
50. Roy P, Rutter M, Pickles A: Institutional care: associations between overactivity and lack of selectivity in social relationships. *J Child Psychol Psychiatry* 45(4):866–873, 2004.
51. Stovall-McClough KC, Dozier M: Forming attachments in foster care: infant attachment behaviors during the first 2 months of placement. *Dev Psychopathol* 16(2):253–271, 2004.
52. Minnis H, Green J, O'Connor TG, et al.: An exploratory study of the association between reactive attachment disorder and attachment narratives in early school-age children. *J Child Psychol Psychiatry* 50(8):931–942, 2009.
53. Green J: Are attachment disorders best seen as social impairment syndromes? *Attach Hum Dev* 5(3):259–264, 2003.
54. Minnis H, Marwick H, Arthur J, McLaughlin A: Reactive attachment disorder—a theoretical model beyond attachment. *Eur Child Adolesc Psychiatry* 15(6):336–342, 2006.
55. Minnis H, Rabe-Hesketh S, Wolkind S: Development of a brief, clinically relevant, scale for measuring attachment disorders. *Int J Methods Psychiatr Res* 11(2):90–98, 2002.
56. Smyke AT, Zeanah CH, Fox NA, Nelson CA: A new model of foster care for young children: the Bucharest early intervention project. *Child Adolesc Psychiatr Clin North Am* 18(3):721–734, 2009.
57. Lieberman AF: The treatment of attachment disorder in infancy and early childhood: reflections from clinical intervention with later-adopted foster children. *Attach Hum Dev* 5(3):279–282, 2003.
58. O'Connor TG, Zeanah CH: Attachment disorders: assessment strategies and treatment approaches. *Attach Hum Dev* 5(3):223–244, 2003.
59. Lieberman AF, Zeanah CH: Contributions of attachment theory to infant–parent psychotherapy and other interventions with infants and young children. *Handbook of Attachment* 555–574, 1999.
60. Lieberman AF, Van Horn P: Child parent psychotherapy. In: Zeanah CH (ed). *Handbook of Infant Mental Health.* New York, Guilford, 239–249, 2009.
61. Lieberman AF, Ippen CG, Van Horn PJ: Child-parent psychotherapy: 6 month follow-up of a randomized controlled trial. *J Am Acad Child Adolesc Psychiatry* 45:913–918, 2006.
62. Cicchetti D, Rogosch FA, Toth SL, Sturge-Apple ML: Normalizing the development of cortisol regulation in maltreated infants through preventive interventions. *Dev Psychopathol* 23(3):789–800, 2011.
63. Toth SL, Rogosch FA, Manly JT, Cicchetti D: The efficacy of toddler-parent psychotherapy to reorganize attachment in the young offspring of mothers with major depressive disorder: a randomized preventive trial. *J Consult Clin Psychol* 74(6):1006–1016, 2006.
64. Dozier M: *Attachment and Biobehavioral Catch-up: An Intervention for Caregivers of Babies who have Experienced early Adversity.* Lexington, MA, Boston Institute for the Development of Infants and Parents, 2006.
65. Bernard K, Dozier M, Bick J, Lewis-Morrarty E, Lindhiem O, Carlson E: Enhancing attachment organization among maltreated children: results of a randomized clinical trial. *Child Dev* 83(2):623–636, 2012.
66. Bick J, Dozier M: The effectiveness of an attachment-based intervention in promoting foster mothers' sensitivity toward foster infants. *Infant Ment Health J* 34(2):95–103, 2013.
67. Dozier M, Peloso E, Lewis E, Laurenceau JP, Levine S: Effects of an attachment-based intervention on the cortisol production of infants and toddlers in foster care. *Dev Psychopathol* 20(3):845–859, 2008.
68. Hoffman KT, Marvin RS, Cooper G, Powell B: Changing toddlers' and preschoolers' attachment classifications: the circle of security intervention. *J Consult Clin Psychol* 74(6):1017–1026, 2006.
69. Cooper G, Hoffman KT, Powell B: *Circle of Security: COS-P Facilitator DVD Manual 5.0.* Spokane, WA, Marycliff Institute, 2009.
70. Powell B, Cooper G, Hoffman K, Marvin RS: Circle of security. In: Zeanah CH (ed). *Handbook of Infant Mental Health.* New York, Guilford, 453–486, 2012.
71. Powell B, Cooper G, Hoffman K, Marvin R: *The Circle of Security Intervention: Enhancing Attachment in Early Parent-Child Relationships.* New York, Guilford Press, 2013.
72. Van Zeijl J, Mesman J, Van Ijzendoorn MH, et al.: Attachment-based intervention for enhancing sensitive discipline in mothers of 1- to 3-year-old children at risk for externalizing behavior problems: a randomized controlled trial. *J Consult Clin Psychol* 74(6):994–1005, 2006.
73. Juffer F, Bakermans-Kranenburg MJ, van IJzendoorn MH: The importance of parenting in the development of disorganized attachment: evidence from a preventive intervention study in adoptive families. *J Child Psychol Psychiatry* 46:263–274, 2005.
74. Klein Velderman M, Bakermans-Kranenburg MJ, Juffer F, van Ijzendoorn MH: Effects of attachment-based interventions on maternal sensitivity and infant attachment: differential susceptibility of highly reactive infants. *J Fam Psychol* 20(2):266–274, 2006.
75. Eyberg SM, Funderburk BW, Hembree-Kigin TL, McNeil CB, Querido JG, Hood K: Parent-child interaction therapy with behavior problem children: one and two year maintenance of treatment effects in the family. *Child Fam Behav Ther* 2001;23:1–20, 2006.
76. Pincus DB, Santucci LC, Ehrenreich JT, Eyberg SM: The implementation of modified parent-child interaction therapy for youth with separation anxiety disorder. *Cognit Behav Pract* 15(2):118–125, 2008.
77. Luby J, Lenze S, Tillman R, Lenze S, Tillman R: A novel early intervention for preschool depression: findings from a pilot randomized controlled trial. *J Child Psychol Psychiatry* 53(3):313–322, 2012.
78. Thomas R, Zimmer-Gembeck MJ: Parent–child interaction therapy: an evidence-based treatment for child maltreatment. *Child Maltreat* 17(3):253–266, 2012.
79. Cline FW: *Hope for High Risk and Rage filled Children.* Evergreen, CO, EC Publications, 1992.
80. Keck GC, Kupecky RM: *Adopting the Hurt Child: Hope for Families with Special-Needs Kids: A Guide for Parents and Professionals.* Evergreen, CO, Pinion Press, 1995.
81. Mercer J: Attachment therapy using deliberate restraint: an object lesson on the identification of unvalidated treatments. *J Child Adolesc Psychiatr Nurs* 14(3):105–114, 2001.
82. Mercer J: *Attachment Therapy: Science and Pseudoscience in Clinical Psychology.* 2nd ed. New York, Guilford, 2013.

CHAPTER 5.15.4 ■ CAREGIVER-FABRICATED ILLNESS IN A CHILD

ANDREA G. ASNES

HISTORICAL NOTE, DEFINITIONAL ISSUES AND THE EVOLUTION OF A NAME

In 1951, Asher first used the eponym Munchausen syndrome to describe adults who consistently fabricate symptoms of illness for themselves, leading to numerous medical investigations and frequently to surgical operations (1). The syndrome was named after Baron von Munchausen of Hanover who lived in the 18th century and was renowned for telling greatly embellished stories about his adventures in the wars against the Turks (2). In 1976, Sneed and Bell used the term "the dauphin of Munchausen" to describe a case in which a 10-year-old boy presented with factitious recurrent urinary calculi and in which the mother was suspected of colluding with the child in fabricating the symptoms (3). The following year, Meadow coined the term "Munchausen syndrome by proxy" in his report of observations of two cases in which parents repeatedly caused their children to be ill (4). Prior to this time, there had been reports in the literature of cases referred to as "nonaccidental poisoning" in which children repeatedly presented as diagnostic dilemmas and were found to have been poisoned by a parent; such cases would today be classified as child abuse (5,6). Subsequent to Meadow's initial report, other suggested names included Meadow syndrome or Polle syndrome, but these gave way to the still frequently used Munchausen syndrome by proxy (7–9). Other terms since used to describe this diagnostic entity have addressed the complexity inherent in making this diagnosis. These include pediatric condition falsification, caregiver fabrication of illness in a child, child abuse in a medical setting, medical child abuse, and factitious disorder by proxy. The most recent version of the *Diagnostic and Statistical Manual of Mental Disorders* (DSM-5) refers to factitious disorder imposed on another, and specifies that deception by the caregiver is a necessary diagnostic feature (10). The range of clinical presentations encountered in practice, however, extends well beyond this relatively narrow definition. Indeed, the diagnosis of caregiver-fabricated or induced illness in a child does not require an understanding of the perpetrator's motive any more than a caregiver's reasons for physically battering a child need to be known in order for a diagnosis of physical abuse to be made (10,11). The evolving name of this diagnostic entity reflects the challenge both of identifying pathologic behavior in one person (the caregiver) and not in another (the child victim), as well as in ascribing (or studiously not ascribing) a motive to the diagnosed person (12).

Initially, Meadow described a caregiver disorder in which a person persistently fabricates symptoms of illness on behalf of another, thereby causing that person to be regarded as ill (4). Meadow subsequently updated and operationalized the syndrome to include a combination of: (1) an illness fabricated in a child by a parent or someone in loco parentis; (2) persistent presentation of a child to medical care while the caregiver denies causing the child's illness; (3) the illness goes away when the child is separated from the perpetrator; and (4) the perpetrator is considered to be acting out of a need to assume the sick role by proxy or as another form of attention-seeking behavior (13). In 1998, a multidisciplinary group convened by the American Professional Society on the Abuse of Children developed definitional guidelines which have since been refined (14,15). These guidelines define the disorder as encapsulating two distinct entities: the maltreatment of a child and the motivation of the adult who perpetrates the maltreatment. The term "pediatric condition falsification" is employed to describe the form of child abuse in which an adult fabricates or directly causes symptoms and/or signs of illness in a child, resulting in a perception of that child as sick (15). The severity of the disorder and extent of the fabrication are variable. In the least severe cases caregivers only report false symptoms, and the physical harm to the children is only that resulting from the unnecessary medical investigations carried out in attempting to diagnose the illnesses. At the other end of the spectrum are instances in which caregivers have caused severe physical harm to or even the death of their children in the continued pursuit of making their children appear ill. Roesler and Jenny emphasize the importance and necessity of singling out the maltreatment of a child in making a diagnosis of what they termed "medical child abuse," particularly for pediatric providers (16). These authors illuminate both the need to diagnose the child with abuse and the lack of necessity to diagnose the caregiver/perpetrator with anything at all. Pediatric providers need not know the motivation of the perpetrators of child abuse in order to diagnose abuse, and attempting to identify such motivation (and, therefore, ascribing a psychiatric diagnosis) is beyond the scope of pediatric expertise. The American Academy of Pediatrics Committee on Child Abuse and Neglect in 2013 settled on the term "caregiver-fabricated illness in a child" and noted that in the setting of multiple definitions and diagnostic terms to describe this form of maltreatment, the essential feature is the "caregiver's falsification and/or inducement of physical or psychological symptoms or signs in a child" (17). The DSM-5 identifies the diagnosis of factitious disorder imposed on another (previously factitious disorder by proxy) and lists the diagnostic criteria as:

A. Falsification of physical or psychological signs or symptoms, or induction of injury or disease, in another, associated with identified deception.
B. The individual presents another individual (victim) to others as ill, impaired, or injured.
C. The deceptive behavior is evident even in the absence of obvious external rewards.
D. The behavior is not better explained by another mental disorder, such as delusional disorder or another psychotic disorder (10).

Notably, this definition excludes caregiver fabrication of or imposition of illness on another for reasons of secondary gain. Caretakers, for example, may invent or induce illness in children to keep them from attending school or falsely allege sexual abuse as a tool in custody battles. In other forms of pediatric condition falsification, the parent falsifies the illness solely to gain help with other problems, such as depression (18). This latter form has been dubbed as "help seeking" and is exemplified by the mother who puts cranberry juice in a child's diaper as a reason to be seen by a doctor, but the behavior ceases once the mother's own psychological needs have been identified and treated (18). Caregivers who abuse a child physically and then invent an organic medical ailment to explain the abuse would not, therefore, be diagnosed with factitious disorder imposed on another, nor would a caregiver who fabricates medical diagnoses for material gain, or malingering, such as would be the case in a caregiver who fabricates a child's illness in order to collect a disability benefit on behalf of the child (15). These motivations have been described by Rogers as being either "criminologic" in nature, as in antisocial behavior, or as "adaptational" as would occur in malingering to secure financial gain when faced with a difficult financial predicament (19). Rosenberg highlights the potential variability in motivation of caregivers by wondering if parents who induce illness in their children are ill themselves or if they simply exhibit "nasty, self-serving cruel behavior" (20). Other entities that must be distinguished from factitious disorder imposed on another are those parents of chronically ill children who are perceived as "difficult" or overly demanding by medical staff, and "overanxious" parents who may display exaggerated concern for their children's health when they feel proper medical attention is not bestowed (18).

Definitional issues also play an important role in the legal aspects of suspected cases of caregiver-fabricated illness. Controversy has played out in courtrooms over whether terms that specify a psychiatric illness in an adult perpetrator may or should be used to prosecute perpetrators of this special form of child abuse. Meadow has suggested that the child victim's diagnosis of this form of maltreatment be used to identify a "collection of features characterizing a particular form of child abuse" and that diagnosing the adult perpetrators is the task of mental health professionals (13). These tensions carry weight when medical professionals are asked to render diagnoses to be used in court. It is self-evident and prudent that pediatric providers are best able to diagnose child abuse and that mental health professionals are best able to diagnose adult psychopathology.

EPIDEMIOLOGY

The true prevalence of caregiver-fabricated illness is unknown. Active reporting of cases in a prospective study conducted over a 2-year period in the United Kingdom and Republic of Ireland established an annual incidence of 0.5/100,000 children aged under 16 years, and the peak incidence of 2.8/100,000 children in the first year of life (21). A prospective study from Italy that evaluated all patients admitted to a pediatric ward over a period of 28 months found a prevalence of what the investigators termed Munchausen syndrome by proxy in 4 of a sample of 751 patients (0.53%) between the ages of 11 months and 16 years (22).

In 1987, Rosenberg conducted a review of the existing literature and summarized all the published reports (23). These included 117 children in 97 families. Of these cases, the perpetrator was the mother in every case reviewed (98% birth mother and 2% adoptive mother). In 2003, Sheridan conducted a similar review and found 451 cases in which 76.5% of the perpetrators were mothers (20). In Ferrara's study from Italy, of the four cases in which Munchausen syndrome by proxy was diagnosed, mothers were the perpetrators in three, and a grandmother in one of the cases (22). Fathers have previously been found to be only rarely implicated as being the perpetrators or appearing to be complicit in the fabrication of illness, although Meadow published a series of 15 such cases occurring over a 10-year period, and in Sheridan's review, fathers were the perpetrators in 6.7% of the cases (24–27). In a review of cases published outside the United States, Canada, United Kingdom, Australia, and New Zealand, Feldman and Brown reported on 93 cases, and in these the mother was the sole perpetrator in 86% and the father was the sole perpetrator in 4% (24,28). Libow describes the phenomenon of "blended cases" in which a caregiver and a child collude to put forth a false medical presentation (29).

The diagnosis of caregiver-fabricated illness has been made in children of all ages from the first month of life to 21 years, with the mean age being reported as 40 months and 49 months in the Rosenberg and Sheridan reviews, respectively (23,24,28). In the prospective British epidemiologic study, however, the median age of diagnosis was 20 months (21). The mean time interval between the onset of symptoms and time of diagnosis was found by Rosenberg to be 15 months, by Sheridan to be 22 months, and by Ferrara to be 10.3 months (22–24). There are reports of instances in which the condition started prior to birth with mothers inducing preterm delivery (30,31). Male and female children are victimized at equal rates (23,24). A fatality rate of 6% to 10% has been identified in two separate studies (21,29).

CLINICAL DESCRIPTION

Medical Presentation

The variety of medical symptoms in children who present with Munchausen syndrome by proxy is extensive and includes practically all organ systems. Generally, the illness appears to be multisystem, and the children may appear to have different types of illness at different times. The four presentations that were among the most common in both Rosenberg's and Sheridan's reviews were seizures, apnea, diarrhea, and fevers. Altogether, Rosenberg listed 68 different presentations or pathologic findings, and Sheridan listed 101, highlighting the striking diversity of possible potential presentations of Munchausen syndrome by proxy cases. The means by which the perpetrators caused the symptoms or abnormal findings are just as diverse and illustrate the severity and horrifying nature of the syndrome: One mother had put bleach in her child's eye, causing the appearance of a periorbital infection; others had repeatedly suffocated their children so as to simulate recurrent apnea or seizures. Other caregivers caused sepsis by putting fecal material into their children's intravenous lines (23,24).

In approximately 40% of cases in Sheridan's review, the perpetrator had simulated an illness but had not actually done anything directly to the child to cause harm (24). These were instances where the perpetrator had done something such as putting drops of her own blood in her child's urine or contaminating the specimen. In these instances, although the perpetrator does not herself physically harm the child, her behavior instigates potentially painful investigations and procedures.

Bools et al. have pointed out that there is a significant amount of comorbidity among cases of caregiver-fabricated illness. In a review of 56 cases, 29% had a history of failure to thrive and 25% had a history of either nonaccidental injury or neglect (32). Siblings also might have a history of such findings or might themselves have been the subjects of fabricated illnesses. This appears to be particularly true among cases that have presented as apnea and which, in fact, are owing to suffocation (32–35). Of note, in Sheridan's sample, apnea was the most common presenting symptom, representing 26.8% of all cases reviewed (24). When children present with apnea, caregiver-fabricated illness should always be considered if there is a history of death of a sibling or if episodes of apnea have occurred only in the presence of one person.

Ayoub et al. reported on a series of five families in which educational disabilities were the presenting symptom in cases ultimately diagnosed as caregiver-fabricated illness. This diagnostic entity has been called educational condition or disability falsification. These cases, unlike those which present with medical problems, are played out within schools, among teachers, guidance counselors and principals, and especially within the special education system (36). Another recently recognized subcategory of caregiver-fabricated illness is that in which a psychiatric or behavioral problem is the presenting complaint. This case has involved repeated outpatient visits and hospitalizations for psychotic disorders, multiple personality disorders, attention-deficit disorders, temporal lobe epilepsy with rage, Tourette disorder, and autistic spectrum disorders (37).

Description of Parents

Mothers are most often associated with perpetration of fabricated illness in children, and often have had prior extensive exposure to the health care system. This, in some instances, has been from past training and work experience as a nurse, medical receptionist, or other health care professional. In Meadow's description of 17 families, nine of the mothers had such a background, and Rosenberg reported that 27% of 97 mothers had a nursing background and another 3% had worked in medical offices (23,38). In other cases, the mother herself has a fabrication disorder and therefore has brought to her experience as a mother, both her own psychopathology and often a vast knowledge of medicine, hospitals, and medical practice acquired from her experiences prior to her child's birth. In a study of covert deaths in infancy, one-half of the perpetrators had some form of abnormal illness behavior such as somatization disorder, and 22% were reported to have Munchausen syndrome, or factitious disorder, and in Sheridan's review, 29% of the perpetrators had some features suggestive of factitious disorder (24,39).

Perpetrating caregivers may be considered exemplary in all their interactions with medical staff, or may be adversarial, especially when challenged about the veracity of reported child symptoms. In spite of having outwardly positive relationships with perpetrators, hospital staff have reported subjective feelings of uneasiness or feeling intrusive in the caregiver's presence (40). Some perpetrators are thought to be motivated by a desire to manipulate or control doctors or other professionals perceived to be powerful. In this case it is the deception of medical staff, rather than a desire to somehow join their ranks or be perceived as an ideal mother, that appears to motivate the perpetrator (14). Recently, attention-seeking behaviors have found a new outlet in online blogs on which caregivers share details of their experiences parenting an "ill" child and where commenters can provide gratifying and immediate messages of support (41). Perpetrating caregivers may be considered model parents who are extremely attentive to their children. They may take over the care of their children to a greater degree than is usual in hospitals and often live in the hospital and remain with the child constantly. It has been noted, however, that the care given to the child can be of an excessive nature; for example, the child may be dressed in inappropriately lavish clothing, or the hospital room may be stocked with an outrageous number of toys (40). Prolonged covert videotaped observation of caregivers, however, has often revealed detached or even directly cruel behavior to children when they are not in the public view (12). One striking quality of a perpetrating caregiver that may be important in recognizing the syndrome is her inappropriate affect when given information about the severity of her child's illness or discussing invasive medical investigations. There is a bland acceptance, rather than obvious distress, and she may appear to be relatively at ease with medical uncertainties (40). In one report, the mother was even described as appearing euphoric as her child became sicker (42).

Besides fabrication of symptoms of illness, these mothers often fabricate extensively about other parts of their lives. An example of this is a mother who made statements that she had just completed a law degree and was working toward a master's degree in Russian history, both of which were false (43). Certainly, an important element of the syndrome is the mother's ability to converse with the medical staff about her child's illness in a very knowledgeable and medically sophisticated manner.

In contrast to the mother's constant presence, a father may have very little involvement in his child's care and sometimes does not even visit the hospital. This is particularly noteworthy considering the severity of the child's illness. In a review of 37 families, 70% of the fathers were described as peripheral or absent from the family system; often the fathers have jobs that keep them away from the family for prolonged periods of time (38,44). The marital relationship between the parents is often poor, although in some instances the child's apparent illness serves to bring the parents closer together.

In rare instances where fathers have been identified as the perpetrators of illness fabrication in a child, their interactions with medical personnel appear quite different than is the case with mothers. Like mothers, the fathers often stay with their children in hospital, but are considered by staff to be demanding, overbearing, and unreasonable, and are often quick to make formal complaints and seek legal redress. It is notable that in Meadow's description of 15 fathers, none were actively employed and 11 had factitious disorders (27).

Description of the Child

There is little in the literature describing the children in this disorder. Older children in particular may collude with their mothers in the ongoing deception. In the original report of Sneed and Bell, it was the 10-year-old boy who was presenting the pebbles as renal calculi (3). Furthermore, these children, like children who have been repeatedly physically abused, may learn to tolerate passively medical procedures. A harrowing look into the experience of a child abused by a mother, a registered nurse, who fabricated illness at one point by tying him/her to a chair and repeatedly beating his/her foot with a hammer can be found in a published account of an adult survivor of the disorder (45). A separate diagnostic entity has emerged from these observations, that of child and adolescent illness falsification. Children who induce or fabricate illness are thought to do so either as a continuation of perpetration of factitious disorder by a parent or covert parent coaching, or because of a strong attraction to the medical world in themselves (46). Other symptoms that have been described include feeding disorders among infants and toddlers and withdrawn, hyperactive, or oppositional behavior among preschoolers (41).

ETIOLOGY

Understanding of the perpetrators of fabricated illness in a child is evolving. Overall, perpetrating caregivers are likely to need or benefit from having a well child being perceived as ill, or a sick child being perceived as more ill than the child actually is (11). Two systematic reviews of perpetrators identified high rates of somatoform disorders, coexisting personality disorders, and a history of self-harm in mothers who fabricated illness in their children (47,48). Adversity in the perpetrator's own childhood also is an important etiologic factor. Family disruption and loss were prominent in Bass and Jones' sample (48). Others have found high rates of physical and sexual abuse in perpetrators (24,44,47). These studies shed light on perpetrator behavior that may be understood as a maladaptive coping strategy in the face of psychic distress, and reveal reasons why children are used as tools for interaction with the medical system (12). An abnormal attachment between the mother and child is postulated to underscore the motivation of perpetrators in caregiver-fabricated illness, possibly in concert with childhood adversity and a personal history of somatization behavior (11). Review of surveillance videos reveals that mothers thought by medical staff to be extremely caring largely ignored their children when alone with them (49,50). In a report by Nicol and Eccles, the mother reported that "she found, in her general practitioner, a source of support and kindness and this reinforced the pattern of very regular attendance at the surgery" (51). Guandolo has commented that "illness is the ticket of admission to a place where understanding and caring relieved the feelings of hopelessness and isolation" (43). Perpetrators also may find a sense of self-worth and importance through interactions with the medical world. Chan and associates described a mother who would visit the intensive care unit just to talk to other mothers, and Meadow has described another mother who had some nursing training and who would help teach nursing students (26,52). In the case discussed by Nicol and Eccles, the mother reported that she liked to feel that she "was being considered by intelligent people" (51). Pathologic lying may be an important comorbidity for perpetrators of fabricated illness. Waller has commented that "the disturbance in thought content and behavior may be a dissociative phenomenon or a form of pseudologia phantastica or pathologic lying in which the parent comes to believe, at least intermittently, the fantasy that the child has a primary rather than a factitious illness" (53). Bass and Jones highlight the importance of pathologic lying in their sample as well, noting that the behavior emerged in the setting of life stress and encompassed other domains of deceit including making hoax telephone calls to the police about invented "harassment" (48).

SPECTRUM OF THE DISORDER

Meadow, in reporting on what he terms mild cases, raises questions regarding the limits of the definition of the disorder. He points out that, at times, caregivers often exaggerate their children's symptoms or may perceive that a problem is present when it is not apparent to the doctor (54). Perpetrators may themselves move along a spectrum by initially exaggerating a real symptom, to fabricating symptoms, to physically inducing symptoms in their child (17). Bass and Glaser frame the spectrum to begin with "erroneous reporting" of medical history, symptoms or signs and progress to "deception by use of hands" which includes falsification of medical records, tampering with specimens of intravenous lines, or induction of illness by, for example, poisoning or suffocation (11).

DIAGNOSIS

The challenge inherent in making a diagnosis of caregiver-fabricated illness cannot be overstated. Pediatric providers are taught to ignore parental concern at their peril; the shift from a partnership with a parent in the care of a child to a relationship in which the parent is suspected of lying about or actively harming a child is a dramatic one. Furthermore, medical providers may become unwitting agents of abuse as they order diagnostic tests and treatments for children based on parental misrepresentations or deceit and this may render these providers even less likely to recognize the pathologic behavior of perpetrating caregivers. The American Academy of Pediatrics suggests that the following three questions be posed when caregiver-fabricated illness is suspected:

1. Are the history, signs, and symptoms of disease credible?
2. Is the child receiving unnecessary and harmful or potentially harmful medical care?
3. If so, who is instigating the evaluations and treatment? (17,55).

A full review of medical records, which can be voluminous, is indicated. Consultation with a child abuse pediatrician may provide needed expertise and objectivity that treating providers will necessarily lack (17). The American Academy of Pediatrics suggests the following as indicators of possible caregiver-fabricated illness:

- Diagnosis does not match the objective findings
- Signs or symptoms are bizarre
- Caregiver or suspected offender does not express relief or pleasure when told that child is improving or that child does not have a particular illness
- Inconsistent histories of symptoms from different observers
- Caregiver insists on invasive or painful procedures and hospitalizations
- Caregiver's behavior does not match expressed distress or report of symptoms (e.g., unusually calm)
- Signs and symptoms begin only in the presence of one caregiver
- Sibling has or had an unusual or unexplained illness or death
- Sensitivity to multiple environmental substances or medicines
- Failure of the child's illness to respond to its normal treatments or unusual intolerance to those treatments
- Caregiver publicly solicits sympathy or donations or benefits because of the child's rare illness
- Extensive unusual illness history in the caregiver or caregiver's family; caregiver's history of somatization disorders (17).

Greiner et al. have piloted a screening tool for early identification of what they term medical child abuse. The authors employ a 15-item checklist for medical record review that had a sensitivity of 0.947 and a specificity of 0.956 ($P < 0.05$) in detecting medical child abuse (56). While covert video surveillance has been proposed as a tool in the diagnosis of caregiver-fabricated illness, it is highly controversial and fraught with ethical concern. A key issue is the need for continuous monitoring of such surveillance in order to allow for immediate intervention in the case of witnessed child harm (57–59). A retrospective review of 41 cases in which covert video surveillance was used to investigate a possible diagnosis of Munchausen syndrome by proxy in one pediatric hospital found that 23 diagnoses were actually confirmed. Of these 23, covert video surveillance was seen as crucial to making the diagnosis in 13 cases (56%) and supportive of the diagnosis in 5 cases (28%) (58). Careful and complete record review (which may be arduous and require collecting data from multiple sources) and in person meetings of all currently involved medical providers are likely the most useful means of detecting caregiver-fabricated illness. Once identified, caregiver-fabricated illness must be promptly reported to child protectiveservices.

TREATMENT

Treating perpetrators of caregiver-fabricated illness is difficult. While some perpetrators admit deceit when confronted, many actively deny it. Schreier has identified the following conditions under which treatment may be successful: (1) the abuser admits to the abuse and has been able to describe specifically how he or she abused the child, (2) the abuser has experienced an appropriate emotional response to his or her behaviors and the harm he or she has caused the child, (3) the abuser has developed strategies to better identify and manage his or her needs to avoid abusing the child in the future, and (4) the abuser has demonstrated these skills, with monitoring, over a significant period of time (60). Challenges inherent in meeting these conditions including the likelihood that the suspected perpetrator has experienced severe adversity in childhood, makes the establishment of both a therapeutic relationship hard and the capacity for self-reflection potentially limited (11). Some mothers have become extremely agitated, acutely psychotic, or depressed and suicidal following the confrontation (61). An assessment may be required regarding the need for psychiatric hospitalization. Child victims of caregiver-fabricated illness may require a variety of treatment strategies including physical rehabilitation, trauma-focused care, and grief support in the wake of being separated from an abusive caregiver. Family-centered care may be crucial for both rehabilitation of offending caregivers and support of nonoffending family members (16).

OUTCOME

The final outcome for child victims of caregiver-fabricated illness is variable and dependent both on the severity of the disorder and treatment provided. The caregiver who has additional psychiatric disorders and who has been involved in the fabrication of symptoms or has suffered from pathologic lying for many years is more difficult to treat than another with a simpler presentation. This is likely true for those caregivers who have factitious disorder themselves, which is often very difficult to treat successfully (62). The child whose symptoms of illness has been caused by a more dangerous activity (e.g., suffocation) is obviously at higher risk of dying than the child whose symptom was owing to less dangerous methods (e.g., a mother's putting blood in her child's urine). In Rosenberg's review of the 117 cases reported in the literature, 9% died and 8% of the survivors had permanent disfigurement or impairment of physical function. The leading causes of death were suffocation and poisoning (23). Children have died even after the diagnosis was made and their mothers confronted, and younger siblings have been abused after older siblings have died. The psychiatric sequelae of caregiver-fabricated illness have been less well described, both for the mother and child. Certainly, some of these children have continued to fabricate illness for themselves, and child victims of fabricated illness may grow up to fabricate illness themselves (54,63). Of the 12 children described by McGuire and Feldman, 11 were described as having adverse effects that included immaturity, abnormal relationships with their mothers, separation problems, and aggressive behavior (41). Some children have expressed fears of poisoning and death, and at least two children have required psychiatric hospitalization (6). Bools et al. described 54 children for whom they obtained information an average of 5.6 years after the event. Thirty of these children continued to live with their biologic mothers, whereas 24 children were with other family members or in substitute care. For 10 of the 30 children living with their mothers there was evidence of further fabrications, and for another 8 there were "other concerns," either about the relationship between the mothers and their children, or about other aspects of the mothers' behaviors. Of these 18 children for whom there were continuing concerns about the family, 12 exhibited psychological symptoms, including somatic complaints, emotional disorders, conduct disorder, and poor functioning at school. Among the 24 children who were no longer living with their biologic mothers, 8 had persistent psychological symptoms, and another 6 children had disorders that had shown signs of gradual improvement. Altogether, the authors of the study concluded that half of the children had outcomes that they considered to be unacceptable, but because of the variability in cases, it was not possible to comment on whether better outcomes were obtained when children remained with their mothers or were separated. However, the authors did conclude that when children remained with their mothers, the outcome appeared improved when there had been a temporary placement in foster care (63). Some children are "quite indifferent" to separation when it does occur, and that they go on to embrace their own wellness and engage with others around them (64). In reporting on the follow-up of cases enrolled in an intensive, inpatient treatment program, Berg and Jones reported greater success. When 16 families were reevaluated at an average of 27 months after treatment, there were no ongoing concerns for nine of the families; the mothers had no mental health problems and had insight into their original condition, and the children had no psychological disorders. There continued to be mild concerns for five families in which the mothers continued to have mild to moderate mental health problems, although these did not impact on their relationship with their children or on the children's development. In only two families were there more serious concerns about the mother's mental health, although they were not overtly abusive. However, the authors stressed that these cases had been selected for treatment on their likelihood of achieving success and that cases considered unsuitable for psychiatric treatment were excluded, usually because of persistent parental denial or the severity of the parent's personality disorder (65).

CONCLUSION

Timely recognition of caregiver-fabricated illness can prevent harm in children. In this condition, perhaps more so than in any other, there needs to be extensive collaboration among all involved medical disciplines. Early involvement of an expert in child abuse pediatrics may be crucial both to the objective evaluation of a case as well to needed coordination among all involved medical providers.

References

1. Asher R: Munchhausen syndrome. *Lancet* 1:339–341, 1951.
2. Raspe RE: *The Singular Campaigns and Adventures of Baron Munchhausen.* London, The Cresset Press, 1948.
3. Sneed RC, Bell RF: The dauphin of Munchhausen: factitious passage of renal stones in a child. *Pediatrics* 58:127–130, 1976.
4. Meadow R: Munchhausen syndrome by proxy: the hinterland of child abuse. *Lancet* 2:343–345, 1977.
5. Lansky SB, Erickson HM Jr: Prevention of child murder: a case report. *J Am Acad Child Psychiatry* 13:691–698, 1974.
6. Rogers D, Tripp J, Bentovim A, Robinson A, Berry D, Goulding R: Non-accidental poisoning: an extended syndrome of child abuse. *Br Med J* 1:793–796, 1976.
7. Lazoritz S: Munchhausen by proxy or Meadow's syndrome? *Lancet* 2:631, 1987.
8. Meadow R, Lennert T: Munchhausen by proxy or Polle syndrome: which term is correct? *Pediatrics* 74:554–556, 1984.
9. Verity CM, Winckworth C, Burman D, Stevens D, White RJ: Polle syndrome: children of Munchhausen. *Br Med J* 2:422–423, 1979.
10. American Psychiatric Association: *Diagnostic and Statistical Manual of Mental Disorders.* 5th ed. Arlington, VA, American Psychiatric Association Publishing, 2013.
11. Bass C, Glaser D: Early recognition and management of fabricated or induced illness in children. *Lancet* 383:1412–1421, 2014.
12. Schreier H: On the importance of motivation in Munchhausen by proxy: the case of Kathy Bush. *Child Abuse Negl* 26:537–549, 2002.
13. Meadow R: Different interpretations of Munchhausen syndrome by proxy. *Child Abuse Negl* 26:501–508, 2002.

14. Ayoub CC, Alexander R: Definitional issues in Munchhausen by proxy. *American Professional Society on the Abuse of Children* 11:7–10, 1998.
15. Ayoub CC, Alexander R, Beck D, et al.; APSAC Taskforce on Munchausen by Proxy, Definitions Working Group: Position paper: definitional issues in Munchhausen by proxy. *Child Maltreat* 7:105–111, 2002.
16. Roesler TA, Jenny C: *Medical Child Abuse: Beyond Munchausen Syndrome by Proxy.* Elk Grove Village, IL, American Academy of Pediatrics Press, 2009.
17. Flaherty EG, Macmillan HL; Committee on Child Abuse and Neglect: Caregiver-fabricated illness in a child: a manifestation of child maltreatment. *Pediatrics* 132:590–597, 2013.
18. Libow JA, Schreier HA: Three forms of factitious illness in children: when is it Munchhausen syndrome by proxy? *Am J Orthopsychiatry* 56:602–611, 1986.
19. Rogers R: Diagnostic, explanatory, and detection models of Munchausen by proxy: extrapolations from malingering and deception. *Child Abuse Negl* 28:225–238, 2004.
20. Rosenberg DA: Munchhausen syndrome by proxy: medical diagnostic criteria. *Child Abuse Negl* 27:421–430, 2003.
21. McClure RJ, Davis PM, Meadow SR, Sibert JR: Epidemiology of Munchhausen syndrome by proxy, non-accidental poisoning, and non-accidental suffocation. *Arch Dis Child* 75:57–61, 1996.
22. Ferrara P, Vitelli O, Bottaro G, et al.: Factitious disorders and Munchausen syndrome: the tip of the iceberg. *J Child Health Care* 17(4):366–374, 2013.
23. Rosenberg DA: Web of deceit: a literature review of Munchhausen syndrome by proxy. *Child Abuse Negl* 11:547–563, 1987.
24. Sheridan MS: The deceit continues: an updated literature review of Munchhausen syndrome by proxy. *Child Abuse Negl* 27:431–451, 2003.
25. Makar AF, Squier PJ: Munchhausen syndrome by proxy: father as a perpetrator. *Pediatrics* 85:370–373, 1990.
26. Meadow R: Fictitious epilepsy. *Lancet* 2:25–28, 1984.
27. Meadow R: Munchhausen syndrome by proxy abuse perpetrated by men. *Arch Dis Child* 78:210–216, 1998.
28. Feldman MD, Brown RM: Munchhausen by proxy in an international context. *Child Abuse Negl* 26:509–524, 2002.
29. Libow JA: Beyond collusion: active illness falsification. *Child Abuse Negl* 26:525–536, 2002.
30. Goss PW, McDougall PN: Munchhausen syndrome by proxy: a cause of preterm delivery. *Med J Aust* 157:814–817, 1992.
31. Porter GE, Heitsch GM, Miller MD: Munchhausen syndrome by proxy: unusual manifestations and disturbing sequelae. *Child Abuse Negl* 18:789–794, 1994.
32. Bools CN, Neale BA, Meadow SR: Co-morbidity associated with fabricated illness (Munchhausen syndrome by proxy). *Arch Dis Child* 67:77–79, 1992.
33. Alexander R, Smith W, Stevenson R: Serial Munchhausen syndrome by proxy. *Pediatrics* 86:581–585, 1990.
34. Light MJ, Sheridan MS: Munchhausen syndrome by proxy and apnea (MBPA): a survey of apnea programs. *Clin Pediatr (Phila)* 29:162–168, 1990.
35. Meadow R: Suffocation, recurrent apnea, and sudden infant death. *J Pediatr* 117:351–357, 1990.
36. Ayoub CC, Schreier HA, Keller C: Munchhausen by proxy: presentations in special education. *Child Maltreat* 7:149–159, 2002.
37. Schreier HA: Factitious disorder by proxy in which the presenting problem is behavioral or psychiatric. *J Am Acad Child Adolesc Psychiatry* 39:668–670, 2000.
38. Meadow R: Munchhausen syndrome by proxy. *Arch Dis Child* 57:92–98, 1982.
39. Meadow R: Unnatural sudden infant death. *Arch Dis Child* 80:7–14, 1999.
40. Zitelli BJ, Seltman MF, Shannon RM: Munchausen's syndrome by proxy and its professional participants. *Am J Dis Child* 141:1099–1102, 1987.
41. Brown AN, Gonzalez GR, Wiester RT, Kelley MC, Feldman KW: Caretaker blogs in caregiver fabricated illness in a child: a window on the caretaker's thinking? *Child Abuse Negl* 38:488–497, 2014.
42. McGuire TL, Feldman KW: Psychologic morbidity of children subjected to Munchhausen syndrome by proxy. *Pediatrics* 83:289–292, 1989.
43. Guandolo VL: Munchhausen syndrome by proxy: an outpatient challenge. *Pediatrics* 75:526–530, 1985.
44. Gray J, Bentovim A: Illness induction syndrome: paper I—a series of 41 children from 37 families identified at the Great Ormond Street Hospital for Children, NHS Trust. *Child Abuse Negl* 20:655–673, 1996.
45. Bryk M, Siegel PT: My mother caused my illness: the story of a survivor of Munchausen by proxy syndrome.*Pediatrics* 100(1):1–7, 1997.
46. Libow JA: Child and adolescent illness falsification. *Pediatrics* 105: 336–342, 2000.
47. Bools C, Neale B, Meadow R: Munchhausen syndrome by proxy: a study of psychopathology. *Child Abuse Negl* 18:773–788, 1994.
48. Bass C, Jones D: Psychopathology of perpetrators of fabricated or induced illness in children: case series. *Br J Psychiatry* 199(2):113–118, 2011.
49. Southall DP, Stebbens VA, Rees SV, Lang MH, Warner JO, Shinebourne EA: Apnoeic episodes induced by smothering: two cases identified by covert video surveillance. *Br Med J (Clin Res Ed)* 294:1637–1641, 1987.
50. Samuels MP, McClaughlin W, Jacobson RR, Poets CF, Southall DP: Fourteen cases of imposed upper airway obstruction. *Arch Dis Child* 67: 162–170, 1992.
51. Nicol AR, Eccles M: Psychotherapy for Munchhausen syndrome by proxy. *Arch Dis Child* 60:344–348, 1985.
52. Chan DA, Salcedo JR, Atkins DM, Ruley EJ: Munchhausen syndrome by proxy: a review and case study. *J Pediatr Psychol* 11:71–80, 1986.
53. Waller DA: Obstacles to the treatment of Munchhausen by proxy syndrome. *J Am Acad Child Psychiatry* 22:80–85, 1983.
54. Meadow R: Management of Munchhausen syndrome by proxy. *Arch Dis Child* 60:385–393, 1985.
55. Stirling J Jr; American Academy of Pediatrics Committee on Child Abuse and Neglect: Beyond Munchausen syndrome by proxy: identification and treatment of child abuse in a medical setting. *Pediatrics* 119(5):1026–1030, 2007.
56. Greiner MV, Palusci VJ, Keeshin BR, Kearns SC, Sinal SH: A preliminary screening instrument for early detection of medical child abuse. *Hosp Pediatr* 3(1):39–44, 2013.
57. Southall DP, Plunkett MC, Banks MW, Falkov AF, Samuels MP: Covert video recordings of life-threatening child abuse: lessons for child protection. *Pediatrics* 100(5):735–760, 1997.
58. Hall DE, Eubanks L, Meyyazhagan LS, Kenney RD, Johnson SC: Evaluation of covert video surveillance in the diagnosis of Munchausen syndrome by proxy: lessons from 41 cases. *Pediatrics* 105(6):1305–1312, 2000.
59. Foreman DM: Detecting fabricated or induced illness in children. *BMJ* 331(7523):978–979, 2005.
60. Schreier H: Munchhausen by proxy. *Curr Probl Pediatr Adolesc Health Care* 34(3):126–143, 2004.
61. Palmer AJ, Yoshimura GJ: Munchhausen syndrome by proxy. *J Am Acad Child Psychiatry* 23(4):503–508, 1984.
62. Mayo JP Jr, Haggerty JJ Jr: Long-term psychotherapy of Munchhausen syndrome. *Am J Psychother* 38:571–578, 1984.
63. Bools CN, Neale BA, Meadow SR: Follow up of victims of fabricated illness (Munchhausen syndrome by proxy). *Arch Dis Child* 69:625–630, 1993.
64. Ayoub CC, Deutsch RM, Kinscherff R: Munchhausen by proxy: definitions, identification, and evaluation. In: Reece R (ed): *The Treatment of Child Abuse.* Baltimore, MD, Johns Hopkins University Press, 213–225, 2000.
65. Berg B, Jones DP: Outcome of psychiatric intervention in factitious illness by proxy (Munchausen's syndrome by proxy). *Arch Dis Child* 81:465–472, 1999.

CHAPTER 5.15.5 ■ CHILDREN EXPOSED TO MASS EMERGENCY AND DISASTER: THE ROLE OF THE MENTAL HEALTH PROFESSIONALS

NATHANIEL LAOR AND LEO WOLMER

INTRODUCTION

Mass disasters, whether natural, technologic or human made, affect individuals, families, and entire communities and impose incalculable physical, psychological, and economic hardships on survivors. In recent years, apparently as a result of increased population density, urbanization, and climatic changes (1), we have been witness to significant growth in the mortality associated with nearly all types of disasters. From 1980 to 2000, about 75% of the world's population lived in areas that were affected at least once by some form of disaster, whether an earthquake, a tropical cyclone, flooding, or drought (2). Each year from 2000 to 2009, 110,000 lives were lost and 255 million people were affected by disasters (3).

In this chapter, we focus on the psychosocial impact of disasters on children. Physical damage is usually easy to identify, but the internal suffering of children can remain hidden even from the most sensitive observers. Therefore, clinicians and researchers have invested efforts in explaining the type, extent, and risks of children's maladaptive responses to mass disaster.

Garmezy and Rutter (4) claimed that children show only a mild response to traumatic conditions. Modern empirical methodologies and clinical observations have refuted this claim, revealing that the adverse psychological effects of such conditions can be severe and long lasting (5–9) and may persist even in the face of apparently normal social functioning (10). Yet according to the Task Force Report of the American Psychological Association, "few psychologists have had specific training for working with children after disasters, and discussions of children's responses to disasters have been rare in texts on psychopathology or issues in normal development" (8).

This chapter has the following objectives: (a) To offer a theoretical perspective of disaster as a systemic social phenomenon; (b) to clarify the role of child mental health professionals in large-scale preparedness and community reactivation under conditions of disaster; (c) to review the major findings on children's responses to disaster; and (d) to propose assessment and intervention models for children, families, and communities exposed to mass disaster.

DEFINITIONS

The literature distinguishes between "traumas" and "disasters." *Traumas* are experiences that threaten the individual's health and well-being, render the individual helpless in the face of intolerable internal or external danger, overwhelm coping mechanisms, violate basic assumptions about survival, and accentuate uncontrollability and unpredictability of the world (11). Traumas may be caused by an isolated, unanticipated, and uncontrolled event or they may be long lasting, the result of repeated exposure to several extreme external events (12).

Disasters are relatively abrupt events that are somewhat delimited by time. They are public events that cause extensive damage to property and lives and that have a total and ongoing disruptive impact on children and families' social networks, basic daily routines, and sense of safety and connectedness (8,13,14). During a disaster, the community's capacity to negotiate the recovery of its individual members is compromised. Matters are often made worse when resources are overextended (1) and the community's infrastructure is affected, often resulting in unemployment, housing and food shortages, poor health, deficient school and mental health services, job absenteeism, and family dysfunction.

Unlike traumas, in disasters victims must face immediate, long-lasting, and repeated exposure to reminders of the event. Disasters usually involve three interconnected types of experiences: terror due to objective and subjective threats to life or exposure to horrifying sights; grief following loss (e.g., human lives, sense of meaning, basic trust, self-esteem); and disruption of normal life (15). On the social level, disasters are accompanied by shock, depression and mourning, confusion and social disarray, rage and blame, the collapse of formal leadership, and social disintegration. Children sense that their family, neighborhood, and school have been disrupted (13). The recovery processes continues long after the disastrous event itself is over. Hence, theoretical, research, and intervention studies should be both all-encompassing and oriented to the long term.

DISASTERS AND THE MENTAL HEALTH SYSTEM

Mass disasters pose a multifaceted challenge to the mental health system (16): (a) *Environmental challenge:* Substantial needs, routinely defined as pathologic, emerge and must be confronted; (b) *Systemic challenge:* Multidisciplinary orientation and multisystemic collaboration are required to counter the impact; (c) *Practical challenge:* Problems to be faced involve resource allocation, extended deployment, organization, dissemination of information, and communications; (d) *Theoretical challenge:* The mental health system lacks a comprehensive and integrative "mass disaster theory" with a general social perspective in addition to the public health perspective (17); and (e) *Professional challenge:* Most programs are not committed to disaster intervention training. Hence, professionals have insufficient knowledge and little resilience in the face of ongoing stress.

DISASTER STAGES

The various models proposed to describe the response to disaster focus mostly on the event perspective (e.g., warning, threat, impact, inventory, rescue, and recovery) (18). The systemic–ecologic model proposes a conceptual framework of disaster that integrates the event, the individual, and the sociocultural reaction, including the mental health response (19). Such a perspective has been called for in the field (20,21). According to such a perspective, a disaster comprises a series of four stages that can start long before the expected event actually takes place (e.g., the months of anticipation preceding the outbreak of a war). This first *pre-disaster stage* includes warning, alert and alarm signs, and a sense of massive threat to communal and personal security. This is the stage in which efforts should be made to build preparedness and resilience.

The *second stage* includes the damaging event itself, the primary disaster, and the attempts to alleviate its effects, i.e., rescuing as many victims as possible and providing basic needs (food, water, and shelter) to the affected population. The *third stage* involves massive changes in societal structure and function (establishment of evacuation centers and tent-cities, movement of refugees), which may lead to a breakdown of societal norms, structures, and functions. This breakdown, reflected in societal regression, may be viewed as the secondary disaster. Life usually stabilizes in due course, generally after 18 to 36 months. At this point, a *fourth stage* of disaster may ensue, wherein the sociocultural losses of the tertiary disaster may threaten the existing cultural matrix and identity, which may be followed by the emergence of extremist ideologies (22,23).

When the severity of the damage evolves gradually and over an extended period of time (e.g., AIDS epidemic in Africa), primary, secondary, and tertiary types of disaster coexist. This gradual pattern allows for preparation and short-term adaptation to minor increments of destruction. Yet it may also prompt habituation (24) within both the affected and the international communities, hence damaging the capacity for long-term forecasting and proper coping.

HOW CHILDREN REACT TO DISASTER: THE DISASTER SYNDROME

A child's protective matrix consists of various dimensions in his or her reality and inner experiences that can be disrupted and rehabilitated, among them political, cultural, social, physical, familial, maternal, and personal dimensions (25). Since disasters affect all these components, unlike posttraumatic syndrome, the disaster syndrome involves all aspects of a child's developing cognitive structures and capacities and poses a more intricate pathologic threat. Children must cope with many different kinds of losses: of people, of support systems, of normal routines, of attachment figures, and of basic assumptions of safety and normalcy. Children may become withdrawn and alienated from the reality they perceive as having betrayed them: nature, parents, society, and technology (20,26,27).

According to Franks (28), disasters impact "moving targets." In other words, children continuously change and mature when disasters strike. Thus, disasters change the context in which child development occurs, and hence change the course of development itself. Franks emphasized the need to approach affected children not only by examining symptom levels but also by focusing on qualitative cognitive and emotional development and age-appropriate functioning.

Disasters may affect children's ability to regulate the intensity of their impulses and unconscious fantasies, consequently jeopardizing their sense of self-efficacy, security and autonomy, the normal maturation of their defensive functioning, object relations, reality testing, and attachment. Structural developments, such as superego consolidation and its behavioral consequences, ideal ego structure formation with its relevance to affiliation and ideology development, and ego functions with their significance in areas of cognition and attention, may also be hampered. Traumatization has a potentially damaging effect on the development of a lasting sense of identity and of the historical continuity of the self that integrates thoughts, images, feelings, and sensations (29).

Preschoolers may exhibit behavioral changes and regressive behaviors, mostly within the normal range. These may include irritability, sleep difficulties, separation problems, fears, nervousness, posttraumatic play, demanding or dependent behavior, whining or temper tantrums (30–34). Furthermore, parents and close individuals seem to play a significant role in preschoolers' responses. As Wolmer et al. (35) found among Israeli preschoolers who endured lasting massive rocket and mortar attacks, those who were more exposed to harsh description of the traumatic event and to severe emotional responses in their close surroundings suffered from more PTSD and impairments in functioning. However, the issue of who impacts whose response in the parent–child dyad remains unclear, as studies show, for example, that more, and not less, maternal emotional sensitivity appears to mediate the development of the child's PTSD (36).

Older children may report disturbances in conscience functioning, although their moral functioning may seem advanced (37), as well as risk-taking behaviors such as substance abuse (34).

Studies suggest that parents and teachers tend to report fewer posttraumatic symptoms (PTS) in children than the children themselves report (21,38–40). Adults may be preoccupied with their own stress and not be attuned to their child's inner emotional states. Children may also be more reliable reporters of internalizing or dissociative symptoms. Thus, clinicians must be careful to assess children's functioning directly and not rely exclusively on external reports (21). They must bear in mind that while the initial response tends to predict later adjustment, initial symptomatic ratings may not correlate with later assessments (41), and posttraumatic responses may have a delayed onset (42), although this does not occur frequently (43). If a disaster is limited and well controlled, most of the pathologic reactions in children will abate within the first year (21,41). If community functioning is substantially disrupted, however, symptoms may persist for years (5,10,21,42).

RESPONSE TRAJECTORIES

For quite a while, research has focused on broad comparisons (i.e., exposed and unexposed populations) or on extreme dysfunction. In the last several years, however, growing interest has focused more closely on the individual (21). For the most part, individuals seem to have intense reactions to an event. Yet, unless the individual is repeatedly challenged, these reactions will likely subside within a month (34). Others may nonetheless experience symptoms later on, peaking approximately within a year, yet recover (44). Among those who continue to experience significant distress, many continue to suffer a great deal longer (43).

On that note, it is important to distinguish resiliency from lack of reaction, or resistance. The term resiliency does not refer to a total absence of psychological distress in the face of adversity but to the ability to remain functional in the face of adversity or to recover and adapt quickly. Resilient individuals consistently present responses, even intense ones, in the short-term postdisaster time frame, yet are able to reassume functioning after a short period of recovery (45).

Different trajectories of responses to disasters seem to exist: resilience (the most common, a mild disruption in functioning followed by a return to baseline within a few weeks or months); recovery (characterized by a more intense response associated with moderate-to-severe levels of distress and disruption of functioning that subsides approximately 1 to 2 years postdisaster); delayed response or "late onset" (a rather mild–moderate levels of distress followed by a rise in dysfunctionality); chronicity (the least optimistic response characterized by an immediate and severe reaction that could last for years if not permanently); and posttraumatic growth (following struggles with acute crises), some people report more meaningful relationships, increased personal strength and appreciation for life, and richer spiritual lives (21,22,46). Some of these trajectories may not be mutually exclusive (e.g., PTS and posttraumatic growth).

POSTDISASTER SYMPTOMS

In response to disasters, children may exhibit a combination of some or many of the following behaviors: posttraumatic stress symptoms, fears, anxiety, behavioral problems, physical symptoms, depression and grief, dissociation, and substance abuse (21,33,47,48). Anthony et al. (49) found that anhedonia, inattention, and learning problems are the most common symptoms after disasters. But rather than being markers of a pathologic reaction, such symptoms reflect the normal disruptive consequences of disasters.

Symptoms of posttraumatic stress disorder (PTSD) are grouped under three domains: intrusion, avoidance/numbing, and arousal. Empirical studies have identified certain symptoms that are specific to children, such as persistent posttraumatic play, omens, separation anxiety, fear of strangers, monsters or animals, and somatic complaints (50,51). Scheeringa et al. (52,53) proposed the following diagnostic criteria for young children. These were integrated into DSM-5 and identify preschoolers' PTSD by a lower threshold for the avoidance and the hyperarousal domains, thereby increasing the prevalence of diagnosed preschoolers following disaster.

Intrusive re-experiencing of the event may be observed in thoughts, feelings, or sensations. Children may retell their experiences over and over, report nightmares, and exhibit repetitive trauma-related play. They may also describe *vivid* traumatic images: visual (mutilated bodies), auditory (sound of the earthquake or screams for help), olfactory (odors of burned bodies), or kinesthetic (feeling as if they were buried under the rubble).

Avoidance of reminders is manifested in the evasion of places, people, thoughts, or activities associated with the disaster. Such avoidance can be both a symptom and a defensive maneuver to reduce internal stress. Nevertheless, persistent avoidance coping is associated with negative mental health outcomes (54). The avoidance may be active (purposeful engagement in thoughts unrelated to the trauma) or passive (not engaging in social interactions) (49).

General psychic numbing may be considered a mild dissociative response and is more difficult to detect in children than in adults (39). Children exposed to disasters may lose interest in activities that were significant in the past, feel estranged from others, exhibit constricted affect, lose recently acquired developmental skills, and express a sense of foreshortened future.

Increased arousal symptoms include irritability, angry outbursts, exaggerated startle response, hypervigilance, difficulty in concentrating, and sleep disturbances such as difficulties in falling asleep or in sleeping alone (55). Although disasters can induce a variety of symptoms, PTS seem to best predict overall distress (56). PTSD following disaster was also found to be directly linked to exposure to the events and to mediate the indirect association between exposure, test anxiety, and depression symptoms (57).

Mass disasters typically induce specific *fears and dependent behavior* in children (32,58). Old fears may be reactivated, current ones may increase, and new fears with a more or less clear relationship to the event may emerge. Fears may lead to dependent and clingy behavior, difficulty separating from caretakers, or refusal to attend school, thereby damaging overall and specifically academic functioning as well as interrupting the separation–individuation process. According to Vogel and Vernberg (8), disasters challenge children's basic assumption that the world is a secure place, leaving them helplessly vulnerable. Empirical support for this hypothesis was provided by the finding that 5 years after a disaster, young children's symptoms still correlated with their mothers' reactions (59).

Children exposed to disasters may exhibit symptoms of *depression and grief*, but these are usually of lesser severity than are PTSD symptoms (8). Since grief and posttraumatic stress symptoms may appear independently, separate diagnostic interviews are required for each domain (21,60). Grief symptoms can further escalate into traumatic/complicated grief, mostly after firsthand exposure to horrifying sights, particularly loss of loved ones (21). The mood symptoms, which have been suggested to be at least partially secondary to the posttraumatic reactions (61) and now are thought to be independent of them (21,48), are the result of different types of loss (home, family members, personal belongings, basic assumptions). The traumatic grief reaction, previously defined for adults (62), is today also defined for children (63).

After the 1999 earthquakes in Turkey, Laor et al. (64) found that children who had seen severely injured or dead people, experienced hunger or lack of sleep after the event, or had undergone more traumatic experiences in the past, reported more depressive/grief symptoms. Furthermore, following hurricane Ike, La Greca et al. (65) showed that more immediate (e.g., relocation) and ongoing (e.g., still living in a house with a leaking roof) hurricane-related loss and disruption significantly predicted depressive symptoms.

Disasters may also be perceived as an overwhelming interruption of human experience, thereby distorting an individual's basic assumptions, both cognitive ("What is real and what is imaginary?") and existential ("Is it happening to me?"). To re-establish well-being, some people define a different "spatial" arrangement of their position relative to the world: "I am not affected because I am elsewhere." This type of distancing is adaptive. Pathologic *dissociation* goes one step further, with manipulation of adverse stimuli through the reconstruction of perception and the splitting up of consciousness: "What is happening to me is not real" or "I, who am experiencing this, am not real" (25).

Dissociative reactions may be manifested by symptoms that reflect a discontinuation of personal experience. Children may have out-of-body experiences, perceive life as a dream or a movie, and "see" or "hear voices" of people who died. Amnesia is apparently less frequent in children than in adolescents. Dissociative mechanisms may provide temporary relief from the overwhelming trauma. If they persist, however, they may engender a long-term alteration in normally integrative functions of identity, memory, and/or consciousness (66).

FACTORS AFFECTING CHILDREN'S RESPONSES TO DISASTERS

Several categories of factors have an impact on the scope of children's symptomatic responses to disaster.

Disaster-Related Factors

Children whose traumatic exposure is more severe tend to react in a more extreme manner (20,21,34,48,57,65,67,68), and these effects can even be transmitted to the next generations (20). This "dose-exposure" effect is apparent, for example, in the child's proximity to the epicenter of an earthquake (69), the impact zone of a hurricane (70), or the site of missile attacks (31). In a 5-year follow-up study after a technologic disaster in the Netherlands, Boer et al. (33) found that compared to children who had not been exposed, exposed children suffered from more physical, behavioral, and emotional symptoms.

More severe responses have been noted in children who were exposed to extremely harsh experiences, such as witnessing severely injured people and mutilated bodies and being faced with a direct threat to their own lives or those of their parents. Subjective perception of threat seems to have a larger impact than objective threat (21,43). Severity of response is also associated with suffering human loss, especially of family members (71,72), as well as sustaining personal injuries (61,73,74). Continuous displacement also predicts the degree of psychological response (10,43,75), and children exposed to several traumatic experiences are more likely to exhibit a greater number of PTS (76,77).

In cases of severe disasters, children need to cope with a massive range of problems: lack of food, water, and shelter; property damage; inadequate housing; violence; lack of medical care; traumatic reminders; bereavement; relocation; separation from parents; impact on caregivers' functioning; and economic crisis. Under such circumstances, their posttraumatic reactions may intensify and interfere with symptomatic recovery as well as with their long-term development (21,29,67,69,71,78). According to a meta-analysis across 96 studies linking disaster and PTS among children (79), exposure was associated with greater distress when involving greater loss of life in general, closer proximity to the event, greater perceived threat, and personal loss.

Child-Related Factors

Age

Due to methodologic limitations and variations both in subject age and in symptom domains as examined by different studies, generalization needs to be considered with caution. Younger children appear more vulnerable (21,24,80) because at the time disasters strike they are still developing (81). Behavioral problems, specific fears, regressive symptoms, sleeping problems, separation problems, and PTSD appear to be more characteristic of young children, whereas depression and anxiety are more characteristic of older children and adolescents (21,33,67,82).

It should be noted, however, that while older children are less vulnerable, they are more exposed to the disasters and their impact on their communities. They are more aware, mobile, and exposed to the media and social networks (68,83).

Gender

Results regarding gender differences are more consistent, though still call for cautious interpretation. Girls appear to be more likely to suffer from greater distress and PTSD than boys (20,21,34,65,79,81). While some studies reported no gender differences (10,31,70), most found that girls tend to report more internalizing symptoms (anxiety, depression, fears) and PTS, while boys exhibit more externalizing behavior (acting out, aggression) (69,74,82,84). Girls are also more prone to utilize maladaptive and emotion-focused coping strategies (20). It has been suggested that girls experience more objective trauma, prior trauma, and postdisaster stressors (85), which consequently lead to their more intense response.

Gender and age differences need to be studied further, especially considering most data are collected via adult reports and often with no comparison groups (20,21,68).

Vulnerabilities and Resiliency

Children with prior pathology, particularly anxiety and learning difficulties (54,74,75), those who have suffered more traumatic events in the past (34,77,86) or must cope with disabilities (87), and children with negative affectivity (57) are more prone to severe symptoms months after a disaster. By contrast, resilient children are those who have the support of caring adults during and after major stressors, as well as those who are good learners, good problem solvers, able to engage with other people, and possess an internal locus of control (88). These children have areas of competence and are perceived to have high efficacy (89,90). Resiliency in children is also associated with secure attachment, better cognitive skills, overall predisaster functioning, self-regulation, faith, and hope (20,34,68). Moreover, Asarnow et al. (54) found that children's reactions to the Northridge earthquake, a mild-to-moderate stressor, showed that the role of heritable biology was minor compared to the role of the children's subjective appraisals of stress and past psychopathology.

Coping Skills

A child's coping skills also mediate between exposure severity and response. More immature coping/defensive strategies for dealing with stress (blaming others, anger) are associated with greater symptomatic persistence over time (55,91). Coping has a bidirectional association with a child's distress. The distress following disasters elicits the use of coping strategies, which later affect the distress, with appraisal processes playing a key role (81).

Biologic Factors

One of the most innovative frontiers in disaster research is the role of psychobiology in disaster response. For example, it was found that possessing a certain gene associated with the Met allele of the brain-derived neurotrophic factor (BDNF) moderates how disaster exposure is linked to PTSD and depression levels, with a stronger association found among those in possession of this gene. This was moderated by children's social support, with a stronger association between exposure and PTSD among those with the allele than among those without it, under conditions of low social support (65). Furthermore, a combination of higher cortisol and sympathetic nervous system activity is associated with potential resilience (92). Variations in the serotonin transporter gene (5-HTT) and variations in genes that regulate the functioning of the hypothalamic–pituitary–adrenal (HPA) axis were also found to be significant in stress response (20).

Socioeconomic Status

Low socioeconomic status (SES) has frequently been found to be a vulnerability factor for severe response to disasters. Lower SES is associated with a higher degree of exposure to the event since lower SES populations tend to inhabit more disaster-prone areas (20). Low SES individuals are also at elevated risk for postdisaster problems (67), possibly due to difficulties in rebuilding their lives, such as resecuring housing, food, finances, and receiving loans. Being a member of a minority group is also associated with poor disaster outcomes (65), probably mostly via lower SES and the challenges related to it (21,93).

Family-Related Factors

Parents' Reactions

The presence of adults caring for a child during and after a major stressor is considered the most important and consistent protective factor (86,89) and the way these adults function can mediate the connection between the disaster and the degree of response to it (34). Indeed, the reaction of parents, especially the mother, to a disaster is generally correlated with the severity of the child's responses, especially among young children (68,94). Researchers found that the reaction of preschool children to the missile attacks during the Gulf War was highly correlated with the reaction of their mothers (10,31,59). This was true for 3 to 4 year olds, but not for 5 year olds, probably owing to the older children's increasing autonomy and the control of psychological buffering systems for development (89). Five years after the war, poor psychological functioning among mothers was associated with heightened symptoms in their children (95).

Parents' ability to contain the anxiety generated by extreme threats of disasters seems to be the most important factor influencing their children's responses (78,96). Parents are critical mediators of stress, mainly owing to their roles in social referencing (pooling information and processing of meaning), responding emotionally, and caring for the child (89).

Family System Role

The family is an important mediating factor, particularly in young children (10,31,97). Families with extreme levels of cohesion—boundaries that are either too loose or too rigid—may not provide the appropriate support or allow the child to withdraw at times in order to process traumatic experiences and reach a constructive resolution of concerns. Caring support, open communication patterns, and sensitivity to the child's needs enable parents and children to regulate dyadic processes and discuss disaster-related issues when necessary. Stressed parents may be preoccupied with their own suffering and may tend to overprotect the child, thus interfering with the healthy process of resolution (78,98,99). Lower parental support and parental overprotectiveness are both associated with child PTSD (100). Findings suggest that stressful experiences during disaster may affect not only the behavior of individuals and culture but also intergenerational transmission of trauma-related biologic vulnerabilities (101,102).

Societal and Cultural Factors

Friendships

Friendships are valuable sources of reciprocal affection and attachment, mutual assistance, emotional security and self-esteem, and nonfamilial contexts for intimacy, thereby contributing to the child's ability to cope with stress (103). Natural sources of friendships—the family, the neighborhood, and the school—may be shattered in times of disaster (21). Friendships may also include supportive relationships with teachers or other adults (38,74). Even the presence of one concerned and caring adult may do much to offset the impact of misfortune in the lives of children (90). And to the contrary, poor child–teacher relationships have been found to increase the risk for child psychopathology following disasters (104). In fact, social support constitutes one of the most important protective factors for children during disasters (105), especially perceived support (21).

Community

The impact of disasters on whole communities and the need to focus on their functioning as a unit in order to improve the well-being of their members are matters of growing concern worldwide (20,21,105). Disasters change the layers of support in the community. Individuals tend to rely more on existing elements despite outside assistance, people perish or move away, and those who stay suffer themselves and thus are less available to support others (21). Communities mobilize at times of disaster by relying on their inner strength and external backup support.

Culture

Cultures define the terms under which symptoms are expressed and set the parameters for expression of personal distress. Some cultures encourage children to express their feelings of distress, while others do not. For example, in some cultures adults may admonish children who were victims of disaster to be prim and proper or to refrain from crying (58,106). Thus, cultural background, with its strengths and its weaknesses, needs to be taken into account by clinicians when planning treatment interventions. In addition, culture also mediates ideology and identity. As the purveyor of the meaning ascribed to disastrous events and consequences, culture regulates the individual's capacity to maintain an active and resilient stance. Yet a traumatically grieving culture may succumb to expressions of mourning and aggression, and when faced with further threats could fuel a cycle of violence. Child soldiers in Africa (107) and adolescents living with ongoing terrorism, war, and intractable political conflict (108,109) are examples of the establishment of a cycle of violence.

Media

The media can play a vital role both during and after disasters, mediating the level of symptoms experienced subsequently (34). News coverage tends to include intensely graphic visual material (21). The extent to which the media can impact the degree of exposure naturally varies depending on media availability (20). In general, exposure through media can be extensive during and after such events (110) and is associated with greater psychopathology and distress, mostly PTSD (111–114). Younger children can be more affected by the media because they do not fully comprehend what they see, are more sensitive to parental reactions, and may not understand that they are watching the same event over and over (28). The general recommendation is to closely monitor children's exposure to the media, especially that of young and sensitive children (20).

CHILD ASSESSMENT UNDER DISASTER CONDITIONS

Children at risk of psychopathology after exposure to disaster should be identified and treated as early as possible. Efforts must also be directed toward reactivating society's childcare systems via existing childcare workers. In a natural setting, assessment (i.e., screening) may be integrated into normal institutional activity (see the section on The School Setting below). Moreover, pediatricians and primary care physicians, who are usually not trained in trauma assessment and care, should be educated and integrated in the process, because on many occasions survivors turn to them first for assessment and treatment (34). For example, through a relatively brief training intervention following 9/11, physicians educated about mental health issues and screening tools were able to assimilate such practices as part of their assessment and test for psychological problems. These physicians subsequently referred fewer patients to mental health professionals (115).

The preferred clinical screening tools are those that directly assess the child rather than relying on external reporters. Such tools should also be simple and quick to administer, accurate, replicable, sensitive, and specific (116,117). The criteria for identifying pathologic cases should be tempered by consideration of the psychological and economic costs of possible false positives and false negatives. The use of cutoff scores may facilitate the decision-making process, but can obscure minor but "real" differences between children with scores slightly above or slightly below threshold. Green (118) suggested that clinicians think in terms of degree of impairment in a given sample rather than in terms of case identification. Moreover, the assessment of a single domain rather than a complex of posttraumatic, dissociative, and grief symptoms may decrease the sensitivity of the battery (116). (For a review of screening tools to assess trauma and its effects, see (119–120).)

Assessment of risk factors deserves special attention. Information should be gathered concerning the child's past functioning (traumatic/stressful experiences such as divorce, hospitalization, birth of a sibling, mental and general health problems) as well as disaster-related events (personal injury, loss of loved ones, witnessing severely injured or dead people, separation from parents, experiencing hunger or lack of sleep). A risk index may prove a useful guide in identifying symptomatic children as well as those requiring special attention (35,64,77,93,121). During screening, mental health professionals should create trusting relationships with parents to enhance commitment and facilitate recovery (122).

CHILD MENTAL HEALTH INTERVENTION PRINCIPLES: THE SYSTEMIC PERSPECTIVE

Mass disasters have an impact on children through the entire sociocultural milieu (20,58,70). To manage this complex challenge, interventions must be formulated from an integrative perspective, focusing on maximizing well-being, self-efficacy and return to normalcy, and minimizing stress and disorganization. Such interventions must help victims find meaning and instill a sense of control without interrupting individuals' and communities' natural processes of resilience (21).

In their approach to public mental health, Pynoos et al. (17) emphasized the need to resolve institutional conflicts over authority and resource allocation, to address teachers' own disaster experiences, and to properly select and train intervention teams to work with severely traumatized victims. Population screening is useful to pinpoint areas that require specific resources and government support.

The effect of mass disasters is extremely devastating because of the concomitant loss of sociocultural regulators, leading to the destruction of basic schemes, values, roles, and structures (family and individual), and leaving the community vulnerable to pain, grief, trauma, and anger. Working in such a milieu, professionals may find themselves embroiled in confusion and red tape from the various social/government systems (medicine, education, welfare, nongovernment organizations [NGOs]) and the intervention teams trying to help. Therefore, a systemic perspective is needed to clarify the picture and to help psychiatrists (a) formulate the newly established needs of child-oriented institutions, (b) transfer knowledge and empower professionals in related fields to resume their role, (c) define their own role and carry out specific interventions, and (d) be familiar with the system within which they operate.

Mental health interventions for children and families exposed to mass disaster should follow the five AREST principles. Specific implementation of these principles will differ according to the particular characteristics of each country (19):

Anticipate: Interventions should provide an integrated vision, foresee different scenarios, and include contingency plans. Professionals and paraprofessionals must be trained, human and economic resources appropriately allocated, and treatment protocols created and exercised. For example, although 95% of 2,137 schools sampled in the United States have emergency evacuation protocols, 30% of them have not practiced them even once (123). Efficient local, national, and international networks need to be developed, including collaboration among agencies (education, police, health), clear command and control chains and communication channels, and the establishment of sponsorship and legitimacy (124).

Redifferentiate: Child psychiatrists should identify the extent of social loss in terms of institutional and role dysfunction. They must plan the process of context-related redevelopment of professional roles within and between systems (health, welfare, education) with the help of multidisciplinary teams. Particular attention should be addressed to reconstituting the roles of parents and teachers.

Empower: Child psychiatrists need to debrief (if necessary), educate, and empower social agents (e.g., teachers) who are in direct contact with children to serve as mental health mediators. They must help these agents restore and adapt their original roles, and delegate some therapeutic responsibilities to them, supplying them with professional vision and positive expectations.

Supervise and Assess: Psychiatrists should define boundaries, provide knowledge, expertise and support to therapeutic agents, assess program development, and identify needs by feedback mechanisms. As leaders, mental health professionals need to encourage creative initiatives among team members and provide them with individualized consideration.

Treat and Follow-up: Treatment focuses on the rehabilitation of individuals and families. Delayed responses should also be considered.

At times of disaster, the priority is basic survival. Safety, shelter, and food, the most immediate and conspicuous needs, are usually within the domain of professional relief teams. Yet team members may themselves suffer from role-related problems because of the disaster-induced collapse of their familiar sociocultural matrix. Therefore, mental health professionals in positions of authority must respond to these needs, both within their own team and in the teams in which they act as mediators (e.g., teachers, school counselors). They must make team members feel cared for and help them develop a sense of belonging and purpose (125).

The ongoing operation of mental health interventions after disasters requires the constant commitment of professionals, leaders, and local agencies. By endorsing a systemic perspective, mental health professionals may overcome repeated adversities and challenges, inadequate professional training, limited resources, and organizational conflicts that tend to characterize the process.

Because parents and teachers tend to underestimate the extent of children's suffering (39), and given that disaster survivors are also often reluctant to seek professional help (126), systematic *outreach* efforts should be made to screen victims at risk. Optimally, this screening should take place 1 to 3 months after the disaster (127). Thereafter, clinical triage protocols can be utilized to match risk groups with intervention programs (15,72,127).

The first step in implementing such programs is to train members of the affected community. The local staff may need constant support and supervision. Such a process may help reduce the ambivalent resistance of traumatized survivors to what might be perceived as a foreign "intrusion" that threatens the "trauma membrane" protecting them from an overload of psychic tension (15,127).

INTERVENTION MODELS

Several issues need to be considered when implementing psychological interventions (20): timing (utilizing a sound, evidenced-based intervention at the wrong time could prove ineffective and harmful); whether the intervention is too intrusive; the empirical support regarding the intervention's effectiveness (20,21); the potential tampering with natural resilience processes (poor implementation of interventions might hinder resilient individuals' ability to recover naturally); and cultural congruence.

Treatments for children in the aftermath of disaster should protect and rehabilitate the secure base of attachment and meaningful relationships, support normalization, and train first responders, including parents and teachers, on relevant developmental issues (68,93). Child intervention programs should aim to restore damaged communal institutions and norms as well as communal functioning (to reclaim communal roles: parent, teacher, worker, leader). In circumscribed mass disasters, effective programs may take 12 to 18 months.

Preparedness Interventions

Disaster preparedness interventions such as training first responders, assigning responsibilities to organizations and improving their communication are of great value (68,88). A plan should be instituted for reuniting families and for maintaining the functionality of all systems, with emphasis on keeping normal routines intact (19,20). Perry and Lindell (128) recommended that preparedness programs be based on accurate knowledge of the threat and of probable responses, encourage appropriate action by emergency personnel, emphasize response flexibility, address inter-organizational coordination, and practice drills.

Appropriate preparedness of a city/country can significantly reduce the consequences of a disaster. For example, the Urban Resilience Program (URP) was implemented in 18 Israeli cities. The URP is based upon special interest in child social services to engage leaders, institutions, and communities to motivate the entire community. The model also recognizes the value of identifying opportunities emerging from communities' failure to meet basic human service needs. As such, the URP focuses on recreating social capital by reconfiguring the relevant human services, so they are accessible and able to provide further training to help the individual, the community, and the system cope with the event. The URP is based on four interrelated resilience components: health and mental health, information, population, and education.

1. Health and mental health resilience are addressed by bestowing the responsibility for these domains under unified and well-controlled municipal coordination. Each city establishes a health headquarters to coordinate emergency medical operations and to integrate community and public health institutions, general and mental health hospitals, as well as private health and mental health agents.
2. Information resilience refers to citizens' urgent need for timely and reliable information that can reduce uncertainty, encourage preparedness, and increase coping among children, parents, families, and communities.
3. The population resilience component is directed at the urban municipality and its emergency preparedness systems, the city's institutional infrastructure, the local authority's psychosocial intervention system for emergencies, and the municipality's communities and inhabitants. The program offers leadership, training protocols, organizational guidelines, emergency simulations, and disaster drills for all urban dimensions, with specific attention to the needs of children and parents.
4. Education resilience is increased by developing teams to handle emergencies and implement preventive programs with children and parents in various educational child programs, from early infancy to adolescence, in collaboration with municipal and emergency bodies. Additionally, the program trains school psychologists as experts in trauma-related interventions and establishes a municipal educational headquarters to integrate between educational programs and security issues.

This model allows the development of a child-oriented URP that integrates all relevant child disaster services under a single command center. Data gathered over the course of 3 years show that the program has indeed increased cities' preparedness on all four components, as evidenced by enquiries conducted with department managers emphasizing actual execution of the program (129–131).

Indeed, the data show positive outcomes of preparedness interventions on risk reduction and resilience enhancement indicators (132). For example, children undergoing such programs frequently exhibit more preparedness knowledge (e.g., what to do in case of an earthquake), more discussions about hazards with others, and more preparedness activities.

Research on preparedness interventions points to four theory-driven ingredients that should be targeted (132): (1) help children increase their knowledge about disaster risk reduction (DRR); (2) encourage them to interact with others regarding their learning; (3) promote experiential activities aimed at DRR; and (4) provide DRR on more than one occasion.

Promoting these interventions at schools with an emphasis on school-wide and local emergency management agency support and providing teachers proper training can improve the chances for implementation (132).

Immediate Interventions—the Event through the First Few Weeks

According to contemporary reviews, interventions implemented immediately after disasters (i.e., 0 to 3 months) should be handled with care, because intervening at this stage could be ineffective and also damaging (20,21). However, as Wang et al. (44) concluded in reviewing 85 studies regarding psychopathology among child disaster survivors, intervening at the early stages of disaster is vital since childhood pathology could have deleterious consequences later in life.

During the acute stage of disasters, the role of the mental health professional needs to be modified because of the limited number of professionals and the masses of individuals requiring help. Large populations need to be screened to identify children at risk. Other important tasks include initiating telephone crisis hotlines, supplying psychological first aid (PFA) for children and families in evacuation centers and hospitals, consulting authorities to assess immediate needs, and planning large-scale public health education programs. At this stage, professionals become aware of the need to acquire new disaster-related skills. Despite their experience with technically formulated protocol-based interventions, such professionals soon discover that mastering new therapeutic techniques and implementing them under disaster conditions require thorough training and ongoing supervision. Such skills can and preferably should be secured before proceeding with the intervention program.

In the following section, we present a brief summary of immediate intervention models and studies conducted to test their effectiveness. Note that studying interventions delivered in the acute aftermath of disasters is immensely challenging due to factors such as the urgency and chaos of the postdisaster environment, ethical concerns regarding withholding treatment and funding issues (21,133,134).

Critical Incident Stress Debriefing

Critical incident stress debriefing (CISD), a common practice of choice, consists of a single session designed to relieve trauma-related distress by providing people the chance to express thoughts and feelings, understand and conceptualize stress responses as normative under the circumstances, and learn about frequent trauma and disaster reactions in supportive settings. Despite the popularity of CISD, however, most studies have found it to be ineffective at best, if not harmful (20,21,134). Following the 2004 tsunami, the World Health Organization (135) recommended that it not be implemented.

Psychological First Aid

PFA is an evidence-informed program developed by disaster mental health experts. It is nonintrusive, applicable across many developmental levels, and culturally sensitive. PFA's focus is on promoting a sense of safety, connectedness, calming, self and community efficacy, and hope. It gives children the freedom to express feelings through storytelling and drawing and to identify areas of need. PFA is also helpful in identifying individuals who may require further assistance. While PFA appears to be a promising component in immediate postdisaster interventions, it still lacks sufficient controlled studies (21,134).

Psychoeducation

Psychoeducation is also recommended, yet also lacks evidence as to its effectiveness. Brochures and fact sheets provide information regarding children's coping in the aftermath of disasters, and children's worries, fears, and security concerns in attempts to normalize their responses. Psychoeducation materials correct misinformation about disaster response and encourage children to express feelings and thoughts, while at the same time motivates them to reassume routine living (21,134).

To summarize, despite the lack of robust evidence the consensus seems to support a general mixture of PFA and psychoeducation materials as a means of action in an effort to assist children at this stage of disaster.

Second and Third Stage Interventions: First Few Weeks through Several Years Postdisaster

Saltzman et al. (136) proposed a public health approach consisting of a screening process and three tiers of mental health school- and community-based interventions after war and terrorism: general and broad-scale psychoeducational activities; manualized trauma/grief focused group psychotherapy for students at risk (see following); and highly specialized traditional treatments in the community for severely distressed and high-risk students.

Few intervention programs have been found to be effective in improving the condition of children survivors of disaster. All, to some extent, entail components taken from CBT (137), the most widely supported approach in this context (133).

The School Setting

Following mass disasters, professionals may need to work within a group format because providing individual assistance is less effective and generally impossible. Since teachers have already established relations of trust with children and parents, and most are ready to be educated and play a therapeutic role, intact school environments are appropriate societal recovery centers for interventions (124,138,139).

Therefore, schools could be utilized as primary settings for intervention with large numbers of children. Schools are familiar, safe places for children and help destigmatize treatment by mental health professionals (34), providing children opportunities for peer support, constructive activities, leadership, self-efficacy, and relationships with competent adults (20). Getting back to normal routine, especially to school, is among the most protective factors against postdisaster pathology (20,68,140). Recommendations emphasize the need to restore the routine operations of schools, monitor the state of the children, supply consultation services to the entire school (including staff), train school faculty to answer children's needs, form support groups, and incorporate the disaster into the syllabus (140).

Teachers should allocate time to deal with traumatic experiences, model children's responses, reinforce emerging coping skills, provide factual information and dispel rumors, facilitate mutual support, identify suffering children, prepare the class for future experiences, and encourage students to become active contributors to their family, school, and community.

For a program to be effective, mental health professionals should ensure that the teachers (a) are not traumatized themselves; (b) are capable of mastering disaster-related educational techniques; and (c) have adapted their view of their role as teachers/educators in the new and harsh reality. To help regenerate the normal school setting after a disaster, the mental health professional needs to meet with teachers, help them process their own disaster experiences, and clearly describe the psychoeducational task at hand.

Based on these principles, Wolmer et al. (77) implemented a three-stage supervision program for the principal and teachers at one school after the 1999 earthquake in Turkey. First, a group session was conducted to normalize responses and enable expression of trauma-related affects (anger, guilt, helplessness, hopelessness). Then, an experiential activity was introduced to help teachers redefine their role *vis-a-vis* the students as educators and leaders. The authors stressed that in times of disaster, teachers were expected to maintain and enhance their role by providing individualized attention, transmitting values, and conveying positive expectations. As part of this role, they were taught to implement a disaster-related classroom activation program (see below). Finally, an ongoing supervision process was begun, led by local professionals, wherein teachers were not only educated but also provided support for each other (141).

Schools can provide excellent settings for preparedness interventions. Wolmer et al. (129) implemented such a program in Israel prior to rocket attacks during Operation Cast Lead. The study included 1,488 students from 12 schools, with half undergoing a 14-session teacher-led intervention 3 months prior to the attacks. Data gathered 3 months after the attacks showed that children in the nonintervention group exhibited more extreme symptoms and 50% more cases of PTSD compared to the study group.

School-based interventions include small-group programs and class activation programs.

Targeted *small-group programs* within the school setting may benefit high-risk children or children who are more agitated and need closer attention than can be provided in the classroom (138,142). Smith et al. (143) formulated a three-session program to teach recovery techniques to small groups of children affected by disaster. The techniques used include psychoeducation, imagery and cognitive techniques, and exposure practice. Each session is dedicated to one domain of the posttraumatic syndrome: intrusion, avoidance, and arousal. The professional may also offer a fourth session for bereaved children and a session with parents, to provide them with information and suggest ways for them to help their children.

Class activation programs may vary in focus, scope, and depth, but all are intended to minimize stigma, encourage normalcy, and reinforce the expectation that the children will soon resume their roles as students (5,124,138). Nevertheless, because teachers themselves may be struggling with severe PTS and personal losses, they may feel unable to help their students. Some may try to avoid dealing with reminders of the event by stressing that children have no need to talk about their traumatic experiences (17).

The teacher-led class activation described in Wolmer et al. (77) began with an initial meeting with the parents to provide information about the program and the children's expected reactions to the disaster and to engage them in the process. The subsequent eight 2-hour meetings of the whole class focused on various aspects of the recovery process (e.g., establishing a safe place, learning about the earthquake, loss and death, dealing with anger, planning the future). The program combined psychoeducational modules, cognitive–behavioral techniques, play activities, and ongoing documentation in personal diaries. The program yielded immediate reductions in PTS and dissociation symptoms. In addition, a 3-year controlled follow-up study showed that children who had participated in the intervention adapted better than nonparticipants in terms of academic, social, and behavioral functioning (144).

CLINICAL INTERVENTIONS

Individual Interventions

Although group interventions are efficient and cost effective, they may not be sufficient for those children who are most affected. Controlled and uncontrolled studies have confirmed the effectiveness of brief cognitive–behavioral treatment in traumatized children (133,145). Other modes have been employed, such as play therapy and psychodynamic psychotherapy, as well as trauma-focused CBT (146). Recently prolonged exposure therapy, including psychoeducation about trauma, recounting scenes from the traumatic events, and in vivo exposures to associated feared stimuli and triggers, has been adapted to toddlers and their parents (147). Particular attention should be directed to prior and current comorbid pathology, as well as to a thorough differential diagnosis (e.g., mania, ADHD).

Another approach is eye movement desensitization and reprocessing (EMDR) (148), devised to process distressing memories by having the child focus simultaneously on the disturbing memory and on a therapist-directed attention stimulus. Although studies on EMDR are scarce and additional research is needed to determine its effectiveness in treating disaster survivors, some evidence exists to support its implementation (149). Another mode of individual intervention involves exposure techniques, often incorporated with relaxation and breathing techniques. In vivo exposure highlights encountering feared stimuli associated with the event, while in vitro exposure highlights mastering traumatic memories (133). Research examining these techniques has yielded data in support of them (e.g., influencing test anxiety and academic performance (150)), yet more study is needed to further validate their efficacy.

Goenjian et al. (141) implemented a brief treatment program combining classroom group psychotherapy and individual sessions that focused on trauma and grief. The sessions, led by therapists, allowed for open discussion of traumatic experiences and associated feelings, assisted the children in solving intra- and interpersonal problems, and offered effective cognitive–behavioral techniques to manage thought distortions, disturbing images, and stress-related sensations. Five years after the event, the PTS of treated adolescents had decreased more significantly that those of untreated adolescents (5).

Group Interventions

Parent–Child Groups

Families have the potential either to protect children and mitigate their postdisaster suffering or to jeopardize how they adjust to and process the event. After disasters, children and parents tend not to discuss their distress, probably to avoid upsetting each other further (7). Yet studies show a significant association between the symptomatic response of children and their parents (particularly their mothers) (10,31,94), which may in turn have a traumatic impact on the parent–child dyad (59).

Based on previous successful application of parent–child group psychotherapy in treating child anxiety disorders (151), and as a second stage of class activation, Laor et al. (106) formulated an eight-session protocol for mothers and children with chronic PTSD. The group addressed dynamic, cognitive, and behavioral aspects of the disaster syndrome, and offered techniques to manage anxiety, relieve, control and transform distressing affects, correct thought distortions, and plan for the future. Special attention was paid to identifying and correcting maladaptive family dynamics and helping mothers and children recover their attachment and roles. Preliminary clinical and empirical results showed significant symptomatic alleviation as well as a dramatic improvement in familial communication and mutual support.

Mothers' Groups

Group interventions with mothers facilitate indirect focusing on preschool children, a population that may not be reached in formal settings, yet can display maladaptive behavioral reactions. Providing structured therapeutic interventions, psychoeducation, and practical suggestions for the children as well as strengthening participants' confidence in their maternal role are important objectives for such groups (152).

POST-DISASTER COMMUNITY-BASED INTERVENTIONS

Disasters affect entire communities, threatening social structures and functions. To be effective, interventions require collaborative efforts among NGOs and formal and informal agencies. Developing a local leadership of committed individuals and empowering these leaders to actively meet the short- and long-term needs of the community provide a valuable source of support (153). If interventions are intended to rebuild and enhance collective resilience, specific efforts need to be made for communities to develop financial resources, minimize resource disparity, and pay special attention to socially vulnerable sectors. Moreover, the local population, including children (140), should be integrated in the planning and execution of such interventions, and connections between different organizations need to be formed. Furthermore, natural social support needs to be enhanced, decision-making and problem-solving abilities need to be developed, and reliable sources of information need to be maintained.

Child psychiatry relief programs need to respond to disasters on three levels: (a) *The family.* Families may suffer from injury, loss, or death of loved ones; relocation and unemployment; loss of boundaries, routine, and values; and loss of esteem and hope. (b) *The neighborhood.* Neighborhoods are subject to physical and economic destruction, loss of routines, boundaries and safety, disintegration of informal networks, and restriction of leisure time activities. (c) *The community.* Communities suffer from a lack of proper leadership and resources, frozen initiatives, dependence on external resources, destruction of social and cultural institutions (schools, community centers, religious centers) and, as a result, a foreshortened sense of a communal future.

Through auxiliary social functions and structures introduced from the outside, as well as through professional clinical and social teams, temporary communities of displaced population can be helped to gradually develop coping and functioning mechanisms. The goal of community-based intervention is to transform evacuated fragments of families and singletons into self-governing communities made up of autonomous individuals and families (16). Since children cannot be fully rehabilitated until their parents resume working and regain income, professionals may also help facilitate the creation of new job resources in the community.

Using the intervention principles described above, child mental health professionals together with child community workers and local leadership can help set up community center programs for young mothers, children, and adolescents. Programs for empowerment and enhancing resilience may include the arts, sports, gardening and decorating, continuing education, job clubs, and volunteer recruitment and training in different areas (154). By *empowerment,* we mean a process of involvement through which individuals and communities supplant their helpless stance by recovering their dignity and self-esteem, enhancing their critical self-awareness, gaining control over resources and objectives, and regaining a sense of personal and collective responsibility and self-efficacy (152,153). Individuals are able to identify specific needs and discover hidden leadership qualities, while communities gain a greater sense of interdependence, cohesion, and cooperation. Professionals may take part in modifying the school curricula to address group mourning and resilience, collective memorials, as well as celebrations of rebirth. The juxtaposition of commemoration and rebirth ceremonies helps individuals gain new meaning in life in the face of profound mourning and leads to integration on both the personal and the communal levels, thus offering children an uninterrupted supportive matrix.

PHARMACOLOGIC INTERVENTIONS

Psychotherapy is widely considered the first-choice treatment for posttraumatic states (155). However, some pharmacologic interventions do exist, though they lack empirical support (137). Nonetheless, reduction of even one disabling symptom (insomnia, hyperarousal) may have a positive ripple effect on a child's functioning (156).

Even in the early stages of intervention, medications can be administered to children with a history of psychopathology; to individuals who do not respond to short-term specific interventions; and to members of families at risk that are overwhelmed by acute symptoms. Medications can be directed at specific symptoms, such as intrusion, hyperarousal and impulsivity (e.g., clonidine), anxiety (SSRIs, benzodiazepines), depression (SSRIs), psychotic symptoms, or severe aggression (antipsychotics) (155).

In a comprehensive review, Donnelly (156) proposed that broad-spectrum agents such as SSRIs are a good first choice because they are effective in treating the core symptoms of PTSD and comorbid symptoms (depression, anxiety). Furthermore, the antiadrenergic agents prazosin and clonidine, the mood stabilizer carbamazepine, and possibly the second-generation antipsychotics risperidone and quetiapine can be helpful, though further investigation is necessary (157,158).

DISASTER RESEARCH

While disaster research is of utmost importance, it is extremely hard to carry out. Most disasters occur unexpectedly, and even those that are predictable have such an overwhelming impact that they exhaust all professional and economic resources. Furthermore, even when professional curiosity is maintained, assessment measures are enlisted, and questions are defined, implementation of such research is met by resistance on the part of both victims and clinicians. Research under such conditions tends to be perceived as hostile, foreign, exploitative, and abusive, and intended to satisfy an alien agenda that is irrelevant to the priorities of disaster relief. These claims have a kernel of truth: The hands that pass out the questionnaires could have been offering bread instead.

Other challenges have contributed to the scarcity of high-value disaster research (20,21,68,133). Apart from the aforementioned issues, disasters cause major devastation and conditions could be dangerous and chaotic, with no research infrastructure. Most disaster research lacks predisaster data. Additionally, it is not easy for researchers to receive funding for such projects, for most funds are logically directed to basic needs such as housing, food, and the like. Moreover, researchers do not always have culturally suitable tools, or are unable to secure good comparison groups (whether due to ethical or pragmatic concerns). In addition, follow-up data are extremely hard to gather and most studies fail to identify the active components of seemingly effective programs.

Research initiatives should be integrated within the systemic intervention program and should rely on direct assessment of the affected population at every stage. In this way, real risks and needs can serve as a basis for rational planning as well as for improvement of existing programs. Professionals are responsible for educating community leaders to take practical advantage of assessment data.

The scene of a disaster as a large-scale natural experiment offers access to communities that constitute different types of research groups and controls. Furthermore, each community may include a large number of entire families whose members were simultaneously exposed and affected in different manners (direct/indirect) and degrees, and for different lengths of time, as well as individuals suffering from losses of varying severity. An important issue in studies of children is the phenomenology and biologic susceptibility to the disaster syndrome, that is, the interplay of traumatic grief, PTS, and dissociation with psychoneuroendocrinologic and psychophysiologic parameters. This particular setting provides a unique opportunity for genetic studies. Special attention also ought to be directed at partial and delayed-onset types of disorder, as well as concurrent psychiatric and medical morbidity.

Another area of interest is the control study and the comparative effectiveness of various interventions, as well as assessment of parameters of community resilience and vulnerability, the long-term sequelae of disaster in terms of the developmental psychopathology of high-risk populations, the transgenerational transmission of trauma and grief, and the development of sociopolitical attitudes. Nevertheless, the search for answers to these questions cannot violate the privacy of the children being studied, and clinicians must be careful to comply with accepted ethical guidelines. Institutional review boards can facilitate the process by offering a fast track for disaster-related research proposals.

CONCLUSIONS

Disasters destroy the space within which children and families thrive, thereby disrupting normal development. The overwhelming nature of such events, combined with the massive extent of the resulting loss, gives rise to a complex clinical and social picture that may be termed the disaster syndrome. Children, families, neighborhoods, and whole communities are affected. Immediate damages can only be partially remedied, and therefore the physical, psychological, and social effects are long lasting.

For effective intervention, child mental health professionals should adopt a comprehensive systemic, social, and mental health perspective in order to develop the appropriate program, team up with the proper authorities, proactively assess needs, and implement intervention based on real-time integrated information systems. The best results can be achieved when communities are prepared. Some interventions are clinical and specific. They may be mediated by educated professionals who work with children in schools and community centers. Other interventions are systemic.

The systemic concepts and principles presented in this chapter (159,160) are reflected in the congressional report investigating the preparation for and response to Hurricane Katrina (161). As the report demonstrates, even when enormous resources are allocated, if authorities do not adhere to theoretical, organizational, and implementation principles of disaster management, disasters exact colossal consequences.

No single community can cope on its own, for adequate coping requires advanced networking on the local, national, and international levels (162). Resilience built on these levels of organization constitute the social capital available to individuals and communities to withstand and recover from disaster (163). Thus, the challenge posed by disasters can be met by our vision of the siblinghood of humanity. A global community committed to children must respond to the challenge.

References

1. Ursano RJ, Fullerton CS, McCaughey BG: Trauma and disaster. In: Ursano RJ, McCaughey BG, Fullerton CS (eds): *Individual and Community Responses to Trauma and Disaster: The Structure of Human Chaos.* Cambridge, Cambridge University Press, 3–27, 1994.
2. Integrated Regional Information Networks: Disaster reduction and the human cost of disaster [Internet]. [Place unknown] 2005 Jun 1 [cited 2016 Jan 24]. Available: http://www.irinnews.org/webspecials/DR.
3. International Federation of Red Cross and Red Crescent Societies: World disasters report-2010 [Internet]. [Place unknown] c2010 [cited Jan 2 2016]. Available: http://www.ifrc.org.
4. Garmezy N, Rutter M: Acute reactions to stress. In: Rutter M, Hersov L (eds): *Child and Adolescent Psychiatry: Modern Approaches.* 2nd ed. Oxford, Blackwell, 152–176, 1985.
5. Goenjian AK, Walling D, Steinberg AM, Karayan I, Najarian LM, Pynoos R: A prospective study of posttraumatic stress and depressive reactions among treated and untreated adolescents 5 years after a catastrophic disaster. *Am J Psychiatry* 162:2302–2308, 2005.
6. Pfefferbaum B: Posttraumatic stress disorder in children: a review of the past 10 years. *J Am Acad Child Adolesc Psychiatry* 36:1503–1511, 1997.
7. Udwin O: Annotation: children's reactions to traumatic events. *J Child Psychol Psychiatry* 34:115–127, 1993.
8. Vogel JM, Vernberg EM: Children's psychological responses to disasters. *J Clin Child Psychol* 22:464–484, 1993.
9. Yule W, Perrin S, Smith P: Post-traumatic stress reactions in children and adolescents. In: Yule W (ed): *Post-traumatic Stress Disorders: Concepts and Therapy.* Chichester, John Wiley & Sons, 25–50, 1999.
10. Laor N, Wolmer L, Mayes LC, Gershon A, Weizman R, Cohen DJ: Israeli preschoolers under Scuds: a thirty-month follow-up. *J Am Acad Child Adolesc Psychiatry* 36:349–356, 1997.
11. Eisen ML, Goodman GS: Trauma, memory, and suggestibility in children. *Dev Psychopathol* 10:717–738, 1998.
12. Terr LC: Childhood traumas: an outline and overview. *Am J Psychiatry* 148:10–20, 1991.
13. Laor N, Wolmer L: Trauma and emergency in child psychiatry: clinical theory and innovative, multidisciplinary and multi-modal interventions. Presented at the 11th International Congress of the European Society for Child and Adolescent Psychiatry, Hamburg, 1999.
14. López-Ibor JJ: What is a disaster? In: López-Ibor JJ, Christodoulou G, Maj M, et al. (eds): *Disasters and Mental Health.* Chichester, John Wiley & Sons, 1–11, 2005.
15. Austin LS, Godleski LS: Therapeutic approaches for survivors of disaster. *Psychiatr Clin North Am* 22:897–910, 1999.
16. Laor N: The role of mental health professionals after mass disasters. *Presented at the Congress on the Promised Childhood,* Tel Aviv, 2001.
17. Pynoos RS, Goenjian AK, Steinberg AM: A public mental health approach to the postdisaster treatment of children and adolescents. *Child Adol Psychiat Clin North Am* 7:195–210, 1998.
18. Raphael B: *When Disaster Strikes: How Individuals and Communities Cope with Catastrophe.* New York, Basic Books, 1986.
19. Laor N, Wiener Z, Spirman S, et al.: Community mental health procedures for emergencies and mass disasters: the Tel-Aviv model. In: Danieli Y, Brom D, Sills J (eds): *The Trauma of Terrorism: Sharing Knowledge and Shared Care, An International Handbook.* New York, Hawarth Press, 681–684, 2004.
20. Masten AS, Narayan AJ: Child development in the context of disaster, war, and terrorism: pathways of risk and resilience. *Ann Rev Psychol* 63:227–257, 2012.
21. Bonanno GA, Brewin CR, Kaniasty K, La Greca AM: Weighing the costs of disaster: consequences, risks, and resilience in individuals, families, and communities. *Psychol Sci Public Interest* 11(1):1–49, 2010.
22. Danieli Y (ed): *International Handbook of Multigenerational Legacies of Trauma.* New York, Plenum Press, 1998.
23. Laor N: Saving the holocaust witness. In: Ariel Y, Biderman S, Rotem O (eds): *Relativism and Beyond.* Leiden, Brill, 265–298, 1998.
24. Solomon Z: *Coping with War-Induced Stress: The Gulf War and the Israeli Response.* New York, Plenum Press, 1995.
25. Laor N: The protective matrix as risk-modifying function of traumatic effects in preschool children: a development perspective. *Presented at the 6th International Psychoanalytic Association Conference on Psychoanalytic Research,* London, 1996.
26. Krystal H: *Massive Psychic Trauma.* New York, International University Press, 1968.
27. Valent P: Disaster syndrome. In: Fink G (ed): *Encyclopedia of Stress,* Vol. 1. San Diego, CA, Academic Press, 706–709, 2000.
28. Franks BA: Moving targets: a developmental framework for understanding children's changes following disasters. *J Appl Dev Psychol* 32(2):58–69, 2011.
29. Pynoos RS, Steinberg AM, Wraith R: A developmental model of childhood traumatic stress. In: Cicchetti D, Cohen DJ (eds): *Developmental Psychopathology. Risk, Disorder, and Adaptation,* Vol. 2. New York, John Wiley & Sons, Inc, 72–95, 1995.
30. Bingham RD, Harmon RJ: Traumatic stress in infancy and early childhood: expression of distress and developmental issues. In: Pfeffer C (ed): *Severe Stress and Mental Disturbance in Children.* Washington, DC: American Psychiatric Association Press, 499–532, 1996.
31. Laor N, Wolmer L, Mayes LC, et al.: Israeli preschoolers under Scud missile attacks: a developmental perspective on risk-modifying factors. *Arch Gen Psychiatry* 53:416–423, 1996.
32. Sullivan MA, Saylor CF, Foster KY: Post-hurricane adjustment of preschoolers and their families. *Adv Behav Res Ther* 13:163–171, 1991.
33. Boer F, Smit C, Morren M, Roorda J, Yzermans J: Impact of a technological disaster on young children: a five-year postdisaster multi-informant study. *J Trauma Stress* 22(6):516–524, 2009.
34. Gurwitch RH, Kees M, Becker SM, Schreiber M, Pfefferbaum B, Diamond D: When disaster strikes: responding to the needs of children. *Prehosp Disaster Med* 19(01):21–28, 2004.
35. Wolmer L, Hamiel D, Versano-Eisman T, Slone M, Margalit N, Laor N: Preschool Israeli children exposed to rocket attacks: assessment, risk, and resilience. *J Trauma Stress* 28(5):441–447, 2015.
36. Scheeringa MS, Myers L, Putnam FW, Zeanah CH: Maternal factors as moderators or mediators of PTSD symptoms in very young children: a two-year prospective study. *J Fam Violence* 5:633–642, 2015.
37. Goenjian A, Stillwell BM, Steinberg AM, et al.: Moral development and psychopathological interference in conscience functioning among adolescents after trauma. *J Am Acad Child Adolesc Psychiatry* 38:376–384, 1999.
38. Vernberg EM, Silverman WK, La Greca AM, Prinstein MJ: Prediction of posttraumatic stress symptoms in children after Hurricane Andrew. *J Abnorm Psychol* 195:237–248, 1996.
39. Yule W, Williams RM: Post-traumatic stress reactions in children. *J Trauma Stress* 3:279–295, 1990.
40. Charuvastra A, Goldfarb E, Petkova E, Cloitre M: Implementation of a screen and treat program for child posttraumatic stress disorder in a school setting after a school suicide. *J Trauma Stress* 23:500–503, 2010.
41. Green BL, Grace MC, Vary MG, Kramer TL, Gleser GC, Leonard AC: Children of disaster in the second decade: a 17-year follow-up of Buffalo Creek survivors. *J Am Acad Child Adolesc Psychiatry* 33:71–79, 1994.
42. Sack WH, Him C, Dickason D: Twelve-year follow-up study of Khmer youths who suffered massive war trauma as children. *J Am Acad Child Adolesc Psychiatry* 38:1173–1179, 1999.
43. McDermott B, Cobham V, Berry H, Kim B: Correlates of persisting posttraumatic symptoms in children and adolescents 18 months after a cyclone disaster. *The Aust NZ J Psychiat* 48(1):80–86, 2014.
44. Wang C, Chan CL, Ho RT: Prevalence and trajectory of psychopathology among child and adolescent survivors of disasters: a systematic review of epidemiological studies across 1987–2011. *Soc Psych Psych Epid* 48(11):1697–1720, 2013.
45. Williams R: The psychosocial consequences for children of mass violence, terrorism and disasters. *Int Rev Psychiatr* 19(3):263–277, 2007.
46. Tedeschi RG, Calhoun LG: Posttraumatic growth: conceptual foundations and empirical evidence. *Psycholl Inq* 15(1):1–18, 2004.
47. Gordon R, Wraith R: Responses of children and adolescents to disaster. In: Wilson JP, Raphael B (eds): *International Handbook of Traumatic Stress Syndromes.* New York: Plenum Press, 561–575, 1993.

48. Lai BS, Auslander BA, Fitzpatrick SL, Podkowirow V: Disasters and depressive symptoms in children: a review. *Child Youth Care Forum* 43(4):489–504, 2014.
49. Anthony JL, Lonigan CJ, Hecht SA: Dimensionality of posttraumatic stress disorder symptoms in children exposed to disaster: results from confirmatory factor analyses. *J Abnorm Psychol* 108:326–336, 1999.
50. Terr LC: Chowchilla revisited: the effects of psychic trauma four years after a school-bus kidnapping. *Am J Psychiatry* 140:1543–1550, 1983.
51. Kar N: Psychological impact of disasters on children: review of assessment and intervention. *World J Pediatr* 5:5–11, 2009.
52. Scheeringa MS, Zeanah CH, Drell MJ, Larrieu JA: Two approaches to the diagnosis of posttraumatic stress disorder in infancy and early childhood. *J Am Acad Child Adolesc Psychiatry* 34:191–200, 1995.
53. Scheeringa MS, Zeanah CH, Myers L, Putnam FW: New findings on alternative criteria for PTSD in preschool children. *J Am Acad Child Adolesc Psychiatry* 42:561–570, 2003.
54. Asarnow J, Glynn S, Pynoos RS, et al.: When the earth stops shaking: earthquake sequelae among children diagnosed for pre-earthquake psychopathology. *J Am Acad Child Adolesc Psychiatry* 38:1016–1023, 1999.
55. La Greca AM: Posttraumatic stress disorder in children. In: Fink G (ed): *Encyclopedia of Stress*, Vol. 3. San Diego, CA: Academic Press, 181–186, 2000.
56. Juth V, Silver RC, Seyle DC, Widyatmoko CS, Tan ET: Post-disaster mental health among parent–child dyads after a major earthquake in Indonesia. *J Abnorm Child Psych* 43:1309–1318, 2015.
57. Weems CF, Scott BG, Taylor LK, Cannon MF, Romano DM, Perry AM: A theoretical model of continuity in anxiety and links to academic achievement in disaster-exposed school children. *Dev Psychopathol* 25:729–737, 2013.
58. Goenjian A: A mental health relief programme in Armenia after the 1988 earthquake: implementation and clinical observations. *Br J Psychiatry* 163:230–239, 1993.
59. Wolmer L, Laor N, Gershon A, Mayes LC, Cohen DJ: The mother-child facing trauma: a developmental outlook. *J Nerv Ment Dis* 188:409–415, 2000.
60. Pynoos RS, Nader K, Frederick C, Gonda L, Stuber M: Grief reactions in school age children following a sniper attack at school. *Isr J Psychiatry Relat Sci* 24:53–63, 1987.
61. Goenjian AK, Pynoos RS, Steinberg AM, et al.: Psychiatric comorbidity in children after the 1988 earthquake in Armenia. *J Am Acad Child Adolesc Psychiatry* 34:1174–1184, 1995.
62. Noaghiul S, Prigerson H: Grieving. In: Fink G (ed): *Encyclopedia of Stress*, Vol. 3. San Diego, CA, Academic Press, 289–296, 2000.
63. Dyregrov A, Dyregrov K: Complicated grief in children—the perspectives of experienced professionals. *OMEGA—J Death Dying* 67(3):291–303, 2013.
64. Laor N, Wolmer L, Kora M, Yucel D, Spirman S, Yazgan Y: Posttraumatic, dissociative and grief symptoms in Turkish children exposed to the 1999 earthquakes. *J Nerv Ment Dis* 190:824–832, 2002.
65. La Greca AM, Lai BS, Joormann J, Auslander BB, Short MA: Children's risk and resilience following a natural disaster: genetic vulnerability, posttraumatic stress, and depression. *J Affect Disorders* 151(3):860–867, 2013.
66. Putnam FW: Development of dissociative disorders. In: Cicchetti D, Cohen DJ (eds): *Developmental Psychopathology. Vol. 2: Risk, Disorder, and Adaptation.* New York, John Wiley & Sons, Inc., 581–608, 1995.
67. Dirkzwager AJ, Kerssens JJ, Yzermans CJ: Health problems in children and adolescents before and after a man-made disaster. *J Am Acad Child Adolesc Psychiatry* 45(1):94–103, 2006.
68. Masten AS, Osofsky JD: Disasters and their impact on child development: introduction to the special section. *Child Dev* 81(4):1029–1039, 2010.
69. Pynoos RS, Goenjian A, Tashjian M, et al.: Post-traumatic stress reactions in children after the 1988 Armenian earthquake. *Br J Psychiatry* 163:239–247, 1993.
70. Shaw JA, Applegate B, Tanner S, et al.: Psychological effects of Hurricane Andrew on an elementary school population. *J Am Acad Child Adolesc Psychiatry* 34:1185–1192, 1995.
71. Husain SA, Nair J, Holcomb W, Reid JC, Vargas V, Nair SS: Stress reactions of children and adolescents in war and siege conditions. *Am J Psychiatry* 155:1718–1719, 1998.
72. Pfefferbaum B, Nixon SJ, Tucker PM, et al.: Posttraumatic stress responses in bereaved children after the Oklahoma City bombing. *J Am Acad Child Adolesc Psychiatry* 38:1372–1379, 1999.
73. Green BL, Korol M, Grace MC, et al.: Children and disaster: age, gender, and parental effects on PTSD symptoms. *J Am Acad Child Adolesc Psychiatry* 30:945–951, 1991.
74. Udwin O, Boyle S, Yule W, Bolton D, O'Ryan D: Risk factors for long-term psychological effects of a disaster experienced in adolescence: predictors of posttraumatic stress disorder. *J Child Psychol Psychiatry* 41:969–979, 2000.
75. Lonigan CJ, Shannon MP, Taylor CM, Finch AJ Jr, Sallee FR: Children exposed to disaster: II. risk factors for the development of post-traumatic symptomatology. *J Am Acad Child Adolesc Psychiatry* 33:94–105, 1994.
76. Thabet AA, Vostanis P: Post-traumatic stress disorder in children of war. *J Child Psychol Psychiatry* 40:385–391, 1999.
77. Wolmer L, Laor N, Yazgan Y: School reactivation programs after disaster: could teachers serve as clinical mediators? *Child Adolesc Psychiatr Clin N Am* 12:363–381, 2003.
78. McFarlane AC: Posttraumatic phenomena in a longitudinal study of children following a natural disaster. *J Am Acad Child Adolesc Psychiatry* 26:764–769, 1987a.
79. Furr JM, Comer JS, Edmunds JM, Kendall PC: Disasters and youth: a meta-analytic examination of posttraumatic stress. *J Consult Clin Psychol* 78(6):765–780, 2010.
80. Garbarino J, Kostelny K: The effects of political violence on Palestinian children's behavior problems: a risk accumulation model. *Child Dev* 67:33–45, 1996.
81. Pfefferbaum B, Noffsinger MA, Wind LH, Allen JR: Children's coping in the context of disasters and terrorism. *J Loss Trauma* 19(1):78–97, 2014.
82. Gleser G, Green BL, Winget C: *Prolonged Psychosocial Effects of Disaster: A Study of Buffalo Creek.* New York, Academic Press, 1981.
83. Becker-Blease KA, Turner HA, Finkelhor D: Disasters, victimization, and children's mental health. *Child Dev* 81(4):1040–1052, 2010.
84. Shannon MP, Lonigan CJ, Finch AJ Jr, Taylor CM: Children exposed to disaster: I. Epidemiology of post-traumatic symptoms and symptom profiles. *J Am Acad Child Adolesc Psychiatry* 33:80–93, 1994.
85. Kimerling R, Mack KP, Alvarez J: Women and disasters. In: Neria Y, Galea S, Norris FH (eds): *Mental Health and Disasters.* New York, Cambridge University Press, 203–217, 2009.
86. Earls F, Smith E, Reich W, Jung KG: Investigating psychopathological consequences of a disaster in children: a pilot study incorporating a structured diagnostic interview. *J Am Acad Child Adolesc Psychiatry* 27:90–95, 1988.
87. Peek L, Stough LM: Children with disabilities in the context of disaster: a social vulnerability perspective. *Child Dev* 81(4):1260–1270, 2010.
88. Brown R: Building children and young people's resilience: lessons from psychology. *Int J Disaster Risk Reduc* 14:115–124, 2015.
89. Masten AS, Best KM, Garmezy N: Resilience and development: contributions from the study of children who overcome adversity. *Dev Psychopathol* 2:425–444, 1990.
90. Cohler BM, Stott FM, Musick JS: Adversity, vulnerability, and resilience: cultural and developmental perspectives. In: Cicchetti D, Cohen DJ (eds): *Developmental Psychopathology. Vol 2: Risk, Disorder, and Adaptation.* New York: John Wiley & Sons, 753–800, 1995.
91. Wolmer L, Laor N, Cicchetti DV: Validation of the Comprehensive Assessment of Defense Style (CADS): mothers' and children's responses to the stresses of missile attacks. *J Nerv Ment Dis* 2001;189:369–376.
92. Vigil JM, Geary DC, Granger DA, Flinn MV: Sex differences in salivary cortisol, alpha-amylase, and psychological functioning following hurricane Katrina. *Child Dev* 81(4):1228–1240, 2010.
93. Wolmer L, Hamiel D, Slone M, et al.: Post-traumatic reaction of Israeli Jewish and Arab children exposed to rocket attacks before and after teacher-delivered intervention. *Isr J Psychiatry Relat Sci* 50(2):165–173, 2013.
94. Winje D, Ulvik A: Long-term outcome of trauma in children: the psychological consequences of a bus accident. *J Child Psychol Psychiatry* 39:635–642, 1998.
95. Laor N, Wolmer L, Cohen DJ: Mothers' functioning and children's symptoms five years after a Scud missile attack. *Am J Psychiatry* 158: 1020–1026, 2001.
96. Bromet EJ, Goldgaber D, Carlson G, et al.: Children's well-being 11 years after the Chernobyl catastrophe. *Arch Gen Psychiatry* 57:563–571, 2000.
97. McFarlane AC: Family functioning and overprotection following a natural disaster: the longitudinal effects of posttraumatic morbidity. *Aust N Z J Psychiatry* 21:210–218, 1987b.
98. Feldman R, Vengrober A, Eidelman-Rothman M, Zagoory-Sharon O: Stress reactivity in war-exposed young children with and without maternal stress hormones, parenting, and child emotionality and regulation. *Dev Psychopathol* 25:943–955, 2013.
99. Nolte T, Guiney J, Fonagy P, Mayes LC, Luyten P: Interpersonal stress regulation and the development of anxiety disorders: an attachment-based developmental framework. *Front. Behav. Neurosci* 5:55, 2011.
100. Bokszczanin A: Parental support, family conflict, and overprotectiveness: predicting PTSD symptom levels of adolescents 28 months after a natural disaster. *Anxiety Stress Copin* 21(4):325–335, 2008.
101. Yehuda R, Daskalakis NP, Lehrner A, et al.: Influences of maternal and paternal PTSD on epigenetic regulation of the glucocorticoid receptor gene in Holocaust survivor offspring. *Am J Psychiatry* 171:872–880, 2014.
102. Dietz DM, Laplant Q, Watts EL, et al.: Paternal transmission of stress-induced pathologies. *Biol Psychiatry* 70:408–414, 2011.
103. Parker JG, Rubin KH, Price JM, et al.: Peer relationships, child development, and adjustment: a developmental psychopathology perspective. In: Cicchetti D, Cohen DJ (eds): *Developmental Psychopathology. Vol. 2: Risk, Disorder, and Adaptation.* New York: John Wiley & Sons, 96–161, 1995.
104. Felix ED, You S, Canino G: School and community influences on the long term postdisaster recovery of children and youth following hurricane Georges. *J Community Psychol* 41(8):1021–1038, 2013.
105. Norris FH, Stevens SP: Community resilience and the principles of mass trauma intervention. *Psychiatr* 70(4):320–328, 2007.

106. Laor N, Wolmer L, Sunar S, et al.: Mother–child short-term group psychotherapy for posttraumatic stress disorder. *Presented at the Congress on the Promised Childhood,* Tel Aviv, 2001.
107. Betancourt TS, Borisova II, Williams TP, et al.: Sierra Leone's former child soldiers: a follow-up study of psychosocial adjustment and community reintegration. *Child Dev* 81(4):1077–1095, 2010.
108. Laor N, Wolmer L, Cohen D: Attitudes toward Arabs of Israeli children exposed to missile attacks: the role of personality functions. *Israel J Psychiat* 41:23–32, 2004.
109. Laor N, Wolmer L, Alon M, Siev J, Samuel E, Toren P: Risk and protective factors mediating psychological symptoms and ideological commitment of adolescents facing continuous terrorism. *J Nerv Ment Dis* 194:279–286, 2006.
110. Comer JS, Kendall PC: Terrorism: the psychological impact on youth. *Clin Psychol Sci Pr* 14(3):179–212, 2007.
111. Ahern J, Galea S, Resnick H, Vlahov D: Television images and probable posttraumatic stress disorder after September 11: the role of background characteristics, event exposures, and perievent panic. *J Nerv Ment Dis* 192(3):217–226, 2004.
112. Bernstein KT, Ahern J, Tracy M, Boscarino JA, Vlahov D, Galea S: Television watching and the risk of incident probable posttraumatic stress disorder: a prospective evaluation. *J Nerv Ment Dis* 195(1):41–47, 2007.
113. Pfefferbaum B, Nixon SJ, Tivis RD, et al.: Television exposure in children after a terrorist incident. *Psychiatr* 64(3):202–211, 2001.
114. Pfefferbaum B, Seale TW, Brandt EN, Pfefferbaum RL, Doughty DE, Rainwater SM: Media exposure in children one hundred miles from a terrorist bombing. *Ann Clin Psychiatry* 15(1):1–8, 2003.
115. Adams RE, Laraque D, Chemtob C, Jensen P, Boscarino J: Does a one-day educational training session influence primary care pediatricians' mental health practice procedures in response to a community disaster? Results from the reaching children initiative (RCI). *Int J Emerg Ment Health* 15(1):3–14, 2013.
116. Cochrane A, Holland W: Validation of screening procedures. *Br Med J* 27:3–8, 1969.
117. Stallard P, Velleman R, Baldwin S: Psychological screening of children for post-traumatic stress disorder. *J Child Psychol Psychiatry* 40:1075–1082, 1999.
118. Green BL: Assessing levels of psychological impairment following disaster: consideration of actual and methodological dimensions. *J Nerv Ment Dis* 170:544–552, 1982.
119. Ohan JL, Myers K, Collet BR: Ten-year review of rating scales. IV: scales assessing trauma and its effects. *J Am Acad Child Adolesc Psychiatry* 41:1401–1422, 2002.
120. Strand VC, Sarmiento TL, Pasquale LE: Assessment and screening tools for trauma in children and adolescents. *Trauma Violence Abus* 6:55–78, 2005.
121. Wolmer L, Hamiel D, Barchas JD, Slone M, Laor N: Teacher-delivered resilience-focused intervention in schools with traumatized children following the second Lebanon war. *J Traum Stress* 24(3):309–316, 2011.
122. Poulsen KM, McDermott BM, Wallis J, Cobham VE: School-based psychological screening in the aftermath of a disaster: are parents satisfied and do their children access treatment? *J Trauma Stress* 28(1):69–72, 2015.
123. Graham J, Shirm S, Liggin R, Aitken ME, Dick R: Mass-casualty events at schools: a national preparedness survey. *Pediatrics* 117(1):e8–e15, 2006.
124. Vernberg EM, Vogel JM: Interventions with children after disasters. *J Clin Child Psychol* 22:485–498, 1993.
125. Bass BM, Avolio BJ: *Improving Organizational Effectiveness Through Transformational Leadership.* Thousand Oaks, CA, Sage Publications, 1994.
126. Schwarz ED, Kowalski JM: Malignant memories: reluctance to utilize mental health services after a disaster. *J Nerv Ment Dis* 180:767–772, 1992.
127. Lindy JD, Grace MC, Green BL: Survivors: outreach to a reluctant population. *Am J Orthopsychiatry* 51:468–478, 1981.
128. Perry RW, Lindell MK: Preparedness for emergency response: guidelines for the emergency planning process. *Disasters* 27(4):336–350, 2003.
129. Wolmer L, Hamiel D, Laor N: Preventing children's posttraumatic stress after disaster with teacher-based intervention: a controlled study. *J Am Acad Child Adolesc Psychiatry* 50(4):340–348, 2011.
130. Hamiel D, Wolmer L, Spirman S, Laor N: Comprehensive child-oriented preventive resilience program in Israel based on lessons learned from communities exposed to war, terrorism and disaster. *Child Youth Care For* 42(4):261–274, 2013.
131. Wolmer L, Gabay A, Spirman S, et al.: Urban disaster preparedness: Baseline assessment and outcomes following a one-year implementation. 2nd Israeli International Conference on Healthcare System Preparedness and Response to Emergencies and Disasters, Tel-Aviv, 15–19, 2012.
132. Ronan KR, Alisic E, Towers B, Johnson VA, Johnston DM: Disaster preparedness for children and families: a critical review. *Curr Psychiatry R* 17(7):1–9, 2015.
133. Pfefferbaum B, Newman E, Nelson SD: Mental health interventions for children exposed to disasters and terrorism. *J Child Adol Psychop* 24(1):24–31, 2014.
134. La Greca AM, Silverman WK: Treatment and prevention of posttraumatic stress reactions in children and adolescents exposed to disasters and terrorism: what is the evidence? *Child Development Perspectives* 3(1):4–10, 2009.
135. World Health Organization: Single session debriefing: not recommended [Internet]. [Place unknown] [cited Jan 2 2016]. Available: http://mhpss.net/?get=242/WHO-on-Debriefing3.pdf.
136. Saltzman WR, Layne CM, Sternberg AM, Arslanagic B, Pynoos RS: Developing a culturally and ecologically sound intervention program for youth exposed to war and terrorism. *Child Adolesc Psychiatr Clin N Am* 12:319–342, 2003.
137. Forman-Hoffman VL, Zolotor AJ, McKeeman JL, et al.: Comparative effectiveness of interventions for children exposed to nonrelational traumatic events. *Pediatrics* 131(3):526–539, 2013.
138. Klingman A: School-based interventions following a disaster. In: Saylor CF (ed): *Children and Disasters.* New York: Plenum Press, 187–210, 1993.
139. Pynoos RS, Nader K: Psychological first aid and treatment approach to children exposed to community violence: research implications. *J Trauma Stress* 1:445–473, 1988.
140. Rush SC, Houser R, Partridge A: Rebuilding sustainable communities for children and families after disaster: recommendations from symposium participants in response to the April 27th, 2011 tornadoes. *Community Ment Hlt J* 51(2):132–138, 2015.
141. Goenjian AK, Karayan I, Pynoos RS, et al.: Outcome of psychotherapy among early adolescents after trauma. *Am J Psychiatry* 154:536–542, 1997.
142. Gillis HM: Individual and small group psychotherapy for children involved in trauma and disaster. In: Saylor CF (ed): *Children and Disasters.* New York, Plenum Press, 165–186, 1993.
143. Smith P, Dyregrov A, Yule W, Gupta L, Perrin S, Gjestad R: *Children and Disasters: Teaching Recovery Techniques.* Bergen, Children and War Foundation, 1999.
144. Wolmer L, Laor N, Dedeoglu C, Siev J, Yazgan Y: Teacher-mediated intervention after disaster: a controlled three-year follow-up of children's functioning. *J Child Psychol Psychiatry* 46:1161–1168, 2005.
145. Perrin S, Smith P, Yule W: Practitioner review: the assessment and treatment of post-traumatic stress disorder in children and adolescents. *J Child Psychol Psychiatry* 41:277–289, 2000.
146. Cohen JA: Practice parameter for the assessment and treatment of children and adolescents with posttraumatic stress disorder. *J Am Acad Child Adolesc Psychiatry* 49:414–430, 2010.
147. Rachamim L, Mirochnik I, Helpman L, Nacasch N, Yadin E: Prolonged exposure therapy for toddlers with traumas following medical procedures. *Cogn Behav Pract* 22:240–252, 2015.
148. Lovett J: *Small Wonders: Healing Childhood Trauma with EMDR.* New York: The Free Press, 1999.
149. Fernandez I: EMDR as treatment of post-traumatic reactions: a field study on child victims of an earthquake. *Educ Child Psychol* 24(1):65–72, 2007.
150. Weems C F, Taylor LK, Costa NM, et al.: Effect of a school-based test anxiety intervention in ethnic minority youth exposed to hurricane Katrina. *J Appl Dev Psychol* 30(3):218–226, 2009.
151. Toren P, Wolmer L, Rozental B, et al.: Case series: brief parent–child group therapy for childhood anxiety disorders using a manual-based cognitive behavioral technique. *J Am Acad Child Adolesc Psychiatry* 39: 1309–1312, 2000.
152. Spirman S, Mizrahi C, Refetov E, et al.: Development and implementation of a community reactivation program after disasters. *Presented at the Congress on the Promised Childhood,* Tel-Aviv, 2001.
153. Rappaport J: Terms of empowerment/exemplars of prevention: toward a theory for community psychology. *Am J Community Psychol* 15:121–145, 1987.
154. Kobasa SC: Stressful life events, personality, and health: an inquiry into hardiness. *J Pers Soc Psychol* 37:1–11, 1979.
155. Shiloh R, Nutt D, Weizman A: *Atlas of Psychiatric Pharmacotherapy.* London, Martin Dunitz, p. 191, 1999.
156. Donnelly CL: Pharmacologic treatment approaches for children and adolescents with posttraumatic stress disorder. *Child Adolesc Psychiatr Clin N Am* 12:251–269, 2003.
157. Strawn JR, Keeshin BR, DelBello MP, Geracioti TD Jr, Putnam FW: Psychopharmacologic treatment of posttraumatic stress disorder in children and adolescents: a review. *J Clin Psychiat* 71(7):e1–e10, 2010.
158. Keeshin BR, Strawn JR: Psychological and pharmacologic treatment of youth with posttraumatic stress disorder: an evidence-based review. *Child Adolesc Psychiatr Clin N Am* 23(2):399–411, 2014.
159. Laor N, Wiener Z, Spirman S, Wolmer L: Community mental health procedures for emergencies and mass disasters: the Tel-Aviv model. *J Aggress Maltreat Trauma* 10(3/4):681–694, 2005.
160. Laor N, Wolmer L, Spirman S, Wiener Z: Facing war, terrorism, and disaster: toward a child-oriented comprehensive emergency care system. *Child Adol Psych Cl N Am* 12:343–361, 2003.
161. Congressional Reports: H. Rpt. 109–377—A Failure of Initiative: Final Report of the Select Bipartisan Committee to Investigate the Preparation for and Response to Hurricane Katrina [Internet]. Washington, DC, House of Representatives; 2006 Feb 15 [cited 2016 Jan 28]. Available: http://www.gpoaccess.gov/serialset/creports/katrina.html.
162. Sippel, LM, Pietrzak RH, Charney DS, Mayes LC, Southwick SM: How does social support enhance resilience in the trauma-exposed individual? *Ecol Soc* 20:10, 2015.
163. Nakagawa Y, Shaw R: social capital: a missing link to disaster recovery. *Int J Mass Emerg Disasters* 22:5–34, 2004.

SECTION VI
TREATMENT

6.1 ■ PEDIATRIC PSYCHOPHARMACOLOGY

CHAPTER 6.1.1 ■ NEUROCHEMISTRY, PHARMACODYNAMICS, AND BIOLOGIC PSYCHIATRY

GEORGE M. ANDERSON AND ANDRÉS MARTIN

INTRODUCTION

Continuing advances in basic neurobiology and psychopharmacology have led to a greatly expanded knowledge of brain functioning and hold the promise of better treatment and fuller understanding of childhood psychiatric disorders (1,2). The recent elucidation of the genetic bases of a number of single-gene childhood psychiatric disorders provides additional hope, and to some extent directions, for tackling the more complex molecular and biologic influences in autism, attention-deficit hyperactivity disorder (ADHD), Tourette syndrome (TS), anxiety, posttraumatic stress disorder (PTSD), depression, and suicide. Identification of causative factors in Parkinson's disease, Huntington's disease, and Alzheimer's disease further encourages the notion that the pharmacology of childhood psychiatric disorders can be made more rational and effective, and the biologic bases of the relevant behaviors ascertained.

The three entwined areas of neurobiology, pharmacodynamics, and biologic psychiatry can be introduced by first considering the basic concepts in the separate realms of inquiry. Relevant neurobiology includes findings in the areas of neuronal circuitry, neural transmission, and intracellular signaling. Pharmacodynamics concerns the short- and long-term effects of drugs on neuronal function and structure. Insights and serendipitous findings from psychopharmacology reciprocally inform basic neuroscience and also have often been central to the hypotheses pursued in biologic psychiatry. Recognition of the importance of genetics and complexity of psychiatric disorders is changing in fundamental ways how biologic psychiatry is approached. Whether the field is termed molecular psychiatry, biologic psychiatry, or clinical neuroscience, an increased focus on genetic influences and on behavioral components or endophenotypes has been prompted by a better appreciation of the scope and complexity of the endeavor.

GENERAL CONSIDERATIONS OF CNS FUNCTIONING

Overview

Neuronal circuitry, synaptic neurotransmission, and intracellular information processing constitute three major levels of central nervous system (CNS) functioning critical to understanding mechanisms of psychotropic drug action and the biologic basis of cognitive and behavioral processes.

Neuronal circuitry to a large extent defines and reflects the functional activity and organization of the CNS. Neuronal communication via neurotransmitter release is a fundamental mechanism of brain function. The release of neurotransmitters and neuromodulators, their mechanisms of action, and their effect on target neurons are complex and still not fully understood; however, despite the diversity of neurotransmitters and receptors in the human brain, all forms of neural communication have the common goal of modulating neuronal activity. This is achieved by changing either the electrical or biochemical properties of the cell. The balance of intracellular and extracellular ions characterizes the electrical properties of the neuron. At rest, there are more negatively charged ions inside than outside the cell, thereby creating a negative resting membrane potential. Decreasing the resting potential leads to excitation, increasing it, to inhibition. The more enduring properties of the neuron are determined by longer-term processes regulating the expression of specific genes, the production of proteins, and the creation of a distinct metabolism.

Neuronal Circuitry

The adult human cerebral cortex has about 100 billion neurons; each neuron establishes about a 1,000 to 10,000 connections to

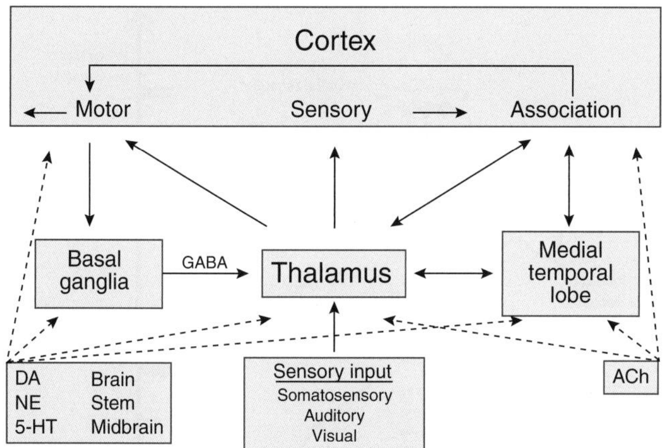

FIGURE 6.1.1.1. Neuronal circuitry. Basic scheme of information processing in the human brain. *Straight arrows* indicate glutamatergic pathways. The BG–thalamus projection is GABAergic. The *broken arrows* indicate the widespread, neurotransmitter-specific projections arising from the basal forebrain (ACh) and brain stem (DA, NE, 5-HT). A1, primary auditory cortex; ACh, acetylcholine; BG, basal ganglia; DA, dopamine; 5-HT, serotonin; see text for further details.

other neurons. Neurons are arranged in distributed networks that play critical roles in the expression of human behavior (3). This involves the collection of sensory information through perceptual modules, the creation of a representation, and the production of a response. Here we focus on four major anatomic systems that are crucial for these three steps of information processing: the cortex, thalamus, basal ganglia, and medial temporal lobe (Figure 6.1.1.1).

1. The thalamus is the gateway to cortical processing of all incoming sensory information, here represented by the three major systems: somatosensory, auditory, and visual (Figure 6.1.1.1). Primary sensory cortices receive information from the appropriate input modules (sensory organ + thalamus).
2. The association cortex integrates information from primary cortices, subcortical structures, and brain areas affiliated with memory to create an internal representation of the sensory information.
3. The medial temporal lobe (including the hippocampus and amygdala) serves two major functions in the brain: to integrate multimodal sensory information for storage into and retrieval from memory, and to attach limbic valence to sensory information (e.g., pleasant or unpleasant, fight or flight).
4. The basal ganglia are primarily involved in the integration of input from cortical areas. The basal ganglia modulate cortical activity via a cortico-striato-pallido-thalamo-cortical (CSPTC) loop. The most prominent projections to the striatum arise from the motor cortex.

All major projections (solid lines) in this basic circuitry (Figure 6.1.1.1) are glutamatergic (using the amino acid neurotransmitter glutamate), except for the projections from the basal ganglia toward the thalamus, which are GABAergic (employing γ-aminobutyric acid). The glutamatergic neurons within each of the major components or regions of the circuit are under inhibitory control by GABAergic interneurons. In addition, four groups of densely packed neurons provide diffuse projections to all areas of the brain to modulate their functions: cholinergic neurons in the basal forebrain and brain stem, dopaminergic neurons in the substantia nigra (SN) and ventral tegmental area (VTA), noradrenergic neurons in the locus coeruleus (LC), and serotonergic neurons in the raphe nuclei. The broken arrows in Figure 6.1.1.1 indicate the four neurotransmitter-specific projection systems. The relay of information from one neuron to another in these various circuits is usually affected by synaptic neurotransmission.

General Aspects of Synaptic Neurotransmission

Dendrites create a network of fibers providing the cell body of the neuron with input from other cells (Figure 6.1.1.2). The cell integrates these different inputs through modulation of the membrane potential, changes in second messenger systems, and at the level of the nucleus (regulation of gene expression). The cell body is also the site of synthesis of nearly all cell-specific proteins, including transporters, receptors, and the enzymes needed for neurotransmitter production.

The axon is the output station of the neuron. The axon can be short (local circuit neuron) or long (projection neuron). If a deviation from the resting membrane potential is above a certain threshold, an action potential is created and travels downstream rapidly. The nerve terminal is the widened terminal part of the axon. It provides a small area of close contact with dendrites of communicating neurons: the synapse. Variations of this typical scheme include synapses between two terminals, two dendrites, and neurotransmitter release in medial parts of the axon.

As seen in Figure 6.1.1.2, the presynaptic neuron releases the vesicular stored neurotransmitter into the synapse and can express two types of proteins that affect synaptic communication: Presynaptic membrane-bound receptors can bind the intrinsic neurotransmitter (at autoreceptors) or transmitters of neighboring neurons (at heteroreceptors) and affect the cell via intracellular messengers. One response, for example, is the modulation of neurotransmitter release (4). Presynaptic membrane-bound reuptake transporters pump the released neurotransmitter back into the cell (5). The released transmitter can undergo intracellular, extracellular metabolism (4B), or be repackaged in vesicules for rerelease.

The neuron receiving the input (postsynaptic cell) can be modulated via two different types of receptors (Figure 6.1.1.2). In the case of fast-acting, class I (ionotropic) receptors, the neurotransmitter binds to the receptor protein and within milliseconds, this leads to a change in the permeability of the associated ion channel, allowing the influx of ions such as Ca^{2+}, Na^{+}, K^{+}, or Cl^{-}. In contrast, with slow-acting, class II (G-protein–coupled) receptors, the binding of the neurotransmitter to the receptor protein leads to a change in the protein conformation. This change is relayed to an associated G-protein, so called because it binds guanidine triphosphate (GTP) in order to be activated. G-proteins regulate two major classes of effector molecules: ion channels and second messenger generating enzymes. This general pattern and form of synaptic neurotransmission is repeated across the six major neurotransmitters. However, the differences seen across the glutamatergic, GABAergic, dopaminergic, noradrenergic, serotonergic, and cholinergic systems are intriguing, form the bases of specific psychopharmacologic effects, and underlie still prevailing neurobiologic theories of biologic psychiatry.

INTRACELLULAR INFORMATION PROCESSING

Our understanding of how neurons relay information between each other has moved beyond the role of synaptic transmission and into that of processes that take place within cells. Each neuron is the target of many projections from local and distant neurons. These influences are integrated at the level

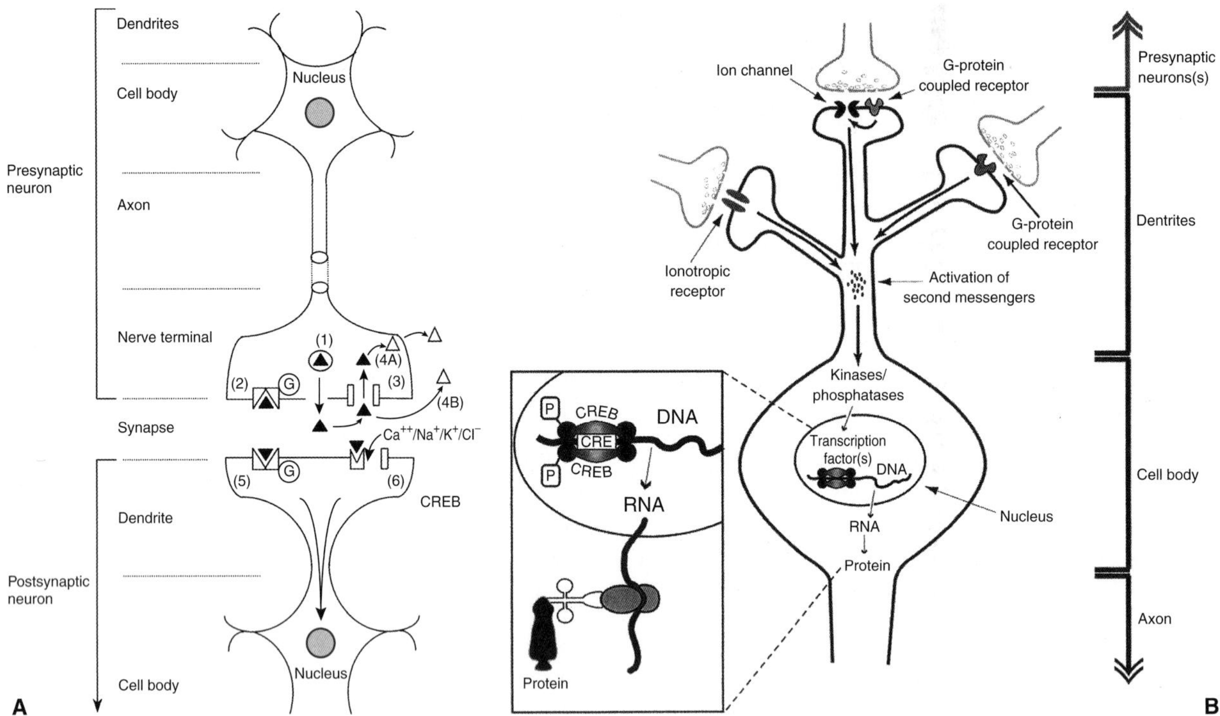

FIGURE 6.1.1.2. A: Anatomy of the neuron with major aspects of typical pre- and postsynaptic neurons labeled. Also depicted are six major mechanisms of synaptic neurotransmission: (1) release of neurotransmitter stored in vesicles; (2) binding of transmitter to presynaptic autoreceptor; (3) clearance of transmitter by reuptake; (4) A-intracellular metabolism of transmitter, B-extracellular metabolism of transmitter; (5) binding of transmitter to G-protein–coupled receptor; (6) binding of transmitter to ion channel coupled receptor; see text for details. **B:** Intracellular information processing. Neurotransmitters released from the presynaptic neuron activate receptors at the postsynaptic neuron. Second messengers either enter the neuron (e.g., Ca^{2+} through ligand-gated ion channels) or are newly synthesized inside the neuron (e.g., G-protein–coupled receptors stimulate adenylate cyclase and the synthesis of cyclic AMP). Neurons usually have multiple receptor types and are able to integrate information from a variety of synaptic inputs. Second messengers stimulate protein kinases and protein phosphatases to control the state of phosphorylation of various proteins inside the neuron. Transcription factors such as CREB are regulated by kinases and phosphatases. A high level of discrimination is observed, although some transcription factors integrate information from different second messenger pathways. Thus, kinases and phosphatases regulate groups of genes under the control of specific transcription factors. **Inset:** Phosphorylation of CREB stimulates the transcription from DNA into RNA, which is transported out of the nucleus and translated (with ribosomes and tRNA) into protein.

of the cell membrane and cell nucleus. The neurotransmitter-mediated activation of ion channels in the cell membrane can lead to an increase or decrease of the resting membrane potential. This may lead to the creation of an action potential. At the level of the cell nucleus, the various receptors and ion channels expressed on the cell membrane may influence gene and protein expression.

Gene expression is regulated by transcription factors that bind to specific sequences of the DNA in the nucleus (Figure 6.1.1.2B); therefore, membrane-bound receptors or ion channels in distal parts of the neuron must be able to activate intraneuronal signal transduction pathways that can span long distances and translocate to the nucleus. Because proteins assemble the neuron and determine neuronal properties, gene expression regulates neuronal function and may cause malfunction. Many psychopharmacologic agents with delayed therapeutic effects are thought to produce their therapeutic benefits through modulation of gene expression (6,7).

Release of neurotransmitters from the presynaptic neuron into the synapse activates receptors on the postsynaptic neuron (see Figure 6.1.1.2B). Ions such as calcium enter the cell and act as second messengers on activation of inotropic receptors. Activation of G-protein–coupled receptors facilitates the opening of neighboring ion channels or the synthesis of second messengers such as cyclic AMP. Second messengers (calcium, cyclic AMP) regulate the activity of protein kinases (proteins that transfer phosphate groups to a substrate protein) and phosphatases (proteins that remove phosphate groups from a substrate protein). In all cases investigated to date, the activation of neurotransmitter receptors changes the state of phosphorylation of neuronal proteins.

The transcription factors are one group of proteins regulated by phosphorylation. Transcription factors operate by recruiting the transcription initiation complex and RNA polymerase to particular genes. The RNA polymerase then transcribes the DNA template into an RNA molecule, which is translated into protein outside the nucleus.

Among the best-studied transcription factors in the brain is the Ca^{2+}- and cyclic AMP-responsive element binding protein (CREB). The study of CREB has provided us with an insight into the complex consequences of transcription factor activation and gene expression on higher brain function. A variety of signal transduction pathways are integrated into CREB-mediated gene expression, such as those activated by Gs-proteins, inotropic receptors, or growth factors. Cyclic AMP-responsive element binding protein is activated by phosphorylation and regulates the expression of several target genes (e.g., genes for peptide neurotransmitters, enzymes involved in neurotransmitter synthesis, and growth factors). The discovery that CREB plays a vital role in processes such as learning and memory provided a link between gene regulation and cognitive function.

Small but persistent abnormalities in neurotransmission can have far-reaching consequences because neurotransmitters and receptors influence gene and protein expression in the brain. An understanding of signal transduction pathways and transcription factors such as CREB may be instrumental in providing new therapeutic avenues in psychopharmacology.

Pharmacodynamics Overview

Pharmacodynamic principles are concerned with the biochemical and physiologic effects of drugs at their active sites, that is, with their specific mechanisms of action. Stated succinctly, "pharmacokinetics describes what the body does to a drug; pharmacodynamics what a drug does to the body" (see Chapter 6.1.2 (Oesterheld, Shader, & Martin)). The effects of a medication may change during development, as brain regions or neurotransmitter systems develop and mature. Most psychopharmacologic agents exert their effects by interacting with specific protein targets—receptors, ion channels, transporters, or enzymes. Each of the major neurotransmitter systems has, therefore, a number of routes by which they can be manipulated (as are delineated in subsequent sections). The nature of the drug effect depends upon the site targeted while the selectivity of action is often a function of the relative affinity of the agent for the target site versus its other, often multiple, sites of interaction. Adverse drug effects are often the result of relatively nonselective agents and can severely limit their clinical utility.

Biologic Psychiatry Overview

Research in biologic psychiatry has made it increasingly clear that the genetics and biology of the common disorders are complex, in that multiple genes appear to contribute to the syndromes (Chapters 3.3.2 (Fernandez, Gupta & Hoffman) and 3.3.3 (Tomasi, Lennington, Leckman, & Lombroso)). This is not surprising given the complex and diffuse nature of the neural systems that subserve the relevant brain processes (8). The genetic complexity is further multiplied by the wealth of variation arising from gene–environment interactions: Illuminating the complexity will require the application of new and appropriate genetic methods (9–11).

An emerging overarching theme is that all biologic, neuropharmacologic, and behavioral investigation needs to be performed in a genetic context. There is also a greater focus on components or domains of behavior and a greater interest in quantifying the traits or variables of interest. The rationale for examining what have been referred to as elementary units of psychological dysfunction (12), core or candidate symptoms, quantitative phenotypes (13), endophenotypes (14), or core psychopathologic processes (15,16) is becoming more and more compelling.

One formulation of the interrelated aspects of biologic psychiatry is presented in Figure 6.1.1.3. The mutual interacting influences of genetic and environmental factors are shown determining the neurobiologic systems that, in combination, form the substrate of relevant behaviors. The field of biologic psychiatry has traditionally emphasized neurochemical and neuroendocrinologic approaches. Other fields and approaches that are now proving critical to advancing an understanding of brain neural transmission in psychiatry include neurophysiology, neuropsychology, neuroimaging (17) pharmacogenetics (18), and network analysis (19). Elucidation of the bases of the childhood disorders can be expected to proceed through an iterative process involving mutually beneficial relationships among all of the perspectives (20). It is clear that one should be ever mindful of the developmental context when studying childhood psychiatric disorders (21,22).

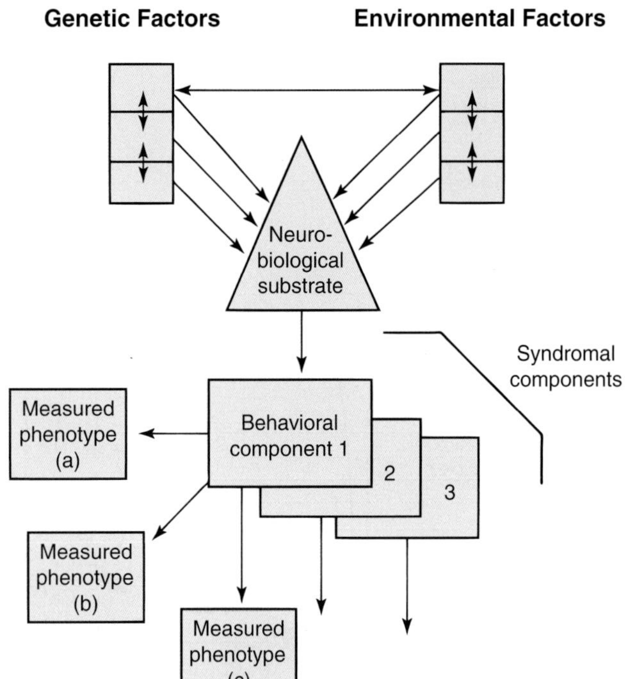

FIGURE 6.1.1.3. Schematic of the interrelated factors underlying biologic psychiatry. The mutual interacting influences of genetic and environmental factors are shown determining the neurobiologic systems that combine to form the substrate of relevant behaviors. The behaviors can be assessed through a range of measured phenotypes (**A–C**). The multiple behavioral components of most syndromes and disorders are depicted by the receding additional behavioral components (1–3).

NEUROTRANSMITTER SYSTEMS

Overview

The major neurotransmitter systems can be divided into two groups based on their anatomic distribution. The first group comprises the serotonergic, dopaminergic, noradrenergic, and cholinergic neurons. These four systems originate from small groups of neurons, densely packed in circumscribed areas of the forebrain or brain stem, and project to their target areas typically by long-ranging projection fibers. The second group includes the glutamatergic and GABAergic systems. Their neurons are by far the most prevalent and widely distributed types in the human brain. As mentioned, a number of similarities and parallels are apparent across the neurotransmitter system. Each system will be considered from the standpoint of its anatomy and neural transmission mechanisms, its pharmacodynamics or psychopharmacology, and the relevant biologic psychiatry investigation.

SEROTONERGIC SYSTEM

Serotoninergic Neural Transmission/ Neuroanatomy

Most serotonergic cells overlap with the distribution of the raphe nuclei in the brainstem. A rostral group (B6–8 neurons) projects to the thalamus, hypothalamus, amygdala, striatum, and cortex (23). The remaining two groups (B1–5 neurons) project to other brainstem neurons, the cerebellum, and the

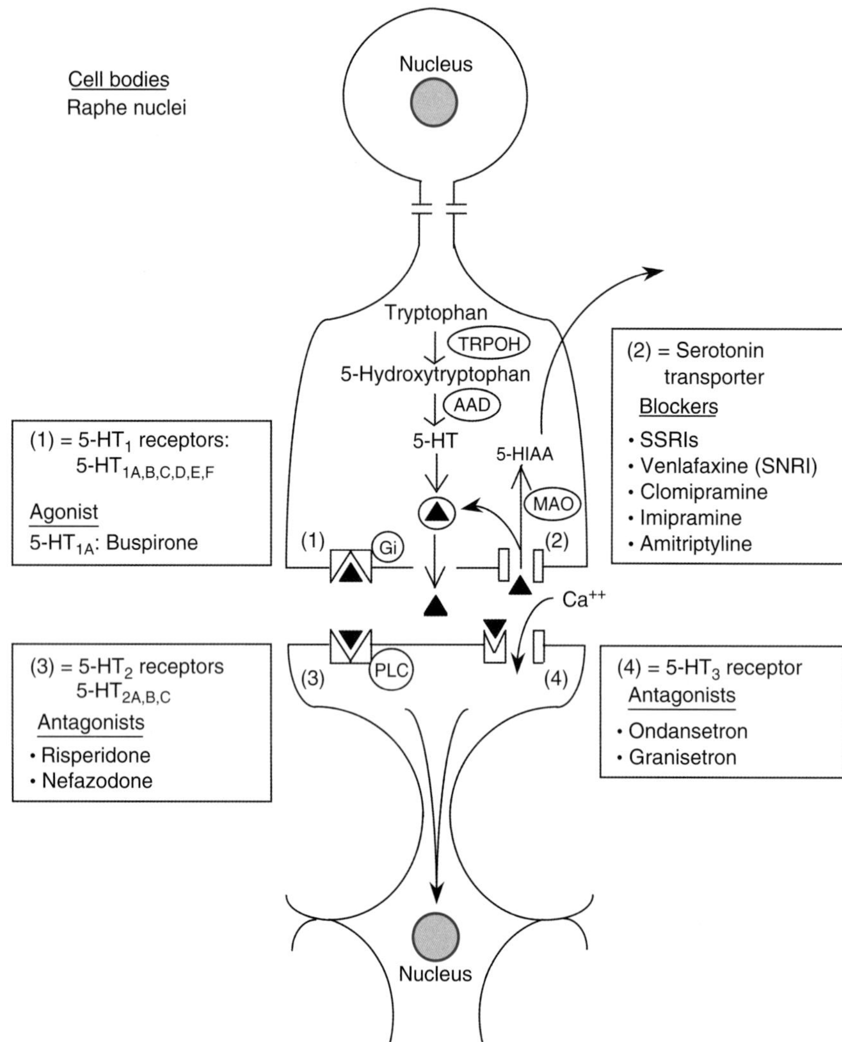

FIGURE 6.1.1.4. Serotonergic neurotransmission. Diagrammatic illustration of a serotonergic neuron. Serotonin (5-HT) synthesized from tryptophan (TRP) by the rate-limiting enzyme tryptophan hydroxylase (TRPOH) can be taken up by the vesicular monoamine transporter (VMAT2) and stored in vesicles for subsequent release or metabolized by the mitochondrial enzyme MAO. Released 5-HT can interact with presynaptic or postsynaptic receptors, diffuse to extrasynaptic sites, or be taken up by neuronal or glial membrane 5-HT transporters (5-HTTs). Inhibition of the 5-HTT by selective serotonin reuptake inhibitors (SSRIs) results in higher levels of synaptic and extracellular fluid 5-HT, leading to greater 5-HT receptor stimulation.

spinal cord. A schematic diagram of a serotonergic neuron and the metabolism of serotonin (5-HT) are depicted in Figure 6.1.1.4. Serotonin is produced after hydroxylation and decarboxylation of the essential amino acid tryptophan. Serotonin produced can be taken up by the vesicular monoamine transporter (VMAT2) and stored in vesicles for subsequent release or metabolized by the mitochondrial enzyme monoamine oxidase (MAO). Once released, 5-HT can interact with presynaptic or postsynaptic receptors, diffuse to extrasynaptic sites, or be taken up by neuronal or glial membrane 5-HT transporters (5-HTTs).

Serotonin acts at two different classes of receptors: at an inotropic receptor (5-HT$_3$ receptor) or at slower acting receptors, coupled either to phospholipase C (5-HT$_2$ receptors) or to G-proteins (5-HT$_{1,4–7}$ receptors) (24). The 5-HT$_1$ receptors (5-HT$_{1A,B,C,D,E,F}$) (Figure 6.1.1.4) are coupled to G$_i$ and lead to a decrease of cyclic AMP. The 5-HT$_{1A}$ receptor is also directly coupled to a K$^+$ channel leading to increased opening of the channel. The 5-HT$_1$ receptors are the predominant serotonergic autoreceptors. 5-HT$_2$ receptors (5-HT$_{2A-C}$) are coupled to phospholipase C and lead to a variety of intracellular effects (mainly depolarization). Three receptors (5-HT$_{4,6,7}$) are coupled to G$_s$ and activate adenylate cyclase. The 5-HT$_3$ receptor is the only monoamine receptor coupled to an ion channel, and is found in the cortex, hippocampus, and in the area postrema, where it mediates nausea and emesis. It is typically localized presynaptically and regulates neurotransmitter release.

Serotonergic Pharmacodynamics

Serotonin is linked to many brain functions because of the widespread serotonergic projections and heterogeneity of the serotonergic receptors (23,25). For example, modulation of serotonergic receptors and the reuptake site is beneficial (among others) in the treatment of anxiety, depression, obsessive–compulsive disorder, and schizophrenia (26). Interest in central 5-HT functioning derives from 5-HT's important role in processes as diverse and important as sleep, mood, appetite, perception, and hormone secretion (25), as well as its critical role in neurodevelopment (27).

Blockade of the serotonin transporter by selective serotonin reuptake inhibitors (SSRIs), such as fluoxetine (Prozac), results in higher levels of synaptic and extracellular fluid 5-HT and leads to greater pre- and postsynaptic 5-HT receptor stimulation. The serotonin transporter is the primary target site for several antidepressants, including the SSRIs, venlafaxine, and tricyclic antidepressants such as clomipramine and, to a lesser extent, imipramine and amitriptyline (Figure 6.1.1.4). Recent work in nonhuman primates has indicated that the increase in functionally active 5-HT occur within hours and is relatively constant over the course of treatment.

The atypical neuroleptics, such as risperidone, ziprasidone, and olanzapine, all act as antagonists at 5-HT$_2$ receptors, as well as having blocking properties at dopamine receptors. The beneficial antipsychotic effects of the drugs appear to be at least partly mediated through their effects at cortical 5-HT_{2A} receptors. In particular, it appears that 5-HT_{2A} receptors on apical dendrites of cortical pyramidal cells may be especially important in gating sensory input. The critical role of the 5-HT_{2A} receptor in perception is underscored by a consideration of the effects of the 5-HT_{2A} agonist lysergic acid diethylamide (LSD). Adverse effects of the atypical neuroleptics on appetite and the associated weight gain appear to be at least partly due to effects at the 5-HT_{2C} receptor, while the substantial and enduring hyperprolactinemia frequently observed is a consequence of the dopamine D_2 receptor blockade in the pituitary.

Other serotonergic agents include the atypical anxiolytic buspirone, which acts as an agonist at the 5-HT_{1A} receptor. Newer antimigraine drugs such as sumatriptan have agonist effects at arterial 5-$HT_{1B/D}$ receptors, while the antiemetic odansetron acts to antagonize 5-HT_3 receptor sites in the intestine and perhaps in the brain.

Biologic Psychiatry of Serotonin

Autism

Initial interest in a role for 5-HT in autism stemmed in part from the powerful effects of serotonergic agents, such as LSD, on perception. Research in the area was further stimulated by early reports of elevated 5-HT in the blood of autistic children (28,29). Beneficial effects of treatment with serotonin reuptake inhibitors (30) and exacerbation observed after tryptophan depletion (31) have also heightened interest in the role of 5-HT in autism. Although most of the 5-HT-related research has focused on the hyperserotonemia of autism, a number of studies of CSF 5-HIAA and several neuroendocrinologic studies of central 5-HT functioning have been reported (32). CSF studies are in general agreement that few or no differences exist between autistic and control groups' mean levels of 5-HIAA (33). A series of studies have provided converging evidence that 5-HT_{2A} receptor function and expression may be altered in autism. In 1989, McBride and colleagues (34) reported that central and peripheral 5-HT_{2A} receptor functioning appeared reduced in autism. Thus, a diminished 5-HT_{2A}-mediated neuroendocrine response was paralleled by a reduced 5-HT_{2A}-mediated platelet aggregation response and lower platelet 5-HT_{2A} receptor binding in autism. Alterations in platelet 5-HT_{2A} binding indices were also reported by Cook et al. (35), with 5-HT_{2A} receptor measures inversely related to platelet 5-HT levels. These reports are paralleled by two neuroimaging studies reporting reduced 5-HT_{2A} receptor density in cortical regions (36).

TS/OCD

A role for 5-HT has been hypothesized because of the close connection between TS and obsessive–compulsive disorder (37). Effective treatment of obsessive–compulsive symptoms in patients with TS with the serotonergic uptake inhibitors, fluvoxamine and fluoxetine, has further stimulated research on the connection. The largest study of the 5-HT metabolite, 5-hydroxyindoleacetice acid (5-HIAA), found similar levels in patients with TS, OCD, or TS plus OCD, and the normal control group (38). No studies of 5-HT receptor functioning have been carried out in patients with TS, and early reports of benefit from the immediate 5-HT precursor, 5-hydroxytryptophan, have not been replicated. Research examining postmortem brain tissue has found decreases in 5-HT, 5-HIAA, and tryptophan across nearly all cortical and subcortical areas in TS (39,40). Further postmortem research is necessary in order to replicate the findings; however, the results tend to increase the possibility that 5-HT may be a factor in the symptomatology of TS.

Attention-Deficit Hyperactivity Disorder

Interest in a role for 5-HT in ADHD was stimulated by early reports of decreased platelet 5-HT in affected children. Subsequent studies have not replicated this finding and have found normal levels of platelet and urine 5-HIAA, as well as normal numbers and affinities of platelet imipramine-binding sites in subjects with ADHD. In addition, studies of CSF 5-HIAA have not found differences between ADHD and control subjects. On the whole, the neurochemical research and the minimal treatment response to serotonergic agents have made it seem less likely that a 5-HT alteration is etiologic. Even so, it appears that the role of 5-HT in disruptive behaviors, particularly with respect to impulse control, deserves further consideration.

DOPAMINERGIC SYSTEM

Dopaminergic Neural Transmission/ Neuroanatomy

Dopaminergic neurons can be divided into three major groups based on the length of their efferent fibers: (a) ultra-short systems in the retina and olfactory bulb; (b) intermediate-length systems originating in the hypothalamus and projecting to the pituitary gland; and (c) wide-ranging systems originating from two areas, the SN and the VTA. The SN neurons (also called A9 neurons) project to caudate and putamen, whereas the VTA neurons (also called A10 neurons) project to limbic areas such as nucleus accumbens and amygdala (i.e., mesolimbic projections) and several cortical areas such as frontal, cingulate, and entorhinal cortex (i.e., mesocortical projections).

The metabolism of the catecholamine dopamine (DA) is shown in Figure 6.1.1.5. DA is synthesized from tyrosine, after hydroxylation to dihydroxyphenylalanine (DOPA) and decarboxylation by aromatic acid decarboxylase (AAAD), and is found in the highest concentration in the midbrain, although extensive cortical projections also occur. Dopamine has been shown to be critical in reward, modulating movement, and cognition. Dopamine is released into the synapse from vesicles (Figure 6.1.1.5) and subsequently removed from the synapse by two mechanisms. First, catechol-O-methyltransferase (COMT) degrades intrasynaptic DA. Second, the dopamine transporter (DAT), an Na^+/Cl^--dependent neurotransmitter transporter, transports DA out of the synaptic cleft (Figure 6.1.1.5). Parenthetically, and of relevance to the action of stimulants, the transporter can actually function in either direction, depending on the concentration gradient. Free intracellular DA can either be taken back up into vesicles or metabolized by mitochondrial MAO.

Dopamine acts at two different classes of dopamine receptors in the CNS, the D_1 and D_2 receptor families (Figure 6.1.1.5) (41). The D1 receptor family includes the D_1 and D_5 receptors. Both are coupled to Gs (G-stimulating) and lead to an increase of cyclic AMP. The D_2 receptor family includes the D_2, D_3, and D_4 receptors. All are coupled to G_i (G-inhibitory) and lead to a decrease of cyclic AMP. There is a predilection of the different dopamine receptors for expression in specific brain areas (e.g., D_1 receptors are found in the striatum and cortex, D_2 receptors in the striatum and pituitary gland, and D_3 receptors in the nucleus accumbens). Presynaptic dopaminergic receptors are typically of the D_2 type and found on most portions of the dopaminergic neuron (as autoreceptors). They regulate DA synthesis and release, as well as the firing rate of DA neurons. Autoreceptors are 5 to 10 times more sensitive to DA agonists than postsynaptic receptors.

Dopamine affects several brain functions primarily by modulation of other neurotransmitter systems (42). Dopaminergic neurons of the SN project to the striatum and modulate the

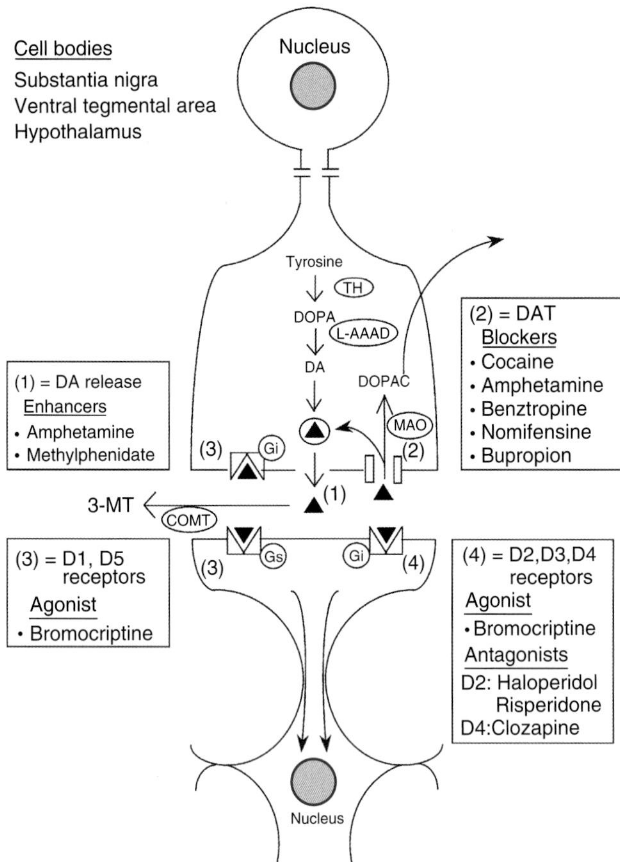

FIGURE 6.1.1.5. Dopaminergic neurotransmission. Diagrammatic illustration of a dopaminergic neuron. Dopamine (DA) synthesized from tyrosine by the rate-limiting enzyme tyrosine hydroxylase (TH) can be taken up by the vesicular monoamine transporter (VMAT2) and stored in vesicles for subsequent release, or metabolized by the mitochondrial enzyme monoamine oxidase. Released DA can interact with presynaptic or postsynaptic receptors. Inhibition of the DA transporter (DAT) by DA reuptake inhibitors (DAT blockers) results in higher levels of synaptic and extracellular fluid of DA and leads to greater DA receptor stimulation.

function of striatal GABAergic interneurons. Dopaminergic projections of the VTA to limbic structures such as the nucleus accumbens are known to be involved in reward behavior and the development of addiction to drugs such as ethanol, cocaine, nicotine, and opiates (43,44). Dopaminergic projections from the VTA to the cortex play a role in the fine-tuning of cortical neurons (i.e., modulation of signal-to-noise ratio) (45).

Dopaminergic Pharmacodynamics

Dopamine receptor blockade, particularly at D_2 sites in the frontal cortex, is a major mechanism of action of most antipsychotic drugs (Figure 6.1.1.5). Both the older typical neuroleptics like the phenothiazines (e.g., chlorpromazine) and butyrophenones (e.g., haloperidol), as well as newer atypical neuroleptics including risperidone, ziprasidone, and olanzapine, have antagonist effects at D2 receptors. The most recently introduced atypical antipsychotic drug, aripiprazole, appears to work by serving as a partial agonist at both pre- and postsynaptic dopamine receptors. By so doing, aripiprazole may moderate dopaminergic function, reducing presynaptic dopamine release while modestly stimulating postsynaptic receptors.

Dopamine is released into the synapse from vesicles (Figure 6.1.1.5) and this process is facilitated by the stimulants methylphenidate and amphetamine. Stimulant drugs such as amphetamine and cocaine also potently block the DAT. The euphoriant properties of the stimulants appear to be principally mediated through their enhancement of dopaminergic transmission in the striatum (specifically, the nucleus accumbens).

Biologic Psychiatry of Dopamine

Attention-Deficit Hyperactiviy Disorder

The symptomatology of ADHD includes inattention, distractibility, and impulsivity, with or without hyperactivity (46). The remarkable effects of stimulants on children with ADHD have led to a longstanding and continuing interest in the role of DA. Family and twin studies have strongly supported the idea that there are inherited components to the disorder (47).

A large number of neurobiologic studies have been carried out; the majority involves the measurement of neurotransmitter metabolites in blood and urine, either at baseline or after pharmacologic perturbation. An increasing number of brain imaging studies have been reported (48). These studies have tended to focus attention on the frontal cortex and midbrain DA nuclei and their projection areas. The well-replicated genetic findings of an association between ADHD symptomatology and alleles of the DAT and D4 DA receptor genes (18) have further increased interest in DA. Although the neurochemical investigation has been extensive and includes studies of dopamine and its principal metabolite, homovanillic acid (HVA), in CSF, plasma, and urine, it has failed to establish definitive alterations in ADHD. Neuroendocrine studies in ADHD are limited and also provide no definite information regarding possible group differences.

Tourette Syndrome

Neuroanatomic and neuropharmacologic considerations have prompted a number of neurochemical studies with a focus on the monoamines DA, 5-HT, and NE in TS (49,50). A role for DA is suggested by the amelioration of tics by neuroleptics, exacerbation of symptomatology after administration of stimulants, and importance of DA pathways in modulating basal ganglia output (51). The measurement of the DA metabolite HVA in CSF has not revealed consistent differences between mean levels in TS and control groups (38). Studies of postmortem brain from a small number of patients with TS have yielded conflicting results. Singer and colleagues (50,52) have found increased densities of the DA transporter in basal ganglia regions and suggested that the increased densities are a reflection of increased DA innervation within the striatum; however, observations of the normal striatal levels of DA, HVA, and tyrosine hydroxylase do not support this idea (39,40). Although an initial imaging study reported higher striatal DA transporter binding in Tourette patients, subsequent studies have not confirmed this elevation (50). Interest in possible alterations in relative densities of brain D2 and D1, DA receptors has increased following a report of a relationship between density and tic severity in twins (53).

Autism

A case for altered DA functioning in autism can be made, based on its clear role in mediating motoric disturbances (e.g., stereotypies) and the observation that DA blockers are effective in treating some aspects of autism. The majority of relevant neurochemical studies have examined levels of HVA (32). The concentration of HVA in CSF does not appear to be altered (54). Measurements of HVA in urine have been inconsistent and the only study of plasma HVA reported similar levels in autistic and control subjects (55). Other relevant measures

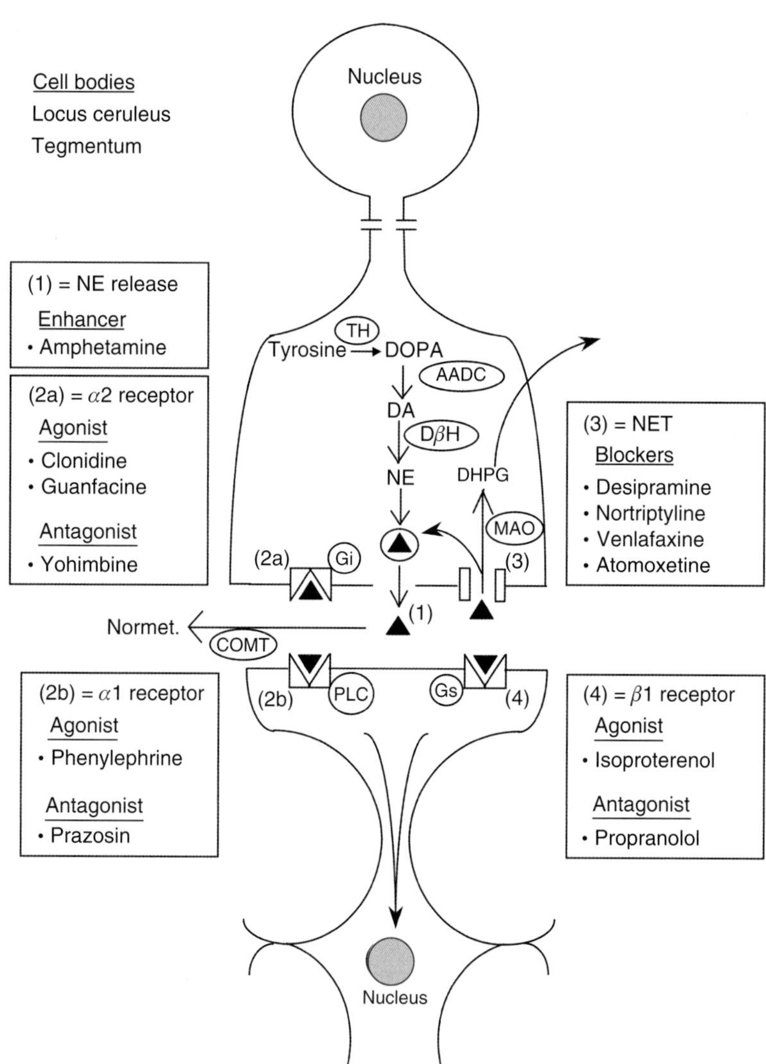

FIGURE 6.1.1.6. Noradrenergic neurotransmission. Diagrammatic illustration of a noradrenergic neuron. Norepinephrine (NE) synthesized from dopamine by the enzyme dopamine-β-hydroxylase (DBH) can be taken up by the vesicular monoamine transporter (VMAT2) and stored in vesicles for subsequent release or metabolized by the mitochondrial enzyme monoamine oxidase. Released NE can interact with presynaptic or postsynaptic receptors. Inhibition of the norepinephrine transporter (NET) by NE reuptake blockers results in higher levels of synaptic and extracellular fluid of NE and leads to greater NE receptor stimulation.

include urinary DA, reportedly normal in autism, and plasma prolactin, which also has been reported to be normal in autistic subjects (55). Taken together, the studies suggest that central dopaminergic functioning, to the extent it can be assessed by the measures employed, is normal in autism.

NORADRENERGIC SYSTEM

Noradrenergic Neural Transmission/Neuroanatomy

About half of all noradrenergic neurons (i.e., 12,000 on each side of the brain stem) are located in the LC. They provide the extensive noradrenergic innervation of the cortex, hippocampus, thalamus, cerebellum, and spinal cord. The remaining neurons are distributed in the tegmental region. They innervate predominantly the hypothalamus, basal forebrain, and spinal cord. Norepinephrine (NE) is released into the synapse from vesicles; amphetamine facilitates this release (Figure 6.1.1.6). NE acts in the CNS at two different types of noradrenergic receptors, α and β.

Adrenergic α-receptors can be subdivided into α_1-receptors, which are coupled to phospholipase and located postsynaptically, and α_2-receptors, which are coupled to G_i and located primarily presynaptically (Figure 6.1.1.6). Adrenergic β-receptors in the CNS are predominantly of the β_1 subtype. β_1-receptors are coupled to G_s and lead to an increase of cyclic AMP. NE is removed from the synapse by catabolism by COMT and through uptake by the norepinephrine transporter (NET), a Na^+/Cl^--dependent neurotransmitter transporter. Once internalized, NE can be degraded by the intracellular enzyme MAO; metabolic end products include 3-methoxy-4-hydroxyphenylethleneglycol (MHPG) and vanillylmandelic acid (VMA).

Noradrenergic projections modulate sleep cycles, appetite, mood, and cognition by targeting the thalamus, limbic structures, and cortex. Also, the LC receives afferents from the sensory systems that monitor the internal and external environments. The widespread LC efferents lead to an inhibition of spontaneous discharge in the target neurons. Stress responses, central and peripheral arousal, and learning and memory are all critically modulated by noradrenergic neurons (56,57). The critical role of the noradrenergic system in the stress response is shown in Figure 6.1.1.7. The extensive interaction of the central/peripheral NE system with the hypothalamic–pituitary–adrenal (HPA) axis is evident and is summarized in the review of Chrousos and Gold (58).

Noradrenergic Pharmacodynamics

Noradrenergic agents function through a variety of mechanisms. Monoamine oxidase inhibitors (MAOIs) act to increase

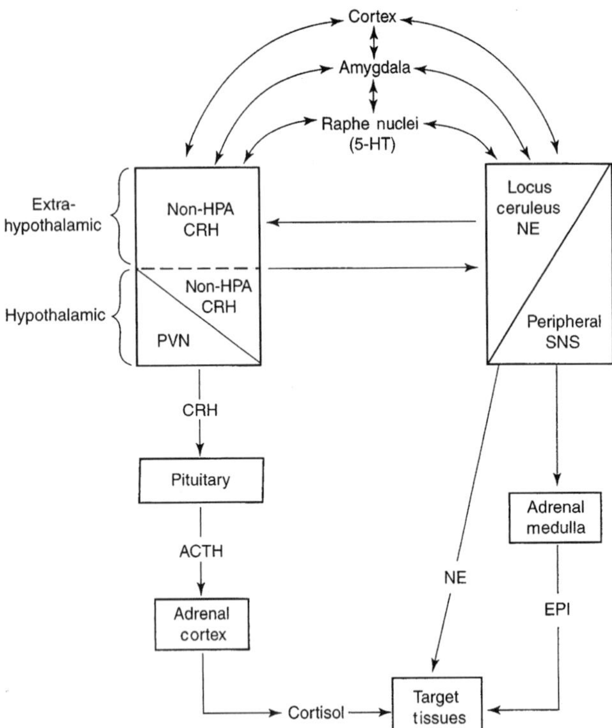

FIGURE 6.1.1.7. Stress response system. Diagram of the two major components of the stress response system: the central noradrenergic/sympathoadrenomedullary system and the hypothalamic–pituitary–adrenal (HPA) axis. The extensive interaction of the central/peripheral norepinephrine systems with the HPA axis is evident. Not shown are the extensive hormonal and neuronal inputs and feedback occurring from the periphery to the central nervous system.

intra- and extracellular NE by inhibiting enzymatic catabolism by MAO. A number of antidepressant drugs, including desipramine, nortriptyline, atomoxetine, and venlafaxine, increase extracellular NE via blockade of the NET (Figure 6.1.1.6) (59). Clonidine and guanfacine are potent α_2-receptor agonists and tend to decrease noradrenergic tone by stimulating presynaptic α_2-autoreceptors in the locus coeruleus. This can lead to sedating and hypotensive effects. However, their actions at postsynaptic α_2-receptors in the cortex may be important to their apparent beneficial effects on attention and impulse control (57). The other major class of adrenergic receptors consists of the β_1 and β_2 adrenergic receptors. The β_1 subtype is found in the cerebral cortex, while both types are found in peripheral vasculature. While the more lipophilic β-blockers (e.g., propranolol) can antagonize both central and peripheral β-receptors, peripheral blockade affected by less lipophilic agents (e.g., nadolol) may be sufficient to have behavioral effects.

Biologic Psychiatry of Norepinephrine

Given the apparent importance of stress and trauma in affecting the onset, expression, and severity of various forms of psychopathology, it is not surprising that NE has been extensively investigated in biologic psychiatry. Certainly, central NE and the noradrenergic sympathetic nervous system (SNS) play a central role in arousal and the stress response.

Tourette Syndrome

The importance of noradrenergic projections from the LC in controlling states of arousal, as well as reports of symptom amelioration after treatment with the α_2-agonist clonidine (60), are suggestive evidence for altered noradrenergic functioning in TS. There are several reports of lowered urinary excretion of MHPG in TS; however, this finding has not been consistently replicated. Assessment of the SNS by measurement of autonomic cardiovascular measures has not revealed any substantial differences in the TS group (61). However, studies of plasma, urinary, and CSF stress hormones before and after a lumbar puncture clearly suggest that at least some patients with TS have an increased stress response (62,63). This conclusion is consistent with the results of the largest study of NE and MHPG in CSF, which found that, although MHPG levels were normal, concentrations of NE were elevated nearly twofold (38). Given the much shorter half-life of NE compared to MHPG, the results are indicative of normal basal stress response functioning and increased acute stress responsivity.

Attention-Deficit Hyperactivity Disorder

Arousal mechanisms almost certainly play an important part in ADHD-associated symptoms of hyperactivity, impulsivity, distractibility, and inattention (64,65). The crucial role of the central noradrenergic system and SNS in regulating arousal, together with noradrenergic effects of stimulant medication, has led to hypotheses of noradrenergic involvement in ADHD (66,67). Treatment studies employing the noradrenergic-specific agents clonidine and guanfacine, as well as an increasing appreciation of the role of central NE in attention and cognition (56,57,68), have served to maintain interest in the role of NE in the symptoms of ADHD.

Baseline measurements of NE in serum and MHPG in plasma have not revealed differences between ADHD and control subjects. The data with respect to MHPG and NE in urine are less consistent, with MHPG excretion, for instance, decreased, unchanged, or increased in ADHD (69). Research establishing a positive association between classroom performance and epinephrine (EPI) excretion (70), along with reports of stimulant-induced EPI release and longstanding observations of cognitive enhancing effects of systemically administered EPI, suggest a possible role for EPI in attention. Several reviews have discussed how altered interaction of the adrenergic and noradrenergic systems might contribute to symptoms of ADHD (66,67,71). Although studies of baseline EPI excretion have not found differences between ADHD and control groups, three studies (72–74) have found substantially lower rates of EPI excretion during cognitive testing in ADHD patients compared to normal controls. In studies examining the effects of amphetamine or methylphenidate in patients with ADHD, both drugs increased EPI excretion, but relatively smaller adrenomedullary responses were seen in patients compared to controls following acute (75) or chronic (76) dosing. A similar reduced adrenomedullary response was observed in children with ADHD during hypoglycemic challenge when plasma levels of EPI were measured. Thus, the finding of a blunted EPI response in ADHD has been seen consistently across a number of situations. In the most recent study (72), the blunted response appeared to be specific to the inattention component or domain of ADHD. Further work in this area appears warranted: It would not be surprising if genetically determined variations in the functioning of each of the catecholamines contributed some part to one or more of the component behaviors of ADHD.

Autism

As one of the two major components of the stress response system (58), the sympathetic/adrenomedullary system has been of interest in autism owing to the hyperarousal, hyperactivity, and overreaction to novel situations often seen in autism. It should be mentioned that the HPA axis, the other major component of the stress response (Figure 6.1.1.7), has also been well studied in autism. The functioning of the sympathetic/adrenomedullary system has been assessed through measurements of NE and EPI in plasma or urine. In addition, plasma and urine levels of the major NE metabolites, MHPG, and VMA have been determined. Serum levels of dopamine-β-hydroxylase—the synthetic enzyme secreted along with NE from sympathetic neurons—also have been studied (77). In nearly all cases, indices that reflect basal functioning of the sympathetic/adrenomedullary system were found to be normal in patients with autism. On the other hand, most of the studies measuring indices of acute stress response have found elevations in patients with autism when they are exposed to the stress of a venipuncture or neuropsychological test. Taken together, the data support the idea that stress response systems are hyperresponsive when individuals with autism are stressed, but that autistic patients are not in a chronic state of hyperarousal. Findings from studies of HPA axis function are consistent with the sympathetic/adrenomedullary results, and support the same conclusions.

The apparent increased response to stressors could result from a difference in the level of perceived stress, an overelicitation of the physiologic response, or an abnormality in the stress response systems themselves. It will be difficult to determine whether the individual with autism experiences a greater threat, if the response to the threat is less well regulated, or both. Despite the difficulties encountered in stress response research in autism, further research in this area is warranted, given the clinical relevance and possible etiologic nature of alterations in this area.

GLUTAMATERGIC SYSTEM

Glutamatergic Neural Transmission/ Neuroanatomy

Glutamatergic neurons are widely distributed throughout the brain (see Figure 6.1.1.1). Prominent glutamatergic pathways are the cortico-cortical projections, connections between thalamus and cortex, and projections from cortex to striatum (extrapyramidal pathway) and to brain stem/spinal cord (pyramidal pathway) (78).

Glutamate acts at three different types of inotropic receptors (Figure 6.1.1.8) and at a family of G-protein–coupled (metabotropic) receptors (79,80). Binding of glutamate to the inotropic receptor opens an ion channel allowing the influx of

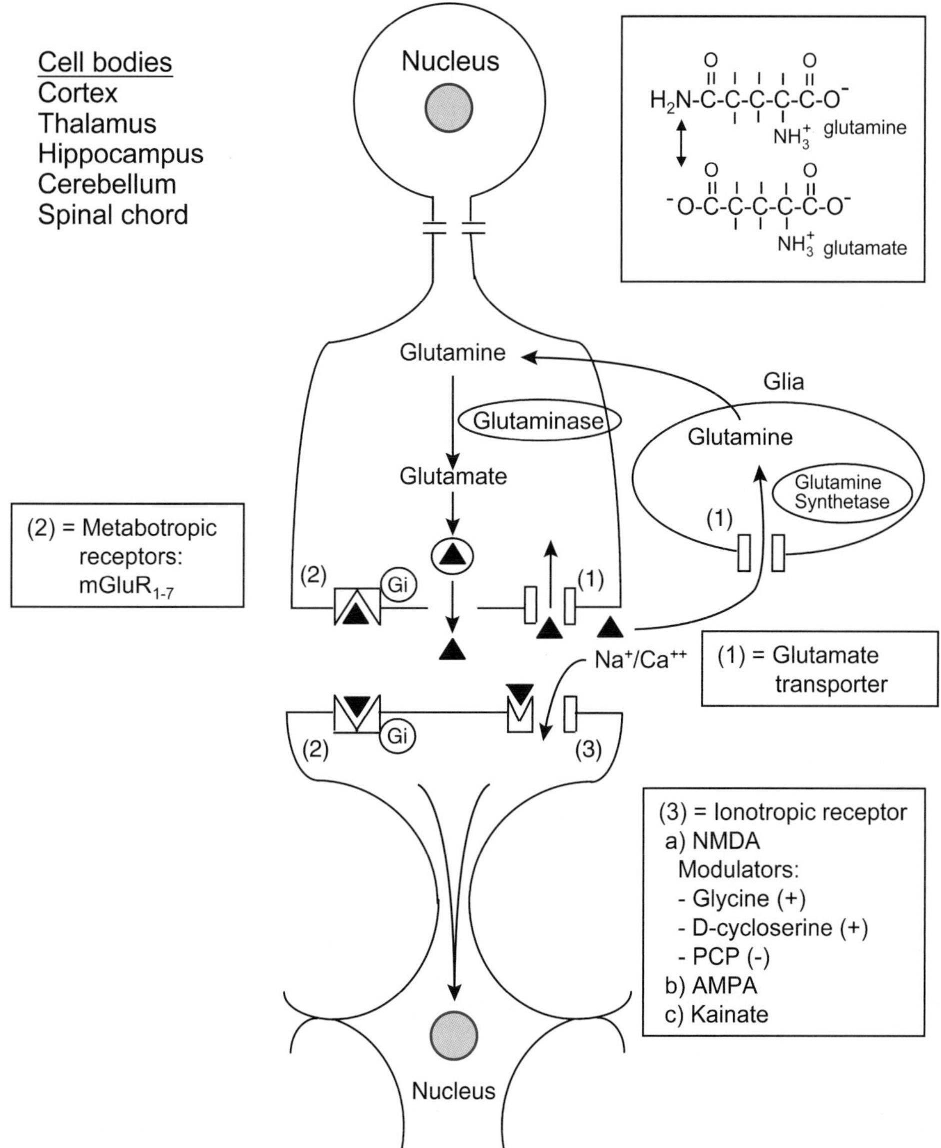

FIGURE 6.1.1.8. Glutamatergic neurotransmission. Diagram of the glutamatergic neuron with the pertinent processes of neural transmission and metabolism depicted. Intraneuronal glutamate is taken up into vesicles by the vesicular glutamate transporter. Released glutamate can stimulate pre- and postsynaptic receptors and be taken up by the membrane glutamate transporter (1). The glutamate–glutamine shunt through glial cells is an importance source of releasable glutamate. An **inset** depicts the interconversion of glutamate (glutamic acid) and glutamine.

Na^+ and Ca^{2+} into the cell. NMDA receptors bind glutamate and *N*-methyl-D-aspartate. The receptor is comprised of two different subunits: NMDAR1 (seven variants) and NMDAR2 (four variants). The NMDA receptor is highly regulated at several sites. For example, the receptor is virtually ineffective unless a ligand binds to the glycine site and it is blocked by binding of ligands (e.g., ketamine and phencyclidine [PCP]) to the PCP site inside the channel. AMPA receptors bind glutamate, AMPA, and quisqualic acid, whereas kainate receptors bind glutamate and kainic acid.

The metabotropic glutamate receptor family includes at least seven different types of G-protein–coupled receptors (mGluR1–7). They are linked to different second messenger systems and lead to the increase of intracellular Ca^{2+} or the decrease of cyclic AMP. The increase of intracellular Ca^{2+} leads to the phosphorylation of target proteins in the cell. Glutamate is removed from the synapse by high-affinity reuptake; two transporter proteins are expressed in glial cells and one in neurons (Figure 6.1.1.8). After uptake into glia, glutamate is converted to glutamine by glutamine synthetase. Glutamine can then diffuse back into the neuron to replenish neuronal glutamate after hydrolysis by mitochondrial glutaminase completing this cycle, termed the glutamine–glutamate shunt.

Glutamate has an effect on many brain functions. For example, glutamatergic neurons and NMDA receptors in the hippocampus are important in the creation of long-term potentiation, a crucial component in the formation of memory (81). Excess stimulation of glutamatergic receptors, as seen in seizures or stroke, can lead to unregulated Ca^{2+} influx and neuronal damage (82–84). Decreased glutamatergic function is thought to be involved in the creation of psychotic symptoms.

GLUTAMATERGIC PHARMACODYNAMICS

Glutamate appears ineffective at the NMDA receptor unless glycine or serine is bound at the strychnine-insensitive glycine modulatory site. PCP and ketamine can block the activity of the NMDA receptor by binding to the PCP site within the NMDA-associated ion channel. Ketamine and PCP can induce psychotic symptoms, though ketamine may prove to be useful therapeutically in certain circumstances. Conversely, serine, *d*-cycloserine, glycine, or inhibitors of glycine uptake have been reported to be useful in decreasing psychotic and/or negative symptoms in schizophrenia (85–87); however, more recent trials have not been impressive in this regard (88).

Antagonists at the AMPA receptor are being studied as possible therapeutic agents in infantile seizures, while ampakines or positive modulators of the receptor complex may offer a fruitful approach in schizophrenia. Investigation of various ways to manipulate glutamatergic functioning in schizophrenia will remain an active area of research (89) and advances may have relevance to autism and early-onset psychosis.

Biologic Psychiatry of Glutamate

Schizophrenia

Although a hypoglutamatergic theory of schizophrenia has been widely touted, the theory is based mainly on consideration of the opposing interrelationships between the dopaminergic and glutamatergic systems and on the psychotomimetic effects of glutamatergic agents, including PCP and ketamine. Postmortem brain research has yet to yield consistent findings with respect to glutamatergic markers in schizophrenia.

Tourette Syndrome

In the one study of central excitatory amino acids in TS, postmortem brain levels of glutamate were lowered in the three projection areas of the subthalamic nucleus (40); it was hypothesized that this might lead to disinhibition of the thalamocortical circuit. This would tend to place TS in the group of hyperkinetic movement disorders, including Huntington's disorder and hemiballismus. As reviewed by Swerdlow and Young (90), further research is needed to clarify basal ganglia functioning in TS. Imaging studies (91) and postmortem research have provided interesting leads to consider with respect to the functioning of cortico-striato-pallido-thalamocortical pathways.

GABAergic SYSTEM

GABAergic Neural Transmission/ Neuroanatomy

GABAergic neurons can be divided into two groups (Figure 6.1.1.1): (a) short-ranging neurons (also called interneurons or local circuit neurons) in the cortex, thalamus, striatum, cerebellum, and spinal cord; and (b) medium- and long-ranging neurons in the basal ganglia, septum, and substantia nigra.

GABA acts at two types of receptors, the $GABA_A$ and $GABA_B$ receptors. The $GABA_A$ receptor is a receptor–channel complex comprised of five subunits (92). Activation leads to the opening of the channel, allowing chloride ions to enter the cell, resulting in decreased excitability. Five distinct classes of subunits and multiple variations in the composition of the $GABA_A$ receptor are known. The receptor can be modulated by benzodiazepines (BZs) at the BZ subunit and by barbiturates and ethanol near the chloride channel (Figure 6.1.1.9). The BZ site is further subclassified into α_1, α_2, and α_3 and four types.

The $GABA_B$ receptor is a G-protein–coupled receptor with similarity to the metabotropic glutamate receptor (93,94). The $GABA_B$ receptor is linked to G_i (decreasing cyclic AMP and opening of K+ channels) and G_o (closing Ca^{2+} channels). GABA is removed from the synapse by a sodium-dependent GABA uptake transporter (Figure 6.1.1.9). Cortical and thalamic GABAergic neurons are crucial for the inhibition of excitatory neurons.

GABAergic Pharmacodynamics

Positive modulation of $GABA_A$ receptors is beneficial in the treatment of anxiety disorders, insomnia, and agitation—most likely because of a general inhibition of neuronal activity. The benzodiazepines, including lorazepam, clonazepam, and midazolam, are widely used to treat anxiety despite problems with tolerance and dependence. Somewhat more α_1-specific agents such as zolpidem (Ambien) and related compounds are useful in reducing sleep latency and increasing overall time asleep, and appear to do so without tolerance or rebound effects even after long-term treatment. Furthermore, GABAergic agonists such as benzodiazepines or barbiturates are efficacious in the treatment and prevention of seizures (95). The wide and age-old use of alcohol for self-medication of a number of life's problems is an enduring testament to the importance of the GABAergic system.

GABAergic Biologic Psychiatry

The importance of GABA in basal ganglia neural transmission has led to treatment studies of GABAergic agents (96) in TS. However, studies of CSF GABA have not found group differences in patients with TS and studies of postmortem tissue have not revealed alterations in GABA concentrations. A

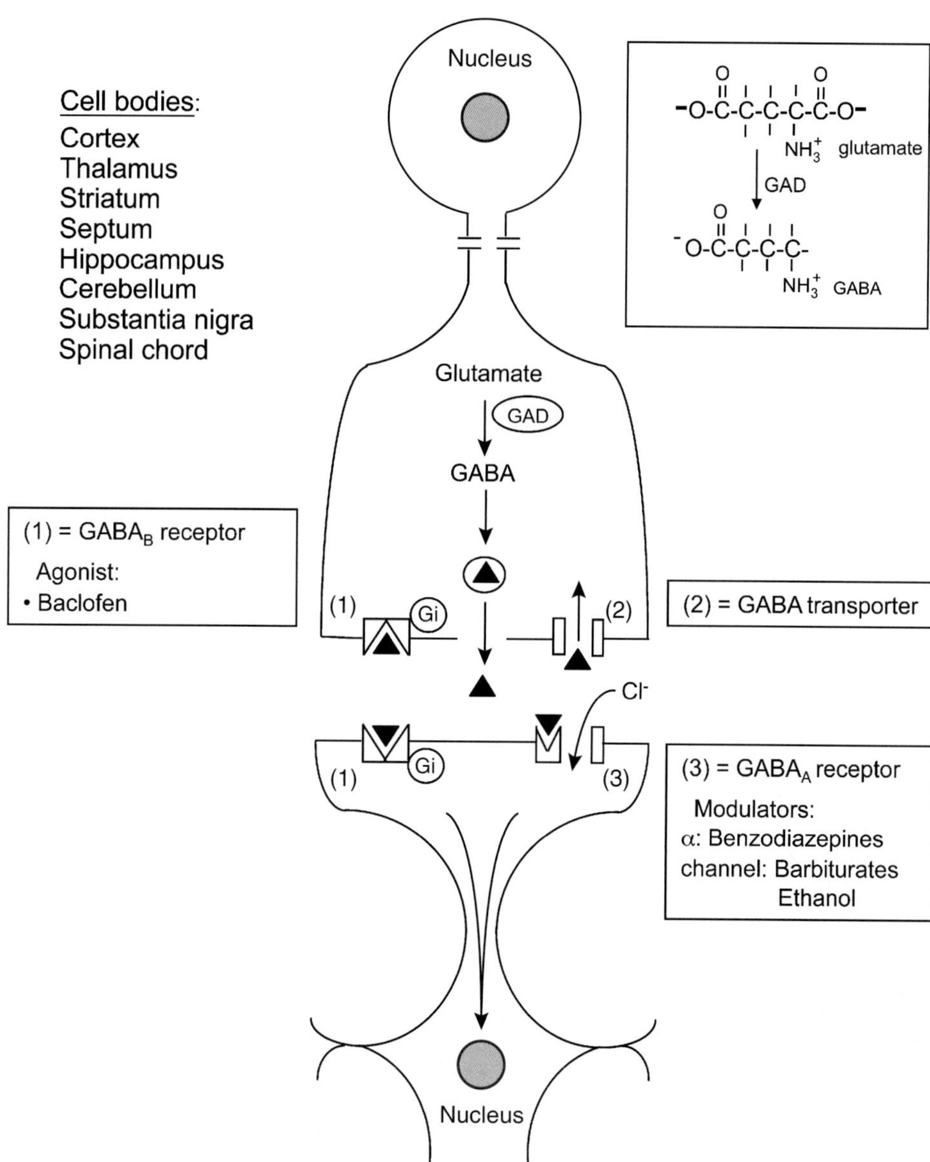

FIGURE 6.1.1.9. GABAergic neurotransmission. Diagram of the GABAergic neuron with the pertinent processes of neural transmission and metabolism depicted. Glutamate serves as the major precursor for GABA, with conversion to GABA occurring through the action of glutamic acid decarboxylase (GAD). An **inset** depicts the conversion of glutamate (glutamic acid) to GABA. Released GABA can stimulate pre- and postsynaptic receptors and be taken up by the membrane GABA transporter (2).

series of recent studies have indicated that cortical GABA may be reduced in depression and that levels may normalize during treatment with antidepressants (97,98).

CHOLINERGIC SYSTEM

Cholinergic Neural Transmission/ Neuroanatomy

Cholinergic neurons in the CNS are either wide-ranging projection neurons or short-ranging interneurons. Projection neurons in the basal forebrain (septum, diagonal band, nucleus basalis of Meynert) project to the entire cortex, hippocampus, and amygdala, and projection neurons located in the brain stem project predominantly to the thalamus. Cholinergic interneurons in the striatum modulate the activity of GABAergic striatal neurons.

Acetylcholine (Ach) acts at two different types of cholinergic receptors. Muscarinic receptors bind ACh as well as other agonists (muscarine, pilocarpine, bethanechol) and antagonists (atropine, scopolamine). There are at least five different types of muscarinic receptors (M1–5). All have slow response times and can be coupled to G-proteins and a variety of second messenger systems. When activated, the final effect can be to open or close channels for K^+, Ca^{2+}, or Cl^- (99).

Nicotinic receptors are less abundant than the muscarinic type in the CNS. They bind ACh as well as agonists such as nicotine (Figure 6.1.1.10) or antagonists such as *d*-tubocurarine. The fast-acting, ionotropic nicotinic receptor allows influx of $Na^+ > K^+ > Ca^{2+}$ into the cell. ACh is removed from the synapse through hydrolysis into acetyl CoA and choline by the enzyme acetylcholinesterase (AChE).

ACh modulates attention, novelty seeking, and memory via the basal forebrain projections to the cortex and limbic structures. Anticholinergic delirium and Alzheimer's disease are examples of a cholinergic-deficit state (100,101). Furthermore, cholinergic interneurons modulate striatal neurons by opposing the effects of dopamine.

Cholinergic Pharmacodynamics

Stimulation of the fast-acting, ionotropic nicotinic receptor with nicotine leads to improvements in attention; however,

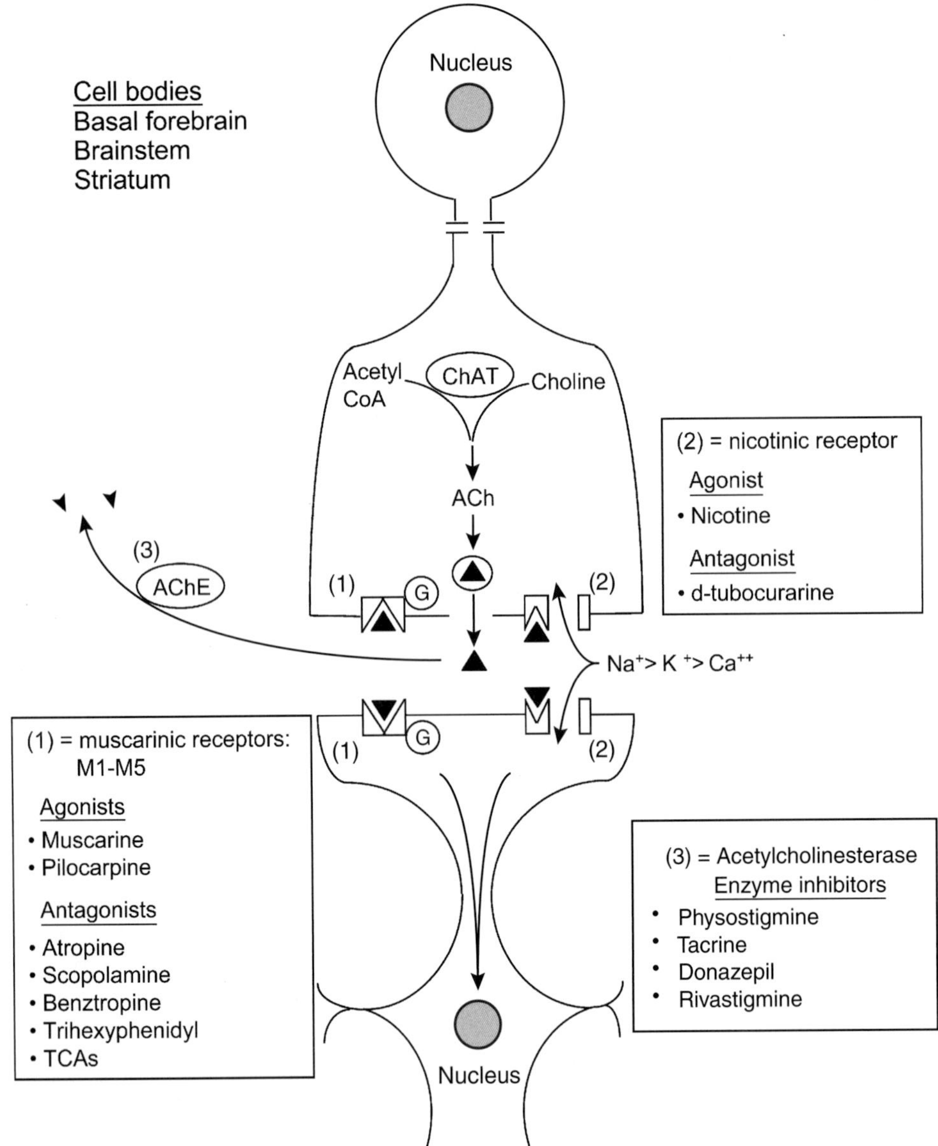

FIGURE 6.1.1.10. Cholinergic neurotransmission. Diagram of the cholinergic neuron with the pertinent processes of neural transmission and metabolism depicted. Acetylcholine (Ach) is formed by the action of choline acetyltransferase (ChAT), and is metabolized after release by the enzyme acetylcholine esterase (AChE) (3).

the addictive properties of nicotine have greatly restricted its use in attentional problems. The acetylcholinesterase inhibitors (AChEIs) are widely used to increase cholinergic function in a more general manner. The AChEIs are most often used to treat the dementia of Alzheimer's; benefits have also been reported in Parkinson and Down syndromes. Like Alzheimer's, the latter disorder appears to have an associated cholinergic deficit. It remains to be seen whether AChEIs like rivastigmine and donepezil will prove of use in treating attention deficits in ADHD and autism.

Cholinergic Biologic Psychiatry

Autism

Studies of peripheral cholinergic markers in autism are limited. However, several studies have reported decreased nicotinic receptor binding in postmortem brain tissue despite relatively normal levels of the presynaptic markers choline acetyltransferase (ChAT) and AChE, and normal muscarinic receptor binding (102). Thus, epibatidine binding to the $a4\beta_2$ nicotinic receptor was reported to be markedly lower throughout the cortex in brain of subjects with autism. Replication of the finding is necessary, but the results to date raise intriguing issues about the possible etiologic role of altered cholinergic functioning during development and the possible therapeutic effects of early manipulation of the cholinergic system.

Attention-Deficit Hyperactivity Disorder

The cholinergic system has been hypothesized to be involved in ADHD, based on its important role in attention and cognition, the high rate of smoking in ADHD (possible self-medication phenomenon), high rates of gestational exposure to maternal smoking, the enhancing effects of nicotine on catecholaminergic systems, and the limited data available on therapeutic effects of nicotinic agents in ADHD. It is not clear whether cholinergic agents, including the AChEIs, will prove to be useful in treating ADHD-related problems.

Tourette Syndrome

The importance of ACh in basal ganglia neural transmission has led to treatment studies using choline and other cholinergic agents (103,104). However, studies of CSF acetylcholinesterase have not found group differences. Though reports of increased red blood cell choline have appeared (105) and muscarinic receptor binding in white blood cells has been reported to be drastically lowered in TS (106), neither observation can be considered definitive.

ACKNOWLEDGMENT

The authors thank Dr. Stephan Heckers of Vanderbilt University for his contributions to an earlier version of this manuscript, and for allowing them to modify and use some of the figures presented.

References

1. Andreasen NC: Linking mind and brain in the study of mental illnesses: a project for a scientific psychopathology. *Science* 275(5306):1586–1593, 1997.
2. Kandel ER, Squire LR: Neuroscience: breaking down scientific barriers to the study of brain and mind. *Science* 290(5494):1113–1120, 2000.
3. Mesulam MM: *Principles of Behavioral Neurology.* New York, Oxford University Press, 2000.
4. Langer SZ: 25 years since the discovery of presynaptic receptors: present knowledge and future perspectives. *Trends Pharmacol Sci* 18(3):95–99, 1997.
5. Lester HA, Cao Y, Mager S: Listening to neurotransmitter transporters. *Neuron* 17(5):807–810, 1996.
6. Duman RS, Heninger GR, Nestler EJ: A molecular and cellular theory of depression [see comments]. *Arch Gen Psychiatry* 54(7):597–606, 1997.
7. Hyman S: Mental illness: genetically complex disorders of neural circuitry and neural communication. *Neuron* 28(2):321–323, 2000.
8. Heninger GR: Special challenges in the investigation of the neurobiology of mental illness. In: Charney DS, Nestler EJ, Bunney BS (eds): *Neurobiology of Mental Illness.* New York, Oxford University Press, 1999, pp. 89–99.
9. Burmeister M: Basic concepts in the study of diseases with complex genetics. *Biol Psychiatry* 45(5):522–532, 1999.
10. Collier DA, Curran S, Asherson P: Mission: not impossible? Candidate gene studies in child psychiatric disorders. *Mol Psychiatry* 5(5):457–460, 2000.
11. Petronis A, Gottesman, II, Crow TJ, et al.: Psychiatric epigenetics: a new focus for the new century. *Mol Psychiatry* 5(4):342–346, 2000.
12. van Praag HM: Over the mainstream: diagnostic requirements for biological psychiatric research. *Psychiatry Res* 72(3):201–212, 1997.
13. Leckman JF, Zhang H, Alsobrook JP, Pauls DL: Symptom dimensions in obsessive-compulsive disorder: toward quantitative phenotypes. *Am J Med Genet* 105(1):28–30, 2001.
14. Almasy L, Blangero J: Endophenotypes as quantitative risk factors for psychiatric disease: rationale and study design. *Am J Med Genet* 105(1):42–44, 2001.
15. Krueger RF: The structure of common mental disorders. *Arch Gen Psychiatry* 56(10):921–926, 1999.
16. Wittchen HU, Hofler M, Merikangas K: Toward the identification of core psychopathological processes? *Arch Gen Psychiatry* 56(10):929–931, 1999.
17. Hendren RL, De Backer I, Pandina GJ: Review of neuroimaging studies of child and adolescent psychiatric disorders from the past 10 years. *J Am Acad Child Adolesc Psychiatry* 39(7):815–828, 2000.
18. Anderson GM, Cook EH: Pharmacogenetics: promise and potential in child and adolescent psychiatry. *Child Adolesc Psychiatr Clin N Am* 9(1): 23–42, viii, 2000.
19. Cramer AO, Waldorp LJ, van der Maas HL, Borsboom D: Complex realities require complex theories: refining and extending the network approach to mental disorders. *Behav Brain Sciences* 33:178–193, 2010.
20. Bailey A, Phillips W, Rutter M: Autism: toward an integration of clinical, genetic, neuropsychological, and neurobiological perspectives. *J Child Psychol Psychiatry* 37(1):89–126, 1996.
21. Dawson G, Ashman SB, Carver LJ: The role of early experience in shaping behavioral and brain development and its implications for social policy. *Dev Psychopathol* 12(4):695–712, 2000.
22. Skuse DH: Behavioural neuroscience and child psychopathology: insights from model systems. *J Child Psychol Psychiatry* 41(1):3–31, 2000.
23. Jacobs BL, Azmitia EC: Structure and function of the brain serotonin system. *Physiol Rev* 72(1):165–229, 1992.
24. Julius D: Molecular biology of serotonin receptors. *Annu Rev Neurosci* 14:335–60, 1991.
25. Lucki I: The spectrum of behaviors influenced by serotonin. *Biol Psychiatry* 44(3):151–162, 1998.
26. Murphy DL, Andrews AM, Wichems CH, Li Q, Tohda M, Greenberg B: Brain serotonin neurotransmission: an overview and update with an emphasis on serotonin subsystem heterogeneity, multiple receptors, interactions with other neurotransmitter systems, and consequent implications for understanding the actions of serotonergic drugs. *J Clin Psychiatry* 59(Suppl 15):4–12, 1998.
27. Rubenstein JL: Development of serotonergic neurons and their projections. *Biol Psychiatry* 44:145–150, 1998.
28. Hanley HG, Stahl SM, Freedman DX: Hyperserotonemia and amine metabolites in autistic and retarded children. *Arch Gen Psychiatry* 34(5): 521–531, 1977.
29. Schain RJ, Freedman DX: Studies on 5-hydroxyindole metabolism in autistic and other mentally retarded children. *J Pediatr* 58:315–320, 1961.
30. McDougle CJ, Naylor ST, Cohen DJ, Volkmar FR, Heninger GR, Price LH: A double-blind, placebo-controlled study of fluvoxamine in adults with autistic disorder. *Arch Gen Psychiatry* 53(11):1001–1008, 1996.
31. McDougle CJ, Naylor ST, Cohen DJ, Aghajanian GK, Heninger GR, Price LH: Effects of tryptophan depletion in drug-free adults with autistic disorder. *Arch Gen Psychiatry* 53(11):993–1000, 1996.
32. Anderson GM, Hoshino Y: Neurochemical studies of autism. In: Cohen DJ, Donnellan AM (eds): *Handbook of Autism and Pervasive Developmental Disorders.* 2nd ed. New York, Wiley, 166–191, 1997.
33. Anderson GM: Studies on the neurochemistry of autism. In: Bauman ML, Kemper TL (eds): *The Neurobiology of Autism.* Baltimore, Johns Hopkins University Press, 227–242, 1994.
34. McBride PA, Anderson GM, Hertzig ME, et al.: Serotonergic responsivity in male young adults with autistic disorder: results of a pilot study. *Arch Gen Psychiatry* 46(3):213–221, 1989.
35. Cook EH Jr, Arora RC, Anderson GM, et al.: Platelet serotonin studies in hyperserotonemic relatives of children with autistic disorder. *Life Sci* 52(25):2005–2015, 1993.
36. Murphy DG, Daly E, Schmitz N, et al.: Cortical serotonin 5-HT2A receptor binding and social communication in adults with Asperger's syndrome: an in vivo SPECT study. *Am J Psychiatry* 163(5):934–936, 2006.
37. Grad LR, Pelcovitz D, Olson M, Matthews M, Grad GJ: Obsessive-compulsive symptomatology in children with Tourette's syndrome. *J Am Acad Child Adolesc Psychiatry* 26(1):69–73, 1987.
38. Leckman JF, Goodman WK, Anderson GM, et al.: Cerebrospinal fluid biogenic amines in obsessive compulsive disorder, Tourette's syndrome, and healthy controls. *Neuropsychopharmacology* 12(1):73–86, 1995.
39. Anderson GM, Pollak ES, Chatterjee D, Leckman JF, Riddle MA, Cohen DJ: Brain monoamines and amino acids in Gilles de la Tourette's syndrome: a preliminary study of subcortical regions. *Arch Gen Psychiatry* 49(7):584–586, 1992.
40. Anderson GM, Pollak ES, Chatterjee D, Leckman JF, Riddle MA, Cohen DJ: Postmortem analysis of subcortical monoamines and amino acids in Tourette syndrome. *Adv Neurol* 58:123–133, 1992.
41. Baldessarini RJ, Tarazi FI: Brain dopamine receptors: a primer on their current status, basic and clinical. *Harv Rev Psychiatry* 3(6):301–325, 1996.
42. Missale C, Nash SR, Robinson SW, Jaber M, Caron MG: Dopamine receptors: from structure to function. *Physiol Rev* 78(1):189–225, 1998.
43. Diana M: Drugs of abuse and dopamine cell activity. *Adv Pharmacol* 42:998–1001, 1998.
44. Koob GF: Circuits, drugs, and drug addiction. *Adv Pharmacol* 42:978–982, 1998.
45. Goldman-Rakic PS: The cortical dopamine system: role in memory and cognition. *Adv Pharmacol* 42:707–711, 1998.
46. Carey WB: A suggested solution to the confusion in attention deficit diagnoses. *Clin Pediatr (Phila)* 27(7):348–349, 1988.
47. Faraone SV, Doyle AE: The nature and heritability of attention-deficit/hyperactivity disorder. *Child Adolesc Psychiatr Clin N Am* 10:299–316, 2001.
48. Castellanos FX, Giedd JN, Marsh WL, et al.: Quantitative brain magnetic resonance imaging in attention-deficit hyperactivity disorder. *Arch Gen Psychiatry* 53(7):607–616, 1996.
49. Cohen DJ, Leckman JF: Developmental psychopathology and neurobiology of Tourette's syndrome. *J Am Acad Child Adolesc Psychiatry* 33(1):2–15, 1994.
50. Singer HS, Wendlandt JT: Neurochemistry and synaptic neurotransmission in Tourette syndrome. *Adv Neurol* 85:163–178, 2001.
51. Leckman JF, Riddle MA: Tourette's syndrome: when habit-forming systems form habits of their own? *Neuron* 28(2):349–354, 2000.
52. Singer HS, Hahn IH, Moran TH: Abnormal dopamine uptake sites in postmortem striatum from patients with Tourette's syndrome. *Ann Neurol* 30(4):558–562, 1991.
53. Wolf SS, Jones DW, Knable MB, et al.: Tourette syndrome: prediction of phenotypic variation in monozygotic twins by caudate nucleus D2 receptor binding. *Science* 273(5279):1225–1227, 1996.
54. Narayan M, Srinath S, Anderson GM, Meundi DB: Cerebrospinal fluid levels of homovanillic acid and 5-hydroxyindoleacetic acid in autism. *Biol Psychiatry* 33(8–9):630–635, 1993.
55. Minderaa RB, Anderson GM, Volkmar FR, Akkerhuis GW, Cohen DJ: Neurochemical study of dopamine functioning in autistic and normal subjects. *J Am Acad Child Adolesc Psychiatry* 28(2):190–194, 1989.
56. Aston-Jones G, Chiang C, Alexinsky T: Discharge of noradrenergic locus coeruleus neurons in behaving rats and monkeys suggests a role in vigilance. *Prog Brain Res* 88:501–520, 1991.
57. Arnsten AF: Catecholamine regulation of the prefrontal cortex. *J Psychopharmacol* 11(2):151–162, 1997.
58. Chrousos GP, Gold PW: The concepts of stress and stress system disorders: overview of physical and behavioral homeostasis. *JAMA* 267(9):1244–1252, 1992.

59. Charney DS: Monoamine dysfunction and the pathophysiology and treatment of depression. *J Clin Psychiatry* 59(Suppl 14):11–14, 1998.
60. Leckman JF, Hardin MT, Riddle MA, Stevenson J, Ort SI, Cohen DJ: Clonidine treatment of Gilles de la Tourette's syndrome. *Arch Gen Psychiatry* 48(4):324–328, 1991.
61. van Dijk JG, Koenderink M, Kramer CG, den Heijer JC, Roos RA: Non-invasive assessment of autonomic nervous function in Gilles de la Tourette syndrome. *Clin Neurol Neurosurg* 94(2):157–159, 1992.
62. Chappell PB, Leckman JF, Scahill LD, Hardin MT, Anderson G, Cohen DJ: Neuroendocrine and behavioral effects of the selective kappa agonist spiradoline in Tourette's syndrome: a pilot study. *Psychiatry Res* 47(3):267–280, 1993.
63. Chappell PB, McSwiggan-Hardin MT, Scahill L, et al.: Videotape tic counts in the assessment of Tourette's syndrome: stability, reliability, and validity. *J Am Acad Child Adolesc Psychiatry* 33(3):386–393, 1994.
64. Halperin JM, Newcorn JH, Koda VH, Pick L, McKay KE, Knott P: Noradrenergic mechanisms in ADHD children with and without reading disabilities: a replication and extension. *J Am Acad Child Adolesc Psychiatry* 36(12):1688–1697, 1997.
65. Ornitz EM, Gabikian P, Russell AT, Guthrie D, Hirano C, Gehricke JG: Affective valence and arousal in ADHD and normal boys during a startle habituation experiment. *J Am Acad Child Adolesc Psychiatry* 36(12):1698–1705, 1997.
66. Mefford IN, Potter WZ: A neuroanatomical and biochemical basis for attention deficit disorder with hyperactivity in children: a defect in tonic adrenaline mediated inhibition of locus coeruleus stimulation. *Med Hypotheses* 29(1):33–42, 1989.
67. Pliszka SR, McCracken JT, Maas JW: Catecholamines in attention-deficit hyperactivity disorder: current perspectives. *J Am Acad Child Adolesc Psychiatry* 35(3):264–272, 1996.
68. Arnsten AF, Steere JC, Hunt RD: The contribution of alpha 2-noradrenergic mechanisms of prefrontal cortical cognitive function. Potential significance for attention-deficit hyperactivity disorder. *Arch Gen Psychiatry* 53(5):448–455, 1996.
69. Baker GB, Bornstein RA, Douglass AB, Van Muyden JC, Ashton S, Bazylewich TL: Urinary excretion of MHPG and normetanephrine in attention deficit hyperactivity disorder. *Mol Chem Neuropathol* 18(1–2): 173–178, 1993.
70. Frankenhaeuser M: Behavior and circulating catecholamines. *Brain Res* 31(2):241–262, 1971.
71. McCracken JT: A two-part model of stimulant action on attention-deficit hyperactivity disorder in children. *J Neuropsychiatry Clin Neurosci* 3(2):201–209, 1991 Spring.
72. Anderson GM, Dover MA, Yang BP, et al.: Adrenomedullary function during cognitive testing in attention-deficit/hyperactivity disorder. *J Am Acad Child Adolesc Psychiatry* 39(5):635–643, 2000.
73. Hanna GL, Ornitz EM, Hariharan M: Urinary epinephrine excretion during intelligence testing in attention-deficit hyperactivity disorder and normal boys. *Biol Psychiatry* 40(6):553–555, 1996.
74. Pliszka SR, Maas JW, Javors MA, Rogeness GA, Baker J: Urinary catecholamines in attention-deficit hyperactivity disorder with and without comorbid anxiety. *J Am Acad Child Adolesc Psychiatry* 33(8):1165–1173, 1994.
75. Rapoport JL, Mikkelsen EJ, Ebert MH, Brown GL, Weise VK, Kopin IJ: Urinary catecholamines and amphetamine excretion in hyperactive and normal boys. *J Nerv Ment Dis* 166(10):731–737, 1978.
76. Elia J, Borcherding BG, Potter WZ, Mefford IN, Rapoport JL, Keysor CS: Stimulant drug treatment of hyperactivity: biochemical correlates. *Clin Pharmacol Ther* 48(1):57–66, 1990.
77. Minderaa RB, Anderson GM, Volkmar FR, Akkerhuis GW, Cohen DJ: Noradrenergic and adrenergic functioning in autism. *Biol Psychiatry* 36(4):237–241, 1994.
78. Ozawa S, Kamiya H, Tsuzuki K: Glutamate receptors in the mammalian central nervous system. *Prog Neurobiol* 54(5):581–618, 1998.
79. Nakanishi S: Molecular diversity of glutamate receptors and implications for brain function. *Science* 258(5082):597–603, 1992.
80. Nakanishi S, Nakajima Y, Masu M, et al.: Glutamate receptors: brain function and signal transduction. *Brain Res Brain Res Rev* 26(2–3):230–235, 1998.
81. Wilson MA, Tonegawa S: Synaptic plasticity, place cells and spatial memory: study with second generation knockouts. *Trends Neurosci* 20(3):102–106, 1997.
82. Coyle JT, Puttfarcken P: Oxidative stress, glutamate, and neurodegenerative disorders. *Science* 262(5134):689–695, 1993.
83. Loscher W: Pharmacology of glutamate receptor antagonists in the kindling model of epilepsy. *Prog Neurobiol* 54(6):721–741, 1998.
84. Dingledine R, McBain CJ, McNamara JO: Excitatory amino acid receptors in epilepsy. *Trends Pharmacol Sci* 11(8):334–338, 1990.
85. Farber NB, Newcomer JW, Olney JW: Glycine agonists: what can they teach us about schizophrenia? *Arch Gen Psychiatry* 56(1):13–17, 1999.
86. Goff DC, Tsai G, Levitt J, et al.: A placebo-controlled trial of D-cycloserine added to conventional neuroleptics in patients with schizophrenia. *Arch Gen Psychiatry* 56(1):21–27, 1999.
87. Heresco-Levy U, Ermilov M, Lichtenberg P, Bar G, Javitt DC: High-dose glycine added to olanzapine and risperidone for the treatment of schizophrenia. *Biol Psychiatry* 55(2):165–171, 2004.
88. Lane HY, Chang YC, Liu YC, Chiu CC, Tsai GE: Sarcosine or D-serine add-on treatment for acute exacerbation of schizophrenia: a randomized, double-blind, placebo-controlled study. *Arch Gen Psychiatry* 62(11): 1196–1204, 2005.
89. Moghaddam B: Targeting metabotropic glutamate receptors for treatment of the cognitive symptoms of schizophrenia. *Psychopharmacology (Berl)* 174(1):39–44, 2004.
90. Swerdlow NR, Young AB: Neuropathology in Tourette syndrome: an update. *Adv Neurol* 85:151–161, 2001.
91. Peterson BS: Neuroimaging studies of Tourette syndrome: a decade of progress. *Adv Neurol* 85:179–196, 2001.
92. Lüddens H, Korpi E: GABAA receptors: pharmacology, behavioral roles, and motor disorders. *Neuroscientist* 2:15–23, 1996.
93. Bettler B, Kaupmann K, Bowery N: GABAB receptors: drugs meet clones. *Curr Opin Neurobiol* 8(3):345–350, 1998.
94. Kaupmann K, Huggel K, Heid J, et al.: Expression cloning of GABA(B) receptors uncovers similarity to metabotropic glutamate receptors. *Nature* 386(6622):239–246, 1997.
95. Bazil CW, Pedley TA: Advances in the medical treatment of epilepsy. *Annu Rev Med* 49:135–162, 1998.
96. Mondrup K, Dupont E, Braendgaard H: Progabide in the treatment of hyperkinetic extrapyramidal movement disorders. *Acta Neurol Scand* 72(3):341–343, 1985.
97. Sanacora G, Mason GF, Krystal JH: Impairment of GABAergic transmission in depression: new insights from neuroimaging studies. *Crit Rev Neurobiol* 14(1):23–45, 2000.
98. Sanacora G, Mason GF, Rothman DL, Krystal JH: Increased occipital cortex GABA concentrations in depressed patients after therapy with selective serotonin reuptake inhibitors. *Am J Psychiatry* 159(4):663–665, 2002.
99. Bonner TI: The molecular basis of muscarinic receptor diversity. *Trends Neurosci* 12(4):148–151, 1989.
100. Geula C: Abnormalities of neural circuitry in Alzheimer's disease: hippocampus and cortical cholinergic innervation. *Neurology* 51(1 Suppl 1): S18–S29; discussion S65–S17, 1998.
101. Giacobini E: Cholinergic foundations of Alzheimer's disease therapy. *J Physiol Paris* 92(3–4):283–287, 1998.
102. Perry EK, Lee ML, Martin-Ruiz CM, et al.: Cholinergic activity in autism: abnormalities in the cerebral cortex and basal forebrain. *Am J Psychiatry* 158(7):1058–1066, 2001.
103. Dursun SM, Hewitt S, King AL, Reveley MA: Treatment of blepharospasm with nicotine nasal spray. *Lancet* 348(9019):60, 1996.
104. Stahl SM, Berger PA: Physostigmine in Tourette syndrome: evidence for cholinergic underactivity. *Am J Psychiatry* 138(2):240–242, 1981.
105. Sallee FR, Kopp U, Hanin I: Controlled study of erythrocyte choline in Tourette syndrome. *Biol Psychiatry* 31(12):1204–1212, 1992.
106. Rabey JM, Lewis A, Graff E, Korczyn AD: Decreased (3H) quinuclidinyl benzilate binding to lymphocytes in Gilles de la Tourette syndrome. *Biol Psychiatry* 31(9):889–895, 1992.

CHAPTER 6.1.2 ■ CLINICAL AND DEVELOPMENTAL ASPECTS OF PHARMACOKINETICS AND DRUG INTERACTIONS

JESSICA R. OESTERHELD, RICHARD I. SHADER, AND ANDRÉS MARTIN

OVERVIEW

In the first part of this chapter, the concept of pharmacokinetics is differentiated from pharmacodynamics, and basic clinical pharmacokinetic principles that are shared by children, adolescents, and adults are reviewed, including therapeutic drug monitoring (TDM). Next, the pharmacokinetic differences that distinguish pediatric populations from adults are examined, highlighting the ontogeny of individual cytochromes P450 (CYPs), intestinal and hepatic influx and efflux transporters, and UDP-glucuronosyltransferases (UGTs). Finally, since one of the more clinically relevant applications of pharmacokinetic principles is in helping to understand (and at times to predict) important drug interactions, emphasis has been placed on presenting basic principles that underlie drug interactions and the real-world strategies to prevent them. This chapter serves as a complement to the following and related chapter, in which specific drug classes and individual agents are discussed in detail.

PHARMACOKINETICS AND PHARMACODYNAMICS

Pharmacokinetic principles relate to the handling and disposition of drugs within the body (i.e., those biologic processes that lead to changes over time in drug concentration in body tissues and fluids). In general, drug concentration in a target organ determines how long a drug's therapeutic and adverse effects will last. Changes during development in the processes of drug absorption, distribution, metabolism, and excretion may have an impact on the delivery of drug to target tissues. By contrast, pharmacodynamic principles are concerned with the biochemical and physiologic effects of drugs at their effect sites, with their specific mechanisms of action. Stated succinctly, pharmacokinetics refers to what the body does to a drug and pharmacodynamics to what a drug does to the body (Figure 6.1.2.1). The effects of a medication may change during development, as brain regions or neurotransmitter systems develop and mature at different rates. These developmental changes in neurochemical systems (pharmacodynamic systems) can influence both therapeutic response and side effect profile. For example: (1) Compared to adults, adolescents have a higher risk of dystonic reactions to conventional antipsychotics agents (1,2); (2) prepubertal children appear to be at a higher risk for the activating side effects of the serotonin selective reuptake inhibitors (SSRIs) (3); and (3) developmental differences in the maturation of noradrenergic pathways may explain, at least in part, why tricyclic antidepressants are less effective in children with depression as compared to adults (4). Taken together, these findings suggest that major neurochemical systems that are altered by psychotropic drug treatments (e.g., dopaminergic, serotonergic, and noradrenergic, respectively) are subject to age-related effects.

BASIC PRINCIPLES

An understanding of pharmacokinetic principles is important for safe and effective patient care. Pharmacokinetic factors are often critical in a variety of clinical decisions, such as choosing between agents within a same drug class, switching between different medication preparations, adjusting dosages, preventing drug interactions, or correctly utilizing and interpreting therapeutic drug levels.

Pharmacokinetics can be conceptualized as having four functionally distinct phases: absorption, distribution, metabolism, and excretion. Absorption and distribution are primarily responsible for determining the speed of onset of drug effect, while the processes of metabolism and excretion terminate the action of the pharmacologic agent by removing the active form of the drug from the body. Taken together, these four phases help to determine the duration of drug activity (5).

Once a drug gains entry to the bloodstream, it is diluted in the plasma and bound at varying degrees to plasma proteins. The drug, usually protein bound, is then either excreted by the kidneys or carried to the liver and transformed to a more water-soluble (and usually inactive) metabolite, which

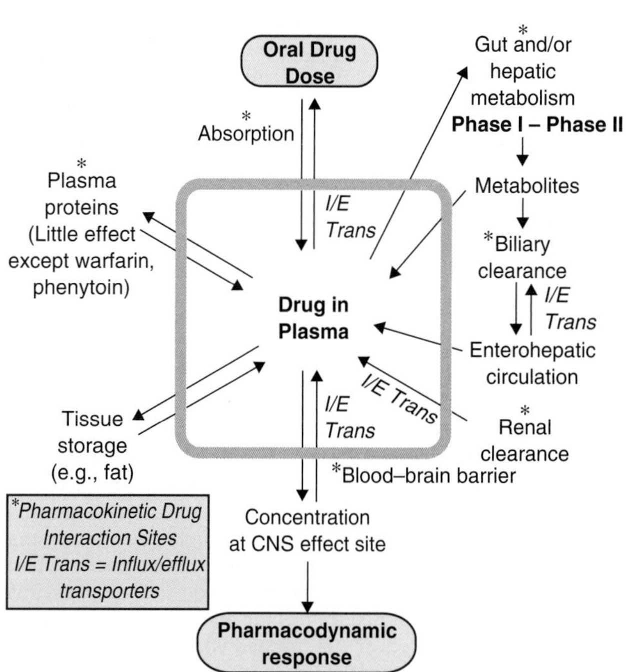

FIGURE 6.1.2.1. Pharmacokinetics and pharmacodynamics of a CNS drug.

can then be excreted in urine or bile. This complicated and interdependent series of events is designed to reduce the effect of foreign molecules, with the ultimate goal of eliminating the drug from the body (Figure 6.1.2.1). If the dose of a drug is sufficiently large to withstand this "pharmacokinetic assault," then a fraction of a psychoactive drug will cross the blood–brain barrier and endure to produce its pharmacodynamic effect (5). The last step of this process presumes that the drug in question is not a substrate for blood–brain barrier transport proteins that keep certain entities from reaching the brain.

LINEAR AND NONLINEAR PHARMACOKINETICS

A basic working knowledge of key pharmacokinetics principles is relevant to the clinical practice of pediatric psychopharmacology to understand the fate of administered drugs. Some psychotropic medications follow *first-order* (or *linear*) *kinetics,* in which the amount of drug eliminated is proportional to its amount circulating in the bloodstream. Once alterations during absorption have taken place, first-order kinetics provide close to a one-to-one relationship between changes in dosage and in plasma concentration. Such a linear association generally allows for clinically relevant predictions of the impact of a dose change on circulating drug levels (bupropion SR (6), oxcarbazepine (7)). By contrast, *zero-order* (or *nonlinear*) *kinetics* prevail when metabolizing or eliminating mechanisms are exceeded or saturated. This results in a fixed amount of drug being eliminated per unit of time, regardless of the plasma level. Certain drugs (paroxetine (8), nefazodone (9)) demonstrate zero-order kinetics at clinically relevant doses, making the relationship between dose changes and subsequent plasma levels much less predictable.

Vignette 1

A 12-year-old boy with a diagnosis of obsessive–compulsive disorder is not responding to 10 mg of paroxetine. Would an increase to 20 mg be appropriate? When the dosing of paroxetine is increased from 10 to 20 mg per day in children and teens, the plasma concentration can increase nearly sevenfold instead of a predicted twofold if the drug's kinetics were linear (8). Paroxetine inhibits its own catabolic pathway (CYP 2D6) and interferes with its own elimination. It could be prudent to increase the dose to 12.5 mg per day.

MULTIPLE DOSING TO AVERAGE STEADY-STATE CONCENTRATION

For drugs that follow first-order kinetics, the concepts of elimination half-life and of steady-state concentration are relevant for the practicing clinician. The elimination half-life ($t_{1/2}$) is the time required for the concentration of drug to decrease by one-half. This term is also referred to as the beta-phase half-life or the biologic half-life. We prefer the term elimination half-life since it makes this concept distinct from the half-life of absorption and the half-life of biologic activity. In clinical practice, this parameter is usually assessed by measuring the decay of plasma or serum drug concentration and is referred to as the plasma or serum half-life. Plasma half-life values can be useful when determining dosing intervals. At consistent dosing intervals, it is the plasma half-life that determines the average plasma *steady-state concentration* (C_{SS}). C_{SS} is reached when there is an equilibrium between the amount of drug ingested and the amount of drug eliminated, resulting in no net change in plasma concentration over time, and it is attained after four to five half-lives.

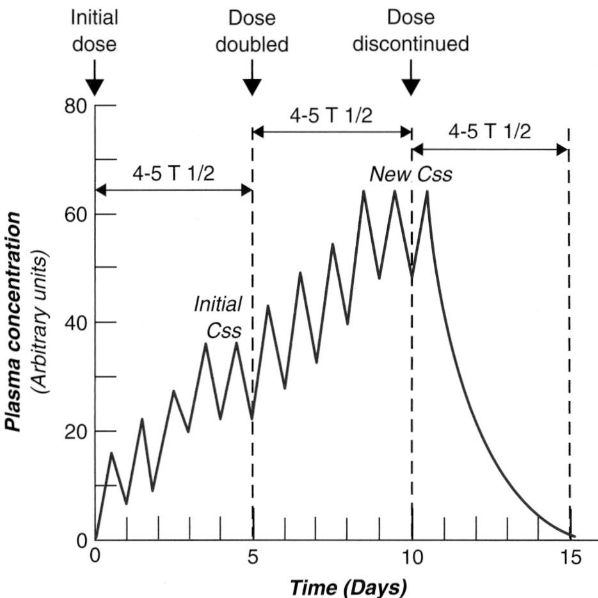

FIGURE 6.1.2.2. Multiple drug dosing leads to steady-state concentration.

The same time is necessary for reaching a new C_{SS} if daily dosing is increased or decreased or for complete elimination after drug intake is abruptly stopped (Figure 6.1.2.2). Most of the drugs commonly used in child psychiatry reach C_{SS}. However, in extensive CYP 2D6 metabolizers, neither psychostimulants nor atomoxetine does because of very short half-lives and therapeutic effectiveness at low concentrations. Carbamazepine, which induces its own metabolism, may take a much greater time to reach C_{SS}.

Vignette 2

A 14-year-old girl with major depression has failed a trial of fluoxetine, and she has been treated with 150 mg of twice-daily bupropion SR for 2 weeks. She has developed adverse cognitive effects. The clinician wishes to know if he discontinues the drug, how long before the adverse effects are likely to diminish. The half-life of bupropion SR in youth is approximately 12 hours (6), and in four to five half-lives or 2 to 3 days, it will be eliminated. This is an approximate answer because certain side effects may have a different concentration–response relationship from the main therapeutic effects.

THERAPEUTIC DRUG MONITORING

C_{SS} is sometimes misunderstood by clinicians to imply an absence of daily peak and trough concentrations. Peak and trough concentrations exist within each dosing interval, and when maximum and minimum drug concentrations are the same with two or more successive doses, C_{SS} is reached (Figure 6.1.2.2). Dosing some drugs once a day because they have a sufficiently long half-life may lead to excessive peak concentrations that can be associated with toxicity or increased adverse effects (e.g., clozapine is dosed twice daily because of potential for seizures at peak concentration). As Figure 6.1.2.3 shows, if the initial dose is doubled and dosed once daily, the peak concentration exceeds the desired concentration to toxicity, but if the original dose is doubled but given twice daily, the concentration is above the plasma concentration that is likely to produce a clinical effect, the minimal effective

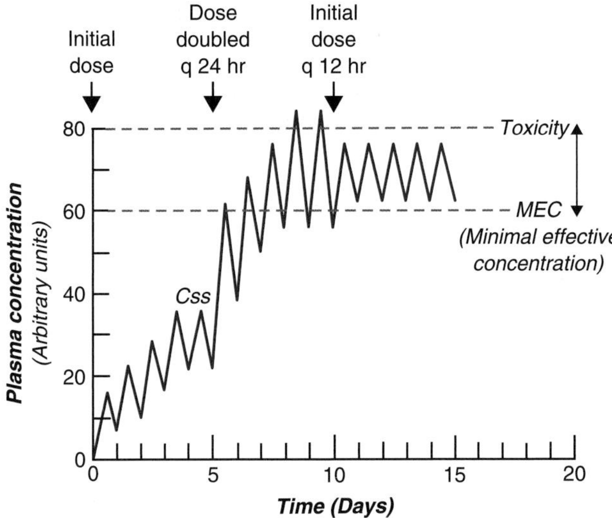

FIGURE 6.1.2.3. Changes in plasma concentration with changes in amount of drug or frequency of dosing.

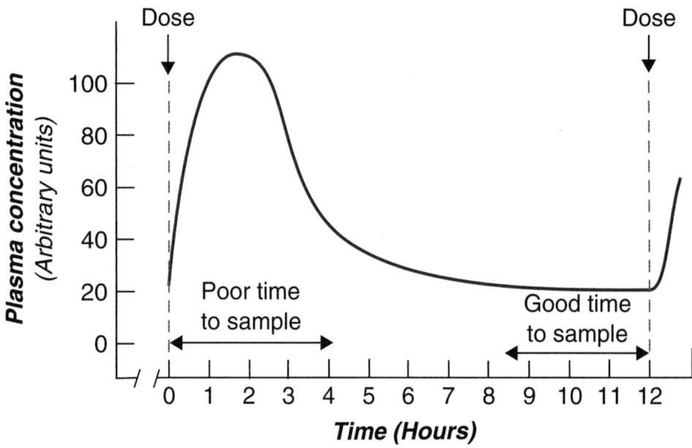

FIGURE 6.1.2.4. Idealized plasma curve.

concentration (MEC), but below toxic levels, the maximal tolerable concentration.

Clinicians must tailor drug dosing and frequency to maximize the probability of drug efficacy and to minimize toxicity. Some drugs (lithium, valproate, carbamazepine, and nortriptyline) that have narrow therapeutic indices, significant consequences associated with toxicity, wide interpatient variability, and no clinical endpoint to guide drug dosing, are candidates for TDM. A final requirement must be met: The concentration of a drug must have a proportional relation to the concentration and the pharmacologic action at the receptor site (10). Ranges of concentrations have been established for drugs that meet these requirements, and values for psychotropic drugs used by child psychiatrists are given in Chapter 6.1.2.

The range between subtherapeutic and toxic doses, or *therapeutic range* (sometimes called the therapeutic window) is a misnomer of sorts, since even when drug concentration is within the range, not every youth will respond to the drug, and a percentage will experience toxicity. For some drugs, there are data only on the MEC. TDM can reveal individuals with unusual metabolism (see the Metabolism section), uncover nonadherence, demonstrate increased or decreased concentration with the addition of other drugs (see Drug Interaction section), and confirm toxicity. TDM provides information that supplements clinical assessment.

There are two common errors in using TDM: not waiting for C_{SS} to occur before drawing a blood sample, and not drawing the blood sample at trough level.

As Figure 6.1.2.4 shows, sampling at "trough," or just before the next dose, offers the flattest part of the curve. For drugs given two or three times daily, sampling blood concentration *before the* am *dose in the morning* is recommended, and for drugs given once daily, sampling *before the next dose* is suggested.

Vignette 3

A 17-year-old girl with bipolar disorder has been maintained on 600 mg of lithium carbonate twice daily. A trough level of lithium of 0.8 mEq/L has been maintained for 8 months, with reduction in her symptoms. Parents phone the clinician because their daughter is nauseated and vomiting. As previously instructed, the teen has not been given her morning medication. The finding of a trough level of 1.4 mEq/L initiates careful inquiry and reveals that friends have been giving her ibuprofen for menstrual cramps. By inhibiting prostaglandins, NSAIDs affect renal blood flow and thus the renal clearance of lithium (11).

PHARMACOKINETICS IN CHILDREN AND ADOLESCENTS

There are many pharmacokinetic similarities between adults and children and adolescents. Indeed, age-independent genetic influences on metabolism can be more salient than those influences attributable to age and developmental change. Nonetheless, children and adolescents do display unique pharmacokinetic parameters. Premature infants, neonates, toddlers, children, and adolescents are not a homogenous group in terms of drug distribution patterns (12). These differences can be especially dramatic both at the neonatal stage and around the time of puberty, when the release of gonadal hormones can strongly influence plasma drug concentrations (13).

FACTORS AFFECTING DRUG DISPOSITION

Absorption and Bioavailability

Drugs gain entry into the body through a variety of portals. The *bioavailability* of a medication in the systemic circulation—the amount of unbound drug available to exert a biologic effect on target tissues—is determined by its absorption and, for orally administered medications, by *presystemic clearance (first pass effect)* from intestinal and hepatic transporters, metabolism, and conjugation (see Intestinal Influx and Efflux Transporters and Intestinal Metabolism section) and protein binding. Drugs have variable *first pass effects*. Some drugs are metabolized very efficiently on first pass (60% to 70%) and others less so (less than 30%). Bioavailability measures the completeness of drug absorption, and it is determined in reference to intravenous dosing. Oral administration is by far the most common portal of entry but often the most unpredictable in terms of final bioavailability. Some drugs are given to children as tinctures or in alcohol-based syrups. Although drugs like penicillin G are absorbed in the stomach, most psychotropic medications are absorbed in the proximal small intestine.

Little information is available regarding the effect of age on the absorption of psychotropic medications, although there are several theoretical considerations regarding the influence of this process in children and adolescents. A major factor influencing gastrointestinal absorption is pH-dependent diffusion. In infants, the gastric pH is nearly neutral in the first week after birth. It slowly reaches adult values by age 3 (14). In toddlers, stomach contents tend to be less acidic than in adults, causing weakly acidic drugs to be more highly ionized. Because it is the unionized fraction that is absorbed from the stomach, weakly acidic drugs may be absorbed more slowly in children. This process theoretically could affect phenobarbital and other anticonvulsants, amphetamines, and antidepressants (15).

Other factors that could reduce overall absorption are gastric and intestinal transit time. Gastric transit time is likely increased in neonates and infants, and the age of maturation is not known (14). Intestinal transit time is increased and the absorptive surface area of the intestine is reduced in young children, suggesting that drugs with a long phase of absorption (e.g., carbamazepine) and some sustained-release preparations may be incompletely absorbed (16). It is important to remember that although the rate at which many drugs are absorbed is slower in neonates and infants, there are no data indicating a generally reduced absorption of orally administered drugs in prepubertal children or teenagers (17).

Intestinal Influx and Efflux Transporters and Intestinal Metabolism

Until 10 to 15 years ago, it was believed that the first pass effect was limited to the hepatic metabolic enzymes and conjugation, and that diffusion was the only mechanism involved in absorption in the small intestine. It was known that lipid-soluble drugs passively diffuse through the apical membrane of the small intestine, that some small hydrophilic ionized drugs squeeze through intracellular junctions, and that both types of drugs cross the cytosol and exit the basolateral membrane into the portal circulation (18). It is now known that non–lipid-soluble drugs are also actively transported (both imported and exported) across these liminal boundaries by members of the solute carrier family of transporter proteins that currently include 43 subfamilies and 298 transporter genes (19,20) (Figure 6.1.2.5). Several names exist for each transporter especially in the earlier literature.

The best characterized of these influx transporters is the peptide transporter 1 (PEPT1). This transporter uses the intestinal–cellular proton gradient as a source of energy to ferry dipeptides and tripeptides across the apical membrane. Hundreds of peptides and other molecules are possible substrates (betalactam antibiotics, ACE inhibitors, thrombin inhibitors, acyclovir, sulpiride, and others). After crossing to the cytosol, these drugs are shepherded across to the portal circulation by a second peptide transporter embedded in the basolateral membrane (Figure 6.1.2.5) (21). Although the development of SLC15A1 has been studied in mice and rats, there is no information about when it matures in humans. Targeting the peptide transport system represents a new strategy for drug delivery of poorly absorbed drugs. Acyclovir, a polar antiviral drug, is poorly absorbed from the intestine, but if the L-valyl ester prodrug valacyclovir is given, it is transported by SLC15A1, and therapeutic levels can be obtained. The ester drugs like methylphenidate are also hydrolyzed by plasma esterases. In the case of methylphenidate, the inactive metabolite ritalinic acid is formed. In the case of acyclovir, an active metabolite is formed.

Efflux transporters are also embedded in both of the intestinal membranes. Members of a superfamily of transporters that use ATP as an energy source (ATP-binding cassette transporters or ABC transporters) (20) can flip compounds which have entered the cytosol back into the intestinal lumen on the apical side and from the cytosol into the portal system on the basolateral side (Figure 6.1.2.5). Efflux transporters act not only to limit drug absorption and bioavailability in the intestine, but they efflux compounds into the biliary system and the kidney, protect "sanctuaries" such as the brain (Figure 6.1.2.1), and are responsible in part for resistance to cancer drugs.

About 30 years ago, Juliano and Ling (22) noted that after initial efficacy, many oncologic drugs stopped being effective at the same time; they named this phenomenon multiple drug resistance (MDR). A gene on chromosome 7 (MDR1) was found to encode a glycoprotein (P-glycoprotein [P-gp]) that pumps out compounds from cells. Multiple drugs were affected at the same time because all of them were P-gp substrates.

P-gp is now numbered 1 of subfamily B of superfamily ABC (ABCB1). Other members of this family involved in efflux drug transport are in subfamily C (Figure 6.1.2.5). There is an avalanche of in vitro data on what compounds are substrates of these transporters, and how other drugs, foods, or genetic variations can affect ABCB1. Since ABCB1 is saturable in vivo, only drugs that are therapeutic in low doses can be shown to be affected (digoxin, talinolol, fexofenadine (23)). Drugs that affect ABCB1 either through inhibition or induction represent a new form of drug interaction. For example, quinidine, an inhibitor of ABCB1, blocks the efflux of digoxin in the kidney, and more digoxin will be absorbed and enter the circulation ((23); see Drug Interaction section).

In the intestine, both ABCB1 and CYP 3A4 are located in the endoplasmic reticulum. There is a considerable overlap in compounds that are substrates of both (dexamethasone, diltiazem, and vincristine).

ABCB1 and CYP 3A4 act together as an intestinal defense tag team to protect against exogenous compounds: ABCB1 provides a barrier to absorption and any remaining compound is converted by CYP 3A4 to less active metabolites ((24); see Metabolism section and Drug Interaction section). Levels of both ABCB1 and CYP 3A4 are higher in the intestine than in the liver, and there is a growing awareness of the importance of these intestinal proteins as compared to hepatic ABCB1/CYP 3A4 in first-pass metabolism. There is no coordination between the duodenal and the hepatic tag teams, and in each organ there is a different ontogeny of CYPs and ABCB1 ((25);

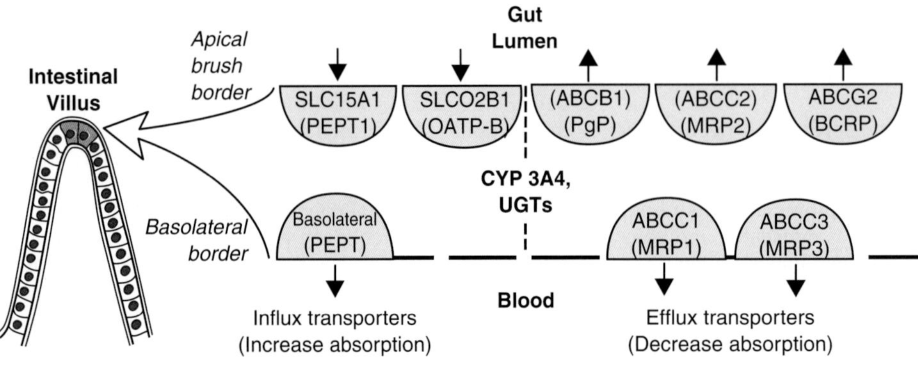

FIGURE 6.1.2.5. Intestinal transporters.

see Metabolism section). ABCB1 is also found in the blood–brain barrier, in the prostate, and in the placenta.

Drug Distribution and Plasma Proteins

Following absorption, drugs are distributed into intravascular and various extravascular spaces. Numerous physical factors can influence the distribution of a drug throughout the body: the size of body water compartments and adipose tissue depots, cardiac output, regional blood flow, organ perfusion pressure, permeability of cell membranes, acid–base balance, and binding to plasma and tissue proteins (13). Each of these factors may change during development, resulting in changes in the distribution of a drug and, subsequently, in its pharmacologic effect.

Drugs are transported in the general circulation in two forms that are in dynamic equilibrium with each other: bound to plasma protein (acidic drugs to albumin and basic drugs to alpha 1-acid glycoproteins) and unbound (free). Only the unbound drug is usually available to pass across membranes and to have pharmacologic effects. Although albumin and alpha 1-acid glycoproteins are reduced in the neonate and infant, this does not appear to be an important developmental factor in older children and adolescents (14,17).

Two important factors affecting distribution that change substantially during development are fat stores and the relative proportion of total body water to extracellular water. The relationship between the amount of drug absorbed (D), also referred to as the concentration at time zero, plasma concentration (Cp), and volume of distribution (Vd) can be summarized by the simple equation: Cp = D/Vd. Note that the larger the Vd, the smaller the Cp. The proportion of body fat is highest in the first year of life, followed by a steady decrease until an increase occurs prepubertally (12,26). The adipose tissue of infants has a lower ratio of lipid to water (17). The relative volume of extracellular water is high in children and tends to decrease with development. For example, total body water decreases gradually from about 85% of body weight in a small premature infant to about 70% in the full-term newborn to about 60% in the 1-year-old infant, a level that is generally maintained throughout adulthood. Similarly, extracellular water decreases gradually from about 40% to 50% of body weight in the newborn to about 15% to 20% by age 10 to 15 years (27). Thus, if weight-based drug administration is utilized, infants will tend to have lower drug plasma levels (17). Drugs that are primarily distributed in body water (lithium) can be expected to have a lower plasma concentration in the pediatric population compared with that in adults because the volume of distribution is higher in children and early adolescents.

Another consideration in distribution of drugs in preterm newborns and infants is the relative permeability of the blood–brain barrier when compared with that in children and adults (14). The blood–brain barrier is formed by capillary endothelial cells that have very tight junctions. Paracellular passive diffusion of hydrophilic substances is blocked, and only low–molecular-weight lipophilic agents can cross the blood–brain barrier. The increased permeability of the blood–brain barrier in infants could result in increased bioavailability of drugs within the central nervous system (CNS), as with anticonvulsants (28).

Compounds can also gain entry into the CNS via solute carrier family transporters (blood to brain (29)). Efflux transporters (especially ABCB1 and ABC subfamily C) in astrocytes and brain capillary cells guard entry to the brain by "flipping" out substrates (amitriptyline, quetiapine, and risperidone) (30). Although the ontogeny of ABCB1 is incompletely understood, there is a suggestion that premature infants may have reduced levels (31).

HEPATIC INFLUX AND EFFLUX TRANSPORTERS AND METABOLISM

Influx and Efflux Transporters

After absorption, drugs are carried to the liver via the portal system. Many drugs are able to passively enter hepatocytes, but large or ionized drugs need active transport. They are transported across the membrane by a variety of solute family carriers, and they are exposed to cytosol CYPs and glucuronide conjugates. Bile acids are similarly transported via specialized influx transporters (the sodium/bile acid cotransporter, NTCP, SLC10A1).

Drugs can be effluxed from hepatocytes into the bile canaliculi via ABC transporters (ABCB1 and ABCC2 transporters), while bile salts have their own unique carrier (bile salt export pump, BSEP, ABCB11). Other ABC efflux transporters can pump out drugs back into the venous circulation (32).

Hepatic Metabolism

Most psychotropic drugs are lipid soluble, which is usually a necessary requirement for absorption, distribution, and availability at receptor sites. To be effectively excreted, however, *lipophilic* drugs need to be metabolized to more polar or *hydrophilic* forms (having a greater affinity for water). Although some drugs are renally excreted unmetabolized (lithium, gabapentin), most undergo extensive biotransformation in the intestine and the liver (Figure 6.1.2.6) (33).

Phase-1 metabolic reactions, including *hydroxylation, reduction,* and *hydrolysis,* convert drugs to forms more suitable for elimination. Intestinal and hepatic CYPs are the most important enzyme systems responsible for phase-I reactions, and others include plasma esterases that metabolize methylphenidate, flavin-containing monooxygenases, and aldehyde oxidase (Figure 6.1.2.6). The products of phase-I reactions, collectively referred to as *metabolites,* are usually less active and less toxic than their parent compounds. Notable exceptions of clinical significance are desipramine, the demethylated active metabolite of imipramine, and norfluoxetine, the demethylated long-lived active metabolite of fluoxetine. These metabolites have comparable toxicities to their parent compounds and comparable therapeutic activity.

In *phase-II reactions, conjugation* of metabolites generated in phase I takes place with glucuronic acid, sulfate, or others. Conjugated compounds are then readily excreted in urine or other body fluids. It is clinically important to note that some drugs

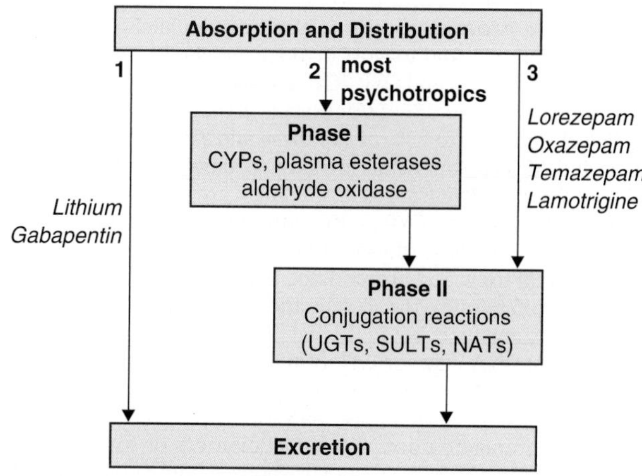

FIGURE 6.1.2.6. Phase I and II.

are never metabolized in a phase-I reaction and instead simply undergo conjugation by phase-II enzymes (Figure 6.1.2.6). Drugs such as the 3-hydroxybenzodiazepines (lorazepam, oxazepam, and temazepam) are conjugated by glucuronidation, and they are rapidly cleared at equal rates regardless of age as long as renal function is normal (34). These drugs are preferred in instances of liver insufficiency because other benzodiazepines depend on cytochromes for metabolism, which may be more influenced by hepatic dysfunction than is glucuronidation.

Cytochromes (CYPs)

CYPs are heme-containing enzymes, located principally in the intestine and liver that metabolize two types of substrates: endogenous (the body's own steroids, lipids, and fatty acids) and exogenous (toxins, drugs). CYPs that metabolize exogenous compounds are located in the endoplasmic reticulum. The sequencing of CYP amino acids has led to a classification system based on similarity (35): Arabic numbers 1 to 4 designate family members, letters A to E label subfamily members, and Arabic numbers note specific enzymes (isoform, gene). CYP 3A4, for example, is a member of family 3, subfamily A, and enzyme 4. The CYPs that are near each other on the same gene and are related are grouped together (CYP 3A4, CYP 3A5, and CYP 3A7) and referred collectively as CYP 3A. It is the major CYP family involved in human hepatic drug metabolism, handling about half of psychotropic drugs. CYP 3A constitutes 30% of total CYP hepatic content and 70% of intestinal CYP content, and it serves as a high-capacity reservoir. The other clinically relevant CYPs include 1A2, 2B6, 2C9, 2C19, 2D6, and 2E1.

Most psychotropic drugs undergo both phase-I and phase-II reactions (Figure 6.1.2.6). A few drugs are metabolized by only one CYP (desipramine via CYP 2D6, triazolam via CYP 3A). Some others undergo phase-II conjugation only (lorazepam, oxazepam, and lamotrigine are glucuronidated only). However, most drugs require multiple CYPs to be completely metabolized. As examples, sertraline is N-demethylated via six different pathways (36), and clomipramine (CMI) demethylated by CYP 1A2, CYP 2C19, and CYP 3A to desmethylclomipramine (DCMI), an active metabolite that is then hydroxylated by CYP 2D6. In addition, CMI is directly hydroxylated by CYP 2D6.

CYP-based metabolism of drugs is influenced by genetic factors. Seven percent to 10% of Caucasians have a genetic deficiency of CYP 2D6 and are thus less efficient at metabolizing CYP 2D6 substrates, including many psychotropic agents. For these "slow metabolizers," blood levels of drugs metabolized by 2D6 may increase considerably as unmetabolized drug enters the blood. Some Asian individuals have a 2D6 variant that causes them to be "somewhat slow" metabolizers, and they require lower dosing of relevant drugs to achieve therapeutic blood levels. Some African Americans also have an allelic variant of CYP 2D6 that is linked to slow or poor metabolism of CYP 2D6 substrates. CYP 2C9 and CYP 2C19 are also genetically polymorphic. One percent to 3% of Caucasians are slow metabolizers of CYP 2C9, and 18% to 23% of Japanese and 2% to 3% of Caucasians and African Americans are slow metabolizers of CYP 2C19 (37). Fewer than five Caucasians in 1,000 are slow metabolizers of both CYP 2D6 and CYP 2C19, putting them at particular risk for high levels of substrates that are metabolized by *both* pathways (certain tricyclics, propranolol, and citalopram).

It has been possible to ascertain the CYP genetic status of individuals for some time, but in the last year, the FDA has approved a diagnostic DNA chip for CYP 2D6 (27 variants) and CYP 2C19 (two variants) (38). Clinicians can consider testing youth who have adverse effects with substrate CYP 2C19 or CYP 2D6 drugs at usual therapeutic doses (poor metabolizers or intermediate metabolizers) or who have poor responses with substrate CYP 2D6 drugs at usual therapeutic doses (ultrarapid metabolizer) (39).

UDP-Glucuronosyltransferases

Located close to the CYPs in the endoplasmic reticulum, UGTs are a superfamily of membrane-based enzymes that catalyze the transfer of glucuronic acid to endogenous or exogenous compounds. They are considered to be the principal phase-II system by virtue of the number of different types of compounds they conjugate, as well as their superior quantity compared to other phase-II enzymes. The nomenclature of UGTs is similar to CYPs, being designated by family, subfamily, and gene (UGT 1A1, UGT 2B7).

There are two families of UGTs, UGT 1 and UGT 2, and three subfamilies (UGT 1A, UGT 2A, and UGT 2B). The subfamily of UGT 1A shares exons two to five in common, and they are distinguished by a unique exon one. UGT 1A1 is the most abundant UGT 1 in the liver (40). UGT 2A and UGT 2B are encoded by separated genes. Like CYPs, individual UGTs have both unique and overlapping substrates (Table 6.1.2.1), and they have tissue-specific patterns of expression and genetic variations.

Unlike CYPs, UGTs handle both endogenous and exogenous compounds. Thus, deficient glucuronidation as a result of genetic polymorphism or UGT inhibition can lead to increased levels of both endogenous and exogenous substrates. For example, UGT 1A1 is the only conjugative pathway for bilirubin. Gilbert syndrome (in which UGT 1A1 activity is reduced by about 70%) is characterized by a benign fluctuating bilirubinemia in association with illness or stress. Individuals with Gilbert syndrome can also develop toxic levels of SN-38, the active metabolite of the cancer chemotherapy agent, irinotecan, because UGT 1A1 is an important conjugative pathway for SN-38. The influence of polymorphisms of individual UGTs has been shown to correlate with clinical outcomes of psychotropic drugs such as clozapine, imipramine, and cyproheptadine (UGT 1A4, 41), with levels of the active enantiomer of oxazepam (UGT 2B15, 42), and with intolerance to morphine (UGT 2B7, 43). A new rapid genetic test for UGT 1A1 has been approved by the FDA (44).

The clinical application of knowledge about UGTs has lagged at least a decade behind CYPs, but it may become increasingly clinically relevant. At present, clinicians must understand UGT-based drug interactions to appropriately use lamotrigine, olanzapine, and others (see Drug Interaction section).

Ontogeny of Hepatic CYPs and Phase-II Enzymes

In the neonate, activities of hepatic CYP-mediated metabolism and the phase-II reactions, UGTs, glutathione conjugation (GST), and acetylation (NAT) are decreased, but some types of sulfate conjugation function efficiently. Since sulfation is a major conjugative pathway of acetaminophen, individuals have speculated that this is the reason why young children are more resistant to the toxic effects of this drug (45).

Neither CYPs nor phase-II enzymes come "on line" at the same time, and each has a unique ontogeny. CYP 3A7 is the predominant fetal CYP. In the first few weeks after birth, CYP 3A4 gradually appears and increases as CYP 3A7 peaks at 2 weeks and fades (46). CYP 3A5 is variably present in some individuals, and it appears to be under genetic control. CYP 2D6, CYP 2C9, and CYP 2C19 become active in the first weeks of life. CYP 2E1 gradually develops over the first 3 months (47). CYP 1A2 is the last CYP to appear at the fourth or fifth month (48). Clinicians must take account of these changes in dosing premature infants and neonates. For example, clinicians must decrease the dosing of midazolam, a CYP 3A4 and CYP 3A5 substrate, as infants are increasing their ability to metabolize it (49).

TABLE 6.1.2.1

UGT TABLE

	UGT1A1	UGT1A3	UGT1A4	UGT1A6	UGT1A9	UGT2B7	UGT2B15
Chromosome	2	2	2	2	2	4	4
Genetic variation	Yes	Yes	Yes	Yes	Yes	Yes	Yes
Some endogenous substrates	Bilirubin Estriol	Estrones	Androsterone Progestins	Serotonin	Thyroxine	Androsterone Bile acid	Dihydrotestosterone
Some substrate drugs	Acetaminophen Buprenorphine Ethinyl Estradiol Ibuprofen Irinotecan Mb-SN-38 Nicotine Phenytoin	Buprenorphine (chlorpromazine) (clozapine) Cyproheptadine Diphenhydramine Doxepin (ibuprofen) (valproate)	(amitriptyline) Chlorpromazine Clomipramine Clozapine Diphenhydramine Cyproheptadine Doxepin Imipramine Lamotrigine Loxapine Olanzapine Phenytoin Trifluoperazine	Acetaminophen Phenytoin Valproate	Acetaminophen Ethinyl estradiol Ibuprofen Phenytoin Valproate	Carbamazepine Ibuprofen Lamotrigine Lorazepam Morphines Propranolol Sertraline Valproate Zidovudine	Desloratadine S-oxazepam S-lorazepam
Possible inducers	Dexamethasone Phenobarbital Phenytoin		Carbamazepine Ethinyl estradiol (oxcarbamazepine) Phenobarbital Phenytoin Rifampin	Dexamethasone	Phenobarbital	Phenobarbital Phenytoin Rifampin	
Possible inhibitors	Ketoconazole Probenecid	Imipramine Probenecid	Probenecid	Probenecid	Probenecid Ketoconazole Valproate	Codeine Diazepam Ketoconazole Morphine Probenecid Valproate	Ibuprofen Ketoconazole Probenecid Valproate

(), minor pathway.

Each CYP has a unique development. CYP 2C19 levels are highly variable from 5 months to 10 years, and levels approach adult values by 10 years of age (50). CYP 2D6 matures to adult levels by 10 years or earlier (46). There is some evidence that levels of CYP 3A4 are actually lower in youth aged 5 to 15 years than in adults (51). CYP 2C9 gradually increases over the first 5 months (and as many as half of individuals may reach adult values), exceeds adult activity in youth from 3 to 10 years, and achieves adult activity after puberty (50). CYP 1A2 activity in childhood exceeds adult levels until after puberty (girls, Tanner stage 2; boys, Tanner stage 4) (52).

There is less known about the development of hepatic phase-II enzymes. The bilirubinemia of premature infants occurs because of the immaturity of hepatic UGT 1A1. Low levels of neonatal UGT 2B7 are responsible for the toxicity of chloramphenicol, the so-called *gray baby syndrome*. Both of these UGTs reach adult values by 3 to 6 months (53), but in some individuals, full maturation may not be reached until 30 months (46). Two UGTs start to develop only after the second year of life: UGT 1A9 and UGT 2B4 (54). It has been speculated that the immaturity of UGTs in young children is partially responsible for their increased risk of valproate hepatotoxicity, and they may produce higher concentrations of a hepatotoxic metabolite of valproate, 4-ene valproic acid (45). Individual enzymes of other phase-II proteins (sulfotransferases [SULTs], N-acetyl transferases [NATs]) have unique stagger-step developments, but most achieve adult levels by 2 to 4 years of age (46).

Plasma Clearances of Liver-Metabolized Drugs by Prepubertal Children

Children under 10 years require larger, weight-adjusted doses of most hepatically metabolized medications than do adults in order to achieve comparable blood levels and therapeutic effects (12,17). The reason for this is not obvious. Originally, it was proposed that the greater liver-to-body mass ratio of children compared to adults and other developmental changes in youth were responsible. However, it has been subsequently shown even when liver volume is normalized, that systemic clearance of a nonspecific CYP substrate (antipyrine) is higher in children when compared to adults (55). It also had been speculated that children have more efficient CYPs, but when individual hepatic CYPs were evaluated in vitro, no differences in maximal activities were found in children when compared to adults (56). Finally, as outlined above, during development, CYPs and phase-II conjugates have *not* been shown to be uniformly increased in prepubertal children.

Renal Excretion

The kidney is an important organ for drug excretion. Three mechanisms are involved in the renal excretion of drugs: glomerular filtration through which drugs not bound to plasma proteins are "filtered," active tubular secretion in the proximal convoluted tubule, and passive reabsorption from the tubule.

Adult values of glomerular filtration are reached by 3 months in full-term infants, and if weight adjusted, they can exceed adult values thereafter (14). Although in infants, tubular secretion is believed to develop more slowly than glomerular filtration, the efficacy of both mechanisms may be greater in children and teens than in adults (14). There is less information available about the ontogeny of tubular reabsorption, but it may not mature fully until adolescence (14).

Increased glomerular filtration and changes in tubular reabsorption, as well as increased body water in children, are responsible for the fact that children from 9 to 12 years can have greater clearance and shorter elimination half-life of lithium (57). Newer anticonvulsants that are primarily or entirely handled by the kidney (gabapentin, levetiracetam, and topiramate) may also require higher weight-adjusted dosing in prepubertal children (58–60).

DRUG INTERACTIONS: FOCUS ON CYPs

Given the increasing recourse to medication combinations, augmentation strategies, and polypharmacy as an accepted and thoughtful (61) or sometimes as a controversial and potentially problematic (62) practice in child psychiatry, astute clinicians need to be aware and clinically suspicious of potential drug interactions. For children concurrently treated with nonpsychiatric drugs (including seemingly innocuous over-the-counter agents), the degree of oversight needs to be particularly heightened.

Time Courses of CYP-Based Drug Interactions

Drugs that interact with CYPs can inhibit, induce, or have no effect on CYP activity. Drugs with a *low presystemic clearance* (little of the drug is metabolized and conjugated in *the first pass* through the intestine and liver) are more susceptible to CYP induction or inhibition because they have *more unused metabolic capacity.* If a CYP is inhibited, more unmetabolized drug will enter the circulation, leading to increased levels of the drug (similar to a phenotypic slow metabolizer). Since inhibition requires blocking *existing* pathways, inhibition occurs rapidly for drugs that have a *high presystemic clearance.* The time course of the occurrence of the drug interaction is not changed if a *victim* drug is added to a *perpetrator* inhibitor drug or if a *perpetrator* inhibitor drug is added to a *victim* drug (see Figure 6.1.2.7). When a *perpetrator* inhibitor drug is added to a victim drug, the time to achieve a new C_{SS} is longer than the initial C_{SS} because the half-life has been prolonged, and the full effect of the interaction may not be evident until the *perpetrator* inhibitor reaches C_{SS}. Further, as illustrated by Figure 6.1.2.7, if the *perpetrator* drug is discontinued, the drug interaction will resolve as the concentration of the *perpetrator* drug falls to zero.

By contrast, if a drug has a *low presystemic clearance,* then the drug interaction will be evident only after both drugs have had several passes through the circulation and the *victim* drug reaches C_{SS}. Therefore the drug interaction will be clinically evident after some time.

Vignette 4

> An 18-year-old woman has generalized anxiety disorder for which she has been prescribed daily triazolam for the past year. She develops a significant bacterial infection and clarithromycin is added. The next day, she develops signs of benzodiazepine toxicity. Triazolam is discontinued, and after 5 days, alprazolam is substituted. The toxicity reemerges 5 days later (63). In this vignette, triazolam has a high presystemic clearance and alprazolam has a low presystemic clearance (even though both are CYP 3A substrates).

If a CYP is induced, additional enzyme will be available for metabolism (similar to a phenotypic ultrarapid metabolizer), leading to lower drug levels. Induction takes some time to start (3 to 10 days) or stop (5 to 12 days), as protein synthesis must first occur and then cease.

The time course of the occurrence of the drug interaction is different if a *victim* drug is added to an already present *perpetrator inducer* drug than if *the perpetrator inducer* drug is added to an already present victim drug. In the first example, the drug interaction will take place quickly because the CYPs are already induced, but in the second, it will occur only after new or additional protein synthesis is initiated. In either case, however, if the perpetrator inducer is discontinued, it will take time for protein synthesis to cease and for the concentration of the perpetrator inducer to decrease. The drug interaction will persist over several days despite the absence of the perpetrator inducer. If both drugs are discontinued at the same time, the half-life of the victim drug will determine the persistence of the drug interaction only if it is less than the time necessary for protein synthesis to cease (see Figure 6.1.2.8).

UGT and Transporter Drug Interactions

Although there are significantly less data, UGTs are also susceptible to inhibition and induction (Table 6.1.2.1). For example, lamotrigine is handled only by glucuronidation (probably UGT 1A4 and UGT 2B7), and the addition of valproate (a UGT

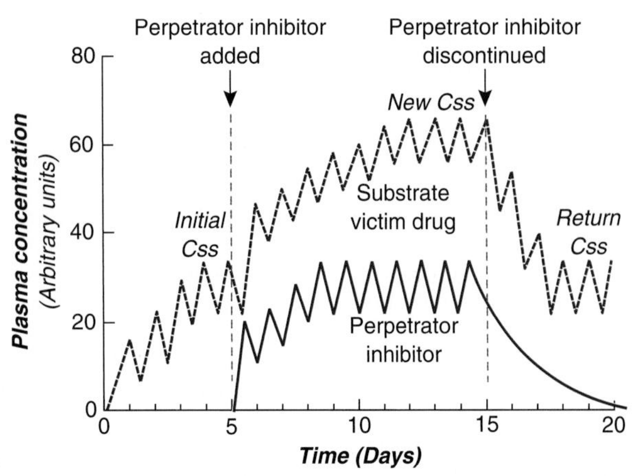

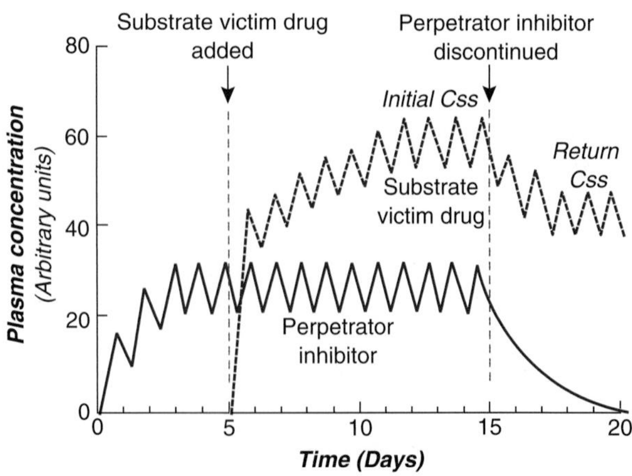

FIGURE 6.1.2.7. A, B: Pharmacokinetics of substrate to inhibitor and inhibitor to substrate.

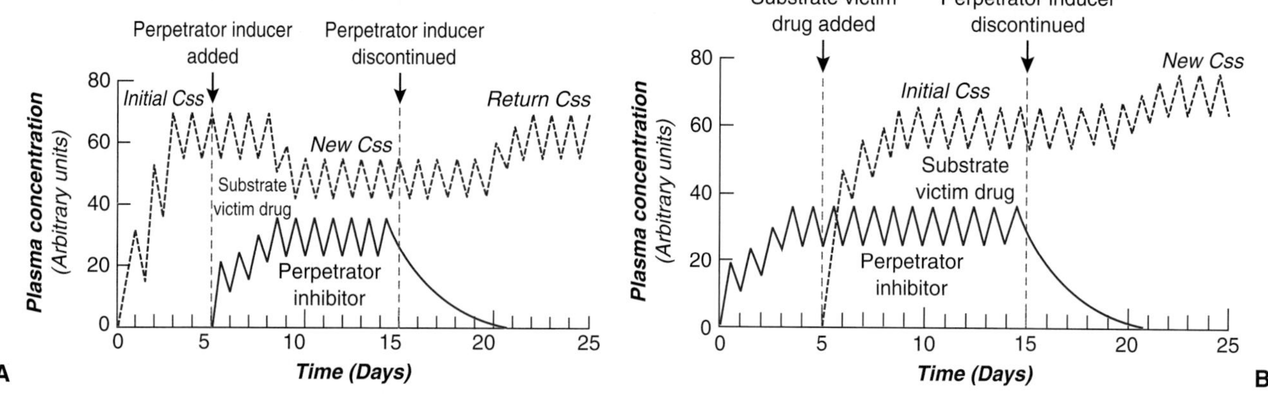

FIGURE 6.1.2.8. A, B: Pharmacokinetics of substrate to inducer and inducer to substrate.

2B7 inhibitor) can significantly elevate lamotrigine levels, and increase the likelihood of the development of life-threatening Stevens–Johnson syndrome (64). The prescribing information of lamotrigine details dosage recommendation for this combination and for other anticonvulsants that induce or inhibit UGTs (65). It is less well known that when coadministered with lamotrigine, ethinyl estradiol (present in oral contraceptives), an inducer of glucuronidation, can reduce levels of lamotrigine up to 50% (66). There are only a few drug interactions involving transporters that are unquestionably tied to a specific transporter and are clinically significant because it is difficult to clearly separate out the effects of transporters from phase-I and phase-II effects and because a drug can have multiple transporters. The best known drug interactions involving efflux transporters are those of digoxin: For example, quinidine inhibits the ABCB1 uptake of digoxin in the kidney, leading to increase in digoxin levels (67). Although the current information about these drug interactions is still meager, as information grows, clinicians will need to keep abreast.

Clinical Aspects of Drug Interactions, Additional Resources

Vignette 5

A 14-year-old girl has diagnoses of major depressive disorder and attention-deficit hyperactivity disorder (ADHD). The depressive symptoms have responded well to fluoxetine at 10 mg per day, but difficulties with attention and impulsivity continue. Because she has had failed trials of methylphenidate and dextroamphetamine, she is begun on nortriptyline. Unaware of a possible drug interaction, the clinician begins treatment with a low dose of nortriptyline and plans to gradually increase dosing. The clinician is surprised to find that after 5 days of 10 mg twice daily of nortriptyline a trough blood level is 85 ng/mL. Fluoxetine is a potent CYP 2D6 inhibitor, and the level of victim CYP 2D6 substrate nortriptyline is already within therapeutic range.

Vignette 6

A 17-year-old youth with a diagnosis of bipolar 1 disorder has failed lithium, valproate, and several atypical antipsychotics. Her manic symptoms are well controlled on carbamazepine. She is sexually active and has been on low-dose oral contraceptives for 1 year without any side effects. The clinician is unaware that carbamazepine is an inducer of CYP 3A4. The patient begins to experience breakthrough bleeding for the first time.

The six most relevant CYPs and selected common psychotropic and other pediatric drugs and herbs metabolized by them are shown in Table 6.1.2.2. Common potent inhibitors and inducers of CYPs are grouped alphabetically by CYP.

The table can be used to anticipate CYP-based drug interactions and to prevent some of the unexpected outcomes depicted in the previous vignettes. If one drug is an inducer or inhibitor and it is listed on the same vertical axis as a substrate (the same CYP), a drug interaction is possible. However, *possible* is not the same as *likely* or *clinically significant.* A drug interaction is more likely to be clinically evident when a new drug is added or an existing drug is discontinued. Three other drug characteristics should help raise a clinician's drug interaction antennae. A drug interaction is especially likely to occur and can be significant if the victim drug has *one major* metabolic pathway (nortriptyline, desipramine, and ethinyl estradiol). Many of the most serious drug interactions occur when a CYP inhibitor or inducer is added to a substrate with a narrow therapeutic index, as exemplified in Vignette 5. Finally, clinicians should be alert if a *perpetrator* inhibitor or inducer is *potent,* as shown in Vignette 6. Potent inhibitors and inducers are marked in bold in Table 6.1.2.2.

Although clinicians can glean important information from this table and from UGT Table 6.1.2.1 to predict drug interactions, they must utilize additional resources. They should know the metabolic characteristics and common drug interactions of medications they frequently prescribe. Clinicians can research these and other coprescribed over-the-counter and recreational drugs and herbs by using any common search engine on their computer to locate a drug's product insert and to review the "Metabolism" and "Drug Interaction" sections. Alternatively, clinicians can use PubMed to find the metabolic characteristics of a drug by entering the drug name and metabolism. They also can uncover clinical studies or case reports of known drug interactions involving pertinent drugs by entering the names of the drugs and the term drug interaction.

Clinicians need to amass trusted references: books such as Ciraulo's *Drug Interactions in Psychiatry* (68), Cozza's *Drug Interaction: Principles for Medical Practice* (69), articles such as Sandson's *An Overview of Psychotropic Drug-Drug Interactions* (70), websites such as Flockhart's CYP table (71), or Oesterheld's P-glycoprotein, ABCB1 table (72), and UGT table (73). A collegial relationship with a clinical pharmacologist, especially one who is hospital based, should be treasured, since they have access to pharmaceutical references not readily available to clinicians. A patient's primary medical provider and his/her family should be educated to the common drug interactions with prescribed psychotropics and encouraged to be vigilant for their possibility. Drug interaction computer programs can be useful, but they are rarely complete (lacking influx and efflux transporters and phase-II

TABLE 6.1.2.2

P450 CYTOCHROME TABLE

	CYP1A2	CYP2B6	CYP2C19	CYP2C9	CYP2D6	CYP3A4/5/7
Substrates	Psychotropics Clozapine Duloxetine Fluvoxamine Imipramine Melatonin (Mirtazapine) (Olanzapine) Propafenone (Propranolol) Ramelteon Others Acetaminophen Caffeine Naproxen (Phenacetin) R-warfarin Theophylline	Bupropion Meperidine Nicotine Methadone Sertraline	Psychotropics Amitriptyline Citalopram Clomipramine Diazepam (Fluoxetine) Imipramine (Sertraline) Anticonvulsants Mephenytoin Phenobarbital Phenytoin Others Progesterone Propranolol (Ranitidine) R-warfarin	Psychotropics Fluoxetine (Sertraline) Valproate NSAIDs (Diclofenac) Flurbiprofen Ibuprofen Indomethacin Meloxicam (Naproxen) Piroxicam Suprofen Hypoglycemics Glipizide <Glucotrol> Glimepiride <Amaryl> Glyburide <DiaBeta> Nateglinide <Starlix> Rosiglitazone Tolbutamide Others Celecoxib Phenobarbital Phenytoin Progesterone Sulfa drugs Tetrahydrocannabinol S-warfarin Zafirlukast <Accolate>	Psychotropics Amitriptyline Aripiprazole Benztropine Chlorpromazine (Citalopram) Clomipramine Desipramine Doxepin Duloxetine Fluoxetine Fluvoxamine Haloperidol Imipramine Mirtazapine Nortriptyline Paroxetine Perphenazine Risperidone (Sertraline) Thioridazine Venlafaxine Others Antihistamines Chlorpheniramine Diphenhydramine Hydroxyzine <Atarax> Anti-ADHD Amphetamines Atomoxetine Cough Medicines MDMA <ecstasy> Opiates Codeine pro-drug Hydrocodone pro-drug (Oxycodone) Tramadol Phenacetin Propranolol (Ranitidine <Zantac>) Tolterodine <Detrol>	Psychotropics Alprazolam Amitriptyline Aripiprazole Carbamazepine Citalopram (Clomipramine) (Clozapine) (Diazepam) Estazolam Eszopiclone <Lunesta> Fluoxetine Haloperidol Midazolam Nefazodone Pimozide Quetiapine Risperidone (Sertraline) Trazodone Triazolam Zaleplon <Sonata> (Ziprasidone) Zolpidem <Ambien> Drugs of abuse/treatment Buprenorphine Cocaine Hydrocodone pro-drug Ketamine Methadone Oxycodone Phencyclidine <PCP> Antibiotics/Antifungal Macrolides Itraconazole Ketoconazole Telithromycin Anticonvulsants Carbamazepine Ethosuximide Felbamate Tiagabine zonisamide Antihistamines Desloratadine <Clarinex> Fexofenadine <Allegra> Loratadine <Alavert, Claritin> Asthma Medication Fluticasone <Flovent> Salmeterol <Serevent> Zileuton <Zyflo> Calcium Channel Blockers Hormones/Steroids/ Immune Modulators Cortisols Desogestrel (pro-drug) Ethinyl estradiol <oral contraceptives> Progestins and progesterone Others Nateglinide <Starlix> Omeprazole Pioglitazone <Actos> Tolterodine <Detrol>

TABLE 6.1.2.2

(CONTINUED)

	CYP1A2	CYP2B6	CYP2C19	CYP2C9	CYP2D6	CYP3A4/5/7
Inhibitors	Caffeine Cimetidine **Ciprofloxacin** Echinacea **Enoxacin** **luvoxamine** Oral contraceptives Zileuton <Zyflo>	**Paroxetine** Fluoxetine Fluvoxamine PCP <phencyclidine> Sertraline	Cimetidine Felbamate Fluconazole (Fluoxetine) **Fluvoxamine** Gestodene Ketoconazole Modafinil Omeprazole **Oral contraceptives** Oxcarbazepine (Sertraline) Topiramate	Cimetidine **Fluconazole** Fluoxetine Isoniazid Sulfinpyrazone Valproate (Zafirlukast)	(Amitriptyline) **Bupropion** Celecoxib Chlorpheniramine Chlorpromazine Cimetidine (Citalopram) Clomipramine Cocaine (Desipramine) Diphenhydramine Doxepin Duloxetine (Fluvoxamine) Haloperidol (Hydroxyzine) Imipramine Methadone Metoclopramide **Paroxetine** **Quinidine** (Ranitidine) (Sertraline) **Terbinafine** Thioridazine	(Cimetidine) Ciprofloxacin **Diltiazem** Doxycycline Echinacea Enoxacin **Clarithromycin** Fluvoxamine **Grapefruit juice** **Itraconazole** **Ketoconazole** **Nefazodone** Star fruit **Telithromycin** **Verapamil**
Inducers	Carbamazepine Charbroiled meat Cigarette smoke Cruciferous vegetables Insulin Marijuana smoke Modafinil Phenobarbital	Carbamazepine Phenobarbital Phenytoin	Carbamazepine Glucocorticoids Phenobarbital	Barbiturates Glucocorticoids	Dexamethasone Rifampin	Barbiturates Carbamazepine Felbamate Glucocorticoids Modafinil (Oxcarbazepine) Phenytoin Primidone St. John's wort pioglitazone Topiramate at >200 mg/day

(), minor pathways or modest inhibitor or modest inducer; bold, potent inhibitors.

proteins) or up to date. Barron's *Evaluation of Personal Digital Assistant Software for Drug Interactions* (74) places iFacts and Lexi-Interact as the best, and ePocrates Rx as the worst. Although computer programs cannot factor in patient's characteristics such as genetic CYP status or developmental age, some are invaluable because they can sum the effects of multiple drugs if patients are taking many drugs or herbs at the same time (e.g., GenemedRx, 75).

In evaluating *suspected* drug interactions that may have already occurred, clinicians can use these resources to determine the metabolic characteristic of the involved drugs. They also should determine the time course between the initiation of the drugs and the development of adverse effects to help evaluate the likelihood of the suspected interaction. Does it fit the time courses that have been previously described? Does it fit the immediate development of adverse effects, as exemplified by the addition of a perpetrator inhibitor added to triazolam in Vignette 4, or the delayed timeline of a perpetrator inducer drug added to an oral contraceptive, as in Vignette 6?

CONCLUSION

Understanding the pharmacokinetic and drug interaction principles discussed in this chapter can be useful in clinical practice. It is hoped that readers will find the information in this chapter useful in improving the quality of care of their patients.

References

1. Aguilar EJ, Keshavan MS, Martinz-Quiles MD, Hernández J, Gómez-Beneyto M, Schooler NR: Predictors of acute dystonia in first-episode psychotic patients. *Am J Psychiatry* 151:1819–1821, 1994.
2. Rodnitzky RL: Drug-induced movement disorders in children and adolescents. *Expert Opin Drug Saf* 4:91–102, 2005.
3. March J; AACAP Committee on Quality Issues (CQI): Practice parameters for the assessment and treatment of children and adolescents with obsessive-compulsive disorder. *J Am Acad Child Adolesc Psychiatry* 37(10 Suppl):27S–45S, 1998.
4. Martin A, Kaufman J, Charney D: Pharmacotherapy of early-onset depression: update and new directions. *Child Adolesc Psychiatr Clin N Am* 9:135–157, 2000.
5. Paxton JW, Dragunow M: Pharmacology. In: Werry JS (ed): *Practitioner's Guide to Psychoactive Drugs for Children and Adolescents.* New York, Plenum, 23–55, 1993.
6. Daviss WB, Perel JM, Rudolph GR, et al.: Steady-state pharmacokinetics of bupropion SR in juvenile patients. *J Am Acad Child Adolesc Psychiatry* 44:349–357, 2005.
7. May TW, Korn-Merker E, Rambeck B: Clinical pharmacokinetics of oxcarbazepine. *Clin Pharmacokinet* 42:1023–1042, 2003.
8. Findling RL, Reed MD, Myers C, et al.: Paroxetine pharmacokinetics in depressed children and adolescents. *J Am Acad Child Adolesc Psychiatry* 38:952–959, 1999.
9. Findling RL, Preskorn SH, Marcus RN, et al.: Nefazodone pharmacokinetics in depressed children and adolescents. *J Am Acad Child Adolesc Psychiatry* 39:1008–1016, 2000.

10. Greenblatt DJ, Shader RI: *Pharmacokinetics in Clinical Practice.* Philadelphia, PA, WB Saunders Company, 1985.
11. Ragheb M: The clinical significance of lithium-nonsteroidal anti-inflammatory drug interactions. *J Clin Psychopharmacol* 10:350–354, 1990.
12. Jatlow PI: Psychotropic drug disposition during development. In: Popper C (ed): *Psychiatric Pharmacosciences of Children and Adolescents.* Washington, DC, American Psychiatric Press, 29–44, 1987.
13. Morselli PL, Pippenger CE: Drug disposition during development. In: Moyer TP, Boeckx RL (eds): *Applied Therapeutic Drug Monitoring.* Washington, DC, American Association of Clinical Chemistry, 63–70, 1982.
14. Strolin Benedetti M, Baltes EL: Drug metabolism and disposition in children. *Fundam Clin Pharmacol* 17:281–299, 2003.
15. Taylor E: Physical treatments. In: Rutter M (ed): *Child and Adolescent Psychiatry.* Cambridge, Blackwell Scientific, 880–899, 1994.
16. Gilman JT, Duchowny M, Campo AE: Pharmacokinetic considerations in the treatment of childhood epilepsy. *Paediatr Drugs* 5:267–777, 2003.
17. Kearns GL, Abdel-Rahman SM, Alander SW, Blowey DL, Leeder JS, Kauffman RE: Developmental pharmacology—drug disposition, action, and therapy in infants and children. *N Engl J Med* 349:1157–1167, 2003.
18. Chan LM, Lowes S, Hirst BH: The ABCs of drug transport in intestine and liver: efflux proteins limiting drug absorption and bioavailability. *Eur J Pharm Sciences* 21:25–51, 2004.
19. Steffansen B, Nielsen CU, Brodin B, Eriksson AH, Andersen R, Frokjaer S: Intestinal solute carriers: an overview of trends and strategies for improving oral drug absorption. *Eur J Pharm Sci* 21:3–16, 2004.
20. Website of HUGO Genome Nomenclature Committee at University College London. Available at: http://www.hugo-international.org/HUGO-Gene-Nomenclature. Accessed August 01, 2016.
21. Terada T, Inui K: Peptide transporters: structure, function, regulation and application for drug delivery. *Curr Drug Metab* 5:85–94, 2004.
22. Juliano RL, Ling V: A surface glycoprotein modulating drug permeability in Chinese hamster ovary cell mutants. *Biochim Biophys Acta* 455:152–162, 1976.
23. Fischer V, Einolf HJ, Cohen D: Efflux transporters and their clinical significance. *Mini Rev Med Chem* 5:183–195, 2005.
24. Kivisto KT, Niemi M, Fromm MF: Functional interaction of intestinal CYP3A4 and P-glycoprotein. *Fundam Clin Pharmacol* 18:621–626, 2004.
25. Fakhoury M, Litalien C, Medard Y, et al.: Localization and mRNA expression of CYP3A and P-glycoprotein in human duodenum as a function of age. *Drug Metab Dispos* 33:1603–1607, 2005.
26. Hattis D, Ginsberg G, Sonawane B, et al.: Differences in pharmacokinetics between children and adults–II. Children's variability in drug elimination half-lives and in some parameters needed for physiologically-based pharmacokinetic modeling. *Risk Anal* 23:117–142, 2003.
27. Fetner HH, Geller B: Lithium and tricyclic antidepressants. *Psychiatr Clin North Am* 15:223–241, 1992.
28. Painter MJ, Pippenger C, Wasterlain C, et al.: Phenobarbital and phenytoin in neonatal seizures: metabolism and tissue distribution. *Neurology* 31:1107–1112, 1981.
29. Kusuhara H, Sugiyama Y: Active efflux across the blood-brain barrier: role of the solute carrier family. *NeuroRx* 2:73–85, 2005.
30. Carson SW, Ousmanou AD, Hoyler SL: Emerging significance of P-glycoprotein in understanding drug disposition and drug interactions in psychopharmacology. *Psychopharmacol Bull* 36:67–81, 2002.
31. Tsai C, Ahdab-Barmada M, Daood MJ, et al.: P-glycoprotein expression in the developing human central nervous system: cellular and tissue localization. *Pediatr Res* 47(Suppl 436A abstract), 436a, 2001.
32. Plass JRM: Function and regulation of the human bile salt export pump. Available at: http://dissertations.ub.rug.nl/faculties/medicine/2005/j.r.m.plass/. Accessed March 01, 2006.
33. Janicak PG, Davis JM, Preskorn SH, et al. (eds): Pharmacokinetics. In: *Principles and Practice of Psychopharmacotherapy.* Baltimore, MD, Williams & Wilkins, 59–79, 1993.
34. Janicak PG: The relevance of clinical pharmacokinetics and therapeutic drug monitoring: anticonvulsant mood stabilizers and antipsychotics. *J Clin Psychiatry* 54:35–41, 1993.
35. Nelson DR, Koymans L, Kamataki T, et al.: P450 superfamily: update on new sequences, gene mapping, accession numbers and nomenclature. *Pharmacogenetics* 6:1–42, 1996.
36. Greenblatt DJ, von Moltke LL, Harmatz JS, Shader RI: Human cytochromes mediating sertraline biotransformation: seeking attribution. *J Clin Psychopharmacol* 19:489–493, 1999.
37. Bertilsson L: Geographical/interracial differences in polymorphic drug oxidation: current state of knowledge of cytochromes P450 (CYP) 2D6 and 2C19. *Clin Pharmacokinet* 29:192–209, 1995.
38. CDRH Consumer Information Website. Available at: http://www.fda.gov/cdrh/mda/docs/k042259.html. Accessed June 01, 2006.
39. de Leon J, Armstrong SC, Cozza KL: Clinical guidelines for psychiatrists for the use of pharmacogenetic testing for CYP450 2D6 and CYP450 2C19. *Psychosomatics* 47:75–85, 2006.
40. Wells PG, Mackenzie PI, Chowdhury JR, et al.: Glucuronidation and the UDP-glucuronosyltransferases in health and disease. *Drug Metab Dispos* 32:281–290, 2004.
41. Mori A, Maruo Y, Iwai M, et al.: UDP-glucuronosyltransferase 1A4 polymorphisms in a Japanese population and kinetics of clozapine glucuronidation. *Drug Metab Dispos* 33:672–675, 2005.
42. Court MH, Hao Q, Krishnaswamy S, et al.: UDP-glucuronosyltransferase (UGT) 2B15 pharmacogenetics: UGT2B15 D85Y genotype and gender are major determinants of oxazepam glucuronidation by human liver. *J Pharmacol Exp Ther* 310:656–665, 2004.
43. Ross JR, Rutter D, Welsh K, et al.: Clinical response to morphine in cancer patients and genetic variation in candidate genes. *Pharmacogenomics J* 5:324–336, 2005.
44. Food and Drug Administration: FDA News. Available at: http://www.fda.gov/bbs/topics/NEWS/2005/NEW01220.html. Accessed June 01, 2006.
45. Johnson TN: The development of drug metabolizing enzymes and their influence on the susceptibility to adverse drug reactions in children. *Toxicology* 192:37–48, 2003.
46. Blake MJ, Castro L, Leeder JS, Kearns GL: Ontogeny of drug metabolizing enzymes in the neonate. *Semin Fetal Neonatal Med* 10:123–138, 2005.
47. Johnsrud EK, Koukouritaki SB, Divakaran K, Brunengraber DK, Hines RN, McCarver DG: Human hepatic CYP2E1 expression during development. *J Pharmacol Exp Ther* 307:402–407, 2003.
48. Oesterheld JR: A review of developmental aspects of cytochrome P450. *J Child Adolesc Psychopharmacol* 8:161–174, 1998.
49. de Wildh SN, Kearns GL, Hop WC, Murry DJ, Abdel-Rahman SM, van den Anker JN: Pharmacokinetics and metabolism of oral midazolam in preterm infants. *Br J Clin Pharmacol* 53:390–392, 2002.
50. Koukouritaki SB, Namro JR, Marsh SA, et al.: Developmental expression of human hepatic CYP2C9 and CYP2C19. *J Pharm and Exp Ther* 307:402–407, 2003.
51. Stevens JC, Hines RN, Gu C, et al.: Developmental expression of the major human hepatic CYP3A enzymes. *J Pharm and Experimental Ther* 307:573–582, 2003.
52. Lambert GH, Schoeller DA, Kotake AN, Flores C, Hay D: The effect of age, gender, and sexual maturation on the caffeine breath test. *Dev Pharmacol Ther* 9:375–388, 1986.
53. de Wildt SN, Kearns GL, Leeder JS, van den Anker JN: Glucuronidation in humans. Pharmacogenetic and developmental aspects. *Clin Pharmacokinet* 36:439–452, 1999.
54. Strassburg CP, Strassburg A, Kneip S, et al.: Developmental aspects of human hepatic drug glucuronidation in young children and adults. *Gut* 50:259–265, 2002.
55. Murry DJ, Crom WR, Reddick WE, Bhargava R, Evans WE: Liver volume as a determinant of drug clearance in children and adolescents. *Drug Metab Dispos* 23:1110–1116, 1995.
56. Blanco JG, Harrison PL, Evans WE, Relling MV: Human cytochrome P450 maximal activities in pediatric versus adult liver. *Drug Metab and Dispos* 28:379–382, 2000.
57. Vitiello B, Behar D, Malone R, Delaney MA, Ryan PJ, Simpson GM: Pharmacokinetics of lithium carbonate in children. *J Clin Psychopharmacol* 8:355–359, 1988.
58. Armijo JA, Pena MA, Adin J, Vega-Gil N: Association between patient age and gabapentin serum concentration-to-dose ratio: a preliminary multivariate analysis. *Ther Drug Monit* 26:633–637, 2004.
59. Vigevano F: Levetiracetam in pediatrics. *J Child Neurol* 20:87–93, 2005.
60. Battino D, Croci D, Rossini A, Messina S, Mamoli D, Perucca E: Topiramate pharmacokinetics in children and adults with epilepsy: a case-matched comparison based on therapeutic drug monitoring data. *Clin Pharmacokinet* 44:407–416, 2005.
61. Wilens TE, Spencer T, Biederman J, Wozniak J, Connor D: Combined pharmacotherapy: an emerging trend in pediatric psychopharmacology. *J Am Acad Child Adolesc Psychiatry* 34:110–112, 1995.
62. Woolston JL: Combined pharmacotherapy: pitfalls of treatment. *J Am Acad Child Adolesc Psychiatry* 38:1455–1457, 1999.
63. Greenblatt DJ, Wright CE, von Moltke LL, et al.: Ketoconazole inhibition of triazolam and alprazolam clearance: differential kinetic and dynamic consequences. *Clin Pharmacol Ther* 64:237–247, 1998.
64. Anderson GD, Yau MK, Gidal BE, et al.: Bidirectional interaction of valproate and lamotrigine in healthy subjects. *Clin Pharmacol Ther* 60: 145–156, 1996.
65. GlaxoSmithKline: Prescribing information, Lamictal. Available at: https://www.gsksource.com/pharma/content/dam/GlaxoSmithKline/US/en/Prescribing_Information/Lamictal/pdf/LAMICTAL-PI-MG.PDF
66. Sabers A, Ohman I, Christensen J, Tomson T: Oral contraceptives reduce lamotrigine plasma levels. *Neurology* 61:570–571, 2003.
67. Ding R, Tayrouz Y, Riedel KD, et al.: Substantial pharmacokinetic interaction between digoxin and ritonavir in healthy volunteers. *Clin Pharmacol Ther* 76:73–84, 2004.
68. Ciraulo DA, Shader RI, Greenblatt DJ, Creelman WL: *Drug Interactions in Psychiatry.* 3rd ed. Philadelphia, PA, Lippincott Williams & Wilkins, 2005.
69. Cozza KL, Armstrong SC, Oesterheld JR: *Drug Interaction: Principles for Medical Practice.* 2nd ed. Washington, DC, American Psychiatric Publishing, 2003.
70. Sandson NB, Armstrong SC, Cozza KL: An overview of psychotropic drug-drug interactions. *Psychosomatics* 46:464–494, 2005.
71. Flockhart D: Drug interactions. Available at: http://medicine.iupui.edu/flockhart/table.htm. Accessed June 01, 2006.
72. Oesterheld J: Pgp table. Available at: http://www.mhc.com/PGP/PgpTable.HTML. Accessed March 01, 2006.
73. Oesterheld J: UGT table. Available at: http://www.mhc.com//Cytochromes//UGT//UGTTable.HTML. Accessed March 01, 2006.
74. Barrons R: Evaluation of personal digital assistant software for drug interactions. *Am J Health Syst Pharm* 61:380–385, 2004.
75. Patterson R, Oesterheld J: GenemedRx drug interaction program. Available at: http://www.genemedrx.com. Accessed June 01, 2006.

CHAPTER 6.1.3 ■ GENERAL PRINCIPLES AND CLINICAL PRACTICE

ANDRÉS MARTIN, JESSICA R. OESTERHELD, MICHAEL H. BLOCH, CHAD BEYER, AND LAWRENCE SCAHILL

INTRODUCTION

The now famous clinical trial conducted by Charles Bradley (1) is often cited as the beginning of pediatric psychopharmacology. In that study, the racemic mixture of levo- and dextroamphetamine (benzedrine) was administered openly to a group of 30 children with mixed behavioral and emotional symptoms. Bradley observed that the children characterized as "noisy, aggressive and domineering" were calmer and more manageable. In the same issue of the *American Journal of Psychiatry*, Molitch and Eccles (2) reported what may be the first placebo-controlled study in child psychiatry. Ninety-three boys described as juvenile delinquents were randomly assigned to gradually escalating doses of benzedrine or placebo. The benzedrine group showed dose-related improvements across a range of measures on learning, motor control, and short-term memory that exceeded the improvements in the placebo group. Since this pioneering work, the field of pediatric psychopharmacology has made steady progress.

Despite clear progress in some areas, there are important gaps between research and clinical practice. For example: (1) there have been over 100 placebo-controlled studies on the efficacy of methylphenidate in the treatment of attention-deficit hyperactivity disorder (ADHD), yet only a few studies have evaluated its long-term effects (3,4); (2) for serious psychiatric disorders such as autism, empirical support for the use of medication remains meager, leaving clinicians and families with limited guidance on appropriate treatment of affected children; (3) despite the demonstrated efficacy and safety of selective serotonin reuptake inhibitors (SSRIs) in the treatment of children and adolescents with obsessive–compulsive disorder (OCD), little is known about the appropriate duration of treatment; (4) while, the empirical foundations for pediatric psychopharmacology are not yet fully anchored, prescribing of psychotropic medications to pediatric population has increased dramatically over the last two decades. Data from the National Ambulatory Care Survey show that in adolescents between 14 and 18 years, the percent of visits to a doctor's office that resulted in a psychopharmacologic prescription rose from 3.4% in 1994–1995 to 8.3% in 2000–2001 (5). Additionally, in 2003–2004 approximately 2 million or 1% of all office visits by children and adolescents involved prescriptions for an antipsychotic (6). Over the past decade, however, there have been several initiatives that are having a substantial impact on the pace of progress in the field.

The purpose of this chapter is to present general principles of clinical psychopharmacology in pediatric populations. Following the discussion of seven overarching principles, this chapter reviews the major classes of psychotropic medications and current approaches to their use in children and adolescents. Drugs within the major classes are considered in terms of their pharmacology, adverse effects, clinical applications and management, and available empirical support. Pharmacokinetic aspects, including drug interactions, as well as mechanisms of action and other pharmacodynamic issues, will be considered only briefly here. Throughout this chapter, the reader is referred to the interspersed tables, in which the most salient information for each drug class and its specific agents are summarized.

Seven Guiding Principles

1. *The Role of Development.* There is a general recognition that development can have a major impact on pharmacologic effects (7). Thus, children and adults may show divergent responses to psychotropic drugs. The sources of these differences, as elaborated in the preceding chapter, are manifold. First, children often metabolize and eliminate drugs from the body more quickly than adults, resulting in shorter drug half-lives. This is apparently due to a larger liver-to-total body ratio and more efficient glomerular filtration rate in children as compared to adults. One practical implication of these pharmacokinetic differences is that in order to achieve therapeutic serum levels for some drugs when compared to adults, children may require higher weight-adjusted (mg/kg) dosages. In addition to pharmacokinetic considerations, because the central nervous system undergoes substantial developmental change during childhood, there can be age effects on drug action as well. For example, activating side effects of SSRIs and other antidepressants (8), and developmental differences in the maturation of noradrenergic pathways may explain, at least in part, why tricyclic antidepressants are less effective in children with depression as compared to adults (9). Taken together, these findings suggest that the three major neurochemical systems that are manipulated by psychotropic drug treatments (dopaminergic, serotonergic, and noradrenergic, respectively) are subject to age effects.

   In recognition of these developmental influences, federal policy initiatives have been instituted to promote studies specific to pediatric populations. First, in 1997 Congress passed the Food and Drug Administration Modernization Act (FDAMA), which offers pharmaceutical companies an additional 6 months of market exclusivity for products that are evaluated in children. For some drugs, this 6-month extension represents a powerful financial incentive. A second policy initiated by the Food and Drug Administration (FDA) requires pharmaceutical companies to evaluate new products in children if they are likely to be used in this population when released into the marketplace (10). A third and related development was the previous commitment of federal funds by the National Institutes of Health to establish research networks capable of conducting large-scale, multisite studies in pediatric populations (3,11–13). The combined impact of these initiatives has led to rapid growth in the knowledge base of pediatric psychopharmacology and its incorporation into clinical practice.

2. *The Limits of Categorical Diagnoses and Occurrence of Multiple Disorders as the Norm.* The second principle acknowledges the limitations of psychiatric diagnoses and of the current nosologic system of classification. Most psychiatric disorders in childhood are probably heterogeneous with respect to etiology. This presumption is supported by the high cooccurrence of psychiatric disorders in children—both in clinical (14) and in community samples (15). The extent to which these mixed syndromes represent a variant of a given disorder is often unclear, but may be relevant to drug response; for example, tics are a common cooccurring feature in OCD. The presence of tics may signal a different form of OCD and may be associated with a lower probability of positive response to monotherapy with an SSRI in OCD (16,17), and improved response to antipsychotic augmentation (18). Along the same lines, hyperactivity and impulsiveness are common complaints for children with pervasive developmental disorders (PDDs). Results from a multisite study in children with PDDs accompanied by hyperactivity, impulsiveness, and distractibility showed a lower rate of positive response to stimulants compared to what is observed in typically developing children with ADHD. In addition, children with PDDs appear to be at higher risk for adverse events with stimulant treatment (19). Thus, etiologic heterogeneity may explain differences in clinical response. These issues underscore the importance of large treatment studies to identify clinically meaningful subgroups and predictors of positive and negative response.
3. *Target Symptoms and the Integration of Data from Multiple Informants.* This principle concerns the importance of pretreatment assessment and the identification of target symptoms. Given the common occurrence of multiple psychiatric disorders in children, the identification of target symptoms for pharmacologic intervention may be easier said than done. One of the practical challenges in child psychiatry is the requirement of gathering information from multiple sources, including the child and parents at a minimum, and in many cases, the child's teacher, or another caregiver as well. Obtaining data from multiple sources can be aided by the use of behavioral checklists, child self-reports, and clinician ratings. Behavioral checklists completed by parents and teachers permit comparison of the current patient to a normative sample. Clinician-rated instruments can assist with establishing a pretreatment baseline of symptom severity. Some checklists and clinician-rated instruments can also be used to measure change over time. Although checklists and rating instruments can be extremely useful in the evaluation phase and to measure change over time, they cannot replace the clinical interview and direct observation of parent and child. A closely related challenge is the integration of all available information, in order to identify the most pressing target symptoms and select the most appropriate medication in combination with other needed interventions. The joint agreement on relevant target symptoms by caregivers and clinicians can be useful in monitoring therapeutic outcomes, but may also lead to greater consumer satisfaction with treatment (20).
4. *Adverse Effects: Monitoring Risks and Benefits.* The dramatic increase in the availability of new psychotropic drugs, their expanded use in pediatric populations, and their uncertain impact on development underscore the importance of ongoing assessment of adverse effects. At present, there is no clear consensus on the best method of eliciting information about adverse events that occur in the context of pharmacotherapy. This lack of consensus is not limited to child psychiatry; it extends to adult psychiatry as well as other areas of medicine. Three approaches have been described: the use of an open-ended general inquiry; the use of general inquiry augmented by a set of drug-specific queries or checklist; or the use of a detailed review of body systems (21). At the center of this debate are concerns about sensitivity, specificity, and efficiency.

   The use of a detailed review of systems by an experienced clinician is unlikely to miss adverse effects of medication (high sensitivity). However, some experts express concern that this method may produce an unacceptably high number of false-positive responses. If true, this low specificity would come at a great cost in clinician time, and contribute to a greater number of unnecessary medication changes.

   On the other hand, the open-ended general inquiry gives the parent and child an opportunity to express any concern that may have emerged since starting the medication or since the last visit. Based on the assumption that parents and children will notice important changes in behavior and/or health status, responses to the open-ended inquiry are likely to be clinically meaningful—even if they are not drug related. Because parents and children may not detect subtle adverse effects, the high specificity may result in missed adverse events (low sensitivity).

   A multisite study compared general inquiry, drug-specific queries, and review of systems approach in 60 children on various medications. The study showed that the review of systems approach did indeed identify adverse effects that the other methods missed. Moreover, in approximately a third of cases, the identified adverse effect from the review of systems interview led to an alteration in dose. Nonetheless, the review of systems used in the study was time-consuming and unlikely to be adopted in busy clinical practice (22). Thus, appropriate clinical practice entails the use of open-ended questions, followed by drug-specific queries. In the pages that follow, we list the adverse effects associated with each of the medications presented. Additional safety concerns are also presented in the tables. Other fundamental issues to be covered in contemporary medication management of children include questions about concomitant medications, concurrent illness, and other medical contacts since the previous visit. The need for vital signs, height, and weight monitoring, for neurologic examination, electrocardiogram, laboratory tests, and drug levels, are medication specific and described in the appropriate sections below.
5. *The Role of Caregivers and the Meaning of Medication.* Collaboration and successful engagement of the child's family are critical to the success of treatment interventions, pharmacologic or otherwise. A detailed discussion with the parents and the child concerning the recommended medication, and an examination of the alternative treatments are prerequisites for initiating psychopharmacologic treatment. In addition, the family and the child should be (to the extent possible) active partners in the treatment process (23). Once chosen, the dose schedule, potential adverse effects, anticipated magnitude of response on target symptoms as well as the time to effect warrant explicit review. This discussion gives an opportunity to evaluate and temper unrealistic expectations about the medication. Depending on the medication, it may be necessary to establish a contingency plan to manage specific adverse effects prior to their occurrence, such as being prepared to start benztropine

for a child who develops dystonia when started on a potent antipsychotic such as haloperidol, or to discontinue medication if excessive weight gain is experienced on an atypical antipsychotic. Children, and to some lesser extent adolescents, are dependent on their parents to administer medications, so that parental endorsement of the treatment plan is both ethically sound and practical. Failure to involve parents in the decision-making process may threaten treatment compliance, which in turn may undermine the success of the intervention. Attention should also be paid to the meaning that taking medication has for the child and family (24), in the context of their cultural beliefs and attitudes toward medication. Consideration and exploration of these aspects may reveal a sense of failure on the part of the child or family. Some children may express concern that having to take medication implies that they are crazy or "weird." These issues should be identified and addressed prior to initiating treatment. Even when handled prior to treatment, however, these issues often reemerge and require attention over the course of treatment.

6. *Psychopharmacology in Context, and the Combination of Therapeutic Modalities.* Psychotropic medications, no matter how effective, are often but one element in a multimodal treatment plan that includes other individually tailored interventions. This guiding principle, which may seem self-evident to clinicians accustomed to using various therapeutic approaches in their practice, has become a focal point for research and practice guidelines. For example, practice parameters often provide guidance of selection and sequence of interventions, such as when to use one modality (behavioral therapy or medication) versus a combined medication approach. Several cognitive-behavioral treatments have proven efficacy and should not be overlooked in the treatment of children and adolescents with major psychiatric conditions (25). Three large-scale, National Institute of Mental Health (NIMH) sponsored, multisite studies in pediatric samples with ADHD (3), depression (13), and OCD (26) have been completed and provide some insight into the use of combined treatments (see following).
7. *Empirically Informed, Evidence-Based Clinical Decision-Making.* A final principle is that treatment plans should be grounded on available empirical evidence. As the database of pediatric psychopharmacology expands, the value of this principle will become even more pressing and places a higher demand for clinicians to stay apace of research findings. The International Association for Child and Adolescent Psychiatry and Allied Professions provides levels of evidence for efficacy of psychotropic medications in children (<18 years) (27). The strength of the evidence relates to the following: type I (strong evidence from at least one systematic review of multiple well-designed randomized controlled trials); type II (strong evidence from at least one properly designed randomized controlled trial); type III (evidence from well-designed trials without randomization, single group, pre–post, cohort, time series or matched case-control studies); type IV (evidence from well-designed nonexperimental studies from more than one center or research group); type V (opinions of respected authorities, based on clinical evidence, descriptive studies, or reports of expert committees) (28). As examples relevant to pediatric psychopharmacology, type I evidence exists in the case of: methylphenidate and dexmethylphenidate, amphetamines, atomoxetine, clonidine, guanfacine for ADHD; clonidine, haloperidol, risperidone, and pimozide for Tourette disorder; fluoxetine and escitalopram for major depression; sertraline for OCD, generalized anxiety disorder (GAD), and social phobia (SP); fluvoxamine for GAD and SP; risperidone for bipolar disorder; risperidone and aripiprazole for agression. Type II evidence exists in the case of: fluoxetine, fluvoxamine, and clomipramine for OCD; fluoxetine for GAD and SP; sertraline and citalopram for major depression; haloperidol for psychosis; risperidone, quetiapine, aripiprazole, olanzapine for schizophrenia; quetiapine, aripiprazole, olanzapine, valproate for bipolar disorder; lithium and valproate for aggression. Type III evidence exists in the case of lithium for bipolar disorder. Type IV evidence is not well represented in psychopharmaceuticals for children. Type V evidence exists in the case of carbamazepine, oxcarbazepine for bipolar disorder; lamotrigine for bipolar depression, and venlafaxine for major depression.

This ranking system clearly reflects the state of the science at a particular point in time. Given the rapid pace of development in pediatric psychopharmacology, clinicians have a responsibility to remain up to date with the empirical evidence to ensure the best possible match between target symptoms and treatment options.

References

1. Bradley C: The behavior of children receiving benzedrine. *Am J Psychiatry* 94(3):577–585, 1937.
2. Molitch M, Eccles AK: The effect of benzedrine sulfate on the intelligence scores of children. *Am J Psychol* 94(3):587–590, 1937.
3. MTA Cooperative Group: A 14-month randomized clinical trial of treatment strategies for attention-deficit/hyperactivity disorder. Multimodal Treatment Study of Children with ADHD. *Arch Gen Psychiatry* 56(12):1073–1086, 1999.
4. MTA Cooperative Group: National institute of Mental Health Multimodal Treatment Study of ADHD follow-up: changes in effectiveness and growth after the end of treatment. *Pediatrics* 113(4):762–769, 2004.
5. Chen LY, Crum RM, Strain EC, Alexander GC, Kaufmann C, Mojtabai R: Prescriptions, nonmedical use, and emergency department visits involving prescription stimulants. *J Clin Psychiatry* 77(3):e297–e304, 2016.
6. Aparasu RR, Bhatara V: Patterns and determinants of antipsychotic prescribing in children and adolescents, 2003–2004. *Curr Med Res Opin* 23(1):49–56, 2007.
7. Vitiello B, Jensen PS: Developmental perspectives in pediatric psychopharmacology. *Psychopharmacol Bull* 31(1):75–81, 1995.
8. Martin A, Scahill L, Anderson GM, et al.: Weight and leptin changes among risperidone-treated youths with autism: 6-month prospective data. *Am J Psychiatry* 161(6):1125–1127, 2004.
9. Kaufman J, Martin A, King RA, Charney D: Are child-, adolescent-, and adult-onset depression one and the same disorder? *Biol Psychiatry* 49(12):980–1001, 2001.
10. FDA Modernization Act (FDAMA) of 1997: *Wiley Encyclopedia of Clinical Trials.* Wiley-Blackwell, 2008.
11. Walkup JT, Labellarte MJ, Riddle MA, et al.: Fluvoxamine for the treatment of anxiety disorders in children and adolescents. *N Engl J Med* 344(17):1279–1285, 2001.
12. McCracken JT, McGough J, Shah B, et al.: Risperidone in children with autism and serious behavioral problems. *N Engl J Med* 347(5):314–321, 2002.
13. March J, Silva S, Petrycki S, et al; Treatment for Adolescents With Depression Study (TADS) Team: Fluoxetine, cognitive-behavioral therapy, and their combination for adolescents with depression: Treatment for Adolescents With Depression Study (TADS) randomized controlled trial. *JAMA* 292(7):807–820, 2004.
14. Biederman J, Newcorn J, Sprich S: Comorbidity of attention deficit hyperactivity disorder with conduct, depressive, anxiety, and other disorders. *Am J Psychiatry* 148(5):564–577, 1991.
15. Angold A, Costello EJ, Erkanli A: Comorbidity. *J Child Psychol Psychiatry* 40(1):57–87, 1999.
16. Scahill L, Riddle MA, King RA, et al.: Fluoxetine has no marked effect on tic symptoms in patients with Tourette's syndrome: a double-blind placebo-controlled study. *J Child Adolesc Psychopharmacol* 7(2):75–85, 1997.
17. Scahill L, Kano Y, King RA, et al.: Influence of age and tic disorders on obsessive-compulsive disorder in a pediatric sample. *J Child Adolesc Psychopharmacol* 13(Suppl 1):S7–S17, 2003.
18. Bloch MH, Landeros-Weisenberger A, Kelmendi B, Coric V, Bracken MB, Leckman JF: A systematic review: antipsychotic augmentation with treatment refractory obsessive-compulsive disorder. *Mol Psychiatry* 11(7):622–632, 2006.

19. Research Units on Pediatric Psychopharmacology Autism Network: Risperidone treatment of autistic disorder: longer-term benefits and blinded discontinuation after 6 months. *Am J Psychiatry* 162(7):1361–1369, 2005.
20. Arnold LE, Vitiello B, McDougle C, et al.: Parent-defined target symptoms respond to risperidone in RUPP autism study: customer approach to clinical trials. *J Am Acad Child Adolesc Psychiatry* 42(12):1443–1450, 2003.
21. Greenhill LL, Vitiello B, Riddle MA, et al.: Review of safety assessment methods used in pediatric psychopharmacology. *J Am Acad Child Adolesc Psychiatry* 42(6):627–633, 2003.
22. Greenhill LL, Vitiello B, Fisher P, et al.: Comparison of increasingly detailed elicitation methods for the assessment of adverse events in pediatric psychopharmacology. *J Am Acad Child Adolesc Psychiatry* 43(12):1488–1496, 2004.
23. Rawat DS, Joshi MC, Joshi P, Atheaya H: Marine peptides and related compounds in clinical trial. *Anticancer Agents Med Chem* 6(1):33–40, 2006.
24. Pruett KD, Joshi SV, Martin A: Thinking about prescribing: the psychology of psychopharmacology. In: Martin A, Scahill L, Kratochvil CJ (eds): *Pediatric Psychopharmacology: Principles and Practice*. 2nd ed. New York, Oxford University Press (OUP), 422–433, 2010.
25. Weisz JR, Kazdin AE (eds): *Evidence-Based Psychotherapies for Children and Adolescents*. 2nd ed. New York, The Guilford Press, 602, 2011.
26. Pediatric OCD Treatment Study (POTS) Team: Cognitive-behavior therapy, sertraline, and their combination for children and adolescents with obsessive-compulsive disorder: the Pediatric OCD Treatment Study (POTS) randomized controlled trial. *JAMA* 292(16):1969–1976, 2004.
27. Vitiello B: Principles in using psychotropic medication in children and adolescents. In: Rey JM (ed): *IACAPAP e-Textbook of Child and Adolescent Mental Health*. Geneva, International Association for Child and Adolescent Psychiatry and Allied Professions, 2015.
28. Gray J: *Evidence-Based Healthcare: How to Make Health Policy and Management Decisions*. New York, Churchill-Livingstone, 1997.

6.1.4 SPECIFIC MEDICATION TREATMENTS

CHAPTER 6.1.4.1 ■ ADHD: STIMULANT AND NONSTIMULANT AGENTS

MICHAEL H. BLOCH, CHAD BEYER, ANDRÉS MARTIN, AND LAWRENCE SCAHILL

STIMULANTS

Clinical Applications and Empirical Support

The stimulants, especially the short- and long-acting forms of methylphenidate and various preparations of amphetamine, are first-line treatments for attention-deficit hyperactivity disorder (ADHD). In its classic form, ADHD is characterized by inattention, impulsiveness, and hyperactivity, though current convention includes primarily inattentive and impulsive/hyperactive subtypes (1). Epidemiologic studies indicate that ADHD is relatively common in childhood, affecting 2% to 10% of school-age children (2,3). Boys are affected more often than girls. It persists into adolescence in a majority of cases (4), and into adulthood in as many as 30% to 40% of cases (5). Studies of clinical populations indicate that the symptoms of ADHD are among the most common reasons for referral of children to mental health agencies (6). Nonetheless, there is also a substantial number of affected children who do not receive treatment (7). Given the high prevalence of ADHD in school-age children, the potential for long-term functional disability and the high health-related costs associated with the disorder (8), ADHD is a major public health concern. To ensure fewer children with ADHD are missed, the DSM-5 states that several of the ADHD symptoms must be present prior to 12 years of age, compared to 7 years of age in the DSM-IV. This is in keeping with there being no clinical difference found between children identified before or after age 7 years in terms of course, severity, outcome, or treatment response.

The most commonly used stimulants for the treatment of ADHD include methylphenidate, dextroamphetamine, and the mixed preparation of D,L-amphetamine and their derivatives. Table 6.1.4.1.1 outlines the characteristics of psychostimulant medications commonly used to treat ADHD. The empirical basis for the use of stimulants in children with ADHD rests on findings from hundreds of short-term, randomized, placebo-controlled studies conducted over the past 30 to 40 years. Results from controlled studies over the last decade provide additional information about dose response, similarities and differences in response across stimulant preparations, and the importance of regular clinical monitoring to achieve optimal response. Rapport et al. (9) conducted a dose–response study in 76 subjects (66 boys and 10 girls) between the ages of 6 and 11. The 5-week study used four dose levels of methylphenidate (5, 10, 15, and 20 mg given bid) and placebo given in random order in a cross-over design. All dose levels of active medication were superior to placebo. In addition, there was a clear linear trend, such that classroom behavior and the number of completed assignments improved with each increase in dose. However, the incremental improvement was smaller as the dose moved above the 10-mg dose level. Meta-analysis shows in parallel-group and cross-over trials participants in the active treatment group, compared with the control group, were more likely to report trouble sleeping, report a decrease in appetite and weight, weigh significantly less and have a lower body mass index, and have a higher pulse, have tics or nervous movements, compulsive acts, obsessive thinking, and overly meticulous behavior. They were less likely compared with the control group to report anger, behavioral complaints, or an increase in appetite (10).

In order to compare methylphenidate and D-amphetamine, a placebo-controlled cross-over study was conducted in 48 boys between 6 and 12 years of age (11). Subjects were treated with methylphenidate, D-amphetamine, or placebo in random order for 3 weeks in each treatment condition. During each condition, the dose was increased on a weekly basis (e.g., methylphenidate doses for children under 30 kg of body weight were 12.5, 20, and 35 mg at breakfast and lunch time for the respective weeks). Based on a global rating of response, there were similar levels of response between the two stimulant classes, with 79% of the subjects showing a positive response to methylphenidate and 88% showing a positive response to

TABLE 6.1.4.1.1

STIMULANT MEDICATIONS FOR ATTENTION-DEFICIT HYPERACTIVITY DISORDER

Drug Name (Brand)	Active Ingredient	Onset of Action	Duration of Effect	Required Number of Doses/Day	Suggested Dosing and Titration
Short Acting					
Ritalin® Methylin® Focalin® Metadate®	Methylphenidate	20–60 min Peak effect: 2 hrs	3–6 hrs	2–3 doses; occasionally 4 doses	Start with one 5-mg tablet (2.5 for Focalin®) 2–3× a day. Increase by 5 mg (or 2.5 mg for Focalin®) until target behavior controlled
Dexedrine® Dextrostat®	D-amphetamine	20–60 min Peak effect: 1–2 hrs	4–6 hrs	2–3 doses	Start with one 5-mg tablet 2–3× per day[a]
Adderall®	D,L-amphetamine	30–60 min Peak effect: 1–2 hrs	4–6 hrs	2–3 doses	Start with one 5-mg tablet 2–3× per day[a]
First Generation: Long Acting					
Ritalin SR® Metadate ER® Methylin ER®	Methylphenidate	60–90 min Peak effect: 8 hrs	5–8 hrs	1–2 doses	Start with one 10-mg tablet 1–2× per day[a]
Dexedrine Spansules®	D-amphetamine	60–90 min Peak effect: 8 hrs	6–8 hrs	1–2 doses	Start with one 5-mg capsule 1–2× per day[a]
Second Generation: Long Acting					
Concerta®	Methylphenidate	30 min–2 hrs	12 hrs	1 tablet	Start with one 18-mg tablet once per day[a]
Metadate CD® Ritalin LA®	Methylphenidate	30 min–2 hrs	6–8 hrs	1–2 capsules	Start with one 10-mg capsule once per day[a]
Daytrana®	Methylphenidate	20–60 min Peak effect: 10 hrs after single application, 8 hrs after repeat applications	8–12 hrs	1 patch	Start 10-mg patch worn 9 hrs daily. Maximum dose: 30 mg patch worn 9 hrs daily
Focalin XR®	Dexmethylphenidate	1–4 hrs	8–12 hrs	1 capsule	Start with one 5-mg capsule once per day[a]
Quillivant XR®	Methylphenidate	30 min Peak effect: 5 hrs	8–12 hrs	1 liquid dose	Start with 20 mg liquid suspension once per day[a]
Adderall XR®	D,L-amphetamine	1–2 hrs	10–12 hrs	1 capsule	Start with one 5- or 10-mg capsule once per day[a]
Vyvanse®	L-lysine-dextroamphetamine	2 hrs Peak effect: 3–4 hrs	10–12 hrs	1 capsule	Start with one 30-mg capsule once daily[a]

[a]Titrate upward until target behavior controlled.

D-amphetamine. Only 2 of the 48 subjects failed to respond to either stimulant.

Pelham et al. (12) compared the extended-release methylphenidate product, Concerta, to immediate-release methylphenidate and placebo in a cross-over trial. Sixty-eight children between 6 and 12 years were assigned to receive placebo, immediate-release methylphenidate, or the extended-release methylphenidate in random order. All children were on methylphenidate prior to enrollment. Thus, each child was assigned to a dosage level that was similar to the pretrial dose. The three dose levels for immediate-release methylphenidate were 5 mg three times per day, 10 mg three times per day, or 15 mg three times per day. Each dose level of immediate-release methylphenidate was matched to a similar, though slightly higher, dose of extended-release. Specifically, the dose levels of extended-release were 18, 36, and 54 mg given as a single morning dose. Each treatment (immediate release, matching dose of extended-release, or placebo) was given in random order for 1 week. Both active treatments were superior to placebo, with approximately 50% improvement on both parent and teacher measures of ADHD symptoms. There were no detectable differences between immediate- and extended-release methylphenidate preparations with respect to efficacy or adverse effects.

There are few studies examining long-term use of stimulants (6). A longitudinal cohort from birth to a mean age of 17.2 analyzed 379 children with research-identified ADHD. Of these children, 283 were treated with stimulants, with an average duration of treatment of 33.8 months (13). Nearly 75% of treatment episodes involving stimulants were associated with a favorable response (74.6% for methylphenidate (MPH) and 74.9% for dextroamphetamine). 22.3% of the 283 children experienced at least one side effect during treatment, with gender not being significantly associated with likelihood to develop side effects. Treatment episodes with dextroamphetamine were significantly more likely to be associated with a side effect compared to methylphenidate (10.0% vs. 6.1%; OR, 1.8; 95% CI, 1.1–3.0; $p = 0.034$). The occurrence of side effects of dextroamphetamine was independent of dose, while the occurrence of side effects with MPH showed dose dependence. Additionally, side effects occurred most frequently at either tail end of age distribution with both MPH and dextroamphetamine.

With its sample size of 576 children, the Multimodal Treatment Study of children with attention-deficit/hyperactivity disorder (MTA) provides convincing evidence for the long-term benefits of methylphenidate. In the MTA study, children between 7 and 10 years of age were randomly assigned to one of four treatment groups: medication management ($N = 144$; primarily methylphenidate administered in a systematic fashion with close monitoring); an intensive behavioral treatment program ($N = 144$); combined medication management and the same behavioral treatment program ($N = 145$); or community care, which served as the control group ($N = 146$). The MTA research sites provided treatment to three of these groups, including the medication management group, the behavioral therapy-only group, and the combined medication plus behavioral therapy group. The community care group received treatment from self-selected practitioners. In most cases (84 of 146, or 58%), community care consisted of methylphenidate given on a twice-daily schedule. After 14 months of treatment, all four groups showed improvement compared to baseline. Comparisons across the four groups showed that the combined treatment group and the medication management group did significantly better than the community care group and the behavioral treatment-only group across a range of outcomes.

Several potentially important differences emerged when community care was compared to medication management provided by the MTA sites. First, community practitioners most often administered methylphenidate on a twice-daily schedule, compared to three times per day in the MTA-treated groups. Second, among the children randomly assigned to community care, 33% ($N = 48$) stopped taking medication during the study period. Not surprisingly, this group showed the least improvement on the primary outcome measures. By contrast, only 3% ($N = 18$) of the research medication management groups (both medication-only and medication plus behavioral treatment) discontinued medication during the study. Third, in the MTA medication management groups, follow-up visits were more frequent and parent and teacher ratings were used in a systematic way to inform clinical decision-making. Fourth, methylphenidate in general was dosed lower in the community care group compared to the medication management groups in MTA, suggesting that most community prescribers may be underdosing the stimulants.

Taken together, the results of these studies suggest that stimulants are effective for short- and long-term treatment of children with ADHD. When considering group effects, stimulants appear to be equally beneficial, but individual patients may respond better to one preparation over another. The modest effectiveness of stimulants observed in the community care group of the MTA suggests that close clinical monitoring with dose adjustments based on systematic assessment of therapeutic and side effects contributes to compliance and optimal results.

Mechanism of Action

Although stimulants have become the standard treatment for ADHD, their mechanism of action is not clearly understood. In addition, the mechanism of action for amphetamines and methylphenidate may be slightly different (14). Methylphenidate promotes the release of stored dopamine and blocks the reuptake of dopamine at presynaptic dopamine transporter sites. Amphetamines also block dopamine reuptake at the transporter, but appear to promote the release of newly synthesized dopamine more selectively. These combined effects enhance dopamine function in the striatum and, at least indirectly, in the prefrontal cortex (PFC). It is also clear that both methylphenidate and the amphetamines affect the norepinephrine (NE) system (15). For example, both compounds decrease the neuronal firing rate in the locus coeruleus (LC), although amphetamine appears to be more potent in this action. Whether the effect on the NE system is facilitatory or inhibitory is not clear at present. Nonetheless, these combined effects appear to be essential to the clinical effects of the stimulants, as drugs with more selective action (guanfacine or desipramine) tend to have smaller clinical effects.

Pharmacokinetics

The pharmacokinetics of all individual currently available stimulant medications for ADHD is outlined in Table 6.1.4.1.1. Immediate-release formulations of methylphenidate, dextroamphetamine, and the combined levo- and dextroamphetamine preparation are readily absorbed and show behavioral effects 30 to 60 minutes after ingestion. The peak level of immediate-release methylphenidate occurs approximately 90 to 150 minutes after ingestion and the clinical effects last 3 to 5 hours. The immediate-release amphetamine products achieve peak levels between 1 and 3 hours, with duration of action of 5 to 7 hours. Based on blinded studies in a research classroom setting, the D,L-amphetamine preparation appears to have a slightly longer duration of action than standard D-amphetamine (16). Methylphenidate and amphetamine are metabolized in the liver, but by quite different pathways (see previous chapter for more details). For the immediate-release formulations of these stimulants, the parent compound and metabolites are excreted in the urine within 24 hours. Several sustained-release (SR) products have been introduced, offering a range of options for clinical management of children and adolescents with ADHD, often with once-a-day dosing. These extended-release formulations have been increasingly utilized based on convenience rather than improved efficacy.

Specific Stimulants and Clinical Management

There has been considerable debate over whether stimulant dose should be weight based or a fixed dose (17). At least in part, this controversy can be traced to early research suggesting that lower doses, such as 0.3 mg/kg/dose, were optimal for enhancing cognitive performance, whereas higher doses (0.6 mg/kg/dose or higher) were more effective for behavioral control (18). Subsequent studies have not supported this view. For example, a convincing linear dose–response was demonstrated across a range of outcomes in a placebo-controlled, cross-over study involving 76 children and four dose levels of methylphenidate (9). Nonetheless, individual children may indeed show variability in response across a range of dose levels. Other children may show an orderly dose–response up to a threshold, above which there is little additive benefit. Thus, the mg/kg calculation can be used as a crude guide to calculate the starting dose of 0.3 mg/kg/dose and to a usual ceiling dose (e.g., 0.8 mg/kg/dose). Thereafter, the dose can be increased to establish an optimal response. For example, school-age children can be started on 5 mg tid (just before breakfast, just before lunch, and 3 to 4 pm). The dosage may be increased to 10 mg bid (morning and noon) and 5 mg after school after 5 to 7 days. Subsequent increases are based on clinical response and emergence of adverse effects. The third dose typically remains half (or even less) of the first and second doses so as to minimize *rebound* effects and possible interference with sleep (17).

To determine the optimal daily dose of methylphenidate, it is essential to get feedback from both parents and teachers. In the MTA study, children were seen weekly when starting the medication to monitor progress and side effects. The study used daily ratings to assist with the assessment of response. Although this is not always feasible in clinical practice, clinicians may elect to pace dose increases with the collection of parent and teacher ratings. For example, in the first month of treatment, clinicians may increase the dose on a weekly basis. Collection of parent and teacher ratings prior to each increase would allow comparisons across dose levels. This information could be integrated with side-effect data in order to select the optimal dose.

A similar approach can be used with D-amphetamine and D,L-amphetamine. The dosing of these two drugs is similar and both have approximately twofold greater effect compared to methylphenidate. Thus, the amphetamines are administered at half the methylphenidate dose. Moreover, due to their slightly longer duration of action, the amphetamines are typically given twice a day—morning and noon. The initial dosage may be a single 2.5-mg dose in younger children or a 5-mg dose in older children. After 5 to 7 days, the medication may be raised 5 mg bid in younger children and 10 mg bid in older children. Thereafter, the dosage may be raised every 5 to 7 days to a total of 15 to 20 mg/day in younger children, and 40 mg/day in older children.

Several extended-release products—formulated with methylphenidate (Concerta, Aptensio, Daytrana transdermal patch, Metadate CD, Metadate ER, Methylin ER, Ritalin LA, Ritalin SR, Quillivant XR; Focalin XR [dexmethylphenidate]) and amphetamine (Adderall XR [dextroamphetamine], Dexedrine-Spansule [dextroamphetamine sulfate], Evekeo [amphetamine sulfate], Vyvanse [lisdexamfetamine]) are available. These longer-acting preparations are as effective as the immediate-release compounds and show similar side-effect profiles (13,19,20). The advantage of the long-acting preparations is that children do not need to take a dose in school, which may enhance compliance. The longer-duration formulations may minimize the behavioral rebound often seen with immediate-release formulations. Originally developed for children who could not swallow pills, Daytrana (methylphenidate transdermal patch) has been tested clinically on youth from 7 to 16 years, with the patch adhered to intact skin, and it appears as effective as oral preparations.

Adverse Effects

Growth retardation, presumed to be secondary to stimulant-induced appetite suppression, has been a common concern among clinicians and families alike. Based on data from a large cohort of clinic cases treated with stimulants, Spencer et al. (21) contend that slowed growth may be temporary, and that children with ADHD may be shorter than their age mates before puberty, but "catch up" in adolescence. Follow-up data from the MTA study show that children who remained on medication from the end of the 14-month study to the 24-month follow-up did not gain as much in height or weight when compared to the children who were never started stimulant medication. The group that did not receive medication ($N = 106$) was about 1 cm taller and 1 kg heavier at the 24-month follow-up than the group ($N = 222$) that was treated with stimulant medication for the entire 2-year period (22). Appetite suppression can often be managed by giving stimulant medications with food, or immediately after meals. Height and weight should be monitored regularly in children treated with stimulants, and tracked during long-term maintenance on growth charts.

Other common side effects include sleep disturbance, depressed mood, stomach aches, headaches, overfocusing on details, tics and mannerisms, and picking at skin. Insomnia can be difficult to sort out, as many children with ADHD have sleep difficulties prior to receiving stimulant medications. Rebound effects associated with stimulant withdrawal may compound pre-existing sleep problems. Thus, the child's sleep history should be documented prior to treatment and monitored throughout. As noted, it is common practice for the third dose of methylphenidate to be lower than the first two in order to minimize a possible rebound effect. The use of clonidine as an aid for sleep has been proposed, yet remains a controversial practice (23). A multisite trial conducted by the Tourette Syndrome Study Group (24) showed that complaints of insomnia were indeed lower in subjects randomly assigned to combined treatment with methylphenidate and clonidine compared to methylphenidate alone.

Results from case reports and controlled studies suggest that exposure to stimulants can be associated with the emergence of tics (25) or the worsening of pre-existing tics (26). However, several studies have also shown that tics do *not* worsen when children with ADHD and comorbid tic disorders are treated with stimulants (and in fact about one-third get better) (24,27,28). Meta-analysis suggests that stimulants are just as effective at reducing ADHD symptoms in children with comorbid tics compared to those without (29). Furthermore, meta-analysis of randomized controlled trials of stimulants for children with ADHD suggests no increased risk of tics with stimulant medication, and that over 6% of subjects reported tics as a side effect of study medication regardless of whether they received stimulants or placebo (30). Exacerbation of existing tics or de novo tics that occur during stimulant use appear to be much more likely to be coincidental than causative.

Nonstimulant Treatments of ADHD

Atomoxetine (Strattera)

Atomoxetine was originally developed for the treatment of depression, but it has never been marketed as an antidepressant. Atomoxetine is a selective NE reuptake inhibitor, a property that it shares in common with desipramine. Unlike desipramine, atomoxetine does not appear to be associated with an increase in QTc interval. Given the efficacy of desipramine for the treatment of ADHD, atomoxetine was evaluated for the same indication. Following the completion of several placebo-controlled trials (31,32), atomoxetine was approved by the FDA as a safe and effective treatment for children and adolescents with ADHD. Atomoxetine may also be useful in the treatment of comorbid oppositional defiant disorder (33,34).

The pharmacokinetics of all nonstimulant medications used to treat ADHD is presented in Table 6.1.4.1.2. The serum half-life of atomoxetine is approximately 4 hours, which implies that the drug would be given at least twice a day. Indeed, initial studies used a twice-daily regimen, but subsequent trials evaluated the efficacy of once-a-day dosing (31,32) and, both dosing strategies have been shown to be superior to placebo and show similar therapeutic benefit (31,32). The improvement of ADHD symptoms is not as robust as with stimulants (35). The total daily dose should fall between 0.8 and 1.2 mg/kg. Doses greater than 1.2 mg/kg/day have no therapeutic advantage (34). Clinicians should start with once-a-day dosing with gradual titration of dose. If the child encounters adverse effects or the benefits are inadequate, a twice-a-day dosing schedule can be considered.

Common side effects of atomoxetine include dyspepsia, nausea, vomiting, fatigue, decreased appetite, weight loss, mood swings, headache, constipation, insomnia, and dizziness

TABLE 6.1.4.1.2

NONSTIMULANT MEDICATIONS FOR ATTENTION-DEFICIT HYPERACTIVITY DISORDER

Medication	Drug Name	Frequency	Daily Dose Range
Atomoxetine	Strattera®	Daily or twice daily	0.5–1.2 mg/kg/day (<70 kg) 40–80 mg/day (≥70 kg)
Clonidine	Clonidine IR®	Twice daily to 4× per day	0.05–0.4 mg/day
	Clonidine ER (Kapvay®)	Daily	0.1–0.4 mg/day
Guanfacine	Guanfacine IR®	Twice daily to 4× per day	0.5–0.4 mg/day
	Guanfacine ER (Intuniv®)	Daily	1–4 mg/day
Desipramine	Norpramin®	Twice daily to 3× per day	2–5 mg/kg/day
Bupropion	Wellbutrin®	Twice daily	50–150 mg

(36). Decreased appetite, vomiting, and weight loss are more likely to occur early in treatment and may be attenuated by slow titration of dose. Black box warnings on this drug include hepatitis, increased aggression and hostility, and suicidal thinking (37). Atomoxetine is metabolized by the cytochrome P450 2D6 and thus it is vulnerable to interaction from drugs that inhibit 2D6, such as paroxetine or fluoxetine.

Bupropion (Wellbutrin)

Bupropion is unrelated to all other available antidepressants. Although its mechanism of action is unclear, it appears to have both dopaminergic and noradrenergic effects. It is approved for the treatment of depression and smoking cessation in adults. Although bupropion has not been studied for depression in children or adolescents, it has been evaluated in controlled studies for the treatment of ADHD. A placebo-controlled trial of bupropion in 72 children with ADHD showed its superiority over placebo, although the treatment effect was smaller than that usually seen with stimulants (38). The dose of bupropion (3 to 6 mg/kg/day) ranged from 50 to 200 mg/day in divided doses. The findings of this study are consistent with previous placebo-controlled studies, and a direct comparison-study with methylphenidate (39). In an open-label study conducted in 24 adolescents (ages 11 to 16) with ADHD and depression, sustained-release bupropion was associated with improvements in both conditions in 58% (N = 14), in depression only in 29% (N = 7), and in ADHD alone in 4% (N = 1), suggesting that further studies of this monotherapy appear warranted for patients with these commonly co-occurring conditions (Table 6.1.4.1.2) (40).

Side effects of bupropion include agitation, insomnia, skin rashes, nausea, vomiting, constipation, and tremor. Bupropion may also reduce the seizure threshold in a dose-dependent fashion. The seizure liability of bupropion was first described in a group of female patients with bulimia nervosa. Because of this, regardless of diagnosis, it is recommended that daily doses not exceed 300 mg in children, and no single dose should exceed 150 mg and should not be used in comorbid eating disorders. Bupropion (Wellbutrin) is available in 75- and 100-mg tablets, in 100- and 150-mg SR tablets, and 150- and 300-mg bupropion XL tablets. Treatment is usually on a tid basis for the immediate-release formulation, given the agent's short half-life; bid dosing is possible with the SR preparations and once daily is recommended with XL preparations.

ALPHA-2 ADRENERGIC AGENTS

Clonidine (Catapres, Kapvay) and Guanfacine (Tenex, Intuniv)

The short-acting alpha-2 adrenergic agents (clonidine and guanfacine) have been used in the treatment of ADHD and tics for well over two decades, but were only FDA approved for use in adults with hypertension. More recently, extended-release forms of both clonidine (Kapvay) and guanfacine (Intuniv) were approved for the treatment of children with ADHD. These long-acting formulations have the advantage of once-a-day dosing and a specific FDA indication for ADHD compared to the short-acting formulations, but represent a significant cost increase compared to the off-patent shorter medications (especially with regard to clonidine).

Clinical Applications and Empirical Support

Meta-analysis has demonstrated that alpha-2 agonists are effective for the treatment of ADHD as monotherapy or as an add-on treatment to stimulants (41). Meta-analysis of 12 randomized controlled trials (including nine monotherapy trials and three add-on trials) demonstrated that alpha-2 agonist monotherapy significantly reduced overall ADHD symptoms (effect size = 0.59), hyperactivity/impulsivity (effect size = 0.56), inattention (effect size = 0.57), and oppositional defiant disorder (ODD) symptoms (effect size = 0.44) or alpha-2 agonists as add-on treatment to stimulants also significantly reduced overall ADHD symptoms (effect size = 0.36), hyperactivity/impulsivity (effect size = 0.33), and inattention (effect size = 0.34) (41). But, not surprisingly, effect sizes were lower for the use of alpha-2 agonists as add-on treatments to stimulants as compared to monotherapy trials (41). Meta-analysis has further suggested that alpha-2 agonists (restricted to short-acting formulations) have a similar effect in reducing ADHD symptoms in children with comorbid tic disorders (effect size = 0.61) (29). Alpha-2 agonists have been demonstrated to significantly reduce tics in meta-analysis of randomized controlled trials (effect size = 0.31). However, there is some evidence to suggest that alpha-2 agonists may be particularly effective in reducing tics in children with comorbid ADHD (effect size = 0.68) and have a much smaller benefit in reducing tics in children without comorbid ADHD (effect size = 0.15) (42). There is no evidence to suggest that there is any difference in efficacy between guanfacine and clonidine derivatives or for that matter, short- or long-acting forms of either medication (29,41,42).

Mechanism of Action

The traditional view is that clonidine regulates central noradrenergic activity through its agonist effects on presynaptic alpha-2 receptors in the locus coeruleus. Clonidine is indeed 10 times more potent than guanfacine in reducing locus coeruleus firing and inhibiting NE release. In addition to weaker presynaptic effects, accumulated data from studies in primates show that guanfacine has direct stimulating effects on postsynaptic alpha-2A receptors located in the PFC (43,44). These animal studies have established that this pharmacologic mechanism improves PFC function. Given the fundamental role of the PFC in attention and working memory, this action is likely to be relevant for the treatment of ADHD.

Clinical Management

Clonidine comes in 0.1-, 0.2-, and 0.3-mg tablets. In school-age children, the starting dose is typically 0.05 (1/2 of a 0.1-mg tablet) at bedtime. The dose is then increased in 0.05 mg increments every 3 to 5 days as tolerated to a maximum of 0.2 mg/day (0.05 mg qid) in prepubertal children, and 0.3 mg in teenagers. To ensure even behavioral effects and thus blood levels across the entire day, clonidine is typically given three to four times per day. Clonidine transdermal patches (Catapres TTS) delivering 0.1, 0.2, and 0.3 mg/day are also available. Extended-release formulations of clonidine (Kapvay) are available in doses of 0.1, 0.2, or 0.3 mg and can be given once per day. However, it is generally recommended to give daily doses of greater than 0.2 mg divided into two doses daily. The typical starting dose of guanfacine is 0.5 mg at bedtime, with 0.5 mg increases every 3 to 5 days to a total of 1.5 to 4.0 mg/day into two divided doses. Guanfacine ER can be given once per day in similar total daily doses (2 to 4 mg) to short-acting guanfacine and titrated in a similar rate (every 3 to 5 days). Guanfacine ER is available in doses of 1, 2, 3, or 4 mg.

Adverse Effects

The adverse effects of clonidine and guanfacine are similar, though guanfacine appears to be better tolerated. The most common side effects include sedation, dizziness, irritability (especially when the medication wears off), and midsleep awakening. Hypotension is generally not a problem with either drug in children and adolescents, but warrants monitoring, particularly in the dose-adjustment phase. A related concern with clonidine is the well-documented phenomenon of rebound hypertension following precipitous withdrawal (45). In adults with high blood pressure, however, abrupt discontinuation of guanfacine did not result in rebound hypertension (46). Nonetheless, abrupt discontinuation of either drug should be avoided.

References

1. American Psychiatric Association: *Diagnostic and statistical manual of mental disorders*. 5th ed. Washington, DC, Author, 2013.
2. Costello EJ, Angold A, Burns BJ, et al.: The Great Smoky Mountains Study of Youth. Goals, design, methods, and the prevalence of DSM-III-R disorders. *Arch Gen Psychiatry* 53(12):1129–1136, 1996.
3. Wolraich ML, Hannah JN, Baumgaertel A, Feurer ID: Examination of DSM-IV criteria for attention deficit/hyperactivity disorder in a county-wide sample. *J Dev Behav Pediatr* 19(3):162–168, 1998.
4. Biederman J, Faraone S, Milberger S, et al.: Predictors of persistence and remission of ADHD into adolescence: results from a four-year prospective follow-up study. *J Am Acad Child Adolesc Psychiatry* 35(3):343–351, 1996.
5. Faraone SV, Biederman J, Spencer T, et al.: Attention-deficit/hyperactivity disorder in adults: an overview. *Biol Psychiatry* 48(1):9–20, 2000.
6. The MTA Cooperative Group: A 14-month randomized clinical trial of treatment strategies for attention-deficit/hyperactivity disorder. Multimodal Treatment Study of children with ADHD. *Arch Gen Psychiatry* 56(12):1073–1086, 1999.
7. Scahill L, Schwab-Stone M, Merikangas KR, Leckman JF, Zhang H, Kasl S: Psychosocial and clinical correlates of ADHD in a community sample of school-age children. *J Am Acad Child Adolesc Psychiatry* 38(8):976–984, 1999.
8. Leibson CL, Katusic SK, Barbaresi WJ, Ransom J, O'Brien PC: Use and costs of medical care for children and adolescents with and without attention-deficit/hyperactivity disorder. *JAMA* 285(1):60–66, 2001.
9. Rapport MD, Denney C: Titrating methylphenidate in children with attention-deficit/hyperactivity disorder: Is body mass predictive of clinical response? *J Am Acad Child Adolesc Psychiatry* 36(4):523–530, 1997.
10. Storebø OJ, Ramstad E, Krogh HB, et al.: Methylphenidate for children and adolescents with attention deficit hyperactivity disorder (ADHD). *Cochrane Database Syst Rev* (11):CD009885, 2015.
11. Elia J: Stimulants and antidepressant pharmacokinetics in hyperactive children. *Psychopharmacol Bull* 27(4):411–415, 1991.
12. Pelham WE, Gnagy EM, Burrows-Maclean L, et al.: Once-a-day concerta methylphenidate versus three-times-daily methylphenidate in laboratory and natural settings. *Pediatrics* 107(6):E105, 2001.
13. Barbaresi WJ, Katusic SK, Colligan RC, Weaver AL, Leibson CL, Jacobsen SJ: Long-term stimulant medication treatment of attention-deficit/hyperactivity disorder: results from a population-based study. *J Dev Behav Pediatr* 35(7):448–457, 2014.
14. Solanto MV: Neuropsychopharmacological mechanisms of stimulant drug action in attention-deficit hyperactivity disorder: a review and integration. *Behav Brain Res* 94(1):127–152, 1998.
15. Biederman J, Spencer T: Attention-deficit/hyperactivity disorder (ADHD) as a noradrenergic disorder. *Biol Psychiatry* 46(9):1234–1242, 1999.
16. Swanson JM, Wigal S, Greenhill LL, et al.: Analog classroom assessment of Adderall in children with ADHD. *J Am Acad Child Adolesc Psychiatry* 37(5):519–526, 1998.
17. Greenhill LL, Abikoff HB, Arnold LE, et al.: Medication treatment strategies in the MTA Study: relevance to clinicians and researchers. *J Am Acad Child Adolesc Psychiatry* 35(10):1304–1313, 1996.
18. Sprague R, Sleator EK: Methylphenidate in hyperkinetic children: differences in dose effects on learning and social behavior. *Science* 198(4323):1274–1276, 1977.
19. Biederman J, Lopez FA, Boellner SW, Chandler MC: A randomized, double-blind, placebo-controlled, parallel-group study of SLI381 (Adderall XR) in children with attention-deficit/hyperactivity disorder. *Pediatrics* 110(2 Pt 1):258–266, 2002.
20. Wigal SB, Wigal TL: The laboratory school protocol: its origin, use, and new applications. *J Atten Disord* 10(1):92–111, 2006.
21. Spencer T, Biederman J, Wilens T: Growth deficits in children with attention deficit hyperactivity disorder. *Pediatrics* 102(2 Pt 3):501–506, 1998.
22. MTA Cooperative Group: National Institute of Mental Health Multimodal Treatment Study of ADHD follow-up: changes in effectiveness and growth after the end of treatment. *Pediatrics* 113(4):762–769, 2004.
23. Wilens TE, Spencer TJ, Swanson JM, Connor DF, Cantwell D: Combining methylphenidate and clonidine: a clinically sound medication option. *J Am Acad Child Adolesc Psychiatry* 38(5):614–619, 1999.
24. Tourette's Syndrome Study Group: Treatment of ADHD in children with tics: a randomized controlled trial. *Neurology* 58(4):527–536, 2002.
25. Borcherding BG, Keysor CS, Rapoport JL, Elia J, Amass J: Motor/vocal tics and compulsive behaviors on stimulant drugs: is there a common vulnerability? *Psychiatry Research* 33(1):83–94, 1990.
26. Law SF, Schachar RJ: Do typical clinical doses of methylphenidate cause tics in children treated for attention-deficit hyperactivity disorder? *J Am Acad Child Adolesc Psychiatry* 38(8):944–951, 1999.
27. Castellanos FX, Giedd JN, Elia J, et al.: Controlled stimulant treatment of ADHD and comorbid Tourette's syndrome: effects of stimulant and dose. *J Am Acad Child Adolesc Psychiatry* 36(5):589–596, 1997.
28. Gadow KD, Sverd J, Sprafkin J, Nolan EE, Ezor SN: Efficacy of methylphenidate for attention-deficit hyperactivity disorder in children with tic disorder. *Arch Gen Psychiatry* 52(6):444–455, 1995.
29. Bloch MH, Panza KE, Landeros-Weisenberger A, Leckman JF: Meta-analysis: treatment of attention-deficit/hyperactivity disorder in children with comorbid tic disorders. *J Am Acad Child Adolesc Psychiatry* 48(9): 884–893, 2009.
30. Cohen SC, Mulqueen JM, Ferracioli-Oda E, et al.: Meta-analysis: risk of tics associated with psychostimulant use in randomized, placebo-controlled trials. *J Am Acad Child Adolesc Psychiatry* 54(9):728–736, 2015.
31. Michelson D, Faries D, Wernicke J, et al; Atomoxetine ADHD Study Group: Atomoxetine in the treatment of children and adolescents with attention-deficit/hyperactivity disorder: a randomized, placebo-controlled, dose-response study. *Pediatrics* 108(5):E83, 2001.
32. Michelson D, Allen AJ, Busner J, et al.: Once-daily atomoxetine treatment for children and adolescents with attention deficit hyperactivity disorder: a randomized, placebo-controlled study. *Am J Psychiatry* 159(11):1896–1901, 2002.
33. Hazell P, Zhang S, Wolańczyk T, et al.: Comorbid oppositional defiant disorder and the risk of relapse during 9 months of atomoxetine treatment for attention-deficit/hyperactivity disorder. *Eur Child Adolesc Psychiatry* 15(2):105–110, 2006.
34. Newcorn JH, Spencer TJ, Biederman J, Milton DR, Michelson D: Atomoxetine treatment in children and adolescents with attention-deficit/hyperactivity disorder and comorbid oppositional defiant disorder. *J Am Acad Child Adolesc Psychiatry* 44(3):240–248, 2005.
35. Wigal SB, McGough JJ, McCracken JT: A laboratory school comparison of mixed amphetamine salts extended release (Adderall XR) and atomoxetine (Strattera) in school-aged children with attention deficit/hyperactivity disorder. *J Atten Disord* 9(1):275–289, 2005.
36. Kratochvil CJ, Heiligenstein JH, Dittmann R, et al.: Atomoxetine and methylphenidate treatment in children with ADHD: a prospective, randomized, open-label trial. *J Am Acad Child Adolesc Psychiatry* 41(7):776–784, 2002.
37. Meinel C, Sack H: *WWW: Kommunikation, Internetworking, Web-Technologien*. *Springer Science+Business Media*, 805–883, 2004.
38. Conners CK, Casat CD, Gualtieri CT, et al.: Bupropion hydrochloride in attention deficit disorder with hyperactivity. *J Am Acad Child Adolesc Psychiatry* 35(10):1314–1321, 1996.

39. Barrickman LL, Perry PJ, Allen AJ, et al.: Bupropion versus methylphenidate in the treatment of attention-deficit hyperactivity disorder. *J Am Acad Child Adolesc Psychiatry* 34(5):649–657, 1995.
40. Daviss WB, Bentivoglio P, Racusin R, Brown KM, Bostic JQ, Wiley L: Bupropion sustained release in adolescents with comorbid attention-deficit/hyperactivity disorder and depression. *J Am Acad Child Adolesc Psychiatry* 40(3):307–314, 2001.
41. Hirota T, Schwartz S, Correll CU: Alpha-2 agonists for attention-deficit/hyperactivity disorder in youth: a systematic review and meta-analysis of monotherapy and add-on trials to stimulant therapy. *J Am Acad Child Adolesc Psychiatry* 53(2):153–173, 2014.
42. Weisman H, Qureshi IA, Leckman JF, Scahill L, Bloch MH: Systematic review: pharmacological treatment of tic disorders—efficacy of antipsychotic and alpha-2 adrenergic agonist agents. *Neurosci Biobehav Rev* 37(6):1162–1171, 2013.
43. Arnsten AF: Catecholamine regulation of the prefrontal cortex. *J Psychopharmacol* 11(2):151–162, 1997.
44. Avery RA, Franowicz JS, Studholme C, van Dyck CH, Arnsten AF: The alpha-2A-adrenoceptor agonist, guanfacine, increases regional cerebral blood flow in dorsolateral prefrontal cortex of monkeys performing a spatial working memory task. *Neuropsychopharmacology* 23(3):240–249, 2000.
45. Leckman JF, Ort S, Caruso KA, Anderson GM, Riddle MA, Cohen DJ: Rebound phenomena in Tourette's syndrome after abrupt withdrawal of clonidine. Behavioral, cardiovascular, and neurochemical effects. *Arch Gen Psychiatry* 43(12):1168–1176, 1986.
46. Wilson MF, Haring O, Lewin A, et al.: Comparison of guanfacine versus clonidine for efficacy, safety and occurrence of withdrawal syndrome in step-2 treatment of mild to moderate essential hypertension. *Am J Cardiol* 57(9):43E–49E, 1986.

CHAPTER 6.1.4.2 ■ ANTIDEPRESSANTS

MICHAEL H. BLOCH, CHAD BEYER, ANDRÉS MARTIN, AND LAWRENCE SCAHILL

The antidepressants include a group of chemically diverse compounds that have been shown to be effective in the treatment of adults with major depression. Some of these medications have been used, and are effective, in the treatment of a variety of other disorders, including obsessive–compulsive disorder (OCD), anxiety disorders, premenstrual dysphoric disorder (PMDD), and posttraumatic stress disorder (PTSD). Antidepressants can be classified according to (1) chemical similarity (such as tricyclic compounds, and within these, secondary or tertiary amines); (2) primary mode of action (such as the selective serotonin reuptake inhibitors [SSRIs], selective norepinephrine reuptake inhibitors [SNRIs], or monoamine oxidase inhibitors); and (3) miscellaneous, newer antidepressants (such as bupropion, vortioxetine, trazodone, vilazodone, or mirtazapine). The SSRIs are by far the most extensively used antidepressant class in children and adolescents, and the class with the best empirical support.

SELECTIVE SEROTONIN REUPTAKE INHIBITORS

The SSRIs are a group of chemically unrelated compounds that potently inhibit the reuptake of serotonin into presynaptic neurons. Currently marketed SSRIs include fluoxetine, sertraline, paroxetine, fluvoxamine, citalopram, and escitalopram. In contrast to tricyclic agents such as desipramine which inhibit the reuptake of both norepinephrine and serotonin, these compounds are far more selective for serotonin.

Clinical Applications

All of the SSRIs in current use are approved for use in the treatment of adults with OCD. With the exception of fluvoxamine, the SSRIs are also approved for use in adults with major depression. Table 6.1.4.2.1 depicts the current FDA-approved antidepressants for use in the pediatric population. In general, the use of antidepressants in children has not been limited to their FDA-approved uses as lack of FDA approval is typically indicative of lack of research in the area rather than lack of efficacy. Furthermore, there is limited data to suggest at least within antidepressant classes that individual medications differ in efficacy.

Empirical Support

The introduction of the SSRIs, starting with fluoxetine in the late 1980s, has had a dramatic impact on the practice of pediatric psychopharmacology. Compared to the tricyclic antidepressants (TCAs), monotherapy with the SSRIs is relatively simple. As a group, these medications are generally well tolerated, with a superior side effect profile to TCAs, with less anticholinergic action can typically be given once a day, do not prolong the QTc interval, therefore require blood-level monitoring or ECGs and, unlike TCAs, are not fatal in overdose (1,2). Following the early clinical trials with clomipramine and fluoxetine in children and adolescents (3–5), several large placebo-controlled clinical trials with sertraline (6) and fluvoxamine (7) in OCD; with fluoxetine (8) and paroxetine (9) in depression; and with fluvoxamine in non-OCD anxiety disorders (10) have been conducted in pediatric populations. In each of these studies, the SSRI was superior to placebo in the primary outcome measure of interest. Trials comparing the relative efficacy of SSRIs, cognitive behavioral therapy (CBT), and their combination have been completed with fluoxetine for depression (11), and with sertraline for OCD (12).

Obsessive–Compulsive Disorder

Clomipramine was the first agent approved by the FDA for use in pediatric OCD in 1989. Several SSRIs have been approved since for the treatment of OCD, following multisite, randomized, placebo-controlled trials. These include sertraline, fluvoxamine, fluoxetine, and paroxetine (7,13–15), with highly significant pooled effects versus placebo, and an overall effect size of 0.46 which correlates with a difference in score of 4 points on the Children's Yale-Brown Obsessive–Compulsive Disorder Scale (CYBOCS). Additionally, pairwise comparison in meta-analysis reported clomipramine as having a significantly greater standard–mean difference than the SSRI

TABLE 6.1.4.2.1

FDA-APPROVED INDICATIONS FOR USE OF ANTIDEPRESSANT MEDICATIONS

<table>
<tr><th rowspan="2"></th><th colspan="12">Age (Years)</th></tr>
<tr><th>5</th><th>6</th><th>7</th><th>8</th><th>9</th><th>10</th><th>11</th><th>12</th><th>13</th><th>14</th><th>15–17</th><th>Adult</th></tr>
<tr><td colspan="13">Selective Serotonin Reuptake Inhibitors</td></tr>
<tr><td>Citalopram</td><td colspan="11">NONE</td><td>D</td></tr>
<tr><td>Escitalopram</td><td colspan="7">NONE</td><td colspan="4">D</td><td>D, G</td></tr>
<tr><td>Fluoxetine</td><td colspan="2">NONE</td><td>O</td><td colspan="8">O, D</td><td>O, D, N</td></tr>
<tr><td>Fluvoxamine</td><td colspan="3">NONE</td><td colspan="8">O</td><td>O</td></tr>
<tr><td>Paroxetine</td><td colspan="11">NONE</td><td>O, D, P, G, S, N</td></tr>
<tr><td>Sertraline</td><td>NONE</td><td colspan="10">O</td><td>O, D, P, S, N</td></tr>
<tr><td colspan="13">Serotonin Norepinephrine Reuptake Inhibitors</td></tr>
<tr><td>Venlafaxine</td><td colspan="11">NONE</td><td>D, G, S, N</td></tr>
<tr><td>Duloxetine</td><td colspan="2">NONE</td><td colspan="9">G</td><td>D, G</td></tr>
<tr><td>Desvenlafaxine</td><td colspan="11">NONE</td><td>D</td></tr>
<tr><td colspan="13">Atypical Antidepressants</td></tr>
<tr><td>Bupropion</td><td colspan="11">NONE</td><td>D</td></tr>
<tr><td>Mirtazapine</td><td colspan="11">NONE</td><td>D</td></tr>
<tr><td>Vilazodone</td><td colspan="11">NONE</td><td>D</td></tr>
<tr><td>Vortioxetine</td><td colspan="11">NONE</td><td>D</td></tr>
<tr><td>Trazodone</td><td colspan="11">NONE</td><td>D</td></tr>
<tr><td colspan="13">Tricyclic Antidepressants</td></tr>
<tr><td>Clomipramine</td><td colspan="5">NONE</td><td colspan="6">O</td><td>O</td></tr>
<tr><td>Desipramine</td><td colspan="11">NONE</td><td>D</td></tr>
<tr><td>Nortriptyline</td><td colspan="11">NONE</td><td>D</td></tr>
<tr><td colspan="13">Abbreviations: O, obsessive-compulsive disorder; D, major depressive disorder; P, posttraumatic stress disorder; G, generalized anxiety disorder; S, social anxiety disorder; N, panic disorder.</td></tr>
</table>

(p = 0.002, chi-square test), which remained significant when the year of study was accounted for (16). The four SSRIs did not differ from one another in efficacy compared to placebo.

Taken together, these data suggest that the SSRIs are effective for the treatment of OCD in children and adolescents. However, some children with OCD may show only a partial response to an adequate trial of an SSRI. For example, approximately 40% of the subjects in the multisite sertraline study showed less than a 25% improvement in obsessive–compulsive symptoms (6). This observation indicates that clinicians should remind parents and patients not to have unreasonably high expectations for SSRI treatment and the importance of combined treatment with CBT. The problem of partial response raises questions about whether to switch to another SSRI or clomipramine, or to embark on one of several medication augmentation strategies. Although not well studied in children (17), two studies have shown that the addition of low-dose haloperidol (18) or risperidone (19) to an SSRI can be effective in adults with refractory OCD. A recent meta-analysis provides support for augmentation of SSRIs with haloperidol and risperidone in the treatment of adults with OCD (20). In light of the inadequate support for combined pharmacotherapy in children with refractory OCD, other interventions should be considered, particularly CBT.

Indeed, the Pediatric Obsessive Compulsive Treatment Study (POTS) (21) showed the combination of CBT and SSRI treatment to be superior over either monotherapy alone. In that study, 112 children (mean age approximately 11.5 years, with 56 boys and 56 girls) with OCD across three treatment sites were randomly assigned to sertraline, CBT, their combination, or pill placebo. Statistical analyses on the CYBOCS indicated a significant advantage for CBT alone (p = 0.003), sertraline alone (p = 0.007), and combined treatment (p = 0.001) compared with placebo. Combined treatment showed a 53% improvement on the CYBOCS compared to 46% for CBT alone, 30% for sertraline alone and 15% for placebo. These results suggest that CBT, if readily available, may be the preferred first treatment for OCD, either alone or in combination with an SSRI. The two groups who were treated with active medication each started on a dose of 25 mg/day with gradual increases to a maximum of 200 mg/d. The combined treatment group received an average of 133 mg/day compared to 170 mg/day for the sertraline-only group.

Based on the demonstrated efficacy and safety of the SSRIs in children and adolescents with OCD, these medications are commonly used to reduce repetitive behavior in pervasive developmental disorders (PDDs) (22). Despite their common use in clinical practice, however, the SSRIs have not been well studied in children with PDD. Moreover, the best available evidence indicates that the SSRIs may only be moderately effective for this indication.

Obsessive–Compulsive Behavior in Autism Spectrum Disorders

Evidence is at best mixed for the efficacy of SSRIs for the treatment of obsessive-compulsive symptoms and repetitive behaviors in children with autism spectrum disorders (ASD).

King et al. (23) of the STAART group conducted an NIH-sponsored, multisite study comparing citalopram to placebo in a 12-week parallel group study. One hundred and forty-nine patients with ASD and high levels of repetitive behavior were randomized to either receive citalopram or placebo. They reported no significant difference in the proportion of CGI-I responders at 12 weeks between the citalopram and placebo groups. Additionally, they reported no significant difference in score reduction on the children's yale-brown obsessive-compulsive scale–pervasive developmental disorders from baseline in either the citalopram or placebo treatment groups.

Carrasco et al. (24) conducted a meta-analysis examining the efficacy of serotonin reuptake inhibitors (clomipramine, citalopram, fluoxetine) in the treatment of repetitive behaviors in ASD. They found a small, but significant efficacy of SRIs in the treatment of repetitive behaviors in ASD that was likely attributable to publication bias in the literature. They reported no significant effect of type of medication, age of participant; while dosing of SRI and trial methodologic quality were significantly associated with efficacy. Furthermore, they subsequently conducted a meta-analysis examining fluoxetine, fluvoxamine, fenfluramine, and citalopram in the treatment of participants with ASD and repetitive behaviors after a few additional trials were published (25). They reported no evidence of effect of SSRIs in children with autism and no remaining evidence of publication bias.

Depressive Disorders

Fluoxetine, sertraline, paroxetine, and citalopram have each been studied for the treatment of depression in children and adolescents. The landmark fluoxetine study by Emslie et al. (8) was the first to show superiority of an antidepressant over placebo for the treatment of depression in children and adolescents and was subsequently followed by a replication study (26). A placebo-controlled, multicenter trial comparing paroxetine, imipramine, and placebo (27) indicated that paroxetine was superior to placebo, achieving a 63% response rate, compared to 46% in the placebo group. By contrast, the response rate in the imipramine group was 50%, although this did not reach statistical significance. Imipramine was associated with common TCA side effects and with a high rate of premature discontinuations. Two identical, industry-sponsored trials of sertraline showed superiority over placebo when combined into a single report (28), but failed to differentiate from placebo when analyzed separately. A randomized clinical trial of citalopram has also shown superiority over placebo.

Since these initial trials, there have been several additional studies conducted on a variety of SSRI medications. Overall, there seems to be compelling evidence for the efficacy of SSRIs in the treatment of depression in children. And although meta-analysis has not been able to identify significant differences in efficacy between SSRI agents, fluoxetine appears to have the best evidence of efficacy. Whittington et al. (29) in 2004 reported a favorable risk–benefit profile for some SSRIs, while cautioning that fluoxetine is the only SSRI that they could conclude with certainty as having a beneficial risk–benefit ratio (although there is no evidence of a significant difference in treatment benefit between SSRIs). Hetrick et al. (30) in 2012 also suggested caution in their conclusions, although in keeping with the risks of untreated depression, they recommend fluoxetine as the first choice. Varigonda et al. (31) in 2015 added that treatment gains in pediatric major depressive disorder were greatest early in treatment, and advocate for a minimum of 4 weeks of SSRI treatment, while they did not report a difference between particular SSRI agents. Cipriani et al. (32) in 2016 examined 14 antidepressants, rating the quality of evidence as very low in most comparisons, and that only fluoxetine was statistically significantly more effective than placebo. In addition, fluoxetine was superior to duloxetine and imipramine in terms of tolerability, while imipramine, venlafaxine, and duloxetine had more discontinuations due to adverse effects than in placebo. They caution that the risk–benefit profile of SSRIs is not clearly advantageous with children and adolescents, and emphasize that fluoxetine appears to be the best option.

The largest and most important study to date in this area is the Treatment for Adolescents with Depression Study (TADS) (11). In it, 439 adolescents 12 to 17 of age were randomly assigned to fluoxetine alone, CBT alone, their combination, or pill placebo. They were followed for 12 weeks in the acute phase and for a 6-month extension. Results of the acute phase (12-week trial) showed that combined treatment had the highest rate of positive response (71% for the combined treatment, compared to 61% for medication alone, 43% for CBT alone, and 35% for placebo). The combined treatment group also had a slightly lower rate of suicidal ideation (5.6%) compared to the fluoxetine-only group (8.3%). Fluoxetine alone and fluoxetine with CBT were both superior to placebo. However, combined treatment with fluoxetine and CBT was not significantly better than medication only and CBT alone was not superior to placebo.

Concerns over the increased risk of suicidality among children treated with SSRIs became paramount, initially garnering substantial attention in the media and lay press, and following extensive review by British and American regulatory agencies, eventually led to their temporary removal (in the United Kingdom) and the introduction of an FDA-mandated *black-box warning* (in the United States) in 2004. The history and full implications of this series of concerns are explored in detail in a review (33) and continue to be a source of controversy, shifting policy, and clinical recommendations. In the context of this general overview of pediatric psychopharmacology, the following are important high points of the discussion to date: (1) A review of all clinical trials (both published and unpublished) using SSRIs in the treatment of children and adolescents with depression and other indications (N > 4,400 subjects, across 26 controlled trials, 16 of them for depression) was commissioned by the FDA. It revealed an increased risk in new onset spontaneously reported suicidal ideation between SSRI- and placebo-treated individuals (occurring at respective rates of 4% and 2%), for a risk ratio of 1.95 (95% confidence interval, 1.28 to 2.98) (34), although there was no increase in suicidal ideation when assessed systematically as an item on depression rating scales; (2) all reported events referred to suicidal *ideation,* rather than suicidal attempt or completed suicides; (3) there is compelling pharmaco-epidemiologic data to suggest that paralleling the widespread use of SSRIs in the United States, the suicide rate among those ages 15 to 19 fell from about 11 per 100,000 in 1990 to 7.3 per 100,000 in 2003 and synchronous with the FDA black-box warning on antidepressants and the likely reduction in antidepressant usage in 2004, the suicide rate climbed 14% for those younger than 20, from 1,737 deaths to 1,985 (35); and (4) based on these data, it is important to recommend close monitoring during the initial period after an antidepressant is started. When treatment with an SSRI is opted for, fluoxetine may be generally recommended as the first-line agent because of its FDA indication for depression and a lower reported rate of incident suicidal ideation. Guidelines from the FDA and the American Academy of Child and Adolescent Psychiatry (AACAP) call for intensive monitoring during the early phases of treatment: weekly for the first 4 weeks, once other two weeks for the next month, and monthly thereafter. While such recommendations are clinically sensible, they may actually contribute to increased suicide rates in children and adolescents, in that practitioners may hesitate in using these agents if they are unable to provide the intensive monitoring recommended. This has become especially problematic in underserved areas, where nonspecialists are resource restricted and therefore may be reluctant to prescribe antidepressants to this population.

Non-OCD Anxiety Disorders

Sertraline has been FDA approved for the treatment of generalized anxiety disorder and social phobia, as research in the Children and Adolescents Anxiety Multimodal Treatment study (CAMS) showed it to be effective, especially in combination with CBT, for the treatment of non-OCD anxiety disorders (36). In this randomized, placebo-controlled trial, 488 children between the ages of 7 and 17 years old with separation anxiety disorder, generalized anxiety disorder, or social phobia were randomized to receive CBT, sertraline up to 200 mg/day, a combination of CBT and sertraline, or placebo for 12 weeks. This study showed 80.7% of participants receiving CBT and sertraline combination therapy improved on the CGI-I scale; 59.7% improved on CBT alone and 54.9% improved on sertraline alone. In this study, they began with 25 mg/day and uptitrated to a daily maximum of 200 mg by week 8. Fluvoxamine has shown efficacy on the Pediatric Anxiety Rating Scale (PARS), although it is *not* FDA approved for non-OCD anxiety disorders in children. In a multisite study sponsored by the National Institute of Mental Health (10), 128 subjects between the ages of 6 and 17 years were randomly assigned to placebo or fluvoxamine after a 3-week psychoeducational intervention. The primary outcome measure was the PARS, a new scale developed specifically for the trial. After 8 weeks of treatment, children in the fluvoxamine group showed a 52% improvement (mean decrease in PARS from 18.7 to 9.0, $p < 0.001$) compared to 16% improvement (mean decrease from 19.0 to 15.9, $p < 0.001$) for the placebo group. The dose began at 25 mg/day, titrated upwards by 25 mg twice a day after 4 days and can continue to be uptitrated in 25-mg increments every 4 to 5 days as tolerated, to a maximum of 200 mg/day. The findings from this study provide support for the efficacy and large effect size of fluvoxamine in the treatment of generalized anxiety disorder, social phobia, and separation anxiety.

Mechanism of Action

The SSRIs inhibit the reuptake of serotonin into the presynaptic neuron by the serotonin transporter located on presynaptic nerve terminals. Over time, this blockade leads to a desensitization of the serotonin autoreceptors, which typically exert an inhibitory influence on serotonin release. With continued receptor antagonism at the transporter, pharmacodynamic tolerance develops as the desensitized autoreceptors do not exert their usual inhibitory influence and an increased receptor firing rate leads to more serotonin being released. Based on a series of animal studies, Blier et al. (38) suggest that the main location of the enhanced serotonergic function appears to be the hippocampus in depression, and the orbital frontal cortex in OCD.

Pharmacokinetics

The pharmacokinetic parameters of antidepressant medications are depicted in Table 6.1.4.2.2. Most SSRIs have relatively long half-lives, permitting single daily dosing. Fluvoxamine, which has the shortest half-life, is given on a twice-daily schedule. A recent pharmacokinetic evaluation of paroxetine showed that children metabolize the medication faster than adults (38). Despite the shorter half-life in the pediatric population, these investigators still recommend once-daily dosing for paroxetine. At low doses of sertraline, 50 mg/day or less, children may require twice-daily dosing (39). The pharmacokinetic profiles of the other SSRIs in pediatric populations have not been documented. In adults, fluoxetine (48 to 72 hours), citalopram (36 hours), and escitalopram (30 hours) have the longest half-lives of available SSRIs, compared with sertraline (24 hours), paroxetine (24 hours), and fluvoxamine (15 hours). in addition, fluoxetine has an active metabolite (norfluoxetine) with an elimination half-life of 7 to 14 days. Both fluoxetine (primarily norfluoxetine) and paroxetine are potent inhibitors of CYP2D6, which is particularly concerning as the activity of CYP2D6 is decreased in children younger than 12 years of age. As paroxetine and fluoxetine are 2D6 substrates, they inhibit their own metabolism, resulting in nonlinear kinetics at higher

TABLE 6.1.4.2.2

CLINICAL GUIDANCE FOR ANTIDEPRESSANT MEDICATIONS UTILIZED IN PEDIATRIC PRACTICE

	Pediatric		Adult		
	Starting Dose (mg/day)	Typical Dose Range (mg/day)	Starting Dose (mg/day)	Typical Dose Range (mg/day)	Half-Life
Selective Serotonin Reuptake Inhibitors					
Citalopram	10	20–40	20	40	20 hrs
Escitalopram	5	10–40	10	20–40	27–32 hrs
Fluoxetine	10–20	20–80	20	20–80	4–6 days
Fluvoxamine	25–50	5–0	100–300	100–300	16 hrs
Paroxetine	10	20–60	10–20	40–60	21 hrs
Sertraline	25–50	100–200	50	150–250	26 hrs
Serotonin Norepinephrine Reuptake Inhibitors					
Venlaflaxine	37.5	150–225	37.5–75	75–375	10 hrs
Duloxetine	40	40–60	20–60	20–80	12.5 hrs
Desvenlafaxine	10	10–100	50	50–400	11 hrs
Atypical Antidepressants					
Bupropion	100	150–300	100–150	150–300	21 hrs
Mirtazapine	7.5	15–45	15	15–45	20–40 hrs
Vilazodone	Not studied		10	10–40	25 hours
Vortioxetine	Not studied		10	10–80	66 hours
Trazodone	25–50	100–150	150	150–300	3–9 hrs
Tricyclic Antidepressants					
Clomipramine	25	50–200	25	100–250	32 hrs
Desipramine	25	50–200	100–200	150–300	12–27 hrs
Nortriptyline	30–50	30–150	100	75–150	18–44 hrs

doses. Fluvoxamine primarily inhibits CYP1A2 and CYP2C19, but also inhibits CYP2C9 and CYP3A4 to a lesser extent, and CYP2D6 to the least extent. Due to the metabolism of fluvoxamine through oxidative demethylation and oxidative deamination by CYP2D6 and CYP1A2, both of which it inhibits, it also displays nonlinear pharmacodynamics.

Treatment gains in the treatment of pediatric major depressive disorder are greatest earlier in treatment, while minimal after 4 weeks of SSRI treatment (31). Additionally, higher doses of SSRIs appear to be more effective in the treatment of major depressive disorder (MDD) in adults, with a plateau of the benefit at 250 mg of imipramine equivalents (50 mg of fluoxetine) (40). Treatment of pediatric OCD shows a similar trend in that the greatest incremental treatment gains are early in treatment with an SSRI, in this way the CYBOCS improvement has a greater rate of improvement between 0 and 2 weeks, in comparison with the lowest rate of improvement between 8 and 10 weeks of treatment (41). In this way, the best-fitting model of SSRI therapeutic response in the treatment of pediatric OCD is logarithmic. The effect of treatment effect by log (week + 1) from the final model was 1.51 (95% CI: 1.14 to 1.87; $p < 0.001$) (42).

Clinical Management

The dosing recommendations for each individual antidepressant medication are depicted in Table 6.1.4.2.2. Each SSRI in also discussed individually in the following section.

Fluoxetine (Prozac) is available in a 10-mg scored tablet, a 20-mg capsule, and in a liquid preparation (20 mg per 5 mL). A typical starting dose for school-age children is 10 mg/day. Given its long half-life, fluoxetine should be titrated slowly (weekly or even at 2-week intervals) to avoid "overshooting" the optimal dose. The usual dose range for children and adolescents is 20 to 40 mg/day, though some children and adolescents may require higher doses (43).

Sertraline (Zoloft) is available in 25-, 50-, and 100-mg tablets that can be easily broken in half; it is also available as an oral suspension (20 mg per 1 mL). Treatment might start with a 12.5 to 25 mg dose, with similar weekly titration to a range between 50 and 150 mg in children. Doses in excess of 50 mg/day may be required in older adolescents due to moderate levels of platelet reuptake inhibition at 50 mg/day. Clinicians should review therapeutic response while titrating the medication to determine whether additional increases are needed, rather than using an automatic dose schedule.

Fluvoxamine (Luvox) is available in 25-, 50-, and 100-mg scored tablets. Treatment usually begins at 25 mg/day and can be titrated by 25 to 50 mg on a weekly basis. The typical dose range is 50 to 200 mg/day. Although a double-blind trial in children and adolescents with OCD used a rapid dose escalation with increases every 3 days (7), the more recent Research Unit in Pediatric Psychopharmacology anxiety study used a slower upward adjustment (10). This study started with 25 mg/day and titrated to 25 mg twice a day within the first week. Thereafter, the dose was titrated in 25-mg steps each week as tolerated, to a maximum of 200 mg/day in children less than 11 years of age. Adolescents may require doses up to the adult maximum of 300 mg/day, whereas female children may achieve therapeutic effect in lower doses.

Paroxetine (Paxil) is available in 10-, 20-, and 30-mg tablets that can be broken in half, as well as in an oral suspension (10 mg per 5 mL). The typical starting dose is 10 mg/day, with weekly increases to a total daily dose of 10 to 40 mg. As paroxetine is neither safe nor effective in children and adolescents, it should not be used in these populations.

Citalopram (Celexa) is available in 10-, 20-, and 40-mg scored tablets, as well as in a liquid preparation (40 mg per 1 mL). In children less than 12 years of age, citalopram should be started as 10 mg/day, with titrating up by 5 mg/day every 2 weeks to a max of 40 mg/day; in children over 12 years of age, citalopram should be started at 20 mg/day, with titrating up by 10 mg/day every 2 weeks to a maximum of 40 mg/d. In both cases, dosages above 40 mg/day increase the risk of QT prolongation so should be avoided.

Escitalopram (Lexapro) is available in 10- and 20-mg scored tablets, and has type I evidence of efficacy in MDD, although it is not recommended in younger children. In the treatment of adolescents, the recommended dose is 10 mg once daily, with the possibility of increasing to a maximum dose of 20 mg after 3 weeks of treatment.

Adverse Effects

As a group, the SSRIs are generally well tolerated, and potentially serious side effects such as alterations in cardiac conduction times or seizures have not often been reported in the usual dose range. In addition to their propensity for cytochrome P450–based drug interactions, common side effects of the SSRIs in children and adolescents appear to be behavioral activation and GI complaints such as nausea or diarrhea. Signs of behavioral activation include motor restlessness, insomnia, impulsiveness, disinhibited behavior, and garrulousness. These may occur early in treatment, with dose increases (44) or following the addition of drugs that inhibit the metabolism of the SSRIs (e.g., cimetidine inhibiting CYP2D6 leading to toxicity of CYP2D6 substrates such as fluoxetine or paroxetine). The potential for behavioral activation early in the treatment underscores the importance of starting at low doses and moving upward slowly. As with other antidepressants, hypomania and mania have also been reported, and peripubertal children may be at especially heightened risk (45). Other adverse effects include diarrhea, nausea, heartburn, decreased appetite, and fatigue. Sexual side effects, such as erectile dysfunction, delayed ejaculation, or anorgasmia, all of which are relatively common in adults, should also be considered in adolescents.

Despite the FDA black-box warning regarding the risk of increased suicidal ideation and behavior in children treated with antidepressants, there is actually fairly modest evidence regarding worsening suicidal ideation or behavior with SSRI that is confined to spontaneous reporting of symptoms rather than systematic assessment of suicidality. As with all antidepressants, particularly when treating depression, clinicians should interrogate and monitor for morbid thought, suicidal ideation, and behavior; as well as the potential risk for these in any child or adolescent treated with an SSRI. In the most recent update on the use of SSRIs and SNRIs in children and adolescents by Garland et al. (46), they draw from five high-quality studies to conclude that SSRI significantly decreases suicidal ideation and suicide attempts in young people; additionally, another two high-quality reviews are drawn on to show that population studies demonstrate an inverse correlation between antidepressant use and youth suicide, and an analysis of over 15,000 postmortems in two separate studies have failed to show a relationship between SSRI use and youth suicide.

The incidence of sexual dysfunction as a side effect of SSRI treatment can range between 15% and 80% in adult studies (47) with citalopram decreasing libido in 54%, having delayed orgasm in 36% and erectile dysfunction in 37% of males in the STAR*D study (48). There is a scarcity of research into adolescent sexual dysfunction in the treatment with SSRIs, with a meta-analysis finding that although nonsexual SSRI-induced adverse effects seem to be similar in adult and adolescent populations, sexual dysfunction is poorly reported in the literature. In 11 years, only eight MedWatch reports regarding SSRI-induced sexual dysfunction in adolescents have been filed (49). In adults, meta-analyses have shown bupropion to be associated with a lower rate of treatment-emergent sexual dysfunction than seen with escitalopram, fluoxetine, paroxetine, or sertraline (50) and that mirtazapine is less likely to cause sexual side effects than other antidepressants (51).

SSRI Discontinuation Syndrome and Duration of Therapy

A flu-like syndrome characterized by dizziness, moodiness, nausea, vomiting, myalgia, and fatigue is common following the withdrawal or acute discontinuation of shorter acting SSRIs (or SNRIs) such as paroxetine, fluvoxamine, venlafaxine, and sertraline (52). Recently, a controlled discontinuation study in 220 adults compared the withdrawal effects of fluoxetine, paroxetine, and sertraline: Paroxetine and sertraline were associated with irritability, agitation, fatigue, insomnia, confusion, dizziness, and nervousness upon abrupt withdrawal, but fluoxetine was not (53). The long half-life of norfluoxetine presumably results in a gradual "auto-taper," even when the oral dose is stopped abruptly. Based on these results, a slow withdrawal of the shorter-acting SSRIs is warranted. Citalopram has a 33-hour half-life, with active metabolites such as desmethylcitalopram and evidence of mild and transient (54) adverse effects following abrupt withdrawal, sudden discontinuation of citalopram should be avoided, but it is unlikely to elicit a full discontinuation syndrome if this occurs.

Another clinical issue that often arises in the course of treating children and adolescents with an SSRI is the duration of treatment required for continued remission of symptoms. Treatment of MDD should have three distinct phases with different aims. The Acute Phase of treatment, wherein remission is induced (minimum of 6 to 8 weeks in duration), is followed by the Continuation Phase wherein remission is preserved and relapse prevented (usually 16 to 20 weeks in duration), ending in the Maintenance Phase wherein susceptible patients are protected against recurrence or relapse (the duration of this phase will vary with the frequency of previous episodes). A basic approach would aim for 1-year total treatment time for a first episode, 2 years if a relapse occurs, and lifelong treatment is likely to be required for MDD that relapses recurrently in the setting of optimal treatment and management. For OCD and anxiety disorders, however, the number of treatment sessions, their length, and the duration of an adequate trial have not been established, but expert consensus recommends 13- to 20-weekly sessions as an adequate trial in most patients (55). A review on OCD suggests discontinuation after a relatively symptom-free period of 8 to 12 months (56). A long-term follow-up study of children and adolescents with OCD ($N = 54$) found that 70% ($n = 39$) remained on medication for more than 2 years (57) and persistence of OCD through late adolescence and into adulthood is estimated to occur in about 40% of subjects (58). Given the potential for chronicity in OCD, children and parents should be informed that symptoms may return following a therapeutic reduction or discontinuation of the SSRI.

Drug Interactions

Due to their multiple clinical applications, ease of use, and perceived safety, the SSRIs are increasingly common in clinical practice. In addition, the use of combined psychotropic medications seems to be on the rise. These trends underscore the importance of discussing and monitoring for drug–drug interactions in clinical practice. SSRIs vary in their potential for such interactions at particular P450 cytochromes. In this way, cimetidine can inhibit CYP2D6 enhancing the therapeutic or adverse effects of CYP2D6 substrates such as fluoxetine or paroxetine. The inverse example is also true, with oculogyric crises and other dystonic reactions occurring after risperidone is added to ongoing treatment with paroxetine. This is understood as being due to paroxetine's inhibition of CYP2D6, a major pathway of risperidone metabolism (59).

Serotonin and Norepinephrine Reuptake Inhibitors

Venlafaxine (Effexor)

Venlafaxine is not FDA approved for the treatment of children and adolescents. Additionally, the evidence for its efficacy is Type V (opinions of respected authorities, based on clinical evidence, descriptive studies, or reports of expert committees: the lowest possible type of evidence). Venlafaxine is an agent that selectively inhibits serotonin reuptake at lower doses (less than 150 mg/day) and inhibits both norepinephrine and serotonin reuptake at doses above 150 mg/day. Meta-analysis of six clinical trials analyzing venlafaxine for MDD in children and adolescents was inconclusive with respect to safety and efficacy, in the context of serious selection and publication bias (60). Venlafaxine is available in 25-, 37.5-, 50-, 75-, and 100-mg tablets, and in 37.5-, 75-, and 150-mg extended release (ER) capsules. Dosing is started with the smallest dose given at bedtime, and with attention to early sedation and dizziness, before moving to a twice-daily regimen. At higher doses (>150 mg/d), venlafaxine can be associated with diastolic hypertension, an effect that is clearly dose dependent in nature, and due to the lack of evidence for efficacy and concerns over safety it should not be recommended in this population

Desvenlafaxine (Pristiq)

Desvenlafaxine is not FDA approved for the use in children or adolescents for any indication. Desvenlafaxine has not been studied in randomized, double-blind, placebo-controlled trials, only in an open-label trial wherein doses between 10 and 100 mg/d in children and 25 to 200 mg/d in adolescents were considered "generally safe and well tolerated" (61). Treatment-emergent adverse effects in the desvenlafaxine group included upper abdominal pain, headache, somnolence, and nausea. In light of the lack of high-quality treatment studies proving a favorable risk–benefit ratio, desvenlafaxine should not be recommended for this population.

Duloxetine (Cymbalta)

Duloxetine is not FDA approved for the use in children or adolescents for any indication. Two recent child and adolescent clinical trials of duloxetine examined fixed doses of duloxetine of 20, 40, and 60 mg against placebo in the treatment of MDD. The trial results were inconclusive while treatment-emergent adverse effects in the duloxetine-treated group included suicidal ideation, with patients receiving duloxetine reported two cases of intentional overdose, nonsuicidal self-injurious behavior, hallucinations, and depression (62). A flexible dose trial had similar findings of inconclusive results, and adverse effects in the duloxetine group including worsening suicidal ideation and suicidal behavior (63). In the context of these results, duloxetine should not be recommended for use in this population.

Tricyclic Antidepressants

Clinical Applications and Empirical Support

TCAs have been used to treat several psychiatric disorders of childhood over the past three decades, including depression, ADHD, OCD, separation anxiety disorder, and enuresis. Although TCAs have been used frequently in clinical practice, evidence for their efficacy in treating children with these psychiatric disorders is inconsistent. For example, a series of carefully conducted controlled trials have consistently failed to show the superiority of any TCA over placebo in the treatment of child- and adolescent-onset depression (64). This poor track record stands in stark contrast to results in adult depression (65). The use of TCAs in non-OCD anxiety is inconclusive. One study found imipramine superior to placebo in the treatment of separation anxiety (66) while another failed to replicate this efficacy (67). Double-blind, placebo-controlled studies have demonstrated the efficacy of desipramine in children with ADHD (68–70). Double-blind, placebo-controlled studies have demonstrated clomipramine to be effective in the treatment of OCD in children and adolescents (3). It is also FDA approved for this treatment in children of 10 years and older. Tricyclic agents continue to have a role in the treatment-refractory ADHD and OCD (Table 6.1.4.2.1). TCAs are considered *third-line* therapy for enuresis, only to be considered if the child has failed alarm therapy and/or desmopressin. In this case, imipramine or desipramine, and in some cases amitriptyline, can be considered.

Mechanism of Action

To varying degrees, all TCAs inhibit the reuptake of norepinephrine and serotonin at presynaptic neurons. Over time, this pharmacologic effect *is presumed* to enhance noradrenergic neurotransmission. Among the TCAs, desipramine is the competitive antagonist with the highest affinity for the presynaptic norepinephrine receptor. This plays a role in desipramine's efficacy in ADHD and was the impetus for research into other compounds, such as atomoxetine, which also has high affinity for the presynaptic receptors that leads to the inhibition of reuptake of norepinephrine (71). While concerns of a prolonged QTc interval has been demonstrated with desipramine, it appears less likely with atomoxetine. Clomipramine is unique among the TCAs in that it is a more potent inhibitor of serotonin reuptake, which explains its superiority over desipramine in the treatment of OCD.

Tertiary amine TCAs such as imipramine (or amitryptiline, rarely used in psychiatry, but useful in medicine for the treatment of peripheral neuropathy and posttherpetic neuralgia) have highly anticholinergic profiles. Because of this, they are less often used as a first-line intervention, with the exception of enuresis, for which imipramine continues to be used in clinical practice. By contrast, the secondary amine TCAs, desipramine and nortriptyline (derived from their parent compounds, imipramine and amitryptiline, respectively), are less likely to cause orthostatic hypotension, constipation, or urinary retention, and are thus generally preferred in clinical practice.

Pharmacokinetics

Cytochrome P450 2D6 (CYP2D6) is the enzyme responsible for the metabolizing of TCAs. This enzyme demonstrates considerable variation in efficiency and amount between individuals. In this way, patients with greater efficiency or amount of CYP2D6 will metabolize TCAs quickly (termed ultra-rapid metabolizers), while patients with lower efficiency or amount of CYP2D6 will metabolize TCA slowly (termed poor metabolizers). Due to this variation, serum levels of TCAs can show wide variation between different patients even if they are taking the same oral dose. For this reason, therapeutic levels are not well established for TCAs in pediatric populations. Serum levels may be useful, however, to identify children who may be poor metabolizers or ultra-rapid metabolizers, and to rule out toxicity, and assess compliance. A useful metric is that blood levels (ng/mL) of nortriptyline should be close in absolute value to daily oral dosage (mg/day), assuming the patient is neither a poor nor ultra-rapid metabolizer. In this way, 75 mg/day would be expected to yield a steady-state trough level of ~75 ng/mL. When major discrepancies are seen with this pattern, the clinician can further interrogate potential noncompliance, CYP2D6 induction, or ultrafast metabolism (in the case of low levels), or CYP2D6 inhibition, or poor metabolism (in the case of high levels).

Clinical Management

An ECG, pulse, and blood pressure should be obtained prior to starting any of the TCAs. If the patient was taking a monoamine oxidase inhibitor (MAOI), there needs to be at least a 2-week washout period before initiating treatment with TCAs. A medical and family history that focuses on symptoms associated with syncope, such as dizziness, light headedness, or palpitations in the child, as well as interrogating episodes of syncope or sudden death in first-degree relatives should be completed. Evidence of a normal physical examination (including a full cardiovascular and neurologic assessment) within the past year should also be documented. The typical dose range for TCAs in children is up to 5 mg/kg/day for imipramine, 2.5 mg/kg/day for nortriptyline, and up to 3 mg/kg/day for clomipramine. Imipramine may be started at a dosage of 25 mg and titrated every 4 to 6 days in similar increments to between 100 and 150 mg/day. In younger children, nortriptyline is typically introduced with a 10 mg dose, with titration every 4 to 6 days to a range between 50 and 75 mg/day in divided doses. Clomipramine is usually started at a dose of 25 mg, with gradual titration every 4 to 6 days up to a maximum of 100 mg/day in children younger than 10 years and 3 mg/kg/day or 200 mg (whichever is the smaller dose) in older children. For all of the TCAs, repeat vital signs and ECGs should be obtained, in addition to discussion and investigating potential adverse effects, during the dose adjustment phase and when the maintenance dose has been achieved. As part of the informed consent process, potential cardiac effects and other side effects, as well as reason for repeat ECG monitoring should be discussed with the family and with the child in a manner appropriate for their developmental level. A corrected QT interval (QTc) above 450 ms, a QRS complex longer than 120 ms, or a PR interval greater than 200 ms (72) may warrant dose reduction, or changing to a less cardiotoxic medication, followed by a repeat ECG, if the ECG still shows abnormalities, then reconsider the treatment, and perhaps consider discontinuation. For cases showing clinical benefit and persistent ECG abnormalities, consultation with a pediatric cardiologist is in order.

Adverse Effects

The TCAs have fallen out of favor in pediatric psychiatry due to the increased availability of alternate medications with superior efficacy and tolerability. The TCAs are associated with a range of (largely anticholinergic-based) adverse effects, including sedation, dizziness, dry mouth, excessive sweating, weight gain, urinary retention, tremor, and agitation. In addition to these, TCAs can have dose-dependent adverse effects on cardiac conduction (which can be tracked with an expectable dose-dependent prolongation of the QTc). TCAs also lower the seizure threshold, with clomipramine showing the highest risk. To avoid this, dose and potential drug interactions need to be monitored closely, especially with clomipramine.

For most adverse effects, lowering the dose, changing dose schedules, switching from a tertiary to a secondary amine, or switching out of the TCA class entirely, can often help manage symptoms. For example, to deal with sedation, the medication could be given twice a day, with the higher dosing in the evening. Switching between TCAs can be helpful at times: For example, imipramine can be changed to nortriptyline in an effort to minimize sedation or constipation. Despite the evidence, of varying quality and reproducibility, showing the efficacy of clomipramine for OCD (FDA approved in children 10 years and older) and desipramine for ADHD (not FDA approved for any indication in childhood), the TCAs appear to be declining in use. This trend is largely due to their side-effect profile and the potential for serious adverse effects, with the rare possibilities of sudden death related to torsade de pointes deteriorating into ventricular fibrillation. Originally reported in cases treated with desipramine, the series of case reports that accrued over ensuing years, and the increased availability of more effective, less dangerous, alternatives has prompted many experts to recommend avoiding TCAs in the pediatric population (73). The selective use of TCAs in nonresponders to first-line agents provides a rational basis for keeping these compounds as potential treatment options, with the following provisos: (1) titration must be stepwise within clear weight-adjusted margins and clearly defined time intervals; (2) careful ECG monitoring must be performed before increasing dose and after reaching maintenance dose; (3) the risk–benefit ratio must be fully disclosed and discussed in the treatment planning process.

Interactions

As with most other psychotropic drugs, the TCAs are metabolized by hepatic enzymes in the cytochrome P450 system (primarily CYP2D6). Several psychotropic (fluoxetine, fluvoxamine, paroxetine), nonpsychotropic drugs (ketoconazole, cimetidine, clarithromycin), and even grapefruit, inhibit the action of one or more of these hepatic enzymes. Inhibition of the enzyme specific for metabolizing the TCA (CYP2D6) can result in toxicity.

Other Antidepressant Medications

Trazodone (Desyrel)

Trazodone is a potent 5-HT2a postsynaptic antagonist and inhibits both serotonin and norepinephrine reuptake. This novel mechanism of action initially raised interest in these compounds, but poor efficacy results in adults, coupled with rare but serious adverse effects (priapism) has led to the selective use of trazodone as an adjunct for insomnia. Trazodone is available in 50-, 100-, 150-, and 300-mg pills, and is prescribed in nighttime dosing for insomnia.

Mirtazapine (Remeron)

Mirtazapine is an alpha-2 adrenoceptor antagonist, which also elicits norepinephrine presynaptic and serotinergic postsynaptic receptor antagonism with a characteristic side-effect profile, consisting of drowsiness, increased appetite, and weight gain. Mirtazapine is mainly used in anxious and agitated depression with associated sleeping problems, as it has been shown in systematic review to have a positive effect on depressive symptomatology, including insomnia in adults (74). Mirtazapine may be started at 15 mg and titrated slowly to 45 mg in a single dose per day. Pediatric research on this compound is limited.

References

1. Barbey JT, Roose SP: SSRI safety in overdose. *J Clin Psychiatry* 59(Suppl 15): 42–48, 1998.
2. Isbister GK, Bowe SJ, Dawson A, Whyte IM: Relative toxicity of selective serotonin reuptake inhibitors (SSRIs) in overdose. *J Toxicol Clin Toxicol* 42(3):277–285, 2004.
3. Deveaugh-Geiss J, Moroz G, Biederman J, et al.: Clomipramine hydrochloride in childhood and adolescent obsessive-compulsive disorder—a multicenter trial. *J Am Acad Child Adolesc Psychiatry* 31(1):45–49, 1992.
4. Leonard HL: Treatment of obsessive-compulsive disorder with clomipramine and desipramine in children and adolescents: a double-blind crossover comparison. *Arch Gen Psychiatry* 46(12):1088–1092, 1989.
5. Riddle MA, Scahill L, King RA, et al.: Double-Blind, crossover trial of fluoxetine and placebo in children and adolescents with obsessive-compulsive disorder. *J Am Acad Child Adolesc Psychiatry* 31(6):1062–1069, 1992.
6. March JS, Biederman J, Wolkow R, et al.: Sertraline in children and adolescents with obsessive-compulsive disorder: a multicenter randomized controlled trial. *JAMA* 280(20):1752–1756, 1998.
7. Riddle MA, Reeve EA, Yaryura-Tobias JA, et al.: Fluvoxamine for children and adolescents with obsessive-compulsive disorder: a randomized, controlled, multicenter trial. *J Am Acad Child Adolesc Psychiatry* 40(2):222–229, 2001.
8. Emslie GJ, Rush AJ, Weinberg WA, et al.: A double-blind, randomized, placebo-controlled trial of fluoxetine in children and adolescents with depression. *Arch Gen Psychiatry* 54(11):1031–1037, 1997.
9. Keller MB, Ryan ND, Birmaher B: *Paroxetine and Imipramine in the Treatment of Adolescent Depression. Program and Abstracts on New Research from the 151st Annual Meeting of the American Psychiatric Association.* Toronto, American Psychiatric Association, NR206, 1998.
10. Walkup JT, Labellarte MJ, Riddle MA, et al.: Fluvoxamine for the treatment of anxiety disorders in children and adolescents. The Research Unit on Pediatric Psychopharmacology Anxiety Study Group. *N Engl J Med* 344(17):1279–1285, 2001.
11. March J, Silva S, Petrycki S, et al.: Fluoxetine, cognitive-behavioral therapy, and their combination for adolescents with depression: treatment for adolescents with depression study (TADS) randomized controlled trial. *JAMA* 292(7):807–820, 2004.
12. Pediatric OCD Treatment Study (POTS) Team: Cognitive-behavior therapy, sertraline, and their combination for children and adolescents with obsessive-compulsive disorder: The Pediatric OCD Treatment Study (POTS) randomized controlled trial. *JAMA* 292(16):1969–1976, 2004.
13. Geller DA, Hoog SL, Heiligenstein JH, et al.: Fluoxetine treatment for obsessive-compulsive disorder in children and adolescents: a placebo-controlled clinical trial. *J Am Acad Child Adolesc Psychiatry* 40(7):773–779, 2001.
14. March JS, Biederman J, Wolkow R, et al.: Sertraline in children and adolescents with obsessive-compulsive disorder: a multicenter randomized controlled trial. *JAMA* 280(20):1752–1756, 1998.
15. Geller DA, Wagner KD, Emslie GJ, et al.: *Efficacy of Paroxetine in Pediatric OCD: Results of a Multicenter Study.* Washington, DC, Annual Meeting New Research Program and Abstract, 2002.
16. Geller DA, Biederman J, Stewart SE, et al.: Which SSRI? A meta-analysis of pharmacotherapy trials in pediatric obsessive-compulsive disorder. *Am J Psychiatry* 160(11):1919–1928, 2003.
17. Fitzgerald KD, Stewart CM, Tawile V, Rosenberg DR: Risperidone augmentation of serotonin reuptake inhibitor treatment of pediatric obsessive compulsive disorder. *J Child Adolesc Psychopharmacol* 9(2):115–123, 1999.
18. McDougle CJ, Goodman WK, Leckman JF, Lee NC, Heninger GR, Price LH: Haloperidol addition in fluvoxamine-refractory obsessive-compulsive disorder: a double-blind, placebo-controlled study in patients with and without tics. *Arch Gen Psychiatry* 51(4):302–308, 1994.
19. McDougle CJ, Epperson CN, Pelton GH, Wasylink S, Price LH: A double-blind, placebo-controlled study of risperidone addition in serotonin reuptake inhibitor—refractory obsessive-compulsive disorder. *Arch Gen Psychiatry* 57(8):794–801, 2000.
20. Bloch MH, Landeros-Weisenberger A, Kelmendi B, Coric V, Bracken MB, Leckman JF: A systematic review: antipsychotic augmentation with treatment refractory obsessive-compulsive disorder. *Molecular Psychiatry* 11(7):622–632, 2006.
21. Weisz JR, Kazdin AE, (eds): *Evidence-Based Psychotherapies for Children and Adolescents.* 2nd ed. New York, The Guilford Press, 2011.
22. Aman MG, Buican B, Arnold LE: Methylphenidate treatment in children with borderline iq and mental retardation: analysis of three aggregated studies. *J Child Adolesc Psychopharmacol* 13(1):29–40, 2003.
23. King BH, Hollander E, Sikich L, et al.: Lack of efficacy of citalopram in children with autism spectrum disorders and high levels of repetitive behavior: citalopram ineffective in children with autism. *Arch Gen Psychiatry* 66(6):583–590, 2009.
24. Carrasco M, Volkmar FR, Bloch MH: Pharmacologic treatment of repetitive behaviors in autism spectrum disorders: evidence of publication bias. *Pediatrics* 129(5):e1301–1310, 2012.
25. Williams K, Brignell A, Randall M, Silove N, Hazell P: Selective serotonin reuptake inhibitors (SSRIs) for autism spectrum disorders (ASD). *Cochrane Database Syst Rev* (8), 2013.
26. Emslie GJ, Heiligenstein JH, Wagner KD, et al.: Fluoxetine for acute treatment of depression in children and adolescents: a placebo-controlled, randomized clinical trial. *J Am Acad Child Adolesc Psychiatry* 41(10): 1205–1215, 2002.
27. Keller MB, Ryan ND, Strober M, et al.: Efficacy of paroxetine in the treatment of adolescent major depression: a randomized, controlled trial. *J Am Acad Child Adolesc Psychiatry* 40(7):762–772, 2001.
28. Wagner KD, Ambrosini P, Rynn M: Efficacy of sertraline in the treatment of children and adolescents with major depressive disordertwo randomized controlled trials. *JAMA* 290(8):1033–1041.
29. Whittington CJ, Kendall T, Fonagy P, Cottrell D, Cotgrove A, Boddington E: Selective serotonin reuptake inhibitors in childhood depression: systematic review of published versus unpublished data. *Lancet* 363(9418):1341–1345, 2004.
30. Hetrick SE, McKenzie JE, Cox GR, Simmons MB, Merry SN: Newer generation antidepressants for depressive disorders in children and adolescents. *Cochrane Database Syst Rev* (11), 2012.
31. Varigonda AL, Jakubovski E, Taylor MJ, Freemantle N, Coughlin C, Bloch MH: Systematic review and meta-analysis: Early treatment responses

of selective serotonin reuptake inhibitors in pediatric major depressive disorder. *J Am Acad Child Adolesc Psychiatry* 54(7):557–564, 2015.
32. Cipriani A, Zhou X, Del Giovane C, et al.: Comparative efficacy and tolerability of antidepressants for major depressive disorder in children and adolescents: a network meta-analysis. *Lancet* 388(10047):881–890, 2016.
33. Rey JM, Martin A: Selective serotonin reuptake inhibitors and suicidality in juveniles: review of the evidence and implications for clinical practice. *Child Adolesc Psychiatr Clin N Am* 15(1):221–237, 2006.
34. Hammad TA, Laughren TP, Racoosin JA: Suicide rates in short-term randomized controlled trials of newer antidepressants. *J Clin Psychopharmacol* 26(2):203–207, 2006.
35. Hamilton BE, Minino AM, Martin JA, Kochanek KD, Strobino DM, Guyer B: Annual summary of vital statistics: 2005. *Pediatrics* 119(2):345–360, 2007.
36. Walkup JT, Albano AM, Piacentini J, et al.: Cognitive behavioral therapy, sertraline, or a combination in childhood anxiety. *N Engl J Med* 359(26):2753–2766, 2008.
37. Blier P, de Montigny C: Possible serotonergic mechanisms underlying the antidepressant and anti-obsessive–compulsive disorder responses. *Biol Psychiatry* 44(5):313–323, 1998.
38. Findling RL, Reed MD, Myers C, et al.: Paroxetine pharmacokinetics in depressed children and adolescents. *J Am Acade Child Adolesc Psychiatry* 38(8):952–959, 1999.
39. Axelson DA, Perel JM, Birmaher B, et al.: Sertraline pharmacokinetics and dynamics in adolescents. *J Am Acade Child Adolesc Psychiatry* 41(9):1037–1044, 2002.
40. Jakubovski E, Varigonda AL, Freemantle N, Taylor MJ, Bloch MH: Systematic review and meta-analysis: dose-response relationship of selective serotonin reuptake inhibitors in major depressive disorder. *Am J Psychiatry* 173(2):174–183, 2016.
41. Varigonda AL, Jakubovski E, Bloch MH: Systematic review and meta-analysis: early treatment responses of selective serotonin reuptake inhibitors and clomipramine in pediatric obsessive-compulsive disorder. *J Am Acad Child Adolesc Psychiatry* 55(10):851–859.e852, 2016.
42. Issaria Y, Jakubovski E, Bartley CA, Pittenger C, Bloch MH: Early onset of response with selective serotonin reuptake inhibitors in obsessive-compulsive disorder: a meta-analysis. *J Clin Psychiatry* 77(5):e605–e611, 2016.
43. Heiligenstein JH, Hoog SL, Wagner KD, et al.: Fluoxetine 40–60 mg versus fluoxetine 20 mg in the treatment of children and adolescents with a less-than-complete response to nine-week treatment with fluoxetine 10–20 mg: a pilot study. *J Child Adolesc Psychopharmacol* 16(1–2):207–217, 2006.
44. King RA, Riddle MA, Chappell PB, et al.: Emergence of self-destructive phenomena in children and adolescents during fluoxetine treatment. *J Am Acad Child Adolesc Psychiatry* 30(2):179–186, 1991.
45. Martin A, Scahill L, Anderson GM, et al.: Weight and leptin changes among risperidone-treated youths with autism: 6-month prospective data. *Am J Psychiatry* 161(6):1125–1127, 2004.
46. Jane Garland E, Kutcher S, Virani A, Elbe D: Update on the use of SSRIs and SNRIs with children and adolescents in clinical practice. *J Can Acad Child Adolesc Psychiatry* 25(1):4–10, 2016 Winter.
47. Michael Hirsh, Birnbaum RJ: Sexual dysfunction caused by selective serotonin reuptake inhibitors (SSRIs): management. 9 January 2016 [cited 2016 15 November]; Available from: https://www.uptodate.com/contents/sexual-dysfunction-caused-by-selective-serotonin-reuptake-inhibitors-ssris-management?source=see_link#H49290360
48. Perlis RH, Laje G, Smoller JW, Fava M, Rush AJ, McMahon FJ: Genetic and clinical predictors of sexual dysfunction in citalopram-treated depressed patients. *Neuropsychopharmacol* 34(7):1819–1828, 2009.
49. Scharko AM: Selective serotonin reuptake inhibitor-induced sexual dysfunction in adolescents: a review. *J Am Acad Child Adolesc Psychiatry* 43(9):1071–1079, 2004.
50. Gartlehner G, Hansen RA, Morgan LC, et al.: Comparative benefits and harms of second-generation antidepressants for treating major depressive disorder: an updated meta-analysis. *Ann Intern Med* 155(11):772–785, 2011.
51. Watanabe N, Omori IM, Nakagawa A, et al.: Mirtazapine versus other antidepressive agents for depression. *Cochrane Database Syst Rev* (12): Cd006528, 2011.
52. Black K, Shea C, Dursun S, Kutcher S: Selective serotonin reuptake inhibitor discontinuation syndrome: proposed diagnostic criteria. *J Psychiatry Neuroscience* 25(3):255–261, 2000.
53. Rosenbaum JF, Fava M, Hoog SL, Ascroft RC, Krebs WB: Selective serotonin reuptake inhibitor discontinuation syndrome: A randomized clinical trial. *Biol Psychiatry* 44(2):77–87, 1998.
54. Markowitz JS, DeVane CL, Liston HL, Montgomery SA: An assessment of selective serotonin reuptake inhibitor discontinuation symptoms with citalopram. *Int Clin Psychopharmacol* 15(6):329–333, 2000.
55. American Psychiatric Association: *Practice Guideline for the Treatment of Patients with Obsessive-Compulsive Disorder.* Arlington, VA, Author, 2007.
56. Grados MA, Riddle MA: Obsessive-compulsive disorder in children and adolescents. *CNS Drugs* 12(4):257–277, 1999.
57. Leonard HL, Swedo SE, Lenane MC: A 2- to 7-year follow-up study of 54 obsessive-compulsive children and adolescents. *Arch Gen Psychiatry* 50(6):429–439, 1993.
58. Deveaugh-Geiss J, March J, Shapiro M, et al.: Child and adolescent psychopharmacology in the new millennium: a workshop for academia, industry, and government. *J Am Acad Child Adolesc Psychiatry* 45(3):261–270, 2006.
59. Lombroso PJ, Scahill L, King RA, et al.: Risperidone treatment of children and adolescents with chronic tic disorders: a preliminary report. *J Am Acad Child Adolesc Psychiatry* 34(9):1147–1152, 1995.
60. Courtney DB: Selective serotonin reuptake inhibitor and venlafaxine use in children and adolescents with major depressive disorder: a systematic review of published randomized controlled trials. *Can J Psychiatry* 49(8):557–563, 2004.
61. Findling RL, Groark J, Chiles D, Ramaker S, Yang L, Tourian KA: Safety and tolerability of desvenlafaxine in children and adolescents with major depressive disorder. *J Child Adolesc Psychopharmacol* 24(4):201–209, 2014.
62. Emslie GJ, Prakash A, Zhang Q, Pangallo BA, Bangs ME, March JS: A double-blind efficacy and safety study of duloxetine fixed doses in children and adolescents with major depressive disorder. *J Child Adolesc Psychopharmacol* 24(4):170–179, 2014.
63. Atkinson SD, Prakash A, Zhang Q, et al.: A double-blind efficacy and safety study of duloxetine flexible dosing in children and adolescents with major depressive disorder. *J Child Adolesc Psychopharmacol* 24(4):180–189, 2014.
64. Hazell P, O'Connell D, Heathcote D, Henry DA: Tricyclic drugs for depression in children and adolescents. *Cochrane Database Syst Rev* (2):CD002317.2002.
65. Martin A, Kaufman J, Charney D. Pharmacotherapy of early-onset depression: update and new directions. *Child Adolesc Psychiatr Clin N Am* 9(1):135–157, 2000.
66. Bernstein GA, Borchardt CM, Perwien AR, et al.: Imipramine plus cognitive-behavioral therapy in the treatment of school refusal. *J Am Acad Child Adolesc Psychiatry* 39(3):276–283, 2000.
67. Klein RG, Koplewicz HS, Kanner A: Imipramine treatment of children with separation anxiety disorder. *J Am Acad Child Adolesc Psychiatry* 31(1):21–28, 1992.
68. Biederman J, Baldessarini RJ, Wright V, Knee D, Harmatz JS: A double-blind placebo controlled study of desipramine in the treatment of ADD: I. Efficacy. *J Am Acad Child Adolesc Psychiatry* 28(5):777–784, 1989.
69. Singer HS, Brown J, Quaskey S, Rosenberg LA, Mellits ED, Denckla MB: The treatment of attention-deficit hyperactivity disorder in Tourette's syndrome: a double-blind placebo-controlled study with clonidine and desipramine. *Pediatrics* 95(1):74–81, 1995.
70. Spencer T, Biederman J, Coffey B, et al.: A double-blind comparison of desipramine and placebo in children and adolescents with chronic tic disorder and comorbid attention-deficit/hyperactivity disorder. *Arch Gen Psychiatry* 59(7):649–656, 2002.
71. Kratochvil CJ, Vaughan BS, Harrington MJ, Burke WJ: Atomoxetine: a selective noradrenaline reuptake inhibitor for the treatment of attention-deficit/hyperactivity disorder. *Expert Opin Pharmacother* 4(7):1165–1174, 2003.
72. Blair J, Taggart B, Martin A: Electrocardiographic safety profile and monitoring guidelines in pediatric psychopharmacology. *J Neural Transm (Vienna)* 111(7):791–815, 2004.
73. Werry JS. Resolved: cardiac arrhythmias make desipramine an unacceptable choice in children. *J Am Acad Child Adolesc Psychiatry* 34(9):1239–1241, 1995.
74. Taurines R, Gerlach M, Warnke A, Thome J, Wewetzer C: Pharmacotherapy in depressed children and adolescents. *World J Biol Psychiatry* 12(Suppl 1):11–15, 2011.

CHAPTER 6.1.4.3 ■ ANTIPSYCHOTICS

MICHAEL H. BLOCH, CHAD BEYER, LAWRENCE SCAHILL, AND ANDRÉS MARTIN

CLINICAL APPLICATIONS AND EMPIRICAL SUPPORT

Antipsychotic agents have become increasingly utilized to treat a variety of mental health conditions in children in recent years including psychosis, bipolar disorder, tic disorders, irritability, and aggression. Although proven efficacious for a number of conditions, antipsychotic use in children is often a difficult treatment decision given the substantial side-effect burden association with these agents. Table 6.1.4.3.1 depicts the current U.S. Food and Drug Administration (FDA)-approved indications for the existing antipsychotics.

Antipsychotics were introduced to adult psychiatry in the early 1950s and began to be used in children shortly thereafter. The antipsychotics can be classified according to chemical family, such as phenothiazines or butyrophenones. Alternatively, they may be classified according to the relative potency of their dopamine blockade. Chlorpromazine and thioridazine are low-potency drugs, in that relatively high doses are required to achieve usual therapeutic effects. By contrast, haloperidol and fluphenazine are high-potency dopamine-blocking drugs. With the introduction of clozapine and a short list of newer compounds, it is becoming commonplace to classify antipsychotics as typical or atypical.

In this section, we will broadly address the variety of FDA-approved and off-label uses that have emerged for antipsychotics in children. More details regarding the dosing of each specific antipsychotic medication will be found in Table 6.1.4.3.1 as well as their approved FDA indications (Table 6.1.4.3.2) and their comparative side effect (Table 6.1.4.3.4). The empirical data supporting the use of each individual antipsychotic medication will be further discussed later in the chapter after the evidence regarding the efficacy of antipsychotic medications as a class are reviewed.

Psychosis

Antipsychotic medications are the first line of treatment for psychosis across the life span. Until the late 1990s, there were very few randomized controlled trials (RCTs) on the treatment of adolescents with psychosis. Most of the treatment guidelines for adolescents with psychosis were derived from data on adults. There is now substantial data demonstrating the efficacy of antipsychotic medications for the treatment of psychosis in

TABLE 6.1.4.3.1

FDA-APPROVED INDICATIONS FOR USE OF ANTIPSYCHOTIC MEDICATIONS

<table>
<tr><th rowspan="2"></th><th colspan="9">Age (Yrs)</th></tr>
<tr><th><1</th><th>1–2</th><th>3–4</th><th>5</th><th>6–9</th><th>10–11</th><th>12</th><th>13–17</th><th>Adult</th></tr>
<tr><td colspan="10">Second-Generation (Atypical) Antipsychotics</td></tr>
<tr><td>Risperidone</td><td colspan="3">NONE</td><td colspan="2">I</td><td colspan="2">I, M</td><td>I, M, S</td><td>M, S</td></tr>
<tr><td>Aripiprazole</td><td colspan="4">NONE</td><td>I</td><td colspan="2">I, M</td><td>I, M, S</td><td>M, S</td></tr>
<tr><td>Quetiapine</td><td colspan="5">NONE</td><td colspan="2">M</td><td>M, S</td><td>M, S</td></tr>
<tr><td>Olanzapine</td><td colspan="5">NONE</td><td colspan="2">D, M</td><td>D, M, S</td><td>D, M, S</td></tr>
<tr><td>Ziprasidone</td><td colspan="8">NONE</td><td>M, S</td></tr>
<tr><td>Clozapine</td><td colspan="8">NONE</td><td>S</td></tr>
<tr><td>Paliperidone</td><td colspan="5">NONE</td><td colspan="3">S</td><td>S</td></tr>
<tr><td>Lurasidone</td><td colspan="8">NONE</td><td>S</td></tr>
<tr><td>Asenapine</td><td colspan="5">NONE</td><td colspan="3">M</td><td>M, S</td></tr>
<tr><td>Iloperidone</td><td colspan="8">NONE</td><td>S</td></tr>
<tr><td colspan="10">First-Generation (Typical) Antipsychotics</td></tr>
<tr><td>Haloperidol</td><td colspan="2">NONE</td><td colspan="6">H, P, S, T</td><td>S, T</td></tr>
<tr><td>Molindone</td><td colspan="6">NONE</td><td colspan="2">S</td><td>S</td></tr>
<tr><td>Pimozide</td><td colspan="6">NONE</td><td colspan="2">T</td><td>T</td></tr>
<tr><td>Chlorpromazine</td><td>NONE</td><td colspan="6">B</td><td>NONE</td><td>M, S</td></tr>
<tr><td>Perphenazine</td><td colspan="6">NONE</td><td colspan="2">S</td><td>S</td></tr>
<tr><td>Fluphenazine</td><td colspan="8">NONE</td><td>S</td></tr>
<tr><td>Thioridazine</td><td colspan="4">NONE</td><td colspan="4">S</td><td>S</td></tr>
</table>

Abbreviations: B, severe behavioral problems marked by combativeness and/or explosive behavior and short-term treatment of hyperactive children who show excessive motor activity with accompanying conduct disorders; D, acute depressive episodes associated with bipolar I disorder (along with fluoxetine); H, hyperactivity; I, irritability associated with autism disorder; M, manic or mixed episodes associated with bipolar I disorder; P, psychosis; S, schizophrenia; T, Tourette syndrome.

TABLE 6.1.4.3.2

CLINICAL GUIDANCE FOR ANTIPSYCHOTIC MEDICATIONS UTILIZED IN PEDIATRIC PRACTICE

	Pediatric			Adult		
	Starting Dose (mg/day)	Typical Dose Range (mg/day)	Number of Daily Doses	Starting Dose (mg/day)	Typical Dose Range (mg/day)	Number of Daily Doses
Second-Generation (Atypical) Antipsychotics						
Risperidone	0.5–2	1–6	1–2	2	2–6	1–2
Aripiprazole	2–5	5–30	1	5–15	10–30	1
Quetiapine	25–50	100–800	2–3	50–100	150–800	2–3
Olanzapine	2.5–5	5–20	1	5–10	5–20	1
Ziprasidone	5–20	40–160	2	40–80	80–160	2
Clozapine	12.5–50	300–900	2	25–50	300–900	1–2
Paliperidone	3	3–12	1	3–6	3–12	1
Lurasidone	20	20–160	1	20–40	20–160	1
Asenapine	5	5–20	2	10–20	10–20	2
First-Generation (Typical) Antipsychotics						
Haloperidol	1–10	2–30	2–3	2–15	2–50	2–3
Molindone	25–75	50–225	3–4	50–75	50–225	3–4
Pimozide	0.5–2	1–6	1–2	1–2	2–10	1–2
Chlorpromazine	30–75	50–200	4	30–75	200–400	3–4
Perphenazine	6–12	12–32	2–4	12–24	16–32	2–4
Fluphenazine	1–10	2.5–20	3–4	2–10	10–40	3–4
Thioridazine	25–50	25–200	2–4	150–300	200–800	2–4

children. However, fairly few RCTs of antipsychotic medications exist because of ethical concerns regarding the use of placebo medications in this severely ill population. That being said, the RCTs that do exist show a strong benefit of antipsychotic medications compared to placebo (1–3). Meta-analysis has not been able to demonstrate a difference in efficacy between different antipsychotic agents for the treatment of pediatric psychosis. Kumar et al. (4) conducted a meta-analysis involving 13 RCTs and a total of 1,112 participants, between 13 and 18 years of age. They found that no convincing evidence that atypical antipsychotics are more effective, at treating the symptoms of psychosis, than typical antipsychotics (4). Given the lack of differences in efficacy between different antipsychotic agents, choice of medication should be primarily made based on the quality of available data as well as the side-effect profile of these medications in combination with patient preference.

Further supporting the absence of evidence in a difference in efficacy between antipsychotic agents for schizophrenia came from the Treatment of Early-Onset Schizophrenia Study (TEOSS) (5). TEOSS was a double-blind multisite trial which randomly assigned pediatric patients (8 to 19 years) with schizophrenia and schizoaffective disorder to treatment with either olanzapine (2.5 to 20 mg/day), risperidone (0.5 to 6 mg/day), or molindone (10 to 140 mg/day, plus 1 mg/day of benztropine) for 8 weeks. TEOSS demonstrated no difference in the primary efficacy measure between the three antipsychotic medications. However, the atypical antipsychotics, especially olanzapine, were associated with significantly greater gain. The magnitude of weight gain with olanzapine (6.1 kg over the 8-week trial) was so significant that the olanzapine arm was discontinued early for safety reasons (5).

Bipolar Disorder

Multiple randomized, placebo-controlled trials have demonstrated that atypical antipsychotics are more effective than placebo for children with bipolar disorder experiencing manic or mixed episodes. Furthermore, a large, multicenter, NIH-funded, head-to-head trial comparing an atypical antipsychotic, risperidone, with two mood stabilizers (lithium and valproic acid) demonstrated the superiority of risperidone over these two mood stabilizers for the treatment of manic symptoms in pediatric bipolar disorder (6). An earlier smaller trial comparing risperidone to valproic acid similarly found greater improvement in the risperidone group although not to the degree of statistical significance. Similarly, these results were reconfirmed when risperidone was demonstrated to be superior to valproic acid for the treatment of manic symptoms in younger children aged 3 to 7 years (7). After the findings from these two important clinical trials antipsychotic medications have become the initial treatment of choice for pediatric mania often in conjunction with mood stabilizers in severe cases.

Tic Disorders

Meta-analysis of RCTs of antipsychotic agents has suggested that they are likely the most effective pharmacologic intervention currently available to treat children with tic disorders (8). Specifically, meta-analysis of five randomized, placebo-controlled trials involving 167 participants demonstrated that antipsychotics had a modest effect size (ES = 0.58) in reducing tic symptoms. Both stratified subgroup analysis and head-to-head trials failed to demonstrate a difference in efficacy between antipsychotic agents. Haloperidol, risperidone, aripiprazole, and pimozide have specific evidence of efficacy compared to placebo for the treatment of tics (9).

Irritability and Aggression

RCTs of atypical antipsychotics have demonstrated a benefit compared to placebo for irritability and aggression in children with and without ASD (10,11). In these RCTs, atypical antipsychotic treatment has been shown to be effective as monotherapy or as an adjunct to evidence-based behavioral treatment. Risperidone and aripiprazole have been the primary atypical antipsychotics examined for the treatment of aggression and irritability in pediatric populations.

Treatment-Refractory Obsessive–Compulsive Disorder

There exist no randomized, placebo-controlled trials of antipsychotics for treatment-refractory obsessive–compulsive disorder (OCD) in pediatric populations. However, antipsychotic augmentation remains an available treatment option for children with severe OCD that has not improved sufficiently on selective serotonin reuptake inhibitor (SSRI) pharmacotherapy and cognitive behavioral therapy. Meta-analysis of nine RCTs involving 278 participants demonstrated a significant benefit (absolute risk difference (ARD) in favor of antipsychotic augmentation of 0.22 [95% confidence interval (CI): 0.13 to 0.31]) compared to placebo. The subgroup of OCD patients with comorbid tics appears to have a particularly beneficial response to antipsychotic augmentation, ARD = 0.43 (95% CI: 0.19, 0.68) (12). Meta-analysis also demonstrated no significant differences in efficacy between individual antipsychotic agents. Based on the currently available data, antipsychotic augmentation should only be attempted following a treatment failure of 10 to 12 weeks of SSRI pharmacotherapy of adequate dose and duration (13). Further, antipsychotic treatment should be discontinued if there is no treatment improvement within 6 to 12 weeks of treatment.

Treatment-Refractory Depressive Disorders

Similar to OCD, there exists no randomized, placebo-controlled trials examining the efficacy of antipsychotic augmentation in treatment-refractory depression. Meta-analysis has demonstrated the efficacy of atypical antipsychotics as an augmentation strategy for treatment-refractory major depression and persistent depressive disorder in adults. Meta-analysis of 16 randomized, placebo-controlled trials with 3,480 subjects demonstrated that adjunctive atypical antipsychotics were significantly more effective than placebo (response: odds ratio = 1.69, 95% CI: 1.46 to 1.95) (14). Meta-analysis also demonstrated no evidence of difference in efficacy between antipsychotics studied. Antipsychotics should be used with extreme caution in children with major depression (even as compared to OCD) as there exists a larger number of potential therapeutic options beyond SSRIs with evidence of efficacy in adults. These alternative pharmacologic options have a lower side-effect burden than antipsychotics.

Atypical Antipsychotics

The dosing recommendations for each individual antidepressant medication is depicted in Table 6.1.4.3.2. Antipsychotics commonly used in pediatric populations are also discussed individually in the following section. The relative side-effect profiles of different antipsychotic agents are also depicted in Table 6.1.4.3.3.

Risperidone (Risperdal)

Large multisite studies in adults with schizophrenia have shown that risperidone is an effective antipsychotic with lower risk of neurologic side effects compared to traditional antipsychotics such as haloperidol (15). Unlike clozapine, it is associated with an increase in prolactin suggesting more potent D_2 blockade. At doses above 6 mg/day, the risk of neurologic side effects increasesin a dose-dependent manner. This apparent dose-threshold effect may be due to protective effects of 5HT2 receptors to which the atypical antipsychotics (AAPs) appear to bind preferentially. In this model, as the dose of the antipsychotic medication increases, 5HT2 receptors become saturated, which is followed by an increase in D_2 binding (16). Alternatively, the protective role of 5HT2 may be less important than D_2 occupancy. Occupancy is influenced by rate of association (binding to the receptor) and the rate of dissociation (release from the receptor). As pointed out by Kapur and Seeman (17), AAPs have lower affinity to D2 receptors because they are more easily displaced by endogenous dopamine. The result of this "fast off" property of the AAPs is that at usual doses these drugs remain under the D_2 occupancy threshold that is associated with neurological side effects. For example,

TABLE 6.1.4.3.3

SIDE EFFECT PROFILE OF COMMONLY PRESCRIBED ANTIPSYCHOTIC MEDICATIONS

	Extrapyramidal	Sedation	Weight Gain	Hyperglycemia	Anticholinergic	Orthostatic Hypertension
Second-Generation (Atypical) Antipsychotics						
Risperidone	++	++	++	++	–	++
Aripiprazole	+	+	+	–	–	+
Quetiapine	+	+++	++	+++	++	++
Olanzapine	+	+++	+++	+++	+++	+
Ziprasidone	+	++	+	+	+	++
Clozapine	+	+++	+++	+++	+++	++
Paliperidone	+	+	+	–	–	+
Lurasidone	+++	+++	–	–	–	–
Asenapine	+	+	+	+	–	+
First-Generation (Typical) Antipsychotics						
Haloperidol	+++	+	++	++	+	+
Molindone	++	–	–	–	+	+
Pimozide	+++	++	Not Reported		++	+
Chlorpromazine	++	+++	+++	+++	+++	+++
Perphenazine	++	++	Not Reported		+	+
Fluphenazine	+++	+	+	+	+	+
Thioridazine	+	++	+	+	++	++

Key: + ≥20% incidence; **10–20% incidence, *1–10% incidence; –minimal evidence of effect.

65% D2 occupancy is the estimated threshold for antipsychotic activity compared to 80% occupancy for neurologic side effects (17). At usual doses, risperidone and olanzapine do not exceed the 80% threshold, but haloperidol does (17).

Risperidone is the best studied AAP in pediatric populations. An emerging body of evidence from short-term, placebo-controlled, randomized clinical trials shows that risperidone is safe and effective for serious behavioral problems in children with autism (18,19); severe disruptive behavior (20–23); and Tourette syndrome (TS) (23,24). A few studies have also shown that short-term gains endure over the intermediate term (23,25).

Risperidone (1 to 3 and 4 to 6 mg/day) has been demonstrated to be more effective than placebo in a 12-week RCT of 160 adolescents schizophrenia (2). Interestingly, there was no evidence of a difference in efficacy between the low (1 to 3 mg) and high (4 to 6 mg) dosing strategies for risperidone (2). The TEOSS study examined olanzapine, risperidone, or molindone; found that only 12% of youths with early-onset schizophrenia spectrum disorders continued on their originally randomized treatment at 52 weeks (26). Risperidone showed significantly greater weight gain than molindone but less than olanzapine.

Risperidone has been shown effective at daily doses of 0.5 to 2.5 and 3 to 6 mg for the treatment of acute mania in adolescents with bipolar disorder (27). Consistent with the trials of adolescent schizophrenia, higher doses of risperidone showed no greater efficacy in treating acute mania but were associated with a worse side-effect profile, while the 0.5 to 2.5 mg exhibited a better side-effect profile (27). The Treatment of Early Age Mania (TEAM) trial demonstrated that risperidone was more efficacious than lithium and divalproex sodium for the initial treatment of childhood mania but had potentially serious metabolic effects, including an increased risk for weight gain, increased BMI, and increased prolactin levels. A smaller trial in preschool children with manic symptoms demonstrated a benefit of risperidone compared to both placebo and valproic acid (7).

Risperidone has been shown to be more effective than haloperidol in the treatment of behavioral symptoms, impulsivity, language skills, and impaired social relations in children with ASD (28). The Research Unit in Pediatric Psychopharmacology Autism Network completed an 8-week, placebo-controlled study of risperidone in 101 children with autism accompanied by tantrums, aggression, and self-injury (18). At an average dose of 1.8 mg/day, the risperidone group improved 57% on a parent-rated scale measuring the target symptoms of tantrums, aggression, and self-injury compared to 14% in placebo. Similarly, blinded clinicians rated 75% of children in the risperidone group as much improved or very much improved compared to 12% for the placebo group. Children initially randomized to placebo who showed no improvement were offered treatment in an 8-week open-label trial using the same dosing schedule that was used in the double-blind trial. Sixty-three who showed a positive response to risperidone (in the double-blind or the open-label trial) were followed forward for an additional 4 months to evaluate the stability of gains and continued safety (25). Finally, at the 6-month mark, children were randomly assigned to remain on risperidone or to gradual withdrawal from active medication by placebo substitution over a 4-week period. This study showed that the short-term gains of risperidone were stable over time and that it was not necessary to increase the dose of medication to maintain the observed benefits. Thirty-two children entered the double-blind, placebo-controlled discontinuation phase. Ten of 16 children assigned to discontinuation showed a return of symptoms compared to two of 16 children who remained on risperidone who met prespecified criteria for relapse.

Aman et al. (20) conducted a 6-week, randomized, placebo-controlled risperidone trial in 118 children with disruptive behavior. The subjects ranged in age from 5 to 12 years; many were functioning in the intellectually disabled range (IQ 36 to 84). After 6 weeks of risperidone, the active treatment group showed nearly a 16-point improvement on the parent-rated Nisonger Child Behavior Rating Form compared to a 6-point improvement in the placebo group. The average dose of risperidone was 1.16 mg/day. This finding was replicated in a separate trial using an identical design and similar inclusion criteria (23). Both studies included a 12-month extension phase, which showed that gains were stable (23). There is also emerging data to suggest risperidone may be an effective treatment for irritability in children without ASD. An RCT of risperidone in children with severe aggression related to ADHD demonstrated that risperidone had added benefit when added to a combination of parent training and stimulant treatment (29).

In a placebo-controlled study of risperidone that included both children and adults, risperidone was superior to placebo for the treatment of tics in Tourette syndrome (24). Thirty-four subjects (26 children and 8 adults) were randomly assigned to placebo or risperidone. After 8 weeks of treatment with doses ranging from 1 to 2 mg/day in the pediatric sample, risperidone was associated with a 36% improvement on a clinician-rated measure of tic severity, which was significantly better than the 9% in the placebo group ($p < 0.01$). No neurologic side effects were observed in this study. Weight gain averaged 2.8 kg in the active treatment group compared to 0.7 kg in the placebo group ($p < 0.05$). Treatment-emergent social phobia was observed in two cases in the risperidone group, which has been reported by others (30).

Risperidone has also been compared to pimozide in a randomized, double-blind trial (31). In that study, risperidone and pimozide were similar in their positive effects, with reductions in tic severity of 44% and 47%, respectively. Not surprisingly, the pimozide group reported more neurologic side effects. Weight gain was greater in the risperidone group (4.5 kg compared to 2.7 kg). Dose ranges were similar, up to 6 mg/day for each drug. The study included 50 subjects in total, but only 17 were in the pediatric age group. Results in the pediatric sample were not reported.

In many of these studies, the drug was initiated at 0.5 mg/day (0.25 in younger children) and increased by 0.5 mg every 5 to 7 days to a range of 1 to 2.5 mg/day in a single dose or two divided doses. Studies by Aman et al. (20), Snyder et al. (23), and Findling et al. (22) used single-daily dosing. Not surprisingly, the average dose in these studies was lower than the studies that used a twice-daily dosing schedule. Taken together, these data suggest that twice-a-day dosing may be better tolerated, though single-day dosing may be considered if the total daily dose is low (less than 1.5 mg/day).

Aripiprazole (Abilify)

Aripiprazole is a third-generation antipsychotic due to its novel mechanism of action. Aripiprazole is classified as a partial dopamine agonist. This term refers to the fact that aripiprazole binds with presynaptic dopamine receptors, which is purported to turn down the dopamine system in brain regions with increased dopaminergic tone. In addition, like the other AAPs, aripiprazole has serotonin-blocking properties at the five HT2 receptor sites. Aripiprazole has been evaluated in pediatric populations for many of the same target symptoms described earlier for risperidone.

Aripiprazole at doses of 10 and 30 mg/day has been demonstrated to be superior to placebo for the treatment of adolescents with schizophrenia (1). Symptom improvement and remission rates were higher (but not statistically significantly so) in the 30 mg compared to the 10-mg aripiprazole group. Similarly, aripiprazole has been demonstrated to be effective compared to placebo for the treatment of acute mania or maintenance treatment for adolescent bipolar disorder (32). Similar to its benefits in adolescent psychosis, aripiprazole demonstrated efficacy for acute bipolar manic and mixed episodes in adolescence with greater (though again not statistically significant benefits observed in the 30-mg treatment arm compared to the 10-mg treatment arm (33)). For maintenance treatment of adolescents with bipolar disorder started on aripiprazole, subjects randomized to aripiprazole had a longer time to the their next mood episode and lower likelihood of medication discontinuation than subjects randomly assigned to placebo (32). In comparison with placebo, aripiprazole showed greater efficacy, was well tolerated, and safe in the short-term treatment of children and adolescents with Tourette's disorder (34). Several placebo-controlled trials have demonstrated the superiority of aripiprazole for the treatment of irritability in children with ASD (35,36). In a double-blind, randomized, placebo-controlled, parallel-group study, 218 children (6 to 17 years) with irritability and aggression symptoms were randomized to aripiprazole (5, 10, or 15 mg/day) or placebo for 8 weeks. All doses of aripiprazole were more effective than placebo with a clear dose–response pattern (36). Aripiprazole and risperidone are the only FDA-approved medications for treating irritability in autistic disorder, a head-to-head study, demonstrated that aripiprazole as well as risperidone lowered aberrant behavior checklist scores during 2 months, and that while the safety and efficacy of aripiprazole (mean dose 5.5 mg/day) and risperidone (mean dose 1.12 mg/day) were comparable, the rates of adverse effects were not significantly different between the two groups (37).

Quetiapine (Seroquel)

Quetiapine is a second-generation antipsychotic that is gradually being shown to be effective and safe for treatment or augmentation in a variety of pediatric conditions. In a 6-week study of adolescent patients, doses of 400 and 800 mg/day provided significant improvements in symptoms associated with schizophrenia in adolescent patients (primarily the Positive and Negative Syndrome Scale total score change) (3). Quetiapine was generally well tolerated with a profile broadly similar to that reported in adult and adolescent populations (3). A head-to-head study of quetiapine and risperidone was conducted into the treatment of the often comorbid bipolar II and conduct disorder (3,38). Both treatments showed similar efficacy in reducing manic symptoms and aggression. In BD type II, CD comorbidity, quetiapine, and monotherapy may be effective and relatively safe (38). Quetiapine demonstrated efficacy in reducing manic symptoms of bipolar disorder in a large, placebo-controlled trial of bipolar mania (39) but not for bipolar depression (40).

Ziprasidone (Geodon)

This atypical antipsychotic medication has also been shown to be effective in adults with schizophrenia (41). Like risperidone, it is a potent blocker at the D_2 and 5-HT_2 sites. Compared to risperidone, however, much larger doses are required to achieve an antipsychotic effect. For example, the usual dose of risperidone in adults with schizophrenia is 6 mg/day. By contrast, the dose of ziprasidone is typically in the range of 40 to 160 mg/day or higher, given in two divided doses (42). In the first trial, 28 children (age 7 to 17 years) with TS or chronic motor tic disorder were randomly assigned to placebo (N = 12) or ziprasidone (N = 16) under double-blind conditions. The mean dose of ziprasidone was approximately 30 mg/day given in divided doses. Using the same outcome measure mentioned for the risperidone study in TS, ziprasidone was associated with a 35% improvement in tic severity, compared to a 7% decline in the placebo group ($p < 0.05$) (43). Common side effects included moderate sedation (one subject), mild sedation (11 subjects), insomnia (four subjects), and akathisia (one subject). There were no changes in laboratory values, cardiac conduction times, or body weight in the ziprasidone group. Although we now know that ziprasidone is associated with greater QTc prolongation compared to other atypical antipsychotic agents.

While generally well tolerated, with an overall neutral weight and metabolic profile, ziprasidone failed to separate from placebo in a 6-week randomized, placebo-controlled trial in 283 adolescents with schizophrenia (44). By contrast, a 4-week, randomized, double-blind, placebo-controlled multicenter trial examining the efficacy of ziprasidone in 237 adolescents with bipolar disorder demonstrated significant benefit compared to placebo for manic symptoms (45).

Olanzapine (Zyprexa)

Olanzapine is another agent with atypical features that are preserved only in the lower dose range (<20 mg/day in adults). In a randomized, double-blind, placebo-controlled trial, olanzapine was superior to placebo, and has been approved by the FDA for the acute treatment of bipolar I depression in patients 10 to 17 years of age. Benefits should be weighed against the risk of adverse events, particularly weight gain and hyperlipidemia (46). While olanzapine was as effective as other antipsychotics in the TEOSS study, the olanzapine treatment arm was terminated early due to concerns about excessive weight gain (47). This weight gain was an average of 6.1 kg in 8 weeks in the olanzapine arm. Because of the excessive weight gain associated with olanzapine, olanzapine is generally not recommended unless children have failed other antipsychotic medications.

Asenapine (Saphris)

Asenapine is an atypical antipsychotic given in sublingual formulations that has FDA approval for the treatment of schizophrenia and acute manic or mixed episodes of bipolar disorder in adults. Asenapine was recently FDA approved for the treatment of adolescents (ages 10 to 17 years) experiencing acute manic or mixed episodes of bipolar disorder. This approval was based on a 3-week randomized, placebo-controlled trial of adolescents with bipolar disorder I (48). All three doses of asenapine (2.5, 5, and 10 mg bid) showed benefit compared to placebo on reducing manic symptoms on the Young Mania Rating Scale. Side effects associated with asenapine treatment included somnolence, sedation, oral numbness, and increased appetite/weight gain. Asenapine is noted to have less anticholinergic and cardiovascular side effects than many other available antipsychotics and its sublingual formulations may be of use in younger children with difficulty swallowing pills (although such use in younger children is off-label and has not supported with adequate research).

Clozapine (Clozaril)

Clozapine was the first AAP agent to be developed and entered into the marketplace. It is a dibenzodiazepine derivative and chemically unrelated to any of the typical antipsychotic drugs. Soon after it was introduced in 1960, its effectiveness in treatment-resistant patients with schizophrenia was recognized, but initial enthusiasm waned following the report of fatal agranulocytosis in a series of cases in Europe. Two open studies (49,50) and one controlled comparison with haloperidol (51) have been carried out in pediatric populations. Collectively, these studies included 53 patients from ages 6 to 18 years. Clozapine was effective in 30 of 53 (56%) of these patients. This figure is impressive considering that this was a group of treatment-resistant patients. In the controlled trial, doses ranged from 125 to 525 mg/day given in divided doses. Although there were no reports of extrapyramidal symptom (EPS), several serious adverse effects were observed, most notably seizures (N = 1) and hematopoietic abnormalities

($N = 4$). Weight gain was a frequently observed complication of clozapine treatment. Due to differences in the duration of the studies, however, it is not possible to aggregate data across them. Additional longitudinal studies of clozapine use in children have continued to suggest a promising short-term and longer-term response. However, these studies also suggest that the rates of neutropenia may be higher in children treated with clozapine compared to adults (52).

Typical Antipsychotics (Antipsychotics)

Chlorpromazine (Thorazine)

Chlorpromazine is an aliphatic agent, and was the first antipsychotic used in children with severe behavioral disturbances. With the introduction of newer agents, the use of chlorpromazine has declined, although it is still routinely used for the acute management of agitation or aggression, where it can be administered through either oral or intramuscular (IM) routes. When used IM, careful caution must be paid to vital signs, as significant hypotension can occur even at seemingly low doses (e.g., <25 mg).

Molindone (Moban)

Molindone is a first-generation antipsychotic over which, second-generation antipsychotics have not proven efficacy. Molindone was the typical antipsychotic comparator in the TEOSS trial (5). No significant differences were found among treatment groups in response rates although molindone had the highest absolute response rate (molindone: 50%; olanzapine: 34%; risperidone: 46%) and magnitude of symptom reduction (53). Molindone was associated with a significantly higher rate of akathisia and lower amount of weight gain compared to olanzapine and risperidone.

Haloperidol (Haldol)

A butyrophenone that is structurally unrelated to the phenothiazines represents the prototype of a high-potency typical antipsychotic. Since its introduction in the early 1960s, it has been used to treat children with psychosis, aggressive behavior, tics, and behavioral dyscontrol associated with autism (54,55).

Compared to the low-potency antipsychotics, haloperidol is much more likely to cause EPS, but it is less sedating. The dose of haloperidol varies according to the target symptoms. For example, in school-age children with tics or severe behavioral dyscontrol associated with autism, the dose is typically in the range of 0.75 to 2.5 mg/day (43,56). By contrast, doses in the range of 10 mg/day may be used to deal with an acute psychotic episode (57).

Fluphenazine (Prolixin)

Fluphenazine, a piperazine phenothiazine, is not approved for children under the age of 12 years, and has not been well studied in pediatric populations. At low dosages (0.04 mg/kg/day), fluphenazine decreased aggression, hyperactivity, and stereotypies in an open-label study of 12 children with PDD (58). At a mean dose of 7 mg/day in divided doses (range, 2 to 15 mg/day), fluphenazine reduced tics and was favored over haloperidol by most patients (59). This open-label trial of 21 patients with TS included both children and adults, but results were not separately reported by age group.

Thiothixene (Navane)

A thioxanthene derivative, this mid-potency agent is structurally unrelated to the phenothiazines or the butyrophenones. It is approved for the treatment of psychosis in children over the age of 12 years. The available evidence in children under age 12 indicates that thiothixene is less sedating than low-potency antipsychotics, and that it may have a lower risk of EPS than high-potency antipsychotics such as haloperidol (60).

Pimozide (Orap)

A diphenylbutylpiperidine, pimozide it is not related to the phenothiazines or to haloperidol. It is a potent blocker of dopamine at the D_2 postsynaptic receptors, and it is used to treat tics in TS. In placebo-controlled studies involving both children and adults, pimozide has been shown to be superior to placebo in reducing tics (61). It has also been evaluated in head-to-head trials with haloperidol. These studies suggest that pimozide is equivalent to haloperidol with respect to tic suppression, and that it has a more favorable side-effect profile (55,62).

Mechanism of Action. The principal therapeutic action of the traditional antipsychotics is to block postsynaptic D2 receptors (17). The observed differences across traditional antipsychotics may be related to the regional specificity of the D_2 blockade (striatum vs. limbic structures), and the effects on other neurotransmitter systems. By contrast, the atypical antipsychotics block both dopamine and serotonin postsynaptic receptors to varying degrees. The addition of postsynaptic 5-HT blockade may lower the risk of neurologic side effects and perhaps of tardive dyskinesia (TD) as well. As noted previously, the protective role of 5HT2 may be less important than D_2 occupancy. Occupancy is influenced by rate of association (binding to the receptor) and the rate of dissociation (release from the receptor). Because the AAPs are more easily displaced by endogenous dopamine, the occupancy at D_2 receptors is lower than the traditional antipsychotics of similar potency. The result of this "fast-off" property of the AAPs is that at usual doses these drugs remain under the D_2 occupancy threshold and less likely to produce neurologic side effects.

Antipsychotic medications may also have anticholinergic and antihistamine effects, as well as adrenergic-blocking effects. These additional pharmacologic properties probably do not contribute to the therapeutic effects of the antipsychotic drugs, but do have an impact on side-effect profiles. For example, low-potency antipsychotics such as chlorpromazine and thioridazine cause more sedation, dry mouth, and constipation, presumably due to antihistamine and anticholinergic effects. Their propensity to cause hypotension may be related to alpha-adrenergic blockade.

Adverse Effects. Neurologic side effects such as dystonic reactions, rigidity, and akathisia are more common with the high-potency antipsychotics. In addition to these neurologic side effects, adverse effects of the typical antipsychotic drugs in children and adolescents can include weight gain, increased risk of diabetes, elevated prolactin levels with possible emergence of gynecomastia in boys, and galactorrhea or amenorrhea in girls. Drowsiness is a common side effect with the low-potency antipsychotic agents, but may occur in the high-potency antipsychotics as well. Anticholinergic side effects such as dry mouth, constipation, and blurred vision should also be monitored. As noted, thioridazine, pimozide, ziprasidone, and other antipsychotics can prolong cardiac conduction times (63). Recommendations on whether to obtain ECGs at baseline and how often to monitor cardiac conduction times when using antipsychotics in children and adolescents are not consistent. For example, electrocardiograms at baseline and during maintenance treatment with antipsychotics are recommended in one guideline (64) but not in others (65). The explanation for this inconsistency is not clear, but may simply reflect the incomplete state of current evidence. Thioridazine has largely fallen out of use. Expert opinion in published guidelines for the use of antipsychotics in TS indicates

TABLE 6.1.4.3.4

MONITORING RECOMMENDATIONS FOR USE OF ANTIPSYCHOTIC MEDICATIONS IN PEDIATRIC AND ADULT PATIENTS

	Baseline	4 Wks	8 Wks	12 Wks	Annually	Reassess
Weight (BMI)	X	X		X	X	3 mo
Waist Circumference	X				X	Annually
Blood Pressure	X			X	X	3 mo for 1 yr, then annually
Fasting Glucose	X		X		X	3 mo for 1 yr, then annually
Fasting lipid profile	X			X	X	Annually

that when using pimozide or ziprasidone in children and adolescents, an ECG should be obtained prior to treatment, during the dose adjustment phase and periodically thereafter (66). One important difference in considering treatment with pimozide or ziprasidone is their relative vulnerability to drug–drug interaction. Pimozide is a substrate for the CYP 3A4 pathway and will show a dramatic rise in serum level following the addition of a potent 3A4 inhibitor such as erythromycin. Case reports indicate that this type of interaction may have serious consequences (67). Ziprasidone, on the other hand, does not appear to be vulnerable to drug–drug interaction due to its use of multiple metabolic pathways (68).

Although the atypical antipsychotics are less likely to cause neurologic side effects, they are not free of adverse effects. Clozapine is associated with a low risk of agranulocytosis and toxic megacolon. For this reason, it is only used in treatment-resistant schizophrenia.

Other adverse effects of clozapine include lowered seizure threshold and tachycardia. An adverse effect of the AAPs that has emerged as a clinically important concern is increased appetite and weight gain. Several reports in pediatric samples across several diagnostic groups have shown that clozapine, olanzapine, quetiapine, and risperidone are associated with excessive weight gain (18,20,24,51,69–72). The weight gain associated with olanzapine reported in two trials ranged from 4 to 6 kg over 6 to 12 weeks' duration (70,73). Table 6.1.4.3.3 depicts the relative risk of weight gain between antipsychotic agents. Generally, aripiprazole and ziprasidone are considered relatively weight neutral but still associated with some weight gain with olanzapine and clozapine causing a large risk of weight gain. Table 6.1.4.3.4 depicts the currently recommended monitoring parameters for antipsychotic medications in pediatric populations. Longitudinal studies examining the trajectory of weight gain with AAP treatment in children and adolescents suggest that the rate of weight gain is greatest in the first 2 months of treatment, with some leveling thereafter. The health consequences of obesity can be significant, including increased serum cholesterol, triglycerides, and drug-induced type II diabetes (74).

The risk of TD increases as a function of dose and duration, but it may occur with brief exposures as well. TD has been reported in pediatric patients (75). Thus, children and adolescents treated with antipsychotics should be monitored for abnormal movements. The largest systematic study to date (76) raises questions regarding the difficulty in distinguishing between TD and withdrawal dyskinesia (77). In that study, 30% of children between the ages of 2 and 8 years showed persistent dyskinetic movements for up to 3 months of follow-up after a planned withdrawal from haloperidol.

Questions of how and when to discontinue antipsychotic medication are critical ones, but data to guide clinical decisions are limited. To minimize TD, dose reductions should be done gradually while evaluating changes in symptom severity. In autism and tic disorders, discontinuation may be considered annually for cases in which good control has been achieved. If symptoms persist, the maintenance dose of the antipsychotic should be reduced to the lowest possible one sufficient to maintain symptomatic control and minimize overall exposure (78). Based on the collective experience with clozapine, the newer atypicals may also have a lower risk of TD. More study, such as long-term follow-up of clinical samples treated with atypical antipsychotics and careful postmarketing surveillance of these agents in pediatric populations, is needed.

Neuroleptic malignant syndrome (NMS) is a rare adverse effect due to antipsychotic medications. NMS is characterized by high fever, autonomic instability, and muscle breakdown (reflected by elevated CPK titers) and is potentially life threatening. The mortality rate may be as high as 9% in children and adolescents (79). Discontinuation of the medication is usually all that is required, highlighting the importance of early identification of the condition. In severe cases, IV fluids are needed, and some authors have advocated the use of dantrolene or bromocriptine to hasten recovery.

Treatment of Antipsychotic-Associated Adverse Effects: Emphasis on Anticholinergic Agents

Among the many potential side effects associated with the traditional antipsychotics, neurologic side effects represent some of the most common and ones likely to be treated with additional pharmacotherapy. Acute neurologic side effects include dystonia, torticollis, or oculogyric crisis. Chronic side effects include parkinsonism, tremor, rigidity, mask-like faces, or festinant gait. These adverse effects can be prevented or reversed with the judicious use of anticholinergic agents. Given that all of these adverse effects are associated with unchecked D_2 receptor blockade, it follows that they are most common with high-potency traditional agents (such as haloperidol or fluphenazine) and least common with low-potency compounds (such as chlorpromazine). Although less common with atypical antipsychotics, the risk of neurologic side effects increases at higher dose levels of risperidone, olanzapine, or ziprasidone. In most instances, the anticholinergics discussed here are used in combination with high-potency agents, and they should rarely (if at all) be used in combination with lower-potency drugs. Not only are the low-potency agents less likely to cause neurologic side effects, the addition of anti-parkinsonian mediations may exacerbate the inherent anticholinergic properties of low-potency antipsychotics. This point is of more than academic interest: The additive effects of combining agents with anticholinergic or anti-histaminergic effects can rapidly lead to behavioral toxicity, including paradoxical agitation, confusion, or full-blown delirium.

The two most commonly used agents in this category are diphenhydramine (Benadryl) and benztropine (Cogentin). The antihistamine diphenhydramine is best used in acute situations, both given its ready availability (in household medicine cabinets and crash carts alike), as well given its side-effect profile. However, the sedation induced by diphenhydramine can be intense, so this agent should be used sparingly as a maintenance intervention. Alternatively, such sedation can be exploited therapeutically in the acutely agitated patient. By contrast, the purely anticholinergic compound benztropine is preferred for longer-term management of neurologic side effects, as it does not induce somnolence. Diphenhydramine is usually dosed in the 12.5 to 50 mg range (single or repeat dose, administered orally or by IM injection), while benztropine is used in 0.5-, 1-, or 2-mg doses, usually given orally in a bid regimen. The long-term use (>1 month) of anticholinergic agents should be avoided if at all possible, particularly in younger children, for whom the resulting Sjögren-like iatrogenic syndrome can lead to widespread cavities. The slow upward adjustment of antipsychotics, coupled with time-limited (as opposed to regular) use of these agents, can avert unnecessary longer-term use.

References

1. Findling RL, Robb A, Nyilas M, et al.: A multiple-center, randomized, double-blind, placebo-controlled study of oral aripiprazole for treatment of adolescents with schizophrenia. *Am J Psychiatry* 165(11):1432–1441, 2008.
2. Haas M, Unis AS, Armenteros J, Copenhaver MD, Quiroz JA, Kushner SF: A 6-week, randomized, double-blind, placebo-controlled study of the efficacy and safety of risperidone in adolescents with schizophrenia. *J Child Adolesc Psychopharmacol* 19(6):611–621, 2009.
3. Findling RL, McKenna K, Earley WR, Stankowski J, Pathak S: Efficacy and safety of quetiapine in adolescents with schizophrenia investigated in a 6-week, double-blind, placebo-controlled trial. *J Child Adolesc Psychopharmacol* 22(5):327–342, 2012.
4. Kumar A, Datta SS, Wright SD, Furtado VA, Russell PS: Atypical antipsychotics for psychosis in adolescents. *Cochrane Database Syst Rev* (10):Cd009582, 2013.
5. Sikich L, Frazier JA, McClellan J, et al.: Double-blind comparison of first- and second-generation antipsychotics in early-onset schizophrenia and schizo-affective disorder: findings from the treatment of early-onset schizophrenia spectrum disorders (TEOSS) study. *Am J Psychiatry* 165(11): 1420–1431, 2008.
6. Geller B, Luby JL, Joshi P, et al.: A randomized controlled trial of risperidone, lithium, or divalproex sodium for initial treatment of bipolar I disorder, manic or mixed phase, in children and adolescents. *Arch Gen Psychiatry* 69(5):515–528, 2012.
7. Kowatch RA, Scheffer RE, Monroe E, Delgado S, Altaye M, Lagory D: Placebo-controlled trial of valproic acid versus risperidone in children 3–7 years of age with bipolar I disorder. *J Child Adolesc Psychopharmacol* 25(4):306–313, 2015.
8. Weisman H, Qureshi IA, Leckman JF, Scahill L, Bloch MH: Systematic review: pharmacological treatment of tic disorders—efficacy of antipsychotic and alpha-2 adrenergic agonist agents. *Neurosci Biobehav Rev* 37(6):1162–1171, 2013.
9. Yang C-S, Huang H, Zhang L-L, Zhu C-R, Guo Q: Aripiprazole for the treatment of tic disorders in children: a systematic review and meta-analysis. *BMC Psychiatry* 15:179, 2015.
10. Loy JH, Merry SN, Hetrick SE, Stasiak K: Atypical antipsychotics for disruptive behaviour disorders in children and youths. *Cochrane Database Syst Rev* (9), 2012.
11. Ching H, Pringsheim T: Aripiprazole for autism spectrum disorders (ASD). *Cochrane Database Syst Rev* (5), 2012.
12. Bloch MH, Landeros-Weisenberger A, Kelmendi B, Coric V, Bracken MB, Leckman JF: A systematic review: antipsychotic augmentation with treatment refractory obsessive-compulsive disorder. *Mol Psychiatry* 11(7): 622–632, 2006.
13. Bloch MH, Storch EA: Assessment and management of treatment-refractory obsessive-compulsive disorder in children. *J Am Acad Child Adolesc Psychiatry* 54(4):251–262, 2015.
14. Nelson JC, Papakostas GI: Atypical antipsychotic augmentation in major depressive disorder: a meta-analysis of placebo-controlled randomized trials. *Am J Psychiatry* 166(9):980–991, 2009.
15. Marder SR, Meibach RC: Risperidone in the treatment of schizophrenia. *Am J Psychiatry* 151(6):825–835, 1994.
16. Kapur S, Remington G, Zipursky RB, Wilson AA, Houle S: The D2 dopamine receptor occupancy of risperidone and its relationship to extrapyramidal symptoms: a pet study. *Life Sci* 57(10):PL103–PL107, 1995.
17. Kapur S, Seeman P: Does fast dissociation from the dopamine d(2) receptor explain the action of atypical antipsychotics? A new hypothesis. *Am J Psychiatry* 158(3):360–369, 2001.
18. McCracken JT, McGough J, Shah B, et al.: Risperidone in children with autism and serious behavioral problems. *N Engl J Med* 347(5):314–321, 2002.
19. Shea S: Risperidone in the treatment of disruptive behavioral symptoms in children with autistic and other pervasive developmental disorders. *Pediatrics* 114(5):e634–e641, 2004.
20. Aman MG, De Smedt G, Derivan A, Lyons B, Findling RL, Risperidone Disruptive Behavior Study Group. Double-blind, placebo-controlled study of risperidone for the treatment of disruptive behaviors in children with subaverage intelligence. *Am J Psychiatry* 159(8):1337–1346, 2002.
21. Buitelaar JK, van der Gaag RJ, Cohen-Kettenis P, Melman CT: A randomized controlled trial of risperidone in the treatment of aggression in hospitalized adolescents with subaverage cognitive abilities. *J Clin Psychiatry* 62(4):239–248, 2001.
22. Findling RL, McNamara NK, Branicky LA, Schluchter MD, Lemon E, Blumer JL: A double-blind pilot study of risperidone in the treatment of conduct disorder. *J Am Acad Child Adolesc Psychiatry* 39(4):509–516, 2000.
23. Snyder R, Turgay A, Aman M, Binder C, Fisman S, Carroll A, Risperidone Conduct Study Group: Effects of risperidone on conduct and disruptive behavior disorders in children with subaverage IQs. *J Am Acad Child Adolesc Psychiatry* 41(9):1026–1036, 2002.
24. Scahill L, Leckman JF, Schultz RT, Katsovich L, Peterson BS: A placebo-controlled trial of risperidone in Tourette syndrome. *Neurology* 60(7): 1130–1135, 2003.
25. Research Units on Pediatric Psychopharmacology Autism Network: Risperidone treatment of autistic disorder: longer-term benefits and blinded discontinuation after 6 months. *Am J Psychiatry* 162(7):1361–1369, 2005.
26. Findling RL, Johnson JL, McClellan J, et al.: Double-blind maintenance safety and effectiveness findings from the treatment of early-onset schizophrenia spectrum (TEOSS) study. *J Am Acad Child Adolesc Psychiatry* 49(6):583–594; quiz 632, 2010.
27. Haas M, Delbello MP, Pandina G, et al.: Risperidone for the treatment of acute mania in children and adolescents with bipolar disorder: a randomized, double-blind, placebo-controlled study. *Bipolar Disord* 11(7):687–700, 2009.
28. Miral S, Gencer O, Inal-Emiroglu FN, Baykara B, Baykara A, Dirik E: Risperidone versus haloperidol in children and adolescents with AD: a randomized, controlled, double-blind trial. *Eur Child Adolesc Psychiatry* 17(1):1–8, 2008.
29. Aman MG, Bukstein OG, Gadow KD, et al.: What does risperidone add to parent training and stimulant for severe aggression in child attention-deficit/hyperactivity disorder? *J Am Acad Child Adolesc Psychiatry* 53(1): 47–60.e1, 2014.
30. Hanna GL, Fluent TE, Fischer DJ: Separation anxiety in children and adolescents treated with risperidone. *J Child Adolesc Psychopharmacol* 9(4):277–283, 1999.
31. Bruggeman R, van der Linden C, Buitelaar JK, Gericke GS, Hawkridge SM, Temlett JA: Risperidone versus pimozide in Tourette's disorder: a comparative double-blind parallel-group study. *J Clin Psychiatry* 62(1): 50–56, 2001.
32. Findling RL, Youngstrom EA, McNamara NK, et al.: Double-blind, randomized, placebo-controlled long-term maintenance study of aripiprazole in children with bipolar disorder. *J Clin Psychiatry* 73(1):57–63, 2012.
33. Findling RL, Nyilas M, Forbes RA, et al.: Acute treatment of pediatric bipolar I disorder, manic or mixed episode, with aripiprazole: a randomized, double-blind, placebo-controlled study. *J Clin Psychiatry* 70(10): 1441–1451, 2009.
34. Yoo HK, Joung YS, Lee JS, et al.: A multicenter, randomized, double-blind, placebo-controlled study of aripiprazole in children and adolescents with Tourette's disorder. *J Clin Psychiatry* 74(8):e772–e780, 2013.
35. Owen R, Sikich L, Marcus RN, et al.: Aripiprazole in the treatment of irritability in children and adolescents with autistic disorder. *Pediatrics* 124(6):1533–1540, 2009.
36. Marcus RN, Owen R, Kamen L, et al.: A placebo-controlled, fixed-dose study of aripiprazole in children and adolescents with irritability associated with autistic disorder. *J Am Acad Child Adolesc Psychiatry* 48(11):1110–1119, 2009.
37. Ghanizadeh A, Sahraeizadeh A, Berk M: A head-to-head comparison of aripiprazole and risperidone for safety and treating autistic disorders, a randomized double blind clinical trial. *Child Psychiatry Hum Dev* 45(2):185–192, 2014.
38. Masi G, Milone A, Stawinoga A, Veltri S, Pisano S: Efficacy and safety of risperidone and quetiapine in adolescents with bipolar ii disorder comorbid with conduct disorder. *J Clin Psychopharmacol* 35(5):587–590, 2015.
39. Pathak S, Findling RL, Earley WR, Acevedo LD, Stankowski J, Delbello MP: Efficacy and safety of quetiapine in children and adolescents with mania associated with bipolar I disorder: a 3-week, double-blind, placebo-controlled trial. *J Clin Psychiatry* 74(1):e100–e109, 2013.
40. Findling RL, Pathak S, Earley WR, Liu S, DelBello MP: Efficacy and safety of extended-release quetiapine fumarate in youth with bipolar depression: an 8 week, double-blind, placebo-controlled trial. *J Child Adolesc Psychopharmacol* 24(6):325–335, 2014.
41. Bagnall A, Lewis RA, Leitner ML, Kleijnen J: Ziprasidone for schizophrenia and severe mental illness. *Cochrane Database Syst Rev* (2):CD001945, 2000.

42. Tandon R: Introduction. Ziprasidone appears to offer important therapeutic and tolerability advantages over conventional, and some novel, antipsychotics. *Br J Clin Pharmacol* 49(Suppl 1):1S–3S, 2000.
43. Sallee FR, Kurlan R, Goetz CG, et al.: Ziprasidone treatment of children and adolescents with tourette's syndrome: a pilot study. *J Am Acad Child Adolesc Psychiatry* 39(3):292–299, 2000.
44. Findling RL, Cavus I, Pappadopulos E, et al.: Ziprasidone in adolescents with schizophrenia: results from a placebo-controlled efficacy and long-term open-extension study. *J Child Adolesc Psychopharmacol* 23(8):531–544, 2013.
45. Findling RL, Cavus I, Pappadopulos E, et al.: Efficacy, long-term safety, and tolerability of ziprasidone in children and adolescents with bipolar disorder. *J Child Adolesc Psychopharmacol* 23(8):545–557, 2013.
46. Detke HC, DelBello MP, Landry J, Usher RW: Olanzapine/Fluoxetine combination in children and adolescents with bipolar I depression: a randomized, double-blind, placebo-controlled trial. *J Am Acad Child Adolesc Psychiatry* 54(3):217–224, 2015.
47. McClellan J, Sikich L, Findling RL, et al.: Treatment of early-onset schizophrenia spectrum disorders (TEOSS): rationale, design, and methods. *J Am Acad Child Adolesc Psychiatry* 46(8):969–978, 2007.
48. Findling RL, Landbloom RL, Szegedi A, et al.: Asenapine for the acute treatment of pediatric manic or mixed episode of bipolar disorder. *J Am Acad Child Adolesc Psychiatry* 54(12):1032–1041, 2015.
49. Frazier JA, Gordon CT, McKenna K, Lenane MC, Jih D, Rapoport JL: An open trial of clozapine in 11 adolescents with childhood-onset schizophrenia. *J Am Acad Child Adolesc Psychiatry* 33(5):658–663, 1994.
50. Siefen G, Remschmidt H: [Results of treatment with clozapine in schizophrenic adolescents]. *Z Kinder Jugendpsychiatr* 14(3):245–257, 1986.
51. Kumra S, Frazier JA, Jacobsen LK: Childhood-onset schizophrenia: a double-blind clozapine-haloperidol comparison. *Arch Gen Psychiatry* 53(12):1090–1097, 1996.
52. Sporn AL, Vermani A, Greenstein DK, et al.: Clozapine treatment of childhood-onset schizophrenia: evaluation of effectiveness, adverse effects, and long-term outcome. *J Am Acad Child Adolesc Psychiatry* 46(10):1349–1356, 2007.
53. Sikich L, Frazier JA, McClellan J, et al.: Double-blind comparison of first- and second-generation antipsychotics in early-onset schizophrenia and schizo-affective disorder: findings from the treatment of early-onset schizophrenia spectrum disorders (TEOSS) study. *Am J Psychiatry* 165(11):1420–1431, 2008.
54. Anderson LT, Campbell M, Adams P, Small AM, Perry R, Shell J: The effects of haloperidol on discrimination learning and behavioral symptoms in autistic children. *J Autism Dev Disord* 19(2):227–239, 1989.
55. Shapiro E, Shapiro AK, Fulop G: Controlled study of haloperidol, pimozide, and placebo for the treatment of gilles de la tourette's syndrome. *Arch Gen Psychiatry* 46(8):722–730, 1989.
56. McDougle CJ, Epperson CN, Pelton GH, Wasylink S, Price LH: A double-blind, placebo-controlled study of risperidone addition in serotonin reuptake inhibitor—refractory obsessive-compulsive disorder. *Arch Gen Psychiatry* 57(8):794–801, 2000.
57. Spencer EK, Kafantaris V, Padron-Gayol MV, Rosenberg CR, Campbell M: Haloperidol in schizophrenic children: early findings from a study in progress. *Psychopharmacol Bull* 28(2):183–186, 1992.
58. Joshi PT, Capozzoli JA, Coyle JT: Low-dose neuroleptic therapy for children with childhood-onset pervasive developmental disorder. *Am J Psychiatry* 145(3):335–338, 1988.
59. Goetz CG, Tanner CM, Klawans HL: Fluphenazine and multifocal tic disorders. *Arch Neurol* 41(3):271–272, 1984.
60. Realmuto GM, Erickson WD, Yellin AM, Hopwood JH, Greenberg LM: Clinical comparison of thiothixene and thioridazine in schizophrenic adolescents. *American Journal of Psychiatry* 141(3):440–442, 1984.
61. Shapiro AK, Shapiro E: Controlled study of pimozide vs. placebo in tourette's syndrome. *J Am Acad Child Psychiatry* 23(2):161–173, 1984.
62. Sallee FR, Sethuraman G, Rock CM: Effects of pimozide on cognition in children with Tourette syndrome: interaction with comorbid attention deficit hyperactivity disorder. *Acta Psychiatrica Scandinavica* 90(1):4–9, 1994.
63. Blair J, Taggart B, Martin A: Electrocardiographic safety profile and monitoring guidelines in pediatric psychopharmacology. *J Neural Transm (Vienna)* 111(7):791–815, 2004.
64. Gutgesell H, Atkins D, Barst R, et al.: AHA scientific statement: cardiovascular monitoring of children and adolescents receiving psychotropic drugs. *J Am Acad Child Adolesc Psychiatry* 38(8):1047–1050, 1999.
65. Pappadopulos E, Macintyre JC, Crismon ML, et al.: Treatment recommendations for the use of antipsychotics for aggressive youth (TRAAY). *Part ii. J Am Acad Child Adolesc Psychiatry* 42(2):145–161, 2003.
66. Scahill L, Erenberg G, Berlin CM, et al.: Contemporary assessment and pharmacotherapy of Tourette syndrome. *NeuroRX* 3(2):192–206, 2006.
67. Desta Z, Soukhova N, Flockhart DA: In Vitro inhibition of pimozide N-dealkylation by selective serotonin reuptake inhibitors and azithromycin. *J Clin Psychopharmacol* 22(2):162–168, 2002.
68. Obach RS, Walsky RL: Drugs that inhibit oxidation reactions catalyzed by aldehyde oxidase do not inhibit the reductive metabolism of ziprasidone to its major metabolite, s-methyldihydroziprasidone. *J Clin Psychopharmacol* 25(6):605–608, 2005.
69. Delbello MP, Schwiers ML, Rosenberg HL, Strakowski SM: A double-blind, randomized, placebo-controlled study of quetiapine as adjunctive treatment for adolescent mania. *J Am Acad Child Adolesc Psychiatry* 41(10): 1216–1223, 2002.
70. Malone RP, Cater J, Sheikh RM, Choudhury MS, Delaney MA: Olanzapine versus haloperidol in children with autistic disorder: an open pilot study. *J Am Acad Child Adolesc Psychiatry* 40(8):887–894, 2001.
71. Ratzoni G, Gothelf D, Brand-Gothelf A, et al. Weight gain associated with olanzapine and risperidone in adolescent patients: a comparative prospective study. *J Am Acad Child Adolesc Psychiatry* 41(3):337–343, 2002.
72. Sikich L, Hamer RM, Bashford RA, Sheitman BB, Lieberman JA: A pilot study of risperidone, olanzapine, and haloperidol in psychotic youth: a double-blind, randomized, 8-week trial. *Neuropsychopharmacol* 29(1): 133–145, 2003.
73. Kemner C, Willemsen-Swinkels SH, de Jonge M, Tuynman-Qua H, van Engeland H. Open-label study of olanzapine in children with pervasive developmental disorder. *J Clin Psychopharmacol* 22(5):455–460, 2002.
74. American Diabetes Association; American Psychiatric Association; American Association of Clinical Endocrinologists; North American Association for the Study of Obesity: Consensus development conference on antipsychotic drugs and obesity and diabetes. *Obes Res* 12(2):362–368, 2004.
75. Riddle MA: Tardive dyskinesia following haloperidol treatment in tourette's syndrome. *Arch Gen Psychiatry* 44(1):98, 1987.
76. Campbell M, Armenteros JL, Malone RP, Adams PB, Eisenberg ZW, Overall JE: Neuroleptic-related dyskinesias in autistic children: a prospective, longitudinal study. *J Am Acad Child Adolesc Psychiatry* 36(6): 835–843, 1997.
77. Wagner KD, Weller EB, Carlson GA, et al.: An open-label trial of divalproex in children and adolescents with bipolar disorder. *J Am Acad Child Adolesc Psychiatry* 41(10):1224–1230, 2002.
78. McClellan J, Werry J: Practice parameters for the assessment and treatment of children and adolescents with schizophrenia. *J Am Acad Child Adolesc Psychiatry* 33(5):616–635, 1994.
79. Silva RR, Munoz DM, Alpert M, Perlmutter IR, Diaz J: Neuroleptic malignant syndrome in children and adolescents. *J Am Acad Child Adolesc Psychiatry* 38(2):187–194, 1999.

CHAPTER 6.1.4.4 ■ MOOD STABILIZERS

MICHAEL H. BLOCH, CHAD BEYER, LAWRENCE SCAHILL, AND ANDRÉS MARTIN

MOOD STABILIZERS

The prototype for the chemically unrelated group of mood stabilizers is lithium, which has been used in the treatment of bipolar illness for over 50 years. It is the only mood stabilizer with two FDA-approved indications for acute mania and maintenance therapy of bipolar disorder in youth (older than 12 years). Other mood stabilizers include valproate (VPA), carbamazepine (CBZ), lamotrigine, oxcarbazepine (OXC), and topiramate. Of these, only VPA, CBZ, and lamotrigine have been carefully studied in adults. The anticonvulsants, CBZ, and VPA have been FDA approved for the treatment of acute mania in adults with bipolar disorder but currently have no FDA indication in children. Lamotrigine only has FDA approval for maintenance treatment of bipolar disorder in adults. In addition to bipolar-spectrum conditions, the mood stabilizers are commonly used in pediatric psychopharmacology for the management of aggressive outbursts and intense emotional lability. Although the empirical database for these indications (including bipolar disorders) is modest, Table 6.1.4.4.1 depicts the varying characteristics, indications, and dosing recommendations for mood stabilizers with evidence of efficacy in pediatric populations.

As discussed in an earlier section of this chapter, several atypical antipsychotics have demonstrated efficacy and approval for treatment of mania and mixed episodes as well as maintenance treatment in pediatric bipolar disorder. A multicenter, randomized clinical trial comparing the efficacy of risperidone to valproic acid and lithium for the treatment of children and adolescents with acute mania has dramatically shifted the evidence base away from mood stabilizers in recent years. The Treatment of Early Age Mania (TEAM) trial demonstrated that risperidone was superior to lithium and divalproex sodium for the initial treatment of childhood mania in terms of both likelihood of response and overall symptoms of mania. The response rate for acute mania was significantly higher with risperidone (65%) than with lithium (36%) or valproic acid (24%) (1). Similarly, a smaller trial in preschool children 3 to 7 years old with manic symptoms of bipolar disorder further demonstrated a benefit of risperidone compared to both placebo and valproic acid in younger children (2). After the results of these two informative trials, the use of mood stabilizers in bipolar disorder is generally reserved for simultaneous treatment with atypical antipsychotics for acute mania or mixed episodes or as the treatment for bipolar depression (or maintenance treatment).

Complicating the evidence surrounding the treatment of pediatric bipolar disorder is the relative controversies surrounding the diagnostic criteria for pediatric populations in recent years. The inconsistent diagnoses and treatment of those with bipolar disorder that are handed down to children often change the patient's view of themselves irrevocably. The prevalence of childhood bipolar disorder has shown a steep increase (40 × increase over the past 10 years) (3). Recent research suggests that episodic versus persistent irritability justifies two distinct disorders, with the latter more suited to a diagnosis of DMDD than bipolar disorder in the DSM-5 (4). The sorting out of treatment algorithms for pediatric patients with more classical symptoms of bipolar disorder as compared to symptoms that are more likely to now be diagnosed as DMDD remains a challenge.

Lithium (Lithobid, Eskalith)

Clinical Applications and Empirical Support

The efficacy of lithium in the acute and maintenance treatment of and prophylaxis of children and adolescents with classic bipolar disorder has been demonstrated in case reports, open trials, and retrospective naturalistic studies (5–9). Geller et al. (10) conducted the first placebo-controlled study of lithium in children including 25 adolescents with various forms of bipolar illness and comorbid substance abuse. Although lithium was associated with improvements in overall functioning and a lower rate of substance abuse relapse, there was no difference between active and placebo groups on measures of manic or depressive symptoms. In children and teens with a BP-1 or BP-2 diagnosis and first treated with a combination of lithium and VPA, maintenance treatment with lithium was equal to VPA (11). As discussed earlier, the TEAM study demonstrated that risperidone was more effective than lithium for the treatment of mania in pediatric bipolar disorder (1). In this way currently atypical antipsychotics are first line treatment of acute mania in pediatric bipolar disorder but lithium is often used in combination with them (12,13). Taken together with the studies cited above, these data provide class B support for the use of lithium for the short-term or maintenance treatment of bipolar illness in children and adolescents. The presence of ADHD in children and teens with Bipolar Disorder (BD) may be a factor that leads to a diminished response either to lithium or VPA (14–16), although this was not shown in another study (17). After relapse on either lithium or VPA of youth with either BP-1 or BP-2, a prospective open study showed that 90% of youth responded to combination treatment (18). The treatment of acute depression in BP-1 in hospitalized teens with lithium is supported by a single open study with a response rate of 50% and a remission rate of about 30% (six youths with psychosis responded to lithium without AAPs) (19).

Other Clinical Applications

Aggression, a study comparing haloperidol, lithium, and placebo in 61 treatment-resistant aggressive children (5 to 13 years) found that after 4 weeks of inpatient treatment, both haloperidol and lithium were superior to placebo in reducing aggressive behavior, and was associated with fewer side effects (20). Lithium was found to be superior (16 out of 20 responders) when compared to placebo (6 out of 20) in the treatment of aggressive behaviors in hospitalized children with conduct disorder (21). In contrast, a study of only 2 week duration failed to demonstrate efficacy in teens with conduct disorder (22).

TABLE 6.1.4.4.1

CLINICAL GUIDANCE ON MOOD STABILIZERS USED IN PEDIATRIC PRACTICE

Drug	Mechanism of Action	Main Indications and Clinical Uses	Dosage	Schedule	Adverse Effects	Comments
Lithium	Inhibition of phosphatidylinositol and protein kinase C signaling pathways; Enhancement of serotonergic transmission	Bipolar disorder, manic; prophylaxis of bipolar disorder; MDD aggressive behavior/conduct disorder; adjunct treatment in refractory MDD	10–30 mg/kg/day, dose adjusted to serum levels in the range of 0.6–1.1 mEq/l	bid/tid	Polyuria, polydipsia, tremor, ataxia, nausea, diarrhea, weight gain, drowsiness, acne, hair loss; possible effects on thyroid and renal functioning with long-term administration; children prone to dehydration are at higher risk for acute lithium toxicity; lithium levels >2 mEq/L can be life threatening	Therapy requires monitoring of lithium levels, thyroid and renal function
Divalproex	Inhibition of catabolic enzymes of GABA and of protein kinase C signaling	Bipolar disorder; aggressive behavior; conduct disorder; seizure disorders	15–60 mg/kg/day, dose adjusted to serum levels in the range of 50–125 mcg/L	bid/tid	Sedation, nausea, liver toxicity (requires baseline and close monitoring), thrombocytopenia, pancreatitis	Polycystic ovarian disorder has been reported during long-term use for seizure control
Carbamazepine	Inhibition of glial steroidogenesis; inhibition of alpha 2 receptors; blocks sodium	Bipolar disorder; complex partial seizures	10–20 mg/kg/day, dose adjusted to serum levels in the range of 4–14 mcg/L	bid	Bone marrow suppression (requires baseline and close monitoring of blood counts); dizziness, drowsiness, rashes, nausea, liver toxicity, especially under 10 yrs of age	Potent inductor of CYP3A4, leading to auto-induction requiring periodic dose adjustment
Oxcarbamazepine	Channels block glial calcium influx	Seizure disorders	Maintenance dose of 18.5–48 mg/kg/day, not to exceed 2,100 mg/day		No reports of bone marrow suppression more benign drug interaction profile compared to carbamazepine; no blood level monitoring necessary	No empirical data available for children and adolescents
Lamotrigine	Weak 5HT3 inhibition; release of aspartate and glutamate	Bipolar depression and maintenance therapy; seizure disorders	75–300 mg/day	qd	Potentially life-threatening rash; Stevens–Johnson syndrome (dose-[direct] and age-[inverse] related event rates)	Slow dose titration (12.5 mg qo wk) may reduce risk of skin reactions

The Cochrane, Oxford team of Cipriani, Hawton, Stockton, and Geddes (23), conducted a meta-analysis to assess whether lithium has a specific preventive effect for suicide and self-harm in adults with unipolar and bipolar mood disorders. They reported that lithium is an effective treatment for reducing the risk of suicide in people with mood disorders, and this antisuicidal effect may relate to reduction in relapse of mood episodes. A additional mechanisms should also be considered, because there is some evidence that lithium decreases aggression and possibly impulsivity, which may be another pathway mediating its antisuicidal effect.

Mechanism of Action

Lithium affects several neurochemical systems, including serotonin, norepinephrine, and dopamine. However, its main actions appear to be mediated by effects on intracellular signaling processes, specifically of the phosphatidylinositol and protein kinase C pathways (24).

Pharmacokinetics and Drug Interactions

Lithium is readily absorbed from the gastrointestinal tract, and peak levels occur 1 to 4 hours after oral ingestion, depending on the formulation. Lithium carbonate is available in tablet and capsule, in two extended-release formulations (Eskalith CR, Lithobid), and a liquid form (lithium citrate). The liquid has the shortest T_{max}, and the sustained-release formulations have slower absorption and lower plasma peaks. Lithium is not metabolized in the liver, nor does it bind to plasma proteins, and approximately 95% of the ingested drug is excreted in the kidneys. The half-life in adults is approximately 24 hours, slightly longer than the 18 hours reported in children (25). This shorter half-life has the practical implication that reliable blood levels can be obtained in children after just 4 days (or approximately 5 × 18 hours), rather than the traditional 5 days required in adults. The shorter half-life in children is due to faster glomerular filtration rates in the young. Because of their higher total body water, prepubertal children require higher weight-adjusted dosage than adults to achieve similar serum levels. Magnetic resonance spectroscopy has revealed that children have lower brain-to-serum concentrations of lithium as compared to adults, and they may require higher serum levels to achieve comparable brain levels (26).

Drug interactions occur at the level of the kidney. When given concomitantly, nonsteroidal anti-inflammatory drugs, tetracyclines, and thiazide diuretics can decrease urinary clearance of lithium and increase lithium levels and should therefore be used cautiously. By contrast, theophylline and caffeine promote lithium excretion, resulting in lower serum levels.

Clinical Management

Prior to initiating a trial of lithium, a child should have a physical examination, including screening laboratory tests such as a complete blood count, electrolytes, blood urea nitrogen, creatinine, and thyroid indices. In outpatient settings, dosing may be initiated at 300 mg twice a day for children and 600 mg twice a day for adolescents.

Weller (27) has developed a useful guide to approximate daily lithium dosing. For children under 12 years of age, dosages in the range of 10 to 30 mg/kg/day are typical. Thus, a 30-kg child would receive 900 mg/day in divided doses. Older adolescents are likely to be treated in the range of 1,200 to 1,800 mg/day during acute mania. Maintenance doses are typically lower.

Due to its narrow therapeutic index, lithium levels should be monitored closely. The optimal serum level range is in the range of 0.6 to 1.1 mEq/L. Serum levels should be drawn on average 4 days after a dose adjustment to ensure that a steady state has been achieved and 12 hours after the previous dose to ensure a trough reading (28). When used to treat bipolar illness, the clinical benefit of lithium may be evident within 10 to 14 days of reaching therapeutic serum level in some cases, although as many as 4 to 6 weeks of treatment may be required (29). Current recommendations include repeat laboratory tests at 6-month intervals. An increased white count in the range of 12,000 to 15,000 cells/mm (30) is common and without clinical significance. Thyroid-stimulating hormone (TSH) levels may increase in association with higher lithium levels and a higher baseline TSH (31), but thyroid hormone replacement is not generally recommended unless T4 levels start to decrease, or if clinical symptoms of hypothyroidism appear. Lithium levels should also be obtained when the patient's clinical status changes, if adverse effects occur, and routinely at 3- to 6-month intervals.

Adverse Effects and Toxicity

Lithium appears to be generally well tolerated in children and adolescents. Common side effects include fatigue, nausea, diarrhea, abdominal distress, tremor, ataxia, aggravation of acne, cognitive dulling, and weight gain. Because lithium is excreted by the kidneys, it is generally not recommended in children with compromised renal function. The risk of glomerular damage with long-term lithium treatment appears to be minimal, but polyuria and polydipsia are relatively common due to lithium's effect on tubular reabsorption. Lithium-induced polyuria can generally be managed conservatively, either by reducing the total daily dose (when possible), by switching from a short- to a long-acting preparation, or by the addition of a low dose of a potassium-sparing diuretic such as amiloride. In a few cases, nephrogenic diabetes insipidus can occur, which may warrant discontinuation of lithium.

Signs of lithium toxicity can occur even at "normal serum levels." In mild forms, symptoms include nausea, diarrhea, impaired concentration, and muscle weakness. At serum levels above 2.5 mEq/L, multiple organs may be affected and toxicity may prove fatal. Because dehydration can increase lithium levels and may induce toxicity, parents and children should be educated about the importance of adequate fluid intake. Lithium has been associated with a small increased occurrence of tricuspid valve abnormalities and transient neurodevelopmental deficits in exposed newborns (32). Contraception should be encouraged in adolescents and treatment of a pregnant mother with lithium should weigh possible fetal effects against the adverse outcomes of an untreated mood disorder (33).

Valproate (Depakote, Depakene)

Clinical Applications and Empirical Support

Valproate is an anticonvulsant that has been shown to be an effective mood stabilizer in adults. Clinicians have utilized VPA in the treatment of a range of problems in children and adolescents, including bipolar illness and aggression associated with conduct disorder or oppositional defiant disorder. There are case reports and open studies that support the use of VPA in youth with conduct disorder, explosive behaviors, or impulsive aggression (34–37), and there are two small randomized clinical trials that support VPA efficacy in this population (38). There is less evidence supporting the use of VPA in acute or maintenance therapy of bipolar disorder in youth; two open studies showed a response rate of 50% to 60% (29,39) and a study in teens with mixed mania showed more than a 70% response (40). Studies involving VPA with atypical antipsychotics have yielded response rates of 80% or higher for the combination therapy (41,42). However, multiple clinical trials in pediatric and even preschool-age populations have suggested that risperidone is more effective than valproic acid as a treatment for acute pediatric mania (1,2). Treatment of ADHD after manic symptoms treated with VPA in children and teens showed that a mixed salt amphetamine did not worsen manic symptoms (43). In conclusion, these emerging data provide a modest level of support for the use of VPA in the treatment of children and adolescents with bipolar disorder (class C support).

Mechanism of Action

VPA has multiple pharmacologic effects decreased dopamine turnover (decreased *N*-methyl-D-asparate currents, decreased release of asparate) (44), and the details of its therapeutic actions are not fully known. VPA enhances GABA-ergic inhibition through increased synthesis and release. Given the inhibitory role of GABA in the brain, this effect may account for the drug's anticonvulsant and antimanic effects. VPA also directly affect neurons by inhibiting sodium influx and increasing potassium influx (45). Additional research has found that it upregulates the FGF21 gene expression and promotes process elongation in glia by inhibiting HDAC2 and 3. This may further explain its mood-stabilizing and anticonvulsant effects (46).

Pharmacokinetics and Drug Interactions

There are three formulations of VPA: valproic acid (Depakene, capsule, and syrup), delayed-release divalproex (a combination of valproic acid and sodium valproate, Depakote, capsule, and sprinkle), and extended-release divalproex (Depakote ER). All formulations release the valproate ion in the gastrointestinal tract, and this moiety is responsible for the pharmacologic action. Absorption is more rapid in the liquid form, and it can be delayed in the enteric forms. The sprinkle form has a lower C_{max} and may have fewer gastrointestinal side effects. Slightly higher dosing (8% to 20%) is needed when shifting from VPA to the extended-release formulation (47). VPA has very complex metabolism. It is, therefore, not surprising that VPA has been noted to interact with medications of all classes. As monotherapy, VPA is metabolized mostly by beta-oxidation or conjugated via glucuronidation. Only 10% to 20% is metabolized via P450 cytochromes (CYP 2C9 and CYP2 A6). Children under the age of 10 years excrete less VPA-glucuronide and metabolize more VPA through the P450 cytochromes (48). When a potent CYP inducer (CBZ, phenobarbital, phenytoin) is added, more VPA shuttles through CYPs and more toxic metabolites are produced. Children under the age of 2 years who are on multiple inducing anticonvulsants, or who have congenital metabolic disease or organic brain syndromes, are more susceptible to developing hepatic failure. VPA is a moderate inhibitor of epoxide hydrolase, CYP 2C9, and some UDP-glucuronylsyltransferases (UGTs). It inhibits the glucuronidation of lamotrigine at UGT 2B7, increasing its blood levels and the risk of developing Stevens–Johnson syndrome (49, 50). In addition, VPA exhibits saturable protein binding (it has nonlinear pharmacokinetics), and it competes with many drugs for protein-binding sites (aspirin can displace it, VPA displaces CBZ).

Clinical Management

Prior to initiating therapy, a physical examination should be completed and laboratory screening studies including a complete blood count, liver function tests, and a pregnancy test for female teens should be obtained. Dosing in outpatient adolescents could start with 250 mg twice daily, and increased every 3 to 5 days in 250- to 500-mg increments to a target dose of 20 mg/kg/day in two to three divided doses. Younger children might start with half the starting dose used in adolescents and move up in 125- to 250-mg increments. Trough levels should be checked after steady state is achieved (3 to 5 days), and target serum levels are in the range of 45 to 125 μg/L. Clinical management involves monitoring weight, appetite, energy level, evidence of bruising or clinical symptoms of pancreatitis, and of androgenism in girls. Liver enzymes and a CBC should be obtained within the first month of treatment and periodically during chronic treatment (51). Reductions in platelets and white blood count can occur and should be carefully evaluated.

Adverse Effects and Toxicity

Gastrointestinal complaints, sedation, and (rarely) transient hair loss may accompany the initiation of treatment and may subside with continued dosing. Other adverse effects include increased appetite and weight gain, postural tremor, dizziness, asthenia, and cognitive dullness. Rare idiosyncratic effects can occur. VPA has also been associated with hepatic failure, and in children under the age of 2, with fatal hepatitis (see Pharmacokinetics and Drug Interactions). Early in the treatment, there is also a small risk of pancreatitis. Agranulocytosis is extremely rare. In women treated for seizure disorders, there have also been reports of polycystic ovary disease manifested clinically by hyperandrogenism, accelerated weight gain, and menstrual and lipid profile irregularities (52). The role of VPA in these adverse endocrine effects is unclear and a matter of some debate, especially among teenage girls. Studies in adult women with bipolar disorder have shown high rates of pre-existing menstrual abnormalities and increased testosterone levels with chronic VPA treatment (53). Clearly, monitoring weight and menstrual cycles are an essential component of clinical care in adolescent and adult females treated with VPA. VPA toxicity can be life threatening and may begin with increased tremor and confusion. It is associated with hyperammonemia, respiratory depression, and multiorgan failure (54).

VPA is associated with a variety of major and minor malformations in babies born to mothers taking VPA during pregnancy, including a 20-fold increase in neural tube defects, cleft lip and palate, cardiovascular abnormalities, genitourinary defects, and others (55). These effects appear to be dose-dependent (especially evident at doses above 800 to 1,000 mg/day) (56). Prior to initiating treatment with VPA in sexually active female adolescents, a negative pregnancy test and a reliable method of contraception should be documented.

Carbamazepine

Clinical Application and Empirical Support

CBZ is an anticonvulsant that has been used in adults for a variety of neurologic and psychiatric disorders, including seizures, trigeminal neuralgia, and bipolar disorder. It has demonstrated efficacy since the 1980s for the treatment of acute mania and prophylaxis of mania and depression in adults, but it was not until 2004 that it received FDA approval for the treatment of acute mania and mixed bipolar states in adults. Case series and open-label studies in children have included bipolar disorder (29,57,58), aggression (59), and treatment-resistant ADHD (60). To date, however, the one controlled CBZ trial in children failed to show its superiority over placebo for the treatment of aggression among 5- to 12-year-old inpatients diagnosed with conduct disorder (61).

Joshi et al. (62) conducted an 8-week, open-label trial of extended-release CBZ, as monotherapy in children with bipolar disorder. Of the 27 participating children with BD, 16 (59%) completed the study. CBZ-ER treatment was associated with statistically significant, but modest levels of improvement in mean YMRS scores (−10.1 ± 10.2, $p < 0.001$) with end-point mean YMRS score (21.8 ± 12.2) suggesting a lack of complete resolution of mania. They reported that open-label CBZ-ER treatment was beneficial for the treatment of BD in children. Weisler et al. (63) used pooled results from two randomized, double-blind, placebo-controlled trials into the use of extended-release CBZ capsules as monotherapy in bipolar disorder, to further reaffirm that CBZ-ERC is effective in the treatment of bipolar I disorder patients with either acute manic or mixed episodes.

Mechanism of Action

The mood-stabilizing effects of CBZ are not well understood: It decreases sodium influx and the release of glutamate; it inhibits adenosine A1 and dopaminergic activity; but it may also affect several types of calcium channels (64).

Pharmacokinetics and Drug Interactions

CBZ is available as an immediate-release formulation in tablets, chewables, and suspension, as well as in sustained-release formulations: an osmotic pump tablet (Tegretol-XR) and beaded extended-release capsules (Carbatrol, Equetro). CBZ is involved in an innumerable number of drug interactions, both as a victim substrate vulnerable to CYP inhibition and as an active inducer of CYPs and UGTs. As a substrate of CYP 3A4 and CYP 2C8, potent 3A4 inhibitors can affect CBZ (erythromycin). As an inducer of CYP 1A2, CYP 3A4, and glucuronidation, CBZ can induce its own metabolism and perhaps decrease the efficacy of the drug. The active metabolite, CBZ 10,11 epoxide, can also be increased or decreased via drug interactions and can contribute to efficacy and toxicity. CBZ's free fraction can be displaced from plasma proteins by aspirin and NSAIDs, leading to toxicity. VPA can inhibit the epoxidation and glucuronidation of CBZ 10,11 epoxide.

Clinical Management

CBZ is slowly absorbed, and peak plasma concentration is achieved within 2 to 8 hours following oral administration. As an anticonvulsant, the initial dose of the immediate and extended-release formulation for children ages 6 to 12 years is 100 mg daily, and it can be increased at weekly intervals by 100 to 200 mg. The usual maintenance dose is 10 to 20 mg/kg/day, administered in divided doses (bid for extended, or tid for immediate formulations). Given the drug's short half-life following the induction of its own metabolism, frequent dose adjustments, especially in the first few weeks of treatment, are common. Pretreatment physical examination and laboratory studies should be completed, including complete blood count, liver function tests, and creatinine. Although there is scant evidence for an increase in major congenital anomalies in babies exposed to CBZ monotherapy in the first trimester of pregnancy (65), until further evidence is available, a pretreatment pregnancy test should be obtained in sexually active girls. They should receive counseling about appropriate contraception (as CYP 3A4 substrates, ethinyl estradiol, and progestins can be reduced through CBZ's induction of CYP 3A4). The clinical utility of therapeutic plasma levels for children with mood disorders is unclear. Trough plasma concentrations for anticonvulsant effect can be drawn after 4 to 5 days, and they may be maintained in the range of 4 to 14 μg/mL. These guidelines may be useful during dose adjustment and in order to prevent toxicity. CBCs and LFTs should be followed periodically. Sedation, gastrointestinal effects, and rash may occur. Leukopenia is common and rarely progresses to agranulocytosis. Very rarely, other bone marrow toxicities, liver toxicity, and inappropriate antidiuretic secretion syndrome may develop. Given the lack of controlled studies, the multiple drug–drug interactions, and its potentially serious adverse effects, CBZ should be considered as a third-line mood stabilizer in the treatment of children and adolescents and may be particularly useful as an alternative if there is morbid weight gain associated with lithium, VPA, or atypical antipsychotics.

Oxcarbazepine (Trileptal)

OXC is a CBZ prodrug metabolized through noncytochromal pathways to an active metabolite, monohydroxy derivative (MHD). In turn, MHD is minimally metabolized through CYP 3A4, and it is mostly glucuronidated and subsequently excreted in the urine. As a result, OXC does not show the auto-induction observed with CBZ, nor is it vulnerable to potent 3A4 inhibitors, but like CBZ, it does possess a moderate ability to induce CYP 3A4 and some UGTs and to potently inhibit CYP 2C19. OXC may act through inhibition of voltage-sensitive sodium channels and modulation of potassium conductance and high voltage-activated calcium channels. OXC does not require the frequent blood monitoring associated with other mood stabilizers. However, a large multicenter, randomized, placebo-controlled trial of 116 subjects with pediatric mania failed to show any sign of improvement of OXC over placebo (66). In epilepsy trials, common adverse events include somnolence, headache, nausea and vomiting, dizziness, and rash (67). Like CBZ, there have been reports of inappropriate secretion of antidiuretic hormone (ADH) and Stevens–Johnson syndrome. Since OXC can induce CYP 3A4 and there is little information about fetal abnormalities, pretreatment pregnancy testing and appropriate contraceptive counseling are needed. According to the prescribing information, the recommended initial dose for youth 4 to 16 years of age with seizures is 8 to 10 mg/kg/day bid not to exceed 600 mg daily, and as monotherapy, a maintenance dose of 18.5 to 48 mg/kg/day not to exceed 2,100 mg/day (see product insert for dosing range by weight) but its use for pediatric mental health conditions should be minimal.

Lamotrigine (Lamictal)

In adults, lamotrigine has been shown to be effective in the treatment of BP-1 depression, to stabilize mood in rapid cycling BP-2 patients, and to provide prophylaxis for depression in BP-1 patients (68). In youth, a recently completed large, multi-center, placebo-controlled trial of lamotrigine for maintenance treatment for pediatric bipolar disorder failed to show statistically significant benefit of lamotrigine compared to placebo on the primary end point but did show some evidence of benefit on secondary outcomes. After initial open-label stabilization with lamotrigine subjects were randomly assigned to placebo or continued lamotrigine treatment, during the randomized phase the mean time to occurrence of a bipolar event (mania, depression, or mixed episode) for lamotrigine (as compared to placebo) was 155 versus 50 days for a depressive episode, 163 versus 120 days for mania/hypomania, and 136 versus 107 days for mixed episodes. The primary end point stratified log-rank analysis of time to bipolar event was not statistically significant; lamotrigine seemed particularly beneficial for adolescents with bipolar disorder rather than children in this trial. Lamotrigine has diverse actions on many neurotransmitters: It inhibits serotonin, norepinephrine, glutamate, and dopamine receptors, blocks calcium ion influx in N- and P-type channels, and stabilizes presynaptic neural membranes through sodium channels (69). Lamotrigine's pharmacokinetics are linear, and most of it is conjugated by the UGTs (UGT 1A4 and UGT 2B7). VPA inhibits its glucuronidation and decreases its clearance by about 50%. Conversely, UGT inducers (CBZ, ethinyl estradiol) can lower lamotrigine levels by 50% (69). Lamotrigine is well documented to cause skin rashes that are usually mild and seen within the first months of treatment, but full-blown Stevens–Johnson syndrome (a potentially fatal condition associated with widespread skin sloughing) can

TABLE 6.1.4.4.2

CLINICAL GUIDANCE ON ANTIENURETIC AGENTS USED IN PEDIATRIC PRACTICE

Drug	Mechanism of Action	Main Indications and Clinical Uses	Dosage (mg/d)	Schedule	Adverse Effects
Desmopressin[a]	Antidiuretic hormone analogue	Enuresis	10–40 meg	qhs/bid	Headache Nausea Hyponatremia and water intoxication at toxic doses
Oxybutynin	Antimuscarinic agents		5.0–15	bid/tid	Anticholinergic side effects
Tolterodine			1–2	bid	Less anticholinergic effects, less sedation

[a]Can be useful for acute situations (e.g., sleepaways).

develop. Rapid dose escalation and co-administration with VPA are risk factors, especially for children. A 10% rate for all rashes is commonly reported in adults (70). A recent review in adults suggests that slow dose titration and dermatologic precautions (limited antigen exposure) may reduce this rate (70). There are data suggesting a higher risk of major congenital abnormalities in babies exposed to lamotrigine in doses higher than 200 mg/day, and pending further studies, pretreatment pregnancy tests and contraceptive counseling should be made available to all pubertal girls (65). Toxicity is associated with lethargy, vomiting, ataxia, vertigo, and tachycardia, but only rarely is the outcome serious (71).

Topiramate (Topamax)

Topiramate is a glutamate-release antagonist, a GABA reuptake inhibitor, and it reduces activity at sodium and calcium channels (72). Most of topiramate is excreted unchanged through the kidney, and therefore, plasma levels will be lower in younger children because of their higher glomerular filtration rates. About 30% is handled by the CYPs and UGTs, and these pathways can be induced when the potent-inducing antiepileptics (CBZ) are added, leading to a doubling of topiramate's clearance. Topiramate modestly inhibits CYP 2C19, and when combined with higher doses of phenytoin, the concentration of the latter drug can be significantly increased. At topiramate doses at or above 200 mg/day, the concentrations of ethinyl estradiol and/or progestins in oral contraceptives can be decreased. Topiramate has been shown to be ineffective in acute mania in adults (73), and as a result, research efforts in youth with mania were largely discontinued (72). Decreased appetite and nausea appeared as the most common adverse events in a discontinued trial in pediatric mania, as did weight loss, especially in some overweight subjects (72). Based on this observation, there has been additional clinical trial data suggesting that topiramate may be effective in reducing antipsychotic associated weight gain (74). Topiramate may be associated with cognitive blunting and word retrieval difficulties. Its use in bipolar disorder in youth as monotherapy cannot be endorsed.

Gabapentin (Neurontin)

This agent undergoes virtually no hepatic metabolism, and it is excreted largely unaltered by the kidneys. Despite a benign side-effect profile among adults, aggressive behavior and worsening hyperactivity have been reported among 12 children receiving gabapentin for the treatment of seizure disorders (51). Studies in adults as monotherapy in bipolar disorder have not demonstrated efficacy. Consequently, its use as a mood stabilizer for children cannot be recommended.

ANTIENURETIC AGENTS

Desmopressin, Oxybutynin, and Tolterodine

Table 6.1.4.4.2 depicts the pharmacologic characteristics of medications used for enuresis. Desmopressin (DDAVP) is a synthetic ADH, a powerful inhibitor of the production of urine. It can be administered orally or via intranasal spray. One review suggested that desmopressin helps approximately 25% of children who use it, with minimal risk of adverse effects (75). Although desmopressin is usually well tolerated, the beneficial effects often do not endure over time. The most effective treatment for enuresis is the use of behavioral interventions, such as a "pad and buzzer" or a "moisture alarm." However, DDAVP can be a useful short-term adjunct, as in the facilitation of sleepovers or overnight camp stays. For longer-term pharmacologic management of enuresis, usually in cases unresponsive or only partially responsive to behavioral interventions, antimuscarinic agents can occasionally be useful. Alternatives to the time-tested use of low (25 to 50 mg HS) (76) or regular dose imipramine include oxybutynin (Ditropan) or the less sedating tolterodine (Detrol). As is the case of other pharmacologic interventions for enuresis, beneficial effects usually disappear rapidly upon drug discontinuation (Table 6.1.4.4.2).

References

1. Geller B, Luby JL, Joshi P, et al: A randomized controlled trial of risperidone, lithium, or divalproex sodium for initial treatment of bipolar I disorder, manic or mixed phase, in children and adolescents. *Arch Gen Psychiatry* 69(5):515–528, 2012.
2. Kowatch RA, Scheffer RE, Monroe E, Delgado S, Altaye M, Lagory D: Placebo-controlled trial of valproic acid versus risperidone in children 3–7 years of age with bipolar I disorder. *J Child Adolesc Psychopharmacol* 25(4):306–313, 2015.
3. Friedman N, Sadhu J, Jellinek M: DSM-5: implications for pediatric mental health care. *J Dev Behav Pediatr* 33(2):163–178, 2012.
4. Regier DA, Kuhl EA, Kupfer DJ. The DSM-5: classification and criteria changes. *World Psychiatry* 12(2):92–98, 2013.
5. McKnew DH, Cytryn L, Buchsbaum MS, et al: Lithium in children of lithium-responding parents. *Psychiatry Res* 4(2):171–180, 1981.
6. Younes RP, DeLong GR, Neiman G, Rosner B: Manic-depressive illness in children: treatment with lithium carbonate. *J Child Neurol* 1(4):364–368, 1986.
7. Delong GR, Aldershof AL: Long-term experience with lithium treatment in childhood: correlation with clinical diagnosis. *J Am Acad Child Adolesc Psychiatry* 26(3):389–394, 1987.
8. Strober M, Morrell W, Lampert C, Burroughs J: Relapse following discontinuation of lithium maintenance therapy in adolescents with bipolar I illness: a naturalistic study. *Am J Psychiatry* 147(4):457–461, 1990.

9. Carlson GA, Rapport MD, Pataki CS, Kelly KL: Lithium in hospitalized children at 4 and 8 weeks: mood, behavior and cognitive effects. *J Child Psychol Psychiatry* 33(2):411–425, 1992.
10. Geller B, Cooper TB, Sun K, et al.: Double-blind and placebo-controlled study of lithium for adolescent bipolar disorders with secondary substance dependency. *J Am Acad Child Adolesc Psychiatry* 37(2):171–178, 1998.
11. Findling RL, McNamara NK, Youngstrom EA, et al.: Double-blind 18-month trial of lithium versus divalproex maintenance treatment in pediatric bipolar disorder. *J Am Acad Child Adolesc Psychiatry* 44(5):409–417, 2005.
12. Kafantaris V, Dicker R, Coletti DJ, Kane JM: Adjunctive antipsychotic treatment is necessary for adolescents with psychotic mania. *J Child Adolesc Psychopharmacol* 11(4):409–413, 2001.
13. Kafantaris V, Coletti DJ, Dicker R, Padula G, Kane JM: Adjunctive antipsychotic treatment of adolescents with bipolar psychosis. *J Am Acad Child Adolesc Psychiatry* 40(12):1448–1456, 2001.
14. Strober M, DeAntonio M, Schmidt-Lackner S, Freeman R, Lampert C, Diamond J: Early childhood attention deficit hyperactivity disorder predicts poorer response to acute lithium therapy in adolescent mania. *J Affect Disord* 51(2):145–151, 1998.
15. State RC, Frye MA, Altshuler LL, et al.: Chart review of the impact of attention-deficit/hyperactivity disorder comorbidity on response to lithium or divalproex sodium in adolescent mania. *J Clin Psychiatry* 65(8):1057–1063, 2004.
16. Masi G, Perugi G, Toni C, et al.: Predictors of treatment nonresponse in bipolar children and adolescents with manic or mixed episodes. *J Child Adolesc Psychopharmacol* 14(3):395–404, 2004.
17. Kafantaris V, Coletti DJ, Dicker R, Padula G, Pollack S: Are childhood psychiatric histories of bipolar adolescents associated with family history, psychosis, and response to lithium treatment? *J Affect Disord* 51(2): 153–164, 1998.
18. Findling RL, McNamara NK, Stansbrey R, et al.: Combination lithium and divalproex sodium in pediatric bipolar symptom restabilization. *J Am Acad Child Adolesc Psychiatry* 45(2):142–148, 2006.
19. Delbello MP, Kowatch RA, Adler CM, et al.: A double-blind randomized pilot study comparing quetiapine and divalproex for adolescent mania. *J Am Acad Child Adolesc Psychiatry* 45(3):305–313, 2006.
20. Campbell M: Behavioral efficacy of haloperidol and lithium carbonate. *Arch Gen Psychiatry* 41(7):650–656, 1984.
21. Malone RP, Delaney MA, Luebbert JF, Cater J, Campbell M: A double-blind placebo-controlled study of lithium in hospitalized aggressive children and adolescents with conduct disorder. *Arch Gen Psychiatry* 57(7):649–654, 2000.
22. Rifkin A, Karajgi B, Dicker R, et al.: Lithium treatment of conduct disorders in adolescents. *Am J Psychiatry* 154(4):554–555, 1997.
23. Cipriani A, Hawton K, Stockton S, Geddes JR: Lithium in the prevention of suicide in mood disorders: updated systematic review and meta-analysis. *BMJ* 346:f3646, 2013.
24. Manji HK, Lenox RH: Lithium: a molecular transducer of mood-stabilization in the treatment of bipolar disorder. *Neuropsychopharmacology* 19(3):161–166, 1998.
25. Vitiello B, Behar D, Malone R, Delaney MA, Ryan PJ, Simpson GM: Pharmacokinetics of lithium carbonate in children. *J Clin Psychopharmacol* 8(5):355–359, 1988.
26. Moore CM, Demopulos CM, Henry ME, et al.: Brain-to-serum lithium ratio and age: an in vivo magnetic resonance spectroscopy study. *Am J Psychiatry* 159(7):1240–1242, 2002.
27. Weller EB, Weller RA, Fristad MA: Lithium dosage guide for prepubertal children: a preliminary report. *J Am Acad Child Psychiatry* 25(1):92–95, 1986.
28. Geller B, Luby J: Child and adolescent bipolar disorder: a review of the past 10 years. *J Am Acad Child Adolesc Psychiatry* 36(9):1168–1176, 1997.
29. Kowatch RA, Suppes T, Carmody TJ, et al: Effect size of lithium, divalproex sodium, and carbamazepine in children and adolescents with bipolar disorder. *J Am Acad Child Adolesc Psychiatry* 39(6):713–720, 2000.
30. A 14-month randomized clinical trial of treatment strategies for attention-deficit/hyperactivity disorder. The MTA Cooperative Group. Multimodal Treatment Study of Children with ADHD. *Arch Gen Psychiatry* 56(12):1073–1086, 1999.
31. Gracious BL, Findling RL, Seman C, Youngstrom EA, Demeter CA, Calabrese JR: Elevated thyrotropin in bipolar youths prescribed both lithium and divalproex sodium. *J Am Acad Child Adolesc Psychiatry* 43(2):215–220, 2004.
32. Kozma C: Neonatal toxicity and transient neurodevelopmental deficits following prenatal exposure to lithium: another clinical report and a review of the literature. *Am J Med Genet* 132A(4):441–444, 2005.
33. Eberhard-Gran M, Eskild A, Opjordsmoen S: Treating mood disorders during pregnancy. *Drug Saf* 28(8):695–706, 2005.
34. Kastner T, Finesmith R, Walsh K: Long-term administration of valproic acid in the treatment of affective symptoms in people with mental retardation. *J Clin Psychopharmacol* 13(6):448–451, 1993.
35. Papatheodorou G, Kutcher SP, Katic M, Szalai JP: The efficacy and safety of divalproex sodium in the treatment of acute mania in adolescents and young adults: an open clinical trial. *J Clin Psychopharmacol* 15(2):110–116, 1995.
36. Donovan SJ, Susser ES, Nunes EV, Stewart JW, Quitkin FM, Klein DF: Divalproex treatment of disruptive adolescents. *J Clin Psychiatry* 58(1):12–15, 1997.
37. Barzman DH, McConville BJ, Masterson B, et al: Impulsive aggression with irritability and responsive to divalproex: a pediatric bipolar spectrum disorder phenotype? *J Affect Disord* 88(3):279–285, 2005.
38. Donovan SJ: Divalproex treatment for youth with explosive temper and mood lability: a double-blind, placebo-controlled crossover design. *Am J Psychiatry* 157(5):818–820, 2000.
39. Wagner KD, Weller EB, Carlson GA, et al: An open-label trial of divalproex in children and adolescents with bipolar disorder. *J Am Acad Child Adolesc Psychiatry* 41(10):1224–1230, 2002.
40. Pavuluri MN, Henry DB, Carbray JA, Naylor MW, Janicak PG: Divalproex sodium for pediatric mixed mania: a 6-month prospective trial. *Bipolar Disord* 7(3):266–273, 2005.
41. DelBello MP, Kowatch RA, Warner J, et al.: Adjunctive topiramate treatment for pediatric bipolar disorder: a retrospective chart review. *J Child Adolesc Psychopharmacol* 12(4):323–330, 2002.
42. Kowatch RA, Sethuraman G, Hume JH, Kromelis M, Weinberg WA: Combination pharmacotherapy in children and adolescents with bipolar disorder. *Biol Psychiatry* 53(11):978–984, 2003.
43. Scheffer RE, Kowatch RA, Carmody T, Rush AJ. Randomized, placebo-controlled trial of mixed amphetamine salts for symptoms of comorbid ADHD in pediatric bipolar disorder after mood stabilization with divalproex sodium. *Am J Psychiatry* 162(1):58–64, 2005.
44. Rana M, Khanzode L, Karnik N, Saxena K, Chang K, Steiner H: Divalproex sodium in the treatment of pediatric psychiatric disorders. *Expert Rev Neurother* 5(2):165–176, 2005.
45. Czapinski P, Blaszczyk B, Czuczwar S. Mechanisms of action of antiepileptic drugs. *Curr Top Med Chem* 5(1):3–14, 2005.
46. Leng Y, Wang J, Wang Z, et al.: Valproic acid and other HDAC inhibitors upregulate FGF21 gene expression and promote process elongation in glia by inhibiting HDAC2 and 3. *Int J Neuropsychopharmacol* 19(8):pii: pyw035, 2016.
47. Dutta S, Zhang Y: Bioavailability of divalproex extended-release formulation relative to the divalproex delayed-release formulation. *Biopharm Drug Dispos* 25(8):345–352, 2004.
48. Reith DM, Andrews J, Parker-Scott S, Eadie MJ: Urinary excretion of valproate metabolites in children and adolescents. *Biopharm Drug Dispos* 21(8):327–330, 2000.
49. Kanner AM: When thinking of lamotrigine and valproic acid, think "pharmacokinetically"! *Epilepsy Curr* 4(5):206–207, 2004.
50. Rowland P, Blaney FE, Smyth MG, et al.: Crystal structure of human cytochrome p450 2d6. *J Biol Chem* 281(11):7614–7622, 2005.
51. Kowatch RA, Strawn JR, Danielyan A. Mood stabilizers: lithium, anticonvulsants, and others. In: *Pediatric Psychopharmacology*. New York, Oxford University Press (OUP), 297–311, 2010.
52. Isojarvi J, Laatikainen TJ, Pakarinen AJ, Juntunen K, Myllyla VV: Polycystic ovaries and hyperandrogenism in women taking valproate for epilepsy. *N Engl J Med* 329(19):1383–1388, 1993.
53. Rasgon NL, Altshuler LL, Fairbanks L, et al.: Reproductive function and risk for PCOS in women treated for bipolar disorder. *Bipolar Disord* 7(3):246–259, 2005.
54. Eyer F, Felgenhauer N, Gempel K, Steimer W, Gerbitz K-D, Zilker T: Acute valproate poisoning: pharmacokinetics, alteration in fatty acid metabolism, and changes during therapy. *J Clin Psychopharmacol* 25(4):376–380, 2005.
55. Alsdorf R, Wyszynski DF: Teratogenicity of sodium valproate. *Expert Opin Drug Saf* 4(2):345–353, 2005.
56. Perucca E: Birth defects after prenatal exposure to antiepileptic drugs. *Lancet Neurol* 4(11):781–786, 2005.
57. Hsu LK: Lithium-resistant adolescent mania. *J Am Acad Child Psychiatry* 25(2):280–283, 1986.
58. Woolston JL: Case study: carbamazepine treatment of juvenile-onset bipolar disorder. *J Am Acad Child Adolesc Psychiatry* 38(3):335–338, 1999.
59. Kafantaris V, Campbell M, Padron-Gayol MV, Small AM, Locascio JJ, Rosenberg CR: Carbamazepine in hospitalized aggressive conduct disorder children: an open pilot study. *Psychopharmacol Bull* 28(2):193–199, 1992.
60. Silva RR, Munoz DM, Daniel W, Barickman J, Friedhoff AJ: Causes of haloperidol discontinuation in patients with Tourette's disorder: management and alternatives. *J Clin Psychiatry* 57(3):129–135, 1996.
61. Cueva JE, Overall JE, Small AM, Armenteros JL, Perry R, Campbell M: Carbamazepine in aggressive children with conduct disorder: a double-blind and placebo-controlled study. *J Am Acad Child Adolesc Psychiatry* 35(4):480–490, 1996.
62. Joshi G, Wozniak J, Mick E, et al.: A prospective open-label trial of extended-release carbamazepine monotherapy in children with bipolar disorder. *J Child Adolesc Psychopharmacol* 20(1):7–14, 2010.
63. Weisler RH, Hirschfeld R, Cutler AJ, et al.: Extended-release carbamazepine capsules as monotherapy in bipolar disorder : pooled results from two randomised, double-blind, placebo-controlled trials. *CNS Drugs* 20(3):219–231, 2006.
64. Schmidt D, Elger CE: What is the evidence that oxcarbazepine and carbamazepine are distinctly different antiepileptic drugs? *Epilepsy & Behav* 5(5):627–635, 2004.

65. Morrow J, Russell A, Guthrie E, et al.: Malformation risks of antiepileptic drugs in pregnancy: a prospective study from the UK Epilepsy and Pregnancy Register. *J Neurol Neurosurg Psychiatry* 77(2):193–198, 2006.
66. Wagner KD, Kowatch RA, Emslie GJ, et al.: A double-blind, randomized, placebo-controlled trial of oxcarbazepine in the treatment of bipolar disorder in children and adolescents. *Am J Psychiatry* 163(7):1179–1186, 2006.
67. Bourgeois BF, D'Souza J: Long-term safety and tolerability of oxcarbazepine in children: a review of clinical experience. *Epilepsy Behav* 7(3):375–382, 2005.
68. Gao K, Calabrese JR: Newer treatment studies for bipolar depression. *Bipolar Disord* 7(Suppl 5):13–23, 2005.
69. Fung J, Mok H, Yatham LN: Lamotrigine for bipolar disorder: translating research into clinical practice. *Expert Rev Neurother* 4(3):363–370, 2004.
70. Ketter TA, Wang PW, Chandler RA, et al.: Dermatology precautions and slower titration yield low incidence of lamotrigine treatment-emergent rash. *J Clin Psychiatry* 66(05):642–645, 2005.
71. Lofton AL, Klein-Schwartz W: Evaluation of lamotrigine toxicity reported to poison centers. *Ann Pharmacother* 38(11):1811–1815, 2004.
72. Delbello MP, Findling RL, Kushner S, et al.: A pilot controlled trial of topiramate for mania in children and adolescents with bipolar disorder. *J Am Acad Child Adolesc Psychiatry* 44(6):539–547, 2005.
73. Powers PS, Santana C: Available pharmacological treatments for anorexia nervosa. *Expert Opin Pharmacother* 5(11):2287–2292, 2004.
74. Narula PK, Rehan HS, Unni KE, Gupta N: Topiramate for prevention of olanzapine associated weight gain and metabolic dysfunction in schizophrenia: a double-blind, placebo-controlled trial. *Schizophr Res* 118(1–3): 218–223, 2010.
75. Thompson S, Rey JM: Functional enuresis: is desmopressin the answer? *J Am Acad Child Adolesc Psychiatry* 34(3):266–271, 1995.
76. Werry JS, Dowrick PW, Lampen EL, Vamos MJ. Imipramine in enuresis–psychological and physiological effects. *J Child Psychol Psychiatry* 16(4): 289–299, 1975.

6.2 ■ PSYCHOTHERAPIES

CHAPTER 6.2.1 ■ PSYCHOTHERAPY FOR CHILDREN AND ADOLESCENTS: A CRITICAL OVERVIEW

V. ROBIN WEERSING, PAULINE GOGER, AND KATE L. CONOVER

The study of psychotherapy in youth dates back to the dawn of therapy itself—to the anxieties of Little Hans (1) and young Peter (2)—and to the beginning of both psychoanalysis and behaviorism. Since these first, seminal case reports, research in child and adolescent therapy has morphed considerably in form and the scale of research has grown exponentially. Over time, the dominant method for investigating therapy effects has become the clinical trial—in essence a psychotherapy experiment including manualization of the "independent variable" of therapy, randomization to treatment conditions, and use of standardized symptom-focused outcome assessments. At last review, thousands of these randomized studies had been conducted (3), and the youth therapy research base grows markedly with every passing year.

In this overview chapter, we aim to provide a brief summary of the main findings across this large literature, focusing on three main questions. First, *can* psychotherapy work? That is, under ideal, experimental conditions, is psychotherapy *efficacious* for youth and families? Second, *does* psychotherapy work? That is, in real-world clinical settings and samples, do we have evidence that psychotherapy is, in fact, *effective* in practice? And third, *how* does psychotherapy work? That is, do we have any substantive evidence on the underlying *mechanisms* of action of therapy effects? Our treatment of the questions of efficacy, effectiveness, and mechanism will be necessarily broad and is designed to highlight progress to date and critical areas for further research.

CAN PSYCHOTHERAPY WORK? THE QUESTION OF EFFICACY

A Historical Overview

The first summary review of the effects of youth psychotherapy appeared over 60 years ago. The author, Eugene Levitt, reviewed the existing evidence base of 18 studies treating "neuroses" in youth and came to a startling conclusion: There was little to no empirical evidence to suggest that psychotherapy was beneficial, and, indeed, the recovery rate for child and adolescent psychotherapy might be marginally worse than the simple improvement observed with the passage of time. In combination with the Eysenck (4) review of adult therapy, the Levitt (5) review and follow-up report (6) produced intense debate in the field. Many of the critiques focused on the methodologic weaknesses of the psychotherapy studies that served as a basis for the author's negative conclusions. Early therapy efficacy studies typically: (a) failed to randomly assign youths to treatment and control conditions; (b) used nonequivalent comparison groups, such as therapy dropouts, as control conditions; (c) failed to specify what therapy procedures were used in the intervention being tested; (d) allowed therapists or other nonmasked raters to assess outcome; and (e) enrolled very heterogeneous samples of youth in terms of diagnoses and developmental level (see Kazdin (7) for review). These characteristics of early efficacy research substantially weakened the internal validity of the designs and made it difficult to impossible to interpret results, whether positive or negative.

In response to these critiques, the design of the prototypical therapy efficacy study evolved into that of the experimental *clinical trial,* characterized by explicit inclusion and exclusion criteria, random assignment, blinded and standardized diagnostic assessment, and manualized treatments. Within two decades, the evidence base of 18 studies available to Levitt had expanded to include over 100 clinical trials, and this explosion of therapy research coincided with the advent of modern meta-analytic methods for summarizing research findings. Together, these two developments provided a unique opportunity to revisit the conclusions of Levitt (5,6), and beginning in the 1980s several major meta-analyses were published on the efficacy of therapy in youth.

Evidence from Meta-Analysis

In *meta-analysis,* traditional narrative reviews of a research area are supplemented by a quantitative analysis of empirical findings across studies. As in a narrative review, meta-analysis begins with an exhaustive, well-documented literature search, with predetermined criteria for study inclusion and exclusion (e.g., requiring a minimum sample size). Following this collection of studies, researchers develop a coding scheme to capture the critical characteristics of each study, establish the reliability of the system, and code the findings from each investigation. Next, the empirical results of each investigation are transformed into a common metric of *effect sizes,* and these effect sizes form the unit of analysis for subsequent statistical tests. Statistical analyses range from simple estimates of a population effect size in a set of homogeneous studies to multivariate models designed to explain variability in effect sizes across a complex literature.

In psychotherapy meta-analyses, the most common effect size metric is Cohen's *d* (8). If the relevant summary statistics are reported in the published study, *d* is very simply calculated by taking the mean of the treated group on a measure of interest (e.g., depression symptoms at posttreatment), subtracting it from the mean of the control group, and then dividing this difference by the standard deviation of the control group (see Smith et al. (9) for other estimation techniques). This process creates a score indicating how "far apart" in outcomes a therapy condition is from a control group, expressed in standard deviation units. By convention, a *d* of 0.2 is considered a small effect size, while a *d* of 0.8 is a large effect (10).

Casey and Berman (11) were the first to apply meta-analytic methods of this kind to the child psychotherapy literature in 1985. They reviewed and coded 64 controlled studies of therapy for youth (age 12 and under) and found that the average effect size for psychotherapy was a very respectable 0.71.

Since the Casey and Berman (11) report, four additional major meta-analyses have been published (12–15), with the most recent of these spanning 50 years of intervention research and including 447 clinical trials (15). Across these meta-analyses, youth therapy had medium to large effects on symptoms, with results similar in magnitude to effect size evidence from the adult literature (9). Furthermore, the confidence intervals around these population estimates did not cross zero, suggesting that, as a whole, psychotherapeutic interventions for youth were more efficacious than control conditions (typically a waitlist or no treatment control). The most recent and comprehensive meta-analysis by Weisz et al. (15) estimated the overall effect of youth psychotherapy to be 0.46 at posttreatment, with effects maintained over follow-up. This effect size is the most modest of the major meta-analyses, notably smaller than the effect reported in the original Casey and Berman paper. Further, Weisz et al. probed for moderators that might predict this apparent decrease in effect size in the literature over time. Of the candidate moderators, it appeared most likely that this decrease may be a function of more modern methods of calculating effect size, using a sample size correction to weight Cohen's *d* (see 16); recalculation of effect sizes from a 1995 meta-analysis also by Weisz using this method yielded a very similar effect size (0.54 vs. 0.71 for an unweighted effect size (14)).

While these broad-based meta-analyses have been consistent in their finding of an overall positive effect for youth psychotherapy, findings have been more mixed on whether therapy is efficacious across types of problems, treatments, and youth and family characteristics. Throughout the 1990s, type of youth problem did not emerge from these analyses as being significantly related to the magnitude of therapeutic improvement (12,14). In these analyses, youth problems were typically categorized into two broad bands—internalizing problems such as depression, anxiety, and somatic complaints and externalizing problems including disruptive behavior, delinquency, conduct problems, and attention/impulsivity. In the more recent Weisz et al. (15) analysis, these broad syndromes were decomposed into the four primary presenting problems seen in outpatient care of youth—anxiety, depression, conduct problems, and ADHD—with an additional category of "multiple problems" also coded. In this analysis, problem type emerged as a powerful predictor of a study's effect size. Trials testing psychosocial treatments for anxiety had significantly larger effect sizes (mean ES = 0.61) than studies targeting any other problem type. Effects for ADHD and conduct problems had the next largest effect sizes, with depression trials having the smallest effects of any of the "big four" problem areas (mean depression ES = 0.29). Studies targeting multiple problems reported even smaller ES values, with the mean effect size estimate for this category of studies not significantly deviating from zero.

Interestingly, although problem type was found to significantly impact effect size, other person-level factors have not been consistently supported as moderators of efficacy in meta-analyses. In the large Weisz et al. (15) pool of studies, treatment did not seem to be differentially beneficial for children versus adolescents, girls versus boys, or Caucasians versus minorities—with the caveat that only 12% of the studies consisted of a non-Caucasian majority sample. The need for more diverse samples in clinical trial research is well documented. In a 2005 review of the methodological characteristics of youth treatment research, fewer than half of the investigations identified the race or ethnicity of study participants and only 25% reported on participant socioeconomic status (16).

In terms of treatment type, the five broad-based meta-analyses do support the overall conclusion that behavioral interventions produce significantly larger effects than nonbehavioral interventions. Some analyses suggest an unqualified superiority of behavioral therapies (14), while others suggest that the heightened value youth-focused behavioral interventions lies in the consistency of positive effects found across reporters (e.g., youth, parents teachers) compared to interventions with more variable effects across reporters. In the meta-analyses probing treatment type, "behavioral treatments" typically include such direct behavioral techniques as teaching parents more effective discipline styles or exposure for youth anxiety, as well as cognitive-behavioral techniques (CBT), such as helping depressed youth to label and correct unrealistically negative thinking and self-talk. Nonbehavioral psychotherapy has been conceived as a broad category including traditional psychodynamic-based approaches, client-centered therapies, and discussion groups. Notably, this division does not characterize well several treatment programs of fairly recent vintage that have significant empirical support, such as interpersonal therapy (IPT) for adolescents with depression (17) or Multisystemic Therapy (MST), a behavioral-family systems approach for juvenile justice-involved youth (18). Also note that some treatment modalities used with youth, such as family therapy (e.g., Multidimensional Family Therapy, 19) or group therapy could be characterized as either behavioral or nonbehavioral depending on the content of the intervention.

Not surprisingly, the finding of superior outcomes for behavioral treatments has been hotly contested, and a host of alternate explanations proposed (20). Differences between treatment types have previously been robust in analyses controlling for other potentially confounding differences between behavioral and nonbehavioral studies that might spuriously produce this effect, such as differences in problem type, severity of symptoms, or methodology (see Weiss and Weisz (21) for discussion). While many posit that behavioral treatments are superior, there are two critiques of this position that cannot be tested in the current clinical trial literature base and remain as possible alternate explanations of this effect: (a) far more clinical trials of behavioral therapies have been published, and additional research on nonbehavioral therapies may yet yield more positive results; and (b) nonbehavioral therapies have been used as control conditions in some studies by investigators, and these treatments may not have been implemented with the same care and vigor as the main behavioral treatment being tested by the study, artificially lowering estimates of nonbehavioral therapy effect sizes (22). These possibilities speak to the chapter (Ritvo/Psychodynamic Principles in Practice) on psychoanalysis and psychodynamically informed psychotherapies, and the growing efforts within the analytic research community to conduct high-quality clinical trials of insight-oriented therapeutic approaches (23,24). However, psychoanalysis and other nonbehavioral therapies may have a high hill to climb, given the volume of research on behavioral treatments and the consistency of positive effects. Evidence appears particularly strong for exposure-based treatments for the anxiety disorders (25–27), behavioral parent training for child oppositional behaviors (28; note that a major evidence-based update review of this literature is in progress (29)), and behavioral parent training and multisystemic treatments with strong behavioral components for adolescent conduct problems (29). The hill also may have been made steeper by the trend in the early 1990s for professional organizations in the mental health field to move beyond broad examination of the efficacy of therapy to begin identifying specific *evidence-based treatment* (EBT) programs for targeted diagnostic clusters.

The Movement toward Evidence-Based Treatment

In the early 1990s, evidence-based medicine was broadly defined as the practice of weighing the available scientific evidence when making decisions regarding clinical care (30). At around the same time, the Society of Clinical Psychology (American Psychological Association [APA] Division 12) formed a task force charged with "educating clinical psychologists, third-party payers, and the public about effective psychotherapies" (31). This effort resulted in a series of reports identifying evidence-based psychosocial treatments (EBT) for adults (31–33). Parallel efforts by the Society of Clinical Child and Adolescent Psychology (APA Division 53) and the Society of Pediatric Psychology (APA Division 54) led to the publication of major EBT reviews for children and adolescents (34,35). Indeed, the practice guidelines of major medical associations also have broadened their focus to consider, evaluate, and include psychosocial interventions into the standard-of-care for emotional and behavioral problems, sometimes as a first-choice intervention (36). In addition to these efforts driven by professional organizations, research groups have endeavored to define and identify EBTs for psychological problems (25,36–39).

As reviewed by Tolin (40), different groups use varying criteria when evaluating the strength of the support for an intervention's efficacy. In general, however, treatments are considered a well-established EBT if they have shown positive effects in a series of carefully controlled, prospective studies by independent teams of investigators. Most often, this is defined as clinical trials in which: (a) participants were randomly assigned to conditions, and (b) treatment was compared to a placebo or other established treatment. However, some groups consider a large series of well-controlled single case studies to be sufficient for the designation of EBT. A second class of EBTs, identified as "probably efficacious" (33), is supported by scientific evidence but has been subjected to less rigorous tests (e.g., comparison to a wait-list control group). Most recently, the Board of Directors of APA Division 53 argued that the previous practice of updating the evidence base roughly every 10 years was not sufficient in light of a fast-exploding youth psychopathology literature, and called for a more continuous practice of updates, addressing different problem types in nearly every issue of Division's 53 journal (41). Accordingly, criteria required to classify the level of an EBT were standardized for this purpose, and included important additions such as a "treatments of questionable efficacy" level—warning clinicians and clients of treatments that were indeed tested but which do not work (41). This showed a greater emphasis on methodologic sophistication, and the attempt to not only identify *if* treatments work, but *how* they work (see Figure 6.2.1.1 for illustration (41)).

Based on these criteria, EBTs have been identified for a wide range of social, emotional, and behavioral difficulties commonly experienced by children and adolescents. To date,

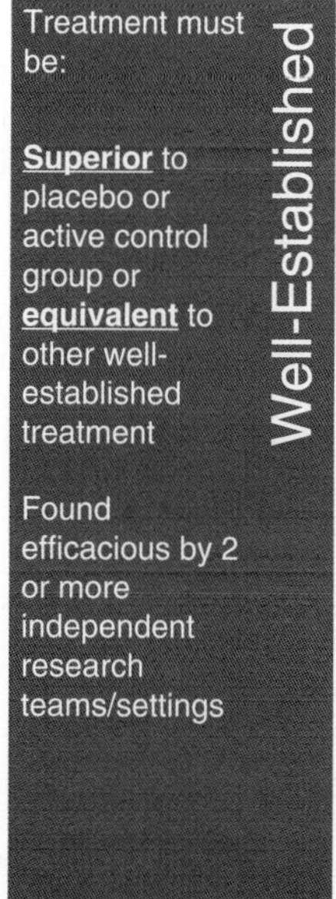

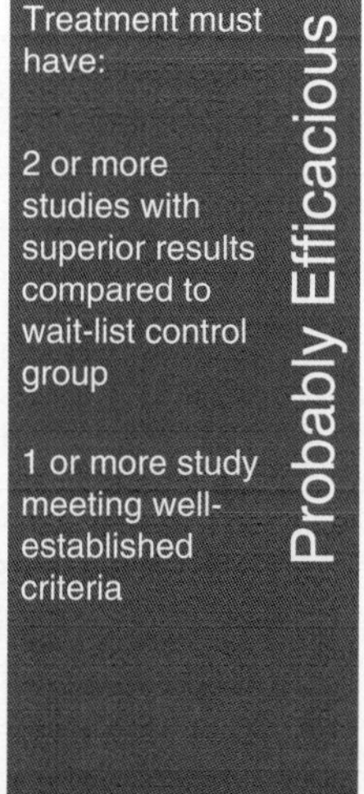

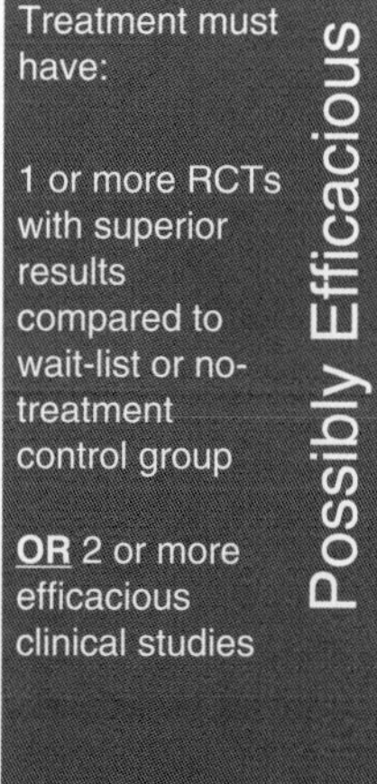

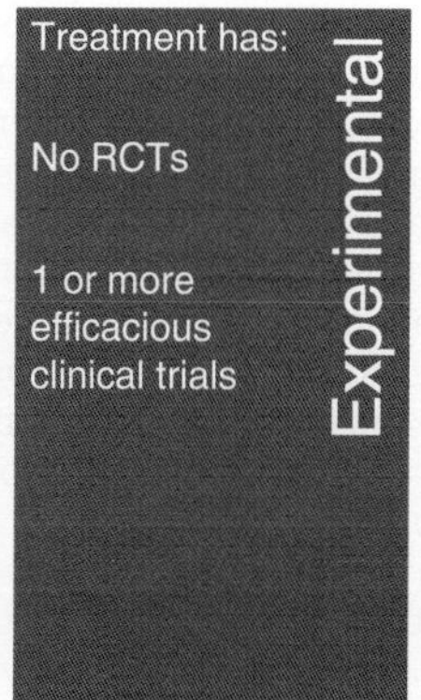

FIGURE 6.2.1.1. Categories of evidence-based psychosocial treatment. (Adapted from Southam-Gerow MA, Prinstein MJ: Evidence base updates: the evolution of the evaluation of psychological treatments for children and adolescents. *J Clin Child Adolesc Psychol* 43(1):1–6, 2014.)

well-established psychosocial interventions have been developed for adolescent depression (42), obesity (43), posttraumatic stress disorder (PTSD); (44), ADHD (45), substance abuse (46), eating disorders (47), disruptive behaviors (28,29), autism (48), enuresis (49), and anxiety (27), and probably efficacious EBTs have been identified for OCD (50), bipolar (51), self-harm (52). As discussed in the section on meta-analysis, behavioral treatments are 8 to 10 times more likely to be tested systematically than nonbehavioral approaches (16), and it is not surprising that the majority of EBTs identified by the various work groups are behaviorally, or cognitive-behaviorally, focused. Although the majority of therapeutic interventions focus on the child, many efficacious programs target the systems in which youths function (53), such as their families (functional family therapy; (54)) or the juvenile justice system (MST; (18)).

Currently, the EBT movement has reached beyond the professional exercise of identifying therapies with promising outcomes and moved into the domain of policy, by funding and shaping the content of youth mental health care in practice. Policymakers at the national (55–57) and international (58) levels have endorsed the importance of evidence-based mental health care, and US federal funding has been made available to clinical care providers to support the training of community therapists in EBT programs (59,60). However, even when providers in community settings intend to select evidence-based interventions, they often fail to identify evidence-based practices as such and may also incorrectly identify label treatments as empirically supported (61). Family and patient organizations have begun to advocate for access to mental health interventions with demonstrated effectiveness (62), and states have developed initiatives to support the use of EBT services (63). Research efforts, too, have increasingly begun to focus not simply on the *efficacy* of psychotherapy in controlled trials and laboratory environments, but also on building an evidence base for the actual *effectiveness* of therapy in practice.

DOES PSYCHOTHERAPY WORK? THE QUESTION OF EFFECTIVENESS

The news, thus far, has appeared good for those concerned with providing quality psychological services to youth and families. Psychotherapy for youth has effects of a reasonable magnitude and progress has been made in identifying specific treatments most likely to be beneficial for particular problems and diagnoses. However, limitations in the conduct of psychotherapy research have left core questions unanswered, including whether the research that supports the benefits of youth therapy and forms the base of the process of identifying EBTs is applicable to everyday clinical practice. As explicated in seminal papers by Weisz et al. (64,65), the majority of therapy clinical trials take place under conditions substantially different from community treatment as usual (TAU). For example, clinical trials typically are based in university clinics, academic medical centers, and research laboratories with copious resources and support staff. Families are usually recruited to participate in the study and screened to identify the primary target problem under investigation. Therapists in a research study may receive extensive pre-therapy training in the treatment protocol, be closely supervised on protocol adherence, and carry a small caseload of homogeneous clients. Psychotherapy may be free, or clients may be paid to participate in the research therapy. And, as discussed earlier, clinical trials are far more likely to utilize behavioral treatments than nonbehavioral therapies, the latter of which are heavily used in typical clinical practice (66,67). These differences between psychotherapy research and community TAU may dim the rosy outlook on the benefit of child and adolescent therapy in two major ways.

The Effects of Community Treatment as Usual

First, clinical care may not currently be as effective as the psychotherapy clinical trial literature suggests. Very few of the thousands of studies of child and adolescent therapy have examined the effectiveness of the therapy program of a functioning service-oriented clinic. In the early 1990s, Weisz et al. searched the youth treatment outcome literature for studies of "real-world" psychological services (68). They found only nine studies of clinic TAU. Results of this small body of research stood in stark contrast to those of the hundreds of typical psychotherapy clinical trials included in meta-analyses. Whereas clinical trials reported consistently beneficial effects of therapy for youth, the mean effect size of the TAU studies was near zero.

Consistent with this pattern, Weiss et al. (69) found minimal effects of TAU delivered to disturbed school-aged youths by therapists hired through a local community clinic. TAU therapists were free to use whatever techniques and dose of treatment they viewed as best, and they averaged 60 individual sessions, 18 parent sessions, and 13 school consultations per treated youth. After this substantial dose of therapy, TAU youth outcomes were equivalent to the outcomes of youth who had been randomized to receive only academic tutoring. At 2-year follow-up, the authors were able to contact 95% of their original sample of participants ($N = 112$), and the outcomes of the two groups remained quite similar (70), arguing against a longer-term preventive benefit or "sleeper effect" for community TAU.

Similarly, large scale effectiveness studies of TAU in mental health care systems have yielded ambiguous results at best. In the massive Fort Bragg investigation, efforts to boost the effectiveness of youth mental health care by coordinating TAU services did not lead to improved outcomes over uncoordinated care (71–73). One explanation of this finding is that the original community TAU elements were not effective to begin with and, thus, synergies between these services impossible to achieve (74). Dose of care also was unrelated to outcome in the sample, further suggesting that the original TAU elements may not have been potent (75,76). In contrast, the longitudinal Great Smoky Mountains Study (77) found that community TAU appeared to deflect the worsening trajectory of already impaired youth, a result interpreted as evidence of effectiveness of services.

These modest findings have reinforced calls by many (78) for a broad effort to reform mental health care practice by exporting EBTs from clinical trials into the community. This prescription relies on the assumption that it is differences in treatment type that account for the superior outcomes of psychotherapy in clinical trials compared to therapy in practice. Certainly, evidence from meta-analyses suggests that this assumption is plausible and that behavioral EBTs may perform robustly in the samples and settings of real-world clinical care. However, this hypothesis has only been tested within the last 15 years, and there are reasons to suspect that the effects of EBT may be attenuated in practice.

The Effectiveness of Research Treatments in Practice

The second implication of the differences between clinical trial research and typical clinical care is that promising EBTs may not work as well when tested under conditions more closely approximating real life. In addition to difference in treatment type, clinical trials and community care may vary along a number of sample and setting factors. For example, clinical trials for youth depression historically have included: (a) youth either "at risk" for depression or exhibiting only mild depression symptoms (79,80); (b) youth recruited from schools and newspaper advertisements rather than ascertained through clinical referral routes (81); and (c) youth carefully screened to possess a minimal number of comorbid psychiatric problems (82)—a sample of young patients *not* representative of community mental health practice (83). Preliminary investigations of patient factors related to depression treatment outcome have suggested that these three characteristics of research samples may predict therapy success (84), and, thus, treatment effects for more severe, comorbid clinical samples of depressed youth may not be as positive as clinical trial data would suggest. There may be a similar level of mismatch between the samples of youths enrolled in clinical trials of anxiety disorders compared to anxious youths in community clinics (85). Clinical trial research on disruptive behavior problems may fare better in terms of research-practice sample comparability, in part because of the efforts of many investigators to recruit research participants from settings such as juvenile justice (53) and foster care (86).

Again, meta-analysis has proved a useful tool to generate hypotheses about the "robustness" of EBTs if transported to practice. Shadish et al. reanalyzed data from several previously published meta-analyses on the effects of psychotherapy in a mega-analysis of the adult and child literature (87,88). Studies were coded in terms of "clinical representativeness"—the extent to which the therapists, setting, and sample of the investigation were similar to active clinical practice. The authors clustered studies into tiers of representativeness and explored whether effect sizes for clinical trials decreased as study characteristics became closer and closer to real-world conditions. Overall, the authors found that effect sizes were constant across levels, but they also found only one study that fulfilled all of their clinically representative criteria. Interestingly, all of the studies included in the Weisz et al. (68) analysis of community TAU were screened out of the Shadish meta-analysis (87) on methodologic grounds, further highlighting the paucity of strong research probing the effectiveness of TAU compared to less active control conditions (e.g., a waiting list).

In a parallel analysis to their major broad-based meta-analytic report (15), Weisz et al. searched their pool of clinical trials for investigations that included (a) an active treatment condition utilizing an identified EBT from the Division 53 list of treatments, and (b) a community TAU comparison condition. They identified 52 trials that met these criteria and conducted a separate meta-analysis of this subgroup of studies to directly test the relative value of EBTs versus TAU (89). Overall, the EBT-TAU effect size was significantly different from zero and favored EBT (mean ES = 0.29). In this pool of studies, effect size did not significantly vary by problem type, although effect sizes were larger in studies of youths selected for having clinically elevated symptoms compared to studies where youths met diagnostic criteria for disorder.

In parallel, community agencies and governmental bodies have begun to systematically move EBT programs into practice. In the internalizing disorders, the greatest efforts and most progress have come in the dissemination and evaluation of treatments for PTSD. There has been a concerted effort to disseminate trauma-focused cognitive-behavioral therapy (TF-CBT) both nationally and internationally. The National Child Traumatic Stress Network (90) was established by the US Congress in 2000 and has grown to over 150 network centers located nationwide in university and community-based organizations. A major focus of the network has been the dissemination of EBT information and partnering with treatment researchers to provide certification in TF-CBT practices, including access to online training materials (91). In a recent review, it was reported that TF-CBT had been formally disseminated in 19 states and several nations (92), with recent trials reporting positive effects of TF-CBT over TAU services in Norway (93) and Zambia (94), and positive effects using TF-CBT in a group format in a clinical trial in the Democratic Republic of the Congo (95). These dissemination efforts built on the base of clinical trials of TF-CBT that have long included elements of effectiveness research. From the very first trials of the intervention, active alternate treatments were used as a comparator, either usual community services or research conditions modeled on the content of typical community TAU for the disorder (see (96) for review).

In comparison, effectiveness and dissemination research in youth depression have been both more modest and less successful. Efforts to disseminate CBT for depression to community mental health settings have yielded negative (97,98) or weak results (99). EBT depression treatments have fared better when exported and tested in health settings, with IPT-A faring well in a trial based in school health clinics (17) and CBT for adolescent depression separating from usual care when delivered as part of a collaborative care model in primary care (100–102).

Efforts to probe the effectiveness of interventions for externalizing behavior problems are significantly more advanced. For many years, treatment researchers interested in disruptive behavior problems have turned to community agencies to ascertain their samples, and randomized effectiveness trials testing the effects of parent management training (PMT) and multisystemic therapy (MST) have been built on this community foundation. Studies testing the effectiveness of PMT in practice have been occurring on both the national and international levels, with accumulating evidence for the clinical and cost-effectiveness of this EBT compared to clinic TAU (103). In one of the most ambitious projects to date, Marion Forgatch and colleagues at the Oregon Social Learning Center partnered with the U.S. National Institute on Drug Abuse and the Norwegian Center for Studies on Behavioral Problems and Innovative Practice to study the adoption, adaptation and implementation of PMT in every community in Norway (104). The project aimed to evaluate adherence to the PMT model and assess whether fidelity to the core PMT treatment elements would prevent negative youth outcomes, such as substance abuse. In addition to these within-PMT analyses, agencies that were selected for PMT training were compared against matched control agencies in terms of therapeutic practices and child outcomes. These efforts were broadly successful, with youths treated with PMT evidencing greater behavioral change than TAU youths, and the intervention operating along the hypothesized mediational pathways specified in the PMT model (e.g., improved discipline, enhanced compliance (105)). Further analyses suggested that these PMT dissemination efforts maintained a similar magnitude of effects as original trials under more controlled conditions (106). The Norway implementation has become an exemplar of successful PMT dissemination and led to additional efforts and research projects in the Netherlands, Iceland, and Michigan (107).

In a similar large-scale fashion, Henggeler, Schoenwald, and the MST research team have conducted a series of community-based effectiveness studies and formed a nonprofit consulting company (MST services) to aid in the implementation and evaluation of MST in real-world service agencies across the United States. MST was developed originally as an ecologic treatment for serious juvenile delinquency. Treatment is home based, targeted at the youth, family, and the surrounding environment, and the techniques employed draw heavily from behavioral and family systems theories (53) (see Adnopoz/Intensive Home-Based Family Preservation Approaches, Including Multisystemic Therapy). Initial efficacy outcomes were very promising, with statistically and clinically significant improvements in "hard outcomes," such as arrests and days in jail, compared to a variety of community TAU control conditions, including traditional juvenile justice services (108–110). MST also has been adapted and tested by the investigators as an intervention for substance-abusing youth, juvenile sex offenders, maltreated youths, and youths at risk for inpatient hospitalization due to serious emotional disturbance (111,112). Unsurprisingly, MST was a prime candidate for dissemination and had been transported into the service systems of 30 states and 8 nations by 2004 (113). The resulting body of program evaluation studies provides a unique dataset in which to examine the generalizability of EBT effects to a wide variety of practice settings and also to probe the sustainability of the intervention, when divorced from the original research team.

In a 2004 meta-analysis, Curtis et al. (114) reviewed 7 studies of MST, enrolling a total of 708 youth, and coded the extent to which the investigations more closely resembled efficacy research or a true effectiveness trial, embedded in real-world practice. Again, all youths in these studies were drawn from real-world referral sources, and the major indicator of the efficacy–effectiveness distinction was the identity of therapists and the mode of supervision. Three investigations utilized graduate student therapists, supervised by MST treatment developers, with extensive weekly reviews and feedback on audio or videotapes of sessions. In contrast, the effectiveness studies used community mental health providers who received initial training in MST but little ongoing supervision (by design, as sustainability of the program was a research question under investigation) (113). Effect sizes were significantly larger in studies utilizing graduate students as therapists ($d = 0.81$) than in studies with therapists from the community ($d = 0.26$). This meta-analytic result maps onto work done by the MST team examining the dissemination of the program to 45 sites, 400 therapists, and 2,000 treated youths, in which adherence to the MST model and strong quality assurance procedures are correlated with positive youth outcomes (115–117). Studies published after these reviews continue to support the likely effectiveness of MST in practice. In a recent trial in Sweden, MST provider adherence predicted client outcomes in MST, consistent with previous findings (118). Importantly, MST effects were recently replicated in an effectiveness trial by a research team that did not include the MST treatment developers. In this independent replication, MST was compared to services as usual for adolescents in the United States drawing from a sample of youths placed in self-contained behavioral management classroom, separate from the general school population (119).

Taken together, results of these studies suggest that EBTs can be successfully delivered in community clinical contexts and often produce similar effect sizes as in the original efficacy trials. This first wave of effectiveness and dissemination research is transitioning to questions focusing on broader outcomes than symptom change (e.g., functioning, cost-effectiveness) and factors related to the initial uptake and sustainability of dissemination efforts in service settings (e.g., willingness to adopt new models, training and turnover, supervision; see (120) for a review focused on trauma treatment).

HOW DOES PSYCHOTHERAPY WORK? THE QUESTION OF MECHANISM

In our final section, we turn to the question of mechanism. Given evidence that psychotherapy for youth *can* work and that, under some conditions, it *does* actually work in practice, is there evidence on *how* psychotherapeutic interventions achieve their effects?

The brief answer to this query is no, due in large part to the content of most therapy manuals for youth and the design of most clinical trials. The majority of research therapies consist of multicomponent treatment packages. For example, a CBT manual for youth anxiety likely includes several of the following components: (a) teaching the child how to identify and label different emotions; (b) working to correct anxious self-talk and thinking; (c) teaching relaxation skills; (d) guiding desensitization of imagined feared objects; (e) participating in role-plays of coping skills; and (f) coaching the youth in real-life exposure to anxiety-provoking stimuli. From a design perspective, if a treatment utilizing a package of these techniques is compared to a waiting-list control and found to be more effective on global measures of anxiety, it is not clear whether every component of the treatment is necessary to produce therapeutic change. Additionally, in this hypothetical design, underlying pathogenic processes have not been assessed (e.g., shifts in anxious cognitions), nor tests conducted to determine if changes in these mechanisms mediate the impact of treatment on anxious symptomatology.

This example is intended as an illustration, yet it describes a fair proportion of the existing youth clinical trial literature. In 2002, Weersing and Weisz reviewed psychosocial clinical trials for anxiety, depression, and disruptive behavior cited in the Society of Clinical Child and Adolescent Psychology EBT reports (34). In this review of 67 studies, only 10% included an attempt to measure treatment processes and test whether change in these processes mediated therapy effects (121). Furthermore, these six investigations (122–127) suffered from significant methodologic limitations, such as failing to show that change in the proposed treatment mechanism actually occurred before change in outcome, and one of the studies did not demonstrate mediation (123). While formal tests of mediation were very rare, simple measurement of possible mediators was much more common in the literature. Nearly every study of parent training assessed whether treatment impacted parenting behaviors, and the majority of depression studies included at least one measure of a potential treatment process (79%) (121). Overall, when EBT studies included these measures, investigators found that treatment significantly changed the process, at least when the process was assessed at posttreatment, along with the other general symptom measures of outcome. This pattern of findings is consistent with mediation of treatment by theoretically specific intervention processes, but it does not preclude other interpretations of results. For example, finding that parent training impacts both positive parenting behavior and child noncompliance may imply that changing parenting improves youth behavior; it also may be that improved youth behavior makes it easier to be a positive parent, and an alternate mediating process was responsible for changing youth noncompliance.

Unfortunately, in the 14 years since this last review, the literature appears to have moved very little. A recent volume by Maric et al. (128) sought to provide a comprehensive report of empirical evidence for moderators and mediators of youth treatment outcome. In our own contribution to this work on youth depression (129), we noted that only two additional mediation studies had appeared in the literature since last review (121), and these studies suffered from the same flaws as previous research in the area—effects of "mediators" measured primarily at posttreatment, inconsistent effects across different measures of mediators and outcomes, and over-reliance on self-report scales. Across disorders, mixed findings for putative statistical "mediators" were quite common (e.g., for anxious self-talk as a cognitive mediator of CBT (122,130)), and the problem of temporal precedence remained a central issue in interpreting even positive results (e.g., (131)).

As treatment mechanism research moves forward, it would seem valuable for psychotherapy investigators to employ more rigorous designs and to move beyond the traditional self-report, parent report, and behavioral observation rating scales that have long characterized assessment of youth therapy processes and outcome. It is notable how little the youth psychotherapy literature appears to have been informed by modern advances in developmental psychopathology, including the explosion of research on biologic bases of behavior (132). In the Weersing and Weisz review (121), the only studies to include putatively "biologic" mediators were early investigations of behavioral treatments for anxiety that measured indices of physiologic habituation such as galvanic skin response and heart rate. This is a far cry from mechanism studies assessing shifts in cortisol, brain activation, or the buffering effect of social support programs on genetic vulnerability to acute stress reactions (133), and a biologically based mediator of psychosocial treatment effects has yet to appear in the depression, anxiety, PTSD, disruptive behavior, or ADHD literatures (128). In the next 50 years of youth psychotherapy research, it seems likely that these sorts of tests will move from conjecture to reality and substantially enhance our knowledge of why therapy is therapeutic.

CONCLUSIONS AND FUTURE DIRECTIONS

In sum, the available evidence suggests that (a) psychotherapy for youth can produce positive effects and is generally efficacious in research studies; (b) there may be a need to improve on the effects of typical community mental health care for youth; and (c) we may have the means to do so, through the careful dissemination and implementation of efficacy-tested EBT programs in practice. However, these general conclusions come with caveats. The number of rigorous studies of community TAU is quite small, and there is still a gap in efficacy research focusing on the insight-oriented and eclectic approaches typically used in practice. The body of EBT effectiveness trials is growing and outcomes appear promising, but coverage of internalizing problems is thin, and results from the better developed externalizing literature suggest that effect sizes of EBTs in practice may be moderated by adherence and quality control of interventions and therapist and organizational factors.

In addition, we still know remarkably little about how psychotherapeutic interventions work. This lack of precision is unsatisfying scientifically and may make the task of transporting these multicomponent research treatments into clinical settings more difficult than need be. If only one or two techniques of a complicated treatment package are producing change, then time spent training and providing the rest of the treatment package is wasted effort. Lack of understanding of mechanism also hampers our ability to develop new treatments that efficiently target core processes of disorder—a critical task, given evidence that the effect sizes for interventions in practice may be halved from efficacy estimates (114). In the next generation of psychotherapy research, a better understanding of why therapy works would seem to be of paramount importance.

References

1. Freud S: Analysis of phobia in a five-year-old boy. In: *Standard Editions of the Complete Psychological Works of Sigmund Freud*. Vol 10. London, Hogarth, pp. 3–149, 1955.
2. Jones MC: A laboratory study of fear: the case of Peter. *Pedagog Sem* 31:308–315, 1924.
3. Kazdin AE: Child and adolescent psychotherapy. In: Friedman HS (ed): *Encyclopedia of Mental Health*. 2nd ed. Oxford, Academic Press, 2016.
4. Eysenck HJ: The effects of psychotherapy: an evaluation. *J Consult Psychol* 16:319–324, 1952.
5. Levitt EE: The results of psychotherapy with children: an evaluation. *J Consult Psychol* 21:189–196, 1957.
6. Levitt EE: Psychotherapy with children: a further evaluation. *Behav Res Ther* 1:45–51, 1963.
7. Kazdin AE: *History of Behavior Modification: Experimental Foundations of Contemporary Research*. Baltimore, MD, University Park Press, 1978.
8. Cohen J: *Statistical Power Analysis for the Behavioral Sciences*. New York, Academic Press, 1977.
9. Smith ML, Glass GV, Miller TI: *The Benefits of Psychotherapy*. Baltimore, MD, Johns Hopkins, 1980.
10. Cohen J: A power primer. *Psychol Bull* 112:155–159, 1992.
11. Casey RJ, Berman JS: The outcome of psychotherapy with children. *Psychol Bull* 98:388–400, 1985.
12. Weisz JR, Weiss B, Alicke MD, Klotz ML: Effectiveness of psychotherapy with children and adolescents: a meta-analysis for clinicians. *J Consult Clin Psych* 55:542–549, 1987.
13. Kazdin AE, Bass D, Ayers WA, Rodgers A: Empirical and clinical focus of child and adolescent psychotherapy research. *J Consult Clin Psych* 58:729–740, 1990.
14. Weisz JR, Weiss B, Han SS, Granger DA, Morton T: Effects of psychotherapy with children and adolescents revisited: a meta-analysis of treatment outcome studies. *Psychol Bull* 117:450–468, 1995.
15. Weisz JR, Kuppens S, Ng MY, et al.: What five decades of research tells us about the effects of youth psychological therapy: a multilevel meta-analysis and implications for science and practice. *Am Psychol* 72:79–117, 2017.
16. Weisz JR, Doss AJ, Hawley KM: Youth psychotherapy outcome research: a review and critique of the evidence base. *Annu Rev Psychol* 56:337–363, 2005.
17. Mufson L, Dorta KP, Wickramaratne P, et al.: A randomized effectiveness trial of interpersonal psychotherapy for depressed adolescents. *Arch Gen Psychiat* 61:577–584, 2004.
18. Henggeler SW, Schoenwald SK, Borduin CM, Rowland MD, Cunningham PB: *Multisystemic Treatment of Antisocial Behavior in Children and Adolescents*. New York, Guilford Press, 1998.
19. Liddle, HA: A multidimensional model for treating the adolescent who is abusing alcohol and other drugs. In: Snyder M, Ooms T (eds): *Empowering Families, Helping Adolescents: Family-Centered Treatment of Adolescents with Alcohol, Drug Abuse and Other Mental Health Problems*. Washington, DC: United States Public Health Service; 1991.
20. Shirk SR, Russell RL: A reevaluation of estimates of child therapy effectiveness. *J Am Acad Child Psy* 31:703–709, 1992.
21. Weiss BH, Weisz JR: Relative effectiveness of behavioral and nonbehavioral child psychotherapy. *J Consult Clin Psych* 63:317–320, 1995.
22. Westen D, Novotny CM, Thompson-Brenner H: Empirical status of empirically supported psychotherapies: assumptions, findings, and reporting in controlled clinical trials. *Psychol Bull* 130:631–663, 2004.
23. Lieberman AF, Van Horn P, Ippen CG: Toward evidence-based treatment: child-parent psychotherapy with preschoolers exposed to marital violence. *J Am Acad Child Adolsec Psychiatry* 44:1241–1248, 2005.
24. Toth SL, Maughan A, Manly JT, Spagnola M, Cicchetti D: The relative efficacy of two interventions in altering maltreated preschool children's representational models: implications for attachment theory. *Dev Psychopathol* 14:877–908, 2002.
25. Compton SN, March JS, Brent DA, Albano AM 5th, Weersing R, Curry J: Cognitive-behavioral psychotherapy for anxiety and depressive disorders in children and adolescents: an evidence-based medicine review. *J Am Acad Child Psy* 43:930–959, 2004.
26. Ollendick TH, King NJ: Empirically supported treatments for children with phobic and anxiety disorders: current status. *J Clin Child Psychol* 27:156–167, 1998.
27. Higa-McMillan CK, Francis SE, Rith-Najarian L, Chorpita BF: Evidence base update: 50 years of research on treatment for child and adolescent anxiety. *J Clin Child Adolesc Psychol* 45(2):91–113, 2016.
28. Brestan EV, Eyberg SM: Effective psychosocial treatments of conduct-disordered children and adolescents: 29 years, 82 studies, and 5,272 kids. *J Clin Child Psychol* 27:180–189, 1998.
29. McCart MR, Sheidow AJ: Evidence-based psychosocial treatments for adolescents with disruptive behavior. *J Clin Child Adolesc Psychol* 45(5):529–563, 2016.
30. Hamilton J: The answerable question and a hierarchy of evidence. *J Am Acad Child Adolesc Psychiatry* 44:596–600, 2005.
31. Task Force on Promotion and Dissemination of Psychological Procedures. Training in and dissemination of empirically validated psychological treatments: report and recommendations. *Clin Psychol* 48:3–24, 1995.
32. Chambless DL, Sanderson WC, Shoham V, et al.: An update on empirically validated therapies. *Clin Psychol* 49:5–18, 1996.
33. Chambless DL, Baker MJ, Baucom DH, et al.: Update on empirically validated therapies, II. *Clin Psychol* 51:3–16, 1998.
34. Lonigan C, Elbert J, Johnson SB: Empirically supported psychosocial interventions for children: an overview. (Special issue on empirically supported psychosocial interventions for children.) *J Clin Child Psychol* 27:138–145, 1998.
35. Spirito A (ed): Special series on empirically supported interventions in pediatric psychology (Series of special issues). *J Pediatr Psychol* 24:2–4, 6, 1999.
36. Cheung AH, Zuckerbrot RA, Jensen PS, Ghalib K, Laraque D, Stein RE; GLAD-PC Steering Group: Guidelines for Adolescent Depression in Primary Care (GLAD-PC): II. Treatment and ongoing management. *Pediatrics* 120(5):e1313–e1326, 2007.
37. Roth A, Fonagy P: *What Works for Whom? A Critical Review of Psychotherapy Research*. New York, Guilford, 1996.
38. Farmer EM, Compton SN, Burns BJ, Robertson E: Review of the evidence base for treatment of childhood psychopathology: externalizing disorders. *J Consult Clin Psychol* 70:1267–1302, 2002.
39. Weisz JR, Kazdin AE (eds): *Evidence-Based Psychotherapies for Children and Adolescents*. New York, Guilford Press, 2003.

40. Tolin DF, McKay D, Forman EM, Klonsky ED, Thombs BD: Empirically supported treatment: recommendations for a new model. *Clin Psychol-Sci Pr* 22:317–338, 2015.
41. Southam-Gerow MA, Prinstein MJ: Evidence base updates: the evolution of the evaluation of psychological treatments for children and adolescents. *J Clin Child Adolesc Psychol* 43(1):1–6, 2014.
42. Weersing VR, Jeffreys M, Do MT, Schwartz KT, Bolano C: Evidence base update of psychosocial treatments for child and adolescent depression. *J Clin Child Adolesc Psychol* 1–33, 2016.
43. Altman M, Wilfley DE: Evidence update on the treatment of overweight and obesity in children and adolescents. *J Clin Child Adolesc Psychol* 44(4):521–537, 2015.
44. Dorsey S, McLaughlin KA, Kerns SE, et al.: Evidence base update for psychosocial treatments for children and adolescents exposed to traumatic events. *J Clin Child Adolesc Psychol* 1–28, 2016.
45. Evans SW, Owens JS, Bunford N: Evidence-based psychosocial treatments for children and adolescents with attention-deficit/hyperactivity disorder. *J Clin Child Adolesc Psychol* 43(4):527–551, 2014.
46. Hogue A, Henderson CE, Ozechowski TJ, Robbins MS: Evidence base on outpatient behavioral treatments for adolescent substance use: Updates and recommendations 2007–2013. *J Clin Child Adolesc Psychol* 43(5):695–720, 2014.
47. Lock J: An update on evidence-based psychosocial treatments for eating disorders in children and adolescents. *J Clin Child Adolesc Psychol* 44(5):707–21, 2015.
48. Smith T, Iadarola S: Evidence base update for autism spectrum disorder. *J Clin Child Adolesc Psychol* 44(6):897–922, 2015.
49. Chambless DL, Ollendick TH: Empirically supported psychological interventions: controversies and evidence. *Annu Rev Psychol* 52:685–716, 2001.
50. Freeman J, Garcia A, Frank H, et al.: Evidence base update for psychosocial treatments for pediatric obsessive-compulsive disorder. *J Clin Child Adolesc Psychol* 43(1):7–26, 2014.
51. Fristad MA, Macpherson HA: Evidence-based psychosocial treatments for child and adolescent bipolar spectrum disorders. *J Clin Child Adolesc Psychol* 43(3):339–355, 2014.
52. Glenn CR, Franklin JC, Nock MK: Evidence-based psychosocial treatments for self-injurious thoughts and behaviors in youth. *J Clin Child Adolesc Psychol* 44(1):1–29, 2015.
53. Henggeler SW, Lee T: Multisystemic treatment of serious clinical problems. In: Weisz JR, Kazdin AE (eds): *Evidence-Based Psychotherapies for Children and Adolescents*. New York, Guilford Press, 2003.
54. Alexander JF, Parsons BV: *Functional Family Therapy: Principles and Procedures*. Carmel, CA, Brooks/Cole, 1982.
55. National Institute of Mental Health: Blueprint for change: research on child and adolescent mental health. In: *Report of the National Advisory Mental Health Council's Workgroup on Child and Adolescent Mental Health Intervention Development and Deployment*. Rockville, MD, Department of Health and Human Services, 2001.
56. Office of the Surgeon General: *Mental Health: A Report of the Surgeon General*. Rockville, MD, Department of Health and Human Services, 1999.
57. President's New Freedom Commission on Mental Health: *Achieving the Promise: Transforming Mental Health Care in America*. Final report. Rockville, MD, Department of Health and Human Services, 2003.
58. National Institute for Health and Clinical Excellence: Published Clinical Guidelines, 2006. Available at: www.nice.org.uk/page.aspx?o=guidelines. Accessed July 3, 2006.
59. Department of Health and Human Services: National Training and Technical Assistance Center for Child and Adolescent Mental Health Cooperative Agreement (SM 04–002). 2004. Available at: http://alt.samhsa.gov/grants/2004/nofa/sm04–002infNTTAC.asp. Accessed March 17, 2006.
60. Department of Health and Human Services: State Implementation of Evidence-Based Practices II—Bridging Science and Service (RFA-MH-05–004). 2004. Available at: http://grants1.nih.gov/grants/fuide/rfa-files/RFA-MH-05–004.html. Accessed June 7, 2006.
61. Allen B, Gharagozloo L, Johnson JC: Clinician knowledge and utilization of empirically-supported treatments for maltreated children. *Child Maltreat* 17(1):11–21, 2012.
62. National Alliance for the Mentally Ill: An update on evidence-based practices in children's mental health. *NAMI Beginnings*. Issue 3, Fall 2003.
63. National Association of State Mental Health Program Directors: NASMHPD website listings: Available at: www.nasmhpd.org. Accessed July 3, 2006.
64. Weisz JR, Weiss B: Assessing the effects of clinic-based psychotherapy with children and adolescents. *J Consult Clin Psych* 57:741–746, 1989.
65. Weisz JR, Donenberg GR, Han SS, Weiss B: Bridging the gap between laboratory and clinic in child and adolescent psychotherapy. *J Consult Clin Psych* 63:688–701, 1995.
66. Weersing VR, Weisz JR, Donenberg GR: Development of the therapy procedures checklist: a therapist-report measure of technique use in child and adolescent treatment. *J Clin Child Adolesc Psychol* 31:168–180, 2002.
67. Kazdin AE, Siegel TC, Bass D: Drawing on clinical practice to inform research on child and adolescent psychotherapy: survey of practitioners. *Prof Psychol Res Pr* 21:189–198, 1990.
68. Weisz JR, Weiss B, Donenberg GR: The lab versus the clinic: effects of child and adolescent psychotherapy. *Am Psychol* 47:1578–1585, 1992.
69. Weiss B, Catron T, Harris V, Phung TM: The effectiveness of traditional child psychotherapy. *J Consult Clin Psych* 67:82–94, 1999.
70. Weiss B, Catron T, Harris V: A 2-year follow-up of the effectiveness of traditional child psychotherapy. *J Consult Clin Psych* 68:1094–1101, 2000.
71. Bickman L: A continuum of care: more is not always better. *Am Psychol* 51:689–701, 1996.
72. Bickman L, Noser K, Summerfelt WT: Long-term effects of a system of care on children and adolescents. *J Behav Health Serv Res* 26:185–202, 1999.
73. Bickman L, Lambert EW, Andrade AR, Penaloza RV: The Fort Bragg continuum of care for children and adolescents: mental health outcomes over 5 years. *J Consult Clin Psychol* 68:710–716, 2000.
74. Weisz JR, Han SS, Valeri, SM: More of what? Issues raised by the Fort Bragg study. *Am Psychol* 52:541–545, 1997.
75. Andrade AR, Lambert W, Bickman L: Dose effect in child psychotherapy: outcomes associated with negligible treatment. *J Am Acad Child Adolesc Psychiatry* 39:161–168, 2000.
76. Bickman L, Andrade AR, Lambert EW: Dose response in child and adolescent mental health services. *Ment Health Serv Res* 4:57–70, 2002.
77. Angold A, Costello JE, Burns BJ, Erkanli A, Farmer EM: The effectiveness of nonresidential specialty mental health services for children and adolescents in the "real world." *J Am Acad Child Adolesc Psychiatry* 39:154–160, 2000.
78. Bickman L: The death of treatment as usual: an excellent first step on a long road. *Clin Psychol Sci Pr* 9:195–199, 2002.
79. Clarke GN, Hawkins W, Murphy M, Sheeber LB, Lewinsohn PM, Seeley JR: Targeted prevention of unipolar depressive disorder in an at-risk sample of high school adolescents: a randomized trial of a group cognitive intervention. *J Am Acad Child Adolesc Psychiatry* 34:312–321, 1995.
80. Weisz JR, Thurber CA, Sweeney L, Proffitt VD, LeGagnoux GL: Brief treatment of mild-to-moderate child depression using primary and secondary control enhancement training. *J Consult Clin Psych* 65:703–707, 1997.
81. Butler L, Miezitis S, Friedman R, Cole E: The effect of two school-based intervention programs on depressive symptoms in preadolescents. *Am Educ Res J* 17:111–119, 1980.
82. Lewinsohn PM, Clarke GN, Hops H, et al.: Cognitive-behavioral treatment for depressed adolescents. *Behav Ther* 21:385–401, 1990.
83. Hammen C, Rudolph K, Weisz J, Rao U, Burge D: The context of depression in clinic-referred youth: neglected areas in treatment. *J Am Acad Child Adolesc Psychiatry* 38:64–71, 1999.
84. Brent DA, Kolko D, Birmaher B, et al.: Predictors of treatment efficacy in a clinical trial of three psychosocial treatments for adolescent depression. *J Am Acad Child Adolesc Psychiatry* 37:906–914, 1998.
85. Southam-Gerow MA, Weisz JR, Kendall, PC: Youth with anxiety disorders in research and service clinics: examining client differences and similarities. *J Clin Child Adolesc Psychol* 32:375–385, 2003.
86. Chamberlain P: *Treating Chronic Juvenile Offenders: Advances Made through the Oregon Multidimensional Treatment Foster Care Model*. Washington, DC, American Psychological Association, 2003.
87. Shadish WR, Matt GE, Navarro AM, et al.: Evidence that therapy works in clinically representative conditions. *J Consult Clin Psych* 65:355–365, 1997.
88. Shadish WR, Matt GE, Navarro AM, Phillips G: The effects of psychological therapies under clinically representative conditions: a metaanalysis. *Psychol Bull* 126:512–529, 2000.
89. Weisz JR, Kuppens S, Eckshtain D, Ugueto AM, Hawley KM, Jensen-doss A: Performance of evidence-based youth psychotherapies compared with usual clinical care: a multilevel meta-analysis. *JAMA Psychiatry* 70(7):750–761, 2013.
90. National Child Traumatic Stress Network: Child trauma home. Available at: http://www.nctsn.org. Accessed November 18, 2016.
91. National Crime Victims Research and Treatment Center: Department of Psychiatry and Behavioral Sciences, Medical University of South Carolina. TF-CBT Web: a web-based learning course for Trauma-Focused Cognitive Behavioral Therapy. Available at: https://tfcbt.musc.edu/. Published 2005. Accessed November 20, 2016.
92. Sigel BA, Kramer TL, Conners-Burrow NA, Church JK, Worley KB, Mitrani NA: Statewide dissemination of trauma-focused cognitive-behavioral therapy (TF-CBT). *Child Youth Serv Rev* 35:1023–1029, 2013.
93. Jensen TK, Holt T, Ormhaug SM, et al.: A randomized effectiveness study comparing trauma-focused cognitive behavioral therapy with therapy as usual for youth. *J Clin Child Adolesc Psychol* 43(3):356–369, 2014.
94. Murray, LK, Skavenski, S, Kane, JC, et al.: Effectiveness of trauma-focused cognitive behavioral therapy among trauma-affected children in Lusaka, Zambia: a randomized clinical trial. *JAMA Pediatr* 169:761–769, 2015.
95. O'Callaghan P, McMullen J, Shannon C, Rafferty H, Black A: A randomized controlled trial of trauma-focused cognitive behavioral therapy for sexually exploited, war-affected Congolese girls. *J AmAcad Child Adolesc Psychiatry* 52(4):359–369, 2013.
96. De arellano MA, Lyman DR, Jobe-Shields L, et al.: Trauma-focused cognitive-behavioral therapy for children and adolescents: assessing the evidence. *Psychiatr Serv* 65(5):591–602, 2014.
97. Kerfoot M, Harrington R, Harrington V, Rogers J, Verduyn C: A step too far? Randomized trial of cognitive-behaviour therapy delivered by social workers to depressed adolescents. *Eur Child Adolesc Psychiatry* 13(2):92–99, 2004.
98. Goodyer I, Dubicka B, Wilkinson P, et al.: Selective serotonin reuptake inhibitors (SSRIs) and routine specialist care with and without cognitive behaviour therapy in adolescents with major depression: randomised controlled trial. *BMJ* 335(7611):142, 2007.

99. Weisz JR, Southam-gerow MA, Gordis EB, et al.: Cognitive-behavioral therapy versus usual clinical care for youth depression: an initial test of transportability to community clinics and clinicians. *J Consult Clin Psychol* 77(3):383–396, 2009.
100. Asarnow JR, Jaycox LH, Duan N, et al.: Effectiveness of a quality improvement intervention for adolescent depression in primary care clinics: a randomized controlled trial. *JAMA* 293:311–319, 2005.
101. Richardson LP, Ludman E, McCauley E, et al.: Collaborative care for adolescents with depression in primary care: a randomized clinical trial. *JAMA* 312(8):809–816, 2014.
102. Clarke GN, Debar L, Lynch F, et al.: A randomized effectiveness trial of brief cognitive-behavioral therapy for depressed adolescents receiving anti-depressant medication. *J Am Acad Child Adolesc Psychiatry* 44:888–898, 2005.
103. Van De Weil NM, Matthys W, Cohen-Kettenis P, Van Engeland H: Application of the Utrecht Coping Power Program and care as usual to children with disruptive behavior disorders: a comparative study of cost and course of treatment. *Behav Ther* 34:421–436, 2003.
104. CRISP (Computer Retrieval of Information on Scientific Projects): Implementing parent management training in Norway (5R01DA016097). 2006. Available at: http://crisp.cit.nih.gov. Accessed July 3, 2006.
105. Ogden T, Hagen KA: Treatment effectiveness of Parent Management Training in Norway: a randomized controlled trial of children with conduct problems. *J Consult Clin Psychol* 76(4):607–621, 2008.
106. Tommeraas T, Ogden T: Is there a scale-up penalty? Testing behavioral change in the scaling up of parent management training in Norway. *Adm Policy Ment Health* 2015.
107. Forgatch MS, Kjøbli J: Parent management training-Oregon model: adapting intervention with rigorous research. *Fam Process* 55(3):500–513, 2016.
108. Borduin CM, Mann BJ, Cone LT, et al.: Multisystemic treatment of serious juvenile offenders: long-term prevention of criminality and violence. *J Consult Clin Psychol* 63:569–578, 1995.
109. Henggeler SW, Melton GB, Smith LA: Family preservation using multisystemic therapy: an effective alternative to incarcerating serious juvenile offenders. *J Consult Clin Psychol* 60:953–961, 1992.
110. Henggeler SW, Rowland MD, Pickrel SG, et al.: Investigating family-based alternatives to institution-based mental health services for youth: Lessons learned from the pilot study of a randomized field trial. *J Clin Child Psychol* 26:226–233, 1997.
111. Henggeler SW, Pickrel SG, Brondino MJ: Multisystemic treatment of substance-abusing and dependent delinquents: outcomes, treatment fidelity, and transportability. *Ment Health Serv Res* 1:171–184, 1999.
112. Henggeler SW, Rowland MD, Randall J, et al.: Home-based multisystemic therapy as an alternative to the hospitalization of youth in psychiatric crisis: clinical outcome. *J Am Acad Child Adolesc Psychiatry* 38:1331–1339, 1999.
113. Henggeler SW: Decreasing effect sizes for effectiveness studies—implications for the transport of evidence-based treatments: comment on Curtis, Ronan and Borduin (2004). *J Fam Psychol* 18:420–423, 2004.
114. Curtis NM, Ronan KR, Borduin CM: Multisystemic treatment: a meta-analysis of outcome studies. *J Fam Psychol* 18:411–419, 2004.
115. Schoenwald SK, Sheidow AJ, Letourneau EJ: Toward effective quality assurance in evidence-based practice: links between expert consultation, therapist fidelity, and child outcomes. *J Clin Child Adolesc Psychol* 33:94–104, 2004.
116. Schoenwald SK, Sheidow AJ, Letournea EJ, et al.: Transportability of multisystemic therapy: evidence for multilevel influences. *Ment Health Serv Res* 5:223–239, 2003.
117. Henggeler SW, Schoenwald SK, Liao JG, Letourneau EJ, Edwards DL: Transporting efficacious treatments to field settings: the link between supervisory practices and therapist fidelity in MST programs. *J Clin Child Adolesc Psychol* 13:155–167, 2002.
118. Lofholm CA, Eichas K, Sundell K: The Swedish implementation of multisystemic therapy for adolescents: does treatment experience predict treatment adherence. *J Clin Child Adolesc Psychol* 43:643–655, 2014.
119. Weiss B, Han S, Harris V, et al.: An independent randomized clinical trial of multisystemic therapy with non-court-referred adolescents with serious conduct problems. *J Consult Clin Psychol* 81(6):1027–1039, 2013.
120. Kolko DJ, Hoagwood KE, Springgate B: Treatment research for children and youth exposed to traumatic events: moving beyond efficacy to amp up public health impact. *Gen Hosp Psychiatry* 32(5):465–476, 2010.
121. Weersing VR, Weisz JR. Mechanisms of action in youth psychotherapy. *J Child Psychol Psychiatry* 43:3–29, 2002.
122. Treadwell KR, Kendall PC: Self-talk in youth with anxiety disorders, content specificity and, treatment outcome. *J Consult Clin Psych* 64:941–950, 1996.
123. Kolko D, Brent D, Baugher M, Bridge J, Birmaher B: Cognitive and family therapies for adolescent depression: Treatment specificity, mediation and moderation. *J Consult Clin Psych* 68:603–614, 2000.
124. Patterson GR, Forgatch MS: Predicting future clinical adjustment from treatment outcome and process variables. *Psychol Assessment* 7:275–285, 1995.
125. Eddy MJ, Chamberlain P: Family management and deviant peer association as mediators of the impact of treatment condition on youth antisocial behavior. *J Consult Clin Psych* 68:857–863, 2000.
126. Huey SJ, Henggeler SW, Brondino, MJ, Pickrel SG: Mechanisms of change in multisystemic therapy: reducing delinquent behavior through therapist adherence and improved family and peer functioning. *J Consult Clin Psych* 68:451–467, 2000.
127. Guerra NG, Slaby RG: Cognitive mediators of aggression in adolescent offenders: 2. Intervention. *Dev Psychol* 26:269–277, 1990.
128. Maric M, Prins PJ, Ollendick TH: *Moderators and Mediators of Youth Treatment Outcomes.* USA, Oxford University Press, 2015.
129. Weersing VR, Schwartz KT, Bolano CA: Moderators and mediators of treatments for youth with depression. In: Maric M, Prins PJM, Ollendick TH (eds): *Moderators and Mediators of Youth Treatment Outcomes.* USA, Oxford University Press, 2015.
130. Kendall PC, Cummings CM, Villabø MA, et al.: Mediators of change in the child/adolescent anxiety multimodal treatment study. *J Consult Clin Psychol* 84(1):1–14, 2016.
131. Kendall PC, Treadwell KR: The role of self-statements as a mediator in treatment for youth with anxiety disorders. *J Consult Clin Psychol* 75(3):380–389, 2007.
132. Caspi A, Sugden K, Moffitt TE, et al.: Influence of life stress on depression: moderation by a polymorphism in the 5-HTT gene. *Science* 301:386–389, 2003.
133. Kaufman J, Yang B, Douglas-Palumberi H, et al.: Brain-derived neurotrophic factor-5-HHTLPR gene interactions and environmental modifiers of depression in children. *Biol Psychiatry* 59:673–680, 2006.

CHAPTER 6.2.2 ■ COGNITIVE AND BEHAVIORAL THERAPIES

MENDY BOETTCHER MINJAREZ, RACHEL A. MONTAGUE, EMILY A. FOX, AND JOHN PIACENTINI

INTRODUCTION

Cognitive-behavioral therapy (CBT) is one of the most widely researched and evidence-based forms of psychotherapy today. Although CBT technically refers to a group of therapeutic interventions employing an integrated approach to both behavior and cognition, this chapter also covers interventions addressing each of these domains in a relatively isolated fashion (behavior therapy and cognitive therapy, respectively; all collectively referred to hereinafter as CBT). CBT can be differentiated from other psychotherapeutic approaches by its historical roots in experimental and learning psychology and by its ongoing emphasis on experimental validation of efficacy and treatment mechanisms. Over the past decades, CBT has rapidly progressed from a specialized intervention to a mainstream therapeutic approach that is now a mandated part of psychiatric residency training in the United States (1–3). This widespread acceptance is due in no small part to the fact that CBT is, by design, a problem-based, short-term, and contextually relevant treatment approach.

BACKGROUND AND HISTORY

Cognitive Therapy Foundations

Cognitive therapies are based on the notion that it is not events, but people's interpretations of events, that cause psychological disturbance. As such, therapy from a cognitive perspective focuses on identifying and changing people's cognitions as a way of changing their feelings and reducing psychological distress.

Behavior Therapy Foundations

When working within a purely behavioral framework, overt behavior is typically the primary concern or symptom. "Overt behavior that one can see" (4) is targeted through a variety of intervention strategies, and behavioral changes are thought to influence thoughts and feelings. Setting concrete goals and measuring specific behaviors is an integral part of this approach and is considered the primary means of evaluating progress and outcomes.

Cognitive-Behavior Therapy Foundations

Behavioral difficulties and other symptoms of disorders often result from a complicated interaction among thoughts, feelings, and behaviors. As such, treatment will often include both cognitive and behavioral techniques. For example, when trying to understand a behavior, it is possible that antecedents and consequences are covert, rather than overt. Covert variables are often internal and consist of cognitions or emotions. Thorough analysis of a behavior that involves covert variables will require that the clinician obtain detailed information about the patient's thoughts and feelings before and after the observable behavior. It has also been noted that while traditional behaviorists believe that changes in behavior result in changes in thoughts and feelings, this relationship can be reversed, such that changes in thoughts and feelings result in behavioral changes (4). As such, many symptoms and disorders are more thoroughly addressed by the combination of cognitive and behavioral techniques that is known as CBT.

COGNITIVE-BEHAVIORAL MODEL

Escape or Avoidance Conditioning

Much of CBT is based on gaining an understanding of why negative thoughts and beliefs persist and why behavioral cycles do not get broken over time. For example, it has been proposed that avoidance, escape, and safety-seeking behaviors (5) maintain anxiety because the individual does not have the opportunity to disconfirm beliefs by experiencing that the anticipated negative outcome does not occur when avoidance or escape is not allowed. Instead, they are led to believe that they did not experience danger because they made a good decision to avoid or escape. People who do not avoid situations may engage in other types of behaviors (safety-seeking behaviors) that allow them to believe that danger was avoided. For example, individuals who engage in compulsions in obsessive-compulsive disorder (OCD) are led to believe that their obsessive thought did not result in a negative outcome because they engaged in the compulsive behavior. Similarly, individuals who "take it slow" to prevent a heart attack in panic disorder believe that they did not have a heart attack because they modified their activity level. In these examples, individuals erroneously believe they prevented the feared situation from occurring by engaging in certain behaviors. Through this cycle, the preventative behaviors are reinforced, which confirms in the individual's mind that the anxiety was legitimate.

Attention-Related Factors

It has also been proposed that attentional factors play a role in disorders that can be treated using a cognitive-behavioral model. For example, individuals with anxiety disorders, depression, and other disorders that involve disturbance in cognitions often selectively attend to cues that confirm or exacerbate their condition (6–8). For example, individuals with social phobia may be overly attentive to negative cues from others at the expense of positive cues, and individuals with panic disorder may attend closely to bodily sensations, which they then interpret as dangerous.

Cognitive Images

Cognitive images are often examined when viewing a disorder from a cognitive-behavioral perspective. Images of distressing events are common among all individuals; however, in individuals with pathology, these images are interpreted as signs of danger. For example, individuals with OCD may believe that thinking about hurting someone increases the likelihood that it will happen. As a result, they believe that something must be done to prevent the danger. Similarly, in posttraumatic stress disorder (PTSD), intrusive memories may frequently occur and are interpreted as a sign that recurrence of the trauma is likely.

Memory Processes

Memory processes may also play a role in disorders. For example, anxious individuals may have a tendency to recall situations that confirm their anxiety, such as a person with social phobia who recalls situations in which he or she performed poorly, but not those where he or she performed successfully. Finally, rumination may perpetuate and enhance fear (5). That is, thinking about an event may lead to the interpretation that the event is more likely to occur. Further, selective attention for negative past events may lead to the perception that they are more likely to happen again in the future. In contrast to some forms of cognitive treatment that involve reliving an event through imagery, rumination does not focus on constructive reprocessing of events. Rather, it focuses on elaboration that makes the event more abstract and, therefore, threatening. For example, an individual with PTSD may persistently ruminate about the event, while asking, "What else could I have done?" without realistically considering the limits of what a person is capable of doing.

Behavioral Conditioning

Many symptoms are also conceptualized as being caused or maintained by behavioral conditioning. Two types of conditioning may occur. In *classical conditioning* (9), a stimulus (unconditioned stimulus) that elicits a reflexive response (unconditioned response) is paired with a stimulus (conditioned stimulus) that initially elicits no response, but, over repeated trials, comes to elicit the same response as the original unconditioned stimulus (e.g., Pavlov's classic study where dogs learned to salivate in response to a bell that had been paired with the smell of meat powder (9)). Phobias typically develop through a classical conditioning paradigm, as stimuli, which were previously neutral, are paired with a traumatic event, leading to future avoidance of stimuli related to that event. The subsequent avoidance behavior does not allow extinction to occur, thus, the phobia is maintained.

The classical conditioning paradigm is often used to explain other phenomena, such as emotional responses, addictions, and psychosomatic disorders. As a result, many treatments for these disorders are based on the notion of classical extinction. Extinction occurs once the connection between the conditioned stimulus and the response has been established and the conditioned stimulus is then presented repeatedly without the unconditioned stimulus (e.g., the bell is presented without the meat powder). When this occurs, the conditioned response will decay over time because the reflexively reinforcing stimulus is no longer available. Therapy techniques that are associated with classical conditioning and classical extinction include counterconditioning, systematic desensitization, covert sensitization, and exposure and response prevention (ERP).

Principles of *operant conditioning* are based on the work of B.F. Skinner (10,11), who demonstrated that new behaviors could be shaped through reinforcement (a behavior followed by a positive consequence is likely to occur again) and its subsequent removal (when reinforcement is removed, the behavior will decline, or extinguish, over time). Principles of operant conditioning also often maintain symptoms (e.g., negative behaviors that are reinforced by maladaptive parenting cycles in attention-deficit hyperactivity disorder [ADHD] and behavioral disorders; food restriction is reinforced by weight loss in eating disorders). These principles are also often used in cognitive-behavioral treatment, as reinforcement can be used to increase or strengthen positive or adaptive behaviors, while punishment and extinction can be used to decrease negative or maladaptive behaviors.

CLINICAL CONSIDERATIONS IN USE OF CBT WITH CHILDREN AND ADOLESCENTS

Generally speaking, the patient–therapist relationship in CBT treatment has been referred to as one of "collaborative empiricism" (12–15). This relationship is characterized by a high degree of collaboration and a "scientific attitude" (13,16,17) toward testing the validity and accuracy of the patient's cognitions and behaviors. That is, the cognitive-behavioral therapist typically works as a team with the patient to examine and understand thoughts, feelings, and behaviors. This is done by developing hypotheses about thoughts and behaviors, collecting data on those thoughts and behaviors, examining patterns, and generating alternative, more adaptive, ways of thinking and behaving.

When working with children and families, however, certain factors must be taken into consideration with regard to this model. For example, children may have difficulty reporting on their thoughts, feelings, and behaviors. Further, parent and family thoughts, feelings, and behaviors may influence those of the child. As a result, the following areas are briefly examined with regard to engaging in cognitive-behavioral treatments with children and families.

Developmental Perspective

Adopting a developmental perspective when working with children and adolescents is critical for effective intervention planning. Several developmental considerations are suggested for use when doing CBT with children. First, the child's level of autonomy and independence must be taken into consideration. The child's autonomy is important both in terms of giving older children and adolescents enough autonomy in setting and following through with their treatment goals, and in making sure that younger children have enough support from parents and other involved individuals. As such, it is also important to consider what other individuals or systems are involved in the child's life and what their role should be in therapy. Further analysis of how other individuals and other family or systems variables may be maintaining the child's difficulties is an important clinical consideration. That is, families, schools, and other systems may have adapted to a child's symptoms in ways that actually maintain, rather than decrease, the difficulties. Parent, teacher, and other adult-focused training is often necessary in addition to individual therapy sessions with the child (4). Involvement of these individuals may also facilitate practice and generalization in the natural environment, which produces more rapid and enduring effects than treatment that only occurs during therapy sessions.

Adapting CBT treatment concepts to the appropriate developmental level is important as well. For example, efforts to address the cognitive biases and distortions underlying a number of psychiatric disorders (e.g., anxiety, depression) can be complicated by the lack of strong abstract thinking skills in most young children. To address this limitation, multiple strategies have been developed to concretize target cognitions and abstract concepts (18). For example, symptoms can be characterized as persona that the child can relate to, such as the "Bad Thought Monster" who must be conquered (19). Similarly, obsessions in OCD can be understood as external and can be blamed on a pesky bug, named "OC Flea" (20), whose ideas must be resisted. Children can also be encouraged to play the role of detective or to team up with a detective in testing assumptions and beliefs (19). These types of developmentally appropriate adaptations assist children in understanding concepts that are otherwise verbally explained in therapy with adults, which may exceed the developmental capacity of children.

With very young children, cognitive-behavioral play therapy (CBPT) may be indicated, as it embeds cognitive-behavioral strategies into play-based interactions (21,22). As young children may have difficulty understanding concepts in CBT, CBPT allows teaching and therapeutic work to occur in play. The primary mechanism for teaching concepts is modeling, which has been shown to be effective in teaching new behaviors (23). Many different CBT concepts can be modeled with puppets or other toys, such as demonstrating that a puppet gets over his fear gradually the more he enters into a situation. CBPT also involves some adult administration of CBT concepts, such as scheduling activities for a withdrawn child.

Other developmental considerations include the child's age, language level, cognitive ability, and the intensity, duration, and frequency of the symptoms. It has been suggested that younger children benefit more from behavioral techniques than cognitive ones, especially because they often have difficulty reporting cognitions that accompany symptoms and behaviors. Cognitive techniques that younger children have benefited from include relaxation training, imagery, and positive self-talk. Children over the age of 9 are thought to have increased capacity for reporting and understanding cognitions and may begin to benefit from more sophisticated cognitive aspects of treatment. Each child must be individually evaluated, however, as other factors, such as language level, may cause cognitive techniques to be difficult for older children, as well.

Family-Related Factors

The Role of Families and Other Systems in Cognitions and Behaviors

Because CBT interventions place an emphasis on antecedents and consequences of behaviors, avoidance behaviors that maintain symptoms, and other factors that may be affected by the environment, the role of family and other relevant systems is critical in assessment and treatment planning in CBT (24,25). Depending on the nature of the symptoms, it is likely that others in the child's life are making accommodations that support and maintain, rather than discourage, the maladaptive behaviors (26). For example, in a child with OCD, the family may tolerate extensive rituals that interfere with daily routines to avoid temper tantrums that might result from setting limits on ritualistic behavior (27,28). As such, careful analysis of the child's symptoms within family, school, and other relevant contexts is critical for CBT treatment planning with children and adolescents.

Parent/Family Involvement in Therapy

Families play a pivotal role in therapy for children in several ways. First, it is often important to have information about family context and parental cognitions, emotions, and behaviors to better understand the child's symptoms within a cognitive-behavioral framework. Changes in family routines, dynamics, and discipline practices may be critical in facilitating changes in individual child-focused symptoms. Young children, in particular, may need ongoing assistance from parents and other relevant adults to follow through with treatment goals and homework. Moreover, with older children, families may need to learn to allow the child or adolescent to take responsibility for treatment goals and homework, which may require the family to decrease their level of involvement. These factors must be considered when deciding whether to work with a child individually, a parent individually, or with the child in conjunction with family members.

Older children and adolescents often attend therapy sessions individually, and parents are informed during the latter portion of the session about session content and subsequent homework that is to occur between sessions. It is sometimes necessary to work individually with parents, however, especially with young children who are having behavioral difficulties.

Finally, the child's symptoms are often a significant source of family stress and parent–child conflict. In these cases, it can be beneficial to work individually with the child and/or the parents. It is sometimes helpful to instruct that parents not remind their child about therapy homework and treatment goals, rather that performance be evaluated by the child and the therapist during sessions. This tactic can be useful in decreasing negative parent–child interactions, especially with adolescents, until symptoms have decreased.

GENERALIZATION AND MAINTENANCE

Three types of generalization are important to consider in CBT interventions with children. These are (a) generalization across settings; (b) generalization across functional domains (behavior, cognitions); and (c) generalization over time, which is termed maintenance. Generalization and maintenance must be considered with regard to intervention strategies, as well as improvements in functioning. That is, for successful change, the patient must use the techniques learned in session across settings, learn to apply them to a variety of domains, and continue to use them over time for as long as necessary. Similarly, when change begins to occur, it is important that the change is observed across settings (not just in the therapy setting), that change in multiple domains occurs, and that the change is maintained over time.

Kendall and Lochman (29) propose several strategies for promoting generalization and maintenance of improvements in functioning when using CBT strategies with children. First, rewarding behavior change using attainable goals that are applied across an increasing number of settings over time may be useful. These goals should be reinforced in each successive setting, and reinforcement should only be faded when the behavioral change appears stable and lasting.

Treatment length is also an important consideration in programming for maintenance of changes made in therapy. A period of 3 to 6 months is most common (13); however, it has been suggested that 6 months or longer may be most effective. It has also been suggested that length of treatment over time may be more important than the number of sessions (30), and intensity may be an important factor, as well (31). Thase et al. (13) suggested that unsuccessful therapy should generally not continue beyond 12 to 16 weeks for outpatients. Use of behavioral rehearsal (e.g., role playing) to emphasize use of techniques in specific situations has also been proposed as an important mechanism for generalization of skills. That is, once a child has learned the concept of a skill, the likelihood that the skill will be used outside therapy in an actual situation is increased if the child has had opportunities to practice it under low demand, low stress circumstances. Role-plays can then be used to assist the child in refining skills to fit increasingly specific situations.

Finally, generalization is promoted when the child is taught skills that apply to multiple behaviors and situations, such as problem-solving processes, rather than specific behaviors. For example, self-instruction training has been proposed as a means of promoting generalization of skills, especially across settings and behaviors. Because self-instruction training involves having the child learn a series of steps in self-instruction of positive decision-making, this skill is considered more flexible than a series of specific steps that apply to a specific situation. In this way, the child can apply the steps to multiple problems in multiple settings.

Although these techniques may be helpful in generalizing skills across settings and over time, long-term data on such procedures are limited, especially with children. The mean duration of follow-up data is 5 to 7 months' posttreatment (32–35), with little available data to indicate outcomes over longer periods of time.

COURSE OF THERAPY

General Characteristics of CBT Treatment Plans

Some general aspects of treatment are characteristic of CBT regardless of diagnosis, age, developmental level, or other individual qualities, and are important for the patient to understand at the outset of treatment. According to Thase et al. (13), these are (1) the patient will be an active participant in trying new strategies; (2) the patient will be expected to complete homework; (3) therapy outcomes will be measured via data collection, and techniques will be modified if they are unsuccessful; (4) the therapist will actively guide treatment; (5) therapy will be time-limited; and (6) treatment strategies will be empirically based. When working with children, families may need to be incorporated in these treatment components. For example, it may be that the child and the parents must be active participants, rather than the patient alone.

CBTs are generally characterized by three phases of treatment. In the initial stage, the nature of the patient's presenting problem is assessed, rapport is established, and psychoeducation (described later) occurs to prepare the patient for the active phase of treatment. Once the symptoms, related variables, and cognitive and emotional characteristics have been identified, a treatment plan is developed. This plan typically begins with psychoeducation of the patient about symptoms, cognitive behavioral understanding of those symptoms, and rationale for treatment. In the middle phase, active treatment occurs, which involves the acquisition, application, and mastery of cognitive-behavioral treatment strategies. This phase involves regular treatment sessions, as well as consistent homework. Over the course of treatment, goals and hypotheses about symptoms are re-evaluated and modified, as necessary, on an ongoing basis. The middle phase tapers off when symptomatic relief has occurred and the patient appears ready for maintenance and relapse prevention.

The final phase focuses on generalization and maintenance of techniques and relapse prevention. During this phase, the treatment schedule is thinned and the patient assumes greater responsibility for implementation of techniques on an ongoing basis. Finally, as necessary, "booster sessions" may occur after treatment has been completed to ensure that long-term changes are maintained.

Frequency and Duration of Treatment

CBT sessions typically occur once or twice per week in an outpatient setting. Generally speaking, it is important that enough time elapses between sessions for homework exercises to be meaningful. In inpatient settings, sessions may occur as frequently as once per day; however, the severity of illness is generally proportional to the frequency of sessions in such cases (i.e., the child is significantly ill to warrant daily monitoring and practicing of techniques). In general, it is recommended that the therapist decide on a case-by-case basis whether sessions should occur any more than once per week, as with any type of therapeutic intervention.

With some exceptions, CBT typically occurs over a 3- to 6-month period, with some type of tapering period near the final termination of therapy (13). Using clinical judgment, it is generally recommended that a tapering strategy be used in termination due to the need for generalization of techniques learned in therapy. That is, once termination has occurred, patients will be required to continue using strategies learned in therapy. Tapering the therapy can be a helpful way to monitor the patient's success in using the techniques on an ongoing basis over increasing periods of time.

It is not uncommon for patients to require a brief "booster" session(s) after termination has occurred. In such cases, patients' use of previously learned CBT techniques may have declined, or new unanticipated situations may have arisen that have resulted in a reoccurrence of symptoms. Frequently, patients do not require an additional full course of therapy; rather, they can benefit from one or several sessions to "refresh" their skills or to assist them with application of their skills to new problems.

Assessment for Treatment Planning

CBT treatment for any disorder must begin with a thorough assessment of the patient's cognitive, behavioral, and emotional symptoms. Assessments should address detailed information about the patient's symptoms (chief complaint) and identification of maintaining factors. Normalization of the patient's problems can be an important therapeutic aspect of the assessment phase, which may lead to immediate symptomatic relief. The goal of this phase should be to develop a cognitive-behavioral model of the presenting problem that can be used to guide treatment. Depending on the chief complaint, the initial assessment may include the following types of information:

- Descriptions of when the symptoms occur (time, place, circumstances, antecedents, consequences)
- Cognitions that accompany each symptom (may be different for different symptoms)
- Behaviors that accompany each symptom (may be different for different symptoms)
- Emotions that occur with each symptom (may be different for different symptoms)
- If cognitions and behaviors relieve symptoms, detailed description of how this occurs
- Information about factors that help or exacerbate the symptoms
- Maintaining variables: avoidance, escape, safety behaviors, attention/focus, dysfunctional/faulty beliefs, automatic thoughts
- Overall beliefs (cognitive schemas) that lead to cognitions, behavior, and feelings
- Previous treatment and treatment outcome
- Onset: including any possible causal factors that are not maintaining factors (e.g., traumatic event in PTSD, negative situation paired with stimuli in specific phobias)

It may be helpful to have the patient describe a recent event in detail, while asking specific questions to elicit information about thoughts, feelings, and behaviors (e.g., "What were you thinking when that happened?" or "How did your body feel at that moment?"). Sometimes it is difficult to elicit enough explicit information from children during a session, and homework is required as part of the assessment phase. Such homework might include writing down thoughts, feelings, and behaviors when certain events occur if the patient has difficulty reporting in session. It might also include having the patient or parent self-monitor the frequency of symptoms and associated variables. Once this initial assessment is complete, the patient's symptoms can be framed and described in terms of a cognitive-behavioral model and treatment can begin with psychoeducation.

Psychoeducation

Cognitive-behavioral interventions typically begin with some form of psychoeducation, which often continues throughout treatment. Psychoeducation is particularly important because many of the techniques utilized in CBT are driven by theoretical or empirical underpinnings that, when understood, allow the patient to better grasp *why* such techniques are being used and *how* change will occur, thus increasing motivation and follow-through. When working with children and adolescents, psychoeducation often occurs separately for children and their parents. This way, parents can have a more in-depth understanding of their child's treatment plan and children's psychoeducation can be developmentally appropriate to their age and cognitive level.

Psychoeducation may be conducted using a variety of procedures. Symptoms and related variables may be explained to individuals, and basic concepts may also be demonstrated. For example, when in the early stages of teaching patients that thoughts do not increase the likelihood of events occurring, *behavioral experiments* to demonstrate this point may be helpful (e.g., have the patient think about making someone else in the room stand up to demonstrate that the thought does not cause the event to occur). Bibliotherapy and Cognitive-Behavioral Play Therapy techniques may also be helpful, with young children in particular, to illustrate concepts and to educate about symptoms. These techniques may be particularly useful for young children who are resistant to change, as the focus is initially on the symptoms of the characters in the story or play, as opposed to the patient.

Psychoeducation often covers a variety of topic areas, as well. For many disorders, it is important to educate the individual about *physiologic* symptoms, which can lead to an immediate reduction in anxiety as they learn that such symptoms are normal and do not represent serious health or physical risk. Education about *cognitive* symptoms is typically relevant, as well, such as teaching a patient with PTSD that intrusive memories are normal reactions to traumatic experiences, or teaching patients with OCD that intrusive thoughts are common in the general population. Education about the *connection between thoughts and events* may also be relevant during this phase. Patients who have specific beliefs about the connection between thoughts and events need to begin to learn that such connections do not exist. Thought–action fusion (TAF), an OCD-related phenomenon characterized as the belief that thinking about a despicable act is as morally wrong as actually doing it, is one example of the kinds of irrational cognitions that need to be addressed in treatment (36). Behavioral experiments (discussed above) may be helpful when educating about this topic. Psychoeducation may also include identification of past experiences that disprove the patient's dysfunctional beliefs. Finally, once the patient is educated about symptoms, education about the rationale and plan for treatment must occur. Understanding the connection between the cognitive behavioral model of the symptoms and the rationale for treatment can be particularly important, as it can have an important effect on motivation and follow-through in treatment.

Middle Phase of Treatment

Once assessment and psychoeducation are complete, the middle, and the most active, phase of treatment begins. This phase typically involves ongoing active participation in therapy, as well as homework. Homework often must be completed on a daily basis. Goals and content of therapy sessions during this phase will vary widely depending on the chief complaint. Some general CBT techniques commonly utilized during this phase are discussed later in this section. More information about the active phase of treatment can also be found under the discussion of specific disorders. During the active phase of treatment, significant symptom reduction should occur.

Termination and Relapse Prevention

Once symptoms are substantially reduced, therapist and patient must begin planning for termination. This phase of therapy involves concrete planning in several areas when using CBT. First, programming for generalization and maintenance must be considered, as discussed earlier. Ideally, active phase intervention was planned to target generalization of skills. The schedule of therapy sessions is also often thinned during this time to promote maintenance of therapeutic changes with decreasing therapist support. Finally, relapse prevention must be addressed to ensure that changes endure over time. Relapse prevention strategies may include a cognitive framework for thinking about brief relapses (37,38), such as helping patients to identify antecedents to relapse behaviors and to think about them in ways that do not lead to total loss of treatment gains. Another common relapse prevention strategy is the use of "booster sessions." Should previous symptoms return or new ones emerge, one or a small number of sessions is often enough to assist the patient in returning to their termination level of functioning.

CBT TECHNIQUES

Cognitive Restructuring

Cognitive strategies are the primary components of CBT interventions (39). Commonly used cognitive strategies focus on restructuring dysfunctional cognitions and intervening on automatic thoughts and their underlying schemas. Automatic thoughts are defined as "cognitions that stream rapidly through an individual's mind" (13). Such thoughts can be spontaneous or in response to stimuli, a situation, or other antecedent. Individuals with automatic thoughts typically do not question them for believability. That is, individuals believe that because the thoughts are present they are true or valid. Such thoughts occur with increased intensity and frequency in disorders such as anxiety, depression, and OCD. Automatic thoughts may be valid worries (e.g., about events that have happened or actually could happen) or they may contain cognitive errors or distortions. Common cognitive errors are identified and described in Table 6.2.2.1.

The following cognitive strategies are commonly used to assess and intervene in automatic thoughts and cognitive errors in CBT.

Identifying Automatic Thoughts

Assessment of automatic thoughts does not always rely on interview techniques, especially with children, who may have difficulty understanding and reporting specific thoughts. Techniques such as imagery and role playing can be helpful in identifying automatic thoughts because they set the scene for an event or situation in which specific questions can be asked. For example, when asked to role play a situation, a child can be asked while acting out the scenario what he or she is thinking, feeling, etc. Such exercises are less hypothetical for children, which often help them generate important information that they cannot report during an interview.

Thought recording is another technique that can be used in a similar fashion. This technique is a form of self-monitoring in which events, thoughts, and feelings are recorded on a daily basis. Self-monitoring is a helpful way to assess automatic thoughts, as it does not rely on recollection of thoughts in a specific situation; rather, it requires that the individual record thoughts as they occur or immediately following an event. Although children often require reminders and assistance from adults to keep this type of data on a daily basis, this technique can be developmentally appropriate, as it does not rely on children's memories to assess cognitions.

Socratic Questioning/Examining the Evidence

Socratic questioning is discussed as an important part of CBT, and is one of the main components of cognitive restructuring. This technique involves questioning the patient with the goal of eliciting automatic thoughts and calling their validity into question. During this process, thoughts are considered to be hypotheses, rather than truths, and the patient is taught to determine and evaluate evidence for and against automatic thoughts. This technique is an important way to begin

TABLE 6.2.2.1

COMMON COGNITIVE ERRORS TO TARGET IN COGNITIVE RESTRUCTURING

Cognitive Error	Description	Example
Catastrophizing	Placing unrealistic importance on thoughts and events and assuming terrible negative outcomes will occur as a result	"I got a C on my report card, so I will never get into college and I will fail in life."
Magnifying/minimizing	Placing an inaccurate amount of importance on thoughts, feelings, events (either too much or too little)	Believing getting caught doing drugs is not important because the implications of having a drug problem are too anxiety provoking (minimizing)
Absolutism (black and white thinking)	All events and experiences are thought of in extreme categories, rather than moderately	"I will *never* lose any weight because I just ate a cookie."
Personalization	Attributing responsibility for external events to the self with no basis for the attribution	"It is my fault that my parents are getting divorced."
Selective abstraction	Taking information out of context and ignoring relevant details	Thinking "my soccer coach hates me" when the coach did not play the child, even though the child has been played first during the last three games
Arbitrary inference	Making arbitrary conclusions contrary to or without evidence	Believing homework is too hard when in fact the child completed the same work that day in class
Ignoring evidence	Leaving out important information when forming thoughts about events	Believing there is high probability of a home invasion, in spite of the fact that this has never occurred, and all doors in the house are locked
Overgeneralization	Believing the outcome of one situation applies in many situations, when it may not	"All my teachers hate me" when one teacher yelled at the child at school
Attending to negative features of events	Placing greater cognitive importance on negative features of events and ignoring positive features	Focusing on one poor grade when all others were good

teaching children that thoughts are not true simply because they occur. This technique may be especially helpful with distorted thoughts because rational consideration of evidence increases the patient's awareness that such thoughts are not grounded in reality.

Once automatic thoughts have been called into question, the therapist and patient can begin to revise them based on evidence and reality, and can generate new coping thoughts that are more accurate. Examining the evidence can be helpful when combined with self-monitoring because it forces the patient to examine the evidence each time they have a maladaptive thought. This repetition is often helpful in changing a patient's beliefs over time, as thoughts are constantly being challenged and new coping thoughts can be generated throughout the day.

Correcting Misinterpretations

Socratic questioning may also be helpful in correcting misinterpretations. Individuals with anxiety and depression, in particular, may misinterpret events, the behavior of others, thoughts, feelings, and other stimuli. Calling into question an individual's interpretation and noting how it impacts thoughts, feelings, and behaviors can be an important aspect of cognitive restructuring, as well.

For example, a client may say, "I had a horrible day, I messed up my class presentation, and everyone thinks I'm stupid." A clinician may respond by asking, "What evidence supports your report? Are you basing your interpretation on your classmates' facial expressions? Did they boo you off the stage? Is it possible there are other explanations for what you saw? Could your classmates have been smiling during your presentation because they wanted to encourage you, rather than to make fun of you? Could someone who looked bored really just be sleepy at the end of a long day? What evidence can you come up with that disproves your interpretation of the events or that people think you are stupid? Weren't you just picked to be the math club captain? How can you, on the one hand, be a leader and, on the other, be stupid?"

Modification of Imagery

Anxious patients, in particular, often have cognitive imagery associated with their symptoms (e.g., imagery associated with a feared or traumatic event). Such patients may benefit from modification of such imagery, such as by identifying aspects of it that are exaggerated. Patients may also benefit from learning to continue the image through to a positive outcome. That is, negative or anxiety-producing images often stop at the height of the crisis in a patient's mind (5), and never come to a positive or adaptive resolution. For example, the images end when the patient has passed out, embarrassed himself in public, or helplessly experienced the traumatic event. Therefore, helping the patient continue the image to a positive resolution (e.g., getting up off the floor after fainting, making statements to others when embarrassed, modifying the outcome of a traumatic event) can be an important exercise in decreasing anxiety and catastrophic thinking. Role-playing exercises may serve a similar role, as they allow the patient an opportunity to understand an event in a new way, with the assistance of a therapist, and then to experience a new, more adaptive, outcome (known as behavioral rehearsal).

Altering Core Beliefs

In addition to identifying automatic thoughts, CBT focuses on the more complex task of identifying the core beliefs, or cognitive schemas, that underlie those thoughts. That is, the thought is typically generated because the individual has an underlying belief about him/herself, which is typically maladaptive. For example, a child who has to complete homework perfectly for fear of being thought stupid may have the automatic thought, "If I don't write that sentence with perfect handwriting, everyone will know I am stupid." Core beliefs that may underlie such a thought could include, "I am stupid" or "Stupid kids are unlovable; therefore, no one loves me." Understanding these core beliefs is important for relapse prevention in particular, as modification of automatic thoughts will generally be temporary if the underlying belief or schema is not addressed.

Modification of the child's existing cognitive structures or schemas is an important way to decrease automatic thoughts and cognitive distortions, increase adaptive thoughts, and promote coping (13,29). Through use of many of the cognitive techniques described in the earlier section, therapy must result in a reduction of support for dysfunctional schemas. As such, a primary goal of CBT when addressing thoughts and schemas is the acquisition and use of a coping template through modification of schemas.

It is important to note that identification of underlying cognitive schemas can be a complicated process, which relies on insight, self-awareness, ability to articulate thoughts, and cognitive ability. As such, this level of cognitive intervention is not always appropriate for all ages and ability levels when working with children. Although adolescents can have difficulty articulating themselves, identifying core beliefs may be more successful with this age group than with younger children.

Mindfulness-Based Stress Reduction

Mindfulness is attending to and accepting the present experiences, thoughts, behavior, and feelings without engaging in judgmental thoughts about them (40,41). Mindfulness-Based Stress Reduction (MBSR) (42) was developed to teach people how to practice mindful presence with an accepting, nonjudgmental manner in all areas of their lives (43). MBSR has been shown to improve a variety of psychiatric conditions in adults with a moderate effect size (44). MBSR has been adapted for adolescent populations in a group therapy format (MBSR-T) (45), and has been shown to effectively reduce anxiety, depression, somatization, and obsessive compulsive symptoms, as well as improve self-esteem and interpersonal sensitivity (46). MBSR-T involves skills in attending to somatic states (body scan), learning meditation skills and practicing those skills across a variety of tasks (homework, walking, eating), and practicing yoga (45).

Mindfulness-Based Cognitive Therapy (MBCT) (47,48) uses elements of MBSR, but the focus is on the reduction of maladaptive behavioral and cognitive patterns that are common in individuals with depressive disorders and has been shown to reduce symptoms in chronically depressed patients (49). Research has shown that MBCT improves symptoms of attention and externalizing and internalizing problems in adolescents with externalizing problems (50), and symptoms of inattention, conduct problems, peer relations, and parenting stress in adolescents with ADHD (51). MBCT has also improved attention, hyperactivity, parenting stress, and mindfulness practice for elementary age children with ADHD (52).

Dialectical Behavior Therapy

Dialectical behavior therapy (DBT) was developed by Dr. Marsha Linehan in the 1970s to treat chronically suicidal adults with borderline personality disorder (53). DBT is delivered in individual and group therapy settings with goals of improving interpersonal effectiveness, developing emotion regulation skills, learning distress tolerance techniques, and using mindfulness strategies to learn to accept intense emotions and feelings. DBT has been modified for use with adolescents to treat depression, suicidal behavior and self-harm, and emotion dysregulation (54–56). DBT with teens includes developmentally and cognitively appropriate modifications to the core elements of DBT, with the additions of caregiver skills training and a family-based module (Walking the Middle Path) to help teens and parents see each others' views, and to learn to effectively validate, negotiate, and compromise (56). DBT targets emotions and behaviors that occur in many psychological conditions and has been found to be effective in the treatment of adolescents with suicidal and nonsuicidal self-injury, eating disorders, bipolar disorder, externalizing disorders, substance use, and PTSD (55,57–59). A universal, school-based DBT program has also been developed for improving social–emotional skills for middle and high school students (60).

Physiologic Techniques

CBT also relies on many physiologic techniques for modifying thoughts, feelings, and behavior. These techniques are particularly useful when treating anxiety disorders, as a core component of such disorders can be misinterpreting and catastrophizing physical symptoms and bodily sensations. These techniques can also be particularly useful with children, as they do not rely on cognitive ability to the same extent as cognitive techniques. Regulated breathing, relaxation training, and interoceptive exposure are all examples of physiologic techniques used in CBT.

Regulated Breathing

Breathing control exercises are often taught in CBT, especially in the treatment of anxiety. These exercises are helpful in two ways. First, they are physically effective for counteracting hyperventilation, reducing physical tension, and decreasing physical sensations associated with anxiety. Second, uncovering the patient's understanding of the physiology behind them is helpful in decreasing their fears of bodily sensations. This change in perception thereby interrupts the vicious cycle in which patients believe that physical symptoms are a sign of danger, thus increasing anxiety. Although understanding how to physically interrupt this cycle may be beyond the cognitive capacity of young children, learning regulated breathing is nonetheless effective without this understanding. Regulated breathing is most effective when practiced during low-stress circumstances on a regular basis to acquire the skill. This technique can then be applied to increasingly stressful situations.

Relaxation Training

Relaxation training is another commonly taught physiologic technique in CBT. This technique incorporates regulated breathing, but also involves progressively tensing and relaxing individual muscle groups in the body until the entire body is relaxed. When doing muscle relaxation with children, it may be necessary to focus on large muscle groups (arms, stomach, legs, whole body at once) such that the progression does not take too long and to ensure that children have adequate muscle control (it may be difficult for children to isolate small muscles). It has been suggested that this technique is helpful for treatment of insomnia (61). Relaxation training is also often incorporated into anger management treatment protocols (62,63), so that children may learn physiologic techniques for calming down. The goal of relaxation in this context is to reduce disruptive behaviors that accompany anger, especially in impulsive children.

Interoceptive Exposure

Interoception refers to the ability to sense physiologic body signals. With interoceptive exposure, individuals purposefully induce and practice experiencing simulated somatic symptoms such as increased heart rate, breathlessness, and lightheadedness. Interoceptive exposure aims to desensitize patients to these body sensations and to decrease catastrophic beliefs about physiologic arousal, as the patient experiences these sensations without having a feared outcome (e.g., if my legs fatigue I will collapse and blackout in front of this crowd). This technique is most commonly used for panic symptoms, phobias, and OCD.

Behavioral Experiments

Many different types of behavioral experiments may be helpful when using CBT, especially during the psychoeducation phase. These "experiments" are exercises that a patient can complete in session, which demonstrate errors in thinking in a concrete manner.

For example, patients are often taught during psychoeducation that attempts at thought suppression actually lead to increased thinking about distressing topics. To demonstrate this principle, the patient may be asked to engage in an exercise where he or she is told to not think of a specific topic (e.g., pink elephants) for a period of 2 minutes. Inevitably, patients find during such an exercise that, in fact, they were unable to avoid thinking about the forbidden topic no matter what it was. This behavioral thought experiment allows patients to learn that an increase in the frequency of a thought is a typical consequence of thought suppression. Instead of trying to suppress thoughts, patients are encouraged to observe their thoughts as they "come and go" without trying to suppress them. This technique typically results in a reduction in intrusive thoughts.

Exposure Techniques

Exposure therapy is based on the premise that patients with anxiety symptoms engage in avoidance or "safety behaviors" that do not allow them to experience that their fears will not be realized if they put themselves in feared situations (64). As such, exposure involves developing a progressive hierarchy of feared situations. The patient then engages in a graded series of exercises whereby these situations are experienced or recreated in order to trigger an increase in fear or anxiety sufficient to facilitate subsequent inhibition of the conditioned fear in response to the triggering stimulus or situation. Anxiety typically decreases during exposure exercises, as the patient has the experience that the feared outcome will not occur (e.g., if I think about death, it will not actually cause someone to die). Although historically, repeated exposure to fear triggers was thought to completely extinguish anxiety through the process of habituation, this is not typically the case. Although a significant reduction in fear and anxiety is common, more recent conceptualizations of exposure also emphasize enhancing patients' ability to tolerate or manage their fear and resist the avoidance behaviors most associated with functional interference and distress (65).

Cognitive techniques can also be used to enhance exposure, although care must be taken to avoid inadvertently reducing anxious arousal during the actual exposure trial. For example, rather than just practicing putting oneself in a feared situation and experiencing that the worst does not happen, thus resulting in a decrease of anxiety over time, this exercise might also include specific discussion of what the patient *thought* would happen, whether it actually did happen, reasons for the outcome, etc. With children, this cognitive component may be more difficult depending on developmental level. Exposure therapy is still effective, however, as anxiety reactions extinguish over time with repeated exercises even without this level of insight.

Exposure techniques are often used in treatment of fears and phobias and research supports their efficacy (66). For example, children with specific phobias can be gradually and systematically exposed to situations that increasingly resemble or represent their fear. Over time, they come to realize that the feared outcome does not occur which can lead to reduced fear and/or enhanced fear management abilities.

In the treatment of OCD, the compulsive behaviors are the "safety behaviors" that prevent bad things from happening as a result of the obsessive thoughts. Therefore, exposure exercises in these cases involve having the patient think about or experience their obsessions, which are often urges accompanied by a worry, without engaging in compulsions. This process, termed exposure and response prevention (ERP), facilitates the repeated experience that their feared outcome does not occur (e.g., have the patient experience that if they do not check the door, a robber will not enter the house).

Flooding is similar to exposure, with the exception that it does not utilize a hierarchy, thus, exposure to the target stimuli is not graded and begins by eliciting the full-blown fear response. While flooding may work more quickly than standard exposure, the treatment response is usually less durable. In addition, given the questionable ethics of exposing youth to significantly distressing levels of distress, flooding is no longer recommended or used with children and adolescents.

Exposure can also be used to challenge core beliefs. When used this way, it is known as cognitive response prevention. Cognitive response prevention entails giving the patient homework assignments that involve behaving in a manner inconsistent with the pathologic or problematic belief. This exercise allows the patient a real-life opportunity to cope with thoughts that accompany behavior. For example, a child who thinks, "I am stupid and a terrible student" if homework is not perfect will be assigned to do homework with some imperfections while thinking coping thoughts (e.g., "A couple of mistakes does not make me stupid."). Similarly, an adolescent who must exercise a certain amount of time per day to prevent thoughts such as, "I am fat" will be assigned to exercise for a shorter period of time and see that his or her pants still fit and weight has not changed.

Self-Monitoring/Self-Management

Self-monitoring is an important part of assessing and intervening on automatic thoughts. This technique can be used in other ways, as well, such as to keep track of moods and plan for pleasant events in the treatment of depression, to increase awareness and train competing responses in habit disorders (Tourette disorder, trichotillomania [TTM]), to assess and modify eating and exercise habits in the treatment of eating disorders, and to track use of breathing and relaxation procedures in the treatment of anxiety disorders.

Extending from self-monitoring techniques are interventions in which the child not only self-monitors behavior, but is also responsible for administration of a behavior intervention plan. Such techniques, known as self-management procedures, are also used in the treatment of a variety of disorders (e.g., disruptive behaviors, communication disorders, developmental disabilities, anxiety disorders). These interventions have been successful in improving a variety of skill areas (play skills, on-task responding, social skills; (67–71)), as well as in decreasing undesirable behaviors (off-task responding, disruptive behaviors, aggression; (69,72,73)).

Activity Scheduling

Activity scheduling is commonly used in the treatment of depression. Models of depression suggest that part of the disorder can be accounted for by a lack of reinforcement in the individual's life (74,75). One cause of this lack of reinforcement is decreased engagement in previously enjoyed activities due to decreased motivation and interest. As such, treatment may include strategies to increase the individual's participation in reinforcing daily activities. In activity scheduling, the patient and therapist agree upon homework assignments to engage in activities that result in pleasurable feelings, feelings of competence/mastery, or other similar positive emotional and cognitive outcomes. Patients begin to monitor their activity and keep daily mood diaries. Using this technique, a change in behavior often results in improvements in emotional functioning.

Applied Behavior Analysis

Applied behavior analysis (ABA) applies operant conditioning techniques to increase desirable behaviors and to decrease undesirable behaviors (76). ABA primarily relies on the use of contingent reinforcement to teach skills (i.e., increase desirable behaviors) and manipulation of antecedents and consequences to decrease challenging (i.e., undesirable) behaviors (e.g., tantrums, noncompliance, avoidance, etc.). In ABA, challenging behaviors are addressed using functional assessment or analysis procedures (76,77) in order to determine the function or "why" of a behavior. Function-based interventions are then developed, which are considered more effective for reducing challenging behaviors than interventions not based on behavioral function (77). Many specific therapeutic techniques that treat a variety of disorders are based on these principles. Several principle techniques specific to ABA therapy are outlined below.

Schedules of Reinforcement

Reinforcement occurs on multiple schedules, which have different impacts on behavior. Schedules of reinforcement are either continuous or intermittent. A continuous schedule is best for initially teaching a new behavior because the behavior is reinforced each time it occurs. Once the behavior is established, it is best to then decrease the ratio of reinforcement to responses (called *thinning* the schedule of reinforcement) so that the individual does not become satiated, leading to decreased motivation. When thinning a continuous schedule of reinforcement, there are four types of intermittent schedules that can be used. These are (1) fixed interval (the individual is reinforced on a fixed time interval), (2) variable interval (the individual is reinforced after varying time intervals), (3) fixed ratio (the individual is reinforced after a fixed number of responses), and (4) variable ratio (the individual is reinforced after a variable number of responses). The variable ratio schedule is the most effective schedule when trying to maintain a behavior because it creates relatively high steady rates of responding.

Many therapy techniques are associated with the principles of operant conditioning. Some common techniques can be found in Table 6.2.2.2. Therapies that use multiple techniques based on operant conditioning include ABA programs for children with autism and various types of behavior management programs, such as Parent Management Training (PMT) (78,79) and Problem-Solving Skills Training (PSST) (4). These therapies will be discussed in detail elsewhere in this chapter.

Extinction

Extinction occurs when reinforcement that was previously available is withheld in order to decrease or eliminate that behavior. That is, a behavior that was previously followed by positive consequences can be eliminated by withholding those positive consequences. When using extinction as an intervention, it is important to understand the phenomenon of an extinction burst. An extinction burst occurs immediately after removal of previously available reinforcement. When reinforcement is initially removed, the individual will engage in higher, more intense rates of behavior before learning that the behavior no longer results in reinforcement. Once this learning has occurred, the behavior will gradually decrease. Understanding this classically characteristic pattern can be important for intervention, as the initial increase in behavior often leads therapists and patients alike to believe that the intervention is not working. In fact, if the reinforcement is consistently not available during this time, the burst will occur and the behavior will decline.

TABLE 6.2.2.2

COMMON THERAPY TECHNIQUES ASSOCIATED WITH PRINCIPLES OF OPERANT CONDITIONING

Type and Technique	Description
Reinforcement to Increase Behaviors	
Token economy	Reinforcing target behavior with tokens (stickers, points, poker chips) that can then be traded in for reinforcement once multiple tokens have been earned.
Differential reinforcement of incompatible (DRI) or alternative behavior (DRA)	Reinforcement behaviors that are *incompatible* with or serve the same function (*alternative*) as the inappropriate behavior. Best used in conjunction with extinction of inappropriate behavior.
DRO (Differential reinforcement of other behavior)	Providing reinforcement for the absence of problem behavior.
Shaping	Reinforcing gradual approximations of a behavior.
Punishment to Decrease Behaviors	
Overcorrection	Applied consequence that involves engaging in a series of retribution steps that are related to the inappropriate behavior (washing soiled clothes after toileting accident).
Response cost	Removal of previously earned reinforcement as consequence of negative behavior. Used especially in conjunction with token economy when tokens are removed.
Time out	Removing all sources of reinforcement for allotted period of time. Typically involves placing the individual in a location where access to reinforcing activities, including social attention, is not available.
Extinction to Decrease Behaviors	Removing previously available reinforcement from an inappropriate behavior to decrease the probability that the behavior will occur in the future.

Counterconditioning

Counterconditioning techniques are used to decrease specific maladaptive behaviors, such as anxiety-related behaviors. Use of such techniques requires pairing a maladaptive behavior with an incompatible behavior in order to eliminate the maladaptive behavior. Counterconditioning techniques are based on the work of Wolpe (80), who stated, "If a response antagonistic to anxiety can be made to occur in the presence of anxiety-evoking stimuli so that it is accompanied by a complete or partial suppression of the anxiety responses, the bond between these stimuli and the anxiety response will be weakened." For example, in one of the earliest demonstrations of counterconditioning, Jones (81) cured a child's phobia of a rabbit by systematically exposing the child to the rabbit while pairing the exposures with eating preferred food when the child's hunger impulse was high. Over time, this conditioning led to a reduction of the fear response to rabbits.

Systematic Desensitization

Systematic desensitization (80) is perhaps the most commonly used counterconditioning technique. It involves training relaxation techniques to be used in conjunction with an anxiety hierarchy for the purpose of reducing fear and anxiety over time. The four stages of systematic desensitization are (1) relaxation training, (2) constructing the anxiety hierarchy, (3) desensitization in imagination, and (4) in vivo desensitization. Specifically, this technique uses an imaginal or in vivo exposure hierarchy paired with progressive muscle relaxation techniques to reduce the anxiety/fear reaction to specific situations. This treatment is typically done first through visualization, followed by in vivo training.

Originally, this technique was based on the premise of counterconditioning; that is, pairing the feared stimulus with relaxation to counter the fear reaction, which results in decreased anxiety. Evidence suggests, however, that the exposure exercises may be the active ingredient in this treatment (13,82), rather than the counterconditioning.

Systematic desensitization is supported in the literature for use with children; however, studies that demonstrated efficacy typically targeted specific, subclinical fears. Little research has been conducted on its use with more generalized anxiety (29) in children. This technique may have limited use with children under age 9 because younger children often have difficulty understanding the notion of a hierarchy, and they often have problems using visual imagery (29,83).

Aversive Counterconditioning

Aversive counterconditioning is another related technique, based on principles of classical conditioning. This technique pairs the target behavior or stimulus associated with it (conditioned stimulus) with a stimulus (unconditioned) that naturally elicits an unpleasant response. As a result, the maladaptive behavior is increasingly avoided in order to avoid the negative outcome. This technique is most commonly used in the treatment of addictions and problematic sexual fetishes. For example, the use of medications such as disulfiram (Antabuse) that cause an individual to be physically ill when consuming alcohol relies on principles of aversive counterconditioning to reduce the patient's drinking behavior. While these techniques may be periodically relevant in the treatment of adolescents, they rarely apply to treatment with children.

Covert Sensitization

Covert sensitization relies on the same principles as aversive counterconditioning; however, the individual *imagines* an aversive condition while imagining engaging in maladaptive behavior, rather than actually experiencing the negative stimuli.

Habit Reversal Training

Habit reversal procedures are most commonly used in the treatment of Tourette's and other tic disorders, as well as hair pulling (e.g., TTM), skin picking disorders, and related body-focused repetitive behaviors (e.g., nail biting) (84). Habit reversal involves three components: (1) Awareness training (e.g., increasing awareness of the urges, sensations, or other phenomena that trigger the target behavior; (2) Competing response (e.g., implementing a behavioral response physically incompatible with the target behavior immediately following the triggering event); and (3) Social support training (e.g., teaching a parent or other responsible individual to monitor and praise correct use of the first two components).

INDICATIONS AND EFFICACY

A wide variety of disorders are commonly treated using cognitive-behavioral treatment strategies. These are outlined in this section with a cognitive-behavioral model of each disorder, followed by a description of the application of CBT to its treatment.

ANXIETY DISORDERS

Cognitive-Behavioral Model

CBT for anxiety "focuses on dysfunctional cognitions and their implications for the child's subsequent thinking and behavior" (4).

Similar to adults, cognitive distortions are thought to play a major role in the development of anxiety in children and have been defined as "information processes that lead to misperceptions of oneself or the environment" (4). The primary cognitive distortion in patients with anxiety disorders is overestimation of the danger associated with certain situations, bodily sensations, or even thoughts (85). Distortions or overestimations may include inaccurate estimates of (1) the likelihood of an event, (2) the severity of an event, or (3) one's coping skills and the availability of help, support, or escape (5). Individuals with anxiety may also tend to interpret events from a negative and, therefore, inaccurate perspective, especially with regard to beliefs about self. For example, an individual with anxiety may have negative thoughts in specific situations when anxious (e.g., kids don't want to play with me because I am stupid, vs. kids don't want to play with me because they all like soccer and I don't).

The two-factor learning theory (86) has been proposed to explain the development and maintenance of fearful behavior. This theory proposes that an anxiety reaction is initially elicited via *classical conditioning* when a feared stimulus or event is experienced. As a result, the individual avoids the situation in the future to avoid experiencing the anxiety again. The avoidance behavior is then reinforced under an *operant conditioning* paradigm when distress is avoided as a result. The individual does not have an opportunity to learn that exposure to the stimuli is unlikely to result in the traumatic outcome again. For example, if a child encounters a scary dog while walking outside, he or she might come to believe that going outside is dangerous (classical conditioning). As a result, staying inside reinforces this notion, as the child does not experience anxiety unless he or she goes outside (operant conditioning). Therefore, until the child can learn that going outside does not result in negative outcomes, the anxiety reaction will continue to be reinforced. Similarly, Clark (5) has proposed that reflexively elicited somatic and cognitive symptoms of anxiety become problematic when they are misinterpreted as indicating danger is present (I'm going crazy). Such an interpretation can lead to further increased physiologic arousal, which then serves to confirm the initial incorrect hypothesis.

Symptoms of anxiety in children may be physiologic, behavioral, and/or cognitive (29,87). For example, physiologic symptoms may include shaky voice, rigid posture, perspiration, abdominal pain, flushed face, need to urinate, trembling, and increased heart rate. Physiologic symptoms, especially ongoing somatic complaints, are often the most common anxiety symptoms in children, as their cognitions may not be as clear and identifiable as those of adults. Behavioral symptoms may include nail biting, avoidance, thumb sucking, crying, toileting accidents, and others. Cognitions may include thoughts of being hurt or scared, thoughts of danger, self-critical thoughts, preoccupation with evaluation by self and others, worries about likelihood of severe negative consequences, ruminative thoughts, and intrusive images or sounds. These can be difficult to determine in anxious children who may not be accurate reporters or who may not have enough self-awareness to understand their thoughts clearly (88). Distorted information processing is another cognitive area that may be involved in anxiety. For example, distorted/biased views of social or environmental cues, preoccupation with evaluation by self and others, preoccupation with likelihood of negative consequences, or misperception of demands in the environment (29) are common distortions.

Treatment

Treatment strategies for anxiety in children must target cognitive, behavioral, physiologic, and emotional aspects of the disorder. Kazdin (4) suggested that these strategies must "help the child develop new skills, provide new experiences for the child to test dysfunctional as well as adaptive beliefs, and assist the child in processing new experiences." Treatment strategies can be divided into several categories, based on which symptom area they address.

Physiologic Treatment Strategies

In CBT for childhood anxiety, physiologic symptoms are typically targeted first, given the high rate with which these symptoms occur in this age group and the difficulty many young children have in identifying and changing cognitions (25). The most common methods for addressing the physiologic symptoms of anxiety are relaxation training and systematic desensitization. Relaxation training for children typically involves a combination of progressive muscle relaxation, deep breathing, and pleasant imagery, which the child and therapist develop prior to starting the training. In systematic desensitization, relaxation techniques are paired with a fear hierarchy to countercondition the fear response. Studies of efficacy for systematic desensitization have generally shown efficacy with otherwise nonclinical samples who have specific fears (89). As systematic desensitization requires the child to report levels of anxiety in relation to various stimuli on a hierarchy, it may be difficult for young children (under age 9). Relaxation training, however, has been used with younger children, although they may not acquire the skill as well as older children.

It has been suggested that young children may have more difficulty with systematic desensitization for two reasons. They appear to have difficulty acquiring the skill of muscle relaxation and may not be able to clearly visualize the fear-producing stimuli (90). Therefore, in vivo desensitization may be more effective with younger children (91). Using developmentally appropriate imagery may help remediate this difficulty, however, such as in a case example by Jackson and King (92). In this example, a child was taught to imagine that Batman (a preferred cartoon character for this child) was accompanying him to view the feared stimulus (the dark and shadows). After four sessions, the child no longer evidenced fear of the dark.

Behavioral Treatment Strategies

Children may also benefit from strategies that address learning new behaviors, such as coping skills. For example, modeling has been used to demonstrate desired coping behaviors for use in a feared situation. The child is then reinforced for engaging in these behaviors and can be provided with feedback (93). The therapist is often used as the coping model (94). For example, the therapist can place him/herself in an anxiety-producing situation and model self-talk in front of the patient. In group settings, children may be models for one another, as well. Role-plays have also been used, particularly with younger children who have difficulty describing anxiety-provoking events. The role play itself may allow the therapist to observe when the child becomes anxious and may help facilitate a more in vivo discussion about the child's cognitions at that time (29). Role-plays may also serve an important behavioral rehearsal function, which allows children to practice new skills under less stressful circumstances before being required to use them in the actual anxiety-provoking situation. Children can also be taught problem-solving steps, such as the ones proposed by Spivak and Shure (95). These include (1) problem identification, definition, and formulation; (2) generation of alternative solutions; (3) choosing a new strategy; (4) implementing the new strategy; and (5) evaluating the new strategy. These types of steps are often the foundation for skills training curriculums for children, both in group and individual therapy.

Cognitive Strategies

Children with anxiety disorders often require assistance in identifying their dysfunctional thoughts and beliefs, which they then must learn to modify. Several strategies are suggested for modification of cognitions and the cognitive and behavioral processes that maintain them. First, psychoeducation is used to increase children's awareness about their cognitive processes and to help them understand how their thoughts maintain anxiety symptoms. An extension of psychoeducation is refocusing the child's attention on less negative aspects of situations, less negative self-evaluation, and less negative interpretations of events. Self-talk is also used to identify maladaptive thoughts (e.g., those that are anxiety-provoking) and internal dialogue, and then to dispute or correct misinterpretations or biases (29,96). For example, children can be taught to think about evidence for and against negative thoughts when they have them. This method of questioning thoughts typically leads the child to the conclusion that the "evidence" does not support their thinking. Similarly, when children have intrusive thoughts, images, or ongoing internal dialogue, they can be taught thought-stopping techniques to interrupt the cycle, such as thinking about yelling, "Stop!" while picturing a large stop sign in their head.

Combined Strategies

Many CBT treatment plans combine physiology, learning new behaviors, and changing cognitions. For example, in vivo exposure and exposure with response prevention combine cognitive and behavioral strategies to reduce anxiety related to specific stimuli or symptoms of OCD. A series of waitlist controlled studies by Kendall et al. (97,98) has demonstrated the efficacy of a combined CBT approach in treating generalized, separation, and social anxiety disorders, with gains maintained up to 7 years posttreatment (98).

OBSESSIVE-COMPULSIVE DISORDER

Cognitive-Behavioral Model

The cognitive-behavioral model of OCD involves "intrusive and distressing thoughts, impulses, or images about possible harm coming to oneself or others" (5), which must then be neutralized through counter-thoughts or behaviors to prevent harm or negative consequences from occurring. Many people have intrusive thoughts of this nature; however, individuals with OCD are thought to interpret them differently. That is, they assume that such thoughts are a sign that something terrible will actually happen and they will be responsible for the outcome. As a result, they engage in all types of neutralizing, undoing, and compensatory behaviors (e.g., checking, washing, ordering, meaningless rituals, self-statements) in order to prevent negative outcomes. As the distressing thoughts in OCD typically have a low likelihood of actually occurring, the individual comes to believe that their neutralizing behaviors (compulsions) successfully prevented the feared outcome. As such, the individual never comes to realize that they are unnecessary. In addition, and perhaps more importantly, reduction in distress and anxiety contingent on performance of the ritual creates a negative reinforcement cycle, which serves to further strengthen the perceived benefits of the ritual (the so-called OCD cycle) (99).

Treatment

Numerous studies support exposure-based CBT, known as exposure and response prevention (ERP), as an effective and appropriate first-line treatment for pediatric OCD, either alone or in conjunction with medication (100,101). ERP begins with the development of a hierarchy of obsessions and compulsions, listed in order from least to most distressing (Table 6.2.2.3). Once this hierarchy is developed, exposure begins with the least distressing item on the hierarchy. Depending on the nature of the obsession, exposure involves either exposing the individual to the actual stimuli or having him/her imagine or think about it. As the symptom pattern in OCD involves compulsions that are tied to obsessions, the exposure will elicit a desire to perform the compulsion. Thus, it is important that the patient refrain from engaging in their compulsive response (response prevention), or at least delaying the response for a period of time, if treatment is to be successful. Repeated exposure to the anxiety (the obsession) in the absence of the neutralizing response (the compulsion) results in inhibitory learning whereby the child's anxiety response to the exposure target decreases. Although some decrease in anxiety is often observed before moving the patient to the next hierarchy item, increasing the amount of time the child is in a state of heightened arousal is thought to enhance inhibitory learning and to lead to better outcomes.

A better understanding of the inhibitory learning processes underlying exposure has led to recommendations designed to increase the efficacy and durability of the treatment (102). These recommendations, which focus on enhancing the generalizability of the underlying inhibitory learning, include greater focus on violating expectancies (e.g., having a child who believes he or she can refrain from washing for only 2 minutes stay in the exposure for 3 minutes) and eliminating safety signals (e.g., using multiple therapy settings or removing parent from the room). In addition, once the child has some experience and success with exposures, selecting exposures randomly from the hierarchy and conducting exposures to multiple hierarchy items simultaneously can also potentially lead to more durable treatment gains (103). At times, booster sessions may be required if obsessions begin to provoke anxiety again.

Numerous studies support both individual and group-administered exposure-based CBT as an effective and appropriate first-line treatment for pediatric OCD, either alone or in combination with medication (100,101). The Pediatric OCD Treatment Study (POTS) (104), the largest pediatric trial of CBT for OCD to date, compared CBT alone, selective serotonin reuptake inhibitor (SSRI) alone, and combined CBT + SSRI to pill placebo in a sample of 128 youngsters drawn from three treatment sites. Overall, CBT + SSRI was found to be the most effective treatment, yielding illness remission in 54% of youngsters, followed by CBT alone (39% remission), SSRI alone (21% remission), and placebo (3% remission). At one site, however, CBT alone was found equally efficacious as CBT + SSRI, leading the researchers to conclude that either CBT or CBT + SSRI should be considered the first line of treatment in children with OCD.

Randomized comparative trials have also demonstrated ERP to be more efficacious than relaxation training in both elementary-aged children and teens (105) and younger children (106).

TABLE 6.2.2.3

SAMPLE OCD SYMPTOM HIERARCHY

OCD Ritual	SUDS Rating
Mom needing to say "okay, goodnight" three times at bedtime	9
Washing hands when feel contaminated	8
Turning light switch on/off three times	7
Turning TV on and off three times	6
Erasing and rewriting math homework	6
Rereading sentences in history book until feels right	5
Rereading sentences in pleasure books until feels right	4
Needing to brush teeth at bedtime three times	3
Saving old school homework	2

SUDS, subjective units of distress scale; SUDS rating, degree of distress associated with not being able to complete each listed ritual.

PHOBIAS

Cognitive-Behavioral Model

As noted earlier, the two-factor learning theory (86) has been used to explain the development and maintenance of phobic behavior, in that repeated avoidance of the feared situation or object does not allow for disconfirmation of distorted harm beliefs and, in fact, is reinforced by the patient's belief that such avoidance is keeping him/her safe. As a result, treatment involves breaking this operant conditioning cycle and teaching the individual that the feared situation is unlikely to occur again even when it is not avoided.

Treatment

Several CBT strategies have demonstrated efficacy in the treatment of phobias. Graded exposure, systematic desensitization, participant modeling, and relaxation training (80,107) have all been effective treatment strategies. Exposure treatment of phobias is much like that described above in the treatment of OCD. In the case of phobias, the individual is exposed to increasingly difficult versions of the feared stimuli, and is prevented from escaping contact with the situation or object. Over time, the individual learns that the feared stimulus or situation does not result in the expected danger, and is, in fact, safe. Long-term treatment success is dependent on the patient retrieving this new learning when they later encounter the fear stimulus. Initially, treatment involves imaginal exposures and then later in vivo exposure exercises.

An intensive form of exposure therapy whereby youth complete one session treatment (OST) has promising outcomes (108). OST utilizes in vivo exposure, cognitive challenges, participant modeling, reinforcement, and psychoeducation (109). An additional promising component for augmenting exposure-based treatment of phobias is the addition of Attention Bias Modification Training (ABMT). ABMT involves using a computerized task to train the patient to quickly shift attention away from threatening stimuli toward a neutral or positive stimuli. This approach has a stronger effect for children with higher threat vigilance (rather than avoidance behavior), as the goal of ABMT is to reduce biases to preferentially attend to fear stimuli, which is thought to maintain anxiety for a subset of anxious children (110,111).

Treatment of social phobia may involve additional components, most notably social skills training (112–114). This combination of CBT with social skills training (called Social Effectiveness Therapy for Children or SET-C) was found to be efficacious for children and adolescents with social phobia (112), with gains maintained at 3-year and 5-year follow-up (113,114). SET-C is a behaviorally oriented intervention where children are taught social skills and coached to complete exposures with nonanxious children. Similarly, Spence et al. (115) found that CBT with strong social skills training, as well as parent involvement in treatment, improved social anxiety symptoms in approximately 80% of youth to the subclinical range, with gains maintained at 12-month follow-up (115). SET-C components have been incorporated into a school-based group treatment called Skills for Academic and Social Success (SASS), with 67% of treatment subjects no longer meeting criteria for social anxiety compared to waitlist controls (116–118). Treatment gains were maintained at 5-year follow-up (119).

Although cognitive-based interventions are not as utilized with children compared to behavior-based intervention, Melfsen et al. (120) demonstrated that cognitive-based intervention with no habituation component for socially anxious youth significantly decreased social anxiety symptoms and negative feelings of self-worth compared to waitlist controls, with 30% of patients no longer meeting criteria for social anxiety. The cognitive-behavioral treatment focusing on cognition involved "(a) using the child's own thoughts, images, attentional strategies, safety behaviors, and symptoms, (b) systematic manipulation of self-focused attention and safety behaviors, (c) systematic training in externally focused attention, (d) techniques for restructuring distorted self-imagery, and (e) behavioral experiments in which a habituation rationale was not used" (120). Although the percentage of treatment participants who no longer met criteria for social anxiety disorder did not reach the range that is typical for CBT treatments (54%), this cognitive-focused intervention showed promising results (121).

SELECTIVE MUTISM

Cognitive-Behavioral Model

Selective mutism is closely related to social anxiety and it is characterized by persistent failure to speak in public situations where speaking is expected, despite speaking in other situations (122). In recent history, selective mutism was thought to be a manifestation of oppositional behavior (123), but research has shown that selective mutism is related to anxiety, shyness, and social anxiety. Developmental delays, speech articulation, and communication problems are also very common comorbid conditions (124–126). Onset of selective mutism is often at a very young age. When a child does not speak, and, by consequence, they can still function or get their needs met (e.g., an adult speaks for them, another child answers the question, they avoid aversive instructions), the child escapes the demand that is feared (speaking aloud), and, thus, the avoidance behavior is maintained.

Treatment

Selective mutism is typically treated using behavioral methods that begin with a functional assessment to evaluate antecedents of the child's failure to speak and the consequences following the behavior (127,128). Based on the observed patterns, shaping and systematic desensitization with gradual exposure to speaking situations are used to increase the frequency with which the child verbalizes (129–131). Cunningham et al. (131) proposed two types of fading: situational and individual. In situational fading, the child and a person he or she is willing to talk to are gradually and systematically moved from a location where speech occurs to one where it does not. In individual fading, new individuals are gradually and systematically introduced into situations in which the child already speaks. When these systematic shaping procedures are paired with reinforcement of speaking, the child gradually learns to speak to an increasing number of individuals in an increasing number of settings.

Bergman et al. (132) developed a novel behavioral intervention for treatment of selective mutism and functional speech (Integrated Behavior Therapy for Selective Mutism [IBTSM]) and found increased functional speaking behavior as rated by parents, teachers, and blind independent raters and reduction in social anxiety symptoms as rated by parents (132). Oerbeck et al. (133) developed a home- and school-based cognitive behavioral treatment for selective mutism involving defocused communication (e.g., sitting beside instead of across from a child, creating joint attention by looking at preferred item, wondering aloud rather than directly speaking to the child, accepting speech in neutral manner, and continuing to talk even if the child does not speak) and behavioral techniques of stimulus fading in the clinic setting, followed by the school setting. The study found that the treatment groups had significantly improved speaking ratings compared to baseline, and half of the participants no longer met criteria for selective mutism posttreatment (133). Treatment effects were maintained at 1-year follow-up and were especially robust for the youngest participants (134).

PANIC DISORDER

Cognitive-Behavioral Model

Panic disorder is characterized by a fear of impending disaster, which is confirmed by physiologic and cognitive symptoms. Individuals with panic disorder often misinterpret their symptoms as confirmation that their anxiety represents real danger, which results in more anxiety, leading to further symptoms, and so on. This loss of control over those symptoms leads to further anxiety, which is a maintaining factor in panic attacks. Individuals with panic disorder typically fear having panic attacks in certain situations and begin altering their behavior as a result. For example, in agoraphobia, individuals may resist leaving the house due to anxiety about the social or interpersonal consequences of having an attack in public. The distinguishing factor between panic disorder and other phobias, however, is that the precipitating factor in the attack is a fear of having one, rather than a fear of a specific stimulus. Therefore, in differential diagnosis of these disorders, an individual who has a panic attack in an elevator because he or she does not like small, enclosed spaces would be diagnosed with a specific phobia, whereas an individual who has a panic attack in an elevator and subsequently refuses to use elevators for fear of having an attack there would be diagnosed with panic disorder.

Treatment

Treatment of panic disorder involves cognitive and physiologic strategies, as well as exposure therapy (135). The patient must learn to interpret bodily cues more accurately and often may benefit from learning to place less emphasis on such cues altogether. Understanding the physiology of the cycle is critical, as well, as the patient can then learn to intervene to decrease physiologic anxiety symptoms. Interoception refers to the ability to sense body signals. Hypervigilance to body sensations and catastrophic beliefs about possibly having somatic sensations are common for individuals with panic. Thus, patients can learn to decrease catastrophic beliefs about physiologic arousal by practicing interoceptive exposure (tolerating somatic sensations). For example, patients can purposely increase their heart rate, induce dizzy sensations, sweat, or simulate feeling out of breath and learn that presence of these sensations do not result in a panic attack (136).

Self-control and relaxation exercises (controlled, deep breathing; muscle relaxation) are important in preventing and controlling panic attacks and their associated symptoms. Cognitive strategies are important, as well, as patients must learn to decrease their exaggerated thinking patterns. Cognitive restructuring, Socratic questioning, and other related strategies are important in decreasing the catastrophizing and ongoing worry that accompany the panic attacks in this disorder. Exposure therapy is often used in the treatment of panic, as well, as the individual has come to avoid certain situations over time due to fear of having an attack. As such, once the individual learns physiologic and cognitive strategies for avoiding and reducing the severity of attacks, he or she may require exposure therapy to learn that previously avoided situations can now be managed. Exposure exercises are conducted on a hierarchy as described above, and, over time, the individual learns that panic attacks will not occur and that situations are therefore no longer to be feared.

Hoffman and Mattis (137) adapted an adult Panic Control Treatment for Adolescents (PCT-A). PTC-A consists of psychoeducation and correcting misinformation about panic attacks, cognitive restructuring, breathing, interoceptive exposures, and graduated exposure to feared stimuli or avoided situations. Pincus et al. (138) later tested PTC-A (also known as Master of Anxiety and Panic for Adolescents: Riding the Wave) compared to self-monitoring waitlist control and found large treatment effects in the reduction of clinician-reported clinical severity to below clinical threshold, as well as decreased self-reported anxiety sensitivity, and general anxiety and depressive symptoms. Gains were maintained at 3-month posttreatment, and an additional reduction in panic symptoms was found at 6-months posttreatment (138).

POSTTRAUMATIC STRESS DISORDER

Cognitive-Behavioral Model

PTSD is diagnosed when a constellation of anxiety-related symptoms manifests after the occurrence of a traumatic event. Many individuals experience symptoms of PTSD after a traumatic event, including intrusive, unwanted distressing thoughts and memories, avoidance, hypervigilance, and hyperarousal. Individuals who then develop PTSD, however, do not adequately cope with these symptoms, and they persist or worsen as a result. Over time, many other cognitive aspects of anxiety may then manifest in individuals with PTSD. For example, they may begin to misinterpret the recurrent, intrusive thoughts as a sign that something terrible will happen again, as described above in the development of OCD. They may also develop anxiety about their symptoms that perpetuates the anxious state (similar to panic disorder), such as, "I can't control my recurrent memories so I must be going mad." As such, while PTSD has an etiology very different from other anxiety disorders, its treatment is quite similar, as misinterpretation of thoughts, avoidance, and other anxiety symptoms must be addressed.

Trauma reactions may appear somewhat different in very young (under age 6) children (122,139). Scheeringa et al. (139) proposed an alternative set of diagnostic criteria for preschool-aged trauma victims [PTSD-AA] (139). Scheeringa's modifications to the previous DSM-IV criteria focused on behavioral symptoms, rather than on thoughts and emotions, and also provided a developmental lens from which to interpret much of the criteria for young children. PTSD-AA modifications included, (1) the individual does not have to be able to report the anxiety reaction, as many young children are incapable of doing so; (2) recurrent recollection of the event may manifest in repetitive, trauma-related play themes; (3) recurrent distressing dreams do not have to include trauma-related content, but must be distressing; (4) flashbacks may be behavioral in nature, with no accompanying verbal description; (5) diminished interest in significant activities may present as constriction of play; (6) a feeling of detachment or estrangement may manifest as withdrawal; (7) loss of developmental skills may occur; and (8) increased arousal may manifest as tantrums and outbursts.

Most of the PTSD-AA modifications were later incorporated into the *Diagnostic and Statistical Manual of Mental Disorders* (DSM-5; 5th ed.) (122). In addition to incorporating nearly all of the PTSD-AA modifications, the DSM-5 removed criterion for "response of fear, helplessness or horror," split the former avoidance/numbing criteria into avoidance and negative alterations in mood, and now only requires one symptom in this avoidance criterion for young children instead of three. Furthermore, two symptoms were removed under avoidance criterion, including (1) sense of foreshortened future and (2) inability to recall aspects of the event, and the increased frequency of negative emotional states was added. Finally, the DSM-5 clarified that avoidance of people, conversations, and interpersonal situations may also be present for young children. Evidence suggests that the new DSM-5 criteria for young children are now more diagnostically sensitive (140).

Treatment

Research suggests that CBT approaches are the most effective treatment for PTSD in children (141–147). Exposure is the primary focus in treatment of PTSD (146,148), although other CBT strategies, such as cognitive restructuring and relaxation, are also often used (146,149–151). The literature proposes that the forced thinking about the traumatic incident involved in imaginal exposure may be especially important because studies have shown that avoidance of thoughts associated with the traumatic event is predictive of persisting PTSD (5,152–154).

Studies using CBT to treat PTSD in children and adolescents are somewhat limited; however, several controlled studies have demonstrated clinically significant reductions in symptoms (142,155–158). Additional randomized controlled trials (RCTs) are available for specific populations, such as victims of sexual abuse (159–161).

Trauma-focused cognitive-behavioral therapy (TF-CBT), which is based on the basic principles of CBT, has been shown to be effective in reducing PTSD symptoms in children exposed to trauma (148,162,163), as well as comorbid depressive and internalizing symptoms, with treatment gains maintained at 1 to 2 years posttreatment (162,164). TF-CBT actively involves both parents and children, and includes psychoeducation; the development of relaxation, affective regulation, and coping skills; the creation of a trauma narrative (TN); and parent–child treatment sessions (162,165,166). Gradual exposure to trauma reminders takes place throughout treatment (148).

The formation of the TN is a key component of TF-CBT. Over the course of treatment, children develop a narrative of the traumatic experience by describing the event in detail and by sharing their "thoughts, feelings, and physiologic reactions" (148).

Exposure therapy in the treatment of PTSD is well validated with adults and is also used with children. Exposure therapy in PTSD typically involves repeated, imaginal re-experiencing of the traumatic event until the anxiety associated with these exposure exercises diminishes. Therapists coaching their patients through exposure exercises typically try to elicit as much detail as possible about the patient's experience of the event, including thoughts and feelings that were experienced at the time. This level of detail and focus on thoughts and feelings results in decreased anxiety over time (167,168). Alternative exposure strategies are sometimes used with children, such as writing or illustrating a book about the event in gradual, systematic steps (160), or having them experience the event via play. In vivo exposure may also be helpful in situations where it is possible for the client to be exposed to the location of the trauma or other related variables.

Individuals with PTSD may also benefit from anxiety management training (141,146,167,169) or stress inoculation techniques (149,160,170), which may include cognitive restructuring of thoughts about the event, relaxation, positive imagery and self-talk, thought stopping, self-monitoring, and other physiologic strategies to decrease hyperarousal (151,171). Cognitive restructuring in PTSD involves altering the distorted cognitions that play a role in the development and maintenance of the disorder. For example, young children often experience serious misattributions about the traumatic event, such as self-blame (160). Anxiety management training may also involve application of learned skills in role-plays and in vivo exposure exercises. Research in this area is limited; however, existing studies appear promising (172).

Parent participation in treatment is often important when working with children and adolescents. Pine and Cohen (160) suggest that parents may participate in exposure exercises with their children, and that they may benefit from learning behavior management techniques.

DEPRESSION

Cognitive-Behavioral Model

Seligman (173) noted that depression in children and adolescents lends itself to a cognitive-behavioral intervention model (when developmentally appropriate), as these individuals tend to exhibit high rates of intrusive negative thoughts (e.g., selective ruminations about past unpleasant events, hopelessness about the future, and helplessness about improving their situation). Consistent with Beck's model (74), adolescents have been shown to attribute positive outcomes to external, unstable, and specific factors (174) and to lack self-efficacy with regard to these outcomes. Individuals with depression may also experience cognitive distortions in attributions, self-evaluation, and perception of past and present events (175,176). Similarly, they may engage in overgeneralization, catastrophizing, taking responsibility for negative outcomes, and attending to negative features of events (175,177,178). These distortions can be thought to result from "pathologic information processing" (17,179), which leads to symptoms of depression.

Children with depression often have low self-esteem, low perceived academic competence, and low perceived social competence (180), and may have poor problem-solving skills, especially regarding interpersonal problems (29). Kazdin (4) also noted that depression in children and adolescents is associated with "restricted behavioral repertoires" (limited participation in pleasant activities, few experiences of reinforcement in the environment), thereby lending itself to the behavioral aspects of treatment.

Treatment

CBT has been found to be effective for the treatment of depression in adults across a variety of studies (179,181) and treatment delivery models (individual CBT, CBT in conjunction with medication, group CBT, marital CBT). Research also shows CBT to be effective in treating depression in adolescents (182–184). In a study by Clark et al. (182), youth who received brief CBT, in addition to self-selected treatment as usual (e.g., outpatient mental health, antidepressants, school counseling), exhibited significantly better rates of recovery from major depression compared to those adolescents randomized to the treatment-as-usual control condition (182). Another study examining the use of CBT as a continuation-phase treatment after an antidepressant treatment found that those children who received CBT in addition to medication management had a significantly lower risk of relapse, as compared to those individuals in the medication management only group (184).

As symptoms of depression are both cognitive and behavioral in nature, a variety of strategies are employed depending on individual patient symptoms. Cognitive restructuring is often used to address negative thought patterns associated with depression. Socratic questioning, in which the patient examines evidence for and against distorted perceptions, is one strategy for intervening on such thought patterns. Patients may also benefit from self-control strategies, including learning more positive self-consequation (reinforce one's self more, punish one's self less), adaptive self-monitoring (increasing attention to positive actions, events, accomplishments), and more accurate and realistic self-evaluation, such as learning to set less perfectionistic standards for one's self. One kind of adaptive self-monitoring includes monitoring pleasant events and associated moods. This type of procedure encourages the child to engage in reinforcing activities, while simultaneously increasing focus on the resulting positive affective change. Charts such as the one in Figure 6.2.2.1 are easily used with older children and adolescents for this type of intervention.

Skills training is also often involved in the treatment of depression, especially for children and adolescents. Types of skills training may include assertiveness training, conflict management skills training, relaxation training, and social skills training. Social skills training, in particular, may be important for children and adolescents, as poor social relationships are predictive of many psychological and emotional difficulties. Further, interpersonal conflicts with peers are the most common antecedent to adolescent suicide attempts (185). Social skills training involves different components and skill sets depending on the model; however, the focus is generally on teaching skills for initiating and maintaining social interactions (186,187). Social skills interventions may also focus on handling

Pleasant Events and Mood Monitoring							
Name:							
Week of (dates):							
Chart filled out by:							
	Monday	Tuesday	Wednesday	Thursday	Friday	Saturday	Sunday
Pleasant events:							
Mood rating:							

DIRECTIONS:

Note pleasant events for each day.

Give each day a rating of 0–5 to indicate overall mood for that day.

If mood changes significantly within a day, it is fine to give that day two separate ratings.

0 = sad, no energy at all, unmotivated
5 = very happy, nonstop busy, very motivated

FIGURE 6.2.2.1. Mood monitoring chart for treatment of depression.

interpersonal conflicts. Other behavioral interventions, such as activity scheduling/monitoring, and tracking pleasant events and associated moods, are also often part of changing behaviors, gaining skills, and increasing self-administered reinforcement.

The Adolescent Coping with Depression Course (CWD-A) (188–191) is a classroom-based group treatment program for treating adolescents with depression. This program first involves increasing the patient's awareness of negative cognitions, followed by learning new, more constructive ones. Strategies to increase positive reinforcement in the patient's life are then used, such as increasing activities associated with positive reinforcement and teaching social skills associated with increased reinforcement. The final component of the program is parent education, which is designed to facilitate practicing skills learned in session at home with parental support. Ongoing research has demonstrated the efficacy of this model (188,190–193), and further examination of various treatment mediators suggests that a reduction in negative thinking may be the primary mechanism involved in reduction of depressive symptoms (189).

DBT, while originally developed to treat individuals with borderline personality disorder (194), has been shown to be effective in treating other disorders and behaviors, including depression, in both adults and adolescents (57,195,196). For adults, there is an evidence that DBT improves self-reported depression symptoms and promotes remission in patients treated with a combination of medication and DBT, in comparison to adults only treated with medication (196). DBT also seems to be effective for treatment-resistant depression in adults (195). In a meta-analysis that examined the research on modified DBT with adolescents, posttreatment results indicated that adolescents who had participated in a DBT intervention engaged in less nonsuicidal self-injury and experienced a reduction in depressive symptoms (57). While these findings are encouraging, further research on modified DBT for adolescents is needed.

AUTISM SPECTRUM DISORDER

Cognitive-Behavioral Model

Previously termed "pervasive developmental disorders" in the DSM-IV (197), individuals who meet criteria for any of these disorders (autistic disorder, Asperger's disorder, or pervasive developmental disorder, not otherwise specified [PDD-NOS]) are now diagnosed with autism spectrum disorder (ASD) under DSM-5 (122). ASD is characterized by deficits in social communication skills (i.e., social reciprocity, nonverbal communication behaviors, and age-appropriate peer relationships) and the presence of restricted interests, repetitive behaviors/speech, insistence on sameness, and unusual patterns in sensory processing (122). Individuals with ASD are often conceptualized as having a core disability in social interaction skills and motivation (198). This inherent difficulty in interacting with others, combined with a lack of social motivation, may result in severe learned helplessness over time. The lack of motivation and learned helplessness that children with autism frequently experience requires that alternative methods of motivating learning be used. Therefore, treatment of autism is primarily behavioral and focuses on finding ways to motivate socially appropriate communication, social, and play skills, as well as behavior, to recruit reinforcement that is meaningful to the child.

Treatment

The treatment of ASD involves the use of operant procedures in applied settings, otherwise known as applied behavior analysis (ABA). ABA utilizes operant conditioning procedures (10,11) to target development of functional behaviors that will make a meaningful difference in quality of life for the individual. Behaviors must be observable and measurable, and data on target behaviors must be collected on a regular and ongoing basis in order to evaluate whether observed changes in behavior are the result of treatment implementation. ABA treatment programs are designed to address any developmental domain in which delays are present, including, but not limited to, communication, social, play, cognitive, adaptive, and motor skills. It is also often necessary to focus on the reduction of challenging behaviors (e.g., tantrums, aggression, self-injury, property destruction), which result from a lack of appropriate skills.

In ABA therapy, the antecedent-behavior-consequence (A-B-C) contingency is used to both teach skills and to reduce challenging behaviors. This framework assumes that antecedents (A) cue or lead to the behavior (B), which is followed by consequences (C) that will either increase or decrease the probability of future behavior. When teaching skills, antecedents and consequences are purposefully introduced in order to create learning trials. For example, an adult might hold a child-preferred object out of reach (antecedent) to cue the child to make a verbal request (behavior), and then reinforce the child's appropriate response (consequence) by providing access to the item. When trying to reduce challenging behaviors, the A-B-C contingency is already in place, as natural factors are typically eliciting (antecedent) and maintaining (consequence) the behavior. As such, these factors must be identified through functional assessment or analysis and altered in order to reduce undesirable behavior.

In ABA therapy, reinforcement is used to teach explicit target behaviors, such as making verbalizations, imitating the actions of others, engaging in appropriate toy play, and following directions. The antecedent-behavior-consequence (A-B-C) contingency is purposefully introduced and manipulated to set up teaching trials to teach skills. Behavioral goals are set for the child at the outset of therapy and progress is tracked through ongoing data collection. Depending on the target behavior, data may be collected using various strategies; however, the most common methods are to collect data on frequency or duration of a behavior. Intensity of a behavior may also be measured, depending on what behavior is being targeted. For example, with severe self-injury, frequency is important, but if the behavior is severely self-injurious, information about the severity of a single incident may also be important. Target behaviors are chosen based on the child's developmental level and current skill set, and are operationally defined for clarity of deciding when reinforcement has been earned and tracking the child's progress.

It is typically recommended that strategies used in the reduction of inappropriate behaviors be selected based on behavioral function. Functional assessment (77) or analysis (76) procedures are used in devising behavior plans for children with autism, as it is necessary to determine the function of the behavior prior to deciding on an intervention plan. Common functions of behavior include behaviors to gain attention, escape/avoid tasks, and obtain tangibles. Once a functional assessment has been completed, interventions can be developed at the antecedent, behavior, or consequence level. Antecedent interventions are typically focused on strategies to prevent the behavior, such as prompts, reminders, and environmental modifications. Replacement behaviors are also taught to ensure the individual is gaining more appropriate skills to meet the same functional need the behavior was serving. Consequence strategies are used to alter how others are responding to the behavior to ensure inappropriate behavior is not being reinforced. Using functional assessment or analysis ensures that the disruptive behavior will be reduced and a positive replacement behavior will be taught in its place. Behavior plans may include many strategies such as those outlined in Table 6.2.2.2.

There are many types of ABA treatment models, such as discrete trial teaching [DTT] (199), pivotal response training [PRT] (198), and incidental teaching (200,201). Some models are structured and require the child to work one-on-one with a therapist [DTT] (199,202), while others embed behavioral teaching trials into developmentally appropriate interactions in the child's natural environment, such as during play-time, while at school, and within family routines (e.g., PRT) (68,203). Interventions that involve structured one-on-one work between a therapist and the patient (e.g., DTT) are often criticized for limitations in generalization effects. That is, targeted behaviors that are successfully elicited in therapy may not be demonstrated by the child in natural settings. As such, a strong program will address both the need for structured, behavioral teaching interactions to teach certain behaviors, as well as the need for opportunities to promote use of skills across settings, behaviors, and social partners (204). This goal is often achieved through training individuals who regularly interact with the child (parents and teachers) in the use of intervention strategies so that target behaviors may be prompted in a variety of natural settings and interactions. Many specific techniques are used in ABA therapy. Some examples of these are outlined in Table 6.2.2.4.

Recently, there has been increased focus in the literature on treatment models that combine ABA therapy techniques and developmental science (e.g., Naturalistic Developmental Behavioral Interventions [NDBI]; (205)). ASD treatment models, such as the Early Start Denver Model (ESDM; (206)); Joint Attention, Symbolic Play, Engagement and Regulation (JASPER; (207)); and Project IMPACT (Improving Parents As Communication Teachers; (208)), focus on embedding ABA teaching strategies in the natural environment, as well as using developmental methods such as imitation of the child to enhance motivation and use of positive affect to foster shared enjoyment. While many ASD treatment models have focused on embedding behavioral teaching trials in the natural environment, use of natural reinforcement, and use of incidental teaching methods for some time (e.g., Pivotal Response Treatment), most recently, the field is moving away from the focus on individual treatment models and toward the identification of core components that are considered effective in teaching children with ASD (205). Many of these models include or are solely focused on training parents to deliver parent-mediated interventions (208).

Behavioral treatments for children with autism have substantial empirical support (199,204). In one of the earliest intervention studies, Lovaas (199) provided intensive behavioral programming to young children with autism, including the use of operant techniques in a one-on-one therapy setting as well as across individuals (parents, teachers). After 2 years of intensive (40 hours per week) therapy, the children had made substantial gains, including improvements in IQ and less restrictive school placements, such as mainstream classrooms. Other studies have suggested that 40 hours of one-on-one therapy is not necessary; rather, children can be taught throughout the natural course of their day (68,203,205) by embedding behavioral trials in natural interactions. Whatever the format for teaching, research clearly supports that behavioral strategies are most effective for teaching children with autism.

Several large-scale projects have attempted to conduct exhaustive reviews of the literature and to categorize treatments according to efficacy criteria. For example, the National Standards Project ((209); nationalautismcenter.org) conducted a literature review based on specific criteria, and classified treatments as "Established," "Emerging," or "Unestablished," based on previously developed criteria. Interventions falling into the "Established" category are primarily behavioral or cognitive-behavioral in nature, as are many in the "Emerging" category. Few, if any, in the "Unestablished" category are behavioral or cognitive-behavioral. As the body of literature in this area continues to grow, increasing emphasis is being placed on the use of RCT to demonstrate efficacy of behavioral

TABLE 6.2.2.4

ABA TECHNIQUES USED IN INTERVENTION FOR CHILDREN WITH AUTISM

Technique	Description	Example
Providing a cue	Providing the child with an indication that a target behavior is expected	Holding up an item and waiting expectantly for the child to request it
Prompting	Providing the child with the assistance that is needed to complete a desired behavior	Providing a model of the word he or she is expected to use to request an item if the child does not say the word spontaneously
Fading	Making prompts less explicit over time, such that the child more independently engages in a behavior	Move from verbally modeling words to waiting for the child to initiate language independently
Shaping	Providing reinforcement for successive approximations of a target behavior, rather than initially expecting the child to perform the behavior fully	Providing reinforcement for saying, "ba" in reference to a ball and reinforcing better approximations of the word over time until the child can say "ball"
Task analysis	Breaking a complex task down into its simpler parts and reinforcing the child for correctly performing each step individually	Teaching getting dressed by reinforcing the child after each step (e.g., after putting on a shirt, after putting on pants, etc.)
Backward chaining	Teaching a complex behavior by starting with reinforcement for correct performance of the last step and working successively backward to the beginning until the child is being reinforced for performing the whole behavior	Teaching putting on your coat by first reinforcing the child for zipping the coat (the final step in the process) while helping with the preceding steps, then requiring the child to pull the coat onto his shoulders, then requiring him to put his arms in the sleeves, then requiring him to complete the sequence from the beginning without help

interventions in autism. While these are still limited in the literature, they are becoming more commonplace, with recent trials supporting ESDM (206), PRT (210), and JASPER (207). As RCTs have been slow to emerge, the field continues to rely on 25+ years of single-case and uncontrolled designs, which demonstrate efficacy of behavioral interventions, especially those that are delivered through early intensive behavioral intervention (EIBI; (211,212)) models.

DISRUPTIVE BEHAVIOR

Children with externalizing problems can present with a range of disruptive behaviors including noncompliance, tantrums, verbal aggression, or more serious behaviors like physical aggression, property destruction, stealing, or other antisocial behaviors (213). Children with externalizing disorders such as conduct disorder and oppositional defiant disorder are at risk for dropping out of school, adult disruptive behaviors, trouble with the law, antisocial personality, anxiety and mood disorders, substance use, interpersonal problems, marital disruption, and poor physical health (214–216).

Cognitive-Behavioral Model

A cognitive-behavioral model of conduct problems suggests that disruptive behavior develops and is maintained by maladaptive parent–child interactions, specifically those that are coercive (217). Coercive interactions involve the child engaging in disruptive behavior and the parent reinforcing it via inadequate and misguided discipline practices.

Distortions or deficiencies in cognitive processes are often present in individuals with behavioral and conduct problems (4). It has also been suggested that cognitive problem-solving skills play a specific role in the prediction of social and behavioral adjustment (4). Other experts in this area (218–221) have suggested that a variety of cognitive distortions may contribute to risk of conduct problems. Milich and Dodge's (219) information processing model suggests that aggressive children make cognitive and attributional errors in processing information related to interactions with others. Specifically, they recall high rates of hostile cues present in social stimuli (218,219), are prone to attribute ambiguous behavior to hostile intentions (218,220), and ignore some cues in their interpretation of the behavior of others (221). These children also have distorted perceptions of their own behavior, such as perceiving their level of aggression as less than it is and taking less responsibility for conflict than other children (222). Similarly, other models have suggested that children with conduct problems have different outcome expectations and social goals than other children. Specifically, they may expect that aggressive solutions will decrease aversive reactions/behaviors of others and believe that aggressive solutions will result in positive outcomes (223). Adolescents have been shown to believe aggression will increase their self-esteem, decrease negative images, and will not cause suffering in victims (224). Finally, children with conduct problems often value the social goals of dominance and revenge more than affiliation (225). As a result, they tend toward action-oriented and aggressive, rather than verbal, solutions to social problems (226–228).

Treatment

Cognitive-behavioral interventions with aggressive children are indicated to address attributional processes, problem-solving, schemas for social goals, and expectations regarding the outcome of behavior. Further, behavioral contingencies are often used to motivate use of adaptive, rather than maladaptive skills once alternative strategies have been taught. CBTs have been shown by several meta-analytic studies to effectively reduce externalizing behavior problems for children and adolescents with moderate to large effect sizes depending on initial problem severity and age of the target child (229,230).

It has been suggested that four types of therapeutic changes are required in the treatment of conduct and related disorders (231). These are (1) ecologic, (2) operant methods, (3) medication, and (4) behavioral parent training (BPT). Specifically, ecologic changes include manipulation of environments to reduce antecedents and increase opportunities for learning more appropriate and adaptive behaviors. Operant methods include reinforcing appropriate behaviors across settings, such as home and school. Medication has been suggested as a helpful addition to behavioral programming and other interventions (232,233). Clinicians are cautioned, however, against using medication alone without engaging in a detailed analysis and behavioral treatment of the child's behavior problems. Finally, BPT (sometimes called PMT; (78,79)) is designed to decrease negative and increase positive interactions between parents and children. It also teaches parents behavior management and problem-solving techniques to improve skills in managing behaviors. BPT is considered more effective than any other treatment approach for disrupting the maladaptive parent–child interactions that lead to and maintain child disruptive behavior (234) and has a larger effect size (in the moderate range) than child-focused or school- or community-based interventions (235).

Components of intervention that are typically included in CBT-based programs for reducing externalizing behavior problems include self-monitoring, affect-labeling or emotion awareness, perspective-taking, social problem-solving, relaxation, anger management, and goal-setting (225,236). Self-monitoring, affect-labeling, or emotion awareness training is taught to monitor arousal state, to learn to label the accompanying emotions, and to learn to recognize trigger situations. Self-instruction includes learning to use inhibitory self-talk (e.g., "Stop and think!"). Perspective-taking involves increasing awareness of nonhostile cues in social situations and teaching children to find alternate explanations for the behaviors of others besides negative ones. In social problem-solving, children are taught to identify a problem and then a variety of choices for responding (such as compromising or yelling) and the associated consequences before choosing a response that will have a favorable outcome. Anger management includes becoming aware when anger levels are rising and to manage it early using relaxation, diverting attention, and coping self-talk. Skills training often involves practice of these alternatives to promote competent enactment when real situations arise. These skills are often most helpful when children learn to "insert" them between the antecedent and the impulsive behavior. In this way, they become preventative and are effective positive coping strategies. Goal-setting is used to establish short- and long-term goals that will help improve functioning (e.g., use calm body during circle time) and is best used in conjunction with an associated rewards system (225,228,236).

Several BPT programs have been developed to target decreasing disruptive behavior. Examples of programs that incorporate the principles outlined above include the Anger Coping Program and Coping Power Program (237–239), Incredible Years (IY) (240), PSST (241), and others (236). Many programs are based on one of two research groups based in the United States: Constance Hanf (Oregon Health Sciences University) and Gerald Patterson (Oregon Social Learning Center) (242,243). Hanf-model BPT programs include Parent-Child Interaction Therapy (PCIT) (244), IY (240), Helping the Noncompliant Child (HNC; (245)), Barkley's Defiant Children (246) and, later, Defiant Teens (247,248).

PCIT (244) is based on Baumrind's (249) developmental theory of parenting and social learning theory whereby parents are taught authoritarian parenting style through direct coaching while interacting with their child. PCIT aims to enhance the parent–child relationship while using social attention, limit-setting, and enhancing communication. IY (250) is a cognitive behavioral intervention for young children, ages 3 to 8, focusing on problem-solving and social skills for children. IY includes both parent management and teacher behavior management skills. It has been shown to reduce problem behavior and conduct problems with parents, and to increase self-regulation, social competence, and compliance. It has also been shown to increase parent positive affect and to replace harsh discipline techniques with effective limit-setting and to improve family communication and monitoring (240).

HNC (245) involves two clinician-coached phases: teaching parents to provide differential attention (ignore negative behavior and provide attention and social praise to appropriate behavior), and then compliance training (provide instruction, then praise for compliance or setting limits for noncompliance). Adjunctive interventions can be added including teaching parents self-control (including monitoring their adherence to HNC techniques), teaching parents about social learning theory, family-related factors including parent support and relationships, and a self-administered version that includes audio and videotapes (245). Defiant Children (246) teaches parents similar strategies to those used in HNC. Barkley later adapted these intervention principles for adolescents in his Defiant Teens program (247).

Kazdin's PMT (78,79) is a widely used model based on Patterson's (217) coercive model of parent–child interactions. The goal of PMT is to alter the interaction patterns between the child and parent, such that "prosocial, rather than coercive, behavior is directly reinforced and supported within the family" (4). Specific parent behaviors that are shaped in sessions over time include (1) establishing clear rules for the child to follow, (2) providing positive reinforcement for appropriate behavior, (3) implementing mild punishments to deter inappropriate behavior, and (4) negotiating compromises. These skills are shaped in treatment sessions through practice, feedback, role-plays, and review of in-home implementation with parents on a regular basis. Intervention also sometimes includes coordination with teachers and other service providers. Parent Management Training-Oregon Model (PMTO) (251,252) is a similar manualized clinic-based parent training program based on social interaction learning theory that involves replacing coercive parenting practices with effective parenting practices. It has shown efficacy with a variety of populations including children of divorced mothers (253), and chronically offending youth (254).

Other CBT-based treatments that have been found effective for the treatment of disruptive behavior include Positive Parenting Program (Triple P; (255)). Triple P targets prevention of behavior and emotional problems of elementary children in the general population, offers advice or brief therapy for parents of children with mild disruptive behavior, and includes intensive programming or enhanced intensive programming for parents of children with more severe behavior problems (255).

PSST (4,241) is an approach designed to develop interpersonal cognitive problem-solving skills in children with conduct problems. PSST begins with a focus on understanding the thought processes involved in how the child approaches situations. Patients are then taught step-by-step processes that guide them through solving interpersonal problems. The PSST therapist plays an active role in modeling behaviors, cueing and prompting skills, giving feedback, and praising and reinforcing correct use of skills.

Problem-Solving Communication Training is a behavioral family-systems model of parent–adolescent conflict (PSCT; (256)) where parents are taught how to understand and respond to developmental changes that their adolescents experience during puberty, with the goal of reducing adolescent–parent maladaptive interaction patterns and increasing effective problem-solving skills. Studies have shown that when comparing PSCT to PSCT plus BMT, both treatments show a decrease in parent–child conflicts with no difference between groups (257).

A primarily cognitive-based approach to reducing oppositional behavior involves reframing parents' cognitive explanations for oppositional and disruptive behavior (Collaborative Problem Solving [CPS]) (258). CPS encourages parents to view their child's disruptive behavior as a cognitive skill deficit, rather than as willful disobedience, and teaches parents how to solve problems in a collaborative way while showing empathy, defining the problem from the child's viewpoint, and inviting the child to help solve the problem (258–260). Compared to Barkley's parent training, CPS treatment resulted in equivalent improvement or better outcomes, such as lower rates of ODD symptoms and higher clinician ratings of improvement than parent training alone (259,261).

ATTENTION-DEFICIT HYPERACTIVITY DISORDER

Cognitive-Behavioral Model

In addition to the inattentive, hyperactive, and impulsive symptoms that characterize the various forms of this disorder, children with ADHD have poor self-monitoring and self-evaluation skills, may have difficulty with receptive and expressive language, and suffer from associated executive functioning deficits, such as disorganization, poor problem-solving skills, and difficulty utilizing the appropriate behavior at the correct time. The symptoms of inattention, hyperactivity, and impulsivity associated with ADHD require that patients learn self-control strategies to improve functioning. These self-control strategies typically target cognitions that accompany behavior, as well as the behaviors themselves.

Treatment

Treatment with stimulant medications is the most well-supported and commonly used intervention for ADHD. Stimulant medication shows significant benefits for improving core symptoms of ADHD, as well as secondary improvements in academic performance, and family and peer relationships (262). Risk of developing comorbid psychiatric conditions is also decreased with stimulant treatment (262). Studies show, however, that side effects may not be tolerated or acceptable (263). In addition, previous symptoms of inattention, hyperactivity, and impulsivity typically return to premorbid levels when medication is terminated (264,265). A recent meta-analysis of between-group effects of behavioral treatments for ADHD implemented in the home, school, or peer setting revealed a comparable or greater effect size (Cohen's $d = 0.74$, approaching the large effect size range) than previous studies have shown (266). Regarding timing of treatment approaches, the addition of stimulant medication after completion of a group parent-training intervention has been shown to result in fewer classroom rule-breaking behaviors and better therapy attendance, as well as lower cost, than starting with a medication-only regimen and adding behavioral treatment (267). Therefore, combination pharmacologic and behavioral treatments are considered more desirable in the treatment of this disorder (268,269), especially when potential side effects associated with long-term stimulant use are considered (265).

Behavioral or cognitive behavioral interventions in the treatment of ADHD are warranted, and have demonstrated efficacy in increasing learning, improving academic performance, reducing impulsivity, and improving attention and concentration. As criteria for ADHD diagnosis require pervasive symptoms across settings, it is generally accepted that the most effective way to implement CBT in treating ADHD is to program in the home and school, as well as through direct intervention with the individual child (268). Meta-analytic studies have supported BPT, school-based classroom management, and behavioral-based peer interventions (especially in the context of recreational summer programs; (270–272)) as effective psychosocial treatments for symptoms of ADHD (272–274). There is some variability in findings, however, with some meta-analyses not demonstrating support for parent behavioral training as a method for clearly reducing ADHD behaviors, although they did result in improvements in parent confidence and stress, and general child behavior (275). Newer research also supports organization training as an evidence-based treatment for ADHD (274,276,277).

Programming at home involves parent education, which typically consists of psychoeducation around symptoms of ADHD, behavioral observation and measurement, and behavior management skills (269). Parents are first taught to observe and measure behavior, including basic functional assessment skills. They are also often required to increase awareness of their own parenting behaviors during this time, through exercises such as monitoring statements made to their child during a 15-minute period, or being required to practice making only positive statements to their child for a specified time period. Behavior management skills are taught to reward appropriate behavior and to extinguish inappropriate behavior. Specifically, parents learn to use positive reinforcement to increase appropriate behaviors (independent play, compliance, prosocial interactions) and mild punishment to decrease negative behaviors (time out, response cost). Recent adaptations to BPT techniques have included shorting intervention periods, phone-only intervention (278), treatment enhancement, including having single mothers observe clinicians implementing behavior management and incentives (Strategies to Enhance Positive Parent Training [STEPP] (279)), or specifically attracting fathers (e.g., Coaching Our Acting-out Children: Heightening Essential Skills [COACHES] (280)). Parent Friendship Coaching targets improvement of social skills by having parents impose contingencies in the context of playdates to improve social skills (281).

School intervention emphasizes behavior management, as well as additional techniques specific to school settings. The use of a daily report card, or other daily management system, in which current goals are evaluated is a recommended component of school-based interventions (268). The daily report card facilitates communication between home and school and allows the child to be reinforced at home for good days at school. Environmental and curricular modifications, such as preferential seating in the classroom and shortened assignments, are also often made for children with ADHD. Coordination of goals across contexts (home, school, other activities) is extremely important to ensure consistency of approach. School-based intervention has also expanded to include behavioral classroom management techniques in the special education setting (282). In addition, social acceptance has been targeted using behavioral classroom management with the addition of teacher-delivered praise, attention, and messages of acceptance (Making Socially Accepting Inclusive Classrooms [MOSAIC] (281)).

A long-term goal in ADHD treatment is to gradually fade the adult control to child-driven self-management. This is one of several key procedures taught to the child individually in ADHD treatment packages. Individuals can learn to self-manage a variety of behaviors such as staying on task, compliance, attention, and suppression of disruptive behaviors. Individuals with ADHD also often need social skills intervention, including instruction in self-evaluation skills and understanding how to choose the appropriate behavior for the context. Hinshaw (268) recommended that these skills be taught in groups so that children may benefit from the inherent social context. They recommend that groups be structured with clear limits and reward systems for appropriate behavior. Further, they suggest that teaching methodologies include discussion of target behaviors and goals, modeling, behavioral rehearsal, rewards for correct performance, and feedback. Structured dyadic behavior therapy (283) is a proposed method of socially mediated behavioral therapy whereby behavioral principles are delivered with the emphasis on the process of instruction, modeling, rehearsal, and feedback to develop self-regulation and behavior management skills in a peer dyad.

Organizational interventions, which typically involve teaching children and adolescents to organize their materials and track assignments have recently shown strong evidence for improving symptoms of ADHD (274) both in the clinic setting (Organization Skills Training [OST] (277)), school (Homework, Organization Planning Skills [HOPS] (276)), and home (Plan My Life; (284)).

It has been suggested that cognitive-behavioral strategies are best for treating impulsivity, specifically (29). Teaching step-by-step problem-solving skills, including learning to anticipate the consequences of actions, is often key in the treatment of this symptom. Problem-solving strategies may be taught in a variety of formats, including coping modeling and role-plays (285). For example, in self-instruction training, children are taught to internalize the steps involved in effective problem-solving (286,287); specifically, they are taught steps such as how to recognize the problem, reflect on solutions, make a decision, and take action (286).

EATING DISORDERS

Cognitive distortions have been described in the literature as the core psychopathology of eating disorders (288,289), with other symptoms being driven by and secondary to cognitive factors. For example, Bruch (290) noted the "relentless pursuit of thinness" in patients with anorexia, and Russell (291) discussed the bulimic patient's "morbid fear of becoming fat." These patients often judge their self-worth almost solely based on weight and shape, leading to related emotional difficulties, such as low self-esteem, and cognitive distortions, such as perfectionism (especially in anorexia). The cognitive distortions are then thought to underlie all other eating disorder symptoms, such as dieting and compensatory behavior, arbitrary rules imposed upon oneself about eating (e.g., lists of allowed and forbidden foods, times of day that one is allowed to eat), and extreme negative reactions to breaking the rules because of the implications for the patient's dysfunctional belief system (breaking a rule means I have no self-control). Anorexia and bulimia will be discussed separately below, as their cognitive models and treatment differ from one another.

Bulimia

Cognitive-Behavioral Model

In bulimia, the patient is caught in a vicious cycle of bingeing and purging. This cycle originates and is maintained as a result of the mistaken view that compensatory behaviors (vomiting, laxative use, diuretics, over-exercising) are effective means of weight control. This belief causes the barrier against binge eating to be removed and the cycle begins. That is, the individual binges because he or she believes before doing so that there is a means of controlling the outcome. This belief is especially salient with vomiting because it is easier to vomit when the stomach is very full. In this cycle, however, vomiting leads to intense self-hatred, which decreases self-esteem, and exacerbates the notion that weight control will lead to more positive self-evaluation. As a result, the cycle is maintained. This binge–purge cycle is also associated with the antecedent of negative affect, which may lead to overeating and begin the cycle. As a result, cognitive and emotional interpretations of a negative event can significantly exacerbate the bulimic cycle and must be a focus in therapy and relapse prevention.

Treatment

Treatment research for bulimia in children and adolescents is somewhat sparse, with most approaches drawing heavily from the adult literature. The most important issues to address in treatment of this disorder include binge eating and purging behaviors, dieting behaviors, and concerns about shape and weight (288). Motivation for treatment is typically less of a problem in bulimia than in anorexia, as bulimic patients are typically distressed by the binge–purge cycle. While traditional CBT approaches to treat bulimia have been shown to result in a reduction of symptoms, only about 40% of individuals with bulimia recover with traditional CBT treatment, and the relapse rate at follow-up is high (292). Thus, to improve treatment outcomes, enhancements (E) have been made to the standard CBT model, and the new model, CBT-E, has shown greater efficacy (293). In CBT-E, processes maintaining an individual's eating disorder are identified, and that information is used to create a personalized treatment approach (294). Additional modules have also been added to the traditional CBT model that address perfectionism, mood, interpersonal problems, and low self-esteem (295). There are two main forms of CBT-E: the "focused" version (CBT-Ef) and the "broad" version (CBT-Eb). The focused version of CBT-E targets eating disorder psychopathology and is appropriate for most patients (296). The broad approach addresses external obstacles, in addition to eating disorder psychopathology, and should be used with those patients who present with additional maintenance mechanisms (perfectionism, low self-esteem, interpersonal difficulties; (296)).

CBT-E follows four main stages. The main goals of the first stage are "to engage the patient in treatment and change, to derive a personalized formulation (case conceptualization) with the patient, to provide education about treatment and the disorder, and to introduce and implement two important procedures: collaborative "weekly weighing" and "regular eating" (294,296). Self-monitoring of eating and related behaviors is also introduced in this stage and is practiced throughout treatment.

To jointly create the formulation, the therapist and the patient work together to identify the processes that are maintaining the eating disorder, and the patient learns that these mechanisms can be changed. The purpose of the education component is to challenge the patient's misconceptions about body weight and methods of weight control and to inform the patient of the adverse physical and psychological effects of eating disorders. The weekly weigh-in is also used as an opportunity for education, as the therapist helps the patient to understand the number on the scale. Patients are encouraged not to weigh themselves at other times, in order to address excessive body checking.

Establishing a schedule of "regular eating" (planned meals and snacks) is essential in the first stage, as it provides the patient with structure and limits opportunities for binge eating (296). Normalization of the eating pattern typically leads to a reduction in bingeing, which automatically leads to a reduction in purging. As such, it may not be necessary to separately address purging behavior. Patients agree not to eat outside of this schedule and to not engage in compensatory behaviors (e.g., vomiting, laxatives, diuretics).

The second stage is brief and is considered a transitional stage (294). In this stage, the therapist and the patient review progress; identify any obstacles to change; revise the formulation, as needed; and plan for stage three (296).

Stage three consists of the main treatment. The goal of this stage is to address those mechanisms that are maintaining the disorder. The first step is to help the patient explore the concept of self-evaluation, and attention is drawn to the patient's over-evaluation of shape and weight. The therapist helps the patient to see how other aspects of life are neglected when their priority is their shape and weight, with the goal being to increase the importance of other aspects of life and to decrease the importance of shape and weight (294).

The patient's reliance on dietary rules is also addressed in this stage. The therapist helps the patient to identify the beliefs that are the basis of those rules, and then supports the patient in breaking the rules and challenging their beliefs (296). The goal is for the patient to learn that "the feared consequences that maintain the dietary rule (typically weight gain or binge eating) are not an inevitable result" (296).

In the last stage of CBT-E, the focus is on developing a plan to maintain progress and to reduce the chances of relapse (296).

Preliminary studies suggest that CBT-E can be helpful for younger patients with eating disorders (292,295). Fairburn (294) proposes several guidelines for adapting CBT-E for use with children and adolescents. These include, (1) helping the child/adolescent to develop autonomy and to take personal responsibility, (2) using age-appropriate language and visual aids, (3) assisting the child with social-communication skills to improve peer relationships, (4) involving the school and family in the treatment plan, and (5) intervening early with treatment to mitigate the medical complications associated with eating disorders.

DBT may also be helpful for adolescents with eating disorders since its focus is on improving emotion regulation, which is often an area of challenge for patients with eating disorders (297). Research on DBT for treating adolescent eating disorders is limited to case series (298) and studies with small sample sizes (297), but results suggest that adolescents engaged in a DBT program experience significant reductions in behavioral (e.g., binging/purging) and cognitive symptoms (e.g., over-evaluation of shape and weight, rigidity, guilt) of eating disorders (297,298). Further research is warranted in this area.

Anorexia

Cognitive-Behavioral Model

The primary cognitive distortion in anorexia is that most patients do not believe they have a problem (294); rather, they believe that they are fat and truly need to lose weight. Therefore, the restricting behaviors of a patient with anorexia are reinforced when they result in weight loss. This egosyntonic viewpoint differs from the view of patients with bulimia, who view their bingeing and purging behavior as aversive, leading to negative self-evaluation and motivation to change. The interaction of dysfunctional cognitions and starvation are important maintaining factors in anorexia (288). For example, preoccupation with food and eating exaggerates the concerns about eating, and lowering of mood due to starvation intensifies negative self-evaluation, thus leading to increased efforts to restrict food to control weight. An additional cognitive distortion that may exist involves "an extreme need for self-control upon which shape and weight concerns are superimposed" (288). This notion suggests that cognitive distortions regarding perfectionism, need for control, and rigidity need to be addressed in treatment.

Treatment

Issues that must be addressed in treatment include concerns about shape and weight, dieting behavior, and lack of motivation to change (288). The first goal of anorexia treatment is typically weight gain, especially in severe cases. Since eating disorders share many clinical features, some of the treatment components outlined in the treatment of bulimia may apply; however, several additional components may be necessary to treat anorexia (294,299). Specifically, clinicians treating anorexic patients must address the patient's lack of motivation. Intervention procedures, such as self-monitoring and meal planning, must be introduced slowly, as the patient is likely to resist them initially.

In trying to alter the lack of motivation in anorexia, the patient's viewpoint must be validated, followed by a review of the advantages and disadvantages of the disorder versus change. It may also be helpful to identify clinical features that the patient might view as problematic to increase motivation, which may be accomplished through psychoeducation about the effects of starvation on the patient's health.

Similar to treatment for bulimia, CBT-E has been shown to be a promising treatment for adults and adolescents with anorexia, with some modifications (16,292,299). Treatment for anorexia using a CBT-E approach includes the following stages.

In stage one, the intent is to help the individual realize the need for weight gain and to agree to this as a treatment goal (299). Establishing the therapeutic alliance and engaging the individual in treatment are particularly important in this initial stage, as these patients are typically unmotivated in treatment (299,300). For treatment with adolescents, the therapist works with parents to identify any family factors that may interfere with treatment.

In stage two, individuals work to regain weight to a healthy level, and eating disorder psychopathology is addressed. Weight gain can be facilitated through psychoeducation regarding issues such as starvation, symptoms of the disorder, and the principles of treatment (294,299,300). Eating disorder psychopathology is addressed by targeting the individual's concerns about shape and weight, addressing restrictive eating and dietary rules, helping the individual learn how to self-monitor and to cope with setbacks, and continuing to emphasize weight gain.

In stage three, the focus is on helping the patient maintain their healthy weight and on "ending the treatment well" (294,299), with a focus on helping the patient to accept and appreciate their new body. The therapist and the patient "end well" by creating a personalized plan that identifies any lingering issues and that anticipates potential setbacks to recovery (299). The goal of this plan is to maximize the chances that advances will be maintained and to minimize the risk of relapse (294).

While the use of CBT-E to treat adolescents with anorexia still needs further research, family therapy with a behavioral focus (FT-B) is considered a well-established treatment for anorexia in adolescents (295). In FT-B, parents are considered a resource in treatment, rather than as having caused or maintained the disorder. Like CBT-E, FT-B has three main stages. In the first stage, parents are encouraged to manage their children's weight restoration via interventions such as food exposure, which targets food anxiety and dietary rigidity (301). Once a healthy weight has been reached, families move on to stage two, in which the child or adolescent slowly begins to take control over their eating. Finally, stage three focuses on relapse prevention. The success rate of FT-B in treating adolescents with anorexia is strong: 60% to 90% of adolescents with anorexia who receive a family-based treatment approach maintain recovery or partial recovery at follow-up (292). New research shows that this treatment may be effective in children with restrictive eating disorders under the age of 12 years, as well (301).

TOURETTE SYNDROME

Cognitive-Behavioral Model

Tourette syndrome and other transient tic disorders are characterized by the presence of vocal and/or motor tics. Although often described as involuntary, research suggests that tics are not analogous to other involuntary movements, such as choreas or dystonias (302). Instead, it appears to be the *urge* to engage in the movement that is involuntary, with the movement behavior itself being "irresistible" as a result of the urge. This conceptualization of tics suggests the role of negative reinforcement (dissipation of the urge upon performance of the tic) as a contributing factor in the shaping and maintenance of tic expression (303) and supports the use of cognitive-behavioral treatments aimed at disrupting the urge–tic relationship (304).

Treatment

The treatment literature strongly supports the efficacy of habit reversal training (HRT), alone or in combination with other behavioral techniques for Tourette's and other tic disorders (305). HRT is designed to disrupt the relationship between the premonitory urge and tic expression in analogous fashion to the role of ERP in disrupting the obsession-compulsion relationship in OCD. More recently, HRT has been combined with a functional assessment/intervention (FAI) procedure and manualized as the Comprehensive Behavioral Intervention for Tics (CBIT; (306)). Based on the positive results from a multisite controlled trial (307), CBIT is considered the first-line treatment for youth with tic disorders (308).

CBIT treatment encompasses a number of steps. During the initial assessment phase, problematic tics are identified and are hierarchically ranked according to how bothersome they are. Self-monitoring is then used to provide information regarding tic frequency across different settings, along with serving to enhance child and parent awareness of the tics. During awareness training, the targeted tic is first operationally defined, and the patient is trained to identify the occurrence of each tic and the sensations that precede it. This procedure is completed through several steps including (1) describing the tic and its associated preceding sensations in detail, (2) observing therapist simulations of the tic, and (3) observing and acknowledging one's own simulated or actual tics. These procedures result in a heightened awareness of the tic that is critical for successful implementation of the habit reversal procedures (306).

After awareness training is complete, competing response training, the primary treatment component for habit reversal, is implemented. Competing responses are incompatible behaviors to be performed instead of the tic, contingent on the urge to tic. Competing response training involves determining the competing behavior, clinician demonstration of the competing response, and patient demonstration of the competing response with feedback from the clinician. The clinician continues to provide feedback until it is clear that the patient is performing the competing response correctly (306). Once competing response training for a given tic is implemented in session, the child is instructed to use the competing response as often as possible, and ideally every time, he or she experiences the premonitory urge or other trigger for the targeted tic. It is also important to note that although the urge often reduces in intensity with treatment, complete disappearance is uncommon. As such, HRT may be more accurately characterized to patients and their families as a tool for managing, but not eliminating tics. See Table 6.2.2.5 for sample tic, urge, and competing response form.

Social support training is the final component of HRT and involves having someone else (usually a parent when working with children and adolescents) support the implementation of the procedures outside the session. The role of the support person involves praising and acknowledging correct use of the competing response, and prompting its use when necessary (when a tic is observed without use of the competing response). The supportive individual should be trained in session through modeling and behavioral rehearsal how to provide both types of feedback. When working with children, it may also be necessary to have a teacher's social support, as the child may spend a substantial period of the day away from parents.

Implemented concurrently with HRT, the FAI procedure is used to identify any environmental variables serving to trigger (antecedents) or maintain (consequences) tics. Although neurologic in origin, multiple studies have demonstrated the sensitivity of tics to environmental factors (309). Therefore, understanding how contextual and socially mediated positive and negative reinforcement play a role in triggering and maintaining tics can be critical to successful treatment. The most common situational antecedents associated with tic exacerbation include playing videogames, home after school, in the car, and doing homework. Tic consequences are classified as either social (e.g., teasing, being told to stop, other negative reaction, positive attention from parent, or other) or escape

TABLE 6.2.2.5

SAMPLE TIC, URGE, AND COMPETING RESPONSE FORM

Name of Tic	Definition	Tic Signals (Premonitory Urge)	Competing Response
Head bobbing	Chin goes down toward the chest and then goes up toward the sky as the top of the head goes back	Tense feelings in neck	Tensing neck muscles gently while facing eyes and head forward
Head turning	Neck jerks or turns side to side repeatedly	Pressure builds in sternocleidomastoid muscle	Hold chin to chest with shoulders gently back
Eye blink	Eyelids open wide and squint repeatedly	Pressure builds around the eye socket	Gently focus on spot a few feet in front while gently/softly closing and then opening eyes
Arm flinch	Arms fly horizontally outward from body or swing back and forth	Deltoid muscle tightens and pressurizes	Hold elbows tight to belt loops with shoulders back
Mouth opening	Jaw opens widely, slight wide eye opening	Pressure builds around the lips	Slight smile with lips closed
Lip pursing/nose scrunch	Lips tightly close and move toward nose; muscle moves nose up and nostrils flare widely	Pressure builds up slightly on the nasalis muscle and then loosens and reduces muscular resistance on the nose. Urge is to reset.	Pinch nasalis muscle/upper nose cartilage with medium pressure as to sense "pulling nose the long way"
Tongue thrusting	Tongue sticks out through lips	Pressure builds inside tongue itself	Touch tongue to hard palate while gently pursing lips closed

from responsibility (e.g., leaving the classroom or dinner table, or not having to complete homework or other aversive tasks). Once identified, these variables are addressed using behavioral or other relevant techniques.

Multiple small studies have demonstrated the efficacy of HRT for Tourette's and other tic disorders in children (304); however, broader acceptance of the behavioral treatment of tic disorders only occurred after publication of the multisite CBIT trial (307). A total of 126 children, ages 9 to 17 years, with Tourette's or chronic tic disorder were randomized to eight sessions over 10 weeks of either CBIT or a manualized version of psychoeducation plus supportive therapy (the most common psychotherapy for youth with pervasive tic disorders at that time). Youth randomized to CBIT had significantly higher response rates (53% vs. 19%) and greater reductions in both tic severity and functional impairment. Treatment gains were largely durable over a 6-month follow-up period. Importantly, the between-group effect size for CBIT ($d = 0.68$) was relatively similar to those found in similarly designed pharmacologic studies with the important benefit being that, unlike pharmacologic treatments for Tourette's, CBIT treatment was absent significant side effects.

TRICHOTILLOMANIA

Cognitive-Behavioral Model

TTM is characterized by chronic hair pulling, which results in noticeable hair loss, most commonly on the scalp, eyebrows and lashes, facial hair, and pubic hair (310). Hair loss may result in distress and stigmatization that leads to avoidance of social situations. Similar to tic disorders, the individual typically experiences an urge or increasing sense of tension prior to pulling that is released when the behavior occurs (311). TTM is categorized in the DSM-5 under obsessive-compulsive and related disorders (122). The cognitive-behavioral conceptualization of TTM suggests that hair pulling behaviors are maintained by a negative reinforcement paradigm similar to OCD and tic disorders, as tension is reduced when the hair-pulling behavior occurs (311).

Treatment

Unfortunately, the empirical database is quite sparse with regard to the treatment of pediatric TTM; however, the only randomized controlled treatment study in this area provides strong support for the efficacy of HRT (312). In treatment of TTM, awareness training involves becoming aware of the tension or urge that precedes the pulling, as well as becoming aware of the behavior itself. Awareness training is followed by competing response training and social support, as in tic disorders. The most common competing responses involve engaging the child's hands in a manner incompatible with pulling (e.g., making a fist, squeezing a soft ball, sitting on hands or putting them in one's pocket). HRT is commonly augmented with other treatment techniques including stimulus control, FAI, and anxiety management (313). Stimulus control techniques such as putting bandages on the pulling fingers and/or wearing gloves or other hand coverings enhance awareness of pulling and picking and make these behaviors more difficult. Functional assessment is used to identify settings and other pulling and picking triggers (e.g., sensory, emotional, etc.), as well as maintaining consequences which are then addressed using behavioral or other strategies (e.g., instructing family members to refrain from telling the child to stop pulling). Relaxation training or other anxiety reduction techniques are commonly employed to reduce stress and anxiety, a common symptom trigger (311).

OTHER CLINICAL PROBLEMS

Enuresis

The night alarm has often been cited as the most effective treatment for nocturnal enuresis (314–316). This device electronically signals the child with an alarm when it becomes wet with urine, thereby providing a prompt to create an active avoidance response when the urinary need occurs, to inhibit urination, and to avoid setting off the alarm (317,318). This procedure has been found to be effective 75% to 80% of the time, with relapse rate at 6 months between 15% and 30% (315,319–322). Alarm training is often packaged with adjunctive treatment components. Full Spectrum Home Training (323) combines alarm training with overlearning (having child purposefully drink water before bed to practice avoidance response at night) and has been shown to decrease relapse rate for alarm-only treatments (318). Dry Bed Training (324) augments alarm training with positive practice (practicing being asleep then rapidly waking and going to the bathroom), waking the child during the night to prompt voiding, self-correction (requiring the child to change the bed and their clothes after a toileting accident, appropriate to their developmental level), self-recording successes and failures, and reinforcing the child for successful nighttime toileting behaviors using tangible and social rewards. This combination treatment lasts 4 weeks, with approximately a 40% relapse rate, and is thought to be more effective than the night alarm alone in relapse prevention (321,325–327). Friman and Jones (328) created an optimal treatment plan for nighttime enuresis by combining the urine alarm with adjunctive treatment components.

Children who have diurnal enuresis are often treated behaviorally, whereby they are prompted to use the bathroom on a regular schedule (e.g., once per hour) and are then reinforced for trying as well as for actually urinating in the toilet (329,330). Over time, prompts can be faded such that the child learns to initiate using the toilet independently. This process may also be accompanied by overcorrection or positive practice. For example, when the child has a toileting accident, he or she may be prompted to return to the scene of the accident and to go through all the steps involved in going to the toilet (e.g., walk to the toilet, pull down pants, sit down, wipe, stand up, etc.) multiple times to practice the positive behavior.

Encopresis

Fecal incontinence often occurs when children become constipated or when there is bowel retention, which can lead to physiologic changes such as decreased ability of the muscle groups to engage in a bowel movement and reduction in the sensation needed to trigger a bowel movement (331). It has been proposed that the pain of having a bowel movement when constipated causes children to become avoidant of doing so due to aversive conditioning and can result in toileting resistance, withholding, and incomplete voiding (231,332,333). Therefore, treatment of encopresis often consists of a combination of laxative prescription, dietary changes, and behavioral methods (334). For example, children are often given laxatives to ensure regular, pain-free bowel movements and are then rewarded for having a movement in the toilet (335–337).

In addition to laxative therapy and dietary changes, behavioral interventions include skills training, establishing a toileting routine, reinforcing the child for sitting on the toilet for a short period of time on a systematic schedule (in the morning, after school, and before bed), and increasing motivation (320). In addition to reinforcement for taking bathroom trips, differential reinforcement can be used if a bowel movement actually occurs. In this way, adaptive toileting behaviors are taught in addition to training actual bowel movements. These procedures may also be complemented with regular pants checks, with clean pants resulting in reinforcement, as well. Overcorrection procedures are sometimes used in conjunction with pants checks, in which the child is required to wash the soiled clothing and to take a bath (337). These procedures must be modified developmentally, as they may result in significant resistance from young children, thereby making the training experience more negative than is necessary. A recent review of behavioral treatments for encopresis with constipation supported behavioral treatments in conjunction with laxative therapy for reducing soiling accidents and author-defined successful resolution of fecal incontinence compared to laxative therapy alone (338).

Stuttering

Direct treatment of stuttering involves working on the speech of the child, while indirect treatment involves changing elements in the environment. While in the past, there was an attitude that addressing stuttering would make the condition worse, by the 1970s, indirect treatments involving manipulation of the environment around the child prevailed. More recently the focus has shifted to direct treatment of the child with the involvement of the parent. Relaxation training is often cited as the most common treatment for stuttering. Often when children are encouraged to slow down their speaking, to take deep breaths, and to relax, their stuttering decreases. Habit reversal is used to treat stuttering when relaxation training is paired with awareness training and psychoeducation about the nature of the disorder. Contingency management may be helpful, whereby a child is reinforced for slowing down and speaking in a more relaxed fashion.

The Lidcombe Program, an operant conditioning (direct treatment) approach, was designed by researchers in Australia. In this program, parents are trained to provide verbal contingencies in one or two 10- to 15-minute conversations per day with their child using predetermined responses for stutter-free and stuttered speech (339,340). The Lidcombe Program has demonstrated efficacy in decreasing stuttering by 9 months posttreatment (341). The Lidcombe Program was compared to another indirect treatment approach (based on the Demands and Capacities Model; RESTART-DCM; (342)) and both treatments showed a high response rate, with 76% and 71% of children classified as nonstuttering at 18 months' posttreatment, respectively (343). Stuttering has a high rate of spontaneous recovery, at nearly 63% by 3 years' postsymptom onset, which makes it difficult to determine treatment effectiveness (344).

References

1. Accreditation Council for Graduate Medical Education (ACGME): *ACGME Program Requirements for Graduate Medical Education in Psychiatry*, 2016.
2. Albano A: Cognitive-behavioral psychotherapy for children and adolescents. In: Sadock B, Sadock V (eds): *Comprehensive Textbook of Psychiatry*. 8th ed. Philadelphia, PA, Lippincott Williams & Wilkins, 3332–3342, 2005.
3. Sudak DM, Goldberg DA: Trends in psychotherapy training: a national survey of psychiatry residency training. *Acad Psychiatry* 36(5):369–373, 2012.
4. Kazdin A: Cognitive-behavior modification. In: Weiner J, Dulcan M (eds): *Textbook of Child and Adolescent Psychiatry*. Arlington, VA, American Psychiatric Publishing, Inc., 985–1006, 2004.
5. Clark D: Cognitive-behavior therapy for anxiety disorders. In: Gelder M, Lopez-Ibor J, Andreasen N (eds): *New Oxford Textbook of Psychiatry*. New York, Oxford University Press Inc., 2000.
6. Beck A: *Depression: Causes and Treatment*. 5th ed. Philadelphia, PA, University of Pennsylvania Press, 1977.
7. Beck A, Clark D, Alford A: *Scientific Foundations of Cognitive Theory and Therapy of Depression*. New York, Wiley, 1999.
8. Beck A, Rush A, Shaw B, Emery G: *Kognitive Therapie der Depression*. Weinheim, Germany, PVU, 1994.
9. Pavlov I: *Conditioned Reflexes*. Oxford, Clarendon Press, 1927.
10. Skinner B: *The Behavior of Organisms*. New York, Appleton-Century-Crofts, 1938.
11. Skinner B: *Science and Human Behavior*. New York, Free Press, 1953.
12. Dattilio FM, Hanna MA: Collaboration in cognitive-behavioral therapy. *J Clin Psychol* 68(2):146–158, 2012.
13. Thase ME, Wright JH, Friedman ES, Russ E: Cognitive and behavioral therapies. In: Tasman A, Kay J, Lieberman JA, First MB, Riba MB (eds): *Psychiatry*. 4th ed. West Sussex, England, Wiley Blackwell, 1836–1858, 2015.
14. Clark D, Beck A, Alford B: *Scientific Foundations of Cognitive Theory and Therapy of Depression*. Hoboken, NJ, John Wiley, 1999.
15. Wright J, Beck A: Cognitive therapy. In: Hales R, Yudofsky S, Talbott J (eds): *American Psychiatric Press Textbook of Psychiatry*. Vol 13. Washington, DC, American Psychiatric Press, 1083–1114, 1994.
16. Dalle Grave R, Calugi S, Doll HA, Fairburn CG: Enhanced cognitive behaviour therapy for adolescents with anorexia nervosa: an alternative to family therapy. *Behav Res Ther* 51(1):R9–R12, 2013.
17. Friedman E, Thase M, Wright J: Cognitive and behavioral therapies. In: Tasman A, Kay J, Lieberman J (eds): Psychiatry. 2nd ed. West Sussex, England, John Wiley & Sons, Ltd., 1753–1777, 2003.
18. Piacentini J, Bergman R: Developmental issues in cognitive therapy for childhood anxiety disorders. *J Cogn Psychother* 15:165–182, 2001.
19. Leahy R: Cognitive therapy of childhood depression: developmental considerations. In: Shirk S (ed): *Cognitive Development and Child Psychopathology*. New York, Plenum, 187–204, 1988.
20. Moritz E, Jablonsky J: *Blink, Blink, Clop, Clop: Why Do We Do Things We Can't Stop*. Plainview, NY, Childswork/Childsplay, 1998.
21. Knell S, Dasari M: Cognitive-behavioral play therapy for anxiety and depression. In: Reddy L, Files-Hall T, Schaefer C (eds): *Empirically Based Play Interventions for Children*. 2nd ed. Washington, DC, American Psychological Association, 77–94, 2016.
22. Knell S: Cognitive behavioral play therapy. In: Schaefer C (ed): *Foundations of Play Therapy*. Hoboken, NJ, John Wiley & Sons, Inc., 177–191, 2003.
23. Bandura A: *Social Learning Theory*. Englewood Cliffs, NJ, Prentice Hall, 1977.
24. Kendall P: *Child and Adolescent Therapy: Cognitive-Behavioral Procedures*. 4th ed. New York, Guilford Publications, 2012.
25. Kendall P, Suveg C: Treating anxiety disorders in youth. In: Kendall P (ed): *Child and Adolescent Therapy*. 3rd ed. New York, Guilford Press, 243–294, 2006.
26. Herren J, Freeman J, Garcia A: Using family-based exposure with response prevention to treat obsessive-compulsive disorder in young children: a case study. *J Clin Psychol* 72(11):1152–1161, 2016.
27. Albert U, Bogetto F, Maina G, Saracco P, Brunatto C, Mataix-Cols D: Family accommodation in obsessive-compulsive disorder: relation to symptom dimensions, clinical and family characteristics. *Psychiatry Res* 179(2):204–211, 2010.
28. Piacentini J, March J, Franklin M: Cognitive-behavioral therapy for youngsters with obsessive-compulsive disorder. In: Kendall P (ed): *Child and Adolescent Therapy: Cognitive-Behavioral Procedures*. New York, Guilford, 297–321, 2006.
29. Kendall P, Lochman J: Cognitive-behavioral therapies. In: Rutter M, Taylor E, Hersov L (eds): *Child and Adolescent Psychiatry*. Oxford, Blackwell Scientific Publications, 844–857, 1994.
30. Lochman J: Modification of childhood aggression. In: Hersen M, Eisler R, Miller P (eds): *Progress in Behavior Modification*. Vol 25. Newbury Park, CA, Sage, 47–85, 1990.
31. Kazdin A: *Conduct Disorder in Childhood and Adolescence*. Newbury Park, CA, Sage, 1987.
32. Weisz JR, Kazdin AE: The present and future of evidence-based psychotherapies for children and adolescents. In: Weisz JR, Kazdin AE (eds): *Evidence-Based Psychotherapies for Children and Adolescents*. 2nd ed. New York, The Guilford Press, 557–572, 2012.
33. Schmidt SJ, Schimmelmann BG: Evidence-based psychotherapy in children and adolescents: advances, methodological and conceptual limitations, and perspectives. *Eur Child Adolesc Psychiatry* 22(5):265–268, 2013.
34. Durlak J, Wells A, Cotton J: Analysis of selected methodological issues in child psychotherapy research. *J Clin Child Psychol* 24:141–148, 1995.
35. Kazdin A, Bass D, Ayers W, Rodgers A: The empirical and clinical focus of child and adolescent psychotherapy research. *J Consult Clin Psychol* 58:729–740, 1990.
36. Rachman S: Obsessions, responsibility, and guilt. *Behav Res Ther* 31(2): 149–154, 1993.
37. Curry S, Marlatt G, Gordon J: Abstinence violation effect: validation of an attributional construct with smoking cessation. *J Consult Clin Psychol* 52(2):145–149, 1987.
38. Curry S, Marlatt G, Gordon J, Baer J, Schneiderman N: A comparison of alternative theoretical approaches to smoking cessation and relapse. *Health Psychol* 7(6):545–556, 1988.

39. Kendall P: *Child and Adolescent Therapy: Cognitive-Behavioral Procedures.* 3rd ed. New York, Guilford Press, 2006.
40. Brown KW, Ryan RM: The benefits of being present: mindfulness and its role in psychological well-being. *J Person Soc Psychol* 84(4):822–848, 2003.
41. Brown KW, Ryan RM, Creswell JD: Mindfulness: theoretical foundations and evidence for its salutary effects. *Psychol Inquiry* 18(4):211–237, 2007.
42. Kabat-Zinn J: *Full catastrophe living: the program of the Stress Reduction Clinic at the University of Massachusetts Medical Center.* New York, Dell, 1990.
43. Shapiro SL, Carlson LE, Astin JA, Freedman B: Mechanisms of mindfulness. *J Clin Psychol* 62(3):373–386, 2006.
44. Grossman P, Niemann L, Schmidt S, Walach H: Mindfulness-based stress reduction and health benefits. *J Psychosomat Res* 57(1):35–43, 2004.
45. Biegel G: *The Stress Reduction Workbook for Teens: Mindfulness Skills to Help You Deal with Stress.* Oakland, CA, New Harbinger Publications, Inc., 2009.
46. Biegel GM, Brown KW, Shapiro SL, Schubert CM: Mindfulness-based stress reduction for the treatment of adolescent psychiatric outpatients: a randomized clinical trial. *J Consult Clin Psychol* 77(5):855–866, 2009.
47. Teasdale JD, Segal ZV, Williams JM, Ridgeway VA, Soulsby JM, Lau MA: Prevention of relapse/recurrence in major depression by mindfulness-based cognitive therapy. *J Consult Clin Psychol* 68(4):615–623, 2000.
48. Segal Z, Williams J, Teasdale J: *Mindfulness-Based Cognitive Therapy for Depression: A New Approach to Preventing Relapse.* New York, Guilford Press, 2002.
49. Cladder-Micus M, Vrijsen J, Becker E, Donders R, Spijker J, Speckens A: A randomized controlled trial of Mindfulness-Based Cognitive Therapy (MBCT) versus treatment-as-usual (TAU) for chronic, treatment-resistant depression: a study protocol. *BMC Psychiatry* 9(15):275–283, 2015.
50. Bögels S, Hoogstad B, van Dun L, de Schutter S, Restifo K: Mindfulness training for adolescents with externalizing disorders and their parents. *Behav Cogn Psychother* 36(2), 2008.
51. Haydicky J, Shecter C, Wiener J, Ducharme JM: Evaluation of MBCT for adolescents with ADHD and their parents: impact on individual and family functioning. *J Child Fam Stud* 24(1):76–94, 2015.
52. van der Oord S, Bogels S, Peijnenburg D: The effectiveness of mindfulness training for children with ADHD and mindful parenting for their parents. *J Child Fam Stud* 21(1):139–147, 2012.
53. Linehan M: *Cognitive-Behavioral Treatment of Borderline Personality Disorder.* New York, Guilford Press, 1993.
54. Miller A, Rathus J, Linehan M, Wetzler S, Leigh E: Dialectical behavior therapy for suicidal adolescents. *J Pract Psychiatry Behav Health* 3:78–86, 1997.
55. Miller A, Rathus J, Linehan M: *Dialectical Behavior Therapy with Suicidal Adolescents.* New York, Guilford Press, 2007.
56. Rathus J, Miller A: *DBT Skills Manual for Adolescents.* New York, Guilford Press, 2015.
57. Cook NE, Gorraiz M: Dialectical behavior therapy for nonsuicidal self-injury and depression among adolescents: preliminary meta-analytic evidence. *Child Adolesc Ment Health* 21(2):81–89, 2016.
58. Salbach-Andrae H, Bohnekamp I, Bierbaum T, et al.: Dialectical behavior therapy (DBT) and cognitive behavioral therapy (CBT) for adolescents with anorexia and bulimia nervosa in comparison. *Child Dev* 18(3):180–190, 2009.
59. Ritschel LA, Lim NE, Stewart LM: Transdiagnostic applications of DBT for adolescents and adults. *Am J Psychother* 69(2):111–128, 2015.
60. Mazza J, Dexter-Mazza E, Miller A, Rathus J, Murphy H, Linehan M: *DBT® Skills in Schools: Skills Training for Emotional Problem Solving for Adolescents (DBT STEPS-A).* New York, Guildford Press, 2016.
61. Lichstein KL, Taylor DJ, McCrae CS, Thomas SJ: Relaxation for insomnia. In: Perlis M, Aloia M, Kuhn BR (eds): *Behavioral Treatments for Sleep Disorders: A Comprehensive Primer of Behavioral Sleep Medicine Interventions.* 1st ed. Amsterdam; Boston, MA, Academic, 45–54, 2011.
62. Lochman J, Wells K, Karen L: *Treatments that Work: Coping Power: Child Group Facilitator's Guide.* Oxford, Oxford University Press, 289, 2008.
63. Kellner M: *In Control: A Skill-Building Program for Teaching Young Adolescents to Manage Anger.* Champaign, IL, Research Press, 2001.
64. Piacentini J, Roblek T: Exposure plus response prevention. In: Ollendick T, Schroeder C (eds): *Encyclopedia of Pediatric and Child Psychology.* New York, Kluwer Academic, 222–223, 2003.
65. Craske M, Treanor M, Conway C, Zbozinek T, Vervliet B: Maximizing exposure therapy: an inhibitory learning approach. *Behav Res Ther* 58:10–23, 2014.
66. Götestam K: One session group treatment of spider phobia by direct or modelled exposure. *Cogn Behav Ther* 31(1):18–24, 2002.
67. Southall CM, Gast DL: Self-management procedures: a comparison across the autism spectrum. *Edu Train Autism Dev Dis* 46(2):155–171, 2011.
68. Koegel R, Frea W: Treatment of social behavior in autism through the modification of pivotal social skills. *J Appl Behav Anal* 26:222–223, 1993.
69. Koegel L, Harrower J, Koegel R: Support for children with developmental disabilities in full inclusion classrooms through self-management. *J Posit Behav Inter* 1(1):26–34, 1999.
70. Ninness C, Fuerst J, Rutherford R, Glenn S: Effects of self-management training and reinforcement on the transfer of improved conduct in the absence of supervision. *J Appl Behav Anal* 24(3):499–508, 1991.
71. Stahmer A, Schreibman L: Teaching children with autism appropriate play in unsupervised environments using a self-management treatment package. *J Appl Behav Anal* 25(2):447–459, 1992.
72. Singh NN, Lancioni GE, Joy SD, et al.: Adolescents with conduct disorder can be mindful of their aggressive behavior. *J Emot Behav Disord* 15(1):55–63, 2007.
73. Gregory K, Kehle T, McLoughlin C: Generalization and maintenance of treatment gains using self-management procedures with behaviorally disordered adolescents. *Psychol Rep* 80:683–690, 1997.
74. Beck A: *Depression: Clinical, Experimental, and Theoretical Aspects.* New York, Harper and Row, 1967.
75. Beck A, Rush A, Shaw B: *Cognitive Therapy of Depression.* New York, Guilford Press, 1979.
76. Hanley G, Iwata B, McCord B: Functional analysis of problem behavior: a review. *J Appl Behav Anal* 36:147–185, 2003.
77. Roane HS, Fisher WW, Carr JE: Applied behavior analysis as treatment for autism spectrum disorder. *J Pediatr* 175:27–32, 2016.
78. Kazdin A: *Behavior Modification in Applied Settings.* 6th ed. Belmont, CA, Wadsworth/Thomson Learning, 2001.
79. Kazdin A: Parent Management Training: evidence, outcomes, and issues. *J Am Acad Child Adolesc Psychiatry* 36(10):1349–1356, 1997.
80. Wolpe J: *Psychotherapy by Reciprocal Inhibition.* Stanford, CA, Stanford University Press, 1958.
81. Jones M: The elimination of children's fears. *J Exp Psychol* 7(5):382–390, 1924.
82. Kazdin A, Wilcoxin L: Systematic desensitization and nonspecific treatment effects: a methodological consideration. *Psychol Bull* 83(5):729–758, 1976.
83. Morris RJ, Kratochwill TR, Schoenfield G, Auster ER: Childhood fears, phobias, and related anxieties. In: Morris RJ, Kratochwill TR (eds): *The Practice of Child Therapy.* 4th ed. Routledge, 93–140, 2012.
84. Woods D, Miltenberger R: *Tic Disorders, Trichotillomania, and Other Repetitive Behavior Disorders: Behavioral Approaches to Analysis and Treatment.* Norwell, MA, Kluwer Academic Publishers, 2001.
85. Beck A: *Cognitive Therapy and the Emotional Disorders.* New York, International Universities Press, 1976.
86. Mowrer O: Two-factor learning theory: versions one and two. In: Mowrer O (ed): *Learning Theory and Behavior.* Hoboken, NJ, John Wiley & Sons, Inc., 63–91, 1960.
87. Barrios B, Hartman D: Fears and anxieties. In: Mash E, Terdal L (eds): *Behavioral Assessment of Childhood Disorders.* 2nd ed. New York, Guildford Press, 196–264, 1988.
88. Francis G: Assessing cognitions in anxious children. *Behav Modif* 12:115–130, 1988.
89. Deffenbacher J, Kemper C: Systematic desensitization of test anxiety in junior high students. *School Couns* 22:216–222, 1974.
90. Rosenstiel S, Scott D: Four considerations in imagery techniques with children. *J Behav Ther Exp Psychiatry* 8:287–290, 1977.
91. Hatzenbuehler L, Schroeder H: Desensitization procedures in the treatment of childhood disorders. *Psychol Bull* 85:831–844, 1978.
92. Jackson H, King N: The emotive imagery treatment of a child's trauma-inspired phobia. *J Behav Ther Exp Psychiatry* 12:325–328, 1981.
93. Ollendick T, Francis G: Behavioral assessment and treatment of childhood phobias. *Behav Modif* 12:165–204, 1988.
94. Kendall P, Chansky T, Kane M: *Anxiety Disorders in Youth: Cognitive-Behavioral Interventions (Psychology Practitioner Guidebooks).* Needham Heights, Allyn and Bacon, 1992.
95. Spivak G, Shure M: *Social Adjustment of Young Children: A Cognitive Approach to Solving Real-Life Problems.* San Francisco, CA, Jossey-Bass, 1974.
96. Kanfer F, Karoly P, Newman A: Reduction of children's fear of the dark by competence-related and situational threat-related verbal cues. *J Consult Clin Psychol* 43:251–258, 1975.
97. Kendall P, Flannery-Schroeder E, Panichelli-Mindel S, Southam-Gerow M, Henin A, Warman M: Therapy for youths with anxiety disorders: a second randomized clinical trial. *J Consult Clin Psychol* 65(3):366–380, 1997.
98. Kendall P, Flannery-Schroeder E, Safford S, Webb A: Child anxiety treatment: outcomes in adolescence and impact on substance use and depression at 7.4-year follow-up. *J Consult Clin Psychol* 72:276–287, 2004.
99. Piacentini J, Langley A, Roblek T: *Overcoming Childhood OCD: A Therapist's Guide.* New York, Oxford University Press, 2007.
100. Freeman J, Garcia A, Frank H, et al.: Evidence base update for psychosocial treatments for pediatric obsessive-compulsive disorder. *J Clin Child Adolesc Psychol* 43:7–26, 2014.
101. McGuire JF, Piacentini J, Lewin AB, Brennan EA, Murphy TK, Storch EA: A meta-analysis of cognitive behavior therapy of CBT and medication for child obsessive-compulsive disorder: moderators of treatment efficacy, response, and remission. *Depres Anxiety* 32:580–593, 2015.
102. Arch J, Abramowitz J: Exposure therapy for obsessive–compulsive disorder: an optimizing inhibitory learning approach. *J Obses Compuls Relat Disord* 6:174–182, 2015.
103. McGuire J, Orr S, Essoe JK, et al.: Extinction learning in childhood anxiety disorders, obsessive compulsive disorder and posttraumatic stress disorder: implications for treatment. *Exp Rev Neurotherapeut* 16(10):1155–1174, 2016.
104. Team POTS: Cognitive-behavior therapy, Sertraline, and their combination for children and adolescents with obsessive-compulsive disorder. *J Am Med Assoc* 292:1969–1976, 2004.
105. Piacentini J, Bergman RL, Chang S, et al.: Controlled comparison of family cognitive behavioral therapy and psychoeducation/relaxation

training for child obsessive-compulsive disorder. *J Am Acad Child Adolesc Psychiatry* 50:1149–1161, 2011.

106. Freeman J, Sapyta J, Garcia A, et al.: Family-based treatment of early childhood obsessive-compulsive disorder: the Pediatric Obsessive-Compulsive Disorder Treatment Study for Young Children (POTS Jr)—a randomized clinical trial. *JAMA Psychiatry* 71(6):689–698, 2014.
107. Wolpe J: *The Practice of Behavior Therapy.* New York, Pergamon Press, 1982.
108. Ollendick TH, Öst L-G, Reuterskoild L, Costa N, Cederland R: One session treatment of specific phobias in youth: a randomized clinical trial in the United States and Sweden. *J Consult Clin Psychol* 77:505–516, 2009.
109. Davis TE III, Ollendick TH, Reuther ET, Muson MS: One-session treatment: principles and procedures with children and adolescents. In: Davis TE III, Ollendick TH, Öst LG (eds): *Intensive One-Session Treatment of Specific Phobias.* New York, Springer, 19–42, 2012.
110. Eldar S, Apter A, Lotan D, et al.: Attention bias modification treatment for paediatric anxiety disorders: a randomised control trial. *Am J Psychiatry* 169:213–220, 2012.
111. Bar-Haim Y, Morag L, Glickman S: Training anxious children to disengage attention from threat: a randomized control trial. *J Child Psychol Psychiatry Allied Discipl* 52:861–869, 2011.
112. Beidel D, Turner S, Morris T: Behavioral treatment of childhood social phobia. *J Consult Clin Psychol* 68:1072–1080, 2000.
113. Beidel D, Turner S, Young B, Paulson A: Social effectiveness therapy for children: three-year follow-up. *J Consult Clin Psychol* 73:721–725, 2005.
114. Beidel DC, Turner SM, Young BJ: Social effectiveness therapy for children: five years later. *Behav Ther* 37:416–425, 2006.
115. Spence SH, Donovan C, Brechman-Toussaint M: The treatment of childhood social phobia: the effectiveness of a social skills training-based cognitive-behavioural intervention, with and without parental involvement. *J Child Psychol Psychiatry Allied Discipl* 41(6):713–726, 2000.
116. Masia C, Beidel D, Albano A, Rapee R, Turner S, Morris T: *Skills for Academic and Social Success.* Available from Carrie Masia-Warner, PhD, New York University School of Medicine, Child Study Center, 215 Lexington Avenue, 13th floor, New York, 100161999.
117. Masia C, Klein R, Storch E, Corda B: School-based behavioral treatment for social anxiety disorder in adolescents: results of a pilot study. *J Am Acad Child Adolesc Psychiatry* 40:780–786, 2001.
118. Masia Warner C, Klein R, Dent H, et al.: School-based intervention for adolescents with social anxiety disorder: results of a controlled study. *J Abnorm Child Psychol* 33:707–722, 2005.
119. Garcia-Lopez LJ, Olivares J, Beidel D, Albano AM, Turner S, Rosa AI: Efficacy of three treatment protocols for adolescents with social anxiety disorder: a 5-year follow-up assessment. *J Anxiety Disord* 20(2):175–191, 2006.
120. Melfsen S, Kühnemund M, Schwieger J, et al.: Cognitive behavioral therapy of socially phobic children focusing on cognition: A randomised wait-list control study. *Child Adolesc Psychiatry Ment Health* 5(5):1–12, 2011.
121. Cartwright-Hatton S, Roberts C, Chitsabesan P, Fothergill C, Harrington R: Systematic review of the efficacy of cognitive behaviour therapies for childhood and adolescent anxiety disorders. *Br J Clin Psychol* 43:421–436, 2004.
122. American Psychiatric Association. *Diagnostic and Statistical Manual, Fifth Edition (DSM-5).* Washington, DC, American Psychiatric Association, 2013.
123. Paez P, Hirsch M: Oppositional defiant disorder and elective mutism. In: Kestenbaum C, WIlliams D (eds): *Handbook of Clinical Assessment of Children and Adolescents.* New York, University Press, 800–811, 1988.
124. Steinhausen H-C, Juzi C: Elective mutism: An analysis of 100 cases. *J Am Acad Child Adolesc Psychiatry* 35(5):606–614, 1996.
125. Kristensen H: Selective mutism and comorbidity with developmental disorder/delay, anxiety disorder, and elimination disorder. *J Am Acad Child Adolesc Psychiatry* 39(2):249–256, 2000.
126. Cohan SL, Chavira DA, Shipon-Blum E, Hitchcock C, Roesch SC, Stein MB: Refining the classification of children with selective mutism: a latent profile analysis. *J Clin Child Adolesc Psychol* 37(4):770–784, 2008.
127. Schill M, Kratochwill T, Gardner W: An assessment protocol for selective mutism: analogue assessment using parents as facilitators. *J School Psychol* 34:1–21, 1996.
128. Reed G: Elective mutism in children: a reappraisal. *J Child Psychol Psychiatry* 4:99–107, 1963.
129. Bergman L: *Treatment for Children with Selective Mutism. An Integrative Behavioral Approach.* New York, Oxford University Press, 2013.
130. Bergman R, Piacentini J: Selective mutism. In: Kaplan H, Sadock B (eds): *Comprehensive Textbook of Psychiatry.* 8 ed. Philadelphia, PA, Lippincott Williams & Wilkins, 3302–3306, 2005.
131. Cunningham C, Cataldo M, Mallion C, Keyes J: A review and controlled single case evaluation of behavioral approaches to the management of elective mutism. *Child Fam Behav Ther* 5(4):25–49, 1983.
132. Bergman RL, Gonzalez A, Piacentini J, Keller ML: Integrated behavior therapy for selective mutism: a randomized controlled pilot study. *Behav Res Ther* 51(10):680–689, 2013.
133. Oerbeck B, Stein M, Wentzel-Larsen T, Langsrud Ø, Kristensen H: A randomized controlled trial of a home and school-based intervention for selective mutism—defocused communication and behavioural techniques. *Child Adolesc Ment Health,* 2014: doi: 10.1111/camh.12045.
134. Oerbeck B, Stein MB, Pripp AH, Kristensen H: Selective mutism: follow-up study 1 year after end of treatment. *Eur Child Adolesc Psychiatry* 24(7):757–766, 2015.
135. Addis M, Hatgis C, Krasnow A, Jacob K, Bourne L, Mansfield A: Effectiveness of cognitive-behavioral treatment for panic disorder versus treatment as usual in a managed care setting. *J Consult Clin Psychol* 72(4):625–635, 2004.
136. Stewart SH, Watt MC: Introduction to the special issue on interoceptive exposure in the treatment of anxiety and related disorders: novel applications and mechanisms of action. *J Cogn Psychother* 22:291–302, 2008.
137. Hoffman E, Mattis S: A developmental adaptation of Panic Control Treatment for panic disorder in adolescence. *Cogn Behav Pract* 7(3):253–261, 2000.
138. Pincus DB, May JE, Whitton SW, Mattis SG, Barlow DH: Cognitive-behavioral treatment of panic disorder in adolescence. *J Clin Child Adolesc Psychol* 39(5):638–649, 2010.
139. Scheeringa M, Zeanah C, Myers L, Putnam F: New findings on alternative criteria for PTSD in preschool children. *J Am Acad Child Adolesc Psychiatry* 42:561–570, 2003.
140. Gigengack MR, van Meijel EP, Alisic E, Lindauer RJ: Comparing three diagnostic algorithms of posttraumatic stress in young children exposed to accidental trauma: an exploratory study. *Child Adolesc Psychiatry Ment Health* 9(14):1–8, 2015.
141. Dowd H, McGuire BE: Psychological treatment of PTSD in children: an evidence-based review. *Irish J Psychol* 32(1–2):25–39, 2011.
142. Kowalik J, Weller J, Venter J, Drachman D: Cognitive behavioral therapy for the treatment of pediatric posttraumatic stress disorder: a review and meta-analysis. *J Behav Ther Exp Psychiatry* 42(3):405–413, 2011.
143. Wethington HR, Hahn RA, Fuqua-Whitley DS, et al.: The effectiveness of interventions to reduce psychological harm from traumatic events among children and adolescents: a systematic review. *Am J Prev Med* 35(3):287–313, 2008.
144. Cohen JA: Practice parameter for the assessment and treatment of children and adolescents with posttraumatic stress disorder. *J Am Acad Child Adolesc Psychiatry* 49(4):414–430, 2010.
145. Cohen J, Berliner L, March J: Treatment of children and adolescents. In: Foa E, Keane T, Friedman M (eds): *Effective Treatments for PTSD.* New York, Guilford Press, 106–138, 2000.
146. Feeny NC, Foa EB, Treadwell KR, March J: Posttraumatic stress disorder in youth: a critical review of the cognitive and behavioral treatment outcome literature. *Prof Psychol Res Pract* 35(5):466–476, 2004.
147. Donnelly C, Amaya-Jackson L: Post-traumatic stress disorder in children and adolescents. *Pediatric Drugs* 4(3):159–170, 2002.
148. Dorsey S, Briggs EC, Woods BA: Cognitive-behavioral treatment for posttraumatic stress disorder in children and adolescents. *Child Adolesc Psychiatr Clin N Am* 20(2):255–269, 2011.
149. Kar N: Cognitive behavioral therapy for the treatment of post-traumatic stress disorder: a review. *Neuropsychiatr Dis Treat* 7:167–181, 2011.
150. Hembree E, Rauch S, Foa E: Beyond the manual: the insider's guide to prolonged exposure therapy for PTSD. *Cogn Behav Pract* 10(1):22–30, 2003.
151. Perrin S, Smith P, Yule W: Practitioner review: the assessment and treatment of post-traumatic stress disorder in children and adolescents. *J Child Psychol Psychiatry* 41(3):277–289, 2000.
152. Hassija CM, Gray MJ: Are cognitive techniques and interventions necessary? A case for the utility of cognitive approaches in the treatment of PTSD. *Clin Psychol Sci Pract* 17(2):112–127, 2010.
153. Bryant R, Harvey A: Avoidant coping style and post-traumatic stress following motor vehicle accidents. *Behav Res Ther* 33(6):631–635, 1995.
154. Ehlers A, Mayou R, Bryant B: Psychological predictors of chronic posttraumatic stress disorder after motor vehicle accidents. *J Abnorm Psychol* 107(3):508–519, 1998.
155. Smith P, Yule W, Perrin S, Tranah T, Dalgleish T, Clark DM: Cognitive-behavioral therapy for PTSD in children and adolescents: a preliminary randomized controlled trial. *J Am Acad Child Adolesc Psychiatry* 46(8):1051–1061, 2007.
156. Cohen J, Mannarino A: A treatment outcome study for sexually abused preschool children: initial findings. *J Am Acad Child Adolesc Psychiatry* 35(1):42–50, 1996.
157. Cohen J, Mannarino A: Interventions for sexually abused children: initial treatment outcome findings. *Child Maltreat* 3(1):17–26, 1998.
158. Deblinger E, Lippmann J, Steer R: Sexually abused children suffering posttraumatic stress symptoms: initial treatment outcome findings. *Child Maltreat* 1(4):310–321, 1996.
159. Foa EB, McLean CP, Capaldi S, Rosenfield D: Prolonged exposure vs supportive counseling for sexual abuse-related PTSD in adolescent girls: a randomized clinical trial. *JAMA* 310(24):2650–2657, 2013.
160. Pine S, Cohen J: Trauma in children and adolescents: risk and treatment of psychiatric sequelae. *Biol Psychiatry* 51(7):519–531, 2002.
161. McDonagh A, Friedman M, McHugo G, et al.: Randomized trial of cognitive-behavioral therapy for chronic posttraumatic stress disorder in adult female survivors of childhood sexual abuse. *J Consult Clin Psychol* 73(3):515–524, 2005.
162. Cary CE, McMillen JC: The data behind the dissemination: a systematic review of trauma-focused cognitive behavioral therapy for use with children and youth. *Child Youth Servic Rev* 34(4):748–757, 2012.

163. Scheeringa MS, Weems CF, Cohen JA, Amaya-Jackson L, Guthrie D: Trauma-focused cognitive-behavioral therapy for posttraumatic stress disorder in three-through six year-old children: a randomized clinical trial. *J Child Psychol Psychiatry* 52(8):853–860, 2011.
164. Mannarino AP, Cohen JA, Deblinger E, Runyon MK, Steer RA: Trauma-focused cognitive-behavioral therapy for children: sustained impact of treatment 6 and 12 months later. *Child Maltreat* 17(3):231–241, 2012.
165. Cohen J, Mannarino A, Deblinger E: *Treating Trauma and Traumatic Grief in Children and Adolescents.* New York, Guilford Press, 2006.
166. Foster JM: Supporting child victims of sexual abuse: implementation of a trauma narrative family intervention. *Family J* 22(3):332–328, 2014.
167. Foa E, Rothbaum B, Riggs D, Murdock T, Beutler L: Treatment of posttraumatic stress disorder in rape victims: a comparison between cognitive–behavioral procedures and counseling. *J Consult Clin Psychol* 59(5):715–723, 1991.
168. Marks I, Lovell K, Noshirvani H, Livanou M, Thrasher S: Treatment of posttraumatic stress disorder by exposure and/or cognitive restructuring: a controlled study. *Arch Gen Psychiatry* 55(4):317–325, 1998.
169. Foa E, Dancu C, Hembree E, Jaycox L, Meadows E, Street G: A comparison of exposure therapy, stress inoculation training, and their combination for reducing posttraumatic stress disorder in female assault victims. *J Consult Clin Psychol* 67(2):194–200, 1999.
170. Meichenbaum D: *Stress Inoculation Training.* New York, Pergamon Press, 1985.
171. Flaxman PE, Bond FW: A randomised worksite comparison of acceptance and commitment therapy and stress inoculation training. *Behav Res Ther* 48(8):816–820, 2010.
172. Farrell S, Hains A, Davies W: Cognitive behavioral interventions for sexually abused children exhibiting PTSD symptomatology. *Behav Ther* 29(2):241–255, 1998.
173. Seligman M: *Helplessness: On Depression, Development, and Death.* San Francisco, CA, W.H. Freeman, 1975.
174. Curry J, Craighead W: Attributional style in clinically depressed and conduct disordered adolescents. *J Consult Clin Psychol* 58(1):109–115, 1990.
175. Rubenstein LM, Freed RD, Shapero BG, Fauber RL, Alloy LB: Cognitive attributions in depression: bridging the gap between research and clinical practice. *J Psychother Integr* 26(2):103–115, 2016.
176. Rehm L, Carter A: Cognitive components of depression. In: Lewis M, Miller S (eds): *Handbook of Developmental Psychopathology.* New York, Plenum Press, 341–351, 1990.
177. Leitenberg H, Yost L, Carroll-Wilson M: Negative cognitive errors in children: questionnaire development, normative data, and comparisons between children with and without self-reported symptoms of depression, low self-esteem, and evaluation anxiety. *J Consult Clin Psychol* 54(4):528–536, 1986.
178. Kendall P, Reber M, McLeer S, Epps J, Ronan K: Cognitive-behavioral treatment of conduct-disordered children. *Cogn Ther Res* 14(3):279–297, 1990.
179. Friedman E, Thase M, Wright J: *Cognitive and Behavioral Therapies.* John Wiley & Sons, Ltd., 2003.
180. Kaslow N, Rehm L, Siegel A: Social-cognitive and cognitive correlates of depression in children. *J Abnorm Child Psychol* 12(4):605–620, 1984.
181. Elkin I, Shea M, Watkins J, et al.: National Institutes of Mental Health treatment of depression collaborative research program: general effectiveness of treatments. *Arch Gen Psychiatry* 46(11):971–982, 1989.
182. Clarke G, DeBar LL, Pearson JA, et al.: Cognitive behavioral therapy in primary care for youth declining antidepressants: a randomized trial. *Pediatrics* 137(5), 2016.
183. David-Ferdon C, Kaslow NJ: Evidence-based psychosocial treatments for child and adolescent depression. *J Clin Child Adolesc Psychol* 37(1): 62–104, 2008.
184. Kennard B, Emslie G, Mayes T, et al.: Sequential treatment with fluoxetine and relapse-prevention CBT to improve outcomes in pediatric depression. *Am J Psychiatry* 171(10):1083–1090, 2014.
185. Hovey J, King C: The spectrum of suicidal behavior. In: Marsh DT, Fristad MA (eds): *Handbook of Serious Emotional Disturbance in Children and Adolescents.* Hoboken, NJ, John Wiley & Sons, Inc., 284–303, 2002.
186. Kendall PC, Peterman JS, Cummings CM: Cognitive-behavioral therapy, behavioral therapy, and related treatments in children. In: Thapar A, Pine DS, Leckman JF, Scott S, Snowling MJ, Taylor E (eds): *Rutter's Child and Adolescent Psychiatry.* 6th ed. Chichester, West Sussex; Ames, Iowa, Wiley, 496–509, 2015.
187. Frame C, Matson J, Sonis W, Fialkov M, Kazdin A: Behavioral treatment of depression in a prepubertal child. *J Behav Ther Exp Psychiatry* 13(3):239–243, 1982.
188. Lewinsohn P, Clarke G, Rohde P, Hops H, Seeley J: A course in coping: A cognitive-behavioral approach to the treatment of adolescent depression. In: Hibbs ED, Jensen PS (eds): *Psychosocial Treatments for Child and Adolescent Disorders: Empirically Based Strategies for Clinical Practice.* Washington, DC, American Psychological Association, 109–135, 1996.
189. Kaufman NK, Rohde P, Seeley JR, Clarke GN, Stice E: Potential mediators of cognitive-behavioral therapy for adolescents with comorbid major depression and conduct disorder. *J Consult Clin Psychol* 73(1):38–46, 2005.
190. Clarke G, Lewinsohn P, Hops H: *Leader's Manual for Adolescent Groups: Adolescent Coping with Depression Course.* Eugene, OR, Castalia, 1990.
191. Clarke G, DeBar L, Lewinsohn P: Cognitive behavioral group treatment for adolescent depression. In: Kazdin A, Weisz J (eds): *Evidence-Based Psychotherapies for Children and Adolescents.* New York, Guilford Press, 120–134, 2003.
192. Garvik M, Idsoe T, Bru E: Effectiveness study of a CBT-based adolescent coping with depression course. *Emot Behav Diff* 19(2):195–209, 2014.
193. Garvik M, Idsoe T, Bru E: Motivation and social relations in school following a CBT course for adolescents with depressive symptoms: an effectiveness study. *Scan J Educ Res* 60(2):219–39, 2016.
194. Linehan MM, Armstrong HE, Suarez A, Allmon D, Heard HL: Cognitive-behavioral treatment of chronically parasuicidal borderline patients. *Arch Gen Psychiatry* 48(12):1060–1064, 1991.
195. Harley R, Sprich S, Safren S, Jacobo M, Fava M: Adaptation of dialectical behavior therapy skills training group for treatment-resistant depression. *J Nerv Ment Dis* 196(2):136–143, 2008.
196. Lynch TR, Morse JQ, Mendelson T, Robins CJ: Dialectical behavior therapy for depressed older adults: a randomized pilot study. *Am J Geriatr Psychiatry* 11(1):33–45, 2003.
197. American Psychiatric Association. *Diagnostic and Statistical Manual, Fourth Edition Text Revision (DSM-IVTR).* Washington, DC, American Psychiatric Association, 2000.
198. Koegel R, O'Dell M, Koegel L: A natural language teaching paradigm for nonverbal autistic children. *J Autism Dev Disord* 17(2):187–200, 1987.
199. Lovaas O: Behavioral treatment and normal educational and intellectual functioning in young autistic children. *J Consult Clin Psychol* 55(1):3–9, 1987.
200. McGee G: What's incidental about incidental teaching? Part I. *Autism-Asperger's Digest.* May–June, 10–13, 2003.
201. McGee G: What's incidental about incidental teaching? Part II. *Autism-Asperger's Digest.* July–August, 20–24, 2003.
202. McEachin J, Smith T, Lovaas O: Long-term outcome for children with autism who received early intensive behavioral treatment. *Am J Ment Retard* 97(4):359–372, 1993.
203. Koegel L, Koegel R, Carter C: Pivotal responses and the natural language paradigm. *Semin Speech Lang* 19(4):355–372, 1998.
204. National Research Council: Committee on Educational Interventions for Children with Autism. *Educating Children with Autism.* Washington, DC, National Academy Press, 2001.
205. Schreibman L, Dawson G, Stahmer AC, et al.: Naturalistic developmental behavioral interventions: empirically validated treatments for autism spectrum disorder. *J Autism Dev Disord* 45(8):2411–2428, 2015.
206. Dawson G, Rogers S, Munson J, et al.: Randomized, controlled trial of an intervention for toddlers with autism: the Early Start Denver Model. *Pediatrics* 125(1):e17–e23, 2010.
207. Kasari C, Gulsrud A, Paparella T, Hellemann G, Berry K: Randomized comparative efficacy study of parent-mediated interventions for toddlers with autism. *J Consult Clin Psychol* 83(3):554–563, 2015.
208. Ingersoll B, Dvortcsak A: *Teaching Social Communication to Children with Autism: A Practitioner's Guide to Parent Training.* New York, Guilford Press, 2010.
209. National Autism Center. *Findings and Conclusions: National Standards Project, Phase 2.* Randolph, MA, Author, 2015.
210. Hardan AY, Gengoux GW, Berquist KL, et al.: A randomized controlled trial of Pivotal Response Treatment Group for parents of children with autism. *J Child Psychol Psychiatry* 56(8):884–892, 2015.
211. Eikeseth S, Klintwall L, Jahr E, Karlsson P: Outcome for children with autism receiving early and intensive behavioral intervention in mainstream preschool and kindergarten settings. *Res Autism Spectr Disord* 6(2):829–835, 2012.
212. Hayward D, Eikeseth S, Gale C, Morgan S: Assessing progress during treatment for young children with autism receiving intensive behavioural interventions. *Autism* 13(6):613–633, 2009.
213. McMahon R, Frick P: Conduct and oppositional disorders. In: Mash E, Barkley R (eds): *Assessment of Childhood Disorders.* 4th ed. New York, Guilford Press, 132–183, 2007.
214. Kazdin A: *Treatment of Antisocial Behavior in Children and Adolescents.* Homewood, IL, Dorsey Press, 1985.
215. Patterson G, DeBarysh B, Ramsey E, Vandenbos G, Horowitz F, O'Brien M: A developmental perspective on antisocial behavior. *Am Psychol* 44(2):329–335, 1989.
216. Reef J, Diamantopoulou S, van Meurs I, Verhulst FC, van der Ende J: Developmental trajectories of child to adolescent externalizing behavior and adult DSM-IV disorder: results of a 24-year longitudinal study. *Soc Psychiatry Psychiatr Epidemiol* 46(12):1233–1241, 2011.
217. Patterson G: *Coercive Family Processes.* Eugene, OR, Castalia Publishing Co., 1982.
218. Dodge K, Pettit G, McClaskey C, Brown M: Social competence in children. *Monograph Soc Res Child Dev* 51(2):1-85, 1986.
219. Milich R, Dodge K: Social information processing in child psychiatric populations. *J Abnorm Child Psychol* 12(3):471–489, 1984.
220. Dodge K, Price J, Bachorowski J, Newman J, Mineka S: Hostile attributional biases in severely aggressive adolescents. *J Abnorm Psychol* 99(4):385–392, 1990.
221. Dodge K, Newman J, Buchwald A: Biased decision-making processes in aggressive boys. *J Abnorm Psychol* 90(4):375–379, 1981.
222. Lochman J, Kazdin A: Self and peer perceptions and attributional biases of aggressive and nonaggressive boys in dyadic interventions. *J Consult Clin Psychol* 55(3):404–410, 1987.

223. Perry D, Perry L, Rasmussen P: Cognitive social learning mediators of aggression. *Child Dev* 57(3):700–711, 1986.
224. Slaby R, Guerra N, Parke R: Cognitive mediators of aggression in adolescent offenders: 1. Assessment. *Dev Psychol* 24(4):580–588, 1988.
225. Lochman J, Meyer B, Rabiner D, White J: Parameters influencing social problem-solving of aggressive children. In: Prinz R (ed): *Advances in Behavioral Assessment of Children and Families*. Vol 5. London, Jessica Kingsley Publishers, 31–63, 1991.
226. Richard B, Dodge K, Garfield S: Social maladjustment and problem solving in school-aged children. *J Consult Clin Psychol* 50(2):226–233, 1982.
227. Asarnow J, Callan J, Kazdin A: Boys with peer adjustment problems: social cognitive processes. *J Consult Clin Psychol* 53(1):80–87, 1985.
228. Lochman J, Lampron L: Situational social problem-solving skills and self-esteem of aggressive and nonaggressive boys. *J Abnorm Child Psychol* 14(4):605–617, 1986.
229. Robinson T, Smith S, Miller M, Brownell M: Cognitive behavior modification of hyperactivity-impulsivity and aggression: A meta-analysis of school-based studies. *J Educ Psychol* 91(2):195–203, 1999.
230. Sukhodolsky DG, Kassinove H, Gorman BS: Cognitive-behavioral therapy for anger in children and adolescents: a meta-analysis. *Aggres Viol Behav* 9(3):247–269, 2004.
231. Herbert M: Behavioral methods. In: Rutter M, Taylor E, Hersov L (eds): *Child and Adolescent Psychiatry Modern Approaches*. 3rd ed. Oxford, Blackwell Scientific Publications, 858–879, 1994.
232. Barkley R. *Hyperactive Children: A Handbook for Diagnosis and Treatment*. New York, Guilford Publications, 1981.
233. Campbell M, Cohen I, Perry R, Small M: Psychopharmacological treatment. In: Ollendick T, Hersen M (eds): *Handbook of Child Psychopathology*. New York, Plenum Press, 1989.
234. Chorpita B, Daleiden E, Ebesutani C, et al.: Evidence-based treatments for children and adolescents: An updated review of indicators of efficacy and effectiveness. *Clin Psychol Sci Pract* 18(2):154–172, 2011.
235. Beelmann A, Raabe T: The effects of preventing antisocial behavior and crime in childhood and adolescence: results and implications of research reviews and meta-analyses. *Eur J Dev Sci* 3(3):260–281, 2009.
236. Lochman J, Powell N, Boxmeyer C, Jimenez-Camargo L: Cognitive-behavioral therapy for externalizing disorders in children and adolescents. *Child Adolesc Psychiatr Clin N Am* 20(2):305–318, 2011.
237. Lochman JE, Wells KC: The Coping Power Program for preadolescent aggressive boys and their parents: outcome effects at the 1-year follow-up. *J Consult Clin Psychol* 72(4):571–578, 2004.
238. Lochman J, Wells K: Contextual social-cognitive mediators and child outcome: a test of the theoretical model in the Coping Power Program. *Dev Psychopathol* 14:971–993, 2002.
239. Larson J, Lochman J: *Helping Schoolchildren Cope with Anger: A Cognitive Behavioral Intervention*. New York, Guilford Press, 2002.
240. Webster-Stratton C, Reid M: The Incredible Years Parents, Teachers and Children Training Series: A multifaceted treatment approach for young children with conduct problems. In: Kazdin AE, Weisz JR (eds): *Evidence-Based Psychotherapies for Children and Adolescents*. 2nd ed. New York, Guilford Press, 194–2010, 2010.
241. Kazdin AE: Problem-solving skills training and parent management training for oppositional defiant disorder and conduct disorder. In: Weisz J, Kazdin A (eds): *Evidence-Based Psychotherapies for Children and Adolescents*. New York, Guilford Press, 211–226, 2010.
242. Reitman D, McMahon J: Constance "Connie" Hanf (1917–2002): The mentor and the model. *Cogn Behav Pract* 20:106–116, 2013.
243. Patterson G: The next generation of PMTO models. *Behav Ther* 28:27–33, 2005.
244. Eyberg S, Robinson E: Parent-child interaction training: effects on family functioning. *J Clin Child Psychol* 11:130–137, 1982.
245. McMahon R, Forehand R: *Helping the Noncompliant Child: Family-Based Treatment for Oppositional Behavior*. 2nd ed. New York, Guilford Press, 2003.
246. Barkley R: *Defiant Children: A Clinician's Manual for Assessment and Parent Training*. 3rd ed. New York, Guilford Press, 2013.
247. Barkley R, Robin A: *Defiant Teens, 2nd Edition: A Clinician's Manual for Assessment and Family Intervention*. New York, Guilford Press, 2014.
248. Kaehler J, Jacobs M, Jones D: Distilling common history and practice elements to inform dissemination: Hanf-model BPT programs as an example. *Clin Child Fam Psychol Rev* 19(3):236–258, 2016.
249. Baumrind D: Effects of authoritative parental control on child behavior. *Child Dev* 37(4):887–907, 1966.
250. Webster-Stratton C, Reid J: The Incredible Years Program for children from infancy to preadolescence: prevention and treatment of behavior problems. In: Murrihy R, Kidman A, Ollendick T (eds): *Clinician's Handbook for the Assessment and Treatment of Conduct Problems in Youth*. Springer Press, 117–138, 2010.
251. Patterson G, Chamberlain P, Reid J: A comparative evaluation of a parent-training program. *Behav Ther* 13:638–650, 1982.
252. Forgatch M, Patterson G: *Parent Management Training–Oregon Model: An Intervention for Antisocial Behavior in Children and Adolescents*. New York, NY, Guildford Press, 2010.
253. Forgatch MS, Patterson GR, Degarmo DS, Beldavs ZG: Testing the Oregon delinquency model with 9-year follow-up of the Oregon Divorce Study. *Dev Psychopathol* 21(2):637–660, 2009.
254. Bank L, Marlowe J, Reid J, Patterson G, Weinrott M: A comparative evaluation of parent-training interventions for families of chronic delinquents. *J Abnorm Child Psychol* 19(1):15–33, 1991.
255. Sanders MR: Development, evaluation, and multinational dissemination of the triple P-Positive Parenting Program. *Annu Rev Clin Psychol* 8:345–379, 2012.
256. Robin A, Foster S: *Negotiating Parent-Adolescent Conflict*. New York, Guilford Press, 1989.
257. Barkley R, Edwards G, Laneri M, Fletcher K, Metevia L: The efficacy of Problem-Solving Communication Training alone, Behavior Management Training alone, and their combination for parent-adolescent conflict in teenagers with ADHD and ODD. *J Consult Clin Psychol* 69(6):926–941, 2001.
258. Greene R: *The Explosive Child: A New Approach for Understanding and Parenting Easily Frustrated, Chronically Inflexible Children*. 5th ed. New York, Harper Collins, 2014.
259. Greene RW, Ablon JS, Goring JC, et al.: Effectiveness of collaborative problem solving in affectively dysregulated children with oppositional-defiant disorder: initial findings. *J Consult Clin Psychol* 72(6):1157–1164, 2004.
260. Greene R, Ablon J: *Treating Explosive Kids: The Collaborative Problem-Solving Approach*. New York, Guilford Press, 2005.
261. Wolff JC, Greene RW, Ollendick TH: Differential responses of children with varying degrees of reactive and proactive aggression to two forms of psychosocial treatment. *Child Family Behav Ther* 30(1):37–50, 2008.
262. Kaplan G, Newcorn JH: Pharmacotherapy for child and adolescent attention-deficit hyperactivity disorder. *Pediatr Clin North Am* 58(1): 99–120, xi, 2011.
263. Peterson K, McDonagh MS, Fu R: Comparative benefits and harms of competing medications for adults with attention-deficit hyperactivity disorder: a systematic review and indirect comparison meta-analysis. *Psychopharmacology (Berl)* 197(1):1–11, 2008.
264. Group MC: National Institute of Mental Health multimodal treatment study of ADHD follow-up: 24-month outcomes of treatment strategies for attention-deficit/hyperactivity disorder. *Pediatrics* 113(4):754–761, 2004.
265. Group MC: National Institute of Mental Health multimodal treatment study of ADHD follow-up: changes in effectiveness and growth after the end of treatment. *Pediatrics* 113(4):762–769, 2004.
266. Fabiano GA, Pelham WE Jr., Coles EK, Gnagy EM, Chronis-Tuscano A, O'Connor BC: A meta-analysis of behavioral treatments for attention-deficit/hyperactivity disorder. *Clin Psychol Rev* 29(2):129–140, 2009.
267. Pelham WE Jr., Fabiano GA, Waxmonsky JG, et al.: Treatment sequencing for childhood ADHD: a multiple-randomization study of adaptive medication and behavioral interventions. *J Clin Child Adolesc Psychol* 45(4):396–415, 2016.
268. Hinshaw S: Attention-deficit/hyperactivity disorder: The search for viable treatments. In: Kendall P (ed): *Child and Adolescent Therapy: Cognitive-Behavioral Procedures*. 2nd ed. New York, Guilford Press, 88–128, 2000.
269. Rapoport J, Inoff-Germain G: Tourette syndrome: medical and surgical treatment of obsessive-compulsive disorder. *Neurol Clin* 15(2):421–428, 1997.
270. Pelham W, Greiner A, Gnagy E: *Summer Treatment Program Manual*. Buffalo, Comprehensive Treatment for Attention Deficit Disorders, Inc., 1997.
271. Sibley MH, Pelham WE, Evans SW, Gnagy EM, Ross JM, Greiner AR: An evaluation of a summer treatment program for adolescents with ADHD. *Cogn Behav Pract* 18(4):530–544, 2011.
272. Pelham WE Jr., Fabiano GA: Evidence-based psychosocial treatments for attention-deficit/hyperactivity disorder. *J Clin Child Adolesc Psychol* 37(1):184–214, 2008.
273. DuPaul G, Eckert T, Vilardo B: The effects of school-based interventions for attention deficit hyperactivity disorder: a meta-analysis 1996–2010. *School Psychol Rev* 41(4):387–412, 2012.
274. Evans S, Owen J, Bunford N: Evidence-based psychosocial treatments for children and adolescents with attention-deficit/hyperactivity disorder. *J Clin Child Adolesc Psychol* 43(4):527–551, 2014.
275. Zwi M, Jones H, Thorgaard C, York A, Dennis J: Parent training interventions for attention-deficit/hyperactivity disorder (ADHD) in children aged 5–18 years. *Cochrane Database Syst Rev* (12):CD003018, 2011.
276. Langberg J, Epstein J, Becker S, Girio-Herrera E, Vaughn A: Evaluation of the Homework, Organization, and Planning Skills (HOPS) intervention for middle school students with Attention Deficit Hyperactivity Disorder as implemented by school mental health providers. *School Psychol Rev* 41(3):342–364, 2012.
277. Abikoff H, Gallagher R, Wells K, et al.: Remediating organizational functioning in children with ADHD: immediate and long-term effects from a randomized controlled trial. *J Consult Clin Psychol* 81(1):113–128, 2013.
278. McGrath P, Lingley-Pottie P, Thurston C, et al.: Telephone-based mental health interventions for child disruptive behavior or anxiety disorders: randomized trials and overall analysis. *J Am Acad Child Adolesc Psychiatry* 50(11):1162–1172, 2011.
279. Chacko A, Wymbs BT, Wymbs FA, et al.: Enhancing traditional behavioral parent training for single mothers of children with ADHD. *J Clin Child Adolesc Psychol* 38(2):206–218, 2009.
280. Fabiano GA, Pelham WE, Cunningham CE, et al.: A waitlist-controlled trial of behavioral parent training for fathers of children with ADHD. *J Clin Child Adolesc Psychol* 41(3):337–345, 2012.
281. Mikami AY, Lerner MD, Griggs MS, McGrath A, Calhoun CD: Parental influence on children with attention-deficit/hyperactivity disorder: II.

Results of a pilot intervention training parents as friendship coaches for children. *J Abnorm Child Psychol* 38(6):737–749, 2010.

282. Fabiano G, Vujnovic R, Pelham W, et al.: Enhancing the effectiveness of special education programming for children with attention deficit hyperactivity disorder using a daily report card. *School Psychol Rev* 39:219–239, 2010.
283. Curtis D: Structured dyadic behavior therapy processes for ADHD intervention. *Psychotherapy* 51(1):110–116, 2014.
284. Kuin M, Boyer BE, Van der Oord S: *Zelf Plannen [Plan My Life]*. Houten, Uitgeverij Lannoo-Campus, 2013.
285. Kendall P, Braswell L: *Cognitive Behavioral Therapy for Impulsive Children*. New York, Guilford Press, 1985.
286. Meichenbaum D, Goodman J, Peterson D: Training impulsive children to talk to themselves: a means of developing self-control. *J Abnorm Psychol* 77(2):115–126, 1971.
287. Ghasabi S, Tajrishi M, Zamani S: The effect of verbal self-instruction training on decreasing impulsivity symptoms in ADHD children. *J Iran Psychol* 5(19):209–220, 2009.
288. Fairburn C: Cognitive-behavior therapy for eating disorders. In: Gelder M, Lopez-Ibor J, Andreasen N (eds): *New Oxford Textbook of Psychiatry*. New York, Oxford University Press, 1388–1393, 2000.
289. Cooper Z, Fairburn CG: The evolution of "enhanced" cognitive behavior therapy for eating disorders: learning from treatment nonresponse. *Cogn Behav Pract* 18(3):394–402, 2011.
290. Bruch H: *Eating Disorders: Obesity, Anorexia Nervosa, and the Person Within*. New York, Basic Books, 1973.
291. Russell G: Bulimia nervosa: an ominous variant of anorexia nervosa. *Psychol Med* 9(3):429–448, 1979.
292. Mairs R, Nicholls D: Assessment and treatment of eating disorders in children and adolescents. *Arch Dis Child* 1–8, 2016.
293. Fairburn CG, Cooper Z, Doll HA, et al.: Transdiagnostic cognitive-behavioral therapy for patients with eating disorders: a two-site trial with 60-week follow-up. *Am J Psychiatry* 166(3):311–319, 2009.
294. Fairburn CG: *Cognitive Behavior Therapy and Eating Disorders*. New York, Guilford Press, 2008.
295. Lock J: An update on evidence-based psychosocial treatments for eating disorders in children and adolescents. *J Clin Child Adolesc Psychol* 44(5):707–721, 2015.
296. Murphy R, Straebler S, Cooper Z, Fairburn CG: Cognitive behavioral therapy for eating disorders. *Psychiatr Clin North Am* 33(3):611–627, 2010.
297. Fischer S, Peterson C: Dialectical behavior therapy for adolescent binge eating, purging, suicidal behavior, and non-suicidal self-injury: a pilot study. *Psychotherapy (Chic)* 52(1):78–92, 2015.
298. Salbach-Andrae H, Bohnekamp I, Pfeiffer E, Lehmkuhl U, Miller A: Dialectical behavior therapy of anorexia and bulimia nervosa among adolescents: a case series. *Cogn Behav Pract* 15(4):415–425, 2008.
299. Dalle Grave R, El Ghoch M, Sartirana M, Calugi S: Cognitive behavioral therapy for anorexia nervosa: an update. *Curr Psychiatry Rep* 18(1):2, 2016.
300. Garner D, Vitousek K, Pike K: Cognitive behavioral therapy for anorexia nervosa. In: Garner D, Garfinkel P (eds): *Handbook of Treatment for Eating Disorders*. 2nd ed. New York, Guilford Press, 94–144, 1997.
301. Campbell K, Peebles R: Eating disorders in children and adolescents: state of the art review. *Pediatrics* 134(3):582–592, 2014.
302. Leckman J, Bloch M, King R, Scahill L: Phenomenology of tics and natural history of tic disorders. In: Walkup J, Mink J, Hollenbeck P (eds): *Advances in Neurology: Tourette Syndrome*. Vol 99. Philadelphia, PA, Lippincott Williams & Wilkins, 1–16, 2006.
303. Piacentini J, Chang S: Behavioral treatments for tic suppression: Habit reversal therapy. In: Walkup J, Mink J, Hollenbeck P (eds): *Advances in Neurology: Tourette Syndrome*. Philadelphia, PA, Lippincott Williams, & Wilkins, 227–233, 2006.
304. Himle M, Woods D, Piacentini J, Walkup J: Brief review of habit reversal training for Tourette syndrome. *J Child Neurol* 21(8):719–725, 2006.
305. McGuire J, Piacentini J, Brennan E, et al.: A meta-analysis of habit reversal training for chronic tic disorders. *J Psychiatry Res* 50:106–112, 2014.
306. Woods D, Piacentini J, Chang S, et al.: *Managing Tourette Syndrome: A Behavioral Intervention for Children and Adults*. New York, Oxford University Press, 2008.
307. Piacentini J, Woods D, Scahill L, et al.: Randomized trial of behavior therapy for children with Tourette's disorder. *J Am Med Assoc* 303(19):1929–1937, 2010.
308. Scahill L, Woods D, Himle M, et al.: Current controversies on the role of behavior therapy in Tourette syndrome. *Mov Disord* 28:1179–1183, 2013.
309. Conelea C, Woods D: The influence of contextual factors on tic expression in Tourette's syndrome: a review. *J Psychosom Res* 65:487–496, 2008.
310. Franklin M, Flessner C, Woods D, et al.: The Child and Adolescent Trichotillomania Impact Project (CA-TIP): exploring phenomenology, comorbid symptoms, functional impairment, and treatment utilization. *J Dev Behav Pediatr* 29:493–500, 2008.
311. Franklin M, Tolin D: *Treating Trichotillomania: Cognitive-Behavioral Therapy for Hairpulling and Related Problems*. New York, Springer Science, 2007.
312. Franklin M, Edson A, Ledley D, Cahill S: Behavior therapy for pediatric trichotillomania: a randomized controlled trial. *J Am Acad Child Adolesc Psychiatry* 50:763–771, 2011.
313. Goldfinger Golumb R, Vavrichek S: *The Hair Pulling 'Habit' and You: How to Solve the Trichotillomania Puzzle*. Washington, DC, Writer's Cooperative of Greater Washington, 2000.
314. Glazener C, Evans J, Peto R: Treating nocturnal enuresis in children: review of evidence. *J Wound Ostomy Continence Nurs* 31(4):223–234, 2004.
315. Doleys D, Hernstein R: Behavioral treatments for nocturnal enuresis in children: a review of the recent literature. *Psychol Bull* 84(1):30–54, 1977.
316. Mowrer O, Mowrer W: Enuresis: a method for its study and treatment. *Am J Orthopsychiatry* 8(3):436–459, 1938.
317. Mellon M, Scott M, Haynes K, Schmidt D, Houts A: EMG recording of pelvic floor conditioning in nocturnal enuresis during urine alarm treatment: a preliminary study. Sixth Florida Conference on Child Health Psychology; University of Florida, 1997.
318. Houts A: Commentary: treatments for enuresis: criteria, mechanisms, and health care policy. *J Pediatr Psychol* 25:219–224, 2000.
319. Butler RJ: Childhood nocturnal enuresis: developing a conceptual framework. *Clin Psychol Rev* 24(8):909–931, 2004.
320. Friman P: Evidence-based therapies for enuresis and encopresis. In: Steele R, Elkin T, Roberts M (eds): *The Handbook of Evidence-Based Therapies for Children and Adolescents: Bridging Science and Practice*. New York, Springer Press, 311–333, 2008.
321. O'Leary K, Wilson G: *Behavior Therapy: Application and Outcome*. 2nd ed. Englewood Cliffs, NJ: Prentice Hall, 1987.
322. Doleys D: Enuresis and encopresis. In: Kazdin A (ed): *Handbook of Clinical Behavior Therapy with Children*. Homewood, IL, Dorsey Press, 412–440, 1985.
323. Houts A, Liebert R: *Bedwetting: A Guide for Parents*. Springfield, IL, Thomas, 1985.
324. Azrin N, Sneed T, Foxx R: Dry-bed training: rapid elimination of childhood enuresis. *Behav Res Ther* 12(3):147–156, 1974.
325. Glazener C, Evans J, Peto R: Complex behavioral and educational interventions for nocturnal enuresis in children. *Cochrane Database Syst Rev* 1:1–99, 2009.
326. Said J, Wilson P, Hensley V: Primary versus secondary enuresis: differential response to urine-alarm treatment. *Child Family Behav Ther* 13(2):1–13, 1991.
327. Ronen T, Wozner Y, Rahav G: Cognitive intervention in enuresis. *Child Family Behav Ther* 14(2):1–14, 1992.
328. Friman P, Jones K: Behavioral treatment for nocturnal enuresis. *J Early Intens Behav Interv* 2(4):259–267, 2005.
329. Dunlap G, Koegel R, Koegel L: Continuity of treatment: toilet training in multiple community settings. *J Assoc Person SeverHandicaps* 9(2):134–141, 1984.
330. Azrin N, Foxx R: *Toilet Training in Less Than a Day*. New York, Simon & Schuster, 1974.
331. Partin J, Hamill S, Fischel J, Partin J: Painful defecation and fecal soiling in children. *Pediatrics* 89(6):1007–1009, 1992.
332. Blum N, Taubman B, Osborne M: Behavioral characteristics of children with stool toileting refusal. *Pediatrics* 99(1):50–53, 1997.
333. Blum N, Taubman B, Nemeth N: During toilet training, constipation occurs before stool toileting refusal. *Pediatrics* 113(6):e520–e2, 2004.
334. Doleys D: Assessment and treatment of enuresis and encopresis in children. In: Hersen M, Eisler R, Miller P (eds): *Progress in Behavior Modification*. New York, American Press, 85–121, 1978.
335. Ashkenazi Z: The treatment of encopresis using a discriminative stimulus and positive reinforcement. *J Behav Ther Exp Psychiatry* 6(2):155–157, 1975.
336. Wright L, Walker C: Behavioral treatment of encopresis. *J Pediatr Psychol* 35–37, 1976.
337. Young I, Goldsmith A, Gendlin E: Treatment of encopresis in a day treatment program. *Psychotherapy Theory Res Pract* 9(3):231–235, 1972.
338. Freeman KA, Riley A, Duke DC, Fu R: Systematic review and meta-analysis of behavioral interventions for fecal incontinence with constipation. *J Pediatr Psychol* 39(8):887–902, 2014.
339. Harrison E, Onslow M: The Lidcombe Program for preschool children who stutter. In: Guitar B, McCauley R (eds): *Treatment of Stuttering: Established and Emerging Interventions*. Baltimore, MD, Lippincott Williams & Wilkins, 118–140, 2009.
340. Onslow M, Menzies R, Packman A: An operant intervention for early stuttering: The development of the Lidcombe Program. *Behav Modif* 25(1):116–139, 2001.
341. Jones M, Onslow M, Packman A, et al.: Randomised controlled trial of the Lidcombe programme of early stuttering intervention. *BMJ* 331(7518):659, 2005.
342. Franken M, Putker-de Bruijn D: RESTART-DCM Method. Treatment protocol developed within the scope of the ZonMW project Cost-effectiveness of the Demands and Capacities Model based treatment compared to the Lidcombe programme of early stuttering intervention: randomised trial. 2014.
343. de Sonneville-Koedoot C, Stolk E, Rietveld T, Franken M-C: Direct versus indirect treatment for preschool children who stutter: the RESTART Randomized Trial. *PLoS ONE* 10(7):e0133758, 2015.
344. Månsson HP: Childhood stuttering: Incidence and development. *J Fluency Disord* 25(1):47–57, 2000.

CHAPTER 6.2.3 ■ INTERPERSONAL PSYCHOTHERAPY

LAURA MUFSON AND JAMI F. YOUNG

INTRODUCTION

Interpersonal psychotherapy (IPT) is a brief, time-limited psychotherapy that was developed in the late 1960s for the treatment of nonbipolar, nonpsychotic, depressed adult outpatients (1). The underlying assumption of IPT is that the quality of interpersonal relationships can cause, maintain, or buffer against depression. This view is similarly articulated in interpersonal theories of depression (2–4). When one is depressed, it affects one's interpersonal relationships. The quality and stability of the relationships in turn affects one's mood. IPT assumes that if one improves the relationships, one can actually change the course of the depressive episode. IPT educates individuals about the link between their mood and problems that are occurring in their relationships, and teaches them how improving their interpersonal skills and addressing these relationship problems can lead to recovery from their depression.

The emphasis on the connection between relationships and mental health has its origin in the work of Adolf Meyer (5) and Harry Stack Sullivan (6). Meyer postulated that mental illness was a result of the difficulties a person had in attempting to adapt to his environment, including his relationships. Sullivan stated that mental disorders were in part affected by inadequate communication and lack of understanding of one's behavior within relationships. In addition to these theories, IPT has its roots in Bowlby's attachment theory, specifically in its emphasis on the importance of relational bonds with other people. When there are conflicts or losses of the important bonds, the outcome is emotional distress, and specifically depression (7). Accordingly, IPT focuses on teaching individuals ways to decrease conflict and to cope with other changes in their relationships, including actual losses of relationships due to death, which can affect a person's mood.

BACKGROUND

Basic Principles

The two main goals of IPT are to: (1) decrease depressive symptoms and (2) improve social functioning within significant relationships. The strategies for achieving these goals include: (1) identifying a specific problem area; (2) identifying effective communication and problem-solving techniques to use with the problem area; and (3) practicing in session, and eventually experimenting outside the session, with the use of these techniques in the context of significant relationships. Clinical depression is conceptualized in IPT as consisting of three components: (1) symptom formation, (2) social functioning, and (3) personality (1). IPT is conceptualized as intervening in symptom formation and social functioning and less in personality, given its short duration.

Modifications for Use with Adolescents

IPT has been selected for use with adolescents due to its developmentally relevant focus on relationships and skill-building. Interpersonal Psychotherapy for Depressed Adolescents (IPT-A) is active, structured, and includes a large psychoeducational component. As treatment progresses, the adolescent takes more control and develops a more active, action-oriented way of problem-solving (8) that is consistent with appropriate developmental changes in their approach to problem-solving (9). IPT-A emphasizes interpersonal competencies and skills training. Treatment works by addressing the difficulties and enhancing the strengths of the individual, with the goal of increasing independence and interdependence on a support system. Thus, IPT-A supports the task of individuation and increased autonomy that is so important to adolescents and therefore makes the treatment attractive to them.

Several alterations have been made to the IPT manual to increase the model's appropriateness for the treatment of adolescent depression. Although the overall goals and problem areas of IPT are employed in IPT-A, the latter also includes a discussion, within the problem area of role transitions, about transitions that are due to family structural change (e.g., divorce, separation, remarriage). This discussion of a specific type of transition is included given the frequency with which it occurs for adolescents, the empirically demonstrated connection to depressive symptoms, and the interpersonal challenges and difficulties that are associated with family transitions (10). A second adaptation is the addition of a parent component to the treatment protocol. Although IPT-A is an individual treatment, some degree of involvement on the part of the parent or guardian is needed to promote the wellbeing of the adolescent and to facilitate the success of the treatment. Parent involvement in IPT-A is flexible, though it should minimally include involvement in the initial phase of treatment so as to provide education about the disorder and its treatment. The parent may also be involved as needed in the middle phase to work on specific relationship strategies and it is best if the parent attends a final session to review his child's progress in treatment and future treatment needs. The role of the parent or guardian in treatment is presented for each phase of the treatment in the manual (11).

The objectives of treatment have been altered slightly to take into account developmental tasks including individuation, establishment of autonomy, development of romantic relationships, coping with initial experiences of death and loss, and managing peer pressure. Second, the techniques employed in the treatment for working toward the goals of decreasing depressive symptoms and improving interpersonal functioning have been geared toward adolescents. Techniques employed with adolescents include giving them a rating scale from 1 to 10 to rate their mood, which is concrete and makes it easier for them to monitor improvement; doing more basic social skills work; conducting explicit work on perspective-taking skills to counteract adolescent black-and-white thinking about solutions to problems; and learning how to negotiate parent–child tensions. Additional strategies have been identified to address special issues that arise in the treatment of adolescents, such as school refusal, physical or sexual abuse, suicidality, aggression, and involvement of a child protective service agency.

Overview of Efficacy

IPT-A meets four conditions that permit its inclusion as an efficacious treatment: (1) the treatment is manual based (1,11); (2) the sample characteristics are detailed; (3) the treatment has been tested in randomized clinical trials (12–16); and (4) at least two different investigator teams demonstrated the intervention's effects (17–19). In addition, IPT-A has been evaluated and included as an efficacious treatment in SAMHSA's National Registry of Evidence-Based Programs and Practices. The efficacy and effectiveness of IPT-A for reducing adolescents' depressive symptoms have been examined in five randomized controlled clinical trials (12–16). Depressed adolescents treated with IPT-A demonstrated fewer depressive symptoms, better social functioning, and better global functioning at the completion of treatment than adolescents in control conditions, although in one study (15), IPT did not show as much improvement as CBT.

The efficacy clinical trial conducted by Mufson et al. (12) included adolescents who met DSM-III-R criteria for major depression. The study showed that IPT-A ($N = 24$) was superior to clinical management ($N = 24$) (monitoring of symptoms) with respect to decreasing depressive symptoms, rates of recovery from depression, and rates of retention in the treatment for depressed adolescents. In addition, adolescents who received IPT-A demonstrated significant improvement in certain areas of social functioning and interpersonal problem-solving skills compared to adolescents who received clinical management.

Rosselló and Bernal (13), who used a different modification of the adult IPT manual (20), provided independent replication in their study that showed that both IPT ($N = 23$) and CBT ($N = 25$) were superior to waitlist control ($N = 23$) for the treatment of depressed adolescents ($N = 71$) who met DSM-III criteria for major depressive disorder, dysthymic disorder, or both. They also found that IPT was significantly better than the waitlist condition at increasing self-esteem and improving social adaptation. They found that 82% of the adolescents receiving IPT compared to 52% of the adolescents receiving CBT met recovery criteria by the end of treatment. In a second study, Rosselló et al. (15) conducted a randomized controlled trial comparing the efficacy of group versus individual IPT, and group and individual CBT for adolescents with depression (either diagnosis or significant severity of symptoms) and reported no significant differences between individual and group formats. On most measures, there were no significant differences in outcomes between IPT and CBT treatments. However, CBT produced significantly greater decreases in depressive symptoms than IPT. It is important to note that there was low fidelity adherence to the IPT treatment in this study, which may explain the weaker results for IPT.

Recently, another research group compared the efficacy of group to individual IPT-A for a primary diagnosis of major depressive disorder (16). Thirty-nine adolescents, aged 13 to 19 years, were randomly assigned in blocks to either group or individual delivery of IPT. Treatment was adapted for group delivery taking into account the recommendations of Mufson et al. (21) and Wilfley et al. (22). There were significant improvements in depression, anxiety, and global functioning from pre- to posttreatment for the sample and no significant differences in outcome between group and individual formats of delivery (16). In secondary data analyses, adolescents showed significant improvements in interpersonal functioning and changes in attachment style following treatment (23). This study provides additional empirical support for IPT-A in both an individual and group format for the treatment of depression. Although tests of mediation were not possible in this sample, their findings suggest that improvements in interpersonal relationships are a possible mechanism of the intervention.

Additional empirical investigations of IPT-A aim to reach a broader range of depressed adolescents by either providing treatment in community-based practice settings or serving more severe populations. For instance, an effectiveness study compared IPT-A to treatment as usual (TAU) in the school-based health clinics in New York City for depressed adolescents with a broader diagnostic picture including major depression, dysthymia, depression disorder NOS, and adjustment disorder with depressed mood (14). In addition, adolescents were included with comorbid diagnoses including anxiety disorders, ADHD, and oppositional defiant disorder. School-based clinicians delivered both treatments. TAU consisted mostly of individual supportive counseling, typical of care delivered in the schools prior to initiation of the study. Adolescents treated with IPT-A compared to TAU showed greater symptom reduction, significantly better social functioning, and greater decrease in clinical severity of depression and improvement in overall functioning. In addition, the study demonstrated the ability to train community clinicians to deliver IPT-A effectively using an abbreviated therapy training program, thereby demonstrating the transportability and effectiveness of IPT-A from the university laboratory to the community setting (24).

Another study was conducted in a high school comparing intensive IPT-A (IPT-A-IN) to TAU (supportive counseling) for depressed adolescents with suicidal risk, although adolescents at imminent risk for suicide were excluded and referred for a higher level of care (25). The treatment was modified; IPT-A-IN consisted of two 50-minute face-to-face sessions weekly and a 30-minute phone follow-up weekly for a total of three clinical contacts per week. Due to the increased frequency of sessions and desire to intervene quickly, the duration of treatment was also shortened to 6 consecutive weeks instead of 12 weeks. The students were identified in school through depression screenings using self-report measures and then evaluated by a psychiatrist for depression and suicide severity by a psychiatrist using a structured diagnostic interview. The sessions were delivered by well-trained school counselors and treatment targeted both the depression and suicidal ideation linking these symptoms to problems in the students' relationships, consistent with IPT-A. Intensive school-based IPT-A-IN was shown to be effective in reducing the severity of depression, suicidal ideation, anxiety, and hopelessness in depressed adolescents with suicidal risk (25).

The efficacy and effectiveness studies demonstrate IPT-A's acceptability, efficacy and effectiveness for a broad cultural population of adolescents from impoverished urban Latinos to adolescents in Japan, Australia, and Puerto Rico (12–15,16,25). IPT-A appears effective both with lower income as well as middle class populations. Age and severity of illness were identified as moderators of IPT-A outcome in the effectiveness study. Older adolescents (15 to 18 years.) and those who were more severely ill showed a greater benefit of being treated with IPT-A than TAU (14). Depressed adolescents with comorbid anxiety who received IPT-A had a better treatment outcome than those who were treated with TAU (26). Finally, IPT-A has been shown to be particularly effective for adolescents with high levels of parent–adolescent conflict (27). To date, there are no identified mediators of IPT-A outcome, in part due to the smaller sample sizes of the IPT-A studies, however the recent study by Spence et al. (23), suggests that change in interpersonal functioning is one possible mediator. Further research is needed to better understand the moderators and mediators of IPT-A. Based on the empirical support for treatment efficacy, IPT-A meets the American Psychological Association Division 12 criteria for a "well-established" psychotherapy for depression in youth (19).

Who Is Suitable to Treat with IPT-A?

An integral part of the assessment process is determining an adolescent's suitability for IPT-A based upon diagnosis, severity of illness and impairment, as well as an assessment of the family environment and willingness to engage in treatment. Based on our clinical experience, the following characteristics of an adolescent make IPT-A a good treatment choice: (1) the adolescent's willingness to work in a one-to-one therapeutic relationship in a time-limited therapy; (2) recognition by the adolescent that there seem to be difficulties of an interpersonal nature that may be causing problems at this time; and (3) a family willing to support the therapy or at least allow the adolescent to participate in treatment.

An adolescent is felt to be suitable for treatment first and foremost if he is willing to acknowledge the depression and is willing to discuss the impact the depression is having on his relationships. An adolescent who is willing to discuss feelings and problems, and explore connections among feelings, events and relationships, is a particularly good candidate for IPT-A. IPT-A is probably most effective with adolescents who have had an acute onset of depressive symptoms and historically have not had chronic and severe interpersonal problems with friends or family. The acute onset increases the likelihood of being able to identify an interpersonal precipitant to the depression and/or exacerbation of a longer-standing interpersonal problem. IPT-A may also be helpful to adolescents with long-standing interpersonal problems, but the goals for improvement may need to be more circumscribed.

IPT-A is designed for use with adolescents, ages 12 to 18 years, who have an acute onset of major depression or other milder forms of depression such as dysthymia, an adjustment disorder with depressed mood or depression not otherwise specified. Adolescents are suitable for the treatment if they are of normal intelligence, and are not actively suicidal. Many of the treated adolescents report suicidal ideation consisting of passive thoughts about wanting to be dead but they typically do not report intent to die or a specific plan to harm themselves. The therapist must feel that once-a-week therapy is sufficient and safe for the adolescent's current level of depression. Tang et al.'s study (25) suggests that twice-a-week therapy may be an effective model for those with elevated suicide risk. Depressed adolescents with psychotic symptoms or primary diagnoses of bipolar disorder, substance abuse, or conduct have not been treated with IPT-A. Initial studies have examined the efficacy of treating bipolar adolescents with Interpersonal and Social Rhythms Therapy for adolescents (IPSRT-A) (28). However, depressed adolescents with comorbid anxiety disorders, attention-deficit disorder, and oppositional defiant disorder have been treated successfully with IPT-A. If the adolescent has comorbid disorders, a decision should be made confirming that the depression is the appropriate disorder upon which to focus treatment initially.

Prior to the initiation of IPT-A, a thorough diagnostic evaluation of the adolescent should be undertaken to gather information on current symptoms as well as previous psychiatric, family, developmental, medical, social, and academic history. The goals of the diagnostic assessment are to: (1) make a current clinical diagnosis using DSM-5 diagnostic criteria; (2) ascertain the adolescent's level of psychosocial functioning and pinpoint areas of interpersonal problems; and (3) assess which treatment would be most appropriate for the adolescent. This evaluation should be conducted by an intake clinician and/or the IPT-A therapist prior to initiating treatment. Such information should be gathered during the evaluation from the adolescent, parents and other family members, teachers and other school personnel, and other caretakers such as pediatricians and clergy to facilitate an informed decision about the treatment of choice for the teen (11).

INITIAL PHASE OF THERAPY

IPT-A is divided into three phases: initial, middle, and termination. There are three main components of IPT-A that are evident in the three phases of treatment (Table 6.2.3.1). The initial phase focuses primarily on the first component of psychoeducation with some attention to affect identification. The middle and termination phases focus more directly on affect identification and interpersonal skill building techniques and prevention of relapse.

Psychoeducation about Depression and IPT-A

There are several tasks to be accomplished during the first session of IPT-A. These include: (1) explaining the nature of depression in adolescents; (2) assigning the limited sick role in treatment; and (3) introducing the basic principles of IPT-A. It is preferable to involve the parents in the first session by dividing the initial IPT-A session into a combination of meetings with the adolescent and parent together, adolescent alone, and parent alone as was done in the pretreatment evaluation. At the conclusion of the initial session, the adolescent and parent(s) should know that the depression symptoms are (a) time limited, (b) reflective of a disorder which can be treated successfully, and (c) that the adolescent will likely be able to function better with treatment.

Explaining the Nature of Depression in Adolescents

An important task of the first session is to impart information about the course of depression and its treatment to both

TABLE 6.2.3.1

INTERPERSONAL PSYCHOTHERAPY: PRIMARY COMPONENTS OF TREATMENT

Education	Affect Identification	Interpersonal Skills Building
• Psychoeducation • Limited sick role • Interpersonal inventory • Treatment contract	• Labeling emotions • Clarification of emotions • Facilitating expression of emotions • Monitoring emotions	• Modeling • Use of therapeutic relationship as sample of interpersonal interaction • Communication analysis • Perspective-taking • Interpersonal problem solving • Role-playing

adolescent and family. This should include a discussion about the symptoms of depression, their impact on functioning, and the prevalence rates of depression in adolescents. It is important for the adolescent and family to know that the prognosis for recovery is good. The adolescent and the parent(s) also need to be informed that there are other treatment options available, including other forms of psychotherapy and/or medication if for some reason IPT-A is not sufficiently effective for this adolescent.

Giving the Adolescent a Limited "Sick Role"

The purpose of the limited sick role is to allow the adolescent some relief from the pressure of performing his usual social role at the same level as prior to being depressed, and to receive some extra support for his efforts without punishment for the quality of the work while he recovers. The adolescent and his family are encouraged to think of him as in treatment and as having an illness that affects his motivation and the quality of his performance. Nonetheless, the adolescent is encouraged to maintain the usual social roles in the family, at school, and with friends. Specifically, he needs to get up every morning and get to school, participate in his usual school activities, complete homework, and perform his chores around his house to the best of his abilities. The parent is advised to be supportive, less punitive, and to encourage the adolescent to engage in as many normal activities as possible, while recognizing that the adolescent may have difficulty performing up to par. The assignment of the sick role and psychoeducation can help family members to respond more positively toward the adolescent and shift the blame for difficulties in fulfilling his social roles from the adolescent to the illness (11).

Education about IPT-A

At this point in the session, it is a good idea to introduce the basic structure of IPT-A to the adolescent. The therapist restates that the focus of treatment will be on reducing the depression symptoms he is experiencing and improving relationship difficulties that seem most connected to his depression. The therapist and adolescent together will identify and practice strategies and skills to improve the targeted relationships and in turn improve his mood. Most of the sessions will occur with the therapist and adolescent alone, but they may talk about inviting parents or significant others into a session or two in the middle phase if it looks like it might be helpful.

Interpersonal Inventory

In the remainder of the initial phase, the therapist conducts the interpersonal inventory, which is a detailed review of the adolescent's significant relationships, both current and past. To conduct the interpersonal inventory, it is helpful for the therapist to use the Closeness Circle (Figure 6.2.3.1). This is a series of concentric circles with the adolescent's name in the center. The goal is to place the adolescent's significant relationships within the appropriate circles of closeness/importance in the teenager's life. The result is a picture of the significant people orbiting the adolescent's life and the emotional valence associated with their position in the adolescent's life.

Once the circle has been completed, the therapist asks detailed questions about each relationship. Examples of questions from the inventory are: "What is your relationship with X like?" "What do you like about X? What don't you like? What types of things do you do with X? Do you ever argue?" The therapist should use these questions to facilitate the adolescent's telling the story of his current life as played out in his significant relationships. It is important when conducting the interpersonal inventory to obtain information about relationships that illustrate interpersonal strengths as well as those that illustrate deficits or areas of weakness.

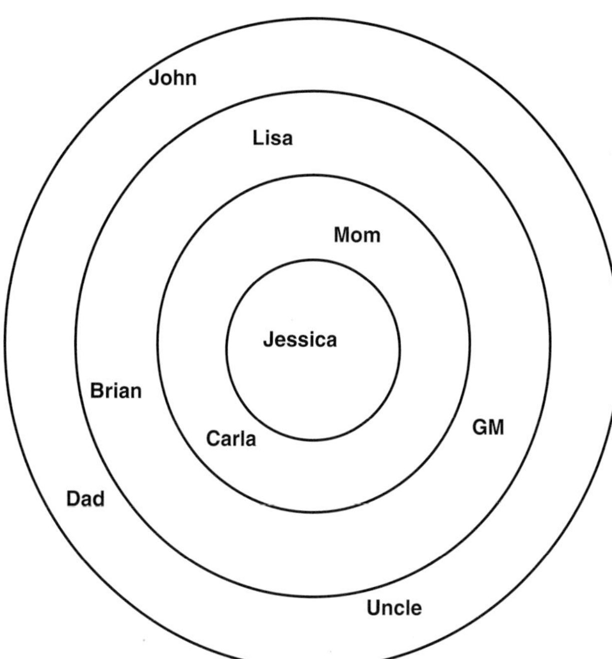

FIGURE 6.2.3.1. Example of a closeness circle.

The interpersonal inventory facilitates the adolescent and the therapist's understanding of the interpersonal context of the depression. The therapist gathers information about events that may have precipitated the depressive episode, the reasons for seeking treatment now, and what has been happening in these significant relationships that may be associated with the onset of symptoms. Although the emphasis is on current relationships, obtaining a complete picture of the adolescent's social relationships including some information about past relationships and interpersonal functioning is helpful in understanding his overall patterns of interaction and communication in his relationships. The therapist can think of it as the diagnostic assessment of interpersonal symptoms to parallel the completed assessment of depression symptoms. This inventory provides the necessary interpersonal data to select one of the four problem areas for focus in the middle phase.

Formulation of Problem Area and Making a Treatment Contract

By the end of the fourth session, the therapist will have completed a comprehensive interpersonal assessment and will conclude the session with an interpersonal formulation linking the adolescent's interpersonal situation with his depressed mood and placing the formulation within the framework of one of the four problem areas. The problem area formulation should occur as a natural outgrowth of the recent discussions. It is helpful for the therapist to weave the narratives of each relationship into one larger interpersonal narrative for the adolescent, pointing out any noticeable patterns across relationships. The therapist should seek the adolescent's opinion of the formulation, giving the adolescent the opportunity to acknowledge the issues, show understanding, and have the opportunity to disagree.

As in the adult version of IPT, there are four identified problem areas in IPT-A upon which the therapy can be focused: (1) grief due to death; (2) interpersonal disputes with friends, teachers, parents, and siblings; (3) role transitions such as changing schools (elementary to junior high or junior high to high school), entering puberty, becoming sexually active, birth of another sibling, becoming a parent, parental divorce, illness of a parent; and/or (4) interpersonal deficits such as difficulty initiating and maintaining relationships and communicating about feelings (11). Grief is defined in IPT-A as loss through death. The grieving process can be abnormal by being delayed, distorted, or by becoming a chronic reaction. Interpersonal disputes are conceptualized as a situation in which the adolescent and other parties have diverging expectations of a situation and this conflict is severe enough to lead to significant distress. Role transitions are situations in which the adolescent is having difficulty adapting to a change in life circumstances. These may be developmental crises or adaptations following life events or relationship dissolutions. Finally, interpersonal deficits is identified as the problem area when an adolescent has impoverished interpersonal relationships in both number and quality of the relationships. When there seem to be two problem areas, the therapist should identify a primary and possibly a secondary problem area to work on in treatment.

Setting the treatment contract involves outlining the adolescent's and parents' roles in the treatment, identifying treatment goals, clarifying expectations for treatment, and outlining the nuts and bolts of treatment. Both the improvement in interpersonal functioning and reduction of symptoms are equally important achievements and most frequently will co-occur. Therapist and adolescent should set goals that are likely to be attainable within the brief treatment so that the adolescent can feel the goals were achieved and can have a sense of progress throughout the treatment. The culmination of this discussion is a specific verbal treatment contract.

MIDDLE PHASE OF THERAPY

Following agreement on the treatment contract and the identified problem area, the middle phase of treatment begins. Typically this occurs by session 5 and continues through session 9. Session 9 is a transitional session in which the work of the middle phase continues while the therapist begins to discuss concluding the treatment in several weeks. The middle sessions focus on the problem area identified in the initial sessions as a means toward achieving recovery from depression. The objectives of the middle phase of treatment for all adolescents include: (1) further clarification of the problem area; (2) identification of effective strategies to attack the problem; and (3) implementation of interventions to bring about resolution of the problem. The therapist's general tasks associated with the middle phase of treatment are as follows: (1) monitoring depression symptoms and the need to consider adjunctive therapy such as medication if there is no improvement or a worsening of symptoms; (2) facilitating the adolescent's self-disclosure of his affective state; and (3) keeping in contact with parents to support and participate in treatment as necessary (11).

During the middle phase of treatment, the therapist and adolescent continually assess the accuracy of the initial formulation of the problem to maximize the amount of change that can be accomplished in the treatment. The therapist must keep the adolescent's discussions relevant to the identified problem areas. The therapist helps generate strategies and suggests the application of techniques that will lead to clarification and resolution of the adolescent's problem. This includes illuminating the process of identifying problems, clarifying the issues, generating strategies, applying strategies for problem resolution, and acquiring skills that result in increased interpersonal self-confidence and improved functioning.

Work on the Identified Problem Area

The therapist and adolescent work to resolve the identified problem area during the middle phase of treatment. In the case of grief, the IPT-A therapist helps by reconstructing the adolescent's relationship with the deceased, addressing unresolved issues in the relationship, linking the depression to the feelings for the deceased, providing empathic listening to help facilitate the mourning process, and assisting the adolescent in establishing new relationships. The IPT-A therapist can use these strategies to similarly help adolescents who are suffering while in the midst of the normal grieving process. In cases where interpersonal disputes are the identified problem area, IPT-A aims to define how intractable the dispute is, the specific stage of the dispute, and identify sources of misunderstanding via faulty communication, poor perspective-taking, and invalid or unreasonable expectations. The therapist aims to intervene by using communication training, problem-solving, or other techniques that facilitate change in the situation.

In the middle phase of treatment, IPT-A for role transitions aims to help the adolescent to reappraise the old and new roles, to identify sources of difficulty in the new role, identify skills and strategies that would make it easier to adapt to the new role, and to develop skills and implement solutions for these difficulties in their significant relationships. Finally, in the case of interpersonal deficits, the adolescent and therapist will need to focus upon old relationships as well as the relationship with the therapist during the middle phase. In the former, common themes should be identified and linked to current circumstances. In using the therapeutic relationship, the therapist aims to identify problematic processes, such as deficits in initiating or maintaining relationships, and to modify these processes by practicing approaches to developing new relationships. By practicing the interpersonal skills with the therapist, the therapeutic relationship can serve as a template for other relationships that the adolescent will be striving to develop.

Therapeutic Techniques

During the middle phase of the treatment, the therapist teaches the adolescent specific strategies that can help him deal with his interpersonal difficulties within one or two of the problem areas. The therapeutic relationship in IPT-A provides a forum in which skills can be practiced and feedback can be given in a nonthreatening environment (11). IPT-A techniques include exploratory techniques, encouragement of affect, communication analysis, behavior change techniques (including decision analysis and role plays), use of the therapeutic relationship and adjunctive techniques such as interpersonal experiments. Exploratory techniques can be either directive or nondirective. Directive exploratory techniques include targeted questioning and interviewing. The nondirective techniques include supportive acknowledgment, and extension of the topic being discussed by the adolescent (11). Encouragement of affect involves facilitating discussion of painful feelings about events or issues and helping the adolescent use his affective experiences to better understand the link between mood and relationships and eventually to make interpersonal change.

Communication analysis is a thorough investigation of a specific dialogue or argument that occurred between an adolescent and another person. Communication analysis identifies ways in which the adolescent's communication is ineffective and fails to achieve the goal of the communication. In conducting the communication analysis, the therapist can illustrate how changing one phrase can change the entire feeling about the interaction and the other person. Decision analysis is employed by the therapist to help the adolescent consider a range of alternative actions that he can take and the possible consequences associated with each of those actions. In role-playing, the therapist and adolescent act out the skills that the adolescent is learning in the treatment in a nonthreatening way. The therapist can model many useful interpersonal skills such as affective expression, effective communication, and decision-making strategies. Adjunctive techniques include work assignments to be done at home between the sessions. The assignments usually involve practicing specific skills that were the focus of the sessions. They are referred to as "interpersonal experiments" or "work at home."

TERMINATION PHASE

A termination date is set with the adolescent and family at the beginning of treatment and the adolescent is reminded of the number of weeks remaining until the end of treatment. Twelve weeks is the time frame chosen for the clinical trials assessing the efficacy of IPT-A. It is a reasonable duration for adolescents who are reluctant to stay in treatment for any significant length of time. The time period can be modified in either direction. The important issue is to retain the treatment's time-limited nature by setting the initial treatment contract for the number of weeks that seem most appropriate for that adolescent.

Tasks of Termination

The termination phase includes clarification of the adolescent's warning symptoms of future depressive episodes, identification of successful strategies that were used in the therapy, generalization of skills to future situations, emphasis on mastery of new interpersonal skills, and discussion of the need for further treatment (11). The therapist needs to balance the tasks of the termination phase with concluding work on the identified problem area. It is crucial to devote a major portion of the termination phase to reviewing interpersonal strategies used during the middle phase and to applying these strategies to ongoing and future situations. This may help reduce relapse and recurrence, which are common in adolescent depression, improve social self-confidence, and enable the adolescent to negotiate successful endings of other relationships at future points in his life.

Throughout the treatment and termination, the therapist should identify the changes that she observes in the adolescent: improved communication and ability to see another person's perspective, attempts made to negotiate a dispute, increased awareness about his own feelings associated with a relationship, successful mourning of the loss and/or the establishment of new relationships. The therapist and adolescent together highlight how specific strategies have enabled him to make improvements within his identified problem area, in specific relationships, and most importantly in his mood.

Terminating treatment with an adolescent also means terminating treatment with the family. Ideally, the therapist will conduct a final termination session with the adolescent alone and then have another joint termination session for the adolescent and family. The therapist also may see the parents alone if necessary or if the adolescent prefers it that way. The goals of the final session for the family are similar to those of the adolescent's final session: a review of the adolescent's presenting symptoms, initial goals for the therapy, achievement of these goals, and a discussion of the changes in the family interactions and functioning as a result of the therapy. The termination phase enables both the adolescent and parent to participate in the review of accomplishments and the identification of areas that would benefit from further treatment. It is important to discuss with the family the possible recurrence of mild symptoms shortly after termination, the need for further treatment if it is indicated, and management of future recurrent episodes of depression.

There are adolescents for whom there has been some improvement, but who are still moderately symptomatic at the conclusion of treatment. Further treatment may be necessary under certain circumstances when the symptoms have not fully remitted or when there are other more chronic problems contributing to the adolescent's impairment. This information is utilized by the family, adolescent, and therapist to make decisions about the need for further treatment and the type of additional treatment that may be needed.

SPECIAL ISSUES

Working with Parents

Due to high divorce rates as well as increases in single-parent families, adolescents often live in nonnuclear families, including homes of other relatives and foster or group homes. As with the parents, these people are important in the adolescent's daily life and must be educated about the nature of depression, ways to support the adolescent's recovery and, if necessary, participate in the treatment to facilitate changes in the home environment that will play a role in the adolescent's recovery.

Awareness and understanding of the mental health status of an adolescent's parent or guardian is critical to understanding the adolescent's depression and developing the most effective treatment plan. In cases where the parent is depressed, it is often necessary for the adolescent's therapist to help the adolescent by first helping the parent find an appropriate referral for her own treatment. It is important to explain that in the IPT-A framework, depression affects the parent's as well as the teen's interpersonal functioning. Any alleviation of parental depression is likely to reduce the stress the adolescent is facing.

Depressed parents often model a depressive interpersonal style that can range from ineffective communication and conflict negotiation skills to social withdrawal and helplessness. Therefore, when these adolescents try to practice new interpersonal skills at home, they face an uphill battle. In such cases, the therapist and adolescent will need to do more in-session practice of interpersonal strategies as well as have the adolescent identify others in his life with whom he can practice these skills. Enlisting the parent as a "coach" and "collaborator" in the treatment can foster the parent's willingness to support the adolescent's experiments with new skills, both during and outside of the session. Having a good grasp of the role of parental depression in the family allows the adolescent and therapist to develop realistic treatment goals and focus on the relationships that can have the greatest impact on increasing his feelings of support and decreasing his depressed mood (11).

Not all parents, unfortunately, are open to intervention for themselves or their child. In these situations, the therapist should, with the adolescent's approval, attempt to intervene with the parent during an in-person meeting, or over the phone if the parent is unable to attend a session. The therapist, using an empathic and nonjudgmental psychoeducational approach, can sometimes alter the parent's perspective and enjoin them to support the treatment. If the parent continues to be resistant to collaborating in the treatment, the therapist will need to work with the adolescent on a modified treatment plan.

Use of Medication with IPT-A

The use of IPT-A in combination with medication has not been studied in a large clinical trial; however, it is frequently used this way in our general outpatient psychiatry clinics with benefits to the adolescent and we have obtained some initial pilot data supporting combined treatment (29). Most of the clinical trials have included a homogeneous sample of adolescents who typically have a depression disorder with a possible anxiety disorder, and have excluded adolescents with other disorders such as conduct disorder or substance abuse (24). However, in treatment in outpatient clinics, adolescents may present with depression and other comorbid disorders that may require a combination of medication and IPT-A. Antidepressant medication is not contraindicated during IPT-A, and in fact, may be a useful adjunctive treatment for severely depressed adolescents whose symptoms do not remit during the initial phase of treatment. The main goal of any acute phase of treatment, medication or psychotherapy, is to achieve a timely treatment response measured by remission of the depressive symptoms. Therefore, if the adolescent is not responding as well as one would like to the therapy, it is advisable to consider adding an adjunctive treatment.

Our guidelines are to consider antidepressants if there is little or no remission of symptoms after 4 weeks of IPT-A. Experience treating adolescents suffering from a more chronic depression (either dysthymia or chronic major depression) suggests that medication might be beneficial from the outset of treatment to help alleviate the hopelessness and listlessness that often characterize these adolescents and prevent them from more actively engaging in psychotherapy (11). The clinician should discuss with the adolescent and his parents the reasons for considering medication: that the adolescent is still showing significant signs of depression or significant anhedonia and lethargy, and that in such instances medication can often be beneficial. These guidelines evolved from our clinical experience using IPT-A to treat depressed adolescents. Recently, a pilot study examining the feasibility and acceptability of delivering a stepped care model of IPT-A in pediatric primary care which included a combined IPT-A and medication arm was completed. This study suggested that IPT-A and medication, in this case Prozac, can be an acceptable and potentially effective treatment for adolescent depression. It was, however, a small sample that received the combined treatment since a significant number of adolescents showed improvement after 8 weeks of IPT-A alone (29). Thus, more research is needed to assess the efficacy of using both medication and IPT-A to treat adolescent depression and its comorbid disorders.

Crisis Management

Crises are not infrequent during the treatment of a depressed adolescent. A crisis is a major change in the adolescent's living situation, interpersonal relationships, family relationships, or emotional well-being that jeopardizes the adolescent's psychological health and overwhelms the adolescent's capacity to cope with the situation. Examples of crises include: running away, pregnancy, illness in family or friend, involvement with the law, exposure or involvement in violence. The first task facing the IPT-A therapist is to determine the nature and etiology of the crisis by speaking both to the adolescent and other parties involved. In the case of suicidal or homicidal ideation, if an appointment cannot be set up soon enough, the adolescent should be sent to the nearest emergency room to evaluate the need for hospitalization or an increase in the frequency and intensity of the treatment. The therapist's most important decision is whether or not the adolescent can remain in IPT-A or whether the adolescent must receive other types of services either at the same or another facility.

If the adolescent is evaluated as being able to remain in outpatient adolescent treatment, the IPT-A treatment contract should be reexamined and revised as necessary. Items in the contract that may change include the frequency of the sessions, involvement of the family, frequency of phone calls between the therapist and adolescent, and the identified problem area that is the focus of the treatment. At times the crisis may suggest that a significant problem area was overlooked or there may be an interaction between two problem areas, thus requiring a shift in the focus of the sessions. With the new contract, the therapist can move forward to address the new information about the adolescent's interpersonal relationships and the context of the depression.

TRAINING IN IPT-A

In the IPT-A efficacy study, therapists received 2 days of didactics and then treated three cases for training purposes, videotaping every session and receiving 1 hour of supervision for each session. A random selection of these tapes was rated by experts for therapist competency prior to certifying the therapists to participate in the clinical trial. Such an intensive training program is not feasible in effectiveness research due to constraints on the clinicians' time, nor is it realistic for training clinicians to implement the treatment in their practices. Clinicians in community-based settings routinely have pressing clinical demands competing for their time so that the training program in the effectiveness study was abbreviated to one full day of didactics and the practice cases characteristic of the efficacy trials were eliminated. Even with this briefer training, clinicians were able to learn IPT-A and deliver it with enough fidelity to obtain good outcomes (24). Such support for briefer training and supervision models is needed in order to be able to disseminate and implement treatment in the community in a cost-effective manner.

Nonetheless, when it comes to training and certifying clinicians as IPT-A therapists, the intensity of the efficacy model of therapist training is still believed to produce the best adherence and competence in IPT-A. In addition, to be considered for training to be an IPT-A supervisor and trainer of other clinicians, at least another two treatment cases with supervision (total = 5) are typically required, along with consultation on the supervision of several cases to ensure that the therapist feels confident and can competently train others in the use of the IPT-A model. The International Society for Interpersonal Psychotherapy (ISIPT) is currently working to settle upon guidelines for the training and certification of IPT therapists.

CONCLUSIONS

IPT for depressed adolescents (IPT-A) is an evidence-based psychotherapy that is based on the premise that depression occurs in an interpersonal context. The goals of treatment are to improve the adolescent's interpersonal relationships and his depression symptoms. IPT-A is defined in a treatment manual that is adapted to address the developmental needs of adolescents and their families in a time-limited approach (11). IPT-A is unique in that it has been demonstrated to be effective both in the laboratory and community setting and when delivered by expert and community clinicians (12–16,25). Furthermore, IPT-A has been demonstrated to be efficacious with an underserved Latino population that typically has less access to treatment services (12,14). Research studies and clinical experiences point to the utility of IPT-A as a treatment for adolescent depression. Clinical experience and a pilot study further suggests the benefits of combining IPT-A with medication for adolescents with more severe depression. However, a larger controlled clinical trial is needed to further examine this question.

References

1. Weissman MM, Markowitz JC, Klerman GL: *A Comprehensive Guide to Interpersonal Psychotherapy*. Albany: Basic Books, 2000.
2. Coyne JC: Toward an interactional description of depression. *Psychiatry* 39:28–40, 1976.
3. Hammen C: The emergence of an interpersonal approach to depression. In: Joiner T, Coyne J (eds): *The Interactional Nature of Depression: Advances in Interpersonal Approaches*. Washington, DC, American Psychological Association, 22–36, 1999.
4. Joiner T, Coyne J, Blalock J: On the interpersonal nature of depression: overview and synthesis. In: Joiner T, Coyne J (eds): *The Interactional Nature of Depression: Advances in Interpersonal Approaches*. Washington, DC, American Psychological Association, 3–20, 1999.
5. Meyer A: *Psychobiology: A Science of Man*. Springfield, IL, Charles C. Thomas, 1957.
6. Sullivan HS: *The Interpersonal Theory of Psychiatry*. New York, W.W. Norton & Co., 1953.
7. Bowlby J: Attachment theory and its therapeutic implications. *Adolesc Psychiatry* 6:5–33, 1978.
8. Mufson L, Dorta KP: Interpersonal psychotherapy for depressed adolescents: Theory, practice, and research. *Adolescent Psychiatry* 25:139–167, 2000.
9. Marx EM, Schulze CC: Interpersonal problem-solving in depressed students. *J Clin Psychol* 47:361–370, 1991.
10. Hetherington EM, Bridges M, Insabella GM: What matters? What does not? Five perspectives on the association between marital transitions and children's adjustment. *Am Psychol* 53:167–184, 1998.
11. Mufson L, Dorta KP, Moreau D, Weissman MM: *Interpersonal Psychotherapy for Depressed Adolescents*. 2nd ed. New York, Guilford Publications, Inc., 2004.
12. Mufson L, Weissman MM, Moreau D, Garfinkel R: Efficacy of interpersonal psychotherapy for depressed adolescents. *Arch Gen Psychiatry* 56:573–579, 1999.
13. Rosselló J, Bernal G: The efficacy of cognitive-behavioral and interpersonal treatments for depression in Puerto Rican adolescents. *J Consult Clin Psychol* 67:734–745, 1999.
14. Mufson L, Dorta KP, Wickramaratne P, Nomura Y, Olfson M, Weissman MM: A randomized effectiveness trial of interpersonal psychotherapy for depressed adolescents. *Arch Gen Psychiatry* 61:577–584, 2004.
15. Rosselló J, Bernal G, Rivera-Medina C: Individual and group CBT and IPT for Puerto Rican adolescents with depressive symptoms. *Cult Divers Ethn Min* 14:234–245, 2008.
16. O'Shea G, Spence SH, Donovan CL: Group versus individual interpersonal psychotherapy for depressed adolescents. *Beh Cogn Psychoth* 43:1–19, 2015.
17. Chambless DL, Hollon SD: Defining empirically supported therapies. *J Consult Clin Psychol* 66:7–18, 1998.
18. Chorpita BF: The frontier of evidence-based practice. In: Kazdin AE, Weisz JR (eds): *Evidence-Based Psychotherapies for Children and Adolescents*. New York, Guilford Press, 2010:42–59.
19. David-Ferdon C, Kaslow NJ: Evidence-based psychosocial treatments for child and adolescent depression. *J of Clin Child Adolesc Psychol* 37:62–104, 2008.
20. Klerman GL, Weissman MM, Rounsaville BJ, Chevron ES: *Interpersonal Psychotherapy of Depression*. New York, Basic Books, 1984.
21. Mufson L, Gallagher T, Dorta KP, Young JF: Interpersonal psychotherapy for adolescent depression: adaptation for group therapy. *Am J Psychoth* 58:220–237, 2004.
22. Wilfley DE, Mackenzie KR, Welch RR, et al.: *Interpersonal psychotherapy for group*. New York, Basic Books, 2000.
23. Spence SH, O'Shea G, Donovan CL: Improvements in interpersonal functioning following interpersonal psychotherapy (IPT) with adolescents and their association with change in depression. *Behav Cogn Psychother* 44(3):257–272, 2016.
24. Mufson LH, Dorta KP, Olfson M, Weissman MM, Hoagwood K: Effectiveness research: transporting interpersonal psychotherapy for depressed adolescents (IPT-A) from the lab to school-based health clinics. *Clin Child Fam Psychol Rev* 7:251–461, 2004.
25. Tang T, Jou S, Ko C, Huang S, Yen C: Randomized study of school-based intensive interpersonal psychotherapy for depressed adolescents with suicidal risk and parasuicide behaviors. *Psychiatry Clin Neurosci* 63:463–470, 2009.
26. Young JF, Mufson L, Davies M: Impact of comorbid anxiety in an effectiveness study of interpersonal psychotherapy for depressed adolescents. *J Am Acad Child Adolesc Psychiatry* 45:904–912, 2006.
27. Gunlicks-Stoessel M, Mufson L, Jekal A, Turner B: The impact of perceived interpersonal functioning on treatment for adolescent depression: IPT-A versus treatment as usual in school-based health clinics. *J Consult Clin Psychol* 78:260–267, 2010.
28. Hlastala SA, Kotler JS, McClellan JM, McCauley EA: Interpersonal and social rhythm therapy for adolescents with bipolar disorder: Treatment development and results from an open trial. *Depression and Anxiety* 27(5):457–464, 2010.
29. Mufson L, Rynn M, Yanes-Lukins P, Choo TS, Wall M: *A stepped care treatment model for depressed adolescents. Paper presentation at the Academy of Child and Adolescent Psychiatry Annual Meeting*; 2014 October 26; San Diego, California.

CHAPTER 6.2.4 ■ PARENT TRAINING

KAREN BEARSS, T. LINDSEY BURRELL, VALENTINA POSTORINO, AND LAWRENCE SCAHILL

INTRODUCTION

Child disruptive behaviors such as whining, crying, tantrums, aggression, and noncompliance are common concerns among parents. When these behaviors reach levels of clinical significance, children may qualify for *Diagnostic and Statistical Manual*—Fifth Edition (DSM-5) diagnoses of oppositional defiant disorder (ODD) and conduct disorder (CD) (childhood onset, adolescent onset, unspecified onset). ODD and CD fall under the category of disruptive behavior disorders (DBDs) and are broadly characterized by problems in behavioral and emotional self-control. When these challenging behaviors persist and impair functioning in the home, school, and community, intervention is warranted. With over half of all referrals to community child mental health clinics focused on oppositional or aggressive behaviors, DBDs are one of the most frequent treatment referrals (1,2). The prognosis for children with significant disruptive behavior problems is poor, with pervasive and unremitting aggression and conduct problems in childhood reliably predicting delinquent, aggressive, and risky behaviors in adolescence (3,4). Adults who exhibited conduct problems in childhood are more likely to have a range of psychiatric disorders and to engage in "life-course–persistent" antisocial behavior, including crime, drug abuse, domestic violence, and child abuse (5–7).

In child mental health services, parent training (PT), also referred to as "parent management training," describes a group of treatments that target disruptive and noncompliant behavior in children and adolescents. Parents are trained to implement specific procedures designed to improve parent–child interactions (8), decrease problematic behaviors, and increase prosocial behaviors (9) by (a) attending to the child's prosocial behaviors, (b) ignoring the child's inappropriate behaviors, (c) decreasing the use of punitive and coercive discipline strategies, and (d) increasing the use of effective, appropriate, *noncoercive* child management strategies to improve parent–child interactions.

PT sessions are structured and treatment is short term, averaging 10 to 12 weekly sessions. Programs vary to some degree in content presented (e.g., knowledge of typical child development, parental self-efficacy, communication skills, discipline or behavior management strategies) (10) and can be conducted in a variety of settings (home, community clinic) and formats (group, individual) (11–13). Delivery techniques used to engage parents and teach relevant content include didactics, modeling, role play, and live action coaching of techniques, and assignment of homework (10).

EVIDENCE-BASED PARENT TRAINING PROGRAMS

With over 40 years of controlled studies proving benefits in reducing disruptive behavior in youth from preschool to adolescence, PT is among the most well-established evidence-based treatments in child mental health (12,14). This body of evidence has influenced international dissemination of PT and prompted several clinical practice guidelines in the United States, United Kingdom, and elsewhere in an effort to raise standards of mental health care for youth (15,16).

Although the primary targets of PT include disruptive and noncompliant behavior, programs have also been shown to promote other positive outcomes such as improved parental warmth, decreased parental hostility, increased parental knowledge, and reduced parent stress (10,17). There also is evidence suggesting that parental self-efficacy and mental health problems, such as maternal depression, improve with PT (18–23). Finally, research on PT extends beyond efficacy trials to investigations of positive effects when delivered in "real-world" community clinic settings (14).

The largest body of evidence for PT supports application in children ages 3 to 12 years with disruptive behavior and average intelligence. There is growing evidence that PT can also be effective for targeted clinical populations (child maltreatment, postdivorce adjustment) (24–26) as well as other diagnostic conditions (separation anxiety) (27). Disruptive behavior is common in children with autism spectrum disorder (28,29). Emerging literature indicates that that PT is effective in this population (30).

THEORETICAL FOUNDATIONS OF PARENT TRAINING

The conceptual framework and theoretical underpinnings of most evidence-based PT programs for behavior problems are based on a combination of Diana Baumrind's work on parenting styles (31,32), Hanf's two-stage operant behavior model (33), Patterson's coercion model (21), and operant and social learning theory.

Baumrind (31,32) described three models of parental control: permissive, authoritarian, and authoritative. Permissive parenting involves acceptance of the child's behaviors and employs collaborative decision-making between the parent and child, while placing few demands and expectations on the child. Authoritarian parenting sets defined rules on child behavior, holds standards against which the child's behaviors are evaluated, and implements strategies to teach obedience. Finally, authoritative parenting directs the child's activities while allowing the child to provide input into decision-making (31,32). The authoritative parenting style also allows for nurturance between parent and child, while also setting appropriate limits on child behavior. PT is consistent with the combined and balanced parenting approach of authoritative parenting. It includes strategies explicitly designed to promote warmth between parent and child, but also defines boundaries and expectancies for child behavior.

Hanf's two-stage operant model provides the foundation to teach effective authoritative parenting, as described by Baumrind. The first stage involves the use of differential reinforcement (providing positive social attention and praise to appropriate prosocial behaviors while removing attention for inappropriate or disruptive behaviors) in order to build the relationship between the parent and child. The second stage promotes the use of direct commands followed by immediate consequences (e.g., time-out for noncompliance; praise for compliance). This model provides the foundation to Parent–Child Interaction Therapy (34) as well as other PT models described in this chapter (9,35,36).

Patterson's coercion model demonstrates the cycle that persists in the relationship between a parent and child that exacerbates the child's disruptive and defiant behavior (21). Patterson's model emphasizes the influence of the parent's behavior on the child and the impact of the child's behavior on the parent. In some families, parent–child relationships are characterized by aversive patterns of negative interactions (e.g., parent yells at the child and, in turn, the child whines or yells back at parents) and the tendency to handle problems in a coercive, negative manner (e.g., resorting to spanking as a discipline strategy). In addition to having negative interaction patterns, there are generally lower rates of positive parent–child interactions and children tend to model their parents' physical and verbally aggressive behaviors (e.g., yelling). A parent who is unsuccessful in using noncoercive parenting strategies, such as redirection when managing the child's behavior, frequently resorts to aversive control strategies, which sets up a pernicious pattern of parent–child interaction (37).

Understanding the development and maintenance of behavior problems has also been aided by social learning theory (38) and operant conditioning (39). Social learning theory describes the process in which people learn through direct experience, observation, and modeling. This framework provides insight into the way children may learn to engage in specific behaviors that they have observed. For example, a child may hit another child on the playground in order to gain access to a ball based on the observation that aggression was successful when used by another child. This process of observing and imitating a model also occurs in the family. Rather than implying that the child or the parent is independently responsible for the child's maladaptive behavior, social learning theory directs attention to the interactions between family members as a source of child behavior difficulties.

A child may initially engage in disruptive behavior through observation and imitation of others. Whether or not the child *continues* to engage in that behavior can be explained through principles of operant conditioning. The organizing principle of operant conditioning is that a behavior can be modified (increased or decreased) through the manipulation of its antecedents and/or consequences. An antecedent is the stimulus that cues an organism to perform a behavior. When an organism perceives an antecedent stimulus, it behaves in a way that is designed to maximize the reinforcing consequences and minimize punishing consequences. A consequence is the event that immediately follows the behavior. The consequences of reinforcement and punishment are the core tools through which operant behavior is modified. Positive reinforcement (e.g., providing praise for cleaning up toys) and negative reinforcement (e.g., taking an aspirin to "remove" a headache) increase the probability of a behavior. By contrast, positive punishment (e.g., scolding for not following directions) and negative punishment (e.g., removing a favorite toy for hitting) reduce the probability of a behavior that it follows.

Operant conditioning is a core component of applied behavior analysis (ABA), which is classically defined as the systematic application of interventions based upon the principles of learning theory. The aim of ABA is to promote socially appropriate behavior, reduce maladaptive behavior, and demonstrate that the interventions employed are responsible for the improvement in behavior (40). ABA formulates that, by understanding a behavior's antecedents and consequences, one can determine its purpose, or *function*. Common functions of disruptive behavior include access to a tangible item (food or a favorite toy), attention from others (positive reinforcement), escape from a demand or an aversive stimuli (negative reinforcement), or sensory or other internal stimulation (automatic reinforcement) (41). By understanding the function of the behavior problem, parents learn to change their usual response in order to teach the child a more appropriate behavior (42). For example, a child may learn that a tantrum will result in escape from a routine demand (e.g., household chore). In such a case, the parent can be taught to (1) ensure the child is not allowed to escape from the routine demands, and (2) implement strategies to promote compliance (e.g., a reward for completing chores).

COMPONENTS OF PARENT TRAINING

Clinicians can now choose from one of several well-established, structured PT programs, including Webster–Stratton's Incredible Years (36), Kazdin's Parent Training (9), Sanders' Triple P-Positive Parenting Program (43), and Eyberg's Parent–Child Interaction Therapy (34) (see Table 6.2.4.1 for key features of commercially available evidence-based PT programs). Although there is variability across these programs in the targeted age range and use of particular behavioral management strategies, common components include *Assessment, Psychoeducation, Prevention Strategies, Consequences, Generalization, and Maintenance.*

Assessment

As with any intervention, treatment should be initiated after completion of an assessment that provides an understanding of the child, family, and broader systems in which the child operates. Multimodal (parent, teacher, other caregiver), multimethod (interview, observation, rating scales) assessment will provide the widest range of information that can be used in treatment planning (95). Information gathered from multiple informants is preferred, as perspectives between parents as well as parents and teachers are often divergent (96,97).

Child and Family History

Information about the child should include collation of the child's development, including prenatal/postnatal complications, medical conditions that may affect the child's development or family functioning, as well as educational history, including special educational services. This information provides a foundation for guiding the family on the application of PT strategies. For example, compliance to commands is clearly tied to the child's receptive language (RL), with an RL threshold of 12 to 18 months required for the child to understand simple, one-step commands. Thus, if a child is identified as having notable developmental delays, family expectations regarding the child's ability to understand and comply with commands will need to be adjusted.

Family history, including psychiatric conditions in immediate and extended family, as well as current medical conditions in family members that may affect caregiving should be evaluated. Individuals involved in caregiving and the network of caregiving (mother, father, extended family members, other caregivers) will inform the family support structure and *who should be included* in treatment planning and implementation. For example, it may not be effective if the parent attending PT is not the primary caregiver for the child. Knowledge of the family structure may also help identify barriers to the application of PT strategies. For example, although the mother may be the primary caregiver, she may be unable to attend sessions due to her work schedule. In such a case, the best option may be to suggest that the grandmother attends the PT sessions. This arrangement could work if the grandmother is able and willing to relay information and implementation plans to the primary caregiver. This solution follows from the principle that, whenever possible, it is strongly preferred that the same caregiver attends each session to ensure continuity.

Current Parenting Practices

Assess the use of current parenting practices, including parental perception of strategies that work versus the strategies that do not work. This will identify what approaches will be new to the parent versus those that may be part of the parent's repertoire. Even techniques that are in a parent's repertoire, however, may need modification. For example, many parents report they have tried time out and are convinced that it does not work. In many instances, however, parents misapply time out (e.g., ending the time out while the child is still upset; conducting time out in front of the television; using time out for an escape-maintained behavior). Effective PT involves educating parents about the use of new techniques and correcting ineffective application of particular strategies.

A focus of the assessment also should be on general parenting perspectives: Is the parent overly harsh (oriented to the authoritarian parenting approach, with an emphasis on punitive discipline strategies) or permissive (appropriate warmth in the parent–child relationship, but ineffective limit-setting and inadequate follow-through with consequences). It may also be informative to discuss the parental understanding of what is "driving" the child's behavioral problems. This discussion may delve into parental perceptions on locus of control (LOC), which is the degree to which the parent feels he or she has the ability to influence the child's behavior and development. Parents with an *internal* LOC acknowledge their impact on the child's behavior. Prior to initiating treatment, these parents may recognize their role in the child's behavior (e.g., "I know I don't follow through"). Conversely, a parent with an *external* LOC may attribute the child's behavior to environmental or biologic factors, with the implication that the parent has little influence on the child's behavior. Research suggests that an internal LOC is associated with higher maternal esteem, parental satisfaction, and fewer child behavioral problems (98–100). Implementation of PT strategies may be especially challenging with parents who describe feeling like the child's behaviors is due to external circumstances (e.g., "he was born that way," "he's just like his father," "it doesn't matter what I do, nothing works"). By contrast, parents who feel responsible, but *at a loss* on how to manage their child's behavior, may be more open and motivated to learn and implement PT techniques.

Topography Target Behaviors

Identification of target behaviors and function of those behaviors can occur through informal discussion with the family, parent ratings, and behavioral observations. Initial discussion should include delineation of the target behaviors that the parent hopes to address in treatment. The parent should be guided to describe the problems in behavioral terms: frequency of occurrence, duration, amplitude, actual appearance of the behavior, immediate aftermath, and impact on

TABLE 6.2.4.1

EVIDENCE-BASED PARENT TRAINING PROGRAMS FOR DISRUPTIVE BEHAVIOR

Program	Format	Target Age	Key Components	Clinical Populations
Defiant Children (DC) (35,44–48)	Individual: Ten 1-hr sessions Group (6–10 families): Ten 2–2.5 hr sessions	2–12	*10-Step Program:* *Step 1*—Why children misbehave *Step 2*—Attending to appropriate behaviors *Step 3*—Increasing compliance and independent play *Step 4*—Implementing sticker and point charts *Steps 5 and 6*—Time out *Step 7*—Targeting behavior in public places *Step 8*—Targeting school behaviors *Step 9*—Handling future problems *Step 10*—Booster session Strategies: psychoeducation, positive attention, positive reinforcement, planned ignoring, compliance training, token economy systems, time out, generalization, and maintenance	• ODD • CD • ADHD • ASD • Juvenile-onset BD • Aggressive behavior • Mild ID • Tourette syndrome • Postdivorce adjustment
Helping the Noncompliant Child (HNC) (49–53)	Individual: Eight to ten 60-90 min sessions	3–8	*Differential Attention (Phase I):* • Promote positive parent–child relationship • Increase social attention • Ignore minor inappropriate behaviors *Compliance Training (Phase II)*: • Use direct, concise instructions • Set appropriate consequences for noncompliance • Establish "standing rules" • Implement techniques outside the home Strategies: positive attention, positive reinforcement, planned ignoring, compliance training, time out, generalization, and maintenance	• ODD • ADHD
Incredible Years (IYS) (36,54–65)	*IYS for Parents:* Groups of 8–12 parents BASIC: • Baby: 9–12 sessions • Toddler: 12 sessions • Preschool: 18–20 sessions • School-Age: 12–16+ sessions ADVANCED: 9–12 sessions SCHOOL READINESS (adjunct to Preschool): 4–6 sessions *IYS for Teachers*: Groups of 12–14 teachers *IYS for Children*: Groups of 5–6 children; 18–22 sessions	Baby/Toddler: 0–2.5 Preschool: 3–5 School Age: 6–12 Teacher: 3–8 Classroom: 3–8 Small Group: 4–8	*IYS for Parents:* BASIC • Enhance positive interactions • Establish proactive discipline ADVANCED • Enhance effective communication • Manage anger and depression • Promote problem solving • Support networks/teacher partnerships *IYS for Teachers*: • Establish proactive discipline • Promote positive teacher–student relationships • Promote social skills and emotional regulation • Promote positive teacher–parent partnerships *IYS for Children*: • Increase emotional, social and academic competencies Strategies: psychoeducation, prevention, positive attention, reinforcement, planned ignoring, compliance training, house rules, time out, token economy	• ODD • ADHD • CD • At risk for CD, delinquency and substance abuse • Aggressive behavior • Anxiety disorders • Depression • High-risk populations (low income, abuse/neglect) • Risk reduction (abuse/neglect) • Foster parents • Postdivorce adjustment • ASD

TABLE 6.2.4.1

(CONTINUED)

Program	Format	Target Age	Key Components	Clinical Populations
Parent–Child Interaction Therapy (PCIT) (25,27,34,66–80)	Individual: Twelve to fourteen 60–90 min sessions Group: 3–6 families Sixteen 1.5–2 hr sessions	2–8	*Phase 1 (Child-Directed Interaction):* • Improve the quality of the parent–child relationship • Use the PRIDE Skills during "special time": Praise, Reflection, Imitation, Behavioral Description, Enjoyment *Phase 2 (Parent-Directed Interaction):* • Establish a structured and consistent approach to discipline Strategies: positive attention, planned ignoring, compliance training, time out, generalization and maintenance	• ODD • CD • ADHD • Posttrauma • Risk reduction (abuse/neglect) • Separation anxiety • Depression • SIB • Postdivorce adjustment • ASD
Parent Management Training (PMT) (9,81–85)	Individual: Twelve to sixteen 45–60 min sessions	2–14	*Four components:* 1. Conceptualize how to change social, emotional and behavioral problems 2. Implement techniques that follow from that conceptual view 3. Develop parent skill through active methods of training 4. Integrate assessment in treatment decision-making Strategies: psychoeducation, positive reinforcement, compliance training, time out, planned ignoring, token economy	• ODD • CD • ADHD • TS • Aggression • ASD • ID • LD
The Community Parent Education Program (COPE) (86–88)	15–25 families Six to eight 2-hr sessions	3–18	• Encourage positive behavior and improving parent–child relationships (positive reinforcement) • Balance family relationships • Avoid conflicts • Manage transitions • Increase compliance • Improve self-regulation • Decrease antisocial behavior • Advanced strategies: set up point systems • Coordinate child management plans Strategies: positive reinforcement, planned ignoring, time out, token economy, compliance training, generalization and maintenance	• ODD • ADHD
Triple P-Positive Parenting Program (24,43,89–94)	5 levels of intervention: *Level 1 (Universal):* Population-based informational media campaign *Level 2:* Individual: One to two 20 min sessions Group: 3, 90-min seminars *Level 3 (Primary Care):* Children with specific, mild to moderate behavioral issues	2–16	*Five core positive parenting principles:* 1. Ensure a safe, engaging environment 2. Create a positive learning environment 3. Use assertive discipline 4. Have realistic expectations 5. Take care of oneself as a parent Strategies: positive attention, behavioral contingencies, token economy, compliance training, planned ignoring, time out	• ODD • ADHD • CD • High-risk populations (low income, maternal depression, relationship conflict, single parent) • Risk reduction (child abuse/neglect) • ASD

(continued)

TABLE 6.2.4.1

(CONTINUED)

Program	Format	Target Age	Key Components	Clinical Populations
	Level 4 (Standard): High-risk children Individual: Ten 1 hr sessions Group-: Five 2-hr sessions with 10–12 families Self-directed: 10 sessions *Level 5, Enhanced:* children with complex behavioral issues and concurrent family issues			

ADHD, attention-deficit hyperactivity disorder; ASD, autism spectrum disorder; BD, bipolar disorder; CD, conduct disorder; ID, intellectual disability; LD, learning disability; ODD, oppositional defiant disorder; SIB, self-injurious behavior; TS, Tourette syndrome.

the family. These descriptions of behaviors promote a common understanding of the child's target problems and provide useful information on severity. For example, tantrums that occur one to two times a week lasting 5 minutes would be less severe than four to five tantrums per day each lasting 30 minutes. Tantrums that involve throwing objects, property destruction, or self-injurious behavior would be more severe than tantrums characterized by yelling and screaming. Parents may describe feeling on "pins and needles" in the immediate aftermath—apprehensive that the child may "go off again." Frequent and severe tantrums in a child may lead to reluctance to set limits in an effort to avoid future outbursts.

Finally, discussion of where and with whom the behavioral problems occur can be informative when planning treatment. The presence or absence of behaviors in specific settings or with particular people also can inform whether PT is the appropriate course of treatment. For example, treatment may be difficult with a parent who reports that behavioral problems are only present at school. If this an accurate report, it may be that the teacher needs guidance on behavior management. In some cases, disruptive behaviors are occurring both at school *and* home, but the parent may be underreporting and perhaps has become tolerant of the child's behavior. In such cases, parents may need help to recalibrate appropriate behavior before initiating PT. Particularly challenging cases involve parents who underreport problem behavior in the home and have little motivation to modify his or her parenting approach. A positive indicator for PT is when a parent reports behavioral problems in the home that are less prominent at school. This suggests that the child has some ability to regulate behavior at school and may prompt the parent to seek help in managing the child's behavior.

Assessment Methods

Behavioral Observation

Direct observations by parents, teachers, and clinicians permit prospective data collection rather than reliance on recall of past events. Standardized observational approaches have been developed to examine the child's behavior and child–caregiver response in semi-structured parent–child interaction-scenarios. For example, the Dyadic Parent–Child Interaction Coding System uses a structured, 15-minute observation with three conditions: child-led play; parent-led play; clean up to ascertain rates of noncompliance, parent use of inappropriate discipline strategies, as well as the general parent–child interactional style (e.g., disengaged, overly directive or harsh, passive with limit-setting, and level of warmth) (101).

Following an ABA framework, observation of child behavior also may take the form of a functional analysis or descriptive functional assessment (102). Functional analysis involves direct observation and manipulation of environmental events that precede (antecedents) and follow (consequences) the behavior of interest in the clinical setting in order to determine the function maintaining the behavior (103). Thus, functional analysis identifies the purpose of the disruptive behavior in a controlled setting. However, this approach requires specialized training, is time consuming, and the experimental conditions may not completely mimic naturalistic settings (102). For these reasons, functional analysis is not common in clinical practice (104).

Descriptive functional assessment uses caregiver report and observation in naturalistic settings (e.g., classroom or home) to determine the purpose or function of the behavior and the environmental response that is maintaining the behavior. In so far as this method relies on information from the natural environment, caregivers can be taught to record observations and contribute to the interpretation of findings and development of specific strategies (105,106). Descriptive functional assessment is less expensive and time consuming than formal functional analysis and thus is easier to utilize in clinical practice (107,108). To date, however, descriptive functional assessment has not been carefully studied. Indeed, systematic reviews have identified only a few studies, and interventions based on this assessment method may be less successful than those based on functional analysis (109).

Informant-Based Methods

The Child Behavior Checklist (CBCL) is a well-established, reliable, and valid parent rating covering a wide range of internalizing and externalizing behaviors. There are two versions of the CBCL: The preschool checklist (CBCL/1½–5) contains 100 questions for children aged 18 months to 5 years, and the school-age version (CBCL/6–18), which contains 120 questions for youth aged 6 to 18 years. There are also CBCL versions for teachers, daycare providers, and a youth self-report (110,111). Responses are recorded on a Likert scale: 0 = Not True, 1 = Somewhat/Sometimes True, 2 = Very True/Often True. Items are summed to produce subscale and syndrome scores, internalizing and externalizing problem scales, as well as a total score derived from all questions. Each syndrome, problem scale, and the total score yields a T score (population mean of 50 and a standard deviation of 10). Scores of 65 or greater on a given scale are considered clinically significant.

The 36-item, parent-rated Eyberg Child Behavior Inventory (112) (ECBI), and the 38-item, teacher-rated Sutter–Eyberg Student Behavior Inventory (113) (SESBI), focus on disruptive behavior problems. The SESBI contains two factors—oppositional behaviors and attention problems—that may be used to track these behavior categories in the classroom.

The Behavioral Assessment System for Children (114) (BASC) is a multi-method, multidimensional approach to evaluating behavior and self-perception of children ages 2 years 6 months to 18 years. It includes teacher (TRS) and parent (PRS) rating scales, a self-report of personality (SRP), a structured developmental history (SDH), and a student observation system (SOS). The PRS is used to measure both adaptive behavior and behavior problems in the community and home setting. Parents or caregivers can complete forms at three age levels—preschool (ages 2 to 5), child (ages 6 to 11), and adolescent (ages 12 to 21). The PRS contains 134 to 160 items and uses a four-point scale ranging from "Never" to "Almost Always." The TRS measures adaptive behavior and behavior problems in the preschool or school setting. Teachers can complete the 100 to 139 items depending on age level (preschool [ages 2 to 5], child [ages 6 to 11], and adolescent [ages 12 to 21]).

The Disruptive Behavior Rating Scale–Parent Version (115) (DBRS-PV) is a brief (26-item) rating scale used to assess inattention, hyperactivity–impulsivity, and oppositional defiant behavior among school-aged children. The DBRS is an expanded version of the Attention-Deficit Hyperactivity Disorder (ADHD) Rating Scale–IV (116) (ADHD-IV). Parents rate how often symptoms occurred in the past 6 months using a four-point Likert scale. The DBRS-PV also has sections assessing the degree to which the symptoms impair the child.

The Swanson, Nolan, and Pelham-IV (SNAP-IV) is a 90-item parent- or teacher-report designed to measure behavior problems in children for children 5 to 18 years (117). The first 46 items cover symptoms of ADHD, ODD, and CD.

Psychoeducation on the Principles of PT

Treatment can begin once a family has been deemed appropriate for PT: the child exhibits target disruptive behaviors, a caregiver can consistently attend weekly clinic appointments and is ideally motivated and open to modifying his or her parenting approach. As parents often describe the child's disruptive behavior as "coming out of nowhere," PT often begins with psychoeducation on the reasons why problem behaviors occur.

Why Children Misbehave

Russell Barkley's manual, *Defiant Children* (35), presents four major factors that contribute to the child's misbehavior: (a) *child psychological characteristics* (e.g., child temperament) and *developmental challenges*; (b) *parental characteristics* (i.e., mental, physical health); (c) *situational consequences* that, over time, teach the child that disruptive behavior allows escape from undesirable tasks; and (d) *family stressors* (financial, marital difficulties). Individually and collectively these factors may increase the likelihood of parent–child conflict and hinder the parent's ability to manage the child's behavior.

Young children may have difficulty communicating everyday concerns, wants, and needs. This is clear for children with developmental delays. Even children who do not have developmental delays may have difficulty "using their words" when frustrated or angry. Disruptive behaviors, such as temper outbursts, become inappropriate, but ironically effective ways for the child to communicate needs and demands. Many PT programs encourage parents to consider what the child maybe trying to communicate through the disruptive behavior. A tantrum could be saying "This is too hard." Screaming could mean "Leave me alone." Hitting could be communicating "That's mine. Give it back."

ABA begins with the assertion that the child's disruptive behavior is not a random occurrence. Parents may be eloquent in their description of the child's behavioral problems, but less able to describe the events and situations that increase the likelihood of the behavior. Faced with the occurrence of behavioral problems that they do not understand, parents may inadvertently respond in ways that reinforce the child's misbehavior. The Antecedent–Behavior–Consequence (ABC) model breaks down the sequence to identify the environmental circumstances that may provoke the behavior (antecedents) and the parental responses that maintain the behavior (consequences). This, in turn, facilitates a better understanding of how to then manipulate the environment by modifying the antecedents that trigger and consequences that maintain a behavior.

Education on Child Development

In PT, parents are encouraged to consider the child's development and to keep expectations in accordance with the child's abilities. Behavioral difficulties may emerge if a parent holds unrealistic expectations about the child's skill level. For example, a child with impaired receptive language skills would affect the child's understanding of verbal commands and predictably reduce compliance if commands are too complex. Conversely, parents may have lowered expectations about a child's abilities and refrain from placing appropriate demands on the child. Although lower demands on the child may reduce noncompliance, lower demands may also interfere with the acquisition of new skills and the regular performance of current skills. Thus, effective PT finds a balance between increasing parental demands or expectations for the child at a pace that fits with the child's development.

Effective Communication

Parents can avert some behavioral problems by using clear language to convey expectancies and consequences to the child. The goal is to move from vague threats or promises (e.g., "You need to behave and listen or you'll be in trouble."), which may confuse the child, to clear contingencies (e.g., "You need to put your toys away before you can go play outside"). Clarity in verbal direction reduces the likelihood of misunderstanding about expectations and the consequences if the child does not comply. An important principle here is to establish the behavioral expectancy before the behavior occurs and not in response to it.

Consistency and Predictability in Behavioral Management

A final treatment consideration to impart to parents early in PT is the importance of consistent implementation of behavior management strategies. Inconsistency aligns with the behavioral principle of "intermittent reinforcement," in which the behavior is reinforced some—but not all the time. Intermittent reinforcement increases the occurrence of the behavior and teaches the child that the persistence of the challenging behavior will eventually be reinforced. Consistency is not always easy, but it is important. In order for any behavioral management strategy to be effective—following through to completion is key to making it work. In time, the child learns that having a tantrum will no longer result in escape from a routine expectation or that screaming will not work to get the parent's attention. This predictability in parental response sets the stage for a new behavioral expectation.

Prevention Strategies

Prevention (or antecedent management) strategies are designed to avert the occurrence of behavioral problems by modifying the antecedents or triggers of the behavior problems. Parents commonly use prevention strategies for young children, such as putting a baby gate on a staircase to prevent the child from falling down the stairs or putting locks on cabinet doors to block access to household cleaners.

Prevention strategies call on parents to think ahead in order to identify a predictable behavioral sequence (e.g., when told "no" [antecedent], the child has a tantrum). Once the pattern is identified, the parent can implement a strategy to eliminate or modify the antecedent of that behavior. Common antecedent management strategies include the following:

Controlling the Environment

For safety concerns, a parent might place locks on drawers or cabinets that hold dangerous chemicals. To minimize property destruction, a parent may place breakable items from reach. Valuable items may be put in a safe location. To prevent the onset of disruptive behavior, a parent might put certain items "out of sight" (e.g., cookies, a certain toy prone to cause fights between siblings). These environmental controls decrease the likelihood of the child engaging in potentially harmful, dangerous, or disruptive behaviors.

Creating Daily Structure and Routines

Increasing predictability in the child's daily routine (e.g., getting ready in the morning, bedtime routine) can avoid instances in which the child might protest in response to a new demand or transition from a preferred to a nonpreferred activity.

Providing Choices

This can be an effective replacement for saying "no" in everyday situations that trigger misbehavior in the child. Choices create the illusion that the child is in control of decision-making, but the choices are defined by the parent. For example, instead of telling a child "No, you cannot have ice cream for breakfast," the parent can provide the choice "Would you like eggs or cereal for breakfast."

Consequences

PT also includes several consequence-based techniques, including positive social attention, planned ignoring, differential reinforcement, behavioral contingencies, token economy systems, compliance training, and time out.

Positive Social Attention

The goal of positive social attention is to reverse the negative (and cyclical) parent–child interaction described by Patterson (21). This involves an increase in parental awareness and acknowledgment of the child's appropriate behaviors. Specific positive social attention strategies include the use of praise, "catching the child being good," and engaging in child-led play.

Praise involves overt verbal expression to the child following the performance of positive behaviors. Although common praises include "great job," "way to go," or "nice job," parents should also be encouraged to label exactly what the child is doing well (e.g., "Great job putting the dish in the sink"). The use of labeled praise can be especially powerful to highlight "positive opposite" situations. For example, if a child frequently hits his sibling, praise would be used to label moments when the child keeps his hands to himself. If loud screaming in the home is a problem, a parent would be encouraged to praise the positive opposite behavior "thank you for using an inside voice."

Catching a child being good is another example of using labeled praise to point out the moments that the child is engaging in appropriate behavior. A parent may target specific times of the day (e.g., the morning routine) or certain behaviors (e.g., sharing toys with a sibling; compliance to commands) that have been challenging. Parents can also be encouraged to identify and declare, through the use of praise, instances when the child is engaging in appropriate behavior.

In order to promote positive parent–child interactions, the parent is encouraged to follow the child's lead in a brief 5- to 15-minute "child-led play" session. In addition to letting the child lead the play, the parent is reminded to avoid giving commands, asking questions, or setting limits, which take the lead away from the child and set up potential conflicts. Parents should take every opportunity to provide positive attention to the child by describing the child's activities, praising appropriate play, and reflecting appropriate child vocalizations. This play situation is a staple for many PT programs (PCIT, Barkley's Defiant Children). Selected activities depend on the age and interest of the child but may include puzzles, play doh, legos, and arts and crafts.

Planned Ignoring

The partner to providing positive social attention to the child is deliberate ignoring of inappropriate behaviors. Common targets for planned ignoring are socially maintained (attention-seeking) behaviors such as tantrums and whining. Planned ignoring requires complete disengagement (silently turning away, no eye contact or directed affect, no language directed toward the child) until the behavior subsides. When the behavior stops, the parent re-engages with the child. Planned ignoring is best applied when the child's behavior is not dangerous to the child, to others, or to property. Behaviors involving aggression, self-injury, or property destruction are more difficult to ignore and may require the parent to intervene in order to reduce harm. A challenge with the implementation of planned ignoring is the child's behavior often escalates to include behaviors that cannot easily be ignored before it eventually decreases. Parents often need guidance on how to handle situations in which the child engages in potentially dangerous or destructive behaviors. For example, if a child who is being ignored by his parents begins to throw objects, the parent may be coached to continue the use of planned ignoring while physically redirecting the child to a different room. Otherwise, parental anxiety about the child's increasingly provocative behaviors may lead some parents to attend to the child and inadvertently reinforce the behavior.

Differential Reinforcement

This approach combines positive social reinforcement and planned ignoring in order to show that positive parental attention will be received only when the child engages in appropriate behavior. Negative behaviors will no longer receive attention (via the use of planned ignoring). For example, a child who initially makes a request (e.g., for a favorite toy or snack) but does so in a demanding manner would be ignored by the parent until the child's negative behavior subsides. Only when the child asks for the item in an appropriate manner would the parent attend and respond to the child. To bolster this concept, the parent can also praise other instances that the child spontaneously requests items in an appropriate way (e.g., "I like how you asked for the snack in a nice way. I would be happy to give it to you.").

Behavioral Contingencies

Sometimes referred to as "behavioral contracts," behavioral contingencies are designed to create clear expectations for the child about a target behavior and its consequences. A common format for a behavioral contingency is "If/First___Then___" statements. This involves a counterbalance of a specific demand or behavior with a reinforcer ("if you finish your dinner, then you can have ice cream"), natural positive consequence ("first you put your coat on, then you can go outside"), or punishment ("if you hit your sister, then you will go to time out").

Another version of a behavioral contingency is the implementation of a "house rule." This involves explicitly stating that a particular behavior (e.g., hitting a sibling) will be met with a predetermined consequence (e.g., time out or loss of a privilege). Strengths of behavioral contingencies and house rules are two-fold. First, they provide a clear understanding to the child about what behavior is being targeted and what the consequence will be for engaging in that behavior. Second, they establish the rules "ahead of time"—which avoids bickering over what the child may perceive is an arbitrary consequence. This sets up an opportunity for the child to contemplate whether or not to engage in a target behavior because, assuming the parent follows through, the child knows what the ramifications will be.

Token Economy Systems

An expanded version of a behavioral contingency is a token economy system, often implemented as a point or a sticker chart. The child earns points or stickers for engaging in targeted behaviors. Points are accumulated and then can be exchanged for preferred items (access to a favorite toy or preferred activity). Weekly allowance follows this principle, in that a child is required to complete a set number of chores in order to earn a predetermined amount of money. Token economy systems provide an opportunity for the parent and child to work collaboratively to define the target behaviors as well as the desired rewards to be exchanged for the tokens. This collaborative effort promotes compromise between parent and child and fosters engagement on the child's part.

Compliance Training

Teaching children how to comply with commands the first time given starts by teaching a parent how to deliver an effective command: one that is direct, simple, one step, and given only one time. The goal is to establish for the child the importance of immediate compliance with a command to decrease occurrences of escape from the demand. These steps avoid common errors such as repeating a command multiple times before having the child comply, providing a command that is too complex (e.g., multistep), and giving vague instructions or indicating that compliance is optional, such as giving a command with statements such as, "Would you mind...?" "How about you...," or "Let's do...." Once an effective command is given, parents are taught to follow through, in some cases with the use of physical prompting or guidance, to ensure the child completes the demand. Parents are also coached to provide immediate praise as the child completes the command.

Time Out

Time out is a form of planned ignoring where the child is removed from all reinforcing stimuli. Time out can be a very effective approach to targeting challenging, persistent behaviors. Unfortunately, parents often make errors in implementation that render the strategy ineffective. An important component to the effective use of time out includes restricting its use to one or two target behaviors at a time. This helps promote predictability for the child in terms of which behaviors will result in a time out. As time out is more formally known as "time out from reinforcement," parents also must ensure that time out is located in a safe, distraction-free area—not on the couch in front of the television or in the bedroom where the child has free access to toys. In addition, the parent deliberately ignores the child during the time out, thus minimizing the amount of attention (positive or negative) that the child receives while in time out. Parents should choose a predetermined minimum amount of time that the child is to stay in time out. Once the predetermined amount of time has passed and the child is seated quietly (and for the child who is in time out for noncompliance, is willing to complete the command), the time out is over. This sequence avoids the problem of the child "completing" the predetermined time (e.g., 5 minutes) while the child is still very agitated, and thus likely to re-engage in the disruptive behavior. A final challenge involves situations where the child is unwilling to stay in time out. PT programs vary on how this issue is addressed such as using a backup time-out room or removal of a predetermined privilege if the child refuses to sit or stay in time out.

A Note on Spanking

Parents may report some success with physical punishment as a way to stop problematic behavior. There is evidence, however, that spanking is ineffective for reducing disruptive behavior. In fact, physical punishment can lead to increased aggression, antisocial behavior, and physical injury (118). For parents who use spanking as a discipline strategy, a nonjudgmental discussion on alternative approaches along with psychoeducation on the potential ramifications of physical punishment is warranted.

Generalization and Maintenance

A final component of many PT programs considers the strategies needed to promote skill generalization to other contexts and to maintain treatment gains over time. The goal of generalization is to increase the likelihood that positive behavior change extends into different settings and contexts that may not have been initially covered in the PT program. Many parents need preparation on how to apply PT strategies in new situations when conditions vary. For example, although a primary target of treatment may be to improve compliance at home, improvements in compliance in public places, at school, and at family events is also important. Thus behavioral generalization involves the transfer of positive behavior change to situations other than the ones initially targeted in the PT program. Maintenance means that positive behavioral changes will continue even after the end of active treatment.

IMPLEMENTING PARENT TRAINING IN CLINICAL SETTINGS

Although evidence for the efficacy of PT abounds, meta-analytic studies examining moderators to treatment suggest certain clinical subpopulations are less likely to show positive response to treatment. Poor treatment response has been found to be related to low family income and, to a lesser degree, related to low parental education/occupational status and maternal psychopathology (119,120). Other potential moderators, of modest effect, involve including the child in treatment and providing treatment in an individual (vs. group) format (13,121). PT components associated with positive response include in vivo practice with the parent's own child, teaching skills related to emotional communication (e.g., active listening, reducing negative communication), teaching parents to interact positively with their children, and an emphasis on consistent discipline (10).

When initiating PT, parents may initially struggle to understand why they are being asked to attend treatment when their child has the behavioral problems. Indeed, some clinicians may raise the same question. Some parents may also silently wonder if their need for PT implies that the child's behavior is the parent's fault. It is often useful to address these concerns up front. For example, it can be noted that children with prominent disruptive behavior require the application of specific parenting techniques that most other children do not require. The easiest contrast is if the family has multiple children—and how similar parenting strategies may work with one child, but not another. Therapists should also reinforce the notion that, because parents are on the "front line" dealing with the child's behavioral problems, they are attending treatment in order to become the agent of change for the child's behavior. A positive rephrasing of this principle is that the therapist is providing the parent with the skills to change the child's behavior. Finally, teaching parents strategies to manage child behaviors increases opportunities for the parent to implement the intervention strategies across multiple settings (e.g., home, the grocery store, the playground) and contexts (e.g., morning routine, homework, mealtimes, bedtime) and to use the tools learned in treatment to address future behavioral problems. This discussion is all about the delicate balance of engaging the parent in the treatment while at the same time avoiding the suggestion that the parent is to blame for the child's disruptive behaviors.

PT involves teaching behavior management strategies that have been proven to reduce disruptive, noncompliant behaviors in children across a wide age range. The programs listed in Table 6.2.4.1 have solid empirical support. Applying a treatment manual into clinical practice, however, can be challenging. Successful implementation occurs when treatment systematically introduces parents to a range of techniques designed to shift the balance of negative parent–child interactions to positive. Although each program in Table 6.2.4.1 includes a range of strategies that have been effective, not every strategy fits with every child and parent. When it comes to specific PT techniques, what works for one parent and child dyad may not work for another. The goal is to tailor each of the strategies to fit the child and family and to equip the parent with the tools that will work for their family circumstances.

References

1. Handwerk M, Field C, Dahl A, Malmberg J: Conduct, oppositional defiant, and disruptive behavior disorders. In: Sturmey P, Hersen M (eds): *Handbook of Evidence-Based Practice in Clinical Psychology. Vol. 1: Child and Adolescent Disorders.* Hoboken, NJ, John Wiley & Sons, 267–301, 2012.
2. Patterson GR, Dishion TJ, Chamberlain P: Outcomes and methodological issues relating to treatment of antisocial children. In: Giles TR (ed): *Handbook of Effective Psychotherapy.* New York, Plenum Press, 43–88, 1993.
3. Broidy LM, Nagin DS, Tremblay RE, et al.: Developmental trajectories of childhood disruptive behaviors and adolescent delinquency: a six-site, cross-national study. *Dev Psychol* 39:222–245, 2003.
4. Fergusson DM, Horwood LJ, Lynskey M: The childhoods of multiple problem adolescents: 15 year longitudinal study. *J Child Psychol Psychiatry* 35:1123–1140, 1994.
5. Champion LA, Goodall G, Rutter M: Behavioral problems in childhood and stressors in early adult life: a 20 year follow-up of London school children. *Psychol Med* 25:231–246, 1995.
6. Moffit TE, Caspi A, Dickson N, et al.: Childhood-onset versus adolescent-onset antisocial conduct problems in males: natural history from ages 3 to 18 years. *Dev Psychopathol* 8:388–424, 1996.
7. Rutter M: Connections between child and adult psychopathology. *Eur Child Adolesc Psychiatry* 5:4–7, 1996.
8. Wierson M, Forehand R: Parent behavioral training for child noncompliance: rationale, concepts, and effectiveness. *Curr Dir Psychol Sci* 3:146–150, 1994.
9. Kazdin AE: *Parent Management Training: Treatment for Oppositional, Aggressive, and Antisocial Behavior in Children and Adolescents.* New York, NY, Oxford University Press, 2005.
10. Kaminski JW, Valle LA, Filene JH, Boyle CL: A meta-analytic review of components associated with parent training program effectiveness. *J Abnorm Child Psychol* 36:567–589, 2008.
11. Barlow J, Stewart-Brown S: Behavior problem and group-based parent education programs. *J Dev Behav Pediatr* 21:356–370, 2000.
12. Dretzke J, Davenport C, Frew E, et al.: The clinical effectiveness of different parenting programs for children with conduct problems: a systematic review of randomized controlled trials. *Child Adolesc Psychiatry Ment Health* 3:7, 2009.
13. Kumpfer KL, Alvarado R: Family strengthening approaches for the prevention of youth problem behaviors. *Am Psychol* 58:457–465, 2003.
14. Michelson D, Davenport C, Dretzke J, et al.: Do evidence-based interventions work when tested in the "real world?" A systematic review and meta-analysis of parent management training for the treatment of child disruptive behavior. *Clin Child Fam Psychol Rev* 16:18–34, 2013.
15. American Academy of Child and Adolescent Psychiatry: Practice parameter for the assessment and treatment of children and adolescents with oppositional defiant disorder. *J Am Acad Child Adolesc Psychiatry* 46:126–141, 2007.
16. NICE: *Parent-Training/Education Programs in the Management of Children with Conduct Disorders.* London, National Institute for Clinical Excellence, 2006.
17. Thomas R, Zimmer-Gembeck MJ: Behavioral outcomes of parent-child interaction therapy and Triple-P-Positive Parenting Program: a review and meta-analysis. *J Abnorm Child Psychol* 35:475–495, 2007.
18. DeGarmo DS, Patterson GR, Forgatch MS: How do outcomes in a specified parent training intervention maintain or wane over time? *Prev Sci* 5:73–89, 2004.
19. Hutchings J, Bywater T, Williams ME, et al.: Improvements in parental depression as a mediator of child behaviour change. *Psychology* 13:795–801, 2012.
20. McCart MR, Priester PE, Davies WH, Azen R: Differential effectiveness of behavioral parent-training and cognitive-behavioral therapy for antisocial youth: a meta-analysis. *J Abnorm Child Psychol* 34:527–543, 2006.
21. Patterson GR: *Coercive Family Processes.* Eugene, OR, Castalia, 1982.
22. Serketich WJ, Dumas JE: The effectiveness of behavioral parent training to modify antisocial behavior in children: a meta-analysis. *Behav Ther* 27:171–186, 1996.
23. Tonge BJ, Brereton AV, Kiomall MC, et al.: Effects on parental mental health of an education and skills training program for parents of young children with autism: a randomized controlled trial. *J Am Acad Child Adolesc Psychiatry* 45:561–569, 2006.
24. Sanders MR, Pidgeon AM, Gravestock F, et al.: Does parental attributional retraining and anger management enhance the effects of the Triple P-Positive Parenting Program with parents at risk of child maltreatment? *Behav Ther* 35:513–535, 2004.
25. Chaffin M, Silovsky JF, Funderburk B, et al.: Parent-child interaction therapy with physically abusive parents: efficacy for reducing future abuse reports. *J Consult Clin Psychol* 72:500–510, 2004.
26. Dadds MR, Schwartz S, Sanders MR: Marital discord and treatment outcome in the treatment of childhood conduct disorders. *J Consult Clin Psychol* 55:396–403, 1987.
27. Pincus DB, Choate ML, Eyberg SM, Barlow DH: Treatment of young children with separation anxiety disorder using parent-child interaction therapy. *Cogn Behav Pract* 12:126–135, 2005.
28. Hartley SL, Sikora DM, McCoy R: Prevalence and risk factors of maladaptive behaviour in young children with autistic disorder. *J Intellect Disabil Res* 52:819–829, 2008.
29. Kaat AJ, Lecavalier L: Disruptive behavior disorders in children and adolescents with autism spectrum disorders: a review of the prevalence, presentation, and treatment. *Res Autism Spectr Disord* 7:1579–1594, 2013.
30. Bearss K, Johnson C, Smith T, et al.: Effect of parent training vs parent education on behavioral problems in children with autism spectrum disorder: a randomized clinical trial. *JAMA* 313:1524–1533, 2015.
31. Baumrind D: Effects of authoritative parental control on child behavior. *Child Dev* 37:887–907, 1966.
32. Baumrind D: Child care practices anteceding three patterns of preschool behavior. *Genet Psychol Monogr* 75:43–88, 1967.
33. Hanf CL: A two-stage program for modifying maternal controlling during mother-child (M-C) interaction. Paper presented at The Meeting of the Western Psychological Association, Vancouver, 1969.
34. McNeil C, Hembree-Kigin TL: *Parent-Child Interaction Therapy.* 2nd ed. New York, Springer, 2011.
35. Barkley RA: *Defiant Children: A Clinician's Manual for Assessment and Parent Training.* 3rd ed. Guilford Press, 2013.
36. Webster-Stratton C: *The Incredible Years Parents, Teachers, and Children Training Series: Program Content, Methods, Research and Dissemination, 1980–2011.* Seattle, WA, Incredible Years, Inc, 2008.

37. Chamberlain P, Patterson GR: Discipline and child compliance in parenting. In: Bornstein MH (ed): *Handbook of Parenting: Applied and Practical Parenting*. Vol. 4. Hillsdale, NJ, Lawrence Erlbaum Associates, 205–225, 1995.
38. Bandura A: *Social Learning Theory*. New York, General Learning Press, 1971.
39. Skinner BF: Operant behavior. *Am Psychol* 18:503–515, 1963.
40. Baer DM, Wolf MM, Risley TR: Some current dimensions of applied behavior analysis. *J Appl Behav Anal* 1:91–97, 1968.
41. Iwata BA, Worsdell AS: Implications of functional analysis methodology for the design of intervention programs. *Exceptionality* 13:25–34, 2005.
42. Horner R, Carr E, Strain P, Todd A, Reed H: Problem behavior interventions for young children. *J Autism Dev Disord* 32:423–446, 2002.
43. Sanders MR, Markie-Dadds C, Tully LA, Bor W: The Triple-P-Positive Parenting Program: a comparison of enhanced, standard and self-directed behavioral family intervention for parents of children with early onset conduct problems. *J Consult Clin Psychol* 68:624–640, 2000.
44. Barkley RA: Psychosocial treatments for attention-deficit/hyperactivity disorder. *J Clin Psychiatry* 63:36–43, 2002.
45. Barkley RA, Murphy JG: Treating attention deficit hyperactivity disorder: medication and behavior management training. *Pediatr Ann* 20:256–266, 1991.
46. HosainzadehMaleki Z, Mashhadi A, Soltanifar A, Moharreri F, GhanaeiGhamanabad A: Barkley's Parent Training Program, working memory training and their combination for children with ADHD: attention deficit hyperactivity disorder. *Iran J Psychiatry* 9:47–54, 2014.
47. Newby RF, Fischer M, Roman MA: Parent training for families of children with ADHD. *School Psychol Rev* 20:252–265, 1991.
48. Scahill L, Sukhodolsky DG, Bearss K, et al.: A randomized trial of parent training in children with tic disorders and disruptive behavior. *J Child Neurol* 21:650–656, 2006.
49. Abikoff HB, Thompson M, Laver-Bradbury C, et al.: Parent training for preschool ADHD: a randomized controlled trial of specialized and generic programs. *J Child Psychol Psychiatry* 56:618–631, 2015.
50. Honeycutt AA, Khavjou OA, Jones DJ, Cuellar J, Forehand RL: Helping the noncompliant child: an assessment of program costs and cost-effectiveness. *J Child Fam Stud* 24:499–504, 2015.
51. Long P, Forehand R, Wierson M, Morgan A: Does parent training with young, noncompliant children have long-term effects? *Behav Res Ther* 3:101–107, 1994.
52. McMahon RJ, Forehand RL: *Helping the Noncompliant Child Family-Based Treatment for Oppositional Behavior*. 2nd ed. New York, Guilford Press, 2003.
53. Wells KC, Egan J: Social learning and systems family therapy for childhood oppositional disorder: comparative treatment outcome. *Compr Psychiatry* 29:138–146, 1998.
54. Dababnah S, Parish SL: Feasibility of an empirically based program for parents of preschoolers with autism spectrum disorder. *Autism* 20:85–95, 2016.
55. Menting AT, Orobio de Castro B, Matthys W: Effectiveness of the incredible years parent training to modify disruptive and prosocial child behavior: a meta-analytic review. *Clin Psychol Rev* 33:901–913, 2013.
56. Webster-Stratton C: The long term effects of a videotape modeling parent training program: comparison of immediate and 1-year follow-up results. *Behav Ther* 13:702–714, 1982.
57. Webster-Stratton C: Teaching mothers through videotape modeling to change their children's behavior. *J Pediatr Psychol* 7:279–294, 1982.
58. Webster-Stratton C. Randomized trial of two parent-training programs for families with conduct-disordered children. *J Consult Clin Psychol* 52:666–678, 1984.
59. Webster-Stratton C: The effects of father involvement in parent training for conduct problem children. *J Child Psychol Psychiatry* 26:801–810, 1985.
60. Webster-Stratton C: Predictors of treatment outcome in parent training for conduct disordered children. *Behav Ther* 16:223–243, 1985.
61. Webster-Stratton C: Systematic comparison of consumer satisfaction of three cost-effective parent training programs for conduct problem children. *Behav Ther* 20:103–115, 1989.
62. Webster-Stratton C: Enhancing the effectiveness of self-administered videotape parent training for families with conduct-problem children. *J Abnorm Child Psychol* 18:479–492, 1990.
63. Webster-Stratton C: Long-term follow-up of families with young conduct problem children: from preschool to grade school. *J Clin Child Psychol* 19:144–149, 1990.
64. Webster-Stratton C, Spitzer A: Parenting a young child with conduct problems: new insights using qualitative methods. In: Ollendick TH, Prinz RS (eds): *Advances in Clinical Child Psychology*. Vol. 18. New York, NY, Springer, 1–62, 1996.
65. Webster-Stratton C: Parent training with low-income families: Promoting parental engagement through a collaborative approach. In: Lutzker JR (ed): *Handbook of Child Abuse Research and Treatment*. New York, NY, Springer, 183–210, 1998.
66. Chaffin M, Funderburk B, Bard D, et al.: A combined motivation and parent-child interaction therapy package reduces child welfare recidivism in a randomized dismantling field trial. *J Consult Clin Psychol* 79:84–95, 2011.
67. Hakman M, Chaffin M, Funderburk B, Silovsky J: Change trajectories for parent-child interaction sequences during parent-child interaction therapy for child physical abuse. *Child Abuse Neglect* 33:461–470, 2009.
68. Herschell A, Calzada E, Eyberg SM, McNeil CB: Parent-child interaction therapy: new directions in research. *Cogn Behav Pract* 9:9–16, 2002.
69. Herschell A, McNeil C: Parent-Child Interaction Therapy with physically abusive families. In Briesmeister JM, Schaefer EC (eds): *Handbook of Parent Training: Helping Parents Prevent and Solve Problem Behaviors*. 3rd ed. Hoboken, NJ, Wiley Press, 234–267, 2007.
70. Johnson BD, Franklin LC, Hall K, Prieto LR: Parent training through play: parent-child interaction therapy with a hyperactive child. *Family J* 8:180–186, 2000.
71. Masse JJ, Wagner SM, McNeil CB, Chorney DB: Parent-child interaction therapy and high functioning autism: a conceptual overview. *J Early Intens Behav Interv* 4:714–735, 2007.
72. McNeil C, Eyberg S, Eisenstadt T, Newcomb K, Funderburk B: Parent-child interaction therapy with behavior problem children: generalization of treatment effects to the school setting. *J Clin Child Psychol* 20:140–151, 1991.
73. McNeil CB, Filcheck HA, Greco LA, et al.: Parent–child interaction therapy: can a manualized treatment be functional? *Behav Analyst Today* 2:106–154, 2001.
74. McNeil C, Herschell AD, Gurwitch RH, Clemens-Mowrer LC: Training foster parents in parent-child interaction therapy. *Educ Treat Child* 28:182–196, 2005.
75. Niec LN, Hemme J, Yopp J, Brestan E: Parent-child interaction therapy: the rewards and challenges of a group format. *Cogn Behav Pract* 12:113–125, 2005.
76. Nixon RD, Sweeny L, Erickson DB, Touyz SW: Parent-child interaction therapy: a comparison of standard and abbreviated treatments for oppositional defiant preschoolers. *J Consult Clin Psychol* 71:251–260, 2003.
77. Schuhmann EM, Foote R, Eyberg SM, Boggs S, Algina J: Parent child interaction therapy: interim report of a randomized trial with short-term maintenance. *J Clin Child Psychol* 27:34–45, 1998.
78. Tempel AB, Wagner SM, McNeil CB: Parent–child interaction therapy and language facilitation: the role of parent training on language development. *J Speech Lang Pathol Appl Behav Anal* 2:216–232, 2008.
79. Timmer SG, Ware LM, Urquiza AJ, Zebell NM: The effectiveness of parent-child interaction therapy for victims of interparental violence. *Viol Victims* 25:486–503, 2010.
80. Ware F, McNeil C: Parent–child interaction therapy: a promising intervention for abusive families. *Behav Anal Today* 3:375–385, 2003.
81. Kazdin AE: Problem-solving skills training and parent management training for oppositional defiant disorder and conduct disorder. In: Kazdin AE, Weisz JR (eds): *Evidence-Based Psychotherapies for Children and Adolescents*. 2nd ed. New York, Guilford Press, 211–226, 2010.
82. Kazdin AE: Parent management training: evidence, outcomes, and issues. *J Am Acad Child Adolesc Psychiatry* 36:1349–1356, 1997.
83. Kazdin AE: *Parent Management Training: Treatment for Oppositional, Aggressive, and Antisocial Behavior in Children and Adolescents*. New York, NY, Oxford University Press, 2005.
84. Kazdin AE, Siegel TC, Bass D: Cognitive problem-solving skills training and parent management training in the treatment of antisocial behavior in children. *J Consult Clin Psychol* 60:733–747, 1992.
85. Kazdin AE, Whitley MK: Pretreatment social relations, therapeutic alliance, and improvements in parenting practices in parent management training. *J Consult Clin Psychol* 74:346–355, 2006.
86. Thorell LB: The Community Parent Education Program (COPE): treatment effects in a clinical and a community-based sample. *Clin Child Psychol Psychiatry* 14:373–387, 2009.
87. Cunningham CE: COPE: large group, community based, family-centered parent training. In: Barkley RA (ed): *Attention Deficit Hyperactivity: A Handbook for Diagnosis and Treatment*. New York, The Guilford Press, 2005.
88. Cunningham CE, Bremner R, Secord M, Harrison R: *COPE, the Community Parent Education Program: Large Group Community-Based Workshops for Parents of 3 to 18 Year Olds*. Hamilton, ON, COPE Works, 2009.
89. Sanders MR: The Triple P-Positive Parenting Program: a public health approach to parenting support. In Briesmeister JM, Schaefer CE (eds): *Handbook of Parent Training: Helping Parents Prevent and Solve Problem Behaviors*, 3rd ed. Wiley Press, 2007.
90. Nowak C, Heinrichs N: A comprehensive meta-analysis of Triple P-Positive Parenting Program using hierarchical linear modeling: effectiveness and moderating variables. *Clin Child Fam Psychol Rev* 11:114–144, 2008.
91. Sanders MR, Markie-Dadds C, Turner K: *Theoretical, Scientific and Clinical Foundations of the Triple P-Positive Parenting Program: A Population Approach to the Promotion of Parenting Competence*. Brisbane, The Parenting and Family Support Centre, 2003.
92. Connell S, Sanders MR, Markie-Dadds C: Self-directed behavioural family intervention for parents of oppositional children in rural and remote areas. *Behav Mod* 21:379–408, 1997.
93. Bor W, Sanders MR, Markie-Dadds C: The effects of Triple P-Positive Parenting Program on children with co-occurring disruptive behaviour and

attentional/hyperactive difficulties. *J Abnorm Child Psychol* 30:571–587, 2002.
94. Hoath FE, Sanders MR; A feasibility study of Enhanced Group Triple P-Positive Parenting Program for parents of children with attention-deficit/hyperactivity disorder. *Behav Change* 19:191–206, 2002.
95. McMahon RJ, Frick PJ: Evidence-based assessment of conduct problems in children and adolescents. *J Clin Child Adolesc Psychol* 34:477–505, 2005.
96. Korsch F, Petermann F: Agreement between parents and teachers on preschool children's behavior in a clinical sample with externalizing behavioral problems. *Child Psychiatry Hum Dev* 45:617–627, 2014.
97. Youngstrom E, Loeber R, Stouthamer-Loeber M: Patterns and correlates of agreement between parent, teacher, and male adolescent ratings of externalizing and internalizing problems. *J Consult Clin Psychol* 68:1038–1050, 2000.
98. Hassall R, Rose J, McDonald J: Parenting stress in mothers of children with an intellectual disability: the effects of parental cognitions in relation to child characteristics and family support. *J Intellect Disabil Res* 49:405–418, 2005.
99. Jones J, Passey J: Family adaptation, coping and resources: parents of children with developmental disabilities and behaviour problems. *J Dev Disabil* 11:31–46, 2005.
100. Koeske GF, Koeske RD: Parenting locus of control: measurement, construct validation, and a proposed conceptual model. *Soc Work Res Abstr* 28:37–46, 1992.
101. Eyberg SM, Nelson MM, Ginn NC, et al.: *Dyadic Parent-Child Interaction Coding System: Comprehensive Manual for Research and Training.* 4th ed. Gainesville, FL, PCIT International, 2013.
102. Tarbox J, Wilke AE, Najdowski AC, et al.: Comparing indirect, descriptive, and experimental functional assessments of challenging behavior in children with autism. *J Dev Phys Disabil* 21:493–514, 2009.
103. Iwata BA, Dorsey MF, Slifer KJ, et al.: Toward a functional analysis of self-injury. *J Appl Behav Anal* 27:197–209, 1994.
104. Oliver AC, Pratt LA, Normand MP: A survey of functional behavior assessment methods used by behavior analysts in practice. *J Appl Behav Anal* 48:817–829, 2015.
105. Fettig A, Barton EE: Parent-implemented interventions for young children with disabilities: a review of fidelity features. *J Early Interv* 35:194–219, 2013.
106. Frea WD, Hepburn SL: Teaching parents of children with autism to perform functional assessments to plan interventions for extremely disruptive behaviors. *J Posit Behav Interv* 1:112–116, 1999.
107. Floyd RG, Phaneuf RL, Wilczynski SM: Measurement properties of indirect assessment methods for functional behavioral assessment: a review of research. *School Psych Rev* 34:58–73, 2005.
108. Thompson RH, Borrero JC: Direct observation. In: Fisher WW, Piazza CC, Roane HS (eds): *Handbook of Applied Behavior Analysis.* New York, The Guilford Press, 191–205, 2011.
109. Herzinger CV, Campbell JM: Comparing functional assessment methodologies: a quantitative synthesis. *J Autism Dev Disord* 37:1430–1445, 2007.
110. Achenbach T: *Manual for the Youth Self-report and 1991 Profile.* Burlington, VT, University of Vermont, Department of Psychiatry, 1991.
111. Achenbach TM, Rescorla LA: *Manual for the ASEBA School-Age Forms & Profiles.* Burlington, VT, University of Vermont, Research Center for Children, Youth, & Families, 2001.
112. Eyberg S, Pincus D: *Eyberg Child Behavior Inventory & Sutter-Eyberg Student Behavior Inventory-Revised: Professional Manual.* Odessa, FL, Psychological Assessment Resources, 1999.
113. Sutter J, Eyberg SM: *Sutter-Eyberg Student Behavior Inventory.* Gainesville, FL, Authors, 1984.
114. Reynolds CR, Kamphaus RW: *The Behavioral Assessment System for Children: The Clinician's Guide to the Behavior Assessment System For Children.* New York, NY, The Guilford Press, 2002.
115. Barkley RA, Murphy K: *Attention-Deficit Hyperactivity Disorder: A Clinical Workbook.* Vol. 2. New York, Guilford, 1998.
116. DuPaul GJ, Power TJ, Anastopoulos AD, Reid R: *ADHD Rating Scale IV: Checklists, Norms, and Clinical Interpretation.* New York, Guilford, 1998.
117. Bussing R, Fernandez M, Harwood M, et al.: Parent and teacher SNAP-IV ratings of attention deficit hyperactivity disorder symptoms: psychometric properties and normative ratings from a school district sample. *Assessment* 15:317–328, 2008.
118. Smith BL: The case against spanking. *Monitor Psychol* 43:60, 2012.
119. Reyno S, McGrath P: Predictors of parent training efficacy for child externalizing behavior problems—a meta-analytic review. *J Child Psychol Psychiatry* 47:99–111, 2006.
120. Maliken AC, Katz LF: Exploring the impact of parental psychopathology and emotion regulation on evidence-based parenting interventions: a transdiagnostic approach to improving treatment effectiveness. *Clin Child Fam Psychol Rev* 16:173–186, 2013.
121. Lundahl B, Risser JH, Lovejoy MC: A meta-analysis of parent training: moderators and follow-up effects. *Clin Psychol Rev* 26:86–104, 2006.

CHAPTER 6.2.5 ■ PSYCHODYNAMIC PRINCIPLES IN PRACTICE

RACHEL Z. RITVO AND MICHAEL SHAPIRO

HISTORY

The monumental work of Sigmund Freud grew out of a broader historic and epistemic context. The term *dynamic* in the late 19th century as used by Leibniz, Fechner, and the renowned neurologist, Hughlings Jackson, referred to changing states of consciousness and physiologic processes, as opposed to static, anatomic structures. Dynamic included a concept of mental energy. It implied functional rather than fixed organic impairment. In the 20th-century dynamic psychiatry—with its emphasis on the patient's subjective experience, the workings of unconscious psychological processes, and the patient's unique inner life—was contrasted with *descriptive* psychiatry, which strove to categorize patients according to observable behavior. Gabbard (1) describes more recent and wider uses of the term *dynamic* to include newer theories and research such as the "deficit model," object relations theory, attachment theory, and the inclusion of a biopsychosocial formulation which incorporates contemporary advances in neuroscience and genetics.

Sigmund Freud was a research neuroscientist before he turned to the clinical practice of neurology and eventually psychiatry. Although he recognized that the research methods of his time did not allow for a full explication of the neuronal base of psychic events, he endeavored to keep his psychological theories consistent with biology. For instance, Freud conceptualized the mind as the interplay of excitatory (drive) and inhibitory (defense) phenomena. Greatly influenced by Darwinian theory (2), Freud sought to construct a developmental framework for his psychology, an approach that put the psychic phenomena of childhood in the spotlight and paved the way for child psychotherapy. Psychoanalytic psychology as a theory of adaptation of humans to our environment derived from these Darwinian roots. Modern neuroscience offers an opportunity to refine psychoanalytic theory. The growing field of neuropsychoanalysis seeks to integrate the latest findings from cognitive neuroscience with psychoanalytic observations to improve our understanding of the brain substrates of psychoanalytic constructs (3).

Psychodynamic psychotherapy of children began with Freud's publication in 1909 (4) of the case of "Little Hans," a 5-year-old boy with a phobia of horses. Freud's interest was in the centrality of childhood experience in shaping the adult psyche. Although he sought to "reconstruct" childhood experience from the analysis of adults, he encouraged his students to observe children for more direct evidence of infantile sexuality. It was in this context that Freud came to supervise the analysis of Little Hans by Hans' father.

Hermine Von Hug-Hellmuth was the first to undertake psychoanalytic therapy of children and adolescents. Her 1921 paper "On the Technique of Child-Analysis" (5) surveyed technical issues in the psychodynamic treatment of children that are still recognized as core issues to this day. She noted that the child does not come of his own accord. She advises against a judgmental stance or the giving of direct commissions and prohibitions. Hug-Hellmuth engaged the child in "talking over things together." She introduced the use of an educational method founded on psychoanalytic knowledge. She examined the multiple ways in which work with children and adolescents differs from that with adults, including the complexities of the relationship between the analyst and the child's parents. Her observation that the child's spontaneous play could stand in the place of the verbal communications of the adult to reveal unconscious conflict was significant for the development of psychodynamic therapy with children. Further, she observed that fully conscious avowal of analytic understanding was not a prerequisite for therapeutic effect in children.

Hug-Hellmuth's early death limited her impact on the field of child psychotherapy. Melanie Klein (6) and Anna Freud (7) emerged as the founders of child psychoanalysis. Klein coined the term play analysis, emphasizing the child's play as equivalent to free association. Her methods encouraged early, deep interpretations and minimized the analyst's contact with parents and teachers. She developed the position that through play interpretation, children could be analyzed just as adults. Klein extended Sigmund Freud's theories about internal conflict to younger children, and even infants, maintaining that libidinous drives and fear of punishment are evident from an early age. Klein portrayed the experience of the infant as shifting between libidinal and aggressive impulses and experiencing oneself as "good" or "bad" in addition to experiencing the "good breast" that provides nourishment and the "bad breast" which is unavailable and abandoning. This paradigm formed the basis for Klein's *paranoid–schizoid* position: paranoid referring to the fear of harm coming to the "good breast" (or good infant) and schizoid referring to splitting away the hated "bad breast" (or bad infant). The counterpart *depressive position* refers to the infant's realization and subsequent horror and guilt that the "breast," mother, and infant are whole objects and cannot be split into good and bad parts.

Whereas Klein continued to focus on interpretation in work with children, Anna Freud took another approach. Anna Freud's long career, from the 1920s to her death in 1982, allowed for significant evolution in her ideas regarding psychodynamic treatment of children and adolescents. Trained as a teacher, she was interested in the "educative" functions of the analyst in working with children, rather than purely interpretive functions. Her contention was that young children could not handle deep interpretations because of their underdeveloped egos. Anna Freud's work on ego mechanisms of defense (8) led to the development of defense analysis of children and adolescents. Her attention to observing the developmental process in children led her to conceptualize interweaving lines of development (9).

The English psychoanalyst Donald Winnicott, who remained independent from both the Kleinians and the Freudians, brought a pediatrician's perspective to his work, particularly his experience of direct involvement with infants and their mothers. Winnicott was interested in how the infant developed a sense of self, a sense of reality, and a capacity for self-regulation. His work influenced Kohut's development of self-psychology (see below). Gifted at coining evocative terms for his novel concepts, Winnicott gave us: "good enough mother," "transitional object," "holding environment," and "false self." Winnicott is known for his aphorism *"There is no such thing as an infant,* meaning, of course, that whenever one finds an infant one finds maternal care, and without maternal care there would be no infant" (10).

John Bowlby (11–13) was a psychoanalyst who broke with mainstream child psychoanalysis in Britain and America by taking a strong empirical approach to studying psychoanalytic developmental constructs. His focus was on the direct observation of the behavior of infants and their caregivers through prospective studies of the effects of early attachment on relationships and on personality development. Attachment theory has bridged the gap between clinical psychodynamic theory and developmental psychology. In the early 21st century, of particular interest to attachment researchers has been the elucidation of the impact of attachment history on patients' capacity for *mentalization,* also referred to as *reflective functioning,* and defined as "the ability to take account of one's own and others' mental states in understanding why people behave in specific ways" (14). An example of treatments developed by drawing on this research is Bleiberg's Mentalization-Based Treatment of Adolescents (MBT-A) for emerging borderline personality disorder (BPD) (15).

Emigrant analysts fleeing the Holocaust brought this rich array of psychoanalytic thought to America. Child analytic training took root in the United States, allowing child psychoanalysts to play a major role in the training of child and adolescent psychiatrists throughout the mid- and late 20th century. A distinctly American therapeutic tradition also contributed to the field of dynamic psychotherapy with children, particularly play therapy. Homegrown American psychodynamic therapists such as Frederick Allen of the child guidance movement (16) and Carl Rogers, author of client-centered therapy (17), sought to counteract the impact of the American behaviorist tradition. Allen objected strongly to the behaviorists' belief that a child was born a blank slate who could be formed by parents into anything the parent wanted. Allen believed this behaviorist stance "created a distortion of a parent's sense of responsibility... [and a] failure to appreciate the nature of growth and the participation of both child and parent in the child's development" (16). Addressing the therapist/patient relationship, Allen regarded the child as a person in his own right, a human being with a capacity to change who should be respected as a an active participant in the therapy (16). The child's exercise of free expression, a here-and-now focus, and rapport in the relationship between patient and therapist were emphasized as an American school of "non-directive" therapy developed through the work of Axline (18) and Dorfman (19).

PSYCHODYNAMIC PSYCHOLOGY

Psychodynamic psychotherapy aims at bringing about change in psychological processes that are largely unconscious but can be inferred from observable phenomena, such as actions or speech. The processes determining the inner world of subjective experience are of particular interest. The plethora of unconscious processes of which the human brain is capable allows for great diversity of focus for dynamic psychotherapy.

Psychodynamic therapy requires as a foundation a theory of the functioning of the unconscious mind and the internal experience of the individual as well as a theory of the psychological impact of human relationships.

In dynamic theory, the mind is not seen as a blank slate at birth but rather as endowed with the biologic potential to develop psychic structure given an adequate environment. *Internalization* denotes the process by which experiences with the external world, usually in the realm of relationships, form stable intrapsychic structures or capacities. Once a process is internalized it no longer requires an external stimulus for its function to be executed. *Identification*, the psychological process by which one individual becomes like another, is a familiar mechanism of internalization.

Unconscious psychological processes may be considered as primary determinants of the inner world of subjective experience. The individual's total subjective experiential world, including thoughts, feelings, and fantasies, as well as perceptions of the external world, regardless of whether they accurately reflect the external world as viewed by another observer, has been termed *psychic reality*. The dynamic therapist attempts to grasp the patient's psychic reality and convey to the patient an interest in understanding his experience of himself.

A primary tenet of psychoanalysis is *psychic determinism* (20), the principle that nothing in the mind happens by chance or in a random way. All psychic acts and events have meanings and causes and can be understood in terms of earlier psychic events. The mind retains experiences and is shaped by them. Conscious thoughts and overt behaviors provide observable clues to their underlying unconscious psychic determinants. A corollary hypothesis, *overdeterminism* or *multideterminism*, states that a psychic event (e.g., a symptom) is typically caused by more than one factor and may serve more than one purpose in the psychic framework. The multidetermined nature of symptoms provides the psychodynamic therapist with more than one way to approach a symptom.

The concept of multideterminism is further refined in dynamic theory by the observation that the multiple determinants of a particular observable psychic phenomenon are frequently in opposition or *conflict* with one another. Psychodynamic theorists have identified several types of psychic conflict. *External conflict* denotes the conflicts that arise between the child and the environment, the consequent frustration demanding management by the child's psyche. External conflicts are most evident in early childhood when the infant or toddler has little internal restraint and struggles with the caretaker over such matters as bedtime or playing with an electrical plug. As prohibitions become internalized, the conflicts become *internal*. Not all conflicts are caused by prohibitions. Conflicts may arise between competing urges, thereby creating ambivalence. For example, conflicts arise between urges toward passive-dependence and active-mastery. An external conflict may or may not become a fully *internalized conflict*. An internalized conflict is conceptualized as continuing in the individual's psyche when environmental forces that triggered the initial internal conflict no longer exist.

Psychodynamic therapy capitalizes on the observation that human beings are psychologically changed by relationships with other human beings. Psychodynamic technique utilizes two aspects of human relationships to achieve its mutative effects, transference, and the real relationship.

Particular attention is paid to *transference*, the unconscious displacement onto the therapist of patterns of feelings, fantasies, attitudes, and behavior originally experienced in relation to significant figures during childhood. Additionally, transference is frequently used as a general term for the patient's attitudes and behavior toward the therapist and as such includes *externalizations*, which Anna Freud specifies as:

> ...processes in which the person of the analyst is used to represent one or the other part of the patient's personality structure....The child thus re-stages his internal (intersystemic) conflicts as external battles with the analyst, a process which provides useful material (9).

Brenner points out that the phenomenon of transference is not unique to the therapeutic relationship but rather "*every* object relation is a new edition of the first, definitive attachments of childhood" (21). In essence, psychodynamic theory proposes that psychologically significant relationships contribute to the individual's perceptions, thoughts, fantasies, feelings, attitudes, and behavior in all future relationships.

A portion of the therapeutic action of psychodynamic therapy rests in the experience of the *real relationship* with the therapist. The child even more than the adult has receptivity for new experiences. The psychodynamic therapist provides the child or adolescent with a new object for internalization. The therapist strives to cultivate specific qualities, some of which may be novel to the child. These include a respectful attitude toward the child, particularly toward the child's thoughts and feelings, as well as the protection of the child's confidences from intrusion by parents or teachers. The therapist strives to be reliable and predictable in the arrangements made for meeting with the child (22). Most significantly, the psychodynamic therapist establishes a relationship with the child that is largely unilateral in its focus so that the events of the therapy evolve primarily from the child. Unlike the relationship with parents or peers, in which there is a necessary and healthy reciprocity, the focus on the child in the relationship with the psychodynamic therapist allows the internal world of the child to dominate their interactions (23). The therapist as an interested and thoughtful observer becomes a model for the child's development of the capacity for self-observation, a capacity termed *observing ego*. For children who have deficits in reflective functioning, the therapist's respect for the child's mental life and implied recognition that it is uniquely the child's is important in helping the child to develop this capacity.

Although the primary focus in the patient–therapist relationship is tipped toward the patient, psychodynamic theory does address the therapist's experience of this relationship. *Countertransference* refers specifically to intrapsychic conflicts stirred in the therapist by the patient. Generically, countertransference refers to all the reactions of the therapist to the patient or the parents, and is a valuable source of information about a patient's internal world, in addition to sometimes interfering with treatment (1). Marshall (24) operationalizes the definition of countertransference into two categories: (a) reactions arising from the therapist's unresolved internal conflicts; and (b) natural reactions to a patient's provocative behavior. Winnicott (25) dubbed this second-type *objective* countertransference, objective in the sense that virtually everyone would find the patient's behavior provocative. The challenge to the therapist when the objective countertransference is recognized is to construct a response that is both honest and therapeutic.

Treatment alliance and *working alliance* are terms used to refer to "all the factors that keep a patient in treatment and which enable him to remain there during phases of resistance and hostile transference" (26). *Resistance* is a conceptualization of the psychological mechanisms that cling to the intrapsychic status quo and seek to prevent change. In essence, resistance is a defense against affects, undesirable self-representations, or unwanted drive derivatives that are stirred and moved toward awareness by the therapeutic process. Inherent in the treatment alliance is the patient's awareness of internal difficulties and an acceptance of the need to be helped. Children with very fragile self-esteem may balk at entering into therapy because they cannot tolerate the recognition of their difficulties.

In child and adolescent treatments, the establishment and maintenance of the alliance are more complex than in adults because of the dependence on parents to bring the child to treatment. A positive alliance with the parents sustains the child's engagement in treatment even when the child's resistance is strong. Since parents can subtly oppose the child's wish to come to treatment or collude with the child's resistance, the therapist must establish and maintain a working alliance with the parents sufficient to keep the therapy going. Novick and Novick (27) reach beyond this minimum. They view the therapeutic alliance with the parents as a transformative task "designed to help parents gain or regain some feeling of competence as parents and love for their child as a separate person."

Defense mechanisms are unconscious, automatic, psychological processes. The individual does not consciously choose to institute a defense; however, an individual can learn to recognize defensive activity as it occurs (28). Anna Freud's classic *The Ego and the Mechanisms of Defense* (8) enumerated several patterns of defense already in the analytic literature: regression, repression, reaction formation, isolation, undoing, projection, introjection, turning against the self, reversal, and sublimation. To these she added: turning passive to active, denial, intellectualization, displacement, identification with the aggressor, and altruistic surrender. Following that publication, effort was devoted to developing a comprehensive catalog of defense mechanisms. Clinical observation eventually led to the conclusion that any aspect of ego functioning may be used in the service of defense and the attempt to delineate a comprehensive list of specific mechanisms was impossible and potentially misleading in its reductionism. Nonetheless, children use certain mechanisms with sufficient frequency that it is of value to psychodynamic child therapists to be able to recognize them in the clinical situation (Table 6.2.5.1).

Controversy exists both within dynamic child psychiatry and between dynamic and descriptive psychiatry regarding the degree to which defensive activity and internal conflict involve such *autonomous* ego functions as perception, motility (walking, eye–hand coordination), intention, intelligence, logical thought, speech, and language. Autonomous ego functions are conceptualized by Heinz Hartmann (30) to be relatively resistant to disturbance by intrapsychic conflict. It is clear that many disturbances in this area have their origins in individual differences in brain functioning. However, it is also clear from clinical material that in many children and adults, these presumed autonomous functions are impacted by conflict and defense. This is no surprise to psychiatrists familiar with the way cognitive function is impaired by defensive denial. The challenge to the child and adolescent psychodynamic therapist is in the differential diagnosis. Psychological testing by a professional skilled in elucidating this distinction can be very useful.

TABLE 6.2.5.1

DEFENSES COMMONLY EXHIBITED BY CHILDREN IN PSYCHODYNAMIC THERAPY

Denial	The disavowal of intolerable external reality factors or of thoughts, feelings, wishes, or needs that are apparent to an observer
Displacement	The transfer of emotions, ideas, or wishes from the original object to a more acceptable substitute
Externalization	The attribution of internal conflicts to the external environment and a search for environmental solutions. In therapy, the person of the therapist is used to represent one or the other part of the patient's personality structure
Reaction formation	The adoption of affects, ideas, or behaviors that are the opposites of impulses harbored either consciously or unconsciously
Repression	The exclusion of unacceptable ideas, fantasies, affects, or impulses from consciousness or the keeping out of consciousness what has never been conscious. Repressed material emerges in disguised form in thought, speech, and actions
Suppression	The conscious effort to control and conceal unacceptable impulses. Suppression is the exception to the rule that defenses are unconscious processes
Somatization	The transfer of tension from drives or affects into disturbances of bodily functions or rhythms
Turning passive to active	The management of affects and impulses stirred by a passive experience with an active, more powerful "other" by playing out in action or story the active "other's" role. This includes the process of identification with the aggressor

From Edgerton J, Campbell RJ (eds): *American Psychiatric Glossary*. Washington, DC, American Psychiatric Press, 1994; Freud A: *The Ego and Mechanisms of Defense*. New York, International Universities Press, 1936; Freud A: *Normality and Pathology in Childhood: Assessments of Development*. New York, International Universities Press, 1965.

SCHOOLS OF PSYCHOANALYTIC THOUGHT

The 20th century witnessed the growth of an extensive body of psychoanalytic observations and theories from which three major schools of psychoanalytic thought emerged: ego psychology, object relations theory, and self-psychology. The dawn of the 21st century has seen the emergence of mentalization-based approaches that draw on the findings of the other schools but develop a new focus. Practitioners often specialize in one school's approach but borrow from the others depending on the features of the clinical situation.

EGO PSYCHOLOGY

Freud realized that a conceptual tool was needed to provide a framework for clinical data and hypotheses about unconscious phenomena and subjective experience. He termed such a tool "metapsychology." Different models evolved as he strove to accommodate all his data. The most lasting of Freud's metapsychological frames is a structural theory, the *tripartite model*, which divides mental functions into *id*, *ego*, and *superego*. Ego psychology developed from this tripartite model.

Id is a concept that encompasses the mental representations of the instinctual drives (31). *Drive* is a term applied to a stimulus arising within the individual that arouses the mind and incites mental activity. Drives may be thought of as genetically endowed motivational states. Commonly we think of these as urges, needs, wishes, and desires.

Feelings are internal stimuli very familiar to the average person. Because emotions arise from physiologic response patterns, they are an early, although in psychoanalytic theory not primary, step in the pathway to arousal and mental activity. In psychoanalytic theory, affects serve a signal function triggering ego efforts to manage drives.

Classical Freudian theory works with a dualistic system of drives, an aggressive and a sexual drive. The sexual or *libidinal* drive includes affiliative and pleasure-seeking urges. A child who desires to be bathed by the parent and have his or her naked body admired is displaying a derivative of the libidinal drive. The pleasure the child takes from the sensuous

TABLE 6.2.5.2

EGO FUNCTIONS

Affect regulation
Capacity for play
Cognition
Defense
Impulse control
Internal representation
Judgment
Language
Memory
Motility
Object relations
Perception
Reality testing
Self-esteem regulation
Self-observation
Stimulus regulation
Symbolization

From Auchincloss, E, Samberg, E, eds: *Psychoanalytic Terms and Concepts*. New Haven, Yale University Press, 2012; Cabaniss DL, Cherry S, Douglas CJ, Schwartz A: *Psychodynamic Psychotherapy: A Clinical Manual*. Oxford, UK, Wiley-Blackwell, 2011.

experience of the water would also be a libidinal drive derivative. While aggression has primarily referred to hostile urges, contemporary analysts have extended it to include assertive, constructive behaviors directed toward mastery, ambition, and fairness (32). Because pleasures sought in response to libidinal drive inevitably run into some requirement for delay or other frustration in the real world, ego mechanisms must develop to regulate aggressive drives if libidinal drives are to be satisfied.

Ego includes all the mental capacities available to the individual for regulation of the internal milieu and adaptation to external reality. Ego's task is to optimize pleasure and gratification of wishes and needs while maintaining internal equilibrium, the health of the body, good relations with the external world, and peace with superego.

Ego is often defined in terms of its numerous functions such as cognition, perception, memory, motility, language, symbolization, reality testing, judgment, impulse control, affect regulation, internal representation, object relations, self-observation, and defense (Table 6.2.5.2). Work with children requires examining each of these functions in the context of the child's age and developmental accomplishments. Therapy is aimed at facilitating the child's progressive development of mature ego functions so the child can better manage situations and internal conflicts that are causing symptoms.

Superego, the moral agency in the tripartite model, encompasses conscience, morality, critical self-observation, self-punishment, and upholding of personal ideals (34). Although available to consciousness as moral precepts and ideals, superego functions are predominantly unconscious. Superego is built out of the child's desire to please adults and the fear of displeasing adults and thereby losing their love and care. It grows from experiencing consequences in the physical and social world and from identification with the models of self-control and moral values presented by important adults. There is continuing development of a set of standards, *ego ideal*, epitomizing the individual's beliefs of what is right, good, or desirable. Superego can be effective in controlling behavior in conformance with this ideal only to the degree that ego capacities have developed to be deployed in thwarting and channeling unacceptable impulses.

When misbehavior is the presenting complaint about a particular child, the clinician must evaluate whether the behavioral expectations of the adults are age appropriate and within the capacity of this child's ego. The clinician also pays attention to the meaning of the behavior in the context of the child's anxieties and conflicts over drive derivatives. When thought and behavior conform to the internalized standards of the developing ego ideal, the child shows pleasure in performance of daily tasks, self-esteem, happiness, or contentment. The child displays signs of humiliation, shame or guilt, and low self-esteem when thought and behavior disappoint the strictures of internalized standards of superego. The child fears losing the love of the adults the child depends upon. Children frequently externalize blame as a defense against painful affects when a sense of being bad is unbearable. Unfortunately, when the child lies or blames others, adults may assume that the child does not know he was naughty, whereas it may be that the child does know but cannot tolerate the knowing. Children frequently express their guilt through actions in which their behavior brings about a punishment. For example, a child struggling with urges to injure a new sibling may become accident-prone.

OBJECT RELATIONS AND ATTACHMENT THEORY

Object relations theory grew out of Freud's emphasis on early experience in relationships as a source of both psychopathology and transference. The interest this stimulated in the earliest relationships of the human infant and the observational studies of young children that it spawned (35–37) have reaped extensive benefit for our understanding of the mental health needs of children. Although loosely anchored in the tripartite model of the mind, psychoanalytic object relations theories as defined by Kernberg are "those that place the internalization, structuralization, and clinical reactivation (in the transference and countertransference) of the earliest dyadic object relations at the center of their motivational (genetic and developmental), structural, and clinical formulations" (38).

Whereas Anna Freud and ego psychologists focused more on intrapsychic conflict, object relations theorists shifted their focus to internalized dyads and interpersonal relationships. Whereas the ego psychologists focused on the child's adjustment to the triadic relationships of the oedipal phase, object relations theorists focused on the dyadic preoedipal experiences.

Object relations theorists use a metapsychology organized around the concept of an *internal representational world*, which is gradually constructed in the course of development (39). It is useful to make a distinction between object representations and images. An object representation is an enduring schema constructed from a multitude of images, each derived from a multitude of experiential impressions. Sandler (39) gives the example of a child who experiences many images of his or her mother—mother feeding, mother talking, mother dressing the child, and so on—out of which gradually is created the mother representation encompassing the entire range of mother images, all bearing the label "mother." A *self-representation* is similarly formed from the accumulation of experiences of one's own subjectivity.

Identification is the coalescence of a *self-representation* with an *object representation*. En route to a stable identification are temporary identifications and imitations with transitory changes in self-image. The object representation used as a model in identification may be based to a degree on fantasy rather than wholly on real attributes of the person from whom it derived. Identification, with its duplication of the object representation within the self-representation, is seen as a step in the loosening of the dependency tie to the object.

Object relations theory looks closely at the child's development of the cognitive awareness that a person, such as the parent, still exists even when not present. This awareness is termed object permanence. With *object permanence* the child gains greater tolerance of absence of the caregiver. A second stage of object development is *object constancy*, a term coined by Margaret Mahler (40), the capacity to maintain love for the object in the face of disappointment and anger. Following this developmental line, psychoanalytic observations reveal how fear of the loss of the caretaker generates a need for defensive maneuvers. With development the fear shifts from fear of loss of the object itself to fear of loss of the object's love and with further development to fear of loss of body integrity, often referred to as castration anxiety. Finally, as superego functions and ego ideals develop fear of loss of love generates unpleasant affects of shame, guilt, and remorse to stimulate restraint.

Attachment research has further informed object relations theory and therapeutic practice. Bowlby surmised that infants were born with a drive toward forming a relationship with the caregiver, an attachment that was not only to gain food and love but also to be protected from danger, to gain security. Ainsworth developed methods, particularly the Strange Situation Interview, to measure and categorize the attachments of young children. Secure attachment to a primary caregiver was seen to positively affect psychological development and resilience whereas disorganized attachments were a risk factor for psychopathology. Mary Main's efforts to measure attachment experience in adults, through the Adult Attachment Interview, has led the way for a life span understanding of the impact of early object relations and of intergenerational transmission of mental health and illness.

The object relations school stimulated the development of dyadic therapies where the caregiver and child are both in the session and their relationship is the focus of the treatment.

SELF-PSYCHOLOGY

Self-psychology grew out of the work of Heinz Kohut, who found that classical transference interpretations were counterproductive when treating adults with maladaptive narcissistic tendencies. He developed an approach of sustained empathic immersion in the patient's subjective reality (41). Moving away from the tripartite model of ego psychology and the focus on internalized objects of object relations theory, Kohut considered the development of the self as a core element of mental well-being. The self, a subjective sense of "I", is in self-psychology "a predominantly unconscious structure at the core of the personality" (32). A healthy self has cohesion, continuity over time, initiative and agency, and self-esteem. Kohut recognized the importance of normal narcissism in children. Kohut theorized that children require a caregiver who reflects and affirms a child's subjective experiences of accomplishment and agency in the world. This experience manifests in therapy as a *mirroring transference*, while identifying with the caregiver as a "powerful other" whom the child can look up to and bond with manifests as an *idealizing transference*. The need for human connection and sense of togetherness manifests in a *twinship transference*. Miller (42), applying Kohut's self-psychology to children, proposes three primary drives: the drive toward internal integration, the will to do, and the need for others. Kohut postulated that children eventually learn from the realities of relationships to be flexible in their expectations of themselves and their parents and to navigate normal disappointments of daily experience. Ideally, the child learns to tolerate these frustrations, soothes the self, and builds internal structure and resilience, a process which Kohut termed *transmuting internalization*. But a range of conditions in the caregiver, the child or the environment may derail this development. Self-psychology differs from classical psychoanalysis in that Kohut found interpretation of these transferences to be unhelpful, even counterproductive, if the patient felt demoralized or defeated. Kohut's process allows for transferences to flourish. After allowing the transference to deepen, the patients will develop a more cohesive, resilient self through tolerance of normal daily frustration with the analyst and internalization of the analyst's strength. "The child who is swooping around the living room in his cape needs to have his exuberance enjoyed, not have his fantasies interpreted as grandiose" (41).

MENTALIZATION-BASED TREATMENT

Mentalization is defined as the capacity to understand the behavior of others and one's own behavior as an expression of mental states such as beliefs, memories, and emotions. Reflective function is the operationalization of this ability to recognize mental states in oneself and others. Mentalization as a focus of psychodynamic therapy developed in the 1990s through the work of Fonagy and colleagues (43–45) who brought together ego psychology, attachment theory, and developmental research on children's emerging theory of mind. The developmental researchers demonstrated that mentalization was required for children to have the capacity to take the perspective of another, to distinguish fantasy from reality and to participate in fantasy play. Fonagy and Bateman (43,44) recognized that deficits in mentalization were found in BPD and developed a dynamic treatment for BPD based on improving mentalization, empirical tests of which are promising.

Child analysts recognized that a mentalization focus with children would move away from seeking to make the patient aware of the "whys" of their difficulties and focus instead on building the child's awareness of inner states and the child's ability to speculate on the inner experience of others. This can be done through play and through the direct experiences shared with the therapist without requiring verbal interpretation (32).

Whichever conceptual framework is utilized, dynamic psychotherapy sees the individual's motivations, impulses, and desires as important determinants of subjective experience, mental functioning, and behavior.

CLINICAL APPROACH

The clinical application of psychodynamic theory to the treatment of children and adolescents is broad, and can be combined with other treatment modalities. Individual psychodynamic therapy, based largely on psychoanalysis but drawing as well on American client-centered therapy and the child guidance model, can be used to demonstrate the fundamental techniques and practices of dynamic psychotherapy.

The line between psychoanalysis and psychodynamic psychotherapy is not distinct but in the United States rests primarily on whether the therapist trained as a psychoanalyst and on the frequency of sessions, with psychoanalytic cases requiring at least four sessions per week, whereas psychodynamic psychotherapy tends to be once or twice per week. In terms of technique, psychodynamic psychotherapy has been more focused on facilitating the child's adaptation to their environment and improving functioning, while psychoanalysis focused more on the transference as a tool to alter the child's internal psychic structure. This distinction has been somewhat eroded, as the current emphasis on psychodynamic psychotherapy has shifted from interpretation and unconscious conflict to placing more value on intrapsychic growth in the hear-and-now relationship with the therapist.

Indications and Goals

The indications for psychodynamic psychotherapy are not diagnosis specific (22). The recommendation for individual psychodynamic therapy derives from the formulation of the intrapsychic component of the child or adolescent's condition within a developmentally attuned biopsychosocial model of dysfunction. Formulation goes beyond the simple descriptive categories of diagnosis to include life events related to the emergence of psychopathology, the pathophysiology of symptoms and problematic behaviors, and the developmental status, leading conflicts, and defense mechanisms of the child (29,46,47). Individual psychodynamic therapy is most clearly indicated in cases where the patient's difficulties are the product of intrapsychic conflict and adherence to defensive solutions or object representations that are developmentally regressive. Frequently, a child's difficult behaviors are externalizations of intrapsychic conflict. Psychodynamic therapy is indicated in cases where the etiologic factors in the social environment have resolved but the child's defenses have become fixed. In contrast, when the patient's difficulties lie in the environment or the child's own constitution, such as blindness or multiple learning disabilities, intensive individual work may be important but is unlikely to bring the youth to health without environmental interventions such as appropriate school placement.

Intensive, individual psychodynamic therapy is contraindicated in cases of severe constitutional deficits such as severe autism spectrum disorder or moderate-to-severe intellectual disability, particularly to the degree that these disorders affect capacity for self-observation and receptive language function. Intensive treatment is contraindicated when circumstances within the family or the treatment facility cannot sustain the continuity and integrity of the therapy, especially if disruption of the therapy repeats previous traumas of abandonment and unpredictability for the child.

The goals of therapy extend beyond symptom relief. A primary goal is to restore psychological development to a normal path of management of anxiety, enhanced affect regulation, improved self-esteem and frustration tolerance, age-appropriate autonomy, greater capacity for pleasure and satisfaction in school work and play, and healthy relationships with peers. Additional goals are to enhance the child's resilience and decrease the likelihood of relapse by developing the child's capacity for understanding his or her own feelings, thoughts, and the connection between feelings and behavior. The child or adolescent comes to a more sophisticated understanding of other people's thoughts, feelings, and behaviors by learning to know and observe his own mental functions. This contributes to improved interpersonal relationships.

Opening Phase

The challenge and gratification provided by the practice of psychodynamic therapy stems in part from the requirement that the practitioner pursue diagnostic and therapeutic goals simultaneously. Thus, the psychodynamic child and adolescent psychiatrist seeks to establish a psychodynamic treatment stance from the very first contact with the adult caregiver and patient. The clinician acts in a manner that respects the parental functions of the caregiver as well as the developmentally appropriate autonomy and inner experience of the child.

The First Visit

With adolescents, particularly older adolescents, the clinician may meet with the patient for one or several sessions before meeting with the parents. This allows the adolescent to explore issues of trust with the clinician and demonstrates that the clinician's primary relationship is to the adolescent. For younger children, it is typical for the parents to meet with the psychiatrist to provide background data and to establish their own trust and confidence in the psychiatrist so that they can assure the child of the appropriateness of this undertaking. It is important to explore with parents how they will prepare the child for the first visit. If the child has expressed distress over a particular symptom, the parent may explain that the doctor is there to help with that symptom. In language appropriate to the child's age, the parents ought to tell the child that the doctor is someone who helps children with their feelings and worries by talking and playing with them.

Structuring the Psychodynamic Therapy for the Child or Adolescent

The intention in individual therapy is for the therapist and child to work together separately from the parents. The child may have difficulty leaving the parent, either because for a preschooler this is within the range of age-appropriate behavior or for an older child because of underlying conflicts. Such separation difficulties require an adaptation of technique and preliminary work with the child and parent to understand and work through the issue. The idea behind working with the child without the parent in the room is to create a zone of confidentiality and psychic safety within which the child and therapist can explore feelings, thoughts, and behaviors. If the parent is present, the child's spontaneity is affected by the possible reaction from the parent. When the child is seen alone, the therapist is in a better position to see how the child has internalized the authority of the parents.

The psychiatrist should clarify to both the parents and the child that, although he or she meets with the child's parents on a regular basis, the confidentiality in this therapy is a "one-way street" which allows the psychiatrist to tell the child what the parents have said but precludes the psychiatrist reporting to the parents what the child has said or done. Children, particularly at the beginning of therapy, frequently will not report to the therapist current events that provide a context for understanding the child's talk and play within the session because children are very oriented in the present moment and are defensive against the affect the reporting might stir up. A meeting or phone call from the parents is important if the therapist is to know about these events. The "one-way street" implies that the therapist will share these communications from the parents with the child as clinically indicated. The child's understanding of the purpose of the therapist's meetings with parents develops as the therapy continues. It is the therapist's task through word and deed to help the child understand that, although the therapist tries to help the parents understand their role as parents of a child of this age and with these problems, the therapist cannot control the parents and will not take sides in a specific struggle between the child and parents. On the other hand, particularly with older children and adolescents, it can be pointed out that the parent has a responsibility to the child for assuring that the therapist is doing a responsible job and thus needs some report from the therapist on the progress of the work.

There are several other elements the psychodynamic therapist uses to create a special person, place, and time for dealing with feelings and worries in addition to creating a zone of confidentiality. The therapist deals with the child in a nonjudgmental and nondirective manner such as that described by Virginia Axline (18) in her classic text, *Play Therapy*. In intensive individual psychodynamic therapy, the therapist strives to relate to the child in the style McConville (48) has described as the "empathic participant" who approaches the child with the wish to know "what's it like to be you." The therapist and child explore together rather than doing something *to* or *for* the child. Eventually the therapist is *with* the child as the child examines and explores his own thoughts, feelings, and conflicts. If doctor–patient relationships are conceived of as either prescriptive, collaborative, or facilitative, the psychodynamic therapist eschews the prescriptive, choosing to be collaborative and facilitative.

The office must be suitably sturdy and equipped in a manner age-appropriate to the patients who will be treated. A separate playroom is advantageous when working with young children who are struggling to control intensely messy or aggressive impulses. Children's activities in a play therapy tend to fall into the following categories: games with rules, physical activities, creative projects, solo imaginary play, and imaginary play with the therapist as a participant. It is helpful to have age-appropriate toys and games readily available in the office. A family grouping of animals or small dolls is useful.

The issue of limit setting will arise no matter how appropriately the office or playroom is outfitted. Common-sense limitations are necessary to protect the room, therapist, and child from physical damage. One way to understand the limits is to say, "When we are done I have to be able to clean up and have you, me, and the office/playroom back the way it was." This creates in the child's world of expression through action the same safety from real-world consequences the adult analyzes and on the couch enjoys when expressing himself or herself verbally. Frequently, the therapist is able to address the impulse toward an unacceptable action while redirecting its aim. Thus one might say, "You may not cut my dress when you feel like attacking but you may cut this paper I will hold. I can see you feel strong and safe when you are doing the cutting. You let me feel how scary it is to have someone attacking." If the child cannot be redirected, the therapist tries to prevent the dangerous action without creating a physical struggle. It is important that the therapist not become angry, blaming, or punitive while commenting on the child's struggle over the destructive wish. The therapist may comment on being maneuvered into the role of the "policeman who must keep us and the office safe." It is also appropriate for the therapist to remind the child that "We must try to find words for these feelings so you can tell me about it without things getting broken." The implementation of a set starting and ending time is the most frequently imposed limitation, as Axline (18) points out. The therapist's adherence to routine in keeping the time and dates of appointments on a predictable schedule is a necessary part of creating reliability and boundaries in the therapeutic relationship. The child's reaction to waiting in the waiting room for the appointed starting time and dealing with leaving the therapist at the end of the session can serve to reveal the particular child's conflicts and defenses.

The Interpretive Session: Structuring the Therapy for the Parents

It is important that the therapist and parents meet in an interpretive session or two to review the formulation of the child's diagnosis and prognosis in dynamic and developmental terms, and to discuss the recommendation for treatment and make the necessary arrangements. Parents understand that frequency of practice enhances the outcome when trying to learn a foreign language or master a musical instrument. In psychodynamic therapy, the child undertakes learning a new "psychological language" and developing new skills to master feelings and impulses. The patient must be helped to counteract the resistance to change that is a natural mechanism for maintaining stability. When possible, twice per week sessions are desirable but clinicians find once per week can also be effective. Less than that may make it difficult to establish the relationship and continuity needed for successful treatment.

The wise therapist is cautious in predicting the duration of treatment unless a specifically time-limited brief treatment technique is being undertaken (22). Much depends on the stability of the environment and degree of current destabilizing stresses. What are the burdens and constraints on the parents in terms of effort and expense that might limit the duration of treatment? Parents should be told that intensive individual psychodynamic therapy is generally measured in months to a year or two. The therapist can work with the parents from the start to generate termination criteria focused on the resumption of progressive development, renewed pleasure in the child's own functioning and in the relationship with the parents (27).

The frequency and purpose of parent sessions also must be discussed. The parents and therapist need to meet to maintain an alliance and avoid undermining splits and competition for the child. Helping parents to make necessary changes in parenting techniques facilitates recovery of a healthy developmental trajectory. Frequently the therapist will need to use his or her dynamic understanding to comprehend the parents' difficulties and conflicts that interfere with their parenting (49).

Beginning the Process of Interpretation

Interpretation is the process whereby the therapist, by expressing in words what he or she has come to understand about the patient's mental life, helps the patient to observe and understand his or her inner life in a new and more complete way (20). The therapist engages the child or adolescent in the act of observation by making *attention statements* (50), comments that draw the patient's conscious attention to the content of his actions or verbalizations. Beginning with nonthreatening content, the therapist provides verbal commentary on the child's play, or enactments within the play, to reflect the child's defenses, judgments, wishes, or anxieties. As the therapeutic alliance develops, the therapist begins to draw the patient's attention to coincidences, paradoxes, and remarkable absences of affects, topics, or persons who ought to be central to the child's experience.

Middle Phase

Whereas the opening and termination phases of therapy may last several weeks to months, the middle phase of treatment lasts months to years. Intrapsychic structure is created or remodeled, new defenses are developed, and old patterns of response are relinquished during the middle phase.

The Child in the Middle Phase

The middle phase begins when the patient has taken in the structure of the treatment: the therapist's nonjudgmental attitude, regularity of appointment times, and maintenance of confidentiality. The patient implicitly knows that a goal of the treatment is to understand the way she or he feels and behaves, that everything she or he says or does can be considered in the therapy. The child's play or the older child's conversation and behavior are part of the associative process revealing the patient's intrapsychic state. The transition in late childhood and early adolescence from playing in therapy to sitting and talking reflects a developmental move from expression through action to enhanced verbal communication. Often in this transitional stage, the patient will fiddle with objects in the office; draw or play cards; or bring in homework, magazines, or a pocket full of gadgets to allow an action outlet that is non-threatening in its pullback toward child's play. In this period, the therapist needs to allow the patient to establish a comfortable blend of action and verbal expression while being alert for the ways in which either might be used as a resistance.

Resistance is an inevitable aspect of a psychodynamic therapeutic process. Lewis and Blotcky (51) describe three categories of resistance: active, passive, and compliant. The actively resistant patient expresses overt objections to the treatment, such as opposition to coming to appointments and complaints about interference in his or her life. The passively resistant youth may be stubbornly silent, withholding, and plead boredom. The compliant patient is described as eager to do the right things, to give lip service but without emotional engagement. These may be thought of as "macroresistances," appearing as an overarching response to treatment. One also finds "microresistances," moment-to-moment rejections of the therapist's offered interpretations. The child may demonstrate these by shutting down, a sudden shift of focus or behavior, or an eruption of disinhibited behavior. By observing these microresistances, the therapist can measure the intensity of the superego in opposing awareness of the mental contents the therapist was seeking to bring to the patient's conscious awareness or the weakness of the ego when it loses control of the drive.

The patient continues to develop a relationship with the therapist during this middle phase. A true transference occurs when the patient experiences in the current relationship with the therapist fixated conflicts, superego projections, and object representations that stem from previous experiences with the parents. The transference is affected and modified by the developmental achievements or delays of the patient. The child patient differs from the adult patient because the child is still living with the parents, who continue to exert influence over the patient. The patient may make a simple, current displacement of the parents onto the therapist rather than a deep transference to the therapist. In addition to the emerging transference, the quality of the real relationship with the therapist is important. The child is not the social equal of the therapist because the child is still a child relating to the therapist as a child to an adult (52). The youth's experience with an adult who respects the child or adolescent's inner life and demonstrates an approach to understanding and managing that inner life contributes significantly to the therapeutic outcome of individual psychodynamic therapy.

It is important not to underestimate the contribution to the therapeutic process of the child's play and verbal self-expression. The play and verbalizations, by expressing heretofore-unconscious mental contents in conscious communications of speech and action, make meaning and offer an opportunity for active mastery of components of the patient's problems apart from the effect of the specific interventions of the therapist (53).

The Therapist's Mental Process

The gap between the therapist's theoretical understanding of the moment-to-moment content of the therapy sessions and what it is possible to do or say at the developmental level of the child is more evident in child psychotherapy than in work with adults. Lewis describes the multistep process by which the therapist, while keeping up the play with the child, takes "mental distance," places the immediate observations into an ongoing formulation, develops an interpretation, brings the interpretation back, and presents it to the child in the context of the play or conversation (52). For many years, interpretation was seen as the *sine qua non* of psychodynamic treatment. Recently, attention has been given to ways in which the therapist may offer developmental help or assistance rather than an interpretation (54). The choice of interpretation versus developmental assistance will be made on the basis of the formulation, particularly the assessment of ego development as age appropriate or lagging in development.

The therapist's interest is neither limited to nor primarily focused on the factual content of the patient's productions in the session. Even when a patient in late childhood or adolescence presents a narrative of an external event, the therapist listens for the defensive regulation of affect and drive in the narrative as well as the accuracy or potential distortions in the presentation of relationships. The therapist also assesses the patient's ability or inability to see multiple sides of the story. Referencing earlier material, the therapist considers what patterns emerge. The therapist may begin to formulate a reconstruction by thinking about how these patterns reflect a repetition of defenses and attitudes fixated by past trauma. The psychodynamic therapist continually monitors the patient's utilization of the therapist. Is the transference being manifested or is the patient turning passive into active and letting the therapist know what it feels like to be on the receiving end? Non-narrative material is as useful in psychodynamic therapy as is narrative. In non-narrative play, the therapist observes where shifts and disruptions in the play occur in response either to frustration or the emergence of strong emotions or thoughts the child finds unacceptable.

The Therapist's Interventions

The basic process of constructing interpretations was laid out by Loewenstein (55) and is explored comprehensively by Lewis in "The therapeutic relationship and the technique of interpretation: The use of play in psychodynamic therapy" (52). Interpretations may be classified as *clarifications, defense interpretations, and reconstructions. Clarifications* bring the patient's attention to bear on his or her characteristic patterns of action and interaction but do not imply a reason for the pattern. A *defense interpretation* picks up on the drive derivative (e.g., rivalry as an aggressive drive derivative) and points out that a defense has been instituted. The drive derivative has been changed in a way that makes it manageable and acceptable to the superego (rivalry becomes the avoidance of competition). The therapist should address the defense before addressing the drive derivative when making a defense interpretation (8). The defense is acceptable to the patient. It is ego-syntonic. Drawing the patient's attention to the defense reminds the patient that he or she has a way to manage the affect or drive derivative. The patient will be more likely to tolerate looking back at the intolerable drive or affect from this position of strength.

A *reconstruction* is an interpretation that explains current feelings, thoughts, and behaviors in terms of critical past events in the patient's life or fantasies from an earlier stage of development. Reconstructions are only offered late in the therapy process. The clinical decision to offer a reconstruction to a child or adolescent requires weighing the patient's capacity to use it to "make sense" of perplexing feelings and behaviors (56). A reconstruction can be helpful to a child when it clarifies an essentially correct perception by the child at the time of the trauma that has subsequently undergone distortion (52). The therapist must consider whether a reconstruction is premature. A child too close to the trauma will reject the reconstruction in order to defend against the affects and drives the reference stirs. A reconstruction may be intellectualized or rejected because it arouses unmanageable shame or guilt.

Developmental help or assistance is a technique of psychodynamic psychotherapy with children and adolescents that has been used for decades but is only being written about and defined recently. Developmental assistance may be seen as a precursor needed to build ego capacities that will eventually allow the patient to use the play process and interpretation to gain self-understanding. Yanof (54) describes working with 7-year-old Robert, who lacked perseverance and frustration tolerance leading to poor performance in school where he had difficulty learning to read. Through much of the treatment he could use imaginative play to express his feelings of anger and unlovableness. As the summer break in treatment approached Robert had undertaken to build Lego models:

> Whenever Robert came to something difficult, he began to complain that he could not do it—that he was not smart enough to do it. He immediately demanded that I do it for him. I made a technical decision not to do it for him but to support his plan to build the object. I did not interpret conflict, but I told him that learning how to do things was hard work and it made everyone feel like giving up. At times I gave him strategies. Much of the time he was angry at me for not doing enough. However, when he finally finished the project, he was elated (54).

Yanof was aware that Robert was lagging behind in his ability to join in his peers' pursuits and function competently. She used her skills to help him increase his frustration tolerance and experience a new competence.

The psychodynamic therapist must select the optimal context in addition to the level of interpretation. In play therapy, the therapist decides whether to work within the play utilizing the defensive protection displacement affords or to comment more directly to the child (53). The relationship between the child and therapist is a context for interpreting transference or externalization, clarifying the real, nontransference, relationship, and offering developmental assistance. Working in the play or in the patient–therapist relationship focuses the work on events inside the treatment setting, but the focus could be extended to events outside the treatment setting. The patient and therapist can discuss issues or experiences with family, peers, or school. Finally, the temporal focus may be on the past, present, or future.

Work with Parents in the Middle Phase

Success of an individual psychodynamic therapy with a child or adolescent often rests on the therapist's skill in the collateral work with the parents. The therapist must come to understand the parents' fantasies and fears about therapy, their child, and themselves as parents. Parents may come with the attitude that the therapist will redeem them from past transgressions that have affected the child, or hope that the therapist will rescue the child. Alternatively, parents may see the therapist as a rival for the child's affection or as an authority figure seeking to find fault or blame the parent. Even with the most dysfunctional parent, the therapist seeks to ally with the parent's wish to be a good parent and supports the parent in those efforts. Many parents find referral for their own individual treatment beneficial. Where there is marital conflict the therapist tactfully explores its role in the child's difficulties. If marital therapy is indicated the parents should be referred to an appropriate clinician in order to maximize the parents' effectiveness in their parenting role, minimize the possibility that the marital conflict will disrupt the child's treatment, and protect the therapist's primary relationship with the child.

In "Problems of termination in child analysis," Anna Freud (57) lists parental reasons for terminating treatment sooner than the Hampstead Child-Therapy Clinic recommended. Parents may be satisfied when presenting symptoms have resolved but the therapist is aware that the underlying pathologic conflicts are not stabilized. Or the parents cannot tolerate transitory oppositional behaviors of the child whose therapeutic developmental gains lead to a newly achieved autonomy.

Parent work in the middle phase has the tasks of (a) facilitating the flow of information from the parents about the child; (b) counseling and educating parents both about sensitive issues in parenting and the particular child's diagnosis, strengths, and vulnerabilities; and (c) assisting parents in advocating for the child and in case management (58).

The therapist must always plan interventions with parents in the context of what the therapist knows of the parents' own issues and needs. Suggestions must be given with cautious awareness that parents may resist giving up a parenting behavior or pattern of relationship with the child either because it is gratifying for the parent or represents a parental defense against negative or aggressive impulses. If such resistances are present or the parent's own conflicts can be shown to destabilize the child's progress in the therapy, the therapist has the additional task of skillfully counseling and educating the parent (27) or assisting the parent to undertake therapy for herself or himself.

In line with more recent innovations in attachment theory and mentalization, Novick and Novick (49) have developed a novel and acclaimed psychoanalytic framework for working with parents. They list the tasks and challenges for parents across different developmental stages, the parents' conflicts around those tasks, and the defenses that are used in managing those conflicts, which the therapist addresses with defense analysis, interpretation, and the use of transference. This allows the parents to work through what is interfering with aspects of their psychological parenting. Each phase of treatment presents parents with new tasks, the accomplishment of which consolidates progressive psychological development in the parents and the child. Both the child and the parents learn to internalize the therapeutic alliance in ways that foster their alliance with each other, which helps the parents view the child through a developmental lens (59).

Closing Phase

The closing phase presents two distinct tasks: the decision to conclude the treatment and the *termination process* by which the treatment is ended. The psychiatrist's ability to maintain the working alliance with the patient and parents consolidates the patient's therapeutic gains and enables the patient or family to seek help in the future if needed.

The Decision to Stop Treatment

Because intensive psychodynamic therapy with children and adolescents is a three-way contract (60) between therapist, child, and parents, the conclusion may be initiated by any one, two, or all three of the parties. The optimal termination situation is for all three to concur that the goals of treatment have been met. Premature terminations occur when there is a decision to end the therapy before the treatment goals have been met. There are two types of premature termination: disruption and interruption. Disruption refers to the decision to end the treatment because of external factors affecting any of the three parties. For example, the family may be moving or the therapist may be leaving the treatment facility. Interruption refers to a unilateral decision by one of the parties to end the treatment based on intrapsychic factors such as parents' unexamined intrapsychic conflicts aroused by the therapy. In all terminations, and particularly in the case of premature terminations, the therapist must be alert to the patient's fantasies about the reasons for ending the treatment so that they can be worked on during the termination process.

In initiating the termination process, the therapist considers the patient's ability to maintain the gains of treatment and grow in the family despite parental difficulties, the extent to which "developmental forces have been set free again and are ready to take over," (57) and the progress the patient has made in internal consolidation of intrapsychic changes. The process of consolidation of intrapsychic changes is called *working-through* (52,61). Psychoanalysis strives for a therapeutic process based on self-observation, self-awareness, and insight. Insight, according to Anna Freud, "does not occur without a working-through process," defined as the elaboration and extension into different contexts and directions of relevant interpretations. The tracing of anxieties resulting from the child's infantile perception of the world and correction of distortions of perception that were caused by the immaturity of the child's cognitive apparatus are included in her concept of working-through (26).

The Termination Process

All psychotherapies have a termination phase regardless of theoretical orientation (51). Psychoanalysts give particular attention to this phase of treatment. The understanding gained of the meaning and psychological challenges to the patient inherent in "saying goodbye" are useful to the clinician in managing the conclusion of any doctor–patient relationship.

At the theoretical level, termination is conceptualized as an experience of separation and loss. The patient, parents, and therapist bring their own characteristic approaches to separation and loss to the process. Although the therapist's attention is primarily on the patient, countertransference reactions may be triggered by the loss of the patient as a real-life object. It is essential to evaluate and address the parents' needs in the face of the impending loss of the therapist as an ally.

The intrapsychic tasks for the patient are the resolution of the transference relationship and relinquishing of the real relationship with the therapist. The transference reaction to termination is colored by the patient's previous experiences with separation and loss. Ego functions may regress and symptoms recur. The therapist works to help the child verbalize feelings and ideas about the impending change and work through these reactions in light of the patient's current capacities, those appropriate to the patient's developmental level, and those gained in therapy. As the patient relinquishes the real relationship with the therapist, the therapist aids the patient to internalize the therapist's functions so that the patient may carry on in developing self-understanding, particularly an ability to tolerate and examine internal conflicts and ambivalence.

The technical and practical approaches to termination are designed to promote the theoretical goals. The therapist engages the patient in *active* planning and execution of the termination seeking to avoid repetition of *passive* experiences of loss (e.g., loss of parental attention with the birth of a sibling). First, the reasons for concluding the treatment must be acknowledged and the treatment goals, child's achievements, and remaining concerns reviewed, allowing the clinician, patient, and parents to gauge the patient's reaction to the impending loss. Typical reactions of children and adolescents faced with the proposition of ending therapy are (a) fear, anger, aggression, or depression; (b) return of symptoms; (c) recapitulation of the themes of the therapy; (d) adoption of the "plan" presented; and (e) a bid not to end the therapy (51).

Next, logistics of termination are addressed. Logistics include setting the date for the last session, deciding whether to make a clean break or a gradual diminution in the frequency of sessions, and clarifying follow-up plans. General guidelines for these decisions are tailored to the needs of the particular patient.

The clinician works to avoid precipitous endings without enough time to say goodbye and work through the patient's reactions. Optimally, the patient chooses the date by working with the therapist to understand why the patient feels one date is more suitable than another. A date at a natural time of separation, such as the end of the school year or the Christmas vacation, tends to downplay the reality of the termination. This may be desirable in some circumstances but may compromise a full working-through of the termination.

Following the model of adult psychoanalysis, many clinicians assume that therapy should be continued at the established intensity until the final session and stopped with no planned follow-up or contact. Anna Freud seriously questioned this approach with children and adolescents (26). She observed that, when normal development is achieved, the child detaches himself or herself in the course of time, just as children move on from teachers and even friends. Therefore, she recommended allowing the child to reduce the frequency of visits or schedule a follow-up visit.

Classical adult psychoanalysis leaves follow-up contact up to the patient. Early follow-up is regarded as evidence of the patient's failure to resolve the transference relationship. With children and adolescents who are in psychotherapy, not analysis, one must be aware that one is working two steps removed from classical adult analysis. In conditions of significant ongoing pathology, either constitutional in the child or endemic in the family, one is well advised to establish a follow-up plan. Even in less severe cases, follow-up offers several potential benefits: reinforcement of treatment gains, assessment of any possible deterioration, maintenance of the therapist–patient relationship, as well as providing valuable communication between parents, clinicians, and teachers (51). Follow-up is also beneficial for the clinician to learn more about the effectiveness of the treatment. Whether or not the clinician initiates follow-up contact, it is important for the patient to feel free to return.

RESEARCH

It is perhaps in the area of research that psychodynamic psychotherapy with children and adolescents has made the greatest gains in the past 20 years. Child psychotherapy began with the advent of psychoanalysis and the observation of children used to clarify the developmental origins of adult psychopathology, namely with Freud's 1909 publication of the case most commonly known as "Little Hans" (4). As important as this interest in developmental origins was, the research method Freud applied to the study of mental disturbances has important shortcomings by today's standards. Born out of the 19th-century Darwinian tradition of naturalistic observation, Freud's methods permitted independent evaluators to compare their findings and accumulate a remarkable and revolutionary body of theories of mental functions and their connections to behavior and to symptoms. However, in the current era of evidence-based medicine, this discipline could not continue to ignore the need for a vibrant research community to test its clinical practices and underlying assumptions.

Moving away from the case report, the emphasis in psychodynamic research has shifted to empirical research. Yet psychodynamic research retains an emphasis that is true to its underlying theoretical base. The perception that evidence-based research supporting psychodynamic psychotherapy has lagged behind other fields has likely developed from an important core discrepancy between psychoanalytic and psychodynamic research compared to research in other psychotherapy modalities: treatment interventions are designed to assess and change psychic structure and overall well-being, not only symptoms and behaviors which are easier to tangibly measure. Additionally, the focus of treatment is frequently relational, whether in the child–parent dyad or the patient–therapist dyad. Much of psychodynamic research has been aimed at those who struggle with adversity in a psychosocial context rather than with specific diagnoses. This is in keeping with the holistic trend in psychodynamic psychiatry that favors a biopsychosocial model over a more narrowly biomedical disease model for clinical formulations. Although in recent years the advance in short-term manualized treatments has shown improvement in specific symptom reduction, it is important to keep in mind that at its heart, psychoanalysis and psychodynamic psychotherapy cannot always be boiled down to improving symptoms of specific diagnoses.

The Case Report

The case report will likely continue to have a role in the development and dissemination of psychodynamic psychotherapy practice for the treatment of children and adolescents. This is not just because of the deep attachment of psychodynamic psychotherapists to reporting their findings in this manner, but also because it is much less expensive than mounting multisubject studies that aim to achieve statistical significance. The strengths of the case report are its ability to portray the subject in all its complexity in a manner that is compelling to clinicians and lends itself to comparison with the clinicians' own cases.

A major disadvantage of case reports is the difficulty accounting for the bias introduced by the subjectivity of the clinician's perceptions, memory, and interpretation of the clinical data. There is also the concern that the clinician's awareness of an intention to write about the case will influence how the clinical material is heard. Further distortion may be introduced by attempts to disguise the case or otherwise protect the patient's confidentiality. Increasingly, patient permission is sought for publication of case material, but this practice also constrains what the clinician is willing to write.

Evidence-Based Outcome Studies

In the 1950s and 1960s, researchers reviewing the available studies of psychotherapy questioned whether outcome was affected by treatment at all. Partially in response to this challenge, overall research methodology improved, with better specification of the therapies through manualization and clearer definition of patient characteristics. With these improvements, the data support the basic tenet that psychotherapy improves outcome. Examination of the results of four meta-analyses of youth treatment outcomes published between 1985 and 1995 concluded that "the average treated youth scored better than more than three-fourths of control group youths on outcome measures at the end of treatment" (62). However, very few of the treatments deemed psychodynamic in these studies met basic criteria for that label. Many lacked an established psychodynamic theoretical framework or trained therapists. For the very few that did truly warrant designation as psychodynamic, the effect sizes were comparable with those for cognitive–behavioral treatments (63).

The Anna Freud Centre, formerly the Hampstead Clinic, has promoted psychoanalytic research since its founding in 1940. The Hampstead Indexing Project (64) established a charting requirement that had clinicians record the clinical data along several constructs critical to psychoanalysis, producing charts unmatched for their quantity and quality of clinical information. In the early 1990s, Mary Target and Peter Fonagy conducted a retrospective chart review of 763 cases, representing 90% of the cases treated at the Centre. Although the study is limited by its retrospective design, it is unlikely ever to be matched for the size of its sample, and represents one of the earliest evidence bases for psychodynamic and psychoanalytic therapy for children and adolescents.

These studies shed some light on which children might be expected to benefit from long-term psychodynamic psychotherapies. Focusing on anxious or depressive disorders, they found 352 charts (65). Seventy-two percent of those youths treated for at least 6 months showed reliable, clinically significant improvement in adaptation. Only 24% of cases had a diagnosable disorder at termination. Children under the age of 11 were significantly more likely to be well at the end of treatment than were older children. More frequent sessions led to greater improvement, independent of the child's age or length of treatment. Intensive treatment, defined as four or five times per week psychoanalysis, was significantly more helpful for children who presented with more severe disturbance, multiple diagnoses, or pervasive impairment affecting social, emotional, or cognitive functioning. Looking at demographic factors, those who were most likely to improve had higher IQ, younger age, longer treatment, good peer relations, poor overall adjustment of mother, anxiety symptoms in the mother, and absence of history of maternal antisocial behavior.

The Anna Freud Centre retrospective chart review compared four to five times per week psychoanalysis with one to three time per week psychodynamic psychotherapy. Either intensity of treatment was undertaken with an open-ended approach to length of treatment. Children under 12 benefited more from the four to five times per week treatments than from those of lesser intensity. However, adolescents, particularly neurotic adolescents, did better with the less intense therapy. In this study, 72% of children with emotional disorders who stayed in treatment for more than 6 months showed reliable, clinically significant improvement in adaptation (66). Further study of the effects of intensity and duration of treatment is necessary if we are to apply resources in a cost-effective manner.

An important question generated by outcome studies on psychodynamic psychotherapies is whether there is a "sleeper effect." Do patients continue to improve on outcome measures months to years after the cessation of the treatment? Continued accrual of benefit is seen in studies of adults treated with psychodynamic psychotherapy (67,68), and psychodynamic psychotherapy can lead to improvements in the long-term outcome of adults with treatment-resistant depression in regards to self-reported depression scores, observer-based ratings, and measures of social adjustment (69). Psychodynamic researchers and clinicians find in the sleeper effect support for the assumption that addressing underlying psychological processes and moving a patient to a more mature and adaptive level of function will bring lasting benefit, while removing target symptoms may bring only transitory relief. Furthermore, demonstration of continued return on the investment made in a therapy directed at deeper structures can support the cost-effectiveness of treatments that may take considerable investment in therapist training at the front end.

Reviews and Meta-Analyses

Beginning in the 21st century, the obvious need for evidence-based practices helped spur further research in operationalizing and manualizing psychodynamic therapy. As is typical for research, new studies started with adults, culminating in Jonathan Shedler's 2010 paper, 'The Efficacy of Psychodynamic Psychotherapy' in *The American Psychologist* (70). This helped pave the way for similar research in the child and adolescent population. Previously, there had been insufficient studies to perform a meta-analysis of psychodynamic psychotherapy in children and adolescents. Midgley and Kennedy, in 2011 (71), were among the first to show an increasing evidence base for psychodynamic work in children and adolescents. Their review yielded 34 studies focusing on the efficacy and effectiveness of individual child and adolescent psychodynamic psychotherapy, including 9 randomized controlled trials (RCTs) focusing on anorexia, PTSD, disruptive disorders, depression, BPD, and mixed diagnoses. Their conclusion was that although there was some evidence to support the effectiveness of psychoanalytic and psychodynamic psychotherapy in young people, the studies have been of limited scale and number. One exception was studies evaluating time-limited or short-term psychodynamic psychotherapy (STPP), particularly for depression, which had an increasing body of evidence to test increasingly precise hypotheses, likely due to the repeatability of time-limited interventions. Midgley and Kennedy's review also yielded support for the sleeper effect phenomenon, noting that a pattern of more gradual, but sustained and continued improvement was noted with children receiving psychodynamic psychotherapy compared to those receiving cognitive-behavioral therapy (CBT).

Abbass et al. (72) focused on STPP for children and adolescents in their meta-analysis published in *JAACAP*. After review and selection, 11 randomized trials or RCTs met the inclusion criteria, published between 1989 and 2010, 9 of them in 1999 or later. Three studies focused on anxiety disorders; another three focused on personality or behavior problems; one investigated mood disorders; and the remaining four studies included participants with mixed mental disorders. STPP was compared to a total of 13 comparator conditions: 7 studies compared STPP to another type of psychotherapy; 3 studies compared STPP to standard care; and 3 studies compared STPP to minimal contact or waitlist controls. The mean treatment dose in the STPP conditions ranged from 10 to 40 sessions. STPP for children and adolescents yielded large effects overall, which was consistent over almost all outcome domains with the largest effects being for general and somatic complaints, medium to large effects for anxiety, mood, and personality/personality conditions, and only small effects for interpersonal problems. However, the diversity of conditions studied may be a better reflection of real-world outcomes, and speaks to the potentially broad utility of the approach. As previously suggested, follow-up analyses revealed a "sleeper effect," in that effects increased after termination of treatment in each outcome domain, suggesting further accrual of gains over time. This again supports the notion that changes made by psychodynamic and psychoanalytic interventions are persistent over time.

Depression and Anxiety

The work of Muratori et al. (73) uses an active treatment versus community services model to examine the short- and long-term effects of time-limited psychodynamic psychotherapy for children meeting criteria for depressive or anxiety disorders. There was no difference on the C-GAS between the experimental group and the comparison group at baseline. No group differences emerged on the CBCL in the first 6 months, whereas at 2-year follow-up only the experimental group improved significantly in all summary scales. The authors describe this continued improvement as a sleeper effect, as previously mentioned, an emerging phenomena in the study of psychodynamic psychotherapies. The authors also noted that patients who received psychodynamic psychotherapy were significantly less likely to seek further treatment than were the community-treated comparison patients. This finding suggests that savings on future treatment may offset costs over time for the psychodynamic therapy group.

Zhou et al. (74) performed a meta-analysis comparing efficacy and compatibility of various forms of psychotherapy for depression in children and adolescents. Only prospective RCTs with manualized or structured psychotherapies were included, regardless of the duration of treatment. The meta-analysis concluded that psychodynamic therapy was not significantly more effective than waitlist at reducing depressive symptoms. However, there are several limitations to this meta-analysis. Among almost 4,000 patients who participated in 50 RCTs, only 35 patients received psychodynamic therapy, and they all represented one study. Additionally, this study followed patients for 9 months of treatment, whereas all of the other studies, such was with CBT and interpersonal psychotherapy (IPT), were conducted in a range of 4 to 16 weeks.

The singular study representing psychodynamic psychotherapy included in the Zhou meta-analysis was the 2007 study by Trowell et al. (75) which compared psychodynamic psychotherapy to family therapy for depression in children ages 9 to 15. Treatment was conducted over 9 months, with 72 patients separated to either 16 to 30 50-minute individual therapy sessions, or 8 to 14 90-minute family therapy sessions. The individual psychodynamic psychotherapy was based on STPP as described by Davanloo (76). In both treatment arms, 75% of patients no longer met criteria for depression when treatment ended. However, at follow-up 6 months later, 100% of the individual therapy patients no longer met criteria for depression, compared to 80% in the family therapy group. Additionally, 11% of the family therapy group was lost to follow up, compared to zero in the individual therapy group. This data supports the aforementioned sleeper effect, suggesting that individual psychodynamic therapy continues to elicit an ongoing response even following completion of the therapy. The authors suggest that those who participated in individual therapy experienced further improvement that followed the end of the treatment, which may be more clinically relevant that treatment gains achieved in only the first 4 to 16 weeks as in the other studies.

Midgley's group, moving on from their aforementioned review of clinical trials (71), are in the process of steering a large-scale clinical trial in the United Kingdom, the Improving Mood with Psychoanalytic and Cognitive-Behavioral Therapy (IMPACT) Study (77). This study aims to be the largest clinical trial examining psychodynamic psychotherapy with children and adolescents, and is an RCT based on the authors' treatment manual for STPP for adolescents with moderate to severe depression, which is currently in press (78).

The *Manual of Panic-Focused Psychodynamic Psychotherapy* (PFPP) developed by Milrod et al. (79) at Cornell University Medical College is a 12-week, 24-session individual psychodynamic psychotherapy emphasizing unconscious thought, free association, and the centrality of transference. The hypothesis underlying PFPP is that common psychodynamic conflicts in panic disorder involve difficulties with separation and independence as well as recognition and management of anger and sexual excitement. These issues are addressed as they arise in the sessions and particularly as they arise in the transference under the pressure of impending termination. Looking separately at the results for patients 18 to 21 years of age showed that these late adolescents, or young adults, did well with PFPP (80). The research team has developed a manual for the treatment of adolescents (PFPP-A) (81). The major changes from the adult version focus on a psychodynamic approach to the work with the adolescent's family and the particular countertransference issues adolescents generate.

Child and Adolescent Anxiety Psychodynamic Psychotherapy (CAPP) is a newer, manualized, twice weekly treatment for children ages 8 to 16 with primary diagnoses of generalized anxiety disorder, social anxiety disorder, or separation anxiety disorder. Much akin to the traditional psychoanalytic process, treatment is broken down into three phases encompassing up to 24 sessions. This approach assumes that anxiety symptoms represent psychological meanings that can be identified by exploring fantasies and feelings related to the symptoms (82).

A German group at the University of Leipzig manualized a short-term psychodynamic treatment program for 4- to 10 year olds with anxiety disorders, Psychoanalytic Child Therapy

(PaCT) (83). PaCT comprises 20 to 25 weekly sessions during which therapist, parents, and child collaborate to identify and modify core conflicts underlying the child's symptoms and family dysfunction. In their pilot study of 30 children randomized to PaCT or wait list, two-thirds of the treatment group were in full remission after treatment (average 40 weeks) compared to zero in the waitlist. After the waitlist families received the treatment, the team collected follow-up data from 25 families after 6 months, 22 of which showed complete diagnostic remission.

Medical Illnesses

In the early 1990s, Moran and Fonagy (84) used success of diabetic control, as manifested in HbA1C levels and other physiologic tests, as an outcome measure for the efficacy of a brief, intensive psychoanalytic psychotherapy for adolescents with insulin-dependent diabetes. Both the treatment and control groups manifested significant psychiatric symptoms on psychological assessment. The treatment group showed considerable improvement in diabetic control on HbA1C, both at the 3-month and 1-year follow-ups, while the control group returned to pretreatment levels. The most interesting aspect of this study from the perspective of psychotherapy efficacy measurement is its use of a physiologic marker for the measurement of outcome. In this way, the investigators sidestepped debates about the relevance to psychoanalytically oriented treatments of currently available psychological measurements of change. More clinical research projects are underway aimed at addressing parental traumatic stress and strengthening mentalization capacities to increase the parents' emotional availability to their medically ill children (85).

Trauma

Like the diabetes study, the work of Trowell et al. (86) on psychodynamic psychotherapy for sexually abused girls focuses on youths struggling with a significant life stress rather than treatment for a specific psychiatric diagnosis. However, psychiatric disorder was common among the total of 81 girls who were assessed at baseline: posttraumatic stress disorder in 73%, major depression in 57%, generalized anxiety disorder in 37%, and separation anxiety disorder in 58%. Seventy-one girls, ages 6 to 14 years, who had experienced sexual abuse were enrolled as they presented for treatment at two clinics in London. Random assignment was made to the study treatment of an individual psychodynamic psychotherapy or a comparison group therapy that combined psychotherapeutic discussion of relationships with psychoeducational topic-focused sessions. The psychotherapy consisted of weekly sessions of manualized, nondirective, psychodynamic psychotherapy. The child's or adolescent's caregiver was seen about every 2 weeks for support and guidance. Both treatment groups showed a substantial reduction in psychopathological symptoms and an improvement in functioning, but with no evident difference between individual and group therapy. However, individual therapy led to greater improvement in severity of PTSD and "persistent avoidance of stimuli" measures on the PTSD scales.

Attachment Difficulties in Mother-Infant Dyads

The dyadic treatment of mothers and their preschool children is an area in which research on psychodynamic interventions is moving forward. This research brings together the work of Bowlby, Ainsworth, and Main on the quality of attachment of infants and toddlers to their caregivers with the work of Selma Fraiberg and her collaborators on the intergenerational transmission of internal representations, aggressive conflicts, and negative self-representations (87). The work of Toth et al. (88) at the University of Rochester testing preschooler–parent psychotherapy (PPP) and of Lieberman, Van Horn, and Ippen at the University of California–San Francisco evaluating child–parent psychotherapy (CPP) are fine examples of this active area of research.

Toth et al. (88) took as their study population maltreated preschoolers and their mothers. Mothers and their preschoolers receiving PPP were seen for weekly, 60-minute, dyadic sessions with a trained therapist, usually at the treatment center but with occasional home visits. The interventions focused on the mother's reflective functioning—the mother's capacity to make sense of her child's internal experience and to understand the child's internal mental states. Increased capacity for reflective functioning allows the mother to anticipate and react appropriately to her child. By using observations and empathic comments, the therapist assists the mother in recognizing how her internal representations are enacted during her interactions with her preschooler. Although the therapist's interactions with the child may provide a model of adult–child interaction, no effort is made to be didactic or explicitly instructive. The therapist seeks to respond to maternal utterances and interactional patterns, linking current maternal conceptualizations of relationships to mothers' own experience of care in childhood.

Lieberman, Van Horn, and Ippen's CPP (89) also takes the mother–child dyad, rather than an individual child patient, as the treatment unit. As with PPP, CPP, a treatment developed for preschoolers exposed to marital violence, draws on attachment theory and the work of Fraiberg. CPP consists of weekly parent–child sessions for 1 year, during which the therapist's interventions are guided by the unfolding child–mother interactions and by the child's free play with developmentally appropriate toys selected to encourage social interaction and to elicit trauma play. The therapist seeks to guide the mother and child in creating a joint narrative of the traumatic events they experienced. Additionally, the therapist seeks to change maladaptive behaviors and support developmentally appropriate interactions between mother and child. Children assigned to CPP improved significantly more than children receiving the community treatment. Children in the test treatment demonstrated decreased total behavioral problems and decreased traumatic stress disorder. Newer attachment-based treatment programs, such as the Mothers and Toddlers Program (a 20-week intervention for substance-abusing mothers) and the Peaceful School Project are good examples of contemporary attachment-based psychodynamic interventions helping children and families in specific clinical or environmental contexts. There is a growing evidence base to support dyadic, parent–child implementation of psychodynamic psychotherapy for a wide range of contexts (90).

Eating Disorders

Although family-based therapeutic treatments have long been the treatment of choice, and perhaps the gold standard of treating adolescents with eating disorders, there is some evidence to suggest that psychodynamic psychotherapy can be effective. In the treatment of 12 to 19 year olds with anorexia nervosa, psychodynamic psychotherapy was found to be comparable to family-based treatment after 12 to 18 months in regards to achieving target weight. An independent study comparing psychodynamic psychotherapy to family-based therapy showed that age was a significant moderator, with older patients benefiting more from individual therapy and younger patient benefiting more from family-based therapy, in both short- and long-term follow-up (91). Psychodynamically informed therapies, including family-based therapies, represent an important option for young people, although further research is needed (92).

Mentalization-Based Treatment of Adolescents (MBT-A) and Emerging Borderline Personality Disorder

As previously discussed, mentalization refers to the ability to understand human behavior as it relates to internal feeling states. Mentalization links psychodynamic and attachment theory with developmental and neuroscientific research. An inability to mentalize may be linked to disordered self-experience and incapacity to understand and relate with others in socially and emotionally meaningful ways. Neuroimaging studies have shown that the capacity to mentalize can be affected by stress and arousal in the context of attachment relationships (15). A growing body of literature suggests that disruptions in mentalizing are a core feature in adolescents' increased susceptibility to developing affective dysregulation, impulsivity, and instability in relationships and self-image that are much akin to the clinical syndrome of BPD. Mentalizing-Based Treatment for Borderline Personality Disorder (MBT-BPD) in adults now has a substantial literature base; that for MBT-A is preliminary, but promising (15). The objective in all mentalization-based treatments is for patients and families to discover how they think and feel about themselves, others, and their relationships, how thoughts and feelings give meaning to behavior and actions, and how disruptions in this process lead to maladaptive behavior and unstable relationships. As often is the case, assisting families in this process alongside the adolescents may be crucial, as a coercive, nonmentalizing interactions in families can reinforce maladaptive behavior in these adolescents.

MBT-A has been evaluated in adolescents who meet criteria for BPD, engage in self-harm or other self-destructive behaviors. Rossouw and Fonagy (45) manualized a year-long treatment program with weekly individual and monthly family sessions aimed at enhancing mentalizing abilities; a 3- to 12-week version for inpatient and partial-hospital programs was also developed by Bleiberg and Williams (93).

Regulation-Focused Psychotherapy for Children (RFP-C) is a manualized psychodynamic approach to children with externalizing behaviors who may be considered to be in the emerging borderline personality category (94). RFP-C is derived from ego psychological approaches to psychodynamic therapy addressing the disruptive behaviors in these poorly regulated children as defenses against affect. This treatment is just beginning pilot studies but is very close to the treatments that did well for children with disruptive behavior in the Anna Freud Centre retrospective studies (95).

Trends and Future

A review by Palmer et al. (90) of RCTs shows a growing body of evidence supporting the use of psychodynamic psychotherapy implemented in family-based contexts, rather than just the more traditional individual therapy, as the family-based treatment may produce quicker results. This is particularly true with children with internalizing disorders. It is likely that family- and parent-focused psychodynamic therapies may make their way to the forefront, and perhaps it is in this mode that psychodynamic psychotherapy may be most at home in the future. Additionally, some suggest that adopting different target measures of improved outcome, such as performance on cognitive activities or physiologic indices, may yield larger effect sizes, and that psychological symptoms are not the only target of psychodynamic psychotherapy.

With technologic advances and increased focus on biomarkers for psychiatric disease and treatment, one wonders if treatment outcomes and predictors for psychodynamic psychotherapy may be discovered through genetic research or neuroimaging. To date, several studies have shown that patients with various psychiatric disorders have improved or normalized neuroimaging findings after psychodynamic psychotherapy (96). Perhaps similar findings are over the horizon.

Furthering the evidence base is designed to inform clinicians in routine practice regarding treatments that offer the best outcomes. Therefore, despite the call for growing numbers of RCTs and meta-analyses, observational studies in the clinic may still play an important role in showing the power of psychodynamic psychotherapy. Edlund and Carlberg of Sweden (97) present results of 218 patients ages 14 to 24 seen from 2002 to 2009 at an institute providing outpatient psychodynamic psychotherapy, using ratings of global functioning from either the therapists or the patients. Improvement was seen across the board. What appears to be most likely is that researchers must follow current trends of what is considered the highest grade evidence to continue proving what is already known: the effectiveness of psychodynamic and psychoanalytic therapies for children, adolescents, and their families for a wide variety of conditions. It appears that future research, growing the body of literature showing that psychodynamic psychotherapy is an effective treatment in children and adolescents, is on the horizon if not already upon us.

References

1. Gabbard G: *Psychodynamic Psychiatry in Clinical Practice.* 4th ed. Washington, DC, American Psychiatric Press, Inc., 2005.
2. Ritvo LB: *Darwin's Influence on Freud: A Tale of Two Sciences.* New Haven, Yale University Press, 1990.
3. Panksepp J, Solms M: What is neuropsychoanalysis? Clinically relevant studies of the minded brain. *Trends Cogn Sci* 16:6–8, 2012.
4. Freud S: Analysis of a phobia in a five-year-old boy. In: Strachey JE (ed): *The Standard Edition of the Complete Psychological Works of Sigmund Freud.* Vol X. London, Hogarth Press, 3–149, 1955.
5. Von Hug-Hellmuth H: On the technique of child analysis. *Int J Psychoanal* 2:287–305, 1921.
6. Klein M: *The Psychoanalysis of Children.* London, Hogarth Press, 1932.
7. Freud A: *The Psycho-analytical Treatment of Children.* London, Imago Publishing, 1946.
8. Freud A: *The Ego and the Mechanisms of Defense.* Vol II. 1966 ed. New York, International Universities Press, Inc., 1936.
9. Freud A: *Normality and Pathology in Childhood: Assessments of Development.* New York, International Universities Press, Inc., 1965.
10. Winnicott DW: *Through Paediatrics to Psycho-analysis.* New York, Basic Books, Inc., 1975.
11. Bowlby J: *Attachment and Loss. Vol 1: Attachment.* New York, Basic Books, Inc., 1969.
12. Bowlby J: *Attachment and Loss. Vol 2: Separation: Anxiety and Anger.* New York, Basic Books, Inc., 1973.
13. Bowlby J: *Attachment and Loss. Vol 3: Loss: Sadness and Depression.* New York, Basic Books, Inc., 1980.
14. Weinberger J, Levy KN: Chapter 30: Psychology. In: Person ES, Cooper A, Gabbard G (eds): *Textbook of Psychoanalysis.* Washington, DC, American Psychiatric Publishing, Inc., 463–477, 2005.
15. Bleiberg E: Mentalizing-based treatment with adolescents and families. *Child Adolesc Psychiatric Clin N Am* 22:295–330, 2013.
16. Allen FH: *Psychotherapy with Children.* New York, Norton, 1942.
17. Rogers CR: The developing character of client-centered therapy. In: Rogers CR (ed): *Client-Centered Therapy: Its Current Practice, Implications, and Theory.* Boston, MA, Houghton Mifflin Company, 3–18, 1951.
18. Axline VM: *Play Therapy.* New York, Ballantine, 1947.
19. Dorfman E: Play therapy. In: Rogers C, (ed): *Client-Centered Therapy.* Boston, MA: Houghton Mifflin, 235–277, 1951.
20. Moore BE, Fine BD: *Psychoanalytic Terms and Concepts.* New Haven, Yale University Press, 1990.
21. Brenner C: *The Mind in Conflict.* New York, International Universities Press, 1982.

22. Kernberg PF, Ritvo R, Keable H; American Academy of Child an Adolescent Psychiatry (AACAP) Committee on Quality Issues (CQI): Practice Parameter for Psychodynamic Psychotherapy with Children. *J Am Acad Child Adolesc Psychiatry* 51:541–557, 2012.
23. Lewis O: Integrated psychodynamic psychotherapy with children. *Child Adolesc Psychiatric Clin N Am* 6:53–68, 1997.
24. Marshall R: Countertransference in the psychotherapy of children and adolescents. *Contemp Psychoanal* 15:595–629, 1979.
25. Winnicott D: Hate in the counter-transference. *Int J Psychoanal* 30:69–74, 1949.
26. Sandler J, Kennedy H, Tyson R: *The Technique of Child Psychoanalysis: Discussions with Anna Freud.* Cambridge, MA, Harvard University Press, 1980.
27. Novick KK, Novick J: *Working with Parents Makes Therapy Work.* Lanham, MD, Jason Aronson, 2005.
28. Gray P: *The Ego and Analysis of Defense.* Northvale, NJ, Jason Aronson Inc., 1994.
29. Edgerton J, Campbell RC, eds: *American Psychiatric Glossary*, 7th ed. Washington, DC, American Psychiatric Press, Inc., 1994.
30. Hartmann H: Comments on the psychoanalytic theory of the ego. *Psychoanal Study Child* 5:74–96, 1950.
31. Ritvo S, Solnit AJ: Instinct theory. In: Moore BE, Fine BD (eds): *Psychoanalysis: The Major Concepts.* New Haven, Yale University Press, 327–333, 1995.
32. Auchincloss E, Samberg E, eds: *Psychoanalytic Terms and Concepts.* New Haven, Yale University Press, 2012.
33. Cabaniss DL, Cherry S, Douglas CJ, Schwartz A: *Psychodynamic Psychotherapy: A Clinical Manual.* Oxford, UK, Wiley-Blackwell, 2011.
34. Compton A: Objects and object relationships. In: Moore B, Fine B (eds): *Psychoanalysis: The Major Concepts.* New Haven, Yale University Press, 433–449:1995.
35. Mahler M: Thoughts about development and individuation. *Psychoanal Study Child* 18:307–324, 1962.
36. Provence S, Ritvo S: Effects of deprivation on institutionalized infants. *Psychoanal Study Child* 17:189–205, 1961.
37. Spitz R: Hospitalism: an inquiry into the genesis of psychiatric conditions in early childhood. *Psychoanal Study Child* 1:53–74, 1945.
38. Kernberg O: Psychoanalytic object relations theories. In: Moore B, Fine B (eds): *Psychoanalysis: The Major Concepts.* New Haven, Yale University Press, 450–462, 1995.
39. Sandler J, Rosenblatt B: The concept of the representational world. *Psychoanal Study Child* 17:128–145, 1962.
40. Mahler MS, Pine F, Bergman A: *The Psychological Birth of the Human Infant: Symbiosis and Individuation.* New York, Basic Books, Inc., 1975.
41. Mitchell SA, Black MJ: *Freud and Beyond: A History of Modern Psychoanalytic Thought.* New York, Basic Books, Inc., 1995.
42. Miller J: *Using Self Psychology in Child Psychotherapy: The Restoration of the Child.* Northvale, NJ, Jason Aronson, 1996.
43. Bateman A, Fonagy P: 8-year follow-up of patients treated for borderline personality disorder: mentalization-based treatment versus treatment as usual. *Am J Psychiatry* 165:631–638, 2008.
44. Bateman A, Fonagy P: Randomized controlled trial of outpatient mentalization-based treatment versus structured clinical management for borderline personality disorder. *Am J Psychiatry* 166:1355–1364, 2009.
45. Rossouw TI, Fonagy P: Mentalization-based treatment for self-harm in adolescents: a randomized controlled trial. *J Am Acad Child Adolesc Psychiatry* 51:1304–1313, 2012.
46. Jellinek MS, McDermott JF: Formulation: putting the diagnosis into a therapeutic context and treatment plan. *J Am Acad Child Adolesc Psychiatry* 43:913–916, 2004.
47. Winters NC, Hanson G, Stoyanova V: The case formulation in child and adolescent psychiatry. *Child Adolesc Psychiatric Clin N Am* 16:111–132, 2007.
48. McConville B: An overview of diagnosis and treatment planning. In: Klykylo W, Kay J, Rube D (eds): *Child Psychiatry.* Philadelphia, PA: W.B. Saunders, 85–103, 1998.
49. Novick KK, Novick J: A new model of techniques for concurrent psychodynamic work with parents and child and adolescent psychotherapy patients. *Child Adolesc Psychiatric Clin N Am* 22:331–350, 2013.
50. Lewis M: Interpretation in child analysis. *J Am Acad Child Adolesc Psychiatry* 13:32–53, 1974.
51. Lewis JM, Blotcky MJ: *Child Therapy: Concepts, Strategies, and Decision Making.* Washington, DC, Brunner/Mazel, 1997.
52. Lewis M: Chapter 79: intensive individual psychodynamic psychotherapy: the therapeutic relationship and the technique of interpretation: the use of play in psychodynamic therapy. In: Lewis M (ed): *Child and Adolescent Psychiatry: A Comprehensive Textbook.* 3rd ed. Philadelphia, PA: Lippincott Williams & Wilkins, 984–992, 2003.
53. Yanof JA: Play technique in psychodynamic psychotherapy. *Child Adolesc Psychiatric Clin N Am* 22:261–282, 2013.
54. Yanof JA: Technique in child analysis. In: Person ES, Cooper A, Gabbard G (eds): *Textbook of Psychoanalysis.* Washington, DC, American Psychiatric Publishing, Inc., 267–280, 2005.
55. Loewenstein R: The problem of interpretation. *Psychoanal Q* 20:1–14, 1951.
56. Kennedy H: Problems in reconstruction in child analysis. *Psychoanal Study Child* 26:386–402, 1971.
57. Freud A: *Problems of termination in child analysis (1970 [1957]). The Writings of Anna Freud.* Vol VII. New York, International Universities Press, Inc, 3–21, 1971.
58. Sperling E: The collateral treatment of parents with children and adolescents in psychotherapy. *Child Adolesc Psychiatric Clin N Am* 6:81–95, 1997.
59. Malberg NT, Mayes LC: The contemporary psychodynamic developmental perspective. *Child Adolesc Psychiatric Clin N Am* 22:33–49, 2013.
60. Novick J: Comments on termination in child, adolescent, and adult analysis. *Psychoanal Study Child* 45:419–436, 1990.
61. Freud S: Remembering, repeating and working-through (Further recommendations on the technique of psycho-analysis II) (1914). In: Strachey JE (ed), Strachey J (trans): *The Standard Edition of the Complete Psychological Works of Sigmund Freud.* Vol XII. London, Hogarth Press, 145–156, 1957.
62. Weisz JR, Hawley KM, Doss AJ: Empirically tested psychotherapies for youth internalizing and externalizing problems and disorders. *Child Adolesc Psychiatric Clin N Am* 13:729–815, 2004.
63. Fonagy P, Target M, Cottrell D, Phillips J, Kurtz Z: *What Works for Whom? A Critical Review of Treatments for Children and Adolescents.* New York, Guilford Press, 2005.
64. Sandler J: Research in psycho-analysis: the Hampstead Index as an instrument of psycho-analytic research. *Int J Psychoanal* 43:287–291, 1962.
65. Target M, Fonagy P: Efficacy of psychoanalysis for children with emotional disorders. *J Am Acad Child Adolesc Psychiatry* 33:361–371, 1994.
66. Target M: The problem of outcome in child psychoanalysis: contributions from the Anna Freud Centre. In: Leuzinger-Bohleber M, Target M (eds): *Outcomes of Psychoanalytic Treatment: Perspectives for Therapists and Researchers.* New York: Brunner-Routledge, 240–251, 2002.
67. Sandell R, Blomberg J, Lazar A, Carlsson J, Broberg J, Schubert J: Varieties of long-term outcome among patients in psychoanalysis and long-term psychotherapy: a review of the findings in the Stockholm Outcome of Psychoanalysis and Psychotherapy Project (STOPPP). *Int J Psychoanal* 81:921–942, 2000.
68. Bateman A, Fonagy P: Treatment of borderline personality disorder with psychoanalytically oriented partial hospitalization: an 18-month follow-up. *Am J Psychiatry* 158:36–42, 2001.
69. Fonagy P, Rost F, Carlyle JA, et al.: Pragmatic randomized controlled trial of long-term psychoanalytic psychotherapy for treatment-resistant depression: the Tavistock Adult Depression Study (TADS). *W Psychiatry* 14:312–321, 2015.
70. Shedler J: The efficacy of psychodynamic psychotherapy. *Am Psychol* 65:98–109, 2010.
71. Midgley N, Kennedy E: Psychodynamic psychotherapy for children and adolescents: a critical review of the evidence base. *J Child Psychother* 37:232–260, 2011.
72. Abbass AA, Rabung S, Leichsenring F, Refseth JS, Midgley N: Psychodynamic psychotherapy for children and adolescents: a meta-analysis of short-term psychodynamic models. *J Am Acad Child Adolesc Psychiatry* 52:863–875, 2013.
73. Muratori F, Picchi L, Bruni G, Patarnello M, Romagnoli G: A two-year follow-up of psychodynamic psychotherapy for internalizing disorders in children. *J Am Acad Child Adolesc Psychiatry* 42:331–339, 2003.
74. Zhou X, Hetrick SE, Cuijpers P, et al.: Comparative efficacy and acceptability of psychotherapies for depression in children and adolescents: a systematic review and network meta-analysis. *W Psychiatry* 14:207–222, 2015.
75. Trowell J, Joffe I, Campbell J, et al.: Childhood depression: a place for psychotherapy: an outcome study comparing individual psychodynamic psychotherapy and family therapy. *Eur Child Adolesc Psychiatry* 16:157–167, 2007.
76. Davanloo H: *Basic Principles and Techniques in Short Term Dynamic Psychotherapy.* New York, Spectrum Publications, 1978.
77. Goodyer IM, Tsancheva S, Byford S, et al.: Improving mood with psychoanalytic and cognitive therapies (IMPACT): a pragmatic effectiveness superiority trial to investigate whether specialized psychological treatment reduces risk for relapse in adolescents with moderate to severe unipolar depression: study protocol for a randomized controlled trial. *Trials* 13:175, 2011. doi: 10.1186/1745-6215-12-175.
78. Cregeen S, Hughes C, Midgley N, Rhode M, Rustin M: *Short-Term Psychoanalytic Psychotherapy for Adolescents with Depression: A Treatment Manual.* New York, Karnac, in press.
79. Milrod B, Busch F, Cooper A, Shapiro T: *Manual of Panic-Focused Psychodynamic Psychotherapy.* Washington, DC, American Psychiatric Press, Inc., 1997.
80. Milrod B, Busch F, Shapiro T: A pilot study of psychodynamic psychotherapy for 18 to 21 year old patients with panic disorder. *Ann Am Soc Adolesc Psychiatry* 29:289–314, 2005.
81. Milrod B, Busch F, Shapiro T: *Psychodynamic Approaches to the Adolescent with Panic Disorder.* Malabar, FL, Krieger Publishing Company, 2004.
82. Silver S, Shapiro T, Milrod B: Treatment of anxiety in children and adolescents using child and adolescent psychodynamic psychotherapy. *Child Adolesc Psychiatric Clin N Am* 22:83–96, 2013.
83. Gottken T, White LO, Klein AM, von Klitzing K: Short-term psychoanalytic child therapy for anxious children: a pilot study. *Psychotherapy* 51:148–158, 2014.

84. Moran G, Fonagy P, Kurtz A, Bolton A, Brook C: A controlled study of the psychoanalytic treatment of brittle diabetes. *J Am Acad Child Adolesc Psychiatry* 30:926–935, 1991.
85. Schwab A, Rusconi-Serpa Schechter DS: Psychodynamic approaches to medically ill children and their traumatically stressed parents. *Child Adolesc Psychiatric Clin N Am* 22:119–139, 2013.
86. Trowell J, Kolvin I, Weeramanthri T, et al.: Psychotherapy for sexually abused girls: psychopathological outcome findings and patterns of change. *Br J Psychiatry* 180:234–247, 2002.
87. Fraiberg S, Adelson E, Shapiro V: Ghosts in the nursery: a psychoanalytic approach to the problems of impaired mother-infant relationships. *J Am Acad Child Adolesc Psychiatry* 14:387–421, 1975.
88. Toth S, Maughan A, Manly JT, Spagnola M, Cicchetti D: The relative efficacy of two interventions in altering maltreated preschool children's representational models: Implications for attachment theory. *Dev Psychopathol* 14:877–908, 2002.
89. Lieberman AF, Van Horn P, Ippen CG: Toward evidence-based treatment: child–parent psychotherapy with preschoolers exposed to marital violence. *J Am Acad Child Adolesc Psychiatry* 44:1241–1248, 2005.
90. Palmer R, Nascimento LN, Fonagy P: The state of the evidence base for psychodynamic psychotherapy for children and adolescents. *Child Adolesc Psychiatric Clin N Am* 22:149–214, 2013.
91. Fonagy P: The effectiveness of psychodynamic psychotherapies: an update. *W Psychiatry* 14:137–150, 2015.
92. Dancyger I, Krakower S, Fornari V: Eating disorders in adolescents: review of treatment studies that include psychodynamically informed therapy. *Child Adolesc Psychiatry Clin N Am* 22:97–117, 2013.
93. Bleiberg E, Rossouw T, Fonagy P: Adolescent breakdown and emerging borderline personality disorder. In: Bateman A, Fonagy P (eds): *Handbook of Mentalizing in Mental Health Practice*. Washington, DC, American Psychiatric Publishing, 463–509, 2012.
94. Hoffman L, Rice T, Prout T: *Manual of Regualtion-Focused Psychotherapy for Children (RFP-C) with Externalizing Behaviors: A Psychodynamic Approach*. New York, Routledge, 2016.
95. Fonagy P, Target M: The efficacy of psychoanalysis for children with disruptive disorders. *J Am Acad Child Adolesc Psychiatry* 33:45–55, 1994.
96. Protopopescu X, Gerber AJ: Bridging the gap between neuroscientific and psychodynamic models in child and adolescent psychiatry. *Child Adolesc Psychiatric Clin N Am* 22:1–31, 2013.
97. Edlund JN, Carlberg G: Psychodynamic psychotherapy with adolescents and young adults: outcome in routine practice. *Clin Child Psychol Psychiatry* 21:66–80, 2016.

CHAPTER 6.2.6 ■ GROUP THERAPY

NANCY E. MOSS, GARY R. RACUSIN, AND CORINNE MOSS-RACUSIN

INTRODUCTION

Group treatment stands as a powerful intervention available to professionals serving the child and adolescent population. The aim of this chapter is to provide an intellectually informed clinical guide to implementation of this modality of treatment. The chapter begins by placing group therapy in a historical context and considering aspects of group development. A theoretical framework for group treatment is then discussed, followed by examination of the many pragmatic issues to be managed in offering a therapeutic group. Parent involvement and leadership functions are then considered. A description follows of special applications of group treatment for HIV-affected youngsters and individuals on the autism spectrum. Indications and contraindications for group treatment, as well as training and supervision needs, are then examined. The chapter concludes with a discussion of the efficacy of group treatment and the status of research in the field.

Group treatment with children and adolescents has a long history (1–6). At the end of the 19th and beginning of the 20th century, early efforts were designed to rehabilitate particular medically affected populations (7). Group homes that included intensive attention to group process were organized to treat adolescents with severe behavior disorders (8). Heavy use was made of psychodrama in treating a variety of problems in a group context (9). Related to the settlement house movement, groups were offered to youngsters from lower socioeconomic strata to expose them to aspects of more affluent, mainstream culture (10). The hope of this last type of group was that such exposure would elevate the group members' overall functioning, improve their behavior, and facilitate their moving into productive adulthood.

As the 20th century continued, many groups for children and adolescents were offered under the auspices of child guidance centers and community mental health centers. Activity groups for children became prominent, based on the premise that participation in age-appropriate play activity would promote better mental health. Later in the 20th century, groups based on the principles of behavior modification were conducted to treat numerous psychiatric problems. As the 20th century closed and the 21st century began, social skill groups and manual-based psychoeducational groups designed to impart specific curricula assumed greater prominence (6).

Just as the broad field of group therapy with children and adolescents has developed over time, many clinicians and researchers involved in child and adolescent group therapy have formulated the developmental stages through which each individual group moves over the course of its operation (11–14). Generally, groups move through an initial phase during which the foundation is laid for group cohesion. The group then often has a relatively euphoric period when the members have great hope and feel relief at having become part of the group. This period may then be followed by a more discouraged period as the full impact of the presenting problems becomes more evident. With good leadership, the group is then able to move into a more realistic, hardworking phase of its life. Ultimately, the group must go through the termination phase, during which members need help in internalizing and consolidating the gains made and in preparing to separate from the group.

Stages of group development take on different contours in both open-ended and shorter-term, time-limited groups. The relevance of group development to leadership interventions varies greatly depending on the type of group offered. In groups intended to be long term but with a planned ending date, correct interpretations of group behavior should rest on a sound understanding of the stage at which a group is operating. In contrast, in open-ended groups, members are admitted and discharged as dictated by their clinical needs. The group as a whole remains in a hardworking developmental stage as it incorporates new members and disengages from departing ones. Finally, in briefer, time-limited groups, group developmental stages become less relevant. The group tackles its specific tasks, knowing throughout that termination is close.

THEORETICAL UNDERPINNINGS OF GROUP THERAPY

Amid the daily pressures of clinic life and professional practice, therapeutic groups are often designed and implemented without a foundation of theoretical knowledge. Rather than being derived from comprehensive theory, many groups reflect professionals' efforts to manage time and caseload constraints. Such an atheoretical approach limits severely the range and effectiveness of group interventions. Without a theory for guidance, group leaders must rely more purely on intuition and moment-to-moment creativity in responding to the ongoing demands of group life.

Theory-based group practice allows for much more coherent intervention and thereby capitalizes most fully on the potential impact of a group treatment. A theoretical foundation allows group leaders to offer a range of group treatments that address group structure, procedures, and leadership style. When issues of structure, procedure, and essential leadership skills are mastered, they can be applied to any clinical population or specified problem. A guiding theory is also invaluable in navigating any single meeting of a group. Since each group meeting generates a wealth of clinical data and information, myriad decisions face the group leaders regarding intervention choices. A theoretical basis provides a map for leaders to discriminate among levels of information and thereby determine the most appropriate responses and interventions at any point in time.

A variety of theories have been used to guide group practice. Cognitive behavioral, psychodynamic, and gestalt theories are prominent among those that have been mined for group practice (15). Choice of a theoretical guide should be at the discretion of the leaders. Designation of a comprehensive theory and its full utilization are much more important than which particular theory is chosen.

While many theories can be helpful in group leadership, Bion's group-as-a-whole is a powerful theory available to group leaders (16–21). Originated in Britain by Wilfred Bion and his psychiatric/psychoanalytic colleagues to assist the British military during World War II, the theory posits that group structure and strong leadership are critical variables in group practice. Essential features of this body of theory are discussed below.

Consistent with its name, this theory asserts that the group as a whole is greater than the sum of its parts. The group as a whole is the "organism" to be considered. Individuals are believed to participate in the group life as dictated by their singular needs and capacities, in interaction with shared group needs and capacities. Individual behavior is therefore always understood as conveying information not only about that individual but about issues that require the group's attention. Individual behavior displayed in a group context is always believed to be a necessary expression by the group and to have relevance for the group. To have the greatest therapeutic impact, then, interpretations of behavior and interventions should be aimed at the group level.

The theory posits further that a group must be distinguished from a more casual collection of individuals. This distinction rests on identification of the group's shared task. The fundamental task of the group becomes the bedrock on which the group's life is based. As the group proceeds, practice decisions and behavioral interpretations should always be evaluated by their fidelity to the fundamental task of the group.

There is a range of tasks that can be addressed in therapeutic groups for children and adolescents. These tasks fall in roughly five categories. Traditionally, many groups were organized to provide formal, insight-oriented, psychodynamic psychotherapy. The task of such a group is to use both talk and play, as appropriate, to help make the unconscious conscious, presumably leading to greater psychological health characterized by intentionally chosen appropriate behaviors. While such formal psychotherapeutic groups still exist, briefer and more behaviorally oriented types of group work with children are now offered more widely. This broadening of the kinds of groups offered can be understood as a response to increased financial constraints in the mental health field. A second type of group offered to children and adolescents is the social skills group. The task of this type of group is to increase the members' repertoire of age-appropriate social skills, thereby enhancing the members' interpersonal relationships overall and improving their peer relationships, in particular. The task of a third type of group, a support group, is to acknowledge a traumatic experience or set of circumstances common to all group members and to provide clinically informed support aimed at facilitating good coping skills. Some groups are more formally didactic, taking on the task of imparting knowledge and teaching skills relevant to a particular psychoeducational problem. Finally, a fifth type of child/adolescent group is a goal-focused group. This group has the task of marshalling internal and external resources to allow the members to attain a specified, tangible goal or create a tangible product.

For groups to be effective, leaders must begin with a clear conceptualization of the group's task. Leaders must be vigilant about remaining true to the task, carrying out actions relevant to the designated task and foregoing actions that would actually be aimed at an alternate one. To take on task-irrelevant issues essentially makes an offer to the group that can't be delivered fully and thereby threatens the integrity of the leadership and the group as a whole.

Members' conceptualization of the group task operates differently than the leaders'. Members must hear a clear statement of the group's task as they enter the group. Otherwise, they would be justifiably confused about the nature of their participation and expectations for them to work would be unfair. It is often true, however, that group members develop a full understanding of the task only as they participate in the life of the group. Many times, the nature of the task is so difficult that the task itself only becomes truly understandable psychologically as the group begins to have some initial success in task accomplishment and develops greater capacity to tolerate the tension involved in group participation.

Once the group begins, its activity can be defined in two ways, rational work and/or basic assumption life. Rational work is defined as any activity that moves the group further toward accomplishment of its task. For groups of children and adolescents, it is essential to note that rational work will be expressed in developmentally determined forms. For young children, this might be a variety of play activities. For older children and adolescents, more conversation might be used. Thus, a firm grasp of normative child/adolescent development is necessary to allow group leaders to recognize and interpret accurately the members' behavior.

This body of theory presumes, however, that carrying out rational work is extremely arduous. By definition, the task of a therapeutic group is difficult. If the task were an easy one, creation of the therapeutic group and its dedication to ongoing effort would be unnecessary. Formal psychotherapy groups lead members to confront some of their most basic unmet needs and deficits. Social skill groups highlight fundamental interpersonal impairment. Support groups focus on specific traumas that engender significant distress. Didactic groups require substantial cognitive growth, typically regarding emotionally charged topics. Goal-focused groups elicit disturbing emotions about the necessity for reaching the specified goal. In addition to particular group characteristics, group membership itself is understood as a psychologically challenging transaction. Each member must relinquish enough individuality to join fully with the group as a whole. At the same time, each member must retain a firm hold on a singular identity. Balancing of these requirements requires considerable psychological energy and strength.

When the difficulties posed by rational work become too great, groups are assumed to feel that their continued existence is threatened. To defend themselves, they retreat to basic assumption life. Basic assumption life is defined as a variety of defensive postures, each expressing a fundamentally irrational notion of how the group may avoid the perils of rational work and thereby continue to exist. It is incumbent upon the leaders to recognize basic assumption life and to interpret it appropriately. Group-as-a-whole theory states that such interpretation and exploration of the group's reaction are instructive for the group and ease the group back into a rational work mode.

Group-as-a-whole theory was developed as a compelling, comprehensive approach to group operation and leadership primarily appropriate for adults. Considerable group experience has demonstrated that, with appropriate developmental modifications, the theory is equally useful with children and adolescents (21,22). Embedded as the theory is in group and organizational life, it takes the fullest therapeutic advantage of the group treatment modality.

PRAGMATICS IN THE OPERATION OF GROUP THERAPY

Along with theoretical underpinnings, a number of pragmatic considerations have a significant impact on the usefulness of group treatment. Many of these considerations are explored by Lomonaco et al. (3), Schamess (23), Schectman (24), and Slavson and Schiffer (25). Relevant considerations are discussed below.

Recruitment of Members

The main goal of the recruitment phase of group treatment is to identify members who need to accomplish the designated task of the group and who are able to work together toward that task accomplishment. Such identification requires sufficient clinical knowledge about each prospective group member. Several concrete steps facilitate the identification and recruitment process. First, group leaders must communicate clearly and broadly with all potential referral sources in an enthusiastic and welcoming manner. Referrals should be encouraged by conveying an eagerness and willingness to be helpful to colleagues and potential group members. Once a referral has been suggested, group leaders need to determine whether the child or adolescent has been fully evaluated. If a psychiatric evaluation or psychological assessment has been completed recently, the results of the evaluation should be reviewed carefully to assess compatibility with the designated group. If no recent evaluation has been done, group leaders either need to obtain in-depth clinical information about the prospective member from a clinician with ongoing knowledge about the member, or the leaders need to carry out a relevant evaluation. An in-depth, clinical understanding of each prospective group member is necessary to ensure appropriate group composition. Should the group leaders then determine that the prospective group member is inappropriate for the designated group, alternative treatment options or experiences should be suggested to the child or adolescent and his/her family. Should the group leaders conclude that the referral is appropriate, the leaders should meet with the group member's parents to describe the group in detail, to plan for the child's or adolescent's course in the group treatment, and to answer parent questions. The leaders should then meet with the prospective group member to again describe the group, make certain that the member appears to fit admission criteria, and to answer the child's or adolescent's questions. At times, actually meeting with the prospective group member raises particular concerns about potential group membership. These concerns should be taken up with parents and referring clinicians to allow for confident admission decisions. If all are then agreed and comfortable, a date should be set for entrance into the group.

Diagnostic Composition

The question arises often about the relative merits of diagnostic homogeneity or heterogeneity in a group. This question should be resolved in relation to the proposed task of the group. A group designed to address specific, diagnosis-related issues would clearly demand diagnostic homogeneity. Thus, for example, a psychoeducational group for children with diabetes would, by definition, require that all members have diabetes. Similarly, a support group for HIV-affected youngsters would require that all members had direct experience with HIV infection. In contrast, a group with a developmental or psychotherapeutic task would thrive on diagnostic heterogeneity. Mirroring the diversity to be encountered in naturalistic environments, such group heterogeneity would bring differences in perspective, observational capacity, and interpersonal relatedness that would allow for spirited, mutually beneficial interactions among members and leaders. To illustrate, a social skills group would do best if members all displayed impaired social functioning but did so for widely different reasons. In such a group, a socially inhibited, depressed member might be able to give very age-appropriate social feedback to an idiosyncratic member on the autism spectrum, while an impulsive, acting-out member might be able to challenge the inhibited member toward more vigorous, instrumental interaction.

One important caution should always be considered in regard to diagnostic composition of the group. To the greatest extent possible given real-life contingencies, a group should not contain only one representative of any critical attribute or category. A solitary representative of any salient classification—racial, religious, ethnic, gender, or level of diagnostic severity—invites isolation and hinders significantly the potentially useful interventions implemented by the leaders. For example, a group for psychotic youngsters could be extremely beneficial, offering them evidence that they were not fully alone in their disorganization, and teaching them pragmatic coping strategies. Placement of a single psychotic child or adolescent into a group of more realistically functioning members, however, intensifies the psychotic member's sense of isolation, highlights his/her impairment, deprives that member of appropriate group interventions, and frightens the group as a whole. In forming a group or admitting new members to an ongoing group, then, every effort should be made to include members who share important, relevant attributes with at least one other member.

Group Size

Therapeutic groups for children and adolescents should be big enough to generate multiple, challenging interpersonal interactions and to allow for both dyadic, triadic, and whole-group activities. At the same time, the groups should be small enough to permit a sense of intimacy and close personal attention. Groups composed of 4 to 6 members are ideal for most therapeutic tasks. While not overwhelming to individuals, groups of this size can continue to work productively even with occasional absences due to member illness, vacation, or other reasons.

Gender

As with the issue of diagnostic consistency, the question of same-sex versus mixed-sex groups is often debated and should be resolved in reference to the group's task. Traditionally, therapeutic groups were offered to single-sex populations. More currently, common practice has changed. For most tasks in groups of children and adolescents, mixed-sex groups prove to be most useful, since interacting with others of both sexes again parallels most closely real-life experience. Group members derive benefits directly applicable to the demands and challenges of daily life. There are, however, some groups that should remain single-sex groups. These are the groups designed to address sensitive issues related to sexuality, aggression, and/or sexual abuse. The need for comfort, trust, and empathy in such groups is difficult enough to satisfy but would be even more difficult in a mixed sex group.

Age Range

In actual clinical life, age ranges are rarely absolute. Developmental and school grade levels tend to influence and sometimes extend the age range of a group. Still, a general age range of 2 to 3 years is most appropriate. It is important, too, that the span of years be contained within one developmental phase of life. This type of clustering allows for the necessary commonality of experience and capacity to benefit from group interventions.

Setting

A space should be dedicated to the group on a consistent, reliable basis. Two conditions are most important in identifying a group setting. First, the setting must be private for the duration of each group meeting. Intrusions by individuals not associated with the group are very destructive of the group process. Second, the setting must be furnished and equipped in a developmentally appropriate manner. While leaders should work hard to limit damage to the physical space, some wear and tear in the environment must be a realistic expectation in working with children and adolescents. It would be too difficult to carry out the work of the group if leaders were faced with constant worry about protecting a more adult-oriented room that contained objects or interior decorations of great value. If these conditions are met, groups can adapt to many different kinds of spaces of varying sizes.

Materials

When embarking on group treatment for children or adolescents, leaders are often tempted to amass a large collection of tempting, exciting, attractive play materials. In actuality, a big, tempting array is usually over stimulating to a group and leads to excessively active, disorganized interactions. A modest amount of developmentally appropriate materials facilitates much more productive group interaction. For adolescents, some decks of cards, a few advanced board games, and some limited art materials would likely be sufficient. Groups at this adolescent level tend to engage more in conversation than activity. Younger groups rely more heavily on activity as the vehicle of their clinical work. Thus, for elementary and middle schoolchildren, it would be best to provide decks of cards, a larger number of simpler board games, limited art materials, some building toys such as Legos, and something that allows the group to engage safely in an indoor large-motor activity, for example, a soft, inflatable beach ball or a plastic indoor bowling set. Preschool groups do best with a small amount of building toys, some drawing materials, a few very simple board and card games, and materials that promote fantasy play such as a dollhouse or dress-ups. Whatever the age of the group, it would always be best to do with fewer rather than more materials.

Food

In carrying out group treatment with children and adolescents, the challenge of group participation should always be remembered. Management of the self in relation to the group as a whole is daunting, in addition to the difficulty of the actual therapeutic work. In recognition of the challenges faced by group members, it is helpful to provide a snack as a tangible support to the group. In addition to its nurturing aspects, time spent eating together as a group promotes more intimate, relaxed interactions that often help with task accomplishment. The logistics of providing food in the group are important, as well. The exact food and accompanying drink to be provided should be very simple and should be decided by the group leaders. Accommodations should be made to any specific dietary requirements of group members. The group should be told that a set amount of snack will be offered to each member. Group protest should be expected no matter what the designated amount of snack is. Such protest should be understood as part of the group establishing and maintaining its trust in the group leadership. Leaders should adhere to the snack plans set forth at the outset of the group. The only useful exceptions to these snack plans involve either essential dietary restrictions on the part of individual members or special occasions. In regard to dietary restrictions, parental report sometimes indicates that a child cannot tolerate a food or drink for medical reasons. At other times, religious or cultural beliefs dictate acceptable versus unacceptable food. These specific needs should be accommodated by the entire group, whenever possible. If group-as-a-whole accommodations are impractical or impossible, the individual member should be cared for appropriately with a simple explanation offered to the group. In regard to special occasions, from time to time the group may observe a holiday if such observance is consistent with the task of the group. On these occasions, it is helpful to have the group plan together about food and drink, with the leaders retaining veto powers if the plans get too lavish to be practical.

Duration

Length of each meeting and lifespan of the group should both be considered. Regarding meeting length, 1 to 1½ hours is an optimal amount of time for a group meeting. Less than 1 hour deprives the group of sufficient time to enter fully into work on its task. Instead of concentrating on the work, both leaders and members feel the constant pressure of time and spend most of their energy hurrying to finish. More than 1½ hours is simply too exhausting. Many groups meet for 1¼ hours and find that duration to be very comfortable. In public school settings, the demands of the school day often dictate that groups must meet for only 20 minutes to ½ hour. Under such conditions, leaders should work hard to design group agendas that can be implemented realistically. Regarding group lifespan, professional preference and practical realities of organizational life in many settings lead to decisions to offer time-limited groups. In such settings, constraints on professional availability, organizational resources, theoretical outlook, and regulations of third-party payers may all require a time-limited group. In other settings and under different conditions, long-term, open-ended groups are still offered, as they were more routinely in earlier years. It should be understood that time-limited versus long-term groups offer different possibilities for meaningful work and can accomplish different tasks. Time-limited groups are best for teaching specific, discrete skills, or imparting well-specified information. They can also be very useful for individuals who could not tolerate the intensity of long-term interpersonal interaction. Brief groups may also lend themselves more readily to empirical research designs. In contrast, long-term, open-ended groups are best for facilitating more fundamental, broader changes in designated areas of personal functioning. To carry out formal, intensive psychotherapy in a group format, to engender genuine change in naturalistic social functioning, to provide support with some life-threatening situations, there is no substitute for a long-term, open-ended group experience.

MEETING PROTOCOL MODEL

To allow the group members to rely fully on the structure of the group, group meetings should always follow the same protocol. The exact amount of time allotted to each portion of the agenda may vary based on the leaders' appraisal of the group work in any particular meeting. What should never vary is inclusion of each segment of the meeting protocol in each meeting. Omission of any segment, regardless of how justified such an omission might seem by the events of the moment, will always diminish the group's trust in its leaders and in the structure of the group and will, therefore, impede the work of the group. A useful protocol follows.

Gathering of Members

A comfortable place for the group to go to on arrival at the clinic, school, or private therapy office should be designated. It should be communicated clearly that parents or substitute caregivers retain responsibility for behavior management in the arrival area. Exactly at the time for the group to begin, the leaders should go to the arrival area to greet the members and bring them to the group meeting room. Acceptable behavioral standards and full physical safety should be maintained as the group is escorted to the meeting room. In some behaviorally challenging groups, members may need to be escorted in subgroups if moving as a whole group is too stimulating. In public schools, this gathering of members may need to be modified to include bringing the group members from their classrooms. Once in the group meeting room, members should be guided to settle into their designated places, putting away any personal belongings as directed. Overall, the purpose of this period is to welcome the group members and help them settle back into being together.

Talking Time

The group should be seated so that everyone can see each other. In most groups, a circular, square, or rectangular seating arrangement on the floor or single chairs is appropriate. In some groups for more psychologically disorganized individuals, the informality and intimacy of such an arrangement might be overwhelming. Such groups should be seated around a table for more formality and support. The first purpose of talking time is to allow the leaders to make any necessary announcements regarding member absences, upcoming events, or other practical issues. The leaders may also use this time to lead the group in discussion of a particular occurrence or ongoing situation that requires the group's consideration. The second purpose of talking time is to promote sustained, verbal interaction among the group members. Each member is encouraged to tell the group something of significance, if they choose to do so. In older, more mature groups, this part of talking time might be fairly informal. To the extent that the members can manage themselves, the leaders might be able to allow for free conversation. In younger, less mature groups, members' participation in talking time has to be managed much more carefully by the leaders. A helpful model is to have each child/adolescent talk to the group about one or two topics of importance and then turn to the next child/adolescent and elicit a question or comment about what was just related. This model teaches group members about listening to one another, staying on topic, responding to someone else, and about distinguishing between questions and comments. In psychotherapy and clinical support groups, talking time may become quite lengthy as the group moves more deeply into its work. In social skill groups, leaders should limit talking time to approximately 10 minutes to allow for sufficient opportunities to engage the group members in fuller social interaction. Leaders should always be the ones to announce when talking time is completed.

Activity Times

The group activity times are periods of the group meeting devoted to developmentally appropriate board or card games, role-playing, projects, arts and crafts, physically active indoor games, and other forms of play. These activity times are intended to enhance age-appropriate, multifaceted interpersonal interaction aimed at accomplishing the group's task. The activity periods are divided between group activity and free activity or play time. The group activity time is a period during which all the members must engage in a whole group activity. In psychotherapy groups, the groups should be free, within parameters specified by the leaders, to choose this whole group activity. The process of choosing and entering into the activity is as important to the work of the group as the activity itself. In social skill and more didactically oriented support groups, the group activities should be designed by the leaders based on adult observations of areas of need in the group. First and foremost, the leader-designated activities should be enjoyable for group members. Beyond the pleasure of the interaction, each activity should incorporate critical variables that teach aspects of the group task. The free activity time is a period during which members are allowed to choose their own forms of play, again within parameters set forth by the leaders and using acceptable play materials. During this period, the leaders are involved directly only as needed and as invited by the members. When not playing directly, the leaders are active observers, moving among the members to interpret or facilitate interactions. Leaders are able to teach a great deal about adaptive behavior in this relatively naturalistic situation. The free activity period is thus intended as a time for members to learn more about spontaneous interactions and the issues engendered by such informality in relationships. For some very young, very impaired groups of children, a free activity time is too overwhelming and disorganizing. Children with extremely deficient play skills, for example, severely affected children on the autism spectrum, experience a free choice playtime as painfully bewildering. Such a lack of structure leads mainly to very maladaptive behaviors as group anxiety increases in the face of ambiguity. For such groups, a leader-guided play time is a good substitute. Each coleader leads a separate, developmentally appropriate game or activity for a portion of the group. The group members alternate between the leaders' activities, according to a schedule designated by the leaders. Disorganized youngsters find this type of adult-centered play much more reassuring and enjoyable. As a result, they are able to learn much more than they would otherwise.

Snack Time

Once cleanup from the activity periods is completed, the group should have snack time. Each member should be assigned an ongoing "job" to help with snack, handing out napkins, spreading a tablecloth. The intention of snack time is to provide tangible support to the group, to promote more relaxed interaction and reflection among group members, and to teach members about appropriate informal behavior. Once the food and drink are passed around, the group journal should be brought out. The journal is a written record of the group's work. Members dictate and the leader writes in the journal. Each member is able to contribute what he/she would like to remember about the current group meeting. Leaders are free to add comments. The combined entries are then read back to the group. Afterward, the journal is circulated among members and leaders for each person's signature. In groups too young to write comfortably and quickly, individualized stamps or hand tracings can replace signatures. The journal provides a wonderful written record of the life of the group. Periodically, members refer to earlier entries to answer questions about the chronology of events or the tenure of various members. At other times, members sign nicknames or add comments to express feelings about themselves, previous group members who are missed, or particular occurrences in group. As time permits in the snack period, groups tend to focus back on their task in a variety of ways. A social skills group, for example, might use the time to tell jokes and rate the humorous value and social comedic skill involved in each joke.

Dismissal

Once snack time is cleaned up, it is time to dismiss the group. This period of the group is typically very tense and overwrought. Having participated in the intense interaction of the group meeting, it is difficult for the members to prepare themselves for separation and return to their individual pastimes. Leaders need to be actively involved in helping the members ready themselves, in maintaining order in the group, and in being reassuring about when the group will meet again. Leaders can help members learn more adaptive ways to manage the ending transition by instituting additional group rituals, providing "social scripts," and modeling appropriate departure behavior. When ready, group members should be returned to their parents or caregivers. In particularly active or disorganized groups, it might be necessary to return the members in shifts separated by 1 or 2 minutes rather than all at once. Leaving in subgroups of two to three members is often more manageable for parents/caregivers and less chaotic in a professional office or clinic setting.

BEHAVIOR MANAGEMENT

Leaders must respect the enormous impact of the particular form of psychopathology, trauma, or skill deficit common to the group members. In dedicating the group to work on grappling with fundamental psychopathology, overcoming significant trauma, or building much-needed skills, the leaders must understand the extreme challenge facing the group as a whole. While every effort should be made to create a group structure that can facilitate accomplishment of a challenging group task, the group should still be expected to falter at times. Through inappropriate behavior, child and adolescent groups often manifest not only their possible presenting problems but also their reaction to the demanding nature of task accomplishment. Because inappropriate behavior is so intimately related to the fundamental clinical core of the group, efforts to manage this behavior should likewise be thoughtfully intertwined with sound, clinical reasoning. Without a comprehensive approach to behavior management, no amount of clinical acumen, theoretical sophistication, or leadership skill will be sufficient to ensure the group's safety, organization, and productivity. Crawford-Brolyn and White (26) and Soo (27) supported the need for careful behavior management in groups for children and adolescents. The five-level approach to behavior management discussed below represents an effort to implement both therapeutic understanding and realistic practicality in managing behavior in a child or adolescent group.

Consideration by Leaders

In the face of difficult, inappropriate behavior, leaders should first think carefully about the communicative intent and underlying meaning of the undesirable behavior. Almost invariably, leaders can either link such negative behavior to the basic problems that led to group admission in the first place or can understand the negative behavior as an expression of the difficulty experienced by the group in attempting to respond to leader interventions. Well-reasoned understanding of the negative behavior constitutes the best foundation possible for effective response by the leadership. As important as this thoughtful consideration is, it should be understood that, on relatively rare occasions, some negative behavior is displayed in group that demands immediate intervention to maintain safety. Quick action should be taken to protect group members and property. Fuller consideration of the meaning of the behavior should follow.

Structural or Procedural Change

Once the behavior has been understood, the leaders should explore the possibility of a structural or procedural change that could address the need being expressed in the negative behavior. A structural change might involve switching from a free activity period to a leader-guided play activity to help the group feel more supported and secure, thereby containing acting-out behavior among very impaired young children. A procedural change might involve escorting group members to and from group in subgroups, rather than in the group as a whole, to reduce stimulation and allow for more organized behavior under closer leader supervision. In most appropriately constructed outpatient or community-based therapeutic groups, most negative behavior can be contained using these two levels of intervention. Realistically, however, not all inappropriate behaviors can be managed so readily. The remaining intervention levels are intended to address greater levels of need.

Verbal Interpretation

Should negative behavior persist despite clear understanding by the leaders and any appropriate structural or procedural accommodation, it is helpful to interpret aloud the meaning of the unwanted behavior. Such verbal interpretation operates in groups much as it does in a dynamically oriented individual psychotherapy. The verbal clarification of the negative behavior illuminates that behavior's communicative intent and/or significance. That intent or significance can then be discussed or acted upon appropriately, relieving the group of the need for continued negative behavioral acting out. Discussion and decisions for group action have the greatest impact if multiple members are involved. Reactions and opinions from the group as a whole have much more motivational power than input solely from group leaders. Again, in most groups, behavior management usually does not move beyond this level.

Verbal Limit

When undesirable behavior does continue despite taking the above steps, a limit is required. If preliminary levels of intervention have been tried and have been inadequate, leaders should not hesitate to set a verbal limit, reminding the group about appropriate behavior and directing members to remain within acceptable behavioral parameters. It is always most effective to phrase verbal limits in positive terms. Group members will respond best when told what *to do* as opposed to what *not to do.*

Physical Limit

On infrequent occasions, inappropriate behavior persists despite all efforts. On such occasions, a physical limit is mandatory to guarantee the group's safety. For example, unacceptable materials should be taken from members, members may have to move to less desirable physical locations within the group meeting room, or members may have to take a time out. The group should be well informed ahead of time of what limits will be implemented, depending on the need. In the most extreme circumstances, a member might pose such a danger to the group due to uncontrolled acting out or some other condition that he/she must be removed permanently from the group. Such a step should be explained clearly and concisely to the group. This step should be taken only if the danger to the group is pronounced and if no alternative is available. Reluctance in removing a group member is recommended because there is always irreparable damage to the group when a member is removed, regardless of the justifications for the removal. The group usually experiences the loss of a member as an aggressive act by the leaders. Remaining group members worry permanently about potential ramifications and implications of that act. Members scrutinize and inhibit their own behavior because they are afraid that they too will be expelled. Members feel angry toward the leaders and guilty about any negative feelings that they may have had toward the lost member. While explanation and reassurance by the leaders is helpful, the leaders should be prepared to deal with reactions to and memories of the removal of the group member for as long as the group continues to meet.

PARENT INVOLVEMENT

For child and adolescent groups to succeed, parent knowledge and support of the group are essential (28). The nature of parent involvement in group treatment for children and adolescents varies greatly, however, depending on the population served and on whether the group is in an outpatient or inpatient/residential program setting. For inpatient/residential program groups, parent involvement is relatively distant. Parents are typically informed periodically about their youngster's progress in the hospital or residential treatment program as a whole.

In contrast, because attendance in the outpatient group generally requires parent assistance with transportation and because the outpatient group tends to represent a singular investment of family time, effort, and finances, parents are much closer to outpatient group experiences. Various approaches to including parents in the group therapeutic work have been discussed elsewhere (29). It is most useful to consult closely with the parents in making group admission decisions. A thorough understanding of parental concerns and perspective is necessary to ensure that the group experience, as constructed, is capable of addressing those concerns. Following admission to the group, parent involvement should be managed in accord with the developmental level of the group members. As appropriate, periodic meetings should be held with parents to keep them informed about group progress and the progress of their individual child. Written correspondence is a good alternative to face-to-face meetings to keep parents informed about the group's work. Whenever possible, suggestions based on knowledge gained in the group should be offered to parents to enhance functioning in all the spheres of the child or adolescent's life.

In addition, parents should be encouraged to contact the group leaders at any time with questions or concerns. Group members should be fully aware of the parents' access to the leaders. Managed correctly, this parent-group leader communication is very beneficial to the child and adolescent group members. Members will often request for direct specific communications between the adults to address particular issues. Adult communication should occur outside of the group meeting times, however. In line with the discussion below about boundary management regarding information, parents should be helped to see that direct parental input into the group meetings would likely interfere with the ongoing group process.

LEADERSHIP FUNCTIONS

Group leaders' fulfillment of their role requirements is essential for the group to accomplish its task (30). The group should be able to rely as heavily as necessary on the consistent strength and good judgment of the leaders as it engages in rational work and struggles to pull itself out of more defensive, irrational functioning. Several leadership functions are of paramount importance.

Safety

The single most important leadership function is to ensure the safety of the group as it works toward task accomplishment. The group leaders must demonstrate a fundamental commitment to physical and emotional safety in the group. A coherent approach to behavior management, such as the one outlined earlier, should be implemented to ensure group safety. Without such a guarantee, it would be unfair to maintain expectations for intensive therapeutic work of any type.

Primacy of Cotherapy Relationship

From a clinical perspective, to ensure physical safety, mainly in groups of younger or more disturbed individuals, to process adequately the enormous amount of clinical information generated in each group meeting, and to have a dyad within the group that can be used as a model of a functional interpersonal relationship, it is always advisable for a group to be led by two coleaders. Dies (31) underscored, however, that empirical support was lacking for the benefits of group cotherapy. In view of the fact that cotherapy is utilized widely regardless of the status of empirical support, both Dies (31) and Riva et al. (30) emphasized the need for careful management of the cotherapy relationship to enhance group functioning. If the group is to reap the benefits of the cotherapy relationship, however, this relationship must be fostered and supported carefully.

The coleaders must communicate openly and honestly regarding their work together. This communication should occur both during regularly scheduled formal meetings as well as in more informal moments while the work proceeds. The leaders should choose a mutually acceptable way of sharing the leadership work. There are many possible, equally productive choices available. Leaders should make a choice based on the task of the group, differential leadership skills, individual preferences, interpersonal style, and relative professional status/responsibilities. One commonly made choice is for one leader to assume managerial responsibilities, that is, setting the agenda, being the most vocal, leading activities, introducing topics, while the other leader remains quieter, focusing intently on emotional reactions within the group and articulating those as appropriate. While no one choice is correct for all coleader pairs, a successful choice must be genuinely acceptable to both leaders and must be made based on leadership strengths rather than weakness or fear of carrying out specific leadership functions.

Leaders should know that they always have the freedom and responsibility to speak directly to one another regarding group matters in the presence of the group. To gain needed support in the face of challenging group interactions, to articulate an issue relevant to the group's work, to ensure full knowledge and cooperation between the leaders regarding a particular intervention, to resolve differences, and to model reciprocity between people, there is no better method than public communication between leaders. Even when the group may appear to be ignoring the leaders' conversation, the group in fact often listens intently and makes productive use of the interaction. Unlike genuine points of disagreement or difficulty in coleading, coleaders will sometimes become embroiled in disagreements or stuck in generalized tension between themselves but be unable to identify the actual source of the problems. Such disagreements and tension should be understood as unspoken, empathic responses to the group. The coleadership relationship often becomes the vehicle for expression of group conflicts, wishes, or needs that the group cannot yet verbalize directly. When the coleader pair finds itself in such a quagmire, first it is best to discuss the problem fully within the pair. Then, it is most useful to offer a developmentally attuned interpretation to the group and go on to help the group identify, understand, and grapple with the issue facing it. Without such exploration between the leaders, it becomes all too easy for the negativity between the coleaders to become so firmly and unpleasantly entrenched that all the work of the group is stalled.

Protection of Group Structure and Boundaries

To provide the group with sufficiently strong support in approaching its task, the third most important function for the leaders is to safeguard the structure within and boundaries around the group (31–34). The members need to be able to rely on predictability and reliability in the group's life if they are to be able to muster the strength to continue with rational work. The leaders must make sure that the group agenda is adhered to at each meeting, that limits are set and implemented in a consistent fashion, and that appropriate material resources are available to the group. The leaders must also maintain firm time, space, informational, and membership boundaries around the group. Group meetings must begin and end promptly, regardless of extraneous demands/events or enticing clinical material that is presented in the last few moments of a group's scheduled meeting. The group must have a dedicated space, in which the group's privacy can be respected for the duration of each group meeting. Leaders should take care to conduct the group's business only within the group's designated space. Entering into group discussion or play in a waiting room or hallway, no matter how critical or tantalizing the material may seem to be, weakens the group's potential reliance on the leader because the work cannot be pursued adequately in a more public and therefore less reliable setting. As the group becomes a meaningful entity for its members, the group should set a policy about how information will flow into and out of the group. Salient facets of this policy include member responsibilities to maintain group confidentiality, procedures for taking up information communicated by parents, and procedures to be followed by leaders in introducing essential issues that members might be uncomfortable about bringing up themselves. In firmly led discussions, groups are usually well able to make rational policy decisions about the flow of information. Leaders always retain veto power should policy decisions be inappropriate. Finally, the leaders must maintain clear distinctions between who belongs to the group and who does not. For both clinically relevant and for defensive reasons, members and their families often invite leaders to allow other people to attend group meetings or to join in group activities. These invitations should be declined politely but firmly in the interests of maintaining the group's integrity and reliability.

Distinction between Leader and Member Roles

Groups that are led with sufficient strength and reassurance are rarely democracies. To provide adequate support and guidance, leaders should retain authority and responsibility while continuing to convey respect and appropriate clinical sensitivity toward the group members. An important aspect of such authority and responsibility is maintenance of the distinction between the roles of members as opposed to leaders. Leaders should reserve the right to make the physical environment as comfortable as necessary to allow them to concentrate fully on their leadership tasks. Decisions about self-disclosure, participation in activities, and behavioral demands should be made in relation to the task of the group rather than to any notion of "fair play" or assumed obligation to do "themselves" whatever is asked of the group members. While such a distinction between leader and member roles may seem autocratic in the abstract, in clinical practice this type of distinction serves very well the clinical work of the group. Group members understand that they can rely heavily on the leaders; they do not feel oppressed by them.

Management of Relationship between Group and Organizational Base

Many clinical groups for children and adolescents are offered under the auspices of a clinic, hospital, or child guidance center. In such settings, factors such as billing practices, physical space, interaction with organizational staff and other patients/clients, attendance policies, privacy, personnel, material resources, and the tone of the organizational atmosphere all have a potential impact on the life of the group. It is the responsibility of the leaders to manage this relationship between the group and its surrounding organization. Although the group leaders rarely if ever have the authority to control the larger organization in the interest of their group, the leaders can and should articulate the needs of the group within the larger organization, advocate strongly for the necessary resources of all types, intervene if there are potentially disruptive interactions between group members and/or their parents and representatives of the organization, and facilitate the group members' transactions within the larger organization. When group leaders abdicate this managerial aspect of their leadership responsibilities, premature departure of members and group dysfunction are common outcomes. Fulfillment of these leadership responsibilities, on the other hand, helps to further protect the group and models adaptive behavior for the group members.

Support through Group Transitions

Some of the most challenging experiences in groups involve major transitions. Changes in coleadership, new members joining a group, either planned or abrupt terminations of an individual's membership in the group, or changes in meeting location are examples of common transitions through which groups must sometimes navigate. At such times, leaders must be very conscious, deliberate, visible, and direct in providing adequate, developmentally attuned information about what the group should expect, reassuring the members about continued leadership and support available to the group, and helping the group articulate their reactions and concerns regarding the transitions. As at all other times in the life of the group, leaders should facilitate the group's movement through any given transition in a manner consistent with the task of the group. The group should be encouraged to marshal skills consistent with its task as it manages the transition.

SPECIAL APPLICATIONS

As discussed throughout this chapter, group treatment can be directed at a wide variety of issues facing children and adolescents. Two particularly useful special applications of this treatment modality involve provision of support for youngsters contending with HIV/AIDS in their families (35,36) and teaching of social skills to youngsters on the autism spectrum (37).

HIV/AIDS Support Groups

In the early days of the HIV/AIDS pandemic, many children faced the rapidly worsening illness and imminent deaths of parents and other loved ones in their families. As medical treatments improved, many children had to learn to contend with HIV/AIDS as a more chronic illness in their families. At any time, supportive group experiences structured and operated in the manner discussed above offer a great deal to children affected by HIV/AIDS. The basis for admission to such a group has to be some family acknowledgment that HIV/AIDS has touched the family. Group members must be able to tolerate learning that the group is designed for youngsters who are facing HIV/AIDS in one or more loved ones. Almost always, youngsters are already aware of the presence of HIV/AIDS in their families even before direct adult acknowledgment is made. Their awareness and understanding are often covert and incomplete, however. Open recognition and admission to the group help to give an honest name to what has often been a burdensome, quasisecret in the family. Participation in the group facilitates a fuller understanding of the facts and implications of HIV/AIDS in the family. Without the burden of secrecy, children and adolescents can feel less afraid to learn how to cope with their situation.

Beyond naming a previously known but unacknowledged phenomenon, membership in an HIV/AIDS support group challenges the sense of isolation that frequently accompanies dealing with a devastating illness. In the case of HIV/AIDS, this isolation often stems from shame and guilt about the nature of the illness itself. The group's existence testifies to the fact that many individuals share the problems associated with HIV/AIDS. Such testimony diminishes individual shame and guilt, thereby relieving the loneliness of coping with the disease, and assists the members as they tackle each difficult phase of HIV/AIDS with their loved ones.

A third benefit of an HIV/AIDS support group is that it offers the members a set of reliable interpersonal relationships that are not endangered by the disease. The group offers closeness and intimacy that are invaluable for the members' sense of interpersonal relatedness. In doing so, the group provides a framework in which more normative psychosocial development can proceed.

Finally, the group experience also reminds members that there is life beyond HIV/AIDS. The group demonstrates that life events and transitions can relate to a host of factors, both positive and negative, unrelated to HIV/AIDS. One particularly striking example involves leadership changes. As with any clinical endeavor, HIV/AIDS support groups must contend with the departure of leaders from time to time due to career changes, assignment of different responsibilities, pregnancies, etc. In this type of support group, members are often shocked when a farewell is prompted by something other than illness and/or death. Enduring the sadness of a parting but knowing that the missed person is going onto another satisfying life stage opens up countless possibilities for the members themselves as they begin to contemplate their own futures.

HIV/AIDS support groups for children and adolescents present two main challenges to leaders. First, leaders must be able to tolerate extremely sad information. Without resorting to defensive minimization or avoidance, leaders must accept and be comfortable exploring devastation in the lives of the group members. Often, to demonstrate concern and to provide assistance, carefully modulated participation in sad events, such as funerals in the families of group members, is also required as part of full group leadership.

Second, leaders must learn to cope with often dramatic acting-out behavior in the group. In many instances, the family's experience of HIV/AIDS is part of a constellation of psychosocial problems. Together with the stress of HIV/AIDS, this constellation of problems contributes frequently to the development of significant behavior problems that challenge the safe operation of the treatment group. Leaders must learn a variety of strategies to meet such behavioral challenges. Relevant strategies have been discussed in Gossart-Walker and Moss (35,36).

Autism Spectrum Social Skill Groups

Social, communication, and peer relationship problems are the core deficits of individuals with diagnoses on the autism spectrum. Accordingly, group treatment is an ideal setting in which to teach social, interpersonal skills to be implemented in real-life situations (38). The group serves as a microcosm in which all the social demands of everyday life come into play. Unlike everyday life, however, leaders of the social skills group are present to instruct and to orchestrate helpful peer interactions.

Social skill groups for individuals with autism spectrum disorders are usually one of two types. The first is curriculum based. Such a group is generally time limited and follows a set plan for teaching discrete social skills. Such a group is excellent for lower-functioning individuals on the autism spectrum. For such group members, learning such skills as how to greet another person or to say thank you when appropriate is an impressive accomplishment.

The second type of social skill group is more naturalistic. Such a group is generally long term or open ended. While structure remains essential, as discussed above, this type of group capitalizes on the naturally occurring interpersonal interactions within the group as the source and object of instruction. Naturalistic social exchanges are used to teach about more fluid social functioning. Given its more interactive nature, this second type of group is better suited to higher-functioning individuals with autism spectrum disorders.

Regardless of level of functioning or type of group, two characteristics are essential if a social skill group is to be useful for autism spectrum members. First, group leadership and instruction have to be concrete, blunt, direct, and down to earth. Subtler, inquiring, insight-oriented forms of leadership and instruction would be far too vague and bewildering for individuals with autism-related disorders. While professional standards demand that leaders refrain from being rude, leaders in this sort of social skill group should understand that their responsibility is to use their own individual behavior, their interaction with one another, judicious self-disclosure, and all of their teaching skill to provide the most direct instruction possible. As a leader in a group for autism spectrum individuals, it is impossible to be too blunt or too concrete.

Second, for the group to be of maximum benefit, it should include exposure to peers who are not on the autism spectrum. Only with some diversity is it possible to provide socially grounded, realistic reactions to and modeling for the members on the autism spectrum. If composed solely of individuals on the autism spectrum, the group risks having no counterbalance to the social idiosyncrasy that characterizes autistic disorders. In turn, those on the spectrum can often bypass defensive behavior on the part of other members and speak directly to the problems that brought them to the group. Exposure to diverse individuals can be accomplished by admitting members with a range of diagnoses to the group. While their diagnostic status can vary, with only some of them on the autism spectrum, all of the group members should have social deficits. This exposure can also be accomplished by admitting only members on the spectrum but incorporating the services of typical peers as role models for the group members. Minimal training should be given to typical peers so as to maximize their capacity to model true-to-life peer behavior rather than pseudoadult, therapist-like behavior. Typical peers should receive enough basic information about the autism spectrum to feel reasonably comfortable, followed by encouragement to behave as naturally as possible.

Social skill groups are capable of facilitating significant improvement among children and adolescents with autism spectrum disorders. Many of the group members are able to fit in much better at school, develop a social life suited to their particular needs and wishes, and display much more socially appropriate general behavior. Enthusiasm about the groups must be realistic, however. Social skill groups are not powerful enough to change the fundamental organization of an autism spectrum disorder. Even successful members may remain idiosyncratic.

INDICATIONS AND CONTRAINDICATIONS FOR GROUP THERAPY

The issue of who would best benefit from group treatment is tied intimately to the identified task of the specific group. Appropriate admissions are those individuals in need of work on the group's task. Beyond this relatively simple statement at the level of group content, however, there are also broader concepts that should guide admission decisions. Group treatment would be indicated for reasons and under conditions such as those discussed directly below.

First, some mental health difficulties and aftereffects of traumatic experience burden affected individuals with a sense of isolation and culpability. Affected individuals may feel somehow to blame for calling down on themselves damaging experiences that paradoxically confirm negative self-assessments. Individual or family treatments in such situations, regardless of how expertly implemented, rely on discussion or other indirect methods to challenge the negative personalization. In contrast, by definition and by its very existence, a treatment group combats the isolation that so often oppresses children and adolescents struggling with developmental, psychological, and behavioral disorders (39). Inclusion in a group with others who are grappling with similar difficulties challenges individual self-blame and invites the individual to join with peers in shared, instrumental attempts to cope and overcome.

Second, whether due to innate personality characteristics, acquired interpersonal experience, or the cumulative effect of multiple therapeutic relationships, some people have the capacity to maintain excessive psychological distance between themselves and an individual therapist. Such individuals can insulate themselves from true consideration of even the best therapeutic overtures, plans, or interpretations. It is much more difficult, however, to ward off the power of an entire group process. Varied input from fellow group members often spurs this type of individual on toward greater therapeutic progress. Conversely, some more psychologically fragile individuals find the intimacy of one-to-one or even family therapy to be overwhelming. The shared relationships of a group treatment dilute the intimacy sufficiently so that therapeutic input becomes tolerable (40).

Third, some problems that are presented to mental health practitioners not only benefit from but also require the presence of more than a therapist–patient dyad for the most efficacious intervention. Most prominent among such problems are deficits in social/peer functioning, such as those that afflict individuals on the autism spectrum, and conditions requiring psychoeducational support (chronic medical illness, family disruption). Unlike more intrapsychic problems or personal psychopathology that often play themselves out in a dyadic therapeutic relationship, thereby lending themselves to psychological interpretation and redirection, peer difficulties and psychoeducational support needs may rarely be as evident in a one-to-one setting. As a result, a therapist–patient dyad would be reduced to talking *about* rather than experiencing immediately the most relevant situations. In contrast, tackling problems with peer relationships in the social environment of the group allows for enactment of and immediate intervention in the problems that interfere with the group member's more optimal functioning in the real world. Addressing needs in the group for guidance regarding logistical organization, social embarrassment, and fear about the future offers maximum support to group members in need of coping assistance. Both the fundamental experiences of group membership, as well as the content of the group's work, have a beneficial effect.

There are three main principles that argue against inclusion of an individual in a group. First, while group treatment can be helpful to impulsive children and adolescents, no individual should be permitted to join a therapeutic group if that individual poses a substantial threat to the basic safety or health of the other group members. Thus, impulsive children and adolescents whose poorly controlled acting-out takes the form of extremely aggressive or excessively risk-taking behavior, are inappropriate candidates for group therapy. This contraindication needs to be taken very seriously since, as noted earlier, physical and psychological safety is the fundamental guarantee that group leaders must provide to the group if any meaningful work is to occur. Prospective members who pose a safety threat to the group should be referred to other treatment modalities or for consultation, as appropriate. Many times, addition or modification of psychiatric medication can alter sufficiently the troubling behavior and thereby allow for reconsideration of an individual's group admission.

The removal of a group member by the group leaders is a related issue that merits attention in the context of indications and contraindications for group treatment. Often, leaders focus on one child or adolescent as the primary source of difficulty in a group. Typically, this is the group member that presents the greatest challenges in behavior management. Many times, leaders wish or proceed to remove this group member in the interests of more meaningful group work. For two main reasons, such a removal is almost never successful. First, as stated before, remaining members become angry and anxious about the possibility that they, too, will be required to leave. Behavior in the group is impacted as the remaining members enact their angry anxiety in the forms of limit testing, excessive inhibition, or open accusations directed against the leaders. Second, theoretical principles argue that the offending member was carrying out a function or making a communication relevant to the group's work, regardless of how seemingly inappropriate that function or communication seemed. As a result, it is usually the case that a previously well-functioning group member takes over the ousted member's more provocative role. The difficult behavior subsides only when the group has dealt with its meaning, in ways discussed above, and then moves onto new aspects of its task.

From time to time, though, the decision to remove a group member is actually clinically indicated. This comes about most often when new, more disturbing diagnostic information becomes manifest as the group proceeds or when an individual's status changes in such a way that poses a risk to the group. Then, the leaders have no choice but to carry out a planned termination in the most open, thoroughly discussed, and fully anticipated way possible. Regardless of the reasons for member removal, the group's negative reaction to removal of a member persists for a substantial amount of time, in some instances for the remainder of the life of the group. Even when the subject is dropped temporarily from discussion, it resurfaces at stressful times in the group's work. Leaders must be prepared to work through the issue of the member's removal on multiple occasions. Partly because removal of a member is so devastating to a group, admission decisions should be made as carefully as possible to do everything possible to avoid the necessity of member removal.

Second, as mentioned previously, groups do not operate effectively if there is only one member representing a key variable (one female in a group of males, one member of a particular race or ethnicity in another homogenous group, one psychotic individual in a group in which no one else's diagnosis involves impairments in reality testing). A single representative along a key dimension promotes loneliness, isolation, and scapegoating. Should an individual be an appropriate admission on other inclusion criteria, admission should be deferred until a similar member can be admitted at the same time.

Third, there are some children and adolescents who need and would benefit from work aimed at the stated task of a given group but who have never before identified or explored their relevant needs. Abused children and adolescents who have never acknowledged the abuse in any way would be examples of this type of prospective group member. While group participation at some point might be the treatment of choice for such children and adolescents, a group is too large, interpersonally diffuse, and unpredictable to be the setting in which an individual takes the first step toward confronting their traumatic history. These children and adolescents should receive more individualized services first to ready them for group participation, as needed and as appropriate.

TRAINING AND SUPERVISION OF GROUP THERAPISTS

Many authorities have addressed training needs as they relate to group therapy practitioners (3,41–43). Azima (44) also addressed the impact of group work on the therapist's own functioning. The foundation of training as a child/adolescent group therapist is the same as the foundation of training for any mental health clinician. Regardless of discipline, the practitioner should have thorough knowledge of child/adolescent development, psychopathology, and a range of therapeutic interventions. The therapist should be comfortable with a wide variety of individuals and diagnostic categories. With this type of foundation, an interested mental health professional would be well able to pursue more specialized training in group approaches. Ideally, the training should be three-pronged. Simultaneously, the practitioner should receive didactic training in the history, theory, and practice of group therapy with children and adolescents, colead a group with an advanced group leader, and receive ongoing clinical supervision of the cotherapy. The didactic experience places the group work in an intellectual and historical context that deepens and solidifies the work, distinguishing clinical group endeavors from more casual group experiences for young people. The coleadership provides immersion in and illustrations of the material discussed in the didactic setting. Finally, the ongoing supervision articulates the nuances of the group life and of the cotherapy relationship, enhancing the trainee's learning and extending his/her clinical skills. When ready, the trainee can assume greater independence in group leadership. In this regard, MacLennan (45) delineated specific training required to conduct groups at particular age and developmental levels while Soo (43) called for strengthening fundamental clinical skills to facilitate successful group leadership.

It should be noted that group supervision/consultation is often very helpful even for well-established, talented group therapists. The supervision can, of course, assist with therapeutic questions and problematic group issues. Beyond the immediate resolution of treatment problems, however, expert group supervision can elevate the leaders' understanding of the group's life. In the press of day-to-day group management demands and the challenges posed by diverse diagnostic needs among group members, it is often understandably easy for group leaders themselves to lose sight of the group historical context or the theoretical concepts that underlie current group experiences. Consultation and guidance from an expert who is somewhat removed from the meeting-to-meeting stimulation can have a clarifying, instructive effect for the group leaders. Critical variables and best practice recommendations regarding supervision of group leadership are well summarized by DeLucia-Waack and Fauth (46).

EFFICACY AND CURRENT RESEARCH

For a long time, there has been a broad consensus that group treatment is beneficial for specified populations of children and adolescents (47). To a great extent, this consensus rested originally on clinical observations and professional experience. Early research efforts were qualitative, narrative reports. While often rich in clinical insight and technique, such efforts were subject to criticism regarding validity, reliability, relevance to larger populations, and cost effectiveness. Mirroring broader psychotherapy research efforts and to address such criticism, group therapy research attempted to move more in the direction of sound, empirical studies (48). A number of studies and reviews demonstrated comparable effectiveness of group and individual therapies (33,49–51). Effective application of group therapeutic techniques to a wide variety of populations has been documented (24).

Yet many questions remain. The full potential efficacy of cotherapy needs to be explored (30,31). The most useful integration and application of theoretical perspectives need to be articulated (6). In addition, the complex interaction among group structure, process, leadership style, and outcome needs further study. Precise linkage of the most curative processes in group therapy with specific populations of children and adolescents stands as most prominent among current research and clinical questions (24,28). New instruments measuring such variables as group cohesion have been developed to facilitate comparability across more rigorous research studies. Leaders in the field have called for shared use of these new instruments to promote comparability across studies (48). While a great deal remains to be done, strong interest in and need for group therapy with children and adolescents exist throughout the medical and mental health communities (52). It would be reasonable to expect a body of research to emerge that expands greatly our knowledge of group treatment, integrates standards for sound empirical research with recognition of clinical complexity, and thereby guides efforts in efficacious ways.

References

1. Anthony J: Comparison between individual and group psychotherapy. In: Kaplan HI, Sadock BJ (eds): *Comprehensive Group Psychotherapy.* Baltimore, MD, Williams & Wilkins, pp. 104–117, 1971.
2. Barlow SH, Burlingame GM, Fuhrman A: Therapeutic application of groups: from Pratt's "thought control classes" to modern group psychotherapy. *Group Dynamics: Theory, Research, and Practice* 4:115–134, 2000.
3. Lomonaco S, Scheidlinger S, Aronson S: Five decades of children's group treatment: an overview. *J Child Adolesc Group Ther* 10:77–96, 2000.
4. Scheidlinger S, Schamess G: Fifty years of AGPA, 1942–1992: an overview. In: MacKenzie MR (ed): *Classics in Group Psychotherapy.* New York, Guilford Press, pp. 1–24, 1992.
5. Scheidlinger S: The group psychotherapy movement at the millennium: some historical perspectives. *Int J Group Psychother* 50:315–339, 2000.
6. Scheidlinger S: Group psychotherapy and related helping groups today: an overview. *Am J Psychother* 58:265–280, 2004.
7. Kraft IA, Riester AE: Past as prologue to the future in child group psychotherapy practice. In: Riester AE, Kraft IA (eds): *Child Group Psychotherapy: Future Tense.* Madison, Connecticut, International Universities Press, pp. 3–8, 1986.
8. Rachman AW, Raubolt RR: The pioneers of adolescent group psychotherapy. *Int J Group Psychother* 34:387–413, 1984.
9. Moreno JL: The ascendancy of group psychotherapy and the declining influence of psychoanalysis. *J Sociopsychopathol Soc* 3:121–141, 1950.
10. Ettin MF: "By the crowd they have been broken, by the crowd they shall be healed": The advent of group psychotherapy. *Int J Group Psychother* 38:139–167, 1988.
11. Dies K: The unfolding of adolescent groups: a five phase model of development. In: Kymmissis P, Halperin D (eds): *Group Therapy with Children and Adolescents.* Washington, DC, American Psychiatric Press, 1996.
12. Dies K: Adolescent development and a model of group psychotherapy: effective leadership in the new millennium. *J Child Adolesc Group Ther* 10:97–111, 2000.
13. Garland JA: The establishment of individual and collective competency in children's groups as a prelude to entry into intimacy, disclosure, and bonding. *Int J Group Psychother* 42:395–405, 1992.
14. Garland J, Jones H, Kolodny R: A model for stages of development in social work groups. In: Bernstein S (ed): *Explorations in Group Work.* Boston, MA, Milford House, pp. 17–71, 1973.
15. Yalom I: *The Theory and Practice of Group Psychotherapy.* 4th ed. New York, Basic Books, 1995.
16. Agazarian Y: Group-as-a-whole systems theory and practice. *Group* 13:131–154, 1989.
17. Agazarian Y: Contemporary theories of group psychotherapy: a systems approach to the group-as-a-whole. *Int J Group Psychother* 42:177–203, 1992.
18. Bion WR: *Experience in Groups and Other Papers.* New York, Basic Books, 1961.
19. Pines M: *Bion and Group Psychotherapy.* London, Routledge & Kegan Paul, 1985.
20. Rioch MJ: The work of Wilfred Bion on groups. *Psychiatry* 33:56–66, 1970.
21. Schamess G: Reflections on a developing body of group-as-a-whole theory for children's therapy groups: an introduction. *Int J Group Psychother* 42:351–356, 1992.
22. Racusin GR, Moss NE: Rational work and basic assumption life in a psychotherapy group for preschool victims of abuse: a case study. *J Child Adolesc Group Therapy* 2:3–15, 1992.
23. Schamess G: Differential diagnosis and group structure in the outpatient treatment of latency age children. In: Riester AE, Kraft I (eds): *Child Group Psychotherapy: Future Tense.* Madison, CT, International Universities Press, pp. 29–70, 1986.
24. Schectman Z: Group counseling and psychotherapy with children and adolescents. In: De-Lucia-Waack JL, Gerrity DA, Kalodner CR, Riva MT (eds): *Handbook of Group Counseling and Psychotherapy.* Thousand Oaks, CA, Sage Publications, Inc., pp. 429–444, 2004.
25. Slavson SR, Schiffer M: *Group Psychotherapy for Children.* Madison, CT, International Universities Press, 1975.
26. Crawford-Brolyn J, White A: A two-stage model for group therapy with impulse-ridden latency age children. In: Riester AE, Kraft I (eds): *Child Group Psychotherapy: Future Tense.* Madison, CT, International Universities Press, pp. 123–135, 1986.
27. Soo ES: Strategies for success for the beginning group therapist with child and adolescent groups. *J Child Adolesc Group Ther* 1:95–106, 1991.
28. Slavson SR: *Child Centered Group Guidance for Parents.* New York, International Universities Press, 1950.
29. Arnold LE, Rowe M, Tolbert HA: Parents groups. In: Arnold LE (ed): *Helping Parents Help Their Children.* New York, Brunner-Mazel, 114–125, 1978.
30. Riva MT, Wachtel M, Lasky GB: Effective leadership in group counseling and psychotherapy. In: DeLucia-Waack JL, Gerrity DA, Kalodner CR, Riva MT (eds): *Handbook of Group Counseling and Psychotherapy.* Thousand Oaks, CA, Sage Publications, Inc., pp. 37–48, 2004.
31. Dies RR: Therapist variables in group psychology research. In: Fuhriman A, Burlingame GM (eds): *Handbook of Group Psychotherapy: An Empirical and Clinical Synthesis.* New York, NY, Wiley, pp. 114–154, 1994.
32. Bednar RL, Melnick J, Kaul TJ: Risk, responsibility, and structure: a conceptual framework for initiating group counseling and psychotherapy. *J Couns Psychol* 21:31–37, 1974.
33. Burlingame GM, Fuhriman A: Epilogue. In: Fuhriman A, Burlingame GM (eds): *Handbook of Group Psychotherapy: An Empirical and Clinical Synthesis.* New York, Wiley, pp. 559–562, 1994.
34. Gazda GM, Ginter EJ, Horne AM: *Group Counseling and Group Psychotherapy.* Boston, MA, Allyn & Bacon, 2001.
35. Gossart-Walker S, Moss NE: Support groups for HIV-affected children. *J Child Adolesc Group Ther* 8:55–69, 1998.
36. Gossart-Walker S, Moss NE: An effective strategy for intervention with children and adolescents affected by HIV and AIDS. *Child Adolesc Psychiatr Clin N Am* 9:331–345, 2000.
37. Volkmar F, Klin A, Paul R (eds): *Handbook of Autism and Pervasive Developmental Disorders.* Hoboken, NJ, John Wiley & Sons, 2005.
38. Krasny L, Williams BJ, Provencal S, Ozonoff S: Social skills interventions for the autism spectrum: essential ingredients and a model curriculum. *Child Adolescent Psychiatr Clin N Am* 12:107–122, 2003.
39. Mishna F, Muskat B: "I'm not the only one!" Group therapy with older children and adolescents who have learning disabilities. *Int J Group Psychother* 54:455–476, 2004.
40. Pfeifer G: Complementary cultures in children's psychotherapy groups: conflict, co-existence, and convergence in group development. *Int J Group Psychother* 42:357–368, 1992.
41. Rosenthal L: Qualifications and tasks of the therapist in group therapy with children. *Clin Soc Work* 5:191–199, 1977.
42. Soo ES: Training and supervision in child and adolescent group psychotherapy. In: Riester AE, Kraft I (eds): *Child Group Psychotherapy: Future Tense.* Madison, CT, International Universities Press, pp. 157–171, 1986.
43. Soo ES: Is training and supervision of children and adolescent group therapists necessary? *J Child Adolesc Group Ther* 8:181–196, 1998.
44. Azima F: Countertransference. In and beyond child group psychotherapy. In: Riester AE, Kraft I (eds): *Child Group Psychotherapy: Future Tense.* Madison, CT, International Universities Press, 139–155, 1986.
45. MacLennan BW: Fifty years of training and supervision for group psychotherapy with children and adolescents. *J Child Adolesc Group Ther* 8:169–170, 1998.
46. DeLucia-Waack JL, Fauth J: Effective supervision of group leaders. In: DeLucia-Waack JL, Gerrity DA, Kalodner CR, Riva MT (eds): *Handbook of Group Counseling and Psychotherapy.* Thousand Oaks, CA, Sage Publications, Inc., pp. 136–150, 2004.
47. Anthony EJ: The history of group psychotherapy. In: Kaplan HI, Sadock BJ (eds): *Comprehensive Group Psychotherapy.* Baltimore, MD, Williams & Wilkins, pp. 4–31, 1971.
48. Burlingame GM, Fuhriman AJ, Johnson J: Current status and future directions of group therapy research. In: DeLucia-Waack JL, Gerrity DA, Kalodner CR, Riva MT (eds): *Handbook of Group Counseling and Psychotherapy.* Thousand Oaks, CA, Sage Publications, Inc., pp. 651–660, 2004.
49. Dagley JC, Gazda GM, Eppinger SJ, Stewart EA: Group psychotherapy research with children, preadolescents, and adolescents. In: Fuhrman A, Burlingame GM (eds): *Handbook of Group Psychotherapy.* New York, Wiley, 1994.
50. Hoag MJ, Burlingame GM: Evaluating the effectiveness of child and adolescent group treatment: a meta-analysis review. *J Clin Child Psychol* 26:234–246, 1997.
51. Kulic KR, Dagley JC, Horne AM: Prevention groups with children and adolescents. *J Specialists Group Work* 26:211–218, 2001.
52. Taylor NT, Burlingame GM, Kristensen KB, Fuhriman A, Johansen J, Dahl D: A survey of mental health care provider and managed care organization attitudes toward, familiarity with, and use of group interventions. *Int J Group Psychother* 51:243–263, 2001.

CHAPTER 6.2.7 ■ FAMILY THERAPY

G. PIROOZ SHOLEVAR

INTRODUCTION

Since the publication of the last volume of this textbook, family therapy has continued to expand its scientific base and theoretical evolution. Evidence-based programs primarily delivered as home-based, family-centered interventions in the community have continued to produce impressive results with adolescents with conduct disorders and substance abuse. Family interventions also have been applied systematically in controlled studies to a very broad range of clinical disorders of children and adolescents.

The fundamental theoretical concepts and technical interventions developed by pioneers in family systems and psychodynamic therapy have been adopted by the contemporary generation of family therapists who apply them in a multidimensional and ecologic manner, incorporating the characteristics of the children, their peer group, community, and broader culture. This broad framework has allowed the incorporation of other treatment modalities, such as cognitive-behavior therapy (CBT) and pharmacotherapy, which has significantly enhanced treatment effectiveness. A more flexible approach to involving parents has enhanced engagement in treatment, retention, and treatment outcome. Partly in response to these developments, NIMH has encouraged the use of family interventions in investigative projects; more than half of NIMH-funded intervention proposals and programs include a family component (1).

DEFINITION

Family theory focuses on human behavior and psychiatric disturbances in the context of interpersonal relationships (2–4). This theory forms the basis of family therapy, which is an umbrella term for a number of clinical practices that treat psychopathology within the context of family systems rather than individuals. Interventions are designed to effect change in family relationships rather than in an individual (2,5). This approach is based on observations that symptomatic behavior appears in individuals involved in certain dysfunctional processes within their families or with other significant persons. Conversely, positive family interactions such as effective parenting practices, emotionally nurturing family environments, and secure attachment relationships are associated with normative child development, healthy functioning, and serve as protective factors against emotional disorders (6).

Family theory considers the family as an interpersonal system with cybernetic qualities. The relationships among the components of the system are nonlinear (or circular); the interactions are cyclical rather than causative. Complex interlocking feedback mechanisms and patterns of interaction among the members of the system repeat themselves sequentially. Any given symptom can be viewed simply as a behavior functioning as a homeostatic mechanism that regulates family interactions (7).

The family system is nonsummative and includes the assets and dysfunctions of the individuals as well as their interactions (8). A person's problems cannot be evaluated or treated apart from the context in which they occur and the functions that they serve. It is assumed, therefore, that an individual cannot be expected to change unless the family system changes (8). Treatment addresses the behavioral dysfunctions as a manifestation of disturbances within the entire family relational system; the role of the total family in aiding or in sabotaging treatment is the focus even when a distinct diagnosable psychiatric illness is present in one of the family members.

The goals of family therapy as a psychotherapeutic approach are as follows (3):

- Explore the interactional dynamics of the family and their relation to psychopathology.
- Mobilize the family's internal strength and functional resources.
- Restructure the maladaptive interactional family styles.
- Strengthen the family's problem-solving behavior.

The term *family therapy* has been expanded to include family intervention, a broader array of procedures. It subsumes a large number of clinical practices based on a variety of theoretical concepts with explicit focus on altering the interactions among family members and subsystems with the goal of improving the functioning of the family as a unit, its subsystems and members. Treatment of disturbed individuals as well as dysfunctional relationships can be achieved through family interventions (3,4). Improved functioning in parental and parent/child subsystems is a fundamental goal in treatment of children and adolescents.

HISTORY

Family therapy and conjointed treatment of families emerged in the late 1940s and early 1950s. The towering figures in the field were Nathan Ackerman, Gregory Bateson, Murray Bowen, Bell, Theodore Lidz, Don Jackson, Jay Heley, and many others. Family therapy with a focus on children and adolescents was introduced by Carl Whitaker, Salvadore Minuchin and more recently by David and Jill Scharff, Joan Zilbach, and others. A detailed description of the history can be found in recent literature (9,10).

In the late 1960s, Minuchin in collaboration with Montalvo and Haley established the Structural School of Family Therapy. The structural approach reached its height in theoretical development by defining the term *psychosomatic families*—the families of patients with anorexia nervosa and other psychosomatic disorders (11). The structural approach has been applied extensively to families of children with behavior disorders (12).

An underappreciated approach to family therapy with adolescents and children was attempted by the Multiple Impact Therapy group (MIT) in Galveston, Texas (13). The novel intervention by this group included 2 days of family therapy by a number of professionals who alternated their work with different family members during the therapeutic encounter. They classified the families according to the disorders of the adolescents and children, mostly oppositional/defiant and conduct disorders.

INDICATIONS AND CONTRAINDICATIONS

An apparent and clear indication for family therapy is open and stressful conflicts among family members, with or without symptomatic behaviors in one or more members. Family therapy also can be applicable when there are covert problems within the family, which can give rise to dysfunctional behavior in one or more family members, or when other family members covertly support and perpetuate the disorder. Recognizing covert family interactional problems coexisting with overt dysfunctions in one or more family members is the specific contribution of the field of family therapy. Recently, family interventions have been used extensively with externalizing adolescent disorders and substance abuse.

Contraindications to family therapy are relative rather than absolute. They include discussing long dormant, charged, or explosive family issues with the whole family before the family commits seriously to treatment. Another relative contraindication is discussing stressful situations with the family when one or more members are severely destabilized and require hospitalization. Insufficient expertise in family therapy relative to a high level of resistance and defensiveness in the family can result in a counterproductive treatment course. Lack of knowledge of child development and psychopathology can render family intervention with children and adolescents equally unproductive and result in missed therapeutic opportunities.

MODELS OF FAMILY THERAPY

The diversity of models of family therapy raises questions about the common ground among family therapies. The pioneers in family therapy focused on different dimensions in the family system, and to some degree, these different focuses reflected unrecognized differences among patient populations treated by the early family therapists. Although family therapists adopted divergent paths, they ignored the likely conclusion that different approaches to family therapy are closely linked to family characteristics commonly observed in different disorders.

Different models of family therapy are applicable to various patient populations. The intergenerational family therapy models are particularly applicable to families whose members have longstanding disorders and have not negotiated adequate separation and differentiation between the generations (14,15). Structural and strategic family therapies are particularly applicable to families encountering a crisis situation in which there has been adequate separation from previous generations and a reasonably satisfactory precrisis adjustment in the nuclear family. Behavior family therapy is particularly applicable to marital problems and children with chronic conduct disorders. Psychodynamic and experiential family therapies are helpful to family members with narcissistic vulnerability and a broad range of personality and neurotic disorders who have maintained a relatively adequate level of functioning but find little enjoyment in their lives. An emerging array of family-based interventions attempt to reverse the disintegrative processes in chronically and seriously disordered families effected by abuse, neglect, and placement of the children outside of the family.

Each model of family therapy includes different theoretical concepts and techniques. Some models of family therapy can be grouped based on their similarities. The major models of family therapy, their core concepts, goals, and approaches and techniques, are summarized in Table 6.2.7.1.

Structural Family Therapy

Structural family therapy was developed by Minuchin in collaboration with Montalvo and Haley and applied to children and adolescents with acute behavioral problems and eating disorders. The foundational theoretical concept in structural family therapy is boundary. Clear and flexible boundaries are characteristic of functional families. Enmeshed and disengaged boundaries describe families with excessive intrusiveness or unavailability to one another, respectively.

Structural family interventions emphasize establishing boundaries within the family through the decisive and sensitive actions of the therapist. Family tasks and homework assignments further enforce this process. Methods of "joining" the family allow the therapist to join the family and shift family members' positions to disrupt dysfunctional patterns and strengthen parental hierarchies. Clear and flexible boundaries are established in the session, and the family is encouraged to search for alternative interactional patterns.

Structural family therapy has been used to treat eating disorders, particularly anorexia nervosa in children and adolescents. Its effectiveness in treating psychosomatic disorders and behavioral problems has been proven through numerous case reports and observations, as well as family outcome studies (11).

Strategic Family Therapy

Strategic family therapy emphasizes the need for a strategy developed by the family therapist to intervene in a family's efforts to maintain homeostasis by adhering rigidly to dysfunctional family patterns and symptoms. Strategic family therapy, like psychodynamic family therapy, has a well-articulated approach to address the resistance within family systems. Dealing with resistance, particularly in the family's response to the therapist's interventions, requires innovative methods. One technique, paradoxical intervention, attempts to reduce resistance and enhance change in the family structure and interactions by discouraging change. Paradoxical interventions facilitate the therapist's joining the family with minimal resistance to restructure the family's interactional system.

Strategic interventions are based on identifying a family's "rules"—the metacommunicational patterns that underlie symptomatic behaviors. These interventions are applied through directives and homework assignments practiced between sessions. The homework can be a logical, straightforward approach to the behavior or a seemingly illogical, paradoxical approach such as "prescribing the symptom," a technique requiring family members to do and acknowledge what the family has been doing all along to undermine interactional patterns by supporting the family's communicational pathways. Family life-cycle passages are considered important because they reveal inflexibility in the family's structure that makes the familial response to internal and developmental demands difficult.

The strategic approach of Haley (8) and Madanes (16) emphasizes the importance of strengthening the parental alliance to deal effectively with the symptomatic and challenging behavior of the children. Power struggles between family members and subsequently between the therapist and the family are the focus of treatment.

TABLE 6.2.7.1

MODELS OF FAMILY THERAPY

Model of Family Therapy	Core Concepts	Goal	Strategies/Techniques
Structural Family Therapy Minuchin et al.	• Generational hierarchy • Boundaries and Subsystems • Flexibility of system for: a. Autonomy and interdependence b. Continuity and adaptive restructuring to fit changing internal and external demands	• Symptoms result from current family structural imbalance: • Enmeshed or disengaged styles • Maladaptive reaction to changing demands (developmental, environmental) • Defuse generational hierarchy and boundaries	• Intervene in family interactions • Reorganize family structure • Shift members' relative positions to balance interactional patterns • Strengthen parental hierarchy • Reinforce clear, flexible boundaries • Mobilize more adaptive alternative patterns
Strategic Family Therapy Milton Erickson Jay Haley Cloe Madanes Paul Waltzlawick John Weakland	• Repeated patterns of interaction • Power/control struggles • Flexibility • Large behavioral repertoire for: a. Problem-solving b. Life-cycle passage	• Symptom is a communication embedded in interaction pattern • Problems; symptoms are maintained by: a. Unsuccessful problem-solving attempts b. Impasse at life-cycle transition c. Rigid view; paucity of alternatives	• Resolve presenting problem through: • Specific strategies/ objecti ves • Interrupt rigid feedback cycle: change symptom-maintaining sequences • Shift perspective to empower positions • Paradoxical instructions
Solutions-focused Steve de Shazar et al.	• Focus on solutions, not problems • Disregard "resistance" • Inattention to origin of problems	• Creation of solutions • Presolve presenting problems	• "Exception" questions • "Miracle" questions • Coping questions • Client empowerment
Bowen Family Systems Murray Bowen, Micheal Kerr, Philip Guerin	• Differentiation of self • Triangulation • Transmission of symptoms across generations • Family emotional system • Emotional cutoffs	• Increased differentiation • Detriangulation • Improved ability to manage anxiety • Resolution of cutoff	• Use of genogram • Therapist as coach • Education about Multigenerational family processes
Psychodynamic-Psychoanalytic Nathan Ackerman David and Jill Scharff Helm Steirlin Emotionally focused Therapy Susan Johnson Leslie Greenburg	• Projective identification • Interlocking conflicts and defenses observation • Object relations • Projective identification • Splitting • Scapegoating problem • Attachment disorders	• Enhance awareness and self • Enhance empathy • Improve insight • Disentangle interlocking alliance pathologies and resistances • Interpretation • Differentiation of Attachment vs. defensive feelings	• Transference, resistance, and countertransference analysis • Creation of holding environment • De-emphasize presenting • Emphasis on therapeutic alliance
Evidence-Based Family Therapies **Parent Management Training (PMT)** Patterson et al. Forehand, McMahon et al.	• Negative reinforcement of maladaptive behaviors • Ineffective/unskilled Parent management Interventions • Coercive family processes	• Establishment of effective parent management techniques • Promotion of prosocial behaviors in children • Reduce coercive interactions	• Parent management training with parents • Behavior management training with parents • Problem-solving and communication training • Intensive home-based
Functional Family Therapy (FFT) Alexander et al. Sexton T	• Defensive interactions • Lack of supportive interaction • Nonfunctional Dysfunctional/ family patterns	• Address the function of symptoms in family interaction • Enhance supportive interactions • Reduce defensive interactions	• Enhance support and other functions in the family
Multisystemic Therapy (MST) Henggeler et al.	• Multisystemic dysfunctions on family, peer group, school and community level	• Multisystemic problem-solving	• Intensive home-based intervention • Train and empower family to problem solve in multiple systems

TABLE 6.2.7.1

(CONTINUED)

Model of Family Therapy	Core Concepts	Goal	Strategies/Techniques
Multidimensional Family Therapy (MDFT) Liddle et al.	• Multidimensional/multisystemic dysfunctions on family, individual, school, community levels	• Multisystemic/multidimensional intervention on family, individual, peer group and community level	• Structural, systemic, strategic, group therapy, behavioral intervention techniques • Multidimensional/multi-component problem-solving
Behavioral Patterson et al. Forehand et al. Falloon	• Adaptive behavior is rewarded; maladaptive behavior is not • Exchange benefits outweigh costs; reciprocity • Communication and problem-solving ability • Flexibility	• Family attention and reward • Alter deficient exchanges (e.g., coercive, skewed) • Correct communication deficits	• Change contingencies of social reinforcement • Reward adaptive behavior, not maladaptive • Communication, problem-solving skills training
Psychoeducational McFarlane Carol Anderson	• Successful coping and mastery of developmental challenges: a. Caregiving in chronic illness b. Skill in family relationships and community living skills • Stress-diathesis model of Biologically based disorders	• Reduction in normative and nonnormative stresses (e.g., in couples; relationships, parenting, remarriage, adverse life events)	• Information, coping skills and social support for: a. Family management of chronic illness b. Stress and stigma reduction c. Mastery of family adaptational challenges

Partially adopted and significantly revised from Steinglass P: Family therapy. In: Kaplan P, Saddack B (eds): *Comprehensive Textbook of Psychiatry*. 6th ed. Baltimore, MD, Williams & Wilkins Publishers, pp. 1838–1847, 1995; and Gurman A, Lebow J: Family and couple therapy. In: Saddock B, Saddock V (eds): *Comprehensive Textbook of Psychiatry*. 7th ed. Lippincott Williams & Wilkins, Baltimore, MD, pp. 2157–2167, 2000.

SOLUTION-FOCUSED THERAPY

Solution-focused therapy concentrates on the "exceptional solution" repertoire already practiced by the patients to deemphasize their problem-saturated outlook and enlarge the application of such solutions. The therapeutic effectiveness is enhanced by shifting the focus to the "solution" rather than the "problems" (10,17).

PSYCHODYNAMIC FAMILY THERAPY

Psychodynamic family therapy emphasizes individual maturation, personality development, early childhood experiences, and resolution of symptoms and conflicts in the context of the family system. Common theoretical concepts of psychodynamic family therapy include projective identification, shared unconscious conflicts and defenses, intrafamilial transference reactions, dyadic and triadic family transferences in treatment, and a host of object relations psychoanalytic concepts, such as holding environment and empathy.

BEHAVIORAL FAMILY THERAPY

Behavioral family therapy applies the principles of positive and negative reinforcement to the family unit with the goal of enhancing reciprocity and minimizing coercive family processes. Coercive family processes generally are in the form of punishment, avoidance, and power play. Enhancing communication and problem-solving skills in the family is emphasized and punishment is discouraged.

Contemporary behavior family therapy is based on social learning theory and has been applied in the form of parent management training (PMT). The parents and children are taught environmental contingencies (positive and negative reinforcement, reward and punishment) which shape behavior. Strong attention is paid to enhancing prosocial behavior.

Behavior family therapy can be combined with communication and problem-solving training.

PSYCHOEDUCATIONAL FAMILY INTERVENTION

Psychoeducational family intervention based on stress-diathesis theory attempts to enhance family adaptation primarily through informing the family and patient about the nature of psychopathology in psychiatric disorders. The family and patient also receive detailed information about the treatment process and outcome. Psychoeducational intervention has been applied extensively in treating major mental illnesses such as schizophrenia, depression, alcoholism, and anxiety disorders. It consists of a series of in-depth and expert instructional sessions on the phenomenology, etiology, and diagnosis of the disorders. Clinical research findings are explained and made user friendly for the family. Information is also provided about social institutions and systems involved in the care of the patient. Psychoeducational family therapy can be easily combined with other treatment modalities, particularly pharmacotherapy and crisis intervention. The psychodynamic and exploratory psychotherapies are postponed to the later phases of treatment, when the patient and the family are stabilized.

Psychoeducational approaches make extensive use of empirical findings on expressed emotion (EE), communication deviance, affective styles, and problem-solving. This reduces the stressful family processes, recurrence in illness and rehospitalization.

The application of psychoeducational model to childhood depression and suicidality has been particularly productive. The model has been applied preventively to a range of stressful and potentially pathogenic situations for the children such as pediatric cancer, death, and dying. A model for prevention of depression in children of depressed parents has been empirically tested by Beardslee and Schwoeri (18) in the past decade with positive outcomes.

THE FAMILY LIFE CYCLE

The term *family life cycle* proposes that the family moves through a series of developmental stages. Carter and McGoldrick defined critical emotional issues for the family at different stages of the life cycle (19). Haley (8) applied the family life-cycle concept to understanding the clinical problems of families by relating their dysfunctions to the difficulties they have in moving from one developmental stage to another.

Marriage is considered the first stage of the family life cycle (20). The expectable seven stages of the family life cycle are (1) beginning family, (2) childbearing family, (3) family with school age children, (4) family with teenagers, (5) family as a launching center, (6) family in its middle years, and (7) aging family. Combrinck-Graham (21) proposed the family life spiral, with overlapping development issues for different generations.

FAMILY THERAPY WITH CHILDREN AND ADOLESCENTS: OVERVIEW

The conceptional and technical differences between the fields of child psychiatry and family therapy can be summarized in the following way. Child psychiatrists have accused systemic family therapists of lack of appreciation for the individual child's unique developmental characteristics and intrapsychic life (22,23). According to child psychiatrists, family therapists were oblivious to biologic vulnerabilities and pharmacotherapy. Conversely, family therapists have accused child psychiatrists of lacking understanding of the interpersonal dimensions of the child's life, the multiple sources of stress in contemporary family life, and preoccupation with minute developmental deviations and past events at the expense of present-life realities.

In the 1980s, the two camps approached reconciliation. Recognition of family therapy's limitations with certain populations forced many family therapists to reach "beyond family therapy" and address peer group, psychological (intrapsychic and cognitive), and social dimensions of behavior disorders. Teaching family therapy has been a requirement in child and adolescent, as well as general, psychiatric residency programs for the past 20 years. The integrative approach in treating major mental illnesses has resulted in the consolidation of a true field of family psychiatry (10,24). Psychodynamic and object relations family therapies have demonstrated the many advantages of recognizing the interrelationships between interpersonal and intrapsychic processes (25–27).

We briefly summarize the application of family therapy to multiple disorders of children and adolescents and refer the reader to the references listed for more information.

THEORETICAL CONCEPTS

All schools of family therapy are founded on theoretical concepts that are specifically applicable to family therapy with children and adolescents. In enmeshed families, there is not sufficient distance and objectivity among family members to allow differentiation of the children through the separation and individuation processes. The children have significant difficulties in school and social relationships, further curtailing their maturity. Overinvolvement between a child and a parent, projective family mechanisms, and triangulation as described by Bowen are major impediments to differentiation and maturity, which can transfer across generations.

Projective identification describes the unconscious processes of projection of unresolved parental conflicts onto a child, who assumes an identity based on a historically assigned role. Assumption of this role interferes with the child's appropriate identity formation. Traumatic events such as child neglect and physical or sexual abuse in the early history of the family can result in the repetition of such traumatic situations in subsequent generations. "Parentification," another impediment to the child's development, assigns a parental role to a child and deprives him or her of age-appropriate experiences.

Although many schools of family therapy recognize the significance of the separation–individuation process for adolescent family members, few of them describe the intricate network of developmental failures within the family and the adolescent that undermine the separation–individuation process. Stierlin (28) proposed that binding, delegating, and expulsion are three ways that families negotiate a pathologic separation to overcome the fear of prolonged fusion. In the binding mode, the excessive binding of the family to the adolescent can force the growing adolescent into psychotic or suicidal behavior to free himself or herself from the family unit. In the intricate delegating mode, the family allows the adolescent to depart from the family unit "on a long leash" to return periodically to share the tales of his or her exploits in order to compensate for the restricted life of the parents. In the expulsion mode, the adolescent is rejected by and extruded from the family to free him or her from the family unit.

TECHNIQUES

The literature on family therapy with children describes the clinical process and office arrangements that are most welcoming toward the children. The office should be equipped with toys that are conductive to imaginative play; paper and crayons provide unlimited possibilities for drawing and expression of fantasies. A special attempt should be made to include the children in the treatment process by using age-appropriate methods of communication for the child. Long and complex discussions discourage children from participating and should be avoided. The observational data on families with young children are especially significant. Techniques for family therapy with children have been described by Zilbach (29) and Chasin and White (30). Sholevar has described in detail the process of initial and diagnostic family interview (31).

Often, family therapy with children can disclose physical or emotional child neglect. When family support is potentially available, family intervention can mobilize and rehabilitate family resources to provide the necessary nurturance to resume the child's developmental progress. When such resources are not present, enabling the family to search for an alternative living situation with the help of social agencies may be necessary (31,32).

FAMILY INTERVENTION WITH ATTENTION-DEFICIT HYPERACTIVITY DISORDER

Family interventions have been employed to reduce the core symptoms of attention-deficit hyperactivity disorder (ADHD). The reduction in negative interaction between the parents and children has been enhanced when parent therapy and family interventions were provided as a primary or adjunctive treatment (33–35). Parent training allows the parents to enhance the capacity of the ADHD child to focus, remain on task, solve problems, act prosocially with peers, and reduce impulsivity and aggression through cognitive processing. These are effective tools to strengthen the positive parent–child bonds and the ADHD child's fragile self-esteem by reducing negative and counterproductive parental behavior and enhancing skillful and goal-directed intervention by parents in potentially conflictual situations.

Multimodal Treatment Study of Children with ADHD is a comprehensive psychosocial treatment package of 30 parent training sessions, school visits, and teacher training with or without medication (33,36). The combined treatment exhibited the best results in control of ADHD core symptoms.

FAMILY THERAPY AND CONDUCT DISORDERS

Paterson et al. (37) described "coercive family processes" by which the parents, who generally lack management skills, initiate overly punitive and aggressive actions toward their children but withdraw in the face of strong opposition by the children. The coercive processes result in a high level of aggressive and uncontrollable behavior in the children. Subsequent research by Patterson et al. (37) focused on the relationship between aggressive behavior in children and depression in parents, particularly single mothers.

Other researchers also have studied the families of children with conduct disorders. Alexander, Barton, and Parsons (38–40) examined the function of aggressive behavior in the family and attempted to change the family's interactions from defensive to supportive interactions through functional in order to undermine conduct problems.

Functional family therapy (FFT), PMT, and multisystemic therapy (MST) have produced very encouraging therapeutic results with conduct disorders.

Parent Management Training

Forehand and Kotchick (41) and Patterson et al. in 1982 have produced extensive and empirically based interventions in PMT. Their approach has been applied in multiple settings by independent teams of investigators and has proved beneficial in altering oppositional/defiant behavior and conduct disorders, and enhancing prosocial behavior in children at home and in school. The preventive effect on younger siblings of children with conduct disorders also has been noted (37,41). PMT addresses the deficient parental management skills that are intimately correlated with antisocial behavior and arrested socialization in children. It teaches the parents to interact proactively and more productively with their children by reinforcing prosocial behavior rather than inadvertently rewarding deviant behavior (42–44).

The basic principles of PMT are accurate labeling of the child's behavior, emphasis on prosocial behavior, de-emphasis of disruptive behavior, administration of tangible reinforcers, use of nonviolent methods of "punishment" and anticipation/resolution of problems. The keystone targeted behavior of the child is noncompliance.

The interventions are based on positive reinforcement of prosocial behavior, use of time out, guidelines for attending/ignoring, shaping the desirable behavior (successive approximation of terminal behaviors), and enhancement of problem-solving, negotiations, and compromise formations. Coercive family processes (37) are identified and resolved through effective reinforcement.

Extensive research by numerous independent investigators in different settings has demonstrated the effectiveness of PMT over the control groups by generalization of therapeutic results in different settings, short-term and long-term beneficial outcomes. There has been a lowering of parental (maternal) depression and subsequent referral of younger siblings for antisocial behavior. The treatment has been less effective with "insular mothers" who are socially isolated, depressed, and have economic problems (45). A range of behavioral and cognitive interventions, enlargement of the social network, and medication in the case of parental depression can all help to enhance maternal functioning.

In response to the large number of delinquent children placed out of home, PMT has been applied to children in foster care. Oregon Treatment Foster Care (OTFC) is a family- and home-based treatment model that teaches effective parenting practices through close monitoring and limiting contact with deviant peer groups (46,47). This intervention has produced a reduction in rearrests, detention center placement, runaway behavior and improved relationships with biologic families in comparison to adolescents placed in conventional foster care.

FUNCTIONAL FAMILY THERAPY

FFT developed by Alexander et al. (38,40) attempts to alter defensive family interactions to supportive ones in families of delinquent children through an integration of behavioral, structural/strategic techniques.

MULTISYSTEMIC THERAPY: MOVING BEYOND FAMILY THERAPY

In the past two decades, there have been many attempts to broaden the scope of family interventions to include multiple other systems. The MST of Henggeler et al. (48,49) is the most widely recognized and empirically validated intervention system of its kind. The target of the family-based intervention has been chronic, violent, or substance-abusing juvenile offenders at high risk for out-of-home placement. The intervention is based on the premise that the individual with CD is nested within a complex network of interconnected systems that encompass individual, familial, and extra-familial (peer, school, neighborhood) factors. The goal of MST is to empower parents with the skills and resources needed to raise their teenage children and to empower the youth to cope with family, peer, school, and neighborhood problems. The therapeutic approach provides support and skill building in the family and the youth to achieve this goal. It emphasizes building youth and family strength (protective factors) on an individualized and comprehensive basis to attenuate risk factors. The home-based model enhances service access and family retention in treatment. It has been applied with male and female African American and white adolescents between the ages of 12 and 17 years. The therapists have a low caseload and strong system of supervision supplemented by consultation to allow intensive intervention. The approximate length of the treatment is 4 months.

MST has produced strong evidence for program effectiveness in multiple controlled and randomized clinical trials with violent and chronic juvenile offenders.

They have demonstrated the following findings:

- Reduction in long-term rate of criminal offences
- Reduced rates of out-of-home placement
- Reduced rates of drug use and drug-related offenses
- Improvement in family functioning
- Decrease of other mental health problems
- A lower level of rearrest, reincarceration, and reduction in the days of out-of-home placement

MST as an alternative to psychiatric hospitalization at the time of crisis has produced an 85% reduction in days of hospitalization.

FAMILY INTERVENTION AND DEPRESSION

Depressed patients tend to be aversive to others and also feel victimized by them. They frequently engage in escalating negative exchanges. Depressed patients and their family members tend to verbalize negative, subjective feelings more frequently than nondepressed couples, whose communications are more task oriented (50–54). The marriages of depressed women (or men) are characterized by friction, poor communication, a lack of affection, withdrawal, and a tendency for the nondepressed spouse to view his or her spouse as accusatory (50,52).

Children of depressed parents are at risk for many diagnosable psychological problems, a rate as high as 40% to 50% (52). The risk to children is increased if (1) the depressed person's spouse becomes depressed or is unavailable to the child, (2) there are marital problems or divorce (52), and (3) there is no supportive relationship with another adult.

Family-based interventions with depressed patients are based on an integration of family systems theory psychoeducational model, psychodynamic theory and attachment theory within a developmental model (53). The role of nondepressed parent in enhancing the coping capacity of the family is crucial (53).

Brent et al. (55) have reported that CBT is more effective than structural family therapy with depressed adolescents at the end of treatment but equally effective in 2-year follow-up. When methodologic issues are put aside, structural family therapy as practiced by the group may not have addressed crucial family issues for depressed adolescents such as poor attachment and low affective involvement between the parents and children. Beardslee and Schwoeri's (18) comprehensive preventive model to reduce the likelihood of transmission of depression from the parents to the children remains dominant in the field.

ANXIETY DISORDERS

A number of family variables have been implicated in anxiety disorders. They include overprotective and overly controlling parenting styles, parents modeling or reinforcing anxious and avoidant behaviors, and parental perception of excessive threats (56). CBT and behavioral family therapy have been compared in treatment of childhood anxiety disorders (57). The family therapy component included communication and problem-solving techniques and anxiety management methods for parents. The combination of CBT and BFT was significantly more effective than CBT alone, particularly with younger children and girls. In addition to a reduction in anxiety, there was an improvement in general functioning and enhancement in parental competence.

FAMILY THERAPY AND "PSYCHOSOMATIC" DISORDERS

Minuchin et al. (11) described several common characteristics among families with children and adolescents who have a range of "psychosomatic" disorders such as anorexia nervosa. "Psychosomatic families" were enmeshed, overprotective, rigid; avoided conflict; and used the child's problems to detract attention from parental. The treatment corrects defensive interactional patterns to enhance separation and autonomy in the child. They demonstrated the impressive impact of structural family therapy on families with younger adolescents who have eating disorders and other psychosomatic reactions. However, the utility of the model with older patients who have bulimia has not been established (58).

Behavioral family therapy and psychoeducation also have been applied to eating disorders and anorexia nervosa. They address risk factors for eating disorders such as parental intrusive, critical, and overcontrolling behavior and low family cohesion (59).

Eisler et al. (60) argue that parallel treatment of the parents and anorexic adolescents is highly effective when there is a high level of maternal criticism. Application of family therapies is effective in bringing about weight gain, but has also increased the level of overt family conflict, which supports the observation that conflict avoidance and denial is a significant characteristic of families of adolescents with eating disorders (61).

FAMILY THERAPY AND ADOLESCENT SUBSTANCE ABUSE

Family therapy with adolescent substance abuse has been described by multidimensional family therapy and MST. Liddle (62) and Liddle and Dakof (63) have applied multidimensional, multicomponent, and multisystemic comprehensive family intervention to substance abusing adolescents. They have investigated the links between changes in parenting and reductions in adolescents' drug abuse, improving the therapist-adolescent alliance and addressing cultural and gender issues in treatment. Their preliminary findings are supportive of effectiveness of family interventions in comparison with other treatment modalities.

MST (48,49,64) has been applied to treatment of substance abuse in adolescents with very encouraging results. It has been effective in reducing drug use, rearrests, and the number of days in placement.

FAMILY INTERVENTION IN RESIDENTIAL TREATMENT CENTERS

Research has identified the lack of a meaningful conceptual framework guiding intervention with families as the major factor limiting the effectiveness of residential treatment (65). Family intervention in a residential treatment center should be guided by two variables: (1) the state of disintegration of the family unit and (2) the level of availability of the family as a potential care provider or participant in psychiatric treatment. Based on assessment of these variables, families of patients in a residential treatment center can be divided into four groups: (1) available families, (2) potentially available families, (3) partially available families, and (4) totally unavailable families (32,65).

Available Families

The available family is forced to institutionalize the child after family confrontations at the height of negatively escalated interactions. The family and child are strongly bonded and depend on one another to the point that they cannot live with or without each other. Such families are available for home visits, participation in family sessions, and eventual family reunification.

Potentially Available Families

The potentially available family has lost its immediate ability to care for the child because of a loss of functional capacity in the nuclear or extended family. A history of divorce, remarriage, physical or psychiatric illness, or death should alert the treatment team to the loss of family resources and capacity. The therapeutic task is to recognize the limitations in the functional and caretaking capacity of these families and protect them from any unrealistic and premature demands. The functional capacity of the family should be increased by resolving intergenerational conflicts, improving the functional and economic capacity of the parents, and activating the parents' social networks.

Partially Available Families

The partially available family interacts with the child through erratic telephone calls, occasional visits, or irregular attendance in treatment sessions. A major clinical finding in such families is the extreme nature of parental incapacity in managing life tasks. A realistic treatment strategy is to maintain the family's connection with the child psychologically while making realistic living plans for the child after discharge from the residential treatment center. The family can continue to remain as a resource to the group home or foster family after the child's discharge from the residential treatment center.

Totally Unavailable Families

The totally unavailable family is characterized by loss of contact with the child many years before his or her admission to a residential treatment center. There is usually a distorted and unrealistic expectation of a potential reunion between the family and the child. Such distorted fantasies should be discussed immediately and continuously throughout residential treatment. It would be helpful if the families could be located early in the course of residential treatment to verify—either in person or by telephone—their inability to take care of the child. This strategy would help resolve some of the child's dormant fantasies and conflicts and facilitate his or her future adaptation to other living possibilities.

RECENT DEVELOPMENTS IN FAMILY THEORY AND THERAPY

In the past decade, the field of family therapy has moved toward more empirically derived measures, such as EE, and away from theoretically driven constructs. There has been a close adherence to the stress-diathesis model (66–68) and the Finnish adoption studies (67), particularly in reference to major mental illnesses. This model recognizes the presence of reasonably convincing evidence for a strong genetic predisposition to a number of major mental disorders, such as schizophrenia, bipolar disorders, and alcoholism, which, in interaction with various intercurrent life events within and outside of the family, can affect the risk for emerging or recurring disorder in a family member. Contemporary family therapy also clearly recognizes the efficacy of psychopharmacology in schizophrenia and depression.

Stress-Diathesis Theory

Stress-diathesis or stress-vulnerability theory was first proposed by Rosenthal in 1970 and further refined by Zubin and Spring (68). Stress-diathesis theory regards the disorder as a product of two sets of variables: (1) vulnerability and (2) stressors. Vulnerability can be the result of genetic and psychobiological factors, although psychological and interpersonal vulnerability can function in a similar fashion. Genetic factors have been studied in schizophrenia, depression, and alcoholism. Stress can be caused by external factors or as a result of stressful psychological mechanisms or interpersonal patterns. The perspective of stress-diathesis theory is that illness is the result of heightened vulnerability and stress, and can be best prevented, managed, and treated by altering both sets of factors. Psychotropic medications function by reducing vulnerability, family interventions focus on lowering interpersonal sources of stress, and enhancing coping and problem-solving capacities.

Finnish Adoption Studies

The Finnish adoption studies (67) have produced data supporting the combined and interconnected role of genetic and familial variables in schizophrenia and other mental disorders. Researchers studied the level of family functioning, adaptability, and organization of adoptive families and dividing them into five groups from "optimally functioning" to "inadequately functioning." Although all families adopted children with comparable genetic vulnerability to schizophrenia, the outcome of the children was significantly correlated with level of family functioning. There were no psychotic or borderline children in the two groups of families with optimal or close to optimal functioning. In contrast, there was a preponderance of schizophrenic and borderline patients in the two groups with the lowest level of functioning. The Finnish study strongly supports the notion that genetic risk can be enhanced or decreased according to the level of functioning and adequacy of the family.

FAMILY VARIABLES IN DEVELOPMENTAL PSYCHOPATHOLOGY; SCHIZOPHRENIA

A significant change has occurred in conceptualizing the family dimension of schizophrenia. The family is viewed as a major resource whose availability to the patient can make a crucial difference in positive outcome. Negative interaction between the patient and family now is seen as largely reactive to the patient's symptoms rather than causative. Blaming family interactions (double blind) or the parents (schizophrenogenic mother) has become obsolete.

Family studies based on the stress-vulnerability model have investigated variables that can differentiate families of schizophrenic patients from families of nonschizophrenic patients. Studies of indicators of risk have focused particularly on three variables: (1) EE, (2) communication deviance, and (3) affective style (69,70).

Expressed Emotion

In 1962, Brown et al. reported that male patients with chronic schizophrenia who had returned to live with their families following psychiatric hospitalization were more prone to rehospitalization than patients who went to other living arrangements (71). He proposed the term *expressed emotion*, a composite variable with the values of high and low, as an index of the family's criticism of and overinvolvement with the patient. EE refers to negative emotional attitude. A number of subsequent British and American studies have indicated that the rate of relapse in schizophrenic and depressed patients in families with high EE is four times higher than that in families with low EE (72). The interventions with families having high EE, with specific goals for reducing familial hostility and over involvement, have provided experimental evidence that a decrease in the level of EE results in a decrease in the occurrence of relapse (72). Vaughn and Leff (73) have suggested that families who blame the illness rather than the patient for the behaviors typically accompanying psychiatric impairment are likely to be supportive or have low EE. Families with high EE, in contrast, seem more inclined to attribute the causes of deviant behavior to the patient.

Communication Deviance

Wynne and Singer (1963) posed the concept of communication deviance to describe nonschizophrenic patients (74,75). A lack of clarity in communication and disturbances in maintaining attention in the parents of schizophrenic patients in comparison to nonschizophrenic patients. Subsequent studies have indicated that communication deviance is related to the severity of psychopathology in the offspring, although some of the disturbances are nonschizophrenic in nature. Communication deviance may represent a cross-generational shared vulnerability in the parents and children affecting attention, perception, and information processing. Longitudinal studies of communication deviance have shown a high risk for psychopathology in children of parents with high communication deviance, particularly if there is concomitant high EE and negative affective style.

FAMILY CLASSIFICATION AND DIAGNOSIS

Family therapists have described different types of families: undifferentiated, enmeshed, disengaged, and psychosomatic. DSM-IV has rekindled the interest in an empirically based family classification and diagnostic system. A family classification system has been proposed by the family committee of the Group for the Advancement of Psychiatry (GAP) (76). They have proposed a document consistent with DSM-IV to specify diagnostic criteria for family and couple relational disorders. The committee's criteria focus on specific family problems such as sexual or physical abuse, divorce, failure to thrive, and separation anxiety (77).

The Global Assessment of Relational Functioning Scale (GARF) developed by Endicott and Spitzer (76) has been used by the GAP committee to evaluate the level of a family's dysfunction, analogous to the axis V rating of global functioning of the individual DSM-III-R. Other authors have proposed a second classification system of family relational disorders (71,78).

FAMILY INTERVENTION IN PSYCHIATRIC HOSPITALS

The goals of the family-oriented model of inpatient intervention are to prevent rehospitalization, strengthen fragile ties between the family and the patient, and help the family and patient reach the highest functional level. This approach is psychoeducationally oriented, and emphasizes the rehabilitation of the family for a successful reunion when the patient returns home. Inpatient family intervention focuses on treating the patient's illness while recognizing the importance of family variables. It places the relatively causative biologic factors in perspective with the familial and environmental influences. Medication is considered a natural ally of family intervention (10,79,80).

The multiple functions of the psychiatric hospital in regard to the family include addressing problems that are disturbing the family's homeostasis, assisting other disturbed but resistant family members, and helping the family to regain a "lost," severely dysfunctional family member. The family is considered the most important resource, and as such deserves support and respect rather than criticism and blame (81). The relationship between the family and the psychiatrist should be collaborative on behalf of the patient. A variety of family therapy approaches have been used in treating hospitalized patients. The psychoeducational model of family intervention is most effective for families with a member who has been hospitalized for schizophrenia or an affective disorder.

Sholevar (80) has described an "institutionalization process" by which a dysfunctional family in a crisis situation attempts to extrude a vulnerable adolescent to reestablish homeostasis. A variation of the institutionalization process is a multiple hospitalization syndrome, whereby the family insists on returning the child home prematurely to reinvolve him or her in the family's conflicts. Institutionalization process can be countered through conjoint family therapy evaluation and treatment of the whole family by the hospital staff. The family should be involved in the treatment process before the patient's admission to the hospital.

RESEARCH IN FAMILY THERAPY

Progress in family therapy research has been apparent in the past two decades. The question of whether family therapy is effective has been further refined by examining the effect of specific treatment formats and strategies on specific family problems, individual diagnoses, and mediating therapeutic goals. Studies comparing family therapy with other treatment modalities or combining family therapy with other treatment approaches have focused on the level of responsiveness of different problems to different treatment modalities including family therapy (82).

Studies on child and adolescent disorders, particularly the treatment of conduct disorders and delinquency, have produced encouraging results. PMT (33,41) and FFT (38) have proved very effective. In addition to their favorable effect on targeted behaviors of adolescent patients, they have produced beneficial results with siblings and parents. Research on family intervention with substance abuse has demonstrated effectiveness with subgroups of substance abusers, possibly with younger abusers still living at home. There has been surprisingly less interest in the efficacy of family therapy in treating patients with eating disorders. The recent findings (60) suggest that nonchronic eating disorders in young patients who live at home with their parents are amenable to family interventions.

There have been a number of studies that clearly define symptomatic behavioral problems in children. The most impressive result has been reduced aggressive behavior in children and adolescents (83). Family therapy was effective in reducing specific problematic child behaviors, as well as in reducing anxiety and depression in the parents, and contributing to parenting skills.

A very promising recent study by Reiss et al. (84) examines the role of genetic and environmental factor in a wide range of family types. The differential impact of shared and nonshared environments on child development can have far-reaching impact on family investigations and treatment in coming decades due to dramatic ongoing changes in family composition.

CONCLUSION

A field of family psychiatry has emerged based on the treatment of disorders with relatively clear genetic components, namely, schizophrenia, depression, and alcoholism. Recent elaboration of stress-diathesis theory has led to new developments in family psychiatry, especially the focus on genetic vulnerability of different family members to stress and on methods for reducing it. Psychoeducational family intervention has been used extensively to enhance family adaptation, without the risk of increasing stresses in the family by stimulating charged conflictual issues.

Family therapy, in collaboration with the broader field of psychiatry, should better define the family variables of different disorders and their responses to single or combined treatment modalities or a particular family therapy approach. Considering the advances made in biologic psychiatry and mapping human genomes, the interactional and psychological correlates of biologic vulnerability and dysfunction present family therapists with an exciting challenge.

References

1. Hibbs ED, Jensen PS: *Psychosocial Treatments for Child and Adolescent Disorders: Empirically Based Strategies for Clinical Practice*. Washington, DC, American Psychological Association, 1996.
2. Minuchin S: *Families and Family Therapy*. Cambridge, MA, Harvard University Press, 1974.
3. Steinglass P: Family therapy. In: Kaplan P, Saddack B (eds): *Comprehensive Textbook of Psychiatry*. 6th ed. Baltimore, MD, Williams & Wilkins Publishers, pp. 1838–1847, 1995.
4. Gurman A, Lebow J: Family and couple therapy. In: Saddock B, Saddock V (eds): *Comprehensive Textbook of Psychiatry*. 7th ed. Lippincott Williams & Wilkins, Baltimore, MD, pp. 2157–2167, 2000.
5. Shapiro R: Psychodynamic family therapy with children and adolescents. In: Sholevar GP (ed): *Treatment of Emotional Disorders in Children and Adolescents*. Jamaica, NY, SP Medical and Scientific Books, pp. 135–159, 1986.
6. Cicchetti D, Toth SL: The development of depression in children and adolescents. *Am Psychol* 53:221–241, 1998.
7. Jackson DD: The question of family homeostasis. *Psychiatr Q* 31(Suppl): 79–90, 1965.
8. Haley J: *Strategies of Psychotherapy*. New York, Grune & Stratton, 1963.
9. Sholevar GP: Family therapy. In: Jerry Weiner, Mina Dulcan (eds): *Textbook of Child and Adolescent Psychiatry*. 3rd ed. Washington, DC, APPI Press, Chapter 53, pp. 1001–1027, 2002.
10. Sholevar GP: Introduction. In: Sholevar GP, Schwoeri L (eds): *Textbook of Family and Marital Therapy*. Washington, DC, American Psychiatric Press, pp. 1–33, 2003.
11. Minuchin S, Rosman B, Baker L: *Psychosomatic Families: Anorexia Nervosa in Context*. Cambridge, MA, Harvard University Press, 1978.
12. Stanton MD: Systems approaches to family therapy. In: Sholevar GP, Jamaica NY (eds): *Treatment of Emotional Disorders in Children and Adolescents*. SP Medical and Scientific Books, pp. 159–180, 1986.
13. MacGregor R: Multiple impact psychotherapy with families. *Fam Process* 1:15–29, 1962.
14. Bowen M: *Family Theory in Clinical Practice*. New York, Jason Aronson, 1978.
15. Boszormenyi-Nagy I, Spark GM: *Invisible Loyalties*. New York, Harper & Row, 1984.
16. Madanes C: *Strategic Family Therapy*. San Francisco, CA, Jossey-Bass, 1981.
17. Browning S, Green RJ: Constructing therapy. In: GP Sholevar (ed). *Textbook of Family and Marital Therapy*. Chapter 3. Washington, DC, APPI Press, 2002.
18. Beardslee W, Schwoeri LD: Preventive intervention with children of depressed parents. In: Sholevar GP, Schwoeri LD (eds): *Transmission of Depression in Families and Children*. Northvale, NJ, Jason Aronson, Inc., pp 285–318, 1994.
19. Carter E, McGoldrick M (eds): *The Family Life Cycle*. New York, Gardner Press, 1980.
20. Zilbach J: The family life cycle: Framework for understanding children in family therapy. In: Combrinck-Graham L (ed): *Children in Family Context*. New York, Guilford, pp. 46–66, 1989.
21. Combrinck-Graham L: A developmental model for family systems. *Fam Process* 24:139–150, 1985.
22. Malone CA: Observations on the role of family therapy in child psychiatric training. *J Am Acad Child Psychiatry* 13:437–458, 1974.
23. McDermott JF, Char WF: The undeclared war between child and family therapy. *J Am Acad Child Psychiatry* 13:422–436, 1974.
24. Malone CA: Child psychiatry and family therapy: an overview. *J Am Acad Child Psychiatry* 18:4–21, 1979.
25. Scharff D, Scharff JS: *Object Relations Family Therapy*. Northvale, NJ, Jason Aronson, 1987.
26. Lansky MR: Family therapy. In: Kaplan HI, Sadock BJ (eds): *Comprehensive Textbook of Psychiatry*. 5th ed. (Vol 2). Baltimore, MD, Williams & Wilkins, pp. 1535–1541, 1989.
27. Ravenscroft K: Family therapy. In: Lewis M (ed): *Child and Adolescent Psychiatry*. Baltimore, MD, Williams & Wilkins, pp. 850–869, 1991.
28. Stierlin H: *Separating Parents and Adolescents*. New York, Quadrangle/New York Times Book Company, 1974.
29. Zilbach J: *Young Children in Family Therapy*. New York, Brunner/Mazel, 1986.
30. Chasin R, White T: Family therapy with children: A model for engaging the whole family. In: Sholevar GP, Schwoeri L (eds): *Textbook of Family and Marital Therapy*. Washington, DC, American Psychiatric Press, 59, 2002.
31. Sholevar GP: Initial and diagnostic family interview. In: Weiner JM, Dulcan MK (eds): *Textbook of Child and Adolescent Psychiatry*. 3rd ed. Washington, DC, APPI Press, pp. 125–136, 2004.
32. Sholevar GP: Family intervention with conduct disorders. In: *Conduct Disorders in Children and Adolescents*. Washington, DC, APPI Press, pp. 193–209, 1995.
33. Diamond G, Sigueland L: Current status of family intervention science. In: Josephson AM (ed): *Current Prospectives on Family Therapy, Child and Adolescent Psychiatric Clinics of North America*. Philadelphia, PA, WB Saunders Co. (vol 10, number 3), 2001.
34. Pelham WE, Wheeler T, Chronus A: Empirically supported psychological treatments for attention deficit hyperactivity disorder. *J Clin Child Psychol* 27:190–205, 1998.
35. Barkley RA: *Hyperactive Children: A Handbook for Diagnosis and Treatment*. New York, Guilford Press, 1981.
36. Hinshaw SP, Owens EB, Wells KC, et al.: Family processes and treatment outcomes in the MTA: Negative/ineffective parenting practices in relation to multimodal treatment. *J Abnorm Child Psychol* 28:555–568, 2000.
37. Patterson GR: *A Social Learning Approach to Family Interventions: III. Coercive Family Process*. Eugene, OR, Castalia, 1982.
38. Alexander J, Barton D, Walfron H: Beyond the technology of family therapy: The anatomy of an intervention model. In: Craig K, McMahon R (eds). *Advances in Clinical Behavior Therapy*. New York, Bronner/Mazel, pp. 48–73, 1983.
39. Alexander JF, Parsons BV: *Functional Family Therapy*. Monterey, CA, Brooks/Cole, 1982.
40. Sexton TL, Alexander JF: Functional family therapy: An empirically supported, family-based intervention model for at-risk adolescents and their families. In: Kaslow FW (ed): *Comprehensive Handbook of Psychotherapy: II: Cognitive-Behavioral Approaches*. New York, Wiley, pp. 117–140, 2002.
41. Forehand R, Kotchick BA: Cultural diversity: A wake-up call for parent training. *Behav Ther* 27:187–206, 1996.
42. Kazdin AE, Siegel TC, Bass D: Cognitive problem-solving skills training and parent management training in the treatment of antisocial behavior in children. *J Consult Clin Psychol* 60:733–747, 1992.
43. Mabe PA, Turner MK, Josephson AM: Parent management training. In: Josephson AM (ed): *Child and Adolescent Psychiatric Clinics of North America: Current Perspectives on Family Therapy* (vol 10). Philadelphia, PA, WB Saunders Co, pp. 451–464, 2001.
44. Sholevar E: Parent management training. In: Sholevar P (ed): *Textbook of Family and Couples Therapy*. Washington, DC, pp. 403–417, 2008.
45. Wahler RG, Cartor PG, Fleishman J, et al.: The impact of synthesis teaching and parent training with mothers of conduct-disordered children. *J Abnorm Child Psychol* 21:425–440, 1993.
46. Chamberlain P, Mihalic S: *Blueprints for Violence Prevention. Book Eight: Multidimensional Treatment Foster Care*. Boulder, CO, Center for the Study and Prevention of Violence, 1998.
47. Chamberlain P, Reid JB: Comparison of two community alternatives to incarceration for chronic juvenile offenders. *J Consult Clin Psychol* 66:624–633, 1998.
48. Henggeler SW, Schoenwald SK, Borduin CM, et al.: *Multisystemic Treatment of Antisocial Behavior in Children and Adolescents*. New York, Guilford Press, 1998.
49. Henggeler SW, Rowland MD, Randall J, et al.: Home-based multisystemic therapy as an alternative to the hospitalization of youth in psychiatric crisis: clinical outcomes. *J Am Acad Child Adolesc Psychiatry* 38:1331–1339, 1999.
50. Haas G, Glick I: Inpatient family intervention: a randomized clinical trial. II: results at hospital discharge. *Arch Gen Psychiatry* 35:1169–1177, 1988.
51. Hinchcliffe M, Hooper D, Roberts F: *The Melancholy Marriage*. New York, Wiley, 1978.
52. Coyne JC: Depression, biology, marriage, and marital therapy. *Fam Process* 24:131–151, 1985.
53. Schwoeri L, Sholevar GP: A social learning family model of depression and aggression: Focus on the single mother. In: Sholevar GP, Schwoeri L (eds): *The Transmission of Depression in Families and Children*, Northvale, NJ, Jason Aranson, pp. 145–166, 1994.
54. Sholevar GP, Schwoeri L, Jardin H: Family therapy with depression. In: Sholevar P (ed): *Textbook of Family and Couples Therapy*. Washington, DC, APPI Press, pp. 619–637, 2003.
55. Brent DA, Holder D, Kilko D, et al.: A clinical psychotherapy trial for adolescent depression comparing cognitive, family, and supportive therapy. *Arch Gen Psychiatry* 54:877–885, 1997.
56. Siqueland L, Kendall PC, Steinberg L: Anxiety in children: perceived family environments and observed family interaction. *J Clin Child Psychol* 25:225–237, 1996.
57. Barrett PM, Healy-Farrell L, March JS: Cognitive behavioral family treatment of childhood obsessive-compulsive disorder: a controlled trial. *J Am Acad Child Adolesc Psychiatry* 43:46–62, 2004.
58. Russell GFM, Szmukler GI, Dare C, et al.: An evaluation of family therapy in anorexia nervosa and bulimia nervosa. *Arch Gen Psychiatry* 44:1047–1056, 1987.
59. Robin AL, Siegel PT, Moye AW, Gilroy M, Dennis AB, Sikand A: A controlled comparison of family versus individual therapy for adolescents with anorexia nervosa. *J A, Acad Child Adolesc Psychiatry* 38:1482–1489, 1999.
60. Eisler I, Dare C, Hodes M, Russell G, Dodge E, Le Grange D: Family therapy for adolescent anorexia nervosa: the results of a controlled

comparison of two family interventions. *J Child Psychol Psychiatry* 41:727–736, 2000.
61. Berkowitz RI, Lyke JA, Wadden TA: Treatment of child and adolescent obesity. In: Johnston FE, Foster GD (eds): *Obesity, Growth and Development*. London, Smith-Gordon, pp. 169–184, 2001.
62. Liddle HA: Family-based therapies for adolescent alcohol and drug use research contributions and future research needs. *Addiction* 99:76–92, 2004.
63. Liddle HL, Dakof G: Family-based treatment for adolescent drug use: State of the science. In: Rahdert E (ed): *Adolescent Drug Abuse Assessment and Treatment*. Rockville, MD, NIDA, pp. 218–254, 1995.
64. Henggeler SW, Cligempee WG, Brondino MJ, Pickrel SG: Four-year follow-up of multisystemic therapy with substance-abusing and substance-dependent juvenile offenders. *J am Acad Child Adolesc Psychiatry* 41:868–874, 2002.
65. Sholevar GP: Family intervention with conduct disorders. In: Josephson AM (ed): *Child and Adolescent Psychiatric Clinics of North America: Current Perspectives on Family Therapy*. Philadelphia, PA, W.B. Saunders Co. (vol 10), pp. 501–518, 2001.
66. Rosenthal D: *Genetic Theory and Abnormal Behavior*. New York, Brunner/Mazel, 1970.
67. Tienari P, Lahti I, Sorri A, et al.: The Finnish adoptive study of schizophrenia: possible joint effects of genetic vulnerability and family interaction. In: Halweg K, Goldstein M (eds): *Understanding Major Mental Disorder: The Contribution of Family Interaction Research*. New York, Family Process Press, pp. 33–54, 1987.
68. Zubin J, Spring B: Vulnerability: a new view of schizophrenia. *J Abnorm Psychol* 86:103–126, 1977.
69. Goldstein MJ: Family interaction patterns that antedate the onset of schizophrenia and related disorders: A further analysis of data from a longitudinal prospective study. In: Halweg K, Goldstein MJ (eds): *Understanding Major Mental Disorder: The Contribution of Family Interaction Research*. New York, Family Process Press, pp. 11–32, 1987.
70. Miklowitz D, Thompson M: Family variables in schizophrenia. In: Sholevar GP (ed): *Textbook of Family and Couples Therapy*. Washington, DC, APPI Press, pp. 585–618, 2003.
71. Brown GW, Monck EM, Carstairs GM, Wing JK: Influence of family life on the course of schizophrenic illness. *Brit J Prev Soc Med* 16: 55–68, 1962.
72. Halweg K, Neuchterlein K, Goldstein MJ, et al.: Parental expressed emotion attitudes and intrafamilial communication behavior. In: Halweg K, Goldstein MJ (eds): *Understanding Major Mental Disorder: The Contribution of Family Interaction Research*. New York, Family Process Press, pp. 156–175, 1987.
73. Vaughn C, Leff J: The influence of family and social factors on the course of psychiatric illness: a comparison of schizophrenic and depressed neurotic patients. *Br J Psychiatry* 129:125–137, 1976.
74. Wynne LC, Singer MT: Thought disorder and family relations of schizophrenics. I: a research strategy. *Arch Gen Psychiatry* 9:191–198, 1963.
75. Wynne LC: Family variables in the University of Rochester Project. In: Halweg K, Goldstein J (eds): *Understanding Major Mental Disorder: The Contribution of Family Interaction Research*. New York, Family Process Press, pp. 55–73, 1987.
76. Group for the Advancement of Psychiatry: *The Family, the Patient, and the Psychiatric Hospital: Toward a New Model*. New York, Brunner/Mazel, p. 24, 1985.
77. Endicott J, Spitzer R: Use of research diagnostic criteria for affective disorders and schizophrenia to study affective disorders. *Am J Psychiatry* 136:52–56, 1979.
78. Clarkin J, Miklowitz D: Diagnosis of family relational disorders. In: Sholevar GP, Schwoeri L (eds): *Textbook of Family and Marital Therapy*. Washington, DC, American Psychiatric Press, 2000.
79. Glick I, Clarkin J, Spencer J Jr, et al.: A controlled evaluation of inpatient family intervention. I: Preliminary results of the six month follow-up. *Arch Gen Psychiatry* 42:882–886, 1985.
80. Sholevar GP: Family therapy with hospitalized and disabled patients. In: Trexler M (ed): *Helping Families with Special Problems*. Northvale, NJ, Jason Aronson, pp. 15–35, 1983.
81. Hatfield A: The family as partner in the treatment of mental illness. *Hosp Community Psychiatry* 30:338–340, 1986.
82. Clarkin J, Carpenter D: Family therapy process and outcome research. In: Sholevar GP, Schwoeri L (eds): *Textbook of Family and Marital Therapy*. Washington, DC, American Psychiatric Press, 2003.
83. Sayger T, Horne A, Walker J, et al.: Social learning family therapy with aggressive children: treatment outcome and maintenance. *J Fam Psychology* 1:261–285, 1988.
84. Reiss D, Neiderhisser JM, Hetherington EM, et al.: *The Relationship Code: Deciphering Genetic and Social Influences on Adolescent Development*. Cambridge, MA, Harvard University Press, 2000.

6.3 ■ THE CONTINUUM OF CARE AND LOCATION-SPECIFIC INTERVENTIONS

CHAPTER 6.3.1 ■ DESIGNING EMERGENCY PSYCHIATRIC SERVICES FOR CHILDREN AND ADOLESCENTS

JENNIFER F. HAVENS, RUTH S. GERSON, AND MOLLIE MARR

CHALLENGES TO EFFECTIVE PSYCHIATRIC EMERGENCY CARE

Child and adolescent mental health–related emergency has risen steadily over the last 20 years (1) with the percentage of youth emergency department (ED) visits for mental health issues increasing from 4.4% of all visits in 2001 to 7.2% in 2011 (2). A recent study reveals that the number of child psychiatric ED visits for children under age 17 rose from 500,536 discharges in 2006 to 605,208 discharges in 2011, a 21% increase, while the numbers of nonmental health–related ED visits remained stable (3). Strikingly, Torio et al. (3) report large increases in mental health–related ED visits for children aged 1 to 4 (20.6% increase), for children 5 to 9 (31.4% increase), and for children 10 to 14 (36.2% increase). Studies drawing from older data indicate the largest increase in mental health–related ED visits was for nonemergent issues and may reflect difficulty in access to outpatient mental health treatment (1). However, the latest available study reveals significant increases for visits related to suicide and self-injury in all age ranges, including children aged 1 to 9 (3).

Youth mental health ED visits create considerable burden for largely unprepared ED providers, with longer lengths of stay, higher rates of ED boarding, inpatient admissions and transfers, and higher rates of restraints when compared with nonmental health–related visits. These findings have been reported in single-site studies (4–6), in multicenter collaborations (7–9) and in the analysis of large data sets tracking ED utilization (3,10). There is also evidence that the lengths of stay associated with these visits have increased over time (6,10).

Despite the well-covered crisis of psychiatric patients of all ages in EDs across the country (11), the emergency management system has been slow to evolve to address the needs of young patients. The overwhelming majority of youth in psychiatric crisis are managed either in medical EDs or psychiatric EDs designed to serve adults. These settings generally lack access to round-the-clock child mental health clinicians, let alone child and adolescent psychiatrists (12). Medical ED settings lack access to psychiatric nursing staff and the facilities to safely manage suicidal or aggressive patients. The priority for inadequately staffed ED providers in these setting is triage rather than treatment. Frequently young patients are admitted for inpatient care because they require immediate care, which could be provided on an outpatient basis if appropriate services were available. With the overall constriction in the public and private inpatient care system (13), the need for inpatient admission can be associated with significant delays and boarding in ED settings (4,10,14). All of this translates into alienating and sometimes traumatizing experiences for children and their families and only serves to reinforce the stigma associated with psychiatric illness.

The crisis in the management of psychiatric emergencies in youth must be understood in the broader context of the challenges in the overall children's mental health service system. Persistent reductions in the number of inpatient psychiatric beds as well as the shift in the inpatient model of care to one of brief stabilization has led to youth at higher acuity being managed in the community. The national average length of stay for youth in inpatient care is now 7 days (3); youth are discharged when they are no longer acutely dangerous, not when they are well. Access to intermediate levels of care (partial hospital programs, intensive outpatient programs) is limited and varies significantly across the country. The children's outpatient care continuum has historically been limited in its capacity to provide acute care and access to child and adolescent psychiatry represents a significant national challenge. These system factors have been noted to be associated with increasing mental health visits to ED, particularly nonemergent visits (1,15,16).

Several structural issues contribute to the challenges EDs face in meeting the mental health needs of youth. First overall volumes tend to be low when compared to adult patients so the ED psychiatry workforce is likely to lack child and adolescent competencies. Severe national shortages of child and adolescent psychiatrists also exacerbate this problem. Second, the psychiatric consultation model in EDs significantly impacts reimbursement, particularly when caring for publicly insured patients. Hospital systems have little incentive to support child mental health clinicians in low-volume, low-reimbursement settings (12,15–18).

These challenges have resulted in a system of ED care which commonly fails to meet the needs of youth in mental health crisis. In 2013, suicide was the second leading cause of death in 15 to 24 year olds and the third leading cause of death in 10 to 14 year olds (19). Unintentional injury is the first leading cause of death in youth (19) and there are reasons to believe that the national system of reporting unintentional injury understates the "overall magnitude of fatalities arising from deliberate, self-destructive behaviors" (20). Deliberate self-harm has been clearly established as a risk factor for youth suicide (21) and yet in 2009 only 39% of self-harming youth covered by Medicaid presenting to EDs received a mental health assessment and only 43% received follow-up outpatient care (22).

MODELS OF EFFECTIVE CRISIS INTERVENTION

Across the United States and in Canada, a number of models have been implemented that address the many challenges to the provision of effective care for young people in psychiatric crisis (18,23,24). Janssens et al. provided a particularly thoughtful and comprehensive overall of both the theoretical and structural underpinning of available crisis intervention models, which have been applied across a broad range of settings, including community and home-based settings, clinics, and EDs. Several have evidence supporting their effectiveness (23,25,26) but it is clear there is a need for more rigorous study in this area (23,27). All of the models require resource allocation to allow for immediate access to child and adolescent mental health clinicians that support children and families through the crisis period; all program models share reductions in inpatient utilization and improvement in quality of care. Several ED models which support after-ED discharge connections have been shown to improve linkage to outpatient services for high-risk patients. These programs are detailed below.

Community-Based Models

Homebuilders and Multisystem Therapy are examples of well-established models that have been adapted to serve children during a psychiatric emergency. Both are evidence-based models centered on intensive community-based care. Initially developed for child welfare populations in order to support family preservation (28,29), the Homebuilders model has been successfully applied in the prevention of psychiatric admissions in children and adolescents (30,31). The New York State Office of Mental Health has invested in the Homebuilders model, now called Home-Based Crisis Intervention, and supports this program throughout New York City. The Home-Based Crisis Intervention provides short-term services (6 to 12 weeks) in the home as well as linkage to outpatient services for youth identified as at-risk for psychiatric hospitalization. In addition to successfully diverting over 90% of young people from psychiatric admission, this model has also been found to successfully manage youth at the same acuity level as patients admitted to inpatient psychiatric services (32).

Multisystemic therapy (MST) has also been adapted for children and adolescents at risk of psychiatric hospitalization. In randomized clinical trials, this MST adaptation was shown to be safe and effective in the management of these at-risk youth (33). Like the Homebuilders model, MST provides home-based services, but the intensity is dependent on the needs of family and is therefore variable. Generally, the length of treatment in MST is longer (average of 4 months) compared to the Homebuilders model. MST is a strength-based model designed to help families identify and leverage resources and strengths to enact change through a combination of family, behavioral, and psychosocial interventions. In order to address the unique needs of families with a child in psychiatric crisis, child and adolescent psychiatrists were added to the treatment team and the development of comprehensive crisis plans was incorporated in the MST adaptations (33–35). A randomized controlled trial of MST versus hospitalization in patients following a psychiatric emergency showed a 57% reduction in hospitalization for those enrolled in MST (36) as well as a reduction in suicide attempts among youth referred for hospitalization following threats of harm to self or others or suicidal ideation or attempt (37).

Mobile crisis services is another community-based model with a growing evidence base. Mobile crisis teams provide on-site evaluation at the place of crisis (home, school, community) and determine what services the child needs. Services are dependent on what is available in the community or region, but may include referral to a higher level of care, referral and linkage to outpatient services, respite care for parents, or short-term wraparound services. Mobile crisis teams are also used to contact high-risk patients with recent ED visits or hospitalizations who fail to attend scheduled appointments or to facilitate linkage to outpatient or supportive services (38). In Milwaukee,

Wisconsin, the ability of mobile crisis teams to facilitate transfers for inpatient treatment and provide access to crisis respite beds has decreased inpatient admissions (39). In New York, a similar program demonstrated a reduction in ED visits and prevented out-of-home placements (39). Further study of the effectiveness of these programs in youth is warranted as the use of this model is expanding; Connecticut has developed a statewide program supported through government funds and New York City has expanded the mobile crisis response model for youth across all five boroughs of the city.

Hospital-Based Models

These models provide hospital-based services on a walk-in basis or as an adjunct to ED visits, often through specialized crisis intervention teams. Frequently, these programs are co-located with other clinical services and thus able to provide rapid access to clinical teams with expertise in crisis management (40). The development of this model represents an evolution in outpatient care to address the growing demand for acute care capabilities and is highly applicable to existing clinical services. One example is the use of specialized teams in outpatient clinics to provide rapid access and intensive case management to patients in crisis, allowing for a briefer ED stay and preventing the hospitalization of those patients who can be safely managed in an outpatient setting. This model requires access to child psychiatric services, and generally works best in an academic setting with trainees. Maimonides Medical Center in Brooklyn, NY has developed an innovative model to actively link local public schools to their outpatient clinic. Schools are able to send students to the clinic for urgent evaluations on a walk-in basis every day of the work week, preventing school referrals to the ED.

Emergency Department-Based Models

ED-based models extend existing emergency services and provide interventions and support beyond the traditional psychiatric consult model. Although there is variability in how the services are integrated and delivered within a given ED, there are three broad approaches currently in use: providing an enhanced evaluation and facilitated referral, delivering therapeutic interventions during the ED visit, and supporting dedicated psychiatric staff within the ED.

In the enhanced evaluation and referral model ED staff provide facilitated referral to outpatient services, create a verbal contract with the patient, review expectations, provide crisis phone support, and call families to remind them of upcoming appointments and to facilitate connection with these services (23,41). The enhanced evaluation and referral model and the therapeutic intervention model have been evaluated with high-risk patients, typically patients who were seen in the ED for suicidal ideation or following self-inflicted injury, and have shown some promise. One example of the therapeutic intervention model is family-based crisis intervention. The goal of the family-based crisis intervention is to help the child and parents to reframe the crisis, communicate more effectively, identify ways to establish and maintain safety, and address attitudes about engaging in mental health care (42,43). The therapeutic approaches to achieve these goals vary, but may include brief family systems therapy, cognitive-behavioral therapy, or a combination of therapeutic techniques. In one study, staff provided linkage calls to support families and increase compliance with scheduled outpatient appointments (43). This study, as well as others, found improved linkage and greater compliance with outpatient referrals following the use of ED-based therapeutic interventions (42,43).

The Child Guidance Model (44) is an example of a specialized team available to provide immediate psychiatric services within the ED. The team evaluates children with psychiatric complaints and includes a psychiatric social worker and a child psychiatrist. The psychiatric social worker is available to perform psychiatric assessments and provide comprehensive disposition planning in the ED 24 hours a day. A study of this model found a reduction in the length of stay in the ED as well as a reduction in costs (44). Additional studies of specialized child psychiatric teams in the ED providing evaluation and disposition planning found reductions in inpatient admissions and return visits to the ED (27).

Specialty Psychiatric Emergency Programs

The New York State Comprehensive Psychiatric Emergency Program (CPEP) model mandates a comprehensive range of services, including comprehensive psychiatric and psychosocial evaluation, extended observation beds for brief stabilization (up to 72 hours), immediate access to outpatient clinic services though an interim crisis clinic and mobile crisis services. This model was implemented in New York State in the late 1980s and provided the first statewide model of the implementation of regulated and organized emergency psychiatric services (45). The first dedicated Children's Comprehensive Psychiatric Emergency Program (C-CPEP) in New York State (at New York Presbyterian Hospital) reduced inpatient psychiatric admissions in Northern Manhattan from 35% to under 10%, but was closed when inadequate volume and reimbursement did not support program costs, reflecting to the reimbursement challenges inherent in operating dedicated psychiatric units for youth. These types of programs, which are becoming more common for adults across the country, require considerable capital investment and institutional commitment to develop and implement as they are expensive to build and operate and require a critical mass of child psychiatry staffing. The second dedicated C-CPEP in New York State (at Bellevue Hospital Center) serves both Bellevue Hospital and as well as several other public hospitals in the New York City Health and Hospitals Corporation that lack child and adolescent inpatient services. The C-CPEP includes six extended observation beds staffed 24 hours a day/7 days a week with child psychiatry, child psychiatric nursing and social work. The service also provides Interim Crisis Clinic services, which follow patients discharged from the C-CPEP for up to three visits. This combination of immediate access to outpatient follow-up and brief stabilization prevents longer admissions except when necessary; only 20% of children and adolescents evaluated in Bellevue C-CPEP are admitted to inpatient psychiatry units. A similar specialized program opened at the Institute of Living in Hartford, Connecticut (the CARES Unit) in 2009, in response to the dramatic increase in young people in psychiatric crisis in medical EDs in that state. Recently, another brief stabilization unit opened in Geneva Switzerland, at the Children's Hospital of Geneva Hospitals.

ROLE OF QUALITY STANDARDS IN IMPROVING PSYCHIATRIC EMERGENCY CARE

The range and variety of psychiatric emergency services for youth across the country reflect the lack of quality standards as well as significant challenges to fiscal sustainability (15,16,24). One significant barrier to the broader implementation of community-based models is the requirement for ongoing public funding to support program costs. Despite the clear cost-savings from hospital diversions, these types of services are generally not covered by insurance providers. Strategic collaboration with insurers (both commercial and public) is essential to the successful dissemination of these program models, which have clear potential to reduce inpatient utilization. More rigorous study of the cost-effectiveness of commonly used community-based models (home-based crisis intervention, mobile crisis services) would be helpful to support the uptake of these services by private insurers.

Increasingly, public sector funding also supports mental health services delivered to youth in EDs. The overall share of ED visits supported by Medicaid increased from 45% in 2006 to 53% in 2011 (3). This represents an opportunity to leverage the increasing focus on quality and outcome demonstrated in public sector funding streams to develop nationwide standards for children's psychiatric emergency care. This would serve to reduce the variability and improve the quality of services children receive; improve the linkage of high-risk youth to aftercare services and potentially change the trajectory of completed adolescent suicide, now trending in the wrong direction (19).

Canada has taken a step in this direction, with the development and implementation of an ED care pathway for youth mental health visits (46). This pathway dictates structured screening to be implemented by all ED staff to identify high-risk youth, the 24/7 availability of a specialized child and adolescent clinician to evaluate identified patients and structured collaboration with community-based providers to provide facilitated and immediate access for high-risk patients and rapid access for lower-risk patients requiring follow-up. This pathway has also standardized documentation and transfer of treatment information across care providers. Evaluation of the pathway is underway.

In the United States, extensive advocacy will be necessary on a national level to force the development of standards of care and insure adequate reimbursement for pediatric psychiatric emergency care. Following the path of emergency medicine and accrediting and designating centers of child and adolescent psychiatric emergency care is one approach to improving the accessibility of quality care, facilitating patient transfer and linkage, and creating an infrastructure for innovation, research, and training. As developed by the Illinois Emergency Medical Services for Children program, the pediatric emergency medicine facility designation process in the area of pediatric trauma care led to the development of statewide standards and protocols for the provision of emergency medical care to children and engaged providers across service systems including EMS, schools, rehabilitation centers, poison control centers, and hospitals (47). They have been able to leverage the partnerships formed as part of the designation process to advance disaster preparedness, develop a surveillance system, implement and evaluate system-wide quality improvement projects, and address workforce, equipment, or space shortages. Their designation process encompasses three levels of pediatric trauma care, based on the ability of hospitals to provide optimal pediatric care. EMS diversion protocols are used to decrease ambulance transport to hospital without adequate care capacity. Hospitals must have transfer guidelines in place, especially those centers unable to provide specialized pediatric care. The system facilitates medically necessary pediatric transfers both through the requirement of current policies and interagency agreements, but also by maintaining up-to-date information on the location and availability of transportation teams, specialized centers of care, and pediatric beds.

Given the workforce constraints in child and adolescent psychiatry, specialization and designation are essential to support centralized settings serving regional areas with adequate staffing and space to manage child and adolescent psychiatric emergencies. The C-CPEP at Bellevue Hospital Center/NYU provides such a model, with the C-CPEP supporting the transfer of patients across New York City from both the public and private sector hospitals. This model is feasible in a well-developed child and adolescent psychiatry department with an adequate psychiatry work force to provide 24/7 coverage and where there is institutional commitment to meeting the mental health needs of children and adolescents. Children's hospitals, who across the country struggle with increasing ED mental health volumes, represent a natural setting for the expansion of the specialized model. Accrediting and designating centers of child and adolescent psychiatric emergency care is an important next step in assuring access to high-quality care, and providing the infrastructure to evaluate and improve the existing service system and support the development of new models of care.

MANAGEMENT PRINCIPLES AND PRACTICE

Safety in the ED

Setting

The first priority of any emergency psychiatric assessment of a child or adolescent is safety. The patient (and others) must be safe in the ED itself, which may be difficult due to space constraints and the staffing challenges described above. Despite these challenges, children and adolescents presenting to the ED in psychiatric crisis should be kept in safe and quiet areas of the ED, both for the evaluation and while awaiting evaluation, transfer or discharge. Particularly for agitated youth or those who present to the ED for self-injury or aggression, the physical space is key to maintaining safety without requiring restraint or seclusion. The area should be free from items that can be utilized for self-harm or to harm others (such as sharps, cords, or IV poles); should allow for continuous observation of the patient by staff (while still providing privacy); and should have a minimum of bright lights, beeping monitors, and other irritations to decrease risk of overstimulation. Ideally the patient will be made comfortable with a place to lie or sit down and given access to food or drink, particularly if there will be a delay before evaluation will commence. Staff should introduce themselves and provide clear expectations as to the procedure for evaluation, the wait time, the rules of the ED, and the interventions and consequences that will be given should the child become agitated, aggressive, or destructive. These steps will reduce, but not eliminate, the risk of a child or adolescent becoming agitated. ED staff need to be trained in engaging, calming and de-escalating the patient, and sufficient additional trained personnel should be available if needed to provide containment, medication, or restraint for acutely dangerous behavior. Protocols and response plans should be designed, in compliance with federal, state, local, and hospital regulations, for response to an agitated child or adolescent, and when and how medication or restraint will be utilized. Staff should be familiar with these protocols, and with how to call other staff for support, where to find and how to utilize restraints safely.

Staffing

Children and adolescents are, in general, extremely sensitive to the tone and approach of the adults they meet. In the ED setting, front-line staff who feel comfortable with children and who can maintain a calm, respectful tone will often be able to diffuse even very tense or hostile situations. The initial triage or preliminary assessment of a youth in the ED is key, particularly if there will be a delay before the full clinical evaluation commences. The initial triage can identify risk of medical comorbidity or complications (such as cases of suicidal youth who have overdosed, or intoxicated youth), and any information needed to respond safely in cases of agitation or medical emergency (such as vital signs, allergies, medications prescribed, medical illnesses, and history of abuse or trauma if possible). Structured screening tools such as the Columbia Suicide Severity Rating Scale (C-SSRS) (48), the Ask Suicide-Screening Questions (ASQ) (49), or the Suicide Assessment Five-Step Evaluation and Triage (SAFE-T) (50) can be useful as part of the initial triage to assist in or supplement the assessment of suicidality. If youth are identified to be at immediate risk for self-harm, suicide or harm to others, staff must be made available for continuous observation; ideally, continuous or 1:1 observation should not be done by uniformed officers, which can frighten young children and risks agitating adolescents indisposed to authority figures.

Many EDs lack trained clinical staff to provide psychiatric evaluation and risk assessment for the growing number of youth in psychiatric crisis passing through their doors. This deficit leaves youth vulnerable to the acute and chronic dangers of untreated mental illness, and EDs potentially liable for negative outcomes. The ideal ED assessment of a child will include a child psychiatrist (or a child psychologist in concert with a pediatrician or psychiatrist) and a psychiatric social worker, if not leading the direct assessment then providing consultation and direction to the clinical team.

COMPREHENSIVE ASSESSMENT OF YOUTH IN PSYCHIATRIC CRISIS

The psychiatric evaluation of a child or adolescent in the ED should be guided by three main priorities: assessing safety, identifying, and addressing both medical and social/systemic causes of behavioral disturbance, and providing a therapeutic initial intervention.

Risk Assessment

Assessing safety of a child or adolescent in psychiatric crisis requires determining acuity and imminence of risk, to ascertain whether a youth with chronic risk factors (such as history of harm to self or others, abuse history, family history of suicide, chronic psychosocial stressors, or substance abuse, among others) can be stabilized sufficiently for safe discharge or requires inpatient hospitalization. Acute risk and protective factors in the mental status, information from available collateral, prior and recent behaviors, engagement with community supports or treatment, and the response to the therapeutic interview and initial treatment will inform the determination of risk (Table 6.3.1.1).

TABLE 6.3.1.1

RISK AND PROTECTIVE FACTORS IN THE CHILD PSYCHIATRIC EVALUATION

	Risk Factors	Protective Factors
Mental status examination	Agitation, paranoid psychosis, insomnia, or anhedonia Refusal to speak or engage, or superficial engagement with interview Currently homicidal or suicidal Unable to talk about the acute events or precipitants Guilt or shame, particularly around recent disclosure of family or sexual abuse Positive expectancies around death (relief of suffering or burdensomeness, joining deceased family members)	Future-oriented (hopeful or curious) Emotionally appropriate when talking about stressors, but able to maintain composure Broad, congruent, and reactive affect No currently suicidal or homicidal ideation (or contingently suicidal, such as, suicidal if made to attend school) No suicidal or homicidal intent or plan
Information from collateral	No available collateral Collateral expresses significant safety concerns Collateral (e.g., parent/guardian) unconcerned despite severe symptoms or acute presentation	Collateral who knows child well understands significance of child's presenting thoughts or behaviors but does not have acute safety concerns
Prior and recent dangerous behaviors	Recent high-lethality suicidal attempt or behavior, escalating suicidal or self-injurious behaviors, or severe aggression Researching death or violent means Longstanding or escalating nonsuicidal self-injurious behavior Believed suicidal behavior would be fatal (regardless of true lethality) Access to sharps, weapons, pills, or other lethal means	Self-aborted attempt to hurt self, called for help, or threatened self-harm or suicide in presence of others Impulsive, low-lethality suicide attempt Minor aggression or property destruction without true intent to harm others High supervision, no access to dangerous objects or lethal means
Engagement with supports or treatment	No outpatient treatment or refusal to attend treatment Poor social supports Limited interest in school, friends, family Recent suicide in peer group, or family history of suicide	Good alliance with outpatient providers Connected to staff and peers at school Supportive family
Response to therapeutic interview and treatment	Does not respond to therapeutic support, remains agitated/suicidal/paranoid/etc. Refuses to engage with therapeutic interview	Responds to therapeutic support and/or medication for psychosis, mania, impulsivity secondary to ADHD, or other acute symptoms Child has successfully coped with similar stressors in the past

Evaluating and Addressing Medical and Psychosocial Causes of Behavioral Disturbance

The second priority of the emergency psychiatric evaluation of a child or adolescent is to determine whether the behavioral disturbance or symptoms are due primarily to psychiatric illness, or a manifestation of either medical illness or social/systemic pathology.

While most children are healthy, a variety of medical illness can masquerade as psychiatric symptoms. While most of these medical illnesses in isolation are rare, together they are a significant (though often missed) cause of psychiatric presentations to the ED. Infections (particularly tropical diseases and encephalitis), neoplasms (both brain tumors and paraneoplastic syndromes), seizures (including temporal lobe and absence seizures), autoimmune diseases (including autoimmune encephalitis as well as systemic autoimmune disorders), and head trauma can present with hallucinations, behavioral dysregulation, and other mental status changes. Undiagnosed genetic syndromes, metabolic disorders, and porphyria can manifest with psychosis or behavioral changes, while youth with undiagnosed sickle cell disease can be dismissed as drug-seekers. Delirium due to drug intoxication, self-poisoning (including accidental ingestions, suicide attempts, or substance misuse), or toxicity from psychotherapeutic agents such as lithium may be missed by parents or medical providers, particularly in adolescents with a history of psychosis or conduct problems. Symptoms that are concerning for possible medical etiology include:

- atypical onset or clustering of psychiatric symptoms (such as acute onset of psychosis in a child with no prior psychiatric history)
- abnormal vital signs
- waxing and waning mental status
- clouding of consciousness
- disorientation
- memory impairment

Medical illness can also complicate treatment of psychiatric illness, due to the frequency of comorbidity and the adverse effects of psychiatric medications. All children and adolescents presenting to the psychiatric emergency room should undergo medical clearance, and if a medical etiology or comorbidity is suspected, an appropriate medical workup should be completed. This may include a full physical examination; monitoring of serial vital signs; diagnostic studies including laboratory work (chemistries including glucose and electrolytes, complete blood count with differential, thyroid tests, liver function tests, urine drug screen, serum drug levels if applicable, blood alcohol level if applicable, and cerebrospinal fluid tests if encephalitis is suspected); an electrocardiogram; and if seizures or brain neoplasm are suspected, brain imaging and electroencephalogram (Table 6.3.1.2).

Children with acute medical illness or significant medical comorbidity (such as injury due to suicide attempt, severe intoxication or withdrawal, or drug toxicity) will benefit from medical admission for stabilization prior to psychiatric hospitalization.

When acute or severe medical illness is not present, the ED clinician should also remember that minor physical ailments such as ear infections, hunger, fatigue, headaches, constipation, tooth aches, and the normal developmental changes of puberty can all trigger behavioral disturbances in children. Children with communication difficulties, such as young children and youth with intellectual or developmental disabilities such as autism, can be particularly vulnerable to acting out in response to physical discomfort.

TABLE 6.3.1.2

COMMON MEDICAL CAUSES OF PSYCHIATRIC DISTURBANCE IN CHILDREN AND ADOLESCENTS

Fever	Sickle cell disease
Nonconvulsive status epilepticus	Substance intoxication
Temporal lobe seizures	Withdrawal from illicit substances
Absence seizure	Anticholinergic delirium
Encephalitis	Steroid psychosis or steroid-induced mania
Cerebral systemic lupus erythematosus	Central nervous system neoplasm or other occult malignancy
Childhood confusional migraine	Medication adverse effects such as akathisia from risperidone or irritability from levetiracetam
Head trauma or postconcussive syndrome	
Porphyria	

Psychosocial crisis can also trigger acting out in children and adolescents, and even classically psychiatric symptoms such as hallucinations or anxiety can be engendered by acute stress such as domestic violence, parental mental illness, or abuse. The clinician should be observant, during the course of the therapeutic interview, for signs of distress or pathology in the family or social system. If the child is the "identified patient" while the true cause of distress is in the family or social context, treating the child alone risks giving the child the message that the problem lies in him, not in the abuse, neglect, or other toxic context in which he finds himself. Even if the child has true psychiatric illness, the presenting issue may be family conflict, parental stress or systems failure that worsen the child's symptoms or hobble the caregivers' ability to manage them. Divorce, parental illness, loss of a grandparent or other secondary caretaker, or even summer vacation (with the loss of structure and routine of school) can hinder a parent's ability to contain a behaviorally difficult child. Removal from parents by child protective services can worsen symptoms of anxiety, depression, or aggression, while placing the child with a foster parent who does not know what triggers or soothes the child. Such situations are common precipitants for an ED visit, yet the crises here are not psychiatric per se. Instead, it is a psychosocial crisis leading to breakdown of the caretaking system. Safe discharge in such cases will depend on identification of caretaking supports as much as provision of psychiatric follow-up.

COMPONENTS OF COMPREHENSIVE EMERGENCY PSYCHIATRIC ASSESSMENT FOR A CHILD OR ADOLESCENT

To stabilize the crisis, the initial interview must be therapeutic in itself. An empathic, open, and curious stance in approaching the child and collateral will help to establish rapport, while direct and clear communication regarding rules and expectations indicate mutual respect. Many agitated, angry or anxious youth can be quickly de-escalated by an adult approaching with empathy and sincere desire to understand what has upset them, rather than with judgment and punishment (Table 6.3.1.3).

The interviews with the child, the parent, and any other collateral sources should ideally be conducted in a quiet, private space free from interruption. If the child or parent is agitated, the clinician should solicit other staff to remain nearby, and should sit between the patient/parent and the door to

TABLE 6.3.1.3

COMPONENTS OF A COMPREHENSIVE ASSESSMENT

Identifying information	Social history including trauma and child welfare involvement
Chief complaint	Developmental and educational history
History of present illness	Family history
Past psychiatric history	Legal history
Current medications and medication history	Mental status examination including cognitive examination when indicated
Past medical history	Medical clearance including physical examination if indicated
Substance use history	
Trauma history	

allow unhindered escape from the room if the patient/parent becomes violent. The child and parent should each be interviewed alone, and in general it is best to interview adolescent patients before their parents or guardians, to demonstrate respect and build rapport with the patient.

Interviewing a Child in Psychiatric Crisis

The first moments of interaction with a child can be rich with information for the diagnostic assessment. Observation of the child's mental status, behavior, attitude toward the parent or accompanying adult and then toward the interviewer, language and social skills, and response to questions all inform preliminary hypotheses about the symptoms or stressors that have precipitated the child's arrival to the ED, and facilitate building rapport and calming agitated or anxious patients.

The interview with the child or adolescent should focus on understanding their perspective, their experience of their symptoms or the reasons behind their behavior, and what they perceive as triggers or protective factors, while observing their mental status. Open-ended questions will be more effective than a "checklist" approach. Specific questions must be asked about suicidal and homicidal ideation, with the recognition that children and adolescents often minimize such acute symptoms once in the ED for fear of being hospitalized or upsetting parents. Asking about suicidal and homicidal ideation at different points in the interview, with phrasing that echoes the child's own words, may be more effective in getting an honest response. Questions about hallucinations and delusions should also be approached directly but phrased carefully, as young children and youth with intellectual or developmental disabilities may misinterpret the questions and give false-positive responses, while those youth who are truly experiencing psychosis may deny such symptoms due to paranoia and anxiety. Finally, the clinician should also observe carefully and query directly for the presence of internalizing symptoms such as depression, anxiety, and trauma-related symptoms, as these are often missed or underreported by parents and other adults (51). If children are very young, have limited expressive language (such as those with autism or intellectual disability [ID]), or are severely uncooperative, the clinician should still attempt a thorough mental status examination using parallel or reciprocal play and observation. The clinician can observe the child's interactions with others, ability to follow commands and express needs (though words or gestures), fine and gross motor skills, hyperactivity, distractibility, frustration tolerance, and attachment to (or fear of) the parent or guardian. Even if the child cannot voice what is wrong, the clinician's observations will nonetheless inform diagnosis, risk assessment and treatment recommendations.

Informants

Thorough assessment of a child in psychiatric crisis requires more information than can be obtained from the patient alone. Collateral from the parent, guardian, and/or other accompanying adult is crucial to understanding the facts of the situation that the child cannot give due to cognitive or emotional immaturity. Other informants will also provide critical information about the child's functioning at home and at school, medical issues and history, prior psychiatric treatment, developmental history, substance use, family history, legal history, social history including trauma exposure, academic history, and current stressors.

The most important collateral information will be obtained from the parent, guardian, foster parent, or other caregiver. This can be complicated, however, as parents and other caregivers whose child is in the ED are often exhausted, frightened, or distraught about the child's illness or behaviors. They may be upset about missing work or afraid about paying the ED or ambulance bill, confused about the nature or source of the child's symptoms, or angry about the child's risky or oppositional behaviors or about the delays in the ED evaluation. Approaching the caregiver with the same empathic, therapeutic stance that is used for the patient can help the parent to calm down and articulate their fears and frustrations. Calming the parent or caregiver will also reduce the child's anxiety or agitation. When the clinician empathizes with how difficult it is to bear a child's illness, to access treatment or services, or to wait for evaluation in the ED, it can also help the parent to be more open to understanding the child's perspective, changing their own parenting behaviors, or in obtaining treatment.

When the child is brought to the ED by someone other than their parent (such as EMS, police, school staff, or child welfare workers), the parent should be contacted as quickly as possible to provide consent for and to participate in the evaluation of the child (52). If the parent or guardian cannot be reached, most state regulations on emergency services allow clinicians to initiate evaluation and treatment of the child without parental consent in cases of truly life-threatening emergencies. In situations that are not immediately life-threatening, staff should make reasonable efforts to contact the parent, and should document these attempts in the medical record, before providing treatment. If the evaluation or treatment must be started before parental consent is obtained, staff should continue to endeavor to reach the parent. If an adolescent insists that parents not be contacted, the clinician should comply with state and local laws regarding adolescents' rights to seek mental health care without parental consent or notification. While many states do allow adolescents to access such care without their parents' knowledge, in general youth should be encouraged to include their parents in the evaluation and treatment, and often the support and facilitation of the ED clinician can produce a rapprochement between the parent and child.

In addition to the parent or guardian, other collateral contacts can provide information that is crucial to the diagnostic evaluation and risk assessment. Adolescents often disclose things to counselors, teachers, therapists, or psychiatrists that they have kept hidden from their parent or guardian. Even if the youth is very open with their parent, teachers, and guidance counselors may be aware of behaviors or social or academic issues at school and can evaluate the child's cognitive abilities and social skills. The pediatrician or case worker can provide an assessment of the family's strengths and vulnerabilities, the child's developmental progression, and any medical issues, issues with compliance, or concerns about abuse or neglect.

The parent should provide consent before any of these individuals are contacted, however in potentially life-threatening situations such as concern for child abuse or suicidality, the safety of the child outweighs the risks of breaching confidentiality. Most states allow for exception to confidentiality rules to ensure the safety of the patient, allowing ED clinicians to have contact with outside individuals and providers in emergency situations (52).

After collecting information from the patient and necessary collaterals, the ED clinician must integrate the perspectives provided into a cohesive formulation. The ED clinician will often find that descriptions of symptoms or behaviors (or even awareness of their existence) and explanations for and interpretations of such will vary widely between informants. Parents and other adults often miss or underestimate the severity of internalizing symptoms and over-estimate externalizing behaviors. Parents may be unaware of substance use, stressors at school, or the impact of family stress (such as domestic violence or parental illness) on the child's mental state. Differences in reporting can also stem from real differences in the child's functioning or behavior in different settings, such as at home versus at school. Discrepancies in reporting can also reflect secret or hidden pathology in the family or system, such as abuse, parental mental illness, or substance use. The clinician may never be certain where the truth lies between discrepant reports, but understanding these sources of variance is necessary for the creation of an effective formulation and treatment plan.

MANAGING THE AGITATED PATIENT

Aggression and agitation are among the most common reasons youth are brought to the ED. Calming agitated youth is key to ensuring that the ED evaluation and treatment is therapeutic, not traumatizing. One in fifteen youth in the ED for psychiatric complaints are restrained due to agitated, aggressive, or otherwise unsafe behavior (53). Restraints can be frightening and confusing for a child or adolescent; afterward they often report feeling afraid of and angry at staff, and their perception of time can become skewed such that they perceive themselves as having been in restraints for much longer than actually occurred (54). Many restraints in the ED can be avoided through proactive steps to prevent agitation and avoid escalation and through judicious use of psychopharmacology.

Most agitation in the ED is, on some level, preventable. Irritants such as excessive noise, overcrowding, lack of privacy, long and unpredictable wait times, uncertainty about process and outcome, and an overall tense atmosphere can agitate even normally quiet children (or adults). This is particularly problematic for youth who are vulnerable to agitation, particularly those with impulse control problems, trauma history, autism, or psychosis. ED staff should be vigilant in observing for early signs of agitation in these youth. Children and adolescents who are prone to agitation or violence can escalate quickly, but even they generally manifest small shifts in their tone or mannerisms, their way of interacting with their family or accompanying adults, or their body language (such as pacing or engaging in repetitive or self-stimulating behaviors). De-escalation strategies are most effective if used in response to these early signs of distress. First, the child should be moved to a safe and quiet area, away from other patients. For children for whom the parent or accompanying adult is a comfort, they should be rejoined with the adult; for those for whom the adult is an agitating or distressing presence (such as police officers or an anxious or critical parent), the adult and child should be separated. If the parent's anger, anxiety or agitation is triggering the child, staff should speak separately with the parent to understand and address their concern, be it about the time or cost of the ED evaluation, feeling blamed or responsible for their child's illness, concern about stigma or fear of their child being "taken away."

To avoid the agitated child feeling threatened or overstimulated, one member of the staff should serve as point-person for the patient, while others are close by for support. Staff can offer the child food, water, juice, or basic entertainment (such as TV) to calm and distract them. Offering choices (such as water or juice, or which TV channel) can help the child feel respected and in control, and thus help them to calm down. The staff member should approach the child with open-ended, nondirective questions to understand the child's complaint or concern and encourage them to express their needs. If the child is able to verbalize their concerns, these should be met with empathy and validation. Often children who become agitated are worried about the ED process, the possibility of hospitalization, or their parents' reaction. Others may be paranoid, may have experienced trauma or abuse that has led to hyperreactivity to perceived threat, or may be hungry or in pain. As the child is able to express their concerns and make incremental steps to calm down, staff should praise these positive efforts and make it clear that staff intend to help, not to give judgment or punishment. At the same time, the youth must understand that violence will not be tolerated and that staff will work to ensure everyone is safe.

The child's response to these interventions will inform next steps as well as contribute to the preliminary differential diagnosis. Agitation or violent behavior in the ED is usually multifactorial. Youth can be vulnerable to agitation due to a range of symptoms and psychosocial factors. Some are chronically irritable, due to temperament, severe anxiety, or upbringing in chaotic, neglectful or violence-prone families or communities. Others have poor frustration tolerance due to cognitive deficits, developmental delays, autism, or upbringing (including exposure to abuse), or misinterpret neutral or benign interactions as hostile or aggressive. Youth who are impulsive, due to ADHD, hypomania, or conduct disorder, are also at risk for aggressive behavior. All of these youth may be able to respond to verbal de-escalation, particularly with validation, positive reinforcement of safe behavior, and coaching around collaborative strategies for solving conflicts or ameliorating anxieties. Youth who are psychotic, manic, delirious, or disorganized, may be less responsive to calming techniques and require medication.

If the patient is not responsive to verbal de-escalation and continues to escalate, oral medications should be offered. Oral medication should always be offered before injectable (IM) medication. Many youth are afraid of needles and may become more violent when approached with an injection. Many youth who refuse an oral medication initially will accept it if given the choice between an oral or injectable dose. Offering such a choice allows the child an opportunity to demonstrate self-control and avoids the potentially traumatic experience of restraint and injectable medication.

The preliminary differential diagnosis inferred from the mental status examination and any information gleaned from the initial interviews, as well as any information about the child's prior diagnoses and current medications (if any), will inform the choice of medication. For example, an adolescent with schizophrenia or bipolar disorder already on medication may require an additional dose of their antipsychotic medication. A young child with a history of abuse who is agitated after separation from the parent, who has never been on medication, may be more safely calmed with diphenhydramine. An adolescent with severe anxiety may benefit from a small dose of a benzodiazepine, while for a child with autism or ID, such medications can cause disinhibition and paradoxical agitation. Medications should be chosen carefully and dosed cautiously, to avoid adverse effects. Youth who are antipsychotic naïve, particularly those who are not psychotic or manic, can be at particularly high risk for adverse effects when given high-potency neuroleptics for agitation.

If all de-escalation techniques have failed, and the child has either refused or not responded to oral medication and is engaging in violent or acutely dangerous behavior, an injectable medication may be required. Depending on the nature of the patient's illness, the medication may be pharmacologic management of the patient's underlying illness in the same way that oral medications would be used (e.g., a dose of antipsychotic given intramuscularly in an agitated psychotic patient who has refused his oral antipsychotic). Alternatively, acute chemical restraint may be required. Given the risks of polypharmacy in children, the medication used should be chosen carefully based on the child's age, size, standing medications (or other recent medication administration), medical conditions, current symptoms, and (if known) the psychological cause of their agitation. For young children, those who are medication naïve, and those whose agitation and aggression are based in trauma or extremely poor self-regulation skills, diphenhydramine (Benadryl) IM may be preferred as it is sedating and generally well tolerated. High or repeat doses of diphenhydramine can cause disinhibition, confusion or delirium, so the total daily dose must be monitored. If diphenhydramine is not tolerated or is insufficient, a sedating lower-potency antipsychotic such as chlorpromazine (Thorazine) may be safe and effective, though higher doses can risk orthostatic hypotension and tachyarrhythmias. Adolescents who are agitated due to anxiety may respond well to IM benzodiazepines such as lorazepam (Ativan), while young children and those with autism or developmental disabilities are more likely to experience paradoxical agitation or disinhibition if given benzodiazepines. Adolescents who are agitated due to paranoid psychosis or mania will likely require haloperidol or another high-potency antipsychotic. If high-potency antipsychotics are administered the patient should concurrently be given diphenhydramine or benztropine (Cogentin) to reduce the risk for dystonic side effects. Adding diphenhydramine to haloperidol (or to a low-potency antipsychotic such as chlorpromazine) can also enhance the sedating effect for youth who are extremely agitated or aggressive. Dosing of injectable medications should generally be half of the oral dose that would be used, and caution should be used before considering typical adult doses of medications for chemical restraint in youth.

In most cases of chemical restraint, a physical hold, restraint or seclusion is also required for the safety of the child and those around him. State and local governmental and oversight agencies, hospital policies, and the regulatory standards set by the Center for Medicare and Medicaid Services and The Joint Commission dictate for which patients a hold, restraint or seclusion is appropriate (55). Physical hold, restraint or seclusion should only be used to prevent serious harm to self or others, but a different intervention will be most therapeutic for the child based on their individual history. Seclusion may be safer for youth with a history of abuse, whereas restraint could be experienced as re-traumatizing. For a young child, a therapeutic hold may be more appropriate, while seclusion could be deeply frightening for the child. The patient in hold, restraint or seclusion should be monitored continuously by staff, and the physician must monitor the child's physical health and comfort and ensure the child is safe. Staff should also explain to the child the reason for the restraint or seclusion and what the child must do to demonstrate that he is safe to be released. The child should be removed from restraint as soon as he is in control, and restraint should never exceed the limits mandated by The Joint Commission, the Health Care Financing Administration, and individual hospital policies. Once the child is released from restraints, the clinician should meet with the child for a debriefing discussion to help the patient to process what has happened and understand the reason for restraint and how to prevent similar incidents in the future. For youth prone to agitation or aggression, the debriefing is an important therapeutic opportunity for the youth to understand his own feelings and behavior with an adult who is empathic and validating, not judgmental or punitive.

SPECIFIC PSYCHIATRIC EMERGENCIES IN YOUTH

Suicidal and Self-Injurious Behavior

Risk Assessment

When children and adolescents present to the ED after an episode of self-harm, it can be difficult to determine whether the self-injury was deliberate or accidental, and whether it was made with suicidal intent. The child's self-report of suicidal intent and current suicidal thinking is not sufficient to determine risk for future suicidal behavior. Many patients who go on to attempt suicide deny suicidal thoughts to clinicians but speak to family members about their suicidal thoughts (56), and in an ED especially youth may be motivated to minimize their suicidal thoughts or intent due to fear of hospitalization, upsetting family members, or other perceived consequences. Thus the ED clinician should speak with collateral regarding any recent statements of suicidal ideation or intent, hopelessness, anhedonia, or command auditory hallucinations to harm self; history of prior suicide attempts or ideation, substance use, prior psychiatric diagnoses (depression, substance use, bipolar disorder, and conduct disorders confer increased risk for suicide); family history of suicide or recent suicide in the peer group or media; and access to firearms or other dangerous means. The context of the self-harm or suicide attempt is also important, and both the collateral and the patient should be asked whether the patient wrote a suicide note or made other preparation for death, made efforts to hide their attempt or ensure no one would find or help them, or if they experienced regret or ambivalence after the attempt and immediately called for help. The ED clinician should ask the child about their intentions and planning leading up the attempt, the anticipated lethality (or if the child thoughts someone would discover or rescue them), and triggers for suicidal thoughts including perceived burdensomeness, social isolation, or rejection (57). During this discussion the clinician should be vigilant for cues in the mental status examination that suggest acute risk, such as hopelessness, perceived worthlessness, preoccupation with death, severe depression, and command hallucinations, as these are more difficult for a child to hide or minimize. Affective disengagement or superficial discussion of serious suicidal behavior is also a red flag that the patient is minimizing the severity of risk.

If the child or adolescent denies suicidal intent and collateral sources corroborate this, it is important not to dismiss self-injurious behaviors as attention-seeking or reflecting personality disorder, as might be done in adult patients. Repeated self-injury in youth is a risk factor for later suicide attempts (21) and youth who cut themselves or engage in other self-harming behaviors without suicidal intent (or with ambivalent intent) can inadvertently hurt themselves, due to misjudgment or impulsivity. Other youth may engage in clearly nonfatal behaviors (such as superficial self-cutting, or taking double the recommended dose of a vitamin or over-the-counter painkiller) but with suicidal intent; clinicians should not dismiss these youth as "dramatic" or attention-seeking as if their intent is to die, their next attempt may be of higher lethality.

Management

Inpatient hospitalization is likely necessary if the patient is at high risk, such as (but not limited to) those youth with:

- persistent, intense suicidal ideation or intent
- serious, high-lethality suicidal behavior or attempt (regardless of whether current or persistent suicidal thoughts are endorsed)
- suicidal thinking or behavior in the context of command auditory hallucinations to harm self, severe depression, hopelessness, self-blame, severe social isolation, or poor supports (family rejection or abuse, no outpatient treatment)
- suicidal thinking or behavior in the context of profound psychosocial stressor, such as recent sexual trauma or disclosure of abuse, severe bullying, or relationship loss

If the patient does not require hospitalization, a safety plan should still be determined for discharge. This includes not only connection with treatment providers (with prompt follow-up, ideally within a week, for reassessment and stabilization), but also identification of supports and coping strategies if suicidal thoughts return, and the triggers for suicidal thoughts. A safety plan is also necessary for youth who present with nonsuicidal self-injurious behavior, with the focus being coping with urges to self-harm rather than suicidal thoughts. The clinician should also help the youth to identify the function of the self-harming behaviors, such as relief of numbness or strong negative emotions, attention from peers or family, or release from conflicts or overwhelming stressors. Self-injurious behaviors in youth with anxiety disorders, childhood maltreatment, or autism may function to allow escape from hyperstimulating or otherwise challenging environments (such as a classroom that is too loud or academically too difficult). Identifying the function of self-injurious or parasuicidal behaviors allows the clinician to identify situations that overwhelm a child's ability to cope or communicate distress and areas where skill-building and support is needed.

Aggression

Risk Assessment

Many youth presenting to the ED for aggression are agitated, irritable, or aggressive on arrival. As noted above, the patient's response to de-escalation techniques over time will inform both diagnosis and risk assessment. Once the patient is calm enough to engage with the interview, the clinician should attempt to understand the aggressive behavior. Aggressive behavior is rarely random and the clinician should endeavor to understand the child's perspective as to the reason for the aggression. Such an approach is therapeutic for the patient and helps to identify specific risk for future aggression. Impulsive, reactive aggression may be triggered by psychological insults such as humiliation or teasing by peers, frustration or rage when limits are set by authority figures, or intense anxiety related to a trauma reminder in a child with PTSD or a change in routine in a youth with autism or ID. "Cold," planned or instrumental aggression may be in response to narcissistic injury, a hostile attribution bias, or a belief (often ingrained by family or peer group) that aggression is an appropriate means to obtain a desired object or assert power. Approaching the child with curiosity and a desire to take his perspective without judgment increases the likelihood that the patient will be honest and forthcoming, and also the patient's response to this approach is revealing. A youth who despite this approach is superficially engaged or insincere, deflects responsibility or minimizes the severity of his behavior, likely has little motivation to change or engage in treatment. Paranoid or disorganized thinking, persistent anger or hostility, and specific homicidal ideation or intent are also indicators of greater risk.

In speaking with collateral sources, the ED clinician should be attentive to different perspectives on the episode, history of severe or escalating violence, evidence of premeditated aggression or homicidal intent, and use of weapons all demonstrate elevated risk. Understanding the context of the aggressive behavior is particularly important for young children and those with autism, ID, or language impairments who may be unable to explicitly identify the trigger for their behavior.

Management

Risk for future violence, and the treatment that may mitigate that risk, depends on the child's underlying psychiatric illness and the nature of the aggressive behavior. Premeditated or instrumental aggression can be seen in youth with conduct disorder or substance use, or in youth with gang involvement or other societal risk factors unrelated to psychiatric illness. Effective treatment of instrumental aggression requires setting clear consequences and promoting prosocial behaviors through programs such as MST, described above. Reactive aggression is more common in youth with mental illness. Treatment for reactive aggression involves identifying and treating the underlying symptoms and deficits in self-regulation that predispose the child to aggression, then identifying triggering situations and teaching coping skills to manage those situations without aggression. Whether such treatment must happen on an inpatient unit or can be safely administered in the community depends on the nature of the underlying illness, the severity of aggression, and the availability of appropriately intensive community supports and treatment. For patients to be discharged from the ED, the clinician should create a safety plan, similar to that for suicidal behaviors, to identify how the child can cope safely with situations that typically trigger aggression (Table 6.3.1.4).

If the aggressive behavior is not rooted in psychiatric illness and inpatient hospitalization or treatment is unlikely to be helpful, the ED clinician may need to coordinate with parents to identify other supports to contain the youth's behavior, or with law enforcement if the behavior is criminal in nature.

TABLE 6.3.1.4

PSYCHIATRIC DISORDERS AND TREATMENT OF ACUTE AGGRESSION

Illness/Symptom	Treatment Focus
ADHD	Address impulsivity
ODD	Set clear limits, reinforce positive behaviors
Psychosis	Treat command hallucinations/ paranoia that are triggering aggression
Mania	Stabilize mania to address impulsivity/irritability
Anxiety or OCD	Identify and address triggers (such as being blocked from completing compulsions)
PTSD	Identify trauma reminders, promote safe coping behaviors
Autism	Promote verbal problem solving and other coping behaviors
Conduct disorder	Set clear consequences for antisocial behaviors and reinforce positive behaviors
Substance use	Increased supervision, motivation enhancement techniques to reduce use

Psychosis

Risk Assessment

The onset of psychotic illness in a child or adolescent is a true psychiatric emergency, but ED clinicians should be mindful that chronic psychotic disorders such as schizophrenia are rare in children, so a broad differential and careful assessment is important. Young children and those with IDs can describe ego-dystonic or shameful thoughts or urges as "voices," or may have difficulty distinguishing intense fears, anxiety-driven illusions, trauma flashbacks, or even imaginary friends from visual hallucinations. Children and adolescents with mood disorders may also experience nonpsychotic hallucinations that are congruent with their mood as well as grandiose, nihilistic, or shameful delusions. OCD can present with thinking that appears psychotic, particularly in youth whose obsessions and compulsions are all internal (with compulsive thoughts rather than behaviors). Other youth who are sent to the ED for "bizarre behavior" or "responding to internal stimuli" have autism or ID; this may be undiagnosed, or the child with known autism may have a change in behavior that is perceived as psychotic but is actually related to a physical ailment or other stressor the child cannot articulate. Information about the child's functioning at home and school, history of symptoms and treatment, recent and prior stressors or traumas is important to obtain from collateral contacts to elucidate the clinical picture.

If the child is truly psychotic, organic causes must be ruled out either before psychiatric treatment begins or concurrently to psychiatric stabilization. The medical workup should include a complete physical examination, serum tests including complete blood count, electrolytes, and liver, kidney, and thyroid tests. Toxicology screening should be completed if there is any chance of substance use or accidental ingestion, and other tests such as lyme, erythrocyte sedimentation rate, rapid plasma regain, brain imaging, lumbar puncture for cerebrospinal fluid analysis (for cases of suspected encephalitis) should be obtained, in collaboration with pediatric and neurology consultation, depending on the patient's history and current symptoms.

Management

Youth with psychosis, related to schizophrenia, bipolar disorder, depression, or OCD, can rarely be stabilized in a few hours in the ED and generally require inpatient hospitalization for stabilization. Whenever possible, treatment should begin as quickly as possible (in the ED if necessary) as psychotic patients can act erratically and because untreated psychosis is terrifying to patients and their families (58). If the psychosis is secondary to drug intoxication or accidental ingestion, the psychosis may clear in hours or days, though youth who have abused newer designer drugs such as synthetic cannabinoids and substituted cathinones may have persistent psychotic symptoms and require hospitalization for stabilization.

If the "voices" or other reported psychotic symptoms are due to anxiety, trauma, or grief, or a manifestation of ID or immaturity, the patient may be safe to return home with community treatment for their underlying disorder. The ED clinician should reassure the child and family while at the same time emphasizing the importance of follow-up psychiatric care.

Youth with Autism and Intellectual Disability

Risk Assessment

Youth with autism spectrum disorder (ASD) are nine times more likely than their neurotypical peers to go to the ED in psychiatric crisis (59). Youth with ASD and/or ID are difficult for ED clinicians as they are often medically and psychiatrically complicated, and because ED staff often lack training in working with such patients. Children and adolescents with ASD or ID are often brought to the ED for behavioral symptoms such as aggression, self-injury, inappropriate sexual behaviors, sleep cycle reversal, or running away. In the ED these children may be aggressive or agitated due to hyperstimulation from the noise and light of the ED and the stress of an unfamiliar and unpredictable environment.

The clinician should look for changes in the environment (school vacation, changes in caregivers or environment) or physical/medical problems (constipation, dental problems, seasonal allergies, ear infections, akathisia from antipsychotic medication, fatigue due to polypharmacy, onset of puberty, or subtle seizure activity) that may be triggering behavioral symptoms. Self-stimulating, aggressive or self-injurious behaviors can be a response to frustration, anxiety, or discomfort that the child cannot communicate verbally. Considering the child's cognitive and developmental age is also crucial when evaluating problematic behaviors. For example, an adolescent boy with severe autism and moderate ID who touches a peer's breasts without permission may have little understanding of why this behavior is intrusive and offensive; hypersexuality related to mania is much less likely the cause. If environmental, medical and developmental causes can be ruled out, the clinician should consider new onset of psychiatric disorder such as mood or anxiety disorder.

Management

Awareness of techniques to work with youth with ASD and ID and small modifications to the ED milieu can help make the ED a safe and therapeutic space for patients with ASD/ID. If available, child life specialists, OT and other allied health professionals can be extremely helpful in engaging and soothing youth with ASD/ID. If such staff are not available, replicating where possible what works for the child at home or at school (such as preferred caregivers, toys or activities; soothing techniques and preferred sensory tools; and communication tools such as "baby sign language" or picture communication tools) can be very helpful. Youth with ASD/ID are often sensitive to physical intrusions, so blood draws, injections, vital signs monitoring, and other procedures should be consolidated when possible and eliminated if not necessary to the medical workup.

Medication should be used cautiously for sedation in ASD and ID patients in the ED, as they often have paradoxical reactions to medications such as benzodiazepines and diphenhydramine and often have little positive response to injectable antipsychotics. Behavioral interventions and relief of the etiology of their stress (such as effective pain control, dental care, resolution of constipation or adverse effects from polypharmacy) can lead to rapid relief and stabilization. Once the underlying problem is resolved, patients who had been extremely difficult to manage can become calm and cooperative enough to be safely discharged, particularly if the ED clinician can assist family in identifying community respite and home-based services for additional support.

Child Abuse or Maltreatment

Risk Assessment

Often when children present to the ED for psychiatric evaluation, the crisis lies not in the child alone, but in the psychosocial context. Cases of child abuse or maltreatment are unfortunately common and are very challenging for the ED clinician to identify and manage. Poverty, single parent households, large family size, social isolation, parental substance use, personal history of abuse in the parent, and psychiatric and developmental disorders in the child all increase risk for child abuse. Maltreatment also increases a child's vulnerability to psychiatric illness. Children rarely freely admit to abuse, parental substance abuse, domestic violence, or other crises in the family. The ED clinician must be vigilant to subtle physical signs of abuse or neglect; externalizing behaviors such as aggression, hoarding or stealing food, running away, regression in toileting, and school refusal; internalizing symptoms such as PTSD, depression, inattention, or withdrawal; and discrepancies in the child's or adults' reports that suggest that the family is actively concealing a family secret.

Management

Safety is the first priority in cases of maltreatment; if the child is being abused, if the parent is severely mentally ill and unable to care for the child, or if there is extreme violence in the home, then child protective services should be notified. The ED clinician should simultaneously work with the child, family, and any available services and supports to identify strengths in the family system that can help to stabilize the crisis. Often allowing both the child and parent to articulate the crisis and access individual and family treatment will reduce both the child's distress and the strain on the family, and increase everyone's openness to treatment.

CONSENT, CONFIDENTIALITY, AND LEGAL CONSIDERATIONS

The ED clinician should be knowledgeable about the federal, state, and institutional regulations that govern emergency psychiatric treatment and hospitalization, particularly those that dictate the emergency evaluation and treatment of minors. As mentioned for consent above, each state has specific statues governing psychiatric hospitalization for minors, generally allowing for parents or guardians to admit minor children on a voluntary basis, and also allowing for involuntary, emergency, or diagnostic admissions (51). Some states allow adolescents above a certain age, or if emancipated, to consent to their own hospitalization. Clinicians should familiarize themselves with their state statues for hospitalization of minors, as well as their institutional policies for hospitalization and consent for treatment (especially consent for psychiatric medication).

ED clinicians must also be mindful of state and local regulations and statues regarding mandated reporting for child abuse or maltreatment, institutional abuse reporting (such as schools or residential programs), duty to third parties (also known as "Tarasoff" duties), and confidentiality of mental health, substance use and sexual health information for minors. Many states allow adolescents some degree of confidentiality vis-à-vis their parents, though if the child is in imminent danger or a danger to others, the parent should be notified. Often the child wishes to keep treatment secret from their parent or guardian due to fear of the parent's reaction, and with the clinician's support, may be able to safely disclose and include the parent in treatment.

Clinicians working in emergency settings often fear litigation and malpractice in settings of adverse outcomes. While there may be pressure to practice defensive medicine, the best defense is to practice excellent medicine that is well documented and supported by clinical science and best practices. Being transparent, compassionate and collaborative with patients and families can also reduce the risk of litigation.

References

1. Sills MR, Bland SD: Summary statistics for pediatric psychiatric visits to US emergency departments, 1993–1999. *Pediatrics* 110(4):e40, 2002.
2. Simon AE, Schoendorf KC: Emergency department visits for mental health conditions among US children, 2001–2011. *Clin Pediatr (Phila)* 53(14):1359–1366, 2014.
3. Torio CM, Encinosa W, Berdahl T, McCormick MC, Simpson LA: Annual report on health care for children and youth in the United States: national estimates of cost, utilization and expenditures for children with mental health conditions. *Acad Pediatr* 15(1):19–35, 2015.
4. Wharff EA, Ginnis KB, Ross AM, Blood EA: Predictors of psychiatric boarding in the pediatric emergency department: implications for emergency care. *Pediatr Emerg Care* 27:483–489, 2011.
5. Mapelli E, Black T, Doan Q: Trends in pediatric emergency department utilization for mental health-related visits. *J Pediatr* 167:905–910, 2015.
6. Sheridan DC, Sprio DM, Fu R, et al.: Mental health utilization in a pediatric emergency department. *Pediatr Emerg Care* 31:555–559, 2015.
7. Santiago L, Tunik M, Foltin G, Mojica M: Children requiring psychiatric consultation in the pediatric emergency department: epidemiology, resource utilization, and complications. *Pediatr Emerg Care* 22(2);85–89, 2006.
8. Grupp-Phelan J, Mahajan P, Foltin GL, et al.: The Pediaitrc Emergency Care Applied Research Network: Referral and resource use patterns for psychiatric-related visits to pediatric emergency departments. *Pediatr Emerg Care* 25:217–220, 2009.
9. Mahajan P, Alpern ER, Grupp-Phelan J, et al.: Epidemiology of psychiatric-related visits to emergency departments in a multicenter collaborative research pediatric network. *Pediatr Emerg Care* 25(11):715–720, 2009.
10. Case SD, Case BG, Olfson M, Linakis JG, Laska EM: Length of stay of pediatric mental health emergency department visits in the United States. *J Am Acad Child Adolesc Psychiatry* 50:1110–1119, 2011.
11. Treatment Advocacy Center: *Trends and Consequences of Closing Public Psychiatric Hospitals*. 2012. Available at: http://www.treatmentadvocacy-center.org/trends-and-consequences-of-closing-public-psychiatric-hospitals-2012/consequences. Accessed on March 21, 2017.
12. Baraff LJ, Janowicz N, Asarnow JR: Survey of California emergency departments about practices for management of suicidal patients and resources available for their care. *Ann Emerg Med* 48:452–458, 2006.
13. Case BG, Olfson M, Marcus SC, Siegel C: Trends in the inpatient mental health treatment of children and adolescents in US community hospital between 1990 and 2000. *Arch Gen Psychiatry* 64:89–96, 2007.
14. Bender D, Pande N, Ludwig M: *A Literature Review: Psychiatric Boarding*. Washington, DC, U.S. Department of Health and Human Services, 2008.
15. Chamberlain JM, Krug S, Shaw KN: Emergency care for children in the United States. *Health Affairs* 32(12):2109–2115, 2013.
16. Thomas LE: Trends and shifting ecologies: Part I. *Child Adolesc Psychiatr Clin N Am* 12(4):599–611, 2003.
17. Woolston JL: The administration of hospital-based services. *Child Adolesc Psychiatr Clin N Am* 11:43–65, vi, 2002.
18. Havens J. Making psychiatric emergency services work better for children and families. *J Am Acad Child Adolesc Psychiatry* 50(11):1093–1094, 2011.
19. National Vital Statistics System, National Center for Health Statistics, Center for Disease Control: 10 leading causes of death by age group, United States–2013, WISQARS, 2013.
20. Rockett IR, Caine ED: Self-injury is the eighth leading cause of death in the United States: is it time to pay attention? *JAMA Psychiatry* 72:1069–1070, 2015.
21. Olfson S, Gameroff MJ, Marcus SC, Greenberg T, Shaffer S: Emergency treatment of young people following deliberate self-harm. *Arch Gen Psychiatry* 62:1122–1128, 2005.
22. Bridge JA, Marcus SC, Olfson M: Outpatient care of young people after emergency treatment of deliberate self-harm. *J Am Acad Child Adolesc Psychiatry* 51(2):213–222, 2012.
23. Janssens A, Hayen S, Walraven V, Leys M, Deboutte D: Emergency psychiatric care for children and adolescents: a literature review. *Pediatr Emerg Care* 29(9):1041–1050, 2013.
24. Havens J, Marr M: Models of emergency psychiatric care for children and adolescents. In: Haddad F, Gerson R (eds): *Helping Kids In Crisis: Managing Psychiatric Emergencies in Children and Adolescents*. Arlington, VA, American Psychiatric Publishing, 191–200, 2014.
25. Shepperd S, Doll H, Gowers S, et al.: Alternatives to inpatient mental health care for children and young people. *Cochrane Database Syst Rev* (2):CD006410, 2009.
26. Pumariega AJ, Winters NC: Trends and shifting ecologies: Part II. *Child Adolesc Psychiatr Clin N Am* 12(4):779–793, 2003.
27. Hamm, MP, Osmond M, Curran J, et al.: A systematic review of crisis interventions used in the emergency department: recommendations for pediatric care and research. *Pediatr Emerg Care* 26(12):952–962, 2010.
28. Kinney JM, Madsen B, Fleming T, Haapala DA: Homebuilders: keeping families together. *J Consult Clin Psychol* 45(4):667–673, 1977.
29. Forsythe P: Homebuilders and family preservation. *Child Youth Serv Rev* 14(1):37–47, 1992.

30. Evans ME, Boothroyd RA, Armstrong MI: Development and implementation of an experimental study of the effectiveness of intensive in-home crisis services for children and their families. *J Emotion Behav Disorders* 5(2):93–105, 1997.
31. Evans ME, Boothroyd RA, Armstrong MI, Greenbaum PE, Brown EC, Kuppinger AD: An experimental study of the effectiveness of intensive in-home crisis services for children and their families program outcomes. *J Emotion Behav Disorders* 11(2):92–102, 2003.
32. Lyons JS: *Redressing the Emperor: Improving our Children's Public Mental Health System.* Westport, CT, Praeger, 2004.
33. Henggeler SW, Rowland MD, Randall J, et al.: Home-based multisystemic therapy as an alternative to the hospitalization of youths in psychiatric crisis: clinical outcomes. *J Am Acad Child Adolesc Psychiatry* 38(11):1331–1339, 1999.
34. Henggeler SW, Rowland MD, Hallisay-Boykins C, et al.: One-year follow-up of multisystemic therapy as an alternative to the hospitalization of youths in psychiatric crisis. *J Am Acad Child Adolesc Psychiatry* 42(5): 543–551, 2003.
35. Huey SJ, Henggeler SW, Rowland MD, et al.: Multisystemic therapy effects on attempted suicide by youths presenting psychiatric emergencies. *J Am Acad Child Adolesc Psychiatry* 43(2):183–190, 2004.
36. Schoenwald SK, Ward DM, Henggeler SW, Rowland MD: Multisystemic therapy versus hospitalization for crisis stabilization of youth: placement outcomes 4 months postreferral. *Ment Health Serv Res* 2(1):3–12, 2000.
37. Huey SJ, Henggeler SW, Rowland MD, et al.: Multisystemic therapy effects on attempted suicide by youths presenting psychiatric emergencies. *J Am Acad Child Adolesc Psychiatry* 43(2):183–190, 2004.
38. Currier GW, Fisher SG, Caine ED: Mobile crisis team intervention to enhance linkage of discharged suicidal emergency department patients to outpatient psychiatric services: a randomized controlled trial. *Acad Emerg Med* 17(1):36–43, 2010.
39. Shulman DA, Athey M: Youth emergency services: total community effort, a multisystem approach. *Child Welfare: J Policy, Practice, Program* 72:171–179, 1993.
40. Blumberg SH: Crisis intervention program: an alternative to inpatient psychiatric treatment for children. *Ment Health Serv Res* 4(1):1–6, 2002.
41. Newton AS, Hamm MP, Bethell J, et al.: Pediatric suicide-related presentations: a systematic review of mental health care in the emergency department. *Ann Emerg Med* 56(6):649–659, 2010.
42. Wharff EA, Ginnis KM, Ross AM: Family-based crisis intervention with suicidal adolescents in the emergency room: a pilot study. *Soc Work* 57:133–143, 2012.
43. Rotheram-Borus MJ, Piacentini J, Cantwell C, Belin TR, Song J: The 18-month impact of an emergency room intervention for adolescent female suicide attempters. *J Consult Clin Psychol* 68(6):1081–1093, 2000.
44. Mahajan P, Thomas R, Rosenberg DR, et al.: Evaluation of a child guidance model for visits for mental disorders to an inner-city pediatric emergency department. *Pediatr Emerg Care* 23(4):212–217, 2007.
45. 2012 Annual Report to the Governor and Legislature of New York State on Comprehensive Psychiatric Emergency Programs. New York State Office of Mental Health. Available at: www.omh.ny.gov/omhweb/statistics/cpep_annual.
46. Provincial Council for Maternal Child Health: Final Report of the Child and Youth Advisory Committee's Emergency Department Clinical Pathways for Youth with mental Health Conditions/Addictions Work Group, January, 2012. Available at: www.pcmch.on.ca/health-care-providers/paediatric-care/pcmch-strategies-and-initiatives/ed-clinical-pathways/.
47. Department of Emergency Medicine. Illinois Emergency Medical Services for children. Available at: http://ssom.luc.edu/emergency-medicine/children. Accessed March 21, 2017.
48. Posner K, Brown GK, Stanley B, et al.: The Columbia Suicide Severity Rating Scale: initial validity and internal consistency findings from three multisite studies with adolescents and adults. *Am J Psychiatry* 168(12):1266–1277, 2011.
49. Horowitz LM, Bridge JA, Teach SJ, et al.: Ask Suicide-screening Questions (ASQ): a brief instrument for the pediatric emergency department. *Arch Pediatr Med* 166(12):1170–1176, 2012.
50. SAFE-T National Suicide Prevention Lifeline Wallet Care: Learn the Warning Signs—U.S. Department of Health and Human Services: Substance Abuse and Mental Health Services Administration. National Suicide Prevention Lifeline. Available at: http://store.samhsa.gov/product/National-Sucide-Prevention-Lifeline-Wallet-Card-Sucide-Prevention-Learn-the-Warning-Signs/SVP-13-0126. Accessed March 21, 2017.
51. Velting DM, Shaffer D, Gould MS, Garfinkel R, Fisher P, Davies M: Parent–victim agreement in adolescent suicide research. *J Am Acad Child Adolesc Psychiatry* 37:1161–1166, 1998.
52. Fortunati FG Jr, Zonana HV: Legal considerations in the child psychiatric emergency department. *Child Adolesc Psychiatr Clin N Am* 12(4):745–761, 2003.
53. Dorfman DH, Mehta SD: Restraint use for psychiatric patients in the pediatric emergency department. *Pediatr Emerg Care* 22(1):7–12, 2006.
54. Regan K: Trauma informed care on an inpatient pediatric psychiatric unit and the emergence of ethical dilemmas as nurses evolved their practice. *Issues Ment Health Nurs* 31:216–222, 2010.
55. Masters KJ, Bellonci C, Bernet W; The Workgroup on Quality Issues: Practice parameter for the prevention and management of aggressive behavior in child and adolescent psychiatric institutions, with special reference to seclusion and restraint. *J Am Acad Child Adolesc Psychiatry* 41(2 Supplement):4S–25S, 2002.
56. Fawcett J, Scheftner W, Fogg L, et al.: Time-related predictors of suicide in major affective disorder. *Am J Psychiatry* 147:1189–1194, 1990.
57. Van Orden KA, Cukrowicz KC, Witte TC, Joiner TE: Thwarted belongingness and perceived burdensomeness: construct validity and psychometric properties of the interpersonal needs questionnaire. *Psychol Assess* 24(1):197–215, 2012.
58. Gerson R, Booty A, Wong C, et al.: Families' experience with seeking treatment for recent onset psychosis. *Psychiatr Serv* 60:812–816, 2009.
59. Kalb LG, Stuart EA, Freedman B, Zablotsky B, Vasa R: Psychiatric-related emergency department visits among children with an autism spectrum disorder. *Pediatr Emerg Care* 28(12):1269–1276, 2012.

CHAPTER 6.3.2 ■ MILIEU-BASED TREATMENT: INPATIENT AND PARTIAL HOSPITALIZATION, RESIDENTIAL TREATMENT

JOSEPH C. BLADER AND CARMEL A. FOLEY

INTRODUCTION

Because they subordinate nearly all aspects of a person's life to external control, inpatient and residential psychiatric treatments are among the most intrusive in health care. Autonomy and privacy may not be abundant in childhood, but their loss in these treatment settings is still nearly total. Separation from home under difficult circumstances and the substitution of strangers as caregivers and peers are confusing and frightening experiences for both patients and families. While admission is typically a last resort and provides some relief, parents look to clinicians for help with their own misgivings and emotional turmoil.

At the same time, the uniqueness and potency of out-of-home treatment may profoundly affect the course of illness and functioning for many youth. The leadership roles that child and adolescent psychiatrists assume in these settings therefore entail not just great responsibility for the children now in their physical custody but great opportunity as well. This chapter's goal is to orient readers: (a) to the mission of milieu-based services in today's system of care; (b) to the development and implementation of the multifaceted programming these services provide; and (c) to contextual issues bearing on leadership, administration, and quality assurance in these complex settings.

EVOLUTION OF MILIEU-BASED TREATMENTS

Confinement of the Mentally Ill

Centers that provided compassionate and humane care for the mentally ill flourished intermittently in Europe and the Arab world since classical times. Healing temples offered care and serenity, at least for the elite of these societies. In some places priests, perhaps exploiting a person's delusions, impersonated gods to provide patients with reassurance or to command changes in behavior (1). Ancient Greek physicians were probably the first to offer physiologic explanations for behavioral disturbances to replace supernatural ones. They devised various somatic therapies to rebalance or promote proper circulation of bodily fluids or "humors." While these treatments were available to the more privileged groups who could afford them, the ancients did have a protoscientific concept of mental disorder.

Nevertheless, for most of Western history, the treatment of people with psychiatric illness rates among the more ignominious of human activities. One influential Roman, Aulus Cornelius Celsus (25 BCE to 50 AD), advocated a calm environment and encouragement for the melancholic in addition to specific herbal remedies (2). However, for agitated behavior he called for punitive measures:

> "If however, it is the mind that deceives the madman, he is best treated by certain tortures. When he says or does anything wrong, he is to be coerced by starvation, fetters and flogging... To be thoroughly frightened is beneficial in this illness." (p. 303)

This strain of thought sanctioned a range of odious practices toward people with severely disordered behavior for centuries to come. In medieval times, demonic explanations for aberrant behavior and thought resurged and motivated the confinement, persecution, shackles, and harsh and neglectful treatment that dominated until the late 18th century.

The contemporary model of the psychiatric hospital originates with reforms during the 1790s in Britain (William Tuke, founding the York Retreat, which in turn influenced Benjamin Rush in America), France (Philippe Pinel at Bicêtre and Salpêtrière asylums), and Italy (Vicenzo Chiarugi at Florence's Hospital of Bonifazio). All three men's writings contributed to the modern nosologic approach to mental illness based on lucid descriptions of symptoms and observed course. In the United States and Britain, facilities for the care of those with chronically debilitating mental illness became a function of local government.

This wave of reform and the infusion of public investment, along with an optimistic view that more humane treatment would also cure patients, helped stimulate a significant growth of institutions for the mentally ill beginning in the early 1800s. Many facilities were set in locations removed from the main population centers from which their residents came. It was almost inevitable, though, that the burdens of increasing urbanization and migration, economic dislocation, and the infectious epidemics of subsequent eras, along with the fact that more humane care was not necessarily curative, combined to strain these resources. Underfunding, public discouragement, and a growing patient population degraded many publicly supported facilities into quite dismal places well into the 20th century. However, the deinstitutionalization movement enabled by the Community Mental Health Act (CMHA) of 1963, the development of more effective treatments, and a generally prosperous economy, led to a major reduction in the census of large long-term hospitals. Inpatient psychiatric treatment gradually came to be seen as another health service, rather than a custodial one, and acute units developed in general hospitals where relatively short stays for episodic crises became the norm. Nevertheless, the ambitious aims of the CMHA were never fully funded and it is unlikely that adequate outpatient supports exist to offset the historically low availability of inpatient beds for those with severe mental illness.

The larger historical context of psychiatric hospitalization, and enduring apprehensions about the people who need it, continue to imbue inpatient psychiatry with arguably the most negative stigma among medical treatments today.

Children's Inpatient Treatment

Both before and after the reforms of the early 1800s, we know that disturbed children and adolescents were at times placed in these facilities along with adults. Beyond a few scholarly reports that documented the occurrence of severe mental illness in the young as scientific curiosity, little is known about the care and outcomes of children in asylums. The first dedicated child psychiatric inpatient units as such in the United States were created in 1920s and 1930s, mostly as custodial services for children with postencephalitic brain disorders. The prevailing philosophies of these settings and their successors are discussed below.

By the mid-1970s, inpatient services for children and adolescents proliferated, chiefly in private sector general and specialty psychiatric hospitals. The U.S. Supreme Court's 1985 decision in *Massachusetts vs. Metropolitan* (3) supported mental health coverage by insurance plans, and earlier the *Parham vs. J.R.* decision affirmed that parents' could compel admission to psychiatric inpatient care for an unwilling minor, much as any other necessary medical treatment (4). Lengths of stay were rather extensive, standards for admission were liberal, and many inpatient settings adopted rather high, if subjective, criteria for judging wellness to warrant discharge. Direct-to-consumer advertising by these facilities, aimed at parents worried about their sullen or unruly teenagers, became commonplace. Inpatient care also served an evaluative purpose, with some referrals made for diagnostic clarification.

However, by the early 1990s this trend rapidly reversed. Scandals plagued certain for-profit facilities. Managed care established increasingly strict criteria in order to justify inpatient admission. The *Parham* decision was partially blamed for the ease with which parents could have their adolescents psychiatrically hospitalized, often for rebellious or obnoxious behavior alone. Lengths of stay plummeted, though actual rates of admission for young people have increased (5).

In the public sector, policy makers also recognized that a disproportionate amount of the mental healthcare dollar was spent on very costly inpatient care that could be redirected to less expensive community-based options that were more appropriate for many children.

Child advocates who had earlier called for more community-based resources to help impaired children remain at home (6,7) found that cost concerns were also aligning policy makers' interests toward less restrictive alternatives. "Continuum-of-care" principles by federal, state, and county mental health agencies increased the array of community-based programming. Such services included in-home and out-of-home respite services, supportive case management, therapeutic after school programs, innovative programs based on "blended funding" from several agencies, etc., all aimed at avoiding or reducing hospitalizations and optimizing a child's opportunities for successful and safe life in their communities. Localities, though, still vary widely in the availability and quality of these resources. Moreover, some evaluation projects raised the prospect that such enhanced services do not necessarily produce more favorable outcomes, although families do find them preferable to service systems that lack them (8).

At the present time, inpatient psychiatric treatment in the United States is regarded, properly, as an expensive resource to be used sparingly and as a last resort for the most ill of youngsters. Comparatively few children now depend on long-term psychiatric inpatient settings to receive care, and acute-care lengths of stay are shorter. Current concerns in children's mental health are almost mirror images of older ones. Worries about excessive use and long stays have been replaced by concern that stays are too short to enable satisfactory transitions of children back home and the dearth of outpatient and supportive services in many areas cause facilities to discharge very fragile youngsters into a void unable to provide an appropriate level of care.

Evolution of Treatment Philosophy

The first children's units were essentially custodial in emphasis due to the mostly organic impairments of the patient population (9). Most would be regarded today as intellectually disabled, whether by congenital or acquired (usually infectious) factors.

By the mid-20th century, psychoanalytic thinking dominated child and adolescent psychiatry. Child psychoanalytic theories emphasized the primacy of interpersonal experience in development and emotional disturbances. Early attachment, nurturance, attunement, and gradual promotion of autonomy provide the template for personality development (10). Separation of the child from his or her supposedly pathogenic home environment, now regarded as a necessary evil, was then felt "to be the first requirement for successful treatment... since he is comparatively helpless to reorder his own surroundings or change them to better suit his needs" (11). Inpatient and residential settings for disturbed children had the premise that a more capable caregiving environment offered corrective experiences that would allay basic insecurities and foster ego development. Residential settings also were thought to provide an empathic surrogate "holding environment" (12) that would help the child manage his or her destructive urges or disorganized behavior. There was no particular expectation that this would be a rapid or easy process and long stays were common.

In the 1960s and 1970s, learning theories from experimental psychology, especially its neobehaviorist schools, acquired greater traction in clinical psychology. Environmental manipulation to modify behavior, known broadly as behavior modification or behavior therapy, gained wider application in facilities for developmentally impaired and chronically mentally ill adults. Approaches based on *operant conditioning* principles defined adaptive behaviors for which the individual had a deficit, and sought to promote them with rewards or reinforcers. Likewise, efforts to eliminate (or "extinguish") problematic behaviors involved withholding the consequence thought to reinforce it (such as attention or avoidance of a demanding situation) or by applying an aversive consequence. Offering patients explicit training and practice in specific behavioral skills, such as assertiveness, anger control, and social interaction, were also undertaken in a variety of formats. Influential reports showed dramatic improvements in the social engagement and activities of daily living among chronically ill adults, the acquisition of some language by autistic children, and reductions in self-abusive behavior by those with intellectual disability (13–16).

Settings that provided round-the-clock care seemed ideal for treatments that required consistent monitoring of behavior and systematic manipulation of the consequences. "Token economies" in which patients earned various privileges for prespecified behaviors, became widespread, and influenced the point or level systems common in today's inpatient and residential settings. The appeal of these systems may derive partly from their implementation on a unit-wide basis, in that many patients will share similar behavioral objectives and thus offer a common template for the whole service. In contrast, classical conditioning and applied behavioral analytic approaches are highly idiographic and the staffing of most psychiatric settings seldom permits such intense staff training and individualized implementation efforts on a routine basis. The obvious availability of a peer group also enables on-the-spot opportunities to develop and practice social and other skills. Behavioral interventions are devised to yield dividends in weeks, or at least that is the period for evaluating the usefulness of a particular treatment plan.

However, the intensity of specialized out-of-home settings that facilitates ecologic interventions of these types also reduces the likelihood that behavior changes will generalize to other settings. It is therefore desirable to involve families as much as possible to enable continuity of factors that promote behavioral stability in the hospital. Family-focused treatment did not assume a major role in the treatment of psychiatrically hospitalized children until the 1980s. In 1980, the most common type of treatment received across all settings was individual therapy, received by 89%, while family therapy was provided to only 38% (17). At that time, some settings had programs where entire families were admitted and under constant observation. Inpatient treatment had in many places evolved to involve parents and other caregivers more actively, and had included time spent off the unit at home to practice and troubleshoot alternate ways of interaction intended to foster more adaptive behavior. More recently, as short lengths of stay became the norm and payers declined reimbursement if the child spent outside of the hospital, these practices have waned.

Pharmacotherapy now plays a prominent role in the psychiatric treatment of youth. The 1980 NIMH report indicated that 42% of child and adolescent inpatients were treated with standing psychotropic medication. It is now the rare youngster whose inpatient or residential treatment does not include medication (18–20). Initiation of medication trials is more readily approved by insurance reviewers as a justification for continuing hospital care than other interventions. The combined effect is that the role of the child psychiatrist in these settings has increasingly focused, perhaps to the detriment of other areas, on which preadmission agents were doing any good, which were potentially making things worse, and what to try next, all in the context of constrained lengths of stay with a possibly more treatment-refractory patient group.

In hospital settings, daily rounds now typically begin with the question, "Why does this child need to be in the hospital"? All hospitalizations covered by managed care plans are constantly monitored by the insurance companies' reviewers. Publicly funded care is also subject to retroactive denial of payments if inspection of the medical record is judged to lack sufficient justification for inpatient care. Although minimizing the time a child spends in a hospital is not a controversial goal, a widespread sentiment is that aggressive cost containment may have compromised care. For instance, payers often regard as inertia the observation of a child after withdrawing preadmission medications, which biases the system toward initiating new, possibly superfluous pharmacotherapy. This is another area deserving more systematic study.

OVERVIEW OF TYPES OF MILIEU SETTINGS AND THEIR PURPOSE IN A SYSTEM OF CARE

Inpatient Care

Inpatient care is now only deemed appropriate when less restrictive alternatives have been considered, have failed, or are not available. The most common reason for admission is behavior that places the child or others in danger. This may translate to suicidal ideation, intent, or attempt, or may reflect sufficient threat of aggression or actual aggression such that the caretaking system, school or home, is concerned and unable to handle the youth. It is difficult nowadays to get authorization from payers to admit for a purely diagnostic assessment. Indeed, many components of such evaluations, say, can generally be secured on an outpatient basis, and payers seldom find the value of inpatient observation a cogent rationale for admission.

The majority of short-stay psychiatric treatment is provided in units located in freestanding psychiatric hospitals or in psychiatric units in general medical/surgical hospitals. These settings generally serve children of ages 5 to 18 years. Very few programs serve a preschool population in an inpatient setting. It is common to have separate inpatient settings for children up to age 12 or 13 and for adolescents up to age 18. Some inpatient units treat children and adolescents together, or those over the age of 16 may be admitted to adult settings, but these practices derive more from necessity than philosophy. Youth inpatient settings not embedded within a medical facility often cannot admit, or decline to admit those with substantial medical needs or who are likely to require specialist consultations as part of their assessments. This can be disadvantageous in many areas of the country where only few providers of inpatient psychiatric care are not a part of a larger medical service.

Municipal and county facilities often have a public mandate to serve the local court system. Judges have the authority to mandate assessments in such units frequently for defined time frames (21 days is common). A complete assessment of the child's mental condition, including psychological testing, and a psychosocial assessment of the child's family, school, and community culminate in an advisory report to the court. This population is considered to be massively underserved with respect to psychiatric illness, the prevalence of which is now known to be quite high. To the extent that mental health services variously exist within the juvenile justice systems residential programs, they constitute another version of a psychiatric inpatient provider system for incarcerated youth.

Inpatient units can be subspecialized for the care of unique psychiatrically impaired populations. Eating disorder services are one example, which enable the more intensive medical management these youth require initially with the specialized psychiatric care that does most of the heavy lifting toward recovery adequate for the resumption of outpatient treatment. Special psychiatric units for the deaf, the blind, and for youth with co-occurring developmental disabilities, also exist. A few units exist for the treatment of chronic pain, in which psychiatric and psychological care have a prominent role. There are also numerous residential centers for adolescent substance abuse, but the involvement of psychiatrists is highly variable.

Partial Hospitalization and Day Treatment

Of the varieties of noninpatient programs, partial hospitalization is the most intensive. The clinical challenge for this level of care is the provision of short-term, crisis stabilization as an alternative to inpatient care or as a step down from inpatient care.

Partial hospital programming may be provided on an inpatient unit. Some refer to this as "unit-based aftercare." It allows the patient to continue working with the same treatment team and the same peer group rather than forcing a change for a short period of time. Partial day hospital licenses require treatment to be no longer than 6 weeks and the provision of daily medical record documentation of progress much like an inpatient setting. However, most inpatient units have a high inpatient census and staffing is not necessarily easily expanded to cope with "day patients," so the model has obvious practical limitations.

More typically, partial hospital programs have their own staff, space, and school. Managed care review generally constrains the actual duration of the patient's involvement to only days or a couple of weeks. Since the setting is generally open, and regulation does not allow restraint or seclusion, but does permit therapeutic hold and use of a quiet room (no locked door), there are practical limitations on the degree of psychopathology for which these settings are suitable. Programmatically, the range of therapeutic services are similar to inpatient settings, and include, individual, group, and family therapies, recreation and rehabilitation therapies, medical care, and psychopharmacology.

Day treatment, sometimes referred to as "continuing day treatment," differs from partial hospitals in several ways. Length of stay is much longer, often driven by the school year's calendar. In some locations, children attending day treatment that is in a clinical facility rather than one run by the educational authority, require approval of that level of care by the home school district, since depending on state law, these authorities assume the cost of the program's educational component. Some localities oblige the home district to provide transportation to these clinical settings within a certain radius, while in others families have to make their own arrangements.

Day treatment settings usually resemble schools more than hospitals, with the addition of outpatient psychiatric care and nursing staff to help manage the setting are provided. When a psychiatric facility houses a day treatment program, it may be chartered to operate its own school. More often, the facility is partnered with a local education systems' special education division. The school service may therefore have some independence from rest of the facility. The psychiatric staff should be aware of this and maintain good rapport with all those involved in the children's care.

Since most commercial payers generally only cover acute short-term care, it is Medicaid that more commonly covers the cost of day treatment, with eligibility based upon either family's precarious finances or the child's own chronic disability. Some day treatment programs are funded entirely by units of state and local government and are therefore available regardless of means.

Partial and continuing day hospital programs occupy "open" settings, and these programs tend to be rather selective in whom they admit. Imminent danger to self or others, elopement risk, and bringing contraband to the program, all preclude successful treatment in such settings. To date, limited treatment effectiveness research suggests that partial/day treatment is a cost-effective approach for some children in crisis in lieu of hospitalization and/or as step down for inpatients (21).

Residential Treatment

Residential treatment services can resemble boarding school-like settings where the child lives, goes to school, receives therapeutic services, and all necessary medical care and psychiatric medicines in one location. The prototype for residential treatment is the "cottage" model. This model, in turn, derives from the heritage of many of these facilities as turn-of-the-century orphanages or shelters for children of destitute families, especially in the Eastern United States. The explicit goal was to emulate family living, complete with live-in "cottage parents," to the extent possible. Child guidance clinics were established at some of these facilities. The Child Welfare Act of 1915 provided widows with at least minimal support, after which the orphanage population began to decline. During the Great Depression, these same charitable entities partnered with the states and could draw down public funding to provide a wide array of services, which included care for emotionally troubled youth. Later in the 20th century, support for foster care, adoption, and small group homes eclipsed large congregate care for the parentless. The coming decades essentially completed the transformation of many of these facilities into therapeutic schools reliant on public funding.

Residential treatment facilities (RTFs) are typically licensed by state departments of mental health, and have the mission of caring for the severely psychiatrically impaired youth who do not need the constraints of an inpatient setting. By contrast, residential treatment centers (RTCs) generally come under the auspices of state departments of social service. The setting and range of services are similar, but the RTC population is generally less psychiatrically impaired and would probably be suitable for outpatient treatment were it not for adverse psychosocial circumstances that make community living inadequately supportive. Reasons may include absent or mentally ill family members or seriously damaged parent–child relationships. In some cases, an RTF may be collocated as a cottage within an RTC but with different staffing and capability for managing behavioral crises, including specialized staff training and a "quiet room."

One of the more controversial aspects of admission to RTCs has been the requirement in many states that parents relinquish custody of their children. Having parents make this wrenching decision seems intended to prevent parents fobbing off care of their children for economic reasons alone, but family advocates point to the family-blaming reasoning and discriminatory infliction of pain on the families of mentally ill children that relinquishing custody entails. Consequently, several state have abandoned this requirement.

REFERRAL AND ADMISSION

Admission Policies

Each setting has to have a realistic appraisal of its limitations since no useful purpose is served by making commitments that diminish the service's overall quality of care or safety.

Acute inpatient services tend to be the least "selective," consistent with their mission to be accessible ports of last resort in a crisis. Nevertheless, difficult situations still present themselves. For instance, many units cannot readily accommodate those with severe developmental disabilities experiencing acute behavioral disturbances, especially those lacking language, or at least needing skillful 1:1 staffing and special milieu accommodations to serve them. That level of care often means diverting available staff to the needs of one patient, rather than obtaining an addition to the staff complement for the child's stay.

Without the pressure to address acute crises, long-term inpatient, partial, day, and residential programs can be more selective, and, as less secure settings, are obliged to be. Policies vary widely as a function of facilities, resources, expertise, and availability of alternatives in the region. Facilities weigh, to varying degrees, factors like histories of substance abuse, fire setting, sexual misconduct, running away and truancy, criminal involvement, developmental needs, medical needs, prospects for family involvement, and so forth to judge appropriateness. These are not always straightforward determinations and sometimes can cause facilities, their payers, and those making referrals to collide. There has been increased vigilance by public agencies to "cherry picking" of children with less complex situations, and to the potential for some of these policies to discriminate against particular ethnic communities.

Preauthorization

This refers to the process by which the patient's insurer, accepts or rejects the referral source's clinical information. This is intended to substantiate the need for inpatient care. Sometimes, rejection by the initial reviewer leads to an immediate doctor-to-doctor review of the circumstances. Because of the time consuming nature of the authorization exercise, hospitals may employ "resource management" nurses or social workers, whose sole job is to interface with insurers or their affiliated mental health care management companies.

Parents are often unaware of their mental health benefits until a crisis develops. Only in the emergency room is it suddenly determined that the insurance plan has a unique contract for the provision of psychiatric inpatient care with one particular facility that may be geographically remote from the patient's home, to the upset of already stressed parents.

A symptom picture that puts the child or others at imminent risk of harm, failure, or lack of available alternative services often tip the balance in favor of hospitalization. Approval for a hospital stay of one to a few days allows the admission to proceed. "Concurrent review" refers to subsequent conversations between the managed care company's reviewer and the resource management/or physician staff about the child's progress and readiness for discharge.

Engaging and Supporting Families

Some units, when time permits, allow parents to come and view the unit and discuss the program with staff in advance of a child's admission. Written informational material provides useful information about visiting, phone calls, clothing, and laundry considerations, how a child's education will be managed, how medical problems will be addressed, as well as rules about forbidden items, such as lighters, matches, cigarettes, pocket knives, drugs, etc. The same or an additional document will describe the unit's points or levels system (usually a version of a token economy program) and how aggression to self and others may be dealt with. It is important that caregivers appreciate that the safety of all is paramount and that seclusion or restraint may be needed if someone is out of control or in imminent danger of losing control. The role of the members of the interdisciplinary team and who to contact for different concerns must be made clear.

While units may administer any medication in an emergency circumstance, it is commonplace to seek separate permission for the administration of standing medications. Justifications differ in whether this permission must be via a special consent form or an oral discussion but the discussion, including the indication for the medication, and the risks and benefits is documented in the patient record.

Every effort to join families as allies in helping the child to cope with whatever is believed to have led to hospitalization is essential to a good ongoing working relationship. The availability of chaplaincy services and interpreter services when needed can be a considerable consolation to parents. It had been customary for units to run parent management training groups, general support groups, discharge preparation groups, disorder-specific psychoeducation groups, medication education groups, as well as traditional individual family therapy meetings. Shortened lengths of stay has in many instances reduced the viability of these services, and the clinical staff who had provided them are more engaged in discharge planning and liaison.

Realistic Expectations

Given the brevity of a hospital stay, caregivers and those making referrals need to be educated that the focus of treatment on acute units is acute stabilization of the presenting problems, rather than resolution of all difficulties a child may have. Where it is suspected that a child will require a different type of school placement upon discharge, the child will rarely be able to remain on an inpatient unit while the school district deliberates the options according to its own time guidelines. Expectations for parental involvement in treatment all need to be spelled out.

Children in Surrogate/Foster Care

A foster parent has no legal standing beyond securing emergency medical care, and therefore a representative of the foster care agency, who in turn is acting as the agent of the State Department of Social Services must be available to sign admission papers. Even after admission, consent must be obtained again for the administration of standing psychotropic medications. Many placements in foster care are voluntary, that is, a court proceeding has not terminated a parent's rights, in which case the foster care agency must make reasonable efforts to obtain the parent's consent. This can be extremely difficult for hospital units with very ill, dyscontrolled children, who without appropriate consent, cannot get on with needed treatment. If a parent refuses consent, the agency may have to go to court to override the refusal.

It sometimes becomes clear, once the child is hospitalized that the foster placement has irretrievably broken down. It is often difficult to secure a new foster home, and carry out the necessary courtship process between the child and the new foster parent on the time schedule of most inpatient units. Clarity of communication as to the limits of the stabilization role of the hospital and the agency's ongoing responsibilities to provide suitable domicile for the child should be extensively documented, prior to admission, if possible. The disordered and compromised attachments of these children are often reenacted in the inpatient setting, either with guarded, mistrustful, or unengaged behavior. Other patterns include traumatic reenactments or angry aggression meted out indiscriminately.

MULTIDISCIPLINARY ASSESSMENT

Diagnostic, Psychosocial/Developmental, Family, and Academic Assessments

Beyond the rather generic principles of good clinical practice in psychiatric assessment, we should note some special aspects of evaluation in milieu settings. Barring a true first-episode of psychosis, usually in an adolescent patient, children coming to inpatient or residential care tend to have extensive prior psychiatric histories because the conditions themselves are often chronic with early onset. Nonetheless, it is important to clarify whether the crisis at hand represents a *major departure* from a prior level of difficulties or whether it is an intensification of the same ongoing difficulties. Indeed, a behaviorally dyscontrolled youngster may be no worse symptomatically relative to the past few years, but admission is indicated just because he or she is now much larger and so now exceeds the caregivers' capacity to provide containment. Abrupt changes, especially if linked to a current stressor, may dispose to a better postdischarge prognosis.

Some settings use standardized rating scales as part of initial assessments. Behavioral rating scales have parent, teacher, and often, self-report versions. We strongly recommend the acquisition of teacher input, which staff can obtain via fax with appropriate parental consent, when possible. Severe dysfunction in the school setting has to be a factor in discharge planning.

Psychological testing was at one time nearly routine, but now is performed only as indicated. One tangible benefit in particular involves the elucidation of academic skills difficulties related to an unidentified learning disorder. School failure is at times wrongly attributed to poor effort or emotional disturbance, when in fact neuropsychological deficits are the main culprit.

Beyond these aspects of psychiatric assessment, each discipline will probably do their own assessment. Hospital charts and RTC records are often chock full of separate initial evaluations by nursing, social work, rehabilitation, school, speech and language, and so on.

Prior Treatment History

Previous trials of medications should be inquired about with respect to target symptoms, compounds used, optimum doses utilized, characterization of the medication trials, and patient responses. Parents are not always able to provide the necessary details, so consent to speak with previous prescribers should be sought.

Previous psychosocial treatments, including type duration, therapeutic targets, and response should similarly be ascertained. Parent past psychiatric history, substance use/abuse history, past and present treatment, and current mental functioning are highly relevant to parental capacity to care for a now ill child.

Prior placement, why it came about, duration, ability of the parent to stay involved with the child during the period of placement, the perspectives of child and parent regarding the placement, the status of reunification plans, and/or actual efforts, all provide a picture of the stability or its lack in the rearing environment. Such history also sheds light on discharge options also.

Quality of Relationships with Family and Peers

Unfortunately, psychopathology among young people is often associated with quite corrosive relationships with their caregivers. By the time of inpatient admission, some families have come to see extrusion of the child as the solution to many of their problems. While this does not bode well, it is important to understand this level of antagonism at the front end. On the other hand, children whose caregivers acknowledge feeling quite stressed and worried by their child's problems seem less hostile, and there is some evidence that they experience better outcomes (22).

It is always appropriate to inquire about preferred activities, perceived strengths and talents, and with whom the child socializes, but these take on special significance in inpatient or residential settings. This information can serve practical purposes for treatment planning, as in the development of incentive plans, or by identifying prosocial activities in which the youth can develop improved peer relations. Among young children, how many friends they have and keep is important. Many of our patients cannot report one out-of-school relationship and parents often relate that the child's behavior hampers development of friendships and deters the parents of their peers. Adolescents, on the other hand, usually identify with some peer group, and it is important to learn whether these youth are prone to troubles of their own, are they invested in school, how much risk-taking behavior they engage in, etc. A lot of progress can be undone if a youngster gravitates back toward a problematic peer group, so alternative social venues that enable the child to gain status and recognition through some strength or talent are important aspects of discharge planning.

The ubiquity of Internet-linked devices poses special challenges to inpatient and residential settings. They are a frequent form of contraband, and quite significant for their potential to breach the privacy of other patients.

Observation in Setting

Unit staff are in a unique position to assess how children tolerate the necessary separation from family, as well as how parents and children interact at visiting time, during on-ground passes, phone contact, etc. The inpatient unit provides a ready-made peer group that allows for some assessment of a given child's ability to share, form relationships, assert themselves appropriately, play, and to solve conflicts.

The unique capacity of staff across multiple domains of functioning from getting up in the morning to going to bed at night provides a rich tapestry upon which historical data and presenting symptoms are confirmed or refuted. Such observational data help detangle purely "situational pathology" from inherent dysfunction in the child him- or herself. Strengths and weaknesses observed, as well as the precise context and patterning of behavioral difficulties form the basis for individualized behavioral therapeutic plans.

However, there is evidence for a "honeymoon" type of phenomenon, where the child looks nearly asymptomatic for a time and then begins to display more difficulties (23). Shorter lengths of stay may permit staff to observe only the period of suppressed behavioral difficulty.

PROGRAMMING

General Principles

Special Factors in Milieu Settings

One of the risks of congregate care for youth with psychiatric disorders is they will not bring out the best in each other, and instead may mutually reinforce self-defeating or antisocial conduct (24). Young children, for the most part, are still motivated more by adult approval and esteem than by that of their peers. By adolescence, though, this preference largely inverts, even in nonclinical groups, and those who challenge the adult-established order and provide their peers with vicarious pleasure may enjoy high status. Psychiatrically involved youngsters can rightly claim more than their fair share of misfortune, and it is well known that misery loves miserable company. However, little good comes when resentment leads to rejection of available treatment and help. An important goal for any milieu setting is to create and sustain a culture that recognizes and values progress toward therapeutic goals while dimming the allure of defeatism that often masquerades as rebellious grandstanding.

Another key milieu feature that requires vigilance concerns the treatment of more vulnerable patients, especially those with cognitive disabilities, odd behavior, or other stigmata who are incapable of sticking up for themselves. Peer harassment of these individuals is of course bullying and cannot be tolerated.

Multidisciplinary Therapeutic Components

Specific disciplines often are associated with specific treatments. It is important to be respectful and collegial with the team members who provide them. For instance, taking a patient out of another therapeutic activity for individual therapy is not only disruptive to the child, but implicitly devalues the work of a colleague. Ideally, there should be a consistent policy about when such interruptions are appropriate. When scheduling makes such conflict unavoidable, the other staff member should be alerted ahead of time. In staff meetings, everyone has an implicit theory about why a child is or is not getting better, and it is wise to recognize such perspectives. The child psychiatrist may correlate improvement with a medication change, for instance, while another therapist may emphasize a particular development in family therapy. Good leaders try to educate without being dismissive of other perspectives, and take into account reasonable attributions beside one's own.

Maintaining Social Development in an Atypical Environment

Treatment settings that segregate youth from usual community and home-living experiences for extended periods also pose a risk of institutionalization. Most facilities' programming therefore includes community trips and other off-campus activities. In fact, many RTCs provide greater opportunities for athletic and cultural enrichment (pools, gymnasia, art studios, music lessons) with skillful supervision than would otherwise be available to many youth in their homes. A careful balance has to be struck between appropriate supervision and allowing a youngster to develop age typical skills, such as going to the store, traveling independently, and making choices about leisure time, purchases, etc. Often, excursions and other related activities are considered privileges that have to be earned, but a case can be made that at least some exposure should be contingent only on the current behavioral control to manage the outing successfully.

Milieu Management

Policies and Staff Training. Nearly all regulatory and accrediting authorities mandate that inpatient services have a written procedures and policies manual. In addition, it is very useful to have a written description for parents that orients them to the unit and its procedures. A separate version for patients will usually depict, as appropriate to age, the rules for the unit.

Service-Wide Behavioral Programs. Milieu-based therapeutic programs based on behavior modification principles are nearly ubiquitous, and go by various names, such as level, point, token economy, or behavioral systems, and we mentioned some of their underlying principles earlier. These types of programs can serve at least three purposes. First, as a means of direct therapy they can be an efficient means of promoting target behaviors that are applicable to a large number of patients and can readily incorporate some individualized behavioral goals as well.

Second, they can help provide the unit with structure, through establishment of a basis for rules to aid in the management of the service. Therefore, not only may such programs benefit a child's own difficult behavior, they also offer a form of "governance" that includes consistency and fairness. Many patients, especially younger ones, need to better restrain retaliatory impulses following provocations by peers. This goal is easier when the child can count on other ways to address their grievances, including consequences for the other child's misbehavior.

Third, these procedures have the potential to provide quantitative information on the nature and extent of patients' problems, their progress while in the hospital, and their response (or lack of) to different treatments. These data can supplement other types of clinical information and at times they serve to correct overly broad and exaggerated reports based on global narratives, such as when one recent difficult day obscures the improvements evident on those that preceded it.

As with any good behavioral therapy program, the consistency of feedback is paramount, especially praise and recognition which should be abundant but sincere. This would in many cases, accompany assignment of points or tokens for achieving the positive behavioral goals of the activity or time of day, which is well-defined. In addition, each patient has up to three or so individualized goals for which he or she obtains praise, encouragement, corrections, as well as points earned. The actual privileges or rewards toward which points accrue can involve some that are earned daily (i.e., video game time) and some that accumulate over several days (i.e., privilege level). The former enable the patient to start each day with a "new start" and to benefit accordingly.

Overall "generic" programs of this sort may require further individualization or tailoring for the developmental or cognitive needs of patients. Modifications might include reducing exposure to triggers of upset or behavioral dyscontrol, having expectations more commensurate with current capabilities, prompts and consequences that are more tangible/visual/frequent and that are individually meaningful. Ideally, each milieu-based behavioral plan would, of course, be individualized and informed by thorough functional assessment of the problem behaviors that takes account of antecedents, consequences, and the context of these difficulties. On the other hand, it is extremely difficult to maintain consistency with a large number of staff attempting to implement even one plan, and many permutations may vitiate the whole endeavor further. With short lengths of stay, the effort is perhaps better directed toward helping families to develop behavioral support strategies most appropriate for their particular situations and working to promote generalization from hospital to community. Nonetheless, the overall point is that the rigidity of an exclusive "one-size-fits-all" approach and the infeasibility and possible inconsistencies in highly idiographic programming can each have detrimental extremes.

Safety

Because the potential for harm to oneself or others as a result of one's psychiatric illness is the chief reason for admission, the safety of patients and staff are paramount concerns. Training in early detection and proactively calming people who show developing agitation, de-escalation techniques, and the safe handling of patients when physical contact is needed are often required for those working in these settings. Measures that restrict an individual's movement to curb potential violence, such as restraints of seclusions, have to follow protocols that adhere to legal standards for their implementation. Statutes and agency directives specify the situations warranting these measures, who can order them, their duration, continuous monitoring, and so forth. The standards for youth typically differ by shorter durations for each order. These events are stressful, even traumatic, for both patients and staff. A substantial literature discusses various approaches to minimizing restraints and seclusions, and quality improvement projects focused on this goal are commonplace in psychiatric units (25,26). These often involve constant retraining of staff in de-escalation techniques, monitoring noneffective decisions, making about use of PRN medications versus changes in standing pharmacologic agents (27–29).

ORGANIZATION

The role of the psychiatrist varies considerably from one setting to the next. A child psychiatrist is often the nominal director of a hospital inpatient unit, although his or her authority and responsibility for nonphysicians depends on local practice. There are often parallel supervision structures within nursing, social work, etc. Regardless of discipline, the individual in charge of the unit must take the lead in galvanizing team members to work in a cohesive and coordinated way. In hospital settings, the psychiatrist's level of involvement in the program also varies widely. In some places, he or she participates in many therapeutic activities with patients, while in others effort is narrowly aimed at physician-specific responsibilities such as medication management and has less involvement in the milieu. Each setting responds to its unique demands and resources, and there is no basis for claiming superiority of one arrangement over another. However, when the psychiatrist's role and visibility on the unit is more limited, residents and other trainees tend to gravitate toward activities they perceive as the things the "doctors do." They should, however, be directed to attend and observe the full range of patient activities, therapies, and experiences. Otherwise, they miss the valuable opportunities for professional growth and patient understanding these settings afford.

CONCLUSIONS

The structure and the form of milieu-based treatments in child and adolescent psychiatry have shown remarkable changes in recent decades. Decreasing reliance on the institutional forms of care that prevailed in earlier erase is certain a welcome development. Nevertheless, demand and utilization for inpatient settings to manage crises have remained stable or grown for all patient groups but the elderly. The current challenge with shorter lengths of stay and thus more rapid discharge planning is aligning inpatient and residential settings with outpatient and other supportive services that can provide ongoing care for youth with this level of psychiatric severity. Postdischarge services are seldom under the control of hospital-based clinicians, but readmissions that result from the shortage of these resources are nevertheless dispiriting to families, staff, and patients themselves. The coming years will show whether we have the rigor and vision to innovate and enhance still further the quality of the children's inpatient, residential, and other hospital-based day treatments that constitute such a formidable responsibility for our discipline.

References

1. Murray DJ: *A History of Western Psychology.* Englewood-Cliffs, NJ, Prentice-Hall, 1983.
2. Celsus AC: *De Medicina. Spencer WG, trans.* Cambridge, MA, Harvard University Press, 1935 (orig. c. 38 AD).
3. Metropolitan Life Insurance Co. v. Massachusetts. US Sup Ct: Supreme Court of the United States; 1985. p. 724.
4. Parham v. J.R. US Sup Ct: U.S. Supreme Court; 1979. p. 584.
5. Blader JC: Acute inpatient care for psychiatric disorders in the United States, 1996 through 2007. *Arch Gen Psychiatry* 68:1276–1283, 2011.
6. Knitzer J: *Unclaimed Children: The Failure of Public Responsibility to Children and Adolescents in Need of Mental Health Services.* Washington, DC, Children's Defense Fund, 1982.
7. Stroul BA, Friedman RM: *A System of Care for Severely Emotionally Disturbed Children and Youth.* Washington, DC, CASSP Technical Assistance Center, Georgetown University Child Development Center, 1986.
8. Bickman L, Guthrie P, Foster EM, et al.: *Evaluating Managed Mental Health Services: The Fort Bragg Experiment.* New York, Plenum Press, 1995.
9. Barker P: *The Residential Psychiatric Treatment of Children.* London, Crosby Lockwood Staples, 1974.
10. Hughes JM: *Reshaping the Psychoanalytic Domain: The Work of Melanie Klein, WRD Fairbairn, and DW Winnicott.* Berkeley, CA, University of California Press, 1989.
11. Saxe E, Lyle J: The function of the psychiatric residential school. *Bull Menninger Clin* 4:163–171, 1940.
12. Winnicott DW: The theory of the parent-infant relationship. In: Buckley P (ed): *Essential Papers on Object Relations.* New York, New York University Press, 233–253, 1986.
13. Azrin NH: A strategy for applied research: learning based but outcome oriented. *Am Psychol* 32:140–149, 1977.

14. Lovaas OI, Schreibman L, Koegel RL: A behavior modification approach to the treatment of autistic children. *J Autism Child Schizophr* 4:111–129, 1974.
15. Bellack AS, Hersen M, Turner SM: Generalization effects of social skills training in chronic schizophrenics: an experimental analysis. *Behav Res Ther* 14:391–398, 1976.
16. Hersen M, Bellack AS: A multiple-baseline analysis of social-skills training in chronic schizophrenics. *J Appl Behav Anal* 9:239–245, 1976.
17. Milazzo-Sayre LJ, Benson PR, Rosenstein MJ, Manderscheid RW: *Use of inpatient psychiatric services by children and youth under age 18, United States, 1980.* Mental Health Statistical Note 175. Report No.: DHHS-ADM-86-1451. Rockville, MD: National Institute of Mental Health, Survey and Reports Branch. 1986 (April).
18. Blader JC: Pharmacotherapy and postdischarge outcomes of child inpatients admitted for aggressive behavior. *J Clin Psychopharmacol* 26:419–425, 2006.
19. Martin A, Leslie D: Psychiatric inpatient, outpatient, and medication utilization and costs among privately insured youths, 1997–2000. *Am J Psychiatry* 160:757–764, 2003.
20. Connor DF, Ozbayrak KR, Kusiak KA, Caponi AB, Melloni RH Jr: Combined pharmacotherapy in children and adolescents in a residential treatment center. *J Am Acad Child Adolesc Psychiatry* 36:248–254, 1997.
21. Kiser LJ, Heston JD, Paavola M: Day treatment centers/partial hospitalization settings. In: Petti TA, Salguero C (eds): *Community Child and Adolescent Psychiatry: A Manual of Clinical Practice and Consultation.* Washington, DC, American Psychiatric Publishing, 189–203, 2006.
22. Blader JC: Symptom, family, and service predictors of children's psychiatric rehospitalization within one year of discharge. *J Am Acad Child Adolesc Psychiatry* 43:440–451, 2004.
23. Blader JC, Abikoff H, Foley C, Koplewicz HS: Children's behavioral adaptation early in psychiatric hospitalization. *J Child Psychol Psychiatry* 35:709–721, 1994.
24. Dishion TJ, Dodge KA: Peer contagion in interventions for children and adolescents: moving towards an understanding of the ecology and dynamics of change. *J Abnorm Child Psychol* 33:395–400, 2005.
25. Gaskin CJ, Elsom SJ, Happell B: Interventions for reducing the use of seclusion in psychiatric facilities: review of the literature. *Br J Psychiatry* 191:298–303, 2007.
26. Valenkamp M, Delaney K, Verheij F: Reducing seclusion and restraint during child and adolescent inpatient treatment: still an underdeveloped area of research. *J Child Adolesc Psychiatr Nurs* 27:169–174, 2014.
27. Donovan A, Plant R, Peller A, Siegel L, Martin A: Two-year trends in the use of seclusion and restraint among psychiatrically hospitalized youths. *Psychiatr Serv* 54:987–993, 2003.
28. Richards D, Bee P, Loftus S, Baker J, Bailey L, Lovell K: Specialist educational intervention for acute inpatient mental health nursing staff: service user views and effects on nursing quality. *J Adv Nurs* 51:634–644, 2005.
29. Measham TJ: The acute management of aggressive behaviour in hospitalized children and adolescents. *Can J Psychiatry* 32:199–203, 1995.

CHAPTER 6.3.3 ■ INTENSIVE IN-HOME PSYCHIATRIC TREATMENT APPROACHES

KATHLEEN M.B. BALESTRACCI, JEAN A. ADNOPOZ, MELISA D. ROWLAND, SAMANTHA J. MOFFETT, AND JOSEPH L. WOOLSTON

THE ORIGINS OF IN-HOME SERVICES

In 1982, Jane Knitzer reported the nationwide failure to meet the mental health needs of children with serious emotional disturbance (SED). Despite enthusiastic contemporary support for treatment in the least restrictive environment (and legal policy mandating it), Knitzer found that two-thirds of SED children and adolescents were either underserved or unnecessarily institutionalized (1). In addition to these primary findings regarding the dearth of non-institutional treatment options, Knitzer added that "it is not enough to develop a range of nonresidential…services for children. These services must be organized so that individual children can move easily from one to another," in short, that the mental health service sector should operate as coordinated "systems of care" (SOC) (1).

In 1984, to encourage states to address the gap between mental health needs of children and the availability of appropriate services, Congress appropriated funds for the National Institute of Mental Health's (NIMH's) Child and Adolescent Service System Program (CASSP). The aim of CASSP was to espouse core principles for the treatment of children with SED and guide states to develop programs which were adherent to them (2). CASSP forwarded the philosophy that programs should be strength based, individually tailored, developmentally appropriate, family-focused, culturally competent, community-based, and systematically coordinated (3). By 1992, every state had received CASSP planning grants to design local SOC that incorporated CASSP principles and offered a broad selection of interconnected services (4). The movement stimulated the development of community-based services, many of them in the home, and placed emphasis on the centrality of the family in decision making and treatment planning processes (5,6).

INTENSIVE IN-HOME SERVICES: AN INTRODUCTION

Intensive in-home services, also known as intensive home-based or family-based services, have been developed largely independent of one another (7). They vary regionally, with differing durations, provider qualifications, intensity, and the presence or absence of a theoretical basis. The majority of these programs share CASSP's guiding principles. These programs recognize the importance of context and ecology to a child's development, and appreciate the degree to which children are profoundly influenced by the family system in which they live (8). They target not only the child's problematic behaviors, but also the issues present in the family system which influence the child's ability to function and may perpetuate the target behaviors (9–11). In accordance with CASSP principles, treatment plans are expected to be individualized and adapted to each child and family's assessed strengths and needs. Treatment is expected to flexible, responsive to the family's schedule, easily accessible, in the home or in the community, and may include members of the family's extended networks. Interventions aim to improve the child's functioning within all relevant systems, including school and neighborhood, and all existing providers are expected to collaborate so that services are coordinated, reasonable and understood by family members. To defer hospitalization or removal from home or community, services may also provide 24/7 crisis intervention or have access to these services. Finally, consistent with their multisystemic treatment targets, in-home services have multiply determined outcomes (12). These outcomes consist not only of reductions in out-of-home placement and symptomatology, the most common and measureable goals of intensive in-home programs, but also of improvements in measures such as child functioning, progress towards goals, family satisfaction with treatment, parent stress, academic functioning or school attendance, and involvement with the legal system (13,14).

Beyond sharing common aims and their unique treatment venue, in-home interventions share a common genesis: the original model from which they have been adapted. The child welfare system was the first to employ intensive in-home interventions as a means of preventing out-of-home placements and promoting a safe environment within the child's home. The earliest intensive, in-home model was the 4-week Homebuilders program implemented in the 1970s (15,16). Homebuilders© sparked the development of a range of home-based service models, many designed to serve targeted populations. Multisystemic therapy (MST), functional family therapy (FFT), and multi-dimensional family therapy (MDFT), all 3- to 6-month interventions, were designed to reduce antisocial behavior (substance use and criminal recidivism) among adolescents (17–19). Together, these four frequently replicated, manualized, interventions have exerted influence on the development of other in-home interventions for emotionally disturbed youth. However, while there are similarities between in-home interventions for delinquent youth and for youth with SED in duration, intensity, and multisystemic focus, there are differences in the treatment population, methods, and targets for change (20).

It is worth noting a distinction between intensive in-home treatment models and other in-home interventions such as wraparound, a care coordination intervention that may be conducted within the home (21,22). Wraparound assesses needs and connects families to concrete resources and therapeutic services, but is not, itself, therapeutic.

IN-HOME INTERVENTIONS FOR CHILDREN WITH SED: A GROWING FIELD

In-home psychiatric interventions have been developed and funded since the mid-1980s (23,24). As of 1999, 35 states offered some form of intensive in-home service to children with SED (25). However, the provider landscape has continuously shifted with funding and legislation. For example, in 1997, the Robert Wood Johnson Foundation funded the implementation of the Mental Health Services Program for Youth (MHSPY) in eastern Massachusetts, which was supported thereafter by pooling portions of Medicaid and other state agencies' budgets (26). MHSPY was a home-based program designed to provide highly coordinated, individualized mental health and pediatric care to children with the most acute emotional and behavioral disturbances. Youth received services for an average of 17 months and showed clinically significant functional improvements. The cost of providing MHSPY was less than other available treatment services for this population (27). However, due to the level of oversight and interagency collaboration required on each case, enrollment was limited. In 2001, nine plaintiffs brought a class action lawsuit against the Commonwealth of Massachusetts (the "Rosie D." case), alleging that a "lack of intensive in-home services" contravened Medicaid's rehabilitation mandate (28). The plaintiffs cited MHSPY as a model program, but were concerned about its limited geographic range and accessibility. The judge ruled for the plaintiffs in 2006, and the court ordered an immediate expansion of in-home treatment programs (29). But without a clear strategy for implementation of the court order, no single model of home-based treatment was selected for implementation and eventually the MHSPY program lost its funding.

The in-home services field continues to grow as national policy increasingly encourages home- and community-based services (HCBS) (30). In 2003, President Bush's New Freedom Commission on Mental Health submitted a report recommending an expansion of these services to reduce the reliance on psychiatric residential treatment facilities (31). In 2005, Congress provided support for the recommendations by allocating $218 million to the development of these services in 10 states: Alaska, Florida, Georgia, Indiana, Kansas, Maryland, Mississippi, Montana, South Carolina, and Virginia. Florida was unable to secure matching state funds, however, and withdrew. Between 2007 and 2012, the remaining 9 projects enrolled more than 5,000 children at risk of out-of-home placement (32). Mississippi enrolled nearly 1,500 children, alone, in its intensive in-home intervention, Mississippi Youth Program Around the Clock (MYPAC). MYPAC enrolls SED youth up to 21 years of age, for between 3 and 9 months of services (33). Children are assigned a master's-level therapist and a wraparound care coordinator, and receive at least three visits per week between these two providers. MYPAC-enrolled youth are also connected with a psychiatrist every 4 to 6 weeks; due to the shortage of local psychiatrists, this treatment is often delivered via videoconference (K. Plotner, personal communication, 12/8/2015). Other state in-home interventions range in duration from 3 to 6 months, with an average intensity of three visits per week. Most do not report following a specific model, but use therapists trained in various evidence-based treatments. Caseloads vary, from a low of 6 to as many as 12 cases, and programs differ in provider qualifications.

Home-based interventions have also been developed by private providers. The nonprofit organization Youth Villages delivers an in-home model (Intercept) to more than 4,500 SED youth per year across 9 states. Intercept does follow a model with a theory of change, and is unique among programs in that it collects long-term follow-up data for each participant 2 years postdischarge (34) (S. Hurley, personal communication, 1/29/2016). The for-profit Virtual Residential Program (VRP) is available in 7 states. It provides in-home step-down treatment, with an initial intensity that can range between 20 and 50 hours (35).

Home-based interventions appeal to states not only for their adherence to CASSP principles, but also for their cost effectiveness. There is considerable evidence that in-home treatment is less expensive to deliver than more restrictive services, and may realize long-term cost savings (7,27,36,37). Even so, the amount expended on home-based family therapy annually is considerable. In fiscal year 2015, Mississippi spent $17.9M delivering MYPAC to more than 840 youth (V. Donaho, personal communication, 1/7/2016) and Virginia spent $108M for in-home services delivered to an average 5,000 youth per month (B. Campbell, personal communication, 1/4/2016). In 2014, Michigan spent $59M on in-home services for 7,700 children (38). As home-based therapies continue to expand, their growth threatens to outpace their research base. Variations in delivery by state, coupled with these high expenditures, speak to the need for additional evaluation (39).

STATE OF THE EVIDENCE FOR INTENSIVE IN-HOME SERVICES

Although programs designed to treat children and youth with SED have proliferated throughout the country, the literature reports few rigorous studies of their effect. The limited number of evidence-based models may be due in part to the funding required to test existing clinical models and the challenges of monitoring fidelity and adherence in the real world. This has led to the implementation of untested interventions which have been driven by assumptions rather than data and experience. In spite of growing enthusiasm and support, some programs have been criticized for lack of structure, failure to articulate a coherent theory of change, limited knowledge of the mechanisms expected to bring about the desired change, lack of specification of active ingredients, and little or no regular evaluation for quality control (40,41). As more program developers attempt to address this challenge by implementing rigorous evaluation or randomized controlled trials that test targeted outcomes, discover the relative value of program components and evaluate the hypothesized mechanisms through which these outcomes are achieved, we will know better which models are most likely to achieve the outcomes desired by their funders. To the extent that these interventions are multisystemic and individualized, thorough and detailed data collection on the process and content of service delivery is necessary. Likewise, efforts must be made to record and account for concurrent receipt of any other mental health services. Multiple sequential studies may be required to meet multi-tiered study aims.

One trial of an intensive in-home service for children with SED randomly assigned 279 youth to 3 different active treatment conditions, 2 of which were iterations of a 4- to 6-week home-based crisis intervention program (HBCI); the third condition was intensive care coordination (42). Six months after discharge, youth from all three conditions showed reductions in internalizing and externalizing behaviors, reductions that were not present at discharge, but there were no significant differences between the three interventions. Families receiving HBCI showed increases in family cohesion between intake and discharge, but these gains were not maintained at 6-month follow-up. The authors suggest that these changes in child and family functioning may require periodic reinforcement (42).

In an experimental study in Canada, youth were assigned to an intensive in-home intervention with a cognitive-behavioral treatment model (n = 38, after attrition) or a 5-day per week residential program utilizing solution-focused brief therapy (n = 27, after attrition) (43). Both treatments lasted 3 months and included family-focused work. On average, youth improved considerably and comparably on internalizing, externalizing, and social competence measures, both at discharge and 1-year follow-up, according to parent report. When reliable change index analyses were applied to each youth on each subscale, however, the study found that a significantly greater percentage of youth in the in-home treatment showed improved ADHD symptomatology (63% vs. 22%). Youth in the in-home arm also showed significantly greater 1-year reductions in anxiety (24% vs. 3%) and depression (26% vs. 11%). By contrast, participants in the residential program were more likely to experience increases in internalizing symptoms (43). However, the covariance of treatment environment with therapeutic modality render the findings difficult to interpret, and while the author reported random assignment of subjects, assignment was dependent on treatment slot availability and limited by cases prohibited from being waitlisted.

MST OVERVIEW

MST is one of the few models that has developed an evidence base. MST Psychiatric is recognized as an evidence-based practice by the Substance Abuse and Mental Health Services Administration (SAMHSA) National Registry of Evidence-Based Programs (NREPP) and by the National Institute of Justices searchable database, Crime Solutions.gov. MST is an intensive home-based family therapy, originally developed in the 1980s to treat delinquent youth at risk of out-of-home placement due to incarceration. Since its inception, this model has been evaluated by 55 published outcome, implementation, and benchmarking studies. Thirty-four of the 55 studies have been conducted by independent researchers and 25 are randomized clinical trials (17). While initial MST treat model development and research focused on serious juvenile offenders and adolescents with serious conduct problems, success with these populations led to the development and evaluation of several adaptations of the model. MST adaptations have been created and empirically evaluated for: delinquents with diagnosed comorbid substance abuse and dependence; juvenile sex offenders; families at risk of disruption due to maltreatment; adolescents with chronic health care conditions; and youths presenting with SED. This section of the chapter will focus on the later adaptation, MST Psychiatric (44).

MST PSYCHIATRIC DESCRIPTION

MST Psychiatric is an adaptation of MST specifically designed to serve families with youth at imminent risk of out-of-home placement due to serious psychiatric symptoms. Often these symptoms are comorbid with behavioral and substance use problems. Specifically, the intervention targets youth ages 9 to 17 years at imminent risk of out-of-home placement in a mental health or correctional mental health treatment facility due to serious behavioral problems and co-occurring mental health symptoms such as drug use/abuse, thought disorder, bipolar affective disorder, depression, anxiety and/or suicidal behaviors. The goal of MST Psychiatric is to diminish substance use, improve behavioral problems, mental health symptoms, suicidal behaviors, and family relations while increasing the amount of time youth spend going to school and living in home-based placements.

MST PSYCHIATRIC TRAINING AND COMPONENTS

MST Psychiatric clinicians receive standard MST training and ongoing quality assurance (QA) support (17) as well as supplemental trainings designed to address: (a) safety risks associated with suicidal, homicidal, and psychotic behaviors in youth and family members; (b) integration of evidence-based psychiatric and psychopharmacologic interventions for youth and caregivers; (c) treatment of adolescent and caregiver substance use/abuse utilizing an evidence-based treatment, contingency management or CM (45); and (d) evidence-based assessment and treatment of youth and caregiver mental illness including anxiety disorders, depression, bipolar affective disorder, thought disorders, attention-deficit hyperactivity disorder, impulse control difficulties, and symptoms of borderline personality disorder.

This adaptation of MST has been modified to incorporate a part-time child psychiatrist (20% FTE) and a full-time bachelor's level crisis caseworker. Otherwise, the team configuration mirrors routine MST with one or two teams of three to four full-time masters-level therapists, working with a full-time experienced MST supervisor serving caseloads of four families for 4 to 6 months. MST has an extensive training and QA protocol which includes intensive well-specified weekly team supervision plus weekly consultation and quarterly booster trainings with an MST expert consultant. All trainings are manualized and the QA process includes routine monitoring of therapist adherence to treatment utilizing evidence-based adherence measures based on caregiver report of therapist behavior as well as supervisor, and consultant adherence monitoring (17).

MST PSYCHIATRIC—ADAPTATION DEVELOPMENT AND RESEARCH HISTORY

As described by lead researchers in the field of mental health services research (46), the development and dissemination of evidence-based practice often follows a series of defined stages. As a rule, evidence-based treatment programs are developed and evaluated first in ideal or university-based settings (*efficacy trials*). Those that are promising move into real-world settings for evaluation (*effectiveness trials*), followed by replication in real-world settings in which the model developers are less involved (*transportability pilots*). If all goes well for the evidence-based practice in each of these stages, it emerges, often more than 20 years after the initial trial, sustainable, replicable and ready for *mature transport* into community-based settings without the need for direct developer involvement. The next section of this chapter will highlight the key outcomes for MST Psychiatric, which more than 20 years since its first evaluation, is on the border between the *transportability pilots* and *mature transport* stages.

RANDOMIZED CONTROLLED TRIAL 1, EFFICACY STUDY, MST AS AN ALTERNATIVE TO PSYCHIATRIC HOSPITALIZATION

MST Psychiatric was first developed and evaluated in a randomized clinical trial funded by the NIMH. The clinical portion of this study was conducted from 1994 to 1999 and included 156 Medicaid or crisis-funded families with youth accepted for inpatient admission into a university psychiatric hospital. Half of these youth received MST while half were admitted to the psychiatric hospital and received routine care after discharge. Findings from this trial are described in four publications (20,47–49). In summary, there was one statistically significant finding favoring youth in the control condition. These youth demonstrated higher self-esteem based on the Family Friends and Self Measure (50) at the time they were discharged from the hospital than their counterparts in MST at approximately 2 weeks from intake (20). Analyses of data collected at 4 months or posttreatment for MST (20,47) revealed that MST caregivers and teachers reported significant improvements in youth externalizing symptoms on the Child Behavior Checklist or CBC (51) compared the control condition. MST youth and caregivers also reported significantly improved family functioning on the Family Adaptability and Cohesion Scale (52) and improved youth and caregiver satisfaction relative to usual services families. Other important significant findings posttreatment for MST included reduced hospitalization (73%) reduced days in other out-of-home placements (49%), and increased time spent in school. One of the most important findings for the trial came approximately 16 months after intake, at 1-year follow-up (48) when youth that had received MST reported a significant reduction in suicide attempts on the Youth Risk Behavior Survey (53) relative to youth in the control condition. Analyses of other data from this time period (16 months from intake) reveal (49) that: (a) across treatment conditions and respondents psychopathology symptoms improved to subclinical range by 12 to 16 months; (b) groups reached improved symptoms with significantly different trajectories (MST improved more rapidly); (c) during treatment (4 months), MST was significantly better at promoting youths functional outcomes such as time in school and living at home, yet these improvements were not maintained posttreatment. At 1-year follow-up (16 months), both groups had similar rates of school attendance and out-of-home placements. Outcomes from this trial let to the next study.

RANDOMIZED CONTROLLED TRIAL 2, EFFECTIVENESS STUDY, HAWAII CONTINUUM OF CARE PROJECT

Funded by the Hawaii Department of Health and Adolescent Mental Health Division, the Annie E. Casey Foundation and the National Institute on Drug Abuse, this randomized clinical trial was designed to determine if an MST-based continuum of mental health treatments spanning from home-based to foster care and inpatient services would be more effective than routine services provided in Hawaii's newly created continuum of care. MST Psychiatric was the model of MST utilized for this project which served families with youth ages 9 to 17 at imminent risk of out-of-home placement due to comorbid serious mental health and behavioral problems. The study was terminated early due to difficulties obtaining adequate participants and an inability to foster the development of a true continuum of services. Data from the 31 youth and families completing treatment and 6-month follow-up measures reveal the following significant findings favoring MST over youth in the control condition (54): (a) decreased externalizing symptoms by youth report on the Achenbach Youth Self Report or YSR (55); (b) decreased internalizing symptoms by youth report on the YSR (55); (c) decreased youth self-reported minor delinquency on Elliott's Self-Reported Delinquency Scale (56); (d) decreased days (68%) in out-of-home placement; (e) increased days (42%) in regular school setting; (f) marginally significant improvements in youth criminal activity based on arrest records; and (g) marginally significant improvements in caregiver satisfaction with social supports. Experience with this effectiveness study led to the next trial of MST Psychiatric, again in a community-based setting serving youth within a continuum of care.

RANDOMIZED CONTROLLED TRIAL 3, EFFECTIVENESS STUDY, PHILADELPHIA CONTINUUM OF CARE PROJECT

Funded by the City of Philadelphia's Department of Health and Behavioral Health System and the Annie E. Casey Foundation, this randomized clinical trial was designed to evaluate the effectiveness of an MST continuum of services in treating juvenile offenders, ages 10 to 16 with a mental health diagnosis, at imminent risk of out-of-home placement due to comorbid psychiatric and/or substance use problems. All youth in the control condition were admitted to a residential treatment center and the majority of these were still in placement at 6 and 12 months postintake. Sixty-three youth reached 6-month follow-up and 44 reached 12-month follow-up before funding sources for the project ended. While results of this trial have not been published in a peer-reviewed journal, findings are outlined in a report submitted to the Annie E. Casey Foundation (57). Statistically significant findings at 6 months postrecruitment (n = 63) favoring MST in this study include: (a) decreased internalizing symptoms by youth and caregiver report on the CBC (51,55); (b) decreased caregiver self-report of alcohol use on the Personal Experience Inventory (58); (c) increased family cohesion by youth report (52); and (d) increased days in community-based placements (home- and MST-based therapeutic foster care). Meanwhile, youth in the usual services condition spent significantly more days in residential placement. In fact, since most youth in the usual services condition did not return home during the study, it was difficult to obtain accurate measures of family functioning and caregiver reports of youth functioning for these families at 6- and 12-month follow-up. However, studies of the relationship between adherence to the MST treatment protocol and clinical indicators at 6 and 12 months revealed significant findings. Specifically, caregiver report of therapist adherence on the MST Therapist Adherence Measure or TAM (17) predicted: (a) improved discipline at 6 and 12 months and (b) a trend toward improved family cohesion (52) at 12 months. Importantly, independent observer ratings of MST adherence on audiotaped sessions predicted decreased caregiver psychiatric symptoms on the Brief Symptom Inventory or BSI (59) at 12 months.

TRANSPORTABILITY PROJECT, ARROW PROGRAM (2010–PRESENT)

Funded by the Robin Hood Foundation, the Arrow Program, housed within the New York Foundling Agency, is designed to provide MST Psychiatric treatment across three boroughs (Manhattan, Queens, Brooklyn) for families served by New York City, Administration for Children's Services' (ACS) Juvenile Justice Initiative (JJI) and Family Assessment Program (FAP) when the youth or caregivers have psychiatric service needs that are too intense for routine MST or the other home-based models provided by these initiatives. JJI youth are delinquents court-ordered to out-of-home placement due to criminal behavior. The FAP program serves families that have filed with ACS to have their children removed from the home due to unruly or unmanageable behavior. This project does not have an experimental design, yet substantial data are collected at pre- and posttreatment for all families served. From the project's inception in March 2010 through December 2013, data were collected on 112 families. Highlights of these outcomes are described in an annual report provided to the Robin Hood Foundation in 2013 (60). Statistically significant findings for MST Psychiatric youth based on data collected at pre- and posttreatment (4 to 6 months) revealed: (a) reductions in total problem behaviors, externalizing and internalizing behaviors by caregiver report on the CBC (51); (b) caregiver self-reports of improved levels of psychological distress, interpersonal sensitivity, depression, paranoid ideation, psychoticism, somatization, hostility, and fewer overall symptoms on the BSI (59); (c) caregiver reports of improved family cohesion (52). In summary, the Arrow project is an example of a standalone MST Psychiatric team working effectively with children and families that represent some of the highest-end users of child welfare (ACS) and juvenile justice resources in New York City.

BLUE SKY CONTINUUM OF CARE PROJECT 2007–PRESENT

Building from prior experience in Hawaii and Philadelphia, this project takes a different approach to providing a continuum of services for delinquent youth at risk of placement. In this study, MST Psychiatric has joined forces with two other evidence-based practices, FFT and Multidimensional Treatment Foster Care (MTFC) to create an integrated treatment continuum of services. Youth slated for out-of-home placement due to criminal behavior, often with comorbid psychiatric symptoms, are referred to the Blue Sky Continuum of Care by the legal system. Within this continuum, the three models work together to provide seamless, integrated clinical services based on the needs of the youth and family. This project has been up and running since early 2007 and has served more than 650 families to date. Of these, approximately 234 have received MST Psychiatric either alone or in conjunction with MTFC and/or FFT. A randomized clinical trial of this model has just been completed with 100 youth and their families. Data from this trial are currently being evaluated.

AN ESTABLISHED, STATEWIDE IN-HOME SERVICE: IICAPS

In a climate of rapid change and little empirical evidence, few programs have been able to establish firm statewide footholds. Among those that have been broadly accepted within a single state is the Intensive In-Home Child and Adolescent Psychiatric Services (IICAPS), which has operated in Connecticut for more than a decade. This chapter provides a closer examination of this model which was founded upon a partnership between the state's child mental health authority, the state's primary funding agency for Medicaid, and the Yale Child Study Center.

IICAPS is a comprehensive home-based treatment designed, disseminated, and monitored by faculty of the Yale Child Study Center (61). IICAPS was developed at Yale in 1997 as an intensive, psychiatric intervention for children and adolescents with serious emotional and behavioral problems at risk of requiring institutional-based care, unable to be discharged from such care without intensive services, or unable to access or benefit from standard, community-based outpatient treatment (62). The IICAPS model is structured and manualized and integrates concepts and findings from developmental psychopathology to understand the multiple determinants that contribute to the presenting problems of the child and family. Interventions are grounded in three broad sets of constructs: developmental psychopathology, psychology of motivation, action and problem-solving and SOS philosophy, all of which further case conceptualization and inform treatment planning. Although IICAPS is customarily delivered by a two-person team composed of master's and bachelor's level clinicians, in some cases two master's level clinicians may compose the team. Teams carry eight cases for an expected length of stay of 6 months, although a 1-month extension can be granted for special situations. Each team is expected to hold three sessions per week; one with the child, one with the parent(s) or caregivers, and one with the family, which both members of the team attend. Other sessions involve only one team member who is either the child or the parent-specific clinician. The services provided by the team include assessment and evaluation, individual child psychotherapy, family treatment, couples counseling, service coordination, and advocacy. Supervision and training are essential elements of the model. All individuals working in IICAPS must complete 15 hours of initial training; booster trainings occur regularly throughout the year to address model delivery concerns and/or to provide topic-specific instruction and guidance. Weekly team supervision is provided by a senior mental health clinician. In addition to acting as Medical Director, child psychiatrists serve in multiple roles within each IICAPS program as rounds leaders, supervisors, and members of the administrative group. All teams are required to attend a weekly rounds group co-led by a child psychiatrist and an IICAPS coordinator or supervisor. Each case is presented at rounds every 3 weeks, IICAPS tools are used to structure the rounds presentation and assure compliance with all billing requirements.

Fidelity to the IICAPS model is measured by clinician adherence to the IICAPS tools. Evidence supporting the continuous and simultaneous use of the treatment and QA tools throughout all phases of treatment is required of all IICAPS programs if they are to retain their status as authorized IICAPS sites. This designation qualifies IICAPS providers to bill Medicaid for the negotiated IICAPS reimbursement rate. IICAPS intervention outcomes are monitored with the help of a web-based data collection system which is managed by IICAPS services, the training, data collection, and data analytic arm of the IICAPS program.

IICAPS STRUCTURE

IICAPS treatment is delivered in three phases: Assessment & Engagement, Work & Action, and Ending & Wrap-Up and targets four domains: child, family, school, and community. A safety plan, with contingencies for 24/7 crisis management, is set in place during the first meeting. A primary task of the clinical team from the first phase of treatment to the last is to build the therapeutic alliance which although not sufficient to guarantee treatment effectiveness is essential to the process. Treatment planning begins with the co-construction of the Main Problem, the child's behavior which is likely to lead to psychiatric hospitalization. Co-construction requires the IICAPS team to join with the family in the process of identifying and rating the frequency of the problematic behaviors that concern them. Main Problems are stated in the language of the family and must refrain from being jargonistic. This process, which includes the completion of IICAPS tools and measures is followed by the establishment of goals and action steps in the four domains, which, when completed, lead to the Work & Action treatment phase.

IICAPS uses two unique tools to structure engagement and help families to recognize the possible etiology of the problems which the child presents. The Cycle of the Main Problem is a pictorial representation of the child's Main Problem, the action(s) which trigger the behavior, the feelings which these actions evoke, those things which maintain or reinforce the behavior and the possible strengths or coping mechanisms which ameliorate it. The team administers the ICE, a 20-item adaptation and enhancement of the 10-item Adverse Childhood Experiences questionnaire (63). The ICE has added 10 additional caregiver resiliency factors to the standard 10 questions that are now in common use as a means of capturing protective factors in childhood, as well (64). In addition the team constructs a genogram with each family, to explore relational patterns, important life events, and significant relationships and ruptures over three family generations (65).

Work & Action is the central phase of treatment during which the family and the team work together to implement the treatment plan and improve the child's functioning in all targeted domains. In addition to their regularly scheduled treatment sessions, Teams are likely to observe the child in school, attend medication appointments, and work collaboratively with other providers. IICAPS' theory of change emphasizes the importance of "quality of fit" between a child and caregivers, particularly regarding family members' perceptions of a child's functioning and severity (61,62).

Treatment concludes with Ending & Wrap-Up. Teams prepare families to disengage from treatment by strengthening the bond between youth and caretakers, reflecting on progress, and connecting youth to the next appropriate level of care. In addition to obtaining final ratings of the Main Problem and treatment goals, discharge measures are administered. These assess child severity, functioning, school attendance, service utilization, and caretaker satisfaction at discharge. It is expected that children referred for IICAPS level of care will continue to require mental health treatment following discharge. Connections to post-IICAPS services are made prior to the end of the IICAPS intervention. In many instances the IICAPS team accompanies the child and family to their intake appointments with the next provider to ensure continuity of care.

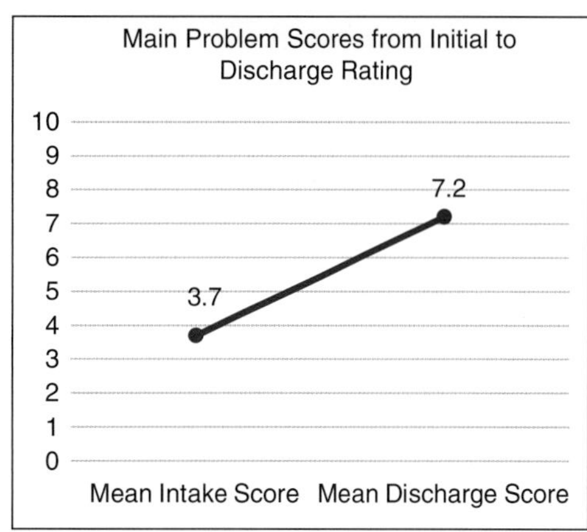

FIGURE 6.3.3.1. Paired T-test result of main problem scores from intake to discharge: IICAPS treatment completers, July 1, 2009 to June 30, 2015 (n = 7,240).

IICAPS EVALUATION DATA

Systematic evaluation of the IICAPS intervention as delivered in all 20 sites throughout Connecticut is conducted quarterly for QA, feedback to IICAPS providers for continuous quality improvement, and for submission to state partners at the Connecticut Department of Children and Families (DCF) and to the Court Support Services Division (CSSD), the state juvenile justice organization. Between July 1, 2009 and June 30, 2015, 11,472 IICAPS episodes of care (EOCs) were closed and evaluated. The identified children served by IICAPS during this 6-year period were 59.9% male, averaged 11.6 years of age, and were racially/ethnically diverse: 14% African-American, non-Hispanic, 42% Caucasian, non-Hispanic, 37% Hispanic, and 7% multiracial or of another race. Almost all of the children receive state health care coverage through Medicaid, as private health insurance companies typically do not pay for in-home psychiatric treatment, and limited funds are available through DCF to provide IICAPS to uninsured or privately insured children and families. They were referred to IICAPS by a range of sources, including DCF, CSSD, psychiatric hospitals, outpatient clinics, other community service providers, and schools. Of these closed cases, 7,883 (68.7%) completed IICAPS treatment. Outcomes for these completed cases are presented in Tables 6.3.3.1 through 6.3.3.3 and Figure 6.3.3.1.

TABLE 6.3.3.1

TOTAL PSYCHIATRIC HOSPITAL STAYS, HOSPITAL DAYS, AND EMERGENCY DEPARTMENT VISITS: IICAPS TREATMENT COMPLETERS, JULY 1, 2009 TO JUNE 30, 2015 (n = 7,883)

SUQ Event	# During 180 Days prior to IICAPS	# During IICAPS EOC (Mean Duration = 178 Days)	% Change
Psychiatric inpatient admissions	2,748	1,251	–54.5%
Psychiatric inpatient days	38,099	12,997	–65.9%
Emergency department visits	3,635	2,294	–36.9%

TABLE 6.3.3.2

McNEMAR'S TEST COMPARING CHILDREN WITH AT LEAST ONE PSYCHIATRIC HOSPITAL STAY OR EMERGENCY DEPARTMENT VISIT PRIOR TO IICAPS VERSUS DURING IICAPS: IICAPS TREATMENT COMPLETERS, JULY 1, 2009 TO JUNE 30, 2015

	During IICAPS[a]		
	At Least One Hospital Admission ($n = 953$)	No Admissions ($n = 6,724$)	McNemar's Test
Prior to IICAPS			
At least one hospital admission ($N = 2,061$)	489	1,572	$X^2 = 603.0, 1, p < 0.001$
No admissions ($N = 5,816$)	464	5,352	
	During IICAPS[a]		
	At Least One ED Visit ($n = 1,560$)	**No ED Visits ($n = 6,321$)**	**McNemar's Test**
Prior to IICAPS			
At least one ED visit ($N = 2,550$)	826	1,724	$X^2 = 398.7, 1, p < 0.001$
No ED visits ($N = 5,331$)	734	4,597	

[a]Missing hospital data = 6; missing ED visit data = 2.

Psychiatric Hospitalization and Emergency Department Use: Table 6.3.3.1 provides data on psychiatric hospital admissions, length of hospital stay, and emergency department visits during the 180 days prior to IICAPS intake and for the duration of the IICAPS intervention (mean duration = 178 days) for children with completed EOCs. There were considerable decreases in the total number of psychiatric inpatient admissions, the total number of psychiatric inpatient days, and the total number of emergency department visits for behavioral health reasons among treatment completers during IICAPS from the 180-day period prior to IICAPS. The decrease in psychiatric inpatient admissions was 54.5%, the decrease in psychiatric inpatient days 65.9%, the decrease in emergency department visits was 36.9%. Table 6.3.3.2 provides results from McNemar's test for differences in the number of children with at least one psychiatric inpatient admission or emergency department visit in the 180 days prior to IICAPS intake and during IICAPS. These data indicate statistically significant reductions in both the number of children with a psychiatric hospitalization and the number of children with an emergency department visit during IICAPS.

Ohio Scales Outcome Data: The Ohio Youth Problem, Functioning, and Satisfaction Scales (the "Ohio Scales") (66) were developed for clinical assessment and outcome measurement, and allow for report of child problem severity and functioning from three sources: the parent/primary caretaker of children ages 5 to 18 years, the worker/clinician providing treatment to a child ages 5 to 18 years, and youth between the ages of 12 and 18 years. Additionally, questions for measuring parent and youth hopefulness and satisfaction are included in the parent report and youth report Ohio Scales forms. In IICAPS, the Ohio Scales are administered to a parent/primary caregiver and youth 12 years and older at intake and discharge; likewise, a clinician on the IICAPS Team fills out the form at these two times.

Table 6.3.3.3 provides mean intake and discharge scores and mean differences for each Ohio Scales domain per each reporter. Data indicate statistically significant changes in all domains per parent, youth, and worker report. The Problem Severity mean difference scores per parent report (–12.6) and worker report (–12.3) surpass the Reliable Change threshold identified by the

TABLE 6.3.3.3

PAIRED T-TEST RESULTS OF OHIO DOMAIN SCORES AT INTAKE AND DISCHARGE: IICAPS TREATMENT COMPLETERS, JULY 1, 2009 TO JUNE 30, 2015

Domains		*N*	Mean Intake Score	Mean Discharge Score	Mean Difference (s.d.)	t-value
Parent report	Problem severity	7,278	33.5	20.9	–12.6 (15.5)	–69.4[a]
	Hopefulness[b]	7,276	12.9	10.0	–2.9 (4.5)	–54.0[a]
	Satisfaction[b]	7,253	8.4	5.5	–2.8 (4.5)	–53.6[a]
	Functioning	7,266	39.7	49.1	9.4 (14.8)	542[a]
Youth report	Problem severity	3,721	26.1	16.8	–9.3 (14.7)	–38.7[a]
	Hopefulness[b]	3,707	11.0	9.3	–1.7 (4.2)	–25.2[a]
	Satisfaction[b]	3,700	10.0	7.5	–2.5 (5.1)	–30.1[a]
	Functioning	3,715	52.6	58.4	5.8 (14.5)	24.4[a]
Worker report	Problem severity	7,490	32.1	20.0	–12.3 (13.8)	–75.2[a]
	Functioning	7,490	38.1	48.3	10.2 (13.4)	65.8 [a]

[a]$p = <0.001$
[b]Decreasing scores in the hopefulness and satisfaction domains indicate increasing hopefulness and satisfaction, respectively.

Ohio Scales developers[1] and mean discharge scores are within one point of the nonclinical range (per parent report) and at the nonclinical range (per worker report) for this domain (a score below 20). Mean differences for scores in the Functioning domain per parent report (9.4) and worker report (10.2) also surpass the Reliable Change threshold for that domain[1]; mean Functioning scores at discharge are two to three points shy of reaching the nonclinical range at discharge (above 51 points per parent and worker report, and above 60 per youth report).

In the Hopefulness domain, there are statistically significant changes indicated per parent and youth report (a 2.9 point improvement in parent Hopefulness and a 1.7 point improvement in youth Hopefulness). Likewise, both parent and youth mean scores indicate improved Satisfaction with IICAPS over mental health services received by the child prior to IICAPS (a 2.8 point improvement per parent report and a 2.5 point improvement per youth report).

Main Problem Outcome: The Main Problem is rated on a 10 point scale from 1 (indicating that the child is at imminent risk of injury to self or others and is gravely disabled) to 10 (no behavioral disturbance). Figure 6.3.3.1 provides data on changes in the Main Problem rating from the initial rating (or in absence of an initial rating, the baseline rating) to the discharge rating. Among closed cases completing treatment, the mean difference in the Main Problem rating from intake to discharge was 3.5 points ($t = 127.6$, $p < 0.001$), indicating considerable improvement in child behavior as identified in the Main Problem.

These data, indicating reduced use of psychiatric hospital care, decreasing problem severity and increasing child functioning at the completion of IICAPS provide support for this intervention among children with SED and their families. Ongoing systematic evaluation of these data, and data on model fidelity: completion of the model-specific IICAPS tools, establishment and rating of the Main Problem and of treatment goals and action steps, and adherence to model duration of care and service intensity expectations, has provided important information for monitoring delivery of the model throughout Connecticut and identifying the positive results of this intensive in-home intervention.

Additional analyses conducted with data from 7,169 youth and their families participating in IICAPS with cases closed between July 2006 and June 2012 used a "Multi-Informant, Latent Consensus" (MILC) approach to examine Ohio Scales data per youth, parent, and worker report (67). Data from the IICAPS sample were compared to a community benchmark estimated from data published by the Ohio Scales developers and colleagues (68), indicating that the Ohio Scales Functioning (MILC score) for the IICAPS youth was dramatically lower (over 3 standard deviations) than the community benchmark, and the Ohio Scales Problem Severity was dramatically higher (over 1.5 standard deviations) than the community benchmark. Mean estimates of Functioning and Problem Severity assessed at discharge from IICAPS were much closer to the community benchmarks with an average increase in Functioning of approximately one standard deviation and a decrease in Problem Severity of nearly the same size.

Confirming these evaluation findings with a control group and identifying the mechanisms by which these positive results are obtained is the aim of a randomized controlled trial of IICAPS undertaken in May 2011. Randomized to either IICAPS or a home-based care coordination model, children and families were followed for 12 months: during the delivery of the study treatment for 6 to 7 months and for a 5- to 6-month posttreatment follow-up period. Data on child behavior, mental health symptoms, and mental health service utilization, parenting practices and parental perception of the child, family problem solving, and parent mental health symptoms were collected at enrollment, following study treatment, and at the end of the posttreatment follow-up from a parent/primary caregiver. Data were requested from schools on absences, suspensions, and other disciplinary actions taken with the identified child, and as was teacher data on child behavior. Analysis of these data is underway to determine the effectiveness of IICAPS as compared to the control in reducing psychiatric hospitalization and decreasing out of control behavior, and identify the influence of parenting practices, parental perception, and family problem solving on these outcomes.

CONCLUSION

In-home treatment does not signify a treatment modality, rather it locates the site at which some type of service which is likely to be consistent with CASSP principles is provided. Over the past three decades interventions which are delivered in the home and purport to offer mental health treatment for children and youth with SED and their families have proliferated most often without regard to their effectiveness and at a significant cost to the federal, state and local funding sources that support their implementation.

MST Psychiatric stands out as an evidence-based practice which has evolved over 20 years in a manner consistent with research on the development and implementation of evidence-based practice (46). The earliest trial was an efficacy study which allowed for the testing and development of clinical protocols and procedures under the relatively more controlled setting provided by the university hospital and university-based therapists. Successful outcomes in this setting allowed for movement of the model into real-world settings working with increasingly difficult populations served by therapists in community-based agencies. Along the way, collection and evaluation of outcomes has played a significant role in ensuring the viability of the model as changes have been made to better meet the needs of the youth and families served.

Systematic evaluation of the delivery of IICAPS across the state of Connecticut has shown consistently positive outcomes for children with SED: reductions in psychiatric hospital admissions and days, decreased problem severity, and increased functioning. Data derived from continuous attention to QA have been used to inform programmatic improvements in the service of providing effective clinical care. Analysis of the data collected during a recently completed randomized controlled trial of IICAPS will help determine the effectiveness of this model compared to a home-based care coordination model in reducing psychiatric hospitalization and decreasing out of control behavior, and identify the influence of parenting practices, parental perception, and family problem solving which may serve as mediating variables on these outcomes.

The well-documented challenges of doing randomized, controlled trials in real-world settings characterized by multigenerational, community-wide adversity has constrained the number of existing evidence-based treatment models. The paucity of proven models has resulted in the proliferation of untested programs which claim to be effective by virtue of belonging to a class of services delivered in the home. Multiple sources of evidence, as described above, give support to the effectiveness of in-home programs in reducing the use of institutional care, improving child and family functioning and reducing symptom severity. However, beyond the programs described above, few programs utilize a manualized protocol, provide intensive training, employ QA measures, and conduct systematic evaluations using outcome and process measures to assess the degree to which they have reached their intended programmatic goals. Importantly, the mechanisms of therapeutic action by which positive changes

[1]Reliable Change = change that cannot be attributed to random measurement error; per Ohio Scales developers, Ben Ogles et al.: Reliable Change for the Problem Severity domain = 10 and for the Functioning domain = 8. Available at: http://mha.ohio.gov/Portals/0/assets/Planning/Outcomes Research/reports/quarterly-12.pdf

for children and families occur have not been thoroughly investigated. Identification of the mediators and moderators of the changes which in-home psychiatric services promise to families and funding sources alike would lead to the establishment of universal, modal practice standards with required, tested components. Movement in this direction will help practitioners, program developers, public policy makers, and funders to make clinically and fiscally sound decisions regarding this class of service and lead to much needed standardization and accountability.

References

1. Knitzer J: *Unclaimed Children: The Failure of Public Responsibility to Children and Adolescents in Need of Mental Health Services.* Washington, DC, Children's Defense Fund, 1982.
2. Kutash K, Duchnowski AJ, Friedman RM: The system of care 20 years later. In: Epstein M, Kutash K, Duchnowski A (eds): *Outcomes for Children and Youth with Emotional and Behavioral Disorders and Their Families: Programs and Evaluation Best Practices.* Austin, TX, Pro-Ed, Inc., 3–22, 2005.
3. Stroul BA, Friedman RM: *A System of Care for Severely Emotionally Disturbed Children and Youth.* Washington, DC: Georgetown University Child Development Center, 1986.
4. Davis M, Yelton S, Katz-Levy J, Lourie I: Unclaimed children: the status of state children's mental health service systems. *J Ment Health Adm* 22:147–166, 1995.
5. Pires SA, Stroul BA, Roebuck L, Friedman RM, McDonald BB, Chambers KL: *Health Care Reform Tracking Project: Tracking State Health Care Reforms as They Affect Children and Adolescents with Emotional Disorders and Their Families. The 1995 state survey.* Tampa, FL, University of South Florida, Florida Mental Health Institute, 1996.
6. Pumariega AJ, Winters NC, Huffine C: The evolution of systems of care for children's mental health: forty years of community child and adolescent psychiatry. *Community Ment Health J* 32:399–425, 2003.
7. Hinkley EC, Ellis WF: An effective alternative to residential placement: home-based services. *J Clin Child Psychol* 14:209–213, 1985.
8. Bronfenbrenner U: *The Ecology of Human Development: Experiments by Design and Nature.* Cambridge, MA, Harvard University Press, 1979.
9. Patterson GR, Reid JB: Social interactional processes in the family: The study of the moment by moment family transactions in which human social development is embedded. *J Appl Dev Psychol* 5:237–262, 1984.
10. Minuchin S: *Families and Family Therapy.* Cambridge, MA, Harvard University Press, 1974.
11. Farmer T, Farmer E: Developmental science, systems of care, and prevention of emotional and behavioral problems in youth. *Am J Orthopsychiatry* 71:171–181, 2001.
12. Hoagwood K, Jensen PS, Petti T, Burns BJ: Outcomes of mental health care for children and adolescents: a comprehensive conceptual model. *J Am Acad Child Adolesc Psychiatry* 35(8):1055–1063, 1996.
13. Slattery JM, Knapp S: In-home family therapy and wraparound services for working with seriously at-risk children and adolescents. In VandeCreek L, Jackson T (eds): *Innovations in Clinical Practice: A Sourcebook 21.* Sarasota, FL, Professional Resource Press, 2003, 135–149.
14. Yorgason JB, McWey LM, Felts L: In-home family therapy: indicators of success. *J Marital Fam Ther* 31(4):301–312, 2005.
15. Kinney JM, Madsen B, Flemming T, Hapala D: Homebuilders: keeping families together. *J Consult Clin Psychol* 45(4):667–673, 1977.
16. Kinney JD, Haapala D, Booth C: *Keeping Families Together: The Homebuilders Model.* New York, Aldine De Gruyter, 1991.
17. Henggeler SW, Schoenwald SK, Borduin CM, Rowland MD, Cunningham PB: *Multisystemic Treatment for Antisocial Behavior in Children and Adolescents.* 2nd ed. The Guildford Press, New York, 2009.
18. Alexander JF, Robbins MS: Functional family therapy. In: Murrihy RC, Kidman AD, Ollendick T (eds): *Clinical Handbook of Assessing and Treating Conduct Problems in Youth.* New York, Springer, 2011, 245–271.
19. Liddle HA, Rodriguez RA, Dakof GA, Kanzki E, Marvel FA: Multidimensional family therapy: a science-based treatment for adolescent drug abuse. In Lebow J (ed): *Handbook of Clinical Family Therapy.* New York, John Wiley & Sons, 2005, 128–163.
20. Henggeler SW, Rowland MD, Randall J, et al.: Home-based multisystemic therapy as an alternative to the hospitalization of youths in psychiatric crisis: clinical outcomes. *J Am Acad Child Adolesc Psychiatry* 38:1331–1339, 1999.
21. Burns BJ, Goldman SK (eds): *Promising Practices in Wraparound for Children with Serious Emotional Disturbance and Their Families.* Washington, DC: Center for Effective Collaboration and Practice, American Institute for Research, 1998 Series, 1999.
22. Bruns EJ, Walker JS, Zabel M, et al.: Intervening in the lives of youth with complex behavioral health challenges and their families: The role of the wraparound process. *Am J Community Psychol* 46:314–331, 2010.
23. Woods LJ: Home-based family therapy. *Social Work* 33(3):211–214, 1988.
24. Heying KR: Family-based, in-home services for the severely emotionally disturbed child. *Child Welfare* 64(5):519–527, 1985.
25. Koyanagi C: *Making Sense of Medicaid for Children with Serious Emotional Disturbance.* Washington, DC, Bazelon Center for Mental Health Law, 1999.
26. Grimes KE, Mullin B: MHSPY: a children's health initiative for maintaining at-risk youth in the community. *J Behav Health Serv Res* 33:196–221, 2006.
27. Grimes KE, Schulz M, Cohen S, Mullin B, Lehar S, Tien S: Pursuing cost-effectiveness in mental health service delivery for youth with complex needs. *J Ment Health Policy Econ* 14:73–86, 2011.
28. Rosie D. v. Swift, 01-CV-30199-MAP (U.S. Dist. Court of Mass, 2001). Complaint. Available at: www.rosied.org/resources/documents/complaint.final.doc
29. Rosie D. v. Romney. (2006). 410 F. Supp. 2d 18, 2006 U.S. Dist., D. Mass.
30. Ng T, Harrington C, Musumeci M, Reaves EL: *Medicaid Home and Community-Based Services Programs: 2012 Data Update.* Washington, DC, Kaiser Commission on Medicaid and the Uninsured, 2015.
31. New Freedom Commission on Mental Health: *Achieving the Promise: Transforming Mental Health Care in America.* Rockville, MD, Final Report. DHHS Pub. No. SMA-03-3832, 2003.
32. Department of Health and Human Services: Report to the President and Congress. *Medicaid Home and Community-Based Alternatives to Psychiatric Residential Treatment Facilities Demonstration.* Washington, DC, 2013.
33. Young J, Plotner K, Damon JD, Hight TL: State mental health policy: overview and goals of the Mississippi youth programs around the clock (MYPAC). *Psychiatr Serv* 59:836–838, 2008.
34. Youth Villages: *Intercept programs: Information from July 2006 through March 2015.* Memphis, TN, 2015.
35. Bailey C, Sampson A: Virtual Residential Program© Outcome Summary 2002–2011. *Providence Service Corporation,* 2012.
36. Burns BJ, Schoenwald SK, Burchard JD, Faw L, Santos AB: Comprehensive community-based interventions with severe emotional disorders: multisystemic therapy and the wraparound process. *J Child Fam Stud* 9(3):283–314, 2000.
37. Crane DR, Hillin HH, Jakubowski SF: Costs of treating conduct disordered Medicaid youth with and without family therapy. *Am J Fam Ther* 33(5):403–413, 2005.
38. Michigan Department of Health and Human Services. Section 404 (2)(c) Part 3 total CMHSP cost by category and CMHSEP, Fiscal Year 2014. Children with serious emotional disturbance. Available at: http://www.michigan.gov/documents/mdch/x_-_Section_404_2c_-_Part_3_500174_7.pdf
39. Hoagwood K, Burns BJ, Kiser L, Ringeisen H, Schoenwald SK: Evidence-based practice in child and adolescent mental health services. *Psychiatr Serv* 52(9):1179–1189, 2001.
40. Farmer EMZ, Dorsey S, Mustillo SA: Intensive home and community interventions. *Child Adolesc Psychiatr Clin N Am* 13:857–884, 2004.
41. Waddell C, McEwan K, Hua J, Shepherd C: *Child and Youth Mental Health: Population Health and Clinical Service Considerations A Research Report Prepared for the British Columbia Ministry of Children and Family Development Mental Health Evaluation &Community Consultation Unit, Department of Psychiatry, Faculty of Medicine.* Vancouver, British Columbia, The University of British Columbia, 2002.
42. Evans ME, Boothroyd RA, Armstrong MI, Greenbaum PE, Brown EC, Kuppinger AD: Effectiveness of in-home crisis services for children and their families: program outcomes. *J Emot Behav Disord* 11(2):92–102, 2003.
43. Wilmshurst L: Treatment programs for youth with emotional and behavioral disorders: an outcome study of two alternate approaches. *Ment Health Serv Res* 4(2):82–96, 2002.
44. Henggeler SW, Schoenwald SK, Rowland MD, Cunningham PB: *Serious Emotional Disturbance in Children and Adolescents: Multisystemic Therapy.* New York, Guilford Press, 2002.
45. Henggeler SW, Cunningham PB, Rowland MD, Schoenwald SK, and Associates: *Contingency Management for Adolescent Substance Abuse: A Practitioner's Guide.* New York, The Guilford Press, 2012.
46. Fixsen DL, Blase KA, Metz AJ, Naoom SF: Producing high levels of treatment integrity in practice: A focus on preparing practitioners. In: Hagermoser Sanetti LM, Kratochwill TR (eds): *Treatment Integrity: A Foundation for Evidence-Based Practice in Applied Psychology.* Washington, DC, American Psychological Association, 2014, 185–201.
47. Schoenwald SK, Ward DM, Henggeler SW, Rowland MD: MST vs. hospitalization for crisis stabilization of youth: placement outcomes 4 months post-referral. *Ment Health Serv Res,* 2(1):3–12, 2000.
48. Huey SJ, Henggeler SW, Rowland MD, et al.: Multisystemic therapy effects on attempted suicide by youth presenting psychiatric emergencies. *J Am Acad Child Adolesc Psychiatry* 43:183–190, 2004.
49. Henggeler SW, Rowland MD, Halliday-Boykins C, et al.: One-Year follow-up of multisystemic therapy as an alternative to the hospitalization of youths in psychiatric crisis. *J Am Acad Child Adolesc Psychiatry* 42:543–551, 2003.
50. Simpson DD, McBride AA: Family Friends and Self (FFS) assessment scales for Mexican American Youth. *Hisp J Behav Sci* 14:327–340, 1992.
51. Achenbach TM: *Manual for the Child Behavior Checklist and 1991 Profile.* Burlington, University of Vermont Department of Psychiatry, 1991.
52. Olson DH, Portner J, Lavee Y: *FACES-III.* St Paul, Minnesota, University of Minnesota, Department of Family Social Sciences, 1985.
53. Kolbe LJ, Kann L, Collins JI: Overview of the youth risk behavior surveillance system. *Public Health Rep* 108:2–10, 1993.
54. Rowland MD, Halliday-Boykins CA, Henggeler SW, et al.: A randomized trial of multisystemic therapy with Hawaii's Felix Class youths. *J Emot Behav Disord* 13(1):13–23, 2005.

55. Achenbach TM: *Manual for the Youth Self Report and 1991 Profile.* Burlington, University of Vermont Department of Psychiatry, 1991.
56. Elliott DS: *Youth Violence: An Overview.* Boulder, Colorado, University of Colorado, Center for the Study and Prevention of Violence, Institute for Behavioral Sciences, 1994.
57. Schoenwald SK, Rowland MD, et al.: MST-Based Continuum of Care in Philadelphia, unpublished results developed for a report to the Annie E. *Casey Foundation, 2004, Author Communication.*
58. Winters KC, Henly G: *The Personal Experience Inventory.* Los Angeles, Western Psychological Services, 1989.
59. Derogatis LR: *The Brief Symptom Inventory: Administration, Scoring and Procedures Manual.* Baltimore, Clinical Psychometric Research, Johns Hopkins, 1992.
60. Rowlands S, Rowland MD, et al.: Multisystemic Therapy Psychiatric Adaptation Program: New York Foundling's Final Report to the Robin Hood Foundation Summary of Outcomes for 2013, unpublished.
61. Woolston JL, Adnopoz JA, Berkowitz SJ: *IICAPS: A Home-based Psychiatric Treatment for Children and Adolescents,* New Haven, CT, Yale University Press, 2007.
62. Adnopoz JA, Woolston J, Balestracci KB: IICAPS: A treatment model for delinquent youths with co-occurring mental health disorders. In: Grigorenko EL (ed): *Handbook of Juvenile Forensic Psychology and Psychiatry.* New York, Springer, 357–369, 2012.
63. Felitti VJ, Anda RF, Nordenberg D, et al.: The relationship of childhood abuse and household dysfunction to many of the leading causes of death in adults. The Adverse Childhood Experiences (ACE) study. *Am J Prev Med* 14(4):245–258, 1998.
64. Rutter M: Psychosocial resilience and protective mechanisms. *Am J Orthopsychiatr* 57(3):316–331, 1987.
65. McGoldrick M, Gerson R, Shellenberger S: *Genograms: Assessment and Intervention,* 2nd ed. New York, NY, W.W. Norton & Company, 1999.
66. Ogles BM, Melendez G, Davis DC, Lunnen KM: *The Ohio Youth Problem, Functioning, and Satisfaction Scales: Technical manual.* Athens, Ohio University, 2000.
67. Barbort B, Bick J, Bentely MJ, et al.: Changes in mental health outcomes with the intensive in-home child and adolescent psychiatric service: a multi-informant, latent consensus approach. *International Journal of Methods in Psychiatric Research* July (3rd Quarter/Summer) 15, 2015.
68. Ogles BM, Dowell K, Hatfield D, Melendez G, Carlston DL: The Ohio scales. In: Maruish M (ed): *The Use of Psychological Testing for Treatment Planning and Outcomes Assessment.* Mahwah, NJ, Lawrence Erlbaum Associates, 275–304, 2004.

CHAPTER 6.3.4 ■ COMMUNITY-BASED TREATMENT AND SERVICES

ANDRES J. PUMARIEGA AND NANCY C. WINTERS

HISTORY AND CHALLENGES IN CHILDREN'S COMMUNITY MENTAL HEALTH SERVICES

The early origins of mental health services for children in the United States emphasized a community and even a systems orientation. In the 1890s, the United States, much as today, was undergoing rapid sociocultural changes due to immigration, industrialization, and urbanization. These social strains and their impact on children and families led to marked increases in juvenile crime and status offenses. Enlightened reformers saw the need for detaining young offenders separately from adults and adjudicating them in a separate court system (juvenile courts) that emphasized rehabilitation. Thus, the new juvenile courts in Chicago and Boston established clinics that comprised the first child mental health services in the nation (1).

Their success led the Commonwealth Foundation to commission a study in the 1920s (and later provided start-up funding) to develop child guidance clinics throughout the United States, staffed with interdisciplinary teams of professionals to serve children and their families. These clinics were first primarily staffed by social workers, but later attracted psychosocially oriented pediatricians, psychologists, and later psychoanalysts (as they emigrated from Europe) and psychiatrists (as the specialty grew and developed). These clinics later served as the bases of the first child psychiatry programs in the nation. They were removed from the specialty-oriented, hospital-based medical system evolving at tertiary medical centers. They provided low cost services oriented to the needs of children and families, with treatment modalities evolving to include individual psychodynamic psychotherapy, family therapy, crisis intervention, and even day treatment programs. Many have survived to this day, and they even served as the model for the community mental health centers implemented by the Kennedy administration throughout the United States in the 1960s (1). The "medicalization" of psychiatry, starting in the 1970s and 1980s, served to move child and adolescent psychiatric services toward a more hospital-based, tertiary care setting. This left the child guidance clinics, and the community mental health centers that followed them, without significant child psychiatric input, adding to the relative neglect of the development of children's services. Many of the children previously served in these clinics were served in inpatient or residential facilities, or placed in foster care or juvenile detention facilities if they lacked third-party payment.

The modern era of community-based systems of care for children was ushered by the publication of Jane Knitzer's (2) groundbreaking book, *Unclaimed Children,* which exposed the aforementioned consequences of neglecting community-based mental health services for children and their families. Her advocacy and that of others led to the development of the Child and Adolescent Service System Program (CASSP), which assisted all 50 states in the development of an infrastructure for publicly funded community-based services. The CASSP initiative was supported by the conceptual work of Stroul and Friedman (3), which coined the term "community-based system of care for seriously emotionally disturbed children and their families" and enunciated the principles behind such systems of care. Stroul and Friedman's work spurred the development of various innovative community-based treatment modalities, as well as a number of model demonstration programs in different parts of the United States using these modalities within the context of organized interagency programs. In the early 1990s, the Robert Woods Johnson Foundation established eight pilot demonstration community systems-of-care programs in different parts of the country that demonstrated the viability of the system-of-care model, demonstrating cost savings as well as less restrictive levels of care. Starting in 1994, the CASSP program was transformed into the Child and

Adolescent Branch of the Center for Mental Health Services of the Substance Abuse and Mental Health Services Administration, which established the Comprehensive Community Mental Health Services for Children and Their Families Program (4). This program has funded over 180 community systems-of-care grant sites throughout the nation in widely diverse communities and American Indian communities, with over 100,000 children and families served by them, with many included in a national evaluation. The Surgeon General's Report on mental health (5) focused many of its recommendations in the area of children's mental health around the system-of-care model and its benefits for service system reform and community-based, individualized care.

INTERFACE OF CHILD MENTAL HEALTH SERVICES WITH OTHER CHILD-SERVING SYSTEMS

A number of health and human service agencies (schools, social welfare agencies, child protective agencies, juvenile justice, and public health) have experienced the increasing impact of psychosocial morbidity experienced by children and youth. These agencies typically address pieces of the service system puzzle, with little to no coordination with other agencies often serving the same youth (6).

Juvenile Justice

In spite of the similarities in their populations, the juvenile justice and mental health systems have significant differences in their service orientations and philosophies. The juvenile justice system has faced a recent split in its orientation, between those who still promote the principles of rehabilitation advocated by its original founders, versus those who promote a more purely punitive and public safety approach. The latter viewpoint, with its push for longer sentences and even waivers into adult courts and prisons, gathered currency as the nation witnessed a major increase in juvenile crime since the 1980s (largely in poor inner city and rural areas), as well as the long list of school shootings starting at Columbine, Colorado, in 1999 to this day. This often clashes with the treatment and services orientation of the mental health system, though the latter suffers due to the lack of focus on behavioral containment and long-term follow-up. The focus in the juvenile justice system shifted toward detention/containment, either in juvenile detention facilities or residential programs with some mental health programming and services (7).

The pressures to detain and incarcerate juveniles have led to overcrowded conditions and poor services in juvenile detention and incarceration facilities that violated several federal mandates. Chief among them is the Civil Rights of Institutionalized Persons Act (CRIPA), which mandates that states provide adequate health, mental health, and human/social services to people detained on a long-term basis under state custody. Other mandates, such as the Individuals with Disabilities Education Act, also apply to such youth. There have been well over 20 class action lawsuits involving juvenile justice systems all across the nation (7,8).

A number of studies have documented high rates of serious emotional disturbance (SED) among youth in the juvenile justice system, with estimates of approximately 50% to 70% (9,10). Youth are referred to juvenile justice due to their propensity to display aggressive or disruptive behaviors, drug offenses, and/or multiple disciplinary interventions in schools. They have similar histories as described for youth in child welfare, and were often previously served by that system. However, these youth typically have underutilized mental health services over their lifetime when compared to cohorts in other systems (11,12). There is also disproportionate representation of minorities in the population of youth served by juvenile justice, especially of African Americans and Latinos. This is both due to the poverty and adversity faced by these youth, as well as the lack of culturally competent services in mental health and other agencies. The poor level of services within juvenile justice facilities also deprives them of adequate services, with racial/ ethnic bias further preventing access to services (7,13). A mandate to reduce disproportionate minority confinement, requiring that states implement efforts to reduce such disparities, existed in federal law up until the late 1990s, but it was discontinued in spite of this serious continuing trend (7).

The trend toward the juvenile justice system becoming the "mental health system of last resort" for juveniles, as well as the public support for crime prevention, has led to increasing funding for services for juvenile offenders, including mental health services. They are leading either to the development of closer alliances between juvenile justice and mental health, or at times to the development of separate mental health services within the juvenile justice system. The latter trend may increase the access and control over these services for juvenile justice, but may result in unnecessary and costly duplication of services (7).

Areas of natural collaboration between these systems are in the prevention of entry into juvenile justice, particularly into detention/incarceration, and the treatment of youth with SED into the juvenile justice system. Multisystemic Therapy (MST), Functional Family Therapy (FFT), Multidimensional Treatment Foster Care, and Brief Strategic Family Therapy have been tested extensively with youth at risk of detention and incarceration, and have resulted in significant reductions in out-of-home placement, externalizing criminal behaviors, substance abuse, rates of arrest and incarceration, and treatment costs (14). The significant reduction of arrests and incarceration by the Center for Mental Health Services (CMHS) system-of-care demonstration sites also support the value of the system-of-care model in addressing the needs of this population of youth (4,15). The Surgeon General's report on youth violence (16) also reviews a number of effective preventive interventions for youth violence and delinquency.

Child Welfare

The original mission of the child welfare system was to provide custodial care for children and youth abandoned or abused by their families, typically through the operation or support of orphanages in years past, and foster homes and group homes in later years. There has been greater recognition in recent years that children in the child welfare system have extremely high mental health needs, with prevalence rates estimated at about 50%, but are significantly underserved by mental health services (17). Already traumatized by the abuse and neglect that led to removal from their parents' care, children placed in foster care are confronted with the additional traumas of the loss of their parents, multiple relocations, uncertainty about their future, the difficult task of establishing positive attachments to new parent figures and foster siblings, and risk of abuse in foster homes. This chronic traumatization not only places them at higher risk of posttraumatic and attachment disturbances, but also disruptive disorders. They have greater difficulties in functioning at home, school, and in their communities, placing them at high risk for additional failed placements and need for residential treatment (17).

These needs led to the proliferation of residential treatment centers focused on the custodial and at times treatment needs of children in custody, particularly adolescents. Many of these facilities provide quality therapeutic and support services, but others in many states are largely unregulated in terms of the level or quality of service provision. The legal and social structures responsible for the care of children in state custody further complicate the situation for children in the child welfare system. The courts may make decisions supporting reunification that compromise the child's physical and/or emotional safety. Ninety percent of children in foster care are returned to their biologic parents (18), and mental health services needed to support the reunification process are often inadequate. These factors have led to a rapid increase in the number of children and youth cared for within such facilities for extended periods of time. Serious problems in the delivery of their care, such as indiscriminate polypharmacy, overuse of seclusion and restraints, and abuse at the hands of direct care staff, continue to hamper the system in spite of Knitzer's (2) original admonitions in the early 1980s (17,19).

When children are in foster care, there are unique challenges to establishing effective services coordination. The child- and family-centered system-of-care model works best when the child's parents are very invested. This may be difficult for foster parents, who are often caring for multiple high-need children and are not able to commit emotionally to a child who may live with them for a short period. Foster parents also suffer from inadequate training, support (including respite services and ongoing mental health consultation), and reimbursement for the care of children, particularly those who are seriously emotionally disturbed.

Another serious problem is the child welfare system being used by families in many states as a way to access intensive mental health services for children with inadequate insurance benefits. In recent years, the expansion of Medicaid to children above the poverty line, and particularly secondary Medicaid for children with mental illness and serious emotional disturbance, has reduced this burden on the child welfare system and served to keep affected children unified with their parents. The Early Periodic Screening Detection and Treatment mandate covers periodic health and mental health screening for covered children and medical necessity authorization of treatments and services to address abnormal findings, a benefit that prevents out of home placement and is increasingly included in managed Medicaid plans (8). Another arbitrary constraint within mental health systems that increase the risk of children being placed in foster care is the lack of needed parenting support services for individuals with mental illness, while states will fund the placement of these children in foster care. A different challenge is presented by the Welfare to Work law, which requires low-income parents to return to work to maintain some of their benefits. For some parents of at-risk children, this requirement makes it exceedingly difficult to spend the time needed to address the child's emotional or behavioral problems (17).

Children in foster care and those at risk for being placed in foster care are ideal candidates for the system-of-care model, which can prevent out-of-home placement, support the strengths of the child and family, and use natural supports in the community. Wraparound programs, intensive case management programs, and therapeutic foster care are community-based interventions that have demonstrated effectiveness with this population of children and families (17). The American Academy of Child and Adolescent Psychiatry (AACAP) and the Child Welfare League of America (20) have developed specific screening, evaluation, and service standards to address the unique needs of children in the child welfare system. There is also a growing evidence base for psychosocial interventions for children with trauma-related disorders (21). Another positive trend is that of supporting foster care within a kinship network (extended family), allowing for relationships with family members to be sustained. More states are allowing families to retain custody of their children while they are in state-supported residential care (Oregon is one example); such changes to existing laws are usually accomplished only through significant advocacy by parent groups (also, see Chapters 5.15.1, 5.15.4, and 7.3).

Education

The educational system faces the impact of increased educational demands for average students due to the increased technologic and informational demands on our society. In addition, the increasing needs of children with learning disorders and serious emotional disturbances are placing added burdens on schools. This occurs in the context of the underfunding of school districts due to downward pressures on property taxes (as exemplified by laws like Proposition 13 in California) and other unequal means of funding education and special education services. Many school districts struggle to meet the mandates of federal laws such as the Individualized Disability Education Act (IDEA) and Section 504 (which outlines services for mentally ill/emotionally disturbed children), often underidentifying children with covered disabilities and temporizing their needs informally through the services of regular classroom teachers so as to prevent added service commitments (22).

An important area of interagency systems of care is that of school-based services. These go beyond traditional school mental health consultation services and involve the colocation of health and mental health professionals within schools to provide a wide array of direct and indirect/preventive health and mental health services. School-based mental health services serve as an ideal core service for a children's system of care, providing an excellent accessible portal of entry which is nonstigmatizing, and a naturalistic setting to observe behavior and integrate interventions into a child's environment. These services are often funded through blended Medicaid fee-for-service and managed care funding augmenting limited school funding. A number of models have been implemented in communities such as Baltimore, Maryland, New York City, rural South Carolina, the state of Hawaii, and Charlotte, North Carolina, with documented success in reducing adverse morbidity and increasing access to needed services (23,24). Innovative approaches through legislation to ensure interagency collaboration in IDEA-mandated services have been promoted in California through legislation that mandates interagency collaboration in the development and implementation of individualized educational plans when these involve domains outside of educational services (25; also, see Chapter 7.3).

Developmental Disabilities

Children and youth with developmental disabilities have significant mental health and social service needs. The prevalence of comorbidity of developmental disorders and behavioral/emotional disturbances is estimated to be quite high. In addition to mental health services, the service needs of children and youth with developmental disorders are often wider ranging, including educational services, medical services (including general pediatric, neurologic, and genetic), child welfare and social supports (with high rates of abuse and abandonment), and even juvenile justice services. The latter need is highlighted by the high prevalence of youth with Asperger disorder found in juvenile justice populations (26). However, there is little recognition of these multiple service needs in the developmental disabilities service sector, much less adequate resources to meet them. Most state governments assign responsibility for serving children with developmental disabilities to the educational system under IDEA and ignore interagency collaborative approaches for their care. However, this system is overwhelmed in meeting its educational mission and dealing with more straightforward learning disabilities. States with developmental disabilities agencies or divisions tend to underfund them, and assign similar levels of mental health benefits as for people without such disabilities in spite of their higher risks and special service needs. The adult developmental disabilities sector is also moving rapidly to deinstitutionalize individuals currently in state training schools or facilities to community care, including the few youth in such programs. The behavioral support resources and staffing needed for successfully moving such individuals to community care are very limited, leaving them functioning at lower levels than their potential, and at risk of frequent utilization of psychiatric emergency services, hospitalization, and overmedication. This has led to many states experiencing class action lawsuits over the access and quality of care for its developmentally disabled citizens (26).

Primary Health Care

Primary care providers (including pediatricians, family physicians, some internists, and primary nurse practitioners) are the first line of mental health services for children in our nation, especially in rural and underserved areas. Studies (27) have demonstrated a high prevalence of mental health need among children and youth seen in primary care practices and settings. This role is even more critical in the Medicaid-covered population, where the EPSDT benefit includes the requirement for annual screening, referral, and treatment for mental, emotional, and developmental disorders as well as physical illness. However, primary care providers receive little to no training in child mental health and mental illness in their preservice or residency training. They are generally not trained to use the increasing number of evidence-based tools for effective screening and identification of youngsters with such needs. Access to specialist child mental health consultants and collaborators is hampered by problems with access and reimbursement. The reimbursement mechanism for the direct delivery of entry-level mental health services by primary care practitioners is shrouded in mystery and bureaucracy, as if in an effort to reduce access to such services. The carve-out model primarily used for mental health benefits under managed Medicaid keeps "medical" and "mental health" sources of funding artificially separated (28). However, primary care has the potential to be the most important system (besides the educational system) in any effective effort to prevent the developmental morbidity of undetected and untreated mental illness in our children and youth (28).

In recent years, in response to increasing challenges in access to mental health care, a strong movement toward developing clinically and cost-effective integrative and collaborative care models has gathered momentum. It is demonstrating results in greater participation by primary care in the care of people with mental health needs. In pediatric primary care, the model has primarily been a collaborative one, with pediatricians accessing pediatric mental health consultation (especially child psychiatric consultation) from collaborative "hubs" serving practices and practitioners in defined regions. These "hubs" are staffed by child and adolescent psychiatrists (CAPs), psychologists, and social workers, and provide a gamut of consultative services, including case management referral to treatment resources (particularly for psychotherapy but also intensive services), diagnostic consultation, and psychopharmacologic consultation. The consultations are mostly telephonic (between the primary care practitioner and mental health professional), but can be live evaluations of the child and family face to face or via televideo. Some of these models also include the use of systematic behavioral health screening for all children served by the participating practices, the use of secondary screening and diagnostic tools, as well as formal training of pediatric primary care providers in psychiatric diagnostic and treatment skills within their practices.

The original model program of this kind was in the state of Massachusetts, starting with a regional model and eventually expanding to cover 97% of all children in the state. The Massachusetts model, now 10 years in operation started with state funding but now includes private third-party funding as part of its funding base. The project had provided over 35,000 encounters over its first 5 years, and served over 14,000 children and adolescents with the full range of psychiatric disorders and needs. The overwhelming majority of pediatric primary care practitioners rated the services highly in terms of access and overall satisfaction (29,30). A National Network of Child Psychiatry Access Programs has been constituted, comprising programs representing 20 states throughout the United States, with many of these programs being statewide (as in New York State and Washington State), or in the process of becoming statewide (such as New Jersey).

COMMUNITY-BASED SYSTEMS OF CARE: AN INTEGRATIVE MODEL

The CASSP principles, now referred to as community systems-of-care principles, are based on a flexible and individualized approach to service delivery for the child and family within the context of his/her home and community as an alternative to treatment in out-of-home settings, while attending to family and systems issues that impact such care. The key principles include: access to a comprehensive array of services, treatment individualized to the child's needs, treatment in the least restrictive environment possible, full utilization of family and community resources, full participation of families as partners in services planning and delivery, interagency coordination, the use of case management for services coordination, no ejection or rejection from services due to lack of "treatability" or "cooperation" with interventions, early identification and intervention, smooth transition of youth into the adult service system, effective advocacy efforts, and nondiscriminating, culturally sensitive services (3). More recently, services quality, cost-effectiveness, and outcomes and integration of evidence-based practices have received greater emphasis within community-based systems-of-care programs. Psychiatry, which was central in the traditional model, has only recently reengaged itself as a discipline in this new model. Psychiatrists continue to face challenges in establishing their position within this model and integrating their developing clinical and scientific knowledge and skills base (3).

Another important principle inherent in this approach is that of the targeting of services to children designated as "seriously emotionally disturbed," defined as having a diagnosis under the diagnostic and statistical manual of the American Psychiatric Association (31), as well as resulting impairment in function in at least one of his/her life domains (school, home, socially with peers). This definition reflects the difficulty in accurately diagnosing many children with serious functional problems, the bias against disruptive disorders (and failure to identify comorbid serious mental illness), and the lack of clarity and validity in clinical child diagnosis. Studies also suggest that the level of care received by children is only partially accounted by their clinical diagnosis, while level of function and psychosocial stressors are stronger predictors (32).

Implementation at the Clinical Level

Family-driven care is a cornerstone of the system-of-care approach and has had a significant influence on national policy for both child and adult mental health (33–35). The child and family drive the clinical planning process through determining the goals and desired outcomes of services, selecting the composition of the interagency service planning team, evaluating the effectiveness of services, and having a meaningful role in all decisions, including those that impact funding of services. The interagency planning team typically has representatives from all the agencies involved with the child, and the team process facilitates interagency and interdisciplinary collaboration. The complementary contributions of various team members function synergistically in identifying system and community resources to promote better outcomes.

Some children and youth enter the system of care with discrete problems that can be addressed by a specific and/or time-limited service. For children with complex problems involved in multiple child-serving agencies, assessment and treatment planning should be accomplished through interdisciplinary clinical teams. These teams bring together different clinical and support resources to address the child's needs to supporting him or her and their family in their community environment. However, funding constraints due to legally mandated categorical limits could leave some needs of a child unfulfilled. Also, many families can be well served by such interagency collaborative efforts, but often a parent or a youth surrounded by a team of professionals finds the experience intimidating and has trouble feeling that they are full participants in the planning process (36).

The wraparound process is a specific model of a child- and family-driven team planning process that has been empirically tested within systems of care. Wraparound is a definable, integrated planning process that results in a unique set of community services and natural supports that are individualized for a child and family to achieve a set of positive outcomes. The wraparound process builds on the strengths of the child and family, is community based (using a balance of formal and informal supports), is outcome driven, and provides unconditional care (37). Use of a strength-based orientation and discussion of needs rather than problems promotes more active engagement of families in service planning activities. Interventions designed to reinforce strengths of the child and family may include nontraditional therapies such as specific skills training or mentored work experiences that remediate or offset deficits. These interventions generally are not included in traditional categorical mental health funding and may require flexible funds that are not assigned to specific service types (38). For example, a youth at risk for substance abuse might receive funding for prosocial activities such as a health club membership or computer training. It has been noted that services are more likely to be effective if the wraparound process is informed by comprehensive clinical assessment addressing diagnostic and treatment issues and if the specific interventions are evidence based (39,40).

Central to this process is the development of a child and family team (CFT). Such teams are composed primarily of nonprofessional members led by the consumer family, usually a parent. In cases of older youth as consumers, and with no parents available, the youth may serve as team leader. Empowering youth and families to assume a central role in outlining treatment goals and planning requires the involvement of specially trained individuals who can guide such families to develop such goals. Family advocates, partnering with professionals, provide the backbone of such a process. The goals for team development are to mobilize the natural support system for the family, including extended family, friends, neighbors, and natural helpers in communities. CFTs may include professionals to whom families have come to feel close, but the general rule is that teams should comprise of no more than 50% professionals. Teams should have access to professional advisors, including CAPs, who can offer advice on services, how best to access them, and on the various agencies in which the child is involved (34).

CFTs collaborate with professionals in agencies providing services. The CFT creates an overall care plan, including a crisis plan. The clinical team then negotiates their role in the crisis and care plans. This negotiation further educates families about how their child's needs could be addressed through treatment, and enables professionals to learn about the realities faced by the family. In this model, the role of the case manager is supplanted by the CFT, which is responsible for maintaining and modifying the overall care plan, with the assistance of family advocates. The most complete evolution of a system of care that supports family-centered care involves agencies blending funds and undoing categorical constraints on the use of funds, with CFTs having control over the expenditure of such funds for services they deem needed and relevant. This radically alters the relationships of service providers to consumer families, enabling poor families to have control similar to middle- or upper-class families in their child's care and encouraging programs to develop new types of resources based on the common needs of families in that community (34).

A number of studies of wraparound in different communities with diverse populations of at-risk children and families have reported positive outcomes in reduction of externalizing behavioral problems, improvement of children's level of function, reduction in out-of-home placement, improved family management skills and function, and increased consumer/family satisfaction (39,41,42). There have been recent efforts to operationalize wraparound as a *planning* model, as there has been some confusion about whether wraparound refers to the services themselves or the planning process. Recent studies on wraparound have incorporated measures such as the Wraparound Fidelity Index to ensure fidelity to the model (43).

Integration of services is fundamental to the community systems-of-care philosophy and approach. Service integration can be implemented in a variety of ways. The most fundamental is the interagency planning team, in which representatives from each agency involved with the child meet as a team to collaborate on the child and family's behalf and develop a single, integrated service plan. Integrated treatment models allowing mental health services to be provided in schools, juvenile justice, or child welfare settings have become more prevalent. Another integration strategy is to colocate providers from different agencies in a single facility to enhance their collaboration and simplify the usually onerous task for families of accessing services from multiple agencies. Equally important in achieving service integration is the combining of funds from different agencies to form "blended" or "braided" funds to pay for services. This allows for the sharing of clinical and fiscal responsibility among agencies and decreases the likelihood of uncoordinated efforts driven by separate funding "silos" (44).

New Professional, Family, and Consumer Roles

Given the complexity of systems of care, the skills and roles that psychiatrists must display go far beyond clinical roles that are usually circumscribed and limited. Besides serving as front-line clinicians, these roles include clinical consultation and collaboration with other professionals, collaboration with family advocates and consumers, clinical team leadership, administrative leadership in a delivery organization/system, quality assurance/improvement consultation, consultation to interagency teams, and outcome evaluation/research in systems of care. CAPs, given their broad biopsychosocial and developmental perspectives, should be best able to integrate and coordinate community-based treatment delivered by multiple professionals with diverse skills. They have played critical roles in supporting some model blended funding programs, and assuring that family-driven systems of care incorporate the most recent scientific advances in child and adolescent mental health. However, given the emphasis on tertiary care models of care in the training of most CAPs, they often have not developed many of the skills needed to serve as effective members, collaborators, and leaders of these new systems (45).

There is also a need for different professional roles for other disciplines and professionals. Social workers and other masters' level professionals assume a different type of care management role in addition to their therapy roles. These new functions involve collaborating and sharing roles with family advocates, and a new approach to partnering with consumer families. Psychologists are involved in the implementation of newer evidence-based practices, such as cognitive behavioral therapy, functional behavioral analysis, and systematic measurement of behavior and strengths along with their psychodiagnostic and therapeutic roles. They may have new roles in program evaluation and quality assurance systems, working collaboratively with families in their design. Nurses are involved in a number of important roles, including greater involvement as psychiatric extenders (or, in some states, as primary psychiatric providers), and liaison roles to pediatric and health systems. Community systems of care also have important roles for educators, formalizing their role as mental health coproviders involved in detection, triage, and behavioral interventions. Recreational and occupational therapists also have greater community involvement in schools and nonpsychiatric settings, rather than more traditional institutional settings. These roles require greater preprofessional training on development, psychopathology, and behavioral approaches (45).

The scope of family and consumer empowerment has been extended beyond the treatment setting to include their participation in a number of other roles within systems of care. These include providing case management and support services to other families, serving in quality assurance and consumer satisfaction assessment, participating in governance over system-of-care programs, and advocating for the maintenance and expansion of these programs. Organizations such as the Federation of Families for Children's Mental Health and other advocacy groups are helping to move the family and youth advocacy agenda (34).

Implementation at the Intervention Level

The President's New Freedom Commission goals and recommendations for a transformed mental health system included the dissemination of evidence-based practices as one of six major goals (46). This has provided the impetus for many states to legislate requirements around the use of evidence-based interventions. The system-of-care approach has provided a context for development of an evidence base for community-based interventions that provides alternatives to intensive treatment traditionally delivered in more restrictive settings, such as hospitals and residential treatment centers. These have been classified under the categories of community-based residential interventions (including therapeutic foster care and group homes), multimodal interventions (such as MST and FFT), service coordination and facilitation (including wraparound and intensive care management), and auxiliary and supportive services (including family education and support, mentoring, and respite services) (42). The evidence supporting these interventions will be described below, according to the schema proposed by Hoagwood et al. (47) for determining the level of evidence for mental health interventions, which includes efficacy, fidelity, and transportability, as well as Kazdin's (48) proposed levels of evidence: (1) not evaluated; (2) evaluated but unclear effects, no effects, or possible negative effects; (3) promising (some evidence); (4) well established (criteria by one system used for identifying evidence-based practice); and (5) better/best treatments (studies shown to be more effective than one or more other well-established techniques).

The treatment foster care (TFC) model was developed by Chamberlain (49) at the Oregon Social Learning Center to address problematic behaviors in children with multiple mental disorders. It includes training of foster parents, in-home therapists, and skills builders, and uses a specific model of behavior modification involving consistency, discipline, and careful monitoring of behavior and consequences (42). Results of several studies indicate that TFC can reduce institutionalization, bring about more rapid improvement, and involves lower costs than other residential placements (49). In contrast to TFC, group homes involve creating a structured family environment for six to eight youths at a time, and the treatment model relies on the peer group milieu rather than parent–child interaction as the mediator of change. Group homes appear to be more common in the child welfare literature and have a less substantial literature than TFC (42). There have been questions about the potential for negative effects of grouping youth with similar problems together, though a robust therapeutic program can provide some efficiencies (50). MST is regarded as among the most robust evidence-based community interventions for youth with disruptive disorders (14). It combines home-based, wraparound, and cognitive-behavioral interventions that are individualized to the youth's ecologic systemic context. Its developers have paid significant attention to manualizing MST and ensuring that it is applied with adequate fidelity in their research sites. It has been evaluated in eight randomized trials, including youth at risk of detention or incarceration and youth at risk of psychiatric or substance abuse hospitalization. It has shown significant results in reducing out-of-home placement, reducing externalizing behaviors, reducing rates of recidivism, and lowered costs of treatment (14,51,52). FFT has been identified as one of the emerging evidence-based intervention programs for at-risk youth and their families. FFT can be conducted in the home or the office, and its techniques are highly specific, with its developers also having paid much attention to manualization, therapist adherence, and treatment fidelity. FFT has an established record of outcome studies that demonstrate its efficacy with a wide variety of adolescent-related problems including youth violence, drug abuse, and other delinquency-related behaviors (14,53; also, see Chapter 6.3.3).

Case management as an intervention has some overlap with wraparound, as both incorporate an assigned coordinator who participates in developing an individualized array of services and supports. Case management includes a variety of functions existing on a continuum from utilization management (or "gate-keeping"), brokering or providing access to services, coordination of services, services monitoring and evaluation, advocacy, assessment, direct family support, and direct therapeutic service provision (36). In four randomized trials and a quasiexperimental study, case management has been compared to other interventions. The more intensive case management models (closer to direct service on the continuum) generally compare favorably with other interventions in reducing out-of-home placements and other functional outcomes, but the more common "broker" model shows primarily changes in service use as opposed to better individual outcomes (42).

In the family support area, the most well-examined intervention is mentoring. Mentoring programs have become fairly widespread. Dubois et al. (54) reviewed 55 mentoring programs, finding that better results were associated with greater number of best practices, which include having more explicit structure and monitoring of expectations, screening and training of mentors, parent involvement, and youth with more limited risk factors as opposed to serious mental health problems. Respite services involve providing temporary care to provide relief to caregivers of individuals with various disabilities. With the increased emphasis in systems of care on keeping children with serious disturbances at home, families have a greater need for relief to diminish caregiver burden. There has only been one quasiexperimental study on respite, which did show decreased caregiver strain and greater optimism, fewer out-of-home placements, and improvement of children's behavioral problems in the community (55). Although the rationale for respite is responsiveness to the needs of overburdened families to support keeping children at home is not disputed, more research is needed to demonstrate its effectiveness.

The Surgeon General reports on mental health (5) and on youth violence (16) point to research evidence supporting a number of community-based interventions for children and youth, such as intensive case management, therapeutic foster care, partial hospitalization, and intensive in-home wraparound interventions. Other community-based interventions that show promise include school-based interventions, mentoring programs, family support and education programs, wilderness programs, crisis mobile outreach teams, partial hospitalization, time-limited hospitalization with coordinated community services, and family support services (39,56). Studies involving these modalities have demonstrated significantly better outcomes than traditional outpatient or residential services. These include reduced levels of externalizing and internalizing symptoms, improved family functioning, reduced utilization of more restrictive services, and improved cost-effectiveness.

One of the challenges facing community systems of care serving youth is the integration of evidence-based psychotherapeutic modalities, especially well tested, manualized interventions with demonstrated efficacy. Such interventions hold promise as broadly applicable interventions that could help address the considerable gap between mental health problems in children and the services needed to address these problems. However, there is still much work to be done in evaluating these interventions in real-world or community-based settings (39,57). Psychosocial interventions having the most empirical support include cognitive-behavioral therapy, interpersonal therapy, parent management training, parent–child interactive therapy (PCIT), and psychoeducational and cognitive-behavioral family interventions (56). Many newer systems-of-care demonstration programs are integrating such interventions into their programs, along with community-based interventions.

Pharmacotherapy in Systems of Care

Psychopharmacology has become increasingly prevalent in community settings as newer and more effective psychotropic agents have become available. These agents play an important role in the treatment of children with serious emotional and behavioral disturbance who have high rates of psychiatric comorbidity, psychosocial adversity, involvement with multiple agencies, and who are at highest risk for placement in restrictive settings (58). Advances in pharmacotherapy have engendered increased expectations that medications can help stabilize and improve the functioning of this high-risk, high-need population. It is important for systems of care to integrate effectively and fully prescribing practitioners into interdisciplinary teams and integrate pharmacologic therapies into children's wraparound plans (38). Effective use of pharmacotherapy includes systematic assessment of target symptoms, behaviors, function, and adverse effects by the whole team (including both synergistic and interfering side effects and issues such as optimal administration and dosing schedules). Ideally the team would also participate in the assessment of the efficacy of medications and interactions between pharmacotherapy and other treatment modalities and strength-based activities.

Effective pharmacotherapy requires that prescribing physicians have access to the inherent resources in a system of care, such as multiple informants to evaluate the child's symptom patterns and function in different contexts, and child and family education and support for treatment adherence. Lack of adequate contact of the children and families with the prescribing physician or medical practitioner often leads to children and families feeling uninformed, disempowered, and mistrustful of pharmacologic therapies. Pharmacotherapy in systems of care should focus on functional improvement as well as on symptomatic relief. It should also include collaboration and psychiatric consultation around medication management with other prescribing medical professionals (58). Prescribing physicians in systems of care should promote use of evidence-based systematic assessment and symptom-rating tools and become actively involved in quality improvement around pharmacologic decision-making (38,59). Attention to ethnic and cultural factors in diagnosis, metabolism of different agents, consent procedures, and attitudes toward medications are also important (60; also, see Chapters 6.1.3 and 6.1.4.1).

The national evaluation of the Comprehensive Mental Health Services Program for Children and Their Families included a substudy on the prescription of psychotropics for children in this program. One-half of the children and youth (52.6%) took at least one medication for their emotional or behavioral symptoms. The majority (85.7%) had their medications prescribed by mental health care prescribers, with the remainder (14.3%) receiving medications from primary care providers. Children and youth whose medications were prescribed by mental health care prescribers had higher levels of internalizing and externalizing symptoms at intake and at 6 months than children and youth whose medications were prescribed by primary care providers. However, the symptoms of all children and youth who received medication improved at the same rate (4).

Implementation at the Programmatic and Service Delivery Level

Following CASSP, several early demonstration projects were initiated to develop systems of care, including those in Ventura County in California (61) and Vermont (62) and the continuum of care established by the Department of Defense CHAMPUS program at Fort Bragg, North Carolina. From 1990 to 1995, the Robert Wood Johnson Mental Health Services Program for Youth funded eight national demonstration programs. More recently, the CMHS Comprehensive Community Mental Health Services Program for Children and Their Families has funded more than 80 demonstration projects in diverse communities throughout the nation to implement systems of care. The goals of these programs have been to implement CASSP values, reduce out-of-home placements, reduce service fragmentation, and promote earlier mental health intervention to reduce functional morbidity. The latter phases of the grant program have focused on culturally diverse populations, early childhood populations, and specialized sectors such as child welfare and juvenile justice (4).

The Fort Bragg program evaluation was an early effort to perform a comparative study between a system-of-care oriented program and services as usual. It demonstrated that system coordination produced improved access to and satisfaction with services and also reduced restrictive forms of care, though costs of care were equivalent across the two models (63). However, the fact that the system-of-care group showed clinical and functional outcomes similar to those of the traditional services group contributed to a shift toward more interest in the interventions themselves (64). More positive findings have been reported in other studies. A longitudinal study of the Vermont system of care concluded that the model was cost-effective and resulted in reduced rates of out-of-home placement (65). Attkisson et al. (61) reported reduced group home and foster care expenditures in three California counties using system-of-care approaches as compared with three counties that had more traditional services. Rosenblatt (66) reviewed results of 20 community-based system-of-care studies, concluding that there were improvements in most domains assessed, including clinical status, cost, and use of restrictive placements. The multisite national evaluation of the Comprehensive Mental Health Services Program for Children and Their Families has shown improved child and family functioning, increased stability of living situation, and reduced cost of care when cost offsets in education, juvenile justice, child welfare, and general health are considered (4,15,67). It has also included a matched comparison evaluation of outcomes from system-of-care programs to treatment as usual, with significantly better functional and cost outcomes, as well as correlation of outcomes to a systems-of-care fidelity measure (4,68,69).

However, questions remain about the effectiveness of community-based interventions and systems-of-care models in comparison to more traditional systems, which outcomes are most meaningful to measure in evaluating the model, and what the active ingredients are that produce desired outcomes. Conducting research in complex systems of care is challenging because of the difficulty of identifying comparison groups and the near impossibility of using randomized assignment since the model has been embraced nationally and to offer less would be perceived as unethical. As a result, the focus has shifted from measuring system-level outcomes to measuring clinical and functional outcomes of individual children (69).

A number of system-of-care demonstration programs that were originally grant funded have been successfully sustained. One such program with unique features is Wraparound Milwaukee in Milwaukee, Wisconsin. In existence since 1995, Wraparound Milwaukee was initially a CMHS-funded system-of-care grant. It evolved into a sustainable publicly operated care management organization that focuses on providing a range of mental health, substance abuse, social, and other supportive services to children and adolescents who are identified by child welfare or juvenile justice as being at immediate risk of placement in a residential treatment center or psychiatric hospital based on emotional, behavioral, or mental health needs (70). Wraparound Milwaukee serves approximately 600 youth during a fiscal year using a CFT process overseen by a care coordinator. Services are purchased from a blended pool from all the contracting agencies. Some of the unique features of Wraparound Milwaukee include the use of a mobile urgent treatment team that has dramatically reduced psychiatric hospital admissions, use of informal services and natural supports, and wraparound resource teams that provide specialized consultation for clinically complex youth (44). Wraparound Milwaukee receive a commendation from the President's New Freedom Commission for its effectiveness in promoting interagency services integration and individualized treatment planning with youth and family participation (46).

CHALLENGES FOR COMMUNITY-BASED SYSTEMS OF CARE

Governmental Policy Imperatives

The Surgeon General's report on mental health in 1999 (5) was a watershed event in children's mental health, as it documented emerging evidence for a variety of psychopharmacologic, psychotherapeutic, and community-based interventions. It also provided support for systems reform according to CASSP principles. This was followed by the President's New Freedom Commission on Mental Health report (46), which was charged with conducting a comprehensive study of the US mental health service delivery system and providing recommendations to the President for improving the system. The report documented pervasive fragmentation and disorganization and called for a fundamental transformation of the nation's approach to mental health care. The report presented six major goals and recommendations for a transformed mental health system: (1) Americans understand that mental health is essential to overall health; (2) mental health is consumer and family driven; (3) disparities in mental health care are eliminated; (4) early mental health screening, assessment, and referral are common practice; (5) excellent mental health care is delivered and research is accelerated; and (6) technology is used to access mental health care and information (46). This report contains elements consistent with the system-of-care model for children with serious emotional disturbance (consumer-driven care, emphasis on resilience and recovery rather than pathology, early intervention), but applies them to all of mental health care in the United States. The President's New Freedom Commission report has provided a strong impetus for states to develop comprehensive state mental health plans containing fundamental changes in adult and children's mental health. Such changes include wide implementation of initiatives toward consumer-driven care, treatment models promoting recovery and resilience, expanded prevention efforts and increased funding for early childhood mental health, and legislation of evidence-based practices.

Funding Challenges

As a result of the growth in mental health expenditures, the resources available to fund child mental health and human services are increasingly strained. Medicaid, the public insurance program for the poor and disabled, funds a significant proportion of child mental health services in the United States. Approximately 37% of children and adolescents 18 years of age and under are enrolled in the Medicaid program. The great majority of these children and youth are poor, underserved children of ethnic minority backgrounds. Children from these populations experience higher levels of stressors, such as poverty, discrimination, immigration, acculturation stress, and exposure to violence and trauma, and are likely to have higher levels of need for services. While children receiving behavioral health services comprise less than 10 of all children on Medicaid, they account for 38% of expenditures. However, the cost of serving these populations of children and adolescents is in contrast to the high cost of the psychosocial morbidity they contend with, including lost productivity and the costs of welfare dependency and institutionalization (6,71,72).

These trends have increased pressures on public child mental health and social service agencies to demonstrate improved clinical and cost-effectiveness, increasingly turning to managed care approaches to finance and organize mental health and social services. Well over half of children who are Medicaid beneficiaries are under managed care plans (72). However, most managed care methods were developed with adult and private sector populations in mind, and are usually accompanied by the privatization of services. Managed care methodology has been implemented increasingly within Medicaid-funded children's mental health services with the aim of reducing utilization and costs, including approaches such as restrictive formularies, level of care criteria, and restrictive case rates. When applied to public child mental health services, these approaches have often resulted in fragmentation of care and the shifting of the burden of services and cost to the other child-serving agencies and systems, with the potential for significantly increased morbidity (73). Such methodology is also being used to manage services funded by the child welfare system and juvenile justice systems, with significant impact on access and quality of care. However, work continues to address the intersection between managed care methodology and systems-of-care principles (71,74,75).

Mental Health Disparities and Needs of Culturally/Ethnically Diverse Populations

The United States is becoming increasingly culturally and ethnically diverse. More than 36% of all children and youth in the United States are from non-European racial and ethnic backgrounds, and this figure is expected to rise to more than 50% by the year 2030. Children and youth from non-European backgrounds and their families face many adversities, including language barriers, social discrimination, and socioeconomic and educational disparities. The Surgeon General's supplement on culture, race, ethnicity, and mental health (76) has highlighted the serious racial/ethnic disparities in child mental health and social services in our nation, which continues to this day. Today Latino and African-American youth are at higher risk for suicidality than its Caucasian cohorts (77,78).

Children and families from ethnically diverse cultures are distinctly different from those of European origins, with different beliefs, values, normative expectations for development and adaptive behaviors, parenting practices, relationship and family patterns, symptomatic expressions of distress, and explanations of mental illness (77). Consequently, they have specific mental health needs with respect to treatment approaches, modalities, and support services. Studies support the presence of significant racial and ethnic disparities in a number of areas relating to children's mental health, including access to community-based services, accurate diagnostic assessment, access to evidence-based interventions, increasing rates of various forms of psychopathology in some populations, and significantly higher rates of out-of-home placements and institutionalization with equal psychiatric morbidity (particularly in child welfare and juvenile justice). In addition, there is evidence of subtle differences in the metabolism of psychopharmacologic agents in diverse populations, related to both genetic and environmental (dietary) factors (77,79).

There is an increasing consensus that culturally informed approaches to care are needed to address the special mental health needs of diverse populations. This must be accomplished through addressing both clinician-related factors (such as acquiring knowledge, skills, and attitudes that enable them to serve populations different from their own) and system factors (such as reviewing and changing policies and practices that present barriers to diverse populations, staff training around cultural competence, and the recruitment of diverse staff and clinicians for planning service pathways and delivering care). This model also calls for the use of natural strengths and resources in concert with professional services that are protective and support children and families in diverse communities and cultures dealing with emotional disturbance. It also includes the adoption of culturally specific therapeutic modalities (such as use of native healers or cultural mediators), the use of culturally adapted mainstream modalities evaluated with diverse populations, and the appropriate use of language interpreters (77).

The cultural competence model has been operationalized in consensus health and mental health cultural competence standards, such as the AACAP Practice Parameter for Culturally Competent Child Psychiatric Practice (77) and the Center for Mental Health Services standards (80). These standards address cultural adaptations and modifications in clinical processes (such as assessment, treatment planning, case management, and linguistic support) and system processes (such as staff training and development, access protocols, governance of service systems, quality assurance and improvement, and information management). There is beginning evidence that adopting such practices results in improved access to services and retention in treatment (77; also, see Chapter 2.2.1).

Prevention and the Problems of the Very Young

One of the guiding principles of CASSP is to promote early identification for children with emotional disturbances, and therefore communities bear responsibility to assign some of their resources to prevention efforts (3). Examples of vulnerable populations include children experiencing violence, abuse, neglect, or other trauma, and children showing signs of depression or other mental health problems in the school or childcare setting. The integration of mental health services into schools, child welfare, and juvenile justice settings provides early intervention opportunities for children and youth with early symptoms of mental health disorders.

The early childhood population (generally aged 0 to 5 years, defined by their preschool-aged status) is a particularly vulnerable group of children for whom it has been shown that environmental risks can have significant long-term developmental impact, and that early intervention has the potential to be very beneficial over the long term (76). Until CMHS recently started funding of system-of-care projects for 0 to 6 year olds, the early childhood age group had not benefited from system-of-care reform (81). Since many agencies are involved with young children, the system-of-care model that promotes integrated planning and service strategies is extremely suitable for this age group. System-of-care integrated service strategies may include such activities as providing mental health consultation to Head Start, early intervention, primary care practitioners, community health nurses, and childcare workers; and providing mental health services to adults whose children are at risk of out-of-home placement. Examples of effective preventive approaches include nurse home visiting (82), referral to early intervention services, advocacy for stable placement, support for prenatal care, provision of substance abuse and mental health services and parenting supports to parents of infants at risk for abuse (83), and early mental health services for children at risk for psychiatric disturbance (84).

Barriers to these efforts persist, however, some of which are related to funding and eligibility for services. Mental health agencies may be unable to provide services to children who do not yet meet the full criteria for a mental health diagnosis, and addressing the parents' mental health or substance abuse issues may not be possible if they are uninsured. To address this issue, the state and local funding agencies need to adopt alternative eligibility criteria for services, have contractual agreements with other child-serving agencies that obviate the need for formal diagnosis, or allow the parent to be the recipient of services. For young children who are already showing some early symptoms of disorder, use of a more age-appropriate Diagnostic System for Zero to Three, Revised (DC:0–3R; 85) is more likely to identify conditions making them eligible for services. A crosswalk to ICD-9 diagnoses is needed for billing under the Medicaid system, however. States such as Maine, Florida, Washington, and California have developed crosswalks from DC:0–3 to ICD-9 diagnoses as part of their statewide early childhood plans. The state of Louisiana has developed a statewide program of infant and early childhood services targeted at its child welfare population (83). One barrier is that there are few clinicians trained to diagnose and treat mental health conditions in very young children. States are beginning to invest resources in training to improve the skills of early childhood clinicians.

Challenges in Replication on a Larger Scale

The greatest challenge experienced by system-of-care demonstration programs is how to sustain the model after the grant period ends. Without external funding, the system often reverts to fragmentation and lack of coordination due to the separate funding and organizational structures of mental health, education, juvenile justice, child welfare, developmental disabilities, and substance abuse services. More recent system-of-care projects have benefited from lessons learned as to how to build in sustainability factors early in their projects. Some of the factors supporting sustainability include developing specific targeted outcomes agreed upon by all stakeholders from the outset, developing effective strategies for tracking and reporting those outcomes, and "social marketing," informing the wider community and legislature of successes of the project in socially meaningful terms (15,86,87).

An additional potentially daunting challenge is how to replicate a small demonstration project on a larger scale that addresses an entire population at a community or state level. It is generally not fiscally viable to apply all aspects of the model on a large scale. For example, regular meetings of interagency teams are costly in terms of personnel time, and may not be needed for children at lower levels of severity. Yet, the systems-level data are not robust enough to guide decision as to which elements of the model to select for the larger population. Thus, states have chosen different elements to implement on a larger scale.

The pediatric collaborative access programs previously described are an example of statewide implementation of one element of systems-of-care design. Some states have implemented statewide versions of wraparound planning programs with intensive in-home services as the front-line intervention. An example of larger scale state implementation to address a particular population need is the Tennessee Centers of Excellence for Children in State Custody. This network of consulting centers located at pediatric medical centers throughout the state is dedicated to address the mental health needs of children in state custody and at-risk of entering custody. They collaborate with regional child welfare agencies in providing case consultation on treatment planning (using the wraparound model), diagnostic evaluation, and pharmacotherapy consultation and services. However, as the centers noted the dearth of child evidence-based practices being delivered to children in custody, they took on the challenge of disseminating key evidence-based practices through statewide trainings, such as trauma-focused cognitive behavioral therapy, PCIT, early infant interventions, and interventions for sexually offending youth. The Centers have been highly successful at directly and indirectly serving thousands of children and youth and were awarded the Silver Service Achievement Award by the American Psychiatric Association (88).

Response to Challenges

There has also been active support for system-of-care reform efforts by professional organizations such as the Academy of Child and Adolescent Psychiatry (AACAP), which in 1994 established a Work Group (now Committee) on Community-Based Systems of Care. The AACAP Committee on Community-Based Systems of Care has developed policy guidelines on relevant topics, including structure of Medicaid managed care programs, training and roles of mental health professionals toward systems of care, outcomes in systems of care, and early childhood systems of care. It has developed tools for assessing service intensity need using a community-based paradigm, and systems-based practice educational materials (38,45,74,75,89).

Systems-of-care reforms have also occurred at the state level. Incremental changes have occurred in many states through national trends, such as managed care Medicaid and the advent of Medicaid waivers that have allowed for innovations and more flexible use of treatment dollars (90). However, reforms associated with managed care Medicaid have not always been positive, as privatization of Medicaid has resulted in some instances in attenuation rather than expansion of appropriate community-based services (44). Some states have legislated very expansive systems reform. For example, Hawaii provides an integrated services model through providing mental health services in schools throughout the state. It has also implemented evidence-based interventions on a wide scale, developing its own classification system for levels of evidence for each treatment modality by diagnosis, and analysis of effective components of each treatment model (91). Hawaii also adopted the Child and Adolescent Service Intensity Instrument (CASII) (92) for statewide use as a treatment planning and outcome measure. The CASII is a tool that provides a uniform procedure for assessment and planning intensity of service need using a community-based systems-of-care paradigm.

A more promising model for funding and service organizations is that proposed by the Affordable Care Act (93). Passed by Congress in 2009, it is a large legislative omnibus bill that attempts to address the United States' chronic problem with lack of insurance coverage for a significant portion of its population. It includes two key provisions that address many challenges posed by systems-of-care reform. First, it includes mental health parity, that is, the equivalent coverage of health and mental health services, a goal that has been pursued by advocates for years. Parity includes coverage going beyond the traditional inpatient–outpatient services and includes coverage of intermediate intensity, community-based services. Furthermore, it promotes the development of "accountable care organizations" which, over time, would be incentivized and reimbursed for clinical outcomes and cost-efficiency, and for a covered population's overall health and function. Such reimbursement and organizational models are totally congruent with the community-based system-of-care model and will hopefully help promote its fuller implementation.

CONCLUSION

The CASSP defined a system-of-care approach to providing mental health and related services to children and adolescents with serious emotional and behavioral disturbances. It has had a major influence on community systems of care through extensive federally funded projects, along with state and national initiatives that have embraced CASSP values. The system-of-care model emphasizes that care should be tailored to the individual needs and strengths of the child and family, culturally competent, coordinated, and integrated, and provided in the most community-based and least restrictive setting that meets their needs. Integrated system-of-care approaches to service delivery have produced favorable outcomes in reducing use of residential and out-of-state placements and achieving improvements in functional behavior in youth with severe emotional and behavioral disorders who are served in multiple systems. Family and consumer organizations, now strengthened by youth participation, have made substantial contributions to the reform of mental health care in this country.

In many ways, the CASSP and community system-of-care movement and model has been a forerunner for the population health and accountable care models being promoted by health care reformers and within the Affordable Care Act (93). In this vein, children's community mental health has much to share with the rest of health care around consumer-driven, community-based, and preventive approaches, striking a balance between individual and family health and population health.

References

1. Lourie I: A history of community child mental health. In: Pumariega AJ, Winters NC (eds): *Handbook of Community-Based Systems of Care: The new Child and Adolescent Community Psychiatry.* New York, Jossey-Bass, 2003.
2. Knitzer J, Olson L: *Unclaimed Children: The Failure of Public Responsibility to Children and Adolescents in Need of Mental Health Services.* Washington, DC, Children's Defense Fund, 1982.
3. Stroul BA, Friedman RM: *A System of Care for Severely Emotionally Disturbed Children and Youth.* Washington, DC, Georgetown University Child Development Center, CASSP Technical Assistance Center, 1986.
4. Comprehensive Community Mental Health Services for Children and Their Families Program. Evaluation Findings: Annual Report to Congress. Center for Mental Health Services, Substance Abuse and Mental Health Services Administration, U.S. Department of Health and Human Services, 2011. (Publication No. PEP-13-CMHI2011)
5. U.S. Department of Health and Human Services: *Mental Health: A Report of the Surgeon General.* Washington, DC, Center for Mental Health Services, Substance Abuse and Mental Health Services Administration, U.S. Department of Health and Human Services, 1999.
6. Pumariega A, Nace D, England M, et al.: Community-based systems approach to children's managed mental health services. *J Child Family Stud* 6:149–164, 1997.
7. Heffron W, Pumariega AJ, Fallon T Jr, Carter D: Youth in the juvenile justice system. In: Pumariega AJ, Winters NC (eds): *Handbook of Community-Based Systems of Care: The New Child and Adolescent Community Psychiatry.* New York, Jossey-Bass, 224–249, 2003.
8. Vaughan T, Pumariega AJ, Klaehn R: Systems of care under legal mandates. In: Pumariega AJ, Winters NC (eds): *Handbook of Child and Adolescent Systems of Care: The New Community Psychiatry.* San Francisco, Jossey-Bass, 414–431, 2003.
9. Atkins DL, Pumariega AJ, Montgomery L, et al.: Mental health and incarcerated youth. I: prevalence and nature of psychopathology. *J Child Family Stud* 8:193, 1999.
10. Teplin LA, Abram KM, McClelland GM, Dulcan MK, Mericle AA: Psychiatric disorders in youth in juvenile detention. *Arch Gen Psychiatr* 59:1133–1143, 2002.
11. Pumariega AJ, Atkins DL, Rogers K, et al.: Mental health and incarcerated youth. II: service utilization in incarcerated youth. *J Child Family Stud* 8:205, 1999.
12. Rogers K, Pumariega AJ, Atkins DL, Cuffe S: Factors associated with identification of mentally ill youth in the juvenile justice system. *Community Mental Health J* 42(1):25–40, 2006.
13. Rogers K, Powell E, Zima B, Pumariega AJ: Who receives mental health services in the juvenile justice system. *J Child Family Stud* 10(4):485–494, 2001.
14. Henngeler S, Sheidow A: Empirically supported family-based treatments for conduct disorder and delinquency in adolescents. *Marital Fam Ther* 38(1):30–58, 2012.
15. Holden EW, Santiago RL, Manteuffel BA, et al.: Systems of care model demonstration projects: innovation, evaluation, and sustainability. In: Pumariega AJ, Winters NC (eds): *Handbook of Child and Adolescent Systems of Care: The New Community Psychiatry.* San Francisco, Jossey-Bass, 432–459, 2003.
16. U.S. Department of Health and Human Services: *Youth Violence: A Report of the Surgeon General.* Center for Mental Health Services, Substance Abuse and Mental Health Services Administration, U.S. Department of Health and Human Services, Washington, DC, 2001a.
17. Marx K, Benoit M, Kamradt B: Foster children in the child welfare system. In: Pumariega AJ, Winters NC (eds): *Handbook of Child and Adolescent Systems of Care: The New Community Psychiatry.* San Francisco, Jossey-Bass, 332–352, 2003.
18. Nordhaus BF, Solnit AJ: Foster placement. *Child Adolesc Psychiatr Clin N Am* 7:345–356, 1998.
19. Fontanella C, Warner L, Phillips G, Bridge J, Campo J. Trends in psychotropic polypharmacy among youths enrolled in Ohio Medicaid, 2002–2008. *Psychiatr Serv* 65:1332–1340, 2014.
20. American Academy of Child and Adolescent Psychiatry and Child Welfare League of America: *Joint Policy Statement on Mental Health Screening and Evaluation of Children in Foster Care.* Washington, DC, Author, 2002.
21. Foa EB, Keane TM, Friedman MJ, Cohen JA: *Effective Treatments for PTSD: Practice Guidelines from the International Society for Traumatic Stress Studies.* 2nd ed. New York, NY, Guilford Press, 2009.
22. Porter G, Pearson G, Keenan S, Duval-Harvey J: School-based mental health services: a necessity, not a luxury. In: Pumariega AJ, Winters NC (eds): *Handbook of Child and Adolescent Systems of Care: The New Community Psychiatry.* San Francisco, Jossey-Bass, 250–275, 2003.
23. Flaherty L, Weist M, Warner B: School-based mental health services in the United States: history, current models, and needs. *Comm Ment Health J* 32:341–352, 1996.
24. Stone-Motes P, Melton G, Pumariega AJ, Simmons W: Ecologically oriented school-based mental health services: implications for service system reform. *Psychol in the Schools* 36(5):391–402, 1999.
25. Schacht T, Hansen G: The evolving climate for school mental health services under the Individual with Disabilities Education Act. *Psychol in the Schools* 36:415–426, 1999.
26. O'Malley K: Youth with co-morbid disorders. In: Pumariega AJ, Winters NC (eds): *Handbook of Child and Adolescent Systems of Care: The New Community Psychiatry.* San Francisco, Jossey-Bass, 276–315, 2003.
27. Asarnow JR, Jaycox LH, Duan N, et al.: Depression and role impairment among adolescents in primary care clinics. *J Adolesc Health* 37:477–483, 2005.
28. Grimes K: Collaboration with primary care: sharing risks, goals, and outcomes in an integrated system of care. In: Pumariega AJ, Winters NC (eds): *Handbook of Child and Adolescent Systems of Care: The New Community Psychiatry.* New York, Jossey-Bass, 316–331, 2003.
29. Sarvet B, Gold J, Bostic J, et al.: Improving access to mental health care for children: The Massachusetts Child Psychiatry Access Project. *Pediatrics* 126:1191–1200, 2010.
30. Sarvet B, Gold J, Straus JH: Bridging the divide between child psychiatry and primary care: the use of telephone consultation within a population-based collaborative system. *Child Adolesc Psychiatr Clin N Am* 20(1):41–53, 2011.
31. American Psychiatric Association: *Diagnostic and Statistical Manual for Mental Disorders.* 5th ed. Washington, DC, APA Publishing, 2013.
32. Silver S, Duchnowski A, Kutash K, et al.: A comparison of children with serious emotional disturbance served in residential and school settings. *J Child Fam Stud* 1:43–59, 1992.
33. Osher T, de Fur E, Nava C, Spencer S, Toth-Dennis D: New roles for families in systems of care. In: *Systems of Care: Promising Practices in Children's Mental Health.* Vol I. Washington, DC, Center for Effective Collaboration and Practice, American Institutes for Research, 1998.
34. Huffine C, Anderson D: Family advocacy development in systems of care. In: Pumariega AJ, Winters NC (eds): *Handbook of Child and Adolescent Systems of Care: The New Community Psychiatry.* San Francisco, Jossey-Bass, 35–65, 2003.
35. Federation of families for children's mental health web page: family leadership in systems of care. Available at: www.ffcmh.org/ systems whatis.htm. Accessed January 2006.
36. Winters NC, Terrell L: Case management: the linchpin of community-based systems of care. In: Pumariega AJ, Winters NC (eds): *Handbook of Child and Adolescent Systems of Care: The New Community Psychiatry.* San Francisco, Jossey-Bass, 171–202, 2003.
37. VanDenBerg JE, Grealish EM: Individualized services and supports through the wraparound process: philosophy and procedures. *J Child and Family Stud* 5:7–21, 1996.
38. Winters NC, Pumariega AJ; Work Group on Community-Based Systems of Care; Committee on Community Psychiatry; Work Group on Quality Issues: Practice parameter on child and adolescent mental health care in community systems of care. *J Am Acad Child Adolesc Psychiatry* 46(2):284–299, 2007.
39. Burns BJ, Hoagwood K: *Community Treatment for Youth: Evidence-Based Interventions for Severe Emotional and Behavioral Disorders.* New York, Oxford University Press, 2002.
40. Solnit AJ, Adnopoz J, Saxe L, Gardner J, Fallon T: Evaluating systems of care for children: utility of the clinical case conference. *Am J Orthopsychiatry* 67:554–567, 1997.
41. Burchard JD, Bruns JD, Burchard SN: The wraparound approach. In: Burns BJ, Hoagwood K (eds): *Community Treatment for Youth: Evidence-Based Interventions for Severe Emotional and Behavioral Disorders.* New York, Oxford University Press, 2002.
42. Farmer EM, Dorsey S, Mustillo SA: Intensive home and community interventions. *Child Adolesc Psychiatr Clin N Am* 13:857–884, 2004.
43. Bruns EJ, Burchard JD, Suter JC, Leverentz-Bracy K, Force MM: Assessing fidelity to a community-based treatment for youth: The Wraparound Fidelity Index. *J Emotional Behav Disorders* 12:79–89, 2004.
44. Winters NC, Marx L, Pumariega AJ: Systems of care and managed care: are they compatible? In: Pumariega AJ, Winters NC (eds): *Handbook of Child and Adolescent Systems of Care: The New Community Psychiatry.* San Francisco, Jossey-Bass, 380–413, 2003.
45. American Academy of Child and Adolescent Psychiatry: *Guidelines for Training Towards Community-Based Systems of Care for Children With Serious Emotional Disturbances.* Washington, DC, Author, 1996.
46. U.S. Department of Health and Human Services: *New Freedom Commission on Mental Health: Achieving the promise: Transforming mental health care in America.* Rockville, MD, Department of Health and Human Services, 2003. Available at: http://govinfo.library.unt.edu/mentalhealthcommission/reports/reports.htm
47. Hoagwood K, Burns B, Kiser L, Ringeisen H, Schoenwald S: Evidence-based practice in child and adolescent mental health services. *Psychiatr Serv* 52:1179–1189, 2001.
48. Kazdin AE: Evidence-based treatments: challenges and priorities for practice and research. *Child Adolesc Psychiatr Clin N Am* 13:923–940, 2004.
49. Chamberlain P: Treatment foster care. In: Burns BJ, Hoagwood K (eds): *Community Treatment for Youth: Evidence-Based Interventions for Severe Emotional and Behavioral Disorders.* New York, Oxford University Press, 2002.

50. Dishion T, McCord J, Poulin J: When interventions harm: peer groups and problem behavior. *Am Psychol* 54:755–764, 1999.
51. Henggeler SW, Schoenwald SK, Rowland MD, Cunningham PB: *Multisystemic Treatment of Children and Adolescents with Serious Emotional Disturbance.* New York, Guilford Press, 2001.
52. Henggeler SW, Rowland MD, Halliday-Boykins C, et al.: One-year follow-up of multisystemic therapy as an alternative to the hospitalization of youths in crisis. *J Am Acad Child Adolesc Psychiatry* 42:543–551, 2003.
53. Sexton T, Turner C: The effectiveness of Functional Family Therapy for youth with behavioral problems in a community practice setting. *J Fam Psychol* 24(3):339–348, 2010.
54. Dubois DL, Holloway BE, Valentine JC, Cooper H: Effectiveness of mentoring programs for youth: a meta-analytic review. *Am J Community Psychol* 30:157–197, 2002.
55. Bruns EJ, Burchard JD: Impact of respite care services for families with children experiencing emotional and behavioral problems. *Children's Services: Social Policy, Research, and Practice* 3:29–61, 2000.
56. Rogers K: Evidence-based community-based interventions. In: Pumariega AJ, Winters NC (eds): *Handbook of Child and Adolescent Systems of Care: The New Community Psychiatry.* San Francisco, Jossey-Bass, 149–170, 2003.
57. Weisz JR: Lab-clinic differences and what we can do about them. I. The clinic-based treatment development model. *Clinical Child Psychol Newsletter* 15, 2000.
58. Pumariega AJ, Fallon T: Psychopharmacology in systems of care. In: Pumariega AJ, Winters NC (eds): *Handbook of Child and Adolescent Systems of Care: The New Community Psychiatry.* San Francisco, Jossey-Bass, 120–148, 2003.
59. Zima BT, Hurlburt MS, Knapp P, et al.: Quality of publicly funded outpatient specialty mental health care for common childhood psychiatric disorders in California. *J Am Acad Child Adolesc Psychiatry* 44:130–144, 2005.
60. Lawson W, Lake J, Malik M, Joshi S: Culturally adapted pharmacotherapy and the integrative formulation. *Child Adolesc Psychiatric Clin N Am* 19:791–814, 2010.
61. Attkisson C, Rosenblatt AB, Dresser KL, Baize HR, Clausen JM, Lind SL: Effectiveness of the California system of care model for children and youth with severe emotional disorders. In: Nixon CT, Northrup CA (eds): *Evaluating Mental Health Services: How do Programs for Children Work in the Real World?* Thousand Oaks, CA, Sage, 146–208, 1997.
62. Bruns E, Burchard J, Yoe J: Evaluating the Vermont system of care: outcomes associated with community-based wraparound services. *J Child Family Stud* 4:321, 1995.
63. Bickman L, Summerfelt WT, Noser K: Comparative outcomes of emotionally disturbed children and adolescents in a system of services and usual care. *Psychiatr Serv* 48:1543–1548, 1997.
64. Hoagwood K, Burns BJ, Kiser L, Ringeisen H, Schoenwald SK: Evidence-based practice in child and adolescent mental health services. *Psychiat Serv* 52:1179–1189, 2001.
65. Santarcangelo S, Bruns EJ, Yoe JT: New directions: evaluating Vermont's statewide model of individualized care. In: Epstein MH, Kutash K, Duchnowski AJ (eds): *Outcomes for Children and Youth with Behavioral and Emotional Disorders and Their Families: Programs and Evaluation best Practices.* Austin, TX, Pro-Ed, 55–80, 1998.
66. Rosenblatt A: Assessing the child and family outcomes of systems of care for youth with severe emotional and behavioral disturbance. In: Epstein MH, Kutash K, Duchnowski AJ (eds): *Outcomes for Children and Youth with Behavioral and Emotional Disorders and Their Families: Programs and Evaluation best Practices.* Austin, TX, Pro-Ed, 55–80, 1998.
67. Foster EM, Connor T: Public cost of better mental health services for children and adolescents. *Psychiatr Serv* 56:50–55, 2005.
68. Hernandez M, Gomez A, Lipien L, Greenbaum PE, Armstrong KH, Gonzalez P: Use of the system-of-care practice review in the national evaluation: evaluating the fidelity of practice to system-of-care principles. *J Emotional and Behavioral Disorders* 9:43–52, 2001.
69. Stephens RL, Connor T, Nguyen H, Holden EW, Greenbaum P, Foster EM: The longitudinal comparison study of the national evaluation of the Comprehensive Community Mental Health Services for Children and Their Families Program. In: Epstein MH, Kutash K, Duchnowski AJ (eds): *Outcomes for Children and Youth with Emotional and Behavioral Disorders and Their Families: Programs and Evaluation Best Practices.* Austin, TX, Pro-Ed, Inc., 2005.
70. Kamradt B, Meyers MJ: Curbing violence in juvenile offenders with serious emotional and mental health needs: the effective utilization of wraparound approaches in an American urban setting. *Intl J Adolesc Med Health* 11:381–399, 1999.
71. Pires SA, Grimes KE, Allen KD, Gilmer T, Mahadevan RM: *Faces of Medicaid: Examining Children's Behavioral Health Service Utilization and Expenditures.* Hamilton, NJ, Center for Health Care Strategies, 2013.
72. Paradise J: *Medicaid Moving Forward.* Kaiser Family Foundation, 2013. Available at: http://kff.org/health-reform/issue-brief/medicaid-moving-forward. Accessed March 6, 2016.
73. Heflinger CA, Northrup DA: What happens when capitated behavioral health comes to town? The transition from the Fort Bragg demonstration to a capitated managed behavioral health contract. *J Behav Health Services and Research* 27:390–405, 2000.
74. American Academy of Child and Adolescent Psychiatry: *Best Principles for Measuring Outcomes in Managed Medicaid Mental Health Programs.* Washington, DC, Author, 1998.
75. American Academy of Child and Adolescent Psychiatry: *Best Principles for Managed Medicaid RFP's.* Washington, DC, Author, 1996.
76. Shonkoff J, Phillips D: *From Neurons to Neighborhoods: The Science of Early Childhood Development. Committee on Integrating the Science of Early Childhood Development, Board on Children, Youth, and Families, Commission on Behavioral and Social Sciences and Education, National Research Council and Institute of Medicine.* Washington, DC, National Academy Press, 2000.
77. Pumariega AJ, Rothe E, Mian A, et al.: Practice parameter for cultural competence in child and adolescent psychiatric practice. *J Am Acad Child Adolesc Psychiatry* 52(10):1101–1115, 2013.
78. Kann L, Kinchen S, Shanklin S, et al.: Youth Risk Behavior Surveillance—United States, 2013. *MMWR Suppl* 63(4):1–168, 2014.
79. U.S. Department of Health and Human Services: *Culture, Race, and Ethnicity: A Supplement to Mental Health: A Report of the Surgeon General.* Washington, DC, Center for Mental Health Services, Substance Abuse and Mental Health Services Administration, U.S. Department of Health and Human Services, 2001b.
80. Panels FR: *Cultural Competence Standards for Managed Mental Health Services for Four Underserved/Underrepresented Racial/Ethnic Groups.* Rockville, MD, Center for Mental Health Services, Substance Abuse and Mental Health Administration, U.S. Department of Health and Human Services, 1999.
81. Cooper J, Aratani Y, Knitzer J, et al.: *Unclaimed Children: The Status of Children's Mental Health Policy in the United States.* New York, NY: National Center for Children in Poverty, Columbia University, 2008.
82. Olds DL, Pettitt LM, Robinson J, et al.: Reducing the risks for antisocial behavior with a program of prenatal and early childhood home visitation. *J Community Psychol* 26:65–83, 1998.
83. Zeanah CH, Larrieu JA, Heller SS, et al.: Evaluation of a preventive intervention for maltreated infants and toddlers in foster care. *J Am Acad Child Adol Psychiat* 40:214–221, 2001.
84. Webster-Stratton C, Reid MJ, Hammond M: Treating children with early-onset conduct problems: intervention outcomes for parent, child, and teacher training. *J Clin Child Adoles Psychol* 33:105–124, 2004.
85. Emde RN, Egger H, Fenichel E, Guedeney A, Wise BK, Wright HH: *ZERO TO THREE: Diagnostic Classification of Mental Health and Developmental Disorders of Infancy and Early Childhood.* Rev ed. Arlington, VA, ZERO TO THREE/National Center for Clinical Infant Programs, 2005.
86. Friesen BJ, Winters NC: The role of outcomes in systems of care: quality improvement and program evaluation. In: Pumariega AJ, Winters NC (eds): *Handbook of Community-Based Systems of Care: The New Child and Adolescent Community Psychiatry.* New York, Jossey-Bass, 459–486, 2003.
87. Woodbridge M, Furlong MJ, Casa JM, Sosna TS: Santa Barbara's multiagency integrated system of care. In: Hernandez M, Hodges S (eds): *Developing Outcome Strategies in Children's Mental Health Programs.* Baltimore, MD, Paul Brooke Publishing, 2001.
88. Moser M, Dean K, Todd J, Ebert J, Pumariega AJ: Centers of Excellence: a systems-building model for children in state custody. *Adolescent Psychiatry* 4(4):251–260.
89. Pumariega AJ, Winters NC (eds): *Handbook of Child and Adolescent Systems of Care: The New Community Psychiatry.* San Francisco, Jossey Bass, 2003.
90. Daleiden EL, Chorpita BF: From data to wisdom: quality improvement strategies supporting large-scale implementation of evidence-based services. *Child Adolesc Psychiatr Clin N Am* 14:329–349, 2005.
91. Stroul BA, Pires SA, Armstrong MI: *Health Care Reform Tracking Project: Tracking State Health Care Reforms as They Affect Children and Adolescents with Behavioral Health Disorders and Their Families—2000 State Survey.* Tampa, FL, Research and Training Center for Children's Mental Health, Department of Child and Family Studies, Division of State and Local Support, Louis de la Parte Florida Mental Health Institute,University of South Florida, 2001.
92. American Academy of Child and Adolescent Psychiatry: *Child and Adolescent Service Intensity Instrument.* Washington, DC, Author, 2004.
93. Katon W, Unützer J: Health reform and the Affordable Care Act: the importance of mental health treatment to achieving the triple aim. *J Psychosom Res* 74(6):533–537, 2013.

CHAPTER 6.3.5 ■ TELEPSYCHIATRY WITH CHILDREN AND ADOLESCENTS

KATHLEEN MYERS AND DAVID E. ROTH

OVERVIEW

Telemedicine services are increasingly used to meet the treatment needs of children and adolescents who live in underserved communities (1). The Centers for Medicare and Medicaid Services (CMS) define *telehealth* as the use of telecommunications and information technology (IT) to provide access to health assessment, diagnosis, intervention, consultation, supervision, and information across distance (2). CMS notes that "for purposes of Medicaid, *telemedicine* seeks to improve a patient's health by permitting two-way, real-time interactive communication between the patient, and the physician or the practitioner at the distant site. This electronic communication means the use of interactive telecommunications equipment that includes, at a minimum, audio and video equipment" (3). When telemedicine is used to provide psychiatric—or more generally mental health—services, the terms "telepsychiatry" and "telemental health" (TMH), respectively are used (4–6). As telepsychiatry is not a specialty area but a mode of service delivery, and as the trend nationally is to consider telepsychiatry services equivalent to in-person services, we use the term "provider" to refer to psychiatrists using either mode of service delivery.

DEVELOPMENT OF CHILD AND ADOLESCENT TELEPSYCHIATRY

The Case for Telepsychiatry

The past two decades have brought considerable insights into the early onset of psychopathology, new approaches to pharmacologic treatment, and the development of effective psychotherapies for youth. Yet, most young people with psychiatric disorders do not receive these evidence-based treatments (EBTs), particularly youth living outside of major metropolitan areas (7,8). Furthermore, this discrepancy in access to care is anticipated to grow due to the "aging out effect" of the current psychiatric workforce while fewer medical students choose careers in psychiatry (9,10) and federal mandates have broadened children's eligibility for mental health services (11). According to the United States Bureau of Health Professions, the United States will have only two-thirds of the child and adolescent psychiatrists required to meet needs in 2020 (12).

Federal mandates for mental health care reform have converged with technologic innovations to make telepsychiatry a viable service delivery model for youth who are underserved by traditional models of care. The *Federal Health IT Strategic Plan: 2015–2020* (13) has prioritized the adoption of meaningful health IT with focus on delivery of behavioral health services and reforming payment systems.

The Expansion of Telepsychiatry

As for many other technology-facilitated domains, the practice of telepsychiatry has quickly expanded beyond the intended goal of rectifying disparities for distant communities (14–16). Telepsychiatry services are increasingly offered in diverse settings, including urban and inner city communities (17), mental health centers and other child-serving facilities (15,18,19), correctional settings (20,21), schools (22,23), and the home (24). Telepsychiatry may be a career choice for child and adolescent psychiatrists. For example, those with expertise in treating selected disorders (e.g., obsessive-compulsive disorder [OCD]), cultural/language populations (e.g., Hispanics, Alaska Natives), or relocated groups (e.g., military, refugees, disaster survivors) may seek to export their practices beyond usual constraints of office practice. Other enterprising child and adolescent psychiatrists may enjoy the alternative professional lifestyle that telepsychiatry offers.

THE EVIDENCE-BASED SUPPORTING TELEPSYCHIATRY

The evidence-base supporting telepsychiatry as an effective service-delivery model is well developed with adults and emerging gradually with children and adolescents. Support may be gleaned from reports on the feasibility and acceptability of telepsychiatry with youth, and several outcomes studies, summarized in Table 6.3.5.1, and briefly summarized.

Some providers suggest that telepsychiatry may be especially suited for adolescents who are accustomed to the technology and may respond to the personal space and feeling of control allowed by videoconferencing (22,46) and have decreased concerns about confidentiality as the provider is outside of the local community (27,54).

Multiple studies have demonstrated the feasibility of implementing telepsychiatry services with young people across diverse settings (14–16,19,50,55–59). Youth 2 to 21 years old with a broad range of behavioral health diagnoses and developmental disorders have been evaluated through videoconferencing (15,19,47,49,55). School-aged children comprise the modal age group, and attention-deficit/hyperactivity disorder (ADHD) and depression are the most commonly treated disorders, consistent with in-person care (15,19,25). Children who are uncooperative pose challenges but can be treated with assistance by staff at the patient site. Providers determine the appropriateness of youth for care via telepsychiatry based on developmental considerations, parents' preferences, supports at the patient site, and the provider's resourcefulness.

Diagnostic assessments have been reliably conducted through videoconferencing (15,42,44,47), including disruptive behavior disorders (28), autism and other developmental disorders (49,52), and psychotic disorders (48). Multiple studies

TABLE 6.3.5.1

EVIDENCE-BASED SUPPORTING SERVICES TO CHILDREN AND ADOLESCENTS THROUGH VIDEOTELECONFERENCING (VTC)

Citation	Sample	Assessment	Findings
Randomized Controlled Trials			
Nelson et al., 2003 (25)	28 youth (8–14 yrs) with depression	Diagnostic interview and rating scale	VTC and in-person treatment with comparable improvement of depressive symptoms
Storch et al., 2011 (26)	31 youth (age 7–16 yrs) with OCD	ADIS-IV-C/P, CY-BOCS, COIS, MASC, CDI, Satisfaction with services	VTC superior to in-person on all primary outcome measures
Himle et al., 2012 (27)	20 children (8–17 yrs) with Tic Disorders	YGTS, PTQ, CGI-S, CGI-I	VTC and in-person groups show comparable tic reduction
Myers et al., 2015 (28)	223 youth (5.5–12.9 yrs) with ADHD	DISC-IV, CBCL, VADPRS, VADTRS, CIS	Children in the VTC group with greater parent-rated improvement in ADHD-related behaviors than those in augmented PCP group. Teachers reported improvement in ODD and role performance, but not ADHD
Vander Stoep et al., 2017 (29)	223 caregivers of youth (5.5–12.9 yrs) with ADHD	Caregiver distress measures: PHQ-9, PSI, CSQ, FES	Caregivers of children in the VTC group reported greater improvements in distress measures than caregivers in the augmented PCP treatment group.
Rockhill et al., 2016 (30)	223 youth (5.5–12.9 yrs) and providers	DISC-IV, CBCL, VADPRS, telepsychiatrists', and PCP's prescribing patterns	Telepsychiatrists with high fidelity to protocols and more assertive in achieving 50% reduction in ADHD than PCPs
Tse et al., 2015 (31)	37 youth (5.5–12.9 yrs) of the larger 223 participant sample	VADPRS, PHQ-9, CSQ, PSI, FES, Satisfaction	VTC delivery of caregiver training was comparable to in-person delivery in improving children's ADHD symptoms but not caregivers' distress
Xie et al., 2013 (32)	22 children (6–14 yrs) with behavioral disorders	PCQ-CA, VADPRS, CGAS	Parent training through VTC was as effective as in-person
Pre-Post or Comparison Studies			
Glueckauf et al., 2002 (33)	22 adolescents (15.4 yrs) 36 parents	SSRS, WAI, issue-specific measures of family problems, adherence to treatment	Comparable improvement for intervention through VTC vs. in-person vs. speakerphone; therapeutic alliance high but teens rated alliance lower in VTC
Fox et al., 2008 (34)	190 youth (12–19 yrs) in detention	GAS	Improvement in the rate of attainment of goals associated with family relations and personality/behavior
Yellowlees et al., 2008 (35)	41 children in an e-mental health program	CBCL	A retrospective assessment of 3-mo outcomes found improvements in selected Domains of the CBCL
Reese et al., 2012 (36)	8 children (M = 7.6 yrs)	ADHD	Group Triple P Positive Parenting Program via VTC associated with improved child behavior and decreased parent distress
Satisfaction Studies			
Blackmon et al., 1997 (37)	43 children (2–15 yrs)	12-item Telemedicine Consultation Evaluation	All children and 98% of parents report satisfaction equal to in-person care
Elford et al., 2001 (38)	30 children (4–16 yrs)	Satisfaction Questionnaire	Psychiatrists, children, teens, parents, endorsed high satisfaction with VTC
Kopel et al., 2001 (39)	136 participants (age not specified—refers to "young person")	Satisfaction Questionnaire	High satisfaction by families and rural health workers in New South Wales, Australia
Greenberg et al., 2006 (40)	35 PCPs, 12 caregivers (mean age of children: 9.3 yrs)	Focus groups with PCPs, interviews with caregivers	PCP and caregiver satisfaction with VTC, limitations of local supports
Hilty et al., 2006 (41)	15 PCPs (400 children and adults)	PCP Satisfaction Survey	PCP satisfaction was high and increased over time
Myers et al., 2007 (19)	172 patients (2–21 yrs) and 387 visits	11-item Psychiatrist Satisfaction Survey	High satisfaction of PCPs, pediatricians more satisfied than family physicians
Myers et al., 2008 (16)	172 patients (2–21 yrs) and 387 visits	12-item Parent Satisfaction Survey	High satisfaction and increasing with return visits; lower satisfaction with care for teens than for children

TABLE 6.3.5.1

(CONTINUED)

Citation	Sample	Assessment	Findings
Myers et al., 2010 (42)	701 patients (7–19 yrs) and 190 PCPs	Collection of patient demographics and diagnoses	VTC with youth is feasible and acceptable; services vary with telepsychiatrists' practices
Pakyurek et al., 2010 (43)	5 case studies of youth in primary care	Effectiveness of VTC in treating a range of problems	VTC might be superior to in-person for selected groups
Lau et al., 2011 (44)	45 youth (3–17 yrs)	Description of patients referred for consultation, reason for consultation, treatment recommendations	VTC consultation provides diagnostic and treatment clarifications to a variety of children
Descriptive and Service Utilization			
Myers et al., 2004 (15)	159 youth (3–18 yrs)	Comparison VTC vs. in-person care on demographic and process variables	VTC patients were representative of in-person outpatients demographically, clinically, and by reimbursement
Myers et al., 2006 (21)	115 incarcerated youth (14–18 yrs)	11-item Teen Satisfaction Survey, medication management	Describes large series of incarcerated youth, including medication management
Jacob et al., 2012 (45)	15 children (4–18 yrs)	12-item Parent Satisfaction Survey	Patient satisfaction high and PCPs found recommendations helpful.
Nelson and Bui 2012 (46)	22 youth (M = 9.3 yrs)	Chart review	No factor inherent to the VC delivery mechanism impeded adherence to national ADHD guidelines
Diagnostic Validity			
Elford et al., 2000 (47)	25 children (4–16 yrs) with various diagnoses	Diagnostic interviews	96% concordance between VTC and in-person evaluations; comparable satisfaction
Stain et al., 2011 (48)	11 patients (14–30 yrs)	Diagnostic Interview for Psychosis, DIP	Strong correlation of assessments done VTC vs in-person
Reese et al., 2013 (49)	21 children (3–5 yrs)	ADOS—Module 1, ADI-R, Parent Satisfaction	VTC comparable to in-person for diagnostic accuracy, observations, parents' report of symptoms, and satisfaction
Other Relevant Studies			
Boydell et al., 2007 (50)	100 youth (2–17 yrs)	Chart review and interviews with case managers	Pros and cons of adherence
Shaikh et al., 2008 (51)	99 youth (1–17 yrs)	Review of patient medical records	VTC consultations associated with changes to diagnoses; repeated VTC consultations associated with improved weight-related status
Szeftel et al., 2012 (52)	45 patients (31 under 18 yrs) with developmental disabilities	Chart review—medication changes, frequency of appointments, diagnostic changes, symptom severity and improvement	VTC led to change of psychiatric diagnoses for 70% of patients, changed medication for 82% of patients, helped PCPs with treatment
Davis et al., 2013 (53)	58 youth (5–11 yrs)	Body mass index, 24-hr dietary recall, ActiGraph, CBCL, BPFAS	Two groups included and showed comparable improvements in BMI, nutrition, physical activity, and primary outcomes

ADI-R, Autism Diagnostic Interview—Revised; ADIS-IV-C/P, Anxiety Disorders Interview Schedule—Child/Parent Version; ADHD, attention-deficit/hyperactivity disorder; ADIS-IV-C/P, Anxiety Disorders Interview Scale—DSM-IV-Parent and Child Versions; ADOS, Autism Diagnostic Observation Scale; BPFAS, Behavioral Pediatrics Feeding Assessment Scale; CBCL, Child Behavior Checklist; CDI, Children's Depression Inventory; CGAS, Clinical Global Assessment Scale; CGI-I, Clinical Global Impressions of Improvement Scale; CGI-S, Clinical Global Impressions of Severity Scale; CIS, Columbia Impairment Scale; COIS, Child Obsessive Compulsive Impact Scale; CSQ, Caregiver Strain Questionnaire; CY-BOCS, Child Yale-Brown Obsessive Compulsive Scale; DIP, Diagnostic Interview for Psychosis; DISC-IV, Diagnostic Interview Scale for Children for DSM-IV; BMI, body mass index; FES, Family Empowerment Scale; GAS, Goal Attainment Scale; MASC, Multi-dimensional Anxiety Scale for Children; PCQ-CA, Parent Child Relationship Questionnaire; PTQ, Parent Tic Questionnaire; PCP, primary care provider; PHQ-9: Patient Health Questionnaire-9 Items; PSI: Parenting Stress Index; OCD: obsessive compulsive disorder; ODD: oppositional defiant disorder; SSRS, Social Skills Rating System (teen functioning); VADPRS, Vanderbilt ADHD Parent Rating Scale; VADTRS, Vanderbilt ADHD Teacher Rating Scale; VTC, videoteleconferencing; WAI, Working Alliance Inventory; YGTS, Yale Global Tic Severity Scale.

have demonstrated the acceptability to referring primary care providers (PCPs), parents, and youth of delivering services through videoconferencing (15,16,19,37–41,43–45,52). Satisfaction studies demonstrate the ability to develop a therapeutic alliance with youth and families during a virtual visit (60).

The delivery of pharmacotherapy through telepsychiatry has been described with youth in schools (61), mental health centers and daycare (17), outpatient settings (15,16,19,42), and juvenile justice facilities (20,21). One recent large community-based randomized trial provides solid evidence of the effectiveness of short- term pharmacotherapy for ADHD delivered by child and adolescent providers compared to treatment in primary care (28). Further, providers demonstrated good adherence to guideline-based pharmacotherapy (30).

There is a strong literature supporting the feasibility of conducting psychotherapy with adults through videoconferencing (62–66) and a developing literature supporting outcomes that are comparable to care delivered in-person (63). Most studies of psychotherapy conducted with young people have been descriptive (14,58,65). Nelson and Patton identified 10 psychotherapy studies (65). Intervention approaches varied in focus on the youth or the parent and ranged from feasibility trials to pre-post designs, and a few controlled trials. Findings were overall positive related to feasibility, satisfaction, and outcomes. This review also identified several case reports and small pilot studies on psychosomatic medicine, addressing mental health approaches for youth with acute and chronic medical conditions, including obesity (51,53).

Several randomized trials of psychotherapy are noteworthy. Nelson et al. found comparable reductions for childhood depressive symptoms treated with eight sessions of cognitive-behavioral therapy (CBT) delivered through videoconferencing versus in-person (25). Storch et al. tested the effectiveness of treatment for OCD and found superior outcomes to children treated in-person (26). The behavioral treatment of tics through telepsychiatry has been found to be comparable to in-person treatment (27). Four small randomized controlled trials have demonstrated the effectiveness of providing family interventions (31–33,36). A recent case report describes family-based interventions for eating disorders (67).

LEGAL, REGULATORY, AND ETHICAL ISSUES

Licensure is a complex issue. The 10th Amendment of the United States Constitution grants the individual States control over establishing and enforcing licensure requirements for health care professionals (68). The potential of telepsychiatry to deliver care across boundaries has challenged the limits of the state-based licensure system and stimulated discussion of alternative approaches such as national licensure, specific telemedicine licensure, and reciprocity of licensure (69). However, movement on this issue is slow.

National organizations differ in their policies and guidelines. While the Federation of State Medical Boards requires physicians to be licensed in the state where the patient is located, it supports the creation of an "interstate compact" licensure system (70), while the American Medical Association supports the existing state-based licensure system. The American Telemedicine Association (ATA) guidelines recommend that health professionals comply with all laws and regulations in both the patient's and provider's sites (71). Some states allow reciprocity of license to neighboring states (72). Providers should check with the requirements of the state medical boards where they plan to deliver services.

Location of Telepsychiatry Services vary by state with respect to the physical location of both the patient and the provider. Generally approved sites include medical and mental health facilities. More variably approved are assisted living facilities, schools, other community sites, and the home. Special approvals may be negotiated with payers. There is a trend toward broadening state and federal guidelines for reimbursement for services delivered to schools and removing the requirement of a defined distance from available on-site services (73). Several states require a "presenter," or "telepresenter," to accompany the patient (73,74).

Authentication of the parties involved in a telepsychiatry encounter ensures accuracy of service delivery and protects against fraud. During the initial encounter with a patient, the provider should collect identifying information about the patient, including location (75). If the patient site is a health care facility, the staff may verify the patient's identity. Typically, providers begin the initial session by stating their name, credentials, and location (city and state). Such information is included in the documentation.

Privacy and Security must comply with the Health Insurance Portability and Accountability Act of 1996 (HIPAA) (76). Compliance is not achieved by following a simple checklist of technical requirements. Software vendors enter into a Business Associate Agreement with HIPAA attesting their due diligence to protect patient privacy and data and agree to an audit of patient health information if a security breach occurs. Potential providers should determine whether a technology vendor is compliant with HIPAA requirements and check relevant state privacy laws that may have more stringent requirements.

Informed Consent also involves a process that varies by state regarding the need for specific consent to receive services through videoconferencing (5). Some elements for consent include: confidentiality and the limits to confidentiality when using electronic communications; potential for technical failure, emergency plans; documentation, recording, and storage of information; protocols for coordination of care with other professionals and contact between sessions; and conditions under which services are terminated and a referral for in-person care made (77).

Emergency Care is a highly desired service for underserved communities. Local civil commitment laws, duty to warn/protect requirements, and mandated reporting of child endangerment vary by jurisdiction. Providers and staff prepare a crisis plan with the family and staff share the plan with other members of the patient's system of care. These crisis procedures are discussed at the initial encounter or as part of informed consent (78). The role of the parent in emergency service planning must consider age of consent.

Ethical Issues in telepsychiatry parallel issues encountered in traditional in-person services. The core ethical goal to protect the patient remains paramount (75,79–81).

TECHNICAL ASPECTS OF TELEPSYCHIATRY

Telecommunications technology refers to the technical methods, or protocols, used to establish a synchronous connection (82,83). The visual and auditory quality of the data must be good enough for the provider and patient to feel it has been an authentic medical experience. Selecting the best technology can be a daunting process because the technology is rapidly changing and many vendors offer a wide range of commercial plans.

Start the selection process by prioritizing the features and functions needed to deliver the clinical services. Second, consider the budget, staffing resources, and startup timetable. Third, decide if the program needs to connect to an existing videoconferencing network. The clinical goals of the program should influence the selection of technology, as specific clinical services and populations may require different technologies. For example, diagnosing genetic and neurodevelopmental disorders may require higher-resolution video to see cutaneous abnormalities while group therapy may require multiple microphones, breakout group, and chat functions. Financial factors related to software subscriptions, hardware purchases, Internet service provider (ISP) contracts, space, and staffing play an important role in the selection of telecommunication technology. The provider and remote site staff must realistically consider their technical and financial ability to operate, and maintain the technology. Finally, deciding to extend an existing videoconferencing system or replace it with a cloud-based system will restrict the decision to a smaller number of vendors and technology options. Providers can learn more about buying technology from these commercial vendors and software companies at the ATA's Resource Center & Buyer's Guide website (84).

If the program will build upon an older system, it is likely a standards-based applications/platform, sometimes referred to as "legacy hardware." These proprietary systems offer the highest quality of audio and video, as well as the most stable data connection, giving participants the most life-like or "telepresence" experience. They transmit data over digital subscriber lines (DSL). This telephone company-based end-user connection transmits secure, point-to-point, high-bandwidth (≥1.5 mbps), high-definition video and audio signals over satellite or fiber-optic systems. Typical DSL broadband capacities are 1.5, 3, 5, 10, 12 mbps, which seem small compared to residential ISP plans that offer 300 mbps, but because these systems use a static Internet protocol (IP), they are guaranteed this speed at all times and the connection is more stable than the dynamic IPs used in residential connections. These systems also offer many sophisticated features including the ability to zoom and pan/tilt cameras at both sites, connect to medical devices like stethoscopes, and connect to multiple microphones, and large (and multiple) monitor systems. These features enable the provider to closely examine the patient and control how he/she view the participants in multipoint conferencing. These systems require technical support to operate with other legacy systems. Despite their superior functioning, standards-based systems are predominantly used in medical centers or other large organizations because they require a considerable initial investment and high costs for maintenance, technical staff, and related IT infrastructure.

Consumer-based software platforms transmit data over the Internet and the consumer interface software run on personal computers, tablets, and smartphones. Subscriptions to these cloud-based services are sold based on the number of users or accounts, ranging from free single account packages to enterprise-level subscriptions with hundreds of accounts. Enterprise-level contracts often include an option to purchase the software that would allow the consumer to host the service on its own server. Local hosting can greatly improve the telepresence quality of the videoconference. Software vendors who advertise telehealth solutions must provide appropriate software encryption and sign Business Associate Agreements to comply with HIPAA regulations.

Recent advances in both hardware and software signal compression has enabled these Internet-based systems to deliver the high-quality video and audio signals necessary for clinical work. They are highly flexible, adaptable, and consumer friendly, enabling rapid deployment to a variety of settings with minimal training, startup costs, and fixed costs. Interested purchasers should review their options on unbiased websites, such as the ATA website (http://www.americantelemed.org).

There are disadvantages to conducting telepsychiatry sessions over cloud-based applications that utilize the Internet. The foremost is the highly variable quality and speed of the connection, which impacts the quality of streaming audio and video. The connection quality and speed can be affected by many factors including nearby Internet traffic (for cable–modem connections), inclement weather, network failures, local electrical device interference to WiFi signals, and *Intranet* network traffic at the origination and destination sites. Other disadvantages to these cloud-based platforms include variable customer support from the vendor, a greater chance that end users will inadvertently alter the hardware or software, limited ability to connect peripheral devices such as a stethoscope, and usually no ability to control the camera at the patient's site. They usually do not connect to legacy videoconferencing devices installed in many health care centers, schools, and other organizations. While many systems provide adequate video and audio quality, the purchase of an external camera and microphone (Figure 6.3.5.1) can considerably improve quality of the interaction.

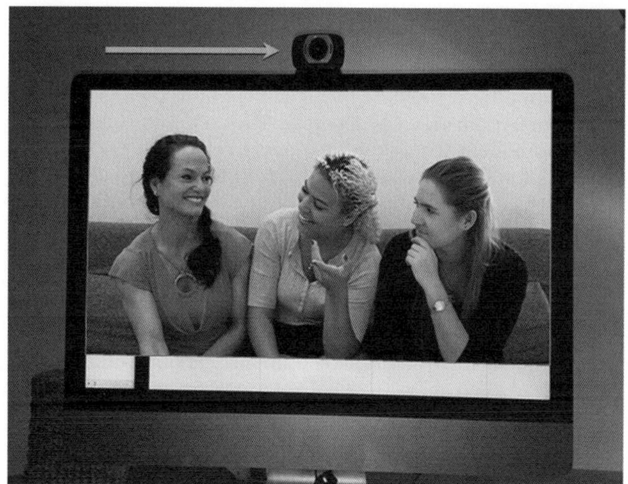

FIGURE 6.3.5.1. External USB cameras improve picture and sound. Photograph courtesy of Dr. Roth, author.

In summary, choosing the best videoconferencing platform is a complicated decision. Providers must consider their budget for initial and ongoing costs, the available bandwidth at all sites, the technical sophistication of users, access to technical support, and the need to control the remote equipment. Other helpful resources are available from the National Telehealth Technology Assessment Resource Center (http://www.telehealthtechnology.org) and the ATA (http://www.americantelemed.org).

ESTABLISHING A TELEPSYCHIATRY PRACTICE

The following is a brief overview of issues for potential providers to address in determining whether telepsychiatry is relevant to their clinical practice. More information can be found through the ATA (http://www.americantelemed.org) and the National Telehealth Technology Assessment Resource Center (http://www.telehealthtechnology.org).

Feasibility and Sustainability of a Telepsychiatry Practice

Telepsychiatry is poised to play an increasingly important role within pediatric health care systems. Services to primary care settings are anticipated to increase with national and state initiatives around the patient-centered medical home (85). Telepsychiatry is one strategy for incorporating mental health treatment into primary care settings and has the added potential for increasing the PCPs' skills in caring for mental health problems.

Determining the feasibility of a telepsychiatry service is based on an accurate needs assessment that identifies the mental health needs of the patient site and determines whether the proposed service is likely to meet those needs and to complement existing services. It is helpful to visit the patient site and meet with local stakeholders for services collaborative problem solving.

Sustainability of a telepsychiatry service is determined within the context of the community's needs. For example, a medical center may not benefit directly from a telepsychiatry service, but there could be financial benefit to the institution if emergency room services decrease. The community as a whole may also benefit from lower expenses related to correctional or educational services for youth. With technology costs lowering and an increasing number of insurers reimbursing telepsychiatry services, sustaining such a service without outside funding is becoming more possible. Telepsychiatry providers are encouraged to review information at the Center for Medicare and Medicaid Services website (www.cms.gov) and the ATA website (http://www.americantelemed.org) prior to any billing to determine any jurisdiction-specific guidelines.

Patient Population and Models of Care

The patients to be served should be identified by the patient site. Patient inclusion and exclusion criteria are based upon judgment of the provider, and resources at the patient site, including the site's ability to attend to acutely suicidal or agitated patients. Exclusion criteria may include factors such as youth without accompanying guardians, patients without a PCP, or patients with a PCP who is uncomfortable resuming care for psychiatric patients. Several models of care have been used to provide telepsychiatry services, including consultation, direct care, or collaboration with another provider (1,86,87). Some programs have developed specific models for consultation to primary care (19,35), including one that moves flexibly between consultation and direct care (42). When ongoing direct care is offered via telepsychiatry, a PCP should be identified to provide care when the provider is unavailable and to resume care when the patient becomes stable.

Private Practice Options

Telepsychiatry programs are no longer solely the purview of major medical centers. Private practice providers have several options (88,89). Those preferring more practice support may choose to work for a company offering a virtual group practice with a spectrum of services ranging from models that provide a high level of structure, including management of the videoconferencing technology and patient referrals, while contracting with providers for the clinical service (83). Providers who are confident with technology and referral sources may contract with a company that simply provides a secure web-based connection (88,89). The independent provider is then responsible for performing the needs assessment to determine whether the telepsychiatry service is needed, feasible, and sustainable, as well as to establish protocols addressing clinical, business, and regulatory issues (88,89).

THROUGH THE LOOKING GLASS: OVERCOMING THE CHALLENGES INHERENT IN CREATING AUTHENTIC PROVIDER–PATIENT RELATIONSHIPS DURING TELEPSYCHIATRY

Like an actor stepping onto the stage, providers must immediately engage patients' attention and convince them that they are trustworthy, competent, empathic, and will be responsive to their needs (90). Providers who naturally create good rapport are instinctually communicating verbally as well as nonverbally. The importance of sending and observing nonverbal communication cannot be overstated; because over two-thirds of communicated meaning can be attributed to nonverbal messages (91). Clear communication is an integral part of good bedside manner and is the key to building and maintaining therapeutic relationships. It is often not what is said, but how it is said, that matters most to patients (92,93). For the purpose of this chapter, nonverbal communication is defined as everything except for the contextual meaning of the spoken words, including: the nature, location, and decoration of the room, the provider's physical appearance, distance between participants, body movements, posture, gestures, facial expressions, eye contact, touch, and the tone, pacing, and volume of the provider's voice.

The nonverbal communication to consider during telepsychiatry includes:

- The nature, location, and decoration of the room
- Physical appearance
- Individuals' distance from one another
- Body movements, posture, and gestures
- Facial expressions
- Touching the other person
- The tone, rate, and volume of the provider's voice

Communicating during telepsychiatry differs from communicating in person. Cameras, microphones, and speakers alter voice and appearance and flatten emotional expressions. Most providers experienced in telepsychiatry slightly enhance their communication style to establish a therapeutic relationship. Many of these enhancements are techniques used by newscasters and actors to communicate authenticity to their audiences.

Providers must command a working knowledge of these nonverbal communication restrictions. The first nonverbal communication is patients' view of the provider as the camera frame limits patients' ability to see the provider and his/her nonverbal communications. They have less access to environmental information to shape their perception of the provider as trustworthy, competent, and empathic. The provider's physical appearance, grooming, uniform/dress, and interactions become a more significant part of how patients' make a first impression (60). If providers' nonverbal communication does not support their verbal communication, the provider seems odd or insincere (94). This weakens the provider–patient relationship (95).

Telehealth technology affects the provider's ability to:

- See the patient
- Be seen by the patient
- Be heard and understood
- Make gestures
- Maintain eye contact
- Touch
- Smell
- Demonstrate usual good bedside manner

Erect and open body posture communicates to patients that the provider is a confident, nonjudgmental, and trustworthy authority figure (96) who is paying attention to their needs (97). Moving toward or away from the camera approximates the effect of interpersonal space during in-person sessions. For example, moving slightly closer to the camera communicates more interest or attention. If the patient seems defensive, moving slightly away from the camera conveys the perception of giving the patient more distance. The picture-in-picture function on the monitor helps providers to monitor how their image is projected and to stay within the frame (Figure 6.3.5.2).

As patients can only see facial expressions, gestures, movements, and activities that fall within the camera frame, providers must replace large gestures with smaller ones that are more easily seen (98). Common gestures like outstretched arms can be replaced with hand gestures or emotionally

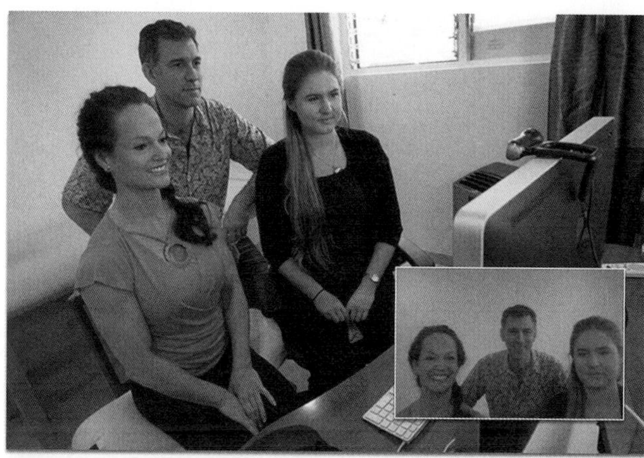

FIGURE 6.3.5.2. Picture-in-picture function monitors screen image. Photograph courtesy of Dr. Roth, author.

congruent facial expressions (99). Hand gestures like waving and the thumbs-up sign can also replace culturally relevant handshakes and fist-bumps that are lost in telehealth.

The provider's tone of voice affects the relationship (100). Without sounding robotic, the provider must sound honest, compassionate and intelligent while speaking slowly, loudly, and clearly enough to be easily heard and understood through the microphone. Many novice providers speak robotically due to performance anxiety or distractions by the electronics (e.g., a medical record that is simultaneously projected onto a monitor during the session). Providers may modulate the pitch of their voice slightly to avoid sounding anxious or robotic, but the challenge then is to avoid seeming theatric. Smiling while speaking makes the provider sound warm and approachable. Placing a smiley face sticker next to the camera is a good reminder for those who often look or sound too serious.

Encouraging patients to speak more is associated with feeling that their needs are fulfilled (101). There is a very brief transmission delay during videoconferencing that affects communication. Therefore, pauses and turn-taking are important for the provider to manage. Giving the patient an extra moment to reply in conversation may seem like a long pause but will replicate a normal pause during in-person conversation. During multi-center sessions, the provider may need to allow for even longer pauses.

Due to the slight audio transmission delay, verbal encouragers (e.g., yes, tell me more, go on) are more difficult to use during telepsychiatry. If the participant has already resumed speaking, he or she stops speaking to listen to the encourager, thereby interfering with communication. Therefore, experienced providers frequently use gestures, such as the thumbs-up gesture, to facilitate the reciprocal exchange of information while maintaining engagement and without interrupting the speaker. The other approach is to nod and smile. After thousands of telepsychiatry sessions, the authors suggest the most important nonverbal rapport-building strategy is to periodically nod and smile while the patient is talking, thereby indicating that the provider is listening and encouraging the patient to continue. Consider placing a sticky note that says, "Nod and smile!" on the monitor until this becomes natural.

OPTIMIZING THE TELEPSYCHIATRY EXPERIENCE

Room Selection

Optimizing the telepsychiatry experience begins with appropriate room selection. In telepsychiatry, the camera is turned on and—boom! The provider is suddenly meeting with the patient. There is no grand hospital architecture, professional décor, or staff interactions to mentally prepare the patient for the clinical encounter. To further complicate matters, the patient site may be a home, school, or another provider's office—all settings the provider cannot control. It is up to the provider to make it an authentic clinical experience. To start, attention is given to selecting, arranging, and appointing the rooms at both the patient and provider sites. Telepsychiatry providers often work with a wide range of rooms, but with the right setup, sessions can be successfully conducted in classrooms, conference rooms, treatment rooms, offices, living rooms, and bedrooms. After the room at the patient's site is selected, it should be appointed to support videoconferences, accommodate the routine number of participants, and maximize participants' focus during the session.

Room selection should ensure that:

- Everyone feels comfortable
- Distractions are minimized
- Everyone is able to see each other
- Everyone is able to hear each other
- The room maintains visual and auditory privacy
- Room size accommodates the clinical encounter
- Décor minimizes camera distortion

Power and Network

One of the most important considerations in room selection for sites using cloud videoconferencing is proximity to the WiFi router to maintain a strong Internet connection. If connecting through a computer, it should be plugged into the router with an Ethernet cable to provide the strongest video and auditory signal. Most software automatically downgrades the picture and sound to match the worst connection, so one slow site compromises the experience for everyone involved. Plugging the router, modem, computer, and monitor(s) into a combination surge protector and battery backup will ensure that the connection will not drop if there is a momentary electrical surge or loss of power.

Room Set-Up

Selecting a room with a camera-friendly color scheme makes it easier for the camera to focus on the participant instead of the background. The camera should be focused on a wall that is painted a soft neutral shade to help the participant's image stand out from the wall. Decorations and patterns that are small, intricate, highly detailed, or cluttered may distort video images and trick the camera into focusing on the background (Figure 6.3.5.3). There should be nothing directly behind the participant's head because the camera's poor depth projection makes them appear to grow out of the participant's head. The decorations in the provider's room should be minimal and professional, reflecting the services delivered.

Cameras

Camera placement will determine framing of the video image. Framing determines who and what is visible on the screen, as well as accurate observation of participants' presentation. Poor placement may detract from the interaction and ultimately whether the clinical experience seems authentic, as shown in Figure 6.3.5.4. Cameras should be positioned at a sufficient distance from the patient to allow visualization of the child's motor abilities and activities but also to allow assessment of facial features and affect.

Participants naturally look at the monitor to relate to one another during videoconferencing. However, the camera is

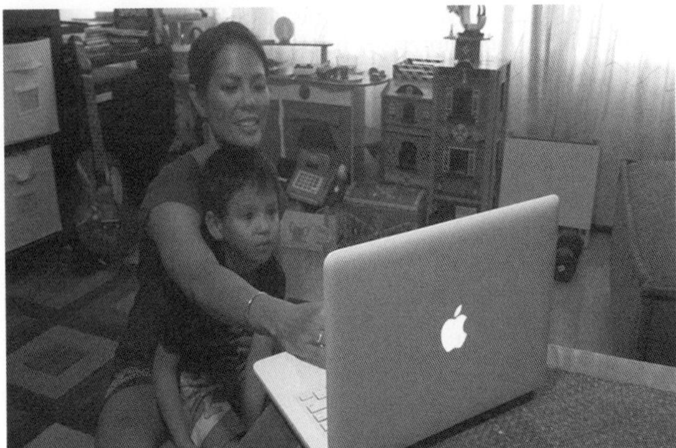

FIGURE 6.3.5.3. Cluttered background and suboptimal lighting interfere with camera's functioning. Photograph courtesy of Dr. Roth, author.

typically placed on top of the screen so that participants appear to be gazing downward. Provider eye contact is significantly related to patients' perceptions of the provider's connectedness and empathy (102). Therefore, providers' cameras should be directly in front of them, positioned at eye level, as shown in Figure 6.3.5.5. This positioning makes the provider gaze toward the camera when looking at the screen. Assessing eye contact is an essential component of the developmental evaluation of children and establishing a therapeutic alliance, particularly during a videoconferencing encounter when there is decreased access to other nonverbal means of communication. The provider should determine whether apparent decreased eye contact represents a technical limitation or a clinical impairment.

If a single participant is using a phone or a tablet, it should be positioned in vertical/portrait orientation. This improves the eye contact between participants because the other participant's eyes are closer to the camera. If the device needs to capture two or more people in the frame, turning the device horizontal/landscape will often create a larger frame that encompasses more of the room.

Medical providers spend 30% of a clinical visit gazing at the electronic medical record (EMR) (103). If the EMR is used during the session and can be projected onto the screen, it should be placed in a vertical window above or below the participants' images. This causes the provider to constantly nod up and down in a positive and affirmative manner when glancing at the participant's EMR. By contrast, if the EMR window were placed lateral to the participant images, the provider would be constantly making negative, head-shaking gestures during the session. Telepsychiatry providers should minimize the time spent looking at the EMR in order to maintain eye contact and rapport with the patient, even if this means charting very little during the session.

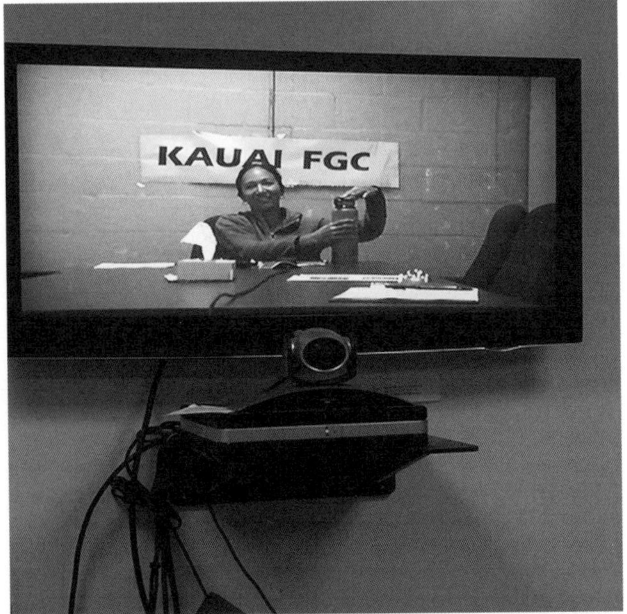

FIGURE 6.3.5.4. Poor framing of video image impedes authentic patient–provider relationship. Photograph courtesy of Dr. Roth, author.

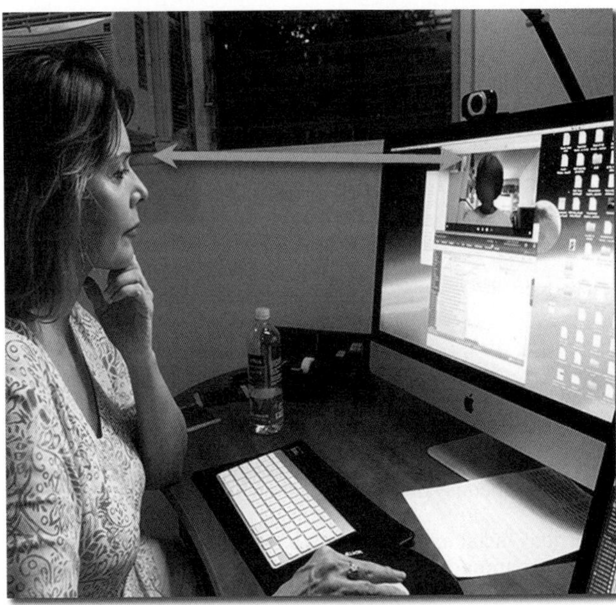

FIGURE 6.3.5.5. Approximate eye contact with proper camera placement. Photograph courtesy of Dr. Roth, author.

Lighting

Lighting affects quality of the videoconferencing session (98). Cameras need more light than human eyes to produce a clear image. An insufficiently illuminated room prevents participants from seeing each other clearly, detecting nonverbal communication, identifying physical signs and symptoms, and detracts from the authenticity of the experience. Backlighting should be avoided. This occurs when a bright light comes from behind the person, such as when seated in front of a window or bright light. The person becomes silhouetted. This issue should be considered early in room selection when the position of the camera is determined. Copious indirect lighting, such as floor lamps that bounce light off the ceiling, is the key to a good lighting plan. It looks natural, softer, and avoids glare or shadows. Removing or covering reflective surfaces that cause glare also helps to optimize the video image.

Privacy

Common sense cures most privacy problems. This is handled at two levels. At the software level, most commercial telehealth vendors advertise whether they meet HIPAA standards. The second aspect of privacy is participation. Sites must ensure that they can restrict access to the videoconferencing room, as well as others' ability to view the session. This may be challenging in very small communities with limited room availability or when providing consultation to a small emergency room. Home-based services provide particular challenges as a space must be large enough to include all participants but not accessible to non-participating family members. Family sessions may be best accommodated in the kitchen or family room, but these are high-traffic areas. Individual sessions, and some parent–child sessions, may be conducted away from other family in a bedroom, office, or porch.

Audio privacy may be the largest obstacle to privacy. If the patient site is a clinical examination room it will already have been soundproofed. However, many times the videoconferencing equipment is set up in a conference room or private office with inadequate soundproofing. Sound privacy may be determined by asking a staff to stand outside the doors and windows during a sham session and report on audibility.

Ways to improve audio privacy

- Close windows
- Block gaps below doors
- Place a white noise machine outside and beside the door to the telehealth room.
- Put carpet or an area rug on the floor
- Add pillows to couches, curtains on windows, and/or tapestries on walls to absorb sound
- When remodeling, use decoupling soundproofing construction techniques
- Consider using a headset microphone

Audio Quality: Distractions and Audio Signal

Audio privacy and comfort also relate to ambient noise that varies across rooms. The microphones are sensitive and amplify sound affecting the volume of participants' speech and quality of the sessions. Common disturbing background sounds are printers, air conditioners, fans, intercoms, animals, lawn equipment, and outside traffic. Rooms should be selected to minimize these common interfering sounds. However, most rooms are not perfectly quiet and the provider should work with staff at the patient site to implement strategies to decrease background noise. If services are provided in the home uninvolved individuals should be forewarned to stay out of the room during the session.

Audio communication depends on the microphone and speakers. Computers, tablets, and phones often have built in microphones and speakers that are adequate for clinical service. However, if providers can add a peripheral device to their system, a quality microphone can filter out background noise and improve communication. If the provider is the only person in the room, he or she could use a headset microphone that eliminates most background sounds, and ensures that participants' voices are not overheard.

Finally, it is important to have a backup plan in case the audio connection fails. Usually, a conference speakerphone can be used to provide an adequate connection while not seriously compromising synchrony with the video signal. The audio device in the videoconference software must be muted to avoid echoes and feedback due to running two microphones simultaneously.

Approaches to minimizing background noise include:

- Close windows and doors
- Turn down/off window and portable air conditioners, fans
- Do not to run other equipment (e.g., printers, fax machines, dishwashers)
- Turn off electronics
- Keep pets out of the room
- Encourage the patient site to only allow quiet toys without multiple parts, such as foam blocks, books, markers, action figures, and dolls

SUMMARY

Effective telepsychiatry providers are able to create authentic provider–patient relationships by augmenting the provider's good bedside manner with a few acting, news casting, and venue staging skills. When these skills, strategies, and techniques are put together well, they make telepsychiatry look easy and the interactions feel authentic to both patients and providers. With sufficient practice, providers can be as effective and comfortable treating patients via telehealth technology as they are in other clinical venues. Additional resources on optimizing the telepsychiatry session are available through the Telemental Health Guide (www.telepsychiatryguide.org), the Telehealth Resource Centers (www.telehealthresourcecenter.org), and ATA (www.americantelemed.org).

INTERVENTIONS

Interventions provided via telepsychiatry to children and adolescents should be consistent with clinical practice guidelines established by the American Academy of Child and Adolescent Psychiatry (AACAP) for specific psychiatric disorders and treatments (104) and should follow guidelines established for TMH service delivery (75,79,105).

The psychiatric assessment of children and adolescents includes spending some time interviewing the youth alone. Older children with good impulse control, adequate verbal skills, and the ability to separate can be interviewed alone. Younger, developmentally impaired or impulsive youth need a modified approach. Traditional play sessions may be challenging. The child may be observed interacting with staff in a structured or free play session. Some limited play with the child may be possible over the telemonitor (e.g., drawing pictures and then discussing them or developing a play scenario with puppets).

Preschoolers should be observed in developmentally appropriate interactions with their parent(s) and, if indicated, with an unfamiliar adult, perhaps a staff member. Many young children will engage in direct interaction with the provider, such as distinguishing colors, pointing to body parts, singing the alphabet, or relating a story.

Pharmacotherapy is a highly desired service. Approaches to medication management depend on the model of care (17,19,106,107). Regardless of the model used, it is important to maintain communication with the PCP about the treatment. Medications that are not regulated by the Drug Enforcement Administration (DEA) can be prescribed consistent with methods used in traditional practice. However, federal legislation regarding the prescription of controlled substances through videoconferencing has implications for telepsychiatry, especially for the treatment of children with ADHD. The Ryan Haight Online Pharmacy Consumer Protection Act of 2008 (108) was designed to expunge illegitimate online pharmacies that dispensed controlled substances without contact with the individual and without physician oversight. The Act placed certain restrictions around the practice of "prescribing by means of the internet." While the Act specifically designates that telemedicine is an exception to the Act, it technically requires that providers conduct at least one face-to-face evaluation of the patient prior to prescribing a controlled substance via telemedicine. Alternatively, patients being treated by and physically located in a hospital or clinic registered with the DEA in the presence of a DEA-registered practitioner may be prescribed controlled substances via telemedicine. The letter of this legislation is difficult to follow and severely dilutes the value of telepsychiatry practice. However, the DEA recently noted that it does not intend to interfere with the legitimate prescribing of controlled substances during telemedicine practice (109). It has further promised to promulgate future rules around telemedicine prescribing and to establish a special telemedicine registration. Unfortunately, these provisions have been left incomplete since 2008. Several states have enacted legislation to allow the prescription of controlled substances through telemedicine practice, particularly for telepsychiatry. Providers should carefully review both federal and state guidelines in establishing their telepractice regarding the prescription of controlled substances and act in the best interests of their patients.

Tracking vital signs, height and weight, obtaining rating scales, monitoring physiologic status, and assessing adverse effects are accomplished with coordination from staff at the patient site. Abnormal movements due to antipsychotic medications can be assessed remotely by the provider using the Abnormal Involuntary Movement Scale (110) or a nurse can be trained to complete the scale in person.

An important aspect of medication management is providing care or assisting staff between sessions. Protocols are needed to provide families clear directions for requesting refills, asking questions, and reporting adverse effects.

Psychotherapy is increasingly provided to families and youth through various devices in multiple settings. In addition to translating evidence-based psychotherapies to the videoconferencing venue, particular attention to cultural context is needed as providers in urban/suburban areas and families in rural areas often differ in their cultural heritage (111). Adolescents' increasing access to mobile device–based (m-health) applications, particularly smart phones, presents a promising opportunity to reach youth in need of services. As of 2014, 58% of the United States population owned a smartphone (112). In underserved populations, rates are 47% for low-income households, 43% for rural areas, and are *higher* for minorities than Caucasians. Moreover, the vast majority of the population will likely own smartphones in the near future as 90% currently own a cell phone and the percentage of smartphones versus traditional cell phones has been rising (112,113). These data suggest that smartphones will be increasingly a convenient medium for reaching individuals of all ethnicities, incomes, and geographic regions. Moreover, m-health applications have a number of capabilities associated with successful interventions utilizing communication technology, including: scheduled reminders to engage in therapeutic exercises (114); point of performance support (115); individually tailored information (116,117); real-time symptom assessment (118); and attractiveness to youth through increased sense of autonomy (119). Such technologic advances may change the face of psychotherapy for both distant and local communities.

EVALUATING A TELEPSYCHIATRY SERVICE

As the demand for telepsychiatry services has outpaced the evidence-based supporting its efficacy, ongoing evaluation of services will help the provider establish best practices. A "lexicon of assessment and outcome measures for telepsychiatry" is available at the ATA website (120). Evaluation may include process variables, such as description of the population served, appointments kept or cancelled, hospitalization, collaboration in the community, types of services provided. Routine measurement of outcomes helps to demonstrate patients' progress and effectiveness of services—particularly important for telepsychiatrists involved with Accountable Care Organizations. Assessment of clinical outcomes may include rating scales obtained from the patient and stakeholders, functional assessments, documentation of adverse events, and adherence to treatment plans. Providers should also consider evaluating caregivers' burden (29). Exploration of the virtual relationship between the patient and provider could help to understand salient mediating factors when delivering care remotely. Kramer et al. (121) have described a model to inform overall telepsychiatry research design and Slone et al. (58) describe additional guidance specific to pediatric research settings.

SUMMARY

The convergence of increasing clinical need, decreasing resources, and technologic advances have made telepsychiatry an attractive approach to deliver evidence-based treatment to youth and families who are not well served by traditional models of care. However, potential telepsychiatrists must keep abreast of technical, financial, and regulatory changes in this rapidly evolving field. Establishing an authentic patient–provider relationship, and a successful practice, requires providers to expand their repertoire of interpersonal relatedness and online presentation to optimize patients' experience. These efforts are increasingly rewarded. Barriers to telepsychiatry are falling as individual states enact parity with in person services, as CMS expands criteria for services, and as research demonstrates the feasibility, acceptability, and effectiveness of telepsychiatry services. Communities are increasingly requesting services. It's time to connect.

References

1. Carlisle LL: Child and adolescent telemental health. In: Myers K, Turvey C (eds): *Telemental Health: Clinical, Technical, and Administrative Foundation for Evidence-Based Practice*. London, Elsevier, 197–221, 2013.
2. Center for Medicare and Medicaid Services: Medicare Telehealth Policy. C.F.R 42 § 410:78, 2011.
3. Center for Medicare and Medicaid Services: Telemedicine. Available at: https://www.medicaid.gov/medicaid-chip-program-information/by-topics/delivery-systems/telemedicine.html. Accessed June 29, 2014.
4. Turvey C, Coleman M, Dennison O, et al.: ATA practice guidelines for video-based online mental health services. *Telemed J E Health* 19(9): 722–730, 2013.
5. Yellowlees P, Shore J, Roberts L: Practice guidelines for videoconferencing-based telemental health—October 2009. *Telemed J E Health* 16(10): 1074–1089, 2010.
6. Shore JH: Telepsychiatry: videoconferencing in the delivery of psychiatric care. *Am J Psychiatry* 170(3):256–262, 2013.
7. Lambert D, Ziller E, Lenardson JD: *Rural Children Don't Receive the Mental Health Care They Need (Research & Policy Brief)*. Portland, ME, University of Southern Maine, Muskie School of Public Service, Maine Rural Health Research Center, 2009.
8. Thomas CR, Holzer CE, 3rd: The continuing shortage of child and adolescent psychiatrists. *J Am Acad Child Adolesc Psychiatry* 45(9):1023–1031, 2006.
9. Association of American Medical Colleges: *AAMC Physician Workforce Policy Recommendations*. 2012.
10. Insel T: Where are we going? 2011; Available at: http://www.nimh.nih.gov/about/director/2011/psychiatry-where-are-we-going.shtml. Accessed February 15, 2015.
11. Patient Protection and Affordable Care Act: Pub. L. No. 111-148. U.S.C., 42 § 2702, 124 Stat. 119, 318–319, 2010.
12. Hyde PS: *Report To Congress on the Nation's Substance Abuse and Mental Health Workforce Issues*. Rockville, MD, U.S. Department of Health and Human Services, Substance Abuse and Mental Health Services Administration, 2013.
13. Office of the National Coordinator for Health Information Technology: *Office of Standards and Technology*. United States, Department of Health and Human Services. Federal Health IT Strategic Plan: 2015–2020, 2015.
14. Duncan AB, Velasquez SE, Nelson EL: Using videoconferencing to provide psychological services to rural children and adolescents: a review and case example. *J Clin Child Adolesc Psychol* 43(1):115–127, 2014.
15. Myers KM, Sulzbacher S, Melzer SM: Telepsychiatry with children and adolescents: are patients comparable to those evaluated in usual outpatient care? *Telemed J E Health* 10:278–285, 2004.
16. Myers KM, Valentine JM, Melzer SM: Child and adolescent telepsychiatry: utilization and satisfaction. *Telemed J E Health* 14:131–137, 2008.
17. Spaulding R, Cain S, Sonnenschein K: Urban telepsychiatry: uncommon service for a common need. *Child Adolesc Psychiatr Clin N Am* 20(1):29–39, 2011.
18. Cain S, Spaulding R: *Telepsychiatry: Lessons from two models of care*. Paper presented at: 53rd Annual Meeting of the American Academy of Child and Adolescent Psychiatry. San Diego, CA, 2006.

19. Myers K, Valentine JM, Melzer SM: Feasibility, acceptability, and sustainability of telepsychiatry for children and adolescents. *Psychiatr Serv* 58:1493–1496, 2007.
20. Kaliebe KE, Heneghan J, Kim TJ: Telepsychiatry in juvenile justice settings. *Child Adolesc Psychiatr Clin N Am* 20(1):113–123, 2011.
21. Myers K, Valentine J, Morganthaler R, Melzer S: Telepsychiatry with incarcerated youth. *J Adolesc Health* 38:643–648, 2006.
22. Grady B, Lever N, Cunningham D, Stephan S: Telepsychiatry and school mental health. *Child Adolesc Psychiatr Clin N Am* 20:81–94, 2011.
23. Stephan S, Lever N, Bernstein L, Edwards S, Pruitt D: Telemental Health in Schools. *J Child Adolesc Psychopharmacol* 26:266–272, 2016.
24. Comer JS, Furr JM, Cooper-Vince CE, et al.: Internet-delivered, family-based treatment for early-onset OCD: a preliminary case series. *J Clin Child Adolesc Psychol* 43(1):74–87, 2014.
25. Nelson E, Barnard M, Cain S: Treating childhood depression over teleconferencing. *Telemed J E Health* 9:49–55, 2003.
26. Storch EA, Caporino NE, Morgan JR, et al.: Preliminary investigation of web-camera delivered cognitive-behavioral therapy for youth with obsessive-compulsive disorder. *Psychiatry Res* 189(3):407–412, 2011.
27. Himle MB, Freitag M, Walther M, Franklin SA, Ely L, Woods DW: A randomized pilot trial comparing videoconference versus face-to-face delivery of behavior therapy for childhood tic disorders. *Behav Res Ther* 50(9):565–570, 2012.
28. Myers K, Vander Stoep A, Zhou C, McCarty CA, Katon W: Effectiveness of a telehealth service delivery model for treating attention-deficit/hyperactivity disorder: a community-based randomized controlled trial. *J Am Acad Child Adolesc Psychiatry* 54(4):263–274, 2015.
29. Vander Stoep A, McCarty CA, Zhou C, Rockhill CM, Schoenfelder E, Myers K: The children's attention-deficit hyperactivity disorder telemental health treatment study: caregiver outcomes. *J Abnorm Child Psychol* 45:27–43, 2017.
30. Rockhill CM, Tse YJ, Fesinmeyer MD, Garcia J, Myers K: Telepsychiatrists' medication treatment strategies in the children's attention-deficit/hyperactivity disorder telemental health treatment study. *J Child Adolesc Psychopharmacol* 26(8):662–671, 2016.
31. Tse YJ, McCarty CA, Stoep AV, Myers KM: Teletherapy delivery of caregiver behavior training for children with attention-deficit hyperactivity disorder. *Telemed J E Health* 21(6):451–458, 2015.
32. Xie Y, Dixon JF, Yee OM, et al.: A study on the effectiveness of videoconferencing on teaching parent training skills to parents of children with ADHD. *Telemed J E Health* 19(3):192–199, 2013.
33. Glueckauf RL, Fritz SP, Ecklund-Johnson EP, Liss HJ, Dages P, Carney P: Videoconferencing-based family counseling for rural teenagers with epilepsy: Phase 1 findings. *Rehabil Psychol* 47(1):49–72, 2002.
34. Fox KC, Conor P, McCullers E, Waters T: Effect of a behavioural health and specialty care telemedicine programme on goal attainment for youths in juvenile detention. *J Telemed Telecare* 15(4):227–230, 2008.
35. Yellowlees PM, Hilty DM, Marks SL, Neufeld J, Bourgeois JA: A retrospective analysis of a child and adolescent eMental Health program. *J Am Acad Child Adolesc Psychiatry* 47:103–107, 2008.
36. Reese RJ, Slone NC, Soares N, Sprang R: Telehealth for underserved families: an evidence-based parenting program. *Psychol Serv* 9(3):320–322, 2012.
37. Blackmon LA, Kaak HO, Ranseen J: Consumer satisfaction with telemedicine child psychiatry consultation in rural Kentucky. *Psychiatr Serv* 48(11):1464–1466, 1997.
38. Elford DR, White H, St John K, Maddigan B, Ghandi M, Bowering R: A prospective satisfaction study and cost analysis of a pilot child telepsychiatry service in Newfoundland. *J Telemed Telecare* 7(2):73–81, 2001.
39. Kopel H, Nunn K, Dossetor D: Evaluating satisfaction with a child and adolescent psychological telemedicine outreach service. *Journal Telemed Telecare* 7(Suppl 2):35–40, 2001.
40. Greenberg N, Boydell KM, Volpe T: Pediatric telepsychiatry in Ontario: caregiver and service provider perspectives. *J Behav Health Serv Res* 33(1):105–111, 2006.
41. Hilty DM, Yellowlees PM, Nesbitt TS: Evolution of telepsychiatry to rural sites: changes over time in types of referral and in primary care-providers' knowledge, skills and satisfaction. *Gen Hosp Psychiatry* 28:367–373, 2006.
42. Myers KM, Vander Stoep A, McCarty CA, et al.: Child and adolescent telepsychiatry: variations in utilization, referral patterns and practice trends. *J Telemed Telecare* 16:128–133, 2010.
43. Pakyurek M, Yellowlees P, Hilty D: The child and adolescent telepsychiatry consultation: can it be a more effective clinical process for certain patients than conventional practice? *Telemed J E Health* 16(3):289–292, 2010.
44. Lau ME, Way BB, Fremont WP: Assessment of Suny Upstate Medical University's child telepsychiatry consultation program. *Int J Psychiatry Med* 42(1):93–104, 2011.
45. Jacob MK, Larson JC, Craighead WE: Establishing a telepsychiatry consultation practice in rural Georgia for primary care physicians: a feasibility report. *Clin Pediatr (Phila)* 51(11):1041–1047, 2012.
46. Nelson EL, Bui T: Rural telepsychology services for children and adolescents. *J Clin Psychol* 66(5):490–501, 2010.
47. Elford R, White H, Bowering R, et al.: A randomized, controlled trial of child psychiatric assessments conducted using videoconferencing. *J Telemed Telecare* 6(2):73–82, 2000.
48. Stain HJ, Payne K, Thienel R, Michie P, Carr V, Kelly B: The feasibility of videoconferencing for neuropsychological assessments of rural youth experiencing early psychosis. *J Telemed Telecare* 17(6):328–331, 2011.
49. Reese RM, Jamison R, Wendland M, et al.: Evaluating interactive videoconferencing for assessing symptoms of autism. *Telemed J E Health* 19(9):671–677, 2013.
50. Boydell KM, Volpe T, Pignatiello A: A qualitative study of young people's perspectives on receiving psychiatric services via televideo. *J Can Acad Child Adolesc Psychiatry* 19(1):5–11, 2010.
51. Shaikh U, Cole SL, Marcin JP, Nesbitt TS: Clinical management and patient outcomes among children and adolescents receiving telemedicine consultations for obesity. *Telemed J E Health* 14(5):434–440, 2008.
52. Szeftel R, Federico C, Hakak R, Szeftel Z, Jacobson M: Improved access to mental health evaluation for patients with developmental disabilities using telepsychiatry. *J Telemed Telecare* 18(6):317–321, 2012.
53. Davis AM, Sampilo M, Gallagher KS, Landrum Y, Malone B: Treating rural pediatric obesity through telemedicine: outcomes from a small randomized controlled trial. *J Pediatr Psychol* 38(9):932–943, 2013.
54. Hilty DM, Shoemaker EZ, Myers K, Snowdy CE, Yellowlees PM, Yager J: Need for and steps toward a clinical guideline for the telemental healthcare of children and adolescents. *J Child Adolesc Psychopharmacol* 26(3):283–295, 2016.
55. Boydell KM, Volpe T, Kertes A, Greenberg N: A review of the outcomes of the recommendations made during paediatric telepsychiatry consultations. *J Telemed Telecare* 13(6):277–281, 2007.
56. Gibson KL, Coulson H, Miles R, Kakekakekung C, Daniels E, O'Donnell S: Conversations on telemental health: listening to remote and rural First Nations communities. *Rural Remote Health* 11(2):1656, 2011.
57. Jones AM, Shealy KM, Reid-Quinones K, et al.: Guidelines for establishing a telemental health program to provide evidence-based therapy for trauma-exposed children and families. *Psychol Serv* 11(4):398–409, 2014.
58. Slone NC, Reese RJ, McClellan MJ: Telepsychology outcome research with children and adolescents: a review of the literature. *Psychol Serv* 9(3):272–292, 2012.
59. Wood J, Stathis S, Smith A, Krause J: E-CYMHS: an expansion of a child and youth telepsychiatry model in Queensland. *Australas Psychiatry* 20(4):333–337, 2012.
60. Glueck D: Establishing therapeutic rapport in telepsychiatry practice. In: Myers K, Turvey C (eds): *Telemental Health: Clinical, Technical, and Administrative Foundation for Evidence-Based Practice*. New York City, Elsevier, 29–46, 2013.
61. Kriechman A, Bonham C: Telemental Health in Primary Care. In: Myers K, Turvey C (eds): *Telemental Health: Clinical, Technical, and Administrative Foundation for Evidence-Based Practice*. London, Elsevier, 2013.
62. Backhaus A, Agha Z, Maglione ML, et al.: Videoconferencing psychotherapy: a systematic review. *Psychol Serv* 9(2):111–131, 2012.
63. Gros DF, Morland LA, Greene CJ, et al.: Delivery of evidence-based psychotherapy via video telehealth. *J Psychopathol Behav Assess* 35(4):506–521, 2013.
64. Hilty DM, Ferrer DC, Parish MB, Johnston B, Callahan EJ, Yellowlees PM: The effectiveness of telemental health: a 2013 review. *Telemed J E Health* 19(6):444–454, 2013.
65. Nelson EL, Patton S: Using Videoconferencing to deliver individual therapy and pediatric psychology interventions with children and adolescents. *J Child Adolesc Psychopharmacol* 26(3):212–220, 2016.
66. Osenbach JE, O'Brien KM, Mishkind M, Smolenski DJ: Synchronous telehealth technologies in psychotherapy for depression: a meta-analysis. *Depress Anxiety* 30(11):1058–1067, 2013.
67. Anderson KE, Byrne C, Goodyear A, Reichel R, Le Grange D: Telemedicine of family-based treatment for adolescent anorexia nervosa: a protocol of a treatment development study. *Int J Eat Disord* 3(1):1–7, 2015.
68. Kramer GM, Mishkind MC, Luxton DD, Shore JH: Managing risk and protecting privacy in telemental health: an overview of legal, regulatory, and risk management issues. In: Myers K, Turvey C (eds): *Telemental Health: Clinical, Technical and Administrative Foundation for Evidence-Based Practice*. London, Elsevier, 83–107, 2013.
69. Center for Telehealth and 2014 e-Health Law: Breaking down telemedicine licensure process: CTeL surveys landscape. 2014. Available at: http://ctel.org/2014/08/breaking-down-telemedicine-licensure-process-ctel-surveys-landscape/. Accessed September 16, 2014.
70. SMART Workgroup: Federation of State Medical Boards: Model Policy for the Appropriate Use of Telemedicine Technologies in the Practice of Medicine. 2014. Available at: http://fsmb.org/Media/Default/PDF/FSMB/Advocacy/FSMB_Telemedicine_Policy.pdf. Accessed March 11, 2017
71. American Telemedicine Association: Core Operational Guidelines for Telehealth Services Involving Provider-Patient Interactions. 2014. Available at: http://www.fsmb.org/Media/Default/PDF/FSMB/Advocacy/FSMB_Telemedicine_Policy.pdf. Accessed March 11, 2017.
72. Interstate Medical Licensure Compact. 2016. Available at: http://www.licenseportability.org. Accessed March 11, 2017.
73. Thomas L, Capistrant G: *50 State Telemedicine Gaps Analysis: Coverage & Reimbursement*. Washington DC, American Telemedicine Association, 2015.
74. Leenknecht CK: The Telepresenting Standards and Guidelines Working Group. Expert Consensus Recommendations for Videoconferencing-Based Telepresenting. 2011. Available at: http://dev.

americantelemed.org/docs/default-source/standards/expert-consensus-recommendations-for-videoconferencing-based-telepresenting.pdf?sfvrsn=4. Accessed March 11, 2017.

75. American Telemedicine Association: Practice Guidelines for Video-Based Online Mental Health Services. 2013. Available at: http://www.americantelemed.org/docs/default-source/standards/practice-guidelines-for-video-based-online-mental-health-services.pdf?sfvrsn=6. Accessed June 29, 2014.
76. Health Insurance Portability and Accountability Act of 1996 (HIPAA). *L. P. No. 104-191, 110 Stat.* 1938.
77. Kramer GM, Luxton DD: Telemental health for children and adolescents: an overview of legal, regulatory, and risk management issues. *J Child Adolesc Psychopharmacol* 26(3):198–203, 2016.
78. Shore JH, Hilty DM, Yellowlees P: Emergency management guidelines for telepsychiatry. *Gen Hosp Psychiatry*. 29(3):199–206, 2007.
79. American Telemedicine Association: *Practice Guidelines for Videoconferencing-Based Telepsychiatry*. 2009. Available at: http://www.americantelemed.org/resources/standards/ata-standards-guidelines/videoconferencing-based-telemental-health. Accessed June 29, 2014.
80. American Academy of Child & Adolescent Psychiatry: Code of Ethics. Approved by Council 9/16/14. Available at: https://www.aacap.org/App_Themes/AACAP/docs/about_us/transparency_portal/aacap_code_of_ethics_2012.pdf. Accessed March 11, 2017.
81. Myers K, Nelson EL, Hilty DM, Rabinowitz T, and the American Telemedicine Association Workgroup on Practice Guidelines: Practice Guideline for Child and Adolescent Telemental Health, *Telemed e-Health*. (in press).
82. Health Resources and Services Administration: Available at: http://www.hrsa.gov/healthit/telehealth/glossary.html.
83. American Telemedicine Association: Available at: http://americantelemed.org.
84. American Telemedicine Association: Resource Center & Buyer's Guide. Available at: http://www.telemedicineresourcecenter.org.
85. Keller D, Sarvet B: Is there a psychiatrist in the house? Integrating child psychiatry into the pediatric medical home. *J Am Acad Child Adolesc Psychiatry* Jan 2013;52(1):3–5.
86. Goldstein F, Myers K: Telepsychiatry: A new collaboration for pediatricians and child psychiatrists. *Pediatr Ann* 2014;43:79–84.
87. Hilty DM, Yellowlees PM, Cobb HC, Bourgeois JA, Neufeld JD, Nesbitt TS: Models of telepsychiatric consultation-liaison service to rural primary care. *Psychosomatics* 47(2):152–157, 2006.
88. Glueck DA: Telepsychiatry in private practice. *Child Adolesc Psychiatr Clin N Am* 20(1):1–11, 2011.
89. Glueck DA: Business aspects of telemental health in private practice. In: Myers K, Turvey C (eds): *Telemental Health: Clinical, Technical, and Administrative Foundation for Evidence-Based Practice*. London, Elsevier, 2013.
90. Riggio RE, Feldman RS (eds): *Applications of Nonverbal Behavioral Theories and Research*. New York, Psychology Press, 2014.
91. Leathers D, Eaves M: *Successful Nonverbal Communication: Principles and Applications*. London, Routledge, 2016.
92. Riess H, Kraft-Todd G: EMPATHY: a tool to enhance nonverbal communication between clinicians and their patients. *Acad Med* 89(8):1108–1112, 2014.
93. Burgoon J, Guerrero L, Floyd K: *Nonverbal Communication*. New York, Routledge, 2016.
94. Knapp M, Hall J, Horgan T: *Nonverbal Communication in Human Interaction*. 8th ed. Boston, MA, Wadsworth, 2014.
95. Henry SG, Fuhrel-Forbis A, Rogers MA, Eggly S: Association between nonverbal communication during clinical interactions and outcomes: a systematic review and meta-analysis. *Patient Educ Couns* 86(3):297–315, 2012.
96. Brugel S, Postma-Nilsenova M, Tates K: The link between perception of clinical empathy and nonverbal behavior: the effect of a doctor's gaze and body orientation. *Patient Educ Couns* 98(10):1260–1265, 2015.
97. Ebner N, Thompson J: @ face value? Nonverbal communication & trust development in online video-based mediation. International Journal of Online Dispute Resolution. 2014. Advanced online publication.
98. Onor ML, Misan S: The clinical interview and the doctor-patient relationship in telemedicine. *Telemed J E Health* 11(1):102–105, 2005.
99. Savin D, Glueck DA, Chardavoyne J, Yager J, Novins DK: Bridging cultures: child psychiatry via videoconferencing. *Child Adolesc Psychiatr Clin N Am* 20(1):125–134, 2011.
100. McHenry M, Parker PA, Baile WF, Lenzi R: Voice analysis during bad news discussion in oncology: reduced pitch, decreased speaking rate, and nonverbal communication of empathy. *Support Care Cancer* 20(5):1073–1078, 2012.
101. Dijkstra H, Albada A, Klockner Cronauer C, Ausems MG, van Dulmen S: Nonverbal communication and conversational contribution in breast cancer genetic counseling: are counselors' nonverbal communication and conversational contribution associated with counselees' satisfaction, needs fulfillment and state anxiety in breast cancer genetic counseling? *Patient Educ Couns* 93(2):216–223, 2013.
102. Montague E, Chen P, Chewning B, Barrett B: Nonverbal interpersonal interactions in clinical encounters and patient perceptions of empathy. *J Particip Med* 5:e33, 2013.
103. Montague E, Asan O: Dynamic modeling of patient and physician eye gaze to understand the effects of electronic health records on doctor-patient communication and attention. *Int J Med Inform* 83(3):225–234, 2014.
104. American Academy of Child & Adolescent Psychiatry: Available at: http://www.aacap.org.
105. American Academy of Child &Adolescent Psychiatry: Practice parameter for telepsychiatry with children and adolescents. *J Am Acad Child Adolesc Psychiatry* 47:1468–1483, 2008.
106. Myers K, Vander Stoep A, McCarty CA: *Effectiveness of treatment provided through telemental health: Outcomes of a randomized controlled trial with multiple under-served communities*. Paper presented at: Annual Meeting of the International Society for Research in Child and Adolescent Psychopathology. Leuven, Belgium, 2013.
107. Cain S, Sharp S: Telepharmacotherapy for children and adolescents. *J Child Adolesc Psychopharmacol* 2016. Advanced online publication.
108. Ryan Haight Online Pharmacy Consumer Protection Act. P. L. No. 110-, H.R. 6353; 2008.
109. James Arnold, Chief, Liaison & Policy Section, Drug Enforcement Administration, United States Department of Justice. *Telemedicine and the Controlled Substances Act*. Presentation at the Short Course, 21st Annual Meeting of the American Telemedicine Association, Minneapolis MN, May 2016.
110. Amarendran V, George A, Gersappe V, Krishnaswamy S, Warren C: The reliability of telepsychiatry for a neuropsychiatric assessment. *Telemed J E Health* 17(3):223–225, 2011.
111. Brooks E, Spargo G, Yellowlees P, O'Neil P, Shore J: Integrating culturally appropriate care into telemental health practice. In: Myers K, Turvey C (eds): *Telemental Health: Clinical, Technical and Administrative Foundation for Evidence-Based Practice*. London, Elsevier, 63–79, 2013.
112. Pew Research Center: Cell Phone and Smartphone Ownership Demographics. *Pew Research Center Internet Project Survey* 2014. Accessed May 2, 2014.
113. Nielsenwire: *Two Thirds of New Mobile Buyers Now Opting For Smartphones*. 2012. Accessed December 18, 2012.
114. Glasgow RE, Bull SS, Piette JD, Steiner JF: Interactive behavior change technology. A partial solution to the competing demands of primary care. *Am J Prev Med* 27(2 Suppl):80–87, 2004.
115. Heron KE, Smyth JM: Ecological momentary interventions: incorporating mobile technology into psychosocial and health behaviour treatments. *Br J Health Psychol* 15(Pt 1):1–39, 2010.
116. Bauer S, de Niet J, Timman R, Kordy H: Enhancement of care through self-monitoring and tailored feedback via text messaging and their use in the treatment of childhood overweight. *Patient Educ Couns* 79(3):315–319, 2010.
117. Burke LE, Conroy MB, Sereika SM, et al.: The effect of electronic self-monitoring on weight loss and dietary intake: a randomized behavioral weight loss trial. *Obesity (Silver Spring)* 19(2):338–344, 2011.
118. Piasecki TM, Hufford MR, Solhan M, Trull TJ: Assessing clients in their natural environments with electronic diaries: rationale, benefits, limitations, and barriers. *Psychol Assess* 19(1):25–43, 2007.
119. Long JD, Littlefield LA, Estep G, et al.: Evidence review of technology and dietary assessment. *Worldviews Evid Based Nurs* 7(4):191–204, 2010.
120. American Telemedicine Association: *Lexicon of Assessment and Outcome Measures for Telepsychiatry*. 2013. Available at: http://www.americantelemed.org/docs/default-source/standards/a-lexicon-of-assessment-and-outcome-measurements-for-telemental-health.pdf?sfvrsn=2. Accessed September 19, 2014.
121. Kramer GM, Shore JH, Mishkind MC, Friedl KE, Poropatich RK, Gahm GA: A standard telemental health evaluation model: the time is now. *Telemed J E Health* 18(4):309–313, 2012.

SECTION VII

INTERFACE AREAS OF CHILD AND ADOLESCENT PSYCHIATRY

7.1 ■ PEDIATRICS

CHAPTER 7.1.1 ■ INTEGRATING BEHAVIORAL SERVICES INTO PEDIATRIC CARE SETTINGS: PRINCIPLES AND MODELS

DAVID J. SCHONFELD AND JOHN V. CAMPO

SCOPE OF THE PROBLEM

Primary care is the label applied to community-based medical settings that offer first-contact personal health care that is comprehensive and longitudinal (1). Most American children make at least one primary care medical visit annually (2), and parents look to pediatric primary care providers (PCPs) as resources for addressing psychosocial problems (3). One important strategy with potential to improve access to pediatric behavioral health services and overcome existing barriers to care is the integration of such services within general medical settings such as primary care. An important concept related to primary care is that of the medical home, which is a model of team-based primary care delivery led by a personal physician that delivers accessible, continuous, comprehensive, coordinated, culturally effective, and patient- and family-centered care (4). The medical home provides or arranges for all of the patient's health needs, including preventive services and chronic illness management. Professional organizations championing the medical home include the American College of Physicians, the American Academy of Family Physicians, and the American Academy of Pediatrics (AAP).

The public health relevance of pediatric mental health (MH) problems is increasingly being appreciated, and their relevance to the medical home should be clear. It is estimated that between 15% and more than 25% of pediatric patients have a MH problem or disorder (5,6). The prevalence of MH problems of concern to pediatricians would be even greater if the MH needs of the parents of pediatric patients (e.g., maternal depression) were considered within the purview of pediatric PCPs (7). Due to the high prevalence of MH concerns in children and adolescents and the frequency of their contact with PCPs, it stands to reason that pediatricians and other PCPs are important resources for identification and early management of common MH problems and disorders.

MH disorders are among the most disabling of pediatric conditions, and are associated with interpersonal difficulties, poor school performance, and school absenteeism, with one-third of all school days missed by adolescents being MH related. It is therefore not surprising that psychosocial problems are the most common chronic conditions presenting during pediatric ambulatory health visits, with a broad range of severity and high rates of comorbidity, comparable to chronic conditions such as asthma and diabetes. Not only are MH disorders highly prevalent across the lifespan, but early onset is more the rule than the exception, with pediatric psychiatric disorder being powerfully predictive of adult disorder and impairment. As demonstrated by the National Comorbidity Study, the onset of approximately half of all MH disorders occurs at or before age 14, with approximately three of four MH disorders beginning by age 24 years (8).

DUALISM IN PEDIATRIC HEALTH CARE

Despite a growing awareness of the biopsychosocial model of health and an appreciation that physical health and MH are inextricably linked, our health care delivery system is split into parallel systems of care depending on whether a problem is conceptualized as physical (general medical conditions) or psychological (MH disorders). While it is true that most professionals, when pressed, will agree that health is a unitary construct that cannot be parsed into physical and mental components, our behavior, the organization of health care, the systems of health care reimbursement, and the behaviors of our patients suggest otherwise. Whether a disorder is conceptualized as physical or mental thus has profound implications for how and where the disorder is cared for, which professionals are expected to bear primary responsibility for care delivery, and how that care is reimbursed. Due to the persistent stigma associated with MH disorders, there are additional societal implications resulting from whether a disorder is considered to be a general medical condition or a MH disorder. In contrast to physical disease, MH disorders are often viewed by our society as being under the voluntary control of the affected individual, the consequence of individual weakness, inadequacy, or moral failing, and thus associated with stigma, shame, and embarrassment.

Physical symptoms are a common presentation of psychiatric disorder in general medical settings, with disorders conceptualized as mental (e.g., anxiety and depressive disorders) commonly presenting to PCPs and medical specialists with very real and disabling physical complaints and distress (e.g., functional abdominal pain and headaches) (9–11). Such patients tend to utilize more health services which can be quite costly to society (12). Potentially serious physical health consequences have also been associated with pediatric MH disorders, most notably increased risks of suicide, violence, and accidental injury, as well as overweight, early pregnancy and alcohol, drug, and tobacco abuse (13–16).

Increasing attention over the past several years to the impact of early childhood adversity on children's emotional and physical health (including serious physical health conditions presenting in adulthood) has underscored not only the growing recognition of the interplay between MH and physical health, but the major public health impact of failure to prevent or mitigate these negative influences (17). Clinical guidance documents from the AAP instructing pediatricians on how to provide psychosocial support to children impacted by disasters and other crises (18) and how to support grieving children and families (19) are recent examples of pediatricians' recognition of not only the need to identify and treat mental illness, but also the necessity to make concerted efforts to promote adjustment and coping for children facing adversity.

It is also well known that physical disease is a significant risk factor for the development of emotional and behavioral problems, with several studies documenting that chronic physical disorder is a risk factor for MH problems and disorders in both community-based and clinical samples across the lifespan (20–23). In part due to the success of modern medicine, chronic physical illness is a growing problem; approximately 1% to 3% of all youth suffer from significant functional impairment resulting from chronic physical illness (21). Physical diseases or injuries that affect the brain (e.g., epilepsy, cerebral palsy, head trauma) are especially potent risk factors for comorbid emotional, behavioral, and learning problems (23,24). The presence of a MH disorder can also influence the course of physical disease, as demonstrated in juvenile diabetes, where comorbid depression has been identified as an independent risk factor for the development of diabetic retinopathy (25), repeat hospitalization (26), overall adaptation to the disease (e.g., adherence to treatment), and possibly metabolic control (27). From this, it should be evident that disorders considered to be mental can have profound physical health consequences and vice versa.

IMPLEMENTING BEST PRACTICES WITHIN PRIMARY CARE SETTINGS

Research has demonstrated the efficacy of a growing number of treatments for common pediatric MH disorders (28), but most affected youth do not receive any treatment (4,29). Of those who do receive services, many are not treated in accordance with available best practices, with considerable gaps existing between research-driven knowledge and routine clinical practices (30,31). Interventions that have been proven efficacious for attention-deficit/hyperactivity disorder (ADHD) (30), anxiety disorders (32–34), and depressive disorders are generally not systematically or effectively applied on the population level, with routine care often falling short of best practices (35). Finding the means to translate advances in treatment efficacy into practical effectiveness strategies will thus be necessary to maximize public health benefits of new advances in therapeutics, and will likely require commitment, multidisciplinary collaboration, and systemic changes in the way that professionals in primary care and specialty MH care work together (36–38). Two examples of such an initiative to improve the quality of care for pediatric MH disorders in pediatric primary care settings are the effort by the AAP to develop practice guidelines for the diagnosis and management of ADHD (39,40) and another initiative involving the AAP in partnership with MH professionals to develop guidelines for PCPs on the diagnosis and management of adolescent depression (41,42).

THE EMERGENCE OF DEVELOPMENTAL-BEHAVIORAL PEDIATRICS

The high prevalence of psychosocial problems in children within pediatric primary care settings was described by Haggerty in 1975 and termed the new morbidity. Due in part to the successes in preventive medicine (e.g., immunizations) and medical therapeutics (e.g., antibiotics), the nature of the pediatric needs of children and their families has changed, resulting in a growing emphasis on developmental and behavioral issues in pediatric care. Much of this alteration in practice pattern was also the result of a changing environment. Major changes in family, school, and neighborhood contexts over the past several decades resulted in an exacerbation and increase in developmental and behavioral problems along with a dramatic decrease in formal and informal social networks that might have in the past provided advice and guidance on their management.

The field of developmental-behavioral pediatrics (DBP) arose from the need to enhance the capacity of pediatricians to identify, manage, and when necessary, refer children with developmental and behavioral concerns and to implement effective prevention approaches. The goal was not to create a cadre of independent clinical subspecialists which might compete with child and adolescent psychiatrists, but to produce academic leaders and researchers that can enhance the training of general pediatricians so that they will be better prepared to address the developmental and behavioral needs of their own patients (43).

DBP focuses on the evaluation and management of common behavioral problems such as temper tantrums or sleep problems and attention-deficit disorders, common developmental disabilities such as autism spectrum disorders or intellectual disabilities, and physical complaints best addressed via a biobehavioral approach, such as recurrent abdominal pain. DBP aims to be eclectic and committed to multidisciplinary collaboration, with developmental-behavioral pediatricians striving to integrate a wide range of complementary theories derived from the medical, biologic, behavioral, and social sciences, and drawing upon clinical skills and research approaches that are otherwise associated with a range of disparate disciplines. As a result, there is significant overlap between conditions appropriate for management by developmental-behavioral pediatricians and other professionals, such as child and adolescent psychiatrists, neurodevelopmental specialists, pediatric neurologists, and child psychologists.

As the field of DBP matured, it became desirable to have a recognized subspecialty so that there could be a core faculty within academic medical programs to organize the teaching of medical students, residents, fellows, and other allied health professionals, to conduct relevant research, and to assist in the delivery of clinical care. The Society for Developmental and Behavioral Pediatrics (initially called the Society for Behavioral Pediatrics) was formed in 1982; it is an international, interdisciplinary organization with over 900 members whose goal is to improve the health of infants, children, and adolescents by promoting research, teaching, and clinical practice in DBP (www.sdbp.org). SDBP has a well-regarded professional journal, *Journal of Developmental and Behavioral Pediatrics* (www.jdbp.org), which is devoted entirely to the developmental and psychosocial aspects of pediatric health care and written for physicians, psychologists, and other clinicians and researchers.

In 1999, the field of DBP was approved as a subspecialty by the American Board of Medical Subspecialties and the first subboard of DBP within the American Board of Pediatrics was established to work with the Residency Review Committee to develop guidelines for subspecialty fellowship training and to develop an examination for certification of subspecialists in DBP. The first application for accreditation of Fellowship Programs in DBP was accepted by the Accreditation Council for Graduate Medical Education in October 2002. Accredited fellowship programs in DBP accept trainees upon completion of an accredited pediatric residency program and are 3 years in duration. The fellowships comprise experiences in patient care to lead to the development of clinical proficiency, involvement in community or community-based activities, and development of skills in teaching, program development, research, and child advocacy. The first board certification examination in DBP was administered in November 2002, with the first certified subspecialists in the field in March 2003.

Both DBP and child and adolescent psychiatry are relatively young fields that share many commonalities. While DBP is firmly identified with traditional medicine by virtue of its subspecialty relationship to pediatrics, and child and adolescent psychiatry typically is considered to fall under the rubric of "mental health," DBP is increasingly integrating the insights offered by modern psychiatry and child and adolescent psychiatry is increasingly acknowledging its medical roots and connections to both pediatrics and psychiatry. The popularity of "triple board" training in pediatrics, psychiatry, and child and adolescent psychiatry, an alternative training pathway that also reflects a growing appreciation of the need to bridge the apparent gap between pediatric physical and MH care, also validates the importance of active collaboration among the disciplines.

SHARING THE CHALLENGE

Although collaboration between pediatrics and psychiatry has been a topic of considerable interest and discussion for at least half a century, the hope of integrating MH services into pediatric general medical settings has yet to be realized. Parallel systems of care for physical and MH problems persist despite governmental recommendations to better integrate existing research-based knowledge into routine clinical practice (37), and existing models of reimbursement (e.g., behavioral health carve-outs) impair rather than facilitate meaningful collaboration. The scope and impact of pediatric emotional and behavioral problems nevertheless dictate that a response limited to the specialty MH sector is unlikely to prove successful in the short or long term, and is particularly unsuited to prevention efforts. Success in addressing the public health challenge presented by pediatric MH disorders will likely depend on multidisciplinary collaboration between child and adolescent psychiatrists, developmental-behavioral pediatricians, general pediatricians, family physicians, and affiliated MH professionals such as nurses, psychologists, and social workers, as well as efforts that span existing parallel systems of physical and MH care and reimbursement.

The public health importance of the primary care setting in the identification and management of common pediatric MH disorders is well recognized (3,38,44). PCPs manage the vast majority of recognized psychosocial problems (4) and prescribe the majority of psychoactive medications to American children and adolescents (37,45). Psychosocial problems are increasingly becoming the major focus of primary pediatric care for school-age children, but surveys of pediatricians suggest that they are among the most time consuming and frustrating problems to deal with in routine practice. PCPs report inadequate training in the management of pediatric MH problems (5,46), and low rates of PCP recognition of youth with MH disorders are the rule rather than the exception (3,44,46). Standardized assessment tools and/or diagnostic criteria are not in common use by PCPs in most clinical settings (47,48).

While pediatricians do identify many MH concerns in their patients (in most cases, identifying far more children in need of treatment than are able to access child MH care), most children with MH needs still go unnoticed. It has been estimated that roughly 20% of children and adolescents have MH problems that are severe enough to warrant treatment (that have a diagnosable mental, emotional, or behavioral disorder), but of this group, less than 20% to 30% receive appropriate MH services in the United States (49). In one study, pediatricians' overall sensitivity for the identification of emotional/behavioral problems among preschool children 2 to 5 years of age was only 21%, while specificity was 93% (50). As a result, just over half (52%) of the children who had an emotional/behavioral problem, based on an independent assessment by two psychologists who performed an evaluation of children who had a positive initial screen, did not receive any counseling, medication, or MH referral from the pediatrician. Pediatricians' assessments tend to have far higher specificity than sensitivity. While they may miss most children with emotional or behavioral problems, they tend not to over-diagnose. Recognition is better in children or adolescents with more severe disturbance and in those with stressful family situations. However, it is likely that early detection, when problems are less severe and less recalcitrant to change, may respond better to less intensive interventions that could be provided in a primary care setting by the pediatrician.

Fortunately, studies have shown that the rate of identification of MH problems by pediatricians in the United States has increased dramatically over the past few decades. In one study, the rates of identification by pediatricians of any MH disorders, psychological symptoms, or social situations warranting clinical attention or intervention increased almost threefold between 1979 and 1996, from 7% to 19% of all pediatric visits among 4- to 15-year-olds (51). Identification, though, represents only the first step in addressing MH needs in children. Pediatricians require additional skills if they are being expected to assist with management of some MH problems. Studies have shown that even when such problems are identified by pediatricians, most are handled through watchful waiting and/or primary care counseling alone; the vast majority of children identified with a MH or psychosocial problem never obtain services from a traditional MH provider, but instead continue to receive services from their PCP (46). Available research suggests that only one in four children with newly recognized psychosocial problems is referred for specialty MH services, with less than half of those referred ever seeing a MH specialist (5). Professional expectations as to the scope of practice are also relevant. While pediatricians have increasingly focused on the evaluation and treatment of common behavioral problems such as ADHD, which is often a major focus of DBP practice, there is considerably more variability in comfort and practice with regard to other problems such as depression and anxiety.

For example, while pediatricians feel an obligation to recognize pediatric depression, many do not consider depression treatment to be a core responsibility (52).

BARRIERS TO CARE

Barriers to MH care can be conceptualized as structural and attitudinal, and stigma likely is responsible for barriers of both types. Structural barriers can be fiscal, such as inability to pay and insurance restrictions. Relatedly, inefficiencies and deficiencies in the operational infrastructure of a health care system that segregates physical and MH care delivery services are important structural barriers to care, as are geography, transportation problems, shortages of competent health and behavioral health professionals, and a maldistribution of clinical services. Serious shortage of pediatric behavioral health specialists exists, and access to specialty behavioral health care is quite limited, particularly for low income, minority, and rural populations (5,46,53). Child and adolescent psychiatrists are particularly in short supply, which is unlikely to improve substantially any time soon given existing trends in training and support (54). Behavioral health specialists tend to cluster in more affluent and populous regions, which contributes to especially poor service access in rural areas and among low income and minority youth (55).

The primary care management of pediatric mental disorders often fails to meet recommended standards for treatment intensity and follow-up, with typically low rates of case recognition, evidence-based treatment, specialty MH referral, and referral completion (2,3,46). For example, PCP management of common disorders such as ADHD often fails to meet recommended standards for treatment intensity and follow-up (30), and PCPs are often uneasy caring for disorders other than ADHD such as depression (52,56,57). Effective care coordination for MH problems is lacking in most pediatric practices, and linkage after specialty MH referral is quite poor, with typically fewer than half of youth referred off-site to specialty behavioral health services receiving any services within the subsequent 6-month period (58–60).

Beyond structural barriers, attitudinal barriers to care such as lack of perceived need for treatment, mistrust of providers, a wish to manage problems within the family, and pessimism about the potential effectiveness of treatment can be quite significant (61). Such attitudinal barriers may be especially relevant for specific patient demographic, ethnic, and cultural groups, including with regard to prescription of psychoactive medications to youth (62), and may be every bit as relevant for providers as for patients and families.

Despite the high prevalence of MH and behavioral concerns in children and the reality that most identification and treatment of these conditions fall to pediatricians and other PCPs, up until fairly recently there was limited training for most pediatricians in this area. In 1978, the Task Force on Pediatric Education of the AAP identified child development and chronic disabling conditions as areas of graduate pediatric education that were in need of enhancement. About that time (and subsequently), surveys completed by primary care pediatricians confirmed that they felt they were not adequately prepared to handle developmental and behavioral problems.

The Residency Review Committee governing pediatric training responded to these concerns by requiring, in 1997, that all accredited pediatric residency programs include at least a 1-month block rotation, as well as additional integrated training experiences, in DBP which are directly supervised by faculty "with training in behavioral-developmental pediatrics." The vast majority of programs are now in compliance with this requirement, yet residency programs have found that providing quality training in DBP can be time-consuming and difficult. The assessment and management of behavioral concerns are highly dependent on the context; there is rarely a simple and direct approach that will work in all situations. Teaching pediatric trainees about the management of behavioral problems therefore requires opportunities for clinical practice under direct supervision and quality faculty who are able to model clinical management, precept the trainee's clinical care, and engage the trainee in a discussion of alternative management approaches, all of which take considerable faculty time and resources. Given the limited number of highly qualified DBP faculty in the country and the low reimbursement rate by health insurers for their clinical services, this poses a significant challenge. In addition, many pediatric training programs provide only limited if any exposure to child and adolescent psychiatry.

Behavioral or MH problems in children may be associated with parent–child, family, or parental problems. Assessment and treatment of the child, the identified patient, often requires assessment and intervention with the parents, yet unlike child and adolescent psychiatrists, pediatricians have very limited training or exposure to the care of adults, particularly adults with serious MH disorders. Despite these barriers, there appears to be a growing recognition among practicing pediatricians of the importance and value of continuing education in DBP and MH topics, which currently are highly prevalent among continuing medical education offerings geared to the practicing pediatrician.

Just as pediatricians may have insufficient training in the diagnosis and treatment of pediatric MH problems, child and adolescent psychiatrists typically have insufficient training on how to establish effective consultative or collaborative relationships with pediatricians and in DBP issues. Child and adolescent psychiatrists often have not been exposed to, or lack sufficient experience with, anticipatory guidance and supportive management of common pediatric concerns and problems (e.g., management of common sleep problems and feeding difficulties), and neurodevelopmental issues have been relatively deemphasized as part of child and adolescent psychiatric training in many venues, at least until more recently. Likewise, developmental-behavioral pediatricians have focused considerably more than psychiatrists on neurodevelopmental issues and on the management of common pediatric problems, but have traditionally been less interested in the assessment and management of youth with serious psychopathology (e.g., bipolar disorder). Differences in training and experience likely have influenced relatively different orientations toward emotional and behavioral problems for child and adolescent psychiatrists and pediatricians, with the former tending to focus on the identification and treatment of MH disorders and the latter more oriented toward promoting overall child developmental health and wellness. One concrete illustration of these perceived differences in orientation was the development of the Diagnostic and Statistical Manual for Primary Care (DSM-PC) (63), which aims to help pediatricians identify and address the full spectrum of psychosocial situations or symptoms, ranging from developmental variations to problems to full disorders, that would benefit from intervention, even if the child's symptoms are not severe enough to meet the criteria for a specific MH disorder within the DSM used by child and adolescent psychiatrists. Furthermore, guild-related issues in these relatively young fields of child and adolescent psychiatry and DBP may not have provided sufficient time for the development of successful collaboration across respective clinical, educational, and research missions.

The traditional isolation and private office orientation of child and adolescent psychiatrists and other MH professionals may also have served to limit and restrict meaningful collaboration with pediatricians. Different expectations about standards of confidentiality in MH and general medical settings can also serve to constrain artificially the sharing of information between PCPs and MH specialists. Current health care practices also undermine efforts to promote collaboration between pediatricians and child and adolescent psychiatrists. Increasing use of behavioral health carve-outs may diminish the willingness and ability of MH providers to establish creative collaborative care models with PCPs. Developmental-behavioral pediatricians who are qualified and interested in providing counseling services may find themselves excluded from behavioral health panels and/or forced to choose between reimbursement for either physical health or MH services, despite being qualified to deliver both and understanding the importance of delivering comprehensive care that integrates both components. Managed behavioral health care organizations usually restrict their focus to specialty MH and substance abuse services and fail to address MH services that are provided in primary care or general pediatric settings. Innovative practices and prevention models that depend on screening, evaluation, and early treatment in primary care for MH needs may not be recognized or reimbursed by either the general managed care company or the managed behavioral health care organization, and obtaining reimbursement for MH services provided in a general medical setting may often seem akin to trying to fit a square peg in a round hole. The escalating productivity demands placed on pediatricians and other PCPs requiring increased throughput of patients, coupled with the historically inadequate reimbursement for MH services provided by pediatricians (and indeed most cognitive services), place enormous time pressure on pediatricians who attempt to deliver such services within their practice setting or to engage in substantive collaborative care with child and adolescent psychiatrists or other MH professionals.

PRIMARY CARE: A BRIDGE TO COLLABORATION

Despite the challenges outlined earlier, the advantages of targeting quality improvement efforts in the primary care setting to address MH needs are quite clear and include familiarity, proximity, and relative acceptability for youth with MH disorders and their families. PCPs remain an important resource for families to address pediatric psychosocial problems, and can deliver services in the context of an established relationship (3). There are many reasons why families might wish to rely on their pediatrician to assess and manage many behavioral and MH problems. Pediatricians are one of the most trusted sources of health information and services and have established relationships with children and their families that often start at the time of the birth of the child, or may even begin during a prenatal visit. The frequent well-child checkups and sick visits, especially during the first few years of life, help to develop the relationship further; the frequent contact promotes both accessibility and convenience. For pediatricians who adopt a biopsychosocial orientation, it is especially clear that it is counterproductive, and indeed impossible, to try to separate the physical and MH care components of pediatric services. Coupled with the limited accessibility to MH providers in many communities and the stigma associated with mental illness, it is understandable why most MH and behavioral concerns present first to the child's pediatrician. A focus on primary care also acknowledges the reality that primary care is the de facto MH care system for most youths with recognized MH disorders (5) and that PCPs prescribe the vast majority of psychoactive medications to youth (37,45). Delivering MH services in primary care powerfully communicates that physical health and MH are inseparable, and may aid in efforts to overcome stigma, improve communication between and among patients, families, and providers, and establish the foundation for meaningful educational and preventive interventions (46). Surveys of patients and families suggest that there is a preference to be seen in primary care for such problems rather than specialty care (1).

While it is recognized that high quality services for emotional and behavioral difficulties in primary care are generally multidisciplinary and collaborative (64), the evidence base necessary to make informed decisions about how to proceed in pediatric primary care is lacking. MH disorders such as ADHD, anxiety, and depression are most often chronic conditions that present with a broad range of severity, are commonly comorbid with other physical and MH disorders, and can exert their impact across the lifespan with a wide range of individual and family implications. Possible quality improvement strategies to address chronic MH problems in primary care settings include expanding the role of PCPs in managing common MH disorders, as well as the use of MH specialists as consultants to support the directed efforts of PCPs and/or to directly provide MH services within primary care (65). Adult depressive and anxiety disorders have been successfully managed in primary care using strategies that employ MH professionals as educators, consultants, supervisors, and/or direct service providers (66–68). Specialist participation in primary care beyond that of traditional off-site referrals can improve communication between PCPs and specialists, improve rates of referral completion, and enhance provider satisfaction (69). The collaborative office rounds model has been one attempt to support small case-oriented discussion groups that focus on MH needs of children presenting to primary care settings; these groups are jointly led by pediatricians and child and adolescent psychiatrists (70). Available research nevertheless suggests that specialist involvement alone is less potent in improving care than are systemic changes in care system design (71–73). A number of studies have used behavioral health specialists colocated in primary care to deliver standardized interventions for emotional disorders such as brief cognitive-behavioral therapy (74,75), interpersonal psychotherapy (76), and internet-based psychotherapy (77). Applications specific to ADHD (78) and pediatric disruptive behavioral problems have also been applied in primary care, including the Incredible Years (79), Parent–Child Interaction Training (PCIT) (80), and the Triple P-Positive Parenting Program (81).

The *chronic care model (CCM)* provides a framework to address the complexities associated with integrating MH services into general medical settings, and shifts the focus of care toward a longitudinal rather than an acute or cross-sectional perspective. Goals include ensuring that a mutually understood and agreed-upon care plan is in place, that patients and families have the skills and confidence necessary to manage the condition, that the most appropriate treatments are available for optimal illness control and the prevention of complications, and that accessible and continuous follow-up care is available (72,82). There are six core elements of the CCM: (1) a *leadership* team composed of organizational partners, with leadership including specialists, generalists, and administrators with accountability for implementing the model; (2) *decision support* for direct care providers in general medical settings, which may include access to MH specialists and evidence-based guidelines to aid in the recognition and management of common MH disorders; (3) improvements in *delivery system design* to promote access to management guidelines and protocols. The use of a *care manager* responsible for coordinating care with PCPs and specialists has been promoted as an especially important element of delivery system design. The goal of a care manager is not to provide a nonphysician substitute for the PCP, but to complement and supplement the PCP's role by delivering services that the PCP does not have the skills or the time necessary to provide, such as formal psychiatric assessment, psychoeducation, and triage (72,73), as well as to facilitate communication among families, PCPs, and supporting specialists (66,73,82). Ideally, the care manager mediates specialty input to the primary care setting (66,71). The use of *patient care registries* to identify, manage, and track affected children can also modify the delivery system; (4) the use of *clinical information systems* to provide the technologic underpinnings necessary to facilitate the roles of PCPs, care managers, and MH specialists; (5) *self-management support* for patients and families that includes materials and processes that promote understanding of common MH disorders and treatment options in order to facilitate patient activation and shared decision-making; and (6) access to *community resources* independent of health care providers to aid patients and families (73,82).

A core value of the CCM is that optimal care is achieved when informed and motivated patients and families interact with a well-prepared and proactive care team that is comprised of a multidisciplinary and diverse group of clinicians who communicate and participate regularly in the care of a defined group of patients (73,82). As an adjunct, a "stepped care" approach emphasizes different levels of care depending on the type of specific disorder, its severity, complexity, and/or persistence in the face of intervention, and acknowledges the need for specialty MH care for selected or treatment refractory patients and families (66,71). For example, a low severity disorder may initially be addressed through discussion of the disorder, basic psychoeducation for the patient and family, and watchful waiting, with higher levels of care being reserved for individuals suffering with the disorder at greater levels of severity and/or complexity. These higher levels of care might include initial management of the disorder in primary care by the PCP, followed by collaborative management in the primary care setting with the assistance of a care manager with specialty MH training, followed by referral for off-site specialty care. The CCM and stepped care approaches acknowledge that high quality illness management is multidisciplinary and collaborative, and a range of services and service delivery settings are indicated based on patient and family needs, since not all MH issues can be practically managed in the primary care setting (71–73,83).

INTEGRATED MENTAL HEALTH SERVICES IN PEDIATRIC PRACTICE

Adult experience with collaborative care approaches to the management of mental problems and disorders in primary care inspired initiatives in pediatric settings, and pediatric experience with this approach is growing (84). Collaborative care interventions have been applied in primary care to disruptive behavioral problems and disorders in children (58–60) and to depression in adolescents (35,84–87). A study of 321 children aged 5 to 12 years with disruptive behavioral problems and disorders used a cluster-randomized design involving 8 primary care pediatric practices to compare a collaborative care intervention known as doctor-office collaborative care (DOCC) to enhanced usual care consisting of psychoeducation and facilitated referral. The study found that the collaborative care intervention (DOCC) was associated with significantly higher levels of treatment initiation and completion, treatment response, consumer satisfaction, and PCP confidence relative to enhanced usual care (60). In the Reaching Out to Adolescents in Distress (ROAD) study, master's level clinicians were deployed as depression care managers and facilitated treatment for adolescent depression in primary care with antidepressant medication, brief cognitive behavioral psychotherapy, or the combination (87). The care managers for the ROAD intervention met weekly with a consulting psychiatrist, psychologist, and pediatrician. Compared to an enhanced usual care condition, adolescents randomized to ROAD were significantly more likely to receive depression treatment consistent with accepted standards (86% vs. 26%), respond to treatment (68% vs. 39%), achieve remission (50% vs. 21%), and report higher levels of satisfaction with care. A recent review and meta-analysis found that collaborative care interventions delivered stronger effects on outcomes than other attempts to provide integrated care, with an effect size of $d = 0.63$ reflecting a 73% probability that a randomly selected child or adolescent struggling with a mental disorder in primary care would experience better outcomes in response to collaborative care than another randomly selected youngster receiving usual care (88).

We have previously described the feasibility of a "real-world" program within a large rural primary care practice in western Pennsylvania that relies on the relationship between PCPs and an on-site collaborative MH care team consisting of an advanced practice nurse (APN) with specialty MH training, a psychiatric social worker, and a child and adolescent psychiatrist (89). In this model, the PCP is the physician of record with responsibilities that include initial case identification, presumptive diagnosis, and ensuring the overall continuity of patient care. The APN serves as the primary liaison between the PCPs and psychiatrist (who is most often off-site), and functions as a bridge between primary and specialty care. The APN works closely with the PCP to complete an initial assessment and to triage each patient with an identified problem, with the goal of determining whether the child might benefit from services, and if so, where and how such services are best delivered. Treatment options include: (1) collaborative management with the PCP in primary care (generally appropriate for relatively straightforward, uncomplicated patients or those on a stable treatment regimen); (2) on-site MH comanagement by the PCP in collaboration with the primary care–based specialty MH team (such an approach might be appropriate for patients who failed earlier treatment by the PCP or patients of intermediate complexity or severity); and (3) off-site specialty MH referral (for patients with more complicated and/or severe disorders and those with psychosocial circumstances likely to render management within the primary care setting unsuccessful).

The APN provides patient and family education, ongoing case management and coordination, school liaison (e.g., requests and obtains teacher reports of patient behavior and performance), and treatment support services (psychopharmacology safety and outcome monitoring; brief psychotherapeutic support and intervention, including parent management training, simple behavior programs, and training in self-management strategies). The psychiatric social worker delivers brief psychotherapy for selected patients and families on-site and the child and adolescent psychiatrist provides MH team leadership, supervision, education, psychiatric consultation for selected cases (diagnostic dilemmas, treatment failures), and will occasionally comanage with the PCP cases requiring input from an experienced psychopharmacologist. Approximately two-thirds of newly evaluated patients are triaged to routine services delivered by the PCP with APN support, 20% are managed on-site by the PCP and MH team, and the remainder is referred to off-site specialty MH services. This rural program has been well received by PCPs, patients, and families, and patient and family compliance with initial assessment and triage visits has been quite high (91%) (89). This collaborative approach allows for MH services to be delivered and supported by blending both general medical and behavioral health funding streams, but other approaches may be even more feasible, such as those built around an APN capable of billing for the assessment and primary care–based management of youth with emotional and behavioral problems via medical funding streams. A stumbling block for collaborative care approaches implemented outside a research setting arises from the practical difficulties of deriving fiscal support for specialist involvement that is not face to face with patients and families.

In response to the need for greater collaboration between pediatric PCPs and child and adolescent psychiatrists, several models using MH specialists to provide brief, focused input to PCPs have evolved, with most relying on the use of the telephone for consultation. Several statewide initiatives have championed this approach, including the Massachusetts Child Psychiatry Access Project (90) and the state of Washington Partnership Access Line (91). In these programs, PCPs can access a child and adolescent psychiatrist for a patient-focused telephone consultation on a broad range of issues, including diagnosis, intervention options, the specifics of management and ongoing monitoring, and determination of the most appropriate level of care. Other approaches have included training PCPs to improve skills related to MH and enhance their willingness and capacity to care for behavioral health problems and disorders by virtue of didactic presentations, group consultation, peer consultation, and clinical practice guidelines for the management of specific disorders. Relatively large-scale efforts focused on PCP training and ongoing practice-based consultation include the REACH Institute (www.thereachinstitute.org) and Ohio Minds Matter (www.ohiomindsmatter.org), a state-sponsored program to aid PCPs in the assessment and management of pediatric mental health problems and disorders with the aim of improving the quality and safety of psychopharmacologic practice.

Unfortunately, novel efforts such as those described above may prove to be "nonstarters" in the real world unless innovations in systems of compensation for the delivery of behavioral health care services are permitted to parallel innovations in care delivery models. Nevertheless, while challenging from a fiscal perspective, collaborative models that flexibly incorporate pediatric MH specialists into primary care appear to be feasible and compatible with the workings of medical practice. Recent health care legislation is beginning to result in shifts in health care financing that encourages an orientation toward promoting the health of a population (rather than exclusively compensating for the treatment of individual illnesses), which in turn has begun to incentivize integrated approaches to behavioral and physical health in order to improve access to high quality behavioral health services, enhance patient outcomes, and decrease overall health care costs. A recent meta-analysis of randomized controlled trials evaluating the benefits of integrated care for children and adolescents has demonstrated positive behavioral health care outcomes when compared to primary care alone, with the greatest effects seen in the area of treatment interventions that used collaborative care models and that targeted MH problems (88).

CONCLUSION

Health is a unitary construct that cannot be effectively parsed into physical health and MH, and thoughtful collaboration between child and adolescent psychiatrists, developmental-behavioral pediatricians, general pediatricians, and other professionals involved in pediatric care is critical to ensure the quality improvement efforts deserved by children everywhere. Integration can help address both structural and attitudinal barriers to behavioral health care delivery and challenge stigma. The familiarity, proximity, and acceptability of the primary care setting builds on established child and family relationships with PCPs. The PCP's attention to MH concerns communicates the powerful message that physical health and MH are inseparable. Equipping PCPs with the requisite knowledge and skills to identify, evaluate, and manage common developmental and behavioral concerns is a major goal of the field of DBP, and child and adolescent psychiatrists are increasingly contributing to such efforts. The integration of MH services into primary care may aid in efforts to overcome previously identified barriers to intervention, such as cost and transportation problems, stigma, and perceptions that treatment is not relevant, and strained relationships with MH service providers (92). Stepped collaborative care approaches that bridge primary and specialty care, as well as traditional medical care and behavioral health care, have the potential to facilitate patient and family access to MH services, improve adherence with initial MH contacts, decrease time between initial MH referral and active treatment, increase the quality of MH services in primary care, reduce stigma, efficiently integrate specialty MH professionals into primary care medical practice, and challenge false dichotomies between physical and MH care and reimbursement strategies. Collaborative care interventions for pediatric mental health problems and disorders have been demonstrated to be feasible and to improve access to behavioral health services, outcomes, and patient and family satisfaction relative to existing care models. Beyond modifying fiscal and regulatory models to accommodate the application of collaborative care interventions in pediatric general medical settings, changes in patient, family, and provider attitudes are likely necessary as well. Research on the successful dissemination of evidence-based collaborative care interventions is needed.

References

1. Kelleher K: Prevention and intervention in primary care. In: Remschmidt H, Belfer M, Goodyer I (eds): *Facilitating Pathways: Care, Treatment and Prevention in Child and Adolescent Mental Health.* Berlin, Springer-Verlag, 2004.
2. Costello EJ, Burns BJ, Costello AJ, Edelbrock C, Dulcan M, Brent D: Service utilization and psychiatric diagnosis in pediatric primary care: the role of the gatekeeper. *Pediatrics* 82:435–441, 1988.
3. Horwitz SM, Leaf PJ, Leventhal JM, Forsyth B, Speechley KN: Identification and management of psychosocial and developmental problems in community-based, primary care pediatric practices. *Pediatrics* 89:480–485, 1992.
4. Croghan TW, Brown JD. *Integrating Mental Health Treatment Into the Patient Centered Medical Home. AHRQ Publication No. 10–0084-EF.* Rockville, MD, Agency for Healthcare Research and Quality, 2010.
5. Rushton J, Bruckman D, Kelleher KJ: Primary care referral of children with psychosocial problems. *Arch Pediatr Adolesc Med* 156:592–598, 2002.
6. Frazer C, Emans SJ, Goodman E, Luoni M, Bravender T, Knight J: Teaching residents about development and behavior: meeting the new challenge. *Arch Pediatr Adolesc Med* 153:1190–1194, 1999.
7. Olson AL, Kemper KJ, Kelleher KJ, Hammond CS, Zuckerman BS, Dietrich AJ: Primary care pediatricians' roles and perceived responsibilities in the identification and management of maternal depression. *Pediatrics* 110:1169–1176, 2002.
8. Kessler RC, Berglund P, Demler O, Jin R, Walters E: Lifetime prevalence and age of onset distributions of DSM-IV disorders in the National Comorbidity Survey Replication. *Arch Gen Psychiatry* 62:593–602, 2005.
9. Campo JV, Bridge J, Ehmann M, et al.: Recurrent abdominal pain, anxiety, and depression in primary care. *Pediatrics* 113:817–824, 2004.
10. Egger HL, Costello EJ, Erkanli A, et al.: Somatic complaints and psychopathology in children and adolescents: stomach aches, musculoskeletal pains and headaches. *J Am Child Adolesc Psychiatry* 38:852–860, 1999.
11. Liakopoulou-Kairis M, Alifieraki T, Protagora D, et al.: Recurrent abdominal pain and headache: psychopathology, life event and family functioning. *Eur Child Adolesc Psychiatry* 11:115–122, 2002.
12. Campo JV, Comer D, Jansen-McWilliams L, Gardner W, Kelleher KJ: Recurrent pain, emotional distress, and health service use in childhood. *J Pediatrics* 141:76–83, 2002.
13. Bernstein G, Shaw K: Practice parameters for the assessment and treatment of children and adolescents with anxiety disorders. *J Am Acad Child Adolesc Psychiatry* 36(10 Suppl):S69–S84, 1997.
14. Birmaher B, Ryan N, Williamson D, et al.: Childhood and adolescent depression: a review of the past 10 years. Part I. *J Am Acad Child Adolesc Psychiatry* 35(11):1427–1439, 1996.
15. Costello EJ, Angold A, Burns BJ, Erkanli A, Stangl DK, Tweed DL: The Great Smoky Mountains Study of Youth: functional impairment and serious emotional disturbance. *Arch Gen Psychiatry* 53:1137–1143, 1996.
16. Lumeng JC, Gannon K, Cabral H, Frank DA, Zuckerman B: Association between clinically meaningful behavior problems and overweight in children. *Pediatrics* 112:1138–1145, 2003.
17. Felitti VJ, Anda RF: The relationship of adverse childhood experiences to adult medical disease, psychiatric disorders, and sexual behavior: implications for healthcare. In: Lanius RA, Vermetten E, Pain C (eds): *The Hidden Epidemic: The Impact of Early Life Trauma on Health and Disease.* Cambridge, Cambridge University Press, 77–87, 2010.
18. Schonfeld DJ, Demaria T; The Disaster Preparedness Advisory Council, and Committee on Psychosocial Aspects of Child and Family Health of

the American Academy of Pediatrics: Providing psychosocial support to children and families in the aftermath of disaster and crisis: a guide for pediatricians. *Pediatrics* 136(4):e1120–e1130, 2015.

19. Schonfeld DJ, Demaria T, Committee on Psychosocial Aspects of Child and Family Health, and Disaster Preparedness Advisory Council: Supporting the grieving child and family. *Pediatrics* 138(3):e20162147, 2016. doi:10.1542/peds.2016-147
20. Dew MA: Psychiatric disorder in the context of physical illness. In: Dohrenwend BP (ed): *Adversity, Stress, and Psychopathology*. New York, Oxford University Press, 177–218, 1998.
21. Gortmaker SL, Walker DK, Weitzman M, Sobol AM: Chronic conditions, socioeconomic risks, and behavioral problems in children and adolescents. *Pediatrics* 85:267–276, 1990.
22. Kovacs M, Goldston D, Obrosky DS, Bonar L: Psychiatric disorders in youths with IDDM: rates and risk factors. *Diabetes Care* 20:36–44, 1997.
23. Rutter M, Tizard J, Whitmore K: *Education, Health, and Behavior.* London, Longman Group, 1990.
24. Max JE, Koele SL, Smith WL, et al.: Psychiatric disorders in children and adolescents after severe traumatic brain injury: a controlled study. *J Am Acad Child Adolesc Psychiatry* 37:832–840, 1998.
25. Kovacs M, Mukerji P, Drash A, Iyengar S: Biomedical and psychiatric risk factors for retinopathy among children with IDDM. *Diabetes Care* 18:1592–1599, 1995.
26. Garrison MM, Katon WJ, Richardson LP: The impact of psychiatric comorbidities on readmissions for diabetes in youth. *Diabetes Care* 28:2150–2154, 2005.
27. Dantzer C, Swendsen J, Maurice-Tison S, Salamon R: Anxiety and depression in juvenile diabetes: a critical review. *Clin Psychol Rev* 23:787–800, 2003.
28. Weisz JR, Jensen PS: Efficacy and effectiveness of child and adolescent psychotherapy and pharmacotherapy. *Mental Health Serv Res* 1:125–157, 1999.
29. Costello EJ, He JP, Sampson NA, Kessler RC, Merikangas KR: Services for adolescents with psychiatric disorders: 12-month data from the National Comorbidity Survey-Adolescent. *Psychiatr Serv* 65(3):359–366, 2014.
30. Jensen PS, Hinshaw SP, Swanson JM, et al.: Findings from the NIMH Multimodal Treatment Study of ADHD (MTA): implications and applications for primary care providers. *J Dev Behav Pediatr* 22:60–73, 2001.
31. Olfson M, Gameroff MJ, Marcus SC, Waslick BD: Outpatient treatment of child and adolescent depression in the United States. *Arch Gen Psychiatry* 60:1236–1242, 2003.
32. Birmaher B, Axelson DA, Monk K, et al.: Fluoxetine for the treatment of childhood anxiety disorders. *J Am Acad Child Adolesc Psychiatry* 42(4): 415–423, 2003.
33. Kendall P, Flannery-Schroeder E, Panichelli-Mindel S, Southam-Gerow M, Henin A, Warman M: Therapy for youths with anxiety disorders: a second randomized clinical trial. *J Consult Clin Psychol* 65:366–380, 1997.
34. Walkup J, Labellart M, Riddle M, Pine D, Greenhill L, Klein R: Fluvoxamine for the treatment for anxiety disorders in children and adolescents. *N Engl J Med* 344:1279–1285, 2001.
35. Asarnow J, Jaycox LH, Duan N, et al.: Effectiveness of a quality improvement intervention for adolescent depression in primary care clinic: a randomized controlled trial. *JAMA* 293:311–319, 2005.
36. Institute of Medicine Committee on Quality of Health Care in America: *Crossing the Quality Chasm: A New Health System for the 21st Century.* Washington, DC, National Academy Press, 2001.
37. Ringeisen H, Oliver KA, Menvielle E: Recognition and treatment of mental disorders in children. *Pediatr Drugs* 4:697–703, 2002.
38. *U.S. Public Health Service Report of the Surgeon General's Conference on Children's Mental Health: A National Action Agenda.* Washington, DC, Department of Health and Human Services, 2000.
39. American Academy of Pediatrics, Committee on Quality Improvement: Diagnosis and evaluation of the child with attention-deficit/hyperactivity disorder. *Pediatrics* 105:1158–1170, 2000.
40. American Academy of Pediatrics, Committee on Quality Improvement: Clinical practice guidelines: treatment of the school-aged child with attention-deficit/hyperactivity disorder. *Pediatrics* 108:1033–1044, 2001.
41. Zuckerbrot RA, Cheung AH, Jensen PS, Stein RE, Laraque D; GLAD-PC Steering Group: Guidelines for Adolescent Depression in Primary Care (GLAD-PC): I. Identification, assessment, and initial management. *Pediatrics* 120(5):e1299–e1312, 2007.
42. Cheung AH, Zuckerbrot RA, Jensen PS, Ghalib K, Laraque D, Stein RE: Guidelines for Adolescent Depression in Primary Care (GLAD-PC): II. Treatment and ongoing management. *Pediatrics* 120(5):e1313–e1326, 2007.
43. Stein RE: Are we on the right track? Examining the role of developmental behavioral pediatrics. *Pediatrics* 135(4):589–591, 2015.
44. Costello EJ, Edelbrock C, Costello AJ, Dulcan MK, Burns BJ, Brent D: Psychopathology in pediatric primary care: the new hidden morbidity. *Pediatrics* 82:415–424, 1988.
45. Kelleher K, Hohmann AA, Larson DB: Prescription of psychotropics to children in office based practice. *Am J Dis Child* 143:855–859, 1989.
46. Kelleher KJ, Childs GE, Wasserman RC, McInerny TK, Nutting PA, Gardner WP: Insurance status and recognition of psychosocial problems: a report from PROS and ASPN. *Arch Pediatr Adolesc Med* 151:1109–1115, 1997.
47. Gardner W, Kelleher KJ, Pajer KA, Campo JV: Primary care clinicians' use of standardized tools to assess child psychosocial problems. *Ambulatory Pediatrics* 3(4):191–195, 2003.
48. Gardner W, Kelleher KJ, Pajer KA, Campo JV: Primary care clinicians' use of standardized psychiatric diagnoses. *Child: Care, Health, and Development* 30(5):401–412, 2004.
49. National Conference of State Legislatures Children's Policy Initiative: *The Consortium on the School-Based Promotion of Social Competence,* 2002.
50. Lavigne JV, Binns HJ, Christoffel KK, Rosenbaum D, et al.: Behavioral and emotional problems among preschool children in pediatric primary care: prevalence and pediatricians' recognition. Pediatric Practice Research Group. *Pediatrics* 91:649–655, 1993.
51. Kelleher KJ, McInerny TK, Gardner WP, Childs GE, Wasserman RC: Increasing identification of psychosocial problems: 1979–1996. *Pediatrics* 105(6):1313–1321, 2000.
52. Olson AL, Kelleher KJ, Kemper KJ, Zuckerman BS, Hammond CS, Dietrich AJ: Primary care pediatricians' roles and perceived responsibilities in the identification and management of depression in children and adolescents.*Ambulatory Pediatrics* 2:91–98, 2001.
53. Blais R, Breton JJ, Fournier M, St-Georges M, Berthiaume C: Are mental health services for children distributed according to needs? *Can J Psychiatry* 48(3):176, 2003.
54. Thomas CR, Holzer CE 3rd: The continuing shortage of child and adolescent psychiatrists. *J Am Acad Child Adolesc Psychiatry* 45:1023–1031, 2006.
55. Gardner W, Klima J, Chisolm D, et al.: Screening, triage, and referral of patients reporting suicidal thought during a primary care visit. *Pediatrics* 125(5):945–952, 2010.
56. Rushton JL, Clark SJ, Freed GL: Pediatrician and family physician prescription of selective serotonin reuptake inhibitors. *Pediatrics* 105(6):E82, 2000.
57. Stein RE, Storfer-Isser A, Kerker BD, et al.: Beyond ADHD: how well are we doing? *Acad Pediatr* 16(2):115–121, 2016.
58. Kolko DA, Campo JV, Kelleher KJ, Cheng Y: Improving access to care and clinical outcome for pediatric behavioral problems: a randomized trial of a nurse-administered intervention in primary care. *J Dev Behav Pediatr* 31(5):393–404, 2010.
59. Kolko DJ, Campo JV, Kilbourne AM, Kelleher K: Doctor-office collaborative care for pediatric behavioral problems: a preliminary clinical trial. *Arch Pediatr Adolesc Med* 166(3):224–231, 2012.
60. Kolko DJ, Campo JV, Kilbourne AM, Hart J, Sakolsky D, Wisniewski S: Collaborative care outcomes for pediatric behavioral health problems: a cluster randomized trial. *Pediatrics* 133(4):e981–e992, 2014.
61. Andrade LH, Alonso J, Mneimneh Z, et al.: Barriers to mental health treatment: results from the WHO World Mental Health surveys. *Psychol Med* 44(6):1303–1317, 2014.
62. Stevens J, Wang W, Fang L, Edwards MC, Campo JV, Gardner W: Parental attitudes towards children's use of antidepressants and psychotherapy. *J Child Adolesc Psychopharmacol* 19:289–296, 2009.
63. Wolraich M, Felice M, Drotar D: *The Classification of Child and Adolescent Mental Diagnoses in Primary Care: Diagnostic and Statistical Manual for Primary Care (DSM-PC), Child and Adolescent Version.* Elk Grove Village, IL, American Academy of Pediatrics, 1996.
64. Pincus H: The future of behavioral health and primary care: drowning in the mainstream or left on the bank? *Psychosomatics* 44:1–11, 2003.
65. Bower P, Garralda E, Kramer T, et al.: The treatment of child and adolescent mental health problems in primary care: a systematic review. *Family Practice* 18:373–382, 2001.
66. Katon W, Von Korff M, Lin E, et al.: Stepped collaborative care for primary care patients with persistent symptoms of depression: a randomized trial. *Arch Gen Psychiatry* 56:1109–1115, 1999.
67. Rollman BL, Belnap BH, Mazumdar S, et al.: A randomized trial to improve the quality of treatment for panic and generalized anxiety disorders in primary care. *Arch Gen Psychiatry* 62(12):1332–1341, 2005.
68. Schulberg HC, Katon WJ, Simon GE, Rush AJ: Best clinical practice: guidelines for managing major depression in primary medical care. *J Clin Psychiatry* 60:19–26, 1999.
69. Forrest CB, Glade GB, Baker AE, Bocian AB, Kang M, Starfield B: The pediatric primary-specialty care interface: how pediatricians refer children and adolescents to specialty care. *Arch Pediatr Adolesc Med* 153:705–714, 1999.
70. Fishman ME, Kessel W, Heppel DE, et al.: Collaborative office rounds: continuing education in the psychosocial/developmental aspects of child health. *Pediatrics* 99:e5, 1997.
71. Katon W, Von Korff M, Lin E, Simon G: Rethinking practitioner roles in chronic illness: the specialist, primary care physician, and the practice nurse. *Gen Hosp Psychiatry* 23:138–144, 2001.
72. Von Korff M, Gruman J, Schaefer J, Curry SJ, Wagner EH: Collaborative management of chronic illness. *Ann Inter Med* 127:1097–1102, 1997.
73. Wagner EH: The role of patient care teams in chronic disease management. *BMJ* 320:569–572, 2000.
74. Weersing VR, Rozenman MS, Maher-Bridge M, Campo JV: Anxiety, depression, and somatic distress: developing a transdiagnostic internalizing toolbox for pediatric practice. *Cogn Behav Pract* 19(1):68–82, 2012.
75. Warner CM, Colognori D, Kim RE, et al.: Cognitive-behavioral treatment of persistent functional somatic complaints and pediatric anxiety: an initial controlled trial. *Depress Anxiety* 28(7):551–559, 2011.
76. Mufson L, Yanes-Lukin P, Anderson G: A pilot study of Brief IPT-A delivered in primary care. *Gen Hosp Psychiatry* 37(5):481–484, 2015.

77. Saulsberry A, Marko-Holguin M, Blomeke K, et al.: Randomized clinical trial of a primary care internet-based intervention to prevent adolescent depression: one-year outcomes. *J Can Acad Child Adolesc Psychiatry* 22(2):106–117, 2013.
78. Epstein JN, Rabiner D, Johnson DE, et al.: Improving attention-deficit/hyperactivity disorder treatment outcomes through use of a collaborative consultation treatment service by community-based pediatricians: a cluster randomized trial. *Arch Pediatr Adolesc Med* 161(9):835–840, 2007.
79. Lavigne JV, Lebailly SA, Gouze KR, et al.: Treating oppositional defiant disorder in primary care: a comparison of three models. *J Pediatr Psychol* 33(5):449–461, 2008.
80. Berkovits MD, O'Brien KA, Carter CG, Eyberg SM: Early identification and intervention for behavior problems in primary care: a comparison of two abbreviated versions of parent-child interaction therapy. *Behav Ther* 41(3):375–387, 2010.
81. Turner KM, Sanders MR: Help when it's needed first: a controlled evaluation of brief, preventive behavioral family intervention in a primary care setting. *Behav Ther* 37(2):131–142, 2006.
82. Rothman AA, Wagner EH: Chronic illness management: what is the role of primary care? *Ann Intern Med* 138:256–261, 2003.
83. Pincus HA, Hough L, Houtsinger JK, Rollman BL, Frank RG: Emerging models of depression care: multi-level ("6P") strategies. *Int J Methods Psychiatr Res* 12:54–63, 2003.
84. Kolko DJ, Perrin E: The integration of behavioral health interventions in children's health care: services, science, and suggestions. *J Clin Child Adolesc Psychol* 43(2):216–228, 2014.
85. Asarnow JR, Jaycox LH, Tang L, et al.: Long-term benefits of short-term quality improvement interventions for depressed youths in primary care. *Am J Psychiatry* 166(9):1002–1010, 2009.
86. Clarke G, Debar L, Lynch F, et al.: A randomized effectiveness trial of brief cognitive-behavioral therapy for depressed adolescents receiving antidepressant medication. *J Am Acad Child Adolesc Psychiatry* 44(9):888–898, 2005.
87. Richardson LP, Ludman E, McCauley E, et al.: Collaborative care for adolescents with depression: a randomized clinical trial. *JAMA* 312(8):809–816, 2014.
88. Asarnow JR, Rozenman M, Wiblin J, Zeltzer L: Integrated medical-behavioral care compared with usual primary care for child and adolescent behavioral health: a meta-analysis. *JAMA Pediatr* 169(10):929–937, 2015.
89. Campo JV, Shafer S, Lucas A, et al.: Managing pediatric mental disorders in primary care: a stepped collaborative care model. *J Am Psychiatr Nurses Assoc* 11:1–7, 2005.
90. Straus JH, Sarvet B: Behavioral health care for children: the Massachusetts child psychiatry access project. *Health Aff (Millwood)* 33(12):2153–2161, 2014.
91. Hilt RJ, Romaire MA, McDonell MG, et al.: The partnership access line: evaluating a child psychiatry consult program in Washington State. *JAMA Pediatr* 167(2):162–168, 2013.
92. Kazdin AE, Holland L, Crowley M: Family experiences of barriers to treatment and premature termination from child therapy. *J Consult Clin Psychol* 65:453–463, 1997.

CHAPTER 7.1.2 ■ PEDIATRIC CONSULTATION LIAISON

LAURIE CARDONA

During the last two decades, there have been dramatic improvements in the treatment of previously life-threatening childhood diseases. The improvements have included: the development of newer vaccines and greater dissemination of immunization programs, improvements in surgical techniques for congenital conditions, advancements in the care of premature infants, broader implementation of prenatal and newborn screening for genetic conditions, and the development of standardized models of medical care, as in the treatment of childhood cancers (1). These medical advances have resulted in significant declines in the incidence and overall impact of childhood diseases. For example, today, the 5-year survival rate for pediatric leukemia is 95%, and there are similar trends with all the major childhood illnesses. Nevertheless, it is estimated that approximately 8% of children have a chronic health condition that affects their daily functioning. Furthermore, data show that children living in poverty are particularly at risk for the development of a chronic health condition (1). Thus, the need for timely mental health assessments and interventions with this population of children becomes of even greater importance.

Children with medical disorders appear to be at increased risk for the development of mental health difficulties in comparison to healthy peers. A 2011 meta-analysis, which integrated the findings from 569 studies, revealed that children and adolescents with a chronic physical condition have higher levels of internalizing problems (somatic complaints, anxiety, depression, social withdrawal) and externalizing problems (aggressive behaviors, delinquent behaviors) in comparison to healthy peers or the test norms (2). There were notable differences across various disease types; for example, there were large elevations in internalizing problems for children with chronic fatigue syndrome and moderate elevations in children with migraine headache, epilepsy, chronic kidney/liver disease, asthma, inflammatory bowel disease, and spina bifida. Moderator effects such as socio-demographic characteristics were also evident. Accordingly, there were stronger elevations of problems in children with chronic illnesses living in developing countries. Gender differences were also evident in the analyses, such that boys exhibited higher rates of externalizing problems.

Families and primary caregivers can also be deeply affected by a child's medical condition. The challenges can vary according to disease, however studies have identified a variety of stressors that confront families including: significant changes in daily routines, increased financial burdens, reduced or loss of employment, social isolation, and marital strain (3). Furthermore, parents of chronically ill children have reported significantly lower health-related quality of life (4); and there is evidence that some parents may develop formal psychiatric symptoms. Parents of childhood survivors of cancer, for example, report posttraumatic stress symptoms associated with the distress of their child's cancer treatments (5). Given the significant burdens of caring for a chronically ill child, the family's level of functioning, coping, and adaptation can become compromised, which will in turn influence child adaptation.

BIOPSYCHOSOCIAL MODEL OF CHILD ADAPTATION TO ILLNESS

Historically, pediatric consultation work has largely focused on assessment and intervention with the child and family. Research has documented, however, that there is a complex

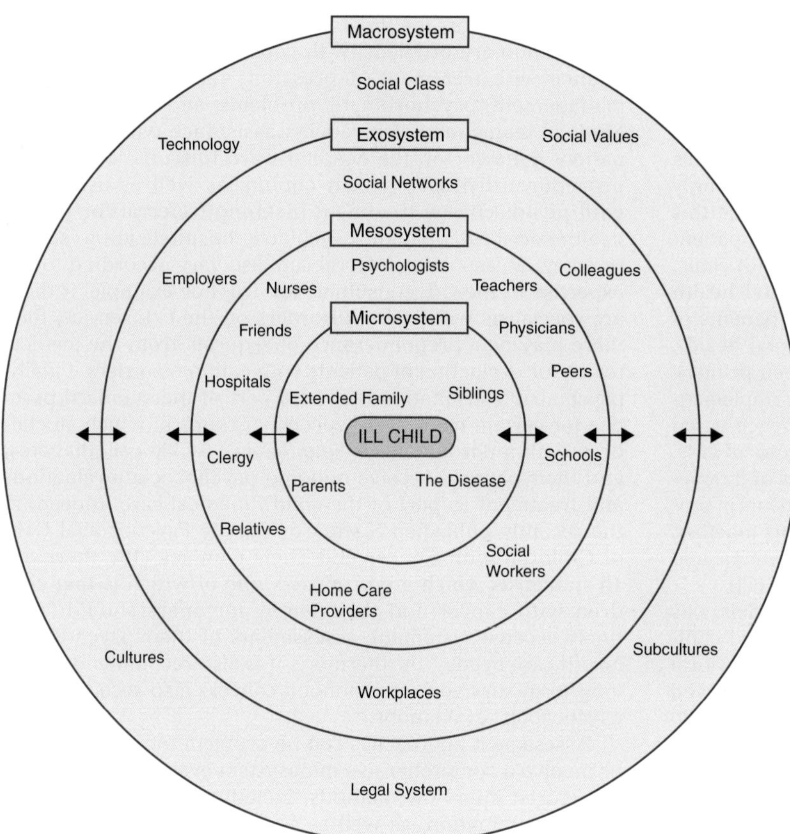

FIGURE 7.1.2.1. A social-ecologic model of children with pediatric illness. (Reprinted from Kazak AE, Segal-Andrews AM, Johnson K: Pediatric psychology research and practice: A family/systems approach. In: Roberts MC (ed): *Handbook of Pediatric Psychology*. 2nd ed. Guilford Press, 1995, p. 88, with permission.)

interplay between child-centered variables, family context, treatment providers and broader systems which can all impact a child's psychological adjustment. Furthermore, there is growing recognition that a child's medical illness also impacts siblings, extended family members, peers, and even community members. Therefore, a biopsychosocial approach to the assessment of a child and family's psychological adjustment provides the most comprehensive framework. Kazak's adaptation (6) of the Brofenbrenner social-ecologic model of child development provides a cohesive overview of the multiple influences on child and adolescent adaptation to medical illness (Figure 7.1.2.1).

Kazak's framework features basic theoretical tenets of (a) multiple layers of influence (nested systems) and (b) bidirectionality of influence on psychological functioning and adjustment. Factors influencing a child's functioning and adaptation are nested within systems that extend from intraindividual (e.g., cognitive functioning) to larger ecologic influences (e.g., medical technology).

As illustrated in Figure 7.1.2.1, systems of influence are nested within one another and represent diminishing causal influences on the patient's adaptation and functioning. The innermost circle is symbolic of the child with pediatric illness and the intraindividual factors that impact the child's psychological adjustment and functioning. Examples of intraindividual variables include a child's level of cognitive functioning, developmental level, temperament, and capacities for coping. These individualistic characteristics can be affected significantly by an array of disease-related variables. Accordingly, disease-related influences that can impact a child's functioning include: restrictions in physical mobility, chronicity of pain, and central nervous system involvement, as in the case of the untoward "late effects" of cranial radiation (7).

The microsystem also involves the patient's most immediate social relationships, including parents, siblings, and extended families. As with healthy children, the role of parental psychological functioning is a significant contributor to child adaptation, particularly to medical illness. Microsystem influences are deemed the most proximal and salient causal influences on the child's adjustment. Mesosystem influences consist of more distal social and ecologic influences on the patient's adaptation, exemplified by peers, school personnel, and an array of medical and mental health providers within the hospital setting and beyond.

Exosystem influences consist of a variety of contexts that impact social relationships and functioning within the mesosystem. Finally, macrosystem influences are those that impact the entire system, such as cultural beliefs, social values, and, particularly relevant to pediatrics, medical technology. These larger systems may have an equally profound impact on the family and child, as in the case of access to health insurance and to specialized medical care, which have become increasingly daunting challenges for many families.

RANGE OF C/L SETTINGS AND ACTIVITIES

Pediatric psychologists and psychiatrists conduct an array of patient-based clinical services. Additionally, they become involved in activities such as development of programs for promotion of health and prevention of health and psychological problems; education programs for pediatricians and family physicians regarding general child development issues; advocacy regarding child health and mental health at the public policy level; and applied clinical research (8).

Roberts (8) described five settings in which pediatric psychology services are most commonly provided: (1) inpatient medical center units, including C/L services for neonatal units, oncology units, respiratory care units, and ICU; (2) outpatient medical clinics such as primary care centers, pediatric oncology clinics, genetics clinics; (3) outpatient clinics providing care for children with psychiatric disorders; (4) specialty facilities such as rehabilitation centers and hospice; and (5) camps or groups such as summer camps for children with diabetes, and support groups for children and their parents.

The American Academy of Child and Adolescent Psychiatry (AACAP) and the American Academy of Pediatrics proposed that mental health services should be increasingly integrated into primary care systems of care (9). While this is a move away from traditional practice models of inpatient consultation or referrals to an outpatient mental health clinic, it is expected that integrated and co-located mental health care will likely increase in the future Act (10). The benefits of co-located care include: improving access to mental health, increased communication and collaboration between primary care providers and psychiatry, and it allows ready implementation of standardized screening measures and evidence-based psychosocial treatments (11). Within a model of co-located care, the mental health clinician can have varying degrees of interaction with the primary care physician, from seeing patients in separate offices within the same facility, to seeing patients together, coordinating case conferences and clinical team meetings, and conducting case-based teaching for primary care staff (11).

The empirical efficacy of collaborative care models was examined through a 2015 meta-analysis of randomized clinical trials that evaluated whether integrated medical-behavioral health care for children and adolescents leads to improved behavioral health outcomes (12). The meta-analysis included 31 studies and found a significant benefit to integrated care, relative to usual care on mental health outcomes. Specifically, the probability was 73% that a randomly selected youth would have a better outcome after receiving collaborative care, than youth receiving usual medical care. The study also concluded that collaborative care had the strongest effect in those treatment trials that included evidence-based medication algorithms plus evidence-based psychotherapy.

Another promising and emerging method of collaborative care has been Telemedicine, in which the use of interactive video technology, web-based support, as well as phone calls, allows patients, pediatricians and mental health providers to work together over large geographic areas. Two such programs, one established in Massachusetts in 2005 (Massachusetts Child Psychiatry Access Project) and the other in Washington State in 2007 (Washington State Partnership Access Line) provide pediatric primary care practices with access to mental health consultation through phone hotlines. A review of the Massachusetts Program (13) indicated that primary care physicians used the service most often for diagnostic questions (34%), identifying community providers (27%), and questions about medications (27%). A review of the Washington State program (14) revealed that 66% of the calls were regarding pharmacologic questions and 87% of the calls resulted in new psychosocial treatment advice.

As pediatric psychologists and psychiatrists become increasingly accessible to patients and families through systems of collaborative care, the challenge is for practitioners to become even more flexible and facile in providing a broad range of assessment and intervention services. In order to do so, they must develop knowledge and practice competencies across a broad range of domains. Content knowledge in the areas of typical child development, child psychopathology, psychological and psychiatric treatment modalities, and consultation with multiple professional disciplines has been identified as prerequisite to effective C/L work (15).

TYPES OF REFERRAL QUESTIONS

Psychiatric assessment of child and family adjustment is a core service provided by mental health consultants. Within inpatient pediatric settings, the most frequent reasons for psychiatric consultation are problems with coping/adjustment, noncompliance with treatment, depression, suicide attempt, pain management, psychosomatic problems, and anxiety (16,17). Medical teams may also request assistance with managing patient behavior on the hospital ward (disruptive behavior, procedural distress), parent coping, as well as assistance with postdischarge treatment planning (referral for mental health services, inpatient psychiatric hospitalization, school re-entry). Reasons for referral can also vary according to the expertise of the C/L consulting service. For example, if there are specialists with eating disorders on the C/L service, then there may be a preponderance of requests from the medical teams for evaluation of patients with eating disorders. Finally, psychiatric consultation may be a part of the standard practice for certain medical subspecialty groups in which all children with a chronic illness (e.g. cancer, sickle cell, diabetes) and their parents, receive ongoing psychosocial evaluations and treatment as part of the child's medical care. Indeed, in the recently published Standards for the Psychosocial Care of Children with Cancer and Their Families (18), there are 15 standards which are proposed, one of which is that children with cancer and their family members should "routinely receive systematic assessments of their psychosocial health care needs." Furthermore, it is also recommended that long-term survivors of childhood cancers also receive yearly psychosocial evaluations.

Assessment approaches can be problem focused in scope, or involve a comprehensive multisystem evaluation approach. Structured interview methods, including the formal mental status examination, as well as standardized behavioral and psychological instruments are typically included in assessment procedures.

EMPIRICALLY SUPPORTED PSYCHOLOGICAL ASSESSMENT AND INTERVENTIONS IN PEDIATRICS

Currently there is a broad range of evidence-based assessment measures that provide standardized methods of evaluating child and family coping along a variety of outcome domains. A Special Issue in the Journal of Pediatric Psychology in 2008 provided a comprehensive review of standardized measures applicable to pediatric mental health (19). These and subsequent measures that have been developed, are rated as "Well Established" if they meet the Chambless criteria endorsed by APA. A complete listing of Evidence Based Assessment Resources is updated annually through the website of Division 54 of the Society of Pediatric Psychology and is available to clinicians as well as researchers (20).

A closer look at the listing of standardized assessment tools reveals that there are evidence-based assessment tools that evaluate numerous domains relevant to pediatric mental health, including: Measures of Family Functioning, Health-Related Quality of Life and Functional Impairment, Adherence to Medical Treatments, Pediatric Pain, Psychosocial Adjustment and Psychopathology, and Stress and Coping. There are also specialized assessment resources for specific pediatric populations, such as Chronic Pain and Functional Impairment; Craniofacial Populations; Obesity; and Pediatric Gastroenterology (20). Given the breath of available measures, evidence-based assessment approaches can thus be readily incorporated into a consulting clinician's routine practice.

Similarly, highly effective, evidence-based psychosocial treatments for chronically ill children can be readily adopted by C/L clinicians. A recent review of psychological interventions for mental health disorders in children with chronic physical illness (21) suggests that cognitive-behavioral treatments for depression, such as those that have been well validated in healthy children, can be of benefit to medically ill children. Interventions for depression typically include elements such as: mood monitoring, problem solving, and behavioral activation. Cognitive-behavioral treatments for anxiety, which include components of cognitive restructuring and exposure exercises, have also been demonstrated to reduce anxiety in pediatric populations. Other reviews have concluded that cognitive-behavioral therapy is a well established treatment for procedure-related pain. These typically include components such as breathing exercises, training in relaxation strategies, self-hypnosis, cognitive coping skills, mental imagery, behavioral reinforcement with rehearsal, and directed coaching by a parent or practitioner in which the child is prompted to engage in coping skills (22).

It is important to note as well, that many cognitive-behavioral treatment programs for medically ill children include a range of modifications such as psychoeducation about the relationship between physical illness and mood; family education sessions; use of simplistic/concrete language; sessions in the homes; and telephone appointments (21). In sum, these findings are quite promising, but much work is still needed to further our knowledge of the most effective treatments for children with medical and psychiatric problems.

FRAMEWORKS FOR CONSULTATION AND LIAISON

Numerous theoretical and practical frameworks have been described to capture the complex nature of the pediatric consultation process (23–26). These models all share the common features of providing guidelines to psychiatric consultants for fostering professional relationships with healthcare providers and patients in order to improve patient care, and to promote the understanding of child and family adjustment to illness or hospitalization (27). The various models of consultation vary with regard to: degree of contact and direct involvement with the patient, degree of involvement with the medical team, the length of time that the consultant remains available to the medical team, and the degree of "shared caregiving" that is established.

Accordingly, the most time-limited model is Resource Consultation (23), also known as Independent Functions consultation (24). In these consultation approaches, the psychiatric consultant addresses a very specific diagnostic question and then offers a set of recommendations to the team and family regarding intervention strategies for the identified problem. Further follow-up and evaluation are generally not offered. In the second type of consultation approach, the Process Educative model (23), the psychiatric consultant offers indirect psychological support to patients by means of advising and educating the medical staff about psychological or pharmacologic treatment strategies. The consultant may not actually have contact with the patient, but instead consults with the pediatrician about their questions. A third consultative approach is the Collaborative Team model (24) in which the psychiatric consultant and the medical team have equal responsibility and decision making in the care of the patient, and is therefore one of "shared caregiving."

CONSULTATION PROCEDURAL GUIDELINES

In 2009, the AACAP published a practice parameter, entitled, "Practice Parameter for the Psychiatric Assessment and Management of Physically Ill Children and Adolescents" (7). This "clinician-oriented" parameter had the aim of delineating important components of assessment and management of physically ill children (Table 7.1.2.1).

TABLE 7.1.2.1

PRINCIPLES FROM THE AACAP PRACTICE PARAMETER FOR THE PSYCHIATRIC ASSESSMENT AND MANAGEMENT OF PHYSICALLY ILL CHILDREN AND ADOLESCENTS (2009)

1:	Mental health clinicians should understand how to collaborate effectively with medical professionals to facilitate the health care of physically ill children.
2:	The reason for and purpose of the mental health referral should be understood.
3:	The assessment should integrate the impact of the child's physical illness into a developmentally informed biopsychosocial formulation.
4:	General medical conditions and/or their treatments should be considered in the etiology of a child's psychological and behavioral symptoms.
5:	Psychopharmacological management should consider a child's physical illness and its treatment.
6:	Psychotherapeutic management should consider multiple treatment modalities.
7:	The family context should be understood and addressed.
8:	Adherence to the medical treatment regimen should be evaluated and optimized.
9:	The use of complementary and alternative medicine should be explored.
10:	Religious and cultural influences should be understood and considered.
11:	Family contact with community-based agencies should be considered and facilitated where indicated.
12:	Legal issues specific to physically ill children should be understood and considered.
13:	The influence of the health care system on the care of a physically ill child should be considered.

Other C/L consultation protocols (28,29) have included specific procedural guidelines in the consultation process such as: (1) defining the referral questions; (2) review of records; (3) interview of primary caretakers; (4) assessment of the patient; (5) referral for additional tests or procedures; (6) assessment of interdisciplinary relationships between medical personnel; (7) collaboration with community agencies or schools; (8) diagnostic feedback and recommendations; (9) intervention phase; and (10) follow-up.

Referral Phase

Initially, the psychiatric consultant should speak directly to the primary physician, and other members of the medical team (primary nurse, residents, or pediatric social worker) to generate a list of concerns or diagnostic questions that are to be addressed during the consultation. It is critical for the consultant to listen for both implicit as well as the explicit messages from the medical team (29). For example, the team may actually have more concerns about parental coping than they do about child psychological adjustment. During the referral phase, it is also important that the consultant take a thorough medical history and current treatment regimen from the referring physician. Finally, it is important that the consultant confirm that the parents and patient have been informed by the medical team about their concerns and that they have agreed to participate with the evaluation (30).

Record Review

Prior to meeting the family and patient, it is important for the consultant to review the medical chart, including prior medical records, for treatment information that may have been omitted by the referring physician. For example, for those patients who have multiple medical subspecialties involved in their care, it is important to review the treatments or consultations provided under their care. Additionally, oftentimes nurses and child life specialists document important observations regarding a child's mental status, mood states, and behavioral functioning that are important sources of data. As part of the record review, it is also critical that the consultant take note of all the medications prescribed to the patient, with particular emphasis on those medications that have psychoactive effects or withdrawal symptoms.

Furthermore, it is useful to obtain additional records or conduct interviews with community-based services such as the child's school (to ascertain information about developmental, cognitive, and academic functioning), community mental health providers and child welfare agencies, if they have been involved with the child and family (30).

Interview with Primary Caretakers

It is usually most informative to begin the evaluation phase with a structured interview with the primary caretakers, which may include biologic parents, foster or adoptive parents. Designated social service agency workers may also need to be contacted in the case of children who are in state custody. During this interview, the consultant should gather information regarding the patient's birth, developmental, social, and educational histories. Of particular importance is the child's history of past psychiatric treatments, history of educational or psychological assessments, and their adherence with ongoing medical care (30).

Additionally, the consultant should inquire about the parents' social and psychiatric histories, parenting styles with the ill child, the marital relationship, sibling relationships, extended family supports, economic and community resources available to the family. To complement a structured interview with primary caregivers, the mental health consultant can also include standardized assessment questionnaires such as The Family Environment Scale (31), the Impact on Family Scale (32), or Coping Health Inventory for Parents (33), along with numerous other measures available for review through the APA Div. 54 Evidence-based Assessment Resources (20).

The interview with the parents should also include a discussion of the family's cultural and religious beliefs regarding the nature of the child's illness, their acceptance of the medical diagnoses and their views about the proposed medical treatments. These views are likely to affect a child and family's acceptance to treatment, as well as help identify potential sources of support for the family and child (7). Thorough assessment of these various family domains is critical because difficulties within any of these areas have been identified as potential risk factors for children with serious medical conditions.

Child and Adolescent Assessment

A comprehensive mental status examination should be conducted with the child, as is permissible given the patient's age and developmental level of functioning. Areas of inquiry may include: the child's understanding of their illness, treatment, and prognosis; the impact of the illness on the child's relationships with their parents, siblings, and peers; the impact of the illness on their school performance; and the child's view of the medical team providers.

Play interviews and observations of the child's behavior during inpatient ward activities are also valuable sources of data. During the evaluation phase, standardized diagnostic procedures such as self-report inventories for depression (e.g., Children's Depression Inventory) (34), anxiety (e.g., Screen for Child Anxiety-Related Emotional Disorders) (35), child health–related quality of life (e.g., Pediatric Oncology Quality of Life Scale) (36), and pediatric pain (e.g., Varni-Thompson Pediatric Pain Questionnaire) (37), may also be included. For those patients with altered states of consciousness, such as possible delirium, repeated serial interviews are necessary. Additionally, use of structured observations, such as nursing ratings with a measure such as the Cornell Assessment of Pediatric Delirium (38), are often critical in order to establish levels of baseline functioning and to explore possible etiologic factors.

Referral for Other Tests or Procedures

Over the course of the evaluation, a range of differential diagnostic questions may arise that will lead the consultant to request additional tests or procedures from the medical team. For example, the consultant may suggest neuroimaging studies or an EEG for a patient with acute changes in mental status. Additionally, neuropsychological testing is often indicated in the context of further clarifying functional capacities for children with central nervous system insults, as in the case of seizure disorders or brain tumors (30).

Systems Assessment

The final components during the assessment phase involve examining the relationships that exist among medical personnel, the child–family system, and relationships among medical personnel and community systems such as schools and social service agencies. The consultant may need to conduct systematic interviews and observations of all these various systems relationships in order to determine whether there are communication or collaboration difficulties contributing to the child's observed difficulties. Clinical researchers such as Kazak (39) suggest that a systems assessment is important because oftentimes family or family–staff interactional factors can play a central role in the child's problematic functioning.

Diagnostic Feedback Phase

Once the consultant has concluded all of the components of the assessment, the next step is to share the diagnostic formulation and set of recommendations with members of the medical team, parents, child, and other systems of care. Typically, consultation findings are summarized within the context of a report placed in the electronic medical chart. It is of paramount importance, however, that the consultant communicates orally with the medical team and family regarding the findings and the recommendations for intervention. Direct discussion of the multiple factors that are contributing to the child's adjustment difficulties can then lead to candid discussions regarding the roles that each member of the medical team or family can assume in promoting improved child adaptation (30). It is important for oral and written communications to be provided in a timely manner, and in language that is concise and free of psychiatric jargon. A developmentally informed feedback discussion with the child and adolescent patient should also be conducted.

Finally, it is equally important for the mental health consultant to communicate the findings and recommendations of the evaluation process to the child's primary care pediatrician, as well as any additional medical specialists responsible for the child's care.

Interventions and Follow-up

Numerous evidence-based treatments have been developed to address child and family coping with acute and chronic illness. For example, there are highly effective cognitive-behavioral treatments such as progressive muscle relaxation and guided imagery training to address pain and anxiety during invasive medical procedures (22). Additionally, there are home-based, manualized, behavioral family therapy treatments targeting issues such as poor medical adherence and family conflict (6). Cognitive-behavioral methods are also useful in addressing more broad-based psychological problems such as anxiety and depression (21). Pharmacotherapy may also become an important component of a medically ill child's treatment regimen. For example, the psychiatric consultant may offer recommendations for medical management of symptoms related to behavioral agitation, delirium, depression, or anxiety. Referrals for occupational therapy, physical therapy, and neuropsychological testing may also be important components of a comprehensive treatment plan.

Additionally, a host of psychosocial interventions may be required. Accordingly, the family may require assistance in securing public assistance, special education services, support groups for children and family members, specialty summer camps, or supportive marital therapy. Some interventions may be possible to introduce within the context of a hospitalization, but oftentimes the psychiatric consultant must provide the family and medical team with suggestions regarding other community-based mental health professionals that can begin to develop a psychological plan of care. If the child will return to the school setting, an important part of consultation should include guidance regarding the child's reentry to school (30).

BARRIERS (AND PROPOSED SOLUTIONS) TO EFFECTIVE CONSULTATION AND LIAISON SERVICES TO PEDIATRICS

Several barriers to effective C/L service to pediatrics have been identified in the literature, such as lack of timely availability of child psychiatry/psychology consultants, time constraints, and contrasts between illness-oriented and biopsychosocial conceptualizations (28). Perhaps the most significant barrier to effective C/L consultation to pediatrics is the difference in the pace of work between the two clinical traditions. The typical psychiatric consultation takes several hours and even days, while the work within pediatric hospital settings moves much more quickly.

Therefore, flexible consultation and treatment approaches have been identified as mechanisms to increase satisfaction and subsequent use of consultation services. Other matters of practical importance involve accessibility of the psychiatric consultant, responsiveness to the consultation request, and minimal time to complete the assessment and share the findings (40). Consultation services are also enhanced with effective communication of assessment findings, collaborative treatment planning, and practical recommendations to both the referring pediatrician and the child and family. For both family and professional audiences, communication should be practical, action-oriented, and free of psychological jargon; for the pediatrician, written communication should be concise.

Improved communication and collaboration can also be facilitated through the consultant's presence during clinical rounds, departmental meetings, and teaching conferences (28). Furthermore, a consultant can demonstrate leadership by offering to develop hospital-based or office-based psychological and behavioral management protocols such as: management plans for eating disorders and other self-harming behaviors, pain management protocols, and end-of-life protocols.

Finally, a consultant that also offers to provide the pediatric team with support and education about common childhood psychiatric conditions and their management, advice about working with challenging children and families, and is available to discuss the professional and personal challenges of caring for medically ill children can then become viewed as an integral member of the health care team.

References

1. Perrin JM, Anderson E, Van Cleave J: The rise in chronic conditions among infants, children and youth can be met with continued health system innovations. *Health Affairs* 33(12):2099–2105, 2014.
2. Pinquart M, Shen Y: Behavior problems in children and adolescents with chronic physical illness: a meta-analysis. *J Pediatr Psychol* 36(9):1003–1016, 2011.
3. Chow MYK, Morrow AM, Cooper Robbins SC, Leask J: Condition-specific quality of life questionnaires for caregivers of children with pediatric conditions: a systematic review. *Qual Life Res* 22:2183–2200, 2013.
4. Hatzmann J, Heymans HSA, Ferrer-i-Carbonell A, et al.: Hidden consequences of success in pediatrics: parental health-related quality of life-Results from the care project. *Pediatrics* 122:e1030–e1038, 2008.
5. Kazak A, Alderfer M, Rourke MT, et al.: Posttraumatic stress disorder (PTSD) and posttraumatic stress symptoms (PTSS) in families and adolescent childhood cancer survivors. *J Pediatr Psychol* 29:211–219, 2004.
6. Kazak A, Segal-Andrews AM, Johnson K: Pediatric psychology research and practice: A family/systems approach. In: Roberts MC (ed): *Handbook of Pediatric Psychology*. 2nd ed. New York, Guilford Press, 1995:84–104.
7. American Academy of Child and Adolescent Psychiatry: Practice parameter for the psychiatric assessment and management of physically ill children and adolescents. *J Am Acad Child Psychiatry* 48:213–233, 2009.
8. Roberts MC, Mitchell MC, McNeal R: The evolving field of pediatric psychology: Critical issues and future challenges. In: Roberts MC (ed): *Handbook of Pediatric Psychology*. 3rd ed. New York, Guilford Press, 2003:3–18.
9. American Academy of Child and Adolescent Psychiatry: Best principles for integration of child psychiatry into the pediatric health home. *Am Acad Child Adolesc Psychiatry* 2012.
10. Burkey MD, Kaye DL, Frosch E: Training in integrated mental health-primary care models: a national survey of child psychiatry program directors. *Acad Psychiatry* 38:485–488, 2014.
11. Cowley D, Dunaway K, Forstein M, et al.: Teaching psychiatry residents to work at the interface of mental health and primary care. *Acad Psychiatry* 38:398–404, 2014.
12. Asarnow JR, Rozenman M, Wiblin J, Zeltzer L: Integrated medical-behavioral care compared with usual primary care for child and adolescent behavioral health: A meta-analysis. *JAMA Pediatrics* 169(10):929–937, 2015.
13. Sarvet B, Gold J, Bostic J, et al.: Improving access to mental health care for children: the Massachusetts Child Psychiatry Access Project. *Pediatrics* 126:1191–1200, 2010.
14. Hilt RJ, Romaire MA, McDonell MG, et al.: The partnership access line: evaluating a child psychiatry consult program in Washington State. *JAMA Pediatr* 167:162–168, 2013.
15. Bronheim HE, Fulop G, Kunkel EJ, et al.: The academy of psychosomatic medicine practice guidelines for psychiatric consultation in the general medical setting. *Psychosomatics* 39:S8–S30, 1998.
16. Shugart MA: Child psychiatry consultations to pediatric inpatients: a literature review. *Gen Hosp Psychiatry* 13:325–336, 1991.
17. Olson RA, Holden EW, Friedman A, et al.: Psychological consultation in a children's hospital: an evaluation of services. *J Pediatr Psychol* 13: 479–492, 1988.
18. Wiener L, Kazak AE, Noll RB, et al.: Standards for the psychosocial care of children with cancer and their families: an introduction to the special issue. *Pediatr Blood Cancer* 62(Suppl 5):S419–S424, 2015.
19. Cohen LL, La Greca A, Blount RL, et al.: Introduction to special issue: evidence-based assessment in pediatric psychology. *J Pediatr Psychol* 33:911–915, 2008.
20. Society of Pediatric Psychology, Division 54. Evidence-Based Assessment Resources. Available at: http://www.apadivisions.org/division-54/evidence-based/assessment-resources.aspx. Accessed March 20, 2017.
21. Bennet S, Shafran R, Coughtrey A, et al.: Psychological interventions for mental health disorders in children with chronic physical illness: a systematic review. *Arch Dis Childhood* 100:308–316, 2015.
22. Powers SW: Empirically supported treatments in pediatric psychology: procedure related pain. *J Pediatr Psychol* 24:131–145, 1999.
23. Stabler B: Pediatric consultation-liaison. In: Routh DK (ed): *Handbook of Pediatric Psychology*. New York, Guilford Press, 1988:538–566.

24. Roberts MC, Wright L: The role of the pediatric psychologist as consultant to pediatricians. In: Tuma J (ed): *Handbook for the Practice of Pediatric Psychology*. New York, Wiley, 1982:251–289.
25. Drotar D: Consulting with Pediatricians: Psychological perspectives. New York, Plenum, 2004.
26. Huszti HC, Walker CE: Critical issues in consultation liaison. In: Sweet JJ, Tovian SM (eds): *Handbook of Clinical Psychology in Medical Settings*. New York, Plenum Press, 1991:165–185.
27. Hamlett KW, Stabler B: The developmental progress of pediatric psychology consultation. In: Roberts MC (ed): *Handbook of Pediatric Psychology*. 2nd ed. New York, Guilford Press, 1995:39–54.
28. Lewis M: The consultation process in child and adolescent psychiatric consultation-liaison in pediatrics. In: Lewis M (ed): *Child and Adolescent Psychiatry: A Comprehensive Textbook*. 3rd ed. Philadelphia, PA, Lippincott Williams & Wilkins, 2002:1111–1115.
29. Smith FA, Querques J, Levenson J, Stern TA: Psychiatric assessment and consultation. In: Levenson J (ed): *Textbook of Psychosomatic Medicine*. Washington, DC: American Psychiatric Publishing, 2005:3–14.
30. Campbell J, Cardona L: The consultation and liaison process to pediatrics. In: Martin A, Volkmar F (eds): *Lewis' Child and Adolescent Psychiatry: A Comprehensive Textbook*. 4th ed. Philadelphia, PA, Lippincott Williams & Wilkins, 2007:912–921.
31. Moos R, Moos B: *Family Environment Scale*. 3rd ed. Palo Alto, CA, Consulting Psychologists Press, 1994.
32. Stein REK, Jessop DJ: The impact on family scale revisited: further psychometric data. *J Dev Behav Pediatr* 24:9–16, 2003.
33. McCubbin HI, McCubbin, MA, Patterson JM, et al.: CHIP—coping health inventory for parents: an assessment of parental coping patterns in the care of the chronically ill child. *J Marriage Fam* 45:359–370, 1983.
34. Kovacs M: The children's depression inventory (CDI). *Psychopharmacol Bull* 21:995–998, 1985.
35. Birmaher B, Khetarpai S, Brent D, et al.: The screen for child anxiety related emotional disorders (SCARED): scale construction and psychometric characteristics. *J Am Acad Child Adolesc Psychiatry* 36:545–553, 1997.
36. Goodwin DAJ, Boggs SR, Graham-Pole J: Development and validation of the pediatric oncology quality of life scale. *Psychol Assess* 6:321–328, 1994.
37. Varni JW, Thompson KL, Hanson V: The Varni/Thompson Pediatric Pain Questionnaire. I. chronic musculoskeletal pain in juvenile rheumatoid arthritis. *Pain* 28:27–38, 1987.
38. Traube C, Silver G, Kearney J, et al.: Cornell assessment of pediatric delirium: a valid, rapid, observational tool for screening delirium in the PICU. *Crit Care Med* 42:656–663, 2014.
39. Kazak A, Simms S, Rourke M: Family systems practice in pediatric psychology. *J Pediatr Psychol* 27:133–143, 2002.
40. Kush SA, Camp JV: Consultation and liaison in the pediatric setting. In: Ammerman RT, Campo JV (eds): *Handbook of Pediatric Psychology and Psychiatry*. NeedhanHeights, MA, Allyn & Bacon, 1998:23–40.

7.2 ■ MENTAL HEALTH ISSUES IN THE MEDICALLY ILL CHILD OR ADOLESCENT

CHAPTER 7.2.1 ■ CANCER

CASEY WALSH AND BRADLEY J. ZEBRACK

The American Cancer Society and the National Cancer Institute estimated that approximately 15,780 new cases of cancer in children and adolescents aged 0 to 19 years were diagnosed in 2014 (1). Approximately 1 in 285 young people in the United States will be diagnosed with cancer before the age of 20 (1). Although childhood cancer is rare, it is the leading cause of death from disease among children aged 1 to 14, resulting in an estimated 1,350 pediatric deaths in the United States in 2014 (1). Among adolescents (ages 15 to 19), there were an estimated 5,330 new cases of cancer diagnosed in 2014, as well as approximately 610 deaths from cancer (1).

Prior to the 1970s and the advent and use of multimodal chemotherapy, children diagnosed with cancer had little hope of long-term survival. However, advances in treatment, including the large-scale coordination of treatment through clinical trials, have greatly increased the long-term life chances of these young people. Notably, mortality rates for all pediatric and adolescent cancers combined have declined steadily from 1975 to 2010 by an average of 2.1% per year, resulting in an overall decline of more than 50% (1). Today, surviving childhood cancer is considered the norm rather than the exception.

Due to successes in treatment, much of the older literature on psychosocial outcomes for children with cancer is no longer relevant to current and future cohorts of patients, survivors, and their family members. Psychosocial studies of children with cancer and their parents were initiated in the 1970s (studies of off-treatment survivors began in the early 1980s with Koocher and O'Malley's (2) groundbreaking work entitled *The Damocles Syndrome*), and occurred at a time when childhood cancer survivors were considered miracle children.

Contemporary trends in the psychosocial literature on childhood cancer encompass some or all of the following elements: (1) a developmental approach in which the issues experienced by children of various ages are treated in the context of their normative physical and psychosocial maturation; (2) a family systems approach emphasizing interactive impacts and responses in families and among family members; (3) a stress-coping framework recently amended with a focus on posttraumatic effects; (4) advancements in web-based technology. The recently published "Standards for Psychosocial Care for Children with Cancer and Their Families" provide evidence-based clinical standards for the psychosocial care of children with cancer and their families from the time of diagnosis through survivorship or end-of-life and bereavement care (3). This incredible resource, developed by an integrated team of leading psychosocial clinicians and researchers, is being released as a special edition of the journal of Pediatric Blood and Cancer, and has been funded by the Mattie Miracle Cancer Foundation (4). For people diagnosed with cancer it is useful to examine their experiences in the context of "survivorship"—the health and life of a person with a history of cancer *beyond* the acute diagnosis and treatment phase (5). Survivorship research seeks to identify, examine, prevent, and control adverse effects of cancer treatment utilizing integrated multi-disciplinary treatment to optimize the psychosocial, physiologic, and functional outcomes for cancer survivors and their families (5).

The research presented in this chapter reinforces the importance of examining the impact of cancer on children of different ages and developmental stages and within the context of family. The chapter also serves to orient the reader to the unique and sometimes subtle psychological, social, and behavioral effects of cancer on children and their families.

DEVELOPMENTAL CONTEXT

The boundaries used by theorists and researchers for classifying a "child" (as opposed to an adolescent or young adult) are varied. Some studies of pediatric cancer patients involve primarily elementary school-age children, while others combine younger school-age children with teenagers. Across this broad age range, the bulk of psychosocial research has been carried out with older school-age children. Very little work has been done with children under the age of 8 or 9 due in part to challenges related to literacy, human subjects' consent, and measurement. The diagnosis and treatment of cancer will be interpreted and experienced differently by children of various ages and life stages. These differences are reflected in the literature presented in this chapter.

FAMILY SYSTEMS

The growth of "family systems theory" (6) has emphasized how childhood illnesses, especially childhood cancer, may place psychological as well as physical strains on the family as a social system (7). In one of the first comprehensive studies of the family impact of childhood cancer, Chesler and Barbarin (8) suggested that childhood cancer is a "family disease" in that it "challenges the life course not only of the ill child but of the entire family." Kazak et al. (9) utilized Bronfenbrenner's social ecologic framework (10); the child is seen within the context of their environments; starting with the child's family, then health care team, extended relatives, schools, neighborhoods, and communities (9). This approach focuses on building a "therapeutic triad," joining the patient, family, and health care team within the larger social system to promote positive outcomes (9). The goal of the health care team in the therapeutic triad is to "join, focus, promote competence, and collaborate" with patients and families (9).

Building upon previous research examining resilience within individual family members, there is emerging research around resilience and family-level processes and outcomes (11). This research supports ongoing monitoring of family functioning, with attention to the cultural and socioecologic contexts of the family (11). Ongoing surveillance of family functioning can increase awareness of opportunities for the health care team to offer family-level supports and services throughout a continuum of care that often lasts months and in some cases (e.g., leukemia) years (11). A subset of parents and siblings of oncology patients may experience increased depression (12), anxiety (13), and posttraumatic stress symptoms (PTSS) (14) compared with parents and siblings of healthy children. Specific sociodemographic factors, such as child age, maternal depression and anxiety, and lower family income have been identified as risk factors for worse cognitive outcomes, increased pain, and increased child depression and anxiety (15–17).

INTELLECTUAL ISSUES

Knowledge about Cancer, Treatment, and Life Threat

At the diagnostic stage, and immediately thereafter, children may experience stress in understanding the seriousness of the situation and in dealing with uncertainty. How do children become aware that they have a condition they ought to worry about? Sometimes parents or staff members tell them directly, but information may not be complete, may be delayed or not presented in a manner appropriate to the developmental stage of the child. Children and family members whose primary language is not English may struggle with simply understanding what hospital personnel are telling them, let alone the complexities and implications of impending medical procedures and treatment. Also, children will astutely draw conclusions from the many cues consciously or unconsciously exhibited by parents, family members, friends and medical staff and by reading between the lines of what is said directly and what is whispered out of earshot. Many children note the rapidity and drama with which they are hospitalized; siblings are allowed to stay home from school in order to be at the hospital; grandparents travel long distances to come to the bedside; friends and relatives visit in large numbers; nurses and doctors visit often; and, almost everyone is extra attentive or looks scared or sad.

Siblings of all ages struggle as well. Recent qualitative research suggests dominant themes of siblings' desire for information and involvement in their sibling's care and support around the changing roles within the family (18). There is need for anticipatory grief, strategies to deal with the emotional "rollercoasters" of hope and disappointment, and effective communication around the sibling's diagnosis (18). Siblings will benefit from social, emotional, and instrumental support (18). Including siblings in family meetings and providing them with age-appropriate information can help keep them informed and connected, *and* provide opportunities to engage with and assess siblings for their own psychosocial needs (19,20).

PRACTICAL ISSUES

The Hospitalization Experience, Including Pain and Painful Procedures

Children with cancer have been found to experience high levels of symptom burden and suffering throughout their illness (21). Early integration of pediatric palliative oncology (PPO) principles by an integrated care team with all high-risk patients and families can help facilitate holistic continuity of care (22). Pediatric cancer treatment often involves multiple administrations of highly aversive medical procedures such as lumbar punctures, bone marrow aspirations, spinal taps, and venipunctures over a prolonged period of time. Surgery, chemotherapy, radiation, repeated hospitalization, tests, and injections all debilitate the child physically and emotionally. According to recent systematic review, the most commonly studied psychological interventions for managing pediatric distress and pain with needle procedures were distraction, hypnosis, and cognitive behavioral therapy (23). Additionally, higher levels of parental self-efficacy around being able to keep their children calm during medical procedures were correlated with lower levels of child distress and increased child cooperation during procedures (24). In addition to pain, the illness and the side effects of treatment may disrupt family life, school attendance, friendships, and social activities. Psychosocial interventions have been developed to support adolescent survivors of childhood cancer and their families. The Surviving Cancer Competently: An Intervention Program (SCCIP) is a 1-day family group intervention that combines cognitive-behavioral and family therapy approaches (25). The goals of SCCIP are to reduce symptoms of distress and to improve family functioning and development (25). Additionally, research around social network development following a child's cancer diagnosis suggests that support is received from pre-existing social connections, as well as new connections with other cancer families (26). Health care professionals served as "network brokers," fostering the development of new connections among families and connecting parents with supportive resources (26).

Managing and balancing family home life and care for a child with cancer are the ultimate challenge for parents. Parental chronic stress has been associated with decreased levels of emotional, physical, and social functioning among pediatric patients (27). Many parents have indicated that uncertainty about their parent role and anticipating their child's distress during medical procedures are primary sources of stress, with uncertainty about the parenting role being associated with other measures of psychological distress (28). Parents may experience loss of control and restriction of their autonomy throughout the process of their child's treatment (29). Parental caregivers have identified that the most helpful action of health care providers was receiving timely, accurate and carefully delivered information about their child, while the most helpful actions of family and friends were gestures of support and understanding (29).

Adherence to Treatment

Nonadherence to prescribed treatments constitutes one of the most frequently encountered impediments to therapy administration in children with cancer, particularly adolescents. Treatment abandonment, defined as the failure to start or complete medically indicated curative therapy (30), is the most common cause of treatment failure for children with cancer in many low- and middle-income countries (31). Recent discussions suggest that the rapport between medical staff, parents, and children may be a key ingredient in overcoming resistance and promoting adherence to medical regimens. Adolescents have indicated a spectrum of preferred decisional roles, which might shift depending upon situational and social contexts, with the most commonly preferred being active involvement, although a shared decision-making approach was still valued (32). Additionally, it is helpful to remember that the cognitive and emotional capabilities of youth are still forming until 25 years old, including their reasoning abilities (33). Adolescents expressed an appreciation of parental presence, clinician guidance, and family insight (32).

Cultural differences between patient, family, and medical staff also may interfere with treatment administration. In our multicultural society, there are varying life experiences, beliefs, value systems, languages, notions of health care, and religions (34). To engage and support families during potentially the most vulnerable time in their lives, we must practice with cultural sensitivity and cultural competence, bridging care and patient need as a vital link in communication with patients and families (34).

School

While most patients are able to resume school activity in early outpatient phases of the treatment, complexities of treatment regimens, frequency of routine follow-up, disease status, neutropenia, and infections can contribute to school difficulties (35). Hospitalizations result in missed school days and often necessitate assistance with schoolwork (obtaining assignments, learning materials, completing homework) (36). Many children's hospitals have inpatient schools where teachers help patients keep up with their schoolwork, often communicating with the child's teachers to obtain assignments.

Barriers to school reentry include changes in the child's appearance, cognitive abilities, emotional status, and physical activity, and misconceptions by peers and school personnel about cancer (37). Childhood cancer survivors as a whole are more likely to utilize special education services when compared to sibling controls, especially those diagnosed at a young age (38,39). Survivors of brain tumors and childhood acute lymphoblastic leukemia (ALL), especially those with a history of cranial radiation, often experience higher rates of neurocognitive dysfunction and educational needs (38,39). They may experience deficits in attention, concentration, memory, handwriting, math, and organizing or sequencing of tasks (40). Recent exploration of neurocognitive assessments of pediatric brain tumor survivors and ALL survivors suggest that brain tumor survivors with deficits exhibited a profile suggestive of global executive dysfunction, while affected ALL survivors tended to demonstrate specific rapid naming deficits (41). Due to the complexities and risks of neurocognitive deficits among survivors, there is increased clinical and research focus on neurocognitive assessment for survivors of pediatric brain tumors (42). A brief neurocognitive screening measure, The Lebby-Asbell Neurocognitive Screening Examination (LANSE), has demonstrated preliminary reliability and validity for youth with brain tumors (42). The advancement of neurocognitive screening tools can help inform late-effects intervention planning (41).

INTERPERSONAL ISSUES

Peer Relationships

Many youth and adolescents experience isolation from peer and family support networks when battling cancer during their formative developmental years (43). Peer support is integral in coping with these challenges, yet cancer treatment can create isolation from friends and family (44). There are many factors that can impact the social functioning of childhood cancer survivors, including biologic effects of treatment, changes in physical appearance and functional impairment, and family factors such as parental overprotection (45). However, there is great heterogeneity in the literature around the social functioning of childhood cancer survivors, with some studies suggesting reduced social engagement while other studies have found no significant differences between childhood cancer survivors and their peers on measures of social functioning (45). Future research around potential strengths in peer relationships or areas of growth in friendships that result from cancer would help better inform the interpersonal impact of cancer in youth (45). Additionally, interventions should be designed and promoted to foster peer engagement and reduce isolation throughout treatment and beyond (45).

EMOTIONAL ISSUES

Distress

As might be expected, children and their families experience and exhibit emotional and behavioral problems during the initial phases of diagnosis and treatment, with investigators reporting behavioral and emotional disturbances manifested in increased anxiety, depression, regression, and withdrawal among children in treatment for cancer. For instance, Cavuşoğlu (46) reports that rates of depression for both males and females aged 9 to 13 and at least 1 year after initial diagnosis were significantly higher than in a healthy age-matched control group and that rates also were significantly higher among patients in treatment than those off treatment and in remission. In contrast, others report few emotional or behavioral problems in children with cancer and demonstrate normal psychosocial functioning during treatment administration (35).

To help monitor distress and proactively support youth and families, brief distress screening tools can be integrated into routine social work and/or nursing intake assessments in multidisciplinary health care settings (47). Review of the literature by Kazak et al. (47) has identified specialized distress screening tools for pediatric cancer: the Distress Thermometer (DT) and the Psychosocial Assessment Tool (PAT). The DT is a very brief unidimensional measure of distress (48) that was developed for screening with adults, and has been adapted for use in pediatrics with a rating scale of faces for 2- to 4-year-old children and with developmentally appropriate words for 4- to 6-year-old children (49). The PAT (50) is a brief parent report measure that screens for key areas of functioning associated with adjustment. The PAT maps onto the Pediatric Preventative Psychosocial Health Model, a conceptual model developed to distinguish among levels of risk (universal, targeted, or clinical risk (51)). With enhanced knowledge of youth and familial risk for adjustment concerns, providers can help to determine what types of supportive care interventions are indicated.

In addition to the research suggesting that for many school-age children emotional problems are either of short duration or not severe, recent work suggests that some children surviving cancer may be emotionally stronger than their healthy peers, and may be significantly more emotionally coherent and centered than they themselves were prior to their cancer treatment. Prior research suggests that some survivors of childhood cancer experience or manifest positive adaptation, or "posttraumatic growth" (52). Barakat et al. studied posttraumatic growth (PTG) following childhood cancer survival, and their findings suggest that the majority of adolescent survivors of childhood cancer and their parents reported PTG, measured as positive changes in self, relationships with others, and plans for the future (53). Families identified multiple positive changes, with endorsement of growth notably high for how they think about their life, how careful they are, their plans for the future, how they treat others and how relatives and others treat them (53). Interestingly, among adolescent survivors, there is a likely interaction between PTG and PTSS and age at diagnosis, such that those who were older than 5 at diagnosis reported more PTG and PTSS than those were under age 5 (53). Adolescent survivors who are better able to remember their treatment experiences appear to appreciate both the challenging and adaptive impacts of cancer on their lives (53).

Among siblings, significant internalizing problems, such as emotional and social withdrawal, anxiety, feelings of guilt, hopelessness, shame and sadness; or externalizing problems, such as anger, noncompliance or other acting-out behavior, have been reported (54). Recent meta-analysis of psychological functioning of siblings in families with chronic health conditions suggest that siblings of children with highly intrusive and/or life-threatening chronic health conditions are at higher risk for psychological concerns (55). Additionally, siblings have been found to be more vulnerable to internalizing problems (55). Siblings also have been found to express fears, worries, and concerns that their brother or sister might not survive their illness (56), and they experience anxiety around a lack of communication within the family (38). Notably, Havermans and Eiser (56) found that siblings in families that scored high on communication also were more likely to report worrying about death of their sibling than did siblings in families scoring low on communication. Over time, impaired psychosocial functioning and quality of life improves for most siblings, although adolescent siblings experience more impaired emotional and social functioning when compared to younger school-age siblings (57). Younger siblings' positive self-attributes also appear to be less negatively affected than older siblings' self-attributes (55).

EXISTENTIAL/SPIRITUAL ISSUES

Uncertainty

Mishel (58) defines uncertainty within the context of illness as the "inability to determine the meaning of illness-related events," which is brought about by "unpredictable and inconsistent symptom onset, continual questions about recurrence or exacerbation, and unknown future due to living with debilitating conditions." While many aspects of cancer and treatment in children remain uncertain (survival, effectiveness of treatment), children may not necessarily characterize themselves or their lives as uncertain. For example, in a study involving 9- to 12-year-old children with a variety of cancer diagnoses, Stewart (59) reports that these children quickly came to view their lives as routine and ordinary despite the unpredictable nature of the course of their illness. They described a process of getting used to cancer that allowed them to keep their focus on the ordinary nature of their everyday lives within the uncertain context of their illness, thus providing important insight into children's psychological adjustment to life-threatening illness. Although children with cancer live with symptoms of treatment on a daily basis, they also suggest that the symptoms are an integral part of overcoming cancer and do not expect complete symptom relief (60). While they suggest that one never gets used to symptoms and that symptoms contribute to discomfort and suffering, there also exists an attitude or belief among some children that they must exchange short-term pain for long-term gain, that they must feel a lot worse before they can feel better (60). This is all part of what Woodgate and Degner (61) theorize and call "keeping the spirit alive."

COPING WITH CANCER

Normalizing the Experience

Children with cancer sometimes feel that they are living between two social worlds, dealing simultaneously with normal social situations and with medical treatment in the hospital environment. Even as children in remission readjust to their social environment, they still need to continually enter the hospital environment for checkups and treatments. Yet, young people with cancer overwhelmingly report that their primary goal is resuming a sense of normalcy in their life as soon as possible. Health care providers can help through providing developmentally appropriate, flexible services that promote a sense of normalcy (62).

Normalizing School, Education, and Social Lives

As children with cancer undergo treatment, they also continue with their lives. For children between the ages of 6 and 18, school attendance is an important part of life, and a vital social and developmental activity. School represents the continuation of children's normal life as well as the primary source of social activity. Yet, parents of youth whose health is seen as fragile may be reluctant to entrust their child's care to the school. Some treatment centers have special programs for school personnel to learn about cancer, while others have members of the treatment team visit the school on request. In other cases, parents become responsible for communicating directly with school personnel.

Normalizing participation in school and social life involves participating in or avoiding social involvement and linking to friendships. Youth may struggle with disclosure of their diagnosis to peers, and fear of acceptance can limit social engagement with peers. Thus, participation in oncology camps, cancer survivor day picnics, and family retreats offer opportunities for life experiences that promote successful achievement of age-appropriate developmental tasks.

Students with cancer or a cancer history whose medical problems adversely affect their educational performance are considered to have a disability—to be "other health impaired," and as such entitled to receive needed special educational services (40). For children whose physical conditions place them at risk of further health problems, homebound education may be called for. Homebound instruction, while often indicated for patients at risk for exposures to infection in public, was recalled by 8- to 17-year-old off-treatment survivors as being academically inadequate and socially isolating (63). Throughout cancer treatment and beyond, youth should be monitored closely to allow for early intervention of support and services to foster educational success (38).

Communicating with Children about Cancer

There is a wide variety of opinion and practice regarding what and how much should be told to a school-age child about their diagnosis, treatment, and prognosis. The Psychosocial Committee of the International Society of Pediatric Oncologists (SIOP) recommends full disclosure to the child, after or during a conference with the parents (64). Current research indicates that both the child's age and their preferences for information are associated with psychosocial outcomes. Children often need to have conversations on their own time frame, and clinicians can foster time for children to share their hopes, expectations, and worries by being attentive and supportive throughout the treatment process (65).

Coping Styles

Questioning, cheerfulness, denial, talkativeness, depression, humor, withdrawal, optimism, and low energy level all may be initial coping responses to therapy in children. These strategies tend to change and alternate over time as children pass through various stages of therapy and off-treatment survivorship (35). Hope theory, as developed by Snyder (66), can be a useful framework to foster positive psychological adjustment in children with cancer through focus on pursuit of goals (67). Hope may influence how stressors are appraised, and clinicians can help guide children with cancer to identify and pursue a variety of goals, to use active coping strategies, and to modify their appraisals of their cancer diagnosis (67). Recent research suggests that increased hope also predicts improved quality of life in children with cancer (67).

Assessment of survivorship needs among young adult survivors of childhood cancer emphasized the need for educational and psychosocial resources, particularly technology-based resources (68). The Children's Oncology Group conducted a review of the psychosocial late effects of pediatric cancer to inform the development of their Long-Term Follow-Up Guidelines (69). Their review suggests that while many survivorship studies continue to specify risk factors for anxiety and PTSS/posttraumatic stress disorder, other outcomes, such as developmental, interpersonal, and familial factors, appear to be emerging in importance (69).

SOCIAL SUPPORT

Many parents seek education and support to help them identify, express, and master the powerful feelings evoked by the difficult events of childhood cancer. Some need only validation of their feelings or that they are managing life adequately given the circumstances. Others need more intensive therapy or emotional support from trained mental health professionals. For many, parental hope is integral to helping parents cope with the illness experience, as is social and family communication (70). Kamihara and colleagues interviewed parents of children with cancer around their hopes for their children in the face of prognostic information (71). Despite concerns about prognosis, parents expressed a wide range of hopes for their children, from hopes related to cure or treatment response, to quality of life, normalcy, love, good relationships, to hopes for their siblings and for better treatment of future children with cancer (71). Many parents were able to acknowledge that their hopes differed from what was likely to happen (71). These findings suggest that clinicians can utilize conversations around hope as a means of joining the family on their journey (71).

Receiving peer support from friends, from other parents of children with cancer and from community-based organizations composed of health professionals or laypersons is critically important (72). Locally organized parent groups exist in over 300 communities and medical sites across the United States. Some are large and formally organized, with bylaws, elected officers and nonprofit legal status, and others are small and informal gatherings. Some include members of the medical staff and others are exclusively parent-led and attended. While not all (nor even a majority) of parents of children with cancer become active members of such groups, those who do report many benefits. The American Childhood Cancer Foundation (formerly Candlelighters) remains the preeminent national clearinghouse and resource for support groups for families of children with cancer (www.acco.org).

Involvement in supportive social networks and having opportunities to express feelings and worries related to cancer may improve parents' adjustment to illness over the long term (73). For example, some parents experience improvements in emotional functioning and adjustment from participating in professionally lead support groups or nonprofessional parent-led self-help groups; supportive programs and interventions appear to offer important coping skills for parents of children in treatment. Current literature also reinforces the importance of support groups and camps for siblings and opportunities for peer involvement with other siblings. Camp facilitates participation in activities that improve knowledge, self-esteem, and social confidence (74).

ADVANCES IN WEB-BASED TECHNOLOGY

Virtual (or online) support communities have become a prevalent mechanism for accessing social support and health care resources, particularly among adolescents and young adults (75). However, factors of access, sociodemographics, computer literacy, and health literacy have been found to significantly impact Internet usage (76). There remains a multitude of questions around Internet usage, such as the opportunities and pitfalls of electronic communication between patients and health care providers, how to measure efficacy of virtual support communities, and overall, how to optimize the positive effect of the Internet without disadvantaging others (76).

There is also a telehealth movement creating change in the way that mental health services are delivered worldwide and reducing environmental and systemic barriers to care, such as geographic isolation and limitations of time and resources (77).

Wakefield et al. in Australia are piloting the use of an online parent-targeted cognitive behavioral intervention, CASCAdE (*C*ope, *A*dapt, *S*urvive: Life after *CA*nc*E*r), to improve the quality of life in families of pediatric cancer survivors (78). Variables such as additional psychosocial support services and peer support are likely to be important in thinking about the efficacy of this intervention and web-based mental health interventions more broadly (78).

CONCLUSION

Cancer impacts youth within and across all systems in their life, including their families, health care teams, schools, neighborhoods, and communities. School-age children diagnosed with cancer enter a world of unfamiliar and threatening people and things, emotional confusion, physical discomfort, and pain. Diagnostic procedures are painful and scary, and the child often exists in the midst of a world of uncertainty—his own and his parents'. This uncertainly is escalated when parents and the medical staff fail to provide the child with information that is adequate, coherent, and tuned to an appropriate developmental level. Even with adequate information, young children often worry about their future, whether they will endure repeated hospitalizations and time away from home. Subsequent hospitalizations, of short or long duration, separate and often isolate the child from peers and schoolmates, as well as from the ordinary routines of family and neighborhood life. In addition, the long-term effects of the disease and treatments may compromise cognitive capacities and social or physical functioning (especially in the case of major surgery or radiation to critical organ systems).

Parents may experience loss of control and restriction of their autonomy throughout the process of their child's treatment. Parents of children diagnosed with cancer typically experience shock and surprise. The stress of having a child diagnosed with a frightening and potentially fatal or disfiguring disease is escalated by the necessary entry into the culture of tertiary care medical facilities and their language, jargon, and status systems. Parents' central role as a parent is to protect their children from harm, and a diagnosis of cancer in a child challenges the core definition of parentage. Parental caregivers have identified that the most helpful action of health care providers was receiving timely, accurate and carefully delivered information about their child, while the most helpful actions of family and friends were gestures of support and understanding.

As all families experience distress in the face of their child's cancer diagnosis, there is increased focus on universal psychosocial screening for youth and families at the time of diagnosis with cancer. Distress screening tools can be integrated into routine social work and/or nursing intake assessments in multidisciplinary health care settings. With enhanced knowledge of youth and familial risk for adjustment concerns, providers can help to determine what types of supportive care interventions are indicated. Parents are often called upon to spend time in the hospital with the ill child, and for many the child's response to the illness raises concern about maintaining normal childrearing practices and discipline. In addition, parents are faced with balancing the competing needs of the ill child, family chores and relationships, and employment requirements. If employers are not responsive to these concerns, the family may face added financial stress. Maintaining normal and satisfying family routines and relationships often is difficult under these circumstances. Siblings often feel left out or overlooked, marital stress may occur (especially when mothers and fathers cope differently and with difficulty) and relationships with parents' parents and friends may also suffer.

Patient experiences need to be understood within the context of survivorship, across the lifespan, to optimize the psychosocial, physiologic, and functional outcomes for cancer survivors and their families. Longitudinal research is indicated to help assess child and family coping over time as the child progresses through different illness stages and developmental levels. The infusion of web-based technology in mental health service delivery may provide opportunities to reduce environmental and systemic barriers to care. Recent research around parental hope suggests that clinicians can utilize conversations around hope as a gateway toward talking about what is possible and as a means of joining the family on their journey. Joining families in their cancer journey has also increased our awareness of resilience and PTG among childhood and adolescent cancer survivors. The future holds great opportunity to support, empower, and enhance the lives of children and youth with cancer during their treatment and beyond.

References

1. American Cancer Society: *Cancer Facts & Figures Special Section: Cancer in Children and Adolescents.* Atlanta, GA, American Cancer Society, 2014.
2. Koocher G, O'Malley J: *The Damocles Syndrome.* New York, McGraw Hill, 1981.
3. Wiener L, Kazak AE, Noll RB, Patenaude AF, Kupst MJ: Standards for psychosocial care for children with cancer and their families: an introduction to the special issue. *Pediatr Blood Cancer* 62(Suppl 5):S419–S424, 2015.
4. Mattie Miracle Cancer Foundation. *Establishing a Minimum Level of Comprehensive Care: Creating Standards for Psychosocial Care for Children with Cancer and their Families.* 2015. Available at: http://www.matti-emiracle.com/#!standards-of-care/c22ij. Accessed November 21, 2015.
5. Aziz NM: Cancer survivorship research: state of knowledge, challenges and opportunities. *Acta Oncol* 46(4):417–432, 2007.
6. Rosenblatt P: *Metaphors of Family Systems Theory* New York, Guilford Press, 1994.
7. Kazak AE, Simms S, Rourke MT: Family systems practice in pediatric psychology. *J Pediatr Psychol* 27(2):133–143, 2002.
8. Chesler M, Barbarin O: *Childhood Cancer and the Family.* New York, Brunner/Mazel, 1987.
9. Kazak A, Segal-Andrews A, Johnson K: Pediatric psychology research and practice: a family/systems approach. In: Roberts M (ed): *Handbook of Pediatric Psychology.* 2nd ed. New York, Guilford, pp. 84–104, 1995.
10. Bronfenbrenner U: *The Ecology of Human Development.* Cambridge, Harvard University Press, 1979.
11. Van Schoors M, Caes L, Verhofstadt LL, Goubert L, Alderfer MA: Systematic review: family resilience after pediatric cancer diagnosis. *J Pediatr Psychol* 40(9):856–868, 2015.
12. Dockerty JD, Williams SM, McGee R, Skegg DC: Impact of childhood cancer on the mental health of parents. *Med Pediatr Oncol* 35(5):475–483, 2000.
13. Vrijmoet-Wiersma CM, van Klink JM, Kolk AM, Koopman HM, Ball LM, Maarten Egeler R: Assessment of parental psychological stress in pediatric cancer: a review. *J Pediatr Psychol* 33(7):694–706, 2008.
14. Ingerski LM, Shaw K, Gray WN, Janicke DM: A pilot study comparing traumatic stress symptoms by child and parent report across pediatric chronic illness groups. *J Dev Behav Pediatr* 31(9):713–719, 2010.
15. Barrera M, Atenafu E, Andrews GS, Saunders F: Factors related to changes in cognitive, educational and visual motor integration in children who undergo hematopoietic stem cell transplant. *J Pediatr Psychol* 33(5):536–546, 2008.
16. Unal S, Toros F, Kutuk MO, Uyaniker MG: Evaluation of the psychological problems in children with sickle cell anemia and their families. *Pediatr Hematol Oncol* 28(4):321–328, 2011.
17. Karlson CW, Smith ML, Haynes S, Faith MA, Pierce J, Elkin DT, Megason G: Risk for psychosocial problems in pediatric cancer: impact of socioeconomics. *Children's Health Care* 42(3):231–247, 2013.
18. Gaab EM, Owens GR, MacLeod RD: Siblings caring for and about pediatric palliative care patients. *J Palliat Med* 17(1):62–67, 2014.
19. CanTeen: Supporting adolescent and young adult siblings of cancer patients: the family context. Research to Practice Paper Sydney: CanTeen, 2011. Available at: https://www.canteen.org.au/health-professionals/research-and-evaluation/best-practice-projects/research-to-practice-paper-issue-1/. Accessed November 20, 2015.
20. Patterson P, Medlow S, McDonald FE: Recent developments in supporting adolescent and young adult siblings of cancer patients. *Curr Opin Oncol* 27(4):311–315, 2015.
21. Wolfe J, Grier HE, Klar N, et al.: Symptoms and suffering at the end of life in children with cancer. *N Engl J Med* 342:326–333, 2000.
22. Kaye EC, Friebert S, Baker JN: Early integration of palliative care for children with high-risk cancer and their families. *Pediatr Blood Cancer* 63(4):593–597, 2015.

23. Uman LS, Birnie KA, Noel M, et al.: Psychological interventions for needle-related procedural pain and distress in children and adolescents. *Cochrane Database Syst Rev* (10):CD005179.
24. Peterson AM, Harper FW, Albrecht TL, et al.: Parent caregiver self-efficacy and child reactions to pediatric cancer treatment procedures. *J Pediatr Oncol Nurs* 31(1):18–27, 2014.
25. Kazak AE, Simms S, Barakat L, et al.: Surviving cancer competently intervention program (SCCIP): a cognitive-behavioral and family therapy intervention for adolescent survivors of childhood cancer and their families. *Fam Process* 38(2):175–191, 1999 Summer.
26. Gage-Bouchard EA, LaValley S, Panagakis C, Shelton RC: The architecture of support: the activation of preexisting ties and formation of new ties for tailored support. *Soc Sci Med* 134:59–65, 2015.
27. Hamner T, Latzman RD, Latzman NE, Elkin TD, Majumdar S: Quality of life among pediatric patients with cancer: contributions of time since diagnosis and parental chronic stress. *Pediatr Blood Cancer* 62(7):1232–1236, 2015.
28. LaMontagne LL, Wells N, Hepworth JT, Johnson BD, Manes R: Parent coping and child distress behaviors during invasive procedures for childhood cancer. *J Pediatr Oncol Nurs* 16(1):3–12, 1999.
29. James K, Keegan-Wells D, Hinds PS, et al.: The care of my child with cancer: parents' perceptions of caregiving demands. *J Pediatr Oncol Nurs* 19(6):218–228, 2002.
30. Mostert S, Arora RS, Arreola M, et al.: Abandonment of treatment for childhood cancer: position statement of a SIOP PODC Working Group. *Lancet Oncol* 12(8):719–720, 2011.
31. Gupta S, Yeh S, Martiniuk A, et al.: The magnitude and predictors of abandonment of therapy in paediatric acute leukaemia in middle-income countries: a systematic review and meta-analysis. *Eur J Cancer* 49(11):2555–2564, 2013.
32. Weaver MS, Baker JN, Gattuso JS, Gibson DV, Sykes AD, Hinds PS: Adolescents' preferences for treatment decisional involvement during their cancer. *Cancer* 121(24):4416–4424, 2015.
33. D'Agostino NM, Penney A, Zebrack B: Providing developmentally appropriate psychosocial care to adolescent and young adult cancer survivors. *Cancer* 117(10 Suppl):2329–2334, 2011.
34. Wiener L, McConnell DG, Latella L, Ludi E: Cultural and religious considerations in pediatric palliative care. *Palliat Support Care* 11(1):47–67, 2013.
35. Die-Trill M, Stuber ML: Psychological problems of curative cancer treatment. In: Holland JC (ed): *Psycho-Oncology*. New York, Oxford University Press, 1998, 897–906.
36. Freeman K, O'Dell C, Meola C: Issues in families of children with brain tumors. *Oncol Nurs Forum* 27(5):843–848, 2000.
37. Peckham VC: Children with cancer in the classroom. *Teach Except Child* 26:26–32, 1993.
38. Mitby PA, Robison LL, Whitton JA, et al.: Utilization of special education services and educational attainment among long-term survivors of childhood cancer: a report from the Childhood Cancer Survivor Study. *Cancer* 97(4):1115–1126, 2003.
39. Ellenberg L, Liu Q, Gioia G, et al.: Neurocognitive status in long-term survivors of childhood CNS malignancies: a report from the childhood cancer survivor study. *Neuropsychology* 23(6):705–717, 2009.
40. Brophy P, Kazak AE: Schooling. In: Johnson FL, O'Donnell EL (eds): *The Candlelighters Guide to Bone Marrow Transplants in Children*. Bethesda, Candlelighters Childhood Cancer Foundation, 68–73, 1994.
41. Winter AL, Conklin HM, Tyc VL, et al.: Executive function late effects in survivors of pediatric brain tumors and acute lymphoblastic leukemia. *J Clin Exp Neuropsychol* 36(8):818–830, 2014.
42. Raiker JS, Manning E, Herrington B, et al.: Brief neurocognitive screening in youth with brain tumours: a preliminary investigation of the Lebby-Asbell Neurocognitive Screening Examination (LANSE). *Brain Inj* 1–7, 2015.
43. Shaw PH, Reed DR, Yeager N, Zebrack B, Castellino SM, Bleyer A: Adolescent and Young Adult (AYA) Oncology in the United States: a specialty in its late adolescence. *J Pediatr Hematol Oncol* 37(3):161–169, 2015.
44. Treadgold CL, Kuperberg A: Been there, done that, wrote the blog: the choices and challenges of supporting adolescents and young adults with cancer. *J Clin Oncol* 28(32):4842–4849, 2010.
45. Katz LF, Leary A, Breiger D, Friedman D: Pediatric cancer and the quality of children's dyadic peer interactions. *J Pediatr Psychol* 36(2):237–247, 2011.
46. Cavuşoğlu H: Depression in children with cancer. *J Int Pediatr Nurs* 16(5):380–385, 2001.
47. Kazak AE, Brier M, Alderfer MA, et al.: Screening for psychosocial risk in pediatric cancer. *Pediatr Blood Cancer* 59(5):822–827, 2012.
48. National Comprehensive Cancer Network: Distress management. Clinical practice guidelines. *J Natl Compr Canc Netw* 1:344–374, 2003.
49. Patel SK, Mullins W, Turk A, Dekel N, Kinjo C, Sato JK. Distress screening, rater agreement, and services in pediatric oncology. *Psychooncology* 20(12):1324–1333, 2011.
50. Kazak AE, Prusak A, McSherry M, et al.: The Psychosocial Assessment Tool (PAT): pilot data on a brief screening instrument for identifying high risk families in pediatric oncology. *Fam Syst Health* 19:303–317, 2001.
51. Kazak AE: Pediatric Psychosocial Preventative Health Model (PPPHM): Research, practice and collaboration in pediatric family systems medicine. *Fam Syst Health* 24:381–395, 2006.
52. Zebrack BJ, Chesler MA: Quality of life in long-term survivors of childhood cancer. *Psychooncology* 11(2):132–141, 2002.
53. Barakat LP, Alderfer MA, Kazak AE: Posttraumatic growth in adolescent survivors of cancer and their mothers and fathers. *J Pediatr Psychol* 31(4):413–419, 2006.
54. Bendor SJ: Anxiety and isolation in siblings of pediatric cancer patients: the need for prevention. *Soc Work Health Care* 14:17–35, 1990.
55. Vermaes IP, van Susante AM, van Bakel HJ: Psychological functioning of siblings in families of children with chronic health conditions: a meta-analysis. *J Pediatr Psychol* 37(2):166–184, 2012.
56. Havermans T, Eiser C: Siblings of a child with cancer. *Child Care Health Dev* 20:309–322, 1994.
57. Houtzager BA, Grootenhuis MA, Last BF: Supportive groups for siblings of pediatric oncology patients: impact on anxiety. *Psychooncology* 10:315–324, 2001.
58. Mishel M: Uncertainty in chronic illness. *Annu Rev Nurs Res* 17:269–274, 1999.
59. Stewart JL: "Getting used to it": children finding the ordinary and routine in the uncertain context of cancer. *Qual Health Res* 13(3):394–407, 2003.
60. Woodgate RL, Degner LF: Expectations and beliefs about children's cancer symptoms: perspectives of children with cancer and their families. *Oncol Nurs Forum* 30(3):479–491, 2003.
61. Woodgate RL, Degner LF: A substantive theory of keeping the spirit alive: the spirit within children with cancer and their families. *J Pediatr Oncol Nurs* 20(3):103–119, 2003.
62. Zebrack B, Mathews-Bradshaw B, Siegel S; LIVESTRONG Young Adult Alliance: Quality cancer care for adolescents and young adults: a position statement. *J Clin Oncol* 28(32):4862–4867, 2010.
63. Bessell AG: Children surviving childhood cancer: psychosocial adjustment, quality of life, and school experiences. *Except Child* 67(3):345–359, 2001.
64. Masera G, Chesler MA, Jankovic M, et al.: SIOP Working Committee on psychosocial issues in pediatric oncology: guidelines for communication of the diagnosis. *Med Pediatr Oncol* 28(5):382–385, 1997.
65. Mack JW, Joffe S: Communicating about prognosis: ethical responsibilities of pediatricians and parents. *Pediatrics* 133(Suppl 1):S24–S30, 2014.
66. Snyder CR: Reality negotiation: from excuses to hope and beyond. *J Soc Clin Psychol* 8:130–157, 1989.
67. Germann JN, Leonard D, Stuenzi TJ, Pop RB, Stewart SM, Leavey PJ: Hoping is coping: a guiding theoretical framework for promoting coping and adjustment following pediatric cancer diagnosis. *J Pediatr Psychol* 40(9):846–855, 2015.
68. Berg CJ, Stratton E, Esiashvili N, Mertens A: Young adult cancer survivors' experience with cancer treatment and follow-up care and perceptions of barriers to engaging in recommended care. *J Cancer Educ* 31(3):430–442, 2016.
69. Bitsko MJ, Cohen D, Dillon R, Harvey J, Krull K, Klosky JL: Psychosocial late effects in pediatric cancer survivors: a report from the children's oncology group. *Pediatr Blood Cancer* 63(2):337–433, 2015.
70. Eapen V, Revesz T: Psychosocial correlates of pediatric cancer in the United Arab Emirates. *Support Care Cancer* 11:185–189, 2003.
71. Kamihara J, Nyborn JA, Olcese ME, Nickerson T, Mack JW: Parental hope for children with advanced cancer. *Pediatrics* 135(5):868–874, 2015.
72. Chesler M, Chesney B: *Cancer and Self-Help*. Madison, University of Wisconsin Press, 1995.
73. Manne S, DuHamel K, Redd WH: Association of psychological vulnerability factors to posttraumatic stress symptomatology in mothers of pediatric cancer survivors. *Psycho-Oncology* 9:372–384, 2000.
74. Hancock L: The camp experience for siblings of pediatric cancer patients. *J Pediatr Oncol Nurs* 28(3):137–142, 2011.
75. Love B, Crook B, Thompson CM, et al.: Exploring the communication of social support online: a content analysis of messages posted to an adolescent and young adult cancer support community. *Cyberpsychol Behav Soc Netw* 15(10):555–559, 2012.
76. Eysenbach G: The impact of the internet on cancer outcomes. *CA Cancer J Clin* 53(6):356–371, 2003.
77. Hilty DM, Ferrer DC, Parish MB, Johnston B, Callahan EJ, Yellowlees PM: The effectiveness of telemental health: a 2013 review. *Telemed J E Health* 19(6):444–454, 2013.
78. Wakefield CE, Sansom-Daly UM, McGill BC, et al.: Online parent-targeted cognitive-behavioural therapy intervention to improve quality of life in families of young cancer survivors: study protocol for a randomised controlled trial. *Trials* 16:153, 2015.

CHAPTER 7.2.2 ■ THE ROLE OF THE CHILD AND ADOLESCENT PSYCHIATRIST ON THE PEDIATRIC TRANSPLANT SERVICE

STEVEN C. SCHLOZMAN AND LAURA M. PRAGER

INTRODUCTION

Both solid-organ and bone marrow transplant procedures have become increasingly successful over the last 30 to 40 years. For example, survival outcomes for pediatric renal transplant are over 95% at 5 years (1). No longer focused solely on the patients' survival, transplant services have begun to recognize the importance of the psychosocial development of those patients whose lives were saved but permanently altered, and their risk for an emotional backlash that parallels the potential for medical complications. In addition, as young transplant recipients live longer, they (like their typically developing peers) struggle with the desire for increasing autonomy from parents and caregivers, a passage that can be fraught with challenges given the possibly life-threatening implications of nonadherence to treatment regimens, experimentation with substance use, or other risky behaviors.

The child and adolescent psychiatrist (CAP) who works with pediatric transplant patients is ideally suited to assess and manage emotional sequelae of transplantation including, among other things, posttraumatic stress disorder (PTSD) from the procedure itself, adjustment to the ongoing risk for infection and/or rejection as well as to the ever-present potential for developing a malignancy, neurocognitive changes, and questions and concerns surrounding sexuality or fertility. The CAP can also help to guide these young, chronically ill patients through the developmental milestones that attend the transition from adolescence to adulthood. Furthermore, as most psychiatric disorders emerge during adolescence and young adulthood, the child and psychiatrist who works on a pediatric transplant service can assist with the diagnosis of emerging psychiatric disorders and devise psychopharmacologic treatment regiments that do not compromise existing immunosuppressive regimens.

In this chapter, we will summarize the psychiatric aspects of pediatric solid-organ and bone marrow transplant patients. We will focus on the evaluation and preparation of patients and their families for the procedure itself, on how to work with the patient and family during and immediately following the procedure, and on the long-term management of these patients as they move forward in their lives. In many ways, pediatric transplant psychiatry epitomizes the fundamental aspects of good consultation–liaison work. The principal challenge for the transplant psychiatrist is balancing the dual role of helping the patient and family maintain a normal developmental trajectory while at the same time assisting the transplant team with the often charged and intense emotions that accompany working with these young patients.

Patients who face either solid-organ transplant or bone marrow transplant are gravely ill and struggling with life and death issues. Transplants are a viable option when other treatment modalities cannot prevent death or progressive, debilitating illness. Depending on the patient's age and developmental stage, he or she will often be acutely aware that organ failure is life threatening, yet unable to weigh the risks and benefits of transplantation. The risks of the surgery itself are even difficult for adults to contemplate, as is the meaning of the commitment to a lifetime of medications with both short- and long-term side effects. Patients and their families will wonder about issues as immediate as whether academic and developmental progress will continue unabated, and as distant as whether or not fertility will be at risk. In this setting, both the patients and their families are usually under enormous stress. Together they must process this complex information and then make a decision about whether or not to proceed with a potentially life-threatening and most certainly life-changing treatment. The CAP on the transplant service can be instrumental in identifying the cognitive and emotional level of the patient based on age and stage, placing the child and his or her needs within the context of a family dynamic, and communicating this information to other members of the team. The CAP can also assist other members of the team to appreciate the families' degree of distress as well as make suggestions for how to discuss potential outcomes with both the child and the parents.

Transplantation is a final common pathway for a group of heterogeneous and not always related conditions. This poses a special challenge to the child psychiatrist working with the transplant team. To be effective, the child psychiatrist must have an understanding of the medical and surgical components of the underlying disease as well as an understanding of the risks and benefits of the transplant itself. He or she must then tailor any treatment to the temperament and pre-existing psychological and developmental challenges facing the child and the family, keeping in mind the inherent limitations posed by both the disease and the treatment. As many patients are quite young, there is the added challenge of balancing the involvement of an extended family and multiple systems of care. The work is complex but immensely rewarding.

IMMUNOSUPPRESSIVE MEDICATIONS

Immunosuppressive medications are still the mainstay of prevention of graft rejection, and many patients experience neuropsychiatric side effects from those medications. The calcineurin inhibitors such as cyclosporine and tacrolimus and the corticosteroids have been associated with anxiety, depression, agitation, delirium, paranoia, cognitive changes, and worsening of pre-existing psychiatric conditions. These effects will be discussed in detail below. The transplant psychiatrist must be aware of the potential for these side effects as well as for the interaction between these agents and psychotropic medications.

Case Illustration 1: Side Effects of Immunosuppression

A 13-year-old boy with a history of autoimmune hepatitis and subsequent hepatic failure received a deceased donor liver transplant at age 12. Before his liver disease and surgery, he carried the psychiatric diagnoses of ADHD and an atypical mood disorder, and was treated with stimulant medications and atypical antipsychotics to prevent his often aggressive outbursts. Given the severity of his psychiatric disorder, his medication was continued throughout his perioperative course. However, after his transplant, he developed significant emotional lability that correlated with the addition of prednisone as a necessary part of his immunosuppressant regimen. This behavior was managed by increasing dosages of his atypical antipsychotic medications. As atypical agents are metabolized in the liver, increased monitoring of his liver function tests was necessary to ensure that the added psychotropics were not further compromising his graft.

Many transplant recipients are on multiple agents, and these may affect each other with significant neuropsychiatric sequelae (refer to Chapter 6.1.1). The transplant psychiatrist may be the member of the team most likely to recognize these interactions given that vigilance regarding drug–drug interactions is a mainstay of psychopharmacology.

Case Illustration 2: Drug–Drug Interactions

An 18-year-old woman who underwent a deceased donor liver transplant for biliary atresia at age 2 presented to the pediatric transplant service for ongoing management of her transplant, as well as for care of her inflammatory bowel disease. Important psychiatric issues included diagnoses of depression and anxiety for which she was prescribed clonazepam and paroxetine. Her history was also significant for recreational marijuana use and a complex partial seizure disorder. Finally, she had persistent difficulties with medication compliance, often stopping her antirejection medications. After her arrest for possession at age 19, she abruptly stopped using marijuana, and almost immediately thereafter experienced another round of graft rejection for which she was admitted to the hospital with the assumption that she had stopped taking her medications. A low tacrolimus level made her insistence that she was indeed compliant all the more puzzling. The transplant service eventually concluded that the sudden withdrawal of marijuana likely increased gastric motility, such that she absorbed her immunosuppressing medication less well than before and thus was not able to maintain her graft without immediate treatment with steroids and a higher overall immunosuppressive regimen. Appropriate adjustments in immunosuppressant dosages adequately addressed the problem, and the patient was able to maintain her graft.

Transplant as Trauma

There is mounting evidence that both bone marrow and solid-organ recipients are at risk for posttraumatic stress syndromes (PTSS) and in some instances will meet full criteria for PTSD. Mental health providers who work on transplant services need to watch for these symptoms, both in patients and in their families. A recent review by Stuber et al. (2) suggested that parental trauma was a strong predictor of patient traumatic reaction among medically ill pediatric cancer patients. Similarly, in pediatric transplant patients, new research stresses that the families' and patients' appreciation of the seriousness of the illness, regardless of how physicians tended to view the severity of the condition, is a potent predictor of pathologic stress reactions (3). There is also evidence to suggest that premorbid parent anxiety predisposes parents of children undergoing transplant to developing PTSD (4). In addition, it is possible that the extent to which parents feel traumatized correlates with the psychological and medical well-being of the pediatric transplant recipient (2,3). Finally, as one might expect, sudden events, such as abrupt rupture of esophageal varices in patients with portal hypertension, are associated with more traumatic responses than insidious serious illnesses, such as slowly progressive cardiomyopathies or a gradual decline in pulmonary function.

Trauma among medically ill children is further complicated by the fact that the child patients may perceive the treaters as perpetrators. This perception can extend to parents, given that parents are often called upon to enforce difficult and painful regimens. This poses a special challenge to the treatment team. Judicious use of anxiolytic medication and psychosocial interventions such as guided imagery and other relaxation techniques have all been useful in helping child patients tolerate difficult procedures and/or participate in their own treatment.

Finally, because avoidance is a core symptom of trauma, patients may be nonadherent with their medications or doctor's visits in order to avoid the negative emotional valence associated with these experiences. This response can occur in both pediatric patients and their parents. The team should be vigilant for trauma as an etiologic factor for nonadherence in this patient population (5).

Graft Rejection

For all patients who undergo transplant procedures, there exists a difficult equilibrium in allowing their children to develop and grow as normally as possible, while remaining constantly vigilant and increasingly anxious about the possibility of graft rejection. Graft rejection is not always obvious, though in some instances it is preceded by a clearly worsening course. In other situations, however, possible graft rejection is discovered in routine laboratory tests, leading to an element of hypervigilance that both patient and parents can experience and that is neither helpful nor healthy. Medication nonadherence is frequent, especially in adolescents, and constitutes one of the most common causes of graft rejection. Studies of barriers to adherence in medication-taking among adolescents have identified that those patients who lack organizational skills have more trouble remembering to take medications, and that those patients with comorbid psychiatric illnesses such as mood disorders, anxiety disorders, or PTSD are also more likely to be nonadherent (6). The transplant psychiatrist can be helpful in identifying, assessing, and managing the risk for nonadherence. His or her unique understanding of transplant medicine may encourage a frank discussion by the patient and family about their heightened concerns about rejection and the ways in which strict adherence to the medication regimen and other recommendations of the treatment team can reduce that risk.

Comorbid Psychiatric Illness

Given the natural epidemiology of childhood psychosocial and psychiatric difficulties, there will inevitably be some children and adolescents who will suffer psychological difficulties not directly related to their transplant, but whose transplant will complicate effective treatment. For these patients, though no clear guidelines exist, keeping in mind drug–drug interactions, the means by which medications are metabolized, and the possible neuropsychiatric side effects of immunosuppressants are all important considerations. In general, one should prescribe psychotropic agents in lower initial dosages and monitor closely both the mental status examination and laboratory values that might suggest adverse drug effects. In addition, one cannot underestimate the effectiveness of supportive, psychodynamic, and behavioral interventions for some patients. Undergoing and living with a transplant is trying at best, and for children and adolescents, the therapist can help them cope with shaping an identity that is informed but not defined by their illness.

BONE MARROW TRANSPLANTATION—SPECIAL CONSIDERATIONS

Patients who require solid-organ transplant (heart, kidney, lung, liver) often see their disease as limited to that organ. Bone marrow transplantation, however, is performed for patients who have an underlying systemic illness, that is, cancer. As cancer itself carries particular emotional valence in our culture, patients receiving transplant procedures for malignancies may require extra attention given the associated stress that the diagnosis and all of its cultural signifiers can entail. Although some pediatric patients may receive solid-organ transplantation for cancer, this is less common than for organ malformation or metabolic and autoimmune diseases. Additionally, the isolation associated with bone marrow transplantation is particularly harrowing for all patients, and attention to the developmental needs of these patients is crucial for their psychological and medical well-being.

THE PRETRANSPLANTATION PSYCHIATRIC EVALUATION

The CAP plays an important and complex role in the evaluation of the child who is approaching transplantation. Initially, the psychiatrist is responsible for conducting a thorough psychiatric evaluation of the patient and family. In addition, the psychiatrist must be familiar with the medical problems facing the patient, both before and after surgery, in order to educate the family about the risks and benefits or transplantation and to assess the family's ability to provide informed consent. The psychiatrist also acts as a liaison between the family and the transplant team. The family will need support, direction, and clarification of the transplant team's expectations and concerns. The team in turn will also need support, direction, and sometimes interpretation of the family's behavior. The psychiatrist may also serve to focus the team's attention on ethical conflicts that may arise, particularly those that involve directed living donation by a related or unrelated donor.

There are no universally accepted guidelines for the psychiatric evaluation of children who are potential candidates for organ transplantation. Some centers routinely offer an open-ended, face-to-face clinical interview with a mental health provider, some require formal psychological testing, and yet others rely on structured or semi-structured interviews. Not all transplant teams have psychiatric consultants. In many centers, psychologists and/or social workers complete psychosocial assessments. There are differences among transplant centers as to what constitutes an acceptable candidate for transplant. Common exclusion criteria include active substance abuse, active psychotic symptoms, suicidal ideation with plan or intent, history of self-injurious behavior or suicide attempts.

As with a standard psychiatric evaluation, the order and style of the interview is dependent on the child's age and developmental stage. With a prepubertal child, it is appropriate, perhaps even necessary, first to meet with the parents in order to get a coherent, longitudinal history. With the adolescent, it is beneficial to interview the child alone before meeting the parents in order to reinforce the primacy of the adolescent's concerns and feelings. At some point, it is imperative to meet with the patient and the parents/caregivers together in order to be sure that all parties hear (and hopefully understand) the same information and that all are in agreement as to how to proceed.

The pretransplantation psychiatric evaluation should be primarily diagnostic but can also be educational and, sometimes, even therapeutic. In addition to the developmental, social, educational, family, and past psychiatric history, the evaluation should address the following aspects:

1. Screening of potential recipients for the presence of significant psychiatric illnesses such as mood, anxiety, or psychotic disorders, as well as potential learning disabilities or frank cognitive impairment
2. History of past or current drug or alcohol abuse, particularly in the adolescent patient

The question of past or ongoing substance abuse in adolescents facing transplant is particularly important and warrants further discussion. In adult liver transplantation programs, ongoing alcohol or addictive drug use is usually a contraindication to transplant (7). Most programs require demonstration of 6 months to 1 year sobriety. With lung transplantation programs, tobacco use is an absolute contraindication to transplant and, again, candidates must demonstrate that they have abstained from cigarettes for over 6 months. Adolescents are less likely than adults to have a longstanding problem with substance abuse but frequently they have tried recreational drugs or alcohol in social situations. Sometimes they drink heavily or smoke marijuana on the weekends with their friends. It can be challenging to help these young people understand that such behavior could jeopardize their eligibility for transplant and could, if it continues after transplant, precipitate failure of the allograft. Individual transplant programs are left to determine what degree of risk they are willing to tolerate.

Indeed, the issue of alcohol use among adolescent transplant recipients and candidates requires special attention. This is of course particularly important when discussing liver transplantation. Although there is ample evidence that many adolescents experiment with alcohol, the use of alcohol by liver transplant patients is potentially extremely dangerous. Because liver failure can be insidious and unpredictable, it is difficult to assess when and to what extent alcohol use is likely to contribute to liver dysfunction. For these reasons, most child psychiatric consultants for liver transplant services feel that they must explicitly convey to their patients the seriousness of alcohol use. However, lecturing to teenagers about the dangers of alcohol use is likely to be met with resistance and defensiveness. Normal adolescent drives toward independence, coupled with the adolescent's unique susceptibility to peer pressure, often lead to alcohol use even among patients who understand intellectually that their liver disease makes this behavior particularly dangerous and unhealthy. At the same time, most transplant services do not view occasional experimentation with alcohol as an absolute contraindication for future transplants in adolescent populations. We have found that frank, developmentally appropriate discussions with adolescent transplant patients about alcohol use are substantially more effective at quelling and preventing experimentation and use of alcohol. While alcohol use is not under any circumstances acceptable, especially in adolescents with liver disease, helping teens to grasp the limitations of their disease in as mature a matter as possible is the best way to ensure healthy behavior.

Adolescents with liver failure are not the only ones vulnerable to the effects of recreational drugs. Adolescents with other forms of end-organ failure are also prone to experimentation, use, and even abuse of alcohol and other drugs. Cigarette smoking is an absolute contraindication to lung transplant, but other drugs that suppress the respiratory drive also have the potential for lethality. As the time for transplant nears, it is often very difficult to know whether the adolescent with substance abuse issues has "reformed" and stopped using simply because he or she has become gravely ill or because he or she has passed through the experimentation phase and recognized the limitations of such behavior. Transplant teams usually hope that the latter is true, but that is not always the case.

Case Illustration 3: Substance Abuse

A recent high school graduate with cystic fibrosis (CF) was hospitalized in the setting of declining pulmonary function for a course of intravenous antibiotics and aggressive chest physical therapy. Her pulmonologist noted that her pulmonary function tests (PFTs) had declined precipitously since her last admission and were not improving with standard medical care. He asked the transplant team to evaluate her for candidacy. On psychiatric evaluation, the patient acknowledged that in the year prior to admission she had developed an addiction to oxycontin (oxycodone). She had had completed a drug treatment program and been "clean" for several months. The transplant team was aware of her difficulty but felt that her drug use was probably adolescent "experimentation." All agreed that she would die without a transplant. She subsequently underwent living donor transplant approximately 9 months later and recovered well following the surgery. However, several months after her transplant she was rushed to the hospital in respiratory distress secondary to inadvertent narcotic overdose. She struggled with intermittent abuse for many months thereafter before finally agreeing to join a methadone maintenance program.

3. Assessment of child's relationship with caregivers
4. Determination of the child and family's motivation for transplant

Because young children do not always have a full understanding of either the gravity of their illness or of the ramifications of transplant, it is their parents and/or other caregivers/guardians who "consent" to the surgery and postoperative care. Nevertheless, a verbal child patient must be able to "assent" to the surgery and be willing to participate actively in the treatment process. Both parent and child must be able to work together toward the common goal of transplant. If parent or child is not fully engaged in the process, then it is difficult for the transplant team to know how best to proceed.

Case Illustration 4: Whose Transplant Is It, Anyway?

An 11-year-old boy with advanced CF and no past psychiatric history was brought by his mother for a living donor pretransplantation psychiatric evaluation. Mother was worried that her son would die before he became ill enough to reach the top of the list for a deceased donor transplant. She herself volunteered to be a living lobar lung donor and she aggressively pursued other potential donors until she found one. On initial interviews, the patient was cheerful and appeared to have a good understanding of why his mother and a neighbor each wished to donate a lung lobe. In his final meeting with the transplant team pulmonologist, however, the patient curled into a ball on the couch, cried quietly, and refused to talk about the impending living donor transplant. Ultimately, the team decided that it was the patient's mother and not the patient who was the motivating force for living donor transplant. The child did not feel ready to have an elective transplant with his mother as a donor. The team reassured the family that the child's situation was not too dire and he could wait until he was ill enough to become eligible for a deceased donor transplant.

5. Evaluation of the child and family's ability to comply with treatment recommendations of caregivers

Candidacy for transplant demands consistent attention to and compliance with the recommendations of the treatment team. Pre- and posttransplant patients must take many medications every day; often they are asked to endure time-consuming and uncomfortable procedures such as chest physical therapy for patients with bronchiectasis or CF. The patient's willingness to adhere to the pretransplant regimen is an important determinant of their readiness for transplant and the complicated posttransplant regimen that follows.

Case Illustration 5: Compliance

A high school girl with end-stage CF met with the child psychiatrist as part of a standard pretransplant evaluation. The patient asked her parents to be present for the entire interview. The young woman was strikingly thin. The transplant psychiatrist asked the patient if her CF doctor had ever suggested that she have a G-tube placed for nutritional supplementation. The patient burst into tears and stated that she could never tolerate a G-tube even though she had been told that she could not gain weight regardless of how many calories she consumed during meals. She acknowledged, also, that she had been instructed to start continuous oxygen but had been unable to do that either because she was too embarrassed to be seen in public with a nasal cannula. The psychiatrist tried to explore with the patient other ways that she might improve her ability to adhere to the recommendations of her doctors but ultimately had to deny her candidacy for transplant based on her history of noncompliance and her inability to adhere to the recommendations of her physicians.

6. Understanding of the social supports available to the family
7. Assessment of psychosocial stressors in the family, such as financial pressures or marital discord
8. Assessment of the patient and family's understanding of the risks and benefits inherent in transplantation
9. Determination of the ability of the patient and family to collaborate with the transplant team with the shared goal of improving the patient's quality of life

PSYCHIATRIC CARE OF THE PATIENT AT THE TIME OF TRANSPLANTATION

For patients undergoing bone marrow or solid-organ transplantation, the stress of the procedure and the resulting hospitalization can be particularly trying. In addition, in cases where deceased donor organs suddenly become available, families find themselves thrown into the hospital with little time to prepare. These aspects of transplantation require special attention by mental health clinicians, especially around the time of admission and during the ensuing hospital stay. However, as with the pretransplant evaluation, there are no clear guidelines detailing the most appropriate intervention. Some centers employ an educational approach, requiring patients and families to undergo orientation to the hospital well before the transplant itself. Other centers focus attention on the patient and family directly after the transplant takes place. We have found that discussing these options with patients and families and allowing them to choose is the best approach. As we have stressed, intervention should focus on individual needs and temperamental differences.

Once the transplant takes place, it is imperative that the transplant psychiatrist be available to the patient, the family, and to the transplant team. Issues such as abrupt mental status changes, acute anxiety, poor medical outcomes, and treatment team stress all are often part of the transplant psychiatrists' responsibilities. These responsibilities are best met by frequent visits with all parties, developmentally appropriate explicit discussion of unfavorable outcomes with the team and with the patient and family, and vigilance for increasing stress and frustration surrounding the posttransplant course. To the extent that families can be made aware of the possibility of difficult postsurgical courses, they will be likely to cope more effectively with whatever outcomes transpire.

WORKING WITH THE TRANSPLANT TEAM

Transplant psychiatrists work with and are part of large multidisciplinary teams. In this setting the psychiatrist who evaluates the child or adolescent for transplant candidacy can sometimes come into conflict with the treatment team. Because many transplant patients endure lengthy hospital admissions, pediatricians (residents and staff), physical therapists, social workers and child-life specialists often form long-term and extremely close relationships with children and adolescents with end-stage organ failure. To these caregivers, referral for transplant evaluation represents an acknowledgment of the failure of current management and, at the same time, a plea for the only viable treatment option.

These children and adolescents may not meet criteria for candidacy for transplant for many reasons. Sometimes, the patient is referred for transplant when they are too close to death and would not be able to tolerate the actual operation. Sometimes, the patient and family may be denied on psychosocial grounds. Regardless of the reason for denial of candidacy, the treatment team may be disappointed and angry with the transplant team. This is particularly difficult when the patient is denied because of a history of nonadherence with medical care in the outpatient setting and/or lack of social supports. Sometimes in these situations, caregivers promise that the patient will "do better" and appeal to the psychiatrist to reevaluate the situation. It is often helpful for the psychiatrist to meet with the treatment team to review the evaluation and to let all involved share their feelings.

Case Illustration 6: Conflict among Caregivers

A high school student with CF was hospitalized frequently on the pediatric service for treatment with antibiotics and chest physical therapy. The patient lived with her mother and her older sister. Her mother was an immigrant who worked long hours and was not home during the day. Her older sister was frequently out of the house as well. The patient spoke English but the mother did not. The patient had a very hard time complying with her outpatient regimen of multiple daily medications, breathing treatments, and chest physical therapy. She had had frequent hospitalizations over the years due to nonadherence with her outpatient self-care. The CF staff had tried many times to effect change in her social situation, without success. When asked why she was not able to take better care of herself, the patient said that she was too embarrassed to go to the nurse during school hours to take her midday medications and that at night she preferred to go out with friends. When the psychiatrist interviewed the patient regarding her interest in and suitability for transplant, the question of compliance took on more importance. The patient insisted that she wanted a transplant and that she would try harder to do all of what the treatment team asked of her. The patient's mother felt that her daughter's health was in God's hands and that she could not do anything more to help her. The transplant psychiatrist, after discussion with the treating pulmonologist, agreed to a trial period of 6 months during which the patient would be monitored carefully on the outpatient basis to assess compliance. Unfortunately, the patient was not able to follow a schedule at home for even a period of a few weeks and was soon readmitted to the hospital in respiratory distress. The transplant team ultimately denied her candidacy.

THE LIVING DONOR TRANSPLANT

As there are many more patients who need organ transplant than there are available organs, living organ donation has become much more widely accepted in the United States. Living donation is a viable option for kidney, lung, and liver transplants. Potential donors also undergo a comprehensive psychological evaluation as well as a medical workup in order to ensure full autonomy, informed consent, and the absence of coercion. In some centers, the child psychiatrist or mental health provider working with the transplant team plays a crucial role in the evaluation of potential living donors. In other centers, the psychiatric screening evaluation of living donors is cursory. Additionally, some centers stress the need for a psychiatrist other than the transplant psychiatrist to evaluate the donor candidate. In all instances, great emphasis is placed on the absence of coercion in these unique situations. Living donors may be biologically related to the recipient, emotionally connected but not biologically related, or unrelated and anonymous. Lung transplantation is unique in that two donors are necessary.

It is very common for a parent to volunteer to donate an organ or part of an organ to a child. In those cases, the issue of benefit to the donor, that is, preservation of the life of a child is incontrovertible. However, the psychiatrist must help the team to consider the well-being of other members of an immediate family if both a child and a parent have surgery simultaneously. The psychiatrist also has an obligation to the patient to ensure that the parents' motivation for transplantation is in the best interest of the child, both physically and emotionally.

Potential donors who are siblings also merit close attention during a screening evaluation. It can be very difficult for a sibling who is blood type identical to refuse to donate, particularly if one or both parents are ineligible. Even though a sibling might deny feeling family pressure, it undoubtedly exists. A lobectomy is a painful and potentially debilitating operation. Siblings who volunteer to be living lobar lung donors must anticipate a 4- or 5-day hospital stay followed by 6 to 8 weeks of recovery before they will be able to resume normal activities.

The screening evaluation of an unrelated but emotionally connected donor or of a donor who has no connection at all with the recipient can present other challenges. Families of transplant recipients often advertise for donors on the Internet or in local community settings. Donors often come with an incomplete understanding of the process and unrealistic expectations for the outcome. Sometimes donors expect payment; sometimes donors are actively struggling with psychiatric illness or substance abuse. Studies of kidney donors have shown that as many as 50% of donors who presented themselves as completely sure that they wanted to donate, expressed ambivalence about donation on self-report questionnaires (6). Again, it is left to the individual transplant center to determine who will make an appropriate, unrelated donor.

NEUROPSYCHIATRIC EFFECTS OF IMMUNOSUPPRESSIVE MEDICATION

The risks of rejection and infection are constants in the life of a posttransplant child or adolescent. All transplant patients are maintained for the rest of their lives on immunosuppressive medications. These medications and their interactions with other agents can have significant neuropsychiatric side effects that can be difficult to distinguish from psychiatric illness and that can complicate any planned psychopharmacologic regimen. It is also important to remember that a child's pharmacodynamics and pharmacokinetics can be different. A child's hepatic metabolic rate is faster than that of an adult and, although pediatric kidney function is similar to that of an adult, children (specifically between the ages of 9 and 12 years) may have a higher glomerular filtration rate as well (see Chapter 6.1.1). Children tend to metabolize common psychotropic medications such as neuroleptics, anticonvulsants, antidepressants, and benzodiazepines more rapidly. However, any psychotropic medication that inhibits the cytochrome P450 IIIA3/4 isoenzyme system can potentially increase the levels of immunosuppressive medication. Conversely, some agents, including the herbal antidepressant St. John wort can be associated with decreased immunosuppressant levels and subsequent graft rejection. Some of the most common neuropsychiatric profiles of immunosuppressant agents are summarized in Table 7.2.2.1.

Cyclosporine (Neoral, Sandimmune) is a polypeptide derived from a fungus and is the mainstay of immunosuppressive therapy. Common adverse effects include nephrotoxicity, hypertension, hypomagnesaemia, hyperkalemia, gastroparesis, and hyperlipidemia. Neuropsychiatric effects are particularly problematic at high serum levels and include delirium, often accompanied by frank psychotic symptoms (auditory and visual hallucinations). These side effects often resolve spontaneously as serum levels decrease, but patients often have a clear memory of their hallucinations. Patients with central nervous system effects sometimes have periventricular white matter changes on MRI. Cyclosporine is metabolized in the liver by the P450 IIIA3/4 system; it is possible that the selective serotonin uptake inhibitors could increase its serum levels through inhibition of the cytochrome system, but this has not been convincingly demonstrated (8). Carbamazepine may decrease its levels through hepatic induction. Patients who undergo bone marrow transplants may be particularly vulnerable to the neuropsychiatric toxic effects of cyclosporine (9).

FK506 (Tacrolimus, Prograf) is a macrolide produced by bacteria, and is also used as a primary immunosuppressive, sometimes as a substitute for cyclosporine. The neuropsychiatric side effects are similar to those of cyclosporine, including delirium, seizures, and akinetic mutism. MRI scans may also reveal white matter changes in patients showing toxicity. Psychotropic medications such as the selective serotonin uptake inhibitors that inhibit the cytochrome P450 IIIA3/4 system can cause increases in serum levels of FK506 and must be used with caution.

Mycophenolate mofetil (Cellcept) suppresses T- and B-cell lymphocyte proliferation and is used as rescue therapy for those patients who cannot tolerate cyclosporine or FK506. It can also sometimes be used as adjunctive immunosuppression

TABLE 7.2.2.1

POTENTIAL PSYCHIATRIC SIDE EFFECTS OF IMMUNOSUPPRESSANT AGENTS

Immunosuppressant Agent	Description	Potential Psychiatric Side Effects	Laboratory Findings
Cyclosporin Neoral *Sandimmune*	Polypeptide fungal product	Delirium, auditory hallucinations, visual hallucinations, other psychotic symptoms	Side effects more prominent at high serum values and tend to resolve as serum levels decrease, SSRIs may increase levels, carbamazepine may decrease levels, herbal agents such as St. John wort may decrease levels, question of increased sensitivity to neuropsychiatric side effects among bone marrow transplant recipients
Tacrolimus *Prograf*	Also called FK506 or 5FK; macrolide antibiotic	Delirium, auditory and visual hallucinations, other psychotic symptoms, seizures, akinetic mutism	Side effects more prominent at high serum values and tend to resolve as serum levels decrease, MRI may reveal white matter changes in toxic patients
Mycophenolate Mofetil *Cellcept*	Suppresses T and B cell proliferation as adjunct immunosuppressant or for patients who cannot tolerate cyclosporine or tacrolimus	Anxiety, depression, sedation	
Muromonab-CD3 *OKT3*	Given immediately postoperatively to prevent rejection, monoclonal antibody that suppresses CD3 T-cell function	Aseptic meningitis, hallucinations during administrations	
Corticosteroids	Mainstay of most transplant regimens, usually started high and tapered over weeks to months, though many patients remain on small dose indefinitely	Increased appetite, anxiety, depression, hypomania, mania, paranoia	Often dose-related and resolve with lowered dose

with cyclosporine. Central nervous system side effects can include anxiety, depression, and sedation.

OKT3 is a monoclonal antibody that is used in the immediate postoperative period to prevent rejection. It can cause aseptic meningitis. Patients can hallucinate during administration, but those symptoms usually abate fairly quickly.

Corticosteroids continue to be a mainstay of treatment for transplant patients. Very high doses in the immediate postoperative period are gradually tapered over several months. Most patients remain on a small daily dose of oral prednisone for the remainder of their lives. Their numerous side effects include weight gain, easy bruising, osteoporosis, hirsutism, affective lability, hypomania, or mania. Some patients can manifest psychotic symptoms at very high doses (10). The neuropsychiatric side effects are sometimes dose related and generally subside with gradual taper of medication. Sudden discontinuation of steroids can result in depression, irritability, or anxiety.

Case Illustration 7: Neuropsychiatric Effects of Immunosuppressives

A young woman with CF underwent bilateral living donor lung transplantation. After a rocky postoperative course, she stabilized and was transferred to the transplant floor. Although her overall condition continued to improve, the nurses often found her crying in her room and the psychiatrist was asked to assess her for a question of depression. On evaluation, the patient's mood was upbeat but she explained that she frequently burst into tears with the smallest stimulus. She felt that she was overreacting to "everything" but she could not help herself. She was embarrassed by how often she cried and puzzled because in between she did not feel sad. When asked about how things had gone for her in general, she reported that she had a vivid memory of her postoperative stay in the intensive care unit. She told the psychiatrist that she had had visions of people she knew coming and going although later her parents had told her that no one was there. She had a picture in her mind of her surgeon as a "prankster," dressed up in a costume. She remembered feeling incredibly fearful of him but also unable to help herself. The patient was relieved to learn that her affective lability was most likely secondary to her high-dose steroids and that her "hallucinations" were also a side effect of the cyclosporine treatment.

LONG-TERM PSYCHIATRIC CARE OF THE PEDIATRIC TRANSPLANT PATIENT

Transplant patients are typically followed closely by the transplant team for the remainder of their lives. They frequently have medical and surgical complications, they sometimes require a second or even a third transplant, and they often suffer significant psychological distress as they attempt to grapple with the long-term implications of their disease. Because of this, the transplant psychiatrist continues to play an important role. Management of all of these issues again calls for the careful reckoning of both psychiatric and nonpsychiatric phenomena. For example, a change in mental status may be secondary to a medication effect, a metabolic encephalopathy, a seizure disorder, a newly presenting psychiatric illness, or a combination of some or even all of these issues. Again, the medical expertise of the CAP makes him or her ideally suited for these complicated issues.

Additionally, as we mentioned above, psychiatric illnesses can occur either as a function of the transplant, or as unrelated conditions and problems such as mood disorders, anxiety disorders, and PTSD more common in pediatric transplant recipients than in their peers who do not suffer from chronic health problems (6).

CONCLUSION

As transplant procedures have become more successful, transplant teams have increasingly embraced the notion that the fundamental goal for young transplant patients is assuming the most normal life possible in spite of the obstacles that their diseases potentially pose. Transplant patients play on soccer teams, go on dates, graduate from school, and often want most of all to be thought of as an ordinary child or adolescent. Empathy for this desire, coupled with the simultaneous vigilance for the numerous problems outlined above, make the job of the pediatric transplant psychiatrist complicated, challenging, and undeniably rewarding.

References

1. LaRosa C, Jorge Baluarte H, Meyers KEC: Outcomes in pediatric solid-organ transplantation. *Pediatr Transplant* 15:129–141, 2011.
2. Stuber ML, Kazack AE, Meeske K, et al.: Predictors of posttraumatic stress symptoms in childhood cancer survivors. *Pediatrics* 100:958–964, 1997.
3. Mintzer LL, Stuber ML, Seacord D, Castaneda M, Mesrkhani V, Glover D: Traumatic stress symptoms in adolescent organ transplant recipients. *Pediatrics* 115(6):1640–1644, 2005.
4. Supelana C, Annunziato RA, Kaplan D, Helcer J, Stuber MI, Shemes E: PTSD in solid organ transplant recipients: current understand and future implications. *Pediatr Transplant* 20:23–33, 2015.
5. McCormick King ML, Mee LL, Futierrez-colina AM, Eaton CK, Lee JL, Blount RL: Emotional functioning, barriers, and medication adherence in pediatric transplant recipients. *J Pediatr Psychol* 90(3):285–293, 2014.
6. Simmons RG, Klein SD, Simmons RL: *Gift of Life: The Social and Psychological Impact of Organ Transplantation*. New York, Wiley-Interscience, 1977.
7. Levinson JL, Olbrisch ME: Psychosocial screening and selections of candidates for organ transplantation. In: Trepacz P, DiMartini A (eds): *The Transplant Patient*. Cambridge, UK, Cambridge University Press, 27–28, 2000.
8. Markowitz JS, Gill HS, Hunt NM, Monroe RR Jr, DeVane CL: Lack of antidepressant-cyclosporine pharmacokinetic interactions. *J Clin Psychopharmacol* 18(1):91–93, 1998.
9. Atkinson K, Biggs J, Darveniza P, Boland J, Concannon A, Dodds A: Cyclosporine-associated central-nervous-system toxicity after allogeneic bone-marrow transplantation. *NEJM* 310(8):527, 1984.
10. Patton SB, Neutel CL: Corticosteroid-induced adverse psychiatric side effects: Incidence, diagnosis and management. *Drug Safety* 22:111–122, 2000.

CHAPTER 7.2.3 ■ PSYCHOSOCIAL ASPECTS OF HIV/AIDS

ROBERT A. MURPHY, KAREN E. O'DONNELL, AND SANDRA GOSSART-WALKER

The epidemic of infection with the human immunodeficiency virus (HIV) and acquired immunodeficiency syndrome (AIDS) continues to be a major world crisis affecting the physical and psychiatric health and well-being of tens of millions of persons. According to estimates from the Joint United Nations Programme on HIV/AIDS; by the end of 2012, approximately 35.3 million people, including children, were living with HIV infection with only 260,000 new infections compared to 600,000 reported in 2005 (1). New HIV infections fell by 33% overall and by 52% for children around the world between 2001 and 2012.

In the United States, 1996 marked a major turning point in the epidemic, when the introduction of new therapies and combination therapy slowed the progression of HIV/AIDS for children and adults and led to an increase in the number of persons living with HIV infection. With successes in the prevention of mother-to-child transmission (PMTCT) in the United States (2) as well as effective drug therapies for those who are infected, HIV/AIDS now disproportionately affects women and minorities who are adolescents and young adults. The 2010 Centers for Disease Control and Prevention report indicated a sharp increase in HIV/AIDS among youth with 26% of new infections in the 13 to 24 age group, accounting for approximately 50,000 new cases annually (3). In the United States, it is estimated that 50% of HIV-infected youth do not know they are infected.

Both HIV-infected and HIV-affected children live in a world of stigma, grief from family deaths, multiple transitions in caregivers, and many other potentially traumatic experiences (4). With the highest incidence globally, adolescents represent a fast-growing population, presenting new needs for their medical and psychological care reflecting the shift from the focus on infants and younger children earlier in the epidemic (5).

PREVENTION OF MOTHER TO CHILD TRANSMISSION

Despite recent advances in PMTCT, early diagnosis in infancy, and effective drug treatments for children and adults that reduce mortality and morbidity from HIV/AIDS, there remains a gap between high (HIC) and low- and middle-income countries (LMIC) in identification, prevention, and treatment successes. The contrast is particularly true for children who, without early identification and treatment, will often die in the first years of life (6–8). Ninety percent of youth with HIV/AIDS live in sub-Saharan Africa, where access to antiretroviral therapy has increased but by less than 20%. Only a small proportion of HIV-infected children in LMIC receive treatment (28% relative to 58% for adults) (1), in part because of persisting low rates of HIV testing and diagnosis (9,10). Between 2011 and 2012, the reach of PMTCT programs increased from 57% to 62%. Areas in which PMTCT programs are readily available and affordable have shown a dramatic decrease in the rate of perinatally infected children, achieving the global goal of 90% by 2015 (11). However, prevention programs in many LMIC countries are still challenged by program access for pregnant women, availability of drug treatments, reluctance to be identified with HIV/AIDS, and adherence to treatment (12,13).

Adolescents and Risk

Throughout the world, there is an increasing focus on children and adolescents who are the age cohort experiencing the highest rate of new infections. When effective treatments are available, children with HIV infection are living into adolescence and adulthood (14) yet, challenges related to illness, medication adherence, and mental health symptoms persist (15). Although some now refer to HIV/AIDS as a chronic illness, youth who are perinatally infected face unique challenges including the association of sexuality and danger, illness, and stigma. Surveillance data indicate that adolescents who were perinatally infected youth are more likely to be from ethnic minority backgrounds, contend with poverty, and live in disadvantaged neighborhoods and communities. They may, along with other family members, struggle with psychiatric and substance abuse problems, and tend to have significantly more school problems (14,16–19).

Newly infected adolescents face stressors that may be different from their perinatally infected peers. Some studies have shown that those infected during adolescence report more frequent and severe stressors, including family financial problems, parental substance abuse and conflict, and family loss and death (20). They are more likely to be acutely ill with a range of psychiatric problems and risk behaviors (e.g., unprotected sexual activity, substance abuse). Living away from home, they may lack the social or financial support of their earlier years (18,21). Due to stigma and secrecy, they may not confide in peers who comprise the majority of their social contacts.

Whether infected perinatally or during adolescence, youth with HIV/AIDS enter adolescence with developmental challenges that are similar to other adolescents, albeit in a context fraught with health risks. As they begin romantic and sexual relationships, their sexual behavior is complicated by their HIV status and the risk of transmitting the virus to others. As the proportion of HIV-infected and noninfected adolescents who are sexually active is similar, it may be that serostatus has little influence on sexual risk behaviors (22). Carter et al. (23) reported that most HIV-positive female adolescents expressed a desire for pregnancy indicating the importance of continued attention to vertical transmission of HIV to the newborn.

HIV-Affected Youth

The uninfected children of HIV-infected parents may have avoided infection due to the mother's antiretroviral treatment or the parent may have contracted the virus when the child was older. In either case, approximately 28% of HIV-infected adults have one or more children younger than 18 years (24). The unpredictable course of HIV/AIDS can limit parents' ability to provide consistent and stable care and perpetuates a sense of anxiety and dread among their children (25). Unlike HIV-infected children who are connected to regular, HIV-specialized care, affected children may have limited opportunities to talk about or receive support for anxieties and worries about their parents. A substantial proportion of HIV-affected children experience significant distress and psychiatric symptoms (26). Stigma due to HIV has been associated with poor psychosocial adjustment and delinquent behavior (27,28).

HIV INFECTED AND AFFECTED ORPHANS

Although new opportunities exist to decrease the number of children infected with HIV, the number of infected adults of childbearing age continues to increase in both HIC and LMIC, resulting in a still increasing number of children orphaned by the epidemic. With 16.6 million HIV orphans worldwide (90% in sub-Saharan Africa) (1), it is recognized that many who have been orphaned by HIV/AIDS do not thrive. Orphaned children in LMIC have high rates of unmet psychological needs (29) and scant access to mental health care (30). When treatment is available, rarely does it have prior evidence of effectiveness (31). Researchers advocate for translating evidence-based treatments (EBTs) from the high-income settings (HIC) in which they were developed to the geographical and cultural environments of resource-limited areas (32,33). World Health Organization guidelines (34) recommend structured interventions for bereavement and cognitive-behavioral therapy (CBT) with a trauma focus for post-traumatic stress (32). One study indicated that children ages 6 through 13 orphaned in a high HIV prevalence area exhibited a high prevalence of maladaptive grief that could be addressed through CBT (6).

Stigma and Disclosure

HIV has been affected by stigma since the early years of the epidemic when fears of contagion were pervasive. Children and youth who experience ignorance and prejudice about HIV may live in isolation, fearing rejection and judgment from others should they disclose their HIV status (35). They likely have few opportunities for the social support that may be offered by connection with similarly infected peers. They may "test" the reactions of others before disclosing by asking general questions or making comments about HIV/AIDS (36). Decisions not to disclose can lead to high-risk sexual behavior and problems with adherence to medical treatment and medication regimens. Often the fear and expectations about stigma can exceed concerns about the disease itself.

The American Academy of Pediatrics has recommended that HIV-infected children be informed of their diagnosis (37). Most protocols suggest that the disclosure should be a dynamic process, involving multiple conversations that are tied to the child's cognitive development and deepen his or her understanding of the HIV infection (38). Although disclosure of other life-threatening illnesses, such as cancer, appears to alleviate anxiety, the social stigma associated with HIV infection may cause some children to experience periods of heightened distress.

Fear, shame, and guilt interfere with disclosure of an HIV diagnosis. Parents may avoid questions about their illness or that of the child due to their own guilt and worry about harming the child emotionally. Some worry about a loss of privacy, including unauthorized disclosure of protected health information (39). They may worry about disrupting a child's sense of normalcy and being like others in this context of illness accompanied by social approbation. In an attempt, albeit an ineffective one, some parents or guardians may make partial disclosures, providing information without naming HIV. A child may be told about having a different, less stigmatizing illness.

Permanency Planning and Transition to Adult Care

As those who were perinatally infected grow into adolescence and young adulthood, the focus on permanency planning during the early years of the epidemic has shifted toward transition to and engagement with adult medical care. In the 1980s and 1990s, permanency planning for children of HIV-infected parents was of paramount concern as HIV/AIDS became the leading cause of death for adults of child bearing age (40). Plans to ensure that the physical and emotional as well as custodial needs for HIV-affected children were at the forefront of concerns to reduce distress in children and improve their coping (37). The urgency of permanency planning has since waned, and in 2012 the American Academy of Pediatrics retired their policy statement regarding planning for children whose parents were dying of HIV/AIDS (41).

Given the longstanding relationships with providers, sometimes since infancy, there can be a great deal of anxiety about transitioning to the adult care system (38). Some fear the loss of their medical home (42). Youth may be ill prepared to take on responsibility for their own medical care, perhaps having little understanding of their HIV disease (HIV literacy) and knowledge of their medical history. Some providers in the adult HIV care setting lack knowledge and experience with this developmental transition or the unique challenges of a long-term survivor. Where pediatric clinics often provide an array of services beyond physicians specializing in pediatric HIV (e.g., social workers, case managers, incentives for medication adherence), adult systems provide fewer ancillary services and provide less active assistance in managing complex medical needs.

NEUROLOGIC AND DEVELOPMENTAL EFFECTS FOR CHILDREN WITH HIV/AIDS

Neurologic, neuropsychological, and developmental manifestations of HIV disease can be the earliest and most devastating markers of infection in children. In fact, neurodevelopmental dysfunction was one symptom of HIV infection that brought children to the attention of a medical community that still saw HIV/AIDS as an adult disease in the early 1980s. Early studies indicated that between 40% and 90% of HIV-infected children had some degree of neurologic involvement (43). These studies, however, were generally conducted in cohorts of children with more advanced disease and before the widespread use of highly active antiretroviral treatment (HAART).

Although early, aggressive, and well-monitored treatment has dramatically reduced HIV/AIDS effects on the central nervous system (CNS), there remain aspects of CNS effects that warrant attention by mental health professionals monitoring and treating the child's psychological status, such as more subtle cognitive and behavioral difficulties that affect learning and social adjustment (44,45). Studies of the CNS as a possible reservoir for HIV and follow-up study of the long-term neurocognitive associations with childhood HIV/AIDS continue to explore the effects of the virus and compromised immune system on child development. Of note, HIV/AIDS in children can be associated with other adverse factors, such as poverty, family disruption, and other perinatal risk factors that also may affect child learning capacity and behavior (46).

An extensive history focusing on developmental milestones and a detailed neurologic examination are important in alerting the mental health clinician to the possibility of the neurodevelopmental and learning effects of HIV/AIDS. A neuropsychological assessment is warranted when there is any suggestion of developmental abnormalities or sign of neurologic disease, which is useful in establishing an initial baseline, monitoring subsequent alterations in cognitive processing secondary to CNS involvement, and devising appropriate developmental or educational interventions.

MEDICAL INTERVENTION FOR HIV INFECTION

The present drug treatment approach to HIV/AIDS referred to as HAART, includes starting treatment early and achieving maximal suppression of viral replication using a combination of at least three different antiretroviral medications. Fortunately, these combination drug protocols have successfully reduced viral load to undetectable levels and preserved immune functioning in as many as one-half of the children who had access to the treatment and who adhered to the protocol (5). Of course, these successes have been documented in wealthy countries in which these expensive treatments are feasible, but less so in low resource countries where HIV/AIDS in children is most prevalent.

A major challenge posed by the advances in therapy of HIV disease has been the need to ensure that patients consistently are able to take all of their medicines. Unfortunately, there is a potential for the virus to develop resistance to antiretroviral medications, particularly when treatment and medication adherence are inconsistent, thereby providing a window for resistant viral strains to replicate, dominate, and increase viral load. In this era of multiple medications for HAART from which to choose, the choices become limited once viral resistance has developed. One study reported a linear association between self-reported adherence and level of HIV viral suppression. Patients taking fewer than 80% of their prescribed doses of antiretroviral medications had a significant increase in viral load measurements compared with those who took more of their medications. Despite this serious risk, adherence is not simple or easy for children and families, and poor adherence is strongly related to mental health (47,48). Treatment regimens often call for a large number of medications, taken at regular intervals each day. Some of the medications are available only as large capsules that are difficult to swallow; others have a particularly bad taste. Important interventions for the care of children with HIV/AIDS include support and strategies for children and families in taking medications on time and more easily.

Psychiatric Effects among Children and Adolescents

Psychiatric symptoms and disorders among HIV infected, affected, and at-risk youth occur at levels above those found in the general population. These include anxiety, depression, posttraumatic stress, and behavior problems (19,49–52). Infected youth contend with chronic, often life-threating illness, complex psychiatric symptoms, and environments marked adversity (51). One study indicated that youth diagnosed with one or more psychiatric disorders were more likely to be sexually active before adulthood, inconsistent in their medication compliance, and involved in alcohol or drug abuse (OR = 2.33) (52). In a study of HIV-infected Tanzanian adolescents, each year increase in age was associated with a 12% increase in depression. The likelihood of depression increased further when youth were female (62%), not attending school (65%), or experienced stigma (9%) (15). After controlling for the severity of mothers' symptoms, results from a 3-year longitudinal study indicated higher levels of internalizing and externalizing symptoms, as well as greater impairments in children's social competence among urban-dwelling, HIV-affected, school-aged children (53). Between 52% and 74% of children who have been orphaned due to parental death from HIV/AIDS experience clinically significant internalizing and externalizing symptoms prior to and following their parent's death when compared to HIV-affected children whose parents remain living and to children of uninfected parents (54).

TRAUMATIC STRESS

Trauma and traumatic stress may serve as a risk factor for contracting HIV, for example, US studies suggest that up to 14.6% of HIV-positive adults have experienced sexual abuse, which in some instances may be the source of HIV infection (55,56). Other studies have suggested that HIV is one among many stressors, albeit a severe one, that can lead to distress and psychiatric symptoms. Stressors that might lead to similar clinical presentations may include multiple caregiver and family losses; responsibility to care for a dying parent; residential, educational, and economic instability; maltreatment; and exposure to violence. Factors that create risk for children contracting HIV (sexual risk taking and drug use in adolescence) (57,58) increase their risk for other negative outcomes. In a study of 1,258 orphaned and abandoned children in five LMICs (59), 98% had experienced at least one traumatic event in addition to the death of a parent due to HIV. Fifty-five percent experienced four or more trauma in addition to parental death. Their traumatic experiences were associated with more prevalent anxiety, conduct problems, and total symptomatology relative to children orphaned for other reasons and children who were not orphans.

Parents and Caregivers

The unpredictable course of HIV/AIDS, marked by multiple episodes of relapse and recovery and a chronic course of illness, may limit HIV-infected parents' ability to provide consistent and stable care and perpetuate a sense of anxiety among their children (51,60,61). In the instance of mother-to-child transmission, parents may contend with guilt at having transmitted the virus, distress and depression secondary to their own illness, and limitations in their capacity for consistent, responsive parenting. Caregiver illness severity, depression, and poor family cohesion, as well as changes in caregivers, have been associated with children's psychiatric status and psychosocial functioning (62,63). From 25% to 74% of adolescents residing with a parent diagnosed with HIV/AIDS consistently have reported high levels of parent–child conflict, academic failure, peer relationship problems, and delinquent behavior (64).

Resilience

Despite the ubiquity of psychiatric problems, many infected and affected youth are resilient and do not develop serious symptoms. Studies of child resilience in the face of HIV have pointed to several factors associated with resilience: positive coping, parent–child relationships, and communication; close parental monitoring; family functioning; and social and peer support (19,49). The complex interplay of resilience and psychiatric status was highlighted in a study of children following the death of an HIV-infected parent. Initially, children who had taken on a parental role during the illness had more distress, behavior problems, and substance abuse. Yet over time, they came to cope and engage social support more effectively and to abuse alcohol and tobacco less often relative to youth who had not taken on this role.

PSYCHOSOCIAL INTERVENTION FOR HIV/AIDS

As with a range of conditions, standards for prevention and psychiatric treatment for HIV infected, affected, and at-risk youth emphasize evidence-based interventions. Although specific criteria for designation as evidence based vary, an expectation of two or more randomized controlled trials (RCTs) showing clinical efficacy is widely accepted (65–68). The number of randomized trials for child and adolescent HIV interventions continues to increase although few are yet supported by a second RCT.

Prevention models typically have been based on psychoeducational and problem-solving approaches to sexual and other risk behaviors. They have demonstrated a range of positive outcomes in HICs and LMICs, including increased condom use, decreased high-risk sexual behavior, increased age at time of first intercourse, and increased discussion of sexual practices between parents and children (69). Secondary prevention and treatment studies have yielded outcomes that include changes in risk behavior, depression, behavior problems, and posttraumatic stress. The growing strength of evidence has not been accompanied by a significant increase in availability of evidence-based interventions.

PRIMARY PREVENTION

Primary (or universal) prevention programs focus on a population of youth rather than a subset selected on the basis of demographics or clinical presentation. Many interventions have demonstrated effectiveness with general populations and some in HIV-specific contexts (70,71). Programs have involved populations of students in a particular grade (i.e., 7th, 10th), including youth from racial and ethnic minorities and from countries other than the United States. Tenth graders in a large Bahamian city were randomized to a youth intervention with and without a parent supplement, as well as to an attention control and a no intervention group (72). Eighteen months later, students in all four groups had improved in HIV/AIDS knowledge, condom use skills, self-efficacy about condom use, and self-reported rates of condom use; youth receiving both youth and parent components derived greater benefit. Native American middle schoolers completing a culturally adapted HIV prevention program had significantly higher HIV-related knowledge at 3-month follow-up relative to control, although effects had dissipated by 12 months. In an RCT involving 7th grade Latino adolescents in the United States, a culturally specific HIV prevention program with and without parent components yielded improvement in family functioning, although not in sexual risk behavior (73).

Kershaw et al. conducted an RCT of the empirically supported Centering Pregnancy program that has been shown to reduce preterm birth and increase medical treatment satisfaction with prenatal care. New mothers received Centering Pregnancy with and without the addition of three sessions focused on HIV prevention education and skills training (74). At 6 and 12 months' postpartum those receiving the HIV supplement used condoms more frequently. At 12 months, frequency of unprotected intercourse was lower, and mothers had more communication with their sexual partners about safe sex practices.

SECONDARY PREVENTION AND TREATMENT

Secondary prevention and treatment select intervention recipients based on risk criteria or clinical need (75–77). An increasingly strong empirical literature supports medium-to-large effects for prevention programs and EBTs for children and adolescents (67,78–80). Some of the interventions are designed for HIV populations; others have strong empirical support but have not been tested with HIV samples.

Project Teens and Adults Learning to Communicate, a well-researched, group-based, cognitive behavioral intervention for parents with HIV and their adolescent children, has been evaluated in two RCTs (81). In the first, the 24-session program addressed cognitive and emotional coping and post-bereavement adjustment and transition. Two years following intervention the adolescents who received the intervention had less psychological distress, including depression, anxiety, and conduct problems. After 4 years, unwanted pregnancies were fewer, as were stressful family events (82). By 6 years, problem and conduct behaviors had increased in both conditions, albeit at a lesser rate in the treatment condition. Those who had received treatment were more likely to be employed or enrolled in school, have better problem-solving skills, and have positive future expectations, and were less likely to receive welfare benefits (83). Another extended follow-up revealed that grandchildren of the HIV-infected mothers had fewer internalizing and externalizing symptoms, higher scores of cognitive development, and better home environments relative to those in the control condition (84). Ten years later, a second, well-designed RCT of a 16-session version did not replicate these positive outcomes, perhaps, although arguably, affected by changes in groups who were HIV infected during the decade between studies (85).

Other studies have yielded equivocal results. A 7-year follow-up from an open trial of an intervention for HIV-infected mothers revealed that maternal functioning exerted a direct effect on child self-concept, which in turn, affected child depression (86) rather than a direct relationship of maternal functioning with child depression. An RCT designed to reduce parenting stress among HIV-infected mothers did not result in differential benefits between intervention and control groups (87).

The focus of studies has shifted to LMICs and, in the process; the feasibility of adapting interventions developed in HICs to LMICs has become evident (6,88–90). South African HIV-infected mothers and their school-aged children were randomized to a 24-session group intervention or services as usual. Although attendance was problematic (54% attended fewer than 16 of the 24 sessions), mothers receiving the intervention reported improvements in their children's externalizing symptoms, communication, daily living skills, and socialization. No intervention benefits were detected for child internalizing symptoms, depression, or adaptive behavior, or for maternal functioning.

A well-validated US intervention was adapted, with feedback from community members and stakeholders, for families with 10- to 13-year-old, HIV-infected youth living in an LMIC. In contrast to the emphasis on verbal and written communication in the US version, the LMIC adaptation used a cartoon-based storyline to facilitate difficult conversations related to HIV. With a dearth of trained mental health professionals in LMICs, trained lay counselors served as interventionists and provided the intervention skillfully. Medication adherence improved among youth, and caregivers reported better communication with their children. Differences in emotional and behavior problems did not occur.

A 12-session, group-based adaptation of Trauma Focused Cognitive-Behavioral Therapy (TF-CBT) for traumatic grief (91) was delivered by rigorously trained lay counselors to HIV/AIDS orphans, ages 7 to 14, in an open trial (6). Children were notably symptomatic at baseline assessment. Three and 12 months following treatment, children self-reported significant improvement in grief (d = 1.36) and posttraumatic stress symptoms (d = 1.87); caregivers reported less traumatic stress among the children (d = 1.15).

CONCLUSIONS

HIV/AIDS continues to be a global health crisis that disproportionately affects youth, who represent the fasting growing group becoming infected. The overall number of new HIV infections has decreased, largely due to the greater availability of highly active antiretroviral treatment, although less so in LMICs. Earlier and effective pharmacotherapies have dramatically reduced mother-to-child transmission, and contrary to expectations during the early years of HIV, youth who were infected perinatally are living into adolescence and adulthood. Treatment successes have been diminished, however, due to problems with medication adherence, resistance to antiretroviral treatment, and insufficient availability of medical care in LMICs. The number of infected adults of childbearing age continues to increase. Large numbers of children and adolescents are affected by parental illness and, in LMICs, orphaned. Youth who are infected with and affected by HIV experience significant psychiatric distress, including anxiety, depression, posttraumatic stress, and behavior problems, and engage in sexual and other behaviors that increase their risk for infection or infecting others (e.g., sex with multiple partners, inconsistent condom use, substance abuse).

Evidence-based prevention and mental health treatment have been effective in mitigating or reducing sexual risk behaviors and improving psychiatric symptoms for HIV infected and affected children and adolescents. The quality of evidence has improved with more RCTs in HICs and LMICs, although results have not been consistently positive. Interventions include those developed specifically for HIV populations and well-validated treatments that have been applied or adapted for HIV populations. Unfortunately, need for effective interventions far outstrips their availability.

Once effectiveness has been established, a next and rarely undertaken step is to study dissemination, implementation, and scale up so that best practices become readily available. Absent a systematic, comprehensive approach to training in evidence-based interventions, they are unlikely to become part of standard care (92). To change practice, researchers, trainers, and clinicians must forego traditional training methods that are ineffective (e.g., seminars) in favor of rigorous methods that assure intervention fidelity among learners, provide case-specific feedback, and offer guidance about barriers to practice change (93–95).

Although effectiveness research is a complex and sometimes daunting endeavor, limitations in emphasis and methods in the existing literature highlight critical areas for future research, including: (1) differentiating psychiatric symptoms that are specific to HIV/AIDS from those that are attributable to other risks and stressors (19,49–51,62), (2) adaptation and study of existing evidence-based interventions to HIV populations, (3) replication studies, (4) control groups consisting of active treatment comparisons, (5) well-validated assessment measures common across studies, (6) assessment of intervention fidelity, (7) duration and clinical significance of outcomes, and (8) better reported study methods and analyses (e.g., sample characteristics, statistical power).

Given the myriad psychosocial stressors encountered by HIV infected and affected children and adolescents, comprehensive and effective medical and mental health services remain crucial for management of the disease and associated psychiatric symptoms. Access to care must be extended to children, adolescents, and families who have traditionally existed at the margins of the health care delivery system. Providers should draw upon the array of evidence-based prevention and treatment models for those conditions that are prevalent among infected and affected children, including depression, posttraumatic stress, and externalizing behaviors. To be maximally effective, psychiatric treatment must address children's well-being through a comprehensive strategy that addresses the medical and mental health needs of individual children, supports family functioning, and addresses transitions from pediatric to adult care.

References

1. Joint United Nations Programme on HIV/AIDS (UNAIDS): *Global Report: UNAIDS Report on the Global AIDS Epidemic*. Geneva, Switzerland, UNAIDS, 2012.
2. Chi BH, Adler MR, Bolu O, et al.: Progress, challenges, and new opportunities for the prevention of mother-to-child transmission of HIV under the US President's emergency plan for AIDS relief. *J Acquir Immune Defic Syndr* 60:S78–S87, 2012.
3. Centers for Disease Control and Prevention, Health Resources and Services Administration, National Institutes of Health, American Academy of HIV Medicine, Association of Nurses in AIDS Care, International Association of Providers of AIDS Care, et al.: *Recommendations for HIV Prevention with Adults and Adolescents with HIV in the United States*. Atlanta, GA, Centers for Disease Control & Prevention, 2014.
4. Gray CL, Pence BW, Ostermann J, et al.: Prevalence and incidence of traumatic experiences among orphans in institutional and family-based settings in 5 low- and middle-income countries: a longitudinal study. *Glob Health Sci Pract* 3(3):395–404, 2015.
5. Brady MT: Pediatric human immunodeficiency virus-1 infection. *Adv Pediatr* 52:163–193, 2005.
6. O'Donnell K, Dorsey S, Gong W, et al.: Treating unresolved grief and posttraumatic stress symptoms in orphaned children in Tanzania: group-based trauma-focused cognitive behavioral therapy. *J Trauma Stress* 27(6):664–671, 2014.
7. Newell ML, Brahmbhatt H, Ghys PD: Child mortality and HIV infection in Africa: a review. *AIDS* 18(Suppl 2):S27–S34, 2004.
8. De Cock KM, Fowler MG, Mercier E, et al.: Prevention of mother-to-child HIV transmission in resource-poor countries: translating research into policy and practice. *JAMA* 283:1175–1182, 2000.
9. O'Donnell K, Yao J, Ostermann J, et al.: Low rates of child testing for HIV persist in high-risk area of East Africa. *AIDS Care* 26(3):326–331, 2014.
10. Kellerman SE, Drake A, Lansky A, Klevens RM: Use of and exposure to HIV prevention programs and services by persons at high risk for HIV. *AIDS Patient Care STDS* 20(6):391–398, 2006.
11. Joint United Nations Programme on HIV/AIDS (UNAIDS): *"15 by 15" A Global Target Achieved*. Geneva, Switzerland, UNAIDS, 2015.
12. Berk DR, Falkovitz-Halpern MS, Hill DW, et al.: Temporal trends in early clinical manifestations of perinatal HIV infection in a population-based cohort. *JAMA* 293(18):2221–2231, 2005.
13. Violari A, Cotton MF, Gibb DM, et al.: Early antiretroviral therapy and mortality among HIV-infected infants. *N Engl J Med* 359(21):2233–2244, 2008.
14. Hazra R, Siberry GK, Mofenson LM: Growing up with HIV: children, adolescents, and young adults with perinatally acquired HIV infection. *Annu Rev Med* 61:169–185, 2010.
15. Dow DE, Turner EL, Shayo AM, Blandina M, Cunningham CK, O'Donnell KO: Evaluating mental health difficulties and associated outcomes among HIV-positive adolescents in Tanzania. *AIDS Care* 28(7):825–833, 2016.
16. Kang E, Mellins CA, Dolezal C, Elkington KS, Abrams EJ: Disadvantage neighborhood influences on depression and anxiety in youth with perinatally acquired human immunodeficiency virus: how life stressors matter. *J Community Psychol* 39(8):956–971, 2011.
17. Koenig LJ, Neshiem S, Abramowitz S: Adolescents with perinatally acquired HIV: emerging behavioral and health needs for long-term survivors. *Curr Opin Obstet Gynecol* 23:321–327, 2011.
18. Lewis JV, Abramowitz S, Koenig LJ, Chandwani S, Orban L: Negative life events and depression in adolescents with HIV: a stress and coping analysis. *AIDS Care* 27(10):1265–1274, 2015.
19. Mellins CA, Elkington KS, Leu CS, et al.: Prevalence and change in psychiatric disorders among perinatally HIV-infected and HIV-exposed youth. *AIDS Care* 24(8):953–962, 2012.
20. Murphy DA, Moscicki AB, Vermund SH, Muenz LR: Psychological distress among HIV+ adolescents in the REACH study: effects of life stress, social support, and coping. The Adolescent Medicine HIV/AIDS Research Network. *J Adolesc Health* 27:391–398, 2000.
21. Tanney MR, Naar-King S, MacDonnel K; Adolescent Trials Network for HIV/AIDS Interventions 004 Protocol Team: Depression and stigma in high-risk youth living with HIV: a multi-site study. *J Pediatr Health Care* 26(4):300–305, 2012.
22. Tassiopoulos K, Moscicki AB, Mellins CA, et al.: Sexual risk behavior among youth with perinatal infection in the United States: predictors and implications for intervention development. *Clin Infect Dis* 56(2):283–290, 2012.
23. Carter MW, Kraft JM, Hatfield-Timajchy K, et al.: The reproductive health behaviors of HIV-infected young women in the United States: a literature review. *AIDS Patient Care STDS* 27(12):669–680, 2013.

24. Schuster MA, Kanouse DE, Morton SC, et al.: HIV-infected parents and their children in the United States. *Am J Public Health* 90(7):1074–1081, 2000.
25. Lester P, Stein JA, Brusch B, et al.: Family-based processes associated with adolescent distress, substance use and risky sexual behavior in families affected by HIV. *J Clin Child Adolesc Psychol* 390(3):328–340, 2010.
26. Murphy DA, Marelich WD, Payne DL: Children affected by maternal HIV/AIDS: feasibility and acceptability trial of the Children United with Buddies (CUB) intervention. *Clin Child Psychol Psychiatry* 20(1):117–133, 2015.
27. Murphy DA, Austin EL, Greenwell L: Correlates of HIV-related stigma among HIV-positive mothers and their uninfected adolescent children. *Women Health* 44(3):19–44, 2006.
28. Cowgill BO, Bogart LM, Corona R, Ryan G, Schuster MA: Fears about HIV transmission in families with an HIV-infected parent: a qualitative analysis. *Pediatrics* 122(5):e590–e598, 2008.
29. Kieling C, Baker-Henningham H, Belfer M, et al.: Child and adolescent mental health worldwide: evidence for action. *Lancet* 378(9801):1515–1525, 2011.
30. Saxena S, Thornicroft G, Knapp M, Whiteford H: Resources for mental health: scarcity, inequity, and inefficiency. *Lancet* 370(9590):878–889, 2007.
31. Patel V, Flisher AJ, Nikapota A, Malhotra S: Promoting child and adolescent mental health in low and middle income countries. *J Child Psychol Psychiatry* 49(3):313–334, 2008.
32. World Health Organization: *Guidelines for the Management of Conditions Specifically Related to Stress.* Geneva, Switzerland, WHO, 2013.
33. Patel V, Chowdhary N, Rahman A, Verdeli H: Improving access to psychological treatments: lessons from developing countries. *Behav Res Ther* 49(9):523–528, 2011.
34. Tol WA, Barbui C, van Ommeren M: Management of acute stress, PTSD, and bereavement: WHO recommendations. *JAMA* 310(5):477–478, 2013.
35. Fielden SJ, Chapman GE, Cadell S: Managing stigma in adolescent HIV: silence, secrets, and sanctioned spaces. *Cult Health Sex* 13(3):267–281, 2011.
36. Close KL, Rigamonti AX: *Psychosocial Aspects of HIV/AIDS: Children and Adolescents.* Houston, TX, Baylor International Pediatric AIDS Initiative, 2006.
37. Disclosure of illness status to children and adolescents with HIV infection. American Academy of Pediatrics Committee on Pediatrics AIDS. *Pediatrics* 103(1):164–166, 1999.
38. Fair CD, Sullivan K, Dizney R, Stackpole A: "It's like losing part of my family": transition expectations of adolescents living with perinatally acquired HIV and their guardians. *AIDS Patient Care STDS* 26(7):423–429, 2012.
39. Thoth CA, Tucker C, Leahy M, Stewart SM: Self-disclosure of serostatus by youth who are HIV-positive: a review. *J Behav Med* 37(2):276–288, 2014.
40. Centers for Disease Control and Prevention: HIV/AIDS surveillance report: HIV infection and AIDS in the United States. Atlanta, GA, US Department of Health and Human Services, Centers for Disease Control and Prevention, 2003.
41. American Academy of Pediatrics Committee on Pediatric AIDS. Disclosure of illness status to children and adolescents with HIV infection. *Pediatrics* 103(1):164–166, 2012.
42. Sharma N, Willen E, Garcia A, Sharma TS: Attitudes toward transitioning youth with perinatally acquired HIV and their family caregivers. *J Assoc Nurses AIDS Care* 25(2):168–175, 2014.
43. Belman AL: HIV-1 infection and AIDS. *Neurol Clin* 3209:983–1011, 2002.
44. Nichols SL, Brummel SS, Smith RA, et al.: Executive functioning in children and adolescents with perinatal HIV infection. *Pediatr Infect Dis J* 34(9):969–975, 2015.
45. Mwaba S, Ngoma MS, Kusanthan T, Menon J: The effect of HIV on developmental milestones in children. *AIDS Clin Res* 6(7):482, 2015.
46. Ad Hoc Committee on Psychology and AIDS: 2014 Annual Report for the Ad Hoc Committee on Psychology and AIDS. Washington, DC, American Psychological Association, 2014.
47. Breet E, Kagee A, Seedat S: HIV-related stigma and symptoms of post-traumatic stress disorder and depression in HIV-infected individuals: does social support play a mediating or moderating role? *AIDS Care* 26(8):947–951, 2014.
48. Lall P, Lim SH, Khairuddin N, Kamarlulzaman A: Review: an urgent need for research on factors impacting adherence to and retention in care among HIV-positive youth and adolescents from key populations. *J Int AIDS Soc* 18(2 Suppl 1):19393, 2015.
49. Betancourt TS, Meyers-Ohki SE, Charrow A, Hansen N: Annual research review: mental health and resilience in HIV/AIDS-affected children—a review of the literature and recommendations for future research. *J Child Psychol Psychiatry* 54(4):423–444, 2013.
50. Brown LK, Lescano CM, Lourie KJ: Children and adolescents with HIV infection. *Psychiatr Ann* 31(1):63–68, 2001.
51. Benton TD: Psychiatric considerations in children and adolescents with HIV/AIDS. *Child Adolesc Psychiatr Clin N Am* 19(2):387–400, 2010.
52. Mellins CA, Brackis-Cott E, Leu C-S, et al.: Rates and types of psychiatric disorders in perinatally human immunodeficiency virus-infected youth and seroreverters. *J Child Psychol Psychiatry* 50(9):1131–1138, 2009.
53. The Family Health Project: a multidisciplinary longitudinal investigation of children whose mothers are HIV infected. Family Health Project Research Group. *Clin Psychol Rev* 18:839–856, 1998.
54. Pelton J, Forehand R: Orphans of the AIDS epidemic: an examination of clinical level problems of children. *J Am Acad Child Adolesc Psychiatry* 44:585–591, 2005.
55. Gutman LT, Herman-Giddens ME, McKinney RE Jr: Pediatric acquired immunodeficiency syndrome: barriers to recognizing the role of child sexual abuse. *Am J Dis Child* 147:775–780, 1993.
56. Lindegren ML, Hanson IC, Hammett TA, Beil J, Fleming PL, Ward JW: Sexual abuse of children: intersection with the HIV epidemic. *Pediatrics* 102:E46, 1998.
57. Brown LK, Lourie KJ, Zlotnick C, Cohn J: Impact of sexual abuse on the HIV-risk-related behavior of adolescents in intensive psychiatric treatment. *Am J Psychiatry* 157(9):1413–1415, 2000.
58. Richter L, Komarek A, Desmond C, et al.: Reported physical and sexual abuse in childhood and adult HV risk behaviour in three African countries: findings from Project Accept (HPTN-043). *AIDS Behav* 18:381–389, 2014.
59. Whetten K, Ostermann J, Whetten R, O'Donnell K, Thielman N; Positive Outcomes for Orphans Research Team: More than the loss of a parent: potentially traumatic events among orphaned and abandoned children. *J Trauma Stress* 24(2):174–182, 2011.
60. Chi P, Li X: Impact of parental HIV/AIDS on children's psychological well-being: a systematic review of global literature. *AIDS Behav* 17:2554–2573, 2013.
61. Mawn BE: The changing horizons of U.S. families living with pediatric HIV. *West J Nurs Res* 34(2):213–229, 2012.
62. Mallee KM, Tassiopoulos K, Huo Y, et al.: Mental health functioning among children and adolescents with perinatal HIV infection and perinatal HIV exposure. *AIDS Care* 23(12):1533–1544, 2011.
63. Holditch-Davis H, Miles M, Burchinal M, O'Donnell K, McKinney R, Lim W: Parental caregiving and development caregiving of infants of mothers with HIV. *Nurs Res* 50:5–14, 2001.
64. Rotheram-Borus MJ, Robin L, Reid HM, Draimin BH: Parent-adolescent conflict and stress when parents are living with AIDS. *Fam Process* 37: 83–94, 1998.
65. Aarons GA, Hurlburt M, Horwitz SM: Advancing a conceptual model of evidence-based practice implementation in public service sectors. *Adm Policy Ment Health* 38:4–23, 2011.
66. Hennessy KD, Finkbiner R, Hill G: The national registry of evidence-based programs and practices: a decision-support tool to advance the use of evidence-based services. *Int J Ment Health* 35(2):21–34, 2006.
67. Kazdin AE: Evidence-based treatment research: advances, limitations, and next steps. *Am Psychol* 66:685–698, 2011.
68. Goldman Fraser J, Lloyd SW, Murphy RA, et al.: A comparative effectiveness review of parenting and trauma-focused interventions for children exposed to maltreatment. *J Dev Behav Pediatr* 34(5):353–368, 2013.
69. Protogerou C, Johnson BT: Factors underlying the success of behavioral HIV-prevention interventions for adolescents: a meta-review. *AIDS Behav* 18:1847–1863, 2014.
70. Daro DA, McCurdy KP: Interventions to prevent child maltreatment. In: Doll LS, Bonzo SE, Mercy JA, Sleet DA (eds): *Handbook of Injury and Violence Prevention.* New York, Springer, pp. 137–155, 2007.
71. Dodge KA, Murphy R, O'Donnell K, Christopoulos C, Dodge KA, Coleman DL: Community-level prevention of child maltreatment: the Durham family initiative. *Preventing Child Maltreatment: Community Approaches.* Duke series in child development and public policy. New York: Guilford Press, pp. 68–81, 2009.
72. Stanton B, Wang B, Deveaux L, et al.: Assessing the effects of a complementary parent intervention and prior exposure to a preadolescent program of HIV risk reduction for mid-adolescents. *Am J Public Health* 105(3):575–583, 2015.
73. Prado G, Pantin HM, Briones E, et al.: A randomized controlled trial of a parent-centered intervention in preventing substance use and HIV risk behaviors in Hispanic adolescents. *J Consult Clin Psychol* 75(6):914–926, 2007.
74. Kershaw TS, Magripies U, Westdahl C, Schindler Rising S, Ickovics J: Pregnancy as a window of opportunity for HIV prevention: effects of an HIV intervention delivered within prenatal care. *Am J Public Health* 99(11):2079–2086, 2009.
75. Olds DL, Holmberg JR, Donelan-McCall N, Luckey DW, Knudston MD, Robinson J: Effects of home visits by paraprofessionals and by nurses on children: follow-up of a randomized trial at ages 6 and 9 years. *JAMA Pediatr* 168(2):114–121, 2014.
76. Prinz RJ, Sanders MR, Shapiro CJ, Whitaker DJ, Lutzker JR: Population-based prevention of child maltreatment: the U.S. Triple p system population trial. *Prev Sci* 10:1–13, 2009.
77. DuMont K, Mitchell-Herzfeld S, et al.: Healthy Families New York (HFNY) randomized trial: effects on early child abuse and neglect. *Child Abuse Negl* 32:295–315, 2008.
78. Washington State Institute for Public Policy Evidence Based Practice Institute. *Updated Inventory of Evidence-Based, Research-Based, and Promising Practices for Prevention and Intervention Services for Children and Juveniles in the Child Welfare, Juvenile Justice, and Mental Health Systems.* Seattle, WA: University of Washington, 2014.
79. Hofmann S, Asnaani A, Vonk IJ, Sawyer AT, Fang A: The efficacy of cognitive behavioral therapy: a review of meta-analyses. *Cognit Ther Res* 36(5):427–440, 2012.

80. Daro D, Barringer E, English B: *Key trends in prevention: Report for the National Quality Improvement Center on Early Childhood.* Washington, DC, Center for the Study of Social Policy National Quality Improvement Center on Early Childhood, 2009.
81. Rotheram-Borus MJ, Lee MB, Gwadz M, Draimin B: An intervention for parents with AIDS and their adolescent children. *Am J Public Health* 91(8):1294–1302, 2001.
82. Rotheram-Borus MJ, Lee M, Leonard N, et al.: Four-year behavioral outcomes of an intervention for parents living with HIV and their adolescent children. *AIDS* 17:1217–1225, 2003.
83. Rotheram-Borus MJ, Lee M, Lin YY, Lester P: Six-year intervention outcomes for adolescent children of parents with the human immunodeficiency virus. *Arch Pediatr Adolesc Med* 158:742–748, 2004.
84. Rotheram-Borus MJ, Lester P, Song J, et al.: Intergenerational benefits of family-based HIV interventions. *J Consult Clin Psychol* 74(3):622–627, 2006.
85. Rotheram-Borus MJ, Rice E, Comulada WS, et al.: Intervention outcomes among HIV-affected families over 18 months. *AIDS Behav* 16:1265–1275, 2012.
86. Murphy DA, Marelich WD, Amaro H: Maternal HIV/AIDS and adolescent depression: a covariance structure analysis of the 'Parents and Children Coping Together' (PACT) model. *Vulnerable Child Youth Stud* 4(1): 67–82, 2009.
87. Johnson ER, Davies SL, Aban I, Mugavero MJ, Shrestha S, Kempf MC: Improving parental stress levels among mothers living with HIV: a randomized control group intervention study. *AIDS Patient Care and STDS* 29(4):220–228, 2015.
88. Mellins CA, Nestadt D, Bhana A, et al.: Adapting evidence-based interventions to meet the needs of adolescents growing up with HIV in South Africa: the VUKA case example. *Glob Soc Welf* 1:97–110, 2014.
89. Murray LK, Familiar I, Skavenski S, et al.: An evaluation of trauma focused cognitive behavioral therapy for children in Zambia. *Child Abuse Negl* 37(12):1175–1185, 2013.
90. O'Callaghan P, McMullen J, Shannon C, Rafferty H, Black A: A randomized controlled trial of trauma-focused cognitive behavioral therapy for sexually exploited, war-affected Congolese girls. *J Am Acad Child Adolesc Psychiatry* 52(4):359–369, 2013.
91. Cohen JA, Mannarino AP, Deblinger E: *Treating Trauma and Traumatic Grief in Children and Adolescents.* New York, Guilford, 2006.
92. Fixsen DL, Naoom SF, Blase KA, Friedman RM, Wallace F: *Implementation Research: A Synthesis of the Literature.* Tampa, FL, University of South Florida, Louis de la Parte Florida Mental Health Institute, the National Implementation Research Network, 2005.
93. Ebert L, Amaya-Jackson L, Markiewicz J, Kisiel C, Fairbank J: Use of the breakthrough series collaborative to support broad and sustained use of evidence-based trauma treatment for children in community practice settings. *Adm Policy Ment Health* 29:187–199, 2012.
94. Markiewicz J, Ebert L, Ling D, Amaya-Jackson L, Kisiel C: *Learning Collaborative Toolkit.* Los Angeles, CA, and Durham, NC, National Center for Child Traumatic Stress, 2006.
95. Herschell AD, Kolko DJ, Baumann BL, Davis AC: The role of therapist training in the implementation of psychosocial treatments: A review and critique with recommendations. *Clin Psychol Rev* 30(4):448–466, 2010.

CHAPTER 7.2.4 ■ EPILEPSY

KAIZAD MUNSHI, CATHERINE BROWNSTEIN, ALEXANDER ROTENBERG, GAUTAMI K. RAO, YANN B. PONCIN, AND JOSEPH GONZALEZ-HEYDRICH

Epilepsy, or recurrent seizures, is one of the more prevalent chronic disorders affecting children, and children and adolescents with epilepsy are at greater risk for psychiatric illness when compared to age-matched patients with other chronic illnesses. Psychiatric disorders are often undiagnosed and poorly managed in these children, despite parent perceptions that the emotional problems are among the more burdensome parts of the illness (1,2). The arrows of directionality go the other way as well: Children with ADHD and adults with major depressive disorder (MDD) are at increased risk for developing epilepsy (3,4). Increasingly, the genetic overlaps between epilepsy and major psychiatric disorders are being recognized. Many identified genetic mutations pleiotropically manifest as epilepsy, autism, psychosis (5–7), and ADHD while each of these clinical entities show great deal of genetic heterogeneity (5). Moreover, some psychiatric medications can worsen seizures, while certain anticonvulsants are useful as treatments for psychiatric disorders. Thus, the study of the pathophysiology of epilepsy may shed light on that of the psychiatric disorders with which it is associated, and vice versa. Child psychiatrists have important contributions to make to the recognition, treatment, and research into the psychiatric repercussions of epilepsy in children. This chapter will provide an overview of epilepsy, its epidemiology, management, and prognosis. Finally, it will also focus on psychiatric disorders associated with epilepsy and offer guiding principles for psychopharmacological management.

DEFINITIONS

A seizure results from a disturbance in the brain's electrical system in the form of an abnormal, hypersynchronous firing of cortical neurons. Its manifestations may be behavioral or sensory and these may be obvious or subtle. An individual seizure may have a variety of causes, such as fever in a young child, hypoxia, hypoglycemia, or infection. Epilepsy is the condition of recurrent seizures in absence of provoking stimuli, or a strong predisposition to recurrent unprovoked seizures as may happen in many genetic syndromes or other diseases of the central nervous system (CNS) (8,9). Nonepileptic seizures (NES), under which psychogenic seizures are classified, may appear similar to epileptic seizures but are not caused by hypersynchronous electrical disruptions in the brain. The time leading up to a seizure, the seizure itself, and the time immediately after a seizure are respectively referred to as the preictal, ictal, and postictal periods. The time in between seizures is called the interictal period. While seizures are the defining and most dramatic manifestation of epilepsy, they are episodic, whereas the brain dysfunction underlying them continues during the interictal periods, as can the associated psychosocial impact. Thus seizures themselves are rarely what is most impairing for children with epilepsy (Table 7.2.4.1).

EPIDEMIOLOGY

While epilepsy is the fourth most common neurologic problem overall (10), it is the most common neurologic condition in the pediatric population (11,12). Among youth in the United States in 2007, it had an estimated lifetime prevalence of 1% and the prevalence of current epilepsy (i.e., point prevalence) was 0.6%, corresponding to 450,000 cases between 0 and 17 years of age. In the United States, in any given year, 1 in 200 children under 15 will have epilepsy (13), or about 326,000

TABLE 7.2.4.1

COMMON CAUSES OF SEIZURES

High fever[a]
Systemic or CNS infection (meningitis, encephalitis, etc.)
Hyperthermia (exogenous)
Congenital disorders of brain development[a]
Perinatal hypoxic/ischemic injury[a]
Tuberous sclerosis
Phenylketonuria
Head trauma[a]
Intracranial hemorrhage
Neoplasm
Metabolic derangements (hypoglycemia, hyponatremia, etc.)
Anoxia
Cardiac disorders
Intoxication (medications, recreational drugs, environmental toxins)
Autoimmune disorders
Lupus, CNS vasculitis, etc.

[a]Most common in children.

children (10). Annually, recurrent unprovoked seizures, or epilepsy, will develop in up to 7 in 10,000 children under the age of 15 years (13), which represents the annual incidence. Across developed countries, the annual incidence is similar (14,15). In US surveys, the incidence of epilepsy is greatest among the very young and the elderly and is generally higher in males, after the age of 5 years (16). Whether the incidence of epilepsy is higher in African Americans or populations with lower socioeconomic status, as reported by some (17,18), is contradicted by others (19,20). Across age groups, in two-thirds of patients the etiology is unknown (16). Populations at special risk for epilepsy are those with a single unprovoked seizure, autism (21), intellectual disability, cerebral palsy (22), and children of parents with epilepsy (23).

PROGNOSIS

Approximately 70% of people with epilepsy will go into remission, defined as 5 or more seizure-free years, whether on or off medication (24). Prognosis will vary according to age and seizure type, with a better prognosis for childhood-onset epilepsy without neurologic or developmental disabilities. A decade's longitudinal follow-up study found that more than one-third of patients with childhood-onset epilepsy with more than 5 years of remission who then stopped their medications relapsed within the next 5 years (25). Approximately 10% of children newly diagnosed with epilepsy will go on to have intractable epilepsy (26). The course and prognosis for the most common psychiatric comorbidities of epilepsy have not been well studied. However, it is clear that for many patients these continue long after seizures have stopped.

INTERTWINING OF EPILEPSY AND PSYCHIATRY: PAST AND PRESENT

The first written records of epilepsy date back to 4000 BC (27). Hippocrates also wrote about epilepsy in 400 BC, describing it as having a natural cause, like other medical conditions, rather than being a divine curse as previously thought. He noted also the association with depression and wrote that *"melancholics ordinarily become epileptics, and epileptics, melancholics: what determines the preference is the direction the malady takes; if it bears upon the body, epilepsy, if upon the intelligence, melancholy"* (28). This coarse link between epilepsy and psychiatric disease continued into the modern era. In mid-19th century England, epilepsy was considered a form of insanity (29). In the late 19th and early 20th centuries, with the advent of neurology as a specialty and the successful use of bromide and barbiturates to suppress seizures, epilepsy became increasingly viewed as a brain disorder, and its social stigma attenuated. However, into the 21st century, large segments of the public continue to have highly negative perceptions of epilepsy (30).

Although epilepsy in modern medicine is not viewed as a simple causal explanation for severe psychiatric illness, the overlap between epilepsy and psychiatry is being increasingly recognized. Seizures can produce alterations in consciousness that can mimic psychiatric symptoms in the ictal and peri-ictal periods, particularly when seizures arise from the temporal lobes (31). There is also a high prevalence of psychiatric comorbidity in the interictal period. Clearly, the presence of epilepsy has neuropsychiatric and psychological associations, if not sequelae. These problems can be conceptualized along two domains: (1) The brain dysfunction causing seizures, the seizures themselves, and adverse effects (AEs) of antiepileptic drugs (AEDs), and their potential contribution to psychiatric pathology, through common physiologic mechanisms, and (2) the psychosocial and psychological consequences of epilepsy or its treatment, irrespective of any biologic overlap.

Regardless of etiology, the psychiatric considerations include the child's concerns about self-image and self-esteem, which can be related to the seizure disorder itself or side effects of drug treatment; intrapsychic issues related to temperament and coping skills; psychosocial issues, such as withdrawal and social isolation in contrast to affiliation; the cognitive impact of seizures or their treatment, including decrements in IQ or other neuropsychological changes; the impact of the disorder or its treatment on daily living (32); and the developmental impact of any or all of these on the individual child in maintaining his or her developmental trajectory.

Learning to live with this chronic, at times severe, disorder while remaining psychiatrically healthy can be a challenge for some children. Child psychiatrists can play an active role in recognizing and treating these psychiatric repercussions or in helping to educate others to do so. With the aim of better helping children who have epilepsy and comorbid psychiatric disorders, it is useful to have a familiarity with the fundamental diagnostic, classification, and treatment considerations in epilepsy. This is reviewed in the following sections, before turning back to psychiatric aspects in more detail.

DIAGNOSIS AND EVALUATION

Most evaluations begin, naturally, with the clinical suspicion that a child is having seizures. These can range from the dramatic, such as tonic–clonic convulsions, to the subtle, such as the brief staring spells of absence seizures. Other common presentations include paroxysmal sensations, repetitive movements, automatic behaviors, or altered consciousness. Most seizures are brief, lasting from a few seconds to several minutes. Afterward, depending on the type of seizure, a person may have a headache, confusion, fatigue, limb weakness, or feel nothing at all. Like all diagnostic evaluations, one begins with a detailed clinical history and a physical (including neurologic) examination. The clinical history is the single most important modality in making a diagnosis, as frequently, neurologic examination and diagnostic testing, including electroencephalogram (EEG)—which may not capture definitive interictal clues of vulnerability to seizure—will not yield any findings. Since the patient himself may have a poor recollection of the event, collateral information is essential. Generally, one wants to know at minimum the time and speed of onset; the presence of abnormal movements; whether bladder control was maintained; whether the patient bit his lips or tongue; how long the episode lasted; and how long it took for the patient to recover after the episode. Details about eye, face, and limb movements are very helpful in the epilepsy history as the lateralization of these can indicate the hemisphere or lobe of seizure origin. The patient can be asked directly how he or she felt after the event and whether or not he or she had any premonitions of the event; these can include aural, visual, tactile, or olfactory sensations, among others. The clinical history and examination will help determine the additional workup needed. The workup almost always includes an EEG as it is among the best predictors of seizure recurrence, unless the examination is suggestive of obvious triggering pathology, such as a high fever in an infant or a headache, vomiting, and focal neurologic findings in a teenager, which indicate the need for urgent neuroimaging and other diagnostics.

GENETICS

Our knowledge of the genetics of the epilepsies has grown exponentially over the past two decades, resulting in a shift in the patient diagnostic journey. The advent of next generation sequencing (NGS), including whole-exome and whole-genome sequencing has improved the rate of detecting etiologically important mutations. The exome is the 1% of the genome that contains the coding region. Therefore, whole-exome sequencing has become the dominant method for defining human genetic diseases as it is powerful as well as economical (33). The advent of more intuitive analysis tools is making NGS more accessible for screening and diagnosing patients. Sequencing studies have defined rare, potentially deleterious mutations within the coding regions of candidate genes for epilepsy (34). A subset can be seen in Table 7.2.4.2.

Other genetic tests that are used to diagnose epilepsy include chromosomal microarray analysis (CMAs) and targeted genetic panels. CMAs evaluate copy number variations. These are duplications or deletions of stretches of a chromosome and typically engulf many genes. CMAs are particularly fruitful when epilepsy occurs alongside developmental delay, dysmorphisms, or intellectual disability. Targeted gene panels are focused on analyzing, in greater depth, a selected set of genes or gene regions that are implicated in a disease. They typically involve NGS, which allows for massively parallel sequencing (many more samples sequenced at once), lowering cost. Another test used in certain situations is genome-wide methylation analysis, which provides a comprehensive view of methylation patterns across the genome and is useful for diagnosing disorders including Prader–Willi and Angelman. The use of more advanced testing including deep sequencing and single-cell sequencing is also being increasingly utilized.

TABLE 7.2.4.2

SELECTED GENETICALLY LINKED EPILEPSY SYNDROMES

Syndrome	Gene Defect
Doose syndrome	SLC6A1, likely others
Epileptic encephalopathies	SCN1A, DNM1, GABBR2, FASN, PCDH19, RYR3, CDKL5, likely others
Angelman syndrome	Maternal deletion or mutation of 15q11–q13 (68%) Uniparental disomy of 15q11–q13 (7%) Methylation defect of 15q11–q13 (imprinting error) (2–4%) UBE3 mutation or deletion (12%) (Inheritance pattern varies with defect)
Rett syndrome	*MECP2*

TABLE 7.2.4.3

TYPICAL FREQUENCIES AND AMPLITUDES OF EEG RHYTHMS

Rhythm	Typical Frequency (Hz)	Typical Amplitude (μV)
Alpha	8–13	20–200
Beta	13–30	5–10
Delta	1–5	20–200
Theta	4–8	10

THE ELECTROENCEPHALOGRAM: BASIC TERMINOLOGY

In the late 19th and early 20th centuries, the EEG was an experimental tool applied to the scalp of animals to examine electrical currents in the brain. In 1929, German psychiatrist Hans Berger published a report on his experiments using it to record the fluctuating electrical potentials of the human cortex (35). He identified the posterior dominant rhythm and called it alpha. Later on, rhythms in other frequency ranges were identified and called beta, gamma, delta, and theta (see Table 7.2.4.3). Soon, the EEG became the prime tool in diagnosing seizures and it remains decades later, now along with neuroimaging, a key instrument in diagnosing epilepsy.

To understand various epilepsy syndromes, one must also be familiar with the basic terminology used to describe EEG tracings. EEGs are traditionally acquired using the 10–20 international electrode placement system, in which electrodes are placed with even spacing over the scalp (36).

The EEG typically starts in wakefulness with the technician asking the patient to close his or her eyes, or in the case of children, placing a hand over the child's eyes. This is done to bring out the occipital alpha rhythm, which is the predominant rhythm of the resting cortex (as is with the occipital cortex when eyes are closed) during wakefulness. Opening the eyes will usually attenuate the alpha occipital alpha rhythm.

As the patient transitions from wakefulness to drowsiness, the background rhythms slow, with theta and delta frequencies becoming most prominent. Paroxysmal EEG activity specific for sleep, such as sleep spindles, appear in this stage and distinguish deeper sleep stages from drowsiness and early sleep.

During the acquisition of the EEG, certain maneuvers are attempted to provoke seizures, including hyperventilation and photic stimulation. The response of the brain to these maneuvers helps the observer to determine if the patient is within the normal range, or may be encephalopathic. For example, an encephalopathic child will have prolonged delta after hyperventilation, and may have a slower-than-normal background at baseline. A patient with absence epilepsy can have an otherwise normal background, but with the onset of hyperventilation, a 3-Hz spike and wave pattern appears along with behavioral arrest. The EEG is also useful because certain epilepsy syndromes have typical and at times, diagnostic EEG patterns.

Several elemental EEG waveforms are presented in Table 7.2.4.3. In most children, an alpha rhythm with an 8-Hz frequency is reached by the age of 3 years.

EPILEPSY: CLASSIFICATION

The 1989 International League Against Epilepsy (ILAE) classification scheme for epilepsy syndromes divided epilepsies into focal- or localization-related syndromes versus generalized ones, and according to etiology. However, due to recent advances in human genomic technology, neuroimaging, and molecular biology (37,38), that scheme is no longer considered adequate. According to the 2010 ILAE proposal, the etiologic terms "idiopathic," "symptomatic," "provoked," and "cryptogenic" that were previously used to describe epilepsy are to be replaced by "genetic," "structural-metabolic," and "unknown" (37,38).

A seizure's manifestations depend on where it starts and where it spreads. Broadly, mechanisms of seizure onset can be classified as generalized (with onset in both hemispheres) or focal. Recalling that the definition of epilepsy is recurrent seizures that occur spontaneously in the absence of provoking stimuli, an isolated seizure is not considered to be epilepsy. An epilepsy syndrome has distinguishing patterns of signs, symptoms, and history. These include the seizure type, whether it starts at an identifiable place or focus in the brain (these can be termed "focal," "partial," or "localization-related" seizures); or whether it has a generalized onset. Partial/focal seizures are further classified according to whether they cause alterations in consciousness (complex partial) or consciousness remains intact (simple partial seizure), and whether they progress to generalized convulsions (with secondary generalization) or not. The definition of an epilepsy syndrome also commonly includes the age of onset, family history, physical examination, EEG findings during and between seizures, etiology, imaging findings, and prognosis.

Common causes of seizures in the first year of life are perinatal complications such as stroke and diffuse hypoxic/ischemic injury, febrile seizures, infections, and metabolic disorders. In adolescents and young adults, common causes are trauma, congenital abnormalities, tumors, and CNS infections. A concern germane to psychiatrists is differentiating paroxysmal nonepileptic events and NES from true epilepsy. Further complicating matters, patients with NES may also have concomitant epileptic seizures. Video EEG monitoring is the ideal modality to differentiate these events.

In the first year of life, generalized seizures are the most common type. The incidence then declines and remains constant throughout childhood and adulthood. Thereafter, partial seizures are the most common type in childhood (39), and the incidence is constant until after age 65, when a precipitous increase occurs attributable to cerebrovascular disease. Absence (what was previously referred to as *petit mal*) seizures, considered in the differential diagnosis of ADHD, rarely occur in the first year, peak from the ages of 5 to 10, and then decline, being quite rare by the age of 30. The incidence of various epilepsy syndromes in newly diagnosed children is described in Table 7.2.4.4, while clinical features and treatment of the various epilepsy syndromes commonly found in children is described in Table 7.2.4.5.

TABLE 7.2.4.4

RELATIVE FREQUENCY OF EPILEPSY SYNDROMES IN A COMMUNITY SAMPLE OF CHILDREN AGED 0 TO 15 YEARS ($N = 613$)

Epilepsy Syndrome	Relative Frequency (%)
Localization-related	58.6
Symptomatic	31.8
Cryptogenic	16.8
Idiopathic	10
Generalized	29
Primary generalized	20.6
Cryptogenic/symptomatic	7
Other syndromes	12.4

Adapted from Berg AT, Shinnar S, Levy SR, Testa FM: Newly diagnosed epilepsy in children: presentation at diagnosis. *Epilepsia* 40(4):445–452, 1999.

BEHAVIORS THAT MIMIC EPILEPSY

Children often have behaviors that are paroxysmal and may be mistaken for seizures. In most cases, these events are easily defined and there is no treatment needed. There are some instances, however, when the only way to differentiate these events from true seizures is to use video EEG to confirm an EEG correlate. To ascertain a true seizure, determining the duration of the event, observing the presence of a postictal

TABLE 7.2.4.5

SELECTED CHILDHOOD EPILEPSY SYNDROMES AND TREATMENTS

Epilepsy Syndromes	Common Clinical Features	Common Treatments
Benign rolandic epilepsy with centrotemporal spikes (BRECTS)	Mouth twitching, drooling, variably GTC; nocturnal predisposition	If indicated (often untreated given favorable prognosis), levetiracetam, oxcarbazepine
Temporal lobe epilepsy	Gastric or olfactory aura, confusion, automatisms, often followed by GTC	Levetiracetam, oxcarbazepine, lamotrigine; zonisamide also helpful
Frontal lobe epilepsy	Hypermotor activity (bicycling, etc.) with change in behavior; often at night; variably with evolution to GTC	Levetiracetam, oxcarbazepine, lamotrigine; zonisamide also helpful
Juvenile myoclonic epilepsy (JME)	Brief myoclonic jerks, GTC	Valproate, lamotrigine, levetiracetam
Childhood absence epilepsy	Staring and brief multiple episodes of behavioral arrest	Ethosuximide (drug of choice), valproate, lamotrigine
Juvenile absence epilepsy	Myoclonic jerks and staring spells with older age of onset	Valproate, ethosuximide, lamotrigine, levetiracetam, topiramate
Epilepsy with GTC	GTC that can occur upon awakening or at any time of day with no partial onset	Levetiracetam, valproate, lacosamide, perampanel

GTC, generalized tonic–clonic seizures.

TABLE 7.2.4.6

BEHAVIORS THAT CAN BE MISTAKEN FOR SEIZURE ACTIVITY

Behavior of Psychiatric or Undefined Origin	Clinical Manifestations
Nonepileptic seizure	May appear very much like a true seizure, but there is no epileptiform activity on EEG. Duration greater than 10 min, the lack of a postictal state, and motor movements incongruent with seizure activity are clues.
Breath-holding	Crying followed by cessation of breathing. Within seconds, cyanosis occurs, followed by loss of consciousness and falling. Quick return to consciousness. No neurologic damage. Triggered by fear, frustration, or minor injury.
Staring	May need to rule out epilepsy, depending on clinical presentation.
Cyclic vomiting	Repeated, spontaneous vomiting lasting days, followed by asymptomatic periods. May have an EEG correlate.
Stereotyped movements	Tics or other stereotypes
Violent attacks	Violence associated with epilepsy is nondirected thrashing. If violence is organized this does not suggest epilepsy.
Shuddering	Shakes and shudders. No loss of consciousness. Lasts seconds.
Jitteriness	Jittering movements in infants. Stopped by holding down the arms.
Head drops	Can be mistaken for infantile spasms, but no EEG correlate.
Behavior Associated with Defined Syndromes	
Syncope	Variably followed by seizure (i.e., convulsive syncope)
Sandifer spasms in children with gastroesophageal reflux	Intermittent contractions of the neck with flexion and syncope.
Chiari malformations	Syncope from increased intracranial pressure. Torticollis, ataxia, opisthotonus, nystagmus.
Cardiac conditions	Lightheadedness, palpitations, pallor. May need EEG with EKG strip running to clarify etiology.
Cataplexy (e.g., of narcolepsy)	Atonia; partial or full loss of tone
Paroxysmal movement disorders resultant from channelopathies	Hard to differentiate at times, but no loss of consciousness.
Episodic ataxia types I and II	Brief attacks of cerebellar ataxia. Type 2 also involves eye movement difficulties.
Paroxysmal kinesigenic dyskinesia	Choreoathetosis or dystonia lasting seconds to minutes triggered by volitional movements such as getting up from chair or out of car.
Paroxysmal exercise-induced dyskinesia	Dystonia occurs 10–15 min after starting exercise.
Benign paroxysmal upgaze of childhood	Spells, lasting hours or days, of intermittent upgaze deviation associated with ataxia; language delay is often present.
Benign paroxysmal torticollis	Starts in infancy with attacks of torticollis lasting minutes or hours.

state, and obtaining a history to uncover any provocative stressors are all useful.

Behavioral events that may appear epileptiform were examined by Kotagal et al. in a retrospective study looking at 134 children and adolescents admitted to their pediatric epilepsy unit. They found that in children less than 5 years, the common diagnoses were parasomnias and sleep jerks. In the older age group, NES were common (40).

Behaviors that can raise the concern for epilepsy but are not epileptiform in etiology are outlined in Table 7.2.4.6.

NONEPILEPTIC SEIZURES IN CHILDREN

NES can be classified as physiologic or psychogenic. Physiologic NES are events that resemble seizures but are not caused by epileptiform discharges; these include, for example, syncopal episodes or hypoglycemia. Psychogenic NES (PNES) refer to behaviors that may resemble seizure activity, but which also are not epileptiform, and are rooted in a psychological etiology. In DSM-5, if they are volitional, NES might be classified as factitious disorder with predominantly psychological signs and symptoms or as malingering if secondary gain is a motive. If the NES are not volitional, conversion disorder with seizures or convulsions is the appropriate diagnosis. PNES are well documented in adult populations, with a prevalence of 2 to 33 per 100,000 (41). In children, NES can be more difficult to delineate from epilepsy as they are not as common. Moreover, children diagnosed with PNES also often carry a diagnosis of EEG-confirmed epilepsy. For example, one study of children with intractable seizures found that one-fifth had NES, and three-quarters of these children also had documented epileptic seizures (42). Kotagal et al. found that 15% of all patients monitored on their pediatric epilepsy unit had PNES; of these, close to half also had epilepsy (40).

The presence of NES in children is attributable to a variety of precipitants, most of which have some identifiable psychological or psychosocial component. In adults, they are frequently attributed to dissociative phenomena (43), posttraumatic stress disorder (44), and mood disorders. In one study designed to study the psychiatric features of children with NES, severe environmental stress and major mood disorders were the most common findings (45). The most common environmental stressor involved the family, including parental divorce, parental discord, or the death of a close family member. Sexual abuse was the second most common environmental stressor, occurring in 32% of children. Separation anxiety with school refusal was found in 24% of the children. Bhatia and Sapra found that school phobias and fear of examinations were the most common precipitating factors (46). Some investigators have found that a family history of epilepsy is commonly found in children with NES (47).

What does PNES look like? Many patients mimic their own seizures (48). Lancman et al. found unresponsiveness with generalized violent and uncoordinated movements or generalized trembling to be the most common manifestations (47). Others have found that tremors, intermittent stiffening, out-of-phase hand movements, and kicking and thrashing of the legs are most common, especially among adolescents; younger children often present less dramatically with staring or closing of the eyes and no responsiveness (49).

Diagnosing NES can be difficult. If a typical nonepileptic event is captured on video without an EEG correlate, there is a greater likelihood that the event is nonepileptic. However, frontal lobe seizures occasionally present without an EEG correlate. Hence, clinical observation is crucial. Generally, an event that has a duration of more than 10 minutes, that does not have a postictal state, and in which the movements are neuroanatomically incongruent with a seizure, is unlikely to be epileptic. Early psychiatric intervention is warranted to address these behaviors and prevent them from becoming more entrenched (50).

INTELLECTUAL DISABILITY AND EPILEPSY

Epilepsy is a common comorbidity in children with intellectual disability, with a direct correlation between the severity of intellectual compromise and the severity of chronic epilepsy. The prevalence of intellectual disability is about 1% of the general population (51), but epilepsy is found in approximately 20% to 40% of children with intellectual disability (52). In addition, about 40% of children with epilepsy have intellectual disability. The age at which epilepsy presents is related to the etiology of the intellectual disability.

Differentiating seizures from paroxysmal behaviors is at times difficult in children with intellectual disability as this population has more frequent repetitive and stereotyped movements and behaviors than the general population. Several such nonepileptic entities include self-stimulation, hyperventilation, Sandifer syndrome, spasticity, clonus, dystonic posturing, and choreoathetosis (53). A study by Donat and Wright examined the most common types of behavior in a sample of 31 girls with intellectual disability. They found 23% had behavioral staring, 40% had abnormal eye movements, and 42% had tonic posturing (54).

Several studies have investigated the age at which seizures present in intellectual disability. One study of 98 children found that the average age of the first seizure was 1.3 years, with an earlier onset in children with severe intellectual disability and a later onset for patients with mild intellectual disability (2). Another study of 151 children with intellectual disability found that 69% had epilepsy by the age of 3 years, without difference between severe and mild intellectual disabilities for onset before or after the age of 3 years. Focal seizures predominated, with 72% of the children having these and 28% having generalized seizures. In this population, as in most studies, a prenatal cause for epilepsy was found in more than 40% of the intellectually disabled children (55). When severe epilepsies occur in infancy, they profoundly impact neuropsychological development (56). They are also usually quite difficult to control with AEDs, with many patients undergoing multiple AED trials before seizure control is improved.

Several epilepsy syndromes can result in significant intellectual disability, including infantile spasms, Lennox–Gastaut syndrome (LGS), and the epileptic encephalopathies. Many genes, including DNM1, GABBR2, FASN, and RYR3 are thought to be involved in these syndromes (57). Infantile spasms, or West syndrome, can be catastrophic. Some patients with infantile spasms will have an MRI lesion, such as cortical dysplasia, hemimegalencephaly, arteriovenous malformation (AVM), stroke, or other lesions. Patients present as neonates with extensor or flexor spasms, or a combination of both. They typically have multiple seizures daily, at times causing profound lethargy. Early diagnosis and treatment are crucial, and carry a more favorable long-term prognosis.

LGS is commonly known as a mixture of seizure types, including tonic, atonic, myoclonic, atypical absence, and generalized tonic–clonic seizures. Patients with LGS are universally intellectually compromised. The majority of children have onset between 3 and 5 years. Most cases have an underlying brain abnormality and are therefore classified as symptomatic. The intracranial pathologies associated with LGS include (but are not limited to) focal cortical dysplasias, diffuse subcortical heterotopias, and the cerebrovascular malformations of Sturge–Weber syndrome. Seizures in LGS occur multiple times daily, especially during sleep. At times, one seizure type predominates over others. In general, tonic seizures are the most common, and can be brief and safe. They may, however, lead to falls and a requirement for patients is to wear a protective helmet. Atypical absence seizures are the second most common type of spell in Lennox–Gastaut, and are associated with some loss of muscle tone, or jerks. Myoclonic jerks are less common. Approximately 50% to 75% of LGS patients will experience nonconvulsive status epilepticus. The intellectual disability in Lennox–Gastaut is severe in most cases, but on occasion, further decline may be halted by controlling the seizures, since the seizures themselves seem to play a role in the cognitive deterioration. Successful treatment with complete seizure control is rare.

Epileptic encephalopathies are conditions in which the epileptiform abnormalities are thought to contribute to progressive cerebral deterioration, which impacts cognition and functioning. These are often associated with nearly continuous spike and wave discharges on EEG, leading to an alteration in consciousness.

Landau–Kleffner syndrome (LKS), also called acquired epileptiform aphasia, involves progressive neuropsychological impairment linked to the appearance of rhythmic EEG activity. Landau and Kleffner first described the correlation between language loss, in previously normally developing children, and paroxysmal EEG discharges in the speech centers (58). Mutations and disruptions (such as translocations) in the GRIN2A gene result in LKS (59,60). LKS is characterized by acquired aphasia and EEG findings that show bilateral, independent temporal spikes that are activated by early sleep. Secondary symptoms include behavioral and psychomotor disturbances. Boys are more affected than girls, with a 2:1 ratio. Children usually present between 3 and 9 years of age. Word deafness is a first sign; the child does not respond to commands from parents. Children with LKS are often referred for audiograms, which are normal. This initial symptom can develop into complete unresponsiveness and impaired communication. The child speaks in a brief, telegraphic manner, and communication may be limited to gestures. In an older child, reading and writing skills can be lost. LKS can also be mistaken for autism. Several important differences are present. Children with autism have language regression before the age of 3, whereas most children in LKS have regression between the ages of 5 and 7 (61). Children with LKS also retain their social skills and do not generally have stereotyped behaviors.

ANTIEPILEPTIC DRUGS: GENERAL CONSIDERATIONS

Patients are rarely started on an AED after a single seizure. Rather, AEDs are started if the seizure recurs or if there are compelling risk factors for recurrence. AED choice depends on evidence of efficacy for that seizure type, AE profile, interactions with other medications, and cost. Treatment is started with a single AED. If that AED is not effective, a second AED is chosen. A drug with a different mechanism of action and lack of drug–drug interaction with the first AED is preferred. The first AED is maintained until the second AED is at a therapeutic dose. Then if seizures are controlled, an attempt to taper off the first one is made. Monotherapy is preferred but some patients will require more than one AED to control their seizures. Use of multiple AEDs simultaneously is associated with a greater likelihood of drug side effects.

The use of animal models and patient-derived induced pluripotent stem cells for functional analysis of genetic mutations has been key in understanding the pathophysiology and mechanisms of many of the epilepsies. However, the pharmacogenomics of antiepileptics is still underdeveloped—screening medications using the patient's own stem cells may, until recently, have sounded unconceivable, but may soon be possible.

Neuropsychiatric Effects of Antiepileptic Drugs

AEDs are of particular interest to psychiatry for three reasons: (1) many have cognitive and behavioral AEs; (2) many have desirable psychotropic effects such as mood stabilization and anxiolysis; and (3) both these sets of effects could provide clues into the pathophysiology of psychiatric disorders.

A number of studies have investigated the cognitive and behavioral side effects of AEDs over the last 40 years. However, there are fewer studies examining the specific side effects of AEDs in children. As a group, AEDs are thought to affect attention, vigilance, and psychomotor speed (62). Attempts to study these effects have been hampered by the difficulties of designing studies in a population with neurologic and developmental heterogeneity. Lack of consensus on how to test for AED effects also limits the power to detect effects, and to generalize from findings, and to compare across studies. The field continues to struggle to develop consistent study designs, testing paradigms, and ways of controlling for confounding variables (63,64). The effect of AEDs on cognition is difficult to disentangle from the effects of seizures and changes in seizure frequency and severity. Importantly, many of the studies on new AEDs are funded by their manufacturers to satisfy FDA requirements for approval. In these studies, efficacy in attenuating seizures is the primary outcome. Measurement of effects on cognition or behavior has received much less scientific attention in these trials. Adequate studies are also lacking that relate potential cognitive and behavioral side effects of AEDs to schooling and social adjustment (65). The impact of AEDs on the developing brain is unclear. While decreasing seizures is expected to have a beneficial effect, some studies have raised concerns. For example, in one study of the developing rat brain, some AEDs have been found to trigger neuronal apoptosis (66).

Several representative studies examine the effects of AEDs as a group on cognition. Williams et al. (67) administered neuropsychological testing to 32 children with newly diagnosed epilepsy, prior to and after initiation of medication monotherapy. They compared this group to a chronic condition comparator group of diabetic children. They found no significant difference between groups on measures of attention, immediate memory, delayed memory, complex motor speed, or behavior problems. Likewise, Mandelbaum and Burack (68) also followed children prospectively and found no cognitive declines directly attributable to AED treatment. The relatively small sample size in both of these studies, however, limits their power to detect anything but large effects. In another study looking at subjective impressions, children and parents differed in their reports of cognitive side effects. Children reported no change in symptoms before and after AED discontinuation, whereas parents found their children to be more alert and active off the AEDs (69).

Despite the lack of conclusive data, it is helpful to examine what is known about the cognitive and behavioral effects of AEDs as a group, and of some individual AEDs that are commonly used in pediatric neurology. A more complete listing of AEDs can be found in Table 7.2.4.7.

With a few notable exceptions such as lamotrigine and felbamate, many AEDs are sedating and their adverse behavioral profile relates to their capacity to induce somnolence and to slow mentation. However, these are not universal and are often dose related. Mitigation and relief of such symptoms can be accomplished by slow titration and use of minimally effective dose. Another common trend is for newer AEDs to produce fewer AEs than the older ones but this is not consistent across all types of AEs. Finally, several concerning reports indicating increased risk of suicidal ideation and suicidal attempts in patients taking AEDs have led the FDA to consider boxed warnings about increased risk of suicidality for essentially all approved AEDs (70). This however, remains controversial, and a recent study found that the association between suicide and epilepsy that exists even before epilepsy manifests, suggesting a common underlying etiology rather than the effects of AEDs (71).

Phenobarbital is among the oldest anticonvulsants and used to treat largely neonatal seizures. In older patients, it is still at times used to manage focal seizures and generalized seizures, except absence seizures, but rarely as a first choice AED. Phenobarbital can have significant AEs on cognition, mood, and behavior. It can also cause hyperactivity, irritability, and depression. Studies have raised the concern that phenobarbital is associated with decreases in IQ, whereas others have not supported this finding (72,73). Cognitive deficits may be reversible with treatment discontinuation, but some published reports indicate that deficits may persist over several years (74). This raises the concern that there exist cumulative impairments that are not completely reversible with extended periods of treatment with some AEDs. Notably, barbiturates (including phenobarbital) are most likely to cause depression and suicidal ideation in patients with a family or personal history of affective disorder (75). Gradual conversion to a nonbarbiturate antiepileptic medication is thus advised for depressed, irritable, or aggressive patients with epilepsy who are on long-term barbiturate therapy.

Phenytoin is effective in treatment of focal and generalized tonic–clonic seizures. It is known to cause a decrease in mental speed and concentration, even at therapeutic ranges in adults (76). In children, there is less literature, but a dose-related slowing in mentation has been observed. It can also cause gingival hyperplasia, hirsutism, and coarsening of facial features. Phenytoin's efficacy varies by patient, partly due to genetic variations in the gene-encoding cytochrome P450 (CYP)2C9 (CYP2C9), which metabolizes the drug (77). Furthermore, the variant allele HLA-B*15:02, encoding human leukocyte antigen, is associated with an increased risk of Stevens–Johnson syndrome and toxic epidermal necrolysis in response to phenytoin treatment (78). Certain ethnicities are more prone to Stevens–Johnson syndrome (78). The Clinical Pharmacogenetics Implementation Consortium (CPIC) guidelines provide information for the interpretation of HLA-B and/or CYP2C9 genotype tests so that the results can guide dosing and/or use of phenytoin.

Carbamazepine had been one of the more commonly used medications in pediatric epilepsy, though in practice it is often replaced by oxcarbazepine. Although carbamazepine is structurally similar to the tricyclic antidepressant imipramine, it does not have antidepressant effects. It is used to treat focal and generalized tonic–clonic seizures, and in psychiatry, to treat mania (79). In recent years, it has been replaced by oxcarbazepine as a first choice for the treatment of focal seizures. Carbamazepine

TABLE 7.2.4.7

COMMON ANTIEPILEPTIC DRUGS (AEDS) AND THEIR MECHANISMS OF ACTION

Drug	Major Mechanism of Action	Clearance	Indications
Carbamazepine	Blocks voltage-gated sodium channels	>95% hepatic	Partial seizures and GTC seizures
Clobazam	1,5 benzodiazepine; facilitates GABA-mediated inhibition	Extensively hepatic	Adjunctive for seizures associated with Lennox–Gastaut syndrome
Ethosuximide	Blocks Ca^{2+} channels	80% hepatic 20% renal	Childhood absence seizures
Ezogabine	Enhances transmembrane potassium current	Mostly hepatic 36% renal	Adjunctive, partial seizures
Felbamate	Unknown; blocks NMDA receptor	50% hepatic 50% renal	Adjunctive for seizures associated with Lennox–Gastaut syndrome
Gabapentin	Unknown; modulates Ca^{2+} channels	100% renal	Adjunctive for partial seizures
Lacosamide	Enhances slow inactivation of voltage-gated sodium channels	95% renal minimally hepatic	Adjunctive for partial seizures
Lamotrigine	Unknown; blocks voltage-gated sodium channels	85% hepatic	Partial seizures, GTC seizures, and seizures associated with Lennox–Gastaut syndrome
Levetiracetam	Unknown; modulates neurotransmitter release	Extensively renal	Adjunctive for partial seizures, GTC, myoclonic seizures (though often used as monotherapy)
Oxcarbazepine	Blocks voltage-gated sodium channels	45% renal 45% hepatic	Partial seizures
Perampanel	Blocks AMPA glutamate receptors	Extensively hepatic	Partial seizures and GTC seizures
Phenobarbital	Barbiturate; facilitates GABA-mediated inhibition	75% hepatic 25% renal	Partial seizures and generalized seizures
Phenytoin	Blocks voltage-gated sodium channels	>90% hepatic	Partial seizures and GTC seizures
Pregabalin	Unknown; modulates Ca^{2+} channel	Extensively renal	Adjunctive for partial seizures
Rufinamide	Unknown; promotes inactivated state of voltage-gated sodium channels	Extensively hepatic	Adjunctive for seizures associated with Lennox–Gastaut syndrome
Topiramate	Unknown; blocks voltage-gated sodium channels, modulates $GABA_A$, NMDA, and AMPA receptors; inhibits carbonic anhydrase	30–50% hepatic 50–70% renal	Partial-onset seizures and GTC seizures
Valproate	Unknown; may increase GABA concentrations; may block voltage-gated sodium channels	>95% hepatic	Partial seizures, GTC seizures, absence seizures, myoclonic seizures
Zonisamide	Unknown; blocks voltage-gated sodium channels	>90% hepatic	Adjunctive, partial seizures

is converted to an active metabolite, carbamazepine epoxide, which also has some associated toxicity. Carbamazepine induces its own metabolism as well as that of several psychotropic agents. It can cause sedation, mild psychomotor slowing, and decreased attention and memory, even within the therapeutic range (80). Studies have demonstrated decreased performances on the continuous performance test (CPT) with carbamazepine exposure (61). However, other studies have found that this initial slowing improves after 1 month of treatment (81).

Oxcarbazepine is structurally similar to carbamazepine and is used for many of the same seizure types. It is not, however, converted to the toxic, epoxide metabolite of carbamazepine and causes less induction of enzymes that metabolize other medications. There has been interest in its use for bipolar disorder but its efficacy, especially in pediatric bipolar disorder, has not been proven in clinical trials (82–85). It has been associated with only mild cognitive impairment.

Valproic acid (commonly administered as divalproex) is a potent broad-spectrum anticonvulsant effective in treatment of absence, generalized tonic–clonic, focal, and myoclonic seizures. Outside of the epilepsy field, it is also used in migraine prophylaxis, and for mood stabilization. It is highly protein bound and can displace other drugs that are protein bound, like phenytoin. It can inhibit the metabolism of phenobarbital. These effects can lead to toxicity. It has a range of potential somatic AEs. Additionally, in therapeutic ranges it has been shown to cause impaired decision making and attention. In children, these effects can be more pronounced. Despite its efficacy in treatment of mania (86), it has also been known to cause aggression, irritability, and hyperactivity in some children in a dose-dependent fashion. In other children, however, it is quite effective in many epilepsy syndromes, and by monitoring AED levels, its side effects can be minimized.

Benzodiazepines, such as lorazepam, diazepam, clonazepam, and clobazam, are used to treat a range of seizures, and are administered as abortive agents to either abort prolonged seizures or to terminate seizure clusters. They can cause profound sedation and impairment. For example, clonazepam has been shown to cause decreased attention, irritability, hyperactivity, and disinhibition (87). Tolerance can develop after 1 to 6 months. These AEs are offset by the excellent efficacy of benzodiazepines in pediatric epilepsy syndromes.

Gabapentin is used for focal seizures, and has some efficacy against anxiety and chronic pain. It has essentially no drug–drug interactions (88). It is not useful for the treatment of mania. It can cause behavioral disinhibition, especially in children with pre-existing behavioral problems or intellectual disability.

Lamotrigine is a broad-spectrum anticonvulsant prescribed for the treatment of both focal and generalized seizures, and is used in bipolar disorder. Its clearance is inhibited by valproic acid and augmented by enzyme-inducing AEDs such as carbamazepine. Lamotrigine has been associated with a high risk of Stevens–Johnson syndrome, but the risk of this serious complication is decreased if lamotrigine is titrated upward slowly. If a rash occurs, the patient should be evaluated right away and serious consideration given to discontinuing the lamotrigine. Lamotrigine has some conflicting evidence linking Stevens–Johnson syndrome and toxic epidermal necrolysis to the HLA-B*15:02 allele (89–92), as do some other AEDs including oxcarbazepine (93). Sedation is not usually a problem with lamotrigine, even on initial titration. Lamotrigine causes little or no cognitive impairment, and as yet has no detectable effect on attention, psychomotor speed, or memory (80). In addition, some authors suggest it may even improve alertness (94). Lamotrigine has stimulant properties, and in a minority of patients, may cause tremulousness, irritability, aggressive behavior, and insomnia (78).

Levetiracetam is also a broad-spectrum anticonvulsant, and in many instances is the first-line treatment for new-onset epilepsy. Approximately 20% of children with epilepsy taking levetiracetam may have behavioral side effects such as irritability, anxiety, or depression. These symptoms are more likely in patients with developmental delay (95). On the other hand, in an open-label study in patients with autism, levetiracetam was found to have a favorable effect on attention, hyperactivity, and mood instability (65).

Topiramate is useful in the treatment of partial and generalized seizures. It is the one newer AED for which there are significant concerns that it adversely affects cognition (96). Specifically, it has been found that it causes declines in word fluency and attention, and poorer attention after 1 month's treatment in young adults (97). Compared to pediatric clinical practice, higher doses and faster titration schedules are used in adult studies. Some suggest that the titration schedule may influence the degree of cognitive AEs. For example, in one such study patients were randomized to the addition of topiramate or valproic acid to already existing carbamazepine monotherapy (98). A slow titration schedule was used. Psychometric testing was done after 8 weeks. There was little difference in cognitive effects between the two drugs. Still, it is advisable to monitor an individual patient's response to topiramate and to monitor school performance. Psychiatric side effects such as depression, paranoia, and acute confusional psychosis have also been reported with topiramate. It can be associated with weight loss. An initial interest in the use of topiramate for bipolar disorder has not been substantiated in controlled trials.

Zonisamide is used to treat focal seizures. There is little sedation associated with this drug. Some patients lose weight because of decreased appetite. A study examining cognition in patients with refractory partial epilepsy before and during zonisamide treatment showed that high zonisamide plasma concentrations were linearly associated with deficits in verbal acquisition, but did not affect psychomotor abilities (99). Another study looked at patients on zonisamide or carbamazepine with phenytoin. There were lower verbal IQ and performance IQ scores in patients on zonisamide compared to carbamazepine (100). Here also, effect increased with dose.

PSYCHIATRIC DISORDERS IN CHILDREN WITH EPILEPSY

General Considerations

Children with epilepsy have high levels of psychiatric comorbidity. In a UK population-based study (101), 80% of children aged 5 to 15 years with active epilepsy were found to meet criteria for either cognitive impairment (IQ less than 85), or a DSM-IV-TR behavioral disorder, or both. In this study, the most prevalent neurobehavioral diagnoses were intellectual disability (40%), ADHD (33%), and autism spectrum disorder (21%).

The Isle of Wight study by Rutter et al. (102) found that children with idiopathic seizures showed a 29% rate of psychiatric disorders. In contrast, the rate for psychiatric disorders was 7% for children in the general population and 12% for those with other physical problems outside the CNS. In a population survey of more than 10,000 children aged 5 to 15 years in the United Kingdom, Davies et al. (103) found similar rates adjusting symptoms to DSM-IV. Psychiatric disorders were 37% in children with epilepsy, 9% in controls, and 11% in the chronic condition comparator, diabetes. More recently, Russ et al. (11) reported that children with current epilepsy had statistically significantly higher incidence of depression (8% vs. 2% in children never diagnosed with epilepsy), anxiety (17% vs. 3%), ADHD (23% vs. 6%), conduct problems (16% vs. 3%), developmental delays (51% vs. 3%), autism spectrum disorder (16% vs. 1%), and headaches (14% vs. 5%). Children with epilepsy also had a higher risk of functional impairment, repeating a school grade, poorer social skills, higher parental aggravation, and frequently did not receive appropriate mental health treatment. Children with prior but not current seizures fared better, with intermediate risk.

Rodenburg et al. (104) conducted a series of meta-analyses, involving 46 studies and 2,434 subjects to examine the types and severity of psychopathology in children with epilepsy. They found a medium to large effect size of psychopathology for children with epilepsy compared to healthy controls. The researchers noted a smaller effect size for psychopathology when comparing children with epilepsy to those with chronic illnesses, leading them to conclude that some, but not all, of the psychopathology in epilepsy is attributable to a "generic feature" of chronic illness. Considering gender, some have found that chronically ill females tend to fare less well emotionally than chronically ill males, and have more suicidal thinking (105). As for treatment, it seems to be underutilized in this population (106). In order to improve recognition and treatment of psychiatric dysfunction in children with epilepsy, it is useful to consider the specific psychiatric disorders associated with epilepsy.

Autism and Epilepsy

The link between autism and epilepsy was first noted by Leo Kanner. The relationship between autism and epilepsy has been controversial. However, it is widely accepted now that there exist underlying brain conditions that predispose an individual to both conditions and frequent seizures can disrupt brain functioning and create autistic symptomatology (107). The incidence of epilepsy in autism has been estimated to range from 5% to over 30%, with a bimodal distribution in the age of onset. The first peak is before 5 years and the other after 10 years. There does not appear to be a gender difference (108). Any seizure type can be associated with autism.

The different subtypes of autism spectrum disorders have different rates of epilepsy. In classic autism, epilepsy has been found to develop in a third of children, with risk linked to intracranial pathology (108). The erstwhile diagnosis of childhood disintegrative disorder carried a risk of 70% for the development of epilepsy. In Rett syndrome, over 90% of patients have epilepsy (109).

A specific EEG pattern that correlates with autism has not been found. About 10% of children with autism have a paroxysmal EEG pattern, such as that found in LKS or with electrical status epilepticus in sleep. EEGs are not routinely requested for patients with autism. A retrospective study by Gabis et al. (110) examined the EEG findings in 56 children with pervasive developmental disorders to examine the value of obtaining an EEG in this patient population. They found that only two children without clinical seizures, or a history of language regression, as in LKS, had an epileptiform EEG. In general, a patient who has autism and displays paroxysmal stereotyped behaviors raises the suspicion of epilepsy. In addition to EEG, home or school videos are helpful to clarify the event. If regression is present, then an EEG should be obtained. A higher index of suspicion is warranted in those patients with autism who are lower functioning or severely impaired, as seizure disorders are more common and more treatment resistant in those with greater intellectual impairment (107,111).

Depression and Anxiety

As in adults, depression and anxiety are commonly found in children with epilepsy. In a study by Vega et al. (112), as compared to healthy matched controls, children aged 6 to 16 years with childhood absence epilepsy (CAE) had higher rates of depression and anxiety symptoms and more general psychosocial difficulties like isolation and low self-esteem. Caplan et al. (113) interviewed 100 children with epilepsy and found that 33% had a depressive or anxiety disorder. Those with mood and anxiety disorders had lower IQ scores. Only 33% of those with identified disorders had received prior mental health treatment, which is surprising given their involvement in the health care system as a result of their epilepsy. Other studies have found depressive symptoms to be the most common psychiatric symptom in children with epilepsy (114).

A variety of factors have been proposed and studied to explain depression in epilepsy, yielding contradictory results. The epilepsy factors include age of onset, duration of epilepsy, seizure type, and seizure severity. Iatrogenic factors include treatment with AEDs and surgery. Psychosocial factors include stigma, discrimination, sense of control, attributional style, and social supports. Ultimately, the likely explanation is multifactorial (115). The etiology of anxiety is less well explored. Some have considered the role of limbic structures, which include the amygdala and hippocampus, as an area of pathogenesis for anxiety (116).

Suicide

In adults, rates of suicide or self-harm in those with epilepsy are thought to be five times that of the general population, with the highest risk for those with temporal lobe epilepsy (117). Lambert and Robertson (115) reviewed studies that examined causes of death in epilepsy and found that the rate of death by suicide was 10 times that of the general population. The data in children also suggest high rates of suicidal thinking or behavior. A chart review of pediatric suicide attempters with epilepsy found a rate 15 times that of the general population (118). In the Caplan study cited above, 20% of the subjects reported suicidal thinking, compared to 9% of controls. Of those with suicidal thinking, 37% had plans. Those with disruptive behaviors, comorbid with depression and anxiety, were 12 times more likely to have suicidal thinking. Duration of illness also corresponded to suicidal thinking.

In a British population-based retrospective cohort study that attempted to estimate the magnitude of the association between suicide and epilepsy, the researchers found that the association exists even before epilepsy manifests, suggesting a common underlying biology rather than the effects of the seizures or AEDs (71).

Psychosis

Psychosis and its relationship to epilepsy have generated a robust literature. Since the mid-19th century, there have been generally two lines of thinking regarding psychosis. In one, epilepsy and active psychosis are thought to be incompatible. ECT for the treatment of psychosis emerged in part from this perspective. The other line of thought views epilepsy as coexisting with or facilitating psychoses (116). The concept of forced normalization and alternative psychoses introduced by Landolt illustrates a reciprocal coexistence (119); patients whose EEGs were abnormal but which normalized with treatment were observed to develop psychopathology. Slater et al. (120) described schizophrenia-like psychoses related to duration of epilepsy and amount of brain damage; this association was especially strong in temporal lobe epilepsy. Support for the relationship of epilepsy and psychosis is found in genes that overlap both conditions (5–7). The concept of kindling as an etiologic theory for epilepsy may also help explain the emergence of psychotic phenomena (121).

Psychotic symptoms have been considered according to their temporal relationship with seizure activity; that is, whether they are preictal, ictal, postictal, or interictal. The psychiatrist is most likely to be concerned with interictal presentations of psychosis, although the hospital-based consultant may be called in during any of the other states. Occasionally, the hospital-based psychiatric consultant may be the first to evaluate a psychotic presentation, before the epilepsy history is revealed through chart records, by a late-arriving family member, or by the patient himself after he recuperates.

There are no epidemiologic studies examining the comorbidity of psychosis and epilepsy in children. Adult studies have methodologic limitations but provide some information. A recent systematic review and meta-analysis by Clancy et al. (122) pertaining to prevalence rates of psychosis in epilepsy concluded that up to 6% of individuals with epilepsy have a comorbid psychotic illness and that such individual with epilepsy have an eightfold increased risk of psychosis. Mendez et al. (123) retrospectively compared outpatients in a neurology clinic with epilepsy or migraine headaches. They found that 9% of the patients with epilepsy had interictal schizophrenia symptoms, versus 1% of the patients with migraine. Shaw et al. (124) found that 3% of patients with temporal lobectomy for intractable seizures developed schizophrenia-like psychoses.

In addition to methodologic issues, studies and descriptions of psychotic states in epilepsy patients have been plagued by matters of semantics in describing both psychotic symptoms and epilepsy. Parnas and Korsgaard (125) observed in 1982 that the descriptions of psychosis seldom fit the bleulerian definition of schizophrenia and advised against the use of the term schizophrenia-like to describe psychoses in epilepsy. With this concern in mind, Kanemoto et al. (126) set out to reexamine the matter of interictal psychoses using DSM-IV criteria definitions of psychotic disorders in conjunction with the ILAE classification criteria. In a retrospective review of all outpatient records from 1984 to 1999 at their regional epilepsy center, they found 132 patients to have interictal psychoses, or 4.5% of all patients. The researches excluded ictal or postictal psychotic phenomenon. Schizophrenia was found in 1.9% of the total sample. Temporal lobe epilepsy made up the vast majority of seizure types with psychosis, accounting for 56% of cases. The patients with schizophrenia were more likely to have had early-onset psychosis (<20 years old) and to have lower IQ. One significant limitation of the study is its retrospective design.

An epidemiologic question mark remains for both adults and children regarding epilepsy and psychosis. The sum of the data suggests that perhaps interictal psychotic states are more commonly seen than would be expected in the general population and that temporal lobe epilepsy seems to be the predominant type accountable for this.

ADHD and Disruptive Behavior Disorders

Symptoms of ADHD in epilepsy syndromes tend to be ones of inattention rather than hyperactivity–impulsivity. Some suggest that ADHD and epilepsy share common risk factors and that both may share common neuropsychological impairments, especially the inattentive type (127). Others have also observed that a number of children with uncomplicated ADHD and without epilepsy have epileptiform discharges (128). In a study on psychiatric disorders and behavioral characteristics of pediatric patients with epilepsy and ADHD, the comorbidity (including anxiety disorders and oppositional defiant disorders) in those patients was similar to that of ADHD without epilepsy (129).

Several studies have examined the prevalence of ADHD in epilepsy populations. In one, a history of ADHD was 2.5 times more common in children newly diagnosed with epilepsy compared to controls (3). In another, Dunn et al. (130) found that 25% to 37% of children and adolescents scored in the clinical range on the attention scale of the Child Behavior Checklist (CBCL); using a symptom inventory which gives symptom profiles according to DSM-IV, they found 24% of children had symptoms consistent with ADHD, predominantly inattentive type, and 11.4% with ADHD, combined type. In the UK population study by Davies et al. (103), the rate of DSM-IV ADHD in complicated epilepsy was 12% and in uncomplicated epilepsy, 0%, suggesting degree of illness may account for ADHD symptoms. As with ADHD symptoms in the general population, these symptoms lessen with age also for patients with idiopathic epilepsy and ADHD, probably because development and brain maturation have a similar positive effect on attentional issues in children with epilepsy (131).

The data for other disruptive disorders are generally embedded in data on ADHD. Caplan et al. (132) found ADHD, oppositional defiant disorder, or conduct disorder in 25% of patients with complex partial epilepsy or generalized primary seizures. Ott et al. (1) found disruptive behavior disorders in up to 23% of those with complex partial epilepsy or primary generalized seizures.

Neuropsychological Functioning and Education

The literature generally suggests that epilepsy negatively impacts cognitive functioning. Although findings are variable, this is related to specific epilepsy syndromes, age of onset, duration, seizure frequency, and number of AEDs.

Williams et al. (133) found that children with epilepsy had a full-scale IQ in the low average to average range. O'Leary et al. (134) also found that children with epilepsy had lower IQs. They administered the WISC-III to 32 child patients with epilepsy, without comorbid conditions and IQ greater than 70, and to matched controls and found a mean difference of one standard deviation on the full-scale IQ, 107 versus 92. Høie et al. (135) studied nonverbal intelligence in 198 children with epilepsy using Raven matrices. Severe nonverbal performance problems were found in 43% of children with epilepsy, compared to 3% of controls. These studies reflect group trends and do not reflect how an individual child will perform; for example, Smith et al. (136) also found IQs in the low to average range, but individual scores ranged from the <1% to >99%.

Regarding IQ stability, Bourgeois et al. (137) prospectively followed children yearly over 4 years, administering their first psychological evaluation within 2 weeks of initial diagnosis. They found that overall IQ did not decrease, but that in a subset of subjects, IQ scores persistently showed a decrease of 10 points or more. This was related to a higher incidence of drug levels in the toxic range, difficulty controlling seizure activity, and an earlier age of seizure onset. Rodin et al. (138) readministered the WISC to children with epilepsy 5 years after initial testing and found that WISC IQ estimates decreased slightly over time; they suggested that decreased mental growth rather than loss of function was responsible.

Regarding education and achievement, Farwell et al. (139) studied 118 children with epilepsy and found they had repeated a grade or been placed in special education at twice the normal rate. In this study, years of seizure activity correlated with lower intelligence. Aldenkamp et al. (140) examined several factors related to achievement and concluded that epilepsy type is the main factor underlying educational achievement. They speculated that since epilepsy type is correlated with intelligence, this may be the primary cognitive factor underlying educational underachievement. Regarding achievement, it seems that only those children with high severity epilepsy have lower school-administered achievement scores compared to national norms, but not those children with inactive or low-severity epilepsy (141). Whether epilepsy (or more generally, the presence of a chronic condition) itself affects achievement has also been studied; those with epilepsy generally do less well (142).

Learning Disorders

Difficulties in reading, writing, and mathematics may be found in one-third of children with epilepsy (143). One study examining children with epilepsy found that academic problems were highest in math, followed by spelling, reading, and comprehension. Children also did less well than expected for age and IQ level (144). Seizure onset in the language-dominant hemisphere is thought to affect reading comprehension, written language, and calculation abilities, more so than seizure onset in the nondominant hemisphere (145).

Family

Rodenburg et al. (146) in a literature review found that compared to control children, families with a child with epilepsy had a lower quality of parent–child relationship, more depression in mothers, and had problems with family functioning. Family factors seem to be stronger predictors of psychopathology than epilepsy-related factors (147).

Quality of Life

Adolescents' perceptions of epilepsy can be highly negative. Cheung and Wirrell (148) interviewed healthy controls and children with chronic conditions. When asked about the physical and social impact of eight chronic diseases (epilepsy, leukemia, HIV infection, Down syndrome, migraine, asthma, diabetes, and arthritis), epilepsy was viewed as having a worse physical impact than all illnesses except Down syndrome. The perceptions included the view that epilepsy commonly causes mental handicap and commonly leads to self-injury and death or injury in others. In addition, healthy controls viewed individuals with epilepsy as less honest, popular, fun, and less adept at sports than healthy teens.

Children with epilepsy often have a poorer self-concept than do those with other chronic conditions (149–151). Older adolescents perceive a greater negative impact on life and general health and have more negative attitudes about epilepsy. Those with severe seizures and female patients seem to have the greatest difficulty (152). Each AED also has its own side-effect profile which may impact self-esteem, such as weight gain. Mitchell (153) argued, however, that family, socioeconomic, and cultural factors are the primary determinants of

TABLE 7.2.4.8

RECOMMENDATIONS FOR COMMONLY USED PSYCHOTROPICS IN THE CHILD WITH A SEIZURE DISORDER

Medication or Class	Recommendations (Low Seizure Risk ≠ Absent Risk)	Key Drug–Drug Interactions with AEDs
First-generation antipsychotics	Use not advised for chlorpromazine and loxapine Use others judiciously Haloperidol has lowest risk	Carbamazepine, phenobarbital, phenytoin, and perhaps oxcarbazepine may reduce levels through cytochrome P450 3A4 induction
Second-generation antipsychotics	Use not advised for clozapine Seizure risk low for others	Risperidone, quetiapine, aripiprazole, and ziprasidone may be reduced by above AEDs through 3A4
SSRIs/SNRIs	Seizure risk low Venlafaxine may have increased risk over others	Fluoxetine and fluvoxamine may increase carbamazepine levels through 3A4 inhibition
Trazodone	Seizure risk low	Substrate of 3A4; above AEDs may reduce
Alpha agonists	Seizure risk low	No known drug interactions with AEDs
Bupropion	Use not advised	Phenytoin and phenobarbital may reduce levels through 2B6 induction
Atomoxetine	Seizure risk unclear. Use judiciously	No known drug interactions with AEDs
Lithium	Use judiciously. Considered proconvulsant	Neurotoxicity with carbamazepine and phenytoin
Stimulants	FDA contraindicates when comorbid seizures are present, but data suggest they can be used judiciously	No known drug interactions with AEDs
TCAs/tetracyclic antidepressants	Use not advised for clomipramine, amoxapine, and loxapine Use others judiciously	Valproate may increase and carbamazepine may decrease TCA levels
Benzodiazepines	Anticonvulsant, but proconvulsant if suddenly discontinued	Alprazolam, diazepam, midazolam, and triazolam are substrates of 3A4

social, academic, and other problems in epilepsy and that medications, seizures, or cognition play a minor role.

Driving restrictions may impact adolescents with epilepsy. Restrictions on driving after a seizure are mandated by law and vary from state to state, usually lasting 3 to 12 months after an index seizure. If no new seizures occur during the restricted time, driving privileges are reinstituted (154).

Examining outcome, Jalava et al. (155) followed a cohort of childhood-onset epilepsy into adulthood with a mean follow-up of 35 years. They found that those with epilepsy and no other neurologic problems did less well than controls in education, employability, marriage rate, and—depending on seizure activity and polypharmacy—satisfaction with present life.

PSYCHOPHARMACOLOGICAL TREATMENT OF CHILDREN WITH EPILEPSY AND COMORBID PSYCHIATRIC DISORDERS

Psychopharmacologic treatment in children with epilepsy should always be embedded in a full biopsychosocial approach to the child's problems. Different domains of dysfunction should be conceptualized and each given treatments specific to that domain. Thus, academic and social skills deficits may require remediation. School failure may require modification of the educational plan. Relationship problems benefit from psychotherapy, as will low self-esteem and coping difficulties. Family and individual misconceptions should be countered with psychoeducation. The primary symptoms of the patient's DSM-5 disorder may, depending on the disorder, benefit from psychotherapy or psychopharmacology, or both.

When the time comes to choose a psychopharmacological agent, four considerations should be borne in mind: efficacy, seizure threshold, interactions, and AEs. Considering efficacy first, for nearly all the psychiatric disorders comorbid with epilepsy, specific randomized controlled trials in children with epilepsy plus that disorder have not been done. Thus clinicians will need to use, as a guide, the efficacy data from children without seizures, but more circumspectly. Similarly, while many psychotropics have been assumed to lower the threshold for having a seizure, randomized controlled data, with the exception of methylphenidate, does not exist for the risk of exacerbating seizures. For most psychotropics, practitioners must rely on the FDA trial data for that agent, by comparing the rate of new-onset seizures in patients receiving active medication to the rate in those receiving placebo (even though patients with epilepsy are excluded from almost all these trials). Other ways to estimate the risk include considering the rate of seizures when the psychotropic has been taken in an overdose and examining the literature for uncontrolled case reports and case series.

Drug–drug interactions between psychotropics and AEDs can be pharmacodynamic (e.g., additive sedation) or pharmacokinetic (e.g., decreased antipsychotic plasma level when the patient is taking carbamazepine). These interactions must be considered when adding or removing an AED or a psychotropic. It is useful to anticipate that the rate of AEs from a psychotropic might be higher in patients with epilepsy than in patients without it. This will result in a frank discussion of risks with the family and "starting low and going slow" with the psychotropic. Table 7.2.4.8 summarizes recommendations for the more commonly prescribed psychotropics when epilepsy is comorbid.

Just as we would not have a patient's seizures go untreated, we and our colleagues in neurology should not overlook the psychiatric and psychological comorbidities commonly present in children with epilepsy, and ensure that these do not go undiagnosed and untreated.

References

1. Ott D, Caplan R, Guthrie D, et al.: Measures of psychopathology in children with complex partial seizures and primary generalized epilepsy with absence. *J Am Acad Child Adolesc Psychiatry* 40(8):907–914, 2001.

2. Steffenburg S, Gillberg C, Steffenburg U: Psychiatric disorders in children and adolescents with mental retardation and active epilepsy. *Arch Neurol* 53(9):904–912, 1996.
3. Hesdorffer DC, Ludvigsson P, Olafsson E, Gudmundsson G, Kjartansson O, Hauser WA: ADHD as a risk factor for incident unprovoked seizures and epilepsy in children. *Arch Gen Psychiatry* 61(7):731–736, 2004.
4. Kanner AM: Depression in epilepsy: prevalence, clinical semiology, pathogenic mechanisms, and treatment. *Biol Psychiatry* 54(3):388–398, 2003.
5. Cappelletti S, Specchio N, Moavero R, et al.: Cognitive development in females with PCDH19 gene-related epilepsy. *Epilepsy Behav* 42:36–40, 2015.
6. Jenkins A, Apud JA, Zhang F, Decot H, Weinberger DR, Law AJ: Identification of candidate single-nucleotide polymorphisms in NRXN1 related to antipsychotic treatment response in patients with schizophrenia. *Neuropsychopharmacology* 39(9):2170–2178, 2014.
7. Rapoport JL, Giedd JN, Gogtay N: Neurodevelopmental model of schizophrenia: update 2012. *Mol Psychiatry* 17(12):1228–1238, 2012.
8. Szabo CA: Patient page. Risk of fetal death and malformation related to seizure medications. *Neurology* 67(3):E6–E7, 2006.
9. Fisher RS, Acevedo C, Arzimanoglou A, et al.: ILAE official report: a practical clinical definition of epilepsy. *Epilepsia* 55(4):475–482, 2014.
10. Epilepsy Foundation: Epilepsy statistics. Available at: http://www.epilepsy.com/learn/epilepsy-statistics. Accessed January 2016.
11. Russ SA, Larson K, Halfon N: A national profile of childhood epilepsy and seizure disorder. *Pediatrics* 129(2):256–264, 2012.
12. Jones JE, Austin JK, Caplan R, Dunn D, Plioplys S, Salpekar JA: Psychiatric disorders in children and adolescents who have epilepsy. *Pediatr Rev* 29(2):e9–e14, 2008.
13. Cowan LD: The epidemiology of the epilepsies in children. *Ment Retard Dev Disabil Res Rev* 8(3):171–181, 2002.
14. Kurtz Z, Tookey P, Ross E: Epilepsy in young people: 23 year follow up of the British national child development study. *BMJ* 316(7128):339–342, 1998.
15. Oka E, Ohtsuka Y, Yoshinaga H, Murakami N, Kobayashi K, Ogino T: Prevalence of childhood epilepsy and distribution of epileptic syndromes: a population-based survey in Okayama, Japan. *Epilepsia* 47(3): 626–630, 2006.
16. Hauser WA, Annegers JF, Rocca WA: Descriptive epidemiology of epilepsy: contributions of population-based studies from Rochester, Minnesota. *Mayo Clin Proc* 71(6):576–586, 1996.
17. Heaney DC, MacDonald BK, Everitt A, et al.: Socioeconomic variation in incidence of epilepsy: prospective community based study in south east England. *BMJ* 325(7371):1013–1016, 2002.
18. Shamansky SL, Glaser GH: Socioeconomic characteristics of childhood seizure disorders in the New Haven area: an epidemiologic study. *Epilepsia* 20(5):457–474, 1979.
19. Annegers JF, Dubinsky S, Coan SP, Newmark ME, Roht L: The incidence of epilepsy and unprovoked seizures in multiethnic, urban health maintenance organizations. *Epilepsia* 40(4):502–506, 1999.
20. Reading R, Haynes R, Beach R: Deprivation and incidence of epilepsy in children. *Seizure* 15(3):190–193, 2006.
21. Tuchman R, Rapin I: Epilepsy in autism. *Lancet Neurol* 1(6):352–358, 2002.
22. Hauser WA, Annegers JF, Kurland LT: Incidence of epilepsy and unprovoked seizures in Rochester, Minnesota: 1935–1984. *Epilepsia* 34(3): 453–468, 1993.
23. Ottman R, Annegers JF, Hauser WA, Kurland LT: Higher risk of seizures in offspring of mothers than of fathers with epilepsy. *Am J Hum Genet* 43(3):257–264, 1988.
24. Annegers JF, Hauser WA, Elveback LR: Remission of seizures and relapse in patients with epilepsy. *Epilepsia* 20(6):729–737, 1979.
25. Sillanpää M, Schmidt D: Prognosis of seizure recurrence after stopping antiepileptic drugs in seizure-free patients: a long-term population-based study of childhood-onset epilepsy. *Epilepsy Behav* 8(4):713–719, 2006.
26. Berg AT, Shinnar S, Levy SR, Testa FM, Smith-Rapaport S, Beckerman B: Early development of intractable epilepsy in children: a prospective study. *Neurology* 56(11):1445–1452, 2001.
27. World Health Organization: *Epilepsy Fact Sheet.* Available at: http://www.who.int/mediacentre/factsheets/fs999/en/. Accessed March 30, 2017.
28. Lewis AJ: Melancholia: a historical review. *J Ment Sci* 1–42, 1934.
29. Roberts A: *The 1844 Report of the Metropolitan Commissioners in Lunacy.* Middlesex University, 1981. Available at: http://studymore.org.uk/4_09.htm. Accessed March 30, 2017.
30. Spatt J, Bauer G, Baumgartner C, et al; Austrian Section of the International League Against Epilepsy: Predictors for negative attitudes toward subjects with epilepsy: a representative survey in the general public in Austria. *Epilepsia* 46(5):736–742, 2005.
31. Mace CJ: Epilepsy and schizophrenia. *Br J Psychiatry* 163:439–445, 1993.
32. Lossius MI, Clench-Aas J, van Roy B, Mowinckel P, Gjerstad L: Psychiatric symptoms in adolescents with epilepsy in junior high school in Norway: a population survey. *Epilepsy Behav* 9(2):286–292, 2006.
33. Yang Y, Muzny DM, Reid JG, et al.: Clinical whole-exome sequencing for the diagnosis of mendelian disorders. *N Engl J Med* 369(16):1502–1511, 2013.
34. Coorg R, Weisenberg JL, Wong M: Clinical neurogenetics: recent advances in the genetics of epilepsy. *Neurol Clin* 31(4):891–913, 2013.
35. Haas LF: Hans Berger (1873–1941), Richard Caton (1842–1926), and electroencephalography. *J Neurol Neurosurg Psychiatry* 74(1):9, 2003.
36. Homan RW, Herman J, Purdy F: Cerebral location of international 10-20 system electrode placement. *Electroencephalogr Clin Neurophysiol* 66(4):376–382, 1987.
37. Berg AT, Scheffer IE: New concepts in classification of the epilepsies: entering the 21st century. *Epilepsia* 52(6):1058–1062, 2011.
38. Korff C, Wirrell E: ILAE classification of seizures and epilepsy. In: UpToDate, Waltham, MA, UpToDate. Accessed on October 20, 2015.
39. Berg AT, Shinnar S, Levy SR, Testa FM: Newly diagnosed epilepsy in children: presentation at diagnosis. *Epilepsia* 40(4):445–452, 1999.
40. Kotagal P, Costa M, Wyllie E, Wolgamuth B: Paroxysmal nonepileptic events in children and adolescents. *Pediatrics* 110(4):e46, 2002.
41. Benbadis SR, Allen Hauser W: An estimate of the prevalence of psychogenic non-epileptic seizures. *Seizure* 9(4):280–281, 2000.
42. Holmes GL, Sackellares JC, McKiernan J, Ragland M, Dreifuss FE: Evaluation of childhood pseudoseizures using EEG telemetry and video tape monitoring. *J Pediatr* 97(4):554–558, 1980.
43. Bowman ES: Why conversion seizures should be classified as a dissociative disorder. *Psychiatr Clin North Am* 29(1):185–211, 2006.
44. Mondon K, de Toffol B, Praline J, et al.: [Psychiatric comorbidity in patients with pseudoseizures: retrospective study conducted in a video-EEG center]. *Rev Neurol (Paris)* 161(11):1061–1069, 2005.
45. Wyllie E, Glazer JP, Benbadis S, Kotagal P, Wolgamuth B: Psychiatric features of children and adolescents with pseudoseizures. *Arch Pediatr Adolesc Med* 153(3):244–248, 1999.
46. Bhatia MS, Sapra S: Pseudoseizures in children: a profile of 50 cases. *Clin Pediatr (Phila)* 44(7):617–621, 2005.
47. Lancman ME, Asconapé JJ, Graves S, Gibson PA: Psychogenic seizures in children: long-term analysis of 43 cases. *J Child Neurol* 9(4):404–407, 1994.
48. Vincentiis S, Valente KD, Thomé-Souza S, Kuczinsky E, Fiore LA, Negrão N: Risk factors for psychogenic nonepileptic seizures in children and adolescents with epilepsy. *Epilepsy Behav* 8(1):294–298, 2006.
49. Kramer U, Carmant L, Riviello JJ, et al.: Psychogenic seizures: video telemetry observations in 27 patients. *Pediatr Neurol* 12(1):39–41, 1995.
50. Brunquell P, Mc Keever M, Russman BS: Differentiation of epileptic from nonepileptic head drops in children. *Epilepsia* 31(4):401–405, 1990.
51. McLaren J, Bryson SE: Review of recent epidemiological studies of mental retardation: prevalence, associated disorders, and etiology. *Am J Ment Retard* 92(3):243–254, 1987.
52. Bowley C, Kerr M: Epilepsy and intellectual disability. *J Intellect Disabil Res* 44(Pt 5):529–543, 2000.
53. Paolicchi JM: The spectrum of nonepileptic events in children. *Epilepsia* 43 Suppl 3:60–64, 2002.
54. Donat JF, Wright FS: Episodic symptoms mistaken for seizures in the neurologically impaired child. *Neurology* 40(1):156–157, 1990.
55. Airaksinen EM, Matilainen R, Mononen T, et al.: A population-based study on epilepsy in mentally retarded children. *Epilepsia* 41(9):1214–1220, 2000.
56. Shields WD: Catastrophic epilepsy in childhood. *Epilepsia*41 Suppl 2:S2–S6, 2000.
57. EuroEPINOMICS-RES Consortium; Epilepsy Phenome/Genome Project; Epi4K Consortium: De novo mutations in synaptic transmission genes including DNM1 cause epileptic encephalopathies. *Am J Hum Genet* 95(4):360–370, 2014.
58. Landau WM, Kleffner FR: Syndrome of acquired aphasia with convulsive disorder in children. 1957. *Neurology* 51(5):1241, 1998.
59. Carvill GL, Regan BM, Yendle SC, et al.: GRIN2A mutations cause epilepsy-aphasia spectrum disorders. *Nat Genet* 45(9):1073–1076, 2013.
60. Endele S, Rosenberger G, Geider K, et al.: Mutations in GRIN2A and GRIN2B encoding regulatory subunits of NMDA receptors cause variable neurodevelopmental phenotypes. *Nat Genet* 42(11):1021–1026, 2010.
61. Tuchman RF, Rapin I: Regression in pervasive developmental disorders: seizures and epileptiform electroencephalogram correlates. *Pediatrics* 99(4):560–566, 1997.
62. Meador KJ: Cognitive outcomes and predictive factors in epilepsy. *Neurology* 58(8 Suppl 5):S21–S26, 2002.
63. Kwan P, Brodie MJ: Neuropsychological effects of epilepsy and antiepileptic drugs. *Lancet* 357(9251):216–222, 2001.
64. Loring DW, Meador KJ: Cognitive side effects of antiepileptic drugs in children. *Neurology* 62(6):872–877, 2004.
65. Rugino TA, Samsock TC: Levetiracetam in autistic children: an open-label study. *J Dev Behav Pediatr* 23(4):225–230, 2002.
66. Bittigau P, Sifringer M, Ikonomidou C: Antiepileptic drugs and apoptosis in the developing brain. *Ann N Y Acad Sci* 993:103–114; discussion 123–124, 2003.
67. Williams J, Bates S, Griebel ML, et al.: Does short term antiepileptic drug treatment in children result in cognitive or behavioral changes? *Epilepsia* 39(10):1064–1069, 1998.
68. Mandelbaum DE, Burack GD: The effect of seizure type and medication on cognitive and behavioral functioning in children with idiopathic epilepsy. *Dev Med Child Neurol* 39(11):731–735, 1997.
69. Aldenkamp AP, Alpherts WC, Sandstedt P, et al.: Antiepileptic drug-related cognitive complaints in seizure-free children with epilepsy before and after drug discontinuation. *Epilepsia* 39(10):1070–1074, 1998.

70. Mula M, Kanner AM, Schmitz B, Schachter S: Antiepileptic drugs and suicidality: an expert consensus statement from the Task Force on Therapeutic Strategies of the ILAE Commission on Neuropsychobiology. *Epilepsia* 54(1):199–203, 2013.
71. Hesdorffer DC, Ishihara L, Webb DJ, Mynepalli L, Galwey NW, Hauser WA: Occurrence and recurrence of attempted suicide among people with epilepsy. *JAMA Psychiatry* 73(1):80–86, 2016.
72. Camfield CS, Chaplin S, Doyle AB, Shapiro SH, Cummings C, Camfield PR: Side effects of phenobarbital in toddlers; behavioral and cognitive aspects. *J Pediatr* 95(3):361–365, 1979.
73. Farwell JR, Lee YJ, Hirtz DG, Sulzbacher SI, Ellenberg JH, Nelson KB: Phenobarbital for febrile seizures–effects on intelligence and on seizure recurrence. *N Engl J Med* 322(6):364–369, 1990.
74. Sulzbacher S, Farwell JR, Temkin N, Lu AS, Hirtz DG: Late cognitive effects of early treatment with phenobarbital. *Clin Pediatr (Phila)* 38(7):387–394, 1999.
75. Brent DA, Crumrine PK, Varma RR, Allan M, Allman C: Phenobarbital treatment and major depressive disorder in children with epilepsy. *Pediatrics* 80(6):909–917, 1987.
76. Gillham RA, Williams N, Wiedmann KD, Butler E, Larkin JG, Brodie MJ: Cognitive function in adult epileptic patients established on anticonvulsant monotherapy. *Epilepsy Res* 7(3):219–225, 1990.
77. Depondt C, Godard P, Espel RS, Da Cruz AL, Lienard P, Pandolfo M: A candidate gene study of antiepileptic drug tolerability and efficacy identifies an association of CYP2C9 variants with phenytoin toxicity. *Eur J Neurol* 18(9):1159–1164, 2011.
78. Caudle KE, Rettie AE, Whirl-Carrillo M, et al; Clinical Pharmacogenetics Implementation Consortium: Clinical pharmacogenetics implementation consortium guidelines for CYP2C9 and HLA-B genotypes and phenytoin dosing. *Clin Pharmacol Ther* 96(5):542–548, 2014.
79. Findling RL, Ginsberg LD: The safety and effectiveness of open-label extended-release carbamazepine in the treatment of children and adolescents with bipolar I disorder suffering from a manic or mixed episode. *Neuropsychiatr Dis Treat* 10:1589–1597, 2014.
80. Meador KJ: The cognitive effects of antiepileptic medication. In: Wyllie AG, Lachhwani DK (eds): *The Treatment of Epilepsy: Principles and Practice.* Philadelphia, PA, Lippincott Williams & Wilkins, 33–62, 2006.
81. Larkin JG, McKee PJ, Brodie MJ: Rapid tolerance to acute psychomotor impairment with carbamazepine in epileptic patients. *Br J Clin Pharmacol* 33(1):111–114, 1992.
82. MacMillan CM, Korndörfer SR, Rao S, Fleisher CA, Mezzacappa E, Gonzalez-Heydrich J: A comparison of divalproex and oxcarbazepine in aggressive youth with bipolar disorder. *J Psychiatr Pract* 12(4):214–222, 2006.
83. Wagner KD, Kowatch RA, Emslie GJ, et al.: A double-blind, randomized, placebo-controlled trial of oxcarbazepine in the treatment of bipolar disorder in children and adolescents. *Am J Psychiatry* 163(7):1179–1186, 2006.
84. Munshi KR, Oken T, Guild DJ, et al.: The use of antiepileptic drugs (AEDs) for the treatment of pediatric aggression and mood disorders. *Pharmaceuticals (Basel)* 3(9):2986–3004, 2010.
85. Vasudev A, Macritchie K, Vasudev K, Watson S, Geddes J, Young AH: Oxcarbazepine for acute affective episodes in bipolar disorder. *Cochrane Database Syst Rev* 12:CD004857, 2011.
86. Bowden CL, Janicak PG, Orsulak P, et al.: Relation of serum valproate concentration to response in mania. *Am J Psychiatry* 153(6):765–770, 1996.
87. Bensch J, Blennow G, Ferngren H, et al.: A double-blind study of clonazepam in the treatment of therapy-resistant epilepsy in children. *Dev Med Child Neurol* 19(3):335–342, 1977.
88. Micromedex® Healthcare Series [Internet database]. Greenwood Village, CO, Thomson Micromedex. Accessed February 2, 2016.
89. An DM, Wu XT, Hu FY, Yan B, Stefan H, Zhou D: Association study of lamotrigine-induced cutaneous adverse reactions and HLA-B*1502 in a Han Chinese population. *Epilepsy Res* 92(2–3):226–230, 2010.
90. Cheung YK, Cheng SH, Chan EJ, Lo SV, Ng MH, Kwan P: HLA-B alleles associated with severe cutaneous reactions to antiepileptic drugs in Han Chinese. *Epilepsia* 54(7):1307–1314, 2013.
91. Hung SI, Chung WH, Liu ZS, et al.: Common risk allele in aromatic antiepileptic-drug induced Stevens-Johnson syndrome and toxic epidermal necrolysis in Han Chinese. *Pharmacogenomics* 11(3):349–356, 2010.
92. Shi YW, Min FL, Liu XR, et al.: Hla-B alleles and lamotrigine-induced cutaneous adverse drug reactions in the Han Chinese population. *Basic Clin Pharmacol Toxicol* 109(1):42–46, 2011.
93. Hu FY, Wu XT, An DM, Yan B, Stefan H, Zhou D: Pilot association study of oxcarbazepine-induced mild cutaneous adverse reactions with HLA-B*1502 allele in Chinese Han population. *Seizure* 20(2):160–162, 2011.
94. Franz DN, Tudor C, Leonard J, et al.: Lamotrigine therapy of epilepsy in tuberous sclerosis. *Epilepsia* 42(7):935–940, 2001.
95. Mula M, Trimble MR, Sander JW: Psychiatric adverse events in patients with epilepsy and learning disabilities taking levetiracetam. *Seizure* 13(1):55–57, 2004.
96. Salinsky MC, Storzbach D, Spencer DC, Oken BS, Landry T, Dodrill CB: Effects of topiramate and gabapentin on cognitive abilities in healthy volunteers. *Neurology* 64(5):792–798, 2005.
97. Martin R, Kuzniecky R, Ho S, et al.: Cognitive effects of topiramate, gabapentin, and lamotrigine in healthy young adults. *Neurology* 52(2):321–327, 1999.
98. Aldenkamp AP, Baker G, Mulder OG, et al.: A multicenter, randomized clinical study to evaluate the effect on cognitive function of topiramate compared with valproate as add-on therapy to carbamazepine in patients with partial-onset seizures. *Epilepsia* 41(9):1167–1178, 2000.
99. Berent S, Sackellares JC, Giordani B, Wagner JG, Donofrio PD, Abou-Khalil B: Zonisamide (CI-912) and cognition: results from preliminary study. *Epilepsia* 28(1):61–67, 1987.
100. Wilensky AJ, Friel PN, Ojemann LM, Dodrill CB, McCormick KB, Levy RH: Zonisamide in epilepsy: a pilot study. *Epilepsia* 26(3):212–220, 1985.
101. Reilly C, Atkinson P, Das KB, et al.: Neurobehavioral comorbidities in children with active epilepsy: a population-based study. *Pediatrics* 133(6):e1586–e1593, 2014.
102. Rutter M, Graham PJ, Yule W: *A Neuropsychiatric Study in Childhood.* London, Heinemann Educational Books, 1970.
103. Davies S, Heyman I, Goodman R: A population survey of mental health problems in children with epilepsy. *Dev Med Child Neurol* 45(5):292–295, 2003.
104. Rodenburg R, Stams GJ, Meijer AM, Aldenkamp AP, Deković M: Psychopathology in children with epilepsy: a meta-analysis. *J Pediatr Psychol* 30(6):453–468, 2005.
105. Suris JC, Parera N, Puig C: Chronic illness and emotional distress in adolescence. *J Adolesc Health* 19(2):153–156, 1996.
106. Ott D, Siddarth P, Gurbani S, et al.: Behavioral disorders in pediatric epilepsy: unmet psychiatric need. *Epilepsia* 44(4):591–597, 2003.
107. Besag FM: Current controversies in the relationships between autism and epilepsy. *Epilepsy Behav* 47:143–146, 2015.
108. Tuchman RF, Rapin I, Shinnar S: Autistic and dysphasic children. II: epilepsy. *Pediatrics* 88(6):1219–1225, 1991.
109. Steffenburg U, Hagberg G, Hagberg B: Epilepsy in a representative series of Rett syndrome. *Acta Paediatr* 90(1):34–39, 2001.
110. Gabis L, Pomeroy J, Andriola MR: Autism and epilepsy: cause, consequence, comorbidity, or coincidence? *Epilepsy Behav* 7(4):652–656, 2005.
111. Volkmar FR, Nelson DS: Seizure disorders in autism. *J Am Acad Child Adolesc Psychiatry* 29(1):127–129, 1990.
112. Vega C, Guo J, Killory B, et al.: Symptoms of anxiety and depression in childhood absence epilepsy. *Epilepsia* 52(8):e70–e74, 2011.
113. Caplan R, Siddarth P, Gurbani S, Hanson R, Sankar R, Shields WD: Depression and anxiety disorders in pediatric epilepsy. *Epilepsia* 46(5):720–730, 2005.
114. Ettinger AB, Weisbrot DM, Nolan EE, et al.: Symptoms of depression and anxiety in pediatric epilepsy patients. *Epilepsia* 39(6):595–599, 1998.
115. Lambert MV, Robertson MM: Depression in epilepsy: etiology, phenomenology, and treatment. *Epilepsia* 40 Suppl 10:S21–S47, 1999.
116. Torta R, Keller R: Behavioral, psychotic, and anxiety disorders in epilepsy: etiology, clinical features, and therapeutic implications. *Epilepsia* 40 Suppl 10:S2–S20, 1999.
117. Harris EC, Barraclough B: Suicide as an outcome for mental disorders. A meta-analysis. *Br J Psychiatry* 170:205–228, 1997.
118. Brent DA: Overrepresentation of epileptics in a consecutive series of suicide attempters seen at a children's hospital, 1978-1983. *J Am Acad Child Psychiatry* 25(2):242–246, 1986.
119. Krishnamoorthy ES, Trimble MR, Sander JW, Kanner AM: Forced normalization at the interface between epilepsy and psychiatry. *Epilepsy Behav* 3(4):303–308, 2002.
120. Slater E, Beard AW, Glithero E: The schizophrenia-like psychoses of epilepsy. *Br J Psychiatry* 109:95–150, 1963.
121. Krishnamoorthy ES, Trimble MR: Forced normalization: clinical and therapeutic relevance. *Epilepsia* 40 Suppl 10:S57–S64, 1999.
122. Clancy MJ, Clarke MC, Connor DJ, Cannon M, Cotter DR: The prevalence of psychosis in epilepsy; a systematic review and meta-analysis. *BMC Psychiatry* 14:75, 2014.
123. Mendez MF, Grau R, Doss RC, Taylor JL: Schizophrenia in epilepsy: seizure and psychosis variables. *Neurology* 43(6):1073–1077, 1993.
124. Shaw P, Mellers J, Henderson M, Polkey C, David AS, Toone BK: Schizophrenia-like psychosis arising de novo following a temporal lobectomy: timing and risk factors. *J Neurol Neurosurg Psychiatry* 75(7):1003–1008, 2004.
125. Parnas J, Korsgaard S: Epilepsy and psychosis. *Acta Psychiatr Scand* 66(2):89–99, 1982.
126. Kanemoto K, Tsuji T, Kawasaki J: Reexamination of interictal psychoses based on DSM IV psychosis classification and international epilepsy classification. *Epilepsia* 42(1):98–103, 2001.
127. Noeker M, Haverkamp F: Neuropsychological deficiencies as a mediator between CNS dysfunction and inattentive behaviour in childhood epilepsy. *Dev Med Child Neurol* 45(10):717–718, 2003.
128. Hemmer SA, Pasternak JF, Zecker SG, Trommer BL: Stimulant therapy and seizure risk in children with ADHD. *Pediatr Neurol* 24(2):99–102, 2001.
129. Gonzalez-Heydrich J, Dodds A, Whitney J, et al.: Psychiatric disorders and behavioral characteristics of pediatric patients with both epilepsy and attention-deficit hyperactivity disorder. *Epilepsy Behav* 10(3):384–388, 2007.
130. Dunn DW, Austin JK, Harezlak J, Ambrosius WT: ADHD and epilepsy in childhood. *Dev Med Child Neurol* 45(1):50–54, 2003.

131. Bechtel N, Weber P: Attention problems in children with epilepsy. How is the long-term outcome? *Eur J Paediatr Neurol* 19(3):383–385, 2015.
132. Caplan R, Arbelle S, Magharious W, et al.: Psychopathology in pediatric complex partial and primary generalized epilepsy. *Dev Med Child Neurol* 40(12):805–811, 1998.
133. Williams J, Griebel ML, Dykman RA: Neuropsychological patterns in pediatric epilepsy. *Seizure* 7(3):223–228, 1998.
134. O'Leary SD, Burns TG, Borden KA: Performance of children with epilepsy and normal age-matched controls on the WISC-III. *Child Neuropsychol* 12(3):173–180, 2006.
135. Høie B, Mykletun A, Sommerfelt K, Bjørnaes H, Skeidsvoll H, Waaler PE: Seizure-related factors and non-verbal intelligence in children with epilepsy. A population-based study from Western Norway. *Seizure* 14(4): 223–231, 2005.
136. Smith ML, Elliott IM, Lach L: Cognitive skills in children with intractable epilepsy: comparison of surgical and nonsurgical candidates. *Epilepsia* 43(6):631–637, 2002.
137. Bourgeois BF, Prensky AL, Palkes HS, Talent BK, Busch SG: Intelligence in epilepsy: a prospective study in children. *Ann Neurol* 14(4):438–444, 1983.
138. Rodin EA, Schmaltz S, Twitty G: Intellectual functions of patients with childhood-onset epilepsy. *Dev Med Child Neurol* 28(1):25–33, 1986.
139. Farwell JR, Dodrill CB, Batzel LW: Neuropsychological abilities of children with epilepsy. *Epilepsia* 26(5):395–400, 1985.
140. Aldenkamp AP, Weber B, Overweg-Plandsoen WC, Reijs R, van Mil S: Educational underachievement in children with epilepsy: a model to predict the effects of epilepsy on educational achievement. *J Child Neurol* 20(3):175–180, 2005.
141. Austin JK, Huberty TJ, Huster GA, Dunn DW: Does academic achievement in children with epilepsy change over time? *Dev Med Child Neurol* 41(7):473–479, 1999.
142. Austin JK, Huberty TJ, Huster GA, Dunn DW: Academic achievement in children with epilepsy or asthma. *Dev Med Child Neurol* 40(4):248–255, 1998.
143. Aldenkamp AP, Alpherts WC, Dekker MJ, Overweg J: Neuropsychological aspects of learning disabilities in epilepsy. *Epilepsia* 31 Suppl 4:S9–S20, 1990.
144. Seidenberg M, Beck N, Geisser M, et al.: Academic achievement of children with epilepsy. *Epilepsia* 27(6):753–759, 1986.
145. Butterbaugh G, Olejniczak P, Roques B, et al.: Lateralization of temporal lobe epilepsy and learning disabilities, as defined by disability-related civil rights law. *Epilepsia* 45(8):963–970, 2004.
146. Rodenburg R, Meijer AM, Deković M, Aldenkamp AP: Family factors and psychopathology in children with epilepsy: a literature review. *Epilepsy Behav* 6(4):488–503, 2005.
147. Rodenburg R, Marie Meijer A, Deković M, Aldenkamp AP: Family predictors of psychopathology in children with epilepsy. *Epilepsia* 47(3): 601–614, 2006.
148. Cheung C, Wirrell E: Adolescents' perception of epilepsy compared with other chronic diseases: "through a teenager's eyes." *J Child Neurol* 21(3):214–222, 2006.
149. Austin JK: Comparison of child adaptation to epilepsy and asthma. *J Child Adolesc Psychiatr Ment Health Nurs* 2(4):139–144, 1989.
150. Austin JK, Huster GA, Dunn DW, Risinger MW: Adolescents with active or inactive epilepsy or asthma: a comparison of quality of life. *Epilepsia* 37(12):1228–1238, 1996.
151. Hoare P, Mann H: Self-esteem and behavioural adjustment in children with epilepsy and children with diabetes. *J Psychosom Res* 38(8):859–869, 1994.
152. Devinsky O, Westbrook L, Cramer J, Glassman M, Perrine K, Camfield C: Risk factors for poor health-related quality of life in adolescents with epilepsy. *Epilepsia* 40(12):1715–1720, 1999.
153. Mitchell WG: Social outcome of childhood epilepsy: associations and mechanisms. *Semin Pediatr Neurol* 1(2):136–143, 1994.
154. Richards KC: Patient page. The risk of fatal car crashes in people with epilepsy. *Neurology* 63(6):E12–E13, 2004.
155. Jalava M, Sillanpää M, Camfield C, Camfield P: Social adjustment and competence 35 years after onset of childhood epilepsy: a prospective controlled study. *Epilepsia* 38(6):708–715, 1997.

CHAPTER 7.2.5 ■ LIFE-THREATENING ILLNESS, PALLIATIVE CARE, AND BEREAVEMENT

JOHN P. GLAZER, MARYLAND PAO, AND DAVID J. SCHONFELD

INTRODUCTION

"Although the world is full of suffering, it is also full of the overcoming of it."

—Helen Keller

While 42,000 infants, children and adolescents died in 2013 (1), an estimated 500,000 children are currently living with life-threatening conditions (2). This reflects evolving medical and technologic advances resulting "in children living longer, often with significant dependence on new and complex technologies (3)." The modern hospice movement began in the 20th century with Dame Cicely Saunders' groundbreaking work at St. Christopher's Hospice, London, on behalf of adults dying of cancer, came to the United States in the 1970s, proliferated rapidly, and more recently was extended to children (2,4).

Over the past two decades pediatric hospice care has broadened so that now the World Health Organization (WHO) (5) defines pediatric palliative care (PPC) as "...the active total care of the child's body, mind and spirit, and also involves giving support to the family. Optimally, the care begins when a life-threatening illness is diagnosed, and continues regardless of whether or not a child receives treatment directed at the underlying illness." This definition differs fundamentally from that traditionally, and currently, applied to adults by the Center for Medicare and Medicaid Services (CMS), which authorizes reimbursement for palliative care services only when a patient's life expectancy is less than 6 months (6). But estimating prognosis for children with life-threatening illness is notoriously unreliable. Increasing recognition of this medical reality, and mounting evidence that children and families are far better served when palliative care services are introduced at the time of diagnosis regardless of predicted outcome, led to the seminal conceptual and clinical advance of section 2302 of the Patient Protection and Affordable Care Act of 2010 (ACA) (7). Under ACA, families and providers of children with life-threatening conditions no longer have to forego curative treatments to qualify for palliative care services under Medicaid.

This chapter addresses the principles and practice of pediatric palliative medicine, bereavement, whether or not in the setting of life-threatening illness, and illustrates the role of the child and adolescent psychiatrist in the context of increasing recognition of the central importance of these issues in clinical practice. Regarding palliative care, the understanding that "palliative care is not all about death" (8) is supported by a growing body of evidence demonstrating the efficacy of

PPC as well as by recent policy positions of leading professional organizations speaking on behalf of children and families, including the American Academy of Pediatrics (AAP) Policy Statement: Pediatric Palliative Care and Hospice Care Commitments, Guidelines, and Recommendations (4), WHO: *Guidelines on the Pharmacological Treatment of Persisting Pain in Children with Medical Illnesses* (9), and the National Hospice and Palliative Care Organization (NHPCO) on Pediatric Palliative Care (10). In addition, "Pediatric Psychosocial Standards of Care for Children with Cancer and their families" was released in December 2015 and includes an evidence-based palliative care standard for children (11). These policy advances recognize both the unpredictability of medical prognosis in children with life-threatening illness, and the role of hope, "the weight of a feather on the side of optimism" as Solnit put it more than 30 years ago (12), noting the denial of hope differs crucially from a realistic appraisal and acceptance of life threat.

Himelstein et al. (2) have proposed the following "essentials" of PPC (Figure 7.2.5.1): (1) physical concerns such as pain assessment and management; (2) psychosocial concerns, including child and family fears, communication and coping styles; (3) spiritual concerns; (4) advanced care planning, including identification of decision-makers, illness trajectory, care goals, and end-of-life care; (5) practical concerns regarding location of care and familiarity with the child and family's community and school environment; and finally, (6) bereavement care for families if the child dies. Communication with and among the ill child and his or her family members and providers, and complex relationships between pain and psychiatric symptom expression, are central to the focus and expertise of the child psychiatrist in a medical setting, as is the grounding of care longitudinally. As such, child and adolescent psychiatry and pediatric palliative medicine are natural partners in the management of children with life-threatening illness.

SCOPE

This chapter addresses psychiatric aspects of pediatric life-threatening illness through review of cognitive-developmental acquisition of concepts of death, pain, and symptom management in the life-limited child, the needs of the parents, siblings and providers of these children, assessment, and management of comorbid psychiatric symptoms and disorders, bereavement, parental loss, and approaches to systems of care. Equally vital is the creation of curricula in medical schools and residency programs to ensure graduates' literacy in this critical dimension of medical practice. "Palliative care" and "bereavement" are meant as inclusive terms: As children with life-limiting illness live longer, with advances in chemotherapy, transplant technology, radiation oncology and other modalities, old distinctions blur. To palliate is to "relieve pain and distress" without cure (13); as already noted, this definition is expanded to include children with life-limiting illness who survive and those who do not. Similarly, bereavement is "a deprivation causing grief and desolation, especially the death or loss of a loved one" (13). In addition to the 40 to 50,000 children and adolescents who will face their own deaths each year in the United States, another 4% of children will lose a parent before age 15 years (14). Professionals responsible for the care of children must address the psychosocial needs of children and families in all of these settings. Speaking to the experience of children and families with life-limiting illness more than 30 years ago, Solnit wrote "the adults and the children don't know whether to prepare for life or for death" (12). The principles discussed here address the universal experience of separation and loss by children, whether they, their parents, or their siblings have a life-limiting illness from which they may recover or die. One other semantic distinction should be mentioned, that of "life-threatening" and "life-limiting"; these have been defined as conditions that potentially threaten life, and those that definitely do. The authors will exclusively use the term life-threatening in the text following to broadly denote both.

CHILDREN'S CONCEPTS OF DEATH

Children experience life-threatening illness in themselves or others through the prism of psychological, physical, and social development. Health professionals must therefore approach such children and their families with expertise in child and adolescent development and family systems (2). Central to this approach is an appreciation of the developmental acquisition of the concepts of death (15,16). The stages in children's understanding of the concepts of death have been well studied (17–21). Four major concepts related to death have been noted consistently: irreversibility, finality (also termed nonfunctionality), causality, and inevitability (also termed universality). Acquisition over time of a mature understanding of each of these concepts inevitably shapes a child's response to life-threatening illness in the child or loved ones. Speece and Brent (20) concluded that most studies found the age of acquisition of the three concepts they reviewed (irreversibility, nonfunctionality, and universality) to occur between 5 and 7 years; earlier studies citing an older age of acquisition were noted to have significant methodologic flaws.

Since infants have been shown to respond to maternal depression with altered feeding patterns and failure to thrive, it is not surprising that they can similarly respond to the affective tone within the household after the serious illness or death of a family member (22). In this way, infants and toddlers are capable of reacting to someone else's death, even if they "understand" little of what has occurred. But once infants have developed object permanence, they are capable of appreciating the permanence of loss. It is therefore probably no coincidence that infants and toddlers engage universally in the game of peek-a-boo (or hide and seek) which has been suggested may be an attempt for children to understand and cope with separation and loss. Indeed, the translation for "peek-a-boo" from Old English is literally "alive-or-dead" (23,24).

Infants, toddlers, and young children generally equate death with disappearance or separation. However, when faced with traumatic events, such as the death of a parent or other family member, some children 2 to 3 years of age or even younger have been able to demonstrate a beginning understanding of some of the concepts of death. In general, the role of personal exposure to the death of others has been controversial; although several studies have shown that such personal experience may promote the acquisition of the concepts of death (25,26), other studies have failed to support this conclusion (27,28). Cross-cultural comparisons (29–31) have illustrated both cultural variations and important cross-cultural consistencies, suggesting that although the underlying developmental framework is likely to be robust across cultures, sociocultural variables may have a significant impact on the rate of acquisition of individual concepts. In addition, developmentally based and conceptually focused education has been demonstrated to have a positive impact on children's rate of acquisition of these concepts (32).

From preschool age to early childhood, children continue to clarify their concepts of death but are still confused at times, remaining prone to misconceptions and literal misinterpretations. Children in this age group with a life-threatening illness have been shown to have a marked awareness of the seriousness of their illness, even if never told that their illness is fatal, and often develop a conceptual understanding of death more typical of an older child (33,34).

During adolescence, reactions to life-threatening illness are influenced both by emerging formal operational cognitive capacities for abstract thought and by intense developmental striving for physical, sexual, social, psychological, and

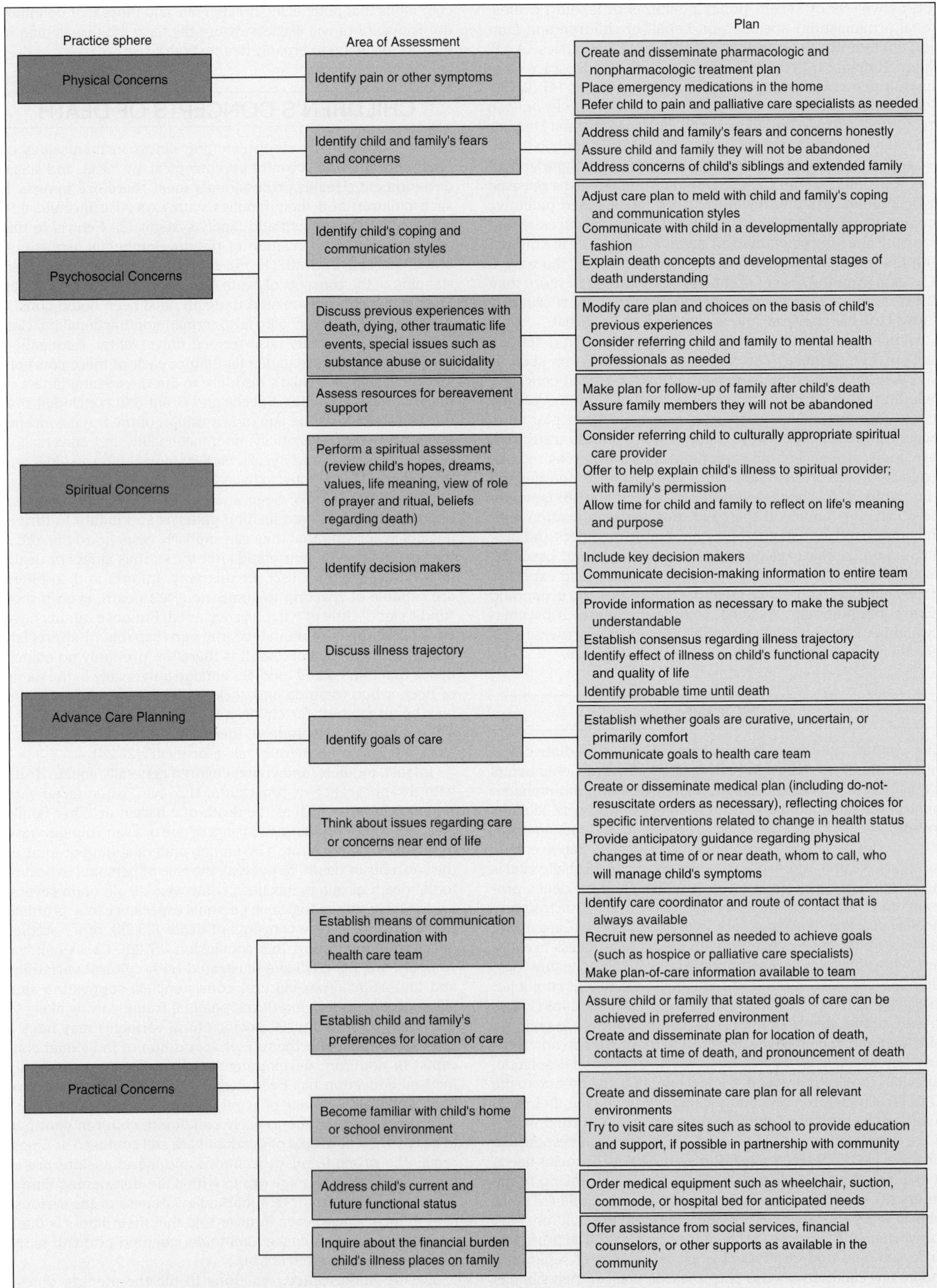

FIGURE 7.2.5.1. Essential elements in the approach to pediatric palliative care. (From Himelstein BP, Hilden JM, Boldt AM, Weissman D: Pediatric palliative care. *N Engl J Med* 350:1752–1762, 2004. With permission.)

intellectual independence and mastery. Life-threatening illness turns this developmental process on its head, bringing physical immobility and dependence rather than independence, isolation from peers rather than the forging of new relationships, and may stop educational progress in its tracks.

PAIN AND SYMPTOM ASSESSMENT AND MANAGEMENT

Cassel's compelling conceptualization of suffering is that of a state of distress specifically and individually linked to a sense that a person's intactness or integrity is threatened or disrupted, that lasts until the threat is gone or intactness restored (35). Fundamental to child and adolescent psychiatry is the notion that when a child's "intactness or integrity" is threatened or disrupted, so is that of the family. Suffering is an apt organizing principle around which pain and symptom assessment and management in children and youth at or near the end of life can be organized diagnostically and therapeutically.

In a cohort of 103 parents of children who died of cancer interviewed a mean of 3.1 years after the child's death, 89% of the children were judged to have suffered "a lot" or "a great deal" from pain, fatigue, or dyspnea while only 27% of parents reported treatment to have been successful (36). Pain may be considered the symptom most often attended to by patients, families, and providers in the palliative care setting. The assessment and treatment of pain in pediatrics and PPC has been extensively investigated, and foundational principles in assessment and treatment have emerged, with a great deal more evidence to guide clinical practice than in the previous edition of this text.

The International Association for the Study of Pain defines pain as "an unpleasant sensory and emotional experience associated with actual or potential tissue damage or described in terms of such damage" (37). Crucially, this definition recognizes that emotional factors are inherent in children's experience and expression of pain, and that its perceived magnitude varies according to factors not limited to the extent of measurable tissue damage.

The historic underrecognition and undertreatment of pain in children and its adverse medical and emotional consequences are well documented (38). Eland's pioneering work in the 1970s (39) found in a chart review of 25 children undergoing major surgery (traumatic amputation, nephrectomy, cleft palate repair) at a major children's hospital, 13 of them received no postoperative analgesia at any point in their hospital stay. Among the 12 children who did receive analgesic drugs, only 24 total doses were given, compared to 372 opioid and 299 nonopioid analgesic doses given to a comparison series of 18 adult postoperative patients. Reflecting prevailing attitudes toward the experience and management of pediatric pain as late as the 1960s, Swafford and Allan reported that just 26 of 180 children (14%) admitted to a pediatric intensive care unit over a 4-month period "required" opioid analgesia, stating "pediatric patients seldom need medication for the relief of pain. They tolerate discomfort well. The child will say he does not feel well or that he is uncomfortable, that he wants his parents but often he will not relate the unhappiness to pain" (40).

Pediatric pain assessment and management have improved dramatically over time, particularly after Anand et al.'s pioneering studies in the 1980s showed that preterm infants undergoing surgery with minimal anesthesia exhibited marked physiologic stress responses, with adverse effects on morbidity and mortality (41). Pain management in children with life-threatening illness continues to be challenging, as reported by Wolfe et al. in the study cited earlier of a cohort of parents whose children had died a mean of 3.1 years prior (36). The authors concluded that while by 2000, PPC had become the standard of care, it was still unclear whether the care of children with cancer met that standard, concluding that treatment (of pain and other end-of-life symptoms) was "seldom successful, even in the case of symptoms that are typically considered to be amenable to treatment." Reflective of advances made since that study was published, a follow-up study by the same authors using a similar design, published 7 years later, after establishment of a formal PPC service at Boston Children's Hospital-Dana Farber Cancer Institute in 1997, found significant improvement in parent beliefs about the efficacy of pain control in their children in the later cohort (42). Since inadequately treated pain is well known to mimic psychiatric symptoms such as anxiety and depressed mood, the role of the child and adolescent psychiatrist is central to assessing the subtle interplay between pain and psychiatric symptomatology to ensure that the appropriate treatment intervention or interventions are employed, whether for psychiatric disorder, pain, or both (43).

Pain Assessment

Pain is common in children in palliative care settings, at a prevalence of 75% in a retrospective chart review study of symptoms in children dying with cancer in Japan (44), comparable to rates found in other studies in the United States (36,45).

Pain assessment in children with life-limiting illness has recently been reviewed (46,47). As noted by Schechter (48), while developmentally appropriate assessment is the "cornerstone" of pediatric pain management, the advent of developmentally sensitive instruments is recent and challenges remain, including the limited capacity of younger children to report pain directly. McCulloch and Collins (46) include the following major factors in clinical pediatric pain assessment: (1) developmental stage, (2) intelligence, (3) personality, (4) temperament, (5) previous pain experience, (6) expectation and acceptance of pain, (7) child and parent coping strategies, anxieties, and cultural background, and (8) prognosis. Clinical studies suggest that most children can identify presence and location of pain by age 2, and pain intensity by age 4 (46,49–51), can participate in formal pain ratings by age 5, and are able to describe the quality of the pain experience by age 8 (46,52–54).

In clinical settings, children age 5 or older are typically able to utilize either a 10-point visual analog scale (VAS) or face-based severity scale (47,55). In Piagetian terms, 8 year and older preadolescent children at a concrete operational level of cognitive development would be expected to have a simple, internalized symbolic capacity to rate pain severity, thus the utility of numeric visual measures (46), and as noted, even younger children appear to be equally capable, perhaps due to cognitive advancement related to being seriously ill itself. Several well-validated measures appropriate for preoperational 3- to 8-year-old children have been developed (55–57). Fortunately, measures specifically applicable to children with cancer as young as age 2 are now available (58,59).

TREATMENT

Pharmacologic

A cornerstone in addressing the pharmacotherapy of pain is the analgesic ladder of the WHO (60) which is applicable to children (60,61). Consistent with the central principles of best practices and evidence-based medicine, the classic "three-step" model has recently been reformulated by the WHO Guideline Review Committee as a two-step model, chiefly due to the "step 2" "weak" opioids codeine and tramadol failing to meet Committee standards. There are no data to support the safe use of codeine in children, and rates of conversion from the prodrug to its active metabolite morphine vary by ethnicity and across individuals depending on "slow," "intermediate," or "rapid" metabolism. Recent concerns about potentially lethal complications of codeine in children led the FDA to issue a warning about its use in children undergoing tonsillectomy (62). There are no robust safety or efficacy data on the use of tramadol in pediatric patients in PPC settings either (63). The change from a "three-step" to a "two-step" model are set down in the *WHO Guidelines on Pharmacological Treatment of Persisting Pain in Children with Medical Illnesses* (9). The WHO analgesic ladder grades pain severity and matches an analgesic category to each level: acetaminophen or NSAIDs, with or without an adjuvant, for mild pain, and potent opioids, morphine being the paradigm, with or without an adjuvant, for severe pain. "Adjuvants" include a broad range of drugs whose primary indication is not pain management but may be efficacious in selected pain syndromes, and may include anticonvulsants, antidepressants, corticosteroids, psychostimulants, and neuroleptics, among others (47).

The WHO guidelines set forth the following principles of analgesic pharmacotherapy (63):

- By the *ladder*, using the new two-step approach
- By the *clock*, using regular dosage intervals and refraining from "PRN" orders
- By the *appropriate route*, preferably oral or other noninvasive routes
- By the *child*, taking the individual child into account

Pain management must also take into account whether the focus of treatment is *somatic or nociceptive* (acute and visceral), where the nervous system is intact, or *neuropathic* pain, when it is not, as different classes of analgesics may be indicated in each. Children in palliative care settings typically exhibit both subtypes, with more robust data available for somatic/nociceptive than for neuropathic pain.

Major strides in empirically supported pediatric pain management principles in the past 5 to 10 years provide new opportunities including the use of different drugs, and novel methods of opioid delivery, including subcutaneous, sublingual, buccal, and intranasal routes (64). New drug classes include the NMDA-receptor antagonist ketamine which may have potential in the treatment of pediatric neuropathic pain (65) and alpha-2-agonists such as clonidine and dexmedetomidine (66–68). The unique selective serotonin/norepinephrine reuptake inhibitors duloxetine and venlafaxine show promise in managing pain in adults, with minimal evidence for pediatric patients.

Challenges in pediatric pain management include limitations of the new WHO guidelines, in the evidence base, and in drug availability worldwide. For example, the WHO guidelines focus on morphine as the opioid of choice, yet it is not available in many parts of the world, whereas Tramadol is widely available and has potential advantages in its oral bioavailability, serotonergic properties, and possibly safety advantages over morphine (63). Despite potential advantages in newer treatments for neuropathic pain, the evidence base remains sparse, even for the popular gabapentinoids gabapentin and pregabalin. Interest in a potential role for psychostimulants such as methylphenidate in improving fatigue in terminally ill patients has been tempered by a recent Australian *N*-of-1 trial in 43 adults failing to demonstrate statistically significant efficacy, though 8 subjects reported "important" improvement (69). Finally, a cautionary note about opioids: with the dramatic rise in opioid-induced deaths in recent years, constituting a public health emergency, and lack of evidence for opioid safety or efficacy in treating chronic, rather than acute, pain, it is critical for physicians caring for children both to be assertive in prescribing opioids for severe, acute pain, and cautious in minimizing risk of overdose and nonefficacy for chronic pain (70).

Psychological and Behavioral

"Health professionals cannot choose to avoid using psychology to treat pain." McGrath and coworkers' formulation (71) provides a useful working model of the role of an array of psychological interventions for managing pediatric pain. The evidence base is limited but growing, and as McGrath (71) notes, "informal psychological interventions accompany every medical intervention . . . our choice is whether to use psychology in a conscious, constructive fashion or to leave the psychological aspect of our interventions to chance." The task of pain management for seriously ill children is to have command of empirically supported psychological and behavioral treatments, integrate them with pharmacologic treatment, and understand the "myths" (71) that needlessly limit them, especially that the need for psychological intervention implies psychopathology.

Historically, empirical support for psychological/behavioral pediatric pain management modalities has been strongest for medical procedures and headache (71). Progressive muscle relaxation, for example, first described by Jacobson (72), in which serial muscle groups are first tensed then relaxed, has demonstrated efficacy in treating pediatric medical procedure pain (73). Patients and parents typically like learning it, and it has no adverse effects, though muscle groups that have been the focus of tissue damage and pain should be avoided. Innovative clinical trials in adults show that training partners in such skills as muscle relaxation has both analgesic efficacy for the patient and enhances a sense of self-efficacy in the partner. Clinical experience suggests similar effects in pediatric pain management where the "partner" is a parent (74,75). Jay et al. (76), using a controlled repeated-measures counterbalanced design, studied a package of cognitive-behavioral (CB) interventions including guided imagery, distraction, and deep breathing in 56 children with leukemia between ages 3½ and 13 years undergoing bone marrow aspiration. Compared to the control condition of 30-minute preprocedure cartoon watching, children in the CB group exhibited significantly less behavioral distress, self-reported pain, and lower heart rate during the procedure. Kuttner and Solomon (77) reviewed the evidence for hypnosis in treating pediatric pain and suggest benefit in children as young as age 3 years (78). More recent reviews (63) cite increasingly robust, empirical support for the use of a spectrum of nonpharmacologic approaches to pediatric pain management including CB (79), guided imagery (80), hypnosis (81), biofeedback (82), and complementary-alternative approaches (83). Many of these more recent studies are not specific to palliative care populations; hopefully, these will be forthcoming. Encouragingly, clinical practice guidelines specific to particular pediatric medical disorders are starting to appear, such as a recently published palliative care curriculum for providers of patients with cystic fibrosis (84). The need to equip physicians-in-training with the requisite skills in pain management is exemplified by an Internet-based pediatric pain management module for medical students (85). Astute clinical judgment, with support in the literature (86), dictates that clinicians become skilled in integrated approaches to pediatric pain management combining pharmacologic and nonpharmacologic methods.

In summary, appropriate use of empirically validated pediatric pain assessment and management tools both pharmacologic and psychological requires that they be embedded "in good clinical pain practice" (71), including the principles that pain is inherently subjective and the child's report of it should be taken at face value; that pediatric pain should be measured and monitored over time; that sick children should be told, in developmentally appropriate terms, what is going to happen to them; and that parents should accompany their children undergoing medical procedures. Dyspnea, somnolence, nausea, and constipation, among other symptoms, must also consistently be addressed to ensure optimal quality of life even at the end of life.

ROLE OF THE CHILD PSYCHIATRIST

Pediatric palliative medicine and PPC clinical services in children's hospitals have undergone explosive growth since the previous edition of this text was published. Feudtner et al.'s recent survey found that from 1997 to 2004, 15 new PPC programs were established in U.S. children's hospitals compared to 52 new programs from 2005 to 2012 (87). Among 162 hospitals responding to the survey, 69% had PPC services. While formal inclusion and funding for child psychiatrists on palliative care teams varies considerably from center to center, Buxton (43) has argued persuasively for the unique contribution child psychiatrists can make to PPC:

> "Because child and adolescent psychiatrists have medical training, they can incorporate the complex biopsychosocial picture of this severely ill population into their diagnostic evaluations...and...their medical understanding of prognostication can help provide more complete psychosocial interventions and treatment recommendations. Without this expertise palliative care providers can misinterpret behaviors and lose opportunities to treat important elements of suffering."

Child psychiatrists' developmental perspective with their understanding that medically ill hospitalized children may regress is critical. Buxton gives the example of an overwhelmed, regressed pre-teen whose pain might better be assessed using a face-based scale rather than VAS; whereas in other patients, cognitive development of concepts of death and dying in children with life-threatening illness may accelerate relative to their healthy-age peers such that children younger than one might expect may want and are able to participate actively in stating their preferences in making advance care planning decisions (43).

Importantly, recent work by Muriel and colleagues (88) presents for the first time a model for the integration, conceptually and in clinical practice, of child psychiatry and palliative care.

Anxiety and Depression

Prevalence

Medical illness is a risk factor for psychiatric comorbidity, particularly anxiety (89) and depression. Anxiety disorders are the most prevalent of all psychiatric disorders of childhood to begin with, with an estimated lifetime prevalence of 15 to 20% (90). Prevalence rises to 20% to 35% in medically ill children (91). Point prevalence of anxiety of 14.3% in children with cancer and up to 63% of children with epilepsy have been reported (92,93). Anxiety symptoms in children with diabetes have been reported in one study to last up to 10 years after diagnosis (94).

While data vary, depression also appears to be more prevalent in medically ill children, as might be expected in a population stressed by life-threat, separation, prognostic uncertainty, and pain. Depression prevalence has been reported to be two to three times greater in children with diabetes than in the general population (95), 16.3% vs 8.6% in youths with asthma (96) and five times the rate in the general pediatric population in children with complex partial or absence epilepsy (93). Atypical clinical presentations in child and adolescent depression relative to adults, important distinctions to be made between depression and end-of-life "existential crises," and the major contribution of intractable pain to mood must all be carefully considered by the child psychiatrist in responding to consultations from pediatric teams to evaluate depression.

Risk of completed suicide in medically ill children has not been systematically compared to that in the general pediatric population. On the other hand, suicidal ideation is reportedly increased in children with epilepsy (93), and adult survivors of childhood cancer (97). No currently validated screening tools for suicidality in medically ill children exist, but thorough, nuanced clinical assessment must be regularly performed. One of us (JG) has treated an adolescent with end-stage liver disease, after two suicide attempts, who went on to liver transplantation after successful treatment for depression, illustrating that treatable psychiatric disorders need not exclude terminally ill pediatric patients from life-saving medical interventions.

Intervention

While the efficacy of behavioral and cognitive approaches to mitigating distress associated with medical procedures in children and youth is well established (98), there are few studies directed at interventions for non–procedure-related anxiety and depression specific to medically or terminally ill children. Advances in treatment for anxious and/or depressed youth in nonmedical settings, however, are relevant to pediatric medical and palliative care. The finding that inflammatory cytokines may be involved in the pathogenesis of both cancer and depression (99) suggests another mechanism whereby children with cancer might be at increased risk for mood disorders and a possible role for antidepressant use in some cases.

Clinicians should be mindful of confounding influences of serious medical illness on the diagnosis of anxiety and depression in youth. Somatic symptoms commonly associated with depression including fatigue, pain, and impaired appetite and sleep are so often caused by the underlying medical illness itself that cognitive symptoms of depression (guilt, feeling like a burden, and hopelessness) are widely considered to be much more useful in medical settings.

De Jong and Fombonne (100) published case reports of four prepubertal children with cancer and "DSM-IV depressive disorder" treated in open-label fashion with citalopram 10 mg. Using child and parent short forms of the Moods and Feelings Questionnaire (SMFQ) and the Hamilton Rating Scale for Depression (HAM-D), the authors report statistically significant mean reductions in depression severity for all three measures at week 12, with initial responses as early as week 2. An earlier pilot study of fluvoxamine in this population came to similar conclusions (92). In nonmedically ill children, the seminal Treatment of Adolescent Depression study (TADS) provides compelling evidence for the tolerability and efficacy of fluoxetine and cognitive-behavior therapy in combination in the treatment of adolescent depression (101). Choice of selective serotonin reuptake inhibitor (SSRI) in medically ill children and adolescents should be guided by relative risk of drug/drug interaction via CY P450, and elimination half-life, for both of which drugs such as escitalopram and citalopram may be preferable to others, particularly fluoxetine. Broad consensus that benzodiazepines can be associated with disinhibition, confusion and worsening of delirium, and antihistamines with cognitive and behavioral impairment due to anticholinergic effects, make these drug classes largely untenable in a medically ill pediatric population. Nonpharmacologic interventions for anxiety and depression in youth with life-threatening illness including expressive psychotherapy, narrative writing and an array of other techniques are central to the treatment of anxious or depressed medically ill youth, and are often first-line interventions prior to consideration of pharmacotherapy, for which the reader is referred to the recent review by Pao and Wiener (91).

SUMMARY

The prevalence of anxiety and depression in medically ill youth, and emerging data documenting the safety and efficacy of both pharmacologic and nonpharmacologic intervention strategies, highlight the central roles to be played by child and adolescent psychiatrists and allied mental health professionals in the comprehensive care of youth with life-threatening illness. Going forward, child psychiatrists will be increasingly essential members of PPC teams, as novel pharmacologic approaches to pain management and intractable depression with such novel agents as ketamine are studied and introduced, and with increasing recognition of the prevalence of and emerging assessment and treatment guidelines for delirium in seriously ill children. Child and adolescent psychiatrists' unique background as physician specialists in child development, family systems, psychodynamics, neurobiology, and psychopharmacology make a compelling case for their role in the growing specialty of pediatric palliative medicine.

BEREAVEMENT

Loss of a Child

Potential Risk Factors

Rando (102) identifies several characteristics of the loss or the mourner that increase the risk of a complicated mourning process for adults. Several factors relate to the nature of the death: sudden, unexpected death, especially when traumatic, violent, mutilating, or random; death resulting from an overly lengthy illness; death of a child; and death the mourner perceives as preventable. If the premorbid relationship with the deceased was marked by anger, ambivalence, or excessive dependence or the mourner has unaccommodated losses or stressors or mental illness, then there is also an increased risk of a complicated mourning process. In addition, complicated mourning is increased if the grief is "disenfranchised" such that the mourner does not perceive adequate social support for grieving because of invalidation of the loss (e.g., early pregnancy losses which are often not met with much overt social support) or the relationship (e.g., death of an ex-spouse).

Anticipatory grieving allows parents and others to experience graduated feelings of grief, while being reassured by the child's continued presence when such feelings become overwhelming. In this manner, anticipatory grieving may allow some of the "work" of grieving to be completed prior to the child's death. Unfortunately, family members (and hospital staff) often engage in anticipatory grieving at a different pace. At times, a parent (or often a hospital staff member) may prematurely disengage from a child who is dying and be seen by others, including the child who is dying, as abandoning the child. Often, unacceptable thoughts arise. For example, parents may find themselves wishing that the child would finally die and relieve everyone of the emotional and financial burden and suffering. Such a wish may horrify a parent and lead to the immediate mobilization of certain defense mechanisms. A common defense mechanism is that of reaction formation whereby the parent becomes extra protective in caring for the dying child. The parent also may feel guilty and express his or her guilt (and anxiety) by asking repetitive questions that require tactful answers. As a chronically ill child nears death, the parents may be filled with remorse and may experience a resurgence of love. Rarely, a denial that death is imminent may remain in force. After the death of a chronically ill child, parents may feel a mixture of relief and guilt, perhaps with feelings of remorse being uppermost (103).

While it is critical to involve parents in decision-making regarding their child's treatment, the health care team should not use this as an excuse to avoid assuming the difficult responsibility of formulating treatment recommendations. In particular, when further treatment is futile and when the child is being maintained on life support, the health care team should convey to the family that the child has died and invite input from the family members about whether they would like to be present when life support is removed and their preferences on timing, without leading them to believe they are being asked whether they believe treatment is likely be effective or whether or not they "wish to allow (their child) to die." Psychiatrists can also guide the medical team on how best to notify members of the family of a child's death and, especially when children are involved, participate in the process as appropriate (103).

Funeral Attendance

Parents should be provided information about the potential benefits for grieving children of attending funerals and participating in other observances and offered advice on how to provide support to children in these settings. Based on clinical experience, it has been shown to be helpful to advise family members to appoint someone, preferably who is not directly impacted by the death, that understands children's developmental needs and that the child knows and trusts to explain in simple terms what should be expected during the funeral or other ritual, to invite the child to participate to the level that he or she is comfortable, and to accompany the child throughout the event(s). This adult can then monitor the child's reactions and allow the child to leave the ceremony whenever desired. Children often can use the funeral rite in the same way adults do, especially if they have adults in attendance who can help them understand their feelings and describe what is taking place. Children who do not wish to attend the funeral should not be made to do so or to feel guilty. Rather, arrangements should be made for them to be in the company of an understanding adult during the time of the funeral. Older children should be encouraged to participate in the rites and rituals with the adults because these practices usually help them to deal with the reality of death and to access comfort and support from family members and friends. If older children choose not to attend the funeral, the reason for the choice should be explored, but if they continue to feel that they do not want to attend, this wish should be respected. Children should not be forced or coerced to participate directly in any portion of the ceremony that they find distressing, such as throwing dirt on the casket or kissing or touching the body of the deceased (16,104).

Advance Care Planning

As noted, comprehensive care of children with life-threatening illness is not limited to dying children. Whether the ultimate outcome is cure, chronic illness, or death, early intervention by the palliative medicine team is crucial: "Until we define the palliative medicine clientele as all children who have a life-limiting condition, even while they are receiving the most aggressive curative therapy possible, we will remain in the untenable position we are in: Palliative medicine teams are allowed in the door for children only when children are very close to death, far too late for the team to forge relationships" (105). Moreover, legal and ethical tensions and uncertainties often complicate end-of-life decision-making and take time to be resolved. Psychiatrists and ethicists may recognize the appropriateness of a competent adolescent to decline aggressive treatment, for example, but state laws may forbid it (2). Himelstein outlines four components to advance planning: (1) identification of the decision-makers; (2) clarification of patient and parents' understanding of the illness and prognosis; (3) establishment of care goals: curative, uncertain, or comfort care; and (4) joint decision-making regarding use or nonuse of life-sustaining medical interventions such as mechanical ventilation, intravenous hydration or phase I chemotherapy (2). Clearly, decisions of this breadth and depth take time. Ideally, palliative care teams become involved early as partners of the primary team: "Palliative care teams work alongside of, not instead of, the primary team. Rather than taking over, they complement that team's efforts. They ease some of the burden of caring for and communicating with the family when complex medical and psychosocial decisions must be made" (105). Advance care planning with adolescents and young adults has been growing in recognition over the past decade including randomized controlled trials of family centered advance care planning in youth and their families with HIV/AIDS (106) and cancer (107). A systematic review has been reported (108). To date only one developmentally appropriate advance care planning guide, *Voicing My Choices,* a seminal collaboration of the National Institute of Mental Health and National Cancer Institute, has been created specifically for adolescents and young adults (109,110), showing great promise in empowering patients to systematically and specifically articulate their uniquely personal wishes regarding end-of-life care.

Special Situations

Parents and Siblings

Parents' response to the death of a child has been addressed in several studies (111). In a study of 21,062 Danish parents with a child who died, mortality from "natural" (cancer, cardiovascular, digestive) and "unnatural" (motor vehicle accidents and suicide) causes was statistically significantly higher 10 to 18 years after childhood death than in control parents who had not lost a child (112). "Persistent Complex Bereavement Disorder" is classified in DSM-5 as a "condition for further study," not a psychiatric disorder per se, though clinical resemblance to major depressive disorder is common (113). Purported differences in symptom expression and impairment in "normal" and "complicated" grief may not be robust (114). Siblings also require clinical attention (115,116). Active outreach to siblings is important prior and subsequent to a child's death; recent clinical guidance from the AAP provides detailed practical advice on how such support can be provided to grieving children and families within a pediatric medical home setting (117). In particular, the impact on older children and adolescents of sibling death is often underappreciated. Parents who are themselves mourning and feeling overwhelmed may be reluctant to appreciate the suffering of the siblings and may in fact turn to them for their own support. It is vital for the medical team, whether hospital-, hospice- or outpatient-based, to provide systematic, clinically sophisticated support and intervention either from a member of the palliative care team or through referrals to community-based psychological, pediatric, school-based (16,30,118) and if appropriate, religious resources. Critical to this process is the palliative care team's active follow-up contact with the family after the child's death.

The psychiatrist can also work with the child's school to offer advice and assistance to peers and school staff after the time of death and to better equip classroom teachers and other school professionals to support grieving siblings (16). A recent survey of educators showed that classroom teachers are well aware of the importance of providing bereavement support to grieving students, but only 7% had ever received any training on this topic and felt that this lack of training was the primary barrier that prevented them from reaching out to their students to offer support. The Coalition to Support Grieving Students, that includes 10 of the major professional associations and unions representing educators, school administrators (including both principals and superintendents), school counselors, nurses, psychologists, and social workers, has recently produced a wide variety of video-based and print materials to address this need, which is freely available at www.grievingstudents.org.

Child's Loss of a Parent

Four percent of children will experience the death of a parent before their 15th birthday (14). Since adults as well as children with life-limiting illness are living longer, needed attention is being paid to the psychosocial needs of these children (117). After a review of the literature on bereavement in childhood, the Institute of Medicine (119) summarized the factors that are associated with an increased risk of psychological morbidity for children after the death of a parent or sibling:

1. Loss in a child younger than 5 years of age, or during early adolescence
2. Loss of a mother for girls younger than 11 years of age, and loss of a father for adolescent boys
3. Premorbid psychological difficulties in the child or lack of prior knowledge about death
4. When the relationship with the deceased had been conflicted or when the parent remarries and there is a poor relationship between the child and the stepparent
5. When the surviving parent is psychologically vulnerable and excessively dependent on the child, or the environment is unstable and inconsistent
6. When there is a lack of adequate family or community supports, or when the surviving parent is unable to access available supports
7. When the death was unanticipated or the result of suicide or homicide

Providers

Hospital staff members also experience anxiety in the presence of a dying child or a grieving parent, and they may tend at times to deal with that anxiety by withdrawal and a conspiracy of silence. These reactions may impair their ability to give the dying child and his or her family the best care possible.

The death of a patient is one of the most stressful personal and professional experiences faced by health care providers. Clinicians need to understand their personal feelings about death in order to be effective in providing support to children who have experienced the death of a loved one, or who are faced with their own impending death. Often this will involve on the part of the physician some introspection about prior personal losses. But perhaps most important, health care providers should remain conscious of the impact that helping children who are dying or grieving has on both their professional and personal lives, and they should seek and establish means of meeting their own personal needs regarding bereavement (117).

Jellinek (120), Frader (121), and others have addressed the special challenges to physicians and allied professionals in the care of seriously ill children, particularly physicians in training. Biologic and psychological patient outcomes, from glucose homeostasis to pain control, are strongly associated with the quality of provider–patient communication. Models for training physicians and allied professionals in patient-centered communication exist, have been evaluated, and are effective (122). Operationalizing provider communications training is challenging, but possible, and is now required in residency training programs by ACGME mandate. An important review on this topic has recently been published (123).

SUMMARY: PALLIATIVE CARE, RELATIONSHIPS, AND MEDICAL EDUCATION

Bowlby's marriage of ethology, neuroscience, and psychoanalysis gave child psychiatry a language for understanding and investigating attachment, separation, and loss (124). This biologic substrate, mediating and mediated by experience, is brought sharply into focus by life-threatening illness. Loss is universal, but the loss of a child—jarring, unexpected, and unnatural—is as severe a stress as the child or the child's parents and siblings can experience. Fortunately, clinical studies demonstrate that gravely ill children and their parents may both endure and even grow under the right circumstances at least some of the time. Hinds et al. (125) evaluated 10- to 20-year olds with advanced cancer within 7 days of one of three decisions: (1) whether to enroll in a phase I clinical trial; (2) whether to support a do not resuscitate order; or (3) whether to limit care to comfort measures and forgo life sustaining treatment. Both children and adolescents in the study understood they were making end-of-life decisions, and strikingly, expressed altruistic motives—the wish to help others unknown to them—in their decision-making, for example, participation in a phase I trial knowing it would not be lifesaving for them but could be for others. Similarly, Mack et al. (126) found in an interview study of parents whose children died of cancer that parent ratings of the quality of the child's care was directly proportional to the quality of physician communication. Parent-reported attributes of "quality communication" by physicians included providing clear information about what to expect at the end of life, conveying bad news sensitively, and including the child patient in discussion when appropriate.

Pediatric palliative medicine is an established, growing multidisciplinary subspecialty. Child and adolescent psychiatrists and allied professionals are uniquely qualified to play key roles on palliative care teams with their special expertise in addressing issues of attachment, separation, and loss universally experienced. Historically, there has been little attention in medical school curricula to training students in the competencies necessary to provide quality communication and caregiving to life-threatened children and their families; as noted, medical educators are recognizing and remediating this. As of this writing, Northwestern and Harvard Medical Schools offer educational programs on palliative care, including pediatrics (127,128). Such efforts must be encouraged, expanded, and their impact on the quality of medical education and clinical care systematically evaluated.

ACKNOWLEDGMENT

The authors wish to acknowledge Melvin Lewis, MB, BS, FRCPsych, DCH for his important contributions to earlier editions of this chapter.

References

1. Osterman MJ, Kochanek KD, MacDorman MF, Strobino DM, Guyer B: Annual summary of vital statistics: 2012-2013. *Pediatrics* 135:1115–1125, 2015.
2. Himelstein BP, Hilden JM, Boldt AM, Weissman D: Pediatric palliative care. *New Engl J Med* 350:1752–1762, 2004.
3. Ullrich C, Duncan J, Joselow M, et al.: Pediatric palliative care. In: Kliegman RM, Stanton B, St. Geme J, Schor N (eds): *Nelson Textbook of Pediatrics*. 20th ed. Philadelphia, PA, Elsevier, 256–267, 2015.
4. American Academy of Pediatrics: Policy statement: pediatric palliative care and hospice care commitments, guidelines, and recommendations. *Pediatrics* 132:966–972, 2013.
5. WHO. *Definition of Palliative Care [Internet]*. Geneva, World Health Organization [cited 2016 March 21]. Available at: http://www.who.int/cancer/palliative/definition/en/.
6. *Memorandum to State Survey Agency Directors*. Baltimore, MD, Centers for Medicare & Medicaid Services; 2012 September 27. Available at: https://www.cms.gov/Medicare/Provider-Enrollment-and-Certification/SurveyCertificationGenInfo/Downloads/Survey-and-Cert-Letter-12-48.pdf.
7. The Patient Protection and Affordable Care Act Appendix 1: *Pub. L. 111-148, 124 Stat. 896 (Mar. 23, 2010), as amended by The Healthcare and Education Reconciliation Act of 2010, Pub. L. 111-152, 124 Stat. 1029 (Mar. 30, 2010).*
8. Hilden JM: *(University of Colorado Cancer Center, Aurora, CO). Personal communication with Glazer JP (Cleveland Clinic Section of Child & Adolescent Psychiatry)*, 2006.
9. WHO: *WHO Guidelines on the Pharmacological Treatment of Persisting Pain in Children with Medical Illnesses*. Geneva, World Health Organization, 2012.
10. *Pediatric Hospice and Palliative Care [Internet]*. Alexandria: National Hospice and Palliative Care Organization; 2012 [cited 2016 March 21]. Available at: http://www.nhpco.org/pediatric.
11. Weaver MS, Heinze KE, Kelly KP, et al.: Palliative care as a standard of care in pediatric oncology. *Pediatr Blood Cancer* 62:S829–S833, 2015.
12. Solnit AJ: Changing perspectives: preparing for life or death. In: Schowalter JE, Patterson PR, Tallmer M, Kutscher AH, Gullo SV, Perets D (eds): *The Child and Death*. New York, Columbia University Press, 3–18, 1983.
13. Stedman TL: *Stedman's Medical Dictionary*. Baltimore, MD, Williams & Wilkins, 1966.
14. Sood AB, Razdan A, Weller EB, Weller RA: Children's reactions to parent and sibling death. *Curr Psychiatry Rep* 8:115–120, 2006.
15. Schonfeld DJ: Talking with children about death. *J Pediatr Health Care* 7:269–274, 1993.
16. Schonfeld DJ, Quackenbush M: *The Grieving Student: A Teacher's Guide*. Baltimore, MD, Brookes Publishing, 2010.
17. Hostler S: The development of the child's concept of death. In: Sahler O (ed): *The Child and Death*. St. Louis, Mosby, 1–25, 1978.
18. Kastenbaum R: The child's understanding of death: how does it develop? In: Grollman E (ed): *Explaining Death to Children*. Boston, MA, Beacon Press, 89–108, 1967.
19. Smilansky S: *On Death: Helping Children Understand and Cope*. New York, Peter Lang, 1987.
20. Speece MW, Brent SB: Children's understanding of death: a review of three components of a death concept. *Child Dev* 55:1671–1686, 1984.
21. Wass H: Concepts of death: a developmental perspective. In: Wass H, Corr CA (eds): *Childhood and Death*. Washington, Hemisphere, 3–24, 1984.
22. Lansky SB, Cairns GF, Stephenson L, Weller E, Cairns GF Jr, Cairns NU: Failure to thrive during infancy in siblings of pediatric cancer patients. *Am J Pediatr Hematol Oncol1* 4:361–366, 1982.
23. Betz CL, Poster EC: Children's concepts of death: implications for pediatric practice. *Nurs Clin North Am* 19:341–349, 1984.
24. Maurer A: Maturation of concepts of death. *Brit J Med Psychol* 39:35–41, 1966.
25. Kane B: Children's concepts of death. *J Gen Psychol* 134:141–153, 1979.
26. Reilly TP, Hasazi JE, Bond LA: Children's conceptions of death and personal mortality. *J Pediatr Psychol* 8:21–31, 1983.
27. Jenkins RA, Cavanaugh JC: Examining the relationship between the development of the concept of death and overall cognitive development. *Omega-J Death Dying* 16:193–199, 1986.
28. Townley K, Thornburg KR: Maturation of the concept of death in elementary school children. *Educ Res Q* 5:17–24, 1980.
29. Florian V, Kravetz S: Children's concepts of death: a cross-cultural comparison among Muslims, Druze, Christians, and Jews in Israel. *J Cross Cult Psychol* 16:174–189, 1985.
30. Schonfeld DJ, Smilansky S: A cross-cultural comparison of Israeli and American children's death concepts. *Death Stud* 13:593–604, 1989.
31. Wass H, Guenther ZC, Towry BJ: United States and Brazilian children's concepts of death. *Death Educ* 3:41–55, 1979.
32. Schonfeld DJ, Kappelman M: The impact of school-based education on the young child's understanding of death. *J Dev Behav Pediatr* 11:247–252, 1990.
33. Clunies-Ross C, Landsdown R: Concepts of death, illness, and isolation found in children with leukemia. *Child Care Health Dev* 14:373–386, 1988.
34. Spinetta JJ: The dying child's awareness of death: a review. *Psychol Bull* 81:256–260, 1974.
35. Cassel EJ: The nature of suffering and the goals of medicine. *New Engl J Med* 306:639–645, 1982.
36. Wolfe J, Grier HE, Klar N, et al.: Symptoms and suffering at the end of life in children with cancer. *N Engl J Med* 342:326–333, 2000.
37. Marskey H, Albe-Fessard DG, Bonica JJ: Pain terms: a list with definitions and notes on usage. *Pain* 6:249, 1979.
38. Schechter NL, Berde CB, Yaster M: Pain in infants, children, and adolescents: an overview. In: Schechter NL, Berde CB, Yaster M (eds): *Pain in Infants, Children, and Adolescents*. Philadelphia, PA, Lippincott Williams & Wilkins, 3–18, 2003.
39. Eland JM, Anderson JE: The experience of pain in children. In: Jacox AK (ed): *Pain: A Source Book for Nurses and Other Health Professionals*. Boston, MA, Little Brown, 453–473, 1977.
40. Swafford LI, Allan D: Pain relief in the pediatric patient. *Med Clin North Am* 52:131–136, 1968.
41. Anand KJ, Hansen DD, Hickey PR: Hormonal metabolic stress response in neonates undergoing cardiac surgery. *Anesthesiology* 73:661–670, 1990.
42. Wolfe J, Hammel JF, Edwards KE, et al.: Easing of suffering in children with cancer at the end of life: is care changing? *J Clin Oncol* 26:1717–1723, 2008.

43. Buxton D: Child and adolescent psychiatry and palliative care. *J Am Acad Child Adolesc Psychiatry* 54:791–792, 2015.
44. Hongo T, Watanbe C, Okada S, et al.: Analysis of the circumstances at the end of life in children with cancer: symptoms, suffering and acceptance. *Pediatri Int* 45:60–64, 2003.
45. McCallum DE, Byrne P, Bruera E: How children die in hospital. *J Pain Symptom Manage* 20:417–423, 2000.
46. McCulloch R, Collins JJ: Pain in children who have life-limiting conditions. *Child Adolesc Psychiatr Clin N Am* 15:657–682, 2006.
47. Collins JJ, Berde CB, Frost JA: Pain assessment and management. In: Wolfe J, Hinds P, Sourkes B (eds): *Textbook of Interdisciplinary Pediatric Palliative Care*. Philadelphia, PA, Elsevier, 284–299, 2011.
48. Schechter NL: The development of pain perception and principles of pain control. In: Lewis M (ed): *Child and Adolescent Psychiatry: A Comprehensive Textbook*. Philadelphia, PA, Lippincott Williams & Wilkins, 408, 2002.
49. Champion GD, Goodenough B, von Baeyer CL, et al.: Measurement of pain by self-report. In: Finley G, McGrath P (eds): *Measurement of Pain in Infants and Children*. Seattle, IASP Press, 5–20, 1998.
50. Hicks CL, von Baeyer CL, Spafford PA, van Korlaar I, Goodenough B: The faces pain scale revised: toward a common metric in pediatric pain measurement. *Pain* 93:173–183, 2001.
51. Hunter M, McDowell L, Hennessy R, Cassey J: An evaluation of the faces pain scale with young children. *J Pain Symptom Manage* 20:122–129, 2000.
52. McGrath PA, Gillespie JM: Pain assessment in children and adolescents. In. Turk DC, Melzack R (eds): *Handbook of Pain Assessment*. 2nd ed. New York, Guilford Press, 97–118, 2001.
53. Shih AR, von Baeyer CL: Preschool children's seriation of pain faces and happy faces in the affective facial scale. *Psychol Rep* 74:659–665, 1994.
54. St-Laurent-Gagnon T, Bernard-Bonnin AC, Villeneuve E: Pain evaluation in preschool children and their parents. *Acta Paediatr* 88:422–427, 1999.
55. Bieri D, Reeve RA, Champion GD, Addicoat L, Ziegler JB: The faces pain scale for the self-assessment of the severity of pain experienced by children: development, initial validation, and preliminary investigation for ratio scale properties. *Pain* 41:139–150, 1990.
56. Beyer JE, Wells N: The assessment of pain in children. *Pediatr Clin North Am* 36:837–854, 1989.
57. Hester NO, Foster RL, Kristensen K: Measurement of pain in children: generalizability and validity of the pain ladder and the poker-chip tool. *Pediatr Pain* 15:79–84, 1990.
58. Gauvain-Piquard A, Rodary C, Rezvani A, Serbouti S: The development of the DEGR(R): a scale to assess pain in young children with cancer. *Eur J Pain* 3(2):165–176, 1999.
59. Marec-Berard P, Gomez F, Combet S, Thibault P, Moine PL, Bergeron C: HEDEN Pain Scale: a shortened behavioral scale for assessment of prolonged cancer or postsurgical pain in children aged 2 to 6 years. *Pediatr Hematol Oncol* 32:291–303, 2015.
60. WHO: *Cancer Pain Relief and Palliative Care*. Geneva, World Health Organization, 1990. Technical Report Series: 804.
61. WHO: *Cancer Pain Relief and Palliative Care in Children*. Geneva, World Health Organization, 1998.
62. Friedrichsdorf SJ, Nugent AP, Strobl AQ: Codeine-associated pediatric deaths despite using recommended dosing guidelines: three case reports. *J Opioid Manag* 9:151–155, 2013.
63. Downing J, Jassal SS, Mathew L, Brits H, Friedrichsdorf SJ: Pediatric pain management in palliative care. *Pain Manag* 51:23–35, 2015.
64. Friedrichsdorf SJ, Nugent AP: Management of neuropathic pain in children with cancer. *Cur Opin Support Palliat Care* 7:131–138, 2013.
65. Taylor M, Jakacki R, May C, Howrie D, Maurer S: Ketamine PCA for treatment of end-of-life neuropathic pain in pediatrics. *Am J Hosp Palliat Care* 32:841–848, 2015.
66. Larsson P, Nordlinder A, Bergendahl HT, et al.: Oral bioavailability of clonidine in children. *Peadiatr Anaesth* 21:335–340, 2011.
67. Mahmoud M, Mason KP: A forecast of relevant pediatric sedation trends. *Curr Opin Anaesthesiol* 29 (Suppl 1):S56–S67, 2016.
68. Roback MG, Carlson DW, Babl FE, Kennedy RM: Update on pharmacological management of procedural sedation for children. *Curr Opin Anaesthesiol* 29 (Suppl 1):S21–S35, 2016.
69. Mitchell GK, Hardy JR, Niles CJ, et al.: The effect of methylphenidate on fatigue in advanced cancer: an aggregated N-of-1 trial. *J Pain Symptom Manage* 50:289–296, 2015.
70. Volkow ND, McLellan AT: Opioid abuse in chronic pain—misconceptions and mitigation strategies. *N Engl J Med* 374:1253–1263, 2016.
71. McGrath PJ, Dick B, Unruh AM: Psychologic and behavioral treatment of pain in children and adolescents. In: Schechter NL, Berde CB, Yaster M (eds): *Pain in Infants, Children, and Adolescents*. Philadelphia, PA, Lippincott Williams & Wilkins, 303–316, 2003.
72. Jacobson E: *You Must Relax*. New York, McGraw-Hill, 1957.
73. Powers SW: Empirically supported treatments in pediatric psychology: procedure-related pain. *J Pediatr Psychol* 24:131–145, 1999.
74. Bauchner H, Vinci R, Bak S, Pearson C, Corwin MJ: Parents and procedures: a randomized controlled trial. *Pediatrics* 98:861–867, 1996.
75. Yaldoo-Poltorak D, Benore E: Cognitive-behavioral interventions for physical symptom management in pediatric palliative medicine. *Child Adolesc Psychiatr Clin N Am* 15:683–691, 2006.
76. Jay SM, Elliot CH, Katz E, Siegel SE: Cognitive-behavioral and pharmacologic interventions for children's distress during painful medical procedures. *J Consult Clin Psychol* 55:861–865, 1987.
77. Kuttner L, Solomon R: Hypnotherapy and imagery for managing children's pain. In: Schechter NL, Berde CB, Yaster M (eds): *Pain in Infants, Children, and Adolescents*. Philadelphia, PA, Lippincott Williams & Wilkins, 317–328, 2003.
78. Felt BT, Mollen E, Diaz S, et al.: Behavioral interventions reduce infant distress at immunization. *Arch Pediatr Adolesc Med* 154:719–724, 2000.
79. Eccleston C, Palermo TM, Williams AC, et al.: Psychological therapies for the management of chronic and recurrent pain in children and adolescents. *Cochrane Database Syst Rev* 5:CD003968, 2014.
80. Petter M, Chambers CT, MacLaren Chorney J: The effects of mindfulness-based attention on cold pressor pain in children. *Pain Res Manag* 18:39–45, 2013.
81. Gulewitsch MD, Müller J, Hautzinger M, Schlarb AA.: Brief hypnotherapeutic-behavioral intervention for functional abdominal pain and irritable bowel syndrome in childhood: a randomized controlled trial. *Eur J Pediatr* 172:1043–1051, 2013.
82. Palermo TM, Eccleston C, Lewandowski AS, Williams AC, Morley S: Randomized controlled trials of psychological therapies for management of chronic pain in children and adolescents: an updated meta-analytic review. *Pain* 148:387–397, 2010.
83. *National Center for Complementary and Integrative Health [Internet]*. Bethesda: U.S. Department of Health & Human Services, National Institutes of Health; [updated 2016 February 22; cited 2016 March 21]. Available at: https://nccih.nih.gov/.
84. Linnemann RW, O'Malley PJ, Friedman D, et al.: Development and evaluation of a palliative care curriculum for cystic fibrosis healthcare providers. *J Cyst Fibros* 15:90–95, 2016.
85. Ameringer S, Fisher D, Sreedhar S, Ketchum JM, Yanni L: Pediatric pain management education in medical students: impact of a web-based module. *J Palliat Med* 15:978–983, 2012.
86. Friedrichsdorf SJ, Kuttner L, Westendorp K, McCarty R: Integrative pediatric palliative care. In: Culbert TP, Olness K (eds): *Integrative Pediatrics*. New York, Oxford University Press, 569–593, 2010.
87. Feudtner C, Womer J, Augustin R, et al.: Pediatric palliative care programs in children's hospitals: a cross-sectional national survey. *Pediatrics* 132:1063–1070, 2013.
88. Muriel AC, Wolfe J, Block SD: Pediatric palliative care and child psychiatry: A model for enhancing practice and collaboration. *Journal of Palliative Medicine* 20:1–7, 2016.
89. Pao M, Bosk A: Anxiety in medically ill children/adolescents. *Depress Anxiety* 28:40–49, 2011.
90. Beesdo K, Knappe S, Pine DS: Anxiety and anxiety disorders in children and adolescents: developmental issues and implications for DSM-V. *Psychiatr Clin North Am* 32:483–524, 2006.
91. Pao M, Wiener L: Psychological symptoms. In: Wolfe J, Hinds PS, Sourkes BM (eds): *Textbook of Interdisciplinary Pediatric Palliative Care*. Philadelphia, PA, Elsevier, 229–238, 2011.
92. Gothelf D, Rubinstein M, Shemesh E, et al.: Pilot study: fluvoxamine treatment for depression and anxiety disorders in children and adolescents with cancer. *J Am Acad Child Adolesc Psychiatry* 44:1258–1262, 2005.
93. Caplan R, Siddarth P, Gurbani S, Hanson R, Sankar R, Shields WD: Depression and anxiety disorders in pediatric epilepsy. *Epilepsia* 46:720–730, 2005.
94. Kovacs M, Goldston D, Obrosky DS, Bonar LK: Psychiatric disorders in youths with IDDM: rates and risk factors. *Diabetes Care* 20:36–44, 1997.
95. Kokkonen J, Taabuka A, Kokkonen ER: Diabetes in adolescence: the effect of family and psychologic factors on metabolic control. *Nord J Psychiatry* 51:165–172, 1997.
96. Katon W, Lozano P, Russo J, McCauley E, Richardson L, Bush T: The prevalence of DSM-IV anxiety and depressive disorders in youth with asthma compared with controls. *J Adolesc Health* 41:455–463, 2007.
97. Recklitis CJ, Lockwood RA, Rothwell MA, Diller LR: Suicidal ideation and attempts in adult survivors of childhood cancer. *J Clin Oncol* 24:3852–3857, 2006.
98. Spirito A, Kazak AE: *Effective and Emerging Treatments in Pediatric Psychology*. New York, Oxford University Press, 2006.
99. Miller AH, Maletic V, Raison CL: Inflammation and its discontents: the role of cytokines in the pathophysiology of major depression. *Biol Psychiatry* 65:732–741, 2009.
100. DeJong M, Fombonne E: Citalopram to treat depression in pediatric oncology. *J Child Adolesc Psychopharmacol* 17:371–377, 2007.
101. TADS Team: The treatment for adolescents with depression study (TADS). *Arch Gen Psychiatry* 64:1132–1144, 2007.
102. Rando TA: *Treatment of Complicated Mourning*. Champaign, Research Press, 1993.
103. Schonfeld DJ: Providing support for families experiencing the death of a child. In: Kreitler S, Ben-Arush MW, Martin A (eds): *Pediatric Psycho-oncology: Psychosocial Aspects and Clinical Interventions*. 2nd ed. Hoboken, John Wiley & Sons, 223–230, 2012.
104. Lewis M, Lewis DO, Schonfeld DJ: Dying and death in childhood and adolescence. In: Lewis M (ed): *Child and Adolescent Psychiatry: A Comprehensive Textbook*. Baltimore, MD, Williams & Wilkins, 1057, 1991.

105. Glazer JP, Hilden JM, Yaldoo-Poltorak D: Pediatric palliative medicine. *Child Adolesc Psychiatr Clin N Am* 15:567–573 xvii–xx, 2006.
106. Lyon ME, Garvie PA, McCarter R, Briggs L, He J, D'Angelo LJ: Who will speak for me? Improving end-of-life decision-making for adolescents with HIV and their families. *Pediatrics* 123:e199–e206, 2009.
107. Lyon ME, Jacobs S, Briggs L, Cheng YI, Wang J: Family-centered advance care planning for teens with cancer. *JAMA Pediatr* 167:460–467, 2013.
108. Lotz JD, Jox RJ, Borasio GD, Führer M: Pediatric advance care planning: a systematic review. *Pediatrics* 131:e873–e880, 2013.
109. Wiener L, Zadeh S, Battles H, et al.: Allowing adolescents and young adults to plain their end-of-life care. *Pediatrics* 130:897–905, 2012.
110. Zadeh S, Pao M, Wiener L: Opening end-of-life discussions: how to introduce Voicing My CHOiCES™, an advance care planning guide for adolescents and young adults. *Palliat Support Care* 13:591–599, 2015.
111. Dyregrov, A: Parental reactions to the loss of an infant child: a review. *Scand J Psychol* 31:266–280, 1990.
112. Li J, Precht DH, Mortensen PB, Olsen J: Mortality in parents after death of a child in Denmark: a nationwide follow-up study. *Lancet* 361:363–367, 2003.
113. American Psychiatric Association: *Diagnostic and Statistical Manual of Mental Disorders: DSM-5*. Washington, American Psychiatric Association, 2013.
114. Ginzburg K, Geron Y, Solomon Z: Patterns of complicated grief among bereaved parents. *Omega-J Death Dying* 45:119–132, 2002.
115. Davies B: *Shadows in the Sun: The Experiences of Sibling Bereavement in Childhood*. Philadelphia, PA, Brunner/Mazel, 1999.
116. Christ G, Bonanno G, Malkinson R, Rubin SS: Bereavement experiences after the death of a child. In: Field M, Behrman R (eds): *When Children Die: Improving Palliative and End-of-Life Care for Children and their Families*. Washington, National Academies Press, 553–579, 2003.
117. Schonfeld DJ, Demaria T: American Academy of Pediatrics, Committee on Psychosocial Aspects of Child and Family Health, Disaster Preparedness Advisory Council. Supporting the Grieving Child and Family. *Pediatrics* 138(3):e2016-e2147, 2016.
118. Newgass S, Schonfeld DJ: School crisis intervention, crisis prevention, and crisis response. In: Roberts A (ed): *Crisis Intervention Handbook: Assessment, Treatment and Research*. 3rd ed. New York, Oxford University Press, 499–518, 2005.
119. Osterweis M, Solomon F, Green M, eds: *Bereavement: Reactions, Consequences, and Care*. Washington, National Academy Press, 1984.
120. Jellinek MS, Todres ID, Catlin EA, Cassem EH, Salzman A: Pediatric intensive care training: confronting the dark side. *Crit Care Med* 21:775–779, 1993.
121. Frader JE: Difficulties in providing intensive care. *Pediatrics* 64:10–16, 1979.
122. Stewart MA: Effective physician-patient communication and health outcomes: a review. *Can Med Assoc J* 152:1423–1433, 1995.
123. Feraco AM, Brand SR, Mack JW, Kesselheim JC, Block SD, Wolfe J:. Communication skills training in pediatric oncology: moving beyond role modeling. *Pediatr Blood Cancer* 63(6):966–972, 2016.
124. Bowlby J: The making and breaking of affectional bonds. I. Aetiology and psychopathology in the light of attachment theory: an expanded version of the fiftieth Maudsley lecture, delivered before the Royal College of Psychiatrists. *Br J Psychiatry* 130:201–210, 1977.
125. Hinds P, Drew D, Oakes LL, et al.: End-of-life care preferences of pediatric patients with cancer. *J Clin Oncol* 23:9146–9154, 2005.
126. Mack JW, Hilden JM, Watterson J, et al.: Parent and physician perspectives on quality of care at the end of life in children with cancer. *J Clin Oncol* 23:9155–9161, 2005.
127. *Welcome to EPEC Program [Internet]*. Chicago: Northwestern University Feinberg School of Medicine Education in Palliative and End-of-life Care; 2006 [updated 2016 February 23; cited 2016 March 21]. Available at: http://www.epec.net/.
128. *PCEP [Internet]*. Boston, MA, Harvard Medical School Center for Palliative Care; [updated 2016 January 20; cited 2016 March 21]. Available at: http://www.hms.harvard.edu/pallcare/PCEP/PCEP.htm.<br clear=all style='page-break-before:always'>

7.3 ■ SCHOOLS

CHAPTER 7.3 ■ SCHOOL CONSULTATION

JEFF Q. BOSTIC AND SHARON A. HOOVER

Schools are among the most valuable sites for child psychiatrists to promote mental health. Almost all children attend schools, where many of their unique needs can be addressed daily by committed professional school staff. Symptoms of psychopathology usually manifest across home and school settings, yet the range of interventions is often much wider in schools where classrooms, school staff, and instructional/behavioral approaches to the child can be configured to optimize the fit between child and school.

As psychiatric hospitalization continues to give way to treatment efforts in more naturalistic settings, schools have become primary venues for management of mental health by child psychiatrists. At one end of the spectrum, the *school psychiatrist* provides *direct* treatment to students or staff. This direct treatment usually occurs on-site at the school and may include face-to-face evaluations of students or staff, individual or group therapy, or medication management. This allows teachers and staff to access the child psychiatrist for specific mental health issues, and allows the child psychiatrist to factor in the school's resources and philosophy in devising interventions. At the other end of the spectrum, the *school consultant* advises school staff, providing *indirect* services to students by assisting school personnel. The consultant may meet with administrators concerned about how best to respond to the death of a teacher, or to provide recommendations to help teachers work with students who have depression, attention or disruptive behavior problems, autism, or other special needs. Child psychiatrists often blend these roles, sometimes treating and advocating for a patient, and sometimes consulting various school staff around complex problems (1).

Child psychiatrists will continue to become essential partners in schooling children, not just those children identified with psychopathology, but all children. The mental health consultant is often able to benefit many more children than would be possible through providing direct service on-site at a school. Of those children with a diagnosable mental health disorder, less than half receive treatment, and over 75% receive this treatment at schools as attrition rates remain high for mental health treatment outside of schools (2,3). Proactive efforts to prevent and diminish psychopathology will continue to supplant reactive, treatment-only approaches employed only in response to crises or emergence of psychiatric disorders. Child psychiatrists will continue to provide input on specific emotional disabilities, and increasingly promote mental health for all students, providing input on programs and principles found effective for everything from combating depression to decreasing bullying, and by working directly with educators to adapt effective treatments to diverse school environments (4).

EMERGENCE OF SCHOOL MENTAL HEALTH SERVICES

Mental health entwined with schools over the last half of the 20th century following significant social movements. After hundreds of thousands of refugee students were displaced at the end of World War II, Gerald Caplan used school-based interventions to assist teachers working with these students. The civil rights movement in the 1960s brought about federal education rights legislation. No longer could schools require students with disabilities to fit into their existing programs. Systematic identification of students with emotional and behavioral disabilities began, accompanied by a need for clinical advice about assessing and treating these students in the least restrictive school settings. Increased social change in the late 1960s and wider recognition of problem behaviors among students, such as substance abuse, unprotected sexual intercourse, and more recently, bullying and school violence, caused schools to turn to mental health clinicians for advice. This increased awareness of student emotional and behavioral health problems was accompanied by language and policy changes, including Eli Bower's research and conceptualization of the "emotionally disturbed" student, which served as a foundation for the initial version of the **Education for Handicapped Children Act** of 1977 (5). This legislation, along with Bower's research and advocacy, are recognized as critical to the establishment of schools as a critical venue for supporting the emotional and behavioral needs of students in order to improve their academic success.

The decrease in the 1990s in psychiatric hospitalizations and residential placements, coupled with the lack of access to mental health care among those most in need, resulted in proliferation of school-based mental health treatment, and delivery of psychiatric services within schools (6). As evidenced in the Dryfoos' (1994) book, *Full Service Schools: A Revolution in Health and Social Services for Children, Youth, and Families,* schools were increasingly recognized as a place where all students, especially students with psychological problems, could receive comprehensive services.

The No Child Left Behind and subsequent legislation required intervention earlier for those students not progressing as expected. The President's New Freedom Commission report of 2003, *Achieving the Promise: Transforming Mental Health Care in America,* emphasized the impacts of mental health on learning and social–emotional development. This report provided recommendations to address gaps in the provision of mental health services to youth, including the expansion of school mental health programs. In 2004, the **Garrett Lee Smith Memorial Act** (P.L. 108–355, October 2004) became the first federal legislation in the United States to provide specific funding for youth suicide prevention and early intervention programs, as well as interventions and treatments for mental and behavioral health problems that can lead to suicide in young people. Most recently, the **Every Student Succeeds Act,** enacted December 2015, requires that states and local education authorities work with diverse stakeholders to develop comprehensive interventions for students at risk of school failure, and that they articulate and measure efforts to improve school climate, including supporting the emotional wellness of students. Psychiatrists and mental health clinicians have become partners with education professionals to respond to traumatic events at schools, such as natural disasters (e.g., surrounding hurricanes or tornados), or catastrophic human events such as murders or war. Increased proactive, resilience-building for students, facing seemingly ever-increasing stress loads, have expanded the range of mental health efforts at school, including social–emotional learning curricula, mindfulness, and executive skill coaching. This chronology, and some important lessons learned over time, are provided in Table 7.3.1.

MODELS OF CONSULTATION

Multiple models of psychiatric consultation to schools have emerged, including the mental health model, the behavioral model, and the organizational model. These models are summarized in Table 7.3.2, as well as differences in their approach to the same problems. Regardless of the specific model, the child psychiatrist role appears broadening as collaborator, expert consultant, and partner in prevention, early intervention, and service delivery efforts (7).

Mental Health Consultation

Mental health consultation (MHC) (8) stresses that the consultant's goals are both to be helpful with the problem at hand and also to provide the consultee new knowledge and skills to handle similar problems in the future. The focus of mental health consultation is usually to understand how a student's mental health functioning impacts his or her school success, and to offer recommendations about school interventions tailored to meet the mental health needs of the student. This type of consultation is frequently "indirect," as the consultant may hear about a troublesome student from a parent or staff, and make recommendations to these staff, sometimes without ever seeing the student. The consultant may be paid by the school district or other entity (e.g., student insurance via a community behavioral health provider), and the consultee is free to follow (or not) the consultant's recommendations.

Behavioral Consultation

Behavioral consultants attempt to change the behavior of teachers and students by focusing on: (a) problem identification, (b) problem analysis, (c) plan implementation, and (d) problem evaluation. During the *problem identification* stage, the consultant and teacher identify a specific problem to address. Usually, a "problem" occurs when the student's observed behavior is not what is desired and expected by the teacher or other school personnel. When a discrepancy exists between current and desired behavior, the consultant and teacher establish goals for the resolution of the problem, formulating the problem in behavioral terms. During *problem analysis,* the consultant and the school staff generate hypotheses about factors that influence the behavior and design a plan to solve the problem. During *plan implementation,* the consultant and school staff enact the plan and also collect data to measure how the problem behavior changes following implementation. During *program evaluation,* the consultant and school staff examine whether the goals have been attained, if new problems have arisen, and how the plan should be continued, modified, or phased out (9–11).

Behavioral consultation has advanced through the *collaborative problem-solving* model described by Greene and Ablon (12). This behavioral approach diverges from preexisting behavioral models by suggesting that students often lack a repertoire of other behaviors to employ when in complex situations, and so revert, almost inflexibly, to primitive or aggressive behaviors in such circumstances. Problem behaviors require adults (teachers or parents) to respond to the "message" attempted by the student's behavior, rather than efforts to immediately stop the behavior or to ignore or tolerate it. Rather than conventional reinforcement when desirable behaviors spontaneously emerge, or punishment when misbehaviors occur, desirable behaviors have to be identified, agreed-upon by the student and teacher, and practiced so that they become familiar parts of the student's repertoire.

Organizational Consultation

Organizational consultation focuses on schools as systems and seeks to facilitate improvement in school functioning through the application of behavioral science concepts and the

TABLE 7.3.1

MAJOR EVENTS IN PSYCHIATRIC CONSULTATION TO SCHOOLS

Social Event	Mental Health Impacts on Schools	Child Psychiatry Response	Lessons Learned
Aftermath of WWII	Displaced orphan students required emotional support to contend with school	Mental health providers worked with educators to manage displaced students	Life events require mindful planning to promote mental health and resiliency in children
Civil rights movement	Equality for all, including those with disabilities, required schools to accept and respond to diverse students	Child psychiatrists identified psychiatric disorders that schools considered as possible educational disabilities	(1) Psychiatric disorders did not necessarily "fit" educational disability categories (2) No consensual or empirical school interventions for identified disorders/disabilities existed
Social change and problem behaviors	Problematic behaviors, and their negative impact on schooling, increasingly evident in the classroom	Child psychiatrists provided input on lifestyle variables influencing quality of life	(1) Little empirical evidence supported child psychiatry recommendations (2) Efforts to identify the prevalence of substance abuse and other problem behaviors helped illuminate mental health issues
Decrease in psychiatric hospitalization	Students managed in non-school environments returned to schools to receive an education appropriate for them, given complex needs	Child psychiatrists focused on discharge planning to provide outpatient treatment, including in school settings	Psychiatrists and educators partnered, by necessity, to address mental health issues impacting children in daily environments
Impacts of mental health on learning	Students with diverse mental health difficulties have similarly diverse struggles at school as well as impact classroom instruction	Embrace broader "RtI" (Response to Intervention) approaches to identify and respond varying degrees and impacts of psychopathology at school	Proactive efforts to screen, recognize and respond to students can enhance school achievement
Resilience to traumatic events at schools	Traumatic events at school illuminated the importance of early detection and intervention for all students	Assist in the development of more sophisticated screening and evidence-based interventions for students at risk	Mental health supports can accelerate recovery from traumatic events
Emphasis on social emotional learning	Increased evidence for the positive impact of universal social–emotional learning on student psychosocial and academic functioning	Consultation on selection of universal mental health promotion and prevention programming and consideration for how brain science can help inform and evaluate this programming	Psychiatrists' knowledge of brain science and etiology and development of psychopathology can support the shift from treatment-only approaches to promotion/prevention activities, and cultivating social skills

involvement of usually multiple system members (e.g., administrators and teachers) in the process of organizational change. Difficulties may emerge because of mismatches between the students and requirements of the educational system. Systemic problems such as communication breakdowns and ambiguity about responsibilities can cause anxiety and frustration among school staff, and impact student progress and behavior. Individual student problems may illuminate school system factors that contribute to the problem, and should be modified. For example, in one suburban elementary school, a large number of students were receiving office discipline referrals. Upon examination of discipline data, it was revealed that the substantial majority of referrals were coming from one out of the five fourth-grade teachers. During consultation it emerged that her referral rates increased following new policies that decreased paraprofessional support while simultaneously increasing the number of students with challenging behaviors in her classroom. In this case, focusing on school policies and practices, rather than solely on the students' individual behaviors, became a priority. Models addressing low-achieving schools, such as the Comer School Development Program precipitated school restructuring and change in school culture and climate, positively impacting student self-esteem, motivation, and achievement (13). The 2015 reauthorization of the **Elementary and Secondary Schools Act** requires states to measure and address organizational factors that may impact student mental health, including school climate, providing increased opportunities for child psychiatry consultants to consider organizational factors that could support students' school success.

THE ROLES OF SCHOOL STAFF WITHIN SCHOOL CONSULTATION

Most commonly, child psychiatrists interact with schools to coordinate treatment for their patients. Whether acting as a school consultant, or communicating with a school to coordinate patient treatment, establishing an effective

TABLE 7.3.2

CONTEMPORARY MODELS OF SCHOOL CONSULTATION

	Consultation Model		
Aspect of the Consultation	**Mental Health Consultation**	**Behavioral Consultation**	**Organizational Consultation**
Initial focus	How mental health impacts student progress	Problematic behaviors exhibited by students/staff	How school contributes to problem
How information is obtained from consultee	Clinical interview with student/parents, review of school data, psychological testing	Direct observation in classroom, counting frequency, length of specified behaviors	Review of school philosophy, curriculum, instructional philosophy, administrative procedures for problem class or group
Objective	Help consultee identify strategies to address mental health problems interfering with school success and strengthen psychological assets	Help consultee measure problem behaviors, alter and shape student responses leading to problem behaviors	Help consultee refine organizational configuration and goals to diminish circumstances
Evaluation of model	Do identified intervention strategies improve student mental health functioning? Does student's school performance improve?	Do specific problem behaviors diminish in frequency/intensity? What does "data collection" reveal?	Does this specific problem illuminate larger problems in policy impacting multiple students? Does the proposed solution benefit everyone?
Example case (17-year-old student who does not attend regularly the year after becoming a teen parent)	Consultee identifies depressive symptoms that occurred postpregnancy, constructs a plan with the student, teachers and family to re-engage student in pleasurable activities, teach cognitive coping, and monitor mood	Consultee keeps track of days/times missed, addresses directly with student, and they construct plan for student to be there on time by having others care for child on certain days; they measure success of plan, and revise as needed	Consultee identifies well-intended but misattuned policies for attendance for current school population, and provide alternative schedule for students with children, course credit that can be completed at home, and course credit shifted to allow parenting study/work to count toward graduation

partnering relationship is critical, particularly if the school is asked to make accommodations for this student. Child psychiatrists often need to be aware of the staff options at a patient's school so that helpful school staff can be accessed and empowered to address the patient's needs.

Roles of School Personnel

As the demands on schools have intensified, staff roles have changed, such that consultants must have realistic expectations about who can perform specific interventions with students. The consultee may be anyone within the school hierarchy, and the consultant must address these needs while being mindful of how the consultation will impact everyone else within the system. The consultant must also consider who is in a position to implement recommendations when providing consultation.

Teachers remain the front-line staff most involved with students. Elementary teachers usually have approximately 25 students for 6 hours each day. By middle school, teachers usually teach in a specific content area, providing instruction to approximately 150 different students each day. *Special education teachers* are credentialed to provide alternative instruction to smaller groups of students with learning disabilities, including dyslexia, nonverbal learning disorders, or emotional disorders that interfere with learning. For students to receive instruction from special education teachers, they must have an individualized education program (IEP). *Aides* often do not possess a 4-year college degree or teacher certification, but may assist a classroom teacher, or work directly with a specific student.

School psychologists are either employed by the school or have a contract with the school to administer and interpret psychological testing and help construct IEPs for students to address their specific learning difficulties. They may also provide individual and group therapy to students. *School counselors* (formerly referred to as guidance counselors) sometimes provide psychotherapy to students, although their primary role in secondary schools is often to assist students in college or vocational planning and academic planning, including class selection. *School adjustment counselors and/or social workers* have been added to school staffs in many locations, where their primary role is to provide psychosocial interventions to students, and sometimes their families.

School nurses address acute health care needs of students, and administer medications to students; however, school nurses sometimes travel between several schools each day so that supporting students' complex or frequent medication regimens become difficult.

Occupational therapists work with students individually or in small groups to help students with basic activities of daily living, and alternative strategies for students who have sensory integration issues to help them learn to cope with various stimuli. *Speech–language therapists* meet with students who have communication and social skills difficulties individually and in small groups.

School administrators liaison between the school and the community. *Principals* manage all services (from teaching to custodial) within their school building, and report to the superintendent. The *superintendent* guides educational activities among all the schools within a school district, and reports to an elected *school board* in public schools, or an appointed board in private, parochial, or charter schools.

ESTABLISHING A RELATIONSHIP WITH A SCHOOL

Schools today face great demands to impart knowledge, to prepare students vocationally, to socialize children to interact with others effectively, and to protect their health and safety. These varied, often competing, agendas impact every intervention proposed by the child psychiatrist, regardless of the child psychiatrist's role "identified" by the school. Moreover, public, private, parochial, and charter schools not only vary widely in their priorities, but also in their system hierarchy and their accountability to the community. Familiarity with each individual school, its priorities, and its staff is a prerequisite to any meaningful consultation.

Evaluating a School

When the child psychiatrist has the opportunity to visit a school, a framework for evaluating the school can help discern the fit between that school and a particular student, as well as better match interventions to the culture of that school. Table 7.3.3 provides a sample approach child psychiatrists can use when entering a school. Awareness of the general reaction the consultant has to the school and its staff helps clarify the likely fit between a school and an identified student. Depending on the needs of the student, the child psychiatrist may employ relevant questions from Box 7.3.1.

TABLE 7.3.3

FRAMEWORK FOR EVALUATING A SCHOOL

School Component	What to Observe	Potential Questions for Staff
School building	Safety/security: Does the building appear safe? Is the building comfortable (temperature, chairs beyond desks, lighting, noisy)? Does the building value students (student art on the walls, recognition of student achievements, evidence of parent–teacher alliance)? Is this a place a child would want to be in?	How does one enter/exit the building? Where do students go if they are having a hard time? Where are students' classwork or projects kept or displayed? What happens after school is over? Do students stay in the building before or after school?
Classrooms	What do classrooms look like? How big is the room? How many students are in this room, and how many adults? How many learning areas are there, and are they separated so children can be in a quiet place within the classroom? How stimulating (visual, auditory, tactile) is this classroom, and do the students appear over/understimulated?	What's the average number of students in each classroom? How are teachers encouraged to set up their classroom? If a student is having a hard time in the classroom, where does he/she go? How did you (teacher) decide what to put up in your classroom?
School atmosphere	How is a stranger greeted? Does the school seem organized for students or for staff? Do most students appear engaged with instruction (are students within classrooms, alert, attentive, answering/asking questions?)? How do students and staff interact (smiling, directives, calm, tense)? Do children thrive here?	Whom should I meet when I enter the building? How do students move between classes/to lunch/recess? What do students do when they've finished classroom assignments? What do staff expect from students here? What do staff most worry about here regarding students?
School Staff		
Administrators	Are administrators present/accessible? What kind of tone/impression does the administrator convey? Do staff appear comfortable around the administrator? Who does this administrator best serve (students, teachers, parents, other administrators)? What led to this administrator being selected for this building (student needs, up/down move for this administrator)?	What kind of interactions does the administrator have with students (discipline, earned reward time, common interests discussed in halls/lunch)? What is the administrator's priority in this building? What do staff seek from the administrator (support, camaraderie, ideas, discipline, avoidance)?
Teachers	Do teachers want to be in this school (eager to be with students or staff)? Do teachers stay in this building? How do teachers engage students (time to work, demonstrate content, model enthusiasm, surprise students)? How often do teachers alter the instructional approach (every 10 min, something different [lecture, student reading, class discussion], or employ different modalities [visual, auditory, tactile]) employed during instruction?	How many teachers left this building last year? Average over the last several (5) yrs? What is the student: teacher ratio? What's the average length of time teachers have been in this district/building? How many teachers here have advanced (masters, doctoral) degrees? What kind of teachers do best in this school (independent, orderly, collaborative, creative)?

TABLE 7.3.3

(CONTINUED)

School Component	What to Observe	Potential Questions for Staff
Special staff	Are other school staff present? How do teachers and other school staff interact (take student out, co-teach, friendly/tense)? How do teachers describe other staff (particularly contributions of special educators)?	What kind of special educational staff work here? How often are they in this building (always, weekly)? What kind of other teachers are in the classroom (parent aides, "paraprofessionals" aides)? Do they work with particular students, with everyone in the classroom...?
Support staff	Are support staff friendly? Do they appear open about discussing the school and students? Do support staff work well with other staff?	What kind of support staff are in this building? How long have most of them been here? How are support staff paired up with other staff?

BOX 7.3.1

School Consultation Framework

The psychiatric school consultant should consider how *micro problems can lead to macro solutions,* that is, how individual student problems can be addressed to improve circumstances for all subsequent students and staff. Five components should be considered in every consultation:

1. Who is the actual **Consultee,** and what are the *confidentiality* parameters?
2. What is the Consultation **Question,** and what is the consultee seeking and wishing will happen?
3. How is the larger **System** experiencing this problem?
4. What **Legal or Ethical Factors** should be considered?
5. How does the consultant understand this problem **Biopsychosocially**?

The Consultee and Confidentiality Parameters

The consultant must establish procedures to clarify who is appropriate to contact or to evaluate. When requested to meet with students, the consultant must obtain parental permission before interviewing any student. If parents refuse for the consultant to evaluate their child, the consultant may still observe, unobtrusively, the student, and consult the staff about their questions on how best to work with this student. Clarification of confidentiality should occur, sometimes recurrently, with staff, students, and parents. Anyone meeting with the consultant should understand how information is shared and whether written clinical information is placed in the student or personnel records.

Clarification of the Consultation Question and Needs/Wishes of the Consultee

Consultants help others define the problem and envision solutions. While consultees may ask for interventions to assist a student, sometimes they actually wish the consultant will address administrators, or recommend the student be removed from this consultee's classroom. Consultants must "read between the lines" to clarify both the consultee's overt request as well as underlying desires. The success of every consultation depends on the consultant understanding the consultee's concerns and wishes, such that both agree on the problem and on realistic goals for any intervention.

The System Reaction to the Problem

The problem will affect various school staff members differently, and each may have different goals for this consultation. Consultants should clarify who requested a consultation, who knows about the consultation, who has consented to the consultation, and who should be informed about the findings for this consultation. The more that differing goals can be aligned, the higher the probability that participants will invest in a proposed solution.

Legal and Ethical Factors

Special educational laws may provide the student different opportunities, yet families or schools may not see the applicability of such laws in a particular case. Similarly, the case may be confounded by ethical dilemmas, particularly in cases of suspected abuse. If abuse is suspected, the consultant may help staff articulate concerns to the appropriate agency, or assist parents and the school in addressing circumstances or staff perceived as abusive. In acutely dangerous situations such as suicidality or homicidality, the consultant can help consultees facilitate emergency treatment or how to warn others who may be at risk. Potential legal and ethical ramifications should be considered for every proposed intervention.

Biopsychosocial Understanding of the Problem

Child psychiatrists consider people's biologic vulnerabilities to psychopathology, their past experiences, and current family, peer, school, or other social stressors in explaining dysfunctional behaviors. These different influences may provide multiple intervention targets for a particular problem and should take into consideration existing services in the school and community. A student may need interventions biologically, psychologically, and socially, such as a referral for a medication evaluation, a behavioral plan at school and home, and connection to social groups such as sports teams, choir or band, or summer camps.

BOX 7.3.2

SCHOOL CONSULTING TECHNIQUES

Ally

(1) *Validate consultees' perceptions before proposing any solutions.*
Validating perceptions cultivates consultee trust that the consultant understands their predicament. If in doubt, ask questions or pose solutions as questions ("What would likely happen if we...?").

(2) *Bind anxiety.*
Everything the consultant does either increases or decreases anxiety within the system. The more people who share the problem, the less anxious each individual will be. While consultants may not know the answer to various problems, thinking through how they would find an answer can diminish consultee's anxiety.

(3) *Create respect for everyone involved.*
Minimizing splitting of staff, students, and parents decreases the probability that individuals will oppose an intervention. The consultant can attempt to separate personalities from the problem by focusing on terms used, by identifying the common goals between parties, and by identifying the circumstances each party uniquely faces.

Align

(4) *Find the good intent gone awry.*
When students or staff act inappropriately, the consultant can back up to the good intention that motivated the person's (mis)behavior so that self-esteem, and thus willingness to attempt different behaviors, is maximized. For example, if a teacher "yells" at students, the consultant can "backtrack" to the diligent efforts by the teacher to get the student's attention and to feel responsible that the student learns the material. Then the consultant is positioned to examine alternatives (visually signal the child, use a very soft voice, etc.), which will seem less critical of the teacher's yelling.

(5) *Help others to see the child (or staff member) differently.*
Maladaptive behaviors may be used to solve problems when no other solution is available (e.g., talking in class may be the only way a student "knows" to slow down instruction or to obtain positive attention from others since the student cannot garner positive attention by doing the academic task).

(6) *Connect others.*
Look for opportunities to connect others to benefit the staff or student, utilizing existing services in the school and in the larger community.

(7) *Appeal to shared values by giving people options they cannot argue with.*
Explore and identify appropriate desires of students and staff so that interventions can be provided to realize those appropriate goals. For example, identifying that a student seeks to attend college, or hold a particular job, provides a "frame" for posed interventions ("You've indicated you want to attend/work at ______, and they require you show up on time so we have to practice going to sleep at 10 PM so that you can be ready the next morning.").

Mobilize

(8) *At every opportunity, expand the consultee's skills.*
Whenever possible, the consultant attempts to assist the consultee in selecting and implementing skills helpful for that situation. The consultant aspires to provide the consultee facility with multiple skills that the consultee can use subsequently independently.

(9) *Use the consultee's own words to frame interventions.*
Framing interventions with terms used by the consultee, by staff, and by students, increases each person feeling heard, and improves the probability of each investing in proposed solutions.

(10) *Identify one step up from the current situation.*
Consultees may need help seeing the steps in a sequence toward appropriate behavior (e.g., Cursing may be "a step up" from physically assaulting others). Even small positive changes generate momentum to achieve greater changes.

(11) *Move toward anticipating problems rather than reacting to them.*
Efforts to help consultees see how problems arise, and how they might be prevented in the future can empower consultees to find and face problems early. More importantly, initial reactions may not represent optimal solutions, but instead create additional conflicts or problems.

THE SCHOOL CONSULTATION PROCESS

The goal of school consultation is to build alliances and to share information that helps the school staff recognize and resolve problems. This process can be broken down into three tasks: (1) *allying with consultees;* (2) *aligning consultee objectives; and* (3) *mobilizing consultees to follow through with interventions* (14). Allying with consultees requires the consultant to empathize with consultees and to decrease their possible resistance. In aligning consultees, the consultant reframes people's comments, behaviors, or positions to establish unifying goals attractive to all participants. Mobilizing consultees to act requires the consultant to invest the participants in solving the problem and to empower consultees with the skills to be successful with the intervention. Consulting techniques helpful in accomplishing these tasks are described in Box 7.3.2.

SPECIAL EDUCATION

Child psychiatrists often identify psychiatric disorders which require changes within the school setting for patients to benefit. The child psychiatrist is expected to identify specific disabilities (disorders) that impact a child's performance in the classroom, and to clarify changes, such as additional time for test-taking for students with attention-deficit hyperactivity disorder (ADHD), or deviations from certain readings for patients with mood disorders, or writing activities in patients with nonverbal learning disorder. Child psychiatrists may recommend services, such as social pragmatics instruction in patients with autism, and may comment on educational settings, although child psychiatrists should not recommend specific placements for their patients. Based on services needed, the child's educational team is obligated to identify the most appropriate site for service delivery. Many options now exist for schools to educate students with psychiatric disorders, so the child psychiatrist must have some familiarity with the special education process, and the legal parameters surrounding educational planning for these students (15).

Special education refers to specialized instruction for students who cannot benefit sufficiently from traditional classroom instruction. Eventually, all students will be appreciated as unique learners, as every child, wherever on the disability spectrum, deserves specialized instruction to optimize his or her potential. Schools continue to become more sophisticated in addressing the needs of all their students, currently propelled by legal efforts to support education of each child in the United States. Legal protections have evolved beyond the equal protection clause of the 14th Amendment to the US Constitution to provide every student with a free, appropriate education. Any child who is not progressing appropriately in school is entitled to an evaluation to determine if a disability is present, whether this disability interferes with school performance, *and* whether specialized teaching and/or other supports are needed. Anyone, including the student, the student's family, school staff, or a clinician (such as a child psychiatrist) can request an evaluation for a student. This eligibility process is summarized in Figure 7.3.1.

The American with Disabilities Act and Section 504 of the Rehabilitation Act of 1973

The **Americans with Disabilities Act (ADA)** prohibits the denial of educational services, programs, or activities to students with disabilities, and prohibits discrimination against all such students once enrolled. If parents suspect their child has a disability, they may request an evaluation to determine if a disability is present and interferes with educational progress. This is usually provided in writing to the school's principal. A child with a suspected disability is usually referred to a student support team at the school to provide accommodations. *Accommodations* refer to classroom changes that help the student meet requirements, without "lowering" academic standards.

Schools may generate an accommodation plan for such a student called a *504 Plan*. These plans derive from **Section 504 of the Rehabilitation Act** (1973), which ensures that all disabled children receive a "free and appropriate public education" (FAPE) in the "least restrictive environment" (LRE). Both ADA and Section 504 are managed by the Office for Civil Rights; the focus of both is to ensure that all students have an equal opportunity to benefit from the educational opportunities available to students in a given school. ADA is broader since Section 504 only pertains to school districts that receive federal funding. Section 504 services apply to any person who has a "physical or mental impairment which substantially limits a major life activity" so schools often attempt a 504 Plan for students with disabilities minimally impacting educational progress. Students qualifying for a 504 Plan may receive special *accommodations* to help them meet educational requirements, usually within regular school classrooms.

The Individual with Disabilities Education Act

For students with more severe psychiatric disorders, additional safeguards have been provided by Public Law 94–142 (1975), revised as the **Individual with Disabilities Education Act (IDEA)**, and most recently reauthorized in 2004 (technically as the Individual with Disabilities **Improvement Act**). IDEA extended a free, appropriate public education to students with disabilities, mandating specialized instruction and related services if necessary to meet these students' unique needs. The IDEA defines "children with disabilities" to mean children with autism; deaf–blindness; deafness; emotional disturbance; hearing impairment; intellectual disability; multiple disabilities; orthopedic impairment; other health impairment (ADHD historically has been included in this category); specific learning disability; speech or language impairment; traumatic brain injury; and visual impairment including blindness. IDEA defines "emotionally disturbed" (previously called "serious emotional disturbance") as a condition having one or more of the following over a long period of time, to a marked degree, and which adversely affect educational performance: an inability to learn that cannot be explained by intellectual, sensory, or health factors; an inability to build or maintain satisfactory interpersonal relationships with peers and teachers; inappropriate types of mood or behavior under normal circumstances; a general mood of unhappiness or depression; or a tendency to develop physical symptoms or fears associated with personal or school problems.

In addition to having a diagnosed disability, to qualify for services under IDEA, the child must require *specialized instruction* (instruction from a special education teacher) because he or she is *not* making effective progress in school (which includes social and interpersonal progress–not just academic progress). If any of the above conditions are *not* met, the child is *not* eligible for IDEA services, but may be eligible for a 504 Plan or for other services.

The evaluation for IDEA eligibility is more comprehensive than for a 504 Plan. A multidisciplinary team of school-based professionals may conduct a comprehensive individual analysis of *all* suspected areas of disability. Usual components include assessment of the student's: (1) cognitive abilities; (2) communication abilities; (3) academic performance; (4) social–emotional status; (5) medical history/health status; (6) vision–hearing screening; and (7) motor abilities. Additional components (specialized evaluations) may be added as deemed necessary, such as intelligence testing, speech–language testing, achievement testing, neuropsychological testing physical examination, occupation–physical therapy evaluations, and psychiatric assessment (4). If the parent feels the evaluation is inaccurate or would like additional input, an independent evaluation may be requested, although the school is *not* "bound" to follow recommendations from an outside evaluator (including the patient's child psychiatrist).

The IDEA provides for educational services to include disabled children under the age of 6, and when necessary, up to the student's 22nd birthday. IDEA ensures that all disabled children receive an *IEP* with parental input and consent, and includes due process guarantees if parents disagree with this IEP or with the student's placement in an alternative setting or school. The IDEA prevented "troublesome" children from being refused admittance or from being ejected from a school because the school contended that it did not offer an appropriate program; instead the school *must* provide a free, appropriate education in the least restrictive setting. IDEA goes beyond Section 504 by allowing *modifications* so that the student does not, depending on that student's disability, have to meet the same academic requirements as students in regular education. For example, just as a wheelchair-bound student would not be required to meet physical education requirements applicable to students without a disability, students with a psychiatric disability might not be required to contend with upsetting curriculum content (posttraumatic stress disorder), or complete the same amount of problems (ADHD),

A. Determining Special Education Eligibility

(1) Does the child have *one or more of the following types of disability* (documented by the medical evaluation/diagnosis, educational/psychological testing, etc.)?

Autism
Developmental Delay
Intellectual Disability
Sensory-Hearing, Vision, Deafness, Blindness
Neurologic
Emotional
Communication
Specific Learning
Other Health

(2) If one or more of these disabilities is present, is the child *making effective progress in school*? If the student is being *reevaluated* to determine if a disability is still impacting the child, would the child continue to make progress in school without the currently provided special education services?

(3) Is the lack of progress a *result of the child's disability*?

(4) Does the child *require specially designed instruction in order to make effective progress in school* or does the child require related services in order to access the general curriculum?

B. School Service Plans for Students with Psychiatric Disorders

Type of School Service Plan	District Service Plan	504 Plan	Individualized Educational Program (IEP)
Purpose	To respond quickly to mild changes in the student's life that impact learning; focus is on mild and/or brief circumstances that may impact learning	To ensure that all students have equal opportunity to learn, even if they have a disability; focus is student's opportunities as compared to other students in that school	To remediate symptoms of a student's disability; student's unique needs are the focus
Criteria to receive this plan	Student has a symptom or disorder that impacts learning	Student has an impairment that limits a major life activity, but may not require specialized instruction	Student has a disability which interferes with educational progress, and which requires specialized instruction
Who develops this plan	Teacher and administrator, usually with parental input	Teacher, administrator (often the school's designated "504 coordinator," school counselor and usually parent, student) (if appropriate)	Educational team, including staff certified in special education; may include evaluations by school psychologist, social worker; parent may bring friends, advocates, own evaluators to be part of team
What is usually provided	Changes within classroom to enable student to perform better	Changes within classroom or school building to enable student to complete curriculum expectations	Changes within classroom setting(s) to provide student different instruction, and may substantially alter what is required of student
Example of what is provided	Student is allowed to sit closer to teacher during instruction; student is met by familiar staff to decrease anxiety	Student is allowed more time to complete tests; Student may be provided device to hear better	Student may leave regular language arts class and receive specialized reading program; student may be exempted from course requirements
Which staff deliver services	Usually regular education staff	Usually regular education staff	Staff with specialized training (special education teachers, speech therapists, occupational therapists, etc.)
Where the student receives services	Regular classroom	Regular classroom with regular peers "to the maximum extent appropriate"	Wide ranging, from regular education classrooms (inclusion) to pullout for special education classrooms, to offsite day school programs, to 24 hr/day residential schools
Review of the plan	As needed	Plan reviewed at least every year	At least every year plan is reviewed, and every 3 yrs the student is retested to see if still qualifies
Disciplinary actions	Usually not applicable	If "manifestation hearing" indicates student's impairment or disability caused misbehavior, then student cannot be suspended/expelled; school is not required to provide free, appropriate education for suspended or expelled students	If "manifestation hearing" indicates student's disability caused misbehavior, then student cannot be suspended/expelled; if student is suspended or expelled, school must still provide free, appropriate education
Appeal recourses	None provided	School may alter 504 Plan immediately should circumstances indicate need; "notice" may be provided verbally; family may appeal to the Office for Civil Rights if perceive school is discriminating against child because of a disability	School must provide "prior written notice" before changes in educational plan or placement are made; family may appeal decisions or plan to local then State departments of education

FIGURE 7.3.1. A: Determining special education eligibility. **B:** School service plans for students with psychiatric disorders.

TABLE 7.3.4

COMPONENTS OF AN INDIVIDUALIZED EDUCATIONAL PROGRAM (IEP)

Component	Example	Comments
Usual Components		
Present level of functioning	Although in the 5th grade, [student] is currently reading at 3rd grade level.	Both strengths and weaknesses should be described, with current functioning identified for each area of need requiring a goal
Educational goals	In normal classroom discussions, [student] will repeat back accurately instructions for a task, 4/5 times daily.	Goals should include: (1) circumstances or setting; (2) observable behavior; and (3) performance measure, as well as staff person responsible for implementing
Educational accommodations and modifications	[Student] will be allowed to take tests verbally or untimed.	Intervention necessary to allow student to access curriculum, or how curriculum will be modified
Special education and related services	[Student] will receive specialized reading instruction 60 min/day for 4 days/wk in the learning center.	Clarification of staff with special expertise to assist student and how that will occur (teaching, consult to teacher, group instruction, etc.)
Placement and participation specifications	[Student] will receive reading, math, and social group instruction in a pullout resource classroom.	Least restrictive environment for student to receive services
Transition services planning	[Student] will work at ______ 2 days/wk starting April 1st.	For all students by age 16, although may start at age 14
Transfer of rights planning	[Student] is aware of right to participate.	Student informed, allowed to participate by age 16, and parental rights transfer when reaches age 18.
Additional Components/Related Services		
Adapted physical education	[Student] will be allowed to ride bicycle for PE requirement in place of group PE.	Changes in physical education requirements based on disability
Behavioral intervention plan	[Student] will access [Staff] and follow de-escalation steps when irritated.	A *Functional Assessment of Behavior* usually includes (1) antecedents to the negative behaviors, (2) specific negative behavior, and (3) consequences (benefits) of this behavior so that interventions can occur at any of these three points
Counseling services	[Student] will receive 30 min of individual counseling per wk.	Counseling is usually to help student function better at school; counseling may include parents or family training
Extended school year services	[Student] will receive tutoring 2 hr/day for 4 wks in Summer.	Extended-year services are required to "prevent regression" rather than to increase new skills throughout the year
Occupational therapy	[Student] will receive keyboarding training.	Often includes additional training in activities of daily living; may also include special cushions, devices, or techniques to address sensory-motor symptoms
Physical therapy	[Student] will practice writing with special paper and pencil.	Includes development of gross and fine motor skills
School health services	[Student] will have blood pressure checked weekly.	Medication administration, vital sign or other check (blood glucose, etc.), or nutritional services may occur
Speech–language therapy	[Student] will receive speech therapy with another student 30 min/wk to develop conversation skills.	Includes social-pragmatic training as well as training for dysarticulation
Transportation services	[Student] will ride a van with an assistant.	May include special vehicles or configurations based on student's needs

or participate in certain class requirements such as speaking in front of the class (social anxiety disorder). The multidisciplinary team devises the IEP, and components of an IEP are provided in Table 7.3.4.

The authority of school officials has increased with subsequent amendments to the IDEA. At this time, administrators may immediately remove and place a student into an alternative setting if the student brings a weapon to school or to a school function, or if the student sells, uses, or attempts to buy drugs at school or at a school function. The alternative placement is decided by an emergency IEP team meeting. The amendments also include a provision for dealing with other conduct considered to be dangerous. School officials can suspend a child for up to 10 days (total within a school year) and in the interim ask for an expedited administrative hearing at which an order changing placement can be obtained on a showing by "substantial evidence that maintaining the current placement of the child is substantially likely to result in injury to the child or to others." This process can be repeated during a formal dispute by parents over the change of placement or of the appropriateness of the alternative placement.

Important protections for students have also emerged with amendments to the IDEA. For students with disruptive behaviors, the school may be required to conduct a *manifestation determination review* to determine if a student's misbehaviors are a result of a disability. For example, a child with Tourette's might not be able to sit still, or quietly, because of tics, or a student with bipolar disorder might not be deemed capable of speaking softly or remaining seated. The educational team must determine whether the student understood that his or her behavior was inappropriate, whether the student could control the behavior, and whether the IEP and placement had been appropriate. If it is determined that the misconduct was not a manifestation of the child's disability, the school may apply the same disciplinary sanctions to that child as apply to children without disabilities. If the conduct is found to be a manifestation of the disability, the school is obligated to continue programming, embodied in an IEP, in the alternative setting. Children subject to discipline, but who have not been evaluated for and/or identified as eligible for special education, but who are suspected of having qualifying disabilities are entitled to the same protections as children already found eligible.

The IDEA provides extensive procedural protections to parents of children with disabilities, including "the right to participate in the development of the IEP, the right to independent evaluations, the right to inspect educational records" and "the opportunity to present complaints with respect to any matter relating to the identification, evaluation, or educational placement of the child, or the provision of a free appropriate public education to such child." Such a proceeding, referred to as a *due process* hearing, requires a neutral adjudicator, a right to counsel at the parent's expense, and the right to present evidence and cross-examine witnesses. If dissatisfied, either party has a right to judicial review in the appropriate state or federal court.

EDUCATIONAL INTERVENTIONS FOR STUDENTS WITH SELECTED PSYCHIATRIC DISORDERS

Psychiatrists may be asked for specific classroom and school environment modifications by the school, the legal system, and/or the parents. The sample interventions in Table 7.3.5, derived from www.schoolpsychiatry.org, may be appropriate for particular students having various psychiatric disorders, depending on the needs of the child and the resources of the school. Such interventions should always be paired with the individual needs of each student rather than categorically applied to every student with that disorder, so interventions addressing several comorbid conditions are often required. Interventions may be adapted to a student's district service plan, 504 Plan, or to an Individualized Educational Program (IEP) as modifications/accommodations, or informally implemented in regular classroom settings. The success or failure of these interventions often helps clarify whether a child can remain in the current school environment or requires a different educational setting. While students are entitled to an education in the least restrictive environment, this parameter may necessitate a student to receive instruction in a regular classroom, receive some instruction outside the regular classroom, receive all instruction in a self-contained special education classroom, go to a program at another site, or attend an off-site 24-hour/day residential school. Accordingly, the psychiatrist's report should clarify diagnoses ("rule-out" diagnoses are not helpful to schools), appropriate accommodations for symptoms that impair school progress, recommendations for services (e.g., social pragmatics training through speech therapy), and program recommendations (e.g., staff trained to work with students with autism spectrum disorders). From these recommendations the student's educational team can identify a specific placement to address the student's unique needs. Evidence-based interventions have been catalogued increasingly, including the elements common to programs and interventions that appear most effective. The following websites emphasize those interventions with the strongest evidence to date:

www.practicewise.com
http://www.ncbi.nlm.nih.gov/pmc/
www.evidencebasedprograms.org
http://autismpdc.fpg.unc.edu/sites/autismpdc.fpg.unc.edu/files/imce/documents/2014-EBP-Report.pdf

Examples of evidence-based interventions for psychiatric symptoms and how these can be applied by school staff are provided in Table 7.3.5.

MENTAL HEALTH SERVICES IN SCHOOLS

Approximately 20% of students aged 6 to 17 years currently suffer from significantly impairing psychopathology (see Chapter 3.2.1). Less than one-fifth of these students receive any treatment for these disorders. Minority groups and the uninsured are less likely to receive mental health services. One-quarter of public schools have no counselors, and over half do not have a social worker, yet schools are being asked to deal with more of the mental health needs of their students (16). In addition, reports of increased bullying and school shootings accent the importance of recognizing and responding to the psychic pain of students.

School psychiatry has expanded to address school violence, bullying, substance abuse, trauma and mental health promotion. The after-school setting as a venue for mental health supports has received increased attention, with increased rates of crime, drug use, and sexual behaviors during the afternoon hours when many youth are without adult supervision. Psychiatrists and other mental health professionals continue to refine child psychiatry's role in schools, incorporating business and educational principles in effecting change and improving system functioning. Modern school consultation focuses more on early identification and intervention at the individual and system levels to help attain short-term educational and behavioral goals and to prevent later long-term negative outcomes.

School-Based Mental Health Services

Although many psychiatrists partner as independent consultants to schools, some work as part of community-partnered school mental health programs. Approximately two-thirds of schools report partnering with community providers, often outpatient community mental health centers, to provide school-based services. Community mental health program partners may include community mental health centers, hospitals, and universities. Such partners are increasingly contracting with schools to provide a full array of tiered services to students in both general and special education, including universal mental health promotion activities, selective prevention, and indicated early intervention services such as clinical assessment and treatment (17).

Prominent in several states (e.g., Hawaii, Maryland, Minnesota, and Ohio), as well as cities (e.g., Baltimore, Dallas, Los Angeles, Nashville), community-partnered (also termed "expanded" or "comprehensive") school mental health programs have continued to proliferate and address the needs of students, particularly when they might otherwise not have access to mental health services. On-site school mental health services provide greater access to youth and their families, with less stigma and the opportunity for early intervention

TABLE 7.3.5

SCHOOL INTERVENTIONS FOR SPECIFIC PSYCHIATRIC SYMPTOMS

SCHOOL-BASED INTERVENTIONS		
	Interventions	**Examples**
Target Symptoms	**To Be Implemented by Teacher/ School Staff**	**To Be Adapted According to Student's Age, Interests, Capabilities**
Anxiety		
Worry	Forewarn the student of transitions, and have "tasks" for the student to focus on during transitions	If the student is worried about a school trip, provide tasks that distract from anxiety, such as checking attendance, or holding the door at the site.
	Devise a desensitization approach agreeable to the student	If the student fears speaking in front of the class, allow the student to: have the speech read by a peer; read the speech into a recorder outside class; do the speech with a peer reading some part.
	Help the student examine other perspectives	The student says "I can't go to the school dance because everyone will notice that I'm nervous." Ask the student: "how would your best friend/ someone you admire handle a situation like this? What does your friend think you should do?"
	Provide the student with competing responses to negative thoughts or behaviors	The student says "I'm afraid I'll start crying in class." Ask the student: "if you start to feel sad, what can you do before you start to cry? Can you distract yourself by doodling?"
Emotionality	Provide specific steps the student can take to relax, or provide a relaxation ritual	Take three deep breaths; tense fingers or toes for 5 s, then relax.
	Provide alternative foci to distract the student from somatic symptoms	Provide the student a phrase to think of or an activity (doing three problems then standing up, 10 problems then walking to the fountain).
Separation difficulty	Provide desirable activity/responsibility for the student upon entering school	Before school begins, allow the student to feed fish, clean boards, play with peers, or discuss music/sports with another student who shares interests.
	Provide times during the school day for the student to convey brief (30 second) messages to his/her family	Have a brief script/message the student can phone to a parent ("Hi Mom, made it through Science—now we're going to make penguins in art class. I love you.); prepare the parent not to overreact to tearful messages.
	Have a parent send notes to the student to read as a reward for staying at school for increasing intervals	Have a parent place a brief note to the student in his/her lunchbox that the student can read at lunchtime ("Dear [name], I know you're at lunch now—enjoy the cupcake. Have a great afternoon, and when I pick you up today we'll get to play soccer. Love, Dad")
Social fears	Allow the student to observe several other students before attempting a task	If the student resists speaking in class, allow the student to observe others, focusing on how they start, how long they speak, where they look, and how they stop
	Have the student rehearse social skills in a smaller or more relaxed setting	In a small group facilitated by a counselor, have students review and role play how to make and keep friends. Give students homework to practice skills in other settings (classroom, playground, home play date, etc.)
Obsessive thoughts	Establish acceptable teacher comments to "unstick" the student when he/she is obsessing	With the student and parents, identify useful statements to break an obsessive cycle ("Move to your seat on 3—1, 2, 3." "Now think about your coach—what would he/she say to your "rut," "stuck moments?")
	Allow the student to dictate or tape record if he/she cannot touch the pencil or paper	Teacher or voice dictation software can "transcribe" the student's ideas to avoid touching/erasing the paper

(*continued*)

TABLE 7.3.5

(CONTINUED)

SCHOOL-BASED INTERVENTIONS

Target Symptoms	Interventions To Be Implemented by Teacher/ School Staff	Examples To Be Adapted According to Student's Age, Interests, Capabilities
Compulsions	Allow the student to alter the work sequence	If the student gets stuck doing problems in a certain way, allow the student to start with even numbers, or start from the end and work backwards to #1
	Have the student identify and substitute less disruptive compulsive behaviors	Allow the student to touch underneath the desk, flex fingers, or do versions of compulsions that are not disruptive to others
Mood Symptoms		
Sad mood	Check in with the student to quantify his/her mood status each day	Allow the student to complete a mood scale (10 = very happy to 1 = very sad) at first check-in time each morning
	Help the student identify "all the evidence" surrounding his/her negative perceptions of self or events	Examine specific events that led to the student's conclusion that "I'm no good." "What happened that led to this conclusion? Did anything happen that disputes your conclusion? What else happened in your other classes that day?
	Help the student identify automatic negative thoughts	The student says "I'm no fun. No one wants to be around/play with me." Ask the student: "What happened that made you think this?" or "what evidence leads you to reach this conclusion?"
	Acknowledge the student's feelings (rather than dispute/argue with feelings)	"It's sad when…," "discouraging," "frustrating" rather than "it's not so bad," or "aw, come on, things will be better soon"
Irritable mood	Model appropriate responses to replace irritable responses	Provide an alternative, appropriate comment: "I know you have something important to say, and I want to hear it, but I can't hear your point when you use sarcasm. It sounds like your point (without sarcasm) is ________." Could you please say your point again without relying on sarcasm?"
	Allow the student to take him/herself out of a situation (self-timeout) when irritability is starting to disrupt others	Provide specific steps for the student to remove him/herself from situations ("I [student)] feel myself getting frustrated, so I am going to leave this kickball game and swing on the swings for 5 min. After I watch others, and think I understand what I'm supposed to do, I'll try kickball again.")
	Provide opportunities for the student to "fix" problems or inappropriate classroom behaviors	Allow the student a chance to "redo" with an appropriate comment or behavior; if the student tears up paper, allow him/her to tape it together.
Manic mood	Allow the student to complete schoolwork or tests in a less stimulating environment	Identify a calm, comfortable area (with limited distractions, noise, and sensory stimuli) where the student can complete work/tests
	Allow the student alternative modes of expression if he/she cannot verbalize in a useful way or is speaking too rapidly	Provide the student with an opportunity to write, dictate, or draw ideas
	Allow the student to have homebound instruction during manic periods	Determine the conditions that warrant homebound instruction (for example, the student is sleeping during the school day while awake at night; the student's fears or delusions are causing conflicts in the classroom). Home instruction may need to be provided by specialized (therapeutically trained) staff.
Appetite changes	Encourage the student to use snacks and/or physical activity to enhance functioning	Provide snack breaks when the student finishes tasks. Encourage the student to be physically active at appropriate times by taking attendance to the office, standing and moving books, etc.

TABLE 7.3.5

(CONTINUED)

SCHOOL-BASED INTERVENTIONS		
Target Symptoms	**Interventions** — **To Be Implemented by Teacher/ School Staff**	**Examples** — **To Be Adapted According to Student's Age, Interests, Capabilities**
	Change food reinforcers to nonedibles	Instead of chips or candy, reinforce the student with stickers, computer time, or points to earn a lunch date with a preferred peer (if increased appetite/weight)
Fatigue; energy loss	Augment classroom instruction with recordings of instruction	Tape-record or videotape lectures and provide recordings to the student
	Identify study partners who can support and assist with assignments	Allow a peer to study with the student and to assist in academic assignments
	Introduce physical activity throughout the day	Provide the student physical responsibilities (taking attendance to the office, emptying trash, putting up class materials) throughout the day to encourage physical activity
	Grade the student based on work completed or attempted (rather than work assigned)	Grade items completed (e.g., even numbers only), and do not count the items the student does not get to (odd items)
Suicidal or self-harm thoughts	Identify appropriate methods for expressing feelings of hopelessness or self-destruction	Encourage the student to draw pictures, write songs or poems, or use sculpting to depict feelings of sadness, anger or despair
	Establish a hierarchy of people for the student and staff to contact if the student has suicidal thoughts	Specify multiple staff and treatment providers, and the order or circumstances for contacting them, when the student is feeling or appearing unsafe
Psychosis Symptoms		
Hallucinations delusions	Identify and avoid the student's exposure to known distressing stimuli	Clarify with the student or family the items, places, or topics that trigger delusional thinking and find alternatives, particularly when the student is stressed or currently experiencing psychosis symptoms
	Allow the student alternative schoolwork or activities to avoid provoking delusions	If the student cannot proceed with a task, provide an alternative, "grounding" task which requires little creativity, such as reading, moving items, or doing rote tasks
	Devise steps to employ when the student is delusional or hallucinating	Employ a series of steps to de-escalate the student when he/she is becoming more delusional (first: change topic, second: change activity, third: change setting, fourth: change staff).
Attention-Deficit Hyperactivity Symptoms		
Inattention	Define classroom expectations in positive terms	"Please sit down, get our your pencils and paper, and let's look at the board to find our first task"
	Problem solving approach	S-A-C-T-A (Situation-Alternatives-Consequences of alternatives-Try best one-Attempt another if first unsuccessful
	Affix materials to the student's desk	Keep regularly needed materials such as pencils attached to the student's desk where they cannot be misplaced
	Provide organizational devices in the classroom	Use colored folders to distinguish math vs. reading vs. social studies work; use a clipboard to hold papers or current activities
	Keep a sample model of a correctly formatted paper for the student to refer to	Keep formatted (even laminated) paper showing where name, date, etc., should appear on the student's assignments
	Have the student repeat directions back to the teacher	After giving directions, have the student repeat back the sequence
	Provide check-in points during lessons	"Raise your hand when you finish the first three problems, and we'll come by to check them."

(continued)

TABLE 7.3.5

(CONTINUED)

SCHOOL-BASED INTERVENTIONS		
	Interventions	**Examples**
Target Symptoms	**To Be Implemented by Teacher/ School Staff**	**To Be Adapted According to Student's Age, Interests, Capabilities**
	Provide untimed or extended time for tests or assignments	Allow the student to work at his/her own pace, even "rest," so he/she can demonstrate all that he/she has learned
	Diminish external distractions	Minimize noise in the classroom by using headphones, tennis balls on chair legs, or rugs
	Use a daily progress book or email between school and parents	Send a small book or email between school and home to keep parents and teacher aware of the student's daily progress, and of any events that might influence the student's attention
Hyperactivity	Clarify volume and movement expectations of the student before unstructured activities	"As we go through the hall, we'll only use our whispering voices if we have to speak, then in the lunchroom we'll remember to use our 'inside' voices"
	Specify acceptable personal space	Clarify space boundaries with visuals such as "each person has the space of four tiles." Put tape on the floor to demonstrate that others stand outside this distance
Impulsivity	Establish a waiting routine	Develop with the student a multistep plan for waiting, such as "count to five then raise your hand and look the teacher in the eyes"
	When behavior is inappropriate, describe what you want (vs. what you do not want) and reinforce	During misbehavior, clarify what you want the student to do rather than describing the misbehavior ("next time you turn in a paper, make sure your name is at the top" instead of "don't turn in a paper without your name at the top")
Autism Spectrum Symptoms		
Communication difficulties	Create situations to motivate language use	Structure situations so that language becomes helpful (choose the flavor of ice cream from a list)
	Allow the student time to process information and respond	Provide sufficient time for the student to understand direction and to respond (wait 10 s for student response)
	Ensure that the teacher is positioned strategically to engage the student's attention	Align at the student's eye level. Touch the student's desk or chair while quietly saying something like, "Look at the —— (checklist or material) and listen. I need you to know……." Pause to give the student time to shift attention.
	Provide choice boards for the student to communicate preferred activities	Show the student different options for tasks (picture of a book [for reading], food [for snack], counting cubes [for math])
	Develop visual cues to reduce sensory overload	Devise visual cues such as hand signals or use of pictures to diminish reliance on verbal and physical prompts
	Use scaffolding techniques to promote spontaneous language	Add "parts" (sentence starters, transition statements to connect ideas) to facilitate conversation with the student
Difficulties with social interaction	Pair the student with a "typical" peer/buddy to help carry out social interactions in structured settings	Team the student with a "typical" peer during a structured recess kickball game to show the student how to kick, run, and catch.
	Divide social skills into successive steps and teach the steps incrementally	Break down social encounters and teach multiple ways to accomplish each part (you can introduce yourself by saying your name, by asking what the other person is doing, by showing the other person an interesting object, by just saying "hi," or by having a friend who already knows someone introduce that person)

TABLE 7.3.5

(CONTINUED)

SCHOOL-BASED INTERVENTIONS		
	Interventions	Examples
Target Symptoms	To Be Implemented by Teacher/ School Staff	To Be Adapted According to Student's Age, Interests, Capabilities
	Provide explicit teaching about how to start conversations, respond to comments, and end conversations	Describe specific phrases and behaviors to create conversations ("stand this far from a person, look at their eyes, say 'hi', ask if they want to play four square with you," "say 'maybe another time' if they say 'no.')
Restrictive routines/interests	Provide alternative tasks, particularly when the student is sensory overloaded	Allow the student several choices within his/her daily tasks. The student can choose the order of tasks, or when/where to take a break.
	Specify the student's routine for asking questions or describing topics when the student seeks or presents information	Explain that the procedure for asking questions is to limit him/herself to two questions, then allow others to ask ("You can ask the two most important questions to begin work.")
Sensory issues Include extreme over-sensitivity or under-responsiveness to sound, light, or other sources of stimulation	To control sensory inputs, allow the student to be first or last in line or to leave class early	Allow the student to change classes 5 min before the other students, or have him/her hold the door open for other students and then join the end of the line as the "caboose"
	Teach students who use distracting vocalizations or other self-stimulating behaviors to employ other intrusive vocalizations or behaviors	Practice humming loudly and softly and have the student role-play appropriate times to hum loudly and appropriate times to hum softly

(18,19). The shared goals of these partnerships emphasize improving student behavior, addressing barriers to learning, increasing access to mental health care, and improving student attendance and academic achievement. This type of programming relies on collaborative partnerships between school systems and community programs so that school-employed mental health professionals are meaningfully supported by community mental health providers (20).

Intervention and Prevention Programs

There are many evidence-based mental health promotion, prevention and early intervention programs that target the full continuum of supports for all students in school, including those at risk and with identified problems. Successful school models integrate the school, family, and community in coordinating services. Common elements in successful intervention and prevention programs include: youth being connected to a trusted adult, access and coordination of appropriate programs and services with ongoing evaluation, program continuity with school support, and emphasis on early identification and intervention. Psychiatrists can help schools identify and implement appropriate programs depending on the needs and resources of the school system. Several repositories have been developed to guide schools and consulting professionals in the selection of programming to meet their student population and target outcomes.

Websites for Evidence-Based Student Interventions

DELINQUENCY/VIOLENCE/AT-RISK BEHAVIORS:

1. **FindYouthInfo.gov:** This program/site features evidence-based programs that prevent and reduce delinquency or other youth problem behaviors (e.g., drug and alcohol use). Programs focus on one of the following problem behaviors: delinquency; violence; youth gang involvement; alcohol, tobacco, and drug use; family functioning; trauma exposure; or sexual activity/exploitation.
2. Promising Practices Network (PPN) on Children, Families and Communities (**http://www.promisingpractices.net/programs.asp**): The PPN site features summaries of programs and practices that improve outcomes for children.
3. Blueprints for Violence Prevention Model Programs Selection Criteria (**http://www.colorado.edu/cspv/blueprints/model/criteria.html**): Blueprints programs have the highest standards by showing evidence of a *deterrent* effect with a strong research design, *sustained* effect, and multiple site *replication*.

SOCIAL–EMOTIONAL LEARNING (SEL):

4. The Collaborative for Academic, Social, and Emotional Learning (CASEL) (**http://www.casel.org/programs/selecting.php**): "CASEL Select" programs provide outstanding coverage in five essential SEL skill areas; have at least one well-designed evaluation study demonstrating their effectiveness; and offer professional development supports beyond the initial training.

MULTITIERED SYSTEMS OF BEHAVIORAL SUPPORT:

5. Positive Behavioral Intervention System (PBIS): **https://www.pbis.org/school/school-mental-health/interconnected-systems:** PBIS provides a school-wide program to enhance positive behavior in the school system.

MENTAL HEALTH AND SUBSTANCE ABUSE

6. The National Registry of Evidence-Based Programs & Practices (NREPP) (**http://www.nrepp.samhsa.gov**): Intervention summaries are provided to help determine whether a particular intervention may meet identified needs.

TABLE 7.3.6

EVIDENCE-BASED MENTAL HEALTH INTERVENTION BY TIER AND TARGET OUTCOME

	Trauma	Anxiety	Depression	Conduct Problems/Aggression	Substance Abuse	Social Skills Building/Other
TIER 1 Universal, whole school/ classroom strategies for promoting positive mental health in ALL students.	• Psychological first aid: listen, protect, connect, model, and teacher • Teacher education to identify and address psychological distress (e.g., Kognito) • School-Side Ecologic Strategies—positive, safe school climate	• Friends • Positive action	• Positive action • SOS—Signs of Suicide	• 4 R's • Al's Pals • Caring school community • Good behavior game (GBG) • High Scope Educational Approach for Preschool • Life Skills Training (LST) • Lion's Quest Skills for Adolescence • Michigan Model for Health • MindUP • Nurturing Parenting Program • Olweus Bully Prevention Program • Open Circle • Peaceworks: Peacemaking Skills for Little Kids • Promoting Alternative Thinking Strategies (PATHS) • PATHS to PAX • Project ACHIEVE • Raising Healthy Children • Resolving Conflict Creatively Program • RULER Approach • Second Step Violence Prevention Program • Social Decision Making/ Problem-Solving Program • Steps to Respect • The Stop and Think Social Skills Program for Schools • Teaching Students to be Peacemakers (Peacemakers) • Tools of the Mind	• Caring School Community • Life Skills Training (LST) • Lion's Quest Skills for Adolescence • Lion's Quest Skills for Action • Michigan Model for Health • Nurturing Parenting Program • PATHS to PAX • Project ALERT • Project TNT: Toward No Tobacco • Raising Healthy Children • The Too Good for Drugs and Violence Programs	• Competent Kids, Caring Communities • Project SUCCESS • Responsive Classroom (RC) • Teen Outreach Program (TOP) • Tribes Learning Communities
TIER 2 Targeted small-group prevention and promotion for at-risk students.	• Bounce Back • Cognitive-Behavioral Interventions for Trauma in Schools (CBITS) • Support for Students Exposed to Trauma (SSET)	• CARE (Care, Assess, Respond, Empower) • The C.A.T. Project • Coping Cat	• CARE (Care, Assess, Respond, Empower)	• Aggression Replacement Training (ART) • CARE (Care, Assess, Respond, Empower) • Coping Power • I Can Problem Solve: Raising a Thinking Child (ICPS) • Incredible Years • Nurturing Parenting Program • Strengthening Families Program (SFP)	• CARE (Care, Assess, Respond, Empower) • Nurturing Parenting Program • Strengthening Families Program (SFP)	• Girls Circle • Primary Project
TIER 3 More intensive, individualized interventions for students experiencing a mental health	• Trauma-Focused Cognitive-Behavioral Therapy (TF-CBT)	• The C.A.T. Project • Coping Cat	• Interpersonal Psychotherapy for Depressed Adolescents (IPT-A)	• Multisystemic Therapy (MST) • Nurturing Parenting Program	• Nurturing Parenting Program	

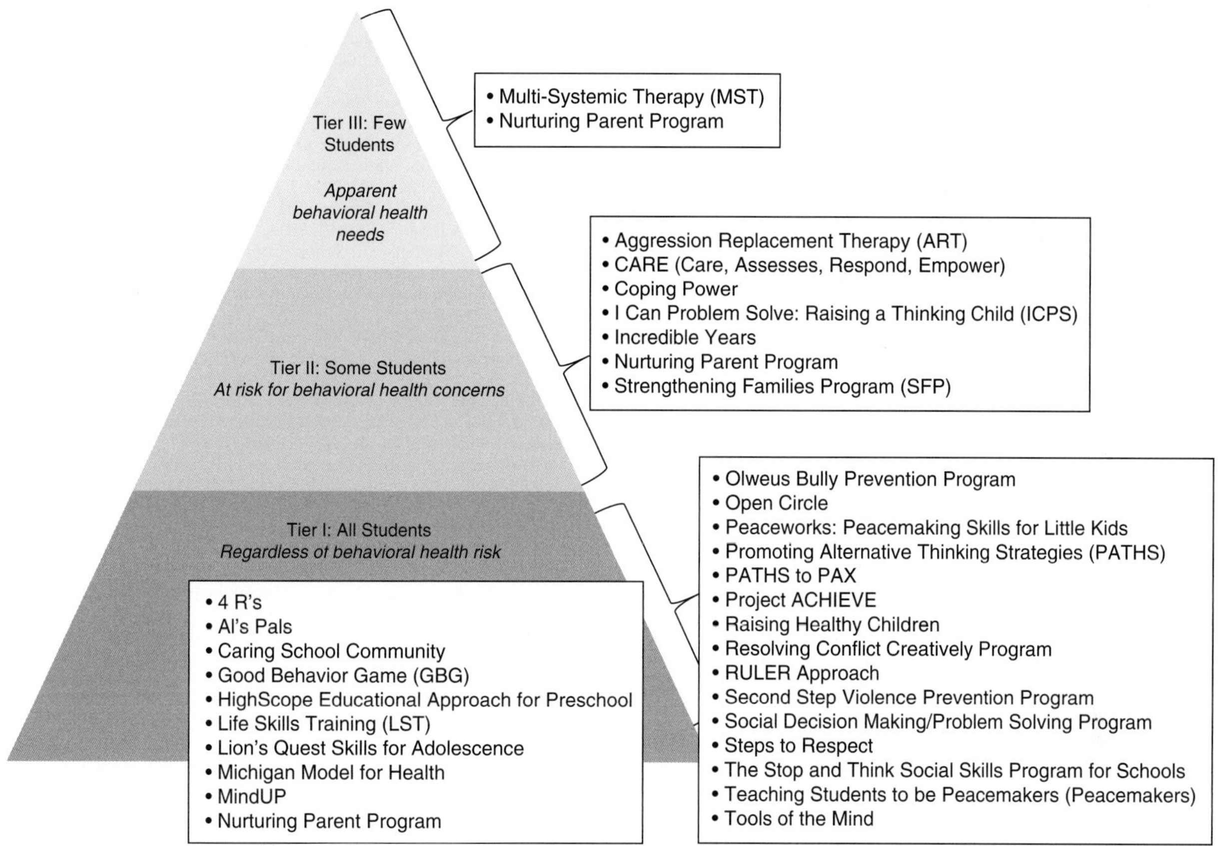

FIGURE 7.3.2. Example of school services to address problems by tier: conduct/aggression.

SUICIDALITY:

7. Suicide Prevention Resource Center: Best Practices Registry (BPR) For Suicide Prevention (**http://www.sprc.org/featured_resources/bpr/index.asp**)

Selection and implementation of school mental health interventions has more recently aligned with the education system's multitiered approach to academic support for all students, termed *Response to Intervention (RtI)*. Essentially, schools use a system of screening and early identification and intervention to identify struggling students and to respond as early as possible with individualized academic supports. Many schools are applying this framework to student mental health, organizing their decision making within a multitiered system of support (MTSS), in which students are identified to receive universal (Tier 1), selected (Tier 2) and/or indicated (Tier 3) supports.

Universal mental health promotion services and supports (Tier 1) are mental health–related activities, including promotion of positive social, emotional, and behavioral skills and wellness which are designed to meet the needs of all students regardless of whether or not they are at risk for mental health problems. About 80% to 85% of students in a school can be successfully addressed through Tier 1 approaches. These activities can be implemented school-wide, at the grade level, and/or at the classroom level. When there is a strong foundation in promoting wellness and positive life skills, concerns or problems can be prevented or significantly reduced. *Selective* services and supports (Tier 2) to address mental health concerns are provided for groups of students, usually between 10% and 15% of students in a school with more complex needs than those who fit in Tier 1, who have been identified through needs assessments and school teaming processes as being at risk for a given concern or problem. When problems are identified early and supports put in place, positive youth development is promoted and problems can be eliminated or reduced. Sometimes these are referred to as mental health "prevention" or "secondary" prevention services. Finally, *indicated* services and supports (Tier 3) are individualized to meet the unique needs of each student who is already displaying a particular concern or problem and displaying significant functional impairment. Tier 3 is usually necessary for approximately 5% of students in a typical school. Sometimes these are referred to as mental health "intervention" or "tertiary" or intensive services. Child psychiatrists are more likely to see patients who may fit in Tiers 2 and 3, where more specialized mental health services are needed.

An example of evidence-based interventions, categorized by tier and target outcome/problem is presented in Table 7.3.6. An example of "tiering" of these evidence-based interventions, is shown in Figure 7.3.2, which is derived from the websites for evidence-based programs described above.

Video Consultation

Video technology has improved alternatives available to schools seeking psychiatric input, particularly those in remote areas with limited access to mental health services. Some of these programs provide indirect service to schools through consultation with school staff provided by a psychiatrist or psychologist around mental health issues impacting students (21). Video consultation can provide individual student evaluations, indirect consultation to teachers and school staff, and opportunities to demonstrate interventions for students whose psychiatric issues impair learning (22). Such technologic advances increase options for collaboration with schools, although new considerations such as billing, confidentiality parameters, providing consultation or treatment across states, receptiveness by staff and students, and potential losses of important observations by not being "in the room" must be anticipated when employing this modality (23). Child psychiatrists have found telepsychiatry in schools to be acceptable, feasible, and an effective vehicle for reducing burden of seeing children across multiple sites (24).

School Consultation Websites

http://www.schoolpsychiatry.org: mental health information for school staff, parents, and clinicians; interventions for psychiatric disorders and symptoms; rating scales to assess disorders and monitor treatments

http://csmh.umaryland.edu: up-to-date information about national school mental health training, practice, research and policy

http://www.schoolmentalhealth.org: a repository of useful resources for school clinicians, educators, families and students on school mental health

http://smhp.psych.ucla.edu: clearinghouse of important mental health, school and education materials

http://ies.ed.gov/ncee/wwc/: information on broad categories of findings of "what works" in schools including academics and mental health

http://www.ldonline.org: information on classroom changes for students with learning disabilities, including ADHD

http://www.ideapartnership.org: up to date information on changes in the IDEA parameters

http://www.wrightslaw.com: information about legal aspects of education, including IDEA 504 Plans

http://www.r14success.org: Response To Intervention school programming across academic and emotional areas

References

1. Bostic JQ, Bagnell A: Psychiatric school consultation. An organizing framework and empowering techniques. *Child Adolesc Psychiatr Clin N Am* 10(1):1–12, 2001.
2. Merikangas KR, He JP, Burstein M, et al.: Service utilization for lifetime mental disorders in US adolescents: results of the National Comorbidity Survey—Adolescent Supplement (NCS-A). *J Am Acad Child Adolesc Psychiatry* 50(1):32–45, 2011.
3. McKay MM, Lynn CJ, Bannon WM: Understanding inner city child mental health need and trauma exposure: implications for preparing urban service providers. *Am J Orthopsychiatry* 75(2):201–210, 2005.
4. Walter HJ, Berkovitz IH: Practice parameter for psychiatric consultation to schools. *J Am Acad Child Adolesc Psychiatry* 44(10):1068–1083, 2005.
5. Cloth AH, Evans SW, Becker SP, Paternite CE: Social maladjustment and special education: state regulations and continued controversy. *J Emot Behav Disord* 22:214–224, 2014.
6. Weist MD, Lever NA, Stephan SH: The future of expanded school mental health. *J Sch Health* 74(6):191, 2004.
7. Erchul WP, Martens BK: *School Consultation: Conceptual and Empirical Bases of Practice*. New York, Plenum, 1997.
8. Caplan G: Types of mental health consultation. *Am J Orthopsychiatry* 33:470–481, 1963.
9. Putnam RF, Handler MW, Rey J, McCarty J: The development of behaviorally based public school consultation services. *Behav Modif* 29(3):521–538, 2005.
10. Stephan SH, Sugai G, Lever N, Connors E: Strategies for integrating mental health into schools via a multitiered system of support. *Child Adolesc Psychiatr Clin N Am* 24(2):211–231, 2015.
11. Kratochwill TR, Albers CA, Shernoff ES: School-based interventions. *Child Adolesc Psychiatr Clin N Am* 13(4):885–903, 2004, vi–vii.
12. Greene RW, Ablon JS: *Treating Explosive Kids: The Collaborative Problem-Solving Approach*. New York, Guilford, 2006.
13. Comer JP, Woodruff DW: Mental health in schools. *Child Adolesc Psychiatr Clin N Am* 7(3):499–513, 1998, viii.
14. Bostic JQ, Rauch PK: The 3 R's of school consultation. *J Am Acad Child Adolesc Psychiatry* 38(3):339–341, 1999.
15. Mattison RE: School consultation: a review of research on issues unique to the school environment. *J Am Acad Child Adolesc Psychiatry* 39(4):402–413, 2000.
16. Waddell C, McEwan K, Shepherd CA, Offord DR, Hua JM: A public health strategy to improve the mental health of Canadian children. *Can J Psychiatry* 50(4):226–233, 2005.
17. Bruns EJ, Walrath C, Glass-Siegel M, Weist MD: School-based mental health services in Baltimore: association with school climate and special education referrals. *Behav Modif* 28(4):491–512, 2004.
18. Benningfield MM, Stephan SH: Integrating mental health into schools to support student success. *Child Adolesc Psychiatr Clin N Am* 24(2):xv–xvii, 2015.
19. Fazel M, Hoagwood K, Stephan S, Ford T: Mental health interventions in schools in high-income countries. *Lancet Psychiatry* 1(5):377–387, 2014.
20. Stephan SH, Weist M, Kataoka S, Adelsheim S, Mills C: Transformation of children's mental health services: the role of school mental health. *Psychiatr Serv* 58(10):1330–1338, 2007.
21. Harper RA: Telepsychiatry consultation to schools and mobile clinics in rural Texas. *Presented at 53rd Annual Meeting of the American Academy of Child and Adolescent Psychiatry*. San Diego, CA, pp. 1–17, October 2006.
22. Stephan S, Lever N, Bernstein L, Edwards S, Pruitt D: Telemental health in schools. *J Child Adolesc Psychopharmacol* 26(3):266–272, 2016.
23. Whitten P, Kingsley C, Cook D, Swirczynski D, Doolittle G: School-based telehealth: an empirical analysis of teacher, nurse, and administrator perceptions. *J Sch Health* 71(5):173–179, 2001.
24. Cunningham DL, Connors EH, Lever N, Stephan SH: Providers' perspectives: utilizing telepsychiatry in schools. *Telemed J E Health* 19(10):794–799, 2013.

7.4 ■ THE LAW

CHAPTER 7.4.1 ■ THE CHILD AND ADOLESCENT PSYCHIATRIST IN COURT

CHRISTOPHER R. THOMAS

This chapter is a guide for child and adolescent psychiatrists on how to work with the legal system; clarifying the complex legal realm and hopefully preparing child and adolescent psychiatrists to be more effective when interacting with the courts. Whether or not a child and adolescent psychiatrist has any interest in forensic work, there may come a time when he or she will have to deal with the legal system. There are many situations in which child and adolescent psychiatrists may become involved with the legal system as part of their practice, including not only forensic testimony, but also legal cases involving their patients. The chapter begins with a brief overview followed by sections that explain the two distinct roles that a child and adolescent psychiatrist may serve within the court. Many of the dilemmas encountered will not

TABLE 7.4.1.1

DEFINITIONS OF LEGAL TERMS

Confidentiality: Secrecy; the state of having the dissemination of certain information restricted.
Cross-examination: The questioning of a witness at a trial of hearing by the party opposed to the party who called the witness to testify. The purpose of cross-examination is to discredit a witness before the fact finder in any of several ways, as by bringing out contradictions and improbabilities in earlier testimony, by suggesting doubts to the witness, and by trapping the witness into admissions that weaken the testimony. The cross-examiner is allowed to ask leading questions but is traditionally limited to matters covered on direct examination and to credibility issues.
Defendant: A person sued in a civil proceeding or accused in a criminal proceeding.
Deposition: A witness's out-of-court testimony that is reduced to writing (usually by a court reporter) for later use in court for discovery purposes.
Direct examination: The first questioning of a witness in a trial or other proceedings, conducted by the party who called the witness to testify.
Expert witness: A witness qualified by knowledge, skill, experience, training, or education to provide a scientific, technical, or other specialized opinion about the evidence or a fact issue.
Fact witness: A witness who may testify only to information that is based on firsthand knowledge.
Guardian ad litem: A caretaker, usually a lawyer, appointed by the court to appear in a lawsuit on behalf of an incompetent or minor party.
Plaintiff: The party who brings a civil suit in a court of law.
Preponderance of evidence: The greater weight of the evidence; superior evidentiary weight that, though not sufficient to free the mind wholly from all reasonable doubt, is still sufficient to incline a fair and impartial mind to one side of the issue rather than the other. It is also referred to as preponderance of proof or balance of probability.
Privilege: A special legal right, exemption, or immunity granted to a person or class of persons; an exception to a duty.
Reasonable doubt: The doubt that prevents one from being firmly convinced of a defendant's guilt, or the belief that there is a real possibility that a defendant is not guilty.
Redirect examination: A second examination, after cross-examination, the scope ordinarily being limited to matters covered during cross-examination.
Subpoena: A writ commanding a person to appear before a court or other tribunal, subject to a penalty for failing to comply.
Subpoena duces tecum: A subpoena ordering the witness to appear and to bring specified documents or records.
Voir dire: A preliminary examination to determine the qualifications of a prospective witness or evidence.

have a clear-cut answer and since factors within any legal situation are complex and often jurisdiction-specific, it is more important for the child and adolescent psychiatrist to not only understand the general guiding principles but also the laws and court procedures where they practice in order to be able to apply these guidelines appropriately (Table 7.4.1.1).

OVERVIEW

The court structure in the United States of America has both state and federal systems. The state and federal courts consist of general trial courts that can have appellate review. That means that at times a case can be decided by a lower court, but a party in the case can later appeal the decision or proceedings to a higher court. General courts in both systems handle criminal and civil cases. Civil cases encompass a wide variety of legal actions ranging from personal injury claims to custody decisions, while criminal courts involve cases brought by the government against a defendant for allegedly committing illegal acts. Psychiatrists are increasingly being called upon to testify in cases involving children and adolescents for varying purposes in both types of legal proceedings.

The state legal systems also provide a series of specialized courts for matters that are better handled in a court of limited jurisdiction. Juvenile court is the type of specialized civil court that is most familiar to many child and adolescent psychiatrists. The creation of the juvenile court in the United States in 1899 focused efforts on the rehabilitation of delinquents rather than their punishment and thus was meant to be different from adult criminal courts. Problems in protecting the rights of youth in the juvenile justice system as well as concerns that it was not effective in preventing recidivism have resulted in court rulings and legal statutes that have made the juvenile justice operate more like the adult criminal court. Over the past few decades what were previously only adult forensic psychiatric evaluations, such as competency examinations, are now being performed in juvenile court.

The extent to which a child and adolescent psychiatrist needs to be familiar with the court system will depend upon their practice. Those who are involved in expert forensic work need to and will be held accountable to have an understanding of the various court systems and different procedures to a much greater extent than the child and adolescent psychiatrist whose only involvement with the court is when subpoenaed as a fact witness.

Many psychiatrists are understandably apprehensive of any contact with the court. Unfamiliarity with the processes and procedures of the judicial system is a major factor in these misgivings and anxieties. Most information child and adolescent psychiatrists have about the judicial system is based on fictional depictions from books, television, and movies, or from news reports about high-profile cases. Imagine the distorted view others have of child and adolescent psychiatry based on the same sources and it is easy to see how unfamiliarity exists on both sides of psychiatry and the law. It is not only the difficulty of dealing with unfamiliar rules, but also very different approaches to evaluating information and making decisions from those used in medicine. While child and adolescent psychiatrists frequently must address conflict in the clinical care of patients, the methods of reaching resolution focus on reducing confrontation through amicable mediation or reconciliation. In contrast, the judicial system relies primarily on an adversarial approach to reach a decision, where opposing parties are allowed the opportunity to present their strongest arguments supporting their position and attacking the other side so that a judge or jury may decide between the two. The aggression of cross-examination can be very intimidating and feel more like a personal attack rather than a dispute of the relevant facts and expert opinions. Medical professionals are often baffled by judicial rulings that go against their opinions or recommendations when they fail to see that the court must consider and balance a wider range of viewpoints or evidence. In addition, the court must follow established procedures and precedent in handling any testimony and evidence it considers. The need to preserve the process over any individual case can appear confusing when certain evidence is removed from consideration. Previous experience with litigious families and rising general concern about medical malpractice also add to misgivings about any contact with the courts for child and adolescent psychiatrists. As in any consultation setting, knowledge and practice can correct most uncertainties and improve the ability of the child and adolescent psychiatrist working with judges and attorneys.

FACT WITNESS

Child and adolescent psychiatrists may be called to testify as a fact witness in a hearing or trial. Fact witnesses provide the most common type of testimony in court, reporting things that they directly saw, heard, or did; in other words, facts.

Process of Involvement

Subpoena

At times, child and adolescent psychiatrists become involved with the legal system by being served a subpoena. A subpoena is a legal summons that requires someone to either appear at a specified proceeding, produce specified documents, or both. In most cases, being served with a subpoena does not mean that the child and adolescent psychiatrist has done something wrong. Generally, it simply means that the recipient possesses information that is relevant to a legal dispute involving other parties. If the child and adolescent psychiatrist works for an organization, be it state or private, they should contact their legal department and inform them of the subpoena as soon as possible. If a recipient is in private practice, he or she may want to discuss the subpoena with an attorney as it may have later implications related to another type of legal claim. The attorney named on the subpoena does not need to be contacted, but may be called to clarify the reason for the issuance of the request. While the child and adolescent psychiatrist may ask the attorney questions about the pending legal case, it is important to remember that attorneys, including those who work for the state or other government agencies, can lack an understanding of privacy laws that direct clinical practice disclosure of information regarding protected health information. It is possible for the child and adolescent psychiatrist to violate the Health Insurance Portability and Accountability Act (HIPAA) Privacy Rule under these circumstances, as subpoenas do not necessarily provide the authority to release confidential personal health information.

Prior to providing any information requested in the subpoena, the child and adolescent psychiatrist needs to ensure that the patient or the guardian, as in the case of a minor child, who controls the privilege to information has consented to the information's release, there has been a judicial determination that the privilege does not apply or privilege has been waived by some action of the patient's, such as making mental health a part of the legal claim. If there has been no waiver by the patient or when it is uncertain who has the ability to consent, such as in custody disputes involving divorced parents, the child and adolescent psychiatrist should contact the issuing attorney to notify him or her that they will not be able to provide any information about the patient without authorization by the patient, the valid representative, or a court order. If the child and adolescent psychiatrist is not provided with any of the above, then he or she must still appear at the court proceeding or deposition and provide information about himself or herself, but when asked information regarding the patient the psychiatrist would respond that the information is confidential and privileged and follow the direction of the judge if in court (1).

There are occasions when the underlying legal dispute may involve, or have the potential to involve, professional liability claims that could expose the practitioner to legal action and would involve different HIPAA regulations that are not covered in this chapter and for which the reader is referred to the chapter on medical malpractice.

As mentioned above, the subpoena could also require the production of all the relevant medical records. Child and adolescent psychiatrists that work for an institution or do contract work are not the legal custodian of the medical records. Any subpoenas requesting copies of medical records should be referred to the department controlling those documents. For clinicians in private practice however, arrangements for the entire medical record that is responsive to the subpoena must be made available.

The child and adolescent psychiatrist may be asked by the family of their patients or the patients themselves to provide legal testimony regarding psychiatric treatment rendered. This may at times be appropriate to agree to as it may offer more flexibility regarding appearance versus a subpoena. However, when the testimony requested is regarding an expert opinion and not a rendition of treatment facts, the requesting party should be informed of the impropriety of the request and that this type of service is best handled by a nontreating psychiatrist. Sometimes a parent might ask for a letter from a psychiatrist providing treatment in support of their fitness in parenting, and it is necessary to explain that such an evaluation has not been part of the treatment, would potentially undermine further care, and is best provided by another psychiatrist. Further information regarding the role of forensic testimony by child and adolescent psychiatrists is detailed in the following section. The child and adolescent psychiatrist should avoid serving as both treating clinician and forensic expert for any given individual.

General Court Procedures

For the child and adolescent psychiatrist who has never been to court before, it is strongly recommended to visit the courthouse prior to testifying. Knowing where to park, where the courtroom in located, where to sit, and the general layout of the courtroom can be helpful to alleviate anxiety and increase the overall comfort level. Juvenile, or family, courts are generally not open to the public and only the parties involved in the current case are allowed attendance without prior permission.

The child and adolescent psychiatrist should dress appropriately for court with either a suit or blazer for both men and women. If bringing files into court they should be contained properly and organized for ease, but avoid unnecessary items to avoid delay with security clearance. Cell phones and pagers are not allowed to be on during court, so other arrangements for coverage will be required. When the physician arrives at court it is important to let the attorneys be aware of the arrival and any time constraints. Although the psychiatrist will be given a specific time for testimony, there is often a significant wait time which is why it is wise to keep the day clear of clinical duties. Many people will bring reading materials to court, but watching the legal process is an interesting way to spend the time as well.

In general, the layout of the courtroom will have a judge presiding on an elevated podium, referred to as a bench, with the court personnel below and to the side of the bench. The attorneys, as there may be several, will be seated at tables facing toward the judge. There will also be a court officer present. If it is an open court, there may be many other people not involved in the case in attendance in the gallery. Depending upon the type of case and the state, a jury may be seated for testimony. When the child and adolescent psychiatrist is called to testify, he or she is sworn in by the officer of the court and then allowed to sit in the witness box which is usually to the side of the judge. The psychiatrist will be asked to state his or her name and business address. It may be helpful to bring a business card to give to the court reporter for difficult spellings, however many courtrooms now do not have court reporters and use audio recording instead. The testimony, either way, will be entered into the official court record. The psychiatrist will be asked to state his or her credentials, training and experience in a process known as *voir dire*.

The psychiatrist may not bill the patient or an insurance company for time spent for testimony or any aspect of the subpoena. In general, there will be no reimbursement for the time spent in court as a fact witness. This may seem unfair for time taken away from practice but still relate to a patient's case. It is best to consider it as part of the unreimbursed activities of clinical care, such as continuing medical education, that are required in order to practice medicine.

Testimony

There may be many lawyers involved in the case and all of them will have an opportunity to question the psychiatrist. There will be initial questioning by the attorney that has asked the fact witness to testify, which is called direct testimony, after which the opposing attorney will ask further questions related to the topic of the earlier testimony or submitted records, referred to as cross-examination. The first attorney then is able to ask the physician further questions if he or she chooses to "redirect" after which the other attorney has the right to again ask questions. The redirect questions can only be about issues raised during the direct and cross-examinations; no new topics can be introduced. The types of questions and the goals of the questioning will vary depending upon the case and the attorney's relationship to it, as each attorney tries to build a logical argument and set of facts for the court to consider in making a decision while attacking the opposing side's argument and evidence. When the witness is finished with his or her testimony, the judge will excuse him or her and the psychiatrist is now free to leave the courtroom. There may be times when the psychiatrist may have to return to court the next day or on a later date. The court will try to work within the physician's schedule, so a prudent physician may wish to bring an appointment book to expedite the process of rescheduling.

When testifying in court, it is important to speak clearly and loudly and allow time to think about a question before supplying an answer. Since the testimony is being recorded or transcribed, all the responses must be verbal. It is important to remain calm and professional regardless of the actions of the attorneys or others involved in the case. The fact witness should give only factual information and not speculate or give any opinion as part of the answer. The simplest and best advice for testifying in court seems to often be the hardest to follow: Answer only the question asked and do not offer further information. If a question is not clear, it is always permitted to say it was not understood and request that it be repeated or rephrased. There will be times when a question cannot be answered as posed and the psychiatrist should feel free to say so to the attorney or presiding judge. This may be the case when the fact witness is asked to give only a yes or no answer to misleading questions, which at times the psychiatrist would be able to clarify if given the opportunity. The psychiatrist does not have to be able to answer each question asked. He or she should feel comfortable saying that aspect was not evaluated or he or she simply does not know the answer to the question. If a question of a fact is asked, the witness has the option, which should be exercised liberally, of checking it against the medical records before responding. The law requires that the fact witness testify according to the best memory or with the aid of written records. This allows the psychiatrist to indicate either uncertainty regarding the answers or no recollection regarding the specific question. Sometimes, attorneys and judges may ask questions regarding the psychiatrist's opinion as an expert. It is very important to not cross the boundary as a clinician testifying as a fact witness and instead become an expert witness, as this can compromise treatment. If this occurs, the psychiatrist can politely raise the issue and express to the judge the problem of providing expert opinion and serving as therapist. Sometimes, questions for expert opinion can be deflected by the fact witness clinician by stating that the question was never addressed or evaluated as part of the routine care of the patient, such as evaluating parental fitness.

Attorneys can raise several types of objections during the course of testimony. The specific legal meaning of each type of objection is beyond the scope of this chapter. The psychiatrist only needs to know that when an objection is made that he or she should either not answer the question or stop speaking if in the middle of a reply. The judge will then make a ruling on the objection and then the psychiatrist will be informed if he or she should answer the question, or the attorney will move on to another line of inquiry.

The physician may be asked if his answer is of "medical certainty," which can be a confusing and misleading term to physicians unfamiliar with the legal system. Most competent physicians are able to acknowledge that there is always the possibility of an incorrect diagnosis, treatment, report, or laboratory result regardless of how unlikely the chances. This may serve the psychiatrist well in a clinical setting and enable them to constantly question and reexamine the diagnosis or treatment plan. However, in a court of law the answer to questions of "reasonable medical certainty" will usually be "yes" if the physician has reached a conclusion or diagnosis and started an appropriate treatment plan. The common legal interpretation of "reasonable medical certainty" is that the physician has sufficient information to be assured that the answer is "more likely than not accurate" (2).

There are some tactics that lawyers may use in their questioning that can be unsettling to the physician who is new to the court process.

1. An attorney will "summarize" the testimony that the physician gave earlier, in direct testimony for example, and then ask the physician if that is correct or use it as an introduction to a question. The physician should be aware of this approach and realize that more often than not the testimony has been altered in some way intentionally. When this occurs, the physician can state that the statement is not entirely correct or have the court record read back.
2. The physician should be aware of any question starting with "Would you agree that . . . ?" This is because there is often a second question after the seemingly innocuous question the physician probably would not agree with and oftentimes the question is intentionally worded to be misleading. This can be done to have the physician answer the question in a way he or she would not have if phrased otherwise. At the same time, the physician does not need to constantly look for traps and try to outmaneuver the lawyer, but instead stick to the basic principles of testifying as a fact witness.
3. Another type of question that may be difficult for physicians to answer in court is: "Is that everything?" It is more likely than not that the physician has forgotten some information and should thus leave the availability of going back to topics at a later time by responding: "That is everything that I recall at this time."

The witness may have to answer questions about previous violations or legal actions in the course of his or her testimony. There may be occasions when a witness may feel harassed by an attorney, but it is not helpful for the child and adolescent psychiatrist to attempt to argue or show his or her anger while on the stand. Ultimately, if the witness either needs to take a break or feels ill they can indicate this to the presiding judge. The judge may either decide to take a short break or adjourn the testimony until another day.

Depositions

Depositions are that part of litigation called discovery and they serve several purposes. They result in both sides showing their hand, they also give attorneys a chance to observe a witness or the types of arguments the other side plans to introduce, which may shape legal strategy in response. Should the case go to trial, a deposition provides a record of answers given by the child and adolescent psychiatrist that, if contradicted in subsequent court testimony, could raise the question of credibility of the practitioner. Deciding to have personal legal counsel present for deposition or testimony depends on the circumstances, but most situations present little or no exposure to the child and adolescent psychiatrist. However, there may be valid reasons why an attorney would prepare and/or accompany a child and adolescent psychiatrist. If the case is volatile or may have further legal implications, it would be prudent to discuss with personal counsel.

If required to by the subpoena and with valid authorization, the psychiatrist may be required to bring the entire clinical file that may be taken by the court, but will be returned later. The psychiatrist can also request to be deposed versus making a courtroom appearance, as a deposition will in general provide more convenience in location and scheduling. The psychiatrist will be sworn in and usually both attorneys will be present along with a court reporter. A deposition usually occurs outside of the courtroom, often at a lawyer's office. One lawyer may object to another lawyer's questions, but the psychiatrist will still be asked to fully answer. At a later time the lawyers may argue the objection in front of a judge and the testimony may be kept or stricken. The psychiatrist should be treated respectfully and allowed to have appropriate breaks. A copy of the deposition transcript may be requested for review and signature by the physician. This is usually helpful in correcting any misspellings of medical terms.

Case Illustration—Subpoena for Custody Case

Dr. Jones has worked with a family for approximately 1 year. The 6-year-old daughter, Anna, has been treated for an anxiety disorder while Dr. Jones also worked with the parents for some behavioral problems. Mrs. Smith was the parent that usually brought Anna to her appointments and Mr. Smith came for the initial evaluation and for two other sessions. The parents during this period have had a breakdown in their marriage and the mother has told Dr. Jones about numerous family problems that are affecting Anna that were discussed in the course of treatment. Dr. Jones has not seen the family for several months and then receives a phone call from Mrs. Smith stating that the parents have decided to divorce, and she asks Dr. Jones to write a letter to the court in support of her having full custody of Anna. She feels that Dr. Jones knows the problems in the family well and would be the best person to explain to the court why she would be the better primary parent for their daughter. Dr. Jones tries to explain that he does not feel comfortable complying with the request and feels that it would be unethical of him to do so. The mother then asks Dr. Jones if she can bring Anna in for a custody evaluation to allow Dr. Jones to feel comfortable writing the letter. Dr. Jones explains that it would be inappropriate for him to change roles from treating psychiatrist to forensic evaluator. Shortly thereafter, Dr. Jones is issued a subpoena duces tecum from Mrs. Smith's lawyer as he feels Dr. Jones' testimony will be helpful to her case. There is also a release of information included from both parents that will allow Dr. Jones to discuss protected health information. Dr. Jones reviews and discusses this request with his attorney. He then blocks his entire clinic day, gathers his case materials, and is in court on the scheduled date and time. During direct examination, the mother's attorney asks Dr. Jones if he thinks the father is emotionally capable of taking care of Anna alone if the parents divorce, and what custody arrangement would be in the child's "best interests" in terms of visitations. Dr. Jones is later asked regarding the child's specific medical treatment rendered and what the long-term prognosis and plan would be for the patient. Dr. Jones has a release to discuss any specifics of the evaluation and treatment of Anna and is required to answer those questions to the best of his ability. However, regarding the earlier questions about the father's capability to raise Anna alone or what type of custody arrangement should be undertaken, Dr. Jones did not perform a custody evaluation and therefore does not have an opinion on those topics relating to Anna and informs the court of this through his answers.

EXPERT WITNESS

Child and adolescent psychiatrists may also contribute to judicial cases as expert witnesses. An expert witness is recognized by the court as being able to offer valuable information based on training and experience. Courts have long recognized that the information provided by individuals with special learning or knowledge can assist in deciding certain cases, such as child custody. A survey of judges and attorneys found that mental health issues were involved in one-third of juvenile cases (3). Unlike the fact witness, the expert witness can provide opinions that the court will treat with the same weight as facts in guiding its decision. Expert witnesses are permitted to testify about conclusions or opinions they have reached based on their professional skills and analysis, as well as provide information about their area of expertise. Serving as an authority for the court is a very different role for child and adolescent psychiatrists from involvement with the legal system on behalf of patients. It is critical for anyone serving as an expert witness to know the procedural, legal, and ethical differences in undertaking evaluations and providing reports for the court from clinical practice with patients and families.

Expert testimony is used in both civil and criminal litigation, two very different judicial settings. It is helpful for any expert appearing in either court to know the differences in the types of cases that are heard and the procedures used in them. Child and adolescent psychiatrists may be called to serve as expert witnesses in civil or family court for custody evaluations, termination of parental rights, or liability claim cases where no one has been charged with a crime. They may also be called to serve as expert witnesses in juvenile or adult criminal court for cases where a minor has been charged with an offense. While juvenile court differs in many aspects from adult criminal court, many of the processes and procedures are the same and the differences have decreased over time. In some states, juvenile courts are referred to as family courts, which can be confusing. Typically in civil or family courts, a plaintiff brings a claim against a defendant for the court to decide. The burden of proof is on the plaintiff and standard for decision is a preponderance of the evidence. In juvenile or adult criminal court, the district attorney brings charges against a minor. The district attorney must meet a much higher standard of proof, where the evidence is beyond a reasonable doubt. In both civil and criminal litigation, the standard for medical expert testimony is a "reasonable medical certainty." Cases in civil and criminal courts may be decided by a judge or by a jury.

Serving as an expert witness ethically requires the avoidance of any potential conflict of interest. A child and adolescent psychiatrist should not provide both therapy and expert testimony for anyone. The impartiality and objective position of the expert witness is undermined by having a therapeutic relationship with a plaintiff or defendant. Likewise, the ability to provide treatment is compromised by also offering expert testimony for any patient. Other potential conflicts of interests for expert witnesses include any outside relationships with any of the parties that create an interest in the outcome of a case, such as serving on the speaker's panel for a drug company involved in a lawsuit.

It is also important to be familiar with the laws and rules concerning expert medical testimony as these may differ from state to state. Some states require licensure within that state in order to conduct an evaluation and testify (4). Some states require specific training or certification in order to perform certain types of forensic exams, such as competency evaluations. Further information and guidelines for conducting forensic evaluations are presented in the American Academy of Child and Adolescent Psychiatry Practice Parameter for Child and Adolescent Forensic Evaluations (5).

Process of Involvement

Child and adolescent psychiatrists are usually contacted directly by the court or by an attorney involved with a case to request expert testimony. The request might also come from a guardian ad litem appointed to represent a minor involved in court litigation or from child protective services pursuing an investigation of a child and family. Sometimes attorneys may have their clients make the initial call seeking expert testimony. This can be confusing as it may appear that the client is seeking clinical evaluation and care as a patient, rather than services from an expert witness. It is best if the initial contact is with the court or the attorneys requesting expert testimony in order to clarify not only the role but also the specific questions to be addressed in any evaluation, as well as details like scheduled trial date. The involvement of an expert witness in a legal case can be required and ordered by a judge, such as a juvenile disposition hearing, or it can be the choice of an attorney in preparing a case, such as a liability claim with emotional injuries for posttraumatic stress disorder. When it is ordered by a judge, it is usually as a court-appointed impartial expert. In this situation, the opposing parties before the court accept that there will be only one expert viewpoint providing testimony, rather than having their own separate or "dueling" experts present.

The first and most important step is to determine the question or questions that prompted the court or attorneys to seek expert testimony, just as in providing any mental health consultation. Sometimes the expectations on what child and adolescent psychiatry can answer or provide are unrealistic, and at other times a request is made for vague or unclear reasons. It is best to clarify the specific request for expert testimony from the start, in order to direct the evaluation and avoid unnecessary complications and confusion later on. This also helps to ascertain the level and extent of expertise required by the case and determines if the child and adolescent psychiatrist is qualified to comment as an expert. Being qualified as an expert for the court does not require that the child and adolescent psychiatrist be recognized as a national authority on the specific area in question, such as posttraumatic stress disorder in a liability claim, but that his or her background include sufficient experience to render a professional opinion. Outlining the specific question or questions for the potential expert will also provide information necessary to judge the relative merits of the case and if the psychiatrist is interested in undertaking the time and effort required to address the issues fully. Finally, along with the details of the parties involved, determining the questions for the expert permits the opportunity to uncover any potential conflicts of interests that might undermine or compromise an objective opinion.

It is also important to determine when and if any court dates have been set. Quite often, expert testimony is the last thing that is arranged as a case develops or a court hearing is scheduled. The psychiatrist must be very clear about the amount of time that will be needed to prepare any evaluation for the court and delays that can be expected in arranging appointments or receiving requested documents. Usually, allowances can be made for the requested evaluations in civil cases and attorneys can request a continuance, but juvenile and criminal courts do not have as much flexibility in their schedules. The child and adolescent psychiatrist should not feel pressured into undertaking cases when adequate time is not permitted to complete a thorough evaluation.

Contract and Payment

Following a decision to take on a forensic evaluation, it is best to have a letter of agreement or service contract outlining the type of evaluation to be performed, rates for fees and related expenses, and how payment will be received. Fees for forensic evaluation will vary from area to area but are typically higher than routine clinical psychiatric services because the nature of the work is more exacting and requires a certain level of expertise. The rates are usually set by the hour rather than a flat fee, since it is impossible to predict how much time any forensic evaluation might take. Charges are for all services, including direct clinical interview of involved parties, review of records, discussion with attorneys, preparation of report, and time spent in deposition or court. There may also be other incurred expenses for travel with certain cases. It is unethical for experts to seek contingent reimbursement based on a percentage of any potential settlement in a civil case. This creates a vested interest in the outcome of the court's decision, undermining the objective position of the expert and compromising the integrity of any opinion expressed. Mental health insurance will not cover the expenses for forensic evaluation. Billing should be directed to those requesting the service, although some attorneys in civil cases may request that it go to the client. Sometimes court appointments for an impartial expert will also define who and what portion of the evaluation will be paid by parents involved in a custody hearing. With any court-ordered forensic evaluation, it is important to request a copy of the order. Quite often, the attorney will request a copy of the child and adolescent psychiatrist's curriculum vitae to be entered in support of the court's determination of expert status. It is important to have an updated curriculum vitae readily handy for court appearance and offer it even when it is not requested in advance.

Evaluation

Forensic evaluations are more complicated than routine clinical evaluations. It is not sufficient to determine if a mental disorder is present or not, but often whether it was present at a specific point in time and what relation it has to the question before the court. For example, the child and adolescent psychiatrist appearing as an expert must be able to say not only that a child has attention-deficit hyperactivity disorder, but also how it might have contributed to his specific behaviors that resulted in charges. For custody evaluations, it is insufficient to just identify the child's developmental needs; there must also be an assessment of both parents' abilities to meet those needs. Questions in a child abuse evaluation must be carefully fashioned to avoid leading the child and suggesting answers. Information must be collected in a fashion that will provide the basis for opinions within reasonable medical certainty.

Offering a psychiatric opinion on anyone requires a thorough evaluation of that individual by the child and adolescent psychiatrist. Interviews should be preceded by obtaining informed consent in which the purpose of the evaluation is made clear, especially that it will serve in preparing a report and who will see it. It is important to remember that those interviewed will probably be influenced in answering any questions by how they desire to see the case decided. Juvenile delinquents may minimize or conceal certain aspects of their life. Parents in custody disputes will want to present themselves favorably. The child and adolescent psychiatrist will want to take this into account and try to obtain the most complete picture by obtaining information from other sources, especially those that are more objective. For example, school records of behavior can be helpful in cases claiming psychiatric trauma, where it is critical to determine exactly when symptoms first appeared in relation to the incident in question. Sometimes evaluations will require interviewing participants opposing each other in court who may not want to cooperate with an interview, such as parents involved in a custody dispute. In those cases, the child and adolescent psychiatrist should inform them that an opinion must be made with or without their participation and that it is in their interest to tell their side of the case.

It is very important to have access to and review of all materials relating to the questions presented by the evaluation. The child and adolescent psychiatrist conducting the examination may need the assistance of the court or attorneys as well as consent of parents in obtaining copies of previous evaluations, school reports, psychological testing, and medical records. Courts or attorneys requesting expert opinion can also be instrumental in arranging clinical interviews with all those necessary to the evaluation. Sometimes, additional consultations or testing may be indicated as part of a forensic evaluation. The recommendation for any referrals should be made to the court or attorney that arranged the initial evaluation.

Report

A written report is usually prepared and submitted prior to any testimony. It is useful to discuss the findings with the retaining attorney or judge prior to composing the report in order to be sure that all questions have been covered. The child and adolescent psychiatrist must not let such conversation influence his or her conclusions unless new facts are presented that had not been previously known. The report should clearly state the psychiatric opinion regarding the legal questions that have been asked and summarize the data on which that opinion is based. It should indicate that all information has been considered, both for and against, and that alternative conclusions have been ruled out. The format is similar to other psychiatric consultative evaluations, but must be more detailed. It should document all sources of information, list all those examined, with both the date and length of interviews, and all records reviewed. The text should be clear and understandable to lay readers, avoiding psychiatric jargon. Pejorative language should not be used. It is important to remember that the opposing side will review any report in detail and unwise language will be brought up in court. Information included in the body of the report should indicate the source, such as "the child described" or "the mother alleged." It is useful to include direct quotations from those interviewed to illustrate specific points. The conclusion should offer a clear formulation from a psychiatric perspective and provide specific responses to all the legal issues raised by the request for expert opinion. If treatment is indicated, an appropriate plan should be outlined and for liability cases it should include the estimated length and costs of all necessary interventions. A well-prepared report sometimes results in reaching a settlement outside of court.

Testimony

The court procedures and advice presented in the section on treatment or fact witness apply to expert testimony as well. Attorneys retaining expert witnesses will most likely want to go over the material that will be presented in court and the questions likely to come up. Depositions are frequently used by attorneys to determine what type of evidence may be presented by an expert witness. Depositions are exactly like courtroom testimony and follow the same procedures in the sequence of examination. Attorneys will object to some questions, but unlike the court, the witness will answer the question and the judge will decide later if the objection will be sustained or overruled. Experts will receive a transcript of the deposition for authentication, and quite frequently it will need correction for medical terms. If followed by later courtroom testimony, statements made in the deposition may be used to challenge the consistency of expert opinion by answers that the expert has made in court.

The process of establishing qualifications may be more detailed if the child and adolescent psychiatrist is appearing for one side of the case and especially if opposing experts might testify. The opposing attorney may try to undermine the value of any subsequent opinion offered by indicating during establishment of qualifications that the child and adolescent psychiatrist is inexperienced, particularly in the areas in question, less worthy than the opposing side's expert, or is just an opinion for sale. The volume of forensic work done by the child and adolescent psychiatrist might be raised not only to challenge experience but also to demonstrate if that is the primary work activity and that the expert is merely a "hired gun."

The process and the advice for handling of direct, cross, redirect, and recross examinations in expert testimony are essentially the same as with fact witnesses. In addition to the qualifications of expertise, the testimony of a child and adolescent psychiatrist is expected to meet the general acceptance rule or Frye test, named after the case of *Frye v. United States* (6). This standard holds that a medical test, procedure, or disorder has been generally accepted in the scientific community. For example, describing a person as suffering from a particular syndrome is unlikely to be considered unless it is included in the *Diagnostic and Statistical Manual of the American Psychiatric Association*. A new standard for scientific opinion in federal cases was set by the U.S. Supreme Court's ruling in *Daubert v. Merrell Dow Pharmaceuticals, Inc.* (7). Unlike the *Frye* standard, *Daubert* states that the judge is the one to determine if the offered evidence is scientifically valid and that it will assist the court in understanding or determining facts relevant to the case. In addition, this assessment by the judge of expert opinion must be made prior to it being presented in court before a jury. Neuroscientific findings are increasingly being introduced as evidence in court cases. It is important to distinguish if the findings from certain tests, such as neuroimaging, refer to a certain disorder or population group in general or if they are regarding the specific individual case. Guidelines have been developed in some instances for the introduction of neuroscientific evidence, such as neuroimaging (8). Sometimes opposing attorneys will object to expert testimony as "hearsay," as evidence based on the statements or experience of those other than the expert witness. Such evidence is permitted for expert witnesses, as the use of others' statements and experience gathered as part of clinical evaluation is a recognized practice in formulating psychiatric opinions. Opposing attorneys may also ask if the child and adolescent psychiatrist accepts or recognizes another professional as an expert in the field or a particular study, paper, or book as authoritative. This is usually in order to present information that may conflict or appear to contradict the evidence presented by the expert witness. It is important to maintain objectivity throughout testimony and avoid the appearance of personal bias. The expert is not a patient advocate in such situations, but presents psychiatric opinion and the data on which it is based.

Specialized Forensic Evaluation

The role and use of psychiatric expert testimony has increased over time and just as the body of knowledge has grown, so have the types of litigation used in court. The specialized topics of child abuse and child custody are handled in separate chapters in this volume. Juvenile justice and tort litigation represent, respectively, the oldest and newest areas of psychiatric expert opinion.

It is understandable that child and adolescent psychiatry be called on to evaluate the problems and needs of youthful offenders in disposition hearings. Child and adolescent psychiatry plays a crucial role in not only understanding antisocial behavior but also in assessing the frequent comorbid and contributing psychiatric disorders of delinquents (9). Beyond the assessment of juvenile delinquents and recommendations for treatment and rehabilitation, child and adolescent psychiatrists are called upon to perform a variety of other assessments for juvenile court. All states permit transfer or waiver of delinquency cases from juvenile to adult criminal court, usually for serious or violent offenses, and many require that a psychological evaluation be performed prior to doing this. The case of *Kent v. United States* (10) established due process and the standards for juvenile transfer. A transfer evaluation usually requires the child and adolescent psychiatrist to assess the amenability to intervention and developmental maturity of the youthful offender. In some cases, state laws require that a minor be tried for certain offenses in adult criminal court, but an appeal can be filed for a "reverse" waiver or transfer back to juvenile court. The same standards regarding maturity and amenability to treatment usually apply in those cases as well. As the juvenile court has become more like adult criminal court, questions have been raised regarding juvenile competency to stand trial and understanding of "Miranda" warning. Evaluation for competency to stand trial is especially relevant for adolescents, as research has shown that few below age 15 meet the adult standard (11). Unlike adults, adolescent incompetency to stand trial is typically due to developmental immaturity rather than mental defect, although adolescents may suffer from mental disorder that impairs cognitive capacity as well. While most states recognize the issue of juvenile competency to stand trial (12), few states have statutes that specify the standards for developmental incompetence, but this is rapidly changing (13). There are instruments that have been developed and tested in assessing an adolescent's competence to stand trial (14), but it will be important to determine what standards are used, if any, in a particular state.

Previously, the only liability cases involving child and adolescent psychiatric expert testimony were claims of malpractice or negligent care. Courts were reluctant to consider any claims for allegations of psychological trauma. The growing scientific understanding of posttraumatic stress disorder and public awareness have resulted in courts considering claims related to psychological trauma (15). Claims for compensation require not only that the child be suffering from posttraumatic stress disorder, but also that the incident in question be a major contributing cause for the symptoms.

Case Illustration—Disposition Hearing for Juvenile Case

Dr. Smith is contacted by the local juvenile court with a request to conduct a transfer evaluation of Jim, a 16-year-old boy currently held in juvenile detention following his arrest for armed robbery. A court hearing has been scheduled but the district attorney and judge agree to reschedule in order to allow time for the completion of the forensic evaluation. Dr. Smith agrees and arrangements are made for billing the court. A copy of the court order, arrest reports, probation record, and psychological testing are sent to Dr. Smith. He contacts the juvenile detention center and arranges times to interview both Jim and his mother, his legal guardian.

Dr. Smith reviews the records and learns that Jim was on probation for possession of a controlled substance (marijuana) when he was arrested for allegedly robbing a pizza delivery boy at gunpoint. No one was injured and apparently the gun was not loaded. He has one other recorded arrest for shoplifting (beer at a convenience store) when he was 13. Psychological testing reveals no current psychiatric complaints other than symptoms associated with his drug use. In addition, it notes that he would be considered competent to stand trial as an adult, although the psychologist expresses the opinion that Jim's needs would be better met by the juvenile court system.

On interview with Jim, Dr. Smith explains that she is preparing a report for the court as it considers sending his case for trial in adult criminal court. Jim understands and agrees to the interview. Jim describes feeling sad since his incarceration but does not have sufficient symptoms for a diagnosis of major depression. He admits to using alcohol and marijuana on almost a daily basis, having begun drinking at age 11 and smoking at age 12. He has drunk until he passed out, but denies blackouts or other symptoms associated with alcohol use. He has had hallucinations associated with marijuana use. He has experimented with cocaine by snorting it on two occasions and has tried ecstasy several times but denies using or trying any other drugs. He also does not think that the marijuana that he uses is laced with other drugs but is not sure. He admits to arrests listed in his criminal record and to having stolen some money from his mother in order to pay for marijuana but denies other antisocial behavior, including physical fights, firesetting, vandalism, cruelty to animals, rape, and involvement with a gang. He states that he had been using both alcohol and marijuana with friends at the time that the pizza delivery boy arrived. He also remembers taking his friend's gun and threatening the delivery boy as a joke, although now he thinks what he did was stupid. His probation officer had made plans to refer him for drug treatment, but that had not taken place at the time of the incident. He also was noncompliant with his probation visits since he did not want to be found in violation with a positive drug screen. He was a student in ninth grade at the time of his arrest, having been held back for failing due to truancy and poor academic performance. He expresses a desire to get his GED and enter a trade school.

His mother also understands the purpose of the interview and agrees to answer Dr. Smith's questions. She reports that she and Jim's father were never married and that they amicably separated when Jim was 3 years old. His father has stayed involved with Jim, taking him every other weekend. She admits that both she and Jim's father have problems with drinking. She currently works evenings cleaning offices and says that it has been hard to supervise Jim. She corroborates Jim's description of his behavior and previous troubles with the law.

Dr. Smith considers that while Jim is mature, his offense was serious and previous probation has not contained his behavior, he does not have a pattern of violent offense and that there has never been a serious effort made to deal with drug use that is central to his antisocial behavior. She calls the district attorney to learn why the request for a transfer hearing was made. The district attorney points out the history of arrests, the appearance of threatening and potentially violent behavior, and that Jim will soon be 17 and beyond the scope of juvenile probation. Dr. Smith asks if the court has the option of deferred or concurrent sentencing, where Jim would be sent for drug treatment by court order and his progress reviewed at age 17, when he would either be released or sentenced as an adult. The district attorney said that was possible but did not know of treatment facilities that would take Jim. Dr. Smith then prepares a report for the court outlining her findings and opinion that Jim should not be transferred because there was no prior rehabilitation for his drug use and the lack of previous violent offenses. She recommends a facility that would accept Jim for drug treatment on court order. The court and district attorney accept Dr. Smith's report and recommendation at the hearing and she does not have to testify.

SUMMARY

There have been numerous changes in the judicial and legal systems in recent years that affect the role of the child and adolescent psychiatrist in court and how the courts deal with children and adolescents (16). The U.S. Supreme Court reviewed neuroscientific research on normal adolescent development in the recent decisions of *Roper v. Simmons* (17), *Graham v. Florida* (18), and *Miller v. Alabama* (19), which overturned the juvenile death penalty and juvenile life without parole (20). Changing laws, judicial rulings, and advancing psychiatric knowledge assure that there will be continued evolution of forensic child psychiatry. It is critical for any professional to keep abreast of these changes, even if forensic child psychiatry is not a part of their clinical practice. Practitioners may not choose to perform custody evaluations, but new laws and judicial decisions regarding custody will affect the children and families they care for. Understanding the judicial process improves the chances of being a more effective advocate for mental health, either as a fact or expert witness.

References

1. Macbeth J: Legal issues in the treatment of minors. In: Schetky DH, Benedek E (eds). *Principles and Practice of Child and Adolescent Forensic Psychiatry*. Washington, DC, American Psychiatric Association Publishing, 2002.
2. Lewin JL: The genesis and evolution of legal uncertainity about "Reasonable Medical Certainty". *Maryland Law Review* 57:380–504, 1998.
3. Mossman D, Kapp MB: "Courtroom whores?"—or why do attorneys call us? Findings from a survey on attorneys' use of mental health experts. *J Am Acad Psychiatry Law* 26:27–36, 1998.
4. Simon RI, Shuman DW: Conducting forensic examinations on the road: are you practicing your profession without a license? *J Am Acad Psychiatry Law* 27:75–82, 1999.
5. Kraus LJ, Thomas CR, Bukstein OG, et al.: Practice parameter for child and adolescent forensic evaluations. *J Am Acad Child Adolesc Psychiatry* 50(12):1299–1312, 2011.
6. *Frye v. United States* 293 F. 1013–1014 D.C. Cir., 1923.
7. *Daubert v. Merrell Dow Pharmaceuticals, Inc.*, 113 S.Ct. 2786, 1993.
8. Meltzer CC, Sze G, Rommelfanger KS, Kinlaw K, Banja JD, Wolpe PR: Guidelines for the ethical use of neuroimages in medical testimony: report of a multidisciplinary consensus conference. *AJNR Am J Neuroradiol* 35:632–637, 2014.
9. Thomas CR, Penn JV: Juvenile justice mental health services. *Child Adolesc Psychiatr Clin N Am* 11:731–748, 2002.
10. *Kent v. United States* 383 U.S. 541, 566–567, 1966.
11. Grisso T, Steinberg L, Woolard J, et al.: Juveniles' competence to stand trial: a comparison of adolescents' and adults' capacities as trial defendants. *Law Hum Behav* 27:333–363, 2003.
12. Soulier M: Juvenile offenders: competence to stand trial. *Psychiatr Clin North Am* 35:837–854, 2012.
13. O'Donnell PC, Gross B: Developmental incompetence to stand trial in juvenile courts. *J Forensic Sci* 57(4):989–996, 2012.
14. Stepanyan ST, Sidhu SS, Bath E: Juvenile competency to stand trial. *Child Adolesc Psychiatr Clin N Am* 25:49–59, 2016.
15. Schetky DH, Guyer MJ: Civil litigation and the child psychiatrist. *J Am Acad Child Adolesc Psychiatry* 29:963–968, 1990.
16. Ash P, Derdeyn AP: Forensic child and adolescent psychiatry: a review of the past 10 years. *J Am Acad Child Adolesc Psychiatry* 36:1493–1502, 1997.
17. *Roper v. Simmons* 543 U.S. 551, 2005.
18. *Graham v. Florida*, 560 U.S. 48, 2010.
19. *Miller v. Alabama* 567 U.S. 460, 2012.
20. Pope K, Luna B, Thomas CR: Developmental neuroscience and the courts: how science is influencing the disposition of juvenile offenders. *J Am Acad Child Adolesc Psychiatry* 51(4):341–342, 2012.

CHAPTER 7.4.2 ■ DIVORCE AND CHILD CUSTODY

MEGAN M. MROCZKOWSKI

INTRODUCTION

Approximately 50% of first marriages in the United States will end in divorce (1–4). Divorce therefore will affect approximately one million children annually in the United States; between 8% and 18% of divorces involve custody litigation (5,6). Thousands of children each year are at the epicenter of often protracted custody battles (1).

As a legal concept, "child custody" is different from "parental rights." Parental rights refers to the legal relationship between the parent and the child (7). This includes the parent's responsibility to provide financial support for the child, the parent's right to custody, to visit with the child, and to make educational, religious, or medical decisions for the child (7). In child custody cases, the court awards one or both parents (joint) legal and physical control of a minor (8). Legal custody refers to parental authority or decision making (9). Joint legal custody means both parents share major decision-making capacity such as education, medical care, and religion (9). Physical custody refers to the time children spend with each parent; joint physical custody indicates children spend time with both parents (9). Split custody refers to arrangements where each parent has sole physical custody of one child (9).

This chapter will highlight the history of child custody disputes, describe practice parameters for custody evaluations and elaborate on important current topics.

HISTORICAL CONTEXT

Beginning in ancient Rome and continuing into the 19th century, children were considered property of their fathers. Therefore, whenever there were custody disputes, children typically were awarded to the father (1). In the 1800s, the courts adopted the principle of *parens patriae*, a moral and legal duty to protect citizens unable to protect themselves. Philosophy evolved into psychology and child development, and the importance of childhood experiences became paramount. Courts followed suit by increasing concern about protecting family members. Courts in Great Britain and the United States became more involved in family disputes, especially when children were involved or at risk (10).

There has been an evolution of models used by judges in custody disputes (11). Psychoanalytic theories highlighting the importance of the mother–infant bond led to the "tender years" doctrine (11). This judicial presumption held that the mother–infant bond is inviolable (11). Barring cases of maternal unfitness, courts awarded custody of young children to the mother (11). The "tender years" doctrine prevailed well into the 20th century.

Within the last century, the prevailing legal test for child custody in all states is the "best interests of the child" (12). This doctrine, first described by Justice Benjamin Cordoza in *Finlay v. Finlay* (12), encompasses the parent–child relationship, the validity of each parent's plans for the child, and puts emphasis on protecting the child's maintenance of bonds with attachment figures (13). It is argued that the benefit of the "best interests of the child" doctrine is to place the judicial focus on the children, making them paramount in the process (1). The concept exemplifies *parens patriae*. Contrary to this, some argue that the use of the word "best" creates an impression that there is a good solution to a particular custody debate, and that the court is responsible for finding this. It has been argued that the terminology should perhaps be changed to "least detrimental alternative," (14) which suggests that all children in custody disputes sustain harm at some level and the best solution is that which causes the least amount of harm (1). Of note, no states have adopted this construct.

The Changing American Family

Same-Sex Marriage

The concept of the American family has grown and evolved. In 2003, in *Goodridge v. Department of Public Health*, Massachusetts became the first state to legalize same-sex marriage (15). In 2013, the U.S. Supreme Court found key provisions of the Defense of Marriage Act (DOMA) unconstitutional (16).

In 2015, the U.S. Supreme Court, in *Obergefell v. Hodges*, extended the right for same-sex couples to marry (17). More specifically, the Court ruled that state bans on same-sex marriage and the refusal to recognize same-sex marriages from another state were both unconstitutional based on the rights of due process and equal protection (17). This case allowed for spouses of the same gender to have the same rights as legally married heterosexual opposite-sex couples including tax relief, emergency medical decision-making power, access to domestic relations laws, spousal benefits (including workers' compensation), inheritance rights, and spousal termination privilege, the ability to divorce (17).

Embryonic Technologies

Recent advances in reproductive endocrinology, including in vitro fertilization (IVF), gamete intra-fallopian transfer, and surrogate embryo transfer, have assisted many couples and individuals achieve pregnancy who may have otherwise been unable to do so (8). During IVF, mature eggs are retrieved from the woman's ovaries, fertilized by sperm in a laboratory, and are implanted into the woman's uterus (18). In gamete intra-fallopian transfer, the sperm and oocytes are directly transferred into the fallopian tube (19). Surrogate embryo transfer involves implanting an embryo into the uterus of a surrogate.

Advances in this technology have led to legal and ethical dilemmas, many of which are not yet covered by state laws. One area of ethical and legal debate is between genetic mother versus gestational mother. In this scenario, one mother donates her egg for fertilization through IVF to another woman for gestation in her uterus. Each of the two women makes a biologic contribution to the creation of the new human life. In *Johnson v. Calvert* (20), the gestational mother filed suit for parental rights of the child that she bore for another couple (8). The court found in favor of the biologic mother and likened the surrogate to a foster parent, standing in for a parent temporarily unable to care for her child.

Surrogacy, impregnation by artificial insemination with the sperm of the husband of a childless couple, carries with it ethical and legal questions. *In Re Baby M* (21,23) the first well-known case of its type, which received notoriety in the lay press, highlights one dilemma. In this case, the surrogate changed her mind after delivering the child and refused to surrender the child (8,23). The court found there was a contract between the parties that was legally enforceable. The surrogate mother appealed her case to the New Jersey Supreme Court, declaring that a surrogacy contract undermines the dignity of human life and cannot be enforced (8). The New Jersey Supreme Court unanimously reversed and invalidated the surrogacy contract, granting custody to the biologic father, with visitation rights to the surrogate (8).

In *Jones v. York* (22), the court ruled that a couple has the right to possession of their embryo (8,22). The Joneses kept one frozen embryo at an IVF program in Norfolk, VA, and when they moved to California, requested the program transport the embryo to an IVF program in CA. The Norfolk program refused to release the embryo citing the signed consent form, legal liability risk, and the demeaning nature of mailing a human embryo. The court ruled for the Joneses and described the embryo as an object rather than a human being. Thus, the embryo was considered property to be returned (8,22).

In *Davis v. Davis* (21,23) a couple cryopreserved seven embryos for possible future use. The couple divorced and the question arose over the possession of the embryos. The husband sought to prevent the release of the embryos to anyone, including his ex-wife, and the wife sought to have the child with the embryos. The court ruled that the seven frozen embryos were "human beings existing as embryos" whose best interests necessitated "they be available for implantation." The judge awarded the wife with the embryos for implantation but reserved the question of child support, custody, and visitation rights until the children were born (8,21). Ms. Davis remarried in Florida and decided to give the embryos for adoption to a childless mother. The husband filed suit and on appeal the higher court reversed and ruled the couple shared an interest in the embryos and in the event they could not agree with what to do, the embryos should remain frozen (8,21).

Fathers

In comparison to issues involving reproductive technologies, the law is clearer regarding the rights of fathers. In *Stanley v. Illinois* (24), Mr. Peter Stanley lived with Ms. Joan Stanley intermittently for 18 years, during which time they had three children. Under Illinois state law, upon the death of a mother, children of unwed fathers become wards of the state. When Ms. Stanley died, the children were declared wards of the state, though their father was never shown to be an unfit parent. When custody of a child is challenged, parents are permitted a hearing in which to demonstrate he or she is a fit parent. The U.S. Supreme Court held that by denying Mr. Stanley a hearing as to his parental fitness, Illinois denied him equal protection of laws under the Fourteenth Amendment (25). The Fourteenth Amendment of the U.S. Constitution forbids states from "denying any person life, liberty or property, without due process of law" or to "deny to any person within its jurisdiction the equal protection of the laws" (26).

In *Michael H. v. Gerald D.* (27), the mother was having an extramarital affair and conceived a child (27). The biologic father filed a "filiation action" in California Superior Court to establish both his paternity and visitation rights. The U.S. Supreme Court held that the genetic father has no legal rights if he became a father through adultery. When a child is born during a marriage, the father is presumed to be the legal father, regardless of the source of the sperm (8,27).

Rights of Third Parties

In 25 states there is statutory law protecting the rights of third parties to maintain a relationship with a child (8). The language of these statutes typically uses the term "significant relationship" in lieu of more specific groups, such as grandparents, stepparents, etc. (8,28).

One example of stepparent's rights is *In Re Ewing* (1974). The court granted custody to the stepfather, who had financially supported the children and with whom the children had lived for 3 years prior to their mother's death instead of their biologic father, with whom they had no contact. Another example of third person rights, in this case grandparents' visitation, is found in *Troxel v. Granville* (29). Following the death of their son, the paternal grandparents filed suit for the right to visit their grandchildren. The U.S. Supreme Court held that the Washington statute, which allows any person to petition for a court-ordered right to see a child over the custodial parent's objection, was unconstitutional. The Court held that even if such visitation was found to be in the child's best interest, it interfered with the fundamental right of a parent to rear his or her children (29).

Divorce—An Update

Short-Term

Conflict within the marriage is a more important predictor of child adjustment than is divorce or postdivorce conflict (30,31). There are three central explanations for why divorce has a negative impact on children's lives: parental absence, economic disadvantage, and family conflict (32). Divorce is associated with a decrease in both quantity and quality of contact between children and their noncustodial parents (32–34). One meta-analysis sought to summarize the effects of parental divorce on children. This study found that compared to children from intact families, children of divorce experience lower levels of well-being, though the effect sizes are weak (32).

Developmental factors dictate how children and adolescents manifest their distress at the time of divorce (35–38). Preschool children may experience regression, intensified anxiety and fears, sleep disturbances, and increased aggression. Middle school–aged children may experience a sense of powerlessness, anxiety, and loneliness. They may also struggle with feelings of responsibility for the divorce, conflicts of loyalty between the parents, and have fantasies of reconciliation. Their school performance and peer relationships may also be negatively affected. Adolescents may experience acute depression, intense anger, and anxiety about their own future relationships. They may also withdraw socially and accelerate their separation and individuation process from the family. In general, this acute response diminishes or disappears over a period of 1 to 2 years (39).

Parental divorce has been shown to be related to an increase in boy's externalizing behaviors in school, especially if the divorce was during middle school (40). Girls externalizing behavior problem trajectories were not affected by parental divorce, regardless of when the divorce occurred (40). Divorce occurring from kindergarten to grade 5 was associated with more adverse effects on internalizing and externalizing problems than divorce occurring between grades 6 and 10 (41). However, divorce occurring between grades 6 and 10 was associated with more adverse effects on grades in school (41).

Long-Term

Dr. Judith Wallerstein conducted a 25-year longitudinal study on the effects of divorce on children (42). She and her colleagues found divorce is a cumulative experience for the child and its impact increases over time and may superimpose a series of difficult tasks on top of normal developmental milestones. There have been several critiques of this study. For instance, it was argued this was not a rigorous study as it included a nonrandom sample, without a comparison group of separating families from the general population of parents with children of similar age (43,44). Additionally, the sample was not a representative sample as it was comprised of mostly white, well-educated parents, a significant proportion of which had psychological problems (43).

One study found divorce was associated with declines in reading scores, positive approach to learning, interpersonal skills, and self-control, and associated with increases in internalizing problems and externalizing problems (45). These results were consistent for younger children and adolescents.

Marital conflict is associated with more depression and psychological disorders in young adults (32). Numerous studies have described that divorced children have been reported to be more aggressive and impulsive and more likely to engage in antisocial behaviors compared to age-matched controls of never-divorced children (46). Divorced children are more likely to use alcohol, cigarettes, and marijuana compared to never-divorced children (46). This is thought to be related to more reliance on peer groups that use substances, less effective coping skills, and impaired parental monitoring (46). Divorce has been associated with lower academic achievement in children, though the effect size is small when socioeconomic controls are utilized (46). It has also been described that children in single-parent families are at higher risk for video game addiction (47).

No "Good" Time

There is no good or ideal time to divorce for children. Rather, there is research that shows the well-being of the children is positively correlated with the postdivorce psychological adjustment of the custodial parent, low parental conflict, and financial security of the mother (48,49). Social functioning of the children is positively associated with custodial mother's reports of extended family support (46). Furthermore, the quality of the relationship between the child and both parents is positively associated with the child's adjustment (49). Several studies show that the well-being of children of divorce improve over time; more specifically, the behavior of boys and girls improved within 2 years following divorce (48).

Etiologies of Divorce

The National Survey of Families and Households (NSFH), a nationally representative sample of adults and their spouses or cohabitating partners, examined the effects of divorce on the couple's attitudes (50). It was found that husbands', but not wives' perceived disagreements was associated with a higher chance of divorce; the couples' marital happiness strongly mediates the effects of the husbands' dissatisfaction (50). Physical violence was found to be the main hardship that causes divorce (50). The findings in this study suggested that relationship instability arises from possibly explosive fights in which very unhappy, dissatisfied partners do not find mutually satisfying solutions (50).

Ways to Avoid Litigation

Collaborative Family Law

In 1990, Mr. Stuart Webb, an attorney in Minnesota, founded a term for a process of alternative dispute resolution called collaborative family law (CFL) (45). CFL consists of attorneys working with couples in four-way settlement conferences in an attempt to settle the divorce amicably and without resorting to the adversarial process in court (51). Prior to settlement conferences, the parties all agree to the basic tenets of collaborative law: to negotiate openly and honestly, motivated by the avoidance of disputes that may arise during discovery (51). Ms. Pauline Tesler, an attorney in California, worked similarly on CFL in San Francisco (51). Collaborative law is also unique in its use of a "participation agreement," a binding contract between counsel and the parties describing collaborative law and encouraging good faith negotiations to avoid litigation (52).

Collaborative law is not without criticism (53). Critics argue that the disqualification requirement is unethical and a violation of the American Bar Association (ABA) Model Rule of Professional Conduct 1.16 because it allows attorneys to withdraw their representation when litigation becomes necessary, which may be when their clients need their help the most (53). Critics also argue that should the collaborative break down, clients will spend more money than they would have in other forms of dispute resolution (53).

Mediation

Mediation provides divorcing couples with a second alternative to the adversarial process in court (46). Research in five countries over two decades has led to the conclusion that custody mediation should be offered widely and should be considered prior to proceeding to court (46). Satisfaction with the process is high, even among those who fail to reach an agreement (46). The outcomes of two types of family mediation, child-focused mediation (focusing on the child's needs without direct involvement of the child) and child-inclusive mediation (includes child interviews), were studied (54). Compared to those in the child-focused mediation, those in child-inclusive mediation had less relitigation (54). Custody mediation leads to settlements in 50% to 85% of cases, and leads to more joint legal custody agreements than litigated cases (55). Some studies have shown that mediation is associated with less postdivorce conflict along with more parental cooperation and communication about children, than parents in adversarial custody disputes (46). Mediation is frequently more efficient and less costly than traditional litigation (52).

There are arguments against mediation (53). Mediation focuses the dispute resolution process on one person, the mediator, instead of the parties and attorneys working together (53). Mediators often emphasize the statutory, common law, and local origins of the suggestions made to clients, which may pressure them to settle due to feeling threatened or overwhelmed (53). Should parties settle through mediation for the wrong reasons, they may pursue additional legal action in the future (53).

Settlement Between Parties

Approximately 90% of child custody disputes are settled out of court (5,56). One survey assessed the perspectives of 59 attorneys regarding child custody evaluations completed by mental health professionals (56). The attorneys were asked their opinions about factors that prompted custody evaluations, expectations regarding evaluation procedures, utility of the resultant report, and the impact of evaluations on litigation. Findings indicate that attorneys are most likely to seek child custody evaluations in the context of questions of parental fitness or allegations of physical or sexual abuse. Attorneys reported they expect a comprehensive evaluation and report. Custody evaluations play a significant role in the decision of whether to negotiate a settlement or proceed to trial (56).

Postdivorce Programs

There are many divorce education programs connected to courts, some of which are mandated by state or local law (46). These programs utilize research about divorce, parental conduct and child adjustment, and some also have sessions for children (46). Typical objectives of divorce education programs include information for parents about how children respond to separation and divorce, information about the potential ill-effects of high conflict divorce on children, illustrate positive parenting responses to help children adapt to divorce, and describing a child's need for continuing relationship with both parents (46). Programs encompassing multimedia approaches including videos, skill-building demonstrations and exercises, discussion, handouts, and some didactics were found to be more effective than single format programs (46).

Examples of postdivorce programs include the PEACE Program, KIDS Program, and Children First (57). One review found limited evidence that these programs achieve their stated goals of improving the quantity of noncustodial parent contact, reducing conflict between parents, improving coparenting, reducing relitigation, or improving outcomes for children (57). The lack of evidence of the programs effects is due to methodologic limitations in the evaluations in that there have not been rigorous evaluations of these programs (57).

Custody Disputes

Why They Happen

Ten percent of divorces involve custody litigation (1). It is important to understand the historical underpinnings of the divorce (58). It has been noted that the adversarial process exacerbates the conditions that create risk for children, and in the process, often undermines efforts of parents to maintain protective conditions for their children following divorce (59). The central failing of the adversarial process in custody disputes are the inherent mechanisms and practices that escalate conflict, decrease the possibility of civil communication between parents, highlight the win–lose atmosphere, and encourages bitterness and irresponsibility of parents (59). Legal strategies focused on winning a custody dispute start early in the adversarial process, and may include parents advised not to speak to the other parent, to search or exaggerate memories of damaging information to build their case (59).

Stress on Parents and Children

Custody disputes can have damaging effects on both parents and children (59). Several studies support the view that children may wish to for their input and concerns to be heard during the divorce process (60).

Positive Effects of Divorce

One study described the positive effects of divorce as perceived by children (61). These included happier mother, happier father, closer relationships with both parents and siblings, and a greater appreciation for siblings (61).

Special Issues in Custody Disputes

Same-Sex Divorce

There are no differences in the development of gender identity and gender role as a function of the sexual orientation of the parent (62). Furthermore, it has not been found that children reared by homosexual parents proportionately identify more as homosexual (63). It is consistently found that children of homosexual parents have no significant differences in separation-individuation, behavior problems, self-concept, moral judgment, school adjustment, or social relationships compared to those with heterosexual parents (64). One recent national, longitudinal, population-based sample described that adult children of same-sex parents were more similar than different from those of heterosexual parents (65). Adult children of same-sex couples were less likely to practice religion and had less contact with their parents than children of heterosexual parents (65). Research findings provide no justification for limiting custody or visitation by homosexual parents (64).

Long-Distance Parenting

As of 2015, at least 37 states had statutes regarding relocation of children following divorce (66). In *Tropea v. Tropea* (67), New York's Court of Appeals, the state's highest court, held "that each relocation request must be considered on its own merits with due consideration of all the relevant facts and circumstances and with predominant emphasis being placed on what outcome is most likely to serve the best interests of the child" (67). Rather than applying the three-step meaningful access exceptional-circumstances analysis, this court held that each relocation request should be based solely on the best interests of the child (67). *In re Marriage of LaMusga* (68), the California Supreme Court held that in parental relocation, the noncustodial parent who opposes the relocation has the initial burden of proof of showing that the relocation would cause detriment to the child (68).

Allegations of Domestic Violence

Child custody decision making in the context of alleged domestic violence is an area both controversial and unpredictable (69,70). The U.S. Department of Justice Office on Violence Against Women (OVW) work led to the National Child Custody Differentiation Project (69). The project's main goals included identifying domestic abuse through screening, understanding the context of the abuse, understanding the implications of abuse, and accounting for the abuse in custody-related decisions (69).

Studies have indicated high rates of intimate-partner violence, ranging from 25% to 50%, in samples of high-conflict divorce (71). Intimate partner violence adds a complicated concern to child custody disputes. Guidance has been provided by experts in the field about assessment, interventions, and visitation centers (72–74). New York Domestic Relations Law 240 requires courts making custody decisions "must consider the effect of such [proven] domestic violence upon the best interests of the child" (75).

Allegations of Sexual Abuse

Child sexual abuse allegations can occur with child custody disputes (75–78). Research has suggested that 50% of allegations made in child custody disputes are unsubstantiated (79,80). There are some best practices that have been described by experts in the area (81). Specifically, when assessing allegations of child sexual abuse, the forensic psychiatrist should gather information from multiple sources, consider all reasonable hypotheses that could explain each facet of the allegation, consider the context of the allegation, and examine and present all evidence that the allegation is true and all evidence that the allegation is false (81).

One Canadian study described that 12% of child abuse investigations were in the context of child custody disputes (82). This study found that 5% of all investigations in child custody disputes involved allegations of sexual abuse; this was not statistically significant from those not involved in a child custody dispute (82).

Drug Use

It is imperative for a child custody evaluator to explore whether either parent abuses drugs or alcohol (1). It is incumbent upon the child custody evaluator to determine the impact of the possible substance abuse on the child (1).

Mental Illness in Parent

A common issue may arise when one parent has a mental illness. The diagnosis itself should not impact the child custody decision; rather, the effect of the psychiatric illness on the parent–child relationship should be explored along with whether the mentally ill parent has insight into his or her illness and is responsible with treatment (1,83). In *Jaffe v. Redmond,* the U.S. Supreme Court held that the Federal Rule of Evidence 501 protects the conversations between a therapist and patient, thereby recognizing a "psychotherapist–patient privilege" (84). Psychotherapy treatment records may be disclosed in a child custody proceeding if the person holding the right to confidentiality, or privilege, voluntarily authorizes disclosure (85). The Health Insurance Portability and Accountability Act (HIPAA) mandates that the authorization for release of protected health information, for example, psychotherapy treatment records, must be voluntary (86).

Child with Special Needs

It is imperative that a child custody evaluator explore the child's physical and mental health (1). The clinician must assess each parent's ability to understand and provide recommended treatment for the child's disorder (1). Examples may include a child with a psychiatric diagnosis such as attention-deficit hyperactivity disorder (ADHD), or neurologic or physical disabilities. The clinician should assess how well each parent can provide specialized care, such as at-home environmental, therapeutic, and behavioral interventions along with ensuring additional services, such as occupational and speech therapy, are obtained if warranted (1).

Grandparent's Rights

The best-interest doctrine is a gender-neutral, child-centered model for decisions of child custody. The landmark case, *Painter v. Bannister* (87), highlights the issue of a custody dispute between a biologic father, Mr. Painter, and biologic maternal grandparents, Mr. and Mrs. Bannister. Immediately following the death of the biologic mother and one child, Mr. Painter, who lived in California, asked his wife's parents, the Bannisters, to care for the surviving child in their home in Iowa. When the biologic father remarried, he sought to return his child to his custody, but his maternal grandparents declined (84). The Iowa Supreme Court awarded custody to the maternal grandparents (87).

Relocation

Many divorced parents seek the court's permission to move with their children away from the other parent (88–90). Relocations may result in substantially less contact with the noncustodial parent. Older children who move following divorce have been shown to have higher levels of maladjustment (91).

Several cases illustrate various courts' differing decisions on this topic. In *Rains v. Rains* (92), the Michigan Court of Appeals held that the party requesting the change of domicile has the burden of establishing by a preponderance of the evidence that the change is warranted (92). The court considered whether the legal residence change had the capacity to improve the quality of life of both the child and relocating parent, the degree to which each parent had complied and utilized his or her time under the current parenting agreement, the degree to which the move would allow continued relationships with both parents, the extent to which the parent opposing the move was motivated by a financial desire to uphold child support, and whether there is a presence of domestic violence (92). In *Tropea v. Tropea* (93), the New York State Court of Appeals, the state's highest court, held that the best interest of the child standard should hold in relocation cases (93).

In contrast to these two cases, the California case, *In re Marriage of Burgess* (94), replaced the best interests of the child standard. In this case, the parent who opposed the move must prove the children would be harmed if they relocated (94). In essence, the best interests if the child standard was replaced by the best interests of the custodial parent standard (88,94). Similarly, in *Baures v. Lewis* (95), the New Jersey Supreme Court held that parents wishing to move must demonstrate good faith and that the move will be in the child's best interests (88,95).

The following factors have been proposed to be considered when determining whether relocation should be permitted (88). First the psychological adjustment and parenting capacities of relocating parents, the psychological adjustment and parenting skills of the nonmoving parents, conflict between parents, economic situation following relocation, and the distance between parents following relocation (88).

Parental Kidnapping

Uniform Child Custody Jurisdiction Act. Parental kidnapping is defined as removal, concealment, detention, or retention of a child from the other parent (96). Before 1968, State courts in the United States could exercise jurisdiction over a child custody case based on the child's physical presence in the state (97). Courts would freely modify sister States' custody orders because the U.S. Supreme Court had never settled the question of whether the Full Faith and Credit Clause of the U.S. Constitution applied to custody decrees, meaning one state must respect the custody decision of another state (95,96). This fostered child abduction and forum shopping (97). The Uniform Child Custody Jurisdiction Act (UCCJA) of 1968 governed the jurisdiction in initial child custody determinations and required States to enforce, not modify, sister States' orders (97,98). The UCCJA established four jurisdictional grounds: home state (child has lived for at least 6 months), significant connection, emergency, and vacuum (applies when no other jurisdictional basis exists (97)). The Uniform Child-Custody Jurisdiction and Enforcement Act (UCCJEA) of 1997, replaced the UCCJA (97). The UCCJEA governs the State courts' jurisdiction to make or modify child custody and visitation orders (97).

Parental Kidnapping Prevention Act. The Federal Parental Kidnapping Prevention Act (PKPA) was signed into law in 1980 to address problems of custody jurisdiction (99). The act provides for full faith and credit for child custody determinations made by the proper state (96,99). The PKPA was drafted to act as a tiebreaker when two states claim they have jurisdiction in a child custody or parental abduction case (96,99). State courts that exercise jurisdiction consistently with the criteria in PKPA are entitled under Federal law to have their custody and visitation orders given full faith and credit in other States (97). Both the UCCJA and PKPA were enacted to prevent jurisdictional gridlock in custody and child abduction cases and to facilitate the interstate enforcement of child custody decisions (96). The UCCJEA, law in all states except Massachusetts, has solved most of the jurisdictional conflicts and ambiguities that remained under UCCJA and PKPA (100).

The Hague Convention and the International Child Abduction Remedies Act. The Hague Convention was signed by the United States in 1981, ratified by Congress in 1986, and implementing legislation was passed in 1988 (101). The Hague Convention accomplishes the same purpose as UCCJA and PKPA on an international level (96,102). The purpose of The Hague Convention is to allow for the prompt return of the parentally abducted or wrongfully retained child to the country of their "habitual residence" (95,101). The International Child Abduction Remedies Act (ICARA) is the implementing statute of the Hague Convention within the United States (103).

Impact on Children. In all 50 states and the District of Columbia, parental child abduction is a crime (104). One study demonstrated parental abduction was associated with an increase in children's conduct problems, learning problems, psychosomatic diagnoses, and anxiety (105,106). Another study reported a high level of posttraumatic stress disorder (PTSD) in children who had been abducted (107). A study of children after abduction found that most reported satisfactory adjustment though a high proportion received mental health services (106). A more recent study corroborates these findings (104). More specifically, abductees were found to have trouble sleeping and concentrating, trouble recalling important aspects of the abduction, trouble making and keeping friends, and loss of trust in the opposite sex (104).

Parental Alienation

In the process of a high-conflict separation or divorce, a child may ally him- or herself strongly with one parent while rejecting another parent. This has been described as parental alienation, a child's strong alignment with one parent without legitimate justification (108). This controversial concept, and the concept of parental alienation syndrome were proposed, but ultimately not included in the *Diagnostic and Statistical Manual of Mental Disorders* (DSM-5) and the *International Classification of Diseases,* Eleventh Edition (ICD-11) (108). Scholars have debated over whether such a syndrome exists, and use of the term has engendered considerable criticism and controversy (109,110).

The Custody Evaluation

Guidelines for evaluating child custody disputes have been published. The American Academy of Child and Adolescent Psychiatry (AACAP) has published Practice Parameters for Child Custody Evaluations (1). The American Academy of Psychiatry and the Law, The American Psychological Association (5,111), The American Psychiatric Association (112), The American Association of Family and Conciliation Courts (113), have all published practice parameters. Several states also have published their own guidelines for custody evaluations (114–123). In addition to these professional organizations and states, several mental health practitioners have also published guidelines (124,125).

The average child custody evaluation takes approximately 21 hours, including time spent completing the following: review of materials, interviews of all relevant parties, observations, collateral contacts, report writing, and sometimes testimony in court (126). The evaluation is composed of several phases: preparing strategy, performing the clinical evaluation, writing the report, and at times, testifying in court (126). The evaluation itself may take 1 to 3 months and it may be over a year before the court hears the case (1).

Referral Process

Section 405 of the Uniform Marriage and Divorce Act states that a court may order a custody evaluation if "a parent or the child's custodian so requests" (127). In several states, for example, New York and California, appointments are court-ordered (1,128). A referral from noncustodial parent, requested while he or she has visitation, should be refused (1). It is both unethical and usually illegal to interview a child without permission of the custodial parent, unless court-appointed and ordered by the judge (1). It is important to accept only cases if the evaluator is court-appointed or agreed-upon by both parties (1). It is better, however, to be court-appointed to come under the court's immunity. The clinician should clarify all questions requested by the judge to determine whether he or she can provide an opinion (1). The fee should cover all clinical interviews, document reviews, consultations by phone, and report writing (1).

Evaluation Structure

The evaluator should request documents, including medical, educational, and psychiatric records (1). In addition to interviewing the parents, children, each parent with the child(ren), and stepparents or significant others who one of the litigants is planning to marry, it may also be helpful, in certain circumstances, to interview extended family, nannies, school teachers, or babysitters (1,129). It is paramount that the clinician inform all interviewees that due to the forensic nature of the evaluation, the interviewee automatically waives their rights to confidentiality (keeping protected health information private) and privilege (the right to keep information private from the court) (1). It may also be helpful to visit one or both homes and to contact school staff and or mental health providers, with consent from parents (1,85).

Interview Structure

The clinician may consider meeting with both parents together, if they are willing, or with each separately (1). During the first session, it is important to explain to each parent the nature of the evaluation. During the next session, or the end of the first, the evaluator should ask what they are seeking from the court as if the clinician had no prior knowledge of the case (1). It is important to obtain a description of each parent's history including family, social, and psychiatric history, each parent's description of the marriage and separation, each parent's perception of his or her relationship with the children, each parent's understanding of and sensitivity to any special needs of the children, and each parent's specific plans for the future if custody is awarded (1). If there is mental illness in either or both parents, it should be fully described as well as its impact on the children.

Interviewing the Child(ren)

It is important to interview the children early in the course of the evaluation. Each child should be seen at least one or two times alone, and should be brought by each parent at least once (1). It may be best to see all siblings together for the first session with each parent for support and to alleviate anxiety (1). Children and parents should be interviewed together, and this should be as unstructured as possible (1).

The Written Report

In preparing the child custody report, the clinician considers a number of factors when making his or her final recommendations. These include: continuity, preference, attachment, sensitivity and respect, parent–child gender, and level of conflict between parents and the impact on the child (1). Reports should be concise but detailed, and without any technical jargon, unless it is explained (1). There should be a list of dates and times of all interview sessions along with a list of all collateral sources of information, including phone calls and review of legal documents (1). The report should contain a "Conclusions and Recommendations" section with the formulation of the case and detailed recommendations as per the order of appointment on custody, visitation, and other recommendations, such as psychotherapy (1).

Testimony

Parents may reach a settlement before, during or after the evaluation, or after the expert's testimony (1). The evaluator should bring all materials to trial (1).

Evaluator Opinions on Child Custody

Forensic assessments in custody disputes often have tremendous weight and can affect the trajectory of the litigation and ultimately the child's life (130). Studies have shown that clinicians' involvement in child custody cases has a high perceived value; courts follow an expert's custody recommendation up to 90% of the time (131–133). There is variability in judges: some judges may request the forensic examiner opine on the ultimate question of custody while others may prefer the forensic evaluator refrain from such opinions.

It has been argued that experts should not testify on the ultimate issue in civil cases, such as custody (132). Tippins et al. argue that evaluators' conclusions on issue of child custody should not be permitted. He argues such opinions exceed the boundaries of the empirical knowledge base of the mental health profession and they implicitly misrepresent the limits of that knowledge base (131). Tippins recommends that clinicians with adequate forensic training can provide very useful and helpful information to the court. For example, admissions regarding disputed questions, descriptions of parenting behavior, and data-based inferences on parenting skills (131). He recommends psychologists and psychiatrists include warnings on reports about the limitations in the capacity to predict the best custody plan. Further, he advises that judges should order specific statements precluding the expert witness from addressing the ultimate issue (131).

The Future

Technologic innovation and sociocultural changes have impacted family structure and functioning, and have driven changes in clinical practice and the law. Child custody cases have evolved significantly from children being considered property of their father to the current "best interests of the child" standard. With further advances in reproductive endocrinology and marriage rights, case law and legislature regarding child custody will further evolve.

References

1. Herman SP: Practice parameters for child custody evaluation. American Academy of Child and Adolescent Psychiatry. *J Am Acad Child Adolesc Psychiatry* 36:57S–68S, 1997.
2. Copen CE, Daniels K, Vespa J, Mosher WD, Division of Vital Statistics: First marriages in the United States: data from the 2006–2010 National Survey of Family Growth. *Natl Health Stat Report* (49):1–21, 2012. Accessed 1 August 2016. Available at: http://www.cdc.gov/nchs/data/nhsr/nhsr049.pdf
3. Goodwin PY, Mosher WD, Chandra A: Marriage and cohabitation in the United States: a statistical portrait based on Cycle 6 (2002) of the National Survey of Family Growth. *Vital Health Stat* 23(28):1–45, 2010. Accessed 1 August 2016. Available at: http://www.cdc. gov/nchs/data/series/sr_23/sr23_028.pdf.
4. Krieder RM, Ellis R: Number, timing and duration of marriages and divorces: 2009. *Current Population Reports.* P70–125. Washington, DC,

U.S. Census Bureau, 2011. Accessed 1 August 2016. Available at: http://www.census.gov/prod/2011pubs/p70125.pdf
5. American Psychological Association: Guidelines for child custody evaluations in divorce proceedings. *Am Psycholt* 49:677–680, 1994.
6. Charlow A: Awarding custody: the best interests of the child and other fictions. *Yale Law & Policy Review* 5(2):3, 2015.
7. Parental Rights: New York State Unified Court System. Accessed 1 August 2016. Available at: https://www.nycourts.gov/courthelp/family/parentalRights.shtml
8. Kermani EE: Issues of child custody and our moral values in the era of new medical technology. *J Am Acad Child Adolesc Psychiatry* 31:533–538, 1992.
9. Emery RE, Otto RK, O'Donohue WT: A critical assessment of child custody evaluations: limited science and a flawed system. *Psychol Sci Public Interest* 6:1–29, 2005.
10. Weithorn LA: *Psychology and Child Custody Determinations.* Lincoln, University of Nebraska, 1987.
11. Kelly JB: The determination of child custody. *Future Child* 4:121–142, 1994.
12. Finlay v. Finlay 240 NY 429, 148 N.E. 624 (1925).
13. Rutter M: Clinical Implications of attachment concepts: retrospect and prospect. *J Child Psychol Psychiatry.* 36:549–571, 1995.
14. Goldstein J, Freud A, Solnit AJ: *Beyond the Best Interests of the Child.* New York, The Free Press, 53–65, 1973.
15. Goodridge v. Dept. of Public Health. 440 Mass. 309, 798 N.E.2d 941 (Mass. 2003)
16. United States v. Windsor, 570 U. S. 12-307 (2013).
17. Obergefell v. Hodges. 135 S.Ct. 2071 (2015).
18. In vitro fertilization (IVF). Mayo Clinic. Accessed 1 August 2016. Available at: http://www.mayoclinic.org/tests-procedures/in-vitro-fertilization/home/ovc-20206838
19. Abramovici HH, Dirnfeld M, Bornstein J, Lissak A, Gonen Y: Gamete intrafallopian transfer. An overview. *J Reprod Med* 38:698–702, 1993.
20. Johnson v. Calvert, Cal. Sup. No. X633190 (October 22, 1990).
21. In Re Baby M., 217 N.J. Sup., 313. (1987).
22. Jones v. York, F. Supp. (E.D. Va., 717F. Supp 421, 1989).
23. Davis v. Davis, 657 S.W.2d 753 (Tenn. 1990).
24. Stanley v. Illinois, 405 U.S. 645, 92 S. Ct. 1208, 31 L. Ed. 2d 551 (1972).
25. Sigal A, Sandler I, Wolchik S, Braver S: Do parent education programs promote healthy postdivorce parenting? Critical distinctions and a review of the evidence. *Fam Court Rev* 49:120–139, 2011.
26. Primary Documents in American History – 14th Amendment to the U.S. Constitution. Accessed 8 August 2016. Available at: https://www.loc.gov/rr/program/bib/ourdocs/14thamendment.html
27. Michael H. v. Gerald D., 491 U.S. 110, 1989.
28. Victor RS, Robbins MA, Bassett S: Statutory review of third party rights regarding custody, visitation, and support. *Family Law Quarterly* 25:19–25, 1991.
29. Troxel v. Granville, 530 U.S. 57 (2000).
30. Buehler C, Krishnakumar A, Stone G, et al.: Interparental conflict styles and youth problem behaviors: a two-sample replication study. *J Marriage Fam* 60:119–132, 1998.
31. Kline M, Johnston JR, Tschann J: The long shadow of marital conflict: a model of children in postdivorce adjustment. *J Marriage Fam* 53:297, 1991.
32. Amato PR, Keith B: Parental divorce and the well-being of children: a meta-analysis. *Psychological bulletin* 110:26–46, 1991.
33. Amato PR: Family process in one-parent, stepparent, and intact families: the child's point of view. *J Marriage Fam* 49:327–337, 1987.
34. Furstenberg FF Jr, Nord CW: Parenting apart: patterns of childrearing after marital disruption. *J Marriage Fam* 47:893–904,1985.
35. Hetherington ME, Kelly J: *For Better or For Worse.* New York, W.W. Norton Company, Inc., 2002.
36. Wallerstein JS, Corbin S: The child and the vicissitudes of divorce. In: Lewis M (ed). *Child and Adolescent Psychiatry: A Comprehensive Textbook.* 3rd ed. Philadelphia, PA, Lippincott, Williams and Wilkins, 1275–1285, 2002.
37. Billick SB, Ciric SJ: Role of the psychiatric evaluator in child custody disputes. In: Rosner R (ed). *Principles and Practice of Forensic Psychiatry,* 2nd ed. Boca Raton, CRC Press, 331–347, 2003.
38. Stahl P: *Complex Issues in Child Custody Evaluations,* Thousand Oaks, Sage Publications, Inc., 1999.
39. Kelly JB, Emery R: Children's adjustment following divorce: risk and resilience perspectives. *Fam Relat* 52:352–362, 2003.
40. Malone PS, Lansford JE, Castellino DR, et al.: Divorce and child behavior problems: applying latent change score models to life event data. *Struct Equ Modeling* 11:401–423, 2004.
41. Lansford JE, Malone PS, Castellino DR, Dodge KA, Pettit GS, Bates JE: Trajectories of internalizing, externalizing, and grades for children who have and have not experienced their parents' divorce. *J Fam Psychol* 20:292–301, 2006.
42. Wallerstein JS, Lewis J: The long-term impact of divorce on children. *Family Court Review* 36:368–383, 1998.
43. Amato PR: Reconciling divergent perspectives: Judith Wallerstein, quantitative family research, and children of divorce. *Fam Relat* 52:332–339, 2003.
44. Ramsey SH, Kelly RF: Assessing social science studies: eleven tips for judges and lawyers. *Family Law Quarterly* 40:367–380, 2006.
45. Amato PR, Anthony CJ: Estimating the effects of parental divorce and death with fixed effects models. *J Marriage Fam* 762:370–386, 2014.
46. Kelly J: Children's adjustment in conflicted marriage and divorce: a decade review of research. *J Am Acad Child Adolesc Psychiatry* 39:963–973, 2000.
47. Rehbein F, Baier D: Family-, media-, and school-related risk factors of video game addiction. *J Media Psychol* 25:118–128, 2013.
48. Amato PR: Children's adjustment to divorce: theories, hypotheses, and empirical support. *J Marriage Fam* 55(1):23–38, 1993.
49. Vanassche S, Sodermans AK, Matthijs K, Swicegood G: Commuting between two parental households: the association between joint physical custody and adolescent wellbeing following divorce. *J Fam Stud* 19(2):139–158, 2013.
50. Sanchez L, Gager C: Hard living, perceived entitlement to a great marriage, and marital dissolution. *J Marriage Fam* 62:708–722, 2000.
51. Heller RJ: *Family Therapy and Collaborative Family Law.* New York, Routledge/Taylor & Francis Group, 265–268, 2013.
52. Vu T: Going to court as a last resort: establishing a duty for attorneys in divorce proceedings to discuss alternative dispute resolution with their clients. *Family Court Rev* 47:586–599, 2009.
53. O'Connell J: Don't settle for the devil you know: the benefits of using collaborative law rather than litigation to resolve employment disputes. *Indiana Law Review* 49(2):533–554, 2015–2016.
54. Rudd BN, Ogle RK, Holzworth-Munroe A, Applegate AG, D'Onofrio BM: Child-informed mediation study follow-up: comparing the frequency of relitigation following different types of family mediation. *Psychology, Public Policy, and Law* 21(4):452, 2015.
55. Kelly JB: A decade of divorce mediation research: some answers and questions. *Fam Conciliation Courts Rev* 34:373–385, 1996.
56. Waller EM, Anasseril DE: Purpose and utility of child custody evaluations: the attorney's perspective. *J Am Acad Psychiatry Law* 33:199–207, 2005.
57. Ayanna A: From children's interests to parental responsibility: degendering parenthood through custodial obligation. *UCLA Women's LJ* 19:1, 2012.
58. Derdeyn AP. Child custody conflicts in historical perspective. *Am J Psychiatry* 133:1369–1376, 1976.
59. Kelly JB: Psychological and legal interventions for parents and children in custody and access disputes: current research and practice. *Va J Soc Policy Law* 10:129, 2002.
60. McIntosh J: Child-inclusive divorce mediation: report on a qualitative research study. *Mediation Q* 1855–66, 2000.
61. Halligan CI, Chang J, Knox D: Positive effects of parental divorce on undergraduates. *J Divorce Remarriage* 55(7):557–567, 2014.
62. Golombok S, Spencer A, Rutter M: Children in lesbian and single-parent households: psychosexual and psychiatric appraisal. *J Child Psychol Psychiatry* 24:551–572, 1983.
63. Tasker FL, Golombok S: *Growing Up in a Lesbian Family: Effects on Child Development.* New York, Guilford Press, 1997.
64. Patterson CC: Children of lesbian and gay parents: psychology, law, and policy. *American Psychol* 64:727–736, 2009.
65. Richards MA, Rothblum ED, Beauchaine TP, Balsam KF: Adult children of same-sex and heterosexual couples: demographic "thriving". *J GLBT Fam Stud* 13:1–15, 2016.
66. Austin WC. Child custody evaluation and relocation, part I of III: forensic guideposts for the evaluator and court. *Am J Fam Law* 29:156–170, 2015.
67. In re Tropea, 87 N.Y.2d 727, 739-40, 665 N.E.2d 145, 150-51 (1996).
68. *In re Marriage of LaMusga,* 32 Cal. 4th 1072, 88 P.3d 81, 12 Cal. Rptr. 3d 356 (2004).
69. Davis G: A systematic approach to domestic abuse-informed child custody decision making in family law cases a systematic approach to domestic violence. *Fam Court Rev* 53:565–577, 2015.
70. Yanni SJ: Experts as final arbiters: state law and problematic expert testimony on domestic violence in child custody cases. *Columbia Law Review* 533–572, 2016.
71. Morrill AC, Dai J, Dunn S, Sung I, Smith K: Child custody and visitation decisions when the father has perpetrated violence against the mother. *Violence Against Women* 11:1076–1107, 2005.
72. Jaffe PG, Crooks CV, Bala N: *Making Appropriate Parenting Arrangements in Family Violence Cases: Applying the Literature to Identify Promising Practices.* Ottawa, Ontario, Canada, Department of Justice, 2005.
73. Jaffe PG, Crooks CV, Bala N: A framework for addressing allegations of domestic violence in child custody disputes. *J Child Custody* 6:169–188, 2009.
74. Parker T, Rogers K, Collins M, et al.: Danger zone: battered mothers and their families in supervised visitation. *Violence Against Women* 14:1313–1325, 2008.
75. Jacquin, Kristine M, Audrey GM: Evaluating allegations of child sexual abuse in custody disputes. In: Goldstein ML (ed). *Handbook of Child Custody.* Switzerland, Springer International Publishing, 163–176, 2016.
76. Brown T, Frederico M, Hewitt L, Sheehan R: Revealing the existence of child abuse in the context of marital breakdown and custody and access disputes. *Child Abuse Neglect* 24:849–859, 2000.

77. Sorensen E, Goldman J, Ward M, Albanese I, Graves L, Chamberlain C: Judicial decision-making in contested custody cases: the influence of reported child abuse, spouse abuse, and parental substance abuse. *Child Abuse Neglect* 19:251–260, 1995.
78. Thoennes N, Tjaden PG: The extent, nature, and validity of sexual abuse allegations in custody/visitation disputes. *Child Abuse Neglect* 14:151–163, 1990.
79. Johnston JR, Lee S, Olesen NW, Walters MG: Allegations and substantiations of abuse in custody-disputing families. *Family Court Review* 43:283–294, 2005.
80. Bala NM, Mitnick M, Trocmé N, Houston C: Sexual abuse allegations and parental separation: smokescreen or fire? *J Family Stud* 13:26–56, 2007.
81. Kuenhle K, Kirkpatrick HD: Evaluating allegations of child sexual abuse within complex child custody cases. *J Child Custody* 2:3–39, 2005.
82. Saini MM, Black T, Fallon B, Marshall A: Child custody disputes within the context of child protection investigations: secondary analysis of the Canadian Incident Study of Reported Child Abuse and Neglect. *Child Welfare* 92:115–137, 2013.
83. Herman SP: Special issues in child custody disputes. *J Am Acad Child Adolesc Psychiatry* 29:969–974, 1990.
84. Jaffee v. Redmond, 518 U.S. 1 (1996).
85. Simon RA, Willick DH: Therapeutic privilege and custody evaluations: discovery of treatment records. *Fam Court Rev* 54.1:51–60, 2016.
86. Pub. L. No. 104-191 (1996).
87. Painter v. Bannister, 140 N.W.2d 152 (Iowa 1966).
88. Kelly JB, Lamb ME: Developmental issues in relocation cases involving young children: when, whether, and how? *J Fam Psychol* 17:193–205, 2003.
89. Austin W: Exploring three functions in child custody evaluation for the relocation case: prediction, investigation, and making recommendations for a long-distance parenting plan. *J Child Custody* 3:63–108, 2006.
90. Atkinson J: The law of relocation of children. *Behav Sci Law* 28:563–579, 2010.
91. McLanahan SS, Sandefur G: *Growing Up with a Single Parent: What Hurts, What Helps*. Cambridge, MA, Harvard University Press, 1994.
92. Rains v. Rains, 836 NW 2d 709 (Mich: Court of Appeals 2013).
93. Tropea v. Tropea, 665 N.E.2d 145 (N.Y. 1996).
94. In re Marriage of Burgess, 913 P.2d 473 (California, 1996).
95. Baures v. Lewis, No. A-135-99 (New Jersey Supreme Court, 2001).
96. Johnston JR, Sagatun-Edwards I: Parental kidnapping. *Child Adolesc Psychiatric Clin N Am* 11:805–822, 2002;.
97. The Uniform Child-Custody Jurisdiction and Enforcement Act. U.S. Department of Justice: Office of Justice Programs. Office of Juvenile Justice and Delinquency Prevention. December 2001. Accessed 1 August 2016. Available at: https://www.ncjrs.gov/pdffiles1/ojjdp/189181.pdf
98. Uniform Child Custody Jurisdiction Act, Prefatory Note: The Full Faith and Credit clause requires that full faith and credit "be given in each state to the public acts, records, and judicial proceedings of every other state" (U.S. Constitution, article IV, § 1).
99. Parental Kidnapping Prevention Act (PKPA). 28 USC, 1738A; 42 USC, 653–655; 663; 18 USC, 1073).
100. Charlow A: There's no place like home: temporary absences in the UCCJEA home state. *J Am Acad Matrimonial Law* 28:25, 2015.
101. Federal Judicial Center International Litigation Guide. The 1980 Hague Convention on the Civil Aspects of International Child Abduction: A Guide for Judges. 2012. Accessed 1 Aug 2016. http://www.fjc.gov/public/pdf.nsf/lookup/hagueguide.pdf/$file/hagueguide.pdf
102. Hague Convention (1988). 42 USC, 11601.
103. International Child Abduction Remedies Act (ICARA). 42 USC, 11601 et seq.
104. Gibbs MJ, Jones WP, Smith SD, Staples PA, Weeks GR: The consequences of parental abduction: a pilot study with a retrospective view from the victim. *Family J* 21(3):313–317, 2013.
105. Forehand R, Long N, Zogg C, Parrish E: Child abduction: parent and child functioning following return. *Clin Pediatr* 28:311–316, 1989.
106. Hegar RL, Greif GL: How parentally abducted children fare: an interim report on families who recover their children. *J Psych Law* 21:373–383, 1993.
107. Terr LC: Child snatching: a new epidemic of an ancient malady. *J Pediatr* 103:151–156, 1983.
108. Bernet WW, Baker AJ: Parental alienation, DSM-5, and ICD-11: response to critics. *J Am Acad Psychiatry Law* 41:98–104, 2013.
109. Kelly JB, Johnston JR: The alienated child: a reformulation of parental alienation syndrome. *Fam Court Rev* 39:249–266, 2001.
110. James Williams J R: Should judges close the gate on PAS and PA? *Fam Conciliation Courts Rev* 39:267–281, 2001.
111. Matthew Bender: *Principles of the Law of Family Dissolution: Analysis and Recommendations*. American Law Institute, 2000.
112. American Psychiatric Association Task Force on Clinical Assessment in Child Custody Disputes: *Child Custody Consultation*. Washington, DC, American Psychiatric Association, 1988.
113. American Association of Family and Conciliation Courts: *Model Standards of Practice for Child Custody Evaluations*. Madison, WI, American Association of Family and Conciliation Courts, 2006.
114. California Rules of Court 5.220. Court-ordered child custody evaluation. 2005.
115. Georgia Psychological Association: *Recommendations for Psychologists' Involvement in Child Custody Cases*. Atlanta, GA, 1990.
116. Judicial Court of California: *Uniform Standards for Practice for Court Ordered Child Custody Evaluations*. San Francisco, CA, 1999.
117. Commonwealth of Massachusetts: The Trial Court, Probate and Family Court Department. Boston, 2005.
118. Louisiana State Board of Social Work Examiners: *Guidelines for Child Custody Evaluations*, 1998.
119. Metropolitan Denver Interdisciplinary committee on Child Custody: *Guidelines for Child Custody Evaluations*, 1989.
120. Nebraska Psychological Association: *Guidelines for Child Custody Evaluations*. Lincoln, NE, 1986.
121. New Jersey State Board of Psychological Examiners. *Specialty Guidelines for Psychologists in Custody/Visitation Evaluations*. Newark, NJ, 1993.
122. Oklahoma Psychological Association. *Ethical Guidelines for Child Custody Evaluations*. Oklahoma City, OK, 1988.
123. Pennsylvania Psychological Association, Clinical Division/Task Force on Child Custody Evaluation: *Roles for Psychologists in Child Custody Disputes*, 1991.
124. Rohrbagh JB. *A Comprehensive Guide to Child Custody Evaluations: Mental Health Perspectives*. New York, Springer Science & Business Media, 2007.
125. Stahl PM. *Conducting Child Custody Evaluations: From Basic to Complex Issues*. Thousand Oaks, CA, SAGE Publications, 2011.
126. Ackerman MJ, Ackerman MC. Custody evaluation practices: a survey of experienced professionals (revisited). *Prof Psychol* 28:137–144, 1997.
127. Herman SP: Child custody evaluations. In: Schetky DH, Benedek EP (eds): *Clinical Handbook of Child Psychiatry and the Law*. Baltimore, MD, Williams & Wilkins, 1992.
128. UMDA § 405(a), 9A U.L.A. 386 (1998).
129. FL-329-INFO Child Custody Evaluation Information Sheet. Accessed 1 August 2016. Available at: http://www.courts.ca.gov/documents/fl329info.pdf
130. Lobel DS. Uses of Collateral Sources of Information in Forensic Child Custody Examinations. In: *Handbook of Child Custody*. Switzerland, Springer International Publishing, 57–64, 2016.
131. Tippins TM, Wittmann JP: Empirical and ethical problems with custody recommendations: a call for clinical humility and judicial vigilance. *Fam Court Rev* 43:193–222, 2005.
132. Bow JN, Quinnell FA: Critique of child custody evaluations by the legal profession. *Fam Court Rev* 42:115–126, 2004.
133. Yanni S J: Experts as final arbiters: state law and problematic expert testimony on domestic violence in child custody cases. *Columbia Law Rev* 116(2):533–572, 2016.

CHAPTER 7.4.3 ■ ADOPTION

RACHEL MARGARET ANN BROWN

Adoption refers to a formal action in which an adult assumes permanent, primary, legal, and other parental responsibility for another person, usually a minor, from the biologic or legal parents. The most recent data available, from 2007 to 2008, indicate that approximately 136,000 children were adopted annually in the United States (1). Despite the psychological significance of the event, it is likely that most of the participants involved in most adoptions never encounter child and adolescent psychiatrists. As our professional pathways intersect the lives of people involved in the adoption process at different places (but almost always at times when there are problems), we see only the fragmented parts of a complex and multifaceted picture. This chapter is directed at providing a cohesive overview of adoption.

HISTORICAL ASPECTS OF ADOPTION

Adoption is an ancient practice, although not a universal one. It was codified more than 4,000 years ago by the Babylonians, and is described in the Bible, for example, in the adoption of Moses by the daughter of Pharaoh. The ancient Romans practiced both the adoption of children and that of adults, in order to provide a suitable heir for the family. Similar practices, with similar motivation, are described in China, in ancient Egypt, Greece, and in the Polynesian societies of Tahiti and Hawaii. Originally, adoption was designed to benefit the adopter, by providing them with a successor, someone to carry out rituals after their death, someone to work on their behalf and support them, or someone to cement a critical power alliance.

Informal adoption has probably always been part of modern American society. In the 19th century, it existed alongside other ways of taking care of orphaned children, including the "boarding out" in foster care of babies from almshouses, the system of apprenticing and indenturing impoverished children, and the practice of sending homeless children from the Northeast by orphan trains to work in farming communities in the Midwest. The world's first adoption statute was implemented by the Commonwealth of Massachusetts in 1851. During the first half of the 20th century, most adoptions in the United States were still informal, and did not guarantee confidentiality for any of the parties. Adoptions were frequently accompanied by the stigma of illegitimacy and fear of the inheritance of defective genes. Throughout the 20th century up to the present day, the states, and later the federal government, have steadily formalized the practice of adoption. Statute now governs the practice, even when it is independently organized by the physicians, lawyers, and families involved. Significant social change has affected the numbers and context in which adoption now takes place. The private adoption of infants was a fairly common practice prior to 1970, when reliable contraception was unavailable and single mothers unsupported and stigmatized. Many unmarried mothers chose (or were pressured to choose) adoption and many healthy infants (mostly white) were placed, often in great secrecy because of the stigma associated with illegitimacy, with unrelated, childless, adoptive parents. The number of nonrelative adoptions increased from about 33,800 in 1951 to 89,200 in 1970. After 1970, the number of children available for adoption, their age and status began to change. The widespread use of birth control, the availability of abortion, and the greater acceptance of single parenthood reduced the availability of infants for adoption by unrelated couples. As a result, the number of unrelated adoptions declined rapidly through the 70s, though it still accounts for nearly half of all adoptions (1). The private adoption of a healthy infant is today an often-expensive undertaking, out of the reach of many middle class couples.

In parallel with the changes affecting the availability of babies for private adoption, two other groups of children became increasingly recognized as suitable for adoptive placements. First, in the mid-1970s, there was a new recognition of the numbers of children living, often in significant instability and for many years, in temporary foster care family placements because of neglect and abuse in their families of origin. In the 1980s, there was a move toward planning for permanency, and an acceptance that children, even older children previously seen as "unadoptable," might benefit from adoptive placement. The Adoption Assistance and Child Welfare Act (1980) was designed to prevent children in foster care from languishing in these temporary situations, and to facilitate adoption for children who could not be reunified with biologic families. Congress passed the Adoption and Safe Families Act (ASFA) in 1997. This legislation requires planning for permanence for children in foster care within a year of removal, and termination of parental rights for children who have been in foster care 15 out of the last 22 months. The Adoption Promotion Act (2003) gave enhanced incentives for adoption of older children. As a result of these shifts in policy and legislation, many children from the foster care system have been placed for adoption, both in unrelated families and with relatives in the so-called "kinship" placements. The statistics on the numbers of children adopted with public child welfare agency involvement are the most reliable and up to date, and rose nationwide from approximately 25,000 in 1995 to around 50,000 in each of the last 5 years (2). For the most part, the focus of policy and professionals working in this area has shifted over the last 100 years or so from a focus on adoption for the psychological or financial benefit of the adults involved toward adoption for the psychological benefit of the child.

The second largest group of children affected by changes in adoption practices has been children adopted from overseas (3,4). These so-called "international" adoptees began arriving in large numbers to the United States and Europe in the aftermath of World War II and the wars in Korea and Vietnam. Many of the first Korean adoptees, who began arriving in 1955, were the offspring of non-Korean military fathers and Korean mothers; however, international adoption from Korea has continued, though in lesser numbers, ever since. More than 150,000 Korean children have been adopted by US parents. American parents have continued to adopt children from other countries, including China, Russia, India, Romania, Guatemala, Colombia, Haiti, Uganda, and Ethiopia. Chinese children, mostly baby girls, have been adopted by American parents in large numbers over the last 30 years (5). For some years, significant numbers arrived from South American countries, including Guatemala and

Columbia (6), and, most recently, larger numbers have arrived from parts of Africa. In the United States and other countries—Sweden, Denmark, and the United Kingdom in particular—this has resulted in a phenomenon known as "visible" adoption: that is, because of the child's and parents' physical appearance, it is obvious that the child is adopted.

Clinicians are likely to encounter the adoption triad of the adopted child, biologic parent(s), and adoptive parent(s), affected by adoption in notably different ways. First, there are children relinquished by their biologic parents, and adopted through private agencies, or independently through attorneys, clergy, or physicians. These account for around 50,000 adoptions a year, a significant decline from the peak of the 1950s and 1960s. Most children adopted by this route are adopted as babies and young infants, either directly from hospital or after short periods in relatively good quality foster homes. Second, the practice of international adoption means that many young children, most between the ages of 3 months and 3 years, arrive in the United States from overseas, after spending time in orphanages, with relatives or in foster homes, where their care may have been less than optimal and about which reliable information may be missing. The adoptive families of many privately adopted US-born and international adoptees are, because of the expense involved, relatively socioeconomically advantaged. Third, about 50,000 children a year are adopted, either by unrelated families who may also have been their foster parents, or by relatives, from the publicly funded child welfare system. More than half of these children are adopted after the age of 6, many of them in adolescence, and they include an over-representation of racial and ethnic minorities. Most have been in foster care for more than 4 years, most often because of significant trauma and neglect. Their adoptive families are somewhat more likely to be older, single parents, and financially less well-off. One notable change in adoption practice over the last 20 years has been the increase in openness in adoption. Openness refers to the degree of contact between the adopted child's families of birth and adoption. The level of contact ranges from the exchange of cards or letters through the placing agency to ongoing personal visits between the two families. Open adoptions have been offered by private agencies since the late 1970s, and increasingly by international adoption agencies. It remains a controversial issue and may be particularly fraught when the adoption follows abuse or neglect in the family of origin. Some authors (7) refer to the adoptive kinship network. This concept sees the child at the center of an extensive family system that includes birth and adoptive relatives and extended family.

Adoption has, therefore, a long history and has impacted many millions of children and adults. Most estimates are that 2.5% to 3.5% of the current US population is adopted. It is a practice that is likely to continue, driven by the needs of orphaned, abandoned, and neglected children worldwide, and by the profound desire of adults to nurture children of their own. Even though the majority of adoptions result in well-adjusted, well-loved children living in contented families, child and adolescent psychiatrists will continue to see all three components of the adoption triad—birth parents, adoptive parents, and adopted children—in their clinical practices. Attempts to answer some of the questions that arise from the natural experiments of adoption will continue to give rise to fascinating and productive research.

NORMAL DEVELOPMENT IN ADOPTIVE FAMILIES

Most adopted children and families appear to fare well, and follow a normal developmental track. Almost all adoptive professionals and families today support telling children early about their origins and the circumstances of their adoption. The increasing numbers of visible adoptions, adoptions of older children, and the practice of increasing openness in domestic infant adoption (8), has had the beneficial effect of lessening secrecy and stigma. Giving children information early, even before they are ready to wholly comprehend the information, leads to a process of understanding governed by the external facts, the child's internal cognitive and emotional development, and the family's ability to talk comfortably about the issues.

At some point in their development, many adopted children will ask difficult questions about their origins. Their adoptive parents will therefore need to find ways to answer honestly and openly, or help their children come to terms with gaps in knowledge. Just as young children whose parents divorce are likely to see themselves as responsible for the divorce, because of their behavior or attitude, so some adopted preadolescent children may assume that they were given for adoption because they were in some way damaged or defective, or unwanted because they were a boy, not a girl, or vice versa. As in other families referred for clinical intervention, it is not uncommon to find that the children have not shared such feelings or thoughts, sometimes because of a wish to protect their parents' perceived vulnerabilities. Although systematic research has not demonstrated it, it is also not uncommon, or surprising, to find adoptive children anxious about being removed from their adoptive families.

Adolescence appears to be a particularly sensitive time for many adoptive families, and possibly a significant stressor for adopted children, for a number of reasons, some inherent to the normal developmental process of adolescence, and some unique to the adoptive situation. The process of developing and focusing self-identity is clearly impacted by the reality of adoption. Some adopted adolescents have little information about their biologic roots and families, and some adoptive parents are made uncomfortable by their child's curiosity. The wish of some adopted adolescents and young adults to search for their biologic family, and meet their first parents, often welcomed by those biologic parents, is, sadly, for some adoptive parents exquisitely painful and may be experienced as rejection, even when the adolescent does not have that intent. Greater satisfaction among family members with the contact that does occur appears to predict better adolescent adjustment (9). Sadly, in some families, this issue becomes focused on the idealization of the biologic parent, and used as a weapon in a war of control around the adolescent's emerging independence.

The challenges of normal parenting are focused in somewhat different ways for some adoptive parents, even when the adoption takes place in infancy. Adoptive parents must relate to children who may not resemble them physically or psychologically, may be placed with them abruptly, and with little preparation, or with whom the legal course of adoption may delay the development of confidence in a future with the child. Moreover, many adoptive couples have already faced the considerable and often prolonged trauma and grief of infertility and its treatment. Research and clinical experience support the view that unresolved grief over the loss of the potential for a natural child may interfere with the emotional availability of new adoptive parents. As their children grow, some adoptive parents may face questions and doubts, from themselves, the child and from others, about their role and abilities in comparison to "real" parents. Some extended families may compare an adopted child negatively with "real" children. Even where such overtly pathologic attitudes are not apparent, it has been suggested that some parents experience difficulties in attaching to, owning, and accepting an adopted child (9).

IS ADOPTION PATHOGENIC?

Even before the recent upsurge in the adoption of children from the welfare system, adopted children were overrepresented in clinical populations. Some of the literature supporting this finding dates from a time when most adopted children were placed in their adoptive families as infants, and many in secrecy. Studies from the 1960s, cited by Durdeyn (9) in a previous edition of this text, establish that adopted children were overrepresented in outpatient settings, and tended to be referred for externalizing behaviors.

More recent studies (10–13) support the conclusion that adopted children are more commonly referred and admitted for inpatient psychiatric treatment when compared to nonadopted children, and for less severe problems (11). Some evidence (12) suggests that differences seen between adopted, foster, and nonadopted children in behavioral problems and rates of referral were the result of a small group of influential cases, rather than a reflection of the group as a whole. Studies of large population samples confirm that being adopted increases the risk for psychiatric illness (14–16). Juffer and van Ijzendoorn (17), in a meta-analysis of a number of studies that included more than 10,000 adoptees, found no differences in self-esteem for international, domestic, same race, and transracial adoptees. However, studies have shown slightly higher rates of externalizing symptoms in adolescence, of self-reported offending and substance abuse (14), higher scores on items reflecting unhappy, anxious behavior, and problems with peer relationships (18), and the suggestion of an increased risk for suicide during adolescence (19). Studies of school and court populations (20) support the finding that problems in psychological and social adjustment are more common in adopted children than in the general population, and are not simply related to increased referral (20). Increased risk for problems does appear to continue into adult life, with recent studies demonstrating increased risk of substance use disorders and personality disorders in adult adoptees (21).

Although these studies demonstrate that adoption for a minority of children appears to be a risk factor for psychopathology, it is only so when adopted children are compared to the general population. When compared to children returned to their families of origin, or to those raised in long-term foster care, adoption is clearly beneficial. For most adopted children, the practice has an overwhelmingly positive outcome, and most adopted children are happy and well adjusted.

The natural experiment of adoption has played an important role in the exploration of the etiology of mental illness, particularly schizophrenia, demonstrating the biologic underpinnings of the disorder (22–25). Studies of adopted children at high risk for schizophrenic illnesses demonstrate that these children exhibit subtle developmental delays, cognitive problems, and poor interpersonal relationships. More recent studies have also examined the contribution of environment, including family environment, to the manifestation of the schizophrenic illness, and support the notion of gene–environment interactions. Using a Finnish sample of children adopted by unrelated parents, Tienari et al. (23) showed that disordered adoptive rearing assessed in the adoptive families predicts schizophrenia-spectrum disorders at 21-year follow-up. The finding was only apparent, however, in adoptees at high genetic risk for schizophrenia, and suggested that adoptees at high genetic risk may be more sensitive to adverse environmental effects in an adoptive rearing environment than were adoptees at low genetic risk. The presumed genotype appears to be "sensitive" not only to dysfunction in the family environment but to protective environmental factors.

Studies like this suggest that adoptive rearing in a quality home environment may be of particular value for those at higher genetic risk. As the possibility that children at high genetic risk for schizophrenia (and other mental illnesses) may be identified in early childhood becomes more realistic, it is possible that adoptive parents, and the psychiatrists working with them, will have new challenges and possibilities in prevention. They, and we, as their psychiatrists, also face the challenge of counseling the children of such high-risk adoptees as they move into the age of risk for onset of schizophrenic disorders.

INTERNATIONAL ADOPTION

Just as the domestic adoption of children of parents with mental illness has shed new light on the etiology of schizophrenia, so has the international adoption brought new insights into the importance of early childhood experiences (1), even when those are relatively brief, as well as an awareness of the relevance of transracial adoption and immigration in the context of already prejudiced and racist societies.

Studies of children recently adopted from overseas show that growth and developmental delays are frequent, particularly where the child is raised in an orphanage rather than in a foster family setting, or with relatives (6). Three-quarters of the Chinese-born adoptees evaluated in a New England adoption clinic (5) had significant developmental delays, with gross motor delays being the most common. Medical problems were also common, some being minor and easily correctable (anemia, elevated lead levels, hepatitis antibodies, parasites, and positive TB skin tests). Others, though less common, were more serious and included hearing loss, syphilis, orthopedic problems, and congenital anomalies. Many internationally adopted children are also inadequately vaccinated (26). Similar findings (6) come from a cohort of children adopted to the United States from Guatemala, though the problems are not as severe as those in the Chinese children. Adopted children were diagnosed with neurologic problems, including hypo- and hypertonia, clonus, intellectual disability and developmental disorders, and with emotional problems, the latter including depression, posttraumatic stress, and eating disorders. They were also commonly seen to exhibit self-comforting behaviors, such as rocking and banging. This study again demonstrates the significant growth and cognitive advantages experienced by children in foster placements rather than orphanages, prior to adoption. Children who were younger at placement also did better, with those younger than 2 being less likely to be developmentally delayed.

After the resolution of initial medical problems most internationally adopted young children appear to adapt well to their new environment (24), and progress satisfactorily during early school age. A large study in Sweden showed that 92% of the internationally adopted girls, and 82% of the boys (27) had no indication of mental health disorders, or maladjustment. It has, however, been of concern to clinicians in a variety of different countries that internationally adopted children appear more commonly in clinical settings than might be expected. Although not all studies are in agreement, most suggest that a larger minority than would be expected do experience significant mental health problems in childhood, adolescence, and early adult life. Dutch studies (28–30) show elevated rates of behavioral problems, anxiety, and depression, especially in the home setting, and especially for boys, with adjustment problems increasing into adolescence, even among those adopted as infants. Evidence from the Swedish national registers for those born in 1970–1979, comparing inter country adoptees to the general population found that the adoptees were more than three times more likely to die from suicide, attempt suicide, or be admitted to a psychiatric hospital, and more than five times more likely to use drugs, twice as likely to use alcohol, and somewhat more likely to commit a crime (29–32). Some evidence supports the view that the problems are not that of the whole sample, but rather a result of small group of significant outliers. Cederblad et al.'s (27) study found that preadoption conditions, rather than age at placement, increased the risk of later maladaptation, and that the rate of children with poor attachments increased if the child had been in an orphanage or foster home for a longer time. The problems of the minority of adoptees at risk do persist into adult life, with identified increased risk of anxiety, mood, and substance abuse disorders as adults (33). Cederblad et al. (27) also found that a substantial number of their subjects had been teased or felt ill at ease because of foreign looks, and two-thirds had been regarded as foreigners. Indicators that the young person was struggling with identity were related to level of symptom load and self-esteem, though most subjects coped well with their "special outsider" status. The issue of transracial adoption has been a sensitive and emotive topic, not only as regards international adoption, but as it pertains to the adoption of (mostly) black children by (mostly) white families in the United States. In a comprehensive review of the issue, Rushton and Minnis (34), in a comprehensive review of the data, acknowledge the highly contentious nature of this subject, and its political and social context. Most empirical research has been done on black infants in white adoptive families in the United States, but other transracial placements include Australasian peoples and gypsies in central Europe. Rushton and Minnis conclude that the available evidence suggests that such placements have satisfactory outcomes in over 70% of placements, comparing favorably with other samples.

Overall, studies of internationally adopted children demonstrate that most fare well, and that it is the minority who experience mental health problems. A number of factors may play a part in increasing the risk. Those factors include being male, being placed with a single parent, or in an adoptive white collar family, older age at placement, and placement in an orphanage rather than a foster home prior to adoption. It is also important to remember that adoptive parents may be, to some degree, super-competent, and that children who fare well in adoptive families may be at genetically higher risk than the general population, but environmentally somewhat protected. These studies also bring forth the subtle, and sometimes not so subtle, challenge of growing up with a distinct and different appearance, in a culture that may not welcome difference, or may even be overtly racist and discriminatory.

Many internationally adopted children come to the United States, and other Western countries, with the assistance of long established international adoption agencies that have worked extensively in the social welfare systems of the countries of origin of the adoptive children, and cooperate with them in providing enhanced orphanage or foster care environments. In contrast, the children adopted into largely middle class American and European families after the fall of the Ceaucescu regime in Romania had experienced extraordinarily deprived orphanage conditions. Their story (35–37) illustrates both the impact of early emotional and social deprivation on child development, as well as the degree of recovery possible in an enhanced family environment. For this group of children, exposed to extreme early global deprivation, duration of emotional deprivation predicted cognitive outcomes at the time of adoption, as well as recovery in the adoptive family. In these studies, the age of "late" adoption was 24 to 42 months—in earlier studies, children placed under the age of 5 are mostly classified as "early" placements; this shift acknowledges the growing understanding in the adoption field of the importance of experiences in the first years of life. Julian's review (37) demonstrates that institutionalization beyond a certain age is associated with lasting difficulties, and that the more severe the deprivation, the earlier the age at which the risk becomes apparent. The Romanian children exposed to longer periods of deprivation were more delayed; those placed at an older age appeared to recover less completely; and, even for those placed at younger ages, the most extensive recovery took place in the first 2 years after placement. Studies of these children as they move into adolescence suggest that a minority, at least, continue to experience particular ongoing problems in social relationships. Some of the behaviors typical of such children when referred for clinical evaluation are described in Stein (38). They include inappropriate social behaviors, attachment problems, odd and bizarre behaviors, language delays, defiance, noncompliance, and anger.

CHILDREN FROM THE WELFARE SYSTEM

For many years, social policy dictated that although babies and young infants could be adopted, children removed from their families by the welfare system or placed by their families after infancy were considered unsuitable for adoption. Social policy shifted significantly, however, in the seventies, as the numbers of children in foster care (and the public expense of their care) grew, and evidence emerged that even older children adopted after adverse care experiences did well after adoption, many better than those who went home to their biologic families (15,16,39,40). It is clear, however, that children adopted older, especially after adverse childcare experiences, have more psychosocial difficulties than those adopted as babies (41,42).

Howe (41) looked at a group of more than 200 adopted children, now young adults, and interviewed their parents. The subjects were baby adoptions, children adopted older who had good care as babies, and children adopted older who had poor care as babies. The latter group was the only one with higher rates of adolescent problems; however, even among that group, no problem behaviors were reported in more than one-fourth. Behavior problems include peer relationship difficulties and the lower likelihood of having a special friend (42). The findings from more recent studies (43), including those of the Romanian orphans, as well as research on the infancy attachment process, suggest that adoption, in most situations, is a potential massive positive intervention in the lives of maltreated children, and demonstrates the plasticity and resiliency of human neurobiologic systems (45). For infants, the timing of placement for permanency (which in most cases means adoption) is a matter of some urgency and that the infant's development (or maldevelopment) proceeds at a pace that is unlikely to be congruent with the timelines of juvenile courts (44). Although the evaluation of potentially abusive families, and the associated legal processes, can be quite lengthy, it is possible and, from a child developmental point of view clearly advisable, for these processes to continue while the child is given the potential for permanence through the so-called "concurrent planning."

It is unlikely that child and adolescent psychiatrists will have extensive involvement with those children adopted from the welfare system who are doing well. However, many clinicians work with the children and families of those who are doing poorly. As a result, clinicians are likely to see adoptive families struggling with children with extreme behavioral and emotional difficulties, especially in relationships within and outside the family, and, at times, be involved in the heartbreaking situations with adoptive families where the placement is disrupted (family breakdown prior to the finalization of the adoption) or dissolved (family breakdown after the adoption is finalized). Breakdown rates of older adoptions are 10% to 50% (46).

CONCLUSION

Adoption touches many lives. Many adults joyfully become parents through adoption, and would be insulted by the suggestion that this is in any way a lesser means of becoming parents. For a minority of adopted children, the process may contribute to, or be associated with, emotional and behavioral problems, and psychiatric disorders. Children at particular risk include those adopted later in life, after early adverse experiences, as well as those at particular genetic risk. However, for most of the babies and children of all ages who find permanent families through this process, adoption has a positive outcome, contributes to positive psychological adjustment, and is clearly protective. It is also important not to neglect, or ignore, the biologic parents and families of children relinquished or removed and placed for adoption. They too may be our patients. Clinicians working with adopted children and their families should be aware of the complexity and variability of the circumstances in which adoption takes place, as well as the meaning of the process for all the individuals involved.

References

1. https://www.childwelfare.gov/pubPDFs/adopted0708.pdf, Accessed December 22, 2015.
2. http://www.acf.hhs.gov/sites/default/files/cb/trends_fostercare_adoption2014.pdf, Accessed December 22, 2015.
3. Tizard B: Intercountry adoption: a review of the evidence. *J Child Psychol Psychiatry* 32:743–756, 1991.
4. http://travel.state.gov/content/dam/aa/pdfs/fy2014_annual_report.pdf, Accessed December 22, 2015.
5. Miller LC, Hendrie NW: Health of children adopted from China. *Pediatrics* 105(6):E76, 2000.
6. Miller L, Chan W, Comfort K, Tirella L: Health of children adopted from Guatemala: comparison of orphanage and foster care. *Pediatrics* 115:e710–e717, 2005.
7. Grotevant HD, Ruetere M, Von Korff, L, Gonzalez C: Post adoption contact, adoption communicative openness and satisfaction with contact as predictors of externalizing behavior in adolescence and emerging adulthood. *J Child Psychol Psychiatry* 52:529–536, 2011.
8. Grotevant HD, Wrobel GM, Von Korff L, et al.: Many faces of openness in adoption: perspectives of adopted adolescents and their parents. *Adopt Q* 10:79–101, 2008.
9. Derdeyn A: Adoption. In: Lewis M (ed): *Child and Adolescent Psychiatry: A Comprehensive Textbook*, 1996.
10. Kotsopoulos S, Cote A, Joseph L, et al.: Psychiatric disorders in adopted children: a controlled study. *Am J Orthopsychiatry* 58:608–612, 1988.
11. Miller BC, Fan X, Grotevant HD, et al.: Adopted adolescents' overrepresentation in mental health counseling: adoptees' problems or parents' lower threshold for referral? *Psychiatry Res* 226:446–450, 2015.
12. Brand AE, Brinich PM: Behavior problems and mental health contacts in adopted, foster and nonadopted children. *J Child Psychol Psychiatry* 40(8):1221–1229, 1999.
13. Keyes MA, Sharma A, Elkins IJ, Iacono WG, McGue M: The mental health of US adolescents adopted in infancy. *Arch Pediatr Adolesc Med* 162(5):419–425, 2008.
14. Fergusson DM, Lynskey M, Horwood LJ: The adolescent outcomes of adoption: a 16 year longitudinal study. *J Child Psychol Psychiatry* 36:597–615, 1995.
15. Hersov L: The Seventh Jack Tizard Memorial Lecture: aspects of adoption. *J Child Psychol Psychiatry* 31:493–510, 1990.
16. Fratter J, Rowe J, Sapsford D, Thoburn J: *Permanent Family Placement: A Decade of Experience*, London, BAAF, 1991.
17. Juffer F, van Ijzendoorn MH: Adoptees do not lack self-esteem: a meta-analysis of studies on self-esteem of transracial, international, and domestic adoptees. *Psychol Bull* 133(6):1067–1083, 2007.
18. Maughan B, Pickles A: Adopted and illegitimate children grown up. In: Robins L, Rutter M (eds): *Straight and Devious Pathways from Childhood to Adulthood*. New York, Cambridge University Press, 1990.
19. Slap G, Goodman E, Huan B: Adoption as a risk factor for attempted suicide during adolescence. *Pediatrics* 108:E30, 2001.
20. Miller BC, Fan X, Christensen M, Grotevant HD, van Dulmen M: Comparisons of adopted and nonadopted adolescents in a large nationally representative sample. *Child Dev* 71:1458–1473, 2000.
21. Westermeyer J, Bennett L, Thuras P, Yoon G: Substance use disorder among adoptees: a clinical comparative study. *Am J Drug Alcohol Abuse* 33:455–466, 2007.
22. Kety SS, Wender PH, Jacobsen B, et al.: Mental illness in the biological and adoptive relatives of schizophrenic adoptees: replication of the Copenhagen Study in the rest of Denmark. *Arch Gen Psychiatry* 51:442–445, 1994.
23. Tienari P, Wynne LC, Sorri A, et al.: Genotype-environment interaction in schizophrenia-spectrum disorder: long-term follow-up study of Finnish adoptees. *Br J Psychiatry* 184:216–222, 2004.
24. Howe OD, McDonald C, Cannon M, Arseneault L, Boydell J, Murray RM: Pathways to schizophrenia: the impact of environmental factors. *Int J Neuropsychopharmacol* 7 Suppl 1:S7–S13, 2004.
25. Wahlberg K-E, Wynne LC, Oja H, et al.: Gene-environment interaction in vulnerability to schizophrenia: findings from the Finnish adoptive family study of schizophrenia. *Am J Psychiatry* 154:355–362, 1997.
26. Hostetter MK: Infectious diseases in internationally adopted children: the past five years. *Pediatr Infect Dis J* 17:517–518, 1998.
27. Cederblad M, Hook B, Irhammar M, Mercke AM: Mental health in international adoptees as teenagers and young adults: an epidemiological study. *J Child Psychol Psychiatry* 40:1239–1248, 1999.
28. Stams GJ, Juffer F, Rispens J, Hoksberger RAC: The development and adjustment of 7 year old children adopted in infancy. *J Child Psychol Psychiatry* 41:1025–1037, 2000.
29. Verhulst FC, Althaus M, Versluis-den Bieman HJ: Problem behavior in international adoptees. I: an epidemiological study. *J Am Acad Child Adolesc Psychiatry* 19:94–103, 1990.
30. Verhulst FC, Versluis-den Bieman HJ: Developmental course of problem behaviors in adolescent adoptees. *J Am Acad Child Adolesc Psychiatry* 34:151–159, 1995.
31. Hjern A, Lindblad F, Vinnerljung B: Suicide, psychiatric illness, and social maladjustment in intercountry adoptees in Sweden: a cohort study. *Lancet* 360:443–447, 2002.
32. Von Borczyskowski A, Hjern A, Lindblad F, Vinnerljung B: Suicidal behavior in national and international adult adoptees: a Swedish cohort study. *Soc Psychiatry Psychiatr Epidemiol* 41:95–102, 2006.
33. Vegt EJ, Tieman W, van der Ende J, Ferdinand RF, Verhulst FC, et al.: Impact of early childhood adversities on adult psychiatric disorders: a study of international adoptees. *Soc Psychiatry Psychiatr Epidemiol* 44: 724–731, 2009.
34. Rushton A, Minnis H: Annotation: transracial family placements. *J Child Psychol Psychiatry* 38:147–159, 1997.
35. Rutter M, Andersen-Wood L, Becket C, et al.: Developmental catch-up, and deficit, following adoption after severe global early privation. *J Child Psychol Psychiatry* 39:465–476, 1998.
36. O'Connor TG, Rutter M, Beckett C, Keaveney L, Kreppner JM: The effects of global severe privation on cognitive competence: extension and longitudinal follow-up. English and Romanian Adoptees Study Team. *Child Dev* 71:376–390, 2000.
37. Julian MM: Age at adoption from institutional care as a window into the lasting effects of early experiences. *J Am Acad Child Adolesc Psychiatry* 39:1504–1511, 2000.
38. Stein M: International adoption: a four-year-old child with unusual behaviors adopted at six months of age. *Dev Behav Pediatrics* 24:63–69, 2003.
39. Hodges J, Tizard B: Social and family relationships of ex-institutional adolescents. *J Child Psychol Psychiatry* 30:77–97, 1989.
40. Seglow J, Pringle MK, Wedge P: *Growing Up Adopted*. Windsor, UK, NFER, 1972.
41. Howe D: Parent reported problems in 211 adopted children: some risk and protective factors. *J Child Psychol Psychiatry* 38:401–411, 1997.
42. Dance C, Rushton A, Quinton D: Emotional abuse in early childhood: relationships with progress in subsequent family placement. *J Child Psychol Psychiatry* 43:395–407, 2002.
43. van Ijzendoorn MH, Juffer F: The Emanuel Miller Memorial Lecture 2006: adoption as intervention. Meta-analytic evidence for massive catch-up and plasticity in physical, socio-emotional, and cognitive development. *J Child Psychol Psychiatry* 47:1228–1245, 2006.
44. Zeanah CH, Larrieu JA, Heller SS, et al.: Evaluation of a preventive intervention for maltreated infants and toddlers in foster care. *J Am Acad Child Adolesc Psychiatry* 40:214–221, 2001
45. Fisher PA: Review: Adoption, fostering and the needs of looked-after and adopted children. *Child Adolesc Ment Health* 20:5–12, 2015.
46. Borland M, O'Hara G, Triseliotis J: Placement outcomes for children with special needs. *Adoption and Fostering* 15:18–28, 1991.

CHAPTER 7.4.4 ■ MALPRACTICE AND PROFESSIONAL LIABILITY

PETER ASH AND BARRY NURCOMBE

Malpractice litigation and other forms of formal legal investigation of medical care, such as state medical licensing board investigations, are society's means of holding physicians to appropriate standards and compensating patients who have been negligently harmed. There are problems with utilizing litigation to achieve these goals: it is an inefficient way of compensating patients, since many who have been harmed do not sue (1), many who have suffered damage and do sue were not harmed by negligence, and the costs of litigation, both financially and emotionally, are very high. Physicians who have been sued describe the process as extremely painful emotionally, even when they prevail (2). Practicing defensive medicine is common (3), though probably less of an issue in child psychiatry than in more technologic medical specialties, and some psychiatrists may avoid taking on the most difficult patients. Physicians understandably hate being sued. In the United States, malpractice premiums have increased markedly over the past 30 years, triggering calls for legislative tort reform. Over half the states now have limits on noneconomic damages (pain and suffering) (4). More systematic reforms of the system have been called for, such as moving to a no-fault system adjudicated administratively, along the lines of the worker's compensation system, but such proposals currently have very limited political support.

Compared to many medical specialties, child and adolescent psychiatry is not high risk. Even when sued, child and adolescent psychiatrists prevail most of the time. While accurate national data are difficult to come by because insurance companies keep much of their loss experience as proprietary information, analysis of the psychiatry dataset of the Physician Insurers Association of America from 1985 to 2000 for child and adolescent patients indicated that only about 14% of claims resulted in a payment, and the average payment was less than the average payment in adult psychiatric malpractice cases (5). These positive outcomes are reflected in the practice of some insurers giving discounted premiums to child and adolescent psychiatrists.

Malpractice litigation is not the only arena in which physicians have professional liability: medical licensing boards investigate complaints, as do ethics committees of professional associations. While such investigations do not directly result in monetary damage payments, in medical licensing investigations the ability of the clinician to practice may be at stake, and findings of fault may later be admitted as evidence in a malpractice case.

THE LAW OF MALPRACTICE

The term *malpractice* refers to an act or omission by a professional in the course of his or her professional duty that causes or aggravates an injury to a patient or client and is the consequence of a failure to exercise a reasonable degree of prudence, diligence, knowledge, or skill. To substantiate malpractice, the plaintiff must establish the following four points, known as the 4 Ds, by a preponderance of the evidence:

1. The clinician had a ***Duty*** *of reasonable care* to the patient
2. There was a ***Dereliction*** *of that duty,* when judged by the standard of the average, prudent practitioner
3. The patient sustained ***Damage,*** a compensable injury or harm
4. The damage was a ***Direct*** *result* of the clinician's failure to exercise a reasonable standard of care

Duty of Care: The Doctor–Patient Relationship

The clinician owes a duty of reasonable care toward a patient when a professional relationship exists between them. This relationship is formed when a clinician explicitly or implicitly agrees to provide care to a patient. The clinician thus enters into a contract that binds him or her to provide a reasonable level of care in return for a valuable consideration (the fee). Unless the clinician has unwisely promised a cure, he or she is not bound to provide more than a reasonable level of care.

The doctor–patient relationship cannot be imposed on a competent patient, nor can a doctor be forced to care for a patient except in special situations, such as an emergency room. Controversial situations arise when it is argued that a relationship has been implied by the physician's actions or words. For example, the discussion of a patient's condition by telephone before transfer to a different hospital has been held to imply a contractual relationship (6). Payment is not necessary; even free advice can create a professional relationship. The clinician should be careful about giving casual advice at cocktail parties and the like, lest it be construed that a contractual relationship has been formed.

Conversely, a physician cannot be forced to treat patients who are unable to pay for services or to use a treatment that he or she is not competent to implement. The physician also has a legal (though perhaps not an ethical) right to refuse to give aid in an emergency. Good Samaritan laws have been enacted to protect from liability those physicians who do render emergency aid, unless they have been grossly negligent (e.g., abandoning a live patient who is still hemorrhaging).

When working with minor patients, it is important to be clear with the family who the patient is. In some types of family work, the "family" is defined as the patient, and the clinician may thereby establish a doctor–patient relationship with each member of the family. When the minor is the identified patient, the physician is not taking on responsibility for treating the parents, and communications from the parent about the child are placed in the child patient's record. However, when advice is given to a parent in a separate parent session (e.g., "Your child would be better off if the two of you divorced"), the physician is likely to be held responsible for the foreseeable consequences of that advice.

The Internet allows doctors to communicate with patients in new ways. Email communications between a patient who is or will be seen in the office clearly fall within an established doctor–patient relationship. Responding to a nonpatient's email with therapeutic advice may establish a doctor–patient relationship, much as if a similar communication was conducted over the telephone (7). Simply responding to a prospective patient's email with a referral to someone in their geographic area does not establish a doctor–patient relationship. While the law is still evolving in this area, the trend is that the medicine is practiced in the state where the patient resides, not where the physician practices (8), so physicians who conduct email treatment with a patient who resides in a state where the clinician does not have a license may be practicing without a license. Prudent risk management dictates that professional email communications with nonpatients that might be construed as therapeutic contain a clear disclaimer that the email does not constitute professional advice and refer the patient to their physician for such advice. Similarly, general information about mental health conditions which a physician may post on his or her website should likewise contain a disclaimer. Professional risk management organizations have developed guidelines for practitioner websites and email practices (9,10).

As psychiatric practice has become more focused on psychopharmacology, collaborative treatment relationships have become more common. The most frequent relationship is one in which the psychiatrist handles medications while another mental health professional conducts psychotherapy. As team medicine and medical homes become more common, another type involves the psychiatrist intermittently seeing the patient but another professional, such as a pediatrician or nurse practitioner, does the bulk of the prescribing. These relationships often leave ambiguous which clinician is responsible for what and how responsibility for care is to be shared. In the event of an adverse outcome, the question of who is potentially liable arises. It is important that the psychiatrist and other professionals are clear on their responsibilities, including what the physician's role will be, who is providing emergency coverage, and the expectations of communication between the collaborating providers. This understanding should be shared with the patient, and the discussion documented.

After the termination of the contract, the physician owes no further obligation to the patient other than that of confidentiality. Physicians who terminate contracts unilaterally and without reasonable cause are at risk of actions for *abandonment*. The physician must give the patient due notice of termination and must ensure that necessary arrangements are made for alternative care. If the patient resists termination, failure to refer to another physician may be construed as negligence. Some risk managers advise that patients be notified at the outset that noncompliance with treatment is deemed a termination of treatment.

Vicarious Liability

In accordance with the doctrine of *respondeat superior* (let the master answer), a physician is legally responsible for the negligent actions of employees or supervisees. Thus, a psychiatrist may be held liable for the negligent or outrageous actions of his secretary and office staff or house officers whom he or she supervises. In malpractice cases involving inpatients, the hospital is often a defendant because of its vicarious liability for the actions of nurses, ward staff, and house officers.

Supervising and Consulting Relationships

Supervisors who provide care, supervise the care of residents, or are the attending physician of record face malpractice exposure for the care they direct, and may be held liable for care they supervise, either as vicariously liable for the actions of a house officer, or as directly liable for inadequate supervision. Consider a suit filed subsequent to an adolescent's suicide after the adolescent was brought to an emergency room and examined by a resident who discharged the patient after discussion with the chief resident but without telephoning the attending child psychiatrist. Assuming the overall care was found negligent, courts may apportion blame differently, depending on local interpretations of whether residents are held to the standard of specialists and the nature of the contract of the on-call attending (who has been found vicariously liable in some cases even when not contacted). If the attending had been called, then the apportioning problem is still complex. At this time there exists no clear standard as to what constitutes reasonable supervision (11,12).

When the physician is asked by another clinician to see a patient, the consulting physician's liability for malpractice is governed by whether a doctor–patient relationship was created. If the consulting physician provides consultation to the treating doctor, but does not write orders or otherwise direct the treatment, then ordinarily no doctor–patient relationship is formed, and the consultant's duty is only to the consultee doctor. However, if the consulting physician writes orders or otherwise directs care, then the court will usually find that a doctor–patient relationship was created.

Clinicians may examine people on behalf of a third party, such as a school or insurer, to whom they owe a contractual duty. However, if the examination causes the examinee harm, for example, by failure to detect suicidality or the possibility of child abuse, the liability risk is ambiguous. Some courts have held that the clinician's duty is to the employer; others have held that, if the person being examined reasonably relied on the examination for diagnosis, a duty may be owed. The physician is advised to inform the examinee that the purpose of the examination is not therapeutic. In court-ordered evaluations, courts typically find that the evaluator is immune as an agent of the court (13).

Fiduciary Relationship

The clinician's obligations toward the patient go beyond the duty to provide reasonable care. The relationship between the psychiatrist and patient is analogous to that between the guardian and ward. The patient has a right to expect the physician to show good faith, that is, to act in the patient's best interest. This, the physician's *fiduciary duty*, is especially onerous in psychiatry, because emotionally disturbed people share their most private experiences with their mental health clinicians and are thus very vulnerable. Improper sexual contact, invasion of privacy, breach of confidentiality, outrageous manipulation of the patient's emotions, and the exploitation of patients for financial gain are all examples of *double agentry* and *breaches of fiduciary trust*. These *intentional torts* are discussed later in this chapter.

Dereliction of Duty: Breach of the Standard of Care

In accordance with the contract inherent in the doctor–patient relationship, the physician is bound to provide a reasonable level of care. In other words, the physician contracts to provide reasonable, prudent, diligent, knowledgeable, and skillful medical care. Unless the clinician has unwisely promised a cure, the contract does not call for exceptional care, only a level of expertise equivalent to that exercised under similar circumstances by the average practitioner in the same field of medicine. *The clinician is not liable for an error of judgment unless the error represented a substandard level of care.* If the clinician exercised reasonable judgment, the clinician is not responsible simply because the patient suffers a bad outcome. If clinicians differ as to how a particular issue should be addressed, it is enough to show that there is a respectable minority who endorse the approach that was taken. The considerable variation among clinicians in methods of treatment has made standards difficult to establish, particularly in regard to psychotherapy where there are many different approaches. The standard is tighter with regard to precautions against suicide or violence or the monitoring of medication.

The standard of care traditionally required that the clinician be judged by the professional standard in the locality. However, the emergence of national standards has caused the courts to move in this direction, with allowance for the paucity of resources in some areas. Since the statute of limitations typically does not begin to toll until a child reaches the age of majority, cases involving children may be filed many years after the alleged malpractice took place. The standard of care is linked to the standard of professional practice at the time of the alleged breach of duty. If a clinician practices medicine in a specialty area for which he or she is not trained, the clinician is likely to be held to the standard applying to that specialty.

Breach of the Duty of Care

Malpractice suits are founded in the legal theories of intentional and negligent torts. An *intentional tort* involves deliberate intent on the part of the wrongdoer or wrongful conduct that the wrongdoer ought to have known was unacceptable (in which case it is known as a *quasi-intentional tort*). Examples of intentional torts are assault, battery, false imprisonment, fraudulent commitment, defamation, invasion of privacy, sexual exploitation, and the intentional infliction of emotional distress. Expert testimony is not required to substantiate an intentional tort, and malpractice insurance may not cover it. A *negligent tort* involves an unintentional error that reflects a failure by the clinician to exercise a reasonable standard of medical care. Expert testimony is required for proof of negligence.

In determining whether treatment fell below the standard of care, the courts may look to a variety of sources, and inquire whether the treatment:

1. Violates a statute (such as the child abuse reporting law or HIPAA regulations)
2. Violates a licensing board regulation or other regulatory agency holdings (such as FDA guidelines)
3. Violates an ethical principle of the profession (such as confidentiality)
4. Violates case law (such as the *Tarasoff* duty to protect)
5. Violates the professional consensus of the community

Professional consensus is the least clear of these elements, and the one about which expert opinion at trial most often differs. When there is no disagreement about what treatment the defendant doctor actually provided, the difficult question is whether that course was reasonable in the specific case at issue. When professional organizations began developing published practice parameters or practice guidelines, clinicians were concerned that such guidelines would create liability by setting the standard of practice. In response to this concern, published guidelines typically contain disclaimers stating the guidelines do not define a standard of practice. Courts frequently allow experts to discuss professional guidelines in their testimony as indicators of standard practice, but acknowledge that they do no set a standard of practice and that approaches may deviate from general guidelines in individual cases (14). Guidelines have often proved useful to defendant doctors by indicating that a range of approaches are acceptable. In day-to-day work, in considering a course of action, a clinician should ask himself, "What would my peers think of this?" and "What would I think if a colleague told me he was going to do this?" If the answer is that the colleague would be concerned, then the physician should consider the approach carefully and document the rationale fully.

Damage, Harm, or Injury

Harm may be physical or psychological. Physical harm or damage resulting from negligence includes, for example, side effects of medication such as tardive dyskinesia, physical injury incurred when a patient is improperly restrained, or homicide or suicide. Psychological damages may be of two types: general pain and suffering, and damages to the patient's mental health. Expert testimony is not needed to establish pain and suffering: the jury can draw its own conclusion as to how much suffering it thinks a normal person would suffer given a particular harm. Psychiatric evidence may be utilized to inform the jury about the impact of an injury on the plaintiff's capacity to enjoy life. Mental health damages typically require expert testimony, as, for example, when a plaintiff alleges that her major depressive disorder has been aggravated by traumatic treatment. Injury to a parent or child may give rise to an action for loss of consortium, that is, loss of the care, comfort, and society of a spouse, parent, or child.

Proximate Cause

The plaintiff must substantiate that the defendant's wrongful act or omission directly caused or aggravated the patient's injury. In other words, it must be proven that, but for the wrongful conduct, the damage would not have occurred, or would not have been aggravated, or that a direct, uninterrupted link or foreseeable chain of events exists between the wrongful conduct and the injury or its aggravation. The legal concept of *cause* is analogous to the psychiatric concept of *precipitation* or *aggravation*.

Some states have comparative or contributory negligence rules that instruct juries to consider whether the plaintiff's negligence, such as failing to inform the clinician of a worsening condition, or failing to cooperate with treatment, contributed to the bad outcome, and reduce damages accordingly. Because a child or adolescent patient's responsibility is generally held to be lower than that of an adult, comparative negligence issues are uncommon in child or adolescent malpractice cases.

Restitutive Payment

If the defendant is found liable, the judge or jury may award damages. Damages are designed to be *compensatory,* that is, to recompense the victim for medical expenses, pain, suffering, loss of enjoyment of life, impairment of capacity, and future loss of earnings and to restore the plaintiff to his or her original position, so far as money is able to do so. If the defendant's behavior has been egregiously outrageous, malicious, or wanton, *punitive* damages may be imposed over and above compensatory damages, but are rare in malpractice cases. By federal law, all payments whether as a result of settlement talks or by trial verdict, are reported to the National Practitioner Data Bank (15).

Managed Care

Although managed care has had considerable impact on clinical practice, it has had rather little impact on malpractice litigation. From the law's perspective, the clinician is responsible for prescribing needed treatment and managed care deals only with payment of fees. In *Wickline v. State of California* (1986) (16), the court affirmed the physician's duty to prescribe care, and suggested that the physician had a duty to appeal adverse decisions made by managed care reviewers. In clinical practice, clinicians routinely take into account the ability of the patient to pay in making treatment recommendations.

A number of states have attempted to pass laws holding managed care entities liable for denying authorization or payment for needed care. However, most managed care contracts are employee benefits, and are covered under the federal Employee Retirement Income Responsibility Act (ERISA). Congress originally passed ERISA to regulate pensions, but it has been interpreted to cover employee health care benefits as well. ERISA has two major prongs that limit the liability of managed care companies: first, it preempts any state law with which it conflicts, and second, it limits the damage for error to the amount of the benefit denied (the cost of treatment). Thus, state laws which assign liability to managed care are voided, and the most the patient can recover for improperly denied care is the cost of the care. The courts have recognized that this leaves patients with little redress (17), but reform, the so-called "patient rights" legislation, requires congressional action.

In malpractice litigation, managed care issues rarely surface: physicians are reluctant to argue that their care, which resulted in a bad outcome, was limited by financial considerations, and plaintiffs are reluctant to assert that they happily would have paid for expensive care out of pocket if only the doctor had recommended it.

COURSE OF A TYPICAL CASE

If a clinician's patient suffers a serious adverse treatment-related event, the clinician should report the matter to his or her insurer and follow their risk management advice. With minor patients, the parents control access to information, so no formal release is necessary to discuss with them what occurred, unlike in cases involving adults. A number of states have passed legislation which prohibits apologies or expressions of sympathy or regret from later being admitted as evidence of physician negligence. Peer-review activities, such as morbidity and mortality conferences, are not discoverable to prove liability in most states. The clinician then enters an uneasy waiting period to see if suit is filed. For minor patients, the statute of limitations (the period during which suit can be filed) typically does not begin to run until the child becomes an adult, so the wait can be quite long. Attorneys for plaintiffs in malpractice actions typically work on a contingency fee basis in which they initially bear the costs of litigation. Attorneys therefore screen cases carefully before making a judgment that spending the time and money to pursue the case is likely to be profitable. In most states, in order to file a malpractice claim, the plaintiff's attorney needs to obtain an affidavit from an expert asserting that the care rendered was below the standard of care. If the physician is served with notice of being sued, the malpractice insurance carrier should immediately be notified.

After suit is filed, the discovery phase begins, which will involve both sides retaining experts and taking depositions, including the deposition of the defendant doctor. Settlement talks also occur in this period. Whether the malpractice insurer can settle without the agreement of the defendant doctor depends on the terms of the insurance contract. If the case does not settle, it progresses to trial. Halleck (18), an experienced forensic psychiatrist who had himself testified in numerous malpractice actions, has described how emotionally wrenching even he found being a defendant. If money is paid to the plaintiff, either as a product of settlement negotiations or a court verdict, the amount and doctor's name are reported to the National Practitioner Data Bank, and the information is available to credentialing bodies, licensing boards, insurers, and managed care entities. This publicity has reduced doctors' willingness to settle a case for "nuisance value."

CIRCUMSTANCES IN WHICH MALPRACTICE IS MOST LIKELY TO OCCUR

While in many ways child and adolescent malpractice cases are similar to adult malpractice cases, only involving younger patients, they differ from adult cases in a number of respects. First, minors are less responsible for their acts, which tends to shift responsibility to the clinician and the parents. Second, minors typically cannot consent to treatment, which introduces a third party decision maker, usually the parents, into the case. Third, parents are often involved as quasi-patients because they receive advice from the clinician. And finally, juries are sympathetic to injured children. While an allegation of malpractice can involve any aspect of practice, the vast majority of cases fall into one of the several areas shown in Table 7.4.4.1.

TABLE 7.4.4.1

COMMON ISSUES IN MALPRACTICE LITIGATION

Area of Practice	Example Plaintiff Allegation
Dangerousness	
Suicide	Weak suicide assessment documentation: "SI–"
Homicide	No violence risk assessment in chart
Failure to protect from danger	Inpatient sexually assaulted by another inpatient
Failure to protect third parties	Dangerous patient escapes from hospital and family not notified
Protecting and releasing information	Confidential information released without authorization
Treatment	
Failure to obtain informed consent	Possible side effects not discussed
Psychotherapy	Implanted memories of sexual abuse
Sex with patient	Therapist had sex with patient
Medication	Girl with bipolar disorder treated with sodium divalproex for 8 mos gives birth to baby with birth defects and there is no documentation of pregnancy status when medication is started
Ending treatment	
Negligent discharge	Patient discharged while still suicidal
Abandonment	Therapist terminated treatment without referral when patient ailed to pay bill

Issues Pertaining to Dangerousness

From a malpractice perspective, the central questions are first, whether the danger was reasonably foreseeable, and second, if it was, whether the clinician took adequate steps to protect the patient and potential victims. Foreseeability focuses on the adequacy of the assessment of risk, and protection focuses on the interventions employed once significant risk is found. While there is general acceptance that psychiatrists lack the ability to accurately predict violence, there is increasing agreement on the standards for assessing the risk of violence.

Suicide

Suicide of a young person is a tragedy. Assessment and treatment of suicidal children and adolescents are covered in detail in Chapter 5.4.3. Assessment of suicidal intent is more difficult in adolescents than it is in adults because the rate of suicidal ideation is so high in middle to late adolescents. The 2013 Youth Risk Behavior Surveillance study found that 17% of high school students had seriously considered suicide in the previous 12 months, 13.6% had made a plan, 8% had attempted suicide, and 2.7% had made an attempt that required medical attention (19). When these rates are compared to the completed suicide rate of approximately 0.007%, it is clear that the ratio of suicidal ideation to completed suicide is very high (over 2,000:1). Assuming that an adequate assessment was conducted, documentation of the assessment is key. The oft-seen suicide assessment note of "SI–" (suicidal ideation negative) does not offer much protection to a defendant psychiatrist because it fails to document the components of the suicide assessment, such as what history was obtained about prior attempts, family history, plan, etc. Where some suicide risk is present, assessment entails weighing risk factors and protective factors. Good documentation of risk and protective factors, and of the physician's reasoning about intervention, is the best protection in the event of an adverse outcome. On an inpatient unit, the psychiatrist should also document his or her review of the assessments of others, such as nurses and house officers. Timely, clear, legible, pertinent, thorough, dated, timed, and signed records are the key to communication and the best proof that the hospital and staff have exercised reasonable care. In *Abille v. United States* (20), after a psychiatrist transferred a patient from a suicidal status to a less dangerous status, the patient committed suicide. The finding of negligence against the defendant hinged on the psychiatrist's failure to keep detailed records that explained his decision to transfer the patient, even though it was conceded that, under the circumstances, the decision may have been reasonable. Finally, it is important to keep in mind that suicide assessment is a process, and for depressed or suicidal youth, repeated assessments need to be documented.

If a physician determines that the patient is at significant risk for suicide, then he or she has a duty to institute reasonable precautions. If the clinician decides not to hospitalize the patient, it is important to document the protective factors and interventions that were employed. For youthful patients, this often involves utilizing the family to monitor the patient's condition, provide some protection, and alert the clinician if the situation deteriorates. The child or adolescent's risk for suicide should be discussed with the parents. If the patient is in the hospital, it is important to document the physician's review of observations of other care providers and to document the reasons when levels of supervision are reduced.

What if the patient refuses to cooperate with the admitting psychiatrist, who consequently does not elicit and diagnose an imminent suicide risk? In *Skar v. City of Lincoln, Nebraska* (21), a recalcitrant patient injured himself in a suicide attempt. The court found for the defendant and held that the patient had a duty to cooperate with his physician as far as he was able. However, it is essential in such a case that the psychiatrist record the questions put to the patient and the patient's responses or failure to respond. Also, with minor patients who cannot legally consent to treatment, courts are likely to apportion less responsibility to the patient.

Failure to Protect or Control a Violent or Sexually Aggressive Patient

Clinicians and hospitals assume a duty of care toward patients with a potential for violence. The psychiatrist must carefully assess the potential for danger and must ensure that the hospital staff take adequate precautions to protect a violent patient from harming others. Past medical records should be scrutinized concerning violence potential, and referring agents and parents should be questioned. In accordance with the imminence of the risk, housing in a secure unit, confinement to a room, close observation, a search of clothing and personal effects, and removal of all dangerous objects (belts, mirrors), may be required. If the patient is medicated, staff members should check that medication is actually swallowed. It is essential that the degree and nature of risk be communicated to all staff who care for the patient.

The prevalence of sexual abuse and its relationship to psychiatric disorder mean that many minors admitted to psychiatric hospitals are at risk of precocious sexual activity and unwanted pregnancy. Suicide and sexual activity involving latency-aged inpatients have been reported to be the most common types of malpractice action brought against child psychiatry training programs (22). These cases may involve two patients cared for by different doctors, and raise complicated confidentiality problems (e.g., can the plaintiff-victim get access to the medical file of the perpetrator?). The central issues are the foresight involving the risk of the activity occurring, and the adequacy of nursing monitoring of patient interaction. Known perpetrators should be closely observed and housed in single rooms, if necessary. However, the closeness of the possible observation decreases if the therapeutic environment is less restrictive, for example, in a residential treatment center.

Negligent Release or Discharge of a Suicidal or Violent Patient

A patient may harm himself or herself or others while on pass in the grounds of the hospital, on leave with relatives or friends, after discharge, or after absconding from hospital. Was the tragedy foreseeable by a reasonably prudent psychiatrist? This is the question that the courts seek to answer. In doing so, they are aware that the safety of the public must be balanced against the need to rehabilitate patients, that reasonable, calculated risks must often be taken, and that *bona fide* errors of clinical judgment are unavoidable (23).

Increasing pressure by managed-care organizations, Medicaid agencies, and insurers has raised the specter of premature discharge against medical advice forced by withdrawal of funding. The clinician should be aware that legal responsibility for any harm that consequently befalls the patient or community will be placed on his or her shoulders. The risk may be so great that the hospital should bear the cost of continued hospitalization.

Wrongful Injury, Assault, and Battery

A patient injured by staff members who use excessive force to subdue him or her may have a claim against the hospital for battery or wrongful injury. Wrongful injury may also be claimed when one patient is harmed by another whom the staff could not control; however, the plaintiff would have to establish that the hospital was derelict in its duty to control the violent patient.

Seclusion and restraint present serious liability risks. They may be legitimate management techniques when the risk of harm is imminent and there are no alternatives; but they should not be used to compensate for understaffing. Physical control should be time limited, and the patient should be examined by a physician if the maximum permissible time (e.g., 1 hour) requires extension. Seclusion and restraint should never be ordered "as needed." Quality assurance tracking is required to ensure that the use of physical controls does not become excessive.

If the person causing the harm is a hospital employee, the hospital may be liable, particularly if it were known that the employee had a propensity for violence or sexual misbehavior (24). The hospital may also be liable for the misbehavior of physicians, agency nurses, or others who work in hospital but who are not employed by it. State institutions may claim *sovereign immunity,* which precludes litigants from suing governmental institutions; however, most jurisdictions have greatly limited or abolished this doctrine.

Failure to Protect Endangered Third Parties

Prior to the first *Tarasoff* decision (25) in 1974, clinicians had duties to their patients, but not to third parties. So, if a patient harmed a third party, the patient might have grounds to sue the clinician for failing to treat or restrain him, but the victim could not successfully sue the clinician. This was in line with general negligence principles which hold that in most situations, one does not have a duty to protect third parties. Thus, if a man sees someone drowning in a river, he has no legal duty to help (although he may have a moral duty). In the clinical situation, it was also thought that the patient's confidentiality prevented notifying a potential victim of threats, and that psychiatrists' inability to accurately predict violence limited their ability to intervene.

The first time the California Supreme Court heard the *Tarasoff* case, it found that clinicians did have a duty to potential victims, and that duty overrode the need for confidentiality, holding "The protective privilege ends where the public peril begins" (*Tarasoff I* at 561). The Court also decided that the duty could be discharged by warning the potential victim, which became known as the "duty to warn."

Concerned by the serious implications for patient confidentiality of this judgment, the American Psychiatric Association pressed the appellate court to reopen the case. In an unusual move, the Court did so, and in *Tarasoff II* (26), the issue of failure to warn was debated. The court decided that there was a *duty to protect* rather than a duty to warn: *if there is a serious danger of violence, the clinician must take reasonable care to protect the foreseeable victim.* The court failed to define what constituted "reasonable care" and how dangerous the patient must be before precautions should be taken.

Following *Tarasoff,* courts and legislatures in other jurisdictions have wrestled with these issues. The key dimensions that need to be decided are:

1. Is there a duty to protect?
2. If there is a duty, who needs to be protected? Only identifiable victims? The general public?
3. What triggers the duty? Is a specific threat required, or only a clinical judgment of risk?
4. How can the duty be discharged? A warning? Calling the police?

Jurisdictions have answered these questions differently, with about half the states finding a duty, a minority holding there is no duty, and some leaving the question unresolved (27). The trend has been toward legislation specifying what the duty is and how clinicians can fulfill it to avoid liability. Clearly, clinicians need to be aware of the law in their own jurisdiction.

Despite the attention paid to *Tarasoff* issues, clinical cases involving a need to breach confidentiality are uncommon with adolescent patients. In the vast majority of cases in which an adolescent is judged an imminent risk to others, the adolescent is hospitalized and kept in the hospital until he or she no longer poses serious risk. Further, in working clinically with dangerous minors, parents control consent to release information, and they will often consent to involving potential victims (as in family treatment), so problems of breaching confidentiality without consent may often be sidestepped. *Tarasoff* situations most commonly arise in two situations: first, when the patient is not available for intervention, as when a therapist hears about a threat over the telephone or the patient escapes from the hospital, and second, in situations of contingent threats ("I think I'll pass, but if that teacher gives me an 'F', I'll shoot her").

What, then, should a clinician do if a patient threatens violence and the situation cannot be managed clinically? First, undertake and document a violence risk–resource analysis. If the risk is serious, take precautions to protect endangered parties, and with minors, discuss the situation with the parents. Second, if the patient is already hospitalized, take precautions against elopement, consider limiting visitation and leave, and do not discharge the patient unless you are convinced that the risk of violence has diminished. Obtain consultation if you are in doubt. Third, if a potentially violent hospitalized patient elopes or fails to return from leave, seek consultation from a colleague and from the hospital's attorney and inform the parents. If the risk of harm is significant, inform the local police and the police department of the area where the patient lives, by telephone and certified letter. If certain people (family, friends, or acquaintances) could be in danger, warn them by telephone, through the police, and by certified letter. Fourth, if you warn a third party by telephone or letter, take care to divulge only as much as necessary to let them know they are at risk. Fifth, involve the patient in the warning process. The patient may agree to having a warning given. If you have control of the patient (i.e., the patient is in the hospital or can be kept in your office), let the patient be present when you telephone the police and the third party, allow him or her to read the contents of the letters sent to the endangered third party and the police, and encourage the patient to discuss his or her reactions to these interventions. Knowing the potential victim has been warned may bolster the patient's own self-control.

If the situation is unclear in the home state, the clinician would be well advised to act as though the broadest interpretation of the doctrine applies. However, as Simon (28) points out, one should not allow concern about *Tarasoff* liability to interfere with sound clinical practice. Instead, the clinician should make reasonable efforts to control potentially violent patients before breaching confidentiality; and if warnings are required, they should be incorporated into treatment whenever possible.

Failure to Report Child Abuse or Neglect

All states have mandatory reporting laws requiring mental health clinicians to report a reasonable suspicion of child abuse or neglect, and failure to do so is malpractice. The statutes immunize a clinician making a good faith report, so a report to protective services that is later deemed unfounded is not a basis for malpractice. However, other interventions taken by the clinician based on a conclusion of abuse may be actionable. In *Montoya v. Bebensee* (29), a clinician advised a mother to withhold visitation from a father who was suspected of abuse. The father sued, and the court held that the report to protective services was immune from suit, even if made negligently, but the advice to the mother fell outside the reporting statute and could be grounds for suit, a holding Guyer (30) characterized as "you can sound an alarm, but you can't form a posse." Litigation over recovered memories has addressed similar issues, and is discussed further below.

Protecting and Releasing Information

The Hippocratic Oath includes a precept regarding confidentiality: "What I may see or hear in the course of the treatment or even outside of the treatment in regard to the life of men, which on no account one must spread abroad, I will keep to myself, holding such things shameful to be spoken about." Confidentiality has always been seen as especially central in psychiatry. The issue is complex in child and adolescent psychiatry because the clinician needs to weigh the child's need for privacy against the parents' right to know by virtue of their legally controlling the release of information until the minor patient becomes an adult. In many jurisdictions, the extent to which an adolescent can enforce a privacy right against the parents' control of the record is legally murky. It is clear that parents have a right to know if the adolescent is involved in a dangerous clinical situation. Many states have allowed minors some control over the record, generally in parallel to the degree that minors in that jurisdiction can consent to treatment. Aside from the legal precedents, children and adolescents value confidentiality in psychotherapy as necessary for feeling comfortable to share sensitive material. While clinicians are advised to be aware of the rules in their jurisdiction, from a clinical perspective, it is important at the outset of treatment to discuss with patients and their parents what information will be shared with parents and under what conditions.

Confidentiality and Privilege

Confidentiality is a duty of the clinician toward the patient that precludes the clinician from divulging private matters revealed by the patient in the context of the doctor–patient relationship. *Privilege* is the patient's legal right to bar the physician from disclosing confidential matters in a court of law. Testimonial privilege derives from statutes in some states, and from court holdings in other states. In *Jaffee v. Redmond* (31) the U.S. Supreme Court held that there was a mental health privilege in federal court. Physicians should consult their local statutes to understand the extent of this privilege and its exceptions. Confusion may occur when a clinician receives a subpoena to appear in court (with or without records). A subpoena merely requires the clinician to appear in court. It does not compel him or her to testify about confidential matters unless the patient has specifically authorized the clinician to do so, or has waived privilege, or unless the clinician is ordered to do so by the judge. Although states vary somewhat in the exceptions allowed to the rule of privilege, the following are the most usual:

1. *Waiver by patient.* The clinician should seek specific written authorization from the patient (or those who legally speak for the patient, such as parents) before disclosing confidential material in court or to other parties.
2. *Evaluation for a reason other than psychiatric treatment.* For example, the psychiatric evaluation of a disputant in a child custody case is not privileged if the evaluation was conducted as part of the case. A similar exclusion applies to evaluations for the purpose of civil commitment.
3. *The patient-litigant exception.* If a patient offers his or her mental health as evidence in litigation, in most states—but not all—he or she generally waives privilege concerning the specific issue in evidence. Similarly, if the patient pleads insanity as a criminal defense, the psychiatric examination conducted to evaluate that matter is not privileged (32).
4. *Duty to protect endangered third parties.* The *Tarasoff* exclusion discussed above applies when the community is endangered.
5. Other limited exceptions authorized by law, such as mandatory reporting of child abuse and civil commitment proceedings.

HIPAA

The Health Insurance Portability and Accountability Act of 1996 (HIPAA) authorized the U.S. Department of Health and Human Services to establish regulations regarding the privacy of medical records, which they did in what is known as the Privacy Rule (33) which went into effect in 2003. The Privacy Rule establishes a federal floor for the protection of protected health information (PHI). In a particular situation, if state law provides for a higher level of privacy protection, then state law controls. For example, some states have statutes that restrict release of mental health records in situations that HIPAA would otherwise allow. The Privacy Rule is complex, and a complete summary will not be attempted here. The Office for Civil Rights in the Department of Health and Human Services provides considerable information on its website regarding the details of the Privacy Rule (34), and many professional organizations provide information and recommendations to their members. Violations of HIPAA and the Privacy Rule can be investigated and prosecuted.

HIPAA has implications for psychiatric practice. First, clinicians covered by the Privacy Rule are required to give patients (or parents) a *Notice of Privacy Practices* at the patient's first appointment. The notice must spell out how clinicians assure privacy and under what conditions and to whom protected health information can be released without obtaining consent. Second, HIPAA gives adult patients the right to see their records (or generally parents, in the case of treatment of children and adolescents), with very limited exceptions. Third, the Privacy Rule restricts third party payer requests for information to the "minimum necessary" information. Previously, insurance companies, relying on the patient's release signed as a condition of obtaining coverage, could, and often did, ask for a copy of the entire chart. The American Psychiatric Association (35) has taken a formal position on what constitutes the minimum necessary information necessary for payment which includes identifying information, diagnosis, treatment plan, and dates of treatment, but excludes much of the detailed material often found in progress notes. Fourth, the Privacy Rule creates a new category of medical record which it terms "psychotherapy notes." Psychotherapy notes, as defined in the Privacy Rule, are notes that are part of the medical record, and so are different from process notes, which the clinician typically holds apart from the medical record and can destroy whenever he or she wishes (except to avoid a subpoena!). However, psychotherapy notes are kept separately from the regular medical record, and can only be released with the consent of the patient, giving such notes substantially greater protection than the regular medical record. Clinicians are permitted, but not required to maintain psychotherapy notes. Psychotherapy notes are the only special category of notes in the Privacy Rule: advocates for AIDS patients and substance abuse patients were unsuccessful in getting special protection for their records. Keeping a second set of records is somewhat cumbersome, and many clinicians do not keep psychotherapy notes, but rather choose not to document highly sensitive fantasy material.

Emailing and Texting Patients

HIPAA has drawn attention to the electronic transmission of information, of which one common form is emailing patients and texting patients. HIPAA requires that electronic transmission of protected health information be encrypted, although many clinicians ignore this when emailing and texting. Even for those who are not "covered providers" under HIPAA, courts increasingly see HIPAA protections as setting a standard of practice. The potential problems with email are that it can be intercepted and may inadvertently be delivered to the wrong person. For emails that involve sensitive information, it is best to use web-based email that is encrypted. For email that simply has to do with arranging appointment times, encryption is probably not necessary. Texting is generally not encrypted unless both clinician and patients use special applications. Emails can be printed and kept in the record; it is more cumbersome to print text messages.

Emailing or texting for administrative matters, such as appointment scheduling, is probably not a liability problem. If a clinician uses email for substantive discussions about treatment, he or she is well advised to have a written policy about emailing that includes how email is to be used and the limits of confidentiality, and includes a consent form signed by the patient. The American Medical Association (9) and some malpractice insurance companies have developed guidelines for professional use of email. Using texting for treatment issues is more problematic, both because of security issues (cell phones can be easily lost or stolen) and because of the difficulty in keeping a record. Novel smartphone applications that involve communicating with a clinician, such as real-time reporting of mood states or other symptoms, will continue to pose novel challenges. Technologic developments in communication are likely to enter clinical practice faster than standards and regulation will keep pace with them. The basic principles in using these new technologies is to assure that confidentiality is preserved, the patient gives informed consent, and the ability to communicate at any time does not create boundary problems for the clinician.

Telepsychiatry

Telemedicine has become an increasingly common method of administering care, especially given the difficulty in many rural areas of locating a child and adolescent psychiatrist. The vast majority of states require that the clinician have a professional license in the state where the *patient*, not the clinician, resides (36). Some states issue special licenses to allow out-of-state clinicians to practice telemedicine. Most states make exceptions for out-of-state consultative examinations done at the request of an in-state clinician, or telemedicine with an established patient who is temporarily out-of-state. Clinicians need to be aware of the licensing laws in effect at their patients' locations.

The standard of care is generally considered to be the same as for in-person care. For example, if the patient is in crisis, the clinician needs to know how to handle the problem at a distance. Professional associations have developed guidelines to assist mental health professionals conduct telepsychiatry competently (37).

Improper Release of Information from Medical Records

The unauthorized disclosure of confidential information from a patient's record could be actionable on the ground of breach of confidentiality and also may constitute a HIPAA violation. Medical records should be kept in a locked place in the ward or medical records department to bar access to unauthorized people. The patient or legal guardian must give consent for the transfer of information to agencies such as attorneys, schools, social welfare departments, and insurance companies. It is generally best to obtain written consent, although if this is impractical, witnessed verbal consent is typically acceptable. State laws vary as to whether information relevant to continuing care can be released to other clinicians or hospitals without consent, but it is generally prudent to attempt to obtain consent even in situations where it is not formally required.

If a subpoena is served unaccompanied by a release from the patient or guardian, the clinician has three alternatives: to seek the patient's consent; to have a motion filed by an attorney to quash the subpoena; or to refuse to testify unless ordered by the judge to do so. If the clinician persists in refusing to testify despite the judge's instruction to do so, he or she may be held in contempt of court (38).

Defamation

Defamation involves communication by one party about a second party to a third party that damages the reputation of the second party. Defamation is most likely to occur in child psychiatry when carelessly written medical records are released to third parties. For example, the patient may have been described in the record as a "psychopath" or "malingerer," labels that could be extremely damaging in the hands of later employers or creditors. Clinicians who gossip about patients over coffee or in elevators put themselves at risk of liability on the grounds of defamation or breach of confidentiality.

Defenses against defamation include *substantial truth* and *conditional privilege*. Conditional privilege allows communication when both parties have a duty and an interest to receive and report such matters. For example, when one doctor refers a patient to another, conditional privilege in most jurisdictions allows the two doctors to discuss the patient's condition. (However, a prudent outpatient practice is to have the referring doctor have the patient sign a release.) No such privilege applies to those who have no such duty and interest. Testimony given in court or provided to the court in documents such as medical reports or medical records attract *absolute privilege* insofar as they refer to the broadly defined matter at issue. *Malice*, if proven, destroys conditional privilege. Malice is substantiated by the author's evident self-interest, excessive distribution of the defamatory material, reckless disregard of the truth, or the vituperative style of the documents involved in the case.

Improper Treatment

Failure to Obtain Informed Consent

The doctrine of informed consent is founded on the constitutional right of the individual to control what is done to his or her own body (39). A patient cannot give informed consent unless he or she has (a) *sufficient information* on which to base a decision, (b) *mental competency* to make a rational decision, and (c) freedom to exercise *voluntary choice*. Almost all states require informed consent, and psychiatrists are also ethically bound to obtain it.

The physician must therefore disclose sufficient information to enable the patient, or the patient's legal representative, to weigh all material pros and cons. How much is that? The earlier "professional" standard (40,41) referred to *what a reasonable medical practitioner would disclose* under similar circumstances. Following two 1972 cases, *Canterbury v. Spence* (42) and *Cobbs v. Grant* (43), some jurisdictions may have adopted the "patient" standard, that is, *as much information as a reasonable patient would require* to make a rational decision under similar circumstances. *Canterbury* and other cases suggest that the physician should discuss the following matters with the patient:

1. The nature of the condition that requires treatment
2. The nature, purpose, and benefits of the proposed treatment, and the probability that it will succeed
3. The risks and consequences of the proposed treatment
4. Alternatives to the proposed treatment (including no treatment) and their attendant risks and consequences
5. The prognosis with and without the proposed treatment

The courts have held that *not all risks need be disclosed—only the material ones.* Unfortunately, there are no clear guidelines concerning what is "material," except to suggest that, even if the likelihood be slight, the more serious the risk, the greater the probability that it should be discussed. *A risk is material when a reasonable person would be likely to attach significance to the risk or cluster of risks.* Risk is linked not only to the procedure but also to the physician and his or her competence to perform the procedure (e.g., if the physician has alcoholism or suffers from human immunodeficiency virus infection). The plaintiff must prove that nondisclosure of material risk caused the injury of which he or she complains. Some courts require that the plaintiff prove that a reasonable person would have refused the procedure had the risks been disclosed.

Therapeutic privilege countervails the clinician's duty to disclose. The physician is obliged to protect a vulnerable patient from the emotional trauma that could be sustained if upsetting risks were prematurely revealed. However, therapeutic privilege should never be invoked merely because the clinician fears that, if apprised of the facts, the patient would reject a desirable treatment. If the clinician proposes to limit disclosure on the ground of therapeutic privilege, clear documentation and expert consultation are required concerning the patient's exceptional sensitivity.

Consent is not required for emergency treatment in which the harm from failure to treat is imminent and outweighs the potential danger of the treatment. However, if possible, a relative's consent should be obtained.

For most children and adolescents, informed consent of a parent or guardian is necessary for psychiatric treatment. In treating a child whose parents are divorced, the clinician should be sure that the parent requesting treatment is legally empowered to give consent. It is generally prudent to keep a copy of the legal custody order in the chart. On a clinical basis, it is generally best to obtain the consent and participation of both divorced parents. Problems can arise if both divorced parents have the power to consent, and one consents but the other refuses. In that case, the clinician should have the requesting parent obtain court authorization for the decision to pursue treatment.

In some cases, minors can consent to treatment on their own behalf. Competence is extended to emancipated minors. When should an unemancipated minor be regarded as sufficiently mature to participate in health care decisions? It depends on the jurisdiction and the condition being treated. All states allow minors to seek treatment for venereal disease. Most allow treatment for substance abuse. Landmark federal decisions (44,45) extended to "mature minors" the right to make health decisions concerning contraception and abortion, and required the availability of a judicial bypass procedure for minors who are not mature, but they left unclear what a mature minor was. Many states have "mature minor" rules which allow "mature" youth to seek treatment on their own. In some jurisdictions, "mature minor" is undefined, while in others it is defined by statute. Some states allow adolescents to seek outpatient psychiatric care. The present situation is very confused, and the practitioner should ascertain the law on the matter in his or her own state. The minor's ability to consent, however, does not generally require the parents to pay for treatment, so youth obtaining psychiatric treatment on their own remains fairly rare. Although it may not be legally required, the desirability of promoting a treatment alliance suggests that it is judicious to promote the understanding and cooperation of all minors mature enough to comprehend. For patients more than 13 years of age, it is prudent to obtain formal assent.

The third element of informed consent, *voluntariness,* is easily compromised. True voluntary consent requires that the patient be free of coercion. However, even a mature minor can be susceptible to threat, cajolement, bribery, or false inducement by parents, physicians, or hospital staff. The inmates of correctional institutions and psychiatric hospitals are particularly vulnerable to therapeutic coercion.

Problems with Admission

A physician who admits a patient to a psychiatric hospital without proper evaluation may be sued for *negligent diagnosis* or *false imprisonment.* A falsely imprisoned plaintiff may recover damages for *loss of dignity* and *emotional distress.* Ignorance of the mental health statutes is no defense; failure to comply with statutory requirements could be actionable. For example, in *Johnson v. Greer* (46), a patient recovered damages after being forcibly detained in hospital for several days beyond the 24 hours permitted on an emergency warrant. Malice, spite, ulterior motive, bad faith, or fraud during involuntary hospitalization could also result in damages for false imprisonment or *malicious prosecution* (47). Parents or guardians may admit unemancipated minors against their will, and health care providers should be able to rely on parental consent (47,48). However, the psychiatric justification for admission should be carefully documented.

Negligent Diagnosis

The physician must distinguish organic disease from functional disorders and, within the latter, must differentiate the major psychoses from each other and from other conditions. The physician who admits patients to a psychiatric hospital must be alert for signs that could indicate a toxic condition. In *Hirschberg v. State* (49), for example, a patient who had taken an overdose of salicylates died after having been hospitalized without adequate physical examination, special investigations, or proper precautions. The hospital was found liable.

The physician who fails to diagnose the patient accurately (e.g., by missing psychosis when it is present or by confusing bipolar disorder with schizophrenia) may found treatment on a false premise and thus may be open to a liability suit. However, there have been few actions on these grounds. Lawyers have been reluctant to pursue such cases in view of the reputedly widely varying expert opinion concerning the most appropriate treatment for different psychiatric conditions. As child and adolescent psychiatry becomes more empirically based, it is likely that such actions will increase in frequency.

Psychotherapy

There are so many schools of psychotherapy that failure to use a particular type of therapy or not conducting psychotherapy very skillfully seldom gives rise to a successful malpractice action for several reasons. There is a lack of consensus in the field as to appropriate methods. It is difficult to prove harm as a result of negligent psychotherapy, because mental injury is hard to substantiate when the plaintiff was already emotionally disturbed before the alleged negligence. In the 1990s, however, suits involving allegations that recovered memories of abuse were "implanted" by therapists became frequent, and some led to large jury verdicts or settlements (50). In the highly publicized *Ramona* case (51) the father of a patient was allowed to sue on his own behalf for damages allegedly flowing from memories implanted in his daughter because the court found that he was a "direct victim" of the psychotherapy. The "direct victim" theory gives rise to many problems, such as who may sue and what the nature of the victim–plaintiff's relationship to the therapist must be (52), and is particularly an issue in child psychiatry because of the therapist's involvement with parents. The direct victim test has not been adopted in many states other than California.

In a variant of this genre, the patient sues the therapist for failing to recognize that dissociative identity disorder is confabulatory or for accepting uncritically the patient's recovered memories of abuse.

Sexual Exploitation and the Tort of Outrage

Expert testimony is not required to substantiate the impropriety of sexually molesting a patient. As an intentional tort, *res ipsa loquitur* ("the thing speaks for itself"), and the burden of proof shifts to the defendant. In *Roy v. Hartogs* (53), the court held that public policy protected patients from such malicious abuses of authority, power, and fiduciary trust. The perpetrator faces criminal sanctions for rape, aggravated assault, or child abuse, as well as civil actions for malpractice or battery (unconsented touching). Most malpractice policies will cover the cost of a defense if the clinician denies that sexual contact occurred, but exclude payment for damages for a sexual relationship with a patient. Liability for improper sexual relations may extend beyond the patient to others involved, such as the spouses of patients so harmed. Residual transference has persuaded courts that cessation of treatment does not open the door to a sexual relationship. Indeed, *negligent management of the transference* is often adopted as the theory behind the action for damages.

The tort of *outrage* refers to the intentional infliction of severe emotional distress on a patient, as a result of reckless and intolerable behavior. For example, in *Abraham v. Zaslow* (54), damages were awarded to a woman who had sustained bruising and renal failure after exposure to "rage-reduction therapy," an intrusive intervention involving several hours of physical restraint, poking, tickling, and verbal insult. Patients have a right to expect that clinicians will adhere to established methods of treatment. If exceptional methods are proposed, full informed consent is required, supportive consultation from a colleague would be advisable, and adequate reference to the scientific literature should be made.

Medication

The points in the medication of a patient at which negligence is most likely to occur are as follows:

1. The diagnosis of the psychiatric disorder
2. The adoption of an appropriate rationale for drug therapy
3. The choice of a particular drug to treat the patient's psychiatric disorder
4. Inquiry concerning a past history of excessive therapeutic response, severe side effects, or allergic reaction to the drug in question or to related drugs
5. The search for coexistent medical conditions that would contraindicate the medication in question or would indicate the need for caution in its use
6. Obtaining informed consent
7. The administration of an appropriate dose of the drug in question, by an approved route
8. The prescription of drugs in combination, or the addition of a drug or drugs to an existing medication regimen
9. The choice of a drug not approved by the U.S. Food and Drug Administration or the use of a drug in a way, or for a purpose, that deviates from that recommended in the package insert or *Physician's Desk Reference* (PDR)
10. Monitoring the therapeutic effect and side effects of the medication
11. Ceasing the medication after a therapeutic effect has been achieved or maintaining long-term medication at the lowest effective dosage

Decision to Medicate

In *Osheroff v. Chestnut Lodge et al.* (55), suit was brought against a private hospital for negligent failure to disclose all treatment alternatives. The plaintiff, who suffered from mixed affective and personality disorder, had been treated for several months with individual psychotherapy. After transfer to a different hospital, he responded to antidepressant medication within a few weeks. Several eminent psychiatrists testified for the plaintiff that antidepressant medication was the treatment of choice, and the plaintiff had had insufficient opportunity to consider it as a treatment alternative. The suit was settled out of court in favor of the plaintiff. Such cases are less common with children because the use of medication is more controversial in this age group.

Inappropriate Rationale for Treatment

Psychotropic drugs are sometimes prescribed to control inmates in correctional or intellectual disability institutions and may be overused in foster care situations where consent is being provided by a protective services worker who is not very familiar with the patient. These situations warrant close scrutiny; the physician may have been induced to medicate the patient by the urgings of harassed staff, rather than by the medical needs of the patient, a practice that has been specifically criticized in at least one class action suit (56) and one malpractice case (57).

Choice of an Inappropriate or Unapproved Drug or Route of Administration

This kind of error occurs when the physician orders a drug that is inadequate to treat the patient's disorder (a benzodiazepine for major depressive disorder) or when the physician prescribes a drug for which there are less risky alternatives (a neuroleptic for anxiety disorder). A different problem arises when the clinician prescribes a drug not approved by the Food and Drug Administration. Undoubtedly, the risk of malpractice is greater if approved guidelines have not been followed. However, because of the great expense of generating data to persuade the FDA to approve an indication for a drug's use in children, more than half of all PDR entries lack labeling with pediatric information (58). Courts generally find that the PDR does not set the standard of practice, and expert testimony is necessary to determine whether a particular use is an accepted treatment. Usage that is more experimental or investigational requires providing considerably more information about benefits, risks, and alternatives to obtain informed consent.

An intravenous or intramuscular route of administration carries an increased risk of excessive or adverse response. This is particularly likely if the patient is predisposed to side effects as a result of hepatic, renal, cardiac, or brain dysfunction. The clinician should be cautious if such conditions are detected. Parenteral administration should generally be reserved for emergencies or long-term depot treatment.

Over the past 5 years, there has been increasing concern that many children in state custody, both in foster care and in juvenile detention facilities, are being overmedicated. The media have highlighted the stories of young children who have received numerous concurrent medications, including multiple antipsychotics, and argued that such medications are being used inappropriately for behavioral control rather than treatment. Attention to this problem has led to calls for increased regulation of prescribing to this vulnerable population. The American Academy of Child and Adolescent Psychiatry (AACAP) has created a practice parameter on the topic (59), and clinicians working with this difficult population are well advised to keep current with their state's regulations and the AACAP guidelines.

Failure to Obtain a Medication History

The patient's past medication history should be ascertained by interview, by review of medical records, and by telephone contact, if required, with other clinicians. The physician may be held liable for excessive side effects, allergic reactions, idiosyncratic responses, or drug interactions, if these had been foreseeable.

Failure to Detect Contraindicative Conditions

The physician may fail to check for conditions or disorders that would render the patient vulnerable to severe side effects. For example, pre-existing hypothyroidism may be overlooked when lithium is prescribed. Different classes of psychotropic drug require different assessments prior to prescribing. If a contraindicative condition is uncovered but the medication is still considered potentially justified, a risk-to-benefit analysis should be documented, expert consultation should be obtained, and specific informed consent should be recorded. Hospitals should mandate, as policy, standard diagnostic workups for all psychotropic drugs. Since a very high proportion of adolescent pregnancies are unplanned and psychotropic drugs cross the placenta, when prescribing medication to an adolescent girl, the clinician should document pregnancy status and use of contraception.

Forcible Administration

The involuntary commitment of a patient to a psychiatric hospital does not permit involuntary medication, except in narrowly defined circumstances, generally having to do with the safety of the patient or others. Forcible medication can place the practitioner at risk of an action for the intentional tort of battery. The legal doctrine most pertinent to this issue, *the right to refuse treatment,* has been most clearly articulated in two convoluted cases, *Rennie v. Klein* (1981) (60) and *Rogers v. Commissioner of Mental Health* (61). In *Rennie,* a New Jersey case, it was determined that the mentally ill had a sufficient liberty interest to require due process before treatment was forcibly administered, but due process was satisfied by an in-hospital review. In considering this case, the U.S. Supreme Court deferred to the professionalization standard articulated in *Youngberg v. Romeo* (1982) (62), in effect declining to uphold a constitutional right to refuse treatment. In *Rogers,* the Massachusetts Supreme Court held that involuntarily committed patients should be presumed competent to refuse treatment except in emergencies. An "emergency" was defined as a situation fraught with the need to prevent violence or associated with the likelihood that the patient's health would significantly deteriorate without treatment. In nonemergency situations, forcible treatment may be administered only after a judicial hearing in which the court approves a "substituted judgment" treatment plan. "Substituted judgment" requires the court to determine what the patient would have decided if he or she were competent.

The failure of the U.S. Supreme Court to clarify this matter means that each state must make its own determination of the boundaries of the right to refuse treatment. The legal situation with regard to children is unclear. The right to refuse treatment apparently extends to the legal guardians of minors, to emancipated minors, and to those minors otherwise empowered to consent. What of the mature minor? Arguably, except in emergencies, the clinician should seek the consent of both mature minor and parent before starting treatment. If the mature minor refuses treatment, and the treatment is regarded vital, a judicial determination of competence should be requested.

Failure to Monitor Treatment

Adequate monitoring of drug effects requires baseline and regular mental status examinations, physical examinations, vital signs, and laboratory testing, in accordance with the pharmacology of the drug and its potential side effects. "Drug holidays" should be considered if long-term medication is required. Physicians run a serious risk if they write "as-needed" orders for potent drugs, if they telephone prescriptions into a pharmacy without examining their patients, or if they provide multiple repeat refills without proper monitoring. In 2004, in response to concerns that SSRIs increase reported suicidal thinking and behavior in some children and adolescents, the FDA issued a "black box" warning, which was then revised in 2007 to say patients started on an SSRI "should be monitored appropriately and observed closely for clinical worsening, suicidality, or unusual changes in behavior" (63). In the event that a child or adolescent commits suicide shortly after beginning an SSRI, a defendant psychiatrist would likely have a difficult time persuading a jury that close monitoring was not necessary. Recent actions by national regulatory agencies in the United States, United Kingdom, and Canada suggest that psychotropic medications are being exposed to increased regulatory scrutiny.

Abandonment

Psychiatrists are most at risk of liability when they terminate the treatment of patients without adequate safeguards, when they are unavailable and either no covering physician is provided or the covering physician has not been given sufficient information, or when adequate steps are not taken to protect endangered third parties.

The physician has the duty to provide continued care, as long as needed, until the doctor–patient relationship is terminated. This relationship may be severed by mutual consent or by the patient. However, unilateral termination of care by the clinician, if abrupt or premature, may put him or her at risk of breach of contract should harm, such as suicide, befall the patient. Failure to provide a telephone number for a disturbed patient to call, failure to provide adequate substitute care during absences, or failure to convey adequate precautionary information to substitute physicians may all be construed as abandonment if the patient is found to have suffered harm as a consequence.

When is the therapist warranted in unilaterally terminating the relationship? Lack of cooperation or threatening behavior may justify termination; failure to pay the bill does not (64). If the clinician does decide to terminate the relationship, the following safeguards are required (28):

1. The reason for the termination should be discussed with the patient and parents. The clinician should give at least 1 month's notice of termination, to allow the patient to locate another therapist.
2. The patient and parents should be provided with the names and telephone numbers of alternative therapists or agencies.
3. The clinician should mail to the patient and parents a certified letter (return receipt requested) reflecting this discussion and containing the reasons for termination. The letter should also convey the names and telephone numbers of alternative clinicians or agencies.

TEACHING, RESEARCH, AND PUBLICATION

The torts of *invasion of privacy, breach of confidentiality,* and *defamation* are the liability risks most commonly incurred by teachers, researchers, and writers.

These torts stem from the ethical, contractual, and (in some jurisdictions) statutory obligation of the clinician not to disclose private information that should be kept within the doctor–patient relationship. In invasion of privacy, the plaintiff alleges that details from his or her private life have been publicized. This may occur, for example, if a clinician publishes an article in which the identity of the subject is insufficiently disguised. It has been held that a patient undergoing psychotherapy cannot give proper informed consent to the publication of a book concerning the treatment (65).

A patient has the right to bar nonessential onlookers when he or she is being examined or treated or when his or her case is discussed. The teacher should seek informed consent before exposing patients to case conferences or discussing cases for teaching purposes. The use of video recordings for teaching necessitates written informed consent, the continuation of which should be requested on a yearly basis.

Research with children poses complex ethical issues over and above issues with adults because of children's vulnerability and lack of legal competence. Federal law includes special protections for children involved in federally sponsored research (66). These include the requirement that, in addition to the parent's consent, the child's assent is required for participation for research that is not expected to benefit the child (assuming the child can give assent). The Privacy Rule authorized by HIPAA carries further requirements for protecting the privacy of actual or prospective research subjects. Institutional review boards (IRB) in universities and most organizations have adopted these principles for all research they review, even if technically the research would not be governed by federal rules. Any practitioner involved in research would be well advised to meet these standards. If research procedures are later questioned, especially if an adverse event befalls a research subject, documentation of approval by an IRB is a crucial component in demonstrating the research was undertaken thoughtfully and with due regard to the well-being of the research subjects.

COMPLAINTS TO OTHER REGULATORY BODIES

Malpractice cases are not the only arena in which care of a child or adolescent may be scrutinized. Complaints may be made to state licensing boards, professional ethics committees, and, for HIPAA violations, to the Office of Civil Rights of DHHS. Unlike in a malpractice case, harm to the patient does not need to be proved for a complaint to be found justified: all that is needed is proof of unethical or incompetent behavior or violation of a regulation. For example, if a clinician is found to have practiced while intoxicated, he can be sanctioned even if his actual care has not been shown to be poor. Furthermore, the range of professional work that can be scrutinized is wider, because a doctor–patient relationship is not necessary for a complaint to go forward. For example, child psychiatrists who conduct child custody evaluations on court order are generally immune from malpractice suit, both because such evaluations, like most forensic evaluations, do not create a doctor–patient relationship, and because the evaluator is an agent of the court and so usually has the immunity of other court personnel. However, disgruntled parents are free to pursue complaints to ethics committees and state licensing boards, and such grievances are not uncommon.

From the perspective of the investigated doctor, complaints to these agencies trigger a process that is similar in many ways to being sued. Sometimes, particularly with ethics committee investigations, the psychiatrist may feel that the whole matter can be disposed of informally by discussion with members of the committee and submitting records for review. Unless the clinician is extremely confident or very familiar with the proceedings, however, he or she is well advised to obtain an attorney before proceeding, rather than run the risk of making admissions that may later prove damaging, or in agreeing to waive due process protections in order to "wrap this up in a hurry." Many malpractice insurance policies cover the cost of attorney representation in licensing board investigations. While money is not at stake directly (although results of these investigations are often admissible in later malpractice actions), the psychiatrist's license to practice medicine may be threatened, and one should proceed cautiously.

RISK MANAGEMENT IN CHILD PSYCHIATRY

Clinical practice is fraught with error, and error can have serious consequences. Confronted by the catalog of litigation in this chapter, even the insouciant may quail. However, defensive psychiatry is no answer, because overly timid treatment can also put the clinician at risk of negligent malpractice. What, then, is the best way to avoid litigation? General risk management principles that apply to adult psychiatry, such as the importance of clear communication with patients and parents and good documentation by the clinician apply to work with children and adolescents as well. Some special considerations that apply to child and adolescent psychiatry are shown in Table 7.4.4.2. The best precaution is to practice careful medicine while fully apprising the patient and family of the diagnosis, treatment plan, and progress of therapy. Many malpractice suits arise from neglect of this simple principle. Hospitals provide many opportunities for failed communication, particularly when the attending physician delegates to other members of the team the responsibility for keeping parents informed of their children's progress. A good therapeutic alliance is the key to good medicine and the avoidance of lawsuits. Used for this purpose, informed consent can be transformed from an empty legalism into the foundation of a true collaboration.

Documentation

The clinician should keep a good record of the rationale for treatment. Progress notes should be timely, regular, dated, and signed. Gutheil, in his classic 1980 article on paranoia and progress notes (67), recommends imagining a plaintiff attorney looking over your shoulder while writing progress notes. Issues that potentially may come to court, such as those described above, should be documented fully. If you disagree with the diagnosis, investigation, or treatment plan in the record, respectfully note that you disagree and insert your amended diagnosis and plan. If you merely sign off on a trainee's notes, you could be concurring with erroneous observations, diagnosis, or treatment. One of the most common errors is to raise a diagnostic question but not follow through by investigating it or, having ordered an investigative test, to not follow up on the results.

Note any discrepancies between the nurses', the therapist's, and the physician's progress notes. If there is such a discrepancy, try to account for it. Do not allow a nursing progress note concerning suicide risk to go unremarked.

If you detect an error in your notes, do not erase it. Draw a line through the error, write "error," and date and sign your correction in the margin. Do not criticize or argue with other professionals or agencies in your notes, and avoid gratuitous or extravagant commentary ("This child has had an appalling home life"). Do not record psychodynamic speculations in the clinical record; those unconscious incestuous strivings may come back to haunt you. You may consider keeping your psychotherapy *process notes* separate from the official record of therapy *progress notes*.

TABLE 7.4.4.2

RISK MANAGEMENT PRINCIPLES

General Principle	Special Consideration in Child and Adolescent Work	Example of Potential Problem
Open communication	Clear understanding of minor's confidentiality and exceptions	Parents have right to see chart Parents need to be told of dangerous situations
Clarity of role definition	Whether the child or the whole family is the patient	In family work, there may be a doctor–patient relationship with each person in the family
Need to obtain informed consent	Assent from minor is useful; consent from parents is usually required	In nontraditional family or postdivorce situations, need to be sure which parent(s) have authority to consent
Appropriate medication use	Much use is off label	Insufficient explanation of possible side effects
Compliance and cooperation with treatment	May be reduced by immaturity or minor's lack of agreement	Jury may see immature child as less responsible than an adult and so attribute more responsibility for safety to the clinician
Documentation of treatment	Documentation of communications with collateral sources (parents, school) is important	Failure to document telling parents that their son had some suicidal symptoms
Careful risk assessment	Risk factors less researched and less predictive than with adults Ratio of suicidal ideation to completed suicide is much higher than with adults	Unforeseen impulsive suicide

Dangerousness Assessment

A risk–resource analysis should be conducted whenever a patient presents a risk of violence to self or others. Such an assessment is most likely to be required in the following circumstances: when the risk of violence is raised during outpatient evaluation or treatment; when a potentially violent patient presents for admission to hospital; when the leave or discharge from hospital of a potentially violent patient is being considered; or when such a patient elopes. Areas of assessment when considering violence toward others commonly cited in the literature are shown in Table 7.4.4.3.

Predatory violence, that is, violence that is planned, is more difficult to assess because the youth has a clear motive to conceal his thinking. In the wake of highly publicized school shootings, many schools have developed the so-called "zero tolerance" policies for direct or implied threats of school violence that may be triggered when a child or adolescent makes a threat, brings a weapon to school, or writes a story that includes violence toward peers. In such situations, schools frequently require a psychological evaluation before allowing a child to return. The clinician should be aware that a single individual assessment alone is of very limited value in these situations, and only tentative conclusions about dangerousness should be drawn. More accurate evaluations require corroborative interviews, especially with friends of the evaluated youth, to assess whether the youth is on a path of escalating interest and planning of hurting others. In such interviews, one is looking not only for direct threats and violent ideation, but for "leakage," a spilling over of preoccupation with violence, such as might be found in diaries, being fascinated with weapons, following prospective victims, drawing plans of the school, etc. (68,69).

Treatment

Before a particular treatment is commenced, be careful to check that the patient harbors no conditions and is taking no drugs that would contraindicate it, and inquire about previous allergic or idiosyncratic reactions to drugs. For drugs with known teratogenic effects in early pregnancy, such as sodium divalproex, the rationale for use in girls should be carefully documented, even for a girl who states she is not planning to become pregnant. Avoid polypharmacy. Monitor the progress of medication regularly. In patients taking long-term medication, "drug holidays" should be considered. Unless there are

TABLE 7.4.4.3

AREAS FOR ASSESSMENT OF RISK OF VIOLENCE TO OTHERS

- Past history of violent threats or actions
- Nature of Threat
  - Direct threat
  - Has potential victim been bullied or provoked patient?
  - Plan for harming the victim
  - Access to lethal weapons?
  - Leakage of preoccupation with violence in journals, web surfing, and writings
  - Taking steps toward action, such as following or stalking victim, obtaining a weapon, rehearsing an attack
  - Threat communicated to others, especially peers
- Past History
  - History of being abused
  - History of alcohol or drug abuse
- Demographic Factors
  - Late adolescent
  - Male
  - Disadvantaged ethnic groups with a cultural tradition of masculine defensiveness
- Psychological Factors
  - Copes with anxiety or hostility by externalizing or projecting it in the form of impulsive, explosive actions, suspicious vigilance, or frank persecutory delusions
  - Command hallucinations that instruct the patient to take violent action or that threaten violence to the patient or his or her family
  - Inner controls against violent actions subjectively or objectively reduced
  - Strong inner urge to be violent
- Social environment
  - Family psychopathology in the form of rejection, neglect, physical or sexual abuse, or family violence

good reasons for departing from them, follow recommended guidelines for dosage and administration. Avoid prescribing medication "as needed" and automatic refills, and be careful of telephone requests for repeat prescriptions. If the suicide risk is serious, only small amounts of a potentially lethal drug should be prescribed. Hospitals should check that potentially suicidal patients are not cheating, concealing, and hoarding medication.

When a patient is admitted to the hospital, the degree of risk of suicide or violence should be assessed, and each degree of risk should be linked to a set of nursing precautions that are automatically activated when the clinician indicates the degree of risk. Every attempt should be made to obtain past records and to scan them for risk factors.

If you are unavailable in case of emergency during treatment, the name of a fully informed substitute physician should be provided to the patient. Do not terminate treatment unilaterally without preparing the patient, giving adequate notice, and providing him or her with the names of other clinicians or agencies that could help.

In outpatient practice, the duty to protect is precipitated when the patient makes a specific threat to harm a specified victim. When possible, incorporate the protection in therapy. Psychotherapy, hospitalization, and medication may be both more protective and more therapeutic than warning the foreseeable victim or alerting the police.

Be vigilant to avoid unauthorized disclosure of confidential information to external agencies, do not gossip about patients, and do not publish articles about patients without adequately disguising their identity. Obtain the parents' consent before releasing reports to external agencies. Blanket consent forms, obtained during the rush of admission, may not hold water legally.

Identified High-Risk Situations

There are often clinical situations in which the physician recognizes a higher than usual risk of an adverse outcome, such as when a chronically suicidal adolescent is to be discharged from the hospital, or standard medications have been tried and failed, and a less tested medication with the potential for serious side effects is being considered. A number of strategies can lessen the liability risk in managing such situations. First, document in more than usual detail the pros and cons of the intervention being considered. Second, be especially attentive to informed consent issues, discuss such issues fully with the parent or guardian, document the discussion, and, if medications are involved, have a parent sign a written consent form. Third, when in doubt, shout! (70) Get a second opinion and have it documented. In case of a malpractice suit, the test will be what a reasonable clinician would have done under the circumstances. A consulting clinician's contemporaneous second opinion will likely carry greater weight than the opinion of a hired expert who wasn't there peering through the retrospectoscope with full knowledge of the subsequent events.

CONCLUSION

When Bellamy (71) examined appellate psychiatric malpractice cases in the 15 years after World War II, he could identify 18 cases, none of which involved child or adolescent patients. The situation is not so rosy today, but defendant doctors still win most cases. The law has no wish to penalize physicians for honest errors. Its purpose is to protect patients from being harmed by reckless, careless, or incompetent clinical practice, and if they have been so harmed, to compensate them for injury. In most successful suits for negligent malpractice, the errors are glaring. Attention to the safeguards described in this chapter will protect clinicians from litigation while allowing them to practice nondefensive psychiatry.

References

1. Studdert DM, Mello MM, Brennan TA: Medical malpractice. *N Engl J Med* 350:283–292, 2004.
2. Charles SC, Wilbert JR, Kennedy EC: Physicians' self-reports of reactions to malpractice litigation. *Am J Psychiatry* 141:563–565, 1984.
3. Studdert DM, Mello MM, Sage WM, et al.: Defensive medicine among high-risk specialist physicians in a volatile malpractice environment. *JAMA* 293:2609–2617, 2005.
4. National Conference of State Legislatures: Medical liability/Medical malpractice laws. Available at: http://www.ncsl.org/research/financial-services-and-commerce/medical-liability-medical-malpractice-laws.aspx. Accessed December 6, 2015.
5. Ash P: Malpractice in child and adolescent psychiatry. *Child Adolesc Psychiatr Clin N Am* 11:869–885, 2002.
6. *O'Neill v. Montefiore Hosp.*, 11 A.D.2d 132; 202 N.Y.S.2d 436 (N.Y. App. 1960).
7. Recupero PR: E-mail and the psychiatrist-patient relationship. *J Am Acad Psychiatry Law* 33:465–475, 2005.
8. Reed J: Cybermedicine: defying and redefining patient standards of care. *Indiana Law Rev* 37:845–877, 2004.
9. American Medical Association: H-478.997 Guidelines for physician-patient electronic mail. Available at: http://hosted.ap.org/specials/interactives/_documents/patient_physician_email.pdf. Accessed April 17, 2017.
10. American Psychiatric Association: The Internet in clinical psychiatry. Available at: http://www.psychiatry.org/psychiatrists/search-directories-databases/library-and-archive/resource-documents. Accessed December 6, 2015.
11. Kachalia A, Studdert DM: Professional liability issues in graduate medical education. *JAMA* 292:1051–1056, 2004.
12. Recupero PR, Rainey SE: Liability and risk management in outpatient psychotherapy supervision. *J Am Acad Psychiatry Law* 35:188–195, 2007.
13. *LaLonde v. Eissner*, 405 Mass 207, 539 N.E.2d 538 (Mass. Sup. Jud. Ct. 1989).
14. Recupero PR: Clinical practice guidelines as learned treatises: understanding their use as evidence in the courtroom. *J Am Acad Psychiatry Law* 36:290–301, 2008.
15. Health Care Quality Improvement Act of 1986, 42 USC §11101 et seq. Title IV (1986).
16. *Wickline v. State*, 239 Cal. Rptr. 810, 819 (Cal. 1986).
17. *Pegram v. Herdrich*, 530 U.S. 211 (2000).
18. Halleck SL: Malpractice in psychiatry. *Psychiatr Clin North Am* 6:567–583, 1983.
19. Kann L, Kinchen S, Shanklin SL, et al.: Youth risk behavior surveillance–United States, 2013. *MMWR Suppl* 63:1–168, 2014.
20. *Abille v. United States*, 482 F. Supp. 703 (N.D. Cal. 1980).
21. *Skar v. City of Lincoln*, Nebraska, 599 F.2d 253 (8th Cir. 1979).
22. Wagner KD, Pollard R, Wagner RF Jr. Malpractice litigation against child and adolescent psychiatry residency programs, 1981–1991. *J Am Acad Child Adolesc Psychiatry* 32:462–465, 1993.
23. *Higgins v. State*, 24 A.D.2d 147, 265 N.Y.S.2d 254 (N.Y. 1965).
24. *Samuels v. Southern Baptist Hospital*, 594 So.2d 571 (La App. 1992).
25. *Tarasoff v. Regents of the University of California* (Tarasoff I), 529 P 2d 553, 118 Cal Rptr 129 (Cal. 1974).
26. *Tarasoff v. Regents of the University of California* (Tarasoff II), 551 P 2d 334, 131 Cal Rptr 14 (Cal. 1976).
27. Johnson R, Persad G, Sisti D: The Tarasoff rule: the implications of interstate variation and gaps in professional training. *J Am Acad Psychiatry Law* 42:469–477, 2014.
28. Simon RI: *Clinical Psychiatry and the Law*. Washington, DC, American Psychiatric Press, Inc., 1987.
29. *Montoya v. Bebensee*, 761 P.2d 285 (Colo. App. 1988).
30. Guyer MJ: Child psychiatry and legal liability: implications of recent case law. *J Am Acad Child Adolesc Psychiatry* 29:958–962, 1990.
31. *Jaffee v. Redmond*, 518 U.S. 1 (1996).
32. *Bremer v. State*, 18 Md.App. 291, 307 A.2d 503 (Md. App. 1973).
33. Standards for Privacy of Individually Identifiable Health Information (the Privacy Rule), 45 CFR Parts 160 and 164 (adopted April, 2001).
34. U.S. Department of Health & Human Services: Summary of the HIPAA Privacy Rule. Available at: http://www.hhs.gov/ocr/privacy/hipaa/understanding/summary/index.html. Accessed December 6, 2015.
35. American Psychiatric Association: Position Statement on Minimum Necessary Guidelines for Third-Party Payers for Psychiatric Treatment. Available at: http://www.psychiatry.org/File%20Library/Learn/Archives/Position-2007-Minimum-Necessary-Guidelines.pdf. Accessed December 1, 2015.
36. Federation of State Medical Boards: Telemedicine policies: Board by board overview. Available at: https://www.fsmb.org/Media/Default/PDF/FSMB/

Advocacy/GRPOL_Telemedicine_Licensure.pdf. Accessed December 8, 2015.
37. American Telemedicine Association: Practice Guidelines for Video-based Online Mental Health Services. Available at: http://www.americantelemed.org/docs/default-source/standards/practice-guidelines-for-video-based-online-mental-health-services.pdf?sfvrsn=6. Accessed December 8, 2015.
38. *In re Lifschutz*, 2 Cal.3d 415, 467 P.2d 557 (Cal. 1970).
39. *Schloendorff v. New York Hospital*, 211 N.Y. 125, 105 N.E. 92 (N.Y. 1914).
40. *Aiken v. Clary*, 396 S.W.2d 668 (Mo. 1965).
41. *Natanson v. Kline*, 350 P.2d 1093 (Kan. 1960).
42. *Canterbury v. Spence*, 464 F.2d 772 (D.C. Cir. 1972).
43. *Cobbs v. Grant*, 8 Cal.3d 229, 502 P.2d 1 (Cal. 1972).
44. Planned Parenthood of Central Missouri v. Danforth, 428 U.S. 52 (1976).
45. *Bellotti v. Baird*, 428 U.S. 132 (1976).
46. *Johnson v. Greer*, 477 F.2d 101 (5th Cir. 1973).
47. *Pendleton v. Burkhalter*, 432 S.W.2d 724 (Tex. Civ. App. 1968).
48. *Parham v. J.R. and J.L.*, 442 U.S. 584 (1979).
49. *Hirschberg v. State*, 91 Misc.2d 590, 398 N.Y.S. 2d 470 (1977).
50. Partlett DF, Nurcombe B: Recovered memories of child sexual abuse and liability: society, science, and the law in a comparative setting. *Psychol Public Policy Law* 4:1253–1306, 1998.
51. *Ramona v. Ramona* (judgment on jury verdict), No. 61898 (Napa [Cal.] Cty. Super. Ct. 1994).
52. Appelbaum PS, Zoltek-Jick R: Psychotherapists' duties to third parties: Ramona and beyond. *Am J Psychiatry* 153:457–465, 1996.
53. *Roy v. Hartogs*, 81 Misc.2d 350, 366 N.Y.S.2d 297 (1975), *affd*, 85 Misc 2d 891, 381 NYS 2d 587 (1976).
54. *Abraham v. Zaslow*, No. 245862 (Santa Clara Cty. Sup. Ct. 1970).
55. *Osheroff v. Chestnut Lodge et al.*, Maryland Health Claims Arbitration (1987).
56. *Nelson v. Heyne*, 355 F.Supp. 451 (N.D. Ind. 1972), *affd*, 491 F 2d 352 (7th Cir), *cert denied*, 417 US 976 (1974).
57. *Clites v. State*, 322 N.W. 2d 917 (Iowa Ct. App. 1982).
58. Sachs AN, Avant D, Lee CS, Rodriguez W, Murphy MD: Pediatric information in drug product labeling. *JAMA* 307:1914–1915, 2012.
59. Lee T, Fouras G, Brown R, American Academy of Child and Adolescent Psychiatry (AACAP) Committee on Quality Issues (CQI): Practice parameter for the assessment and management of youth involved with the child welfare system. *J Am Acad Child Adolesc Psychiatry* 54:502–517, 2015.
60. *Rennie v. Klein*, 720 F.2d 266, 653 F.2d (3rd Cir. 1983), *vacated* 458 U.S. 1119 (1982).
61. *Rogers v. Commissioner of Mental Health*, 458 N.E.2d 308 (Mass. 1983), began as Rogers v. Okin, 478 F Supp 1342 (D Mass 1979), affd in part, revd in part, 634 F 2d 650 (1st Cir 1980), vacated subnom, and was later reviewed by the U.S. Supreme Court as Mills v. Rogers, 457 US 291 (1982).
62. *Youngberg v. Romeo*, 457 U.S. 307 (1982).
63. Food and Drug Administration: Revisions to Product Labeling: Suicidality and Antidepressant Drugs. Available at: http://www.fda.gov/downloads/Drugs/DrugSafety/InformationbyDrugClass/UCM173233.pdf. Accessed December 5, 2015.
64. Smith JT: *Medical Malpractice: Psychiatric Care*. Colorado Springs, Colo., New York, Shepard's/McGraw Hill, 1986.
65. *Doe v. Roe & Poe*, 400 N.Y.S.2d 668 (1977).
66. Protection of Human Subjects—Additional Protections for Children: 45 Code of Federal Regulations [CFR], Subtitle A, Part 46, Subpart D, 10–1–99 Edition.
67. Gutheil TG: Paranoia and progress notes: a guide to forensically informed psychiatric recordkeeping. *Hosp Community Psychiatry* 31:479–482, 1980.
68. Borum R, Fein R, Vossekuil B, Berglund J: Threat assessment: defining an approach for evaluating risk of targeted violence. *Behav Sci Law* 17:323–337, 1999.
69. Federal Bureau of Investigation [FBI]: *The School Shooter: A Threat Assessment Perspective*. Washington, DC, U.S. Department of Justice, 2000.
70. Rappeport JR: *Malpractice Prevention*. Catonsville, MD, Paper presented at: Spring Grove State Hospital Center, May, 1984.
71. Bellamy WA: Malpractice risks confronting the psychiatrist: A nationwide fifteen year study of appellate court cases, 1946 to 1961. *Am J Psychiatry* 118:769–780, 1962.

POSTSCRIPT ■ LOOKING BACK, DREAMING FORWARD: REFLECTIONS ON THE HISTORY OF CHILD PSYCHIATRY

LEON EISENBERG

Anyone willing to write a chapter entitled Looking Back, Dreaming Forward must hesitate on recalling Yogi Berra's quip, "The future ain't what it used to be." However cloudy my vision forward, what I see when I look back (it's 60 years since my graduation) may be instructive for younger readers (by now almost everyone is younger than I am). What I see when I remember the child psychiatry of the 1950s is both ignorance (for which we cannot be blamed) and arrogance (for which we can). As Bertolt Brecht has Galileo say in his play:

> One of the chief causes of poverty in science is imaginary wealth. The purpose of science is not to open the door to an infinitude of wisdom, but to set some limits on the infinitude of error (1).

When I was trained by Leo Kanner, there was no subspecialty certification, and hence no ABPN-approved residencies. In the 1950s, most departments of psychiatry were heavily psychoanalytic in orientation; departments of psychology were behavioristic; the word *neuroscience* had yet to be coined. When I say I was trained by Kanner, I mean that quite literally. I acknowledge that I did gain a great deal of practical knowledge from the one social worker (Barbara Ashenden) and the one psychologist (Charlotte Waskowitz) on the staff, but neither was academic in orientation. When I joined the full-time staff of the Children's Psychiatric Service after completing my training, I effectively doubled the number of psychiatrists.

Leo Kanner was a polymath. If there is such a thing as *eidetic* imagery, he had it. He could picture in his mind the page on which he had read a poem in high school. He recalled the names of teachers who had attended his evening adult education classes at Hopkins when he saw them on the city streets. They were astonished to be remembered by name (and often he added the names of their seatmates) 5 or 10 years after a one-semester course (and I was equally astonished as I looked on!). A graduate of the Sophien-Gymnasium in Berlin who had earned his M.D. from the University of Berlin with a thesis on electrocardiography, he knew classical Greek and Latin (and frequently quoted Homer and Virgil). As a child he had learned Polish, Hebrew, and German, went on to learn English, and had familiarized himself with other languages as well. He was vain enough to display his erudition with multilingual puns that kept a monolingual American (with only remnants of high school Latin and German) hopping trying to figure them out.

His principal mode of teaching was extending to me the privilege of sitting in on his consultations with patients and families. The "price" for the privilege was taking notes and writing up the case report for the formal record (once he had come to trust the fidelity of my accounts). And it was an extraordinary privilege. He was polite and gentle but his questions were penetrating. He listened intently. He was unfailingly courteous, even to the most arrogant and dismissive parents. He charmed children and adolescents alike. His secret psychiatric technique (no longer permissible) was smoking a cigar. He blew lingering smoke rings (in those days, no one knew of the risks of second-hand smoke; those who objected to smoking did so on aesthetic grounds). The children were invariably fascinated. While he saw the parents, the clinic psychologist did a Binet or a WISC on the youngster and provided a brief and usually quite insightful report on her findings before he met the parents again. He wrapped up the 2- to 3-hour sessions with a sagacious review of what he had learned, with what he thought might be helpful to child and family, and with appropriate referrals (his was primarily a consulting practice). Then, he and I would have another 30 minutes together. I was free to pose any questions I wanted. I was encouraged to challenge his conclusions. I often did but usually came around to his position when he mustered the grounds for it.

During the other 4½ days of the week, I saw and treated clinic patients referred from pediatrics and, with the other fellows and occasional rotating pediatric residents, participated in a weekly case conference chaired by Dr. Kanner with the social worker and psychologist in attendance. There was no journal club, no regular supervision. It was catch as catch can with colleagues.

Kanner had come to America in 1924 amid the economic chaos in Berlin for a job in the State Hospital in Yankton, South Dakota (German inflation was on an exponential curve). In this unlikely setting, he found a way to do research and to publish several papers, one of which (on the rarity of general paresis among Native Americans) attracted the attention of Kraepelin, who visited Yankton to meet Kanner. In 1928, he applied for and received a Commonwealth Foundation Fellowship from Adolf Meyer, then the doyen of American psychiatry, at the Henry Phipps Clinic of the Johns Hopkins Hospital. At the completion of the 2-year fellowship, Meyer and Edwards A. Park, the Professor of Pediatrics, chose Leo Kanner to inaugurate a new clinic in pediatrics, charged with "investigating the rank and file of patients in the pediatric clinic for the form(ul)ation of psychiatric problems, the mastery of which should be made accessible to the pediatrician to serve him as the psychopathological principles in dealing with children."

The clinic was initiated in 1930 with support from the Rockefeller Foundation. His office was a small pediatric examining room with a sink and a table. Five years later, based on his intensive study of the world literature and his clinical experience, Kanner wrote the first English-language textbook on child psychiatry (2). Its first edition paid homage to Meyer's psychobiological terminology, but by the second (3), the Meyerian neologisms were abandoned. Kanner's most outstanding and lasting contribution was the identification of the syndrome he called "autistic disturbances of affective contact" (4). On the basis of 11 patients who had been brought to him because of their unusual psychopathology, he formulated the characteristics of a syndrome still identified by these very features. In Michael Rutter's words (5): "Kanner's paper was a model of clarity in its combination of systematic, thorough, and objective observation with deep clinical understanding and appreciation of the personal problems faced by each child, and his family:... Nearly all the basic points made in the original paper have been amply confirmed by other writers."

Kanner had concluded his 1943 article with the statement: "Here we seem to have a pure culture example of an inborn autistic disturbance of affective contact." That conclusion, at a time when child psychiatric disorders were uniformly attributed to psychogenic causes, left him out on a limb and probably delayed widespread acceptance of the syndrome as a clinical entity. His syndrome remains unique.

MENTAL RETARDATION

The very terms in the official classification for the mentally retarded offend today's sensibilities. The terms ran from feebleminded to moron to imbecile to idiot. Down syndrome was still known as Mongolian idiocy, a label reflecting Langdon-Down's belief that it was an atavistic throwback to a more primitive "Mongolian race" (6). We did know that risk increased with the mother's age, but trisomy 21 was not identified until the late 1950s (7,8). That is hardly surprising, given that the correct human chromosome number was not established until 1948! Whatever the terminology and whatever the ignorance about pathophysiology, what remains distressing is that most child guidance clinics of the '50s and '60s screened out retarded children as if retardation excluded treatable psychiatric disorders. A recent study of an epidemiological cohort of almost 600 children with intellectual disability has provided documentation of the substantial and persistent level of psychopathology and the need for effective interventions (9).

Few things epitomize Kanner's personal commitment to the rights of all children more than his concern for the "feebleminded" at a time when most psychiatrists assiduously excluded them from their clinics and offices. The Superintendent of the Maryland State Training School for the Retarded, knowing of Kanner's concern for such patients, appealed to Leo Kanner for help in controlling an appalling problem. Female patients were being removed from the training school by court orders and were being exploited in the community for cheap domestic labor. The superintendent was at his wits' end; he simply didn't know what to do. With the assistance of Miss Mabel F. Kraus, a social worker, Kanner (10) did a followup study on 166 patients who had been released from the school via habeas corpus writs secured by lawyers over the previous two decades. Three-quarters of these releases had been obtained by enterprising attorneys who, for a fee, secured what were essentially indentured domestic servants for affluent Baltimore households; others had been claimed by relatives who suddenly appeared to manipulate estates that had been left them; a few were demanded by parents who, after years of neglect, asserted their "natural rights."

Kanner was able to follow 102, of whom only 13 were making even a modestly satisfactory adjustment in the community at the time of the study; 11 had died of illness and neglect before they reached 30; 17 had tuberculosis, syphilis, or gonorrhea; 29 were prostitutes; 8 had been committed to mental hospitals; and 6 were in prison. In total, these released patients had given birth to 165 offspring, 18 of whom had died from neglect, 30 of whom had been committed to orphanages, and 108 of whom tested at a "feebleminded level" when examined. The customary sequence had been a period of domestic servitude, followed by peremptory release when the young women proved to be inadequate as maids, and then a mournful hegira through the whorehouses and flophouses of the Baltimore slums. Few now remember Kanner's paper in the *American Journal of Psychiatry*, but in 1938, the study had a dramatic impact. The release of the information produced a double row of inch-high headlines across the front page of the April 8th edition of the *Baltimore Sun* and provided the impetus to end an evil practice that had arisen from the collusion of attorneys and judges against the valiant but unsuccessful opposition of the superintendent of the Training School. It is a study worth remembering (10). Clinical precision joined with social conscience in a clinical project with immediate benefit for the lives of a despised minority.

In 1942, amid the war against the Nazis, Foster Kennedy, a well known neurologist, published a paper in the *American Journal of Psychiatry* entitled: "The problem of social control of the congenital defective: Education, sterilization, euthanasia" (11). In it, he proposed that defective children with no future or hope of a worthwhile life "should be relieved of the agony of living," language remarkably similar to the Nazi policy to *end life unworthy of life*. In a vigorous response to Kennedy, Kanner (12) wrote: "Let us try to recall one single instance in the history of mankind when a feeble-minded individual or group of individuals was responsible for the retardation or persecution of humaneness and sciences. They who caused Galileo to be jailed were not feeble-minded. They who instituted the Inquisition were not mental defectives. The great man-made catastrophes resulting in wholesale slaughter and destruction were not started by idiots, imbeciles, morons, or borderlines. The one man, Schicklgruber, whose IQ is probably not below normal, has in a few years brought infinitely more disaster and suffering to this world than have all of the innumerable mental defectives of all countries and all generations combined."

Kanner's revulsion against euthanasia for the severely retarded was not universal; in the same issue of the *Journal* an unsigned editorial argued that the role of psychiatrists should be to persuade parents to agree to release their defective children from "the burden of living" (13). Euthanasia never became official policy, but sterilization was widespread in U.S. institutions for the mentally retarded.

EARLY RESEARCH ON THE HERITABILITY OF EARLY INFANTILE AUTISM

When Leo Kanner (4) first identified infantile autism as a diagnostic entity, he concluded that his patients had:

> ... come into the world with an innate inability to form the usual, biologically provided affective contact with people, just as other children come into the world with innate physical or intellectual handicaps.... [W]e seem to have pure culture examples of inborn autistic disturbances of affective contact (p. 250).

Kanner believed that his emphasis on an "inborn" disturbance delayed the acceptance of early infantile autism as a clinical entity. Recognition of the impact of severe maternal deprivation on child development had brought psychogenesis to the fore (14–16). Psychiatry was dominated by Don Jackson's "schizophrenogenic mother" and Gregory Bateson's "double-bind" (17). When Kanner coined the term "refrigerator mother," the diagnosis of autism became more fashionable; it suggested that a "refrigerator mother" produced a "frozen child" (something he later regretted). Kanner was aware of the frequency of obsessional and schizoid traits among the parents and even suggested that the parents might be "successfully autistic adults." Indeed, in my paper on the fathers of autistic children I suggested that the severe obsessional traits and relative social isolation some displayed might represent a *forme fruste* of the complete entity (18). Thirty years later, Sula Wolff and her colleagues (19) compared the parents of autistic patients with the parents of other child psychiatric patients and confirmed Kanner's observations on the predominance of schizoid and socially gauche characteristics. But neither he nor I seriously pursued the genetic hypothesis. At Kanner's invitation, I reviewed the charts of his first 100 patients and found 131 siblings, of whom 3 were autistic (20). I did not have a clue about the significance of what I had found. All I knew of genetics was Mendelian; it was clear that Mendelian laws were not operative in autism. Autism, I concluded, was not inherited because it was not Mendelian. No one called attention to my error.

In the 1950s, there were no published data on the prevalence of autism; but assuredly we knew it was rare. It was not until 10 years later that modern child psychiatric epidemiology began with the Isle of Wight study by Rutter and his colleagues (21,22). In a total population of 2,200 children, they found only one autistic child, a prevalence similar to the estimate of 4 to 5 per 10,000 published in the same year by Lotter (23). But I didn't understand what finding three autistic children among 131 sibs implied. The rate I observed among siblings was two orders of magnitude greater than expected and established a genetic risk. Not until the mid-1970s did Folstein and Rutter (24) provide unequivocal proof of inheritance by comparing the identical and fraternal cotwins of autistic probands in a total population sample. I call attention to my failure to understand the data I analyzed to remind readers that the prevalent concepts, ideas, and methods of any given era act as blinders to all but the very gifted.

"ADHD" IN THE 1950s

When my professional career began, what is now known as ADHD had not yet been recognized as a diagnostic entity. Symptoms of overactivity and inattentiveness existed, of course, but were allocated to such categories as "behavioral disorder," "minimal brain damage," "minimal brain dysfunction," or "post-encephalitic syndrome" (even though an episode of encephalitis had never been documented). The patients were not of much interest to most child guidance clinics because of the supposition of "organicity." The one symptomatic treatment that seemed to be as effective was dextroamphetamine. It was not in wide use and had never been put to an exacting test. Indeed, when the Psychopharmacology Service Center of the NIMH convened a conference in 1958 on Child Research in Psychopharmacology (25), "there was essentially no research on drugs in children" (26). Randomized controlled trials were being introduced into psychiatry in the late 1950s. Our research group at Hopkins received the first NIMH grant for RCTs on tranquilizers and stimulants for treating hyperkinesis in children (27). Tranquilizers proved to be worse than placebos (28), but stimulants were clearly effective (29), a finding that has been repeatedly confirmed.

What was entirely unexpected was the explosion in the use of these agents in subsequent decades for a condition that had been regarded as uncommon, so uncommon that the first edition of the APA *Diagnostic and Statistical Manual* (DSM I), published in 1952, had no such categories as hyperactivity or attention deficit disorder. In 1967, I participated in a World Health Organization Symposium on Diagnosis and Classification in Child Psychiatry (30). Mike Rutter and I had to argue vigorously for the inclusion of hyperkinesis as a syndrome. The other participants were highly skeptical of the diagnosis hyperkinesis. Most U.K. psychiatrists allocated it to the category "behavior disorder." We won the day, and hyperkinetic reaction of childhood appeared in DSM II in 1968; however, it was not until DSM III (1980) that attention deficit/hyperactivity disorder (ADHD) entered the official lexicon.

It is, of course, not possible to find data on rates before a given disease has entered the official nomenclature. The Centers for Disease Control (31) estimate ADHD population prevalence based on parental reports from the National Survey of Children's Health in 2003 at about 4.4 million American children aged 4–17 years of age. More than 50% of those children (2.5 million) were reported currently to be taking medication for the disorder. The survey reports a remarkably wide difference in the percentage of children with ADHD between

Colorado (~5.1%) and Alabama (~11.2%), with an overall U.S. average of about 7.8%. Can these disparities possibly be valid? Are there localized "epidemics" of ADHD or is it that there are epidemics of diagnosis? Do the variations reflect differences in the availability of specialists, in fashions in diagnosis, and in their administrative consequences in particular communities?

It is useful to recall, in this connection, Judy Rapoport's studies in the late 1970s. At the time, dextroamphetamine was labeled pharmacologically as a stimulant. Because hyperkinetic children responded to the stimulant by slowing down as if it were a sedative, their response was termed paradoxical. When Judy (alone of all of us with the courage to do the study!) put the matter to empirical test by giving dextroamphetamine to normal children (including several of her own), they slowed down just as the patients did (32). The "paradox" was age-related, not "disease"-related. That lesson continues to elude most child psychiatrists. A "therapeutic" response to the drug is taken as "confirmation" of a diagnosis. Are we converting a dimensional spectrum that covers the entire population arbitrarily into a diagnostic category? Have we become carpenters with hammers who see all problems as nails?

WHAT ESTABLISHED AND WHAT ERODED PSYCHOANALYTIC HEGEMONY?

When I completed my training in psychiatry, a half-century ago, psychoanalysis was in and genetics was out. Fifty years later, genetics is in and psychoanalysis is out. What happened? Did the change result from scientific progress? Science had a good deal to do with the blossoming of genetics, but economics proved decisive for practice.

How had an untestable theory and a treatment without proof of effectiveness come to be so dominant a half-century ago? Three characteristics of medicine (*all* of medicine, including psychiatry) in the 1950s help to explain it: treatment recommendations were based on "clinical experience" rather than exacting trials; there were few therapeutic alternatives in psychiatry and no equally comprehensive theory; and, most important of all, psychoanalysis taught psychiatrists to listen to their patients.

As to the first, treatment decisions in all of medicine as well as in psychiatry rested largely upon expert opinion (33). The first randomized clinical trial in medicine (on streptomycin for tuberculosis) was not published until 1948 (34).

As to the second, other than ECT, there were no reliably effective treatments for psychotic patients. Psychiatric patients were being warehoused in state mental hospitals in evergrowing numbers. So desperate was the state of affairs that more than 20,000 frontal lobotomies were performed in the United States in the 20 years following its introduction in 1936! What led to the abandonment of lobotomy was not the moral sensitivity of science, but rather the appearance of the dramatically effective psychotropic drugs that replaced it (35).

No other psychological theory provided as comprehensive an account of the origins of psychopathology. The brain sciences of the era were entirely irrelevant to clinical practice. Diagnosis was unreliable and made little difference for treatment. Psychoanalysis seemed to "explain" the bizarre symptoms patients exhibited. Its very complexity and counterintuitiveness enhanced its allure. It connected the symptoms of mental illness to the psychopathology of everyday life.

As to the third, many patients improved when we listened to them and offered what other specialists derided as "talk therapy." Proof that talk therapies do work had to wait another 30 years. Psychiatry as a profession remained remarkably indifferent to the absence of empirical justification. Warnings that lack of data would threaten our credibility (and likelihood of being reimbursed for our services!) were simply ignored. In the late '60s I wrote (36):

> What is remarkable is how little effect these studies [of psychotherapy outcomes] with their scots verdict of "not proven" have had on professional practice. Surely ... they should have led to ... studies to define the indications for, the best methods of, and the limitations to, psychotherapy rather than what can only be compared to a religious conviction in possessing an exclusive road to salvation.

At the 1962 APA Conference on Psychiatric Training (37), I spoke from the floor at the final plenary session. During the preceding 4 days, there had been general agreement on the importance of further training in newly arising or rediscovered disciplines (psychopharmacology, sociology, anthropology); at the same time, the acknowledged shortage of psychiatrists and the financial burden precluded lengthening residency training. I made the obvious point that something had to go. No one had indicated what should be cut back to make room for the new, even though more sausage could not be squeezed into the same casing. Accordingly, I volunteered a modest proposal: namely, that the time devoted to psychoanalytic theory and practice be sharply reduced. I questioned psychoanalysis as a "science" because its propositions were formulated in such a way that they could not be disconfirmed. A didactic analysis for psychiatric house officers, I added, limited their geographic mobility, necessitated moonlighting to secure supplementary income, prepared them for practice patterns limited to middle- and upper class patients, turned them away from research because they had been fed readymade "answers," and isolated them from public service (38).

I had never before, nor have I ever since, had such an electrifying effect on a professional audience. I was barely able to get out of the way of a veritable stampede of eminent department chairmen who lined up behind the floor microphones to challenge my facts, my conclusions, my credentials, and my lineage! (I say "chair*men*" advisedly; there was not a single chair*woman*.) My modest proposal disappeared with the merest trace: a footnote on page 8 of the Conference Report (37). However, by the 1976 APA Conference on training (39), the influence of psychoanalysis had ebbed markedly, not because of my or other theoretical challenges, but because of the rising tide of psychopharmacology.

REFLECTIONS ON MY CRITIQUE OF PSYCHOANALYSIS

Do I still believe what I said then? My scientific critique is unchanged. The "research" method of psychoanalysis follows none of the accepted scientific principles of prediction, design, control, and quantification. Freud's ideas had been revolutionary in their time, but "the history of science... is replete with instances in which an initially liberating conceptualization, once institutionalized, becomes a barrier to progress" (40).

What I failed to acknowledge was the powerful and lasting contribution psychoanalysis had made to psychiatry by teaching trainees to listen to patients and to try to understand their distress, rather than merely to classify them with a diagnostic algorithm, or snow them with drugs, or lock them away, or release them to homelessness. Basing care on what is unique to the individual patient is central to clinical competence, whether in medicine or surgery or psychiatry. Psychoanalysis made a dynamic psychological approach central to general psychiatry. It emphasized the importance of memory, its vulnerability to distortion, and its centrality to each person's life narrative, the way we explain ourselves to ourselves and to others. Because those narratives can be self-defeating, therapy must be designed to help patients to reconstruct their autobiographies in ways that permit growth. Those principles remain as important in caring for patients today as they were then, but the paymasters of the healthcare marketplace are making time less and less available to patients (41). The economic barriers that hinder psychiatrists in providing psychotherapy have impoverished clinical psychiatry.

Psychoanalysis itself continues to do well in private institutes and conclaves, but it is largely missing from the academic scene in psychiatry, where it was once dominant (42). There has been, however, a sea change in psychotherapy research. Whereas there were no psychotherapies of proven efficacy 50 years ago (36), randomized controlled clinical trials have shown that a number of nonanalytic psychotherapies do work for particular disorders (43). Does the new evidence explain the recession of psychoanalysis? Not at all! Despite proof of efficacy, the provision of any brand of psychotherapy is diminishing. HMOs and insurance companies simply won't pay for more than a soupcon. Psychiatrists now make DSM-IV diagnoses and prescribe drugs. Money is shaping practice (44).

I hope I have persuaded readers of the importance of skepticism toward received wisdom. Psychoanalysis circa 1950 was no more the royal road to salvation than the human genome project is 60 years later. The challenge is the integration of concepts of mind and brain: Can we invent paradigms that will give new meanings to an old term, "psychogenetic?" For that, we will need to provide an education for our successors that will bridge disciplines among the brain, behavioral, and clinical sciences (45). We would do well to heed the admonition of Sir Aubrey Lewis (46), late head of Maudsley Hospital in London:

> The philosophers thought it proper to put not one but two mottoes on the Temple at Delphi: one, the better remembered, was "Know Thyself": but the second, equally imperative, enjoined "Nothing in Excess." It might be worth inscribing that over the Temple of Psychiatry.

DREAMING AHEAD

What are my credentials as a futurologist? I offer a prediction I made 20 years ago (44), which readers can check against the two decades that have followed to make an informed decision about the believability of my dreams.

A PARABLE FOR OUR TIME

I invented a virtual experiment as a metaphor for a clear and impending danger: the threat that reliance on technology would replace concern for the patient and the patient's story (44). The starting point for the studies in our Laboratory of Mental Science was the neurobiological breakthrough by René Descartes, identifying the pineal glad as the seat of the soul (47).

> The part of the body in which the soul exercises its functions immediately is in nowise the heart, nor the whole of the brain, but merely the most inward of all its parts, to wit, a certain very small gland which is situated in the middle of its substance and so suspended above the duct whereby the animal spirits in its anterior cavities have communication with those in its posterior, that the slightest movements which take place in it may alter very greatly the course of these spirits; and reciprocally that the smallest changes which occur in the course of the spirits may do much to change the movements of this gland ... The whole action of the soul consists of this, that solely because it desires something, it causes the little gland with which it is closely united to move in the way requisite to produce the effect which relates to this desire.

Accordingly, our research team grew pineal cells in tissue culture and eluted a unique protein from the supernatant. Against this pineal-specific protein, we prepared a monoclonal antibody made radioactive by incubating the hybridoma cells with oxygen-labeled acetate. Administered parenterally, the tracer molecule, modified to permeate the blood-brain barrier in the region of the pineal body, binds to the gland tightly and specifically. As the positrons emitted by O collide with electrons in the adjacent tissues, the gamma rays produced by particle annihilation are detected and converted by appropriate instrumentation into a visual image. A major step forward occurred when our engineers succeeded in constructing a luminescent screen on which moment-to-moment changes could be displayed. Thus, displacements in the pineal (accompanied, as Descartes had predicted, by ventricular currents) could be correlated with fluctuations in the state of the soul.

That must suffice for an account of the science of the matter. Now consider its economics. The instrument, destined to be patented as *PinealPet®*, can be guaranteed to increase the earning capacity of American psychiatrists handsomely, when they work in a fee-for-service system. Because its immediate imaging properties make it ideal for office use, psychiatrists rather than radiologists can bill for it, and thus attain economic parity with other technology-based disciplines. Because it will no longer be necessary to inquire of the patient about the state of his or her soul, a notoriously time-consuming, uncertain, and altogether messy procedure, time savings will be prodigious; productivity will increase; cost-effectiveness will please both supply side and free market economics. For myself, I intended to ask no profit (other than the Nobel Prize money).

Furthermore, the therapeutic potential of this technological advance will not have escaped notice. It should prove possible, in principle, by a kind of psychochiropractic, to correct the subluxations of the pineal which result in existential *angst*. By means of the piezoelectric effect, the therapist should be able to manipulate the pineal body with pulses of current under direct visual control to align it in such fashion as to produce harmony in the soul.

Yet, at the very point that the device was ready to be marketed, I was afflicted by an acute crisis of conscience, in all probability resulting from *mal de mer* of the pineal. I melted the instrument down; I shredded blueprints and protocols before they could be copied by sinister commercial interests. In the nick of time, I had realized the consequences of my thought experiment. Once at hand, PinealPet, like the endoscope, the stent, and the cardiac catheter before it, would have come to dominate clinical practice through its potential for increasing earnings *and* its capacity to generate nominally objective data. A technology invested with the authority of science is irresistible to patient and doctor alike in reifying disease.

How good was that prediction? Psychochiropractics, of course, have not quite arrived (though brain stimulation techniques are multiplying). There has been an enormous increase in technological capabilities for brain imaging. For an understanding of the brain-mind interface, that bodes only good. For practice, it carries the risk of premature application, as PinealPet did. What the thought experiment left out—until I at the very last moment "melted the instrument down and shredded the blueprints"—is *agency;* that is, the responsibility of physicians committed to patient care to resist and even roll back the tide of reductionism.

Until recently, financial subsidies from industry and uncontrolled access for pharmaceutical sales representatives have been "embedded" in departments of academic medicine much as journalists were with military units in the invasion of Iraq.

The ubiquity of drug company-sponsored meals, lectures, and visits from PSRs during medical residency training represented a very considerable investment by the industry. Reflecting a conviction that this investment pays off, big Pharma has been spending two to three times as much on marketing and administration as it does on research and development (48,49). However, in the past 10 years, leading teaching hospitals have ended "pizza lunches" for house staff and have limited the access of drug detail representatives to faculty and house staff. Academic psychiatry is beginning to assert the primacy of evidence-based medicine and alerting physicians to the risks of seduction by gifts and blandishments.

In a second major step forward, the American Board of Psychiatry and Neurology now requires that residents demonstrate familiarity with and competence in a set of evidence-based psychotherapies, in addition to competence in psychopharmacology. The impact of this requirement depends on progress in developing reliable measures of competence and making these measures a key to accreditation. Once again, it will be up to all of us to assure the achievement of that goal.

A third major deficit in academic psychiatry—the decades-long decline in the number of psychiatrist-investigators—is being addressed in a serious and credible way. In 2003, the Institute of Medicine issued a scholarly document *Research Training in Psychiatry Residency: Strategies for Reform* (50). Among its many excellent recommendations (51) was a proposal that a public-private consortium be created to carry the program forward. With support from NIMH and leading psychiatric societies, precisely such a consortium was created: the National Psychiatry Training Council. In 2005, it completed its work with a report, *Educating a New Generation of Psychiatrist Investigators* (52). Its recommendations include a call for the Residency Review Committee to give greater flexibility to program directors in designing the order of training (so that child and adolescent training within the first 2 years counts toward subspecialty training, for example) and to permit the creation of research tracks by shortening mandated requirements. No less important, it emphasizes that "research literacy" be made the goal for all residents. To reinforce that proposal, the ABPN examination must include questions to demonstrate literacy in assessing methodology and outcome of research protocols. It calls for a "national academy" of senior research mentors to be available on an ad hoc basis to all trainees.

These recommendations have been presented at a number of professional psychiatric meetings; several model child psychiatry research training fellowships have come into being, the most notable being the Albert J. Solnit Integrated Child and Adult Research Residency Pathway at the Yale Child Study Center (53). Once again, how far this effort to recruit a new generation of child psychiatry investigators will proceed will depend upon the support it receives from the old (faculty) as well as the young (students in training). Our fate is in ourselves, not in our stars.

THE FUTURE OF PATIENT CARE: ECONOMICS AND ETHICS

Nothing has shaken my conviction that the superiority of patient-centered, psychologically sensitive, integrative medicine will become ever more evident. Patients as well as physicians will serve as its advocates and assure its ascendancy. In his surrealistic short story, *A Country Doctor*, written early in the last century, Franz Kafka wrote: "To write prescriptions is easy; to come to an understanding with people is difficult." The first part of the aphorism no longer rings quite true; choosing the right prescription for the individual patient at the appropriate moment is a real challenge in an era when we have powerful medications (with powerful side effects) at our command. However, it remains true that coming to an understanding with people is even more difficult and demands more time than writing a script. Time is the essence of good medical care. It is time that is at threat.

I conclude with a passage from Plato's *The Laws*, written about 350 BC (54). An Athenian "Stranger" addresses Cleinias, a Cretan, and Megillus, a Spartan. The Athenian Stranger (in effect, Plato himself) has this to say about "slave" and "free" physicians in Greek society:

> Slaves... are almost always treated by other slaves who either rush about on flying visits or wait to be consulted in their surgeries. This kind of doctor never gives any account of the particular illness of the individual slave, or is prepared to listen to one; he simply prescribes what he thinks best in the light of experience, as if he had precise knowledge, and with the self-confidence of a dictator. Then he dashes off on his way to the next slave-patient, and so takes off his master's shoulders some of the work of attending the sick.
>
> The visits of the free doctor, by contrast, are mostly concerned with treating the illnesses of free men; *his* method is to construct an empirical case history by consulting the invalid and his friends; in this way he himself learns something from the sick and at the same time he gives the individual patient all the instruction he can. He gives no prescription until he has somehow gained the invalid's consent; then, coaxing him into continued cooperation, he tries to complete his restoration to health.
>
> The Stranger asks: "Which of the two methods do you think makes a doctor a better healer...?"

The reader of this textbook will have no difficulty in choosing the preferred option. In return for what that reader has learned, he and she have incurred an obligation: to fight to preserve that option. Commitment to assuring children access to the best professional care is the precondition for child psychiatry to flourish.

References

1. Brecht B (1943): *Life of Galileo*, trans. Willett J. In: Willett J, Manheim R (eds): *Bertolt Brecht: Plays, Poetry and Prose. The Collected Plays* vol. 5, p 1. Methuen, London, 1980.
2. Kanner L: *Child Psychiatry*. Springfield, IL, Charles C Thomas, 1935.
3. Kanner L: *Child Psychiatry*, 2nd ed. Springfield, IL, Charles C Thomas, 1948.
4. Kanner L: Autistic disturbances of affective contact. *Nervous Child* 2: 217–250, 1943.
5. Rutter M: Foreword to *Childhood Psychosis* by Kanner L. Washington, DC, Winston and Sons, 1973, p. viii.
6. Down JLH: Observation on an ethnic classification of idiots. *London Hospital Clinical Lecture Reports* 3:259, 1866.
7. LeJeune J, Gauthier M, Turpin R: Les chromosomes humaines en culture de tissus. *Compte du Rendu Academy of Science* 248:602, 1958.
8. Jacobs PA, Baikie AG, Court Brown. WM, Strong JA: The somatic chromosomes in Mongolism. *The Lancet* 1:710–711, 1959.
9. Einfeld SL, Piccinin AM, Mackinnon A, et al.: Psychopathology in young people with intellectual disability. *Journal of the American Medical Association* 296:1981–1989, 2006.
10. Kanner L: Habeas corpus releases of feebleminded persons and their consequences. *American Journal of Psychiatry* 94:1013–1033, 1938.
11. Foster Kennedy R: The problem of social control of the congenital defective: Education, sterilization, euthanasia. *American Journal of Psychiatry* 99:13–16, 1942.
12. Kanner L: Exoneration of the feebleminded. *American Journal of Psychiatry* 99:17–22, 1942.
13. Editorial: Euthanasia. *Journal of Psychiatry* 99:141–143, 1942.
14. Goldfarb W: Effects of psychological privation in infancy and subsequent stimulation. *American Journal of Psychiatry* 102:18–33, 1945.
15. Spitz RA: Hospitalism: An inquiry into the genesis of psychiatric conditions in early childhood. *Psychoanalytic Study of the Child* 1:53–74, 1945.
16. Bowlby J: *Material Care and Mental Health*. Geneva, WHO Monograph Series, no. 2, 1951.
17. Bateson G, Jackson DD, Haley J, Weakland JH: Toward a theory of schizophrenia. *Behavioral Science* 1:251–264, 1956.

18. Eisenberg L: The fathers of autistic children. *American Journal of Orthopsychiatry* 27:715–714, 1957.
19. Wolff S, Narayan S, Moyes B: Personality characteristics of parents of autistic children: A controlled study *Journal of Child Psychology and Psychiatry* 29:143–154, 1988.
20. Kanner L, Eisenberg L: Follow-up studies in infantile autism. In: Hoch PH, Zubin J (eds): *Psychopathology of Childhood,* New York, Grune & Stratton, 1957, pp. 227–239.
21. Rutter M, Graham P: Psychiatric disorder in ten and eleven year old children. *Proceedings of the Royal Society of Medicine* 59:382–387, 1966.
22. Rutter M, Tizard EJ, Whitmore K: *Education Health and Behavior.* London: Longman, 1970.
23. Lotter V: Epidemiology of autistic conditions in young children: Part I. Prevalence. *Social Psychiatry* 1:124–137, 1966.
24. Folstein S, Rutter M: Infantile autism: A genetic study of 21 twin pairs. *Journal of Child Psychology and Psychiatry* 18:297–321, 1977.
25. Fisher S (Ed.): *Child Research in Psycho-Pharmacology.* Springfield IL: Charles C Thomas Publisher, 1959.
26. Cole J: Introduction. In: Conners CK (ed) In: *Clinical Use of Stimulant Drugs in Children: Proceedings of a symposium held at Key Biscayne, Florida,* March 5–8, 1972. New York, American Elsevier Publishing Co., Inc., pp. xi–xii, 1974.
27. Lipman RS: NIMH—Pre-support of research in minimal brain dysfunction in children. In: Conners CK (ed) *In Clinical Use of Stimulant Drugs in Children: Proceedings of a symposium held at Key Biscayne, Florida,* March 5–8, 1972. New York: American Elsevier Publishing Co., Inc., pp. 202–206, 1974.
28. Cytryn L, Gilbert A, Eisenberg L: The effectiveness of tranquilizing drugs plus supportive psychotherapy in treating behavior disorders of children. *American Journal of Orthopsychiatry* 30:113–129, 1960.
29. Eisenberg L, Lachman R, Molling P, Lockner A, Mizelle J, Conners K: A psychopharmacologic study in a training school for delinquent boys. *American Journal Orthopsychiatry* 33:431–447, 1963.
30. Rutter M, Lebovici S, Eisenberg L, et al.: A triaxial classification of mental disorders in childhood. *Journal of Child Psychology and Psychiatry* 10: 41–61, 1969.
31. Centers for Disease Control and Prevention: Prevalence of diagnosis and medication treatment for attention/deficit/hyperactivity disorder: United States 2003. *Morbidity and Mortality Weekly Reports* 54:842–847, 2005.
32. Rapoport JL, Buchsbaum MS, Zahn TP, et al.: Dextroamphetamine: Cognitive and behavioral effects in normal prepubertal boys. *Science* 199:560–563, 1978.
33. Doll R: Development of controlled trials in preventive and therapeutic medicine. *Journal of BioSocial Science* 23:365–378, 1991.
34. Medical Research Council: Streptomycin treatment of tuberculous meningitis. *Lancet* 1:582–596, 1948.
35. Pressman JD: *Last Resort: Psychosurgery and the Limits of Medicine.* New York, Cambridge University Press, 1998.
36. Eisenberg L: Child psychiatry: The past quarter century. *American Journal of Orthopsychiatry* 39:389–401, 1969.
37. Barton WE, Malamud W (eds): *Training the Psychiatrist to Meet Changing Needs* Washington, DC: American Psychiatric Association; p. 8, 1963.
38. Eisenberg L: If not now, when? *American Journal of Orthopsychiatry* 32:781–793, 1962a.
39. Rosenfeld AH (ed): *Psychiatric Education: Prologue to the 1980s.* Washington, DC, American Psychiatric Association 1976.
40. Eisenberg L: Discussion. In: Hoch PH, Zubin J (eds): *The Future of Psychiatry,* New York, Grune & Stratton, 1962b pp. 251–255.
41. Eisenberg L: Whatever happened to the faculty on the way to the Agora? *Archives of Internal Medicine* 159:2251–2256, 1999.
42. Eisenberg L: The "ecology" of psychiatry and neurology. In: Hagar M. (ed) *The Convergence of Neuroscience, Behavioral Science, Neurology, and Psychiatry.* New York; Josiah Macy Jr. Foundation, 2005.
43. Kazdin AE: Developing a research agenda for child and adolescent psychotherapy. *Archives of General Psychiatry* 57:829–835, 2000.
44. Eisenberg L: Mindlessness and brainlessness in psychiatry. *British Journal of Psychiatry* 148:497–508, 1986.
45. Pellmar T, Eisenberg L (eds): *Bridging Disciplines in the Brain, Behavioral and Clinical Sciences.* Washington, DC: National Academy Press, 2000.
46. Lewis A: Ebb and flow in social psychiatry. *Yale Journal of Biology and Medicine* 35:62–83, 1962.
47. Descartes R: The passion of the soul. In *Philosophical Works (vol. I),* trans. Haldane ES and Ross GRT, New York: Dover, 1649.
48. Angell M: *The Truth About the Drug Companies: How They Deceive Us and What to Do About It.* New York: Random House, 2004.
49. Avorn J: *Powerful Medicines: The Benefits, Risks, and Costs of Prescription Drugs.* Knopf, 2004.
50. Abrams MT, Patchan KM, Boat TF: *Research Training in Psychiatry Residency: Strategies for Reform.* Washington, DC: National Academies Press, 2003.
51. Eisenberg L: Review of Abrams MT, Patchan KM, Boat TF: *Research Training in Psychiatric Residency: Strategies for Reform.* Washington, DC: National Academies Press. *American Journal of Psychiatry* 161: 1930–1931, 2004.
52. *National Psychiatry Training Council: Educating a New Generation of Psychiatrist Investigators,* (unpublished manuscript), Washington, DC, 2005.
53. Martin A, Block M, Pruett K, et al.: From too little too late to early and often: Child psychiatry education during medical school (and before and after). *Child & Adolescent Psychiatric Clinics of North America,* doi:10.1016/j.chc.2006.07.005.
54. *Plato (350 BC) The Laws.* Trans Saunders TJ, London, Penguin Classics, 1970, pp. 181–182.

INDEX